NINTH EDITION

Textbook of
PEDIATRICS

Edited by

WALDO E. NELSON, M.D., D.Sc. (Hon.)

Professor of Pediatrics, Woman's Medical College of
Pennsylvania and Temple University School of
Medicine; Attending Pediatrician, St. Christopher's
Hospital for Children, Philadelphia

Associate Editors

VICTOR C. VAUGHAN, III, M.D.

Professor and Chairman, Department of Pediatrics,
Temple University School of Medicine; Medical
Director, St. Christopher's Hospital for Children,
Philadelphia

R. JAMES McKAY, M.D.

Professor and Chairman, Department of Pediatrics,
The University of Vermont College of Medicine; Chief
of Pediatric Service, Medical Center Hospital of
Vermont, Burlington

WITH THE COLLABORATION OF 78 CONTRIBUTORS

W. B. SAUNDERS COMPANY · Philadelphia · London · Toronto · 1969

W. B. Saunders Company: West Washington Square
Philadelphia, Pa. 19105

12 Dyott Street
London W.C. 1

1835 Yonge Street
Toronto, Ontario 295

Textbook of Pediatrics

To the Child's Physician

and especially

*to those who through their expressed
confidence in past editions of this
book have provided the stimulus for
this revision*

CONTRIBUTORS

S. T. ACHAR, M.D.*
Madras, India.

JOHN A. ANDERSON, M.D., Ph.D.
Professor and Head of Department of Pediatrics, University of Minnesota Medical School, College of Medical Sciences.

JAMES B. AREY, M.D., Ph.D.
Professor of Pathology, Temple University School of Medicine. Pathologist, St. Christopher's Hospital for Children.

VICTOR H. AUERBACH, Ph.D.
Research Professor of Pediatrics (Biochemistry), Temple University School of Medicine. Director of Enzyme Laboratory and Director of Research Chemistry, St. Christopher's Hospital for Children.

LEONARD BACHMAN, M.D.
Professor of Anesthesia, University of Pennsylvania School of Medicine. Director of Anesthesiology, Children's Hospital of Philadelphia.

HENRY W. BAIRD, M.D.
Professor of Pediatrics, Temple University School of Medicine. Attending Pediatrician, St. Christopher's Hospital for Children and Temple University Hospital.

GIULIO J. BARBERO, M.D.
Professor and Chairman of Department of Pediatrics, Hahnemann Medical College and Hospital of Philadelphia.

LEWIS A. BARNESS, M.D.
Professor of Pediatrics, University of Pennsylvania School of Medicine. Chief of Pediatrics, Hospital of the University of Pennsylvania; Senior Physician, Children's Hospital of Philadelphia and Philadelphia General Hospital.

*Deceased.

JOHN B. BARTRAM, M.D.
Professor of Pediatrics, Temple University School of Medicine. Senior Attending Pediatrician, St. Christopher's Hospital for Children and Temple University Hospital.

PAUL C. BEAVER, Ph.D.
William Vincent Professor of Tropical Diseases and Hygiene, Tulane University School of Medicine.

MILDRED J. BENNETT, M.S., Ph.D.
Formerly Lecturer in Nutritional Sciences, University of California. Research Biochemist, Children's Hospital of the East Bay, Oakland, California.

WILLIAM H. BERGSTROM, M.D.
Professor of Pediatrics, State University of New York, Upstate Medical Center at Syracuse. Attending Pediatrician, State University Hospital and Crouse-Irving Memorial Hospital.

JOSEPH B. BILDERBACK, M.D.
Clinical Professor of Pediatrics, University of Oregon Medical School. Attending Pediatrician, Doernbecher Memorial Hospital for Children.

RUSSELL J. BLATTNER, M.D.
Professor and Chairman of Department of Pediatrics, Baylor University College of Medicine. Pediatrician-in-Chief, Ben Taub General Hospital and Jefferson Davis Hospital; Physician-in-Chief, Texas Children's Hospital; Chief of Pediatrics, Hermann Hospital.

WILLIAM L. BRADFORD, M.D.
Professor Emeritus of Pediatrics, University of Rochester School of Medicine and Dentistry; Distinguished Visiting Professor of Pediatrics, University of Missouri School of Medicine. Pediatrician, Strong Memorial Hospital, Rochester, New York; Consultant, Children's Mercy Hospital, Kansas City, Missouri.

CARROLL F. BURGOON, Jr., M.D.
Professor of Dermatology, Temple University School of Medicine. Chief Attending Physician, Skin and Cancer Hospital of Philadelphia.

ELSIE R. CARRINGTON, M.D.
Professor and Chairman of Department of Obstetrics and Gynecology, Woman's Medical College of Pennsylvania.

J. JULIAN CHISOLM, Jr., M.D.
Associate Professor of Pediatrics, Johns Hopkins University School of Medicine. Associate Chief Pediatrician, Baltimore City Hospitals.

AMOS CHRISTIE, M.D.
Professor of Pediatrics, Vanderbilt University School of Medicine.

DAVID B. CLARK, M.D., Ph.D.
Professor and Chairman of Department of Neurology, University of Kentucky College of Medicine. Chairman of Department of Neurology, University of Kentucky Medical Center Hospital.

DAVID F. CLYDE, M.D., Ph.D., D.T.M.&H.
Professor of International Medicine, University of Maryland School of Medicine. Member, Expert Advisory Panel on Malaria, World Health Organization.

CHARLES D. COOK, M.D.
Professor and Chairman of Department of Pediatrics, Yale University School of Medicine. Pediatrician-in-Chief, Yale-New Haven Hospital.

ROBERT E. COOKE, M.D.
Given Foundation Professor of Pediatrics and Chairman of Department of Pediatrics, Johns Hopkins University School of Medicine. Pediatrician-in-Chief, Johns Hopkins Hospital.

ALLEN C. CROCKER, M.D.
Assistant Clinical Professor of Pediatrics, Harvard Medical School. Senior Associate in Medicine, Children's Hospital Medical Center.

EDWARD C. CURNEN, M.D.
Carpentier Professor of Pediatrics, Columbia University College of Physicians and Surgeons. Attending Pediatrician and Director of Pediatric Service, Babies Hospital and Vanderbilt Clinic, Columbia-Presbyterian Medical Center.

ANGELO M. DiGEORGE, M.D., M.S. (Ped.)
Professor of Pediatrics, Temple University School of Medicine. Senior Attending Pediatrician and Director, Division of Endocrine and Metabolic Disorders, St. Christopher's Hospital for Children.

PAUL A. di SANT'AGNESE, M.D., Sc.D. (Med.), Dr. Med. (Hon.)
Clinical Professor of Pediatrics, Georgetown University School of Medicine. Chief of Pediatric Metabolism Branch, National Institutes of Health.

JOHN J. DOWNES, M.D.
Assistant Professor of Anesthesia and Pediatrics, University of Pennsylvania School of Medicine. Senior Anesthesiologist and Director of the Intensive Care Unit, Children's Hospital of Philadelphia.

JOHN M. DUNN, M.D.
Associate Professor in Psychiatry (Child), Temple University School of Medicine. Staff Psychiatrist, St. Christopher's Hospital for Children.

HEINZ F. EICHENWALD, M.D.
William Buchanan Professor and Chairman of Department of Pediatrics, University of Texas Southwestern Medical School in Dallas. Chief of Staff, Children's Medical Center; Chief of Pediatrics, Parkland Memorial Hospital.

ERNEST C. FAUST, Ph.D., LL.D.
Emeritus Professor of Parasitology, Tulane University School of Public Health and Tropical Medicine.

HARRY A. FELDMAN, M.D.
Professor and Chairman of Department of Preventive Medicine, State University of New York, Upstate Medical Center at Syracuse. Attending Physician, State University Hospital.

F. CLARKE FRASER, Ph.D., M.D., C.M., D.Sc. (Acadia), F.R.S.C.
Professor of Human Genetics, Department of Genetics, McGill University. Director of Department of Medical Genetics, Montreal Children's Hospital.

LYTT I. GARDNER, M.D.
Professor of Pediatrics, State University of New York, Upstate Medical Center at Syracuse. Attending Pediatrician, State University Hospital; Consultant Pediatrician, Syracuse Memorial Hospital.

SYDNEY S. GELLIS, M.D.
Professor and Chairman of Department of Pediatrics, Tufts University School of Medicine. Pediatrician-in-Chief, Tufts-New England Medical Center.

ELI GOLD, M.D.
Associate Professor of Pediatrics, Case-Western Reserve University School of Medicine. Pediatrician, Cleveland Metropolitan General Hospital.

ROBERT J. HAGGERTY, M.D.
Professor and Chairman of Department of
Pediatrics, University of Rochester School of
Medicine and Dentistry. Pediatrician-in-
Chief, Strong Memorial Hospital.

SCOTT B. HALSTEAD, M.D.
Professor of Tropical Medicine, University of
Hawaii School of Medicine.

ROBISON D. HARLEY, M.D., Ph.D.
Associate Professor of Ophthalmology, Temple
University School of Medicine. Attending
Ophthalmologist, St. Christopher's Hospital
for Children, Temple University Hospital, and
Atlantic City Hospital.

JEROME S. HARRIS, M.D.
Professor of Pediatrics, Duke University School
of Medicine. Attending Pediatrician, Duke
Hospital.

ROBERT H. HIGH, M.D., M.S. (Ped.)
Chairman of Department of Pediatrics, Henry
Ford Hospital, Detroit.

PAUL H. HOLINGER, M.D.
Professor of Bronchoesophagology, Depart-
ment of Otolaryngology, University of Illinois
College of Medicine. Attending Broncho-
esophagologist, Presbyterian-St. Luke's Hos-
pital; Attending Bronchoesophagologist and
Laryngologist, Children's Memorial Hospital,
University of Illinois Research and Edu-
cational Hospitals, and Illinois Eye and Ear
Infirmary.

JOHN B. ISOM, M.D.
Associate Professor of Pediatrics and Neu-
rology, University of Oregon Medical School.
Pediatric Neurologist, University of Oregon
Medical School Hospital.

CHARLES A. JANEWAY, M.D., M.D. (Hon.)
Thomas Morgan Rotch Professor of Pediatrics,
Harvard Medical School. Physician-in-Chief,
Children's Hospital Medical Center; Con-
sulting Pediatrician, Boston Hospital for
Women and Beth Israel Hospital.

SAMUEL KAPLAN, M.D.
Professor of Pediatrics and Associate Professor
of Medicine, University of Cincinnati College
of Medicine. Director of Division of Cardiology,
Children's Hospital.

ROBERT KAYE, M.D.
Professor of Pediatrics, University of Pennsylvania School of Medicine. Deputy Physician-
in-Chief, Children's Hospital of Philadelphia.

JOHN A. KIRKPATRICK, JR., M.D.
Professor of Radiology, Temple University
School of Medicine. Radiologist, St. Christo-
pher's Hospital for Children.

JOHN W. LACHMAN, M.D.
Professor and Chairman of Department of
Orthopedic Surgery, Temple University School
of Medicine. Staff Orthopedic Surgeon, St.
Christopher's Hospital for Children and First
Assistant Surgeon, Shriners Hospital for
Crippled Children.

THEODORE R. LAMMOT, III, M.D.
Associate Professor of Orthopedic Surgery,
Temple University School of Medicine. Associate Surgeon, Temple University School of
Medicine, Shriners Hospital for Crippled
Children, St. Christopher's Hospital for Children; Chief Orthopedic Consultant to Children's Seashore House, Children's Heart Hospital of Philadelphia, and Children's Aid Society.

WILLIAM E. LAUPUS, M.D.
Professor and Chairman of Department of
Pediatrics, Medical College of Virginia Health
Sciences Division of the Virginia Common-
wealth University. Pediatrician-in-Chief,
Medical College of Virginia Hospitals.

HEROLD LILLYWHITE, Ph.D.
Professor of Speech Pathology, University of
Oregon Medical School.

GEORGE H. McCRACKEN, JR., M.D.
Assistant Professor of Pediatrics, University
of Texas, Southwestern Medical School in
Dallas. Attending Physician, Children's
Medical Center and Parkland Memorial
Hospital.

R. JAMES McKAY, M.D.
Professor and Chairman of Department of
Pediatrics, University of Vermont College of
Medicine. Chief of Pediatric Service, Medical
Center Hospital of Vermont; Attending Pedi-
atrician, De Goesbriand Memorial Hospital.

ROBERT W. MILLER, M.D., Dr. P.H.
Chief of Epidemiology Branch, National
Cancer Institute.

JOHN D. NELSON, M.D.
Associate Professor of Pediatrics, University
of Texas, Southwestern Medical School in
Dallas. Active Attending Physician, Chil-
dren's Medical Center; Senior Attending
Physician, Parkland Memorial Hospital.

WALDO E. NELSON, M.D., Sc.D.
Professor of Pediatrics, Woman's Medical
College of Pennsylvania and Temple University School of Medicine. Attending Pediatrician, St. Christopher's Hospital for Children.

CHARLES M. NORRIS, M.D., F.A.C.S.
Professor and Chairman of Department
of Laryngology and Broncho-esophagology
(Chevalier Jackson Clinic), Temple University
School of Medicine. Consultant in Otolaryn-
gology, Lankenau Hospital.

RICHARD W. OLMSTED, M.D.
Professor and Chairman of Department of Pediatrics, University of Oregon Medical School.

FREDERICK M. PARKINS, D.D.S., M.S.D., Ph.D.
Assistant Professor and Director of Pedodontics, University of Pennsylvania. Dental Consultant, Medical Staff, Children's Hospital of Philadelphia; Consultant in Operative Dentistry, Veterans Administration Hospital.

HOWARD A. PEARSON, M.D.
Professor of Pediatrics, Yale University School of Medicine. Attending Pediatrician, Yale-New Haven Hospital.

LAWRENCE K. PICKETT, M.D.
Professor of Surgery and Pediatrics, Yale University School of Medicine. Attending Surgeon, Yale-New Haven Hospital.

STANLEY A. PLOTKIN, M.D.
Assistant Professor of Pediatrics, University of Pennsylvania School of Medicine. Associate Member, Wistar Institute of Anatomy and Biology; Associate Physician, Children's Hospital of Philadelphia.

DANE G. PRUGH, M.D.
Professor of Psychiatry and Pediatrics, University of Colorado School of Medicine and Dentistry. Chief of Child Psychiatry Division, University of Colorado Medical Center.

W. JOSEPH RAHILL, M.D.
Assistant Professor of Pediatrics, State University of New York at Buffalo School of Medicine. Assistant Attending Pediatrician, Children's Hospital of Buffalo.

FREDERICK C. ROBBINS, M.D.
Professor of Pediatrics and Dean, Case-Western Reserve University School of Medicine. Associate Pediatrician, University Hospital; Pediatrician, Cleveland Metropolitan General Hospital.

HOWARD W. ROBINSON, Ph.D.
Professor Emeritus of Physiological Chemistry, Temple University School of Medicine.

MITCHELL I. RUBIN, M.D.
Professor of Pediatrics, State University of New York at Buffalo School of Medicine. Attending Pediatrician and Head of Renal Division, Children's Hospital of Buffalo.

JANE SCHALLER, M.D.
Assistant Professor of Pediatrics, University of Washington School of Medicine. Director of Pediatric Arthritis Clinic and Attending Physician, University Hospital; Attending Physician, Children's Orthopedic Hospital and Medical Center; Attending Physician, King County Hospital.

THOMAS F. McNAIR SCOTT, M.D.
Professor of Pediatrics, University of Pennsylvania School of Medicine. Senior Physician, Children's Hospital of Philadelphia.

CALVIN F. SETTLAGE, M.D., M.S.
Director of Child Psychiatry and Staff Psychiatrist, Mount Zion Hospital and Medical Center.

HARRY C. SHIRKEY, M.D.
Professor of Pediatrics (Chairman) and Pharmacology, University of Hawaii School of Medicine. Medical Director, Kauikeolani Children's Hospital; Chief of Pediatrics, Leahi (University) Hospital; Consulting Staff, Tripler General Hospital.

CHARLES E. SMITH, M.D.*
Berkeley, California.

DAVID W. SMITH, M.D.
Professor of Pediatrics, University of Washington School of Medicine.

ALEX J. STEIGMAN, M.D., D.Sc. (Hon.)
Professor of Pediatrics, Mount Sinai School of Medicine. Attending Pediatrician, Mount Sinai Hospital.

MARIE A. VALDES-DAPENA, M.D.
Professor of Pathology, Temple University School of Medicine. Associate Pathologist, St. Christopher's Hospital for Children.

VICTOR C. VAUGHAN, III, M.D., F.A.A.P.
Professor and Chairman of Department of Pediatrics, Temple University School of Medicine. Medical Director, St. Christopher's Hospital for Children.

LEWIS W. WANNAMAKER, M.D.
Professor of Pediatrics and Microbiology, University of Minnesota; Career Investigator, American Heart Association, University of Minnesota Medical School. Member of Medical Staff, University of Minnesota Hospital; Attending Physician, Hennepin County General Hospital; Consultant, St. Paul-Ramsey Hospital.

*Deceased.

JOSEF WARKANY, M.D.
    Professor of Research Pediatrics, University of Cincinnati College of Medicine. Fellow, Children's Hospital Research Foundation.

RALPH J. WEDGWOOD, M.D.
    Professor and Chairman of Department of Pediatrics, University of Washington School of Medicine. Director of Pediatric Services, University Hospital; Associate Chief of Pediatric Services, Children's Orthopedic Hospital and Medical Center; Attending Pediatrician, King County Hospital.

WARREN E. WHEELER, M.D.
    Professor and Chairman of Pediatrics, University of Kentucky College of Medicine. Director of Pediatric Service, University of Kentucky Medical Center.

STANLEY W. WRIGHT, M.D.
    Professor of Pediatrics, University of California, Los Angeles School of Medicine. Associate Program Director, Mental Retardation, The Neuropsychiatric Institute (UCLA).

PREFACE

This, the ninth edition of the single volume Textbook of Pediatrics,* has provided the editor his first opportunity to share editing responsibilities with medical colleagues. The relentless progression of time as it applies to the individual is sufficient reason to bring in younger blood to assume responsibility. But there are additional justifications. Chief among these are the great increase in medical knowledge and the potentials for application of it to the medical care of children.

It continues to be our goal to provide in a single volume a synthesis of pediatric knowledge which will be appropriate for the student as an introduction to pediatrics and for the clinician as a useful and competent reference. For the assembly of the text material we are dependent upon the many contributors, the selection of whom constitutes one of the major responsibilities of editorship. It is the final synthesis and shaping of the contributed manuscripts into a text with some semblance of unity and balance in each section and in the book as a whole which constitute the sizable and painstaking task that one should be wise enough to avoid.

Into such a forbidding situation we welcome Drs. Vaughan and McKay. They were not chosen lightly, nor did they come in blindly. Each has been a major contributor to past editions and Dr. Vaughan has given much help with sections other than his own in several editions. Their strengths are well known to the editor. Each has a broad base in pediatrics, each has special interests which are complementary, and each is a competent and stimulating teacher. For the current edition they have shared in the general planning, in the selection of contributors and in editing. At least for the editor it has been a pleasant and an invigorating experience.

No attempt will be made to delineate the changes in this edition; they are recorded and will be apparent in the Table of Contents. We have done our best with the help of the contributors to prepare a pediatric text which depicts the status and provides perspective of current knowledge in a usable manner. The task has been a tremendous one, and we can only hope that in some degree we have measured up. It is not difficult to be humble under such circumstances. There are new contributors for several of the major sections and for a larger number of the shorter ones. To both the old and new contributors we are indebted for the thoroughness with which they have covered their respective subjects and for their generosity in accepting the editing necessary to permit publication in a single volume and to provide a semblance of unity in literary style throughout.

As must be the case in a textbook such as this one, there are many unrecorded contributors who have helped in a variety of ways. Most of the members of our respective departments and many in other departments of our medical schools have provided assistance. It is not possible to acknowledge all of them, but we must give special credit to Drs. Richard Behrman, Mary Coté, Catharine Dacou, George Farrar, Joseph Garfunkel, Warren Grover, Doris Howell, Eleanor Hunt, Jerold Lucey, Demosthenes Pappagainis, Carol Phillipps, Charles Poser, Nancy Huang and J. Viswanathan.

To our publisher, the Saunders Company, we acknowledge not only our continuing indebtedness for their interest and care in providing a suitable format but also for the pleasure of working with them. We must here acknowledge the long and pleasant association of Mr. John Shaw in the editing of our book and wish him all the best in the retirement which he is now looking forward to.

*Griffith-Mitchell ('33, '37, '41), Mitchell-Nelson ('45, '50) and Nelson ('54, '59, '64) Textbook of Pediatrics; there were two 2 volume editions, Griffith, 1919, and Griffith-Mitchell, 1927. Both J. P. Crozer Griffith and A. Graeme Mitchell died in 1941, shortly after publication of the 3rd edition.

For the many tasks involved in the work of the book we have had not only the best but the most pleasant of help. The new members have included Mrs. Vaughan and Mrs. Estelle W. Brown (a former colleague and a long time friend of the senior editor and more recently a colleague of Dr. McKay). And as usual my family has constituted the inside work force: Jane (Mrs. Edward F. Beatty, Jr.), Ann (Mrs. Richard E. Behrman) and Deborah (William's wife).

And as for the final editing there has been no change. I need only repeat a paragraph from the Preface of the fourth edition (my first):

"Finally, the editorial 'we' must be explained. The task of editing has been shared by my wife. No one has made a comparable contribution. She has read and reread every word in this entire book, except those in this paragraph. If there is any evenness and smoothness of construction, much of the credit is hers."

And so with the associate editors and the contributors we trust that this ninth edition will serve effectively for those who are interested in and concerned about the welfare of children.

WALDO E. NELSON

CONTENTS

xiii

11. THE DIGESTIVE SYSTEM

13. THE CARDIOVASCULAR SYSTEM

1.   The Field of Pediatrics

AN INTRODUCTION TO THE MEDICAL PROBLEMS OF INFANTS AND CHILDREN

No field of specialized medicine has a broader scope, greater responsibilities or greater possibilities than has pediatrics. One important fact sets it apart from other divisions of medicine: it is chiefly concerned with the *continued* growth and development of its subjects.

The goal in the medical management of the child is to permit him to come into adulthood at *his* optimal state of development, physically, mentally and socially, so that he can compete at *his* most effective level. The physician who cares for children must of course be familiar with the illnesses and psychologic disturbances peculiar to infants and children and their reactions to them. But he must also know what constitutes adequate achievement at successive age levels for children of different body types and capabilities, with or without obvious physical or mental handicaps. *This, the individualization of the child, is the essence of pediatric practice.*

In the years from birth to maturity, when growth is complete, the physician must deal with a subject who is so different at various stages that it might almost seem he had been several distinct individuals. The characteristics of these stages are not sharply demarcated, but blend from one into the next. Nevertheless the general pattern of each stage is sufficiently different to consider each one separately. These stages, the general characteristics of which are considered in the section on Growth and Development, are (1) the intrauterine period; (2) the neonatal period, the first 4 weeks of life; (3) the period of infancy and of rapid growth, the first 2 years; (4) the preschool period, 2 to 6 years; (5) the period of midchildhood or the early school period, 6 to 10 years for girls and 6 to 12 years for boys; (6) the prepubescent period, 10 to 12 years for girls and 12 to 14 years for boys; and (7) the pubescent and postpubescent period (adolescence), 12 to 18 years for girls and 14 to 20 years for boys. In the strict sense the process of birth should also be considered a separate period, since infection or injury to the infant at this time may have serious and even permanent effects.

A number of factors are responsible for variations in the clinical manifestations of disease caused by identical causative agents in infants or children and in adults. These differences are implied by the phrase that "the child is not a little man" and include variations at the several age levels in anatomic, physiologic, pathologic and immunologic patterns. In most respects there is a direct relation to age: the younger the child, the more notable are the differences.

Anatomic variants, such as the relative thinness of the chest wall, the more horizontal position of the heart, and the open sutures of the cranial bones in infants, are responsible for physical findings which both in health and in disease differ from those related to the same structures in adults.

Physiologically, the relatively greater nutritional needs of infants (calories, proteins, minerals, vitamins and water) reflect the requirements for growth in excess of those for basal functions and physical activity. During illness the infant and the small child have less ability than the adult to maintain homeostasis. For example, the infant with a diarrheal disturbance is in a more precarious position than an older child because of the greater rapidity with which severe disturbances of water and electrolyte metabolism develop.

Pathologically, the differences appear to be related mainly to the effects of injurious agents upon growing tissue in contrast to those upon mature tissue. The distinctly different clinical patterns of vitamin D (rickets) and vitamin C (scurvy) deficiencies in infants in contrast to the manifestations of the same deficiencies in older children or in adults are excellent examples.

Immunologically, the infant is, in general, more susceptible and less resistant to infection. There are exceptions: to a few infections the infant inherits a short-lived immunity from the mother.

Mental development and *psychologic development* provide the most important measures of the adequacy of growth during infancy and childhood. Training, education and molding of the child's personality determine the level of ultimate achievement. Parent education and child and family guidance have become increasingly important in the medical care of children.

Pediatrics as a specialty of medical practice had its inception in this country in the latter part of the nineteenth century. Since then there have been great changes in the medical problems of children and consequently in pediatric practice. In 1900 the death rate for infants under 1 year of age was in the range of 200 per 1000 live births; in 1965 it was 24.7 for the country as a whole, and in some areas significantly lower. The death rates in the subsequent years of childhood have been reduced to an even greater extent. The notable

1

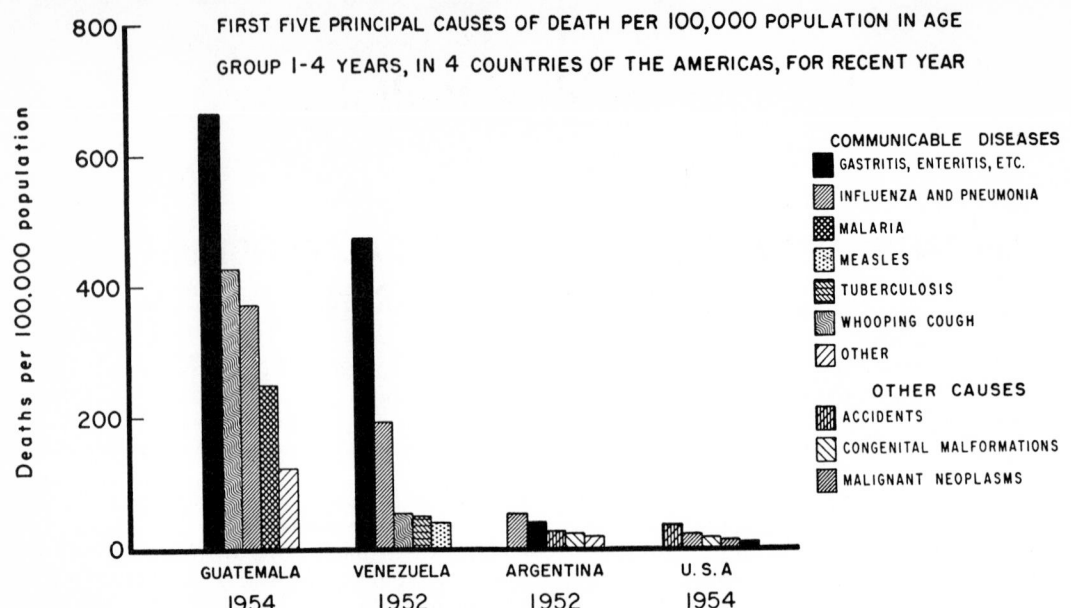

Figure 1-1. Child Mortality in the Americas, March, 1957. (Pan American Sanitary Organization — World Health Organization.)

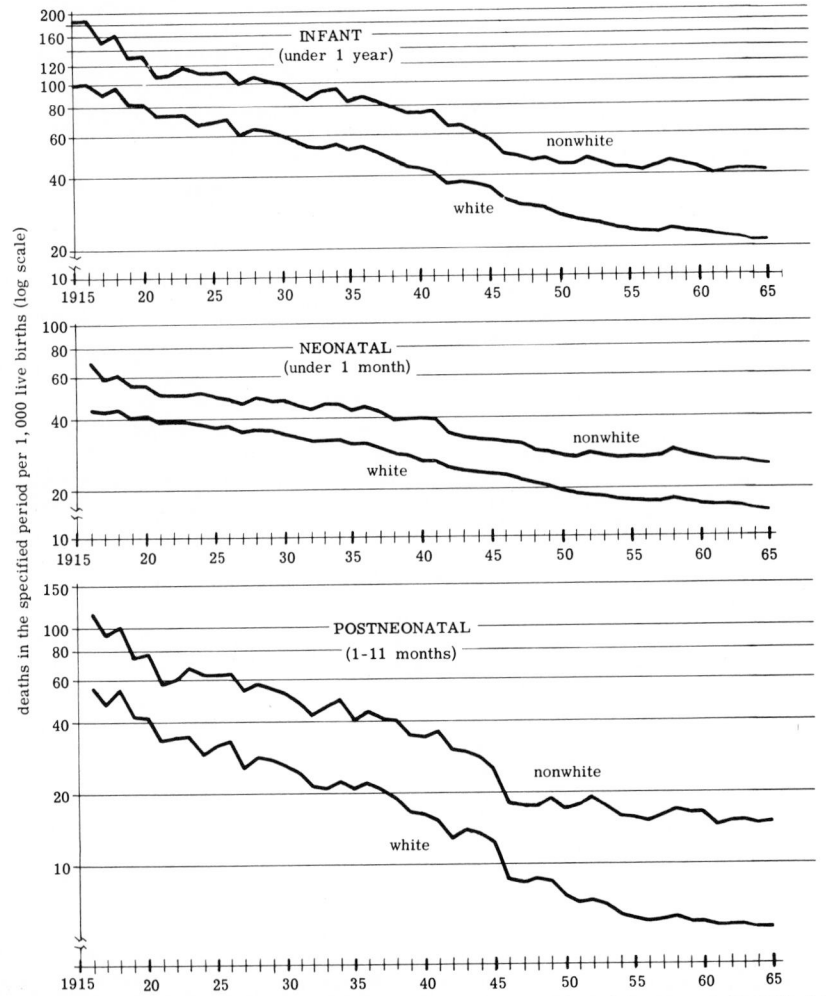

Figure 1-2. Mortality rate of white and of nonwhite infants by age, United States, 1915-1965 (birth registration area). (United States Department of Health, Education, and Welfare, Social and Rehabilitation Service, Children's Bureau. Data from United States Public Health Service, National Center for Health Statistics.)

2

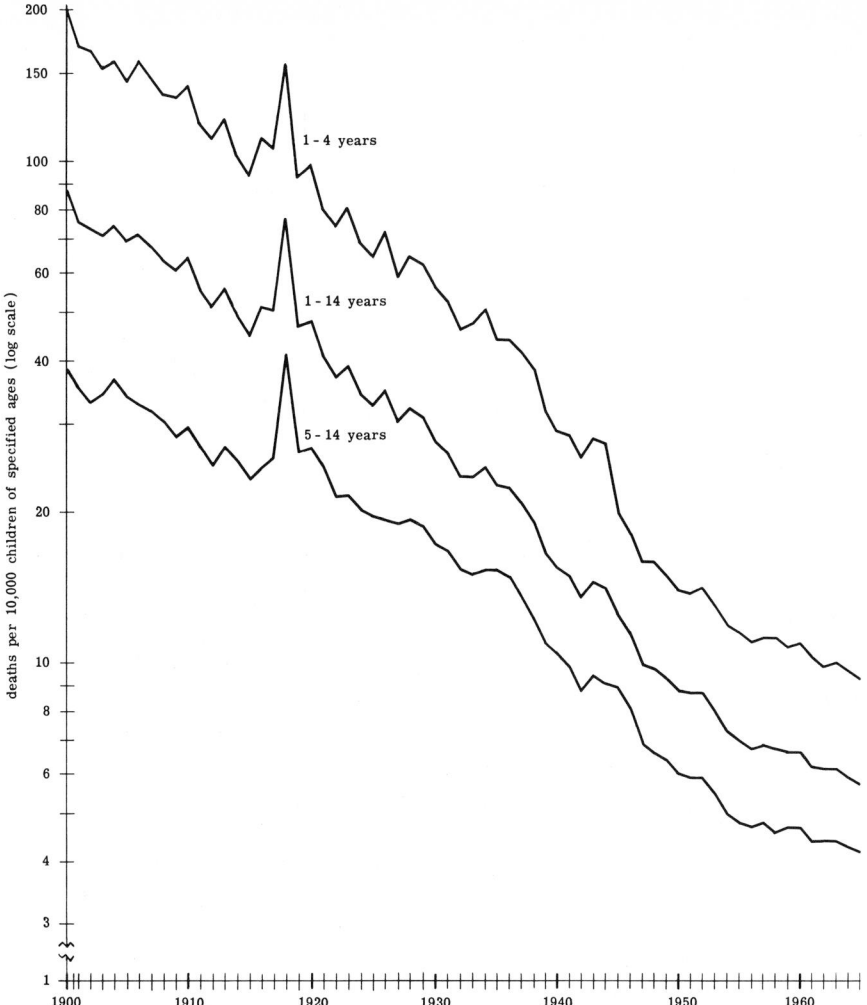

Figure 1-3. Childhood mortality rate by age, United States, 1900-1965 (death registration area). (United States Department of Health, Education, and Welfare, Social and Rehabilitation Service, Children's Bureau.)

reduction in the incidence of serious illness is attributable to a number of factors, some general, some specific. Improvements in the socioeconomic status of population groups as represented by better housing and more adequate diets have been factors in increasing resistance to disease. Specifically, prevention of such diseases as diphtheria, smallpox, poliomyelitis and measles has been accomplished by active immunization. Educational measures have been highly effective in the prevention of other diseases; these include isolation of tuberculous patients and the sterilization of milk formulas for infant feeding. The latter, in preventing diarrheal disease, has been the most important factor in the reduction of infant mortality in the postneonatal period. Within the past 30 years or so the availability of effective antimicrobial agents has made possible successful therapy of many otherwise fatal infections. Such nutritional disturbances as rickets, scurvy, pellagra and nutritional edema have been largely eradicated in this and many other countries by

general and specific health measures. The differences in the mortality rates of infants and small children between countries with variations in living standards are shown in Figures 1-1 through 1-6. Though there have been sharp reductions in morbidity and mortality in many of the developing countries, high rates for both continue in many underprivileged areas, including the slum areas of urban United States (see p. 9).

PEDIATRIC CARE

Certain persons, even some closely connected with medical circles, hold a limited concept of the field of pediatrics. To some the practice of pediatrics is essentially infant feeding; to others it is the management of the ills of the first 2 or 3 years of life; to still others it is the practice of preventive medicine; and to a few it is simply the management of behavior disorders. It is all these and

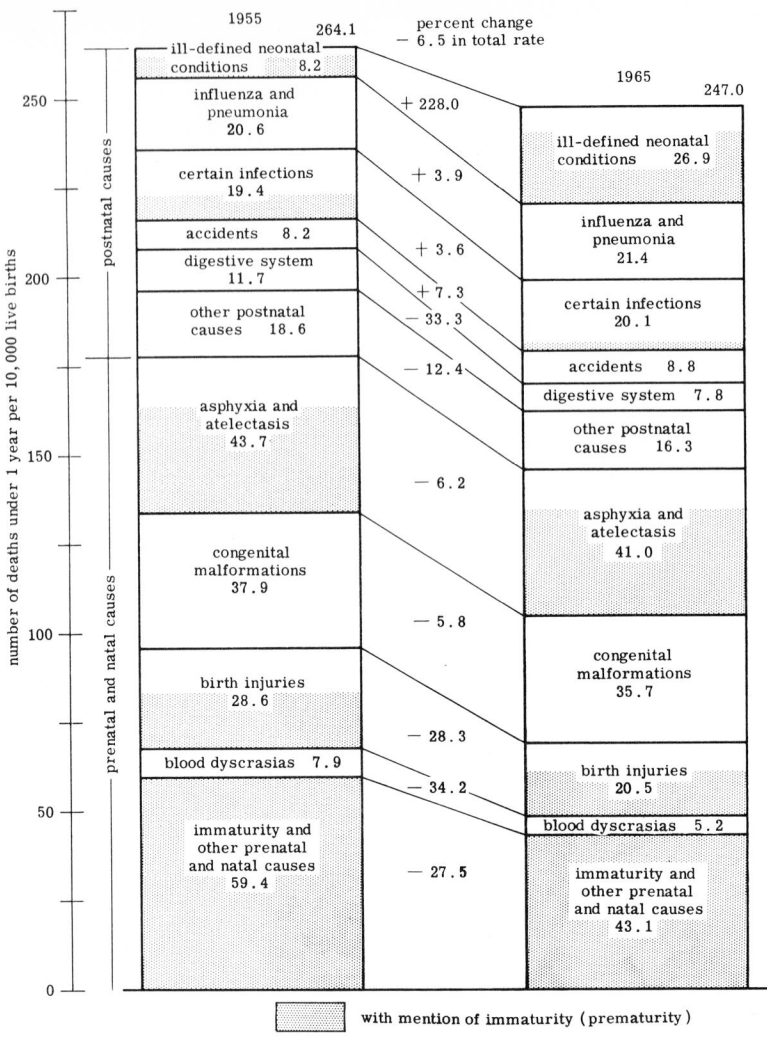

Figure 1-4. Infant mortality rate: main causes by international lists (6th and 7th revisions), United States, 1955 and 1965. (United States Department of Health, Education, and Welfare, Social and Rehabilitation Service, Children's Bureau. Data from United States Public Health Service, National Center for Health Statistics.)

more. Concern for the child must antedate conception and extend through the final phases of growth in the period of adolescence. Care of the unborn child is provided by adequate supervision of the pregnant woman, and obstetric care at the time of delivery is directly reflected in the welfare of the infant. The neonatal period is the most hazardous period of life and presents problems that never arise again. Infancy is the period of most rapid growth. This is the time when the infant is completely dependent on others for all phases of his care; when he is not only more susceptible to infections and nutritional disturbances, but often has a pattern of response to them which differs from that of later years. As infancy is passed and the preschool, prepuberty and adolescent ages are attained, the child assumes increasing responsibility for his own care, but intelligent and understanding pediatric supervision can continue to be an important aid. Surveys of children in all eco-

nomic strata reveal a high incidence of nutritional and physical disturbances and of psychologic difficulties which are remedial and, more important, preventable.

PROBLEMS OF VARIOUS AGE PERIODS

Advisability of Parenthood (see also pp. 121 and 343). Young persons contemplating marriage, and couples who have had one or more defective offspring, often seek advice about the advisability of future parenthood. The increasing tendency for some degree of civil control over physical and mental fitness for marriage and parenthood will probably result in more frequent consultations. The physician who assumes such a responsibility must be well informed in the medical and legal aspects of fitness for parenthood. The problem involves factors related to the genetic

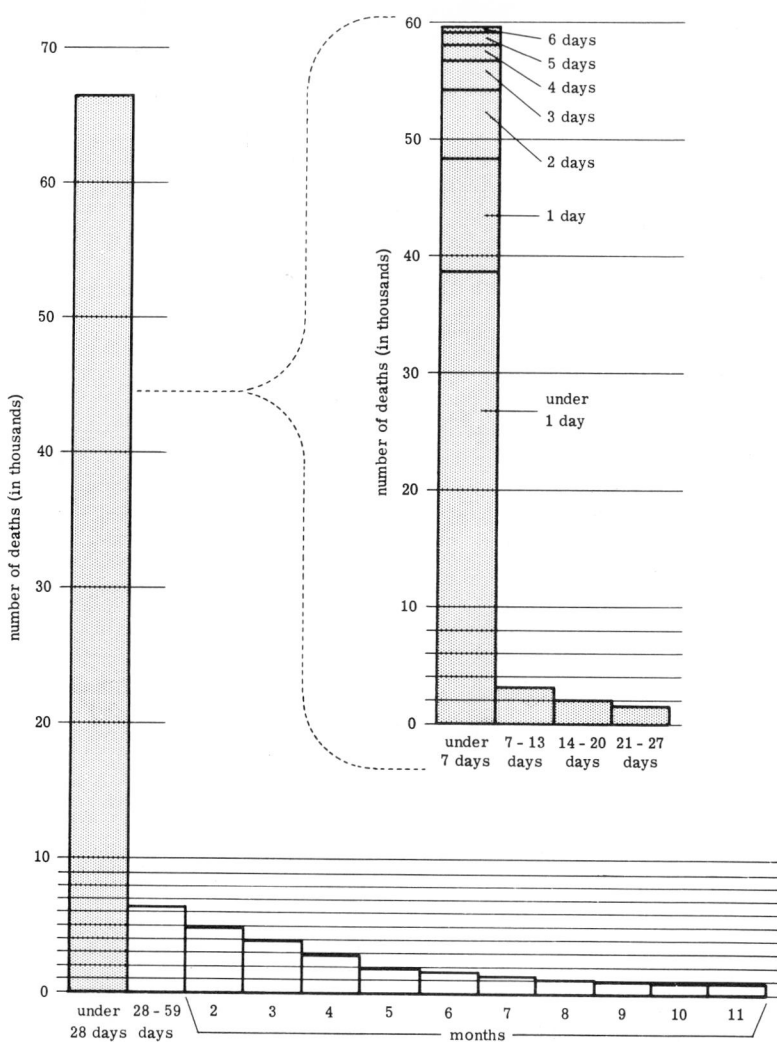

Figure 1-5. Infant mortality by age, United States, 1965. (United States Department of Health, Education, and Welfare, Social and Rehabilitation Service, Children's Bureau. Data from United States Public Health Service, National Center for Health Statistics.)

patterns and to the physical, mental and moral fitness of the prospective parents. Moral fitness constitutes the most difficult problem and, unless legal measures can be taken, is not controllable beyond the cooperation of the prospective parents.

Prenatal Factors (see also pp. 19, 318 and 347). Factors which determine the physical, mental and emotional pattern of the child-to-be are operative in each parent before conception, and medical interest must be directed increasingly at such factors. The pediatrician should recognize his responsibilities for assisting in the preparation of his child-patient for his role as a parent. Here, attention is directed to those factors which determine the survival and health status of embryo, fetus and child.

A variety of antenatal influences may be responsible for stillbirth, premature birth, or retardation of growth in utero with shortened, average or prolonged gestation, and for disease or deformities which are manifest postnatally. In general these factors can be grouped into 3 categories: (1) the effects of one or more abnormal genes, (2) the effects of chromosomal aberrations, and (3) the effects of abnormal intrauterine (environmental) influences. A few examples in each category are listed in Table 1-3; detailed descriptions are provided elsewhere.

Regular prenatal visits to the physician have had a distinct effect in the reduction of both maternal and infant mortality. These visits should also be used to counsel the parents about the care of the newborn infant. Many problems of early infancy could be averted if prospective parents had a better concept of infant care and especially of how simple and natural it can and should be.

Perinatal Factors. Every infant should be delivered by an adequately trained physician. The fact that more than 5000 infant deaths a year are directly attributable to birth injuries and that

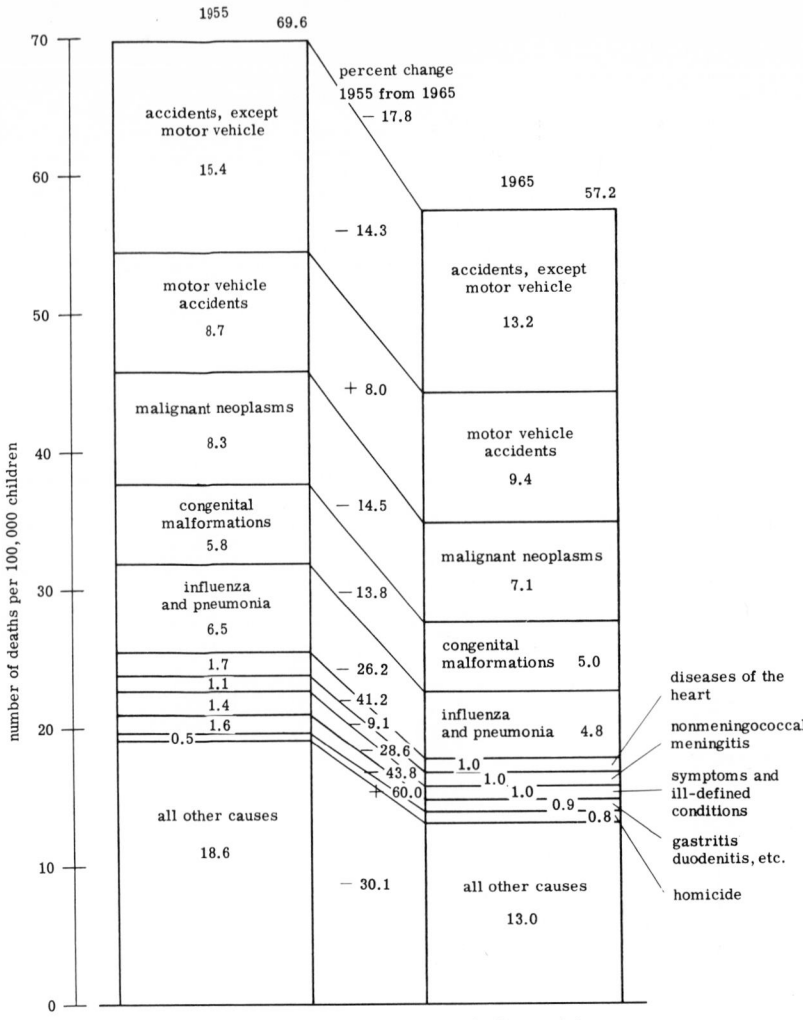

Figure 1-6. Childhood mortality rate, 1-14 years of age, United States, 1955 and 1965: main causes by international lists (6th and 7th revisions). (United States Department of Health, Education, and Welfare, Social and Rehabilitation Service, Children's Bureau. Data from United States Public Health Service, National Center for Health Statistics.)

many other infants are crippled for life illustrates the need for improvement in the technique of obstetric care. The choice and use of sedatives and anesthetics, the mechanics of delivery, including the improper use of forceps as well as failure to use them at appropriate times, and the management of the infant immediately after birth are factors which affect the offspring. Failure to clear the air passages of mucus and amniotic fluid contents, damage resulting from manual and mechanical attempts at resuscitation, failure to prevent chilling the infant, and nonantiseptic technique are also important factors.

The perinatal period (from the beginning of labor or the time of rupture of the amniotic membrane, whichever is first, through the first day of life) is of extraordinary importance. Infections acquired at this time include gonorrheal ophthalmia, oral moniliasis, salmonellosis, herpes simplex,

listeriosis and, most important from the standpoints of frequency and total mortality, pneumonia. The last is usually caused by bacteria, most often of the coliform group, acquired through the vaginal tract, and occurs with particular frequency among infants born after premature rupture of the membranes or traumatic delivery and among those whose birth weights are less than 2500 gm.

Neonatal Factors (see also pp. 20 and 353). During the neonatal period the infant must make adjustments to extrauterine existence. The difficulties are illustrated in part by the exceedingly high mortality rate and by the multiplicity of physical disturbances, many of them characteristic of this period.

Low weight (less than 2500 gm.) at birth has traditionally been identified by the term *prematurity* (pp. 23, 360). Though it has long been recognized that some infants born at term or even

TABLE 1-1. MAIN CAUSES OF DEATH AMONG CHILDREN 1-4 YEARS OF AGE;
UNITED STATES, 1965 AND SPECIFIED YEARS

CAUSE OF DEATH*	RATE PER 100,000 CHILDREN 1-4 YEARS					
	1965	1960	1950	1940	1930	1920
	92.9	108.8	139.4	289.6	563.6	987.2
	72.3	83.6	98.0	198.4	409.7	794.4
	31.8	31.5	36.8	48.7	61.2	80.2
, except motor vehicle	21.3	21.5	25.3	36.3	46.7	71.1
hicle accidents	10.5	10.0	11.5	12.4	14.5	—
and pneumonia	11.4	16.2	18.9	62.5	123.1	283.7
l malformations	10.2	12.8	11.1	10.3	—	—
t neoplasms, including neoplasms of lym- and hematopoietic tissues	8.6	10.8	11.7	—	—	—
is, except meningococcal and tuberculous	2.6	2.8	2.8	—	—	—
, duodenitis, enteritis and colitis, except ea of newborn*	2.4	3.2	5.3	—	—	—
ns and ill-defined conditions	2.4	2.8	—	—	—	—
ococcal infections	1.8	1.4	2.6	—	—	—
tis	1.1	2.1	2.5	—	—	—
Ms	—	—	—	—	21.9	56.4
Tuberculosis, all forms	—	—	6.3	12.3	25.9	45.4
Dea, enteritis, etc.*	—	—	—	30.2	95.6	141.3
Wing cough	—	—	—	9.7	23.4	57.7
Diphtheria	—	—	—	9.0	33.5	90.5
Lises of the ear, nose and throat	—	—	—	8.9	15.2	12.3
Appendicitis	—	—	—	6.8	—	—
Scaret fever	—	—	—	—	9.9	23.2
Dysentery	—	—	—	—	—	12.8
All other causes	20.6	25.2	41.4	91.2	153.9	192.8

*Causes of death listed each year are the 10 main causes in that year. For 1960 and 1965, titles of the causes listed, and inclusions in each cause group, are those of the Seventh Revision, International Statistical Classification of Diseases, Injuries and Causes of Death; for 1950 and 1955, inclusions are those of the Sixth Revision; for 1940, inclusions are according to the Fifth Revision; for 1930, according to the Fourth Revison; and for 1920, according to the Second Revision. Rates are unadjusted for changes in the classification of causes of death in successive revisions of the lists. In 1950 and later years, "Diarrhea of the newborn" was included in "Diarrhea, enteritis, etc."

Department of Health, Education, and Welfare, Social and Rehabilitation Service, Children's Bureau. Based on data from the Public Health Service, National Vital Statistics Division, National Center for Health Statistics.

Symbol: — Class or item not applicable.

always be available when needed and, of equal importance, where confidence and love are continually present. Many of the preventable cases of juvenile delinquency have their inception during these years. It is the wise physician who can assist in the problems of adjustment within the child's various groups—his family, school and playmates.

goal is a physically sound, mentally alert, y adjusted preadolescent child.

escent Factors (see pp. 28 and 71). During this period there are tremendous physical and physiologic changes which in natural situations occasion no difficulties. Unfortunately, al situations" prevail too infrequently. The man who guides a child through the pre- ent years and understands him should have advantages as the medical advisor for escent years. But this can be true only if rstands the problems of this period and necessary time to each of his patients. ysical disturbances include such chronic as dental caries, acne, otitis media, s and nontuberculous pulmonary in- eumatic carditis, osteomyelitis, gonor-

rhea and syphilis; nutritional disturbances which range from undifferentiated malnutrition through the various specific nutritional deficiency diseases; and endocrine disturbances.

The onset of puberty and the rate of development during adolescence vary considerably from child to child. The rapidity of growth at this time makes the child especially vulnerable to detrimental influences, and one may expect physical disturbances to have more significant effects upon growth and development than they do in the years of relatively slower growth between infancy and puberty.

The working adolescent child presents special problems. In part these are being met by special legislation; but many factors center in the home and in recreational and educational facilities, besides those concerned with the type and place of work.

Health education should include adequate sex education; it should have been initiated in the earlier years of childhood and can be effectively reinforced at this age. Behavior and social problems constitute a large part of adolescent care. Though emphasis should be placed on preventive post term may weigh less than 2500 gm., the relative frequency of intrauterine growth retardation has been appreciated only in recent years. At the moment, efforts are being made to find a more suitable term to categorize the low-birth-weight infant. Until such a term is adopted, it will be appropriate in most instances to assume that, when the term "prematurity" is used, it is to identify the low-birth-weight infant irrespective of the length of his gestation.

The enormity of the risks attendant in being born at a weight of less than 2500 gm. is illustrated by the mortality rates of the first year of life and by the high incidence of permanent mental and physical defects among the survivors. Prematurity, immaturity or low-birth-weight should not be considered a cause of death, at least in infants weighing more than 1000 gm. at birth. Careful postmortem examination will reveal the cause of death in the majority of instances. The three principal causes of death in low-birth-weight infants are the pulmonary hyaline membrane syndrome, intraventricular hemorrhage and infection. The first two are rare in term infants, and the mortality rate due to infection in low-birth-weight infants approximates a ratio of 40:1 with that in full-term infants (Temple data). Case fatality death rates within the several weight groupings of low-birth-weight infants and causes of death are listed on page xxx. The smaller the infant, the less is his chance of survival. Unfortunately, United States vital statistics data do not relate first-year mortality rates with birth weight (see Tables 1-1, 1-2, and Figures 1-2, 1-3, 1-4, 1-5, 1-6). Reasonable estimates indicate that about 90 per cent of the more than 90,000 deaths of infants annually in this country occur in the 7 to 8 per cent of infants born at birth weights less than 2500 gm. Of the survivors (low birth weight), it has been estimated that as many as one third have significant mental or motor handicaps.

Though disease acquired during the first month of life is relatively less important as a cause of death in the neonatal period than that acquired during the birth process, it does account for a significant number of deaths in the first year of life. Within hospital nurseries the danger of cross infections of epidemic proportions is a constant one. Infections with *Staphylococcus aureus,* pseudomonas and enteropathogenic *E. coli,* as well as certain viruses, are especially important in this respect.

Infancy Factors. Infancy is the period of most rapid extrauterine growth. Adequate growth and development, both physical and mental, are essential to normal infancy, and the rates of development constitute the best measures available for evaluation of the infant's status. During most of this period the infant is dependent on others for maintenance. Walking and eating alone are usually achieved by the latter part of this period. Nutritional deficiencies are thus particularly likely to be the fault of the person who designs the diet or feeds the infant. Likewise, infec-

tions a
going to
school ye
they make
simpler to a
only more su
disorders, but
to them, and
clinical patterns.
immunity during
for measles, dipht
myelitis if the moth
other common contag
coccal, staphylococcal,
infections.

The mortality rate for ti
months of the first year o
that for the first month alone

Analyses of mortality rate
death rates are consistently hig
for females in all races, higher
than in the white race, and higher
in the winter months than in othe
year. It has been demonstrated
infant mortality rate among familie
nomic status can be reduced by educ
mother in the principles of infant ca
gence, education, housing, and economic
probably more important than racial fact

Preschool Age Factors. This period, t
lier part of which is termed the toddler ag
safer one than infancy. The preschool age i
portant because the health of the child at
period is definitely reflected in the school ye
Emphasis should be placed on normal living, wi
ample opportunity for the child to explore and b
come acquainted with his expanding world. T
"guiding hand," which seems to be a necessit
the complexity of modern living, must lead
restrain (set and maintain limits), but shou
prohibit the child from developing his own n
pattern.

Adequate nutrition, immunization ap
preventable diseases, education in the
of the nonpreventable ones and in the
of accidents, secondary screening for
visual defects (primary screening d
with correction when indicated,
quate medical care for disease, a
family living are the important
is a physically sound, mentall
justed candidate for entrance

School Age Factors. T
period from 5 through 14 y
that for the period of 1 t
ticular interest is the re
the relative positions
diseases and cancer as

The expanding envi
these years provide
portunities for men
parents will permi
determination wit
a haven at home

TABLE 1-2. MAIN CAUSES OF DEATH AMONG CHILDREN 5-14 YEARS OF AGE; UNITED STATES, 1965 AND SPECIFIED YEARS

CAUSE OF DEATH*	RATE PER 100,000 CHILDREN 5-14 YEARS					
	1965	1960	1950	1940	1930	1920
All causes	42.2	46.6	59.8	103.7	171.7	263.9
Main causes	32.8	35.9	44.7	67.6	111.8	196.3
Accidents	18.7	19.2	22.6	28.6	36.1	44.3
Accidents, except motor vehicle	9.8	11.3	13.8	17.1	21.4	31.3
Motor vehicle accidents	8.9	7.9	8.8	11.5	14.7	13.0
Malignant neoplasms, including neoplasms of lymphatic and hematopoietic tissues	6.5	6.8	6.7	3.0	—	—
Congenital malformations	2.8	3.6	2.4	2.1	—	—
Influenza and pneumonia	2.1	2.6	3.2	9.0	18.8	45.1
Vascular lesions affecting central nervous system	0.7	0.7	—	—	—	—
Benign neoplasms and neoplasms of unspecified nature	0.6	0.7	0.8	—	—	—
Homicide	0.6	—	—	—	—	—
Anemias	0.4	0.5	—	—	—	—
Diseases of the heart*	0.4	1.3	3.9	10.6	15.1	21.8
Symptoms and ill-defined conditions	—	0.5	0.8	—	—	—
Acute poliomyelitis	—	—	2.5	—	—	—
Appendicitis	—	—	—	0.8	13.1	—
Tuberculosis, all forms	—	—	1.8	5.5	11.9	22.4
Chronic and unspecified nephritis	—	—	—	1.7	—	3.5
Diphtheria	—	—	—	1.7	8.1	28.0
Typhoid fever	—	—	—	—	4.4	7.1
Meningococcal infections	—	—	—	—	4.3	—
Diarrhea, enteritis, etc.	—	—	—	—	3.0	4.1
Diabetes mellitus	—	—	—	—	—	3.5
All other causes	9.4	10.7	15.1	36.1	59.9	67.6

*Causes of death listed each year are the 10 main causes in that year. For 1960 and 1965, titles of the causes listed, and inclusions in each cause group, are those of the Seventh Revision of the International Statistical Classification of Diseases, Injuries, and Causes of Death; for 1950 and 1955, inclusions are those of the Sixth Revision; for 1940, inclusions are according to the Fifth Revision; for 1930, according to the Fourth Revision; and for 1920, according to the Second Revision. Rates are unadjusted for changes in the classification of causes of death in successive revisions of the lists, but the category "Diseases of the heart" was adjusted to include rheumatic fever for each year specified.

Department of Health, Education, and Welfare, Social and Rehabilitation Service, Children's Bureau. Based on data from the Public Health Service, National Vital Statistics Division, National Center for Health Statistics.

measures in the preadolescent period, many maladjusted children will continue to require treatment. The problem of juvenile delinquency is especially urgent. Special clinics for adolescents are doing much to meet the needs of this age group, and their extension is to be encouraged, as are increased provisions for vocational guidance.

Handicapped Children. Children with physical and mental handicaps present special problems. The term "handicapped" implies a physical or mental defect not compatible with usual activity or expected achievement. Formerly much attention was centered on the orthopedic cripple, but in recent years interest has broadened to include almost all types of defects. Special attention is required for children with hearing, speech and sight defects, with cardiac disease, with tuberculosis, with orthopedic defects of peripheral and central origin, with mental retardation and with psychotic disorders. In addition to specialized medical attention, there is need for special classes, schools and institutions.

Initially, the problem is one of detection. Then the child must be thoroughly evaluated physically, mentally and psychologically. The family situation must also be appraised. All this usually requires a team approach. But the child and his family must have a single physician who assumes overall responsibility and directs the program for the child. "Handicapped" children and their families must be treated realistically. Everything should be done which will provide the child with *his* optimal opportunities, but neither the child nor his family should be led to expect the impossible. Only to the extent that the child can be brought to a stage of independence compatible with his handicap can success be said to have been attained.

Socioeconomic Factors. The health problems of infants and children are distinctly different, both qualitatively and quantitatively, in population groups of low socioeconomic status in contrast to those in groups with higher average annual incomes and greater educational opportunities. These differences are illustrated in part by the comparative infant mortality rates in the United States between white and nonwhite persons: 21.5 and 40.3, respectively, per 1000 live births in 1965 for the country as a whole; the relatively low combined rate of 18.3 for white and nonwhite infants

TABLE 1-3. Examples of Congenitally Acquired Disorders in Each of the 3 Principal Categories: Genetic, Chromosomal and Intrauterine (Environmental)

GENETIC DISORDERS

Spontaneously manifest

  Tay-Sachs disease
  Vitamin D-resistant rickets

Manifestations dependent upon contributing factors

Contributing factors	*Clinical consequence in genetically susceptible persons*
Trauma	Hemorrhage with hemophilia Fractures with osteogenesis imperfecta
Bacterial invasion	Infection in agammaglobulinemia
Ingestion of specific nutrients	
Galactose	Galactosemia
Phenylalanine	Phenylketonuria
Leucine	Hypoglycemia
Fava beans	Hemolytic anemia (G-6-PD deficiency)
Environmental	
Temperature	Hyperpyrexia and dehydration in nephrogenic diabetes insipidus Hyponatremia and shock in fibrocystic disease Hyperpyrexia in anhidrotic ectodermal dysplasia
Drugs and poisons	
Succinyl dicholine	Prolonged apnea in pseudocholinesterase deficiency
Primaquine, naphthalene, sulfonilamide and others	Hemolytic anemia in G-6-PD deficiency
Isoimmunization	Hemolytic disease of the newborn
Solar radiation	Hydroa estivale in congenital porphyria

CHROMOSOMAL ABERRATIONS

Chromosomal aberrations include (1) variations in number, more or less than 46; (2) mosaicism; and (3) structural alterations

Variations in numbers (aneuploidy)

Autosomes	
Down's syndrome (mongolism)	Trisomy 21
D trisomy	Trisomy 13-15
Trisomy 18	
Sex chromosomes	
Turner's syndrome	XO
Klinefelter's syndrome	XXY
Klinefelter variants	XXXY, XXXXY
Others	XXX, XXXX, XXXXX, XYY

Mosaicism of numbers

Autosomes	
Partial trisomy 21	46/47
Sex chromosomes	
Turner's syndrome	XO/XX

Translocations

Autosomes	
Translocation Down's syndrome or translocation carrier ...	15/21 translocation 21/21 translocation 21/22 translocation

Deletions

Autosomes	
Cri du chat syndrome	Deletion of short arm of B chromosome
Deletion of short arm of chromosome 18	
Deletion of long arm of chromosome 18	
Ring chromosomes	Variable clinical expression
Sex chromosomes	
Deletion of X chromosome	

TABLE 1-3. EXAMPLES OF CONGENITALLY ACQUIRED DISORDERS IN EACH OF THE 3 PRINCIPAL CATEGORIES: GENETIC, CHROMOSOMAL AND INTRAUTERINE (ENVIRONMENTAL) *(Continued)*

INTRAUTERINE (ENVIRONMENTAL) FACTORS

Causative factor	*Disorder*
Trauma	
Isolated injury during pregnancy (most unusual)	Varied
Intrauterine pressure (Chapple)	Congenital hip dysplasia (?), micrognathia
Maternal undernutrition, especially preconceptional	Low birth weight Anemia
Irradiation	Unknown with certainty for human beings
Infections	Evident maternal disease Syphilis, tuberculosis, rubella, poliomyelitis
	Nonevident maternal disease Toxoplasmosis, cytomegalic inclusion disease, listeriosis, viral myocarditis, homologous serum hepatitis, pneumonia via amnionitis
Maternal medication	
Aminopterin (as abortifacient)	Gross anomalies
Quinine	Deafness
Dicoumarin	Hypoprothrombinemia
Vitamin K	Hemolytic anemia
Propylthiouracil, Tapazole and iodides	Goiter
Organic iodides, Iophenoxic acid (Teridax)	Prolonged elevation of PBI
Androgens and progestational compounds with androgenic effect	Masculinization of female infant
Intrauterine exsanguination	Intertwin transfusion Fetus-to-mother (transplacental) transfusion
Maternal diabetes	Macrosomia Respiratory distress syndrome
With genetically appropriate mate	Diabetes mellitus
Maternal myasthenia gravis	Transient myasthenia gravis
Maternal thrombocytopenic purpura	Transient thrombocytopenia
Maternal parathyroid adenoma	Transient tetany
Maternal systemic lupus erythematosus	Transient L.E. phenomenon

Some genetic disorders are manifest at birth, some become manifest spontaneously some time after birth, and others become manifest only in conjunction with a contributing or triggering factor.

Genetic disorders may be manifest primarily as metabolic diseases (e.g. diabetes mellitus), as structural disorders (e.g. osteogenesis imperfecta), as mental deficiency (e.g. phenylketonuria), as neoplastic disease (e.g. bilateral retinoblastoma) or as combinations of any or all of these (e.g. tuberous sclerosis). In a broad sense, perhaps all genetic disorders could be classified as metabolic.

for the state of Utah (the lowest state record) and the high one of 36.1 for Washington, D.C. (the highest record for a large urban area); and the total white and nonwhite rate of 39.6 in the poverty areas of Chicago versus that of 24.5 in the nonpoverty areas of the city. The most favorable infant mortality rates are in the small European countries in which there are relatively small differences in socioeconomic status (Sweden, 13.3; Netherlands, 14.4; Norway, 16.4). The United States, with a much more disparate situation, rated fourteenth in 1965 among countries with populations in excess of one million, with vital statistics based on W.H.O. definitions and with a per capita gross product of $710.00 (U.S.) or more in 1964.

In the United States the concentration of low income and untrained and poorly educated families has shifted from rural to urban areas. Although a large proportion of these underprivileged persons are nonwhite, a significant percentage is white. The least favorable premature birth rates and perinatal, neonatal (first 28 days of life) and infant (first year) mortality rates are now to be found in the large cities. To a great extent, the pediatric health problems of cities are emphasized by high rates of low-birth-weight infants, of illegitimate births (many to very young girls) and of juvenile delinquency. For example, in Philadelphia the percentage of infants born at weights less than 2500 gm. was 11.2 in 1963 in contrast to 8.2 for the country as a whole. Within the Philadelphia metropolitan area the differential is considerably greater: in 1963, 19 per cent of infants born at Philadelphia General Hospital weighed less than 2500 gm. in contrast to 5.4 per cent of those born at a representative suburban hospital. It is obvious that data of these sorts must be utilized if planning for adequate health services has any potential to be effective.

The contrasts in health status within the underprivileged or developing countries are even more distinct. Although vital statistics of an accuracy comparable with those of the more developed countries are not available, infant mortality rates well in excess of 100 per 1000 live births obtain in some areas, with comparatively high mortality rates throughout childhood. In these countries major problems are low birth weight and high incidences of infectious diseases and malnutrition —in the main all preventable through known health measures: family planning, prenatal care, improved housing, personal hygiene, public sanitation, active immunization against preventable diseases, health education and increased financial income.

Community Responsibility. Health is a community problem. This does not imply that the individual must not assume personal responsibility or that the practice of medicine should not be a private enterprise. Certain aspects of health, such as control of communicable diseases, become the responsibility of the community merely for the protection of the uninfected. But other aspects are humanitarian ones. In a true democracy, health services should be the right of each child.

In his presentation before the White House Conference on Children in a Democracy in 1940, A. Graeme Mitchell stated the problem simply and clearly; the statement is as applicable today (1969) as it was at that time:

. . . Proper physical and mental health cannot be expected unless there are good housing, proper clothing, satisfactory food, happy family life, facilities for recreation and education. . . . There is an obvious inequality in distribution of medical care in economic groups and in communities.

. . . Some families are able through their own resources to furnish good housing, clothing, food, recreation, education, and medical care to their children. Other families must face . . . unpredictable emergencies . . . which [cause] health as well as other essentials of family life to suffer. Then there is the group who are unable through their own resources to provide even the minimum needs.

. . . These inadequacies and many others constitute failure to protect the children of this democracy. All these inequalities are the concern of all of us—of the local community, the State, and the Nation.

Individuality of the Child. In the enthusiasm of solving a medical problem the physician often fails to recognize that he is dealing with a child who is sick rather than with a physical illness itself. Often the psychic disturbances of illness are as great as or greater than the physical ones. This is as true for infants and children as for adults. Thus in pediatric practice, interest should be primarily in the child and secondarily in his disease. Every disturbance should be viewed from the standpoint of its effect upon the child and his family and why it has such an effect.

The need for such consideration was aptly expressed by the late James S. Plant in material prepared for an earlier edition of this book. An excerpt from it follows:

THE PEDIATRICIAN AND HIS PATIENT

Every child is an actor in a play; each phrase or deed is understood only as a part of his total role, and that role is meaningless except as a part of the total drama.

This role was pressed into his tiny hands long before he stepped upon the stage. Months before he was born, parents, relatives and neighbors "hoped it would be a boy" or "hoped it would be a girl"—lacking the courtesy to wait upon his arrival before deciding the part he must play. Indeed, his role goes farther back to the dreams, the tragedies, the triumphs of the early years of his parents. Who of us has not mended the disappointments of youth and adulthood with the promise that his child "will live it differently"? The role he is to play is often cast down to the last dotting of the "i" or crossing of the "t."

Children as actors differ greatly in what they do with their roles. Many, in comfortable security, accept and play the role given to them. Many are tragically unsuited for the part they are expected to play—of the wrong sex, too intelligent, too retarded, too individualistic, too dependent, too frail for the titanic struggle or too eagerly adventuresome for a part that calls for docility. Some children forever grope in confusion to find the meaning of their roles, whereas others in ritualistic manner grow, go to school, work, marry, have children, amass a fortune, die—without ever having had the slightest idea of what it is all about. The pediatrician must understand these things and carefully assay the child's fitness to do what he is supposed to do.

Time should be taken to think of the family in its total setting. If the parents are overanxious, mere irritation toward them accomplishes nothing. If the child is driven physically and mentally beyond his powers, the answer does not lie in exasperated denunciation, but rather in getting the family to assay its goals and values with more care. Every illness may be complicated—seriously so—by the family's call upon the child to be the Spartan or the dependent one. These compelling attitudes have a natural cause just as surely as do fever and pain.

It is important to know what the child means to each parent. Sometimes anxious concern over his illness is a sort of emergency repair patch for a precariously thin marital situation. Just as often the physician will find a growing jealousy in one parent as the child absorbs the interest of the other. Some carry the care and expense of the child with poor grace; others glory in this and unwisely lavish too much in their joy of self-denial. An endless number of complaints about a child may mean that he has rudely broken in upon a "career" or the building of family fortunes.

The pediatrician may feel that these matters are none of his concern. But they are serious "complications" of every illness, and the basis of all sorts of problems of child rearing that are brought to his office.

The pediatrician must also cultivate the practice of seeing the child alone and having him feel that his confidences are respected. The technique of the "own story" should be developed. This is a brief recapitulation of events, starting well behind the event under consideration. If one asks a child (or adult, for that matter) why he stole or played truant, he usually does not know. Many things we do are inexplicable as we look back upon them, but seemed reasonable when we did them. Thus the pediatrician must approach events as the child approached them. It is only as one sees what an act meant to the child at the time it was carried through that it can be understood.

The language of intelligence is words; the language of the emotions is the psychomotor tensions. One can tell a child that he has a fever; one has to show a child equanimity, courage, faith. The pediatrician cannot anxiously tell the parent to be calm, or hurriedly tell the child to be patient. We depend so much upon the written and spoken word that we fail to realize how utterly inadequate it is in the important field of the emotions. It is in the way that we talk, stand, walk, give advice that we transmit our most important messages.

In order to understand the activities and reactions of a child, the pediatrician must have or acquire three fundamental attributes:

1. *Everlasting patience.* The "ortho" tendency,

the fundamental drive to right the ship, is strong in all of us. Giving the child time and freeing him from adult anxieties and meddlesomeness are extremely important.

2. *Faith in the child's ability to solve his own problem.* Enuresis is the child's problem, as is petty stealing, lying and a legion of other matters that the parents or teachers are feverishly trying to solve for the child. When once the pediatrician has really won the child's confidence, he must persistently show his faith in that child's own ability to work out whatever his problem may be. It is not so much the pediatrician's task to stop the child's temper tantrums as to give him a fair and objective picture of what happens if they are continued.

3. *Ability to see the problem through the child's own eyes.* This is not to excuse—but to understand. Until the pediatrician has seen what the child is trying to do, he is working in the dark. Problem children are not trying to create problems—but to solve them. As fever and pain are normal reactions of normal people to abnormal conditions, so lying and stealing and persistent bed-wetting and temper tantrums may be normal reactions of normal children to unusual or abnormal conditions. In each instance the child is trying in his own way to solve a problem in human relationships.

In all these matters the pediatrician is in a peculiarly difficult position. His age and position of authority lead the child to feel that he is "just another adult." Thus he invites those same reticences, rebellions and bombastic aggressions that forced the parents to bring the child to him. Yet unless he resolutely attempts to approach the problems of childhood on this broader and natural basis, he remains a specialist in the diseases of children, rather than a specialist for children.

WALDO E. NELSON

PROLOGUE

No appraisal of the child is complete which does not assess his developmental status, nor any program of management complete which does not continuously evaluate how illness or treatment may change or distort his pattern of growth or behavior. The thoughtful physician must be concerned also with the ways in which assets or liabilities in the child's family, neighborhood, school or community may facilitate or impede his progress toward healthy and productive adulthood.

The study of the child begins with examination of the patterns of growth of normal children. These must serve as guides to detection, diagnosis and treatment of the disorders of childhood. They will help the physician guide child and parents toward the fulfillment of their roles in satisfying ways. Those caring for children should understand, respect and enjoy them. It is our hope that the pages that follow will contribute to this understanding, respect and enjoyment.

2. Developmental Pediatrics

GROWTH AND DEVELOPMENT

The ripening of a fertilized human ovum through the stages of embryonic and fetal life, infancy, childhood and adolescence has physical, behavioral, intellectual, emotional, social and cultural aspects. Each aspect is the subject of intensive study in its own right and is the focal point of a growing body of knowledge. Growth and development do not take place independently in discrete areas or systems, but represent a continuum of interactions between innate genetic potential on the one hand and the environment on the other.

The degree of realization of biologic potential in the individual is the product of many interrelated factors or forces. *Genetic* factors, which are often thought of as establishing final limits to biologic potential, are inextricably interwoven with the environment. For example, in galactosemia the deleterious effect of abnormal genes may be aborted if the diet of the newborn infant does not contain lactose. *Trauma* may be prenatal or postnatal; it may be chemical as in the distortion of growth by drugs such as thalidomide and abortifacients, or it may be physical, radiant, immunologic, or residual from infection. *Nutritional* factors are fundamental to optimal growth, both prenatally and postnatally; faulty nutrition in the mother, for example, may contribute to increased incidences of stillbirths and premature births and to other conditions such as toxemia of pregnancy, which may present a hazard to the survival of the newborn infant. Nutritional and *socioeconomic* factors are, of course, closely interwoven. *Social and emotional* factors are important modifiers of growth potential. The position of the child in the family, the quality of interaction between child and parent within the first few months of life, the child-rearing patterns and the personal concerns and needs of the parents are profoundly important to the degree of self-realization achieved by the growing child. *Cultural* considerations may limit the child by establishing conventional expectations as to what his behavior will be throughout his life, and may conspicuously alter the time scale for acquisition of skills such as sitting, creeping, standing or walking, which were thought to be almost entirely maturationally determined. Further study is needed to determine the degree to which developmental patterns depend upon genetic, nutritional, emotional, socioeconomic and cultural determinants.

PARAMETERS OF GROWTH AND DEVELOPMENT

The term *growth* has commonly been used for those aspects of maturation which can be reduced to a measurement of size; the term *development* refers to changes in the function of the organism. Because these 2 aspects cannot be sharply differentiated, the term *growth and development* is generally given a unitary meaning implying both the magnitude and quality of maturational changes.

Physical growth and development encompasses changes in the size and function of the organism. Changes in function range from those at the molecular level in fetal life through the activation of enzyme systems in the neonatal period to the complex metabolic changes associated with puberty and adolescence.

Intellectual growth and development is difficult to differentiate from neurologic and behavioral maturation in early infancy. In later infancy or early childhood, intellectual function is increasingly measured by communicative skills and the ability of the child to handle abstract and symbolic material.

Emotional growth and development depends upon the infant's ability to establish effective bonds of feeling with persons who have the greatest meaning for him. The capacity for love and affection, the ability to handle anxieties arising out of frustrations, and the ability to control aggressive impulses are aspects of the emotional life with which each child must learn to cope.

Closely related to emotional growth and development are social and cultural patterns of maturation which, in the final analysis, prove to be the strongest determinants of emotional maturity. The earliest and most basic factors are the relations with parents. These relations are extended during childhood to familial and extrafamilial contacts. As early as 4 to 6 months of age one may expect imitation of a primitive sort, at 8 or 9 months the beginnings of imitative play, and by 3 to 5 years creative play which includes the playing of adult roles.

Learning is an essential aspect of acculturation. Current learning theory suggests that the behavior of the infant is modified both by inner needs

15

and tensions and by contingencies in the environment. If a pattern of behavior is reliably followed by pleasant circumstances such as reduction of need or by intrinsically satisfying stimuli, then that pattern of behavior will tend to occur with increasing probability; if by unpleasant circumstances, then with decreasing probability. The reinforcement of behavior may be positive or negative, according to whether it is pleasant or painful. A reinforcing experience may be *primary,* such as the direct reduction of a need which leads toward restoration of emotional balance, or *secondary,* such as a stimulus associated with primary reinforcement of behavior, but which satisfies another need (e.g. thumb-sucking in the anxious child).

The broad picture of growth and development, then, is an intricate pattern of genetic, nutritional, traumatic, social and cultural forces dynamically affecting the child from conception to adulthood. The pattern is unique for each child and may be profoundly different for individual children within the broad limits which designate "normality." The most obvious differences are those which distinguish male and female. Beyond these the patterns of growth and development may have such variability that they can be adequately expressed only in statistical terms.

VARIABILITY IN HUMAN GROWTH PATTERNS

In biologic data which vary over a range of normal values the largest number tend to cluster about a mean value. When data are plotted on a graph in the manner indicated in Figure 2-1, the resultant curve is often a close approximation of the theoretic bell-shaped curve (Fig. 2-2) which describes the ideal or equal distribution of continuously variable values about a population mean. Statistical treatment of data so arranged may give a number of useful concepts, the most important of which are the *mean* or *average* and the *standard deviation* from the mean.

In a theoretically perfect distribution the average value will be the one most commonly found, i.e. the *modal* or *normal* value (mode or norm) for the population under study. If, on the other hand, a distribution includes a larger number of high values than low, or vice versa, the average value may not be the most representative or modal value for the population studied. Asymmetrical curves of this sort are said to be *skewed.* Figure 2-3, which presents the weights of a group of children, is an example of such a skewed curve.

Occasionally a bimodal curve is found. Under these circumstances it may generally be inferred that not one but 2 groups are being studied, which have some feature differentiating one from the other. When 2 different samples or populations vary with respect to average values for some biologic trait, it is often difficult to evaluate this difference unless the distribution or dispersion of values in each sample is known. When the *standard deviations* of 2 samples are available, then the likelihood can be calculated whether an observed difference between them may have occurred solely as the result of randomly distributed values or whether the variable is a significant differential factor between the 2 groups.

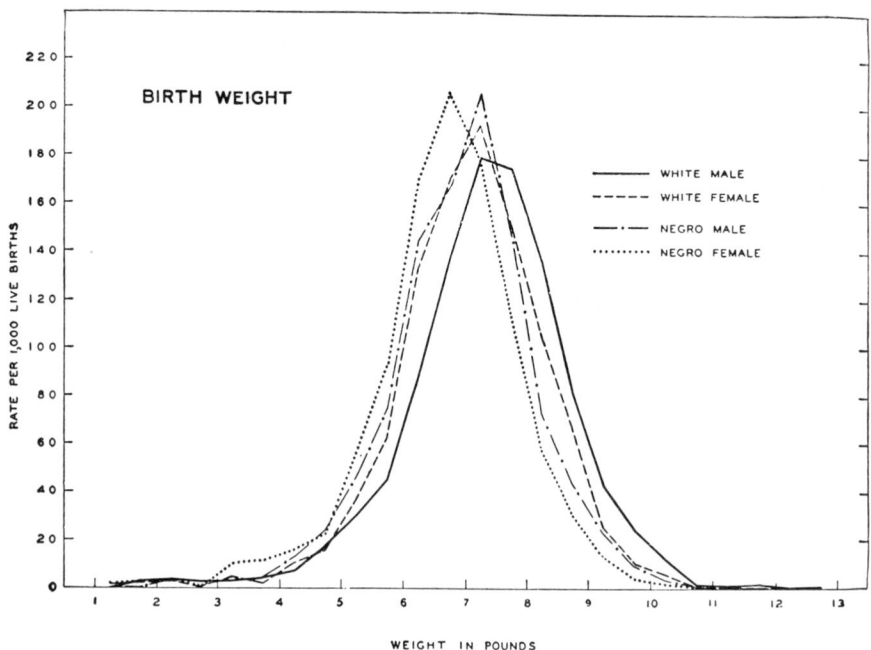

Figure 2-1. Weight at birth; rates by color and sex per 1000 live births. (After Anderson, Brown and Lyon: Causes of Prematurity. III. Influence of Race and Sex on Duration of Gestation and Weight at Birth. *Am. J. Dis. Child.,* Vol. 65.)

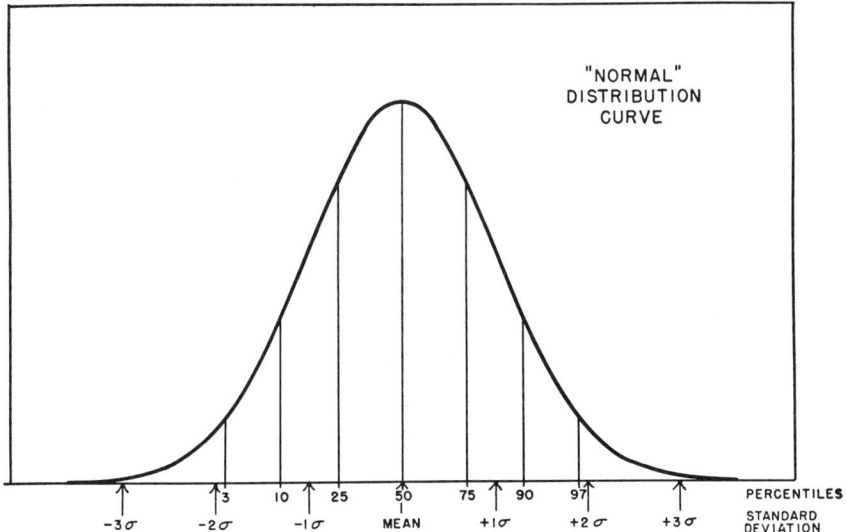

Figure 2-2. "Normal" distribution curve. This theoretical curve represents a type of distribution characteristic of the range of variability between values for many measurements obtained from groups of children at a given age. The percentiles indicate certain positions within this distribution, as do the standard deviations from the mean. Samples of actual distributions of values obtained from children are shown for comparison with this curve in Figures 2-1 and 2-3.

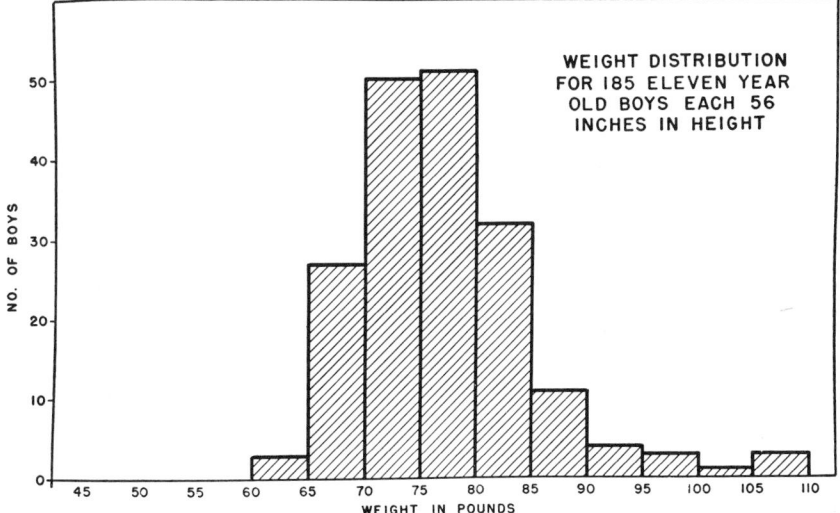

Figure 2-3. Weight distribution of 185 boys. The mean for the distribution of weights is 77.2 pounds, within the range of the column of greatest concentration of values. There is a slight skew to the right of this curve, suggesting the inclusion of a few obese subjects. (Values from Franzen: School Health Research Monograph No. II. New York, American Child Health Association, 1929.)

The *standard deviation* (root mean square or quadratic mean) describes the degree of dispersion of observed values as they deviate from the mean value. The range of values lying between the points one standard deviation below and one standard deviation above the mean value will include about 68 per cent of all values on a theoretic distribution about this mean. The range, *mean plus or minus 2 standard deviations,* will include about 95 per cent of values distributed about this mean, and the range, *mean plus or minus 3 standard deviations,* will include about 99.7 per cent of such values. Such measurements of dispersion are commonly used to locate an individual member of a population with respect to the average member. The growth charts in common use for following the physical development of children make this location easy by showing developmental lines at a number of different positions corresponding to deviations from average values above and below the mean. These are often expressed in terms not of standard deviation, but of *percentile* location in the distribution pattern.

When the items in a set of quantitative data

are arranged in order of ascending or descending magnitude, a value can be found which is called the *median,* above and below which lie half the observed values. In the distribution described by the symmetrical normal curve, the median, the mode and the average fall at the same point. Values may also be designated which divide the data into 2 groups at the *first quartile point,* below which will lie one quarter of the values, the *second quartile point* (which corresponds to median), and the *third quartile point,* below which lie three quarters of the observed values. The *percentile* points in a distribution of ordered data have similar meaning, one tenth of observations falling below the tenth percentile, three tenths below the thirtieth percentile, nine tenths below the ninetieth percentile, and so on.

Although such measures of growth as weight, height, and circumference of head at a particular time do indicate the status of a given child in relation to other children of the same age, only sequential measurements for some months or even years will indicate whether the child is achieving his growth potential. For example, a child below the tenth percentile point in weight for age might be thought of as undernourished, but one in 10 normal children will be below this level. If such a child continues to grow in height and weight within expected limits, he may be considered to be within the normal range in respect to his physical growth status. On the other hand, another child whose height and weight at a given time might approximate the fiftieth percentiles for his age might be significantly below his ideal levels. Thus repeated recording of growth measurements throughout infancy and childhood provides the only certain means available to demonstrate the adequacy of physical growth.

Whenever one aspect of growth differs significantly from other aspects, possible reasons should be sought. For example, if a child's height and bone age place him at the fiftieth percentile for age, one would be concerned to find his weight at the third or ninety-seventh percentile. The differences in *physique* which would be represented by such a child can be readily imagined.

In evaluating the possibility that a growth pattern is deviant, it may also be helpful to examine the physical patterns of other members of the child's family. The small child of small but normal parents seems less out of place than the conspicuously small child of average or large parents. The setting, too, in which apparent growth failure or growth excess (such as obesity) occurs may give clues to its meaning. The tensions, anxieties and cultural goals of parents and children may be intimately involved in potential or actual disturbances of growth. Before such causal relations are assumed, however, the child must be adequately studied clinically to ensure that no chronic disturbance such as renal disease or metabolic disorder is responsible for the abnormal growth pattern.

FETAL GROWTH AND DEVELOPMENT

The potentialities of the individual reside in a unique manner in the genetic substance of the nucleus of the fertilized ovum. The period of intrauterine life may be divided into 2 principal phases, the *embryonic* and the *fetal.* The dividing line is not sharp, but the embryonic period is usually considered to be the first 8 weeks of growth, during which the fertilized ovum differentiates rapidly into an organism which has most of the gross anatomic features which distinguish the human form. Organogenesis does continue beyond 8 weeks in some systems, so that some prefer to designate the embryonic period as the first trimester of pregnancy, or the first 12 weeks. The period after the twelfth week of gestation and through the fortieth week is distinguished by rapid growth and elaboration of function. Before the twenty-eighth week of gestation the fetus is generally considered *previable;* from 28 to about 38 weeks the infant is considered *viable,* with decreasing degrees of prematurity.

Many abnormalities of children have their origins in abnormal genes or chromosomes or derive from disturbances in growth during the embryonic period. During this period the mortality rate is probably higher than at any other time of life. Causes of mortality include abnormalities of genes and chromosomes and alterations of maternal health, and these may at times be interrelated. Advanced maternal age, for example, seems to dispose to chromosomal abnormalities (see p. 325) which may give rise to Down's syndrome, Klinefelter's syndrome or other conditions. Maternal infection during the first trimester of pregnancy may alter the differentiation of the fetus in such a way as to produce congenital anomalies, e.g. those resulting from rubella in the mother during the first 8 weeks of pregnancy. In general, intrauterine environmental factors responsible for defects in differentiation of the newborn infant exert their effects within the first trimester of pregnancy.

Morbidity during the fetal period may result from a variety of intrauterine factors. These include interference with *oxygenation* of the fetus through disturbances of the placenta or umbilical cord, *infections* such as syphilis, toxoplasmosis, cytomegalic inclusion disease and other viral or bacterial conditions, *injury* by radiation, trauma or noxious chemicals, by *immunologic* disorders in which erythrocytes, white blood cells or platelets are altered by isoantibodies or by maternal *nutritional* disturbances (see p. 352).

So far as is known, deficiencies in the maternal diet are more apt to affect the weight and general condition of the human infant than to produce such specific anatomic defects as occur in certain animals. Malnutrition in the pregnant woman leads to a high incidence of stillbirths or premature births, and deficiencies of calcium and of protein in the maternal diet seem to be clearly related to osseous structure and muscular mass in the newborn infant. The brain of the fetus appears to be more resistant to dietary deficiency than is muscle or subcutaneous tissue. Maternal toxemia increases the risk of prematurity and of intrauterine growth failure.

FETAL DEVELOPMENT

The embryo is grossly inert during the first 7 weeks of development, except for the heart beat, which begins by about 4 weeks. The first week of embryologic life is germinal, consisting of active cell division. During the second week the tissues differentiate into 2 layers, entoderm and ectoderm, and during the third week the third layer, mesoderm, is added. During the fourth week the growing organism elaborates the somites and between the fourth and eighth weeks undergoes rapid differentiation into an essentially human form. At 8 weeks of age the fetus weighs approximately 1 gm. and is about 2.5 cm. in length; at 12 weeks it weighs about 14 gm. and is about 7.5 cm. long. By the end of the *first trimester of pregnancy* the sex of the fetus can be distinguished by external examination.

The *second trimester of pregnancy,* ending by about 28 weeks, is characterized by rapid growth in size of the fetus, especially in linear dimensions, and by rapid acquisition of new functions. By the end of the second trimester the fetus weighs approximately 1000 gm. and is about 35 cm. (14 inches) in length. During the *third trimester* the further increase in size of the now viable fetus involves especially subcutaneous tissue and muscle mass.

The *circulatory* system of the fetus attains its final form between the eighth and twelfth weeks of gestation. Blood returning to the fetus from the placenta through the umbilical vein enters the inferior vena cava through the ductus venosus. As it enters the right atrium, this blood tends to be preferentially shunted through the patent foramen ovale into the left atrium. From the left ventricle this blood then enters the ascending aorta and is distributed to the head and the brain. Blood returning from the head by way of the superior vena cava tends to move across the right atrium into the right ventricle, and through the pulmonary artery and ductus arteriosus into the descending aorta, whence it is returned to the placenta by way of the umbilical arteries. In this way the head and brain receive proportionately more oxygenated blood than other parts of the body.

At birth, or shortly thereafter, there is closure of the ductus venosus, the ductus arteriosus, the foramen ovale and the umbilical arteries and vein. Closure of the foramen ovale is very likely functionally complete within the first few minutes after birth, owing to establishment of a lower pressure on the right side of the heart than on the left, after aeration of the lungs. Temporary reversal of

flow through the foramen ovale may occur with crying and lead to mild cyanosis during the first few days of life. Closure of the ductus arteriosus probably occurs somewhat later, though usually within the first 2 or 3 days of life. The stimulus for this closure is very likely the establishment of a high oxygen level in the arterial blood. Umbilical arteries undergo spasm with the cutting of the umbilical cord, and are reduced ultimately to fibrous cords. The changes in blood flow with birth of the infant have the effect of transforming the circulatory system from the fetal one in which the two ventricles act in parallel, with shunts adjusting possible unequal outputs, to a system in which the 2 pumps act in series, which requires that the output of the right and left sides of the heart be equal.

Although *respiratory* movements of the fetus may be seen as early as the eighteenth week of gestation, the development of the alveolar structures of the lung will not generally be sufficient to permit survival until the twenty-seventh or twenty-eighth week. The early respiratory movements of the fetus result in a tidal flow of amniotic fluid into and out of the developing lung and may contribute to pulmonary arborization. Respiratory movements seem to be more active between the eighteenth and twenty-seventh weeks of gestation than in the later fetal period, when there seems to be inhibition of respiratory activity which may be overcome by anoxia. If anoxia and gasping occur late in pregnancy, when amniotic fluid contains a larger number of cells than earlier and may contain meconium and other debris, aspiration may lead to deposition of these materials in the alveoli and to consequent respiratory embarrassment at delivery.

The hemoglobin of the fetus is predominantly fetal in type (hemoglobin F) and differs from that of adults (hemoglobin A) in its greater resistance to alkaline denaturation. Fetal blood is capable of carrying more oxygen at a given oxygen tension than is that of the adult. Adult hemoglobin begins to be produced late in fetal life and represents about 30 per cent of the hemoglobin of the mature newborn infant.

The fetus makes swallowing movements as early as the fourteenth week of gestation; at 17 weeks it may protrude the upper lip on stimulation in the oral area, and by 20 weeks it may protrude both lips on stimulation. At 22 weeks the lips are pursed upon stimulation, and by 28 to 29 weeks the fetus may actively suck in an attempt to gain nourishment.

Bile begins to be formed by about 12 weeks of gestation, and digestive enzymes appear soon thereafter. Meconium, the distinctive intestinal content of the fetus, is present by 16 weeks; it consists of desquamated intestinal cells and intestinal juices, and of squamous cells and lanugo hair swallowed by the fetus in amniotic fluid. Meconium is typically dark green to black and is gelatinous and sticky in consistency.

Neurologic activity in the fetus is first manifest

by about 8 weeks of gestation, when isolated local muscular reactions may be seen in response to stimulation. By 9 weeks contralateral flexion may be followed by ipsilateral flexion (swimming motions), and some spontaneous movements may be seen. In the fetus of 9 weeks' gestation the palms and soles have become reflexogenic; by 13 to 14 weeks graceful flowing movements may be produced by stimulation of all areas except the back, the back of the head and the vertex. At this time the movement of the fetus may first begin to be perceptible to the mother. The grasp reflex is evident by 17 weeks and is generally well developed by 27 weeks. Respiration may occur in the fetus delivered at 18 weeks; at 22 weeks respiratory activity may be accompanied by weak phonation. By 25 weeks the earliest signs of the Moro response (p. 1269) can be elicited.

After the fifteenth to seventeenth week of gestation there is apparently some decrease of fetal activity, the fetus being somewhat sluggish until the time of birth.

It seems clear that the amount of activity differs among fetuses, and there is evidence that fetal activity may be responsive to maternal emotions, possibly as a result of placental transfer of epinephrine or other humoral concomitants of strong feelings. Virtually nothing is known as to how the activity of newborn infants or the quality of the infant's demands during the first few weeks of life may reflect aspects of his gestation which were dependent upon maternal emotional states. The fetus is capable of being conditioned to certain sensory stimuli; e.g. changes in the fetal pulse rate in response to noise transmitted through the mother's abdomen are blunted by repetition of the noise. The comfort derived by some newborn infants from rhythmic motion or rhythmic sound may stem from similar sensations imparted in utero by maternal respiration or heart sounds.

The placenta is the principal avenue of metabolic interchange between mother and fetus. Its most urgent function is to provide for gas exchange between mother and fetus, which requires adequate perfusion on both sides. The placenta is a complex organ, elaborating hormones and enzymes which participate in the regulation of pregnancy, and effecting the selective transfer of nutrients and metabolites between mother and infant. Placental permeability is selective even for such closely related substances as antibodies against viruses and bacteria, the former being more readily transmitted than the latter. The placenta is particularly active in transferring calcium, iron and gamma globulins to the infant in the last trimester of pregnancy, with the result that the infant born prematurely may have unusual needs for calcium and iron and unusual susceptibility to infection.

THE NEWBORN INFANT
(See also p. 353)

The general physical features of the newborn infant differentiate him sharply from the older infant, child or adult in respect to body proportions (Fig. 2-4). The head is relatively large, the face round and the mandible relatively small. The chest tends to be rounded rather than flattened anteroposteriorly; the abdomen is relatively prominent, and the extremities are relatively short. The midpoint of the stature of the newborn infant is approximately at the level of the umbilicus, whereas in the adult it is at the symphysis pubis.

At birth the infant is generally covered with vernix caseosa, a cheesy white substance adherent to the skin. There may be edema of the vertex or other presenting part, or an abnormal shape to the head molded by the forces of labor, with overriding of the bones of the cranial vault.

The predominant posture of the newborn infant is one of partial flexion. It is often possible to establish what the predominant intrauterine position of the infant was by determining the most comfortable pattern into which the extremities can be flexed and adjusted to each other ("folded") so as to make the infant assume a more or less ovoid shape. Sometimes minor, and occasionally

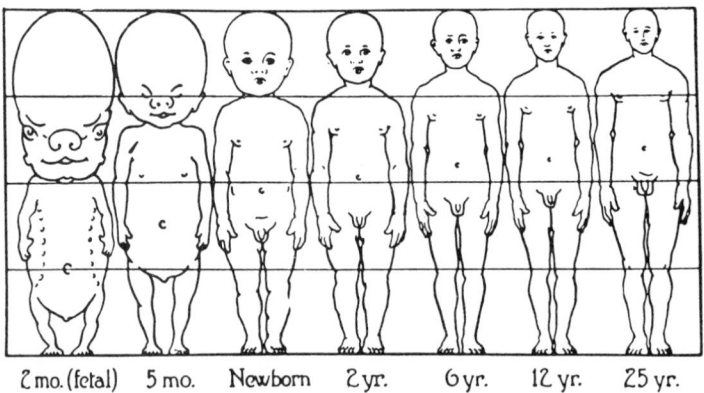

2 mo. (fetal)   5 mo.   Newborn   2 yr.   6 yr.   12 yr.   25 yr.

Figure 2-4.   Changes in body proportions from second fetal month to adulthood. (From Robbins et al.: *Growth.* New Haven, Yale University Press. By permission of publisher.)

major, orthopedic abnormalities reflect the effect of intrauterine posture upon the growing fetus (see also p. 1351).

Localized anatomic variants which may be observed in the newborn infant include telangiectases of the eyelids and of the nape, mongolian spot, milia, phimosis, and the epithelial pearls of the oral mucous membrane. The external auditory canal of the newborn infant is short, and the drum is placed obliquely across the canal. The eustachian tube is short and broad. There is usually a single mastoid cell in the antrum; maxillary and ethmoid sinuses are small, and the frontal and sphenoidal ones undeveloped. The liver and spleen are commonly felt at or just below the costal margins, and the kidneys are often palpable.

An average newborn infant weighs approximately 3.4 kg. (7½ pounds), boys being slightly heavier than girls. Approximately 95 per cent of full-term newborn infants weigh between 2.5 kg. (5½ pounds) and 4.6 kg. (10 pounds). The length averages about 50 cm. (20 inches), approximately 95 per cent of infants being between 45 and 55 cm. (18 and 22 inches). The head circumference averages about 35 cm. (14 inches). (See pp. 23 and 48 to 49.)

The most critical need of the newborn infant is for the establishment of adequate respiratory activity with effective exchange of gases. The rate of established respirations averages 30 to 40 per minute. Other activity useful in respiration includes crying, sneezing, coughing, yawning and stretching.

The cardiac adjustments of the neonatal period are often associated with transient cardiac murmurs. The heart rate ranges from 120 to 160 per minute. The heart of the newborn infant often seems large with respect to the size of the chest when measured by adult standards.

The activity of the newborn infant directed toward meeting his nutritional needs includes crying when hungry, a tendency when hungry to turn his head toward and to "root" about for the nipple or other stimulus placed close to his oral area (rooting reflex) and sucking, gagging and swallowing reflexes. The newborn infant is capable of manifesting nausea and of vomiting.

Breast feeding (p. 144) of the newborn infant will be facilitated if the mother is instructed as to the nature and meaning of the rooting reflex and if she knows that in nursing the infant will draw an unexpectedly large amount of nipple and areola into his mouth and that there will be rhythmic closure of the jaw upon the nipple in such a manner as to empty the postareolar sinus located at the point of confluence of lacteal vessels. Most failures of breast feeding are the result of errors in technique or of an emotional reaction against breast feeding.

The infant initially expresses his hunger at irregular intervals, but during the first week he will fall reasonably comfortably into patterns of feeding at intervals ranging from 2 to 4 or 5 hours.

No schedule of feedings will meet the demands or needs of all infants; if infant and mother are close to each other during the immediate postnatal period, as in a rooming-in arrangement, the opportunities for comfortable meeting of the baby's needs are optimal.

The first stools will generally be passed within 24 hours and will consist of meconium. With the establishment of milk feedings, the meconium stools begin to be replaced on the third or fourth day by *transitional* stools, which are greenish-brown and may contain milk curds. The typical milk stool of the older infant follows after an interval of 3 or 4 days. The frequency of stools in the newborn infant seems closely related to the frequency with which he is fed and the amount of food obtained, averaging between 3 and 5 stools a day by the end of the first week of life. On any given day during the first week about one infant in 50 will have no stool at all; it is not unusual for an infant to have as many as 6 or 7 stools after the second day.

At delivery the infant's body temperature is likely to be virtually the same as his mother's. After delivery there is a transient fall in temperature, which is usually restored within 4 to 8 hours. Under usual environmental circumstances the daily caloric need of the infant to maintain body heat and basal activity is about 55 calories per kg. By the end of the first week the caloric needs will be approximately 110 calories per kg., of which 50 per cent supplies basal metabolic needs, 40 per cent is invested in growth and in activity, 5 per cent is for the specific dynamic action of protein, and 5 per cent is lost in urine and feces or as other caloric loss in excreta.

The newborn infant is well supplied with body water; that in the extracellular compartment may constitute up to 35 per cent of body weight. During the first few days of life there is a loss of excess fluid which, in the absence of unusual oral intake, generally averages about 6 per cent of body weight and may occasionally exceed 10 per cent. When this loss is excessive, there may be so-called dehydration or inanition fever on the third or fourth day.

After the first week of life the need for water will be in the range of 120 to 150 ml. per kg. Approximately half of this will be devoted to formation of urine and the rest to insensible loss by lungs and skin and to other losses. The insensible loss is in a relatively fixed relation to the calories metabolized by the infant (about 40 ml. per 100 calories). Losses in stool are variable; those in sweat, minimal.

The metabolism of the newborn infant favors the anaerobic or glycolytic pathway, so that he is more tolerant of periods of deprivation of oxygen than is the older infant, child or adult. This tolerance for anoxia is only relative, however. If oxygenation of the newborn infant is not quickly established, there may be a rapidly developing metabolic acidosis (owing to the accumulation of lactic acid) and respiratory acidosis (owing to rapid accumulation of carbon dioxide).

Renal function in the newborn infant does not meet the standards of later life. Urine often contains protein in small amounts and during the first week of life may contain an abundance of urates, which may give the diaper a pink stain. Urea clearance is low, and the ability to concentrate urine is limited. There is limited production of ammonium ion and relatively limited clearance of phosphate ion. There may be a transient, slight rise in the blood urea nitrogen level during the first days.

The hemoglobin level of the newborn infant averages around 17 to 19 gm. per 100 ml.; mild reticulocytosis and normoblastemia may be observed for the first day or two of life. Leukocytes number about 10,000 per ml. at birth and generally increase in number for the first 24 hours, with a relative neutrophilia. Occasionally counts as high as 25,000 to 35,000 are encountered. After the first week the white cell count is likely to be below 14,000 with the characteristic relative lymphocytosis of infancy and early childhood. Stressful situations in the newborn infant, including overwhelming infection, may on occasion be associated with little or no leukocytosis and even with leukopenia.

The transition from intrauterine to extrauterine life imposes upon the infant the need to activate a number of functions which have been dormant. Some of them, such as respiratory activity and the maintenance of body temperature, are under usual circumstances quickly achieved. By contrast, there are delays in the development of certain enzymatic, hemostatic and immunologic functions, so that the infant may temporarily be subject to increased risk when exposed to infection or when given certain drugs which he is able to metabolize adequately only some weeks after birth.

There appears to be little or no passive transfer of certain clotting factors from mother to infant. Establishment of normal hemostatic mechanisms depends upon early establishment of normal intestinal flora and elaboration of vitamin K.

Placentally transmitted maternal hormones are responsible for temporary changes in the breasts (enlargement, and production of milk), uterus and possibly other tissues, and the withdrawal of maternal hormones or other metabolites may contribute to temporary hypofunction of the fetal parathyroid. Blood levels of sugar and calcium are normally relatively low in the newborn infant, and further decreases (below about 20 mg. per 100 ml. of sugar or about 7.5 mg. per 100 ml. of calcium) may be responsible for convulsions.

Adjustment to extrauterine life is likely to be prolonged in respect to resistance to infection. The gamma globulin level of the newborn infant (almost entirely IgG) is slightly higher than that of his mother, a fact which suggests that there is an active transport mechanism for gamma globulin. Protection is afforded in some measure against many viral and some bacterial diseases, by antibodies of the IgG variety transferred from mother to infant. Antibodies against certain antigens of gram-negative enterobacteria, on the other hand, like isohemagglutinins, are found in the IgM fraction of immune globulins, which do not cross the placenta in large amounts. IgM antibodies may be formed, however, by the fetus in response to intrauterine infection. IgA antibodies and IgE (reagins) do not generally cross the placenta.

The gamma globulin level of the infant falls to a low level by about 3 months of age, with a subsequent rise to those levels which characterize the older child and the adult. The responses of the newborn infant to immunization are relatively sluggish by the standards of older infants; this sluggishness is accentuated in premature infants. Antibodies belonging to the major blood group system usually appear by the end of the first month of life.

The secretory enzymes of the digestive tract are usually adequate for the diet of the newborn infant, although fat is handled somewhat less well than protein or carbohydrate. At the cellular level, however, a number of deficiencies may have important clinical consequences. The red blood cells of the newborn infant have a relatively low level of reduced glutathione, which may contribute to increased hemolysis of red blood cells under a variety of circumstances. A deficiency in capacity of the liver to conjugate bilirubin with glucuronic acid leads to hyperbilirubinemia, often with no evidence of abnormal hemolysis. When hyperbilirubinemia is severe, kernicterus becomes a threat.

These evidences of metabolic immaturity generally do not persist beyond the first week of life; they may persist longer in premature than in fullterm infants.

The repertory of behavior of the infant at birth is limited. Tensions arising from hunger, cold, pain or other discomfort lead to restlessness or crying. Prompt satisfaction of indicated needs will usually restore the infant's composure. Some infants seem to need more than the usual amount of "mothering" and are comforted by gentle handling, rocking and the like.

Some of the essential ingredients of the relations between certain newborn animals and their parent are obtained through a process which has been given the name *imprinting*. Imprinting occurs when during a *critical period* after delivery an animal is presented with an appropriate stimulus to which it turns for social interactions. The effect of the stimulus is to establish important controls over the interaction between the newborn animal and its environment, with other animals and especially with the parent. Little is known about the occurrence of imprinting in man. If it exists, increasing attention to the circumstances surrounding the delivery of the infant, his care in the hospital and the early weeks at home may lead to substantial revision of some current practices of infant care. In particular, the role of analgesic and anesthetic agents in labor may need to be reviewed, as well as the possible advantages or disadvantages of a rooming-in arrangement for the infant after delivery.

GROWTH AND DEVELOPMENT OF THE INFANT BORN PREMATURELY

(See also p. 364)

The fetus born prematurely has some chance of survival by about 28 weeks' gestation, at which time its weight is about 1000 gm. and its length approximately 35 cm. The specific areas in which the premature infant faces difficulties owing to failure of adequate maturation of enzymatic, renal, metabolic, hematologic and immunologic mechanisms are discussed elsewhere.

The behavioral characteristics of premature infants vary with their gestational age. The heads of infants whose birth weights are 1000 to 1500 gm. tend to be rounded and large in relation to body size, and the skin appears transparent. They tend to be predominantly atonic and to lie in a tonic neck attitude, often with little motion of the extremities. Vocalization is weak, as are the grasp and Moro responses. The sucking responses may also be weak, and these infants may show little evidence of hunger on deprivation of food. It is difficult to tell when they are awake and when asleep, though they can be stimulated to greater alertness.

Somewhat larger infants, those from 1500 to 2000 gm., have more subcutaneous tissue and relatively less enlargement of the head. These infants have good muscle tone when stimulated, more vigorous grasp and complete Moro responses. A sleep pattern is easily discernible, and they are able to fixate visually some objects in their environment. The most vigorous of these babies are able to manage breast feeding.

Infants weighing between 2000 and 2500 gm. at birth generally have the appearance of small full-term infants, from which they cannot usually be differentiated by developmental examination. They have a good cry and sustained muscle tone.

The average premature infant is likely to gain 6 to 7 kg. (13 to 15 pounds) in the first year, which is the average gain for the full-term infant. Although a small premature infant, by the time he reaches his expected date of delivery, may seem more alert and active than a full-term baby born on that day, the actual developmental level which is reached later in the first year will generally be lower than that indicated by his chronologic age. The deficit in attained level tends to correspond to the degree of prematurity. These differences become less conspicuous and will generally have disappeared by the end of the second year of life, so long as no complicating factors occur. Developmental defects are more common in premature infants than in full-term infants and often include impairment of intellectual or motor function.

GROWTH DURING THE FIRST YEAR

Most full-term infants regain their birth weight by the age of 10 days. After this, weight gain averages approximately 20 gm. per day for the first 5 months of life and approximately 15 gm. per day for the remainder of the first year. The full-term infant will generally double his birth weight by 5 months and triple it in 1 year. The length of the normal infant increases during the first year by 25 to 30 cm. or 10 to 12 inches. (The average length at birth is 50 cm., or 20 inches.) There is a conspicuous increase of subcutaneous tissue in the early months of life, which reaches its peak by about 9 months.

The anterior fontanel of the newborn infant may increase in size for several months after birth, but generally diminishes in size after 6 months and may become effectively closed at any time from 9 to 18 months. The posterior fontanel is generally closed to palpation by 4 months.

The circumference of the head, which is 34 to 35 cm. at birth, increases to approximately 44 cm. by 6 months and to 47 cm. by 1 year (Table 2-1). The circumference of the head is somewhat larger than that of the chest at birth, but the two become approximately equal at 1 year.

Deciduous teeth appear in most infants between 5 and 9 months. The first to erupt are the lower central incisors, followed by the upper central and then the upper lateral incisors. The lower lateral incisors follow, the first deciduous molars, canines and second deciduous molars appearing in that order. By the age of 1 year most children have 6 to 8 teeth. Occasionally an infant has as few as 2 teeth at 1 year without other evidence of growth disturbance.

TABLE 2-1. MEDIAN VALUES FOR CIRCUMFERENCE OF HEAD AND OF THORAX AND FOR STEM LENGTH BY AGE IN THE FIRST 5 YEARS OF LIFE

AGE	HEAD CIRCUM-FERENCE		CHEST CIRCUM-FERENCE		STEM LENGTH	
Yr. Mo.	In.	Cm.	In.	Cm.	In.	Cm.
Birth	13.8	35.0	13.0	33.0	—	—
3	15.9	40.4	15.8	40.2	16.0	40.7
6	17.1	43.4	17.1	43.4	17.6	44.6
9	17.8	45.3	18.0	45.7	18.5	47.0
1 – 0	18.3	46.6	18.6	47.3	19.2	48.8
1 – 6	18.9	47.9	19.4	49.2	20.4	51.2
2 – 0	19.3	48.9	19.8	50.4	21.3	54.9
2 – 6	19.5	49.5	20.2	51.4	22.0	56.0
3 – 0	19.6	49.8	20.6	52.2	22.6	57.5
3 – 6	—	—	20.8	52.8	23.2	59.0
4 – 0	19.8	50.4	21.0	53.4	23.9	60.6
5 – 0	20.0	50.8	21.5	54.6	24.8	62.9

From studies at Harvard School of Public Health. For percentile distributions of these measurements by sex, see Tables 2-7 and 2-9 (pp. 48, 52).

THE FIRST THREE MONTHS OF LIFE
(Table 2-5)

With adequate nutrition and mothering the infant will make rapid developmental progress during the first 3 months of life, his principal achievement being an appreciation of and relation to persons and objects in his environment. The newborn infant's range of behavior is limited, but there are qualities of excitation and inhibition and, even at this early age, differences among infants in levels of activity and in intensity of reactivity. Recent studies indicate that the mother elicits specific behavior from the infant, not just in response to the infant's needs, but as a pattern of development in which the infant appears to be seeking an object (the mother) upon which to place certain responses. It is not known whether critical periods exist for this interaction.

When the newborn infant is placed prone upon a firm surface, he is able to avoid suffocation by turning his face from side to side. By 4 weeks of age he is able to lift his head above the surface. By 4 weeks the stiff and rather symmetrical flexed posture of the infant has become more relaxed, and he is likely to lie, when supine, in a tonic neck posture (head turned to one side).

The infant is generally able to fixate a light or bright object in the first hours or days of life, and will be able to follow it with his eyes for a few degrees away from the line of vision. He should be able to follow it through an arc of 180 degrees by the end of the second month.

When the infant within the first 4 to 8 weeks of life is pulled from a supine to a sitting position, the head lags, and with the infant in the upright position, head control is absent. By 12 weeks of age he has some control of his head as he is drawn to a sitting position, but holds the head forward when he is upright; irregular head control results in a bobbing motion.

The grasp reflex persists until the age of about 8 weeks, after which, with growing eye and hand coordination, active grasp becomes more evident; by 12 weeks the infant attempts to make contact with an offered object and will hold it briefly if appropriate contact is made. The coordination of eye and hand implicit in this activity seems to arise in some measure out of the tonic neck attitude.

By 8 weeks most infants will smile when social contact is made with them. The infant who at 4 weeks was able to vocalize small throaty noises and at 8 weeks to produce some vowel sounds will at 12 weeks produce these sounds with evident pleasure on social contact.

The 3-month-old infant is still relatively undiscriminating as to persons in his environment; there is little evidence that various persons are differentiated as individuals. These social responses are important milestones, and the infant who does not have a social smile at the age of 12 weeks should be regarded as deviant with respect either to developmental potential or to quality of antecedent experiences.

Child-rearing practices differ widely in various parts of the world with respect to the attention accorded this age period. Little is known about the specific ways in which differing practices may modify the quality of socialization of the infant in these early months. There is reason, however, to feel that his sense of security will be optimally fostered when he is given care by a mother or mother-figure during this period in a prompt, confident and loving manner.

Both consistency and promptness seem important in the responses of the caretakers to the behavior of infant or child. The timing and quality of maternal responses to the infant, for example, may have powerful motivational impact. In instances of defective mothering the infant's normal or appropriate behavior may not be consistently or reliably rewarded by reduction of tension, or an effective maternal response may come so late and after so much anxiety, or hostility, that the infant cannot associate any specific action of his own with relief of tension. Such infants may come to feel that they have no way to affect their environment through their own actions. Life-long retreat, anxiety or hostility may be the consequences.

THREE TO SIX MONTHS
(Table 2-5)

By the age of 3 months the infant placed prone upon a firm surface is generally able to raise his head and chest from the surface if his arms are extended before him. By 4 months he is able in this position to raise his head to an upright position, and it can be turned easily from side to side. At 5 to 6 months of age the infant begins to roll over, at first from the prone to the supine position and then in the reverse direction.

Between 3 and 4 months of age the infant gradually abandons the tonic neck posture as his predominant posture, and the head is generally maintained in the midline, with the arms and legs in more or less symmetrical positions, and the hands often brought together in the midline or to the mouth. In this position the 4- to 6-month-old infant often develops a bald spot over the occiput. By 4 months the infant becomes more adept in making contact with objects brought within reach and will often bring these to the midline and to the mouth for oral exploration.

When the infant of 4 months is pulled to a sitting position, the head is brought up without lag; in the upright position the head tilts a little forward, but is held steadily without bobbing. The head will be maintained erect and steady by 5 months of age.

By 4 to 5 months the infant will enjoy being supported in an upright posture and becomes increasingly attracted to objects presented on a plane surface. By 6 months of age he is able to change the orientation of the entire body in order to extend a hand toward a desired large object such as a rattle or ring.

At 4 months of age the infant will be able to grasp an object of moderate size, but will have difficulty in visualizing such a small object as a pellet. By 7 months the pellet is promptly seen and may be vigorously pursued by raking motions of the fingers, but the infant is not apt to be able to pick it up.

After 6 months the functions of the hand are increasingly lodged in the structures on the radial side, the thumb being used in conjunction with the palm. By 6 to 6½ months most infants can grasp a large object, such as a rattle, and transfer it from hand to hand.

At 6 to 6½ months the infant is often able to sit alone, leaning forward upon his hands, or with slight support; he will not yet have developed a lumbar lordosis, and the spine will have a gentle kyphotic curve from sacrum to cervical region. At 5 to 6 months the infant can often be pulled from a sitting to a standing position and will support his weight upon extended legs. At 6 to 6½ months, in this same position, he will often flex the knees momentarily and return to a standing posture.

By 3 to 4 months of age the infant ought to have become clearly related to *objects* in his environment and to persons who give him care. By 4 months he is able to *laugh* aloud at pleasurable social contact. Moreover, if a pleasant contact is terminated, he may show displeasure by change of expression, fussing or crying. Between 4 and 7 months the infant begins to be responsive to the emotional tone of his social contacts, and by 7 months he will respond to changes in the facial expressions of those having close rapport with him. By the end of the sixth month the normal infant will show a preference for the person giving him most of his care.

SIX TO TWELVE MONTHS
(Table 2-5)

By 7 months the infant in the prone position is able to *pivot* in pursuit of an object, but if it is not within his reach, he may be unable to attain it. By 9 to 10 months most infants have learned to *creep* or to *crawl*.

The supine infant is able by 6 months or so to lift his head up and becomes increasingly interested in his legs. By 8 to 9 months he is able to assume a sitting position without help and soon is able to maintain this with the back straight. He is often able at 8 months to stand steady for a short while so long as his hands are held and by 9 months may be able to take some steps with both hands held.

Between 6 and 9 months the radial palmar grasp becomes clearly elaborated into movements involving thumb and forefinger. The index finger is used to poke at objects by 9 months, and at this time the thumb and forefinger can be brought into sufficiently accurate apposition to permit a pellet to be picked up with a pincer motion. This movement is apt to be made with the ulnar surface of the hand supported on the same surface upon which the pellet lies. By 12 months the pincer movement will be executed without this ulnar support.

The infant is able to make repetitive vowel sounds at 6½ months and by 8 months is likely to execute repetitive consonant sounds, such as ba-ba, ma-ma, da-da, although not necessarily associating these sounds with objects. The child of 8 or 9 months becomes attentive at the sound of his own name. He may knowingly use 1 word besides ma-ma or da-da by the age of 1 year and may show by his behavior that he knows the names of some objects.

The preference for his mother which was manifested by the 6-month-old infant may, by 8 months, have evolved into a complaint when his mother leaves the room. About this same time a mother may experience difficulty in putting a baby to sleep who always went willingly before. Sometimes a mother whose child is fretful when she leaves the room can comfort him by maintaining vocal contact with him. By 9 to 10 months the infant begins to be less dependent upon the physical presence of his mother, partly because he is increasingly able to follow her around. It can be demonstrated also at this time that, if an object which has attracted his attention is covered with a cloth before he has an opportunity to grasp it, he is able to uncover it and grasp it with the apparent sure knowledge that its being out of sight did not mean that it was not available. Peek-a-boo often becomes a pleasant game about this time.

Between 6 and 12 months one sees the earliest beginnings of imitative behavior. At 6 months, if shown how to tap a table with a pencil, he may crudely imitate this behavior. At 9 months he will wave bye-bye or bring the hands together imitatively; at 12 months a child may enter into very simple games with a toy such as a ball.

At 9 months an infant may be able to release an object upon request, if the object is grasped as the request is made. By 1 year most infants will extend the object and release it into an offered hand.

The demands on mother and infant during the first year are for the development of comfortable interactions which will lead to the infant's movement from a position of dependency to one of independent activity. The satisfactions of the first year of life are gained in large measure through *oral* activity and through bodily contacts of feeding and other care. Failure of achievement of the developmental goals of the first year leads to emotional dissatisfaction or to chronic anxieties on the part of the infant, which may be the root of life-long personality disorders.

GROWTH AND DEVELOPMENT IN THE SECOND YEAR

During the second year of life there is a further deceleration in the rate of growth; the average child will gain about 2.5 kg. (5 to 6 pounds) and about 12 cm. (5 inches). (See pp. 43 and 49.) After 10 months of age there is often a decrease in appetite extending well into the second year. The result is a loss during the second year of some of the subcutaneous tissue which reached its maximal development around 9 months; the plump infant begins to change gradually to the lean and muscular child. The mild lordosis and protuberant abdomen appear which are characteristic of the second and third years of life.

The growth of the brain decelerates during the second year; head circumference, which increased approximately 12 cm. (4+ inches) during the first year, will increase only 2 cm. during the second year. By the end of the first year the brain has reached approximately two thirds, and at the end of the second year four fifths, of its adult size.

Weech suggested a useful set of mnemonics for recalling the height and weight of children during the preschool and school years; a slight modification is given in Table 2-2.

During the second year 8 more teeth erupt, making a total of 14 to 16, including the first deciduous molars and the cuspids. The order of eruption may be irregular; the cuspids commonly appear after the first molars have erupted.

During the second year the infant moves from an awkward upright stance in which he could walk with support to a high degree of locomotor control. By 15 months he is generally able to walk alone, and by 18 months he may run stiffly. At this time he is able to sit down upon a chair of proper height.

At 18 months the infant can climb stairs, with 1 hand held, going 1 step at a time. By 20 months he is able to go downstairs, 1 hand held, and may be able to climb stairs holding to the stair railing. By 24 months he is able to run well and has generally outgrown the tendency to fall. Between 18 and 24 months the child normally enters the "run-about" age. He is able to move quickly from a safe or protected environment into danger and will need constant surveillance.

With the second year the infant enters a period when he will vigorously and imitatively exploit the objects in his environment. He can empty waste baskets, drawers and shelves and may try to examine everything within his reach. Fragile objects and certainly all household poisons, drugs and chemicals must be kept in places inaccessible to him.

The child who at 12 months was able to release a pellet into the hand of a person requesting it will at 15 months generally be able to put the pellet into a small bottle. He may attempt to remove the pellet from the bottle by inserting his finger; by 18 months he will be able to dump a pellet from a glass bottle.

By 15 months the child is able to put a 1-inch cube on top of another in response to a demonstration; by 18 months he is able to make a tower of 3 cubes and by 24 months a tower of 6 cubes. Imitative behavior and conceptual behavior continue to evolve with spontaneous scribbling and with imitation of vertical lines at 18 months; by 24 months the child imitates circular strokes and can make a horizontal line.

The normal infant, who often has 1 word besides ma-ma or da-da by the end of the first year, commonly has a vocabulary of 10 words by 18 months. There is wide variation in the times at which words begin to flow readily; it is not unusual for an entirely normal child to have few or no sounds conveying a definite meaning until 18 months or later. Some children with delay in development of recognizable speech have a rich jargon before communicative sounds appear; this jargon often has many of the intonations and punctuations of human speech, but the sounds otherwise convey no meaning. In those normal children in whom speech is delayed to 18 or 20 months, there is often rapid acquisition of words and meaning after this time, with the result that most normal children by their second birthday are able to put 3 words together.

The 3 words which the child puts together at the end of the second year are likely to be subject, verb and object. This ability appears to reflect

TABLE 2-2. MNEMONICS (WEECH) FOR APPROXIMATE HEIGHT AND WEIGHT OF INFANTS AND CHILDREN

(a) At birth: Weight (W) in lb. = 7 lb. 6 oz. (7.35 lb.)
(b) From 3 to 12 months: W (lb.)   = age (mo.) plus 11
(c) From 1 to 6 years: W (lb.)   = (age [yr.] × 5) plus 17
(d) From 6 to 12 years: W (lb.)   = (age [yr.] × 7) plus 5

Note: (c) and (d) give the same value (47 lb.) at 6 years. 48 lb. is a closer approximation of average. The following mnemonic is suggested: "Up to 5: 5A plus 17. From 7 on: 7A plus 5. At 6: use either one, but add 1."

(e) At birth: *Length* = 20 in.
(f) At one year: *Length* = 30 in.
(g) From 2 to 14 years: *Height* (in.) = (age [yr.] × 2½) plus 30

the growing awareness in the child of his individuality, so that the subject of the short sentence is often "me." Shortly thereafter he is able to use the nominative "I" in an appropriate manner.

During the second year the child becomes highly imitative. He becomes increasingly aware of and responsive to other persons, including siblings. Until the end of the second year, however, the infant's play is generally solitary and consists in active manipulation of objects available to him. During the third year of life he moves increasingly into play activities in which other children are involved. By the end of the fourth year the child is increasingly engaged in activity with other children in which the group begins to enact imaginative roles and activities. This tendency to role-playing will increase into the school years.

By 18 to 24 months most children are able to verbalize their toilet needs and can be helped at this time to follow acceptable social patterns in meeting them. In settings in which the young child has adequate models to follow it seems increasingly evident that toilet training need not become the focus of either emotion-laden educational activity on the part of parents or disciplinary concern.

The need for the child to submit his growing control of his body and of his environment to social and cultural pressures often produces frustration and anger in him. Temper tantrums, breath-holding spells and less dramatic outbursts are common consequences. These episodes respond best to management by a firm and loving parent who is able to set the necessary limits for the child.

GROWTH AND DEVELOPMENT DURING THE PRESCHOOL YEARS

During the third, fourth and fifth years of life gains in weight and height are relatively steady at approximately 2.0 kg. (4.5 pounds) and about 8 to 6 cm. (3½ to 2½ inches) per year, respectively (see Table 2-5, p. 43). Most children are lean relative to their earlier body configuration. The lordosis and protuberant abdomen of late infancy tend to disappear by the fourth year along with the pads of fat which underlie the normal arches of the feet during the earlier years.

By 2½ years the 20 deciduous teeth have usually erupted. During the rest of the preschool period the face tends to grow proportionately more than the cranial cavity and the jaw to widen preparatory to the eruption of permanent teeth.

The refinement of motor skills includes alternation of the feet in ascending stairs by 3 years and alternation in descending stairs by 4 years. By 3 years most children can stand for a short period on 1 foot; by 5 years they are generally able to hop on 1 foot and soon to skip.

By 3 years an infant may be able to imitate crudely the drawing of a cross. By 4 years the cross figure may be copied without previous demonstration, possibly as a 4-element figure. By 5 years the child can make correctly proportionate copies of the figures and for the first time becomes able to handle figures with slanting lines, such as triangles. A diamond-shaped figure may not be accurately and proportionately reproduced until the sixth year.

By 3 years the child is able to count 3 objects correctly; a 4-year-old, four; a 5-year-old, 10 or more.

By 3 years most children can state their ages and whether they are boys or girls. With the increasing awareness that they are destined to become larger children and adults, children in the later preschool period begin to seek adequate models by which to learn and play their future roles. The most accessible models are, of course, the parents and other members of the immediate family. The child's imperfect perception of the realities of his future often engenders conflicting pressures and anxieties. The so-called Oedipus situation may be regarded as the natural setting in which a child of 4, 5 or 6 years assumes those habits of thought, feeling and action which surround his growing perception or fantasy as to his future life. Inside the home the child's fantasies about his further role include playing the part of the parent of the same sex, and he may have an increasing curiosity and concern as to what the realities of this role may be, along with more general questions and fantasies as to the origin of babies, differences between boys and girls, and the like.

Outside the home, concerns and fantasies about future roles are likely to be expressed in play, children assuming the parts of exciting figures ranging in immediate knowledge of them from milkman to jet pilot. The interest of children of this age in sex differences, which often appears as questions inside the home, may appear in the form of sex play among children of each sex. This is so common as to appear to be entirely normal, although neither questions about reproductive or sexual matters nor sex play among small children is likely to be received with equanimity by parents in Western culture.

This is a time when the changing pattern of parent-child interaction and of other relations in and out of the home often leaves elements of hostility or aggression in the child's behavior, thoughts and fantasies. Anxieties may be expressed as nightmares or as fears of separation, death or bodily injury. Children with serious problems may display bedwetting or thumb-sucking, speech or learning difficulties, inability to enter into a comfortable sharing relation with others, temper tantrums or other behavior acquired at earlier developmental levels.

With the development of the child's ability to translate his conception of abstract forms into figures and structures, by the age of 6 he should be ready for formal education.

GROWTH AND DEVELOPMENT DURING THE EARLY SCHOOL YEARS

The early school years are a period of relatively steady growth beginning by about the age of 6 years and ending in a preadolescent growth spurt by about the age of 10 in girls and about 12 in boys. The average gain in weight during these years is about 3 to 3.5 kg. (7 pounds) per year, and that in height approximately 6 cm. (2½ inches) per year. Growth in head circumference is much slower than earlier, the circumference increasing from about 51 cm. (20 inches) to 53 to 54 cm. (21 inches) between the ages of 5 and 12 years. At the end of this period the brain has reached virtually adult size (see pp. 48 to 49).

The school years are a time of vigorous physical activity. The spine becomes straighter, but the child's body is supple, and postural attitudes may be assumed which are often disturbing to parents and to teachers. Mild degrees of knock-knee or flatfoot which may be apparent in the late preschool years tend to correct during the first year or two of the school years. The crude motor activities, such as running and climbing of the earlier years, become increasingly directed to more specialized activities and games requiring particular motor and muscular skills.

The development of the facial bones continues actively during the school years, particularly with enlargement of the sinuses. The frontal sinus has usually made its appearance by the seventh year.

The first permanent teeth, the first molars, most often erupt during the seventh year of life. With these so-called 6-year molars in place, the shedding of deciduous teeth begins, following approximately the same sequence as their acquisition. They are replaced at a rate of about 4 teeth a year over the next 7 years. The second permanent molars are commonly erupted by the fourteenth year; the third molars are irregular in their occurrence and time of eruption and may not appear until the early twenties.

Lymphatic tissues are at the peak of their development during these years and generally exceed the amount of such tissue in the normal adult. The abundance of lymphoid tissue during this time of life bears some relation to the frequency with which tonsillectomy and adenoidectomy are incorrectly recommended (p. 895). Respiratory infections are common during these years, and the response of the child to infection begins to be more like that of the adult than of the infant or young child. The usual number of respiratory infections during the school years is high; as many as 6 or 7 illnesses a year is not uncommon.

With the removal of a large portion of the child's life from the home to the school environment, children begin increasingly to live independently and to look outside the home for goals and for standards of behavior. This shifting of interests is often anxiety-provoking for parents. Needless to say, if earlier problems between parent and child have not been adequately resolved, adjustments to forces outside the home are apt to be difficult.

A large responsibility of the school years is the creation in the child of the senses of duty, of responsibility and of accomplishment. There is a possibility of great frustration for parents and children when the child's achievement does not measure up to parental hopes or expectations. The child unable to meet adequate standards may learn for the first time the sense of *failure* and may react with anxiety and hostility to the school situation or to specific persons. Antisocial behavior may develop through which the child attempts to gain recognition which he cannot attain otherwise.

GROWTH AND DEVELOPMENT IN ADOLESCENCE

Adolescence comprises nearly half of the growing period in man. It has its beginning by about the age of 10 years in girls and 12 in boys. The end of adolescence is not clearly delineated and varies with the physical, emotional, mental, social or cultural criteria which define the adult. The word *puberty* is used to designate an arbitrary point in the continuum of maturation: the menarche in girls, and some less clearly defined event occurring approximately 2 years later in boys. *Pubescence,* which is the time during which secondary changes such as pubic hair are appearing, is not clearly demarcated as to length, but it seems to be about 2 to 3 years. *Prepubescent* changes precede the first secondary sex changes of adolescence and are integral elements of maturation, not simply preparatory ones.

Growth and development in adolescence must be considered separately for boys and girls (see pp. 50 to 51). Some parameters of growth differ in boys and girls from early infancy. Boys on the average are larger than girls from birth to the prepubescent period, and their deciduous teeth erupt somewhat earlier. They have slightly less subcutaneous fat during the middle years of childhood and a slightly higher basal metabolic rate when referred to body surface. Boys and girls have much the same degree of motor activity and coordination until the age of 7 or 8 years, but by 9 years, while still preadolescent, boys move ahead of girls in some motor skills. By contrast, the acquisition of permanent dentition, another preadolescent growth feature, is earlier in girls than in boys.

For both boys and girls there is wide individual variability in the time of onset and rate of acquisition of adolescent changes. Not all the factors are known which contribute to this variability; some certainly are genetic, some nutritional and others socioeconomic. Neither climatic nor racial differences in average rates of adolescent growth seem well established. Growth in height occurs at an accelerated rate in the spring months, growth in weight in the fall of the year.

Individual variability in the progress of events in adolescence is best documented in longitudinal studies which indicate that growth patterns are established early in life and tend to follow a consistent course within set limits for each child. It has been shown, for example, that as early as 2 years of age those children who will be slow to mature at adolescence are smaller than their contemporaries. Girls in whom the menarche occurs early have a greater velocity of growth, but a shorter growth period, during adolescence. Girls who mature early continue to have an increased ratio of weight to height in adult life when compared to those who mature more slowly.

A trend toward increasing height and weight of adults has been evident over the past 100 years and probably longer. This trend can be observed in heights and weights of children as early as the seventh year of life. Concurrently there has been a tendency to earlier appearance of the menarche; in the United States the average age at menarche is now 1 year earlier (just under 13 years) than it was 50 years ago.

PREPUBESCENT AND POSTPUBESCENT PHASES OF MATURATION

The earliest indications of specific preparatory change for adolescence seem to occur by about 7 years of age in both boys and girls; at this time there is an increased production of 17-ketosteroids. Shortly afterward there is a gradual increase in production of estrogen and a little later of androgen in each sex. At the onset of pubescent changes in girls (9 to 11 years) estrogen production becomes greatly increased, attaining the levels for normal adults; similarly, increased androgen production occurs in boys between the ages of 12 and and 14 years. The differences between male and female adult output of 17-ketosteroids become established after 14 to 16 years of age.

The fat in subcutaneous tissue, which showed a steady proportionate decrease in amount from the ages of 1 to 6 years in both sexes, begins to reaccumulate as early as 8 years in girls and 10 years in boys. This reaccumulation will be clinically apparent as a filling out of subcutaneous tissue in most girls and in about two thirds of boys. This increase in fat content will tend to remain in girls, but will be a temporary feature of most boys, much being lost during the adolescent growth spurts in height and weight.

About a year after the increase in fat is first apparent the general growth spurt is initiated; it is concomitant in both sexes with the first signs of secondary sex maturation. Urinary gonadotropins may generally be detected by this time.

The earliest secondary sex changes observed in boys are usually an increase in the size of the testes and scrotum and later of the penis. About a third of boys have some conspicuous swelling of the breasts, often unilateral, and commonly with a small, sometimes tender, lump of tissue centrally located behind the nipple. This may persist for several months. Pubic, axillary and facial hair appears in that order, a sparse growth of downy pubic hair occurring close to the time of early enlargement of the testes and penis, becoming darker and more heavily pigmented within a year's time and, over the next 2 or 3 years, more curly and more extensive until the adult distribution is reached. Axillary hair usually appears about 2 years after pubic hair, along with facial hair. The change of voice occurs gradually, beginning with the early pubescent phase, and nocturnal emissions occur for the first time about a year after the beginning of secondary sex changes. There is some uncertainty as to when fully competent spermatozoa begin to be produced; relative infertility may extend in males to the fifteenth or sixteenth year or later.

In girls the secondary sex changes of pubescence have their onset on the average 2 years earlier than in boys. An increase in the width of the pelvis follows shortly upon the establishment of the secretion of estrogen and is most pronounced during the year of most rapid growth which just precedes the menarche. The first overt sign of pubescence is generally development of the breasts. Occasionally pubic hair will appear first, by as much as a year, and rarely the development of either breasts or pubic hair may anticipate true pubescence by a number of years – premature thelarche or pubarche. Axillary hair appears approximately a year after pubic hair. Along with early breast development, the vaginal secretion changes from alkaline to acid, and Doederlein's bacillus becomes established as the predominant flora.

About 2 years after the first evident pubescent change in the breasts the menarche is likely to occur. It is commonly preceded for several months by a regularly recurrent, clear vaginal discharge. The first few menstrual periods may be anovular, and irregularity is not unusual; this irregularity, sometimes with mild menorrhagia, is sufficiently common to be a normal variant, and generally subsides within a year after menarche. Irregularities after this time will be related more often to factors of general health, such as nutrition, fatigue or emotional tensions, than to primary endocrine or glandular abnormalities.

In both boys and girls the order of events in adolescence is subject to some variability and the time of onset to wide variability. The generally acceptable range of onset of pubescent changes in boys is from 10 to 14 years of age and in girls from 8 to 13 years. The earlier onset of the prepubescent growth spurt in girls decrees that, though boys are generally larger than girls of the same age for the first 11 years of life, between 11 and 13 years they will generally be smaller. The maximum increase in physical growth in girls occurs just before the menarche, at an average age of just under 13 years, with a range from 10 to 16 years. In boys the maximum increase occurs at a less well defined point with respect to the beginning of pubescent changes, about 2 years after the first change.

Radiographic examination of the epiphyses (bone age) gives the best indication of physiologic maturity in adolescence. For example, the standard deviation of chronologic age at menarche in relation to the mean age at menarche is 0.94 year, whereas the standard deviation of osseous age at menarche in relation to the mean chronologic age is only 0.44 year. The closure of the epiphyses occurs rapidly as the general growth spurt subsides (see p. 35).

In the period of rapid growth just preceding the menarche in girls or in the corresponding period in boys, there are increased retentions of nitrogen and calcium which fall to substantially lower levels in the following period of deceleration of growth. The slipped capital femoral epiphysis is particularly likely to appear in tall, heavy children during the active growth period, and vertebral epiphysitis during the following period, when growth of extremities has ceased, but vertebral growth continues a while longer.

The tendency of girls to retain fat accumulated during the prepubescent phase is matched by a tendency on the part of boys and a few girls to expand muscle mass in the later adolescent period. Boys grow rapidly in muscular strength and coordination after the average age of 13 years.

Other differentials between male and female become established during adolescence; these include the lower red blood cell counts and hemoglobin levels characteristic of women, the increased creatinine output in males, stabilization of basal body temperature at a level somewhat higher in females than in males, and a possibly related increased heart rate in girls. The blood pressure and pulse pressure attain normal adult values during adolescence, being slightly higher in boys than in girls. Respiratory rate and volume are higher for boys, as are maximal breathing capacity and alveolar carbon dioxide. This last appears related to the large muscle mass in males and is accompanied by a slightly higher average plasma bicarbonate level.

Social and educational activities for adolescents are set at levels determined by school achievement or chronologic age, rather than by physiologic maturity. The peak of physical differential between the sexes is reached in the eighth grade, when most girls are larger than their male classmates, a fact which gives the school dance and other social activities a mildly grotesque air. The slowly maturing child is often left out of social activities and team sports. By the time he or she matures physically the opportunity may have been lost for self-realization in some of these areas. The emotional integrity of adolescents is threatened by physical and sensory changes, by their changing status at home and in the community and by anxious preoccupation as to the meaning or adequacy of these changes and of their relation to their future roles in society. The physician can often be of great help to the adolescent in interpreting these changes in a friendly and casual way, with reassurance that physical changes are following normal and expected pathways.

The physician will often find himself under pressure to relieve anxiety through action other than reassurance. He may be urged, for example, to give hormones to the small boy to make him larger or to the tall girl to limit her ultimate height. An adequate assessment of growth records and of the present developmental status of the child in respect to chronologic age will generally permit reasonable predictions to be made. A slowly maturing boy of 16 or 17 may need study for hypogenitalism *(q.v.)*, and sometimes a trial of therapy. The long-range effects of using estrogen in tall girls to reduce ultimate height by hastening epiphyseal closure have not yet been assessed adequately.

Medical problems of adolescence include overnutrition and undernutrition, sometimes related to dietary habits determined by social pressure rather than by absence of adequate diet at home. Fatigue is common in adolescence and may be related to protein or iron deficiency, the latter sometimes expressed not so much by anemia as by lessened optimal function of enzyme systems using heme prosthetic groups. During adolescence there is heightened susceptibility to some illnesses and heightened reactivity to others. Myopia commonly has its onset during adolescence, as may some orthopedic conditions leading to kyphosis or scoliosis.

Acne adds to the physical and emotional burdens of adolescents, leading as it does to some disfigurement and accompanied as it is by a complex folklore. Adolescents are often reluctant to discuss their acne with the physician, who often must initiate its management (p. 1413).

The most significant health problem of adolescence is the frequency with which serious accidents occur. These are often directly related to the intense physical activity and emotional strivings of this age, particularly in boys. In the accident-prone child repeated accidents may be related to poorly solved problems of earlier life.

As the adolescent approaches adulthood, his path in Western culture is made difficult by the increasing span of higher education during which he continues to be dependent upon parents and home.

Erikson has listed a number of more or less sequential achievements for the healthy adolescent. The first he called *identification*. If this is achieved, the adolescent is able to plan a realistic future, with goals in education and vocation toward which he can effectively plan. Adolescents who have had difficulties in earlier life in finding adequate models and goals with which to identify will have a resurgence and intensification of their earlier problems.

The second goal is the establishment of a meaningful and healthy personal and social *intimacy,* based upon the capacity to share one's deepest feelings. Intimacy in this sense is established between boys and between girls as well as between boy and girl, or man and woman, and is more than just getting along with people and has much more than sexual connotations. This sharing of feelings is an essential ingredient of the quality of *empathy,* which is the ability to know how others feel and to respond to this feeling understandingly.

Generativity is the name given to the next goal in growth of the adolescent or young adult, not simply in the sense of producing children for another generation, but in the sense of producing something useful for society, with the incidental expectation that essential needs and reasonable wants will be gained or earned in return.

The final stage of growth is *integration.* Erikson visualizes this as the ability "to accept one's individual life cycle and the people who have become significant to it as meaningful within the segment of history in which one lives. . . . Integrity thus means a new and different love of one's parents, free of the wish that they should have been different and an acceptance of the fact that one's life is one's own responsibility. It is a sense of comradeship with men and women of distant times and of different pursuits, who have created orders and objects and sayings conveying human dignity and love."

SPECIAL ASPECTS OF GROWTH

Many structural and functional details of growth and development are inconspicuous for the broad pattern outlined above, but take on significance as they become foci of clinical concern or contribute to the evaluation or management of a clinical problem. The physician who monitors the growth and development of the child will need to known or find the limits of normal variability in these details, not only quantitatively and qualitatively, but also with respect to their interrelations.

VARIABILITY IN BODY PROPORTIONS

Besides the profound changes in general body proportions between fetal life and adult life (Fig. 2-5), there are also individual differences which seem to be the expression of innate growth potential and environmental modifications. These variations in body forms of normal persons may be designated as differences in *physique.* The term *constitution* connotes loosely the potentialities inherent in the individual at the time of birth for the development of a particular physique. Sheldon classified the physical types of man into

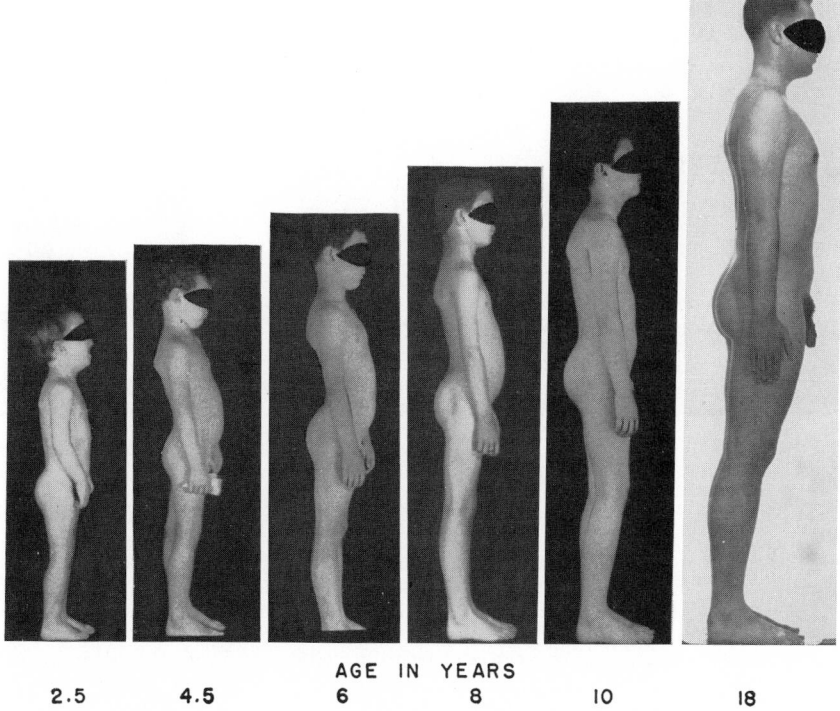

AGE IN YEARS

2.5   4.5   6   8   10   18

Figure 2-5. Lateral photographs which show characteristic developmental changes in body proportions and in erect posture. (From unpublished studies at Harvard School of Public Health.)

3 broad groups: the ectomorphic, the mesomorphic and the endomorphic (Fig. 2-6). The ectomorphic group is characterized principally by relative linearity, relatively light bone structure and relatively small mass in respect to body length. The endomorphic group is characterized by relatively stocky build and relatively large amounts of soft tissue. The pattern of the mesomorph is between that of the ectomorph and the endomorph. A variety of psychic and other functional attributes may be loosely related to constitution and to body type.

Somatotype is sometimes evident in early childhood, and at other times becomes clear only with the termination of the growth period. Somatotype does not seem to be closely related to the ultimate height or weight achieved, but the endomorph appears to mature earlier than the ectomorph. As a result of this early maturation the endomorphic child may have a tendency to be taller than the ectomorphic one in late childhood, the differences being reduced as the ectomorph completes his growth.

Other changes in bodily proportions depend not upon constitution or somatotype, but on different rates of growth of various body parts. The most

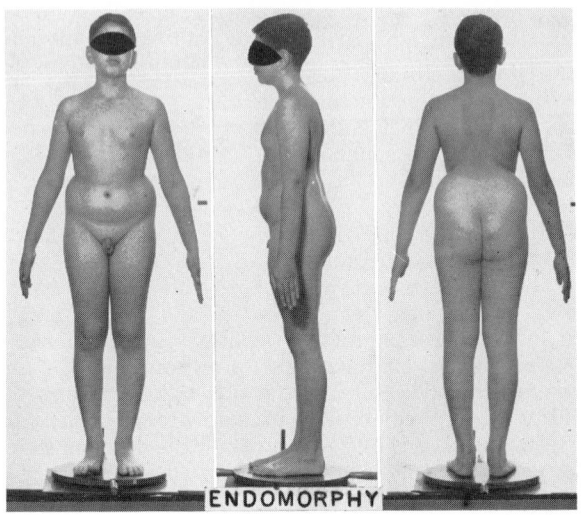

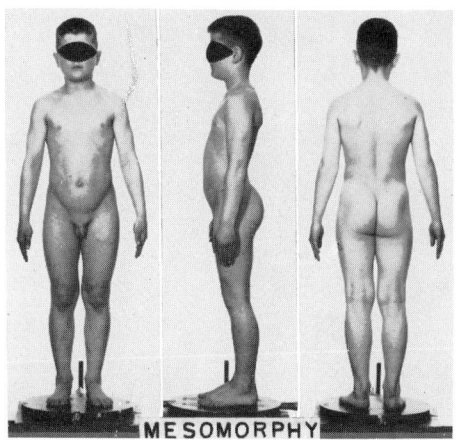
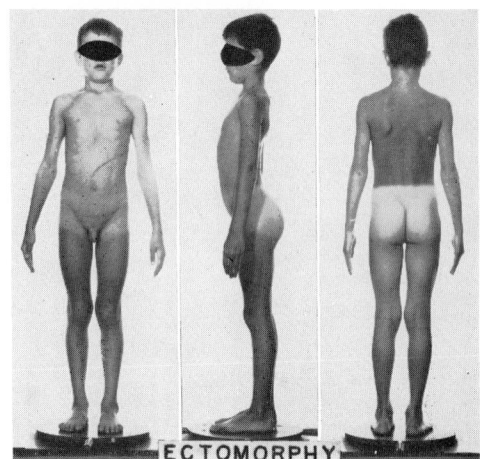

Figure 2-6. Examples of dominance of the 3 types of body build according to somatotype classification of Sheldon.* (Photos provided by E. E. Hunt, Forsyth Dental Infirmary, Boston.)

The principal characteristics of each of the 3 components of bodily constitution, some of which may be recognized in these photographs, are as follows:

Endomorphy—relative preponderance of soft roundness throughout the body, with large digestive viscera and accumulations of fat, usually large trunk and thighs and tapering extremities.

Mesomorphy—relative preponderance of muscle, bone and connective tissue, with heavy, hard physique of rectangular outline.

Ectomorphy—relative preponderance of linearity and fragility, with large surface area and thin muscles and subcutaneous tissue.

*Sheldon: *The Varieties of Human Physique.* New York, Harper & Brothers.

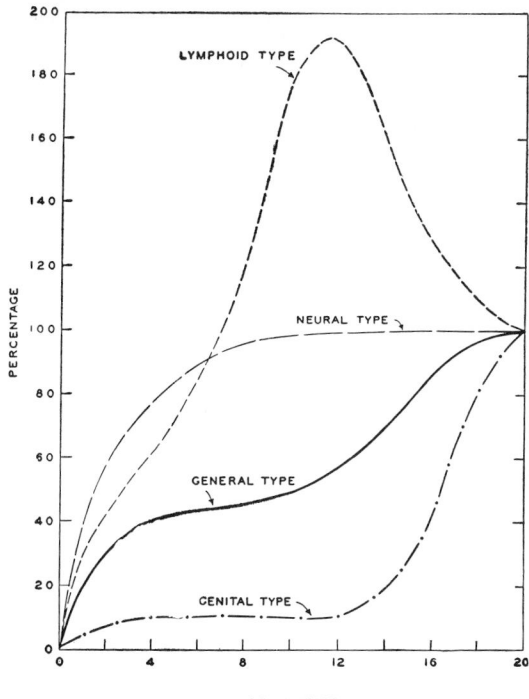

Figure 2-7. Main types of postnatal growth of the various parts and organs of the body. (After Scammon: *The Measurement of the Body in Childhood, The Measurement of Man.* University of Minnesota Press.)

conspicuous changes are in head size relative to body length, and length of the extremities relative to total body length. The size of the brain and cranial cavity approaches adult levels much more rapidly than the size of the face or the length of the legs. This relative preponderance of growth at the cephalad part of the body in fetal life, infancy and early childhood, with corresponding early elaboration of function, followed by the growth of trunk and extremities, has been termed the cephalocaudad progression. One of the last consequences of this for man is that the adolescent may find the extremities growing more rapidly than skills can be developed in their utilization.

Alterations in proportionate sizes of trunk, extremities and head are characteristic of certain disturbances of growth, and may give insight as to the underlying pathophysiologic process. The measurements which are usually most helpful will be sitting and standing heights, span, body weight, and circumference of head. Normally, the sitting height represents about 70 per cent of body length in the newborn infant, but only 57 per cent at 3 years, and about 52 per cent at the time of the menarche in girls and about 15 years in boys. Following this lowest ratio, there is a slight increase of 1 or 2 percentage points, as the trunk continues and the extremities have ceased their growth in the postpubescent period.

Other variations in rapid growth, again correlated with function, are distinctive for a number of body systems. Figure 2-7 illustrates the pro-

portionate rates of growth for several body systems. Standards are available for the weights of organs at various ages, which indicate that organs follow characteristic patterns which may be designated as lymphoid, neural, general and genital. There are a number of deviations. For example, although the ovary and testes follow the designated genital pattern, the uterus and adrenals are relatively large at birth, and show involution in the early weeks of life. The spleen appears to follow the lymphoid pattern, and the liver the general growth pattern. Skeletal muscle follows the general pattern, but is slow to achieve its ultimate

BREADTHS OF SOFT TISSUES IN CALF FROM A-P ROENTGENOGRAMS OF LEG

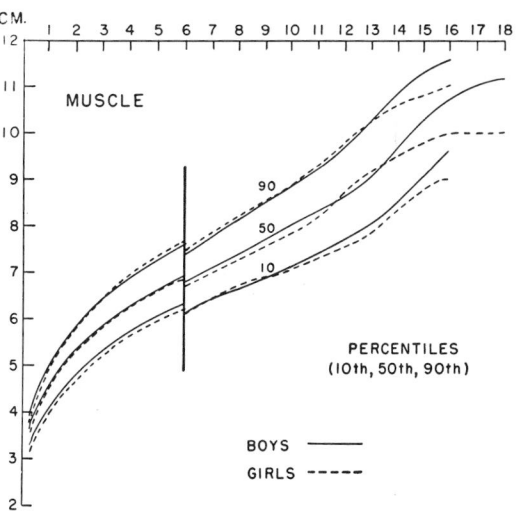

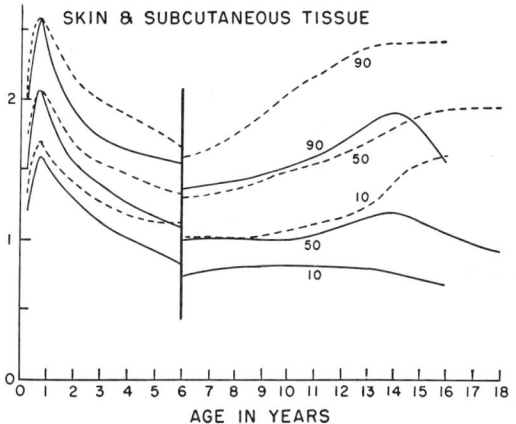

Figure 2-8. Breadths of muscle and of double layers of skin and subcutaneous tissue at greatest width of calf by age and sex from 3 months to 18 years of age.

The graphs reveal the close similarity in pattern of the curves for muscle to those of general growth, but a unique pattern of increase and decrease and a sex difference in the skin and subcutaneous tissue. (For details, see Stuart and Sobel: *J. Pediat.,* Vol. 28, and Lombard: *Child Dev.,* Vol. 21. For distribution of subcutaneous fat in childhood and adolescence, see Reynolds: Monographs Soc. Res. Child Dev., Vol. 15.)

TABLE 2-3. Ages at Onset of Ossification, Recognized by Appearance of Centers in Roentgenograms, Useful as Maturity Indicators During Infancy and Childhood

BOYS Mean Yrs.	Mos.	Standard Deviation* Mos.	NO. CORRESPONDING TO CENTER IN FIG. 2-9	BONE AND OSSIFICATION CENTER	GIRLS Mean Yrs.	Mos.	Standard Deviation* Mos.
Shoulder and Elbow							
3 weeks		—	1	Humerus, head	3 weeks		—
0	7	4	2	Humerus, capitellum	0	4	2
1	1	7	3	Humerus, greater tuberosity	0	6	3
5	5	15	4	Radius, proximal epiphysis	4	1	14
6	1	15	5	Humerus, medial epicondyle	3	7	12
—	—	—	6	Ulna, olecranon, 1	—	—	—
—	—	—	7	Humerus, trochlea	—	—	—
—	—	—	8	Humerus, lateral epicondyle	—	—	—
—	—	—	9	Ulna, olecranon, 2	—	—	—
Hand and Wrist							
0	2	2	1	Capitate	0	2	2
0	3	2	2	Hamate	0	2	2
1	1	5	3	Distal epiphysis, radius	0	10	4
1	4	4	4	Proximal epiphysis, 3rd finger	0	10	3
1	4	4	5	Proximal epiphysis, 2nd finger	0	11	3
1	5	5	6	Proximal epiphysis, 4th finger	0	11	3
1	6	5	7	Epiphysis of metacarpal II	1	0	3
1	7	7	8	Distal epiphysis, 1st finger	1	0	4
1	8	5	9	Epiphysis of metacarpal III	1	1	3
1	11	6	10	Epiphysis of metacarpal IV	1	3	4
1	9	5	11	Proximal epiphysis, 5th finger	1	2	4
2	0	6	12	Middle epiphysis, 3rd finger	1	3	5
2	0	6	13	Middle epiphysis, 4th finger	1	3	5
2	2	7	14	Epiphysis of metacarpal V	1	4	5
2	2	6	15	Middle epiphysis, 2nd finger	1	4	5
2	6	16	16	Triquetral	1	9	14
2	4	6	17	Distal epiphysis, 3rd finger	1	6	4
2	4	6	18	Distal epiphysis, 4th finger	1	6	15
2	8	9	19	Epiphysis of metacarpal I	1	6	5
2	8	7	20	Proximal epiphysis, 1st finger	1	8	5
3	1	9	21	Distal epiphysis, 5th finger	1	11	6
3	1	8	22	Distal epiphysis, 2nd finger	1	11	6
3	3	10	23	Middle epiphysis, 5th finger	1	10	7
3	6	19	24	Lunate	2	10	13
5	7	19	25	Greater multangular	3	11	14
5	9	15	26	Lesser multangular	4	1	12
5	6	15	27	Navicular (hand)	4	3	12
6	10	14	28	Distal epiphysis of ulna	5	9	13
—	—	—	29	Pisiform	—	—	—
12	8	18	30	Sesamoid in adductor pollicis	10	1	13
Hip and Knee							
(Usually at birth)			1	Femur, distal epiphysis	(Usually at birth)		
(Usually at birth)			2	Tibia, proximal epiphysis	(Usually at birth)		
0	4	2	3	Femur, head	0	4	2
3	6	10	4	Femur, greater trochanter	2	5	5
3	9	12	5	Fibula, proximal epiphysis	2	9	11
3	10	11	6	Patella	2	5	7
—	—	—	7	Tibia, tuberosity, 1	—	—	—
—	—	—	8	Tibia, tuberosity, 2	—	—	—

* *Standard deviation* adjusted to nearest month. The range included between minus 1 and plus 1 standard deviation from the mean for any center will usually include about 68 per cent of a population of healthy children.

TABLE 2-3. *(Continued)*

BOYS			NO. CORRESPONDING TO CENTER IN FIG. 2-9	BONE AND OSSIFICATION CENTER	GIRLS		
Mean		Standard Deviation*			Mean		Standard Deviation*
Yrs.	Mos.	Mos.			Yrs.	Mos.	Mos.

Foot and Ankle

Yrs.	Mos.	Mos.	No.	Bone	Yrs.	Mos.	Mos.
2 weeks		—	1	Cuboid	2 weeks		—
0	4	2	2	Tibia, distal epiphysis	0	4	1
0	4	4	3	Lateral cuneiform	0	4	4
1	1	4	4	Fibula, distal epiphysis	0	9	3
1	4	6	5	Distal epiphysis, great toe	0	9	3
1	7	5	6	Proximal epiphysis, 3rd toe	0	11	4
1	8	5	7	Proximal epiphysis, 4th toe	1	1	4
1	9	5	8	Proximal epiphysis, 2nd toe	1	1	4
2	1	10	9	Medial cuneiform	1	4	7
2	4	5	10	Proximal epiphysis, great toe	1	6	4
2	5	5	11	Metatarsal I	1	7	3
2	5	9	12	Middle cuneiform	1	7	7
2	7	13	13	Navicular (foot)	1	9	10
2	7	7	14	Proximal epiphysis, 5th toe	1	8	5
2	10	7	15	Metatarsal II	2	0	5
3	5	8	16	Metatarsal III	2	5	5
3	11	8	17	Metatarsal IV	2	9	7
4	5	10	18	Distal epiphysis, metatarsal V	3	2	8
7	5	11	19	Calcaneus, epiphysis, 1	5	0	11
—	—	—	20	Accessory talus	—	—	—
—	—	—	21	Proximal epiphysis, metatarsal V	—	—	—
—	—	—	22	Calcaneus, epiphysis, 2	—	—	—

AGE AT ONSET OF FUSION IN SKELETAL REGIONS USEFUL AS MATURITY INDICATORS DURING ADOLESCENCE

BOYS	SKELETAL REGION	GIRLS
Modal Skeletal Age in Years*		Modal Skeletal Age in Years*
	Elbow	
13.0 — 13.5	Begins in humerus	11.0 — 11.5
15.0 — 15.5	Completed in ulna	12.5 — 13.0
	Foot and ankle	
14.0 — 14.5	Begins in great toe	12.5 — 13.0
15.5 — 16.0	Completed in tibia and fibula	14.0 — 14.5
	Hand and wrist	
15.0 — 15.5	Begins in distal phalanges	13.0 — 13.5
17.5 — 18.0	Completed in radius	16.0 — 16.5
	Knee	
15.0 — 15.5	Begins in tibial tuberosity	13.5 — 14.0
17.5 — 18.0	Completed in fibula	16.0 — 16.5
	Hip and pelvis	
15.5 — 16.0	Begins in greater trochanter	14.0 — 14.5
after 18.0	Completed in symphysis	17.5 — 18.0
	Shoulder and shoulder girdle	
15.5 — 16.0	Begins in greater tuberosity	14.0 — 14.5
after 18.0	Completed in clavicle	17.5 — 18.0

* Modal skeletal age is given for onset of fusion because satisfactory means and standard deviations are not available for these ages.

Note. The norms in this table present a composite of published data from the Fels Research Institute, Yellow Springs, Ohio (Pyle and Sontag: *Am. J. Roentgenol.*, Vol. 19), and unpublished data from the Brush Foundation, Western Reserve University, Cleveland, Ohio, and the Harvard School of Public Health, Boston, Massachusetts. Compiled by Lieb, Buehl and Pyle.

mass. Cardiac muscle is initially proportionately large to body size and thereafter follows the general growth curve.

The weight of the thymus is labile in childhood, decreasing rapidly during illness. It appears to follow the general pattern of growth during the first 5 years of life, then maintains a relatively steady state, with involution at adolescence.

As indicated earlier, the proportionate mass of subcutaneous tissue is greatest by about 9 months; it then decreases steadily to about 6 years, when the increase begins which presages the "fat spurt" in preadolescence, at which time sex differences become apparent (Fig. 2-8).

EVALUATION OF OSSEOUS MATURATION

The ossification of the skeleton of the fetus begins by about the fifth month and from that time makes considerable demands upon the maternal supply of bone-forming substances. Ossification occurs earliest in the clavicle and membranous bone of the skull, and follows rapidly in long bones and spine. The distal femoral and proximal tibial epiphyses are usually ossified in the normal full-term infant. The fusion of the humeral capitellum with the shaft is said to mark the end of the period of most rapid growth in girls and to predict the menarche within the next year.

There is no better index of general growth than bone age as determined from roentgenograms. This is based (1) on the number and size of epiphyseal centers at a given chronologic age, (2) on the size, shape, density, and sharpness of outline of the ends of bones, and (3) on the distance separating epiphyseal center and zone of provisional calcification or the degree of fusion between these 2 elements. The information gained from

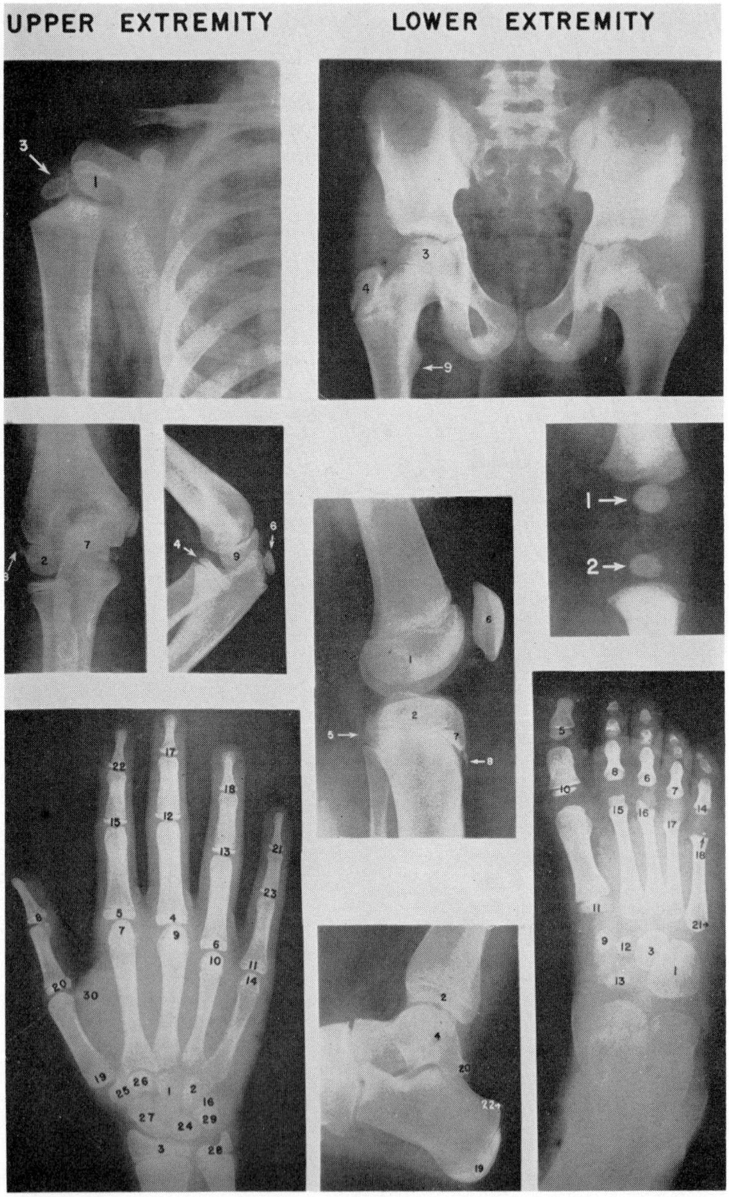

UPPER EXTREMITY   LOWER EXTREMITY

Figure 2-9. Centers of ossification in the extremities for use in referring to Table 2-3.

Roentgenograms of children of different ages selected to show as clearly as possible the epiphyseal centers of interest in each view and to identify them by the numbers which correspond to those in Table 2-3. (Figure prepared by I. Pyle, D. G. Shields, and W. H. Golden.)

the various epiphyseal areas varies with chronologic age. The hand and wrist are useful at all ages of childhood; useful information can also be derived from the lower extremity, especially in early infancy. The most widely used standards are those of Todd, of Greulich and Pyle, and of Vogt and Vickers for the hand. Reynolds and Asakawa have provided useful standards for the lower extremity, head of the humerus, and capitellum in early infancy. Figure 2-9 and Table 2-3 show expected times of appearance of various ossification centers with normal variabilities for each. Since girls are more advanced than boys in skeletal development at all ages, separate standards are necessary.

No interpretation of skeletal age should fail to take into account that 1 normal child in 20 can be expected to have a skeletal age either advanced or retarded by 2 standard deviations from the mean for his chronologic age. Data of Pyle, Reed and Stuart indicate that in boys the standard deviation of bone age (given by the norms of Greulich and Pyle) around chronologic age is about 2 months in the first year of life, and increases to

TABLE 2-4. CHRONOLOGY OF HUMAN DENTITION
Primary or Deciduous Teeth

	CALCIFICATION		ERUPTION		SHEDDING	
	Begins at	Complete at	Maxillary	Mandibular	Maxillary	Mandibular
Central incisors	5th fetal month	18–24 months	6–8 months	5–7 months	7–8 years	6–7 years
Lateral incisors........	5th fetal month	18–24 months	8–11 months	7–10 months	8–9 years	7–8 years
Cuspids (canines)	6th fetal month	30–36 months	16–20 months	16–20 months	11–12 years	9–11 years
First molars..........	5th fetal month	24–30 months	10–16 months	10–16 months	10–11 years	10–12 years
Second molars........	6th fetal month	36 months	20–30 months	20–30 months	10–12 years	11–13 years

Secondary or Permanent Teeth

	CALCIFICATION		ERUPTION	
	Begins at	Complete at	Maxillary	Mandibular
Central incisors..........................	3–4 months	9–10 years	7–8 years	6–7 years
Lateral incisors..........................	Max., 10–12 months Mand., 3–4 months	10–11 years	8–9 years	7–8 years
Cuspids (canines)	4–5 months	12–15 years	11–12 years	9–11 years
First premolars.........................	18–21 months	12–13 years	10–11 years	10–12 years
Second premolars........................	24–30 months	12–14 years	10–12 years	11–13 years
First molars.............................	Birth	9–10 years	6–7 years	6–7 years
Second molars...........................	30–36 months	14–16 years	12–13 years	12–13 years
Third molars............................	Max., 7–9 years Mand., 8–10 years	18–25 years	17–22 years	17–22 years

Adapted from chart prepared by P. K. Losch, who carried out roentgenographic assays of the jaws of 1000 children in metropolitan Boston in 1942 at the Harvard School of Dental Medicine and provided the data for this chart.

4 months during the second year, to 6 months during the third year, and to 10 months by the seventh year. Thereafter, for the rest of the growth period, the standard deviation is about 12 to 15 months. The variability is less for girls than for boys, especially in later childhood. The theoretical percentile points corresponding to such variability can be calculated.

EVALUATION OF DENTAL DEVELOPMENT

The calcification of teeth begins in fetal life about the seventh month. This calcification involves principally deciduous teeth, but shortly before term calcification begins in the permanent teeth which will be first to erupt. Nutritional disorders and prolonged illness in infancy may interfere with calcification of deciduous and permanent teeth.

Such nutritional disturbances, if temporary, may leave defects in the enamel ranging from a line of small pits across the tooth to a broader band of hypoplasia. It is possible at times to date a nutritional disturbance by these bands of hypoplasia.

The formation of healthy tooth structure is fostered by a diet adequate in protein, calcium, phosphate and vitamins, especially C and D, and depends further upon an adequate supply of thyroid hormone. The resistance of teeth to dental caries is significantly increased when fluoride is available in optimal quantities.

Table 2-4 lists the times of eruption of the deciduous and permanent teeth. Delay in eruption of deciduous teeth occurs in hypothyroidism and in other nutritional and growth disturbances, but the normal variability in eruption prevents such delay from being useful as an index of a growth disorder. In some families the children have conspicuously early or late dentition without other signs of retardation or acceleration of growth.

The first permanent teeth to erupt are the 6-year molars; they are often mistaken for deciduous teeth by the uninformed. The first permanent molars serve as focal points in the dental arch and so have a great deal to do with the ultimate shape of the jaw and the orderly arrangement of teeth. Caries or other defects in them should receive prompt attention; these teeth should not be extracted.

SPECIAL ASPECTS OF GROWTH IN THE RESPIRATORY TRACT

Anatomically, the respiratory tract of the newborn infant is distinguished by the lack of well developed accessory sinuses, by the close relation of the nasopharynx to the middle ear through a eustachian tube which is relatively short and broad, and by the absence of well developed mastoid air cells. The maxillary sinus at this time consists of a single cell, the ethmoid sinus of a few cells, and the mastoid only of an antrum. The sphenoidal sinuses appear by about the age of 3 years, and the frontal sinuses between 3 and 7 years of age.

The tympanic membrane in the newborn infant has a more oblique position with respect to the external auditory canal than it will have in later life, and the drum is somewhat thicker and more opaque. The middle ear at birth is filled with a mucoid substance which may be mistaken for exudate of infection if the ear is opened. The shortness and relative wideness of the eustachian tube contribute to the high incidence of otitis media in infancy.

DEVELOPMENTAL ASPECTS OF THE CARDIOVASCULAR SYSTEM

Figures 2-10 and 2-11 show the pulse and respiratory rates for children of various ages and indicate the distinctive differences between boys and girls which become evident at adolescence. See page 964 for other aspects of development of the cardiovascular system.

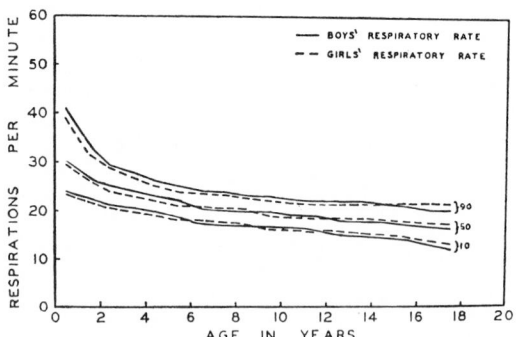

Figure 2-10. Respiratory rates in infants and children.

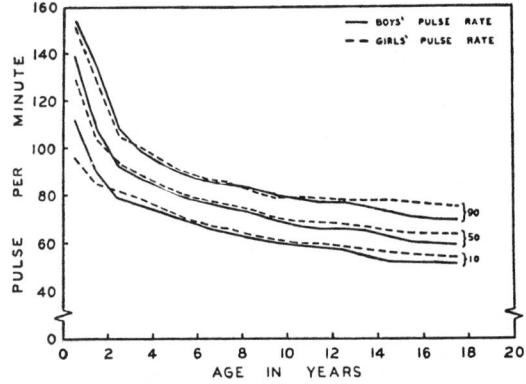

Figure 2-11. Pulse rates in infants and children.

DEVELOPMENTAL ASPECTS OF NUTRITION AND METABOLISM

(See also page 127)

The infant's and child's nutritional requirements increase with growth in size. The parameter of growth with which many of the nutritional factors bear the most nearly constant relation is body surface, which appears to be as closely related to the body's mass of metabolically active tissue as any other simple measurement. Owing, however, to fundamental differences in the metabolic activity of infants and children at various ages, adjustments may be necessary. This is particularly evident with respect to administration of drugs in the neonatal period.

Measurements of body surface which correspond to given heights and weights are available; reasonably accurate estimates of body surface can be obtained from nomograms (p. 236). Cruder estimates of body surface from weight only can be made for children whose physique is average; Lowe's formula is:

$$\text{surface area (M}^2) = \sqrt[3]{\text{Wt.}^2 \text{ (kg.)}} \times 0.1$$

Another crude estimate for children of average physique is given by the simpler formulas:

Approximation of Surface Area (M²) to Weight (kg.)

WEIGHT RANGE	APPROXIMATE SURFACE AREA
1 to *5* kg.	M² = 0.05 × kg. + 0.05
6 to *10* kg.	M² = 0.04 × kg. + 0.10
11 to *20* kg.	M² = 0.03 × kg. + 0.20
21 to *40* kg.	M² = 0.02 × kg. + 0.40

(The figures 5, 10, 20 and 40 are given in italics to indicate a simple mnemonic.)

Examples:
for 7 kg. infant, area (M²) = 0.04 × 7+0.10 = 0.38 M²
for 17-kg. infant, area (M²) = 0.03 × 17+0.20 = 0.71 M²
(estimates of 0.4 M² and 0.7 M² respectively would be reasonable)

(The formula M² = 0.02 × kg. + 40 is reasonably accurate from 21 to 70 kg.)

Basal caloric needs, when referred to body surface, appear to be somewhat lower in premature infants than in full-term ones. They increase during the first year of life from approximately 30 calories per square meter per hour to about 50 by the second year, with a subsequent fall to adult levels of 35 to 40 calories per square meter per hour. The data of Lewis indicate that the rate of fall is slowed during prepubertal and adolescent years, owing to the need for additional energy for accelerated growth.

Needs for water and electrolytes remain roughly constant in their proportion to body surface through most of the growing period; the inevitable variations in intake are met by the capacity of homeostatic mechanisms to adjust to varying conditions of supply and demand. Talbot, Richie and Crawford have outlined the limits within which the body is equipped to adjust to variations in intake and output.

ASSESSMENT OF PHYSICAL GROWTH AND DEVELOPMENT

Appraisal of growth and development in the infant and the child has its greatest usefulness only if it is accurate and continuous in each of the areas in which changes can be observed. In the infant the most useful physical measurements are head circumference, length and weight (Fig. 2-12 and Tables 2-5, 2-6, 2-7). Note should also be made of the nutritional state, dentition, and the size or patency of fontanels. In selected instances measurements of the thickness of subcutaneous tissue or the lengths of body segments may be appropriate.

The record of the child's growth can be kept in a number of ways and according to various standards. This information will be most useful if it is recorded at serial examinations on charts permitting comparisons with standards for each age. The Harvard charts (Fig. 2-12), Iowa charts (Fig. 2-13) and Wetzel grids offer ways in which this may be accomplished. The standards used for these charts reflect the achievement of Caucasian children of predominantly middle class origin and may need revision for other socioeconomic, ethnic or racial stocks. There is growing evidence that ethnic differences depend in largest measure upon differences in prevalence of malnutrition and infectious diseases in different parts of the world. Accuracy of measurement is essential to the reliable interpretation of growth data; slight variations in technique may result in significantly large errors in the placement of children according to percentile rank.

TECHNIQUES OF MEASUREMENT

Height. *Recumbent length* can be more accurately measured than standing height in children under the age of 5 years, after which measurement of standing height is generally more convenient. Recumbent length is measured as the child lies on a firm table which has a measuring stick at least 125 cm. or 50 inches long inserted along one edge. The soles of the feet are held firmly against a fixed upright placed at the zero mark. A movable upright crosses the table above the head and is brought firmly against the vertex. If recumbent length is used after 5 years of age, the value obtained may be reduced by 1 cm. and then considered against the scale for standing height.

Standing height is measured as the child stands erect, his heels, buttocks, upper part of the back

(Text continued on page 54.)

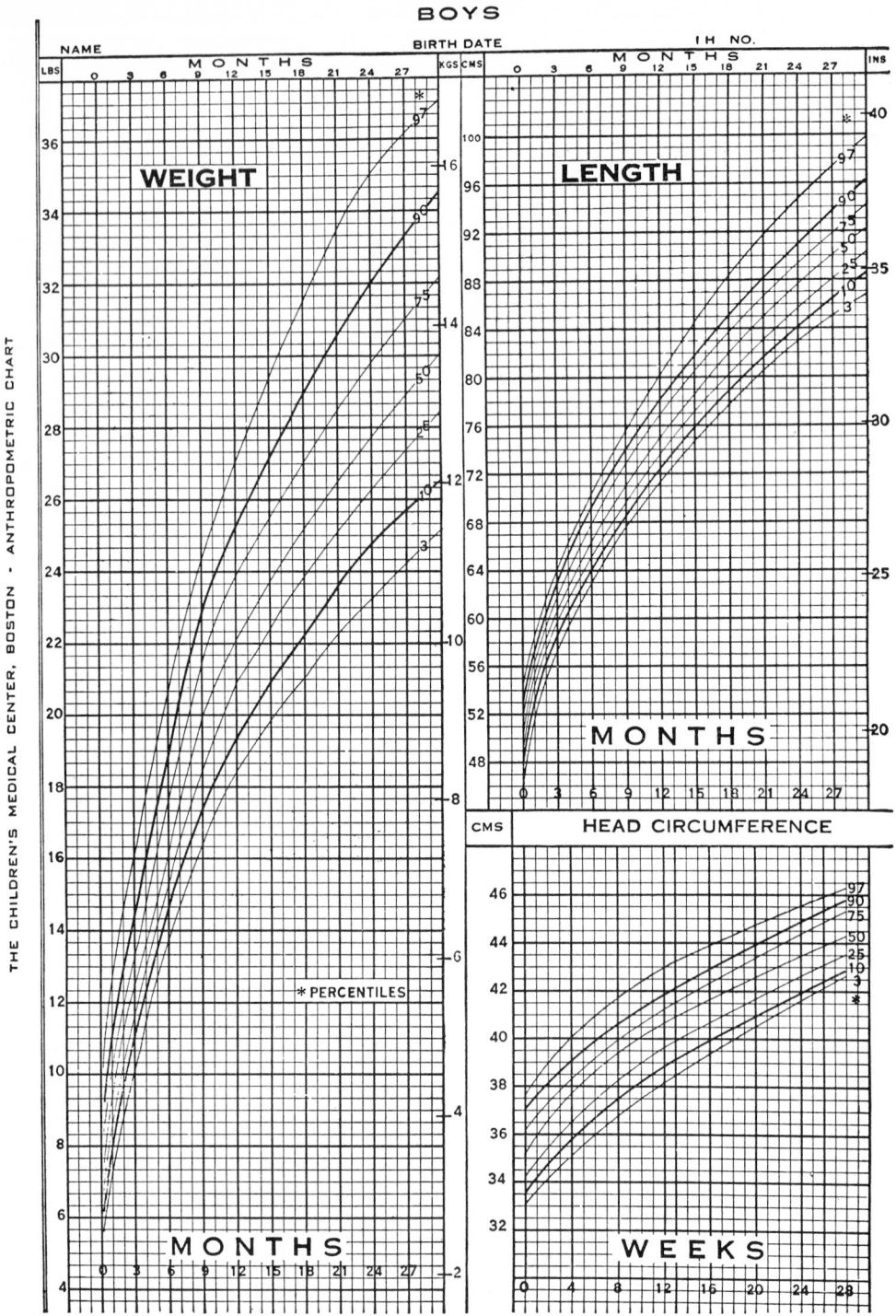

Figure 2-12. Graphs for plotting selected measurements in infancy. These graphs as well as those in Figure 2-13 are based on studies conducted by the Harvard School of Public Health of white children in Boston of predominantly north European stock. Separate charts are used for girls, since norms for the 2 sexes differ appreciably.

These graphs serve for plotting weight and height measurements up to 30 months and head circumference up to 30 weeks. The percentile values on which they are based are given in Tables 2-5 and 2-7.

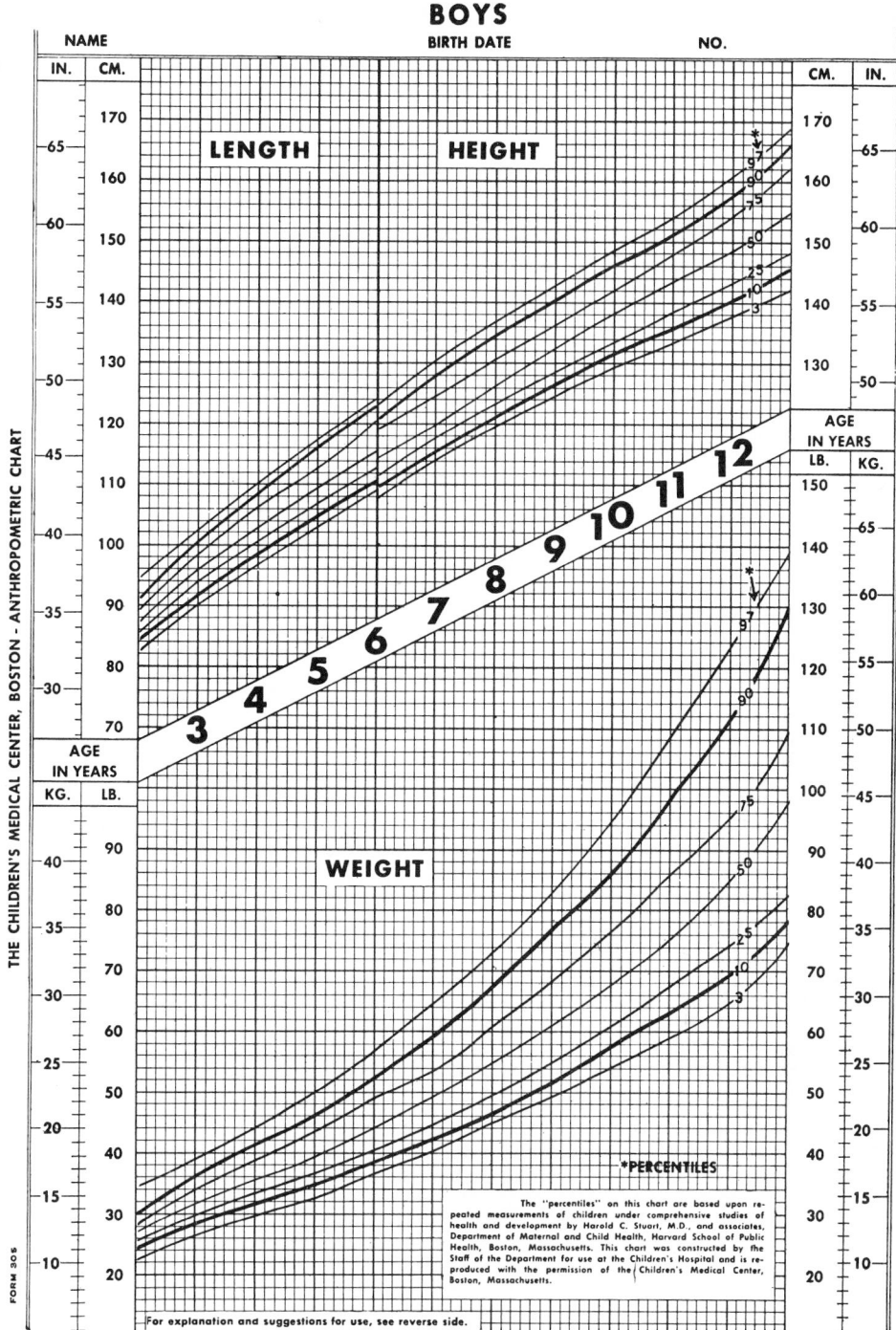

Figure 2-13. Graphs for plotting weight and height in childhood. This graph serves to plot weight and height from 2 to 13 years of age (height is measured in recumbent position to 6 years of age).

Percentile graphs for plotting measurements against chronologic age are not as satisfactory for use after 13 years, owing to the wide age variability in the timing of maximum growth during adolescence. For graphs which extend to 18 years based on the percentile values given in Tables 2-6 and 2-8, see Stuart and Meredith: *Am. J. Pub. Health*, Vol. 36. Other percentile graphs covering various age periods are available from the Iowa Child Welfare Research Station, University of Iowa.

In evaluation of the measurements of the 13-year-old child it is usually possible to recognize by the appearance of secondary sex characters those children who deviate from expected percentile positions because of early or late pubescence.

GROWTH MEAS.

TABLE 2-5. PERCENTILES FOR WEIGHT AND LENGTH—BIRTH TO 5 YEARS

Measurement	Boys 3	Boys 10	Boys 25	Boys 50	Boys 75	Boys 90	Boys 97	Girls 3	Girls 10	Girls 25	Girls 50	Girls 75	Girls 90	Girls 97
Birth														
Weight in Pounds	5.8	6.3	6.9	7.5	8.3	9.1	10.1	5.8	6.2	6.9	7.4	8.1	8.6	9.4
Weight in Kg.	2.63	2.86	3.13	3.4	3.76	4.13	4.58	2.63	2.81	3.13	3.36	3.67	3.9	4.26
Length in Inches	18.2	18.9	19.4	19.9	20.5	21.0	21.5	18.5	18.8	19.3	19.8	20.1	20.4	21.1
Length in Cm.	46.3	48.1	49.3	50.6	52.0	53.3	54.6	47.1	47.8	49.0	50.2	51.0	51.9	53.6
3 Months														
Weight in Pounds	10.6	11.1	11.8	12.6	13.6	14.5	16.4	9.8	10.7	11.4	12.4	13.2	14.0	14.9
Weight in Kg.	4.81	5.03	5.35	5.72	6.17	6.58	7.44	4.45	4.85	5.17	5.62	5.99	6.35	6.76
Length in Inches	22.4	22.8	23.3	23.8	24.3	24.7	25.1	22.0	22.4	22.8	23.4	23.9	24.3	24.8
Length in Cm.	56.8	57.8	59.3	60.4	61.8	62.8	63.7	55.8	56.9	57.9	59.5	60.7	61.7	63.1
6 Months														
Weight in Pounds	14.0	14.8	15.6	16.7	18.0	19.2	20.8	12.7	14.1	15.0	16.0	17.5	18.6	20.0
Weight in Kg.	6.35	6.71	7.08	7.58	8.16	8.71	9.43	5.76	6.4	6.8	7.26	7.94	8.44	9.07
Length in Inches	24.8	25.2	25.7	26.1	26.7	27.3	27.7	24.0	24.6	25.1	25.7	26.2	26.7	27.1
Length in Cm.	63.0	63.9	65.2	66.4	67.8	69.3	70.4	61.1	62.5	63.7	65.2	66.6	67.8	68.8
9 Months														
Weight in Pounds	16.6	17.8	18.7	20.0	21.5	22.9	24.4	15.1	16.6	17.8	19.2	20.8	22.4	24.2
Weight in Kg.	7.53	8.07	8.48	9.07	9.75	10.39	11.07	6.85	7.53	8.03	8.71	9.43	10.16	10.98
Length in Inches	26.6	27.0	27.5	28.0	28.7	29.2	29.9	25.7	26.4	26.9	27.6	28.2	28.7	29.2
Length in Cm.	67.7	68.6	69.8	71.2	72.9	74.2	75.9	65.4	67.0	68.4	70.1	71.7	72.9	74.1
12 Months														
Weight in Pounds	18.5	19.6	20.9	22.2	23.8	25.4	27.3	16.8	18.4	19.8	21.5	23.0	24.8	27.1
Weight in Kg.	8.39	8.89	9.48	10.07	10.8	11.52	12.38	7.62	8.35	8.98	9.75	10.43	11.25	12.29
Length in Inches	28.1	28.5	29.0	29.6	30.3	30.7	31.6	27.1	27.8	28.5	29.2	29.9	30.3	31.0
Length in Cm.	71.3	72.4	73.7	75.2	76.9	78.1	80.3	68.9	70.6	72.3	74.2	75.9	77.1	78.8
15 Months														
Weight in Pounds	19.8	21.0	22.4	23.7	25.4	27.2	29.4	18.1	19.8	21.3	23.0	24.6	26.6	29.0
Weight in Kg.	8.98	9.53	10.16	10.75	11.52	12.34	13.33	8.21	8.98	9.66	10.43	11.16	12.07	13.15
Length in Inches	29.3	29.8	30.3	30.9	31.6	32.1	33.1	28.3	29.0	29.8	30.5	31.3	31.8	32.6
Length in Cm.	74.4	75.6	77.0	78.5	80.3	81.5	84.2	71.9	73.7	75.6	77.6	79.4	80.8	82.8
18 Months														
Weight in Pounds	21.1	22.3	23.8	25.2	26.9	29.0	31.5	19.4	21.2	22.7	24.5	26.2	28.3	30.9
Weight in Kg.	9.57	10.12	10.8	11.43	12.2	13.15	14.29	8.8	9.62	10.3	11.11	11.88	12.84	14.02

TABLE 2-5. *(Continued)*

Length in Inches	34.1	33.3	32.6	31.8	31.1	30.2	29.5	30.5	31.0	31.6	32.2	32.9	33.5	34.7
Length in Cm.	86.7	84.5	82.9	80.9	79.0	76.8	74.9	77.5	78.8	80.3	81.8	83.7	85.0	88.2
2 Years														
Weight in Pounds	34.4	31.7	29.2	27.1	25.3	23.5	21.6	23.3	24.7	26.3	27.7	29.7	31.9	34.9
Weight in Kg.	15.6	14.38	13.25	12.29	11.48	10.66	9.8	10.57	11.2	11.93	12.56	13.47	14.47	15.83
Length in Inches	36.7	35.8	35.0	34.1	33.3	32.3	31.5	32.6	33.1	33.8	34.4	35.2	35.9	37.2
Length in Cm.	93.3	91.0	88.9	86.6	84.7	82.0	80.1	82.7	84.2	85.8	87.5	89.4	91.1	94.6
2½ Years														
Weight in Pounds	38.2	34.6	31.9	29.6	27.4	25.5	23.6	25.2	26.6	28.4	30.0	32.2	34.5	37.0
Weight in Kg.	17.33	15.69	14.47	13.43	12.43	11.57	10.7	11.43	12.07	12.88	13.61	14.61	15.65	16.78
Length in Inches	38.9	37.9	36.9	36.0	35.2	34.0	33.3	34.2	34.8	35.5	36.3	37.0	37.9	39.2
Length in Cm.	98.7	96.4	93.8	91.4	89.3	86.3	84.5	86.9	88.5	90.2	92.1	94.1	96.2	99.5
3 Years														
Weight in Pounds	41.8	37.4	34.6	31.8	29.6	27.6	25.6	27.0	28.7	30.3	32.2	34.5	36.8	39.2
Weight in Kg.	18.96	16.96	15.69	14.42	13.43	12.52	11.61	12.25	13.02	13.74	14.61	15.65	16.69	17.78
Length in Inches	40.7	39.8	38.6	37.7	36.8	35.6	34.8	35.7	36.3	37.0	37.9	38.8	39.6	40.5
Length in Cm.	103.5	101.1	98.1	95.7	93.4	90.5	88.4	90.6	92.3	93.9	96.2	98.5	100.5	102.8
3½ Years														
Weight in Pounds	45.3	40.4	37.0	33.9	31.5	29.5	27.5	28.5	30.4	32.3	34.3	36.7	39.1	41.5
Weight in Kg.	20.55	18.33	16.78	15.38	14.29	13.38	12.47	12.93	13.79	14.65	15.56	16.65	17.74	18.82
Length in Inches	42.5	41.5	40.2	39.2	38.1	37.1	36.2	37.1	37.8	38.4	39.3	40.3	41.1	41.9
Length in Cm.	108.0	105.4	102.0	99.5	96.9	94.2	92.0	94.3	96.0	97.5	99.8	102.5	104.5	106.5
4 Years														
Weight in Pounds	48.2	43.5	39.6	36.2	33.5	31.2	29.2	30.1	32.1	34.0	36.4	39.0	41.4	44.3
Weight in Kg.	21.86	19.73	17.96	16.42	15.2	14.15	13.25	13.65	14.56	15.42	16.51	17.69	18.78	20.09
Length in Inches	44.2	43.1	41.6	40.6	39.5	38.4	37.5	38.4	39.1	39.7	40.7	41.9	42.7	43.5
Length in Cm.	112.3	109.6	105.8	103.2	100.3	97.6	95.2	97.5	99.3	100.8	103.4	106.5	108.5	110.4
4½ Years														
Weight in Pounds	50.9	46.7	42.1	38.5	35.3	32.9	30.7	31.6	33.8	35.7	38.4	41.4	43.9	47.4
Weight in Kg.	23.09	21.18	19.1	17.46	16.01	14.92	13.93	14.33	15.33	16.19	17.42	18.78	19.91	21.5
Length in Inches	45.7	44.7	43.0	42.0	40.8	39.7	38.6	39.6	40.3	40.9	42.0	43.3	44.2	45.0
Length in Cm.	116.2	113.5	109.3	106.8	103.6	100.9	98.1	100.6	102.4	104.0	106.7	109.9	112.3	114.3
5 Years*														
Weight in Pounds	52.8	49.2	44.8	40.5	37.4	34.8	32.1	33.6	35.5	37.5	40.5	44.1	46.7	50.4
Weight in Kg.	23.95	22.32	20.32	18.37	16.96	15.79	14.56	15.24	16.1	17.01	18.37	20.0	21.18	22.86
Length in Inches	46.8	45.4	44.0	42.9	41.6	40.5	39.4	40.2	40.8	41.7	42.8	44.2	45.2	46.1
Length in Cm.	118.8	115.4	111.7	109.1	105.7	103.0	100.0	102.0	103.7	105.9	108.7	112.3	114.7	117.1

From Studies of Child Health and Development, Department of Maternal and Child Health, Harvard School of Public Health.
*The figures for the several percentiles of each measurement at 5 years differ slightly from those given in Table 2-8 for this age because they were obtained from a different population of children.

GROWTH MEAS.

TABLE 2-6.　PERCENTILES FOR WEIGHT AND HEIGHT—5 TO 18 YEARS

	PERCENTILES (BOYS)							PERCENTILES (GIRLS)						
	3	10	25	50	75	90	97	3	10	25	50	75	90	97
5 Years*														
Weight in Pounds	34.5	36.6	39.6	42.8	46.5	49.7	53.2	33.7	36.1	38.6	41.4	44.2	48.2	51.8
Weight in Kg.	15.65	16.6	17.96	19.41	21.09	22.54	24.13	15.29	16.37	17.51	18.78	20.05	21.86	23.5
Height in Inches	40.2	41.5	42.6	43.8	45.0	45.9	47.0	40.4	41.3	42.2	43.2	44.4	45.4	46.5
Height in Cm.	102.1	105.3	108.3	111.3	114.2	116.7	119.5	102.6	105.0	107.2	109.7	112.9	115.4	118.0
5½ Years														
Weight in Pounds		38.8	42.0	45.6	49.3	53.1			38.0	40.8	44.0	47.2	51.2	
Weight in Kg.		17.6	19.05	20.68	22.36	24.09			17.24	18.51	19.96	21.41	23.22	
Height in Inches		42.6	43.8	45.0	46.3	47.3			42.4	43.4	44.4	45.7	46.8	
Height in Cm.		108.3	111.2	114.4	117.5	120.1			107.8	110.2	112.8	116.1	118.9	
6 Years														
Weight in Pounds	38.5	40.9	44.4	48.3	52.1	56.4	61.1	37.2	39.6	42.9	46.5	50.2	54.2	58.7
Weight in Kg.	17.46	18.55	20.14	21.91	23.63	25.58	27.71	16.87	17.96	19.46	21.09	22.77	24.58	26.63
Height in Inches	42.7	43.8	44.9	46.3	47.6	48.6	49.7	42.5	43.5	44.6	45.6	47.0	48.1	49.4
Height in Cm.	108.5	111.2	114.1	117.5	120.8	123.5	126.2	108.0	110.6	113.2	115.9	119.3	122.3	125.4
6½ Years														
Weight in Pounds		43.4	47.1	51.2	55.4	60.4			42.2	45.5	49.4	53.3	57.7	
Weight in Kg.		19.69	21.36	23.22	25.13	27.4			19.14	20.64	22.41	24.18	26.17	
Height in Inches		44.9	46.1	47.6	48.9	50.0			44.8	45.7	46.9	48.3	49.4	
Height in Cm.		114.1	117.2	120.8	124.2	127.0			113.7	116.2	119.1	122.6	125.6	
7 Years														
Weight in Pounds	43.0	45.8	49.7	54.1	58.7	64.4	69.9	41.3	44.5	48.1	52.2	56.3	61.2	67.3
Weight in Kg.	19.5	20.77	22.54	24.54	26.63	29.21	31.71	18.73	20.19	21.82	23.68	25.54	27.76	30.53
Height in Inches	44.9	46.0	47.4	48.9	50.2	51.4	52.5	44.9	46.0	46.9	48.1	49.6	50.7	51.9
Height in Cm.	114.0	116.9	120.3	124.1	127.6	130.5	133.4	114.0	116.8	119.2	122.3	125.9	128.9	131.7
7½ Years														
Weight in Pounds		48.5	52.6	57.1	62.1	68.7			46.6	50.6	55.2	59.8	65.6	
Weight in Kg.		22.0	23.86	25.9	28.17	31.16			21.14	22.95	25.04	27.13	29.76	
Height in Inches		47.2	48.6	50.0	51.5	52.7			47.0	48.0	49.3	50.7	51.9	
Height in Cm.		120.0	123.5	127.1	130.8	133.9			119.5	122.0	125.2	128.8	131.8	

*The figures for the several percentiles of each measurement at 5 years differ slightly from those in Table 2-7 for this age because they were obtained from a different population of children.

TABLE 2-6. *(Continued)*

8 Years

	1	2	3	4	5	6	7		1	2	3	4	5	6	7
Weight in Pounds	48.0	51.2	55.5	60.1	65.5	73.0	79.4		45.3	48.6	53.1	58.1	63.3	69.9	78.9
Weight in Kg.	21.77	23.22	25.17	27.26	29.71	33.11	36.02		20.55	22.04	24.09	26.35	28.71	31.71	35.79
Height in Inches	47.1	48.5	49.8	51.2	52.8	54.0	55.2		46.9	48.1	49.1	50.4	51.8	53.0	54.1
Height in Cm.	119.6	123.1	126.6	130.0	134.2	137.3	140.2		119.1	122.1	124.8	128.0	131.6	134.6	137.4

8½ Years

	1	2	3	4	5	6	7		1	2	3	4	5	6	7
Weight in Pounds		53.8	58.3	63.1	68.9	77.0				50.6	55.5	61.0	66.9	74.5	89.9
Weight in Kg.		24.40	26.44	28.62	31.25	34.93				22.95	25.17	27.67	30.35	33.79	40.78
Height in Inches		49.5	50.8	52.3	53.9	55.1				49.0	50.1	51.4	52.9	54.1	56.5
Height in Cm.		125.7	129.1	132.8	137.0	140.0				124.6	127.3	130.5	134.4	137.5	143.4

9 Years

	1	2	3	4	5	6	7		1	2	3	4	5	6	7
Weight in Pounds	52.5	56.3	61.1	66.0	72.3	81.0	89.8		49.1	52.6	57.9	63.8	70.5	79.1	89.9
Weight in Kg.	23.81	25.54	27.71	29.94	32.8	36.74	40.73		22.27	23.86	26.26	28.94	31.98	35.88	40.78
Height in Inches	48.9	50.5	51.8	53.3	55.0	56.1	57.2		48.7	50.0	51.1	52.3	54.0	55.3	56.5
Height in Cm.	124.2	128.3	131.6	135.5	139.8	142.6	145.3		123.6	127.0	129.7	132.9	137.1	140.4	143.4

9½ Years

	1	2	3	4	5	6	7		1	2	3	4	5	6	7
Weight in Pounds		58.7	63.7	69.0	76.0	85.5				54.9	60.4	67.1	74.8	84.4	
Weight in Kg.		26.63	28.89	31.3	34.47	38.78				24.9	27.4	30.44	33.93	38.28	
Height in Inches		51.4	52.7	54.3	55.9	57.1				50.9	52.0	53.5	55.1	56.4	
Height in Cm.		130.6	134.0	137.9	142.1	145.1				129.4	132.2	135.8	139.9	143.2	

10 Years

	1	2	3	4	5	6	7		1	2	3	4	5	6	7
Weight in Pounds	56.8	61.1	66.3	71.9	79.6	89.9	100.0		53.2	57.1	62.8	70.3	79.1	89.7	101.9
Weight in Kg.	25.76	27.71	30.07	32.61	36.11	40.78	45.36		24.13	25.9	28.49	31.89	35.88	40.69	46.22
Height in Inches	50.7	52.3	53.7	55.2	56.8	58.1	59.2		50.3	51.8	53.0	54.6	56.1	57.5	58.8
Height in Cm.	128.7	132.8	136.3	140.3	144.4	147.5	150.3		127.7	131.7	134.6	138.6	142.6	146.0	149.3

10½ Years

	1	2	3	4	5	6	7		1	2	3	4	5	6	7
Weight in Pounds		63.7	69.0	74.8	83.4	94.6				59.9	66.4	74.6	84.1	95.1	
Weight in Kg.		28.89	31.3	33.93	37.83	42.91				27.17	30.12	33.79	38.15	43.14	
Height in Inches		53.2	54.5	56.0	57.8	58.8				52.9	54.1	55.8	57.4	58.9	
Height in Cm.		135.1	138.4	142.3	146.8	149.7				134.4	137.5	141.7	145.9	149.7	

11 Years

	1	2	3	4	5	6	7		1	2	3	4	5	6	7
Weight in Pounds	61.8	66.3	71.6	77.6	87.2	99.3	111.7		57.9	62.6	69.9	78.8	89.1	100.4	112.9
Weight in Kg.	28.03	30.07	32.48	35.2	39.55	45.04	50.67		26.26	28.4	31.71	35.74	40.42	45.54	51.21
Height in Inches	52.5	54.0	55.3	56.8	58.7	59.8	60.8		52.1	53.9	55.2	57.0	58.7	60.4	62.0
Height in Cm.	133.4	137.3	140.5	144.2	149.2	151.8	154.4		132.3	137.0	140.3	144.7	149.2	153.4	157.4

11½ Years

	1	2	3	4	5	6	7		1	2	3	4	5	6	7
Weight in Pounds		69.2	74.6	81.0	91.6	104.5				66.1	74.0	83.2	94.0	106.0	
Weight in Kg.		31.39	33.84	36.74	41.55	47.4				29.98	33.57	37.74	42.64	48.08	
Height in Inches		55.0	56.3	57.8	59.6	60.9				55.0	56.3	58.3	60.2	61.8	
Height in Cm.		139.8	142.9	146.9	151.4	154.8				139.8	143.1	148.1	152.9	157.0	

GROWTH MEAS.

TABLE 2-6. *(Continued)*

97	90	75	50	25	10	3		3	10	25	50	75	90	97
							12 Years							
127.7	111.5	98.8	87.6	78.0	69.5	63.6	Weight in Pounds	67.2	72.0	77.5	84.4	96.0	109.6	124.2
57.92	50.58	44.82	39.74	35.38	31.52	28.85	Weight in Kg.	30.48	32.66	35.15	38.28	43.55	49.71	56.34
64.8	63.2	61.6	59.8	57.4	56.1	54.3	Height in Inches	54.4	56.1	57.2	58.9	60.4	62.2	63.7
164.6	160.6	156.6	151.9	145.9	142.6	137.8	Height in Cm.	138.1	142.4	145.2	149.6	153.5	157.9	161.9
							12½ Years							
	118.0	104.9	93.4	83.7	74.7		Weight in Pounds		74.6	80.6	88.7	102.0	116.4	
	53.52	47.58	42.37	37.97	33.88		Weight in Kg.		33.84	36.56	40.23	46.27	52.8	
	64.0	62.6	60.7	58.8	57.4		Height in Inches		56.9	58.1	60.0	61.9	63.6	
	162.7	159.1	154.3	149.3	145.9		Height in Cm.		144.5	147.5	152.3	157.2	161.6	
							13 Years							
142.3	124.5	111.0	99.1	89.4	79.9	72.2	Weight in Pounds	72.0	77.1	83.7	93.0	107.9	123.2	138.0
64.55	56.47	50.35	44.95	40.55	36.24	32.75	Weight in Kg.	32.66	34.97	37.97	42.18	48.94	55.88	62.6
66.3	64.9	63.6	61.8	60.1	58.7	56.6	Height in Inches	56.0	57.7	58.9	61.0	63.3	65.1	66.7
168.4	164.8	161.5	157.1	152.6	149.1	143.7	Height in Cm.	142.2	146.6	149.7	155.0	160.8	165.3	169.5
							13½ Years							
	128.9	115.4	103.7	94.6	85.5		Weight in Pounds		82.2	89.6	100.3	115.5	130.1	
	58.47	52.35	47.04	42.91	38.78		Weight in Kg.		37.29	40.64	45.5	52.39	59.01	
	65.3	64.0	62.4	60.8	59.5		Height in Inches		58.8	60.3	62.6	64.8	66.5	
	165.9	162.6	158.4	154.4	151.1		Height in Cm.		149.4	153.1	158.9	164.6	168.9	
							14 Years							
150.8	133.3	119.7	108.4	99.8	91.0	83.1	Weight in Pounds	79.8	87.2	95.5	107.6	123.1	136.9	150.6
68.4	60.46	54.29	49.17	45.27	41.28	37.69	Weight in Kg.	36.2	39.55	43.32	48.81	55.84	62.1	68.31
67.2	65.7	64.4	62.8	61.5	60.2	58.3	Height in Inches	57.6	59.9	61.6	64.0	66.3	67.9	69.7
170.7	167.0	163.7	159.6	156.1	153.0	148.2	Height in Cm.	146.4	152.1	156.5	162.7	168.4	172.4	177.1
							14½ Years							
	135.7	121.8	111.0	102.5	94.2		Weight in Pounds		93.3	101.9	113.9	129.1	142.4	
	61.55	55.25	50.35	46.49	42.73		Weight in Kg.		42.32	46.22	51.66	58.56	64.59	
	66.0	64.7	63.1	61.8	60.7		Height in Inches		61.0	62.7	65.1	67.2	68.7	
	167.6	164.3	160.4	156.9	154.1		Height in Cm.		155.0	159.4	165.3	170.7	174.6	

TABLE 2-6. *(Continued)*

Measurement														
15 Years													
Weight in Pounds	161.6	147.8	135.0	120.1	108.2	99.4	91.3	155.2	138.1	123.9	113.5	105.1	97.4	89.0
Weight in Kg.	73.3	67.04	61.23	54.48	49.08	45.09	41.41	70.4	62.64	56.2	51.48	47.67	44.18	40.37
Height in Inches	71.6	69.6	68.1	66.1	63.9	62.1	59.7	67.6	66.2	64.9	63.4	62.1	61.1	59.1
Height in Cm.	181.8	176.7	173.0	167.8	162.3	157.8	151.7	171.6	168.1	164.9	161.1	157.7	155.2	150.2
15½ Years													
Weight in Pounds		152.6	139.7	124.9	113.5	105.2			139.6	125.6	115.3	106.8	99.2	
Weight in Kg.		69.22	63.37	56.65	51.48	47.72			63.32	56.97	52.3	48.44	45.0	
Height in Inches		70.2	68.8	66.8	64.8	63.1			66.4	65.1	63.7	62.3	61.3	
Height in Cm.		178.2	174.8	169.7	164.7	160.3			168.6	165.3	161.7	158.2	155.7	
16 Years													
Weight in Pounds	170.5	157.3	144.4	129.7	118.7	111.0	103.4	157.7	141.1	127.2	117.0	108.4	100.9	91.8
Weight in Kg.	77.34	71.35	65.5	58.83	53.84	50.35	46.9	71.53	64.0	57.7	53.07	49.17	45.77	41.64
Height in Inches	73.1	70.7	69.5	67.8	65.8	64.1	61.6	67.7	66.5	65.2	63.9	62.4	61.5	59.4
Height in Cm.	185.6	179.7	176.6	171.6	167.1	162.8	156.5	172.0	169.0	165.7	162.2	158.6	156.1	150.8
16½ Years													
Weight in Pounds		161.0	147.9	133.0	121.6	114.3			142.2	128.4	118.1	109.4	101.9	
Weight in Kg.		73.03	67.09	60.33	55.16	51.85			64.5	58.24	53.57	49.62	46.22	
Height in Inches		71.1	69.8	68.0	66.3	64.6			66.6	65.3	63.9	62.5	61.5	
Height in Cm.		180.7	177.4	172.7	168.4	164.2			169.2	165.9	162.4	158.8	156.2	
17 Years													
Weight in Pounds	175.6	164.6	151.4	136.2	124.5	117.5	110.5	159.5	143.3	129.6	119.1	110.4	102.8	93.9
Weight in Kg.	79.65	74.66	68.67	61.78	56.47	53.3	50.12	72.35	65.0	58.79	54.02	50.08	46.63	42.59
Height in Inches	73.5	71.5	70.1	68.4	66.8	65.2	62.6	67.8	66.7	65.4	64.0	62.6	61.5	59.4
Height in Cm.	186.6	181.6	178.1	173.7	169.7	165.5	159.0	172.2	169.4	166.1	162.5	159.0	156.3	151.0
17½ Years													
Weight in Pounds		166.8	153.6	137.6	125.8	118.8			143.9	130.2	119.5	110.8	103.2	
Weight in Kg.		75.66	69.67	62.41	57.06	53.89			65.27	59.06	54.2	50.26	46.81	
Height in Inches		71.6	70.3	68.5	67.0	65.3			66.7	65.4	64.0	62.6	61.5	
Height in Cm.		182.0	178.5	174.1	170.1	165.9			169.4	166.1	162.5	159.0	156.3	
18 Years													
Weight in Pounds	179.0	169.0	155.7	139.0	127.1	120.0	113.0	160.7	144.5	130.8	119.9	111.2	103.5	94.5
Weight in Kg.	81.19	76.66	70.62	63.05	57.65	54.43	51.26	72.89	65.54	59.33	54.39	50.44	46.95	42.87
Height in Inches	73.9	71.8	70.4	68.7	67.0	65.5	62.8	67.8	66.7	65.4	64.0	62.6	61.5	59.4
Height in Cm.	187.6	182.4	178.9	174.5	170.5	166.3	159.6	172.2	169.4	166.1	162.5	159.0	156.3	151.0

The measurements in this table are from studies by and are reproduced by courtesy of Howard V. Meredith, Iowa Child Welfare Research Station, The State University of Iowa.

GROWTH MEAS.

TABLE 2-7. PERCENTILES FOR SELECTED MEASUREMENTS—BIRTH TO 5 YEARS—IN CENTIMETERS

	PERCENTILES (BOYS)							PERCENTILES (GIRLS)						
	3	10	25	50	75	90	97	3	10	25	50	75	90	97
Birth														
Pelvic Breadth	7.1	7.4	7.7	8.1	8.4	8.7	9.0	7.0	7.2	7.4	7.7	8.2	8.5	8.9
Head Circ.	33.0	33.5	34.4	35.3	36.2	37.0	37.5	32.5	33.4	33.9	34.7	35.4	36.0	36.6
Chest Circ.	29.8	30.6	31.8	33.2	34.4	35.7	36.8	30.0	30.8	31.8	32.9	34.0	35.0	36.0
3 Months														
Pelvic Breadth	9.8	10.0	10.2	10.6	11.2	11.5	12.1	9.4	9.6	9.9	10.4	10.9	11.4	12.2
Head Circ.	38.7	39.2	40.0	40.9	41.5	42.1	43.2	37.9	38.5	39.2	40.0	40.8	41.7	42.3
Chest Circ.	37.6	38.3	39.3	40.6	41.6	42.9	44.1	36.5	37.6	38.8	39.8	40.9	42.0	43.0
Abd. Circ.	33.6	35.5	36.8	38.5	39.8	41.4	43.5	32.3	34.4	36.8	38.4	40.4	41.7	42.7
6 Months														
Pelvic Breadth	10.5	10.8	11.2	11.6	12.0	12.4	13.1	10.3	10.5	10.8	11.3	11.8	12.4	13.2
Head Circ.	42.1	42.7	43.3	43.9	44.8	45.4	45.9	40.9	41.4	42.0	42.8	43.6	44.5	45.4
Chest Circ.	40.1	41.6	42.5	43.7	45.0	46.3	47.2	39.4	40.6	41.8	43.0	44.2	45.4	46.6
Abd. Circ.	36.4	38.4	39.8	41.4	43.2	45.0	46.0	36.2	37.9	39.5	41.4	43.5	45.0	46.2
9 Months														
Pelvic Breadth	11.0	11.5	11.9	12.3	12.7	13.1	13.7	11.0	11.3	11.5	12.0	12.5	13.1	13.8
Head Circ.	43.8	44.5	45.1	46.0	46.5	47.1	47.8	42.6	43.2	43.8	44.6	45.4	46.3	47.2
Chest Circ.	42.0	43.7	44.3	46.0	47.5	48.9	49.9	41.7	42.7	44.0	45.4	46.6	47.9	49.2
Abd. Circ.	38.1	40.1	41.7	43.4	45.6	47.6	48.4	38.0	39.9	41.3	43.4	45.7	47.7	49.2
12 Months														
Pelvic Breadth	11.4	11.9	12.4	12.8	13.2	13.7	14.2	11.4	11.7	12.0	12.4	13.0	13.6	14.4
Head Circ.	44.9	45.5	46.5	47.3	47.8	48.4	48.9	43.6	44.3	45.0	45.8	46.7	47.7	48.4
Chest Circ.	43.5	45.1	46.3	47.6	49.3	50.7	51.9	43.1	44.2	45.6	47.0	48.2	49.5	50.9
Abd. Circ.	39.3	41.1	42.9	44.6	47.0	48.9	50.0	38.7	40.9	42.4	44.5	46.9	49.2	51.1
15 Months														
Pelvic Breadth	11.8	12.4	12.8	13.3	13.7	14.2	14.7	11.6	12.1	12.4	12.9	13.5	14.1	14.8
Head Circ.	45.6	46.3	47.1	48.0	48.5	49.2	49.8	44.3	44.9	45.6	46.5	47.4	48.4	49.1
Chest Circ.	44.7	46.1	47.3	48.6	50.1	51.7	52.8	44.1	45.1	46.5	47.9	49.2	50.5	51.9
Abd. Circ.	40.0	41.7	43.5	45.1	47.4	49.3	50.5	39.3	41.5	43.0	45.0	47.3	49.8	51.8

TABLE 2-7. *(Continued)*

Measurement														
18 Months														
Pelvic Breadth	15.2	14.7	14.2	13.7	13.2	12.8	12.1	11.8	12.4	12.8	13.3	13.9	14.5	15.2
Head Circ.	50.6	49.9	49.2	48.7	47.7	47.0	46.2	44.9	45.5	46.2	47.1	48.0	49.0	49.8
Chest Circ.	53.7	52.6	50.9	49.5	48.2	47.0	45.9	45.0	46.0	47.3	48.8	50.2	51.4	52.9
Abd. Circ.	50.9	49.6	47.8	45.5	44.0	42.2	40.6	39.8	42.1	43.6	45.5	47.6	50.3	52.5
2 Years														
Pelvic Breadth	16.1	15.5	15.0	14.4	13.9	13.5	12.8	12.5	13.1	13.5	14.1	14.7	15.3	16.1
Head Circ.	51.7	51.0	50.2	49.7	48.2	48.0	47.0	45.8	46.4	47.2	48.1	49.1	50.1	50.9
Chest Circ.	54.9	53.9	52.2	50.8	49.5	48.4	47.4	46.3	47.4	48.6	50.1	51.8	53.0	54.2
Abd. Circ.	51.5	50.2	48.4	46.2	44.8	43.4	41.6	40.7	42.8	44.4	46.3	48.5	51.4	53.5
2½ Years														
Pelvic Breadth	16.7	16.2	15.7	15.1	14.6	14.2	13.6	13.2	13.7	14.2	14.8	15.4	16.1	16.9
Head Circ.	52.3	51.6	50.9	50.2	49.2	48.5	47.5	46.3	47.0	47.8	48.8	49.8	50.8	51.5
Chest Circ.	55.8	54.9	53.2	51.7	50.3	49.3	48.2	47.3	48.4	49.7	51.2	52.8	54.3	55.5
Abd. Circ.	52.0	50.7	49.1	46.7	45.5	44.0	42.0	41.7	43.6	45.2	47.0	49.4	52.6	54.7
3 Years														
Pelvic Breadth	17.4	16.9	16.4	15.8	15.2	14.8	14.2	13.8	14.3	14.8	15.4	16.1	16.8	17.7
Head Circ.	52.7	51.8	51.3	50.4	49.6	48.9	47.9	46.8	47.5	48.4	49.3	50.3	51.1	52.0
Chest Circ.	57.0	55.8	54.1	52.4	51.0	49.9	48.9	47.9	49.3	50.5	51.9	53.5	55.1	56.7
Abd. Circ.	52.7	51.1	49.6	47.2	46.0	44.6	42.1	42.7	44.5	46.0	47.7	50.2	53.6	55.8
3½ Years														
Pelvic Breadth	17.9	17.4	16.9	16.3	15.7	15.3	14.7	14.4	14.9	15.4	16.0	16.7	17.4	18.3
Chest Circ.	58.0	56.6	54.9	53.1	51.6	50.5	49.6	48.5	50.1	51.2	52.5	54.1	55.8	58.1
4 Years														
Pelvic Breadth	18.5	18.0	17.5	16.9	16.2	15.8	15.2	15.0	15.4	15.9	16.5	17.2	17.9	18.9
Chest Circ.	58.9	57.2	55.5	53.7	52.2	51.1	50.1	49.2	50.7	51.7	53.1	54.7	56.5	59.0
4½ Years														
Pelvic Breadth	19.1	18.5	18.0	17.3	16.6	16.2	15.7	15.5	15.9	16.4	17.0	17.7	18.5	19.4
Chest Circ.	59.3	58.0	56.3	54.4	52.9	51.7	50.7	49.8	51.3	52.3	53.7	55.4	57.3	59.6
5 Years*														
Pelvic Breadth	19.7	19.0	18.5	17.8	17.1	16.7	16.1	16.0	16.3	16.8	17.5	18.2	18.9	19.8
Chest Circ.	60.5	58.8	57.0	55.0	53.5	52.3	51.2	50.4	51.7	52.8	54.2	56.0	57.9	60.2

From Studies of Child Health and Development, Department of Maternal and Child Health, Harvard School of Public Health.
*The figures for the several percentiles of each measurement at 5 years differ slightly from those given in Table 2-10 for this age because they were obtained from a different population of children.

TABLE 2-8. PERCENTILES FOR SELECTED MEASUREMENTS—5 TO 18 YEARS—IN CENTIMETERS

PERCENTILES (BOYS)						PERCENTILES (GIRLS)				
10	25	50	75	90		10	25	50	75	90
					5 Years*					
17.0	17.6	18.3	18.9	19.6	Pelvic Breadth	17.0	17.4	18.0	18.7	19.4
51.6	52.8	54.5	56.2	57.5	Chest Circ.	50.2	51.4	52.9	54.6	56.5
21.0	21.7	22.6	23.6	24.6	Leg Circ.	21.1	21.8	22.8	23.8	24.7
					5½ Years					
17.4	18.0	18.7	19.4	20.1	Pelvic Breadth	17.4	17.8	18.4	19.1	20.0
52.4	53.6	55.3	57.1	58.5	Chest Circ.	50.9	52.2	53.7	55.5	57.4
21.4	22.2	23.1	24.1	25.2	Leg Circ.	21.5	22.3	23.3	24.3	25.3
					6 Years					
17.7	18.4	19.1	19.8	20.5	Pelvic Breadth	17.7	18.2	18.8	19.5	20.5
53.2	54.4	56.1	57.9	59.5	Chest Circ.	51.5	52.9	54.5	56.3	58.2
21.8	22.6	23.6	24.6	25.7	Leg Circ.	21.9	22.7	23.8	24.8	25.8
					6½ Years					
18.1	18.8	19.5	20.2	21.0	Pelvic Breadth	18.1	18.6	19.2	20.0	21.1
54.1	55.3	57.0	58.9	60.6	Chest Circ.	52.2	53.7	55.3	57.2	59.2
22.2	23.1	24.1	25.2	26.3	Leg Circ.	22.3	23.2	24.3	25.4	26.4
					7 Years					
18.5	19.2	19.9	20.6	21.4	Pelvic Breadth	18.4	18.9	19.6	20.4	21.6
54.9	56.1	57.8	59.8	61.6	Chest Circ.	52.8	54.4	56.1	58.0	60.1
22.6	23.5	24.6	25.7	26.9	Leg Circ.	22.7	23.7	24.8	25.9	27.0
					7½ Years					
18.9	19.6	20.3	21.0	21.9	Pelvic Breadth	18.8	19.3	20.1	20.9	22.1
55.8	57.1	58.8	61.0	62.9	Chest Circ.	53.5	55.1	57.0	59.0	61.2
23.1	24.1	25.2	26.3	27.6	Leg Circ.	23.1	24.2	25.3	26.4	27.7
					8 Years					
19.2	19.9	20.7	21.4	22.3	Pelvic Breadth	19.1	19.7	20.5	21.3	22.6
56.7	58.0	59.8	62.1	64.1	Chest Circ.	54.2	55.8	57.8	59.9	62.3
23.6	24.6	25.7	26.8	28.2	Leg Circ.	23.5	24.6	25.8	26.9	28.3
					8½ Years					
19.6	20.3	21.1	21.8	22.7	Pelvic Breadth	19.4	20.1	20.9	21.8	23.1
57.6	59.0	60.8	63.3	65.4	Chest Circ.	54.9	56.5	58.7	60.9	63.5
24.1	25.1	26.3	27.4	28.9	Leg Circ.	23.9	25.0	26.3	27.5	28.9
					9 Years					
19.9	20.6	21.4	22.2	23.0	Pelvic Breadth	19.7	20.5	21.3	22.2	23.5
58.4	59.9	61.8	64.4	66.7	Chest Circ.	55.5	57.2	59.6	61.9	64.7
24.5	25.6	26.8	28.0	29.5	Leg Circ.	24.2	25.4	26.8	28.1	29.5
					9½ Years					
20.2	21.0	21.7	22.6	23.5	Pelvic Breadth	20.1	20.9	21.8	22.8	24.1
59.3	60.9	62.9	65.5	68.1	Chest Circ.	56.2	58.0	60.5	63.2	66.1
24.9	26.0	27.3	28.5	30.1	Leg Circ.	24.7	25.9	27.3	28.6	30.2
					10 Years					
20.4	21.3	22.0	22.9	23.9	Pelvic Breadth	20.5	21.2	22.2	23.3	24.6
60.1	61.8	63.9	66.6	69.4	Chest Circ.	56.9	58.7	61.4	64.4	67.4
25.3	26.4	27.7	29.0	30.7	Leg Circ.	25.1	26.3	27.7	29.1	30.9
					10½ Years					
20.8	21.6	22.3	23.2	24.4	Pelvic Breadth	21.0	21.7	22.9	24.0	25.3
60.9	62.8	64.9	67.7	70.7	Chest Circ.	57.8	59.9	62.8	65.8	69.0
25.7	26.8	28.1	29.5	31.4	Leg Circ.	25.6	26.8	28.3	29.9	31.8
					11 Years					
21.1	21.8	22.6	23.5	24.8	Pelvic Breadth	21.4	22.2	23.5	24.6	26.0
61.7	63.7	65.9	68.8	71.9	Chest Circ.	58.6	61.1	64.2	67.2	70.5
26.0	27.1	28.5	30.0	32.0	Leg Circ.	26.0	27.3	28.9	30.6	32.6

*The figures for the several percentiles of each measurement at 5 years differ slightly from those in Table 2-9 for this age because they were obtained from a different population of children.

The measurements in this table are from studies by and are reproduced by courtesy of Howard V. Meredith, the Iowa Child Welfare Research Station, The State University of Iowa.

TABLE 2-8. *(Continued)*

PERCENTILES (BOYS)						PERCENTILES (GIRLS)				
10	25	50	75	90		10	25	50	75	90
					11½ Years					
21.5	22.2	23.1	24.0	25.3	Pelvic Breadth	21.9	22.8	24.2	25.4	26.8
62.5	64.6	66.9	69.9	73.1	Chest Circ.	59.6	62.5	65.5	68.5	72.2
26.4	27.6	29.0	30.6	32.8	Leg Circ.	26.6	27.9	29.5	31.2	33.2
					12 Years					
21.9	22.6	23.5	24.5	25.8	Pelvic Breadth	22.4	23.4	24.9	26.2	27.6
63.3	65.5	67.8	70.9	74.2	Chest Circ.	60.6	63.8	66.7	69.7	73.8
26.8	28.0	29.5	31.2	33.5	Leg Circ.	27.1	28.5	30.1	31.8	33.8
					12½ Years					
22.3	23.1	24.1	25.1	26.5	Pelvic Breadth	23.0	24.0	25.5	26.8	28.3
64.2	66.5	69.1	72.4	75.8	Chest Circ.	61.8	64.9	67.7	70.9	75.3
27.3	28.6	30.1	32.0	34.2	Leg Circ.	27.7	29.1	30.7	32.4	34.3
					13 Years					
22.7	23.6	24.6	25.6	27.2	Pelvic Breadth	23.6	24.6	26.0	27.4	29.0
65.0	67.4	70.3	73.8	77.4	Chest Circ.	62.9	65.9	68.6	72.0	76.7
27.8	29.2	30.8	32.7	34.8	Leg Circ.	28.2	29.7	31.2	32.9	34.8
					13½ Years					
23.2	24.1	25.2	26.4	27.8	Pelvic Breadth	24.2	25.2	26.5	27.8	29.5
66.3	68.8	72.4	75.8	79.4	Chest Circ.	63.8	66.6	69.3	72.9	77.7
28.5	29.9	31 6	33.4	35.3	Leg Circ.	28.7	30.2	31.6	33.4	35.1
					14 Years					
23.6	24.6	25.8	27.1	28.3	Pelvic Breadth	24.8	25.8	26.9	28.1	29.9
67.6	70.2	74.5	77.8	81.4	Chest Circ.	64.6	67.2	69.9	73.7	78.6
29.1	30.6	32.3	34.1	35.8	Leg Circ.	29.2	30.6	32.0	33.8	35.4
					14½ Years					
24.1	25.1	26.3	27.5	28.7	Pelvic Breadth	25.2	26.2	27.2	28.4	30.3
69.4	72.3	76.3	79.6	83.1	Chest Circ.	65.1	67.7	70.4	74.2	79.2
29.8	31.3	32.9	34.6	36.2	Leg Circ.	29.6	30.9	32.3	34.1	35.7
					15 Years					
24.6	25.6	26.7	27.9	29.1	Pelvic Breadth	25.6	26.5	27.5	28.7	30.6
71.1	74.4	78.0	81.3	84.8	Chest Circ.	65.5	68.1	70.9	74.7	79.8
30.4	31.9	33.4	35.1	36.6	Leg Circ.	29.9	31.1	32.6	34.3	35.9
					15½ Years					
25.1	26.0	27.1	28.2	29.4	Pelvic Breadth	25.9	26.7	27.8	29.0	30.8
72.8	75.8	79.4	82.9	86.3	Chest Circ.	65.8	68.4	71.3	75.1	80.2
30.9	32.3	33.8	35.5	37.0	Leg Circ.	30.1	31.4	32.9	34.5	36.1
					16 Years					
25.6	26.4	27.4	28.4	29.6	Pelvic Breadth	26.1	26.9	28.0	29.2	31.0
74.4	77.2	80.7	84.5	87.8	Chest Circ.	66.1	68.7	71.6	75.4	80.5
31.3	32.7	34.2	35.8	37.3	Leg Circ.	30.3	31.6	33.1	34.6	36.3
					16½ Years					
25.9	26.7	27.6	28.6	29.8	Pelvic Breadth	26.2	27.0	28.2	29.3	31.1
75.4	78.1	81.6	85.4	88.8	Chest Circ.	66.3	69.0	71.9	75.7	80.7
31.5	32.9	34.4	36.1	37.6	Leg Circ.	30.5	31.8	33.3	34.8	36.5
					17 Years					
26.1	26.9	27.8	28.7	29.9	Pelvic Breadth	26.3	27.1	28.3	29.4	31.2
76.4	78.9	82.5	86.2	89.7	Chest Circ.	66.4	69.2	72.1	75.9	80.9
31.7	33.1	34.6	36.3	37.8	Leg Circ.	30.6	31.9	33.4	34.9	36.6
					17½ Years					
26.3	27.0	27.9	28.8	30.0	Pelvic Breadth	26.4	27.2	28.4	29.5	31.3
77.0	79.4	83.0	86.7	90.2	Chest Circ.	66.5	69.3	72.2	76.0	81.0
31.8	33.3	34.8	36.5	38.0	Leg Circ.	30.7	32.0	33.5	35.0	36.7
					18 Years					
26.5	27.1	28.0	28.9	30.1	Pelvic Breadth	26.4	27.2	28.4	29.5	31.3
77.5	79.8	83.4	87.1	90.7	Chest Circ.	66.6	69.4	72.3	76.1	81.1
31.9	33.4	34.9	36.6	38.1	Leg Circ.	30.8	32.1	33.6	35.1	36.8

TABLE 2-9. SITTING HEIGHT (STEM LENGTH) IN CENTIMETERS

PERCENTILES (BOYS)							AGE (YRS.)	PERCENTILES (GIRLS)						
3	10	25	50	75	90	97		3	10	25	50	75	90	97
41.4	42.3	43.4	44.8	46.2	47.4	48.4	0.5	40.0	41.0	42.1	43.3	44.5	45.6	46.8
45.1	46.1	47.4	48.7	50.1	51.2	52.4	1.0	44.2	45.2	46.3	47.5	48.7	49.8	50.9
48.3	49.2	50.3	51.6	52.9	54.1	55.4	1.5	47.1	48.1	49.2	50.4	51.6	52.7	53.9
50.6	51.4	52.5	53.8	55.1	56.3	57.6	2.0	49.2	50.2	51.4	52.7	54.0	55.2	56.4
52.2	53.1	54.2	55.6	56.9	58.1	59.5	2.5	50.9	51.9	53.1	54.4	55.7	57.0	58.3
53.5	54.5	55.6	57.1	58.5	59.7	61.1	3.0	52.2	53.4	54.6	56.0	57.4	58.7	60.0
54.8	55.8	57.0	58.6	60.0	61.2	62.6	3.5	53.6	54.8	56.1	57.5	59.0	60.3	61.6
56.0	57.1	58.3	60.0	61.4	62.6	64.0	4.0	54.9	56.1	57.4	58.9	60.4	61.7	62.1
57.1	58.3	59.6	61.3	62.8	64.0	65.4	4.5	56.1	57.4	58.7	60.2	61.7	63.1	64.5
58.2	59.5	60.9	62.6	64.2	65.4	66.8	5.0	57.3	58.6	59.9	61.4	63.0	64.4	65.9
59.3	60.7	62.1	63.9	65.6	66.8	68.2	5.5	58.6	59.9	61.2	62.7	64.3	65.8	67.3
60.4	61.8	63.3	65.2	66.9	68.2	69.6	6.0	59.9	61.2	62.5	64.1	65.6	67.1	68.7
61.5	62.9	64.5	66.4	68.2	69.6	71.0	6.5	61.2	62.5	63.8	65.4	66.9	68.4	70.0
62.6	64.1	65.8	67.6	69.4	71.0	72.4	7.0	62.5	63.7	65.0	66.6	68.2	69.7	71.3
63.7	65.4	67.0	68.8	70.7	72.3	73.8	7.5	63.6	64.9	66.2	67.8	69.4	70.9	72.6
64.9	66.6	68.2	70.0	72.0	73.6	75.1	8.0	64.6	65.9	67.3	68.9	70.5	72.1	73.8
66.0	67.7	69.3	71.2	73.2	74.8	76.4	8.5	65.5	66.8	68.2	69.8	71.4	73.1	74.9
67.0	68.6	70.3	72.2	74.2	76.0	77.6	9.0	66.3	67.7	69.1	70.7	72.4	74.1	76.0

TABLE 2-9. (*Continued*)

77.1	75.2	73.4	71.7	70.0	68.5	67.1	9.5	78.8	77.1	75.2	73.1	71.2	69.5	67.9
78.3	76.3	74.5	72.8	71.1	69.4	67.8	10.0	79.9	78.1	76.1	73.9	72.0	70.3	68.8
79.6	77.6	75.7	73.9	72.2	70.4	68.6	10.5	80.8	78.9	76.9	74.6	72.7	71.0	69.6
81.2	79.2	77.2	75.3	73.4	71.5	69.6	11.0	81.7	79.8	77.6	75.3	73.4	71.7	70.2
83.2	81.0	78.9	76.8	74.8	72.8	70.7	11.5	82.8	80.7	78.5	76.2	74.2	72.5	70.9
85.1	82.9	80.8	78.7	76.4	74.2	72.0	12.0	84.2	81.9	79.6	77.2	75.0	73.3	71.6
86.8	84.6	82.4	80.3	78.2	76.0	73.7	12.5	86.0	83.4	81.0	78.3	76.0	74.1	72.4
88.2	86.0	83.8	81.8	79.7	77.5	75.2	13.0	88.1	85.4	82.5	79.6	77.0	75.0	73.3
89.1	87.0	85.0	83.1	81.0	78.9	76.6	13.5	89.9	87.4	84.3	81.2	78.4	76.1	74.3
89.8	87.8	85.9	84.0	81.9	80.0	77.9	14.0	91.4	89.3	86.1	82.9	80.0	77.4	75.6
90.2	88.4	86.6	84.7	82.7	80.9	79.1	14.5	92.7	90.7	87.7	84.7	81.7	78.9	77.0
90.4	88.7	87.0	85.2	83.4	81.7	80.0	15.0	93.7	91.9	89.2	86.3	83.4	80.6	78.5
90.5	89.0	87.4	85.6	83.9	82.3	80.7	15.5	94.6	92.8	90.4	87.7	85.0	82.5	80.3
90.6	89.1	87.6	85.9	84.2	82.7	81.2	16.0	95.3	93.6	91.4	88.9	86.4	84.1	82.0
90.7	89.2	87.7	86.1	84.4	82.9	81.4	16.5	95.9	94.2	92.1	89.8	87.5	85.2	83.2
90.8	89.3	87.8	86.2	84.6	83.1	81.6	17.0	96.4	94.6	92.7	90.4	88.4	86.0	83.9
90.8	89.4	87.9	86.3	84.7	83.2	81.7	17.5	96.7	94.9	93.1	90.7	88.8	86.5	84.4
90.8	89.4	87.9	86.3	84.7	83.2	81.7	18.0	96.8	95.0	93.4	90.9	89.0	86.8	84.7

The data were collected 1930–46 on Iowa City boys of northwest European ancestry in attendance at the University of Iowa experimental schools.

Technique for measuring sitting height: The child sits on a horizontal bench about 30 cm. high at the base of a vertical measuring rod. The knees are flexed and spread apart and the ankles crossed, and the sacral, upper thoracic and occipital regions are in contact with the scale. The measurement is taken as in height. This measurement is of value when the question of disproportionate growth is being considered: disproportions will be evident when the percentile positions for standing height and sitting height differ appreciably.

The measurements in this table are from studies by and are reproduced by courtesy of Howard V. Meredith, the Iowa Child Welfare Research Station, the State University of Iowa.

and occiput against a vertical upright; the heels should be close together, and the arms should hang naturally at the sides. The external auditory meatus and the lower border of the orbit should lie in a plane parallel with the floor. A wooden head piece having 2 faces at right angles may be placed firmly on the head against a 2-meter or 6-foot measuring scale attached to the vertical surface against which the child is positioned.

Head Circumference. This measurement is particularly valuable in infants; it need not be taken routinely after 3 years of age. The tape is applied firmly over the glabella and supraorbital ridges anteriorly and that part of the occiput posteriorly which gives the maximal circumference. Difficulties with measurement of head circumference will sometimes arise when the head has an abnormal shape, as in hydrocephalus. Under these circumstances serial measurements of the changing size of the head may best be made through positioning the tape over whatever points on the forehead and occiput give the *maximal* circumference.

Measurements of circumference should be made with steel, cloth or disposable paper tapes. Cloth tapes may stretch with aging and will need to be checked frequently against wooden or steel standards.

Chest Circumference. Measurement of chest circumference is made in midrespiration, at the level of the xiphoid cartilage or substernal notch, in a plane at right angles to the vertebral column. Measurement is made recumbent up to the age of 5 years, the child standing thereafter.

Abdominal Circumference. This measurement is taken to 3 years only and will be of value principally in recognizing and following the course of chronic intestinal disturbances. Measurement is made in the plane of the umbilicus when the infant is recumbent.

Leg Circumference. The maximal girth of the calf is measured with the child standing with his feet several inches apart and his weight equally distributed through both legs.

Pelvic Breadth. Pelvic, bi-iliac or bicristal breadth is the distance between the lateralmost points of the iliac crest of the pelvis, including the overlying soft tissues. Measurement is made on the recumbent infant or young child by spreading or obstetrical calipers. The norms in Table 2-8, for children 5 years and over, were made with a broad sliding caliper applied over the crest of the ilia, the child standing and facing the measurer. The points of spreading calipers should not be pressed deeply into the soft tissue, whereas with sliding calipers the maximal pressure without causing pain should be applied. If these precautions are followed, measurements taken by the 2 instruments will not differ appreciably; otherwise, measurements by spreading calipers will be somewhat smaller in obese children than those made by sliding calipers.

ASSESSMENT OF NEUROLOGIC AND PSYCHOLOGIC DEVELOPMENT

(See also pages 1264 and 57)

The assessment of the functional status of the infant or child is an essential part of each examination, but is all too often uncritical. Only with some knowledge of developmental standards can the physician caring for children be adequately sensitive to deviations which indicate slight or early impairment of development. Moreover, only if he can quickly and confidently compare his observations with the normal developmental schedule will he be able to handle the questions of parents or make appropriate suggestions for further study.

In making the developmental examination an integral part of the routine office visit, the observations made and the techniques used must be appropriate to the age of the infant or child. The physician will often use readily available materials which have not been standardized, but which will usually reveal whether a more comprehensive developmental evaluation is indicated, possibly by a psychologist. The casual examination should be interpreted with caution, particularly when an infant or child who is irritable, hungry or ill fails to perform at his chronologic level. For such patients a future reassessment is in order. For the premature infant an adjustment in chronologic age will need to be made for the degree of prematurity.

In the young infant the examination may begin by observation of the child in the prone and supine positions, note being taken in each position of his spontaneous activity, and then of the manner in which he adjusts to being pulled from a supine to a sitting position and being held in ventral suspension *(Landau response)*. His reaction to moving persons or to objects brought within his sight or grasp can be determined, both for relatively large objects such as a rattle or stethoscope and for such small objects as a pellet. His behavior when standing with support should also be observed.

After the first year of life the child may be given blocks as well as a pencil and paper and his ability observed to mimic or copy the scribblings or figures of the physician. The standard blocks used in construction of various figures are 1-inch red cubes. After 3 years the child can be asked to "draw a man," to draw figures and to count pennies.

Tables 2-10 and 2-11 list expected behavior of infants and children of various ages and circumstances. The data are derived from those of Gesell, Shirley, Provence, Wolf, and others.

A number of relatively simple tests permit the physician or his assistant to make helpful assessments of the intellectual level of older children as part of normal office practice. Such tests include

TABLE 2-10. EMERGING PATTERNS OF BEHAVIOR DURING THE FIRST YEAR OF LIFE

NEONATAL PERIOD (FIRST 4 WEEKS)

Prone:	Lies in flexed attitude; turns head from side to side; head sags on ventral suspension
Supine:	Generally flexed and a little stiff
Visual:	May fixate face or light in line of vision; "doll's-eye" movement of eyes on turning of the body
Reflex:	Moro response active; stepping and placing reflexes; grasp reflex active; Landau response absent

AT 4 WEEKS

Prone:	Legs more extended; holds chin up; turns head; head lifted momentarily to plane of body on ventral suspension
Supine:	Tonic neck posture predominates; supple and relaxed; head lags on pull to sitting position
Visual:	Watches person; follows moving object a few degrees

AT 8 WEEKS

Prone:	Raises head slightly farther; watches moving object; head sustained in plane of body on ventral suspension
Supine:	Tonic neck posture predominates; head lags on pull to sitting position
Visual:	Follows moving object 180 degrees
Social:	Smiles on social contact; listens to voice and coos

AT 12 WEEKS

Prone:	Lifts head and chest, arms extended; head above plane of body on ventral suspension
Supine:	*Tonic neck posture predominates*; reaches toward and misses objects; waves at toy
Sitting:	Head lag partially compensated on pull to sitting position; early head control with bobbing motion; back rounded
Reflex:	Typical Moro response has not persisted; makes defense movements or selective withdrawal reactions
Social:	Sustained social contact; listens to music; says "aah, ngah"

AT 16 WEEKS

Prone:	Lifts head and chest, head in approximately vertical axis; legs extended
Supine:	*Symmetrical posture predominates,* hands in midline; reaches and grasps objects and brings them to mouth
Sitting:	No head lag on pull to sitting position; head steady, held forward; enjoys sitting with full truncal support
Standing:	When held erect, pushes with feet
Adaptive:	Sees pellet, but makes no move to it
Social:	Laughs out loud; may show displeasure if social contact is broken; excited at sight of food

AT 28 WEEKS

Prone:	Rolls over; may pivot
Supine:	Lifts head; rolls over; squirming movements
Sitting:	Sits briefly, with support of pelvis; leans forward on hands; back rounded
Standing:	May support most of weight; bounces actively
Adaptive:	Reaches out for and grasps large object; *transfers* objects from hand to hand; grasp uses radial palm; rakes at pellet
Language:	Polysyllabic vowel sounds formed
Social:	Prefers mother; babbles; enjoys mirror; responds to changes in emotional content of social contact

AT 40 WEEKS

Sitting:	Sits up alone and indefinitely without support, back straight
Standing:	Pulls to standing position
Motor:	Creeps or crawls
Adaptive:	Grasps objects with *thumb and forefinger*; pokes at things with forefinger; picks up pellet with assisted pincer movement; uncovers hidden toy; attempts to retrieve dropped object; releases object grasped by other person
Language:	Repetitive consonant sounds (mama, dada)
Social:	Responds to sound of name; plays peek-a-boo or pat-a-cake; waves bye-bye

AT 52 WEEKS (1 YEAR)

Motor:	Walks with one hand held; "cruises" or walks holding on to furniture
Adaptive:	Picks up pellet with unassisted pincer movement of forefinger and thumb; releases object to other person on request or gesture
Language:	2 "words" besides mama, dada
Social:	Plays simple ball game; makes postural adjustment to dressing

TABLE 2-11. EMERGING PATTERNS OF BEHAVIOR FROM 1 TO 5 YEARS OF AGE

---

15 MONTHS

Motor: Walks alone; crawls up stairs
Adaptive: Makes tower of 2 cubes; makes a line with crayon; inserts pellet in bottle
Language: Jargon; follows simple commands; may name a familiar object (ball)
Social: Indicates some desires or needs by pointing

---

18 MONTHS

Motor: Runs stiffly; sits on small chair; walks up stairs with one hand held; explores drawers and waste baskets
Adaptive: Piles 3 cubes; imitates scribbling; imitates vertical stroke; dumps pellet from bottle
Language: 10 words (average); names pictures
Social: Feeds self; seeks help when in trouble; may complain when wet or soiled

---

24 MONTHS

Motor: Runs well; walks up and down stairs, one step at a time; opens doors; climbs on furniture
Adaptive: Tower of 6 cubes; circular scribbling; imitates horizontal stroke; folds paper once imitatively
Language: Puts 3 words together (pronoun, verb, object)
Social: Handles spoon well; often tells immediate experiences; helps to undress; listens to stories with pictures

---

30 MONTHS

Motor: Jumps
Adaptive: Tower of 8 cubes; makes vertical and horizontal strokes, but generally will not join them to make a cross; imitates circular stroke, forming closed figure
Language: Refers to self by pronoun "I"; knows full name
Social: Helps put things away

---

36 MONTHS

Motor: Goes up stairs alternating feet; rides tricycle; stands momentarily on one foot
Adaptive: Tower of 9 cubes; imitates construction of "bridge" of 3 cubes; copies a circle; imitates a cross
Language: Knows age and sex; counts 3 objects correctly; repeats 3 numbers or a sentence of 6 syllables
Social: Plays simple games (in "parallel" with other children); helps in dressing (unbuttons clothing and puts on shoes); washes hands

---

48 MONTHS

Motor: Hops on one foot; throws ball overhand; uses scissors to cut out pictures; climbs well
Adaptive: Copies bridge from model; imitates construction of "gate" of 5 cubes; copies cross and square; draws a man with 2 to 4 parts besides head; names longer of 2 lines
Language: Counts 4 pennies accurately; tells a story
Social: Plays with several children with beginning of social interaction and role-playing; goes to toilet alone

---

60 MONTHS

Motor: Skips
Adaptive: Draws triangle from copy; names heavier of 2 weights
Language: Names 4 colors; repeats sentence of 10 syllables; counts 10 pennies correctly
Social: Dresses and undresses; asks questions about meaning of words; domestic role-playing

---

After 5 years the Stanford-Binet, Wechsler-Bellevue and other scales offer the most precise estimates of developmental level. In order to have their greatest value, they should be administered only by an experienced and qualified person.

the Peabody Picture Vocabulary Test, the Quick Test, the Raven Matrices, and the Denver Developmental Screening Test.* Occasional or casual testing may be misleading. In using these or other tools for evaluation of performance the tester should become thoroughly familiar with the procedures, their rules for administration, and their limitations. The Draw-a-Man Test, for example, should be given to a child who is comfortably seated; he is given a plain piece of white paper 8½ by 11 inches and a pencil with an eraser, and should be left undisturbed for as long as he needs to complete his drawing. The test may have grossly distorted values when the child uses a ball-point pen to put a hasty drawing on a precription pad, while he stands at a corner of the physician's desk. When doubts exist as to the interpretation of any of these tests, the child should be referred to a qualified psychologist.

VICTOR C. VAUGHAN, III

---

*See page 1551 for description of Denver Developmental Screening Test.

REFERENCES

Barnett, S. A. (Ed.): *Lessons from Animal Behavior for the Clinician.* Little Club Clinics in Developmental Medicine, No. 7 London, National Spastics Society, 1962.

Erikson, E. H.: *Childhood and Society.* New York, W. W. Norton and Co., 1950.

Falkner, F. (Ed.): *Human Development.* Philadelphia, W. B. Saunders Company, 1966.

Frankenburg, W. K., and Dodds, J. B.: The Denver Developmental Screening Test. *J. Pediat.,* 71:181, 1967.

Gesell, A., and Amatruda, C. S.: *Developmental Diagnosis.* 2nd ed. New York, Paul B. Hoeber, Inc., 1947.

Greulich, W. W., and Pyle, S. I.: *Radiographic Atlas of Skeletal Development of the Hand and Wrist.* Stanford, Calif., Stanford University Press, 1950; 2nd ed., 1959.

Iliff, A., and Lee, V. A.: Pulse Rate, Respiratory Rate, and Body Temperature of Children Between Two Months and Eighteen Years of Age. *Child Develop.,* 23:237, 1952.

Illingworth, R. S.: *The Development of the Infant and Young Child, Normal and Abnormal.* Edinburgh, Livingston, 1960.

Illingworth, R. S.: *An Introduction to Developmental Assessment in the First Year.* Little Club Clinics in Developmental Medicine, No. 3. London, National Spastics Society, 1962.

Lewis, R. C., Duval, A. M., and Iliff, A.: Standards for the Basal Metabolism of Children from 2 to 15 Years of Age, Inclusive. *J. Pediat.,* 23:1, 1943.

Meiks, L. T., and Green, M. (Eds.): Symposium on Adolescence. *Pediat. Clin. N. Amer.,* 7:1-226, 1960.

Munn, N. L.: *The Evolution and Growth of Human Behavior.* Boston, Houghton-Mifflin Co., 1955.

Pyle, S. I., Reed, R. B., and Stuart, H. C.: Patterns of Skeletal Development in the Hand. *Pediatrics,* 24:886, 1959.

Reynolds, E. L., and Asakawa, T.: Skeletal Development in Infancy: Standards for Clinical Use. *Am. J. Roentgenol. & Radium Ther.,* 65:403, 1951.

Stuart, H. C.: Normal Growth and Development During Adolescence. *New England J. Med.,* 234:666, 693, 732, 1946.

Talbot, N. B., Richie, R. H., and Crawford, J. D.: *Metabolic Homeostasis: A Syllabus for Those Concerned with the Care of Patients.* Cambridge, Mass., Harvard University Press, 1959.

Tanner, J. M.: *Growth at Adolescence.* Springfield, Ill., Charles C Thomas, 1956.

Todd, T. W.: *Atlas of Skeletal Maturation (Hand).* St. Louis, C. V. Mosby Company, 1937.

Vaughan, V. C., III: New Insights in Social Behavior. *J.A.M.A.,* 198:46, 1966.

Vogt, E. C., and Vickers, V. S.: Osseous Growth and Development. *Radiology,* 31:441, 1938.

Watson, E. H., and Lowrey, G. H.: *Growth and Development of Children.* 5th ed. Chicago, Year Book Publishers, Inc., 1967.

Watson, R. I.: *Psychology of the Child.* New York, John Wiley and Sons, 1959.

Weech, A. A.: Signposts on Highway of Growth. *Am. J. Dis. Child.,* 88:452, 1954.

PSYCHOLOGIC DEVELOPMENT

At birth only a few of the inherited patterns of adaptive behavior of the human infant are sufficiently mature to contribute to his survival. He has inherent rooting, sucking and swallowing reflexes which enable him to find and take nourishment, provided the breast or bottle is within the range of his head movements. He is capable of vocalizing relatively undifferentiated cries of distress, signalling that he is in need. Within a period of days he can make cooing noises and winsome facial expressions which, importantly, evoke feelings of tenderness and warmth in his mother. Except for these rather primitive patterns and certain automatic and homeostatic regulative functions, which are by no means infallible, he is completely helpless and, unless cared for, will die.

More complex behavior patterns, such as the ability to track an object with his eyes or to coordinate visual perception with reaching for and grasping an object, are potentially rather than immediately useful skills. The higher mental abilities such as conscious memory, anticipation, speech, abstract reasoning, and communication by spoken and written language develop at varying intervals after birth.

The infant's prolonged dependency and vulnerability, however, are well compensated by his ultimately greater capabilities. The fact that he inherits so few of the automatic, autonomous and complex patterns of behavior seen in lower animals means that he is much less bound to automatic and rigid ways of adaptation. His inherited abilities mature slowly and in stepwise fashion. Not only are they subject to influence, but their full realization requires appropriate environmental influences. The development of the child's skills, the effectiveness with which he uses them, and the use to which they are put are determined by interaction with his environment.

Out of this interaction the human mind or psyche develops, and takes over the management of the inherited patterns of behavior and the higher mental abilities. The result is man's capacity to alter his environment and adapt it to his needs, instead of having to adapt to it. On the other hand, the fact that his development is so much shaped by experience allows for the possibility of unfavorable influences and accounts in large measure for his susceptibility to emotional and mental illness.

Since psychic or personality development, or *psychologic development* in accordance with the terminology used here, takes place after birth, postnatal experiences are of great importance. The capacity for memory and the related faculty of anticipation have their beginnings in the first months of life and make it possible for earlier experience to influence the reaction to later experience. Significant experiences in the first weeks, months and years of life are especially important because they affect the very foundations of psychologic development.

BASIC CONCEPTS

There is relatively little psychologic functioning in the first weeks of life; however, psychologic factors play an increasing part in subsequent interactions. Psychologic development can be appraised in terms of the interaction of the child's natural endowment and the *environmental factors* which influence it.

BIOLOGIC FACTORS

The role of the child's biologic make-up in his development can be discussed in terms of three different but closely interrelated factors: (1) *endowment,* (2) the predetermined pattern and schedule of *biologic maturation,* and (3) the *energy* necessary for growth, development and functioning.

Endowment. Endowment is the term used for the inherited constitutional patterns, the basic elements being the physical and physiologic make-up of the individual, his potential for intelligence, and his more specific potentials such as talents for music or mathematics.*

In the first months of life a predominant temperament or behavioral pattern is observed in some infants which may persist relatively unchanged through childhood into adulthood. Temperament or personality in infants and children stems from the summation of such relatively independent qualities of behavior as activity level, rhythmicity, adaptability, the tendency to approach or withdraw from new stimuli, intensity of reaction to stimuli, mood, sensory threshold, distractibility, and attention spans. The affectual experiences in mother-infant relations are vital to personality development and have early impact on the infant. The relative importances of heredity or endowment and of environmental-social factors in forming temperament or personality have not been clearly delineated. In any case, degrees of compatibility or incompatibility may exist between the temperament of the child and the attitudes and expectations he meets in his environment, which may contribute either to healthy development and adaptation or to disturbances in behavior.

Endowment is shaped not only by heredity, but also by postconceptional factors. Untoward events occurring during the intrauterine, parturient or postnatal periods, for example, may produce conditions such as cerebral palsy, in which the neurologic defect illustrates that the constitution of the child at birth may be different from what was intended by heredity. Because cerebral palsy is readily perceived, parents and physicians make allowance for this handicap when evaluating the development of the child. When there is alteration in hereditary endowment without clearly demonstrable clinical manifestations, however, the child is not likely to be recognized as constitutionally handicapped, and appropriate allowances will not be made. This situation may cause problems in development because the child lacks the capacity to measure up to expectations. Such subtle handicaps conceivably can result either from damage to anatomic structures or from physiologic malfunctioning. For example, a subclinical lesion in a "silent area" of the cerebral cortex having to do with the coordination of the various elements in the motor speech apparatus can delay development of speech. This could result in anxiety in the parents, which in turn would cause anxiety in the child and a disturbed relationship with his parents.

Since optimum development requires that the child's endowment and parental expectations be in accord, it is important to make careful and continuing appraisals of both the constitutional and environmental factors.

Biologic Maturation. Innate factors, such as those which determine the physical characteristics and the timing of their appearance in the embryo, continue to operate after birth. Thus the times of emergence of the capacity to walk, of puberty and of the ability for abstract reasoning are biologically predetermined. Although the time of appearance of each of these various capacities and functions is fairly predictable, there is considerable individual variation, and, as with organic or constitutional differences, it is important that the environmental expectations be in keeping with the time schedule of the individual child.

Because the child's psychologic and personality development is uniquely tied to the development of his mental abilities, special note must be taken of the biologically predetermined maturation of the nervous system. Maturation of nervous system pathways proceeds gradually and sequentially from the autonomic level, to the spinal cord level of the sensory and lower motor neuron reflex arc,

---

*Evidence suggests that such talents may be due not only to endowment, but also to factors such as early exposure to specific kinds of stimulation and unusually strong interest and motivation, which result in a greater development of potential in particular areas of capability.

to a subcortical level, to the level of the upper motor neuron and cerebral cortex. At birth (except in the case of prematurity) the autonomic nervous system, which participates importantly in the homeostatic regulative functions, normally is functioning and reasonably well integrated. Similarly, the lower motor neuron reflex arcs also are functioning, as is evidenced by response to stimuli.

The integration of sensorimotor reflex pathways with other sensory and motor pathways and with the higher centers is dependent upon continuing maturation of the central nervous system and upon experience. For example, although each eye is capable of receiving light stimuli and transmitting nerve impulses to the brain at birth, the eyes normally operate relatively independently during the first days of life, and coordinated binocular vision is achieved only gradually. Similar maturation and practice are required before the various sensorimotor pathways involved in walking are sufficiently functional and integrated for the child to be able to walk. On a less observable level, there is evidence to suggest that the capability for abstract reasoning appears by about the age of 12 years, when there is a further maturation of the endocrine and possibly of the central nervous systems.

The innately predetermined individual pattern in the timing of sensorimotor maturation also is affected by experience. For example, serious nutritional deficiency can impair physiologic functioning and the rate of physical growth. Under such conditions there may be delayed onset of puberty, which can have important implications for psychologic development. The impact of emotional deprivation during infancy is revealed by studies which suggest that an optimal amount of stimulation is necessary to bring forth innate patterns. Although it has not been established that the imprinting phenomena (see p. 22) described in lower animals also apply to the human being, it does seem that there is a similarity, at least in the sense that certain kinds of stimulation and experience are desirable, or perhaps necessary, at certain times in the development of the organism. A rather extreme illustration is the observation that continuous bandaging of the eyes of chimpanzees during a critical period of visual development results in blindness. Similarly, work with psychotic children suggests that the development of language may be seriously impaired in the child whose mother was emotionally ill and essentially nonvocal while caring for him in his infancy.

Energy. The third biologic factor requiring consideration is that of the energy of life. This is utilized in two related but different ways. On the one hand, it is used for the growth of the child, for the physiologic functions necessary for sustaining life, and ultimately for reproducing life. On the other hand, energy is used for mental and physical activities which are not immediately and directly related to the viability of the individual or to the survival of the species.

Fundamentally, the biologic destiny of man is to reproduce his own kind. Even though capacity for procreation does not appear until puberty, the developmental years are largely concerned with helping the child to become a social being able to get along with people and ultimately to marry, to function sexually and to rear children. Thus, even though much of the activity and behavior of man are not directly sexual, the energy used in other activities serves or is derived from the sexual drive. It is from this viewpoint that Freud spoke of the sexuality of the child and of the adult and described the sexual drive as the central factor in human behavior. His original conceptualizations were misunderstood and met with much resistance, but his ideas, taken in their intended meaning, are essential to an understanding of child development.

The sexual drive in the foregoing sense is basic, and energy derived from chemical processes is utilized by and channeled through it. A normal characteristic of behavioral manifestations of the sexual drive is a quality of pleasure, affection and satisfaction which tends to bring the individual into relation with other people. There are other feelings and activities, however, which have a different quality and are concerned with the overcoming of obstacles and the solution of problems. These behavioral manifestations have been summed up under the term "aggression." Although there continue to be differences of opinion about the number and nature of basic life drives, for practical purposes child development can be adequately understood in terms of these 2 qualitatively different drives: *the sexual drive* and *the aggressive drive*.

Observation of the infant in the neonatal period tends to support this formulation of drives and suggests the order of their emergence. When the infant has recovered from the effects of birth, and assuming that he is healthy and receives care appropriate to his needs, the first observable evidence as to his emotional state suggests pleasure and satisfaction; normally he is relaxed, he coos, he smiles. It is only with frustration of his needs — this being inevitable in spite of the best possible care — that evidence of aggression is observed. If he is improperly fed, restrained or hurt, he cries in a way which suggests anger, and he shows increasingly vigorous, uncoordinated movements which at a later age, when directed and coordinated, undoubtedly would aim at avoidance of or coping with the cause of his discomfort. If, however, his first aggressive actions call forth an environmental response which relieves his frustration, he does not become unduly distressed. Thus it is tenable to think of aggression as normal and constructive.

On the other hand, if his discomfort continues and his tension increases, his behavior takes on a destructive quality. In acute distress he shows the equivalent of rage and hostility. With continuing neglect of his needs the rage subsides, but since he does not have the means for directing his aggression toward solving the problem, the aggression is contained and expressed internally. In more moderate situations this may become manifest in various kinds of physiologic disturbance. In the most extreme case of deprivation of emotional needs the infant exhibits a clinical picture analogous to depression, and without proper treatment there ensues a progressive decline of emotional tone and physiologic functioning.

The developing personality of the child plays an increasingly important role in subsequent development. In early infancy the sexual and aggressive drives readily gain expression, owing to the relative lack of internal organization and means of control. Initially the energy of these drives is utilized largely for physical purposes, but as the mind develops, it is also directed to mental activities and is identified as psychic energy.

The term used for the psychic energy derived from the sexual drive is *libido*. Libido is conceived of as a force or flow of psychic energy which can be controlled and directed toward or away from parts of one's self, other people and tangible or abstract goals, in dynamic and constantly changing ways and amounts. For example, normal stimulation of the sensory endings of the skin of the infant causes libido to be invested in this body area. In this experience the anatomic covering of the body is defined and the development of the body image promoted, helping the child to demarcate himself from the rest of the world. Later, as relationships are increasingly established with other human beings, certain amounts of libido must be directed toward or invested in other persons.

The supply of psychic energy varies with changes in physiologic functioning in different stages of development or in physical illness, but the total amount available at any given time is limited. If too much energy is expended in emotional conflicts rather than in effective action, the individual has a problem. For example, the child whose mental energy is consumed by a conflict between an intense desire to excel and an equally strong fear of failure may not invest sufficient libido in the task of learning, and he may fail in school for this reason rather than because of deficiency in intelligence.

The choice as to investment of libido will determine the basic pattern of the child's development and behavior, and thus is primary. The psychic energy of the aggressive drive is secondary to libido, being used to implement or fulfill the libidinal choices or aims. In a sense, life consists of repeated tension and relief-of-tension patterns. The sexual and aggressive drives can be temporarily held in check, but inevitably they gain expression in healthy or abnormal ways.

One way to evaluate a child's development is to study his use of libido and aggression in relation to others and to himself, comparing his current status with that of his earlier development and with that of the average child of his age and social group.

ENVIRONMENTAL FACTORS

There has been a tendency to believe that unless an experience is consciously remembered, it is of no lasting significance. But the work of Freud demonstrated that experiences can be retained outside of conscious awareness and can significantly influence behavior. This being so, the question is: At what age is the human organism able to retain impressions at conscious or unconscious* levels? The answer is largely speculative. Nevertheless the question needs consideration in view of growing concern that certain clinical practices applied to the infant may have psychologic impact contrary to past interpretations. For example, there is considerable interest in the impact of various aspects of the care of premature infants, including their isolation, upon subsequent personality and cognitive functions. More concretely, the justification for performing circumcision shortly after birth without adequate anesthesia has been based in part on the assumption that the painful experience had no untoward psychologic influence.

One source for data relative to the question of retention of impressions is study of the conditioned reflex. Conditioning can take place outside of conscious awareness and be retained even in the human fetus during the last trimester of pregnancy with persistence after birth. Studies have indicated that the restlessness of infants can be lessened by an instrument reproducing the sound of the mother's heartbeat. And at a few weeks of age infants have been observed to respond to their mother's voice with a lessening of distress and tension, even though the mother was not in direct contact with them, and in spite of simultaneous exposure to the sounds of other voices. It seems probable that impressions can be retained before the capability of conscious memory.

One cannot fail to be impressed with the tremendous capacity of the human being to absorb trauma and survive. Perhaps it is this capacity which, at least in part, has permitted us inappropriately to discount the significance of untoward events in the earliest period of life.

Concern for the psychologic development and future mental health of the child requires that events in the neonatal as well as in any later stage of development be managed in such a way as to keep tension in the child within tolerable limits.

Prenatal Environmental Influences. Physicians do not attribute birthmarks and other physical characteristics of infants and children to acute or chronic emotional upsets in the mother during pregnancy. The probability of such a cause

---

*The term *unconscious* as used in psychology is equivalent to the lay term *subconscious*, and means outside of conscious awareness. It is not to be confused with the physical state of being unconscious or in coma.

and effect is exceedingly unlikely. On the other hand, one cannot be certain that the mental and emotional state of the mother during pregnancy is not reflected in some way in the personality of the child. One may speculate that hormonal influences associated with an acute or chronic state of tension in the mother can be passed through the placental barrier to the fetus. Although such effects might be only temporary, the possibility must be considered that they may have a continuing effect.

Postnatal Environmental Influences. The emotional and attitudinal climate into which a child is born has its beginnings long before his arrival. Even the fantasies about babies and motherhood which the mother had as a little girl and as an adolescent play a role in her functioning as an adult. The extent to which husband and wife agree as to when to have and how to rear children also is important. The experience of the mother during pregnancy, labor and delivery is particularly significant, perhaps because earlier fantasy now is being fulfilled or contradicted by reality. A woman who feels that her husband has withdrawn his love and emotional support from her during the pregnancy may feel conscious or unconscious resentment toward the unborn child. Or, when the child is born, she may "love" it too much, trying to gain from the child the love which she normally should be receiving from her husband. An overt or subclinical depressive reaction in the mother from any cause during the infant's first months of life may produce an infant-mother relationship that is unnatural and lacking in warmth and spontaneity.

A clear need for emotional satisfaction exists in the neonate. This is seen in his pleasure in sucking and clinging, and in "following" his mother with sight and hearing, as well as in the various sensory experiences provided through his mother's ministrations, such as body warmth, cuddling, rocking, bathing, anointing the skin, and her soothing voice. These needs become increasingly strong and meaningful during the first year of life, and ultimately are subsumed under what we call the need for love.

The crowded hospital nursery cannot provide the kind of infant-mother interaction described above. It is difficult even for a trained mother-substitute to give the unique care provided by the infant's own mother. The physical health of the newborn infant must of course be protected during the few days he remains in the hospital after birth, but everything possible should be done to ensure his emotional health as well. Placement of the infant in the mother's hospital room most or all of the time, "rooming-in," provides opportunities for the establishment of better mother-infant relations.

It seems reasonable to generalize that, whenever possible, the newborn infant as well as the sick infant or young child should have a close and continuing relation with his parents.

Owing to the immaturity of the infant's perceptual and motor apparatus, the mother must supplement his undeveloped functions and must meet his needs. Stated in psychologic terms, the *"maternal auxiliary ego"* (René Spitz) complements and takes over for the undeveloped ego of the infant. This places the mother in a unique position which may explain the tendency for some mothers to feel unduly guilty when problems arise in their child's physical or emotional development and for the physician to look particularly to the child-mother relationship in an attempt to understand emotional imbalance in a child. Objectivity requires, however, that one neither excuse the parents from responsibility for the child's psychologic development nor hold them entirely responsible. The physician should attempt to convey an understanding of this to parents.

The infant also needs an optimal amount of frustration and opportunities to bear tension. These needs, although less well recognized, are as important as the need for satisfaction. Thus the mother is both satisfier and frustrator, giving to her child, but also confronting him with the realities of physical and social living. In the first weeks and months of life the primary needs of the infant are satisfaction and relief of tension. In deciding how much the infant should be held, whether he should be permitted to cry himself to sleep, whether he should be fed by "demand" or according to schedule, and a host of other common but important matters, the mother is influenced by her own needs as well as the needs of other people, particularly the father, the immediate family and other relatives. As the infant approaches the end of his first year, both father and mother are expected to begin to present the culturally prescribed limits upon his behavior so that he will develop an adequate personality and character structure.

The sine qua non of successful child-rearing is the achievement of an optimal balance between satisfying the child's needs on the one hand and frustrating and challenging him on the other, so as to stimulate the development of his latent abilities and potentialities.

PSYCHOLOGIC FACTORS

The Id. The normal state of the infant is a dynamic one in which tensions are constantly being built up and relieved. At the beginning of life the tensions are largely due to internal, physiologic processes necessary for the sustenance of life, e.g. the hunger tension. Very early, however, the infant becomes more wakeful, and there are signs of surplus energy. This presages the beginning of mental development. The only element of psychic structure present at this time is the id. *The id can be defined as the inherited reservoir of unorganized drives. It is mostly unconscious, is governed by the pleasure-pain principle, aims at immediate satisfaction of libidinal urges, is unmoral, is illogical and lacks unity of purpose.*

The Ego. Out of the interaction between mother and infant with its repetition of stimulation, tension and relief-of-tension, the ego and mental organization of the infant begin to develop. As his personality and capacities gradually emerge, more is expected of him, and the mother begins to introduce the previously referred to limits and frustrations. The infant responds with his biologically innate tendency to strive for mastery.

The ego can be defined as the integrating or mediating part of personality, which develops out of the interaction of id and environment and controls the tendencies of the id, excluding or modifying those tendencies which are in conflict with reality. It is predominantly conscious or preconscious, and has perception both of the internal self and of the external world.

The ego of the mother complements and supplements the ego of the child. As the child's ego gradually develops, however, she must gradually turn over to the child an increasing amount of responsibility for himself, until one day he is able to function relatively autonomously and independently. For example, though the potential for walking is biologically provided, the development of the capacity to walk is ascribed to the ego as a part of psychologic development.

The skills acquired by the ego and used in the solution of problems and conflicts can be referred to as *ego defenses.* An individual's ego defenses serve the purposes of adaptation and survival and of productive and creative functioning. Certain defenses deal mostly with the external world, e.g. the ability to perceive, to walk and to talk. Other defenses deal more with the internal world of drive, conflict, tension and emotion.

Superego. As we ascend the phylogenetic scale, an increasing amount of energy becomes available for activities other than those directly concerned with sustaining life. Purely pleasurable or play activity is more characteristic of mammals than of other animals. Man, in comparison with other mammals, not only plays, but also is capable of creative activity. Man as a social being has had to develop a system of values for guiding behavior. He makes laws and concerns himself with religion and philosophy. In so doing he develops a conscience or superego. The behavior of man without a conscience does not differ materially from the behavior of the lower animals.

The child is born without a superego. This element of personality structure, like the ego, is developed under the training and influence of the environment. The superego normally develops under the aegis of love. As the child's urges and behavior bring him into conflict with his parents, it is his need to continue receiving their love and approval which causes him to accept their judgments and disciplinary actions, and to internalize their values to form his own superego.

The superego makes value judgments about the individual's urges, impulses and activities, and can be defined as the latest development of the mind (both phylogenetically and ontogenetically), embodying the code of society and including concepts of right and wrong, the value system, and the ideals.

Conscious, Preconscious and Unconscious Areas of the Mind. It appears that conscious perception at birth is exceedingly limited. Even when fully awake, the newborn infant is thought to have no awareness of himself as separate from the rest of the world. As his various sensory systems mature and are repeatedly stimulated, impressions are received on a cortical and conscious level. Conscious awareness is thought to develop gradually during the first year of life.

The conscious mind is defined as that relatively small part of mental life of which the individual is aware at any given time. Although conscious awareness is a continuum during normal waking life, its content is extremely transitory and constantly changing. On the other hand, there is a great deal of the mental life which is available to consciousness through recall or association of ideas. *For purposes of definition, this material, which is readily available to consciousness, is referred to as being preconscious.*

There is still another significant body of material which is *unconscious* and either not available to consciousness at all, or available to it only with special techniques such as the free association technique of psychoanalytic treatment or hypnosis. Certain experiences may be unconscious because their engrams were established before the development of the capacity for conscious memory. One evidence in support of this idea is the "screen" or false memory observed in psychoanalytic treatment, wherein a patient claims to have a memory of some experience occurring in the first year or two of life, at a time when conscious memory normally is not functional. The proposed explanation is that the patient did have an experience which was stored in the nervous system, most likely more in terms of feelings or emotions than in terms of visual or verbal images, and that the patient now fabricates visual and verbal imagery to suit the experience he is attempting to recall.

Experiences may be unconscious for another reason. One of the ways in which the mind attempts to protect itself from unpleasant or intolerable tension is to eliminate the memory of the experience and the associated feelings from conscious awareness. This is known as *repression.* Though the painful thoughts or feelings are no longer in conscious awareness, they are nevertheless still a part of mental life. Within certain limits repression can be a normal and successful way of dealing with tension and conflict. On the other hand, repression is a basis for development of emotional disturbance, since the repressed material continues to be invested with psychic energy and can influence behavior in spite of the person's having no conscious awareness that this is the case. Thus a primary factor in the consideration of normal child development should be the prevention of pathologic repression and the ensuing development of emotional problems.

GENERAL PRINCIPLES GOVERNING CHILD DEVELOPMENT

The sexual and aggressive drives may be increased or decreased by changing conditions of stimulation, physical health, and environment, but they demand fulfillment. The child needs to develop a personality which can control these drives and at the same time obtain sufficient satisfaction of them in keeping with the requirements of social living. Thus the sexual curiosity of a 6-year-old child at times will be satisfied with direct information about sexual matters, but much of the time will be sublimated, his energy being used in the classroom to learn subjects far removed from sex. As a result of the progressive biologic maturation and cultural conditioning the aims of the sexual and aggressive drives are constantly changing. Freud proposed the term *psychosexual development* to characterize the child's progress through what he called the oral, anal, phallic, latency and adolescent stages (see Table 2-12).

Ego Mastery. Erikson has clarified the importance of ego development as the counterpart of the changing focus of sexual and aggressive drives. He lists for each stage of development of the child a certain predominant *ego quality* which is normally acquired during that stage, and results from mastery of the challenges presented and from resolution of the resulting conflicts. For example, at the close of the oral phase the infant normally should have acquired a feeling of trust as a result of his various experiences with his mother, including the experience of being weaned. The infant should derive ego strength from having been able to give up pleasure in sucking the breast or bottle in return for maternal approval.

The child should have the experience of surmounting the various challenges and conflicts presented to him by his own biologic maturation and by his environment in such a way as to develop a sense of ego mastery.

Maturation-Development. The readiness for weaning is usually present toward the end of the first year of life, when the need for sucking seems to have been sufficiently satisfied, and when erupted teeth provide the ability and the motivation for chewing food. Weaning at either 6 or 18 months of age is likely to be out of step with biologic maturation, and such action may cause unnecessary difficulty in development. Similarly, an unexpected biologic deviation, such as the onset of puberty and menstruation in a girl at 9 years of age, may cause difficulty in development because her environment understandably has not prepared her for this event.

Biologic maturation and psychologic development should progress hand in hand and complement each other.

Pleasure-Pain Versus Reality Principle. Early in life the child is governed by what Freud called *the pleasure-pain principle:* he seeks that which is pleasurable and avoids or rejects that which is unpleasurable. At first this behavior is essentially on a reflex level, but as conscious awareness increases and the infant becomes more discerning, his behavior becomes increasingly purposeful. The parents and subsequently society take cognizance of the child's increasing ability to understand and to exercise self-control, and begin to present him with various demands which intrude upon his pleasure. These demands gradually increase throughout the child's development and require him to take on increasing amounts of responsibility for himself and finally for others.

During the course of his development the child learns to postpone and moderate his needs, wants and pleasures in order to function as a responsible member of a society; thus the pleasure-pain principle gradually yields to the reality principle.

Progression-Regression. The child does not find the demands of reality always to his liking, nor is he able to meet and master them easily. Thus, in spite of the inevitability of biologic maturation and the strong innate tendency toward achievement and mastery, the child at times will temporarily retreat in the face of difficult problems and tension-creating conflicts. Within certain limits regression not only is normal, but also may be essential and helpful, since the child is attempting to replenish his emotional energy and prepare himself once again to forge ahead.

Child development normally is characterized by a pattern of progression and regression.

Love and Limits. The early training of the child and his later education constitute his acculturation, and are achieved through the judicious use of approval and disapproval by parents and teachers. Generally speaking, parents readily voice approval and disapproval, but they frequently have difficulty in backing up these attitudes with convincing firmness and consistency. Words alone are not always enough. Thus verbal encouragement given to a 7-year-old child who is having difficulty learning in school may not be sufficiently motivating if the child feels that his relation to his parents is superficial and lacking in emotional support. The toddler who does not respond to repeated verbal admonishments against touching and playing with a forbidden object will tend to be more convinced of the parent's intent when the object is removed.

Just as the use of aggression in overcoming obstacles is normal in the child, the use of aggression in training the child is normal in the parent. Difficulty arises when parents do not have sufficient conviction about the values they present to their child, or when for other reasons they fail to take action sufficiently early. In consequence of mounting anger, their aggression usually bursts out of control in the form of hostility, and their effectiveness is thus diminished. Many parents feel that love and aggression are mutually exclusive and fear that the consequence of aggression toward their child will result in the loss of his love. Firmness on the part of the parent does not alienate the child from the parent; after his temporary negative response to frustration the child tends to identify with the parent, gaining a feeling of confidence and strength from the experience of having his drives controlled. Actually, love requires that the parent do what is best for the child; only by setting and holding limits on the child's behavior will the child develop into a reasonably controlled and social human being. While he is learning to control his drives, the child is acquiring a sense of values. These values come to make up the bulk of his superego, or conscience. Following through on attitudes of approval and disapproval is essential to the development of ego and superego.

Normality. So long as the child is continuing to progress in all aspects and lines of development at a rate reasonably close to the norms for his age and is not lagging too far behind in any particular aspect of development, the probability is that he is developing normally.

AIMS IN CHILD DEVELOPMENT

According to the principles stated above, the broad aims in any given stage of child development can be stated as follows: (1) sufficient gratification of the child's basic needs, both physiologic and emotional, so as to provide feelings of well-being, satisfaction, security and self-esteem; (2) the gradual presentation of the frustrating parental and societal demands, these being properly timed in keeping with the child's rate of biologic maturation and ego development; (3) mastery by the child of these demands and of the accompanying feelings and conflicts, with the twofold result of learning new techniques of managing himself and of gaining feelings of competence and self-confidence. (4) The basic child-parent love bond, however strained, should not be broken, and inevitable incidences of resentment and hostility should be temporary; the desired relation should be reestablished before the limits of the child's tolerance of the threat of loss of love are exceeded. (5) As the child is called upon to yield gradually his earlier modes of satisfaction and his dependency, he is helped to redirect or rechannel his drives into socially approved, preferably constructive outlets.

If these aims are successfully accomplished in each age period, the child will be ready for each succeeding stage of development and eventually for entrance to competent adult life.

STAGES OF PSYCHOLOGIC DEVELOPMENT

The format of Table 2-12 (pp. 65 through 71) facilitates the understanding of sequential development during infancy and childhood. A longitudinal view of child development as a continuum is gained by tracing an aspect of development from page to page through the successive stages. On the other hand, a cross-sectional view of development at a particular age or stage is gained by reading in a vertical direction on each page, noting the principal happenings in all aspects of development. Evaluation of the development of a particular child at a particular time requires careful study of all available data, both current and from the past history, using and correlating the cross-sectional and longitudinal points of view. The reader is referred to the sources listed in the bibliography for more detailed information.

REFERENCES

Aldrich, C. A., and Aldrich, M. M.: *Babies Are Human Beings.* New York, Macmillan Company, 1938.

Bateson, G.: Cultural Determinants of Behavior; in J. McV. Hunt (Ed.): *Personality and the Behavior Disorders.* New York, Ronald Press, 1944, Vol. II, pp. 714-33.

Benedict, R.: *Patterns of Culture.* Boston, Houghton Mifflin Company, 1934.

Bowbly, J.: Maternal Care and Mental Health. Geneva, World Health Organization, 1951.

Brazelton, T. B.: Observations of the Neonate. *J. Am. Acad. Child Psychiat.,* 1:38, 1962.

Brenner, C.: *An Elementary Textbook of Psychoanalysis.* New York, International Universities Press, 1955.

Chess, S., Thomas, T., and Birch, H. G.: Behavior Problems Revisited. *J. Am. Acad. Child Psychiat.,* 6:321, 1967.

English, O. S., and Pearson, G. H. J.: *Emotional Problems of Living.* New York, W. W. Norton & Co., 1945.

Erikson, E. H.: *Childhood and Society.* New York, W. W. Norton & Co., 1950, pp. 219-34.

Escalona, S.: Emotional Development in the First Year of Life; in M. J. E. Senn (Ed.): *Problems of Infancy and Childhood.* New York, Josiah Macy, Jr. Foundation, 1949, pp. 30-51.

Ferenczi, S.: Stages in the Development of the Sense of Reality; in *Contributions to Psychoanalysis.* Boston, Richard C. Badger, 1916.

Freud, A.: *The Ego and the Mechanisms of Defense.* New York, International Universities Press, 1946.

Freud, A.: Some Remarks on Infant Observation; in *Psychoanalytic Study of the Child.* New York, International Universities Press, 1953, Vol. 8.

Freud, A.: Adolescence; in *Psychoanalytic Study of the Child.* New York, International Universities Press, 1958, Vol. 13.

Freud, S.: Three Contributions to the Theory of Sex (1905); in A. A. Brill (Ed.): *The Basic Writings of Sigmund Freud.* New York, Random House (Modern Library), 1938.

Josselyn, I.: Psychosocial Development of Children. New York, Family Service Association of America, 1948.

Josselyn, I.: The Adolescent and His World. New York, Family Service Association of America, 1952.

La Barre, W.: *The Human Animal.* Chicago, University of Chicago Press, 1954.

Mahler, M. S., and Gosliner, B.: On Symbiotic Child Psychosis; in *Psychoanalytic Study of the Child,* New York, International Universities Press, 1955, Vol. 10, pp. 195-212.

Newton, N., and Newton, M.: Mothers' Reaction to Their Newborn Babies. *J.A.M.A.,* 181:122, 1962.

Ribble, M. A.: Infantile Experience in Relation to Personality Development; in J. McV. Hunt (Ed.): *Personality and Behaviour Disorders.* New York, Ronald Press, 1944.

Settlage, C.: Values of Limits in Child Rearing. *Children,* 5: No. 5, September-October, 1958.

Spitz, R.: The Psychogenic Diseases in Infancy; in *Psychoanalytic Study of the Child.* New York, International Universities Press, 1951, Vol. 6.

Waelder, R.: *Basic Theory of Psychoanalysis.* New York, International Universities Press, 1960.

TABLE 2-12. STAGES OF PSYCHOLOGIC DEVELOPMENT

Both pediatric and psychoanalytic terminologies are used to designate the successive stages of development.

1. AGE. The years of growth and development are divided into periods based on both physical and psychologic characteristics. These periods are not sharply demarcated, but each blends imperceptibly into the following one. Furthermore, there are distinct variations in the rates of transition within the range of normality.

2. BIOLOGIC MATURATION. Each stage is characterized by the appearance of certain physical and mental abilities which are innately predetermined.

3. LIBIDO. As the predetermined abilities mature, their proper functioning requires that they become invested with psychic energy (libido).

4. BIOLOGIC AND CULTURAL CHALLENGES. Each new capacity arising out of biologic maturation presents the child with a challenge requiring mastery. Concurrently, certain cultural and familial attitudes and insistences that he give up early forms of gratification and assume gradually increasing responsibility are brought to bear. As he responds to and masters these challenges, his unique physical and psychologic development takes place, and he becomes a social being able to function in his particular culture or subculture.

5. AGGRESSION. Under normal circumstances aggression arises and is expressed in response to the challenges and insistences on renunciation of gratification and as an aid in facing and mastering them.

6. OBJECT RELATIONSHIP. In psychoanalytic psychology the term "object" includes inanimate and animate objects, human and nonhuman, but most commonly refers to people. The establishment and maintenance of relationship require that the object be invested with libido (see 3, above).

7. EGO AND IDENTITY. The ego is that part of personality structure which serves an integrating function in relation to the self and a mediating function between the self and the environment. An important aspect of the ego is the concept of self or of one's own identity which develops gradually throughout childhood. Attention will be called to the *ego qualities* and to the development of the *sense of reality*.

8. SUPEREGO (CONSCIENCE AND IDEALS). The superego arises out of the ego and embodies the code of the parents and of society or, more specifically, concepts of right and wrong and the individual's ideals and aspirations.

9. TYPICAL NORMAL BEHAVIOR. The composite of all aspects of development in any given stage should result in behavior characteristic and normal for that age period.

DEVELOPMENTAL STAGES

TABLE 2-12.   *(Continued)*

NEONATAL AND EARLY INFANCY PERIODS

Oral stage: Normal autistic phase

D
E
V
E
L
O
P
M
E
N
T
A
L   **S**
T
A
G
E
S

1. AGE. Birth to 3 or 4 months.

2. BIOLOGIC MATURATION. After birth the infant must adjust immediately to extrauterine existence. Normally, the basic autonomic and subcortical homeostatic functions are operative at birth, as are the less automatic, sensorimotor reflexes responsible for sucking and crying. Crying is initially an unrefined signal to the mother. The newborn infant is ill equipped to bear tension and has a stimulus barrier, which functions to avoid excessive stress.

3. LIBIDO. Because the infant at birth lacks both conscious awareness and a concept of self, it is conceived that investment of libido in his biologic functions takes place automatically and unconsciously, as each of the various systems is activated. As conscious awareness increases, libidinization becomes increasingly volitional. In the first months of life libidinal investment proceeds sequentially from the internal visceral systems, to the respiratory function, to the oral zone involved in sucking and ingestion, and then to the surface of the body, as the various sensory endorgans mature and receive stimuli from the general physical environment and through the ministrations of the mother.

4. BIOLOGIC AND CULTURAL CHALLENGES. The primary challenges to the infant are the biologic requirements of shifting from intrauterine to extrauterine existence.

Culture generally makes no additional demands upon the infant. It influences this transition, however, through customs and practices such as whether the infant is with the mother from birth or is put in a nursery, whether feeding is by breast or bottle, whether the bottle-fed infant is held by the mother during feeding, and by the amount and kinds of exposure to light, sound, tactile and other stimuli.

5. AGGRESSION. The newborn infant lacks sufficient coordination and ability for effective aggressive acts. But with frustration of his needs and any undue disturbance in his homeostasis, aggression is evidenced in crying and aimless motor activity. The most severe state of distress has been termed infantile rage. Gradually, as a result of the mother-infant interaction, aggressive responses become more purposeful; e.g. the hunger cry has a different quality from the cry of pain.

6. OBJECT RELATIONSHIP. In the same way that he unconsciously and automatically libidinizes his body systems, the infant also libidinizes the mother. During these first few months, while the perceptual-conscious system is still developing, he does not discern his mother as separate from himself, and his experience is truly autistic, as if everything arose from and took place within him. It is necessary also that the mother properly invest her newborn child with her libido.

7. EGO AND IDENTITY. Such functions as sucking and crying can be regarded as rudiments of the ego, since they function to mediate the needs of the infant in relation to the environment. Those ego functions which are not yet developed are provided by the mother (maternal auxiliary ego). The task of the combined mother-infant ego is to meet the needs of the infant, keeping his tensions within tolerable limits.

There is no concept of the self and therefore no identity, but the experiences in these first months presumably are recorded on an unconscious level and can give a feeling of well-being and contribute to the development of feelings of security, confidence and integration or oneness.

8. SUPEREGO (CONSCIENCE AND IDEALS). Superego as such does not exist. The pleasure-pain principle is the basis for the later development of concepts of good and bad and of right and wrong.

9. TYPICAL NORMAL BEHAVIOR. The infant functions in closeness with the mother (in the dual unity), manifesting an alternation of tension, gratification and relief of tension. At the beginning of this stage the most characteristic behavior is brief wakefulness and restlessness, and then sleeping after eating. Gradually, as the periods of wakefulness increase, personality begins to develop.

TABLE 2-12. *(Continued)*

INFANCY PERIOD

Oral stage: Symbiotic phase

1. AGE. 3-4 months to 12-18 months. The *separation-individuation phase* of ego development begins in the latter part of the oral stage and continues through the phallic stage (3 to 6 or 7 years), as the child gradually separates from his mother and becomes increasingly autonomous.

2. BIOLOGIC MATURATION. There is continuing maturation of the end-organs of taste, smell, touch, vision and hearing, and of the nervous pathways permitting development of the first coordinated movements, such as binocular vision and hand-to-mouth integration, and walking begins.

3. LIBIDO. Libidinization of these various organ systems is contributed to by the mother, through nursing, skin contact, being held and rocked, and seeing her facial expressions and hearing her voice.

4. BIOLOGIC AND CULTURAL CHALLENGES. Biologic maturation presents the challenge of coordinated movement and the purposeful use of the perceptual-conscious system, and also the discomfort associated with the eruption of teeth, and subsequently the use of teeth and jaws in mastication.

   Partly in relation to the appearance of teeth, but also partly as a cultural attitude, the infant is weaned from the breast or bottle near the end of the first year of life. The mother allows the infant to bear tension for increasing periods of time; when he is hungry, she will not feed him so promptly as in the first few weeks of life.

5. AGGRESSION. Aggression is manifest in proportion to unpleasant or frustrating experiences such as interference with feeding, excessive stimulation, painful dentition, too early or too abrupt weaning, or separations from the mother.

6. OBJECT RELATIONSHIP. The infant gradually becomes aware of his close relationship with his mother. As his abilities to perceive and to remember develop, he begins to distinguish himself from his mother. The first real awareness of separateness from his mother appears by about 8 months of age; he has severe anxiety when separated. Investment of libido in relationships becomes increasingly volitional and under the control of the ego.

7. EGO AND IDENTITY. The infant's behavior has gradually become more purposeful. His vocal signals are more purposeful, and his mother responds more specifically. His first coordinated movements allow him to begin to do for himself, e.g. to convey food to his mouth. Repeated sensory experiences have enabled him to begin to define the boundaries of his body, laying the foundation for his body-image concept and the feeling of identity. As his ego develops, his mother is able to relinquish some of the ego functions she had to provide for him.

   As a result of optimum experiences in the oral stage, including a satisfactory weaning experience, the infant should have gained the *ego quality* of a feeling of *trust* in his mother and a good feeling about life.

   The infant's *sense of reality* is beginning to develop. Ferenczi postulated that the infant (if he had any concept of self) would have a feeling of *"unconditional omnipotence,"* everything seeming to be self-contained and under his control. In the latter part of the first year the infant begins to be aware that this is not the case, and he attempts to manage his mother and maintain his feeling of omnipotence with *"magical gestures,"* e.g. a smile, a cry or a reaching out with his hand.

8. SUPEREGO (CONSCIENCE AND IDEALS). In many little ways, both verbal and nonverbal, the mother conveys attitudes of approval and disapproval to the infant. The first renunciation is weaning, which requires that the infant give up the pleasure of sucking the breast or bottle and substitute drinking from a glass and eating solid food. This is a precursor of superego, since it implies a value judgment and introduces the idea that one's drives or impulses are to be controlled.

9. TYPICAL NORMAL BEHAVIOR. Throughout the first year of life the infant is dependent, demanding and mostly oral in his orientation. He responds positively to experiences of pleasure or manifestations of love. He normally suffers relatively little hurt or frustration during his first year and therefore has not yet reacted with hostility and other defenses which serve a protective function. As his wakefulness, coordination and motility gradually increase, he explores his own body, parts of his mother, and the environment, using all his sensory organs, but mostly his mouth.

DEVELOPMENTAL STAGES

TABLE 2-12. *(Continued)*

TODDLER YEARS

Anal stage

DEVELOPMENTAL STAGES

1. AGE. 12 to 36 months

2. BIOLOGIC MATURATION. Maturation of nerve pathways from the cerebral cortex to the external sphincters of the bowel and bladder occurs by about 18 months of age and allows for the possibility of volitional control of these organs. There is heightened awareness of pleasurable sensations from the mucosa, skin and musculature of the anal zone, and continuing maturation of neuromuscular systems, most importantly the locomotor system and the speech apparatus.

3. LIBIDO. The principal libidinal investment of a sensual or erotic quality is in the anal (perineal) area. Additionally, and importantly, the speech apparatus, with beginning language formation, and the locomotor and other neuromuscular functions are libidinized.

4. BIOLOGIC AND CULTURAL CHALLENGES. Biologic maturation presents the challenges of sphincter control and such neuromuscular coordination as that involved in walking, running, talking and manipulating objects. Culture requires the child to gain control of evacuation of his bladder and bowel, and to control himself in the pleasure of uninhibited motility and physical exploration of the environment. This last demand typically is conveyed by his mother's oft-repeated "No! no!"

5. AGGRESSION. Aggression increases considerably in response to the first disciplinary experiences. The toddler meets the mother's attempts at training with vocal and physical resistance. He may lash out against his mother or other frustrating objects, or may vent his feelings in a temper tantrum.

6. OBJECT RELATIONSHIP. The child-parent relationship undergoes a decided change. The child's feeling of power and sense of omnipotence are disabused by increasing parental demands and by his ability to recognize his dependence and relative helplessness. His aggressive urges and his need for love and approval are in conflict with each other. He is ambivalent: aggressive, independent, negativistic, and helpless and clinging. From the parental point of view, the child, who has been enjoyable during the oral stage, is now becoming difficult; their concept of him as they fantasied and wished him to be is disturbed. With increasing awareness of himself as a separate being, he is more discerning of people, and begins to exercise choice as to relationships and their intensity.

7. EGO AND IDENTITY. Ego growth is rapid. Control of bowel and bladder and of various motility patterns and learning defensive techniques for managing feelings and impulses are achieved. Locomotion permits active rather than passive separation. The toddler masters his anxiety as he experiments with separation. His motility increases his sphere of contact, and he learns about physical and social realities. His intellect is sufficiently developed that he can learn his language. He plays and fantasies with much trial-acting and make-believe, these being the forerunners of thinking.

He gains the *ego quality* of a feeling of *autonomy,* rather than excessive feelings of shame or doubt. His body-image concept becomes more clearly defined. His identity takes on more meaning in terms of *his* name and *his* family. Parental attitudes convey that he is good or bad, or clean or dirty. He identifies himself as a boy or girl, although the anatomic basis for this differentiation is not entirely clear to him.

This stage is characterized by a tendency to view all objects as alive and animate. In his fantasy play, animals, plants, trucks, and blocks of wood are imbued with qualities of people.

8. SUPEREGO (CONSCIENCE AND IDEALS). Toilet training and the "No! no!" admonitions contribute to superego formation. Value judgments and character traits of giving and taking, responsibility, self-control, cleanliness, orderliness, punctuality, property rights, and right and wrong begin to develop.

9. TYPICAL NORMAL BEHAVIOR. Behavior is characterized by great energy and a desire to be constantly on the go. Interference is resisted to the point of obstinacy, negativism or temper tantrums. Ambivalence with rapidly oscillating feelings of love and anger is characteristic of relationships with people. A concern about power and control, and who bosses whom, is manifest in play activities.

TABLE 2-12. *(Continued)*

Phallic stage

1. AGE. 3-4 to 5-7 years.

2. BIOLOGIC MATURATION. Continuing maturation allows for increased pleasurable sensation in the penis and clitoris. General physical and intellectual maturation continues, but the pace is slackened.

3. LIBIDO. The predominant investment of libido, psychologically, is in the phallic area, i.e. the penis or clitoris.

4. BIOLOGIC AND CULTURAL CHALLENGES. The new biologic challenge is control and moderation of the urge for enjoyment in stimulation of the penis or clitoris. The broader challenge of mastery of the maturing neuromuscular and intellectual systems continues.

   Cultural attitudes focus on phallic pleasure and on sexualized or eroticized play. The incest prohibition is mostly implicit, but may be explicit, e.g. parental interdictions against brother and sister continuing to bathe together or against body-contact play. This same sensual quality enters into the child-parent relationship. A parent feels uncomfortable about close physical contact with the child, and previous practices of hugging, kissing and holding the child upon the lap usually are curtailed or modified. Parents generally react with discomfort and disapproval to masturbatory activity. Even when the parent intellectually regards masturbation as a normal phenomenon of development, he still is likely to *feel* disapproving, and the child, consciously or unconsciously, perceives this disapproval. Fear of injury to the penis or clitoris, or a fantasy that these organs may already have been damaged (particularly in the female), is a universal concern at this age, and is referred to as *castration anxiety.*

5. AGGRESSION. As the previously comfortable, affectionate relation with the parent of the opposite sex is interfered with by genital sexual feelings, the child is confronted with the necessity of giving up the close physical attachment. This mobilizes feelings of resentment and aggression which normally are directed most strongly toward the parent of the same sex. Frequently the aggression is displaced to siblings, teachers or other objects where the fear of the loss of love is less important.

6. OBJECT RELATIONSHIP. Sexual feelings threaten to disrupt the child-parent relationship. As the child feels or imagines disapproval from the parent, his urges and fears conflict with each other. The boy feels that his father is a competitor for his mother's love, and his aggressive fantasies and impulses are directed toward his father. In consequence, he fears punishment or retaliation from his father, usually in the form of injury to the penis. But the boy also loves his father, and needs him and his approval. The conflict is resolved when the boy gives up his sexual urges toward his mother (later directing them toward females outside his own family) and contents himself with tender but asexual feelings toward her. At the same time he identifies more strongly with his father, thus affirming his identity as a male. He thus yields much of his former dependency, particularly upon his mother. The child normally is ready for school by about 5 or 6 years of age.

   The girl too finds her dependent relationship with mother threatened by sexual feelings. Additionally, she may resent having been somehow deprived by her mother of the seemingly more desirable male genital organ. Her initial reaction of envy of the penis is due in part to the fact that the girl at this age is comparing external genitalia only. Both she and the boy have little or no knowledge of the vagina and its significance in relation to internal sexual organs and the childbearing potentiality. The little girl shifts her sexual feelings from mother to father, and then is in a position comparable to that of the boy in relation to his mother. Ultimately she yields her sexualized feelings for her father, retaining feelings of tenderness for him, and identifies with her mother.

   These conflicts, which stem from the triangular relationship of the child and the parents, are known as the *oedipal conflict.*

7. EGO AND IDENTITY. The ego is strengthened by consolidation of the physical skills and intellectual capabilities which have been developing in the preceding stages. Control of sexual urges and repression of incestuous feelings and fantasies also add an increment of ego strength, provided this is achieved with real mastery rather than as a hasty solution amounting only to an avoidance of the conflict. In the latter instance an excessively defensive repression may form the basis for subsequent development of a neurosis.

   The ego quality of *initiative* derives from resolution of the oedipal conflict; guilt and inertia from its persistence. Identity as a male or female is strengthened by identification with the parent of the same sex. Through this identification the child takes on personality traits of the parent of the same sex; the child also identifies with and acquires some of the qualities and traits of the parent of the opposite sex.

   Because of the child's rapidly changing situation and its attendant anxieties, the development of the *sense of reality* again is characterized by a resort to magic for reassurance. This may take the form of *magical words, thoughts and fantasies,* e.g. the gamelike compulsion of touching every pale of a fence, or avoiding the cracks in the sidewalk in order to prevent unforeseen diaster.

8. SUPEREGO (CONSCIENCE AND IDEALS). With resolution of the oedipal conflict, the superego is crystallized into a definite structural component in the psyche. The impetus for this crystallization comes from the urgent necessity of controlling incestuous feelings and from attitudes and value judgments derived from the preceding stages of development.

9. TYPICAL NORMAL BEHAVIOR. Ambivalence toward both parents is common as the child shifts back and forth from one side of his conflicts to the other. Characteristically, there is an alternation of displays of aggressive and regressive behavior. Much of the time the boy appears confident and self-assured, and the girl appears coy and flirtatious. This bold front collapses, however, suddenly and frequently, and the child is easily "crushed." The boy, in particular, is physically active with much aggressive play and fantasy, the latter sometimes cruel and violent in its content.

DEVELOPMENTAL STAGES

TABLE 2-12. *(Continued)*

MIDCHILDHOOD YEARS

Latency stage

1. AGE. 5-7 to 8-10 years.

2. BIOLOGIC MATURATION. There is a continuing, gradual maturation of central nervous system pathways, permitting increasingly skillful and coordinated physical movements and providing greater intellectual capacity.

3. LIBIDO. Some libidinal energy continues to be invested in the phallic zone. Masturbatory activity and conflict and an interest in sexual matters persist to a greater or less degree throughout the latency stage. A large share of libidinal energy, however, is channelled into intellectual curiosity and the development of mental abilities and physical skills.

4. BIOLOGIC AND CULTURAL CHALLENGES. The child is challenged to develop his physical and intellectual skills, even more than in the phallic stage. Culture first of all asks the child to renounce his interest and pleasure in direct sexual activity. Secondly, he is introduced to the requirement of work. This is presented in the home by giving small responsibilities such as picking up his clothes or helping with the dishes, and in school by being expected to give proof of his learning.

5. AGGRESSION. Aggression is mobilized and (hopefully) constructively used to meet the frustrations and challenges of healthy competition in scholastic and physical activities.

6. OBJECT RELATIONSHIP. The pattern of identification with the parent of the same sex, and feelings of tenderness for the parent of the opposite sex, reached at the end of the phallic stage continue. Additionally, the child increasingly turns to other people, particularly to the teacher, as a model for identification.

   Children of latency age tend to form groups and clubs, this being their first experience in a kind of society of their own making. These groups characteristically are limited to members of the same sex.

7. EGO AND IDENTITY. The ego consolidates the technique of sublimation which is so important in learning and in the development of the capacity for thinking.

   The important *ego quality* of *industry* is acquired, rather than the undesirable trait of feelings of inadequacy. Physical and intellectual abilities are further refined.

   Although a certain amount of magical and wishful thinking persists, and likely will persist even in the adult, the child of latency age is capable of *reality adaptation*. His increasing powers of perception and evaluation of what he perceives allow him to test reality. As his dependency on his parents lessens, he begins to see them more realistically. They are no longer seen as "Godlike" figures, all-powerful and all-knowing. The child's disillusionment in his parents is compensated, however, by the satisfaction he gains from pointing out to them their inconsistencies and ineptitudes.

8. SUPEREGO (CONSCIENCE AND IDEALS). The superego becomes more firmly established and serves in aiding adaptation to the external world and in controlling and redirecting the instinctual drives. The superego may be modified if the child discerns that the cultural values of society differ greatly from the values taught him by his parents.

9. TYPICAL NORMAL BEHAVIOR. Continuing concern about controlling sexual and aggressive drives causes sleep disturbances in the latency stage. The nightmares of the phallic stage are likely to be replaced by insomnia, often in association with a conscious fear of death.

   The clubs, with boys, may take on qualities of a "gang" if the aggressive feelings and destructive fantasies get out of hand. This activity is part of the attempt to master and control the sexual and aggressive drives. The girl of latency age is likely to be a year or two ahead of the boy in social and emotional maturity, and perhaps in the capacity to use intellectual abilities.

TABLE 2-12. *(Concluded)*

ADOLESCENCE

Puberty and Adolescence

1. AGE. 10-12 to 16-18 years.

2. BIOLOGIC MATURATION. During the prepubertal and early adolescent years there is a sharp increase in general body growth; and increase in the size of the genital organs; change in body configuration with the development of the secondary sex characteristics; the appearance of menstruation in the female and ejaculation in the male; and the emergence of the capacity for the highest form of abstract thinking and reasoning.

3. LIBIDO. Libido is concentrated in the various changes occurring in the body, particularly in the sexual parts. At the same time there is an actual increase in total energy available, with a resultant strengthening of the sexual and aggressive drives. The greater mental capacity also is highly libidinized.

4. BIOLOGIC AND CULTURAL CHALLENGES. The tremendous physical and physiologic changes of puberty tend to disturb the child. The sexual and aggressive drives pose the threat of inadequate control over impulses. The changes in body size and configuration disturb the body-image concept and require that it be revised. The sexual changes confront the child with the fact that he will shortly be capable of adult sexual functioning. The biologic changes challenge him to accept himself in his new form and to become master of himself.

   The rapid changes and increase in energy and activity of the adolescent cause society to regard him with mixed feelings. Normally he is given greater responsibility, but he is also expected to control his sexual and aggressive impulses and to continue in the role of a child subject to adult authority.

5. AGGRESSION. Aggression is mobilized by the frustrations experienced by the adolescent as he seeks to fulfill his destiny of adulthood under the controls exercised by his parents and society. A certain amount of rebellion is inevitable, but hopefully the aggression is channelled into constructive attempts to gain independence, as well as into healthy competitive activity and productivity.

6. OBJECT RELATIONSHIP. The increased strength of sexual drives causes the adolescent to withdraw even further from parental relationships than was the case in the phallic stage of development. Temporarily and characteristically, the adolescent seeks relationship with other adolescents. He and his peer group stand apart from adult society, and to some extent are in conflict with it. The adolescent often finds satisfactory relationship with adults younger than his parents. His interest in these persons is often intense and may amount to hero worship. If the hero is a good leader and socially responsible, the adolescent is led in the right direction. On the other hand, identification with the wrong kind of hero can result in antisocial behavior, which may become serious because the adolescent is endowed with physical strength and sexual capacity which permit him to carry his thoughts and fantasies into action.

   Also characteristic of adolescence, particularly in the latter half, is the experience of falling in love (normally at least several times) as a preliminary to the eventual choice of a marital partner.

   As the adolescent masters the biologic and cultural challenges, he once again draws closer to his parents. Ultimately he normally takes his place in society as a cooperative and constructive young adult.

7. EGO AND IDENTITY. The increase in sexual and aggressive drives reawakens the conflicts of earlier stages and presents new conflicts. The id-ego-superego equilibrium which had attained a fair degree of stability in the latency stage is disturbed. There is a renewed struggle on the part of the ego to gain mastery over the disturbing forces. In this struggle the ego may run the gamut of its defensive techniques. At times the ego is in alliance with the superego, and its inner needs and impulses are denied and inhibited to the point of asceticism. At other times the superego is ignored, and urges are permitted immediate satisfaction. Temporary regressions to behavior associated with earlier stages of development are common.

   As the revived conflicts are reworked and again solved, and as the adolescent comes to terms with his new sexual and aggressive capacities, the equilibrium is reinstated. The final outcome of the adolescent stage is the attainment of a reasonably clear and stable *identity* which permits the pursuit of educational, occupational and marital goals.

   The *capacity for self-evaluation and introspection increases,* and ideally culminates in a capacity for *insight,* or understanding of oneself.

8. SUPEREGO (CONSCIENCE AND IDEALS). Withdrawal from dependency on the parents results in a weakening of the superego, since originally it is derived largely from the parents. In consequence, the adolescent, more or less consciously, is able to examine and decide for himself about many of the value judgments put forth by his parents. Much of the time it appears as though he had completely rejected everything the parents stand for. This is part of the assessment process, and normally the adolescent returns to the parental value system.

9. TYPICAL NORMAL BEHAVIOR. Particularly in the first half of adolescence, the adolescent is in turmoil with rapidly changing moods and behavior. The feelings of internal disorganization and inadequacy for the most part are denied and covered up by bravado, loudness and expansiveness. The problem of control of drives and feelings is evidenced in unpredictability and impulsiveness. The intense interest in the peer group is evidenced by clothing fads, teen-age heroes, and a taste for a kind of music which generally is abhorrent to the parents. There tends to be considerable falling in and out of love, and much experimenting with extrafamilial relationships, most of which serves the purpose of aiding the definition of the self. As equilibrium is regained, there is a turning toward more intellectual and philosophical interests. The grasp on the peer group is loosened, and the adolescent moves toward taking his place in adult society.

DEVELOPMENTAL STAGES

PSYCHOLOGIC DISORDERS

The factors which account for man's flexibility and great adaptive capacity also account for his susceptibility to emotional and mental illness. Psychic development takes place after birth and is determined by the interaction of the child with his environment. Thus there are possibilities for unfavorable as well as favorable experiences.

PSYCHOPATHOLOGY

Traumatic Experiences. Psychopathology may result from physical or emotional traumatic experiences. It may be evident immediately, or it may remain latent and become manifest under sufficiently stressful conditions. Optimal parental care and rearing cannot foresee and prevent such severely disturbing events as physical illness or injury, hospitalization, loss of or separation from loved ones or other emotional disturbances. Whether such experiences have a lasting psychopathologic effect depends essentially upon whether the child was able to gain mastery over them.

A particular traumatic experience can be viewed as having 3 phases: preparation for the untoward event, management of it, and subsequent mastery of the unfavorable psychologic effects.

Preparation. Obviously no preparation can be made for an accidental traumatic experience. The way in which previous experiences have been handled by the parents or the pediatrician, however, can be helpful to the child in unanticipated experiences. Adults should be honest with the child about unpleasant experiences and give considerable attention to his needs at those times so that he comes to have confidence in adults.

Whenever possible, the child should be forewarned of an unpleasant experience in keeping with his understanding and his ability to bear tension. These capacities constantly change as the child develops. Thus a 4-year-old child is not helped by long and detailed discussion of the anxiety-creating aspects of a forthcoming tonsillectomy; nor is it wise to tell him about it more than a day or so in advance; otherwise his apprehension causes too much tension which must be borne too long. On the other hand, an 11-year-old child is capable of understanding a good deal about such things, and a carefully considered explanation, avoiding discussion of the more dire possibilities, can be extremely helpful in preventing psychologic trauma. He can be told about the event considerably in advance, and he will likely use the intervening time to think and ask questions and to prepare himself.

Parents and physicians may overidentify with the child in his fear of pain and become distressed by his crying and protests in anticipation of the frightening event. For this reason they often rationalize that the child is better off not knowing what is coming. Although this plan may spare both the child and the adults some distress in advance of the event, its consequences are highly undesirable. The child feels betrayed by those whom he must trust and depend upon. In addition, he is deprived of the opportunity to prepare himself for what is to come. The crying and protests of the child at such a time are needed and healthy expressions of feeling and relief of tension.

Management of the threatening event. It is important to try to keep the tension within the child's limits of tolerance. Physically painful and psychologically frightening factors should be kept to a minimum, and the child's relation with his parents should be maintained as the principal source of emotional support and security so far as is possible. If relation with the parents cannot be sustained in a degree adequate to meet the child's needs, a parent-substitute should be provided. The parents should ensure that the child understands that this person is acting on their behalf. Proper preparation for and explanation of procedures and happenings are important also in this phase.

"Working through" or mastery. Children universally and spontaneously re-enact threatening experiences in their play and fantasy. Thus a 3-year-old girl who was given an enema will subsequently administer enemas to her dolls in her play. Similarly, after a visit to the pediatrician for a routine physical examination, the young child most likely will play doctor. This is a normal, innate response which helps the child come to terms with the experience and the feelings associated with it. Perhaps the most helpful factor in this attempt at mastery is the change in role from passive recipient to active doer.

This natural tendency in the child, even when minimally evident, can be called forth and utilized if one is aware that it exists. On a similar basis the child psychiatrist can use the spontaneous play of the child as a means of understanding and helping him. Unfortunately, however, both the laity and the medical profession commonly think that the best remedy for the distress of the child who has undergone a threatening experience is to help him forget it. If this remedy is applied, the child is deprived of the opportunity of playing out and mastering the experience, and, if fantasies and tensions persist, repression may take place. Because the repressed experience continues to be invested with psychic energy (libido), it persists as an active but unconscious force in the psychologic equilibrium, and may provide a basis for subsequent psychologic disorder.

Experiences may be traumatic and leave a psychopathologic imprint for 3 general reasons: (1) the experience may be overwhelming, e.g. loss of the mother to a 6-month-old infant, without replacement with a mother-substitute (René Spitz); (2) there may be environmental inadequacy in helping the child through the 3 phases described above; or (3) because of deficiencies in himself the child may be unable to cope with the experience.

THE CHILD'S ABILITY TO COPE. In order to understand the child's ability to cope with inside and outside forces, it may be helpful to view the progress of his psychic development from the standpoint of homeostasis. This term was originally used by Cannon to designate the tendency of the physiologic bodily processes to maintain a state of equilibrium. Neither physical nor psychologic homeostasis implies a completely stable state, but rather an equilibrium of constantly varying and changing forces. In a state of absolute stability there would be no growth or development, either physical or psychologic.

A parallel can be drawn between physiologic homeostasis and the structural components of personality. Thus the basic biochemical and biophysiologic processes can be conceived of as the prototype of the id; the innate mechanisms which regulate these physiologic processes are the prototype of the ego; and the limits within which, for example, the pH of body fluids and the body temperatures may vary constitute physiologic laws which bear similarity to the attitudes and value judgments which come to compose the child's superego, or conscience.

In the normal autistic stage of psychologic development the neonate is functioning essentially on a physiologic level. In the symbiotic stage the situation changes with beginning maturation and the emotional alliance of mother and infant. The biochemical processes are gradually organized and expressed through the sexual and aggressive drives, which are seen only indirectly through their manifestations in tension and behavior. The id begins to have some meaning on a psychologic level. The physiologic regulatory mechanisms persist, and are added to on a psychologic level by the combination of the "rudimentary" ego of the infant and the ego of the mother (maternal auxiliary ego). The superego, at this stage, is represented by the maternal-familial or cultural value system. Because of the lack of ego capacity in the infant, his mother does most of his coping. He tends to fare well in proportion to her ability to understand and meet his needs for gratification, stimulation and frustration. If the mother misinterprets his needs, or if other circumstances such as illness and hospitalization of the infant or prolonged separation from his mother prevent her from helping him, psychopathology is likely to result.

As the infant begins to separate from his mother and concurrently progresses through the successive stages of psychosexual development, the id drives become more clearly focused in their aims, and their manifestations are increasingly evident. The functions provided by the maternal auxiliary ego are gradually taken over by the child's own

ego. Similarly, the external value system gradually becomes internalized to form the child's superego.

As the child develops, he acquires an increasing array of skills and ego defensive and adaptive techniques, and his psychologic and mental functioning becomes increasingly complex. Thus his first attempts at mastery of a bad experience through play must be fairly primitive, amounting only to a re-enactment on the basis of memory, with little or no elaboration in imagination or fantasy. By the age of 2 or 3 years the child is capable of fantasy which makes his play more varied, although still rather literal and lacking in the quality of make-believe. Once he has gained the rudiments of language and is able to distinguish between what is real and what is pretended, his play begins to serve the purpose of trial-acting (a forerunner of thinking). Ultimately the mastery and working through of bad experiences through play activity tend to be replaced by verbalization, or "talking it out."

Although fantasy and imagination play an important role in the mastery of bad experiences, they can also contribute to the development of psychopathology. Thus, through imagination and fantasy, a child may distort reality and develop fears and conflicts, which in turn may contribute to the development of a psychologic disorder. For example, a child who has been repeatedly warned not to play in the street and is subsequently struck by a car while playing there may interpret the injury as a severe punishment for his disobedience. Such a fantasy could result in excessive reinforcement of his developing conscience, and an ensuing attempt on the part of the ego to inhibit his aggression in order to avoid an even worse fate. In consequence the child may become unduly passive and conforming.

If the child's attempt to master a threatening experience through re-enactment does not succeed, the tendency toward re-enactment persists, but takes the form of disturbed behavior. The term "repetition-compulsion" has been used to characterize this pathologic re-enactment. Thus a child who continues to feel or fantasy himself to be rejected by his parents may be repetitiously provocative to them, as well as to other adults such as teachers. Although the underlying aim is that he should not be rejected, but be loved in spite of his provocativeness, the adult response naturally is likely to be to the provocativeness rather than to the underlying aim. Accordingly he undergoes further rejection and additional reinforcement of his feeling of being unloved.

If one understands the roles of reality distorting fantasy, of anxiety, of repression and of unconscious mental life in the causation of psychopathology, then the importance for the developing child of adequate explanations, of permitting re-enactment in play, of inviting questions and of appropriate discussion becomes clear.

Another concept pertaining to the child's ability to cope with traumatic experiences is that of "phase-specificity," (Hartmann). This concept holds that an experience will be particularly traumatic if it happens to impinge on those developing functions which characteristically are most heavily libidinized in the particular stage during which the child suffers the experience (see under Libido in Table 2-12). For example, a fracture of the jaw in an 11-month-old infant at the time he is being weaned which forces him abruptly to give up his oral gratification could be severely traumatic. On the other hand, the same injury in a child 3 years of age is not likely to have the same effect because he is beyond the oral stage of development. Similarly, an operation performed on a child 5 or 6 years of age, who at that age is normally greatly concerned about injury to his body or his genitals, is likely to have threatening implications which it might not have at the age of 9 or 10 years. It is because of the concept of phase-specificity of trauma that the psychologically oriented physician may advise postponement of certain surgical or medical procedures (provided postponement is not detrimental to health) until the child has entered another stage of development.

In summary, the ability of the child to cope with experience is influenced (1) by the constitutional adequacy of the ego apparatus and functions, (2) by the adequacy of the care provided by the mother or mother-substitute, (3) by the timing of traumatic experience in relation to degree of psychologic development and the adequacy of the ego defensive and adaptive techniques available, and (4) by the timing of the trauma in relation to the particular stage of development in accordance with the concept of phase-specificity.

Kinds of Psychopathology. It is important to understand that a child may have a psychologic disorder without psychopathology having been firmly established within him. Conflict usually begins and exists for a time outside the child before it becomes internalized. Conflict between the child and his environment can cause psychologic disorders which symptomatically appear to be the same as disorders resulting from internal psychopathology. Such disorders, however, respond to early correction of the situation causing the conflict, and direct treatment of the child is usually not necessary.

Psychologic disorders which are manifestations of internal psychopathology are serious and difficult to treat. Conflicts exist within the personality structure, as it has developed out of the interaction of the child and his environment. Through the mental mechanisms of introjection and identification, the attitudes and traits of the parents and other significant persons in the child's life normally become internalized to form parts of the ego and superego. So long as the state of tension or the psychologic equilibrium of the child is kept within reasonable limits and he gains mastery over the disturbing experiences which inevitably occur in the course of development, the internalization tends to take place gradually and results in a reasonably harmonious internal personality structure.

If, however, the infant or young child experiences too much tension, he internalizes the images derived from his experiences too quickly and unselectively. Although this internalization is aimed at regaining psychologic equilibrium, it tends to set up conflicts between the id drives and needs, the ego, and the superego in various combinations. For example, a child who feels that his mother is unduly harsh during toilet training may internalize her punitive attitudes to avoid further conflict with her. These attitudes now become a part of his superego, which as a result is set at odds with his normal aggressive drive and his normal id needs for pleasure and gratification; these features are damaging to his developing self-image and self-esteem, which are in the realm of the ego. Thus what was formerly a conflict with the external world (his mother) has now become an internal or intrapsychic conflict.

On the basis of the time of occurrence of traumatic experiences in relation to the child's position in the stages of psychologic development, it is possible to distinguish 2 major kinds of internal psychopathology. These are designated: *psychoses,* which appear to have their origin from constitutional deficiencies, or from traumatic experiences occurring in the first 2 years or so of life; and *neuroses,* which have their origin from traumatic experiences occurring, for the most part, in the age range from 2 to 6 or 7 years.

The basic images — those of the mother and the self — begin to be established gradually during the symbiotic phase of development. The acute anxiety occurring normally by about 8 or 9 months of age is presumed to be due to the acquisition of sufficiently clear images of mother and self for the infant to realize that his mother is not part of him. It seems probable that it takes a further period, extending well into the period between 12 and 24 months of age, until these first images (both perceptual and emotional) have become sufficiently stable so that the child can call forth a memory of his mother as a kind of reassurance when she is absent from him. Thus he has attained an important step in his psychologic independence. Before these images of mother are available from memory, traumatic experiences tend to be felt as a threat or *fear of loss of the love object,* i.e. the mother. If the traumatic experiences during this period are severe, or if there is unduly prolonged or too frequent separation from the mother, the effect on the child is proportionately severe.

Severe traumatic experiences occurring in this early period of development cause a psychosis at the time of the trauma, or can predispose the infant to the development of a psychotic disorder at a later age.

After the establishment of reasonably stable and constant images of the mother, traumatic experience causes *fear of loss of her love.* This is a lesser threat than the threat of losing the love object itself. Ego development and the establishment of basic identity have had a good beginning; the developing personality is well integrated; the child has confidence in people and seeks to continue receiving love from them; and his good relations with the outside world facilitate his adaptation. Now, when he and his environment are in conflict, his wish to continue receiving love causes him to attempt to control and modify the impulses and feelings which are bringing him into conflict with his parents. But since the traumatic experience has caused an excessive amount of conflict and tension, he cannot manage himself by normal defensive and adaptive techniques, and he exhibits symptoms.

Traumatic experiences occurring after the establishment of stable images and reasonably adequate relations with people either cause neurosis at the time of the trauma, or predispose to the development of a neurotic disorder at a later age.

GENERAL CONSIDERATIONS IN DIAGNOSIS AND TREATMENT

DIAGNOSIS

Diagnostic evaluation requires careful study both of the child and of the persons in his environment. The study of the environment and evaluation of its role in the child's disorder are concerned largely with his relation to his mother in the neonatal and infancy periods; it includes the father and other members of the family during the preschool years and persons outside the family during the middle years and adolescence. Most of the discussion of normal child development and of the causation of psychologic disorders centers about the child's relation with his mother, for the reason that his life begins in closeness with her, and she is most directly concerned with his care and rearing during the early years. On the other hand, this situation does not minimize the importance of the father. Even if he has little to do with the care of his infant or young child in a direct way, his influence is felt indirectly in terms of emotional support of the mother. In the present culture the father shares increasingly in the care of the infant and figures importantly in the life of the young child.

An important concept pertaining to the study of the environment is that of *family dynamics.* The family is conceived to be a unit with a dynamic equilibrium determined by the interaction of all the members of the family. Thus a particular child may acquire a certain role which is important to the equilibrium of the family group, e.g. the good child or the bad child, or the smart child or the dull child. This concept is different from the notion that members of a family function only as individuals. A technique in use in child psychiatry studies family dynamics by bringing all the members of the family together in a discussion with the psychiatrist. The ways in which they relate to each other and the roles they play in the family equilibrium can be observed for diagnostic purposes, and in some instances the observations

can be discussed with the family with therapeutic benefit.

In general terms, the kinds of environmental influence to be considered are (1) understimulation, (2) overstimulation, (3) emotional deprivation, (4) overindulgence, (5) overprotection, (6) too little challenge, (7) undue pressure, (8) inconsistency, in the same parent or between the parents, (9) excessive conflict and tension in the home atmosphere, (10) unconscious approval by the parents of behavior which they consciously disapprove of (the child acts in accordance with the unconscious or true attitude of the parents).

In the study of the child the history of his earlier development is obtained from his parents. The neonatal and infancy periods are carefully reviewed in an attempt to evaluate the role of environmental factors as opposed to factors in the make-up of the child. Environmental influence begins so early that the responses it causes in the child may be misattributed to his innate endowment. Conversely, subtle innate factors may be the cause of environmental responses or attitudes which are falsely viewed as primary and etiologic. The latter possibility needs to be considered in the case of incompatibility between the child's temperament or behavior style and the mother's ministrations or expectations.

The most crucial qualities in the make-up of the child are the following, as suggested by Anna Freud. These important qualities are determined both by constitution and by environmental influence and experience.

Intensity of Drives and Needs. The needs of the undemanding child may go unrecognized and therefore unmet. The overdemanding child, on the other hand, because he is difficult to satisfy and to manage, may cause anxiety or other feelings in the parent, which secondarily will disturb the parent-child relation.

Ability to Tolerate Frustration. The child who can tolerate frustration has less need to resort to the use of pathologic defenses.

Willingness to Accept Substitutes. The child who cannot accept a substitute, whether this is a substitute parent such as a baby-sitter, or substituted food, toys or activities, remains tied to the frustration, and tensions increase.

Ability to Tolerate Anxiety. The ability to tolerate tension and anxiety and to control urges and feelings without repressing them and making them unconscious enables the child to face difficulties, to learn to interpose thought between the urge to act and action, to give and take and to negotiate with his parents and other people.

Evaluation of the child by means of the history is followed by appraisal of his current functioning and behavior. This is done through information supplied by the parents, the school or other sources and through direct observation and study of the child. The young child can be observed during the course of physical examination or other procedures or in a play situation. Such information

about the older child and adolescent can sometimes be gained through conversation with him.
Whether one observes the child at play or engages
him in conversation, the information is gained
through study of his ego defensive and adaptive
behavior. Understanding of other facets of his
personality such as his drives or id and his conscience or superego is deduced from their apparent
effect upon the ego. The inner conflicts and outer
reality problems which motivate his defenses and
behavior are reflected in the defenses and can be
inferred from them.

A complete evaluation of a child and his disorder, sufficient for adequate diagnosis and prognosis, requires consideration of all aspects of each
of the stages of psychologic development (Table
2-12, pp. 65 to 71).

TREATMENT

Treatment must be based upon an adequate
diagnosis of the underlying psychopathology.
Confronted with a patient whose primary symptom is headache, no physician would regard the
headache as an entity. He would feel that he must
diagnose the underlying cause of the headache,
and treat this cause to gain indirect relief of the
headache. Possible treatments would differ considerably, depending upon whether the headache
was caused by tension, fatigue, the toxic effects
of systemic infection or brain tumor.

The same principle holds in the treatment of
psychologic disorders. *It is fallacious to regard
symptoms such as thumb-sucking, temper tantrums, enuresis, masturbation and social ineptitude
as clinical entities, and to expect them to be treatable in and of themselves in some specific way.*
Suggestions can be made for the management of
symptomatic behavior (in the same way that one
can prescribe aspirin for a headache of undetermined origin), but *the real diagnostic and treatment effort must be directed at determining and
remedying the underlying cause.*

If a disorder has its basis in internal psychopathology, its remedy almost always requires
psychotherapy with the child. The aim is to help
him uncover, understand and work through his
inner conflicts and the experiences which produced
them. In order to do this effectively, the physician
as a rule needs to undergo special training in the
theory and technique of psychotherapy. He also
must be able to offer an amount of time and a
regularity of appointment schedule which is difficult for the pediatrician or general physician to
provide. Unless a pediatrician has had special
training in psychotherapy with children, he may
find it difficult to treat a child with a neurosis or
any of the more severe disorders. On the other
hand, the child's physician can and should provide
support to the child and parents while arrangements are being made for further evaluation or

psychotherapy, as well as during psychotherapy.
This support may be primarily verbal, or it may
include the judicious use of sedative or tranquilizer
drugs. The pediatrician's responsibility for the
general well-being of the child continues during
psychiatric treatment; optimum for the child and
parents is a truly cooperative liaison between
pediatrician and child psychiatrist.

The pediatrician is in an ideal position to help
children with psychologic disorders by recognizing potential illness early and by directing therapeutic efforts to the incipient or less severe *developmental* and *situational* disorders (see below).
With relatively little special training and relatively small demands upon his time he may be
quite effective, since the treatment is directed at
resolving conflict between the child and his environment. The child is involved in the conflict,
and his contribution to it needs to be understood,
but the task for the most part consists in working
with the parents. They need to be aided initially
to see what their attitudes, wishes, fears, resent-
ments or guilt feelings are in relation to their
child and how these attitudes are affecting him.
Then they need emotional support and guidance
in changing their attitudes and practices and in
helping each other and their child to resolve the
undesirable conflicts.

NOSOLOGY

Most attempts at classification of psychologic
disorders in children have been based upon description of clinical manifestations and similarity
of mode of expression of symptoms. In accordance
with such a system a clinical pattern may be falsely
regarded as a clinical entity. Thus persistent
thumb-sucking, nail-biting and masturbation
are recognized as habits and are classed as habit
disorders. Stealing, lying and destructiveness of
property are antisocial acts and are categorized
as conduct disorders. Asthma, neurodermatitis
and ulcerative colitis are modes of expression of
dysfunction of the autonomic nervous system and
are grouped together as psychophysiologic disorders.

Although a nosologic system can be constructed
on this basis, it is unsatisfactory. Clinical manifestations and modes of expression of symptoms
are superficial variables which do not permit
valid estimation of prognosis or requirements for
treatment.

The ideal nosologic system would be based primarily upon the underlying psychopathology as
determined by psychogenesis (etiology) and psy-
chodynamics, as well as upon the capacity for
adaptation. The categories presented here are
based upon these more fundamental considerations and are felt to be both simple and understandable. They do not correspond exactly to
other nomenclatures.

CATEGORIES OF PSYCHOLOGIC DISORDERS

Categories of psychologic disorders are listed in order of increasing severity, which depends on psychopathology, prognosis and potential for reversibility with treatment:

1. Developmental disorders
2. Situational disorders
3. Neurotic disorders
4. Neurotic character disorders
5. Psychotic character disorders
6. Psychotic disorders
7. Psychologic disorders associated with organic brain damage

The basic characteristics of the disorders in each category will be considered under the headings of *psychopathology* and *adaptability*. *Psychopathology* will deal with the internal condition of the child. This will be viewed primarily in terms of the child's psychologic equilibrium. *Adaptability* will deal with the child's functioning in relation to his environment. The main subjects commented upon are his relations with people (object relations), his ability to perceive and evaluate the world of external reality, and his performance.

DEVELOPMENTAL DISORDERS

Developmental disorders are due to the inevitable and characteristic conflicts associated with the successive stages of psychologic development. They are usually transitory and within certain limits are to be regarded as phenomena of normal development. They will be discussed in general terms and in relation to the stages of psychologic development (see Table 2-12, pp. 65-71).

Psychopathology. In normal development the conflicts between the child and his environment lead to the establishment of normal adaptive and defensive techniques. This results in a certain amount of conflict within the child between his drives and his methods of self-control. Under usual circumstances the conflict is readily managed by the child and should not be regarded as psychopathologic. If circumstances cause the conflicts to be unduly intense or to persist unduly long, they tend to take on psychopathologic significance. Hence the importance of proper management of developmental disorders should be apparent.

Adaptability. Disturbance in functioning or relationship is minimal, temporary and usually limited to a particular aspect of the total personality.

Treatment. If the conflict and the resulting symptoms become too severe and it is felt that help is needed, the therapeutic effort is directed mainly to the environment. If the parents can be helped to understand the conflict situation, and then to modify those demands and attitudes which exceed the child's capacity, the disorder in the child is indirectly alleviated.

NEONATAL PERIOD (ORAL STAGE: NORMAL AUTISTIC PHASE)

Clinical Manifestations. The first signs of distress are likely to be excessive crying, disturbance in function of the alimentary tract, such as refusal to suck, excessive sucking, excessive regurgitation or vomiting, constipation or diarrhea, and disturbance in the sleep pattern. The intensity and duration of symptoms vary with the severity of the environmental situation.

Differential Diagnosis. The same symptoms may also be caused by temporary disturbances related to the trauma of birth and to postnatal infectious or organic factors.

Treatment. When constitutional or organic factors in the infant have been ruled out, attention must be focused on the environment. Developmental disorders occurring in this period suggest deficiency on the part of the mother or mother-surrogate in meeting the infant's physiologic or emotional needs. The infant needs protection from changes in body temperature and from excessive stimulation by light, sound and handling. On the other hand, as he matures, he has a gradually increasing need for an optimal amount of gentle stimulation of his various sensory end-organs, e.g. through body contact, through bathing and anointing the skin, through being held and rocked, through the sound of mother's voice, and through various objects which he can see, particularly the mother's face. Anxiety or other emotional difficulty in the mother is the most common reason for inability to meet the child's needs in a reasonably adequate manner.

INFANCY PERIOD (ORAL STAGE: SYMBIOTIC PHASE)

Clinical Manifestations. During the latter part of infancy the same kinds of symptoms may be manifest as were described in the neonatal phase. The patterns may become more definite, however, as psychologic development permits more specific expression. Thus crying may occur in relation to a particular experience, or sleep disturbance may be linked to a particular time of day. The observant mother may have noted a cause and effect relation between events and the infant's symptom pattern.

When the infant is capable of distinguishing himself from his mother, he becomes aware of his dependence upon her. A need for love has been added to his physical and physiologic needs. Toward the end of this phase the infant is prone to greater conflict, tension and anxiety because of his awareness that his mother is separate from him, and because of the frustration of weaning.

Severe crying at separation and various disturbances in feeding and bowel function are common.

Differential Diagnosis. It is necessary to distinguish the causes of these clinical manifestations from those in situational disorders, and also to rule out organic causes.

Treatment. Treatment usually consists in working with the parents to help them perceive and change those attitudes or reactions which the child feels are threatening his relations with them. If, for example, a child has the symptom of excessive thumb-sucking as a response to being weaned too quickly, the remedy is to persuade the mother that the weaning should be more gradual.

TODDLER YEARS (ANAL STAGE)

Clinical Manifestations. With the advent of locomotion the child's sphere of contact with his environment is greatly increased. At the same time his parents note his developing coordination and control and his increasing ability to understand, and begin to expect more of him. He is subjected to his first disciplinary experiences. This usually causes a good deal of conflict between the child and his parents.

The child has difficulty in managing his increased aggression. Tantrums are frequent, sometimes severe. Obversely, some children may curb their aggression to the point at which they become unduly passive.

Because speech is developing during this stage, conflicts not uncommonly are reflected in a transient stutter. Sleep disturbances in the form of resistance to going to bed and going to sleep or of night terrors also are common. As the child is falling asleep, ego control over aggressive impulses diminishes, and he is frightened by the feeling that his aggressive fantasies and impulses may be expressed in action. Fear and anxiety on separation from the parents at bedtime or when left with a baby-sitter also are common.

Coercive or even normal toilet training tends to produce problems at this stage. Frustration or anxiety may give rise to symptoms such as messing with food, temporary food dislikes, smearing feces, constipation or diarrhea. Directing aggression toward playmates, siblings, pets or inanimate objects is also common. Thumb-sucking and eating disturbances may be seen in this stage as a consequence of regression to the previous stage with the aim of easing tension through oral gratification.

Differential Diagnosis. The same kinds of problems may also be seen in situational disorders, but usually with greater intensity and persistence. As the child approaches the end of this stage, he normally is beginning to develop some of the precursors of superego. This allows for the possibility of internal conflicts between his impulses and his developing superego. Neurotic disorders therefore may be seen in children at 2 to 3 years of age, but are relatively rare. This diagnosis is suggested by unusually severe or persistent symptoms of the type mentioned above, particularly in a child with precocious psychologic development as evidenced, for example, by unusually good language development.

Treatment. Treatment is aimed at helping the parents to be kindly and sympathetic, but also to be sufficiently firm and controlling so that the child feels protected from external dangers and from his own impulses. The experience of being controlled by his parents, even though he protests it, is reassuring and provides the model for development of self-control. The child may have considerable difficulty if he is given too much freedom in making decisions. The parents must be able to use their aggression in a healthy way in the management of the child. On the other hand, if the parents are too strict and too demanding, this tends to increase the strength of the child's impulses and poses a problem in control and tends to make him feel unloved. The parents are encouraged to ease up and give the child more time to meet their requirements.

PRESCHOOL YEARS (PHALLIC STAGE)

Clinical Manifestations. The problem of control of aggressive impulses continues. There is a heightened awareness of pleasurable sensations in the genital area, and sexual feelings are now added to and complicate the love feelings toward the parents. Fear of loss of love and of punishment persists and tends to be expressed in fantasies of injury to the penis or clitoris. Because of the diminution of ego control during sleep, the intensified sexual aggressive urges and fantasies cause sleep disturbances. At times a nightmare may continue into a semiwakeful state, and the child may be delirious. Phobias also are common, particularly of destructive animals or "bad" men, such as robbers who will break into the house at night. These are the result of an unconscious mental mechanism whereby the child tries to escape his frightening impulses and fantasies by projecting them outside of himself and attributing them to external objects; but this is only a partial solution, for he now fears them as external dangers.

As a result of regression there may be lapses in bladder and bowel control, and various oral symptoms. Some children become excessively clinging and dependent. Symptoms of passivity and conformity in the boy may be the unconscious defensive means of avoiding transgression, which would bring punishment or the imagined threat of castration. The girl may reject her femaleness and behave like a tomboy.

Differential Diagnosis. In addition to distinguishing between developmental and situational disorders, a neurotic disorder must be considered, since its likelihood increases with increase in age and psychic development. There is also the possibility that some of the defenses the child is using are becoming habitual and that he is developing a neurotic character disorder.

Treatment. One of the best guarantees that

the child will successfully resolve the conflicts of this stage is a good sexual and social relationship between the parents. Conversely, if the parents are at odds with each other, the child's fantasies of maintaining intimate relations with the parent of the opposite sex are encouraged.

The child, in controlling his impulses, continues to need firmness, but without excessive threat at this age. It is helpful if the parents begin to introduce the concept of modesty and to exercise more restraint in dressing and undressing and in the use of the bathroom.

For the child with temporary sleep difficulties a small night light, or the parent staying with the child until he goes to sleep, may be helpful. These aids, however, should be regarded as temporary measures; the child's continued requirement of them may indicate a more serious disorder.

The child who awakens frightened from a bad dream should be comforted and returned to his own bed. He often wishes to sleep with one or both of his parents, but this is not to be encouraged. Not only would he literally come between his parents, but also the physical proximity to the parent stimulates his sexual feelings and fantasies. These factors can aggravate his oedipal conflict and delay its resolution.

Owing to the child's preoccupation with sexual difference and its implications, it is reassuring to children to know that in contrast to the externally evident sexual organs of the male, the sexual organs of the female are concealed and internal, and that the female is not simply a damaged or defective male. A specific case requiring help is the boy with an undescended testis. If his condition and the fact that it can be remedied are explained to him, he will be spared much worry as well as potential psychopathology resulting from his own distorted, imaginary explanations.

MIDCHILDHOOD YEARS (LATENCY STAGE)

Clinical Manifestations. The most common cause of problems in these years is failure of resolution of the oedipal conflict. As a result the dependency-independency conflict is unduly troublesome, and the anxieties of the phallic stage persist; symptoms disappear and change as the child tries out different defensive solutions. At one extreme a child may become withdrawn and excessively shy and passive. At the other extreme a child who is unable to ease his tensions and maintain control over his impulses may "act-out" his feelings and conflicts. The latter solution results in a behavior problem, with such symptoms as destructiveness, bullying or stealing.

As in the phallic stage, the child may seek solution by temporarily reversing his identification, so that the boy identifies with the mother, the girl with the father. Phobias, sleep disturbances and problems of bladder control may persist.

The disturbed child often has difficulty in learning in school. His mental energies may be tied up

in his internal conflicts to such a point that he has little energy left for concentration; he may have curbed his aggression so thoroughly that he is unable to use it in a healthy way in asking questions and seeking knowledge; or the fears and fantasies associated with his sexual curiosity may have caused him to inhibit his curiosity.

Differential Diagnosis. As in the earlier age periods, developmental disorders must be distinguished from situational ones. Additionally, the possibility of similar symptoms as a reflection of a more serious neurotic disorder or a neurotic character disorder must be kept in mind.

Treatment. The aims of treatment are essentially the same as in the phallic stage. The child is helped indirectly if the parents can be guided to modify their attitudes and improve their relations to each other. In addition, as the child grows older, healthy identifications may stem from contacts with other adults such as teachers, scout leaders, and from supervised group activities with children.

ADOLESCENT YEARS

Clinical Manifestations. Owing to the tremendous physiologic and psychologic upheaval during these years, problems occur frequently and in great variety. As was true of the child in the phallic stage, the adolescent struggles with strong sexual and aggressive impulses, but now with the important difference of the advent of physical and sexual maturity. Loss of self-control with acting-out of conflicts can result either in antisocial behavior or in behavior detrimental to himself. At the other extreme, control gained by severe inhibition may result in pathologic withdrawal from relations with people. Urges and desires may be so much denied that the adolescent becomes an ascetic. Overintellectualization is resorted to in an attempt to manage feelings and impulses by thought. Overcompensation for feelings of inferiority and inadequacy results in false bravado and acts of daring. Some adolescents remain too dependent and too attached to their parents; others break away too completely.

Commonly the adolescent is upset over sexual and aggressive feelings and fantasies which he feels to be abnormal, since he may not have discussed them with anyone and does not know that they are universal. The great turmoil and feeling of disorganization and the poor self-control are responsible for the common fear of becoming insane.

Precocious puberty is likely to cause at least a developmental disorder, since biologic maturation is ahead of the child's emotional readiness for this event. Some children react to an early onset of puberty by attempting to grow up quickly. These children have a façade of sophistication and a pseudomaturity. Since they have been deprived of some of their childhood years, there may be a more serious disorder later. Other children react to early puberty by regression to an earlier stage of development. If they are subsequently able to face and deal with the changes caused by puberty, their adolescence may be fairly normal.

Psychologic problems also result from a delayed onset of puberty. The child begins to worry about his physical normality and feels undesirably different from his peers. If he is helped to verbalize his fears and is reassured, the development of feelings of inferiority and inadequacy, as well as of social estrangement, may be prevented.

Differential Diagnosis. The average adolescent can temporarily assume rather extreme positions of defense, such as withdrawal, asceticism, overindulgence in oral or other pleasures, or antisocial acting-out. The total personality and functioning of the adolescent therefore must be carefully evaluated before concluding that the behavior pattern is normal and need cause no concern, or that the adolescent is mentally ill. Because similar clinical patterns may be based upon different underlying psychopathologic disturbances, one must consider the possibility of any category of psychologic disorder, including psychotic ones.

Treatment. The adolescent is likely to engender anxiety in his parents, causing them to lose the objectivity and the stability which he so much needs. If this happens, confusion is compounded, tensions rise, and problems increase. It is important that the parents understand the nature of normal adolescence and do not overreact to the typical adolescent behavior with its wide mood swings and changeability.

TABLE 2-13. FACTORS OF ETIOLOGIC SIGNIFICANCE IN SITUATIONAL DISORDERS

Rough handling, excessive handling or differences in handling of the neonate by the mother and father, or by the mother and a nursemaid

Too little handling and stimulation of an infant by a mother who for neurotic reasons fears that her ministrations may be harmful

Incompatibility between the temperament or personality of the infant or young child and that of the parent

Excessive or irritating stimulation from inanimate sources, e.g. from rough fabrics next to the infant's skin

A feeding schedule out of phase with the infant's desires

Self-demand feeding when the mother is unable to distinguish between the various causes of tension and crying and gives the bottle not only for relief of hunger, but also as a panacea for distress of all kinds

Insufficient kinesthetic stimulation as evidenced by the infant who rocks in bed (the rocking chair may be helpful)

Postpartum depression in the mother

Maternal anxiety about breast feeding communicated to the child (breast feeding may be unwise in such a case)

Inconsistent and uncertain care of an infant by a mother who feels unsure of herself and unconsciously avoids responsibility by attempting to follow the advice of other people (the infant may be helped if the pediatrician authoritatively insists that the mother follow only his advice)

Detrimental attitudes by a mother who feels guilty because her child was conceived before marriage, or by a mother who strongly wished that the child be of the other sex. Illness or death of close relatives during the pregnancy or postnatally may upset the mother and make her unable to adequately invest herself emotionally in the relationship with the child. Sometimes she unconsciously may feel that the child's birth was in some way responsible for the death of the loved one

Maternal worry about her own health, the health or the welfare of another child, or about her relationship with her husband

Leaving the infant alone too much of the time

Overeagerness of the parent to get the child to bed and to sleep. The child senses that the parent is pulling away, and resists separation

Attempts to create a favorable situation for sleep by making the child's room quiet and dark. This may be distressing to the infant who finds familiar sounds and objects reassuring, even if they are only in the background

Failure of parents to say goodbye when they are leaving temporarily, because they feel that they are sparing the child distress if they slip away while he is awake or leave after he is asleep

Difficulty of some mothers in letting the child separate and become more independent. Such mothers may either prolong the child's infancy by overprotecting him and meeting his needs too well or deal with their anxiety by pulling away too completely too soon

Too little maternal attention after the next child is born. The child should not be neglected in favor of the new baby, nor should he be overindulged in an attempt to prevent a normal amount of envy

Competition of one parent with the child for the attention of the other parent; this is usually not recognized by the parents

Too early toilet training

A mother who is rejecting of her role as a female, or a father who is passive and not sufficiently masculine; the child has difficulty in development of identity

Teasing, threatening and lecturing to the child

An immature parent who may be unconsciously sexually seductive to the child, overstimulating him and encouraging unhealthy fantasies with ensuing fears

Parental separation or divorce, particularly during the preschool and middle years; the child uses his fantasy ability to give himself explanations which create anxiety or a sense of guilt

High parental expectations for the child with relatively little support in helping him to measure up to the expectations. The parental expectations may be implicit rather than openly expressed. This is a common cause of learning difficulty

Significant differences in the child's family and cultural background from those of most of the other children in his school

Alcoholism in a parent

Too little contact with the father, who is important for the development of both boy and girl. Also, the mother may not feel sufficiently supported in the task of rearing the children, and they sense her resentment

The mother who is a slave to her children and home; entanglements with the children usually develop

Too many outside interests and activities by the mother

In making the transition from childhood to adulthood the adolescent needs opportunities for independent action and decision, and for assuming an increasing amount of responsibility for himself. On the other hand, he is in such inner turmoil and so much at the mercy of his impulses that he also continues to need the guidance and support of his parents, particularly in the setting of limits on his behavior. Characteristically, the adolescent complains that his parents do not care about him if they give him too much freedom, and he resents and rebels against too much restriction.

It is important that adolescents have accurate factual knowledge about the changes in growth and physiologic functions which are occurring in their bodies, particularly those having to do with sexual functioning such as nocturnal emissions and menstruation. Ejaculatory or orgastic experiences associated with masturbation or sexual arousal, although pleasurable, can be frightening and may cause severe guilt feelings. The adolescent needs to know that sexual and aggressive fantasies are common at his age and are a normal part of his attempt to gain mastery over his new capabilities and newly strengthened drives. The physician may be able to help by discussing these matters with the adolescent. Such discussion frequently has not taken place in the family because of mutual embarrassment and discomfiture between parent and adolescent.

SITUATIONAL DISORDERS

Situational disorders stem from environmental situations which are abnormal for a given child at a given age, and with which he is unable to cope. Any of the problems which occur as developmental disorders may also be seen in situational disorders. The latter diagnosis is to be suspected whenever symptoms are severe, persistent and especially clearly defined.

Psychopathology. As with developmental disorders, the conflict initially is between the child and his environment; if this is resolved in time, internal psychopathology can be prevented. Because the abnormal environmental situation interferes with satisfaction of the child's needs, his sexual and aggressive drives are likely to be increased. Regressively, he may attempt to ease his tension through indulgence in libidinal pleasure or self-gratification. The form of indulgence will vary with the age of the child. For example, the 2-year-old who is frustrated by overstrict toilet training may turn to excessive thumb-sucking, and the adolescent whose strivings for independence are unduly frustrated may turn to excessive masturbation. Aggression may also be displayed in severe temper tantrums or in rebelliousness expressed verbally.

Adaptability. The child may evidence difficulty in relations with people by being withdrawn or excessively aggressive toward them. His usual level of mental performance may be lowered.

Environmental Factors. Determination of the pathologic environmental situation is essential to the diagnosis of a situational disorder. Table 2-13 lists situations which can be of etiologic significance.

Treatment. Treatment for the most part consists in alleviation of the unhealthy interaction between the child and his environment. It may be helpful to discuss the problem with the older child or adolescent with the aim of increasing his understanding, easing his anxiety and giving him emotional support. The extent to which discussion with the parents will be helpful is determined by their ability to gain understanding and to change. If there is significant psychopathology in the parents, it may be necessary to refer them for additional psychotherapeutic help.

CLINICAL PATTERNS

Conflicts Between Temperament (Personality) and Environment. Various behavioral patterns can be understood as deriving from incompatibility between the temperament or personality of the infant and those of one or both parents. Regardless of whether temperament or personality is innate or is in part shaped by the earliest life experiences, parent-child interaction should be studied not only for parental influences on the child, but also for the influence of the child's individual characteristics on the parent. With the identification of the pertinent temperamental and environmental issues, the parents can be guided in attempting to modify their interactive pattern with the child in a healthy direction.

A temperamental pattern which carries a high risk for the development of behavior problems combines in the infant or child irregularity in biologic functions, predominantly negative (withdrawal) responses to new stimuli, nonadaptability or slow adaptability to change, frequent negative moods and predominantly intense reactions. As infants, children with this pattern have had irregular sleep and feeding patterns, slow acceptance of new foods, prolonged adjustment periods to new routines, and frequent periods of loud crying. They are not easy to feed, to put to sleep, to bathe or to dress. They respond with initial loud protest or with crying to new places, new activities or strange faces, and frustration characteristically produces a violent tantrum. These children experience as stressful the demands of socialization, such as the demands to conform to the usual patterns of the family, the school and the peer group. Yet, once they learn the rules, they may function easily, consistently and energetically.

The care of these infants makes special requirements upon the parents for unusually firm, patient, consistent and tolerant handling. If new demands are presented inconsistently, impatiently or punitively, negativism is a frequent outcome.

At the opposite end of the temperamental spectrum from the "difficult" child is the child who is regular, responds positively to new stimuli, adapts quickly and easily to change, and shows a predominantly positive mood or mild or moderate intensity. As infants, they develop regular sleep and feeding schedules easily, smile at strangers, and later, as children, they adapt quickly to a new school, accept most frustrations with a minimum of fuss, and learn the rules of new games quickly. The "easy" child, in short, confronts his parents with few if any problems in handling. Although these children do as a rule develop significantly fewer behavior problems than do the difficult infants, their very ease of adaptability may under certain circumstances be the basis for a psychologic disorder. If problems develop, they may occur most typically when there is severe dissonance between the expectations and demands of the family and of the community. When the child is engaged in situations outside the home, such as in peer play and school activities, stress and malfunction may develop if the extrafamilial standards and demands conflict sharply with the patterns learned in the home. For example, pressures for conformity and attentiveness to rule may conflict with need for individuality and freedom of expression. Such conflicts are relatively easily resolved if the parents are willing to modify their attitudes to be more in keeping with the realities of the external world.

Another important temperamental pattern combines negative responses of mild intensity to new stimuli with slow adaptability after repeated contact. These children usually do not have irregularity of function, frequent negative moods, nor intense reactions, and their withdrawal from the new is quiet rather than loud. With the first bath the child lies still and fusses mildly, with a new food he turns his head away quietly and lets the food dribble from his mouth, and when a stranger greets him loudly, he clings to his mother. If given the opportunity to re-experience new situations without pressure, such a child gradually comes to show quiet and positive interest and involvement. A key issue, therefore, is whether parents and teachers allow this child to make an adaptation to the new at his own tempo or insist on immediate positive involvement.

In contrast to the child who is slow to respond is the very persistent child who is most likely to experience stress not with his initial contact with a situation, but whose persistence after the first positive adaptation has been made leads him to resist interference or attempts at subsequent diversion. If the parent or adult interferes arbitrarily or forcefully, tension and frustration tend to mount quickly in these children and may reach explosive proportions.

The foregoing samples of temperamental patterns are not exhaustive. Further careful observation and study will permit other maladaptive interactions to be identified and appropriate management to be determined.

Eating Disorders. *Infantile colic* (p. 160) may be caused by various factors singly or in combination; one of the possible causes is an environmental situation which creates tension in the infant.

Pica, or perverted appetite, occurs most often in the first 3 years of life. A child may ingest any of a large variety of unsuitable substances, such as sand, earth, grass, wool from blankets, broken glass, animal droppings, paint from furniture, coal, ashes, or plaster from the wall.

The crawling infant and the toddler normally put foreign objects into their mouths, partly for exploration of the outside world and partly to satisfy a craving for mouthing experience and sucking. This behavior often accompanies messy play and interest in dirt and feces.

This activity may also be seen in neurotic children, and it is common in mentally defective ones. The possibility of an underlying physiologic or nutritional disturbance must also be considered; the behavior may indicate mineral, vitamin or other deficiency.

Provision for the child to have adequate sucking, biting, chewing and other mouth, lip and tongue pleasures during the oral stage of development may eliminate the need for abnormal continuation of these activities.

Obesity. (See also p. 165.) A child who is unhappy or under tension due to a difficult situation may seek to ease his tensions and give himself pleasure by overeating, consequently becoming obese. If the situation can be changed, the abnormal eating usually subsides. Attention should be directed primarily at the psychologic disorder.

Thumb-sucking and its equivalents, such as sucking of the tongue, fingers, toes, lips, a rubber nipple, pacifier or the corner of a blanket, are common and normal in infancy. Thumb-sucking is one of the first coordinated acts through which the infant can give himself pleasure and become somewhat less dependent upon the environment.

Thumb-sucking that persists beyond infancy, particularly into the preschool years, suggests the possibility of a situational disorder. It is most likely to occur when the child is about to go to sleep, when he is watching television or when he is hungry, sleepless or ill. It may occur if the child feels displaced by a younger child or otherwise senses withdrawal of parental interest from him. In most instances the habit is given up spontaneously, particularly if it has not become an issue between child and parents. If it persists continuously and intensely, it may cause malpositioning of the teeth requiring orthodontia.

In the case of the infant it is important to reassure the parents that the activity is normal. If the infant is taking his feedings too rapidly and has too little sucking pleasure, it is desirable to lengthen the feeding periods.

In older children threats of punishment, shaming and reminders to remove the thumb from the mouth are usually of no avail and tend to reinforce the activity. Applying bad-tasting substances to the thumb and using thumb covers, metal mittens or elbow splints are equally ineffective and may cause additional emotional trauma. Effective treatment is indirect, consisting in correcting an unfavorable situation or, when thumb-sucking is a symptom in a neurotic child, alleviation of his internalized conflicts.

Nail-Biting. Whereas thumb-sucking is primarily a pleasurable and comforting activity, nail-biting is more a manifestation of aggression. It is seen more commonly in the older child and may be an unconscious means of controlling aggressive urges. Nagging and scolding should be avoided. Treatment is aimed at correcting the underlying cause.

Eczema. (See also page 506.) Emotional conflict and tension may be important aggravating factors in infants with eczematous lesions. Treatment for emotional factors is directed at remedying the environmental causes of tension and improving parent-child relations.

Sleep Disorders. In early childhood sleep disturbances are usually a manifestation of separation anxiety, in later childhood more likely fear of loss of control over aggressive impulses. In mid-childhood, fear of aggressive impulses in combination with awareness of the reality of death may cause insomnia. The pathologic environmental situation has the effect of increasing the child's impulses and fears, thereby causing more severe sleep disturbance.

A child needs to be reassured verbally, and at times by the physical presence of the parent. If movies or television shows with a frightening content are connected with a sleep disturbance, they should be eliminated. Effective treatment requires alleviation of the disturbed situation.

Rhythmic movements may be seen in normal, emotionally disturbed or mentally retarded infants.

Head-rolling by the infant lying in bed may be continued until the hair is almost completely worn away from the back of the head. This behavior is most likely in the very young infant. When determined by situational factors, it is usually due to emotional deprivation and may also be seen in undernourished or chronically ill children.

Head-nodding is relatively rare and is the equivalent of head-rolling. It occurs with the child in a sitting position and consists either of a vigorous nodding, or a lateral shaking movement. Head-rolling and nodding may also be seen in spasmus nutans (p. 1303).

Body-rocking may take place in a sitting position or in a semikneeling position, resting on the elbows and knees. It is fairly common in infancy and usually occurs before going to sleep. It usually disappears spontaneously, but may persist into later childhood.

In the severe forms it may occur frequently during the day and may continue for hours at a time. In such instances emotional deprivation is suggested, e.g. inadequate satisfaction of the need for stimulation of kinesthetic sensations through the normal experiences of being held, carried or rocked by the mother.

Head-banging appears to be an extension of rocking, usually in the knee-elbow position. It usually occurs in the latter half of the first year of life. The infant does not seem to experience pain or discomfort; bruising and callus formation may occur. Head-banging suggests a greater amount of tension in the infant, since the aim has shifted from pleasurable self-stimulation (autoerotism) to unpleasant or painful self-stimulation (auto-aggression).

Treatment of these symptom patterns consists in helping the parents to meet the unfulfilled needs. The parent most able to give, or a mother-surrogate, is encouraged to spend more time holding or rocking the infant, or staying with him and soothing him at bedtime. Gentle vocal stimulation through talking or singing, and stroking or rubbing the skin may also be helpful. In the more severe cases serious emotional difficulty in the mother or tension in the home environment is to be considered.

Picking, pulling, and rubbing habits are similar to rhythmic movements, but involve more specific coordination patterns in respect to a particular part of the body. A child may pick at his nose, lips or scabs, or he may pull at his penis or the lobe of an ear. An infant may repetitiously pull his hair (trichotillomania) until large areas of the scalp become bare. In some cases hair is eaten and may produce a hairball in the stomach (p. 796). These activities may be seen in any category of disorder, including psychoses. Contributory factors such as local irritation, fatigue and malnutrition need to be considered.

Nagging or shaming the child is of no avail, and treatment is directed at remedy of the underlying cause.

Breath-holding usually occurs in response to frustration and is similar to a temper tantrum. It may be seen in the young infant when he is startled. He cries, hyperventilates and has a sudden cessation of respiration, followed by cyanosis and rigidity. In severe cases there may be momentary loss of consciousness (syncope), possibly convulsive twitching, pallor or cyanosis and finally general relaxation. Presumably this series of symptoms results from hypoxia.

As in temper tantrum, the child cannot be dealt with during the height of an attack, owing to the temporary loss of object relationship. Understanding and kindness are most effective. Punishing the child is not helpful, and in some instances may precipitate an attack. Measures should be taken to avoid precipitating conditions and to correct faults in the environment.

Teeth-grinding, or bruxism, is observed chiefly during sleep; it may be associated with various acute and chronic disturbances, including disturbing dreams. When determined by emotional or environmental factors, it suggests that the child is having difficulty managing his aggression. It may occur in mental deficiency, and is fairly common in unconscious states due to disease, especially of intracranial origin, e.g. meningitis.

There is no treatment other than to improve

the environmental situation which is creating the conflict and tension in the child.

Bowel and Bladder Disorders. In a child beyond 2½ or 3 years of age, symptoms such as diurnal or nocturnal enuresis (see p. 87), fecal smearing, defecation elsewhere than in the toilet, and fecal soiling suggest a situational disorder. The most common cause is excessive pressure from the parents during toilet training with resultant resentment and rebellion on the part of the child. Occasionally these symptoms indicate that toilet training has not been seriously attempted, usually because the mother cannot manage her own or her child's aggression.

These same symptoms in midchildhood or adolescence suggest a neurotic or more severe disorder. Treatment is directed at correcting the environmental situation.

Masturbation may be performed by manipulation of the genitals, by movement of the thighs or contraction of the perineal musculature, by copulatory movements sometimes with an object such as a pillow between the legs; or an equivalent sensation may be derived from tight clothing or activities such as horseback riding, straddling rails and climbing trees. In the younger child who is not aware of the cultural taboo against masturbation, the parents may observe the activity or the associated signs of intense concentration and excitement. Most children sense parental disapproval, however, and the activity is carried out in privacy. Rarely, the child may masturbate openly, an act which suggests poor awareness of social reality by the child or lack of censorship by the parents. Some well-meaning parents who know that masturbation is a normal activity may inadvisedly encourage it.

Masturbation is normal. In the young child it presents a self-gratification analogous to thumb-sucking. In the older child, particularly the adolescent, it serves the purpose of exploring and experimenting with newly developing sexual capacities and feelings and may aid in gaining control over the sexual urges and becoming less afraid of them.

Masturbation occurs most commonly at bedtime when anxiety is increased, owing to separation or fear of loss of control over sexual and aggressive impulses. For the same reasons the child is most likely to masturbate when he is alone and lonely. This fact leads to the logical, but usually mistaken, assumption that the urge to masturbate is the motive for rather than the consequence of being alone. Masturbation may also be performed, sometimes repetitiously and compulsively, as a reassurance against fear of injury to the private parts. Excessive masturbation suggests some problem or deficiency in object relationships. In some instances it is a symptom of a neurotic or more severe disorder.

It is appropriate for the parent to censor open masturbation and to be concerned about excessive masturbation, but to forbid it absolutely, to shame the child, to threaten punishment or to suggest injury to the genitals not only is ineffective, but also tends to create guilt and additional anxiety which may even increase the activity. The most helpful treatment is to remedy any environmental situation which is interfering with gratification of the child's needs or is causing tension and anxiety. It is important that the child be reassured that masturbation does not cause physical or mental deterioration. The adolescent should be given an explanation of ejaculation, orgasm and menstruation, so that he or she can understand them as normal body functions.

Acting-Out Behavior. During the course of growing up some children act out those tensions and impulses which stem from conflicts in their relations with other people. This acting-out most commonly takes the form of antisocial or "delinquent" behavior which expresses aggressive or sexual urges or admixtures of both. More common manifestations are cruelty to animals, fighting, stealing, destroying property, and sexual activity such as mutual examination of the genitals or mutual masturbation. Such activities may be normal in the early years of childhood, but indicate developmental or situational problems in the later years. In some instances the child may not feel sufficiently loved. If so, the main reason for exercise of self-control and restraint is lacking. In other instances the child may be acting out unconscious wishes or urges in the parents.

In most instances firmness and protection of the child from his impulses by adequate supervision are indicated. Severe punishment or threats do not help, since they tend to increase the strength of the child's impulses and create a greater problem in ego control. Effective treatment requires determination of the underlying cause and correction of the environmental situation.

NEUROTIC DISORDERS (NEUROSES)

Developmental, situational and neurotic disorders can present the same or similar clinical manifestations, and differential diagnosis may be difficult. The child is more likely to suffer a situational disorder when faced with a situation in which the parental problem is gross and can be perceived and identified as such by the child; he is more likely to suffer a neurotic disorder when the parental disorder is less obvious, and unconscious attitudes are masked by seemingly benign conscious attitudes and behavior. The child has difficulty in coping with what is outside his conscious awareness.

If the history indicates severe environmental disruption, the likelihood of a neurotic disorder is increased. The longer the duration of symptoms, the greater the likelihood of a neurosis. A neurotic disorder is seen only infrequently in a child under the age of 4 or 5 years, since the psychic structure before this age is usually not sufficiently developed to permit internal conflict of pathologic significance.

If treatment measures appropriate to developmental and situational disorders do not succeed, or if there is uncertainty about the diagnosis, it is wise to seek psychiatric consultation.

Psychopathology. In neurotic disorders the conflicts are internalized and constitute a definite psychopathologic situation in the child.

It is essential to the definition of neurosis that the internalized conflict, either entirely or in part, be outside the child's conscious awareness. Repression is an automatic and unconscious defense mechanism whereby there is an attempt to escape unpleasant feeling, fantasy or tension by making it unconscious. At times this may be successful, but in a neurosis it fails, and symptoms and difficulty in adaptation result.

Because the trauma occurs after basic ego development has taken place, the personality disturbance in neurotic disorders is only partial, and with proper treatment the child can come to function normally. The earlier the neurotic disorder is diagnosed, the more facilitated will be the treatment.

Adaptability. As is true of the child with a developmental or situational disorder, the child with a neurotic disorder is able to relate well. The fact that his first experiences with people have been reasonably good causes him to value them and seek to continue receiving their love and approval. His perception of the world of external reality, on the whole, is good, although at times it may be distorted by his fantasies or through the use of defense mechanisms such as projection or displacement. His disorder usually interferes with only a relatively small part of his total functioning.

Treatment. Treatment of neurotic disorders requires work with the parents to allay their anxiety, to give them understanding, to gain their cooperation, to acquire additional information about the child's disorder and to alleviate current environmental difficulties. At the same time it is necessary to engage the child in psychotherapy. This is done through regular appointments, usually at no less than weekly intervals, in a setting which offers play or other activity appropriate to the child's age. The aim of the treatment is to ascertain and help the child understand his anxieties and unconscious conflicts, thereby permitting him to re-experience and gain mastery over them.

In successful treatment the child comes to trust the therapist, has some temporary dependence upon him and becomes involved in the treatment both intellectually and emotionally. The unresolved conflicts and problems from the past are transferred into the treatment situation. The conflicts increase in intensity, and if they are not understood and dealt with in an adequate way, symptoms may become aggravated, and the neurotic disorder may be reinforced rather than eliminated. Therapeutic competence based upon adequate theoretical knowledge, and training and supervision in technique are essential.

CLINICAL PATTERNS

Neurotic conflicts may be expressed at various levels: (1) at an ideational level in the form of conscious worries, guilt feelings, irrational fears, or of disturbing wishes, thoughts and fantasies; (2) at the level of sensory or motor functions by either inhibition or exaggeration of activity, such as functional aphonia or blindness, enuresis, disturbance in physiologic functioning; (3) at the level of disturbance in physiologic function, such as peptic ulcer.

Anxiety neurosis is the simplest form of neurosis. The impulses and fantasies which were disturbing when in the child's conscious awareness have been dealt with by repression, without the use of other mental mechanisms. Anxiety is the ego's reaction to the danger that those things which are repressed may re-enter conscious awareness. Technically, anxiety is defined as a state of tension and apprehension wherein the cause is not discerned by the patient. This is in contrast to fear, wherein the danger is consciously recognized. Secondary symptoms may develop as a result of the anxiety, e.g. regression with thumbsucking, overeating with consequent obesity, nailbiting, various fears, and sleep disturbances.

Neurotic anxiety must be differentiated from similar tension due to organic causes such as hypoglycemia, hyperthyroidism and Sydenham's chorea.

Phobia. In phobia diffuse anxiety is replaced by fear of a specific thing or situation. The fear, although real to the child, is not rational, since it is caused by unconscious factors rather than by that to which he attributes his fear. The child, for example, may be preoccupied with a fear of tigers or of robbers in his bedroom at night. In phobia, repression is supplemented by the mechanism *displacement*, whereby fear of a real object, e.g. of the father, is shifted away from the father to another object, or by *projection*, whereby anxiety-creating impulses are falsely attributed to an external object or situation.

Phobias occur normally at certain stages in childhood, and may also be a manifestation of a situational disorder.

In *school phobia* the child appears to be irrationally afraid of going to school. He may say that he is afraid of the teacher or of other students in the school. In some instances what at first appears to be a phobia can be described more accurately as a refusal of school.

The real cause of school phobia is fear of leaving home, or separation anxiety. Careful study as a rule will reveal that the parent also fears separation or is abnormally fearful that something will happen to the child when he is away.

Obsessive-Compulsive Disorder. An obsession is a persistent and repetitive thought, usually recognized by the child as having little or no basis in reality. As an example, a child may be obsessed with the idea that his parent is going to die. A compulsion is a persistent and repetitious act, also recognized as being unrealistic and serving no constructive purpose. For example, a child may not be able to go to sleep unless he first closes the closet door, carefully aligns his shoes, putting the ends of his shoelaces inside of them, and tucks loose ends of the covers beneath the mattress. Obsessive-compulsive behavior is most likely to be seen during the middle years or adolescence. The obsessive-compulsive activity keeps the repressed thoughts and feelings from entering conscious awareness. At times a compulsion becomes ritualistic and serves magically to forestall dangers which usually are not consciously discerned.

Conversion Disorder. In this disorder repressed conflicts are prevented from entering consciousness in recognizable form by being converted to symptoms such as blindness, deafness, paralysis of the arm or leg or various somatic complaints. There is no physiologic disturbance in the affected part. Psychosomatic symptoms due to conversion take place on a psychologic level; these differ from psychophysiologic disturbances, which take place at the level of the autonomic nervous system.

Conversion symptoms are relatively rare in children and are most likely to be seen in the adolescent. Differential diagnosis requires consideration of organic causes.

Dissociative Disorder. This condition is a functional disturbance of consciousness usually shortlived. It is relatively rare in children. It may be manifest as sleepwalking, amnesia or states of confusion resembling delirium. The alteration of consciousness maintains repression and in some instances enables the child to do something which he would not do if he were fully conscious. For example, a child in a confused state may express aggression in some destructive activity or may express forbidden thoughts.

It is necessary to rule out the possibility of organic causes such as infectious illness, drug intoxication and cerebral injury.

Somnambulism. Sleepwalking occurs mainly in midchildhood and in adolescence. The child, although not fully conscious, is able to get out of bed and walk about the house. On occasion he may leave the house or climb out on a roof or window ledge. The eyes are open, but the child either is unresponsive to questions or answers them briefly in a voice devoid of normal modulation and inflection. He usually returns to bed by himself and resumes sleep. Characteristically, there is amnesia for the sleepwalking. If awakened during this state, the child is sometimes frightened, but more usually is puzzled and at a loss to understand his behavior.

Sometimes the activities during sleepwalking may give indication of the underlying problem. For example, the child may walk into the parents' bedroom, thus revealing a desire to be with the parents or perhaps a repressed curiosity as to their activities in the bedroom.

Depression. Neurotic depression is seen most frequently in the adolescent. This in part is due to the fact that depressive feelings in the younger child may be masked by activity or regression.

A fully developed and strict superego is usually a requisite for depression. Most commonly angry feelings and hostile impulses cannot be expressed toward the person causing them because the superego prohibits this. In consequence they are turned toward the self. In other instances the child has a superego or ego ideal which requires him to achieve in accordance with unrealistically high standards. When he does not measure up to these standards, he feels that he has failed and becomes depressed. At the same time he may also have feelings of frustration and anger which are blocked from expression.

Aggression turned toward the self sometimes causes a child to have an unusual number of accidents. Suicidal thoughts are rare in young children, but common in adolescents. Thoughts of suicide are far more numerous than suicidal attempts, but accidents and suicide rank high among the causes of death in adolescents, particularly during late adolescence. Accident proneness and persistent or severe depression require careful evaluation and merit psychiatric consultation.

Acting-Out Disorder. In this disorder the child acts out unconscious conflicts and impulses without awareness of the meaning of his behavior. Stealing, for example, may be an unconscious expression of feelings of rejection and a need for love. Aggressive or sexual impulses are expressed outwardly in destructive or sexual behavior. The impulses may gain expression because they temporarily override the ego controls, or because, although prohibited, they are felt to be justified. Some children may act out repetitiously because the punishment for the misdeeds brings temporary relief from unconscious guilt feelings. Antisocial behavior of this type can be termed neurotic delinquency.

Accident Proneness. One cause of accident proneness is masked depression as described above. Another cause is acting-out behavior. This behavior is sometimes described as counterphobic, because the child attempts to cope with his unconsciously determined fear by exposing himself to the very danger he is afraid of. This child is the type who must take the dare, or who rushes headlong into situations without considering the risks. He often is a tense, high-strung child who seems to be under pressure to be active. In some instances, however, particularly in the older child, the activity may be deliberate, as for example in carrying out a dangerous chemical experiment or making an explosive device.

Learning Problems. As in developmental and

situational disorders, problems in learning may be caused by a severe inhibition of aggression and curiosity because of unconscious fear of the consequences.

Another cause of learning difficulty is excessively high standards. The child characteristically begins each school term with enthusiasm and high ambition. Because he expects so much of himself, however, even a slight or moderate amount of dropping away from "perfect" performance is painful. He becomes unwilling to risk further effort and further investment of libidinal energy, because of the blow to self-esteem which he experiences with failure. He finds it much less painful to fail without having put forth effort, since this kind of failure is not so disappointing and he can rationalize that he could have succeeded if he had wanted to do so.

A child also may have difficulty in learning because of inability to concentrate, owing to the distraction of daydreams. Children with this kind of difficulty sometimes are better able to study with background noise from a radio, which seemingly serves to screen out the fantasies from within.

A child may have a pattern of repeated failures because successful achievement is equated at an unconscious level with the attainment of a forbidden goal. For example, the child who has not resolved his oedipal conflict may unconsciously equate success in school with success in winning his mother's affection from the father.

These are examples of learning difficulties on a neurotic basis. Organically caused intellectual deficiency and inability to acquire basic skills need to be ruled out.

Enuresis. (See also page 1107.) Enuresis is defined as an involuntary discharge of urine occurring beyond the age when control of the urinary bladder should have been acquired. A few children achieve voluntary control as early as 1 year of age. The majority do not begin to gain control before 15 to 18 months of age, and nocturnal control is usually not established until 2 or 3 years of age. Some children may not be dry at night until 4 to 6 years of age. In children who have acquired good control there still may be, for several years, occasional lapses in nighttime control associated with fatigue or emotional turmoil, or even in daytime control at times of excitement, extreme urgency or engrossment in play. In some cases development of bladder control may be delayed because the parent has made no reasonable attempt at toilet training.

Before 5 or 6 years of age, enuresis is usually a manifestation of a developmental or situational disorder. Enuresis as a symptom of neurosis is most likely to be seen in midchildhood (the latency years) or in adolescence. Whereas nocturnal enuresis is fairly common, diurnal enuresis, in the absence of an organic lesion, is rare and usually indicates a more severe pathologic disturbance. Enuresis may be a symptom of nocturnal epilepsy or of lesions of part of the spinal cord or of the genitourinary system. It may also be a symptom of diabetes mellitus or diabetes insipidus.

The most common cause of persistent bedwetting extending from infancy is too vigorous and too early attempts at toilet training, before the age of physiologic readiness (usually 15 to 18 months). The same conflicts which cause enuresis in developmental and situational disorders become established internally and persist as a basis for neurotic enuresis. Enuresis may express (1) a desire to regress and receive the care and attentions associated with earlier childhood, (2) unconscious resentment of the parents, or (3) anxiety caused by an unconscious fear of injury to the genitals. This last fear is frequently associated with feelings of guilt due to sexual fantasies or activities, such as masturbation.

Occasional lapses are indicative of temporarily aggravated emotional conflicts and need cause little concern. If the child sleeps deeply, it is possible that signals from the bladder indicating that it needs to be emptied may not reach consciousness in time for the child to get out of bed and go to the bathroom. The child may be given a little more time to see whether control ultimately is gained. On the other hand, both the deep sleep and the enuresis may be determined by emotional factors.

The primary treatment is psychotherapy for the underlying neurotic disorder. Shaming, nagging and punitive actions by the parents do not help and may aggravate the problem. Contrariwise, if the parents can be helped to become less concerned, this may help the child gain mastery over the problem. The older child may sometimes gain control as he becomes increasingly fearful of humiliation if the condition comes to the attention of his friends, e.g. when he visits at someone's home or goes to summer camp. Disappearance of the symptom under these circumstances does not necessarily mean that the neurotic problem is solved; it may still persist and show itself in another form.

Limiting fluids for a few hours before bedtime and waking the child up so that he may void before he has wet the bed are sometimes helpful. These measures should not be a substitute, however, for direction of attention to the emotional causes.

The use of drugs such as tincture of belladonna, ephedrine, dextroamphetamine or tranquilizers is of doubtful value. Their effectiveness, if any, is often only temporary, and may be more on a psychologic than pharmacologic basis.

It has been assumed by some that the enuretic child has a smaller than average bladder capacity. It is proposed that bladder capacity may be increased by increasing the intake of fluids during the daytime and encouraging the child to suppress the urge to void. This may be worthy of trial. On the other hand, the small bladder capacity and frequent urination may both be a manifestation of tension and anxiety.

Some success is claimed for the conditioning

type of treatment wherein a bell rings and wakens the child when the voided urine completes an electrical circuit in a pad placed beneath the child. This generally is not effective, however, particularly if the enuresis is a symptom of neurosis.

Encopresis. (See also page 782.) Fecal soiling in a child beyond the age of 4 or 5 years may be a manifestation of a neurotic disorder as well as of more severe psychopathologic disturbances. There usually has been serious difficulty in the parent-child relations, most likely having its beginnings during bowel training. Treatment is aimed at remedying the underlying psychopathology.

Peptic Ulcer. Gastric and duodenal ulcers (see p. 797) may occur at all ages of infancy and childhood. In the young child the cause is more likely to be organic, but a severe pathogenic environmental situation should be considered. Chronic peptic ulcers occur more frequently after infancy, the incidence being highest in late childhood. The symptoms are similar to those in adults, and range from vague digestive complaints to severe pain, vomiting and blood in the stools.

The neurotic child with ulcer often presents an external appearance of competence and self-sufficiency, while denying strong dependent and regressive urges. There may be tension, compulsiveness or other signs of maladjustment. Psychiatric evaluation and psychotherapy should be considered.

Peptic ulcer may also be a manifestation of neurotic character disorder.

NEUROTIC CHARACTER DISORDERS

Because the young child is rapidly changing and is in a continuing process of development, his behavior patterns are usually not stabilized or ingrained in his personality. Therefore character disorders are seldom seen in children under 10 years of age. The developmental history of the child with a neurotic character disorder includes traumatic experiences which for the most part are equivalent to those of the neurotic child. Differentiation is made on the basis of the psychopathology and adaptability described below.

Psychopathology. The child with a neurotic character disorder attempts to maintain psychologic equilibrium by using certain defenses in a habitual way. His equilibrium is somewhat more unstable than that of the neurotic child because early relations with people have had a more adverse effect on his psychic development. Owing to greater frustrations, the strength of the drives and impulses is increased. Parental disciplinary attitudes are prematurely internalized in an attempt to control the impulses and to achieve more comfortable relations with the parents. The superego is thus likely to be excessively harsh and incompatible with the drives. For these reasons the ego, which has the task of mediating between the child's needs and the demands of his conscience and external reality, is hard pressed and is relatively weaker than that of the neurotic child.

Because strong aggressive and sexual feelings and fantasies are disturbing, the child with a neurotic character disorder eliminates them from his conscious awareness. He is then cut off from his feelings and fantasies, and because they normally are important to thought and action, this internal isolation has the consequence of further limiting his flexibility, creativity and adaptability.

Another result of this defense is a lack of awareness of anxiety and a lack of insight. Although he may acknowledge that he is having trouble learning in school, the child with a neurotic character disorder is unable to see that this is a consequence of difficulty within himself. He lacks the capacity for self-observation and self-evaluation.

Adaptability. The child with a neurotic character disorder has had more difficulty in his relations with people during the earlier developmental years than has the neurotic or normal child. He values relations with people, but has difficulty in relating to them and they to him. He may be described as excessively shy or quiet or "hard to get to know."

His perception of external reality is fairly adequate, although less so than that of the child with a neurotic disorder. His adaptation is usually considerably more impaired than that of the neurotic child, owing largely to the rigidity of his character structure.

Treatment. The same general considerations described under treatment of neurotic disorders apply to treatment of neurotic character disorders. The treatment is more difficult, however, because of the rigidity of the character structure and the lack of awareness of anxiety, of self-observation and of insight. The first phase of treatment is concerned with establishing a working relationship and making the child aware that he does in fact have internal conflicts, feelings and fantasies which are interfering with his adaptation.

CLINICAL PATTERNS

Many of the clinical patterns discussed under neurotic disorders also occur as neurotic character disorders, but with the differences described above; problems discussed previously will not be taken up under this category.

Passive-Aggressive Character Disorder. The passive-aggressive child is outwardly passive and conforming; he does not display aggression toward others in a direct way. Aggression, when evident, takes the form of such symptoms as uncooperativeness, stubbornness, pouting, procrastination and "passive" obstructionism. Passivity and passive resistance are rigidly used as defenses against aggression.

Impulse-Ridden Character Disorder. This child is almost the direct opposite of the passive-aggressive child. He seemingly makes little or no attempt to control his impulses, and there is no apparent anxiety or appropriate concern when the impulsive actions get him into trouble. The causes of this problem are much the same as those discussed in connection with neurotic acting-out.

Antisocial Character Disorder. This condition is analogous to neurotic delinquency, but the child has little or no anxiety and on the surface appears relatively unconcerned about his deeds.

In some of the more severe cases the child may have had good or reasonably adequate relations with people in infancy, but subsequently may have suffered severe deprivation and abuse. Characteristically, this type of child is "tough," aloof and seemingly disinterested in receiving help. Yet he may be reached through strenuous therapeutic efforts.

Sexual Character Problems. *Reversed sexual identification.* Effeminate tendencies in the boy and tomboyishness in the girl may become habitual patterns of adaptation.

Sexual perversions. Persistent homosexual activity must be considered a perversion and most likely indicates a character disorder. The same is true for persistent transvestism, i.e. dressing up in the clothing of the opposite sex. This is more common in boys and is usually done covertly because of the awareness that the behavior is disapproved.

Stuttering. Stuttering may persist into the later years of childhood and become habitual, being a part of everyday speech or appearing at times of stress. Although stuttering may occur transiently and normally in the toddler, it is a serious problem at later ages, and often is exceedingly difficult to resolve even with thorough treatment of the underlying psychopathology (p. 106).

Tics. Tics are spasmodic, irregular movements of isolated groups of muscles not associated with organic disease. They occur most often in later childhood, but may be seen during the preschool years. On occasion the origin of a tic may be traced to interference with normal motility during early childhood due to illness or artificial restraint such as that imposed by casts or elbow splints.

Tics are of various types and degrees of severity. The movements may be occasional or frequent. They are performed unconsciously, although the child is sometimes able to restrain them for a time. They generally are increased when the child is excited or under stress. The majority of tics involve the facial muscles and consist of twitching or distortion of the mouth, wrinkling of the forehead or winking and blinking of the eyes. Sighing, coughing, sniffling, or jerking movements of the head may be seen. Less often there are jerking movements of the body which may be localized in the hands, arms or shoulders.

Tics also may be seen in neurotic disorders, but when well established they suggest psychopathology more in keeping with neurotic character disorders.

Gilles de la Tourette's disease. This is a relatively infrequent syndrome occurring most often in late childhood or in adolescence. The symptoms are violent twitching or convulsive movements, usually of the muscles of the face and arms, but sometimes of other parts of the body. With the movements there are associated explosive sounds, such as a loud barking cough or indistinct vocal sounds. At times these sounds are enunciated more clearly, and then are discerned to be obscene words.

Since the tic is of unconscious origin, it is of no avail to call attention to it or to pressure the child to control it. Treatment needs to be directed toward the underlying psychopathology.

Anorexia Nervosa. (See also page 774). This syndrome, more common in girls than in boys, is most frequent in adolescence. It is characterized by intense self-starvation, severe loss of weight and at times amenorrhea in the female.

The condition may be precipitated by a relatively small criticism or confrontation with imperfection, such as being called fat or being unable to achieve in some athletic endeavor. The anorexia may be preceded by a conscious and deliberate refusal of food.

These children usually have strict superegos and very high standards for themselves. Distorted fantasies about conception and pregnancy may enter into the determination of the condition. There may be the fear, for example, that impregnation takes place through the mouth and can occur after kissing. In other children the ingestion of food may be associated with frightening aggressive fantasies of devouring or being devoured. These fantasies are usually revealed only during psychotherapy.

The more severe cases may be confused with Simmonds's cachexia, and with malnutrition due to other organic causes. Although the onset of the anorexia may be acute, the associated underlying character disorder develops over a relatively long time.

Treatment consists initially in correction of any electrolyte imbalance and in establishing minimally adequate nutrition. This may require hospitalization and parenteral therapy. Immediate psychiatric consultation should be requested in order to begin psychotherapy promptly. The condition is difficult to treat, and the prognosis is often grave.

PSYCHOTIC CHARACTER DISORDERS

Like neurotic character disorders, psychotic character disorders are seen mostly in the older child and adolescent. In contrast to neurotic character disorders, which are based upon psychopathology similar to that of neuroses, psychotic character disorders are based upon a kind of psychopathology similar to that of psychoses (see Kinds of Psychopathology, p. 74).

Psychopathology. The psychotic character disorder is manifest in habitual patterns of behavior which are even more rigid and less varied than those in neurotic character disorders. The child has had serious difficulty during his early psychologic development, so that his equilibrium is easily disturbed. In his attempt at maintenance of equilibrium he isolates and distorts his perception of his own feelings and fantasies. Because unexpected events or experiences are very disturbing, he avoids them by limiting his activities and contacts with people. Thus his perception of the world around him becomes constricted and his character make-up increasingly rigid. His ability to deal with his drives and impulses, the demands of his conscience and with external reality is inadequate.

Adaptability. The child with a psychotic character disorder appears to place relatively little value on relations with people. Nevertheless he does not withdraw completely. He fails in his adaptation to an even greater extent than does the child with neurotic character disorder, and he is often regarded as "peculiar" or eccentric. He does not adjust well with his peer group, and he has a tendency to isolate himself, either alone or with one or two friends whose make-up is similar to his own. He is likely to perform poorly. He has had difficulty in most aspects of psychologic development. Although his general performance is poor, he may do well in a specific area. For example, an adolescent may be outstanding in academic learning, while failing to achieve in social and physical skills.

Treatment. The psychotherapy is difficult and delicate. Although the patient wishes for relationships, he is afraid of them. The therapist must proceed slowly and cautiously lest he disturb the precarious psychologic equilibrium.

CLINICAL PATTERNS

Psychotic character disorders usually bear little resemblance to neuroses or neurotic character disorders, the symptoms and behavior being more akin to those of psychotic disorders.

Inadequate Character Disorder. A child with an inadequate character is unable to respond adequately to intellectual, emotional, social and physical demands. Although children with this disorder are not mentally or physically defective, they function so inadequately as to suggest that they are. This condition may be due in part to constitutional inadequacy. It can result from severe emotional deprivation with an attempt at adaptation through withdrawal and passivity.

Schizoid Character Disorder. The symptoms and behavior in the schizoid character disorder resemble those seen in schizophrenia. The child is unable to form close relations or to express aggression; his awareness of reality is much constricted. He lives mainly in a fantasy world of his own creating. He may have sufficient capacity to fit into the family routine and to carry out certain specific tasks and activities. In the more serious cases the child may avoid speaking for periods of time, since relationship with people is disturbing to his equilibrium.

Paranoid Character Disorder. This disorder, rare in children, is also characterized by a schizoid type of behavior in which the child's own feelings of inadequacy and hostility are projected onto other people and then are felt to be directed toward himself as accusations from them. This kind of child is excessively suspicious, envious, jealous and prone to project the blame for his failures upon other people or upon inanimate factors.

Dyssocial Character Disorder. The term "dyssocial" connotes a lack of social values and is to be distinguished from the term "antisocial," which suggests values which are against those of society. Although the dyssocial child may have a generally good sense of reality, he lacks conscience and appreciation of social reality. This can result from his having been brought up in a morally abnormal environment or in a subcultural group with values very much different from those of society in general. His dyssocial behavior is based not upon emotional conflicts or traumatic experiences, but upon a difference in his character structure, specifically in the content of his superego. Because he comes into sharp conflict with society and in effect has a character defect, he is classed, somewhat inappropriately, among the psychotic character disorders.

Ulcerative Colitis. Ulcerative colitis (see also p. 799) is characterized by recurrent episodes of diarrhea with loss of appetite, malnutrition and bleeding due to ulceration of the lower bowel. In some instances psychologic factors may play a large role in the illness. The child usually has had difficulty in managing his hostility and aggression since early childhood. Although he relates to people, he prefers to be by himself and is not comfortable with other children. He has ambivalent feelings toward everyone in his environment, and particularly toward his parents. Eating and elimination usually have become very much involved in the child's emotional conflicts. Characteristically he has a strict, punitive superego which forbids the expression of his strong oral needs and of aggression. Outwardly he may appear to be calm, but inwardly he seethes with tension. During the course of psychotherapy primitive and distorted oral and anal fantasies are likely to be revealed. They usually include fantasies of destruction as well as of procreation.

Intense psychotherapy of long duration is usually required to improve the severe psychopathology.

PSYCHOTIC DISORDERS (PSYCHOSES)

Psychotic disorders are the most serious of the psychologic disorders, having comparability to "insanity" in the adult.

Psychopathology. In psychotic disorders difficulty in early psychologic development has resulted in deficiencies in personality development and integration. The young psychotic child often has defects in coordination which are difficult to distinguish from those caused by organic lesions. Language development may be grossly impaired or completely lacking. Thought processes are disorganized, and social reality either is not perceived or is ignored.

Adaptability. Owing to insurmountable difficulties in the early relations with the parents or other adults, the psychotic child has little or no interest in relating to people. He is withdrawn, preferring to live in a fantasy world of his own creation, and usually fails completely in his adaptation.

Treatment. Children with psychotic disorders, particularly in early childhood, are among the most difficult to treat. Even with intensive and prolonged efforts, utilizing individual psychotherapy, supervised group experience, special education, treatment of the parents, and the use of parent substitutes with or without institutionalization, most of these children are unable to achieve a level of functioning anywhere near that of the normal child.

CLINICAL PATTERNS IN EARLY CHILDHOOD

Anaclitic Depression. The term "anaclitic" connotes dependence or leaning upon. This disorder is seen in infants at 4 to 6 months of age after complete separation from the mother. Initially the infant reacts with crying and apprehension, and then by withdrawal of interest in people. Over a period of weeks psychologic development becomes retarded, and there is decreased motility and responsiveness to stimuli (Spitz).

Autistic Childhood Psychosis (Autism). This disorder, originally described by Kanner, is characterized by profound withdrawal from contact with people, including the parents, an obsessive desire for preservation of sameness, a skillful and even affectionate relation to inanimate objects, retention of an intelligent, pensive physiognomy, and mutism or a kind of language development which is not understandable. In rare instances the diagnosis has been made as early as 18 months of age. More often the symptoms, although present, go unrecognized until the age of 4 or 5 years. Parents frequently minimize signs of the condition until the child goes to nursery school or kindergarten, where his difficulties become clearly evident.

In the more severe cases the child may appear extremely regressed. He may sit and rock back and forth incessantly; he may drool, and his only vocalizations may be grunts or other animal-like sounds. Although he may seem aware of people, he makes no attempt to relate to them. He may scratch his skin to the point of excoriation and bite or slap himself when frustrated or intruded upon, without evident awareness of pain. Physical coordination may be poor.

In the less severe cases the child has good physical coordination and sometimes may be skillful in handling his body or manipulating objects. He uses words and on occasion may verbalize a request, but sentence formation and language development are inadequate for his age. He has the capacity for memory, sometimes to a remarkable degree. His level of intelligence is difficult to gauge, but his activities suggest ability to reason and understand cause-and-effect relations. He is interested in and sometimes intensely preoccupied with inanimate objects. Intrusions of other people into his autism are resented, and at first will be ignored or brushed aside. If one persists in the intrusion or attempts to establish a relationship, he becomes upset and has a severe temper tantrum in which he may break things or display aggression toward himself.

In some instances the disorder is felt to be due to constitutional deficiencies, as suggested, for example, by the history of absence of a smiling response or acceptance of cuddling as early as the neonatal period. In other instances the history indicates that the child most likely was severely traumatized through environmental experiences in infancy. For example, serious physical problems in the infant or serious emotional problems in the mother interfered with adequate maternal care. There is often a combination of constitutional and environmental factors.

Differential diagnosis includes consideration of mental retardation, brain injury causing interference with mental functioning, e.g. agnosia or aphasia, deafness and Heller's disease. Heller's disease is a rare progressive degeneration of the central nervous system. It has an acute onset between 18 months and 4 years of age and is characterized by progressive deterioration of all aspects of mental functioning.

Symbiotic Childhood Psychosis. This disorder, described by Mahler, is frequently precipitated by separation or threat of separation from the mother. The child at first may protest with severe crying and then by regression with bizarre behavior, such as attempting to climb into the toilet bowl, taking off all clothing and going out of doors naked, eating in an animal-like fashion, talking or singing in an endless and singsong fashion, and staying awake and moving about aimlessly through the night. During such behavior the child is withdrawn and is unamenable to management by reason or persuasion. The possible causes are similar to those of the autistic childhood psychosis. Careful consideration should be given to the possibility of organic factors.

The acute phase may last for hours or days. It is followed by a chronic phase which may last for months or years. In the chronic phase the child seeks to relate to people, but in an abnormal way. He lacks normal reticence, and family and complete strangers are approached without discrimination. Frequently the child seeks close physical contact, and in some instances behaves as if he would wish to merge with or burrow into the other person. He may be uncommunicative; or language development may appear to be normal, and the child may engage in conversation, but its content is disorganized or monothematic.

CLINICAL PATTERNS IN LATER CHILDHOOD

Whereas the psychoses of early childhood represent failure to achieve psychologic development, the psychoses of later childhood result from a breakdown in personality integration and ego functioning. This type of psychotic disorder is seen occasionally in the prepuberty period, but more often in adolescence. These children usually have had traumatic experiences during their early psychologic development, with a resulting predisposition to psychotic disorder at a later date. Nevertheless they were able to progress in their development, functioning sufficiently well to cause no great concern and to attend school. In some instances the personality of the child before the collapse in functioning resembles that of the child with a psychotic character disorder. The combination of predisposition and the increased emotional stress normally associated with puberty accounts for the onset of psychotic disorder in adolescence. On the other hand, just because emotional stress is normally increased at this age, a psychosis in adolescence often has a less serious prognosis than the same condition occurring either in midchildhood or in adulthood.

The psychoses of later childhood are characterized by (1) withdrawal from relations with people, (2) distorted perception and evaluation of reality, (3) disordered thinking which may include delusions and hallucinations, and (4) general disorganization and regression resulting in bizarre behavior. In some instances the child may be completely withdrawn, uncommunicative and essentially immobile (catatonic). In other instances he may behave in an infantile manner, seemingly without awareness of the cultural mores which he previously had accepted. For example, he eats messily with his fingers, he is careless about his personal appearance and body hygiene, he soils and wets himself, and he may masturbate openly, or he is silly (hebephrenic). In some instances aggressive impulses are expressed in destructive behavior or in serious assault on people. Psychotic disorders in adolescents are similar to schizophrenic and manic-depressive psychoses in adults. The schizophrenic reactions are not sufficiently differentiated in their symptomatic manifestations to warrant classifying them in the adult subtypes of simple (inadequate), hebephrenic, catatonic and paranoid schizophrenia. Psychotic clinical patterns may also be caused by organic brain lesions, such as brain tumor, and by toxic effects of an infectious illness.

When the diagnosis of psychotic disorder has been made or is suspected, immediate psychiatric consultation is indicated. Hospitalization is usually necessary both for the protection of the child and of the family and in order to carry out treatment measures.

PSYCHOLOGIC DISORDERS ASSOCIATED WITH ORGANIC BRAIN DAMAGE

An organic disorder (see also p. 110) may be the principal factor in the origin of a psychologic disorder in some instances, whereas in others an organic and psychologic disorder may exist in the same child with little or no relation in terms of cause and effect. The basis for a diagnosis of a psychologic disorder in this category therefore is the same as in each of the 6 preceding categories, but is complicated by the necessity of having to evaluate the significance of the organic problem as to its possible causative role in the psychologic disorder and its current influence on the child's adaptation and behavior.

An organic defect or problem in the child is likely to stir up latent guilt feelings and neurotic conflicts in otherwise well adjusted parents. They may lose their objectivity and behave unrealistically in their attempt to meet the needs of the child. They may be unnecessarily overprotective and overindulgent, thus interfering with maximum development of the child's potentialities. At the other extreme they tend to deny the reality of the limitations which the organic problem poses and expect of the child achievement which is impossible.

The parents need to have an opportunity to discuss their reactions, feelings and concerns about the child. The perceptive physician can serve an important role in preventing the parents from repressing their feelings and denying reality.

CALVIN F. SETTLAGE

REFERENCES

Burks, H. L., and Harrison, S. I.: Aggressive Behavior as a Means of Avoiding Depression. *Am. J. Orthopsychiat.,* 32:416, 1962.

Chess, S., Thomas, T., and Birch, H. G.: Behavior Problems Revisited. *J. Am. Acad. Child. Psychiat.,* 6:321, 1967.

Cramer, J. B. Common Neuroses of Childhood; in S. Arieti (Ed.): *American Handbook of Psychiatry.* New York, Basic Books, Inc., 1959, Vol. 1, p. 797.

Cutter, A. V., and Hallowitz, D.: Diagnosis and Treatment of the Family Unit with Respect to the Character-Disordered Youngster. *J. Am. Acad. Child Psychiat.,* 1:605, 1962.

Finch, S. M.: *Funadamentals of Child Psychiatry.* New York, W. W. Norton & Co., 1960.

Finch, S. M., and Hess, J. H.: Ulcerative Colitis in Children. *Am. J. Psychiat.,* 118:819, 1962.

Freud, A.: Assessment of Childhood Disturbances; in *Psychoanalytic Study of the Child.* New York, International Universities Press, 1962, Vol. XVII, pp. 149-58.

Hartmann, H.: Psychoanalysis and Developmental Psychology;

in *Psychoanalytic Study of the Child.* New York, International Universities Press, 1950, Vol. V, pp. 7-17.

Johnson, A. M.: Juvenile Delinquency; in S. Arieti (Ed.): *American Handbook of Psychiatry.* New York, Basic Books, Inc., 1959, Vol. 1, p. 840.

Kahn, J. H., and Nursten, J. P.: School Refusal: A Comprehensive View of School Phobia and Other Failures of School Attendance. *Am. J. Orthopsychiat.,* 32:707, 1962.

Kanner, L.: *Child Psychiatry.* 2nd ed. Springfield, Ill., Charles C Thomas, 1948.

Kanner, L.: Early Infantile Autism. *Am. J. Orthopsychiat.,* 19: 416, 1949.

MacKeith, R., and Sandler, J. (Eds.): *Psychosomatic Aspects of Paediatrics.* Pergamon Press, 1961.

Mahler, M. S.: Ego Psychology Applied to Behavior Problems; in N. D. C. Lewis and B. L. Pacella: *Modern Trends in Child Psychiatry.* New York, International Universities Press, 1949, pp. 43-56.

Mahler, M. S., Furer, M., and Settlage, C. F.: Severe Emotional Disturbances in Childhood Psychoses; in S. Arieti (Ed.): *American Handbook of Psychiatry.* New York, Basic Books, Inc., 1959, Vol. 1, pp. 821-4.

Meyer, R., Levitt, M., Falick, M., and Rubenstein, B.: *Essentials*

of Pediatric Psychiatry. New York, Appleton-Century-Crofts, Inc., 1962.

Pearson, G. H. J.: *Emotional Disorders of Children.* New York, W. W. Norton & Co., 1949.

Prugh, D. G.: Investigations Dealing with the Reactions of Children and Families to Hospitalization in Illness: Problems and Potentialities; in G. Caplan (Ed.): *Emotional Problems of Early Childhood.* New York, Basic Books, Inc., 1955.

Ribble, M. A.: *Rights of Infants.* New York, Columbia University Press, 1943.

Settlage, C. F.: Psychoanalytic Theory in Relation to the Nosology of Childhood Psychic Disorders. *J. Am. Psychoanal. Assn.,* 12:776-801.

Spitz, R., Anaclitic Depression; in *Psychoanalytic Study of the Child.* New York, International Universities Press, 1946, Vol. II, pp. 313-42.

Spitz, R.: Hospitalism; in *Psychoanalytic Study of the Child.* New York, International Universities Press, 1945-46, Vols. I and II, Parts I and II.

Toolan, J. M.: Depression in Children and Adolescents. *Am. J. Orthopsychiat.,* 32:404, 1962.

Toolan, J. M.: Suicide and Suicidal Attempts in Children and Adolescents. *Am. J. Psychiat.,* 118:719, 1961.

THE ROLE OF THE PEDIATRICIAN IN EMOTIONAL AND BEHAVIORAL DISORDERS

There are increasing demands on the physician to be knowledgeable about the effects of the child's environment on his psychologic development, yet there often seems to be insufficient time to deal with related complex behavioral problems. If the physician elects to function in this area, it is incumbent that he develop competence in assembling and analyzing diagnostic data and in providing guidance.

PREVENTIVE PSYCHOLOGY

Active immunization of an infant against certain infectious illnesses is an accepted pediatric practice. Though comparable procedures are not so well defined for psychologic problems, there is much pertinent knowledge that each physician should be able to use in a preventive or ameliorative way through advising and working with the child or his parents.

The pediatrician, through periodic well-baby examinations and through his role in childhood illnesses, is usually the first professional person to be consulted by the parents for information and advice on child-rearing practices. Thus he has an unusual opportunity to be a particularly vital, evaluative and educative agent during infancy and the preschool period. A variety of developmental and situational crises will come to his attention which will provide him with background information of the family's patterns and of the child's reactions to them and should enable him to be helpful as a guide and counselor. What follows is an attempt (1) to point out some of the more common and important environmental or situa-

tional factors which may result in untoward deviation of the child's development, (2) to indicate means for securing background information (inquiry), and (3) to suggest some plans for guidance.

Inadequate or Excessive Stimulation. It is assumed that events occurring early in infancy have a strong impact and long-lasting effects on personality organization. For example, postpartum depression in the mother may result in a lack of adequate or appropriate stimulation for the infant during the first weeks of life which will leave a lifelong impact upon his personality. If it is observed during the initial well-baby examination that the mother does not pick up and hold and cuddle the infant or talk or vocalize or give kinesthetic stimuli to him, the pediatrician should look for the cause of these omissions. The temperament of the child also needs to be evaluated. A hypoactive infant born to an undemonstrative mother may urgently require the intervention of the physician to prevent failure to thrive or an autistic pattern. The physician can explain the importance of providing stimuli in a consistent and satisfying way, emphasizing that this is the need of this particular baby so as to avoid creating guilt in the mother. If illness in the mother or other factors such as emotional immaturity or a substandard socioeconomic condition should preclude adequate mother-child interchange, the physician should recommend substitute or supplementary mothering through other means such as a relative, a mother's helper or, in extreme cases, placement in a foster home. A home visit may be necessary to assess the adequacy of stimulation provided by maternal care or to determine who is, in fact, providing mothering, and how.

A more common problem, particularly in the

upper middle-class family, is presented by the infant who is inappropriately or unduly stimulated. This may at times lead to a kind of autistic withdrawal on the part of the infant, but the most frequent pattern is that of a fussy or colicky infant. The infant cannot organize and cope with confusing, excessive or overwhelming stimuli, and he is likely to react to a variety of stimuli such as food, touch, noise and motion with the same general responses of tension and irritability. Here the manner of the pediatrician and the personality of the mother may be vital to successful management. A quiet, authoritative explanation of the child's optimal needs will be effective only if the mother finds this explanation acceptable and supportive. If she is too anxious and disorganized to be "grandmothered" by the physician, both parents should be seen and evaluated. When their capabilities for supportive parental behavior seem borderline or inadequate, a family agency or psychiatrist should be consulted. A fussy baby is often a signal of individual trouble or marital conflict in the parents.

Early and Ill-Timed Separation of the Infant. The achievement of emotional independence and autonomy is a critical continuum in child development. Whereas the infant below 6 months of age is unaware of his separate identity and after an early normal autistic period feels at one with his mother, in the second half of his first year he becomes increasingly aware of his own identity and shows anxiety at separation from the mother or the approach of strangers. With the development of locomotion and speech the child also learns that he as well as his mother can go and come, and he develops rudimentary mastery over separations from her. He does not gain confidence in his mother and environment or in his own autonomy until about age two. If during the period from about 6 to 24 months the infant's mother is absent physically or disconnected psychologically for a significant period of time, the establishment of trust is impaired. Psychologic separation can be mediated through the mother's depressive illness, the transfer of her interest to a new pregnancy or to some external stress. These situations may be sensed by the child as relative separation. If such separation is poorly mastered, there will be pathologic reverberations in subsequent critical separations, e.g. when the child first goes to school and again during adolescence. The pediatrician can advise the mother to avoid undesirable separations during infancy. When the mother is ill or hospitalized or the infant must be hospitalized, supplementary mothering should be arranged. No verbal preparation is of any use for children under the age of 3 years; the child with only rudimentary speech and cognitive functions cannot comprehend the meaning of the separation. When mothering has been shared by another person in the home, the absence of one may be less traumatic than when the child is dependent on a single person.

An important corollary of this concept of prevention of trauma due to separation is that regular and brief separations are necessary for the infant to achieve independence. Mothers should be encouraged to leave their infants at times with a competent substitute and to increase the frequency during the second year of life. The hovering mother may prevent immunization against separation anxiety and end up with a clinging, emotionally immature child. The reasons for such hovering must be sought. Inappropriate concern with the physical health of the child may contribute to the underlying problem and may be reinforced by the physician's failure to differentiate clearly the various needs of the child. For example, during an illness of the infant the anxiety of the parent is an integral part of the total medical problem which requires management by the physician— in this case an adequate explanation of the expected course of the illness. The parents need guidance in providing for the child's sufficient care without being oversolicitous. Otherwise the infant may become conditioned to use unduly psychosomatic means to secure attention for the satisfaction of his usual needs.

Attention should be given to the family's sleeping patterns; they too may militate against the establishment of the infant's autonomy. Parents who constantly accede to their children's bed-hopping are not conveying firmly and clearly the child's basic need to be separate. The parents' ambivalence about the child's nighttime fears may become evident, and parent and child thus mutually reinforce each other's anxieties.

Development of the Child's Self-Control System. If parents commonly complain to the pediatrician about their child's behavior, this reflects the problem of the child's development of an inner control system. The infant and the young child need to develop the capacity to make value judgments (superego) and a sufficient pliability to avoid excessive conflicts between their basic urges and an increasingly internalized system of do's and don't's derived from their parents and others in their environment. Out of rudimentary capacity for understanding the no-yes axis developed by about 1 to 2 years of age, through the establishment of locomotion and sphincter control, the child can develop his own age-appropriate discipline only if the parents are themselves disciplined, and present, consistently, love, firmness and an appropriate system of expectations. Parental discipline, punishment and reward should be administered as nearly as possible in the parents' own natural and comfortable style, but with regularity and within a context of genuine concern and love. The pediatrician can help the parent to interpret behavior as a means of communication which initially is unconscious to the child. Management of unacceptable behavior at the age of one may consist of appropriate conditioning of the infant, whereas by the age of 3 years, with verbalization possible, such behavior must be interpreted in verbal terms so that both the child and his parents understand that he is expressing a wish or anger, or both. Such a plan helps the child achieve increasing control of his actions, since he can accept and understand his anger and find more self-satisfying and acceptable ways of expressing it.

Parents who seem overconcerned with control of behavior are usually too rigid in their own self-expectations. They may not interfere in a developing situation soon enough or effectively enough to make it clear to the child what is expected, and when they do move in, they overreact, thus confusing the child. Another common problem arises when one parent plays the role of disciplinarian, the other that of defender. In such instances the parents may become extremely angry with each other and, without really understanding what is taking place, express their dissatisfaction less toward each other than toward the child. The child then behaves erratically, hoping that someone will explain the situation. A meeting of the pediatrician with both parents can be effective in working out a compromise approach which is practical and satisfactory to both. Some parents seem unduly lackadaisical about providing limits for the behavior of their children. Such patterns often reflect a reaction to their own unduly controlled upbringing. It is essential for the pediatrician to recognize acceptable differences in patterns of child-rearing. Whether a given pattern differs greatly from what the pediatrician might choose for his own family is much less important than the effectiveness and the consistency with which it is communicated and enforced.

Lack of Affectional Play with Siblings and Peers. There are no convincing data which define an optimal size of a family, nor any recognized advantages to an ordinal position within a sibship. Much acquired behavior, however, even in the preschool years, stems from a child's relations with siblings of various ages. The "only child" may require a more nearly optimal relation with parents than when there are sibs that help out. Children commonly unburden a great deal of feeling to their sibs which they cannot direct to their parents. Parents must be able to tolerate rough and tumble play between young children and thus allow them to experiment with aggression and affect within the accepting and safe atmosphere of the family. The child must have confidence that the parent will not let things go too far. Unless sibling rivalry is so intense as to be out of proportion to other aspects of the child's life, it can permit and foster maturation of the child's interpersonal skills.

Several common clinical problems are related to this aspect of the child's development. A mother may complain that her boy (girls seem not to suffer this problem in the same way) has few if any friends, seems shy, almost effeminate in his manner, and yet may be critical and a nag at home. Often it is rationalized that there are no boys in the neighborhood with whom he can play. There may be some physical symptoms or possibly enuresis. Careful listening indicates, in many cases, that the mother clearly communicated her dis-

comfort with the child's early mock fighting behavior. Some shy and undemonstrative parents may themselves be quite uncomfortable with their aggressive or love feelings toward others. The only child, the invalid child or the retarded child may have more need of open, emotive and gregarious parents than the healthy child who has siblings. It may be critically important for the pediatrician to guide the parents in finding supplemental help for the child to learn about exchanging feelings with others. The parents may need to work hard at arranging group experiences for the child even before his entrance into school. They need to appreciate the importance of leaving the child on his own with others and to know that this is not rejection, but an effort to promote healthy growth.

Severe Psychologic Trauma Such as That of Death and Serious Illness. The physician is often the principal support in situations in which a child must suddenly reorganize his life, owing to the death of a parent or sibling or because he himself may have become chronically or seriously ill. The physician must have his own feelings under control and in perspective. During the phase of shock immediately after the loss of a parent or sibling the child's manner of coping with the situation may need to be accepted. Such reactions may be those of denial, apathetic withdrawal or open grief. If disabling symptoms occur, such as hallucinations or insomnia, these can be ameliorated with tranquilizers and quiet support. There follows a transitional phase during which the child begins to adapt to the new situation and to master the overwhelming anxiety created by the trauma. Initially there is a need for basic parental support. If the surviving parent or parents are unable to function because of their own grief, a capable relative, neighbor or homemaker should be brought in. Then the real nature of the event and its causes, so far as they are known, should be explained to the child. This information can be presented by the physician or parent in simple terms and in an increasingly complete perspective. There is no advantage in shielding the child either from information of the event or from the parents' own emotional reactions to it. Such explanation may lessen the universal tendency for the child to assume that he is somehow to blame. He should know the facts so that he can, in time, separate his unrealistic feelings of guilt from his more reasonable reaction of grief.

In addition to the presentation of the facts to the child, he should be encouraged to express his thoughts in words or play. It is of course important not to discourage the expression of the normal feelings of grief. Unless the mourning process takes place, the final phase of re-adaptation is often more or less permanently tinged with behavioral and regressive phenomena such as not learning in school, bedwetting and hypochondriacal concern with his physical well-being. The pediatrician should not hesitate to question the parent or child in subsequent meetings about their feelings regarding the traumatic event. When done supportively, such communication can help the parents understand that the complex of memories can gradually be modified to arouse decreasing anxiety.

Suicide. Before puberty, threats of suicide are infrequent. Depressive feelings are usually masked and expressed indirectly in antiparental behavior. The prepubertal child who threatens suicide is often trying to manipulate his parents, whom he knows to be vulnerable. In such a case the parents need help in providing more effective emotional support, which includes the setting of clear and definite limits without anxiety. With the pediatrician's support they can often do this. The suicidal threat should not be obsessively examined; attention should rather be focused on the causes of unhappiness in the child.

In the adolescent, suicide or its threat occurs with some frequency and is a perplexing problem. The incidence of suicides in the 15- to 19-year age group is the second highest of the 5-year age groupings. The threat must be taken seriously and psychiatric consultation arranged. Here too the threat may have a manipulative aspect, but it is an act of desperation. The adolescent with suicidal intent not only feels emotionally cut off from his parents, which is not unusual, but also, more importantly, has been unable to obtain acceptance from other adults or from his peer group. The physician must try to gain or regain the confidence of the adolescent so that he can provide a verbal and emotional outlet. With the adolescent's permission a joint conference can be arranged with both parents and the patient. If hope can be created for being understood or for some action being taken to improve the situation, suicide is not as likely. When tension is high and parents are not able to give verbal support, hospitalization can provide a period of separation and a chance for the physician to get to know his patient and to secure psychiatric consultation.

Two syndromes related to suicide that need to be understood and managed in much the same manner are accident proneness and a girl's sudden sexual promiscuity. In all three cases the adolescent is expressing anger and loneliness in a self-punitive way. The girl often desires to get pregnant, thinking that this will remove her from an intolerable situation at home. A more subtle and complex variant is academic suicide, wherein the adolescent who has done well scholastically stops studying and sometimes resorts to acting out his anger by associating with a "bad crowd." The physician's role is to reduce anxiety, begin an inquiry, establish communication for the child with someone and re-establish a sense of successful mastery on the part of the child over his environment and a feeling of acceptance by his fellow human beings.

Psychosomatic Illness. Knowledgeable intervention on the part of the pediatrician can be critical for the patient with a psychosomatic illness. His management may accentuate the physical aspect of the illness, lead to a stalemate or ameliorate the disease through reduction of tension. In the first instance the physician and the patient or parents settle for a diagnosis of physical illness, avoiding or failing to recognize the psychic factors responsible for the illness. In the second instance the physician dismisses the patient with, "It's all in the mind" or, "There is nothing the matter with him." Some physicians may order an excessive number of laboratory studies to prove their point. In such situations the stalemate continues or the patient may go to another physician. In the third and desired instance the physician helps the parent and the child to translate the meaning of the symptoms at both psychologic and physiologic levels.

It is important that the child become aware of all his emotions and that he feel free to express them verbally. This capacity to understand and to respond is learned primarily by observing and by imitating parents who are comfortable in expressing their own feelings. The parent who does not want to hear the child's expression of emotional pain inhibits its verbal expression and reinforces its physical counterpart. If a normally tense and anxious child cannot admit that he is angry, he may become more keenly aware of the feelings emanating from hypomotility of the gastrointestinal tract which result in pain and diarrhea or cardiac palpitations or tics and headaches. Parents commonly find the child's anxiety or depression contagious. They identify with the affect and instead of calming the child actually heighten his discomfort. The pediatrician may commonly be used as anxiety reliever with such words as "The doctor is here, everything will be all right." If this statement rings false, it may be prophylactic for the physician to spend a short time with the parents alone, identifying their unrealistic fear for them, supporting them in what they have done and telling them what they can do further after he leaves. It should be added that talking about feelings is not helpful unless it really deals with what the parent and the child are actually feeling. The child who describes a severe pain with a bland affect should have this discrepancy pointed out. He is telling you one thing, but feeling something else.

INQUIRY, DIAGNOSIS AND TREATMENT

Perhaps the greatest area of frustration in managing emotionally and behaviorally disturbed children is the fact that the parent or physician does not know what to do. The physician's training emphasizes management rather than inquiry, and it takes effort to postpone an attempt at a technical solution of a problem until the various aspects have been put into perspective. The patient expects that on presenting a list of symptoms and submitting to a physical examination which includes x-ray and laboratory tests, diagnosis and treatment will readily follow. The patient trusts his physician and has a deeply imbedded need for him to be omniscient.

Inquiry must take these factors into account, but it must not be controlled by them. A proper inquiry will be both goal-directed and supportive. It should not ramble aimlessly, but must convey to the parent and the child that they are expected to be involved in the process. Thoughts and feelings are as important to inquire about as the physical complaint itself.

Model for Inquiry. The child's life may be conceptualized as a cone. The point of the cone locates his conception. Were the parents married? What did they hope for this child? What were the physiologic and psychologic experiences of the mother during her pregnancy? What can we learn about the genetic and constitutional backgrounds? The funnel of the cone widens with increasingly complex experiences and reactions, and counterreactions to them. One can generally identify only major events as remembered and, at times, distorted by the parents; but how the parent feels or felt about what happened may be more important than the event itself. At the wide end of the cone we have a cross section of the child as he is today. There are 4 principal sources of information to help us see what the cross section looks like. First is the parent, second the child, third the physical examination and laboratory tests, and fourth the school report, which may include psychologic testing. Often other sources, such as a minister or a relative, may be helpful. These 4 sources should in turn be equated with 5 segments of the child's life.

The first segment of concern is the place of the *child in the family* and, as an extension of this, perhaps, the family in the community. What sociocultural factors impinge on this child as viewed and interpreted by the family? For example, do the parents present the child with 2 somewhat different value systems from 2 differing subcultures? How is this child seen by the parents? What is his personality like, his role in the family? How does he deal with his parents and his siblings? What are his activities at home, his sleeping and eating patterns? What is the father's occupation, and what does he do at home? Who disciplines the child, how and when? What are his responsibilities? How capable is he of attending to his personal hygiene, and so on?

The second segment represents the *child at school*. Two main areas of interest are his academic achievement and his social and emotional performance. How much discrepancy is there between the parents', the child's and the teacher's view of him? Intelligence quotient and achievement tests can help in estimating whether he is, in fact, learning up to his capacity. By viewing his report card one can determine whether he is letting his teacher know how much he knows. Is he isolated, teased, or an activist at school?

The third segment is the *child at play*. What does he do, think and feel during the time he is not directly engaged with the family or in school? How much independence and self-control can he manifest? In the older child some of this time is taken up with work or other activity that he has chosen or that he has been involved in by his family. Is he hanging out with a bad crowd, is he staying out late at night, and so on? What are the family's rules for management of the social segment of the child's time? Is the child aware of them, are they consistent and are they enforced?

The fourth segment is the *child's inner life*. What does it reveal about his developing personality structure? What does he think about or feel in relation to what he says and does? Is he essentially pleased with himself, or does he have a poor self-image? What, if anything, does he plan for the future, and how realistic is it in terms of his age? To understand these aspects one must understand the cognitive as well as the emotional development of the child. For instance, not until the age of 8 years is a child capable of understanding the concept of death except in a "going away" sort of way, nor can the child before 12 or 13 years really be expected to use abstract reasoning. What are his worries, what makes him sad, and how does he feel about anger and its expression? Does he daydream or remember night dreams? What does he think about as he falls asleep at night? This kind of information cannot be determined for the most part from anyone other than the child. Further, the child must have achieved enough rapport with the physician to permit a conversational interview in order for him to reveal these aspects of himself.

The fifth segment represents the *physical and physiologic dimensions of the child*. Here the physician generally feels at home, but often the relation of this sector to the other four is difficult to elucidate. For instance, to what extent might a petit mal convulsive state be related to a poor capacity for physical or social competition with other children at school? Is the child's "dull attitude" in school related to insufficient sleep, a mild anemia or hypoglycemia or a defense against unmastered anxiety?

Special Problems of Inquiry. Even with such a model as a framework on which to build an understanding of the child, there remains the problem of knowing how to set it up, how to weigh the importance of the information gathered and how to synthesize it into a usable diagnosis. This process is learned through clinical experience, but *even the experienced physician enters the inquiry with certain biases of his own which he should recognize and compensate for.* Many pediatricians, for example, raise an emotional flag at the first evidence of an overprotective mother, whatever that may mean to them. Too early an attempt to separate such a mother from her child may tend to inhibit seeing the part of the child that might stimulate such maternal overconcern. A more organically oriented physician notes the high fever in early life, suspects subclinical encephalitis, and sees in a hyperactive child a postencephalitic syndrome, ignoring the experiential factors leading to the child's behavioral pattern.

A useful method of inquiry is the *family interview*. The pediatrician, either at the patient's home or in his office, sits down with the whole family and discusses the problem and its ramifications. He observes the interaction of the group and identifies patterns of family functioning. Once a beginning has been made toward a psychosocial estimate of the child, seeing him with the whole family can provide information as to how he (the child) is seen by members of the family and how he deals with them. A mother's overprotectiveness may be seen as part of the struggle of wills with a passive or subtly stimulating father. Siblings may reveal a point of view neither parent nor the child patient could admit to. More importantly, this confrontation with each other may be the beginning of a psychotherapeutic experience for the family. First, it shifts the focus from the "mechanics" of examining the child to a view of the whole family's effect on the child and his symptomatology. Secondly, this may be their first experience in sitting down together with a neutral but concerned physician to examine themselves. This can help them clarify how they function and their use of or reaction to illness. For the not too disorganized family, this can be the beginning of a pattern which they can perpetuate themselves.

Another step in the art of acquiring information is *learning to listen to the right material.* With the compulsive talker active interruption and direction must be almost continuous. With the very anxious parent active emotional support and helpful questioning must be supplied by the physician. It is often helpful to interrupt a rather unproductive question-answer dialogue by remarking on the difficulty the parent is having in freely expressing himself. Sometimes behind the superficial content of answers is an unvoiced fear that the child is retarded, has cancer, or will have the social or emotional problems of some relative. If this fear can be overcome, a flow of more meaningful information will ensue.

Shifting from one level of interaction to another is important. If the child is present while the physician and the mother are talking, a sudden question to the child or remark on his nonverbal responses (e.g. his sour look) can often uncover important information. The more free the physician can be in verbalizing his own observations of nonverbal response (for instance, "You're smiling as you tell me that"), the more free will the family be in divulging their thoughts. Such techniques shift the level of interaction from a question-and-answer session to a conversation and therefore to fuller interaction.

The interview with the child deserves special consideration. Adolescents in conflict with parents and struggling for independence are best seen alone as early in the inquiry as possible, perhaps even before the parents are seen. For instance, if the parent calls about acne or a behavioral problem, the physician may suggest that the son or daughter come alone for the examination. Such a visit can help to gain the confidence of the adolescent and convey your respect for and concern with what he or she is feeling. You can then plan with him later contacts with other members of the family. A neutral position in reference to the adolescent and his parents must of course be maintained. When discussing plans for helping with a problem, the adolescent and his parents should be seen together. With the younger child of school age, the interview with the child can be revealing only if the pediatrician can chat with the child about those areas he feels free or enthusiastic to talk about. Focusing on "the problem" is usually unfruitful. The preschool child is usually seen with the parent, and the interactions are noted. A brief separation may help assess the degree of anxiety the child experiences and how he handles it, or how quickly he adapts to being alone with the physician. The mother's difficulty in leaving her child with the physician is also worthy of note.

Diagnosis. The diagnosis should be functional. Conventional psychiatric diagnostic nomenclature is not necessarily helpful for the general physician. In the preceding section a series of diagnostic categories are presented and arranged in accord with the degree of disturbance or disorganization of personality. Identification of the child in one of these categories is intended to help in the synthesis of the information gained through the inquiry, but does not necessarily give a ready guide to management.

There are 4 principal diagnostic categories. These are presented in order of increasing severity: (1) *Reactions to environment and biologic development* (situational and developmental disorders). Here the inquiry reveals problems of relatively short duration which have occurred in relation to obvious environmental disturbances (e.g. the birth of a sibling or concern around a developmental milestone, such as stuttering in a 3-year-old child whose speech is developing normally). (2) *Neurotic disorders*: children with these disorders may be doing well in several sectors of their activities (e.g. in academic and family ones), but they have a circumscribed maladaptation which seems internalized. The antecedents, whatever they may have been, no longer seem evident or indeed necessary for the persistence of such symptoms as a phobia or an obsessive ritual. A large question is whether a neurotic disorder has progressed to the next more serious category. There is a tendency, unless remission occurs, for other areas of the patient's life to become involved in the neurotic process. If a child with a fear of loud noises, for example, begins to avoid playing with peers or feels unduly anxious in school, his social and academic life will suffer. (3) *Character or personality disorders:* The child with a character or personality disorder is no longer aware of his original discomfort, but has developed certain character traits such as passivity or rebelliousness which tend to protect him from his underlying conflicts. Although the child may appear unhappy, and his family and peers certainly are unhappy with him, he now feels that his personality, with its pathologic adaptations, is the way he wants it to be. The child often has a poor self-image, but may see no inconsistency in his self-destructive behavior. The phobic child can see the irrationality of his phobia, whereas the child with a characterologic problem tends to rationalize or to project the blame on others. The more disorganized members of this group operate poorly, use poor judgment and seem quite erratic. They demonstrate inappropriate feeling and behavior. (4) *A psychotic* or *severely disturbed child* is relatively easy to identify by his obviously bizarre behavior. He may have poor appreciation of reality, poor control over his impulses, or be dissociated from people. It is more difficult to determine what factors were involved in the development of this severe disturbance or how one goes about correcting the pathologic state. It is often difficult to know how much of the disturbance is related to genetic factors and how much to environmental mishandling. Regardless of the cause, this group of children tend to have the same pattern of retardation in many areas of ego development: in speech, ability to relate, flexibility, attention span, capacity to withstand frustration, and the like. The younger the child, the more difficult the diagnosis, since some areas of development which appear precocious (e.g. the intellect) may mask the more important basic immaturity in the child's ability to relate socially. The so-called idiot savant is an extreme example of this situation. He can do complex mathematical problems or may have an amazing ability to memorize, yet he has for the most part no capacity for or interest in meaningful human relations.

Treatment. Readers who come initially to this section for therapeutic suggestions for their disturbed patient miss the first step in therapy: the evaluative process. It is well recognized in child psychiatry clinics that many patients improve by the time the evaluation is complete; social workers have called it "the process." Questions which parents and child have been asked, the supportive interest they have been shown, the feeling that someone of competence is overseeing the problem and going to help: all these and other factors have an alleviative, if not a curative, effect. The young physician usually underrates the value of his interest and of his willingness to listen to a confused parent or unhappy, distressful child. He feels that "he is not doing anything," and sometimes finds it difficult to charge a fee for his time in this effort.

If a proper inquiry has been made, not only the child and his mother, but also the father and perhaps the entire family have been seen. The critical question now is: What do you tell the parents and the child?

The playback. Initially the physician restates, in the family's language, the problem as he understands it, and reviews the important factors bearing on its development and perpetuation and allays the worries of the family which are not pertinent to it. For instance, "Your child has no

evidence of neurologic deficit, cancer or defective genes." Such worries may not have been fully evident to the parents and should be identified for them. Further, it is helpful to be objective in admitting gaps in your understanding. This may help the parents to shed further light which they have been loath to bring to bear on the investigation. It helps them achieve the position of co-investigator rather than passive recipient.

Altering the immediate environment. The next step is to make any obvious suggestions which will help re-establish the child's psychologic equilibrium. This is often an *educative maneuver* in that the parents learn something they had not known. For instance, the child's angry behavior may now be interpreted as an obvious request for firmer and more consistent control from parents who can now agree on a pattern of discipline. The parents may have unconsciously resisted providing this control, owing to their own inner conflict or misunderstanding or may have assumed that to be loving is to give in to the child. If the inquiry has properly exposed the parents' mixed feelings toward a wayward child, he may now for the first time begin to understand that his parents really do care, but have not been able to communicate it to him. The child may also begin to appreciate and find that there are better ways to ask for what he needs than what he has been doing.

It may be educative or re-educative to explain how developmental stresses determine the emergence of new problems. For example, a diabetic boy who at puberty suddenly rebels against his disease can be dealt with more understandingly if his desires to be just like the rest of his group and to begin to separate from his parents are recognized. It is important to *stress the positive aspects* of parental behavior as well as the strengths of the child, but without exaggeration or pretense. If the parents feel less guilty and not overwhelmed, they have a more solid position from which to operate. The light touch can often help parents to feel less anxious. For instance, it can be suggested that a mild obsessive ritual may be an effort to control anxiety which to some extent is preferable to poorly controlled behavior. Meanwhile the physician is obligated to continue his search for the origin and nature of the tensions which cause the anxiety.

It is helpful for the parents to understand that *some anxiety is normal in children* and plays a part in forming character. On the other hand, when the family is disabled by anxiety, there are several techniques to reduce it. Some reduction is attained by the physician's supportive interest and reassurance, and subsequent brief visits help the family to maintain this feeling of support. The impulsive, poorly organized child often gains added control from repeated visits to the physician. It is perhaps more anxiety-provoking for a child to have loose parental control than to be rigidly controlled. This point is often poorly understood by parents who need only to be encouraged by the physician to take a firmer stand.

Drugs. The prescription of drugs to lessen anxiety will help most when they are part of a comprehensive approach. Positive expectation on the part of the prescribing physician seems to be helpful. In the more disorganized child and especially the younger one, barbiturates are not reliable; they often promote a paradoxical increase in the child's anxiety and in his disruptive behavior. It is probably best for the physician to become acquainted with one or two of the tranquilizers and use those exclusively. For example, thioridazine (Mellaril) is often helpful in reducing hyperactivity and severe anxiety and may be given in doses of 25 mg. 2 to 4 times a day. Phenothiazines are effective in severely disturbed children. Diphenhydramine (Benadryl) is one of the oldest and safest drugs for control of anxiety with attendant impulsive behavior. It is generally stated that its benefits are more pronounced in children below the age of 10 years. Amphetamine has been used to quiet the impulsive hyperkinetic child; it is found effective by many physicians, though reports as to its general usefulness are conflicting. It is usually given in the morning in a single dose of 5 mg., which may be increased if needed to 10 to 15 mg. per day.

Separation. Separation of a child from his family is never to be taken lightly. There are times, however, when for purely psychosocial reasons, just as for physical illness, anxiety of separation seems to be the lesser of 2 evils. The adolescent in crisis with his parents may need a brief separation from home to become less anxious and more capable of rational planning. He may be admitted briefly to a hospital, particularly if there is a somatic concomitant that needs management, or a brief visit with a friend or relative may be arranged. In either case it is important for the pediatrician to maintain communication between the parents and the adolescent, to provide a working plan with them for reunion and, if necessary, to lay the basis for referral to a psychiatrist.

The child and his mother who are in a deeply embedded conflict which often accompanies a psychosomatic illness can benefit from separation. The physician can use the diagnostic potential of brief hospitalization not just to secure laboratory and x-ray studies, but to observe the child's symptoms in a different and more neutral environment. Wheezing, abdominal pain and diarrhea are often lessened and may disappear or become clearly related to parental visits. This kind of observation can help, if properly used, in explaining to the family the importance of emotion in the psychosomatic state. It can also provide a setting for the psychiatric consultant.

There are times when the disorganization of the family or evidence of willful trauma (the battered-child syndrome) suggests the need for protracted periods of placement of the child in a more nurturant setting. Here the pediatrician should work with a social agency in evaluating the home situation and in identifying possible resources for placement of the child outside the home. All reasonable efforts should be made to rehabilitate the family, particularly since the child's need to maintain identification with his own family is a strong element in his subsequent development. There are times when a severely mentally ill or retarded child needs a special therapeutic setting in order to develop more adequately. In such a case the services of a psychiatrist and a psychologist will be needed to evaluate the child and plan the therapeutic program. There is a trend toward the development of day-care programs for severely disturbed children so that they can remain with their family.

Referral for psychiatric management. As the process of inquiry and management outlined above evolves, psychiatric referral may at any point become an obvious and acceptable necessity. In some cases it may be obvious at the time of the initial inquiry, owing to the severity of the problem. Occasionally, despite the severity of the illness, the family may resist the idea of psychiatric help. In this case the pediatrician must provide interim management. He will have a chance to help the parents develop better understanding of the need for examining all aspects of the child's difficulty and to explain the potential of a psychiatric consultation. As with any referral, it is important to acquaint the consulting psychiatrist, psychologist or psychiatric clinic with the relevant data before the patient's first appointment. In preparing the family for the referral it is helpful to explain that the psychiatrist may wish to talk individually with the parents and the child. The family with appropriate management by the referring pediatrician will not interpret the referral as a rejection, but as a move toward getting specialized help in evaluation and treatment. The referring physician should emphasize his readiness to continue to be helpful in any appropriate way. His continued interest and concern will be supportive for the child and his family in their new relation with the psychiatrist or mental health team.

JOHN MALCOLM DUNN

DISORDERS OF COMMUNICATION

HEARING DISORDERS

Hearing is the principal sensory pathway through which speech and verbal communication develop. Learning and other aspects of maturation are also influenced by hearing. Since impairment of hearing, even of mild degree, may significantly hinder the development of the child, early diagnosis is essential. Impaired hearing, however, may not be obvious, and the child may not express his difficulty; accordingly, the diagnosis is often delayed.

General Considerations of Hearing. The human ear responds to frequencies of sound ranging from 20 to 20,000 hertz (cycles per second), but receives speech and most environmental sounds in the frequency range of 250 to 4000 hertz at varying levels of intensity (loudness). Impairments of hearing affect both the intensity and the frequency of sound as it is perceived through the auditory apparatus.

In some hearing impairments the main deficiency is a reduction in the loudness of sound. If a moderate reduction is even or nearly even throughout the frequency range, speech sounds are muffled, but otherwise are not distorted in clarity and there is little difficulty in discrimination of their meaning.

The clarity of sounds is determined by both their intensity and their frequency spectrum. If certain frequencies are perceived less perfectly than others, speech sounds may be distorted and the discrimination of their meaning is difficult.

The severity of the handicap imposed by a hearing impairment depends upon which components of sound are primarily affected and to what degree. In general the younger the child is affected, the greater is the functional disability.

Measurement of Hearing and Classification of Hearing Disorders. The measurement of hearing acuity is concerned with (1) the intensity level at which sounds are perceived and (2) the ability of the person to discriminate and recognize the meaning of complex sounds, particularly those of speech.

Perception of sound is measured by delivery to the auditory apparatus of pure tones at specific frequencies from a standardized audiometer. Intensity is designated in terms of decibels. The tone is delivered to the external auditory canal to measure air conduction and to the mastoid tip to measure bone conduction. Normally the levels of perception by the 2 routes are equal, as measured by the audiometer. In certain instances, such as when disease involves the middle ear, air conduction will be diminished in comparison with bone conduction. Whenever the air conduction and bone conduction are about equally involved in hearing loss, this finding is suggestive of a sensorineural defect.

For measurement of discrimination between individual sounds, techniques other than pure-tone audiometry must be used. A variety of tests have been developed to measure speech reception threshold (the least intensity level at which words are heard) and speech discrimination (the ability to make fine phonetic discriminations). Other types of hearing tests have been developed to aid in delineation of the exact nature and severity of hearing impairments.

Impairments of hearing are difficult to classify, since many variables are involved. Designations such as "hard of hearing" or "deaf" have led to confusion, both among the public and among physicians. The important consideration must be the effect of a hearing impairment on the functioning of the child as a whole.

If a person perceives sound at hearing levels of 0 to 20 decibels at all the frequencies commonly tested in the human speech range, hearing is considered to be normal. If greater than 20 decibels are required for perception of sound at any frequency level in the speech range (500 to 4000 hertz) or if there is any difficulty in discrimination of sound, hearing is considered abnormal. With losses between 20 and 30 decibels (mild loss) speech reception becomes difficult, and the person must strain to hear. With losses of 40 decibels (moderate) or more, only the loudness peaks of conversational speech can be heard, and speech reception becomes virtually impossible without amplification or lip reading.

Hearing cannot be classified in terms of decibels alone. If certain frequencies are affected more than others, speech sounds are distorted. The high-frequency sounds of speech are most commonly affected, and misunderstanding of words results. The problem becomes not so much that speech cannot be heard, but that it cannot be translated.

Even in the so-called deaf child with the most profound impairment of hearing, some residual hearing is generally present, particularly in the low frequencies. This fact has important implications for the use of amplification and in the education of these children.

Types of Hearing Defects. *Conductive defects.* Conductive defects result most commonly from pathologic changes in the middle ear. These include congenital or acquired abnormalities of the ossicles, the presence of fluid, adhesions or other material in the middle ear, and congenital atresia or other obstructions of the external canal. Conductive defects are the most common of hearing impairments in children. They are most often of mild degree and are amenable to medical or surgical therapy.

In conductive defects, reception of sound at most frequencies is affected to essentially the same degree. The main effect on sound is a reduction in loudness, but clarity is not distorted. Mild conductive losses frequently remain undetected, particularly when the loss is unilateral.

Sensorineural defects. Sensorineural defects result from abnormalities of the inner ear or the auditory nerve. High frequencies tend to be more affected than low tones, but, with more severe involvement, acuity for both high and low tones is involved. In any event, sounds appear distorted and discrimination is impaired.

Sensorineural defects generally result in a greater handicap to communication than do the conductive losses. They are rarely amenable to medical or surgical therapy.

Central auditory defects. Central auditory defects are extremely complex, and their cause and pathogenesis poorly understood. The peripheral auditory apparatus appears to convey stimuli adequately, and the child seems to be aware of sound, but unable to discriminate its meaning.

The incidence of central auditory dysfunction may be increasing as many children survive various formerly fatal perinatal conditions with impairment of certain sensory functions. Moreover, many lifesaving drugs may affect the auditory system. Central auditory defects cause severe problems in communication.

Psychogenic loss of hearing. Apparent loss of hearing of psychogenic origin is not uncommon and is often difficult to differentiate from that due to organic causes. The patient commonly presents exaggerated symptoms of hearing impairment, which may be unilateral or bilateral. There is often a history of prior ear infections or of preexisting organic loss of hearing; the ear thus appears to act as a "shock organ" for localization of the psychic symptoms. It is of the utmost importance that malingering be distinguished from pure psychogenic impairment. Appropriate specialized audiologic techniques combined with careful clinical appraisal can usually make the differentiation possible.

Etiology of Hearing Defects. Hearing defects may be *congenital,* including heritable types, or *acquired.* The conductive and the sensorineural defects have, for the most part, different causations.

Inherited defects. An increasing number of hearing defects, particularly of the sensorineural type, are known to be genetically determined. Despite genetic transmission, the defect may not express itself until late in life. Thorough investigation of families with history of hearing defects is essential. Many defects are associated with other disorders, such as pigmentary defects, or renal or thyroid disease. Some heritable disorders may be associated with abnormalities of the external ear or ear canal which lead to conductive losses.

Prenatal or perinatal factors. Rubella in the early months of pregnancy, and possibly other maternal infections of viral or other origins may affect the auditory system of the fetus. Bilirubin encephalopathy (kernicterus) has a predilection for damage to the auditory system. Premature and other low-birth-weight infants and infants suffering from trauma or hypoxia at birth are at high risk for the development of hearing defects.

Acquired defects. Most conductive defects are acquired, most commonly from the accumulation of fluid in the middle ear. This fluid may result from repeated infections of the middle ear, may be associated with respiratory allergy or may stem from other causes. It may lead to adhesions or even to destruction of the ossicular chain.

Sensorineural defects also may be acquired. Hearing impairment may be a sequel of meningitis, and of certain viral infections and of mumps in particular.

Certain drugs such as dihydrostreptomycin, streptomycin and kanamycin have specific ototoxic effects, which may be greater in infants than in older children, owing to increased susceptibility of the developing auditory system.

Diagnosis of Hearing Impairments. The diagnosis of impaired hearing may be difficult. Children rarely complain of difficulty in hearing, and even those with the most profound impairments compensate for their defects in many ways. Essential to the diagnosis are a high degree of suspicion on the part of the physician, and an awareness that certain children are at high risk for the development of hearing disorders.

In addition to clinical evaluation, the detection of impaired hearing is aided by audiometric screening techniques. The definitive diagnosis of the exact nature and severity of a hearing defect is dependent upon the use of specialized audiologic procedures.

Clinical diagnosis. Conductive defects may be present in infancy, but most commonly they are not manifested until the child is older. The loss of hearing is usually of mild to moderate degree.

In the younger child the presenting complaint is often that the child pays little attention to the parents' commands. A frequent explanation for his behavior is that he is stubborn or that he is "normal and will outgrow it." Conductive defects in the younger age group are undoubtedly more common than is recognized.

In the older child, hearing difficulty may be first suspected by the parents or detected by audiometric screening examination in school or in the office. The signs of a hearing defect are, however, frequently unrecognized by parents or by others. Even on direct questioning the child with a hearing loss may deny difficulty. The presenting symptoms may be scholastic difficulty, inattentiveness, or change in personality. If the loss of hearing remains unrecognized, the symptoms will become more severe, with distressing consequences to the child.

Speech disturbances due to conductive defects are less common than those due to sensorineural losses. If the hearing loss has existed from infancy, however, a speech disorder may result.

Detection of mild to moderate conductive losses

by clinical evaluation alone is difficult. The child's ability to hear speech at close range does not rule out a handicapping hearing loss. For example, a child with only a 20 to 25 decibel loss is able to hear conversational voice in a face-to-face situation. Under other conditions, as in a large classroom, this same degree of loss will prevent him from hearing adequately. Furthermore, the loss of hearing may be unilateral, making its detection even more difficult.

A history of chronic nasal obstruction, of recurrent otitis media or of persistently abnormal appearance of the tympanic membranes suggests the possibility of a conductive defect.

Since sensorineural defects, in general, produce more severe losses of hearing than do the conductive ones, it would seem that their detection should be more obvious, but this is not the case. The sensorineural defects may be of mild to moderate degree and may be unilateral; in such instances the symptomatology and the differential diagnostic considerations are similar to those of the conductive defects.

Because sensorineural losses of hearing may involve only certain frequencies, the child may respond to most sounds at ordinary levels of loudness. He may fail to hear only high-pitched sounds. This kind of loss is least understood by parents and teachers, and it is not uncommon to find high-frequency losses in children previously thought to have normal hearing.

A most important factor in diagnosis of a hearing defect, besides its severity, is its time of onset. If hearing loss of moderate to profound degree is present before the acquisition of speech, the presenting symptom will likely be failure to speak, or delayed or distorted speech. If the loss occurs after acquisition of speech, other symptoms will predominate. In any instance of delayed or distorted speech, however, the presence of an auditory defect must be considered.

A common pitfall in evaluation of losses of hearing in infants is the history that the child said words at one time. Even the deaf child may exhibit reflex babbling in the first months of life. This babbling may include such sounds as "ma ma," "da da" and "ba," which may be interpreted as meaningful words. Babbling tends to decrease if the hearing defect is marked, and the deaf child tends to be relatively silent after the first year of life. There is, however, variability in the amount of sound an individual deaf child makes and in the time at which he becomes more silent. The presence or absence of utterances is not, therefore, an infallible indicator of deafness.

In the older child the onset of a sensorineural defect may be manifest by an obvious decrease in auditory acuity. Commonly, however, the presenting symptoms are a decrease in scholastic achievement or change in personality. Older children with organic defects are frequently considered to be malingerers.

The clinical manifestations of the central auditory disorders may be variable. In general, they are similar to those of the child with a severe sensorineural defect.

Screening audiometry. With increasing frequency mass surveys of hearing are being instituted in the schools of the United States. These surveys utilize audiometers which deliver pure tones under standardized conditions. Children found to have losses of 20 decibels or more in one or more frequencies tested should be suspected of having a significant hearing impairment and be referred for further otologic and audiologic evaluation. Though some of these children prove to have only transient or insignificant hearing losses, these screening programs detect many children with significant losses who otherwise would have remained undetected.

Screening audiometry is also being used with increasing frequency in physicians' offices. It is of particular value in determining whether or for how long hearing loss follows otitis media and for the detection of otherwise unsuspected hearing impairment.

Pure-tone audiometry can be used with relative reliability in children from about the age of 3 years. For screening of younger children, procedures have been developed which use such sound generators as tissue paper for high tones and other appropriate noise-makers for lower tones. These procedures require that the infant's attention be first directed away from the sound source, and then the sound delivered. The infant's response is observed, such as quieting, turning toward the sound, or eye blinking. With experience the physician or a trained assistant can perform these tests with considerable reliability. If obvious responses are repeatedly obtained, it can be assumed that there is no loss of hearing sufficient to interfere with function. If the infant fails to respond, if his responses are variable, or if there is any doubt on the part of the examiner, the patient should be referred for more thorough evaluation.

In newborn and other young infants the responses produced by sound stimuli in the electroencephalogram may be a valuable means for detection of hearing impairment. This procedure has its greatest value in testing of newborn infants who are at high risk of hearing impairment, such as those born to mothers who have had rubella or other infections during pregnancy.

Definitive audiologic evaluation utilizes, besides pure-tone audiometry, speech reception and speech discrimination tests and a variety of other specialized techniques. These procedures require the services of a skilled audiologist.

Treatment. Conductive defects are mainly due to disturbances within the middle ear, and most of them are amenable to medical or surgical therapy. Appropriate treatment of acute infections of the middle ear and the prevention of chronic infections will greatly reduce the incidence of impaired hearing. Serous otitis media is probably the single most common cause. Though its etiology may be imperfectly understood, its impairment of hearing can be ameliorated (p. 899). Appropriate therapy of respiratory allergy will also reduce the incidence of conductive hearing impairments. Other causes of eustachian tube obstruction such as hypertrophied adenoids or anatomic abnormalities, although less common causes of conductive defects, must be evaluated and treated.

For children with sensorineural defects the principal aims of therapy are audiologic and educational. The management of these children requires the services of skilled specialists in many disciplines, particularly in otology, audiology, psychology and special education. Management extends over a long time, and it is essential that someone be identified who will coordinate the efforts of the various specialists involved; preferably this should be the child's physician.

Most children with moderate sensorineural defects will probably need a hearing aid, auditory training, lip reading instruction and language training. The type of amplification required can be determined only after precise audiologic evaluation, best conducted by an audiologist skilled with children. Special educational adjustments will also be required in most instances. Most affected children will be able to attend regular schools, so long as they may have continued access to special speech, language and auditory training, as necessary.

For children with more profound hearing defects special schooling may be required, but even children with profound losses, the so-called deaf children, may have reasonable expectation for achievement of normal education. Full development of this potential, however, is almost totally dependent upon early diagnosis of the hearing defect.

The management of children with central auditory dysfunctions is extremely difficult and requires extensive and prolonged individual therapy with persons especially trained to work with these problems. The prognosis for the development of adequate communication is generally guarded.

RICHARD OLMSTED

SPEECH AND LANGUAGE DEVELOPMENT AND DISORDERS

Disorders of speech and language in childhood are not uncommon. Therapy for them requires understanding of those processes involved in the normal development of speech and language function.

Development of Speech and Language. Development of speech and language skills depends upon a broad range of activities of many organ systems. The first stage, audition, requires an intact peripheral auditory mechanism. The second stage is the transmission of sound from the organs

of hearing to the brain and the organization of the transmitted impulses for a response. The third stage, the verbal response, involves respiration, phonation, resonation and articulation. A high degree of intricate cortical and neuromuscular integration is required for all these activities.

The processes involved in development of speech and language are highly vulnerable, since the organ systems on which they depend have more urgent biologic functions to serve than communication. For example, the basic function of the respiratory apparatus is gas exchange; of the larynx, air control; and of the articulators, mastication of food. These functions take precedence over those of communication, since man can function, albeit inadequately, without being able to hear or speak. Thus illness, trauma and other factors may result in disruption of the "unnecessary" function of communication, either temporarily or permanently. Awareness of this instability of the process of communication is essential to the understanding of speech and language disorders.

Normal speech and language development. Maturation of a child's speech and language normally keeps pace with the maturation of the total organism, and follows a fairly predictable pattern up to the age of about 6 years.

The early stages of speech and language development reflect the child's reception of speech sounds and are revealed by his responses to them. By 4 to 6 months the infant normally demonstrates ability to discriminate among speech sounds by beginning to babble close approximations of a number of the early consonant sounds, principally *m, n, p, b, k, g, t* and *d*. By 6 to 8 months he has learned to enjoy making these sounds, and should exhibit a rather wide repertory of babbling combinations of these consonants with a few vowels such as *ba-ba, ma-ma, da-da, goo,* and so on.

By about 9 months the child further demonstrates his ability to discriminate among various inputs by imitating changes of pitch he hears in voices around him. At the same time he also begins to attempt to imitate facial expressions and formation of sounds on the lips of people who talk to him.

At 10 to 12 months, through these processes of discriminative babbling, changes of pitch and imitation of visual and auditory sound combinations, the child begins to discover that particular combinations repeated often enough will bring about certain desirable ends. Usually among the earliest discoveries is that the combination *ma-ma* will bring his mother to pay some attention to him or to administer to some want.

By 12 months he should be using at least 1 to 3 such combinations meaningfully; i.e. he uses them to gain some specific end—usually food or attention. He will not develop meaningful use of these early combinations, however, unless they have been observed and reinforced by frequent repetition by someone near him, usually his mother.

The entire first year ideally is a "vocal play" period in which the child learns to enjoy making vocal noises, has them pleasantly reinforced, and eventually becomes able to discriminate among and make use of particular combinations for his own benefit. From these early few meaningful combinations vocabulary develops by extension of the process, new meanings being associated with the repetition of other combinations which lead to fulfillment of other needs.

Between 12 and 18 months there is relatively little demonstrated increase in the expressive vocabulary, although the child continues with a great deal of vocal play, and he may learn to use with considerable effectiveness perhaps a dozen more words by the time he is 18 months of age. During this period he is preoccupied with learning to walk and exploring his physical environment and seems not to have much time to devote to the intricacies of language production. He is, however, rapidly expanding his comprehension vocabulary and the number and variety of his responses to meaningful vocalizations of others.

By about 18 months the child has considerable mastery of locomotion and other physical activities, and there is now likely to be an acceleration of the development of speech and language. Between 18 and 24 months he begins to try to put together many of the combinations he has been hearing, and to make some sort of organized system of responses. At this time the relation of meaning to sound symbols begins to become important. Frequently what he utters during the early part of this period is a complicated, largely unintelligible jargon—sometimes so bizarre that parents are frightened by it. If all goes well, however, out of this jargon will develop 2- and 3-word phrases by the age of about 24 months. At this age the child should begin to use connected speech for a purpose, such as *go bye-bye, want cookie,* and so forth.

Comprehension of language develops more rapidly than the ability to verbalize; almost from the very beginning the child is able to understand many more words and more complicated combinations than he can use. This remains true until his adult speech pattern is established.

At the time the child begins to use connected speech, intelligibility becomes important. At 2 years 50 to 60 per cent of his words and phrases should be understood, so long as the general context of his speech effort is known.

Between the second and third birthdays, owing to his limited expressive ability and vocabulary, the child often has difficulty trying to express complicated ideas. During this period he is trying also to develop fluency and some rhythm to his speaking; but so many children are not capable of a stable rhythm until 4 or 5 that the period from 2 to 5 years has often been called the nonfluent period. It is during this time that the child, particularly the boy, may begin to say something and cannot find a word for it, so that he searches for the word, and while doing so repeats effortlessly, "I - I - I - I," or uses some other verbal stopgap. This nonfluency period may last only a few months or it may continue to about the age of 5, but it normally disappears as the child increases his vocabulary and masters syntax, general language structure, and rhythm.

Between the ages of 3 and 4 years the child becomes very conscious of the importance of speech and the power it gives him. Because his speech and language are unstable and he is nonfluent, the process of communicating easily can be interfered with, and speech troubles may have their origin during this period.

By age 3 years the child should have mastered the use of all vowels, and the consonants *w, m, n, p, b, k, g, t* and *d.* At this age he generally is 70 to 80 per cent intelligible, and uses an average of 3 words per speech attempt. At the age of 4 he should be 100 per cent intelligible and use an average of 4 words per response. At 5 years of age he should use an average of 5 words. At 5, also, he should be using some blends, such as *tr, bl, pr, gr,* and use *f, v, r* and *l* generally without error; but these may not be mastered until age 6.

At 4 years the child uses some adjectives, adverbs, prepositions and simple sentences. Articles begin to appear, and he recognizes plurals and sex differences. He generally replaces the pronoun *me* with nominative *I,* when appropriate, and uses a few other personal pronouns.

By age 6 the child's general language structure is stable, the nonfluency has passed, and he has mastered all the consonant sounds with the exception perhaps of the sibilants and sibilant combinations, primarily *s* and *z.* After 6 years, school and other social influences play such a large part in shaping the child's speech and language that it becomes increasingly difficult to relate his performance to innate developmental aspects.

It has become obvious that the preschool years are extremely important to the development of speech and language in the child, especially the first year. Many speech and language problems can be prevented if deviations are detected and treated early. Abnormal development of speech and language in the first year or two, moreover, may be the first clue to other developmental deviations.

Conditions Which May Interfere with Development of Speech and Language. Any condition which seriously impairs or disrupts the normal development of the child, physically, psychologically or socially, may disrupt the development of his speech and language skills. Among such conditions are the following:

1. *Mental retardation* is by far the most frequent associated factor in the child's failure to develop speech and language normally. The child with either generalized or specialized areas of retardation is almost certain to have a delay in achievement of speech and language skills; moreover, when these skills do develop, they may be faulty from a symbolic, structural and articulatory point of view. The degree of delay or distortion in speech and language will generally correlate with the

amount of mental retardation. Even the "educable" retarded child (I.Q. 50 to 70) exhibits relatively severe speech and language deficiencies when compared with children of normal intelligence.

2. *Prematurity* may sometimes affect preverbal achievement levels during the first year of life; but the prematurely born child of normal mentality, and without organic injury, generally begins to attain normal developmental landmarks in speech and language by the age of about 2 years.

3. *Abnormalities of neuromuscular function,* such as cerebral palsy, or *structural inadequacies,* such as cleft palate, may also profoundly distort development of language. Children with cerebral palsy and those with cleft palate are almost universally delayed rather markedly (for the first 2 or 3 years) in speech and language development, even when they have normal mentality. They also may have associated problems of hypernasality, articulation and inadequate voice.

4. *Serious illness or injury* to the child, especially during the first year, may delay or severely distort the development of speech or language. This is especially true of illnesses which require prolonged hospitalization and extensive treatment procedures.

5. *Neurologic dysfunctions,* even when unassociated with the motor disabilities of cerebral palsy, may be associated with retardation in the development of speech and language. When these skills do develop, they may be distorted by disorders of symbolic language of an aphasic nature and also by severe articulatory disorders or by inadequate voice production. The so-called congenital aphasia is typical of this kind of disorder. The child with acquired neurologic damage also may suffer from the same kinds of interference with speech and language development, but the deficiencies are likely to be more limited and localized than with the congenitally affected child.

6. Profound *deafness* always causes communication disorders, but much more frequent and more elusive than severe deafness is mild to moderate hearing loss; it is difficult to recognize, but often results in distortions of both receptive and expressive communicative skills. The child's hearing should always be investigated if there is a problem in the development of speech and language.

7. Some *dysfunction of the tongue* is commonly blamed for speech which is distorted or does not develop. The tongue is rarely responsible, however, unless there is some actual structural damage or paralysis. Tongue-tie accounts only rarely for problems of speech unless there is so much restriction of the tongue-tip that adequate articulation is not possible. In those rare instances in which the tongue, when protruded slightly beyond the lower incisors, is grooved in the middle by a tight frenulum, it may be necessary to free the tip surgically before adequate articulation can be achieved.

8. *Tongue-thrust* is a cause of articulatory problems when the thrust is strong or when the pattern is not reversed by the age of 7 or 8 years. This occurs when the tip of the tongue is forced strongly between the teeth or against the upper incisors during speaking and swallowing. This results in a forward displacement of the upper incisors, causing an interference with sibilant sounds, principally *s* and *z*. The condition can be corrected if detected before the child reaches the age of 7 or 8 years.

9. *Excessive adenoid tissue* may cause a hyponasal quality of the voice, but only rarely interferes with the development of vocabulary and intelligible speech. Equally rarely will the removal of adenoids result in improvement of the child's speech. In fact, removal occasionally may result in hypernasal speech.

10. *Social, psychologic and environmental conditions,* if severe, may interfere with speech or language development. Serious communicative and emotional disturbances such as autism or schizophrenia may result, or less severe adjustment problems involving primarily the child's inability or unwillingness to use ordinary communicative skills. Environmental stresses must be severe to interfere with language development; it is likely that well intentioned parents have often been made to feel unnecessarily guilty by professional persons who blamed them for children's communication problems lying outside their power to influence.

11. The common scapegoats of baby-talk, position in the family, "only" children, sibling rivalry, parental anxiety, or interference with speech, and the child's "not being required to talk" rarely create severe disturbances in the development of speech and language. Parental anxiety and interference may, however, contribute significantly to stuttering.

Stuttering. Stuttering certainly relates to environmental and psychosocial factors, but there are many aspects of stuttering which are not understood. There are strong emotional components in secondary stuttering, but it is not clear that these are basic causes. There is some evidence to suggest that the child who develops stuttering has a less well integrated nervous system, to which are added environmental factors with which he is unable to cope.

Stuttering often begins during the nonfluent period, between the ages of 2 and 5 years, especially in the male. Adverse psychosocial and environmental factors during this period can prolong the nonfluency until it becomes a real dysfluency, and eventually secondary stuttering.

The physician's advice to parents of the preschool child who is said to be stuttering is often to ignore it. This good advice may not be adequate, however, since it may also be necessary to instruct the parents as to *how* to ignore the speech. They must be helped to treat the child as normal, to understand that nonfluency is a normal developmental stage, and to accept the child's speech without hurrying him, without demanding repetition, and without showing concern. They must give the child full attention during his speech attempts. Approximately 99 per cent of children pass through this nonfluency period to develop stable, nonstuttering speech; many who do not would develop adequate speech if handled as described.

When the older child with strong secondary stuttering is presented to the physician, the same kind of help should be given to the parents, but every effort should be made also to refer the child to a speech pathologist or speech clinic.

Assessment and Treatment of Deviations in Development of Speech and Language. When speech or language disorder is suspected, the physician must answer such questions as, "Are the speech and language skills of this child developing within the range of normal? If not, what further studies will disclose the nature of the disorder? What therapy may be needed?" To answer such questions the physician will need to take the following steps: (1) obtain an accurate history of the child's acquisition of developmental landmarks of speech and language; (2) ascertain through tests whether hearing is normal or defective; (3) estimate the child's levels of development in the areas of verbal comprehension, expression, articulation and intelligibility; (4) form an estimate of the child's level of intellectual function; (5) determine through careful physical and neurologic evaluation whether any organic defects are present; (6) make an assessment of the environment to discover any major psychosocial factors which might interfere with the development of communication skills.

In addition to the foregoing rather general screening procedures, the physician may find the following 20 conditions of speech and language development useful as rough guidelines in determining whether a child has a problem, what its nature may be, and whether or not he should be referred to a speech pathologist or audiologist for more detailed evaluation. If any of the following conditions exist, the child should be referred:

1. If the child is not producing any intelligible speech by age 2
2. If speech is largely unintelligible after age 3
3. If there are many omissions of initial consonants after age 3
4. If there are no sentences by age 3
5. If sounds are more than a year late in appearing, according to expected developmental sequence
6. If there is an excessive amount of indiscriminate, irrelevant verbalizing after 18 months
7. If there is consistent and frequent omission of initial consonants at any age
8. If there are many substitutions of easy sounds for difficult ones after age 5
9. If the amount of vocalizing decreases rather than steadily increases at any period up to age 7
10. If the child uses mostly vowel sounds in his speech at any age after 1 year
11. If word endings are consistently dropped after age 5
12. If sentence structure is consistently faulty after age 5
13. If the child is embarrassed and disturbed by his speech at any age
14. If the child is noticeably nonfluent (stuttering) after age 5
15. If the child is distorting, omitting or substituting any sounds after age 7
16. If the voice is a monotone, extremely loud, largely inaudible, or of poor quality
17. If the pitch is not appropriate to the child's age and sex
18. If there is noticeable hypernasality or lack of nasal resonance
19. If there are unusual confusions, reversals or telescoping in connected speech
20. If there is abnormal rhythm, rate and inflection after age 5.

For children with communication disorders, help may be found in university or college speech and hearing clinics, in community speech and hearing centers, with certified speech pathologists or audiologists in private practice or in the special education departments of the public schools. Speech and hearing specialists also may be found in medical schools, child development programs, rehabilitation centers, mental health clinics and child guidance centers. The speech and hearing specialist should hold the Certificate of Clinical Competence in the American Speech and Hearing Association as assurance that he is adequately trained and experienced.

HEROLD LILLYWHITE

READING DISABILITIES

Some facility with spoken language ordinarily precedes the acquisition of reading skills; the basic skill is the decoding of a written symbol.

Learning to read can be considered a 2-stage process. The first stage consists in perceiving written symbols in their proper temporal sequence. The second stage is the obtaining of meaning from these written words. Most poor readers have difficulty with the first stage, not the second.

There is variability in the rates at which normal children mature in certain basic functions required for reading. These include differential perception of various letter and syllabic forms, the ability to associate these symbols with their sounds, and short-term memory sufficient for correct sequential representation of them. Fluency in speech and reading support each other. A critical listening ability is necessary for the development of vocabulary, proper pronunciation, and the rules of grammar and spelling.

A minimal level of visual acuity is necessary for reading, but striking reduction in acuity need not prevent effective reading. Reduction in auditory acuity, if it interferes with the manipulation of symbols in such a way as to impair speech development, may also have an impact upon reading achievement.

In the range of I.Q.'s from 80 to 130 there is some correlation between I.Q. and reading ability in the early grades. This correlation diminishes in the higher grades and is virtually nonexistent in college. Children who score below 80 in I.Q. generally do not read well.

The child's general motivation and his interest in the content of the material being read are powerful determinants of his reading achievement. The attitudes of peers, family members and others also exert profound influences.

A few children can read at 3½ to 4 years of age; most can learn to read easily at 5 to 6 years of age. A few are not ready for reading until 9 or 10; an unknown number never acquire functional reading skill.

It is generally considered that a child with normal or superior intelligence, without significant sensory deficit, who cannot learn to read at his age level in an ordinary school setting has a reading disability or "developmental dyslexia" or "specific reading disability." Children in the primary grades may be considered retarded readers if they are 6 to 12 months below grade placement; at higher grade levels a criterion of 24 months or more below grade placement defines the poor reader.

The term "reading disability" is not limited to a single clinical entity. Among poor readers are children and adults who from their earliest encounters with reading have had difficulties; others have mastered the fundamental skills, but through lack of motivation or opportunity, or because of emotional or socioeconomic stresses, have failed to mature in reading skills to the point at which reading has become an effective tool for them.

Etiology. The causes suggested for reading retardation reflect the prevalent confusion about definitions and understanding. Because so many affected children appear to be unable to master the most elementary reading skills, in spite of normal intelligence, and because impairment of the ability to perceive or register items in an orderly sequence seems to lie at the root of much disability, attention has been focused upon central nervous system dysfunction. So-called brain damage or minimal cerebral dysfunction, inheritance of a specific reading disability, incomplete or crossed or mixed laterality or cerebral dominance, defects in visuomotor coordination, and deficits in spatial perception or directional orientation have all been considered causes of reading disability, as well as such peripheral defects as abnormalities of ocular structure or movement. Support is given the notion of central defect by the common occurrence in affected children of such so-called soft neurologic signs as generalized motor awkwardness, "overflow" of voluntary muscle activity, inability to concentrate, short attention span, hyperactivity and easy distractibility. But these signs are not precisely defined or quantitated, nor is it clear whether they represent organic or functional disorders. Moreover, it is difficult to explain how many children with such severe central disabilities as those associated with athetosis or spastic paraplegia or congenital nystagmus may learn to read well so long as general intelligence is preserved.

Some poor readers make spontaneous improvement late in the first decade of life or early in the second; it is difficult to reconcile this finding with the notion of an organic defect. Such improvement may follow change of residence, of teacher or of system of reading instruction, whether in the regular school or in remedial work.

So far as poor sequencing and visuomotor coordination are concerned, one finds poor readers who read music well, or who can follow diagrammatic outlines to assemble intricate models or devices. The importance of failure of binocular vision, of refractive errors and of oculomotor imbalance as causes of reading disability has been exaggerated. These conditions may discourage reading because of fatigue, but they do not prevent children from developing reading skills.

Many children will not learn to read if presented with dull or difficult reading materials, if they live in home environments which do not encourage or which actively discourage reading, or if they have no opportunity to acquire an adequate vocabulary. These factors may prove stronger than the influence of the school. The poor reader often comes from a disorganized family setting.

Clinical Manifestations. Reading difficulties may come to the physician's attention because of academic failure or for less clearly related reasons such as psychosomatic complaints or behavioral disturbances.

Contrary to widely held opinion, the poor reader does not generally do well in arithmetic, sciences or other fields of study. He has particular difficulty with spelling, with grammar and with rapid retrieval of words required for precise description and exposition. Even if he can learn through audition and perform orally, bypassing reading and writing, he will be increasingly unable to keep up with his classmates, particularly after the third grade. The effectiveness of his style will vary with his intelligence, motivation and emotional strengths.

Observation of the child in the act of reading may show that he does not persevere unless prodded, or that he may lose interest rapidly. Embarrassed by his poor performance, he may try to hide it by dropping his voice, turning his head or covering his mouth. His impairment is magnified by anxiety or fatigue, with pressure of time or with fear of failure. He may brighten perceptibly with encouragement.

Some poor readers do not pause at words they cannot correctly pronounce, nor attempt to phoneticize them. As if to terminate a painful process as quickly as possible, they produce words variously comparable to the one read, which may have a common initial letter or syllable but disparate meaning (*course* for *cause*), different spellings but related meaning (*mother* for *father* or *brother* for *sister*), minor perceptual differences which produce major semantic changes (*humidity* for *humility*), or no relationship, representing blind guesses.

Errors which demonstrate disturbances of serial order or temporo-spatial sequence are substitutions, deletions, additions and faulty juxtaposition of letters, especially consonants. Reversals are common (strophic errors, or strephosymbolia). *Was* for *saw* and *left* for *felt* are two familiar examples. The equivalent of strophic errors in arithmetic can alter the written sequence of digits or lead to the "carrying" of the wrong digit in addition.

Phonic errors include confusion of 2 or more sound values corresponding to the same symbol, such as *kity* for *city* or *seize* for *size*. Other less common errors include inappropriate use of clues from context or accompanying pictures, mispronunciation of words, and incorrect intonation of phrases and sentences. These latter errors are considered secondary results of imperfect reading.

Some poor readers may have poorly performed diadochokinetic movements, clumsy voluntary acts, impaired right-left orientations and other equivocal neurologic signs. These do not correlate closely with the severity of the impairment or with the success of treatment.

After years of scholastic difficulty, repeating of grades, and perhaps much fruitless remedial instruction, the poor reader may progressively restrict his social contacts and extracurricular activities, manifest behavioral and disciplinary difficulties and be intractable to help and unwilling to undertake new ventures because of the fear of failure and the pain of expected frustration.

Many more boys than girls have reading disabilities, for reasons not yet established.

Diagnosis. The adequate assessment of reading disabilities may require neurologic and psychologic examination as well as review by someone with experience in reading disorders. Only rarely does a discrete diagnostic entity account for a relatively isolated reading problem, but the exclusion of organic disease may allay parental fears of some more serious deficit.

Appropriate studies must determine (1) whether a disability actually exists in perceptual abilities, in developing meaningful sequential order from items of sensory input, or in the level of reading achievement by a child with adequate perceptual skills; (2) whether emotional problems may have been responsible for the development of reading difficulties; (3) whether spontaneous improvement can be anticipated or treatment will be needed; and (4) what treatment may be appropriate, if any, and where it can be obtained.

It is usually more difficult to evaluate children in the primary grades than in subsequent ones.

Performance tests exploring short-term memory for serial items are particularly useful and relatively reliable in children by their tenth year. These include the span of retention of memory for a succession of digits, or the ability to reproduce such items of "automatic" memory as one's birth date, name, address, telephone number, days of the week and months of the year. From the age of 9 through 15 years there is an increasing number of children who can perform on these tests at levels comparable to those of normal adults. Children with reading disabilities generally do poorly at these tasks; a good performance casts doubt on the diagnosis of reading disability.

On the whole, poor readers have lower I.Q.'s than average or good readers, though most fall within the normal range. It is characteristic of these children that their scores on the *performance* items of an intelligence scale, such as the Wechsler (WISC), tend to be substantially higher than their *verbal* scores. When the verbal score is relatively high, the child's difficulty may more likely be the result of emotional problems, lack of motivation, or a nonliterary milieu in the home than the result of a "primary" reading disability. Such interpretations become unreliable when the child's I.Q. approaches or is in the retarded range.

If a child has attained the fifth grade in school and his reading achievement tests indicate that he is functioning below a third or early fourth grade level, he will generally not have mastered basic reading skills. These will be the children considered to have "dyslexia," "primary reading retardation" or "specific language disorder." They present a different problem from children in the higher grades whose reading ability is considered to be retarded about 2 years. The latter children have clearly mastered the basic mechanics of reading. Their low levels of achievement are usually attributable to lack of motivation, to culturally impoverished home environments, to limited educational opportunities, and the like. These 2 groups will require different approaches to improvement of reading skills.

Differential Diagnosis. Consultants in problems of "dyslexia" must make sure that the child has a reading problem. In children with learning problems of whatever sort, reading is likely to be involved, but may not be the primary problem. Children may be referred for reading or language problems because their styles in reading or in other academic functions are out of step, or because their classroom behavior is unacceptable. Such children may be awkward, ungainly, slow, socially immature, inattentive or distractible. Careful evaluation may detect causes other than reading disability for their behavior.

Prognosis. It is doubtful whether there are any children with reading disabilities in the context used here who remain totally unable to read, but the degree of impairment may be severe. It is not presently possible to distinguish the relatively small percentage of children with reading disability who will improve spontaneously from those who will not. Well motivated children who are not overwhelmed by their difficulties and who have only mild deficiencies may improve gradually or suddenly and have no lasting impairment. Many remedial programs can be expected to benefit the poor reader, whether they are devoted exclusively to the teaching of reading or coupled with visuomotor and perceptual training procedures. There are, however, no programs of remedial reading which, with high probability and efficiency, will lead to development of normal reading skills in those with significant difficulty. If in the early years of school the reactions of those close to the child are unsympathetic to his poor performance, he may remain a poor reader for emotional reasons.

Poor readers usually have little or no gross motor disability as adults. They tend to seek occupations which require minimal verbal but high mechanical skills. Their imperfections of speech tend to improve. Their ability to reproduce familiar items (names, days of the week, alphabet, and the like) also improves, but difficulty remains for newly presented items (e.g. series of random digits, unrelated words).

Treatment. Two broad categories of therapy are available for children with reading disabilities:

remedial reading for the child with decoding difficulties due to faulty sequencing or other visuoperceptual or integrative disabilities, and *corrective instruction or exercises* for the child or adult whose basic equipment and reading skills may be adequate, but who has lacked motivation to read or has had an arrest in reading development.

The plan for *remedial reading* should be individually designed for a child after careful analysis by appropriately trained specialists. In *corrective instruction or exercises* the primary purpose is to induce greater interest, attention and diligence in school tasks. The child's self-confidence, willingness to risk failure, and motivation for self-directed achievement must be assessed. Some children require the setting of short-term goals with frequent reinforcement of success; others do well with long-range goals and occasional reinforcement. Some children profit more if their errors are pointed out, others if their successes are underscored.

It is important that the older retarded reader achieve some success, however limited, quickly and easily upon beginning remedial work or instruction. The resulting self-esteem enhances interest and creates a desire for further progress.

JOHN ISOM

CEREBRAL DYSFUNCTION
("Brain Damage"; Learning Disorders)

A number of children, estimated to be greater than 10 per cent of the school population, though they are not mentally retarded or defective or do not have readily detectable neurologic defects, have problems in learning and in behaving like other children. This is a heterogeneous group, and there is no single or clear-cut cause of the behavioral deviations, many of which are similar in the affected children.

During the past decade a variety of categorical terms has been proposed for these disorders, based on assumed cause, either intrinsic or environmental, or on manifestations, symptoms or consequence of an apparent learning and behavior disorder. Of the many terms proposed or used, "children with learning disorders" and "minimal cerebral dysfunction syndrome" seem as acceptable as any. To some, minimal brain dysfunction is an unproved presumptive diagnosis without demonstrable physiologic, biochemical or structural alteration in the brain. To others, deviate behavior, developmental lags, learning disabilities and various motor-perceptual irregularities are valid indices of altered brain functions. It seems reasonable to accept as a working basis that these children have some disorganization of their central nervous system and that this factor in some way affects adversely their capacities to learn or to

conform to usual behavioral patterns of their peers.

The term "minimal cerebral dysfunction" is currently used to identify a syndrome in which a child, in spite of average or nearly average intellectual ability, has learning or behavioral disabilities ranging from mild to moderately severe which are attributable to such deviations of cerebral function as impairment in perception, conceptualization, language comprehension or expression, memory, or control of attention, impulse or some motor functions. Similar deviations may at times complicate the more obvious disorders of the central nervous system such as mental retardation (p. 113), seizures (p. 1247), cerebral palsy (p. 1311), behavioral disorders (p. 77), blindness (p. 1432) or deafness (p. 101). It has also been suggested that there may be relations of this syndrome with that of the hyperkinetic child, with primary reading retardation and with the aphasias.

In the majority of instances no specific cause can be determined for the syndrome of minimal cerebral dysfunction, but in some there is an apparent relation with a genetic disorder, birth injury, or prenatal or postnatal illness or injury of the central nervous system.

Clinical Manifestations. In the preschool

child the symptoms may include a variety of relatively minor deviations in behavioral development, and in some in motor development. Among the characteristic manifestations are unpredictable variations of behavior, distractability, short attention span for the age (or the converse—perseveration), hyperactivity, impulsiveness, irritability, low frustration level, perceptual and conceptual difficulties, poor motor coordination, sleep disorders, and abnormal reactions to environmental stimuli.

The school child exhibits, in addition, difficulties in organizing and finishing his work, in comprehending and following instructions, in learning, particularly in the communication skills, and in memory and abstract thinking. All of these contribute to some degree of school failure. Throughout childhood there is usually increasing emotional reaction in being different from one's peers.

None of these disturbances of integrated behavior by itself is of diagnostic significance, but when several are manifest by a child, they suggest a disturbance in cerebral function. The child's behavior may vary from day to day without relation to any recognizable factor and is apparently as unpredictable to himself as to others. His restlessness is frequently marked by running to and fro, by constant physical activity, and by a briefer interest for any one activity than is appropriate for his chronologic age. His enthusiasms may be intense but short. Many of his acts appear to follow no pattern of thought. He tends to react violently to frustration and to other stimuli, and he may be a constant storm center in the family, at play or at school. Although by many tests he has normal, superior or borderline intelligence, he usually has difficulty in numeral concepts, in associating the particular with the general, and in drawing logical conclusions from abstract material. He can think in concrete terms much better than in abstract ones, so that he may do well in rote memory subjects, such as spelling and multiplication tables, as opposed to reading and other areas in which symbols are important. Allied to the problem of handling abstract concepts are deficiencies in perception of environmental situations in their entirety; rather he is apt to direct his attention only to a minimally important part of what he sees or hears with a reaction as confusing and disturbing to others as to himself.

As the child grows older, secondary behavioral manifestations related to his frustrations about how he feels about himself and to his contacts with people may obscure the earlier pattern. In many instances the secondary symptoms are manifest as emotional immaturity, anxieties and fears, inattention, school failure and the like. The results of his impulsive behavior may lead to severe remorse, and he frequently shows an inappropriate display of affection. Some of the symptoms seen in cerebral dysfunction are not readily distinguished from the ones stemming from abnormal infant-mother interactions.

The syndrome might well be suspected in any child with several of the above-mentioned symptoms, particularly if there is clinical evidence or a history of brain damage. There may be a history of some delay in motor development, and there may be considerable variation from time to time in the reported hyperactivity or hypoactivity.

In many instances no abnormalities can be demonstrated by conventional neurologic examination. Many of these children, however, are clumsy in gross or fine motor activities. There may be poor or tardy development of skill in use of scissors or pencil, in bouncing or catching a ball, in hopping or in jumping rope. Handedness may develop late, and there is frequently mixed or confused laterality. Abnormalities may or may not be detected by electroencephalography. Pneumoencephalography and cerebral arteriography usually give normal results, and no laboratory test is specific for the syndrome. Some of the children have mild visual or hearing impairment in addition to the evidence of disorganization.

Psychologic testing will frequently provide clues to and sometimes pinpoint the special learning disabilities of the child with minimal cerebral dysfunction. There are often great variations in performance and specific deficits in conceptual thinking. There also may be problems of perceptual motor adequacy, so that tasks such as copying geometric forms are characterized by particular distortions and other evidences of inadequacy of coordinated function. There may be evidence of impaired discrimination of size, of right to left, of up to down, and of impaired tactile discrimination. There may be evidence of poor spatial orientation, impaired understanding of time and distorted concept of body image. Perceptual reversals in reading and in writing letters and in numbers may be present. There may be difficulty in fusing sensory impressions into meaningful entities. Projective tests, such as the Rorschach, may disclose inadequate emotional controls, excessive impulsivity or impotence, and failure in perception. Intelligence quotients alone often tend to obscure more than they reveal, since these children may have a normal or even superior performance in some areas of functioning, but the overall score may be low as a result of excessively poor ratings in other areas. Such scatter is the rule rather than the exception. It is important for the psychologist to define as accurately as possible the specific assets and liabilities of the child and to define his optimal method of learning. Without such specific help for the child's parents and for his teacher, the diagnosis of this syndrome is a handicap rather than an aid in planning a constructive learning program.

Differential Diagnosis. This syndrome of poorly integrated behavior associated with learning disabilities should be distinguished from mental retardation or mental deficiency, from hearing loss, from behavioral disorders arising principally on an emotional basis, from cultural deprivation, and from specific language disorders.

A careful history of events in the prenatal and perinatal periods and a detailed developmental history will frequently give clues that lead to an understanding of the basic problem and to the separation of the primary manifestations from the secondary behavior or emotional ones. The child with cerebral dysfunction is likely to have a history of slow motor development, such as difficulty in self-feeding, in manipulating buttons, tying shoelaces, or in balancing, whereas the retarded child is more likely to be slow in all achievements. The deprived child may start out with a normal developmental pattern, and at some later time manifest delay in achievement, particularly in language and social skills. Primary delay in speech should suggest a hearing loss.

Treatment. Although the educational psychologist and the teacher in special education have the principal responsibility to develop a program for specific management and treatment, the pediatrician is in a position to help in identifying the child with a learning disability. He should identify and secure corrections of visual and auditory defects, plan and manage the therapy if the child has seizures, and supervise the general health program. He can assist in interpreting the problem to the parents and to professional persons who are also concerned with the care of children. Such children are frequently characterized as "bad" or "lazy" or "nervous," and an explanation of the real problem should relieve pressures and aid in the achievement of academic success and in effective living with others. Parents are frequently put at ease if behavior is explained on the basis of a physical factor rather than as a result of parental incompetence. Since behavior appropriate to the age usually cannot be expected in these children, their erratic behavior and lack of self-control point to the need for establishment of definite limits of conduct and for consistent controls and discipline. Firm, constructive guidance is indicated rather than permissiveness. It is most important that the child be given goals that are obtainable so that he may profit by the feeling of success rather than of continuing frustration and disappointment. Psychiatric treatment may in some instances be helpful in the management of the child and his family.

Medication may at times be a helpful adjunct in the management. Prolongation of the attention span and reduction in behavioral outbursts have been attributed to the amphetamines. Dexedrine (dextroamphetamine sulfate) or Benzedrine (amphetamine sulfate) may be used in doses of 5 mg. in the morning and increased to 20 or more mg. per day if there appears to be benefit. Various tranquilizing agents may lessen irritability and decrease impulsiveness, as may Benadryl (diphenhydramine) in younger children. Anticonvulsive drugs are not, in general, helpful in modifying behavior, and phenobarbital in the usual doses may have an undesirable stimulating effect on children with this syndrome.

The physician should give teachers and others concerned with the child all the information about his behavior and learning that will be helpful in developing an appropriate program for him. An increasing number of private and public schools are providing special classes for children with learning disabilities. Modification of curricula and techniques by placement in smaller classes, by individualized attention, by use of concrete materials in teaching abstractions, by minimizing competition, and by the use of multisensory approaches to reinforce perception are frequently helpful. Since each child's problems, both in behavior and in learning, are individual, ideally the psychologist, the parent, the physician and the teacher should work together in developing a program, individualized for this child and taking into account all facets of his growth and development: physical, mental and social.

Prognosis. The outlook for such children appears to be dependent in part on the attitude and guidance of those who deal with them, on the age at which effective intervention is initiated, and on the degree of success which can be achieved in family living. In conjunction with a planned educational program, desired achievement depends on the extent to which the child develops a feeling of competency within himself. Some children unfortunately become delinquent or are labeled mentally defective or psychotic. Most, however, who can be helped to feel confident in themselves are able to attain a reasonable level of adjustment during adolescence and eventually to achieve a comfortable way of life in relatively competitive activities.

REFERENCES

Birch, H. G.: *Brain Damage in Children: The Biological and Social Aspects.* Baltimore, Williams & Wilkins Company, 1964.

Clements, S. D.: Minimal Brain Dysfunction in Children. Washington, D.C., United States Department of Health, Education, and Welfare, Public Health Service, Publication #1415, 1966.

Golick, M.: Strictly for Parents/A Parents' Guide to Learning Problems. *J. Learning Disabilities,* 1:366, 1968.

Paine, R. S.: Syndromes of "Minimal Cerebral Damage." *Pediat. Clin. N. Amer.,* 15:779, 1968.

MENTAL RETARDATION

Mental retardation, as the term is used diagnostically, implies impairment in intelligence from early in life and inadequate mental development throughout the growth period, which is manifest by slow and incomplete maturation, impaired learning ability and poor social adjustment. In the minority of cases, mental retardation is primarily a medical problem. As a significant cause of lifetime disability and as a complex medical, social, educational and economic problem, mental retardation currently presents a strong challenge to science and to society that defies easy solution.

Mental retardation may well be the most handicapping of all childhood disorders. There are only 4 other significantly disabling conditions – mental illness, cancer, heart disease and arthritis – that have a higher prevalence, but each of these is in greatest measure a problem of adult life. It is estimated that 3 per cent of the population may be identified as mentally retarded at some point in their lives. Of preschool children, approximately 0.5 per cent are retarded. The peak period of recognition is between 6 and 16 years of age, when the pressures of formal schooling seem to identify a larger number, that may reach 10 per cent or more of the school population in some urban deprived areas. Only approximately 1 per cent of adults are considered to be retarded, the percentage having been reduced by death and by successful assimilation of some of the survivors into the general population. Mental retardation appears to be more frequent in boys than in girls: 55 per cent to 45 per cent. This disparity may in part be related to biologic factors (sex-linked genetic disorders) and in part to differences in social expectations for the sexes. At least 75 per cent of the retarded have no obvious physical stigma, although the group as a whole has a higher percentage of sensory defects, language disorders, neuromuscular impairment, seizures and physical anomalies than the general population. The retarded, like other children with handicapping defects, are more vulnerable to emotional problems; conversely, children with emotional problems frequently function at a retarded level.

At present it is estimated that of the probable six million mentally retarded persons in the United States, 200,000 are in institutions, 300,000 are on waiting lists for such care, and an equal number are in general or special hospitals or prisons. More than 85 per cent live at home. Seven out of 10 of these are of school age, and it is estimated that the majority receive only minimal medical care and guidance.

Intelligence is not the result of a single mental process, but includes abstract thinking, visual and auditory memory, causal reasoning, verbal expression, manipulative capacities and spatial comprehension. This multifactor concept is taken into account in the development of mental and psychologic tests. The current inadequate practice of quantitatively identifying intelligence in terms of mental age or of intelligence quotient (I.Q.), which is the ratio of mental age to chronologic age, supplies only averages of the composite attainments in some of these mental abilities. Since it also reflects in part the experience and cultural background of the subject tested, the I.Q. may conceal more than it reveals. The I.Q. is not fixed and may be modified by a number of factors, largely environmental. This method of grading intelligence apparently depicts the status of persons of average or better than average mental ability more accurately than it does that of those of lesser ability. Arrested or inadequate mental development is only rarely equally manifest in the various intellectual spheres. Frequently some mental functions are within normal limits in moderately retarded children.

The importance of this concept in relation to diagnosis of mental deficiency becomes apparent when it is realized that the various mental abilities do not play equal roles in influencing subsequent social or vocational adjustment. Acceptable progress in academic schooling in the main depends on adequate development of such factors as visual and auditory memory, verbal facility, abstract reasoning, and creativity, as well as conformity to existing social standards. Other aspects of intelligence also play a role in school progress, but in general not to the extent as do those mentioned. In contrast, reasonable success in adjusting to many of the simple industrial disciplines in later life depends much more on such aspects of intelligence as those related to visual-manual coordination, spatial relations, and causal reasoning, as well as on acceptable personality characteristics. The relative value of comprehensive psychologic examination is dependent more on these broader concepts of multiple factors in intelligence and their interaction in terms of potential social adaptability than simply on estimates of average mental age. Unfortunately, there is no objective measure or scientific standard of adaptive behavior to differentiate which behavior is a function of inherent or organic inferiority and which is a function of cultural background. This becomes a subjective judgment.

For academic and administrative purposes the intelligence quotient is useful, though inadequate and not infrequently misleading, to help classify mentally subnormal children in regard to the degree of defect.

Persons with an I.Q. between 50 and 75 are considered to be mildly retarded and "educable." This group comprises 85 to 90 per cent of the total. They are usually capable of reaching the fourth or fifth grade level in a conventional school system and can generally make a moderately satisfactory social adjustment. In general, they are self-supporting in times of high employment, particularly in jobs not requiring abstract thought. The majority of this group are recognized in the early school years as a result of poor academic achievement.

Moderately retarded children have an I.Q. approximately in the range of 35 to 50. They are considered "trainable" and can be capable of their own physical self-care. They also, if accepted, can make an adequate social adjustment in the home and the neighborhood, and some will achieve some degree of economic usefulness at home or in a sheltered type of occupation. This group comprises 5 to 10 per cent of the total. They are usually identified during preschool years because of significantly delayed developmental milestones, and many have physical defects.

Persons with an I.Q. below 35 are classified as severely retarded, and those below 20 are considered to be profoundly retarded. They have minimal response to their environment, are generally considered to be "nontrainable," and are usually dependent on others for most of their care. They constitute approximately 5 per cent of the total retarded group. The majority are identified during infancy and have multiple disabilities requiring medical diagnosis and special care.

More than 100 different factors have been identified as being closely or causally related to mental retardation; yet there is not an identifiable biologic or organic cause for 65 to 75 per cent of retarded children. This largest segment of the retarded is probably caused by sociocultural or environmental deprivation, and is a byproduct of poverty. The majority of the mildly retarded children come from the more disadvantaged classes of society characterized by low income, limited educational achievement, unskilled occupations and generally impoverished environment. These children are, in general, poorly nourished, subject to more acute and chronic illness, and receive less medical and dental care than do those from the middle and upper income groups. Children of migrant farm workers and from the ghetto are rarely brought up in homes where there is stimulating conversation, where books are read, where there is an opportunity for good education, or where the intellectual and cultural advantages taken for granted by the children of middle and upper income groups are available. Many come from disadvantaged and broken homes. Many are born to mothers who are poorly nourished and who receive little prenatal, perinatal or postnatal care. Many are unplanned and unwanted children who are frequently born out of wedlock and grow up in homes with absent fathers and with an inconstant or unstable mother figure. They learn to survive, but not to thrive. The premature rate in such environments is two to three times that of the national average. Retardation in these underprivileged children is largely acquired, possibly beginning in utero in many instances, and becomes apparent during the second or third year of life, probably as a consequence of lack of good interpersonal relations, the absence of psychologic stimulation, and an overall sensory, emotional, environmental and nutritional deprivation. In most instances the way of life rather than the genes that are associated with or create mental retardation is inherited. The cycle of dependecy, poverty and frustration of most welfare recipients is a typical example.

Children reared in significantly deprived circumstances arrive at school age equipped with neither experience nor skills necessary for formal learning. They are, in general, behind age level in language development and in ability for abstract thinking necessary for success at school. They perform poorly; this results in negative feelings toward the learning process, and continued failure follows. Frustration, anxiety, low motivation, lack of opportunity, and unstimulating school curricula lead to lack of self-respect, to truancy, to dropouts, and predispose to delinquency. Many as young adults are unemployed and are unable to meet minimum mental or health standards for military service. This large group of the poor whose cultural and psychologic background simply prevents them from performing adequately in middle-class society constitutes 75 to 80 per cent of those considered mentally retarded. In a more fortunate society this group would probably approach the same range of intellectual ability and performance as that shown by the more favored groups. It is frequently difficult to distinguish objectively between the child who functions at a retarded level because of environment and the one who suffers from prematurity, nutritional deprivation, or a variety of medical problems associated with neglect, since both are frequently children of poverty.

In contrast to these symptoms of mild retardation inherent in the lower sociocultural groups, the more severe degrees of retardation appear to be more evenly distributed throughout the population. Some of the medical and biological causative factors which can be identified as significant in over 25 per cent of the cases appear to be increasing. More low-birth-weight babies live because of somewhat better medical care. More infants with intracranial trauma during the perinatal period and more of those with serious infections or poisoning during early childhood survive. Nonfatal accidents in and out of the home are increasing.

The etiologic classification which follows includes only the major causes, which account for approximately 25 per cent of the retarded. Children with these disorders, in general, are the more severely retarded and can usually be identified early in life by the physician. Most of the children so affected have other manifestations of central nervous system defect or damage such as motor handicaps, seizures, sensory defects and learning disabilities, and many have involvement of skeletal, circulatory, endocrine and other systems. Many syndromes are consistently, and others only rarely, associated with mental retardation.

  I. Prenatal
    A. Genetically determined
      1. Disorders of protein, carbohydrate or fat metabolism, e.g. histidinemia, homocystinuria, maple syrup urine disease, phenylketonuria, galactosemia and the cerebral lipidoses
      2. Cerebral demyelinating diseases
      3. Gargoylism
      4. Cranial anomalies: primary microcephaly, craniostenosis and congenital hydrocephalus
      5. Congenital ectodermoses: tuberous sclerosis, neurofibromatosis, cerebral angiomatosis
      6. Chromosomal abnormalities: Down's syndrome, Klinefelter's syndrome, triple X syndrome, hermaphroditism, cri du chat syndrome, trisomy 18, trisomy D_1 and others
    B. Maternal and fetal infections: syphilis, German measles, toxoplasmosis, cytomegalic inclusion disease
    C. Fetal irradiation
    D. Kernicterus
    E. Cretinism
    F. Prenatal unknown or indefinite causes associated with placental abnormality, toxemia of pregnancy, prematurity, maternal medication, poisoning, nutritional deficiency, infection or trauma
  II. Natal
    A. Birth injuries, infection, cerebral trauma, hemorrhage, anoxia, hypoglycemia
  III. Postnatal
    A. Cerebral infections: meningitis, encephalitis, abscess
    B. Cerebral trauma
    C. Poisoning (lead, carbon monoxide, and others)
    D. Cerebral vascular accidents, occlusion and hemorrhage from congenital defects, deficiency diseases, or unknown cause
    E. Postimmunization encephalopathy: pertusis, smallpox, rabies and others

Most of these conditions are discussed elsewhere, and reference should be made to discussions of symptoms, differential diagnosis and specific treatment.

PHENYLKETONURIA

Phenylketonuria is a genetic defect of phenylalanine metabolism, in which mental retardation is the most serious manifestation. It occurs once in approximately 10,000 births in the United States. The disorder was identified by Følling in 1934 and named phenylpyruvic oligophrenia, a term no longer used. Phenylalanine, which is present in all natural proteins, accumulates in the blood at abnormal concentrations in the absence of the enzyme phenylalanine hydroxylase, which normally converts it to tyrosine. Damage to the developing brain almost always results when these abnormal concentrations of phenylalanine and other metabolites persist in the blood. The biochemical mechanism by which this occurs is not clearly understood.

Phenylketonuria is transmitted by an autosomal recessive gene. Approximately 1 in 50 persons is an asymptomatic heterozygous carrier who cannot be identified with certainty, though phenylalanine loading tests may be useful.

The untreated affected child may have clinical evidence of arrested brain development by 4 months of age, and eventually the typical "classic" picture of a moderate to severely retarded child with schizoid-like behavior evolves. Such children are blonder than unaffected siblings, have blue eyes, a musty odor and a tendency to seborrheic eczematous skin lesions. Many have abnormal electroencephalographic patterns, and approximately one third have seizures. There are no consistent neurologic abnormalities, although many of these children are hypertonic or hyperactive and have unsocial behavior.

Infants with phenylketonuria appear to be normal at birth and during the perinatal period. Plasma phenylalanine levels are normal at delivery (0.4 to 2.0 mg. per 100 ml.), and phenylalanine does not appear in the urine until plasma phenylalanine levels rise to about 30 mg. per 100 ml. or higher during the neonatal period. During late infancy and thereafter phenylpyruvic acid may appear in the urine when plasma phenylalanine levels are over 15 mg. per 100 ml. By this time cerebral damage has begun, which probably reaches its maximum at 2 to 3 years of age. Hence dietary treatment should be begun as soon after birth as diagnosis can be established. Though the blood level of phenylalanine rapidly rises to significant values within a few days after birth, the appearance of phenylpyruvic acid in the urine of an affected infant may be delayed for a somewhat longer time.

A screening test, the bacteria inhibition assay method of Guthrie, for detection of abnormal levels of serum phenylalanine in newborn infants is widely used. It requires several drops of capillary blood; plasma concentrations of phenylalanine may not be significantly elevated until the third to sixth day of life or until the infant has had dietary protein for 24 to 48 hours. When this test indicates an elevated level or when the urine reaction is positive at any age, the phenylalanine concentration of the plasma should be determined chemically before the diagnosis of phenylketonuria is considered to be established. Newborn infants whose results are negative should be reappraised with a urine test within 4 to 6 weeks after birth.

The amount of phenylpyruvic acid excreted in the urine varies with the protein intake; on an ordinary diet it is in the range of 0.5 to 2.5 gm. per day. For preliminary diagnostic or screening purposes after the neonatal period, a random urine specimen is usually satisfactory. Phenylpyruvic acid is indicated by the deep bluish-green color produced by a few drops of 10 per cent ferric chloride solution in about 5 ml. of urine or by the use of Phenistix. This color fades within seconds or minutes, depending on the urinary concentration of phenylpyruvic acid. Color changes are also produced by ferric chloride in the urine of patients with other types of aminoaciduria and in those who have ingested aspirin or one of the phenothiazine derivatives. A few drops of this solution on a urine-wet diaper of an affected infant will yield the characteristic color.

The finding of transient, slightly elevated serum levels of phenylalanine in some infants through screening programs has led, in a few cases, to the diagnosis of maternal phenylketonuria. Some of these infants with transient elevations of serum phenylalanine are believed to be heterozygous carriers for the phenylketonuria trait.

Owing to the delayed maturation of the tyrosine oxidizing system, many premature infants and occasionally full-term ones (p. 423) have slightly elevated serum values for phenylalanine, usually in the range of 5 to 15 mg. per 100 ml. These infants also have elevated serum and urinary concentrations of tyrosine and elevated urinary values for parahydroxyphenylacetic acid. The oral administration of ascorbic acid usually corrects this defect promptly (p. 369). There is no similar effect from ascorbic acid on tyrosinosis (p. 423), which is an inherited metabolic disorder of tyrosine metabolism.

As a rule, increased concentrations of phenylalanine in the blood of children or adults are associated with mental retardation. There are, however, several documented instances in which persons with persistently high serum levels of phenylalanine have had normal intelligence. Systematic controlled studies of children in whom phenylalaninemia was demonstrated in early infancy have yet to be reported which would permit clear evaluation of the effects of dietary treatment upon subsequent physical and mental status.

At present, restriction of phenylalanine in the diet appears to be indicated for infants with persistent serum phenylalanine concentrations over 20 mg. per 100 ml. and normal concentrations of tyrosine in serum and with phenylketones in the urine. Those with transient hyperphenylalaninemia probably do not require treatment. Infants with serum phenylalanine concentrations in the range of 10 to 20 mg. per 100 ml. and with normal serum tyrosine values and no phenylketonuria while they are receiving a normal diet, probably need not be treated. If reduction of dietary proteins to 1.2 to 2.0 gm. per kg. per day is not effective in significantly reducing serum concentrations of phenylalanine, restriction of phenylalanine in the diet is indicated. All infants for whom dietary restriction of phenylalanine is prescribed should be placed on a regular diet for 2 to 3 days at periodic intervals to determine whether the metabolic abnormality has persisted and whether there is a need for continued dietary treatment to maintain the plasma phenylalanine level within the desired range. All infants for whom dietary restriction is not undertaken should be followed systematically with developmental evaluations and repeated urine or blood tests to establish the safety of continuing with a nontreatment regimen.

The purpose of the diet is to prevent or minimize brain damage in susceptible children. A milk substitute has been prepared, especially for use in infants, but its use is continued for a variable time into childhood. It is an enzymatic hydrolysate of casein, which contains a very small amount of phenylalanine, but normal amounts of other amino acids, and has added carbohydrate and fat.[*] Other natural foods which are calculated for their phenylalanine equivalents are added gradually after an initial period of feeding limited to this milk substitute. The optimal serum level to be maintained probably lies between 3 and 7 mg. per 100 ml. Since most natural food proteins contain approximately 5 per cent of phenylalanine, their intake must be limited. The administration of the low phenylalanine diet demands close nutritional supervision of the child and frequent monitoring of the serum concentration of phenylalanine. Phenylalanine is not synthesized in the body; hence "overtreatment," particularly in rapidly growing infants, may lead to phenylalanine deficiency, which is manifest by lethargy, anorexia, anemia, skin rashes and diarrhea.

Initiation of dietary treatment at a later age, but before the age of 2 or 3 years, may limit the progress of the brain damage. It does not, however, appear to reverse the process. In older phenylketonuric children there is no apparent improvement of mental capacity from the use of such diets. Lowering of the high concentration of phenylalanine or its metabolites in these children by dietary measures, however, frequently results in improved attention span, less hyperactive behavior, diminution of the number of seizures or changes in the electroencephalographic pattern.

More difficult than the dietary management is the prevention of emotional problems resulting from dietary restriction and abnormal eating habits. The parents have obvious difficulty in controlling the diets of ambulatory children, and they become disturbed by the realization that ingestion of normal amounts of usual foods may increase the mental retardation. The maintenance of such dietary control without psychologic difficulties is rarely, if ever, attained, and it is understandable that parents of these children will need continuous support and guidance.

The birth of mentally retarded children without phenylketonuria to phenylketonuric mothers suggests that cerebral damage of the fetus may be caused by placental transfer of increased amounts of phenylalanine from the maternal circulation. This observation is an indication for identifying the pregnant phenylketonuric woman and for maintaining her on a low phenylalanine diet during gestation; unfortunately, however, a suitable diet has not been devised.

---

[*]Dietary management with this milk substitute is described in a pamphlet: Phenylketonuria—low phenylalanine dietary management with Lofenalac, available from Mead Johnson Laboratories, Evansville, Indiana 47721.

DOWN'S SYNDROME
(Mongolism)

(See p. 331 for chromosomal aberrations.)

Down's syndrome is one of the most common of the clinically classifiable categories of mental retardation. The incidence is estimated at 1.5 per 1000 births. It accounts, frequently inappropriately, for approximately 10 per cent of retardates in institutions. The majority have trisomy 21; a small percentage have partial translocation of chromosomes 15 and 21. The chromosomal abnormality is the most consistent finding and is essential for the etiologic diagnosis.

The clinical diagnosis depends on the presence of mental retardation in association with a variety of manifestations of disordered growth of the skeletal system, particularly of the skull and long bones. Evidence of defective development of other tissues is also usually manifest.

The abnormal development of the skull is responsible for the characteristic facies. The circumference of the head is usually in the third to twentieth percentile, and the head tends to be flattened anteriorly and posteriorly. The bony orbits are smaller than normal. There is a lateral upward slope of the eyes, and an epicanthic fold is present in the younger child which differs from that of Asiatic races by being confined to the inner angle rather than including most of the upper lid. The epicanthus tends to disappear during puberty. Chronic inflammatory changes involving the conjunctivae and lid margins are common. Cataracts are occasionally present; strabismus is common, as are speckling of the iris (Brushfield spots) and sparse, thin eyelashes. The external ears are usually small, and there may be cartilaginous anomalies. The tongue is usually protruded as a result of the smallness of the oral cavity and

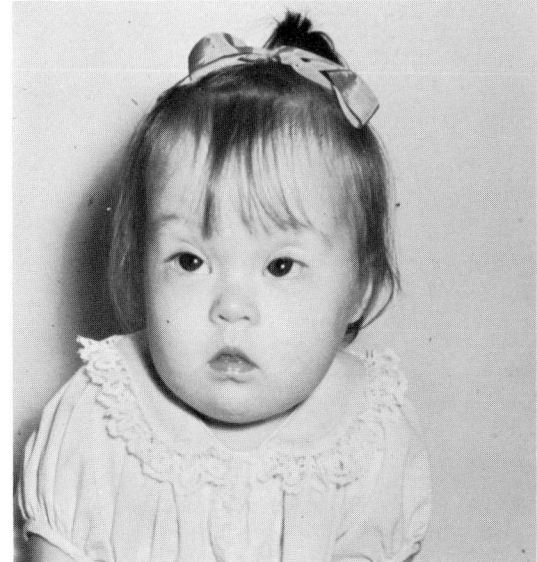

Figure 2-14. Typical facial appearance of young child with Down's syndrome.

hypoplasia of the mandible. The surface may be fissured and furrowed (scrotal tongue) as the result of sucking and mouth-breathing. The nose is short with a flat bridge, resulting from underdevelopment of the nasal bone. The teeth are usually delayed in eruption; they are small and frequently abnormally aligned.

The neck is short and broad, and there is laxity of the skin on the lateral aspects. Generalized hypotonia is usually evident in infancy and becomes less apparent as the child becomes older. In the young child the abdomen is prominent, owing to hypotonia of the abdominal muscles, and there are frequently associated diastasis recti and umbilical hernia.

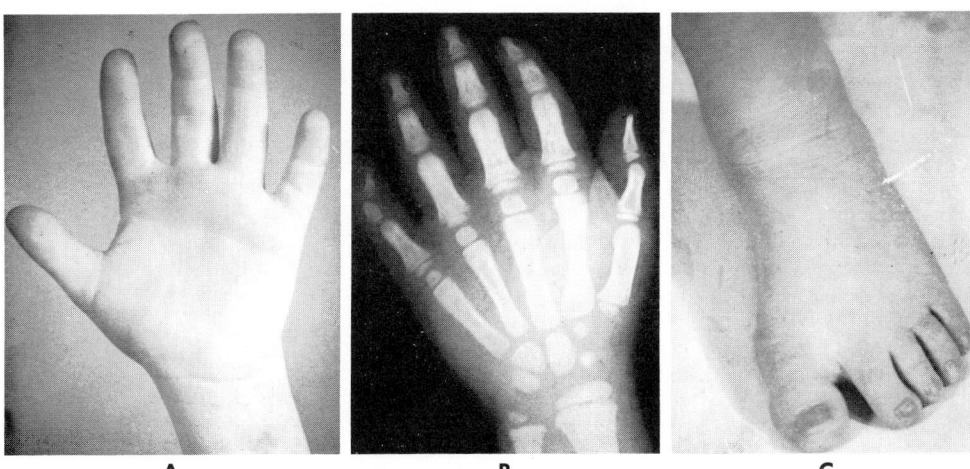

A　　　　　**B**　　　　　**C**

Figure 2-15. *A*, The typical broad, spadelike hand of Down's syndrome in a 12-year-old boy. Note the shortness of all fingers, especially the fifth. The presence of a single transverse palmar crease, instead of the 2 creases normally seen, is well shown. *B*, Roentgenogram of the hand of a 7-year-old girl with Down's syndrome. Note the maldevelopment of the second phalanx of the fifth finger responsible for the shortening and incurving. The metacarpal bones and remaining phalanges also tend to be short and broad. *C*, The typical broad flat foot of Down's syndrome in a 12-year-old boy. Note the wide space between the first and second toes.

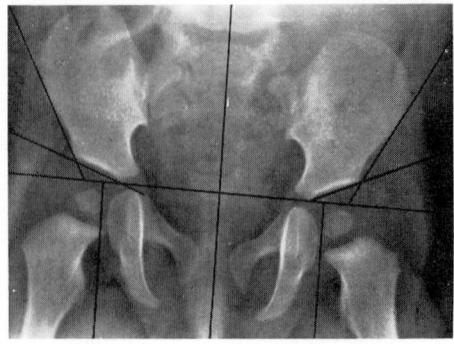 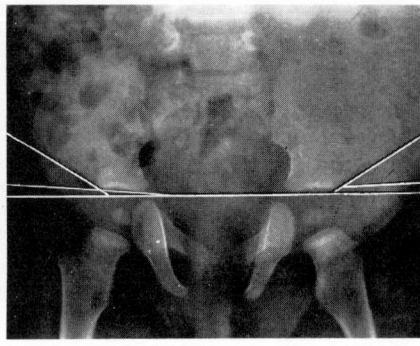

A   **B**

Figure 2-16. *A,* Roentgenogram of pelvis and hips of a normal infant at 9 months of age. *B,* Roentgenogram of pelvis and hips of an infant with Down's syndrome at 7 months of age. The acetabular roofs are almost horizontal, and there is flaring of the ilia. These abnormalities may be measured as illustrated and as described by Caffey.

The extremities are shortened, especially the phalanges, so that the hands and feet tend to be broad, flat and square. The fifth finger is proportionally small and tends to curve inward. The second phalanx of the fifth finger is rudimentary in about 40 per cent of affected children. The spaces between the first and second fingers and toes are increased; in the foot this is frequently associated with a prominent skin crease and with partial syndactyly. The dermal ridge pattern in the hands and feet is frequently abnormal (see p. 329). Frequently there is a single transverse palmar crease instead of the two normally present.

Alterations in the bony pelvis recognizable radiographically in early infancy consist of broad ilia, small acetabular angles and elongated ischia. Cardiac anomalies are more common than in the general population, most often involving the atrioventricular structure. Duodenal atresia is also relatively common. The genitalia are usually poorly developed; secondary sex characteristics are delayed in their appearance, and the pubic hair tends to be straight and to have a silky quality. There are frequently abnormalities of the white blood cells, and the incidence of leukemia in Down's syndrome is 10 to 20 times greater than in the general population (see also p. 1078 re leukemoid reactions). An increase in some of the gamma globulin fractions has also been observed.

There are no pathognomonic changes in the brain or spinal cord. Minor fissural and gyral deviations have been described, and histologically there are minor changes in the ganglion cells, as well as areas of defective myelin formation.

The mental status is usually in the moderate to severely retarded range, though in some instances the rate of development may approach that of normal for the first 3 or 4 years of life and then decelerate. In the absence of serious associated congenital defects, and when the child is given good medical care, the life span can be expected to approach that of normal.

Probably owing to the dryness of the skin with frequent fissuring and cracking during cold weather, furunculosis and other skin infections are more common than in normal children. The child is also more susceptible to acute and chronic infections of the upper respiratory tract, perhaps owing to the decreased anteroposterior diameter of the nasopharynx which contributes to inadequate drainage.

The diagnosis of Down's syndrome in the older child is relatively simple, being based on the combination of the characteristic physical pattern and

TABLE 2-14. DIFFERENTIAL FACTORS IN DOWN'S SYNDROME AND CRETINISM

	DOWN'S SYNDROME	CRETINISM
Recognizable	At birth	After 2–3 months
Body growth	Retarded	Retarded
Head	Brachycephalic	Normal size
Eyes	Upward, outward slant	Puffy
Osseous orbits	Smaller than normal	Normal
Epicanthus	Present at inner angle	Not present
Nose	Small; bridge underdeveloped	Normal
Tongue	Scrotal; may protrude	Thick, large; protrudes
Hands	Short; incurved 5th finger; single palmar crease; dermatoglyphic changes	Short; square
Feet	1st and 2nd toes widely spaced	Short; square
Skin	Occasionally dry	Very dry, pale, coarse
Hair	Variable	Very dry and coarse
Muscle tone	Poor; joint laxity	Unchanged
Constipation	Uncommon	Common
Congenital anomalies	Frequent: heart; eyes; duodenum; leukocytes	Umbilical hernia
Ossification	Slight or no delay	Considerable delay
B.M.R.	Normal	Decreased
Serum iodine	Normal	Decreased
Cholesterol	Normal	Increased
Chromosomal pattern	Abnormal	Normal

mental retardation. In the early weeks of life, however, when most of the signs are not as obvious, it may be less certain. The typical facies, generalized muscular hypotonia, and the dermatoglyphic changes are the most common early findings; the diagnosis is confirmed by chromosomal analysis.

Cretinism, which is not usually manifest at birth, may cause some difficulty in the differential diagnosis. The child with Down's syndrome may, however, also be a cretin. There is no evidence that the course of mongolism is significantly benefited in any way by the use of hormonal or other types of medication.

DIFFERENTIAL DIAGNOSIS OF MENTAL RETARDATION

Diagnosis involves consideration of the most common conditions which may be mistaken for mental retardation or which may so interfere with the capacity to learn as to result in a clinical picture characterized by depressed intellectual function. A critical use of psychologic tests, evaluation of the physical status, and knowledge and understanding of the family and the social background are essential for the diagnosis and an appreciation of the complex contributory factors. Since psychologic tests are, as a general rule, based on the acquisition of learned experiences, the following conditions, by impairing the learning process, may also adversely affect the results of these tests and add to the diagnostic difficulty.

Delayed Educational Maturation. This is a normal variation in the development of motivation or readiness to partake in organized learning experiences, especially those involving academic schooling. It usually becomes evident as a diagnostic problem on entering school if the immaturity is great. Some of these children will catch up and do well if academic competition with their peers is temporarily postponed.

Peripheral Sensory Defects. Screening tests for visual and hearing acuity should be done on all children by at least 3 or 4 years of age. Irreversible changes affecting the learning capacity take place very early in children with critical defects in these sensory mechanisms.

Cerebral Palsy. In infancy, assessment of development is in great part dependent on such motor achievements as holding up the head, sitting, hand manipulations, crawling, standing, walking, and the like. Low developmental quotients based on these considerations may erroneously be attributed to mental retardation in the presence of motor defects such as cerebral palsy. Such motor defects not only interfere with learning opportunities, but also, particularly when language function is involved, prevent effective use of the intellectual capacity.

Language and Speech Disorders. These include disturbances of the cortical mechanisms that control expressive, central and receptive language which, when severely impaired, are manifest clinically as aphasia. Lesser degrees of difficulty may show up as reading disorders, speech disabilities, visual motor or space discrimination disorders, or a variety of learning disabilities involving only one or two of the processes of intelligence. All can seriously affect the learning potential and create diagnostic problems which will require psychologic testing to support the clinical appraisal.

Environmental Deprivation. The absence of adequate learning opportunities, the lack of emotional stimulation and other environmental factors prevent development of intellectual potential and, if not corrected early in life, result in functional or permanent retardation. Quantitatively, within the total population, deprivation factors are largely related to poverty, although broken homes, inadequate parent-child relations, unsatisfactory social environment and lack of motivation are not restricted to any geographic, social, racial or economic group.

Primary Personality Disorders. These include basic personality defects which are believed to be the result of faulty cerebral development; some may be genetically determined. The basic clinical manifestations are failure to relate appropriately to the environment and failure in the development of normal interpersonal relations. There is a spectrum in the disorder which has at one extreme the complete failure of personality development sometimes called infantile autism, and at the other extreme the minor variations in personality structure that blend with normal behavior. Childhood schizophrenia fits into this scheme. Such defects seriously impair the learning capacity and are frequently mistaken for or are associated with mental retardation.

Other factors to be considered in the differential diagnosis include seizure disorders, drug-induced states, some allergies, and nutritional deprivation.

PREVENTION

The complexity of mental retardation defies a single approach to any phase of its management. The prevention of mental retardation in the large group of children who are deprived of the opportunity for optimal development requires a broad, community-wide social, educational and cultural approach. The relatively smaller group of children with associated organic and physical defects tends to be more severely retarded, but fortunately it seems that many of these disorders could be prevented by application of existing biomedical knowledge. The physician must be involved with both groups; in the case of the first group he must support and participate in community activities designed to provide appropriate living and educational opportunities for all children. In the latter group he must provide or secure early diagnostic evaluation and a suitable plan of management for the child and general support for the parents and, when indicated, genetic counseling.

The most important aspects in the prevention of mental retardation are centered in preconceptional and prenatal factors. The best insurance for a healthy physical and mental life is to be born after a wanted pregnancy at term to healthy parents and to be reared in a stable, responsible home. Such a wide variety of factors, genetic, chromosomal and intrauterine environmental ones (see Table 1-3, p. 10), can interfere with mental as well as physical development that they cannot be enumerated here, but they are discussed in the introductory section and in the sections on Growth and Development, Prenatal Factors, Inborn Errors of Metabolism, The Newborn Infant and Infectious Diseases.

An increasing number of disorders related to mental retardation and other disabling conditions that are associated with chromosomal abnormalities are identifiable; a few of these are transmitted. Many of the metabolic disorders are of genetic origin, and in some, such as galactosemia and phenylketonuria, mental retardation can be avoided or lessened by early diagnosis and appropriate management. In some disorders heterozygote carriers can be identified, and genetic counseling, if accepted, can be highly effective in limiting the production of probable defectives. An increasing number of medical conditions which may lead to fetal damage of the nervous system are becoming identifiable through maternal or fetal diagnostic procedures. In such circumstances the advisability of therapeutic abortion must be judiciously considered (see below).

Appropriate use of available immunologic agents to prevent infectious and contagious diseases, prevention and adequate treatment of infections, prevention of poisoning, accidents and child abuse, and an early intervention in the lives of sensorially and otherwise deprived children by provision of appropriate learning experience would eliminate many instances of retardation.

PROGNOSIS

When he has reached his fifth birthday, a retarded child has a good a chance of growing up and probably has about the same life expectancy as do others who receive good medical care, an adequate diet, early and adequate treatment of infections, and the like. For severe and profoundly retarded children with multiple defects the life expectancy is substantially less, though with appropriate care it can be significantly extended.

It must be remembered that intelligence is not a fixed factor and that modification of environment and improvement in learning opportunities and in social acceptance will bring about improvement in almost all retarded children. The degree of improvement is less in the more severely involved child and in the one with multiple handicaps.

TREATMENT AND MANAGEMENT

See also page 121.

The effective management of a retarded child is a complex problem requiring the physician to become involved as a compassionate, understanding, resourceful person who treats the child, supports the family, and communicates effectively with others in the community over a considerable period of time.

As a physician, he is daily involved in the prevention and early recognition of the potential retardate. He, frequently with other professional persons and parents, establishes the fact of the child's slow intellectual development. He identifies and secures treatment, if any is established as effective, for conditions that cause or are associated with decreased effectiveness of learning capacity, such as motor, visual and hearing disorders. These include metabolic disorders of protein, such as phenylketonuria, maple syrup urine disease, hyperglycinuria, leucine intolerance, tyrosinosis and Hartnup disease; abnormal carbohydrate metabolism, such as galactosemia, fructose intolerance and hypoglycemia; pyridoxine dependency; hyperbilirubinemia; plumbism; hypercalcemia; hypothyroidism; hypoparathyroidism; hydrocephalus; craniostenosis; and subdural accumulations. For many identifiable syndromes there is still only symptomatic and supportive treatment.

Unless a specific defect is identified, there is no generally accepted evidence to support the efficacy of a variety of therapies recommended at one time or another, which include the use of glutamic acid, vitamins, hormones, tissue extracts, minerals, drugs of various kinds, surgical procedures, or manipulations to increase cerebral blood flow or to improve neurologic organization.

Retarded children require the same general pediatric care which is desirable for all children. If a good parent-child relation early in life and a home environment providing adequate learning experiences, relative security, love and acceptance as an individual are essential for development of the inherent potential of the normal infant, these factors are even more essential for the development of the retarded child. Efforts to decrease disability and to increase functional capacity are essential at all ages, but are most effective early in life when the child is developing and is most actively using his learning capacity. Developmental gains by the retarded child should be assessed on the basis of his potential and estimated ability to approximate relative independence. During the pediatric age the specific amount of knowledge acquired is perhaps less important than is the development of proper work habits, of sustained interest in an activity, of satisfaction from attainable goals, and of personality factors that make for successful relations with the family, social contacts, and the potential employer.

The family of a retarded child needs support, particularly in the interpretation of the child's problems, in the daily management, in developing and carrying out long-term plans, in the use of community resources, in self-understanding, in the understanding of genetic factors if present, and at times of crisis (see below). The physician must share these responsibilities with the family, the school, the community and the government.

Others may make a greater contribution to the ultimate adjustment of the retarded child than the physician. His ability, however, to understand growing children, to communicate his knowledge to others, and to be realistic in helping set goals may be critical factors. As family advisor, the physician must know what resources are available in the community, help the family use the services which are appropriate, and perhaps help develop services not available in the community. These may include specialized diagnostic facilities, home nursing programs, genetic counseling, specialized nursery and day-care centers, special classes in public and other day schools, religious nurture, camping and other recreational programs, vocational training, sheltered workshops, specialized employment services, income maintenance when necessary, foster homes and emergency care facilities, as well as residential institutions.

Great strides have been made in the field of special education in helping children who have special learning problems. Special classes are becoming available in greater number, and curricula are being developed on an individual basis. Formal and informal learning experiences are being developed for younger children such as the Head Start and Get Set programs.

It is generally agreed that most children with mild to moderate retardation should be kept and cared for within their own homes. Serious emotional and behavior disorders may arise. Foster home care or group living in another community may then be considered. Supportive care away from home for the more severely retarded should be considered only when home care is completely impossible or has proved unsuccessful. The decision for removal of the child from the home is a parental responsibility, but parents should be guided and supported by the physician. The decision depends on the economic status of the family, and the availability of space and an appropriate program in a state-supported or private institution, on reaction of other children in the family, and on the emotional stability of the parents, particularly the mother.

There are certainly defendable medical, genetic, social, economic and moral indications for the voluntary limitation of the number of children in certain families, and for therapeutic abortion under certain circumstances. Sterilization of certain persons can be supported for genetic reasons or because of poor potential for undertaking responsibilities of parenthood. The legal status, personal rights, moral and social acceptability, and practical indications for these procedures are undergoing debate and rapid change. The physician has a large responsibility in discussing and influencing such changes within the community.

Both government and private citizen organizations have accomplished much in developing better services for the retarded. The physician should give guidance and perspective in the areas of his competence to both groups so that realistic programs are developed with appropriate priorities to meet the extensive needs.

REFERENCES

Berry, H. K., and Wright, S.: Conference on Treatment of Phenylketonuria. *J. Pediat.*, 70:142, 1967.

Cravioto, J., DeLicardie, E. R., and Birch, H. G.: Nutrition, Growth and Neurointegrative Development: An Experimental and Ecologic Study. *Pediatrics*, 38 (supp.):319, 1966.

Committee on the Handicapped Child: Selected References on Mental Retardation: An Annotated Bibliography. Evanston, Ill., American Academy of Pediatrics, 1967.

Hurley, R. L.: Poverty and Mental Retardation: A Causal Relationship. State of New Jersey, Department of Institutions and Agencies, Trenton, N.J., April 1968.

Mental Retardation: A Family Crisis—The Therapeutic Role of the Physician. New York Group for the Advancement of Psychiatry, Report No. 56, 1963.

Mental Retardation Abstracts. Washington, D.C., United States Department of Health, Education, and Welfare, Public Health Service, National Institutes of Health, annually, starting 1964.

Mild Mental Retardation: A Growing Challenge to the Physician. New York, Group for the Advancement of Psychiatry, Report No. 66, 1967.

President's Panel on Mental Retardation: Report to the President: A Proposed Program for National Action to Combat Mental Retardation. Washington, D.C., Superintendent of Documents, United States Government Printing Office, October 1962.

Richmond, J. B.: Mental Retardation: A Handbook for the Primary Physician. *J.A.M.A.*, 191:183, 1965.

THE PHYSICIAN AND THE CHILD WITH A PERMANENT HANDICAP

It is increasingly important for the physician who cares for children to become familiar with the special problems of the child who chronically and perhaps permanently deviates from normal because of some congenital or acquired disability. The successful management of such a child depends as often on the social, academic and home adjustments that can be achieved as it does on purely technical and medical procedures.

The Physician. Some physicians are not suited by temperament or training to provide adequate management for the handicapped child and his family. The comprehensive care required is time-consuming, and many of the children as well as their parents are uncooperative. They may disrupt a busy appointment schedule, and much time must be spent with parents whose emotional reactions frequently present greater problems than do those of the child. The physician who extends his responsibility beyond the treatment of the "chief complaint," however, will find rewards in helping the young handicapped patient and his family to live more comfortably and effectively with a long-term disability.

The physician may feel inadequate because the complexity of the problems makes them appear unsolvable or beyond means at his immediate command. He must be aware of his own possible negative attitudes, prejudices and limitations, or these will be reflected in his poor relationships with the child and the family. He must, above all, be able to utilize other professional disciplines to make appropriate referrals and to use other resources in the community while he maintains his own professional relationship as primary physician to the family. Abandonment or rejection of the handicapped child by a physician by failing to provide good pediatric care, by ignoring the real problem, by giving the family false assurances, or by not seeking and using help which is available in the community only compounds everyone's difficulties. The physician may feel inadequate if a specific diagnosis cannot be made or if the evaluation cannot be completed at one visit. Intelligent management should begin at the first meeting with the family with a simple functional appraisal of the child and a simple explanation to the parents.

The physician who cannot be a patient, uncritical listener, who cannot be satisfied with small gains, who cannot project himself into the child's and the parents' position sufficiently to offer intelligent support when a cure or complete recovery is not possible, who clings to outmoded concepts and is not realistically aware of both the possibilities and limitations of habilitation, who cannot communicate and work effectively with others in the community, and who does not provide adequate general pediatric care for the child and an acceptable role for the parents at all times should not complain if others take over where he has failed.

Management of the Child. Through continuing contacts and interest in the child and the family the physician can help in developing and periodically revising a plan that is realistic for all concerned. He should help the child to make use of his abilities as effectively as possible and become as socially acceptable and self-sufficient as his limitations permit. Immediate goals should be realistic so that success is possible and likely, since failure discourages further effort. The physician who is aware that the child with single or multiple handicaps has limited opportunities for normal learning and development will make particular efforts to see that a variety of experiences are available at appropriate ages. Opportunities for learning, for social and group experiences, and for the achievement of self-discipline should be provided. A balance between overprotection and overstimulation must be sought. The child with multiple handicaps is rarely capable of achieving a high degree of independence, so that the physician must interpret the child and his behavior to those who are in regular or occasional contact with him. Every effort should be made to minimize secondary handicaps in personality development so that they do not become more serious than the primary defect. The physician should above all else try to help the child lead a happy life.

The Family's Problems. Since the child's environment and the emotional climate of the home are of equal and sometimes of greater importance than the medical care for the child's eventual adjustment, every effort must be made to assist the family to understand their own feelings and to fulfill their own needs. They must always be given something constructive to do. Parents' reactions to a defective child depend on the extent to which they feel their competency, social standing and anticipated way of life to be threatened by the handicap. Most parents initially attempt to deny the reality of the defect, particularly if it is not obvious physically. This stage is usually followed by one of frustration and disorganization and of self-accusation and questioning in which fears and anxieties about the future become overwhelming. Simple explanation, support and guidance for the family are particularly necessary during this stage. As parents' defenses are organized, denial, hostility, and shifting of responsibility take place. If communication and counseling with the mother and father are not effective, the "no one ever told me anything" reaction sets in and "shopping around" ensues. Establishment of support by communicating a genuine professional interest and concern in the child often spells the difference between active family involvement and rejection of help with subsequent poor adjustment and failure to achieve the maximum potential in the child. Depending on the degree of maturity and emotional resources of the family, they can be helped to accept their problems realistically and to plan constructively for the long-term needs of the child.

The problems are as varied as the people involved. Most parents, regardless of their background, have feelings of guilt which must be resolved lest attitudes of self-sacrifice, excessive overprotection or rejection of the child develop. Most families have ambivalent feelings about the child, varying from overt hostility to gross overindulgence. The child may actually become deprived of normal experiences because of overindulgence or, because of his neglect and deprivation, be inadequately stimulated. The establishment of limits of acceptable behavior and the consistent teaching of discipline which are so important to a child's emotional development may thus be lacking. The handicapped child frequently may be the precipitating factor in marital difficulties which are not basically related to him.

As the child grows older the parents have to accept many roles, and make psychologic adaptations which would otherwise not be necessary, because of the child's prolonged dependency upon them. The problems of social isolation, sexual development and unpleasant behavior become increasingly important to the family as the child grows older.

Family Therapy. Parents in retrospect often complain that the status of the child was not made clear to them, that the diagnosis was based on an incomplete examination or hasty judgment, that poor prognosis was not justified or that their part in helping the child was not explained. It must be remembered that many parents hear, retain and comprehend only in part, and that various interpretations must be given *and repeated* in an acceptable and understandable way to those concerned. Reinforcement of information given the family may be made by other members of the physician's staff or by members of varying disciplines if consultation services are available through a clinic or other community agency.

The initial explanation of the facts about a child with a handicap should be made to the parents *together* in as simple a way as possible. Technical explanations are usually only confusing. Long-term prognosis and planning should be left for a later interview, but emphasis should be on management of immediate problems and symptoms. Questions should be answered simply, reassurance be given to minimize guilt feelings, and the importance of time in determining the developmental ability of the child should be stressed. Attention cannot be given too early to the avoidance of secondary emotional problems in the child and his family. The practical problems of carrying out a reasonable home program can best be appreciated by a visit to the home. Grandparents and other relatives who may be involved in family affairs should be brought into explanations as necessary in order that the parents' efforts with the child will not be negated. The time, expense and effort involved in the evaluation of the handicapped child may be largely wasted if explanation and interpretation to all concerned is not simply and effectively carried out.

A physician who is not aware that the parents' feelings of guilt about the child may be projected to him will be unprepared to act with the necessary understanding and patience and will emerge with a bruised ego. Guidance and support to the family are a continuing affair, and acceptance of the handicapped child is probably never fully accomplished by the parents because the problems change with advancing age.

Care should be taken to assure the siblings an equal share of the parents' time, attention and interest. With inadvertent or intentional neglect their problems may become greater than those of the affected child. Their questions about the abnormal child should be answered simply and honestly. The experience of living with a seriously handicapped brother or sister may be used constructively to teach tolerance, patience and understanding of others. If parents openly accept the child as an individual despite his limitations, and if they accept his failures as inevitably as they do his more limited successes, a good example is set for others in the community. This is the best method of "public education." The converse is also true.

The question of the probable outcome of future pregnancies is frequently raised by parents. If the cause of the disability is clearly an accidental one, it is easy to be reassuring. If it is known to be genetically determined or to arise as a result of circumstances that might be repeated, the physician should explain the facts as simply and clearly as possible and help the parents to make their own decision based on available evidence. When the family has made its decision on grounds that for them are valid, the physician should support them in it

Institutional Care. With a seriously involved child who will always be completely or partially dependent on others for his care, the question of support away from home will arise. The physician should help the family to make their own decision about this by objectively discussing with them the advantages and disadvantages of such care. The decision is the family's and not the physician's, though he may diplomatically initiate the discussion if the family appears reluctant to open the question and if he is convinced that such a solution might be beneficial to all.

The potential value of home care during infancy and early childhood, not only for the child's subsequent development, but also for the family's sense of participation and accomplishment, is emphasized. Even seriously handicapped children can profit by tender loving care at home; it has been shown that children with Down's syndrome have a much greater potential if given good care in the average home than if placed in an institution at birth.

It is sometimes said that defective children should be placed away from home at birth lest the parents become abnormally devoted to them. This is unlikely, and the average family with guidance can handle such children to advantage at home for a few years. Parents in general feel more comfortable about later placement if they gradually gain acceptance of the child's limitations by normally fulfilling their role as parents. Too early placement may lead to doubts and greater feelings of guilt. The physician should be aware of the appropriateness, the cost and the availability of supportive or training facilities away from home before advising their use.

Temporary placement away from home is indicated when the child himself can profit by greater opportunities in a different environment or for a short term when inevitable family emergencies arise or when a vacation is needed by all. If the defective child becomes a serious burden to the physical or emotional health of the parents and siblings, the change should be made. Placement is wrongly used as an escape from the physician's or the family's responsibility. It is usually not wise to encourage brothers and sisters to assume the permanent care of a dependent child.

Use of Community Resources. The physician should help to develop and make effective use of local community resources such as public health nurses, baby-sitters, "home maker" services, day-care centers, special schools, social agencies, voluntary health agencies and temporary boarding homes to give the family a vacation or to tide them over emergencies. The physician often overlooks the support which the church can give to families in time of stress. A religiously oriented parent is better able to accept the burden of a handicapped child than one without such a resource. Better communication between the clergy and the medical profession can lead to more effective family counseling and support.

For less severely affected children the physician should assist the family to get appropriate help from public or private schools that may offer programs for exceptional children. An increasing number of special classes for orthopedically, mentally and emotionally handicapped children, as well as for those with visual, hearing, language and learning defects, is being provided by the public school systems in many areas. The physician is in a unique position to interpret to others in the school, the church and the community center the special problems presented by the child with a handicap. It is incumbent on him to take leadership in this area.

Most communities encouraged by voluntary health agencies and by parents' organizations are developing services for various categories of children with handicaps. These include medical facilities for early diagnosis, evaluation and treatment, social case work, home care by nurses, psychologic evaluation and counseling, baby-sitting or temporary home care, educational and recreational facilities, occupational training and vocational placement, sheltered workshops as well as smaller local residential programs and supportive care. Community centers for mental health and mental retardation are being developed in many areas, and such centers can provide many of the services needed by children with multiple handicaps. Greater use is being made of volunteers and of nonprofessional workers to provide services in a variety of areas. The physician can contribute significantly to the training and orientation of such personnel as well as help in planning community service centers.

Parents' Organizations. Parents' organizations have been outstandingly successful in affording those with common problems an opportunity to share their anxieties, to gain strength and hope through identification with a group, and to bring about effective changes in legislative and community health programs. Efforts in behalf of community education, support of research and voluntary participation in a variety of services are psychologically important to the family of children with handicaps and are constructively helpful to the community.

JOHN B. BARTRAM

THE CARE OF THE CHILD WITH A FATAL ILLNESS

From time to time every physician has the painful duty of caring for a child with a fatal illness. It is then his responsibility to help the family cope with their pain and grief in such ways that the experience may have the best possibility of being growth-promoting, rather than destructive of family integrity or of the emotional well-being of the family members. The physician's acceptance of these goals as realistic and urgently in need of his professional skills will help blunt his own sense of frustration, grief or professional inadequacy.

When the physician is certain of a fatal outcome, there should ordinarily be no equivocation in conveying the diagnosis to the family in a frank, direct and empathic way. If both parents are available, the fact that their child has an illness from which recovery is not expected should be conveyed to them when they are together. The words chosen and the manner of the physician should be gentle and honest, and he should be prepared to meet the parents' anguish or disbelief

with answers to their questions and with information as to what measures will be taken to try to forestall what seems to be inevitable.

The place in which this conversation occurs should be carefully chosen. It should be apart from the other activities of the hospital, and should be available for an adequate, uninterrupted time. The physician should understand that much of the conversation at this time will not be truly heard or registered by the parents of the sick child, and he should plan another session later in the day or on the next day when he can review the information he has given and answer new or recurring questions.

Ordinarily the physician should avoid taking the stand that nothing can be done in a situation which the parents sense as a disaster, but should emphasize the positive steps which he and the parents can take together to surmount the difficulties ahead. He should generally avoid detailed predictions of the course of the illness, emphasizing that in such situations one generally lives from day to day, and that it is usually possible to avoid undue suffering or pain. When the illness may endure for months or years, it may not be inappropriate to hold out the hope that medical research may provide methods of control which are not currently available.

Parents are often reluctant to ask whether some other physician or resources of some other medical center may offer more hope, or even whether the diagnosis may be in doubt. They will need help in expressing these concerns and should be encouraged and helped to seek additional medical opinions, if they wish. These matters should be discussed in such a way that the family should feel no embarrassment, and they should know that they are causing none. They can be helped to understand that medical communication is generally good enough to provide prompt dissemination of any real break-through in the management of the otherwise fatal illness of their child. It is also reasonable to advise them that they may do the ill child and the rest of the family a disservice if they dissipate the family's emotional and other resources in a frantic search for something that is not available.

It is natural and inevitable that parents will ask themselves whether the fatal illness of their child was not in some measure avoidable. Some will seek causes in inadequate medical care, in incompetent physicians or in other environmental circumstances; others will assume a burden of guilt at their own failure to recognize the symptoms of illness or to take action quickly enough so that a cure could have been effected. Each of these reactions may be irrational. When these feelings are implicit in questions or responses of parents, the physician should often make them explicit; he should point out the inevitability of such feelings, and when he can honestly do so, he should reassure the parents that there are no grounds for their shouldering blame for a situation which no one could say might have been averted. The feeling of guilt, or the sense of punishment, may be particularly strong in genetic disorders. Here it may be helpful to encourage the family to regard genetic mutations as tragic accidents, most often beyond the ability of man to avoid.

In the management of the affected child, parents should be encouraged to handle the life situation of the child as normally as possible. This may be difficult for parents, who may think that their usual disciplinary activities may make the child's pain or illness worse. These feelings should be allayed, and the parents should be encouraged to maintain the child in his normal place in the family hierarchy. Special arrangements, such as the celebration of Christmas in the summertime, or other public dramatizations of the child's illness should be discouraged; they may be more anxiety-provoking for the child than fulfilling of some special need. As much as possible, the parents should be encouraged to participate in the care of the child in the hospital, so long as their responsibilities to other children at home are adequately met. They may also need encouragement to take adequate respite from the care of the ill child.

As the physician follows the evolution of a fatal illness in a child, he should observe the manner in which the parents are coping with the situation. He may, for example, see that the parents are increasingly turning their attention to other sick children in the hospital. This is a healthy sign if it is not premature; if it comes too early, it may represent the parents' unresolved burden of guilt or their pain in facing the ill child. This turning away to help other children is healthy, so long as the parents still have adequate resources and strength for the sometimes increasing or diminishing needs of the patient.

At times the guilt of parents is intensified by a wish that the illness were all over, or by an unexpected sense of relief or release at the terminal event itself. The considerate and skillful physician will be on the watch for signs of these reactions and find the right words of reassurance or encouragement that such feelings are normal and that the parents have given everything that could have been expected of them to a situation which they have found very trying and toward which they will forever have sensitive and tender feelings.

What to tell the child who has a fatal illness about his future will vary with the condition and circumstances. Most children do not ask whether they are going to die. They can often be told that they have an illness which may last for some time and which has ups and downs, and that it is important for them to get adequate rest and to be active when they feel up to it. Unrealistic reassurances that they look well and are doing fine will be less helpful than the frank recognition of the child's feeling that being ill is no fun and that having it going on so long is discouraging. This can be accompanied by assurances that the physician will get the child back to school or whatever activity is normal for him as soon as possible. Meanwhile it is supportive, when appropriate, for the child to receive attention from school teachers and play therapists in the hospital who will help blunt the sense of inevitability of worsening illness.

Occasionally, older children, especially adolescents, do come to know that they have a fatal illness, and at times it is appropriate to face this fact with them, with the assurance, more in action than in word, that they are not being abandoned in any sense and that whatever they need will promptly be made available to them. This realistic facing of the future may free all participants in a difficult experience for interaction at new levels of frankness, freedom, tenderness and love.

In dealing with the problems of patient and family around a fatal illness, the physician will often call upon professional persons for help. The family's minister or other spiritual advisor can often be of immense comfort. When family problems are likely to be ameliorated by the use of community resources, the help of skilled social workers may be extremely important. When the family is not intact, owing to the death or previous separation of a parent, the likelihood of emotional difficulties complicating the management of the illness is sufficiently great that social service resources should probably be involved from the time when the diagnosis is known.

In the management of terminal illness the physician should not leave decisions about what is to be done for the child to the parents, but should give positive advice as to what he plans to do. He should be responsive, however, to the suggestions of parents when these represent a helpful and realistic appraisal of the child's needs.

When death is imminent, the patient should be kept comfortable and the parents, as much as possible, close at hand. The physician should be available to both parents and to the patient. Control of his own feelings is important; if he allows his own distress to let him become less involved, the anger of the child or parents at what may be perceived as abandonment of them may make terminal care much more difficult. The continued interest and concern of the physician are important in preventing the emotional situation from deteriorating at this time.

As the moment of death approaches, the child should be in a room where he can be alone, his parents at the bedside or nearby. The sensitive physician will see that the occasion is accorded appropriate dignity and not rendered more frustrating or agonizing by fruitless efforts to prolong vital functions in mechanical ways or in a climate of purposeless hyperactivity.

When death has occurred, the patient, bed and room should be made neat, and the paraphernalia of illness removed. If the parents are not at hand, they should be asked to come to the hospital and be informed of the circumstances. Parents should be given the opportunity to be with the child a little while in the relatively peaceful and un-cluttered setting which has been created. A brief and tender parting may help the parents in the adjustments which they must ultimately make. In the case of a newborn infant, the body can often be taken to the mother or both parents at her bedside or some other point in the hospital, where this contact with her baby may be the mother's only opportunity to establish for herself the reality of the birth and death of her infant, and to adjust toward reality her current or future fantasies as to what might *really* have happened.

A request for postmortem examination should be made by the responsible physician who knows the family best. This is often not the house officer, but the attending physician. The need for postmortem examination should be urged as strongly as conviction permits. It can be emphasized that such examinations are always helpful, that information is gathered and saved which may be extremely useful in years to come in solving similar problems of other children, or in providing definitive answers to questions which other children in the family or their relatives or descendants may have concerning the patient's illness, now or in the future.

Later the physician should describe the important and relevant findings of the gross postmortem examination for the parents in simple terms, and they should be permitted to discuss them as freely as they desire.

VICTOR C. VAUGHAN, III

REFERENCES

Evans, A. E.: If a Child Must Die. . . . *New England J. Med.*, 278:138, 1968.

Hamovitch, M. B.: The Parent and the Fatally Ill Child. City of Hope Medical Center, Duarte, California, 1964.

Howell, D. A.: A Child Dies. *J. Pediat. Surg.*, 1:2, 1966.

3. Nutrition and Nutritional Disorders

NUTRITIONAL REQUIREMENTS

A clear understanding of the fundamentals of nutrition is required for skillful supervision of the health of children. The Food and Nutrition Board of the National Research Council has established a table of Recommended Dietary Allowances as a guide to the attainment of good nutritional status for healthy persons of all ages. In most instances these recommendations include a safety factor of 50 to 100 per cent, providing a margin of sufficiency above minimal needs as compensation for individual variations in utilization and for needs arising from unanticipated daily stresses. Nutrition studies in children are even more complex to perform and interpret than those with adults, and much remains to be learned about human metabolism. It is best to consider the Recommended Dietary Allowances as "educated guesses"; they are not *a priori* optimal levels of intake. Fomon has used the designation "advisable intake" for normal infants to indicate an adequate amount which is greater than the requirement to prevent deficiencies, but less than the Allowances.

Although the range for good nutrition must be accorded considerable variability, it is well to remember that mild excesses of caloric intake may prove to be as undesirable as mild deficiencies. The present evidence is insufficient to permit final conclusions as to the influence of diet in infancy and childhood upon the aging process, atherosclerosis or longevity in adult life, but avoidance of excessive caloric and fat intake would appear to be wise at any age.

WATER

Water is second only to oxygen as an essential for existence; lack of it results in death in a matter of days. The water content of infants is relatively higher (70 to 75 per cent of the body weight) than of adults (60 to 65 per cent). Assuming that water comprises 70 per cent of the body weight, 5 per cent is blood plasma, 15 per cent is interstitial fluid, and 50 per cent is intracellular fluid. Fluids provide the principal source of water; some is obtained from the oxidation of foods (mixed diets yield about 12 gm. of water per 100 calories) as well as of body tissues.

Requirements for water are related to caloric consumption and to the specific gravity of the urine. The infant must consume much larger amounts of water per unit of body weight than the adult, but when calculated per 100 calories of intake, the amounts required are practically the same (see Table 3-1). The daily consumption of fluid by the healthy infant is equivalent to 10 to 15 per cent of his body weight, whereas it is only 2 to 4 per cent in the adult. The natural food of infants and children is high in water content, most of the solid food in the child's diet containing 60 to 70 per cent water, and many of the fruits and vegetables, 90 per cent.

TABLE 3-1. WATER REQUIREMENTS

URINE SP.GR.	INFANT—3 KG. 300 CALORIES INTAKE			ADULT—70 KG. 3000 CALORIES INTAKE		
	WATER INTAKE			WATER INTAKE		
	Gm.	Gm./100 Cal.	Gm./ Kg.	Gm.	Gm./100 Cal.	Gm./ Kg.
1.005......650		217	220	6300	210	90
1.015......339		113	116	3180	106	45
1.020......300		100	100	2790	93	40
1.030......264		88	91	2430	81	35

Little if any water is absorbed directly from the stomach; absorption is through the entire intestinal tract. Some water may go directly into the lymph stream, but most is taken into the bloodstream. The quantity of water in the interstitial compartment changes considerably in order to maintain homeostatic balance within the intracellular and vascular compartments. The interchange of water among these compartments is dependent on their respective protein and electrolyte concentrations. Depending upon the rate of growth, about 0.5 to 3 per cent of the fluid intake will be retained. Fomon has calculated water retentions of the order of 13 to 9 ml. per day for the "male reference infant" in the first year of life.

Water balance depends on such variables as fluid intake, protein and mineral content of diet, solute load presented for renal excretion, metabolic and respiratory rates, and body temperature. Fecal losses are small (3 to 10 per cent of intake). Evaporation from lungs and skin accounts for 40 to 50 per cent of intake (sometimes more), and renal excretion for 40 to 50 per cent or more. The kidney preserves the fluid and electrolyte

TABLE 3-2. RANGE OF AVERAGE WATER
REQUIREMENT OF CHILDREN AT
DIFFERENT AGES UNDER
ORDINARY CONDITIONS

AGE	AVERAGE BODY WEIGHT IN KG.	TOTAL WATER IN 24 HOURS, ML.	WATER PER KG. BODY WT. IN 24 HOURS, ML.
3 days	3.0	250- 300	80-100
10 days	3.2	400- 500	125-150
3 months......	5.4	750- 850	140-160
6 months......	7.3	950-1100	130-155
9 months......	8.6	1100-1250	125-145
1 year	9.5	1150-1300	120-135
2 years.........	11.8	1350-1500	115-125
4 years.........	16.2	1600-1800	100-110
6 years.........	20.0	1800-2000	90-100
10 years.........	28.7	2000-2500	70- 85
14 years.........	45.0	2200-2700	50- 60
18 years.........	54.0	2200-2700	40- 50

equilibrium of the body by varying the osmolar content and volume of urine. Urine usually has a greater osmotic pressure (300 to 1000 milliosmoles per liter) than the internal environment (293 milliosmoles per liter).

CALORIES

The unit of heat in metabolism is the large calorie (Cal.), defined as the amount of heat necessary to raise the temperature of 1 kg. of water from 14.5 to 15.5°C. The production of heat varies with the oxidation of different foods, so that measuring the amount of oxygen consumed is an indirect method for measuring the amount of food oxidized and the heat produced. Estimates of heat production obtained from measurements of the end-products of oxidation, carbon dioxide and water, approximate those obtained by direct calorimetry.

There is great variation in the energy needs of children at different ages and under various conditions (see Fig. 3-1 and Table 3-3). The average expenditure of energy by the child of 6 to 12 years of age is approximately as follows: maintenance of basal metabolism, 50 per cent; specific dynamic action of food, 5 per cent; growth, 12 per cent; physical activity, 25 per cent; and loss by way of feces, about 8 per cent, mainly as unabsorbed fat.

Basal metabolism is measured at room temperature (20°C.) 10 to 14 hours after a meal, with the patient physically and emotionally quiet. For each degree centigrade of fever the basal metabolism is increased approximately 10 per cent. The basal requirement in infants is about 55 calories per kg. per day and decreases to 25 to 30 calories at maturity. The term *specific dynamic action* (SDA) refers to the increase in metabolism over the basal rate brought about by the ingestion and assimilation of food. Protein may increase the metabolism as much as 30 per cent above the basal level, except when it is being deposited in tissues, whereas fat and carbohydrate, which have a "sparing" effect on the specific dynamic action of protein and upon each other, cause an increase of only 4 to 6 per cent, respectively. Practically, the theoretic specific dynamic action is probably never attained. In infants about 7 to 8 per cent of the total caloric intake goes to specific dynamic action, whereas in older children on an ordinary mixed diet it is not likely to be more than about 5 per

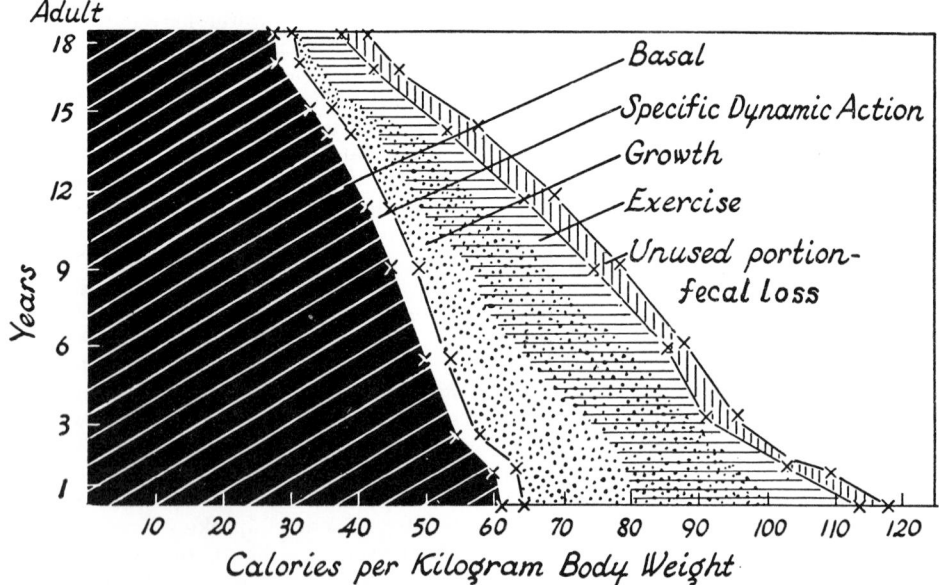

Figure 3-1. Total daily expenditure of calories with approximate distribution among individual factors in relation to age and weight.

TABLE 3-3. APPROXIMATE DAILY REQUIREMENTS OF CHILDREN FOR CALORIES, PROTEIN AND WATER

AGE IN YEARS	CALORIES*		PROTEIN	WATER*	
	Per Kg.	Per Lb.	Gm./Kg.†	Ml./Kg.	Oz./Lb.
Infancy‡..............................	110	50	3.5-2.0	150	2 /4
1-3	100	45	2.5-2.0	125	2-
4-6	90	41	3.0	100	1½
7-9	80	36	2.8	75	1.0+
10-12	70	32	2.0	75	1.0+
13-15	60	27	1.7	50	¾
16-19	50	23	1.5+	50	¾
Adult...................................	40	18	1.0	50	¾

*At least 10 per cent variation.

†To convert gm./kg. to gm./lb., divide by 2 and subtract 10 per cent of the quotient. Thus 4 gm./kg. is equivalent to 1.8 gm./lb.

‡First weeks lower; first 6 months relatively higher than last 6 months.

cent of total intake. The energy necessary to build body tissue *(growth)* is estimated to be the difference between the calories ingested and those expended for other purposes. The average requirement for *physical activity* is 15 to 25 calories per kg. per day, peak utilizations being as high as 50 to 80 calories for short periods of time. The amount of energy-producing food lost in the stools *(unused portion)*, except when absorption is impaired, is not more than 10 per cent of the intake.

Although caloric requirements can best be predicted from the surface area rather than from age or weight, the final criteria for meeting the child's needs depend upon the growth pattern, the sense of well-being and satiety. As indicated in Figure 3-1, the daily requirement is approximately 100 to 120 calories per kg. for the first year of life, with subsequent decreases of about 10 calories per kg. for each succeeding 3-year period. Periods of rapid growth and development near puberty require increased caloric consumption. The average distribution of calories in a well balanced diet is as follows: protein, 15 per cent; fat, 35 per cent; carbohydrates, 50 per cent.

Each gram of ingested protein or carbohydrate provides 4 calories, and 1 gm. of fat provides 9 calories. A continued caloric intake greater or less than the body expenditure will result in an increase or decrease in body fat. Abnormalities or adjustments in body weight will not be discussed here, but, in general, a consistent caloric imbalance of 500 calories a day results in a body weight change of about 1 pound per week.

PROTEINS

Protein, the predominant solid structure of the body, constitutes about 20 per cent of the body weight of the adult. Its amino acids are essential nutrients in the formation of cell protoplasm. It is found principally in the muscular and nervous systems and in the visceral and glandular tissues.

Protein is an integral part of most body fluids and secretions.

The kind, number and arrangement of the amino acids in a protein molecule determine the characteristics of the protein. Twenty-four amino acids have been identified; nine have been found to be essential for infants: threonine, valine, leucine, isoleucine, lysine, tryptophan, phenylalanine, methionine and histidine (necessary only for young infants). New tissue cannot be formed unless all the essential amino acids are present in the diet simultaneously; hence the absence of only one essential amino acid will result in a negative nitrogen balance. The requirements for the individual amino acids are considerably smaller for the school child than for the infant.

Complex protein structures are broken down to proteoses, peptones, simple peptides and finally to amino acids in the digestive process. The hydrochloric acid of the stomach acts upon the protein to form acid metaprotein, which is soluble in an acid medium and can be readily acted upon by rennin and pepsin. Rennin changes casein of milk to paracasein, which pepsin hydrolyzes along with other proteins to proteoses and peptones. In the alkaline medium of the intestine, trypsin from the pancreas hydrolyzes these proteoses and peptones to dipeptides, tripeptides and tetrapeptides and to some amino acids, and peptidase from the intestinal juices carries digestion of these to the amino acid stage.

Minute amounts of certain proteins may be absorbed unchanged, as evidenced by immunologic reactions, but it is the hydrolytic products, the amino acids, which are normally absorbed through the intestinal mucosa. The amino acids are carried to the liver by the portal circulation and from there distributed by the systemic circulation and taken up rapidly by the tissues. Excess amino acids undergo deamination, and the nitrogenous portions are converted to urea in the liver and excreted by the kidneys. The carbon from amino acids is oxidized much as that of carbohydrate or fat, some amino acids being

TABLE 3-4. FUNCTION, EFFECTS OF DEFICIENCY AND EXCESS, REQUIREMENTS AND SOURCES OF WATER, PROTEINS, CARBOHYDRATES AND FATS

FOOD-STUFFS	FUNCTIONS	EFFECTS OF DEFICIENCY	EFFECTS OF EXCESS	REQUIREMENTS	SOURCES
Water	Structure of cells; solvent for cellular changes; medium for ions; transport of nutrients and waste products; regulation of body temperature	Thirst, dryness of tongue, dehydration, anhydremia, high sp. gr. of urine, loss of kidney function (acidosis, uremia, anuria, death)	Abdominal discomfort, headache, cramps (water without salt), intoxication, convulsions, edema and circulatory failure	See Tables 3-1, 3-2 and 3-3 Related to calories consumed; greater in hot weather	Water as such All foods
Proteins	Supply amino acids for growth and repair of tissue cells; sols for osmotic equilibrium; ions in acid-base balance. With prosthetic groups to form hemoglobin, nucleoproteins, glycoprotein and lipoproteins. Enzymes, hormones, cellular respiratory substance, antibodies. Protective structures (nails and hair). Source of energy	Lassitude, abdominal enlargement, edema; depletion of plasma proteins, negative nitrogen balance; (no clinical syndrome due to lack of specific amino acid); kwashiorkor (protein malnutrition); marasmus (protein-calorie malnutrition)	Prolonged high protein intake probably not harmful. Important in certain anomalies involving amino acid and protein metabolism	See Table 3-3	Milk, eggs, meat, fish, poultry, cheese, soybeans, peas, beans, cereals, nuts, lentils
Carbohydrates	Readily available source of energy, antiketogenic, structure of cells, antibodies, source of stored calories (glycogen and fat), conversion to fat, resynthesis of amino acids, roughage	Ketosis if protein intake is less than 15% of calories or in starvation; underweight if total calories are low	Overweight if total calories are high. Various syndromes due to inborn errors of sugar metabolism.	To supply 25 to 55% of calories	Milk, cereals, fruits, sucrose, syrups, starches, vegetables
Fats	Concentrated source of energy; physical protection for vessels, nerves, organs: insulation against changes in temperature; structure of body tissues, cell membranes and nuclei; vehicle for absorption of vitamins (A, D, E and K); appetite appeal; aids satiety (delays emptying time of stomach); avoids necessity of ingestion of large bulk of foods; spares protein, vitamin A and thiamine; supplies linoleic acid	Lack of satiety (craving for fat); underweight; skin changes with intakes very low in linoleic acid	Overweight; abdominal symptoms in familial hyperlipemia; high cholesterol intakes may be harmful	Minimal not known; usually supplies 35% of calories Probably 1-2% of calories as linoleic acid	Milk, butter, egg yolk, lard, bacon, meat, fish, cheese, nuts, vegetable oils Breast milk usually supplies 4-5% of calories as linoleic acid; vegetable oils vary greatly, safflower, corn, soy and others being especially rich

glycogenic, others ketogenic. The absorption of protein is so efficient that little nitrogen is found in the stools.

The total plasma protein in the normal child ranges from 6 to 7.5 gm. per 100 ml., with somewhat lower values in newborn and premature infants. The albumin-globulin ratio is usually 2:1, fibrinogen varying from 0.1 to 0.4 gm. per 100 ml.

Aberrations in the metabolism of protein and the amino acids constitute a significant portion of disease entities in the category of inborn errors of metabolism. Important among these are phenylketonuria, leucine-induced hypoglycemia, maple syrup urine disease, histidinemia, hyperglycinemia, argininosuccinic aciduria and possibly other aminoacidurias, as well as protein-induced (gliadin and others) enteropathies.

There is an abundant protein supply available for infants and children in the United States. But neither the minimal nor the optimal intake is actually known, despite the fact that the supply of protein in many countries is so limited that the greatest need of infants throughout the world is for this nutrient.

CARBOHYDRATES

The greatest portion of the caloric needs of the body is supplied by carbohydrates, which also supply the necessary bulk of the diet. Carbohydrates are stored chiefly as glycogen in the liver and muscles, but probably make up no more than 1 per cent of the body weight. The infant's liver is one tenth that of the adult and the muscle mass one fiftieth; hence the infant has only a small fraction (approximately one twenty-sixth) of the glycogen reserve of the adult.

Carbohydrate is oxidized as glucose (dextrose), but is consumed in various forms: the monosaccharides (glucose, fructose, galactose), the disaccharides (lactose, sucrose, maltose, isomaltose) and the polysaccharides (starches, dextrins, glycogen, gums, cellulose). Pentoses are poorly absorbed.

Through a series of enzymatic and chemical reactions in the digestive tract, complex carbohydrates are split into simpler structures. Salivary and pancreatic amylases are primarily concerned in the breakdown of starch to oligosaccharides (dextrins) and disaccharides, primarily maltose. The disaccharides are absorbed intact into the intestinal brush border cells, where the various disaccharidases in the membrane fraction of the microvilli complete the hydrolysis to the monosaccharides: maltose to 2 molecules of glucose; sucrose to glucose and fructose; lactose to glucose and galactose. The monosaccharides are rapidly absorbed, glucose and galactose being actively taken up against concentration gradients, whereas fructose absorption is passive. During absorption

phosphoric acid radicals combine with hexose sugars in the intestinal mucosa, and the hexose-phosphates formed separate again into their component parts.

Some glucose may be oxidized directly, as in the brain and heart. Most of the absorbed sugar is converted to glycogen in the liver, although glycogenesis also occurs in other tissues of the body. Up to 15 per cent (usually about 10 per cent) of the weight of the liver and 3 per cent of the muscle may be glycogen; there are also small amounts in the skin and in practically all other organs. Glycogenolysis in the liver yields glucose as the chief product, whereas glycogen breakdown in the muscle yields lactic acid. The overall oxidation of glucose has 2 phases, the anaerobic (glycolysis) and the aerobic (tricarboxylic acid cycle). In the former, glucose is broken down to pyruvic acid; in the aerobic cycle pyruvic acid is completely oxidized to carbon dioxide and water. Insulin and the pituitary and adrenal hormones are involved in these processes, and nicotinic acid, thiamine, riboflavin and pantothenic acid take part in the enzymatic reactions. Carbohydrate which is not oxidized or stored as glycogen is converted to fat.

The principal carbohydrate metabolic disorders are diabetes mellitus, glycogen storage disease, galactosemia, fructose intolerance and glucose intolerance; lack of sugar-splitting enzymes in the intestines (lactase, invertase, maltase) is associated with diarrhea and malabsorption resulting from the osmotic effect of the unabsorbed sugar and from fermentation of the carbohydrate by intestinal bacteria.

FATS

Simple lipids are esters of fatty acids with various alcohols. They are the most abundant fats in the body and in food, the most common being triglycerides. *Compound lipids* (lecithin, cephalin, sphingomyelin, cerebrosides, sulfa and amino lipids) contain nitrogen bases, phosphoric acid, sugar, sulfur or amino groups with fatty acids and alcohol. *Derived lipids* from these 2 groups are separated out by hydrolysis; they include cholesterol and saturated and unsaturated fatty acids.

Naturally occurring fats contain straight-chain fatty acids, both saturated and unsaturated, varying in length from 4 to 24 carbon atoms, most of them containing 16 or 18. The degree of absorption varies in general with the melting point and the degree of unsaturation.

Ingested triglycerides are emulsified in the stomach by the continuous shearing action of the gastric muscular contractions. This emulsion passes into the duodenum, where pancreatic lipase hydrolyzes the triglycerides to monoglycerides and fatty acids. Intraluminal solubility is greatly enhanced by the presence of bile salts which form polymolecular micelles with the monoglycerides and fatty acids; the remaining unsplit diglycerides and triglycerides are insoluble even in the presence of bile salts.

Long-chain fatty acids and monoglycerides (those with more than 10 carbon atoms) are presumably absorbed into the mucosal cell by diffusion. Transport across the cell involves re-esterification of these fatty acids and mono-glycerides to triglycerides, which are then "coated" with lipoprotein to form the moiety known as the chylomicron, in which the fat is transported in the lymph system to the venous circulation via the thoracic duct.

Short and medium-chain triglycerides are handled in a somewhat different manner; they are readily hydrolyzed by pancreatic lipase to free fatty acids which are transported through the cell. Even when intraluminal hydrolysis is in-adequate because of pancreatic lipase or bile salt deficiency, these fats will be absorbed and, to some extent, will be hydrolyzed to free fatty acids within the cell by mucosal lipase. With neither esterifica-tion to triglycerides nor subsequent chylomicron formation, these free fatty acids directly enter the intestinal veins and pass to the liver via the portal system.

Linoleic and Arachidonic Acids. Human beings do not synthesize linoleic acid, an 18-carbon atom chain with 2 double bonds (dienoic acid); hence it must be supplied in the diet. Rapidly growing young infants maintained on diets very low in linoleic acid undergo dryness and thicken-ing of the skin with desquamation and intertrigo. These clinical symptoms disappear readily when the diet contains 1 to 2 per cent of the calories as linoleic acid. In patients with linoleic acid defi-ciency the blood serum values for dienoic and tetraenoic acids are less than 5.0 per cent and for trienoic acids greater than 5.0 per cent of the total fatty acids. In healthy infants the levels for these unsaturated fatty acids depend upon the amount of linoleic acid in the diet. For example, in infants 3 months of age receiving an evaporated milk for-mula the values are in the range of 12.0, 2.5 and 8.0 per cent for dienoic, trienoic and tetraenoic acids, respectively; in those receiving breast milk, in the range of 23.7, 1.2 and 12.0, and in those re-ceiving commercial milk preparations, in which certain vegetable oils replace the butterfat, the values are in the range of 32.0, 1.0 and 12.0 per cent of the total fatty acids. An abnormal meta-bolic eicosatrienoic acid accumulates in the blood and tissues when the linoleic acid content of the diet is very low.

Arachidonic acid, which can be synthesized readily if the diet contains linoleic acid, is much less efficient in alleviating the clinical and chemical manifestations of fat deficiency. Diets extremely low in linoleic acid require greater caloric consumption for comparable growth in both experimental animals and in infants.

The relation of dietary fat intake in infancy and childhood to the intimal fat streaking which begins in the major arterial vessels early in life remains to be clarified. Reduction of total fat in-take and an increase in the ratio of unsaturated to saturated fats is associated with significant re-duction in serum cholesterol levels in adults with hyperlipidemia. In the United States polyun-saturated vegetable fats have been widely substi-tuted for the more saturated butterfats in com-mercial milk formulas for many years; it has not yet been established whether atheromatous changes in young human subjects or in other primates are lessened by such substitutions.

MINERALS

Table 3-5 summarizes the physiologic aspects and dietary sources of the principal mineral ele-ments which have nutritional significance.

The ash content of the fetus is low; at birth it constitutes only about 3 per cent of the body weight. It increases continuously throughout childhood, both absolutely and relatively, so that in the adult the mineral content is 40 times greater than in the newborn, whereas the body weight is but 23 times greater. In the adult the ash content is 4.35 per cent of the body weight, 83 per cent of which is in the skeleton and 10 per cent in the muscle. It has been estimated that for each gram of protein retained, 0.3 gm. of mineral matter is deposited. The important electropositive elements (cations) are calcium, magnesium, potas-sium and sodium; the important electronegative ones (anions) are phosphorus, sulfur and chloride. Iron, iodine and cobalt appear in important organic complexes. The trace elements fluoride, copper, zinc and manganese have known metabolic roles; selenium, silicon, boron, nickel, aluminum, arsenic, bromine, molybdenum and strontium are present in the diet and in the body, but their functions have not been clarified.

Selenium. In areas where there is a high con-centration of selenium in the soil and food, ani-mals have severe nutritional disturbances. The significance in man is not known; however, in children in certain parts of Oregon where a high content of selenium has been found in soil and water, the incidence of dental caries and the urinary excretion of selenium are greater than in areas where exposure to selenium is known to be not as great.

Silicon. Silicon is present in all tissues, con-stituting as much as one ninth of the total ash. Because the amount in the skin decreases with age, it is believed to be related to its elasticity. Blood levels in man are as high as 16 mg. per 100 ml. Some silicon is excreted in the urine, but most in the feces. Silicosis has not been known to result from a dietary source.

Boron, Nickel, Aluminum, Bromine, Arsenic. These elements exist in minute traces in man, but have not been shown to be significant in either

(*Text continued on page 136.*)

TABLE 3-5. Physiology and Sources of Nutritionally Important Minerals

MINERAL	FUNCTION	PHYSIOLOGY	EFFECTS OF DEFICIENCY	EFFECTS OF EXCESS	DAILY ALLOWANCE	SOURCES
Calcium	Structure of bone and teeth, muscle contraction, nerve irritability, coagulation of blood, cardiac action, production of milk	Absorbed from upper small intestine: aided by vitamin D, ascorbic acid, lactose, acid reaction; hindered by excesses of dietary oxalic acid, phytic acid, fat, fiber, phosphate. Deposited in bone trabeculae and maintained in dynamic equilibrium with body tissues through action of parathyroid hormone. About 70% excreted in feces, 10% in urine; 15-25% retained, depending on growth rate	Poor mineralization of bones and teeth; osteomalacia; osteoporosis; tetany; rickets; impairment of growth	Unknown	Children under 10 years, 0.5-1.0 gm., depending on size and age; over 10 years, 1.1-1.4 gm., depending on vitamin D and sunlight. FAO-WHO* allowances less (0.5-0.7 gm.)	Milk, cheese, green leafy vegetables, canned salmon, clams, oysters
Chloride	Osmotic pressure; acid-base balance; HCl in gastric juice	Readily absorbed; about 92% of intake is excreted, mainly in the urine, some in feces and sweat; comprises about 2/3 of the blood plasma anions; blood serum level, 99-106 mEq./L.; in intracellular and extracellular fluids; parallels sodium intake and output	Hypochloremic alkalosis may occur in prolonged vomiting or excessive sweating, with the use of parenteral fluids (glucose) without saline; with excessive ACTH therapy and in congenital alkalosis (rare)	Unknown	Probably 0.5 gm.; average diet contains 3-9 gm.	Table salt, meat, milk, eggs
Cobalt	Part of vitamin B_{12} (cobalamin) molecule; contained in erythropoietin	Not utilized for synthesis of cobalamin by man; readily absorbed and excreted	None known	None (dietary); taken medicinally, may be goitrogenic	Unknown	Widely distributed
Copper	Essential for production of red blood cells; catalyst in hemoglobin formation; absorption of iron. Associated with activity of tyrosinase, catalase, uricase, cytochrome C oxidase, delta-aminolevulinic acid dehydrase (porphyrin formation)	Little information on factors affecting absorption; transported in plasma bound to plasma proteins and in ceruloplasmin; present in erythrocytes in a labile form and the more stable hemocuprein; highest concentration in liver and central nervous system (cerebrocuprein); excretion is mainly via the intestinal wall and bile; deranged metabolism in Wilson's disease (hepatolenticular degeneration)	Not established	None (dietary)	Estimated for children, 0.05-0.1 mg./kg.	Liver, oysters, meats, fish, whole grains, nuts, legumes
Fluoride	Tooth and bone structure	Retained when intake above 0.6 mg./day; excreted in urine and sweat; deposited in bones as fluorapatite (dynamic equilibrium)	Tendency to dental caries	Fluorosis: mottling of teeth with intake of more than 4-8 mg./day	0.5-1 mg. Recommended that community water supply contain 1 p.p.m. fluorine	Water, sea foods, plant and animal foods, depending upon content in soil and water

*Food and Agricultural Organization of United Nations.

TABLE 3-5. Physiology and Sources of Nutritionally Important Minerals *(Continued)*

MINERAL	FUNCTION	PHYSIOLOGY	EFFECTS OF DEFICIENCY	EFFECTS OF EXCESS	DAILY ALLOWANCE	SOURCES
Iodide	Constituent of thyroxin and triiodothyronine	Readily absorbed from intestine; circulates as inorganic and organic iodide; selectively concentrated about 25:1 in the thyroid gland, quickly iodized and incorporated into a complex known as thyroglobulin; proteolytic enzymes release thyroxin and triiodothyronine into the blood. Excretion mainly in urine. Antithyroid compounds interfere with iodine metabolism: goitrin of Brassicae; certain drugs	Simple goiter, endemic cretinism	Not harmful (less than 1 mg./day). Medicinally may cause iodism	Children, 0.04-0.10 mg.	Iodized salt, sea food, food grown in nongoitrous areas
Iron	Structure of hemoglobin and myoglobin for O_2 and CO_2 transport; oxidative enzymes: cytochrome C and catalase	Absorbed in ferrous form according to body need, aided by gastric juice and ascorbic acid; hindered by fiber, phytic acid, steatorrhea. Transported in plasma in ferric state bound to transferrin (a beta-1 globulin); stored in liver, spleen, bone marrow and kidney as ferritin and hemosiderin; carefully conserved and reused; minimal losses in urine and sweat; about 90% of intake excreted in the stool	Anemia: hypochromic, microcytic	Hemosiderosis in Bantu people of Africa due to low phosphorus and high iron contents of diet Poisoning by medicinal iron	Infants: 1 mg./kg. Children: ages 1 to 9, −8 to 12 mg.; ages 10 to 18, −15 mg.	Liver, meat, egg yolk, green vegetables, whole grains, legumes, nuts
Magnesium	Structure of bones and teeth; activation of enzymes in carbohydrate metabolism; muscle and nerve irritability. Important intracellular cation, essential to all metabolic processes	Principal cation of soft tissue; location chiefly intracellular; absorption from small intestine varies with level of intake; some urinary excretion, but excellent renal conservation; antagonist to calcium action	Not adequately understood; occurs in malabsorption and deficiency states; may be expressed clinically as tetany	None (dietary); toxicity from intravenous medication	150-300 mg. average intake	Cereals, legumes, nuts, meat, milk
Manganese	Enzyme activation, especially in mitochondria	Poor absorption from intestine; transported in plasma; particularly high turnover rate in mitochondria; excretion mainly via the intestine in the bile	Not known	Not known	Unknown	Legumes, nuts, whole grain cereals, green leafy vegetables
Molybdenum	Component of enzymes: xanthine oxidase for conversion to uric acid and mobilization of ferritin iron in liver, liver aldehyde oxidase	Readily absorbed from intestine; excreted chiefly in urine, some in bile	Not observed in man	Not established	Unknown	Legumes. grains, dark green leafy vegetables, animal organs

TABLE 3-5. PHYSIOLOGY AND SOURCES OF NUTRITIONALLY IMPORTANT MINERALS *(Continued)*

MINERAL	FUNCTION	PHYSIOLOGY	EFFECTS OF DEFICIENCY	EFFECTS OF EXCESS	DAILY ALLOWANCE	SOURCES
Phosphorus	Constituent of bones and teeth; structure of nucleus and cytoplasm of all cells; acid-base balance; key position in energy transformations and transmission of nerve impulses; metabolism of carbohydrate, protein and fat	About 70% of intake absorbed as free phosphorus from intestine; vitamin D implicated in intestinal absorption and kidney retention; excreted in urine and feces; occurs in blood as phospholipids, organic esters and inorganic phosphorus; inorganic phosphorus in blood serum of infants and children, 4-7 mg. 1100 ml.; ratio of inorganic-organic phosphorus in whole blood is about 1:20	Not established; rickets may develop in rapidly growing, very low-birth-weight babies with low intakes of both P and Ca	Possibility of tetany during recovery from rickets or in newborn on formula with low Ca: P (1:1) ratio	At least equal to calcium need; readily met if dietary calcium and protein requirements are met	Milk, milk products, egg yolk, flesh foods, legumes, nuts, whole grains
Potassium	Muscle contraction; nerve impulse conduction; intracellular osmotic pressure and fluid balance; heart rhythm	Primarily intracellular; absorption via intestine; excretion 80% in urine—some in sweat and feces; about 8% retained by growing child; blood serum level 4.0-5.6 mEq./L.	In starvation or in such pathologic conditions as diarrhea, diabetic acidosis, ACTH excess: muscle weakness, anorexia, nausea, abdominal distention, nervous irritability, drowsiness, confusion, tachycardia; deficiency exaggerates effects of sodium	Heart block at serum levels of 10 mEq./L.; important in Addison's disease, renal failure or administration of K-containing salts	1-2 gm. or 1.5 mEq./kg. or 40 mEq./M²	All foods
Sodium	Osmotic pressure; acid-base balance; water balance; muscle and nerve irritability	Readily absorbed from intestine; excreted chiefly in urine (98%); parallels intake; renal excretion controlled by adrenal cortical hormone; extracellular cation, but small amount in muscle and cartilage; blood serum level, 135-145 mEq./L.	Nausea; diarrhea, muscle cramps, dehydration	Edema if inadequate excretion or excessive parenteral fluids	2.0 mEq./kg. or 50 mEq./M² (newborn and prematures less)	Table salt, flesh foods, milk, eggs, sodium compounds as baking soda and powder, glutamate, seasonings and preservatives
Sulfur	Constituent of all cellular protein; cocarboxylase; melanin; mucopolysaccharides of mucous secretions, vitreous humor, synovial fluid, connective tissues, cartilage, heparin; insulin; metabolism of nerve tissue; detoxification mechanisms; tissue metabolism as SH group in coenzyme A, cystothioneine and glutathione	Only sources utilized are cystine and methionine; inorganic forms unavailable to body; excreted as inorganic sulfate or ethereal sulfate via urine and bile	Not known; growth failure from protein deficiency may be due in part to deficiency of S-containing amino acids	Not harmful; excreted in urine as sulfates	Not known; average intake 0.5-1.0 gm.	Protein foods contain about 1%

TABLE 3-5. Physiology and Sources of Nutritionally Important Minerals *(Concluded)*

MINERAL	FUNCTION	PHYSIOLOGY	EFFECTS OF DEFICIENCY	EFFECTS OF EXCESS	DAILY ALLOWANCE	SOURCES
Zinc	Constituent of several enzymes: carbonic anhydrase (in erythrocytes) which is essential for CO_2 exchange; carboxypeptidase of intestine for hydrolysis of protein; dehydrogenase of liver	Found in liver and organs, muscles, bones, red and white cells; higher tissue concentration in young subjects; excreted chiefly from intestine	Dwarfism, iron deficiency anemia, hepatosplenomegaly and hypogonadism in young males in Egypt (Nile Valley) is probably zinc deficiency state	Gastrointestinal upsets (from galvanized iron cooking utensils)	Not known; estimated intake 0.3 or more mg./kg. body weight; slight retention by children, therefore may be required	All foods

human or animal nutrition. Boron is essential for plants; nickel delays insulin hypoglycemia; aluminum in excess may interfere with absorption of phosphorus; and bromine and arsenic are important pharmacologically.

Strontium-90 and other radioactive isotopes are of increasing concern owing to the potential for radiation injury. They should also be studied in respect to their effects on nutrition.

VITAMINS

The word "vitamin" refers to organic compounds which are required in minute amounts to catalyze cellular metabolism essential for maintenance or growth of the organism. They must be supplied wholly or in part exogenously. In general, the B-complex vitamins function as coenzymes in a variety of specific biochemical reactions, whereas the exact modes of action of ascorbic acid and vitamins A, D, E and K are still obscure. Table 3-7 outlines aspects of the individual vitamins pertinent to human metabolism.

The physician should be aware that both vitamin deficiencies and excesses may exist. Hypervitaminosis A and hypervitaminosis D have been recognized for many years. More recently an increased incidence of idiopathic hypercalcemia of infancy in Great Britain was traced to the vitamin D enrichment of cereals and dried milks in addition to normal prophylactic vitamin supplementation. Daily intakes of up to 3000 to 4000 I.U. of vitamin D became common; this is 7 to 10 times the currently recommended allowance of 400 I.U. per day.

MISCELLANEOUS FACTORS

Roughage. Roughage is indigestible vegetable fiber. Amounts as high as 170 to 300 mg. per kg. per day appear to cause no difficulty. Most children who receive average, well balanced diets obtain sufficient amounts of roughage.

Digestibility. The relative amount of a given food available for assimilation is high in most of the common food classes: carbohydrate is 97 per

TABLE 3-6. Recommendations for Daily Intake of Minerals and Vitamins

AGE	MINERALS		VITAMINS						
	Ca*	Fe	A	Thiamine	Riboflavin	Niacin	Ascorbic Acid	D	B_6
	gm.	mg.	I.U.	mg.	mg.	mg.	mg.	I.U.	mg.
Infancy	0.7	6†	1500	0.4	0.6	6	30	400	0.2-0.3
1 to 3 years	0.8	8	2000	0.5	0.8	9	40	400	0.1-0.2
4 to 6 years	0.8	10	2500	0.6	1.0	11	50	400	0.1-0.2
7 to 9 years	0.8	12	3500	0.8	1.3	14	60	400	0.1-0.2
10 to 12 years	1.1	15	4500	1.0	1.4	16	70	400	0.1-0.2
13 to 15 years	1.4	15	5000	1.2	1.8	20	80	400	0.1-0.2
16 to 19 years	1.4	15	5000	1.6	2.0	22	80	400	0.1-0.2

Adapted from recommendations by the Food and Nutrition Board of the National Research Council. Slight variations were made in order to state the amounts necessary for each 3-year period after infancy in direct arithmetic progression. Values in adolescent years are for males.

*Food and Agricultural Organization of United Nations recommends somewhat lower intakes for calcium than those of the National Research Council: e.g. 0-12 mo., 500-600; 1-9 yrs., 400-500; 10-15 yrs., 600-700; 16-19 yrs., 500-600; adults, 400-500; with pregnancy, 1000-1200, and lactation, 1500-2000 mg./day.

†Or 1 mg./kg.

TABLE 3-7. Physical and Metabolic Properties and Food Sources of the Vitamins

NAME AND SYNONYMS	CHARACTERISTICS	METABOLISM	BIOCHEMICAL ACTION	EFFECTS OF DEFICIENCY	EFFECTS OF EXCESS	RECOMMENDED ALLOWANCES	SOURCES
VITAMIN A: An alcohol of high molecular weight attached to a beta-ionone ring *Provitamin A:* The plant pigments, alpha-, beta- and gamma-carotenes and cryptoxanthin	Fat-soluble; water-insoluble; heat-stable at usual cooking temperatures; destroyed by oxidation, drying and very high temperatures	Bile is necessary for absorption of the provitamins. Conversion of provitamins takes place primarily in the walls of the intestine, to some extent in the liver. Vitamin A and provitamins stored in liver. Absorption of both facilitated by the presence of fat, impaired by intake of mineral oil or by defect in fat absorption. Vitamin E minimizes oxidation of both in the intestine	Vitamin A aldehyde is retinene, which combines with specific proteins to form the retinal pigments, rhodopsin and iodopsin, for vision in dim light; bone and tooth development; formation and maturation of epithelia of skin, eye, digestive, respiratory, urinary and reproductive tracts	Nyctalopia, photophobia, xerophthalmia, conjunctivitis, keratomalacia leading to blindness; faulty epiphyseal bone formation; defective tooth enamel; keratinization of mucous membranes and skin; retarded growth	Dietary excess of vitamin A unlikely. Excessive carotene intake may produce carotenemia with xanthosis cutis. Individual variation in sensitivity to high intakes of vitamin A concentrates; 50,000 I.U. taken daily for prolonged periods may be toxic and cause anorexia, slow growth, drying and cracking of skin, enlargement of liver and spleen, swelling and pain of long bones, bone fragility	Up to 1 year, 1500 I. U./ day; 1 to 12 years, 2000 I.U. increasing to 4500 I.U. with age; over 12 years, 5000 I.U./day. These amounts assume that ⅔ comes from the provitamins, which are less efficiently utilized than the vitamin. If only vitamin A is taken, then 900 to 3000 I.U. would suffice	Liver, fish-liver oils, whole milk, milk fat products, egg yolk, fortified margarines. Carotenoids from plants— green vegetables, yellow fruits and vegetables
VITAMIN B COMPLEX: *Cobalamin:* Group of complex coordination compounds of cobalt-vitamin B_{12}; antipernicious anemia factor; Castle's extrinsic factor; animal protein factor (APF)	Slightly soluble in water; stable to heat in neutral solution; labile in acid or alkaline ones; destroyed by light	Castle's intrinsic factor of the stomach, necessary for absorption	Transfer of one-carbon units in purine and labile-methyl group metabolism; essential for maturation of red blood cells in bone marrow; metabolism of nervous tissue	Juvenile pernicious anemia, due to defect in absorption rather than to dietary lack; also secondary to gastrectomy	Unknown	Requirement probably 1 to 2 micrograms/day	Muscle and organ meats, fish, eggs, milk, cheese
Vitamin B_6 3 active forms: pyridoxine, pyridoxal, pyridoxamine	Water-soluble; destroyed by ultraviolet light and by heat	Readily absorbed; phosphorylated in tissue to form coenzyme; intestinal synthesis important	Constituent of coenzymes for amino acid metabolism: decarboxylation, transamination, transsulfuration, conversion of tryptophan to niacin; fatty acid metabolism	Infants: irritability, convulsions, hypochromic anemia; peripheral neuritis in patients receiving isoniazid, which is vitamin B_6 antagonist	Unknown	Estimated requirement: 1 to 2 mg./day. Infants: 0.2 to 0.3 mg./day normally; 2 to 5 mg./day if abnormal B_6 metabolic state exists	Meat, liver, kidney, whole grains, peanuts, soybeans
Folacin: Group of related compounds containing pteridine ring, para-amino benzoic acid and glutamic acid. Pteroylglutamic acid (PGA); folinic acid; citrovorum factor; leucovorin	Slightly soluble in water; labile to heat, light, acid	Excreted in both urine and feces in amounts in excess of intake (intestinal bacterial synthesis). Ascorbic acid is instrumental in the conversion of folic to folinic acid, the biologically active compound	Concerned with formation and metabolism of one-carbon units; hence participates in synthesis of purines, pyrimidines, nucleoproteins and methyl groups	Megaloblastic anemia (infancy, pregnancy); usually occurs secondary to malabsorption disease or to ascorbic acid deficiency	Unknown	Requirement probably 0.05 to 0.1 mg./day	Liver, green vegetables, nuts, cereals, cheese

TABLE 3-7   Physical and Metabolic Properties and Food Sources of the Vitamins *(Continued)*

NAME AND SYNONYMS	CHARACTERISTICS	METABOLISM	BIOCHEMICAL ACTION	EFFECTS OF DEFICIENCY	EFFECTS OF EXCESS	RECOMMENDED ALLOWANCES	SOURCES
Niacin: Nicotinamide; nicotinic acid; antipellagra vitamin	Water- and alcohol-soluble; stable to acid, alkali, light, heat, oxidation	Readily absorbed from small intestine; limited storage; excess excreted in urine as several metabolites; synthesized in the body from tryptophan; vitamin B_6 is essential for conversion	Active constituent of coenzymes I and II, cofactors in a number of dehydrogenase systems	Pellagra: multiple B-vitamin deficiency syndrome. Early symptoms: fatigue, anorexia. weight loss, headache	Nicotinic acid (not the amide) is vasodilator; reactions include skin flushing and itching, circulatory disturbances, increased peristalsis	6.6 mg./1000 calories; children under 10 years, 6 to 14 mg.; over 10 years, 16 to 22 mg./day, depending on caloric intake	Meat, fish, poultry, liver, whole-grain and enriched cereals, green vegetables, peanuts. Protein foods in general, from conversion of tryptophan (60 mg. forms 1 mg. of niacin)
Riboflavin: Vitamin B_2	Sparingly soluble in water; sensitive to light and alkali; stable to heat, oxidation, acid	Absorbed from the intestines; limited storage in tissues; excess excreted in urine; careful economy when intake is low and rapid excretion when intake is high. Absorption impaired in achlorhydria, diarrhea, vomiting. Utilization greater with increased metabolism	Constituent of 2 coenzymes which are components of a number of flavoprotein enzymes important in hydrogen transfer in a variety of reactions: amino acid, fatty acid and carbohydrate metabolism and cellular respiration. Retinal pigment of eye for light adaptation	Ariboflavinosis; early symptoms: photophobia, blurred vision, burning and itching of eyes, corneal vascularization, poor growth. One of the most common dietary inadequacies, often accompanying other B-vitamin deficiencies	Not harmful	0.025 mg./gm. of dietary protein; children under 10 years, 0.6 to 1.4 mg.; over 10 years, 1.4 to 2.0 mg./day, depending on food intake	Milk, cheese, liver and other organs, meats, eggs, fish, green leafy vegetables, whole or enriched grains
Thiamine: Vitamin B_1; antiberiberi vitamin; aneurin	Water- and alcohol-soluble; fat-insoluble; stable in slightly acid solution; labile to heat, alkali, sulfites	Readily absorbed from small and large intestines; combines with phosphate in all cells to form thiamine pyrophosphate (cocarboxylase); limited body stores; excess excreted in urine; destroyed in body by intake of raw fish or clams which contain thiaminases. Poor absorption in persistent GI disturbances	Component of carboxylases, which act in various oxidative decarboxylations, including that of pyruvic acid	Beriberi—early stages: easily fatigued, irritable, emotional instability, anorexia. Later: indigestion, constipation, headache, insomnia, tachycardia after exercise. Late stage: polyneuritis, cardiac failure, edema. Diagnosis: elevated pyruvic acid in the blood after exercise or after intake of standard amount of glucose, in conjunction with low urinary thiamine	None from oral intake	0.5 mg./1000 calories; children under 10 years, 0.4 increasing to 1.1 mg.; children over 10 years, 1.2 to 1.4 mg./day, increasing with caloric requirement	Liver, meats, especially pork, milk, whole-grain or enriched cereals, wheat germ, legumes, nuts
VITAMIN C: *Ascorbic acid:* Vitamin C; antiscorbutic vitamin	Water-soluble; easily oxidized; oxidation is accelerated by heat, light, alkali, oxidative enzymes, traces of copper or iron; fairly stable in acid solution at low temperature	Readily absorbed; blood plasma levels reflect daily intake, whereas concentration in leukocytes reflects tissue level; excess excreted in urine; little tissue storage, but high concentrations in glandular tissues; man, monkeys, guinea pigs cannot synthesize it from glucose; dehydroascorbic acid, first oxidation product, is biologically active	Mechanism of action not known; structure and maintenance of intercellular material in all tissues; facilitates absorption of iron; conversion of folic acid to folinic acid; probably coenzyme in the metabolism of tyrosine and phenylalanine. Contributes to activity of succinic dehydrogenase and serum phosphatase in infants, not in adults	Scurvy; early symptoms are irritability and slow growth; susceptibility to infection; hemorrhagic manifestations; poor wound healing	Not harmful	First year, 30 mg.; 1 to 12 years, 40 mg., increasing to 80 mg.; 13 to 20 years, 80 mg.	Citrus fruits, tomatoes, berries, cantaloupe, cabbage, green vegetables. Cooking has deleterious effect

TABLE 3-7 Physical and Metabolic Properties and Food Sources of the Vitamins (Concluded)

NAME AND SYNONYMS	CHARACTER-ISTICS	METABOLISM	BIOCHEMICAL ACTION	EFFECTS OF DEFICIENCY	EFFECTS OF EXCESS	RECOMMENDED ALLOWANCES	SOURCES
VITAMIN D: Group of sterols having similar physiologic activity. D$_2$-calciferol is activated ergosterol. D$_3$ is activated 7-dehydrocholesterol	Fat-soluble; stable to heat, acid, alkali and oxidation	Absorbed from intestine with fat, bile salts being required. Pro-vitamin D$_3$ is synthesized in the skin and is converted to the vitamin by ultraviolet irradiation and absorbed. Storage is primarily in the liver. Excretory products not known	Mechanism of action not known. Regulates absorption and deposition of calcium and phosphorus, presumably by affecting permeability of intestinal membrane. Regulation of level of serum alkaline phosphatase, which is believed to be concerned with calcium phosphate deposition in bones and teeth	Rickets (high serum phosphatase level appears before bone deformities); infantile tetany, poor growth, osteomalacia	Wide variation in tolerance; in general, 20,000 to 50,000 I.U./day is toxic when continued for weeks (prolonged administration of 1800 I.U./day may be toxic (see Hypercalcemia, p. **0000**). Manifestations are nausea, diarrhea, weight loss, polyuria, nocturia, eventually calcification of soft tissues, including heart, renal tubules, blood vessels, bronchi, stomach	400 I.U./day	Vitamin D-fortified milk and margarine, fish liver oils, exposure to sunlight or other ultraviolet sources
VITAMIN E: Group of related chemical compounds — tocopherols — having similar biologic activity	Fat-soluble; heat-stable in absence of oxygen; unstable to ultraviolet light, alkali; readily oxidized by oxygen, iron, lead, rancid fats. Antioxidant in foods and the body	Absorption may be affected by fat digestion. Some storage in fatty tissues, but not in liver	Mechanism of action unknown (cell maturation and differentiation). Minimizes oxidation of carotene, vitamin A and linoleic acid in the intestine. Possibly related to muscle metabolism and to erythrocyte fragility	Not established; may be involved in red blood cell fragility and muscle cell metabolism	Unknown	Not known	Germ oils of various seeds, green leafy vegetables, nuts, legumes
VITAMIN K: Group of compounds: naphthoquinones, with similar biologic activity	Natural compounds are fat-soluble, but several water-soluble products have been developed (menadione). Stable to heat and reducing agents; labile to oxidizing agents, strong acids, alcoholic alkali, light	Bile salts necessary for intestinal absorption of fat-soluble forms. Limited storage in liver; synthesized by intestinal microorganisms	Mechanism of action unknown; necessary for prothrombin formation, hence normal blood clotting	Hemorrhagic manifestations: result of faulty intestinal synthesis of vitamin K (newborn, prolonged use of sulfonamides and antibiotics), faulty intestinal absorption, or inability to synthesize prothrombin (hepatic damage). Except in the last condition, menadione and bile salts effective. Dicumarol and salicylates act as vitamin K antimetabolites	Not established. Medicinally may produce hyperbilirubinemia in prematures	Not a dietary problem. 1 to 2 mg./day appear to be adequate	Green leafy vegetables, pork liver. Widely distributed

cent; fat, 95 per cent; protein, 92 per cent. Cooking is a factor in digestibility. For example, the boiling of milk reduces the size of the curd and renders it more digestible for infants; by contrast, heating destroys vitamin C activity.

Satiety. The ingestion of a meal should provide a sense of well-being. Whole milk, cream, eggs and fatty foods have a high satiety value; sugar increases the flow of gastric juice and delays emptying of the stomach, thus increasing satiety. Bread and potatoes have relatively low satiety values, as do lean fish, vegetables and many fruits.

Availability. Poverty and lack of practical education in food buying and preparation, and sometimes illness leading to parental neglect, are the main causes of malnutrition in children. Diets of families in the lower income brackets are likely to be deficient in milk, fruits, fresh vegetables and meats. A suggested method for planning low-cost meals is to divide the money available for food into fifths: one fifth each for vegetables and fruits; milk and cheese; meats, fish and eggs; bread and cereals; and fats, sugar and other food adjuncts.

Geographic distribution also influences the availability of foods, the tendency being for a population to consume foods indigenous to its own area.

The effect of geographic factors on deficiency diseases is evidenced in the high incidence of goiter due to a deficiency of iodine in certain areas and by the relation between dental caries and fluoride in communal water supplies.

Bacterial Synthesis. Certain vitamins are synthesized in the human gastrointestinal tract; however, the extent to which they can meet the body needs is uncertain. Once the bacterial flora of the intestinal tract has been established, vitamin K is readily available to the body. Pantothenic acid and biotin play essential roles in human metabolism; bacterial synthesis alone is sufficient to meet the body needs for them. Thiamine, riboflavin, niacin, vitamin B_6, vitamin B_{12} and folic acid are synthesized in some species, but synthesis is limited or does not exist at all in man. The kind of food or nature of intestinal flora may affect vitamin production or availability. For

instance, 3 per cent of the population in Kobe, Japan, were found to harbor intestinal bacteria which split thiamine, and evidences of beriberi appeared in these persons.

Antimicrobial Agents. Administration of antimicrobial agents may influence the nutritional status. Sometimes appetite is impaired sufficiently to precipitate borderline deficiency states. Several antibiotics are known to produce steatorrhea; penicillin and sulfonamide seem to provoke the syndrome only when used together. Neomycin has been shown to produce malabsorption in adults. Orally administered broad-spectrum antibiotics decrease nitrogen balance. Isoniazid combines with pyridoxal phosphate and may produce symptoms of vitamin B_6 deficiency. Antimicrobial compounds may be transmitted in breast milk and may be ingested in foods from animals which have been fed these compounds.

TABLE 3-8. RECOMMENDED FOOD INTAKE FOR GOOD NUTRITION ACCORDING TO FOOD GROUPS AND THE AVERAGE SIZE OF SERVINGS AT DIFFERENT AGE LEVELS

FOOD GROUP	SERVINGS PER DAY	AVERAGE SIZE OF SERVINGS					
		1 year	2-3 years	4-5 years	6-9 years	10-12 years	13-15 years
Milk and cheese .... (1.5 oz. cheese = 1 C milk) (C = 1 cup − 8 oz. or 240 gm.)	4	½ C	½-¾ C	¾ C	¾-1 C	1 C	1 C
Meat group (protein foods)	3 or more						
Egg....................................		1	1	1	1	1	1 or more
Lean meat, fish, poultry .... (liver once a week)		2 Tbsp.	2 Tbsp.	4 Tbsp.	2-3 oz. (4-6 Tbsp.)	3-4 oz.	4 oz. or more
Peanut butter........................			1 Tbsp.	2 Tbsp.	2-3 Tbsp.	3 Tbsp.	3 Tbsp.
Fruits and vegetables	At least 4, including:						
Vitamin C source (citrus fruits, berries, tomato, cabbage, cantaloupe)...........	1 or more (twice as much tomato as citrus)	⅓ C citrus	½ C	½ C	1 medium orange	1 medium orange	1 medium orange
Vitamin A source.................... (green or yellow fruits and vegetables)	1 or more	2 Tbsp.	3 Tbsp.	4 Tbsp. (¼ C)	¼ C	⅓ C	½ C
Other vegetables (potato and legumes, etc.) *or*	2	2 Tbsp.	3 Tbsp.	4 Tbsp. (¼ C)	⅓ C	½ C	¾ C
Other fruits (apple, banana, etc.)		¼ C	⅓ C	½ C	1 medium	1 medium	1 medium
Cereals (whole-grain or enriched)	At least 4						
Bread...................................		½ C	1 slice	1½ slices	1-2 slices	2 slices	2 slices
Ready-to-eat cereals...............		½ oz.	¾ oz.	1 oz.	1 oz.	1 oz.	1 oz.
Cooked cereal (including macaroni, spaghetti, rice, etc.)......		¼ C	⅓ C	½ C	½ C	¾ C	1 C or more
Fats and carbohydrates	To meet caloric needs						
Butter, margarine, mayonnaise, oils: 1 Tbsp. = 100 calories		1 Tbsp.	1 Tbsp.	1 Tbsp.	2 Tbsp.	2 Tbsp.	2-4 Tbsp.
Desserts and sweets: 100-calorie portions as follows: ⅓ C pudding or ice cream 2-3″ cookies, 1 oz. cake, 1⅓ oz. pie, 2 tbsp. jelly, jam, honey, sugar		1 portion	1½ portions	1½ portions	3 portions	3 portions	3-6 portions

Prepared in collaboration with Mildred J. Bennett, Ph.D., from "Four Food Groups of the Daily Food Guide," Institute of Home Economics, U.S.D.A., and Publication #30, Children's Bureau of the United States Department of Health, Education, and Welfare.

Endocrine Factors. Antithyroid substances (goitrogens) have been found in turnips, ruta-bagas, cabbage, soybeans, cobalt-containing foods, food additives and medications; they increase the requirement for iodine. Administration of ACTH or corticosteroids necessitates an increase in protein and calcium and a decrease in sodium intake. Relative hypoparathyroidism with tetany has been observed in the neonatal period after excessive intakes of vitamin D and phosphates.

Radioactivity. Apparently there is little danger from carbon-14, owing to its long half-life. Iodine-131 is removed from milk by aeration or storage. Cesium-137 may be found in meat and milk products and can be counteracted by a high potassium intake or by the use of Diamox. Strontium-90 is filtered out to a large extent by the mammary gland, and only 10 per cent of ingested strontium-90 is found in milk.

Emotional Factors. Along with increased knowledge of the significance of various nutrients there has developed excessive parental and professional concern over the food intake of the individual infant or child. The mother may become so infatuated with statements of so-called experts in nutrition that she develops a sense of fear, even guilt, about her child's eating habits. The result is a battle of wits between mother and child which may have far-reaching effects. The physician who sees children in his practice must be well informed in the fundamentals of nutrition in order to recognize and manage emotional and behavioral problems arising from undesirable dietary practices.

EVALUATION OF DIET

The physician who sees children should have a reasonable knowledge of the properties of various foods so as to be able to take and evaluate a meaningful dietary history, to know which laboratory tests have value for diagnosis, and to be able to interpret therapeutic responses (see Tables 3-8, 3-9, 3-10).

The recall-interview for determining food habits of children is satisfactory under usual circumstances, but for more accurate accounting of food consumption the mother should be instructed to observe the actual food intake. It is best to report the *amount* and *frequency* of food intake in terms of the standard measuring cup or tablespoon, weight or size of pieces. The data may then be converted to "servings" appropriate to the age of the child (see Table 3-8). It is important to include items such as liver, cake and eggs, which may not be consumed daily.

The dietary guide according to food groups (Table 3-8) provides flexibility in cultural, religious and personal preferences and in seasonal, regional and economic availability. The food intake record (Table 3-10), based on selections from the food groups, is helpful in indicating possible nutritional imbalances. An excessive intake of foods of one group may result in a high caloric level and, hence, overweight and may lead to a dangerously low intake of other essential nutrients. A notable example is the overconsumption of milk and the underconsumption of meat and

TABLE 3-9. COMPARISON OF NUTRIENT VALUES OF THE DIETS PRESENTED IN TABLE 3-8 WITH THE RECOMMENDED DIETARY ALLOWANCES

AGE AND WEIGHT (Boys and Girls 25-75th percentiles)	CALORIES*	PROTEIN gm.	CALCIUM gm.	IRON mg.	VITAMIN A I.U.	THIAMINE† mg.	RIBOFLAVIN† mg.	NIACIN† mg.	ASCORBIC ACID mg.	VITAMIN D I.U.
1 year (22 ± 2 lb.)	1020 (1000)	42 (20)	0.6 (0.7)	5.4 (6.0)	2325 (1500)	0.47 (0.4)	1.0 (0.6)	3.4 (6.0)	40 (30)	300 (400)
2-3 years (30 ± 5 lb.)	1320 (1300)	48 (32)	0.8 (0.8)	6.1 (8.0)	3225 (2000)	0.64 (0.5)	1.0 (0.8)	7.3 (9.0)	51 (40)	400 (400)
4-5 years (39 ± 6 lb.)	1720 (1600)	67 (40)	1.0 (0.8)	8.4 (10.0)	4270 (2500)	0.85 (0.6)	1.5 (1.0)	11.7 (11.0)	60 (50)	500 (400)
6-9 years (56 ± 15 lb.)	2130 (2100)	76 (52)	1.1 (0.8)	11.4 (12.0)	5140 (3500)	1.2 (0.8)	2.0 (1.3)	19.3 (14.0)	88 (60)	600 (400)
10-12 years (81 ± 20 lb.)	2480 (2200-2400)	93 (55-60)	1.4 (1.1)	13.0 (15.0)	4590 (4500)	1.4 (1.0)	2.5 (1.4)	23.0 (16.0)	102 (70)	600 (400)
13-15 years (108 ± 27 lb.)	2580-3080 (2500-3000)	100 (62-75)	1.4 (1.4)	14.4 (15.0)	5540 (5000)	1.5 (1.2)	2.5 (1.8)	23.7 (20.0)	107 (80)	600 (400)

Recommended Dietary Allowances, Revised 1968, National Research Council, National Academy of Sciences, and FAO recommendations for calcium requirements.

*Selections from fats and carbohydrate group included for caloric values, but not for other nutrients.

†Based on the following: thiamine, 0.5 mg./1000 calories; riboflavin, 0.025 mg./gm. of protein; niacin, 6.6 mg./1000 calories.

eggs, with the resultant danger of iron deficiency anemia. When certain key foods, such as milk, eggs and citrus fruits, are eliminated for personal or medical reasons, the deficiencies imposed may be compensated by judicious substitutions. Following is a list of the primary nutrient contributions, besides calories, of the food groups:

Milk: high-quality protein, calcium and phosphorus; riboflavin; vitamin A; vitamin D (if fortified)

Meat and eggs: high-quality protein, iron, B vitamins; vitamin A from liver and eggs

Fruits and vegetables: vitamin C; provitamin A from green and yellow ones; trace elements; fiber

Cereals: less expensive and supplementary amounts of protein, minerals, fiber, B vitamins

Suspected dietary insufficiencies may be corroborated by appropriate laboratory tests and clinical evaluation. When malnutrition, either as dietary deficiency or excess, or failure to thrive exists in spite of what appears to be a satisfactory food intake, intense efforts must be made to detect evidences of infection, malignancy, faulty absorption, excretion or utilization, endocrine disorders, parasitic infestation, degenerative disease and especially errors in metabolism.

This section originally prepared for this textbook by Arild E. Hansen.

WILLIAM E. LAUPUS
MILDRED J. BENNETT

TABLE 3-10. DIETARY HISTORY

Food Record of _____

Age _____ Sex _____ Height _____ in. (_____ %ile) Weight _____ lb. (_____ %ile)

FOOD GROUP	AM'T/WK.	AM'T/DAY	SERVINGS/DAY PER GROUP* ACTUAL	RECOM- MENDED
Milk and cheese (1.5 oz. cheese = 1 C milk)				
Milk (indicate whole or skim; include that taken as beverage, on cereal, in cooked foods)	_____	_____		
Cheese	_____	_____		
Total milk equivalents (4 servings)			_____	(4)
Meat group (protein foods)				
Eggs (cooked any way, in custards, etc.)	_____	_____		
Lean meat (beef, veal, pork, ham, lamb, poultry, fish)	_____	_____		
Liver	_____	_____		
Peanut butter	_____	_____		
Total (at least 3 servings)			_____	(3)
Fruits and vegetables				
Vitamin C (orange, grapefruit, berries, tomato, cantaloupe, etc.)	_____	_____		
Green or yellow (leafy vegetables, peas, green beans, carrots, yellow squash, peaches, apricots, etc.)	_____	_____		
Other vegetables (potato, beans, parsnips, turnips, etc.)	_____	_____		
Other fruits (apple, banana, pear, etc.)	_____	_____		
Total (at least 4 servings)			_____	(4)
Cereal group (whole grain or enriched)				
Bread	_____	_____		
Cooked cereal (farina, oatmeal, macaroni, rice, spaghetti, etc.)	_____	_____		
Ready-to-eat	_____	_____		
Total (at least 4 servings)			_____	(4)
Miscellaneous (for calories and satiety)				
Fats—Butter and margarine	_____	_____		
Mayonnaise	_____	_____		
Oils and salad dressing	_____	_____		
Sweets (cake, pie, cookies, candy, soft drinks, sugar, etc.)	_____	_____		
Total			_____	

*See Table 3-8 for sizes of servings for the different ages.

Evaluation and/or recommendations _____

_____

_____

_____

REFERENCES

General

Beaton, G. H., and McHenry, E. W. (Eds.): *Nutrition*. New York, Academic Press, Inc., 1965.

Burton, B. T.: *The Heinz Handbook of Nutrition*. Published for H. J. Heinz Co. Inc., New York, Blakiston Division, McGraw-Hill Book Company, Inc., 1965.

Cheek, D. B.: *Human Growth*. Philadelphia, Lea & Febiger, 1968.

Committee on Nutrition, American Academy of Pediatrics: Water Requirement in Relation to Osmolar Load as It Applies to Infant Feeding. *Pediatrics*, 19:339, 1957.
On the Feeding of Solid Foods to Infants. *Pediatrics*, 21:685, 1958.
Trace Elements in Infant Nutrition. *Pediatrics*, 26:715, 1960.
Composition of Milks. *Pediatrics*, 26:1039, 1960.
Appraisal of Nutritional Adequacy of Infant Formulas Used as Cow's Milk Substitutes. *Pediatrics*, 31:329, 1963.
Factors Affecting Food Intake. *Pediatrics*, 33:135, 1964.
Protection of the Infant Diet: Government and Industry. *Pediatrics*, 36:648, 1965.
Nutritional Management in Hereditary Metabolic Disease. *Pediatrics*, 40:290, 1967.
Obesity in Childhood. *Pediatrics*, 40:455, 1967.

Duncan, G. G.: *Diseases of Metabolism*. 5th ed. Philadelphia, W. B. Saunders Company, 1964.

Everson, G. J.: Bases for Concern About Teenagers' Diets. *J. Am. Diet. A.*, 36:17, 1960.

Falkner, F. (Ed.): *Human Development*. Philadelphia, W. B. Saunders Company, 1966.

Fomon, S. J.: *Infant Nutrition*. Philadelphia, W. B. Saunders Company, 1967.

Food and Nutrition Board: Recommended Dietary Allowances. Washington, D.C., National Research Council, 1968.

Hansen, A. E.: Symposium on Nutrition and Nutritional Problems. *Pediat. Clin. N. Amer.*, 9:877-1045, 1962.

Mitchell, H. S., Rynbergen, H. J., Anderson, L., and Dibble, M. V.: *Cooper's Nutrition in Health and Disease*. 15th ed. Philadelphia, J. B. Lippincott Company, 1968.

Pike, R. L., and Brown, M.D.: *Nutrition: An Integrated Approach*. New York, John Wiley & Sons, 1967.

Stanbury, J. B., Wyngaarden, J. B., and Frederickson, D. S. (Eds.): *The Metabolic Basis of Inherited Disease*. 2nd ed., New York, McGraw-Hill Book Company, Inc., 1966.

Turner, D. (Ed.): *Handbook of Diet Therapy*. 4th ed. Chicago, University of Chicago Press (American Dietetic Association), 1965.

White, A., Handler, P., and Smith, E. L.: *Principles of Biochemistry*. 4th ed., New York, Blakiston Division, McGraw-Hill Book Company, Inc., 1968.

Wohl, M. G., and Goodhart, R. S.: *Modern Nutrition in Health and Disease*. 2nd ed. Philadelphia, Lea & Febiger, 1960.

Protein, Fat and Carbohydrate

Albanese, A. A. (Ed.): *Protein and Amino Acid Metabolism*. New York, Academic Press, Inc., 1959.

Cornblath, M., and Schwartz, R.: *Disorders of Carbohydrate Metabolism in Infancy*. Philadelphia, W. B. Saunders Company, 1966.

Flodin, N. W. (Ed.): Protein Nutrition. *Ann. New York Acad. Sc.*, 69:855-1061, 1958.

Food and Nutrition Board, Division of Biology and Agriculture: Evaluation of Protein Nutrition. Washington, D.C., National Research Council, Committee on Amino Acids, 1959.

Hansen, A. E., Stewart, R. A., Hughes, G., and Soderhjelm, L.: The Relation of Linoleic Acid to Infant Feeding, a Review. *Acta Paediat.*, 51: Suppl., 1962.

Holt, L. E., Jr., Gyorgy, P., Pratt, E. L., Snyderman, S. E., and Wallace, W. M.: *Protein and Amino Acid Requirements in Early Life*. New York, New Press, 1960.

Isselbacher, K.: Biochemical Aspects of Fat Absorption. *Gastroenterol.*, 50:78, 1966.

Sargent, D. W.: An Evaluation of Basal Metabolic Data for Infants in the United States. United States Department of Agriculture. Home Economics Research Report No. 18, 1962.

Vitamins

Committee on Nutrition, American Academy of Pediatrics: Appraisal of the Use of Vitamin B_1 and B_{12} as Supplements Promoted for the Stimulation of Growth and Appetite in Children. *Pediatrics*, 21:860, 1958.
Vitamin K. Compounds and the Water-Soluble Analogues. *Pediatrics*, 28:501, 1961.
Infantile Scurvy and Nutritional Rickets in the United States. *Pediatrics*, 29:646, 1962.
Vitamin E in Human Nutrition. *Pediatrics*, 31:324, 1963.
The Prophylactic Requirement and the Toxicity of Vitamin D. *Pediatrics*, 31:512, 1963.
Vitamin B_6 Requirements in Man. *Pediatrics*, 38:1068, 1966.

FEEDING OF INFANTS

Successful infant feeding requires *cooperative* functioning between the mother and her baby, starting with the initial feeding experience and continuing throughout the child's period of dependency. The close relation between feeding habits and personality patterns begins shortly after birth, and prompt establishment of comfortable, satisfying feeding practices contributes greatly to the infant's emotional well-being. Feeding time should be a pleasant and pleasurable period for both mother and child. Maternal feelings are readily transmitted to the baby and, in large measure, determine the emotional setting in which feeding takes place. Unquestionably, a mother who is tense, anxious, irritable, easily upset or emotionally labile is more likely to experience difficulty in the feeding relationship.

The feeding of infants requires practical interpretation of specific nutritional needs and of the widely varying limits of the normal baby's appetite and behavior with regard to food. The empty-ing time of the infant's stomach may vary from 1 to 4 or more hours; thus considerable difference in desire for food may be expected in the infant at different times of the day, and ideally the feeding schedule should be based on reasonable "self-regulation" by the infant. Variation in the time between feedings and in the amount taken per feeding is to be expected in the first few weeks with such a plan of "self-regulation," but by the end of the first month more than 90 per cent of infants will have established a suitable and reasonably regular schedule.

Most healthy infants will want 6 to 8 feedings a day by the end of the first week of life. The majority will take enough at 1 feeding to satisfy them for approximately 4 hours; some who are smaller or whose gastric emptying time is more rapid will want milk about every 3 hours. Most infants will not awaken for the middle-of-the-night feeding after 3 to 6 weeks of age; some may never need it. The majority will omit the late evening feeding between 4 and 8 months of age and will be satisfied with 3 meals a day by 9 to 12 months.

In helping to provide a schedule guided by the infant's needs and behavior, it is important to establish that he may cry for other reasons than hunger and that *he need not be fed every time he cries*; some infants are placid, some unusually active, some irritable; sick infants are often disinterested in food. Babies who awaken and cry consistently at short intervals may not be receiving enough milk or may have discomfort from some other cause than hunger. Included in the last category are too much clothing; soiled, wet or uncomfortable diapers and clothing; colic; swallowed air ("gas"); uncomfortably hot or cold environment; and illness. Some babies cry to gain sufficient or additional attention, whereas others deprived of adequate mothering become disinterested. Infants who stop crying when they are picked up or held do not usually need food, nor do those who continue to cry when food is offered. The habit of offering frequent, small feedings or of holding and feeding to pacify all crying should not be cultivated.

The advantages to the infant in supplying his needs as they are expressed are several: his physiologic requirements are met promptly; he does not learn to associate prolonged crying and discomfort with feeding; and he is less likely to develop poor eating practices such as gulping his feedings or taking small amounts too frequently. He soon establishes a regular schedule which permits the family to resume normal function. If he does not, individual feedings or the whole day's schedule can be moved ahead or delayed sufficiently to avoid conflicts with necessary family activities.

Some mothers will not understand the goals of "self-regulation" by the infant; some will misinterpret the physician's instructions, and others may not have the capacity to adjust themselves to the regimen of the infant. *The orderly, overanxious and compulsive parent will do better with a more specific outline for the infant's activities.*

The postpartum period is often a time of great anxiety and insecurity for the mother, who may be temporarily overwhelmed by the reality of the responsibilities of motherhood. It is important that the hospital setting and the attitude of the hospital personnel be comforting and supporting while the mother finds and develops confidence in her maternal abilities. Time is rewardingly spent in conferences at the hospital or in the home, where simple procedures are explained and potential problem areas are discussed. *The questions of inexperienced or uncertain mothers will frequently go unanswered unless time is set aside to consider them.*

Fathers and other members of the household should not be neglected by physicians in these anticipatory guidance sessions. Knowledge of the personalities and expectations of both parents is invaluable in helping to avert physical and psychologic problems centered around feeding. Parental misconceptions and confusion concerning the dietary and satiety needs of infants and children are often the bases for abnormal parent-child relations which can be avoided by appropriate counseling. The experienced physician will utilize similar general principles pertaining to infant feeding practices whether the infant is breast- or bottle-fed.

BREAST FEEDING

In the past half century the incidence of breast feeding has significantly declined in the industrially developed countries for a variety of reasons, among which changing social patterns and the development of excellent substitutes for breast milk are most important. Nevertheless breast feeding continues to have practical and psychologic advantages which should be considered when the mother selects the way in which she will feed her baby.

Advantages of Breast Feeding. Human milk is always readily available at the proper temperature wherever the mother may be. No time is required in preparation of the feeding. The milk is always fresh and free of contaminating bacteria, so that the chances of gastrointestinal disturbances are lessened. Although there is little if any difference in mortality rates in formula-fed and breast-fed infants receiving good care, among the lower socioeconomic groups and where sanitary conditions are poor the breast-fed infant continues to have a much greater likelihood of survival.

Feeding difficulties such as "spitting," colic and allergic reactions are fewer and less severe in breast-fed infants. Cow's milk allergy or intolerance is not seen in infants fed human milk. The occurrence of atopic eczema is somewhat more frequent in infants receiving formulas derived from cow's milk.

Stevenson reported a slightly higher incidence of respiratory infections during the second 6 months of life in formula-fed babies. Heiner and others have correlated chronic pulmonary hemosiderosis with the presence of precipitins to milk proteins in the serum of infants and have described improvement when cow's milk is removed from the diet.

The influence of the various bacterial and viral antibodies in human milk on resistance to infection in the infant is probably small. Breast-fed infants of mothers with high antipoliomyelitis titers are relatively resistant to infection by the attenuated live poliomyelitis vaccine viruses, a matter of practical importance in the administration of oral vaccines to these infants. It has also been shown that growth of the mumps, influenza, vaccinia and Japanese B encephalitis viruses can be inhibited by substances in human milk. But in contrast to the situation in calves, few of these ingested antibodies in infants escape digestion; those which remain intact may provide some local gastrointestinal immunity against organisms which enter the body via this route.

Although the stool of the breast-fed infant has a lower pH than that of the infant fed cow's milk, and its bacterial content is predominantly of the lactobacillus group in contrast to preponderance of the coliform group in artificially fed infants, it is not clear that the intestinal flora of infants fed human milk endows special benefits. Gyorgy demonstrated that a strain of *Lactobacillus bifidus* requires a "growth factor" contained in human milk for its propagation; no human nutritional advantage has been attributed to this substance.

Breast milk is the natural food for full-term infants during the first 2 to 3 months of life. Milk from the mother whose diet is quantitatively adequate and properly balanced will supply the necessary nutrients with the exception of vitamin D, fluoride and iron. Iron stores will be sufficient for the first 3 or 4 months in term infants, but should be supplemented after 3 months of age by the addition of cereal and meat to the diet or by administration of one of the ferrous iron preparations. Although the community water supply contains adequate amounts of fluoride, the breast-fed infant may receive little of it, and fluoride should be supplied during the first months of life. Human milk contains sufficient vitamin C for the infant's needs, provided the mother's intake of it is adequate.

The psychologic advantages of breast feeding for the infant and for the mother have been widely proclaimed. Certainly successful breast feeding is a satisfying experience for both. The mother is more personally involved in the nurturing of her baby, gaining both a feeling of essentialness and a sense of great accomplishment. The infant is afforded a close and comfortable physical relationship with his mother. Breast feeding offers increased opportunity for close sensual contact between mother and infant; studies in other mammals suggest that tactile contact and stimulation may be of considerable importance in the "imprinting process" and in determining the quality of mothering which is provided the infant.

The mother who wishes but is unable to nurse her infant need have no less sense of affection for him. Though it has been suggested that the breast-fed infant will be emotionally more stable than the bottle-fed infant, it would seem that the latter, provided he is a "wanted baby," would have adequate contact and affection from his mother. Speculation that emotional instability is likely to be an aftermath of bottle feeding requires confirmation which is not available; until it is, the obvious conclusion that security and affection can be given to the bottle-fed infant deserves strong emphasis.

Disadvantages of and Contraindications to Breast Feeding. For the average healthy full-term infant there are no disadvantages to breast feeding, provided the mother's milk supply is ample and her diet contains sufficient amounts of protein and vitamins. Infrequently, allergens to which the infant is sensitized may be conveyed in the milk. In such instances an attempt should be made to find the specific allergen and to remove it from the mother's diet; the presence of such allergens rarely becomes a valid reason for weaning the baby.

From the standpoint of the mother, there may be temporary or permanent contraindications to breast feeding. Fissuring or cracking of the nipples is an indication for temporary cessation of nursing when the use of a nipple shield is unsatisfactory. Mastitis necessitates discontinuance of nursing, although when treatment is rapidly effective, breast feeding may be resumed after several days. Acute illness in the mother may be considered a contraindication to breast feeding, if the infant does not have the same infection; otherwise there is no need for cessation of nursing unless the condition of either makes it mandatory. When the infant is not affected, and the mother's condition permits, the breast may be emptied and the milk given to the infant after sterilization.

Several disturbances such as septicemia, nephritis, eclampsia, profuse hemorrhage, active tuberculosis, typhoid fever or malaria are permanent contraindications to nursing, as are chronic poor nutrition, debility, convulsive disorders, severe neuroses and postpartum psychoses.

The resumption of menstruation is not a contraindication to continued nursing, although temporary changes in the behavior of mother or baby may call for reassurance. Pregnancy does not necessitate immediate cessation of nursing, but the combined demands of supplying milk to the infant and nutrients to the fetus are formidable and require special attention to maternal diet and nutrition; breast feeding probably should not be continued beyond the first 20 weeks of gestation.

Prematurely born infants weighing 2000 gm. (4 pounds) or more usually thrive well on breast milk. But infants of lesser birth-weight (1000 to 2000 gm.) may have such rapid rates of growth that human milk alone cannot provide sufficient quantities of phosphorus and protein, and possibly calcium for normal growth.

Breast feeding, inadequate maternal nutrition or deprived socioeconomic circumstances, alone or more often in combination, have long been cited in the development of the vitamin K-dependent hypoprothrombinemic variety of hemorrhagic disease of the newborn. The studies of Jewett and Sutherland strongly suggest that the initial period of relative starvation in breast-fed infants and the low vitamin K content of human milk are the important features in this disorder, which they find confined to breast-fed infants receiving no vitamin K prophylaxis. Administration of 1 mg. of vitamin K_1 parenterally at birth is recommended for all infants and appears to be mandatory for those who are breast-fed.

Sporadic occurrence of prolonged unconjugated

hyperbilirubinemia has been reported by Gartner, Arias and others in breast-fed infants. An unusual steroid metabolite of progesterone, pregnane-3 alpha, 20 beta-diol, which inhibits glucuronyl transferase activity in vitro, has been isolated from the milk of mothers of infants with this problem. Cessation of breast feeding leads to prompt decline in the bilirubin level, which reaches normal in 4 to 6 days. Interruption of nursing for 2 to 3 days will usually provide sufficient lowering of the serum bilirubin value to permit safe resumption of breast feeding.

Hemolytic disease of the newborn (erythroblastosis fetalis) is not a contraindication to breast feeding if the infant's general condition warrants it, since antibodies in the mother's milk are inactivated in the intestinal tract and do not contribute to further hemolysis of the infant's red blood cells.

Preparation of the Prospective Mother. Despite the fact that breast milk is the natural food for infants, many receive little or none of it. A few mothers are not good milk producers and are unable to provide an amount sufficient to justify even partial feeding of their infants (combined breast and supplemental milk feedings). Nevertheless most women are physically capable of breast feeding, provided they receive sufficient encouragement and are protected from dispiriting experiences and comments while the secretion of breast milk is becoming established.

The physician interested in aiding the prospective mother to breast feed will discuss the advantages of breast feeding during the midtrimester of pregnancy or whenever the mother becomes naturally concerned with the planning for her baby. Many mothers whose feelings toward breast feeding are ambivalent will be able to nurse successfully if they are given reassurance and support by physicians whose own convictions accord breast feeding a natural and logical place in childbearing and child-rearing. If the mother rejects the suggestion that she nurse her infant, it is probably wise to avoid overpersuasion, which might distort mother-infant relations.

Physical factors conducive to breast feeding include establishing and maintaining a state of good health: proper balance of rest and exercise, freedom from worry, early and sufficient treatment of any intercurrent disease and adequate nutrition. Nutritional deficiencies are contributory factors to inadequate lactation and to infant morbidity.

There appears to be no advantage in the so-called hardening processes designed to toughen the nipples. Such procedures may increase the likelihood of cracking or fissuring. Retracted nipples may be benefited by daily manual or breast pump traction during the latter weeks of pregnancy, but truly inverted nipples are not helped.

The mother may be confidently told that she need not gain or lose weight if her diet is adequate. Both mother and father should be reassured that breast tone will be preserved by the use of a properly fitted brassiere to support the breast, especially before delivery and during the nursing period.

To permit the mother greater freedom of activity outside the home, a daily bottle of formula can be substituted for one of the breast feedings some time before she is ready to resume normal activities.

ESTABLISHMENT AND MAINTENANCE OF MILK SUPPLY

The only known satisfactory stimulus to the secretion of human milk is regular and complete emptying of the breasts. There are many reasons for incomplete nursing, but the principal ones are weakness of the infant and failure of initiation of a natural hunger cycle. When the breasts are not emptied completely by the infant during the early days of nursing, they should be emptied regularly by artificial means. This is sometimes necessary on the fifth day to relieve lacteal overdistention of the breast so that the infant is able to grasp the mother's nipple. A hand breast pump or a water suction pump may be used, or the mother may be taught manual expression. Every effort should be directed toward the early establishment of normal, vigorous nursing by letting the infant empty the breast frequently during the time when colostrum is being formed. The infant should be allowed to nurse when he is hungry whether or not there appears to be any milk.

Breast feeding should be begun as soon after delivery as the condition of the mother and of the baby permits, preferably within 6 to 12 hours. If the infant cannot be fed on demand, he should be brought to the mother for feeding about every 3 hours during the day and every 4 hours during the night. He should be fed from both breasts at each feeding until the supply from one breast is sufficient for his needs. Breast feeding can be successful when delayed for 24 hours or more, but, barring maternal conditions which necessitate such delay, a sufficient supply of milk will generally appear earlier in the mother whose milk supply is stimulated by frequent suckling as soon after birth as is feasible. There would seem to be little justification for routine use of prelacteal feedings of sugar water or formula. To minimize nipple trauma the nursing time can be limited initially and gradually increased as the milk supply increases. In the period before the appearance of colostrum, 5 minutes' suckling at both breasts at each feeding is usually well tolerated and stimulates early milk production. As the condition of the breasts and the supply of milk permit, the nursing time can be gradually increased to 20 minutes, or even longer, if the baby insists. In beginning to nurse, almost all mothers experience some nipple tenderness, discomfort or pain which is greatest during the first part of the feeding. When expected and accepted as an unavoidable but temporary difficulty, anxiety is lessened and milk production is little affected.

The first 2 weeks of the neonatal period are the crucial time for the establishment of breast feeding. Lactogenic hormones have not been shown to be effective in the stimulation of breast secretion of the human being. Too much emphasis has been put on daily weight gains. When early supplemental milk feedings are given to achieve this false goal, attempts at breast feeding are doomed to failure; usually the infant finds that it is easier to get milk from a bottle than from a breast.

Supplemental milk should never be given before the fifth day and rarely before the end of the first week. An exception may be made on the day the mother is discharged from the hospital, particularly if her confinement is limited to 4 or 5 days. By this time lactation may not be well established, and the excitement of going home may not be conducive to an initially successful nursing experience there. A wise physician will foresee this experience and supply the mother with enough isocaloric formula for complementary feedings for the rest of the day and evening, thus avoiding discouragement which might prejudice the success of further nursing. If the effect which such excitement and unusual activity are likely to produce is anticipated, the mother is not likely to be upset when her milk supply is temporarily decreased.

Psychologic Factors. Attention to the details of maternal hygiene is paramount. No factor is more important than a happy, carefree state of mind; worry and unhappiness are the most effective means for decreasing or abolishing breast secretion.

Mothers worry that their babies are abnormal when they cry, are drowsy, sneeze, or regurgitate milk. Mothers are upset by any suggestion that their milk may be lacking in quantity or quality. They are disturbed at the thin appearance of colostrum, at tenderness of the nipples and at the fullness of the breasts on the fifth day. Many mothers cannot feel comfortable when trying to nurse in an open ward or with another person in the room. Mothers worry about what is going on at home while they are hospitalized and about what is going to happen when they arrive home. An alert physician is conscious of these worries, particularly if the baby is a first-born, and by tactful reassurance and explanation he can help prevent or minimize worry, thus contributing to successful breast feeding.

Fatigue. Avoidance of fatigue is important, but the mother should have sufficient exercise to promote a sense of physical well-being.

Hygiene. The nipples should be washed with water before and after each nursing and carefully dried. Cotton balls are useful for this cleansing. Once a day the breasts should be washed with soap and water. Additional care is seldom needed if the nipple area is kept dry. *Boric acid must not be used.* Care should be taken to prevent irritation and

infection of the nipples by prolonged initial nursing, maceration from wetness of the nipple, irritation of clothing, or difficult nursing associated with engorged or overdistended breasts. Serious difficulties can usually be avoided by discontinuing feeding from an affected breast temporarily and expressing the milk manually. Occasionally, nipple shields may be of help. The infant should be returned to breast feeding as soon as the nipple is healed.

A properly fitted brassiere should be worn day and night. An absorbent pad (commercially available) or a clean cloth or handkerchief may be placed inside the brassiere to absorb any milk which leaks out. Change to a clean brassiere should be made at least daily.

Diet. The diet should contain enough calories to compensate for those contained in the secreted milk as well as those required for its production. A diet adequate to maintain weight and relatively high in protein, fluid, vitamins and minerals will suffice, but the mother should have the benefit of more specific instruction in composing her diet. Milk is important, but should not replace other essential foods. When the mother is allergic or has an aversion to milk, 1 gm. of calcium may be added to her daily diet. The fluid intake should approximate 3 quarts daily; urinary output is a good measure of the adequacy of fluid in the daily diet.

There are mistaken ideas that such substances as milk, beer, oatmeal and tea are galactogenic. There is no objection to small amounts of alcoholic beverages if they contribute to the mother's peace of mind. Smoking of cigarettes should be discouraged. Particular foods in the mother's diet seldom have a disturbing influence on the breast-fed infant. Occasionally, however, maternal ingestion of certain berries, tomatoes, onions, members of the cabbage family, chocolate, spices and condiments may cause gastric distress or loose stools in the infant. No food need be withheld from the mother's diet unless it causes distress to the infant. It is better to control maternal constipation by inclusion in the diet of raw and cooked fruits and vegetables, whole wheat bread and an adequate amount of water than by use of laxatives. Certain substances, such as the arsenicals, barbiturates, bromides, iodides, lead, mercurials, salicylates, opium, atropine, sulfonamides, most antimicrobial agents, and cascara, may be transmitted through the milk and exert an effect on the infant.

TECHNIQUE OF BREAST FEEDING

The technical aspects of breast feeding require careful consideration. It is not unusual for breast feeding to be deemed impossible simply because the attending physician fails to recognize that the difficulties are related to the manner of feeding and not to qualitative or quantitative inadequacy of the milk.

The infant should be hungry at feeding time, dry and neither too cold nor too warm. He should be held in a comfortable, semisitting position for his enjoyment and for facilitation of eructation without vomiting. The mother, too, must be comfortable and completely at ease. When she is able to be out of bed, a moderately low chair with armrest is preferable, and a low stool is advantageous for resting her foot and raising her knee on the nursing side. The baby is supported comfortably with his face close to the breast by one arm and hand while the other hand supports the breast so that the nipple is easily accessible to the infant's mouth and yet does not obstruct his nasal breathing. The baby's lips should be well out over the areola of the breast.

Success in infant feeding depends to a great extent upon the adjustments during the first few days of life. Difficulties are likely to result when attempts are made to adapt the infant to the nursing procedure rather than to try to satisfy his natural desires. Rigid adherence to clock schedules and the "assembly line" manner in which babies are handled in many nurseries may contribute to the baby's confusion. Most of the trouble can be avoided by conforming to the infant's spontaneous pattern. If he is put at the breast when there is normal hunger crying and if his appetite is satisfied, the fundamental requirements are met. Aldrich emphasized the natural initial responses to hunger; his account of one of them, rooting reflex, is so well phrased that we have taken the liberty of reproducing it here.

At the time he is born, the normal infant is equipped with several reflexes, or behavior patterns, which are designed to make him a successful feeder from the breast. The most obvious of these reflexes are those concerned with the actual getting of food—rooting, sucking, swallowing, and satiety reflexes.

The *rooting reflex* is the first one of these to come into play. When a baby smells milk, he moves his head around and attempts to find its source. If one cheek is touched by a smooth object, he will turn his mouth toward that object and open it in anticipation of grasping the nipple. This obviously gives a clue as to how milk should be given to the baby. His cheek applied to his mother's breast will start him rooting with his mouth for the nipple.

I can illustrate a mistake made in this regard by telling the . . . experience of a patient in one of our best hospitals. As I was making daily rounds, she said to me: "Your nurses don't know their stuff! . . . They don't know anything about the rooting reflex. They bring my baby in, place her beside me and with their hand on the baby's cheek try to push her head around to meet the nipple. The baby, feeling the pressure of the hand, tries to turn toward the nurse's palm instead of toward my breast. A fight ensues, and usually the natural response is prevented. I always tell the girls to go out of the room; that I can handle this myself if they just lay the baby down beside me. I touch her cheek with my breast and let her do the rest." This experienced mother had learned to respect her baby's ability in these basic matters. This is a highly important lesson for anybody to learn.

Mothers should know that if the infant is not hungry, he will not search for the nipple or suck. Infants are usually sleepy for several days, and most are not initially avid suckers. Particularly on the third day, when there has been some weight loss, mothers are anxious about infants who do not seem particularly interested in eating. It is reassuring for them to know that most healthy babies "wake up" and become good eaters on the fourth day. Kron and Brazleton have reported that infants whose mothers received obstetric sedation during labor sucked at lower rates and pressures and consumed less milk than comparable infants from mothers given no sedation.

Some infants will empty a breast in 5 minutes; others will be more leisurely and nurse well for 20 minutes. The baby should be permitted to suck until he is satisfied. Efforts to wake up a sleepy baby and to "make him" nurse by snapping his feet, pinching or shaking him are rarely successful.

At the end of the nursing period the infant should be held erect over the mother's shoulder to eructate swallowed air; often this "burping" procedure is necessary one or more times during the feeding as well as 5 to 10 minutes after the infant has been put into the crib. It is an essential procedure during the early months, but should not be overdone. When nursing is completed, the infant should be placed in the crib on his abdomen or on his right side to facilitate emptying of the stomach into the intestines and to lessen the chances of regurgitation.

One or Both Breasts per Feeding. The infant should empty at least one breast at each feeding; otherwise it will not be stimulated to refill. If the milk supply seems inadequate, both breasts should be used at each feeding. After the milk supply has been established the breasts may be alternated at successive feedings, and the baby will usually be satisfied with the amount obtained from one. When the secretion of milk is too great, however, both breasts may again be offered at each feeding and incompletely emptied with the intent of securing a partial decrease in lactation.

Determination of Adequacy of Breast Supply. If the infant is satisfied at the completion of the nursing period, sleeps 3 to 4 hours and gains weight adequately, it can be assumed that the milk supply is sufficient; weighing of the infant at other than weekly to monthly intervals is neither necessary nor desirable. But if the infant nurses avidly and is not satisfied after completely emptying both breasts, does not go to sleep or sleeps fitfully and awakens after an hour or two, and fails to gain weight satisfactorily, the milk supply is probably inadequate.

The extent to which the mother's breasts become filled during the intervals between nursing is an additional measure of her capacity to produce milk. The "let-down" reflex, wherein milk flows from one nipple when the baby nurses from the other, is another sign of successful nursing. This milk-ejection reflex is an important part of successful breast feeding. Sucking, or often psychologic stimuli associated with nursing, leads to secretion of the oxytocic principle by the posterior pituitary. As a result, the smooth muscle fibers surrounding the alveoli deep in the breast contract, expelling milk into the larger ducts, where it is more easily available to the sucking infant. This reflex is frequently absent or erratic during the periods of emotional distress, and its malfunction is thought to be responsible for retention of milk in women who are unsuccessful in breast feeding.

Having the mother weigh her baby before and after nursing is a generally unsatisfactory way of judging the adequacy of milk supply. It wrongly focuses attention on how much the infant takes at a given time (normally there may be variations of one to several ounces in the various feedings in a 24-hour period), and the results obtained are readily misinterpreted. Small gains may cause the mother additional worry, and, in turn, her milk supply may diminish. She may soon find it urgent to give the baby a bottle to assure herself that he is getting enough and to see how many ounces he will take. The result of the "test bottle" may so discourage her that subsequent breast feeding becomes impossible, even when she has an adequate supply of milk. Before it is assumed that the mother is unable to produce sufficient milk, 3 possibilities should be excluded: (1) errors in feeding technique responsible for the infant's inadequate progress; (2) remediable maternal factors related to diet, rest or emotional distress; or (3) physical disturbances in the infant which interfere with eating or otherwise with gain in weight.

Supplementary Feedings. One substitute feeding a day, after the first weeks when the mother's milk supply has been adequately established, has the advantage of permitting the mother greater freedom in her activities. If the baby who is otherwise normal and healthy is getting insufficient breast milk, he should be offered additional artificial feedings either immediately after or in place of one or more breast feedings. Any of the milk formulas described under Formula Feeding may be used and should be offered to the baby in amounts sufficient to satisfy him. If formula is to be given after the baby has completed a breast feeding, the bottle should be warmed and handy so that it can be offered immediately after the infant has been given an opportunity to eructate any swallowed air. The holes in the nipples should not be so large that the baby gets this portion of his food without any effort, or he will quickly abandon any efforts to suck adequately at his mother's breast.

A replacement feeding is preferably substituted for the breast when the milk supply is observed to be scanty, usually late in the afternoon. The infant is given as much as he wants of an isocaloric formula. It is frequently accepted better from a person other than the mother from whom he is conditioned to nurse. Combined breast and bottle feedings may be continued as long as seems practical and satisfying to the mother and the infant.

Manual Expression of Breast Milk. This is achieved by 2 movements. The first is compression of the whole breast between the hands, starting at the base and continuing toward the areola. Firm pressure is maintained throughout the movement, which is repeated several times. The purpose is to impel milk to the lacteal sinuses. The second movement empties the sinuses. The breast is supported with one hand while the tissue just behind the areola is repeatedly compressed between the thumb and first finger of the other hand. The direction of the force is backwards toward the center of the breast rather than toward the nipple. The fingers are not moved from this initial position, nor is the skin rubbed over the breast tissue. The procedure should not be painful even though the nipples are sore and cracked.

Weaning. Weaning is usually advisable when the infant is 6 to 9 months of age, but should be avoided, if possible, during extremely hot weather. When a bottle feeding per day has been substituted for one of the breast feedings, as suggested previously, there is no difficulty in weaning. If the infant is not acquainted with the bottle, cup feeding may be tried. Not infrequently the cup is taken as readily as the bottle and the subsequent transfer to cup from bottle feeding is avoided. In any event, when the mother's milk is abundant, the process of weaning should be sufficiently gradual to avoid causing her unnecessary discomfort and to let the baby learn to accept milk from a new source. Initially, one of the breast feedings is replaced by a bottle feeding. After several days another breast feeding is replaced, and so on until the baby is entirely weaned. The total time required is governed by the status of the maternal milk supply.

When weaning is necessary at an earlier age because of illness of the mother or prolonged illness or death of the infant, a tight breast binder may be used and ice bags applied for a day or so. Restriction of the mother's fluid intake is also helpful in decreasing milk production rapidly.

FORMULA FEEDING

Artificial feeding is now viewed as a simple procedure in which complicated calculations and elaborate preparations are not necessary. Cow's milk in the whole state or some modified form is the basis for most formulas. Other milks and milk substitutes are available for infants who cannot tolerate cow's milk. Drastic reduction in the morbidity and mortality from gastrointestinal infections has resulted from sterilization of the formula and refrigeration of it until used. Milk processing (varying from simple boiling in the home to commercial pasteurization, homogenization and evaporation) has so altered the casein that small and readily digestible curds are formed in the stomach, thereby eliminating the principal cause for indigestibility of cow's milk protein.

Though breast feeding is generally considered superior to formula feeding for normal infants, surveys indicate that nearly 80 per cent of infants in the United States receive formula from birth.

Changing social and cultural patterns have contributed in largest measure to this increased reliance on formulas. Many mothers are reluctant to nurse their infants because of employment outside the home or implied limitations on social activities; others refuse because of fear of failure or of worry that loss of physical attractiveness will ensue from gain of weight and loss of breast tone; some do not consider breast feeding socially acceptable. Whatever the mother's reason or combination of reasons, the present popularity of artificial feeding could not have been reached without prior improvements in the safety and quality of the substitute milks.

The superiority of breast milk (as distinct from breast feeding) over the present-day artificial feedings derived from cow's milk has become less apparent with better understanding of milk processing and food chemistry. Objective studies of the state of nutrition in growing infants (rate of growth in weight and length, normality of various constituents in blood, performance in metabolic studies, body composition, and the like) show relatively small, and probably insignificant, differences between infants fed human milk and a variety of cow's milk feedings, although it has been argued that such techniques* may not be sufficiently sensitive to record small but important variations. These investigations attest to the ability of the normal infant to thrive by making satisfactory physiologic adjustments to relatively wide ranges of intake of protein, fat, carbohydrate and minerals.

Conventional whole and evaporated cow's milk formulas provide approximately 3.0 to 4.0 gm. of protein per kg. per day ("high protein" intake with a relatively large excess above the basic need), whereas breast milk and many commercially prepared feedings simulating the composition of breast milk supply 2.0 to 2.5 gm. per kg. per day ("low protein" intake supplying a smaller margin of excess). Other milk products which furnish a protein intake intermediate between the "high" and "low" levels are also marketed.

The basic question as to whether the formula-fed infant should be provided with a higher allowance of protein than the breast-fed one has not been completely resolved. The available evidence, although lacking in many essential details, may be summarized as follows: (1) only minor differences in the nutritional values of protein from human and cow's milk have been demonstrated; (2) the natural and commercial milks for which analyses are available contain at least the minimal amounts, and usually a surplus, of the essential amino acids; (3) the existence of a "protein reserve" similar to that for glycogen and fat, implying the storage of proteins in the body in

excess of current requirements and available to meet stressful situations, is open to question; (4) protein metabolism ("turnover") is closely related to and conditioned by the level of intake; (5) studies relating high and low intakes of protein to resistance to infection are inconclusive; and (6) normal infants receiving low, intermediate or high intakes of protein appear to do equally well clinically.

Fomon has calculated the rate of increase in total body protein mass in the "male reference" term infant to average approximately 3.5 gm. per day in the first 4 months of life. Assuming 0.5 gm. per day nitrogen loss from the skin, total protein need is estimated to be about 4.0 gm. per day during the first 4 months and slightly less during the remainder of the first year.

It seems reasonable to conclude that normal infants can be expected to thrive on dietary intakes within the wide range of protein (2.0 to 3.5 or 4.0 gm. per kg. per day) and of minerals which are provided by the usual daily ingestion of human milk, of the whole and evaporated cow's milk formulas in common use, and of the commercially prepared feedings of low, intermediate and high protein content.

Prematurely born babies appear to require more protein per unit of body weight than term infants. Davidson and associates, using isocaloric 0.8 calorie per ml. formulas in which the protein, fat and ash contents were varied, found that protein intakes of 4.0 gm. per kg. per day were superior to lower intakes (2.0 and 3.0 gm. per kg. per day) and equivalent to higher ones of 6.0 gm. per kg. per day in terms of rate of gain in body weight and serum protein levels; no differences in rates of body weight gain could be attributed to the fat or ash content of these isocaloric diets.

TECHNIQUE OF ARTIFICIAL FEEDING

The setting is similar to that for breast feeding, with the mother in a comfortable position, pleasant, unhurried and free from distractions. The infant should be hungry, fully awake, warm and dry; he should be held as though he were being nursed. The bottle should be held so that milk, not air, is channeled through the nipple. Bottle propping, even with a "safe" holder, should be avoided; propping not only deprives the infant of the physical contact, comfort and security of being held, but also may be dangerous to small infants who may aspirate if unattended.

The bottle of milk is customarily warmed to body temperature, though no harmful effects have been demonstrated from feedings at room temperature or cooler, as when the bottle is taken directly from the refrigerator. The temperature may be tested by dropping milk on the wrist. The nipple holes should be of such size that milk will drop slowly.

Especially during the first 6 or 7 months of life, the eructation of air swallowed during feeding is

---

*For example, the commonly used gain in weight does not differentiate between accumulations in lean body mass and fat stores and may possibly also include increases in body water due to excess solute retention under certain circumstances.

important for avoidance of abdominal discomfort and of regurgitation. Holding the infant upright over the shoulder with or without gently rubbing or patting the back assists in expelling the air. A few babies relieve themselves best after being replaced in the crib. All babies will, at times, regurgitate or "spit up" a small amount of milk after feeding, a fact the mother should know. "Spitting up" occurs more often in the artificially fed than in the breast-fed infants. Aspiration of this milk is less likely if the infant lies on his right side or abdomen, rather than on his back.

A feeding may require from 5 to 25 minutes, depending on the vigor and the age of the infant. Since the appetite varies from feeding to feeding, each bottle should contain more than the average amount taken per feeding. In no instance should the baby be urged to take more than he desires. The excess milk should be discarded, and the bottle and nipple rinsed with cool water.

COMPARISON OF HUMAN AND COW'S MILKS

Average values for the various constituents of human milk and whole fresh and evaporated cow's milk are listed in Table 3-11. Human milk and cow's milk differ during the various stages of lactation, and there are some differences between milks of individual women as well as of cows. The differences in milks from women whose diets are adequate are insignificant.

Colostrum. The secretion of the breasts for the first 2 to 4 days after delivery is termed "colostrum." It has a deep lemon-yellow color, its reaction is alkaline, and its specific gravity is 1.040 to 1.060, in contrast to the average specific gravity of 1.030 for fresh breast milk. The total amount of colostrum secreted daily is not large (10 to 40 cc.). Colostrum contains several times as much protein as breast milk and more minerals, but less carbohydrate and fat. After the first few days of lactation, colostrum is replaced by secretion of a transitional form of milk which gradually assumes the characteristics of mature breast milk by the third or fourth week.

Water. The relative amounts of water and solids in human and cow's milks are about the same, each having a water content of about 87 to 87.5 per cent; the specific gravity of each is in the range of 1.030 to 1.032.

Calories. The energy value of each milk may vary slightly, but for practical purposes each may be assumed to contain 20 calories per ounce.

Protein. There are both qualitative and quantitative differences between the proteins of the 2 milks. Human milk contains only 1.0 to 1.5 (average 1.1) per cent protein in contrast to about 3.3 per cent in cow's milk. The increased protein of cow's milk is almost entirely accounted for by the sixfold higher content of casein. The principal quantitative differences are in the relative amounts of whey proteins and casein. In human milk the protein consists of approximately 60 per cent whey proteins, largely lactalbumins and lactoglobulins, and 40 per cent casein; whereas in cow's milk the ratio is reversed, to 18:82. The proteins of the 2 milks are essentially equivalent for infant nutrition.

Carbohydrate. The sugar of the 2 milks differs only quantitatively, both containing lactose. Human milk contains 6.5 to 7.0 per cent, and cow's milk about 4.5 per cent.

Fat. The fat content of milks is more variable than any other constituent, but the average content is about 3.5 per cent. The amount in human milk varies somewhat with maternal diet; the fat content of milk obtained during a single nursing is higher in the latter portion of the feeding.

The milks of different breeds of cattle vary in fat content. Most market milk in urban areas, however, is pooled, and the fat content is adjusted to a standard level, generally from 3.25 to 4 per cent.

There are qualitative differences between the fats of human and cow's milks. The fats of each are composed principally of the triglycerides, olein, palmitin and stearin. Human milk, however, contains twice as much of the more readily absorbed olein. The volatile fatty acids (butyric, capric, caproic and caprylic) account for only about 1.3 per cent of the fat of human milk, in contrast to about 9 per cent in cow's milk. Hansen called attention to the need for linoleic acid, a dienoic fat, in infant nutrition. Babies fed fat-poor diets deficient in this substance develop thickened, dry and scaly skin and fail to grow normally; the small amount of linoleic acid in most milks is sufficient to prevent deficiency. The normal infant has no difficulty in digesting the fat of cow's milk, whereas the premature or debilitated infant may have steatorrhea after ingesting it. For such infants it is wise to keep the fat content of the milk formula relatively low or to substitute a more readily assimilated vegetable fat.

Minerals. The total mineral content of human milk (0.15 to 0.25 per cent) is considerably less than that of cow's milk (0.7 to 0.75 per cent). With the exception of iron and copper, cow's milk contains considerably more of all the minerals. Neither milk contains an adequate amount of iron; the deficiency is compensated for in the first 4 months or so of life by iron stored in fetal life. Although the need for calcium and phosphorus is relatively great during periods of rapid growth, adequate balances are maintained on breast milk in spite of its comparatively low content of these minerals.

Vitamins. The vitamin content of each milk varies with the maternal intake. Each has relatively large amounts of vitamin A and small amounts of vitamin D. Human milk has more vitamin C except when the maternal intake is deficient in vitamin C-containing foods. Cow's milk contains more thiamine and riboflavin than human milk and about an equal quantity of niacin. It is assumed that each milk contains adequate amounts of vitamin A and the B-complex vitamins

TABLE 3-11. COMPARISON OF HUMAN AND COW'S MILKS

	REPRESENTATIVE COMPOSITION OF MATURE MILKS			VARIATIONS IN COMPOSITION OF UNPOOLED MILK SAMPLES†			
	HUMAN	COW'S	COW'S EVAP.	HUMAN		COW'S	
Components (per cent):							
Water	87.6	87.3	73.0	87.0 -	89.0	83.0 -	88.0
Total solids	12.4	12.7	27.0	8.5 -	15.0	8.5 -	19.0
Proteins	1.2	3.3	7.3	0.7 -	2.0	2.8 -	3.6
Casein	0.4	2.8	6.2	0.14-	0.68	2.1 -	2.8
Whey	0.6	0.6	1.3	0.5 -	1.1	0.3 -	0.6
Lactalbumin	0.3	0.4	0.88	0.14-	0.6	0.27-	0.57
Lactoglobulin	0.2	0.2	0.44			0.14-	0.42
Lactose	7.0	4.8	10.6	5.0 -	9.2	4.0 -	5.5
Fat	3.8	3.7	8.2	1.3 -	8.3	3.1 -	5.2
Minerals (ash)	0.21	0.72	1.6	0.16-	0.27	0.64-	0.75
Minerals (per liter):							
Sodium (mEq.)	7.0	25.0	55.0	2.0 -	13.0	13.5 -	93.0
Potassium (mEq.)	14.0	35.0	77.0	9.5 -	17.5	9.7 -	74.0
Chloride (mEq.)	12.0	29.0	46.0	2.6 -	21.0	27.0 -	40.0
Calcium (mg.)	330.0	1250.0	2750.0	170.0 -	610.0	560.0 -	3810.0
Phosphorus (mg.)	150.0	960.0	2112.0	70.0 -	270.0	560.0 -	1120.0
Magnesium (mg.)	40.0	120.0	264.0	20.0 -	60.0	70.0 -	220.0
Sulfur (mg.)	140.0	300.0	660.0	50.0 -	300.0	240.0 -	360.0
Iron (mg.)	1.5	1.0	2.2	0.2 -	1.8	0.2 -	1.4
Zinc (mg.)	1.2	3.8	8.4	0.17-	3.02	1.9 -	6.6
Copper (mg.)	0.4	0.3	0.66	0.1 -	0.7	0.2 -	0.8
Iodine (mg.)	0.07	0.21	0.46	0.05-	0.09	0.13-	1.8
Amino Acids (mg./liter):							
Histidine	230.0	800.0	1760.0	160.0 -	340.0	700.0 -	1300.0
Isoleucine	860.0	2120.0	4664.0	460.0 -	1020.0	1800.0 -	2900.0
Leucine	1610.0	3560.0	7832.0	720.0 -	1590.0	2400.0 -	3900.0
Lysine	790.0	2570.0	5654.0	530.0 -	1040.0	2200.0 -	3100.0
Methionine	230.0	870.0	1914.0	90.0 -	210.0	600.0 -	900.0
Phenylalanine	640.0	1730.0	3860.0	300.0 -	580.0	1400.0 -	2200.0
Threonine	620.0	1520.0	3344.0	400.0 -	760.0	1200.0 -	2200.0
Tryptophan	220.0	500.0	1100.0	130.0 -	260.0	400.0 -	800.0
Valine	900.0	2280.0	4956.0	480.0 -	1140.0	2100.0 -	2800.0
Calories (approximate):							
Per fluid ounce	20.0	20.0	44.0*	18.0 -	24.0	17.0 -	25.0
Per liter	710.0	690.0	1520.0	600.0 -	790.0	570.0 -	850.0

The data are assembled from a number of sources.

*In practice, commonly regarded as 40 calories.

†Values are taken from several studies; agreement is approximate, but not all components were evaluated in each.

and inadequate amounts of vitamins C and D for the nutritional needs of infants in the first months of life.

Bacterial Content. Human milk is essentially free from bacterial contamination. Pathogenic organisms in significant numbers may gain access to the milk from mastitis. Both tubercle bacilli and typhoid bacilli may be found at times in the milk of women infected with these organisms. Cow's milk is regularly contaminated, but in most instances the bacteria are not especially harmful to man. Cow's milk, however, is a good culture medium for pathogenic bacteria, and many infections are milk-borne. Such infections include streptococcal diseases, diphtheria, typhoid fever, salmonellosis, tuberculosis and brucellosis. Furthermore, certain bacteria which may not affect older children or adults may cause diarrhea in infants. For this reason, in most cities, pasteurization of all marketed whole milk is required. In addition, boiling the milk immediately before mixing the infant's formula or terminal sterilization is advisable.

Digestibility. The emptying time of the stomach is more rapid for human than for whole cow's milk; however, there is no appreciable difference in gastrointestinal passage time during the first 45 days of life between human milk and processed milk formulas. The curd of cow's milk is reduced in size by boiling and is made considerably less tough and much smaller by the heating required in evaporation, by the addition of acid or alkali and by homogenization. In contrast, the curd of breast milk is fine and flocculent and readily broken down in the stomach. The fat of cow's milk is less readily digested than that of breast milk.

FORMS OF COW'S MILK USED IN FORMULAS

Raw Milk. This milk is not advised for infant feeding; it forms large curds in the stomach, is slowly digested, and is easily contaminated with pathogenic organisms. Its sale is forbidden in most urban communities.

Pasteurized Milk. Pasteurization destroys pathogenic bacteria and modifies the casein so that smaller and less tough curds are produced in the stomach. It is accomplished by holding heated milk at a specified temperature for a specific length of time, e.g. at 145°F. (63°C.) for 30 minutes or, more commonly, at 161°F. (72°C.) for 15 seconds followed by rapid cooling to 148°F. (65°C.) or lower (60°C.). Standards for the bacterial content of pasteurized milk vary in different cities, tolerable counts ranging as high as 50,000 nonpathogenic bacteria per cc.; average counts in many cities, however, are as low as 5000 to 10,000. Pasteurized milk should be boiled when used for infant feeding. If allowed to stand in the refrigerator for as long as 48 hours, a significant increase in bacterial count may occur.

Homogenized Milk. The processing of milk so that the fat globules are broken into a homogeneous emulsion of minute particles is termed homogenization. Owing to the decrease in size and dispersion of the fat molecules, the cream does not separate. The principal advantage of homogenized milk lies in the smaller and less tough curd produced in the stomach.

Evaporated Milk. Evaporated milk has many advantages, including almost universal availability. In the unopened can it will keep for months without refrigeration. The casein curd produced in the stomach is softer and smaller than that of boiled whole milk; homogenization of the fat also contributes to smaller curd formation. The lactalbumin appears to be less allergenic than that of fresh milk. The sugar is unchanged. When necessary, evaporated milk can be fed in higher concentrations than whole milk formulas. The standard can contains 14.5 ounces avoirdupois or 13 fluid ounces* (384 cc.). Each fluid ounce is equal to about 44 calories; in practice the value is generally considered to be 40 calories. Whether diluted with an equal quantity of water (13 ounces or 384 cc.) or reconstituted at a ratio of 1:1.2 (15½ ounces or 458 cc.), one can is equivalent to only about 28 ounces (or 828 cc.) of whole milk. Vitamin D is usually added in the processing so that each reconstituted quart contains 400 I.U.

Condensed Milk. About 45 per cent cane sugar has been added in sweetened condensed milk, making the carbohydrate content approximately 60 per cent in the evaporated form before

dilution. The usual dilutions (1:10 to 1:4) are disproportionately high in sugar and low in fat and protein. Although readily digestible, it has no use in infant feeding for more than short periods when a high caloric diet is desired.

Dried Whole Milk. Standard regulations govern the production of dried milk. The fat content of fluid milk is adjusted to 3.5 per cent, and the milk is evaporated with extreme rapidity to powder form by spray-, freeze- or roller-drying. Reconstituted dried milk has most of the advantages of evaporated milk, but does not keep well when exposed to air.

Dried Skim Milk. Available as either nonfat skim milk (fat content 0.05 per cent) or half-skim milk (fat content 1.5 per cent), these milks have limited usefulness: (1) for infants with fat intolerance, (2) for infants convalescing from diarrheal diseases; and (3) for premature infants when diets high in protein and low in fat are prescribed. Many of these products do not contain added vitamin D.

Acid and Fermented Milks. So-called acid milks are prepared by addition of acid or are fermented by bacterial action. Acid milk may be prepared by the addition of lactic acid, U.S.P. (or other acids), to previously boiled and cooled cow's milk formulas; the amount required varies with the fat content, those with higher concentrations requiring more acid. Milks containing 3.5 to 4 per cent fat require about 1½ fluid drams (6 cc.) to the quart. Reconstituted evaporated milk requires about the same amount. The acid is added drop by drop to the cooled milk formula with constant stirring with a wooden spoon to avoid curd formation. Several commercial preparations of dried lactic acid whole and skim milk are also available. Most fermented milks (i.e. buttermilks) are acidified by the addition of lactic acid-producing organisms (*Lactobacillus acidophilus* and *L. bulgaricus*).

These milks require less hydrochloric acid for gastric digestion. The casein is altered so that smaller and less tough curds are formed in the stomach. Their use appears to be limited to the feeding of infants with digestive disturbances and those convalescing from diarrheal disease; currently they are rarely used in infant feeding.

OTHER MILKS USED IN FORMULAS

Goat's Milk. In many countries goat's milk is used extensively for infant feeding; its use in this country is limited to management of cow's milk allergies; because of inconsistent antigenic cross-reaction between cow's and goat's milks it is less popular than the soya "milks" and the formulas derived from lamb and beef and from casein hydrolysis.

Goat's milk is similar in composition to cow's milk; it contains less sodium, more potassium and chloride, and more of the essential linoleic and arachidonic acids; its fat may be more digestible

---

*One fluid ounce is equivalent to approximately 29.57 cc.

TABLE 3-12. Natural Milks, Prepared Milks and Milk Substitutes Used in Infant Feeding

	NORMAL DILUTION		APPROXIMATE PERCENTAGE COMPOSITION IN NORMAL DILUTION (Grams per 100 ml.)				APPROXIMATE ELECTROLYTE COMPOSITION IN NORMAL DILUTION (Milliequivalents per liter)					MILLIGRAMS PER LITER
	Ratio†	Cals./oz.	Protein	Carbohydrate	Fat	Minerals	NA	K	CL	CA	P‡	Fe
Human milk, mature, average	Undiluted	20	1.2	7.0	3.8	0.21	7	14	12	17	9	1.5
Cow's milk, market, average	Undiluted	20	3.3	4.8	3.7	0.72	25	35	29	62	53	1.0
Cow's milk, evaporated, many brands	1:1	22	3.8	5.4	4.0	0.8	28	39	32	65	59	1.0
Cow's milk, powdered:												
Klim, Borden	1:7	20	3.3	4.7	3.5	0.7	22	35	28	58	48	1.0
Commercial premodified milks:												
Infant Formula, Baker*	1:1	20	2.2	7.0	3.3	0.6	17	23	19	42	37	7.9
Bremil with Iron, Borden	1:1	20	1.5	7.0	3.5	0.5	11	16	13	35	18	8.5
Bremil Powder, Borden	1:8	20	1.5	7.1	3.5	0.4	16	36	13	35	18	8.5
Modilac, Gerber	1:1	20	2.2	7.8	2.7	0.4	17	27	19	42	37	10.6
Enfamil, Mead*	1:1	20	1.5	7.0	3.7	0.3	11	19	12	32	32	8.5
Olac, Mead*	1:1	20	3.4	7.5	2.7	0.7	22	41	29	60	58	tr.
Nan Powder, Nestlé	1:7	20	1.6	7.3	3.4	0.3	11	20	11	17	22	—
Lactogen Powder, Nestlé	1:6	20	2.5	8.0	3.6	0.5	11	22	14	34	27	—
Lactogen Powder, Full Protein, Nestlé	1:5.5	20	3.5	8.2	3.0	0.8	16	30	17	47	38	—
Prodieton Powder, Nestlé	1:5	22	3.3	11.0	3.4	0.7	16	32	21	55	37	—
Similac with Iron, Ross**	1:1	20	1.8	6.6	3.4	0.4	12	26	18	34	30	12
Similac Powder with Iron, Ross**	1:8	20	1.8	6.6	3.4	0.5	17	31	17	41	30	12
Similac PM 60/40 Powder, Ross	1:8	20	1.5	7.2	3.4	0.2	7	14	12	17	10	—
SMA S-26, Wyeth*	1:1	20	1.5	7.2	3.6	0.25	7	14	12	21	21	8
Goat's milk, powdered:												
Dale's, Cutter	1:6	20	3.3	4.7	4.1	0.77	18	46	45	61	55	tr.
High protein, low fat powdered milks:												
Dryco, Borden	1:8	16	4.0	5.7	1.5	0.9	27	38	32	65	57	1.0
Alacta, Mead	1:7	14	4.2	5.9	1.5	0.9	26	75	36	75	65	1.2
Probana, Mead	1:7	20	3.9	7.3	2.0	0.6	26	31	28	100	58	3.0
Protein Milk, Mead	1:10	14	3.8	2.7	2.7	0.7	30	30	29	63	57	1.3
Eledon, Nestlé	1:8	14	3.7	4.8	1.7	0.8	16	32	21	55	37	—
Nestogen, Half-Skimmed, Nestlé	1:5.5	22	3.4	10.1	2.0	0.8	18	35	22	55	45	--
Skim milk, many brands	1:10	10	3.5	4.8	0.2	0.7	26	34	32	62	56	0.5
Hypoallergenic milk substitutes:												
Mullsoy Liquid, Borden (Soya)	1:1	20	3.1	5.2	3.6	0.8	16	40	16	60	46	5
Mullsoy Powder, Borden (Soya)	1:8	20	3.1	4.5	4.0	0.7	26	35	13	65	58	4
Neo-Mullsoy, Borden (Soya)	1:1	20	1.8	6.4	3.5	0.5	17	25	6	42	24	8.4
Lambase, Gerber	1:1	20	2.4	7.9	2.4	0.3	24	28	7	46	45	7.9
Meat-base, Gerber	13:19.5	17.4	2.7	4.0	3.1	0.33	12	12	17	52	40	9.7
(Requires added carbohydrate)												
Soyalac Liquid, Loma Linda (Soya)	1:1	20	2.1	5.9	4.0	0.3	14	23	10	21	21	10
Soyalac Powder, Loma Linda (Soya)	1:8	20	2.9	5.9	3.5	0.45	14	34	15	42	21	10
Nutramigen Powder, Mead	1:6	20	2.2	8.5	2.6	0.6	17	26	23	50	52	10
Pro-Sobee, Mead (Soya)	1:1	20	2.5	6.8	3.4	0.5	24	28	7	47	42	8.5
Sobee, Mead (Soya)	1:1	20	3.2	7.7	2.6	0.5	22	33	14	50	32	8.5
Isomil, Ross (Soya)	1:1	20	2.0	6.8	3.6	0.4	13	16	15	35	28	12
Milk substitutes, specialty products:												
Cho-free Formula Base Borden	1:1	20	1.8	6.4	3.5	0.5	17	25	6	47	47	8.4
(12.5% Dextrose added)												
Lofenalac, Mead	1:6	20	2.2	8.5	2.7	0.75	26	38	23	47	47	1.6
Lonalac, Mead	1:6	20	3.4	4.8	3.5	0.6	1.1	27	14	56	57	2.1
Portagen, Mead	1:6	20	2.7	7.7	3.2	0.7	17	33	23	48	46	11.3

Data supplied by processors or assembled from other sources.
*Also available in powdered form with similar composition.
**Also available without iron supplementation.
†Number of ounces of milk to number of ounces of water. (Most powdered milks may also be prepared by adding 1 level tablespoonful or special measuring spoonful of powder to each 2 ounces of water.)
‡Calculated for valence of 1.8.

and its curd tension is lower than cow's milk. It is low in vitamin D, iron and folic acid; infants fed exclusively on goat's milk are prone to megaloblastic anemia due to folate deficiency. The goat is especially susceptible to brucellosis; the milk should be boiled before use. It is commercially available in evaporated and powdered forms.

Prepared Milks. Numerous commercially prepared premodified milks which require only the addition of water are widely used in infant feeding. They are derived basically from cow's milk, and many are available in both liquid and powder forms. The majority have compositions which simulate breast milk in one or more ways: reduced protein content (varying from 1.5 to 2.8 gm. per 100 cc. of reconstituted milk); reduced mineral salts (sodium, potassium, chloride, calcium phosphorus); fat modification by substitution of vegetable fat for butterfat; and addition of carbohydrate (lactose or dextrin-maltose). All are fortified with vitamin D; many contain other vitamins, and some have added iron. In the recommended 1:1 dilution of most of the liquid forms, each can provides 26 ounces (768 cc.) of formula. Table 3-12 lists the varieties of milks and milk substitutes available for infant feeding.

These milks are nutritionally adequate for normal infants, simple to prepare and convenient to use. Their cost is somewhat greater than evaporated milk-carbohydrate-water formulas.

Other prepared milks which may have virtue for special circumstances are now available. Those with very low electrolyte content (mineral content similar to human milk) may be helpful in infants with congestive heart failure, nephrogenic diabetes insipidus and marginal renal function. A low sodium milk, containing about 1 mEq. of sodium per reconstituted quart, is commercially available for use in the management of infants with congestive heart failure. Milks low in phenylalanine content are useful in the management of infants and children with phenylketonuria.

Milk Protein. Powdered protein is used chiefly for increasing the protein content of dilute skim milk or other formulas for feeding during diarrheal conditions, or to premature or debilitated infants.

Milk Substitutes and Hypoallergenic Milks. There are a number of milks and milk substitutes for infants allergic to cow's milk. These include evaporated goat's milk, a preparation in which nutrient nitrogen is supplied as an amino acid mixture (casein hydrolysate), nonmilk foods in which the protein is derived from soybeans, and meat-base formulas (beef and lamb sources). All appear to be nutritionally satisfactory and to have a place in the management of infants who cannot tolerate cow's milk; those which do not contain lactose are useful for infants with galactosemia.

MILK FORMULAS

Most methods for calculating milk formulas result in somewhat similar combinations of milk, water and sugar. No method stands out as definitely superior. Although there has been increasing simplification in the construction of formulas, understanding of the nutritional requirements and eating habits of infants is fundamental for proper guidance of mothers in the feeding of infants and children.

The ingredients of the formula are milk, water and sugar. Some modification of the milk which results in smaller curd formation in the stomach is desirable and is achieved to some extent by boiling raw milk and to a greater extent by boiling previously pasteurized milk. Homogenization and evaporation further alter the milk curd; the addition of acids or alkalis has a similar effect. The choice of milk depends somewhat upon available supplies and upon individual preferences. The formula should contain approximately 20 calories per ounce.

Caloric Requirements. (See also page 129.) The average caloric requirements of full-term infants are about 50 to 55 calories per pound or 110 to 120 calories per kg. during the first few months of life; and about 45 calories per pound, or 100 per kg. (or slightly less), by 1 year of age; individual variations are significant, and for many infants intakes of this order are in excess of caloric need.

Fluid Requirements. (See also page 128.) Fluid requirements are high during infancy.

During the first 6 months of life they range from 2 to 3 ounces per pound, or 130 to 190 cc. per kg., per day. The requirements may be increased during hot weather. As a rule, the infant will regulate his own fluid intake, provided adequate amounts are offered. Most of the fluid requirement is in the formula, but some is supplied in orange juice and other foods and by water between feedings.

Number of Feedings Daily. (See also page 143.) The number of feedings required per day decreases throughout the first year so that by 1 year of age most infants are satisfied with 3 meals a day. The interval between feedings differs considerably among infants, but, in general, ranges from 3 to 5 hours during the first year of life, with an average of 4 hours for full-term, healthy infants. Small and weak infants may prefer feedings at 2- to 3-hour intervals. For the first month or two, feedings are taken throughout the 24-hour period, but thereafter the infant will usually sleep from 10 or 12 p.m. to 6 or 7 a.m. Time of omission of the late evening feeding (10 to 12 p.m.) varies from the third to the eighth month.

Quantity of Formula per Feeding. Although the quantity taken at a feeding will vary with different infants of the same age and with the same infant at different feedings, it is necessary to know the average amounts taken at various ages. A general rule for the estimation of the quantity of the individual feeding to be offered during the first half year of life is to add 3 to the age in months. It is good practice to put more in each bottle than the infant is expected to take. Estimates which more nearly reflect the average infant's intake are shown below. The "rules of thumb" are, at best, guides; each infant must be given the primary responsibility in determining the quantity of his intake. Rarely will an infant want to take more than 7 or 8 ounces of milk at one feeding if his caloric and nutritional needs are adequately supplemented by other foods.

AGE	AVERAGE QUANTITY TAKEN IN INDIVIDUAL FEEDINGS
1st and 2nd weeks	2-3 ounces
3 weeks-2 months	4-5 ounces
2-3 months	5-6 ounces
3-4 months	6-7 ounces
5-12 months	7-8 ounces

TABLE 3-13. AVERAGE NUMBER OF FEEDINGS PER 24 HOURS

AGE	AVERAGE NUMBER OF FEEDINGS IN 24 HOURS
Birth-1 week	6-10
1 week-1 month	6-8
1-3 months	5-6
3-7 months	4-5
4-9 months	3-4
8-12 months	3

Quantity of Milk. The amount of whole milk usually taken daily in the first 6 months of life varies from $1\frac{3}{4}$ to 2 ounces per pound of body weight (evaporated milk, approximately 1 ounce per pound). The relative requirements are somewhat less in the first 2 weeks than in the succeeding 5 or 6 months. After this time milk, though still of great value, has diminishing importance in meeting total nutritional requirements.

Rarely is it necessary to use more than one can (13 fluid ounces) of evaporated milk or a quart of whole milk per day. By the time the infant is taking these quantities, other foods will be added to the diet in increasing amounts.

Water. It is common practice to dilute cow's milk with water for the feeding of infants during the first few months of life. In the 2 weeks or so after birth, dilution of cow's milk will lessen the possibility of tetany by reducing the amount of phosphorus to be excreted. Although it has been demonstrated that infants will tolerate undiluted cow's milk or fully reconstituted (ratio 1:1) evaporated milk after the first few days of life, infants so fed tend to have a moderate elevation of the blood urea nitrogen level and to obligate a large proportion of the ingested water for renal solute excretion. Increased insensible water loss with fever or high environmental temperatures may exceed the narrow margin of safety provided in the solute-to-water ratio of these formulas. Therefore it is helpful to add water and sugar to milk for infants up to 4 or 6 months of age in order to reduce the renal solute load with respect to ingested protein and minerals. With whole and evaporated cow's milk feedings, water should be offered between feedings during periods of high environmental temperature, and additional water will be needed when there are unusual losses as with vomiting or diarrhea.

Sugar. A number of carbohydrates are used in infant feeding, and all seem to be satisfactory. Theoretically it might seem that lactose, the sugar of milk, would be the one of choice; it appears to have little advantage, however, over the others and may even cause an increased amount of flatulence, owing to a greater degree of fermentation. Cane sugar has advantages of universal

availability and low cost. Its only apparent disadvantage is a greater sweetness than the others. There are a number of popular dextrin-maltose preparations whose principal advantages are a slower rate of digestion and absorption and a less sweet taste. Honey is also used, but has no particular advantages. There are several rules for estimating the quantity of sugar. In our clinic $\frac{1}{2}$ ounce of sugar is added to the daily formula during the first week or so of life, and then 1 ounce until about 4 to 6 months, when it is discontinued, usually in 2 equal steps with an interval of a week or so. (See Table 3-14.)

Example of Formula Calculation. The following are formulas for an infant 3 months of age weighing 11 pounds:

$$Cal.$$

1. Total fluid per 24 hours $(11 \times 2\text{-}3)$ = 28 oz.
2. Total whole milk $(11 \times 1\frac{3}{4}\text{-}2)$ 21 oz. 420
3. Water $(28 - 21)$ = 7 oz.
4. Carbohydrate 1 oz. $\underline{120}$
$$540$$

(cal. per oz. = $540 \div 28 = 19+$)
(cal. per lb. = $540 \div 11 = 49+$)

1. Total fluid per 24 hours $(11 \times 2\text{-}3)$ = 28 oz.
2. Total evaporated milk (11×1) = 11 oz. 440
3. Water $(23 - 11)$ = 17 oz.
4. Carbohydrate 1 oz. $\underline{120}$
$$560$$

(cal. per oz. = $560 \div 28 = 20$)
(cal. per lb. = $560 \div 11 = 51$)

5 bottles of $5\frac{1}{2}$ oz. each

These formulas are satisfactory for an initial prescription. Subsequent adjustments of milk and water should be made on the basis of the infant's response as measured by satiety and by the growth curve. It is not necessary to calculate the percentages of the various ingredients of formulas composed on this basis, but for those who may want it, a method of calculation is given below.*

Preparation of formula. UTENSILS. Several more bottles than the required number for feedings are needed for water and orange juice. Bottles should be made of heat-resistant glass, be smooth inside, and marked in ounces. A wide-mouthed bottle is preferable because it is more easily cleaned, and those with adequate protection of the nipple are preferable if the baby is to be fed away from home. There should be several more nipples than the number required for feedings. Rubber caps or a plastic such as Pliofilm held in place by cardboard retainers may be used as bottle covers. The graduate should be made of heat-resistant glass and marked in ounces. A saucepan for heating and mixing the formula, a container for nipples, a glass funnel if narrow-mouthed bottles are used, a large kettle or special bottle sterilizer, a measuring spoon, a can opener, a knife, a standard tablespoon and a strainer complete the list of utensils.

Cleansing of utensils. All utensils required for the mixing and storing of the formula should be sterilized by boiling for 5 to 10 minutes. The rubber nipples and caps should not be boiled more than 5 minutes. After each feeding the bottle and nipple should be thoroughly flushed and the bottle filled with water until washed with water and a detergent.

TABLE 3-14. HOUSEHOLD MEASURES OF SOME COMMONLY USED SUGARS

	TABLESPOONFULS PER OUNCE
Lactose	3
Sucrose (cane)	2
Dextrin-maltose preparations:	
Mead's Dextri-Maltose	4
Karo	2
Cartose	2
Dexin	6

Caloric value of each is 120 calories per ounce, except Dexin, 115.

*Percentage of fat, carbohydrate or protein =

$$\frac{\text{Number of ounces of milk} \times \text{percentage of ingredient in whole or evaporated milk}}{\text{Total number of ounces in formula}}$$

Percentage of carbohydrate from added sugar =

$$\frac{\text{Number of ounces of sugar} \times 100}{\text{(percentage of carbohydrate in sugar)}}$$

$$\overline{\text{Total number of ounces in formula}}$$

METHOD. The hands should be thoroughly scrubbed and the sterilized bottles and utensils arranged on a clean table. If whole milk is used, the bottle is turned so that the contents are mixed, and the top is washed with hot water before the cap is removed. The water for the formula (it is necessary to allow for a slight loss in boiling) is brought to the boiling point in a saucepan; the amount of whole milk ordered is added; and the whole is boiled for 5 minutes. Constant stirring is necessary. The sugar is added while the milk is still warm.

If evaporated milk is used, the top of the can is washed with soap and hot water, rinsed with hot water, and 2 holes punctured in it. The water for the formula is boiled for 5 minutes, and the evaporated milk and sugar are added to it. No further boiling is necessary.

The freshly prepared and sterile formula is poured in appropriate amounts into sterilized nursing bottles. The bottles are capped by aseptic technique and stored in the refrigerator until time for the feedings.

TERMINAL STERILIZATION. This method has practical advantages and does not require presterilization of bottles or utensils. The formula is poured into clean nursing bottles, and the nipples are applied. The nipples are then loosely covered with glass, metal or paper caps and placed in a container with a rack on the bottom and tall enough to prevent the bottles from touching the lid. The container is filled with water to about the midpoint of the bottles, covered and placed over a moderate flame. The water is allowed to boil gently for 25 minutes. The bottles are then removed with tongs and placed in a container of cold water for 10 minutes. The caps are then tightened and the bottles stored in a refrigerator.

Whole Milk. Whole milk or a reconstructed evaporated milk without added carbohydrate may be substituted for the formula when the infant is 4 to 6 months of age. Subsequently most infants will take 1½ pints to a quart of milk a day. There is no advantage in the ingestion of more, and there is the possible disadvantage that other essential foods may be displaced. Some of the milk may be incorporated in the cereal and in the preparation of such foods as custards, soups and sauces.

OTHER FOODS

Vitamins. The diets of breast-fed babies should be supplemented from early in the neonatal period by vitamins C and D and possibly by vitamin A. Almost all artificial milk feedings are fortified with 400 I.U. of vitamin D and often with other vitamins as well. Hence it is essential to know the vitamin content of the milk before prescribing additional vitamins for the bottle-fed baby (see Table 3-15).

Orange and other citrus fruit juices are natural sources of *vitamin C*, but since many young infants do not seem to tolerate them in amounts large enough to supply an adequate vitamin intake, it is preferable to give 25 to 50 mg. of ascorbic acid initially. During the second month of life orange juice diluted with water may be offered; when at least 2 ounces of fresh, frozen or canned orange juice (or equivalent amounts of other sources of vitamin C) are taken daily, the ascorbic acid may be discontinued.

Vitamin D should be started early in the neonatal period with a daily intake of approximately 400 I.U. only if the baby is breast-fed or is taking a formula which does *not* contain vitamin D. A number of preparations are available which in recommended doses contain this amount of vitamin D, 50 mg. of ascorbic acid and 3000 to 5000 I.U. of vitamin A. Concentrates in water-miscible vehicles are desirable to avoid aspiration of oil.

"Solid" Foods. The caloric content of the various prepared baby foods differs widely. Egg yolk, cereals with added milk, meats and puddings have greater caloric density than milk, whereas vegetables and fruits have a similar or lower energy value than milk. Food selection which tends to be poorly discriminating without good advice and supervision plays a significant role in the caloric intake of infants receiving "solid" foods and contributes to obesity in infancy.

Cereal is an excellent food to offer the baby who has a large appetite early in life and is not satisfied with the calories provided by his intake of milk. Fruits, especially bananas and applesauce, are usually well tolerated and may be offered first. There is little evidence that the addition of any of these foods to the normal infant's diet before 3 or 4 months of age contributes in any significant way to his well-being, although many physicians are advocating the introduction of "solid" foods at 3 to 6 weeks of age.

Any new food should be offered initially once a day in small amounts (1 to 2 teaspoonfuls). A demitasse spoon that easily fits the baby's mouth may be used. New foods are generally best accepted if fairly thin or dilute. Food is frequently pushed out rather than back by the tongue because the baby does not yet know how to swallow efficiently. This possibility should be mentioned to the mother, who might otherwise interpret the "spitting-back" of new foods as an idiosyncrasy or dislike. It is usually wise to offer the same food daily until the baby becomes accustomed to it and not to introduce new foods more often than every week or two.

The feeding at which these foods are offered is not particularly important. They should be given when the baby's hunger is no longer satisfied by milk alone and when they logically fit into the daily schedule. There is no reason for persisting with or forcing a particular food that is definitely disliked. The family's dislikes and prejudices for particular foods are contagious and should not be displayed before the infant. The physician should avoid prescribing a definite amount of a given food lest the mother interpret the suggestion too literally. Many infants are overfed by overzealous parents who mistake acceptance of food for appetite. The infant's appetite is the best index of the proper amount, and respect for his wishes will avoid many problems.

Cereal. The various precooked cereals on the market provide in a convenient form a variety of grains excellent for infants. Most contain iron and factors of the vitamin B complex. They are easily prepared by adding boiled milk or formula.

Fruits. Strained or puréed cooked fruits furnish minerals and some water-soluble vitamins and usually have a mildly laxative effect. Raw ripe

TABLE 3-15. VITAMIN CONTENT OF NATURAL MILKS, PREPARED MILKS AND MILK SUBSTITUTES

	VITAMIN CONCENTRATION PER LITER IN NORMAL DILUTION							
	A (I.U.)	D (I.U.)	E (I.U.)	C (mg.)	THIAMINE (µg.)	NIACIN (µg.)	PYRIDOXINE (µg.)	PANTOTHENATE (µg.)	RIBOFLAVIN (µg.)
Human milk, mature, average	1898	21	6.6	43	160	1470	100	1840	360
Cow's milk, market, average	1025	13	1.0	11	440	940	640	3460	1750
Cow's milk, evaporated, many brands	1850	420	1.3	5.5	280	1000	370	3500	1900
Cow's milk, powdered:									
Klim, Borden	1850	423	–	1.9	380	1300	–	–	1900
Commercial premodified milks:									
Infant Formula, Baker	1782	423	–	35	446	7400	297		1102
Bremil with Iron, Borden	2640	423	5.3	53	420	6340	420		1060
Bremil Powder, with Iron, Borden	2640	423	5.3	53	420	6340	420		1060
Modilac, Gerber	1585	423	–	48	528	5300	740		740
Enfamil, Mead	1586	423	–	53	423	4200	317	2100	1000
Olac, Mead	2643	423	–	tr.	–	–	–	–	–
Nan Powder, Nestlé		–	–						–
Lactogen Powder, Nestlé		–	–						–
Lactogen Powder, Full Protein, Nestlé		–	–						–
Prodieton Powder, Nestlé		–	–						–
Similac with Iron, Ross	2640	423	5	53	700	6000	240	2000	1100
Similac Powder with Iron, Ross	2640	423	5	53	700	6000	220	2000	1100
Similac PM 60/40, Ross	2640	423	5	53	700	5300	220	–	1100
SMA S-26, Wyeth	2650	423	8.5	53	710	5300	420	2100	1100
Goat's milk, Powdered:									
Dale's, Cutter	–	–		14	480	2700	70	2900	1140
High protein, low fat powdered milks:									
Dryco, Borden	2640	423	–		500	220			2000
Alacta, Mead		–	3.7						230
Probana, Mead	5285	1057	11	–	–	–	–	–	–
Protein Milk, Mead	–	–	–	–					–
Eledon, Nestlé		–	–						–
Nestogen, Half-Skimmed, Nestlé		–	–						–
Skim milk, many brands	–	None	4.8	–	360	1060	450	3880	1890
Hypoallergenic milk substitutes:									
Mullsoy Liquid, Borden (Soya)	2100	423	10.6	42	530	9500	420	1000	845
Mullsoy Powder, Borden (Soya)	–	None	4	80		3500	235	1000	260
Neo-Mullsoy, Borden (Soya)	2110	423	10.6	53	530	7390	420	2640	1060
Lambase, Gerber	1585	423	5.3	48	420	5300	630		1050
Meat-Base, Gerber	1585	423	5.3	42	420	10600	507		1370
Soyalac Liquid, Loma Linda (Soya)	1584	423	5	32	422	6000	422	–	634
Soyalac Powder, Loma Linda (Soya)	1584	423	5	32	422	6000	422	–	634
Nutramigen, Powder, Mead	1586	423	5.3	32	486	4200	529	3400	1903
Pro-Sobee, Mead (Soya)	1586	423	5	53	530	7400	427	2600	1057
Sobee, Mead (Soya)	1586	423	5	53	530	7400	427	2600	1057
Isomil, Ross (Soya)	1500	423	5	50	600	6000	400	5000	600
Milk substitutes, specialty products:									
Cho-Free Formula Base, Borden	2110	423	10.6	53	530	7390	420	2640	1060
Lofenalac, Mead	1586	423	5.3	32	486	4200	529	3400	
Lonalac, Mead	1015	–	–	–	423	900	–	–	1800
Portagen	3540	284	7	57	850	1140	830	7100	1135

banana is readily digested and enjoyed by most babies. It should be mashed with a fork. Many infants who are slow in accepting new foods seem to prefer fruits.

Vegetables. The various "colored" vegetables are moderately good sources of iron and other minerals and of the vitamins of the B complex. They may be freshly cooked and strained, but many mothers prefer the commercially prepared vegetables because of their convenience. "Colored" vegetables are usually added to the infant's diet by about 4 months of age.

Meats, eggs and starchy foods. Eggs and starchy foods are usually introduced during the second 6 months of life, although some physicians offer egg yolk at an earlier age. The yolk of the egg is used initially and is preferably hard-cooked and then added to cereal or other food. As with all new foods, a small amount (pea-sized) is offered at first with gradual increases up to a whole yolk 2 or 3 times a week. Egg white should be introduced with equal caution to minimize the possibility of allergic manifestations.

Potatoes, rice, spaghetti, bread and similar starchy foods have principally a caloric value. As a rule they are not included in the infant's diet until the more essential foods mentioned above are being taken regularly. Baked potato, mashed with milk and butter, is a favorite. Zwieback, toast or graham crackers may be offered to the infant when he shows an interest in "gumming" on coarser foods (usually 6 to 8 months of age). It is with such foods that he learns to chew and to feed himself.

Meat is an excellent source of protein as well as of iron and vitamins. Ground fresh beef or liver or the strained canned meats may be used initially by about 4 months of age. Meats seem to be more readily accepted when mixed with another food.

The commercial "soups" and meat and vegetable mixtures are relatively high in carbohydrate and are not to be considered optimal sources of iron or protein. Many home-prepared soups are bulky out of proportion to their food value, and much of the vitamin content is lost by overcooking.

Desserts. Puddings, junkets and custards are

good foods for older infants, particularly if they temporarily prefer milk in that form. If, however, such foods are given as a bribe or reward or only after other foods have been finished, poor eating habits are apt to be established. Sweet foods should be offered as casually as the rest of the meal and at any place in the meal that the child desires.

Salt Intake. To increase palatability, salt is usually added to commercially prepared baby foods; soups, cereals, meats, and meat with vegetable mixtures may contain unexpectedly large amounts of salt. Puyau has calculated the sodium intake of 11- to 13-month-old infants to be approximately 60 mEq. per day, equivalent to a daily salt intake of 20 or more gm. in the adult. The significance of these large intakes, which are in the ranges seen in populations with a high incidence of hypertension, is not clear, although the possibility that they might contribute to the development of hypertension later in life cannot be ignored.

FIRST-YEAR FEEDING PROBLEMS

Underfeeding. Underfeeding is suggested by restlessness and crying, and by failure to gain weight adequately in spite of complete emptying of the breast or bottle. Underfeeding may also result from the infant's failure to take a sufficient quantity of food even when offered. In these instances the frequency of feedings, the mechanics of nursing, the size of the holes in the nipple, the adequacy of eructation of air, and the possibility of systemic disease in the baby should be investigated. The extent and duration of underfeeding determine the clinical manifestations. Constipation, failure to sleep, irritability and excessive crying are to be expected. There may be poor gain in weight or an actual loss. In the last instance the skin becomes dry and wrinkled, subcutaneous tissue disappears, and the infant assumes the appearance of an "old man." Deficiencies of vitamins A, B, C and D and of iron and protein may be responsible for characteristic clinical manifestations.

Treatment consists in increasing the fluid and caloric intake, correcting deficiencies in vitamin and mineral intake, and instructing the mother in the art of infant feeding. The physician should anticipate the possibility that some infants will fail to thrive despite the institution of all the recognized corrective measures. In such instances careful clinical search is indicated to determine whether some underlying disorder is responsible for the failure to thrive.

Overfeeding. Overfeeding may be quantitative or qualitative. Regurgitation and vomiting are frequent symptoms of overfeeding. As a rule, infants can be depended upon not to take excessive quantities; but occasionally an infant has postprandial discomfort from eating too much, and he may gain weight excessively. Diets too high in fat delay gastric emptying, cause distention and abdominal discomfort and may cause excessive gain in weight. Diets too high in carbohydrate are likely to cause undue fermentation in the intestine, resulting in distention and flatulence and in too rapid gain in weight. Such diets may be deficient in essential protein, vitamins and minerals. Formulas too high in caloric content in the first week or two of life are likely to result in loose or diarrheal stools.

Regurgitation and Vomiting. The return of small amounts of swallowed food during or shortly after eating is termed "regurgitation" or "spitting up." More complete emptying of the stomach, especially when it occurs some time after feeding, is termed "vomiting." Within limits, regurgitation is a natural occurrence, especially during the first half-year or so of life. It can be reduced to a negligible extent, however, by adequate eructation of swallowed air during and after eating, by gentle handling, by avoidance of emotional conflicts, and by placing the infant on his right side or abdomen for a nap immediately after eating. One should also ensure that the head is not lower than the rest of the body during the rest period.

Vomiting is one of the most common symptoms in infancy and may be associated with a wide variety of disturbances, both trivial and serious. Its cause should always be investigated (see page 777).

Loose or Diarrheal Stools. Acute infectious diarrhea and chronic diarrheal conditions are discussed elsewhere; only milk disturbances of dietary origin will be considered here.

The stool of the breast-fed infant is naturally softer than that of the infant fed cow's milk. From about the fourth to the sixth day of life the stools go through a transitional stage in which they are rather loose and greenish-yellow and contain mucus; within a few days the typical "milk stool" appears. Subsequently the use of laxatives or the ingestion of certain foods by the mother may be temporarily responsible for an infant's loose stools. Excessive intake of breast milk may also increase the frequency and the water content of the stool. Actual diarrhea in a breast-fed infant is unusual and should be considered infectious until proved otherwise.

Though the stools of artificially fed infants tend to be firmer than those of breast-fed infants, under certain circumstances loose stools may result from artificial feeding. In the first 2 weeks or so of life, overfeeding is likely to cause loose, frequent stools. Later, formulas which are too concentrated or whose sugar content is too high, especially in lactose, may be responsible for loose, frequent stools. Many of the temporary diarrheal disturbances in artificially fed infants are the result of contaminations of food which would not disturb an older child and are not serious enough to cause prolonged disturbance in the infant. The ease with which artificially fed infants acquire diarrheal disturbances and the potential seriousness of them are strong arguments for extreme care in providing a food supply free of pathogenic bacteria.

Mild diarrheal disturbances due to overfeeding respond quickly to temporary decrease or cessation of feeding. The withholding of all solid food and of one or several milk feedings, with the substitution of boiled water or 5 per cent glucose in water or in a balanced electrolyte solution, is usually all that is required.

Constipation (see also p. 779). Constipation is practically unknown in breast-fed infants who receive an adequate amount of milk, and is rare in artificially fed infants receiving an adequate diet. The nature of the stool, and not its frequency, is the criterion of constipation. Although most infants have one or more stools daily, an occasional infant will have a stool of normal consistency only at intervals of 36 to 48 hours. Whenever constipation or obstipation is present from birth or shortly thereafter, a rectal examination should be performed. Tight or spastic anal sphincters may occasionally be responsible for obstipation, and correction usually follows finger dilatation performed twice or 3 times a day. Anal fissures or cracks may also cause constipation. If irritation is removed, healing usually occurs quickly. Aganglionic megacolon may be manifest by constipation in early infancy; the absence of stool in the rectum on digital examination suggests this possibility.

Constipation in the artificially fed infant may be due to an insufficient amount of food or fluid. In other instances it may result from diets too high in fat or protein or deficient in bulk. Simply increasing the amount of fluid or sugar in the formula may be corrective in the first few months of life. After this age better results are obtained by adding or increasing the amounts of cereal, vegetables and fruits. Prune juice (½ to 1 ounce) may be given as a temporary measure, but it is better to add foods with some bulk. Enemas and suppositories should never be more than temporary measures. Milk of magnesia may be given in doses of 1 or 2 teaspoonfuls, but should be reserved for emergencies.

Colic. The term "colic" is used to describe a frequent symptom complex of paroxysmal abdominal pain, presumably of intestinal origin, and of severe crying. It usually occurs in infants under 3 months of age.

The clinical pattern is characteristic. The attack usually begins suddenly; the cry is loud and more or less continuous; so-called paroxysms may persist for several hours; the face may be flushed, or there may be circumoral pallor; the abdomen is distended and tense; the legs are drawn up on the abdomen, although they may be momentarily extended; the feet are often cold; the hands are clenched. The attack may terminate only when the infant is completely exhausted, but often there is relief with the passage of feces or flatus.

Certain infants seem to be peculiarly susceptible to colic. The cause of recurrent attacks is usually not apparent, although it may be associated with hunger and with swallowed air which has passed into the intestine. Overfeeding may also cause discomfort and distention, but rarely to the degree seen in colic. Certain foods, especially those of high carbohydrate content, may be responsible for excessive fermentation in the intestines, but only occasionally does a change in diet prevent further attacks of colic. Crying from intestinal discomfort is seen in infants with intestinal allergy, but colic is not limited to this group. Intestinal obstruction or peritoneal infection may mimic an attack of colic. Recurrent attacks are frequent late in the afternoon or evening, suggesting some preceding event in the household routine as a possible cause. Worry, fear, anger or excitement may cause vomiting in an older child, and may result in colic in an infant. Certainly no single causative factor consistently accounts for colic, nor does any method of treatment consistently provide satisfactory relief.

Holding the baby upright or permitting him to lie prone across the lap or on a hot water bottle or heating pad is occasionally helpful. Passage of flatus or fecal material spontaneously or with expulsion of a suppository or enema sometimes affords relief. Carminatives before feedings are ineffective in preventing the attacks. Sedation is occasionally indicated for a prolonged attack, and sometimes over a period of time for parent or child if other measures fail. Temporary hospitalization of the infant, often without resorting to more than a change in the infant's feeding routine and providing a period of rest for his mother, may be helpful in extreme cases. The prevention of attacks should include adequate feeding techniques, including burping, the provision of a stable emotional environment, the search for a possible allergenic food in the infant's or nursing mother's diet, and avoidance of underfeeding. The condition rarely persists after 3 months of age.

FEEDING DURING THE SECOND YEAR OF LIFE

Most infants naturally adapt themselves to a schedule of 3 meals a day by about the end of the first year of life. Though considerable latitude in the diet of the individual infant must be permitted to allow for personal idiosyncrasies and family habits, the mother should be given an outline of the daily basic dietary needs (see Table 3-16).

Reduced Caloric Intake. Toward the end of the first year of life and during the second year, owing to the constantly decelerating rate of growth, there is a gradual reduction in the infant's caloric intake per unit of body weight. In addition, it is not unusual for him to have temporary periods of disinterest in food in general or in certain articles of it. Failure to recognize these features, especially the decreasing caloric needs, results in attempts to force feeding. The natural reaction of the child is rebellion, and feeding problems ensue. Prevention is much more effective than are methods of correction, and the changing

TABLE 3-16. RECORD OF DIETARY HISTORY

TYPE OF FOOD	DAILY CONSUMPTION	RECOMMENDED ALLOWANCE FOR GROWING CHILD
I. Milk.............................	Total......................	$\frac{1}{2}$-$\frac{3}{4}$ qt.
	With meals..........Between..............	
	With cereal..........In cooking...........	
Milk products.........................	Cheese................Cream	
	Others	
II. Eggs	Total......................	2 or 3 a week
	With meals..........In cooking...........	
III. Meats...............................	Total......................	1 serving daily or 5 times a week
(a) Lean..............................	Beef....................Lamb..................	
	Pork ....Others................	
(b) Poultry	Chicken..............Others................	2-3 ounces (varies with age)
(c) Fish..............................	Salmon ....Others................	
(d) Seafood	Shrimp.................Others................	
(e) Liver	Liver	1 serving a week
IV. Vegetables		
(a) Potatoes	Total......................	1 serving daily
	Irish ....Sweet	
(b) Green, leafy......................	Total......................	1 serving daily
	Lettuce ....Spinach..............	$\frac{1}{2}$ cup
	Chard ....Brussels sprouts...	
	Broccoli...............Cabbage..............	
	Others	
(c) Others............................	Total......................	1 serving daily
	Beans...................Peas	$\frac{1}{2}$ cup
	Asparagus ....Corn...................	
	Beets ....Carrots	
	Cauliflower..........Parsnips	
	Squash................Turnips..............	
	Others	
V. Fruits		
(a) Citrus and tomato..............	Total......................	1 serving daily
	Orange...............Lemon	Whole orange
	Grapefruit...........Tomato	$\frac{1}{2}$ grapefruit
(b) Others	Total......................	1 serving daily
	Peach.................Apricot	$\frac{1}{2}$ cup
	Pear ....Apple	
	Fig ....Prunes................	
	Plums ....Berries	
	Pineapple ....Bananas	
	Others	
VI. Breadstuffs and cereals............	Total......................	Varies with caloric needs
(a) Bread..............................	Total......................	1 slice or equivalent with each meal
	Whole grain.........Enriched............	
	Others	
(b) Cereals	Total......................	1 serving daily of whole grain or enriched cereal
	Cooked:	
	Whole grain......Enriched............	
	Macaroni..........Spaghetti	
	Soybean ....Others................	
	Prepared:	
	Whole grain......Enriched............	
	Others	
VII. Fats		
(a) Butter or oleomargarine with vitamin A	Total......................	2 tablespoonfuls daily
	As spread ....In cooking...........	
(b) As source of essential fatty acids..........................	Total......................	Possibly 1 to 2 tablespoonfuls daily
	Lard ....Corn oil	
	Others	

(Concluded on next page)

TABLE 3-16. RECORD OF DIETARY HISTORY *(Concluded)*

TYPE OF FOOD	DAILY CONSUMPTION	RECOMMENDED ALLOWANCE FOR GROWING CHILD
VIII. Vitamin D	Total......................	800-1000 I.U. daily
IX. Iodized salt	....	As desired (in goiter belt)
X. Desserts, sugars and syrups	Total...................... Custards ....Jell-o................... Cake...................Cookies............... Ice cream ....Puddings............. Sugar.................Syrup .... Jam, jelly ....Others	As needed for calories

Courtesy of Arild E. Hansen.

pattern of the infant's food habits during the second year of life should be explained to the mother before its appearance.

Self-Selection of Diet. Though a great variety of foods is not possible at each meal, strong likes or dislikes of children for particular foods should be respected. Spinach is an example of a non-essential food whose virtues have been over-emphasized, conceivably to the point of causing feeding difficulties. When rejected foods consistently include such basic dietary staples as milk and eggs, the possibility of food allergy should be given consideration.

Children, including infants, tend to select diets which over a period of several days assume a balanced nature. Thus the child may be permitted a rather wide choice of foods without concern so long as the eating performance is adequate over the longer period. Under normal circumstances the child should determine the quantity to be eaten with respect to both a given food and to the entire meal. At this age the child should be fed separately from the other children in the family, who otherwise might strongly influence the development of his eating habits by the example of their own food likes and dislikes. Eating patterns and habits developed in the first 2 years of life are likely to persist for several years.

Self-Feeding by Infants. Before the infant is a year of age he should be permitted to participate in the act of feeding himself. By 6 months or so he can hold his bottle. Within another 2 or 3 months he can hold a cup. The introduction of zwieback, graham crackers and bacon by the time he is 7 to 8 months of age gives the infant something which he can hold and thus learn one of the principles of self-feeding. He may use a spoon for feeding himself as soon as he can hold and direct it to his mouth, possibly by 10 to 12 months of age. Mothers often inhibit this learning process because of their objection to the messiness incident to the learning of adequate control.

Acquisition of the ability to feed himself is an important step in the infant's development of self-reliance and of a sense of responsibility. By the end of the second year of life the infant should be largely responsible for his feeding.

In comparison with the supervision commonly maintained over the feeding of infants, the diets of children beyond the age of 2 years are badly neglected. Though it is desirable that children should not be aware of constant supervision of their dietary habits and that they should be given every opportunity to form eating habits naturally, the diets of all children should be supervised. Surveys of dietary habits of children in various economic groups reveal a high incidence of inadequate diets and of malnutrition. Although the nutritional requirements per unit of body weight are constantly decreasing with increasing age (110 calories per kg. in infancy; 50 calories per kg. at 15 years), at all times the need for calories as well as for protein, vitamins and minerals is relatively greater than it is in the adult.

Daily Basic Diet. Parents should be given a daily basic diet for the child from which the family menu can be prepared. It is essential that the entire family partake of the same diet and that the sense of "being on a diet" be avoided. The quantity of the intake after the basic requirements have been met can in most instances be determined by the healthy growing child; the obese child is an exception. A history of the dietary habits of the child is essential for evaluation of his nutritive intake, but such histories are often unreliable. More dependable information can be secured by providing the mother with a number of dietary history blanks such as the one illustrated in Table 3-16, on which she can record the daily intake for several representative days. From such information, corrections in the diet may be made more effectively. This table also contains the recommended daily dietary intake.

Adequate quantities of all the essential classes of foods must be provided in order to avoid specific nutritional deficiencies. The child should know the content of a basic diet and its importance to proper growth and good health, but this information should never be presented as a threat to enforce rigid feeding practices.

The following is a daily menu which will provide all the essential nutrients:

Breakfast: Citrus fruit or tomato juice
　　　　　Cereal — whole grain or enriched
　　　　　Egg
　　　　　Whole-wheat toast
　　　　　Butter
　　　　　Milk

Lunch:　　Sandwich with whole-wheat bread or
　　　　　Casserole dish — containing meat or meat substitute
　　　　　　and starchy vegetable
　　　　　Green vegetable, raw
　　　　　Milk
　　　　　Custard, pudding, cake, ice cream or gelatin dessert

Dinner:　　Meat — fish — liver
　　　　　Potatoes, rice or spaghetti
　　　　　Green vegetable
　　　　　Whole-wheat bread, butter
　　　　　Milk
　　　　　Fruit
Vitamin D (throughout childhood)

Eating Habits. As stated previously, eating habits formed in the first year or two of life have a distinct effect upon those of subsequent years. Feeding difficulties between the ages of 2 and 5 years frequently result from too great parental insistence on eating and too great anxiety when the child does not conform to some arbitrary standard. Negativistic reactions by the child are natural consequences of excessive stress at meal-time, and correction requires improvement in parent-child relations. Other factors which disturb eating are too much confusion at mealtime, insufficient time for eating, either on the part of the adult or of the child, food dislikes of other members of the family, and poorly prepared and unattractively served food. A comfortable chair of proper height with a foot-rest is important for a child's ease at the table.

It is good practice to call the child from play 15 or 20 minutes before mealtimes, allowing time for going to the toilet and washing the hands and face and cooling off from strenuous activity. This is an excellent time especially for younger children to spend with the father, reading or playing quiet games. Mealtimes should be happy. Discussion about the food, except for occasional favorable comments, should be avoided, and the conversation should be on subjects of interest to the entire family. The child should feel that he is part of the family group. The child's appetite should be respected; if his desire for food at times is below average, there should be no persuasion to eat more. Adults should realize that eating habits are taught better by example than by formal explanation.

Lunches Between Meals. During the second year and even for several years thereafter, orange juice or other fruit juice or fruit together with a cracker may be given in either or both of the midmeal periods. For older children midmeal nourishment should be avoided if it reduces the appetite for the following meal. When a snack after school results in greater enthusiasm and energy for play and does not reduce the appetite for the evening meal, it should be encouraged. Fruits are especially recommended for such lunches.

There are differences of opinion about midsession lunches in school. Though in general they are just as well omitted, when a session is relatively long, fruit juice may be advantageous, especially for the younger child.

WILLIAM E. LAUPUS

REFERENCES

Aldrich, C. A.: Ancient Processes in Scientific Age; Feeding Aspects. *Am. J. Dis. Child.*, 64:714, 1942.

Barnes, G. R., Jr., Lethin, A. N., Jr., Jackson, E. B., and Shea, N.: Management of Breast Feeding. *J.A.M.A.*, 151:192, 1953.

Call, J. D.: Emotional Factors Favoring Successful Breast Feeding of Infants. *J. Pediat.*, 55:485, 1959.

Committee on Nutrition, American Academy of Pediatrics: Composition of Milks. *Pediatrics*, 26:1039, 1960.

Committee on Nutrition, American Academy of Pediatrics: Proposed Changes in Food and Drug Administration Regulations Concerning Formula Products and Vitamin-Mineral Supplements for Infants. *Pediatrics*, 40:916, 1967.

Davidson, M., Levine, S. Z., Bauer, C. H., and Dann, M.: Feeding Studies in Low-Birth-Weight Infants. I. Relationship of Dietary Protein, Fat and Electrolyte to Rate of Weight Gain, Clinical Course and Serum Chemical Concentrations. *J. Pediat.*, 70, 695, 1967.

Fomon, S. J.: Comparative Study of Human Milk and a Soya Bean Formula in Promoting Growth and Nitrogen Retention by Infants. *Pediatrics*, 24:577, 1959.

Fomon, S. J.: Comparative Study of Protein from Human Milk and Cow's Milk in Promoting Nitrogen Retention by Normal Full-Term Infants. *Pediatrics*, 26:51, 1960.

Fomon, S. J.: Body Composition of the Male Reference Infant. *Pediatrics*, 40:863, 1967.

Fomon, S. J.: *Infant Nutrition.* Philadelphia, W. B. Saunders Company, 1967.

Gartner, L. M., and Arias, I. M.: Studies of Prolonged Neonatal Jaundice in the Breast-Fed Infant. *J. Pediat.*, 68:54, 1966.

Gordon, H. H., and Ganzon, A. F.: On the Protein Allowances for Young Infants. *J. Pediat.*, 54:503, 1959.

Hewitt, E. S., and Aldrich, C. A.: Poor Eating Habits of the Runabout Child: The Role of Physiologic Anorexia. *J. Pediat.*, 28:595, 1946.

Holt, L. E., Jr.: The Protein Requirement of Infants. *J. Pediat.*, 54:496, 1959.

Holt, L.E., Jr., and Snyderman, S. E.: The Amino Acid Requirements of Infants. *J.A.M.A.*, 175:100, 1961.

Hytten, F. E., and Thomson, A. M.: Clinical and Chemical Studies in Human Lactation. X. The Maintenance of Breast Feeding. *Brit. M. J.*, 2:232, 1955.

Macy, I. G., Kelly, H. J., and Sloan, R. E.: The Composition of Milks. A Compilation of the Comparative Composition and Properties of Human, Cow and Goat Milk, Colostrum and Transitional Milk. Washington, D.C., Publication 254, National Academy of Science–National Research Council, 1953.

Newton, M., and Newton, N.: The Normal Course and Management of Lactation. *Clin. Obst. & Gynec.*, 5:44, 1962.

Newton, N., and Newton, M.: Psychologic Aspects of Lactation. *New England J. Med.*, 277:1179, 1967.

Omans, W. B., Barness, L. A., Rose, C. S., and Gyorgy, P.: Prolonged Feeding Studies in Premature Infants. *J. Pediat.*, 59:951, 1961.

Powers, G. F.: Infant Feeding: Historical Background and Modern Practice. *J.A.M.A.*, 105:753, 1935.

Puyau, F. A., and Hampton, L. P.: Infant Feeding Practices,

1966. Salt Content of the Modern Diet. *Am. J. Dis. Child.,* 111:370, 1966.

Spock, B.: *Baby and Child Care.* New York, Pocket Books, Inc., 1962.

Sutherland, J. M., Glueck, H. I., and Gleser, G.: Hemorrhagic Disease of the Newborn: Breast Feeding as a Necessary

Factor in the Pathogenesis. *Am. J. Dis. Child.,* 113:524, 1967.

Von Sydow, G.: Study of Development of Rickets in Premature Infants. *Acta Paediat. Scand.* (Suppl. 2.), 33:3, 1946.

Woodruff, C. W.: Protein Requirements of Full-Term Infants. *J.A.M.A.,* 175:114, 1961.

NUTRITIONAL DISORDERS

MALNUTRITION

Malnutrition may be due to improper or inadequate food intake or may result from inadequate absorption of food. Deficient supply of food, poor dietary habits and food faddism, and emotional factors may limit intake. Certain metabolic abnormalities may also cause malnutrition. Requirements for essential nutrients may be increased during stress and disease and during the administration of antibiotics or of catabolic or anabolic drugs. Malnutrition may be acute or chronic, reversible or irreversible.

Precise evaluation of nutritional status is difficult. Severe disturbances are readily apparent, but mild disturbances may be overlooked, even after careful physical and laboratory examinations. The diagnosis of malnutrition rests on an accurate dietary history (Table 3-16, p. 161), upon evaluation of present deviations from average height and weight and of past rates of growth in height and weight or of certain organs, and upon evidence of specific clinical deficiencies. Deficiencies of some nutrients may be revealed by low blood levels of them or their metabolites, by observing biochemical or clinical effects of administration of the nutrient or its products, or by giving the patient substantial amounts of appropriate nutrients and noting the rate at which they are excreted.

The most acute nutritional disturbances are those which involve water and electrolytes, especially sodium, potassium, chloride and hydrogen ions. These are discussed elsewhere (p. 203). The more chronic conditions, involving deficits of calories, proteins and vitamins, are discussed here. Clinical malnutrition usually involves deficits of more than a single nutrient.

MARASMUS

(INFANTILE ATROPHY; INANITION; ATHREPSIA)

Severe malnutrition in infants is common in areas with insufficient food, inadequate knowledge of feeding techniques or poor hygiene. The synonyms listed above have been applied to patterns of clinical illness emphasizing one or more features of protein and calorie deficiency.

Etiology. The clinical picture of marasmus is due to general starvation. It stems from an inadequate caloric intake due to insufficiency of the diet, to improper feeding habits such as those of disturbed parent-child relations, or to metabolic abnormalities or congenital malformations. Severe impairment of any body system may result in malnutrition.

Clinical Manifestations. In marasmus there is failure to gain weight, followed by loss of weight until emaciation results, with loss of turgor in skin and subcutaneous tissue; the skin becomes wrinkled and loose as subcutaneous fat disappears. Because fat is lost last from the sucking pads of the cheeks, the face may retain a relatively normal appearance for some time before becoming shrunken and wizened. The abdomen may be distended or thin. The intestinal pattern becomes readily visible. Atrophy of muscles occurs, with resultant hypotonia. Edema may be present.

The temperature is usually subnormal, the pulse may be slow, and the basal metabolic rate tends to be reduced. At first the infant may be fretful, but later he becomes listless, and the appetite diminishes. The infant is usually constipated, but the so-called starvation type of diarrhea may appear, with frequent, small stools containing mucus. Terminally, frank diarrhea is common.

MALNUTRITION IN CHILDREN BEYOND INFANCY

Etiology. Malnutrition in older infants and children may be a continuation of an undernourished state begun in infancy, or it may stem from factors which become operative during childhood. In general, the causes are the same as those responsible for malnutrition in infants. The problem may be complex. Poor dietary habits may be associated with a generally poor hygienic situation, with chronic disease, with finical eating habits of other members of the family, or with disturbed parent-child relations, especially with overanxiety about eating habits.

Poor eating habits in children under the age of 5 or 6 years can often be traced directly to parental factors, of which overconcern about the quantity or quality of the diet is a common one. In children of all ages inadequate rest, insufficient sleep and too much emotional excitement, such as that associated with the movies, radio and television, are important factors. In older children schoolwork and social activities may interfere with securing adequate rest. School-age children often develop irregular or inappropriate eating habits, especially at breakfast and lunch, because sufficient time is not allotted or because the meals may be poorly balanced. During adolescence girls frequently restrict their dietary intake for esthetic reasons. Eating between meals, especially of such items as candy, ice cream and malted milks, is likely to reduce the appetite at mealtime.

Clinical Manifestations. Malnutrition does not invariably result in underweight. Fatigue, lassitude, restlessness and irritability are frequent manifestations. Restlessness and overactivity are frequently misinterpreted by parents as evidences of lack of fatigue. Anorexia, easily induced digestive disturbances and constipation are common complaints, and even in older children the starvation type of mucoid diarrheal stool may be observed. Malnourished children often have a limited span of attention and do poorly in schoolwork. They have increased susceptibility to infections, especially of the gastrointestinal and respiratory tracts. Muscular development is inadequate, and the poor tone of the flabby muscles results in a posture of fatigue, with rounded shoulders, flat chest and protuberant abdomen. Such children often look tired; the face is pale, the complexion is "muddy," and the eyes lack luster. Hypochromic anemia is common. In protracted cases there may be delayed epiphyseal development, irregularities in dentition and delayed puberty.

Evaluation should always include a careful history of dietary habits, physical hygiene and illness, a thorough physical examination, and such laboratory examinations as will establish, whenever possible, the cause or causes of malnutrition.

Treatment. There is a great need for individualization of treatment aimed at correction of the underlying psychologic and physical disturbances. An adequate diet (p. 161) should be outlined; vitamin concentrates may be added and continued for a time after the dietary intake has been adequate. When anorexia is a problem, the essential items of the diet should be provided in as concentrated a form as possible, and the fat content should be low. Between-meal snacks need not be prohibited if they do not interfere with the appetite for the next meal; milk and candy should not be given at such times, but fruit or fruit juices provided. Re-education of the whole family in respect to eating habits may be necessary.

Reasonable regularity in habits without regimentation should be encouraged. Quiet periods of 15 to 20 minutes before meals may abolish the tension which at times interferes with the appetite. Bedtime should be sufficiently early to ensure a full night's sleep, and a nap during the daytime may be helpful. Exciting stories, movies, radio and television should be avoided before bedtime.

Outdoor activity is to be encouraged in sedentary children and group play for those who tend to be seclusive. Every attempt should be made to permit the child to develop natural interests.

OBESITY

There is no exact line of demarcation between normal nutrition and overnutrition; practically, the diagnosis is made from the appearance of the child rather than from an arbitrary excess in weight. Children of the stocky type may have relatively large skeletal frames and more than the average amount of muscular tissue, so that their weight and height as well as their appearance of bigness exceed those of the average child of their age, but they are not to be considered obese. Obesity or overnutrition is a generalized excessive accumulation of fatty subcutaneous tissue.

Etiology. Obesity is usually due to an excessive intake of food compared with its utilization. Concepts of desirable body proportions vary with family, social and cultural factors. Food intake may be responsive to these considerations or to psychic disturbances; or hypothalamic, pituitary or other brain lesions or hyperinsulinism may be responsible for hyperphagia.

In 1901 Frölich reported a boy with a tumor at the base of the brain who presented a picture of obesity accompanied by physical and sexual infantilism. Since then the term "Frölich's syndrome" has been loosely applied, and many preadolescent obese boys are erroneously labeled with this diagnosis (see p. 1229).

Endocrine and metabolic disturbances are rare causes of obesity, though disorders of the thyroid, adrenals, pituitary and gonads may occur in obese persons. Genetic predisposition to obesity occurs in certain animals and may occur in man. In a study of adults, obesity was found to be 7 times more common in the lowest than in the highest social class.

Lack of activity causes obesity in some children whose intake of food may not be unusual.

Clinical Manifestations. Obesity may become evident at any age, but makes its appearance most frequently in late childhood. The child whose obesity is due to excessively high caloric intake is usually not only heavier than his cohorts, but also taller, and bone age is advanced. The facial features often appear disproportionately fine, the nose and mouth being small; there is often a double chin. The adiposity in the mammary regions is often suggestive of breast development, a feature usually embarrassing to the boy. The abdomen tends to be pendulous, and white or purple striae are often present. The external genitalia of boys appear disproportionately small, but actually are of average size; the penis is often nearly submerged in the pubic fat. Puberty may occur early, with the result that the ultimate height of the obese boy may be less than that of his slower-maturing peers. In only a few instances are the genitalia smaller than would be expected for age, with delayed puberty. The development of the external genitalia is normal in the majority of girls, and menarche is usually not delayed. The obesity of the extremities is usually greater in the upper arm and thigh and is at times limited to them. The hands may be relatively small, and the fingers tapering. Genu valgum is common, and coxa vara and slipping of the epiphysis of the head of the femur may occur. Skinfold measurements with calipers placed over the triceps muscle, at the midpoint of the back of the right upper arm flexed at 90 degrees, have been found useful in assessing fatness of children.

Psychologic disturbances are common in obese children. Even in the apparently well adjusted child adequate psychologic evaluation often discloses significant underlying emotional problems. These may have contributed initially to the causes of obesity, and in any event are usually an additive factor.

Prevention and Treatment. Because obesity may be self-perpetuating for psychologic or perhaps physiologic reasons, children of obese parents or obese siblings should be encouraged to adhere to a systematic program of energetic exercise and a balanced diet. Since there appears to be no proved proximate cause for juvenile obesity other than excessive food intake, rational therapy consists in a reduction in the diet and an increase in energy output. Emotional disturbances must be assessed and managed and the child permitted to lead a natural active life. When the dietary habits of the obese child are patterned after those of the family, as is frequently the case, treatment must include the entire family.

In planning the diet, the basic nutritional needs (p. 141) must be met. All the essential dietary needs may be included in a 1000- to 1200-calorie diet for children 10 to 14 years of age for several months. Some children avoid excessive eating after they have been allowed to return to a free choice of diet. The diet should contain as much bulk as possible. At times greater cooperation is secured if small portions of the diet are permitted between meals, especially in the afternoon. If there is reasonable doubt that the daily vitamin intake is adequate, vitamin concentrates may be prescribed. Vitamin D should be included, as for all growing children. Too rapid decreases in weight should not be attempted, and medical supervision should be maintained. There is at best a limited place for drug therapy. A trial with amphetamine in conjunction with dietary restriction and psychotherapy may be justified for children whose habits are sedentary or who have frequent states of depression. Because many obese children become obese adults, the child's motivation for reducing must be persistent. Psychologic support is often an essential element in management.

The *Pickwickian syndrome* is a rare complication of extreme exogenous obesity, in which there is severe cardiorespiratory distress. It is termed "Pickwickian" for the fat boy, Joe, in

TABLE 3-17. 1200-1400 Calorie Diet

BREAKFAST

1 orange, ½ grapefruit or 1 cup of tomato juice
1 egg
1 slice of whole-wheat bread or 1 serving of cereal without sugar
1 teaspoonful of butter
1 cup of whole milk

LUNCH

2 ounces of lean meat, 1 egg or ½ cup of cottage cheese
1 serving of raw vegetable as salad — no dressing
1 slice of whole-wheat bread
1 teaspoonful of butter
1 serving of fresh or unsweetened fruit
1 cup of whole milk

DINNER

2 ounces of lean meat (liver once a week), poultry or fish
2 servings of green, yellow or red vegetables*
1 serving of fresh or unsweetened fruit
1 cup of whole milk
(Part or all of bread and butter from one of the other meals may be included here)
A 1000-calorie diet may be obtained by eliminating the butter or cream from milk. In this case it becomes especially important to add vitamin A to the daily diet.

---

*Does not include Irish or sweet potatoes, parsnips, dried peas or beans, lima beans or corn.

Dickens's *Pickwick Papers*. The extreme obesity causes alveolar hypoventilation, with a decrease in pulmonary, tidal and expiratory reserve volumes. The manifestations include polycythemia, hypoxemia, cyanosis, cardiac enlargement, congestive cardiac failure and somnolence. High concentrations of oxygen may be dangerous in the treatment of the cyanosis, since respiration may depend solely on the stimulatory effect of hypoxia. Reduction in weight is extremely important and should be accomplished as rapidly as feasible.

REFERENCES

Cayler, G. C., Mays, J., and Riley, H. D.: Cardiorespiratory Syndrome of Obesity (Pickwickian Syndrome) in Children. *Pediatrics*, 27:237, 1961.
Mayer, J.: Some Aspects of the Problem of Regulation of Food Intake and Obesity. *New England J. Med.*, 12:662, 1966.
Stunkard, A., and Pestka, J.: The Physical Activity of Obese Girls. *Am. J. Dis. Child.*, 103:812, 1962.

PROTEIN MALNUTRITION

(Hypoproteinemia; Kwashiorkor;
Third-Degree Malnutrition [Gómez];
Prurideficiency Syndrome)

During the period of growth enough nitrogenous food must be consumed to maintain a positive nitrogen balance, whereas adults need only maintain nitrogen equilibrium. Not all protein is equally efficient in the maintenance of nitrogen equilibrium or in the establishment of nitrogen retention. When the diet does not contain adequate amounts of the essential amino acids, nitrogen equilibrium is not maintained, irrespective of the total quantity of protein in the diet.

There is no clinical evidence of human protein malnutrition except when it is well advanced. It may then be revealed in inadequate growth, lack of stamina, loss of muscular tissue, increased susceptibility to infections, and edema.

Etiology. Protein malnutrition may follow deprivation of sufficient quantity or quality of protein foods. It may also be due to impaired absorption of protein, as in chronic diarrheal states. Abnormal losses of protein in proteinuria (nephrosis), infection, hemorrhage or burns, or failure of protein synthesis, as in chronic liver disease, may also result in protein malnutrition.

Clinical Manifestations. Kwashiorkor is a clinical syndrome which results from a severe deficiency of protein with adequate or almost adequate caloric intake. It is the most serious and prevalent form of malnutrition in the world today, especially in technically undeveloped areas. Although deficiencies of calories and other nutrients may complicate the clinical and chemical patterns, the principal symptoms are due to deficiency of protein of good biologic value.

Kwashiorkor refers to the "deposed child," i.e. the child who is no longer suckled; it occurs in children from 4 months to 5 years of age. In areas where kwashiorkor is common the height and weight curves of infants and young children after weaning are below those of children of similar ages in areas where good nutrition is available. Although gains in height and weight are accelerated with treatment, these attainments never equal those of consistently well nourished children.

Edema usually develops early, not necessarily in those receiving the poorest basic diet, but more often in those in whom an added stress has occurred. Infection constitutes the most important added stress, and diarrhea may occur shortly be-

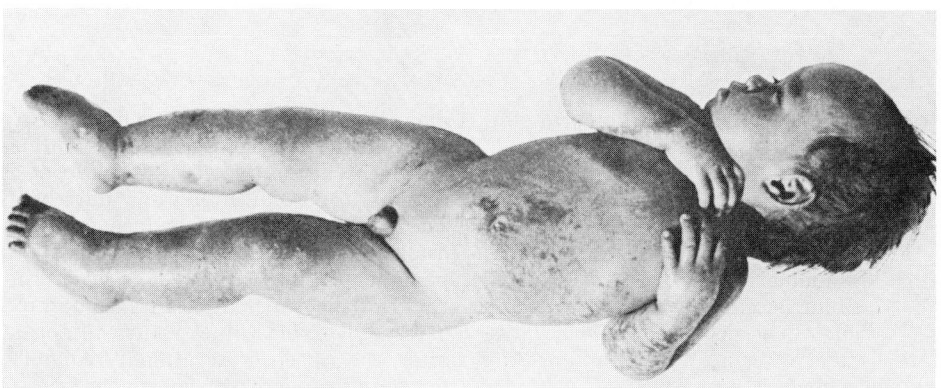

A

Figure 3-2. *A,* Kwashiorkor in a 2-year-old boy. Note the generalized edema, the typical skin lesions and the state of prostration. *B,* Close-up of the same child showing the hair changes and psychic alterations (apathy and misery); the edema of the face and the skin lesions can be seen more clearly. (Photographs made available by the Institute of Nutrition of Central America and Panama [INCAP], Guatemala, C.A., through the courtesy of Dr. Moisés Béhar.)

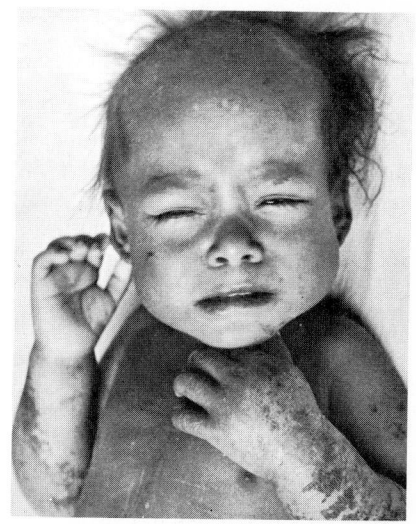

B

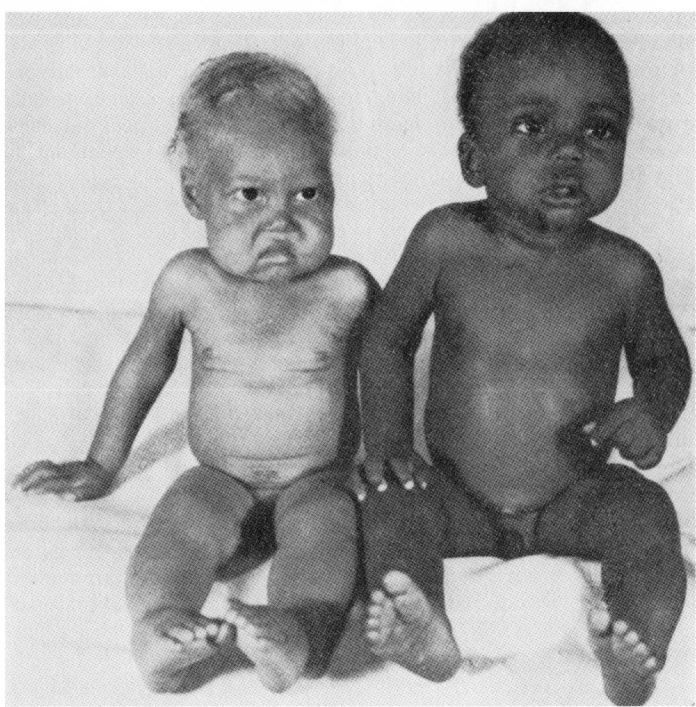

Figure 3-3. Jamaican infants of predominantly African stock. *Left,* Infant with "sugar-baby" kwashiorkor, showing stunting, edema of feet and hands, hepatomegaly with fatty infiltration, moon face, misery and extreme dyspigmentation of the hair (hypochromotrichia) and of the skin generally. *Right,* Normal infant of same racial group. (N.B. The hypochromotrichia here is one of the most extreme examples seen in Jamaica.) (From D. B. Jelliffe: Hypochromotrichia and Malnutrition in Jamaican Infants. *J. Trop. Pediat.,* Vol. 1.)

fore the onset of edema. Ascites and pleural effusions are unusual.

Dermatitis is common. Darkening of the skin appears in areas of irritation, but not in those exposed to sunlight, in contrast to the situation in pellagra. Dyspigmentation may occur in these areas after desquamation; vitiligo may occur elsewhere. The hair is often sparse and thin and loses its elasticity. In dark-haired children, dyspigmentation may result in a streaky red or gray color of the hair.

Infections and parasitic infestations are common, as are anorexia, vomiting and continued diarrhea. The muscles are weak, thin and atrophic, but there may be an excess of subcutaneous fat. Mental changes, especially irritability and apathy, are common.

Liver enlargement is common; biopsy usually reveals fatty infiltration. Necrosis or fibrosis may occur, but cirrhosis is rare. The heart may be small in the early stages of the disease, but is usually enlarged later.

Laboratory Data. The most significant index of protein malnutrition is the lowering of the serum albumin level. In early stages the albumin level may be only slightly reduced; severe lowering of the albumin concentration is one of the factors responsible for nutritional edema.

Ketonuria is common in the early stage of inanition, but frequently disappears in the later stages. Glucose tolerance curves may be diabetic in type. Urinary excretion of hydroxyproline relative to creatinine may be decreased. Levels of essential amino acids in plasma may be decreased relative to unessential amino acids, and there

may be increased aminoaciduria. An absolute and relative potassium deficiency is almost always present. The serum cholesterol level is low; it returns to normal after a few days of treatment. The serum values of amylase, esterase, cholinesterase, transaminase, lipase and alkaline phosphatase are decreased. There is diminished activity of the pancreatic enzymes and of xanthine oxidase. Enzyme values return to normal shortly after the onset of treatment. Anemia may be normocytic, microcytic or macrocytic. Other deficiencies, as of vitamins and minerals, are usually evident. In addition to general slowing of development, bone growth is usually delayed.

Differential diagnosis of protein deprivation includes chronic infections, diseases in which there is an excessive loss of protein through urine and stools, and conditions with a metabolic inability to make protein.

Prevention requires a diet containing an adequate quantity of protein of good biologic quality.

Treatment. Treatment of kwashiorkor requires immediate management of any acute problems presented by diarrhea or shock (see p. 217 for fluid and electrolyte therapy) and ultimately the replacement of missing nutrients. Shock should be treated as an emergency; renal function must be re-established. Gradual increases in the dietary intake of calories and protein should follow. Skim milk, casein hydrolysates or synthetic amino acid mixtures may be used. When high calorie and high protein diets are given too early and rapidly, the liver may become enlarged, and the child improves slowly. Protein hydrolysates, when used alone, may result in hypoglycemia.

Vitamins and minerals, especially potassium, are necessary from the outset of treatment.

Infections must be treated concomitantly with the dietary therapy, whereas treatment of parasitic infestation, if not severe, may be postponed until recovery is under way.

After treatment has been initiated the patient may lose weight for a few weeks, owing to loss of edema. Weight loss may occur even when edema was not previously obvious, and will reflect inapparent edema or unusual distribution of water within body fluid compartments. During recovery, serum and intestinal enzymes return to normal, and intestinal absorption of fat and protein improves.

If impairment of growth and development has been extensive, mental and physical retardation may be permanent. Apparently, the younger the infant at the time of deprivation, the more devastating are the long-term effects.

REFERENCES

Barness, L. A., and Gyorgy, P. G.: Research Advances in Infant Nutrition; in G. Bourne (Ed.): *World Review of Nutrition and Dietetics.* London, Pitman Medical Publishing Co., Ltd., 1962.

Cabak, V., and Najdanoic, R.: Effect of Undernutrition in Early Life on Physical and Mental Development. *Arch. Dis. Childhood,* 40:532, 1965.

Cravioto, J., DeLicardie, E. R., and Birch, H. G.: Nutrition, Growth and Neuro-integrative Development: An Experimental and Ecologic Study. *Pediatrics,* 38:319, 1966.

Garrow, J. S., Fletcher, K., and Halliday, D.: Body Composition in Severe Infantile Malnutrition. *J. Clin. Invest.,* 44:417, 1965.

Hansen, J. D. L.: Protein Malnutrition and Its Prevention and Treatment, with Special Reference to Kwashiorkor and Marasmus; in J. F. Brock: *Recent Advances in Infant Nutrition.* Boston, Little, Brown and Company, 1961, Chap. 23.

Naeye, R. L.: Malnutrition. *Arch. Path.,* 79:284, 1965.

Whitehead, R. G.: Hydroxyproline Creatinine Ratio as an Index of Nutritional Status and Rate of Growth. *Lancet,* 2:567, 1965.

VITAMIN A DEFICIENCY

Carotenes and their derivative, vitamin A, are required in the diets of infants and children. Carotenes of plant origin are readily converted into vitamin A by the liver, in which the vitamin is to a large extent stored, to be released as needed. In infants the vitamin A level of the blood plasma varies between 50 and 100 I.U.; in adults, between 100 and 300 I.U.* In disorders of the liver, in diabetes mellitus and in hypothyroidism the conversion of carotene may be disturbed, and it may appear in unusual amounts in the blood (carotenemia). In children with carotenemia the skin shows a yellow discoloration, but the color of the scleras remains unchanged.

Etiology. The liver at birth has a low vitamin A content which is rapidly augmented, since colostrum and the initial breast milk furnish large amounts of the vitamin. Breast milk and whole cow's milk are satisfactory sources of vitamin A. Other foods (vegetables, fruits, eggs, butter, liver) or vitamin supplements provide vitamin A as the infant's diet is expanded. The loss in cooking is small, and canning and freezing of foodstuffs do not appreciably affect their vitamin A content. Oxidizing agents, however, destroy this vitamin.

The danger of vitamin A deficiency is small in healthy children with varied diets. Deficient diets commonly cause disease by 2 to 3 years of age. Vitamin A deficiency also results from inadequate intestinal absorption or from metabolic disorders; these include chronic intestinal disorders, celiac disease, hepatic and pancreatic diseases, iron deficiency anemia, chronic infectious diseases or chronic ingestion of mineral oil. Low intake of dietary fat results in low vitamin A absorption.

Pathology. In the retina, vitamin A_1 aldehyde (retinal) or vitamin A_2 aldehyde (3-dehydroretinal) forms the prosthetic group of the visual pigments of rods and cones.

Other probable functions of vitamin A include maintenance of lysosomal stability, formation of mucopolysaccharides and synthesis of protein. Characteristic changes in epithelium occur in vitamin A deficiency, including proliferation of basal cells, hyperkeratosis and the formation of stratified, cornified squamous epithelium. Epithelial changes may also occur in the respiratory system, causing bronchiolar obstruction. Squamous metaplasia of the renal pelves, ureters, urinary bladder, enamel organs, and pancreatic and salivary ducts may occur.

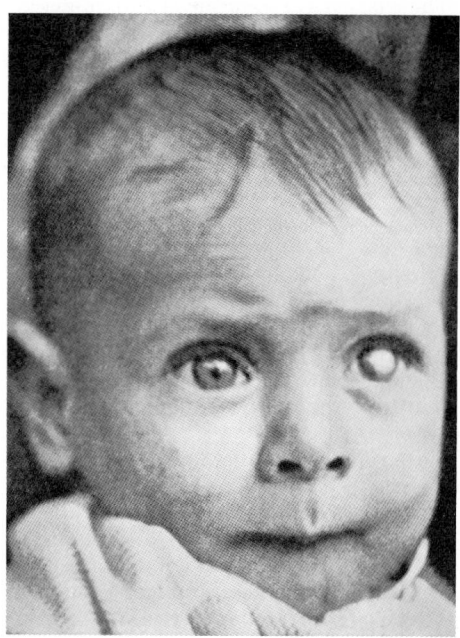

Figure 3-4. Recovery from xerophthalmia, showing permanent eye lesion. (Bloch: *Am. J. Dis. Child.,* Vol. 27.)

---

*One international unit (I.U.) of vitamin A is equivalent to 0.3 microgram of vitamin A alcohol.

In a group of children with protein malnutrition 80 per cent of those who died had evidence of severe deficiency; 15 per cent of the group who were equally malnourished did not have such evidence.

Clinical Manifestations. Ocular lesions develop insidiously. First the posterior segment of the eye is affected, with impairment of dark adaptation and night blindness. Later the anterior segment is affected, with drying of the conjunctiva (xerosis conjunctivae) and of the cornea (xerosis corneae), followed by wrinkling and cloudiness of the cornea (keratomalacia) (Fig. 3-4). Dry, silver-gray plaques may appear on the bulbar conjunctiva (Bitot's spots), with follicular hyperkeratosis and photophobia.

Symptoms of vitamin A deficiency include retardation of mental and physical growth, and apathy. Anemia with or without hepatosplenomegaly is usually present. Night blindness, loss of visual acuity in dim light, may be due to vitamin A deficiency.

The skin is dry and scaly, and at times follicular hyperkeratosis may be found on the shoulders, buttocks and the extensor surfaces of the extremities. The vaginal epithelium may become cornified, and epithelial metaplasia of the urinary tract may contribute to pyuria and hematuria. Hydrocephalus, with or without paralyses of the cranial nerves, is an infrequent manifestation.

Diagnosis. Dark adaptation tests, made carefully and under strictly standardized conditions, may be helpful, but the method is not adaptable to routine clinical practice. If xerosis conjunctivae precedes night blindness, it can be detected by biomicroscopic examination of the conjunctiva. Examination of the scrapings from the eye and vagina has also been recommended as a diagnostic aid. The plasma carotene level falls quickly, but the vitamin A concentration decreases more slowly. An absorption test for vitamin A is available (see p. 805). Low absorption curves are obtained in children with cystic fibrosis, celiac disease, obliteration of the bile ducts, and cretinism.

Prevention. Infants should receive at least 1500 I.U. daily, older children 2000 to 4500 I.U. of vitamin A or carotene, and adults, 5000 I.U. The average diets of infants and children in this country supply enough vitamin A to prevent symptoms of deficiency. If children receive, in addition, one of the vitamin A and D concentrates or a multiple vitamin preparation, most of which contain 3000 to 5000 I.U. of vitamin A per recommended dose, their requirements are more than adequately covered.

Children on a low fat diet for therapeutic reasons should receive supplementary vitamin A. In disorders which result in poor absorption of fat, water-miscible preparations of vitamin A should be administered in amounts equivalent to several times the usual daily requirement. Premature infants, who absorb fats and vitamin A less efficiently than do full-term infants, should also receive water-miscible preparations.

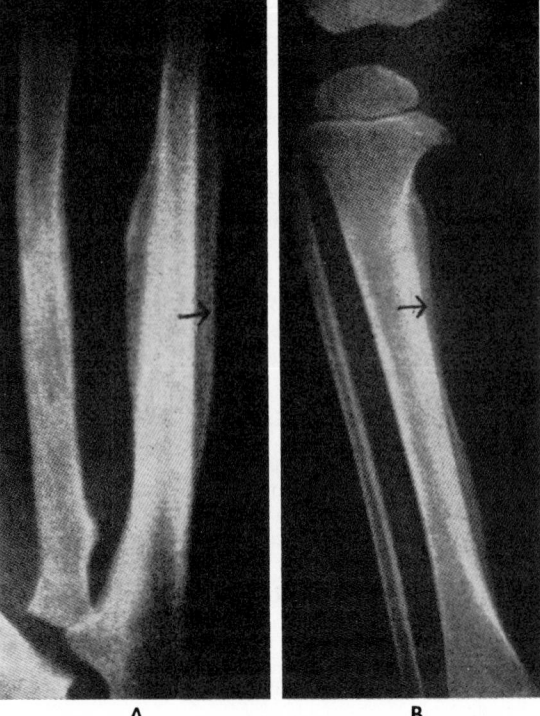

A   **B**

Figure 3-5. Hyperostosis of the ulna and the tibia in an infant 21 months of age, resulting from vitamin A poisoning. *A*, Long, wavy cortical hyperostosis of ulna. *B*, Long, wavy cortical hyperostosis of right tibia; striking absence of metaphyseal and epiphyseal changes. (J. Caffey: *Pediatrics*, Vol. 5. Published by Charles C Thomas, Springfield, Ill.)

Treatment. In cases of latent vitamin A deficiency a daily supplement of 5000 I.U. of vitamin A to the diet is all that is required. For xerophthalmia 5000 I.U. per kg. per day is given orally for 5 days, and then combined with intramuscular injection of 25,000 I.U. of vitamin A per kg. in oil daily until recovery occurs.

Hypervitaminosis. Acute hypervitaminosis A may occur in infants after the ingestion of 300,000 I.U. or more. The symptoms are nausea, vomiting, drowsiness, and bulging of the fontanel. Diplopia, papilledema and other symptoms suggesting brain tumor (pseudotumor cerebri) may also occur.

Chronic hypervitaminosis A appears after ingestion of excessive doses for several weeks or months. The initial manifestations are not specific. The child has anorexia, pruritus and a lack of gain in weight. There are increasing irritability, limitation of motion and tender swellings of the bones. Alopecia, seborrheic cutaneous lesions, fissuring of the corners of the mouth and hepatomegaly may develop. Craniotabes and desquamation of the palms and soles are common. Roentgenograms reveal hyperostosis affecting several long bones; it is most notable at the middle of the shafts. A history of excessive ingestion of vitamin A is helpful in the differentiation of cortical hyperostosis (Caffey's disease, p. 1359). The serum vitamin A level is elevated.

REFERENCES

Brown, P. K., and Wald, G.: Visual Pigments in Human and Monkey Retinas. *Nature*, 200:37, 1963.

Hillman, R. W.: Hypervitaminosis A; Experimental Induction in Human Subject. *Am. J. Clin. Nutr.*, 4:603, 1956.

McLaren, D. S.: Xerophthalmia: A Neglected Problem. *Nutr. Rev.*, 22:289, 1964.

Naiman, J. L., Oski, F. A., and Diamond, L. K.: The Gastrointestinal Effects of Iron-Deficiency Anemia. *Pediatrics*, 33:83, 1964.

Roels, O. A.: Present Knowledge of Vitamin A. *Nutr. Rev.*, 24:129, 1966.

Wolbach, S. B., and Bessey, O. A.: Tissue Changes in Vitamin Deficiencies. *Physiol. Rev.*, 22:233, 1942.

VITAMIN B COMPLEX DEFICIENCY

Vitamin B complex includes a number of factors which vary greatly in chemical composition and function. Several members of the B complex are important constituents of enzyme systems. Since many of these enzymes are closely related functionally, lack of one factor can interrupt an entire chain of normal chemical processes and produce diversified clinical manifestations.

Diets deficient in one factor of the B complex are frequently poor sources of other B vitamins. It is therefore not unusual to find manifestations of several B deficiencies in one patient, and a sharp separation of the symptoms caused by deficiencies of the single factors may be impossible. In the majority of instances it is advantageous to treat a patient with the entire B complex.

Factors such as pantothenic acid, choline, biotin and inositol are of importance for the normal functioning of the human organism, but at present no specific deficiency syndromes can be ascribed to lack of them in the diets of children.

THIAMINE DEFICIENCY

(BERIBERI)

Etiology. Vitamin B_1 (thiamine) is one of the water-soluble vitamins, and as thiamine pyrophosphate or cocarboxylase functions as a coenzyme in carbohydrate metabolism. A deficiency of this coenzyme results in accumulation of pyruvic acid in the tissues. Thiamine is also required for the synthesis of acetylcholine, and deficiency may result in impaired nerve function.

The foods usually given to infants—breast milk or cow's milk, vegetables, cereals, fruits, eggs—are fair sources of thiamine. Mothers with thiamine deficiency produce a milk deficient in thiamine, and infants fed their milk may acquire beriberi. Older children whose diet contains such good sources of thiamine as meats and legumes do not require supplements of this vitamin.

Thiamine is easily destroyed by heat in neutral or alkaline media and is readily extracted from foodstuffs by cooking water. The presence of a destructive enzymatic factor in certain types of fish explains why a diet low in thiamine induces beriberi rapidly when it is supplemented by such fish.

Pathology. In fatal cases of beriberi, lesions are located especially in the heart, peripheral nerves, subcutaneous tissue and serous cavities. The heart is dilated, particularly the right side; the interstitial tissue is edematous; and fatty degeneration of the myocardium is commonly present. Generalized edema or edema of the legs, serous effusions, and venous engorgement of the viscera may be present. The peripheral nerves undergo varying degrees of degeneration of myelin and of axon cylinders; these changes are more likely to be found in chronic deficiency states.

Clinical Manifestations. Infantile beriberi is rare in the United States. Congenital beriberi in infants of mothers with a severe deficiency has been observed, usually within the first 3 months of life. The vague initial symptoms are restlessness, anorexia, vomiting and constipation.

Physical findings distinguish two types. In *dry* beriberi the infant may appear plump, but is pale, flabby, listless and dyspneic; the heart rate is rapid and the liver enlarged. In *wet* beriberi the infants are undernourished, pale and edematous, and have dyspnea, vomiting and tachycardia. Knee and ankle jerks are absent in each type. There is no gain in weight except in infants who have edema, which is usually restricted to the distal parts of the extremities. The skin appears waxy. The urine may be scanty and contain albumin and casts.

The nervous symptoms are caused by changes in the central as well as in the peripheral nervous system. Apathy and drowsiness are common. There may be ptosis of the eyelids and atrophy of the optic nerve. Hoarseness due to paralysis of the laryngeal nerves is a characteristic sign. Paralytic symptoms are rare in infants.

The cardiac signs at first are slight cyanosis and dyspnea. Tachycardia, enlargement of the liver, loss of consciousness, and convulsions may develop rapidly. The heart is enlarged, especially to the right. The heart sounds are rapid, and the second pulmonic sound is accentuated. Gallop rhythm may be present. The roentgenogram shows cardiac dilatation, and the electrocardiogram indicates myocardial damage. Cardiac failure may lead to death in either chronic or acute beriberi. In the latter it may occur with dramatic suddenness in infants previously considered healthy.

Diagnosis. The early symptoms, such as restlessness, anorexia, gastrointestinal disturbances and pallor, are encountered in many types of nutritional disturbances which are not necessarily caused by thiamine deficiency. Since blood lactic and pyruvic acid levels rise in thiamine deficiency, these may be measured after oral administration of glucose or after exercise. The levels should return to normal after ingestion of thiamine. Demonstration of decreased red cell transketolase and increased blood or urinary glyoxylate has been proposed as a diagnostic test of thiamine deficiency. Excretion, after an oral loading dose, of thiamine or its metabolites, thiazole or pyrimidine, may help determine the deficiency state. Clinical response to administration of thiamine remains the best test for thiamine deficiency.

Prevention. Thiamine deficiency in breast-fed infants is prevented by a maternal diet which contains sufficient amounts of this vitamin. The recommended daily dietary allowances of thiamine are 1.8 mg. during pregnancy and 2.3 mg. during lactation. The recommended daily dietary allowance of thiamine is 0.4 mg. for infants and 0.6 to 1.2 mg. for older children. Thiamine requirements are increased with a high carbohydrate diet. Excessive cooking of vegetables or the refining of cereal grains destroys available thiamine.

Treatment. If beriberi occurs in a breast-fed infant, both mother and child should be treated with thiamine. The daily dose for adults is 50 mg., and for children 10 mg. or more. Oral administration is effective unless gastrointestinal disturbances prevent absorption. Thiamine should be given intramuscularly or intravenously to children with cardiac failure. Such treatment is followed by dramatic improvement within 2 hours. Complete cure requires several weeks; the beriberi heart is not permanently damaged. There is often deficiency of other B vitamins in patients with beriberi; for this reason all the vitamins of the B complex should be administered, in addition to large doses of thiamine chloride.

RIBOFLAVIN DEFICIENCY
(ARIBOFLAVINOSIS)

Riboflavin deficiency is rarely encountered without manifestations of other deficiencies of the B complex. Riboflavin is a water-soluble, yellow, fluorescent substance, stable to heat and acids, but destroyed by light and alkalis. The coenzymes flavin mononucleotide (FMN) and flavin adenine dinucleotide (FAD) are synthesized from riboflavin, and form the prosthetic groups of several enzymes important in electron transport. The vitamin occurs in large amounts in liver, kidney, brewer's yeast, milk, cheese, eggs and leafy vegetables. Cow's milk contains about 5 times as much riboflavin as human milk.

Riboflavin deficiency is usually due to inadequate intake, but faulty absorption may be a contributory factor.

Clinical Manifestations. Riboflavin deficiency may manifest itself by cheilosis, glossitis, keratitis and lesions of the skin. Cheilosis begins with pallor at the angles of the mouth, followed by thinning and maceration of the epithelium. Superficial fissures often covered by yellow crusts develop in the angles of the mouth and extend radially into the skin for distances of 1 to 2 cm. Cheilosis (*perlèche*) occurs in epidemics in institutions and in families where the diet is inadequate. In ariboflavinosis the tongue is smooth and shows loss of papillary structure.

Prevention. The daily amount of riboflavin recommended for infants is 0.6 mg.; for children and adults, 1 to 2 mg. Riboflavin deficiency is usually prevented by a diet which contains adequate amounts of milk, eggs, leafy vegetables and lean meats.

Treatment. Treatment consists in the oral administration of 3 to 10 mg. of riboflavin daily. If no response is obtained within a few days, intramuscular injections of 2 mg. of riboflavin in saline solution may be made 3 times daily. The child should also be given a well balanced diet and, temporarily at least, more than the usual requirements of the B complex.

NIACIN DEFICIENCY
(PELLAGRA)

Pellagra (*pellis*, skin; *agra*, rough) probably has existed under certain unfavorable conditions at all times in all parts of the world.

Etiology. Pellagra is a deficiency disease which affects all the tissues of the body. Although it is doubtful whether all its manifestations can be attributed to the deficiency of a single vitamin, the lack of niacin (nicotinic acid) is presumably responsible for most of them.

Niacin forms part of 2 enzymes important in electron transfer and glycolysis: diphosphopyridine nucleotide, or nicotinamide adenine dinucleotide (DPN, NAD), and triphosphopyridine nucleotide, or nicotinamide adenine dinucleotide phosphate (TPN, NADP). Although 60 mg. of tryptophan can be utilized in place of 1 mg. of niacin, exogenous sources of niacin are necessary. Liver, lean pork, salmon, poultry and red meat are good sources of niacin, but most cereals contain only small amounts of it. Pellagra occurs chiefly in countries where corn (maize), a poor source of tryptophan, is used as a basic foodstuff. Milk and eggs, which contain little niacin, are good pellagra-preventive foods, owing to their high content of tryptophan. Because niacin is a stable compound, there are only small losses in cooking if the cooking water is not excessive and not discarded.

The incidence of pellagra is increased in spring and early summer months. This disorder is frequent in women in the postpartum period, since pregnancy and lactation increase the niacin requirement. Pellagra usually does not occur in breast-fed infants.

Pathology. Histologically, there is edema and degeneration of the superficial collagen of the dermis. The papillary vessels are engorged, and there is perivascular lymphocytic infiltration in the dermis. The epidermis is hyperkeratotic and later becomes atrophic.

Changes comparable to those in the skin are present in the tongue, buccal mucous membranes and vagina. These changes may be associated with secondary infection and ulceration. Changes in the nervous system occur relatively late in the disease and consist of patchy areas of demyelinization and degeneration of ganglion cells; demyelinization in the spinal cord may involve the posterior and lateral columns.

Clinical Manifestations. The early symptoms of pellagra are vague. Anorexia, lassitude, weakness, burning sensations, numbness and dizziness may be prodromal symptoms. After a long period of niacin deficiency the characteristic symptoms of pellagra appear. The classic triad consists of diarrhea, dermatitis and dementia. Manifestations in children who have parasites or chronic disorders may be especially severe.

The most characteristic manifestations are the cutaneous ones, which may develop suddenly or insidiously and may be elicited by irritants, particularly by intensive sunlight. They first appear as a symmetrically developed erythema of the exposed surfaces. The erythema resembles sunburn and in mild cases, especially in young children, may easily escape recognition. The lesions are usually sharply demarcated from the healthy skin around them, and their distribution may change frequently. The lesions on the hands sometimes have the appearance of a glove (pellagrous glove) (Fig. 3-6), and similar demarcations are occasionally seen on the foot and leg (pellagrous boot) or around the neck (Casál's necklace). In some instances vesicles and bullae develop (wet type), or there may be suppuration beneath the scaly, crusted epidermis; in others the swelling disappears after a short time and desquamation begins. The healed parts of the skin may remain pigmented.

The cutaneous lesions are sometimes preceded by symptoms in the alimentary tract, such as stomatitis, glossitis, vomiting and diarrhea. Swelling and redness of the tip of the tongue and its lateral margins appear relatively early. Later there may be intense redness of the entire tongue with swelling of the papillae and even ulceration.

Nervous symptoms include depression, disorientation, insomnia and delirium.

The classic symptoms of pellagra are usually not well developed in infants and children. Anorexia, irritability, anxiety and apathy are observed frequently in young children of "pellagra families." They may also have sore tongues and lips, and the skin is usually dry and scaly. Diarrhea and constipation may alternate, and a moderate secondary anemia may occur. Children who have pellagra often have evidences of other nutritional deficiency diseases.

Prevention. The recommended daily allowance of niacin is 6 mg. for infants and 9 to 20 mg. for older children. A well balanced diet containing meat, vegetables, eggs and milk meets this requirement, so that supplements of niacin are necessary only in breast-fed infants whose mothers suffer from pellagra or in children on restricted diets.

Treatment. Children respond rapidly to antipellagral therapy. A liberal and well balanced diet should be supplemented with 50 to 300 mg. of niacin daily; a smaller amount may be given intravenously, or approximately 100 mg. by hypodermoclysis in severe cases or in those patients in whom intestinal absorption is poor. The administration of large doses of niacin is often followed within a half hour by a sensation of increased local heat and flushing and burning of the skin. These unpleasant effects are not produced by niacinamide.

Since vitamin deficiencies are rarely single, it is good practice to supplement the diet with other vitamins, especially with the other members of the B complex. Sunshine should be avoided during the active phase, and the skin lesions may be covered with soothing applications. A blood transfusion may be helpful in cases of severe anemia; the less severe hypochromic ones should be treated

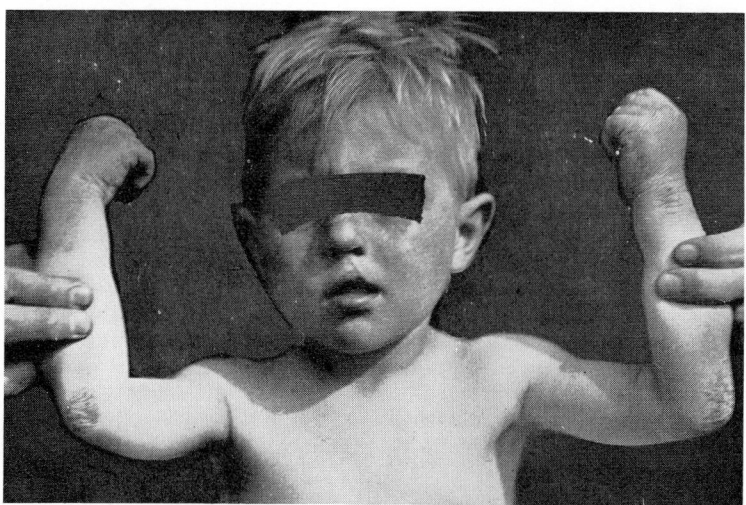

Figure 3-6. Pellagra in a boy 3 years of age, showing lesions on the hands and elbows and an early lesion over the nose and malar eminences.

with iron. The diet of the cured pellagrin should be continuously supervised to prevent recurrence.

REFERENCES

Thiamine Deficiency

Haridas, G.: Infantile Beriberi in Singapore During the Latter Part of the Japanese Occupation. *Arch. Dis. Childhood*, 22: 23, 1947.

Van Gelder, D. W., and Darby, F. N.: Congenital and Infantile Beriberi. *J. Pediat.*, 25:226, 1944.

Riboflavin Deficiency

Najjar, V. A., and Holt, L. E., Jr.: A Riboflavin Excretion Test as a Measure of Riboflavin Deficiency in Man. *Bull. Johns Hopkins Hosp.*, 69:476, 1941.

Sebrell, W. H., and Butler, R. E.: Riboflavin Deficiency in Man. *Pub. Health Rep.*, 53:2282, 1938.

Sydenstricker, V. P., Sebrell, W. H., Cleckley, H. M., and Kruse, H. D.: The Ocular Manifestations of Ariboflavinosis. *J.A.M.A.*, 114:2437, 1940.

Wolbach, S. B., and Bessey, O. A.: Tissue Changes in Vitamin Deficiencies. *Physiol. Rev.*, 22:233, 1942.

Niacin Deficiency

Goldsmith, G. A.: Niacin-Tryptophan Relationships in Man, and Niacin Requirements. *Am. J. Clin. Nutr.*, 6:479, 1958.

Smith, D. T.: Nicotinic Acid Deficiency (Pellagra). *M. Clin. N. Amer.*, 27:379, 1943.

Spies, T. D., Walker, A. A., and Wood, A. W.: Pellagra in Infancy and Childhood. *J.A.M.A.*, 113:1481, 1939.

PYRIDOXINE (VITAMIN B₆) DEFICIENCY

Vitamin B_6 includes pyridoxal, pyridoxine and pyridoxamine. These are converted to pyridoxal-5-phosphate, or pyridoxamine-5-phosphate, which acts as a coenzyme in decarboxylation and transamination of amino acids, e.g. in the decarboxylation of 5-hydroxytryptophan in the formation of serotonin, and in the metabolism of glycogen and fatty acids. Vitamin B_6 is also essential for the breakdown of kynurenine. When this does not occur, xanthurenic acid appears in the urine. Adequate functioning of the nervous system is dependent on pyridoxine; its deficiency results in seizures in man and in peripheral neuropathy. It participates in active transport of amino acids across cell membranes, chelates metals, and participates in the synthesis of arachidonic acid from linoleic acid. If it is lacking, glycine metabolism may lead to oxaluria. It is excreted largely as 4-pyridoxic acid.

Etiology. Though pyridoxine is adequately available in human and cow's milk as well as in cereals, prolonged processing of the latter two may alter its availability. Pyridoxine deficiency was first recognized in infants fed a proprietary formula which had been processed several times. Prolonged heating of milk may cause destruction of the vitamin. Diseases with malabsorption, such as celiac syndrome, may contribute to vitamin B_6 deficiency.

Infants born of women who have received large doses of pyridoxine for the relief of nausea and vomiting in early pregnancy may have an increased requirement of the vitamin. This has been termed *pyridoxine dependency.*

Pyridoxine antagonists, such as isonicotinic acid hydrazide (isoniazid), which is used in the treatment of tuberculosis, increase the requirement for pyridoxine; such deficiency symptoms are not as readily produced in children as in adults.

Cystathioninuria (p. 425) exemplifies the dependency upon vitamin B_6 of a single enzyme, cystathioninase.

Clinical Manifestations. Four clinical disturbances due to vitamin B_6 deficiency have been described in man: convulsions in infants, peripheral neuritis, dermatitis and anemia.

A small percentage of infants fed a formula deficient in vitamin B_6 for 1 to 6 months may exhibit irritability and generalized seizures. Gastrointestinal distress and an aggravated startle response are common.

Infants with so-called pyridoxine dependency have similar seizures, but the cause is believed to be an error in pyridoxine metabolism. The onset is at 1 to 5 days of age.

Peripheral neuropathy may occur during treatment of tuberculosis with isonicotinic acid hydrazide. The neuropathy responds to administration of pyridoxine or to a decrease in the dose of the drug. Administration of isonicotinic acid also may be followed by manifestations of pellagra.

Skin lesions include cheilosis, glossitis, and seborrhea around the eyes, nose and mouth. Microcytic anemia has been described, which fails to respond to therapy until vitamin B_6 is added. There may be a deficiency of pyridoxine and folic acid in refractory normoblastic anemia.

Laboratory Data. Anemia is not common in affected infants. After administration of 100 mg. per kg. of tryptophan, large amounts of xanthurenic acid will be found in the urine of patients with pyridoxine deficiency. In normal persons none is detected. This test result may be normal in patients with "pyridoxine dependency." Serum and red blood cell glutamic oxalacetic transaminase is decreased in experimental B_6 deficiency.

Diagnosis. Infants with seizures should be suspected of having vitamin B_6 deficiency or dependency. If commoner causes of infantile seizures such as hypocalcemia, hypoglycemia and infection can be eliminated as causative factors, 100 mg. of pyridoxine should be injected. If the seizure stops, B_6 deficiency should be suspected, and a tryptophan loading test is indicated.

Prevention. Balanced diets usually contain enough pyridoxine, so that deficiency is rare. Children receiving high protein diets should have vitamin B_6 added. Infants whose mothers have received large doses of pyridoxine during pregnancy should be watched for the development of seizures which may be due to pyridoxine dependency. Any child receiving a pyridoxine antagonist such as isoniazid should be carefully observed for neurologic manifestations. If these develop, either pyridoxine should be administered or the dose of the antagonist decreased. Daily intake of 0.1 to 0.5

mg. in the infant, 0.5 to 1.5 mg. in the child, and 1.5 to 2.0 mg. in the adult prevents deficiency states.

Treatment. For convulsions possibly due to pyridoxine deficiency 100 mg. of the vitamin should be given intramuscularly. One dose should suffice if the diet is adequate. For "pyridoxine-dependent" children 2 to 10 mg. intramuscularly or 10 to 100 mg. by mouth daily may be necessary.

REFERENCE

Scriver, C. R.: Vitamin B$_6$ Deficiency and Dependency in Man. *Am. J. Dis. Child.*, 113:109, 1967.

SCURVY

Scurvy is a manifestation of deficiency of vitamin C (ascorbic acid). Ascorbic acid is a dietary essential for primates and guinea pigs, but can be synthesized by most other species. It is a potent reducing agent, easily oxidized and destroyed by heating. No biologic oxidation system has yet been described in which ascorbic acid is the specific coenzyme.

Premature infants fed high protein diets which contain large amounts of tyrosine excrete p-hydroxyphenyllactic and p-hydroxyphenylpyruvic acids unless given increased quantities of ascorbate. The reduction of folic acid to its tetrahydro derivative apparently requires ascorbate (see p. 137).

Hydroxyproline, which is found only in collagen, is formed from proline in a reaction requiring ascorbic acid. Defects in collagen formation explain most of the effects noted in vitamin C deficiency.

Etiology. The infant is born with adequate stores of vitamin C if the mother's intake has been adequate. The vitamin C content of cord blood plasma is 2 to 4 times greater than that of maternal plasma. As a rule, breast milk contains about 4 to 7 mg. of ascorbic acid per 100 ml., thus forming an adequate source of vitamin C. A deficiency of vitamin C in the mother's diet may result in scurvy in her breast-fed infant. Infants fed artificially must receive vitamin C supplements; such supplements will provide additional protection for the breast-fed infant.

Scurvy may occur at any age, but is extremely rare in the newborn infant. The majority of cases are seen in the latter half of the first and in the second year of life. Apparently all febrile diseases, particularly infectious and diarrheal diseases, increase the need for vitamin C.

Pathology. Collagen formed during vitamin C deficiency is said to be low in hydroxyproline, and formation of collagen and chondroitin sulfate is impaired. The tendencies to hemorrhage, to defective tooth dentin and to loosening of the teeth are due to deficient collagen. Since osteoblasts no longer form their normal intercellular substance, osteoid, endochondral bone formation ceases. The bony trabeculae which have been formed continue to be calcified, but become brittle and fracture easily. The periosteum becomes loosened, and subperiosteal hemorrhages occur, especially at the ends of the femur and tibia.

Clinical Manifestations. Scurvy requires time for its development; after a variable period of vitamin C depletion vague symptoms of irritability, digestive disturbances and loss of appetite appear. The irritability becomes progressively greater, and there is evidence of general tenderness especially noticeable in the legs when the infant is picked up or when the diaper is changed. The pain causes pseudoparalysis, and the legs assume the typical "frog position" (Fig. 3-7), which consists in semiflexion of the hips and knees with the feet rotated outward. Edematous swelling along the shafts of the legs may be present, and in some cases a subperiosteal hemorrhage can be palpated at the end of the femur. The facial expression is apprehensive. Changes of the gums, most noticeable when the teeth are erupted, are characterized by bluish-purple, spongy swellings of the mucous membrane, usually over the upper incisors. The swollen gums sometimes completely conceal the teeth. There may be a "rosary" at the costochondral junctions and a depression of the sternum. The angulation of the "scorbutic beads" is usually sharper than that in the rachitic rosary, since it is produced by a subluxation of the sternal plate at the costochondral junction (Fig. 3-7)

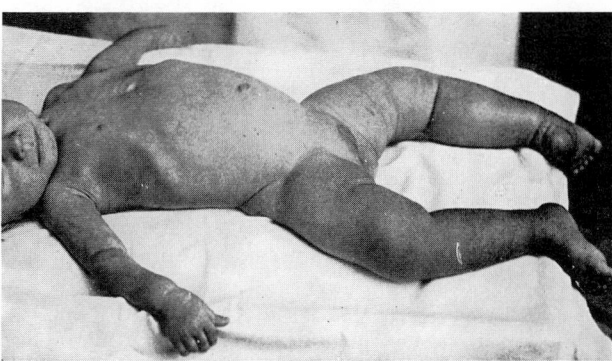

Figure 3-7. Scorbutic rosary, depression of sternum and the so-called frog position.

rather than by widening of the softened epiphyses as occurs in rickets (p. 180).

Petechial hemorrhages may occur in the skin and mucous membranes. Hematuria, melena, or orbital or subdural hemorrhages may be found. Low-grade fever is usually present. Anemia may reflect inability to utilize iron or impaired folic acid metabolism (p. 1046). Wound healing is delayed, and healed wounds may break down.

Roentgenographic Manifestations. The diagnosis of scurvy is usually based on roentgenographic changes in the long bones, especially of their distal ends. Changes are greatest, as a rule, in the area of the knee. In the early stages the appearance resembles that of simple atrophy of the bone. In the shaft the trabeculae cannot be

discerned, and the bone assumes a "ground-glass" appearance. The cortex is reduced to "pencil-point thinness," and the epiphyseal ends are sharply outlined. The white line of Fraenkel, which represents the zone of well calcified cartilage, can be clearly discerned as an irregular but thickened white line at the metaphysis. The epiphyseal centers of ossification also have a ground-glass appearance and are surrounded by a white ring corresponding to the white line of the shaft (Fig. 3-8). At this stage scurvy cannot be diagnosed with certainty from the roentgenogram; if, however, under the white line at the metaphysis the zone of rarefaction becomes apparent, the roentgenogram is diagnostic. The zone of rarefaction is a linear break in the bone proximal and parallel to the

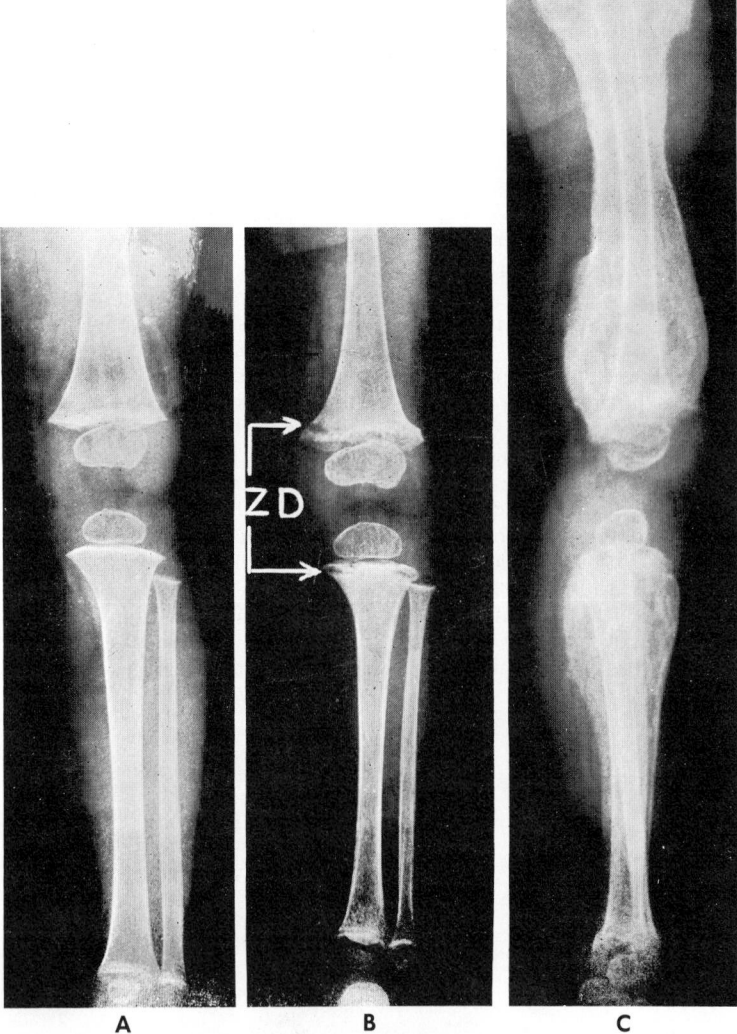

A   B   C

Figure 3-8. Roentgenograms of leg. *A*, Early scurvy: "white line" is visible on the ends of the shafts of the tibia and fibula; rings around epiphyses of femur and tibia. *B*, More advanced scorbutic changes; zones of destruction (*ZD*) in femur and tibia. *C*, Healing scurvy; calcification of subperiosteal hemorrhages.

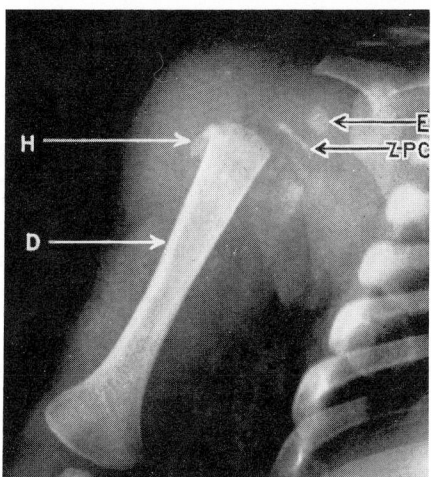

Figure 3-9. "Slipped diaphysis" in scurvy. The epiphysis (*E*) of the humerus and calcified cartilage of the zone of primary calcification (*ZPC*) remained in place and in contact with the glenoid fossa. The diaphysis (*D*) was displaced laterally and separated from the epiphysis. The shadow (*H*) at the proximal end of the diaphysis represents beginning calcification of a subperiosteal hemorrhage.

white line. It often does not traverse the shaft in its entire width and may be seen only in its lateral parts as a triangular defect (Fig. 3-8, *B*). A spur, as lateral prolongation of the white line, may be present. Epiphyseal separation may occur along the line of destruction with linear displacement (Fig. 3-9) or compression of the epiphysis against the shaft. Subperiosteal hemorrhages are not visible roentgenographically in active scurvy. During healing, however, the elevated periosteum becomes calcified and presents a striking picture. The affected bone assumes a dumbbell or club shape, since the hemorrhage occurs at the ends of the bone and elevates the periosteum more at this site than in the middle of the shaft (Fig. 3-8, *C*). As healing progresses, the shadow of the hemorrhage becomes more intense, but diminishes in width; the rings around the epiphyseal centers of ossification become more distinct, and the zone of destruction disappears and is replaced by calcified tissue.

Diagnosis. Diagnosis is based mainly on the characteristic clinical picture, the roentgenographic appearance of the long bones and history of poor intake of vitamin C. Occasionally a mother will have been boiling fruit juices.

Laboratory tests for scurvy are unsatisfactory. A fasting vitamin C level of the blood plasma of over 0.6 mg. per 100 ml. aids in the exclusion of scurvy, but a lower vitamin C level does not prove its presence. A better index of vitamin C deficiency is furnished by the ascorbic acid concentration of the white cell-platelet layer (buffy layer) of centrifuged oxalated blood. A level of zero in this layer indicates latent scurvy, even in the absence of clinical signs of deficiency. The saturation of the tissues with vitamin C can be estimated from the amount of urinary excretion of the vitamin after a test dose of ascorbic acid. During the 3 to 5 hours after the parenteral administration of the test dose 80 per cent of the total 24-hour excretion can be found in the urine. Children with vitamin C deficiency excrete less ascorbic acid under these conditions than normal children with well saturated tissues. A generalized, nonspecific aminoaciduria occurs in children with scurvy, while blood values of amino acids remain normal. After a tyrosine load the scorbutic infant excretes metabolites similar to those of the premature one. These may be detected with Millon's reagent. Tests for capillary fragility, almost always with positive results in scurvy, may give negative results in latent scurvy.

Differential Diagnosis. The tenderness of the limbs and the pain elicited by movement have often led to a false diagnosis of arthritis or acrodynia. The patient's age aids in differentiating scurvy from rheumatic fever, since rheumatic fever is rare in children under 2 years of age. Suppurative arthritis and osteomyelitis occur in young children and infants and should be considered in the differential diagnosis. The pseudoparalysis of syphilis usually occurs at an earlier age than does that of scurvy, and is often accompanied by other signs of syphilis. A roentgenogram aids in the diagnosis. Poliomyelitis causes a true flaccid paralysis, and in infants the exquisite tenderness present in the limbs in scurvy is absent. Henoch-Schönlein purpura, thrombocytopenic purpura, leukemia, meningococcemia or nephritis may be suspected.

Prognosis. Recovery occurs rapidly in cases correctly treated. Pain ceases in a few days, but the swelling caused by subperiosteal hemorrhage may require months to disappear. Body growth is usually quickly resumed. In unrecognized and untreated cases death is likely to occur after a few months from malnutrition, exhaustion, some complication or intercurrent disease. Permanent deformity from scorbutic lesions is uncommon; even when there has been metaphyseal separation, reconstruction is usually good without orthopedic treatment.

Prevention. Scurvy may be prevented by a diet adequate in vitamin C. All infants, even breast-fed ones, should receive ascorbic acid (25 to 50 mg.), orange juice (1 to 2 ounces) or fresh or canned tomato juice (2 to 3 ounces) daily, beginning at 2 to 4 weeks of age. Lactating mothers should take generous amounts of vitamin C; a minimum daily intake equal to 150 mg. of ascorbic acid has been recommended. A daily intake of 25 to 50 mg. of ascorbic acid for infants, 50 mg. for children, and 75 mg. for adults is considered adequate.

Treatment. The administration of 3 to 4 ounces of orange juice or tomato juice daily will quickly produce healing, but ascorbic acid is preferable. The daily therapeutic dose is 100 to 200 mg. or more, orally or parenterally.

REFERENCES

Grevar, D.: Scurvy and Its Prevention by Vitamin C-Fortified Evaporated Milk. *Canad. M.A.J.*, 80:977, 1959.

Hess, A. F.: *Scurvy, Past and Present.* Philadelphia, J. B. Lippincott Company, 1920.

Jonxis, J. H. P., and Huisman, T. H. J.: Aminoaciduria and Ascorbic Acid Deficiency. *Pediatrics*, 14:238, 1954.

Meiklejohn, A. P.: The Physiology and Biochemistry of Ascorbic Acid. *Vitamins and Hormones.* New York, Academic Press, Inc., 1953, Vol. XI.

Park, E. A., Guild, H. G., Jackson, D., and Bond, M.: Recognition of Scurvy, with Especial Reference to the Early X-Ray Changes. *Arch. Dis. Childhood*, 10:265, 1935.

Wolbach, S. B., and Bessey, O. A.: Tissue Changes in Vitamin Deficiencies. *Physiol. Rev.*, 22:233, 1942.

RICKETS OF VITAMIN D DEFICIENCY*

Rickets is a metabolic disorder of bone resulting in bony deformities. In contrast to scurvy, in which the connective tissue is defective, but calcification proceeds, rickets is characterized by formation of normal collagen and matrix and of osteoid with defective mineralization. When ossification improves with administration of vitamin D, the rickets is termed vitamin D-deficient; if no improvement occurs after conventional administration of usual doses of vitamin D, the condition is called vitamin D-resistant or refractory rickets.

Etiology. Appropriate concentrations of calcium and phosphorus in serum and osteoid are essential for mineralization of bone. Vitamin D participates in the regulation of these minerals within the body.

Secretions of the human skin contain 7-dehydrocholesterol, provitamin D_3. Under natural living conditions this provitamin is activated by ultraviolet rays of sunlight (296 to 310 microns) and converted into vitamin D, which is absorbed into the blood and distributed throughout the body.

Sunlight which has passed through ordinary window glass is deprived of its antirachitic potency. As a rule, infants in the temperate and arctic zones escape rickets only when they receive a protective amount of vitamin D in their diet.

The natural diet of infants contains only small amounts of vitamin D; breast milk is a poor source, and cow's milk contains only 5 to 40 I.U. per quart. Sugar, cereals, vegetables and fruits contain only negligible amounts. Egg yolk contains 140 to 390 I.U. per 100 gm.

Many sterol derivatives have antirachitic value, but only two of them, 7-dehydrocholesterol and ergosterol, are of practical importance. The biologic properties of activated 7-dehydrocholesterol resemble those exhibited by vitamin D

preparations of animal origin. Ergosterol is of plant origin and is the sterol found in fungi. Irradiation transforms ergosterol into vitamin D_2 (calciferol), with certain by-products such as tachysterol and lumisterol. There is no vitamin D_1.

Besides lack of vitamin D in the diet or lack of access of skin to ultraviolet irradiation, several factors may predispose to vitamin D deficiency. Rickets or epiphyseal dysplasia may develop during rapid growth, as occurs in premature infants and adolescents.

Negro children are singularly susceptible to rickets. Whether this is due to the pigmentation of their skin or to their living conditions has not been determined. Genetic factors are responsible for vitamin D-refractory rickets (p. 1364), but there is no evidence that they have any role in vitamin D-deficient rickets.

Children with disorders of absorption, such as celiac disease, steatorrhea or cystic fibrosis, may acquire rickets because of failure to absorb vitamin D or calcium, or both. In children with hepatic disease, rickets may develop because of an inability to absorb vitamin D or calcium or because of a specific metabolic defect.

Pathology. Defective growth of bone in rickets results from retardation or suppression of normal growth of epiphyseal cartilage and of normal calcification. These changes are dependent upon a decrease in the calcium and phosphorus salts available in the serum for mineralization. The failure of cartilage cells to complete their normal cycle of proliferation and degeneration and the subsequent failure of capillary penetration occur in a patchy manner. The result is a frayed, irregular epiphyseal line at the end of the shaft.

There is also failure of normal mineralization of osseous and cartilaginous matrix. The zone of preparatory calcification fails to mineralize, and newly formed uncalcified osteoid is deposited. As a result a wide, irregular, frayed zone of nonrigid tissue (the rachitic metaphysis) is produced, composed of noncalcified cartilage and osteoid tissue. This zone is responsible for many of the skeletal deformities. It becomes compressed and bulges laterally, producing flaring of the ends of the bones and the rachitic rosary.

Changes also occur in bone at sites other than the epiphyseal-metaphyseal region. Mineralization is lacking in subperiosteal bone, and a shell of osteoid tissue is formed which surrounds the shaft over its entire length. Pre-existing cortical bone is resorbed in a normal manner, but is replaced by osteoid tissue which fails to mineralize. If this process continues, the shaft loses its rigidity, resulting in softened, rarefied, cortical bone which is readily distorted by stress, and deformities and fractures result.

Healing rickets. With healing, degeneration of cartilage cells occurs along the diaphyseal border of the cartilage, capillary penetration of the resultant spaces is resumed, and calcification takes place in the zone of preparatory calcification.

*Vitamin D-refractory rickets and metabolic bone disorders simulating rickets are described on page 1363.

This calcification occurs approximately at the line at which normal calcification would have occurred had the rachitic process not supervened, and produces a line clearly demonstrable in roentgen films. As healing progresses, the osteoid tissue between this line of preparatory calcification and the diaphysis also becomes mineralized (Fig. 3-10). Osteoid tissue in the cortex and about the trabeculae in the shaft rapidly becomes mineralized. Months or years may be required to repair the deformities, and in extreme instances complete repair may be impossible.

Chemical pathology. In healthy infants the inorganic serum phosphorus concentration is 4.5 to 6.5 mg. per 100 ml., whereas in rachitic infants it is usually reduced to 1.5 to 3.5 mg. The serum calcium level is usually normal, but under certain conditions it too is reduced, and tetany may develop.

The phosphatase level of the serum, which in normal children ranges between 5 and 15 Bodansky units per 100 ml., is elevated in mild rickets to 20 to 30 units per 100 ml. and to 60 units or more in severe cases. As rickets heals, the phosphatase level returns slowly to normal levels.

Though several factors have been isolated which affect serum concentrations of calcium and phosphorus, as well as mineralization, no unified schema explains all the aspects of calcium transport.

Calcium and phosphorus homeostasis depends on dietary calcium and phosphorus. Maximum calcium absorption occurs in man when the relation of calcium to phosphorus in the diet is about 2:1; increase in phosphate decreases absorption of calcium. Acidity of intestinal contents increases absorption of calcium. An increase in calcium absorption occurs with lactose as the dietary sugar. Chelating agents such as ethylene diamine tetraacetic acid (EDTA) or the phytates of cereals may also decrease calcium absorption. Dietary iron may decrease absorption of phosphate.

Parathyroid hormone (p. 1200) decreases renal tubular reabsorption of phosphate; hyperphosphaturia is accompanied by elevation of serum calcium levels through mobilization of calcium and phosphorus from bone. The hormone may increase calcium absorption from the intestine, and probably influences transport of calcium and phosphorus.

Normal serum calcium levels vary from 9 to 11 mg. per 100 ml., but only 5 to 6 mg. is ionic; the remainder is nondiffusible and bound to protein. Both neuromuscular irritability and bone metabolism are related more closely to ionic than to total calcium. Acidosis increases ionic calcium. Decreased levels of serum proteins are accompanied by low levels of serum calcium, but ionic calcium may be normal. Normally, levels of serum calcium and phosphorus have an inverse relation. In hyperparathyroidism, however, both may be elevated, and in rickets, depressed. Calcitonin, citrate and tartrate decrease serum calcium, probably through its deposition in bone. Heparin chelates serum calcium, and its administration may be followed by osteoporosis. Immobilization of the child is followed by mobilization of calcium from the bone and by osteoporosis and hypercalcemia. Osteoporosis may also follow the administration of adrenal cortical steroids; the mechanism is unclear. Magnesium may replace calcium in some biochemical reactions and compete with it in others.

Vitamin D has 3 probable sites of action in the regulation of calcium and phosphorus metabolism: it increases renal tubular reabsorption of phosphate; it increases intestinal absorption of both calcium and phosphorus; and it has a direct effect on deposition in bone.

Vitamin D deficiency is also accompanied by generalized aminoaciduria, a decrease of citrate in bone and increased urinary excretion of it, decreased ability of the kidneys to make an acid urine, phosphaturia and occasionally mellituria. The parathyroid glands hypertrophy in rickets. Hemolytic anemia has been associated.

Clinical Manifestations. After several months of vitamin D deficiency osseous changes of rickets can be recognized. Breast-fed infants whose mothers have osteomalacia may have rickets develop within 2 months. Florid rickets becomes apparent toward the end of the first and during

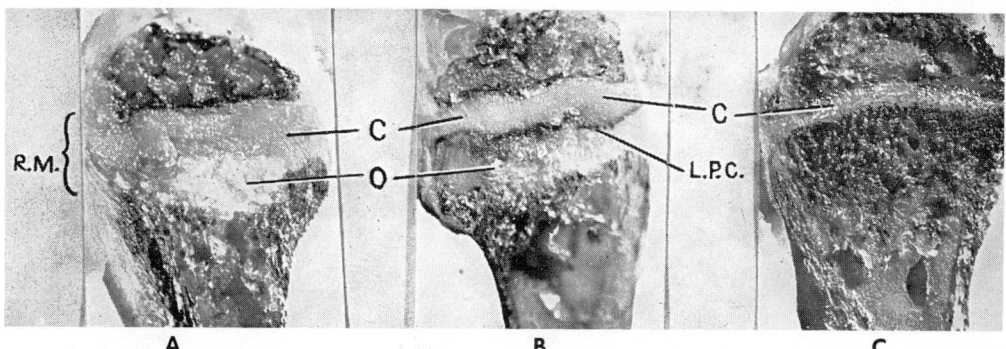

A   **B**   **C**

Figure 3-10. Line tests in rats (proximal end of tibia) (calcified tissue stained with silver appears black.) *A,* Active rickets. The light broad zone between epiphysis and shaft represents the rachitic metaphysis (*R.M.*); *C,* cartilage; *O,* osteoid. *B,* Healing rickets. Line of preparatory calcification (*L.P.C.*) between zone of cartilage (*C*) and osteoid (*O*). *C,* Healed rickets. Cartilaginous disk (*C*) between epiphysis and normal shaft.

the second year of life. In later childhood clinical rickets is rare. In adults, vitamin D deficiency produces osteomalacia.

One of the early signs of rickets is craniotabes. Craniotabes is due to thinning of the inner table of the skull and is detected by pressing firmly over the occiput or posterior parietal bones. A ping-pong ball sensation will be felt. Craniotabes near the suture lines is a normal variant. Premature infants are particularly prone to rickets and to craniotabes. Palpable enlargement of the costochondral junctions (the "rachitic rosary") and thickening of the wrists and ankles are other early evidences of osseous changes.

Advanced rickets. Signs of advanced rickets are easily recognized.

HEAD. Craniotabes may disappear before the end of the first year, though the rachitic process continues. The softness of the skull may result in flattening and, at times, permanent asymmetry of the head. The anterior fontanel is larger than normal; its closure may be delayed until after the second year of life. The central parts of the parietal and frontal bones are often thickened, forming prominences or bosses, which give the head a boxlike appearance (*caput quadratum*). The head may be larger than normal and may remain so throughout life. Eruption of the temporary teeth is sometimes delayed and out of the normal order. There may be defects of the enamel and extensive caries. The permanent teeth which are calcifying may be affected; usually the permanent incisors, canines and first molars show defects of the enamel, especially on the distal portion.

THORAX. In advanced rickets the enlargement of the costochondral junctions may become prominent; in many cases the beading of the ribs is not only palpable, but also visible (Fig. 3-11). The sides of the thorax become flattened, and longitudinal grooves develop posterior to the rosary. The sternum with its adjacent cartilages appears to be projected forward, producing the so-called pigeon breast deformity. Along the lower border of the chest there develops a horizontal depression, Harrison's groove (Fig. 3-12), which corresponds to the costal insertions of the diaphragm. The chest may show a variety of other deformities, and

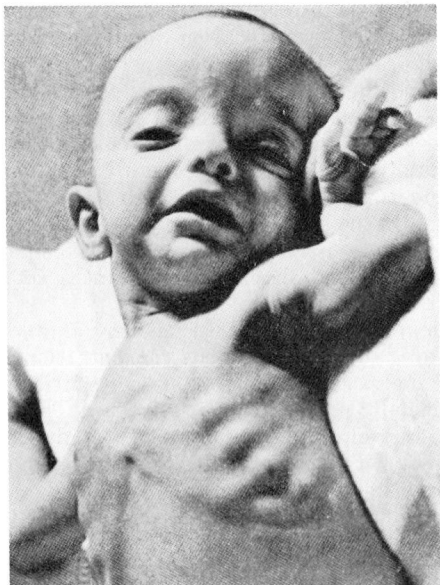

Figure 3-11. Rachitic rosary in a young infant. (Lyons and Wallinger: *Pediatrics and Pediatric Nursing.*)

the bones of the shoulder girdle may also be involved.

SPINAL COLUMN. Slight to moderate degrees of lateral curvature (scoliosis) are common, and a kyphosis may appear in the dorsolumbar region in rachitic children who sit up (Fig. 3-13). Lordosis of the lumbar region may be seen in the erect position.

PELVIS. In children with lordosis there is frequently a concomitant deformity of the pelvis. The pelvis in rickets is small and continues to be retarded in growth. The pelvic entrance is narrowed by a forward projection of the promontory, and the exit by a forward displacement of the caudal part of the sacrum and the coccyx. In the female these changes, if they become permanent, add to the hazards of childbirth and may necessitate cesarean section.

EXTREMITIES. As the rachitic process continues, the epiphyseal enlargements at the wrists and ankles become more noticeable. The enlarged

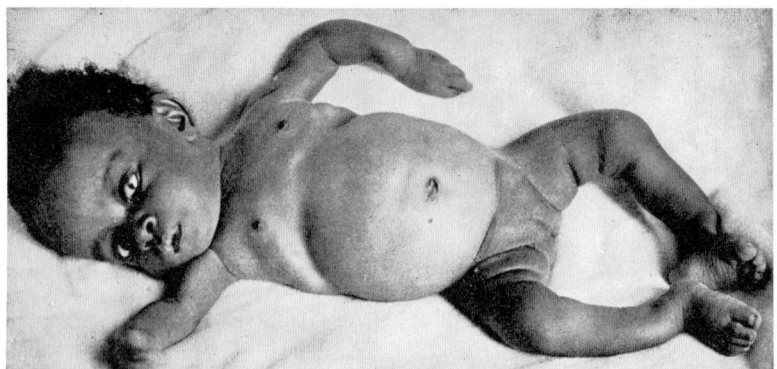

Figure 3-12. Deformities in rickets, showing curvature of the limbs, potbelly and Harrison's groove.

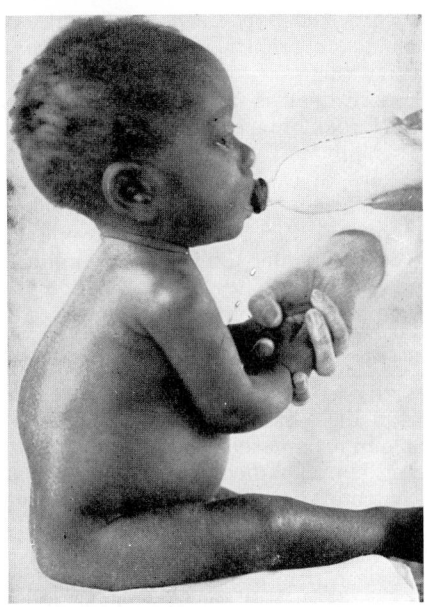

Figure 3-13. Rachitic spinal curvature, well marked when the child is sitting.

epiphyses can be seen (Fig. 3-14) or palpated, but are not distinct in roentgenograms, since they consist of cartilage and uncalcified osteoid tissue. Bending of the softened shafts of the femur, tibia and fibula results in bowlegs or knock knees; the femur and the tibia may also show an anterior convexity. Coxa vara is sometimes the result of rickets. Green-stick fractures occur in the long bones, but seldom cause clinical symptoms.

Deformities of the spine, pelvis and the legs result in reduction in height of the body, *rachitic dwarfism.*

LIGAMENTS. Relaxation of ligaments aids in producing deformities. It partly accounts for the production of knock knees, overextension of the knee joints, weak ankles, kyphosis and scoliosis.

MUSCLES. The muscles are poorly developed and lacking in tone. As a result, children with moderately severe rickets are late in standing and walking. The common condition of potbelly (Figs. 3-12, 3-14) depends to a large extent upon weakness of the abdominal muscles; weakness of the gastric and intestinal walls aids in its production.

Diagnosis. The diagnosis of rickets is based on a history of inadequate intake of vitamin D and on clinical observation, and is confirmed by serum chemical determinations and roentgenographic examination. The serum calcium level may be normal or low, the serum phosphorus level is below 4 mg. per 100 ml., and the serum alkaline phosphatase is usually elevated.

Roentgenographic changes. ACTIVE RICKETS. A roentgenogram of the wrist is best for early diagnosis, since characteristic changes of the ulna and the radius occur at an early stage. The distal ends of the radius and the ulna appear widened, concave (cupping) and frayed, in contrast to the normally sharply demarcated and slightly convex

ends. The distance between the distal ends of the ulna and the radius and the metacarpal bones is increased, since the large rachitic metaphysis, which is not calcified, does not appear on the roentgenogram. The density of the shafts is decreased, but the trabeculae are unusually prominent. In Figure 3-15, *A*, 2 dense areas are seen in the ulna that represent callus formation at sites of healing fractures. The outer contour of the radius appears double and could be mistaken for "periostitis." The double contour represents, however, the layer of osteoid tissue formed by the periosteum, and not an inflammatory process.

HEALING RICKETS. Beginning healing is indicated by the appearance of the line of preparatory calcification (Fig. 3-15, *B*). This line is separated from the distal end of the shaft by a zone of decreased calcification, the zone of the osteoid tissue. As healing progresses and the osteoid tissue becomes calcified, the shaft "grows" toward the line of preparatory calcification (Fig. 3-15, *C*) until it becomes united with it (Fig. 3-15, *D*).

Differential Diagnosis. Nonrachitic craniotabes is sometimes present in the immediate postnatal period, but it tends to disappear before rachitic softening of the skull would become manifest (second to fourth months of life). Craniotabes also occurs in hydrocephalus and osteogenesis imperfecta, but it is not difficult to differentiate these conditions from rickets.

Enlargement of the costochondral junctions occurs in rickets, scurvy and chondrodystrophy. The enlargements in rickets are rounded knobs, whereas in scurvy there is a ledgelike depression with the chondral or sternal portion lower than the osseous. In chondrodystrophy there may be irregular concave outlines of the distal ends of the

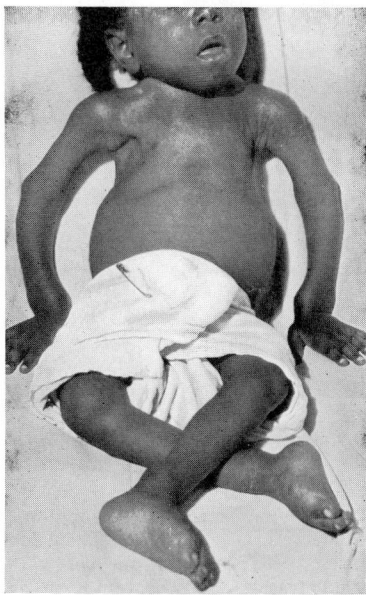

Figure 3-14. Curvature of arms, deformed "violin-shaped" chest, potbelly, enlarged epiphyses in a child 3 years of age.

bones, but there is no roentgenographic evidence of fraying. It is sometimes difficult to distinguish rachitic deformities of the chest from congenital deformities. Bowlegs can be the result of rickets, but may be due to osteogenesis imperfecta, or they may be a familial characteristic. Vitamin D-resistant rickets and other metabolic disturbances with osseous lesions resembling rickets must be differentiated (see p. 1363).

Complications. Respiratory infections such as bronchitis and bronchopneumonia are common in rachitic infants. Pulmonary atelectasis is not infrequently associated with severe deformities of the chest.

Chronic gastroenteric disturbances are common; there may be diarrhea or constipation, or the two may alternate.

Anemia due to iron deficiency or accompanying infections often develops in severe rickets.

Prognosis. Though "spontaneous" healing of mild rickets often occurs from exposure to sunshine, severe cases require more energetic treatment. If sufficient amounts of vitamin D are administered, healing begins within a few days and progresses until the normal bony structure is restored. Recovery, however, from the bony deformities is slow; in many instances the enlargement of the epiphyses and of the rosary and the deformities of the skull disappear only after months or years of treatment. Even rather severe bowing of the legs may correct itself after several years of vitamin treatment, without osteotomies. In advanced cases there may be permanent osseous alterations in the form of bowlegs, knock knees,

curvature of the upper arms, deformities of the chest and spine, rachitic pelvis, rachitic coxa vara, and even dwarfism.

Rickets in itself is not a fatal disease, but complications and intercurrent infections such as tetany, pneumonia, tuberculosis and enteritis are more likely to cause death in rachitic than in normal children.

Prevention. Rickets can be prevented by exposure to ultraviolet light or by oral administration of vitamin D. Sunlight, as a prophylactic agent, can be considered effective in the temperate zones only during the summer months in haze-free areas.

The daily requirement of vitamin D is estimated to be 400 I.U. per day. Much of the whole milk available in urban areas and most, if not all, evaporated milk are fortified by the addition of vitamin D concentrate, so that 1 quart of fresh, whole milk or a can of evaporated milk contains 400 I.U. of vitamin D. It would seem reasonable not to rely upon vitamin D milk alone, but to provide added protection by the administration of 400 I.U. of vitamin D in a concentrate. Vitamin D should be given to breast-fed as well as bottle-fed infants, and full-term as well as premature infants, beginning about 5 to 10 days of age.

Vitamin D should be administered to the pregnant or lactating mother.

Treatment. Natural and artificial light is effective therapeutically, but oral administration of vitamin D is preferred. The daily administration of 1500 to 5000 I.U. (6 to 20 drops of a preparation containing 10,000 units per gm.) will produce

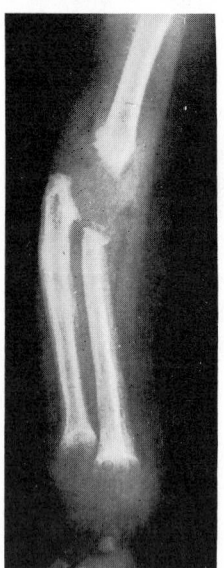 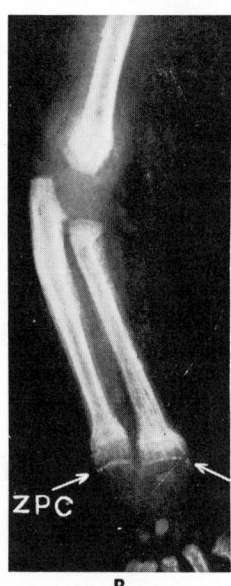 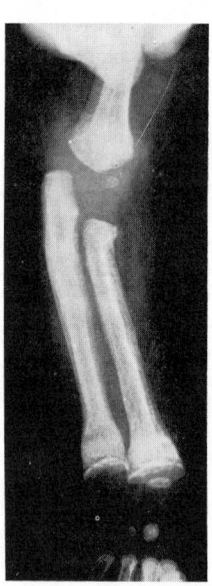 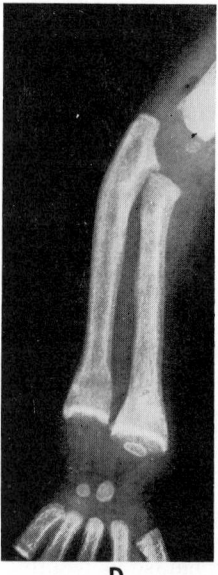

A   B   C   D

Figure 3-15. *A*, Active rickets; cupping and fraying of distal ends of radius and ulna; double contour along lateral outline of radius (periosteal osteoid). The 2 dense zones in the shaft of the ulna are calluses of greenstick fractures. *B*, Healing rickets after 12 days of treatment with vitamin D. Zones of preparatory calcification (*ZPC*); above them in the rachitic metaphyses there is beginning calcification. *C*, Healing rickets after 18 days of treatment. The zones of preparatory calcification are well defined, and the rachitic metaphyses appear well calcified. The epiphysis of the radius has become visible. *D*, Healing rickets after 29 days of treatment. Zones of preparatory calcification, rachitic metaphyses and shafts have become united.

healing demonstrable on roentgenograms within 2 to 4 weeks except in the unusual cases of vitamin D-refractory rickets.

The feeding of 600,000 units of vitamin D in a single dose, and no further vitamin for several months, may be advantageous. This is followed by more rapid healing, possibly prompt differential diagnosis from resistant rickets, and less dependence on the parents. If no healing occurs within 2 weeks, the dose may be repeated once. If still no healing occurs, the rickets is resistant to vitamin D. After healing is complete the dose of vitamin D should be lowered to 400 units daily.

REFERENCES

Follis, R. H., Jr.: *Deficiency Disease*. Springfield, Ill., Charles C Thomas, 1958.

Harrison, H. E., and Harrison, H. C.: Mechanisms of Action of Vitamin D. *Pediatrics*, 14:285, 1954.

Pena, J., Cerquiero, M., Belmonte, V., del Rio, R., and Nestal, A.: Estudios Hematologicos en el Raquitismo Comun. *Rev. Esp. Pediat.*, XX:15, 1964.

Winberg, J., and Bergstrom, T.: Renal Acidification Defects in Infants with Mild Deficiency Rickets. *Acta Ped. Scand.*, 54:139, 1965.

TETANY OF VITAMIN D DEFICIENCY
(INFANTILE TETANY)

Tetany due to deficiency of vitamin D is an occasional accompaniment of rickets. Formerly relatively common, it is now rare, owing to the widespread prophylactic use of vitamin D. Tetany is also an infrequent manifestation of vitamin D-refractory rickets. Occasionally it is observed in association with celiac disease, probably as a result of deficient absorption of both vitamin D and calcium. Tetany of vitamin D deficiency occurs most frequently between the ages of 4 months and 3 years; rarely is it observed before 3 months of age. Acute infections or hepatitis may precipitate an attack of tetany.

Chemical Pathology. When the serum calcium level falls below 7 to 7.5 mg. per 100 ml., there is muscular irritability, apparently due to loss of the inhibitory control which the ionized calcium of the serum exerts upon the neuromuscular junctions. Why serum calcium is decreased in some infants or children with rickets is not clear; failure of the parathyroids to compensate for the low serum calcium level may occur. Tetany also occasionally occurs in infants with rickets shortly after vitamin D treatment has been started. This is assumed to be due to a rapid depletion of serum calcium secondary to increased deposition of calcium in the rachitic osteoid tissue and perhaps also to a decrease in parathyroid activity.

Clinical Manifestations. The symptoms are those of tetany, irrespective of the cause (see p. 1262). Vitamin D-deficient tetany may exist in either a latent or a clinically manifest stage. In practically all instances there are manifestations of rickets.

Latent tetany. There are no evident symptoms, but they can be elicited by means of the Chvostek, Trousseau and Erb procedures (see p. 1262). The serum calcium level is less than 7 to 7.5 mg. per 100 ml.

Manifest tetany. Spontaneous clinical manifestations include carpopedal spasm, laryngospasm and convulsions. The serum calcium level is often well under 7 mg. per 100 ml.

Diagnosis. The diagnosis is based on the combination of rickets, low serum calcium level and the symptoms of tetany. The serum phosphorus level may be low, normal or elevated; the serum phosphatase level is increased. In the differential diagnosis other causes of tetany must be eliminated.

Prognosis. The prognosis is good unless treatment is delayed. Death rarely occurs in tetany, though it may result from laryngospasm and possibly from cardiac dilatation, as so-called cardiac tetany.

Prevention. Prophylactic treatment is identical with that for rickets (p. 182).

Treatment. Active treatment is designed to raise the serum calcium above the tetany level. This level may be attained by administration of calcium chloride in 1 or 2 per cent solution in milk. For the first day or two, 4 to 6 gm. daily may be given in 1-gm. doses, the initial dose being 2 or 3 gm.; smaller doses of 1 to 3 gm. a day should then be continued for a week or two. Calcium chloride in more concentrated solution may cause severe gastric ulceration. Large doses of calcium chloride may cause acidosis. Calcium lactate may be added to milk in doses of 10 to 12 gm. a day for 10 days. When oral medication is impractical, calcium gluconate (5 to 10 ml. of a 10 per cent solution) can be administered intravenously, but not subcutaneously or intramuscularly, because of the dangers of local necrosis.

Oxygen inhalation is indicated during convulsive seizures. When intravenous administration of calcium gluconate does not quickly control the attacks, sodium phenobarbital may be given intramuscularly (p. 1254). Parathyroid hormone in a dose of 10 to 30 units may be given in acute cases, but is rarely necessary and should not be repeated because of its rachitogenic effect. Dihydrotachysterol is contraindicated because of the slowness of its action and because it also is rachitogenic. Prolonged attacks of laryngospasm are usually controlled by sedation and the administration of calcium salts. Intubation is only occasionally necessary. After the acute manifestations have been controlled, administration of vitamin D in daily doses of 2000 to 5000 I.U. should be started and the oral administration of calcium continued (see above). When the rickets is healed, the dose of vitamin D should be decreased to the usual prophylactic one.

HYPERVITAMINOSIS D

Ingestion of excessive amounts of vitamin D results in signs and symptoms similar to those of idiopathic hypercalcemia (p. 1369), which may be due to hypersensitivity to vitamin D. Symptoms develop after 1 to 3 months of large intakes of vitamin D; they include hypotonia, anorexia, irritability, constipation, polydipsia, polyuria and pallor. Hypercalcemia and hypercalciuria are notable. Evidences of dehydration are usually present. Aortic valvular stenosis may occur.

The urine may contain albumin. With continued excessive intake, renal damage and metastatic calcification occur. Roentgenograms of the long bones reveal metastatic calcification and generalized osteoporosis.

Excessive intake of vitamin D may result from inadvertently substituting a concentrated form of vitamin D for a more dilute preparation, from increase of a prescribed dose by a parent ("if a little is good, a lot is better") and from inadequate control of dosage in children receiving large amounts of vitamin D for chronic hypophosphatemic states (p. 1363).

Differential diagnosis includes chronic nephritis, hyperparathyroidism and idiopathic hypercalcemia. All may cause metastatic calcifications, and the latter two are accompanied by hypercalcemia.

Prevention consists in careful evaluation of vitamin D dosage.

Treatment includes discontinuance of vitamin D intake and a decrease in intake of calcium. For severely involved infants, aluminum hydroxide by mouth, cortisone or sodium versenate may be used.

REFERENCE

Winberg, J., and Zetterstrom, R.: Cortisone Treatment in Vitamin D Intoxication. *Acta Pediat.*, 45:96, 1956.

VITAMIN E DEFICIENCY

Vitamin E deficiency leads to varied effects in different animal species. Until recently its role in human nutrition has been nebulous. It is a fat-soluble antioxidant, and may be involved in nucleic acid metabolism. No precise biochemical action of vitamin E (α-tocopherol) has been found; it resembles in many of its actions ubiquinone (coenzyme Q), but is structurally unrelated. Vitamin E is widely present in foods.

Deficiency may occur in malabsorption states such as cystic fibrosis or acanthocytosis. Diets with a high unsaturated fatty acid content increase the vitamin E requirement in premature infants.

When exposed to peroxide, red blood cells of newborn infants are hemolyzed in vitro more readily than those of adults. Hemolysis is greater in the blood of premature than of full-term infants, in Negro than in white infants, and is less in the blood of infants fed human milk than of those fed cow's milk. Hemolysis is rapidly inhibited by ingestion of 50 mg. of vitamin E.

Some patients deficient in vitamin E have creatinuria, ceroid deposition in smooth muscle, focal necrosis of striated muscle and muscle weakness. Some improvement may occur after administration of vitamin E. Vitamin E deficiency has been suggested as a causative factor in the anemia of kwashiorkor. Premature infants may have low serum levels of tocopherol, with development of a hemolytic anemia at 6 to 10 weeks of age which is corrected by administration of vitamin E.

Prevention. Minimal daily requirements of vitamin E are not known; 1 mg. per 0.6 gm. of unsaturated fat in the diet appears adequate. Intake should be increased in children with deficient fat absorption.

REFERENCE

Oski, F. A., and Barness, L. A.: Vitamin E Deficiency: A Previously Unrecognized Cause of Hemolytic Anemia in the Premature Infant. *J. Pediat.*, 70:211, 1967.

VITAMIN K DEFICIENCY

Vitamin K is a naphthoquinone which participates in oxidative phosphorylation. The exact function of vitamin K is uncertain; absence of the vitamin or failure of its absorption from the intestinal tract results in hypoprothrombinemia and decreased hepatic synthesis of proconvertin. Prothrombin (factor II) and proconvertin (factor VII) are important to the second stage of coagulation (see p. 1083). The second stage of coagulation is studied by the one-stage prothrombin time (Quick). Administration of vitamin K to the newborn infant increases levels of prothrombin, proconvertin, plasma thromboplastin component (factor IX, PTC) and Stuart-Prower factor (factor X).

Sources of Vitamin K. Naturally occurring vitamin K is fat-soluble and found in high concentrations in hog's liver, soybeans and alfalfa, and in smaller amounts in some vegetables such as spinach, tomatoes and kale. The natural vitamin, whose formula is 2-methyl-3-phytyl-1,4-naphthoquinone, has been labelled vitamin K_1 to distinguish it from synthetic naphthoquinones with vitamin K activity.

Many bacteria, including normal intestinal flora, are capable of synthesizing quinones with vitamin K activity. Suppression of intestinal bacteria by various antibiotics may be responsible for vitamin K deficiency with resultant diminution of prothrombin. Radiated foods have been related to vitamin K deficiency in animals. Cow's milk has more vitamin K than human milk.

Clinical Manifestations. Deficiency of vitamin K, or hypoprothrombinemia, should be considered in all patients with a hemorrhagic disturbance. The incidence of hemorrhagic disease of the newborn (p. 396) has been markedly decreased by the prophylactic administration of vitamin K. Vitamin K deficiency in childhood is usually due to factors affecting absorption or utilization of fat, or to factors limiting synthesis of vitamin K in the intestine, such as prolonged use of antibiotics. Diseases of the liver may lead to hypoprothrombinemia; in these cases hypoprothrombinemia does not usually respond to administration of vitamin K.

Hypoprothrombinemia may also result from administration of certain drugs. Dicumarol, obtained from spoiled sweet clover, is used specifically for the production of hypoprothrombinemia in the prevention and treatment of venous thrombosis. Dicumarol is thought to prevent the liver from utilizing vitamin K and to have no direct effect on prothrombin. Blood prothrombin is continually destroyed in the body; since Dicumarol prevents its replacement, a fall in prothrombin occurs. If a dangerously low level results, massive doses of vitamin K_1 may be necessary to restore the prothrombin to the normal level; whole blood transfusions may be necessary.

Salicylic acid, a degradation product of Dicumarol, produces hypoprothrombinemia by similar action. The fall in prothrombin resulting from the use of salicylates, however, is only mild as compared with that brought about by Dicumarol. The hemorrhagic manifestations in acute rheumatic fever may be due in some instances to large doses of salicylates. Vitamin K is effective in neutralizing this action of salicylates, and its routine use in children receiving large doses of salicylates is recommended.

Treatment. Mild prothrombin deficiency may be corrected by oral administration of vitamin K. One to 2 mg. daily for an infant will usually suffice. If prothrombin deficiency is severe and hemorrhagic manifestations have appeared, vitamin K_1, 5 mg. daily, should be given parenterally. Large doses of synthetic vitamin K analogues, but not of vitamin K_1, may result in hyperbilirubinemia and kernicterus in the glucose-6-phosphate dehydrogenase (G-6-PD) deficient newborn, and in the premature infant. When hypoprothrombinemia is due to liver damage, vitamin K_1 may be given, but whole blood is usually necessary.

LEWIS A. BARNESS

REFERENCE

Zinkham, W. H.: Peripheral Blood and Bilirubin Values in Normal Full Term Primaquine-Sensitive Negro Infants: Effects of Vitamin K. *Pediatrics*, 31:983, 1963.

4. Preventive Pediatrics and Hygiene

PREVENTIVE PEDIATRICS

Preventive services for children began in the late 1800's with attention to provision of pure milk to combat the most serious problem of childhood at that time—infantile diarrhea. In the 1900's the development of immunization procedures gave further impetus to preventive services. Today the principal goals are detection of presymptomatic illness, the promotion of normal physical development and emotional health and, most recently, guidance to the adolescent. Pediatrics has been more concerned with preventive services than any other clinical specialty, and today about 50 per cent of the time of most practicing pediatricians is spent in preventive services.

Definition. Prevention of illness in children has 5 aspects: (1) promotion of general health (e.g. nutrition, hygiene); (2) prevention of specific diseases (e.g. immunizations); (3) early diagnosis of asymptomatic disease to permit early therapy and prevent sequelae (e.g. screening tests for vision and hearing); (4) early diagnosis and appropriate therapy of symptomatic disease to prevent sequelae (e.g. diagnosis and therapy of streptococcal infections to prevent rheumatic fever); and (5) prevention of unnecessary disability due to established symptomatic disease (e.g. rehabilitation to prevent contractures or emotional crippling in cerebral palsy). The preventive point of view in pediatrics should embrace all of child health care. The general principles of preventive services should apply not only to those visits to the physician for which the main purpose is a preventive service, such as the so-called well-child visit, but also to every contact with a child. During a home visit for an acute illness, for example, if parents are alerted to hazards observed in the home, more can often be done to prevent accidents than by exhortation in the office.

Scope and Goals. To have significant impact, preventive services must be related to the health problems most prevalent in the community. Specific programs will therefore vary from place to place and time to time. Health problems include those that cause death, acute and chronic diseases, functional disabilities of emotional or social nature, or other kinds of distress and dissatisfaction. The principal causes of death and acute and chronic diseases are listed elsewhere (pp. 1-9). Table 4-1 indicates how common the conditions may be which underlie emotional, social and intrafamilial disability and distress. To promote the optimal functioning of each child,

the physician will need to "help parents become capable and self confident, to build good parent relations, and to promote family well being" (Standards, 1967).

Not all preventive health services are best administered by the physician. Many, such as provision of pure water and milk, are community responsibilities. Other preventive services first introduced at the personal level have with time been transferred to the community level (e.g. fluoridation of water supplies) because they can be safely and more efficiently implemented in this way.

Since pediatrics is concerned with the wellbeing of all children, not just those who readily come to physicians, and because there are large deficits in manpower for health services today, it would seem appropriate to transfer certain preventive services to community agencies, especially those that do not depend upon the professional relation between physician and patient for their success. This is made easier by the fact that at certain periods in their life children represent captive populations (e.g. in the neonatal period

TABLE 4-1. SOCIAL ENVIRONMENT OF CHILDREN (NEWCASTLE 1000 FAMILY STUDY BIRTH TO 5 YEARS)

	PER 1000 CHILDREN
Deprivation of Parental Care	452
Permanent loss of one or both parents	74
Temporary loss of one or both parents	105
Mothers working full-time	142
Parents incapacitated by illness	121
Marital instability	137
Deficiency of Care	
Defective diet, cleanliness, supervision	160
Social Dependence	202
Unemployment for more than 3 months	153
National assistance	70
Crime	23
Delinquency, truancy, corrective supervision	53

From F. J. W. Miller, S. D. M. Court, W. S. Walton and E. G. Knox: *Growing up in Newcastle-upon-Tyne.* Nuffield Press, Oxford, 1960.

and in school). At these times all can be reached for certain technical procedures. The individual physician's job should not be to devote his time to tasks that others can perform more efficiently, but he should seek to use his special or unique skills or his relation to individual patients to the fullest and where they are most needed.

Not all children have the same risks of development of a given disease, and to apply all preventive services at the same level of intensity to all children is inefficient. For instance, the mother of a third child in an upper middle-class family who has successfully reared previous children, and whose infant is the result of a normal pregnancy and delivery with no evidence of congenital disease by 6 months of age, will have considerably less need for certain aspects of counseling during the so-called well-child visits than would the mother of a first-born premature infant of lower social class. The increasing shortage of health personnel demands that we be more discriminating in our use of preventive services.

This concept of varying degrees of vulnerability has led to the development of "high-risk" registries in certain areas. These are usually developed at a community level and identify children who at birth have a high risk of disease in subsequent months or years (e.g. premature infants with unfavorable obstetric history, children with anomalies or defects detected during the neonatal period). The physician should build his own high-risk registry in order to give such children more careful attention and to be certain that they are receiving preventive or remedial care.

CONDUCT OF PREVENTIVE CHILD HEALTH SERVICES

Visits for preventive services, so-called well-child visits, constitute 40 to 60 per cent of total visits to pediatricians in the United States. In most other countries these preventive services are carried out in separate physical locations and by personnel different from those who provide care for illness. It is a useful aspect of American pediatrics that both curative and preventive services are provided in one place and by one person or team, since 10 to 30 per cent of children who come for well-child visits are actually sick. Moreover, knowledge of the whole child and his family is more comfortably gained in this setting. This does not mean, however, that many preventive services should not be given by the physician's assistants, or that certain screening tests should not be utilized with large groups of children when possible; it does indicate the advantages of and need for one central responsible source of coordinated medical care for each child. This may be the office of the private physician, of a group practice, or of a clinic providing comprehensive care.

The American Academy of Pediatrics has long recommended the following schedule of well-child visits:

Prenatal—Initial contact with pediatrician urged
Birth—At least 2 examinations in the hospital: one within the first 24 hours, the second at discharge
First 6 months—Monthly visits
Second 6 months—Visits every 2 months
Second year of life—Four visits
Two to 6 years—One or 2 visits a year
After 6 years—Annual visits

For many children the most vulnerable period is the first 4 to 6 weeks of life, and more frequent contact than recommended, at least by phone, may be necessary. Many visits will be for immunizations and simple screening tests that can be accomplished in the low-risk patient by the physician's assistant if she is adequately trained. For some disorders (e.g. those of vision or hearing) diagnosis should be made long before school entry if developmental problems such as amblyopia or speech problems (see pp. 1419 and 104) are to be avoided. The physician is the person principally responsible for such detection during the preschool period, and his preventive services may be critical. In school-age children the mass application of screening tests, such as for vision and hearing, and group psychologic testing, can be done best in the school; but this will lead to therapy for abnormalities that are found only if effective communication is maintained between the physician and the school.

Screening Tests. Screening tests should separate from a large group of apparently healthy persons those with a high probability of having disease. Such tests should be simple to perform and yield few falsely negative responses or falsely positive ones.

The accurate recording of *height* and *weight* on a growth chart (p. 40) constitutes perhaps the most important screening procedure, especially in infancy. During the first year head circumference should also be recorded. Since growth rate is most rapid in the first year and in preadolescence, the frequency of measurements should be greater at these times, but they should be recorded at least annually throughout childhood.

Vision screening (p. 1420) can be done from approximately 3 years of age. Between 5 and 10 per cent of preschool children have some visual impairment; the number increases to 30 per cent at school age. The illiterate E charts, Allen cards* or the "Stycar" set are adequate to screen for visual acuity in the preschool period. After 5 to 6 years of age an ordinary Snellen chart can be used. Good lighting, a 20-foot distance and proper cover for the occluded eye are important technical points. Difficulty in completing a screening test for vision in the child 3 to 6 years of age

---

*Available from Ophthalmix Corporation, LaGrange, Illinois.

should suggest behavior problems or developmental retardation. In addition to tests for acuity, latent squint should be looked for by the cover test.

Screening tests for *hearing* (p. 101) are difficult to do, but since about 1 per cent of young school children have hearing impairments, such screening is important. At 4 to 6 months of age hearing can be tested by having the child sit on his mother's lap, facing another person. The examiner stands behind the child and crackles tissue paper, spins a rattle or utters k-k-k, s-s-s or buh-buh sounds The hearing child will turn toward this sound. After this age the most useful screening tests are the mother's suspicion of hearing loss, a family history of hearing loss, or the repeated turning up in volume of radio or television. Retardation in speech or repeated ear infections always call for evaluation of hearing. Most audiologists recommend a formal hearing test, most offices and clinics being too noisy for confident use of the 3-tone screening audiometer.

Development assessment and diagnosis can be carried out by a variety of tests. The most useful for the pediatrician are the Denver Developmental Test and the Knobloch Developmental Test. After age 5 years the Draw-a-Man Test is a useful screening test, as are the Amman's Quick Test and the Sprigle School Readiness Test. Behavior problems are best identified through an adequate history from the mother or teacher; a simple questionnaire (Standards, American Academy of Pediatrics, 1967) is also useful.

Urinalysis is a traditional screening test, though the number of treatable conditions detected by routine test is certainly low. The "dip stick" tests for protein and glucose are simply performed and are adequate. The justification for microscopic examination as a screening test is debatable; in girls it seems wise at least once during school age to perform a quantitative urine culture rather than rely on microscopic examination for pyuria to exclude bacteriuria.

Tuberculin tests are important, especially as there are increasingly fewer positive reactions, so that early detection of infected children and identification of their contacts are important both for therapeutic and prophylactic reasons. Intradermal O.T. or P.P.D. or tine tests are effective and should be done yearly. The Vollmer patch test is not considered reliable for screening.

The microhematocrit or falling-drop copper sulfate method is an adequate screening test for *anemia* and should be performed in high-risk infants at 9 to 12 months and at 2 years of age.

The only *biochemical abnormality* that is presently tested for routinely is phenylketonuria, through examination of blood or urine of the newborn infant.

Screening for *lead poisoning* is recommended for children of 18 months to 5 years of age living in old or dilapidated housing, where up to 5 per cent of children will have abnormally high lead levels. There is no entirely satisfactory screening test, but children with a history of pica should at least have urine tested for coproporphyrin (p. 466).

PREVENTIVE MEASURES AT DIFFERENT AGE PERIODS
(See sections 2 and 7)

There are general features of preventive services appropriate to each age period of childhood.

Prenatal and Neonatal Periods. No greater benefit to children could occur than the development of effective methods to prevent prematurity (low birth weight) and congenital malformations. Effective prevention starts even before conception; there is evidence that the early life of the mother, her childhood nutrition and her pattern of living are related to her reproductive efficiency. Preventive services to children may do much to prevent problems of the perinatal period for the next generation.

During pregnancy early diagnosis and adequate management of maternal infections, minimal use of radiation, cautious use of drugs, maintenance of good maternal nutrition, Rh determinations, adequate management of maternal diabetes and a safe, atraumatic delivery are largely in the hands of the obstetrician; yet they may have greater impact upon the child's subsequent health than anything the pediatrician can do later. The pediatrician and the obstetrician should establish a close working relation in order to develop the field of perinatology as a joint enterprise. Many pediatricians meet prospective parents at a prenatal visit in order to establish better physician-patient relations, to promote attitudes favoring the mental health of the child, to determine any potentiality for a genetic disease, and to help the family prepare physically and emotionally for the new baby.

After delivery the pediatrician should carry out a careful physical examination within 24 hours, or in the delivery room if complications are expected or develop, and again before discharge from the hospital. Such examinations are aimed at early detection of congenital anomalies, such as congenital heart disease, hip dysplasia and neurologic disorders. Initiation of appropriate feeding, prevention of infection in nurseries, screening tests such as for hereditary metabolic disorders (phenylketonuria), and promotion of a healthy mother-child relation are all aspects of medical care at this time and are described elsewhere (p. 353).

Infancy. The main problems for which some measure of success of preventive measures can be expected during the first year of life are nutritional disorders, infections, developmental problems and deficiencies of maternal care. The physician also seeks to make early diagnosis of congenital anomalies and hereditary metabolic disturbances.

Early detection of solid tumors may improve the prognosis.

At each visit an assessment of *nutrition* should be made. The scientific basis for nutritional advice is given elsewhere (pp. 127, 143). Today in the United States, although general affluence and simplified nutrients should make this advice relatively simple, among certain indigent groups, such as migrant labor, the rural poor, and the disadvantaged of the inner city, deficiencies in calories, vitamins and protein continue to be seen. The chart of height and weight, the dietary history and the physical assessment of the child constitute adequate screening for malnutrition.

All the dietary essentials can be obtained from natural foods except vitamin D, which must be given as a supplement, either in a separate vehicle or in fortified foods, such as cow's milk. Occasionally, supplementation of the diet with other vitamins is necessary to prevent the development of specific deficiencies (p. 136).

In many localities the problem of undernutrition is less common than that of *obesity*. The prevention of overnutrition is properly an objective of preventive pediatrics because of the high morbidity and mortality attributable to this condition in later years. The causes of obesity are many, but the common denominator is the intake of more calories than are needed to balance energy output. Prevention, which is far easier than cure, is dependent upon early detection of those factors in the child's environment or personality which predispose to obesity (p. 165).

The principal nutritional deficiency of infancy is *iron deficiency* in the last half of the first year of life. This is preventable if solid foods, especially the infant cereals which contain added iron, are introduced between 2 and 6 months of age, when most children accept these additions willingly. Weaning from bottle to cup some time between 6 and 12 months of age will often decrease the intake of milk and increase that of solid food. A screening test for anemia should be done on infants at 6 months and at 1 and 2 years of age if they are socioeconomically deprived or if they have a poor dietary intake of iron. The prevalence of iron deficiency anemia ranges from 10 to 20 per cent in the lower socioeconomic groups and is less than 1 per cent among the more advantaged children.

Fluorine can now be considered an essential element in prevention of *dental caries*. It is easiest and best given in the public water supply; where this is not yet available, sodium fluoride drops containing 0.5 mg. of fluoride should be given daily from birth until 10 to 12 years of age. Good dental hygiene and restriction of sugar intake also are important factors in prevention of caries.

The other large difficulties in nutrition during this period involve weaning and feeding problems between mother and child. Almost all babies have a decrease in appetite around 1 year of age as their growth rate slows. Anticipatory guidance by about 10 months should familiarize parents with this fact and prevent many feeding problems.

Infections. Specific prevention is now available against many of the formerly serious infections. Table 4-2 summarizes the schedule of immunizations recommended in the definitive booklet published by the American Academy of Pediatrics (the Red Book, 1966). This booklet should be immediately available to all physicians who treat children. Details of the techniques of administration of the various immunizing agents are given, as are the contraindications to and complications of their use. It is more important that all children receive immunizations than that an arbitrary schedule be followed. Parents should be given a record of the child's immunization, and the physician should also keep a record.

All children should receive immunization against diphtheria, pertussis, tetanus, measles and poliomyelitis during the first year of life, and smallpox in the first part of the second year.

Active immunization against diphtheria (p. 566), *pertussis* (p. 569) *and tetanus* (p. 579) is accomplished by use of a mixture of killed pertussis organisms with alum-precipitated or aluminum hydroxide-adsorbed diphtheria and tetanus toxoids. Most preparations contain in the usual 0.5-ml. dose adequate amounts of diphtheria and tetanus toxoids and 4 N.I.H. units of pertussis vaccine. The minimal course is 3 intramuscular injections of this combined material at about monthly intervals. Immunization is usually started by about 2 months of age.

Injections are given intramuscularly into the lateral thigh of infants or into the deltoid or triceps muscles of older children. It is best to use a different site for each injection. Deep injection and massage after injection reduce the incidence of so-called antigenic cysts. Mild fever often occurs within 12 to 24 hours and is not a contraindication to further injections. Administration of aspirin may make an irritable child more comfortable.

When a convulsion occurs as part of a reaction, further administration of pertussis vaccine is contraindicated. Subsequent immunization may be carried out with diphtheria and tetanus toxoids, beginning with reduced doses (0.05 to 0.1 ml.).

After 6 years of age children should not receive pertussis vaccine; boosters should then consist of "adult" diphtheria-tetanus toxoid to reduce reactions. A Schick test is no longer used routinely, since reactions to "adult" DT are so minimal that it is simpler to give a booster injection than a Schick test. Booster doses are important to maintain immunity and should be kept up for diphtheria and tetanus throughout life.

It is usually unwise to give any immunization during an acute illness, because the fever from the injection may confuse the picture of the illness. Some children who have frequent upper respiratory tract infections may have long delays in completion of immunizations if this policy is over-rigidly followed; mild convalescent or healing infections should not be an absolute contraindication to immunization.

TABLE 4-2. Recommended Schedule for Active Immunization and Tuberculin Testing of Normal Infants and Children

2 months	DTP; trivalent OPV[1, 2]
3 months	DTP[3]
4 months	DTP; trivalent OPV
6 months	Trivalent OPV
12 months	Tuberculin test[4]
	Live measles vaccine[5]
15-18 months	DTP; trivalent OPV; smallpox vaccine[6]
4-6 years	DTP; trivalent OPV; smallpox vaccine
12-14 years	Td; smallpox vaccine; mumps vaccine (see p. 650)
Thereafter	Td every 10 years[7]
	Smallpox vaccine every 3-10 years

From the *Report of the Committee on the Control of Infectious Diseases.* Evanston, Ill., American Academy of Pediatrics, 1969.

Abbreviations: *DTP* is diphtheria and tetanus toxoids combined with pertussis vaccine; *Td* is combined diphtheria and tetanus toxoids (adult type) for those over 6 years of age, in contrast to *DT*, which contains a larger amount of diphtheria antigen; *OPV* is trivalent oral poliovaccine.

[1]Handling and storage of immunizing agents, dosage, sites and routes of administration and courses should follow product (package) information.

[2]Trivalent OPV is recommended, but monovalent OPV may be substituted; the order of administration of monovalent virus is type 1 followed by type 3 and then type 2.

[3]If DTP dose is not given to an infant at 3 months, it should be given at 4 and 6 months of age.

[4]The frequency of repeated tuberculin tests depends on the risk of exposure of children under care and the prevalence of tuberculosis in the population group, annually to biannually.

[5]Live attenuated measles vaccine with or without immune serum globulin (measles) or further attenuated measles vaccine without the simultaneous administration of immune globulin is recommended. Killed measles virus vaccine is not recommended.

Measles vaccine should be given to all children with a positive tuberculin reaction only after initiation of tuberculosis therapy.

[6]Any licensed smallpox vaccine may be used. The reaction should be read and recorded. Combined administration of smallpox vaccine and OPV may be considered if there is a threat of concomitant exposure or if the patient will be inaccessible for completion of the series.

[7]The 10-year interval for tetanus boosters may be calculated from each dose given for prophylaxis (injury). Prophylactic use for wounds is a matter for clinical judgment. Persons who have had the initial series and booster doses may be expected to have adequate protection for at least 1 year after the last dose without receiving an additional booster dose. (See p. 579).

Administration of oral live attenuated *poliomyelitis vaccine* (p. 687) containing the 3 types of virus is the safest of all immunization procedures. Though there may be some competition with other enteric viral infections, it is not recommended that poliomyelitis vaccination be deferred during the summer.

Vaccination against smallpox (p. 644) is performed between 1 and 2 years of age after completion of other procedures and should be repeated every 5 years, or every 3 years for foreign travel. It is contraindicated in children with eczema or other forms of dermatitis and for children who have household contacts with such children. Kempe's new attenuated strain may make vaccination of such children a safe procedure.

Vaccination against measles (p. 626), using an attenuated strain of virus, should be initiated about 9 to 12 months of age. Booster doses of this vaccine have not yet been recommended.

Other immunizations are recommended for various parts of the world. Information on these can be found in the Red Book and in publications of the United States Public Health Service.*

Passive immunization against measles, rubella, infectious hepatitis, varicella and poliomyelitis through the use of gamma globulin has some place, but except for infectious hepatitis and occasionally rubella and varicella *(q.v.)* the use of active immunization is far preferable, even in an epidemic situation.

Quarantine is not generally effective for the control of the contagious diseases of childhood.

Parents commonly seek advice about prevention of other infections for which no specific immunization is available. It is wise not to invite exposure of children to such bacterial infections as impetigo, salmonella or shigella, but it is hardly practical and may even be unwise to try to prevent contact of normal children with the common epidemic viral upper respiratory and gastrointestinal tract infections. Since many asymptomatic children excrete the viruses of these diseases, prevention of contact with only symptomatic children will not be very effective. Moreover, after the first few months of life it is part of the process of growing up to develop immunity to a wide variety of agents through being infected with them. Even if we could prevent infections through isolation techniques, it is questionable whether we should postpone for the healthy child the development of this normal immunity against common infections.

*Superintendent of Documents, Government Printing Office, Washington, D.C. 20402.

Other preventive measures. *Congenital malformations* and *hereditary metabolic disorders* are detected by careful physical examination of the baby in the newborn nursery, again by about 1 to 2 months, and at 6 months of age. These examinations will reveal nearly all the disorders for which treatment has any value, such as hypothyroidism, adrenal hyperplasia and galactosemia. Without new symptoms there is no evidence that a physical examination is necessary at each of the visits during the first year of life. Though this may shock some, and though a careful examination is one way of winning the confidence of mothers, there simply are not enough physicians to justify examination of all babies at each visit, when the yield of treatable disease will be so low. Nurses or medical aides may be trained to perform some screening measures. Perhaps the most useful procedure for each visit is a developmental examination, such as the Denver Developmental Test,* 3 to 5 per cent of children will be found to be abnormal. It is possible to help those suffering environmental deprivation.

At each visit of the infant or child to the physician or some other member of the health team there are 4 areas of service to be considered: *(a)* health promotion, *(b)* specific prevention, *(c)* health appraisal, and *(d)* anticipatory guidance.

Special mention should be made of the principle of *anticipatory guidance,* through which problems may be prevented from developing. It requires knowledge of normal growth and development (p. 15). Some examples: (1) Normal children begin to roll over by about 5 months of age. Anticipatory guidance alerts parents to this possibility by about 3 to 4 months of age and suggests that infants should not be left unprotected on a bassinet or bed. (2) The normal child slows in growth rate by about 10 to 12 months of age, with reduction of appetite. If parents know this, they are reassured that the decrease in intake is normal and they will not force their children to eat. In this way they will avoid a common type of feeding problem.

The following is a general and simple guide to the conduct of health visits during the first 2 years of life. The nurse or some other member of the health team is given more initiative and activity than has been customary. The schedule need not be followed slavishly. For some children more frequent visits are essential; for others less frequent ones are adequate.

AGE	SERVICES
1-3 weeks	A telephone contact is made with the mother. Questions are asked about feeding, stools, color, skin, urinary stream (boys), sleep, and mother's health and concerns
4-6 weeks	Office visit with physician. History as above, and complete physical examination with special attention to weight, length, head circumference, nervous system, vision, heart, abdominal masses (especially kidneys) and hip for dislocation. Immunizations started by nurse, with first DPT-OPV

*See page 1551 for description of Denver Developmental Screening Test.

10 weeks	Office visit. History, which may be taken by nurse, includes illnesses since last visit and any pertinent events in family; length, weight, head circumference and developmental assessment by nurse are adequate screening if no symptoms or complaints. Second DPT-OPV by nurse. Introduction of cereal as tolerated
14 weeks	Office visit, as at 10 weeks. Same screening tests as at 10 weeks. Observe for strabismus. Third DPT-OPV. Begin to add other baby foods
5-6 months	Office visit with physician. History and physical examination; hearing screening; developmental appraisal. Weaning may begin for some
9 months	Office visit with nurse. History, length, weight, developmental appraisal. Hematocrit determination if diet is poor. Anticipatory guidance about change of appetite
12 months	Office visit with physician. Weaning should be complete. Tine test; measles vaccine. Accident prevention discussed
15 months	Office visit with nurse. Height, weight, developmental appraisal. Accident prevention discussed. Smallpox vaccination
18 months	Office visit with nurse. DPT booster, OPV booster. Toilet training may be begun. Accident prevention reinforced
24 months	Office visit with physician. Toilet training is usually progressing. Accident prevention again. Urine test for coproporphyrin in population susceptible to lead ingestion

At each visit inquiry is made into the health of other family members, any family changes such as job changes of father, death or illness of grandparents, and mother's feelings. Perhaps the most useful guide to preventive services which the health team has to offer during this period comes through assessment of the mother's skills in child care. The key processes are the development in the child of trust in the mother during the first year of life and the gradual ability to separate from her and develop his own identity and autonomy during the second year. The physician should assess the progress of these developments and assist the mother to achieve them. Praise for the mother, especially for skills shown in care of her first child, is a valuable way to build her confidence. Since there are many different successful techniques for rearing children, the pediatrician will be wise to refrain from intervention unless he is sure that deleterious effects are seen or expected. Mothers receive bewilderingly different kinds of advice; it is generally best to support and praise a mother for what she is doing well and naturally and to foster her self-confidence rather than try to cast her into one's own image of what a proper mother should be.

Preschool Period. The health problems of the preschool child consist principally of morbidity from acute infections and accidents and of the development of chronic diseases. Deaths are rare; most are due to accidents.

Accident prevention. The magnitude of the problem demands that physicians and others educate parents about the hazards to children, aiming their efforts particularly at the high-risk groups. Age is an important risk factor. Most accidental

TABLE 4-3. Accident Prevention at Various Age Levels

TYPICAL ACCIDENTS	NORMAL BEHAVIOR CHARACTERISTICS	PRECAUTIONS
	First year	
Falls Inhalation of foreign objects Poisoning Burns Drowning	After several months of age can squirm and roll, and later creeps and pulls self erect Places anything and everything in mouth Helpless in water	Do not leave alone on tables, etc., from which falls can occur Keep crib sides up Keep small objects and harmful substances out of reach Do not leave alone in tub of water
	Second year	
Falls Drowning Motor vehicles Ingestion of poisonous substances Burns	Able to roam about in erect posture Goes up and down stairs Has great curiosity Puts almost everything in mouth Helpless in water	Keep screens in windows Place gate at top of stairs Cover unused electrical outlets; keep electric cords out of easy reach Keep in enclosed space when outdoors and not in company of an adult Keep medicines, household poisons and small sharp objects out of sight and reach Keep handles of pots and pans on stove out of reach and containers of hot foods away from edge of table Protect from water in tub and in pools
	2-4 years	
Falls Drowning Motor vehicles Ingestion of poisonous substances Burns	Able to open doors Runs and climbs Can ride tricycle Investigates closets and drawers Plays with mechanical gadgets Can throw ball and other objects	Keep doors locked when there is danger of falls Place screen or guards in windows Teach about watching for automobiles in driveways and in streets Keep firearms locked up Keep knives, electrical equipment out of reach Teach about risks of throwing sharp objects and about danger of following ball into street
	5-9 years	
Motor vehicles Bicycle accidents Drowning Burns Firearms	Daring and adventurous Control over large muscles more advanced than control over small muscles Has increasing interest in group play; loyalty to group makes him willing to follow suggestions of leaders	Teach techniques and traffic rules for bicycling Encourage skills in swimming Keep firearms locked up except when adults can supervise their use
	10-14 years	
Motor vehicles Drowning Burns Firearms Falls Bicycle accidents	There is a need for strenuous physical activity Plays in hazardous places (street, railroad tracks, near rivers) unless facilities for supervised, adequate recreation are provided Need for approval of age-mates leads to daring or hazardous feats	Teach the rules of pedestrian safety Teach bicycling safety Instruct in safe use of firearms Provide safe and acceptable facilities for recreation and social activities Prepare for automobile driving by good example on part of adults and by closely supervised instruction

Adapted from T. E. Shaffer: *Pediat. Clin. N. Amer.,* 1:426, 427, 1954.

poisonings occur in children 2 to 4 years of age, whereas firearm injuries occur mostly in school-age children. Boys have more accidents than girls, and recurrent accidents are more likely in impulsive, acting-out, attention-seeking children. Some parents are too anxious about the risk of accidents; they should learn to foster self-confidence and responsibility in their children. The mildly painful experience of a fall may be far more effective in prevention of future accidents than an attempt at complete protection of the child from all hazards. Table 4-3 outlines the kinds of accidents expected at various ages and precautions that can be taken. It is useful to have pamphlets or printed sheets for parents to remind them of these hazards, but they are not substitutes for personal discussions.

Other preventive measures. *Malignant neoplasms,* including *leukemia,* are the second cause of death in this age period. Aside from a few solid tumors which can be detected early enough to allow successful treatment, no prevention is now available.

Most *congenital anomalies* will have been detected by this age, so that it cannot be expected that physical examinations will identify many unrecognized ones.

Of the acute *infections* common in this period, primary prevention is possible for only a few. Immunization should have been completed by 2 years of age against diphtheria, tetanus, pertussis, poliomyelitis and measles. Prevention of other infections is by avoidance of children with severe infections, such as shigellosis and salmonellosis, community protection of food and water supplies, and early detection and treatment of complications of the common respiratory infections, such as otitis media, meningitis and pneumonia.

The early discovery of chronic disabilities not threatening to life, such as impairment of vision, hearing and development, and the promotion of an emotionally satisfying pattern of living are the main goals of prevention in the preschool period. A simple behavior questionnaire can help select those parents who have most need to discuss problems in these areas.

The following is a guide to preventive measures during this age period.

AGE	SERVICES
2½ years	Office visit. History of behavior, illness and accidents, eating, sleeping, elimination, toilet training, current family situation. Examination: height, weight, development. Tuberculin test. Discussion of accident prevention. Dental referral
3 years	Office visit. History, especially of behavior. Examination: height, weight, development, hearing, vision test. Tuberculin test. Discussion of accident prevention and nursery school
4 years	Office visit. History as for 3-year-old. Examination: height, weight, development. Tuberculin test. Discussion of accident prevention
5 years	Office visit, as for 4-year-old. School readiness screening tests (Sprigle or Frostig) and discussion with parents about child's behavior and development

School Age. School health programs have come under criticism from several aspects. They are often isolated from other medical activities, especially from the care of the child's illnesses, and even from the educational process and from problems related to school activities. Much of this criticism is justified and at least in part identifies ways in which the school can provide health care. Some screening tests, such as vision, hearing and group psychologic, are most efficiently performed in the school. Moreover, the child's relations with peers and teachers and his performance in school are as good a screening assessment for psychologic problems as there is. The child's physician should receive such information from the school and remain the focal point for medical care. The physician should in turn transmit to the school pertinent information about the child, with appropriate recommendations for individual attention.

The important role of the school physician is not in performing physical examinations on children who have a family physician, but in participating in conferences with teachers and school nurses about problem children, in helping to plan curricula in health, including sex education, and in biology, and in interpreting health matters to the school administrators.

Conduct of preventive services for school-age children. It is customary to recommend yearly visits of the child to the physician to maintain a relationship among physician, patient and family. Developmental problems are best indicated by school performance; emotional and learning problems are frequent. Decisions are difficult as to which ones the child's physician will manage himself and which he will refer for psychiatric evaluation. He will be asked for advice on child rearing, discipline, summer camps, sleep, the viewing of television, sports, sex education, dating, school performance, and a host of other matters. To do his job properly, he must be interested in these matters, learn as much as possible about them, avoid extremes of advice, and foster a feeling of confidence in parents that they can make wise decisions.

The annual physical examination provides an opportunity to answer some of the questions which all children have about their developing bodies, and, as adolescence approaches, to help the youngster to realize and accept that his body is normal and can be examined without discomfort or shame. Height and weight remain useful screening tests for significant occult illness and should be recorded yearly. Vision and hearing should be tested and development assessed. The school may be equipped and able to do this through group testing. It is important that innocent heart murmurs be recognized, and that children having them be not referred for cardiac diagnostic studies, so that unnecessary anxiety by the child and his family are avoided.

One of the most important and difficult areas is that of so-called minimal brain damage (see p. 110). School and reading problems are common; reading readiness and school readiness tests are available which may forestall some of these problems through identifying them before they become overlaid by much anxiety, anger and sense of failure on the part of child and family (see p. 107). Progress in school should be under continuous review, and if trouble occurs, an early, full investigation should be made under the direction of the child's regular physician, who should be best able to put together the family history, perinatal experiences and emotional climate of the home in such a way as to make sensible recommendations to the family. Prevention lies in helping parents and children as early as possible to have realistic expectations for achievement.

Booster immunizations are continued during the school period, at the 4- to 6-year intervals indicated in Table 4-2.

Robert J. Haggerty

REFERENCES

Frankenburg, W. K., and Dodds, J. B.: The Denver Developmental Screening Test. *J. Pediat.,* 71:181, 1967.

Harper, P. A.: *Preventive Pediatrics: Child Health and Development.* New York, Appleton-Century Crofts, 1962, p. 798.

Health Supervision of Young Children: A Guide for Practicing Physicians and Child Health Conference Personnel. Revised edition. American Public Health Association, New York, 1960.

Immunization Information for International Travel. U.S. Dept. Health, Education and Welfare, Public Health Service, Publication No. 384, Washington, D.C.

Report of the Committee on the Control of Infectious Diseases (Red Book). American Academy of Pediatrics, P.O. Box 1034, Evanston, Ill., 1966, $1.50.

Report of the Committee on School Health. American Academy of Pediatrics, Evanston, Ill., 1966.

Standards of Child Health Care. Council on Pediatric Practice, American Academy of Pediatrics, Evanston, Ill., 1967.

Wallace, H. M.: *Health Services for Mothers and Children.* Philadelphia, W. B. Saunders Company, 1962, p. 466.

HYGIENE

Child health supervision at selected intervals offers the physician ample opportunity for meaningful guidance to parents who are subjected to and sometimes overwhelmed by advice on the bringing up of children. Magazine articles, syndicated columns in the daily press, advertising and radio and television commentaries are utilized to bring information to this receptive group. Most of the advice is good, but some is contradictory and much is subject to misinterpretation; undue emphasis of minor and unimportant detail is a common failing. Well meant suggestions from family and friends frequently add to the parents' difficulty in selecting a proper course of action. As a result the role of the physician in health education will usually include interpretation of conflicting recommendations and opinions as well as direct instruction.

Habits. The daily practices which promote good health and personal well-being, usually referred to as personal hygiene, are facilitated by the development of habits which begin at birth and continue throughout life. They usually arise from conscious acts reinforced by repetition and frequent use until they function as patterned reactions requiring little or no thought. Generally, habits are considered to be good when they conform to acceptable behavior and bad when they do not. Praise, encouragement, attention and personal satisfaction strengthen them, whereas lack of attention and parental displeasure discourage them; they are easily formed and much less easily changed or eliminated.

Although children appear to do equally well with strict or *laissez-faire* discipline, reasonable expectations and acceptable limits to behavior need to be defined and upheld. When parents appreciate that their responsibility in guiding habit formation is to help the child gain increasing independence at his own optimal rate, much concern over trivia is avoided. Consistency of action by both parents is essential if children are to be helped rather than confused. Personal examples are more important in promoting good habits than what is said, especially when parents do not "practice what they preach." Comparison with others, the setting of too rigid standards and impatience with lack of success lead to frustrations and ten-

sions in both children and their parents. When demands made by the family exceed the ability or readiness of the child, conflicts result which the physician may help to resolve and explain. Children want to conform to what is expected of them, and their well intended efforts toward a goal, as well as successful achievement, merit praise.

Habit formation is usually thought of in relation to establishment of eating, sleeping, and bowel and bladder patterns. Regularity and relatively automatic functioning in these fields are necessary before children are free to progress to more complicated learning.

Eating. Eating habits of infants are discussed on page 159, of older children on page 160.

Sleep. There is considerable variation in the amount of sleep required by different children. Many children get too little rest, and often the symptoms of irritability, lethargy, anorexia, temper tantrums and perhaps increased susceptibility to infection result. Many behavior problems are precipitated by fatigue.

Most infants sleep 16 to 20 hours a day during the first half year; by 6 months of age they sleep through the night and are awake for periods totaling 6 to 8 hours. By 1 year of age the child sleeps an hour or two less and by 2 years of age averages 12 to 14 hours a day. The need for sleep gradually decreases, but rarely becomes less than 10 hours during the pediatric age range. A nap during the day is desirable until school interferes with this routine, and rest periods should have an important place in kindergarten and first and second grade schedules.

Early establishment of regularity of bedtime is most important; nowhere in the field of habit formation is consistency more important. The presleep period should be free of excitement, rushing, scolding and physical activity. Stimulation of children by exciting stories, radio, television, active play or a battle of wills should be avoided. A familiar story, quiet discussion of happy events of the day, a warm bath and reasurance of love and affection are conducive to easy sleep. Children, even when sleepy, normally do not want to stop doing something interesting. The habit of going to bed on schedule and sleeping promptly can be established and maintained by a consistent and understanding approach.

Infants and children should have their own beds and, if possible, their own rooms. The sleeping room should be ventilated, but free of drafts. Bed clothing is frequently too heavy and should be varied with the temperature. Overall sleeping garments for infants who may get uncovered in cold weather are useful. Although position during sleep is relatively unimportant, the position of infants, especially of premature ones, should be changed often enough to prevent moulding of the cranium from constant pressure on one area.

Disturbances of sleep are discussed on page 83.

Elimination. Control of the anal and bladder sphincters is naturally acquired by most children during the second or third year of life. Efforts to "train" a baby before he is ready for voluntary control of his sphincters are usually disastrous and frequently lead to unhappy parent-child relations. He is not ready to use the toilet until he is old enough to understand what it is for and to let his mother know of his needs, until his bowel movements come at fairly regular times, and until he is willing to sit on the toilet. A comfortable seat with a rest for the feet and a strap for safety should be provided. Suppositories or soap sticks have no place in the establishment of regular bowel habits, and coercive methods of any sort are contraindicated.

By about 18 months of age most toddlers have acquired enough bladder control to retain urine for 2 hours or so. At this age they may be encouraged to sit on the toilet and void. It is best to make initial efforts just after meals or naps and when the child is dry and likely to void readily. Other routines or interesting play should not be interrupted for this purpose. Nocturnal control of urination is not usually attained until the third year of life or later.

Exercise. The normal infant or child, in a reasonable environment, will have sufficient muscular activity for good growth and development. The young infant begins to develop his large muscles by kicking, stretching, crying and squirming. He should be allowed to do so several times a day on a safe flat surface, unencumbered by clothes. He should be provided with easily grasped toys to develop hand use. Limits for safety's sake must be provided when he crawls and begins to walk, but his activities at this stage should not be limited to a playpen. This piece of furniture was designed for adult convenience, not to aid the child's development. Toddlers should be provided with safe areas both indoors and outdoors in which to run, climb and explore. They need large blocks, push and pull toys, materials for imitative play, and the privilege of getting dirty and playing with water. Children's toys should, in general, be washable, not easily broken, free of sharp edges and splinters and of removable parts that can be swallowed or aspirated.

Schools should provide an opportunity for universal participation in organized sports. Intramural teams can offer the less well coordinated boy or girl an opportunity to take part in group sports.

Sunlight and Fresh Air. Sunshine and fresh air are essential for the development and maintenance of sound health. Dependence is no longer placed on sunlight for the prevention of rickets, but many other benefits accrue from it. There is no reason, however, to justify making a fetish of exposure of young infants to the sun, particularly in cold weather. Care should always be taken to avoid sunburn. Outdoor play should be encouraged at all ages when the weather permits and clothing is adequate. Fresh air should be provided indoors by adequate ventilation.

Clothing. Tremendous improvements have been made in the functional design and in the materials of infants' and children's clothing. The diaper is still standard equipment, but tapes, drawstrings, many tiny buttons, frilly dresses and bulky winter clothes have largely been replaced by elastic materials, grippers, zippers, a few large buttons, slip-on shirts and pants and by new materials of lighter weight for cold weather. The principles guiding the choice of good clothing for children are attractiveness and color, simplicity in design, ease of use, softness of texture, lightness of weight, washability, relative looseness of fit and freedom from irritation to the skin. Knitted cotton is usually best next to the body. Children should be dressed appropriately for the environment. A universal tendency to overdress children in the winter frequently results in excessive perspiration. Extra water-repellent garments are easily put on a child to secure the warmth and protection needed for outdoor activities, and they should be removed as soon as he re-enters the warm house or schoolroom. The legs should be covered in cold weather.

Layettes are usually too elaborate. Infants need shirts with and without sleeves, nightgowns, diapers, socks or booties, a sweater and an outer garment with a hood for outdoor winter use. Rubber or plastic pants should be loose enough to permit evaporation, but should not be used except for relatively short periods to avoid otherwise troublesome situations. Lightweight cotton blankets are generally preferable to heavy woolen ones; a well made sleeping bag is satisfactory for cold weather.

Children's shoes are discussed on page 1353.

Cleanliness. Certain aspects of cleanliness such as the bath, washing at mealtimes and at toilet time, the use of a handkerchief and of a napkin, brushing the teeth and some responsibility in caring for clothing are essentials that should be reduced to the level of habitual reactions as early in life as possible. Formation of habits of personal cleanliness is encouraged, like all other habits, by the examples of parents, by praise and recognition of effort, by pleasant rather than unpleasant experiences, by consistency and by gradually decreasing assistance on the parents' part. Many parents need help in achieving a perspective on healthy cleanliness, which lies somewhere between asepsis and filth.

A daily bath for infants is a good rule. In warm weather more frequent sponging may be necessary. As soon as the umbilicus has healed, the infant may be immersed in a basin or tub. The room should be comfortably warm; supplies should be ready at hand; a safe flat working surface must be available; care must be taken not to let the infant slip or fall; and the experience should be made a happy, playful one. A regular time for bathing as well as for other routine activities should be established. A nonirritating soap is lathered over the trunk and extremities with care to avoid the eyes and mouth, and the baby is then rinsed with fresh, comfortably warm water. The scalp should be washed as needed. The skin is patted dry, with special attention to the creases.

Oil, powder or lotion is usually not necessary, although their use is sometimes helpful for dry skins and in the diaper area. Caution should be used to avoid inhalation of any powder, and zinc stearate should not be permitted in the nursery (see p. 926).

The face is washed with clear water, except when soap or oil is necessary to remove dried excretions or vomitus.

The external ear may be washed with a soft cloth; dried accretions in the creases may be removed with a cotton-tipped applicator moistened with oil. The ear canal, except at its opening, should not be cleaned by an untrained person.

The eyes usually require no special care. Accumulated secretions in the corner of the eye should be wiped out with a piece of cotton saturated with clear water.

The nose does not need cleaning unless there are dried secretions at the openings of the external nares. Secretions may be removed with a dry or moistened cotton-tipped applicator. Oil should not be used.

Under no circumstances should attempts be made to clean the mouth, since the mucous membrane is easily damaged and is then especially susceptible to infection.

Brushing the teeth is not advised until the third year of life. Before this time they may be cleaned occasionally with a cotton-tipped applicator saturated with saline or sodium bicarbonate solution.

Nails need trimming when they protrude beyond the ends of the fingers or toes. Toenails should be cut straight across without rounding the corners so that ingrowing toenails may be prevented.

The bathing of older children requires no special consideration. In summertime there should be daily baths; in the winter months this is not necessary and, in children with dry skins, should be avoided. In the latter instance, 2 to 4 baths a week are adequate, depending on the state of cleanliness. Baths should be taken preferably at night to lessen the degree of chafing, which is reduced significantly by thorough drying (dry towels and warm air). Anointing the skin with oil or skin lotion helps to avoid chafing of dry and sensitive skins.

The genitals should be washed at bath time. In the uncircumcised male infant the foreskin may be retracted as far as possible without trauma. Adhesions will usually be broken as the child grows older, and no strenuous effort need be made to break them. Smegma may be removed from the vulva with a soft cloth or a cotton pledget saturated with oil. Genitalia of both sexes should be rinsed with clean water at the end of the bath to prevent irritation from soap, which otherwise might dry on the mucous membranes.

WILLIAM E. LAUPUS

5. General Considerations in the Care of Sick Children

CLINICAL APPRAISAL OF INFANTS AND CHILDREN

The pediatrician must be competent in the comprehensive evaluation of both somatic and psychologic components of illness and in the promotion of emotional as well as physical health in the child and his family. Hospital-trained physicians often rely too heavily upon laboratory data in their evaluation of the sick child. In doing so they may fail to take advantage of a variety of clues to be had from careful observation of the behavior of the child and of interactions between child and parent.

Basic principles in the clinical examination of infants and children include the following:

1. Health is more than the absence of disease.

2. Clinical study is based upon a holistic concept of human function; physiology of organs and behavior of the organism cannot be separated.

3. The cause of disease involves multiple factors; whether the disorder is predominantly somatic or psychologic, predisposing, contributory, precipitating and perpetuating forces are involved. Adequate clinical study must include genetic, constitutional, physiologic, psychologic and interpersonal factors.

4. The family is the ultimate epidemiologic unit of clinical study for both infectious and psychologic disturbances.

Since parents cannot assess accurately the competence of the physician, it is his manner which most effectively permits the development of confidence in him. Such a feeling *may* exist whether or not medication or other treatment is provided. Some parents unconsciously endow the physician with almost magical attributes; others are overdependent and cannot take simple and obvious steps without consulting him. Among negative parental attitudes are distrust, suspicion, fear of domination or resentment toward authoritative figures. Parents with such attitudes may be unable to utilize effectively the services of the physician.

The attitudes of children toward the physician are modified by those of their parents and by their own experiences. Most emotionally healthy children are able to overcome their inevitable anxieties and to develop trust in the physician. The child who is acutely ill, however, may regress emotionally and behave like a much younger child even with a physician he knows. Fears of pain or of the unknown and fears of going to the hospital and of being separated from the parents are important at such times.

The wise and experienced physician who works with children develops a capacity to view the behavior of the parent and the child as data revealing their personalities and their interaction, data which form a part of his clinical findings and may be of importance in the approach to management.

HISTORY

The leads which arise in securing the history during the initial interview will determine in part the points of emphasis in the physical examination and the selection of laboratory studies. Of equal importance is the opportunity for the physician to begin the establishment of effective relations with parent and child. The quality of this relationship will influence both the accuracy of the data obtained and the response to therapeutic measures or anticipatory guidance.

In later interviews the physician enlarges and at times revises his initial impression. Different physicians will apply the principles of interviewing in individual ways. The physician should feel comfortable with *his* interviewing technique rather than attempt to imitate too closely that of someone else.

Young children of preschool age are usually seen with the mother. The physician may give the child a toy or other object with which to play. If the parent's concern is the child's behavior, or if the parent talks too freely about the child's personality, the physician may prefer, with the help of a nurse or secretary, to interest the child in some play activity in the waiting room while he talks with the parent.

The physician may learn a good deal in a few moments of casual observation of the young child's play during the interview with the parent. One may obtain impressions of the level of his development from the degree of complexity and organization of his play, the length of his span of concentration and other factors. His attitude toward the physician, often reflecting parental anxiety, may also be apparent in his drawing, play with dolls and his general demeanor.

With older children and young adolescents it is best to see parent and child together at the first interview, since an anxious or suspicious child may fear that the parent is imparting secret in-

197

formation to the physician. If it is necessary to see the parent alone for free discussion of emotional problems, this may be done at a later, separate interview. Occasionally, if the parent wishes to discuss some urgently disturbing aspect of the child's behavior, the initial interview may be without the knowledge of the child; at this time it can be decided whether the child should be seen alone or with the parent. Whenever both parents can be seen together, with or without the child, valuable impressions may be obtained about their relations, their attitudes as parents and their attitudes toward the child and his illness or adjustment.

With the older child verbal data may be much more accurate and voluminous after a positive relationship has been established. In the first contact, school-age children may be inhibited and withdrawn in the face of anxiety, without any deep underlying emotional disturbance or limitation in intellectual capacity. The wise physician will avoid premature judgment of the child's capacity for adjustment or his mental status. With the child who is old enough to talk freely one can and should gain impressions, even in predominantly somatic illness, of the meaning to him of his symptoms or disability, in terms of its effect upon his adjustment at school, his status with his peer group, his attitude toward his own body, and other factors. With frightened or withdrawn children, such data may have to be sought indirectly by asking them for their aspirations, what they wish for most, what they would do if they were well, or even what a hypothetical child might wish for or do in a particular situation.

At the outset of history taking it is important to permit the parent or child to talk freely without significant interruption. Leading questions must be avoided. Even if the physician's time is limited and the parent's initial comments seem confused, too detailed, or irrelevant to the child's obvious condition, the parent should be allowed to talk freely and to set the pace, for at least a brief time. The act of talking helps to discharge initial tensions and assists in overcoming anxiety. A few extra minutes during the initial interview will save much time later. With an unhurried approach it may become apparent that the declared reason for a visit or the stated chief complaint may not be the parent's chief concern. For example, the mother of a mildly obese boy of nine, who seeks guidance about his weight, may indicate with some embarrassment in the course of such a relaxed interview that her real concern is the apparent smallness of his genitalia.

Certain historical data may carry an emotional charge for the parent, and some revelations may be painful and difficult. This is particularly true of the history of familial illnesses and of emotional disturbances in child or parent. For example, some parents of children with seizures may be unable to disclose in the initial interview the presence of epilepsy in close relatives because of their fear that they have been personally guilty of transmitting the illness. Parents also recognize that their feelings about the child may be involved in disturbances of his behavior. Thus in following up leads to possible psychologic problems or in asking questions dealing with behavior, it is important not to adopt too frontal an approach, which the anxious parent may misinterpret as a critical attack. Questions such as, "Did you want this child?", "Does your son masturbate?" or "Was she jealous of the new baby?" are all too frequently doomed, in the initial interview, to receive socially acceptable replies or to be answered with defensive indignation. Such information is important, but must be gathered initially by inference or by the use of less loaded and indirect questions. Nonverbal behavior, such as blushing, nail-biting or neuromuscular tension, may give important clues to be followed up later. Expectant waiting is vital even if the mother appears on the verge of tears. The physician can, with practice, curb his natural social impulse to stem the expression of strong emotion, and might better encourage crying in a tense and troubled mother. The release of such feeling in a sympathetic atmosphere may be of help to the parent and may strengthen the relationship with the physician.

In closing the initial interview it is wise to return to the parent's concern. The physician can then ask questions arising from the leads he has gained up to this point. This kind of termination of the interview indicates to the parent that the physician has fully comprehended her concern and will endeavor to deal constructively with it during further studies.

Observation of Child and Parent. Clues available from careful observation of the child and of the parent-child interaction are frequently overlooked. From the moment parent and child enter his office rich clinical impressions are available to the physician or to an alert nurse or secretary. Some parents cannot permit the child to answer a question independently, manifesting the need to dominate the child or the situation. Other parents constantly correct the child or require him to sit impossibly still, indicating unrealistically high standards of conformity. If the father and the mother are interviewed together, they may disclose disagreements in child-rearing practices. A few parents pay little attention to their children, such as the mother who does not stand close to her infant to prevent his falling off the examining table. Occasionally, disturbed parents unconsciously may need to deny the extent or seriousness of the child's obvious illness and to belittle him or to urge him to act "as if he were well." Even balanced and effective parents may exhibit such behavior at times of anxiety. The wise physician will record such observations and test them against later impressions. Observations of this sort are most readily available to the physician who visits the home and enjoys continuity of contact with the parents and child. The standards of parental care and the pattern of family living are more evident on a home visit than in the office.

Historical Data. The following outline of information to be sought in the pediatric history is modified from the traditional format and is intended only as a guide, not as a check list. A check-list approach in history taking may seriously inhibit the parent's spontaneous and more detailed remarks.

The details of the family's living circumstances, their position as members of a particular minority group, the chronic depression of the father over unsatisfying work experiences, the part-time work of a mother coming just at the child's bedtime, and similar factors may be as relevant to assessment of the child's health as factors relating directly to a physical illness. It is important to determine whether there is or has been familial illness which may be relevant to the child's illness, but the experienced physician will avoid the monotonous listing of all possible illnesses.

In securing details of the child's birth, growth and development, past illnesses and parental child-rearing practices, it must be remembered that the average parent has difficulty in recalling many items with accuracy. Subsequent recollections or other sources of data, such as "baby books," may amplify or correct the initial recollections.

Obviously, not all the potential information listed below can be obtained in the initial interview. In recording the history it is important to list pertinent negative items, in order to indicate that all possible aspects of the problem have been explored.

Identification of Informant: Initial description of parent or informant (if not parent, state relation to patient), manner of giving data, and apparent accuracy. Evaluation of emotional state or other factors which might bear on accuracy of data.
Chief Complaint or Complaints: In terms of parent or child.
Present Illness: Date of onset and initial symptoms. Health prior to onset. Careful description of kind, duration and degree of symptoms. Chronologic progress or change in symptoms, including details of any therapy. Pertinent epidemiologic information (exposure to illness, potential carriers, animal or insect vectors). Effect of illness on behavior or adjustment of patient and family. Pertinent negative data.
Past History
1. *Developmental Survey*
   Prenatal: Health, nutrition, attitudes and emotional state of mother during pregnancy. Illnesses during pregnancy: toxemia, diabetes, cardiac disease, depression. Health and attitudes of father during pregnancy. Pregnancy planned or unplanned. Living circumstances of family during pregnancy. Fetal activity.
   Birth: Date; weight; premature or term; birth order. Nature of birth; presentation; use of forceps; cesarean section; length of labor and delivery; degree of difficulty.
   Neonatal Condition: Spontaneous respiration; difficulty in resuscitation; respiratory distress; degree of activity; jaundice; cyanosis; convulsions; paralysis; hemorrhage; stupor; difficulty in sucking; rash; snuffles; congenital anomalies; intractable crying. Mother's condition; reaction to baby. Blood group incompatibility.
   Feeding
      Infancy: Breast- or bottle-fed; if artificial feeding, why and when started, type, frequency, amount taken; hunger. Infant's response to feeding; regurgitation; mother's feelings about feeding of infant; attitudes and degree of help by father.

Supplementary Vitamins: Age when begun; regularity of administration; amount taken.
Solid Foods: Time of starting various items, infant's response.
Weaning: Breast to bottle or breast or bottle to cup; reason weaned; time started; length of time required; infant's response.
   Childhood: Appetite and intake; food likes or dislikes; feeding difficulties if present; parents' attitudes toward food and feeding.
   Growth and Development
      Psychomotor: Age of control of head; hand-to-mouth coordination; social response; sitting with support or alone; creeping; differentiation between parents and strangers; standing; walking, with support and alone; first words, brief sentences; difficulties in coordination; hyperactivity; speech disturbance, hesitation, stammering, infantile speech, aphasia.
      Growth Patterns: Approximate weights at 1 year, 2 years, 5 years, 10 years; steadiness of gain; growth spurts; age at eruption of first tooth; abnormal dentition.
      Sleep Patterns: Amount of sleep in relation to age; daytime naps, when given up; night terrors, somnambulism, nightmares; disturbances in sleep rhythm; struggles over bedtime.
      Toilet Training: Bowel and bladder; time begun; methods used; age control was achieved; later relapses in control, enuresis or encopresis; parents' attitudes.
      Habit Patterns: Nail-biting, thumb-sucking, rocking, head-banging, pica, rumination, rituals, others.
      Sexual Development: Child's questions about conception, pregnancy, or differences between boys and girls, information given; preparation for menarche, age at onset, girl's reaction; preparation of boy for puberty, secondary sex characteristics, boy's reaction; parents' attitudes; masturbation; difficulties in sexual adjustment, attitudes of child and parents.
      Discipline: Parents' methods; child's acceptance; negativism; tantrums; rebelliousness; aggressive or destructive behavior; withdrawal; running away.
      School Adjustment: Preschool experience; age at entrance into school; adjustment; child's and parents' attitudes toward school program; child's progress.
      Social Adjustment: Early response to separation from mother; child's relation to peers; degree of independence; participation in scouting and other group activities; hobbies, sports and other interests; difficulties in adjustment (aggressive, withdrawn, oversubmissive).
2. *Medical Survey*
   Prophylaxis: Immunizations against smallpox, pertussis, diphtheria, tetanus, poliomyelitis, measles, typhoid fever, yellow fever; age at immunization, number of injections, booster shots, untoward reactions; scar of smallpox vaccination, tuberculin test and serologic tests for syphilis.
   Specific Illnesses:
      Contagious Diseases: Age at illness, complications.
      Other Illnesses: Listed according to system involved; age, severity, treatment, sequelae; hospitalization; reaction to serum, blood or blood derivatives.
      Allergic Reactions: Eczema, asthma, hay fever, urticaria, hypersensitivity reactions to inhalants, food, drugs, contact with cloth, soaps; age at onset; treatment; complications.
      Operations: Dates, nature, results; complications or sequelae; reactions of child and parents.
      Injuries: Dates, frequency, nature and circumstances of accidents, sequelae; nature of study and treatment; reactions of child and parents.
   Review of Regions and Organic Systems of Body
3. *Family Survey*
   Parents: Age; occupation; state of physical and emotional health of each parent or parent-substitutes; if parents not living, age at death and cause; individual attitudes of parents toward patient and toward child-rearing practices; previous pregnancies of mother, outcome; brief summary of family circumstances; backgrounds from which each parent derived; current state of health of grandparents (if not living, age at death, cause); degree of cohesiveness of family, patterns of communication.
   Siblings: Age; where living; state of health (if not living, age at death, cause, nature of symptoms); general school and social

performance; nature of relationship to patient; attitudes of parents toward patient in relation to siblings.

Living Circumstances: Nature of dwelling; sleeping arrangements; number of persons living in home in addition to parents and children; relation of such persons to family members; members of family who work; working hours if unusual; general level of economic independence, support from community agencies if any; neighborhood circumstances; available recreational outlets.

Familial Illnesses or Anomalies: Tuberculosis, syphilis, diabetes, cancer, epilepsy, rheumatic fever, allergy, hereditary blood dyscrasias, mental illness, mental retardation, dystrophies, congenital anomalies, heredo-degenerative diseases.

Summary: A brief recapitulation of the essential features of the present illness or the current state of health if the child is being seen for a health examination; significant correlations between features of past development or illness and significant life events or family circumstances; essentially an organization and synthesis of the historical data into meaningful trends, so far as they can be derived.

The recorded history of the experienced physician may more closely approximate an expanded summary than the basic outline suggested, but for the person in training an outlined plan is essential. With the use of the general approach indicated it is possible to secure psychologic and social data at the same time that somatic factors are explored.

If the child is acutely ill, the physician should take only a brief history relative to the current illness before beginning the physical examination. Subsequently the history should be completed.

PHYSICAL EXAMINATION

Certain basic principles assist in the direct study of the child. Some thought should be given to the appearance of and arrangements in the office or examination room. Children respond favorably to bright colors; white is cold and strange to the small child. Pastel colors achieve a cheerful and familiar effect. The room should contain pictures and other colorful items.

Approach to the Child. The physician will have gained during the taking of the history certain impressions of the child's general physical and emotional state, and of the nature of any illness, as well as of the interaction between child and parent. With this background he may turn to the child at an appropriate point. He can anticipate active participation in the examination by the child, but he should be prepared for resigned submission, passive resistance or, more rarely, active refusal or violent battle. The degree of rapport established with the child and the parent may determine the diagnostic success of the examination. In the seriously ill child the physical examination may be done while the latter portion of the history is taken, to save time and to decrease the suspense of the anxious child and the parent.

The child should ordinarily be undressed by the mother or nurse just before the examination. All clothing should be removed from young children. It is well to remember that refusal by preschool children to remove certain items of clothing may indicate anxiety over being so completely exposed rather than sexual modesty. This initial apprehension should be respected; it is ordinarily soon overcome. Older children may retain their underpants, with temporary dropping for genital examination when they are at ease.

No matter what the circumstances, the physician must have a relaxed and unhurried approach. A few moments spent initially in conversation with the child about a doll or in admiring an item of clothing, using the child's first name or nickname, may save valuable time and considerable struggle, but the physician must avoid being overlong in the initial preparation. Some explanation of each step, as in examining the throat or darkening the room for ophthalmoscopic examination, can be given quietly, using terms the child can grasp. For the physician to be able to relate to the child, he should not lower himself to the level of the child; his behavior must remain adult in the child's eyes. It is imperative that the child be told the truth at his level of understanding whenever uncomfortable procedures are to be performed; any other course will seriously compromise his later trust or cooperation.

The young child may be permitted to explore certain instruments such as the stethoscope before they are used; attempts at listening to themselves or their dolls may be enjoyed and may overcome tension. "Blowing out" the light of the otoscope is a time-honored pediatric detractor for the toddler.

In the latter part of the first year most infants show some fear of the physician, even if they have seen him regularly for health examinations. This change represents the developing capacity of the infant to identify strangers. The physician may offer the mother a throat stick or similar object to give to the infant while he sits in her lap during the interview, permitting him to appraise the physician from a safe vantage point.

The infant often resists examination on his back on an examining table, and it may be best to examine him on his mother's lap, permitting her to hold his head against her shoulder for examination of ears and throat. The nurse may be able to obtain a more positive initial response from the older infant than the less familiar male physician. Anxiety or even terror in the infant need not initially be considered by the physician a sign of failure.

During the latter part of the second and most of the third year the child often exhibits so-called normal negativism, which reflects a healthy drive toward independence and aggressive self-assertion. Asking a child of this age to perform some step in the examination, such as opening the mouth, may result in a firm "No." Patience is of the essence. A stubbornly negativistic child, diverted at this point to some other activity, may later become suddenly able to reverse his previous rebellious stand. Physical battles almost inevitably result in the child's loss of trust in the physician.

The preschool child can ordinarily be examined on a table. Most children at this age are frightened when they are compelled to lie down, and feel less anxious in a sitting position.

With children of school age, as with older preschool children, much can be learned during the physical examination about the child's attitudes toward his own development, his feelings about himself as a developing person, and his concern over minor blemishes or abnormalities. If the child feels secure with the physician, he may himself bring up his fears or misconceptions. At times the parent also will bring up similar concerns during an unhurried examination.

With preadolescents and adolescents, modesty may become apparent during the examination. Such feelings should be respected, and these children should be handled in about the same way as adults. Adolescent boys may have fears about how a growth lag bears upon their ultimate masculinity, or about other real or imaginary deviations. Adolescent girls may be concerned particularly about the onset of the menses and the development of secondary sex characteristics. A nurse should be in the room during the examination of girls of this age.

Approach to the Parent. Some busy or impatient physicians prefer to exclude an anxious mother from the physical examination, recognizing that the child often submits more passively in her absence. This approach carries with it not only the pain of separation for the young child, particularly acute for the overdependent and frightened child of an overanxious mother, but also the implication for the child of punishment by the physician. The parent may react with feelings of guilt and at times with resentment, surmising that the physician believes her to be a poor parent. It is almost always wisest to permit the parent to remain with the infant or young child.

At times a particularly apprehensive parent will ask to leave during the physical examination and should ordinarily be permitted to do so, preferably before rather than during the examination. If the mother leaves the room, it is wise to tell the child where she will be and when she will return. If restraint is indicated under such circumstances, it should be carried out promptly, with a brief explanation of its need.

Method of Examination. It is important that instruments applied to the skin, such as the stethoscope, be warm. It may be of help, with a young or anxious child, to rinse the hands in warm water before beginning the examination, since any coldness to the touch may add to the child's fear or resistance.

The usual order of procedure in the examination of adults is often not appropriate for young children. In general, it is wiser to leave examination of ears and throat to the last. This approach may vary with the age of the patient as well as with circumstances surrounding the examination. For the older infant deep tendon reflexes may be a suitable maneuver for beginning the examination. With the preschool child, listening to the chest may be the appropriate opening move. An occasional child is made more anxious by waiting too long for the anticipated and disliked throat examination, and in such instances it may be wiser to perform it initially. When restraint is required, the need for it should be explained, and then the examination should be made with as much dispatch as is commensurate with gentleness and thoroughness.

Pulse and respiratory rates and blood pressure levels in infants and young children are variable and may be altered by fear or apprehension. Only persistent deviations can be relied upon. In young children, in particular, temperature also may be influenced by emotions or activity. Rectal temperatures may be elevated as much as a degree Fahrenheit immediately after active exercise, whereas the oral temperature usually is not. Oral temperatures may be altered immediately after ingestion of hot or cold substances. Rectal temperature recordings are generally considered to be nearly a degree higher than oral ones, but there is a lesser difference if each recording is made properly. Rectal temperatures are preferable in infants and small children. Preschool children may resist this approach, although not yet able to retain the thermometer safely by mouth. In such a situation an axillary temperature reading may suffice.

Examination of the heart and lungs is complicated in infants and young children by the thinness of the chest wall and the consequent relative loudness of breath sounds. Sounds resembling bronchial breathing are frequently heard over the right upper lobe in normal chests. The physician must learn to listen quickly and accurately during periods of freedom from crying or other vocal activity.

In examining the abdomen considerable time must be spent in putting the child at ease in order to achieve sufficient relaxation of the abdominal musculature. Talking with the child often helps to divert his attention. If the child is old enough to respond to a request to take a deep breath, the pressure of the physician's hand can be increased gently with each inspiration without undue voluntary resistance.

For children beyond early infancy rectal examinations may be disturbing and should be performed with great care and gentleness, and with adequate explanation to the child. Caution should be observed in the vaginal inspection of preadolescent or adolescent girls, since their apprehension and misconceptions about such manipulations may be extreme.

After the examination the child should be given time to ask questions, if he desires, about procedures or instruments used or about any other phase of the examination. The physician should always terminate the interview with a friendly and personal farewell to the child.

LABORATORY DIAGNOSTIC STUDIES

The indications for specific laboratory or other diagnostic tests are discussed in the sections on specific diseases. Routine procedures in the usual clinical examination include hemoglobin level, white blood cell count and differential, urinalysis and a tuberculin test. Routine serologic studies for syphilis have been discontinued in some pediatric clinics. When additional laboratory studies are contemplated, they should be critically selected on the basis of their relevance to the problem at hand. The need for interpreting the indications for laboratory tests to anxious parents is fundamental in any diagnostic approach.

When painful procedures such as throat cultures, venipunctures, blood cell counts, intradermal tests, as well as more involved procedures, are to be performed, it is essential that the child be told briefly what will happen in terms he can understand. The child should be given enough time to ask questions in advance of the procedure. Too long a period of anxious questioning and delay may permit the build-up of excessive anxiety. Sufficient explanation should be given to the parent also, even about brief and simple procedures. If restraint is indicated, the child should be told that his arm or other body part will be held in order to help him hold still so that the procedure will be less painful.

PREPARATION FOR HOSPITALIZATION

Although hospitalization need not be an emotionally traumatic experience, the chances of such an eventuality are great enough that the psychologic aspects of admission and management should not be overlooked. For the child under 4 years of age, and for some older but dependent or definitely disturbed children, the concomitant separation from the mother, often misinterpreted as punishment, is the most anxiety-provoking aspect of the experience.

With the young preschool child, verbal preparation may be of limited value, but should nevertheless be undertaken. Preparation should be discussed by the physician with the parents, who may have questions, often seemingly irrelevant ones, which may reflect their own apprehensions or a tendency toward self-blame in relation to the child's illness. A period of several days is usually sufficient for the preschool child to bring up questions, misconceptions and potential misinterpretations about the coming experience, which parents can then discuss with the child if they themselves have a reasonably clear grasp of the facts involved. Actual explanation to the young child should be couched in simple terms, related to the need for "getting well" or helping the child's "tummy" to stop hurting. Concrete facets of the experience are best explained, such as the dress of physicians

and nurses, the procedures involved in admission, hospital sleeping arrangements, the experience of anesthesia, and the use of bed pans. A nurse or social worker can be helpful in discussing such factors with the parents before elective hospitalization.

The older child can be prepared further in accord with his greater capacities for intellectual understanding and his ability to tolerate, for longer periods of time than the preschool child, the tension involved in the anticipated hospitalization. For preschool and younger school-age children the opportunity to "play out" feelings of fear or resentment is important, both before and after the hospitalization or painful procedures. Opportunity for the use of dolls, doctor kits, and Plasticine or other play materials should be available to the child for this purpose in the hospital. Occupational therapists or recreational therapy personnel can contribute significantly to such constructive and age-appropriate modes of adaptation.

Frequent parental visiting is valuable in preventing disturbed reactions to hospitalization. Overnight stay in the hospital by the mother may be a most effective support for the young or very anxious child, provided the parent feels comfortable in doing so.

IMPLEMENTATION OF RESULTS OF THE CLINICAL EXAMINATION

Once the physician has achieved a balanced diagnostic appraisal of the child in his family setting, his plan of therapy or his approach to well-child care must be communicated effectively to patient and parents. He should repeat in simple language, without recourse to medical terminology, his suggestions for therapeutic plans and write out the detailed or complicated instructions for care. Many parents remain so anxious throughout such a final interview that they may indicate understanding at times when they are too confused to retain details or even to grasp implications. An opportunity for the parents to talk freely about their reactions will bring out many misconceptions or misunderstandings which must be patiently dealt with if therapeutic or preventive measures are to succeed.

The role of the physician dealing with children and their parents is an exceedingly challenging and uniquely satisfying one. Parents are turning with increasing frequency to physicians for guidance. To bring a comprehensive approach to the clinical examination, the physician must have increased knowledge of human biology in its behavioral as well as physiologic aspects. With such knowledge he is in the best possible position for the detection, treatment and prevention of disease and for the positive promotion of healthy development and adaptation.

DANE G. PRUGH

THE PATHOPHYSIOLOGY OF BODY FLUIDS

Clinically, it is necessary to consider the physiology of body fluids from 3 standpoints: (1) the amounts of water and solutes such as electrolytes in the body as a whole; (2) the distribution of these materials in the various compartments of the body; and (3) the concentration of the solutes within each compartment.

The quantities of these substances are the result of the balance between intake and output which, for materials of physiologic significance, are under careful regulation. Many of the controlling mechanisms are extremely complex; those of importance to the clinician will be discussed in some detail. The distribution of water and solutes is of critical importance, and precise regulation requires considerable energy to maintain steady states. Relatively few materials are maintained in simple equilibrium, free of energy-requiring processes.

Alterations in concentrations of substances within the body lead to profound changes in function; this is particularly so in respect to substances of normally low concentration. A physiology dictum entitled "The effect of the low concentration component" states that the rate of percentage change rather than absolute change in concentration is of maximal importance physiologically. The lower the normal concentration, the greater will be the percentage change when there is an absolute loss or gain of a substance. For example, changes in concentration of potassium in the extracellular fluid have far greater effect physiologically on function than do similar changes in intracellular potassium. By contrast, changes in volume are relatively well tolerated, but here, too, rate of percentage change is more critical than absolute change. For example, the loss of 100 ml. of blood in a few minutes in a large adolescent would produce a negligible disturbance, but in a newborn infant it would result in shock. Nevertheless a similar loss in the infant extended over days could be fairly well compensated.

WATER

Body water as a percentage of body weight decreases with age from 78 per cent at birth to the adult value of about 60 per cent at 1 year of age. Since adipose tissue is low in water content, the measurement of body water has been related to the fat-free mass of the body. The lean body mass (LBM) bears a constant relation to total body water (TW), and can be predicted from the equation:

$$LBM = \frac{TW}{0.72}$$

Total body water is best described as a linear function of weight (WT), as shown in Figure 5-1, and is estimated by the equation:

$$TW = 0.611 \, WT + 0.251$$

The intake of water is regulated by the thirst mechanism, localized in the midhypothalamus. The usual stimulus for increased drinking is a rise in osmolality of extracellular fluid in relation to intracellular fluid, e.g. with the infusion of hypertonic saline solution. The infusion of urea which diffuses readily into intracellular fluid produces little sustained change in water intake. Reduction in volume of body fluids, even though they become hypotonic as in salt depletion, may also lead to a sensation of thirst. Diseases of the central nervous system, potassium deficiency and malnutrition may lead to increased drinking, even though the content of body water is greater than usual, and osmolality is decreased. The retention of body water ascribed to inappropriate antidiuretic hormone (ADH) response (see below) suggests that the thirst mechanism and ADH release are interrelated.

Absorption of water takes place by passive diffusion in response to active solute transport from intestinal lumen to interstitial fluid and plasma.

Figure 5-1. Total body water in boys plotted against body weight. The relevant equation is given in the text. The data of Cheek are indicated by X; those of Friis Hansen, by ⊗. (From D. B. Cheek: *Human Growth.* Philadelphia, Lea & Febiger, 1968; and B. Friis Hansen: Changes in Body Water Compartments During Growth. *Acta Paediat.*, 1957.)

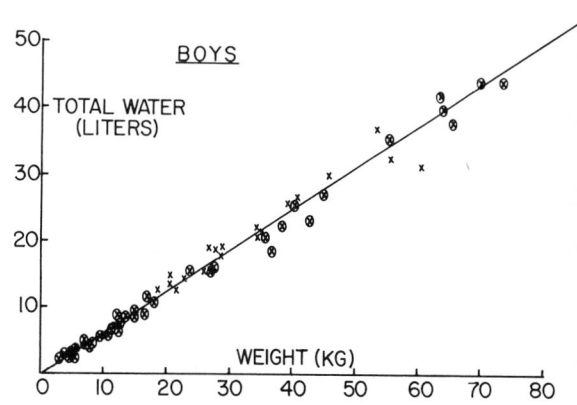

The active transport of sodium is the bulk process responsible for generating the osmotic gradient leading to movement of water. Any inhibition of sodium transport or failure of reabsorption of solute, such as in disaccharidase deficiency, can lead to large volumes of unabsorbed intestinal water and result in diarrhea.

Water is also derived from the oxidation of carbohydrate, fat and protein of exogenous and endogenous origin, and these sources must be considered in the calculation of water requirements during anuria.

Obligatory losses of water occur as evaporative losses from the lungs and skin and depend upon surface area, surface temperature and the partial pressure of water vapor in the environment.

Sweating is controlled by the autonomic nervous system and may be reduced even in heat stress by severe deficits in volume of body fluids or in concentrations of electrolytes. Precise control of the amount of water in the body, however, is dependent upon a finely regulated feed-back system involving the hypothalamus, posterior pituitary and collecting ducts of the nephrons.

Urinary volume is determined by multiple factors such as glomerular filtration rate (GFR), kind and quantity of solute load (dependent upon diet), the state of the renal tubular epithelium, and concentrations of adrenal steroids and particularly of ADH in body fluids. The influence of the central nervous system on the glomerular filtration rate is not large. Changes in the rate are not of importance as regulatory mechanisms of water excretion in man. When large quantities of protein are ingested, the renal solute load may be an important factor in increasing water losses. A neurogenic effect on renal tubular epithelium has not been demonstrated. Deficiency of adrenal corticoids seems to potentiate ADH action, probably by facilitating the back diffusion of water in the distal tubule as a result of a change in membrane permeability.

The action of ADH, a crystalline octapeptide, increases the permeability of the collecting ducts to water, thereby permitting the back diffusion of water into the interstitial tissue and peritubular capillaries in the medulla and pyramids of the kidney. In those regions fluids are hypertonic from the action of a countercurrent exchange system and an active transport system which control the concentrations of sodium and urea.

Secretion of ADH has been localized to the supraoptic-hypophyseal system, interruption of which leads to diabetes insipidus. The axons which descend from supraoptic and paraventricular nuclei through the infundibular stem to the pars nervosa of the posterior pituitary carry a neurosecretory substance which is stored in and released from the terminal arborizations. This material is probably ADH itself. Depletion of the neurosecretory material occurs in animals deprived of water, and storage occurs when water loads are administered.

Control of ADH output in many ways resembles control of water intake. Emotional factors may stimulate or inhibit release of ADH. Such stressful stimuli as pain, mass discharge of peripheral receptors resulting from trauma, burns or surgery increase ADH output and are important considerations in fluid therapy. With the exception of nicotine, which is a potent stimulator of ADH output, most drugs that produce antidiuresis do so by affecting glomerular filtration rate. Morphine and barbiturates are probably antidiuretic in this way, although the results of some experiments are interpreted to the contrary. Anesthesia also reduces urinary flow, probably by altering renal hemodynamics. Alcohol is a potent inhibitor of ADH release, and there is a consistent dose-response relation.

The most important homeostatic mechanism responsible for control of ADH secretion is the distribution and volume of body fluids. The absolute level of osmolality has no effect on ADH release or inhibition. Administration of urea, which produces little shift of water between cells and interstitial fluid, does not evoke consistent antidiuresis. Intravenous injection of an equivalent quantity of hypertonic saline solution evokes intense antidiuresis. Conversely, administration of water which expands intracellular volume inhibits release of ADH.

The distribution of water is determined completely by physical factors, and there is no evidence to support the concept of active transport or secretion of water. Water movement against a concentration gradient has been described in the gallbladder, but here the active transport of sodium and sequestration of water in the wall with subsequent filtration under pressure account for the paradoxical movement of water.

The large compartments of the total body water are plasma water (5 per cent BW), interstitial water (15 per cent BW), transcellular water (5 to 10 per cent BW) and intracellular water (35 to 40 per cent BW) (see Fig. 5-2).

The transcellular compartment is primarily water in gastrointestinal secretion, and the amount is highly variable, depending upon the absorptive and secretory activities of the intestines. It may expand rapidly as in gastrointestinal allergy, in early and severe diarrhea or in paralytic ileus with multiple fluid levels. The plasma, and interstitial and transcellular water make up the extracellular water.

The volume of fluid in the intravascular space (plasma water) is maintained in a steady state by a balance between filtration and oncotic forces. The bulk of the oncotic pressure (effective osmotic pressure) results from the presence of small protein molecules, primarily albumin, that do not readily pass through the capillary pores. Decreases in protein concentration, as in the nephrotic syndrome, or acidosis which alters the association of proteins with cations through the Donnan effect leads to reduction in plasma volume with equiv-

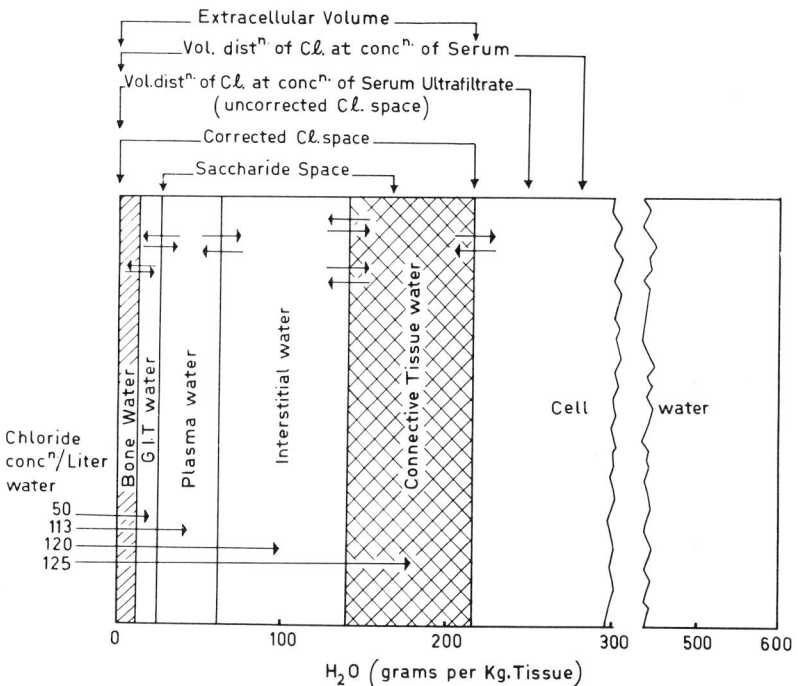

Figure 5-2. The relative sizes of the subcompartments that make up extracellular volume. The diagram is based on experimental data from the rat. Such subdivision is probably similar for all mammals. (From. D. B. Cheek: Extracellular Volume: Its Structure and Measurement and the Influence of Age and Disease. *J. Pediat.*, 58:103, 1961.)

alent increase in interstitial volume. Because plasma volume is only one third of the interstitial volume, reduction in plasma volume through shifts of water to the interstitial space may not be observed clinically as edema, even though circulating volume may be compromised enough to reduce glomerular filtration rate (GFR) and flow to other vital organs.

Any increase in capillary permeability to protein as in angioneurotic edema leads to a rise in protein concentration of the interstitial fluid with a reduction in the oncotic pressure and an increase in interstitial fluid. The increase may be localized, appearing as a wheal or urticaria, or may be generalized.

Alterations in filtration pressure resulting from increase in venous pressure as in heart failure or in retention of sodium with hypervolemia as in glomerulonephritis may increase the interstitial space.

Extracellular volume (ECV) bears a fairly straight-line relation to weight [ECV = 0.239 (WT) + 0.325] and to total body water in normal infants and children. Extracellular volume is larger than the intracellular space in the fetus, but the ratio of extracellular water to intracellular water falls to the adult level of 40/60 by 9 months of postnatal life. The relative loss of extracellular volume is presumably the result of the increasing growth of cellular tissue and a decreasing rate of growth of collagen relative to muscle during the early months of life.

Intracellular volume is the difference between total body water and extracellular water and is maintained in a relatively constant state by osmotic forces operating across membranes freely permeable to water. The maintenance of these forces is dependent upon active transport of sodium out of cells by energy-consuming processes (see below). A disturbance in cellular function can lead to swelling of cells. A rise in extracellular osmolality leads to a fall in cell water. Conversely, with water intoxication a fall in extracellular osmolality leads to an increase in cell volume.

Intracellular volume is related to the excretion of creatinine and body potassium, both of which are closely related to the mass of muscle in the body. A new concept of some importance is that of visceral mass, which is the lean body mass (as determined by potassium measurement from whole-body scintillation counting) minus muscle mass (as determined from creatinine excretion). An approximation of visceral mass can also be obtained by calculation through appropriate geometric formulas of the volumes of head, chest and abdomen. The visceral mass seems to be closely related to oxygen consumption at rest and accounts for the high oxygen consumption of small babies at rest per kg. of lean body tissue, since muscle mass is relatively low and the oxygen consumption of individual tissue such as brain, heart and liver is high per gram of tissue.

The concentrations of the bulk solutes of the extracellular and intracellular fluids are illustrated in Figure 5-3. Although the chemical activity of water (i.e. the tendency of molecules to escape to another compartment) is the same in each compartment because the concentration of solute particles (osmoles) is the same, the weight or volume of water in various spaces or tissues differs considerably.

Variations in water content are of clinical significance only in regard to large changes in plasma water. When plasma solids—proteins and lipids—are elevated as may occur in diabetic ketosis with hyperlipemia, serum water is markedly decreased per kg. or liter of serum. Since electrolytes are dissolved in the aqueous phase, serum electrolyte concentrations as usually determined will be low per liter of serum, though normal per kg. of serum water. Treatment of such a patient on the basis of hypotonic dehydration could be disastrous. Measurement of osmolality by freezing point depression (osmometry) provides true values, since only the activity of water is measured in this determination.

SODIUM

Sodium is the bulk cation of the extracellular fluid and is the principal osmotically active solute responsible for the maintenance of intravascular and interstitial volumes. Its role in intracellular processes seems more as an inhibitor than a stimulant of some intracellular enzymes, although its full role remains to be elucidated.

The quantity of sodium in the body amounts to approximately 58 mEq. per kg., approximately 70 per cent of the total body sodium being exchangeable within 24 to 36 hours. The fetus has a relatively high sodium content, owing to relatively large amounts of cartilage, connective tissue and extracellular fluid in relation to muscle.

The amount of sodium in the body is determined by the balance between intake and output. Dietary intake of sodium has a wide range, depending upon the cultural characteristics of the person. Infants in general have a fairly high intake, since milk is relatively high in sodium.

The regulatory mechanism for sodium intake comparable to the thirst mechanism for water is poorly developed and poorly responsive to other than gross changes. Nevertheless salt craving does occur in some patients with salt-wasting disorders.

Absorption of sodium occurs throughout the gastrointestinal tract, minimally in the stomach and maximally in the jejunum, probably by way of a sodium-potassium activated ATPase system. This transport mechanism is augmented by aldosterone or desoxycorticosterone acetate (DCA).

Excretion of sodium is primarily by way of the kidney, although some regulation of output can be effected through the varying reabsorptive capacity of the sweat ducts. Sweat sodium concentrations ranging from 10 to 200 mEq. per liter have been observed; cystic fibrosis and Addison's disease are examples of diseases in which there are high values, and sodium depletion, acclimatization, hyperaldosteronism are states characterized by low values.

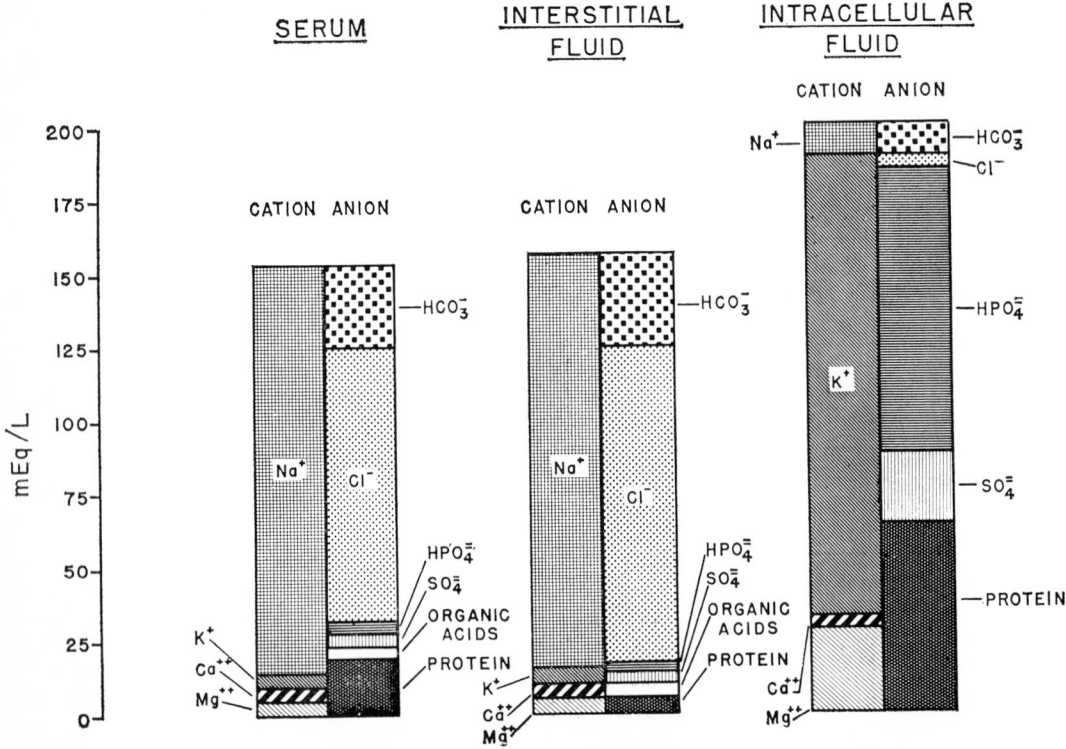

Figure 5-3. Differences in composition of intracellular and extracellular fluids.

The kidney is the principal organ for the facultative regulation of sodium output. The quantity excreted per unit of time is the result of the balance between glomerular and tubular activity. Large reduction in GFR leads to sodium retention unless tubular function is equivalently depressed. This balance is effected in part by extrarenal regulatory mechanisms originating in the macula densa or granular cells of the juxtaglomerular apparatus releasing renin in response to decrease in pressure or in sodium content. Renin converts angiotensin I of the plasma to angiotensin II, which stimulates aldosterone output in addition to producing pressor response. An intrarenal mechanism permits local change in sodium reabsorption independent of the adrenal. Likewise, a rise in GFR increases tubular volume and thereby tubular pressure, which in turn reduces effective filtration pressure and thereby filtration rate—a built-in mechanical feed-back system.

The adrenal cortex plays the large role in regulation of sodium excretion through release of aldosterone in response to changes in volume of body fluids, potassium concentration and ACTH output.

The existence of a sodium-losing hormone originating in the region of the midbrain, or hypothalamic region, which inhibits renal tubular transport of sodium has been demonstrated, but its validity is in question. It is postulated that the elevated concentrations of urinary sodium which occur within water retention, after loading with isotonic saline, or in disease states of the central nervous system or thorax may be the result of the release of this factor.

The measurement of the content of body sodium by radioisotope dilution is complicated by the existence of a sizable pool of slowly exchangeable and nonexchangeable sodium in bone, amounting to as much as 40 per cent of total body sodium, or 25 mEq. per kg. Bone sodium exists as free extracellular sodium, exchangeable sodium adsorbed on bone crystals and nonexchangeable sodium in the crystals. The exchangeable sodium of the body decreases from approximately 85 mEq. per kg. in the fetus to 40 mEq. in the adult. The plasma sodium pool averages 6.5 mEq. per kg.; in interstitial fluid it is 16.8 mEq. Intracellular sodium amounts to only 1.4 mEq. per kg., or 2.4 per cent of total body sodium, and 3.4 per cent of exchangeable sodium. This quantity of sodium may be the result of limitations in the absolute efficiency of the sodium-potassium activated ATPase system which is responsible for the extrusion of sodium from cells. Since cell membranes are relatively permeable to sodium and since sodium concentration is high in extracellular fluid, high intracellular content of sodium accompanied by swelling of the cell is prevented by active transport of sodium outward, potassium remaining intracellularly.

Sodium activation of the enzyme is specific. No other cations can replace sodium in this action, although potassium may be replaced by ammonium, rubidium, cesium and lithium. Magnesium

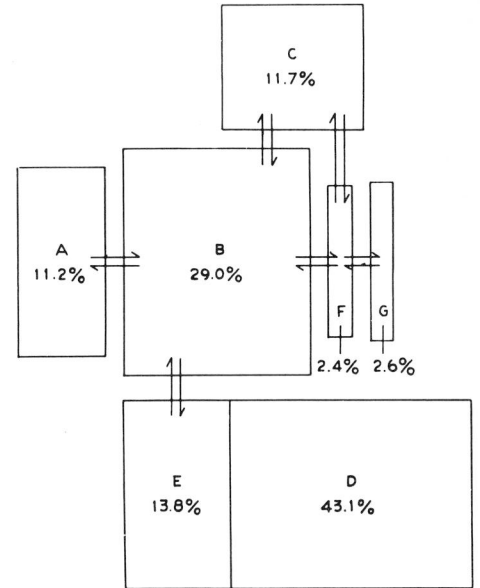

Figure 5-4. Schematic diagram of distribution of sodium within the body of a normal young adult man. *A*, Plasma sodium; *B*, interstitial-lymph sodium; *C*, Dense connective tissue and cartilage sodium; *D*, total bone sodium (including *E*); *E*, exchangeable bone sodium; *F*, intracellular sodium; *G*, transcellular sodium. (From I. S. Edelman and J. Liebman: Anatomy of Body Water and Electrolytes. *Am. J. Med.,* 27:256, 1959.)

is essential for enzyme function at a low level, and calcium inhibits the enzyme, as do ouabain and related cardiac glycosides.

The concentration of sodium in various sites (Fig. 5-4) can be readily calculated from available data on the amounts of sodium and the volume of water in the body compartments. Interstitial sodium concentration is approximately 97 per cent of the plasma sodium value as the result of the Donnan distribution for anionic proteins. The plasma sodium level normally ranges from 142 to 146 mEq. per liter. Intracellular sodium concentration is usually less than 12 mEq. per liter and is a negligible part of the sodium balance, and yet may be critical in modifying certain enzyme activities. Transcellular sodium concentrations vary considerably, indicating that such fluids are not in simple diffusion equilibrium with plasma (Table 5-1).

POTASSIUM

The total potassium content of the adult body approximates 50 mEq. per kg.; exchangeable potassium determined by isotope dilution techniques amounts to 95 per cent of that total. Because potassium is principally intracellular, the change in total potassium content with age and growth is of great interest as an index of cellular mass.

Total body content of potassium is highly cor-

TABLE 5-1. SODIUM, POTASSIUM AND CHLORIDE CONCENTRATIONS IN TRANSCELLULAR FLUIDS

FLUID	SODIUM (mEq./L.)	POTASSIUM (mEq./L.)	CHLORIDE (mEq./L.)
Saliva	33.1 ± 13.4	19.5 ± 3.4	33.9 ± 10.2
Gastric juice	60.4 (9-116)	9.2 (0.5-32.5)	84.0 (7.8-154.5)
Ileal fluid	129.4 (105.4-143.7)	11.2 (5.9-29.3)	116.2 (90-136.4)
Cecal fluid	52.5	7.9	42.5
Pancreatic juice	141.1 (113-153)	4.6 (2.6-7.4)	76.6 (54.1-95.2)
Bile	148.9 (131-164)	4.98 (2.6-12)	100.6 (89-117.6)
Cerebrospinal fluid	140.0 (130-150)	3.3 (2.7-3.9)	126.8 (115.5-132.4)
Aqueous humor (rabbits)	143.0 (141.7-145.0)	4.7	107.9 (106.2-109.5)
Sweat	45.0 (18-97)	4.5 (1-15)	57.5 (18-97)

From I. S. Edelman and J. Liebman: Anatomy of Body Water and Electrolytes. *Am. J. Med.*, 27:256, 1959.

related with body weight and height. Abnormally low amounts of whole body potassium have been demonstrated in a variety of disease states, which include muscular dystrophy, myotonia atrophica, renal tubular disease, and particularly such endocrinopathies as Cushing's disease, aldosteronism and thyrotoxicosis. Increase of total body potassium has not been described and would probably be lethal.

The intake of potassium varies to a large extent with the quantity of food ingested, since it is present in remarkably constant quantities in almost all animal and vegetable tissues. Absorption of potassium is fairly complete in the upper gastrointestinal tract; in the lower tract, potassium from the plasma, however, is exchanged for sodium from the lumen. In this manner sodium is conserved, but large losses of potassium occur in diarrhea, and with chronic catharsis and frequent enemas.

Potassium in sweat varies from 10 to 25 mEq. per liter, possibly being higher in aldosteronism, but losses are not significant.

Excretion by the kidney provides the primary means for regulation of the body's potassium content. Micropuncture studies show that a small but significant fraction of filtered potassium escapes reabsorption. The principal site for excretion is the distal tubule where cellular potassium (transported from plasma potassium) is exchanged for filtered sodium not reabsorbed proximally. Potassium excretion is thus dependent to a large extent on the delivery of sufficient sodium into the proximal tubule for adequate exchange in the distal tubule; a reduction in glomerular filtration will sharply reduce the renal excretion of potassium.

Increase in excretion of potassium may occur during both increased and decreased excretion of sodium. This paradox may be explained by assuming that 2 factors are operative in potassium exchange: (1) the number (and possibly the concentration) of sodium ions reaching the exchange site — "the mass factor"; (2) the degree of substitution of potassium for a given number of sodium ions — "the percentage factor." If sodium diuresis occurs, potassium output increases (unless potassium exchange is blocked as in mercurial diuresis), since the opportunity for contact with exchange sites is greatly increased. If the supply of intracellular potassium is abundant, exchange of potassium increases and effects a decrease in sodium excretion.

Aldosterone plays a large role in potassium regulation in the kidney and in other tissues as well. Aldosterone injected intravenously into a patient with Addison's disease reduces urinary excretion of sodium and increases the excretion of potassium perceptibly, possibly by increasing the permeability of the luminal border of the distal tubule to sodium and increasing the opportunity for exchange of it with intracellular potassium. The control of aldosterone secretion and the feedback mechanisms involved permit immediate and delayed adjustments to electrolyte loads, thereby stabilizing body composition.

When a load of sodium is administered, excretion of potassium increases immediately. The excreted potassium comes from renal tubular cells, which in turn remove potassium from the plasma. The fall in concentration of plasma potassium, as well as the rise in effective circulating volume caused by the intake of sodium, decreases adrenal cortical secretion of aldosterone. If renal tubular permeability to sodium is decreased by a fall in aldosterone levels, exchange of hydrogen ions and potassium for sodium decreases and sodium excretion rises as potassium excretion falls. Likewise, reduced exchange of plasma potassium for sodium in the gastrointestinal tract tends to restore body composition toward normal.

On the other hand, depletion of sodium by extrarenal routes such as in diarrhea leads to reduction in the quantity of sodium reaching exchange sites for potassium in the distal tubules, particularly if the glomerular filtration rate is lowered by concomitant circulatory insufficiency. The fall in extracellular volume and probably the rise in potassium concentration under these circumstances effect an increase in aldosterone secretion. The elevated levels of aldosterone not only permit conservation of sodium, but also facilitate excretion of potassium. Increased gastrointestinal conservation of sodium and excretion of potassium also occur.

When a load of potassium is administered, sodium loss occurs immediately, and depletion of sodium would result except for a rise in aldosterone output. The increase in concentration of plasma potassium resulting from such a load, as well as the reduction in extracellular volume from loss of sodium, stimulates secretion of aldosterone. Elevated levels of aldosterone result in conservation of sodium and facilitate the excretion of potassium by increasing exchange of them in the distal tubule. The action of aldosterone on the gastrointestinal tract limits potassium absorption and conserves body sodium.

Depletion of the body's potassium results in a reduction of aldosterone output, so that potassium exchange in the renal tubule and potassium loss into the gastrointestinal tract are lessened and the body's composition of potassium tends to return toward normal.

Thus the immediate effect of loads of sodium or of potassium is an increase in the urinary excretion of the other ion. Depletion of the ion whose supply is limited is prevented by alterations in the output of aldosterone.

The bulk of body potassium is intracellular, particularly in muscle (Fig. 5-5), amounting to 48 mEq. per kg., whereas extracellular potassium amounts to only 5.5 mEq. per kg. (4 mEq. of which is in bone). The concentration of potassium in cells approximates 146 mEq. per liter of cell water; extracellular concentrations approximate 4 to 5 mEq. per liter. Most of the intracellular potassium is unbound and osmotically active, but sequestration by active transport in subcellular particles such as mitochondria is likely.

The relation of extracellular to intracellular potassium concentration is of vital importance to cell function. External losses of potassium lead to a shift of cellular potassium to the extracellular phase. Intracellular potassium under these circumstances is replaced in part by sodium, hydrogen ions and dibasic amino acids. When the change occurs in the kidney, the excessive loss of intracellular hydrogen in exchange for sodium in the tubular fluid results in paradoxical aciduria and excretion of ammonia. The result is extracellular alkalosis.

Concentrations of potassium in extracellular fluid are affected by alterations in pH. Acidosis (lowered pH) leads to a rise in plasma potassium, and alkalosis causes a decrease of it. Further, alterations in cellular metabolism or in oxygenation may lead to a shift of potassium to the plasma.

Hypokalemia produces functional alterations in the heart, skeletal muscle, smooth muscle, kidney and possibly the brain. The effects on muscle are probably dependent on the rate of percentage change and are manifested by weakness and characteristic electrocardiographic changes (see p. 954).

Potassium deficiency leads to a characteristic vacuolar change in the convoluted tubular epithelium of the kidney and if maintained for a long time contributes to nephrosclerosis, interstitial fibrosis and pyelonephritis. Functionally, nephropathy associated with potassium deficiency is characterized by reduced clearance of free water (TcH_2O); concentrating ability is markedly reduced and diluting capability is somewhat reduced, resulting in polyuria and polydipsia. Bicarbonate reabsorption and hydrogen ion secretion are increased and lead to alkalosis.

Elevations of serum potassium lead to alterations in cardiac function with characteristic changes in the electrocardiogram (p. 954), except in newborn infants, in whom high serum values of potassium may be observed in association with electrocardiographic findings of hypokalemia.

CALCIUM

The metabolism of this divalent ion is discussed in other sections of this book (see Tetany, Rickets, and Metabolic Disorders of Bone). It is considered here briefly because of its interrelations with other electrolytes. Ninety-nine per cent of the body's calcium is in bone at all ages. The bones of infants are less densely mineralized than those of adults; there are approximately 400 mEq. per kg. of calcium in the infant and about 950 mEq. in the adult.

The regulation of body calcium content is primarily by way of the gastrointestinal tract, not the kidney. Through an obscure feed-back mechanism, shortage of bone mineral elicits an increase in intestinal absorption of calcium in the presence of vitamin D. Low calcium intake, pregnancy, vitamin D or parathormone also lead to increased intestinal absorption of ingested calcium. Altera-

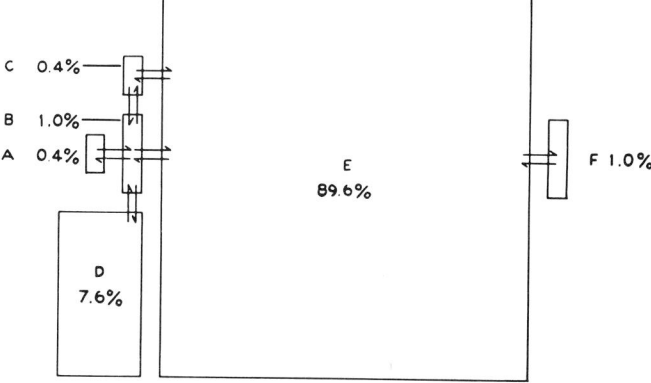

Figure 5-5. Schematic diagram of distribution of potassium within the body of a normal young adult man. *A*, Plasma potassium; *B*, interstitial-lymph potassium; *C*, dense connective tissue and cartilage potassium; *D*, bone potassium; *E*, intracellular potassium; *F*, transcellular potassium. (From I. S. Edelman and J. Liebman: Anatomy of Body Water and Electrolytes. *Am. J. Med.*, 27:256, 1959.)

C 0.4%
B 1.0%
A 0.4%
E 89.6%
F 1.0%
D 7.6%

tions leading to hypercalcemia occur in sarcoidosis, carcinomatosis and multiple myeloma.

Renal excretion of calcium is a small factor in the maintenance of calcium balance. Urinary output increases during hypercalcemia and particularly during chronic acidosis, in which loss of bone salts may produce growth retardation. Parathyroid hormone increases calcium reabsorption by the renal tubules, partially accounting for the elevation of serum calcium in hyperparathyroidism.

Calcium loading increases renal excretion of sodium and potassium and produces a profound reduction in ability to concentrate the urine in association with a diminution of TcH$_2$O.

The remarkable aspect of calcium metabolism is the constancy of the extracellular and plasma calcium pools and the constancy of plasma calcium concentrations despite fairly free exchange with the enormous reservoir of calcium in bone. The concentration of plasma calcium is maintained at 2.5 millimoles per liter (10 mg. per 100 ml.) with 40 to 45 per cent of this calcium bound to protein, so that the calcium level of the protein-free interstitial fluid is about 1.5 millimoles per liter (6 mg. per 100 ml.). The degree of protein binding is influenced by changes in hydrogen ion activity of plasma, but the effects are not clinically significant even in severe acidosis or alkalosis. A pH change of 1.0 unit alters the ionized calcium concentration by only 10 per cent (less than 0.2 millimole per liter or less than 0.5 mg. per 100 ml.).

The balance between deposition and mobilization of calcium in bone determines to a large extent the concentration of plasma calcium. Parathyroid hormone and thyrocalcitonin play opposing roles in modulating changes in the concentration of extracellular calcium.

The concentrations of sodium and potassium play some role in this balance, since treatment of hypernatremia with fluids low in potassium content frequently leads to hypocalcemia.

MAGNESIUM

Magnesium is the fourth most abundant cation in the body, and the key bulk electrolyte affecting cellular enzymatic activity (Fig. 5-6). The total body content of magnesium is about 2000 mEq. in a 70-kg. man. (The contents of calcium, sodium and potassium are approximately 60,000, 5500 and 3000, respectively.) The infant's body contains approximately 220 mEq. per kg.; the adult's, 280 mEq. The intake of magnesium ranges from 10 to 25 mEq. per day, depending on age; more is required during periods of rapid growth.

Approximately 70 per cent of the intake is lost in the feces. Vitamin D increases absorption of magnesium, and increased calcium intake tends to decrease absorption of magnesium. Increased intestinal motility increases stool losses of magnesium.

Urinary excretion of magnesium amounts to about one third of the intake and is increased by calcium loading. Parathyroid hormone increases tubular reabsorption of filtered magnesium, which can be almost complete when the intake of magnesium is very low. Low concentrations of serum magnesium increase the release of parathyroid hormone, thereby decreasing urinary losses of magnesium and elevating plasma concentration of calcium.

Sixty per cent of the body's magnesium is in bone; the remaining portion is intracellular. Extracellular magnesium accounts for only 1 per cent of the total.

Magnesium in red blood cells varies considerably with their age; it is highest in reticulocytes.

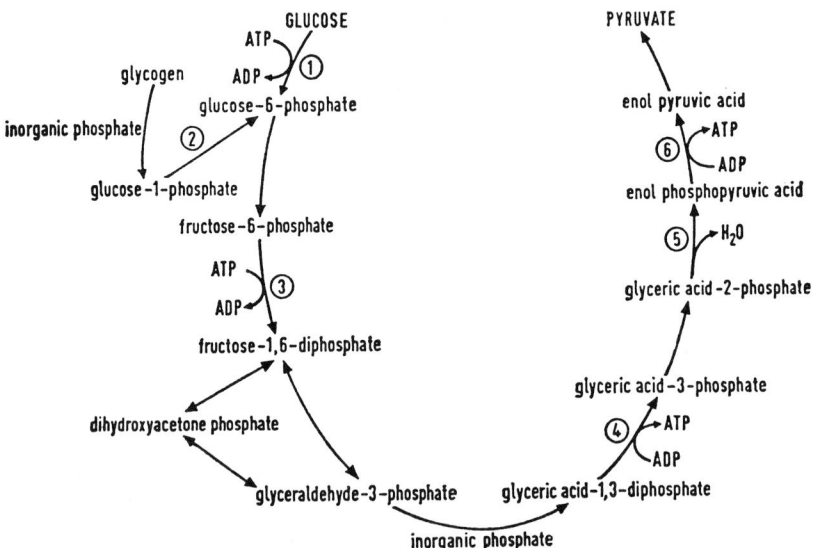

Figure 5-6. Stages of glycolysis activated by magnesium ions. (From I. MacIntyre: Magnesium Metabolism. *Advances Int. Med.,* 13:143, 1967.)

Nucleic acid and lipoproteins bind magnesium, so that in muscle approximately 30 per cent, or 6.8 mEq. per 100 gm., is free. Despite free exchangeability by isotope methods, much of the intracellular magnesium is not free for exchange with plasma magnesium, whereas bone magnesium is. Largely through renal regulation, plasma magnesium is normally maintained at 1.5 to 1.8 mEq. per liter; 60 to 85 per cent of this magnesium is ultrafilterable. Unfortunately, the concentration of magnesium in the plasma is not a reliable indication of magnesium depletion. Reduction in the concentration of plasma magnesium may occur in the absence of appreciable magnesium losses, and conversely the plasma concentration may be normal during magnesium depletion.

Experimental magnesium deficiency leads to hypercalcemia, slight reduction in the content of muscle magnesium (in growing animals the deficiency is severe) and a reduction in the content of muscle potassium. The most prominent pathologic change is calcification of the kidney. Clinically, intense vasodilatation occurs, and audiogenic seizures result.

In human magnesium deficiency, particularly in severe nutritional insufficiency such as kwashiorkor, the content of magnesium in muscle is decreased. Hypomagnesemia occurs in a variety of clinical states, especially in adults with alcoholism, malabsorption syndromes, hypoparathyroidism, diuretic therapy, hypercalcemia, tubular acidosis, primary aldosteronism and prolonged fluid therapy. The symptoms are primarily those of increased neuromuscular irritability, tetany, severe seizures, tremors and occasionally electrocardiographic alterations and changes in cardiac function. Hypermagnesemia with serum levels in excess of 5 mEq. per liter occurs rarely in Addison's disease and in acute renal failure; it is usually iatrogenic in origin from treatment of hypertension or use of magnesium sulfate orally or in enemas for megacolon. Depression of deep tendon reflexes usually antedates respiratory depression, drowsiness and coma. Symptoms are rapidly reversed by intravenous administration of calcium.

HYDROGEN ION

(ACID-BASE BALANCE)

The availability of apparatus for determination of the blood gases in small samples of blood and the demonstration of the clinical significance of acidosis in respiratory distress of the newborn and in cardiovascular surgery have led to increased awareness of clinical problems related to hydrogen ion activity of body fluids. The subject has been obscured over the years by a confusion of terminologies, each with a reasonable but conflicting approach. The older terminology which referred to fixed cations such as sodium and potassium as bases, and chloride and phosphate as anions had value in clinical thought, but alienated students of modern chemistry. The terminology used here is that agreed upon recently under the auspices of the New York Academy of Sciences.

The Brønsted-Lowry terminology puts emphasis in acid-base balance on the hydrogen ion, which is a hydrogen atom with its neutralizing electron removed. An acid is a proton (hydrogen ion) donor; a base, a hydrogen ion acceptor. Sodium, potassium, calcium, magnesium and chloride are "aprotes."

The amount of potential hydrogen ion in the body is very large. The rate of formation and removal also is enormous, but the concentration of free hydrogen ion is very low. Table 5-2 illustrates the quantities of hydrogen ions, potential and free in the body. These quantities are related to size as well as metabolic turnover. The largest part of the hydrogen ion pool of the body is not in free form, but is bound to many buffers of the body—bicarbonate, phosphate and proteins—producing neutral salts and a weak, poorly dissociated acid.

$$\boxed{H+}\ A^- + B^+Buf^- \rightarrow B^+A^- + \boxed{H} \cdot Buf$$

$$\boxed{H+}\ A^- + B^+HCO_3 \rightarrow B^+A^- + \boxed{H} \cdot HCO_3$$

$$\boxed{H+}\ A^- + B_2{}^+HPO_4{}^{--} \rightarrow B^+A^- + B^+ \boxed{H}\ HPO_4$$

$$\boxed{H+}\ A^- + B^+Prot.^- \rightarrow B^+A^- + \boxed{H} \cdot Prot.$$

A buffer is defined as a substance which reduces the change in free hydrogen ion concentration of a solution upon the addition of an acid or base. Since the dissociation constants of the weak acids of the buffer pair are very small, the change in concentration of free hydrogen ion is minimized.

Bound hydrogen ions and buffers are distributed throughout the intracellular and extracellular fluids. Hydrogen ion exchanges with cations such as sodium and potassium in both extracellular and intracellular spaces, thereby speeding the change in hydrogen ion concentration over a large volume and quantity of buffer. The principal buffer of extracellular fluid is the bicarbonate-carbonic acid system. The principal buffer of urine is the inorganic mono- and di-hydrogen phosphate system. The principal buffers of intracellular fluid are various proteins, organic phosphates and other micromolecules. Each is discussed below in relation to regulation of free hydrogen ion concentration.

TABLE 5-2. APPROXIMATE ORDER OF MAGNITUDE OF CERTAIN FACTORS IN HYDROGEN ION METABOLISM IN STANDARD MAN OF 1.73 M^2

Total CO_2 turnover	24,000 mM./24 hr.
Total hydrogen turnover	69 mEq./24 hr.
Total buffer in body	2100 mEq.
Total hydrogen in buffer (max. capacity)	700 mEq.
Total hydrogen in buffer (normal amount)	105 mEq.
Total free H$^+$ in body fluids	0.0021 mEq.

From J. R. Elkington: Hydrogen Ion Turnover in Health and in Renal Disease. *Ann. Int. Med.*, 57:660, 1962.

The daily turnover of hydrogen ions is large, amounting to more than half of the hydrogen ion usually present in the body buffers and one tenth the maximum storage capacity of the buffer. Hydrogen ions are produced from 3 sources:

1. When carbohydrates, fats and organic acids such as pyruvic, lactic, acetoacetic and citric acids are completely catabolized, there is no excess hydrogen ion produced, since water and carbon dioxide are the final reaction products of complete oxidation of these compounds. Incomplete metabolism adds hydrogen ions.

2. Protein is the largest source, resulting primarily from the oxidation of sulfur-containing amino acids yielding sulfuric acid.

3. The oxidation and hydrolysis of phosphoproteins also yield phosphoric acid. Sources 2 and 3 make up the acid ash residues of milk and meat diets, amounting to 50 to 70 mEq. of hydrogen ion per day or 65 per cent of the total. The balance of the hydrogen ion comes from source 1 (Table 5-3).

The disposition of hydrogen ion of metabolic origin is almost entirely by the kidney. With vomiting or gastric drainage, some hydrogen ion could be lost, and in diarrhea some hydrogen acceptors could be lost as well, but the main output is by way of the kidney.

The renal mechanisms for the excretion of potential or free hydrogen ion are highly developed, energy-requiring, active transport processes in contrast to the pulmonary excretion of carbon dioxide, which is by simple passive diffusion (Fig. 5-7).

The renal mechanisms by which hydrogen ion is excreted depend upon exchange of hydrogen ion for filtered sodium. This process is driven by the "sodium pump" in the proximal tubule, hydrogen ion diffusing into the lumen down an electrochemical gradient. Bicarbonate moving transcellularly is derived from carbon dioxide (Fig. 5-8). Hydrogen ion excretion in the distal tubule is by active secretion in exchange for sodium; hydrogen ions and potassium ions probably compete for available sodium within the lumen. The transport of hydrogen ion is limited at this site, not by a Tm or rate of transport, but rather by a concentration gradient or limit of hydrogen ion concentration against which hydrogen ion can be transferred.

Two systems facilitate hydrogen ion transport at this point by reducing the gradient. The first is passive and is due to the presence of phosphate buffer (and other buffers to a lesser extent), which reduces the lowering of hydrogen ion concentration in response to the secretion of hydrogen ion. The second process is active and requires work involving the synthesis of ammonia, a hydrogen ion acceptor or base, from glutamine through the action of glutaminase. Ammonia diffuses through the lipid membrane of cells and reacts with hydrogen ion to form ionized ammonium ion, NH_4^+, which cannot readily diffuse back from luminal fluid.

These 2 processes, by reducing the rise in hydrogen ion concentration, permit an increased exchange of hydrogen ion for sodium in the distal renal tubule.

The failure to add adequate hydrogen ion leads to excretion of bicarbonate without hydrogen ion and a net gain of H^+ ions in the body. Thus the absolute net rate of excretion by the kidney of metabolic hydrogen may be measured by the sum of the excretion rates of titratable acid (TA) plus ammonium ion minus bicarbonate:

$$U\,V_H{}^+ = UV_{TA} + UV_{NH4}{}^+ - uV_{HCO3}{}^-$$

where U represents volume per unit time and V represents concentration of the respective substances.

Reduction in renal function can thereby lead to an accumulation of hydrogen ion of metabolic origin by means of several factors. In predominantly tubular disease, hydrogen ion secretion is reduced because of inability to transport hydrogen ion against a concentration gradient. With the

TABLE 5-3. PREDICTED AND OBSERVED MOIETIES OF PRODUCTION AND EXCRETION OF HYDROGEN ION IN SUBJECTS INGESTING A NORMAL DIET

URINARY EXCRETION	PREDICTED FROM THEORETICAL NORMAL DIET* (mEq./24 hr./1.73 m²)	OBSERVED AVERAGE IN 7 SUBJECTS ON AD LIBITUM NORMAL DIET† (mEq./24 hr./1.73 m²)
Sulfate—80% from diet	38 (55%)	39 (65%)
Organic acids from diet	31	(21)
Total H⁺ from diet	69	60
Total phosphate from diet (mM)	28	28
Acid phosphate from diet at pH 7.4	6	
Acid phosphate from diet at pH 5.8	26	26
Increase in $H_2PO_4^-$	20	
Titratable acidity		30
Ammonium		31
Bicarbonate		1

*Protein (lean beef) 70 gm., fat 190 gm., carbohydrate 250 gm., calories 3100.
†Data from study of author and colleagues, *Am. J. Med.*, 29:554, 1960.
From J. R. Elkinton: Hydrogen Ion Turnover in Health and in Renal Disease. *Ann. Int. Med.*, 57:660, 1962.

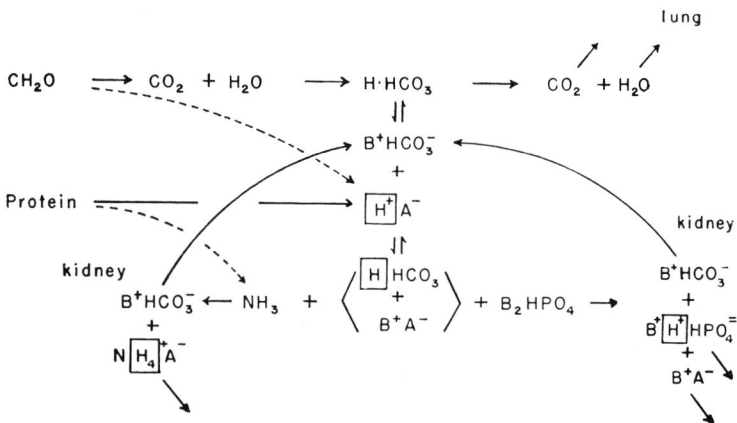

Figure 5-7. Hydrogen ion turnover. Summary of the pathways of metabolic hydrogen production, buffering, transport and excretion. (From J. R. Elkinton: Hydrogen Ion Turnover in Health and in Renal Disease. *Ann. Int. Med.*, 57:660, 1962.)

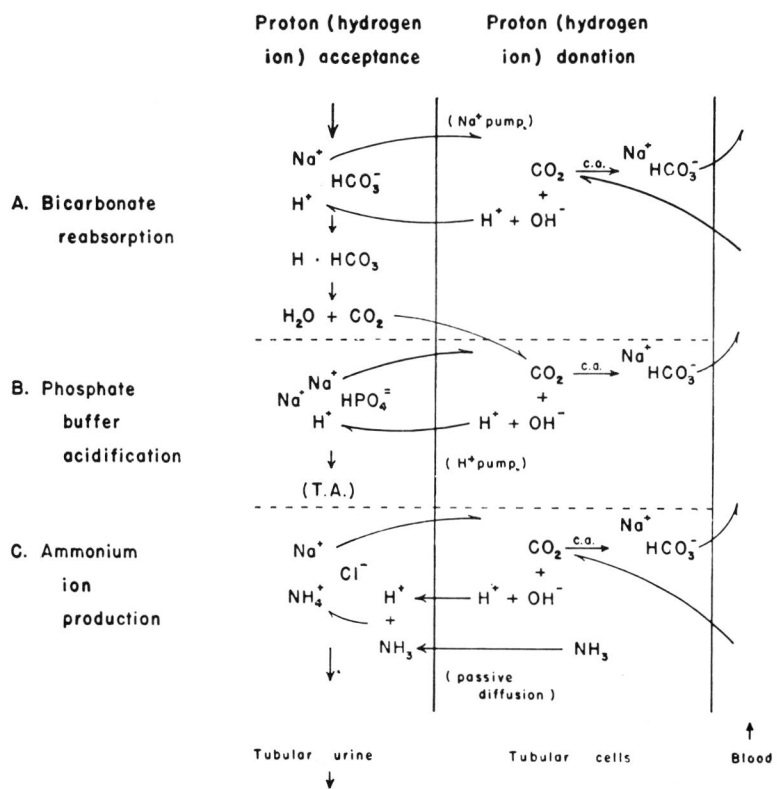

Figure 5-8. Intrarenal processes of hydrogen ion exchange and excretion. (From J. R. Elkinton: Hydrogen Ion Turnover in Health and in Renal Disease. *Ann. Int. Med.*, 57:660, 1962.)

administration of large amounts of phosphate intravenously or by mouth, titratable acid (buffered acid) may be increased with only slight increases in hydrogen ion concentration. Low urine pH (pH less than 5.5) is rarely seen in pure renal tubular acidosis. Rarely reduction in ammonia synthesis, as in the cerebro-oculo-renal syndrome of Lowe, occurs.

Reduction in production of ammonia either as a specific disorder or owing to a loss of nephrons (thereby also reducing the capacity to secrete hydrogen ions) leads to cessation of hydrogen ion secretion because H^+ ion concentration rises rapidly to the level that inhibits further H^+ ion transport.

A low glomerular filtration rate, as in the newborn, limits the renal capacity to excrete hydrogen ion by reducing the filtered load of phosphate. With the bulk of phosphate thereby reabsorbed in the proximal tubule, little is left for buffering of added hydrogen ion in the distal tubule. Hydrogen ion transport is thus reduced by rapid attainment of a maximal concentration gradient in the absence of buffer.

Free hydrogen ion concentration is maintained at a very low but constant level in extracellular fluid (0.00398 mM per liter at pH 7.40) despite the production of hydrogen ion of metabolic origin and the production of enormous quantities of carbon dioxide. This essential homeostasis is the result of the unique properties of the bicarbonate-carbonic acid buffer system and a highly developed respiratory control mechanism. The weak acid of the bicarbonate-carbonic acid system is volatile and has a relatively low solubility coefficient in body fluids.

$$H_2CO_3 = CO_2 + H_2O$$

$$H_2CO_3 = \alpha\, pCO_2$$

where α represents solubility coefficient.

$$H^+ = K \times \frac{H_2CO_3}{HCO_3} \quad \text{by the law of mass action}$$

$$\log H^+ = \log k + \log \frac{H_2CO_3}{HCO_3^-}$$

$$pH = \log 1/H^+$$

$$pK = \log 1/K$$

then

$$pH = pK + \log \frac{HCO_3^-}{H_2CO_3} \quad \text{(Henderson-Hasselbalch equation)}$$

When the rate of pulmonary excretion of carbon dioxide differs from the rate of production of carbon dioxide, the ratio of H_2CO_3/HCO_3^- changes, and the free hydrogen ion concentration changes.

The measurement of free hydrogen ion concentration in various body compartments is extremely difficult. The glass electrode measures hydrogen ion activity; an activity coefficient of 1 is assumed in all calculations. pH can also be calculated if pCO_2 and bicarbonate concentrations are known.

Likewise, pCO_2 can be calculated if pH and HCO_3^- are measured.

The following definitions are helpful in understanding the use of apparatus such as the Astrup and in interpreting laboratory data.

1. *Total carbon dioxide concentration* is the carbon dioxide extractable from a biologic fluid in the presence of a strong acid. This represents the following known chemical species: dissolved carbon dioxide, carbonic acid, bicarbonate ion, carbonate ion, carbamino compounds. Usual units are millimoles per liter.

2. *Partial pressure of carbon dioxide, the carbon dioxide tension of biologic fluids,* is the partial pressure of carbon dioxide in a gas phase in equilibrium with the biologic fluid. The symbols are Pco_2 or pCO_2. Usual units are mm. Hg.

3. *Carbonic acid concentration* is the concentration of the chemical species, H_2CO_3. In biologic fluids the concentration of this species is quantitatively negligible in comparison with dissolved carbon dioxide concentration. Usual units are millimoles per liter.

4. *Dissolved carbon dioxide concentration* is strictly the concentration of the physically dissolved gas, but carbonic acid, H_2CO_3, is usually included. The sum is designated as $S \times Pco_2$, where S is the coefficient relating the sum of the concentrations of dissolved carbon dioxide and H_2CO_3 in millimoles per liter to pCO_2 in mm. Hg. The value of S is temperature-dependent.

5. *Bicarbonate ion concentration.* The strict chemical definition is the concentration of the HCO_3^- ion in a biologic fluid. But in physiologic studies, bicarbonate ion concentration is calculated as total carbon dioxide concentration minus $S \times Pco_2$. Thus the physiologic usage includes carbamino compounds, and carbonate plus bicarbonate, whereas the chemical definition does not.

In the definitions which follow, the term "bicarbonate" is used in the physiologic sense. The error introduced by this approximation is small in plasma and extracellular fluid, but large in intracellular fluid. Units are millimoles per liter or mEq. per liter.

6. *Standard bicarbonate concentration* is the plasma bicarbonate ion concentration in the plasma from whole blood that has been equilibrated to a Pco_2 of 40 mm. Hg at 37°C. (As defined originally by Jorgensen and Astrup, the temperature of equilibration was 38°C.) Units are mEq. per liter.

7. *Carbon dioxide-combining power* is the total carbon dioxide concentration of anaerobically separated plasma equilibrated to a Pco_2 of 40 mm. Hg at room temperature. (This determination is no longer generally used because it is too dependent upon the conditions in the blood when plasma is separated.) Usual units are millimoles per liter.

8. *Buffer base* is, in Brønsted terminology, the sum of concentrations of the buffer anions of whole blood bicarbonate, plasma proteins, hemoglobin. Units are mEq. per liter.

9. *Base excess* is the base concentration in mEq.

per liter of whole blood as measured by titration with strong acid to pH 7.40 at a Pco$_2$ of 40 mm. Hg at 37°C. For negative values of base excess the titration is carried out with strong base. Negative values can be denoted by the term "base deficit." Units are mEq. per liter.

Clinical disturbances in pH can be described in terms of 2 approaches using either the whole blood base excess (Fig. 5-9) or the bicarbonate concentration. The latter is defended strongly by most experts as being the least misleading in the interpretation of physiologic processes.

Fortunately, there is complete agreement that pCO$_2$ is the only adequate measure of the respiratory component. Accumulation of carbon dioxide (pCO$_2$ greater than 40 mm. Hg) is considered respiratory acidosis (tendency of pH to fall). Excessive ventilation leads to rising pH (respiratory alkalosis). Accumulation of hydrogen ion of metabolic origin (without equivalent amounts of bicarbonate) leads to metabolic acidosis. Loss of hydrogen ion (without equivalent amounts of bicarbonate) leads to metabolic alkalosis. The respiratory disturbances may have fairly complete compensation (restoration of pH toward normal) by renal mechanisms, and metabolic abnormalities may be compensated by respiratory changes in pCO$_2$. Mixed disturbances can occur, as in the respiratory distress syndrome, in which metabolic and respiratory acidosis often coexist.

The effects of extracellular acidosis and alkalosis are not yet fully understood. Low pH produces a slight change in the Donnan distribution across the capillary membrane, so that some decrease in oncotic pressure results with reduction in plasma volume. Low pH also seems to reduce myocardial contractility and impairs catecholamine

action and increases the likelihood of arrhythmia, particularly with hypoxia.

The hydrogen ion concentration of the cerebrospinal fluid does not change instantaneously with change in extracellular pH. Increases or decreases in carbon dioxide tension of blood are reflected in similar changes in cerebrospinal fluid. Increases or decreases in bicarbonate concentration in blood lead to only small and delayed changes in the bicarbonate concentration in cerebrospinal fluid, so that pH of each fluid at times may differ significantly, particularly if active respiratory compensation of the metabolic disturbance has occurred. These alterations in cerebrospinal fluid free hydrogen ion concentration may lead occasionally to abnormalities in respiration in acute situations, but rarely in chronic ones.

Intracellular pH is maintained at a lower level (pH 6.8) than that of extracellular fluid, and mitochondrial pH may be even lower. Intracellular changes in hydrogen ion concentration may occur as a result of hypercapnia or hypocapnia. Intracellular alkalosis as measured by the DMO method after hypocapnia is proportional to the degree of extracellular alkalosis, whereas intracellular acidosis after hypercapnia is more marked than the extracellular changes. Likewise, metabolic disturbances lead to an alteration in exchange of sodium and potassium for hydrogen ion, and deficiency of potassium may result in a decrease in the intracellular pH, when extracellular pH is elevated.

Changes in intracellular pH should affect the activities of many enzymes. Decrease in carbohydrate tolerance has been observed in acidosis, and increase in neuromuscular irritability (latent or manifest tetany) occurs in alkalosis. Hypo-

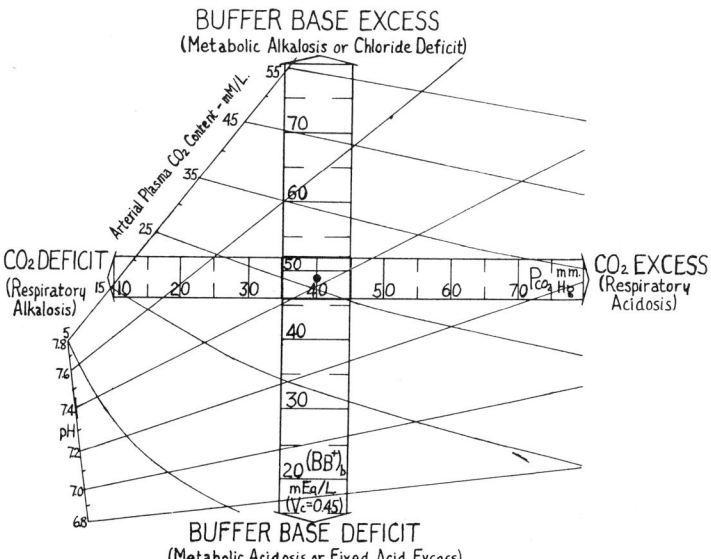

Figure 5-9.   Diagram of disturbances in pH. (From R. B. Singer: A New Diagram for the Visualization and Interpretation of Acid-Base Changes. *Am. J. M. Sc.*, 221:199, 1951.)

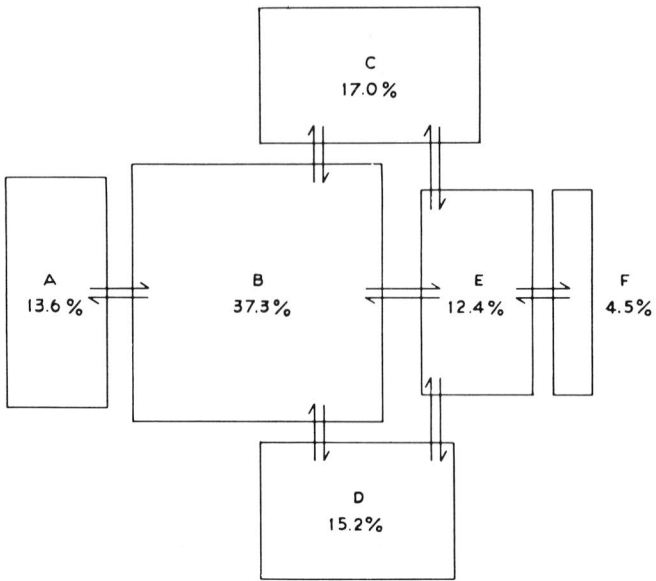

Figure 5-10. Schematic diagram of distribution of chloride within the body of a normal young adult man. *A*, Plasma chloride; *B*, interstitial-lymph chloride; *C*, dense connective tissue and cartilage chloride; *D*, bone chloride; *E*, intracellular chloride; *F*, transcellular chloride. (From I. S. Edelman and J. Liebman: Anatomy of Body Water and Electrolytes. *Am. J. Med.*, 27:256, 1959.)

capnia leads to an increase in blood lactic acid with a decrease in bicarbonate concentration and production of acidosis of metabolic origin.

CHLORIDE

Chloride is the bulk anion of extracellular fluid. As an aprote it is not directly involved in the regulation of free hydrogen ion concentration. Nevertheless, as metabolic adjustments within the kidney are made on the basis of plasma levels of bicarbonate through secretion of hydrogen ions, the concentration of chloride generally changes reciprocally.

Total body chloride amounts to 33 mEq. per kg.; almost all chloride is in the extracellular and transcellular fluid, except for small quantities in red blood cells and connective tissue. Exchangeable chloride as determined by isotope dilution or with bromide is in a fairly straight-line relation to age.

Since chloride concentration is relatively constant with age, extracellular volume bears a close relation to weight, height, age, bone age, lean body mass and other parameters. The distribution of body chloride is presented schematically in Figure 5-10.

The intake and output of chloride parallel those of sodium. The transport of chloride, however, is to a large extent passive and down an electrochemical gradient created in part by sodium transport.

Chloride may be lost in excess of sodium and

potassium in vomitus or gastric drainage. Chloride may be conserved in excess of sodium and potassium by the kidney with the formation of alkaline urine in the renal correction of alkalosis. Chloride may be excreted in excess of sodium and potassium through the substitution of hydrogen ion and ammonium ion for fixed cations in the renal correction of acidosis.

Although chloride is described as playing a secondary role in body physiology, ample evidence exists that correction of alkalosis with or without potassium deficiency requires an abundance of chloride. Renal chloride wasting is excessive in potassium deficiency, and both potassium and chloride should be given in correction of deficits of each.

PHOSPHORUS

Inorganic phosphate is present at relatively low concentrations in extracellular fluid and even lower in intracellular fluid despite massive quantities of it in bone salts. Organic phosphates exist as sources of energy in all cells of the body. The largest quantities exist in muscle as creatine phosphate, ATP and glycogen. The principal sources of phosphorus are milk and meat proteins. Excessive quantities of calcium interfere with intestinal absorption of phosphorus, forming insoluble complexes; likewise, large amounts of phosphorus interfere with absorption of calcium.

The excretion of phosphorus is by glomerular filtration with facultative reabsorption by the proximal tubule. Parathyroid hormone reduces the tubular maximum (TmP) for phosphorus reabsorption, so that there is hyperphosphatemia in hypoparathyroidism. Reduction in the glomerular filtration rate below 25 per cent rapidly leads to an elevated concentration of plasma inorganic phosphate. Vitamin D is necessary for appropriate tubular transport of phosphorus; and hypophosphatemia is characteristic of vitamin D deficiency rickets and of vitamin D-resistant rickets.

In the young infant glomerular filtration (GFR) is low in relation to active cell mass, and the dietary phosphorus intake is high; consequently plasma inorganic phosphorus is high. The premature infant has plasma concentrations ranging from 2.5 to 3.0 millimoles per liter (7.5 to 9.0 mg. per 100 ml.), whereas in the adult the concentration is 1.0 to 1.3 millimoles (3 to 4 mg.). Hence reduction in GFR or relative hypoparathyroidism in infants rapidly leads to very high plasma values of phosphate, with depression of calcium concentration and latent or manifest tetany as a consequence. The plasma deficit of calcium results from its formation into bone salts.

Secondary hyperparathyroidism may occur as the result of reduction in GFR. In rare instances of chronic glomerular insufficiency, the parathyroid hyperfunction may continue unregulated, and so-called tertiary hyperparathyroidism may develop (see p. 1203).

Inorganic phosphorus serves a critical function as the principal urinary buffer in the regulation of free hydrogen ions (see above). Intracellularly it serves as the source of phosphorus for high-energy synthesis of ATP. Lowering of serum phosphorus is observed in the treatment of diabetic ketosis, as carbohydrate is phosphorylated in the formation of glycogen. The clinical significance of this phenomenon is not known, but efforts should probably be made in therapy to minimize this decrease.

REFERENCES

Ad Hoc Committee on Acid-Base Terminology: Report. *Ann. New York Acad. Sc.,* 133:251, 1966.

Bleich, H. L., Berkman, P. M., and Schwartz, W. B.: The Response of Cerebrospinal Fluid Composition to Sustained Hypercapnia. *J. Clin. Invest.,* 43:11, 1964.

Brooks, C. M., Kao, F. F., and Lloyd, B. B. (Eds.): *Cerebrospinal Fluid and the Regulation of Ventilation.* Philadelphia, F. A. Davis Company, 1965.

Cheek, D. B. (Ed.): *Human Growth.* Philadelphia, Lea & Febiger, 1968.

Cooke, R. E. (Ed.): *The Biologic Basis of Pediatric Practice.* New York, McGraw-Hill Book Company, Inc., 1968.

Cooke, R. E., and Ottenheimer, E. J., Jr.: Clinical and Experimental Interrelations of Sodium and the Central Nervous System. *Advances in Pediatrics,* 11:81, 1960.

Darrow, D. C.: *A Guide to Learning Fluid Therapy.* Springfield, Ill., Charles C Thomas, 1964.

Edelman, I. S., and Liebman, J.: Anatomy of Body Water and Electrolytes. *Am. J. Med.,* 27:256, 1959.

Elkinton, J. R.: Hydrogen Ion Turnover in Health and in Renal Disease. *Ann. Int. Med.,* 57:660, 1962.

Kassirer, J. P., Berkman, P. M., Lawrenz, D. R., and Schwartz, W. B.: The Critical Role of Chloride in the Correction of Hypokalemic Alkalosis in Man. *Am. J. Med.,* 38:172, 1965.

Katz, A. I., and Epstein, F. H.: Physiologic Role of Sodium-Potassium-Activated Adenosine Triphosphatase in the Transport of Cations Across Biologic Membranes. *New England J. Med.,* 278:253, 1968.

Leaf, A.: The Clinical and Physiologic Significance of the Serum Sodium Concentration. *New England J. Med.,* 267:24, 1962.

MacIntyre, I.: Magnesium Metabolism. *Advances Int. Med.,* 13:143, 1967.

Metcoff, J.: Regulation of the body fluids; in R. E. Cooke (Ed.): *The Biologic Basis of Pediatric Practice.* New York, McGraw-Hill Book Company, Inc., 1968, pp. 95-134.

Schwartz, W. B., and Relman, A. S.: A Critique of the Parameters Used in the Evaluation of Acid-Base Disorders. *New England J. Med.,* 268:1382, 1963.

Schwartz, W. B., and Relman, A. S.: Effects of Electrolyte Disorders on Renal Structure and Function. *New England J. Med.,* 276:383, 452, 1967.

Sutherland, E. W., Robison, G. A., and Butcher, R. W.: Some Aspects of the Biological Role of Adenosine 3′, 5′-Monophosphate (Cyclic AMP). *Circulation,* 37:279, 1968.

Walser, M.: *Magnesium Metabolism. Reviews of Physiology, Biochemistry and Experimental Pharmacology.* Berlin, Springer and Verlag, 1967.

Winters, R. W.: Studies of Acid-Base Disturbances. *Pediatrics,* 39:700, 1967.

PARENTERAL FLUID THERAPY

The preceding section has outlined the chemical anatomy of body fluids and some mechanisms regulating body composition. This section presents a practical application of such principles to specific problems of fluid therapy.

Fluid therapy has 4 aspects: (1) *deficit therapy,* which is concerned with the normalization of the volume of body fluids and of the concentration of solutes, and supplies water and electrolytes to replace deficiencies resulting from inadequate intake as in thirsting and fasting or from excessive losses as in diarrhea or diabetic acidosis; (2) *maintenance therapy,* which is concerned with administration of water and solutes in quantities approximating those lost from the body under usual circumstances; (3) *the concomitant replacement of abnormal losses,* which supplies water and electrolytes to meet ongoing losses particular to the disease under treatment, whether these occur from the body as a whole (external abnormal losses, such as gastric drainage) or represent sequestration of water or solutes, or both (e.g. pleural effusion may represent an internal loss of regional nature); and (4) *supplemental therapy,* which is concerned with the restoration or the support of a particular physiologic function or with correction of a distorted metabolic situation by such means as alkalinization of the urine or induction of diuresis.

DEFICIT THERAPY

General Considerations. Disturbances in body composition may result from reduced intake in the presence of usual losses or from excessive losses with or without the usual intake. The severity of the disturbance depends on the relation between intake and output and the magnitude of the body reservoirs. Infants frequently exhibit decreased appetite with disease and have limited capacities to reduce the usual loss of water in the urine. On the other hand, the volume of water and the quantity of available sodium and chloride per unit of body weight are greater in the infant than in the adult. Deficit therapy must be based, therefore, on an appraisal of the relative changes in body composition. Such an appraisal must rest largely on clinical evaluation of the patient through an accurate history and careful physical examination. Table 5-4 lists the historical data which constitute the necessary background for decisions involving fluid therapy.

Of particular importance in judging the magnitude of deficits in infants is change in weight. Losses in excess of 1 per cent of the body weight per day represent loss of body water. The exact composition of the infant's feeding mixtures also permits some assessment of the water and electrolyte balance. Homemade electrolyte mixtures for the oral treatment of diarrhea are often responsible for severe hyperosmolality, owing to failure of the mother to follow precisely the directions of the physician. The time and frequency of recent urinations, whether excessive or suppressed, may provide some appreciation of the severity of dehydration. Frequent and excessive urination is suggestive of diabetes mellitus, diabetes insipidus and nephrogenic diabetes. Usual output without increased intake of water in association with physical signs of dehydration suggests a loss in capacity of the kidney to conserve water.

The physical signs of disturbances in body composition are of even greater value than the historical data in the planning of fluid therapy

TABLE 5-4. HISTORICAL DATA REQUIRED IN PLANNING DEFICIT THERAPY

Intake—during period of illness
   Quantity and how given
   Kind: water, electrolyte, protein, drugs

Output—during period of illness
   Quantity
   Kind: urine, vomiting, diarrhea, sweat, drainage

Balance
   Weight change

General medical
   Age
   Cardiovascular, respiratory, renal or central
     nervous system disease

(Tables 5-5, 5-6). Some of the signs listed in Table 5-5 are not specific for dehydration, but are characteristics of shock, which frequently accompanies dehydration. In the well nourished older infant or child, skin turgor may remain fairly normal in the presence of dehydration. The clinical determination of isotonic, hypertonic or hypotonic dehydration is usually not as definitive as may be suggested by Table 5-5. When findings are definite, differentiation may be possible, but borderline findings, such as somewhat dry mucous membranes and somewhat poor skin turgor, cannot be interpreted as confirming the presence of disturbances in osmolality.

The physical findings which characterize variations in the concentration of specific substances in the blood (Table 5-6) require some explanation. The characteristic signs of acidosis are increased depth and rate of respiration, which may, however, be depressed in the presence of severe circulatory insufficiency. The compensatory diminution in breathing associated with alkalosis, though usually absent in adults, is conspicuous in infants with pyloric stenosis. Deficiencies of potassium, calcium or magnesium may exist without obvious physical findings. Hypopotassemia may not always

TABLE 5-5. PHYSICAL SIGNS OF DEHYDRATION

	ISO-OSMOLALITY (LOSS OF WATER AND SALT) ISOTONIC DEHYDRATION	HYPEROSMOLALITY (LOSS OF WATER IN EXCESS OF SALT) HYPERTONIC DEHYDRATION	HYPO-OSMOLALITY (LOSS OF SALT IN EXCESS OF WATER) HYPOTONIC DEHYDRATION
Skin			
Color*	Gray	Gray	Gray
Temperature	Cold	Cold or hot	Cold
Turgor	Poor	Fair	Very poor
Feel	Dry	Thickened	Clammy
Mucous membrane	Dry	Parched	Slightly moist
Eyeball	Sunken and soft	Sunken	Sunken and soft
Fontanel	Sunken	Sunken	Sunken
Psyche	Lethargic	Hyperirritable	Coma
Pulse*	Rapid	Moderately rapid	Rapid
Blood pressure*	Low	Moderately low	Very low

*Signs of shock rather than of dehydration itself.

TABLE 5-6. PHYSICAL SIGNS OF VARIATIONS IN
CONCENTRATION OF SPECIFIC IONS

Acidosis
  Respiration: increased depth and rate
Alkalosis
  Respiration: decreased depth and rate
  Latent or manifest tetany
Hypopotassemia
  Heart: fast or slow; poor quality to heart sounds
  Skeletal muscle: weakness or paralyses; diminished
  reflexes
  Smooth muscle: abdominal distention; ileus
Hyperpotassemia
  Heart: slow or fast; poor quality to heart sounds
  Skeletal muscle: fibrillation; paralyses
Hypocalcemia
  Latent tetany (see p. 1262)
  Manifest tetany (see p. 1262)
Hypercalcemia
  Gastrointestinal: fecal masses
  Hypotonia
Hypomagnesemia
  Latent or manifest tetany
  Muscular twitching
Hypermagnesemia
  Decreased deep tendon reflexes
  Central nervous system depression

be present even when cells are depleted of potassium. Such deficits may be inferred from history alone.

Certain laboratory data (Table 5-7) are helpful in the initial planning of therapy. None is so essential that adequate therapy cannot be initiated without it. The laboratory is of greater importance in assessing the results of deficit therapy and in guiding subsequent maintenance therapy.

The Astrup apparatus has made determinations of pH, pCO_2 and standard bicarbonate concentration increasingly available. These measurements are particularly valuable as guides to assisted or artificial respiration or in appraisal of the severity of metabolic disorders.

TABLE 5-7. LABORATORY DATA USEFUL IN
PLANNING THERAPY

Serum or plasma
  Carbon dioxide content and chloride concentration
  Sodium, potassium and magnesium concentration
  Serum osmolality (freezing point depression)
  Protein concentration
  Serum solids (refractometer)

Whole blood
  pH, pCO_2 and standard HCO_3^- (Astrup)
  Hematocrit
  BUN or SUN or NPN

Urine
  Volume and specific gravity
  Albumin, sugar, acetone
  Sediment

Electrocardiogram

The difference between the sodium concentration and sum of the carbon dioxide content or standard bicarbonate and the chloride concentration is usually 15 ± 5 except in ketosis. The difference is useful in indicating the possibility of a laboratory error in the sodium or chloride determination. The serum (or plasma) sodium level is of particular importance in determining how the loss of water relates to that of electrolytes. Hypernatremia indicates excessive loss of water in relation to electrolytes; hyponatremia indicates excessive loss of electrolytes in relation to water. Serum osmolality is an accurate index of body water content in relation to solute. The serum potassium concentration at the beginning of therapy is not particularly helpful, since it may be elevated because of anoxia, diminished renal function or acidosis, even when there are significant cellular deficits. Measurement of the blood or serum urea nitrogen or nonprotein nitrogen level is helpful in following the progress of therapy, a rising urea nitrogen level indicating either intrinsic renal injury or continuing circulatory insufficiency. The level of plasma protein and the hematocrit value have limited usefulness at the beginning of therapy, but the initial determinations are of considerable help in assessing the effects of therapy. When correlated with physical findings, they may be useful in planning therapy. For example, when there is a low or even normal hematocrit value with signs of dehydration, anemia must be present. Serial determinations of the hematocrit value and of the plasma protein concentration in capillary blood are essential in following the course of patients with burns. Measurements of urinary output, specific gravity, proteinuria, glycosuria and ketonuria are valuable in assessing the degree of renal compensation which may be expected during therapy, as well as in guiding therapy in diabetic acidosis.

Serial electrocardiograms may provide clues to disturbances in concentration of such electrolytes as potassium and calcium. Leads II and aV_5 are particularly useful for this purpose (see p. 954).

The quantities of water and electrolytes which may be lost in various conditions have been estimated by a variety of techniques, such as balance studies, isotope dilution methods, tissue and whole body analyses and animal experiments. The data given in Table 5-8 represent *only an order of magnitude* and serve as a partially quantitative guide rather than as a precise determinant of therapy. It can be seen from Table 5-8 that there is a decided similarity in the magnitudes of deficits, despite the fact that the precipitating conditions vary widely. This is not surprising, since the deficits reflect readjustments as well as the direct losses. Loss of chloride in the vomitus in pyloric stenosis, for example, leads to an increase in excretion of sodium and potassium in the urine. Thus deficits of these cations will result even though the original losses of them in the vomitus were relatively small. Similar compensatory losses are seen in diarrhea and other conditions.

TABLE 5-8. PROBABLE DEFICITS OF WATER AND ELECTROLYTES IN INFANTS WITH MODERATELY SEVERE DEHYDRATION

CONDITION	H_2O ML.	NA mEq.	K* mEq.	CL mEq.
	PER KG. OF BODY WEIGHT			
Fasting and thirsting....................	100-120	5-7	1-2	4-6
Diarrhea				
Isotonic................	100-120	8-10	8-10	8-10
Hypertonic............	100-120	2-4	0-4	−2−−6†
Hypotonic..............	100-120	10-12	8-10	10-12
Pyloric stenosis	100-120	8-10	10-12	10-12
Diabetic acidosis......	100-120	8-10	5-7	6-8

*Converted for breakdown of tissue cells: −1 gm. N = 3 mEq. of K.

†Negative balance of chloride indicates excess at beginning of therapy.

These considerations justify similar therapeutic approaches, with only minor modifications, to a variety of conditions.

In planning deficit therapy the initial step is aimed at improving circulatory dynamics and renal function, since these are of primary importance in the morbidity and mortality of dehydration. Restoration of these functions depends on rapid expansion of extracellular volume with a fluid such as Ringer's lactate, which resembles the extracellular fluid and remains completely in this compartment. Such solutions are preferably administered intravenously, although some improvement may result from subcutaneous injection. Glucose in water or in dilute saline solutions must not be administered subcutaneously. Shock can be precipitated by the rapid migration of salt and water into the subcutaneous pool as glucose slowly diffuses into the vascular compartment. Circulatory insufficiency due to dehydration should not be treated by the immediate administration of blood, owing to the possibility of thrombosis and renal tubular injury from minor degrees of blood incompatibility. Blood should be given for shock associated with dehydration only after the extracellular volume has been rapidly expanded. The *intracellular* deficits of water and electrolytes must be replaced *slowly* and only after improvements in circulation and renal functions have been effected.

DEFICIT THERAPY IN SPECIFIC CONDITIONS

Fasting and Thirsting. One of the most common problems requiring fluid therapy is the initial treatment of the infant or child who has taken little or no water and food for 1 to 5 days. Table 5-8 indicates that such infants are deficient not only in water, which has evaporated from the lungs and skin, but also in electrolytes, particularly sodium and chloride, which have been excreted in the urine. The administration of electrolyte-free solutions under such circumstances leads only to an increase in urine volume with possible increased losses of electrolytes and may actually increase the dehydration. If fasting and thirsting continue beyond 4 or 5 days, urinary output will fall to such a low level that there will be no significant continued loss of electrolytes, and further severe deficiency of water alone will result.

Therapy (Table 5-9) is begun with Ringer's lactate solution to produce rapid and safe expansion of extracellular volume and improvement in renal function. A large part of the remaining deficiency of water and electrolytes may be made up by a solution containing carbohydrate, sodium chloride, some potassium and potential bicarbonate, such as lactate or acetate. Children and adults should be given approximately one fourth to one third less water and sodium per kg. than infants for a given degree of clinical dehydration, owing to the relatively smaller extracellular reservoirs with increasing age. Potassium deficits are relatively the same in infants, children and adults, since they have approximately the same quantity of potassium per kg. When deficit therapy is planned for obese patients, the quantities of water and electrolytes to be given should be based on a weight more nearly approximating the ideal than the actual one. Water, carbohydrate and electrolytes may be administered to the mildly ill patient by mouth. Infants, however, often vomit when they are dehydrated, and for this reason initial therapy is usually given parenterally. After completion of the deficit therapy the patient should be sustained on a maintenance basis as outlined on page 227.

Acute Diarrhea. Despite improved infant care, diarrhea continues to be a serious problem in many areas of the world. The physical signs which result are principally those outlined in Tables 5-5 and 5-6. As indicated in Table 5-8, diarrhea results in large losses of water and electrolytes in varying proportions. In approximately 70 per cent of instances there is isotonic dehydration in which the losses of water and electrolytes are proportionate, so that total solute concentration in body fluids remains fairly normal even though there may be severe acidosis.

Isotonic dehydration. The therapy outlined in Table 5-9 is based upon the principle that initially extracellular volume must be restored in order to improve circulation and renal function. Administration of an approximately isotonic fluid, such as Ringer's lactate solution, for a short time expands extracellular volume effectively and moves solute concentration toward normal, whether the sodium concentration is elevated or low. The balance of the deficit of extracellular water and electrolytes is given and the beginning of correction of the intracellular deficit of potassium and water carried out slowly over a six- to eight-hour period. After this deficit therapy usual maintenance therapy is begun, and in addition enough water, sodium, chloride and potassium are administered to

TABLE 5-9. Deficit Therapy of Infants with Moderately Severe Dehydration and Electrolyte Disturbances

CLINICAL CONDITION	SOLUTION	ML./KG.	TIME SCHEDULE IN HOURS FROM ONSET OF THERAPY	ROUTE
Fasting and thirsting	Ringer's lactate	20	0-1	IV
	5% or 10% invert sugar or glucose in H₂O	60	1-8	IV
	Darrow's K lactate*	20		
Diarrhea				
Isotonic dehydration	Ringer's lactate	20	0-1	IV
	Blood or plasminate†	10	1-2	IV
	5% or 10% invert sugar or glucose in H₂O	40	2-8	IV
	Darrow's K lactate*	60		
Hypotonic dehydration	Ringer's lactate	20	0-1	IV
	Blood or plasminate†	10	1-2	
	5% invert sugar or glucose in Ringer's lactate	40	2-8	IV
	Darrow's K lactate*	60		
Dehydration in malnourished infants	5% invert sugar or glucose in Ringer's lactate	40	0-1	IV
	Blood or plasminate†	10	1-2	IV
	5% invert sugar or glucose in Ringer's lactate	40	2-8	IV
	Darrow's K lactate*	60		
	MgSO₄ · 7H₂O · 50%	0.1		IM
Hypertonic dehydration	Ringer's lactate	20	0-1	IV
	Blood or plasminate†	10	1-2	IV
	5% or 10% invert sugar or glucose in H₂O	60	2-10	IV
	M/6 Na lactate	20		
	K acetate concentrate§	0.5		
	Calcium gluconate‖			
Pyloric stenosis	Isotonic NaCl	20	0-1	IV
	Blood or plasminate†	10	1-2	IV
	5% or 10% invert sugar or glucose in H₂O	40	2-8	IV
	Isotonic NaCl*	40		
	Isotonic KCl*	20		
Diabetic acidosis	Ringer's lactate	20	0-1	IV
	Blood or plasminate†	10	1-2	IV
	5% or 10% invert sugar or glucose in H₂O	50	2-8	IV
	KPO₄ concentrate‡	0.5		
	Darrow's K lactate*	50		

All of above to be followed by maintenance therapy.

*May be given separately subcutaneously.

†For shock not responding to Ringer's lactate.

‡Phosphate concentrate contains 2 mEq. of K per ml.

§K acetate concentrate (Cutter) contains 4 mEq. of K per ml.

‖Total dose, 10 ml. of 10% solution slowly IV.

approximate the continuing abnormal losses in the stool. The deficit therapy outlined for diarrhea does not differ greatly from that for fasting and thirsting, nor from that for diabetic ketosis, and differs only slightly from the therapy for pyloric stenosis. This plan does not represent the only approach to the treatment of diarrhea, but serves as a framework upon which modifications may be made. In young infants, acidosis may not respond readily to the suggested treatment, and additional sodium bicarbonate should be slowly administered (see p. 225).

Hypotonic dehydration. At times, particularly in bacillary dysentery in older infants and young children, large amounts of electrolytes may be lost in the stool. Consequently hypotonic dehydration may result (10 per cent of all cases of diarrhea), and be accentuated if only electrolyte-free fluids are taken by mouth. The serum sodium concentration may fall to less than 130 mEq. per liter. Under these circumstances the basic plan of therapy is modified by administering relatively less glucose in water and relatively more glucose in electrolyte-containing solutions (Table 5-9) so that gradual correction of concentration is accomplished as volume is expanded. No attempt is made to elevate abruptly the sodium concentration by administration of hypertonic saline solution unless symptoms of water intoxication are present, such as convulsions. Delay in administration of potassium is necessary because hyperpotassemia is frequently associated with hyponatremia.

Dehydration from diarrhea in chronically malnourished children. Severe malnutrition complicated by diarrheal dehydration is a common problem of subtropical and tropical countries, and an occasional one in the temperate zones. Therapy must be adapted to meet the specific disturbances in body composition characteristic of the dehydrated malnourished infant. There appears to be an overexpansion of the intracellular space, with extracellular and presumably intracellular hypo-osmolality. Serum sodium, potassium and magnesium levels are low in most cases. Tetany may occasionally result from the magnesium deficiency. The level of serum proteins is frequently less than 3.6 gm. per 100 ml. The sodium content of muscle is high; potassium and magnesium contents are low. The electrocardiogram frequently shows tachycardia, low amplitude, and flat or inverted T waves. Cardiac reserve seems lowered, and heart failure is a common complication.

Despite clinical signs of dehydration and reduced body water, urinary osmolality may be low, owing to failure of tubular water conservation. The glomerular filtration rate is low, resulting in a lesser loss of water than would otherwise be expected. The dilute urine may result from the failure of urea to contribute to a hypertonic fluid in the renal papillae, owing to low protein intake. Renal concentrating ability returns after several days of high protein feedings.

Survival of the malnourished infant with diarrhea is limited by caloric deficit to a greater extent than by water and electrolyte deficit. Reparative calories can be given by slow drip through an indwelling nasogastric tube while electrolyte and water are given parenterally. If appetite is poor and vomiting and gastric distention are absent, feeding is begun early at the level of 30 to 40 calories per kg. per day, given by slow intragastric drip. Increases to 50 to 100 calories per kg. and 1 to 2 gm. of protein per kg. per day are made in a few days. Ad libitum intake should be permitted in the succeeding weeks, up to 250 to 300 calories per kg. per day, with an adequate supply of iron and copper.

Initial parenteral therapy is designed to improve the circulation and to expand extracellular volume. The repair solutions recommended resemble those for hypotonic dehydration. Rate of administration and quantity of fluid should be reduced from recommended levels if edema is present, to avoid pulmonary edema. Blood should be given if the patient is in shock, severely ill, or anemic. Potassium salts can be given early if urine output is good. Controlled trials suggest that survival can be improved by the intramuscular injection of 1.0 to 1.5 ml. of a 50 per cent solution of magnesium sulfate (4.0 mEq. per ml.) every 12 hours for 1 to 3 days. Clinical and electrocardiographic improvement may be more rapid with magnesium therapy, and seizures occurring during recovery from diarrhea complicating severe malnutrition may respond to magnesium.

Hypertonic dehydration. Although this condition is less common (approximately 20 per cent of cases of diarrhea) than isotonic dehydration, it occurs frequently in young infants in whom conservation of water by the kidney is limited, and particularly when the renal solute load is high, as when boiled skim milk is fed to infants with diarrhea. Hypertonic dehydration may also result from administration of solutions of high electrolyte concentration, such as improperly prepared homemade or commercial salt and water mixtures. High environmental temperatures and hyperventilation also significantly increase evaporative losses of water.

Of particular importance in hypertonic dehydration are the cerebral changes which result from severe hyperosmolality. Seizures are the most common clinical manifestation. Widespread cerebral hemorrhages and thromboses may occur. There is usually an elevated protein level in the cerebrospinal fluid. Hypocalcemia has occasionally complicated hyperosmolality (Finberg and Harrison). Severe hypocalcemia may not be encountered if administration of potassium is part of the routine therapy of diarrhea. Cerebral injury from hypertonicity may have permanent effects and be one of the causes of acquired cerebral palsy. Renal tubular injury, with azotemia and loss of concentrating ability, may complicate treatment.

Balance studies reveal a slight deficiency of sodium, an excess of chloride and a relatively minor deficit of potassium. Serum potassium frequently falls to low levels during therapy, however, unless potassium is administered. Characteristically, with treatment consisting of large amounts of water, whether with or without salt, there is expansion of extracellular volume. Significant edema and at times cardiac failure may develop before there is any notable excretion of chloride or correction of the acidosis.

The therapy for hypertonic dehydration (Table 5-9) presents some deviation from the usual therapy of diarrhea. The principles are essentially the same, however: rapid expansion with extracellular fluid to improve circulation, followed by *slow* replacement of intracellular water and electrolytes. The intake of chloride is minimized, and water is administered rather slowly after the initial improvement of circulation and renal function. Intravenous administration of calcium may occasionally be required. Digitalization is indicated at the earliest evidence of cardiac failure. Administration of phenobarbital may minimize the occurrence of seizures. Some investigators have attributed seizures to relative water intoxication even though the serum sodium has been reduced only 5 to 10 mEq. per liter and is still considerably above normal. Such an origin has not been proved.

Nevertheless, if seizures occur which do not respond to usual anticonvulsant therapy and are not the result of hyperpyrexia, 3 per cent sodium chloride (3 to 5 ml. per kg.) may be given intravenously.

General considerations in treatment of diarrhea. In addition to replacement of the deficits of water and electrolytes, efforts must be made to obtain an etiologic diagnosis so that specific chemotherapy may be given if indicated. There are no aspects of chemotherapy that modify fluid therapy except that during the administration of sulfonamides adequate amounts of fluid must be provided for urine formation.

The maintenance of fluid balance in the patient with diarrhea (see above) requires an excess of water and electrolytes for stool formation. The extent of the losses ranges from 40 to 400 ml. per day in infants and 100 to 1000 ml. in children. These losses may be replaced by equal parts of 5 per cent glucose in water and Darrow's K lactate or similar commercially available solutions.

Drugs which inhibit peristaltic activity or methylcellulose derivatives which absorb intestinal contents and produce a more bulky stool have relatively little effect on the course of infantile diarrhea.

Although the net absorption of carbohydrate, fats and proteins may be increased by feeding large amounts of milk during diarrhea, there is unquestionably an increase in the volume of stool which makes the replacement of water and electrolytes exceedingly complicated and extends the need for parenteral fluids over several days.

With complete omission of oral feedings to infants with moderately severe diarrhea, frequency and volume of stools will usually subside rapidly within 48 hours. When this occurs, and if gastric distention and vomiting are absent, oral feeding of glucose, carbohydrate and electrolyte mixtures may be initiated. Commercial mixtures, such as Lytren, are available, or a somewhat similar, less expensive mixture* may be prescribed. It should be strongly emphasized that any such mixture be compounded exactly as prescribed, since hyperosmolality may result from a more concentrated one. When the infant tolerates the carbohydrate and electrolyte mixture by mouth without exacerbation of the diarrhea, the caloric intake may be increased gradually by the substitution of mixtures which also contain fat and protein until the usual dietary intake is achieved in 6 to 8 days. Premature administration of large numbers of calories in the form of milk may induce exacerba-

tion of the diarrhea. In the young infant with a family history of allergy the use of a hypoallergenic feeding mixture, such as Nutramigen or a soybean mixture, is recommended for the recovery phase from diarrhea, since permeability of the gastrointestinal tract to whole protein may be increased during this time.

Therapy of mild diarrhea. Many infants and children with diarrhea do not require parenteral fluid therapy. The decision for the use of oral rather than parenteral therapy rests on clinical appraisal of the patient. If there are signs of circulatory insufficiency, lethargy, vomiting or gastric distention, intravenous therapy must be given. In the absence of these findings and with only mild signs of dehydration, mixtures of sugar and electrolytes as described above may be fed. Parenteral therapy is indicated for infants when amounts in excess of 1.5 liters per day are required to meet continued stool losses. Infants with mild diarrhea have been observed in whom intakes of 2 to 3 liters of electrolyte mixtures orally per day have led to increases in the volume of stools; cessation of oral intake resulted in prompt cessation of the diarrhea. Such instances are sufficiently rare that they do not contraindicate an initial trial with oral carbohydrate and electrolyte mixtures.

Chronic Diarrhea. When diarrhea is severe and prolonged, intravenous administration of amino acids, plasma and alcohol or fat in addition to carbohydrates and electrolytes is required to sustain body reserves. Occasionally, full oral feedings are required during chronic diarrhea in addition to parenteral fluid therapy, especially in severe malnutrition as noted above. Allergy to milk protein or specific disaccharidase deficiencies should be suspected in infants with persistent diarrhea. Acquired disaccharidase deficiency (especially for lactose) may develop as a complication of many chronic disorders of the gastrointestinal or other systems. Hypoallergenic feeding mixtures containing monosaccharides as the sole carbohydrate should be administered until cessation of the diarrhea and improvement in nutrition have occurred. Specific tests of carbohydrate (disaccharide) splitting and absorption and of milk protein sensitivity should then be carried out.

Congenital Alkalosis of Gastrointestinal Origin. Rarely, chronic diarrhea may be due to a congenital defect in the transport of water and electrolytes across the intestinal wall. In contrast to usual diarrhea, the watery stools of such patients have a high content of potassium and chloride, and alkalosis results. The deficit therapy is analogous to that of pyloric stenosis, but must be on a continuing basis and planned in conjunction with an adequate dietary intake of potassium and chloride.

Pyloric stenosis. This condition exemplifies the correction of deficits associated with alkalosis. The therapy (Table 5-9) differs little from that of diarrhea, except for the substitution of solutions which contain relatively more chloride in relation to sodium and potassium (NaCl and KCl); these

---

*Example of a sugar and electrolyte mixture for oral administration:

Final Concentration

Sucrose ......50.0 gm.   Sucrose....... 5 gm.%
NaCl.......... 1.7 gm.   NaCl..........30 mM./L.
$KHCO_3$ ...... 2.0 gm. $KHCO_3$.......20 mM./L.

Dissolve in 1 liter (1 quart) of water.

permit replacement of the relatively larger deficit of chloride and some correction of the alkalosis as volume is expanded. Correction of the hypochloremia by administration of ammonium chloride without correction of the deficit of potassium results in continued dysfunction of renal tubular cells as well as of other cells. Although deficits may be replaced and serum levels returned to normal within 12 hours, operation should not be performed for at least 36 to 48 hours to permit optimal readjustment of body functions, except in very mildly ill infants with no signs of dehydration. Adequate fluid therapy prevents deterioration during this period of preparation, and the stomach may be decompressed by gentle suction. (See page 229 for preoperative, paraoperative and postoperative therapy.)

Diabetic Acidosis (see also p. 1158). The deficit therapy of diabetic acidosis (Table 5-9) approximates that of diarrhea. Extracellular volume is expanded rapidly with Ringer's lactate solution. The balance of the replacement therapy is carried out slowly over a 6- to 8-hour period. The administration of carbohydrate fairly early in therapy permits glycogenation of the liver after response to insulin and reduces the danger of hypoglycemia. In the appraisal of deficits in patients with diabetic ketosis, laboratory studies may be misinterpreted. Hypo-osmolality may be assumed erroneously on the basis of measurement of the serum sodium concentration. Extracellular osmolality may be normal or high even in the presence of a low serum sodium concentration if there is a high concentration of glucose. Blood sugar levels of 1800 mg. per 100 ml. are the equivalent of an additional 50 mEq. per liter of sodium. Elevations of serum lipid and protein concentrations in diabetic acidosis may also reduce the water content of the serum so that sodium concentrations per liter of serum are low while sodium concentrations per liter of extracellular water are normal or high.

Administration of potassium fairly early in therapy of these patients is essential. A rapid fall in potassium concentration occurs shortly after administration of insulin or fructose. Such changes may produce alterations in the functioning of the heart, liver, brain and kidneys, may contribute to gastric distention and may even lead to respiratory paralysis. Changes in serum inorganic phosphate concentration during therapy are likewise striking and parallel those in potassium concentration. This fall is due primarily to cellular uptake of phosphorus as glycogen is formed. Although the clinical significance of such changes has not been established, it is our opinion that serum inorganic phosphorus should be sustained at low normal levels. For this reason some potassium is administered as the phosphate salt. Magnesium levels may be elevated at the beginning of therapy and fall rapidly to below normal in a manner similar to potassium values. No clinical significance has been attributed to these changes.

No specific attempts are made initially to elevate the low carbon dioxide content and pH except by expanding extracellular volume with fluids resembling an ultrafiltrate of normal plasma (Ringer's lactate, see Table 5-9). Such therapy frequently results in a significant reduction in acidosis with symptomatic improvement. If extreme respiratory distress persists, the administration of sodium bicarbonate may be indicated. The dose required may be calculated from the formula on page 225. There is, however, a large reservoir of potential bicarbonate in the form of ketone acids which are metabolized with improvement in carbohydrate utilization after administration of insulin, so that bicarbonate concentration of the serum should not be elevated abruptly to more than 12 to 15 mEq. per liter.

The amount of insulin which can be given during this time varies considerably from one patient to another. Enough crystalline zinc insulin to effect clearing of the ketosis by accelerating the utilization of carbohydrate should be given, with adequate carbohydrate to prevent development of hypoglycemia. An initial dose of approximately 2 units per kg. for severe diabetic ketosis and then subsequent doses at 1- to 3-hour intervals of $\frac{1}{2}$ to 1 unit per kg. are usually appropriate. Half of the initial dose of insulin should be given intravenously. Approximately 1 to 2 gm. of carbohydrate per unit of insulin may be necessary to prevent hypoglycemia. The aim of therapy should be the elimination of ketonemia and ketonuria, since persistence of acetoacetic acid and beta-hydroxybutyric acid indicates diminished operation of the Krebs cycle. Collection of urine at hourly intervals, preferably without resort to catheterization, is essential for modifying the dosage of insulin and carbohydrate as therapy progresses. Only rarely in children will ketones be absent from the urine when the serum level is significantly elevated. Reduction of the blood sugar to a level which avoids excessive glycosuria prevents unusual loss of water in the urine. But reduction of the blood sugar to excessively low levels by administration of insulin without adequate carbohydrate leads rapidly to a return or exacerbation of ketosis and to hypoglycemia.

Fructose is phosphorylated rapidly in the absence of insulin and can be converted to glycogen in the diabetic patient more rapidly than glucose. Fructose, therefore, may be given relatively early in therapy without significantly increasing total blood and urinary sugar levels. Rapid administration of fructose alone, however, produces a profound acidosis as organic acid is transferred to extracellular fluid. Moreover, since fructose is not readily metabolized by the cerebral cortex, symptoms due to hypoglycemia induced by excessive doses of insulin would probably not be relieved by fructose until it was converted to liver glycogen and thence to glucose. Fructose has also been dèmonstrated to produce profound hypoglycemia in the newborn. For these reasons the use of invert sugar is preferred; it provides fructose for rapid increases in glycogen stores, and glucose for the prevention of hypoglycemia.

Parenteral administration of vitamins of the B complex is advised to compensate for the preexisting malnutrition.

THERAPY OF DISTURBANCES IN CONCENTRATIONS OF ELECTROLYTES

Acidosis. In the newborn infant with respiratory distress syndrome, in patients receiving assisted ventilation, and in cardiac surgery, measurements of blood pH and blood gases facilitate active correction of acidosis.

In disorders involving severe respiratory insufficiency, pH may be markedly lowered, primarily as a result of carbon dioxide retention; mild metabolic acidosis may also exist, because hypoxia leads to the accumulation of lactic acid and other organic acids in extracellular fluid. The appropriate treatment of such disturbances is improvement of ventilation by assisted respiration, rather than by large amounts of sodium bicarbonate, which may produce hyperosmolality and cardiac failure.

When metabolic acidosis results from renal maladjustments (hyperchloremia) or from accumulation of organic acids, administration of sodium bicarbonate is indicated if symptoms are evident. Sodium lactate may not be adequately metabolized in lactic acidosis, in glycogen disorders or in circulatory insufficiency and hypoxia. Sodium bicarbonate is the preferred agent for alkalinization. The dosage required is given by the following general formula:

$$(C_d - C_a) \times f_d \times \text{body weight in kg.} = \text{mEq. required.}$$

Here C_d and C_a represent respectively the bicarbonate concentration desired and the one actually present; f_d represents that fraction of the total body weight in which the administered material is apparently (not actually) distributed. This factor varies with the substance administered. The apparent distribution factor for bicarbonate or potential bicarbonate approximates one half to six tenths of the body weight.

Such calculations indicate that 0.5 ml. per kg. of a molar solution of sodium bicarbonate would raise the serum bicarbonate concentration approximately 1 mEq. per liter. There are, however, wide variations in the responses to administered bicarbonate, since administered sodium may be sequestered in bone or muscle or lost in urine. In glomerular insufficiency, caution must be exercised in correcting acidosis; hyperphosphatemia should be corrected by diet and administration of aluminum compounds before elevation of the pH of the blood is attempted.

Hypochloremic Alkalosis. Rarely respiration may be so depressed in infants with severe hypochloremic alkalosis that oxygenation of the blood is diminished. Severe alkalotic tetany may also occur. In such instances the administration of ammonium chloride may effect symptomatic improvement. The dose of ammonium chloride may be calculated from the formula above; the probable f_d is 0.2 to 0.3. Such therapy is for relief of symptoms only and must not be used in place of administration of potassium chloride for repair of intracellular deficits.

Hyponatremia. Sodium chloride is the main solute of extracellular fluid. Hyponatremia, therefore, always indicates hypo-osmolality except in the presence of hyperglycemia and hyperlipemia, as in diabetic acidosis.

A lowered concentration of sodium in the serum may result from a decrease in the amount of sodium in the extracellular space or from an increase in the volume of extracellular water (Table 5-10).

TABLE 5-10. CLINICAL STATES COMPLICATED BY HYPONATREMIA

I. Expansion of extracellular space
   A. Excessive intake
      1. Parenteral fluid therapy—glucose in water
      2. Oral (with diminished output)
   B. Diminished output (usual intake)
      1. Renal
         a. Intrinsic: nephritis, nephrosis, tubular necrosis, prematurity
         b. Extrinsic
            (1) Excess of antidiuretic hormone: acute and chronic central nervous system disease, Pitressin therapy, surgery, pulmonary disease
            (2) Circulatory: heart failure, cardiovascular surgery, malnutrition
      2. Skin: premature infant in high humidity
II. Deficiency of extracellular sodium
   A. Inadequate intake
      1. Low salt diet
      2. Parenteral therapy with glucose in water
   B. Excessive losses
      1. Gastrointestinal: vomiting, salivary, gastric, biliary, pancreatic drainage, diarrhea, resin therapy, enemas (especially megacolon)
      2. Genitourinary
         a. Intrinsic renal disease: chronic nephritis, acute tubular necrosis (recovery phase), nephrosis (diuresis)
         b. Extrinsic influences: mercurial diuretics, Diamox, hypoadrenalism, rare central nervous system disease, expanded volume (Pitressin, excessive water therapy)
         c. Arachnoid: ureterostomy
      3. Skin
         a. Normal sweat
         b. Abnormal sweat: cystic fibrosis, adrenal insufficiency
         c. Burn therapy with silver nitrate (hypochloremia)
      4. Parenteral: thoracentesis, paracentesis, burns
   C. Redistribution
      1. Severe malnutrition
      2. Potassium deficiency
      3. Trauma

Of particular pediatric interest are the disturbances in sodium concentration related to diseases of the central nervous system. They seem to be of 3 types:

1. Patients with diverse lesions such as encephalitis, bulbar poliomyelitis, cerebrovascular accidents, tumors of the fourth ventricle and subdural hematoma may lose large amounts of sodium in the urine. This is evidenced by dehydration, hypotension and azotemia unless large amounts of salt are administered and the intake of water is somewhat limited.

2. Patients with tuberculous meningitis who are severely ill and comatose are frequently hyponatremic, but exhibit no symptoms which can be attributed to hyponatremia. This situation may be analogous to the asymptomatic hyponatremia of severe malnutrition or pulmonary disease. Relatively large amounts of salt may be lost in the urine when attempts are made to correct the hyponatremia by salt loading. It has been postulated that there may be a deficit of intracellular solute which leads to a homeostatic lowering of osmolality. Careful clinical and laboratory observations are essential to ensure that salt depletion and water intoxication do not occur. Potassium should be administered in amounts at least 50 per cent greater than usual maintenance therapy (see p. 228).

3. Patients with acute infections of the central nervous system occasionally have symptoms of acute water intoxication as a manifestation of rapid fall in serum sodium concentration. These patients retain an excessive amount of water and have excessive thirst. Convulsions are severe and resistant to anticonvulsant therapy, but respond to the intravenous administration of hypertonic saline solution. The dose may be calculated according to the formula on page 225. Since there is osmotic equilibrium between cells and extracellular water, changes in osmolality are distributed over total body water, and the value of 0.6 to 0.7 may be used for f_d.

Elevation of the sodium concentration should be effected in small increments (5 to 10 mEq. per liter) over 1 to 4 hours. A dose of 12 ml. per kg. of 3 per cent (M/2) saline solution should raise the concentration of sodium approximately 10 mEq. per liter.[*]

If no symptoms are present, correction of hyponatremia may be accomplished by restriction of water, administration of alcohol to produce a water diuresis or brief substitution of isotonic electrolyte solution for the usual water intake. In the therapy of disturbances in concentration, accurate chemical analyses are essential for confirmation of clinical findings. Therapy must be directed at correction of symptoms, however, and not at laboratory findings. Central nervous system diseases in which *hypernatremia* predomi-

nates must be differentiated; in these situations further limitation of the intake of water would be disastrous.

Salt Poisoning. The accidental ingestion of excessive amounts of sodium chloride leads to such serious residuals that special attention is warranted. The substitution of salt for cane sugar in private homes as well as in institutions occurs with sufficient frequency to justify the routine use of liquid sugars in infant feeding. Hypernatremia resulting from the excessive intake of sodium, in contrast to hypertonic dehydration resulting from diarrhea, is accompanied by increases in total body sodium and in the volume of extracellular water. Severe acidosis results from the shift of organic acids and free hydrogen ions to extracellular fluid. With shift of water from brain cells distention of cerebral vessels occurs, leading to subdural, subarachnoid and intracerebral hemorrhage. The complications and residuals of salt poisoning are similar to, but may be more severe than, hypertonic dehydration. In the former the rapid removal of excess sodium from the body is the principal goal of treatment.

Intravenous fluids should consist of glucose in water, potassium acetate and calcium as needed. Intermittent peritoneal dialysis with glucose solutions can remove large quantities of sodium, correcting the hyperosmolality without the danger of pulmonary edema and heart failure. Approximately 40 ml. per kg. of 7 per cent glucose solution in water can be injected intraperitoneally for severe hypernatremia (serum sodium concentration more than 200 mEq. per liter) and withdrawn 1 hour later. Subsequent dialysis may be carried out using 5 per cent glucose in water as the serum sodium level falls. Exchange transfusion is not a desirable substitute for dialysis because enormous quantities of blood would be required to effect a change in osmolality of total body water. Phenobarbital should be administered to prevent or control seizures. Digitalization may be necessary to counteract heart failure.

Hypopotassemia (Hypokalemia). Disturbances in concentration of potassium in the absence of disturbances of volume of body fluids have been described in primary hyperaldosteronism and in a poorly defined condition termed congenital alkalosis of renal origin, thought by some to be secondary hyperaldosteronism. In these disturbances large amounts of potassium are lost in the urine, resulting in low serum potassium and high serum bicarbonate concentrations. The administration of large amounts of potassium (10 mEq. per kg. per day) and severe restriction of the intake of sodium effect some clinical as well as biochemical improvement. Congenital alkalosis of gastrointestinal origin represents another anomaly of metabolism, in which large amounts of potassium and chloride are lost in the stools (p. 223).

Hypocalcemia and **hypercalcemia** are discussed on pages 133, 1200 and 1260.

Hypomagnesemia. The importance of mag-

---

[*] $(10) \times 0.6 \times 1 = 6$ mEq. per kg. required.
1 ml. 3% NaCl = 0.5 mEq.
Therefore 12 ml. per kg. required.

nesium in fluid and electrolyte therapy has been reviewed earlier (p. 210). The only definitive symptom complex associated with hypomagnesemia (serum magnesium less than 1.8 mEq. per liter) is that of latent or manifest tetany. Convulsions, muscular twitching, disorientation, athetoid movements, carpopedal spasm, and hyperreactivity to mechanical and auditory stimulation have been observed. Lowered serum concentrations and whole body deficits of magnesium are found in chronic diarrhea or vomiting, sprue, celiac disease, prolonged parenteral fluid therapy, and hyperaldosteronism. Harrison observed low serum magnesium levels in infantile tetany, presumably on the basis of transient hypoparathyroidism. The intramuscular injection of 0.1 ml. of a 25 per cent solution of $MgSO_4 \cdot 7H_2O$ (0.2 mEq. per kg.) repeated every 6 hours for 3 to 4 doses produces symptomatic and biochemical improvement. The addition of 3 mEq. of magnesium per liter to maintenance fluids for patients requiring long-term therapy may decrease the chance of serious deficiency.

Hypermagnesemia. Levels of serum magnesium in excess of 10 mEq. per liter are accompanied by drowsiness and occasionally coma. Deep tendon reflexes may also be abolished along with respiratory depression at higher concentrations. Disturbances in atrioventricular and intraventricular conduction may be detected at levels of 5 mEq. per liter. Acute renal failure and Addison's disease are accompanied by significant elevations in magnesium concentrations. Iatrogenic magnesium poisoning can result from its use in the treatment of hypertension; deaths have been reported from the use of magnesium sulfate enemas in megacolon and from oral administration for purging.

The administration of calcium gluconate intravenously as in the treatment of tetany rapidly reverses the depressant effects of magnesium as well as the cardiac abnormalities.

MAINTENANCE THERAPY

This phase of fluid therapy is concerned with supplying the usual requirements of water, electrolytes, protein and calories. Such therapy, by either oral or parenteral routes, directly follows deficit therapy and is continued until the usual dietary intake is re-established.

Deficit therapy is calculated on the basis of body weight. Maintenance requirements, on the other hand, depend upon the rate of metabolic turnover and hence are calculated on the basis of 100 calories metabolized (Darrow and Pratt). The use of such a unit rather than surface area has a sound theoretic basis and does not unduly complicate practical therapy, since the pediatrician commonly thinks in terms of caloric requirements in infant feeding (see Table 5-11).

TABLE 5-11. STANDARD BASAL CALORIES

WEIGHT KG.	CALORIES/24 HOURS MALE AND FEMALE	
3	140	
5	270	
7	400	
9	500	
11	600	
13	650	
15	710	
17	780	
19	830	
21	880	
25	1020	960
29	1120	1040
33	1210	1120
37	1300	1190
41	1350	1260
45	1410	1320
49	1470	1380
53	1530	1440
57	1590	1500
61	1640	1560

Modified from Talbot.
Increments or decrements:
1. Add or subtract 12% of above for each degree C. (8% for each degree F.) above or below rectal temperature of 37.8° C. (100°F.)
2. Add 0 to 30% increments for activity.

Use of ideal weight as obtained from the fiftieth percentile for age and height from the table on page 42 is necessary for obese infants and children. Calculation of the total number of calories metabolized is readily made by the additions or subtractions listed in Table 5-11. Adjustments for temperature and activity must be made to assure optimal intake rather than to depend upon estimations determined from a fixed surface area. Corrections for activity may be approximated by observation of the patient. No increments for activity are needed for patients in coma or under anesthesia. Usual bed activity does not exceed an increment of 20 to 30 per cent. In the first 3 to 5 days of life, activity is low and total caloric expenditure does not usually exceed 50 calories per kg. Increments for growth may be ignored, as may those for specific dynamic action, unless large amounts of amino acids or alcohol are administered.

The usual losses of water and electrolytes from the lungs and skin, in the stool and in the urine are charted in Table 5-12 for each 100 calories metabolized. The amount of water necessary for urine formation is directly related to the concentrating or diluting activities of the kidney and to the renal solute load, which is largely a function of the diet (Fig. 5-11). The approximate solute excretion for patients receiving no electrolyte and adequate carbohydrate to minimize tissue breakdown is 10 to 15 milliosmoles per 100 calories metabolized. Usual electrolyte allowances would increase this value to 20 to 25 milliosmoles per 100

TABLE 5-12. Water and Electrolyte Losses per 100 Calories Metabolized

H₂O ML.	RANGE Na	RANGE K	USUAL H₂O ML.	USUAL Na	USUAL K
	MEQ.			MEQ.	
*Evaporative**					
Lungs 10-60	0	0	15		
Skin 20-100	0.1- 3.0	0.2- 1.5	40		
Total 30-160	0.1- 3.0	0.2- 1.5	55	0.1	0.2
*Stool** 0-50	0.1- 4.0	0.2- 3.0	5	0.1	0.2
*Urine** 0-400	0.2-30.0	0.4-30.0	65	3.0	2.0

*High values may also be considered to represent abnormal losses.

calories. The amount of exogenous water required for maintenance needs is approximately 10 to 15 ml. per 100 calories less than total requirements because of the release of that volume of water during oxidation of endogenous and exogenous carbohydrate, fat and protein. Thus the maintenance supply of water for the average patient ranges from 110 to 120 ml. per 100 calories metabolized. Such an allowance permits excretion of solutes without maximal dilution or concentration of the urine. This volume of fluid is less than that prescribed in usual oral infant feeding (140 ml. per 100 calories of food) because the intake of excretable solute is considerably greater on a milk or other protein-containing diet.

With alterations in body functions, adjustments in water allowances for maintenance must be made. In anuria or extreme oliguria (less than 10 ml. per 100 calories metabolized) only about 45

ml. of exogenous water per 100 calories are required, since only evaporative and stool losses occur. Careful calculation of water of oxidation is particularly important in this condition, and water allowances should be adjusted accordingly. In the presence of excessive release of antidiuretic hormone as in some acute infections, particularly of the central nervous system, the intake should not exceed 80 to 90 ml. per 100 calories. When urinary specific gravity is fixed as in chronic renal disease, water requirements rise to 140 ml. per 100 calories, and in diabetes insipidus of nephrogenic or hypothalamic origin to as high as 400 ml. per 100 calories. In such instances the thirst of the patient and an awareness of the urinary output are usually more reliable than the physician's estimates, and oral feedings should be used if possible. Urinary losses of water must not be replaced on a volume-for-volume basis; the author has observed adult patients who put out daily volumes of urine up to 8 and 10 liters in order to excrete loads of water administered "to balance" urinary losses incident to an initial diuresis of fluid retained during an oliguric phase. In hyperventilation and in heat stress evaporative losses of water may increase as much as 90 and 120 ml. per 100 calories, respectively, and increments in fluid intake should be made accordingly. High humidity, as in incubators, may reduce evaporative losses of water by 20 to 50 per cent, and appropriate decrements in intake should be made.

Although there is great variability in excretion of electrolytes (Table 5-12), the average sodium and potassium requirements for parenteral fluid therapy are 2 to 4 and 2 to 3 mEq., respectively, per 100 calories metabolized. A solution of 5 or 10 per cent invert sugar containing 30 mEq. per liter of sodium and chloride and 20 mEq. per liter of potassium as the lactate, acetate or glutamate salt is an adequate maintenance solution* which meets the usual requirements when given in amounts of 110 to 120 ml. per 100 calories metabolized. Such a solution should be given *only* intravenously at a fairly constant rate throughout the day. If maintenance therapy must be conducted by subcutaneous administration of fluid, owing to technical difficulties, equal parts of 5 per cent glucose or 5 per cent invert sugar in water and Darrow's K lactate may be administered. Glucose in water or in very dilute electrolyte solution should not be given, since diffusion of sodium chloride and water into such an extravascular pool may acutely reduce plasma volume and precipitate shock.

Just as intake of water must be adjusted to meet specific alterations in body functions, so must intakes of electrolytes be individualized. For example, in anuria or oliguria no electrolyte should be administered for maintenance. In congestive heart failure, limitation of sodium intake is as

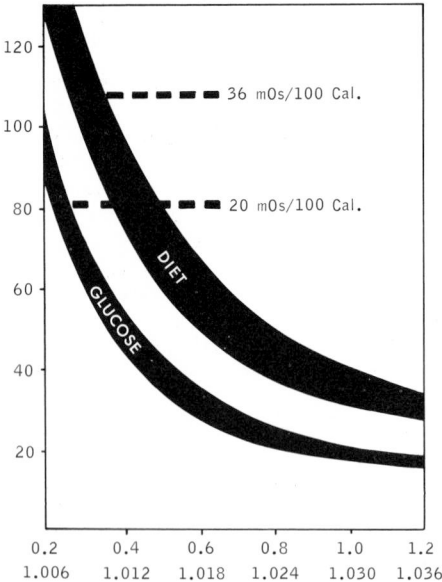

Figure 5-11. Relation of water requirement for urine formation to urinary concentration and dietary renal solute load. (Modified slightly from Darrow and Pratt: *J.A.M.A.*, Vol. 143.)

*5 or 10% invert sugar or glucose in H₂O .... 800 ml.
Isotonic saline.. 200 ml.
Potassium glutamate concentrate (Abbott) .... 10 ml.
              or
Potassium acetate concentrate (Cutter).................... 5 ml.

important in parenteral as in oral therapy. Reduction of sodium intake during fluid therapy of a patient with cardiac failure also demands some limitation of water, since renal solute load is decreased and retention of water may occur.

In parenteral maintenance therapy for extended periods of time, and particularly in malnourished patients, carbohydrate, alcohol and amino acids may be necessary to attain caloric and nitrogen balance. Albumin may be given as a source of preformed protein intravenously in doses of 2 gm. per 100 calories metabolized, particularly when severe malnutrition is present. The addition of a multivitamin preparation is indicated whenever previous nutrition was poor and maintenance therapy is prolonged.

Regardless of the accuracy of planning, periodic analyses of the serum and frequent physical examinations of the patient must be carried out in order to assess alterations in concentration and volume of body fluids as therapy progresses. Measurements of the blood urea nitrogen and the serum sodium, chloride and potassium levels are essential at intervals of 24 to 72 hours, depending on the clinical status of the patient. Such analyses may be performed on capillary blood.

MAINTENANCE THERAPY IN PREOPERATIVE, PARAOPERATIVE AND POSTOPERATIVE CARE

Preoperative preparation of a patient who has no pre-existing deficit or in whom the deficit has been repaired consists mainly in the supply of carbohydrate to ensure adequate storage of glycogen in the liver. The requirements of water and electrolytes for maintenance are similar to those for usual circumstances. Small infants who are not vomiting should receive carbohydrate and sodium chloride mixtures by mouth until 3 hours before operation to prevent postoperative fluid retention. Such fluids are readily absorbed from the gastrointestinal tract and will not produce aspiration pneumonitis if vomited and aspirated.

Preoperative preparation in the newborn involves certain unique hazards. Deficits of water and electrolytes from vomiting or from stasis in intestinal obstruction should be replaced before operation. If aspiration pneumonitis is suspected, it should be treated with kanamycin. Nasogastric suction is frequently inadequate; gastrostomy should then be performed to aid in decompression and in postoperative feeding. In intestinal obstruction conjugated bilirubin may be deglucuronidated by intestinal enzymes. An enterohepatic circulation of unconjugated bilirubin can then lead to very high serum levels and to kernicterus. Hypoprothrombinemia should be prevented by administration of 1.0 mg. of vitamin K_1 oxide.

For the first 24 hours postoperatively, limitation of water and electrolytes is indicated. The water requirements during operation are given in Table 5-13. Additional amounts of blood, plasminate or saline must be given if blood loss or tissue trauma is significant. Owing to the dangers of anoxia and shock, no potassium should be administered during these periods. The water intake should not exceed 85 ml. per 100 calories metabolized, because of antidiuresis resulting from trauma or circulatory readjustment, unless renal insufficiency and limited concentrating capacity are present (e.g. in sickle cell anemia). If the intake of water is not limited, whether given parenterally or by mouth, water intoxication may result. Sodium intake for maintenance should also be low, owing to the low caloric expenditure during anesthesia and postoperatively. During operation, fluid such as blood or plasma must be given to meet large losses into traumatized tissue. The magnitude of such internal abnormal losses is judged best by the experienced surgeon as he operates. Postoperatively, limitation of intake should be maintained for 24 hours. Thereafter usual maintenance therapy is gradually resumed.

TABLE 5-13. APPROXIMATE REQUIREMENTS OF WATER WITHOUT ELECTROLYTES DURING OPERATION

WEIGHT KG.	BASAL CAL./24 HOURS	EVAP. WATER, ML./HR. (90 ML./100 CAL./24 HOURS)*	URINE WATER, ML./HR. (30 ML./100 CAL./24 HOURS)†	TOTAL‡ ML./HOUR
3	150	6	2	8
5	270	10	3	13
7	410	15	5	20
10	550	21	7	28
20	850	32	10	42
30	1100	41	14	55
40	1300	49	16	65

From H. S. Harned, Jr., and R. E. Cooke: *Surg., Gynec. & Obst.,* 104:543, 1957, by permission.
*This value is assumed to be high because of possible sweating and hyperventilation.
†This value is assumed to be low because of probable antidiuresis.
‡Does not include abnormal losses of fluid (hemorrhage, wound edema, suction) which must be replaced by appropriate electrolyte-containing fluids.

TABLE 5-14. COMPOSITION OF EXTERNAL ABNORMAL LOSSES

FLUID	NA	K	CL	PROTEIN GM.%
	mEq./L.			
Gastric	20-80	5-20	100-150	—
Pancreatic	120-140	5-15	90-120	—
Small intestine	100-140	5-15	90-130	—
Bile	120-140	5-15	80-120	—
Ileostomy	45-135	3-15	20-115	—
Diarrheal	10-90	10-80	10-110	—
Sweat:				
Normal	10-30	3-10	10-35	—
Cystic fibrosis	50-130	5-25	50-110	—
Burns	140	5	110	3-5

ABNORMAL LOSSES OF WATER AND ELECTROLYTES

The principles underlying the concomitant replacement of external abnormal losses require little explanation. Such losses depend on the specific clinical disturbance (see Table 5-14). Considerable variation in composition exists from patient to patient and from time to time in the same patient. Although only an approximation can be made, these losses must be replaced, as nearly as possible, volume for volume as they occur in order to prevent physiologic readjustments which may further deplete the body of water and electrolyte. Losses in gastric or intestinal drainage can be replaced satisfactorily by solutions which are isotonic or somewhat hypotonic and contain some excess of chloride over sodium for gastric replacement and sodium over chloride for intestinal replacement. Ten to 20 mEq. per liter of potassium should also be included. Losses of sodium chloride in sweat are of little significance except in adrenal insufficiency and cystic fibrosis. Heat stress should be avoided in such patients.

Burns. Internal abnormal losses of fluids are difficult to quantitate. This phase of fluid therapy is exemplified by the treatment of burns. Unless unusual delay has occurred before a burned child is brought to the hospital, pre-existing deficits are minimal and significant deficits result solely from inadequate or delayed fluid therapy after admission. Maintenance requirements for water are diminished when the large surface area is covered by wet dressings which limit evaporation from the skin; evaporation from the lungs is normal or increased. Urinary output of water is probably limited by some antidiuresis which results from massive stimulation of nerve receptors. Thus the fluid therapy of burns is concerned principally with the replacement of abnormal losses. Some of these losses are external, such as oozing of plasma from the burned surface. In addition, a significant number of erythrocytes are destroyed or damaged by exposure to heat, and their survival time is

shortened. The largest part of the abnormal loss is internal in the form of plasma and plasma ultrafiltrate sequestered around the burn site. The magnitude of this sequestration has been approximated by measurements of the extracellular space in patients with severe burns. Such measurements are partially invalidated, however, by the fact that large amounts of saline solution were administered therapeutically, and true obligatory losses can only be approximated.

Losses of fluids are proportional not to the weight or metabolism of the patient, but to the surface area of the second- or third-degree burn. This area can be approximated by the "rule of nine"* or from appropriate charts of the body surface.

The composition of an ideal replacement solution cannot be fixed. A mixture of 3 parts of plasma, 1 part of blood and 3 parts of a balanced saline solution† is a reasonable replacement fluid which may be given at the rate of 10 liters per square meter of second- or third-degree burned surface area per 48 hours. A third is administered in the first 6 hours, a third in the next 12 hours and a third in the next 30 hours. Such a program can only approximate the actual needs. The progress of therapy must be monitored at 1- to 2-hour intervals by the determination of hematocrit values of capillary blood and of plasma protein levels and by careful measurements of the volume and concentration of urine obtained by an indwelling catheter. Urine volume should be held at 30 to 50 ml. per 100 calories metabolized. A rising hematocrit value and falling urine volume, for example, indicate an inadequate rate of replacement of fluids. After 48 hours fluid therapy should be sharply limited. The sequestered fluid may return at this time to the vascular compartment and produce acute pulmonary edema, particularly if there has been thermal injury to the lungs. Digitalis and diuretics, if there has been no renal injury, or even phlebotomy with removal of plasma and replacement of red blood cells may be helpful.

Abnormal Urinary Losses. In certain conditions occult abnormal losses occur into the urine. Sodium-losing disorders such as pulmonary, cerebral or adrenal "salt wasting" or potassium-losing disorders such as primary hyperaldosteronism or congenital alkalosis of renal origin may be suspected when there are alterations in concentrations of serum electrolytes in the absence of obvious losses. "Wasting" of a particular electrolyte is established when excessive quantities of it are demonstrated in the urine in the presence of restricted intake and a low serum concentration in association with a normal or reduced volume of

---

*Head, arm, one quarter of trunk, one half of leg: each equals 9 per cent of the body surface. The sum of the percentages times total surface area as given by nomogram on page 236 equals the area used in calculating requirements. Infants and small children, owing to relatively larger heads and trunks and smaller extremities, fit more exactly to a "rule of sixes." Arm, one half of head or leg and one eighth of trunk: each equals 6 per cent of the body surface.

†Two parts isotonic saline, 1 part sixth-molar sodium lactate.

TABLE 5-15. COMPOSITION OF COMMONLY USED ORAL AND PARENTERAL SOLUTIONS

ORAL

	CHO Prot.* GM./100 ML.		CALORIES PER L.	Na	K	Cl	HCO₃†	Ca	P‡
						MEQ./L.			
Milk (whole)	4.9	3.5	670	22	36	28	30	60	54
Ginger ale	9.0		360	3.5	0.1		3.6		
Coca-Cola	10.9		435	0.4	13		13.4		
Pepsi-Cola	12.0		480	6.5	0.8		7.3		
Orange juice (sweetened)	14.0		540	0.2	49		50		
Grape juice	18.0		670	0.4	31		32		
Tomato juice (canned salted)	4.3		210	100	59	150	10	3	9
Lytren	7.0		280	25	25	30	19	4	5
H.L.H. mixture	5.0		200	30	20	30	20		

PARENTERAL

	CHO Prot.* GM./100 ML.		CALORIES PER L.	Na	K	Cl	HCO₃†	Ca	P‡
CHO§ in H₂O	5-10		200-400						
Isotonic saline	0-5		0-200	154		154			
½ Isotonic saline	2.5-5		100-200	77		77			
⅓ Isotonic saline	5		200	50		50			
3% (M/2) saline				500		500			
5% Saline				850		850			
2% Ammonium chloride						400			
M/6 Sodium lactate				167			167		
7.5% Sodium bicarbonate				892			892		
Ringer's lactate	0-10		0-400	130	4	109	28	3	
Darrow's KNL				122	35	104	53		
Butler's	5-10		200-400	55	23	45	26		12
Modified Butler's 1	5-10		200-400	25	20	22	23		3
Modified Butler's 2	5-10		200-400	60	25	53	25		12
Talbot's	5-10		200-400	40	35	40	20		15
Ordway's	3.5-10		140-400	26	27	53			
Gastric replacement	0-10		0-400	63	17	150			
Intestinal replacement	5-10		200-400	80	36	63	60	4.6	
Amigen	5-10	5	345-515	30	15	22		5	30
Amigen, dextrose and Ringer's lactate	3.3	3.3	230	65	10	51	10	5	20
Amigen, dextrose and alcohol	5-12	5	670-800	30	15	22		5	30
Dextran 6%	0-5		0-200						
Dextran 6% in saline				154		154			
Plasminate		5		110	2	50	50		
Blood‖		3		95	4	50	40		2
Lipomul IV	4.0		1600						

ADDITIVES

Glucose 50% .... 0.5 gm. per ml.
Sodium chloride .... 4.0 mEq. per ml.
Sodium lactate .... 4.0 mEq. per ml.
Potassium chloride .... 1.0 or 2.0 mEq. per ml.
Potassium phosphate .... 2.0 mEq. per ml.
Potassium acetate .... 4.0 mEq. per ml.
Ammonium chloride .... 4.0 mEq. per ml.
Magnesium sulfate
(MgSO₄ · 7H₂O) 50% .... 4.0 mEq. per ml.

*Protein or amino acid equivalent.
†Actual or potential bicarbonate, such as acetate, lactate, citrate.
‡Calculated according to valence of 1.8.
§Glucose (dextrose), fructose or invert sugar.
‖Red cell contents not included in calculations.

body fluids. "Spot tests" which indicate only the concentration of electrolytes in the urine are inadequate for diagnostic purposes.

SUPPLEMENTAL THERAPY

It is occasionally necessary in fluid therapy to supply an excess of certain substances to effect a particular change in physiologic function or to facilitate excretion of a particular substance. Such therapy in the form of water and electrolytes is given in the absence of specific deficits and above the usual needs.

Salicylate Poisoning. Supplemental therapy is of particular importance in the treatment of salicylate poisoning. The initial effect of a high concentration of salicylate is to sensitize the respiratory center to carbon dioxide, probably by interfering with oxidative phosphorylation. The resultant hyperventilation leads to increased evaporative losses of water and to respiratory alkalosis. The renal compensation for respiratory alkalosis consists in the excretion of large amounts of sodium and potassium bicarbonate. In addition, toxic levels of salicylate may reduce hepatic glycogen. Ketonemia and ketonuria usually result; occasionally there is hypoglycemia, but hyperglycemia and glycosuria are more common. The loss of sodium and potassium in excess of chloride and the accumulation of acetoacetic and beta-hydroxybutyric acids eventually lead to severe metabolic acidosis. In addition, 2 moles of free hydrogen ion (H^+) are derived from each mole of aspirin absorbed and hydrolyzed. A dose of 200 mg. per kg. adds an acute H^+ load of 2 mEq. per kg. Transition from respiratory alkalosis to metabolic acidosis may be relatively rapid. Therapy must be followed by periodic evaluation of the serum carbon dioxide content and the pH of the blood and urine. Early therapy must supply adequate amounts of water, carbohydrate and electrolytes to meet the increased evaporative losses and to permit maximal renal compensation. Maintenance therapy should provide 200 to 250 ml. of water, 15 to 20 gm. of glucose, 6 to 8 mEq. of sodium and 3 to 4 mEq. of potassium per 100 calories metabolized.

The early administration of sodium bicarbonate and potassium acetate or glutamate to maintain an alkaline urine (pH higher than 7.5) will facilitate excretion of salicylate by reducing the back-diffusion of salicylate in ionized form through lipid tubular membranes. The dose of bicarbonate necessary to alkalinize the urine is approximately 2 mEq. per kg., given over 1 hour. An additional 2 mEq. of sodium bicarbonate should be given if urine pH does not reach 7.0. The urinary pH should then be checked every 30 minutes. If the pH falls below 7.0, additional sodium bicarbonate and potassium should be given to avoid renal tubular potassium depletion with paradoxical aciduria. The additional administration of aceta-

zolamide (5 mg. per kg. repeated 2 or 3 times in 24 hours) also increases salicylate excretion, and should be a part of the management of all seriously ill patients. Exchange transfusion, peritoneal dialysis or dialysis by means of the artificial kidney may also be used to remove salicylate loosely bound to plasma proteins in severely ill patients with high blood levels of salicylate. Vitamin K_1 oxide (Konakion) should be given intramuscularly.

Potassium Intoxication. The excretion of potassium may be increased by loading with hypertonic sodium bicarbonate (2 mEq. per kg. in 1 hour as M/2 sodium bicarbonate). Such supplemental therapy may be lifesaving in acute hyperpotassemia, since elevation of serum sodium concentration and pH reduces serum potassium concentration even in the nephrectomized animal. A small amount of invert sugar and 0.2 unit of insulin per kg. may accelerate the shift of potassium from the extracellular to the intracellular space.

Although water loading may be considered a form of supplemental therapy, excretion of solute, such as urea in glomerular insufficiency, is not increased by such a procedure unless pre-existing dehydration is present. Water retention, edema or water intoxication may result.

Urine volume may be increased by the administration of a 1 per cent urea solution, which produces a profound solute diuresis. Clinical situations requiring such a diuresis are rare, but large urine volumes may occasionally be helpful in the treatment or prevention of urinary tract infections.

PARENTERAL SOLUTIONS

Table 5-15 lists various solutions commercially available for use in deficit, maintenance, abnormal loss replacement and supplemental therapy. The large number of carbohydrate and electrolyte mixtures available permits great flexibility and individualization of therapy.

Robert E. Cooke

REFERENCES

Caddell, J. L., and Goddard, D. R.: Studies in Protein-Calorie Malnutrition. I. Chemical Evidence for Magnesium Deficiency. II. A Double-Blind Clinical Trial to Assess Magnesium Therapy. *New England J. Med.*, 276:533, 1967.

Calcagno, P. L., Rubin, M. I., and Singh, N. S. A.: The Influence of Surgery on Renal Function in Infancy: The Effect of Surgery on the Postoperative Renal Excretion of Water—The Influence of Dehydration. *Pediatrics*, 16:619, 1955.

Colle, E., and Paulsen, E. P.: The Responses of the Newborn to Major Surgery: Urinary Electrolyte, Water and Nitrogen Losses. *Pediatrics*, 23:1063, 1959.

Cooke, R. E.: Contributions of the Laboratory to the Practical Management of Disorders of Body Water and Electrolyte. *Pediatrics*, 16:555, 1955.

Cooke, R. E., and Ottenheimer, E. J.: Clinical and Experimental Interrelations of Sodium and the Central Nervous System. *Advances in Pediatrics*, XI:81, 1960.

Danowski, T. S., Greenman, L., Weigand, F. A., and Mateer, F. M.: Acidosis and Coma in Juvenile Diabetics. *Am. J. Dis. Child.*, 93:341, 1957.

Darrow, D. C.: Congenital Alkalosis with Diarrhea. *J. Pediat.*, 25:519, 1945.

Darrow, D. C., and Pratt, E. L.: Fluid Therapy: Relation to Tissue Composition and Expenditure of Water and Electrolyte. *J.A.M.A.*, 143:365, 432, 1950.

Darrow, D. C., Pratt, E. L., Flett, J., Jr., Gamble, A. H., and Wiese, H. F.: Disturbances in Water and Electrolyte in Infantile Diarrhea. *Pediatrics*, 3:129, 1949.

Elliott, G. B., and Crichton, J. U.: Peritoneal Dialysis in Salicylate Intoxication. *Lancet*, 2:840, 1960.

Finberg, L.: Experimental Studies of the Mechanisms Producing Hypocalcemia in Hypernatremic States. *J. Clin. Invest.*, 36:434, 1957.

Finberg, L.: Pathogenesis of Lesions in Nervous System in Hypernatremic States. I. Clinical Observations of Infants. *Pediatrics*, 23:40, 1959.

Gordillo, G., Soto, R. A., Metcoff, J., Lopez, E., and Antillon, L. G.: Intracellular Composition and Homeostatic Mechanisms in Severe Chronic Infantile Malnutrition. III. Renal Adjustments. *Pediatrics*, 20:303, 1957.

Gruskay, F. L., and Cooke, R. E.: The Gastrointestinal Absorption of Unaltered Protein in Normal Infants and in Infants Recovering from Diarrhea. *Pediatrics*, 16:763, 1955.

Harned, H. S., Jr., and Cooke, R. E.: Symptomatic Hyponatremia in Infants and Children Undergoing Surgery. *Surg. Gynec. & Obst.*, 104:529, 1957.

Holliday, M. A., and Segar, W. E.: The Maintenance Need for Water in Parenteral Fluid Therapy. *Pediatrics*, 19:823, 1957.

Kaplan, S. A., Strauss, J., and Yuceoglu, A. M.: Use of a Fat Emulsion Infused Intravenously in Infants and Children. *Pediatrics*, 25:645, 1960.

Leitsen, S. L., and Emmanouilides, G. C.: Use of Exchange Transfusion in Salicylate Intoxication. *J. Pediat.*, 57:715, 1960.

Metcoff, J.: Some Aspects of Renal Structure and Function Concerned with Regulation of the Body Fluids. *Pediat. Clin. N. Amer.*, 6:43, 1959.

Miller, N. L., and Finberg, L.: Peritoneal Dialysis for Salt Poisoning. *New England J. Med.*, 263:1347, 1960.

Nyhan, W. L., and Cooke, R. E.: Symptomatic Hyponatremia in Acute Infections of the Central Nervous System. *Pediatrics*, 18:604, 1956.

Rapoport, S.: Hyperelectrolytemia and Hyperosmolarity in Pathologic Conditions of Childhood. *Am. J. Dis. Child.*, 74:682, 1947.

Sotos, J. F., Dodge, P. R., Meara, P., and Talbot, N. B.: Studies in Experimental Hypertonicity: Pathogenesis of the Clinical Syndrome, Biochemical Abnormalities and Cause of death. *Pediatrics*, 26:925, 1960.

Walser, M.: Magensium Metabolism. *Ergebn Physiol.*, 59:185, 1967.

Whitten, C. F., Kesaree, N. M., and Goodwin, J. F.: Managing Salicylate Poisoning in Children: Evaluation of Sodium Bicarbonate Therapy. *Am. J. Dis. Child.*, 101:178, 1961.

DRUG THERAPY

GENERAL CONSIDERATIONS

The physician's diagnostic ability and skills are ultimately expressed in his ability to treat his patient. Treatment may or may not include drug therapy. The decision as to the form of therapy to be used is the responsibility of the physician and should not be relegated to or dictated by parents or others. Confidence in the physician is an essential part of a successful therapeutic program, and the development of this confidence will depend on the physician's attitude and actions. A resourceful physician will adjust his approach and therapy to each patient as seen in different families and under different circumstances. A young mother is often overwhelmed by the problem of caring for the first coryza of her first infant. A veteran mother of 6 children may take the sixth case of measles too lightly.

Rational therapy depends on (1) precise diagnosis, (2) an understanding of the normal metabolic and emotional processes peculiar to children of different ages, and how these are affected by the disease, (3) knowledge of socioeconomic factors involved, and (4) the therapeutic means available. When a drug is part of the treatment, the physician must have knowledge of the pharmacologic action and metabolism of the drug in the patient. Improper therapy may be due to inadequate diagnosis, poor choice of drug, improper directions for dispensing or administration, faulty storage of the drug, or inadequate evaluation of the total health care situation.

ADVERSE DRUG REACTIONS

Any pharmacologically active drug may cause an undesirable reaction in addition to or instead of the desired action. The risk of an undesired reaction must be evaluated against the potential benefit. There are several types of undesirable reactions:

Reaction to Overdose. Large amounts of most drugs will usually cause toxic manifestations. Some drugs will cause toxic manifestations when the amounts taken represent only small excesses over therapeutic amounts.

Side Effects. Undesirable pharmacologic effects can be expected with predictable frequency with the *usual* doses of certain drugs.

Allergic or Hypersensitive Reactions and Idiosyncrasy. These responses are abnormal reactions of the host and are not exclusively related to the dose or to the pharmacologic action of the drug.

Developmental Aspects of Adverse Drug Reactions. In addition to the above-mentioned reactions which may be expected in persons of any age, certain reactions are intimately or uniquely related to the processes of growth and development. The intensity of such reactions is often dependent on the rapidity of the growth process.

During the *embryonic period* (first 12 weeks or so of gestation) certain drugs taken by the mother may prove to be teratogenic and produce structural malformations. Among these are thalidomide, a sedative which produces phocomelia and other anomalies; some cancer therapeutic agents, such as methotrexate, which profoundly distort the growth pattern; and progestins, testosterone, other androgenic agents, and even stilbestrol, which may cause masculinization of the female fetus. The teratogenic effects of drugs are likely to be both time- and dose-related.

The tragic European epidemic of phocomelia resulting from the use of thalidomide in pregnant women precipitated world-wide reaction; in the United States this included the passage of Federal laws in 1962 which require proof of efficacy of drugs as well as of safety.

During the *fetal period*, drugs administered to the mother may be responsible for modification of growth of a structurally intact fetus. For example, goitrogens, such as the iodides, radioactive iodine, thiouracils and perchlorates, may cause goiters, which may be so large as to interfere with respiration and delivery; tetracyclines may, when deposited in bones and teeth, cause discoloration and distortion of growth; and cancer therapeutic agents may suppress growth and cause congenital anomalies.

Some drugs administered during or shortly before labor may have little effect on the newborn infant; others may cause serious problems. Among the latter are acidifying and adrenergic agents, analgesics (both narcotic and non-narcotic), anesthetics, antibiotics and chemotherapeutic agents, antihypertensives, endocrine products, hypnotics and sedatives, muscle relaxants, tranquilizers, vitamin K and xanthines (aminophylline or theophylline). In addition, the injudicious use of both hypotonic and hypertonic electrolyte solutions in the mother may be reflected by serious disturbances in the newborn infant.

Drugs which can cause difficulty on reaching the fetus through the placenta may cause similar difficulties when administered to the newborn infant, particularly in large or frequent doses. Moreover, certain drugs which will be tolerated in later infancy may cause serious reactions in the neonatal period. Chloramphenicol, for example, is poorly conjugated and excreted, especially by the premature infant, and may cause the "gray syndrome" in infants less than a week of age. At 3 weeks the same dosage may be insufficient to produce effective blood levels.

Physicians prescribing for mothers who are nursing infants must also know that a number of drugs are excreted in breast milk. The amounts are seldom sufficient to yield activity in the infant, but some may cause trouble, and the physician should know which these are.

Each age period after the neonatal one has its special problems related to metabolic and developmental differences. Whenever the use of a drug is considered, its potential for harm must be carefully weighed against its potential value, with a clear understanding of how its use and effects will be reflected by the developmental status of fetus, infant or child.

TYPES OF DRUG THERAPY

Specific Therapy. The action of a drug is said to be specific when it is capable of combating a specific causative agent (e.g. penicillin versus the beta hemolytic streptococcus) or of alleviating a specific symptom for which the pathophysiology is understood (e.g. digitalis for cardiac failure).

Empiric Therapy. When a drug apparently alleviates symptoms or exerts a beneficial effect on a disease process, but the mode of action is not understood, the effect is termed empiric. Such therapy is based on prior experience, which has established the value and hazards involved. In many instances further study will establish whether the value observed is a true pharmacologic effect or a placebo effect.

Therapeutic Trial. Drug therapy may on occasion be diagnostic. The response of rheumatic arthritis to therapy with a salicylate is an example.

Supportive and Symptomatic Therapy. Supportive therapy includes palliative and corrective measures which are not specific in the sense that they directly attack the disease agent or process. They may, however, be as important as specific medication, even when the latter is also available. Supportive and symptomatic measures include correction of fluid and electrolyte imbalance, alleviation of pain, sedation, use of cardiac stimulants, inhalation of oxygen and other therapy. The acquisition of adequate skill in administering such therapy is less readily attained than is competence in the prescription of specific therapy.

Placebo Therapy. There is a place for such therapy in the practice of pediatrics, if it is used thoughtfully. All drugs have some placebo effect added to their pharmacologic activity. The placebo effect is much stronger in some patients and in some families than in others. The physician's attitude can greatly enhance or minimize this effect; it is essential that when he uses a placebo, he keep its true nature in mind. The physician caring for growing children is usually in an excellent position to educate them and their families to rational attitudes toward drug therapy; he should reserve pure placebo therapy for specific indications.

Psychotherapy. Though not a form of drug therapy, psychotherapy is in varying degree an essential part of the care of all patients. The unusual relation between a physician and his patient and the patient's family makes this aspect of therapy especially important. The physician must be able to deal with parental anxiety, grief and guilt, and to assist parents in reaching a realistic acceptance of their child's illness in order to carry out a therapeutic program. It is not only what he does, but also how, that is important. Attention to small details to facilitate home care or to make hospital care more pleasant is essential. So many seemingly little things are important: the kindly smile, the unhurried attitude and, above all, the time for explanation.

INITIATION OF DRUG THERAPY

One of the most severe tests of clinical judgment in pediatrics is selection of the proper time to institute drug therapy. Most diseases of infancy and childhood are self-limited. A few are rapidly fatal if proper therapy is not instituted immediately. If a precise diagnosis can be made, the choice of therapy is apt to be obvious. It if cannot be made, the physician must decide either to withhold therapy until the diagnosis can be made or to institute therapy for selected diagnostic possibilities while waiting for information essential to a precise diagnosis. At times such blind therapy may be lifesaving; at other times it may obscure the diagnosis and lead to serious consequences. In some instances, when a disease has not responded to a therapeutic program, it is wise to discontinue it in order to re-evaluate the initial diagnosis.

CHOICE OF DRUG

If the decision has been made that drug therapy is indicated, several factors should be taken into consideration in choosing the specific drug or drugs. When there is a choice between equally effective drugs, the least toxic one should be selected; when of equal effectiveness and toxicity, the least expensive one should be chosen. No drug should be prescribed except as there is a reason for it. The more drugs used, the greater the chance for undesirable reactions which may confuse the clinical course of the patient. In general, mixtures of several drugs in one vehicle should be avoided, since dosage and times of administration are better controlled when drugs are given separately. We know very little of the synergistic and antagonistic effects of drugs given together.

For any drug prescribed, the physician should know the route and rate of absorption; the rate, method and organ of excretion or detoxification; the pharmacologic action expected and any possible undesirable reactions. It is desirable for a physician to select one or two drugs from each class for general use so that he can gain from personal experience the necessary familiarity with the variations in expected reactions in different patients. It is not possible to acquire such knowledge for a large number of drugs.

ADMINISTRATION OF DRUGS

Clear and explicit directions should be written for the administration of drugs. The route of administration and the prepared form of the drug should be chosen carefully with the age and symptoms of the patient clearly in mind. The drug must be in a form that the attendant can administer to an infant or child. The parenteral administration of drugs is the most reliable route, but it is generally not practical for home use. Table 5-16 lists the possible routes of administration, the different prepared forms and doses of many drugs.

The *oral route* can be utilized for many drugs unless refusal or nausea, vomiting or other disorders of the gastrointestinal tract do not make their use impossible. Children vary in their ability to swallow tablets and capsules. As a rule, liquids should be prescribed for children under 5 years of age. Forced administration of solids or liquids to a struggling child may result in aspiration. If liquid preparations are not available, tablets can often be mashed, or capsules emptied and mixed with syrups, jellies, jams, honey or other vehicles. Unpleasant-tasting drugs should not be put in food that is or should be frequently eaten by the child.

Standardized measuring devices are preferred for measuring dosage. The volume contained by household teaspoons and droppers vary greatly. Calibrated droppers can be obtained for the measurement of smaller doses. The volume prescribed should always be large enough so that minor errors in measurement will not significantly alter the administered dose. When prescribing for infants and children, the physician must keep in mind all possible factors that may interfere with the drug arriving at the desired place in the recommended dose.

The *rectal route* cannot be expected to provide reliable absorption. If this route is chosen for reasons which seem appropriate in a particular situation, the rectum should be prepared by cleansing with an enema of isotonic saline solution. Multiple enemas may create fluid and electrolyte disturbances. The medication should be dissolved or suspended in 10 to 30 ml. of water and gently injected through a catheter or bulb syringe. Then the buttocks should be held together with tape and the catheter withdrawn. Some drugs are incorporated in suppositories; they are poorly absorbed by the dehydrated patient.

The *parenteral routes* are the most reliable ones for the administration of drugs. In severe or potentially severe illness or when vomiting is a factor, parenteral therapy should be utilized. The rate of absorption varies with the site of administration (subcutaneous, intramuscular or intravenous), with the absorbability of the drug or its vehicle and with the adequacy of the circulation. The objections to the parenteral route include the unavoidable trauma of administration, a greater risk of sensitization, and local reactions. Especially in infants there is a risk of sciatic palsy when intramuscular injections are given in the gluteal area.

Necrotizing or sclerosing drugs should be avoided, if at all possible; when necessary, they should be given intravenously with great caution.

Intrathecal therapy is rarely indicated.

The *sublingual* and *buccal* routes can be utilized for certain drugs, but only older children are able to cooperate with this type of therapy.

Topical therapy is often of great value, but requires careful direction and supervision if it is to be effective. Many parents and nurses have difficulty instilling medication in the eyes, ears, nose and mouth of infants and young children. Solutions are usually easier to handle than ointments for use in the eye or ear. The attendant should be instructed to rest the hand holding the dropper on the head, so that it moves with the head. The dose should be expelled rapidly, not by drops. Plastic droppers should be used rather than glass, and should often be calibrated.

Generally, ointments and creams are ineffective when applied to an oozing surface. Topical medication, if toxic when ingested or rubbed in the eyes, should be covered. As a rule, drugs that are commonly used for systemic therapy, such as certain antibiotics or antihistamines, should not be used topically, in order that the possibility of sensitization may be lessened.

Inhalation therapy utilizing aerosol medication is practical only for cooperative older children. With younger children, the aerosol must be given in a small tent, and adequate dosage control is impossible with most drugs.

THE DOSE OF DRUGS

The proper dose of a drug is the amount required to effect safely the desired pharmacologic action. As patients vary in their responses, the average recommended dose may have to be increased to accomplish the purpose or decreased to avoid undesirable reactions. Careful observation of the patient and individualization of therapy are essential. In some instances the dosage should be controlled by serial determinations of the concentration in the blood. Clinical observation and often laboratory measurements are essential to detect early evidence of toxicity, indicating the need to decrease the dose or to discontinue therapy.

Table 5-16 lists the average recommended dose of many drugs. When only the adult dose is known, there are many formulas to calculate the dose for a child. None is entirely satisfactory. Since many physiologic phenomena are more closely related to body surface area than to age, height or weight, the formula utilizing surface area* may be more accurate than others. The West nomogram (Fig. 5-12) can be used to calculate surface area.

Figure 5-13 permits calculation of surface area and the percentage of the adult dose from body weight.

In Table 5-16 the doses of many drugs are related to surface area (M^2) as well as to body weight. The dose for a given patient based on his surface

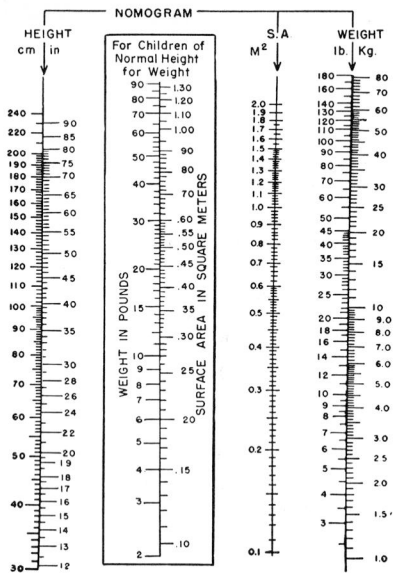

Figure 5-12. Nomogram for estimation of surface area. The surface area is indicated where a straight line which connects the height and weight levels intersects the surface area column; or the patient is roughly of average size, from the weight alone (enclosed area). (Nomogram modified from data of E. Boyd by C. D. West.)

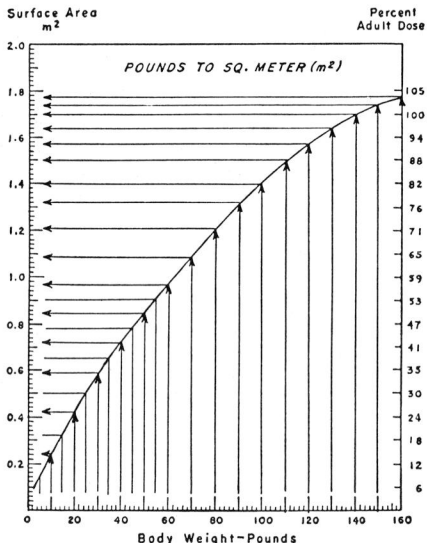

Figure 5-13. Relations between body weight in pounds, body surface area and adult dosage. The surface area values correspond to those set forth by Crawford et al. (1950). Note that the 100 per cent adult dose is for a patient weighing about 140 pounds and having a surface area of about 1.7 square meters. (From N. B. Talbot et al.: *Metabolic Homeostasis—A Syllabus for Those Concerned with the Care of Patients.* Cambridge, Harvard University Press, 1959.)

$$\frac{*\text{Surface area of patient (in square meters)}}{1.7} \times \frac{\text{Adult}}{\text{dose}} = \frac{\text{Approximate dose}}{\text{for patient}}$$

area can be determined as follows:

Surface area of patient (in M²) × dose per M² = approximate dose for patient.

*Clark's Rule** may be used to estimate dosage on the basis of the child's weight in respect to the adult dose of the drug.

These and other formulas provide only an approximate dose which must be adjusted to fit the individual patient. These formulas are highly unreliable when applied to premature infants and more reliable when applied to children over 2 years of age.

HARRY C. SHIRKEY

---

*Clark's rule:

$$\frac{\text{Patient's weight in pounds}}{150} \times \frac{\text{Adult}}{\text{dose}} = \text{Approximate dose for patient}$$

TABLE 5-16. DRUGS AND THEIR DOSES IN PEDIATRIC PRACTICE

Drugs in this table are grouped and listed alphabetically under the following therapeutic or diagnostic categories (the name of each drug also appears in the Index):

DRUGS

TABLE 5-16. DRUGS AND THEIR DOSES IN PEDIATRIC PRACTICE*

DRUG	DOSAGE AND ROUTES	SUPPLIED
Acidifiers		
Ammonium chloride, U.S.P.	75 mg./kg./24 hr. 2 gm./M.²/24 hr. Divide into 4 doses (O) **Caution:** May produce acidosis by continued use; not to be used in liver disease; use with caution in infants	Tablets: 0.3 gm. (5 gr.) Tablets (enteric): 0.5 and 1 gm. (7½ and 15 gr.) Solutions and syrups Vials: 5 mEq./ml.
Ascorbic acid, U.S.P.		
Methionine, N.F. (Amurex, Dyprin, Meonine, Methiocon, Metione, Oradash, Pedameth)	Urinary infections: 250 mg./kg./24 hr. 8 gm./M.²/24 hr. Divide into 3-4 doses (O) Ammoniacal dermatitis 200 mg./24 hr. Single dose (O) **Contraindication:** Liver disease	Powder Tablets: 0.5 gm. Capsules: 200, 250 and 500 mg. Envelopes: 2 gm.
Adrenal steroids *(see* Endocrines, *p. 294)*		
Adrenergic blocking agents *(see* Phentolamine, *p. 289)* *and* Antihypertensives, *p. 281)*		
Adrenergics		
Amphetamine sulfate, N.F. (Benzedrine sulfate) Amphetamine phosphate, N.F. (many trade names)	5-20 mg./24 hr. 15 mg./M.²/24 hr. Divide into 3 doses or as delayed-action single dose (O) 15 mg./M.²/dose (I.M. or slowly I.V.) (analeptic) Repeat p.r.n. **Contraindications:** Agitated prepsychotic patients or those taking monoamine oxidase inhibitors **Caution:** Use with caution in hypersensitivity to sympathomimetics, in severe hypertensive, or cardiovascular disease	Tablets: 5 and 10 mg. Spansules: 15 mg. Ampules: 20 mg./ml.
Dextroamphetamine sulfate, U.S.P. (Dexedrine sulfate and many other trade names)	2-15 mg./24 hr. 10 mg./M.²/24 hr. Divide into 3 doses or delayed-action single dose (O) **Contraindications:** As for amphetamine sulfate **Caution:** As for amphetamine sulfate	Tablets: 5 mg. Spansules: 5, 10 and 15 mg. Elixir: 5 mg./5 ml.

Dosages given in this table are not specifically intended for premature and newborn infants unless so indicated. Dosages prescribed elsewhere in this volume for individual disease entities should take precedence over dosages given in the table. All doses are average doses and are approximate. Variability of response may require alteration of dosage. Doses based on different criteria (e.g. body weight, surface area) frequently do not correspond.

To change the dose per kilogram to the dose per pound, divide the dose by 2.2 (or, more conveniently, by 2). To change the dose in gm./lb., multiply the dose in gm./kg. by 7.

The designations "U.S.P." and "N.F." identify *essential* and *valuable* drugs. Absence of designation does not indicate that a drug is without efficacy or value, but does indicate that it is *not* accepted by the *Pharmacopeia of the United States* or *The National Formulary.*

---

*For individual drugs, see general index.

Key: *M.*, dose per square meter of body surface.   *R*, rectal.
     I.M., intramuscular.   *S.C.*, subcutaneous.
     I.Th., intrathecal.   *Subl.*, sublingual.
     I.V., intravenous.   *T*, topical.
     O, oral.

This table, originally designed for this textbook, has been modified and updated; it is now also published in Shirkey, H. C. (Ed.): *Pediatric Therapy.* 3rd ed. St. Louis, C. V. Mosby Company, 1968; and in other publications by permission (Ed.).

TABLE 5-16. *Continued*

DRUG	DOSAGE AND ROUTES	SUPPLIED

Ephedrine sulfate, U.S.P.	3 mg./kg./24 hr.
	100 mg./M.^{2}/24 hr.
	Divide into 4-6 doses (O, S.C. or I.V.)
	Caution: Insomnia, headache, nervousness, palpitation (arrhythmias on digitalis therapy), precordial pain, nausea, sweating, urinary retention; may potentiate theophylline (aminophylline) toxicity
		Capsules and tablets: 25 and 50 mg.
		Syrups:
		  N.F.: 20 mg./5 ml.
		  Others: 11 and 15 mg./5 ml.
		Ampules: 25 and 50 mg./ ml.

Epinephrine and salts, U.S.P. (Adrenalin and many other trade names)	Asthma or tolerance test:
	  Hydrochloride:
	    1:1000 (aqueous)
	      0.01 ml./kg./dose (maximum 0.5 ml.)
	      0.3 ml./M.^{2}/dose
	      Repeat every 4 hr. p.r.n. (S.C.)
	    1:100 (aqueous) by nebulizer p.r.n.
	  Base:
	    1:200 (suspension,
	      0.004 ml./kg./dose
	      0.125 ml./M.^{2}/dose
	      Repeat every 8-12 hr. (S.C.)
	    1:400 (suspension,
	      Double above dose
	    1:500 (in oil):
	      0.01-0.02 ml./kg./dose
	      0.3-0.6 ml./M.^{2}/dose
	      Daily or every 12 hr. (I.M.)
	Caution: Overdosage (*see* Ephedrine)
		1:1000 (aqueous):
		  Ampules: 1 ml.
		  Vials: 30 ml.
		  Bottles: 30 ml.
		
		1:100 (aqueous);
		  Bottles: 5 ml.
		
		1:200 (Sus-Phrine):
		  Bottles: 5 ml.
		  Ampules: 0.5 ml.
		1:400 (Asmolin):
		  Vials: 10 ml.
		
		1:500 (oil):
		  Ampules: 1 ml.

Isoproterenol hydrochloride, U.S.P. (Isuprel hydrochloride, Norisodrine hydrochloride, Proterenol hydrochloride)	5-10 mg. (Subl. or R)
	Repeat 3-4 times every 24 hr.
	I.V. use, see package insert
	Contraindication: With epinephrine (may produce arrhythmia)
	Caution: Careful dosage adjustment in hyperthyroidism, heart failure or limited cardiac reserve, sensitivity to sympathomimetics
		Hydrochloride:
		  Tablets (Subl. or R):
		    5, 10 and 15 mg.
		  Solution:
		    Vials: 1:200, 1:100
		  Nebulizer: Pressurized mist, 1:400
		  Ampules: 1:5000

Isoproterenol sulfate, N.F. (Isonorin sulfate, Norisodrine sulfate)	1:200 or 1:400: 1-2 inhalations
	Powder by inhalation
	Contraindication: With epinephrine (may produce arrhythmia)
	Caution: Careful dosage adjustment in hyperthyroidism, heart failure or limited cardiac reserve, sensitivity to sympathomimetics
		Sulfate (cartridges):
		  Powder: 10 and 25%
		  Tablets: 10 mg.
		  Solution: 1% (10 mg./ml.)

Levarterenol bitartrate, norepinephrine bitartrate, U.S.P. (Levophed bitartrate)	1 ml. of 0.2% solution (0.1% base) in 250 ml. diluent Drip at 0.5 ml./min. to give 2 μg (base)/min. (I.V.) 2 μg/M.^{2}/min. (I.V.) Titrate dose with blood pressure **Contraindication:** During cyclopropane anesthesia **Caution:** Headache, hypersensitivity, bradycardia; slough results from extravascular leakage Treat extravasated area quickly; infiltrate phentolamine (see p. 289) solution (5-10 mg. in 15 ml. saline solution)	Ampules, 0.2%, 2 mg./ml.

(Table Continues)

**D
R
U
G
S**

TABLE 5-16. *Continued*

DRUG	DOSAGE AND ROUTES	SUPPLIED
Mephentermine sulfate, N.F. (Wyamine sulfate)	0.4 mg./kg. 12 mg./M.² Single dose (O, I.M., or slowly I.V.) Repeat p.r.n. or by slow drip (0.1%) **Contraindications:** Hemorrhagic shock, concealed hemorrhage, phenothiazine hypotension	Tablets (scored): 12.5 and 25 mg. Elixir: 25 mg./5 ml. Vials: 15 and 30 mg./ml. Ampules: 15 mg./ml. Tubex: 30 and 60 mg.
Metaraminol bitartrate, U.S.P. (Aramine bitartrate)	0.1 mg./kg. 3 mg./M.² Single dose (S.C. or I.M.) Intravenous: Single dose: 1/10 of above dose I.V. by drip: 0.4 mg./kg. 12 mg./M.² Dilute each mg. in 25 ml. normal saline solution or 5% glucose; adjust rate to maintain blood pressure **Caution:** Cyclopropane anesthesia; thyroid or heart disease, diabetes	Ampules and vials: 10 mg./ml.
Methoxamine hydrochloride, U.S.P. (Vasoxyl)	0.25 mg./kg. 7.5 mg./M.² Single dose (I.M.) I.V. dose — ⅓ of I.M. (slowly) **Caution:** Severe hypertension, hyperthyroidism	Ampules: 20 mg./ml.
Phenylephrine hydrochloride, U.S.P. (Neo-Synephrine hydrochloride and many other trade names)	0.1 mg./kg. 3 mg./M.² Single dose (S.C. or I.M.) Oral: 1 mg./kg./24 hr. 30 mg./M.²/24 hr. Divide into 6 doses (O) **Caution:** Severe hypertension, cardiac disorders, hyperthyroidism, hyperglycemia	Capsules: 10 and 25 mg. Elixir: 5 mg./5 ml. Ampules: 2 and 10 mg./ml.

Adrenocorticotropin
(see Endocrines, *p. 297)*

Analeptics

Amphetamine sulfate *(see* Adrenergics, *p. 238)*		
Bemegride, U.S.P. (Megimide)	1 mg./kg. 30 mg./M.² Single dose (I.V.) Repeat in 3-5 min. for effect **Caution:** Convulsive (overdosage); keep pentobarbital sodium available	Ampules: 5 mg./ml. Vials: 5 mg./ml.
Caffeine and sodium benzoate, U.S.P.	8 mg./kg./dose (maximum, 500 mg.) 250 mg./M.²/dose Repeat every 4 hr. p.r.n. (S.C., I.V. or I.M.)	Ampules: 0.25 and 0.5 gm. (3¾ and 7½ gr.)

Key: *M.*, dose per square meter of body surface.   *R.*, rectal.
     I.M., intramuscular.   *S.C.*, subcutaneous.
     I.Th., intrathecal.   *Subl.*, sublingual.
     I.V., intravenous.   *T.*, topical.
     O., oral.

DRUGS

TABLE 5-16. *Continued*

DRUG	DOSAGE AND ROUTES	SUPPLIED
	Toxicity: CNS stimulation, convulsions; increase in gastric secretion and urinary excretion; hypotension and cardiac collapse	
Dextroamphetamine sulfate *(see* Adrenergics, *p. 238)*		
Ephedrine sulfate *(see* Adrenergics, *p. 238)*		
Ethamivan (Emivan)	0.5-5 mg./kg. 15-150 mg./M.² Single injection (I.V. slowly) Repeat at 5-min. intervals or follow by continuous I.V.: 0.2 mg./kg./min. 6 mg./M.²/min. Dilute each 4 mg. in 1 ml. fluid Titrate dose to patient **Contraindication:** Epilepsy **Caution:** May cause coughing, sneezing, laryngospasm, twitching, convulsions, pruritus; additive effects with monoamine oxidase inhibitors	Tablets: 20 and 60 mg. Ampules: 50 mg./ml.
Methylphenidate hydrochloride, N.F. (Ritalin hydrochloride)	0.75 mg./kg./dose 20 mg./M.²/dose Repeat in 30 min. if needed (I.M. or slowly I.V.) **Contraindications:** Epilepsy, tension states, glaucoma **Caution:** Use cautiously with pressor agents; may cause gastrointestinal symptoms, headache, rash, angina, cardiac arrhythmia	Tablets: 5, 10 and 20 mg. Vials: 10 mg./ml.
Nikethamide, N.F. (Coramine, Nikorin)	25 mg./kg./dose (maximum, 10 ml.) 0.75 gm./M.²/dose Well diluted (I.V. or I.M.) Repeat as needed	Ampules: 250 mg./ml. Vials: 250 mg./ml. Oral solution: 250 mg./ml.
Pentylenetetrazol, N.F. (Metrazol, Pentrazol)	20 mg./kg./dose (maximum, 10 ml.) 500 mg./M.²/dose Diluted (I.V. slowly) Dose for marked barbiturate depression may be repeated every 15 min. p.r.n. **Caution:** Convulsions (overdosage)	Tablets: 100 mg. Ampules: 100 mg./ml. Liquid: 100 mg./ml.
Picrotoxin, N.F.	Barbiturate poisoning: 0.2 mg./kg. 6 mg./M.² Single dose I.V. or I.M.; repeat in 15 min. **Caution:** Continuous observation; convulsions with overdosage	Ampules and vials: 3 mg./ml.

Analgesics (narcotic) Codeine phosphate, U.S.P.	For pain: 3 mg./kg./24 hr. 100 mg./M.²/24 hr. Divide into 6 doses (O or S.C.) For cough ⅓-½ of dose for pain **Warning:** May be habit-forming	Tablets: Many sizes Cough syrups often contain 10 mg./5 ml.

(Table Continues)

TABLE 5-16. *Continued*

DRUG	DOSAGE AND ROUTES	SUPPLIED
	Caution: Side effects like morphine (large doses) **Toxicity:** CNS depression; convulsions; meiosis; dyspnea	

Meperidine hydrochloride, N.F. (Demerol hydrochloride)
(as preanesthetic, *see* Table 5-17; *p. 314)*
	6 mg./kg./24 hr. (maximum, 100 mg./dose)
	175 mg./M.²/24 hr.
	Divide into 6 doses (O, I.M. or S.C.)
	Contraindications: Intracranial lesions causing increased pressure, atrioventricular flutter, bronchial asthma; potentiation with monoamine oxidase inhibitors, isoniazid or derivatives
	Warning: May be habit-forming; for **overdosage,** *see* Nalorphine, *p. 273*
		Tablets: 50 and 100 mg.
		Elixir: 50 mg./5 ml.
		Ampules (50 mg./ml.):
		  25 mg./0.5 ml.
		  50 mg./1 ml.
		  75 mg./1.5 ml.
		  100 mg./2 ml.
		Vials: 50 and 100 mg./ml.
		Disposable syringes: 75 and 100 mg./ml.
		Tubex (disposable): 25, 50, 75 and 100 mg./ml.
		Powder (vials): 15 gm.

Methadone hydrochloride, U.S.P. (Adanon hydrochloride, Althose, Amidone hydrochloride, Dolophine hydrochloride)	Analgesic dose:
	  0.7 mg./kg./24 hr.
	  20 mg./M.²/24 hr.
	  Divide into 4-6 doses (O or S.C.)
	Antitussive dose:
	  ¼ of analgesic dose (O)
	Warning: May be habit-forming; for **overdosage,** *see* Nalorphine, *p. 273*
	Caution: May cause nausea, vomiting, dizziness, dry mouth, euphoria, depression
		Tablets: 2.5, 5, 7.5 and 10 mg.
		Elixir: 5 mg./5 ml.
		Syrup: 1.66 mg./5 ml.
		Ampules or vials: 5 and 10 mg./ml.

Morphine sulfate, U.S.P. (paregoric contains 0.4 mg. morphine/ml.)	Analgesic dose: General use: 0.1-0.2 mg./kg./dose (S.C.) (maximum, 15 mg.) (preoperative, *see* Table 5-17; *p. 314*	Tablets: 10, 15 and 30 mg. Injection (suitable salts): 10 and 15 mg./ml.
Paregoric, U.S.P. (camphorated opium tincture)	Analgesic dose: 0.25-0.5 ml./kg./dose (O) Smaller dose may be offered initially; increase to analgesic dose as maximum *See* Morphine *above*	Paregoric: 0.4 mg. morphine/ml.

Analgesics (nonnarcotic) and antipyretics

DRUG	DOSAGE AND ROUTES	SUPPLIED

Acetaminophen, *N*-acetyl-*p*-aminophenol, N.F. (Tempra, Tylenol, and many other trade names)	Under 1 yr.: 60 mg.
	1-3 yr.: 60-120 mg.
	3-6 yr.: 120 mg.
	6-12 yr.: 240 mg.
	Single dose repeated every 4-6 hr. (O)
	0.7 gm./M.²/24 hr., divided into 4 or 6 doses (O)
		Tempra:
		  Tablets: 325 mg.
		  Syrup: 120 mg./5 ml.
		  Drops: 60 mg./0.6 ml.
		Tylenol:
		  Tablets (scored): 300 mg.
		  Elixir: 120 mg./5 ml.
		  Drops: 60 mg./0.6 ml.

Aspirin, acetylsalicylic acid, U.S.P. (Empirin)	Antipyretic dose:
	  65 mg./kg./24 hr. (maximum, 3.6 gm./24 hr.)
	  1.5 gm./M.²/ 24 hr.
		Supplied in many forms
		Tablets:
		  30, 60, 75, 300 and 600 mg.
		  (½, 1, 1¼, 5 and 10 gr.)

Key: *M.,* dose per square meter of body surface.   *R.,* rectal.
    I.M., intramuscular.   *S.C.,* subcutaneous.
    I.Th., intrathecal.   *Subl.,* sublingual.
    I.V., intravenous.   *T.,* topical.
    O., oral.

TABLE 5-16. *Continued*

DRUG	DOSAGE AND ROUTES	SUPPLIED
	Divide into 4-6 doses (O or R) Avoid overdosage, particularly in infants To obtain salicylate level of 20 mg./ 100 ml. of blood: 3 gm./M.^{2}/24 hr. (O) **Caution:** Salicylism, especially in infants (see p. 1501)	Suppositories: 60, 200, 300 and 600 mg. (1, 3, 5 and 10 gr.)
Methotrimeprazine (Levoprome) **Note:** Manufacturer does not presently recommend use in children under 12 years of age.	Parenteral: 0.22-0.33 mg./kg. 6-8 mg./M.^{2} Single dose (I.M. [deep] or diluted [saline] slowly I.V.); may repeat every 4-6 hr. **Contraindications:** History of idiosyncrasy to phenothiazines, premature infants, CNS depression (drug), severe cardiac or hepatic disease, hypertension or antihypertensive drugs **Caution:** May cause hypotension (keep supine several hours after use), drowsiness, vomiting (rare), dry mouth, nasal stuffiness, extrapyramidal symptoms (?), dermatitis, local pain (injection site), agranulocytosis (rare), jaundice **Toxicity (overdosage):** Tremor, ataxia, hypotonia, tachycardia, fever, hypotension; treat CNS depression (if necessary) with caffeine or amphetamines (p. 240)	Ampules: 20 mg./ml. Vials: 20 mg./ml.
Salicylamide, N.F. (Amid-Sal, Dropsprin, Liquiprin, Raspberin, Salamide, Salicim, Salrin)	Antipyretic-analgesic dose: 65 mg./kg./24 hr. 1.5 gm./M.^{2}/24 hr. Divide into 6 doses (O) **Caution:** Sensitivity to salicylates: may cause nausea, vomiting, drowsiness, hyperventilation, rash	Tablets: 300 and 600 mg. Suspension: 65 mg./ml.
Anthelmintics Bephenium hydroxynaphthoate (Alcopara)	Under 23 kg.: 1.0-2.5 gm./24 hr. Over 23 kg. and adult: 5 gm./24 hr. Divide into 2 doses (O); bitter taste may be disguised in carbonated beverages, flavored milk, orange juice; withhold food for 2 hr. after use **Caution:** Nausea, vomiting and diarrhea may occur; correct electrolyte imbalance before use; careful use in hypertension	Granules (packets): 5 gm. (equivalent to 2.5 gm. of base)
Diethylcarbamazine citrate, U.S.P. (Hetrazan)	Filariasis: 6 mg./kg./24 hr.	Tablets: 50 mg. Syrup: 120 mg./5 ml.

(Table Continues)

DRUGS

TABLE 5-16. *Continued*

DRUG	DOSAGE AND ROUTES	SUPPLIED

	150 mg./M.²/24 hr.
	Divide into 3 doses (O)
	Treat 7-10 days
	Ascariasis:
	  15 mg./kg./24 hr.
	  500 mg./M.²/24 hr. (O)
	  Single daily dose for 4 consecutive days
	Caution: May cause headache, malaise, weakness, nausea, vomiting; many reactions from filaricidal action	

Gentian violet, methylrosaniline chloride, U.S.P.	Oral moniliasis
	  Aqueous, 0.25%: 3-day courses (T), t.i.d.
	Oxyuriasis (as coated tablets):
	  2 mg./kg./24 hr.
	  50 mg./M.²/24 hr.
	  Divide into 2 or 3 doses/24 hr. (O)
	  Treat 7-10 days
	  Rest 7-10 days
	Caution: Caustic, not to be chewed; may cause nausea, vomiting (purple), diarrhea, abdominal pain; use with caution in cardiac, hepatic, renal or gastrointestinal disease
		Tablets (enteric-coated): 10 and 30 mg.
		Tablets: 15 and 30 mg.
		Solutions: Per cent desired
		Powder

Hexylresorcinol, N.F. (Caprokol)	0.1 gm./yr. of age (maximum, 1 gm.) Single dose (O) May repeat in 3 days **Caution:** Not to be chewed (caustic)	Crystoids: 0.1 and 0.2 gm.

Piperazine (as salts) (piperazine citrate, U.S.P.) (Antepar citrate, Anthalazine hexahydrate, Multifuge citrate, Oxucide citrate, Parazine citrate, Perin calcium edetate, Piperate tartrate, Piperazole phosphate, Pipizan citrate, Vermizine gluconate)	Dosage expressed as hydrous base
	Oxyuriasis:
	  Up to 7 kg.: 250 mg.
	  7-14 kg.: 500 mg.
	  14-27 kg.: 1 gm.
	  Over 27 kg.: 2 gm.
	  1 gm./M.²
	  Once daily before breakfast for 7 consecutive days (O)
	Ascariasis:
	  Up to 14 kg.: 1 gm.
	  14-23 kg.: 2 gm.
	  23-45 kg.: 3 gm.
	  Over 45 kg.: 3.5 gm.
	  2 gm./M.²
	  Once daily for 2 consecutive days (O)
	Contraindications: Patients with predisposition to grand or petit mal epilepsy
	Caution: Large doses: vomiting, blurred vision, muscle weakness, urticaria
		Tablets: 250 and 500 mg.
		Wafers: 500 mg.
		Syrup: 500 mg./5 ml.

Pyrvinium pamoate, U.S.P. (Povan)	5 mg./kg. (as base) 150 mg./M.² Single doses (O) **Caution:** Colors stools red; nausea, vomiting, cramping; suspension and chewed tablets stain; swallow tablets whole	Tablets (coated): 50 mg. (base) Suspension: 50 mg. (base)/5 ml.

Key: *M.,* dose per square meter of body surface.   *R.,* rectal.
      I.M., intramuscular.   *S.C.,* subcutaneous.
      I.Th., intrathecal.   *Subl.,* sublingual.
      I.V., intravenous.   *T.,* topical.
      O., oral.

TABLE 5-16. *Continued*

DRUG	DOSAGE AND ROUTES	SUPPLIED
Quinacrine hydrochloride *(see p. 729)* Tetrachloroethylene, U.S.P.	0.1 ml./kg. (maximum, 5 ml.) 3 ml./M.² Single dose (O) **Caution:** Avoid fats or alcohol (drug vehicle); toxic reactions rare—dizziness, nausea, drowsiness	Capsules: 0.2, 0.5, 1, 2.5 and 5 ml. Veterinary preparation of U.S.P. purity

Thiabendazole (Mintezol)	44 mg./kg./24 hr. (maximum, 3 gm.)
	1.3 gm./M.²/24 hr.
	Divide into 2 doses (O)
	Enterobiasis:
	  Repeat above dose in 7 days
	  If not practical, give above dose on 2 successive days
	Intestinal parasitoses:
	  (Singly or combinations)
	  Above dose—1 day or 2 successive days
	Cutaneous larva migrans:
	  Above dose—2 successive days
	  If active lesions after 2 days, repeat the course
	Trichinosis:
	  Above dose—2-4 successive days
	Caution: Gastrointestinal symptoms, dizziness, headache, fatigue, pruritus; rarely tinnitus, collapse, abnormal ocular sensations, numbness, hyperglycemia, xanthopsia, enuresis, cephalin flocculation and SGOT rises—transitory; odor to urine, crystalluria, transient leukopenia
		Suspension: 500 mg./5 ml.

Antiasthmatics
(see Bronchodilators, p. 279)

Antibiotics and chemotherapeutics
Antibiotics
Ampicillin
(see p. 251)

| Bacitracin, U.S.P.
(1 mg. = 50 units) | Systemic infections:
  Premature infants: 900 units/kg./24/hr.
  Full-term newborn infants to 1 year:
    1000 units/kg./24 hr.
    30,000 units/M.²/24 hr.
  Divide into 2 or 3 doses (I.M.)
  Not longer than 10-12 days
Enteric infections:
  Premature infants: 1000 units/kg./24 hr.
  Older infants and children:
    2000 units/kg./24 hr.
    60,000 units/M.²/24 hr.
  Divide into 4 doses (O)
Caution: Nephrotoxicity, anorexia, nausea, rashes, local irritation; store solution at 4°C.; use within 24 hr. after mixing | Powder (ampules): 2000, 10,000 and 50,000 units
Tablets: 2500 and 5000 units |

TABLE 5-16. *Continued*

DRUG	DOSAGE AND ROUTES	SUPPLIED
Cephaloridine (Loridine)	Mild to moderately severe infections: 30-50 mg./kg./24 hr. (maximum, 4 gm./24 hr.) 0.9-1.5 gm./M.²/24 hr. Divide into 3 doses* Severe infections: 100 mg./kg./24 hr. (maximum, 4 gm./24 hr.) 2.3 gm./M.²/24 hr. Divide into 4 doses* (Store freshly made solutions not more than 96 hr.—refrigeration) **Warning:** Caution in administration of this or other antibiotics to allergic (particularly drugs) patients, give only for absolute necessity; anaphylaxis is rare; doses not to exceed 4 gm./24 hr. (nephrotoxicity); close observation or hospitalization, if known or suspected renal impairment—discontinue drug if impaired renal function develops; not to be used in azotemic patients; with renal impairment: use with caution and reduced dose; casts, proteinuria, falling urinary output, rising BUN or creatinine may indicate renal impairment; use drug with caution when given with other potentially nephrotoxic antibiotics **Contraindications:** Known hypersensitivity to this drug or cephalothin (Keflin), azotemia; not for oral use (poorly absorbed) **Caution:** Protect from light; do not mix with other antibiotics; full 10-day course—streptococcal treatment; darkfield examination of lesions and at least 3-monthly serologic tests in gonorrheal patients; superinfection with resistant organisms may occur; safety for premature infants under 1 month of age not established or recommended; urticaria, skin rash and itching (3% of patients); eosinophil rise (1% of patients), leukopenia, transaminase elevation, alkaline phosphatase rise, acute tubular necrosis, renal failure, and death have occurred (possibility greater in seriously ill given more than recommended dose); rare gastrointestinal symptoms; local pain, phlebitis rare	Ampules: 0.5 and 1.0 gm.

*I.M. deep, usual infection

I.V. by slow push or continuous drip, extremely serious infections.

Note: Not recommended for premature infants or term infants under 1 month of age.

Key: *M.,* dose per square meter of body surface.　　*R.,* rectal.
　　　I.M., intramuscular.　　　　　　　　　　　*S.C.,* subcutaneous.
　　　I.Th., intrathecal.　　　　　　　　　　　*Subl.,* sublingual.
　　　I.V., intravenous.　　　　　　　　　　　*T.,* topical.
　　　O., oral.

TABLE 5-16. *Continued*

DRUG	DOSAGE AND ROUTES	SUPPLIED
Cephalothin sodium (Keflin)	Most susceptible infections: 50 mg./kg./24 hr. 1.5 gm./M.^{2}/24 hr. Divide into 4 doses* Severe infections: May need double above dose. Life threatening infections, lowered resistance: 80-225 mg./kg./24 hrs. (maximum 12 gm.) 2.5-7 gm./M.^{2}/24 hr. Divide into 4 to 6 doses* Moderately severe oliguria: 120 mg./kg./24 hr. (maximum) 3.5 gm./M.^{2}/24 hr. (maximum) Divide into 4 to 6 doses* Anuria: Loading dose: 120 mg./kg. 3.5 gm./M.^{2} Maintenance dose: $\frac{1}{6}$-$\frac{1}{2}$ of loading dose Single dose or divided into 2 doses* or into 2 to 3 doses* if dialysis is performed Peritoneal dialysis: Up to 6 gm./100 ml. of dialysis fluid Store solution in refrigerator not more than 48 hr. Add to I.V. solutions (5% D/W or N.S.) with pH between 4 and 7 **Caution:** May produce neutropenia, eosinophilia, allergic reactions, rash, anaphylaxis, positive Coombs's test in azotemia or in newborn infant if mother treated; positive urinary reducing agents to copper salts; irritating I.M. (pain, induration) and I.V. (phlebitis); overgrowth of nonsusceptible organisms may occur	Ampules: 1 and 4 gm.
Chloramphenicol, U.S.P. (Chloromycetin) and derivatives. *See p. 312 for special warning regarding use in newborn infants.*	Premature and full-term newborn infants (up to 2 wk.): 25 mg./kg/24 hr. Over 2 wk.: Infants: 50 mg./kg./24 hr. Older children: 50 mg./kg./24 hr. 1.5 gm./M.^{2}/24 hr. Double dose for severe infections Divided doses: Intervals: 6 hr. (O) 6 hr. or continuous (I.V.) **Caution:** Adjust newborn infant's dose by frequent blood levels (10-20 μg/ml.) to avoid "gray syndrome" **Warning:** Serious and even fatal aplastic anemia, hypoplastic anemia, thrombocytopenia and granulocytopenia (long- or short-term therapy); blood studies	Capsules: 50, 100 and 250 mg. Suspension (palmitate): 156 mg./5 ml. Powder: (I.V. only) 0.25 gm. 1.0 gm. Ophthalmic: 25 mg. powder for solution Ointment: 1% Otic: 0.5% solution Other topical and parenteral forms available

(Table Continues)

---

*I.M. (deep) or I.V. (slow push or continuous drip)

TABLE 5-16. *Continued*

DRUG	DOSAGE AND ROUTES	SUPPLIED
	during treatment; not to be used when less dangerous agents will be effective; not to be used for trivial infections or to prevent bacterial infections, or in known sensitivity to it; danger of high levels in hepatic or renal disease	
Colistin (Coly-Mycin) *(see p. 255)* Erythromycins Erythromycin and salts, U.S.P. (Erythrocin, Ilotycin, Pediamycin)	Oral: 30-50 mg./kg./24 hr. 0.9-1.5 gm./M.²/24 hr. Divide into 4-6 doses (O) Parenteral: 10 mg./kg./24 hr. 300 mg./M.²/24 hr. Divide into 2 or 3 doses (I.M. [deep] or I.V.) Rheumatic fever prophylaxis: Single dose: 200 mg./24 hr. (O) **Caution:** Hypersensitivity to the drug, overgrowth of nonsusceptible organisms	Tablets: 100 and 250 mg. Tablets (chewable): 125 and 200 mg. Suspension: 200 mg./5 ml. Drops (oral): 100 mg./2.5 ml. (dropperful) 5 mg./1 drop Ampules: 50 mg./ml. (I.M.) Vials: 250, 300, 500 mg., and 1 gm. (I.V.) (powder) 50 mg./ml. (I.M.) Syringes (disposable): 50 mg./ml. (I.M.) Suppositories: 125 mg.
Erythromycin estolate, N.F. (Ilosone)	Moderate infections: Under 11 kg.: 40 mg./kg./24 hr. 11-23 kg.: 500 mg./24 hr. Over 23 kg. and adults: 1 gm./24 hr. 750 mg./M.²/24 hr. Divide into 4 doses (O) Severe infections: Double above doses **Contraindications:** Sensitivity to this drug, pre-existing liver disease **Caution:** Gastrointestinal and allergic reactions, intrahepatic cholestasis (changed hepatic function tests), jaundice may or may not be present), eosinophilia	Tablets (chewable): 125 mg. Capsules: 125 and 250 mg. Liquid: 125 mg./5 ml. Suspension: 125 mg./5 ml. Drops: 5 mg./drop (100 mg./ml.) (calibrated at 25 and 50 mg.)
Kanamycin sulfate, U.S.P. (Kantrex)	Systemic infections: Premature and full-term newborn infants to 1 year: 15 mg./kg./24 hr. Divide into 2 doses (I.M.) Older infants and children: 6-15 mg./kg./24 hr. 150-450 mg./M.²/24 hr. Divide into 2 doses (I.M.) Intestinal infections (all ages): 50 mg./kg./24 hr. 1.5 gm./M.²/24 hr. Divide into 4-6 doses (O) for 5-7 days Inhalation: Add 1 ml. (250 mg./ml.) to 3 ml. normal saline solution	Capsules: 0.5 gm. Vials: 37.5 mg./ml. 250 mg./ml. 333 mg./ml.

Key: *M.*, dose per square meter of body surface.   *R.*, rectal.
      I.M., intramuscular.   *S.C.*, subcutaneous.
      I.Th., intrathecal.   *Subl.*, sublingual.
      I.V., intravenous.   *T.*, topical.
      O., oral.

TABLE 5-16. *Continued*

DRUG	DOSAGE AND ROUTES	SUPPLIED
	Contraindications: Sensitivity to this drug; previous eighth nerve damage from this or other drugs **Caution:** Overgrowth of nonsusceptible organisms, local irritation (I.M.), renal or auditory toxicity, skin reactions; assess kidney function before and during therapy; reduce dose and lengthen interval with impaired function; stop dosage, check hearing with nitrogen retention, tinnitus, subjective or high-frequency loss (audiometry); intraperitoneal use only after recovery from anesthesia	

Lincomycin hydrochloride monohydrate (Lincocin)	Oral (over 1 mo. of age):
	  Mild to moderately severe infections:
	    30 mg./kg./24 hr.
	    0.9 gm./M.²/24 hr.
	    Divide into 3 or 4 doses (O)
	    Nothing but water by mouth 2 hr. before and after administration
	  Severe infections:
	    Double above dose (O)
	Intramuscular (over 1 mo. of age):
	  Mild to moderately severe infections:
	    10 mg./kg./24 hr.
	    0.3 gm./M.²/24 hr.
	    Single dose (I.M.)
	  Severe infections:
	    Repeat dose every 12 hr. (I.M.)
	Intravenous (over 1 mo. of age):
	  10-20 mg./kg./24 hr.
	  0.3-0.6 gm./M.²/24 hr.
	  Divide into 2 or 3 doses (as infusion in glucose or saline) (I.V.)
	Contraindications: Hypersensitivity to this drug, minor bacterial and viral infections, monilial infections, infants under 1 mo. of age
	Caution: Blood cell counts during therapy; liver function tests after 1-2 weeks, gastrointestinal symptoms, rash, urticaria and itching; with severe renal impairment reduce dosage to 25-30% of above dosage
		Capsules: 250 and 500 mg.
		Syrup: 250 mg./5 ml.
		Drops: 250 mg./5 ml.
		Vials: 300 mg./ml.

Methicillin *(see p. 252)*		
Nafcillin *(see p. 253)*		

Neomycin sulfate, U.S.P. (Mycifradin sulfate, Neobiotic)	Premature and full-term newborn infants:
	  50 mg./kg./24 hr.; divide into 4 doses (O)
	  4 mg./kg./24 hr.; divide into 4 doses (I.M.)
	  Limit, 10 days
	Older infants and children:
	  100 mg./kg./24 hr.
	  3 gm./M.²/24 hr.
	  Divide into 4 doses (O)
	  7.5-15 mg./kg./24 hr.
		Tablets: 0.5 gm.
		Oral solution: 125 mg./ml.
		Vials: 0.5 gm. (0.35 gm., base)
		Vials (topical): 5 and 10 gm.

DRUGS

(Table Continues)

TABLE 5-16. *Continued*

DRUG	DOSAGE AND ROUTES	SUPPLIED

	(Not more than 1 gm./24 hr.)
	200-400 mg./M.²/24 hr.
	Divide into 4 doses (I.M.)
	Limit, 10 days
	Peritonitis:
	  (Not more than 20 mg./kg./24 hr.)
	  0.6 gm./M.²/24 hr.
	  Single or divided doses as 0.5-1%
	    solution in normal saline (intra-
	    peritoneal) for no more than 3 days
	Bowel preparation:
	  40 mg./kg./24 hr.
	  1.2 gm./M.²/24 hr.
	  Divide into 6 doses (O)
	  (Not more than 72 hr.)
	Contraindications: Intestinal obstruc-
	tion, ulcerative bowel lesions; discon-
	tinue with signs of renal damage
	Caution: Renal and eighth nerve dam-
	age; concomitant use of other ototoxic
	drugs may add to toxicity; overgrowth
	of nonsusceptible organisms, neomycin
	sensitivity; intraperitoneal-respiratory
	failure (curare-like effect)	

Novobiocin salts, N.F.
  (Albamycin, Cathomycin)
	Newborn and premature infants:
	  20 mg./kg./24 hr.
	  Divide into 2 or 3 doses (O, I.M. or
	    I.V.)
	Older infants and children:
	  20-45 mg./kg./24 hr.
	  0.6-1.2 gm./M.²/24 hr.
	  Divide into 4 doses (O)
	  15-40 mg./kg./24 hr.
	  0.5-1 gm./M.²/24 hr.
	  Divide into 2 doses (I.V. or I.M.)
	Caution: Avoid during first week of life
	if possible (bilirubin elevation); eo-
	sinophilia, rashes and fever
		Capsules: 250 mg.
		Syrup: 125 mg./5 ml.
		Vials: 500 mg.

Oleandomycin phosphate (*see* Triacetyloleandomycin, *p. 258*)		

Paromomycin sulfate (Hu-
matin sulfate)
	Amebiasis (intestinal) (as base):
	  25 mg./kg./24 hr. for 5 days
	  0.75 gm./M.²/24 hr. for 5 days
	  Divide into 3 doses (O)
	Dysentery:
	  Double amebiasis dose up to 7 days;
	    divide into 3 or 4 doses (O)
	  Severe: Up to 4 times amebiasis dose
	Caution: Course of treatment should
	not exceed 10 days; potential neph-
	rotoxicity from absorption, overgrowth
	of nonsusceptible organisms; diarrhea,
	nausea common; headache, vertigo,
	skin rashes, abdominal pain and vom-
	iting may occur
		Equivalent of base:
		  Capsules: 250 mg.
		  Syrup: 125 mg./5 ml.

Key: *M.*, dose per square meter of body surface.   *R.*, rectal.
    I.M., intramuscular.   *S.C.*, subcutaneous.
    I.Th., intrathecal.   *Subl.*, sublingual.
    I.V., intravenous.   *T.*, topical.
    O., oral.

DRUGS

TABLE 5-16. *Continued*

DRUG	DOSAGE AND ROUTES	SUPPLIED

Oxacillin *(see p. 253)*

DRUG	DOSAGE AND ROUTES	SUPPLIED
Penicillins: Ampicillin, anhydrous, tri-hydrate, and sodium (Amcill, Omnipen, Penbritin, Polycillin, Principen)	Under 40 kg.: Moderately severe infections: 50-100 mg./kg./24 hr. Divide into 4 doses (O, I.M. or I.V.) Severe infections: 200 mg./kg./24 hr. Divide into 4 to 6 doses (O, I.M. or I.V.) Over 40 kg. and adults: Moderate infections: 1-2 gm./24 hr. Divide into 4 doses (O, I.M. or I.V.) Severe infections: Up to 8-14 gm./24 hr. Divide into 4 to 6 doses (O, I.M. or I.V.) Parenteral: Use within 1 hr. of reconstitution I.V. direct—over 5 min. I.V. drip—10% loss of activity in 4 hr. **Contraindications:** Serious penicillin sensitivity, penicillinase-producing organisms; infectious mononuclosis (rash) **Caution:** Allergic patients; periodic renal, hepatic and hematopoietic tests; care in newborn use; superinfections with nonsensitive organisms may follow use; skin, gastrointestinal, anaphylactic reactions, SGOT rise, eosinophilia, 2.7 mEq. Na/gm.	Tablets chewable: 125 mg. Capsules: 250 and 500 mg. Oral suspension: 125 and 250 mg./5 ml. Drops: 100 mg./ml. Vials: 125, 250 and 500 mg.; 1 gm.
Penicillin G: Potassium penicillin G, U.S.P. (1 mg. = 1595 units) Sodium penicillin G, N.F. (1 mg. = 1667 units)	Premature and full-term newborn infants: 60,000 units/kg./24 hr. Divide into 2 doses (I.M. or I.V.) Older children: 25,000-50,000 units/kg./24 hr. 0.5-1 gm./M.^{2}/24 hr. Divide into 4-6 doses (O, I.M., I.V. or S.C.) (oral, $\frac{1}{2}$ hr. a.c.) Severe infections (e.g., meningitis): 300,000-400,000 units/kg./24 hr. (I.V.) Rheumatic fever prophylaxis: 200,000 units twice daily (O) (p. 541) **Contraindications:** Sensitivity to this drug **Caution:** Penicillin reactions, allergic, anaphylactic; if either Na$^+$ or K$^+$ effect is feared (large doses I.V.), order the particular salt desired; each million units of potassium penicillin G yields 1.68 mEq. of potassium (65.8 mg.); each million units of sodium penicillin G yields 1.68 mEq. of sodium (38.7 mg.); dilute well and give slowly	Many forms and preparations
Benzathine penicillin G, U.S.P. (Bicillin, Neolin, Permapen) (1 mg. = 1211 units)	0.6-1.2 million units (I.M.) Rheumatic fever prophylaxis: 1.2 million units once a month (I.M.) (p. 541)	In units: Tablets: 100,000 and 200,000 Suspension: 150,000 and 300,000/5 ml. Drops: 150,000/ml. *(Table Continues)*

DRUGS

TABLE 5-16. *Continued*

DRUG	DOSAGE AND ROUTES	SUPPLIED
	Contraindications: As for penicillin **Caution:** As for penicillin	Vials: 300,000 and 600,000/ml. Steraject, Tubex: 600,000 Syringe (disposable): 900,000/1.5 ml. 1,200,000/2 ml. 2,400,000/4 ml.

Cloxacillin, sodium mon-ohydrate (TegoPen)	Up to 20 kg.: 50 mg./kg./24 hr.
	Over 20 kg. and adults:
	  Mild to moderate infections:
	    1 gm./24 hr.
	    0.6 gm./M.²/24 hr.
	  More severe infections:
	    2 gm./24 hr.
	    1.2 gm./M.²/24 hr.
	  Divide into 4 doses (O)
	  Very severe infections:
	    Larger and more frequent doses
	Contraindications: As for oxacillin
	Caution: As for oxacillin
		Capsules: 125 and 250 mg.
		Oral solution: 125 mg./5 ml.

Dicloxacillin (sodium) monohydrate (Dynapen, Pathocil, Veracillin)
 	
Note: Do not use in infections known to be due to penicillinase-producing staphylococci.
	Mild to moderate infections:
	  Adults and children over 40 kg.:
	  500 mg./24 hr.*
	  Children under 40 kg.:
	  12.5 mg./kg./24 hr.*
	Severe infections:
	  Double above doses*
	Contraindications: History of allergy to penicillin or to this drug.
	Caution: In asthma or allergies, may cause skin rash, pruritus, urticaria, drug fever, eosinophilia, gastrointestinal disturbances, elevated SGOT, positive cephalin flocculation test. Long-term therapy—periodically assess hepatic, renal and hemopoietic function
		Capsules: 62.5, 125 and 250 mg.
		Oral suspension: 62.5 mg./5 ml.

Methicillin sodium, dime-thoxyphenyl penicillin sodium, U.S.P. (Dimocillin-RT, Staphcillin)	100 mg./kg./24 hr. 3 gm./M.²/24 hr. Divide into 4-6 doses (I.M. [deep]) **Contraindications:** History of serious allergic reaction to any penicillin **Caution:** In patients with allergies or asthma; may cause skin rash, urticaria, pruritus, overgrowth of non-susceptible organisms, transient neutropenia, bone marrow depression,	Vials (powder): 1, 4 and 6 gm. (1 gm. is equivalent to 900 mg. base)

*Divide into 4 doses (O). (Give 1 hour before or 3 hours after meals.)
Note: Neonatal dosage not established.
Key: *M.*, dose per square meter of body surface.　　　　*R.*, rectal.
　　　I.M., intramuscular.　　　　　　　　　　　　*S.C.*, subcutaneous.
　　　I.Th., intrathecal.　　　　　　　　　　　　*Subl.*, sublingual.
　　　I.V., intravenous.　　　　　　　　　　　　*T.*, topical.
　　　O., oral.

TABLE 5-16. *Continued*

DRUG	DOSAGE AND ROUTES	SUPPLIED
	renal impairment; in prolonged therapy do periodic assessment of renal, hepatic and hematopoietic function; avoid mixing with other drugs	
Nafcillin (Unipen)	Oral: Newborn infants: 40 mg./kg./24 hr. Divide into 4 doses (O) Older infants and children: Scarlet fever and pneumonia: 25 mg./kg./24 hr. 0.75 gm./M.²/24 hr. Divide into 4 doses (O) Staphylococcal infections: Double above doses Parenteral: Newborn infants: 20 mg./kg./24 hr. Divide into 2 doses (I.M.) Older infants and children: 50 mg./kg./24 hr. 1.5 gm./M.²/24 hr. Divide into 2 doses (I.M.) Divide into 6 doses (I.V.) (May need double this dose in severe infections) **Contraindications:** Penicillin sensitivity, trivial infections **Caution:** Gastrointestinal superinfection with nonsusceptible organisms, allergic reactions, gastrointestinal symptoms	Capsules: 250 mg. Oral solution: 250 mg./5 ml. For injection: Reconstituted, 250 mg./ml.
Oxacillin sodium, U.S.P. (Prostaphlin, Resistopen)	Mild to moderately severe infections (O): Premature and full-term newborn infants: 25 mg./kg./24 hr. Under 40 kg.: 50 mg./kg./24 hr. 1.5 gm./M.²/24 hr. Over 40 kg. and adults: 2-3 gm./24 hr. Divide into 4-6 doses (O) (1-2 hr. before meals) Serious infections (O): Under 40 kg.: 100 mg./kg./24 hr. 3 gm./M.²/24 hr. Over 40 kg.: 4-6 gm./24 hr. Divide into 4-6 doses (O) (1-2 hr. before meals) Parenteral (I.M.): Under 40 kg.: 50-100 mg./kg./24 hr. 1.5-3 gm./M.²/24 hr. Depending on severity of infection Divide into 4 doses (I.M.) Over 40 kg. and adults: 1-6 gm./24 hr. Depending on severity of infection Divide into 4-6 doses (I.M.)	Capsules: 250 and 500 mg. Oral solution: 250 mg./5 ml. Vials: 250, 500 mg., and 1 gm.

D
R
U
G
S

(Table Continues)

TABLE 5-16. *Continued*

DRUG	DOSAGE AND ROUTES	SUPPLIED

	Parenteral (I.V.):
	   Follow (I.M.) dosage
	   Well diluted, give slowly (over 10 min.
	     or by drip)
	 Contraindications: Sensitivity to this
	 or other penicillins
	 Caution: Allergy, weigh need against
	 danger; may cause rash, urticaria,
	 pruritus, gastrointestinal symptoms,
	 SGOT rise, hepatic dysfunction, gran-
	 ulocytopenia, leukopenia, thrombo-
	 phlebitis (I.V. use)	

Phenethicillin potassium, N.F. (Alpen, Chemipen, Darcil, Dramcillin-s, Maxipen, Ro-Cillin, Semopen, Syncillin) (125 mg. = 200,000 units)	Same as penicillin V (see below) **Contraindications:** As for penicillin **Caution:** As for penicillin	Tablets (scored): 125 and 250 mg. Syrup: 125 mg./5 ml. Oral solution: 125 mg./5 ml. Drops: 125 mg./0.6 ml.

Phenoxymethyl penicillin,
 penicillin V, N.F.
 (Compocillin V, Pen-Vee,
 V-Cillin)
 (1 mg. = 1695 units)
	25,000-50,000 units/kg./24 hr.
	 0.5-1 gm./M.²/24 hr.
	 Divide into 4 doses daily (O)
	
	 Rheumatic fever prophylaxis: 125 mg.
	   once or twice daily (O)
	 Contraindications: As for penicillin
	 Caution: As for penicillin
		Tablets and capsules:
		   125 mg. (200,000 units)
		   250 mg. (400,000 units)
		   500 mg. (800,000 units)
		 Suspension:
		   90 mg. (150,000 units)/5 ml.
		   125 mg. (200,000 units)/5 ml.
		   180 mg. (300,000 units)/5 ml.
		   250 mg. (400,000 units)/5 ml.
		 Drops:
		   90 mg./ml.
		   125 mg./0.6 ml.
		 Wafers (chewable):
		   125 mg. (200,000 units)
		   250 mg. (400,000 units)

Phenoxymethyl penicillin
 potassium, penicillin V
 potassium, U.S.P.
 (Compocillin-VK, Pen-Vee
 K, V-Cillin K)
 (1 mg. = 1530 units)
	Same as penicillin V
	 Contraindications: As for penicillin
	 Caution: As for penicillin; prolonged
	   high dosage—check renal and hema-
	   topoietic systems
		Tablets:
		   125 mg. (200,000 units)
		   250 mg. (400,000 units)
		   500 mg. (800,000 units)
		 Tablets (long acting): 250 mg.
		   (400,000 units)
		 Liquids (solution and suspen-
		   sions):
		   125 mg. (200,000 units)/5 ml.
		   250 mg. (400,000 units)/5 ml.

Procaine penicillin G,
 U.S.P.
 (1 mg. = 1009 units)
	0.5-1 million units/M.²/24 hr.
	 0.5-1 gm./M.²/24 hr.
	 Single dose (I.M.)
	 Avoid in newborn infants
	 Contraindications: As for penicillin
	 Caution: As for penicillin
		Injection:
		   300,000 units/ml. (0.3 gm./
		   ml.)
		   500,000 units/ml. (0.5 gm./
		   ml.)
		 With aluminum monostearate
		   300,000 units/ml. (0.3 gm./
		   ml.)

Key: *M.,* dose per square meter of body surface.   *R.,* rectal.
    I.M., intramuscular.   *S.C.,* subcutaneous.
    I.Th., intrathecal.   *Subl.,* sublingual.
    I.V., intravenous.   *T.,* topical.
    O., oral.

TABLE 5-16. *Continued*

DRUG	DOSAGE AND ROUTES	SUPPLIED

Polymyxins
  Colistin sulfate and sodium colistimethate, U.S.P., polymyxin E (Coly-Mycin)
	Bacterial enterocolitis:
	  3-5 mg./kg./24 hr.
	  90-150 mg./M.²/24 hr.
	  Divide into 3 doses (O)
	Systemic infections:
	  5 mg./kg./24 hr.
	  150 mg./M.²/24 hr.
	  Divide into 2-4 doses (I.M.)* (not for I.V. or I.Th. use)
	Contraindications: Sensitivity to this drug
	Caution: Neurotoxic (circumoral paresthesias or numbness, tingling or formication of extremities, pruritus, vertigo, dizziness, slurred speech); avoid machinery operation; nephrotoxic – great care in renal insufficiency; overgrowth of nonsusceptible organisms
		Oral suspension: 25 mg./5 ml.
		Vials: 150 mg. (contains dibucaine hydrochloride [Nupercaine])

Polymyxin B sulfate, U.S.P. (Aerosporin sulfate)	Enteric infections:
	  10-20 mg./kg./24 hr.
	  250 mg./M.²/24 hr.
	  Divide into 3 or 4 doses (O)
	Systemic infections:
	  Intramuscular:
	    1.5-2.5 mg./kg./24 hr.
	    (Maximum, 200 mg./24 hr.)
	    (Maximum, 120 mg./M.²/24 hr.)
	    Divide into 4 doses (I.M. [deep])*
	  Intravenous:
	    2.5 mg./kg./24 hr.
	    (Maximum, 200 mg./24 hr.)
	    Single infusion or divided into 2 infusions (give dose in 1-1½ hr.)
	Renal impairment:
	  1.5 mg./kg./24 hr. (I.V. or I.M.)
	Intrathecal (in addition to systemic doses):
	  Under 2 yr.: 2 mg./day for 3-4 days; then 2.5 mg. every other day
	  Over 2 yr. and adults: 5 mg./day for 3-4 days; then 5 mg. every other day (avoid local anesthetic in solution)
	Contraindications: Hypersensitivity to this drug
	Caution: Nephrotoxic, neurotoxic (ataxia, paresthesia, hyperesthesia), fever, rashes; overgrowth of nonsusceptible organisms; stop use if circumoral or peripheral paresthesias or marked dizziness appears; reduce dose with renal damage or nitrogen retention
		Tablets: 50 mg.
		Tablets (soluble): 25 mg.
		Sterile powder: 50 mg./vial
		1 mg. = 10,000 units

Streptomycin sulfate, U.S.P.	Premature and full-term newborn infants:
	  20-30 mg./kg./24 hr.
	  Divide into 2 doses (I.M.)
		Syrup: 250 mg./5 ml.
		Vials (solution): 0.4 and 0.5 gm./ml.
		Vials and ampules: 1 and 5 gm.
		(Table Continues)

*I.M. doses – care to avoid injection into nerves or blood vessels.

TABLE 5-16. *Continued*

DRUG	DOSAGE AND ROUTES	SUPPLIED
	Decrease with decreased urinary output Course: Not more than 10 days General use (older children): 40 mg./kg./24 hr. 1 gm./M.²/24 hr. Divide into 2 doses (I.M.) Up to 10 days Renal depression: give ½-¾ of dose Tuberculosis: 20 mg./kg./24 hr. Single dose (I.M.) Aerosol: 300 mg./2-ml./dose Repeat 4 times daily Intrathecal: 1 mg./kg./day (Diluted to 5 mg./ml.) Intraperitoneal, intrapleural, intra-articular: 50 mg./ml. **Contraindications:** Sensitivity to this drug **Caution:** Observe and test auditory and vestibular function; nephrotoxicity, may cause optic nerve dysfunction, paresthesias of lips and extremities, allergic reactions (skin, eosinophilia, drug fever, blood dyscrasias), CNS depression (stupor, flaccidity, coma, respiratory depression); intrathecal use—cervical pain, headache, malaise, convulsions; reduce dose with renal excretory impairment; overgrowth of nonsusceptible organisms may occur	
Tetracyclines: Chlortetracycline hydrochloride, N.F. (Aureomycin) Chlortetracycline calcium	As tetracycline **Contraindications:** As for tetracycline **Caution:** As for tetracycline	Tablets: 50 mg. Capsules: 50, 100 and 250 mg. Syrup: 125 mg./5 ml. Spersoids: 50 mg./tsp. Powder (surgical): 200 mg./gm. I.V.: 250 and 500 mg.
Demethylchlortetracycline, N.F. (Declomycin)	10 mg./kg./24 hr. 0.3 gm./M.²/24 hr. Divide into 2-4 doses (O) **Contraindications:** As for tetracycline **Caution:** As for tetracycline	Capsules: 75 and 150 mg. Tablets: 150 mg. Film tabs: 75 and 150 mg. Syrup: 75 mg./5 ml. Suspension: 75 mg./5 ml. Drops: 60 mg./ml.
Doxycycline monohydrate and hyclate (Vibramycin)	Less than 45 kg.: Initial: 4.4 mg./kg./24 hr. Divide into 2 doses (O) Maintenance: ½ of above dose Single or divide into 2 doses (O)	Hyclate Capsules: 50 and 100 mg. Monohydrate For oral solution: 25 mg./5 ml.

Key: *M.*, dose per square meter of body surface.   *R.*, rectal.
    I.M., intramuscular.   *S.C.*, subcutaneous.
    I.Th., intrathecal.   *Subl.*, sublingual.
    I.V., intravenous.   *T.*, topical.
    O., oral.

TABLE 5-16. *Continued*

DRUG	DOSAGE AND ROUTES	SUPPLIED
	More than 45 kg. and adults: Initial: 200 mg. Divide into 2 doses (O) Maintenance: ½ of above dose Single or divide into 2 doses (O) **Contraindications:** Sensitivity to this drug **Warning:** Hepatic *toxicity* with excessive dosage or renal impairment with standard dosage (lower dose and do serum level determinations with renal impairment); see tetracycline caution (p. 258) for other dangers—bone, tooth, increased intracranial pressure, photosensitivity **Caution:** Overgrowth of nonsusceptible organisms, gastrointestinal symptoms, vaginitis, dermatitis, glossitis, stomatitis, proctitis, onycholysis, discoloration of nails, elevation of SGOT or SGPT, anemia, neutropenia, eosinophilia may occur; discontinue use with severe adverse reaction	
Methacycline hydro- chloride (Rondomycin)	12 mg./kg./24 hr. 350 mg./M.²/24 hr. Divide into 2-4 doses 2 hr. p.c. **Contraindications:** As for tetracycline **Caution:** As for tetracycline	Capsules: 150 and 300 mg. Syrup: 75 mg./5 ml.
Oxytetracycline, its salts and derivatives, N.F. (Terramycin)	As tetracycline Also: 50 mg./ml. twice daily as aerosol in 10% propylene glycol **Contraindications:** As for tetracycline **Caution:** As for tetracycline	Capsules: 125 and 250 mg. Syrup: 125 mg./5 ml. Pediatric drops: 5 mg./drop I.M. (ampules and vials): 50 and 125 mg./ml. I.V.: 250 and 500 mg.
Rolitetracycline, *N*-(pyr- rolidinomethyl) tetra- cycline (Syntetrin, Velacycline)	15-20 mg./kg./24 hr. 0.45 gm./M.²/24 hr. Single dose or divided into 2 doses (I.M. or I.V.) **Contraindications:** As for tetracycline **Caution:** As for tetracycline	I.M. vials: 150 and 350 mg. I.V. vials: 700 mg.
Tetracycline, its salts, U.S.P., and complexes (Achromycin, Bristacycline, Kesso-Tetra, Panmycin, Steclin, Sumycin, Tetracyn, Tetrex, and others)	Newborn infant (not recommended) 100 mg./kg./24 hr. Divide into 2 doses (O) 10-15 mg./kg./24 hr. Divide into 2 doses (I.V.) Older infants and children: 25-50 mg./kg./24 hr. 0.6-1.2 gm./M.²/24 hr. Divide into 4 doses (O) (1 hr. before feedings) 10-25 mg./kg./24 hr. (Not more than 250 mg./injection) Divide into 2 or 3 doses (I.M.) 10-15 mg./kg./24 hr. Divide into 2 doses (I.V.) Children over 40 kg. and adults: Moderate infections: 1 gm./24 hr. Divide into 4 doses (O) Severe infections: Double above dose (O)	Tablets: 50 and 250 mg. Capsules: 50, 100, 125, 250 and 500 mg. Suspension: 250 mg./5 ml. Syrup: 125 mg./5 ml. Drops: 100 mg./ml. Calibrations: 5 mg./drop, or 25 and 50 mg. Vials: I.M. (local anesthetics added): 100 and 250 mg. I.V.: 100, 250 and 500 mg.

DRUGS

(Table Continues)

TABLE 5-16. *Continued*

DRUG	DOSAGE AND ROUTES	SUPPLIED
	Moderate infections: 　200-300 mg./24 hr. 　Divide into 2 or 3 doses (I.M.) Severe infections: 　500 mg./24 hr. 　Divide into 2 doses (I.M.) Adult: 　1 gm./24 hr. 　Divide into 2 doses (I.V.) (maximum, 2 gm./24 hr.) **Contraindications:** Sensitivity to tetracyclines or additives (see label of container) **Caution:** Overgrowth of nonsusceptible organisms, tooth discoloration and enamel hypoplasia, unites with growing bone, increased intracranial pressure, gastrointestinal symptoms, vaginitis, proctitis, glossitis, stomatitis, skin reactions, photosensitivity (all routes); altered renal function, negative nitrogen balance, outdated drug—tubular damage (Fanconi syndrome) I.M.: Sensitivity to local anesthetic(s) added, irritating to tissues, abscess, slough I.V.: Avoid large doses in presence of renal dysfunction—liver failure I.M. and I.V.: Use only as long as is necessary; oral route generally preferred	
Triacetyloleandomycin, N.F. (Cyclamycin, Tao)	Premature and full-term newborn infants and older infants and children: 30 mg./kg./24 hr. 1 gm./M.^{2}/24 hr. Divide into 4 doses (O) **Contraindications:** Sensitivity to this drug **Caution:** Liver function abnormalities (including jaundice) and hepatocellular changes may occur (not recommended if previous history of above); allergic reactions, possibility of overgrowth of nonsusceptible organisms	Capsules (as base): 125 and 250 mg. Oral suspension (as base): 125 mg./5 ml. Drops: 100 mg./ml. (5 mg./drop) Oleandomycin phosphate available in both I.M. and I.V. dosage forms (vials: 500 mg.)
Vancomycin hydrochloride, U.S.P. (Vancocin)	Premature and newborn infants: 10 mg./kg./24 hr. Divide into 2 doses (I.V.) Older infants and children: 40 mg./kg./24 hr. 1.2 gm./M.^{2}/24 hr. Daily continuous (I.V.) Dose may be divided into 2-4 doses **Contraindications:** Sensitivity to this drug; avoid use in renal insufficiency or previous hearing loss (reduce dose	Ampules: 500 mg. (50 mg./ml.)

Key: *M.*, dose per square meter of body surface. 　　　*R.*, rectal.
　　I.M., intramuscular.　　　　　　　　　　　　　　　*S.C.*, subcutaneous.
　　I.Th., intrathecal.　　　　　　　　　　　　　　　*Subl.*, sublingual.
　　I.V., intravenous.　　　　　　　　　　　　　　　*T.*, topical.
　　O., oral.

TABLE 5-16. *Continued*

DRUG	DOSAGE AND ROUTES	SUPPLIED
	and follow renal function and blood levels of drug, if it must be used) **Caution:** Inject or drip slowly, diluted solutions; rotate veins (thrombophlebitis), extravasation painful; overgrowth of nonsusceptible organisms, chills, fever, rash, urticaria may occur; hearing loss with high blood levels, especially in renal dysfunction; renal toxicity	
Antifungal drugs Amphotericin B, U.S.P. (Fungizone)	Test dose: 0.1 mg./kg./24 hr. (I.V.) in 6 hr., increase to: 1 mg./kg./24 hr. (I.V.) 30 mg./M.²/24 hr. (I.V.) (Give over 6-8 hr. period) Intrathecal: See p. 710 **Contraindications:** Sensitivity to this drug unless condition is life-threatening and amenable only to this drug **Caution:** Use aseptic technique in handling; do not use if a precipitate is present; limit parenteral use to closely observed hospitalized patients; avoid corticosteroids (except to control drug reactions); avoid antibiotics or nitrogen mustard; urinalysis, BUN, hemogram, serum potassium—weekly; intolerance to I.V. therapy in most patients: fever, chills, headache, gastrointestinal symptoms including pain, melena; local venous pain, phlebitis, thrombophlebitis: rarely rash, vertigo, visual difficulties, neuropathy, hypotensive and anaphylactoid reactions; anemia, thrombocytopenia, hepatotoxicity may occur; transient or permanent renal damage may occur	Vials: 50 mg. (mix with 5% dextrose water; pH above 5.0)
Griseofulvin, U.S.P. (Fulvicin, Grifulvin, Griseofulvin-Ayerst)	Double the dose of griseofulvin microcrystalline (see below) **Contraindications:** See below **Caution:** See below	Tablets (scored): 250 and 500 mg. Suspension: 250 mg./5 ml.
Griseofulvin microcrystalline (Fulvicin-U/F, Grifulvin V, Grisactin)	10 mg./kg./24 hr. 300 mg./M.²/24 hr. Divide into 2-4 doses (O) Widespread lesions may require: 450-600 mg./M.²/24 hr., reduce dose to above with response **Contraindications:** Hypersensitivity to this drug, porphyria, hepatocellular failure **Caution:** Prolonged therapy requires blood cell counts at regular intervals and periodic liver and renal function tests; close observation of patient; may cause gastrointestinal symptoms, headache, dizziness, insomnia, fatigue, proteinuria (temporary), peripheral neuritis, mental impairment, photosensitivity, allergic skin reactions, and "serum sickness," overgrowth of nonsusceptible organisms (monilia) (thrush), and leukopenia (discontinue with granulocytopenia)	Tablets (scored): 125, 250 and 500 mg. Capsules: 125 mg.

DRUGS

(Table Continues)

TABLE 5-16. *Continued*

DRUG	DOSAGE AND ROUTES	SUPPLIED
Hydroxystillbamidine isethi-onate, U.S.P. (Stilbamidine isethionate)	See package insert	Ampules: 225 mg.
Nystatin, U.S.P. (Mycosta-tin)	Premature and full-term newborn infants: 400,000 units Divide into 4 doses (O) Older infants and children: 1-2 million units/24 hr. Divide into 3 or 4 doses (O) Oral moniliasis: 4 times daily (T) **Contraindications:** Hypersensitivity to this drug **Caution:** May produce diarrhea and gastrointestinal distress	Tablets: 500,000 units Suspension (O or T): 100,000 units/ml.
Antituberculosis drugs *(see p. 606)* Aminosalicylic acid, p-aminosalicylic acid, PAS, U.S.P. (Pamisyl, Para-Pas, Parasal) Salts of PAS: sodium, potassium, and calcium	0.3 gm./kg./24 hr. 8 gm./M.²/24 hr. Divide into 3 doses p.c. (O) Increase PAS dose by 25% **Caution:** Do not use solutions older than 24 hr. or if darker than when prepared; may cause nausea, vomiting, abdominal pain, diarrhea, goiter (hypothyroidism), electrolyte disturbances, hypersensitivity, albuminuria, hematuria, skin reactions, lymphadenopathy, fever, jaundice, hepatomegaly, eosinophilia, blood dyscrasias, fatal hepatic damage, fever, crystalluria **Note:** 1 gm. of the sodium salt yields 109 mg. of Na. Urine reduces copper reagents	Acid: Tablets: Plain, enteric-coated, effervescent: 0.3, 0.5, 1 and 2 gm. Crystals Powder Resin: 8 gm. Calcium: Tablets: 0.5 gm. Potassium: Tablets: 0.5 gm. Powder Sodium: Tablets: 0.5, 0.69 and 1 gm. Granules: 454 gm. Powder: To be reconstituted, 0.93 and 1 gm./5 ml. Vial (dry): Reconstituted, 100 mg./ml.
Cycloserine (Oxamycin, Seromycin)	Initial dose: 2 wk. 10 mg./kg./24 hr. 300 mg./M.²/24 hr. Divide into 2 doses (O) Maintenance dose: Titrate dose to yield blood level of 20-30 µg/ml. **Contraindications:** Hypersensitivity to this drug, epilepsy **Caution:** Careful evaluation of urinary function; may cause grand or petit mal seizures, drowsiness, hyperreflexia, confusion, dermatitis; pyridoxine may relieve CNS symptoms (anticonvulsants if needed); careful observation	Capsules: 250 mg.
Isoniazid, U.S.P. (many trade names)	Conversion of tuberculin test with no manifest disease and "prophylaxis" (see p. 605)	Tablets and capsules: 50 and 100 mg. Syrup: 50 mg./5 ml.

Key: *M.*, dose per square meter of body surface.
    I.M., intramuscular.
    I.Th., intrathecal.
    I.V., intravenous.
    O., oral.

    R., rectal.
    S.C., subcutaneous.
    Subl., sublingual.
    T., topical.

D R U G S

TABLE 5-16. *Continued*

DRUG	DOSAGE AND ROUTES	SUPPLIED
	15 mg./kg./24 hr. 450 mg./M.²/24 hr. Divide into 2 or 3 doses (O or I.M.) Therapeutic, meningitis (tuberculous), miliary (see also p. 606): 20 mg./kg./24 hr. 0.6 gm./M.²/24 hr. Divide into 2 or 3 doses (O or I.M.) **Caution:** May intensify epilepsy, CNS stimulation, peripheral neuritis rare in children; some persons are genetically "fast inactivators", some "slow"	Ampules: 100 mg./ml.
Streptomycin *(see p. 255)*		
Antiviral drugs Amantadine hydrochloride (Symmetrel)	1-9 yr.: 4-8 mg./kg./24 hr. (Not more than 150 mg./24 hr.) Divide into 2-3 doses (O) 9-12 yr.: 200 mg./24 hr. Divide into 2 doses (O) Known exposure: 10-day course Possible repeated, unknown exposure: 30-day course Possible repeated, uncontrolled and unknown exposure: up to 90-day course **Contraindications:** Not for prophylaxis of any viral infections except for A_2 influenza; not for treatment of any virus or respiratory disease **Warning:** Strict observations when given to patients with CNS disease, especially epilepsy **Caution:** Nervousness, insomnia, dizziness, ataxia, tremors, depression, blurred vision, dry mouth, etc., rash, gastrointestinal symptoms, pollakiuria, nocturia	Capsules: 100 mg. Syrup: 50 mg./5 ml.
Chemotherapeutics Ammonium mandelate	250 mg./kg./24 hr. 7.5 gm./M.²/24 hr. Divide into 4 doses (O)	As chemical for solution and syrups
Furazolidone, N.F. (Furoxone)	6 mg./kg./24 hr. 200 mg./M.²/24 hr. Divide into 4 doses (O) **Contraindication:** Under age 1 mo. **Caution:** Primaquine type hemolytic anemia (genetic); rashes, urticaria; fall in B.P., fever, arthralgia, gastrointestinal symptoms, headache	Tablets (scored): 100 mg. Suspension: 16.7 mg./5 ml.
Methenamine mandelate, U.S.P. (Mandelamine)	0.1 gm./kg./24 hr. initially; then 0.05 gm./kg./24 hr. (Maximum, 3 gm./24 hr.) 3 gm./M.²/24 hr. initially; then 1.5 gm./M.²/24 hr. Divide into 3 doses/24 hr. (O) **Contraindication:** Renal insufficiency **Caution:** Maintain acid urine; gastrointestinal disturbances, skin rash	Tablets: 0.5 gm. Tablets (enteric-coated): 0.25, 0.5 and 1 gm. Suspension: 250 mg./5 ml. Suspension (forte): 500 mg./5 ml.

(Table Continues)

D R U G S

TABLE 5-16. *Continued*

DRUG	DOSAGE AND ROUTES	SUPPLIED
Methenamine hippurate (Hiprex) **Note:** Safe dosage not established for children under 6 years of age.	40 mg./kg./24 hr. 1.2 gm./M.^{2}/24 hr. Divide into 2 doses **Contraindications:** In renal insufficiency, severe hepatic disease, severe dehydration, as sole agent in parenchymal infections with systemic symptoms **Caution:** Maintain urine in acid pH; perform liver function studies periodically; may cause gastrointestinal symptoms, dysuria, rash	Tablets (scored): 1 gm.
Methionine *(see p. 238)*		
Nalidixic acid and sodium salt (NegGram)	Over 1 mo. of age: 50 mg./kg./24 hr. 1.5 gm./M.^{2}/24 hr. Divide into 4 doses (O) **Caution:** Observe for increased intracranial pressure, gastrointestinal symptoms, visual disturbances, confusion, hallucinations, convulsions, photosensitivity, rash, eosinophilia; periodic blood and liver tests for treatment more than 1 wk; use with caution in renal or liver disease; nonglucose copper-reducing substance in urine	Caplets: 250 and 500 mg. (O)
Nitrofurantoin, U.S.P. (Furadantin)	Up to 7 kg.: 6 mg./kg./24 hr. 7-11 kg.: 50 mg./24 hr. 12-21 kg.: 100 mg./24 hr. 22-31 kg.: 150 mg./24 hr. 32-40 kg.: 200 mg./24 hr. 150 mg./M.^{2}/24 hr. Divide into 4 doses (O) Reduce to ½ of above dosage if continued beyond 10-14 days; after another 10-14 days reduce to ¼ of above **Contraindications:** Anuria, oliguria, infants under 1 mo. **Caution:** Presence of marked renal impairment and prolonged therapy requires careful clinical and laboratory evaluation (chemical and cellular evaluations of blood and urine), dose regulated accordingly; may cause peripheral neuritis (discontinue), primaquine-type hemolytic anemia, sensitization (skin rashes and urticaria), pleuropneumonitis with eosinophilia, anaphylactoid reaction, chills and fever, cholestatic jaundice, leukopenia, headache, gastrointestinal symptoms, renal toxicity; dispense in amber bottles	Tablets (scored): 50 and 100 mg. Oral suspension: 25 mg./5 ml. Sterile vials (sodium): 180 mg. (dry)

Key: *M.*, dose per square meter of body surface.
    I.M., intramuscular.
    I.Th., intrathecal.
    I.V., intravenous.
    O., oral.

    R., rectal.
    S.C., subcutaneous.
    Subl., sublingual.
    T., topical.

TABLE 5-16. *Continued*

DRUG	DOSAGE AND ROUTES	SUPPLIED
Phenazopyridine hydrochloride (Pyridium, etc.)	12 mg./kg./24 hr. 350 mg./M.²/24 hr. Divide into 3 doses (O) after meals **Caution:** Renal insufficiency, gastrointestinal disturbances	Tablets: 0.1 gm.
Sulfonamides:	**Caution:** Absorbable sulfonamides are contraindicated in first 2-3 mo. of life.	
Phthalylsulfathiazole, U.S.P. (Sulfathalidine)	Presurgery: Initial: 125 mg./kg./24 hr. Maintenance: 125 mg./kg./24 hr. (maximum, 8 gm./24 hr.) 4 gm./M.²/24 hr. Divide into 3, 4 or 6 doses (O) Ulcerative colitis: 0.05-0.1 gm./kg./24 hr. (maximum, 8 gm./24 hr.) Divide into 3, 4 or 6 doses (O) **Contraindications:** As for sulfadiazine **Caution:** As for sulfadiazine	Tablets: 0.5 gm. Suspension: 1 gm./5 ml.
Salicylazosulfapyridine (Azulfidine)	Initial: (usual) 75-150 mg./kg./24 hr. 2.3-4.5 gm./M.²/24 hr. Divide into 4, 6 or 8 doses (O) Initial: (severe colitis) 37.5-150 mg./kg./24 hr. 1.2-4.5 gm./M.²/24 hr. Divide into 3, 4 or 6 doses (O) Maintenance: 40 mg./kg./24 hr. 1.25 gm./M.²/24 hr. Divide into 4 doses Recurrence of symptoms: Increase to previously effective dose **Contraindications:** As for sulfadiazine **Caution:** As for sulfadiazine	Tablets: 0.5 gm. Tablets (enteric) 0.5 gm.
Succinylsulfathiazole, U.S.P. (Sulfasuxidine)	0.25 gm./kg./24 hr. 8 gm./M.²/24 hr. Divide into 6 doses (O) **Contraindications:** Intestinal obstruction; as for sulfadiazine **Caution:** As for sulfadiazine	Tablets: 0.5 gm. Powder: 454 gm.
Sulfacetamide, N.F. (Sulamyd)	Urinary infections: 60 mg./kg./24 hr. 1.8 gm./M.²/24 hr. Divide into 3 or 4 doses (O) **Contraindications:** As for sulfadiazine **Caution:** As for sulfadiazine	Tablets: 0.5 gm.
Sulfachlorpyridazine (Sonilyn)	Initial: 65 mg./kg. (maximum, 4 gm.) 2 gm./M.² Single dose (O) Maintenance: 130 mg./kg./24 hr. (maximum, 6 gm.) 3.5 gm./M.² Divide into 4 doses (O) **Contraindications:** As for sulfadiazine **Caution:** As for sulfadiazine	Tablets: 0.5 gm.

(Table Continues)

DRUGS

TABLE 5-16. *Continued*

DRUG	DOSAGE AND ROUTES	SUPPLIED

Sulfadiazine, the sodium salt, U.S.P. (or combinations of sulfonamides)	150 mg./kg./24 hr. (maximum, 6 gm./24 hr.)
	4 gm./M.^{2}/24 hr.
	Divide into 4-6 doses/24 hr. (O)
	Initial dose, $\frac{1}{2}$ of 24-hr. dose
	100 mg./kg./24 hr.
	2.25 gm./M.^{2}/24 hr.
	Divide into 3 doses/24 hr. (S.C. 5% solution) or into 4 doses/24 hr. (I.V.)
	Rheumatic fever prophylaxis:
	    Under 30 kg.: 0.5 gm./24 hr. (O)
	    Over 30 kg.: 1 gm./24 hr. (O)
	Contraindications: Sensitivity to sulfonamides; under age 2-3 mo.
	Caution: In renal dysfunction, allergies or asthma, glucose-6-phosphate dehydrogenase deficiency; may cause crystalluria, hematuria, renal shutdown, blood dyscrasias, gastrointestinal symptoms, photosensitivity, hepatotoxicity, jaundice, cyanosis, purpura, CNS and peripheral neuropathy; nephrosis, collagen diseases, allergic skin reactions, including Stevens-Johnson syndrome
		Tablets: 0.5 gm.
		Suspension: 0.325 and 0.5 gm./5 ml.
		Ampules (sodium): 0.25 gm./ml.

Sulfadimethoxine, N.F. (Madribon)	Severe infections:
	  Initial:
	    60 mg./kg. (maximum, 2 gm.)
	    1-2 gm./M.^{2}
	    Single dose (O)
	  Maintenance:
	    $\frac{1}{2}$ of initial dose
	    Single daily dose (O)
	Usual dose (moderate to severe infections):
	  Initial:
	    55 mg./kg. (maximum, 2 gm.)
	    1.1 gm./M.^{2}
	    Single dose (O)
	  Maintenance:
	    $\frac{1}{2}$ of initial dose
	    Single daily dose (O)
	Mild infections:
	    $\frac{1}{2}$ of above dosages
	Contraindications: As for sulfadiazine
	Warning: Fatalities have occurred (Stevens-Johnson syndrome) following use of this drug; observe closely, discontinue with rash; long-lasting blood level — dose smaller than shorter-acting sulfonamides, the use of which should be ruled out before long-acting sulfonamides are given
	Caution: As sulfadiazine
		Tablets (double scored): 0.5 gm.
		Tablets (chewable): 0.25 gm.
		Suspension: 0.25 gm./5 ml.
		Drops: 0.25 gm./ml. (12.5 mg./drop)

D
R
U
G
S

Key: *M.*, dose per square meter of body surface.   *R.*, rectal.
    I.M., intramuscular.   *S.C.*, subcutaneous.
    I.Th., intrathecal.   *Subl.*, sublingual.
    I.V., intravenous.   *T.*, topical.
    O., oral.

TABLE 5-16. *Continued*

DRUG	DOSAGE AND ROUTES	SUPPLIED
Sulfaethidole (Sul-Spansion, Sul-Spantab)	Maintenance dose, moderate infections: 60 mg./kg./24 hr. 1.6 gm./M.²/24 hr. Divide into 2 doses Severe infections: Double maintenance dose Initial dose: Double maintenance dose **Contraindications:** As for sulfadiazine **Caution:** As for sulfadiazine	Tablets: 0.65 gm. Liquid: 0.65 gm./5 ml.
Sulfamethizole, N.F. (Sulfurine, Thiosulfil, Utrasul)	30-45 mg./kg./24 hr. 1.2 gm./M.²/24 hr. Divide into 4 doses **Contraindications:** As for sulfadiazine **Caution:** As for sulfadiazine	Tablets (scored): 0.25 and 0.5 gm. Suspension: 0.25 gm./5 ml.
Sulfamethoxazole (Gantanol)	Initial dose: 60 mg./kg. (maximum, 2 gm.) 1.2 gm./M.² Single daily dose (O) Maintenance: Divide initial dose into 2 doses (O) **Contraindications:** As for sulfadiazine **Caution:** As for sulfadiazine	Tablets (double scored): 0.5 gm. Suspension: 0.5 gm./5 ml.
Sulfamethoxypyridazine, U.S.P., and acetylsulfa-methoxypyridazine (Kynex, Midicel)	Initial: 30 mg./kg. (maximum, 1 gm.) 0.6 gm./M.² Single dose (O) Maintenance: 15 mg./kg./24 hr. (maximum, 0.5 gm.) 0.3 gm./M.²/24 hr. Single daily dose after meals (O) **Contraindications:** As for sulfadiazine **Warning:** As for sulfadimethoxine **Caution:** As for sulfadiazine	Tablets (quarter scored): 0.5 gm. Suspension: 250 mg./5 ml.
Sulfaphenazole (Orisul, Sulfabid)	Initial dose: 65 mg./kg. 1.8 gm./M.² Single dose (O) Maintenance dose: Divide above dose into 2 doses (O) **Contraindications:** As for sulfadiazine **Caution:** As for sulfadiazine	Tablets: 0.5 gm. Suspension: 0.5 gm./5 ml.
Sulfisomidine (Elkosin)	6 mo.-3 yr.: Initial: 1 gm. Single dose (O) Maintenance: 1 gm. Divide into 4 doses (O) 3-10 yr.: Initial: 1.5 gm. Single dose (O) Maintenance: 2 gm. Divide into 4 doses (O) Adults: Systemic infections: Initial: 2 gm. (1.2 gm./M.²) Single dose (O)	Tablets (double scored): 0.5 gm. Suspension: 312 mg./5 ml.

DRUGS

(Table Continues)

TABLE 5-16. *Continued*

DRUG	DOSAGE AND ROUTES	SUPPLIED

	Maintenance:
	  6 gm. (3.5 gm./M.^{2})
	  Divide into 4 doses (O)
	Urinary tract infections:
	  $^1/_2$ of above dose
	Contraindications: As for sulfadiazine
	Caution: As for sulfadiazine	

Sulfisoxazole, U.S.P.
  (Gantrisin and many other
  trade names)
	Oral:
	  Initial:
	    $^1/_3$ of total daily dose
	  Maintenance:
	    180 mg./kg./24 hr.
	    3.6 gm./M.^{2}/24 hr.
	  Divide into 6 doses (O)
	Parenteral:
	  100 mg./kg.
	  2.4 gm./M.^{2}
	  Single dose (I.M. or I.V. drip)
	  Repeat to total 2 or 3 doses/24 hr.
	Contraindications: As for sulfadiazine
	Caution: Dilute to 5% or less concentration for S.C. use
		Tablets (scored): 0.5 gm.
		Suspension: 0.5 gm./5 ml.
		Syrup: 0.5 gm./5 ml.
		Lipogantrisin: 1 gm./5 ml.
		Ampules: 400 mg./ml.

Anticholinergics
(see Cholinergic blocking agents, *p. 286)*

Anticholinesterases
(see Cholinesterase inhibitors, *p. 288)*

Anticoagulants

Heparin sodium, U.S.P.
  (1 mg. = 120 or more U.S.P.
  units)
	Initial dose:
	  50 units/kg. (I.V. drip)
	Maintenance dose:
	  100 units/kg. added and absorbed
	    q. 4 hr. (I.V. drip)
	  20,000 units/M.^{2}/24 hr.
	  Continuous dosage
	  Titrate dose to yield 20-30 min. clotting time or 2-3 times preheparin clotting time
	Antidote: Protamine sulfate (I.V. drip) 1 mg. for each 1 mg. heparin in previous 4 hr.
	Contraindications: Bleeding tendency (hemophilia, purpura, jaundice, postoperative oozing of blood, etc.), subacute bacterial endocarditis, intracranial or hidden hemorrhage, ulcerative lesions (hidden), shock, hypersensitivity to this drug; may cause fever, skin rashes, nasal congestion, asthma, anaphylaxis, alopecia
	Caution: Follow clotting time
		In thousands of units:
		  Ampules and vials: 1, 5, 10,
		    20 and 40/ml.
		  Syringes (disposable): 20/ml.
		  Tablets, sublingual: 1500
		    units (potassium)
		Protamine sulfate:
		  Ampules and vials: 10 mg./ml.

Anticonvulsants
(see p. 1256)
Acetazolamide *(see* Diuretics, *p. 289)*

Key: *M.,* dose per square meter of body surface.
    I.M., intramuscular.
    I.Th., intrathecal.
    I.V., intravenous.
    O., oral.

    R., rectal.
    S.C., subcutaneous.
    Subl., sublingual.
    T., topical.

DRUGS

TABLE 5-16. *Continued*

DRUG	DOSAGE AND ROUTES	SUPPLIED

Amphetamine sulfate *(see* Adrenergics, *p. 238)*
Barbiturates *(for other barbiturates see* Sedatives and hypnotics, *p. 305)*

Mephobarbital, N.F. (Mebaral)	1½-2 times dose of phenobarbital **Contraindications:** As for phenobarbital **Caution:** As for phenobarbital	Tablets: 30, 50, 100 and 200 mg.
Metharbital, N.F. (Gemonil)	Initial dose (O): Infants and small children: 50-100 mg. 1-3 times daily Adults: 100 mg. 1-3 times daily **Contraindications:** As for phenobarbital **Caution:** As for phenobarbital	Tablets (scored): 100 mg.
Phenobarbital, U.S.P. (Luminal)	Sedation: 6 mg./kg./24 hr. 180 mg./M.²/24 hr. Divide into 3 doses (O or R) Anticonvulsant dose: 3-5 mg./kg./dose (I.M.) 125 mg./M.²/dose (I.M.) **Contraindications:** In severe hepatic or renal dysfunction, porphyria, hypersensitivity to barbituric acid derivatives **Caution:** Idiosyncrasy (excitement, pain, hangover, prolonged action), in respiratory depression; may cause rash, gastrointestinal symptoms, vertigo; may be given in dilute solution *slowly* I.V. **Toxicity:** Respiratory, circulatory and renal depression	Tablets: 15, 30, 60 and 100 mg. (¼, ½, 1 and 1½ gr.) Spansules: 60 and 100 mg. Elixir: 20 mg./5 ml. Ampules (sodium): 125 and 300 mg. (2 and 5 gr.)
Bromides, N.F.	Anticonvulsant dose: 50-100 mg./kg./24 hr. 1.5-3 gm./M.²/24 hr. Divide into 3 doses every 8 hr. (O) Maximum blood level, 200 mg.% **Caution:** Acne, rash, granuloma, ataxia, lethargy and psychosis	As chemicals Three bromides tablets (N.F.) Total: 0.45 and 0.9 gm. Bromides syrup (N.F.) Total: 1.2 gm./5 ml. Three bromides elixir (N.F.) Total 1.2 gm./5 ml.

Dextroamphetamine *(see* Adrenergics, *p. 238)*

Diphenhydramine hydro-
chloride (Benadryl) *(see* Antihistaminics, *p. 274)*

Hydantoins

Diphenylhydantoin and diphenylhydantoin sodium, U.S.P. and N.F. (Dilantin and Dilantin sodium, Diphentoin, and many other trade names)	3-8 mg./kg./24 hr. 250 mg./M.²/24 hr. Single dose or divide into 2 doses (O, I.M. or I.V. slowly) **Caution:** Gingival hyperplasia, dermatitis, hirsutism, lymphadenopathy, granulocytopenia, megaloblastic anemia, blood dyscrasias, lupus, fibrosis of lungs, and acute liver damage, motor hyperactivity, nystagmus, arthropathy, skin rashes; overdosages—cerebellar incoordination	Tablets: 50 mg. (¾ gr.) Capsules: 30 and 100 mg. (½ and 1½ gr.) 100 mg. (delayed action) 100 mg. (in oil) Suspension; 30, 100 and 125 mg./5 ml. Vials: 50 mg./ml.

(Table Continues)

D R U G S

TABLE 5-16. *Continued*

DRUG	DOSAGE AND ROUTES	SUPPLIED
Ethotoin, ethyl phenyl-hydantoin (Peganone)	80 mg./kg./24 hr. 2.5 gm./M.²/24 hr. Divide into 4 doses **Caution:** Withdraw therapy with liver damage or marked depression of blood cell count; blood cell counts, urinalyses at onset of therapy and monthly intervals; liver function tests with clinical suggestion of hepatic disorder; caution if given with phenacemide (paranoid symptoms); less gastric distress (nausea, vomiting) when given after meals; may cause fatigue, insomnia, dizziness, headache, diplopia, nystagmus, numbness, rash, fever, diarrhea, chest pain; ataxia and gingival hypertrophy rarely, lymphadenopathy, lupus (remitting on drug withdrawal)	Tablets (scored): 250 and 500 mg.
Mephenytoin, methyl phenylethylhydantoin (Mesantoin)	3-15 mg./kg./24 hr. 100-450 mg./M.²/24 hr. Divide into 3 doses/24 hr. (O) **Caution:** Discontinue use with untoward reaction: (1) skin rash, (2) blood dyscrasia, (3) CNS effects; do WBC, differential (neutrophils) before therapy, at 2 wk. (on low dosage), and 2 wk. (on full dosage), monthly for 1 yr., then every 3 mo.; counts every 2 wk. — if neutrophils drop to 2500-1600; stop drug for count of 1600; instruct patient or parents of symptoms and signs of agranulocytosis; keep under close supervision	Tablets: 100 mg.
Oxazolidines Paramethadione, U.S.P. (Paradione)	Under age 2 yr.: 0.3 gm./24 hr. 2-6 yr.: 0.6 gm./24 hr. Over 6 yr. and adults: 0.9 gm./24 hr. Adjust subsequent doses by response (O) **Contraindications:** As for trimethadione **Caution:** As for trimethadione	Capsules: 150 and 300 mg. Solution: 300 mg./ml.

Trimethadione, U.S.P. (Tridione)	Initial daily dose:
	  Infants: 300 mg.
	  Age 2 yr.: 600 mg.
	  Age 6 yr.: 900 mg.
	  Age 13 yr.: 1200 mg.
	  40 mg./kg./24 hr.
	  1 gm./M.²/24 hr.
	  Divide into 3 or 4 doses (O)
	Contraindications: Not ordinarily to be used with severe hepatic or renal impairment or blood dyscrasias
	Caution: In diseases of the retina or optic nerve; withdraw if the following are encountered — scotomata, persist-
		Capsules: 300 mg.
		Tablets (Dulcet): 150 mg.
		Solution: 163 mg./5 ml.

Key: *M.*, dose per square meter of body surface.   *R.*, rectal.
   I.M., intramuscular.   *S.C.*, subcutaneous.
   I.Th., intrathecal.   *Subl.*, sublingual.
   I.V., intravenous.   *T.*, topical.
   O., oral.

DRUG	DOSAGE AND ROUTES	SUPPLIED
	ent or increasing albuminuria, jaundice or other signs of hepatitis, lupus-like manifestations or lymphadenopathy, total number of neutrophils of 2500 or below, or skin rash; may cause "glare phenomenon" (relieved with dark glasses), drowsiness (relieved with an amphetamine), skin rash, blood dyscrasias (including fatal aplastic anemia), nephrosis, grand mal seizures, hair loss; avoid concurrent use of other drugs known to cause toxic effects or use with extreme caution; strict medical supervision during initial treatment period, laboratory tests of blood and urine—monthly intervals, more frequent when count is less than 3000	

Paraldehyde *(see* Sedatives and hypnotics, *p. 305)*

Phenacemide, phenacetyl-carbamide (Phenurone)	5-10 yr.: Initial dose: 0.25 gm. t.i.d. 2nd week: Add 0.25 gm. on arising 3rd week: May add 0.25 gm. at bedtime **Caution:** Ordinarily should not be used unless other anticonvulsants have been found ineffective; may cause psychic changes, hepatitis, skin rash, gastrointestinal disturbances, nephritis; extreme caution in patients who previously have shown personality disorders (alert patient and family to possibilities of suicide and psychoses and to report same); use with caution if history of liver dysfunction (death reported) or if history of allergy, particularly in association with use of other anticonvulsants; withdraw drug if the following are encountered—severe or exacerbated personality changes, jaundice or other signs of hepatitis, marked depression of blood cell count, abnormal urinary findings; laboratory tests should be performed—complete blood cell counts before use, at monthly intervals for 1 yr., and (if no abnormalities) at extended intervals; (follow total numbers of cellular elements, as leukopenia [4000/mm.[3]], aplastic anemia and death have occurred); liver function tests before and during therapy, urine examinations at regular intervals	Tablets (scored): 500 mg. Enterab: 300 mg.

Phenothiazines *(see p. 308)*

Primidone, U.S.P. (Mysoline)	Week / Adults and children over 8 yr. / Children under 8 yr. 1 250 mg. h.s. 125 mg. h.s. 2 250 mg. b.i.d. 125 mg. b.i.d. 3 250 mg. t.i.d. 125 mg. t.i.d. 4 250 mg. q.i.d. 125 mg. q.i.d.	Tablets (scored): 50 and 250 mg. Suspension: 250 mg./5 ml.

(Table Continues)

TABLE 5-16. *Continued*

DRUG	DOSAGE AND ROUTES	SUPPLIED
	Continue weekly increments; dose not to exceed 2 gm./24 hr. (O) 1.25 gm./M.²/24 hr. Divide into 2-4 doses (O) **Caution:** May cause megaloblastic anemia (rare) (responding to folic acid while continuing drug); minor and infrequent—gastrointestinal symptoms, drowsiness, fatigue, hyperirritability, emotional disturbance, dizziness, ataxia, diplopia, nystagmus, morbilliform rashes; persistent or severe effects—withdraw drug	

Succinamides
  Ethosuximide (Zarontin)
	Initial dose:
	  Under 6 yr.: 0.25 gm./24 hr. (O)
	  Over 6 yr.: 0.5 gm./24 hr.; divide into 2 doses (O)
	Continued dose:
	  Increase only p.r.n.; add 0.25 gm. every 4-7 days
	Warning: Associated with use: aplastic anemia, agranulocytosis, pancytopenia, leukopenia, dermatitis; great caution in hepatic or renal disease; operation of motor vehicles not advised (drowsiness); may increase grand mal attacks; periodic blood tests, routine urinalyses, frequent liver tests advised
	Caution: May cause gastrointestinal, neurologic (headache, dizziness, euphoria, hiccup), psychiatric symptoms, rash, vaginal bleeding, swelling of tongue
		Capsules: 0.25 gm.

Methsuximide, N.F.
    (Celontin)
	Initial dose:
	  0.3 gm./24 hr. for 1 wk. (O)
	Increase:
	  0.3 gm./24 hr./wk. for 3 wk. to 1.2 gm. (O)
	Caution: Observe patient, blood cell counts, and urinalyses at frequent periods; may cause gastrointestinal, CNS symptoms (drowsiness, ataxia, irritability, headache, blurred vision, photophobia, hiccup), psychologic disturbances, skin reactions, eosinophilia, leukopenia, monocytosis, periorbital edema, hyperemia; instruct family to withdraw drug with behavioral alterations
		Capsules: 0.3 gm.

Phensuximide, N.F. (Milontin)	1-3 gm./24 hr. Divide into 2 or 3 doses (O) **Caution:** Evaluate patient, blood and urine studies regularly; when dis-	Capsules: 0.5 gm. Suspension: 313 mg./5 ml.

Key: *M.*, dose per square meter of body surface.   *R.*, rectal.
       I.M., intramuscular.   *S.C.*, subcutaneous.
       I.Th., intrathecal.   *Subl.*, sublingual.
       I.V., intravenous.   *T.*, topical.
       O., oral.

D
R
U
G
S

TABLE 5-16. *Continued*

DRUG	DOSAGE AND ROUTES	SUPPLIED
	continuing drug, do so gradually; may cause gastrointestinal (anorexia, vomiting) and CNS symptoms (drowsiness, dizziness), microscopic hematuria, granulocytopenia, aplastic anemia, skin reactions	

Antidotes

(*see also* Adrenergics, Analeptics, Antihistaminics, Calcium salts, Cholinesterase inhibitors)

Atropine sulfate (*see* Cholinergic blocking agents, p. 286)

DRUG	DOSAGE AND ROUTES	SUPPLIED
Biperiden hydrochloride or lactate (Akineton)	Drug-induced extrapyramidal reactions: 0.04 mg./kg. 1.2 mg./M.^{2} Single dose (I.M.) Repeat in ½ hr. if needed, not more than 4 doses in 24 hr. **Caution:** In glaucoma; may cause dry mouth, blurred vision, drowsiness, decreased urinary flow, disorientation, euphoria, gastric irritation, postural hypotension	Tablets (scored): 2 mg. Ampules: 5 mg./ml.
Calcium disodium edetate, calcium disodium edathamil, EDTA calcium disodium, U.S.P. (Calcium Disodium Versenate) (*see p. 1489*)	Not to exceed: 70 mg./kg./24 hr. 1.7 gm./M.^{2}/24 hr. Divide into 2 doses (I.V.) Dilute to 0.2-0.4% solution Course: Up to 5 days; intervals of 2 days before repeat Repeat course if needed **Caution:** See package insert	Ampules: 200 mg./ml. Tablets: 500 mg.
Charcoal (activated) (*see p. 1492*)		
Deferoxamine mesylate (Desferal mesylate) (*see p. 1499*)	For iron poisoning: Parenteral (only) Initial: 20 mg./kg. 0.6 gm./M.^{2} Repeat ½ of initial dose every 4 hr. (2 doses) Subsequent doses: ½ of initial dose every 4-12 hr. (depending on clinical response) Not to exceed 6 gm./24 hr. (adult) or 3.5 gm./M.^{2}/24 hr. I.M. (preferred) *all patients not in shock* or by slow infusion (I.V.) not to exceed: 15 mg./kg./hr. (I.V.) 0.45 gm./M.^{2}/hr. (I.V.) *Only for patients in cardiovascular collapse* Discontinue and give I.M. as soon as clinical condition permits **Contraindications:** Contraindicated in patients with severe renal disease or anuria, since drug and chelate that it forms with iron are excreted primarily by the kidney	Ampules: 500 mg.

D
R
U
G
S

(*Table Continues*)

TABLE 5-16. *Continued*

DRUG	DOSAGE AND ROUTES	SUPPLIED
	Warning: Long-term administration has been associated with cataracts in dogs and man; no ocular abnormalities by slit lamp in a few patients treated for acute iron intoxication **Caution:** Flushing of the skin, urticaria, hypotension, shock (rapid intravenous injection); *give intramuscularly* or *by slow intravenous infusion;* pain and induration at the site of injection; long-term therapy, allergic-type reactions (cutaneous wheal formation, generalized itching, rash, anaphylactic reaction), blurring of vision, abdominal discomfort, diarrhea, leg cramps, tachycardia and fever	
Dimercaprol, British anti-lewisite, U.S.P. (BAL) *(see p. 1492)*	For arsenic, mercury and gold poisoning (mild): 1st day, 2.5 mg./kg. every 4 hr. (6 inj.) 2nd day, 2.5 mg./kg. every 6 hr. (4 inj.) 3rd day, 2.5 mg./kg. every 12 hr. (2 injection/I.M.) Each of following 10 days (or until recovery), 2.5 mg./kg./24 hr. (1 injection/I.M.) Increase dosage 25% for severe poisoning **Caution:** See package insert	Ampules: 100 mg./ml. (10% in oil)
Disodium edetate, U.S.P. (Endrate disodium)	50 mg./kg. 1.5 gm./M.² Single dose (I.V.), slowly over 3-4 hr. **Caution:** Concentration not to exceed 7 mg./ml.; avoid extravasation; frequent serum calcium levels (ready calcium gluconate solution in syringe), urinalyses; with caution in tuberculosis and metastatic calcification (embolization); may cause hypocalcemic convulsions, cardiac and respiratory collapse, reduced prothrombin time, thrombophlebitis, hypotension, chills, fever, back pain, muscle cramps, vomiting, urinary urgency, gastrointestinal symptoms, genitourinary reactions	Ampules: 150 mg./ml.
Levallorphan tartrate, N.F. (Lorfan)	Newborn infants: 0.02 mg./kg. Single dose (I.V. or I.M.) Repeat if needed Premature infants: 0.05 mg. (I.V. or I.M.) **Caution:** See package insert	Ampules: 1 mg./ml. Vials: 1 mg./ml.
Methylene blue, U.S.P.	Methemoglobinemia: 2 mg./kg./dose 50 mg./M.²/dose Give over 5 min. (I.V.)	Ampules: 10 mg./ml. (1%)

Key: *M.,* dose per square meter of body surface.   *R.,* rectal.
    I.M., intramuscular.   *S.C.,* subcutaneous.
    I.Th., intrathecal.   *Subl.,* sublingual.
    I.V., intravenous.   *T.,* topical.
    O., oral.

TABLE 5-16. *Continued*

DRUG	DOSAGE AND ROUTES	SUPPLIED
Nalorphine hydrochloride, U.S.P. (Nalline)	0.1 mg./kg./dose (I.V. or I.M.) May repeat in 15 min. **Caution:** See package insert; may accentuate depressions	Ampules for neonatal use: 0.2 mg./ml. Ampules and vials: 5 mg./ml.
Penicillamine (Cuprimine)	Infants over 6 mo. and young children: 250 mg. (O) Single dose (in fruit juice) Older children and adults: 1 gm./24 hr. (O) Divide into 4 doses Dose based on urinary copper excretion; may increase to 4-5 gm./24 hr. **Caution:** Routine urinalysis, WBC, differential, Hb, platelet count every 3 days (4 wk.), every 7-10 days (3 mo.), then monthly; frequent liver and kidney function tests; careful observation with renal disease; take temperature nightly first few months; observe skin and mucous membranes for allergic reactions; discontinue drug if fever or reaction in skin occurs or above tests so indicate; reinstitute small dose, gradually increase to full dosage; may need systemic adrenocorticosteroid in **toxicity** (second or third time); discontinue drug with bleeding into skin; may cause nephrotic syndrome, elevated sedimentation rate, liver dysfunctions, eosinophilia, monocytosis and leukocytosis, thrombopenia and leukopenia, fatal granulocytopenia; examine eyes for cataracts before and twice yearly during drug therapy; give pyridoxine (25 mg. daily); discontinue sulfurated potash or resin when iron is administered	Capsules: 250 mg.
Pralidoxime chloride (Protopam chloride)	25-50 mg./kg. 0.6-1 gm./M.^{2} As 5% solution (I.V. slowly [I.M. or S.C. not preferred]) Repeat every 10-12 hr. if needed **Contraindications:** Poisoning by the carbamate insecticide Sevin, in patients receiving morphine, theophylline and derivatives, succinylcholine, reserpine and phenothiazine-type drugs **Caution:** In myasthenia gravis, in patients given large doses of atropine for anticholinesterase poisoning; may cause transient dizziness, blurred vision, diplopia, tachycardia	Tablets: 0.5 gm. Vials: 1 gm.
Protamine sulfate injection, U.S.P.	Heparin antidote: See p. 266	Ampules and vials: 10 mg./ml.

Antiemetics
Antihistaminics *(see p. 274)*

Diphenidol and its salts (hydrochloride and pamoate) (Vontrol)	6 mo. age or 12 kg. or more — not more than: 5 mg./kg./24 hr. 150 mg./M.^{2}/24 hr.	Tablets: 25 mg. Oral suspension: 20 mg./5 ml. Suppositories: 25 and 50 mg. Injection: 20 mg./ml.

(Table Continues)

TABLE 5-16. *Continued*

DRUG	DOSAGE AND ROUTES	SUPPLIED
	Divide into 4 doses (O or R) I.M.: 60% of above **Contraindications:** Anuria, hypotension **Caution:** In glaucoma, pylorospasm or stenosis, obstructing gastrointestinal or genitourinary lesions, sinus tachycardia; drowsiness, dizziness, auditory and visual hallucinations, confusion can occur; avoid operation of machinery; patients under hospital or comparable supervision	
Tranquilizers *(see p. 307)*		
Trimethobenzamide hydrocholoride, N.F. (Tigan)	15 mg./kg./24 hr. 450 mg./M.²/24 hr. Divide into 3-4 doses (O or R) **Caution:** Drowsiness (prohibit motor operation), obscures gastrointestinal diagnoses, sensitivity to "-caine" anesthetics (suppositories), Parkinson-like reactions, hypotension, rare reports of blood dyscrasias, others	Capsules: 100 and 250 mg. Suppositories: 200 mg. Injection: 100 mg./ml.

Antiepileptics
(see Anticonvulsants, *p. 266)*

Antifungal drugs
(see p. 259)

Antihistaminics

	Contraindications: Hypersensitivity to the particular drug **Caution:** All produce undesired effects; be familiar with each drug prescribed, read package insert and pharmacology text; choose and use only a few; may produce many effects—CNS (sedation [avoid motor vehicle operation], excitation, insomnia, nervousness, convulsions, death), autonomic imbalance (dryness of mucous membranes, blurred vision, urinary retention, tachycardia, hypotension), gastrointestinal disturbances (anorexia, vomiting, diarrhea, pain), blood dyscrasias (pancytopenia, agranulocytosis, thrombocytopenia), additive effects with depressant drugs **Toxicity:** CNS depression; children may be stimulated; atropine-like symptoms; gastrointestinal disturbances	
Brompheniramine maleate, parabromdylamine maleate, N.F. (Dimetane)	0.5 mg./kg./24 hr. 15 mg./M.²/24 hr. Divide into 3 or 4 doses (O., S.C., I.M. or I.V.)	Tablets (scored): 4 mg. Extentab: 8 and 12 mg. Elixir: 2 mg./5 ml. Injection: 10, 20 and 100 mg./ml.

Key: *M.,* dose per square meter of body surface.   *R.,* rectal.
    I.M., intramuscular.   *S.C.,* subcutaneous.
    I.Th., intrathecal.   *Subl.,* sublingual.
    I.V., intravenous.   *T.,* topical.
    O., oral.

DRUGS

TABLE 5-16. *Continued*

DRUG	DOSAGE AND ROUTES	SUPPLIED
Carbinoxamine maleate, N.F. (Clistin)	0.4 mg./kg./24 hr. 12 mg./M.²/24 hr. Divide into 3 or 4 doses (O)	Tablets (scored): 4 mg. Tablets (long-acting): 8 and 12 mg. Elixir: 4 mg./5 ml.
Chlorcyclizine hydrochloride, U.S.P. (Perazil)	1.5 mg./kg./24 hr. 45 mg./M.²/24 hr. Divide into 2 doses (O)	Tablets (plain): 25 and 50 mg. Tablets (coated): 25 and 50 mg.
Chlorpheniramine maleate, U.S.P. (Chlor-Trimeton, Teldrin)	0.35 mg./kg./24 hr. 10 mg./M.²/24 hr. Divide into 4 doses (O or S.C.) 0.2 mg./kg. 6 mg./M.² As single dose (long-acting) (O)	Tablets (scored): 4 mg. Repetabs: 8 and 12 mg. Syrup: 2.5 mg./5 ml. Injection: 1-ml ampules (10 mg./ml.) 2-ml. vial (100 mg./ml.) Teldrin Spansules: 8 and 12 mg.
Cyclizine salts, U.S.P. (Marezine)	3 mg./kg./24 hr. 100 mg./M.²/24 hr. Divide into 3 doses (O or I.M.) Rectal dose: 2 times oral or I.M. dose	Tablets (scored): 50 mg. Suppositories: 50 and 100 mg. Ampules: 50 mg./ml.
Cyproheptadine hydrochloride (Periactin hydrochloride)	0.25 mg./kg./24 hr. 8 mg./M.²/24 hr. Divide into 3 or 4 doses (O)	Tablets: 4 mg. Syrup: 2 mg./5 ml.
Dexbrompheniramine maleate (Disomer)	0.17 mg./kg./24 hr. 5 mg./M.²/24 hr. Divide into 4 doses (O)	Tablets: 2 mg. Tablets (prolonged-action): 4 and 6 mg. Syrup: 2 mg./5 ml.
Dextrochlorpheniramine maleate (Polaramine maleate)	0.15 mg./kg./24 hr. 4.5 mg./M.²/24 hr. Divide into 4 doses (O)	Tablets: 2 mg. Repetabs: 4 and 6 mg. Syrup: 2 mg./5 ml.
Dimenhydrinate, U.S.P. (Dramamine)	5 mg./kg./24 hr. (maximum, 300 mg./24 hr.) 150 mg./M.²/24 hr. Divide into 4 doses (O, R or I.M.)	Tablets: 50 mg. Suppositories: 100 mg. Liquid: 15.6 mg./5 ml. Ampules: 50 mg./ml.
Dimethindene maleate (Forhistal maleate) **Note:** Safe dosage not established for children under 6 years.	0.1 mg./kg./24 hr. 3 mg./M.²/24 hr. Divide into 1-3 doses (O)	Tablets: 1 mg. Tablets (long-acting): 2.5 mg. Syrup: 1 mg./5 ml. Oral drops: 0.5 mg./0.6 ml.
Diphenhydramine hydrochloride, U.S.P. (Benadryl hydrochloride)	5 mg./kg./24 hr. (maximum, 300 mg./24 hr.) 150 mg./M.²/24 hr. Divide into 4 doses (O or I.M.)	Capsules: 25 and 50 mg. Tablets (enteric): 50 mg. Elixir: 12.5 mg./5 ml. Ampules: 50 mg./ml. Vials: 10 mg./ml.
Doxylamine succinate, N.F. (Decapryn succinate)	2 mg./kg./24 hr. 60 mg./M.²/24 hr. Divide into 4-6 doses (O)	Tablets (scored): 12.5 and 25 mg. Syrup: 6.25 mg./5 ml.
Methapyrilene hydrochloride, N.F. (Dozar, Histadyl, Semikon, Thenylene, and many other trade names)	5 mg./kg./24 hr. (maximum, 300 mg./24 hr.) 150 mg./M.²/24 hr. Divide into 5 doses (O) ¼ to ⅓ oral dose (S.C. or I.M.)	Capsules: 25 and 50 mg. Syrup: 20 mg./5 ml. Ampules and vials: 20 mg./ml.
Methdilazine and methdilazine hydrochloride (Tacaryl and Tacaryl hydrochloride)	0.3 mg./kg./24 hr. 10 mg./M.²/24 hr. Divide into 2 doses (O) **Caution:** Phenothiazine derivative; *see* Chlorpromazine Hydrochloride, *p. 308*	Hydrochloride: Tablets (scored): 8 mg. Syrup: 4 mg./5 ml. Base (chewable tablets): 3.6 mg.

(Table Continues)

TABLE 5-16. *Continued*

DRUG	DOSAGE AND ROUTES	SUPPLIED
Promethazine hydrochloride *(see* Tranquilizers, *p. 311)*		
Pyrrobutamine phosphate, N.F. (Pyronil)	0.6 mg./kg./24 hr. 20 mg./M.²/24 hr. Divide into 2 doses (O)	Tablets (scored): 15 mg.
Trimeprazine tartrate (Temaril)	Under 2 yr.: 3.75 mg./24 hr. (maximum) 3-12 yr.: 7.5 mg./24 hr. 6 mg./M.²/24 hr. Divide into 3 doses (O) **Caution:** Phenothiazine derivative; *see* Chlorpromazine Hydrochloride, *p. 308*	Tablets: 2.5 mg. Capsules (Spansules): 5 mg. Syrup: 2.5 mg./5 ml.
Tripelennamine citrate and hydrochloride, U.S.P. (Pyribenzamine citrate and hydrochloride)	5 mg./kg./24 hr. (maximum, 300 mg./24 hr.) 150 mg./M.²/24 hr. Divide into 4-6 doses/24 hr. (O)	Plain tablets (scored): 50 mg. Tablets (coated): 25 mg. Tablets (delayed-action): 50 and 100 mg. Elixir: 25 mg./5 ml. Ampules: 25 mg./ml.
Triprolidine hydrochloride (Actidil)	Under 2 yr.: 1.25 mg. Over 2 yr.: 2.5 mg. 4 mg./M.²/24 hr. Divide into 2 or 3 doses (O)	Tablets (scored): 2.5 mg. Syrup: 1.25 mg./5 ml.
Antihypertensives *(see* Cardiovascular drugs, *p. 280)*		
Antimalarials *(see p. 743)*		
Antineoplastics Adrenal steroids *(see* Endocrines, *p. 294)*	See package insert for Contraindications and Caution	
Busulfan (Myleran)	0.06 mg./kg./24 hr. 1.8 mg./M.²/24 hr. Titrate dosage to yield about 20,000 WBC/mm.³ (chronic myelogenous leukemia)	Tablets (scored): 2 mg.
Chlorambucil, U.S.P. (Leukeran)	0.1-0.2 mg./kg. 4.5 mg./M.²/kg. (O) Single daily dose or divided dose	Tablets: 2 mg.
Cyclophosphamide, N.F. (Cytoxan)	Initial dose: Relatively susceptible neoplasms: 2-3 mg./kg./24 hr. 60-90 mg./M.²/24 hr. Daily O or I.V. dose for 6 or more days (or total of 7 days' dosage [I.V.] once weekly) Oral: Divided doses Subsequent dose regulated by WBC, platelet count, and response Relatively resistant neoplasms: 4-8 mg./kg./24 hr. 125-250 mg./M.²/24 hr.	Tablets: 50 mg. Vials: 100, 200 and 500 mg.

Key: *M.,* dose per square meter of body surface.   *R.,* rectal.
    I.M., intramuscular.   *S.C.,* subcutaneous.
    I.Th., intrathecal.   *Subl.,* sublingual.
    I.V., intravenous.   *T.,* topical.
    O., oral.

TABLE 5-16. *Continued*

DRUG	DOSAGE AND ROUTES	SUPPLIED
	Daily O or I.V. dose for 6 days (or total of 7 days' dosage [I.V.] once weekly) Oral: Divided doses Subsequent dose regulated by WBC, platelet count, and response Maintenance dose: 2-5 mg./kg. twice weekly (O) 50-150 mg./M.² twice weekly (O)	
Dactinomycin, actinomycin D (Cosmegen)	15 µg/kg./24 hr. Divide into 4 or 5 doses (I.V.) Repeat daily dose for 5 days or 2400 µg/M.² over wk. period (I.V.)	Vials: 0.5 mg.
Mechlorethamine hydrochloride, nitrogen mustard, U.S.P. (Mustargen)	0.4 mg./kg. Single dose (I.V.) or divide into 2 or more doses with interval of 1-2 days or 1-2 wk.; or as 4 daily doses (0.1 mg./kg.)	Ampules: 10 mg.
Mercaptopurine, 6-mercaptopurine, U.S.P. (Purinethol)	2.5 mg./kg./24 hr. 70 mg./M.²/24 hr. Single dose (O)	Tablets (scored): 50 mg.
Methotrexate (formerly amethopterin), U.S.P.	0.12 mg./kg./dose 3 mg./M.²/dose Daily dose (O or I.M.) 0.25-0.5 mg./kg./24 hr. (I. Th.); may have systemic effect	Tablets: 2.5 mg. Ampules: 5 and 50 mg.
Vinblastine sulfate (Velban)	0.1-0.2 mg./kg. 3-6 mg./M.² Single *weekly* dose (I.V.) See Vincristine below	Ampules: 10 mg. dry powder (reconstituted, 1 mg./ml.)
Vincristine sulfate (Oncovin)	0.05-0.15 mg./kg. 1.5-4.5 mg./M.² Single *weekly* dose Use dry needle technique (I.V.)	Ampules: 1 and 5 mg.
Antiprotozoan drugs Carbarsone phosphate	Amebiasis: 10 mg./kg./24 hr. (maximum, 500 mg./24 hr.) 300 mg./M.²/24 hr. Divide into 2 or 3 doses (O) for 10 days **Contraindications:** Hypersensitivity to arsenic; kidney or liver disease (amebic hepatitis or abscess) **Caution:** Arsenic (cumulative), interrupted therapy; discontinue if following occur—vomiting, increasing diarrhea, pulmonary congestion, neuritis, dermatitis, pruritus, hepatosplenomegaly, albuminuria; **overdose:** treat with BAL for arsenic poisoning (p. 0000)	Tablets: 0.25 gm. Capsules: 0.25 gm. Suppositories (vaginal): 130 mg. Vials (powder): 2 gm.
Chloroquine phosphate (Aralen phosphate) *(see p. 750)*		
Diiodohydroxyquin, U.S.P. (Diodoquin and many other trade names)	Amebiasis (for 21 days): 40 mg./kg./24 hr. (maximum, 1.95 gm./24 hr.) 1.2 gm./M.²/24 hr. Divide into 3 doses (O)	Tablets: 650 mg.

(Table Continues)

TABLE 5-16. *Continued*

DRUG	DOSAGE AND ROUTES	SUPPLIED
	Contraindications: Liver damage and iodine sensitivity **Caution:** Dermatitis, chills and fever	

Quinacrine hydrochloride, U.S.P. (Atabrine hydrochloride)	Giardiasis (5 days):
	  8 mg./kg./24 hr. (maximum, 300 mg./24 hr.)
	  250 mg./M.²/24 hr.
	  Divide into 3 doses (O)
	Tapeworm:
	  15 mg./kg. (maximum, 800 mg.)
	  0.5 gm./M.²
	  Divide into 2 doses (O) 1 hr. apart
	  Saline purge 2 hr. after last dose
	Caution: See package insert
		Tablets: 100 mg.

Antipruritics
Antihistaminics *(p. 274)*

Cholestyramine resin (Cuemid, Questran)
 	
  Note: Safe dosage not established for children under 6 years.
	240 mg./kg./24 hr.
	7 gm./M.²/24 hr.
	Divide into 3 doses (O); give as slurry with water, pulpy fruit juice, applesauce, etc.
	Contraindication: Complete biliary obstruction
	Warning: Supplement vitamins A, D and K
	Caution: Increased bleeding (hypoprothrombinemia); this responds to parenteral vitamin K; administer any other drugs 1 hr. prior to this drug; may cause hyperchloremic acidosis (prolonged use), constipation, diarrhea, gastrointestinal distress, vomiting, distention, perianal rash, tongue or skin irritation
		Powder:
		  Packets: 4 gm.
		  Bottles: 216 gm.

Tranquilizers *(see p. 307)*		

Antipyretics
(see Analgesics [*nonnarcotic*] and antipyretics, *p. 242)*

Antispasmodics
(see Cholinergic blocking agents, *p. 286)*

Antituberculosis drugs
(see p. 260)

Antitussives

Benzonatate (Tessalon, Ventussin)	8 mg./kg./24 hr. 250 mg./M.²/24 hr. Divide into 3-6 doses (O) **Caution:** Not to be chewed; dermatitis, nasal congestion, constipation, sedation, hypersensitivity	Capsules: 50 and 100 mg.
Chlophedianol hydrochloride (Ulo)	2 mg./kg./24 hr. 60 mg./M.²/24 hr. Divide into 4 doses (O)	Syrup: 25 mg./5 ml.

DRUGS

Key: *M.,* dose per square meter of body surface.   *R.,* rectal.
    I.M., intramuscular.   *S.C.,* subcutaneous.
    I.Th., intrathecal.   *Subl.,* sublingual.
    I.V., intravenous.   *T.,* topical.
    O., oral.

TABLE 5-16. *Continued*

DRUG	DOSAGE AND ROUTES	SUPPLIED
	Caution: May cause hyperexcitability, nightmares, hallucinations, dry mouth, nausea, vomiting, drowsiness; cautious use with other drugs that stimulate or depress CNS	
Codeine phosphate U.S.P. *(see p. 241)*		
Dextromethorphan hydrobromide, N.F. (Romilar hydrobromide)	1 mg./kg./24 hr. 30 mg./M.²/24 hr. Divide into 3 or 4 doses (O) **Caution:** Do not mix together with penicillins, tetracyclines, salicylates, sodium phenobarbital, iodides; may cause nausea, dizziness	Syrup: 15 mg./5 ml.
Dimethoxanate hydrochloride (Cothera)	2 mg./kg./24 hr. 60 mg./M.²/24 hr. Divide into 3 or 4 doses (O) **Caution:** See package insert	Syrup: 25 mg./5 ml.
Hydrocodone bitartrate, dihydrocodeinone bitartrate, N.F. (Dicodid, Hycodan)	0.6 mg./kg./24 hr. 20 mg./M.²/24 hr. Divide into 3 or 4 doses (O) **Caution:** Addicting	Tablets: 5 mg. Syrup: 12.5 mg./5 ml.
Levopropoxyphene napsylate (Novrad)	6 mg./kg./24 hr. 200 mg./M.²/24 hr. Divide into 6 doses (O) **Caution:** Rash, drowsiness, jitteriness, dizziness; **overdose**—muscle tremor, agitation, vomiting, sedation	Capsules: 50 and 100 mg. Suspension: 50 mg./5 ml.
Methadone hydrochloride U.S.P. *(see p. 242)*		
Pipazethate hydrochloride (Theratuss)	2 mg./kg./24 hr. 50 mg./M.²/24 hr. **Caution:** *See* chlorpromazine, *p. 308*	Tablets: 10 and 20 mg.

Barbiturates
(see Sedatives and hypnotics, *p. 305)*

Blood derivatives (proteins)

DRUG	DOSAGE AND ROUTES	SUPPLIED
Albumin, normal serum (human), U.S.P.	2 ml./kg./dose 60 ml./M.²/dose	Vials: 250 mg./ml. (25%) Bottles: 50 mg./ml. (5%)
Immune serum globulin, gamma globulin, U.S.P. *(see p. 484)*	**Caution:** I.M. only	Vials: 165 mg./ml. (16.5%)

Bronchodilators

DRUG	DOSAGE AND ROUTES	SUPPLIED
Aminophylline, theophylline with ethylenediamine (85% theophylline), U.S.P.	12 mg./kg./24 hr. 0.4 gm./M.²/24 hr. Divide into 4 doses (I.V. or I.M.) Rectal dose: Same as above **Caution:** Poisonous by all routes in **overdosage:** rectal absorption unpredictable *(see* Theophylline *below)*	Ampules: 25 mg./ml. (I.V.) 250 mg./ml. (I.M.) Suppositories: 0.125, 0.25 and 0.5 gm. (R)
Diphylline, glyceryl theophylline (Iphyllin) (71% theophylline)	14 mg./kg./24 hr. 0.45 gm./M.²/24 hr. Divide into 3 doses (O) **Caution:** As for theophylline	Tablets: 100 and 200 mg. Elixir: 33 mg./5 ml. Ampules: 250 mg./ml.

Ephedrine sulfate *(see* Adrenergics, *p. 238)*

(Table Continues)

DRUGS

TABLE 5-16. *Continued*

DRUG	DOSAGE AND ROUTES	SUPPLIED
Epinephrine hydrochloride *(see* Adrenergics, *p. 238)*		
Isoproterenol *(see* Adrenergics, *p. 238)*		
Oxtriphylline (Choledyl) (64% theophylline)	15 mg./kg./24 hr. 0.5 gm./M.²/24 hr. Divide into 4 doses (O) **Caution:** As for theophylline	Tablets: 100 and 200 mg.
Pseudoephedrine hydro-chloride (Sudafed)	4 mg./kg./24 hr. 125 mg./M.²/24 hr. Divide into 4 doses (O) **Caution:** In hypertension	Tablets (scored): 60 mg. Tablets (coated): 30 mg. Syrup: 30 mg./5 ml.
Theophylline, N.F.	10 mg./kg./24 hr. 0.3 gm./M.²/24 hr. Divide into 2 or 3 doses (O) **Caution:** In giving other xanthines (aminophylline, caffeine, theobromine); may be contraindicated in peptic ulcer; care with cardiac, renal or hepatic disease, glaucoma, hyperthyroidism **Toxicity:** All routes *(see* Caffeine, *p. 240)*	Tablets: 100 and 200 mg. Elixir: 27 and 50 mg./5 ml.
Calcium salts Calcium chloride, U.S.P. (27% calcium)	0.3 gm./kg./24 hr. 8 gm./M.²/24 hr. Give as 2% solution Divide into 4 doses every 6 hr. (O) and rarely I.V. **Caution:** Acidifying; give 2-3 days, then change to another calcium salt (newborn); gastric irritation, well diluted and slowly I.V.; local necrosis with leakage from vein; avoid scalp; bradycardia	Supplied as solution of desired strength (O) Ampules: 100 mg./ml. (10%) I.V. only
Calcium gluconate, U.S.P. (9% calcium)	0.5 gm./kg./24 hr. 12 gm./M.²/24 hr. Divided doses (O or I.V. diluted and slowly) **Caution:** Bradycardia; local necrosis with leakage from vein; avoid scalp	Powder (O) Ampules: I.V. use only. 100 mg./ml. (10%)
Calcium lactate, N.F. (13% calcium)	0.5 gm./kg./24 hr. 12 gm./M.²/24 hr. Divided doses (O)	Powder (O) Tablets: 0.3, 0.5 and 0.6 gm. Wafers: 0.5 and 1 gm.
Cardiovascular drugs *Antiarrhythmics (cardiac depressants)*		
Procainamide hydrochloride, U.S.P. (Pronestyl hydro-chloride)	50 mg./kg./24 hr. 1.5 gm./M.²/24 hr. Divide into 4-6 doses/24 hr. (O) See package insert for Cautions and Contraindications	Capsules: 0.25 gm. Vials: 100 mg./ml.

Key: *M.*, dose per square meter of body surface.   *R.*, rectal.
    I.M., intramuscular.   *S.C.*, subcutaneous.
    I.Th., intrathecal.   *Subl.*, sublingual.
    I.V., intravenous.   *T.*, topical.
    O., oral.

TABLE 5-16. *Continued*

DRUG	DOSAGE AND ROUTES	SUPPLIED
Propranolol hydrochloride (Inderal)	Adults: Oral (preferred route): Arrhythmias: 10-30 mg. (single dose) 3-4 doses/24 hr. (Before meals and at bedtime) Hypertrophic aortic stenosis: 20-40 mg. (single dose) 3-4 doses/24 hr. (Before meals and at bedtime) Pheochromocytoma: Preoperatively: 60 mg./24 hr. Divided doses for 3 days (with alpha-adrenergic blocking agent) Inoperable or metastatic tumor: 30 mg./24 hr. In divided doses Intravenous (ECG monitoring): 1-3 mg. Rate not to exceed 1 mg./min. Repeat dose, if needed, after 2 min. No additional dosage within 4 hr. (Oral dosage as soon as possible) For excessive bradycardia (atropine, p. 286): 0.5-1 mg. (I.V.) For **warning** and **caution** see package insert	Tablets: 10 and 40 mg. Ampules: 1 mg./ml.
Quinidine sulfate, U.S.P.	Test dose: 2 mg./kg. 60 mg./M.² (O, IV. or I.M.) Therapeutic dose: 30 mg./kg./24 hr. 900 mg./M.²/24 hr. Divide into 5 doses/24 hr. (O, I.V. or I.M.) **Caution:** See package insert	Tablets: 100, 200 and 300 mg. Capsules: 100, 200 and 300 mg. Ampules (other salts): 40, 65, 80, 200 and 600 mg./ml.

Antihypertensives and vasodilators
(see also Diuretics, *p. 289)*

DRUG	DOSAGE AND ROUTES	SUPPLIED
Chlorisondamine chloride (Ecolid)	1st day: 10 mg./M.² in morning (O) 2nd day: 10 mg./M.² in morning (O); 10 mg./M.² at night (O) Increase 10 mg./M.² to gain effect Add hydralazine or reserpine for maximal control with minimal side effects **Caution:** Renal disease with increasing nitrogen retention, cerebral complications, encephalopathy; potentiated by anesthetics; effects of ganglionic block—blurred vision, dry mouth, constipation (lower dose, give laxatives); postural hypotension (weakness, dizziness), nausea, photophobia	Tablets: 10, 25 and 50 mg. Ampules: 5 mg./ml.

Chlorthalidone (Hygroton) *(see* Diuretics, *p. 289)*

DRUG	DOSAGE AND ROUTES	SUPPLIED
Guanethidine sulfate, U.S.P. (Ismelin)	0.2 mg./kg./24 hr. 6 mg./M.²/24 hr. Single dose (O) Increase every 7-10 days by above dose as added increment	Tablets (scored): 10 and 25 mg.

(Table Continues)

D
R
U
G
S

TABLE 5-16. *Continued*

DRUG	DOSAGE AND ROUTES	SUPPLIED
	Effective dose may be 5-8 times initial dose **Contraindications:** Monoamine oxidase inhibitors, pheochromocytoma **Caution:** In renal disease with increasing nitrogen retention, encephalopathy, in increased parasympathetic tone (peptic ulcer, etc.), incipient heart failure (edema); discontinue 2 wk. before surgery; periodic blood cell counts and liver function tests; side effects of sympathetic blockade—hypotension, weakness, dizziness, increased bowel activity, bradycardia, urinary incontinence, nasal congestion, many others	
Hydralazine hydrochloride, N.F. (Apresoline hydrochloride)	Initial (oral): 0.75 mg./kg./24 hr. 25 mg./M.^{2}/24 hr. Divide into 4 doses (O) Increase over next 3-4 wk. to as much as 10 times above dose if necessary Parenteral (with reserpine): 0.15 mg./kg. 4 mg./M.^{2} Single dose every 12-24 hr. (I.V. or I.M.) Given alone: 1.7-3.5 mg./kg./24 hr. 50-100 mg./M.^{2}/24 hr. Divide into 4-6 doses (I.V. or I.M.) **Caution:** In reduced renal function; follow blood pressure more closely; cardiovascular, neurologic, gastrointestinal, hematologic (including agranulocytosis and purpura) and skin reactions; lupus-like and arthritis-like reactions	Tablets: 10, 25, 50 and 100 mg. Ampules: 20 mg./ml.
Magnesium sulfate *(see* Laxatives, *p. 302)*		
Mecamylamine hydrochloride, U.S.P. (Inversine hydrochloride)	Adult dose (initial): 2.5 mg. twice daily p.c. (O) Increase 2.5 mg. at intervals of 2 or more days to response Average total adult dose: 25 mg./24 hr. 1.5 mg./M.^{2}/24 hr. (initial) Divide into 2 doses p.c. (O) Increase to 15 mg./M.^{2}/24 hr. **Caution:** In compromise of renal, cerebral or coronary blood flow; may cause dryness of mouth, blurred vision, diarrhea, constipation (avoid), urinary retention, vomiting, weakness, sedation, syncope, paresthesias, tremor, mental disturbances, postural hypotension	Tablets: 2.5 and 10 mg.

Key: *M.,* dose per square meter of body surface.　　*R.,* rectal.
　　I.M., intramuscular.　　*S.C.,* subcutaneous.
　　I.Th., intrathecal.　　*Subl.,* sublingual.
　　I.V., intravenous.　　*T.,* topical.
　　O., oral.

TABLE 5-16. *Continued*

DRUG	DOSAGE AND ROUTES	SUPPLIED
Methyldopa (Aldomet)	Oral: 10 mg./kg./24 hr. 300 mg./M.²/24 hr. Divide into 2 or 3 doses (O); increase or decrease to effect Increase at 2-day or more intervals to not more than: 65 mg./kg./24 hr. 2 gm./M.²/24 hr. Intravenous (crises): 20-40 mg./kg./24 hr. 0.6-1.2 gm./M.²/24 hr. Divide into 4 doses (I.V.) Continue same dosage orally when controlled **Contraindications:** Active hepatic disease, pheochromocytoma **Caution:** In hepatic disease (history); may cause sedation, headache, weakness, dizziness, cardiovascular insufficiency, orthostatic hypotension, bradycardia, nasal stuffiness, gastrointestinal symptoms, edema, heart failure, dark urine (in air), psychic changes, fever, abnormal liver function tests, jaundice, BUN rise, hemolytic anemia, positive Coombs's test, granulocyte depression, spurious high urinary catecholamines; do hepatic function tests and WBC and differential counts at intervals, first 6-8 weeks of treatment or with fever (unexplained)	Tablets: 250 mg. Solution (injection): 50 mg./ml.
Papaverine hydrochloride, N.F.	6 mg./kg./24 hr. 200 mg./M.²/24 hr. Divide into 4 doses/24 hr. (I.V. or I.M.) **Caution:** Large doses—quinidine-like effect	Tablets: 30, 60, 100 and 200 mg. Ampules: 30 mg./ml. Vials: 30 mg./ml.
Pentolinium tartrate (Ansolysen tartrate)	Initial dose: 1 mg./kg./24 hr. 30 mg./M.²/24 hr. Divide into 3 doses, waking hours Initial dose (S.C. or I.M.) ⅕ of above dose **Caution:** Check B.P. frequently in initial and increasing use	Tablets: 20, 40 and 100 mg. Vials: 10 mg./ml.
Phenoxybenzamine hydrochloride (Dibenzyline)	Initial: 0.2 mg./kg./24 hr. 6 mg./M.²/24 hr. Single dose (O) Maintenance: Increase by above dose as increments at intervals of not less than 4 days to effect; range—12-36 mg./M.²/24 hr. Single or divided doses (O) **Contraindications:** Compensated heart failure, when hypotensive effect is undesirable **Caution:** In renal damage; may cause nasal congestion, postural hypotension, tachycardia	Capsules: 10 mg.

DRUGS

(Table Continues)

TABLE 5-16. *Continued*

DRUG	DOSAGE AND ROUTES	SUPPLIED
Reserpine, U.S.P. (Eskaserp, Raurine, Reserpoid, Sandril, Serfin, Serpasil, Serpate, and many other trade names)	General: 0.02 mg./kg./24 hr. 0.6 mg./M.²/24 hr. Divide into 1 or 2 doses/24 hr. (O) Hypertension: 0.07 mg./kg./dose 2 mg./M.²/dose With hydralazine every 12-24 hr. (I.M.) **Caution:** Nasal stuffiness, including newborn infant of mother treated, diarrhea, and increased gastric acidity; discontinue 2 wk. or more before elective surgery	Tablets: 0.1, 0.25, 0.5, 1, 2, 3, 4 and 5 mg. Elixir: 0.25 and 1.25 mg./5 ml. Ampules: 2.5 mg./ml. Vials: 2.5 mg./ml.
Thiazides *(see* Diuretics, *p. 289)*		

Cardiotonics

DRUG	DOSAGE AND ROUTES	SUPPLIED
Digitalis type preparations *(see p. 1032)*	Individualize digitalizing and maintenance doses *for each patient*	
Deslanoside, desacetyllanatoside C, N.F. (Cedilanid D)	Digitalizing dose: Premature and full-term newborn infants, reduced renal function and myocarditis: 0.022 mg./kg. 0.3 mg./M.² Age 2 wk. to 3 yr.: 0.025 mg./kg. 0.75 mg./M.² After age 3 yr.: 0.0225 mg./kg. 0.75 mg./M.² Divide into 2-3 doses (I.V. or I.M.) with 3-4 hr. between doses Emergency: Single dose (I.V. or I.M.) **Caution:** Patient should not have had digitalis or long-acting derivatives for 2 wk. or more; give slowly, I.V.; watch ECG; redigitalize with digoxin in 12-24 hr. (with care)	Ampules: 0.2 mg./ml.
Digitalis (leaf), U.S.P.	Digitalizing dose: Under age 1 yr.: 0.045 gm./kg. 1-2 yr. 0.04 gm./kg. Over 2 yr.: 0.03 gm./kg. 0.75 gm./M.² Divide total dose into 3, 4 or more portions with 6 hr. or more between doses (O, I.V. or I.M.) **Caution:** Patient should not have had digitalis or long-acting derivatives for 2 wk. or more; lower dose with renal failure or myocarditis Maintenance dose: Give ¹⁄₁₀ of digitalizing dose daily	Tablets: 60, 85 and 100 mg. Pills: 30, 50, 60 and 100 mg. Tincture: 1 ml. = 0.1 gm. Ampules: Variety of preparations

Key: *M.*, dose per square meter of body surface.   *R.*, rectal.
        I.M., intramuscular.   *S.C.*, subcutaneous.
        I.Th., intrathecal.   *Subl.*, sublingual.
        I.V., intravenous.   *T.*, topical.
        O., oral.

DRUGS

TABLE 5-16. *Continued*

DRUG	DOSAGE AND ROUTES	SUPPLIED

Digitoxin, U.S.P. (Crysto-digin, Digitaline nativelle, Purodigin) *(see p. 1033)*	Digitalization:
	Individualize for each patient
	Premature and full-term infants, reduced renal function, and myocarditis:
	    0.022 mg./kg.
	    0.3-0.35 mg./M.²
	After age 2 wk.:
	    Under age 1 yr.: 0.045 mg./kg.
	Age 1-2 yr.: 0.04 mg./kg.
	    Over age 2 yr.: 0.03 mg./kg.
	    0.75 mg./M.²
	Divide total dose into 3, 4 or more portions with 6 hr. or more between doses (O, I.V. or I.M.)
	Caution: Patient should not have had digitalis or long-acting derivatives for 2 wk. or more
	Maintenance dose:
	    Give ¹⁄₁₀ of digitalizing dose
		Tablets (scored): 0.05, 0.1, 0.15 and 0.2 mg.
		Solution:
		  1 mg./ml.
		  0.02 mg./drop
		Ampules:
		  0.2 mg./ml.

Digoxin, U.S.P. (Lanoxin) *(see p. 1033)*	Premature and full-term infants (reduced renal function, and myocarditis):
	  Digitalizing dose:
	    0.03-0.05 mg./kg. (I.V. or I.M.)
	    0.75 mg./M.² (I.V. or I.M.)
	  Maintenance dose:
	    ¹⁄₁₀-¹⁄₅ of digitalizing dose
	Infants age 2 wk. to 2 yr.:
	  Digitalizing dose (O):
	    0.06-0.08 mg./kg.
	    1.5 mg./M.²
	  Digitalizing dose (I.V. or I.M.):
	    0.04-0.06 mg./kg.
	  Maintenance dose (O):
	    ¹⁄₅-¹⁄₃ of digitalizing dose
	  Maintenance dose (I.V. or I.M.):
	    ¹⁄₁₀-¹⁄₅ of digitalizing dose
	Children over 2 yr.:
	  Digitalizing dose (O):
	    0.04-0.06 mg./kg.
	    1.5 mg./M.²
	  Digitalizing dose (I.V. or I.M.):
	    0.02-0.04 mg./kg.
	Caution: Patient should not have had digitalis or long-acting derivatives for 2 wk. or more
	  Maintenance dose (O):
	    ¹⁄₅-¹⁄₃ of digitalizing dose
	  Maintenance dose (I.M. or I.V.):
	    ¹⁄₅ of digitalizing dose
	Divide total dose into 3, 4 or more portions with 6 hr. or more between doses
		Tablets (scored): 0.25 and 0.5 mg.
		Elixir (calibrated dropper): 0.05 mg./ml.
		Ampules: 0.25 mg./ml.

Lanatoside C, N.F. (Cedilanid) *(see p. 1033)*		
Ouabain, G-strophanthin, U.S.P.	0.01 mg./kg. 0.3 mg./M.² ¹⁄₂ dose stat (I.V.) Then fractions of dose every 30 min. until response or total dose given (I.V.) **Caution:** Not to be given if a long-acting digitalis type of drug given in preceding 2 wk.	Ampules: 0.2 and 0.25 mg./ml.

(Table Continues)

TABLE 5-16. *Continued*

DRUG	DOSAGE AND ROUTES	SUPPLIED
	Redigitalize with long-acting drug 12 hr. after onset of treatment Check patient and ECG before each dose	

Cathartics
(see Laxatives, *p. 302)*

Chemotherapeutics
(see Antibiotics and chemotherapeutics, *p. 261)*

Cholagogues and choleretics

Dehydrocholate sodium, N.F. (Decholin sodium)	Under 4 kg.: 400 mg. Over 4 kg.: 1 gm. Slowly and dilute I.V. 3 times in 1 wk. **Contraindications:** Complete obstruction of common duct **Caution:** Preliminary skin test, cholinergic action	Ampules: 200 mg./ml.
Ketocholanic acids (Ketochol)	Under 4 kg.: 125 mg./feeding Over 4 kg.: 250 mg./feeding Until jaundice disappears or 3 wk. (if no effect)	Tablets: 250 mg.

Cholinergic blocking agents

Atropine sulfate, U.S.P.
(As preanesthetic, *see* Table 5-17, *p. 314)*
	General use:
	    0.01 mg./kg./dose (maximum, 0.4 mg.)
	    0.3 mg./M.²/dose
	May repeat every 4-6 hr. (S.C.)
	Contraindications: Glaucoma, hypersensitivity
	Caution: May cause dryness of mouth, blurred vision (motor vehicle warning), photophobia, anhidrosis (fever), constipation (completing partial gastrointestinal obstruction), urinary retention, bronchial plugging, major CNS signs, milder (dizziness, restlessness, fatigue, tremor), hypersensitivity reactions [rash, exfoliation], leukocytosis
	Toxicity: Tachycardia, hyperpyrexia, erythema, dilated pupils, delirium, urinary retention
		Tablets: Several sizes
		Ampules and vials: 0.4 and 0.5 mg. (¹/₁₅₀ and ¹/₁₂₀ gr.)/ml.

Belladonna tincture, U.S.P.	0.1 ml./kg./24 hr. (maximum, 3.5 ml./day) 2.5 ml./M.²/24 hr. Divide into 3 or 4 doses (O) **Contraindications and caution:** As for atropine sulfate **Toxicity:** As for atropine	Tincture: About 0.3 mg. of atropine (¹/₂₀₀ gr.)/ml.
Methantheline bromide, N.F. (Banthine bromide)	6 mg./kg./24 hr. 150 mg./M.²/24 hr. Divide into 4 doses (O or I.M.)	Tablets (scored): 50 mg. Ampules: 50 mg.

Key: *M.*, dose per square meter of body surface.   *R.*, rectal.
    I.M., intramuscular.   *S.C.*, subcutaneous.
    I.Th., intrathecal.   *Subl.*, sublingual.
    I.V., intravenous.   *T.*, topical.
    O., oral.

TABLE 5-16. *Continued*

DRUG	DOSAGE AND ROUTES	SUPPLIED
	Contraindications: Glaucoma, severe cardiac disease **Caution:** Dry mouth, blurred vision (motor vehicle operation warning), mydriasis, constipation, urinary retention, central nervous stimulation, tachycardia	
Methscopolamine bromide, N.F. (Ampyrox, Lescopine bromide, Pamine bromide, Proscomide, Scoline, Tropane)	0.2 mg./kg./24 hr. 6 mg./M.²/24 hr. Divide into 4 doses p.c. and h.s. (O) **Contraindication:** Glaucoma **Caution:** In cardiac disease, pyloric obstruction; may cause dry mouth, blurred vision (motor vehicle operation warning), constipation, dysphagia, urinary retention, dizziness, flushing of skin, nausea	Tablets: 2, 2.5 and 5 mg. Capsules: 7.5 mg. Syrup: 1.25 mg./5 ml.
Oxyphenonium bromide (Antrenyl bromide)	0.8 mg./kg./24 hr. 25 mg./M.²/24 hr. Divide into 4 doses (O) **Contraindications:** Glaucoma, pyloric obstruction **Caution:** May cause dryness of mouth (motor vehicle operation warning), urinary retention, constipation, weakness, drowsiness, vomiting, tachycardia, skin rash, flushing, urticaria	Tablets (scored): 5 mg.
Propantheline bromide, U.S.P. (Pro-Banthine)	1.5 mg./kg./24 hr. 40 mg./M.²/24 hr. (O) Divide into 4 doses p.c. and h.s. **Contraindications:** As for methantheline bromide **Caution:** As for methantheline bromide	Tablets (coated): 7.5 and 15 mg. Long-acting: 30 mg. Ampules: 30 mg.
Scopolamine hydrobromide, U.S.P. (Hyoscine hydrobromide)	0.006 mg./kg. 0.20 mg./M.² As single dose (O or S.C.) **Contraindications, caution and toxicity:** As for atropine	Tablets: 0.3, 0.4 and 0.6 mg. (1/200, 1/150 and 1/100 gr.) Vials: 0.5 mg. (1/120 gr.)/ml. Ampules: 0.3, 0.4, 0.6 and 0.8 mg. (1/200, 1/150, 1/100 and 1/75 gr.)/ml.

Cholinergics (parasympathomimetics)

DRUG	DOSAGE AND ROUTES	SUPPLIED
Bethanechol chloride, U.S.P. (Urecholine chloride)	0.6 mg./kg. 20 mg./M.² Divide into 3 doses (O) 1/3 to 1/4 of above dose (S.C.) Sweat chloride test: Add 1 ml. (5 mg.) to 3 ml. 5% glucose in water: Under 1 yr.: 0.4 ml. (0.5 mg.) Over 1 yr.: 0.8 ml. (1 mg.) (Intradermally) Avoid I.M. or I.V. use **Contraindications:** Bronchial asthma, intestinal or bladder neck obstruction **Caution and toxicity:** Have atropine sulfate syringe immediately available; may cause muscular cramps and weakness, flushed skin, sweating, asthma, hypotension, circulatory collapse, abdominal cramps, vomiting, diarrhea (bloody), shock, bradycardia, cardiac arrest	Tablets: 5 and 10 mg. Ampules: 5 mg./ml.

(Table Continues)

TABLE 5-16. *Continued*

DRUG	DOSAGE AND ROUTES	SUPPLIED
Methacholine salts, N.F. (Mecholyl salts)	Parenteral: 0.1-0.4 mg./kg. 3-12 mg./M.² Single dose (S.C.) Oral: Start with 10 times above dose **Contraindications, caution and toxicity:** As for bethanechol	Ampules (chloride): 25 mg. Tablets (bromide): 0.2 gm.
Pilocarpine hydrochloride, U.S.P.	0.1 mg./kg. 3 mg./M.² Single dose (I.M. or S.C.) **Contraindications, caution and toxicity:** As for bethanechol	Tablets (hypodermic): 15 mg.
Cholinesterase inhibitors Ambenonium chloride (Mytelase chloride)	Individualize dose: Initial dose: 0.3 mg./kg./24 hr. 10 mg./M.²/24 hr. Maintenance dose: Increase to 1.5 mg./kg./24 hr. 50 mg./M.²/24 hr. Divide into 3 or 4 doses (O) **Contraindications:** Intestinal or urinary tract obstruction; extreme caution in bronchial asthma **Caution:** May cause muscarinic effects (salivation, sweating, bronchial constriction, vomiting, abdominal cramps, diarrhea, hypotension, etc.) and nicotinic effects (muscle cramps, fasciculations, muscle weakness)	Tablets: 10 and 25 mg.
Edrophonium chloride, U.S.P. (Tensilon chloride)	Myasthenia gravis test: 0.2 mg./kg. 6 mg./M.² Single dose: Give ⅕ of dose slowly (I.V.) in 1 min.; if tolerated, give remainder Premature infants: 1 mg. single dose (I.M. or S.C.) **Warning:** When testing, keep atropine sulfate syringe ready; with caution in bronchial asthma, cardiac dysrhythmias **Caution:** May cause cholinergic reactions *(see Bethanechol, p. 287)*	Ampules: 10 mg./ml.
Neostigmine bromide, U.S.P. (Prostigmin bromide)	2 mg./kg./24 hr. 60 mg./M.²/24 hr. Divide into 6-8 doses (O) **Contraindications, caution and toxicity:** As for bethanechol	Tablets: 15 mg.
Neostigmine methylsulfate, U.S.P. (Prostigmin methylsulfate)	Myasthenia gravis test: 0.04 mg./kg./dose (I.M.) 1 mg./M.²/dose (I.M.) ½ of above dose (I.V.)	Ampules: 0.25 and 0.5 mg./ml. (1:4000 and 1:2000) Vials: 0.5 and 1 mg./ml. (1:2000 and 1:1000)

Key: *M.*, dose per square meter of body surface.   *R.*, rectal.
    I.M., intramuscular.   *S.C.*, subcutaneous.
    I.Th., intrathecal.   *Subl.*, sublingual.
    I.V., intravenous.   *T.*, topical.
    O., oral.

D R U G S

TABLE 5-16. *Continued*

DRUG	DOSAGE AND ROUTES	SUPPLIED
	Contraindications: Intestinal and urinary obstruction **Caution:** In asthma; keep atropine sulfate syringe and antishock therapy ready (large doses) **Toxicity:** As for bethanechol	
Pyridostigmine bromide, U.S.P. (Mestinon bromide)	7 mg./kg./24 hr. 200 mg./M.²/24 hr. Divide into 5 or 6 doses **Contraindications:** As for ambenonium chloride **Caution:** Difficulty in differentiation of muscle weakness (including respiratory muscles and death) of cholinergic crisis from **overdosage** and myasthenic crisis; may cause side effects (see Ambenonium above), bromide rash **Toxicity:** As for bethanechol; atropine may mask signs of **overdosage**	Tablets (scored): 60 mg. Timespan: 180 mg. Syrup: 60 mg./5 ml.

Decongestants (nasal)
(see Bronchodilators, *p. 279)*

Diagnostic agents
Edrophonium chloride *(see* Cholinesterase inhibitors, *p. 288)*

Iodized oil, N.F. (Lipiodol)	Oral (40%):
	    Infants: 5 ml.
	    10-20 kg.: 0.5 ml./kg. (maximum, 10 ml.)
	Caution: Do not use if dark in color; alters PBI test; iodine sensitivity (urticaria, skin eruptions)
		Ampules (40% I): 1, 2, 3, 5 and 10 ml.
		Vials: 20 ml.

Neostigmine methylsulfate *(see* Cholinesterase inhibitors, *above)*

Phentolamine mesylate, U.S.P.; hydrochloride, N.F. (Regitine mesylate and hydrochloride)	Pheochromocytoma test:
	    Adult dose: 5 mg.
	    Child:
	        0.1 mg./kg.
	        3 mg./M.²
	    Single dose (I.V.)
	Therapeutic:
	    5 mg./kg.
	    150 mg./M.²
	    Divide into 4-6 doses (O)
	Caution: May cause tachycardia, weakness, dizziness, flushing, orthostatic hypotension, nasal stuffiness, gastrointestinal disturbances
		Ampules (mesylate): 5 mg.
		Tablets (hydrochloride): 50 mg.

Diuretics
Acidifiers
(see p. 238)

Aldosterone inhibitor
(see Endocrines, *p. 297)*

Carbonic anhydrase inhibitor

Acetazolamide, U.S.P. (Diamox)	Diuretic:
	    5 mg./kg./24 hr.
	    150 mg./M.²/24 hr.
	    Single daily dose (O, I.M.)
	Epilepsy or glaucoma:
	    8-30 mg./kg./24 hr.
		Tablets (scored): 250 mg.
		Vials (sodium salt): 500 mg.

(Table Continues)

DRUGS

TABLE 5-16. *Continued*

DRUG	DOSAGE AND ROUTES	SUPPLIED
	300-900 mg./M.²/24 hr. Divide into 3 or 4 doses (O) **Contraindications:** With depression of serum Na or K, marked hepatic or kidney disease or dysfunction, adrenal failure, hyperchloremic acidosis **Caution:** Increasing dose may increase drowsiness or paresthesia; may cause sulfonamide type reactions (fever, rash, crystalluria, renal calculus, blood dyscrasias); polyuria, drowsiness, confusion, urticaria, melena, hematuria, glycosuria, hepatic insufficiency, paralysis, convulsions; acidosis (long-term therapy)	
Mercurials (see p. 1032)		
Meralluride, U.S.P. (Mercuhydrin)	Below 3 kg.: 0.125 ml. 3-7 kg.: 0.25 ml. 8-15 kg.: 0.5 ml. 16-25 kg.: 0.75 ml. 26-35 kg.: 1 ml. 1 ml./M.²/dose (I.M.) Once or twice weekly; no more frequently than once daily **Contraindications:** Acute nephritis, intractable oliguria **Caution:** Idiosyncrasy (gastrointestinal disturbances, vertigo, fever, skin reactions); observe for electrolyte imbalance, renal function; use only clean, dry, sterile syringe	Ampules and vials: 1 ml. contains equivalent of 39 mg. Hg and 48 mg. theophylline
Mercaptomerin sodium (Thiomerin sodium)	Dosage: Same as for meralluride injection **Contraindications:** Nephritis (acute and subacute), ulcerative colitis, dehydration, mercurial sensitivity **Caution:** Maintain sufficient Na intake, instruct patient or parents in symptoms of salt depletion; sensitivity may occur (flushed face, fever, chills, gastrointestinal disturbances, skin eruptions, pruritus, urticaria)	Vials: Solution and dry form (1.4 and 4.2 gm.), 1 ml. equivalent to 40 mg. Hg Suppositories: 0.5 gm. equivalent to 165 mg. Hg
Thiazides Bendroflumethiazide (Benuron, Naturetin)	Edema: Initial, up to: 0.4 mg./kg. 12 mg./M.² Single or divided into 2 doses (O) Maintenance: ⅛ to ¼ above dose Single dose (O) Hypertension: Initial: ¼ to full edema initial dose Single or divided into 2 doses (O)	Tablets: 2.5 and 5 mg.

Key: *M.,* dose per square meter of body surface.   *R.,* rectal.
    I.M., intramuscular.   *S.C.,* subcutaneous.
    I.Th., intrathecal.   *Subl.,* sublingual.
    I.V., intravenous.   *T.,* topical.
    O., oral.

TABLE 5-16. *Continued*

DRUG	DOSAGE AND ROUTES	SUPPLIED
	Maintenance: $^1\!/_8$ to $^3\!/_4$ initial edema dose Single or divided into 2 doses (O) Dose given with morning meal **Contraindications:** In anuria; discontinue if azotemia and oliguria occur during treatment of severe renal disease **Warning:** May precipitate or increase azotemia; avoid cumulation in impaired renal function **Caution:** In hepatic cirrhosis; decrease dose of other antihypertensive drugs; bowel ulcerations (stenosis) associated with thiazides and enteric-coated K salts (care in administration, discontinue with symptoms); observe and test for fluid and electrolyte imbalance (serum and urinary electrolyte determinations), symptoms (dry mouth, thirst, weakness, muscle pains, hypotension, oliguria, tachycardia, gastrointestinal); avoid hypokalemia and low salt syndrome; hypokalemia may develop with ACTH, steroid or cirrhosis; hypokalemia dangerous with digitalis treatment; discontinue 48 hours before elective surgery; insulin requirements may change; may cause hyperglycemia and glycosuria, blood dyscrasias, jaundice, paresthesias, neonatal thrombocytopenia, glomerulonephritis, pancreatitis, and jaundice (hyperbilirubinemia), weakness, dizziness	
Benzthiazide (Exna, formerly NaClex)	1-4 mg./kg./24 hr. 30-120 mg./M.²/24 hr. Divide into 3 doses (O) Reduce dose as needed **Contraindications and caution:** As for bendroflumethiazide	Tablets (scored): 50 mg.
Chlorothiazide, N.F. (Diuril)	20 mg./kg./24 hr. 600 mgm./M.²/24 hr. Divide into 2 doses (O) **Contraindications and caution:** As for bendroflumethiazide	Tablets (scored): 250 and 500 mg. Syrup: 250 mg./5 ml. Vials (sodium) (I.V.): 500 mg.
Cyclothiazide (Anhydron)	0.02-0.04 mg./kg./24 hr. 0.6-1.2 mg./M.²/24 hr. Single dose in morning (O) Reduce dose as needed **Contraindications and caution:** As for bendroflumethiazide	Tablets (scored): 2 mg.
Hydrochlorothiazide, U.S.P. (Esidrix, HydroDiuril, Oretic)	$^1\!/_{10}$ of chlorothiazide dose **Contraindications and caution:** As for bendroflumethiazide	Tablets (scored): 25 and 50 mg.
Hydroflumethiazide (Saluron)	1 mg./kg./24 hr. 30 mg./M.²/24 hr. Single dose (O) Increase or reduce as needed **Contraindications and caution:** As for bendroflumethiazide	Tablets (scored): 50 mg. Syrup: 50 mg./5 ml.

DRUGS

(Table Continues)

TABLE 5-16. *Continued*

DRUG	DOSAGE AND ROUTES	SUPPLIED
Methyclothiazide (Enduron)	0.05-0.2 mg./kg./24 hr. 1.5-6 mg./M.²/24 hr. Single dose (O) **Contraindications and caution:** As for bendroflumethiazide	Tablets (scored): 2.5 and 5 mg.

Polythiazide (Renese)	Initial dose (O):
	  0.02-0.08 mg./kg./24 hr.
	  0.5-2.5 mg./M.²/24 hr.
	Maintenance dose (O):
	  Adjust to need
	Contraindications and caution: As for bendroflumethiazide
		Tablets (scored): 1, 2 and 4 mg.

Trichlormethiazide (Naqua, Metahydrin)	0.07 mg./kg./24 hr. 2 mg./M.²/24 hr. Single or divided dose (O) **Contraindications and caution:** As for bendroflumethiazide	Tablets (scored): 2 and 4 mg.

Other diuretics
Chlorthalidone (Hygroton)
	Initial dose:
	  2 mg./kg.
	  60 mg./M.²
	Single dose, repeat 3 times a week
	Maintenance dose:
	  Adjust to need
	Contraindications: Hypersensitivity to this drug, severe renal or hepatic disease
	Warning: Enteric-coated K salts (alone or with thiazide or other diuretics) may be associated with bowel ulcerations
	Caution: Use with care with ganglionic blocking agents, other antihypertensives or curare; periodic BUN, stop drug if rising or if aggravated liver dysfunction; observe for K, Na depletion (muscle weakness, cramps, gastrointestinal symptoms, lethargy, confusion); supply sufficient dietary salt; hypokalemia may develop with ACTH, steroid, digitalis treatment or cirrhosis; nausea, weakness, headache, dizziness, hypotension, myopia, dysuria, skin reactions, purpura, hyperglycemia, glycosuria, hyperuricemia, blood dyscrasias, pancreatitis, jaundice, paresthesias may occur
		Tablets (scored): 100 mg.

Ethacrynic acid and sodium ethacrynate (Edecrin)	Children only:
	Initial: 25 mg.
	  Single dose (O)
	Maintenance:
	  Increase by 25-mg. increments to effect
	  Maintain on alternate daily schedule or alternate therapy periods with rest periods
		Tablets (scored): 25 and 50 mg.
		Vials (sodium): 50 mg.

Key: *M.*, dose per square meter of body surface.   *R.*, rectal.
    I.M., intramuscular.   *S.C.*, subcutaneous.
    I.Th., intrathecal.   *Subl.*, sublingual.
    I.V., intravenous.   *T.*, topical.
    O., oral.

TABLE 5-16. *Continued*

DRUG	DOSAGE AND ROUTES	SUPPLIED
	Contraindications: Anuria, increasing azotemia or oliguria during treatment **Caution:** Follow electrolytes and B.P.; care in cirrhosis, digitalized patients; weakness, muscle cramps, paresthesias, hyponatremia, hypokalemia, hypotension, shock, hypouricemia, hypoglycemia, gastrointestinal symptoms, jaundice, agranulocytosis, purpura, CNS symptoms, rash may occur; no dose for infants available	
Glycerin	1.0-1.5 gm./kg. 40 gm./M.² Single dose (O) in water or milk; repeat in 4-8 hr. **Caution:** Nausea, diarrhea, headache; local caries-pain	As the chemical (U.S.P.) or Solution (flavored): Osmoglyn (50%)
Mannitol, N.F. (Osmitrol)	Oliguria, anuria: Test dose: 0.2 gm./kg. 6 gm./M.² Single dose given within 3-5 min (I.V.) Edema, ascites: As 15-20% solution 2 gm./kg. 60 gm./M.² Given over 2-6 hours (I.V.) Cerebral or ocular: As above dose in 30-60 min. Intoxication: As 5-10% solution 2 gm./kg. 60 gm./M.² Continued as needed or until this dose is reached (I.V.) **Caution:** Circulatory overload, electrolyte imbalance, tremors and convulsions (hyponatremia), headache; nausea, chills, dizziness, tachycardia, intraocular hemorrhage, death in organic CNS disease, pulmonary hypertension; do not mix with infused blood	Injection: 50, 100, 150, 200, and 250 mg./ml. (5, 10, 15, 20, and 25%)
Spironolactone (Aldactone) *(see p. 297)*		
Triamterene (Dyrenium)	Initial dose: 2-4 mg./kg./24 hr. (maximum, 300 mg./24 hr.) 60-120 mg./M.²/24 hr. Divide into 1 or 2 doses p.c. or every other day (O) **Contraindications:** Severe or progressive kidney disease or dysfunction (except possibly nephrosis), severe hepatic disease, hypersensitivity to this drug, patients with pre-existing hyperkalemia, or who develop hyperkalemia while on this drug; avoid potassium supplements (drug or diet) **Warning:** Observe regularly for blood dyscrasias, liver damage, other idiosyncrasies; do periodic BUN and serum K determinations **Caution:** Tends to conserve K, can cause hyperkalemia; withdraw use with	Capsules: 100 mg.

DRUGS

(Table Continues)

TABLE 5-16. *Continued*

DRUG	DOSAGE AND ROUTES	SUPPLIED
	elevated serum K; after prolonged use withdraw gradually; may aggravate electrolyte imbalances in heart failure, renal disease, cirrhosis; may cause low salt syndrome with salt restriction, nitrogen retention; observe for hypotension—may potentiate other antihypertensive drugs; may cause gastrointestinal symptoms, weakness, headache, dry mouth, anaphylaxis, photosensitivity, rash	
Urea, U.S.P.	Cerebral and ocular: 1-1.5 gm./kg./dose 35 gm./M.²/dose As solution I.V. over 30 min. Diuretic: 0.8 gm./kg./24 hr. 25 gm./M.²/24 hr. Divide into 3 doses (O) In juice, jellies, jam, etc. **Contraindications:** In severe renal or hepatic dysfunction, marked dehydration, intracranial bleeding **Caution:** May cause headache (relieved by narcotics and phenothiazines) from dehydration, arm pain, phlebitis, skin blebs, slough (local injection sites) *(prevent extravasation)*; thrombosis; too rapid drip increases reactions—nausea, vomiting, confusion, nervousness, hyperthermia, tachycardia	Powder 16% solution; 40 gm./250 ml. (Ureaphil); 30% solution (in 10% invert sugar) (Urevert): 40 and 90 gm. (120 and 270 ml.)

Xanthines *(see* Bronchodilators, *p. 279)*

Emetics

| Apomorphine hydrochloride, N.F. | 0.1 mg./kg.
3 mg./M.²
Single dose (S.C.)
Caution: Do not use solution if green (decomposed) | Tablets: 6 mg. |
| Ipecac syrup, U.S.P. | Over 1 yr.: 15 ml. (O); follow with water; repeat once within 20 min. if needed
Caution: Recover doses (lavage) if not vomited; include complete name —ipecac syrup—in ordering | Syrup |

Endocrines

Adrenal cortex—glucocorticosteroids and synthetics

| | *For drugs of this group:*
Contraindications: In serious fungal, viral or bacterial infections for which adequate therapy is lacking, peptic ulcer, recent intestinal anastomosis
Caution: Large pharmacologic doses for prolonged periods of time may be associated with adverse reactions varying with the particular drug used; the re- | |

Key: *M.,* dose per square meter of body surface. *R.,* rectal.
    I.M., intramuscular. *S.C.,* subcutaneous.
    I.Th., intrathecal. *Subl.,* sublingual.
    I.V., intravenous. *T.,* topical.
    O., oral.

TABLE 5-16. *Continued*

DRUG	DOSAGE AND ROUTES	SUPPLIED
	actions follow—edema, moon facies, acne, hirsutism, striae, bruising, prominent fat pads, increased appetite, headache, weakness, vertigo; more serious ones: growth retardation, osteoporosis, myopathy, hyperglycemic effects (increased insulin requirements), reduced resistance to infection, pseudotumor cerebri, papilledema, headache, vomiting, peptic ulcer, adrenal cortical atrophy, increased intravascular clotting, glaucoma, cataracts, CNS stimulation (euphoria, psychotic episodes); with great caution in healed tuberculosis; see individual diseases for uses; may need to give supplemental K and restrict Na	
Betamethasone acetate and disodium phosphate, N.F. (Celestone)	$1/40$ of cortisone dose	Tablets (scored): 0.6 mg. Syrup: 0.6 mg./5 ml. Injection (Soluspan): 6 mg./ml.
Cortisone acetate, N.F. (Cortivite, Cortogen acetate, Cortone acetate)	Physiologic replacement dose: 0.7 mg./kg./24 hr. 20 mg./M.^{2}/24 hr. Divide into 3 doses (O) I.M. dose (once daily): $1/3$-$1/2$ of oral dose Adrenocortical virilism: 1.75 mg./kg./24 hr. 50 mg./M.^{2}/24 hr. Divide into 3 or 4 doses (O) I.M. dose: Same as oral dose every third day or $1/3$-$1/2$ once daily Pharmacologic dose varies with disease: 2.5-10 mg./kg./24 hr. 75-300 mg./M.^{2}/24 hr. Divide into 3 or 4 doses (O) I.M. dose: $1/3$-$1/2$ oral dose every 12-24 hr.	Tablets: 5, 10 and 25 mg. Injection (suspension): 25 and 50 mg./ml.
Dexamethasone, N.F. (Decadron, Deronil, Dexameth, Gammacorten, Hexadrol, Maxidex)	$1/30$ of cortisone dose	Tablets (scored): 0.5 and 0.75 mg. Elixir: 0.5 mg./5 ml. Injection (sodium phosphate): 4 mg./ml.
Fluprednisolone (Alphadrol)	$1/10$ of cortisone dose	Tablets: 0.75 and 1.5 mg.
Hydrocortisone and salts, U.S.P.	$4/5$ of cortisone dose	Tablets: 5, 10 and 20 mg. Oral suspension: 10 mg./5 ml. Topical: 1 and 2.5% Vials: 100 mg. (dry) 50 mg./ml. For dilution I.V.: 100 mg./ 20 ml. Mix-O-Vial: 100 and 250 mg. Intra-articular: 50 mg./5 ml.
Methylprednisolone, N.F. (Medrol)	$1/6$ of cortisone dose	Tablets (scored): 2 and 4 mg. Capsules (sustained release): 2 and 4 mg. I.M. (Depo): 20 and 40 mg./ml.

(Table Continues)

DRUGS

TABLE 5-16. *Continued*

DRUG	DOSAGE AND ROUTES	SUPPLIED
Paramethasone acetate, fluoromethylprednisolone acetate (Haldrone)	$\frac{1}{12}$ of cortisone dose	I.V. (sodium succinate): 40 and 125 mg./ml. Tablets (scored): 1 and 2 mg.
Prednisolone, U.S.P. (Delta-Cortef, Hydeltra, Meti-cortelone, Paracortol, Prednis, Sterane, Sterolone) Acetate, U.S.P. (Nisolone, Sterane)	$\frac{1}{5}$ of cortisone dose (O, I.M. or I.V.)	Tablets (scored): 1, 2.5 and 5 mg. Aerosol spray (T): 16.6 and 50 mg. in 50 gm. Cream (T): 0.5% Aqueous suspension and vials: 25 mg./ml. (I.M. and intra-articular)
Butylacetate (Hydeltra-T.B.A.)		Suspension: 20 mg./ml.
Sodium phosphate (Hydeltrasol)		Suspension: 20 mg./ml.
Sodium succinate (Meticortelone soluble)		Powder: 50 mg. (I.V.)

Prednisone, U.S.P.
 Deltasone, Deltra, Lisacort, Metasone, Meticorten, Paracort)
	General: $\frac{1}{5}$ of cortisone dose
	 Nephrosis (initial dose/24 hr.):
	  18 mo.-4 yr.: 30-40 mg.
	  4-10 yr.: 60 mg.
	  Older: 80 mg.
	  Divide into 4 doses (O)
	 Rheumatic carditis (p. 539); leukemia (p. 1077):
	  2 mg./kg./24 hr.—2-3 wk.
	  60 mg./M.²/24 hr. for 2-3 wk.
	  1.5 mg./kg./24 hr. for 4-6 wk.
	  45 mg./M.²/24 hr. for 4-6 wk.
	  Divide into 4 doses (O)
	 Tuberculosis (p. 606)
	  2 mg./kg./24 hr.—2 mo.
	  60 mg./M.²/24 hr. for 6-8 wk.
	  Gradual withdrawal
	  Divide into 4 doses (O)
		Tablets (scored): 1, 2.5 and 5 mg.

Triamcinolone, U.S.P. (Aristocort, Kenacort)	$\frac{1}{6}$ of cortisone dose	Tablets (scored): 1, 2, 4, 8 and 16 mg. Capsules (extended-action): 5 mg. Syrup (diacetate): 4 mg./5 ml. Suspension (intralesional): 10, 25 and 40 mg./ml.
Adrenal cortex—mineralocorticoids Desoxycorticosterone acetate, U.S.P., and pivalate (trimethylacetate), N.F. (Cortate, Cortinaq, Decortin, Decosterone, Descotone, Doca acetate,	1-5 mg./24 hr. 1.5-2 mg./M.²/24 hr. Single dose in oil (I.M.) **Caution:** Observe for edema, cardiac failure, hypertension, lowered serum K (weakness, ECG changes)	Tablets (buccal, lingual): 2 and 5 mg. Pellets: 75 and 125 mg. In oil: 5 mg./ml. Repository: 25 mg./ml. Aqueous: 5 mg./ml.

Key: *M.*, dose per square meter of body surface.   *R.*, rectal.
     I.M., intramuscular.   *S.C.*, subcutaneous.
     I.Th., intrathecal.   *Subl.*, sublingual.
     I.V., intravenous.   *T.*, topical.
     O., oral.

TABLE 5-16. *Continued*

DRUG	DOSAGE AND ROUTES	SUPPLIED
Percorten, Steraq, and others)		

Adrenal medulla
Epinephrine hydrochloride *(see* Adrenergics, *p. 238)*
Levarterenol bitartrate *(see* Adrenergics, *p. 238)*

DRUG	DOSAGE AND ROUTES	SUPPLIED
Aldosterone inhibitor Spironolactone, U.S.P. (Aldactone)	Diagnostic test (primary hyperaldosteronism): 125-375 mg./M.²/24 hr. Divided doses (O) Edema and ascites: 60 mg./M.²/24 hr. Divide doses (O); readjust dose after 5th day; may need to triple dose; restrict to 1 mo. **Contraindications:** Acute renal insufficiency (lower nephron nephrosis) **Caution:** Judiciously with elevated serum K (K therapy not indicated unless glucocorticoid is given); discontinue drug use with hyperkalemia; may cause drowsiness, confusion, rash, androgenic effect, gynecomastia	Tablets: 25 mg.
Anabolic steroids Norethandrolone (Nilevar)	0.5 mg./kg./24 hr. 15 mg./M.²/24 hr. Daily dose (O) **Caution:** Androgenicity, liver disease, and sodium and water retention; check bone age and liver function with prolonged use; preferably limited to 7-21 days	Tablets: 10 mg. Drops: 0.25 mg./drop Ampules: 25 mg./ml.
Oxymetholone (Adroyd)	0.175 mg./kg./24 hr. 5 mg./M.²/24 hr. Single dose (O) **Caution:** As for norethandrolone	Tablets (scored): 2.5, 5 and 10 mg.
Stanozolol (Winstrol)	0.1 mg./kg./24 hr. 3 mg./M.²/24 hr. Divide into 3 doses **Caution:** As for norethandrolone; voice changes and hirsutism may be irreversible	Tablets (scored): 2 mg.
Pancreas Glucagon, U.S.P. (1 U.S.P. unit = 1 mg. U.S.P. Reference Standard)	0.025 unit/kg. Single dose (S.C., I.M. or I.V.) May repeat in 20 min. if needed	Ampules: 1 and 10 units
Pituitary, anterior Corticotropin, U.S.P., adrenocorticotropic hormone, ACTH (1 unit = 1 mg.)	1.6 units/kg./24 hr. 50 units/M.²/24 hr. Aqueous: Divide into 3 or 4 doses (I.V. most effective, or I.M. or S.C.) Gel: 0.8 unit/kg./24 hr. 25 units/M.²/24 hr. Single dose or divide into 2 doses **Contraindications:** Absolute: acute psychoses, Cushing's syndrome,	Aqueous: Vials: 10, 20 and 40 units Ampules: 10 units/ml. Dry: 10, 25 and 40 units Gel: Vials: 20, 40 and 80 units/ml. Cartridge: 40 units/ml. Zinc: 40 units/ml.

(Table Continues)

D
R
U
G
S

TABLE 5-16. *Continued*

DRUG	DOSAGE AND ROUTES	SUPPLIED
	active tuberculosis or peptic ulcer, congestive heart disease except rheumatic fever **Caution:** Use with greater care in hypertension, diabetes; see also **contraindications** and **caution** for glucocorticosteroids, p. 294	

Pituitary, posterior

DRUG	DOSAGE AND ROUTES	SUPPLIED
Posterior pituitary, U.S.P.	Diabetes insipidus: Nasal insufflation p.r.n. (T)	Capsules (powder): 40 mg.
Vasopressin injection, U.S.P. (Pitressin)	Aqueous: 1-3 ml. (S.C.) Divide into 3 doses Tannate in oil: 0.2 ml./dose (I.M.); increase to 1-2 ml. 0.25-0.5 ml./M.² (I.M.) Daily, twice daily, or every 2-3 days (p.r.n.)	Vasopressin injection, Aqueous: 20 units/ml. Pitressin tannate in oil: 5 units/ml.; *shake well*

Thyroid

DRUG	DOSAGE AND ROUTES	SUPPLIED
Sodium dextrothyroxine (Choloxin)	Initial: 0.05 mg./kg./24 hr. 1.5 mg./M.²/24 hr. Single dose (O) Increase the above dose at monthly intervals to maintenance Maintenance: Recommended: Double initial dose (maximum, 8 times initial dose) **Contraindications:** Euthyroid patients with organic heart disease, hypertensive, hepatic or renal disease, history of iodism, hyperthyroidism **Caution:** Potentiates coumarin type anticoagulants, decreases other clotting factors; particular care for surgical and diabetic patients, increases PBI, metabolism, hyperthyroid symptoms and signs, rashes; assess growth	Tablets (scored): 2 and 4 mg.
Sodium levothyroxine, U.S.P. (Letter, Levoid, Synthroid sodium) (0.1 mg. = 65 mg. thyroid, U.S.P.)	0.006 mg./kg./24 hr. 0.15 mg./M.²/24 hr. Not less than 0.1 mg./24 hr. under 1 yr. (cretinism) Single dose daily (O) **Contraindications and caution:** As for sodium dextrothyroxine	Tablets (scored): 0.025, 0.05, 0.1, 0.2, 0.3 and 0.5 mg. Injection: 0.05 and 0.1 mg./ml.
Sodium liothyronine, sodium L-triiodothyronine, U.S.P. (Cytomel)	Initial dose: Under 7 kg.: 2.5 μg/24 hr. (O) Over 7 kg.: 5 μg/24 hr. (O) 5 μg increments Weekly intervals p.r.n. (O) Maintenance dose: 15-20 μg/24 hr. (O)	Tablets: 5 and 25 μg

Key: *M.*, dose per square meter of body surface.
    I.M., intramuscular.
    I.Th., intrathecal.
    I.V., intravenous.
    O., oral.

    R., rectal.
    S.C., subcutaneous.
    Subl., sublingual.
    T., topical.

TABLE 5-16. *Continued*

DRUG	DOSAGE AND ROUTES	SUPPLIED
	Contraindications and caution: As for sodium dextrothyroxine	
Thyroid (U.S.P.), desiccated thyroid	4 mg./kg./24 hr. 100 mg./M.²/24 hr. Not less than 60 mg./24 hr. under 1 yr. (cretinism) Single daily dose (O) **Contraindications and caution:** As for sodium dextrothyroxine	Tablets: Many sizes
Thyroid inhibitors Methimazole, U.S.P. (Tapazole)	Initial dose: 0.4 mg./kg./24 hr. 12 mg./M.²/24 hr. Maintenance dose: ½ of initial dose Divide into 3 doses (O) **Contraindications:** Hypersensitivity or idiosyncrasy to this drug **Caution:** Agranulocytosis, pancytopenia, exfoliative dermatitis, hepatitis, neuropathy, CNS stimulation or depression, headache, fever, arthralgia, pruritus, edema, hypothyroidism	Tablets: 5 and 10 mg.
Potassium iodide, U.S.P.	Thyrotoxicosis: 0.9 ml. of saturated solution (equals 0.9 gm. KI/24 hr.) Divide into 3 doses (O)	Solution (N.F.): "Saturated": 1 gm./ml.
Propylthiouracil, U.S.P.	Initial dose: 6-10 yr.: 50-150 mg./24 hr. 10 yr. and over: 150-300 mg./24 hr. 150 mg./M.²/24 hr. Divide into 3 doses every 8 hr. (O) Maintenance dose: 50 mg. b.i.d. when euthyroid **Contraindication:** Hypersensitivity to this drug **Caution:** Agranulocytosis, fever, lymphadenopathy, hepatoxicity, purpura, and dermatitis	Tablets: 50 mg.
Enzymes Pancreatic enzymes (Cotazym, Panteric granules, Viokase), pancreatin, N.F., pancrelipase	Granules: ¼-½ tsp. with meals (O) Tablets: 1-2, whole or crushed with meals (O) Capsules: Contents of 1-3 with meals (O) Gauge dose by quality of stool **Caution:** Hypersensitivity to hog or beef products	Granules: 1 and 4 oz. Tablets: 0.3 gm. Capsules: 2000 units (lipase) Powder
Streptokinase-streptodornase (Varidase)	Buccal tablets: 1-4 daily Topical and local: To be individualized: Intramuscular: 10,000 units divided into 2 doses **Contraindications:** Reduced plasminogen or fibrinogen levels **Caution:** Allergic and pyrogenic reactions, gastrointestinal symptoms, skin rash; not for use in closed cavities without adequate drainage. Not for intravenous administration.	Oral and buccal tablets: 10,000 units of streptokinase and 2500 units of streptodornase Local-topical: Ampules: 100,000 units of streptokinase and 25,000 units of streptodornase I.M. ampules: 20,000 units of streptokinase and 5000 units of streptodornase

(Table Continues)

TABLE 5-16. *Continued*

DRUG	DOSAGE AND ROUTES	SUPPLIED

Ganglionic blocking agents
(*see* Cardiovascular drugs, antihypertensives, *p. 281*)

Hematologic Agents
Immunosuppressive agents
(*see* Antineoplastics, *p. 276*)

Iron salts and complexes
(*For toxicity of iron preparations, see p. 1499*)

DRUG	DOSAGE AND ROUTES	SUPPLIED
Iron requirements (elemental iron)	Prophylaxis: 1 mg./kg./24 hr. (single or divided dose) Treatment: 6 mg./kg./24 hr. Divide into 3 doses	
Dextriferron (Astrafer) (20 mg. Fe/ml.)	Initial treatment: 0.03 ml./kg. 1 ml./M.² Increase by like amount daily to: 0.1 ml./kg./24 hr. 3 ml./M.²/24 hr. Single dose (I.V. slowly) **Contraindications:** In all anemias except iron deficiency, liver damage **Caution:** Sensitivity (flushing of face, body warmth), abdominal pain, vomiting, wheezing, pharyngeal or facial edema, hypotension, collapse, local pain, and brown stain of skin (avoid extravasation)	Ampules: 5 ml. (20 mg./ml.)
Ferrocholinate, iron choline citrate (Chel-Iron, Ferrolip) (12% Fe)	**Caution:** Less reliable than ferrous sulfate	Tablets: 333 mg. (40 mg. Fe) Syrup: 166 mg. (20 mg. Fe)/5 ml. 417 mg. (50 mg. Fe)/5 ml. Liquid: 50 mg. Fe/5 ml. Drops (Pediatric): 25 mg. Fe/ml.
Ferroglycine sulfate complex (Ferronord) (40 mg. elemental iron per tablet or ml.)	**Caution:** Less reliable than ferrous sulfate	Tablets: 40 mg. Fe/tablet Liquid: 40 mg. Fe/ml.
Ferrous fumarate, U.S.P. (Firon, Fumiron, Hemoton, Ircon, Toleron) (33% Fe)		Tablets: 200 and 325 mg. Tablets (chewable): 200 mg. Suspension: 100 mg./5 ml.
Ferrous gluconate, N.F. (Fergon, Irox, Nionate) (12% Fe)		Tablets: 300 and 325 mg. Elixir: 60 mg./ml.
Ferrous lactate (Ferro drops) (36% Fe)		Drops: 25 mg./ml.
Ferrous sulfate, U.S.P. (20% Fe)		Tablets and capsules: 200 mg. (40 mg. Fe) 300 mg. (60 mg. Fe)

Key: *M.*, dose per square meter of body surface.   *R.*, rectal.
    I.M., intramuscular.   *S.C.*, subcutaneous.
    I.Th., intrathecal.   *Subl.*, sublingual.
    I.V., intravenous.   *T.*, topical.
    O., oral.

TABLE 5-16. *Continued*

DRUG	DOSAGE AND ROUTES	SUPPLIED
		Spansules (capsules): 225 mg. (45 mg. Fe) Syrup (N.F.): 200 mg. (40 mg. Fe)/5 ml. Elixir (Feosol): 200 mg. (40 mg. Fe)/5 ml. Fer-in-Sol: 75 mg. (15 mg. Fe)/0.6 ml. 125 mg. (25 mg. Fe)/ml.
Iron dextran injection (Imferon) (2% Fe)	Surface area in $M.^2 \times 55$ $\times$ (13.5 − patient's Hb. in gm. %) = mg. of iron needed (Formula useful under age 3-4 yr.) *or* Wt. (kg.) $\times$ (13.5−patient's Hb. in gm. %) $\times$ 2.5 = mg. of iron needed *or* Wt. (lb.) $\times$ (13.5 − patient's Hb. in gm. %) = mg. of iron needed Add 10-50% to above for stores **Contraindications:** Hypersensitivity to this drug, in all anemias except iron deficiency **Warning:** Has been associated with fatal reactions, allergic and anaphylactic **Caution:** Do not give if sensitive to test dose (0.5 ml.); inject only I.M. by Z technique; may stain skin or cause urticaria, arthralgia, lymphadenopathy, nausea, headache, fever	Ampules and vials: Equivalent to 50 mg. Fe/ml.
Polyferose, iron-carbohydrate complex (Jefron) (45% Fe)	**Caution:** Less reliable than ferrous sulfate	Tablets: Equivalent to 100 mg. Fe Elixir: Equivalent to 100 mg. Fe/5 ml.
Other hematologic agents Aminocaproic acid (Amicar)	Initial dose: 100 mg./kg. 3 gm./M.^{2} (O) or by infusion (I.V.) slowly Maintenance dose: $1/3$ of above dose hourly to achieve plasma level of 13 mg.% Not more than 18 gm./M.^{2}/24 hr. **Contraindications:** Active intravascular clotting **Side effects:** Gastrointestinal symptoms, nasal and ocular suffusion, tinnitus, headache, rash; hypotension, bradycardia or arrhythmia by rapid infusion	Tablets: 500 mg. Syrup: 1.25 mg./5ml. Injection: 250 mg./ml.
Cyanocobalamin (vitamin B$_{12}$ *(see p. 1049)*		
Folic acid *(see p. 1046)*		

Hormones
(see Endocrines, *p. 294)*

(Table Continues)

TABLE 5-16. *Continued*

DRUG	DOSAGE AND ROUTES	SUPPLIED
Hypertensives *(see* Adrenergics, *p. 238)*		
Hypnotics *(see* Sedatives and hypnotics, *p. 305)*		
Immunosuppressive agents *(see* Antineoplastics, *p. 276)*		
Iron preparations *(see* Hematologic agents, *p. 300)*		
Laxatives		
Bisacodyl (Dulcolax)	0.3 mg./kg. 8 mg. /M.² Single dose (O) 6 hr. before desired action or procedure Bowel preparation: Add rectal dose 2 hr. before procedure Under age 2 yr.: 5 mg. (R) Over age 2 yr.: 10 mg. (R) **Caution:** Usual laxative precautions; avoid rectal use—rectal fissures and ulcerations; avoid chewing tablets	Tablets (enteric): 5 mg. Suppositories: 10 mg.
Cascara sagrada, aromatic fluidextract, U.S.P.	Infants: 1-2 ml./dose Children: 2-8 ml./dose 5 ml./M.²/dose Increase dose p.r.n. for effect (O)	Aromatic fluidextract (liquid)
Castor oil, U.S.P.	Infants: 1-5 ml./dose (O) Children: 5-15 ml./dose (O) 15 ml./M.²/dose (O)	Oil or tasteless emulsion
Magnesium citrate, N.F.	4 ml./kg./dose 120 ml./M.²/dose Flavored solution ready for use (O)	Solution: 200 and 350 ml.
Magnesium sulfate, U.S.P. (Epsom salt)	Cathartic: 0.25 gm./kg./dose (O) 8.0 gm./M.²/dose (O) Hypertension: Intramuscular—50% solution: 0.2 ml./kg./dose 5 ml./M.²/dose Repeat every 4-6 hr. p.r.n. (I.M.) Intravenous—1% solution (10 mg./ml.) Maximum: 100 mg./kg./dose	Crystals Ampules: 100 mg., 250, and 500 mg./ml. (10, 25 and 50%)

Key: *M.,* dose per square meter of body surface.
    I.M., intramuscular.
    I.Th., intrathecal.
    I.V., intravenous.
    O., oral.
    R., rectal.
    S.C., subcutaneous.
    Subl., sublingual.
    T., topical.

TABLE 5-16. *Continued*

DRUG	DOSAGE AND ROUTES	SUPPLIED
	10 ml./kg./dose 3 gm./M.²/dose 300 ml./M.²/dose Slowly (I.V.); check blood pressure carefully Hypomagnesemia: see p. 0000 **Caution:** Respiratory depression; keep calcium gluconate available for use (I.V.)	
Milk of magnesia, U.S.P., magnesium hydroxide suspension	0.5 ml./kg./dose (O) 15 ml./M.²/dose (O)	U.S.P. magma (milk): Contains 8% magnesium hydroxide
Phenolphthalein, N.F. (many trade names)	1 mg./kg./dose (O) 30 mg./M.²/dose (O)	Various solid and liquid preparations
Senna, N.F.	Powder: 40 mg./kg./dose 1.2 gm./M.²/dose Fluidextract: 0.04 ml./kg./dose 1.2 ml./M.²/dose Syrup: 0.15 ml./kg./dose 4.5 ml./M.²/dose Syrup—flavored ready for use (O) Fluidextract and powder to be mixed with hospital or household flavors	N.F. monographs: Powder, fluidextract and syrup
Sodium phosphate, N.F. (dihydrogen sodium phosphate)	80 mg./kg./dose 2.5 gm./M.²/dose Dilute in flavored vehicle (O)	N.F. chemical
Sodium sulfate (Glauber's salt)	0.3 gm./kg./dose 9 gm./M.²/dose Dilute in flavored vehicle (O)	N.F. chemical

Muscle relaxants
(see also Tranquilizers, p. 307)

Carisoprodol (Soma)	25 mg./kg./24 hr. 0.75 gm./M.²/24 hr. Divide into 4 doses (O) **Contraindications:** Hypersensitivity or idiosyncrasy to this drug **Caution:** With sensitivity to similar drugs (meprobamate) may cause weakness, dizziness, ataxia, tremor, agitation, headache, gastrointestinal symptoms, respiratory depression, flushed face, eosinophilia, pancytopenia, leukopenia, allergic reactions	Tablets (coated): 350 mg. Tablets (scored): 350 mg. Capsules: 250 mg.
Chlorzoxazone (Paraflex)	20 mg./kg./24 hr. 0.6 gm./M.²/24 hr. Divide into 3 or 4 doses (O) **Caution:** In patients with known drug allergies, observe for liver damage (withdraw use); may cause gastrointestinal symptoms, drowsiness, dizziness, overstimulation, rashes, petechiae, ecchymoses, angio-edema, anaphylaxis	Tablets (scored): 250 mg.

Diazepam (Valium) *(see Tranquilizers, p. 309)*

(Table Continues)

TABLE 5-16. *Continued*

DRUG	DOSAGE AND ROUTES	SUPPLIED

Mephenesin, N.F. (Tolserol and many others) and mephenesin carbamate	175 mg./kg./24 hr.
	5 gm./M.²/24 hr.
	Divide into 3-5 doses (O)
	Intravenous (2% solution):
	  1-3 ml./kg.
	  30-90 ml./M.²
	  Single dose (I.V.) slowly injected or by slow drip
	Caution: May cause weakness, nystagmus, paresthesia, euphoria, diplopia, muscular incoordination, hemolysis, hemoglobinuria, blurred vision, hypotension; avoid with renal impairment
		Tablets: 0.25 and 0.5 gm.
		Capsules: 0.25 gm.
		Elixir: 0.5 gm./5 ml.
		Ampules: 20 mg./ml.
		Carbamate:
		  Tablets: 0.5 gm.
		  Oral suspension: 1 gm./5 ml.

Methocarbamol (Robaxin)	Usual dose:
	  60 mg./kg./24 hr.
	  2 gm./M.²/24 hr.
	  Divide into 4 doses (O, I.V. or I.M.)
	Contraindications: Hypersensitivity to this drug; renal disease if by injection (vehicle)
	Caution: Inject slowly I.V. (1.8 ml./M.²/min.); special caution in epilepsy, avoid extravasation; tetanus, not more than 18 ml. (100 mg./ml.)/M.²/24 hr. for 3 consecutive days; may cause dizziness, drowsiness, gastrointestinal symptoms, skin rash, conjunctivitis, nasal congestion, fainting, collapse
		Tablets (scored): 500 and 750 mg.
		Ampules: 100 mg./ml.

Neostigmine (Prostigmin) *(see p. 288)*		

Parasiticides
(see Anthelmintics, p. 243)

Parasympatholytics
(see Cholinergic blocking agents, p. 286)

Parasympathomimetics
(see Cholinergics, p. 287)

Renal tubular depressants
Probenecid (Benemid)
	Initial dose:
	  25 mg./kg.
	  0.7 gm./M.²
	Maintenance dose:
	  40 mg./kg./24 hr.
	  1.2 gm./M.²/24 hr.
	Divide into 4 doses (O)
	Contraindications: In children under 2
		Tablets: 0.5 gm.

Key: *M.*, dose per square meter of body surface.   *R.*, rectal.
     I.M., intramuscular.   *S.C.*, subcutaneous.
     I.Th., intrathecal.   *Subl.*, sublingual.
     I.V., intravenous.   *T.*, topical.
     O., oral.

DRUGS

TABLE 5-16. *Continued*

DRUG	DOSAGE AND ROUTES	SUPPLIED
	yr., patients with hypersensitivity to this drug, those with blood dyscrasias or uric acid kidney stones **Caution:** Determine sulfonamide levels when used with sulfonamides; urinary copper-reducing substance; may cause headache, gastrointestinal symptoms, increased urinary frequency, flushing, dizziness, anaphylactoid reactions, hemolytic anemia, aplastic anemia, nephrotic syndrome, hepatic necrosis	

Sedatives and hypnotics
(see also Anticonvulsants, *p. 266)*

Barbiturates

Amobarbital and amobarbital sodium, U.S.P. (Amytal and sodium Amytal)	Sedation: 6 mg./kg./24 hr. 180 mg./M.²/24 hr. Divide into 3 doses (O or R) Anticonvulsant dose: 3-5 mg./kg./dose (I.M.) 125 mg./M.²/dose (I.M.) See below for (I.V.) use **Contraindications:** In severe hepatic dysfunction, porphyria, hypersensitivity to barbituric acid derivatives, uncontrolled pain **Caution:** Idiosyncrasy (excitement, pain, hangover, prolonged action), in respiratory depression; may cause rash, gastrointestinal symptoms, vertigo; I.V. rate must not exceed 1 ml./min. (0.6 ml./M.²/min.) (10% solution) **Toxicity:** See p. 267	Amobarbital: Powder, ½ and 4 oz. Tablets: 16, 32, 50 and 100 mg. (¼, ½, ¾ and 1½ gr.) Elixir: 20 and 40 mg./5 ml. Amobarbital sodium: Powder: ½ oz. Capsules: 65 and 200 mg. (1 and 3 gr.) Suppositories: 0.2 gm. (3 gr.) Ampules: 65, 125, 250 and 500 mg. and 1 gm. (1, 1⅞, 3¾, 7½ and 15 gr.)
Butabarbital sodium, N.F. (Butisol sodium and many others)	Same as amobarbital above **Contraindications and caution:** As for amobarbital **Toxicity:** See p. 267	Tablets (scored): 15, 30, 50 and 100 mg. (¼, ½, ¾ and 1½ gr.) Capsules: 100 mg. (1½ gr.) Elixir: 30 mg. (½ gr.)/5 ml.
Pentobarbital sodium, U.S.P. (Napental, Nembutal sodium, Pental)	Same as amobarbital above (As preanesthetic, see Table 5-17, p. 314) **Contraindications and caution:** As for amobarbital above **Toxicity:** See p. 267	Capsules: 30, 50 and 100 mg. (½, ¾ and 1½ gr.) Long-acting Gradumet: 50 and 100 mg. Suppositories: 30, 60, 120 and 200 mg. (½, 1, 2 and 3 gr.) Elixir: 20 mg./5 ml. Ampules: 50 mg./ml. Vials: 50 mg./ml.
Phenobarbital (see p. 267)		
Secobarbital and secobarbital sodium, U.S.P. (Seconal and Seconal sodium, Evronal)	Same as amobarbital above	Tablets (coated): 50 and 100 mg. Capsules: 30, 50 and 100 mg. (½, ¾ and 1½ gr.) Suppositories: 30, 60, 125 and 200 mg. (½, 1, 2 and 3 gr.) Elixir: 22 mg./5 ml. Ampules and vials (sodium): 50 mg./ml.

(Table Continues)

D R U G S

TABLE 5-16. *Continued*

DRUG	DOSAGE AND ROUTES	SUPPLIED
Nonbarbiturates		
Chloral betaine (Beta Chlor)	Chloral hydrate dose × 1.75 = chloral betaine dose **Contraindications and caution:** As for chloral hydrate	Tablets: 870 mg. (equivalent to 500 mg. chloral hydrate)

Chloral hydrate, U.S.P. (many trade names)	Hypnotic dose:
	   50 mg./kg./24 hr. (maximum, 2 gm./ dose)
	   1.5 gm./M.²/24 hr.
	   Divide into 3 or 4 doses (O or R)
	Sedative dose:
	   ½ of hypnotic dose
	Contraindications: Marked hepatic or renal impairment, hypersensitivity or idiosyncrasy
	Caution: Avoid large doses in cardiac disease; may cause gastric irritation, excitement, delirium
		Oral use: In solution
		Rectal use: In cottonseed oil
		Suppositories: 0.3, 0.5, 0.6 and 1 gm.
		Capsules: 250 and 500 mg.
		Syrup: 250, 500 and 600 mg./ 5 ml.
		Elixir: 267 mg./5 ml.

Paraldehyde, U.S.P..	Sedative dose:
	   0.15 ml./kg./dose
	   6 ml./M.²/dose
	   (O, R or I.M.)
	   Oral: With flavor (iced)
	   Rectal: With equal parts of cotton-seed oil
	Hypnotic and anticonvulsant dose:
	   May double sedative dose (O and R)
	Caution: Use fresh supply, discard bottles opened *more* than 24 hr.; avoid in hepatic and pulmonary disease; avoid plastic syringes or containers (use glass)
	   Oral: Irritating—dilute well
	   Overdose: Respiratory and cardiac depression
		U.S.P. (liquid) (dark bottles)
		Capsules: 1 gm.
		Ampules: 2 ml.

Steroids (adrenal cortical)
(see Endocrines, *p. 294)*

Stimulants (central nervous system)
(see Analeptics, *p. 240)*

Aminophylline *(see* Bronchodilators, *p. 279)*

Amphetamine sulfate *(see* Adrenergic, *p. 238)*

Dextroamphetamine sulfate *(see* Adrenergics, *p. 238)*

Diphylline *(see* Bronchodilators, *p. 279)*

Ephedrine sulfate *(see* Adrenergics, *p. 238)*

Methylphenidate *(see* Analeptics, *p. 240)*

Oxytriphylline *(see* Bronchodilators, *p. 279)*

Key: *M.,* dose per square meter of body surface.   *R.,* rectal.
   I.M., intramuscular.   *S.C.,* subcutaneous.
   I.Th., intrathecal.   *Subl.,* sublingual.
   I.V., intravenous.   *T.,* topical.
   O., oral.

TABLE 5-16. *Continued*

DRUG	DOSAGE AND ROUTES	SUPPLIED

Theophylline *(see* Bronchodilators, *p. 279)*

Stool softeners

Dioctyl sodium sulfosucci-nate, N.F. (Aquatyl, Colace, Diovac, Doxinate Doxol, Molofac)	5 mg./kg./24 hr. 150 mg./M.²/24 hr. Divide into 3 or 4 doses (O) Enema: Add 50-100 mg. to enema (R)	Capsules: 50, 60, 100 and 240 mg. Solution: 10 and 50 mg./ml. Syrup: 10 and 20 mg./5 ml.
Poloxalkol (Polykol)	Under age 3 yr.: 100-200 mg. Over age 3 yr.: 200 mg. Single dose 1-3 times/24 hr. (O)	Capsule: 250 mg. Solution: 1 gm./5 ml.

Sulfonamides
(see Antibiotics and chemotherapeutics, *p. 263)*

Sympatholytics
(see Adrenergic blocking agents, *pp. 281, 289)*

Sympathomimetics
(see Adrenergics, *p. 238)*

Tranquilizers

Acetophenazine maleate (Tindal)	0.8-1.6 mg./kg./24 hr. (maximum, 80 mg./ 24 hr.) 25-50 mg./M.²/24 hr. Divide into 3 doses (O) **Contraindications and caution:** As for chlorpromazine hydrochloride; aceto-phenazine maleate is a piperazine type phenothiazine **Toxicity:** As for chlorpromazine	Tablets (coated): 20 mg.
Chlordiazepoxide hydro-chloride (Librium)	Children over 6 yr.: 0.5 mg./kg./24 hr. 15 mg./M.²/24 hr. Divide into 3 or 4 doses (O or I.M.) **Caution:** *Injection*: keep under observa-tion for 3 hr. (preferably in bed); do not permit vehicle operation; avoid in coma or shock. *Oral and injection*: Avoid concomitant use of other psychotropic drugs; special care with MAO inhibitors or phenothi-azine, with renal or hepatic impair-ment, and in emotional depression; may cause excitement, stimulation (hyperactive children and psychiatric patients), drowsiness, ataxia, confu-sion, syncope, skin eruptions, edema, gastrointestinal symptoms, blood dys-crasias, jaundice and hepatic dysfunc-tion, changes in EEG patterns; with protracted treatment, do periodic blood cell counts and liver function tests; not indicated for children under 6 yr.	Capsules: 5, 10 and 25 mg. Ampules: 100 mg.
Chlormezanone (Trancopal)	12 mg./kg./24 hr. 350 mg./M.²/24 hr. Divide into 3 or 4 doses (O) **Caution:** May cause rash, flush, dizzi-ness, drowsiness, weakness, chole-static jaundice (reversible)	Tablets (scored): 100 and 200 mg.

(Table Continues)

TABLE 5-16. *Continued*

DRUG	DOSAGE AND ROUTES	SUPPLIED
Chlorpromazine hydro-chloride, U.S.P. (Thorazine hydrochloride)	General use: 2 mg./kg./24 hr. 60 mg./M.²/24 hr. Divide into 4-6 doses (O) Chorea Initial dose: 50 mg. Increase 12.5 mg./dose every 6-8 hr. for control (O) Maintenance dose: Usual dose, 300-400 mg./24 hr. for 10-14 days; reduce dose by 12.5 mg. as possible (O) **Contraindications:** Hypersensitivity to phenothiazines, in bone marrow depression, psychic depression or depression by CNS drugs (barbiturates, narcotics, analgesics, antihistamines, alcohol) **Cautions for phenothiazine drugs:** Extrapyramidal symptoms often with phenothiazines (especially in children); dimethylaminopropyl derivatives (chlorpromazine, promazine [Sparine] and triflupromazine [Vesprin]) more likely — parkinsonian symptoms (tremors, postural abnormalities, mask facies, salivation, akinesia, rigidity, shuffling gait); piperazine derivatives (acetophenazine [Tindal], carphenazine [Proketazine], fluphenazine [Permitil, Prolixin], perphenazine, prochlorperazine, trifluoperazine [Stelazine] and thiopropazate [Dartal]) more likely — dyskinetic symptoms, especially in children; oculogyric crisis, torticollis, hyperextension of neck and trunk, mask facies, protrusion of tongue, perioral spasms, sweating, pallor, fever, catatonic positions while conscious; symptoms resemble tetanus; use cautiously with convulsive history (grand or petit mal), may precipitate grand mal convulsions; may cause skin reactions, cholestatic jaundice, blood dyscrasias (most common with dimethylaminopropyl and piperidyl groups); incidence of leukopenia, granulocytopenia and agranulocytosis, purpura, and pancytopenia are low, but mortality rate high; discontinue drug with symptoms, do appropriate blood tests and cell counts, discontinue with bilirubinuria or jaundice; avoid use in liver disease; may cause drowsiness (motor vehicle), dizziness, fatigue, sedation, potentiation of CNS depressants (reduce dosage); antiemetics may obscure nausea or vomiting of organic	Tablets: 10, 25, 50, 100 and 200 mg. Spansules: 30, 75, 150, 200 and 300 mg. Syrup (store in dark bottle): 10 mg./5 ml. Oral concentrate: 30 mg./ml. Ampules: 25 mg./ml. Vials: 25 mg./ml. Suppositories: 25 and 100 mg.

Key: *M.*, dose per square meter of body surface.   *R.*, rectal.
    I.M., intramuscular.   *S.C.*, subcutaneous.
    I.Th., intrathecal.   *Subl.*, sublingual.
    I.V., intravenous.   *T.*, topical.
    O., oral.

TABLE 5-16. *Continued*

DRUG	DOSAGE AND ROUTES	SUPPLIED
	diseases; adrenergic blocking action may cause hypotension (orthostatic) (epinephrine contraindicated in treatment of hypotension), potentiation of antihypertensives, may alter EEG (resembling hypopotassemia or quinidine) (caution in heart disease), anticholinergic action (intraocular tension rise, flushed face, heat prostration, dry mouth, urinary retention, constipation); photosensitivity, skin pigmentation, ocular pigmentation and cataracts, melanosis of internal organs may occur; chlorpromazine is a dimethylaminopropyl phenothiazine	
Diazepam (Valium)	0.12-0.8 mg./kg./24 hr. 3.5-24 mg./M.^{2}/24 hr. Divide into 3 or 4 doses (O) 0.04-0.2 mg./kg. 1.2-6 mg./M.^{2} Single dose I.M. (deep, slowly) or I.V. (slowly) May repeat in 1-4 hr. (Not more than 18 mg./M.^{2} in 8 hr. period) **Contraindications:** In infants under 6 mo. of age, glaucoma, sensitivity to drug **Caution:** Prolonged use—blood cell counts and liver function tests; avoid abrupt cessation of use; do not dilute or add to parenteral fluids; not for psychotic, severely depressed, comatose patients, or patients in shock; avoid use of other CNS depressants or operation of machinery; multiple symptoms in many organ systems; EEG changes See package insert	Tablets (scored): 2, 5 and 10 mg. Ampules: 2, 5 and 10 mg./ml.
Hydroxyzine hydrochloride, N.F. (Atarax) Hydroxyzine pamoate (Vistaril)	2 mg./kg./24 hr. 60 mg./M.^{2}/24 hr. Divide into 4 doses (O) Preoperative dose: ½ of above dose (I.M.) Antiemetic: Under 6 yr.: 50 mg./24 hr. Over 6 yr.: 50-100 mg./24 hr. 45-225 mg./M.^{2}/24 hr. Divide into 4 doses (O) Preoperative and postoperative—antiemetic: 1 mg./kg. 30 mg./M.^{2} Single dose (I.M.) **Contraindications:** Hypersensitivity to this drug; do not inject subcutaneously or intra-arterially **Caution:** May potentiate barbiturates and meperidine (Demerol)—reduce dosage of hydroxyzine when used with CNS depressants; may cause drowsiness (vehicle operation), dryness of mouth, tremor, convulsions; avoid	Hydrochloride: Tablets: 10, 25, 50 and 100 mg. Syrup: 10 mg./5 ml. Vials: 25 and 50 mg./ml. Pamoate: Capsules: 25, 50 and 100 mg. Oral suspension: 25 mg./5 ml. Vials: 25 and 50 mg./ml. Ampules: 50 mg./ml.

D
R
U
G
S

(Table Continues)

TABLE 5-16. *Continued*

DRUG	DOSAGE AND ROUTES	SUPPLIED
	extravasation of intravenous drug, inject slowly (not more than 15 mg./M.²/min. or 60 mg./M.²/single dose to prevent phlebitis) and diluted (to prevent hemolysis)	
Imipramine hydrochloride (Tofranil) **Note:** Not presently recommended by manufacturer for use in children under 12 years of age.	Initial: 1.5 mg./kg./24 hr. 45 mg./M.²/24 hr. Divided into 3 or 4 doses (O or I.M.) **Contraindications:** Glaucoma, monoamine oxidase inhibitors **Caution:** Perspiration, CNS and gastrointestinal symptoms, eosinophilia and skin reactions, leukopenia, jaundice (liver function and blood cell counts for extended use), heart block, hypotension, atropine-like reactions (dry mouth, tachycardia, constipation, visual disturbances, ileus) **Toxicity:** Depression, irregular respiration, ataxia, convulsions and death	Tablets: 10 and 25 mg. Injection: 12.5 mg./ml.
Meprobamate, N.F. (Equanil, Miltown, Viobamate)	25 mg./kg./24 hr. 0.7 gm./M.²/24 hr. Divide into 2 or 3 doses/24 hr. (O) Tetanus, initial, parenteral: (Oral dosage when possible) Infants: 600 mg./24 hr. Divide into 4 doses (I.M.) (Not for I.V. use) Older: 50-70 mg./kg./24 hr. (maximum, 3.2 gm./24 hr.) 1.5-2 gm./M.²/24 hr. Divide into 6-8 doses (I.M.) (Not for I.V. use) **Contraindications:** Previous allergic or idiosyncratic reactions to this drug **Caution:** Dependency may follow prolonged use; sudden withdrawal may precipitate anxiety, insomnia, vomiting, ataxia, tremors, twitching, convulsions; may cause drowsiness (motor vehicles), grand mal attacks in patients prone to grand or petit mal epilepsy, ataxia, urticaria, rash, bullous dermatitis, nonthrombocytopenic purpura, leukopenia, edema, chills, fever, bronchial spasms, hypotension, anaphylaxis, stomatitis, proctitis, fast EEG activity	Tablets: 200 and 400 mg. Extended action capsules: 200 and 400 mg. Suspension: 200 mg./5 ml. Ampules: 80 mg./ml.
Methdilazine and methdilazine hydrochloride (Tacaryl and Tacaryl hydrochloride *(see p. 275)*		

Key: *M.*, dose per square meter of body surface.   *R.*, rectal.
   I.M., intramuscular.   *S.C.*, subcutaneous.
   I.Th., intrathecal.   *Subl.*, sublingual.
   I.V., intravenous.   *T.*, topical.
   O., oral.

TABLE 5-16. *Continued*

DRUG	DOSAGE AND ROUTES	SUPPLIED
Perphenazine (Trilafon)	1-6 yr.: 4 mg./24 hr. 6-12 yr.: 6 mg./24 hr. Over 12 yr. (lower adult dose): 6-12 mg./24 hr. 7 mg./M.²/24 hr. Divide into 3 doses (O) Rectal: ½ of oral dose **Contraindications and caution:** As for chlorpromazine hydrochloride; perphenazine is a piperazine type phenothiazine **Toxicity:** As for chlorpromazine	Tablets: 2, 4, 8 and 16 mg. Repetabs: 8 mg. Syrup: 2 mg./5 ml. Concentrate (graduated dropper): 16 mg./5 ml. Suppositories: 2, 4 and 8 mg. Injection (ampules and vials): 5 mg./ml.
Prochlorperazine edisylate or maleate, U.S.P. (Compazine) **Note:** Not recommended for use in children under 10 kg. in weight.	0.4 mg./kg./24 hr. 10 mg./M.²/24 hr. Divide into 3 or 4 doses (O or R) I.M. dose: ½ of oral dose **Contraindications and caution:** As for chlorpromazine hydrochloride; prochlorperazine is a piperazine type phenothiazine **Toxicity:** As for chlorpromazine	Tablets: 5, 10 and 25 mg. Spansules: 10, 15, 30 and 75 mg. Suppositories: 2.5, 5 and 25 mg. Syrup: 5 mg./5 ml. Ampules: 5 mg./ml. Vials: 5 mg./ml. Concentrate: 10 mg./ml.

Promethazine hydrochloride, U.S.P. (Phenergan hydrochloride)	0.5 mg./kg./dose
	15 mg./M.²/dose (O, R or I.M.)
	Antihistaminic dose:
	  Full dose at night, ¼ dose a.m. or p.r.n.
	Nausea and vomiting:
	  ½ to full dose every 4-6 hr.
	Preoperative dose:
	  Full or double dose
	Motion sickness:
	  Full dose, repeat 12 hr. p.r.n.
	Caution: As for chlorpromazine
		Tablets (scored): 12.5, 25 and 50 mg.
		Syrup:
		  6.25 mg./5 ml.
		  25 mg./5 ml. (Fortis)
		Injection:
		  Ampules: 25 mg./ml. (I.M. or I.V.)
		  Tubex: 25 mg./ml. (I.M. or I.V.)
		  Vials: 50 mg./ml. (I.M. only)
		  Tubex: 50 mg./ml. (I.M. only)
		Suppositories: 25 and 50 mg.

Reserpine *(see Cardiovascular drugs, antihypertensives, p. 284)*

DRUG	DOSAGE AND ROUTES	SUPPLIED
Thioridazine (Mellaril) **Note:** Not recommended for use in children under 2 years of age.	1 mg./kg./24 hr. 30 mg./M.²/24 hr. Divide into 3 or 4 doses (O) **Contraindications and caution:** As for chlorpromazine hydrochloride; thioridazine is a piperazine type phenothiazine less likely to cause extrapyramidal reactions or jaundice **Toxicity:** As for chlorpromazine	Tablets (coated) (hydrochloride): 10, 25, 50, 100 and 200 mg. Oral concentrate (hydrochloride): 150 mg./5 ml.

Trimeprazine tartrate
  (Temaril) *(see p. 276)*

Uricosurics
(see Renal tubular depressants, *p. 304)*

Urinary antiseptics
(see Antibiotics and chemotherapeutics, *p. 245)*

Vasodilators
(see Cardiovascular drugs, antihypertensives, *p. 281)*

(Table Continues)

TABLE 5-16. *Continued*

DRUG	DOSAGE AND ROUTES	SUPPLIED
Vasopressors *(see* Adrenergics, *p. 238)*		
Vitamins *(see Table 3-7, p. 137)*		

Vitamin K
  Synthetic:
    Menadiol sodium diphosphate, U.S.P., vitamin K analogue Kappadione, Synkayvite)
	Hemorrhagic disease of newborn:
	  Prophylaxis: 1 mg. (I.M.)
	Caution: See p. 185
		Tablets: 5 mg.
		Ampules:
		  1 and 2.5 mg./0.5 ml.
		  5 and 10 mg./1 ml.
		  75 mg./2 ml.

Menadione sodium bisulfite N.F. (Hykinone) (5 mg. = 2.6 mg. menadione)	Hemorrhagic disease of newborn:
	  Prophylaxis: 1 mg. (I.M.)
	Caution: See p. 185
		Tablets: 5 mg.
		Ampules:
		  2.5 mg./0.5 ml.
		  5 mg./1 ml.
		  10 mg./1 ml.
		  72 mg./10 ml.

Natural K_1:
  Phytonadione, U.S.P.
    (AquaMephyton, Konakion)
	Hemorrhagic disease of newborn:
	  Prophylaxis: 1 mg. (I.M.)
	  Treatment: 5-10 mg. (I.V.)
	    (Konakion for I.M. use only)
	Other prothrombin deficiencies:
	  Infants: 2 mg. (O)
	  Older infants and children: 5-10 mg. (O)
	    Aqueous: (I.M., I.V. or S.C.)
	Contraindications: Repeated doses in liver disease if responses unsatisfactory
	Caution: Avoid rapid intravenous injection (not to exceed 3 mg./M.²/min. or total 5 mg.); may cause flushing, alteration of taste, dizziness, weak pulse, sweating, hypotension, cyanosis, pain, and swelling at injection site, allergic hypersensitivity, anaphylaxis; dosage guided by prothrombin times; hyperbilirubinemia of the newborn after 25 mg.
		Tablets: 5 mg.
		Ampules (emulsion): 10 and 50 mg./ml.
		
		Ampules (aqueous):
		  10 mg./ml.
		  2 mg./ml.
		Vials (aqueous): 10 mg./ml.

TOXICITY OF CHLORAMPHENICOL IN NEWBORN INFANTS

The Gray Syndrome. In newborn infants, especially premature ones, usual doses of chloramphenicol, because of reduced rates of conversion to glucuronide and of renal excretion, may lead to toxic levels of the drug in the blood. Toxicity appears, usually on the third or fourth day of continued treatment, as regurgitation of feedings followed by abdominal distention and refusal to suck. If the drug is not discontinued, cardiovascular collapse follows, manifest as respiratory distress, flaccidity and an ashen color from which the syndrome derives its name. In fatal cases, death occurs 24 to 48 hours after onset of symptoms. There are no characteristic findings at autopsy. The gray syndrome has also been observed in older infants and children who have received excessive doses of chloramphenicol.

In view of the seriousness of this condition, the use of chloramphenicol should be avoided, especially in premature and newborn infants. If used, the dose should not be over 25 mg. per kg. per 24 hours, and the drug should be discontinued at the first appearance of symptoms suggestive of toxicity.

PREOPERATIVE AND POSTOPERATIVE CARE AND CARDIOPULMONARY RESUSCITATION

Pediatric anesthesiology encompasses not only the administration of anesthesia in children undergoing operation, but also closely related aspects of intensive care and cardiopulmonary resuscitation.

To provide safe and effective anesthesia for infants and children, a physician must thoroughly understand the basic principles of modern anesthetic practice and the pharmacology of the drugs given. He must recognize the ways in which pediatric patients differ from adults in anatomy, physiology and response to drugs; he must understand the emotional reactions to anesthesia and surgery encountered in the various pediatric age groups. And in each instance he must be thoroughly familiar with and understand the physical status of the patient, the surgical lesion and the operation to be performed.

With these factors in mind, the anesthesiologist can make a preoperative evaluation, produce the desired degree of preanesthetic sedation, and select the least hazardous anesthetic agents and techniques that will produce satisfactory operating conditions. He should determine the appropriate modes of monitoring various vital functions and provide for maintenance of an adequate circulating blood volume as well as fluid, electrolyte and acid-base equilibrium.

PREOPERATIVE EVALUATION

Information provided by the parents and the child's physician enables the anesthesiologist to plan the management of anesthesia and the post-anesthetic period with greater effectiveness. The parents must be questioned about the following:

Recent upper respiratory tract infection
Exposure to the exanthems
Previous laryngotracheobronchitis (croup)
History of asthma or wheezing during respiratory infections
Bleeding tendencies
Abnormal weight loss
Exercise tolerance
Reactions to drugs
Blood transfusion reactions
Prior administration of corticosteroids
Medications currently being given
Emotional reactions of the child to the proposed operation
When and what the child last ate

A history of frequent croup will require special airway management during anesthesia; a familial history of abnormal response to muscle relaxants might indicate a genetically abnormal pseudocholinesterase which the anesthesiologist must take into consideration when selecting a muscle relaxant; infants and children receiving cortisone, antiepileptic and sedative drugs may have altered responses to anesthetic agents; a patient with a full stomach risks aspiration during induction of anesthesia.

The physical examination should emphasize the heart, the lungs and the upper airways. The presence of heart murmurs, rales in the chest or wheezing requires a complete cardiac or pulmonary evaluation before the anesthesiologist proceeds. Small, narrow nares filled with secretions, large tonsils and adenoids that necessitate open mouth-breathing, or a small, underdeveloped mandible with a protruding maxilla predispose to upper airway obstruction after sedation or induction of anesthesia. Tracheal intubation may be difficult if the larynx lies anterior to its normal position. *Before proceeding with an operation the physician should decrease excessive fever, correct dehydration, compensate for acidosis, and restore a depleted blood volume.*

The laboratory tests required prior to anesthesia include a hemoglobin or hematocrit determination, a white cell count and a urinalysis. In patients with serious systemic disease or those about to undergo extensive surgery, a preoperative roentgenogram of the chest, arterial $Paco_2$, pH, serum electrolytes and blood urea nitrogen will provide essential data.

The American Society of Anesthesiologists' classification provides a useful numerical scale of physical status:

Class 1. No organic, physiologic, biochemical or psychiatric disturbance
Class 2. Mild to moderate systemic abnormalities caused either by the disease to be treated surgically or by another pathophysiologic process
Class 3. Severe systemic abnormality from any cause
Class 4. Immediately life-threatening, severe systemic disorder
Class 5. Moribund patient who is submitted to operation in desperation
Emergency Operation (E). Any patient in one of the classes listed above who is operated upon as an emergency receives the letter "E" beside the numerical classification, such as "2E."

PREOPERATIVE PREPARATION AND SEDATION

Children are frightened by leaving the security and familiarity of home, especially those between 1 and 4 years of age who are unable to understand the purpose of hospitalization. Terrifying experiences during induction of anesthesia or in the immediate postoperative period can produce disabling psychologic changes such as night terrors, enuresis and temper tantrums. Certain steps will minimize the psychologic trauma: (1) For the child over 3 years of age, the parents should explain the purpose of the proposed operation in simple terms, and inform him of the probable sequence of events as well as any discomfort that may be involved. (2) Parents must be encouraged to display confidence and cheerfulness, since their tension and anxiety is readily transmitted to the child. (3) The anesthesiologist should visit the child prior to operation, in the presence of the parents whenever possible, so that the child will regard the anesthesiologist as a sympathetic friend who will be caring for him. (4) Preanesthetic sedation should permit the child to be transported to the operating room lightly asleep, allow induction of anesthesia without awakening, and provide some analgesia during postanesthetic recovery.

A wide variety of drugs are used for preanesthetic sedation. Studies have shown that a barbiturate in combination with an opiate and belladonna alkaloid produces suitable preanesthetic sedation in most children. Table 5-17 lists appropriate drugs and dosages for various age groups. Atropine provides more effective abolition of vagal reflexes than does scopolamine and, therefore, is preferred in infants under 1 year of age, in whom vagal reflexes tend to be more active. Scopolamine provides better drying of airway secretions in addition to a sedative effect, and may be used in patients over 1 year of age.

Although the child's stomach should be free of solids prior to anesthesia, it is important not to interrupt fluid intake longer than necessary. No milk or solids should be given less than 12 hours prior to anesthesia. Clear fluids with glucose, however, ought to be given up to 4 hours prior to induction of anesthesia in infants from day 1 to age 6 months; 6 hours prior to induction from 6 months to 3 years; and 8 hours prior to induction over 3 years. Children to be operated on in the afternoon should receive clear liquids in the morning 4 to 6 hours prior to scheduled time for induction of anesthesia.

The febrile, dehydrated child who requires emergency surgery, such as appendectomy, should receive at least partial rehydration rapidly (see

TABLE 5-17. PREOPERATIVE MEDICATION

AGE (MONTHS)	DRUGS
0-6	Atropine only
6-12	Atropine + pentobarbital
Over 12	Atropine (or scopolamine) + pentobarbital + morphine (or meperidine)

Dosage:

Atropine or scopolamine:	0.02 mg./kg. — minimum 0.15 mg., maximum 0.60 mg.
Pentobarbital:	3.0-4.0 mg./kg. — maximum 120 mg.
Morphine:	0.05-0.10 mg./kg. — maximum 10 mg.
Meperidine:	1.0-2.0 mg./kg. — maximum 100 mg.

p. 229), along with correction of any concomitant metabolic acidosis by intravenous sodium bicarbonate (2.0 to 3.0 mEq. per kg.). General endotracheal anesthesia with neuromuscular blockade and controlled ventilation followed by surface cooling with water mattresses on the anterior and posterior body surfaces can then be instituted. Cooling should be continued until the colonic or esophageal temperature is under 38°C. The anterior water mattress can be removed when the body temperature is below 39°C. (102.2°F.), and the operation safely started.

Newborn infants who require immediate operation and who have made little or no recovery from birth asphyxia or who have a body temperature below 35°C. (95°F.) require oxygen, intravenous sodium bicarbonate (3 to 5 mEq. per kg.), and elevation of body temperature toward 37°C. (98.6°F.). Analysis of arterial blood for pH, $PaCO_2$, PaO_2, electrolytes, glucose and hematocrit eliminates the guesswork inherent in clinical estimates of ventilation and metabolic status and should be regarded as essential initial monitoring.

INTRAOPERATIVE MANAGEMENT

All of the common inhalation agents have been used in children, but in recent years halothane, cyclopropane, and nitrous oxide with d-tubocurarine for neuromuscular blockade have replaced diethyl ether as the preferred agent. For induction, most anesthesiologists prefer to use gravity flow of cyclopropane or nitrous oxide over the face, with application of a face mask only after the child has lost consciousness. Regional anesthesia has limited application in infants and small children because of their fears and apprehension.

Experience has shown that the nondepolarizing muscle relaxants, especially d-tubocurarine, can be used with effectiveness and safety even in the newborn infant. Tracheal intubation and controlled ventilation provide optimal gas exchange, and neostigmine restores neuromuscular transmission at the conclusion of anesthesia.

Tracheal intubation is indicated in (1) operations about the head and neck, (2) intrathoracic and intraperitoneal procedures, (3) operations in the prone position, (4) most procedures in infants under 1 year of age, and (5) emergency procedures when there is some uncertainty about the contents of the stomach. Ventilation should be controlled manually or mechanically in all intrathoracic procedures, intraperitoneal operations, and when the patient is in the prone position.

During anesthesia, monitoring of heart tones with a precordial stethoscope, continuous measurement of rectal temperature with a thermistor probe, and assessment of arterial pressure by the Riva-Rocci method or oscillotonometry are mandatory in all age groups. For children in poor physical condition (classes 3 to 5) or when extensive surgery is required, a lead II electrocardiogram should be displayed on an oscilloscope, and continuous direct measurement of intra-arterial and right atrial pressures may be indicated.

Although the infant's heart and peripheral vasculature have a remarkable capacity to compensate for hypovolemia, decompensation occurs suddenly and cardiac arrest ensues rapidly. An awareness of the infant's approximate blood volume (90 ml. per kg. in the newborn, 75 ml. per kg. in the older infant) and immediate replacement of losses exceeding 10 to 15 per cent of that volume can prevent hypovolemic shock. Rapid transfusion with cold bank blood can produce cardiac arrest. Blood for infusions should be warmed to 30°C. 15 minutes before use. When the anticipated losses exceed one third of the patient's estimated blood volume, blood less than 4 days old should be used because older blood becomes extremely acidotic (pH 6.5 to 6.7) and hyperkalemic (K− 15 to 25 mEq. per liter). Even fresh A.C.D. blood, in conjunction with the decreased tissue perfusion that occurs with hemorrhage, produces a transient but severe acidosis. Intravenous administration of sodium bicarbonate, 1 to 2 mEq. per 100 ml. of blood given, may provide sufficient buffer to keep arterial pH above 7.30.

In modern air-conditioned operating rooms inadvertent hypothermia (colonic temperature under 35°C., 95°F.) which develops frequently in small infants undergoing laparotomy or thoracotomy is associated with ventilatory depression, peripheral vasoconstriction, and a moderate metabolic acidosis in the immediate postanesthetic period. Malignant hyperpyrexia, the abrupt and unexplained rise in body temperature above 41°C. (105.8°F.) during administration of inhalation anesthesia, occurs in children over 2 years and in young adults. The overall mortality rate exceeds 75 per cent. Successful management demands immediate recognition and cessation of anesthesia and hyperventilation with oxygen. Management also includes packing the patient in ice, ice-water gastric lavage, rapid infusion of intravenous fluids at 5 to 10 times the maintenance rate, intravenous administration of sodium bicarbonate (4 to 7 mEq. per kg.), and peripheral vasodilatation with chlorpromazine by intermittent injection (up to a total of 0.1 to 0.2 mg. per kg.).

POSTANESTHETIC RECOVERY

Recovery room facilities and nursing must be available to provide the constant surveillance of airway patency, adequacy of ventilation, and circulatory stability. Children with a history of repeated episodes of infectious laryngotracheitis may have stridor after tracheal intubation. A high humidity environment and light sedation with rectal chloral hydrate (25 mg. per kg.) for 8 to 12 hours will often relieve partial airway obstruction. In more resistant patients parenteral administration of a corticosteroid and orotracheal intubation followed by tracheostomy may be required to guarantee an adequate airway. Malignant hyperpyrexia can occur in the immediate postanesthetic period so that careful monitoring of temperature remains important.

Intensive Care. The following are necessary elements of intensive care: (1) nursing and paramedical personnel specially trained in the care of the critically ill, (2) monitoring and alarm systems for continuous assessment of vital functions, (3) respiratory therapy and resuscitation equipment and drugs, (4) physician specialists in anesthesiology, pediatrics and surgery immediately available for intensive care responsibilities, (5) a 24-hour laboratory service for routine hematologic studies, and rapid, precise determination of blood pH and gas tensions. The total objective is to provide maximal surveillance and care to patients with acute but temporary life-threatening impairment of pulmonary, cardiovascular, renal or nervous system functions.

Commercially available monitoring systems are adequate for continuous monitoring and have appropriate alarms for respiratory rate (impedance pneumograph), heart rate, arterial and central venous pressures and body temperature (thermistor probes) in small infants and children. Umbilical artery catheterization in the critically ill newborn infant permits continuous pressure monitoring and frequent blood sampling for pH and gas tensions. In older infants and children, cannulation of a peripheral artery can be utilized. Continuous measurement of ambient oxygen concentrations with high and low alarm devices represents a major advance in oxygen therapy of the small infant. Incubators equipped with servo-controlled heating units regulated by the infant's surface temperature enable the physician to prevent thermal stress.

Patients with existing or impending respiratory failure require intensive respiratory therapy. Respiratory failure exists when the impairment of ventilation poses an immediate threat to life.

An acute rise in $PaCO_2$ over 65 mm. Hg or PaO_2 under 100 mm. Hg at an inspired oxygen concentration over 95 per cent indicates life-threatening impairment of ventilatory function. Successful respiratory therapy requires artificial airway (nasotracheal intubation or tracheostomy) (Table 5-18), continuous humidification of inspired gases and sterile tracheobronchial toilet at 1- to 3-hour intervals. Infants and children with severe acute lung disease can recover good pulmonary function in a minimum of time when chest percussion, vibration and postural drainage are also utilized.

In an intensive care unit precise administration of intravenous fluids can be provided by mechanical syringe pumps. Total or partial caloric requirements are infused parenterally in infants able to tolerate a hyperosmolar infusion into a major vein.

Cardiopulmonary Resuscitation. Cessation of *effective* ventilation or circulation calls for immediate treatment. The cardinal signs of respiratory arrest are apnea and cyanosis. Circulatory arrest results in absence of heart tones and of carotid and femoral pulses. Primary respiratory

TABLE 5-18. PEDIATRIC OROTRACHEAL TUBE SPECIFICATIONS

AGE	FRENCH SIZE	INTERNAL DIAMETER (I.D. in mm.)	LENGTH (cm.)	15 mm. MALE CONNECTOR SIZE (mm. I.D.)
Newborn (<1.0 kg.)............................11-12		2.5	10	3
Newborn (>1.0 kg.)............................13-14		3.0	11	3
1-6 months.......................................15-16		3.5	11	4
6-12 months 17-18		4.0	12	4
12-18 months...................................19-20		4.5	13	5
18-36 months...................................21-22		5.0	14	5
3-4 years...23-24		5.5	16	6
5-6 years...25		6.0	18	6
6-7 years...26		6.5	18	7
8-9 years...27-28		7.0	20	7
10-11 years......................................29-30		7.5	22	8
12-14 years......................................32-34		8.0	24	8

Clear polyvinyl-chloride endotracheal tubes which satisfy the Armed Forces standard implant test and lightweight nylon connectors are recommended.

arrest can be caused by airway obstruction, central nervous system depression or neuromuscular paralysis. The 3 types of circulatory arrest that occur are asystole, ventricular fibrillation, and cardiovascular collapse associated with extreme arterial hypotension. If the diagnosis of cardiopulmonary arrest is doubtful, proceed with artificial ventilation and closed-chest massage.

Successful resuscitation must progress in a rapid but orderly sequence, with priority given to coordinated ventilation of the lungs and compression of the heart.

Airway. A clear airway must be obtained immediately. Vomitus and secretions should be aspirated or removed with fingers and a handkerchief. Soft tissue obstruction can be overcome by extension of the occipito-atlantal joint and forward displacement of the mandible.

Ventilation. Inflation of the lungs with air or oxygen can be accomplished effectively by mouth-to-mouth or mouth-to-nose insufflation, or by bag and mask devices. A good fit of the mask on the face with minimal or no leaks is essential. The hallmark of adequate lung inflation is thoraco-abdominal motion. The lungs should be inflated rapidly with a breath interposed between each 3 or 4 cardiac compressions.

Circulation. An effective cardiac output in the newborn or small infant can be produced by applying maximum pressure over the middle third of the sternum while the vertebral column is firmly supported. In larger infants and children the pressure is applied over the sternum opposite the fourth interspace, and compression is applied by the heel of the right hand. In large children the heel of the left hand is placed over the right hand to provide the strength of both arms and shoulders. If the maximum compression is held for a fraction of a second, a larger stroke volume will be ejected. The usual rate in infants is 100 compressions per minute, in children approximately 80 per minute.

When ventilation and massage are effective, carotid and femoral pulses become palpable, pupils constrict, and the color of mucous membranes improves.

Open thoracotomy and direct cardiac massage are not indicated outside the operating room.

Drugs. When artificial ventilation and cardiac massage become effective, drug therapy with sodium bicarbonate and epinephrine becomes the next important step (Table 5-19). The drugs can be given intravenously or directly into the heart. Sodium bicarbonate compensates for the extreme metabolic acidosis which develops rapidly after

TABLE 5-19. DRUGS FOR RESUSCITATION

DRUG	CONCENTRATION USED	INTRAVENOUS DOSE	INTRACARDIAC DOSE	FREQUENCY OF DOSE
Sodium bicarbonate...........1 mEq./ml.		2.0-4.0 mEq./kg., up to 200 mEq.	1.0-2.0 mEq./kg., up to 20 mEq.	5-10 minutes
Epinephrine ....1:10,000 (0.1 mg./ml.)		0.01 mg./kg., up to 0.5 mg.	0.05-0.01 mg./kg., up to 0.5 mg.	3-5 minutes
Isoproterenol ....0.2-0.4 mg. in 100 ml. of isotonic solution		Continuous infusion		Continuous infusion
Calcium chloride...............10% (100 mg./ml.)		0.2 ml./kg., minimum, 1.0 ml., maximum, 10.0 ml.	Same as intravenous	10 minutes (if effective)

TABLE 5-20. PEDIATRIC RESUSCITATION KIT: RECOMMENDED CONTENTS

Airway equipment
1. Bag and masks (infant, child, adult) with nonrebreathing valve that has universal 15-mm. female adaptor for male 15-mm. endotracheal tube connectors
2. Oropharyngeal airways (Guedel sizes 0, 1, 2, 3, 4)
3. Orotracheal tubes (complete sterile set with connectors) (see Table 5-18)
4. Aspiration equipment:
    Metal tonsil suction tip
    Disposable sterile plastic suction catheters sizes (Fr.) 5, 8, 10, 14
5. Laryngoscope:
    Standard handle
    Blades: Miller—newborn
            Wis-Forreger—1½
            Flagg—child
            Macintosh—adult (no. 3)
    2 extra batteries
    1 extra light bulb for each blade

Drugs

Sodium bicarbonate	1 mEq./ml.	4	50-ml. vials
Epinephrine	1 mg./ml.	4	1-ml. vials
Isoproterenol	0.2 mg./ml.	2	2-ml. vials
Calcium chloride	100 mg./ml. (10%)	2	10-ml. vials
Dextrose	500 mg./ml. (50%)	1	20-ml. vial
Pentobarbital	50 mg./ml.	1	30-ml. vial
Heparin	1000 u./ml.	1	10-ml. vial
Saline (for dilution)	0.9 N	2	30-ml. vials

Miscellaneous
Intracardiac needles: 20 and 22 gauge, 6-8 cm. length
Syringes (plastic disposable): 2, 5, 10 ml., 2 each
Needles: 3 each, 18, 20, 22, 25 gauge regular
         2 each, 19, 21, 23, 25 gauge scalp vein

Other:
Tongue blades
Sterile 4 × 4 gauze sponges
Alcohol swabs (packaged individually)
Sterile hemostat
Sterile scissors

---

cessation of circulation. Epinephrine, which increases the myocardial contraction force without producing a decrease in systemic vascular resistance, should be given when artificial ventilation, cardiac massage and sodium bicarbonate have not restored spontaneous, effective circulation within 3 minutes.

Defibrillation. An electrocardiogram should be obtained and run continuously as soon as possible after the diagnosis of circulatory arrest to detect ventricular fibrillation. External defibrillation can be achieved with an appropriate electric shock, 100 watt-seconds in infants, 200 to 300 watt-seconds in older children, and 400 watt-seconds in adults.

Postresuscitation care includes vigorous treatment of the cause of the collapse and monitoring and regulation of the electrocardiogram, arterial pressure and arterial pH and gas tensions.

Successful resuscitation cannot be achieved without careful preplanning and a coordinated team effort (Table 5-20).

JOHN J. DOWNES
LEONARD BACHMAN

REFERENCES

Downes, J. J., and Nicodemus, H.: Preparation for and Recovery from Anesthesia. Pediat. Clin. N. Amer., 16: August, 1969 (in press).
Dripps, R. D., Eckenhoff, J. E., and Vandam, L. D.: *Introduction to Anesthesia.* 3rd ed. Philadelphia, W. B. Saunders Company, 1967.
Goodman, L. S., and Gilman, A.: *Pharmacologic Basis of Therapeutics.* 3rd ed. New York, Macmillan Company, 1965, pp. 43-100.
Smith, R. M.: *Anesthesia for Infants and Children.* 3rd ed. St. Louis, C. V. Mosby Company, 1968.

Intensive Care

Bachman, L., Downes, J. J., Richards, C. C., and Coyle, D.: Organization and Function of an Intensive Care Unit in a Children's Hospital. *Anesthesia and Analgesia,* 48:570, 1967.
Smith, R. M.: Op. cit., Chaps. 28, 29, pp. 466-95.

Resuscitation

Cardiopulmonary Resuscitation: Statement by the ad hoc committee on cardiopulmonary resuscitation (NAS-NRC). *J.A.M.A.,* 198:372, 1966.
Downes, J. J.: Resuscitation and Intensive Care in the Newborn. *International Anesthesiology Clinics,* March, 1969.
Thaler, M. M., and Stobie, G. H. C.: An Improved Technique of External Cardiac Compression in Infants and Young Children. *New England J. Med.,* 269:606, 1963.

6. Prenatal Disturbances

PRENATAL FACTORS IN DISEASES OF CHILDREN

GENETIC FACTORS

The interplay of many factors determines health or disease of children. The physician who observes many persons exposed to equal traumas, infections or deficiencies notices that they react differently to injuries of the same type and intensity. Such differences are conveniently explained as due to varying "constitutions." It may be useful to attempt an analysis of latent or remote factors underlying this differential behavior. Some of these factors were at work before the child was born, and obviously it is difficult to study them. Nevertheless their remoteness or latency does not make them less real, and they deserve as much study and, if possible, treatment as the factors which finally elicit the disease.

The Fertilized Ovum. The child's life begins with fertilization of the ovum. The structure and composition of the fertilized egg (zygote) determine the potential somatic and mental traits of the new individual, but a favorable environment is also indispensable for coordinated embryonic differentiation and growth. Abnormalities of the elements of the zygote as well as prenatal environmental disturbances may result in congenital defects or "points of minor resistance" in the new organism. Congenital deviations are often at the root of chronic and intractable diseases of children.

Abnormalities of the chromosomes and genes, contained in the nucleus of the fertilized ovum, cause many defects in children. In addition, injurious environmental factors are capable of altering the development of an otherwise healthy zygote and are thus responsible for the production of abnormalities. Such factors should be more accessible to preventive measures than other prenatal pathogenic factors.

Injurious Factors. Injurious genetic and prenatal environmental factors will be discussed separately, although they are often difficult to distinguish in practice. Prenatal development is regulated by a continuous interaction of genes with their surrounding cytoplasm, the latter reacting in turn with the intramaternal and extramaternal environments. This continuous process is a chain of complicated physicochemical reactions, which may be interrupted or diverted by genetic or environmental interference. Genetically determined abnormalities may be imitated by environmental disturbances and result in nonhereditary "phenocopies" of hereditary defects.

Chromosomes. The essential genetic material of the chromosomes is the threadlike intranuclear structures which carry the genes, deoxyribonucleic acid, or DNA. In man, the sperm and the egg (gametes) each carry a set of 23 chromosomes; the fertilized egg and the somatic cells derived from it by mitosis therefore contain 2 such sets, or a total of 46 (44 somatic and 2 sex) chromosomes. The gametes are thus said to be *haploid,* and the somatic cells *diploid.*

The haploid gametes for the next generation are derived from the diploid cells of the gonad by a reduction division, or *meiosis,* in which the homologous chromosomes pair and then separate, one member of the pair going to one pole of the dividing cell, and the other to the opposite pole. Thus the 2 new cells each have a set of 23 chromosomes to contribute to the next generation. When the homologues separate, it is a matter of chance whether the maternal or the paternal member of the pair goes to a particular pole, so that any germ cell contains a random mixture of maternal and paternal chromosomes. This provides the physical basis for the segregation of genes.

Genes. Protein structure and function are genetically determined. A protein is composed of polypeptides, which are chains of amino acids. The sequence of amino acids in the polypeptides determines the shape, and therefore the physicochemical properties, of the protein. For each polypeptide being synthesized there is a corresponding region of a chromosome in which the structure of the DNA determines the amino acid sequence. That particular area of the DNA is said to be the gene for the corresponding polypeptide. This concept was first suggested by observations in sickle cell anemia, where a single gene difference was shown to be associated with a difference in the beta chain of the hemoglobin molecule; the sixth amino acid from the C-terminal end is a glutamic acid in the normal beta chain, whereas it is a valine in the sickle cell beta chain. This and other evidence led to the concept of a gene that determines the amino acid sequence of the beta chain, another for the alpha chain, and in fact one gene for every kind of polypeptide chain.

The basic structure of the DNA molecule can be likened to a rope ladder, in which the ropes are made up of alternating deoxyribose and phosphate molecules, and each rung consists of 2 of 4 nucleotide bases: guanine *(G),* cytosine *(C),* adenine *(A)* and thymidine *(T)* — the whole structure being twisted into a double helix. The physicochemical requirements are such that guanine always pairs with cytosine, and adenine with thymidine.

The sequence of bases in the DNA constitutes a code that determines the amino acid sequence of the corresponding protein, a triplet of 3 bases corresponding to one amino acid. For instance, it appears that the triplet CTT, at a particular place in the DNA, determines that there will be a glutamic acid molecule at a particular place on the corresponding polypeptide.

The genetic information is carried from the chromosomal gene to the cytoplasmic protein-synthesizing site, the ribosome, by a labile type of RNA called messenger RNA. (RNA is like a single-stranded rope with ribose instead of deoxyribose, and uridine instead of thymidine.) The messenger RNA is synthesized on the DNA strand, with the same requirements of complementary pairing as the 2 DNA strands; thus the CTT triplet of the DNA will result in a GAA triplet in the RNA. The messenger RNA migrates from the nucleus to the ribosomes, where it acts as a mold, or template, on which the amino acids are assembled into polypeptide chains in the following way.

A third type of RNA, the transfer RNA, exists in the cytoplasm in 20 different varieties, one for each amino acid. Each type is characterized by a specific base triplet, which corresponds in some still unknown way to its particular amino acid. Thus a variety of transfer RNA, with a specific triplet CUU at a specific attachment site on the molecule, can attach itself (with the aid of a specific enzyme) to a glutamic acid molecule at the other end. This is an oversimplification; the code is redundant, and several different transfer RNA's may code for the same amino acid.

If the transfer RNA-amino acid complex approaches the messenger RNA template, it can attach itself to the template at any point where there is a triplet corresponding to its own specific triplet. Thus a transfer RNA carrying glutamic acid at one end and a CUU triplet at the attachment site will fit in wherever there is a GAA triplet in the messenger RNA. Similarly, a transfer RNA carrying valine has a specific CAU triplet and will fit in anywhere where there is a GUA triplet on the template. In this way the amino acids are lined up on the template in an order specified by the sequence of triplets in the messenger RNA, which in turn was specified by the sequence of triplets in the DNA. These findings, coming mainly from microbial genetics, are the basis for the modern concept of a gene — a sequence of base pairs in the chromosomal DNA which determines the sequence of amino acids in a polypeptide.

An alteration in a gene will result in an alteration in the corresponding polypeptide and in the protein of which the polypeptide is a part. This change may lead to altered function of the protein and to a corresponding variation in the development or function of the organism, as in persons with sickle cell hemoglobin.

Since each cell carries the genes for all peptides, but only synthesizes some of them, it follows that a given gene is active only in certain cells. Evidence from microorganisms shows that the activity of groups of functionally related genes is regulated by other genes, through the production of cytoplasmic repressors. Systems of genetically controlled regulation of gene activity are being demonstrated in mammals.

For most genetically controlled variations in man the underlying biochemical change has not been identified, and one may think of the gene simply as a locus on a chromosome that carries an instruction regarding a particular characteristic or trait of the organism. Since the chromosomes are paired, the genes also are paired, and the 2 members of a pair may carry similar or different instructions regarding the trait which they determine, such as 5 or 6 fingers, presence or absence of melanin, or presence or absence of red-cell antigen A or B. If the members of a gene pair are the same, the person is said to be *homozygous* for the gene pair. If the members of a gene pair carry different instructions, the person is *heterozygous*. In this case the resulting trait may be determined by only one member of the pair, in which case the gene that is expressed is said to be *dominant*, and the one that is not manifested is *recessive*. The outward appearance, or array of physical traits, is called the *phenotype*, and the underlying genetic constitution is called the *genotype*. Because of recessive genes, as well as other irregularities to be mentioned later, one cannot always deduce the genotype from the phenotype.

It now appears that in the normal female one X chromosome replicates its DNA during mitosis later than the other chromosomes, remains condensed and physiologically inactive in the interphase cell, and forms the sex-chromatin *(Barr body)* characteristic of female somatic nuclei. Thus the female, like the male, has only one functioning X chromosome. If more than 2 X chromosomes are present, as in the XXX female, or XXXY male, the extra X's are also inactivated; thus the number of Barr bodies is always one less than the number of X chromosomes in the diploid complement *(the Lyon hypothesis)*.

Either the maternal or the paternal X may be inactivated in different cells of the same female, so that a woman who is heterozygous for any gene on the X chromosome will be mosaic, with one allele active in some cells and the other allele in other cells.

DOMINANT PATHOLOGIC TRAITS

Because dominant abnormal traits are relatively rare, a person who has such a trait is usually heterozygous. The heterozygote has one dominant, pathologic gene *(P)* and one recessive, normal gene *(p)* for the trait in question. The person shows the pathologic trait, since the abnormal gene expresses itself *(Pp)*. The heterozygote usually mar-

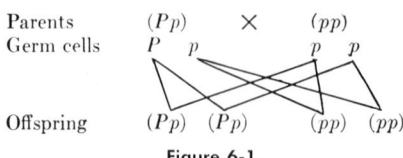

Parents (Pp) × (pp)
Germ cells P p p p

Offspring (Pp) (Pp) (pp) (pp)

Figure 6-1.

ries a person who is free of the same pathologic trait and has 2 normal recessive genes *(pp)* for the character in question. The abnormal person forms 2 kinds of germ cells in equal numbers, those containing the gene *P* and those containing the gene *p*. All the germ cells of the normal mate contain the gene *p*. Figure 6-1 illustrates the results to be expected from such a mating: half of the offspring *(Pp)* can be expected to exhibit the pathologic trait, but the other half *(pp)* will be entirely free of it. Unless it represents a new mutation, a dominant abnormality appears in every previous generation of a kinship, and each offspring of an affected parent has an equal chance of being affected or unaffected. If one of these affected children marries a normal person, he must expect to see the trait in about half of his offspring. Those children who do not show the trait will have entirely normal offspring if their mates are normal.

Figure 6-2 presents a pedigree in which a pathologic trait, multiple exostoses, is inherited as a dominant factor. The abnormal trait is transmitted from affected parents to approximately half of their children, while the other members who are free of the trait have only healthy offspring. Although each child of an affected parent has exactly a 1:1 chance of inheriting the abnormal gene, the proportion of affected to nonaffected children in any one family may deviate from the 1:1 ratio, within the limits of random variation.

A number of pathologic conditions may be inherited as dominant traits. These include achondroplasia, aniridia, diabetes insipidus (ADH-deficient), ectodermal dysplasia (hydrotic), elliptocytosis, epidermolysis bullosa simplex, epiloia,

hemorrhagic telangiectasia, Huntington's chorea, hyperelastosis cutis, keratosis follicularis, multiple exostoses, multiple polyposis, muscular dystrophy (facioscapulohumeral), myotonia congenita, myotonia dystrophica, neurofibromatosis, night blindness (without myopia), osteogenesis imperfecta, peroneal atrophy, polycystic kidney disease (adult type), sicklemia, spherocytosis, split hands or feet and thalassemia minor (see McKusick for a more complete list). It should be emphasized that in some instances the same clinical pattern may be produced in more than one way, e.g. by a mutant gene or an environmental agent. Thus inheritance of a pathologic trait in one or several pedigrees does not imply that the trait in question is always hereditary, nor that it is always inherited in the same manner.

Modification of Hereditary Traits. *Skipping of a generation.* Contrary to the rule developed, a dominant trait may occasionally skip a generation. Thus the abnormal trait may not appear in a person who has inherited the abnormal gene and transmits it to half of his offspring. This behavior may be due to reduced *expressivity* of the gene, which may result in only a slight abnormality not obvious to the casual observer. In some instances the abnormality may be found in a mild form (microform). In some cases of hereditary malformations, such as brachydactyly or exostoses, apparent skipping can be explained by roentgenographic demonstration of the abnormality in a mild form in an apparently normal parent who transmitted the anomaly to some of his children. In other instances chemical or hematologic methods reveal that the transmitting person carries the basic hereditary anomaly (hyperuricemia, spherocytosis) without clinical manifestations (gout, hemolytic jaundice).

In other instances no expression of the abnormal gene can be detected. Skipping of a generation in this manner is attributed to reduced *penetrance* (the percentual frequency with which a heterozygous dominant or a homozygous recessive gene

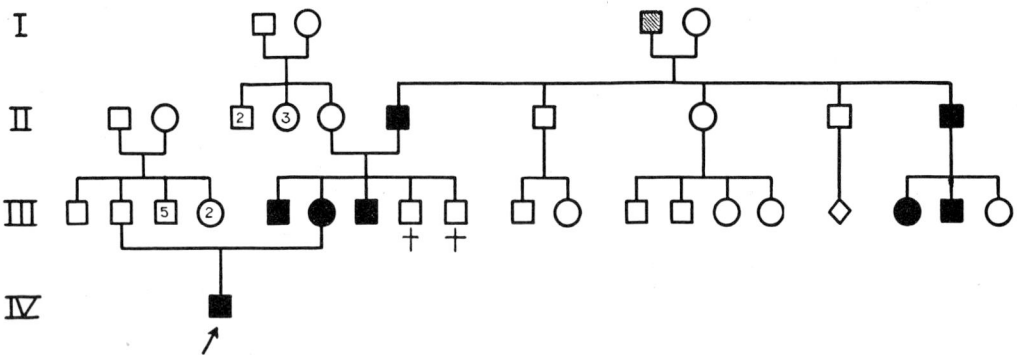

Figure 6-2. Pedigree of a sibship in which multiple exostoses occurred in several members. The abnormal condition was transmitted by the affected members to part of their offspring, but the children of the unaffected members remained free. This suggests a dominant mode of inheritance. The pedigree was drawn according to the report of the mother of the propositus (↗), a 4-year-old patient of the Children's Hospital, Cincinnati, Ohio.
■● Male and female with multiple exostoses.
▨ Man with a "bone disease" considered tuberculous (?).
See Figure 6-3 for explanation of other symbols.

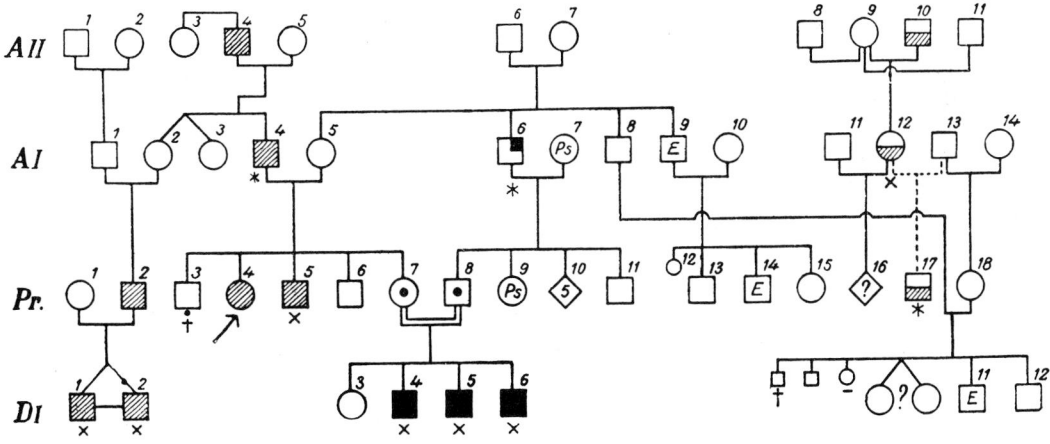

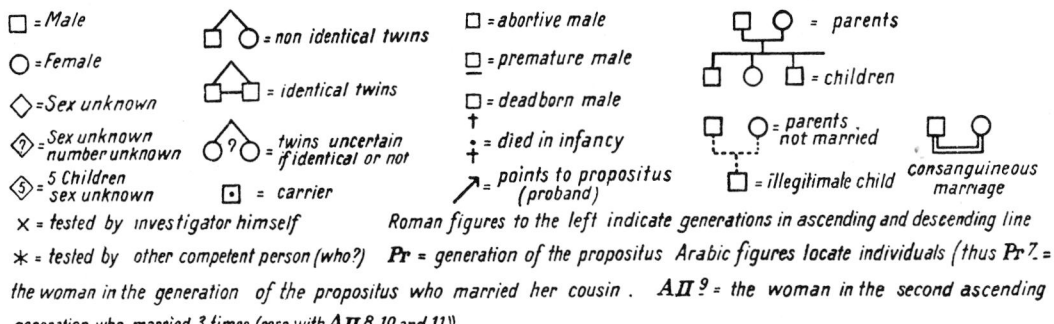

EXPLANATION OF SYMBOLS

A. Standard for all Pedigree-Charts:

□ = Male

○ = Female

◇ = Sex unknown

◈ = Sex unknown, number unknown

⬙ = 5 Children, sex unknown

× = tested by investigator himself

∗ = tested by other competent person (who?)

⬠ = non identical twins

△ = identical twins

⬡ = twins uncertain if identical or not

⊡ = carrier

□ = abortive male

⬓ = premature male

⬓ = deadborn male

† ⬓ = died in infancy

↗ = points to propositus (proband)

□ □ ○ ⬓ = parents

□ ○ □ = children

□┈○ = parents not married

⬓ = illegitimate child

□ ○ = consanguineous marriage

Roman figures to the left indicate generations in ascending and descending line

Pr = generation of the propositus   Arabic figures locate individuals (thus Pr 7 =
the woman in the generation of the propositus who married her cousin.   AII 9 = the woman in the second ascending
generation who married 3 times (resp with AII 8, 10 and 11)).

B. Especially devised or selected for this particular pedigree-chart:

▨ ⊘ = polydactyly   ■ ● = deafmuteness   ⬓ = deafness   Ps = psychopathic   E = epileptic.

⬓ ⊖ = strongly curled hair.   Other symbols may be used and added.

Figure 6-3.   Standard symbols for pedigree charts. (Bureau of Human Heredity, London.)

manifests itself). Other genetic or environmental factors may be responsible for the varied expression of the abnormal trait.

Environmental effects.   Environment plays an important role in the prenatal or postnatal manifestation of hereditary disease, in which often only a "tendency" is genetically transmitted. The disease may be manifest in a person with the abnormal tendency only if he encounters certain environmental conditions. Thus the inherited deficiency in glucose-6-phosphate dehydrogenase in red blood cells produces a hemolytic anemia only if the affected person ingests substances which have oxidant properties, such as fava beans, primaquine or sulfonamides.

The basis for such pathologic tendencies may be anatomic, histologic or functional deviations from the normal which often are not manifest clinically. Thus reduced diameter and spherical shape of the red blood corpuscles (spherocytosis) can be observed in certain families as a dominant hereditary trait. Some carriers of spherocytes are completely unaware of their abnormal trait, whereas in others there is an increased hemolysis of the abnormal cells, with resultant anemia, jaundice, spleno-

megaly and other manifestations. The clinical patterns of those with manifest disease vary, and occasionally members of an affected family may have no symptoms in common. Thus spherocytosis, inherited as a simple dominant, may cause a confusing variety of clinical symptoms (pleiotropism), which may not be recognized as being related without hematologic studies. Patients with hemolytic jaundice can be freed of their disturbing symptoms by splenectomy. This shows that a hereditary disease can be effectively treated postnatally and refutes the false but widely accepted opinion that "nothing can be done about hereditary diseases." Splenectomy, however, does not change the patient's genetic make-up, and he can transmit the abnormal trait to half of his offspring.

Another example of multiple symptoms of one dominant hereditary trait is represented by a *mesenchymal dysplasia,* which manifests itself in bluish scleras and long, gracile bones. Such bones may fracture with the slightest trauma. Some affected persons have a tendency to dislocations of joints, some to otosclerosis. In taking a history of the sibship of an affected person one may learn that one member suffered from deafness and mul-

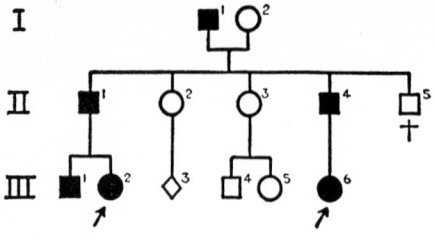

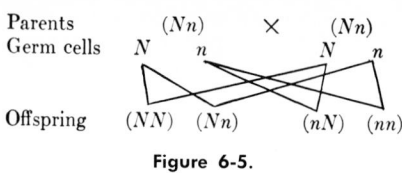

Figure 6-5.

■ ● Persons with blue scleras.

Figure 6-4. Pedigree of a family in which blue scleras occurred in several members. In addition, the following associated symptoms were seen by the recorder or reported by a member of the family (II₄): III₁: long, gracile bones in roentgenograms; II₂: multiple fractures (osteopsathyrosis); III₆: multiple fractures; II₁: multiple fractures; II₄: multiple dislocations, otosclerosis.

The abnormal condition which manifested itself in various symptoms was transmitted as a dominant trait.

tiple dislocations, and that other members were subject to multiple fractures (Fig. 6-4). Unless the observer knows the disease entity, he will not recognize the dominant inheritance of the underlying trait.

Incompatibility of Parental Genetic Factors. The degree of complexity with which genetic factors may interact with other factors in the causation of disease is well illustrated in erythroblastosis fetalis (hemolytic disease of the newborn, p. 1060). In this condition the interaction of *normal* genes of parents and child is associated with a pathologic condition in the fetus or newborn infant which stems directly from these normal genes.

RECESSIVE PATHOLOGIC TRAITS

A person with an abnormal recessive gene paired with a normal dominant gene appears normal and produces normal offspring with a mate who has 2 normal genes for the trait in question. If, however, such a heterozygous person marries a person who is similarly heterozygous, then each child has one chance in four of being homozygous and of having the pathologic trait. In Figure 6-5 the 2 apparently normal but actually heterozygous parents are represented by *(Nn)*, N representing the normal dominant and n the pathologic, recessive gene.

The abnormal offspring has the genetic constitution *(nn)*. Three fourths of the offspring appear phenotypically normal, but only one fourth *(NN)* is genotypically normal. One half of the children *(Nn)* are heterozygous, like the parents; they appear normal, but carry the pathologic gene. Since such carriers of one recessive abnormal gene appear normal, there is the possibility that they may marry unknowingly a carrier of the same pathologic trait. The chances of such a mating are related to the frequency of the pathologic gene in the general population. Consanguineous marriages favor the appearance of recessive traits. If a recessive gene is rare in a population, a homozygous, affected person may appear only once in a pedigree. *Thus the lack of a pathologic trait in the traceable genealogy does not exclude its genetic determination* (Fig. 6-6).

If a homozygous person with a pathologic trait caused by recessive genes *(nn)* marries an apparently normal person who is actually a heterozygous carrier of the same pathologic gene *(Nn)* (Fig. 6-7), half of the children will appear normal and the other half will exhibit the pathologic trait. To the observer such a family will appear like the

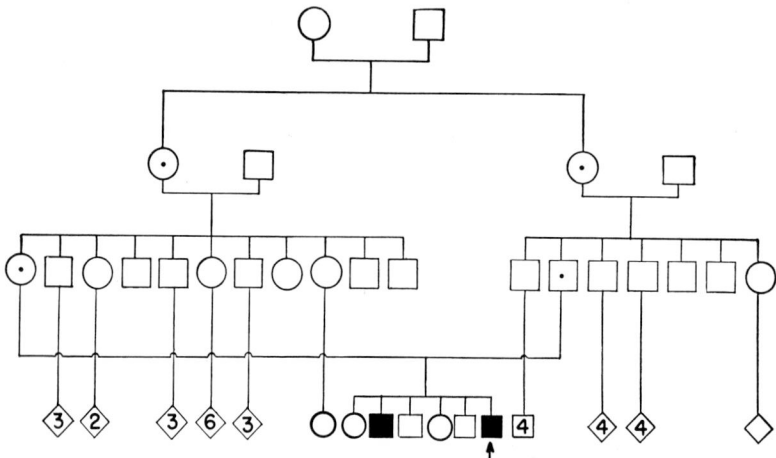

Figure 6-6. Transmission of a recessive pathologic gene by heterozygote parents. Werdnig-Hoffmann muscular atrophy (■) occurring in offspring of a consanguineous marriage. The disease does not appear in the collateral close relatives, but because the recessive disease-producing gene was received by both parents from one of their common ancestors, each of their offspring has one chance in four of being homozygous *(nn)* for it and having the disease.

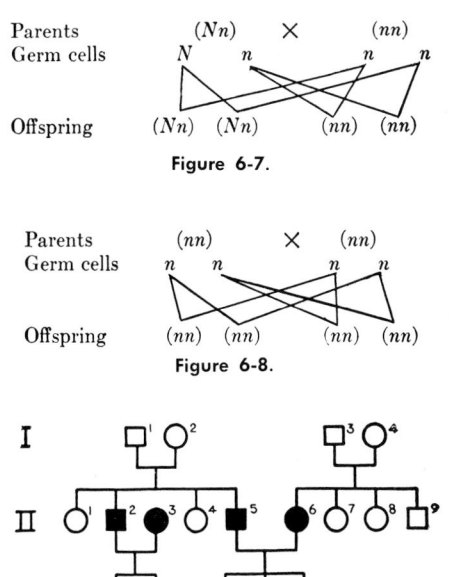

Figure 6-7.

Figure 6-8.

Figure 6-9. Deaf-mutism (■●) in a pedigree recorded by Albrecht, inherited as a recessive trait. The deaf-mutism of all the affected persons is genetically determined with the exception of that of II$_3$, who acquired deafness as a sequel of scarlet fever in infancy. (After Blacker.)

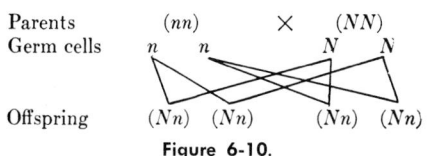

Figure 6-10.

one represented in Figure 6-1, where an abnormal person, heterozygous for a dominant pathologic gene *(Pp),* married a normal person *(pp).* In both cases one of the parents and half of the children show the defect, but the genetic make-up of the children is different. In the case of the dominant pathologic trait the unaffected children are genetically normal. They neither show nor carry the abnormal gene. In the case of the recessive abnormal character the children who appear normal carry the pathologic gene and transmit it to half of their children, who will also appear normal.

Thus a family history which includes only the parents and their children is insufficient to determine whether an inherited pathologic trait is dominant or recessive.

If 2 persons who exhibit an abnormal recessive trait and are therefore homozygous *(nn)* marry, the expectation is that all their offspring will be abnormal (Fig. 6-8). Such matings occur sometimes with deleterious effects among hereditary deaf-mutes. On the other hand, there is no objection to the marriage of persons whose deaf-mutism is acquired and not genetically determined. Figure 6-9 presents a pedigree in which 2 marriages of deaf-mutes occurred: II$_5$ and II$_6$ suffered from hereditary deaf-mutism, and all children were deaf-mutes. The marriage of II$_2$ and II$_3$ resulted in the birth of 2 normal children. Though II$_2$ was genetically a deaf-mute, II$_3$ was genetically normal and acquired deafness as a sequel of scarlet fever in infancy. Only normal children, all carriers of the pathologic trait, will be expected from such a marriage (Fig. 6-10). It is also possible that 2 deaf-mute parents who are affected by different genes for deaf-mutism may have normal children.

Pathologic conditions that may show autosomal recessive inheritance include the adrenogenital syndrome, albinism, alcaptonuria, amaurotic idiocy (Tay-Sachs), chondrodystrophia calcificans congenita, chondroectodermal dysplasia, cystinuria, cystinosis, dysautonomia (Riley's), deaf-mutism (several types), epidermolysis bullosa (severe type), familial goitrous cretinism (several types), Friedreich's ataxia, cystic fibrosis, galactosemia, gargoylism, glycogen storage disease (several types), Hartnup disease, hepatolenticular degeneration (Wilson's disease), hereditary spastic paraplegia, hypophosphatasia, Laurence-Moon-Biedl syndrome, microcephaly, Morquio's disease, muscular dystrophy (limb girdle and occasionally Duchenne), progressive spinal muscular atrophy (Werdnig-Hoffmann), Niemann-Pick disease, peroneal atrophy, phenylketonuria, retinitis pigmentosa, sickle cell anemia, thalassemia major and xeroderma pigmentosum (see McKusick for a more complete list). Again it is emphasized that the same clinical disease may result from different mutant genes, and may therefore show different patterns of inheritance in different families. Thus a number of clinical entities may be inherited as either dominant or recessive traits.

X-LINKED RECESSIVE PATHOLOGIC TRAITS

Of the 46 chromosomes of human cells, only 44, the somatic ones, can be arranged in 22 homologous pairs. The remaining pair are the sex chromosomes. In males this pair consists of 2 chromosomes of unequal size: a large submetacentric X chromosome and a small acrocentric Y chromosome. In females there are 2 X chromosomes. Thus every somatic cell of the male organism contains 22 pairs of homologous chromosomes (autosomes) plus one X and one Y chromosome, and every somatic cell of the female organism contains 22 pairs of autosomes and 2 X chromosomes. Reduction division, which leads to the formation of germ cells, produces 2 types of sperm cells: one containing 22 autosomes and a Y chromosome and another containing 22 autosomes and an X chromosome. All the germ cells produced by the female contain 22 autosomes and an X chromosome. Fertilization may result, therefore, in the formation of one of 2 types of zygotes: one which receives an X chromosome from both father and mother, the resulting offspring being female (XX), and another which receives a Y chromosome from the father and an X chromosome from the mother, the offspring being male (XY). The X chromosome carries many genes; the Y chromosome appears to be mainly concerned with determining maleness. The genes of the X chromosome of the male are, therefore, in an exceptional position because they are not matched by corresponding genes of the Y chromosome. If a mutant gene is located in the X chromosome of the male, it can manifest itself even if it is recessive, since its effects are not masked by a normal gene of the homologous chromosome. A similar recessive mutant gene in the X chromosome of a female may be kept in check, however, by a normal gene in the other X chromosome. In this manner certain hereditary pathologic traits may appear in the males of a family without becoming manifest in the females. Hemophilia A, Christmas disease, color blindness, Hunter type of gargoylism, progressive muscular dystrophy (Duchenne type), peroneal atrophy, night blindness with myopia, and the anhidrotic type of ectodermal dysplasia are such sex-linked traits (see McKusick for a more complete list).

Figure 6-11 illustrates the transmission of a recessive pathologic gene located in an X chromosome (n_X). There is no corresponding gene in the Y chromosome (O_Y). The affected father's pair of genes is represented by the formula $(n_X \ O_Y)$. If the mother has 2 normal dominant genes in her X chromosomes $(N_X \ N_X)$, the following results are to be expected: The sons $(N_X \ O_Y)$ are all normal, having received their normal X chromosome from their mother. All the daughters $(N_X \ n_X)$ appear normal, but carry a recessive pathologic gene (n_X) in one of their X chromosomes. If such a carrier-daughter marries a normal man $(N_X \ O_Y)$, half of her sons $(n_X \ O_Y)$ will show the abnormal trait of the maternal grandfather, and half will be genetically normal $(N_X \ O_Y)$. Half of the daughters will be genetically normal $(N_X \ N_X)$, and half $(N_X \ n_X)$ will carry the pathologic trait in one X chromosome (Fig. 6-12).

Figure 6-13 shows the sex-linked recessive inheritance of progressive muscular dystrophy in a sibship. This type of pathologic trait appears chiefly in males, but in rare cases females will also have it. If an affected man $(n_X \ O_Y)$ marries a carrier $(N_X \ n_X)$, half their daughters $(n_X \ n_X)$ will have the disease and half will be carriers $(N_X \ n_X)$; half their sons will be affected $(n_X \ O_Y)$, and half will be genetically normal $(N_X \ O_Y)$ (Fig. 6-14).

PATHOLOGIC TRAITS WHICH DEPEND ON MULTIPLE GENETIC FACTORS

The hereditary traits discussed so far are attributable to one gene or one pair of genes. Hereditary characters, however, may depend on the combined action of several genes. If these genes are located in different chromosomes, they associate and dissociate in different matings according to the laws of chance. Obviously, the greater the number of independent genes involved in determining a given trait, the more complicated the pattern of inheritance will be, and the less it will resemble the mendelian patterns described above. Furthermore, such a group of genes may determine only a predisposition, which may or may not produce a clinical disease or defect, depending on the environment in which the individual develops. There is evidence that a number of familial conditions that do not conform to the mendelian patterns of inheritance, such as cleft lip and cleft palate, congenital hypertrophic pyloric stenosis

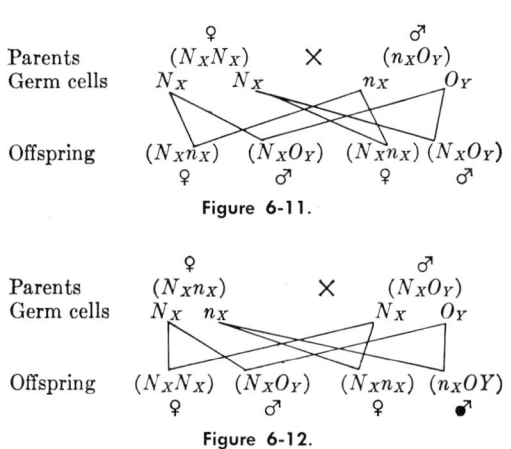

Figure 6-11.

Figure 6-12.

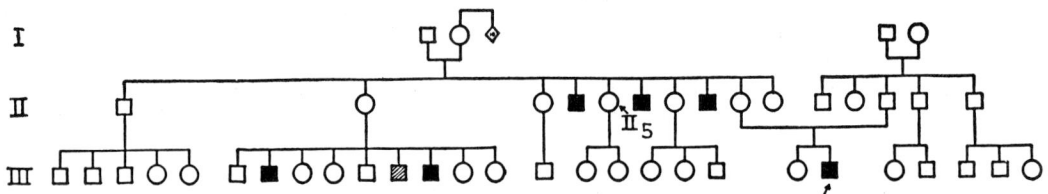

Figure 6-13. Pedigree in which progressive pseudohypertrophic muscular dystrophy was transmitted as a sex-linked recessive trait. The pedigree was drawn according to the report of the mother of the propositus (↗), a 5-year-old patient in the Children's Hospital, Cincinnati, Ohio.

The maternal grandmother of the patient was obviously a carrier of the abnormal trait, which was transmitted to 3 of her sons. A fourth son, who did not inherit the disorder, had 5 normal children. Of 5 daughters (generation II), 2 transmitted the muscular disorder to a part of their sons. Since this pedigree was drawn the daughter marked II₅ had 2 sons; both have progressive muscular dystrophy.

■ Patients with progressive muscular dystrophy.

▧ Patient with a mild case of muscular dystrophy who recovered, according to the reporter.

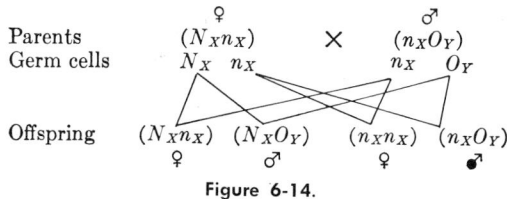

Figure 6-14.

and congenital dislocation of the hip, may fall into this category.

LETHAL TRAITS

A gene or a combination of genes may lead to developmental defects incompatible with life. Severe defects cause intrauterine death; the responsible genes are called "lethal genes." Milder defects may cause death soon after birth; responsible genes are termed "sublethal."

Lethal genes may produce only slight effects, or none at all, in a heterozygous person, but may cause death in the homozygote. For example, a dominant gene is known which, in heterozygous subjects, leads to brachyphalangia, a shortening of the second phalanx of the second fingers and toes. Such a defect is of no practical importance to the affected person. If, however, 2 heterozygous persons with this defect marry, one fourth of their offspring may be homozygous. Such a homozygous person may have no fingers and toes and may have other defects incompatible with postnatal life.

Congenital ichthyosis is an example of a disorder which appears in children homozygous for a recessive sublethal gene. The parents of such children appear normal, but carry the abnormal gene, and some of their offspring have hyperkeratosis incompatible with life.

JOSEF WARKANY
F. CLARKE FRASER

REFERENCES

Ballantyne, J. W.: *Manual of Antenatal Pathology and Hygiene. The Embryo.* Edinburgh, W. Green and Sons, Ltd., 1904.

Corner, G. W.: *Ourselves Unborn.* New Haven, Yale University Press, 1945.

Goldstein, L., and Murphy, D. P.: Etiology of Ill Health in Children Born After Maternal Pelvic Irradiation; Defective Children Born After Postconception Pelvic Irradiation. *Am. J. Roentgenol.*, 22:322, 1929.

Gregg, N. M.: Congenital Cataract Following German Measles in the Mother. *Tr. Ophth. Soc. Australia*, 3:35, 1942.

Hale, F.: Relation of Vitamin A to Anophthalmos in Pigs. *Am. J. Ophth.*, 18:1087, 1935.

Hartman, P. E., and Suskind, S. R.: *Gene Action.* Englewood Cliffs, N. J., Prentice-Hall, Inc., 1964.

Mall, F. P.: Pathology of the Human Ovum; in F. K. J. Keibel and F. P. Mall: *Manual of Human Embryology.* Philadelphia, J. B. Lippincott Company, 1910.

McKusick, V.: *Mendelian Inheritance in Man.* Baltimore, Johns Hopkins Press, 1966.

Potter, E. L., and Adair, F. L.: *Fetal and Neonatal Death.* Chicago, University of Chicago Press, 1940.

Taussig, H. B.: A Study of the German Outbreak of Phocomelia. The Thalidomide Syndrome. *J.A.M.A.*, 180:1106, 1962.

Thompson, J. S., and Thompson, M. W.: *Genetics in Medicine.* Philadelphia, W. B. Saunders Company, 1965.

Weller, T. H., and Hanshaw, J. B.: Virologic and Clinical Observations on Cytomegalic Inclusion Disease. *New England J. Med.*, 266:1233, 1962.

CHROMOSOMAL ABNORMALITIES IN MAN: THE AUTOSOMES
(ABNORMALITIES OF SEX CHROMOSOMES, PP. 1227-1235)

The remarkable demonstration by Tjio and Levan in 1956 of the normal chromosome number and morphology in human fetal lung tissue marked the beginning of a new era in human genetics. Techniques were quickly developed for chromosomal analysis of peripheral blood lymphocytes, bone marrow cells, and fibroblasts and applied to the study of persons with congenital malformations and disorders of sexual differentiation. These studies led to the association of specific chromosomal abnormalities with clinical syndromes. About one of 150 newborn infants has a gross chromosomal alteration; identification of these patients is important for prognosis and genetic counseling.

THE HUMAN KARYOTYPE

Methods. The cell most commonly used for study of the *mitotic* chromosomes is the small lymphocyte of peripheral blood; bone marrow and fibroblast tissue cultures also may be studied. The lymphocytes are grown in a nutrient medium; at 72 to 96 hours, colchicine is added to stop cell division in metaphase. The cells are swollen by application of a hypotonic solution which separates the chromosomes from each other; they are then placed on a glass slide and stained. The chromosomes from well spread metaphases are photographed, cut out, and arranged into 7 groups according to the length of the chromosome and position of the centromere. This systematized arrangement of chromosomes from a single cell is called a karyotype (Fig. 6-15, Table 6-1). Types of metaphase chromosomes are shown in Figure 6-16. Morphologic identification can usually be made for chromosomes no. 1, 2, 3, 16, 17, 18, and the Y chromosome. Other features of the normal karyotype may include satellites on the acrocentric chromosomes of groups D and G, as well as variation in the length of their short arms and differences in the length of the Y chromosome.

Autoradiography may be useful in identification of some chromosome pairs. During replication each

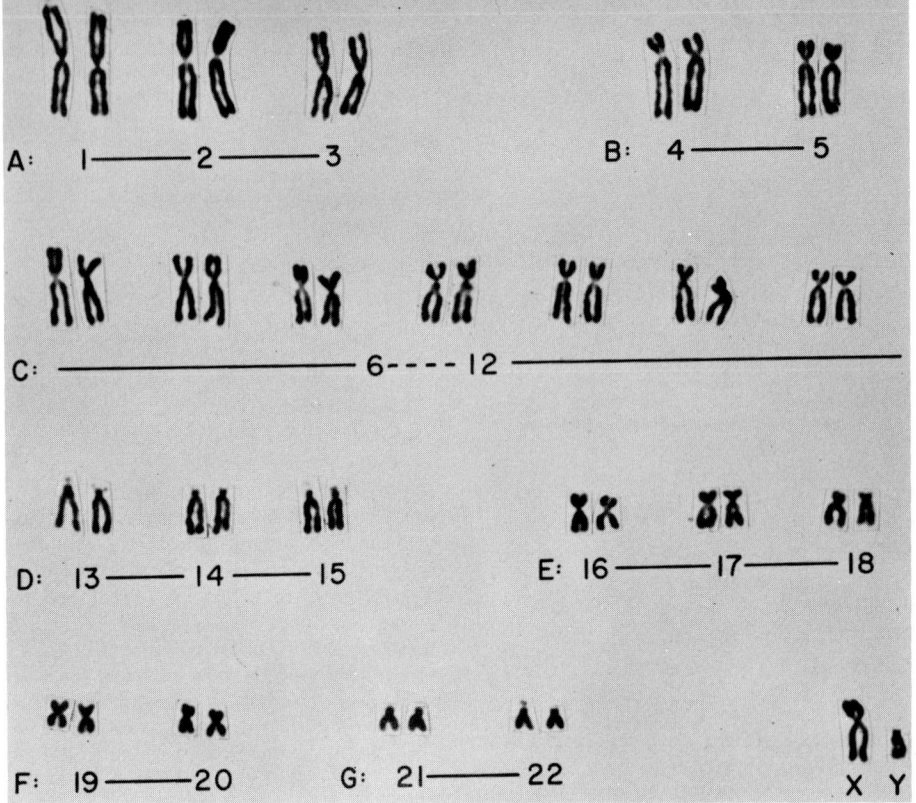

Figure 6-15. Normal male karyotype.

chromosome pair is synthesizing new deoxyribonucleic acid (DNA) at a different time in the mitotic cycle. These differences will be reflected in the amount of radioactive thymidine that is incorporated into newly synthesized DNA; the amount incorporated is demonstrated by autoradiography. With this technique, chromosomes no. 4, 5, 13, 14, 15 and one X chromosome in the female may be identified. The technique is difficult, and presently is not available for routine use. Chromosomes no. 6-12, 19, 20, 21, 22, the X in the male and one X in the female cannot be distinguished morphologically or by autoradiography.

Techniques are now being developed for the

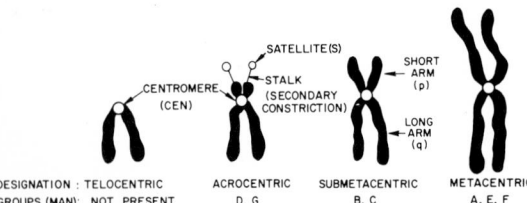

Figure 6-16. Types of metaphase chromosomes. Designations are based on position of the centromere. The stalk and satellites on acrocentric chromosomes are not always visible. No normal chromosome in man is telocentric. The Y chromosome in man is acrocentric, but does not have satellites on the short arms. The X chromosome is submetacentric. The notations are according to the Chicago Conference (1966).

identification of chromosomes in fetal cells obtained by amniotic puncture. The results will be useful in instances in which induced abortion is being considered because of a high risk of a chromosomal abnormality in the fetus.

Visualization of the chromosomes during *meiosis* is limited to investigations of spermatogenesis. Satisfactory techniques for such study are still being developed and when available will provide information on both normal and abnormal rearrangements of chromosomes in the sperm. Clinically, this information should prove to be of value for genetic counseling.

Nomenclature. The current nomenclature for designation of the karyotype is that proposed at the Chicago Conference; Table 6-2 gives the designations for representative karyotypes.

The normal or *diploid* number of chromosomes in man is 46 (2n), and the *haploid* set present in the gametes is 23 (n). The *modal count* is that chromosome number with the greatest frequency of occurrence when cells from the same culture are counted; other counts are termed nonmodal. Numerical abnormalities include *polyploidy*, the presence of additional sets of chromosomes, e.g. 69 (3n) or 92 (4n); *aneuploidy*, the presence or absence of an additional chromosome(s), e.g. trisomy, $2n + 1 = 47$; monosomy, $2n - 1 = 45$; and *mosaicism*, the presence of two or more cell lines with different modal counts or morphology (Table 6-2).

TABLE 6-1. ARRANGEMENT OF HUMAN MITOTIC CHROMOSOMES

Group 1-3 (A)	Large chromosomes with approximately median centromeres (metacentric chromosomes). The 3 chromosomes are readily distinguished from each other by size and centromere position. In some cells a secondary constriction is observed in the proximal region of the long arm of no. 1
Group 4-5 (B)	Large chromosomes with submedian centromeres (submetacentric chromosomes). The 2 chromosomes are difficult to distinguish, but chromosome 4 is slightly longer
Group 6-12 and X (C)	Medium-sized chromosomes with submedian centromeres. The X chromosome resembles the longer chromosomes in this group, especially chromosome 6, from which it is difficult to distinguish. This group is the one which presents most difficulty in identification of individual chromosomes
	Four of the C group autosomes are comparatively metacentric. They are usually numbered 6, 7, 8 and 11. The X chromosome belongs to this subgroup
	Three chromosomes are submetacentric and are usually numbered 9, 10 and 12. A secondary constriction is found in the proximal part of the long arm of at least one of the pairs, and this is usually designated as no. 9. In normal female cells one chromosome characteristically incorporates isotopically labeled thymidine over most of its length later than the others in the group. This chromosome is believed to be an X
Group 13-15 (D)	Medium-sized chromosomes with nearly terminal centromeres (acrocentric chromosomes). All 3 pairs have satellites which are variably detectable
Group 16-18 (E)	Rather short chromosomes with an approximately median centromere in chromosome 16 and submedian centromeres in 17 and 18. A secondary constriction has been frequently seen in the proximal part of the long arm of no. 16
Group 19-20 (F)	Short chromosomes with approximately median centromeres
Group 21-22 and Y (G)	Very short, acrocentric chromosomes. Satellites are variably present on 21 and 22. The Y chromosome is similar, but tends to have somewhat more parallel long arms which vary in size from individual to individual. It is usually larger than 21 or 22

Adapted from Chicago Conference: Standardization in Human Cytogenetics. Birth Defects: Original Article Series, II:2, 1966. The National Foundation, New York.

TABLE 6-2. KARYOTYPE NOTATION, CHICAGO CONFERENCE (1966)

PHENOTYPE	DESIGNATION
Normal male	46,XY
Normal female	46,XX
Klinefelter's syndrome	47,XXY
Turner's syndrome	45,X
Down's syndrome (trisomy 21, mongolism), male	47,XY,21+
Down's syndrome (D/G translocation), male	46,XY,D−,t(Dq21q)+
Down's syndrome (mosaic), male	46,XY/47,XY,21+
Trisomy 18 (trisomy E), male	47,XY,18+
Trisomy 13 (trisomy D_1), male	47,XY,13+
Cat-cry syndrome, male	46,XY,Bp− (or 5p−)
No. 18 deletion (long arm), male	46,XY,18q−
No. 18 deletion (short arm), male	46,XY,18p−

X, Y = sex chromosomes.

As suggested at the Chicago Conference, the total number of chromosomes is given first, e.g. 45, 46, 47, etc., followed by the sex chromosome complement, e.g. X, XX, XY, XXY, etc. The autosomal abnormality is then specified; a numerical alteration is indicated by a + or − after the number of the trisomic or monosomic chromosome, respectively. The short arm of the chromosome is designated "p," the long arm "q." A + or − indicates an increase or decrease, respectively, in length of the arm. For example, a deletion of the short arm is indicated as "p−," and of the long arm "q−." A translocation is indicated by "t" followed by the chromosomes involved in the translocation, and listed in alphabetical or numerical sequence. (See also Figure 6-19.)

NUMERICAL ABNORMALITIES

Trisomy, the presence of a third homologue to a pair of chromosomes (2n + 1), is the most commonly observed aneuploid state in man. This alteration may arise from *nondisjunction* (Fig. 6-17) or from *anaphase lag* (Fig. 6-18) at either meiotic or mitotic cell division. Three syndromes associated with autosomal trisomy have been documented: Down's syndrome (trisomy 21), trisomy 18 and trisomy 13 (D_1 trisomy). Rarely, patients with trisomy of other chromosome pairs have been reported; however, associations with specific clinical syndromes have not been established. The failure to identify a trisomic syndrome in live births for the other autosomes may reflect the lethality of trisomy in the gamete, zygote or embryo; e.g. there is a high frequency of chromosomal abnormalities in spontaneous abortuses (see this section). *Monosomy,* the absence of one of a pair of chromosomes (2n − 1), is consistently found in Turner's syndrome (45, X). Complete loss of an autosome in all cells is almost always lethal, and even the loss of a small portion of an autosome (deletion) may be associated with severe malformations.

Mosaicism has been observed for each of the autosomal trisomy syndromes and for several of the X chromosome syndromes. As shown in Figure 6-18, it may result from abnormal chromosome distribution at mitotic division. Cell lines with differing modal numbers are produced, e.g. in

MEIOTIC DISJUNCTION - NON DISJUNCTION

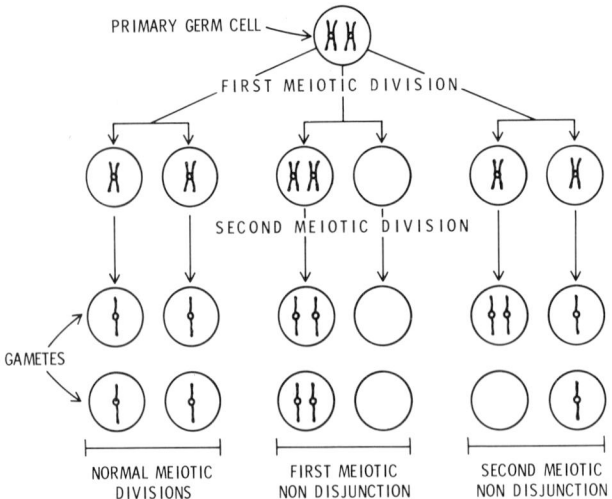

Figure 6-17. Diagram of the 2 meiotic stages in man shown for 1 pair of homologous chromosomes. In the primary germ cell, replication, condensation and pairing of the chromosomes have already occurred. At the left is shown the normal sequence of events in which each gamete contains the haploid number (23). Nondisjunction occurring at the first or second stages of meiosis is shown in the center and right-hand diagrams, respectively. These gametes may have an extra chromosome (23 + 1) or are deficient in one chromosome (23 − 1). Fertilization by a normal gamete will produce a trisomic or monosomic zygote, respectively.

Down's syndrome mosaic (46,XX/47,XX,21+), or with differing structural changes. Mosaicism can arise at the first cleavage division in the zygote or at any subsequent cell division; it can involve multiple tissues or be localized to a single tissue; hence its demonstration may depend on sampling of different tissues, e.g. peripheral blood and skin.

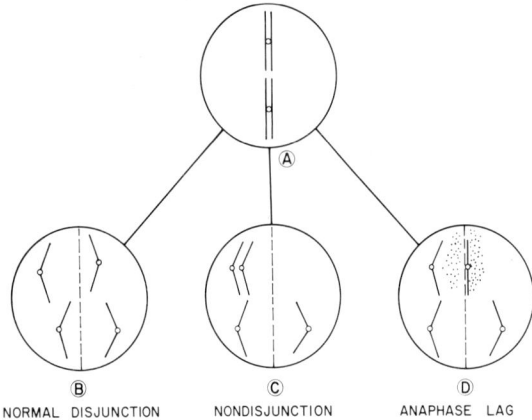

NORMAL DISJUNCTION   NONDISJUNCTION   ANAPHASE LAG

Figure 6-18. Diagram showing normal *mitotic* disjunction, nondisjunction and anaphase lag. *A,* Two homologous chromosomes which have already replicated themselves are shown in metaphase. *B,* The centromeres have divided, and normal separation of chromosomes occurs, producing 2 cells each of which is genetically identical. *C,* One of the pairs has failed to separate (or disjoin) during anaphase, giving rise to one trisomic and one monosomic cell. *D,* Anaphase lag of one chromosome with failure of inclusion in either of the daughter cells. Note that the events shown in *C* and *D* could produce a mosaic chromosome pattern, since the other cells are dividing normally.

STRUCTURAL ALTERATIONS

The most commonly observed structural abnormality of the autosomes is a *translocation;* it involves breakage and exchange of genetic material between 2 chromosomes. Most translocations involve the acrocentric chromosomes in the D and G groups, e.g. D/D, D/G and G/G, but they have also been described involving chromosomes of all groups. The sequence of events which follows a translocation between a D and a no. 21 chromosome is shown in Figure 6-19. Note that the person with the genotype "translocation Down's syndrome" is trisomic for the genetic material of the long arm of the no. 21 chromosome, although the total number of chromosomes is normal.

Deletions of chromosomal material producing a *partial monosomy* result from breakage and loss of a segment of genetic material. Autosomal deletions have been found in association with the cri du chat (cat-cry) syndrome due to partial deletion of a no. 5 chromosome (Bp-, or 5p-), and in syndromes associated with loss of a portion of the long arm or short arm of a no. 18 (18q-, or 18p-, respectively). If both ends of a chromosome are lost, the broken ends may fuse to form a *ring* (r) *chromosome.*

Isochromosomes (i) result from horizontal rather than longitudinal division of the centromere (Fig. 6-20). They have been demonstrated only in X chromosome abnormalities.

More complex structural abnormalities undoubtedly occur, but are often difficult to demonstrate. These include partial trisomies (additions), pericentric inversions, and insertions.

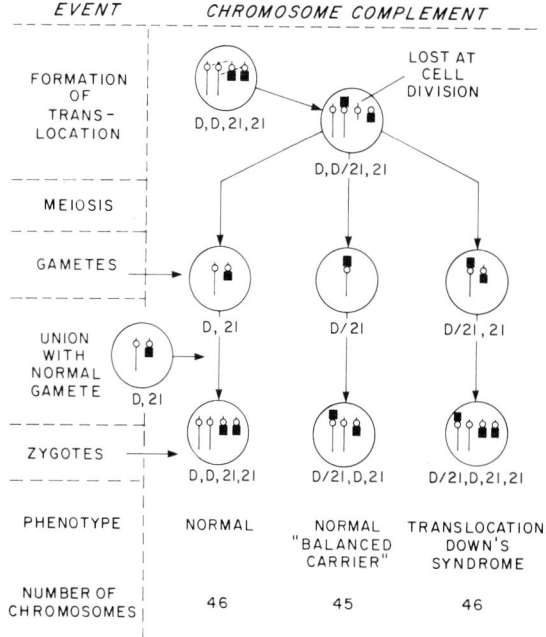

EVENT   CHROMOSOME COMPLEMENT

FORMATION OF TRANS-LOCATION

D,D,21,21

LOST AT CELL DIVISION

D,D/21,21

MEIOSIS

GAMETES

D, 21   D/21   D/21,21

UNION WITH NORMAL GAMETE

D,21

ZYGOTES

D,D,21,21   D/21,D,21   D/21,D,21,21

PHENOTYPE   NORMAL   NORMAL "BALANCED CARRIER"   TRANSLOCATION DOWN'S SYNDROME

NUMBER OF CHROMOSOMES   46   45   46

Figure 6-19. Sequence of events and observed phenotypes in D/21 translocation Down's syndrome. The diagram shows one possible mechanism for production of a translocation between a D and a no. 21 chromosome. The cause of the 2 chromosome breaks (upper left) is not known. Only 3 types of gametes are shown in the diagram to be produced at "meiosis." Three zygotes are produced from fertilization by the "normal gamete," and their chromosome complements are shown. Other complements are possible, but have not been observed; possibly this is because a large loss or addition of genetic material occurs and is lethal to the zygote.

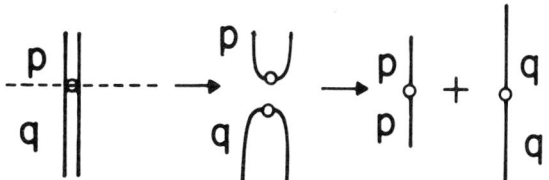

Figure 6-20. Formation of isochromosome by misdivision of the centromere. "p" is short arm, "q" long arm. Note that if a gamete containing only the long arms is fertilized by a normal gamete, the zygote will be trisomic for the long arms, and monosomic for the short arms.

DERMATOGLYPHIC PATTERNS

Characteristic changes in the dermatoglyphic patterns occur in the 3 autosomal trisomy syndromes (see below); less specific changes are found in the other chromosomal syndromes. Identification of these changes may be useful as a screening measure for chromosomal alterations; the presence of normal patterns, however, does not exclude a chromosomal abnormality. Dermal patterns are fully determined by the fourth fetal month and do not change thereafter. Hereditary factors, probably polygenic, play a large role in their deter-

mination. The description of the patterns is based on the following 4 features:

Fingers. Three basic patterns are found: loops, whorls and arches (Fig. 6-21). The number of triradii formed by the junction of 3 sets of parallel ridges determines the type of pattern. An arch is *simple* if it has no triradius and *tented* if there is a centrally placed triradius. A loop has one triradius, laterally placed, and a whorl has 2 triradii. A loop may open to the radial or ulnar side of the hand. Ridge counts represent the number of dermal ridges lying between a triradius and the center of the pattern. There is no count for an arch pattern. The total ridge count is the sum of counts on the 10 fingers and averages 145 in males and 127 in females.

Palms. The main topographic areas are shown in Figure 6-22. These include the interdigital areas, determined by the triradii at the distal end of each metacarpal, and the hypothenar and thenar areas. The normal main axial triradius, usually designated *t*, is proximal on the palm and just distal to the most distal wrist crease.

The position of the *t* triradius determines the *atd* angle, i.e. the angle formed by lines from the *t* triradius to the first (*a*) and fourth (*d*) digital triradii. Normally the angle is less than 58 degrees. The terms *t'*, *t"* refer to axial triradii that are displaced more distally than *t*. Their *atd* angles are about 66 and 81 degrees, respectively, and they frequently are associated with hypothenar patterns. The *t* triradius also may be specified by its position on a line drawn from the crease at the base of the middle finger to the first flexion crease on the wrist. The *t* triradius is within the proximal 35 per cent of this line.

Soles. The topographic areas are similar to those of the palms. Usually only the hallucal area is studied. Whorls or large distal loops are seen commonly in normal persons.

Flexion creases. These represent attachment of the skin to the underlying structures. Normal findings are shown in Figure 6-22.

The patterns can be seen by direct observation, with a magnifying lens or with an otoscope lens. Direct prints can be made for permanent records. This is difficult in newborns and young infants because of indistinct patterns.

Dermatoglyphic patterns of patients with *Down's syndrome* reveal a high frequency of the following: ulnar loops on the fingers, a high or distal axial triradius, designated *t"*, a loop in the third interdigital area, hypothenar patterns, a single palmar crease, and a single crease on the fifth finger. These characteristics are shown in Figure 6-23. They are one part of the clinical pattern of Down's syndrome; their presence or absence alone does not establish or preclude the diagnosis. Over 90 per cent of patients with *trisomy 18* have arch patterns on at least 6 fingers (Fig. 6-21): this number of arch patterns is found in only 2 per cent of the normal population. In conjunction with the other clinical signs it supports the diagnosis of trisomy 18. In *trisomy 13*

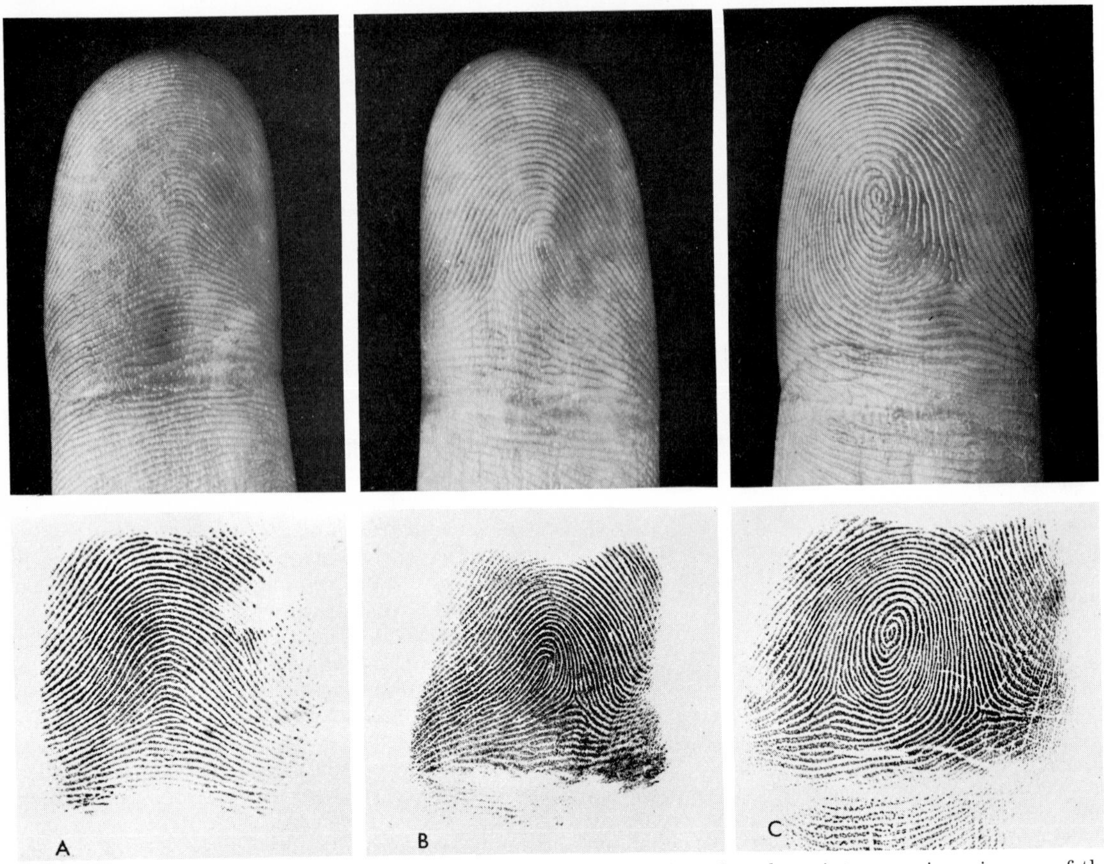

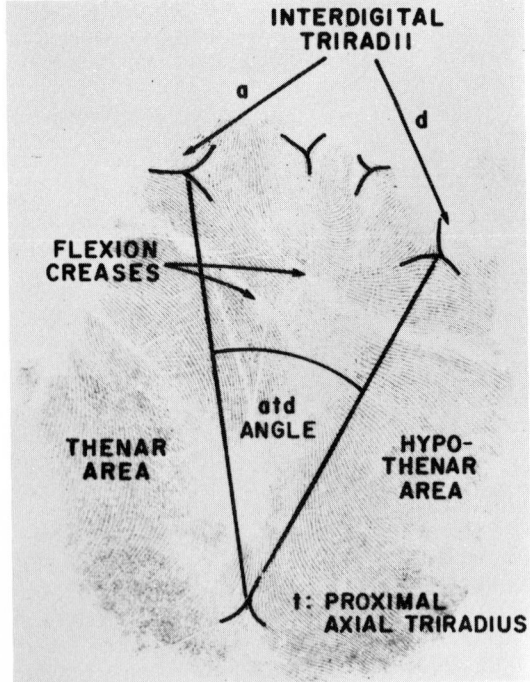

Figure 6-21. Examples of 3 basic types of fingerprint patterns. Note that the prints are mirror images of the dermal ridge patterns of the fingers. *A*, Simple arch (no triradius). *B*, Loop (one triradius, on the right where 3 ridges meet). *C*, Whorl (2 triradii). (From J. R. Miller & J. Giroux; *J. Pediat.*, 69:302, 1966.)

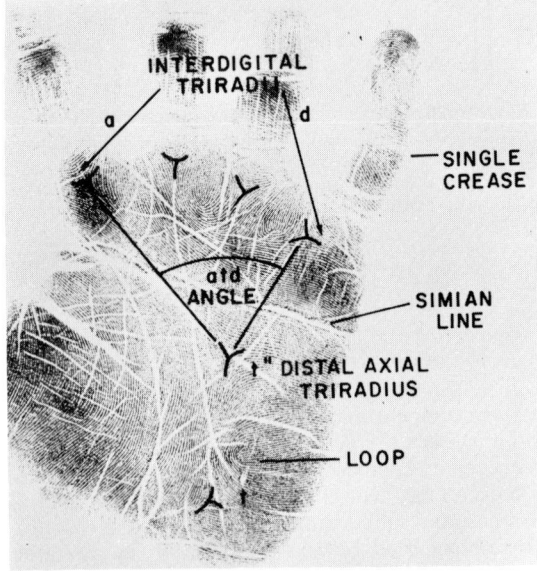

Figure 6-22. Normal palm print showing principal areas.

Figure 6-23. Palm print of child with Down's syndrome, showing typical dermatoglyphic features.

the axial triradius is distal, as in Down's syndrome, and single palmar creases may be present.

Pattern variations have been described in other chromosome and nonchromosome disorders. These patterns show less specificity; they include the Smith-Lemli-Opitz syndrome, broad thumb and great toe syndrome, Turner's syndrome, Klinefelter's syndrome, rubella syndrome and cri du chat syndrome. Distorted patterns are often found in patients with malformations of the extremities, e.g. polydactyly, syndactyly and ectrodactyly.

CONGENITAL SYNDROMES

Down's Syndrome (Mongolism, Trisomy 21). For clinical description of Down's syndrome, see p. 331.

The majority of children with Down's syndrome have 47 chromosomes and are trisomic for a G-group chromosome; arbitrarily this is designated the no. 21 chromosome. The additional no. 21 chromosome is presumed to be the result of nondisjunction during the meiotic process in a parental, usually the maternal, gamete (Fig. 6-17). Theories about the causes of chromosomal nondisjunction in Down's syndrome center about the effects on the ovum of aging, radiation, viruses and thyroid disorders. A "clustering" of births of infants with Down's syndrome has been observed in relation to epidemics of infectious hepatitis and of rubella; these associations have not been confirmed by other investigators. Although viruses are known to cause chromosomal breakage, there is no evidence that they will produce an aneuploid state in vivo. Young mothers of infants with Down's syndrome are reported to have an increased frequency and higher titer of antibodies against thyroglobulin in their serums than do control mothers with normal offspring. The significance of these findings in relation to aneuploidy is not known.

A smaller group of patients with Down's syndrome have 46 chromosomes and carry a chromosomal translocation, as shown in Figure 6-19. No clinical differences have been found between affected persons with regular trisomy or trisomy due to a translocation.

Translocations in Down's syndrome are mainly of 2 types: (1) those of the D and G groups, designated as a D/21 translocation; and (2) those of the G group, designated as G/21 translocation. The term "G/21" identifies a 21/21 or 21/22 translocation; these may be differentiated only through family studies.

Translocations are classified further into (1) inherited, i.e. the translocation can be identified in a phenotypically normal parent; this is the "balanced translocation" or "balanced normal" person as shown in Figure 6-19; and (2) sporadic, or de novo, i.e. the parents have normal karyotypes and it is assumed that the translocation occurred in one parental gamete and represents a new mutational event. It is important for genetic counseling that the translocation be identified as inherited or sporadic; inherited translocations carry an increased risk for recurrence; sporadic translocations have a low recurrence rate.

The frequencies of trisomy and of inherited and sporadic translocations in patients with Down's syndrome are given in Table 6-3; the data are correlated with maternal age at birth of the affected child. The frequencies and proportions of

TABLE 6-3. RESULTS OF CHROMOSOMAL STUDIES ON 1382 PATIENTS WITH DOWN'S SYNDROME (SUMMARY FROM 20 PUBLICATIONS)

MATERNAL AGE (YEARS)	NO. OF PATIENTS	TRISOMY 21 AND MOSAICS (%)	TRANSLOCATIONS (%)
< 30	722	91.1	8.9
> 30	660	97.9	2.1

From S. W. Wright et al.: *J. Pediat.,* 70:420, 1967.

TABLE 6-4. FREQUENCIES AND PROPORTIONS OF INHERITED AND SPORADIC TRANSLOCATIONS IN DOWN'S SYNDROME

	D/G21 TRANSLOCATION		G/G21 TRANSLOCATION	
	SPORADIC	INHERITED	SPORADIC	INHERITED
Maternal age < 30				
Number	16 (59%)	11 (41%)	23 (92%)	2 (8%)
	Sporadic translocations = 39/52 = 75 per cent			
	Inherited translocations = 13/52 = 25 per cent			
Maternal age > 30				
Number	5 (71%)	2 (29%)	6 (100%)	0 (0%)
	Sporadic translocations = 11/13 = 84.6 per cent			
	Inherited translocations = 2/13 = 15.4 per cent			

From S. W. Wright et al.: *J. Pediat.,* 70:420, 1967.

TABLE 6-5. RECURRENCE RISK FIGURES IN DOWN'S SYNDROME

	MATERNAL AGE						
	15-19	20-24	25-29	30-34	35-39	40-44	45-49
General population risk for Down's syndrome (live births)*	1/1850	1/1600	1/1350	1/800	1/260	1/100	1/50
Observed recurrence risk if chromosome studies not done on affected child**	30-50× increased over general population risk		5× increased			As above	
Recurrence risks: if chromosome studies on affected child reveal:							
1. Trisomy	Recurrence risk low: probably only slightly greater than general population risk (see above, 1st row)						
2. Translocation: inherited	Observed risk will depend on type of translocation and sex of parental carrier (see Table 6-6)						
3. Translocation: not inherited	Recurrence risk not known, but estimated as less than 1-2%						

*Adapted from C. O. Carter and K. A. Evans: *Lancet,* 2:785, 1961.

**Ibid. Risk is based on maternal age at birth of first affected (index) patient rather than maternal age at succeeding pregnancy.

inherited versus sporadic translocations are shown in Table 6-4. If the affected patient was born at a maternal age of less than 30 years, the *chance* of finding a translocation on chromosome analysis is about 9 per cent. About one fourth of these are inherited from a carrier parent (Table 6-4). Thus the overall probability for an inherited translocation is about 2 per cent (0.09×0.25), or one in 50. Among infants born to mothers 30 years or older, an inherited translocation would be found in about one in 333 affected infants. These estimations do not apply if there is a history of familial Down's syndrome, when chromosomal analysis is necessary before adequate counseling can be given.

In families with 2 affected sibs, about three quarters of the sib groups will have regular trisomy, and the remainder will have inherited translocations or mosaicism. The explanation for recurrence of an affected child with regular trisomy is not known; in some families it may represent a random risk; in others unknown genetic or environmental factors may be operating to cause repeated nondisjunction.

Recurrence risks as determined by chromosomal analysis are summarized in Table 6-5. If the patient has regular trisomy, the risk for recurrence is slightly higher than the risk in the general population. If the patient has a sporadic translocation and the parents have normal karyotypes, the risk of recurrence is probably low. If the translocation is inherited from one parent, the observed recurrence risk varies, depending on the type of translocation and the sex of the parent carrying it; these risks are summarized in Table 6-6. The differences in observed types of offspring produced by maternal and paternal "balanced" carriers are unexplained.

Mosaicism has been reported in 2 to 3 per cent of patients with Down's syndrome. There is some suggestion that there are fewer stigmata and a milder degree of impairment of intelligence in patients with mosaicism. Recurrence risks in mosaicism probably are small; data are insufficient to warrant definite conclusions.

For estimation of recurrence risks it is advisable to identify the karyotypes of children with Down's syndrome. If the child has regular trisomy, i.e. 47 chromosomes, and the parents are phenotypically normal, it may be presumed that the parental karyotypes are normal. If the child has a translocation, the parental karyotypes must be determined before counseling can be given.

Trisomy 18 Syndrome (E Trisomy). Clinical and pathologic features in this syndrome are summarized in Table 6-7 and Figure 6-24. The clinical picture is characteristic and is recognizable

TABLE 6-6. OBSERVED RISKS FOR OFFSPRING OF PHENOTYPICALLY NORMAL PARENTS WITH BALANCED COMPLETE TRANSLOCATIONS

		OBSERVED OFFSPRING		
TRANSLO-CATION	PARENT	NORMAL	"BALANCED" CARRIER	DOWN'S SYNDROME
D/21*	Mother	40%	40%	20%
	Father	50%	50%	< 2%
21/22**	Mother	33%	33%	33%
	Father	50%	50%	< 2%
21/21	Either	0%	0%	100%

*From T. W. Hustinx.

**From F. A. Hecht (unpublished observations).

TABLE 6-7. CLINICAL AND PATHOLOGIC FINDINGS IN TRISOMY 18 (E) SYNDROME

I. Present in 80% or more of patients:
   Polyhydramnios; female sex; small placenta; birth weight < 6 pounds; single umbilical artery; low-set, malformed ears; micrognathia and narrow palatal arch; overlapping of fingers (usually second over third), six or more digital arch patterns; death 0-6 months of age; failure to thrive; mental defect and muscular hypertonicity

II. Present in 50-80% of patients:
   Prominent occiput; short or dorsiflexed big toe; short sternum; small pelvis; limited hip abduction; cardiac murmur; inguinal or umbilical hernia

III. Present in 10-50% of patients:
   Metopic suture; cleft lip ± palate; minor external ocular anomalies; simian crease, hypoplasia of fingernails, ulnar or radial deviation of hand; "rocker-bottom" feet, equinovarus; widely spaced nipples; webbed neck

Additional lesions demonstrable at necropsy:
Ventricular or atrial defects, patent ductus; renal malformations; Meckel's diverticulum and heterotopic pancreatic tissue; diaphragmatic anomalies

Adapted from D. W. Smith: *Am. J. Obst. & Gynec.,* 90:1055, 1964; and A. I. Taylor: *Develop. Med. & Ch. Neurol.,* 9:78, 1967.

in the nursery by attention to the obstetrical history and physical examination. The frequency of the syndrome is estimated at 1:6500 live births. Recognition is important because of specificity of diagnosis and anticipation of a poor prognosis. The majority of patients die in early infancy.

Unusual clinical features have been described in trisomy 18; these include severe central nervous system malformations, e.g. myelomeningocele, cebocephaly, hydrocephalus and microcephaly, as well as ocular defects, polydactyly, cleft lip and palate, and others. These indicate the wide variety

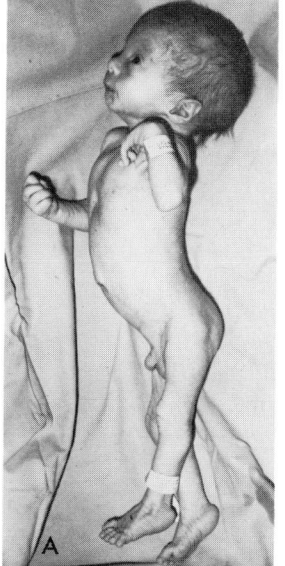

Figure 6-24. *A,* Photograph of male infant with trisomy 18, age 4 days. There are prominent occiput, micrognathia, low-set ears, short sternum, narrow pelvis, prominent calcaneus, and flexion abnormalities of the fingers. (Courtesy of Robert E. Carrel.) *B,* Several of the common anomalies in the 18 trisomy syndrome, including the unusual position of the fingers with hypoplasia of fifth fingernail; the simple arch pattern on the fingers; and the dorsiflexed hallux with hypoplasia of toenails. (From D. W. Smith: *Am. J. Obst. & Gynec.,* 90:1055, 1964.)

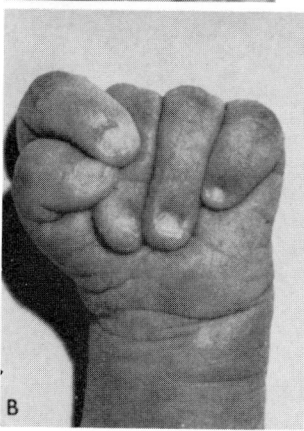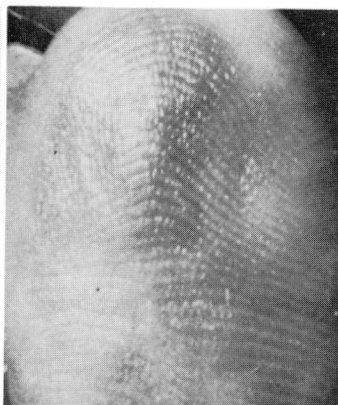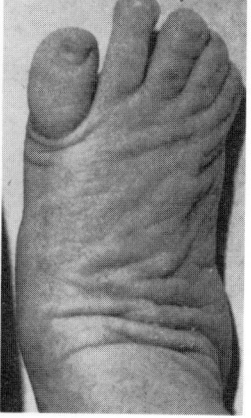

TABLE 6-8. CLINICAL AND PATHOLOGIC FINDINGS IN TRISOMY 13 (D₁) SYNDROME

I. Present in 80% or more of patients:
   Apneic spells; microcephaly; cleft lip ± palate; malformed ears; single palmar crease, distal axial triradius, fibular S-shaped hallucal arch, long hyperconvex fingernails; undescended testes

II. Present in 50-80% of patients:
   Seizures; microphthalmos, colobomata; capillary hemangiomas; polydactyly; flexion deformity of fingers; prominent calcaneus

III. Present in 10-50% of patients:
   Single umbilical artery; shallow supraorbital ridges, absent eyebrows, micrognathia, localized scalp defects; retroflexible thumb

Additional lesions demonstrable at necropsy:
Agenesis of corpus callosum, cerebellar hypoplasia; arhinencephaly, agenesis of olfactory lobes; cardiac malformations, including septal defects and anomalies of heart valves and great vessels; polycystic renal cortex, hydronephrosis; bicornuate uterus

---

Adapted from D. W. Smith: *Am. J. Obst. & Gynec.*, 90:1055, 1964; and A. I. Taylor: *Develop. Med. & Ch. Neurol.*, 9:78, 1967.

of malformations that may accompany the additional genetic material present in a trisomy syndrome.

Trisomy 13 (D₁ Trisomy). This syndrome is associated with an additional chromosome in the D group; autoradiographic studies suggest that it is a no. 13 chromosome. Clinical and pathologic features are shown in Table 6-8 and in Figure 6-25. The clinical picture is one of severe malformations centering about the facial structures and central nervous system. Incidence is estimated at 1:4600 live births. Seventy to 80 per cent of patients die within 6 months after birth.

Several interesting biochemical and hematologic changes occur in D₁ trisomy. An embryonic hemoglobin, Gower II, consisting of 2 alpha and 2 epsilon chains, is found in some patients at birth,

and an abnormal persistence of fetal hemoglobin has been described. The relation of these findings to gene loci on the chromosome has been suggested. A high proportion of polymorphonuclear leukocytes in the affected newborn infant has sessile or pedunculated nuclear projections with a "hooklike" appearance; some observers feel that these projections may have diagnostic value in trisomy 13.

A smaller number of patients with the clinical signs of trisomy 13 have been shown to have a D/13 translocation. Only rarely is this inherited from a "balanced carrier" parent. Mosaicism also has been described.

Cri du Chat (Cat-Cry) Syndrome. The cri du chat syndrome is characterized by a partial deletion of the short arm of a no. 5 chromosome (5p-);

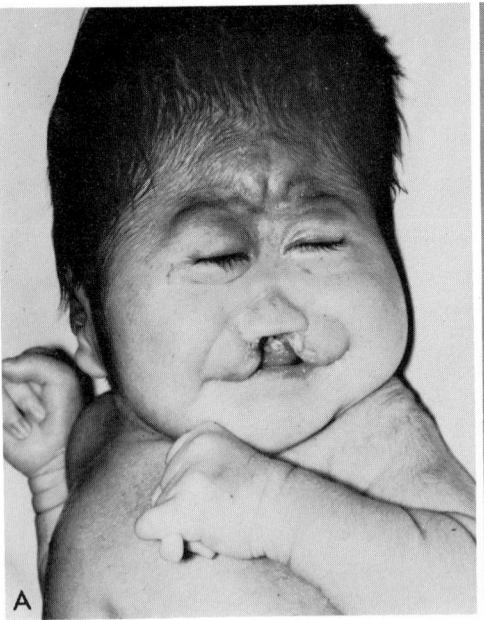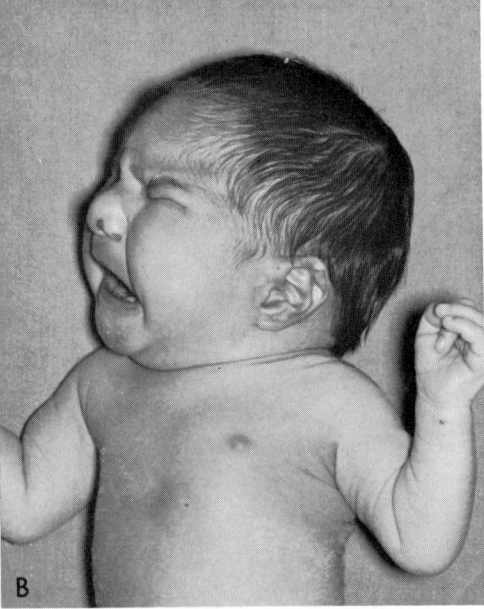

Figure 6-25. *A*, Female infant with trisomy 13 syndrome. There is a midline cleft of the lip and palate, microcephaly, hypotelorism, microphthalmus and polydactyly. *B*, Female infant with trisomy 13 syndrome. There is microcephaly, microphthalmus, bulbous nose, overlapping of fingers, and scalp defects (not shown). (Courtesy of Miriam G. Wilson.)

thus the patient is monosomic for a portion of the short arm. Although many patients have been reported, the incidence is not known; some patients may not be recognized, since the characteristic cry may disappear in early childhood.

Females are affected more frequently than males; there is no relation to maternal age; gestational age is normal; the mean birth weight is 2570 gm.; and the case fatality rate is low. Clinical findings are not as characteristic as those of the trisomic syndromes. The most frequent sign is the peculiar cry due to a small epiglottis and larynx. The cry is similar to that of a kitten and is characterized by a high-pitched, tense phonation. Other findings include small body size, moon face, microcephaly, severe mental retardation, a downward slant to the palpebral fissures, epicanthal folds, hypertelorism, divergent strabismus, abnormal ear canals, minor skeletal malformations and congenital heart disease (Fig. 6-26). As with the trisomic syndromes, patients with the cat-cry syndrome have strong facial resemblances to each other in infancy and early childhood.

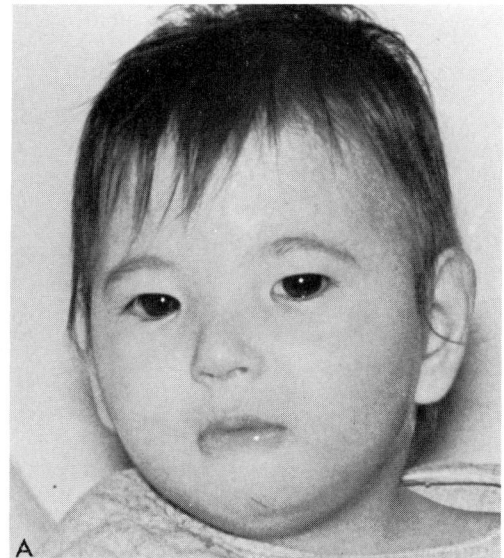

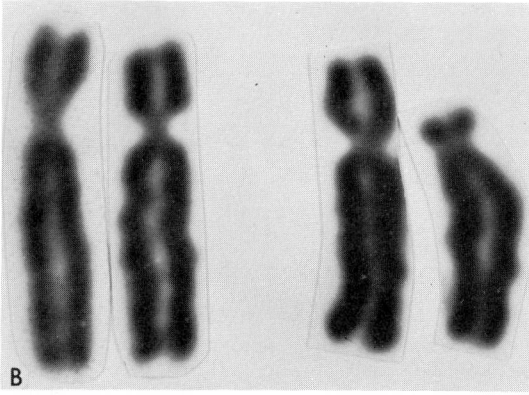

Figure 6-26. *A,* Male infant with cat-cry syndrome. (Courtesy of J. de Grouchy.) *B,* Group-B chromosomes showing partial deletion of short arm of no. 5.

In about 10 per cent of these patients the deletion is inherited from a normal "balanced carrier" parent. Thus chromosomal analysis of the parents must be carried out in order to estimate recurrence risks. If the parental karyotypes are normal, recurrence risks are probably low.

Clinical Syndrome Associated with a Deletion of the Short Arms of No. 4 (4 p-). This clinical syndrome presents several similarities with the cat-cry syndrome (5 p-), including mental retardation, oblique palpebral fissures, microcephaly, hypertelorism and strabismus. Distinguishing features include hypospadias (males), sacral dimple, seizures, underdeveloped dermal ridges, cleft palate, preauricular sinus, simple ear configuration, a beaklike nose, ptosis, and absence of a catlike cry (Fig. 6-27).

Clinical Syndrome Associated with a Deletion of the Long Arms of No. 18 (18q-). Clinical manifestations include severe mental retardation, midfacial hypoplasia, atretic or hypoplastic ear canals, prominent antihelices, absent labia minora, subacromial dimples, subcutaneous nodules at corners of the mouth, long tapering fingers, cataracts, and growth failure (Fig. 6-28).

Clinical Syndrome Associated with a Deletion of the Short Arms of No. 18 (18p-). Characteristic clinical features are lacking except that in 3 recorded patients there were severe malformations of the midface and brain, including cyclopia or cebocephaly. Mental retardation, strabismus, flattened nose, large and floppy ears, shield type of chest and cubitus valgus have been noted in some patients.

Clinical Syndrome Associated with an Extra, Acrocentric Chromosome, Which Is Slightly Smaller than a G Chromosome. In its complete form this syndrome consists of colobomata, imperforate anus, mental retardation, congenital heart disease, urinary tract malformations and preauricular fistula. The disorder is rare, and phenotypic manifestation may show considerable variation (see Schmid-Fraccaro syndrome, p. 1519).

Clinical Syndrome Associated with a Deletion of a D-Group Chromosome ("Ring D"). This syndrome is characterized by absence of the thumbs, mental retardation and other malformations. The chromosomal abnormality involves the no. 14 chromosome.

Other Congenital Malformations. A bewildering number of numerical and structural abnormalities of the autosomes has been described in association with a wide range of malformations. In most instances chromosomal analyses are normal in patients with odd facies, mental retardation, multiple anomalies and growth failure. Patients with single major malformations, e.g. congenital heart disease, rarely have a chromosomal alteration.

Spontaneous Abortions. Fifteen to 20 per cent of pregnancies terminate as spontaneous abortions; of these, about 30 per cent in the first trimester and 10 per cent in the second trimester are associated with chromosomal aneuploidy in the

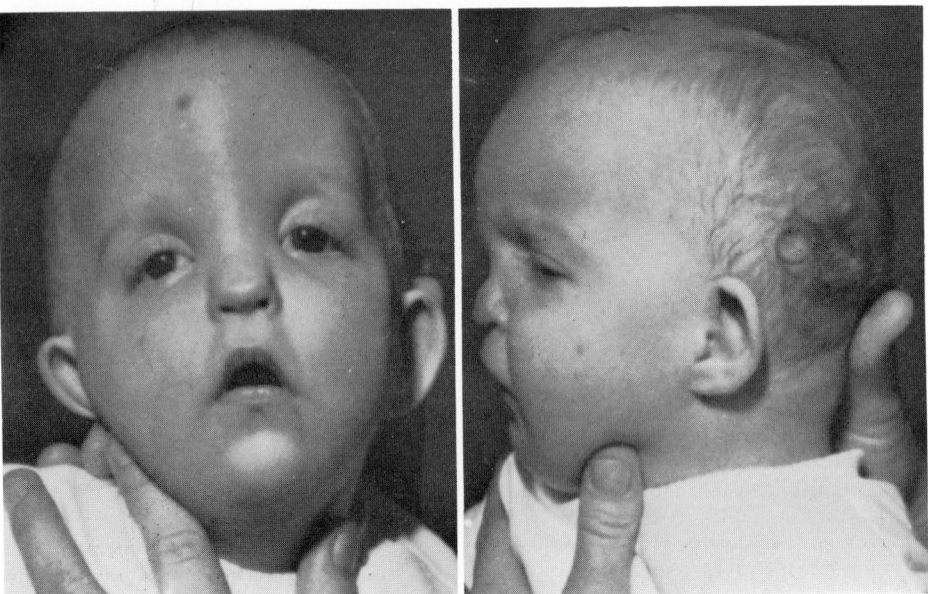

Figure 6-27. A 1-year-old male infant with deletion of the short arm of a no. 4 chromosome (4 p-). (Courtesy of W. R. Breg.)

fetal tissues or amnion. Thus about 5 per cent of conceptuses have a demonstrable chromosomal abnormality; fortunately the majority are aborted.

Most chromosomal alterations in abortuses can be divided into 3 categories: 45,X complements, autosomal trisomies, and triploidy or tetraploidy (Table 6-9). The most frequent alterations involve the autosomes and include abortuses with trisomy for groups A, B, C, D, E, F or G.

ACQUIRED CHROMOSOMAL ABNORMALITIES

An increasing number of agents, including viruses, radiation and chemicals, have been found to induce structural abnormalities of the chromosomes such as breaks, fragments, dicentrics and rings. Similar changes are found in several genetic diseases, as well as in leukemia and other malignancies. Interest in these agents and diseases centers about the relation of the chromosomal aberrations to teratogenetic and neoplastic dis-

orders. In addition, chromosomal analysis may provide a basis for evaluation of the safety of radiation and drugs.

Viral Infections. The inoculation into a tissue culture system of measles, herpes simplex, chickenpox, rubella, cytomegalic inclusion disease or certain tumor-producing viruses is followed by the appearance of chromosomal breaks. Only measles, chickenpox and possibly mumps viruses are known to be associated with chromosomal damage during or following human infections. The relation of these chromosomal changes to subsequent oncologic or morphologic events in tissues is still to be determined.

Radiation. Chromosomal breakage has been observed in the lymphocytes of persons who have received therapeutic radiation or have been exposed to nuclear accidents. The majority of these cells are eliminated after one cellular division, since they are not viable. A few cells with abnormal chromosomes may persist for some years. Though the susceptibility of the genetic materials

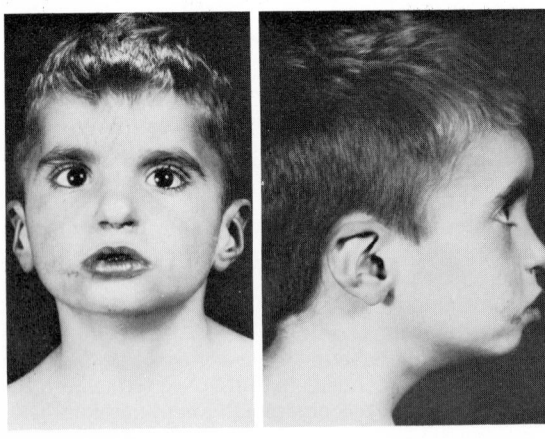

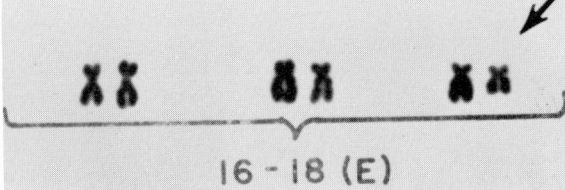

16 - 18 (E)

Figure 6-28. Patient with deletion of the long arms of a no. 18 chromosome (inset). There is midfacial dysplasia with carp-shaped mouth, prominent forehead and prominent antihelices. Narrowing of the ear canals and proximal implantation of the thumb were present. (Courtesy of Park S. Gerald and Wladimir Wertelecki.)

TABLE 6-9. Frequency of Chromosomal Abnormalities in Spontaneous Abortions and Live Births

CONDITION	FREQUENCY/1000 SPONTANEOUS ABORTIONS	FREQUENCY/1000 LIVE BIRTHS	RATIO OF VIABLE: INVIABLE FETUSES
X monosomy (XO)	40	0.4	1:100
Autosomal trisomies	80	2.0	1:40
Triploidy, tetraploidy	43	Very rare	—

From *Bulletin of World Health Organization*, 34:765, 1966.

to radiation is apparent, a causal relation between radiation, chromosomal damage and malignancy remains to be determined.

Leukemia and Other Neoplasia. Numerical and structural changes are seen frequently in the chromosomes of leukemic cells. The critical event leading to a clone of cells of different chromosomal constitution is not known; the same event which produced the chromosomal change may also have initiated the leukemic process. The chromosomal aberration is demonstrated by direct examination of blast cells in the bone marrow; it is not found in cultures of peripheral lymphocytes or of fibroblasts. A normal karyotype may be found during remissions. In acute leukemia of children the type of aneuploidy is consistent for a given patient, but varies among patients.

The only specific karyotypic change is in chronic myelogenous leukemia; in most patients there is a deletion of a portion of the long arm of a G-group chromosome (Gq-), which is designated the Philadelphia (Ph[1]) chromosome. It can be found in myeloblasts, erythroblasts and megakaryocytes at all stages of the disease; in peripheral blood it is present only in myeloblasts. The relation of the chromosomal deletion to the leukemic state is not known. Since myelogenous leukemia is rare in children, there are few reports of a Ph[1] chromosome in this age group.

Chromosomal changes are also found in the cells of some solid tumors, e.g. lymphosarcoma, Hodgkin's disease and chorioepithelioma. No chromosomal abnormality has been found to be specific for the type of malignancy.

Other Diseases. Chromosomal breakage has been described in 3 autosomal recessive disorders: in Bloom's syndrome or congenital telangiectatic erythema, in Fanconi's anemia with pancytopenia and multiple congenital malformations, and in ataxia-telangiectasia. The development of leukemia or other malignancies is common in these patients.

Drugs. A number of mutagenic chemicals, which include alkylating agents and nucleic acid analogues, as well as streptonigran, mitomycin C and chlorpromazine, may induce chromosomal abnormalities. Current interest has focused on the hallucinogen, lysergic acid diethylamide (LSD-25). Some observers have reported an increased frequency of chromosomal breaks among some users of LSD-25 as well as among some children and infants who were exposed in utero to the drug; these results have not been confirmed in other studies. Although LSD may produce congenital

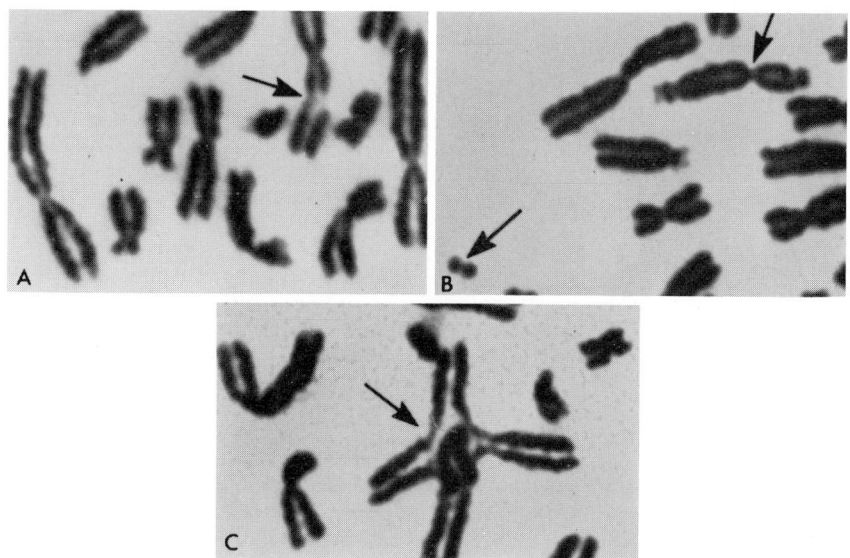

Figure 6-29. Human mitotic chromosomes with chromosome breakage. *A,* Single chromatid break, *B,* Top arrow, tricentric chromosome; other arrow, acentric chromosome fragment. *C,* Quadriradial formation. (Courtesy of R. S. Sparkes.)

malformations in some mammalian species, there is no confirmed evidence at present to indicate that it is teratogenic to the human fetus.

STANLEY W. WRIGHT

REFERENCES

Batalos, M., and Baranki, T. A.: *Medical Cytogenetics.* Baltimore; Williams & Wilkins Company, 1967. (For extensive listing of reference material.)

Carr, D. H.: Chromosome Studies in Spontaneous Abortions. *Obst. & Gynec.,* 26:308, 1965.

Cohen, M. M., Hirschhorn, K., and Frosch, W. A.: In Vivo Chromosomal Damage Induced by LSD-25. *New England J. Med.,* 277:1043, 1967.

Day, R. W.: The Epidemiology of Chromosome Aberrations. *Amer. J. Human Genet.,* 18:70, 1966.

de Grouchy, J.: Genetic Diseases, Chromosome Rearrangements and Malignancy. *Ann. Int. Med.,* 65:603, 1966.

Ferguson-Smith, M. A.: The Techniques of Human Cytogenetics. *Am. J. Obst. & Gynec.,* 90:1035, 1964.

Fialkow, P. J.: Thyroid Antibodies, Down's Syndrome and Maternal Age. *Nature,* 214:1253, 1967.

Huehns, E. R., Hecht, F., Keil, J. V., and Motulsky, A. G.: Developmental Hemoglobin Anomalies in a Chromosomal Triplication: D_1 Trisomy Syndrome. *Proc. Nat. Acad. Sc.,* 51:89, 1964.

Hustinx, T. W. J.: Cytogentisch onderzock bij enige families. Thesis Nijmegen. Drukkerij-Uitgeverij Brakkenstein, 1966.

Migeon, B. R.: Short Arm Deletions in Group E and Chromosomal "Deletion" Syndromes. *J. Pediat.,* 69:432, 1966.

Miller, J. R., and Dill, F. J.: The Cytogenetics of Mongolism. *Internat. Psychiatry Clinics,* 2:127, 1965.

Nichols, W. W.: The Role of Viruses in the Etiology of Chromosomal Abnormalities. *Am. J. Human Genet.,* 18:81, 1966.

Reisman, L. E., Mitani, M., and Zuelzer, W. W.: Chromosome Studies in Leukemia. I. Evidence for the Origin of Leukemic Stem Lines from Aneuploid Mutants. *New England J. Med.,* 270:591, 1964.

Schmickel, R.: Chromosome Aberrations in Leukocytes Exposed in Vitro to Diagnostic Levels of X-rays. *Am. J. Human Genet.,* 19:3, 1967.

Sparkes, R. S., Carrel, R. E., and Wright, S. W.: Absent Thumbs with a Ring D-2 Chromosome: A New Deletion Syndrome. *Am. J. Human Genet.,* 19:644, 1967.

Tjio, J. H., and Levan, A.: The Chromosome Number of Man. *Hereditas,* 42:1, 1956.

Valentine, G. H.: *The Chromosome Disorders. An Introduction for Clinicians.* London; William Heinemann Medical Books, Philadelphia; J. B. Lippincott Company, 1966.

Wertelecki, W., Schindler, A. M., and Gerald, P. S.: Partial Deletion of Chromosome 18. *Lancet,* 2:641, 1966.

Yunis, J. J.: *Human Chromosome Methodology.* New York; Academic Press, 1965.

INTRAUTERINE AND ENVIRONMENTAL FACTORS

In mammals prenatal development is protected, since it takes place in the uterus, but this protection is not complete. Mechanical, actinic, chemical, nutritional and infectious agents may cause prenatal injury. Such agents are called *teratogens.*

Intrauterine life may be divided into an *embryonic period* (approximately the first trimester) and a *fetal period* (from the twelfth week to birth). This division is arbitrary, but it distinguishes the period in which organogenesis takes place from the period which is devoted chiefly to growth.

Severe injuries lead to prenatal death; milder injuries may result in changes compatible with life. Environmental interference during the embryonic period leads to arrest of development and to malformations. A noxious agent may be harmless at certain stages of this period and deleterious at others, since the various organs are sensitive to noxious agents at periods of rapid differentiation and less sensitive in resting stages. Since biochemical differentiation precedes morphologic differentiation, the period sensitive to interference by a teratogen may precede the stage of visible change. It can be assumed that agents responsible for malformations act early in prenatal life, probably within the first 2 or 3 months of gestation. Later, during the fetal period, injuries result in changes which more closely resemble those of postnatal damage, such as scars and mutilations.

Mechanical Injuries. Mechanical injuries may result in fetal death. External, intra-abdominal or intrauterine pressure has been said to lead to malformations, but only a few specific possibilities are seriously considered. In extrauterine pregnancies the fetus is often deformed. The deformity cannot be attributed to mechanical causes alone, however, since an ectopic embryo is embedded in an abnormal decidua, and faulty nutrition may be the cause. Malformations in a twin have been attributed to pressure exerted by the other twin. It is often asserted that intrauterine malposition of the fetus leads to malformations; it seems just as reasonable, however, to consider malposition secondary to the malformation. There is a possibility that a deformed fetal part which assumes an abnormal position impairs the normal development of another part and thus causes secondary deformities (mutilations). Amniotic bands are sometimes associated with malformations, but there is no proof that they are the cause of the deformities.

Chemical Injuries. Certain chemicals are capable of destroying the embryo, and malformations can be produced in animals by adding toxic substances to the environment. Alcohol, benzol, nicotine, lead, mercury and iodine have been suspected as injurious agents, but experimental results have been contradictory. Quinine taken by the mother during pregnancy may cause congenital deafness in her child.

A number of drugs have been found to be teratogenic in animals. Antimetabolites such as galactoflavin or x-methyl-folic acid have been used successfully to induce congenital malformations in rodents. The folic acid antagonist 4-amino-folic acid (aminopterin) has caused congenital malformations in human embryos whose mothers used the drug in attempted abortion. Thalidomide, alpha (N-phthalimido) glutarimide, a hypnotic and antiemetic, can induce severe malformations in human embryos if ingested by the mother in the first weeks of pregnancy. The incidence of malformations is highest if the drug is taken between the thirty-fifth and fiftieth days after the last menstrual period. Amelia, phocomelia, acheiria

(p. 1333) and other limb defects may result from the embryo's exposure to this drug. In addition, congenital hemangiomas, ear and eye defects, cardiac malformations and atresias of the gastro-intestinal tract have been caused by this chemical compound. These observations have demonstrated that the embryos of man are just as susceptible as other mammalian embryos to chemical injurious agents. Other drugs which may damage the embryo or fetus are dicumarol (fetal bleeding); progestational agents, estrogens and androgens (masculinization of female fetus); thiouracil derivatives, iodine and iodides (goiter). Since it is difficult to be sure that any drug is not harmful to an embryo, drug intake during pregnancy should be restricted to those clearly necessary to the mother's health.

Nutritional Disturbances.   Nutritional disturbances may adversely influence the embryo. Faulty implantation of the ovum and degeneration of the chorion may interrupt the nutrition of the embryo and disturb its development. Malformation in fetuses derived from ectopic pregnancies is mentioned above. Deficiencies of nutritional constituents of the maternal diet and deficiency of oxygen have been responsible for defective offspring in animal experiments, but there is no proof that these observations can be applied to human beings. In many regions of Europe, Asia and South America endemic goiter of the parents is associated with endemic cretinism of the children. The serious mental and physical retardation of the offspring is usually attributed to a lack of iodine in the maternal diet. Other, unknown goitrogenic factors may also contribute to this anomaly, however.

Extensive studies have shown a relation between the diet of pregnant women and the physical condition of newborn infants. Stillborn, premature and functionally immature children are born more often to mothers whose diet is poor prior to or during pregnancy than to mothers whose diet is adequate. General starvation, as in war or famine, leads to a sharp fall in the conception rate, associated with amenorrhea.

Injuries from Infection.   Severe maternal infections during early pregnancy often result in abortion. Mothers who have had German measles during the first 2 or 3 months of pregnancy may give birth to infants with a variety of defects and widely disseminated infection (see p. 630). Cytomegalic inclusion disease and toxoplasmosis are examples of inapparent maternal infections which can cause extensive damage in the fetus; each may be responsible for microcephaly and hydrocephalus as well as widespread disease.

Infections of the fetus during the latter stages of prenatal life cause manifestations which more closely resemble those of postnatal life. Smallpox has been observed in fetuses older than 3 months; the fetus may recover and be born with scars. Rare cases of fetal measles and scarlet fever have been reported. Placental transmission of typhoid and tubercle bacilli occurs occasionally, and that of *Treponema pallidum* is common in infected, untreated mothers.

Actinic Injuries.   Roentgen rays and radium rays are capable of arresting embryonic development and producing malformations. Microcephaly, mental retardation, spina bifida and deformities of the extremities have been ascribed to such intrauterine injuries.

Other Factors.   In addition to the pathogenic environmental factors considered, there may be others still unrecognized. The possibility that abnormal endocrine factors influence the development of the embryo deserves consideration. Diabetic mothers treated with insulin often have abortions and stillbirths, and the neonatal death rate of their infants is high. Some children of treated diabetic mothers are born with defects of the sacrum or femora. Cortisone injected into pregnant mice or rabbits may induce cleft palate and other malformations in the fetus. Administration of progestins to a woman during pregnancy can result in masculinization of a female fetus.

Advanced parental age may play a role in the origin of congenital defects such as achondroplasia. Advanced maternal age is a factor in Down's syndrome (p. 331).

CONGENITAL MALFORMATIONS

More deaths occur in the first month of life than in the remaining months of the first year. This is not surprising if neonatal mortality is regarded in part as a continuation of the process of "natural selection" which eliminates defective embryos and fetuses throughout the preceding intrauterine period.

Structural anomalies of the embryo play a leading role in the mortality of the first trimester of intrauterine life. Most abnormal embryos die early, but structural anomalies may be compatible with intrauterine life. Shortly before and after birth (perinatal period) the fetus must adjust to the profound physiologic changes associated with the onset of extrauterine life. Many abnormal fetuses are incapable of doing so and die. They contribute considerably to the peak of mortality, which occurs in the perinatal period. About 20 per cent of deaths in the third trimester of gestation and about 15 per cent in the neonatal period are attributed to gross congenital malformations. Although the elimination of deformed children decreases after the first month of postnatal life, the process of natural selection continues throughout infancy and childhood. The relative importance of congenital malformations as a cause of death is

depicted graphically and numerically in the introductory section, The Field of Pediatrics.

Many children with congenital malformations
are permanently disabled. Malformations such as
clubfoot, dislocation of the hip and spina bifida
are among the leading causes of crippling in childhood.

The role of congenital malformations in the
causation of diseases of children is difficult to
evaluate. Some defects, such as those of the osseous system, the heart and the intestinal tract,
are well recognized, but many malformations may
go unnoticed for years. The affected organs, e.g.
malformed kidneys, may function for some time,
but fail when faced with increased demands. Congenital malformations are often predisposing
factors to disease because they represent points
of inadequate resistance; organs can be damaged
by minor infections, toxins or traumas which are
usually tolerated by the normal organism without
serious consequences. Diseases resulting from
such a combination of circumstances may be attributed to the eliciting factor, while the underlying malformation is overlooked.

For example, the primary cause of so-called
renal rickets may be a congenital obstruction of
the urinary tract. Dwarfism, malnutrition, osseous
changes, polyuria, polydipsia, renal insufficiency,
chemical changes of the blood, infections of the
urinary tract or other symptoms may dominate
the clinical picture. Obviously treatment of the
symptoms enumerated will not meet with success,
whereas early detection and removal of the congenital obstruction may lead to permanent cure.

Congenital defects need not be grossly demonstrable, but may be anomalies of histologic structure. The role of misplaced cells in the genesis
of certain tumors is well known. Some disorders
of the nervous system or the endocrine glands
must be attributed to histologic congenital defects.
Spherocytosis is a congenital anomaly. The intimate relation of certain forms of anemia to malformations is indicated by their association in
syndromes. For example, in some forms of aplastic
anemia, association with congenital defects of
the skeleton, heart and genital tract points to
the developmental origin of the disorder (e.g.
Fanconi's anemia).

Etiology and Pathogenesis. With respect to
etiology, congenital malformations can be considered in 4 major categories: gene mutations,
chromosomal aberrations, adverse intrauterine
environmental factors, and a group in which the
malformation results from a combination of many
factors, both genetic and environmental, no single
one of which may be detectable (see Table 1-3,
p. 10).

It has been roughly estimated that about 10
per cent of congenital malformations result from
mutant genes. These are inherited according to
mendelian laws, and relatively precise predictions
can be made about the probability of occurrence
in the patient's sibs, his offspring, and other relatives. Theoretically, such malformations should

have an underlying biochemical defect. In a few
cases structural malformations are associated
with inborn errors of metabolism, e.g. adrenogenital syndrome, but in most congenital malformations transmitted by mendelian inheritance no
biochemical defect has been identified.

Animals often inherit congenital malformations with great
regularity of pattern, and it is possible by systematic examination of their embryos of different ages to ascertain step by step
the deviations from normal development. In this way the action
and mechanism of the abnormal gene can be investigated and
the development of the finished character observed.

Perhaps about 1 per cent of malformations present at birth and 20 per cent or more of early spontaneous abortions have abnormal chromosomal
constitutions (see section on chromosomal abnormalities). Relatively few congenital malformations can be attributed to specific environmental
teratogens. Maternal rubella in the first trimester
of pregnancy, toxoplasmosis, cytomegalic inclusion disease, exposure to therapeutic levels of
radiation and the ingestion of certain drugs have
been mentioned elsewhere in this section.

The embryo requires adequate nutrition for normal growth and differentiation. Interruption of
nutrition results in death of the embryo, and minor
disturbances of the metabolic exchanges between
mother and embryo may lead to malformations of
the developing organism. The chorion of pathologic
embryos is frequently diseased, but it is difficult
to decide whether the chorionic changes are
responsible for the abnormal development or
whether an inherent anomaly of the fetus incompatible with life leads to secondary changes of
the chorion.

Experimental observations indicate that chemical changes of the environment can alter the
development of the embryo; at certain stages
minor abnormal stimuli can produce severe anomalies. Maternal diseases and hormonal disturbances can change the chemical environment of the
human embryo.

As previously noted, severe infections of the
mother in early pregnancy often result in abortion,
and relatively mild infections with the rubella
virus in the first trimester of gestation may result
in a variety of congenital anomalies of the fetus.

Perhaps the majority of congenital malformations are the result of a combination of genetic
and environmental factors. Malformations such
as congenital hypertrophic pyloric stenosis, cleft
lip and cleft palate, congenital dislocation of the
hip and talipes equinovarus probably fall into this
group. They tend to be familial, but do not have
mendelian patterns of inheritance. Most have no
demonstrable chromosomal anomaly and no identifiable abnormal prenatal environmental factors.
Probabilities of recurrence can be estimated em-
pirically from observation of affected families,
and used for counseling.

Teratogenic factors are not specific, and the
lack of specificity manifests itself in 2 ways. An
injurious agent may cause various abnormalities,

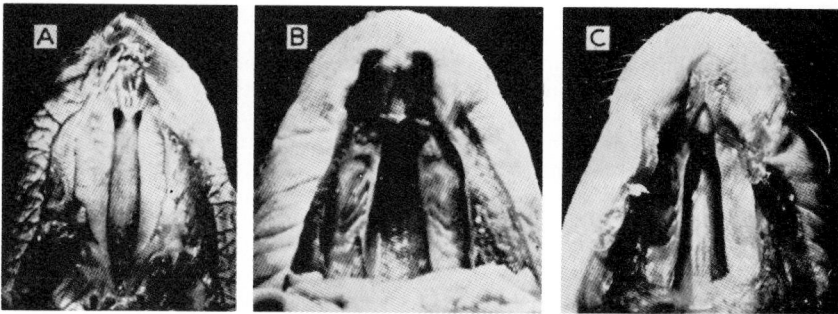

Figure 6-30. Cleft palates of different etiology. *A*, Mouse, derived from strain in which harelip and cleft palate were hereditary (Steiniger: *Ztschr. f. menschl. Vererb.-u. Konstit.*, Vol. 23); *B*, rat whose mother was deficient in riboflavin; *C*, rat whose mother was exposed to roentgen rays on day 15 of gestation.

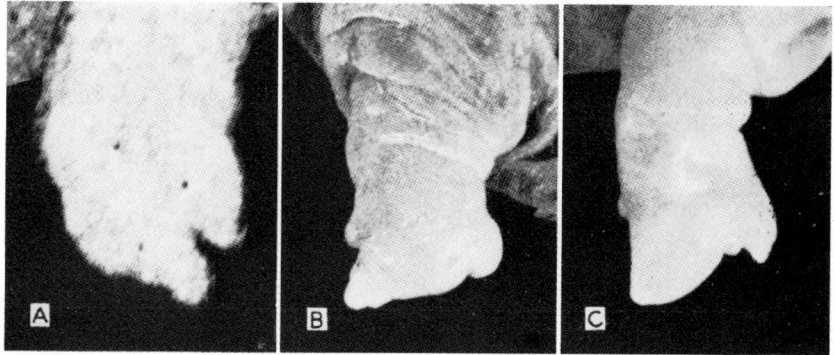

Figure 6-31. Syndactylism of different etiology. *A*, Mouse, derived from strain with hereditary congenital defects (Bagg: *Am. J. Anat.*, Vol. 43); *B*, rat whose mother was deficient in riboflavin; *C*, rat whose mother was exposed to roentgen rays on day 13 of gestation.

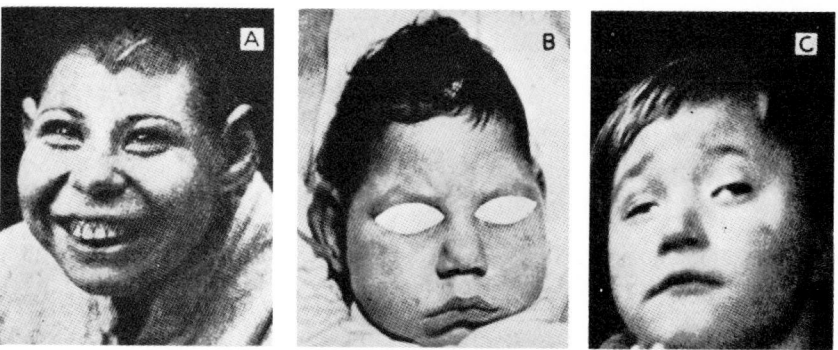

Figure 6-32. Microcephaly of different etiology. *A*, In a child who had 2 siblings with microcephaly and 3 normal siblings and a paternal granduncle who was mentally deficient (Goldblatt: *Arch. f. Psych.*, Vol. 70); *B*, in a child with toxoplasmosis (Levin and Moore: *J. Pediat.*, Vol. 21); *C*, child of a mother irradiated with roentgen rays during the second and third months of pregnancy (Engelking: *Klin. Monatschr. f. Augenh.*, Vol. 94).

(Figures 6-30, 6-31 and 6-32 from Warkany; in *Advances in Pediatrics.* Interscience Publishers, Inc., Vol. 2.)

according to the time or intensity of its action, as illustrated by the wide variety of congenital anomalies induced by maternal rubella. Maternal roentgen-ray irradiation results in abnormalities in the offspring which vary with the dose applied and the gestational period in which the exposure took place. An abnormal gene may manifest itself in various abnormalities and exercise a pleiotropic effect. Conversely, a specific type of malformation may be caused by different etiologic factors, and hereditary anomalies may resemble each other. For example, each of the 3 pathologic conditions illustrated in Figures 6-30, 6-31 and 6-32 can be attributed to 3 different causes.

In spite of the variability of syndromes, it is of definite value to study and record combinations of defects frequently encountered. A knowledge of such syndromes is an aid in diagnosis and prognosis, particularly if one keeps in mind that the association of defects may vary. Two examples will suffice: Night blindness may be due to a deficiency of vitamin A, but it is also a symptom of retinitis pigmentosa, a degenerative process of the retina which is a constituent of the Laurence-Moon-Biedl syndrome. Night blindness in a child with polydactylism, obesity and mental retardation assumes, therefore, a different aspect from that in an otherwise normal child. The diagnosis of mental retardation is difficult in the neonatal period. The presence of epicanthal folds, slanting eyes and other somatic anomalies makes possible, however, the diagnosis of Down's syndrome, with all its prognostic implications, immediately after birth.

Besides such well established syndromes, many combinations of congenital defects are encountered which have not been described or named. Thus, in children with congenital heart disease, conditions such as cleft palate, polydactylism, malformations of the kidney, atresia ani, encephalocele and hydrocephalus are more frequent than in the average child population. The occurrence of external and skeletal defects in children with mental deficiency is well known. Such visible defects have been considered "stigmata of degeneration." Though this term is ill chosen, it is correct that malformations are found more often in patients with mental deficiency of prenatal origin than in mentally normal children. It is useful to keep this principle of multiplicity of malformations in mind when there is doubt whether one is dealing with a congenital or a postnatally acquired disorder. The finding of one or several additional malformations makes prenatal origin of the disorder more likely.

Malformations may occur sporadically or repeatedly in a sibship (p. 320). Identical malformations, such as cleft palate, may be found in several members of a pedigree. In other instances the same cause may produce different malformations; e.g. one member may have microphthalmus and another glioma retinae. Entire syndromes may recur in families, e.g. gargoylism or the Laurence-Moon-Biedl syndrome. But the various symptoms of a syndrome may also be dissociated in a family; one member may have one abnormal manifestation or one group of anomalies, and other members may have another part of the syndrome. Thus one child may have the entire Laurence-Moon-Biedl syndrome, while another child of the same family is mentally retarded and obese and a third child has mental retardation and polydactylism. In spite of such irregularities, the family history is often a great aid in the diagnosis and prognosis of the disease of an individual patient.

Whenever environmental or genetic factors are unfavorable for reproduction, various manifestations of reproductive failure are observed. The most unfavorable conditions result in sterility. Between this extreme and the favorable one which leads to normal reproduction there may be abortion, stillbirth, premature birth or neonatal death. Malformations contribute to all degrees of reproductive failure and are a substantial cause of abortions in the first trimester. Deformed fetuses which reach the end of the normal gestational period and die in the perinatal period or survive birth represent a relative reproductive "success" when compared with sterility or early abortion. This possibility makes it understandable that an improvement of reproductive conditions may result in a higher incidence of congenital malformations. It explains why the true incidence of malformations cannot be estimated without a thorough examination of aborted and stillborn fetuses.

One can produce congenital malformations in animals by planned creation of adverse conditions or by applying injurious agents which damage the embryo without killing it. Starvation, severe infection of the mother or traumatic injury of the embryo may result in death before malformations develop. In genetically determined malformations, death may occur in utero. Between this lethal state and normality there is a wide range of congenital malformations which are compatible with a limited life span or with a normal expectancy for life, with or without functional deficits. These examples illustrate how closely related are the causes of congenital malformations to other forms of reproductive failure.

GENETIC COUNSELING

If a person or one of his close relatives suffers from a congenital defect, he may ask his physician whether he should have children; or parents who have had a defective child may ask whether they should have more offspring. Such questions can rarely be answered adequately, but a knowledge of the facts discussed in the foregoing pages may serve as a guide.

In general it is preferable to give the parents all the available facts about the cause, the theoretical chance of transmission of the disorder, and its clinical course rather than advise them whether or not to have children. Many nonmedical factors enter into such a decision, such as the parents' desire to have children, the size of the family, economic circumstances and religious convictions.

It is important to ascertain whether a given defect or disorder is hereditary or not, since the prognosis will differ greatly in cases of genetic origin from those of postconceptional damage. In certain instances such a differentiation can be made without difficulty; in many it may not be possible. Before a statement is made about the heredity of a trait the following considerations should be taken into account.

Not all congenital anomalies and defects are hereditary, and not all hereditary anomalies are congenital. The defects produced in the fetus by maternal rubella or toxoplasmosis are congenital, but not genetically determined and, therefore, not hereditary. On the other hand, hereditary traits such as Friedreich's ataxia, Huntington's chorea, diabetes mellitus, retinitis pigmentosa and many others are not congenital, but develop in postnatal life. The terms "congenital" and "hereditary" are not synonymous.

The widespread belief that anomalies which occur repeatedly in a family are hereditary, whereas those which appear sporadically are not, is not necessarily correct. A defect may be genetically determined, although only one known member of the kindred shows the trait. The defective person may be the first to manifest a genic mutation. In the case of a dominant hereditary trait, his ancestors and siblings are free of the trait, but each of his children has a 1:1 chance to have the anomaly and to pass it on to half of their children. This illustrates that sporadic occurrence of a congenital anomaly does not assure normal offspring to the (first) affected member. Similarly, genetically determined defects may appear sporadically if they depend upon recessive factors or if a limited pedigree does not include other defective members. The repeated occurrence of a defect in a pedigree does not prove, however, that it is genetically determined, since several members of a sibship may be exposed to the same pathogenic environmental factors. Thus endemic goiter, rickets, pellagra, and the like, are often familial, but they are usually not hereditary and may be prevented by a change of dietary habits. "Familial" and "hereditary" are not synonymous terms.

Differentiation between hereditary and nonhereditary anomalies is further complicated by the fact that the clinical picture of a nonhereditary modification may resemble closely that of a hereditary mutation. Thus congenital cataract is hereditary in some families, but cataract in an infant whose mother had German measles during the first 2 months of pregnancy is of environmental origin. Similarly, syndactyly, cleft palate, microcephaly, spina bifida, microphthalmus and many other congenital defects may be due to genetic mutation, to environmental modification, or to a combination of the two.

The history of pregnancy should include a description of the mother's state of health during the early weeks of pregnancy and of any roentgen-ray or drug therapy. Organogenesis is finished at approximately 12 weeks of gestation, and most structural anomalies such as congenital heart disease, spina bifida, colobomas of the eye and cleft palate are determined by that time. Anomalies arising during the remaining 6 months represent trauma, disease or interference with growth of structurally complete organs. Hydrocephalus, microphthalmus, chorioretinitis and malposition of the extremities are examples. Threatened abortions, diseases and traumas of the mother should be recorded.

The birth history may indicate that physical and mental anomalies can be attributed to injuries received during delivery.

Taking the family history is a time-consuming but necessary procedure. The mother's and the father's ages should be recorded, and the parents should be asked whether they are blood-related (consanguineous). It is sometimes useful to make a pedigree chart (p. 321), but this is usually impractical in a busy clinic. At least there should be a statement whether there is any condition similar to the patient's disease or defect in other members of the family. If there is, and a pedigree is to be constructed, the medical history of the patient (propositus) is recorded, then that of his brothers and sisters. Miscarriages, stillbirths and causes of deaths of siblings are also recorded. Healthy persons as well as defective ones must be included in the family history. Next the medical histories of the grandparents, their siblings and siblings' offspring, and so on, are obtained until the pedigree is traced backwards and collaterally as far as the information is reasonably reliable.

If a pathologic trait known to be usually dominant appears in a family, and if the pedigree of that family suggests dominant inheritance, it is possible to give a genetic prognosis. An affected parent who marries a mate normal for the character in question can be told that his children have a 1:1 chance to be normal. But if the parent comes from a family affected by a dominant pathologic trait, but does not have it he can be assured that he will not transmit the trait to his offspring. Before such assurance is given it should be established that the inherited trait has complete penetrance and expressivity (p. 320), since otherwise a person may appear normal, but transmit the trait. In case of variable expressivity a person may appear normal on superficial examination, but reveal the abnormal trait in a mild form when subjected to special examinations.

For example, multiple exostoses (p. 1346) are usually well developed in affected males, but in affected females may be so small that the carriers may not be conscious of them. If roentgenograms of the prospective mother reveal slight osseous excrescences in places where exostoses usually occur, she is likely to transmit the disorder, and her sons could be severely affected.

At times laboratory tests can aid in detecting carriers of an abnormal trait with low expressivity. A member of a family affected with hemolytic jaundice may be clinically well, but have spherocytosis and increased fragility of the red cells which is revealed only by special tests. "Carriers" of gout can be discovered by chemical demonstration of hyperuricemia. In addition, before a member of an affected family is declared free, one must be sure that he has reached an age after which the onset of the disease is unlikely. Since cerebellar ataxia may not begin before the fourth decade, no member of an affected family should be considered normal before reaching the age of 40 years. These examples demonstrate that even in dominant inheritance a genetic prognosis must be made with caution.

Analysis and prognosis of a recessive trait are more difficult. A recessive gene can be carried in the heterozygous form through many generations without causing visible effects, and then the abnormal trait can appear in about one fourth of the children of normal parents who are both heterozygous carriers. Such traits are sometimes so sporadic that their distinction from nonhereditary similar conditions (phenocopies) may be impossible. On the other hand, if a homozygous person who has the trait marries a heterozygous carrier who appears normal, the children have a 1:1 chance to be homozygous and to exhibit the trait. Such a pedigree simulates that of a family in which a dominant trait is transmitted through 2 generations. When 2 persons homozygous for a recessive trait marry, all the children must be expected to be abnormal.

Deaf-mutism is sometimes determined by a recessive gene. A deaf-mute is homozygous for the trait. If 2 persons of this type marry, one can predict that all their children will be deaf-mutes (see Fig. 6-8). If, however, a person with such hereditary deafness marries a normal mate or a person with acquired deafness, all the children can be expected to have normal hearing, though they will be carriers of the abnormal trait (Figs. 6-9, 6-10). If 2 carriers who have an abnormal (homozygous) child ask about the chances of a second child, they must be told that the following child has again one chance in four to be affected. The chances that 2 heterozygous carriers of the same recessive mutant gene will meet are increased by consanguineous marriages. Heterozygous carriers of the

abnormal recessive gene for a number of inborn errors of metabolism can be identified by appropriate biochemical tests (see secton on Inborn Errors of Metabolism).

A man who manifests a sex-linked recessive trait will—with a normal wife—have sons who neither show nor transmit the trait, but all his daughters will be carriers. The sons of such female carriers will have a 1:1 chance of showing the abnormal trait; those sons who do not manifest the disorder do not transmit it. All the daughters will appear normal, but have a 1:1 chance of being carriers like their mother. There is usually no way to distinguish the carrier daughters from their normal sisters unless their offspring reveal their heterozygous state.

Calculation of Carrier State (Gene Frequency). It is sometimes useful, in the case of recessively inherited diseases, to know the frequency of heterozygous carriers of the gene. Consider the case of an albino man (aa) who wants to know what the probability is that his children will be albinos. The possibility of procreating an albino child depends on the chance of marrying a heterozygote, Aa, which (provided he does not marry a relative) depends on the frequency of heterozygotes (Aa) in the population.

To estimate this frequency, one must think of the genes on a population, rather than a family, basis. If one in every 100 genes at the "A" locus is a, and the other ninety-nine are A, and if mating is at random, the probability that one individual will draw 2 a genes and be an albino is $1/100 \times 1/100$, or $1/10,000$. That is, the frequency of homozygotes in the population is the square of the frequency of the gene. In practice, the known quantity is the frequency of the disease, $1/10,000$, and one can estimate the frequency of the gene as the square root of this number, or $1/100$.

The probability that a person will be a heterozygote is dependent on obtaining an a gene from one parent and an A from the other, which, based on the incidence of albinism, is $1/100 \times 99/100$ plus $99/100 \times 1/100$, or roughly $2/100$. Thus there is a 2 per cent probability that the albino's (unrelated) wife will be a heterozygote; the probability that the first child will be albino is half of this rate, or 1 per cent.

Formally stated, the relation between gene frequencies and genotype frequencies is known as the Hardy-Weinberg rule, which states that, if mating is random with respect to genotype, and if p is the frequency of an allele A and q the frequency of a, the frequency of genotypes AA, Aa and aa will be p^2, 2 pq, and q^2, respectively. The relation is also useful in calculations involving the effects of selection, mutation, and the like, on gene frequencies.

Hereditary traits may be transmitted differently in different sibships. It was mentioned before that polydactylism, achondroplasia, glioma retinae and many other anomalies are sometimes inherited in a dominant and sometimes in a recessive manner. Progressive muscular dystrophy, peroneal atrophy and cataract are transmitted in some families as dominant, in some as recessive, and in others as sex-linked recessive traits.

If a congenital anomaly was caused by an environmental accident, the prognosis for a subsequent pregnancy will depend upon the kind of interfering agent. If the child's anomalies are due to maternal rubella or toxoplasmosis, to administration of therapeutic doses of roentgen rays or toxic drugs, and a repetition of the faulty treatment can be avoided, the prognosis for a second child is good.

When neither a definite genetic nor a known environmental factor can be shown to be responsible for a congenital defect, the chances for the outcome of a subsequent pregnancy cannot be stated precisely.

When possible, it is helpful to indicate to parents the approximate chances for normal or abnormal children. Such empirical risk figures have been worked out for congenital disorders such as epilepsy, diabetes mellitus, cardiac malformations, facial clefts, clubfoot and others. Since such disorders are of heterogeneous origin, empirical risk figures represent merely average risks for the disorder, which should be used only when actual risk figures cannot be had.

If, for instance, normal parents have a child with harelip (with or without cleft palate), the average risk for another child having a similar malformation is about 5 per cent. If the parents have had 2 affected children, the risk of having still another is about 10 per cent. If one parent has the anomaly, the average risk for a child is 5 per cent. If, however, one parent and one child of a family are affected, the risk for other children being affected is about 15 per cent. The risk figures are fairly similar for cleft palate without harelip. If the parents are unaffected, but one child has cleft palate, the risk of having this malformation is about 3 per cent for subsequent children. If one parent has the anomaly, the risk for a child is said to be 7 per cent, but this estimate is questionable, since it is derived from a small sample. If one parent and one child are affected, the risk for other children is said to be 17 per cent.

Such risk figures are better than none at all, but they should be considered merely provisional estimates.

Protection of the Mother. Eugenic measures and advice are not restricted to the genetic aspects of prenatal life. The normal development of the fetus should be assured as far as possible by protection of the expectant mother from adverse environmental influences. Roentgen-ray treatment must be avoided whenever there is the possibility of a pregnancy. It is of great importance to point out that the first 3 months of pregnancy are decisive in the formation of the organs of the child, and that the embryo in its early stages is more vulnerable than the fetus.

Josef Warkany
F. Clarke Fraser

REFERENCES

Carter, C. O.: The Inheritance of Common Congenital Malformations. *Progress in Medical Genetics,* 4:59, 1965.

First International Conference on Congenital Malformations. Philadelphia, J. B. Lippincott Company, 1961.

Fraser, F. C.: Genetic Counselling in Some Common Paediatric Diseases. *Pediat. Clin. N. Amer.,* 5:475, 1958.

Fraser, F. C.: Taking the Family History. *Am. J. Med.,* 34:585, 1963.

Fraser, F. C.: Some Genetic Aspects of Teratology; in J. G. Wilson and J. Warkany (Eds.): *Teratology.* Chicago, University of Chicago Press, 1964, Chap. 2.

McKusick, V.: *Mendelian Inheritance in Man.* Baltimore, Johns Hopkins Press, 1966.

Warkany, J., and Kalter, H.: Congenital Malformations. *New England J. Med.,* 265:993, 1961.

7. The Fetus and the Newborn Infant

The neonatal period is arbitrarily considered to be the first 4 weeks of life. Fetal and neonatal life is a continuum during which the growth and development of the human organism are affected by genetic and by intrauterine and extrauterine environmental factors (see Table 1-3, p. 10), the latter are modified by social, economic and cultural influences. For example, low economic status is one of the factors most frequently associated with low birth weight (premature birth), which in turn is associated with high rates of morbidity and mortality, not only in the neonatal period, but also throughout infancy. Social as well as economic factors are reflected in the much higher (50 per cent) neonatal mortality rate of nonwhite infants in the United States than of white ones. The difference in the mortality rates of these groups is even more impressive for the entire first year of life (Fig. 1-2; Table 7-1). Although social influences such as the unwillingness of physicians and their families to live in areas of social and economic poverty affect the availability of medical care to those most in need of it, the failure of many mothers in these areas to make effective use of prenatal and other preventive medical care, even when it is available to them, also contributes to fetal and infant morbidity and mortality. Social factors leading to illegitimate births and cultural practices, including the use of drugs which may damage the fetus, also increase the incidence of fetal and neonatal death and disease.

Neonatal mortality is highest during the first 24 hours of life (Fig. 1-5) and has shown little change in rate in the United States since 1955. The lack of success in combating diseases which result from factors acting during gestation and at delivery, as opposed to diseases arising as a result of postnatal factors, has led to the establishment of increasing interest in fetal and neonatal physiology and in the noxious factors which influence them. The term *perinatal mortality* has been adopted to identify fetal and neonatal deaths influenced by prenatal conditions and circumstances surrounding delivery. In practice, perinatal mortality has been defined in 3 ways: (1) deaths of fetuses and infants weighing 1000 gm. or over which occur from the twenty-eighth week of gestational life through the twenty-eighth day of neonatal life; (2) deaths of fetuses and infants from the twenty-eighth week of fetal life through the seventh day after birth; (3) deaths of fetuses and infants from the twentieth week of gestational life through the twenty-eighth day after birth. The last definition is being used with increasing frequency, but a significant body of data exists based on each of the first 2 definitions.

Emphasis on perinatal mortality, initiated by obstetricians, has been the greatest single factor in bringing about a team approach, involving obstetricians, pathologists, pediatricians, public health officials and nurses, to the problems of fetal and neonatal life. Fetal and neonatal deaths contribute about equally to perinatal mortality; the key position of the obstetrician in the reduction of perinatal mortality is obvious. Because of the high incidence of permanent handicaps, especially neurologic ones, among surviving infants with a history of low birth weight, anoxia, birth injury or malformations, it is apparent that research and public health efforts should be directed primarily at determination and elimination of the causes of low birth weight, of obstetric injury and of malformations.

Perinatal and infant mortality rates vary from country to country; they are lowest in the Scandinavian countries and The Netherlands and highest in the so-called underdeveloped countries. Even though socioeconomic, cultural and perhaps geographic factors may be the most important influences which determine perinatal mortality, autopsy findings on a series of live-born infants without eliminating any because of assumption of "previability" indicate that there are potentials for further reductions in perinatal mortality by prophylactic health measures (Table 7-2).

The high incidence of disease and excessive mortality rate during the first few days of life (Fig. 1-5) emphasize the need to identify as early as possible those fetuses and infants who are at greatest risk. Both the obstetrician and pediatrician should be aware of and heed all the untoward prenatal and natal factors which may affect the newborn infant; they must likewise maintain effective communication so that problems may be anticipated and preventive and therapeutic measures taken promptly.

Of equal importance with the need to lower the perinatal mortality rates is the need to lower the incidence of handicapping conditions resulting from untoward prenatal and natal factors. Since

TABLE 7-1. DEATH RATES PER 1000 LIVE BIRTHS FOR INFANTS IN THE UNITED STATES IN 1965, ACCORDING TO COLOR

AGE	WHITE	NONWHITE
Less than 28 days	16.1	25.4
Under 1 year	21.5	40.3

Vital Statistics of the U.S. 1965, Vol. II – Mortality, Part A, Section 2 – Infant Mortality.

346

TABLE 7-2. MAJOR AUTOPSY FINDINGS ON 501 NEWBORN INFANTS (1960-1966)

	110-1000 gm.	1001-2500 gm.	2501 gm. +	TOTAL
Number of Infants	253	192	56	501
Pulmonary hyaline membrane	59	106	9	174
Inflammatory lesions (infection)	66	50	17	133
Intraventricular hemorrhage	86	43	1	130
Undetermined (over 500 gm.)	35	14	3	52
Congenital anomalies	1	28	20	49
Immaturity (less than 500 gm.)	47	0	0	47
Fetal anoxia	13	6	6	25
Trauma	0	3	4	7
Hemolytic disease of the newborn	1	2	4	7
Infants of diabetic mothers	2	1	3	6
Idiopathic hydrops	0	1	1	2
Tumor	0	0	1 (thyroid)	1
Totals	310	254	69	633*

Based on data from Temple University Health Sciences Center, Philadelphia, supplied by Drs. Marie Valdés-Dapena and J. B. Arey.
*Some infants had more than one major finding at autopsy.

both mortality and permanent neurologic sequelae are in large measure caused by the same or similar disturbances, it would seem that measures directed at reduction in perinatal mortality would also reduce the incidence of handicapping conditions. That this assumption has limitations is illustrated by the high incidence of mental retardation among infants who required vigorous and prolonged resuscitation at birth and of retinal and pulmonary damage among those who had prolonged exposure to high concentrations of oxygen in the immediate postnatal period.

THE FETUS

Fetal life as differentiated from embryonic life begins with the completion of organogenesis, which is about the twelfth week of gestation. Genetic and environmental influences, however, which affect the fetus are at work even before conception. The genetic material contained in the chromosomes from each parent plays an important role not only in fetal development, but even in fetal survival; recognizable chromosomal abnormalities are 20 to 30 times more frequent among spontaneously aborted embryos and fetuses than among liveborn infants. Environmental factors may influence the selection and propagation of genes transmitted to the infant, as well as be responsible for mutations of parental genes.

The father's health may affect the motility of the spermatozoon and its ability to penetrate the ovum. Likewise the mother's health and state of nutrition may affect ovulation, the viability of the ovum and the zygote, and the availability of an adequate site for implantation; women who suffer from malnutrition or debilitating illness have diminished fertility and often diminished frequency of menstruation. Exposure of the zygote or embryo to drugs, chemicals, infectious diseases and other noxious influences may affect cell division and result in structural malformations. The general health and nutrition of the mother, and possibly her emotional health, during pregnancy also affect the fetus; the infants of malnourished mothers weigh less and are somewhat shorter at birth than those of mothers with adequate nutri-

tion. Illness of the mother during pregnancy may result in fetal death, abortion or premature delivery. Infectious diseases of the mother may also affect the fetus.

From the practical standpoint, major emphases in fetal medicine at this time should be in 4 directions: (1) fetal effects of maternal disease; (2) fetal effects of drugs administered to the mother; (3) identification of fetal disease, particularly that of genetic origin; and (4) treatment of fetal disease. In time it is reasonable to expect that increasing knowledge of fetal physiology may pave the way for practical approaches to problems of adaptation of the newborn infant, particularly of the premature one. Unfortunately much of our knowledge of fetal physiology has been obtained from animals and often is not directly applicable to man; the increasing use of primates for fetal studies should provide physiologic information more applicable to the human fetus. A number of the known aspects of human fetal growth and development are summarized on pages 18 through 20.

Maternal Disease and the Fetus. *Infections.* Almost any maternal infection with severe systemic manifestations may result in abortion, stillbirth or premature labor. Whether these results are due to infection of the fetus or are secondary to the stress imposed on the mother by the infection is not always clear. Certain agents, however, do infect the fetus more or less regularly without relation to the severity of the maternal infection, and frequently with a disastrous effect on life or development. Certain infections, such as rubella, may also produce congenital malformations if they occur during the period of organogenesis. Infections which are known to cause disease in the fetus or the newborn infant include *chickenpox* or *herpes zoster* (p. 638), *Coxsackie* B viruses (p. 673), *cytomegalovirus* (p. 663), *hepatitis* (p. 834), *herpes simplex* (p. 634), *listeriosis* (p. 408), *malaria* (abortion, premature delivery), *mumps* (fetal death and possibly endocardial fibroelastosis), *poliomyelitis* (abortion, congenital paralysis or poliomyelitis), *rubella* (p. 630), *rubeola* (abortion, prematurity, fetal measles, ? congenital malformations), *smallpox* (fetal smallpox), *syphilis* (p. 615), *toxoplasmosis* (p. 745), *tuberculosis* (congenital tuberculosis), *vaccinia or vaccination* (fetal vaccinia), *vibrio fetus* (abortion, prematurity, meningitis) and *Western equine encephalitis* (encephalitis).

Noninfectious diseases. *Maternal diabetes* usually results in hypertrophy and hyperplasia of the islets of Langerhans of the fetus, a finding also present in erythroblastosis fetalis. Most of the increase is due to increase in number and size of the beta cells. There is a high incidence of intrauterine death after the thirty-sixth week of gestation (see also disturbances of newborn infants of diabetic mothers, p. 402). *Toxemia* of pregnancy is responsible for small size of the fetus for gestational age and for intrauterine death. These effects are probably due to placental insufficiency secondary to infarction. Uncontrolled *hypothyroidism* or *hyperthyroidism* in the mother is responsible for relative infertility, a tendency to abortion, premature labor and fetal death. The offspring even of treated hypothyroid mothers frequently have low intelligence quotients. Untreated maternal *phenylketonuria* results in abortion, congenital malformations and injury to the brain of the non-phenylketonuric fetus. *Placental tumors* may interfere with placental function and result in low birth weight for gestational age.

Maternal Medication and the Fetus. The effects of drugs taken by the mother vary considerably, but especially in relation to the time in pregnancy when they are taken. Abortion or congenital malformations result from maternal ingestion of teratogenic drugs during the period of organogenesis. Maternal medications taken later, especially during the last few weeks of gestation or during labor, tend to affect the function of specific organs or enzyme systems and to exert their chief adverse function on the neonate rather than on the fetus (Tables 7-3, 7-4). The teratogenic effects of drugs on the embryo may be limited to a specific period of gestation (40 to 60 days after the last menstrual period for thalidomide), and there may be genetically determined differences in susceptibility to some, if not to all, drugs. It is also conceivable that some drugs may be synergistic with others in their teratogenic effects.

In view of the limited state of current knowledge of fetal effects from maternal medication, it should be clear that no drugs should be prescribed during pregnancy without weighing the maternal need against the risk of fetal damage.

Identification of Fetal Disease (Intrauterine Diagnosis). The term "intrauterine diagnosis" is applicable to diagnostic procedures for the identification of disease in the fetus when interruption of the pregnancy is under consideration

TABLE 7-3. Maternal Medications Which May Adversely Affect the Fetus and Newborn Infant

DRUG	EFFECT ON FETUS	DEPENDABILITY OF EVIDENCE
Adrenal corticosteroids	Cleft palate	Suggestive
Aminopterin	Abortion, malformations	Conclusive
Busulfan (Myleran)	Stunted growth, corneal opacities, cleft palate, hypoplasia of ovaries, thyroid and parathyroids	Doubtful
Chlorambucil	Renal agenesis	Suggestive
Chloroquine	Deafness	Doubtful
Chlorothiazide	Thrombocytopenia	Conclusive
Cigarette smoking	Low birth weight for gestational age	Suggestive
Dicumarol	Fetal bleeding and death	Conclusive
Insulin shock	Death	Conclusive
Lysergic acid diethylamide (LSD) or impurities in commercial preparations	Skeletal defects / Chromosome damage	Doubtful / Suggestive
Meclizine (Bonine)	Congenital malformations	Doubtful
Mepivacaine	Bradycardia, death	Conclusive
Methimazole	Goiter	Conclusive
Methyltestosterone	Masculinization of female fetus	Conclusive
17-Alpha-ethinyl-19-nortestosterone (Norlutin)	Masculinization of female fetus	Conclusive

TABLE 7-3. MATERNAL MEDICATIONS WHICH MAY ADVERSELY
AFFECT THE FETUS AND NEWBORN INFANT (Continued)

DRUG	EFFECT ON FETUS	DEPENDABILITY OF EVIDENCE
Phenmetrazine (Preludin)	Defect of diaphragm	Doubtful
Potassium iodide	Goiter	Conclusive
Progesterone	Masculinization of female fetus	Suggestive
17-Alpha-ethinyl testosterone (Progestoral)	Masculinization of female fetus	Conclusive
Propylthiouracil	Goiter	Conclusive
Quinine	Abortion, thrombocytopenia	Conclusive
	Deafness	Doubtful
Radioactive iodine (I[131])	Destruction of fetal thyroid	Conclusive
Stilbestrol	Masculinization of female fetus	Suggestive
Streptomycin	Deafness	Suggestive
Tetracycline	Retarded skeletal growth	Suggestive
	Pigmentation of teeth, hypoplasia of enamel	Conclusive
	Cataract, limb malformations	Doubtful
Thalidomide	Phocomelia, other malformations	Conclusive
Tolbutamide	Congenital malformations	Doubtful
Vitamin D	Supravalvular aortic stenosis, hypercalcemia	Doubtful

in the interest of the mother or of the baby, and in instances in which direct treatment of the fetus may be possible. In a broader context it might be applied also to those aspects of the family history, reproductive history of the mother, and course of the pregnancy which lead to the nonspecific diagnoses of "high-risk pregnancy" or "high-risk infant" (p. 351).

Amniocentesis, the withdrawal of amniotic fluid during pregnancy for diagnostic purposes, is most frequently done to determine the need for fetal transfusion or the timing of delivery of fetuses with erythroblastosis fetalis (p. 1060). It is also done to determine the sex of the baby when the mother is known to carry a severe X-linked recessive trait such as hemophilia or progressive muscular dystrophy. Cells from the amniotic fluid can be stained and examined for the presence or absence of the sex chromatin (Barr) body; absence of Barr bodies in the stained nuclei indicates male sex and a child with a 50 per cent chance of having the disease in question. Cells from amniotic fluid withdrawn as early as the tenth to fourteenth weeks of gestation may be grown in tissue culture and used for chromosomal analysis as, for example, when one of the parents is the carrier of a known transmittable chromosomal abnormality. Enzyme defects involving all cells of the body, such as deficiency of glucose-6-phosphate dehydrogenase, may be identified by enzymatic analysis of cells cultured from amniotic fluid as tissue culture and microassay techniques become more sophisticated. Adrenal cortical hyperplasia has been diagnosed before birth through demonstration of higher than normal levels of pregnanetriol and 17-ketosteroids in amniotic fluid. A decrease, particularly as the

fetus nears term, in the normal 3:1 ratio of creatinine in amniotic fluid as compared to that of the maternal serum may result from diminished fetal renal function and be an indication for early delivery to prevent intrauterine death of infants of diabetic mothers.

Although amniotic puncture can be carried out with little discomfort to the mother, there is, even in experienced hands, some risk of direct damage to the fetus, of placental puncture and bleeding with secondary damage to the fetus, and of stimulating premature labor. The earlier in gestation amniotic puncture is done, the greater the risk to the fetus. Therefore the procedure should be limited to those cases in which it is estimated that the value of the findings will outweigh the risk.

Roentgenologic examination of the fetus may be useful in certain situations. Since it is desirable, however, not only for genetic reasons, but also for reasons of possible interference with the development of the fetus, to keep fetal exposure to irradiation at a minimum, roentgenologic diagnosis of the fetus should probably be used only when therapeutic action is contemplated before spontaneous delivery is expected. Skeletal abnormalities may be detected after ossification of the part has occurred; these include hydrocephalus, anencephaly, achondroplasia, infantile cortical hyperostosis, osteogenesis imperfecta, and, in addition, meconium peritonitis. The edematous thickening of the scalp in fetal hydrops may be apparent as a halo around the fetal cranium, but a more constant sign is complete or partial obliteration of the black "fat line" which normally outlines the fetal subcutaneous tissue. Other signs of edema are a froglike position of the legs and

TABLE 7-4. Maternal Medications Which May Adversely Affect the Newborn Infant

DRUG	EFFECT ON NEWBORN
Adrenal corticosteroids	Adrenocortical failure
Ammonium chloride	Acidosis (clinically inapparent)
Caudal anesthesia with mepivacaine (accidental introduction of anesthetic into scalp of baby)	Bradypnea, apnea, bradycardia, convulsions
CNS depressants (narcotics, barbiturates, tranquilizers) during labor	Central nervous system depression
Cephalothin	Positive direct Coombs test reaction
Hexamethonium bromide	Paralytic ileus
Intravenous fluids during labor, e.g. salt-free solutions	Electrolyte disturbances Hyponatremia
Lysergic acid diethylamide (LSD) or impurities in commercial preparations	Convulsions (?) Chromosome damage (?)
Morphine and its derivatives (addiction)	Withdrawal symptoms (poor feeding, vomiting, diarrhea, restlessness, yawning and stretching, dyspnea and cyanosis, fever and sweating, pallor, tremors, convulsions)
Naphthalene	Hemolytic anemia (in glucose-6-phosphate dehydrogenase [G-6-PD]-deficient infants)
Nitrofurantoin	Hemolytic anemia (in G-6-PD-deficient infants)
Primaquine	Hemolytic anemia (in G-6-PD-deficient infants)
Reserpine	Drowsiness, nasal congestion
Sulfonamides (long-acting)	Interfere with protein binding of bilirubin: kernicterus at low levels of serum bilirubin
Vitamin K (excessive amounts)	Hyperbilirubinemia

abduction of the arms. The ribs may be elevated because of enlargement of the liver and spleen.

Amniography, carried out by first withdrawing 50 to 75 ml. of amniotic fluid and then injecting a like amount of 50 per cent Hypaque or other suitable contrast medium into the amniotic sac through the same needle, is also useful. The soft tissue swelling of fetal hydrops and of myelomeningoceles may be identified, and esophageal and other upper intestinal atresias may be diagnosed by the failure of the radiopaque material to traverse the gastrointestinal tract within 12 to 24 hours after injection. Failure of the fetus to swallow contrast medium at all within this time is usually indicative of fetal death. Other *roentgenologic signs of fetal death,* in approximate order of reliability, are gas in the fetal circulatory system, fetus rolled into a ball, overriding of the cranial bones (Spalding's sign), accentuation of the lumbosacral curve in the lateral projection, and constant position of the fetal bones in serial films.

Saling has devised an endoscopic technique for obtaining blood samples from the fetal scalp or breech through a slightly dilated cervix. Measurements of fetal pH and of oxygen and carbon dioxide tension, especially during labor, may be made in this manner and be utilized to determine whether operative delivery is indicated. Saling has also used endoscopy for the detection of fetal distress by noting the appearance of meconium-staining of the amniotic fluid.

The *excretion of estriol in maternal urine* usually rises to 12 to 50 mg. per 24 hours during the third trimester of pregnancy. Values between 4 and 12 mg. per 24 hours have been interpreted as indicative of fetal jeopardy in cases of maternal diabetes, hypertension or toxemia. Values below 4 mg. have usually been associated with fetal death, particularly when such values represent a documented fall from the normal range. A high incidence of neurologic defect has been documented in one series of infants whose mothers had low (2.6 to 7.5 mg.) levels of estriol excretion. Nevertheless the use of maternal estriol excretion as a reliable index of fetal jeopardy remains to be proved. Estriol values in maternal plasma have been less than 2.6 micrograms per 100 ml. in all cases of fetal death in which they have so far been studied, but neither estriol levels nor their serial determination appears to be of value in judging fetal jeopardy.

Fetal electrocardiography has shown some promise in the diagnosis of cardiac arrhythmia and for monitoring the fetal heart rate during labor. *Pulsed ultrasound* has been used for determinations of the biparietal diameter of the fetal head as a measure of fetal growth. *Fetal phonocardiography and electroencephalography* have been performed with limited success and application.

The use of *fiberoptics* to see the fetus directly is under development. None of these diagnostic procedures has so far reached the level of simplicity, accuracy and standardization which would make them appropriate for routine clinical use.

Treatment of Fetal Disease. The successful treatment of disease in the fetus at present is more of a challenge than an accomplishment. Before it can be a reality there must be great advances in accuracy of diagnosis, in fetal pharmacology and immunology, in the availability of drugs effective against infectious (particularly viral) agents, and in diagnostic and therapeutic surgical procedures.

Syphilis provides a model for the successful treatment of a fetal disease. Involvement of the fetus is nearly universal in the presence of active, untreated maternal syphilis. Unfortunately, syphilis is virtually the only disease of the fetus the presence of which can be accurately diagnosed and that can be treated effectively, safely and inexpensively. Most infectious diseases with specific adverse effects on the fetus are of viral origin and, aside from the difficulties of diagnosis, await the development of effective and safe antiviral pharmacologic agents. Thus the main thrust in the area of combating infectious disease of the fetus is prevention through effective immunization of the mother prior to pregnancy, and this is limited to only a few diseases.

Surgical treatment of the fetus is currently limited to the management of severe erythroblastosis fetalis. Intrauterine transfusions (p. 1062) have been carried out on many infants with varying degrees of safety, depending on the skill and experience of the operators. A few intrauterine exchange transfusions have been done through blood vessels in fetal legs exposed by hysterotomy and amniotomy, or via extra-amniotic placental veins.

Maternal hyperventilation, advocated by some to treat apparent fetal distress before and during delivery, may produce an unexplained and undesirable acidosis of the fetus.

HIGH-RISK PREGNANCIES

See also The High-Risk Infant (p. 360). Pregnancies in which factors exist which increase the likelihood of abortion, fetal death, premature delivery, low birth weight, disease, congenital malformations, mental retardation or other handicapping conditions are termed high-risk pregnancies. Some of these factors, such as ingestion of a teratogenic drug in the first trimester, bear a causal relation to the risk; others, such as hydramnios, are associations which merely serve to alert the physician to the existence of the risk or risks.

The identification of high-risk pregnancies is important not only because it is the first step toward prevention, but also because in many instances therapeutic steps may be taken to reduce the risks to the fetus or to the neonate, if the physician is alerted to the increased possibility of difficulty. Identification and optimum management of high-risk pregnancies are dependent on careful attention to the family history, reproductive history of the mother, course of the pregnancy, and the delivery, *together with close and continuing personal communication between the physician caring for mother and fetus and the physician who will care for the infant after birth.*

Genetic Factors. The occurrence of chromosomal abnormalities, congenital anomalies, inborn errors of metabolism, mental retardation or indeed of any familial disease in blood relatives increases the risk of the same condition in the infant. Because many parents are not aware of the name or existence of these genetically determined diseases, but only of one or more of their manifestations, specific inquiry should be made about any disease affecting more than one blood relative. (See the following sections: Prenatal Factors in Disease; Inborn Errors of Metabolism; Jaundice in the Newborn; Metabolic Disorders; Diseases of the Blood; Mental Retardation; The Bones and Joints; The Muscles; The Skin; The Eye; Allergy; Abnormalities of the Chromosomes; and the sections on each of the systems of the body.)

Maternal Factors. The lowest neonatal mortality rate (about 2 per cent) occurs in infants of mothers 20 to 30 years of age; it is almost doubled if the mother is 40 to 45 years, and quadrupled if she is 45 or over. The neonatal mortality rate is also high if the mother is less than 15 years of age.

Maternal illness (p. 347) increases the risk to a pregnancy; the degree varies with the illness and its severity. The dangers of incompatibility between maternal and fetal blood groups are discussed on page 1060. Certain diseases in the mother may be transiently manifest in and constitute a risk to her newborn infant. Platelet antibodies may be transferred across the placental membrane to cause temporary platelet deficiency in the infant. Likewise myasthenia gravis and hyperthyroidism may be manifest for a few weeks in the infants of mothers with these diseases. Maternal hyperparathyroidism may result in tetany of the newborn. Certain drugs (Tables 7-3, 7-4) increase the risk to the pregnancy when administered to the mother during its course. Maternal toxemia, diabetes mellitus and blood group incompatibilities may increase the risk to the pregnancy by influencing obstetric management as well as through direct effects on the fetus. Lactation tends to be less successful in the toxemic woman. Prematurity, stillbirth and neonatal death are twice as frequent in infants born to toxemic mothers as in those born to healthy ones. Maternal malnutrition may lead to small size of the baby for gestational age. Multiple pregnancies, particularly those involving monochorionic twinning, are at risk when compared to single pregnancies (p. 364).

Polyhydramnios is associated with various congenital malformations (Table 7-5) and is present in approximately 80 per cent of infants with trisomy 18 (p. 332). Atresias of the upper intestinal tract presumably interfere with the reabsorption into the circulation of swallowed amniotic fluid; faulty fetal formation or release of antidiuretic hormone is postulated as the mechanism of hydramnios in fetuses with anomalies of the central nervous system. Conversely, congenital aplasia or hypoplasia of the fetal kidneys is often accompanied by a reduced amount of amniotic fluid *(oligohydramnios),* presumably because fetal urine has not been formed. Oligohydramnios from whatever cause before the last few weeks of pregnancy may result in mechanically induced abnormalities of the fetal limbs, such as genu recurvatum (p. 1353). Intrauterine amputations or other malformations due to local constriction during fetal growth may result from amniotic bands or fibrous strings, presumably formed as a result of rupture of the fetal membranes early in gestation.

Obstetric factors are of understandable importance when one considers that neonatal mortality is greatest during the first 24 hours after delivery. Rupture of membranes earlier than 24 hours before delivery carries a risk of infection of the intrauterine contents. Prolonged and difficult labors increase the risks of mechanical and hypoxic damage. The risk of neonatal deaths in uncomplicated labors lasting 24 hours or less is approximately 0.3 per cent; it increases sixfold in labors lasting over 24 hours, and to 6 per cent (twentyfold) in those over 30 hours. A tumultuous short labor, with a precipitate delivery, increases the risk of intracranial hemorrhage. Placental separation at any time prior to delivery, and abnormal implantation or compression of the cord, increase the possibility of brain damage from fetal anoxia; brown or muddy amniotic fluid at the time of rupture of the membranes or of prior endoscopic examination suggests that meconium has been passed during an episode of fetal anoxia. Likewise, the occurrence of a transient unusual increase of fetal movement suggests fetal distress due to anoxia.

Although the relative danger of any type of delivery depends upon the skill of the obstetrician, an increased hazard accompanies certain methods (Table 7-6). Obviously, this results not only from the method, but also from the circumstances which dictated its use. Neonatal deaths following deliveries by mid and high forceps, breech extraction and version are likely to be related to intracranial injury; those following other forms of delivery are more apt to be due to anoxic disturbances.

Infants born by cesarean section present problems which may be related to the unfavorable

TABLE 7-5. CONGENITAL ABNORMALITIES IN 287 INFANTS WITH MATERNAL HYDRAMNIOS

Anencephaly	59
Other central nervous system abnormalities	14
Cleft palate and harelip	8
Esophageal atresia	7
Fetal hydrops	6
Achondroplasia	5
Defects or hernia of diaphragm	4
Other	15
Total	118 (41%)

Adapted from K. A. Rahimtulla: Hydramnios in Relation to Foetal Mortality. *Arch. Dis. Childhood,* 36:418, 1961.

obstetric circumstance which necessitated the operation or to prolonged maternal anesthesia. The impression prevails, however, that even in the absence of these factors, delivery through the abdomen carries a greater risk than delivery through the birth canal. Though the neonatal mortality rate from elective cesarean section performed at term by a skilled obstetrician with an experienced anesthetist is extremely low, occasional deaths do occur. Idiopathic respiratory distress syndrome (p. 381) is the condition most frequently associated with an unfavorable outcome. Moreover, perhaps 5 per cent of infants so delivered have some degree of respiratory difficulty for a day or two after birth.

Anesthesia and analgesia affect the fetus as well as the mother. Skilled use of either consists in avoiding severe fetal narcosis while securing the benefits of gentle and unhurried delivery. Even skilled use often results in a mildly depressed infant whose crying and breathing may be delayed a minute or two and who may be somewhat inactive for several hours. Such infants are of less concern than those in whom an apparently similar status has been produced by central nervous system impairment from anoxia or trauma. When anesthesia and analgesia are carelessly used, or when their milder effects are added to already unfavorable fetal circumstances such as prematurity, anoxia or trauma, the result may be catastrophic.

TABLE 7-6. NEONATAL MORTALITY RATE PER 1000 LIVE-BORN INFANTS BY VARIOUS METHODS OF DELIVERY

Spontaneous vertex delivery	24.7
Low forceps	7.9
Mid and high forceps	29.7
Cesarean section	35.7
Breech extraction	39.6
Version and extraction	118.2
Total mortality rate by all methods of delivery	21.5

From Bundesen, Potter et al.: *J.A.M.A.,* 148:907, 1952.

THE NEWBORN INFANT

The *newborn* or *neonatal* period, the first 28 days of life, is a highly vulnerable time during which it is assumed that many of the physiological adjustments required for extrauterine existence are completed. Its importance is attested by the high morbidity and mortality rates; in the United States over two thirds of the deaths in the first year of life occur in the first 28 days after birth (Fig. 1-5, p. 5). In turn, deaths during the first year of life occur at an annual rate not again reached until the seventh decade.

The transition from intrauterine to extrauterine life requires many biochemical and physiologic changes. Removal from dependence on the maternal circulation via the placenta imposes the necessity of activation of pulmonary function for purposes of exchange of oxygen and carbon dioxide, of gastrointestinal function for absorption of food, of renal function for excretion of wastes and maintenance of chemical homeostasis, of liver function for neutralization and excretion of toxic substances, and of function of the immunologic system for protection against infection. The cardiovascular and endocrine systems also undergo adaptations necessitated by removal from maternal and placental support. Many of the special problems of the newborn infant are related to interference with or failure of these biochemical and physiologic adjustments, as by premature birth, anatomic abnormalities or adverse environmental influences, either intrauterine or arising at or after birth.

THE HISTORY IN NEONATAL PEDIATRICS

The medical history of the neonate should (1) be aimed at early identification of diseases in which disability or mortality may be prevented by prompt treatment, (2) lead to anticipation of conditions which may be of later importance, and (3) uncover possible causative factors which may help explain any pathologic condition regardless of its immediate or future significance. Ideally, a detailed family history, including the mother's current and past pregnancies, should be elicited and recorded for every newborn infant (see also High-Risk Pregnancy).

PHYSICAL EXAMINATION OF THE NEWBORN INFANT

The purposes of the initial examination of the newborn as soon as possible after delivery are twofold: to detect abnormalities and to establish a baseline for subsequent examinations. Since examination in the mother's presence affords an ideal opportunity for initiating the anticipatory guidance which should be an integral part of all periodic health examinations, a second one should be performed when she has had a chance to rest from the rigors of her labor. At this time even minor anatomic variations which seem insignificant should be explained, because the mother may be disturbed if she has to point them out or if the physician does not appear to give them adequate consideration. This procedure carries the possibility of unduly alarming otherwise unworried parents unless it is carefully and skillfully done. No infant should be discharged from the hospital without a final examination, since certain abnormalities, particularly heart murmurs, frequently appear or disappear in the immediate neonatal period, or there may be evidence of acquired disease. Pulse and respiratory rates, weight, length, head circumference, and dimensions of any visible or palpable structural abnormality should be recorded.

Many of the physical and behavioral characteristics of the newborn infant are described on page 20; that section should be consulted before reading this one.

The examination of the newborn infant requires patience, gentleness and flexibility in routines of procedure. Thus, if the infant is quiet and relaxed when first approached, palpation of the abdomen or auscultation of the heart should be performed before other, more disturbing manipulations.

General Appearance. Physical activity may be absent in the relaxation of normal sleep or depressed by illness or drugs; the infant may be lying with motionless extremities because all his energies are conserved for the effort of difficult breathing, or he may be vigorously crying with accompanying activity of arms and legs. Coarse, tremulous movements with ankle or jaw clonus are more common and of less significance in newborn infants than at any other age. Such movements tend to occur when the infant is active, whereas convulsive twitching usually occurs in an otherwise quiet state. Nutritional status is evidenced by weight and length and by wrinkling or smoothness of the body surfaces. An appearance superficially suggesting good nutrition may be produced by edema. There may or may not be pitting after pressure, but the fingers and toes will lack the normal fine wrinkles over the knuckles because they are puffed out with fluid. Edema of the eyelids is a common result of irritation from silver nitrate. Generalized edema may be an accompaniment of prematurity. It may also result from hypoproteinemia secondary to severe erythroblastosis fetalis (hydrops fetalis), congenital nephrosis, Hurler's syndrome or unknown cause. Localized edema suggests a congenital malformation of the lymphatic system; when confined to one or more extremities of a female infant, it may be the presenting sign of Turner's syndrome (p. 1231).

Skin. Vasomotor instability and sluggishness of peripheral circulation are revealed by deep redness or purple lividity in the crying infant, whose color may darken profoundly with closure of the glottis preceding a vigorous cry, and by harmless cyanosis of the hands and feet, especially when these are cool. Mottling is another example of general circulatory instability. An extraordinary division of the body from forehead to pubis into a red half and a pale half has been aptly named a *harlequin color change.* This is transient, apparently harmless, and inadequately explained. Significant cyanosis may be masked by pallor in circulatory failure; on the other hand, the relatively high hemoglobin content of the first few days and the thin skin may combine to produce an appearance of cyanosis when the arterial oxygen saturation is adequate. Localized cyanosis is differentiated from ecchymosis by the momentary pallor which follows pressure. The same maneuver is also helpful in demonstrating icterus, which may be of considerable degree, but pass unnoticed if the skin is suffused with blood. *Pallor* may represent anoxia, anemia, shock or edema. Early recognition of anemia may lead to a life-saving diagnosis of erythroblastosis fetalis, rupture of the liver, subdural hemorrhage, or fetal-maternal or inter-twin transfusion. Postmature infants tend to have whiter skin than do term or premature ones.

The vernix and lanugo hair are described elsewhere (p. 1375), as are the common transitory capillary hemangiomas of the eyelids and neck (p. 1381). Slate-blue, well demarcated areas of pigmentation are seen over the buttocks, back and sometimes other parts of the body in about half of Negro infants and occasionally in white ones. These have no known anthropologic significance in spite of their designation as *mongolian spots;* they tend to disappear within the first year. The vernix, skin and, especially, the cord may be stained a brownish yellow if the amniotic fluid has been colored by passage of meconium during or before birth, usually because of intrauterine anoxia. The skin of the premature infant is thin and delicate and tends to be deep red; in extreme degrees of prematurity the appearance is almost gelatinous. The nails are rudimentary at very premature birth; conversely, they may protrude beyond the fingertips in infants born past term. Such infants also tend to have a peeling, parchment-like skin (Fig. 7-9, p. 371); a severe degree of parchment-like skin suggests ichthyosis congenita (p. 1389).

The *skull* may be molded, particularly if the infant is the first-born and if the head has been engaged for a considerable time. The parietal bones tend to override the occipital and the frontal bones. The head of an infant born by cesarean section or from a breech presentation is identified by its characteristic roundness. The suture lines and the size and tension of the anterior and poste-

rior fontanels should be determined digitally. There is much variation in the size of the fontanels at birth; if small, the anterior fontanel usually tends to increase during the first few months of life. Soft areas *(craniotabes)* are occasionally found in the parietal bones at the vertex near the sagittal suture; they are usually inconsequential, but, if they persist, should be differentiated from other causes of craniotabes (p. 180). Soft areas in the occipital region suggest the irregular calcification and wormian bone formation associated with osteogenesis imperfecta, cleidocranial dysostosis, cretinism and occasionally Down's syndrome. Transillumination of the skull in a dark room will rule out hydranencephaly (p. 1293) or porencephaly (p. 1276).

The *face* may be asymmetric from fetal posture (p. 752), when the jaw has been held against a shoulder or an extremity during the intrauterine period, the mandible may deviate strikingly from the midline. The skull of the premature infant may suggest hydrocephalus because of the relatively larger brain growth as compared to that of other organs. The *eyes* are often opened spontaneously if the infant is held up and tipped gently forward and backward. This is undoubtedly a result of labyrinthine and neck reflexes. This maneuver is more successful than that of forcing the lids apart to inspect the eyes. Focus and equality of pupils are normally established some weeks after birth. Conjunctival and retinal hemorrhages do not by themselves have serious significance. Deformities of the pinna of the *ears* are seen occasionally. Unilateral or bilateral preauricular papillomas occur fairly frequently; if pedunculated, they can be ligated tightly at the base, and dry gangrene and slough will result. The tympanic membrane is easily visualized otoscopically through the short, straight external auditory canal and is normally dull in appearance. There may be a slight obstruction of the *nose* from an accumulation of mucus in the narrow nostrils. The *mouth* may rarely show precocious dentition, with supernumerary teeth in the lower incisor position or aberrantly placed; these teeth are shed before the deciduous ones erupt. Premature eruption of deciduous teeth is even more unusual. On the hard palate on either side of the raphe may be temporary accumulations of epithelial cells called Epstein's pearls. Retention cysts of similar appearance may also be seen on the gums. Both disappear spontaneously, usually within a few weeks of birth. Clusters of small white or yellow follicles or ulcers on an erythematous base may be found on the anterior tonsillar pillars, most frequently on the second or third day of life. Their cause is unknown, and they clear without treatment in 2 to 4 days. There is no active salivation. The *tongue* appears relatively large; the frenulum may be short, but rarely, if ever, is this a reason for cutting it. Occasionally the sublingual mucous membrane forms a prominent fold. The *cheeks* have a fullness on both the buccal and the external aspects due to the accumulation of fat which makes up the sucking pads. These pads, as well as the labial tubercle on the upper lip, disappear when the suckling days are over.

The *throat* of the newborn infant is hard to see because of the arch of the palate; this, however, should be clearly seen because of the possibility of easily missed clefts of the posterior palate or uvula. The small tonsils give no clue to the size to be attained during later lymphoid tissue growth.

The *neck* appears relatively short. Abnormalities are not common; they include goiter, cystic hygroma, branchial cleft rests and lesions of the sternocleidomastoid muscle, which are presumably traumatic (p. 1317). Redundant skin or webbing in a female infant suggests Turner's syndrome (p. 1231).

Almost as much can be learned about the *lungs* by observation of breathing as by auscultation and percussion. Variations in rate and rhythm are characteristic. The rate may vary from 20 to 100 per minute in normal infants, fluctuating according to physical activity, state of wakefulness or presence of crying. Because fluctuations are rapid, counting of the respiratory rate should be done for a full minute with the infant in the resting state, preferably asleep. Under these circumstances the usual rates for normal term infants are 30 to 40 per minute; for premature infants they are higher and fluctuate more widely. Rates which are consistently over 60 per minute during periods of regular breathing usually indicate cardiac or pulmonary insufficiency. Miller divides newborn infants into 3 groups, depending on the trend of their resting respiratory rates (Table 7-7). The premature infant may normally breathe with a Cheyne-Stokes rhythm, known as periodic respiration, or with complete irregularity. Periodic respiration is rare in the first 24 hours of life. At any stage of maturity irregular gasping, sometimes accompanied by spasmodic movements of the mouth and chin, strongly indicates serious impairment of respiratory centers. The breathing of newborn infants is almost entirely diaphragmatic, with the result that the soft front of the thorax is commonly drawn inward during inspiration and the abdomen simultaneously protruded.

If the baby is quiet, relaxed and of good color, this "paradoxical movement" is not necessarily a sign or an evidence of insufficient ventilation. On the other hand, labored respiration is important evidence of abnormal pulmonary ventilation, pneumonia or other mechanical disturbance of the lungs. The intercostal tissues are usually drawn in during inspiration when the mechanical difficulty is either too much or too little air in the lungs, so that the differentiation between atelectasis and emphysema must be made from the size and shape of the chest, the percussion note and roentgenographically. The weak groaning or whining cry which often accompanies expiration in severe disturbances of respiration is a most unfavorable prognostic sign. A method of "retraction scoring" which, along with the respiratory rate and the presence or absence of cyanosis, affords a convenient gauge of respiratory difficulty in newborn infants is illustrated in Figure 7-1. This method, which is applicable an hour or two after birth, is not be confused with the Apgar scoring system, which is used to evaluate the infant in the minutes immediately after birth.

Percussion may be more informative than auscultation, because in the small total area of the lungs breath sounds from an adjoining region may be heard as though directly under the stethoscope. Normally, the breath sounds are bronchovesicular. Suspicion of diminished breath sounds should always be verified by inducing deeper breathing and, if a local area is suspicious, altering the position of the infant's head and body before final decision. This latter maneuver also applies to suspected percussion dullness. The fine, crackling rales of early pneumonia in the newborn may at times be heard only at the end of the deep inspirations induced by crying.

The size of the *heart* is estimated with some difficulty, owing to normal variations in the size and shape of the chest. There may be transitory murmurs; conversely, congenital malformations may not at once produce the murmur which will be present later. According to Richards, there is only a 1:12 chance that a murmur heard at birth represents congenital heart disease. Evaluation

TABLE 7-7. First-Week Deaths According to Birth Weight and Respiratory Group

| RESPIRATORY GROUP | BIRTH WEIGHT — GM. | | | | | | | |
| | 1001-1500 | | 1501-2000 | | 2001-2500 | | TOTAL | |
	BORN	DIED	BORN	DIED	BORN	DIED	BORN	DIED
I	2	0	20	0	104	0	126	0
II	2	0	30	0	90	0	122	0
III	31	11	42	10	29	2	102	23

Group I: Infants who, while quiet, breathe approximately 40 times per minute from birth on without fluctuations greater than 15 per minute.

Group II: Infants whose respiratory rates are high (usually over 60 per minute) the first hour, show no significant increase after the first hour and subsequently decrease to normal levels, usually within 4 to 48 hours after birth.

Group III: Infants whose respiratory rates show a significant increase (15 per minute or more over the mean for the first hour) during the first 48 hours.

Infants with major anomalies or with hemolytic disease of the newborn were excluded.

Adapted from H. C. Miller: Studies of Respiratory Insufficiency in Newborn Infants. *Pediatrics,* 20:817, 1957.

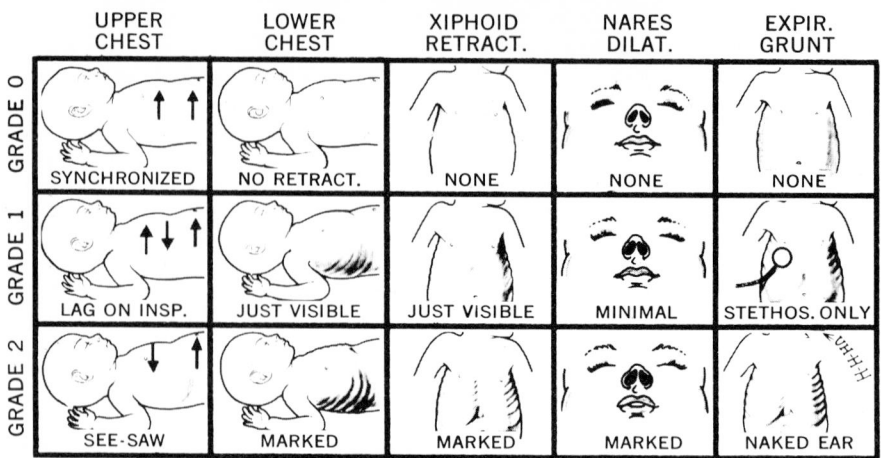

	UPPER CHEST	LOWER CHEST	XIPHOID RETRACT.	NARES DILAT.	EXPIR. GRUNT
GRADE 0	SYNCHRONIZED	NO RETRACT.	NONE	NONE	NONE
GRADE 1	LAG ON INSP.	JUST VISIBLE	JUST VISIBLE	MINIMAL	STETHOS. ONLY
GRADE 2	SEE-SAW	MARKED	MARKED	MARKED	NAKED EAR

Figure 7-1. Criteria of respiratory distress. Grade 0 for each criterion indicates no respiratory distress; grade 2 for each criterion indicates severe respiratory distress. *Abbreviations:* DILAT., dilatation; EXPIR., expiratory; INSP., inspiratory; RETRACT., retraction; STETHOS., stethoscope. (Courtesy of Mead Johnson & Company, Evansville, Ind.; adapted from Silverman and Andersen: *Pediatrics* 17:1, 1956.)

of the heart by roentgenogram and electrocardiogram is desirable when the possibility of significant lesions exists. The pulse may vary normally from 70 per minute in relaxed sleep to 180 during activity. The still higher rate of paroxysmal tachycardia may be counted better on an electrocardiogram than by ear. Premature infants, whose resting heart rate is usually 140 to 150, may have a sudden onset of sinus bradycardia, not infrequently associated with nodal escape. The rate may fall as low as 32 beats per minute. Extrasystoles also occur with some frequency, and sinus arrest with nodal escape may be observed during continuous electrocardiographic monitoring. These arrhythmias are most frequently observed during drowsiness or deep sleep, but a significant number occur during gastrointestinal stimulation (defecation, regurgitation, insertion of a rectal thermometer, insertion of a gavage tube). Many are accompanied by a "startle" reaction. Immaturity of the autonomic nervous system has been postulated as the basic reason for the occurrence of these arrhythmias; a causative relation to sudden unexpected death among premature infants has also been proposed.

Blood pressure measurements, though technically difficult, are sometimes a valuable diagnostic aid (see p. 948). The *auscultatory method* can often be used satisfactorily, provided the stethoscope head is small enough. Other methods are the *palpatory method,* in which the systolic blood pressure is taken to be the point at which the pulse distal to the cuff becomes palpable in the course of deflation, and the *flush method,* in which the extremity is first compressed to render it relatively bloodless below the cuff followed by deflation of the cuff with the systolic pressure recorded at the point flushing appears in the arm and hand below the cuff. Each has the disadvantage that the pulse pressure is not obtained and that the reading lies between the systolic and diastolic pressures obtained by the auscultatory method. Vari-

ations of the palpatory method utilize oscillometry or a loose cuff at the wrist, connected to a pulse indicator.

In the *abdomen* the liver is usually palpable, sometimes as much as 2 cm. below the rib margin. Less commonly, the spleen and kidneys may be felt. Unusual masses should be investigated immediately by "flat film" of the abdomen, followed by intravenous pyelography and exploratory laparotomy if their innocent nature cannot be established. Urinary tract anomalies, renal embryoma, ovarian cysts and intestinal duplications are the commonest masses encountered. Abdominal distention at or shortly after birth suggests perforation of the gastrointestinal tract, which is often due to meconium ileus. Later it suggests lower bowel obstruction or peritonitis. Scaphoid abdomen in the newborn suggests diaphragmatic hernia. At no period of life is the air content of the gastrointestinal tract so varied in amount, nor may it be so relatively great under normal circumstances. The abdominal wall is normally weak (especially in premature infants), and diastasis recti and umbilical hernias are common, particularly among Negro infants.

The *genitalia* and *mammary glands* normally respond to transplacentally obtained maternal hormones to produce enlargement and secretion of the breasts in both sexes and prominence of the female genitalia, often with considerable nonpurulent secretion. These are transitory manifestations requiring observation but no interference. The scrotum is relatively large; its size may be increased by the trauma of breech delivery and also by a transitory hydrocele, which is distinguished from a hernia by palpation and transillumination. The testes may be in the scrotum or palpable in the canals, or may not be felt until they descend spontaneously, which may not occur until later infancy. The male Negro infant usually has dark pigmentation of the scrotum before the rest of the skin assumes its permanent color.

TABLE 7-8. Evaluation of the Newborn Infant

SIGN	0	1	2
Heart rate	Absent	Below 100	Over 100
Respiratory effort	Absent	Slow, irregular	Good, crying
Muscle tone	Limp	Some flexion of extremities	Active motion
Response to catheter in nostril (tested after oropharynx is clear)	No response	Grimace	Cough or sneeze
Color	Blue, pale	Body pink, extremities blue	Completely pink

Sixty seconds after the complete birth of the infant (disregarding the cord and placenta) the 5 objective signs above are evaluated, and each is given a score of 0, 1 or 2. A total score of 10 indicates an infant in the best possible condition.

Modified from Virginia Apgar: *Current Researches in Anesth. & Analg.,* 32:260, 1953.

The prepuce of the newborn infant is normally so tight and adherent that no information can be obtained as to later need for circumcision. Apparent hypospadias or epispadias should always arouse suspicion of abnormality of the sex chromosomes (p. 1226) or that the infant is actually a masculinized female with enlarged clitoris, since this may be the first evidence of the adrenogenital syndrome (p. 1215). Erection of the penis is common and has no significance. Urine is usually passed during or immediately after birth; there may then normally follow a period without voiding, unusually as long as 24 hours.

Some passage of *meconium* usually occurs within the first 12 hours after birth, but may be delayed until the third or fourth day. Imperforate *anus* is not always visible and may require evidence obtained by the examiner's little finger or a rectal thermometer. The dimple or irregularity of skinfold often normally present in the sacrococcygeal midline may be mistaken for an actual or potential pilonidal sinus.

In examining the *extremities* the effects of fetal posture (p. 1351) should be noted if for no other reason than that their cause and usual transitoriness can be explained to the mother. The suspicion of a fracture or nerve injury associated with delivery is more commonly aroused by observing the extremities in spontaneous or stimulated activity than by any other means.

Neurologic Examination. See page 1267.

ORDINARY CARE OF THE NEWBORN INFANT

The basic requirements of the newborn infant are immediate assistance at birth, when needed, for the *establishment of respiration* and subsequent assistance in obtaining *adequate nutrition,* in maintaining a *normal body temperature* and in *avoiding contact with infection.* These requirements should be met in an environment which not only provides constant nursing and medical alertness for any sign of specific illness, but also reduces separation of the infant from his mother to a necessary minimum. The care of full-term and premature infants differs only in the degree of

emphasis on each of the 3 general factors listed above (see p. 367).

Care in the Delivery Room. The infant should be suspended head downward immediately after delivery until the mouth, pharynx and nose have been cleared of fluid, mucus, blood, and amniotic debris by gravity and gentle suction with a bulb syringe or soft rubber catheter. Wiping the palate and pharynx with gauze may lead to abrasions and the development of thrush, pterygoid ulcers (Bednar's aphthae) or, rarely, to tooth bud infection with maxillary osteomyelitis and retrobulbar abscess formation. If the infant appears to be in satisfactory condition, he should then be placed on his side, head downward, in a bassinet tilted at an angle of about 30 degrees to promote drainage from the respiratory tract for 4 to 8 hours. When there is a possibility of intracranial hemorrhage following difficult delivery, the reverse position may be indicated. As a guide to prognosis and the need for particularly close observation or care in the delivery room and nursery, Apgar has devised a method of scoring which is of practical value (Table 7-8). The score is a more accurate index of likelihood of death (Figs. 7-2, 7-3) or neurologic residual (Table 7-9) if it is taken at 5 minutes instead of 1 minute after delivery; *it should be taken at 1 minute as an index of asphyxia and of the need for assisted ventilation.* Infants with prolapsed cord or delayed delivery and evidence of intrauterine asphyxia should receive prompt resuscitation (p. 380). For reasons not clear, the stomachs of infants delivered by cesarean section may contain more fluid than those

TABLE 7-9. Neurologic Abnormality at 1 Year of Age, by Birth Weight and 5-Minute Apgar Score

FIVE-MINUTE APGAR SCORE	BIRTH WEIGHT		
	1001-2000 GM.	2001-2500 GM.	2501 GM. OR OVER
0-3	19%	13%	4%
4-6	14%	5%	4%
7-10	9%	4%	1%

Adapted from J. S. Drage and H. Berendes: Apgar Scores and Outcome of the Newborn. *Pediat. Clin. N. Amer.,* 13:635, 1966.

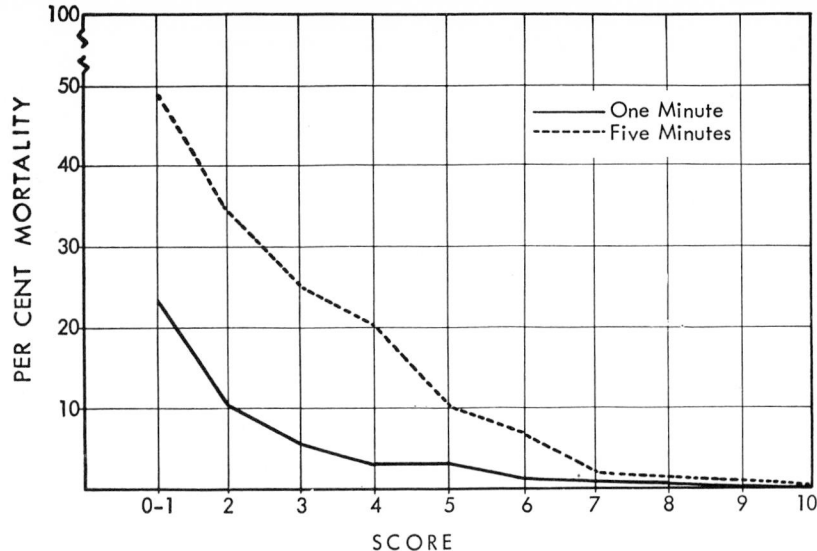

Figure 7-2. Percentage of infants with various Apgar scores dying during first 28 days of life: comparison of outcome according to scores recorded at 1 minute and at 5 minutes. (From J. S. Drage, and H. Berendes: Apgar Scores and Outcome of the Newborn. *Pediat. Clin. N. Amer.,* 13:635, 1966.)

of infants delivered normally. It is recommended that the stomach be emptied, preferably before the first breath is taken, in order to prevent possible aspiration of gastric contents.

Maintenance of body heat. Relative to body weight, the body surface of the newborn infant is approximately 3 times that of the adult, and the insulating layer of subcutaneous fat is thinner, particularly in infants with low birth weight. The rate of heat loss in the newborn is estimated to be approximately 4 times that of an adult. Under conditions usual in hospital delivery rooms skin temperature falls approximately 0.3°C. and deep body temperature approximately 0.1°C. (corre-

sponding to a heat loss of approximately 200 calories per kg.) per minute during the period immediately after delivery, resulting usually in a cumulative loss of 2° to 3°C. in deep body temperature. Oxygen consumption in the newborn infant appears to be correlated with the gradient between skin and environmental temperatures; it is least when the gradient is less than 1.5°C. Overheating of the infant increases oxygen consumption, even at slight increases in body temperature. The newborn infant also tends to have metabolic acidosis which is compensated by elimination of carbon dioxide; this compensation is more difficult for depressed infants, and progres-

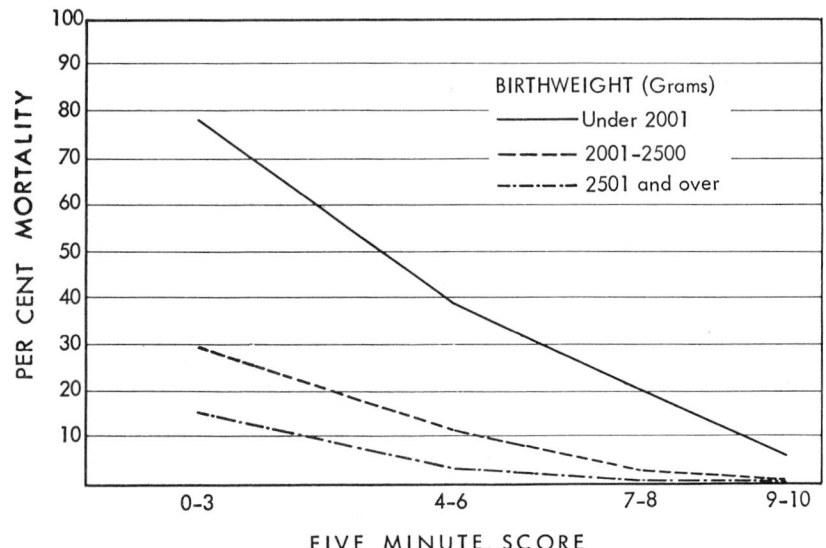

Figure 7-3. Mortality (percentage) during first 28 days of life of infants with various Apgar scores recorded at 5 minutes, arranged according to birth weight. (From J. S. Drage, and J. Berendes: Apgar Scores and Outcome of the Newborn. *Pediat. Clin. N. Amer.,* 13:635, 1966.)

sive metabolic acidosis may result from prolonged exposure to usual room temperatures. In view of these factors it is desirable to protect the infant from heat loss within seconds after birth. This is traditionally done by wrapping with blankets, a procedure which is not infrequently overlooked in the bustle of the delivery room, especially during resuscitation. Since placement of the infant in a preheated closed incubator makes it difficult to carry out resuscitative measures, an open-ended incubator or simply a heat light suspended above the bassinet for immediate reception of the baby may be used.

Antiseptic skin and cord care. In order to reduce the incidence of skin and periumbilical infection, the entire skin and cord should be cleansed in the delivery room, if possible, or upon admission to the nursery, with sterile cotton soaked in a warm detergent solution containing 3 per cent hexachlorophene, such as pHisoHex. A cotton-tipped applicator can be used to cleanse thoroughly the creases where the cord meets the umbilicus. The infant may or may not be rinsed with water at body temperature, if care is taken to avoid chilling. The baby is then wrapped in sterile blankets and taken to the nursery. To lessen the chance of carrying pathogenic organisms into the nursery, the outer blanket can be discarded at the nursery door. Subsequent daily bathing in the nursery or any other necessary washing should be done with the same cleanser, since soap or alcohol will wash away the protective coating of hexachlorophene. If detergent containing 3 per cent hexachlorophene is not available, blood or vernix should be wiped from the face (largely for esthetic reasons) after arrival in the nursery and initial and daily painting of the umbilical cord stump with a bactericidal dye (p. 406) may be used until hospital discharge in an attempt to reduce bacterial colonization.

Other measures. The *eyes* of all infants must be protected against gonorrheal infection. Although numerous methods of ophthalmic prophylaxis with sulfonamide or antibiotic preparations have been advocated, the instillation of 1 per cent silver nitrate drops remains the best-proved and only universally lawful method. Prompt subsequent irrigation of the eyes with isotonic saline solution is said to reduce the incidence of chemical conjunctivitis without affecting the prophylactic efficacy.

Though hemorrhage in the newborn (p. 396) may be due to factors other than vitamin K deficiency, an intramuscular injection of 1.0 mg. of water-soluble vitamin K_1 can be justified for all infants immediately after birth in order to correct any coagulation defect related to vitamin K deficiency and to prevent the usual neonatal decrease in plasma prothrombin level. Larger amounts may predispose to the development of hyperbilirubinemia and kernicterus and should be avoided. Administration of vitamin K to the mother during labor is less dependable.

Nursery Care. Infants not in the "high-risk" category (p. 360) may be taken after examination in the delivery room to the "regular" newborn nursery, or may be placed in the mother's room if the hospital has a rooming-in arrangement.

The bassinet should be easily and frequently cleaned and preferably be of plastic material to allow easy visibility. All care should be given in the bassinet; this includes physical examination, change of clothing, temperature-taking, skin cleansing and other procedures which, if performed elsewhere, establish a common point of contact and provide a channel for cross infection. The clothing and bedding should be the minimum needed for the infant's comfort. Maintenance of a fairly constant temperature in the nursery at approximately 75°F. will simplify problems of clothing. The temperature of the infant may be taken by rectum or, if properly done, in the axilla. The interval depends on many circumstances, but need not be less than 4 hours during the first 2 or 3 days and 8 hours thereafter. Axillary temperatures of 96° to 99°F. are considered within normal limits.

Skin care has been described above. Clothing can be put on the bathed or unbathed baby. Vernix is spontaneously shed within 2 to 3 days; much of it will adhere to the clothing, which should be completely changed daily. The diaper should be checked before and after feeding and when the baby cries. When wet or soiled, it should be changed. Meconium or feces should be cleansed from the buttocks with sterile cotton moistened with sterile water. The foreskin of the male infant should not be retracted.

Little is gained by frequent *weighing* of the healthy infant. Weighing at birth and on alternate days thereafter is sufficient, and even less frequent weighing is satisfactory for the majority of infants.

The problems of staphylococcal infections in the nursery are discussed on page 405.

Feeding. Only the initiation of feeding will be considered here (see p. 143 for other details). More mistakes are made by feeding the infant too much or too early than too little or too late. Inadequate fluid intake, particularly in hot weather, may, however, result in "dehydration fever"; feedings are customarily instituted gradually, beginning 12 to 24 hours after birth. Satisfactory progress is being made if the infant is no longer losing weight by the seventh day and is gaining by the fourteenth. Many infants are unnecessarily fed artificially merely because the physician did not acquaint the mother with the delays normally encountered in establishing breast feeding.

If the principles of feeding are understood by the mother and the nursery staff, fixed routines will have little applicability. The schedule is less important than the principle of unhurried beginning and patient assistance and instruction by the nurse who takes the infant to the mother. But since some general plan may be useful from the standpoint of the hospital, the following is suggested: During the first 12 hours after birth no feeding is given. The infant is taken to the mother for his first feeding at 10 a.m. or 6 p.m., whichever is nearer the end of the 12-hour period of postnatal rest. Subsequent feedings are given every 4 hours day and night except for the first 2 nights, when no 2 a.m. feeding is given. Artificially fed infants

should receive 5 per cent glucose or water for the first feeding, since regurgitation and aspiration of these liquids are not likely to cause significant irritation of the respiratory tract. There is no clear need for complicating neonatal care by the addition of vitamins until the infant is at least 2 weeks of age.

The High-Risk Infant

(See also High-Risk Pregnancies p. 351).

In order to improve care and to decrease neonatal morbidity and mortality, it is useful to single out those live-born infants who are at particular risk during the first few days and weeks of life. The term "high-risk infant" has come into common usage to designate infants who should be under close observation by the most interested and experienced nurses available and visited frequently by a physician until such time as complications arising from the circumstances leading to the increased risk may no longer reasonably be expected. The duration of such observation is usually a few days, but may be only a few hours or several weeks. Large institutions may find it advantageous to provide a special "high-risk nursery" for the care of high-risk infants in the hospital.

Infants considered to be in the high-risk category include those (1) born prematurely, at low or very high weight for gestational age or of multiple pregnancy; (2) delivered operatively or with any unusual obstetric complication; (3) who required resuscitation in the delivery room; (4) born to mothers with infections or with a history

of any illness during pregnancy listed on page 348, with premature rupture of the membranes, with toxemia or diabetes mellitus or other metabolic diseases, with a history of serious illness or death of previous infants during the neonatal period, with a history of drug addiction or of taking any of the medications listed in Tables 7-3 and 7-4 during pregnancy, or with hydramnios; (5) who have a single umbilical artery, or any important malformation or suspicion of one; (6) who are being observed for blood incompatibility disease; or (7) who were delivered more than 3 weeks after expected confinement.

With or without the other conditions mentioned, the majority of high-risk infants are either born prematurely or have low weight for gestational age. Generally speaking, for any given duration of gestation, the lower the birth weight, the higher the neonatal mortality; as a group the smallest infants with the shortest gestation for their birth weight have the highest neonatal mortality (Table 7-10). The highest risk of neonatal mortality is among infants who weigh less than 1000 gm. at birth and whose gestation was less than 30 weeks. The lowest risk of neonatal mortality is among

TABLE 7-10. Neonatal Mortality Rates by Birth Weight and Gestational Age, New York City, 1957-1959 (Single White Live-Born Infants)

GESTATION (WEEKS)	≤ 1000	1001- 1250	1251- 1500	1501- 1750	1751- 2000	2001- 2250	2251- 2500	2501- 3000	3001- 3500	3501+	TOTAL
0-27	944.8	800.0	615.9	305.6	147.1	219.5	111.1	73.2	41.7	83.3	674.2
28	887.3	645.6	594.3	517.2	218.8	74.1	58.8	34.5	20.0	–	400.0
29	833.3	476.9	471.7	442.3	160.7	161.3	68.2	12.0	22.2	27.8	291.0
30	862.1	526.3	474.5	407.4	383.7	137.3	39.0	25.4	–	15.2	207.1
31	772.7	518.5	362.6	274.0	375.0	179.5	73.7	16.7	4.1	20.6	166.9
32	866.7	590.9	400.0	252.3	190.3	109.9	98.7	25.2	23.7	6.1	112.6
33	800.0	294.1	509.4	287.7	142.9	102.6	92.5	16.4	5.0	4.3	70.6
34	750.0	400.0	342.1	205.9	128.3	63.6	46.7	24.5	11.4	13.6	41.6
35	777.8	333.3	285.7	250.0	107.0	57.3	28.1	20.6	10.8	13.0	28.4
36	777.8	125.0	416.7	127.7	84.1	47.3	23.8	13.8	5.0	7.7	17.1
37	714.3	333.3	474.5	156.9	91.8	56.6	18.9	9.3	5.4	9.2	12.0
38	666.7	666.7	71.4	239.1	111.1	39.0	12.2	6.0	4.1	5.0	6.7
39	500.0	400.0	277.8	303.0	68.8	37.0	19.0	4.3	3.3	3.6	4.8
40	428.6	500.0	222.2	178.6	76.3	49.0	16.0	5.8	4.0	3.1	4.7
41-42	714.3	333.3	476.2	350.0	149.1	47.9	21.1	9.6	3.6	4.0	5.7
43+	1000.0	666.7	500.0	230.8	139.5	77.8	41.3	12.3	7.6	8.0	10.4
Total	917.0	613.9	464.8	283.4	151.9	61.6	24.8	8.1	4.3	4.5	14.1

From J. Yerushalmy: The Classification of Newborn Infants by Birth Weight and Gestational Age. *J. Pediat.,* 71:164, 1967.

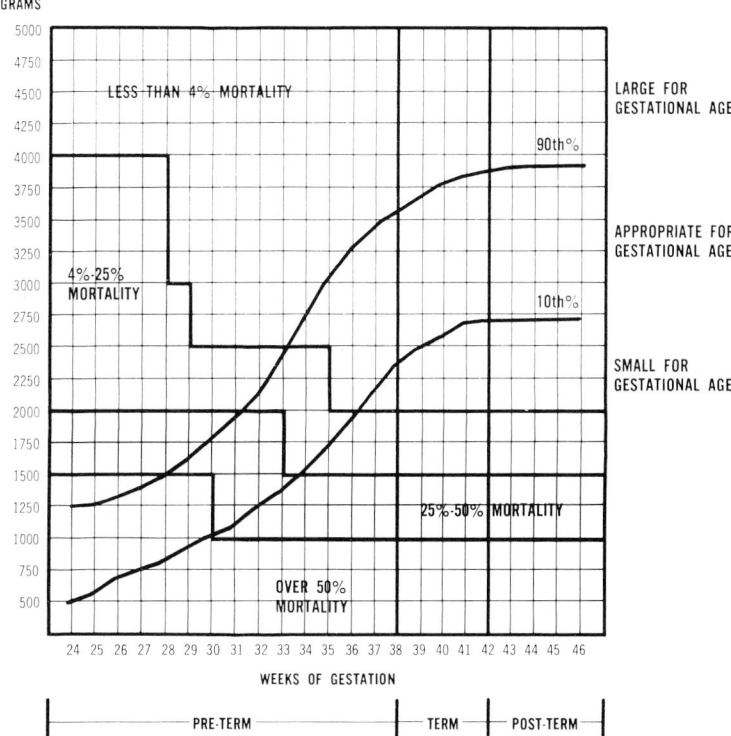

Figure 7-4. Estimated risks of neonatal mortality according to birth weight and gestational age. (From F. C. Battaglia and L. O. Lubchenco: A Practical Classification of Newborn Infants by Weight and Gestational Age. *J. Pediat.*, 71:159, 1967.)

infants with birth weights of 3000 to 4000 gm. and whose gestational age was 38 to 43 weeks. Neonatal mortality rates rise sharply for infants whose birth weight is over 5000 gm. and for those whose gestational period was 43 weeks or more.

Infants with a birth weight of 2500 to 3000 gm. and with gestational periods of 28 to 29 weeks have approximately 5 times the perinatal and neonatal mortality rate as do those of similar weights born after 37 to 39 weeks of gestation.

Figures 7-4 and 7-7 are useful for rapid identification of high-risk infants according to birth weight and gestational age.

MULTIPLE PREGNANCIES

Incidence. The reported incidence of twins is highest among Negroes and East Indians, followed by whites of northern European extraction, and lowest among the Mongolian races. In the United States twins occur in approximately 1 of 86 pregnancies; other ratios are as follows: Belgium, 1:56; United States Negroes, 1:70; United States whites, 1:88; Italy, 1:86; Greece, 1:130; Japan, 1:150; and China, 1:300. Differences in the incidence of twins exist mainly in fraternal (polyovular) twins; the frequency of identical (monovular) twins is about the same in all racial and ethnic groups. It is roughly estimated that triplets occur in 1 of 86^2 pregnancies and quadruplets in 1 of 86^3 pregnancies in the United States. Quintuplets, sextuplets and septuplets are very rare. The incidence of females increases with the number of fetal products of a multiple pregnancy, reaching approximately 53.5 per cent for quadruplets, as opposed to approximately 48.5 per cent among single births.

Causes. The occurrence of monovular twins appears to be independent of genetic or environmental influences. Such births constitute 25 to 33 per cent of twins. Polyovular pregnancies, on the other hand, are more frequent beyond the second pregnancy, in older women and in families with a history of polyovular twins. They may result from simultaneous maturation of multiple ovarian follicles, but follicles containing 2 ova have been described as a genetic trait leading to twin pregnancies. Polyovular pregnancies occur in approximately 50 per cent of women treated for infertility with human pituitary or menopausal urinary gonadotropins. Approximately 1 out of 3 such pregnancies results in twins, and 1 out of 5 in triplets or more; 1 instance of septuplets has been reported.

Monovular twinning is believed to result from a retardation of growth in the early stages of development. But since it is known that binucleated ova may occur, the possibility of "monovular" but genetically nonidentical twins from the union of 2 spermatozoa with such an ovum cannot be ruled out. Likewise twinning as the result of fertilization of a polar body as well as of the ovum cannot be excluded as a possibility. When more than 2 fetuses coexist in the uterus, each may be derived from a separate ovum, all may come from the same ovum, or they may result from combined monovular and polyovular twinning.

Conjoined twins (Siamese twins) are probably the result of relatively late monovular twinning, as is the presence of 2 embryos in one amniotic sac. The latter condition has a high fatality rate, owing to obstruction of the circulation secondary to intertwining of the umbilical cords. The prognosis for conjoined twins depends on the possibility of surgical separation.

Superfecundation, the fertilization of an ovum by an insemination which takes place after one ovum has already been fertilized, has occasionally been advanced as the cause of differences in size and appearance of twins. *Superfetation*, the fertilization and subsequent development of an ovum when a fetus is already present in the uterus, has been proposed as a reason for differences in size of certain twins at birth, but evidence to support this theory is lacking.

Monozygotic Versus Dizygotic Twins. The identification of twins as monozygotic or dizygotic (monovular or polyovular) is of importance because the study of monozygotic twins is a useful scientific tool in determining the relative influence of heredity and environment on human development and disease. It is obvious that twins who are not of the same sex are heterozygotic. Among twins of the same sex, zygosity should be determined and recorded at birth through careful examination of the placenta, or later through comparison of physical characteristics, detailed blood typing or even trial of tissue transplant from twin to twin, if the determination is of critical importance. It is desirable to furnish the parents with a written report of the results of such examinations.

Examination of the Placenta. An *accurate, carefully recorded* examination of the placenta is the simplest and best way of differentiating between monovular and polyovular twins. It may also reveal information of more immediate clinical importance.

Inspection of the placenta is carried out with knowledge of the sex and birth of the twins and with identification of the cords as belonging to twin 1 or to twin 2. If one twin is male and the other female, they are obviously dizygotic. If the placentas are separate, they are always dichorionic, but the twins are not necessarily dizygotic, since initiation of monovular twinning at the first cell division or during the morula stage may result in 2 amnions, 2 chorions, and even 2 placentas. Therefore twins of the same sex, if not monochorionic, should be re-evaluated between the ages of 2 and 4 years, when physical criteria for identification of monovular twins tend to be most valid. At this time differences caused by inequalities of intrauterine existence have been largely erased and differences created by extrauterine environmental factors have not yet become notable. If there are important physical differences by 2 to 4 years of age, dichorionic twins may be presumed to be dizygotic. If they are physically identical, detailed blood grouping studies should be carried out in an attempt to determine their zygosity.

An apparently single placenta may be present with either monovular or polyovular twins. Yet inspection of the polyovular placenta reveals for each fetus a separate chorion which crosses the placenta between the attachments of the cords. Separate or fused dichorionic placentas may be disproportionate in size. The fetus attached to the smaller placenta or portion of placenta is then usually smaller than its twin, or is malformed. Monochorionic twins may be presumed to be monovular. They are usually diamnionic. Monoamnionic twins have a high rate of stillbirth of one or both twins because of interference with one or both fetal circulations because of extensive intertwining of the umbilical cords.

Placental vascular anastomoses are seen with high frequency in monochorionic twins, and the resulting exchange of blood proteins and cells may have as much to do with later homograft tolerance between monovular twins as does their common genetic make-up. Vascular anastomoses between dichorionic twins have not been described, although the possibility may be inferred from the reported existence of blood group chimeras in heterosexual twins. The female members of such human twin pairs are reproductively competent, phenotypically normal women rather than freemartins as seen in bovine heterosexual twin pairs. Such twins also appear to tolerate reciprocal skin homografts almost as if they were autografts.

The vascular anastomoses in monochorionic placentas may be artery-to-artery, vein-to-vein or artery-to-vein. Usually they are fairly well balanced so that neither twin suffers. In rare cases one umbilical cord may arise from the other after leaving the placenta. In such instances the twin attached to the secondary cord is usually malformed or dies in utero. Table 7-11 lists the more frequent changes associated with a large uncompensated arteriovenous shunt from the placenta of one twin to that of the other (Fig. 7-5); twins of widely discrepant size are usually monochorionic.

Maternal hydramnios in a twin pregnancy should always lead to suspicion of the "fetal transfusion syndrome." Anticipation of this possibility

TABLE 7-11. Characteristic Changes in Monochorionic Twins with Uncompensated Placental Arteriovenous Shunts

	TWIN ON
ARTERIAL SIDE	VENOUS SIDE
Oligohydramnios	Polyhydramnios
Small premature	Large premature
Malnourished	Well nourished
Pale	Plethoric
Anemic	Polycythemic
Hypovolemic	Hypervolemic
Shock	Cardiac failure
Microcardia	Cardiac hypertrophy
Glomeruli small or normal	Glomeruli large
Arterioles thin-walled	Arterioles thick-walled

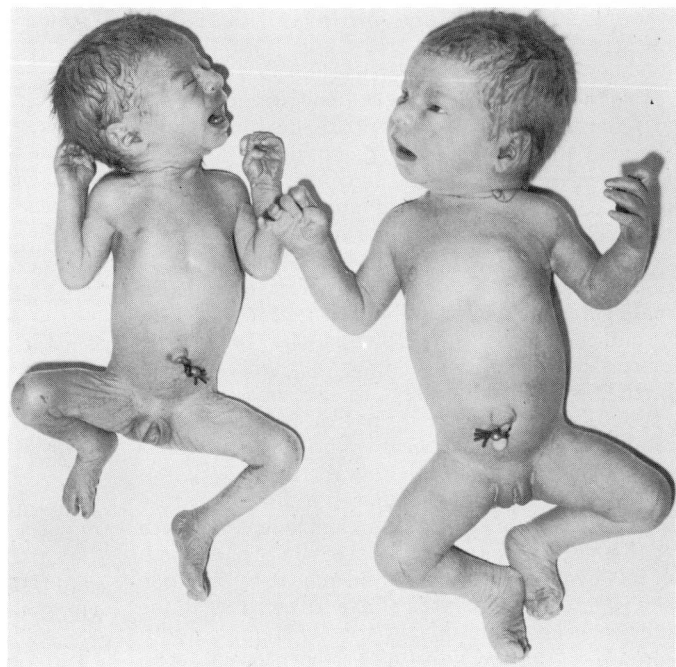

Figure 7-5. Slightly premature mono-chorionic "identical" twins at birth. Twin 1 at left weighed 3 pounds 12 ounces, and twin 2 at right weighed 5 pounds 15 ounces. Note appearance of dehydration in groin of smaller twin. (From K. Benirschke: Twin Placenta in Perinatal Mortality. *New York State J. Med.,* 61:1499-1508, 1961.)

may lead to lifesaving readiness to give a transfusion to the donor twin or to bleed the recipient twin. The additional cardiac load as evidenced by arteriolar hypertrophy (Fig. 7-6) in a distressed recipient twin suggests that digitalization might be indicated. Death of the donor twin in utero may result in generalized fibrin thrombi in the smaller arterioles of the recipient twin, possibly as the result of transfusion of thromboplastin-rich blood from the macerating donor fetus.

Postnatal Identification. *Physical criteria* for determining monovular twins are as follows: (1) both must be of the same sex; (2) their features, including ears and teeth, must be obviously alike (but they need not resemble one another more than the lateral halves of one individual); (3) their hair must be identical in color, texture, natural curl and distribution; (4) their eyes must be of the same color and shade; (5) their skin must be of the same texture and color (nevi may be differently apportioned and distributed); (6) their hands and feet must be of the same conformation and of similar size; and (7) their anthropometric values must show close agreement. Dermatoglyphics are of limited use in the diagnosis of zygosity; though prints of monozygous twins may have similar patterns, they are not identical and may be quite dissimilar.

Although *detailed blood typing* can offer absolute proof only that twins are dizygotic, with currently available methods a reasonable presumption of monozygosity may be made if no blood group discrepancies can be demonstrated between twins. Smith and Penrose calculated that in twins

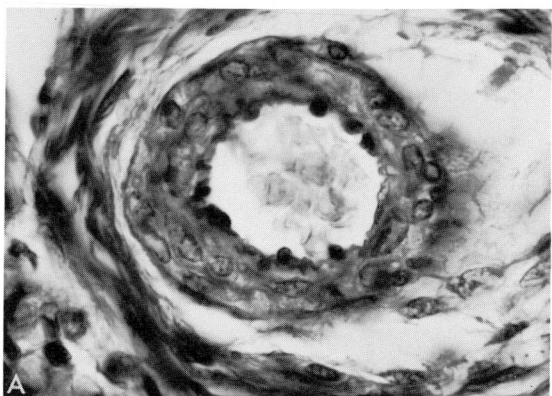
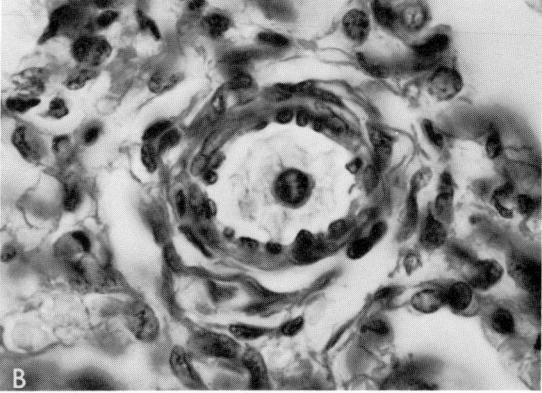

Figure 7-6. *A,* Pulmonary muscular artery from the recipient member of a newborn twin pair with the fetal transfusion syndrome. The medial muscle mass is increased for the gestational age of 29 weeks. *B,* Pulmonary muscular artery from the donor member of a newborn twin pair with the fetal transfusion syndrome. The medial muscle mass is subnormal.

who are alike in sex, and in ABO, MNSs, P, Rh, Lutheran, Kell, Lewis, Duffy and Kidd factors, the chance of dizygosity is 0.0116.

Prognosis. Most twins are born prematurely, and maternal complications of pregnancy are more common than with single pregnancies. There is no significant difference between the neonatal mortality rates of twin and single births in comparable weight groups. Yet since most twins are premature by weight, their overall mortality is higher than that of single births. The incidence of malformations incompatible with life is greater in multiple than in single pregnancies. In general, mortality rates of twins do not vary with order of birth if macerated fetuses are excluded. If one of the fetuses is macerated, the live twin is usually delivered first. Theoretically, the second twin is more subject to anoxia than is the first because of the possibility that the placenta may separate after the birth of the first twin and before the birth of the second. Notable differences in size at birth of monovular twins usually disappear by the time the infants are 6 months of age. In contrast to the aforementioned lack of statistically significant difference in the mortality of live-born twins when compared with live-born single births in comparable weight groups, Benirschke has shown (Table 7-12) that there appears to be a significant increase in perinatal mortality among monochorionic twins.

Management. The obstetrician and the pediatrician should be alert, particularly in hydramniotic twin pregnancies, to the possibility of the "fetal transfusion syndrome." One should be prepared to perform an immediate blood transfusion on a severely anemic "donor twin." Decisions of whether to bleed or digitalize the "recipient twin" must be based on clinical judgment.

TABLE 7-12. PERINATAL MORTALITY OF TWINS ACCORDING TO PLACENTATION

TYPE	BABIES	DEATHS	%
Monoamnionic-monochorionic	6	3	50
Diamnionic-monochorionic	120	28	23
Diamnionic-dichorionic, fused	126	6	5
Diamnionic-dichorionic, separated...	148	14	9
Total monochorionic	126	31	25
Total dichorionic	274	20	7

Adapted from K. Benirschke: Twin Placenta in Perinatal Mortality. *New York State J. Med.,* 61:1499, 1961.

PREMATURITY AND LOW BIRTH WEIGHT

Definition. Live-born* infants delivered before 37 weeks from the first day of the last menstrual period are considered to have a shortened gestational period and are termed *premature.* Infants who weigh 2500 gm. or less at birth are considered to have had either a shortened gestational period, a less than expected rate of intrauterine growth, or both, and are termed *infants of low birth weight.* Prematurity and low birth weight are usually concomitant, particularly among infants weighing 1500 gm. or less at birth, and both are associated with increased neonatal morbidity and mortality.

*Live birth is defined by the World Health Assembly (1950) as "the complete expulsion or extraction from its mother of a product of conception . . . which, after such separation, breathes or shows any other evidence of life such as beating of the heart, pulsation of the umbilical cord, or definite movement of the voluntary muscles, whether or not the umbilical cord has been cut or the placenta is attached." This definition is approved by the American Public Health Association.

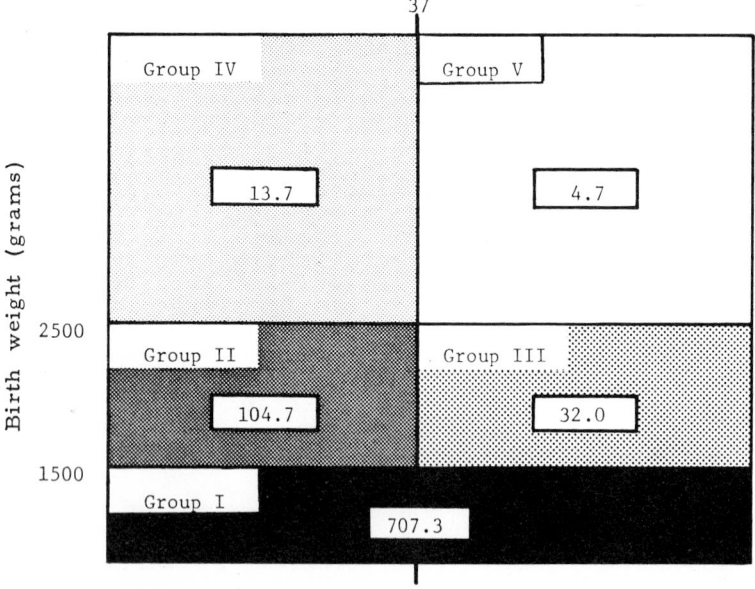

Figure 7-7. Graphic presentation of the division of newborn infants in 5 groups by birth weight and gestational age, and the neonatal mortality rate in each group (based on data for a 3-year period in New York City). (From J. Yerushalmy: The Classification of Newborn Infants by Birth Weight and Gestational Age. *J. Pediat.,* 71:164, 1967.)

TABLE 7-13. Percentage Distribution of Live Births by Birth Weight Group and Color, United States, 1965

	500 GM. OR LESS	501-1000	1001-1500	1501-2000	2001-2500	2501-3000	3001-3500	3501-4000	4001-4500	4501-5000	OVER 5000 GM.
White	0.1	0.4	0.6	1.3	4.8	18.3	38.5	27.1	7.4	1.3	0.2
Nonwhite	0.2	0.9	1.2	2.7	8.8	26.2	37.3	17.8	3.9	0.9	0.1
Total	0.1	0.5	0.7	1.6	5.5	19.6	38.3	25.6	6.8	1.2	0.2

From U.S. Vital Statistics: Natality, 1965.

Since the length of the normal gestational period is essentially the same for all human populations, the foregoing definition of prematurity is considered to be universally applicable. Yet the range of birth weights of infants born at term varies from one population group to another. Hence, ideally the definition of low birth weight would be set for individual populations which are genetically and environmentally as homogeneous as possible.

History. For statistical purposes in the United States, since 1935, a premature infant has been defined as a liveborn infant weighing 2500 gm. (5 pounds 8 ounces) or less at birth. This definition was also adopted by the World Health Organization in 1950, but its Expert Committee on Maternal and Child Health in 1961 recommended that the term "premature" be replaced by the more appropriate term "low birth weight" and that the term "premature" be used only for infants born less than 37 weeks after the beginning of the mother's last menstrual period. The American Academy of Pediatrics has adopted these recommendations.

Since most of the statistical data of the last 30 years have not related low birth weight to gestational age, many concepts about "prematurity" may have to be changed as statistics based on this relationship are evaluated. Figures 7-4 and 7-7 and Table 7-10 indicate observed variations in neonatal mortality based on birth weight in respect to gestational age.

Incidence of Prematurity. Because statistical emphasis on gestational age as well as on birth weight is recent, the incidence of prematurity (short gestation) has not been adequately determined. Nevertheless in a largely Caucasian population with a 6.7 per cent incidence of low-birth-weight infants (1000 to 2500 gm.), Usher found that approximately half of the low-birth-weight infants had a gestational age of 37 weeks or more. About 4 per cent of the infants who weighed over 2500 gm. had gestational ages less than 37 weeks, and the number of premature births among the larger infants was greater than in the low-weight group.

Incidence of Low Birth Weight. In the United States (1965) 7.2 per cent of white live-born infants and nearly 14 per cent of nonwhite ones weighed 2500 gm. or less (Table 7-13); the incidence varies from 6 to 16 per cent in different areas and populations. Since such variability exists throughout the

world (Table 7-14), it will be necessary to develop for individual countries and population groups correlation of birth weight and gestational age with risks of neonatal morbidity and mortality. Black, Indian and other South Asian infants tend to weigh less at birth than white and North Asian infants of the same gestational ages; the incidence of birth weight of 2500 gm. or less is greater among blacks than among whites in the United States. The perinatal and neonatal mortality rates in each low-weight group, however, are lower for black infants than for white ones.

Factors Related to Premature Birth or Low Birth Weight. Because of failure until recently to record both gestational age and low birth weight in the compilation of birth statistics, it is rarely possible to separate factors associated with prematurity from those associated with low birth weight. Even reports in which some attempt has been made to consider both gestational age and low birth weight have exhibited a confusing tendency to use the terms "prematurity" and "low birth weight" synonymously.

In general, *premature birth* is associated with conditions in which there is inability of the uterus to retain the fetus, artificial interference with the course of the pregnancy, premature separation of the placenta, or a stimulus to effective uterine contractions prior to term. *Low birth weight for*

TABLE 7-14. Comparative Percentages of Infants Weighing Less than 2500 Grams Among Live Births in Various Populations

POPULATION	PER CENT WEIGHING LESS THAN 2500 GM.
Netherlands	3.5
Denmark	4.6
New Zealand	5.6
Norway	5.7
United States (white)	7.2
Bantu (South Africa)	11.6
United States (nonwhite)	13.8
Indian (South Africa)	18.3
Indian (Calcutta)	34.7

From L. J. Verhoestrate and R. R. Puffer: Challenge of Fetal Loss, Prematurity and Infant Mortality—World View. *J.A.M.A.*, 167:950, 1958; U.S. Vital Statistics, 1965; and others. (This table is a composite. Data for the United States are for the year 1965, others chiefly from figures gathered in the early 1950's. Despite some variations in the reporting of live births, the basic comparisons seem valid.)

gestational age is associated with conditions which interfere with the circulation and efficiency of the placenta, with the development or growth of the fetus, or with the general health and nutrition of the mother.

There is a positive correlation of both premature birth and low birth weight with low socioeconomic status. In such families there are relatively high incidences of maternal undernutrition, anemia and illness, inadequate prenatal care, obstetrical complications, and maternal histories of reproductive inefficiency (relative infertility, abortions, stillbirths, premature or low-weight infants). Other, less clearly associated factors such as illegitimacy, working mothers and mothers who have borne more than 4 previous children are also encountered more frequently in families living in poor economic conditions. Owing to the difficulties in assigning cause and effect in most instances of premature birth or of low birth weight at present, it would seem logical in planning studies to determine causes of them to approach the problems in population groups of low economic status through evaluation of general health measures such as nutrition, infection, housing, overwork, fatigue and family planning. By contrast, such studies in population groups of better socioeconomic status in which the incidence of low-birth-weight infants is relatively low (5 to 6 per cent) would be directed at the presumed specific causes of reproductive inefficiency which appear to exist in spite of good general health measures.

Assessment of Gestational Age at Birth. Certain physical and neurologic signs may be useful in estimating gestational age at birth. Until 36 weeks of gestation there are only 1 or 2 transverse skin *creases on the sole of the foot* anteriorly. By 37 or 38 weeks more creases have appeared, and by 40 weeks there is a complex series of crisscrossed creases covering the entire sole. The *size of the breast nodule* correlates generally with gestational age. It is usually not palpable at 33 weeks, is usually not over 3 mm. in diameter at 36 weeks, and is usually 4 to 10 mm. in term infants. The scalp hair tends to be short and fuzzy up to 37 weeks, but to consist mainly of silky strands by 40 weeks. The *cartilaginous development of the ear lobe* which makes the folds of the helix and antihelix stand out occurs chiefly between 36 and 40 weeks. At 36 weeks the testes are usually not completely descended, and the scrotal rugae are limited to the anterior and inferior aspects of the scrotum; by 40 weeks the testes are usually descended, and rugae cover the entire scrotal surface. Table 7-15 lists some measures for neurologic assessment of fetal age.

Pathology in Low-Birth-Weight Infants. Neonatal deaths among premature and term infants result from the same general group of pathologic disturbances (Table 7-2), the principal differences being in the distribution of the causes of death. When the cause of death is sought by careful macroscopic postmortem examination, it is found in a high percentage of instances. Prematurity itself should not be considered a cause of death in an infant born alive. The principal causes of death among premature as well as term infants are anoxia, birth injuries (principally cerebral), malformations, idiopathic respiratory distress syndrome ("hyaline membrane disease"), bronchopneumonia, septicemia and other infections.

Pulmonary hyaline membranes associated with "resorption atelectasis" are found at autopsy in 40 to 50 per cent of low-birth-weight infants dying 1 hour to 4 days after birth, and rarely in larger infants born at or near term except those delivered by cesarean section or born to diabetic mothers.

Hemorrhage (see p. 396), whether associated with trauma, anoxia, infection, or defect of clotting mechanism, is frequent and often severe. Subcutaneous ecchymoses, bleeding into the choroid plexus, and subependymal and intraventricular hemorrhages are frequent in premature infants and are presumably due to "increased capillary fragility." Sudden shock and collapse during the first few days of life are often due to intraventricular hemorrhage. Fatal hemorrhage into the lungs may also occur without clear cause.

Retrolental fibroplasia (see p. 1425) is a retinopathy of premature infants which results from too great an exposure to atmospheres with increased oxygen content. Before this effect of oxygen administration was appreciated, partial or complete blindness was reported in 5 to 25 per cent of surviving infants whose birth weights were below 4 pounds (1800 gm.); the condition has replaced

TABLE 7-15. REFLEXES OF VALUE IN ASSESSING GESTATIONAL AGE

REFLEX	STIMULUS	POSITIVE RESPONSE	WEEKS OF GESTATION IF REFLEX IS	
			ABSENT	PRESENT
Pupil reaction	Light	Pupil contraction	< 31	29 or more
Glabellar tap	Tap on glabella	Blink	< 34	32 or more
Head-turning	Diffuse light from one side	Head-turning to light	Doubtful	32 or more
Traction	Pull up by wrists from supine	Flexion of neck or arms	< 36	33 or more
Neck-righting	Rotation of head	Trunk follows	< 37	34 or more

Note: Time measured is from the first day of the last menstrual period. If there is a conflict between 2 results, the reflex placed higher in the Table is more likely to give the true gestational age.
Adapted from R. J. Robinson: Assessment of Gestational Age by Neurological Examination. *Arch. Dis. Childhood,* 41:437, 1966.

gonococcal ophthalmia as the commonest cause of blindness in children. The practice of administering oxygen only in such amounts and at such times as are absolutely necessary for relief of respiratory distress and cyanosis has nearly but not completely eradicated the disease.

Kernicterus associated with hyperbilirubinemia (see p. 1278) is seen in 2 to 20 per cent of autopsies of premature infants. Incidences of kernicterus approaching the latter figure are probably the result of procedures used locally in the care of premature infants, such as administration of large amounts of vitamin K analogues to mothers in labor or to newborn infants, and use of sulfisoxazole as chemoprophylaxis (see p. 395).

Immaturity, as a measure of the relative inability of the premature infant to survive, is a reflection of inadequately developed anatomic, physiologic and biochemical functions. Deficiencies in these functions affect the infant's ability to withstand demands that do not exist for him in the protective environment of intrauterine life, such as control of body heat, pulmonary function, nutrition, disposal of metabolic waste, immunologic function, and detoxification and excretion of toxic substances. The shorter the period of gestation, the more likely is the infant to be unprepared to meet the rigors of extrauterine life. Though general immaturity may not permit survival in some very small newborn infants, it is desirable that it not be considered a cause of death. To do so at this time carries the risk of detracting from a careful search for explicit causes of all prenatal and postnatal deaths. When cause of death is not identified, it should be listed as *undetermined* (see Table 7-2).

Naeye has described 2 groups of infants of low birth weight for gestational age on the basis of pathologic observations.

One group has anatomic changes similar to those found in infants with postnatal alimentary malnutrition: diminished subcutaneous fat and small organs, particularly the adrenals, liver, spleen and thymus. The small size of organs is due chiefly to a subnormal amount of cytoplasm in individual cells rather than to a diminished number of cells. The adrenal cortex is reduced in size relatively more than the medulla, and the exocrine part of the pancreas more than the endocrine part. Naeye postulates the possibility of a deficiency of production of the adrenal corticosteroids which facilitate gluconeogenesis, as well as the possibility of relative hyperinsulinism. The reduced cytoplasmic mass of individual cells also suggests the possibility that deficient antenatal storage of glycogen may contribute to the neonatal hypoglycemia to which these infants are prone. This group of infants with apparent fetal malnutrition includes infants of toxemic mothers, multiple pregnancies and prolonged pregnancies, or with placental abnormalities which might interfere with intrauterine nutrition.

The other group of infants of low birth weight for gestational age has a reduced number of cells in various body organs, but with a normal amount of cytoplasm per cell. This "hypoplastic" group includes infants with chromosomal abnormalities, congenital heart disease (except transposition of the great arteries), congenital rubella, and cytomegalovirus infection.

Complications. Infants with intrauterine malnutrition, especially males, tend to have significant and symptomatic neonatal hypoglycemia (p. 403). There is also an increased incidence of neonatal respiratory distress, particularly in infants born with meconium-stained amniotic fluid, in whom it is presumably secondary to aspiration of meconium. Infants with cellular hypoplasia are subject to the neonatal and later problems to which the associated pathologic conditions predispose them.

Care. At birth the same measures for clearing of airway, initiation of breathing, and care of the cord and of the eyes are required as for infants of normal birth weight or maturity. Additional considerations are (1) need for incubator care, (2) need for increased oxygen, and (3) details of feeding. Safeguards against infection and against careless or inefficient nursing can never be relaxed. Finally, the need of instructing the mother for the care at home and the question of prognosis for later growth and development require special consideration.

Incubator care. Modern incubators conserve body heat through provision of a warm atmospheric environment and standard conditions of humidity. They also provide a regulated oxygen supply and reduced atmospheric contamination. The latter aim is accomplished only if they are scrupulously cleaned. On the basis of current experience the optimal incubator temperature is that which will maintain the axillary temperature of the infant at approximately 36°C. or 96.8°F. This is usually an air temperature of approximately 31.7°C. (89°F.) for infants over 1000 gm., but may be higher for smaller infants. Maintenance of a relative humidity between 60 and 70 per cent aids in keeping the body temperature up and stable as well as in preventing the drying effect of low atmospheric humidity on the linings of the respiratory passages. It also serves to reduce the irritant effect of administered oxygen. Supersaturation of the atmosphere of the incubator to create a mist reduces insensible water loss from the lungs, but it has not been shown to affect favorably the prognosis of the infant, nor has the addition of surface-tension-reducing agents to the nebulized water.

Owing to the risk of retrolental fibroplasia, the use of increased atmospheric oxygen as a general supportive measure should be avoided. Oxygen should be used only when there are such definite indications as cyanosis or dyspnea. The atmospheric concentration of oxygen should be kept at the lowest level providing adequate relief for the infant, and its administration should be discontinued as soon as possible. The practice of limiting the atmospheric concentration of oxygen delivered to anoxic infants to an empiric maximum may be undesirable, since the incidence of retrolental fibroplasia is most likely related to the pO$_2$ of the baby's blood rather than to the atmospheric concentration of oxygen.

If an incubator is not available, the general conditions of temperature and humidity control outlined above can be attained by the intelligent use of blankets and warm water bottles and by control of the temperature and humidity of the room.

The infant should be removed from the incubator only when the gradual change to the atmosphere of the nursery is not accompanied by a significant change of his temperature, color or activity. The removal may be only a day or two after birth for some infants, or at more than a month of age for less mature ones.

Feeding. There is a variety of techniques for the feeding of premature infants. There is general agreement on the importance of avoiding fatigue and the aspiration of food during feeding or by regurgitation. No method of feeding will avoid these risks unless the person using it has been well trained in the process.

Large premature infants can often be fed by bottle or at the breast. Since the effort of sucking is usually the limiting factor, breast feeding is least likely to be successful. In bottle feeding, effort may be reduced by use of special small, soft nipples with large holes. Infants as small as 3 pounds at birth are occasionally vigorous enough for bottle feedings. Smaller or less vigorous infants should be fed by gavage; a soft plastic tube of no. 5 French external and approximately 0.05 cm. internal diameters with a rounded atraumatic tip and 2 holes on alternate sides is preferable. The tube is passed through the nose until approximately 1 inch of the lower end should be in the stomach. The free end of the tube is then placed under water. If bubbles appear with each expiration, the catheter is in the trachea and must be reinserted into the proper position. The free end of the tube has an adapter into which the tip of a glass syringe is fitted, and the measured amount of feeding is allowed to flow in by gravity. Such tubes may be left in place for 3 to 7 days before replacement by a similar tube through the alternate nostril. The tubes may be cleaned, sterilized and reused, but are usually discarded after one use. An occasional infant has enough local irritation from an indwelling tube that troublesome secretions gather around it in the nasopharynx. In such instances a sterile no. 10 French catheter may be passed through the mouth by a skilled person and removed at the end of each feeding. Change to bottle or breast feeding may be instituted gradually as soon as the infant displays general vigor adequate for oral feeding without fatigue.

The so-called Breck feeder, with which food is forced into the infant's mouth, is unsafe. Premature infants can be fed successfully and safely with a rubber-tipped medicine dropper by a nurse skilled in the procedure.

The value of gastrostomy as an adjunct to the feeding of premature infants is not established.

Initiation of feeding. The main principle in the feeding of premature infants is to proceed cautiously and gradually. Comparative inactivity, low heat production if body heat is artificially conserved, and, perhaps, relatively large body water content at birth all reduce the immediate need for calories, water and electrolytes. Proponents of "late" feeding point to an increased mortality rate due to aspiration of vomitus among premature infants fed a milk formula within 8 hours of birth, but others have shown that early feeding of glucose or saline solutions tends to reduce the incidence of hypoglycemia and hyperbilirubinemia without added risk, provided the presence of respiratory distress or other disorder is considered an indication for withholding oral feedings and administering electrolytes, fluids and calories intravenously.

As soon as the infant has recovered from the stress of delivery and appears active and in no distress, oral feedings may be instituted. This interval is usually 2 to 12 hours, but may be 5 to 7 days in sick infants who will require intravenous feeding in this interim. If the infant is vigorous and making sucking movements, oral feeding may be attempted, though most infants under 1500 gm. and many larger ones require tube feeding. A suggested schedule is to begin with 1.0 ml. of a sterile solution of 5 per cent glucose in water for infants under 1000 gm.; 4 ml. for infants between 1000 and 1500 gm.; and 8 ml. for infants over 1500 gm. If the beginning amount is 1 ml., feedings may be given hourly for the first 8 hours, increasing the amount by 1 ml. at every other feeding. Feedings may then be given every 2 hours, with an increment of 2 ml. at every other feeding until 12 ml. is reached. This amount may be continued every 2 to 3 hours for 24 to 48 hours, at which time a mixture of 8 ml. of 5 per cent glucose in water and 4 ml. of a half-skim milk formula containing 0.67 calorie per ml. (20 calories per ounce) may be substituted for 2 feedings, then 4 ml. of 5 per cent glucose in water and 8 ml. of formula for 2 feedings, and then the full-strength formula. Amounts of formula may then be gradually increased so that the intake is approximately 150 ml. per kg. per 24 hours. If the infant still seems hungry or fails to gain weight, the amounts should be further increased. Certain infants with small gastric capacities fail to gain on tolerated amounts of formula containing 0.67 calorie per ml. In such instances more frequent feedings may be given in order to increase the total daily intake, or the caloric content may be increased to as high as 1 calorie per ml. (30 calories per ounce).

To infants of 1000 to 1500 gm. the glucose and water feedings may be given every 2 to 3 hours with 4-ml. increments at every other feeding until feedings of 16 ml. are reached, at which point formula may be gradually substituted. With infants over 1500 gm. the interval may be 3 to 4 hours with 8-ml. increments up to 32 ml., at which point formula is substituted gradually.

The occurrence of regurgitation or vomiting in the early stages of the feeding schedule should arouse suspicion of intestinal obstruction; later it is an indication to drop back in the schedule and increase subsequent feedings slowly. Gain in weight may not be achieved for 10 or 12 days, and a daily intake as high as 130 to 150 calories per kg. may be necessary for some infants.

When tube feeding is used, the contents of the stomach should be aspirated before each feeding. If only air or small amounts of mucus are obtained, the feeding is given as planned. If any of the previous feeding is obtained, it is a signal to reduce the amount of the feeding and to proceed more gradually with subsequent increases.

The digestive enzyme systems of premature infants seem to be mature enough to permit efficient absorption of protein and carbohydrate. Fat is less well absorbed; unsaturated fats and the fat of human milk are absorbed better than that of cow's milk. Weight gain of infants weighing 1500 gm. or more at birth is adequate with a protein intake of 2 gm. per kg., but some smaller infants require more; Levine and Gordon have shown that better weight gain can be achieved with formulas made with half-skim milk than with human milk, which has a higher fat and lower protein and mineral content. Nitrogen retention of premature infants can be increased by feeding large amounts of protein. The high protein and mineral contents of balanced cow's milk formulas of high caloric content, however, constitute an extra excretory load for the kidney, a fact which at least has importance in the maintenance of water balance in the infant with diarrhea or fever. The exact importance to the premature or term infant of the secretory immunoglobulins contained in human milk remains to be evaluated.

There is need for an increased intake of vitamins C and D. Intermediary metabolism of phenylalanine and tyrosine is incomplete unless ascorbic acid is provided. Moreover, any tendency to loss of fecal fat involves loss of fat-soluble vitamins and calcium. Approximately 50 mg. of ascorbic acid and 1000 I.U. of vitamin D daily begun during the second and third weeks, respectively, appear to be ample. Since intakes of vitamin D in excess of 1500 I.U. per day may cause the syndrome of idiopathic hypercalcemia in certain infants (p. 1369), the total intake of vitamin D from all sources should not exceed that amount. Supplementation with other vitamins has not been shown to be necessary, though anemia may develop in premature infants severely deficient in vitamin E. The addition of iron to the diet is discussed on page 1050.

The properly fed premature infant may have from 1 to 6 stools of semisolid consistency daily; sudden increase in number or a change to a watery consistency is reason for more concern than any arbitrarily stated frequency. He should not vomit or regurgitate. He should be satisfied and relaxed after a feeding, but may normally show the activity of hunger shortly before the next one.

Prevention of Infection. Prevention is accomplished by safeguarding the infant's food and the few objects which come in contact with him, reducing his direct and indirect contacts with nursery personnel (including other infants) and preventing contamination of the air he breathes. No one with an infection has a responsibility toward a premature nursery as essential as staying out of it. Gowns, caps, masks and hand-scrubbing techniques do not guarantee safety of the infant if an infected person enters the nursery.

Prevention of transmission of infection from infant to infant is difficult because frequently neither term nor premature newborn infants manifest clear clinical evidence of infection. If the unit admits infants born outside the hospital, it should be assumed that they are infected until a week or more of observation in a special nursery or an incubator with an individual air supply proves otherwise.

Perhaps the most important factor in the successful care of premature infants is the skill, experience and number of the *nursing* staff. It is the responsibility of the physician to insist upon expert nursing.

General Considerations of Disease. Prematurity tends to increase the severity and to reduce the clinical manifestations of all neonatal diseases. Subcutaneous and intracranial hemorrhage, "primary" atelectasis, respiratory distress syndrome, pneumonia, bacteremia, hypoglycemia and hyperbilirubinemia occur more frequently among premature than among term infants. Retrolental fibroplasia is seen almost exclusively in premature infants.

Drugs. Renal clearances for almost all substances excreted in the urine are diminished in

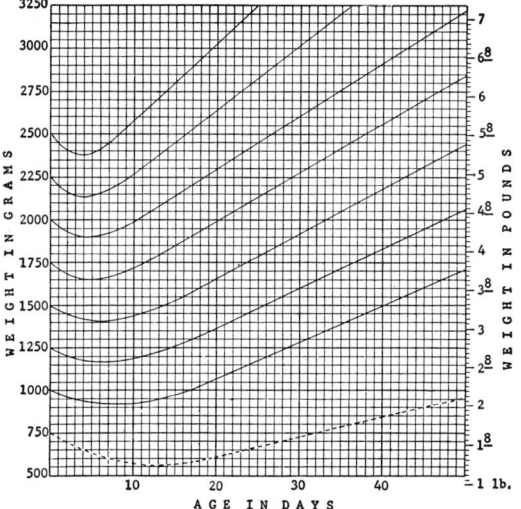

Figure 7-8. Grid for recording weights of premature infants. The average weight increments are indicated on the basis of weight at birth. (J. Dancis et al.: *J. Pediat.,* Vol. 33.)

all newborn infants, and perhaps more so in premature ones. Half or less of the customary dose of any drug excreted chiefly by the kidney is usually adequate to maintain a therapeutic level, even when given at longer than the customary interval between doses. For instance, highly satisfactory levels of penicillin and streptomycin are maintained on doses given at 12-hour intervals. Drugs detoxified in the liver or requiring chemical conjugation before renal excretion should also be given with caution and in smaller than usual doses. Intramuscularly administered broad-spectrum antibiotics are absorbed less well than penicillin and streptomycin, presumably owing to the severity of local tissue reaction and to relative circulatory inadequacy. Broad-spectrum antibiotics are also poorly absorbed from the intestinal tract unless administered in dilute form. Decision as to the administration of antibacterial agents to possibly infected infants should be made on an individual rather than on a routine basis, owing to the dangers of (1) development of infections with organisms resistant to antibacterial agents, (2) destruction or inhibition of intestinal bacteria which manufacture significant amounts of essential vitamins (e.g. vitamin K and thiamine), and (3) possible deleterious interference in important metabolic processes (e.g. the role of sulfisoxazole in hyperbilirubinemia).

Since pure food and drug laws and regulations are based on toxicity studies on adult animals and human beings, apparently "safe" drugs may not be so for newborn infants, especially premature ones. Oxygen, vitamin K analogues, sulfisoxazole (Gantrisin), chloramphenicol and novobiocin, all presumably "safe" drugs, have proved to be toxic to newborn premature infants in amounts not harmful to term infants. Thus administration of any drug to newborn infants, particularly in large doses, should be done with care and with risk weighed against potential benefit.

Gamma globulin levels of premature infants at birth are significantly lower than those of their mothers at the time of delivery or those of term infants; since they undergo the usual "physiologic" decrease during the first months of life, the routine administration of gamma globulin on discharge from the hospital and at intervals during the first year of life has been advocated as a prophylactic measure. No adequate evaluation of this procedure is available.

Prognosis. Neonatal mortality rates for low-birth-weight infants are shown in Figures 7-4 and 7-10, and causes of death in Table 7-2. The mortality rate of low-birth-weight infants who survive to be discharged from the hospital is approximately 3 times that of full-term infants during the first 2 years of life. Many of these deaths are attributable to infection and are, therefore, at least theoretically preventable.

Congenital anatomic anomalies are present in approximately 25 per cent of live-born infants with birth weights less than 1500 gm., in approximately 12 per cent with birth weights between 1500 and 2500 gm., but in only 6 per cent with birth weights of 2500 gm. or more. They are more common among low-birth-weight infants who are small for gestational age than among those whose weight is appropriate for gestational age.

In the absence of congenital abnormalities, physical growth tends to overtake that of term infants during the second year; this occurs earlier in premature infants of larger size at birth. Premature birth in itself may prejudice later development, but there is also a greater frequency of other obstetric factors, such as intrauterine anoxia and intracranial hemorrhage, than would occur in infants born at term. Follow-up studies of surviving premature infants reveal a discouragingly high incidence of handicaps among small premature infants (Table 7-16). These data also indicate the double role played by socioeconomic factors: mothers of low socioeconomic status are more apt to have low-birth-weight babies, and such infants reared under low socioeconomic conditions tend to develop less well than do those in better environments.

Behavior and personality problems also appear to be common in children born prematurely. The circumstances of nursery care in early infancy and of home care thereafter conspire against a normal relation between the prematurely born infant and his family. The extent to which understandable parental anxiety and overprotectiveness may foster an abnormal emotional environment for the growing infant should be greatly reduced by avoiding unnecessarily prolonged hospitalization and by encouraging parental visiting and participation in the care of the infant while in the nursery.

Home Care. While the infant is in the hospital the mother should be instructed for her responsibilities when the baby is discharged. This program will include at least one visit to her home by a person capable of evaluating domestic arrangements and of advising as to improvements, if needed. Premature infants are usually sent

TABLE 7-16. OBSERVATIONS ON 72 INFANTS WITH BIRTH WEIGHTS OF 3 LBS. (1360 GM.) OR LESS FOLLOWED UP 5 YEARS OR MORE

	CHILDREN
Below 5th percentile in weight	25 (35%)
Below 5th percentile in height	33 (46%)
Below 5th percentile in weight and height	20 (28%)
I.Q. under 100 (66 tested)	60 (91%)
Uneducable in normal school because of physical or mental handicap	26 (36%)
Require special treatment in normal school	25 (35%)
Slower than all siblings (51 had sibs)	39 (76%)
Behavior problem present	51 (71%)
Physical defect	38 (53%)
Physical defect and/or mental retardation	55 (76%)

Data drawn from C. M. Drillien: *The Growth and Development of the Prematurely Born Infant.* Edinburgh and London, E. & S. Livingstone, Ltd., 1964.

home when they reach 5½ pounds (2500 gm.) in weight, but many may go before that time, while others should be kept longer.

POSTMATURITY

The term *postmaturity* is used for infants whose gestation exceeds the normal by 7 days or more. Large size of the infant does not correlate well with late delivery, but does tend to correlate with large size of either parent, multigravidity, diabetes mellitus, or the prediabetic state in the mother and possibly also in the father.

The *placental dysfunction syndrome* is often associated and frequently confused with postmaturity.

Approximately 25 per cent of all pregnancies end on or after the 287th day of gestation (usual, 280 days), 12 per cent on or after the 294th day, and 5 per cent on or after the 301st day. The cause of postmaturity will presumably remain unknown until the mechanism of onset of labor is fully understood.

Clinical Manifestations. The appearance and behavior of the postmature infant approximate those of an infant 1 to 3 weeks of age. He tends to have absence of lanugo, long nails, abundance of scalp hair, white skin and an increased alertness. The skin may be parchment-like with desquamation, as the result of diminution of vernix caseosa beyond term.

Prognosis. When postmaturity exceeds 3 or more weeks, there is a significant increase in mortality, which in some series has approximated 3 times that of a control group of infants born at term; the fetal mortality exceeds that of the neonatal period. Each has been lowered markedly through improved obstetric management. Primiparity and maternal age over 25 years appear to increase the mortality rates.

Treatment. The induction of labor before the cervix is soft and dilated is felt by most obstetricians to be a greater risk than postmaturity itself. A possible exception is the performance of cesarean section on elderly primigravidas who go more than a week or two beyond term, particularly if there is evidence of fetal distress.

PLACENTAL DYSFUNCTION SYNDROME

Incidence and Etiology. The incidence of some clinically recognizable form of placental dysfunction has been estimated to be as high as 12 per cent of all births. The incidence of the clearly recognizable form of the syndrome, with yellow staining of the vernix and skin, is approximately 1.2 per cent of all births. *Only about 20 per cent of infants with placental dysfunction syndrome are postmature.* Premature infants and infants of toxemic mothers, elderly primigravidas and women with

"reproductive inefficiency" often associated with small or poorly attached placentas account for most of the rest. This syndrome has been postulated to be the result of degenerative changes in the placenta resulting in progressive reduction of oxygen and nourishment for the fetus.

Clinical Manifestations. Infants who are born prematurely at weights lower than expected for gestational age are discussed on page 365. Those who are born past term in association with presumed placental dysfunction have been categorized in 3 groups by Clifford: *stage I*—infants with the usual signs of postmaturity, which are desquamation, long nails, abundant hair, white skin and alert facies and loose skin, especially around the thighs and buttocks, giving the appearance of recent loss of weight; *stage II*—infants with the changes of stage I plus meconium-stained amniotic fluid, skin, vernix, umbilical cord and placental membranes, possibly a manifestation of fetal anoxia; *stage III* (Fig. 7-9)—infants with the signs of stages I and II, except that their nails and skin are stained a bright yellow and the umbilical cord yellow-green.

Prognosis. Stage I infants have no known

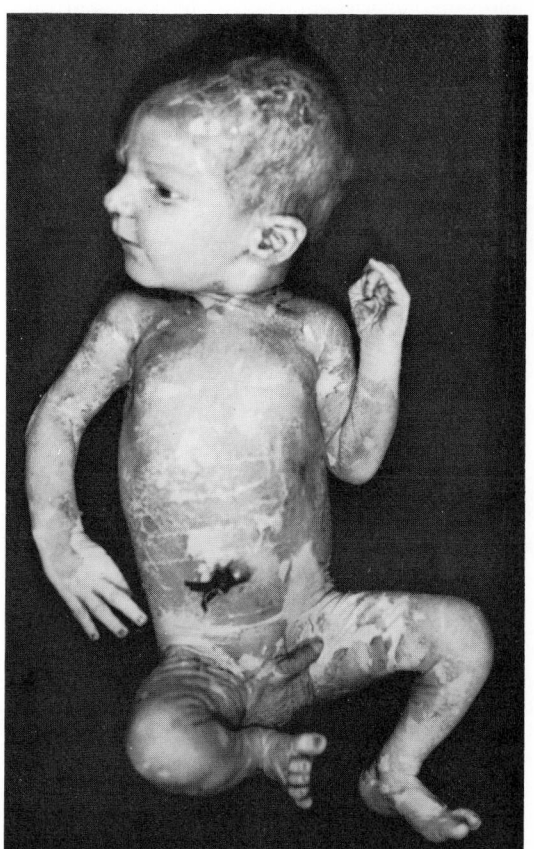

Figure 7-9. Placental dysfunction syndrome, stage III. Note long, thin infant with loose, peeling, parchment-like skin, alert expression, staining of skin and nails. (From Clifford: *Advances in Pediatrics*, Vol. 9. Yearbook Publishers, Inc.)

mortality associated with the syndrome, though up to one third of them have been reported as showing some evidence of respiratory distress or central nervous system irritation. Stage II infants are born at the height of intrauterine anoxia. About two thirds of them have severe respiratory symptoms, apparently resulting from the aspiration of meconium-containing amniotic fluid. A smaller number have clinical signs of anoxic cerebral damage. The overall mortality rate is estimated to be about 35 per cent. Live-born stage III infants have presumably survived the acute anoxic phase of stage II; they have the same clinical problems, but with a lower morbidity, and a mortality rate of approximately 15 per cent. See also Figures 7-4 and 7-7 and Table 7-2.

Treatment. See also Prematurity and Low Birth Weight (p. 364). The treatment of placental dysfunction lies chiefly in preventing the conditions which predispose to it. It therefore constitutes an obstetric and perhaps a genetic and social problem. Aspiration pneumonia and cerebral anoxia are treated symptomatically.

Diseases of the Newborn Infant:
Premature and Full Term

It is essential that the child's physician have an appreciation of the wide variety of disorders which may have their origin in utero, during birth or in the immediate postnatal period, and of the need to distinguish them etiologically in respect to their time and place of origin.

Disorders which have their origin in utero may represent genetic mutations, chromosomal aberrations or acquired diseases (see Table 1-3, p. 10, which deserves careful study). Some of these disorders are described in this section under Birth Injury, Disturbances of Organ Systems, Metabolic Disturbances and Infections; others are described in other sections, which include Inborn Errors of Metabolism, Immunologic Deficiency Disorders, Nutritional Disorders, Infectious Diseases, and the various systems of the body.

CLINICAL MANIFESTATIONS OF DISEASE DURING THE NEONATAL PERIOD

Recognition of disease in the newborn infant is dependent upon knowledge and appraisal of a limited number of relatively nonspecific clinical signs and symptoms.

Cyanosis usually indicates respiratory insufficiency, which may be due to pulmonary conditions or may be secondary to intracranial hemorrhage. If it is due to the former, respirations tend to be rapid and may be accompanied by retraction of the thoracic cage. If it is due to the latter, respirations tend to be irregular and weak and often slow. Cyanosis persisting for several days, when unaccompanied by obvious signs of respiratory difficulty, is suggestive of cyanotic congenital heart disease or methemoglobinemia. Episodes of cyanosis may be the presenting sign of hypoglycemia, bacteremia or meningitis.

In addition to anemia or hemorrhage, *pallor* should suggest hypoxia, hypoglycemia, sepsis, shock or adrenal failure.

Convulsions (see also page 1247) usually point to a disorder of the central nervous system and suggest intracranial hemorrhage, cerebral anomaly, subdural effusion, meningitis, tetany or, rarely, pyridoxine dependency or hypoglycemia. They may also be the first sign of bacteremia or other severe infection and may occur as a nonspecific sign in any severe illness. Rapid or striking changes in serum electrolyte concentrations may also cause convulsions, as may "withdrawal changes" in infants of mothers addicted to narcotics (see p. 401).

Lethargy may be a manifestation of anoxia, of sedation from maternal analgesia or anesthesia, of cerebral defect, of severe infection and, indeed, of almost any severe disease. Lethargy appearing after the second day should in particular suggest infection.

Irritability may be a sign of discomfort accompanying intra-abdominal conditions, meningeal irritation, infections, or any condition producing pain. Toward the latter part of the neonatal period, as in later infancy, the eardrums should always be examined as a possible source of pain.

Hyperactivity, especially of the premature infant, may be a sign of hypoxia, pneumothorax, emphysema, hypoglycemia, hypocalcemia or central nervous system damage.

Failure to feed well is seen in most sick newborn infants and should always occasion a careful search for infection and other abnormal conditions.

Fever may be the result of too high an environmental temperature due to hot weather, overheated nurseries or incubators, or too many clothes or bedclothes. It is also seen in "dehydration fever" of newborns. If these causes of fever can be eliminated, serious infection (pneumonia, bacteremia, meningitis) must be ruled out. On the other hand, serious infections often occur without provoking any febrile response in newborn infants; an unexplained *fall in body temperature* may accompany infection or other serious disturbance of the metabolic processes of the neonate.

Periods of *apnea,* particularly in the premature

infant, suggest metabolic as well as respiratory or central nervous system disturbance. They have been described in association with hyponatremia and hypoglycemia.

Jaundice during the first 24 hours of life should be considered due to erythroblastosis fetalis until proved otherwise. Cytomegalic inclusion disease, the congenital rubella syndrome and toxoplasmosis should also be considered.

Jaundice after the first 24 hours may be "physiologic," due to any of the foregoing causes, or to septicemia, hemolytic anemia, galactosemia, hepatitis, congenital atresia of the bile ducts, inspissated bile syndrome following erythroblastosis fetalis, syphilis or herpes simplex.

Vomiting during the first day of life suggests obstruction in the upper digestive tract or increased intracranial pressure. Anteroposterior and lateral *upright* films of the abdomen are indicated, followed by barium studies if the diagnosis remains in doubt. Later, although it still points to the central nervous system or gastrointestinal tract, vomiting may be a nonspecific symptom of an illness such as septicemia. It is also a common manifestation of overfeeding, pyloric stenosis, milk allergy, duodenal ulcer, stress ulcer, adrenal insufficiency and a reflection of a "nervous" or apprehensive mother, or of an actual emotional upset in the parents. Infants placed in body casts for orthopedic treatment often vomit transiently, apparently as a manifestation of frustration of physical movement. Vomitus containing dark blood is usually a sign of terminal illness, whatever the cause.

Diarrhea may be a symptom of overfeeding, acute gastroenteritis or a nonspecific symptom of infection *(parenteral diarrhea)*. It may be seen in conditions accompanied by compromised circulation of part of the intestinal or genital tract such as strangulated hernia, intussusception, and torsion of the ovary or testis.

Abdominal distention, usually a sign of intestinal obstruction or an intra-abdominal mass, may also be seen in infants with enteritis or with temporary ileus accompanying sepsis or respiratory distress.

Failure to move an extremity or part of it suggests fracture, dislocation or nerve injury. It is also seen in osteomyelitis and other infections which cause pain on movement of the affected part.

CONGENITAL ANOMALIES

Congenital anomalies are important as a cause of stillbirths and neonatal deaths, but are perhaps even more important as causes of physical defects and metabolic disorders. (Anomalies are discussed in general on page 339 and specifically in the sections on the various systems of the body. For congenital mental defects, see page 113; for congenital metabolic and chemical disorders, see page 413; and for immunologic deficiency disorders, see page 477.) Recognition of anomalies as early as possible is desirable. For some, such as tracheo-esophageal fistula or intestinal obstruction, immediate medical and surgical therapy is mandatory for survival. In all instances early diagnosis permits a planned approach and an explanation to parents, who are likely to be assailed by anxiety and guilt when they become aware of the existence of a congenital anomaly.

BIRTH INJURY

The term *birth injury* is used to denote avoidable and unavoidable mechanical and anoxic trauma incurred by the infant at birth. Most lay persons interpret *birth injury* as meaning avoidable trauma incurred through lack of medical skill or attention. In order to prevent later misunderstandings, recriminations and self-recriminations on the part of parents of a child who has residuals from birth trauma, anoxia or disease, it is important that the physician take time to inform them about the broad use of the term "birth injury" and the fact that trauma or anoxia may, in our present state of obstetric knowledge and skill, be unavoidable during the process of birth.

CRANIAL INJURIES

Caput succedaneum is a diffuse, edematous swelling of the soft tissues of the scalp involving the portion presenting during delivery. General or localized ecchymotic discoloration may be present. The edema disappears within the first few days of life. Analogous swelling, discoloration and distortion of the face are seen in face presentations. *Molding* of the head and overriding of the parietal bones are frequently associated with caput succedaneum and become more evident after the caput has receded, but disappear during the first weeks of life.

Erythema, abrasions, ecchymoses and *subcutaneous fat necrosis* (p. 1378) may be seen after forceps deliveries. Their location depends upon the area of application of the forceps. Ecchymoses may be seen after manipulative deliveries and occasionally in premature infants for no discernible reason.

Subconjunctival hemorrhages are frequent, and *petechiae* of the skin of the head and neck are not uncommon. Generalized ecchymotic suffusion of the head and neck is rare. All are probably secondary to a sudden increase in intrathoracic pressure during passage of the chest through the birth canal. Parents should be assured that they are temporary and the result of *normal* hazards of delivery.

Cephalhematoma (Fig. 7-10) is a subperiosteal hemorrhage, hence always limited to the surface of one cranial bone. Other points of distinction from caput succedaneum are that there is no dis-

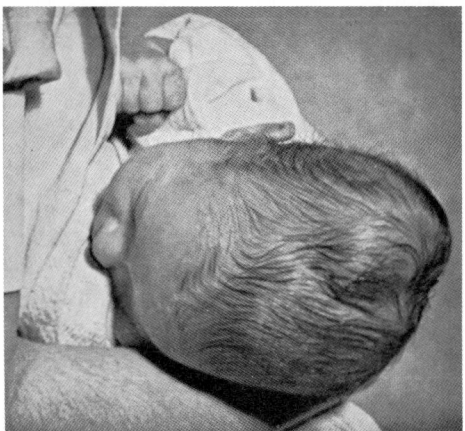

Figure 7-10. Cephalhematoma of the right parietal bone.

plication, incision or aspiration is contraindicated.

Fractures of the skull may occur as result of pressure from forceps or against the maternal symphysis pubis, sacral promontory or ischial spines. Linear fractures are the most common. They cause no symptoms and require no treatment. Depressed fractures are usually indentations of the calvarium similar to a dent in a ping-pong ball. It is advisable to elevate such depressions surgically to prevent cortical injury from sustained pressure. Fracture of the occipital bone with separation of the basal and squamous portions almost invariably causes fatal hemorrhage, owing to disruption of the underlying sinuses. It may result from traction on the hyperextended spine of the infant with the head fixed in the maternal pelvis during breech deliveries.

coloration of the overlying scalp due to subcutaneous hemorrhage and that swelling usually is not visible until several hours after birth, since subperiosteal bleeding is a slow process. In approximately 25 per cent of cephalhematomas there is an underlying skull fracture. It is rarely of the depressed type, although a sensation of central depression suggesting underlying fracture or bony defect is usually encountered on palpation of the organized rim of a cephalhematoma. Cranial meningocele may be differentiated from cephalhematoma by pulsation, increased pressure on crying and the roentgenographic evidence of bony defect. Cephalhematomas begin to calcify by the end of the second week.

Most are resorbed during the first 6 weeks of life. A few remain as bony protuberances for years and are detectable roentgenographically as widening of the diploic space; cystlike defects may persist for months or years. Despite these residuals, cephalhematomas require no treatment. Since the introduction of infection is the only serious com-

Intracranial Hemorrhage

Intracranial hemorrhage may result from trauma or anoxia and, rarely, from a primary hemorrhagic disturbance or congenital vascular anomaly. Traumatic hemorrhage is especially likely when the fetal head is large in proportion to the size of the mother's pelvic outlet; when for other reasons the labor is prolonged; in breech deliveries; in precipitate deliveries; or when there is injudicious mechanical interference with delivery. On the other hand, the proper use of forceps is thought to decrease the incidence of intracranial bleeding in prolonged, hard labors. Intracranial hemorrhage may occur in infants, especially premature ones, delivered spontaneously without apparent trauma. In premature infants subependymal, subarachnoid, intracerebral and intraventricular hemorrhages are common (Fig. 7-11). Spontaneous intraventricular hemorrhage in which no physical damage to the tentorium, falx or other structures is found at autopsy is practi-

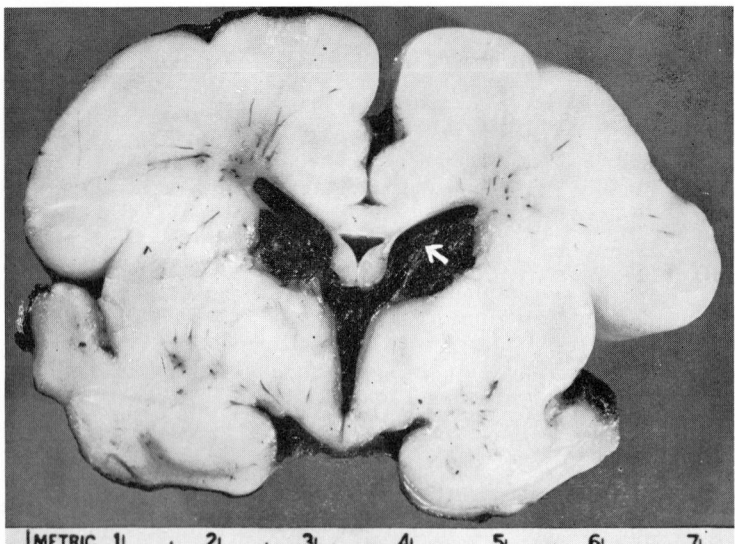

Figure 7-11. Bilateral subependymal and intraventricular hemorrhage in a premature infant. The floor of the lateral ventricle is marked by an arrow, outside of which is a large subependymal hemorrhage. (From Arey and Dent., *J. Pediat.,* Vol. 42.)

METRIC 1   2   3   4   5   6   7

cally limited to premature infants. Conversely, massive subdural hemorrhages, often associated with tears in the tentorium cerebelli or less frequently in the falx cerebri, are encountered more often in full-term than in premature infants.

Hemorrhage due to anoxia tends to be petechial, and subarachnoid and intracerebral in distribution. There is usually only mild extravasation of erythrocytes, and symptoms and sequelae are dependent more on anoxia than on hemorrhage. Primary hemorrhagic disturbances usually give rise to subarachnoid hemorrhage, and vascular anomaly to subarachnoid or intracerebral hemorrhage.

Clinical Manifestations. Symptoms of intracranial hemorrhage may be present at birth or may not appear for a variable time after delivery. The commonest symptoms soon after birth are a general failure to move normally, diminished or absent Moro reflex, lethargy and somnolence. Great irregularity of respirations in the absence of other signs of respiratory distress is often a sign of severe hemorrhage. Periods of apnea, pallor, cyanosis or cyanotic attacks, failure to suck well, forceful vomiting, anxiety and restlessness, a high-pitched, shrill cry, muscular twitchings, convulsions or paralyses may be the first indications that intracranial hemorrhage is present. The fontanel *may* be tense and bulging, and an adder-like protrusion of the tongue may be seen. Retinal hemorrhage, ocular palsies, inequality in size and failure of the pupils to react to light, or nystagmus may be observed.

Diagnosis is based chiefly on the history of delivery, the clinical manifestations and the course. Since nonlocalizing signs of intracranial hemorrhage are identical with those caused by cerebral edema or anoxia, before carrying out any diagnostic procedure the chance of helping the patient should be weighed against the risk. Subdural taps are usually unrewarding, even in the presence of subdural hemorrhage, since it is likely that the blood will have clotted; on the other hand, they are occasionally lifesaving. Trephining is rarely indicated, owing to the remoteness of the possibility that it will be either diagnostically or therapeutically efficacious. For similar reasons ventricular taps are rarely done even when there is suspicion of intraventricular hemorrhage. Lumbar puncture is indicated in the presence of signs of increased intracranial pressure to identify gross subarachnoid hemorrhage, to rule out the possibility of bacterial meningitis, and possibly to relieve pressure on vital structures.

Since a small amount of bleeding often occurs in the course of normal and even cesarean deliveries, small numbers of red blood cells or slight xanthochromia in subarachnoid fluid is not necessarily indicative of significant intracranial hemorrhage. Bilirubin may produce a yellowish discoloration of the cerebrospinal fluid in jaundiced infants; conversely, the subarachnoid fluid may be absolutely clear with severe subdural or intracerebral hemorrhage when there is no communication with the subarachnoid space.

Prognosis. Intrapartum death may occur in the more severe cases; postnatally, fatalities usually occur within the first 3 days and result from respiratory failure. If an infant survives, recovery may be complete, or there may be permanent residuals mainly in the category of cerebral palsy. Presumably some of the membrane-enclosed subdural effusions observed in later infancy may have their origin in subdural hemorrhage at birth. Statistics on incidence and prognosis of intracranial hemorrhage in the newborn are not available, since autopsy material is the only source and since one can rarely be certain of the diagnosis in the surviving patient.

Because the majority of parents are aware of and fear the possibility of cerebral residuals following intracranial hemorrhage or cerebral anoxia, it is probably wisest to give them an opportunity to air their anxiety in a frank discussion of the problem, during which their questions should be invited rather than suppressed or evaded. As optimistic an attitude as possible, consistent with the physician's opinion of the prognosis of the individual case, should be maintained.

Prevention. Prophylactic measures include continuing improvements in obstetric management; many instances of intracranial hemorrhage are avoidable.

Treatment. The infant should be handled as little and as gently as possible. He is best kept in an incubator which allows good temperature control, continuous observation, and easy administration of oxygen for cyanosis. Sodium phenobarbital (8 mg. [$^1/_8$ grain]), administered intramuscularly, or other anticonvulsant drugs in appropriate doses, may be used to control convulsive movement. A small dose of vitamin K or, preferably, K_1 oxide should be administered (see Hyperbilirubinemia, p. 394). A small (5 ml. per pound) transfusion of fresh blood is indicated in the presence of hemorrhagic disease of the newborn. There is lack of agreement about the advisability of spinal punctures for the relief of increased intracranial pressure and to remove gross blood in order to reduce its irritant effect on the cerebral cortex and to prevent possible interference with the normal resorptive mechanisms for cerebrospinal fluid. In our opinion such punctures are indicated, particularly in the presence of grossly bloody spinal subarachnoid fluid.

Neurosurgical procedures are of doubtful advantage; most of them aim at relieving pressure, a goal which is usually readily accomplished by withdrawal of spinal fluid at lumbar puncture.

Cerebral edema may result in any or all of the clinical signs produced by intracranial hemorrhage. Trauma and anoxia are the usual causative factors. Treatment is directed toward relieving increased intracranial pressure by lumbar puncture, restriction of fluid intake to 800 ml. per square meter per 24 hours, and parenteral administration of 10 mg. of dexamethasone per square meter followed by 5 mg. per square meter every 6 hours (20 mg. per square meter per 24 hours). Mannitol may be used intravenously with caution, if necessary. Three or 4 days of therapy usually suffice.

SPINE AND SPINAL CORD

Strong traction exerted when the spine is hyperextended or when the direction of pull is lateral may produce fracture and separation of the vertebrae. Such injuries are rare and are most likely to occur when difficulty is encountered in delivering the shoulders in cephalic presentations and the head in breech presentations. The injury is most commonly at the level of the seventh cervical and first thoracic vertebrae. Transection of the cord may occur, but hemorrhage and edema may produce neurologic signs indistinguishable from those of transection, except that they are not permanent. There is complete paralysis of voluntary motion below the level of injury, though the persistence of a withdrawal reflex mediated through spinal centers distal to the area of injury is frequently misinterpreted as representing voluntary motion. Severe spinal cord injuries usually cause death soon after birth. In the survivors there is often permanent injury. In compression from a fracture or dislocation the prognosis is related to the time elapsing before the compression is removed.

PERIPHERAL NERVE INJURIES

Brachial Palsy. Injury to the brachial plexus may cause paralysis of the upper arm with or without paralysis of the forearm or hand. Such an injury occurs when traction is exerted on the head during delivery of the shoulder.

In *Erb-Duchenne paralysis* the injury is limited to the fifth and sixth cervical nerves. The infant loses the power to abduct the arm from the shoulder, to rotate the arm externally and to supinate the forearm. The characteristic position consists in adduction and internal rotation of the arm with pronation of the forearm. The power of extension of the forearm is retained, but the biceps reflex is absent. The Moro reflex is absent on the affected side (Fig. 7-12). There may be some sensory impairment on the outer aspect of the arm. The power in the forearm and the hand grasp are preserved unless the lower part of the plexus is also injured; the presence of the hand grasp is a favorable prognostic sign. When the injury includes the phrenic nerve, alteration of the diaphragmatic excursion may be observed fluoroscopically.

Klumpke's paralysis is a rarer form of brachial palsy; injury to the seventh and eighth cervical nerves and the first thoracic nerve produces a paralyzed hand, and ptosis and miosis if the sympathetic fibers of the first thoracic root are also injured.

The mild cases may not be detected immediately after birth. Differentiation must be made from cerebral injury, from fracture, dislocation or epiphyseal separation of the humerus, and from fracture of the clavicle.

The *prognosis* depends upon whether the nerve was merely injured or was lacerated. If the paralysis was due to edema and hemorrhage about the nerve fibers, there should be a return of function within a few months; if due to laceration, permanent damage may result. The involvement of the deltoid is usually the most serious; dropping of the shoulder may result from muscular atrophy.

Treatment consists in relaxation of the paralyzed muscles by preventing the antagonistic pull of the nonparalyzed muscles. While the infant is in his crib, the wrist can be held by a clove-hitch to the head of the bed so that the arm is maintained abducted and rotated externally, with the elbow flexed. If the hand is paralyzed, padding should be placed in the fist. Later an airplane splint may be used to hold the arm in proper position. Physical therapy is a necessary adjunct to the treatment. If the paralysis persists, because of laceration of the nerve fibers, for 2 or 3 months, neuroplasty offers hope for partial recovery.

Phrenic Nerve Paralysis. Phrenic nerve injury with diaphragmatic paralysis must be con-

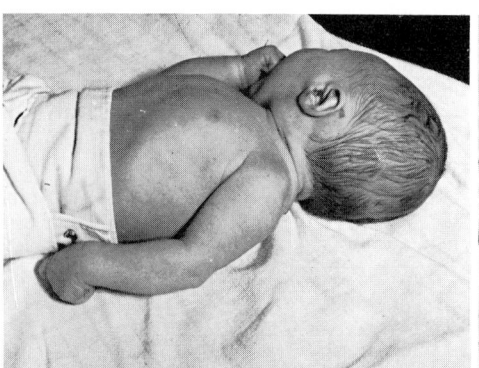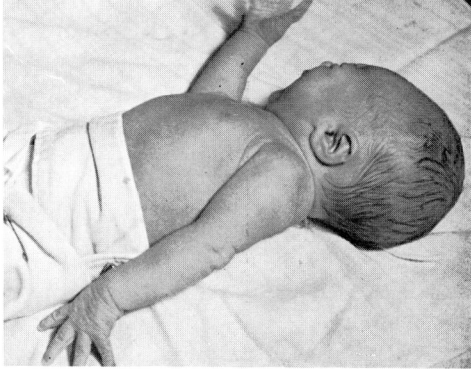

Figure 7-12. Brachial palsy of the left arm (asymmetric Moro reflex).

sidered when cyanosis and irregular and labored respirations develop. Such injuries are usually associated with a brachial palsy. Breathing is thoracic in type, so that there is no bulging of the abdomen with inspiration. Breath sounds are diminished on the affected side. The *diagnosis* is established by fluoroscopic examination, which reveals the elevation of the diaphragm on the paralyzed side (Fig. 7-13) and seesaw movements of the 2 sides of the diaphragm during respiration.

There is no specific *treatment;* the infant should be placed on the involved side; oxygen therapy may be necessary. Feeding by gavage often saves the infant's energy for maintenance of the labored respiratory movements. Recovery usually occurs. Pulmonary infections are a serious complication.

Facial Nerve Palsy. Rarely facial palsy is nonobstetric, resulting from nuclear agenesis of the facial nerve. Usually, however, the paralysis is peripheral and results from pressure over the facial nerve in utero, during labor, or from forceps during delivery. When the infant cries, there is movement on only one side of the face, and the mouth is drawn to that side. On the affected side the eye cannot be closed and the nasolabial fold is absent. The *prognosis* depends upon whether the nerve was injured by pressure or whether the nerve fibers were torn. Improvement will occur within a few weeks in the former instance. Care of the exposed eye is essential. Faradic stimulation is probably of no benefit, but neuroplasty may be indicated when the paralysis is persistent.

Other Peripheral Nerves. Other nerves are

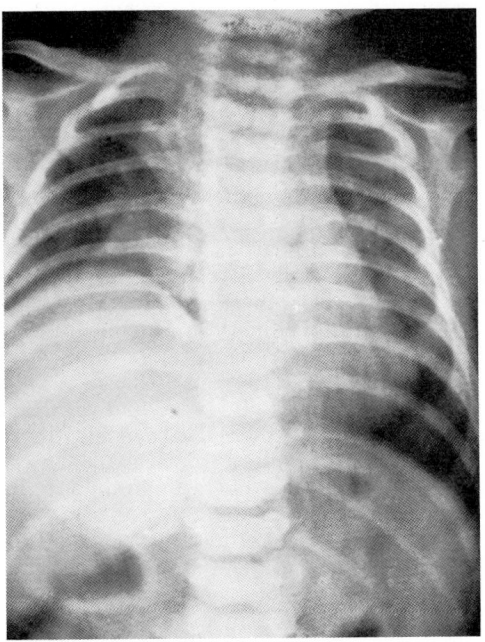

Figure 7-13. Phrenic paralysis in a newborn infant. The right leaf of the diaphragm is elevated, owing to injury to the right phrenic nerve. Fluoroscopically, the right and left leaves of the diaphragm moved in a seesaw manner. There were also fractures of both clavicles and a right brachial palsy.

seldom injured at birth, except as they are involved in fractures or hemorrhages.

VISCERA

The *liver* is the only internal organ, other than the brain, injured with any frequency during birth. The damage usually occurs from pressure on the liver during delivery of the head in breech presentations. Overzealous manual attempts to apply artificial respiration or extrathoracic cardiac massage are less frequent causes. The injury is rupture of the liver with formation of a subcapsular hematoma. The hematoma may be large enough to cause anemia. Shock and death occur if the hematoma breaks through the capsule, reducing pressure and allowing fresh hemorrhage from the liver. Alertness to the possibility of this condition in infants delivered by breech presentations and in infants who receive manual resuscitation should make it possible to save some of them and to prevent the condition in others.

Rupture of the spleen may occur in association with rupture of the liver. The causes, complications, treatment and prevention are similar.

Although *adrenal hemorrhage* occurs with some frequency, especially after breech delivery, it is not known whether it is due to trauma, anoxia or severe stress, as in overwhelming infections. In older infants old calcified central hematomas of the adrenal have been identified at autopsy, suggesting that not all adrenal hemorrhages are fatal. The diagnosis is usually made at postmortem examination. The symptoms are profound shock and cyanosis. If adrenal hemorrhage is suspected, the treatment is the same as for acute adrenal failure (p. 1210).

INJURY OF THE STERNOCLEIDOMASTOID

A firm mass 1 to 2 cm. in diameter is occasionally noted in the midportion of the sternocleidomastoid muscle about the second week of life, although it may be present shortly after birth. It is believed by some to be a small hematoma from injury to the muscle at birth, by others to be a fibromatous malformation of the muscle. It usually but not always is responsible for torticollis on the affected side (see p. 1317).

FRACTURES

Clavicle. The clavicle is fractured more frequently than any other bone and is particularly vulnerable when there is difficulty in delivery of the shoulder. The infant characteristically fails to move, or to move freely, the arm on the affected side, and crepitus may be elicited. The Moro reflex is absent on the affected side, and there is spasm of the sternocleidomastoid muscle with obliteration of the supraclavicular depression at the site

of the fracture. In greenstick fractures there may
be no limitation of movement and the Moro reflex
may be present. Fracture of the humerus or brachial palsy may also be responsible for limitation
of movement of an arm and the absence of a Moro
reflex on the affected side. The *prognosis* is excellent. *Treatment,* if any, consists in immobilization
of the arm and shoulder on the affected side. A
remarkable degree of callus develops within a
week at the site of the fracture. This may be the
first evidence of a fracture.

Extremities. In fractures of the long bones
spontaneous movement of the extremity is usually
absent. The Moro reflex is absent from the involved extremity. The possibility of associated
nerve involvement must be considered. Satisfactory results for a fractured humerus are obtained
by strapping the arm to the chest or applying a
Velpeau bandage, and later an airplane splint or
a shell cast. For fracture of the femur, good results
are obtained with Buck's extension. Splints are
effective for treatment of fractures of the forearm
or leg. Healing is usually accompanied by excess
callus formation.

Dislocations and *epiphyseal separations* rarely
result from birth trauma. The upper femoral epiphysis may be separated by forcible manipulation
of the infant's leg as, for example, in breech extraction or after version. There is swelling, slight
shortening, limitation of active motion, painful
passive motion, and external rotation of the leg.
The diagnosis is established roentgenographically.
The prognosis is good for the milder injuries, but
coxa vara frequently results from extensive displacement.

Nose. The most prevalent injury of the nose is
a dislocation of the cartilaginous portion of the
septum from the vomerine groove and the columella. The infant may have difficulty in nursing
and some impairment in nasal respiration. Treatment should be instituted immediately.

ANOXIA

Anoxia is not a clinical entity, but a term
loosely applied to indicate the end-result of lack
of oxygen from a number of primary causes.
Separate consideration will be accorded it, however, since it is the leading immediate, though
not basic, cause of perinatal death or permanent
damage to central nervous system cells which is
manifest later as cerebral palsy or mental deficiency. Its prevention and treatment are essentially those of the basic conditions which cause it,
although death and disability may sometimes be
prevented through symptomatic treatment with
oxygen or artificial respiration.

Fetal anoxia may result from (1) inadequate
oxygenation of maternal blood as in hypoventilation during anesthesia, cardiac failure or carbon
monoxide poisoning, (2) low maternal blood pressure as in the hypotension that may complicate

spinal anesthesia, (3) inadequate relaxation of the
uterus to permit placental filling as in uterine
tetany caused by administration of Pituitrin or
Pitocin, (4) inadequate attachment of the placenta
as in premature separation of the placenta, (5)
impedance to the circulation of blood through the
umbilical cord as in compression or knotting
of the cord, and (6) placental inadequacy from
numerous causes, including toxemia and postmaturity.

After birth, anoxia may result from (1) anemia
severe enough to lower the oxygen content of the
blood to a critical level as in severe anemia due
to hemorrhage or hemolytic disease, (2) shock
severe enough to interfere with the transport of
oxygen to vital cells as in adrenal hemorrhage,
ventricular hemorrhage, overwhelming infection
or massive blood loss, (3) poisoning of tissue cells
so that they are unable to use oxygen as in narcosis
from barbiturates or other drugs, (4) a deficit in
arterial oxygen saturation from failure to breathe
adequately postnatally, owing to narcosis or cerebral defect or injury, and (5) failure of oxygenation
of an adequate amount of blood as in severe forms
of cyanotic congenital heart disease or deficient
pulmonary ventilation.

Studies have failed to show any close correlation
between oxygen content of cord or arterial blood
immediately after birth and later intellectual
development. Most of the deaths and cerebral
damage which result from anoxia are probably
related to fetal or postnatal periods of anoxia. The
known resistance to anoxia demonstrated by newborn infants may be related to oxygen-saving
short-cuts in essential metabolic pathways. It is
possible that these factors are absent or diminished in some infants as a result of deficiency of
specific enzymes.

Clinical Manifestations. The signs of anoxia
in the *fetus* are usually noted a few minutes to a
few days before delivery. There is a sudden increase in activity as if the baby were struggling
in utero, which may be followed by diminished
activity. The fetal heart rate slows, and the beat
may become weak and irregular. Particularly in
the infant near term, these are signs which should
lead to immediate delivery to avoid death or central nervous system damage.

At the *time of delivery* the presence of yellow,
meconium-stained amniotic fluid and vernix caseosa is a warning that there has been fetal distress,
probably anoxic. Pallor, cyanosis, apnea, slow
heart rate, unresponsiveness to stimulation, and
muscular flaccidity are definite signs of anoxia.

After delivery anoxia is due to respiratory failure
and will be discussed under that heading.

Pathology. The pathologic changes which result from anoxia are principally those caused by
congestion and increased capillary permeability.
Congestion and petechiae are found in all organs,
but are especially noticeable in the pleura, pericardium, thymus, adrenals, brain and meninges.
Cerebral edema is common. Gross subarachnoid,
intraventricular or adrenal hemorrhage may be

present without demonstrable tear of blood vessels. Histologic study of the brain and liver, particularly the right lobe, may reveal cellular degenerative changes similar to those produced experimentally by anoxia. Fetal anoxia is characterized pathologically by the additional finding of large amounts of amniotic debris in the respiratory passages. Pathophysiologically, the development of metabolic acidosis within minutes of onset of anoxia is probably a large factor leading to shock and cardiovascular collapse.

PEDIATRIC EMERGENCIES IN THE DELIVERY ROOM

The most common and immediately most important emergencies related to the newborn infant in the delivery room are failure to initiate respiration and to maintain satisfactory respirations. Less frequent, but having potentially serious import, are severe anemia, plethora and convulsions.

Respiratory Distress and Failure. Disorders of respiration in the newborn infant can be categorized in 2 general groups (Table 7-17), one representing failure of the respiratory center (central nervous system failure) and the other interference with the alveolar exchange of oxygen and carbon dioxide (peripheral respiratory difficulty). Cyanosis occurs in both central nervous system failure and peripheral respiratory difficulty. The respiratory problems encountered in the delivery room are most frequently those of central nervous system failure and the accompanying absence of adequate respiratory effort.

Respiratory distress in the presence of good respiratory effort should lead to an immediate consideration of peripheral causes; *respiratory distress is an indication for a roentgenographic examination of the chest* if this is at all possible without undue stress for the infant.

If respiratory movements are made with the mouth closed, but the infant fails to move air in and out of the lungs, bilateral *choanal atresia* (p. 883) or other obstruction of the upper respiratory tract should be suspected. The mouth should be opened and the tongue pulled forward. If this maneuver is successful in allowing air exchange, nasal obstruction may be assumed; an oropharyngeal airway should be inserted and the source of the obstruction sought immediately, but in an unhurried manner. If effective respiratory flow is not produced by opening the infant's mouth, laryngoscopy is indicated. With obstructive malformations of the epiglottis, larynx or trachea an endotracheal tube should be inserted and tracheotomy performed at the earliest opportunity.

Hypoplasia of the mandible (p. 753) with posterior displacement of the tongue may result in symptoms similar to those of choanal atresia; they may be temporarily relieved by pulling the tongue forward. A scaphoid abdomen suggests *hernia or eventration of the diaphragm,* as do asymmetry of contour or movement of the chest or shift of the apical impulse of the heart; these latter manifestations are also compatible with tension pneumothorax.

Causes of peripheral respiratory difficulty are discussed below under Disturbances of the Respiratory Tract.

Failure to Initiate or Sustain Respiration. Failure to initiate or sustain respiratory effort originates in the central nervous system; immaturity in itself is seldom a causative factor.

Narcosis results from heavy doses of morphine, Demerol, barbiturates, reserpine or tranquilizers to the mother shortly before delivery or from maternal anesthesia, especially if prolonged, during delivery. The infant is cyanotic at birth and slow to cry or breathe; when respiration is established, it is extremely slow.

Narcosis is rarely excusable and should be avoided by appropriate analgesic and anesthetic practices.

TABLE 7-17. RESPIRATORY DISTRESS AND FAILURE IN NEWBORN INFANTS

TYPE	MANIFESTATIONS	CLINICAL ENTITY
Central nervous system failure	Apnea Slow, irregular, gasping respiratory efforts	Narcosis Prenatal or perinatal anoxia Intracranial hemorrhage or trauma CNS anomalies
Peripheral respiratory difficulty	Rapid respiratory rate Increasing respiratory rate Chest lag Intercostal retraction Xiphoid retraction Chin tug Expiratory grunt Frothing at lips	Primary atelectasis Congestive pulmonary failure Idiopathic respiratory distress (hyaline membrane) syndrome Aspiration of amniotic fluid containing formed elements Pneumonia Diaphragmatic hernia Lung cysts Lobar emphysema Pneumothorax Aspiration of food or mucus

Treatment consists of physical stimulants such as frequent snapping of the soles of the feet to stimulate crying and deeper breathing, or insertion of a catheter through the nostril into the nasopharynx to produce reflex irritation and breathing. Caffeine with sodium benzoate, U.S.P., 0.5 ml. intramuscularly, may be used as often as every 20 to 30 minutes, if necessary and effective in stimulating the infant. If narcosis is due to morphine or its derivatives, n-allyl normorphine (Nalline), 0.1 mg. per kg., should be injected intravenously. This drug is a respiratory depressant and should be used only for this specific indication. Oxygen should be administered as long as cyanosis is present, and some form of artificial respiration may be necessary until a regular and adequate respiratory pattern is established.

Prenatal or *perinatal anoxia*, whatever the cause, if sufficiently severe, will produce a central nervous system type of respiratory failure. Death is due to apnea and may be prevented by resuscitation, provided the basic cause of the anoxia can be eliminated within a reasonable time and while artificial respiration, if necessary, is being carried out. Hypothermia as a means of temporarily reducing metabolic needs for oxygen during the period of oxygen want has not proved to be of practical value. Extensive subcutaneous fat necrosis with calcification has been reported following the induction of hypothermia to combat neonatal asphyxia.

Intracranial hemorrhage and trauma are discussed on page 374.

Central nervous system anomalies may be responsible for respiratory failure.

Resuscitation. Failure to breathe spontaneously within 1 minute of birth is an indication for some method of resuscitation. If the central mechanism can be revived, the infant will usually be more effective in ventilating his lungs than will any available machine. When the need for resuscitation results from failure of peripheral rather than central mechanisms, as in "previable" premature infants, most of whom demonstrate adequate initial function of the respiratory center, present resuscitative measures are notably ineffective.

After the upper and central airway has been cleared as adequately as possible by removal of accumulated liquid contents, resuscitation should start with some method of simple, gentle physical stimulation such as snapping the soles of the feet with a finger or repeatedly passing a nasal catheter. If this is unsuccessful in initiating satisfactory respiration, the upper respiratory passage should be suctioned again and a small plastic or metal airway inserted to lift the tongue off the posterior pharyngeal wall. If the infant has an Apgar score of 1 or less (p. 357), or if the pulse rate is less than 80 beats a minute, some method of artificial respiration or pulmonary inflation is usually indicated. If a gentle flow of oxygen at pressures up to 25 cm. of water, administered either steadily or in puffs through a small mask,

does not produce improved color and tone followed by spontaneous respiratory movements, direct laryngoscopy or direct endotracheal intubation with suctioning of the lower respiratory passages and an attempt to inflate the lungs through the application of short bursts of oxygen at higher pressures or through use of a positive-pressure respirator is indicated. Maintenance of the circulation through closed cardiac massage at a rate of 100 or more per minute is an important adjunct to artificial respiration in infants in circulatory collapse with slow, weak heart beats. Laryngoscopy, intubation and cardiac massage should be carried out by personnel skilled in the techniques, of whom there should be one (usually the anesthetist) in every delivery room. Negative intrathoracic pressures between 20 and 70 cm. of water have been recorded during the first few breaths; positive pressure much lower than 20 cm. of water is unlikely to introduce oxygen into the lungs. Pressures of 25 cm. may rupture the lung if only a small area is being expanded. On the other hand, positive pressures of 40 cm. have been safely applied by using a resuscitator which automatically limits the inspiratory phase to 0.1 second and provides an expiratory phase of 5.9 seconds.

The elementary procedure of mouth-to-mouth breathing has presumably been successful in resuscitating some infants, but may have been harmful to others by introducing infection or alveolar rupture from uncontrolled pressures. Even if safety devices are interposed, the gas thus applied is less effective than oxygen. Manual compression of the soft thorax is unlikely to be followed by enough rebound expansion to produce air movement.

If the infant is making feeble but spontaneous respiratory movements, their effectiveness will be increased by raising the partial pressure of oxygen at the nose and mouth, even without any change in atmospheric pressure. Oxygen administration, particularly to premature infants, should always be discontinued as soon as the baby can get along without it.

No drug advocated as a respiratory stimulant has proved to be of definite value; moreover, most of them may be convulsant if given in doses slightly greater than those supposed to stimulate breathing.

Severe *edema* noted at birth in infants should be considered to be due to erythroblastosis fetalis until proved otherwise; blood group incompatibilities not detected by routine Rh screening of the parents are not infrequent. The concentrations of hemoglobin and serum bilirubin and a Coombs test should be determined from a sample of umbilical cord blood, and a unit of blood should be cross-matched with the mother's blood in case transfusion or exchange transfusion should be necessary.

Edema and *convulsions* may result from intravenous administration of large amounts of hypotonic solutions to the mother shortly before and during delivery. Determination of the level of sodium in the infant's serum is indicated, followed by administration of appropriate amounts of 3 or 5 per cent sodium chloride solution by vein, if indicated.

Pallor noted at birth may be due not only to hypoxia, but also to loss of blood from intrauterine hemolysis, bleeding into or from the placenta, ruptured liver or spleen, or even cephalhematoma. If there is respiratory distress which can be assumed to be due to the anemia, immediate cautious transfusion of group O, Rh-negative blood may be lifesaving. A careful search for a source of hemolysis or bleeding should be instituted immediately and appropriate remedial measures taken.

Shock noted at birth may be due to brain injury, hemorrhage, or an intra-abdominal condition such as rupture, perforation or gangrene of a viscus. Excessive abdominal distention should be considered an emergency, and managed accordingly.

Disturbances of Organ Systems

DISTURBANCES OF THE RESPIRATORY TRACT

Disturbances of respiration which are manifest in the immediate postnatal period may have had their origin in utero, in the delivery room or in the nursery. A wide variety of pathologic lesions may be responsible, and differential diagnosis is often difficult. There are, however, characteristic manifestations for many of them which the student must learn and the physician should come to know from experience. These are described, some in this section, others in appropriate ones of the text. The most common and among the most serious of the pulmonary lesions are the idiopathic respiratory distress syndrome and pneumonia. Other lesions include choanal atresia, hypoplasia of the mandible with posterior displacement of the tongue, macroglossia, malformation of the epiglottis, malformation or injury of the larynx, tracheo-esophageal fistula, evulsion of the phrenic nerve, hernia or eventration of the diaphragm, congenital heart disease, intracranial lesions and metabolic disturbances (see Table 7-17 for a listing of intracranial and pulmonary lesions). *Any sign of postnatal respiratory distress* (Fig. 7-1; Tables 7-7, 7-17) *is an indication for a roentgenogram of the chest.*

ATELECTASIS

Atelectasis is almost constantly present in infants dying shortly after delivery. It is no longer considered an adequate explanation for death; careful postmortem examination usually reveals a cause for persistent atelectasis.

Primary atelectasis (failure of initial alveolar expansion), common among premature infants without other apparent abnormality at autopsy, is regarded as due to immaturity of the diaphragm and other respiratory muscles, hypermobility of the thoracic cage, or to other defects of the peripheral respiratory mechanism. It is also seen as a result of brain injury.

Secondary atelectasis (alveolar collapse after initial expansion by air) may occur as a gross or microscopic lesion in all types of pulmonary disease in the newborn.

Pathology. In the stillborn infant the lungs have a uniformly beefy red appearance. Histologically, the interstitial tissues are congested, and the alveoli present the appearance of a crumpled sac. The degree of crumpling varies inversely with the amount of expansion of the alveoli by fluid, presumed to be amniotic. With sudden anoxia in utero there may be more vigorous inspiratory movements than usual, with an increase in aspiration of amniotic fluid and its contents. The later in pregnancy this takes place, the more likely is one to find squamous epithelial cells and debris in the alveolar spaces.

If an infant has breathed, the lungs may show beefy red areas alternating with lighter, aerated, raised portions. Histologically, the red areas are congested, and the alveolar spaces may be filled with varying amounts of blood or edema fluid. In lighter, aerated portions there are varying degrees of distention of alveoli. If there has been vigorous inspiration, either natural or artificial, one may find irregular areas of overdistention of alveoli. Some of these may have ruptured with resultant interstitial emphysema and, at times, pneumomediastinum and pneumothorax.

Clinical Manifestations. Cyanosis and poor respiratory exchange on auscultation of the chest are the cardinal signs of extensive atelectasis, which may be confirmed roentgenographically.

Prevention and Treatment. Prevention of premature labor, fetal and neonatal anoxia, intracranial hemorrhage, the respiratory distress syndrome and pneumonia would presumably eliminate most of the causes of atelectasis. Treatment should be aimed at early recognition and proper management of the underlying condition.

IDIOPATHIC RESPIRATORY DISTRESS SYNDROME
(Hyaline Membrane Disease)

The terms given above are those most widely used to describe a syndrome of neonatal respiratory distress in which pulmonary hyaline membranes with atelectasis are the principal findings at autopsy. It is by far the commonest cause of death among premature infants, but is also seen with significant frequency among infants of diabetic mothers, among infants born by cesarean section, and occasionally among infants in whom no predisposing factor is apparent. The incidence among premature infants is given in Table 7-18.

TABLE 7-18. INCIDENCE OF IDIOPATHIC RESPIRATORY DISTRESS SYNDROME* AND MORTALITY PER CLINICAL CASE AND PER LIVE BIRTH AMONG PREMATURE INFANTS

		IDIOPATHIC RESPIRATORY DISTRESS SYNDROME				
	LIVE			MORTALITY DUE TO H.M.D.		
BIRTH WEIGHT	BIRTHS	NO.	PER CENT	NO.	PER CASE	PER BIRTH
≤ 1000 gm. (2 lb. 3 oz.)	13	2	15%	2	100%	15%
1000-1500 gm. (2 lb. 3 oz.-3 lb. 4 oz.)	23	13	57%	8	62%	24%
1500-2000 gm. (3 lb. 4 oz.-4 lb. 6 oz.)	90	14	16%	4	29%	4.5%
2000-2500 gm. (4 lb. 6 oz.-5 lb. 8 oz.)	206	15	7%	6	40%	3%
All prematures	332	44	13%	20	45%	6%

Data from Boston Lying-In Hospital, 1959 (infants of diabetic mothers excluded).
*The term "idiopathic respiratory distress syndrome" is used to designate the clinical syndrome in which no other cause of respiratory distress than hyaline membrane formation was discoverable.
From S. G. Driscoll and C. A. Smith: Neonatal Pulmonary Disorders. *Pediat. Clin. N. Amer.,* 9:325, 1962.

Etiology. During fetal life most of the venous blood passes from the venous to the arterial circulation through the foramen ovale and ductus arteriosus, thus bypassing the lungs, which at this time have a high vascular resistance. With the onset of breathing, pulmonary vascular resistance is greatly reduced, resulting in a corresponding increase in pulmonary blood flow. Left atrial pressure increases as a result of increased pulmonary venous return, so that the foramen ovale closes. The ductus arteriosus possibly closes because of the constricting effect on its muscular wall of the increased tension of oxygen in the systemic arterial blood which passes through it after breathing has begun.

In the idiopathic respiratory distress syndrome, pulmonary vascular resistance is high, probably because of constriction of peripheral pulmonary arterioles. As a result, pressure rises on the venous side of the circulation and blood is shunted to the arterial side without passing through the lungs; hypoxia, cyanosis and respiratory distress result. A high proportion of infants who later have the respiratory distress syndrome have had periods of asphyxia before or immediately after birth. The pH of the blood drops rapidly, and carbon dioxide tension rises in the hypoxic fetus or newborn infant; resuscitative measures frequently lead to chilling, a physiologic change to which premature infants are particularly susceptible because of their lack of insulating body fat, low thermal stability and small energy stores. Hypoxia, acidemia, increased carbon dioxide tension and chilling all have a vasoconstrictive effect on the pulmonary arterioles, which leads to hypoperfusion of the lungs and shunting of blood past the lungs. Atelectasis and alveolar effusion add to the problem by reducing gas exchange with the blood which does pass through the alveolar capillaries. This "hypoperfusion theory" of the origin of hyaline membrane disease, for which there is experimental support, is illustrated in Figure 7-14. Infants with severe respiratory distress also have

systemic hypotension, cutaneous vasoconstriction, oliguria and ileus.

Cheek and Rowe have suggested that the biochemical and physiologic changes in the respiratory distress syndrome might be explained on the basis of overactivity of the sympathetic nervous system in response to stress, particularly the stress of hypoxia and hypercapnia. They point out that deficiency of the enzyme catechol-o-methyl transferase, which destroys epinephrine, might contribute to sustained overaction of the sympathetic nervous system, resulting in constriction of peripheral arterioles, diminished blood volume, leakage of fluid and protein into the interstitial compartment, increased venous pressure, and cardiac failure, all of which are present in the respiratory distress syndrome.

The hyaline membranes observed at autopsy of

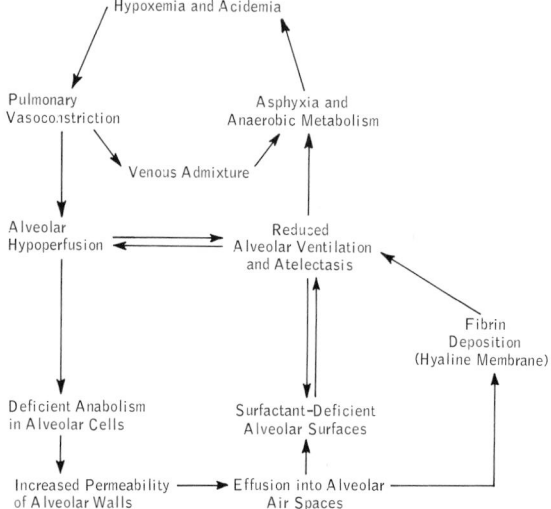

Figure 7-14. Hypoperfusion theory of hyaline membrane disease. (Adapted from J. Chu, et al.: The Pulmonary Hypoperfusion Syndrome. *Pediatrics,* 35:733, 1965.)

infants dying with idiopathic respiratory distress syndrome are probably only a secondary manifestation of the pathophysiology of the disease. They contain fibrin, and are the result of (1) effusion from the pulmonary circulation, (2) conversion of fibrinogen in the effusion fluid to fibrin (possibly increased by the thromboplastic activity of aspirated amniotic fluid), and (3) syneresis of the fibrin to form a membrane.

Deficiency of a surface-tension-reducing film of lipoprotein (surfactin) normally present in the alveoli may also be a factor in the pathogenesis of this disorder. The deficiency is presumably produced by an inhibiting substance derived from damaged pulmonary tissue or inhaled with amniotic fluid.

Pathology. The lungs appear deep purplish-red and are liver-like in consistency. Microscopically, there is extensive atelectasis with engorgement of the interalveolar capillaries, and a number of the alveolar ducts, alveoli and respiratory bronchioles are lined with acidophilic, homogeneous or granular membranes. Amniotic debris, intra-alveolar hemorrhage, pneumonia and interstitial emphysema are additional but inconstant findings (Fig. 7-15). The characteristic hyaline membranes are rarely seen in infants dying earlier than 6 to 8 hours after birth. Intracranial hemorrhages are common, but are probably associated with anoxia or prematurity rather than the idiopathic respiratory distress syndrome.

Clinical Manifestations. The idiopathic respiratory distress syndrome begins with rapid, shallow respirations which usually increase to 60 or more per minute within 2 hours of birth. It is often preceded by a need for resuscitation at birth. Rapid

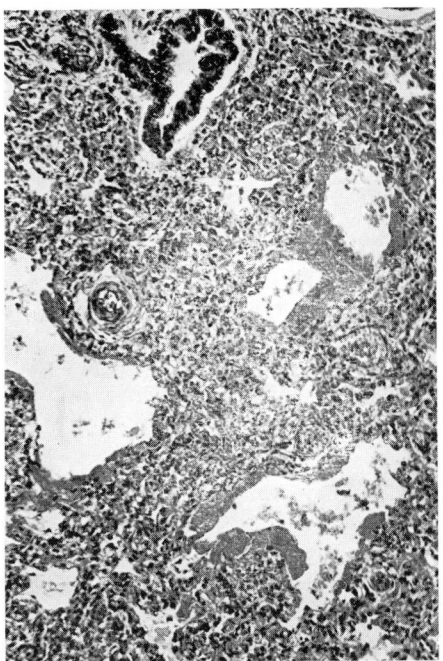

Figure 7-15. Pulmonary hyaline membranes lining the air spaces of the lung in a premature infant.

breathing beginning later suggests conditions other than hyaline membrane disease. Other symptoms are listed in Table 7-17 and illustrated in Figure 7-1. Intercostal retractions and an expiratory grunt are prominent symptoms, and the course is characterized by increasing evidence of air hunger and fatigue from excessive respiratory effort. On auscultation, air exchange may seem to be normal or diminished. On deep inspiration fine rales are often heard, especially over the lung bases, posteriorly. Roentgenographically (Fig. 7-16), the lungs have a reticulogranular appearance which is characteristic but not pathognomonic. The condition may progress to death within a few hours, but in milder cases the symptoms reach a peak within 3 days, after which gradual improvement sets in. Death is rare after 3 days, except among infants in whom the natural course of the disease has been altered by the use of a respirator, particularly of the positive-pressure type.

Prognosis. Although the diagnosis is established with certainty only at autopsy, the currently high correlation of clinical diagnoses with postmortem ones does permit estimation of mortality rates (Table 7-18). The mortality rate is lower among mature infants with the disease. When recovery occurs, the prognosis is generally good, although persistent pulmonary disease does occur in a small percentage of infants and may possibly be related to oxygen therapy (see below). Neurologic residuals are probably related more to intracranial hemorrhage, hypoglycemia, hyperbilirubinemia and other complications of immaturity than to the respiratory distress syndrome.

Prevention. The prevention of prematurity, avoidance of unnecessary cesarean section, and careful management of the diabetic mother are the most important factors in the prevention of the respiratory distress syndrome. If the hypoperfusion theory is correct, measures designed to minimize pulmonary vasocontriction at birth seem logical. Avoidance of maternal hypoxia, acidemia and systemic hypotension (with decreased uterine blood flow) are indicated, and intervals of diminished umbilical blood flow should be minimized so far as possible. Chilling, as well as hypoxia, of the newborn infant results in acidemia and pulmonary vasoconstriction; both should be avoided. Prompt treatment or prevention of severe acidemia through intravenous administration of sodium bicarbonate solution may be helpful. Clamping of the umbilical cord after the second breath rather than before remains to be confirmed as an effective preventive measure. Differing definitions of what constitutes "early" or "late" clamping have helped to obscure the results of studies of this feature, but current consensus appears to be in favor of "late" clamping.

Treatment. Regardless of whether this syndrome is due to pulmonary vascular constriction and shunting, atelectasis, hyaline membranes or some combination of them, the basic defect which requires treatment is inadequate pulmonary ex-

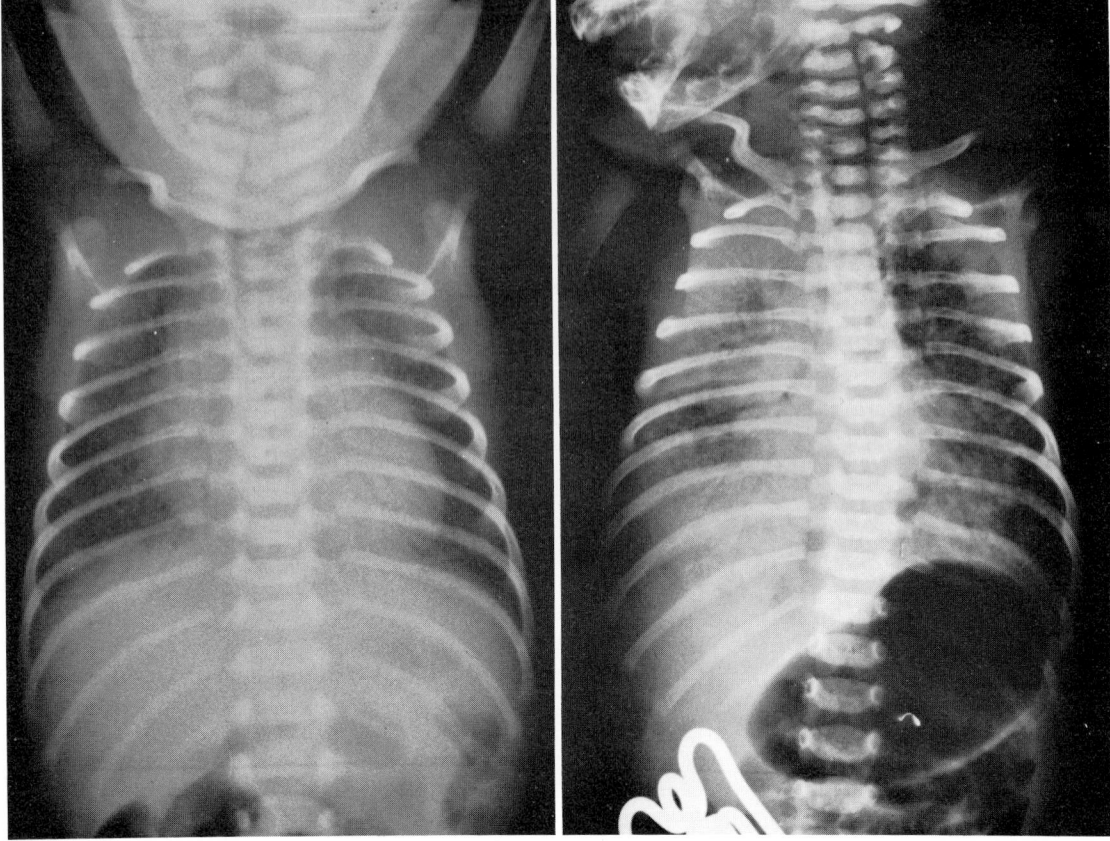

Fig. 7-16.   Fig. 7-17.

Figure 7-16. Respiratory distress syndrome. A diffuse reticulogranular pattern is evident throughout the lungs. The air-containing bronchi are visible by virtue of surrounding nonaerated lung, particularly on the left.

Figure 7-17. Fetal distress syndrome.

Figures 7-16 and 7-17 show the contrasting radiographic pictures seen in infants with neonatal respiratory distress. Figure 7-16 shows the uniform reticulogranular pattern consistently seen in, but not pathognomonic of, the respiratory distress syndrome (hyaline membrane disease). The apparent cardiac enlargement is also characteristic. Figure 7-17 shows the coarsely granular pattern with irregular aeration typical of fetal distress from aspiration of materials such as vernix caseosa, epithelial cells and meconium contained in amniotic fluid.

change of oxygen and carbon dioxide; metabolic acidosis is a secondary manifestation. The infant tries to overcome his ventilatory problem by increasing the rate and depth of respiration. Grunting, formerly thought to be merely a sign of respiratory distress, serves the physiologic purpose of increasing alveolar ventilation; the insertion of an endotracheal tube makes grunting impossible and results in a fall in arterial oxygen tension in the distressed infant.

The infant may be aided in his efforts by the avoidance of chilling, which causes pulmonary vasoconstriction and increases the metabolic need for oxygen and the production of carbon dioxide. Since hypoxia and acidemia both result from and cause pulmonary vasoconstriction (Fig. 7-14), the administration of oxygen and a buffer constitutes rational treatment. Intravenous feeding is a convenient way to administer the buffer solution and also allows the infant to receive fluid and calories

without fatigue from oral feeding. Mechanical assistance in breathing *may* be required in order to increase alveolar ventilation directly. The application of these methods is best carried out in a specially staffed and equipped hospital unit, the *intensive care nursery.* The facilities of the intensive care nursery may also appropriately be used for the care of other sick newborn infants and for the initial observation of "high-risk" infants (p. 360).

Chilling is avoided and oxygen consumption of premature infants is minimal when abdominal skin temperature is kept between 36 and 37° C.; apneic spells are said to be less frequent if it is nearer 36 than 37° C. Temperature control is best accomplished by special thermoregulating equipment controlled by a thermistor taped to the skin of the abdomen. If such equipment is not available, an incubator temperature between 32 and 34° C. at a relative humidity of 80 to 90 per cent is usually necessary to maintain thermal stability of the infant. Relative humidity of 30 to 60 per cent is adequate when special thermoregulating equipment is being used, but in its absence heat loss is less at a relative humidity of 80 to 90 per cent. *Nebulized water mist* offers no advantage over proper humidification, except when the nose is bypassed, as with the use of tracheal intubation or tracheostomy. In such instances, if an ultrasonic nebulizer is used, care must be taken lest too much water be inhaled into the lungs.

Periodic monitoring of oxygen and carbon dioxide tension and of the pH of arterial or capillary blood is an important part of the management; if assisted ventilation is being used, it is essential. Arterial oxygen tension is conveniently measured in blood drawn from the temporal artery or from an indwelling plastic catheter threaded through one of the umbilical arteries so that its tip lies just above the bifurcation of the aorta. Carbon dioxide tension and pH may also be measured from arterial blood obtained by these methods, and the umbilical arterial catheter may be used for administration of fluids and drugs.

In order to attain an environment with a high, constant oxygen content, it is necessary to use a plastic hood constructed so that it is just large enough to accommodate the infant's head, and through which oxygen flow can be maintained and adjusted. Even so, periodic measurements of the oxygen content of the atmosphere within the box are necessary. The air flow in commercially available incubators is such that it is impossible to maintain a high or constant atmosphere of oxygen, particularly when the infant is receiving direct care by nurse or physician.

Reasonable indications for *assisted ventilation* would appear to be (1) failure to maintain respiration without assistance, (2) cyanosis while breathing 100 per cent oxygen, or (3) arterial oxygen tension under 50 mm. Hg, or (4) arterial carbon dioxide tension over 70 mm. Hg when measured after the infant has breathed 100 per cent oxygen for 15 minutes. In a group of infants who did not receive assisted ventilation and who had arterial oxygen tensions below 100 mm. Hg during the first 10 hours of life while breathing 100 per cent oxygen, Boston noted a case fatality rate of 80 per cent.

The simplest method of assisted ventilation is intermittent use of a mask and bag resuscitator for 5 minutes out of every 20 minutes, or another time regimen adapted to the needs of the individual infant. A patient-cycled positive-pressure respirator with a nasotracheal tube in place has been widely used, but its use has been accompanied by a disturbing incidence of complications. Those related to trauma from the intratracheal tube may be avoided in most cases by substituting a well fitting anesthetic gas mask. Negative-pressure respirators have the advantage of requiring neither a mask nor endotracheal tube, and their use has so far been virtually free of accompanying oxygen toxicity to the lungs, which appears to be a serious drawback to prolonged use of the positive-pressure type of respirator.

Monitoring of *aortic blood pressure* through an umbilical arterial catheter and *central venous pressure* by a catheter passed through the umbilical vein may provide useful guides to management of the shocklike state which is common for the first hour or so after premature birth.

Owing to the frequency of pneumonia accompanying the respiratory distress syndrome and of infection complicating assisted ventilation and indwelling vascular catheters, the routine administration of antibacterial agents is advocated by some, but rejected by those who are more fearful of upsetting bacterial ecology. If they are to be used, penicillin or ampicillin with kanamycin is suggested. Appropriate doses are 25,000 units of penicillin or 50 mg. of ampicillin, and 7.5 mg. of kanamycin per kg. every 12 hours until recovery seems assured.

The use of acetylcholine or adrenergic inhibitors, though a logical approach to the problem of pulmonary vasoconstriction, has not been shown to be therapeutically effective.

Usher confirmed the correlation, previously noted by others, of low plasma pH values and death in infants with idiopathic respiratory distress. He also pointed out that infants with a venous blood pH below 7.15, a carbon dioxide tension above 70 mm. Hg or a plasma bicarbonate level of less than 18 mEq. per liter rarely survive without treatment of their acidosis. He further pointed out that the plasma potassium concentration of such infants rises, and that hyperkalemic electrocardiographic conduction disturbances appear. He therefore recommends that all infants with idiopathic respiratory distress receive a continuous intravenous infusion containing varying concentrations of glucose, insulin and sodium bicarbonate, depending on the results of repeated determinations of blood pH and carbon dioxide content, and of serum potassium. Infants with severe hyperkalemia are given 20 per cent glucose in water containing 1 unit of insulin for each 3 gm. of glucose for several hours to correct the hyperkalemia. The infusion is given at the rate of 65 ml. per kg. per 24 hours. It is then continued at the same rate, using 10 per cent glucose in water with sodium bicarbonate added in concentrations which depend on the current blood pH of the infant, as shown below.

pH VENOUS BLOOD	pH CAPILLARY OR ARTERIAL BLOOD	CONCENTRATION OF SODIUM BICARBONATE
Over 7.20	Over 7.30	5 mEq. or 0.42 Gm. per 100 ml.
7.10-7.20	7.20-7.30	10 mEq. or 0.83 Gm. per 100 ml.
7.00-7.10	7.10-7.20	15 mEq. or 1.25 Gm. per 100 ml.

Other investigators have advocated the correction of acidemia by rapid and repeated small-volume infusions of amounts of sodium bicarbonate calculated to correct the acidosis present at the time of infusion. This regimen may result in hypernatremia. Liver necrosis may be caused by rapid infusion of concentrated solutions of sodium bicarbonate through an umbilical catheter into the portal vein, and by tris-hydroxymethyl aminomethane (THAM), which has also been used to combat the acidosis of asphyxia and of the respiratory distress syndrome. Since circulatory stasis at the time of rapid infusion of concentrated solutions seems to contribute to their toxicity, caution should be taken to maintain an adequate blood pressure, by careful external cardiac massage if necessary, while they are being given.

Complications of Intensive Care. The most serious complication of nasotracheal intubation is cardiac arrest during intubation or suctioning. Other complications include bleeding from trauma during intubation, difficult extubation requiring tracheotomy, ulceration of the nares due to pressure from the tube, permanent narrowing of the nostril due to tissue damage and scarring from irritation of infection around the tube, evulsion of a vocal cord, laryngeal ulcer, papilloma of a vocal cord, subglottic stenosis, and persistent hoarseness, stridor or edema of the larynx.

Measures to reduce the incidence of these complications include use of polyvinyl endotracheal tubes that do not contain tin, which is toxic to cells; use of a tube of the smallest practicable size in order to reduce local ischemia and necrosis; avoidance of frequent changes of the tube; avoidance of motion of the tube in situ; avoidance of too frequent or vigorous suctioning; and avoidance of infection through meticulous cleanliness and frequent sterilization of all apparatus attached to or passed through the tube. The personnel inserting and caring for the endotracheal tube should be experienced and skilled. The use of an anesthetic gas mask instead of an endotracheal tube has been shown to be practical and to avoid the foregoing complications; care must be taken to avoid damage to the eyes and skin from pressure, if a mask is used. The use of a negative-pressure respirator eliminates the need for either tube or mask, but has the drawback of being less easy to regulate than are patient-cycled positive-pressure machines.

The incidence of serious *complications of catheterization of the umbilical artery* observed at autopsy is about 2 per cent. Transient blanching of the leg occurs in approximately 5 per cent of patients. It is usually due to reflex arterial spasm, the incidence of which can be diminished by use of the smallest available catheters, particularly in very small infants. Occasionally the spasm can be relieved by warming the opposite leg; if this is unsuccessful after 15 to 20 minutes, the catheter should be removed. Accidental lodgment of the catheter in a smaller artery so as to block it completely or cause unrecognized local vascular spasm may result in gangrene of the organ or area supplied by the vessel. To prevent this complication the catheter should be removed promptly if blood cannot be obtained through it; it is advisable to use a radiopaque catheter whose position is checked roentgenographically after insertion. Serious hemorrhage on removal of the catheter is rare; its incidence may be reduced by not removing the catheter for 6 hours after any heparin has been pushed through it. Thrombi may form in the aorta or in the catheter; their incidence is lowered by use of a smooth-tipped catheter with a hole only at its end, and by rinsing the catheter with a small amount of saline solution containing 10 units of heparin per ml. Some prefer to use the umbilical artery for blood sampling only, leaving the catheter filled with heparinized saline between samplings. The best position for the tip of the catheter is just above the bifurcation of the aorta or above the renal arteries and celiac axis. Dunn has found that the distance from the umbilical ring to the bifurcation of the aorta is approximately half the distance between the top of the shoulder over the lateral end of the clavicle and a point vertically beneath it and level with the center of the umbilicus, and that the distance from the umbilical ring to the diaphragm is approximately the same as this "shoulder-umbilicus length." The later hazards of catheterization of the umbilical artery or umbilical vein, particularly when it has been traumatic, are as yet unknown, but may well exist. An umbilical arterial or venous catheter should be removed at the earliest possible moment, and its placement and supervision should be by skilled and experienced personnel.

The toxicity to the retina of high concentrations of oxygen administered for prolonged periods has been amply demonstrated; retrolental fibroplasia is probably secondary to partial pressures of oxygen above the normal range in the blood and is rare with concentrations of less than 40 per cent in the inspired air. The oxygen tension of the blood under normal circumstances while breathing air is approximately 100 mm. Hg; while breathing 40 per cent oxygen it is usually 140 to 150 mm. Therefore the partial pressures of oxygen in the arterial blood should be monitored in the pink infant receiving oxygen and kept preferably below 100 mm. Hg; the oxygen tensions in cyanotic infants are well below 100 mm. Hg.

Oxygen has been demonstrated to be toxic to the lung, particularly if administered by means of a positive-pressure respirator. Instead of showing improvement on the third or fourth day, consistent with the natural course of the disease in survivors, some infants who have been on prolonged intermittent positive-pressure breathing using high concentrations of oxygen have roentgenographic evidence of worsening of their pulmonary condition (Fig. 7-18, *A*), and they continue to be cyanotic without oxygen in high concentration. The chest roentgenogram is described as gradually changing from a picture of almost complete opacification with air bronchogram to one of small, round, lucent areas alternating with areas of irregular density resembling a sponge (Fig. 7-18, *B*). This picture is similar to that seen in the "bubbly-lung syndrome" of Wilson and

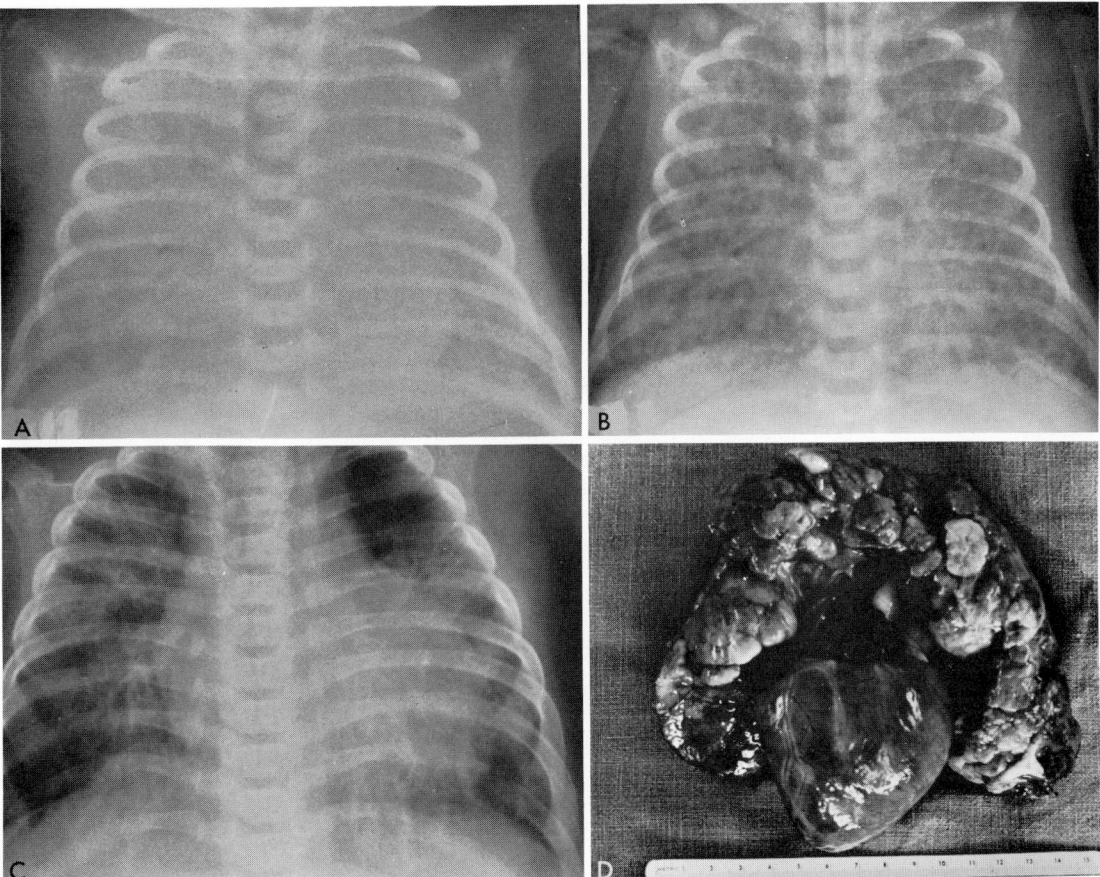

Figure 7-18. Pulmonary changes in 4 infants who were treated in the immediate postnatal period for the clinical syndrome of idiopathic respiratory distress with prolonged, intermittent positive-pressure breathing with air containing 80 to 100 per cent oxygen. In all infants there was persistent respiratory disease. Nine of 13 infants lived beyond 2 weeks of age; 5 of the 9 died, and all had right-sided congestive heart failure. The remaining 4 were described as having chronic pulmonary disease. *A,* A 5-day-old infant with nearly complete opacification of lungs. *B,* A 13-day-old infant with "bubbly lungs" simulating the roentgenographic appearance of the Wilson-Mikity syndrome. *C,* A 7-month-old infant with irregular, dense strands in both lungs, and cardiomegaly. *D,* Large right ventricle and cobbly, irregularly aerated lung of an infant who died at 11 months of age; this infant also had a patent ductus arteriosus. (From W. H. Northway, Jr., R. C. Rosan and D. Y. Porter: Pulmonary Disease Following Respirator Therapy of Hyaline-Membrane Disease. Bronchopulmonary Dysplasia. *New England J. Med.,* 276:357, 1967.)

Mikity (p. 390). In the histologic picture at this stage (10 to 20 days after beginning oxygen therapy) there is less evidence of hyaline membrane formation, progressive alveolar coalescence with atelectasis of surrounding alveoli, interstitial edema, coarse focal thickening of the basement membranes and widespread bronchial and bronchiolar mucosal metaplasia and hyperplasia. In the series studied, respiratory difficulty persisted in the 4 of 13 infants who survived (see legend of Fig. 7-18). Postmortem studies in those who died revealed cardiac enlargement and pulmonary changes consisting of focal areas of emphysematous alveoli with hypertrophy of the peribronchial smooth muscle of the tributary bronchioles, some perimucosal fibrosis and widespread metaplasia of the bronchiolar mucosa, and thickening of basement membranes and separation of the capillaries from the alveolar epithelial cells.

It is suggested that oxygen tension in the ar-

terial blood be kept in the range of 60 to 100 mm. Hg when assisted ventilation is being used. A question has also recently been posed regarding the possible toxicity of oxygen for cerebral blood vessels. *The principle of using as little oxygen as possible for the shortest possible time must be rigidly adhered to in the therapy of infants.*

Another iatrogenic complication of intensive care is *anemia secondary to frequent withdrawal of blood samples.* The cumulative amount of blood withdrawn should be carefully recorded. Replacement by transfusion is indicated if more than 10 to 15 per cent of estimated total blood volume is removed.

Results of Intensive Care. Evaluation of the efficacy of intensive care of infants with hyaline membrane disease or other respiratory problems is clouded by the following factors: (1) the criteria for its application vary from one institution to another; (2) the definition of what constitutes intensive care varies from one institution to another; (3) the infants to whom it is applied do not represent a homogeneous group from the standpoints of origin or of severity of their respiratory problem; (4) external factors (race, transport, admitting and referral practices) may bias the findings when one compares sequential results in the same institution as well as results between institutions; (5) it is difficult to attribute good results to methodologic changes in care because of the increased interest and intensity of nursing care which almost always accompanies a methodologic change; and (6) follow-up studies are not yet adequate to determine whether intensive care increases or decreases the absolute or relative numbers of surviving infants with neurologic residuals. There is a general impression, however, that intensive care of high-risk newborn infants reduces the mortality of those whose respiratory problems are not secondary to intracranial hemorrhage or to irremedial congenital malformations.

Other Aspects of Intensive Care. The concept of intensive care of the newborn implies attention to problems other than respiratory ones. Many of these, such as hypoglycemia and hyperbilirubinemia, are common among infants who are candidates for intensive care because of respiratory difficulties associated with asphyxia or prematurity. The satisfactory management of these problems, like those of respiratory distress, requires a high degree of mutual interest and coordination among anesthetist, obstetrician and pediatrician and pathologist. The continuous night and day availability of interested and skilled laboratory personnel is essential.

PNEUMONIA

Histologic evidence of pneumonia is a frequent finding at autopsy in newborn infants, particularly among those who die after signs of respiratory distress of whatever cause. Its role as a cause of death is not always clear in such instances, and the clinical manifestations may merge indistinguishably with those of the primary disturbance. Perhaps about 10 per cent of neonatal deaths are primarily attributable to pneumonia.

Etiology. There are 2 main types of neonatal pneumonia. The first, sometimes termed *congenital pneumonia,* occurs during the first few days of life. It is particularly common when there has been premature rupture of the membranes, prolonged labor, premature labor, maternal fever or fetal distress. The presence of chorioamnionitis in most instances suggests aspiration of infected amniotic fluid as its cause. Aspiration of vaginal secretions during delivery may also be a cause. The second type of pneumonia, beginning after the first few days of life, is usually acquired through contact with adults or children with respiratory infections, or through bacteremia. Coliform organisms and *Staphylococcus aureus* are the most frequent causative organisms for either type of

pneumonia. Enterococci, Klebsiella, Pseudomonas, Proteus and Salmonella also tend to be more frequent pathogens in the newborn than are Pneumococcus, *H. influenzae* and beta hemolytic streptococcus, the commonest acute pulmonary pathogens of older infants and children. The relative incidence of viral pneumonitis in the neonatal period is not adequately defined.

Pathology. Pneumonia in early infancy is usually bronchopneumonic in type, occasionally interstitial or lobar.

Clinical Manifestations. The first signs of pneumonia in the newborn are usually nonspecific. They include loss of appetite, listlessness, poor color which may or may not be definable as cyanosis, a rise or sudden fall in body temperature, abdominal distention, sudden loss or gain in weight, and a general impression on the part of the nurse or mother that the baby is doing less well. Cough is inconstant, but almost always means pneumonia when present. A significant increase in respiratory rate, usually to about 80, is a constant and early finding. Flaring of the alae nasi, accentuation of the normal irregularity of breathing, and respiratory distress may be present.

Diagnosis. Often no physical signs are elicited; although careful auscultation may reveal fine, crackling rales, most commonly in the perihilar areas posteriorly, they may be localized in any portion of the lungs. It is important to auscultate the chest with the baby crying as well as quiet, since frequently rales are heard only at the end of the deep inspirations which come only with crying in the newborn. Areas of hyperresonance may indicate compensatory emphysema. Roentgenograms of the chest are often helpful. Nasopharyngeal and blood cultures are helpful in making an etiologic diagnosis.

Aspiration of Foreign Material ("Fetal Anoxia"; "Fetal Distress Syndrome"; "Aspiration Pneumonia") (see also p. 926). During prolonged labors and difficult deliveries infants often attempt to breathe in utero, owing to interference with the supply of oxygen via the placenta. Under such circumstances the infant aspirates amniotic fluid containing such debris as vernix caseosa, epithelial cells, meconium or material from the birth canal. This debris blocks the smallest airways and interferes with alveolar transmission of oxygen and carbon dioxide. Pathologic bacteria frequently accompany the aspirated material. When this is the case, pneumonia is apt to ensue, but even in the noninfected cases there are respiratory distress and usually roentgenographic evidences of aspiration (Fig. 7-17).

Other situations in which pulmonary aspiration of foreign material may contribute to serious consequences in the newborn infant include tracheo-esophageal fistula, esophageal and duodenal obstructions, improper feeding practices, the administration of medicines and improper handling and placement of infants in their cribs.

The contents of the stomach should always be aspirated through a soft rubber catheter just

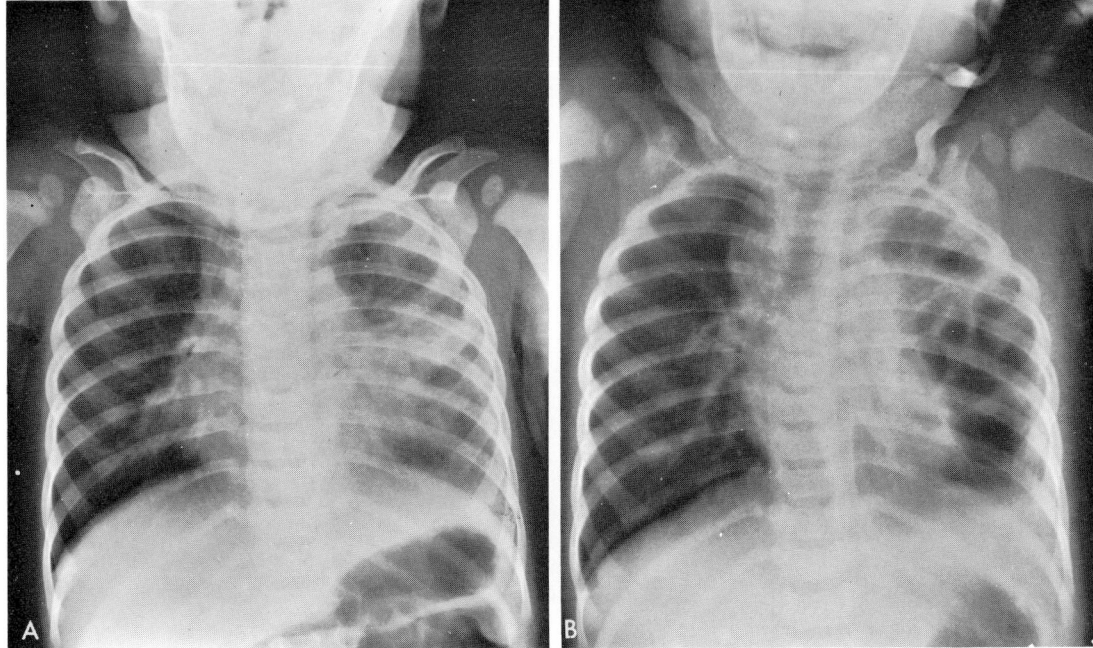

Figure 7-19. Staphylococcal pneumonia in an infant 7 months of age. *A*, The diffuse inflammatory process involving the left lung and pleura is evident. *B*, Five days later, just before death, there are multiple air-containing cavities in the lung and pleura.

before operation or other procedures requiring anesthesia. Procedures which may significantly disturb the infant, and particularly those which interfere with changing the infant to the head-down position, such as jugular and femoral punctures, lumbar puncture and subdural taps, should be performed at least 2 hours after a feeding.

Staphylococcal pneumonia should be suspected in any infant who shows even slight and nonspecific untoward signs and who has been exposed to staphylococcal skin infections. Empyema and pneumothorax are frequent complications. The latter constitutes such an immediate threat to life that infants with staphylococcal pneumonia must be watched closely for acute onset of respiratory distress, so that treatment by closed thoracotomy drainage can be carried out without delay.

Treatment. See pages 406 and 919.

PNEUMOTHORAX AND PNEUMOMEDIASTINUM

Asymptomatic pneumothorax, either unilateral or bilateral, is estimated to occur in as many as 1 per cent of all newborn infants; symptomatic pneumothorax and pneumomediastinum are less common.

Etiology. Since pneumothorax is frequent among newborn infants who have been subjected to resuscitative measures, it seems likely that the most common cause is overinflation and resulting alveolar rupture. If the ruptured alveoli are on the pleural surface, pneumothorax without pneumomediastinum occurs. If they are not, pulmonary interstitial emphysema results. If the volume of

escaped air is great enough, it is believed to follow the vascular sheaths to the mediastinum, causing mediastinal emphysema. In turn, the mediastinal air may "break" into the pleural space to cause pneumothorax, or into the subcutaneous tissues of the neck and chest to cause subcutaneous emphysema. Ball-valve types of bronchial or bronchiolar obstruction resulting from aspiration may also cause alveolar overinflation which, if mild, produces local emphysema, but, if severe, results in alveolar rupture and pulmonary interstitial emphysema, pneumomediastinum or pneumothorax.

Pneumothorax may also result from direct trauma such as puncture from a broken rib or from rupture of a lung abscess associated with staphylococcal pneumonia. It also occurs from rupture of pulmonary cysts. It occurs rarely as a result of alveolar rupture in lobar emphysema.

Clinical Manifestations. Localized areas of emphysema frequently seen in roentgenograms of the chest of newborn infants may represent ball-valve bronchial obstruction, pulmonary interstitial emphysema or emphysematous blebs (cysts). The physical findings of asymptomatic pneumothorax are hyperresonance and diminished breath sounds over the involved side of the chest.

Symptomatic *pneumothorax* is characterized by respiratory distress which varies from only an increased respiratory rate to severe dyspnea and cyanosis. The onset may be sudden or gradual. The chest may appear asymmetric with increased anteroposterior diameter and bulging of the intercostal spaces on the affected side, and there are hyperresonance and diminished or absent breath

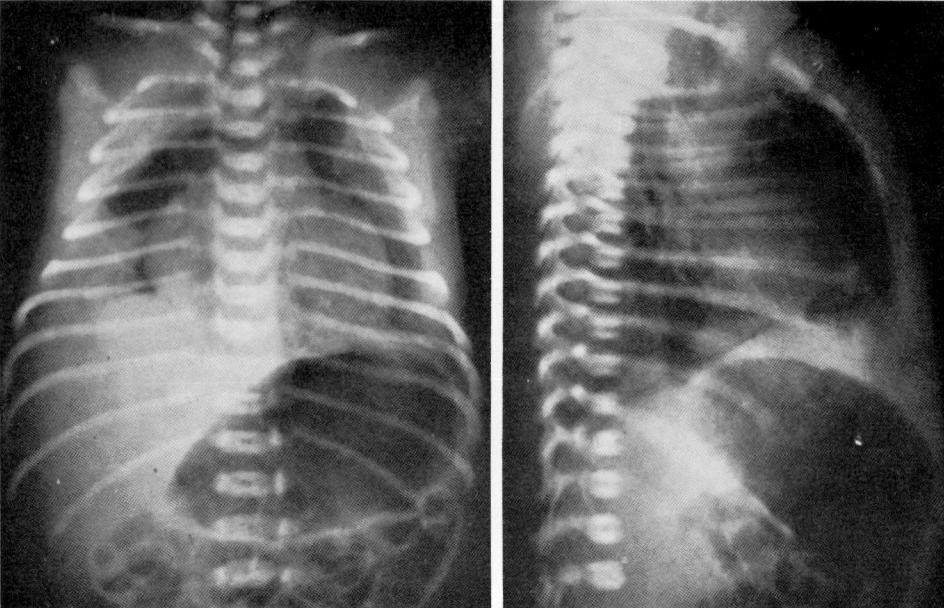

Figure 7-20. Pneumomediastinum in a newborn infant. Anteroposterior view demonstrates compression of lungs and the lateral view bulging of the sternum, each resulting from distention of the mediastinum by trapped air.

sounds. The heart is displaced toward the unaffected side, and the diaphragm is displaced downward, as is the liver with right-sided pneumothorax. Since both sides may be affected, symmetry of findings does not rule out pneumothorax.

With *pneumomediastinum* the degree of respiratory distress is again dependent on the amount of trapped air. If it is great, there is bulging of the midthoracic area, the neck veins are distended, and the blood pressure is low. The last 2 findings are the result of blockage of the circulation by compression of the systemic and pulmonary veins. Subcutaneous emphysema in the newborn infant is almost pathognomonic of pneumomediastinum.

Diagnosis. Pneumothorax and pneumomediastinum should be suspected in any newborn infant with respiratory distress; the diagnosis is established roentgenographically (Fig. 7-20).

Treatment. Asymptomatic pneumothorax or pneumomediastinum requires no treatment. If severe respiratory or circulatory embarrassment is present, needle aspiration is indicated. If this is unsuccessful in maintaining relief of distress, closed thoracotomy is indicated with the tube connected to a water trap so that air may escape, but not enter the chest.

INTERSTITIAL PULMONARY FIBROSIS OF PREMATURITY
(Wilson-Mikity Syndrome; Bubbly-Lung Syndrome; Pulmonary Dysmaturity)

Wilson and Mikity have described a pulmonary syndrome of premature infants, usually of gestational age less than 32 weeks and birth weights below 1500 gm., which is characterized by insidi-

ous onset of hyperpnea and cyanosis during the first month of life. Cough, wheezing and rales may develop, but fever occurs only with concomitant infection. Abdominal distention, vomiting and loose, frothy stools may be present, and eosinophilia has been reported. Stress fractures of the ribs may occur as a complication of the dyspnea and coughing, and collapse of a lobe or a lung has been observed; re-expansion usually occurs within a few days. Right-sided heart failure is a serious complication.

The *cause* of the Wilson-Mikity syndrome is unknown; it has been speculated that the disease may be a manifestation of the stresses imposed by respiration on immature respiratory structures or response to respiratory disease or to some aspect of treatment. The roentgenographic findings resemble some of those attributed to oxygen therapy utilizing an intermittent positive-pressure apparatus (p. 386). The histologic picture of emphysema with wide, cellular alveolar septa with mononuclear infiltration and fibrosis, however, does not correspond.

Roentgenographically (Fig. 7-21), there is a rather characteristic diffuse, coarse, streaky infiltration with small areas of emphysema which may create a "bubbly" appearance.

Diagnostically, this condition must be differentiated from interstitial plasma cell pneumonia due to *Pneumocystis carinii,* cystic fibrosis and possibly pulmonary damage from oxygen therapy (see p. 386). Since its cause is unknown, purposeful prevention is not possible, and *treatment* consists of such supportive measures as oxygen for cyanosis and digitalization for cardiac failure. About one quarter of the identified infants have died of cardiac or respiratory failure within a few

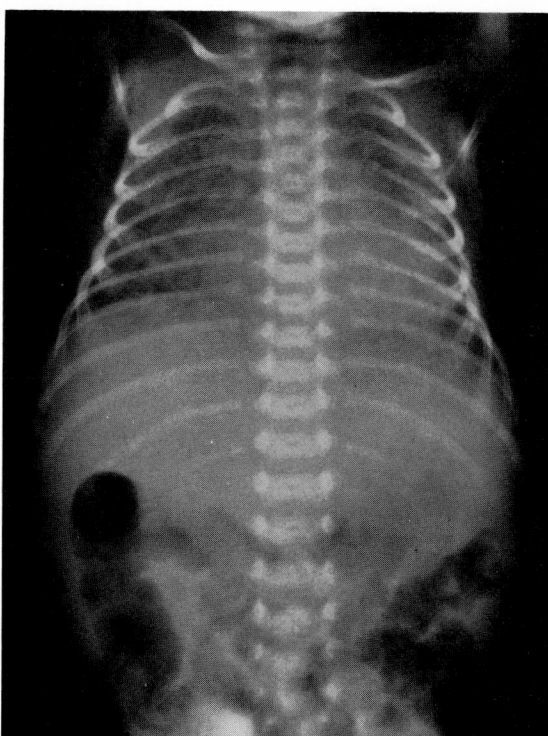

Figure 7-21. Interstitial pulmonary fibrosis of prematurity.

months of onset; the remainder tend to show gradual improvement and resolution of the pulmonary disease.

LOBAR EMPHYSEMA

See page 933.

LUNG CYSTS

Most lung cysts observed during the neonatal period are acquired as the result of rupture of alveoli from overinflation or by infection, often staphylococcal; congenital cysts are rare. They may be solitary or multiple, air-containing or filled with fluid, and are believed to result as a developmental anomaly of the bronchial buds (see p. 910). Air-filled cysts on the surface of the lung, whatever their origin, sometimes rupture and cause pneumothorax. This is particularly true of multicystic disease. Since most cystic areas discovered by roentgenologic examination will disappear spontaneously, treatment, which is surgical removal, should be reserved for those which cause severe respiratory distress.

PULMONARY HEMORRHAGE

Massive pulmonary hemorrhage is present in about 15 per cent of premature infants and 45 per

cent of mature infants who come to autopsy in the first 2 weeks of life. The reported incidence at autopsy varies from about 1 to 4 per thousand live births. About three fourths of the patients weigh less than 2500 gm. at birth.

Most infants in whom pulmonary hemorrhage is demonstrated at autopsy have had symptoms of respiratory distress that are indistinguishable from those of so-called hyaline membrane disease. About one fourth of them have had obvious hemorrhage from the nose or mouth. Roentgenographic findings are varied and nonspecific.

The cause of massive pulmonary hemorrhage is unknown, but a possible relation to hyaline membrane disease has been proposed. It does not seem likely that there is a single cause, but rather that such hemorrhage may be a response to a variety of abnormal factors. Although in the majority of instances bleeding into other organs is observed at autopsy, bleeding other than through the nostrils and mouth is relatively rare during life. Bleeding is predominantly alveolar in about two thirds of cases, predominantly interstitial in the rest.

Since most of the available knowledge about pulmonary hemorrhage in the newborn has been obtained by retrospective study of the records of patients in whom the diagnosis has been made at autopsy, there is little information about the prognosis of infants who bleed through the mouth or nostrils, except that it is extremely poor. Death occurs in the first 48 hours of life in two thirds of the infants who come to autopsy. Treatment is supportive.

DISTURBANCES OF THE DIGESTIVE SYSTEM

Vomiting. Infants at times vomit mucus, often blood-streaked, in the first few hours after birth. This vomiting infrequently persists after the first few feedings; it may be due to irritation of the gastric mucosa by material swallowed during delivery. If the vomiting is protracted, gastric lavage with physiologic saline solution may relieve it.

Vomiting is a relatively frequent symptom during the neonatal period. In the majority of instances it is simply regurgitation from overfeeding or from failure to permit the infant to eructate swallowed air. When vomiting occurs shortly after birth and is persistent, the possibilities of increased intracranial pressure and of intestinal obstruction must be considered.

Obstructive lesions of the digestive tract occur most frequently in the esophagus (p. 768) and intestines (p. 787). Vomiting from esophageal obstruction occurs with the first feeding. The diagnosis of *esophageal atresia* can be suspected if there is unusual drooling from the mouth and if resistance is encountered in the attempt to pass a catheter into the stomach. There is considerable advantage in establishing the diagnosis before the infant chokes on oral feedings and endangers himself to aspiration pneumonia. *Cardiospasm* is a rare cause of vomiting in the newborn infant; it is demonstrable roentgenographically by obstruction at the cardiac end of the esophagus, without organic stenosis. Regurgitation of feedings due to continuous relaxation of the esophageal-gastric sphincter, *chalasia,* is an infrequent cause of vomiting, which can be controlled by keeping the infant in a semi-upright position. Vomiting from obstruction of the small intestine usually begins on the first day of life and is frequent, persistent, usually nonprojectile, copious and, unless the obstruction is above the ampulla of Vater, bile-stained; it is associated with abdominal distention, visible deep peristaltic waves, and reduced or absent bowel movements. Upright roentgenographic films of the abdomen will show the distribution of air in the intestine and often aid in the location of the site of the obstruction; the use of contrast material for these studies is usually unnecessary. Normally, air can be demonstrated roentgenographically in the jejunum by 15 to 60 minutes, in the ileum by 2 to 3 hours, and in the colon by 3 hours after birth. Persistent vomiting may occur with congenital hernia of the diaphragm (p. 823) when the viscera are crowded. The vomiting of *pyloric stenosis* may begin any time after birth, but does not assume its characteristic pattern before the second or third week. Vomiting may occur with many other disturbances which do not obstruct the digestive tract, such as celiac disease, milk allergy, adrenal hyperplasia of the salt-losing variety, septicemia, meningitis and other infections. It is common with urinary tract infections.

Thrush (Oral Moniliasis). Thrush of the mouth (p. 763) is mentioned here to emphasize its importance in newborn infants. At this age healthy infants may be infected; later, the infection is rare except in debilitated infants and children and those receiving antibiotic therapy.

There is a positive correlation between maternal vaginal and infantile oral moniliasis. The maternal source appears to be the principal primary means of infection in healthy newborns. Secondary cases develop in the hospital nursery, presumably by contact with infected infants and contaminated supplies.

Occasionally a heavy coat forms on the tongue, but its appearance is not that of thrush, nor do cultures from it reveal *Candida albicans.* It can be removed by 1 or 2 applications of 1 per cent aqueous solution of gentian violet.

Oral thrush in an otherwise healthy infant is usually a self-limited infection, but treatment is advised (see p. 763).

Diarrhea. See pages 373, 405 and 407.

Constipation. More than 90 per cent of newborn infants pass meconium within the first 24 hours, and most of the remainder do so within 36 hours. The possibility of intestinal obstruction should be considered in any infant who does not pass meconium within that time. Intestinal atresia or stenosis (p. 788), congenital aganglionic megacolon (p. 791), meconium ileus or meconium plugs should be suspected. Constipation not present from birth, but appearing during the first month of life, suggests congenital aganglionic megacolon, cretinism or anal stenosis. It must be kept in mind that infrequent bowel movements do not necessarily mean constipation (p. 779). Breast-fed infants may rarely go as long as a week without a bowel movement and without evidence of discomfort, and then pass a large but otherwise normal stool.

Meconium Plugs. Anorectal plugs (Fig. 7-22) of lower water content than normal may be a cause of intestinal obstruction in newborn infants. Rarely a firm mass of meconium may form elsewhere in the intestine and cause intrauterine intestinal obstruction and meconium peritonitis unrelated to cystic fibrosis. Likewise, anorectal plugs may cause intestinal ulceration and perforation. The plug may require irrigation with isotonic sodium chloride solution or half-strength hydrogen peroxide for evacuation. After removal of a meconium plug the infant should be observed closely for the possible presence of congenital aganglionic megacolon.

Meconium Bodies. These light yellow particles are usually no more than 1 mm. in diameter, but may rarely be large enough to cause distortion of the intestine. They are occasionally associated with intestinal atresia.

Meconium Ileus. Impaction of meconium is a relatively rare cause of intestinal obstruction in the newborn infant. It is associated with cystic fibrosis. The depletion or absence of the pancreatic ferments prohibits normal digestive activities in the intestine, and meconium is left in a viscid, mucilaginous state. It clings to the intestinal wall and is moved with difficulty or not at all by intestinal peristalsis. The inspissated and impacted meconium fills the intestinal canal, but is most concentrated in the lower ileum.

Clinically, the pattern is that of congenital intestinal obstruction with or without intestinal perforation (see Meconium Peritonitis). Abdominal distention is prominent, and persistent vomiting soon occurs. Infrequently, one or more inspissated meconium stools may be passed shortly after birth.

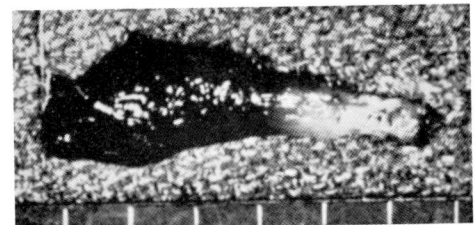

Figure 7-22. Anorectal plug, from child who had not passed meconium for 2 days after birth, is indistinguishable from normal plug. Pale end was adjacent to anus. (From J. L. Emery: Abnormalities in Meconium of Foetus and Newborn. *Arch. Dis. Childhood,* Vol. 32.)

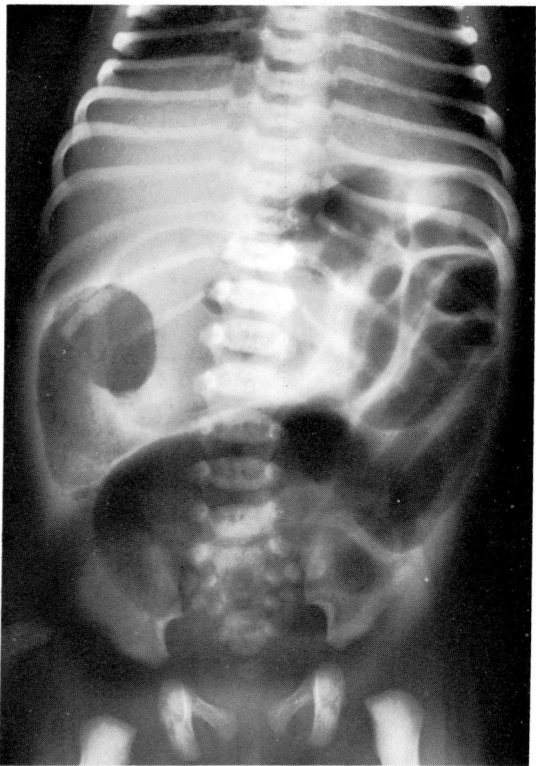

Figure 7-23. Meconium ileus. Impacted meconium with small amounts of air interspersed throughout it in loops of intestine on the right side of abdomen; intestinal loops above this impaction are greatly distended.

The *differential diagnosis* involves other causes of intestinal obstruction; an exact diagnosis cannot be made except by laparotomy. A presumptive diagnosis can be made on the basis of a history of cystic fibrosis in a sibling, by palpation of doughy or cordlike masses of intestines through the abdominal wall and by the roentgenographic appearance. In contrast to the generally evenly distended intestinal loops above an atresia, the loops may vary in width and not be as evenly filled with gas. At points of heaviest meconium concentration the infiltrated gas may create a granular appearance (Figs. 7-23, 7-24).

The case fatality rate is high, but a number of infants have survived the neonatal period; their subsequent *prognosis* is dependent upon the basic disturbance, cystic fibrosis.

Treatment is surgical. It consists basically in opening the ileum at the point of greatest diameter of the impaction and removing the inspissated meconium by gentle and patient irrigation with warm isotonic sodium chloride solution introduced through a fine catheter which may be passed between the impaction and the bowel wall.

Meconium Peritonitis. Perforation of the intestine may occur in utero or shortly after birth. The tear may be sealed by natural processes relatively quickly with only a small amount of meconium escaping, or the meconial contents may largely be emptied into the peritoneal cavity. Such

perforations occur most often as a complication of meconium ileus in infants with cystic fibrosis, but occasionally the perforation is due to a meconium plug, meconium bodies or intestinal obstruction of whatever cause.

When the intestinal perforation is spontaneously sealed and only a small amount of meconium has escaped, the event may never be known, except as some of the meconial particles become calcified and are subsequently discovered fortuitously on roentgenograms of the abdomen. Otherwise the clinical picture is dominated by the signs of intestinal obstruction or peritonitis. Characteristically, there are abdominal distention, vomiting and absence of stools. The treatment is primarily elimination of the intestinal obstruction and drainage of the peritoneal cavity.

JAUNDICE IN THE NEWBORN INFANT

Etiology. Before it can be excreted in bile or urine, lipid-soluble bilirubin (indirect-reacting) must be converted to a water-soluble ester glucuronide of bilirubin (direct-reacting). This conversion appears to require adequate amounts of an enzyme, bilirubin glucuronyl transferase. The enzyme is present either in small amounts or in an inactive state in newborn infants, particularly in premature ones. Therefore any factor which increases the load of bilirubin to be metabolized by the liver (erythroblastosis fetalis, other hemolytic anemias, infection), any factor which may damage or reduce the activity of the enzyme (anoxia, infection, possibly hypothermia and thyroid deficiency), any factor which may compete for or block the enzyme (drugs and other substances requiring

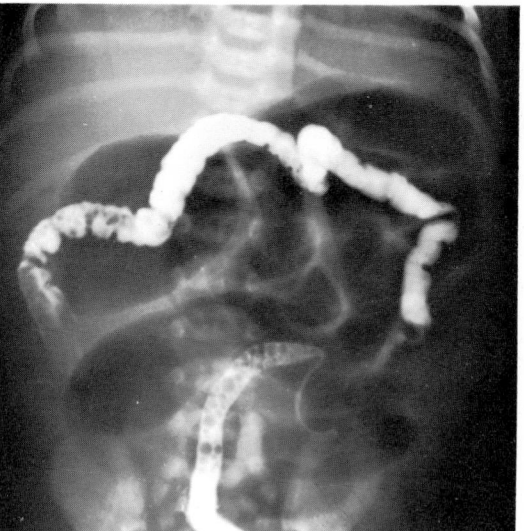

Figure 7-24. Meconium ileus. The colon, outlined by contrast material, is small because meconium has not reached it. The small, circumscribed radiolucencies in the colon represent air injected with the contrast material and mucus present in the colon.

glucuronic acid conjugation for excretion) or any factor leading to absence or decreased amounts of the enzyme (genetic defect, prematurity) may be expected to cause or increase the degree of jaundice.

Clinical Manifestations. Jaundice may be present at birth or may appear at any time during the neonatal period, depending on the condition responsible for it. *Its intensity bears no dependable relation to the degree of hyperbilirubinemia.* Jaundice resulting from deposition of indirect bilirubin in the skin tends to appear bright yellow or orange; jaundice of the obstructive type (direct bilirubin), a greenish or muddy yellow. This difference is usually apparent only in severe jaundice. The infant may be lethargic, feed poorly and become dehydrated.

Differential Diagnosis. Jaundice present at birth or appearing within the first 24 hours of life should be considered due to erythroblastosis fetalis (p. 1060) until proved otherwise; cytomegalic inclusion disease, rubella and congenital toxoplasmosis are other infrequent possibilities. Jaundice which first appears on the second or third day is usually "physiologic," but may represent the more severe form now called hyperbilirubinemia of the newborn. Familial nonhemolytic icterus also is seen initially on the second or third day. *Jaundice appearing after the third day and within the first week should suggest septicemia as the most likely cause*; it may be due to other infections, notably syphilis, toxoplasmosis and cytomegalic inclusion disease.

Jaundice initially noted after the first week of life suggests septicemia, congenital atresia of the bile ducts, homologous serum hepatitis, herpetic hepatitis, idiopathic dilatation of the common bile duct, galactosemia, congenital hemolytic anemia (spherocytosis) or possibly the crises of other hemolytic anemias such as thalassemia, sickle cell disease, hereditary nonspherocytic anemia or hemolytic anemia due to idiosyncrasy to drugs or other substances, as in congenital deficiency of the enzyme glucose-6-phosphate dehydrogenase. Jaundice secondary to extensive ecchymoses has been reported.

Persistent jaundice during the first month of life suggests the so-called inspissated bile syndrome, which may follow hemolytic disease of the newborn, hepatitis, cytomegalic inclusion disease, syphilis, toxoplasmosis, familial nonhemolytic icterus, congenital atresia of the bile ducts, idiopathic dilatation of the common bile duct, or galactosemia. Rarely, physiologic jaundice may be prolonged for several weeks, as in infants with hypothyroidism or pyloric stenosis.

Physiologic Jaundice (Icterus Neonatorum). The usually slight degree of jaundice which is clinically visible on the second or third day in about two thirds of full-term newborn infants and ordinarily disappears between the fifth and the seventh days of life is termed physiologic jaundice. It is dependent on a rise in serum bilirubin level which is believed to be the result of breakdown of fetal red cells combined with transient deficiency of bilirubin glucuronyl transferase in the liver. Among premature infants this rise in serum bilirubin tends to be a little slower and of longer duration, resulting in generally higher levels, the peak being reached between the fourth and seventh days; peak levels in term infants usually occur on the second or third day of life.

Hyperbilirubinemia of the Newborn. When total serum bilirubin levels reach 15 to 20 mg. per 100 ml. during the first week of life, bilirubinemia beyond "physiologic" bounds (hyperbilirubinemia) is considered to be present. This may occur as an exaggeration of "physiologic" jaundice, particularly in premature infants, or as a result of excessive hemolysis, as in erythroblastosis fetalis. The term *hyperbilirubinemia of the newborn*, however, should be reserved for those infants whose primary problem is a deficiency or inactivity of bilirubin glucuronyl transferase rather than an excessive load of bilirubin for excretion. Serum bilirubin may rarely reach the alarming level of 60 to 70 mg. per 100 ml. in the absence of any blood group incompatibility.

The *significance* of hyperbilirubinemia lies in the high incidence of kernicterus associated with serum bilirubin levels over 18 to 20 mg. per 100 ml. The correlation between serum bilirubin levels and kernicterus in infants with erythroblastosis fetalis (Table 7-19) probably holds for premature infants without blood group incompatibilities, except that they may have kernicterus at serum values somewhat below 18 mg. per 100 ml.

The *incidence* of hyperbilirubinemia among term infants without blood group incompatibility is about 5 per cent and among premature infants without blood group incompatibility is significantly higher. Because the incidence of kernicterus varies from 2 to 16 per cent in all autopsies done on premature infants, there is little doubt that factors other than the initial unavailability of bilirubin glucuronyl transferase play a role. Excessive doses of vitamin K analogues and moderate doses of novobiocin may be associated with hyperbilirubinemia. It is also observed with some frequency in infants of diabetic mothers and in those with prolonged neonatal cyanosis or bacteremia. (For relation to sulfisoxazole, see Kernicterus below.) Certain mothers appear to

TABLE 7-19. RELATION OF MAXIMUM TOTAL SERUM BILIRUBIN CONCENTRATION TO INCIDENCE OF KERNICTERUS

MAXIMUM BILIRUBIN CONCENTRATION (Mg./100 Ml.)	KERNICTERUS
10-18	0
19-24	7%
25-29	30%
30-40	70%

Adapted from Mollison and Cutbush: *Recent Advances in Paediatrics.* London, J. & A. Churchill, Ltd., 1954, p. 112.

have elevated serum levels of an inhibitor substance, probably a progestin, against the enzyme, bilirubin glucuronyl transferase. Such women may repeatedly have infants with significant hyperbilirubinemia in whose serum elevated levels of the inhibitor substance can also be demonstrated. Negro infants appear to be less susceptible, but studies to date deal only with babies premature by weight, and it is well known that Negro infants tend to weigh less than white infants of the same gestational age. Since hyperbilirubinemia is related to short gestational age rather than to low birth weight, the supposed difference between white and Negro infants may be more apparent than real.

The absence of significant hemolysis in many infants with hyperbilirubinemia associated with ABO blood group incompatibility or glucose-6-phosphate dehydrogenase deficiency suggests that genetic factors which affect the incidence of hyperbilirubinemia may operate through mechanisms which are as yet unidentified.

Neonatal Hyperbilirubinemia Associated with Breast Feeding. Arias and Gartner identified unconjugated hyperbilirubinemia among breast-fed infants during the second week of life due to pregnane-3 (alpha), 20 (beta)-diol in the mother's milk. This substance inhibits conjugation of bilirubin. Upon discontinuance of breast feeding, the serum bilirubin values return to normal within about 5 days.

"Inspissated Bile Syndrome." Rarely in infants with hemolytic disease of the newborn with hyperbilirubinemia, the icterus persists and is associated with a significant and increasing elevation of direct as well as of indirect bilirubin. The nature of this lesion is not known, and most pathologists would discard the term. Among the hypotheses is the suggested possibility that the hepatic cells have been damaged by the primary disease. The jaundice clears spontaneously within a few weeks to months.

Neonatal Hepatitis. See page 834.

Congenital Atresia of the Bile Ducts. See page 851.

Kernicterus. The pathology and clinical manifestations of kernicterus, one of the principal causes of neurologic abnormalities, are described on pages 1060 and 1278. Most studies suggest that kernicterus results from deposition of indirect-reacting bilirubin in brain cells. This rarely occurs with serum levels of indirect bilirubin under 20 mg. per 100 ml., and it appears that such levels must be maintained for at least 24 hours for kernicterus to occur.

The extent of binding of unconjugated bilirubin by serum albumin, the permeability of the walls of brain cells to bilirubin, and varying susceptibility of the brain cells to the toxic effects of bilirubin are factors which influence the development of kernicterus at a given level of serum bilirubin. Sulfonamides, salicylates, antibiotics, heparin, hematin and fatty acids are capable of displacing bilirubin from its binding sites on serum albumin, although only sulfisoxazole (Gantrisin) has been proved to increase susceptibility of the infant to kernicterus at relatively low (12 to 15 mg. per 100 ml.) levels of bilirubin in the serum. Hypoproteinemia, with reduction of the amount of albumin available for binding bilirubin, may also contribute to the occurrence of kernicterus at levels of total bilirubin below 18 to 20 mg. per 100 ml. of serum. Conversely, a high level of serum albumin may provide extra binding sites, so that a higher level of bilirubin may be tolerated. Anoxia, low pH of the blood, hemolytic disease and hypoglycemia may increase susceptibility to kernicterus by increasing the permeability of brain cells to bilirubin, or by rendering them more susceptible to its toxic effects.

Prevention of Hyperbilirubinemia and Kernicterus. The decolorizing effect of sunlight and artificial light reduces the concentration of bilirubin in solution, apparently without producing toxic byproducts. When premature infants are exposed, uncovered except for the eyes, to artificial blue light continuously during the first 6 days of life, hyperbilirubinemia may be avoided or lessened. In other infants jaundiced from factors which do not cause a rapid rise of serum bilirubin, the elevations in the serum may also be limited by exposure to light. The effect is insufficient to offset increases in the level of serum bilirubin caused by rapid hemolysis. Dark color of the skin does not interfere with the effect of light on the level of bilirubin in the serum.

Aside from preventing and treating hyperbilirubinemia, prevention of kernicterus includes measures to prevent and treat hemolytic disease of the newborn, avoidance of the use of sulfisoxazole, novobiocin and high doses of vitamin K, and avoidance of anoxia and premature birth, and probably of other as yet unknown factors. In populations with a known high incidence of glucose 6-phosphate dehydrogenase deficiency, pregnant women and nursing mothers as well as susceptible infants should avoid exposure to substances known to cause hemolysis in persons deficient in glucose 6-phosphate dehydrogenase (p. 1055).

Treatment of Hyperbilirubinemia. Jaundice requires treatment when bilirubinemia reaches levels at which kernicterus is a risk. Exchange transfusion (p. 1062), repeated as frequently as necessary to keep indirect bilirubin levels in the serum under 20 mg. per 100 ml., has been the most widely accepted treatment. A variety of factors as mentioned, may, however, alter this criterion in either direction in an individual case. Appearance of clinical signs suggesting kernicterus is indication for exchange transfusion at any level of serum bilirubin. Healthy full-term infants tend to tolerate bilirubin concentrations somewhat higher than 20 mg. per 100 ml. with no apparent ill effect, whereas sick premature infants sometimes acquire kernicterus at levels which are significantly lower. A level approaching that considered critical for the individual infant may indicate exchange transfusion during the first day or two of life when a further rise is to be anticipated, but not on the fourth day in term infants or on the seventh day in premature infants, when an imminent fall may be anticipated as the conjugating mechanism becomes more effective. Liberal use of phototherapy for newborn infants jaundiced from whatever cause may reduce the frequency of need for exchange transfusion. The use of phenobarbital to induce activity of bilirubin glucuronyl transferase or to expand the smooth endoplasmic reticulum of the liver to promote excretion of bilirubin is currently under investigation.

DISTURBANCES OF THE BLOOD

Anemia in the Newborn Infant. *Anemia at birth* is manifest by pallor or shock. It is usually caused by hemolytic disease of the newborn (p. 1060), but may also be the result of tearing or cutting of the umbilical cord during delivery or of hemorrhage from the fetal side of the placenta. The last may be caused by accidental incision of the placenta in the course of cesarean section or by so-called transplacental hemorrhage. Anemia at birth may also be seen in one of twins with conjoined placental circulation, in which case the anemic twin "bleeds into" the other twin.

Transplacental hemorrhage, with bleeding from the fetal into the maternal circulation is probably more common than is generally recognized, but is usually not sufficient to cause clinically apparent anemia at birth. The cause of transplacental hemorrhage is not clear, but its occurrence has been proved by demonstration of significant amounts of fetal hemoglobin and red cells in the maternal blood on the day of delivery.

Anemia appearing in the first few days after birth is also most frequently the result of hemolytic disease of the newborn. Other causes are hemorrhagic disease of the newborn, bleeding from an improperly tied or clamped umbilical cord, large cephalhematomas, intracranial hemorrhage or subcapsular bleeding from rupture of the liver. Rapid decreases in hemoglobin or hematocrit values during the first few days of life may be the initial clue to either of the 2 last-named conditions.

Later in the neonatal period delayed anemia from hemolytic disease of the newborn, with or without exchange transfusion, may be seen. Vitamin K (as Synkayvite) in large doses may cause anemia in premature infants characterized by inclusion bodies (Heinz bodies) in the erythrocytes. Congenital hemolytic anemia (spherocytosis) occasionally makes its appearance during the first month of life, and hereditary nonspherocytic hemolytic anemia has been described during the neonatal period secondary to deficiency of such enzymes as glucose 6-phosphate dehydrogenase and pyruvate kinase. Bleeding from hemangiomas of the upper gastrointestinal tract or from ulcers caused by aberrant gastric mucosa in a Meckel's diverticulum or duplication is a rare source of anemia in the newborn.

Since a further "physiologic" decrease in erythrocytes and in hemoglobin content is to be expected in all newborn infants (Table 14-3, p. 1043), treatment of any significant anemia (less than 8 gm. of hemoglobin per 100 ml.) present at or shortly after birth consists not only in eliminating its cause, if it is still present, but also in small transfusions of packed red blood cells (10 to 15 ml. per kg.; 2 ml. per kg. raises hemoglobin about 1 gm. per 100 ml. There is inconclusive evidence that early feeding of red meats or intramuscular administration of iron is effective in enabling anemic infants to increase rather than decrease their erythrocyte and hemoglobin concentrations before the second or third month of life.

Plethora in the Newborn Infant. Plethora or apparent cyanosis associated with abnormally high erythrocyte, hemoglobin and hematocrit values has been reported in association with and without clinical findings suggestive of placental dysfunction syndrome (p. 1067), plus anorexia, lethargy, cyanosis and convulsions appearing on the second and third days of life. The pathophysiology of the condition is not clear. Plethora may also be due to a "placental transfusion" in the recipient twin of monozygotic twins with parabiotic placental circulations (p. 362). Plethora as the result of transfusion from the maternal to the fetal circulation has not been described.

The *treatment* of symptomatic plethora of the newborn has been by bleeding and replacement with plasma. A partial exchange transfusion would appear to be a technically simpler and therapeutically more effective approach.

Hemorrhage in the Newborn Infant. *Hemorrhagic disease of the newborn.* Between the second and fifth days of life spontaneous and prolonged bleeding due to an accentuation of multiple coagulation deficiencies normally present in newborn infants is seen rarely among term infants and more frequently among premature infants. Two forms of hemorrhagic disease may be distinguished on the basis of the clinical pattern and the response to prophylactic and therapeutic measures.

The first form appears to be due to *vitamin K deficiency*, which presumably exists until the infant's intestinal flora is sufficiently established to supply the normal needs of this substance, or until normal hepatic function is established. It is characterized by prolongation of the blood coagulation time and of the plasma recalcification time and by low one-stage prothrombin activity, with depletions of factor VII complex and true prothrombin. The bleeding time is normal, as are factor V, capillary fragility, platelets and clot retraction. There is also a decided alteration of the first stage of coagulation which appears to be due to deficiencies of factor IX and the Stuart-Prower factor. The most frequent sites of bleeding are the gastrointestinal tract, the nose and the subgaleal region. Either vitamin K (1 to 10 mg.) or fresh whole blood (10 mg. per kg.) brings about rapid improvement in all the coagulation defects and cessation of bleeding within a few hours. This form of hemorrhagic disease of the newborn is not seen among infants who have received vitamin K prophylaxis, and the mortality rate is low among treated cases. (Also see p. 1084.)

The other form of bleeding, clinically indistinguishable from hemorrhagic disease of the newborn, occurs chiefly among premature infants and is neither prevented by nor successfully treated with vitamin K. Nearly all the infants have had hypoxia or infection; the most frequent sites of bleeding are the lungs and central nervous system. The prognosis is poor regardless of therapy. The coagulation defects are less severe than in the previously described form of the disease, but most patients have increased capillary fragility and prolongation of the bleeding time. Factor V is usually diminished, and a few patients have thrombocytopenia. There may be overlap of these 2 forms of hemorrhagic disease.

Since a clinical pattern identical to that of hemorrhagic disease of the newborn may result from any of the congenital defects in blood coagulation (p. 1082), infants with central nervous system or other bleeding constituting an immediate threat to life should receive a small transfusion of fresh, compatible whole blood or plasma, as well as vitamin K, as soon as possible after blood has been drawn for coagulation studies.

The so-called *swallowed blood syndrome*, in which blood or bloody stools are passed, usually on the second or third day of life, may be confused with hemorrhage from the gastrointestinal tract. The blood may be swallowed during delivery or from a fissure in the mother's nipple. Differentiation from gastrointestinal hemorrhage is based on the fact that the infant's blood contains mostly fetal hemoglobin, which is alkali-resistant, whereas swallowed blood from a maternal source contains adult hemoglobin, which is promptly changed to alkaline hematin upon the addition of alkali. Apt devised the following test for this differentiation:

(1) Rinse a bloodstained diaper or some grossly bloody stool with a suitable amount of water to obtain a distinctly pink supernatant hemoglobin solution. (2) Centrifuge the mixture. Decant the supernatant solution. (3) To 5 parts of the supernatant fluid add 1 part of 0.25 normal (1 per cent) sodium hydroxide. Within 1 to 2 minutes a color reaction takes place: a yellow-brown color indicates that the blood is maternal in origin; a persistent pink, that it is from the infant. A control test with known adult or fetal blood, or both, is advisable.

Widespread *subcutaneous ecchymoses* in premature infants at or immediately after birth are apparently a result of fragile superficial blood vessels rather than of a coagulation defect. In any event, vitamin K administration to the mother during labor seems to have little effect on their incidence. An occasional infant is born with petechiae or a generalized bluish suffusion limited to the face, head and neck. These are probably the result of venous obstruction caused by sudden increases in intrathoracic pressure during delivery. It may take 2 to 3 weeks for such suffusions to disappear.

Neonatal thrombocytopenic purpura. See p. 1087.

DISTURBANCES OF THE GENITOURINARY SYSTEM

See also section on The Urinary System.

One or both kidneys are often easily palpable in the newborn infant. When both are palpable, there is usually no particular diagnostic problem, but when only one kidney can be felt, it frequently gives the impression that it is larger than normal or represents or is displaced by an intrinsic or extrinsic mass. Fetal lobulation may contribute to the impression of abnormality. Usually the problem resolves itself as the kidney becomes progressively less easily palpable during the early months of life. Since palpable enlargement or displacement of the kidney in the newborn may rarely be due to hydronephrosis, an embryoma or a cystic malformation, an abdominal scout film or intravenous urograms are indicated if there is serious question about the palpable mass. Owing to the poor concentrating ability of the neonatal kidney, relatively large amounts of contrast material (10 to 20 cc. of Diodrast) must be injected to get satisfactory films. Elevations of blood urea nitrogen may occur during the neonatal period in association with polycystic disease and hydronephrosis without necessarily implying a poor prognosis.

During the neonatal period moderate elevation of the blood urea or nonprotein nitrogen does not necessarily signify renal disease. The urine may also contain casts and cellular elements simply as a manifestation of dehydration.

Bilateral Renal Agenesis. Infants with bilateral renal agenesis have a characteristic facies: a general appearance of premature senility, a mild increase in width between the eyes, with a prominent fold of skin arising at the inner canthus and extending downward and laterally below the eyes to form a wide semicircle, and unusual flattening and slight broadening of the nose, a recession of the chin, and large, low-lying ears with incomplete cartilaginous development. There is usually a diminished quantity of amniotic fluid, presumably due to lack of urine formation. At autopsy there is no evidence of the ureters or kidneys. Pulmonary hypoplasia has also been observed. The anomaly has occurred predominantly in male infants. In some of the female infants there has been failure of development of the uterus and the vagina, the gonads and the fallopian tubes being present. In male infants the prostate, seminal vesicles, ductus deferens and testes are normally formed. The bladder is a tubelike structure with little musculature. The rudimentary adrenal glands are normal. The outlook is hopeless, the infant dying during labor or shortly after birth.

Urinary Tract Infection. In contrast to the sex distribution in later infancy, pyuria may occur as frequently in the male as in the female newborn infant. The causative agent is usually the colon bacillus, although it may be any of the urinary tract pathogens.

The symptoms may be vague; on occasion they are predominantly gastrointestinal. Fever, difficulty in feeding and failure to gain weight are commonly encountered; jaundice and meningismus are occasional features. There may be urinary suppression.

For diagnosis and treatment see page 1121.

Thrombosis of the Renal Vein. See page 1149.

DISTURBANCES OF THE CRANIUM

See also Anencephaly, Microcephaly, Craniosynostosis and Hydrocephalus.

Craniotabes (Congenital Cranial Osteoporosis). Palpation of the skull of the newborn infant may reveal areas of softening along the suture lines, especially in the parietal area, which indent from pressure of the fingers with the resilience of a ping-pong ball. This phenomenon is demonstrated more frequently in premature infants, but occurs in 10 to 35 per cent of all newborn infants. Failure to observe it in breech presentations has led to an assumption that it may be due to intrauterine pressure against the maternal pelvis. This condition is a harmless and physiologic result of incoordination between the rapid growth of the brain and the calcification processes in the vertex in the last month of gestation and is associated with a generalized osteoporotic process in the newborn infant. Differentiation must be made from the craniotabes of rickets, from lacunar skull, in which honeycombed areas of porotic bone create a characteristic appearance in the roentgenogram of the skull, and from osteogenesis imperfecta.

DISORDERS OF THE SKIN

See section on the Skin of the Infant (p. 1375).

Mastitis Neonatorum. Engorgement of the breasts is physiologic in newborn infants. Infection may be abetted by undue manipulation of the breasts and is manifest by redness, local heat, swelling and pain. Fever and other general symptoms may also be present. The prognosis is favorable unless septicemia develops. Prophylaxis consists in avoidance of manipulation or other trauma of the engorged breasts. Treatment includes systemic antibiotic therapy and hot compresses applied locally. If an abscess develops, it should be incised and drained.

Sequels from scar formation include impairment of the secreting power of the mammary gland in later life and distortion of the nipple.

DISTURBANCES OF THE EYE

See the section beginning on page 1419.

THE UMBILICUS

Umbilical Cord. The cord contains the 2 umbilical arteries, the vein, the rudimentary allantois, the remnant of the omphalomesenteric duct and a gelatinous substance called the jelly of Wharton. The sheath of the umbilical cord is derived from the amnion. The arteries have a strong contractile capacity, whereas that of the vein is less; as a result it retains a fairly large lumen after birth. When the cord sloughs, portions of these structures remain in the base. The blood vessels are functionally closed, but are patent anatomically for 20 to 25 days. The arteries become the lateral umbilical ligaments; the vein, the ligamentum teres; and the ductus venosus, the ligamentum venosum. During this interval the umbilical vessels are potential portals of entry for infection.

Only a *single umbilical artery* is present in about 5 of 1000 births; the frequency is about 35 per 1000 infants born of twin births. Approximately one third of infants with a single umbilical artery have congenital abnormalities, usually more than one, and many such infants are born dead or die shortly after birth. Trisomy of chromosome 18 is one of the more frequent abnormalities associated with single umbilical artery. Otherwise the defects tend to involve the genitourinary tract, the gastrointestinal tract, the skeleton, the cardiovascular system and the central nervous system. Since many of these abnormalities are not apparent on gross physical examination, it is important that at every delivery the cut cord and the maternal and fetal surfaces of the placenta be inspected. The number of arteries present should be recorded as an aid to the early suspicion and identification of abnormalities in such infants.

Types of Navel. There are 3 types of navels: normal, amniotic and the skin or cutis navel. When the skin of the abdominal wall meets the umbilical cord at the level of the abdomen, there remains only a small amount of skin at the base when the cord sloughs, and a *normal* umbilical cicatrix results. If the skin does not extend to the base of the cord and the amniotic membrane must cover the skin surface adjacent to the base, a small superficial ulcer will result which closes in by granulation and leaves the flat scar of the *amniotic* navel. When the skin extends up the sides of the cord, a protruding stump, the *skin* navel, remains after the cord has sloughed. The protrusion of the skin or cutis navel must be differentiated from a postnatal hernia, with which, of course, it can be associated; a skin navel does not have a defect in the abdominal wall and therefore is not exaggerated when the infant strains or cries. Usually the skin navel becomes less prominent with age.

Anomalies. *Patency of the omphalomesenteric duct* may be responsible for an intestinal fistula, prolapse of the bowel, polyp or a Meckel's diverticulum (p. 790).

A *persistent urachus* (urachal cyst) is due to failure of closure of the allantoic duct. Patency should be suspected if there is a clear, light yellow, urine-like discharge from the umbilicus (p. 1152).

Congenital Omphalocele. An omphalocele is a herniation or protrusion of abdominal contents into the base of the umbilical cord. In contrast to the more common umbilical hernia, the sac is covered merely with peritoneum without overlying skin. The size of the sac which lies outside the abdominal cavity depends upon its contents. It has been estimated that there is herniation of intestines into the cord in about 1 of 5000 births and of liver and intestines in 1 of 10,000 births. The abdominal cavity is proportionately small, owing to deficient impulse to grow and develop. Immediate surgical repair, before infection has taken place and before the tissues have been damaged by drying or the sac has ruptured, has been generally considered to be essential for survival. Promising results have been reported in the treatment of omphalocele by "tanning" the sac with a 2 per cent aqueous solution of Merthiolate, applied 2 or 3 times daily. Epithelization as well as intra-abdominal containment of the viscera has been attained by this method.

Tumors. Tumors of the umbilicus are rare; they include angioma, enteroteratoma, dermoid cyst, myxosarcoma and cysts of urachal or omphalomesenteric duct remnants.

Hemorrhage. Hemorrhage from the umbilical cord may be due to trauma, to inadequate ligation of the cord or to failure of normal thrombus formation. Hemorrhage may also be an evidence of hemorrhagic disease of the newborn, septicemia or local infection. The infant should be observed frequently during the first few days of life so that, if hemorrhage does occur, it will be detected promptly.

Granuloma. The umbilical cord usually dries and separates within 6 to 8 days after birth. The raw surface becomes covered by a thin layer of skin, scar tissue forms, and the wound is usually healed within 12 to 15 days. The presence of saprophytic organisms delays separation of the cord and increases the possibility of invasion by pathogenic organisms. Mild infection may result in a moist granulating area at the base of the cord with a slight mucoid or mucopurulent discharge. Good results are usually obtained by cleansing with alcohol several times daily.

The persistence of exuberant granulation tissue at the base of the umbilicus is not uncommon. The tissue is soft, vascular and granular, dull red or pink, and may have a seropurulent secretion. The *treatment* is cauterization with silver nitrate; it should be repeated at intervals of several days until the base is dry.

Umbilical granuloma must be differentiated from umbilical *polyp*, a rare anomaly resulting from persistence of all or part of the omphalomesenteric duct or the urachus. The tissue of the polyp is firm and resistant and bright red, and has a mucoid secretion. If there is a communication with the ileum or bladder, small amounts of fecal material or urine may be discharged intermittently. Histologically, the polyp consists of intestinal or urinary tract mucosa. Treatment is surgical excision of the *entire* omphalomesenteric or urachal remnant.

Infections. Inflammation in the umbilical region, which may be caused by any of the pyogenic bacteria, is especially serious because of the danger of hematogenous spread or extension to the liver or peritoneum. The general manifestations may be minimal even when septicemia or hepatitis has resulted. Prevention of infection depends upon maintenance of a clean umbilical field. Daily hexachlorophene baths or daily application of triple dye to the umbilical stump and surrounding skin may reduce the incidence of umbilical infection. *Treatment* includes prompt antibacterial therapy and, if there is abscess formation, surgical incision and drainage.

UMBILICAL HERNIA

Umbilical hernia is due to an imperfect closure or weakness of the umbilical ring and is often associated with diastasis recti. It is common in all races, but especially in the Negro. It appears as a soft swelling covered by skin which protrudes during crying, coughing or straining and can be reduced easily through the fibrous ring at the umbilicus. The hernia consists of omentum or portions of the small intestine. The size of the defect varies from less than a centimeter in diameter to as much as 5 cm., but large ones are rare.

Treatment. Few medical problems have given rise to more contradictory opinions and practices than has the management of umbilical hernia in infancy. Most umbilical hernias which appear before the age of 6 months will disappear spontaneously by 1 year of age. Even large hernias (5 to 6 cm. in all dimensions) have been known to disappear spontaneously by 5 or 6 years of age. Strangulation is extremely rare. There is considerable agreement that "strapping" is ineffective as usually practiced. At least one study indicates that any form of strapping has a deleterious rather than a beneficial effect. Other evidence has been interpreted that careful strapping, in which the hernia is reduced by finger pressure and the defect closed by drawing each side of the adjacent abdominal wall toward the midline by means of interlocking straps of broad adhesive tape, increases the incidence of closure of hernias over 6 mm. in diameter or in protrusion. Unfortunately, lack of comparability of data between various studies and, particularly, lack of a careful, long-term study of the natural history of umbilical hernias do not permit establishment of a logical basis for either strapping or surgery. Avoidance of surgery is advised unless the hernia persists to the age of 3 to 5 years, causes symptoms, becomes strangulated, or becomes progressively larger after the age of 1 or 2 years.

Metabolic Disturbances

Hyperthermia in the Newborn (Transitory Fever of the Newborn; Dehydration Fever). Elevations of temperature (100 to 104°F.) are occasionally noted on the second or third day of life in infants whose clinical course has been otherwise satisfactory. This disturbance is especially likely to occur in breast-fed infants whose intake of supplementary fluids such as glucose water or water has been particularly low or in infants exposed to high environmental temperatures, either in the nursery or in a bassinet near a radiator or in the sun. The lack of consistent relation with the extent of weight loss or inadequacy of fluid intake may be a reflection of variation in initial stores of body water. The rise in temperature is associated with an increase in concentration of the serum protein; the fall, with an increase in plasma water. The rapid alleviation of symptoms by oral or parenteral administration of fluids can leave no doubt as to the cause.

The infant may be restless, and there may be a precipitous drop in weight. The urinary output and frequency of voiding diminish. The skin may lose some of its elasticity, and the fontanel may be depressed. The infant appears unhappy and takes fluids avidly. The usual apparent vigor of the infant is in contrast to the usual appearance of "being sick" in the presence of infection.

Oral administration of fluids leads to prompt reduction of the fever.

A more severe form of neonatal hyperthermia occurs among both newborn and older infants when they are bundled up against an outside low temperature which does not exist in their immediate indoor environment. The diminished sweating capacity of the newborn infant is a contributing factor. Bundled-up infants left near stoves or radiators, travelling in well heated automobiles or left with bright sunlight shining directly on them through the windows of a closed room or automobile are likely victims. Overclothing in hot weather, especially when the infant is left in the sun, is a less common cause. Body temperature is often as high as 106 to 111°F. (41 to 44°C.). The skin is hot and dry, and initially the infant usually appears flushed and apathetic. This stage may be followed by stupor, grayish pallor, coma and convulsions. Hyperelectrolytemia may contribute to the convulsions. The mortality and morbidity rates (brain damage) are high. Prevention is by provision of clothing suitable for the temperature of the *immediate* environment. In the newborn infant exposure of the body to usual room temperature or immersion in tepid water usually suffices to bring the temperature back to normal levels. Older infants may require cooling for a longer time by repeated immersions or by use of a water-cooled mattress or other apparatus for induction of hypothermia. Attention to possible fluid and electrolyte disturbance is essential.

Neonatal Cold Injury. Neonatal cold injury usually occurs among infants in inadequately heated homes during damp cold spells when the outside temperature is in the range of freezing. The presenting features are apathy, refusal of food, oliguria and coldness to touch. The body temperature is usually between 85 and 94°F. (between 29.5 and 35°C.), and there is immobility, edema, and redness of the extremities, especially of the hands, feet and face. The facial erythema frequently gives a false impression of health, delaying recognition that the infant is ill. Local hardening over areas of edema may lead to confusion with sclerema. Rhinitis is common, as are serious metabolic disturbances, particularly hypoglycemia. Hemorrhagic manifestations are frequent, and massive pulmonary hemorrhage is a common finding at autopsy. Treatment consists in *gradual* warming with scrupulous attention to recognition and correction of metabolic imbalances, particularly hypoglycemia. Prevention consists in provision of adequate environmental heat. The mortality rate is about 25 per cent; about 10 per cent of the survivors have evidence of brain damage.

Edema. Generalized edema occurs in association with the most severe forms of Rh isoimmunization, with homozygous alpha thalassemia, and in the offspring of diabetic mothers. Some premature infants may have considerable puffiness for no apparent reason. Edema of the face and scalp may result from pressure from the umbilical cord around the neck, and transient localized swellings of the hands or feet may similarly be due to intrauterine pressures. Edema may be present with heart failure due to congenital cardiac lesions, even in the absence of a murmur; a lag in renal excretion of electrolytes and water may result in edema when there has been a sudden large increase in intake of electrolytes, particularly with feeding of concentrated mixtures of cow's milk. It is difficult to show a relation between low serum protein or low hemoglobin and the occurrence of edema in older premature infants, but occasionally the therapeutic response to plasma or blood transfusion is prompt. Rarely *"idiopathic hypoproteinemia"* with edema lasting weeks or months is observed in term infants. The cause is unclear, and the disturbance is benign. Persistent edema of one or more extremities may represent congenital lymphedema (Milroy's disease) or, in females, *Turner's syndrome*. Generalized edema with hypoproteinemia may be seen in the neonatal period with congenital nephrosis and, rarely, with Hurler's syndrome. Scleredema is described on page 1378.

Tetany. Tetany unrelated to a deficiency of vitamin D occurs occasionally in newborn infants, usually within the first week of life. The increased neuromuscular irritability stems from a decrease in serum calcium associated with an increase in serum phosphate (see p. 1260). The serum phosphatase level is normal. Transient physiologic hypoparathyroidism, diminished ability of the kidney to excrete phosphate, and a high phosphate load from undiluted cow's milk formulas have all been considered contributory.

Irritability, muscular twitchings, tremors and convulsions are the symptoms. Laryngospasm and carpopedal spasm are less common. Since a positive Chvostek's sign is frequently observed in normal newborn infants, it cannot be interpreted as a sign of tetany of the newborn. The level of the serum calcium is regularly reduced below 7 or 8 mg. per 100 ml., and that of the serum phosphate is elevated; an absolute diagnosis cannot be made in the absence of these chemical findings. The favorable response of symptoms to administration of calcium is not sufficient in itself to make the diagnosis, since calcium may act nonspecifically. Furthermore, symptoms such as irritability and tremors may subside spontaneously, and convulsions resulting from cerebral edema, anoxia or injury may not be repeated during the neonatal period. The good prognosis of hypocalcemic convulsions and the guarded to poor prognosis for convulsions from other causes in the neonatal period make establishment of the diagnosis by lumbar puncture (meningitis; intracranial hemorrhage) and by chemical examination of the blood (tetany) desirable. When there is associated albuminuria, pyuria or a persistently high blood urea level not associated with dehydration, urologic studies are indicated.

The response to calcium therapy is dramatic, convulsions being controlled by the intravenous administration of 5 to 10 ml. of calcium gluconate in 10 per cent solution. Intramuscular injection of calcium is contraindicated because local induration and necrosis may occur. Calcium should be given orally for approximately a week, preferably as calcium chloride (1.0 gm. a day, divided in 3 or more doses) or calcium lactate (2 to 3 gm. a day, divided in 3 or more doses) in 10 per cent solution. The use of parathyroid extract or of dihydrotachysterol is not indicated; vitamin D is not effective.

Hypomagnesemia. Hypomagnesemia in the newborn infant may occur as a result of exchange transfusion with citrated blood or as a result of an unknown defect in intestinal transport of magnesium or in magnesium homeostasis. Infants of diabetic mothers tend to have serum magnesium levels which are lower than the normal mean. The clinical manifestations of hypomagnesemia are indistinguishable from those of tetany and may, in fact, be secondary to the accompanying hypocalcemia.

The normal range of serum magnesium levels in the newborn infant is 1.2 to 1.8 mEq. per liter, with a mean of 1.5 mEq. per liter. During exchange transfusion with citrated blood which is low in magnesium ion, owing to binding by citrate, the serum magnesium drops about 0.5 mEq. per liter; approximately 10 days are required for magnesium to become unbound from the citrate and for the level of magnesium ion in the serum to return to normal. In hypomagnesemia which is not iatrogenically induced the serum magnesium may be less than 0.5 mEq. per liter. The serum calcium in either instance is usually at levels seen in hypocalcemic tetany, but the serum phosphorus value is normal. *Hypomagnesemia should, therefore, be suspected in any infant with tetany and a normal level of phosphorus in the serum.* Since the hypocalcemia accompanying hypomagnesemia is inadequately corrected by administration of calcium, hypomagnesemia should also be suspected in any patient with tetany not responding to calcium therapy. Almost all the spontaneously occurring cases thus far reported have been in males.

Immediate *treatment* consists in the intramuscular injection of magnesium sulfate. For newborn infants 0.2 ml. per kg. of a 50 per cent solution daily usually suffices. The accompanying hypocalcemia usually corrects itself as the hypomagnesemia is relieved. In most cases the metabolic defect is transient and treatment can be discontinued after 2 to 3 weeks. A few patients appear to have a permanent form of the disease which requires continuous oral supplementation with magnesium in order to prevent the recurrence of hypomagnesemia. As with hypocalcemic tetany, there appears to be no residual damage to the central nervous system.

Hypermagnesemia. Hypermagnesemia with serum levels as high as 15 mEq. per liter may occur in newborn infants of mothers treated with magnesium sulfate for eclampsia. At these levels there is depression of the central nervous system and total paralysis of the skeletal musculature, so that artificial respiration is required to maintain life. Exchange transfusion has been used as a means of rapid removal of magnesium ion from the blood. Recovery appears to be complete.

Other Metabolic Diseases. A number of inborn errors of metabolism may be manifest during the neonatal period; these include phenylketonuria, galactosemia and hyperglycinemia. Pyridoxine deficiency and dependency are considered on page 174.

Narcotic Addiction and Withdrawal. Physiologic addiction to narcotics exists in most infants born to actively addicted mothers. It may be manifest even before birth by unusual activity of the fetus at times when the mother feels the need for the drug. Morphine and its derivatives are the drugs most frequently involved.

Withdrawal symptoms usually appear within 24 hours after birth and include various combinations of tremors, hyperactivity, muscular hypertonicity, hyperreflexia, irritability, poor feeding, shrill cry, vomiting, diarrhea and fever. Yawning, sneezing, respiratory depression, apneic attacks, cyanosis, flushing alternating rapidly with pallor, twitching, convulsions, stuffy nose, lacrimation and sweating are less common. The *diagnosis* is made by establishing the history of maternal drug addiction. *Treatment* has been successful using various combinations of narcotics, sedatives and hypnotics. Mild cases may respond to sedation for a few days with ordinary doses of phenobarbital; patients with severe autonomic symptoms may require gradually diminishing doses of morphine, paregoric, chloral hydrate or chlorpromazine for 2 to 10 weeks. Chlorpromazine is recommended in a starting dose of approximately 1.0 mg. per kg. every 6 hours (4 mg. per kg. per 24 hours). Paregoric at a beginning dose of 3 to 5 drops every 3 to 6 hours, depending on the size and response of the infant, is an acceptable alternative. The dose and duration of therapy may be adjusted according to the clinical response. Parenteral administration of fluids may be necessary to prevent aspiration or dehydration until the symptoms are brought under control. Current mortality is not over 10 per cent; with early recognition and treatment the prognosis is good. *Prognosis* for normal development is good, except as affected by the environment to which the infant is returned after recovery.

Disturbances of the Endocrine System

Details of diagnosis and management of the endocrinopathies are covered in the section on The Endocrine System. The purpose of this section is merely to call attention to those endocrine disturbances which may be identified at birth or during the first month of life.

Pituitary dwarfism is usually inapparent at birth, the infant being of normal size. Conversely, constitutional dwarfs usually demonstrate length and weight consistent with prematurity when they are born after a normal gestational period and otherwise have the physical appearance of infants born at term.

Thyroid deficiency may be apparent at birth in genetically determined cretinism or in infants of mothers treated with thiouracil or its derivatives during pregnancy. Constipation, prolonged jaundice, lethargy or poor peripheral circulation as manifest by persistently mottled skin or cold extremities should always rouse suspicion of *cretinism.* Temporary *hyperthyroidism* may be seen at birth in the infants of mothers with hyperthyroidism or of those who have been receiving thyroid medication. *Congenital goiter* is discussed on page 1194.

Transient *hypoparathyroidism* may be manifest as tetany of the newborn.

The *adrenal gland* is subject to numerous disturbances which may be manifest and require lifesaving treatment during the neonatal period. Acute adrenal *hemorrhage* and failure may be seen after breech or other traumatic deliveries or in association with overwhelming infection. Phallic or clitoral enlargement apparent at or soon after birth may be the clue to *adrenal cortical hyperplasia.* Signs of deficiency of salt and water hormone are vomiting, diarrhea, dehydration, convulsions or shock. Since the condition is genetically determined, newborn siblings of patients with the salt-losing variety of adrenal cortical hyperplasia should be observed closely for manifestations of adrenal insufficiency. *Congenitally hypoplastic adrenal glands* may also give rise to adrenal insufficiency during the first few weeks of life. A syndrome clinically indistinguishable from adrenal insufficiency has been identified as a rare manifestation of cow's milk allergy in the first month of life.

Anomalies of the *gonads* may be apparent at birth. Of particular interest is gonadal dysgenesis (Turner's syndrome). Female infants with webbing of the neck, lymphangiectatic edema, hypoplasia of the nipples, cutis laxa, low hairline at the nape of the neck, deep-set ears, high-arched palate, deformities of the nails, cubitus valgus and other anomalies should be suspected of having gonadal dysgenesis (see p. 1231).

Transient *diabetes mellitus* (p. 1163) of unknown origin is occasionally and only seen in the newborn. It usually presents as dehydration, loss of weight, or acidosis. *Hypoglycemic convulsions* may occur during the first few days of life in infants of diabetic mothers, and especially in low-birth-weight infants of mothers with toxemia of pregnancy.

INFANTS OF DIABETIC MOTHERS

The successful control of diabetes with insulin has led to the survival and fertility of increasing numbers of diabetic women who in many instances seem almost to accept the disease as a challenge to their biologic competence. Their infants and the infants of women who later have diabetes share certain morphologic characteristics. In addition to their distinctive physical characteristics, infants of diabetic mothers have a high incidence of associated hydramnios and of intrauterine deaths after the thirty-sixth week of gestation, and a high neonatal mortality rate. Infants of prediabetic women have a lesser, but increased, neonatal mortality rate.

Pathology. Aside from the characteristic gross morphologic changes, autopsied infants of diabetic mothers show only hypertrophy of the pancreatic islets and their beta cells, with an increased insulin content of the islet tissue. In infants dying shortly after birth there is also a high incidence of the idiopathic respiratory distress syndrome. Fetal hyperinsulinism in response to maternal hyperglycemia has been postulated as the cause of the large size of these infants, but does not explain the large size of the infants of prediabetic women. Increased secretion of maternal corticotropin has also been postulated as contributing to the large size and "cushingoid" appearance of the infants. On the other hand, the increased body weight appears to be due to fat rather than to fluid and electrolyte retention. The currently suspected role of pituitary growth hormone in the production of diabetes could account not only for the maternal diabetes, but also for the hypertrophy of the islets and "gigantism" of the infant. The usual neonatal hypoglycemia is exaggerated among infants of diabetic mothers, particularly if the mother is insulin-dependent. Hypocalcemia is also common, and there is an increased incidence of renal vein thrombosis. *Physiologically*, infants of diabetic mothers have an increased rate of disposal of exogenous glucose, increased plasma insulin-like activity after a glucose load, and suppressed levels of free fatty acids during periods of hypoglycemia.

Clinical Manifestations. The infants of diabetic and prediabetic mothers bear a surprising resemblance to each other (Fig. 7-25). They tend to be large and plump with a puffy, plethoric facies resembling that of patients who have been receiving corticotropin or a corticosteroid. They have a bloated appearance and tend to be "jumpy" or "trembly" after the first 24 hours of life. Unexplained cyanotic attacks and the idiopathic respiratory distress syndrome (see p. 381) are common.

Convulsions associated with severe hypoglycemia, which respond clinically to the intravenous injection of glucose, are occasionally observed. The "jitteriness" which is common on the second and third days of life appears as likely to be related to hypocalcemia as to hypoglycemia.

Although an increased incidence of congenital malformations is commonly ascribed to infants of diabetic mothers, adequate data are lacking.

Prognosis. Fetal loss is lowest among diabetic women whose diabetes has been under good control during pregnancy and who have had adequate antenatal obstetric care. Although cesarean delivery near the thirty-sixth week of gestation reduces the fetal mortality rate during the last weeks of pregnancy, there is disagreement as to whether this procedure reduces overall fetal loss, owing to an increase in neonatal deaths resulting from the addition of problems associated with cesarean section and prematurity to those of the infants of diabetic mothers.

Treatment. The blood sugar of infants of diabetic mothers should be monitored about 2 hours

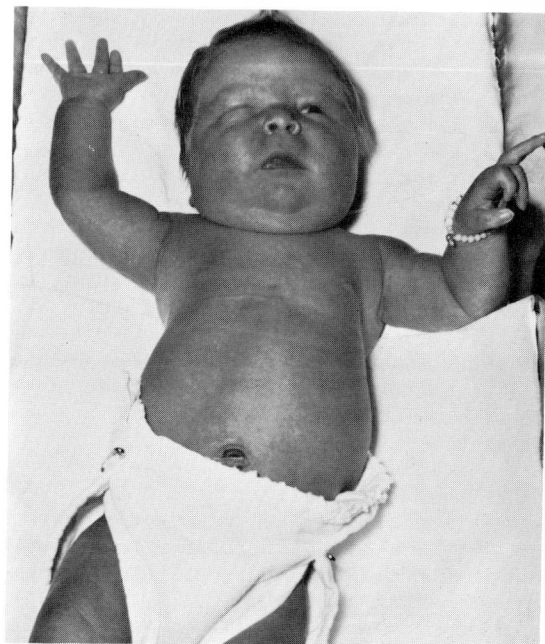

Figure 7-25. Large, plump, plethoric infant of a prediabetic mother. Baby was born at 38 weeks of gestation, but weighed 9 pounds 11 ounces (4408 gm.). Mild respiratory distress was the only symptom other than appearance.

after birth, when it is likely to be lowest in apparently well infants. Values under 20 mg. per 100 ml. should probably be treated even in asymptomatic infants, who will respond to the parenteral administration of 300 micrograms of glucagon per kg. Sick or symptomatic infants with hypoglycemia will not respond to glucagon, presumably because of depletion of their glycogen stores (see below). It seems logical to begin oral feedings 2 or 3 hours after birth, though there is no evidence that this significantly reduces hypoglycemia. Likewise, the feeding of a formula of low phosphate content might be expected to lessen the likelihood of hypocalcemia (supporting evidence is lacking). Sick infants of diabetic mothers are more apt to have severe hypoglycemia, which may be symptomatic or asymptomatic, than are apparently well infants. The management of hypoglycemia in sick or symptomatic infants is discussed in the following section on hypoglycemia. Infants with symptoms pointing to the central nervous system should have diagnostic lumbar puncture to rule out meningitis, cerebral hemorrhage or cerebral edema. The treatment of tetany of the newborn is outlined on page 401, and the management of the respiratory distress syndrome on page 383.

HYPOGLYCEMIA

Symptomatic hypoglycemia may occur among infants of nondiabetic as well as diabetic mothers. It is most common among male infants of low birth weight for their gestational age, and is particularly likely among the smaller of twins discordant for birth weight. The relative frequency among infants of toxemic mothers appears to be related less to the toxemia than to inadequate stores of hepatic glycogen secondary to intrauterine malnutrition, and to an abnormally sensitive insulin release mechanism after birth.

Symptomatic and asymptomatic hypoglycemia may occur with erythroblastosis fetalis before or after exchange transfusion, as well as among infants of low birth weight who are sick for any reason. In such instances it is difficult to tell whether the symptoms attributed to hypoglycemia are due to it or to the underlying disturbance, which may be the cause of both the symptoms and the hypoglycemia.

The onset of symptoms has been observed from a few hours to a week after birth. Normal blood sugar levels have been demonstrated subsequently in the hypoglycemic infants. The symptoms in approximate order of frequency are tremors, episodes of cyanosis, apathy, convulsions, apneic spells or respiratory distress, weak or high-pitched cry, limpness, difficulty in feeding, and eye-rolling. The role of the frequently accompanying hypocalcemia or polycythemia as causes of the symptoms is not clear.

Treatment consists in administration through a peripheral vein of 1 to 2 ml. per kg. of 50 per cent glucose solution for immediate relief of symptoms, followed by continuous intravenous infusion of 10 per cent glucose solution until blood glucose levels have stabilized, when it should be discontinued. If available, the use of fructose instead of glucose for the continuous infusion has the advantages of not stimulating the release of insulin and of gradual conversion to glucose in the body. The addition of corticotropin (ACTH), 4 units every 12 hours, or hydrocortisone, 5 mg. every 12 hours, may be necessary to maintain blood sugar at normal levels and to eliminate the symptoms. The use of diazoxide (3-methyl-7-chloro-1,2,4-benzothiadiazine-1,1-dioxide) in the treatment of transient neonatal hypoglycemia remains to be investigated. Treatment is usually necessary for a few days up to several weeks, after which it should gradually be discontinued. Recurrences are relatively rare, but have been reported as late as the age of 8 months.

Prognosis for life is good in the absence of congenital anomalies severe enough in themselves to be lethal. Prognosis for normal intellectual function must be guarded, since the incidence of apparent intellectual defect approaches 20 per cent.

Hypoglycemia with Macroglossia. Beckwith and Combs and their co-workers recently described a syndrome of neonatal hypoglycemia occurring in infants with macroglossia, large size, visceromegaly, mild microcephaly and umbilical abnormalities. The visceromegaly involves chiefly the liver and the kidneys, in which there is a non-cystic hyperplasia. Some of the infants are also polycythemic. Treatment is that of idiopathic hypoglycemia, as described above.

Infections of the Newborn

The reader is referred to other sections for discussion of specific diseases which may be particularly important in the newborn infant. See, in particular, Congenital Rubella Syndrome, Syphilis, Tetanus, Cytomegalic Inclusion Disease, Toxoplasmosis.

Infections of the newborn infant may be caused by any pathogenic bacterial or viral agent. He is particularly susceptible, however, to organisms which are usually nonpathogenic for older children and for adults outside of the geriatric age group, in whom such infections are again seen with relatively greater frequency. The Pneumococcus, beta hemolytic streptococcus and *H. influenzae*, common pathogenic agents in later infancy, are relatively uncommon causes of infection in the first few weeks of life. At this time coliform organisms and *Staphylococcus aureus* are the most frequent causes of severe infections; other relatively common bacterial pathogens are enterococci, Klebsiella, Pseudomonas, Proteus and Salmonella. Nursery epidemics caused by any organism with antibiotic susceptibility may be managed in a manner similar to that to be described for the prevention of epidemics of staphylococcal infection (see below).

The most frequent serious infections of the newborn are pneumonia, septicemia, diarrhea, meningitis and peritonitis. Of these, pneumonia and septicemia are common; diarrhea has become relatively uncommon in the United States, but has a high incidence in individual epidemics; meningitis is present in approximately 25 per cent of cases of septicemia; and peritonitis is relatively rare as a well developed clinical entity.

In pneumonia, septicemia and meningitis the prognosis is heavily influenced by early diagnosis and institution of specific treatment with appropriate antibacterial agents. *All three are distinguished by their lack of specific signs or symptoms in the early stages* (see Clinical Manifestations of Disease in the newborn, p. 372, and Pneumonia on p. 388. In the absence of dehydration or high environmental temperature they are the commonest causes of body temperatures over 100°F. in the newborn infant. Frequently, however, there is no elevation of temperature, or the temperature may be subnormal, and failure to feed well, lethargy, irritability, vomiting or episodes of cyanosis may be the only evidence of any one of these major infections. The onset of icterus after the second or third day of life is especially suggestive of septicemia. The classic signs of meningitis in the small infant (bulging fontanel, high-pitched cry, vomiting and convulsions) are late signs, and the diagnosis must be made before they appear in order to reduce the mortality of the disease. Acute meningitis caused by gram-negative bacilli, in particular, frequently becomes chronic, with a high incidence of permanent residuals. Clinical detection of pneumonia, septicemia or meningitis is dependent on liberal indications for securing a roentgenogram of the chest and a blood culture and for performing a spinal puncture in infants who "are not doing well." Premature infants are especially prone to serious infections with few or no clinical manifestations.

Histologic examination of amniotic smears and frozen sections of the umbilical cord for bacteria and inflammatory cells has been advocated as a means of early identification of infection in the infant at birth. The lack of correlation between the inflammatory changes in these tissues and disease in the infant, however, does not permit diagnostic deductions. Another deterrent is the observation that hypoxia without infection may be responsible for the infiltration of inflammatory cells in the placenta and cord. These techniques at best have limited clinical application and none beyond emphasizing the need for careful observation of the infant in the first postnatal days for evidence of disease.

Infections which may be responsible for neonatal morbidity and mortality may be acquired during the embryonic, fetal or neonatal period. From the standpoints of prevention, recognition and management, it is helpful to know as much as possible of the pathogenesis of each of these diseases; one important aspect is knowledge of the time of acquisition. The following tabulation lists the more important infections which may occur during gestation, during birth (perinatal period) and during the neonatal period. They are arranged on the basis of preventability in relation to current knowledge. It is important to recognize that a number of these infections may be transmitted by the mother even though she has had no clinical evidence that she is a carrier.

Infections acquired during gestation

Preventable	*Nonpreventable**
Syphilis	Toxoplasmosis
Tuberculosis	Cytomegalic inclusion disease
Residuals of rubella	Listeriosis
Vaccinia	Myocarditis, viral
Poliomyelitis	Hepatitis, homologous serum
Pneumonia**	Varicella
Sepsis**	Herpes simplex
	Vibrio fetus infection

Infections acquired during birth† (immediate perinatal period)

Preventable	*Nonpreventable*
Gonorrheal ophthalmia	Herpes simplex
Oral moniliasis	Listeriosis
Salmonellosis	
Pneumonia‡	
Sepsis‡	

---

* On basis of current knowledge.

** Usually secondary to premature rupture of membranes or to interference with placental circulation.

†Most often from the mother, who may be infected or may be a carrier.

‡Usually secondary to premature rupture of membranes, to interference with placental circulation, or to prolonged or traumatic delivery.

Infections acquired after birth in the neonatal period

Staphylococcal infections
  Carrier state, skin lesions, pneumonia, otitis media, meningitis, osteomyelitis, diarrhea, generalized sepsis
E. coli infections
  Septicemia, omphalitis, pneumonia, diarrhea, and others
Salmonella infections
  Septicemia, meningitis, osteomyelitis, and others
Beta hemolytic streptococcal infections
  Occasionally responsible for disease in this age period
Pneumococcal and H. influenzae infections
  Less frequent pathogenic agents than in subsequent months
Tetanus
Tuberculosis
Viral infections
  Upper respiratory tract infections, pneumonitis, myocarditis, generalized infections

Escherichia Coli Infections. The commonest *etiologic agent* of all serious infections (pneumonia, septicemia, meningitis and diarrhea) of the newborn is *E. coli*. Ten serologic types of *enteropathogenic E. coli* have been linked to individual epidemics of diarrhea of the newborn, types 0111:B4, 055:B5, 026:B6 and 0127:B8 being the most common. The relation of these particular strains of *E. coli* to infections other than diarrhea has not been clearly defined; they have not been shown to produce epidemic disease other than diarrhea.

Systemic infections caused by *E. coli* are best treated with kanamycin in dosage of 15 mg. per kg. per day divided into 2 equal doses administered intramuscularly at 12-hour intervals. Ampicillin is also effective against many strains of *E. coli* and may be used in combination with kanamycin. In intestinal infections neomycin is effective (see p. 408).

STAPHYLOCOCCAL INFECTIONS

Second in frequency to *E. coli* as a cause of infection in the newborn, *Staphylococcus aureus* assumed relatively greater importance between 1950 and 1960, owing to the frequent occurrence of epidemic nursery infections with strains resistant to most of the commonly used antibacterial agents.

Although staphylococcal pneumonia, septicemia or enteritis may occur without warning in the newborn infant, each is frequently preceded by apparent skin infections of the infant or of contacts which may consist of small pustules or furuncles, or of large furuncles, cellulitis, bullous impetigo or breast abscess. Osteomyelitis and meningitis are relatively frequent complications of septicemia. Staphylococcal meningitis without bacteremia suggests the presence of a communication (dermal sinus) between the skin and the subarachnoid space. A leaking meningocele is an obvious portal of entry. The umbilicus, a circumcision wound or other surgical incision may serve as a route for staphylococci to reach the bloodstream, as may any abrasion of the skin.

Nursery epidemics of staphylococcal infection usually begin with increasingly frequent appearance of small pustules. More severe infections of the skin, septicemia or enteritis are usually seen next. Although the initial infection is acquired in the nursery, these and other serious manifestations may not make their appearance for weeks or even months after the baby has been discharged. Therefore the existence of an epidemic of serious proportions may not be suspected unless the infants are followed up carefully after discharge and unless all cases of furuncles, breast abscess, pneumonia and other less frequent staphylococcal infections during the first months of life are reported to the nursery where the infants were born. A high incidence of small pustules may be the only evidence in the nursery of an epidemic which is resulting in major staphylococcal infections among discharged infants and other members of their families.

Investigations suggest that epidemics are due to certain strains of hemolytic *Staphylococcus aureus* which appear to have unusual pathogenicity. One such strain (phage type 80/81) has perhaps been the most frequently identified in severe hospital epidemics. The pathogen is undoubtedly introduced initially into the nursery by personnel or by an infant who acquires it through contact with his mother. Once the organism has been introduced, the infants in the nursery, as well as adult carriers, constitute the reservoir of infection, and it spreads from baby to baby. Anatomic areas of the infant which constitute particular reservoirs are the skin, the anterior nares and the umbilical cord stump.

Prevention. All persons with skin infections should be excluded from the nursery and from contact with the infant after discharge. Mothers with staphylococcal infections should be isolated and treated while their infants remain in an isolation nursery out of contact with them or with other newborn infants. Use of soap or detergent containing hexachlorophene tends to reduce the bacterial population on the skin of nursery personnel. The latter should also be specifically instructed that the anterior nares constitute the chief reservoir in carriers. Initial and daily bathing of the infants with a soap or detergent containing hexachlorophene reduces the incidence of skin infection with staphylococci, but such infants may acquire pustules due to *E. coli*. Daily painting of the umbilical cord stump with bactericidal dyes* reduces the incidence of nasal and skin colonization of staphylococci, provided all infants in the nursery are so treated. Avoidance of overcrowding in the nursery is important. Since the infants themselves appear to be the chief reservoir of staphylococcal infection in nursery epidemics, it is desirable to have multiple nurseries each accommodating 4 to 6 infants, so that, once a nursery is filled, no new babies need be admitted until all

its previous occupants have been discharged and the nursery has been cleaned. This will serve to break any baby-to-baby cycle of infection.

Once an *epidemic* of staphylococcal infection has started, there appear to be only 2 effective ways of stopping it. The preferable method is to admit all new babies to newly established nurseries staffed by separate, uninfected personnel in a different area of the hospital. Admission of new infants to the regular nurseries is resumed only after all their infant occupants have been discharged, after any staphylococcal carriers have been identified and excluded, and after the nurseries have been thoroughly cleaned and disinfected. The second and less preferable method is the routine administration to each infant in the nursery from the day of admission through the day of discharge of full therapeutic doses of an antibiotic effective against the strain of staphylococci responsible for the epidemic. For this purpose erythromycin or one of the synthetic penicillins is usually the drug of choice, owing to the greater potential toxicity of chloramphenicol, novobiocin, bacitracin or kanamycin. Maintenance of this regimen for 3 weeks is ordinarily sufficient to control an epidemic, provided the usual measures of tightening up on nursery techniques in general and the exclusion of personnel who are carriers of the pathogenic strain are also taken.

Artificial colonization of the nose and umbilical cord stump with a nonpathogenic strain of coagulase-positive *Staphylococcus aureus* has been demonstrated to interfere with colonization by pathogenic strains. The application of this phenomenon to the prevention and interruption of nursery epidemics of staphylococcal infection is in the experimental stage and should be done only by experienced investigators under carefully controlled conditions

Treatment. The treatment of staphylococcal infections is best accomplished by systemic administration of an antibiotic effective against the particular strain of the organism involved.

Because many, if not most, strains of staphylococci infecting newborn infants are producers of penicillinase, the drug to be used should be effective against such strains, and if the organism is isolated, it should be tested for its in-vitro susceptibility to several of the synthetic penicillins and other antibiotics effective against penicillin-resistant staphylococci. In our clinic oxacillin is the antibiotic currently in use for severe staphylococcal infections prior to receipt of information from the laboratory of the in-vitro susceptibilities of the bacterium. It is administered parenterally in a dose of 25 mg. per kg. every 12 hours. After the first 5 days of life the same dose should be given every 6 to 8 hours. This dose may be doubled for severe infections. Should the organism be known to be sensitive to penicillin G, it is the drug of choice in a dose of 50,000 units per kg. every 12 hours for the first 5 days of

---

*"Triple-dye": Acriflavine, 1.14 gm.
Gentian violet, 2.29 gm.
Brilliant green, 2.29 gm.
Distilled water, 1000 ml.

life, and every 6 hours thereafter. The combination of penicillin G or ampicillin (50 mg. per kg. every 12 hours for the first 5 days and every 6 hours thereafter) and kanamycin in a dose of 7.5 mg. per kg. every 12 hours by the intramuscular route has been effective against many strains of staphylococci and has the advantage, in cases in which the organism is presumed, but not proved, of effectiveness against *E. coli* and a number of other gram-negative organisms.

Tests of antibiotic sensitivity in vitro should always be done and the medication changed accordingly if the drug being used is not producing a satisfactory clinical response. In the presence of an obviously good clinical response a shift of medication on the basis of the results of sensitivity tests in vitro should be questioned.

In addition to systemic therapy, bathing with soaps or detergents containing hexachlorophene and the local application of bacitracin ointment will aid in eradicating skin lesions. Accumulations of pus, wherever encountered, should be drained surgically.

PSEUDOMONAS INFECTIONS

See also page 592.

Currently, perhaps owing to several factors such as measures to eliminate staphylococci from hospital nurseries and the common use of complicated equipment that is difficult to sterilize or that includes water reservoirs, gram-negative and ordinarily nonpathogenic bacteria have become increasingly important as a cause of infections acquired in the newborn nursery. As the population of gram-positive bacteria is reduced by use of hexachlorophene soaps and detergents, there has been a corresponding increase of gram-negative organisms. Unfortunately, these organisms are less susceptible to antibiotics than are the gram-positive ones.

The pseudomonas group of organisms, which are normal inhabitants of water and soil, have come to be of considerable importance as causes of nursery infections, but the klebsiella, aerobacter and proteus groups are also involved. Pseudomonas has become an important cause of mortality from bacteremia, pneumonia and meningitis in premature and intensive care nurseries, where the debilitated infant population is particularly susceptible to infection. The use of such equipment as endotracheal and other indwelling tubes further promotes the proliferation of these organisms through interference with clearance of respiratory secretions.

Preventive measures include careful and frequent cleansing and sterilization of equipment used for respiratory therapy, avoidance of equipment or procedures which promote stasis of respiratory secretions, and use of a bactericidal agent effective against pseudomonas in the humidification pans of incubators. Sophisticated methods of filtration and exchange of the air circulating in the nursery are probably of little avail against organisms which are constantly reintroduced from the skin of nurses and other personnel who care for the infants. Water in humidification pans of incubators may be sterilized by the addition of 50 micrograms of silver nitrate per liter of water. Distilled water must be used, since chlorine in water will precipitate the silver out as the insoluble and nonbactericidal chloride. Plastic pans should be used, because silver nitrate disappears rapidly from solution in metal pans. The bacterial population in the reservoirs of nebulizers may be kept down by frequent changes of *sterile* distilled water, and mist from ultrasonic nebulizers tends to be less contaminated than mist from mechanical nebulizers.

Treatment of infections with the pseudomonas group of bacteria is unsatisfactory; the organisms are rarely sensitive to bacterial agents other than polymyxin B or polymyxin E (colistin). The dose of polymyxin B is 1.5 to 2.5 mg. per kg. every 12 hours by the intramuscular route. The dose of colistin is 2 to 4 mg. per kg. every 12 hours by the intramuscular route. Because of poor diffusion into the spinal fluid in cases of meningitis, polymyxin B should be given intrathecally in a dose of 1 mg. daily until the infection is under control. Colistin should not be administered intrathecally.

DIARRHEA IN THE NEWBORN

A scourge of all nurseries because of its great contagiousness and high morbidity and mortality rates, epidemic diarrhea of the newborn is fortunately now a relatively infrequent but still serious problem in the United States.

Etiologically, it is not an entity. A number of bacterial and viral agents have been identified as the causative or probable causative agents in individual epidemics. With the exception of enteropathogenic strains of *E. coli* and occasional viruses causing respiratory or oral infections in adults, they do not differ significantly from the usual causative agents of diarrhea (p. 782). On the basis of present evidence it would appear that certain types of *E. coli* (p. 405) are responsible for a high percentage of nursery epidemics of diarrheal disease. The specificity and severity of the disease are related principally to the host factors of low immunity, small metabolic reserve of water and electrolytes, and poorly developed homeostatic mechanisms. The large, changing, crowded and susceptible population in almost any newborn nursery is also an ideal environmental situation for a contagious disease to become epidemic. Premature or debilitated infants are especially susceptible. Sporadic cases are also seen; they usually occur in the home after exposure to an older sibling or adult with an enteric infection.

Clinical Manifestations. The incubation period is most commonly 1 to 3 days. At onset the infant usually becomes listless or fretful, nurses less well than usual, fails to gain or may actually lose weight. Vomiting is an inconstant symptom, as is abdominal distention. The temperature is usually normal, but may rise to 100 to 104°F. When the diarrhea starts, the stools tend to be watery, yellowish (later greenish) and acid enough to produce irritation of the skin of the buttocks within a few hours. They are usually frequent and passed explosively. On the other hand, an occasional infant may go into shock and die from water and electrolyte loss into the intestinal lumen before a diarrheal stool is passed. Mucus, pus and macroscopic blood are usually not evident or at least not prominent. As the diarrhea progresses the infant becomes increasingly restless with a frequent, short and feeble cry. With progressive dehydration, thirst may give way to refusal to feed, and the infant becomes drowsy and, finally, comatose. In the final stages of dehydration the eyes are deep-sunken, the skin takes on a grayish cast, and there is circumoral cyanosis and an apparent state of shock. Hyperpnea is frequently absent in spite of acidosis with carbon dioxide levels as low as 2 mEq. per liter. There is hemoconcentration, and protein, white cells and casts are found in the urine in considerable quantities. The severity and the clinical manifestations vary greatly from patient to patient.

The clinical course varies from a few days to several weeks. Exacerbations are common. Complications include otitis media, bronchopneumonia, bacteremia, peritonitis from perforation of an intestinal ulcer, and renal vein and cerebral sinus thrombosis.

Prevention. The hospital nursery technique should be designed to eliminate chances of infection or cross infection among the infants. This involves adequate floor area to avoid overcrowding, complete individual bassinet units and equipment for each infant, careful supervision of the preparation of formulas, and well trained, conscientious personnel who are numerically adequate.

Any direct or indirect contact with persons with intestinal disease or direct contact with any with respiratory infections must be avoided. This means the exclusion from the nursery of all personnel who have had even mild diarrhea or vomiting within 48 to 72 hours, and of all personnel having more than the most fleeting contact with active cases of diarrhea either professionally or at home. In nurseries a high index of suspicion must be maintained, especially since the onset of an epidemic may be so insidious that the possibility is not considered until several infants have diarrhea. A frequent cause of this situation is the discharge from the nursery of the initial case or cases before definite signs of the disease have appeared, but after the contagious state is already present. Therefore it is essential that the development of diarrhea in an infant after discharge be reported immediately to the person in charge of the newborn nursery. Immediate reporting to local or state health officials is equally important.

Nursery personnel must be constantly on the alert for abnormal stools among their charges. Differentiation must be made between diarrhea and the loose and frequent movements characteristic of transitional stools. The breast-fed infant may have more frequent and more liquid stools than the bottle-fed infant, and may be affected by the dietary or medicinal intake of his mother. Overfeeding, high carbohydrate content of the formula, intestinal intolerance to cow's milk or the use of soybean or protein hydrolysate formulas may be responsible for loose stools in the bottle-fed infant. Aganglionic megacolon may be manifest initially as diarrhea. Once a baby in a nursery for newborns is identified as having diarrhea, he should be isolated in a separate nursery and cared for by personnel who do not have contact with the remaining infants. The latter and those discharged from the exposed nursery must be watched closely for any untoward signs. New infants should not be admitted to the nursery from the time of recognition of the second case until it has been cleared of its current population. It should then be thoroughly scrubbed and aired before admissions are resumed.

Prognosis. The fatality rate in epidemics of recent years has been about 40 per cent. With presently available treatment it should be lower, and in a few epidemics all affected infants have survived. The subsequent course of surviving infants is, in general, uneventful, although chronic intestinal disturbances are an uncommon sequel.

Treatment. Except for those epidemics due to bacteria against which effective specific antibacterial agents are available, treatment is symptomatic and supportive. It does not differ from that of diarrheal disturbances in later infancy (pp. 220, 782). Neomycin has been effective in breaking nursery epidemics due to most of the enteropathogenic types of *E. coli*. For this purpose 50 mg. of neomycin per kg. per day may be administered orally in divided doses to all infants in the nursery up to the time of discharge of the last infant present at the time the medication is started. Nursery personnel should also be cultured, since they may be asymptomatic carriers of enteropathogenic strains of *E. coli*. Any carriers discovered should be relieved of duty and treated with neomycin until the organism has been eradicated from their intestinal tracts.

INFECTION DUE TO LISTERIA MONOCYTOGENES

Of the human infections caused by *Listeria monocytogenes*, that of purulent meningitis is the one most commonly recognized (p. 571), but a generalized *miliary granulomatosis* in stillborn fetuses and newborn infants is unique. The incidence is not known, probably because the infection is most often not identified.

The fetus is apparently infected transplacentally and usually dies before birth. In those born alive manifestations may be apparent from the time of birth or may be delayed a week or so. The clinical pattern is not characteristic. There is often brownish discoloration of the amniotic fluid. When the onset is shortly after birth, the principal signs are those of cardiorespiratory distress. Diarrhea and vomiting are common. When the onset is delayed, the course may be gradual, but is progressive and is usually characterized by bronchopneumonia. Meningitis is not uncommon. Granulomas appearing as dark red or livid papules are infrequently present on the oropharynx and the skin.

Pathologically, there are microscopic to pinhead-sized nodules in many organs, viz., liver, spleen, adrenals, lungs, pharynx, gastrointestinal tract, brain and meninges and skin.

The diagnosis is established by identification of the organism in the urine or blood of the infant, and suggested by similar identification in the mother. High agglutinative titers may be observed for a short time after the infection.

Most of the available antibiotic agents are effective against *L. monocytogenes*; penicillin is probably the agent of choice.

VIBRIO FETUS INFECTION

Vibrio fetus, a small, gram-negative motile rod with frequent spiral forms, which grows best in an anaerobic medium, is a leading cause of abortion in sheep and cattle. A number of human infections have been identified. Those reported have been in pregnant women, suggesting venereal transmission, as is the case in animal-to-animal transmission. In men the infection is believed to be acquired largely through contact with infected animal tissue.

The usual clinical picture of infection of the newborn infant with the *Vibrio fetus* is one of fulminating meningoencephalitis. The placenta often has a necrotic appearance; abortion and premature delivery are common, and suggest transplacental infection of the fetus. "Related vibrios" have been isolated from stools and blood of older infants, with a relatively mild diarrheal illness in which the stools contain blood and mucus. The bacterium may be *Vibrio jejuni*, the causative agent of winter dysentery in cattle.

Treatment of infections with *Vibrio fetus* in the newborn has not been satisfactory. Chloramphenicol and streptomycin have been suggested as drugs of choice. Data on the use of ampicillin are not available.

COXSACKIE VIRUS INFECTION

See also page 673.

An acute, fulminating febrile illness may re-sult from infection of newborn infants with Coxsackie virus group B. It may be associated with minor respiratory or other infection in the mother shortly before delivery or be contracted after birth. At autopsy the characteristic finding is diffuse myocarditis; other organs, especially the central nervous system, may be involved.

HERPES SIMPLEX

Severe and usually fatal generalized infection of the newborn infant may be caused by the virus of herpes simplex (see p. 634).

R. JAMES MCKAY

REFERENCES

Benirschke, K.: Twin Placenta in Perinatal Mortality. *New York State J. Med.,* 61:1499, 1961.

Boston, R. W., Geller, F., and Smith, C. A.: Arterial Blood Gas Tensions and Acid-Base Balance in the Management of the Respiratory Distress Syndrome. *J. Pediat.,* 68:74, 1966.

Brown, A. K.: Bilirubin Metabolism, with Special Reference to Neonatal Jaundice; in S. Z. Levine (Ed.): *Advances in Pediatrics.* Chicago, Year Book Publishers, Inc., 1962, Vol. XII, p. 121.

Cheek, D. B., and Rowe, R. D.: Aspects of Sympathetic Activity in the Newborn, Including the Respiratory Distress Syndrome. *Pediat. Clin. N. Amer.,* 13:863, 1966.

Combs, J. T., Grunt, J. A., and Brandt, I. K.: New Syndrome of Neonatal Hypoglycemia. Association with Visceromegaly, Macroglossia, Microcephaly and Abnormal Umbilicus. *New England J. Med.,* 275:236, 1966.

Craig, W. S.: Intracranial Irritation in Newborn: Immediate and Long-Term Prognosis. *Arch. Dis. Childhood,* 25:325, 1950.

Driscoll, S. G., and Smith, C. A.: Neonatal Pulmonary Disorders. *Pediat. Clin. N. Amer.,* 9:325, 1962.

Dunn, P. M.: Localization of the Umbilical Catheter by Postmortem Measurement. *Arch. Dis. Childhood,* 41:69, 1966.

Eichenwald, H. F., and Shinefield, H. R.: Viral Infections of the Premature and Newborn Infant; in S. Z. Levine (Ed.): *Advances in Pediatrics.* Chicago, Year Book Publishers, Inc., 1962, Vol. XII, p. 249.

Farquhar, J. W.: The Child of the Diabetic Woman. *Arch. Dis. Childhood,* 34:76, 1959.

Forfar, J. O., Gould, J. C., and MacCabe, A. F.: Effect of Hexachlorophene on Incidence of Staphylococcal and Gram-Negative Infection in the Newborn. *Lancet,* 2:177, 1968.

Graham, C. G., Barness, L. A., and Gyorgy, P.: Serum Calcium and Inorganic Phosphate in the Newborn Infant, and Their Relation to Different Feedings. *J. Pediat.,* 42:401, 1953.

Greenman, G. W., Gabrielson, M. O., Howard-Flanders, J., and Wessel, M. A.: Thyroid Dysfunction in Pregnancy: Fetal Loss and Follow-up Evaluation of Surviving Infants. *New England J. Med.,* 267:426, 1962.

Grossman, M.: Antimicrobial Therapy in the Newborn Infant. *Pediat. Clin. N. Amer.,* 15:157, 1968.

Harris, J. R., and Schick, B.: Erythema Neonatorum. *Am. J. Dis. Child.,* 92:27, 1956.

Harrison, V. C., Heese, H. de V., and Klein, M.: The Significance of Grunting in Hyaline Membrane Disease. *Pediatrics,* 41:549, 1968.

Herbst, A. L., and Selenkow, H. A.: Hyperthyroidism During Pregnancy. *New England J. Med.,* 273:627, 1965.

Hill, R. M., and Desmond, M. M.: Management of the Narcotic Withdrawal Syndrome in the Neonate. *Pediat. Clin. N. Amer.,* 10:67, 1963.

Illingworth, R. S.: Cyanotic Attacks in Newborn Infants. *Arch. Dis. Childhood,* 32:328, 1957.

James, L. S. (Ed.): Symposium on the Newborn. *Pediat. Clin. N. Amer.*, 13:573-1205, 1966.

Jellard, J.: Umbilical Cord as Reservoir of Infection in a Maternity Hospital. *Brit. M.J.*, 1:925, 1957.

Kendall, N., and Woloshin, H.: Cephalhematoma Associated with Fracture of the Skull. *J. Pediat.*, 41:125, 1952.

Kumar, D.: Intra-uterine Diagnosis, Indices of Fetal Jeopardy and Intra-uterine Therapy: in Barnes, A. C., (Ed.): *Intra-Uterine Development*. Philadelphia, Lea & Febiger, 1968, p. 477.

Levine, S. Z., and Gordon, H. H.: Physiologic Handicaps of the Premature Infant. I. Their Pathogenesis. II. Clinical Applications. *Am. J. Dis. Child.*, 64:274, 1942.

Light, I. J., Sutherland, J. M., Cochran, M. L., and Sutorius, J.: Ecologic Relation Between Staphylococcus Aureus and Pseudomonas in a Nursery Population. *New England J. Med.*, 278:1243, 1968.

McCann, M. L., and others: Effects of Fructose on Hypoglucosemia in Infants of Diabetic Mothers. *New England J. Med.*, 275:1, 1966.

Moffett, H. L., Allan, D., and Williams, T.: Survival and Dissemination of Bacteria in Nebulizers and Incubators. *Am. J. Dis. Child.*, 114:13, 1967.

Nachtigall, L., Bassett, M., Hogsander, U., and Levitz, M.: Plasma Estriol Levels in Normal and Abnormal Pregnancies: An Index of Fetal Welfare. *Am. J. Obst. & Gynec.*, 101:638, 1968.

Nichols, W., Jr., and Wooley, P. V., Jr.: Listeria Monocytogenes Meningitis. *J. Pediat.*, 61:337, 1962.

Northway, W. H., Jr., Rosan, R. C., and Porter, D. Y.: Pulmonary Disease Following Respirator Therapy of Hyaline-Membrane Disease. Bronchopulmonary Dysplasia. *New England J. Med.*, 276:357, 1967.

Potter, E. L.: *Pathology of the Fetus and the Infant*. 2nd ed. Chicago, Year Book Publishers, Inc., 1961.

Raiha, C. E.: Prevention of Prematurity; in S. Z. Levine (Ed.): *Advances in Pediatrics*. Chicago, Year Book Publishers, Inc., 1968, Vol. XV, p. 137.

Reardon, H. S., Wilson, J. L., and Graham, B. D.: Physiologic Deviations of the Premature Infant, with Summary of Principles of Care. *Am. J. Dis. Child.*, 81:99, 1951.

Robinson, R. J.: Assessment of Gestational Age by Neurologic Examination. *Arch. Dis. Childhood*, 41:437, 1966.

Rosenfeld, G. B., and Bradley, C.: Childhood Behavior Sequelae of Asphyxia in Infancy: With Special Reference to Pertussis and Asphyxia Neonatorum. *Pediatrics*, 2:74, 1948.

Rowe, S., and Avery, M. E.: Massive Pulmonary Hemorrhage in the Newborn. II. Clinical Considerations. *J. Pediat.*, 69:12, 1966.

Saling, E.: Amnioscopy and Foetal Blood Sampling: Observations on Foetal Acidosis. *Arch. Dis. Childhood*, 41:472, 1966.

Shaffer, T. E., Baldwin, J. N., and Wheeler, W. E.: Staphylococcal Infections in Nurseries; in S. Z. Levine (Ed.): *Advances in Pediatrics*. Chicago, Year Book Publishers, Inc., 1958, Vol. X, p. 243.

Shinefeld, H. R., Ribble, J. C., Boris, M., and Eichenwald, H. F.: Bacterial Interference: Its Effect on Nursery-Acquired Infection with Staphylococcus Aureus. I. Preliminary Observations on Artificial Colonization of Newborns. *Am. J. Dis. Child.*, 105:646, 1963.

Silverman, W. A.: *Dunham's Premature Infants*. 3rd. ed. New York, Paul B. Hoeber, Inc., 1961.

Silverman, W. A., and Sinclair, J. C.: Temperature Regulation in the Newborn Infant. *New England J. Med.*, 274:92, 146, 1966.

Smith, C. A.: *The Physiology of the Newborn Infant*. 3rd ed. Springfield, Ill., Charles C Thomas, 1959.

Standards and Recommendations for Hospital Care for Newborn Infants, Full-Term and Premature. Evanston, Ill., American Academy of Pediatrics, Committee on Fetus and Newborn.

Takeuchi, A., and Benirschke, K.: Renal Venous Thrombosis of the Newborn and Its Relation to Maternal Diabetes. Report of 16 Cases. *Biol. Neonat.*, 3:237, 1961.

Torpin, R.: Amniochorionic Mesoblastic Fibrous Strings and Amniotic Bands: Associated Constricting Fetal Malformations or Fetal Death. *Am. J. Obst. & Gynec.*, 91:65, 1965.

Van Leeuwen, G., Behringer, B., and Glenn, L.: Single Umbilical Artery. *J. Pediat.*, 71:103, 1966.

Wheeler, W. O., and Wainerman, B.: The Treatment and Prevention of Epidemic Infantile Diarrhea Due to E. Coli 0-111 by the Use of Chloramphenicol and Neomycin. *Pediatrics*, 14:357, 1954.

Wilson, M. G., and Mikity, V. G.: A New Form of Respiratory Disease in Premature Infants. *Am. J. Dis. Child.*, 99:489, 1960.

Wood, J. L.: Plethora in the Newborn Infant Associated with Cyanosis and Convulsions. *J. Pediat.*, 54:143, 1959.

8.   Sudden Unexpected Death in Infancy

Sudden and unexpected death during early infancy in apparently healthy infants which is not explained by careful postmortem studies has become a serious pediatric problem. Comparatively recently it was thought that painstaking postmortem examinations would provide the explanation for the majority of such deaths, and it was postulated that acute pulmonary infection would be found to be the most frequent cause. Subsequent experience has not supported this assumption. At present only 15 to 20 per cent of such deaths are explained at necropsy. Among the identified causes of such deaths are endocardial fibroelastosis, viral myocarditis and septicemia. Whether most of the sudden unexpected deaths are due to a common cause or to a common combination of factors is not known, but such possibilities have been postulated.

Sudden unexplained deaths occur most often in infants 2 to 4 months of age, seldom in the first or after the sixth month of life, and more often in males than in females. Many more infants die suddenly and unexpectedly between midnight and 9:00 a.m., than during the remainder of the day, and during the colder months of the year than at other times.

There are no reliable data to document the frequency of such deaths in infants for any country as a whole, but there are some data from several large urban areas of the United States indicating that the incidence may be as high as 2 or 3 deaths per thousand live births.

Such deaths occur much more often among the impoverished than among the well-to-do, with a disproportionately high frequency in the slums and depressed areas of cities. The smaller the infant at birth, the greater is the probability of sudden unexpected death. In Steele's series 16.2 per cent of affected babies weighed less than 2500 gm. at birth at a time and in a locale where only 6.8 per cent of all live-born infants had weighed less than 2500 gm. One in approximately every 70 sudden deaths is a recurrence within a family.

At necropsy the majority of infants who have died suddenly and unexpectedly appear to be well developed and well nourished. The thymus often appears large, but its weight is within the limits of the accepted normal range. It would appear that the thymus has simply not been depleted by prolonged illness or by undernutrition. Petechiae are often present in the thymus, the pleura and the epicardium; and occasionally in the brain and meninges.

In about half of the infants studied, histologic sections of the larynx reveal a moderate degree of subacute inflammation, but rarely, if ever, does this process seem sufficient to account for death. The lungs are expanded and may be moderately congested; histologic sections often reveal some edema and occasional scattered areas of hemorrhage. The adrenals are small and rather flat, but this pattern may be normal for the age.

One school of thought proposes that most of these presently unexplained deaths will eventually be found to be due to a common pathogenetic mechanism; certain aspects such as the predictable pathologic changes support this contention. Others doubt whether there is a common cause, but rather think that there are many causes, not yet discovered, such as overwhelming infection with as yet unrecognized viruses, unknown inborn errors of metabolism, or disorders of neurologic mechanisms such as might lead to laryngospasm or failure of cardiac conduction.

There is no evidence that mechanical suffocation, either by a large thymus or by bed clothing, accounts for these deaths. Overwhelming bacterial sepsis has not been demonstrated to play a role in more than about 3 per cent of instances, and bacterial pneumonias may account for about the same percentage. The results of attempts to isolate viruses have been inconsistent, and there is as yet no proof that overwhelming viral infection plays an important role. This possibility is under intensive investigation.

There is no evidence that hypogammaglobulinemia or dysgammaglobulinemia is responsible for these deaths. Hypersensitivity to cow's milk has been suggested as a cause. It was postulated that the susceptible infant might become reactive to the proteins in cow's milk during the first few months of life. Milk regurgitated from the gastric contents and aspirated while sleeping might then lead to sudden death from anaphylaxis. Subsequent studies have cast doubt on the importance of such a mechanism.

Because of the suddenness of the death and the paucity of findings at autopsy, the possibility has been considered that some rapidly developing malfunction of a basic physiologic mechanism such as of the respiratory or cardiac system might be at fault. It has been suggested, for example, that the so-called cardio-auditory syndrome is responsible for at least some of these deaths. Patients with this syndrome have congenital perceptive deafness with syncopal attacks and characteristic electrocardiographic abnormalities. It has been proposed that the irregularity of the heart rate might eventuate in cessation of its beat.

Another neural mechanism to which interest has been directed is the so-called diving reflex, the physiologic adjustment of seals and pearl divers during submersion, in which apnea and bradycardia are associated with other cardiovascular adjustments. Excessive stimulation of the limbic area of the brain has been shown to result in similar bradycardia and apnea, and fear or anxiety can trigger the reflex without contact with water. Arrhythmias are known to accompany the "diving reflex" or limbic stimulation. It has been suggested that an infant who has rolled his face into a pillow might develop an arrhythmia eventuating in ventricular fibrillation as a result of this so-called diving reflex.

Another suggestion is that the critical event may be laryngospasm at the end of expiration. No mechanism leading up to a fatal spasm has been elucidated, however, nor has the spasm itself been confirmed. There is no evidence that absence of parathyroid function or any other form of tetany is an important cause of sudden death.

When adequate postmortem examination yields no explanation for sudden and unexpected death, it is important that the obscure nature and the relative frequency of this entity be fully conveyed to the family. They should be confidently reassured that a careful evaluation leaves no reason for them to feel that they could in any way have been responsible, by either commission or omission, for the infant's death. In particular, they should be told that neither suffocation nor infection is an explanation and that there is nothing to suggest that greater vigilance on their part would in any way have prevented the event.

M. A. VALDÉS-DAPENA

REFERENCES

Peterson, D. R.: Sudden Unexpected Death in Infants. An Epidemiologic Study. *Am. J. Epid.,* 84:478, 1966.

Steele, R., Kraus, A. S., and Langworth, J. T.: Sudden Unexpected Death in Infancy in Ontario. I. Methodology and Findings Related to the Host. II. Findings Regarding Season, Clustering of Deaths on Specific Days and Weather. *Canad. J. Pub. Health,* 58:359, 1967.

Valdés-Dapena, M. A.: Sudden and Unexpected Death in Infancy: A Review of the World Literature 1954-1966. *Pediatrics,* 39:123, 1967.

Wedgwood, R. J., and Bendit, E. P.: Sudden Death in Infants. Proceedings of the Conference on Causes of Sudden Death in Infants, Seattle, Wash., Sept. 9 and 10, 1963.

9. Inborn Errors of Metabolism
(The Enzymopathies)

Many disorders have their origin in mutational events which alter the genetic constitution of an individual and disrupt normal function. The number of human hereditary biochemical disorders, named "inborn errors of metabolism" by Garrod at the turn of the century, has grown from the four originally described by him into hundreds. New ones are being discovered each year.

Modern biochemical genetics has provided a conceptual scheme to describe how genetic information is translated into the synthesis of proteins with specific metabolic or structural properties. Within the nucleus of each cell, genetic information resides in the chromosomes, encoded in deoxyribonucleic acid (DNA) molecules. The code is made up of combinations of 2 purine and 2 pyrimidine bases arranged on the DNA helix. The genetic information contained in DNA is transcribed to messenger ribonucleic acid (m-RNA), which is free to leave the nucleus. Proteins are synthesized from individual amino acids in the cytoplasm, where the information carried by the m-RNA is translated into the linear array of amino acids comprising the polypeptide chain.

A mutation may alter the structure of a protein by introducing an error into the sequence of amino acids through substitution of one amino acid for another. If the region of substitution is necessary for function, then, depending on the nature of the alteration, part or all of the normal function of this protein may be lost. Alternatively, an amino acid substitution may render the protein very labile, and it may be destroyed as rapidly as it is synthesized. Another mutation might affect the different set of genes which control the rate of synthesis of a normally structured protein. Such a mutation can result either in lowered rate of synthesis of an enzyme or in its complete lack. In drug-induced hemolytic anemia, for example, erythrocyte glucose-6-phosphate dehydrogenase is synthesized, but it is altered structurally so that it cannot carry out its normal function, whereas, in analbuminemia, plasma albumin is either not synthesized at all or is made in an altered and unstable form.

Much of what is known of human biochemical genetics has been garnered from studies of the hemoglobin molecule and the genetic factors which determine its chemical and physical properties. Information so obtained has been applied to the study of many other proteins and of the disease processes caused by their malfunction. Hemoglobin serves as a model substance because, unlike most enzymes, it is freely obtainable and can be separated from other protein contaminants with ease. Certain changes in structure are revealed by alteration of electrophoretic mobility, and other analytic techniques can reveal the exact amino acid sequence of the polypeptide chain.

The predominant normal hemoglobin is hemoglobin A, which consists of 2 pairs of polypeptide chains (alpha and beta). Alpha and beta chains, as well as the less common delta and gamma chains (p. 1040), differ only slightly in the composition or sequential arrangement of their component amino acids. The composition of each polypeptide chain is under genetic control, and the sequential arrangement of the amino acids corresponds to the order of bases on the deoxyribonucleic acid molecule.

Studies of many varieties of hemoglobin, some of which are discussed elsewhere (p. 1040), indicate that approximately half of the alpha chains and half of the beta chains are synthesized under the control of a gene obtained from the father, and the other half by a gene obtained from the mother. If a gene for an abnormal hemoglobin is obtained from only one parent, then only half of the hemoglobin molecules will be affected (heterozygous). For all the hemoglobin to be affected (homozygous), the same gene must be obtained from each parent. It is essential to recognize, however, that more than one defect can occur within the same polypeptide chain; there can be at least as many defects as there are positions for amino acids in the molecule. Within the same chain, different defects may occur at the same amino acid locus. Thus within the beta chain of hemoglobin at a point which is normally occupied by glutamic acid, one mutation results in its replacement by valine (hemoglobin S), and another mutation results in replacement by lysine (hemoglobin C). Thus if parents carry different abnormal genes at the same locus, e.g. one parent hemoglobin S, the other hemoglobin C, then all the hemoglobin in the offspring inheriting each parent's abnormal gene will be abnormal. Approximately half of this child's hemoglobin will be hemoglobin S, and the other half, hemoglobin C (so-called hemoglobin SC disease).

A genetic defect in hemoglobin structure may or may not have clinical significance, depending on how it affects the ability of the hemoglobin molecule to function. As indicated, each mutation of a gene manifests itself as a chemically unique structure. In the case of sickle cell hemoglobin (hemoglobin S), the heterozygote (hemoglobin A plus hemoglobin S) is identified clinically as having the sickle cell trait, but has little or no evidence of any disorder related to it, whereas the homozygote (all hemoglobin S) has sickle cell disease and is seriously affected. In certain types of methemoglobinemia, on the other hand, the heterozygote (hemoglobin A plus hemoglobin M) has a significant clinical disorder. At the other extreme of the spectrum of hemoglobinopathies, alterations in hemoglobin structure are not reflected in functional disorders. This, for example, is the case in a homozygote for hemoglobin G, in which all hemoglobin is made up of this abnormal variety.

Although the terms "recessive" and "dominant," as well as "incompletely recessive," "incompletely dominant," "penetrance" and "expressivity," describe the patterns of inheritance (see p. 318), it should be understood that alteration of a structural gene always leads to abnormal protein formation, even in the heterozygote without evidence of clinical disorder.

The mutations just described predominantly affect the amino acid composition of protein; other mutations alter the rate at which protein will be synthesized. Mutations of the second type may be responsible for the thalassemias (p. 1058). In these anemias there may be decreased synthesis of either alpha or beta chains of hemoglobin A. In the latter instance, synthesis of fetal hemoglobin (2 alpha plus 2 gamma chains) and hemoglobin A_2 (2 alpha plus 2 delta chains) may continue; when synthesis of the alpha chain is not possible, hemoglobin molecules with only beta chains (4 beta, hemoglobin H) or only gamma chains (4 gamma, Bart's hemoglobin) may appear.

Although hemoglobin has been used as a model for the discussion of genic action, the principles apply to all proteins, including enzymes. In evaluating enzyme function, the biochemist measures only the activity of the enzyme. For most enzymatic defects it is not known whether the enzyme is altered in such a way as to have no activity, or is not synthesized in normal quantities.

Other generalizations are germane to a discussion of hereditary defects. It should be appreciated that the absence of activity of a specific enzyme may have one or more of several effects:

1. The end-product is not made. If this is a substance essential to life, the result is lethal.

2. Precursor substances may accumulate. If they are toxic, specific dysfunction results.

3. Minor metabolic pathways may become manifest or more heavily utilized, and normal metabolites may accumulate or be excreted in unusual quantities.

Some enzyme functions may not be fully developed at birth, but mature later, e.g. glucuronide transferase (p. 831). These are not to be confused with true enzymopathies in which function will never develop, e.g. Crigler-Najjar disease (p. 832).

These new tools of modern biochemistry have permitted some disorders, such as the abnormal accumulation of glycogen in glycogen storage disease, once thought to be due to the absence of a single enzyme (glucose-6-phosphatase), to be resolved into a number of different clinical entities, each associated with dysfunction of a different enzyme. All of the involved enzymes, however, have roles in glycogen and glucose metabolism.

Even in those disorders in which only one enzyme is involved there is evidence that different mutations result in different degrees of enzyme activity which in turn result in a spectrum of phenotypic effects. As in the case of the hemoglobinopathies, the possibility exists that for a given enzyme protein at least as many different abnormalities may exist as there are amino acids in the protein chain. Although this number is large, as in the case of the hemoglobinopathies, only mutations which affect enzyme activity sufficiently to produce clinical disease need concern us.

Enzymopathies may have their important clinical effects in almost any body system and be manifest in most aspects of pediatric medicine. A listing of the various inborn errors of metabolism appears in Table 9-1. Discussions of the following defects will be found in other chapters of this book where the clinical considerations are germane to the system being discussed: the hemoglobinopathies (p. 1056), disorders of clotting mechanisms (p. 1079), the lipidoses (p. 453), disorders of pigment metabolism (p. 461), the mucopolysaccharidoses (p. 1337), defects of cellular transport (p. 1146), defects of hormone synthesis (p. 1212), and defects of immunoglobulin synthesis (p. 471). In general, the disorders listed in Table 9-1 and not followed by page references will be discussed in this chapter; these are mainly the disorders associated with defects of metabolism of amino acids, carbohydrates, purines and pyrimidine, and other disorders not easily categorized. Attention is given only to those which have clinical significance.

TABLE 9-1. Inborn Errors of Metabolism*

I. **Defects of protein metabolism**
  A. Defects in plasma proteins*
   1. Factors associated with clotting of blood* (11 types) (p. 1082)
   2. Immunoproteins (> 6 types) (p. 483)
   3. Other plasma proteins*
    a. Analbuminemia**
    b. Haptoglobin deficiency
    c. Ceruloplasmin deficiency (Wilson's disease) (cf. XII, A, 1)
    d. Abeta-lipoproteinemia (acanthocytosis) (cf. VII, C, 1)
    e. Analpha-lipoproteinemia (Tangier disease) (cf. VII, C, 2)
    f. Absence of transferrin (cf. XII, B, 2)
    g. Deficiencies of complement factors
     (1) C'-l esterase inhibitor (angioneurotic edema)
     (2) Other complement factors (p. 474)
    h. Alpha-trypsin inhibitor (pulmonary emphysema)
    i. Thyroid-binding globulin (p. 1188)
    j. Leukocyte-opsonizing factor
  B. Defects of enzymes found in plasma
   1. Pseudocholinesterase
    a. Deficiency (3 types)
    b. Increased activity
   2. Hypophosphatasia (p. 1371)
   3. Lecithin-cholesterol acyltransferase deficiency (cf. VII, B)
   4. Carnosinase deficiency (cf. IV, J, 4)
  C. Defects of proteins of other tissues
   1. Duchenne's muscular dystrophy (p. 1326)
   2. DNA-repairing enzymes (xeroderma pigmentosum)
   3. Proteins in pancreas
    a. Lipase deficiency
    b. Trypsinogen deficiency
    c. Amylase deficiency
  D. Defects in hemoglobin*
   1. Amino acid substitutions (sickle cell anemia and at least 64 others) (p. 1056)
   2. Defects of total synthesis (alpha and beta thalassemias) (p. 1058)
   3. Primary familial erythrocytosis
II. **Defects in erythrocyte metabolism**
  A. Hereditary methemoglobinemia (p. 468)
   1. Methemoglobin reductase (2 types)
   2. Hemoglobin M diseases (many types)
  B. Drug-induced hemolytic anemia (p. 1055)
   1. Glucose-6-phosphate dehydrogenase

  C. Hereditary hemolytic anemias (p. 1054)
   1. Glucose-6-phosphate dehydrogenase
   2. 6-Phosphogluconate dehydrogenase
   3. Hexokinase
   4. Glucose phosphate isomerase
   5. Aldolase
   6. Triosephosphate isomerase
   7. Phosphoglyceric acid kinase
   8. 2, 3-Diphosphoglyceric acid mutase
   9. Pyruvic acid kinase
   10. Glutathione reductase
   11. Glutathione peroxidase
   12. Glutathione synthetase
   13. Adenosine triphosphatase
  D. Other erythrocyte enzymes
   1. Catalase (acatalasia) (2 types)
   2. True cholinesterase
   3. Elevated ATP production
   4. Carbonic anhydrase deficiency
   5. Nicotinamide adenine dinucleotide nucleosidase deficiency
   6. Glutathione reductase (increased activity – gout)
III. **Defects in other formed elements of blood*** (p. 1085)
  A. Platelet defects (several thrombocytopathies and thrombocytasthenias involving metabolic or membrane defects)
  B. Granulocyte defects (defective oxidation following phagocytosis) (chronic granulomatous disease)
IV. **Defects of amino acid metabolism**
  A. Phenylalanine
   1. Phenylketonuria (PKU)
    a. Phenylalanine hydroxylase (absent, deficient or delayed maturation)
   2. Phenylalaninemia
    a. Phenylalanine hydroxylase (deficient)
    b. Phenylalanine transaminase (absent, deficient or delayed maturation)
    c. p-Hydroxyphenylpyruvic acid oxidase (delayed maturation)
  B. Tyrosine
   1. p-Hydroxyphenylpyruvic acid oxidase
    a. Delayed maturation
    b. Tyrosinosis (Medes)
    c. Tyrosinosis (Sakai)
   2. Tyrosine transaminase
    a. Tyrosinemia
   3. Albinism (tyrosinase) (3 types) (cf. VIII, E, 1)

---

*Disorders followed by an asterisk (*) are those in which determination of enzyme activity or specific protein content of blood leads directly to diagnosis or in which the underlying defect is in some other tissue, but demonstrable also in erythrocytes or leukocytes.
**Polymorphisms without clinical significance such as bisalbuminemia or the multiple forms of haptoglobin are not listed separately.

TABLE 9-1 *(Continued)*

4. Alcaptonuria (homogentisic acid oxidase)
5. Goitrous cretinism (p. 1192)
C. Methionine
   1. Methioninemia
   2. Methionine malabsorption
   3. Homocystinemia (2 types)
   4. Cystathioninemia
D. Cysteine
   1. Cystinuria (3 types)
   2. Cystinosis* (p. 1367)
   3. Sulfite oxidase deficiency
   4. β-Mercaptolactate cysteinuria
E. Tryptophan
   1. Hartnup disease (p. 426) (cf. IX, C, 1)
   2. Tryptophanemia (cf. IX, C, 2)
   3. Kynureninuria
   4. Kynureninase defects
     a. Hydroxykynureninuria
     b. Pyridoxine dependency (xanthinuria)
   5. Indicanuria (blue diaper syndrome)
   6. Hydrindicuria
F. Valine, leucine, isoleucine
   1. Maple syrup urine disease* (2 types)
   2. Valinemia*
   3. Isovaleric acidemia*
   4. Leucine-induced hypoglycemia (p. 1168)
G. Proline
   1. Prolinuria
   2. Prolinemia (2 types)
   3. Hydroxyprolinemia
   4. Glycylprolinuria
H. Glycine
   1. Glycinemia* (4 types)
   2. Sarcosinemia
   3. Glycinuria
   4. Glucoglycinuria
   5. Primary oxaluria and oxalosis
     a. L-Glyceric aciduria
     b. Glycolic aciduria
I. Urea cycle
   1. Hyperammoniemia (2 types)
   2. Citrullinemia
   3. Argininosuccinic acidemia*
J. Histidine
   1. Histidinemia (3 types)
   2. Histidine and folic acid (cf. IX, B)
   3. Imidazole aciduria
   4. Carnosinemia (cf. I, B, 4)
K. Alanine
   1. Alaninemia
L. Beta amino acids
   1. β-Alaninemia
   2. β-Aminoisobutyric aciduria
M. Lysine
   1. Lysinemia (2 types)
   2. Saccharopinemia
   3. Lysine intolerance
V. **Defects of carbohydrate metabolism**
A. Defects in absorption of carbohydrate (p. 811)
   1. Lactose
     a. Lactosuria (lactose intolerance)

     b. Malabsorption of lactose (alactasia)
     c. Malabsorption of glucose and galactose
   2. Malabsorption of sucrose and isomaltose
   3. Renal glycosuria
B. Defective mucopolysaccharide metabolism
   (p. 1337)
   1. Hurler's disease
   2. Hunter's disease
   3. Sanfilippo's disease
   4. Morquio's disease
   5. Scheie's disease
   6. Maroteaux-Lamy disease
   7. Farber's disease (cf. VII, E, 10)
   8. Marfan's syndrome
   9. Fucosidosis (cf. V, D, 2)
   10. Mannosidosis (cf. V, D, 3)
   11. Other unclassified types
C. Defects of monosaccharide metabolism
   1. Diabetes mellitus (p. 1155)
   2. Scurvy
   3. Essential benign pentosuria (xylulosuria)
   4. Essential benign fructosuria (kinase defect)
   5. Fructose intolerance (aldolase defect)
     (p. 1166)
   6. Galactosemia* (uridyltransferase defect)
     (3 types)
   7. Galactosemia* (galactokinase defect)
     (galactose diabetes)
D. Miscellaneous aspects of carbohydrate
   metabolism
   1. Blood group substances*
     a. N-acetylgalactosamine transferase
       (absent in non-A group)
     b. Galactose transferase (absent in non-B group)
     c. Fucose transferase (absent in non-secretors)
   2. Fucosidosis (cf. V, B, 9)
   3. Mannosidosis (cf. V, B, 10)
   4. Aspartylglycosaminuria
   5. Methylmalonic acidemia* (2 types)
   6. Leigh's encephalomyelopathy (pyruvic
     acid carboxylase defect)
   7. Sialic acidemia
E. The glycogenoses: disorders of glycogen
   metabolism (glycogen storage disease)
   1. Involving principally liver
     a. Types Ia and Ib (von Gierke)
       (hepatorenal)
     b. Types IIIa, IIIb and IIId* (Forbes)
       (Cori) (limit dextrinosis)
     c. Type IV* (Andersen) (amylopectinosis)
     d. Type VI* (Hers) (liver phosphorylase
       or phosphorylase kinase)
     e. Type O (glycogen synthetase deficiency)
   2. Involving principally heart
     a. Type IIa* (Pompe)
   3. With muscular involvement
     a. Type IIb* (Pompe)
     b. Types IIIa, IIIc and IIId* (limit
       dextrinosis)

c. Type V (McArdle)
d. Type VIII* (phosphofructokinase deficiency)
e. Type VIII (phosphoglucomutase deficiency)

VI. **Defects of pyrimidine and purine metabolism**
  A. Pyrimidines
    1. Orotic aciduria*
  B. Purines
    1. Xanthinuria
    2. Hyperuricemia* (gout) (3 types)
    3. Lesch-Nyhan disease* (hypoxanthine-guanine phosphoribosyl transferase)
    4. Pseudouridinuria

VII. **Defects of lipid metabolism**
  A. The hyperlipoproteinemias (5 types) (p. 458)
  B. Lecithin-cholesterol acyltransferase deficiency (cf. I, B, 3)
  C. The hypolipoproteinemias
    1. Abeta-lipoproteinemia (acanthocytosis) (cf. I, A, 3, d)
    2. Analpha-lipoproteinemia (Tangier disease) (cf. I, A, 3, e)
  D. Steroid metabolism
    1. Congenital adrenal hyperplasia (p. 1212)
      a. Defect of 11-hydroxylase
      b. Defect of 21-hydroxylase
      c. Defect of 3-beta-hydroxydehydrogenase
    2. Defect of 17-hydroxylase (p. 1219)
    3. Selective defects of aldosterone synthesis (p. 1208)
      a. Defect of 18-hydroxylase
      b. Defect of 18-OH-corticosterone dehydrogenase
  E. The lipidoses (p. 453)
    1. Gaucher's disease* (cerebroside lipidosis) (3 types)
    2. Niemann-Pick disease* (sphingomyelin lipidosis) (2 types)
    3. Tay-Sachs disease* (ganglioside lipidosis) (3 types)
    4. Norman's disease (generalized gangliosidosis) (β-galactosidase defect)
    5. Metachromatic leukodystrophy* (sulfatide lipidosis)
    6. Krabbe's disease (globoid leukodystrophy) (sulfate transferase defect)
    7. Wolman's disease
    8. Refsum's disease (phytanic acid lipidosis)
    9. Fabry's disease (glycolipid lipidosis)
    10. Farber's disease (lipogranulomatosis) (cf. V, B, 7)
    11. Fucosidosis (absent α-fucosidase) (cf. V, D, 2)
    12. Mannosidosis (cf. V, D, 3)
  F. Miscellaneous
    1. Sweaty-feet syndrome (butyric and hexanoic acidemia)

VIII. **Defects of pigment metabolism**
  A. Porphyrin metabolism (p. 461)
    1. Congenital erythropoietic porphyria

2. Intermittent acute porphyria
3. Porphyria variegata
4. Erythropoietic protoporphyria
5. Erythropoietic coproporphyria
  B. Methemoglobinemias (p. 468)
    1. Methemoglobin reductase*
    2. Hemoglobin M disease* (many types)
  C. Primary hemochromatosis (p. 469)
  D. Glucuronide conjugation (p. 831)
    1. Crigler-Najjar disease
    2. Dubin-Johnson disease
    3. Gilbert's disease
    4. Rotor's syndrome
  E. Melanin metabolism
    1. Albinism (cf. IV, B, 3)
    2. Chediak-Higashi syndrome (p. 1074)
    3. Waardenburg's syndrome (p. 1435)

IX. **Defects of vitamin metabolism**
  A. Ascorbic acid (scurvy)
  B. Folic acid
    1. Formiminotransferase defect*
    2. Cyclohydrolase defect*
    3. N^5-methyltransferase defects*
  C. Niacin
    1. Hartnup disease (p. 426) (cf. IV, E, 1)
    2. Tryptophanemia (cf. IV, E, 2)
    3. 3-Hydroxykynureninuria

X. **Primary defects of renal tubular transport mechanism**
  Many different disorders, e.g. nephrogenic diabetes insipidus, renal glycosuria, Fanconi's syndrome (p. 1146)

XI. **Genetic defects resulting in intestinal malabsorption**
  A. Carbohydrates (cf. V, A)
  B. Amino acids (cf. IV, C, 1; D, 1; E, 1; J, 3)
  C. Lipids (cf. VII, c)
  D. Proteins
    1. Cystic fibrosis (p. 856)
    2. Pancreatic enzyme defects (cf. I, C, 3)
    3. Gluten-induced enteropathy (p. 807)

XII. **Defects involving mineral metabolism**
  A. Copper
    1. Wilson's disease (cf. I, A, 3, c)
  B. Iron
    1. Hemochromatosis (p. 469)
    2. Absence of transferrin* (cf. I, A, 3, f)
  C. Potassium
    1. Periodic paralysis (2 types) (p. 1324)
  D. Phosphorus
    1. Hypophosphatemic-resistant rickets (p. 1364)
  E. Iodine
    1. Defects of iodine transport (p. 1192)
    2. Defects of thyroid hormone formation (4 types) (p. 1192)

XIII. **Defects about which the biochemical aberration is unknown**
  Many different disorders, e.g. achondroplasia, Ehlers-Danlos disease and osteogenesis imperfecta

DEFECTS OF PROTEIN METABOLISM

Defects in the immunoproteins and in the proteins involved in the clotting of blood are discussed elsewhere (pp. 483 and 1082), respectively.

In not describing genetic alterations without clinical significance we have omitted consideration of the subject of polymorphism. As an example of this phenomenon the various forms of *bisalbuminemia* may be given. Although most persons produce only one form of serum albumin, which migrates electrophoretically as a single band, some persons demonstrate 2 albumin bands, one normal, and, depending on the genetic situation, one either faster or slower than normal. Such persons are heterozygous for an amino acid substitution involving albumin. Persons homozygous for a variant form of albumin have also been described.

Polymorphic variation probably occurs for all proteins and has been extensively studied in erythrocyte acid phosphatase, haptoglobin, transferrin and beta-lipoprotein. These variations are of more interest to the population geneticist than to the clinician.

Defects in Plasma Proteins

Analbuminemia. Plasma albumin has 2 main functions: (1) to maintain the oncotic pressure of blood and (2) to serve as a vehicle for the transport of many normal blood constituents, such as free fatty acids. A few persons have been observed in whom no circulating albumin could be demonstrated. Some were asymptomatic; others exhibited only slight edema. The first cases reported were siblings whose parents were double second cousins, suggesting that the disorder is genetic in nature. Periodic administrations of albumin result in disappearance of edema, but usually no treatment is necessary.

It may be speculated that lack of symptoms in analbuminemia depends on lifelong compensations in fluid dynamics which patients with such disorders as nephrosis or protein-losing enteropathy are unable to make in the face of their acutely lowered oncotic pressure.

Haptoglobin Deficiency. Haptoglobin is an alpha-2-globulin which binds free hemoglobin. There are numerous phenotypic variations (polymorphism) in the types of haptoglobins among normal persons. These are demonstrable by starch gel electrophoresis and are under genetic control. In the presence of severe hemolytic anemia, haptoglobin levels may be greatly decreased or absent. Healthy persons also have been found who have no demonstrable circulating haptoglobin, on a genetic basis, without any apparent ill effects.

Ceruloplasmin Deficiency (Wilson's Disease) (see p. 842). Ceruloplasmin, a blue-colored alpha-2-globulin containing 8 copper atoms per molecule, constitutes 0.5 per cent of the total plasma proteins. The average normal serum concentration is 25 mg. per 100 ml. (range, 16 to 33 mg.). Low levels are found in newborn infants and in patients with active nephrosis, in whom ceruloplasmin is lost in the urine. Wilson's disease, or hepatolenticular degeneration, is a hereditary disorder transmitted by an autosomal recessive gene, in which low serum levels of ceruloplasmin are characteristic; they average 5 mg. per 100 ml. (range, 0 to 14 mg.). Several unequivocal cases, however, have been observed with normal levels of ceruloplasmin. It is not certain whether the structure of the ceruloplasmin found in blood of affected subjects is similar to that of normal persons. Although at one time it appeared likely that the primary genetic defect in Wilson's disease was in the synthesis of ceruloplasmin, this is no longer certain. The ability of other proteins to bind copper may be increased, producing an abnormal pattern of copper metabolism.

Increased amounts of copper are absorbed from the intestinal tract and are present in tissue and urine, though levels in blood are typically decreased. Injury to parenchymatous organs (kidney, liver and brain), whether anatomic or functional, seems related to elevated concentrations of copper. The presence of the pathognomonic eye sign, Kayser-Fleischer rings, is also secondary to copper deposition.

Renal copper intoxication is presumably the cause of increased excretion of amino acids, uric acid, polypeptides, glucose and phosphate in urine. The disorder can be detected while it is still latent by ascertainment of the ceruloplasmin level, and therapy can be initiated with drugs that lower the body content of copper.

Abeta-Lipoproteinemia (Acanthocytosis). Abeta-lipoproteinemia (see pp. 812, 1302), a defect in synthesis of beta-lipoprotein, is characterized by bizarrely shaped erythrocytes with thornlike projections (acanthocytes) and steatorrhea in infancy, followed by the development of ataxic neuropathy in childhood and retinitis pigmentosa in early adulthood. Characteristic pathologic changes have been observed in the intestinal mucosa; the columnar epithelium is filled with globules containing lipids. Plasma cholesterol, phospholipid and triglyceride levels are sharply reduced. Beta-lipoprotein and chylomicra are absent. The disorder is transmitted in an autosomal recessive manner.

Analpha-Lipoproteinemia (Tangier Disease). Tangier disease is a rare congenital metabolic defect first described in siblings residing on Tangier Island in Chesapeake Bay. This disorder is characterized by enlarged tonsils which have a distinctive orange color. Other clinical manifestations may include enlargement of the liver, spleen and lymph nodes.

Although plasma levels of cholesterol and phospholipids are moderately reduced, there is storage of large amounts of cholesterol esters in reticuloendothelial tissues, including the tonsils.

The basic defect is absence in serum of alpha-lipoprotein (high-density lipoprotein). The disease is inherited in an autosomal recessive manner. Heterozygotes have about half the normal concentrations of high-density lipoprotein, but are asymptomatic.

Absence of Transferrin. Transferrin, or siderophilin, is a plasma protein of molecular weight 90,000, with the electrophoretic mobility of a beta-2 globulin. It is assumed that it has a prominent role in the transport of iron. In the only recorded instance of a congenital absence of transferrin, anemia sufficiently severe to require multiple transfusions was present at birth. Iron was absorbed from the intestinal tract and transported to the tissues. The patient, a girl, was physically retarded and had hepatomegaly and splenomegaly. The anemia did not respond to any of the antianemic agents used. Her erythrocytes were hypochromic, and the marrow contained many immature erythroblasts. Liver biopsy revealed cirrhosis and siderosis. Immunochemical studies revealed complete absence of transferrin. Antibodies to transferrin developed after multiple transfusions. Sudden death at 7 years of age was attributed to hemosiderosis. The disease may be inherited in an autosomal recessive manner; both parents had lower than normal amounts of transferrin.

C'-l Esterase Inhibitor. Reduced levels of C'-l esterase inhibitor, an alpha globulin, are associated with hereditary angioneurotic edema (giant urticaria). The protein is an inhibitor of the esterase activity of the complement component designated C'-l. The esterase rises to high concentrations during an attack and is thought to be responsible for increased capillary permeability. Prednisolone has been used successfully to treat the condition; during its administration the inhibitor becomes demonstrable and the enzyme activity decreases. Affected persons are apparently heterozygous for the condition and manifest their fluctuating levels of the inhibitor as episodic edema. No homozygous persons with the condition are known.

Alpha$_1$-Antitrypsin Protein Deficiency. Normal persons produce a circulating protein which in in-vitro assays inhibits trypsin activity. This inhibitor is not made by persons who are homozygous for a mutant gene. Many persons without alpha$_1$-antitrypsin protein suffer pulmonary emphysema as they grow older, and significant numbers of patients with emphysema can be shown to lack this protein. It has been speculated that the protein inhibits bacterial proteinase which would otherwise destroy alveolar architecture.

Defects in Plasma Enzymes

Pseudocholinesterase. Pseudocholinesterase is found in plasma, liver and neural tissue; its physiologic function is poorly understood.

Numerous presumably allelic forms of the altered enzyme are known. Some with reduced enzyme activity are characterized by the extent of inhibition by dibucaine or fluoride, whereas a "silent" form has no activity. Homozygotes for each form and mixed heterozygotes are known. About one in 25 persons is heterozygous for one or another of these defects.

The one person in 3000 who is homozygous for one of these genes is asymptomatic. The defect was discovered because the enzyme participates in the destruction of a commonly used muscle relaxant, succinylcholine. In the normal person this drug is rapidly destroyed by pseudocholinesterase and therefore has a transient effect. Persons homozygous for mutant pseudocholinesterase split the drug abnormally slowly or not at all, and apnea results, lasting for hours. Artificial respiration is required, preferably through an endotracheal tube; the period of apnea can be shortened by transfusion with normal plasma.

Another genetic alteration of pseudocholinesterase has been described which leads to *increased* enzyme activity and hence to resistance to the pharmacologic effects of succinylcholine. These observations demonstrate how unusual sensitivity or resistance to the pharmacologic effects of drugs may be predetermined by the genetic constitution of the person. The study of such interactions is known as pharmacogenetics. Other well studied examples are primaquine sensitivity and variation in response to isoniazid.

Lecithin-Cholesterol Acyltransferase Deficiency. Three sisters with corneal opacity, normochromic anemia and proteinuria have been reported who were shown to have the following abnormal blood chemical findings: decreased alpha-lipoprotein and prebeta-lipoprotein, increased concentration of free cholesterol, almost absent esterified cholesterol and, in 2 cases, hyperlipidemia. There were none of the changes of the tonsils seen in analpha-lipoproteinemia. The defect was demonstrated to be an almost complete absence of lecithin-cholesterol acyltransferase, a plasma enzyme which normally esterifies cholesterol; lecithin is the source of the fatty acid.

Defects of Proteins of Other Tissues

Primary Familial Erythrocytosis. The disorder is characterized by increased synthesis of normal hemoglobin and results in high hematocrit values; it may result from an increase of erythropoietic levels or from depression of a hemoglobin controller gene. Although this disorder is usually benign, one of 2 affected siblings has been reported to have pulmonary hypertension and easy fatigability which responded to phlebotomy.

Myoglobin. Myoglobin, a heme protein found in muscle, is responsible for the intracellular transport of oxygen. Two different variants of myoglobin have been identified by starch gel electrophoresis. Changes in amino acid sequence producing myoglobinopathies are analogous to the changes responsible for the hemoglobinopathies. In each of 2 families observed, mother and son were heterozygous for the normal and for the aberrant molecules. Each family had a distinctive aberrant molecule. Neuromuscular diseases were not found in these families.

Spectrophotometric analyses of myoglobin from a number of patients with various neuromuscular diseases have revealed consistent changes in those with the sex-linked form of pseudohypertrophic muscular dystrophy (Duchenne) and the persistence of fetal myoglobin in one patient with facioscapulohumeral dystrophy. Fetal myoglobin has also been found in a patient with recurrent myoglobinuria. The myoglobin isolated from patients with progressive spinal muscular atrophy and the limb-girdle type of muscular atrophy appears to be normal by this method. Females who carry the defect for the Duchenne type of muscular dystrophy have moderately elevated serum levels of creatine phosphokinase and, on biopsy, small areas of dystrophic muscle fibers intermingled with the normal muscle fibers. The genetic form of muscular dystrophy of mice responds therapeutically to the vitamin-like substance coenzyme Q, suggesting that perhaps one of the human forms of the disease may involve a derangement of the synthesis of coenzyme Q.

Xeroderma Pigmentosum. Extreme dermal sensitivity to sunlight or ultraviolet light and the development of skin cancers which metastasize and lead to death are characteristic of this rare recessive disease (p. 1402). It has recently been shown in skin fibroblasts grown in tissue culture that there is a defect of the enzymatic mechanism for repair of DNA. In normal persons the rupture of one strand of DNA in the double helical form by a mutagenic agent such as ultraviolet light is rapidly repaired by a set of specific enzymes which ensure integrity of the genetic material. Persons with xeroderma pigmentosum lack one of these enzymes and are therefore subject not only to skin damage by what would normally be small doses of radiation, but also to the immediate potentially carcinogenic effects of other unrepaired breaks in DNA.

Pancreatic Enzyme Deficiencies. Malabsorption due to pancreatic dysfunction is a cardinal feature of the genetic disease cystic fibrosis (p. 856), but it is fairly certain that the *basic* genetic defect is not an inability to synthesize one or another of the pancreatic enzymes. A number of patients have been described in whom malabsorption appears to result from a specific enzymopathy involving a pancreatic enzyme or proenzyme. They have none of the pulmonary or electrolyte abnormalities of cystic fibrosis. A syndrome with inability to produce trypsin, lipase and amylase in conjunction with hematologic evidence of bone marrow dysfunction has also been described, but in this case, as in cystic fibrosis, pancreatic dysfunction is presumed to be secondary to an underlying defect (p. 868).

Lipase deficiency. Four children have been described with congenital inability to form active pancreatic lipase (two formed none, and two synthesized small amounts). They had malabsorption of lipids and fatty, and sometimes malodorous, stools. Treatment with pancreatin was effective.

Trypsinogen deficiency. A number of children with severe malnutrition, growth failure and hypoproteinemic edema resembling kwashiorkor have been shown to lack the ability to synthesize pancreatic trypsinogen. As a result, chymotrypsin and carboxypeptidase activities are also low, since these enzymes need to be formed from the corresponding proenzymes by trypsin activity. Treatment with a protein hydrolysate diet and exogenous pancreatic enzymes is recommended.

Amylase deficiency. Less defined deficiencies of pancreatic amylase activity have been described in at least 2 children with malabsorption who were shown not to have cystic fibrosis. One of the children also had reduced trypsin activity.

These observations indicate the need to investigate pancreatic function in children with malabsorption in whom the causative factors are unknown; these disorders may be more common than is indicated by the relatively few cases reported.

DEFECTS IN ERYTHROCYTE METABOLISM

Genetic defects are known for many of the enzymes involved in the catabolism of glucose in the erythrocyte, in both the Embden-Myerhof and the pentose phosphate pathways. Many of these disorders present as hemolytic anemias and are discussed elsewhere (p. 1054). In one of these there is a deficiency of the enzyme pyruvate kinase which leads to decreased intracellular concentrations of ATP. Other persons are known who have inherited an increased activity of the same enzyme and have higher than normal ATP concentrations, but with no clinical manifestations. These defects are limited to the red blood cell. There are many other conditions in which more generalized defects may be reflected in red cell abnormalities, e.g. galactosemia.

Erythrocyte acid phosphatase occurs in many genetically determined forms, none of which has any clinical significance. Erythrocyte carbonic anhydrase activity also exhibits genetic polymorphism; a patient with grossly deficient carbonic anhydrase activity is known who also has persistence of fetal hemoglobin, changes in red cell morphology and nonspecific clinical findings. Absence of erythrocyte niacinamide adenine dinucleotide nucleosidase has been demonstrated in the Negro, and a variant of glutathione reductase with increased activity has been shown to be associated with one form of primary gout.

Acatalasia. Catalase is found in most tissues, including the erythrocytes. Persons with decrease of catalase activity in all tissues, to less than 1 per cent of normal, can be detected by the demonstration that blood placed in contact with hydrogen peroxide turns brown and does not produce the oxygen bubbles usually seen. The disorder is heterogeneous; some instances appear to be mutations of the controller gene, whereas others are alterations of the structural gene. In all instances the mode of inheritance is autosomal recessive; the heterozygote can be detected by quantitative catalase assays. Of the 2 main types, the Japanese variants have oral gangrene (*Takahara's disease*), whereas the Swiss variants are asymptomatic. A genetic strain of mice with acatalasia is known; catalase encapsulated in semipermeable membranes has been used successfully in their treatment.

True Cholinesterase. True cholinesterase, an enzyme essential for neural and muscular function, is also found in erythrocytes, where its function is unknown. A brother and a sister have been observed whose erythrocyte cholinesterase activity was decreased to about one third of normal. They appeared to be homozygous for the condition, and their parents and 2 siblings appeared to be heterozygous. There were no associated clinical manifestations. It has been suggested that a deficiency of true cholinesterase at the neuromuscular endplate may account for the defect in myotonia congenita (Thomsen's disease, p. 1323).

DEFECTS IN METABOLISM OF AMINO ACIDS

Disorders are considered here which are produced by defects in enzymes responsible for steps in the catabolism of amino acids, the so-called aminoacidopathies. Disorders of cellular transport of amino acids by intestinal mucosa or renal tubule are discussed elsewhere (e.g. methionine malabsorption, Hartnup disease, cystinuria). Aminoaciduria secondary to some other genetic defect is also considered elsewhere (e.g. Wilson's disease, galactosemia). Aminoacidopathies are characterized by elevated levels in plasma of the involved amino acid, with overflow into the urine of the amino acid or related metabolites.

PHENYLALANINE

Phenylketonuria (PKU). Phenylketonuria (see also p. 115) is a disorder of phenylalanine metabolism resulting from absence of the hepatic enzyme, phenylalanine hydroxylase, which converts phenylalanine to tyrosine. The dietary phenylalanine which is not required for protein synthesis is degraded via the tyrosine pathway (see Fig. 9-1). In phenylketonuria, owing to the enzymatic defect in this pathway, phenylalanine accumulates and is transaminated to phenylpyruvic acid, which can then be converted to other metabolites. These metabolites and the excess phenylalanine are excreted in the urine.

In untreated phenylketonuria, blood levels of phenylalanine rise rapidly in the neonatal period and may reach 60 to 80 mg. per 100 ml. In most patients these levels of phenylalanine lead to urinary excretion of large amounts of phenylpyruvic acid and its metabolites. The peculiar musty or mouselike odor characteristic of untreated patients has been attributed to the presence of phenylacetic acid. The frequency with which persons with this disorder are fair-skinned, blue-eyed blondes is due in part to inhibition of the enzyme responsible for melanin formation (tyrosine) by phenylalanine or its metabolites. The mechanism of the mental retardation, the most important consequence of phenylketonuria,

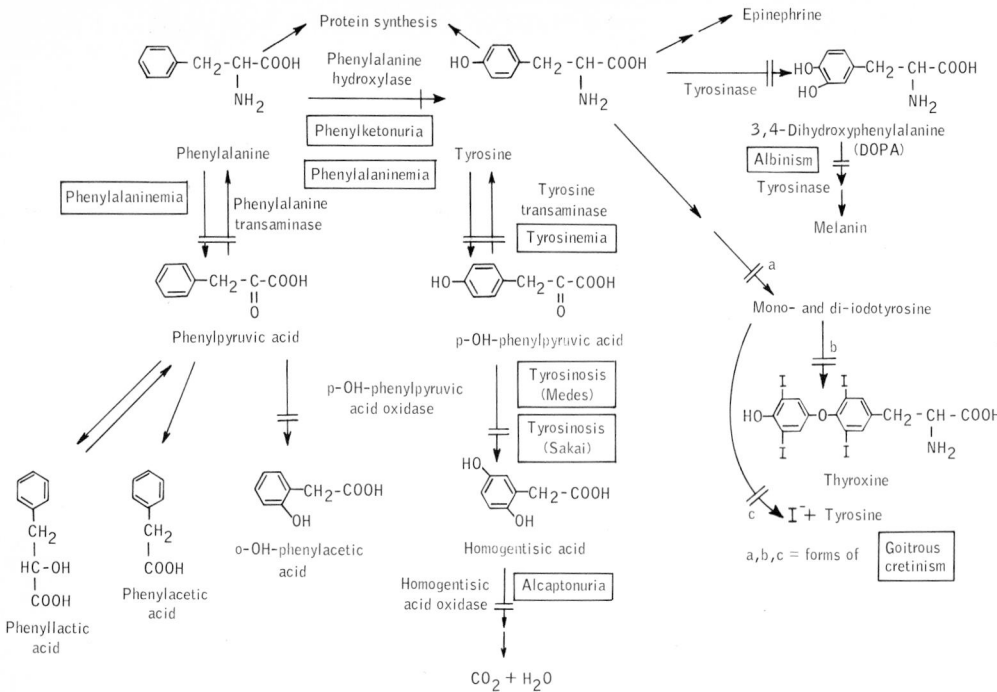

Figure 9-1. Pathways in the metabolism of phenylalanine and tyrosine. In this and subsequent figures the structural formulae and the names of various metabolites are shown. Inborn errors are depicted as bars crossing the reaction arrow or arrows and the name of the associated defect or defects is given within the nearest box. In some figures the name of the enzyme is given in association with the reaction arrow.

is not known. An occasional patient escapes mental retardation for reasons equally obscure. Dietary management of this condition has been more extensive and successful than with any of the other aminoacidopathies and allows for nearly normal mental development in many affected subjects when instituted early in life.

Atypical Phenylketonuria. Whereas classic phenylketonuria is caused by the absence of phenylalanine hydroxylase activity in affected persons, atypical phenylketonuria occurs when the genetic mutation produces an altered phenylalanine hydroxylase with substantially reduced activity. Although such infants are detected by the Guthrie bacterial inhibition assay, levels of phenylalanine in the blood are not as high as in the usual phenylketonuric child. Phenylpyruvic acid is present in urine. Treatment is the same as for the child with classic phenylketonuria.

Other Phenylalaninemias. Occasionally in affected infants the blood levels of phenylalanine are only slightly elevated and are insufficient (less than 15 to 20 mg. per 100 ml.) to result in the excretion of phenylpyruvic acid. These infants presumably also have an altered phenylalanine hydroxylase enzyme, but one which has retained much of its activity. Such infants are detected by screening tests in the neonatal period and usually appear to develop normally without special dietary treatment.

Moderately elevated levels of phenylalanine occur secondarily to the transient tyrosinemia in the newborn infant (see below). When the infant's ability to oxidize tyrosine matures, the elevated levels of tyrosine and phenylalanine return to normal.

Absence of or delayed maturation of the enzyme phenylalanine transaminase can also produce phenylalaninemia if the infant is being fed milk with a high protein content. Such infants cannot produce much phenylpyruvic acid even when their blood levels of phenylalanine approach 30 mg. per 100 ml.; they have normal blood levels when fed milks with the usual content of protein.

Delayed maturation of phenylalanine hydroxylase activity has been observed on a few occasions. It is recommended that infants on a restricted phenylalanine diet be tested periodically (every 3 months) to rule out this possibility. Delayed maturation of phenylalanine transaminase can occur concurrently with classic or atypical phenylketonuria. The absence of phenylpyruvic acid in the urine of such patients presents difficulty in the diagnosis of phenylketonuria. Phenylalanine tolerance tests are rarely of value in the differential diagnosis of the various conditions causing elevated levels of phenylalanine.

TYROSINE

The hepatic enzyme para-hydroxyphenylpyruvic acid oxidase is necessary for the conversion of para-hydroxyphenylpyruvic acid to homogentisic acid (Fig. 9-1). The excretion of tyrosine and para-hydroxyphenylpyruvic, -lactic and -acetic acids in patients with deficiency of this enzyme is referred to as *tyrosyluria*. Deficiency of this pivotal enzyme occurs in a variety of clinical conditions. The deficiency is most often transitory, owing to delayed maturation of the enzyme, and occurs commonly in premature infants and occasionally in full-term infants. The levels of tyrosine in the blood (usually less than 2 mg. per 100 ml.) may be as high as 40 mg. per 100 ml.

A secondary increase in the plasma level of phenylalanine is a common occurrence in neonatal tyrosyluria and must be taken into account in the differential diagnosis of causes for phenylalaninemia.

The defect is promptly corrected by the administration of vitamin C. Since vitamin C is necessary for optimal functioning of para-hydroxyphenylpyruvic acid oxidase, it is not surprising that tyrosyluria occurs in scurvy. Deficiency of the enzyme also may occur because of malnutrition or hepatic disease.

Tyrosinosis (Medes).   In 1932 Medes reported studies of an adult male who had a defect in tyrosine metabolism. No symptoms could be related to the metabolic defect. The presence of para-hydroxyphenylpyruvic acid in urine (greater than 1 gm. per day) and the excretion of other oxidation products of tyrosine indicated that catabolism of tyrosine was blocked at the level of its keto-acid derivative. Medes proposed that the tyrosyluria was due to virtual absence of activity of para-hydroxyphenylpyruvic acid oxidase (see Fig. 9-1). Although this patient also had myasthenia gravis, this was believed to be unrelated to the defect in tyrosine metabolism.

Tyrosinosis (Sakai).   Another clinical disorder associated with a defect in para-hydroxyphenylpyruvic acid oxidase and occurring in infants and children was first described by Sakai.

Clinical manifestations.   The onset is usually between 1 and 6 months of age. Failure to thrive, irritability, fever and hepatomegaly are the most frequent manifestations. Anorexia, vomiting, diarrhea and abdominal distention are common. Bleeding manifestations such as melena, hematemesis, hematuria and ecchymoses occur early and may be serious. Ascites, jaundice, lethargy, coma and death ensue soon thereafter. Some patients appear to survive the acute hepatic decompensation and undergo chronic hepatic and renal disease. In such children hepatoma may be found at autopsy. The urine has the peculiar odor of methionine.

Laboratory data.   Glycosuria may be present. Generalized aminoaciduria and tyrosyluria are constant findings. Plasma amino acids are elevated, particularly tyrosine and methionine, which may be 5 to 10 times normal levels. Tyrosine crystals have been found in bone marrow. Direct and indirect serum bilirubin values are increased; those of alkaline phosphatase and total cholesterol are markedly decreased. Hypoproteinemia and hypoprothrombinemia are common; transaminases (SGOT and SGPT) are only slightly increased. Variable degrees of hypoglycemia and rachitic changes are common. Pathologically, the principal findings are cirrhosis and dilation of the renal tubules.

Although para-hydroxyphenylpyruvic acid oxidase activity is absent in this disorder, it is still not clear whether this is the primary defect. Reasons for doubt are based upon the following considerations: (1) Patients with delayed maturation of this enzyme or with isolated defect of it (Medes type) have no clinical manifestations. (2) Levels of another enzyme in the tyrosine pathway (tyrosine transaminase) are also low in this disorder. (3) Elevated levels of methionine in plasma indicate a defect in enzymes involved in methionine catabolism, and indeed methionine-activating enzyme and cystathionine synthetase levels in liver are low. Whether these findings are caused by a primary defect in amino acid metabolism (tyrosine or methionine) or whether they are secondary to some yet undefined hepatic disorder is unsettled. Nor has it been convincingly demonstrated that all such patients have the same disorder.

The disorder (or disorders) is inherited in an autosomal recessive manner. Early results with diet therapy indicate that the restriction of phenylalanine and tyrosine (and perhaps also of methionine) intake is beneficial.

Tyrosinemia.   Blood levels of tyrosine as high as 70 mg. per 100 ml. and excretion of para-hydroxyphenylpyruvic acid have been reported in a child with congenital malformations and mental retardation. In this instance the defect was shown to be the absence of the soluble fraction of tyrosine transaminase. Mitochondrial tyrosine transaminase is present and produces the para-hydroxyphenylpyruvic acid found in urine. Presumably para-hydroxyphenylpyruvic acid oxidase is inhibited by the high levels of tyrosine.

Albinism.   Generalized albinism (see also p. 1392), one of Garrod's 4 inborn errors of metabolism, is a defect in the formation of the pigment melanin. The albino has normal numbers of pigment-forming cells (melanocytes) in the basal layer of the skin. Owing to the absence of activity of the copper-containing enzyme, tyrosinase, the cells do not form melanin. Recent evidence suggests that the tyrosinase molecule is normal, and a variety of reasons have been proposed to explain its inadequate function.

Albinism occurs in all races, varying in incidence from 0.7 per cent in the San Blas Indians of Panama to one in 100,000 in France. In the United States the rate is approximately one in 20,000. It is transmitted as an autosomal recessive characteristic. Different allelic forms of generalized albinism are presumed to occur, since normal children have been born to a couple both of whom had albinism.

In addition to the extremely fair skin and fine silky hair, albinos have numerous ocular abnormalities. Although traces of pigment may occur on the uveal borders, it is absent from the iris, sclera and fundus, and the iris appears pink or blue. Refractive errors, strabismus, nystagmus and photophobia are common.

Other forms of albinism. Partial albinism is characterized by localized areas of skin and hair devoid of pigment. In some instances a white forelock or a patch of depigmented hair elsewhere may be the sole manifestation. This form of albinism is inherited as a dominant trait.

In albinism limited to the eye, the depigmentation may be limited to the retina or may also involve the iris. Visual acuity is decreased, and there is nystagmus. This defect is sex-linked.

In Waardenburg's syndrome (p. 1435) and in the Chediak-Higashi syndrome (p. 1074) defective pigment metabolism contributes to the clinical pattern, and each must be taken into account in the differential diagnosis of partial albinism. Each of these disorders is genetically transmitted.

Alcaptonuria. Alcaptonuria is a disorder of phenylalanine-tyrosine metabolism characterized by accumulation in the body and excretion in the urine of homogentisic acid (2,5-dihydroxyphenylacetic acid) (see Fig. 9-1) and its oxidation products. This disorder was one of 4 inborn errors of metabolism described by Garrod. More than 600 cases have been recorded. The disorder is transmitted by an autosomal recessive gene. It is estimated that there are about 5 alcaptonuric persons per million population, and that one person in 200 is a heterozygous carrier of the recessive gene. Defective activity of the enzyme, homogentisic acid oxidase, arrests the catabolism of tyrosine, and large amounts of homogentisic acid are excreted in the urine.

Urine from affected patients becomes black on standing, owing to oxidation and polymerization of the homogentisic acid. In infants, staining of the diaper may lead to detection of the defect. The darkness of the stain increases with continued exposure to air, a dried diaper having a pitch-black stain. Although the abnormality is usually noted in infancy, in some instances the dark urine has not been observed until the second or third decade of life. The slow accumulation of the black polymer of homogentisic acid in cartilage and other mesenchymal tissues produces a black discoloration (*alcaptonuric ochronosis*) of the cheeks, nose, sclerae and ears which becomes evident by mid-adult life. Degeneration of pigmented cartilage leads to arthritis in about half of the older patients with alcaptonuria. These changes are sufficiently characteristic to have permitted recognition of alcaptonuria in an ancient Egyptian mummy by radiography. The defect is otherwise asymptomatic.

The urine has reducing properties; it produces a positive reaction with Fehling's or Benedict's reagent and reduces an ammoniacal solution of silver nitrate in the cold. Homogentisic acid does not react with glucose oxidase. The dark urine of phenol poisoning and that associated with melanotic tumors do not have reducing properties.

Hyperaminoaciduria is found in phenol intoxication, but not in alcaptonuria.

There is no effective treatment for the disorder.

METHIONINE

Methioninemia. Abnormally elevated levels of methionine in plasma are observed in a number of disorders, including liver disease, tyrosinosis and homocystinemia. Some believe that a disturbance of methionine metabolism may be the primary defect in one form of tyrosinosis; others that it is not responsible for any clinical manifestations. Transient methioninemia, presumably due to delayed maturation of an enzyme, has also been reported in an otherwise healthy premature infant.

Malabsorption of Methionine. A mentally retarded girl with diarrhea, convulsions, tachypnea and a peculiar odor has been found to have a defect in the intestinal absorption of methionine and of other amino acids. Methionine is fermented by intestinal bacteria to alpha-hydroxybutyric, alpha-ketobutyric and alpha-aminobutyric acids, which are absorbed and excreted in urine, where they produce the unusual odor. Treatment with a diet low in methionine has shown some promise. Alpha-hydroxybutyric acid has been found also in the urine of a child with phenylketonuria; this combination of findings is referred to as *oasthouse disease*, the name suggested by the odor of urine.

Homocystinemia. Homocysteine, an intermediary in the production of cysteine, results when the methyl group of methionine is removed (see Fig. 9-2). It is ordinarily not found in plasma or urine. Approximately 100 patients have been reported who excrete large amounts of homocystine (the dithiol of homocysteine) in the urine and have detectable amounts of both homocysteine and homocystine in the blood. The methionine level of plasma is often elevated, and other unusual thiol compounds are excreted. The biochemical defect has been shown to be a deficiency of the enzyme cystathionine synthetase, which condenses homocysteine with serine to form cystathionine. Normal brain contains large amounts of cystathionine; the brain of a patient who died with homocystinuria was shown to be devoid of this compound, indicating a possible causal relation to the patient's mental retardation.

Many of the patients originally described were mentally retarded, but approximately half of the newly found affected persons are intellectually normal. The disease, or at least the principal variant form, is characterized clinically by ectopia lentis, an appearance resembling Marfan's syndrome, malar flush, osteoporosis, and sticky platelets which lead to thromboembolic episodes. Homocystine can be readily detected in urine by the use of the cyanide-nitroprusside reagent. The effect of dietary restriction of methionine has not been adequately assessed. Some patients have biochemical improvement when fed large doses of vitamin B₆. Pyridoxal phosphate increases the activity of cystathionine synthetase in liver specimens. Blood folic acid levels are often low, owing to increased conversion of homocysteine to methionine; treatment with large doses of folate has been advocated.

Cystathioninemia. Cystathionine is an intermediate in the conversion of methionine to cysteine; it is not normally found in plasma or urine. Cystathioninuria occurs in patients with neuroblastoma, other neural tumors, hepatoblastoma or liver disease, particularly when due to galactosemia. Cystathioninuria in association with cystathioninemia is inherited in an autosomal recessive manner; affected persons have an aberrant form of the enzyme cystathioninase which normally splits cystathionine to homoserine and cysteine (see Fig. 9-2). The binding site for its coenzyme, pyridoxal phosphate, is altered on the affected enzyme molecule. It has been shown both in vitro and in vivo that an increase in function of the enzyme occurs on addition of vitamin B₆ or of its coenzyme form.

About a dozen patients with the disease have been studied, one of whom also had phenylketo-

nuria. Clinical manifestations have been variable and perhaps coincidental; 3 patients are mentally retarded; one had convulsions; 2 sisters had mitral regurgitation, and one had thrombocytopenic purpura and renal calculi. Therapy with vitamin B₆ has led to decreased urinary and blood levels of cystathionine, but its further clinical effects are unknown.

Latent cystathioninuria has been described in 2 mentally retarded brothers who excreted large amounts of cystathionine only when loaded with excess methionine, but not when fed normal diets. They do not appear to be heterozygotes for the usual form of cystathioninemia, since another sibling and their mother excreted small amounts of cystathionine after methionine loading. Cystathioninuria has also been observed in a patient as a transient phenomenon secondary to hepatic disease. This patient later proved to be a heterozygous carrier for cystathioninemia.

Recently a 2-year-old boy and his 8-year-old sister were found by chance to be homozygous for cystathioninemia. Both were clinically normal. These observations again point out that abnormal clinical manifestations observed in the first few cases of a newly discovered inborn error of metabolism may or may not be related to the enzymatic defect.

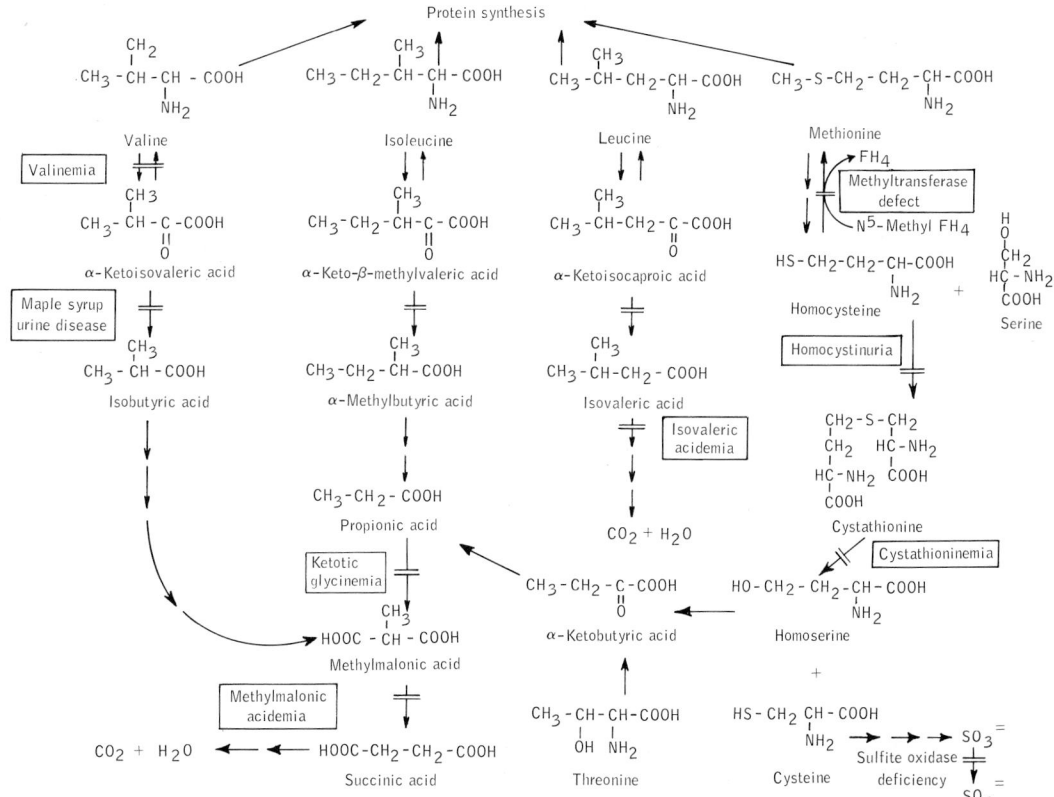

Figure 9-2. Pathways in the metabolism of the branched chain and sulfur containing amino acids. See legend for Fig. 9-1. (Actually, many of the intermediates in these pathways are metabolized *via* their coenzyme A derivatives.)

CYSTINE

Cystinuria. The term "cystinuria" (see p. 1148) is applied to at least 3 closely related disorders, all of which are inherited in an autosomal recessive manner. The homozygotes all have excessive urinary loss of cystine and of 3 other dibasic amino acids: arginine, lysine and ornithine. The urinary loss of cystine has been recognized for many years through the formation of renal calculi. This defect was one of the 4 disorders on which Garrod based his hypothesis of inborn errors of metabolism.

Recently the 3 forms have been distinguished from each other on the basis of (*a*) the pattern of excretion of dibasic amino acids in the clinically normal heterozygote, and (*b*) the nature of the defect in active intestinal transport in affected homozygous persons. The disorder is more fully described elsewhere with other disorders of the renal tubules.

Isolated cystinuria has been reported in a brother and a sister and appears to be inherited as an autosomal recessive.

Cystinosis. In this syndrome (see p. 1367) there is excessive storage of cystine crystals in the reticuloendothelial system and parenchymatous organs. The enzymatic defect is unknown. The disorder is transmitted as an autosomal recessive, and heterozygous carriers can be detected by the elevation of intracellular free cystine in peripheral leukocytes or in fibroblasts grown in tissue culture.

Sulfite Oxidase Deficiency. In the final step of cystine catabolism, inorganic sulfate is formed and excreted in the urine. Absence of inorganic sulfate in the urine has been reported in a mentally retarded child with dislocated lenses who died at 3 years of age. Three siblings (out of seven) died in infancy with neurologic abnormalities. It was proved that the patient lacked sulfite oxidase activity. As a consequence, he excreted large amounts of sulfite, thiosulfate and S-sulfo-L-cysteine in his urine. The defect is presumably inherited as an autosomal recessive.

β-Mercaptolactate-Cysteine Disulfiduria. β-Mercaptolactate-cysteine disulfide is a derivative of cystine in which one of the 2 amino groups is replaced by a hydroxyl group. This substance has been found in high concentration in the urine of a mentally retarded patient who was the product of a sibling mating. There were no other amino acid abnormalities. It was detected by the nitroprusside test while screening for cystinuria.

TRYPTOPHAN

Hartnup Disease. Hartnup disease, an eponymic reminder of the affected English family in whom the disease was discovered, is a rare hereditary molecular disease in which there is a defect in the transport of tryptophan by intestinal mucosa and renal tubules.

There is massive aminoaciduria. Plasma amino acid concentrations are normal, so that the aminoaciduria must be due to faulty tubular reabsorption. The single exception to this generalization is the amino acid tryptophan; characteristically, levels of it in plasma are abnormally low. Impaired intestinal absorption of tryptophan results in its bacterial decomposition to various indole and indoxyl derivatives which are absorbed, detoxified, and excreted in the urine in abnormally large amounts.

Clinical manifestations of cutaneous photosensitivity are seen early in most affected children. Unprotected areas of skin become rough and red after moderate exposure to the sun. With greater exposure, a rash identical with that seen in pellagra develops. Patients with Hartnup disease may also have a neurologic syndrome which consists of cerebellar ataxia with evidences of involvement of the pyramidal tracts. During a febrile illness, ataxia may develop without a rash. The clinical course is variable; severe cutaneous and nervous disturbances may alternate with periods of complete remission over many years. Mental deficiency was apparently an incidental finding in the original kindred and has not been observed in other cases. The disease is transmitted by an autosomal recessive gene. It is clear that Hartnup disease should be considered in the differential diagnosis of pellagra.

The impaired intestinal absorption and urinary loss of tryptophan result in decreased synthesis of nicotinic acid. It is not surprising, therefore, that large doses of nicotinamide may cause a sustained remission of the neurologic and cutaneous aspects of the disorder. Such remissions, however, may occur without any therapy. The aminoaciduria and urinary excretion of indole compounds are not suppressed by such therapy, nor do they decrease during spontaneous remissions. It has been suggested that high protein diets compensate for the loss of amino acids.

Tryptophanemia. In contrast to Hartnup disease, in which there is impaired absorption of tryptophan, the catabolism of tryptophan (presumably in its conversion to kynurenine) is involved in this disorder (see Fig. 9-3). The patient was a mentally retarded child with dwarfism who had the same pellagra-like rash seen in Hartnup disease. There were tryptophanemia and tryptophanuria without generalized aminoaciduria or indicanuria. Parental consanguinity and the suspicion of a similar disorder in 2 cousins indicate an autosomal recessive inheritance.

Kynureninuria. An abnormality of tryptophan metabolism consistent with a partial block of the enzyme kynurenine hydroxylase has been reported in 4 generations of a family. Although the propositus had scleroderma, the other members of the kindred were healthy. Abnormal amounts of kynurenine and other tryptophan metabolites proximal to hydroxykynurenine (Fig. 9-3) are excreted in the urine both before and after administration of tryptophan. Pyridoxine did not affect the excretion

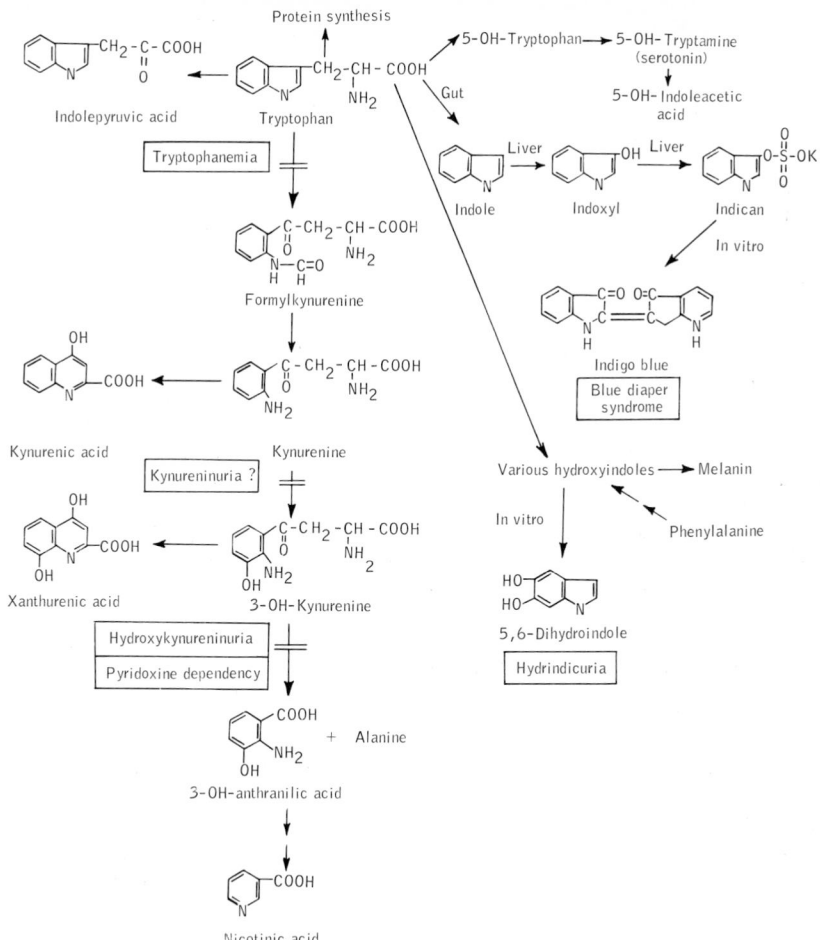

Figure 9-3. Pathways in the metabolism of tryptophan. See legend for Fig. 9-1.

pattern of tryptophan metabolites. The affected persons appear to be heterozygous for the condition.

Kynureninase Defects. *Hydroxykynureninuria.* A defect has been described in the tryptophan pathway which is consistent with lack of activity of the enzyme kynureninase. In this disorder large amounts of kynurenine, 3-hydroxykynurenine and xanthurenic acid are excreted (see Fig. 9-3). Signs and symptoms of nicotinic acid deficiency develop in the absence of added dietary nicotinic acid; affected persons cannot synthesize it from tryptophan. A patient was mildly mentally retarded and complained of migraine headaches. Treatment with pyridoxine did not alter the excretion pattern of the tryptophan metabolites, but did relieve the headaches.

Pyridoxine dependency (xanthinuria). Children with pyridoxine dependency have convulsions and are mentally retarded (p. 174). After tryptophan loading they excrete the same metabolites of tryptophan, mainly xanthurenic acid, as are seen without tryptophan loading in hydroxykynureninuria. These metabolites are also excreted by persons who are deficient in pyridoxine. Pyridoxal phosphate is the coenzyme for many

enzymes involved in amino acid metabolism, including kynureninase. Whereas low doses of the vitamin correct the abnormalities in the deficiency state, high doses are required to treat the dependent state. In pyridoxine dependency it has been shown in vitro that there is a defect of the enzyme kynureninase which affects its ability to bind with the coenzyme form of the vitamin.

Indicanuria. Indicanuria arises when tryptophan is poorly absorbed from the gastrointestinal tract and is converted there by bacterial action to indole. Indole is absorbed, oxidized, sulfated and excreted as an indican (see Fig. 9-3). Indicanuria is commonly observed whenever there is stasis in the bowels such as in constipation or the "blind loop syndrome"; it also occurs in Hartnup disease, in which tryptophan is poorly absorbed, and in phenylketonuria. The *blue diaper syndrome*, a familial disorder characterized by hypercalcemia, nephrocalcinosis and indicanuria, derives its name from the fact that indican is oxidized to indican blue on exposure to air.

Hydrindicuria. Indole pigments related to both tryptophan and phenylalanine metabolism have been found in the urine of a mentally retarded child who had a persistent metabolic acidosis, presumably caused by carboxyindole derivatives. Laboratory manipulation of urine containing abnormal urinary indoles converts them to 5,6-dihydroxyindole (hydrindic acid); hence the name of the disorder (see Fig. 9-3). Prolonged administration of antibiotics in an effort to halt indole formation in the gut had no effect upon indole excretion, and loading tests showed an increase in urinary hydrindic acid after administration of phenylalanine and tryptophan, but not of tyrosine.

VALINE, LEUCINE, ISOLEUCINE

Maple Syrup Urine Disease. This recessive disorder is characterized by the excretion of urine with an odor of maple syrup and by central nervous system manifestations appearing within the first weeks of life. In the neonatal period there is difficulty in feeding, and the beginning of progressive neurologic and mental deterioration. Death usually occurs within the first few months of life.

The blood and urine contain increased amounts of the 3 branched-chain amino acids, valine, leucine and isoleucine. The urine characteristically also contains increased amounts of the keto-acid derivatives of these amino acids. The defect is known to be in oxidative decarboxylation of the keto-acids (see Fig. 9-2). There is some disagreement at present whether the 3 keto-acids are decarboxylated by 3 separate enzymes or by 2 enzymes, one of which can act upon two of the acids. The concentration in the blood of allo-isoleucine, a stereo-isomer of isoleucine formed by way of the keto-acid, is also increased.

The enzymatic defect can be demonstrated in leukocytes in vitro; this method also serves to detect heterozygotes. Treatment with a diet low in the branched-chain amino acids has been successfully used to arrest the progressively downhill course of the disease. Variable degrees of central nervous system manifestations may persist, depending upon adequacy of treatment and amount of damage present prior to its institution.

Intermittent branched-chain ketonuria is a variant of maple syrup urine disease. Children who are apparently healthy suddenly become ill, present the odor of maple syrup, exhibit neurologic symptoms, and excrete leucine, isoleucine and valine and the corresponding keto-acids in urine. The disorder is genetically transmitted as an autosomal recessive. Activity in leukocytes of branched-chain decarboxylase is reduced, but not to the extent as in the more common form of the disorder.

Valinemia. A child has been observed with elevated levels of valine in plasma and urine, and with mental deficiency and growth failure, but without the characteristic urinary odor or excretion of keto-acids of maple syrup urine disease. Transamination of valine is impaired; the defect can be demonstrated in leukocytes in vitro.

Isovaleric Acidemia. Another defect in leucine catabolism results in the accumulation of isovaleric acid (Fig. 9-2). Two affected siblings had mild retardation, severe acidosis, vomiting and coma, and the peculiar odor of sweaty feet. They had an aversion to protein foods. The defect, which has been demonstrated in leukocytes, is in the oxidation of isovaleric acid to beta-methylcrotonic acid.

What may be a more severe form of the disorder was reported in an infant who died within a week of birth in acidosis. Isovaleric acidemia should be distinguished from the defect of green acyldehydrogenase (p. 450), which leads to the accumulation of butyric and hexanoic acids (*odor of sweaty feet syndrome*).

Leucine-Induced Hypoglycemia. Hypoglycemia occurs after the feeding of protein to patients who are hyperresponsive to leucine. In the normal person, leucine elicits a small but significant hypoglycemic effect. In either case hypoglycemia results from the release of insulin. The defect is not in the metabolism of leucine, but probably resides in aberrant pancreatic receptor sites. See also page 1168.

PROLINE AND HYDROXYPROLINE

Proline and hydroxyproline are found in high concentration in collagen. Neither of these amino acids is normally found in urine in its free form except in early infancy. "Bound" hydroxyproline (dipeptides and tripeptides containing hydroxyproline) is excreted whenever there is rapid turnover of collagen such as may occur in such disorders as rickets and hyperparathyroidism.

Prolinuria. A defect in renal tubular transport of proline is inherited as an autosomal recessive. Since proline, hydroxyproline and glycine are all transported by a common mechanism, patients with familial prolinuria also excrete the other 2 amino acids in abnormal amounts; the concentrations of these amino acids in serum are, however, normal. Many of the affected persons are mentally retarded and also have impaired intestinal transport of proline.

Prolinemia. Two distinct types of prolinemia are known in which excessive amounts of proline are present in both blood and urine. Hydroxyproline and glycine are also excreted in abnormal amounts in the urine, owing to the inhibition of the common tubular reabsorption mechanism. In the first type of prolinemia the enzymatic defect involves proline oxidase (Fig. 9-4). In the second type the defect is presumed to be in the enzyme of the next step, a dehydrogenase, since pyrrolidine carboxylic acid, as well as proline, accumulates abnormally. Type I prolinemia has been associated with mild mental retardation, renal abnormalities, nerve deafness and photogenic epilepsy. Whether there is a causal relation, however, is uncertain, since both types of prolinemia appear to be in-

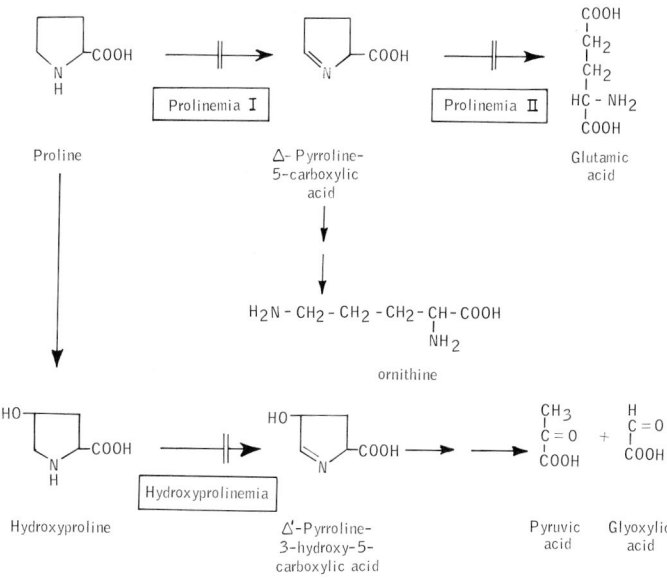

Figure 9-4. Pathways in the metabolism of the imino acids. See legend for Fig. 9-1.

herited on an autosomal recessive basis, and the other abnormalities were dominantly inherited. Type II prolinemia was observed in a young child who had only mild mental retardation.

Hydroxyprolinemia. This disorder has been described in a severely retarded girl. Excessive hydroxyproline was found in serum and urine. In hydroxyprolinemia, in contrast to prolinemia, excessive urinary excretion of the other 2 amino acids (proline and glycine) which share the same transport mechanisms does not occur. The defect is in the enzyme hydroxyproline oxidase (Fig. 9-4). This enzyme is distinct from the corresponding enzyme which acts upon proline. The disorder is presumed to be inherited as an autosomal recessive; the association with mental retardation may be fortuitous.

Glycylprolinuria. Glycylproline has been found in the urine in 2 syndromes. In the first syndrome, though various other proline dipeptides were found in urine, only glycylproline was demonstrated in serum. The patient had hepatosplenomegaly and a peculiar face, but no bone disease. The electron microscopic appearance of collagen was similar to that seen in lathyrism. In the second syndrome, glycylproline could not be demonstrated in serum, but appeared in large amounts in urine. The patients, 2 sisters, had thickened bone cortices, macrocranium and frequent fractures.

GLYCINE

Glycinemia with Ketosis. Abnormal plasma levels of glycine are found in what appear to be 3 separate disorders, each inherited as an autosomal recessive. In the classic form of this disorder there is increased accumulation of glycine in blood (over 10 mg. per 100 ml.) and excessive excretion in urine. Moderate increases in the plasma levels of other amino acids (serine, alanine, isoleucine and valine) also are found, but only glycine is excreted in unusual amounts. The disease has its onset in infancy, and the nature and severity of the clinical course suggest that an occasional unexplained death in infancy may be due to this disease. The defect is in the conversion of propionate to methylmalonate (see Fig. 9-2).

The earliest recognized clinical manifestations are severe acidosis and ketonuria within the first few days of life, so severe as to require administration of sodium bicarbonate. Subsequently there are recurrent episodes of metabolic ketosis and acidosis, mental and physical retardation, osteoporosis and periodic thrombocytopenia and neutropenia. The episodes of vomiting, ketosis and acidosis appear to be related to the quantity of protein in the diet; reduction in the dietary intake of protein has been associated with decreased frequency and severity of the clinical attacks and increase in circulating neutrophils. It is interesting that the individual administration of methionine, threonine, valine, leucine or isoleucine produces ketosis. The ketosis is unusual in that ketone bodies, presumably derived from the branched-chain amino acids (2-butanone and to a lesser extent pentanones and hexanones), appear in large amounts in addition to acetone. This is in contrast to the finding that acetone accounts for nearly all the ketones in the more usual forms of ketosis.

Treatment with a diet low in glycine, methionine, threonine, leucine, isoleucine and valine may prove effective in lessening or preventing mental retardation.

Glycinemia without Ketosis. In three other forms of glycinemia the blood levels of this amino

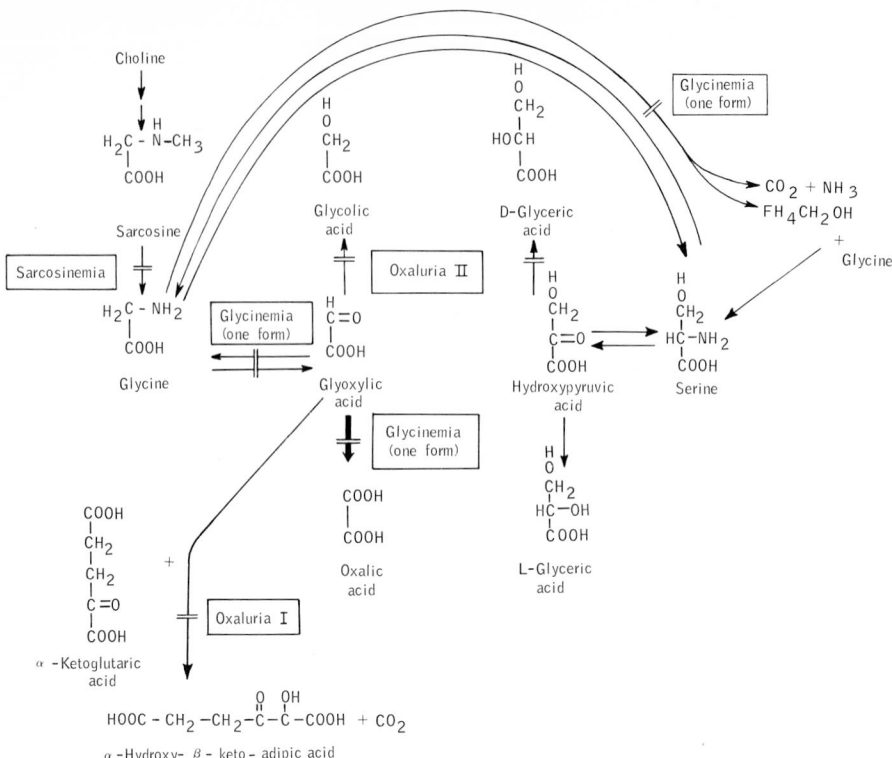

Figure 9-5. Pathways in the metabolism of glycine. See legend for Fig. 9-1.

acid average about 5 mg. per 100 ml.; acidosis and ketosis are not clinical features. Some infants with this form of glycinemia excrete decreased quantities of oxalic acid in urine due to a defect in one or the other of two enzymes which convert glycine to oxalic acid. Other infants with normal oxalic acid excretion have a defect in the first of two enzymes which convert two molecules of glycine to serine, ammonia, and carbon dioxide via hydroxymethyltetrahydrofolic acid (see Fig. 9-5).

Glycinemia with Methylmalonic Acidemia. In the third condition, glycinemia, glycinuria and acidosis occur in conjunction with methylmalonic acidemia. This entity is described on page 439.

Sarcosinemia. Increased concentrations of sarcosine (N-methylglycine) have been observed in both blood and urine in 2 siblings, one of whom was mentally retarded, had difficulty in swallowing, failed to thrive and died at 14 months of age. Loading tests in other family members suggest that this is a recessively inherited inborn error probably involving sarcosine dehydrogenase, the enzyme which converts sarcosine to glycine (Fig. 9-5). A third patient with hepatosplenomegaly and fatty metamorphosis of the liver has been described with this disorder, who at 8 months of age was apparently developing normally.

Glycinuria and Glucoglycinuria. Glycinuria and glucoglycinuria have been identified as separate disorders of the renal tubules. Glycinuria is also observed in prolinemia and prolinuria, since there exists a common transport system for proline, hydroxyproline and glycine, in addition to the specific renal transport system for glycine alone.

Primary Oxaluria and Oxalosis. Oxalic acid is a 2-carbon dicarboxylic acid which is derived mostly from the oxidation of the amino acid glycine via glyoxylic acid (Fig. 9-5). A storage disease, *oxalosis*, is characterized by the deposition of calcium oxalate crystals throughout the body tissues. In a milder form, *oxaluria*, there are excessive urinary excretion of oxalic acid, renal and vesical lithiasis, and nephrocalcinosis. Clinical manifestations appear in childhood, and death occurs in early adulthood. Although the clinical disorder has long been known, the biochemical defect has only recently been delineated. It is now known that primary oxaluria comprises 2 distinct disorders, each caused by a different enzymatic deficit.

In the first type, which is the common form and the more severe, there is usually excess excretion of *glycolic acid* and glyoxylic acid as well as oxalic acid. The missing enzyme, α-ketoglutarate-glyoxylate carboligase, normally removes glyoxylic acid to form α-hydroxy-β-ketoadipic acid. In the absence of this enzyme the glyoxylic acid floods the pathways leading to glycolic and oxalic acids.

In the second type of hyperoxaluria, *L-glyceric acid is also excreted* in the urine in large amounts. This acid, which is not produced by normal persons, arises from the reduction of hydroxypyruvic acid (the keto-acid of serine) by lactic dehydrogenase. Ordinarily, hydroxypyruvic acid is reduced to D-glyceric acid by the specific enzyme D-glyceric acid dehydrogenase. This enzyme is also capable of reducing glyoxylic acid to glycolic acid. In its absence hydroxypyruvic acid is converted to and excreted as L-glyceric acid, and glyoxylic acid is converted to and excreted as oxalic acid.

UREA CYCLE

Catabolism of amino acids results in the production of free ammonia, a compound highly toxic to the brain. Ammonia is catabolized further to urea by a series of reactions known as the Krebs-Henseleit or urea cycle (see Fig. 9-6). A number of enzymatic defects are known which involve the urea cycle. In each instance the affected persons exhibit mental retardation presumably resulting from intoxication with ammonia. In some instances a deficiency of an enzyme in the urea cycle has been directly demonstrated in biopsy material; in other instances the defect in urea synthesis is only postulated. Since most patients with defects of the urea cycle excrete normal amounts of urea, it is presumed that the defect is either not present in all tissues or that other pathways exist for synthesis of urea. A new pathway for urea synthesis involving guanidosuccinic acid has been postulated recently, based upon the finding of this acid in the urine of patients with uremia.

Hyperammoniemia. Mental retardation and failure to thrive, apparently related to greatly increased levels of ammonia in the blood, have been described in a few children, two of whom were first cousins. The urine was persistently alkaline, and virtually all the excreted hydrogen appeared as ammonium ions. Some of the children had an increase of glutamine in the urine which accounted for most of the excess alpha-amino nitrogen. Examination of liver tissue obtained by biopsy in one child revealed normal activity of carbamyl phosphate synthetase and a significant deficiency in activity of the enzyme ornithine transcarbamylase. Loss of activity of ornithine transcarbamylase leads to failure of incorporation of ammonia into urea and to elevated plasma concentrations of ammonia (0.5 to 1.0 mg. per 100 ml.). There is still some question about the enzymatic defect in this condition, since in one patient both ornithine transcarbamylase and carbamyl phosphate synthetase were decreased.

Citrullinemia. Three patients with citrullinemia have been described. The first, a mentally retarded child with seizures, whose parents were first cousins, had high levels of citrulline in plasma, spinal fluid and urine. No other amino acids were excreted in unusual amounts. The blood level of ammonia rose sharply after feeding. Since the level of urea in blood was normal, it is probable that the urea cycle in the liver functioned normally. The second patient was a mentally retarded boy who died in status epilepticus before other studies could be obtained. The third patient was a microcephalic girl 21 months of age who presented with vomiting and seizures. Examination of urea cycle enzymes in fibroblasts grown in tissue culture revealed that some argininosuccinic acid syn-

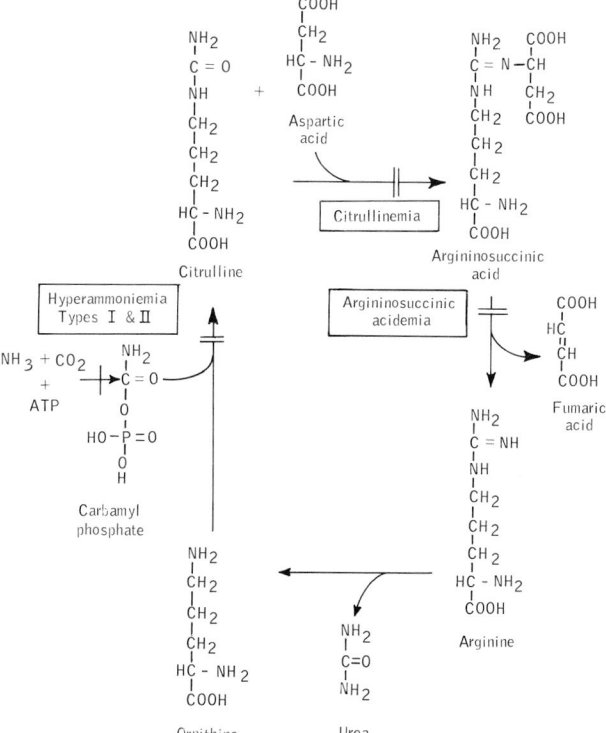

Figure 9-6. Pathways in the metabolism of ammonia and in the urea cycle. See legend for Fig. 9-1.

thetase activity was present, but kinetic studies suggested the presence of a mutant enzyme.

Argininosuccinic Acidemia. Children with argininosuccinic acidemia and aciduria have usually been mentally retarded, and some have had abnormally friable hair (trichorrhexis nodosa). Not all patients with this type of hair abnormality, however, have argininosuccinic acidemia. The defect is in argininosuccinase, the enzyme which splits argininosuccinic acid to arginine and fumaric acid. The defect can be demonstrated in erythrocytes; heterozygotes have lower than normal activity. The disorder is transmitted as an autosomal recessive. Levels of argininosuccinic acid are higher in the cerebrospinal fluid than in the blood; concentrations of urea in the blood and urine are normal. The defect in the urea cycle in these patients may be limited to the brain.

HISTIDINE

Histidinemia. In histidinemia the activity of the enzyme histidase, which normally converts histidine to urocanic acid, is deficient in liver and skin. As a result, histidine is transaminated to imidazolepyruvic acid, which appears in the urine along with excessive amounts of histidine (see Fig. 9-7). Imidazolepyruvic acid, like phenylpyruvic acid, reacts with ferric chloride to produce a blue-green color. Most patients with histidinemia have been detected in screening tests for phenylketonuria, and some cases have been mis-

diagnosed as such. Demonstration of elevation in plasma levels of histidine is necessary for definitive diagnosis of this disorder.

Some of the affected persons have had impaired speech, a few were retarded in growth, and some were mentally retarded. The relation of these defects to histidinemia is unknown. The metabolic defect is transmitted as an autosomal recessive character; in some families the heterozygous state can be identified by demonstration of decreased histidase activity in skin obtained by biopsy.

There is some evidence for genetic heterogeneity in histidinemia. In some but not in all affected children, plasma levels of alanine as well as of histidine were elevated. The reason for this association is unknown. In some families with histidinemia the level of histidase in skin is normal, and perhaps the defect in enzymatic activity is limited to the liver.

Histidine and Folic Acid Metabolism. After histidine has been converted to urocanic acid it is further metabolized to formiminoglutamic acid (FIGLU). The formimino group of this compound is normally transferred to folic acid with the concomitant production of glutamic acid (see Fig. 9-7). Measurement of the urinary excretion of FIGLU after loading with histidine has been used as a method for the detection of folic acid deficiency states. Both FIGLU and urocanic acid are excreted by patients with megaloblastic anemia. Urocanic acid is found in the urine of children with kwashiorkor.

A group of mentally retarded infants have been described in Japan who have defects in folic acid

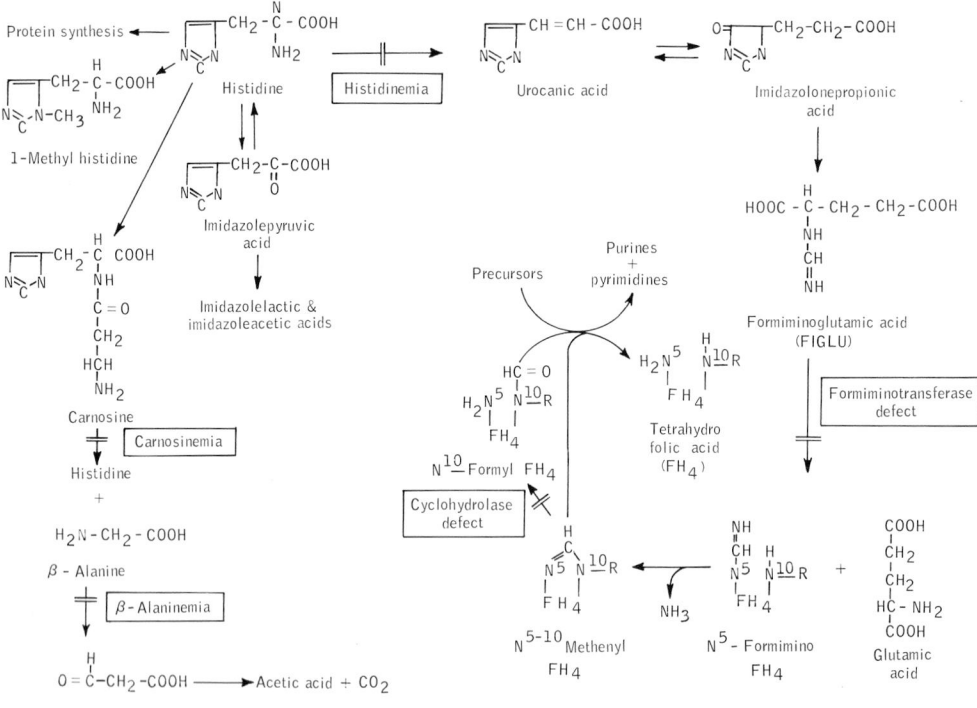

Figure 9-7. Pathways in the metabolism of histidine, beta amino acids and folic acid. See legend for Fig. 9-1. FH$_4$ is an abbreviation for tetrahydrofolic acid.

metabolism. Microcephaly and electroencephalographic abnormalities were frequent findings. Three distinct defects have been delineated, in each of which the blood values of folic acid are elevated. In the first, formiminoglutamic acid is increased after administration of histidine; the enzyme formiminotransferase is deficient. In the second disorder FIGLU is not excreted even after an oral load of histidine; the defect is in the enzyme cyclohydrolase. The third disorder is further down the metabolic pathway and involves a defect in the enzyme which normally transfers the methyl group of N^5 methyl tetrahydrofolate to homocysteine-forming methionine (Fig. 9-2, p. 425).

Dipeptides of Histidine. Carnosine (β-alanylhistidine) and anserine (β-alanyl-1-methyl histidine) are dipeptides of histidine found in muscle, where their function is unknown. These peptides, as well as 1-methyl histidine derived from anserine, have been found in urine of normal persons, particularly after the ingestion of large amounts of turkey and chicken. In the disorders described below the findings of the dipeptides of histidine in urine have been specific and independent of dietary intake.

Imidazole Aciduria. Excessive excretion of carnosine, anserine and occasionally of homocarnosine (γ-amino butyryl histidine), as well as of histidine and 1-methyl histidine, has been reported in a number of patients with a form of cerebromacular degeneration resembling juvenile Tay-Sachs disease. The use of labeled histidine provided some evidence for increased synthesis of the dipeptides. The genetic basis of the disorder is not clear; in the 3 families studied the cerebromacular degeneration was inherited on a recessive basis, whereas the histidine peptiduria appeared to be transmitted on a dominant one.

Carnosinemia. Two unrelated children with severe mental retardation and myoclonic seizures have been found who excreted large amounts of carnosine. One child had persistent carnosinemia on a dietary regimen free of carnosine; both had a tenfold increase of homocarnosine in cerebrospinal fluid. The defect is in the enzyme carnosinase, which normally hydrolyzes carnosine to histidine and β-alanine and can be assayed in plasma. The disorder appears to be inherited as an autosomal recessive.

ALANINE

Alaninemia. Alaninemia has been described in conjunction with one form of histidinemia (see above).

A child with lactic acidosis, mild mental retardation and growth failure has been described who had abnormally high plasma levels (9 mg. per 100 ml.) and increased urinary excretion of alanine, and some elevation of plasma pyruvate (up to 2 mg. per 100 ml.). A second child with similar chemical findings has had optic atrophy and recurrent cerebellar ataxia. The nature of the defect is not known; the alaninemia may be secondary to an increase in pyruvate and result from transamination of the keto-acid to its amino form. The relation of this disorder to Leigh's encephalomyelopathy is unknown (see p. 1302).

BETA AMINO ACIDS

Beta-Alaninemia. An infant with lethargy, somnolence and grand mal seizures who died at 5 months of age was found to have persistent β-alaninemia, at a concentration 2 to 4 times that of normal. Beta-alanine is derived from the hydrolysis of certain dipeptides and by the degradation of uracil. It is normally further metabolized by transamination to malonic acid, then to acetate and carbon dioxide. Preliminary evidence suggests a block in the transamination of this compound. Two interesting features of the disorder are the increased concentrations of β-aminoisobutyric acid and taurine as well as of β-alanine in urine. These findings have been used in support of the concept of a common renal transport mechanism for the β-amino acids. The affected child also had increased concentration of γ-amino butyric acid in cerebral spinal fluid, plasma, and urine. The neurologic symptoms have been attributed to the increase in β-alanine and the decrease in γ-amino butyric acid within the brain.

Beta-Aminoisobutyric Aciduria. Excessive excretion of β-aminoisobutyric acid (BAIB) is a genetic variant in metabolism in a small percentage of the population; there are racial and geographic variations in incidence. In addition, β-aminoisobutyric aciduria occurs in a variety of illnesses in which there is tissue destruction, and deoxyribonucleic acid is catabolized excessively. Beta-aminoisobutyric acid is a normal metabolite of both valine and thymine. Normal persons fed large amounts of β-aminoisobutyric acid have the ability to excrete it rapidly, which indicates that the renal tubular excretion of this compound is an adaptive process secondary to an increased plasma level. In any case, increased excretion of β-aminoisobutyric acid is not evidence of a renal tubular defect, since reabsorption in the tubules does not occur.

Affected persons with the congenital form are asymptomatic; they excrete 100 to 300 mg. of β-aminoisobutyric acid daily in contrast to 10 to 40 mg. in other persons. The condition is transmitted by a single recessive gene.

LYSINE

Lysine is an essential amino acid which shares a common renal transport mechanism with other

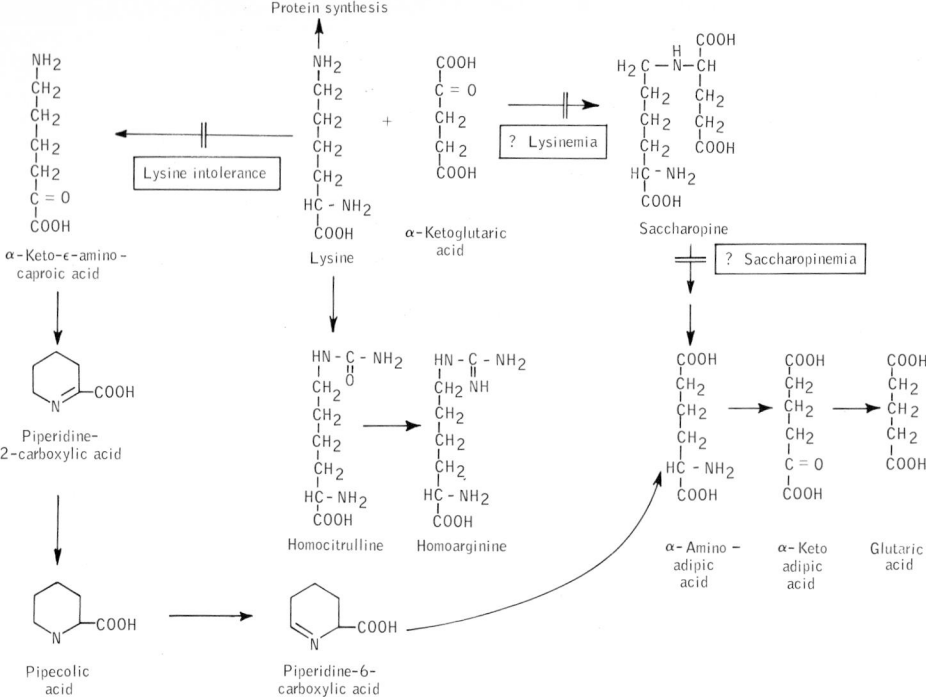

Figure 9-8. Pathways in the metabolism of lysine. See legend for Fig. 9-1.

dibasic amino acids. Lysinuria has been observed in some children with malnutrition. There are at least 3 enzymopathies in which elevations of plasma lysine occur.

Lysinemia. Persistent lysinemia and lysinuria have been observed in 6 children studied by 3 groups of investigators. One group studied 2 siblings who had severe mental retardation and muscle weakness. Another group studied 3 children (2 siblings and a third cousin) with even higher plasma lysine levels than in the first cases, but only one of the siblings was retarded. The third group reported a child in whom mental retardation may have been coincidental, since the mother and some unaffected siblings were also mentally retarded. In none of these children has a metabolic defect been delineated. A theory that lysine was not incorporated into muscle protein has been abandoned. There is an unexplained difference in the findings of two of the groups: in 1 patient almost no labeled carbon dioxide appeared in expired air after administration of carbon-labeled lysine, whereas in another one oxidation to carbon dioxide was unimpaired. These observations suggest at least 2 different biochemical defects.

Study of these patients has added to knowledge of the pathway of lysine degradation in man (see Fig. 9-8). One of the main routes of catabolism appears to be the condensation of lysine with alpha-keto-glutaric acid to form a compound known as saccharopine. A defect at this locus is presumed responsible for at least one form of lysinemia. Minor pathways for lysine degradation have been shown; homocitrulline and homoarginine, ε-N-acetyl-L-lysine and alpha-N-acetyl-L-lysine are formed and excreted.

Saccharopinemia. A short, mentally retarded woman has been described who had lysinuria, citrullinuria, homocitrullinuria and saccharopinuria. These compounds were also elevated in the serum, and saccharopine was found in high concentrations in cerebrospinal fluid. The locus of the metabolic block is not as yet known, but is presumably at the degradation of saccharopine (see Fig. 9-8).

Congenital Lysine Intolerance. This disorder has been observed in a 3-month-old infant who had episodes of ammonia intoxication. With normal intake of protein, blood levels of lysine and arginine were normal, but when the protein intake was raised to 2.5 to 3 gm. per kg. per day, plasma lysine, arginine and ammonia levels increased to at least double their control values. The increases in arginine and ammonia were thought to be due to inhibition of arginase by lysine, with consequent inability to detoxify ammonia by the formation of urea. The administration of lysine orally depressed erythrocyte arginase activity, and led to an increase of blood ammonia to 680 μg. per 100 ml., and coma. There was a diminution in the activity of lysine dehydrogenase in liver; this enzyme converts lysine to alpha-keto-ε-amino caproic acid (Fig. 9-8).

DEFECTS IN METABOLISM OF CARBOHYDRATES

DEFECTS IN ABSORPTION OF CARBOHYDRATES

A variety of syndromes have been described in infants and children characterized by defective intestinal absorption and hydrolysis of monosaccharides and disaccharides. These patients have diarrhea as a presenting symptom. Absorption of monosaccharides and disaccharides takes place in the small intestine. It is important to remember that digestion of disaccharides involves at least 2 steps: absorption into the mucosal cells and splitting within the cells. Glucose, galactose and perhaps lactose are absorbed against a concentration gradient (active transport) by what appears to be the same mechanism. Fructose and, probably, sucrose are absorbed by passive diffusion.

Hydrolysis of the disaccharides occurs within the mucosal cells, and the resultant monosaccharides are released into the circulation. Lactase (beta-galactosidase) is responsible for the hydrolysis of lactose to glucose and galactose. Sucrase (invertase) hydrolyzes sucrose to glucose and fructose and also splits maltose into 2 glucose molecules, but at a slower rate. Isomaltase splits isomaltose and other 1-6 linked glucose residues; isomaltase also has some activity against maltose. In addition to these enzymes, the intestinal mucosa contains maltases which are specific for the disaccharide maltose.

Lactase is an inducible enzyme whose activity is greatest during infancy and may disappear in adulthood, when *lactosuria* may follow heavy ingestion of disaccharide. *Sucrosuria* is also a common finding in normal adults and children after a sucrose load. Severe diarrhea in children may lead to inability to hydrolyze disaccharides, which in turn prolongs the diarrhea if disaccharides are ingested.

A number of conditions are described on page 811 in which inability to absorb or hydrolyze monosaccharides or disaccharides is due to abnormal genes. Treatment always consists in removal of the offending carbohydrate from the diet.

DEFECTS IN MUCOPOLYSACCHARIDE METABOLISM

The mucopolysaccharidoses are discussed elsewhere (p. 1337). Other disease processes also involve metabolism of mucopolysaccharides. In cystic fibrosis, in which yet undefined changes take place in mucus-secreting tissue, fibroblasts from both homozygous and heterozygous persons, grown in tissue culture, stain metachromatically, indicating an underlying abnormality of mucopolysaccharide metabolism.

Some increase in urinary excretion of normal mucopolysaccharides occurs in systemic lupus erythematosus, rheumatoid arthritis, leukemia, lymphoma and multiple myeloma.

There is some overlapping in classification between the mucopolysaccharidoses and the lipidoses. Farber's disease (p. 457) and generalized gangliosidosis (p. 457) involve deposition of both classes of compounds. This is also the case in a newly described disorder (p. 439) in which the enzyme defect is absence of α-fucosidase.

DEFECTS IN MONOSACCHARIDE METABOLISM

The most common clinical disorder involving monosaccharides is diabetes mellitus (p. 1155).

Defective Pentose Metabolism. The pentose D-ribose is a constituent of many coenzymes and of ribonucleic acid; deoxyribose is a constituent of deoxyribonucleic acid. These pentoses are not derived directly from dietary sources, but are synthesized as needed from glucose via the pentose-phosphate pathway. Pentoses are absorbed slowly from the intestine, and renal tubular reabsorption of filtered pentose is also poor. Normal persons excrete up to 100 mg. of pentose per day in the urine, and twice this amount when the intake of pentose-containing fruits is excessive. In such instances the urinary pentoses are xylose and arabinose.

Scurvy. The formation of ascorbic acid from gulonic acid, through pentoses, requires a highly specific enzymatic transformation. Most species have this ability and are able to synthesize ascorbic acid (vitamin C). On the other hand, man, some monkeys, the guinea pig, the Indian fruit bat and the red-vented bulbul have a defect in this enzyme system and require exogenous vitamin C to prevent death from scurvy. It is appropriate to think of scurvy as an inborn error of monosaccharide metabolism which is limited to certain species. The administration of vitamin C to prevent this disorder exemplifies the ease with which certain enzymatic defects can be circumvented.

Essential benign pentosuria (L-xylulosuria). This rare anomaly, transmitted on an autosomal recessive basis, is characterized by excessive excretion of L-xylulose (1 to 4 gm. per day), regardless of diet. Found almost exclusively in Jewish families, it has an incidence of about one in 50,000. Most cases are not detected until adult life; however, it has been encountered in a 19-month-old infant. The heterozygous carrier can be detected by measurements of L-xylulose in serum or urine after the oral administration of D-glucuronolactone. Homozygous persons with pentosuria, unlike normal persons, cannot convert L-xylulose

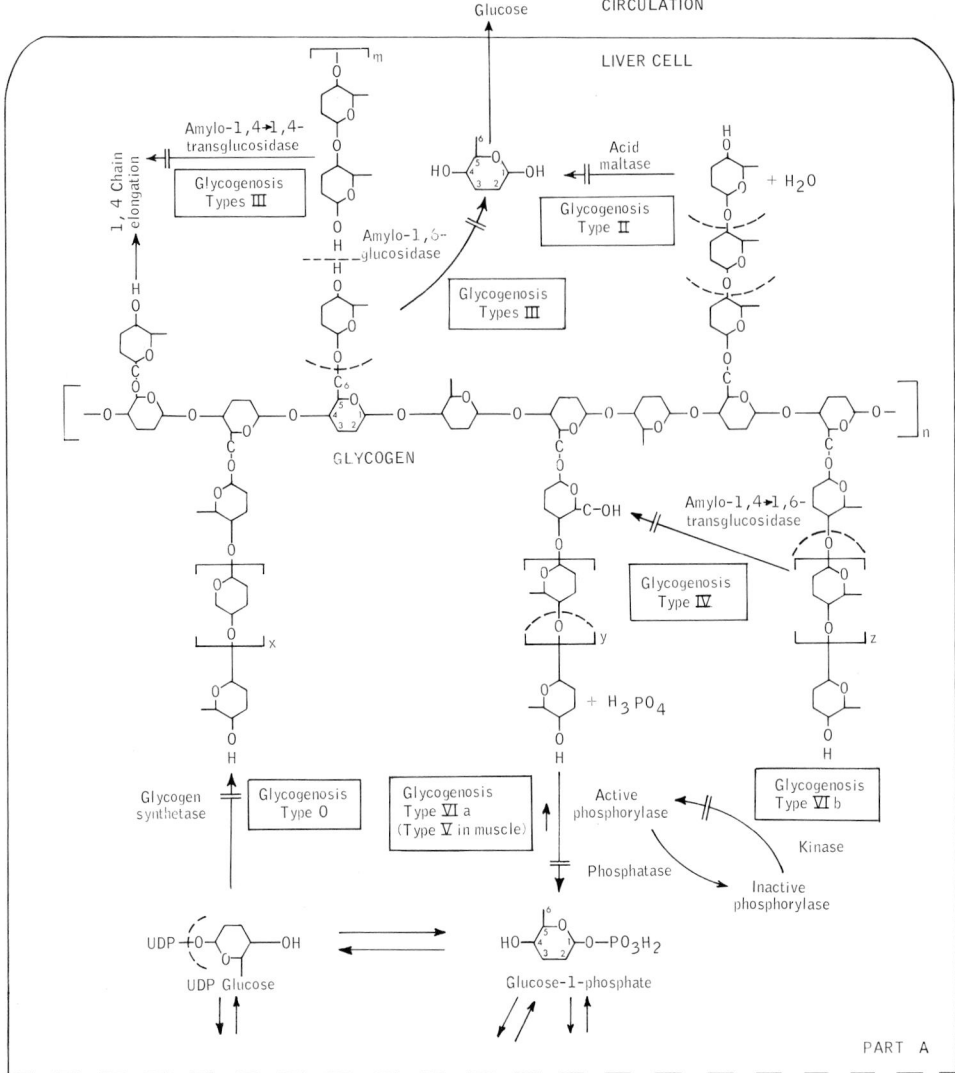

Figure 9-9 A. Pathways in the metabolism of glycogen. Stereospecificity of bonds and correct lengths of chains are not shown.

back to glucose from which it was originally formed via glucuronic acid. The defect is in the same metabolic pathway as the one leading to scurvy.

L-xylulosuria is usually harmless and symptomless. It is ordinarily discovered by urinalysis. Because L-xylulose reduces Benedict's and Fehling's solutions, it may be confused with glucosuria. It does not react with glucose oxidase.

Essential (Benign) Fructosuria. This rare and benign defect is characterized by the presence of fructose (levulose) in the urine. It results from an inability to metabolize fructose. Fructose occurs as a monosaccharide in many fruits and vegetables and in honey. It is also derived from the intestinal hydrolysis of sucrose and of complex polysaccharides in certain vegetables.

From 10 to 20 per cent of ingested fructose is excreted in the urine of patients with the defect. Inherited as a recessive trait, essential fructosuria occurs in less than one in 100,000 persons. The cause of the fructosuria is a defect in fructokinase, the enzyme which converts fructose to fructose-1-phosphate (see Fig. 9-9, B).

Fructose reduces Benedict's and Fehling's solutions, but does not react with glucose oxidase. Other causes of fructosuria must be eliminated before it can be designated as genetic in origin. In acquired hepatic disorders with severe cellular damage such as infectious hepatitis, cirrhosis and syphilitic hepatitis, fructose is occasionally found in the urine. Since the loss of dietary fructose in the urine is apparently harmless, dietary restriction is not indicated.

Fructosemia (Fructose Intolerance). Absence of the hepatic enzyme fructose-1-phosphate aldo-

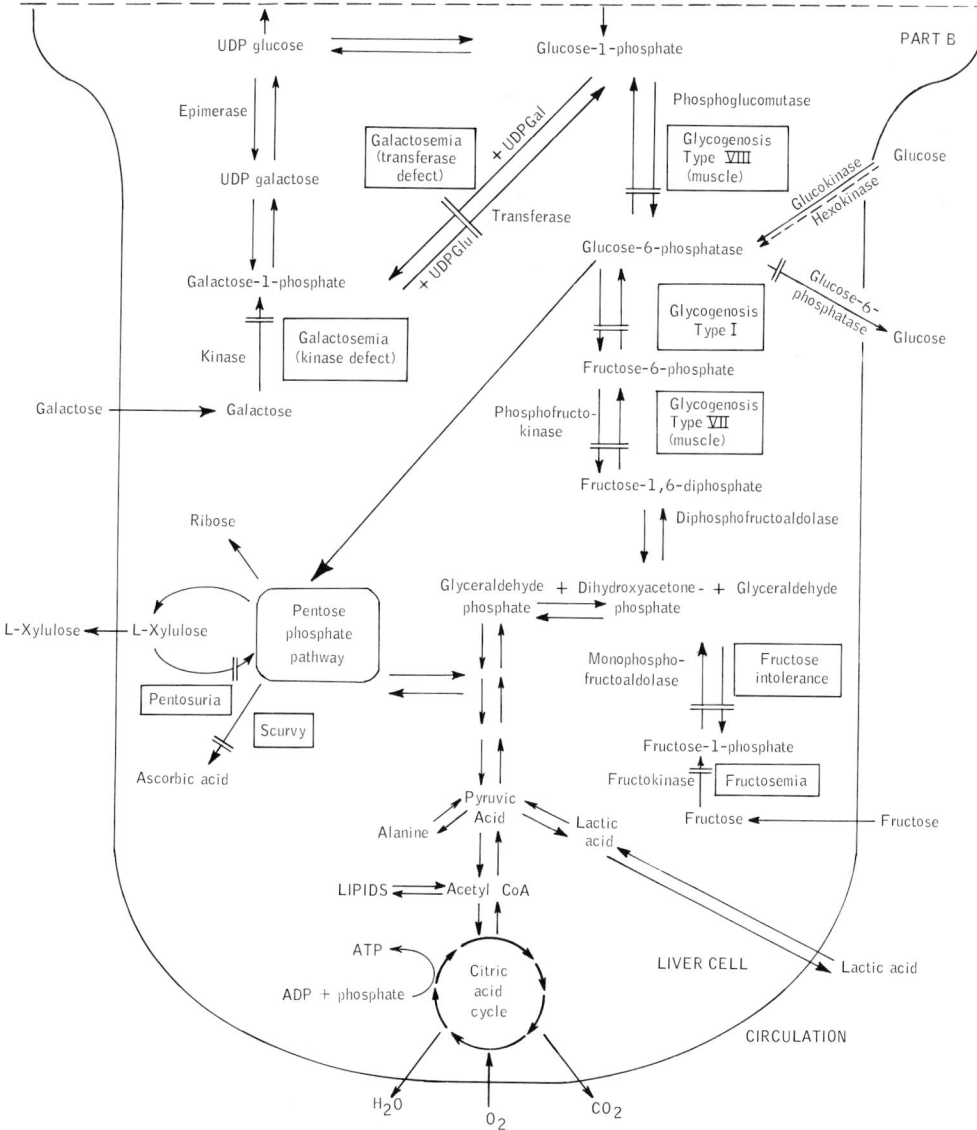

Figure 9-9 B. Pathways in the metabolism of hexoses and pentoses. See legend for Fig. 9-1.

lase activity has been found in patients with fructosemia. Systemic effects include severe hypoglycemia (see p. 1166).

GALACTOSE

Abnormal elevations of the concentration of galactose in blood result from defects in its metabolism. Two different enzymatic defects are known to produce galactosemia, but the ensuing clinical manifestations of each one are distinct. In the more common form there is almost complete deficiency of galactose-1-phosphate uridyl transferase activity, and the disorder is a serious one leading to death in infancy or to mental retardation in those who survive. The other disorder, in

which there is a deficiency of galactokinase, is rare and, in contrast, relatively benign, being characterized clinically only by the presence of cataracts. Patients with the transferase defect have been further classified into several subtypes depending largely upon the degree of enzymatic deficiency and the tissues involved. Each of the defects and variants represents distinct genotypes, and each is inherited in an autosomal recessive manner.

Galactosemia: Transferase Defect. When galactose is absorbed, it is phosphorylated in the tissues to galactose-1-phosphate. This compound reacts with uridine diphosphoglucose (UDPGlu) in the presence of the enzyme galactose-1-phosphate uridyl transferase to form uridine diphosphogalactose (UDPGal); glucose-1-phosphate is liberated. The UDPGal is then converted directly to UDPGlu by an epimerase; the new UDPGlu may again liberate glucose-1-phosphate on reaction with another molecule of galactose-1-phosphate (see Fig. 9-9, B). If the transferase activity is absent, galactosemia results. This enzyme is normally found in liver, leukocytes and erythrocytes. Sufficiently sensitive enzyme assays have been devised to allow not only for diagnosis of the homozygote, but also for the accurate detection of the heterozygote. The clinically normal heterozygote has approximately half of normal transferase activity.

CLINICAL MANIFESTATIONS. Infants appear normal at birth, but in most instances symptoms appear soon after milk feedings have been instituted. Listlessness, feeding difficulties, vomiting and weight loss are the earliest manifestations. Jaundice is common and may seem to be a prolongation of the neonatal physiologic jaundice; this symptom is caused by early hepatic damage or interference with glucuronidation of bilirubin. Hepatomegaly and occasionally splenomegaly appear early in the untreated patient and may be accompanied by signs of portal obstruction; lenticular cataracts may appear about the same time. With the onset of hepatic failure, hemorrhages, due to prothrombin deficiency, occur in skin and mucous membranes, and generalized edema and ascites may develop. Hypoglycemic symptoms may result from the low blood glucose levels even in the presence of normal or elevated *total* blood sugar concentrations. The symptoms rapidly progress to emaciation, hypotonia and death from infection or severe hepatic failure.

Occasionally the manifestations of galactosemia evolve more slowly and are milder, and the diagnosis may not be suspected until later infancy or even early childhood. The presence of hepatomegaly and retarded physical and mental development, particularly in association with cataracts, should suggest the diagnosis. A significant degree of mental retardation occurs in most infants when diagnosis is delayed beyond the first month of life.

LABORATORY DATA. Galactosuria is a constant finding when milk is fed; it rapidly disappears, however, when milk feedings are replaced by oral or parenteral administration of glucose solution. Galactose will reduce copper (Fehling's or Benedict's solution), but will not be detected by Testape or Clinistix, each of which is impregnated with glucose oxidase and reacts specifically with glucose.

There is generalized aminoaciduria resulting from damaged tubular reabsorption. Cystathioninuria may occur secondarily to the hepatic disease. Proteinuria is present in all untreated infants and may amount to 1 gm. per day. These findings are the result of the toxic effects of galactose-1-phosphate upon the kidney and disappear when galactose is removed from the diet.

Hepatic involvement is manifest by elevated levels of bilirubin and alkaline phosphatase, prolonged prothrombin time and positive cephalin flocculation test results. Blood levels of galactose are elevated, and galactose tolerance test results are abnormal. Galactose loading may result in sudden depression of glucose concentration and produce clinical manifestations of hypoglycemia. For this reason and because more specific diagnostic tests are available, galactose tolerance tests should not be performed.

The definitive diagnosis of galactosemia can be made by measurements of the specific enzyme in erythrocytes.

TREATMENT. Withdrawal of milk from the diet and substitution of a galactose-free diet result in cessation of galactosemia and galactosuria and, when done early in the clinical course, in disappearance of the abnormal clinical findings. Cataracts which persist require surgical treatment. The small quantities of galactose (less than 0.1 per cent) present in milk substitutes made with casein hydrolysates do not raise the blood galactose level high enough to cause galactosuria and are well tolerated by affected infants. Strict avoidance of milk, milk products containing galactose and such unsuspected sources as lactose-containing tablets and prepared dessert foods is essential. Galactose is an essential component of many brain lipids. Biosynthesis of these galactolipids uses UDPGal, which the body can make as needed from UDPGlu through the action of epimerase, even when the diet contains no galactose. Absence of transferase is irrelevant to this synthesis.

Dietary lapse should be suspected as a cause of an illness in a treated infant, especially if hepatomegaly or jaundice develops. In the absence of galactosuria, aminoaciduria is a sensitive indicator of the presence of galactose in the diet.

Transferase Variants. Most patients with the classic form of galactosemia cannot metabolize galactose to carbon dioxide, as demonstrated by administration of labeled galactose. A few patients, however, can metabolize galactose to a limited degree, even in the presence of clinical manifestations of galactosemia and proved absence of transferase activity in erythrocytes. All such patients thus far studied have been Negro, and it is presumed that they have an anomalous distribution of enzyme activity, and that the liver contains some transferase enzyme, although there is none in the red blood cells. This situation is in contrast to the usual one, in which the enzyme is inactive in all tissues. It is of interest that some untreated Negro infants with absent erythrocyte transferase activity have mild clinical manifestations or none at all.

In another variant of the transferase defect the affected person is completely asymptomatic. In such persons the defect is in the same enzyme, but at a different locus. The defect was discovered during a survey designed to determine the frequency of heterozygosity of the classic form of galactosemia in the general population. *The*

Duarte variant, as it is known, is characterized by a reduction of erythrocyte transferase activity to 75 per cent of normal in heterozygous persons and consequently to 50 per cent of normal activity in persons who are homozygous for this variant gene. Persons who are heterozygous for both the classic and Duarte variants have also been detected.

Galactosemia: Galactokinase Defect. A patient was described in the 1930's as having "galactose diabetes." Recent reinvestigation of this patient and observations on several new patients have revealed a deficiency of galactokinase, the enzyme responsible for the initial phosphorylation of galactose. The disease is characterized by galactosemia, galactosuria and cataracts, without mental retardation or aminoaciduria. In contrast to the transferase-deficient type of galactosemia in which both galactose-1-phosphate and dulcitol (galactitol) accumulate, in the kinase type of galactosemia only dulcitol accumulates. These observations and animal experiments suggest that the cataracts in both forms of galactosemia are caused by the abnormal accumulation of dulcitol, whereas damage to the developing brain and the renal tubules in the transferase-defect variety results from the accumulation of galactose-1-phosphate.

MISCELLANEOUS ASPECTS OF CARBOHYDRATE METABOLISM

Blood Group Substances. The immunologic differences in blood groups are complicated. The distinguishing features of the ABO system depend on the structures of *glycoproteins*, which form the blood group substances within the red cell membrane and within body fluids. The differences in the glycoproteins are referable to the presence or absence of an N-acetylgalactosamine residue or a galactose residue. For example, in persons who have the A gene, N-acetylgalactosamine is combined with the basic "O" substance through the action of the specific enzyme N-acetyl-D-galactosaminyl-transferase. Persons who lack the A gene do not have this enzyme and have blood group B or O. Persons who carry the B gene (types AB or B) have the enzyme galactosyl transferase, which adds a galactose residue to the basic blood group glycoprotein to form B substance.

Persons who have blood type substance in soluble form in various body fluids, and particularly in saliva, are called "secretors." The quality of being a secretor resides in an enzyme, fucosyltransferase, which adds the monosaccharide fucose (6 deoxy-L-galactose) to the basic blood group glycoproteins of the ABO system. Those homozygous or heterozygous for this enzyme activity are "secretors." "Nonsecretors" cannot form fucosyltransferase. They have blood group substances only on the surface of their erythrocytes. The incidence of nonsecretors varies from about 40 per cent in American Negroes to 25 per cent in Caucasians and to near 0 per cent in American Indians.

Fucosidosis (Absence of α-Fucosidase). Three children have been described with the clinical appearance of Hurler's syndrome, with progressive cerebral degeneration and mental retardation. Vacuoles described as "balloon or pseudogargoyle cells" were found in the lymphocytes and hepatic cells. Chemical analysis of tissues revealed increased amounts of mucopolysaccharides and the accumulation of 2 unusual glycolipids, in which hydrolysis revealed an elevation of fucose. The lysosomal enzyme α-fucosidase was shown to be absent in liver, brain, lung and kidney.

Mannosidosis (Deficient α-Mannosidase Activity). A boy who died at 4 years of age with signs and symptoms similar to those seen in Hurler's syndrome has been described in whom it was shown that the mannose content of tissue was abnormally high. The lysosomal enzymes which hydrolyze sugars were all present; α-mannosidase activity was markedly deficient, while the other activities, including α-fucosidase, β-galactosidase and β-glucuronidase, were abnormally elevated.

Aspartylglycosaminuria. The compound 2-acetamido-1 (β-L-aspartamido)-1,2 dideoxyglucose (AADG) is a substituted hexose which forms one of the linkage points between the carbohydrate moiety and the amino acid groups of many glycoproteins. Large quantities of AADG have been found in the urine of 2 mentally retarded siblings; one had petit mal seizures; the other, a manic-depressive psychosis. The defect of glycoprotein metabolism is in the lack of the enzyme, normally demonstrable in seminal fluid, which hydrolyzes AADG to glucosamine and aspartic acid.

Methylmalonic Acidemia. Methylmalonic acid is a structural isomer of succinic acid. The two are normally readily interconvertible in their coenzyme A forms with the aid of the enzyme methylmalonyl CoA isomerase, which requires cobamide. In vitamin B_{12} deficiency states increased amounts of methylmalonic acid are excreted in urine. Methylmalonic acid is normally derived from propionic acid and therefore from the catabolism of isoleucine, methionine and threonine and directly from valine (see Fig. 9-2). It is probably by way of these routes that methylmalonic acid appears in excessive amounts in one of the forms of glycinemia (p. 429).

Methylmalonic acidemia and massive methylmalonic aciduria were first described in 2 unrelated children who failed to thrive and exhibited bouts of severe metabolic acidosis from the time of birth. One died at 2 years of age in acute acidosis; the other, a 6-year-old girl, was treated with alkalinization and despite episodes of vomiting and acidosis had normal physical and mental development. She had had a brother who died in infancy after vomiting and failure to thrive. Loading tests with protein, valine or propionic acid led to hypoglycemia and ketosis as well as to slight increases in the excretion of methylmalonic acid. About 8 additional patients with this disorder are now known; in each of these patients in whom glycinemia was looked for, it also was present (see p. 429).

Methylmalonic acid exists in 2 stereoisomeric forms, a and b, which are interconverted through the action of a specific racemase; only the b form can be converted to succinic acid, through the action of a specific isomerase. The precise defect in methylmalonic acidemia has recently been shown to be in the isomerase. An unspecified defect in this pathway can be demonstrated in leukocytes. Some, but not all, patients with methylmalonic acidemia respond to the administration of massive doses of vitamin B_{12}, indicating that 2 forms of the defect exist, one affecting the cofactor binding site and the other a different locus.

Leigh's Encephalomyelopathy (Pyruvic Acid Carboxylase Defect). This disorder, also known as infantile subacute necrotizing encephalomyelopathy, is a progressive encephalopathy of early childhood. The onset may be in the first weeks of life or be delayed for a year or so. Clinical manifestations are variable; most patients have failure to thrive and progressive mental retardation; some have seizures, vomiting and respiratory difficulty. Most patients have bulbar symptoms and die by 4 years of age; a few have survived into the adolescent years. Postmortem examination reveals symmetrical necrosis of the basal ganglia and brain stem. The disorder is familial and appears to be inherited as an autosomal recessive.

Children with Leigh's encephalomyelopathy have been noted to have acidosis and hyperlacticacidemia and pyruvicacidemia. In one patient, assay of liver tissue did not reveal any activity for pyruvic carboxylase. This enzyme converts pyruvic acid to oxaloacetic acid, which can then either be oxidized in the citric acid cycle or participate in gluconeogenesis. The high blood levels of lactic acid have fallen temporarily in response to administration of lipoic acid, the cofactor required for the conversion of pyruvic acid to CoA. Lipoic acid is effective in reducing the lacticacidemia by aiding in the removal of excess pyruvate via the acetyl CoA pathway. It is not known whether patients with the recently described disorder of alaninemia and lactic acidosis (see p. 433) have Leigh's encephalomyelopathy, whether patients with this disorder also have alaninemia or whether the 2 conditions are identical.

Sialic Acidemia. Neuraminic acid is a condensation product of pyruvic acid and mannosamine. The N-acetyl derivative is known as sialic acid and is widely distributed in the body mucopolysaccharides, mucoproteins and brain lipids such as gangliosides. Massive excretion in urine (5 to 7 gm. per day) and elevated blood level of sialic acid have been reported in a 4-year-old boy who was retarded, and had a peculiar facial appearance and hepatomegaly. The nature of the defect is unknown.

GLYCOGENOSES: DISORDERS OF GLYCOGEN METABOLISM
(GLYCOGEN STORAGE DISEASES)

A variety of disorders result from derangements of either the synthesis or degradation of glycogen and of its subsequent utilization. This group of disorders has been known as the glycogen storage diseases, but this name is not sufficiently inclusive to encompass those disorders in which accumulation of glycogen is deficient or in which there is synthesis of glycogen with an abnormal structure. For this reason the collective term "glycogenoses" has been adopted.

In Table 9-2 the various recognized entities are grouped for clinical purposes on the basis of the principal organ or systems involved. In the first group the liver is the principal organ affected, and the symptomatology can include hypoglycemia, ketosis, acidosis, hepatomegaly and failure to thrive. In the second group, cardiomegaly is the most prominent manifestation, and patients usually die from cardiac failure in infancy, but there is also massive accumulation of glycogen in most other tissues. In the third group skeletal muscle is principally involved, and the main complaints are easy fatigability and muscular cramps. The glycogenoses have been assigned numbers (see under Type in Table 9-2) in the order in which the enzymatic defect was delineated, irrespective of clinical distinctions. Thus when the Coris discovered diminished activity of the enzyme glucose-6-phosphatase in a patient with what was then known as von Gierke's disease, the disorder became known as type I glycogen storage disease.

Chemical and physiologic understanding of each of the known glycogenoses is far from complete. Uncritical acceptance of an arbitrary classification may unwittingly convert hypotheses to truths. These in turn may be perpetuated, and an apparently suitable working classification may actually hinder rather than help comprehension of this group of diseases. It is essential for the physician or student to know that he will encounter clinical patterns which do not fit in all details into any of the present categories and that ultimately some apparent variants may be found to be entities in their own right. Furthermore, one cannot always predict the nature of the enzymatic defect from the clinical pattern. Though it is assumed that all these disorders are genetically determined, some patients have been observed with more than one type of defect, and several different types have been noted within a single kindred. To add further uncertainty, some patients have a clinical pattern with metabolic derangements simulating one or the other of the glycogenoses without having any demonstrable enzymatic defect. All these features make it essential that any categorical scheme be recognized for what it is—an arbitrary arrangement of currently available data.

Glycogen is a branched polysaccharide of high molecular weight (range three to ten million) which is present in most animal tissues. It is composed entirely of glucose units linked together by alpha 1-4 and alpha 1-6 bonds; in this respect it resembles the starches of plants. Both muscle and liver store glucose in the form of glycogen, and both can degrade glycogen to glucose and then to pyruvic and lactic acids via the Embden-Meyerhof pathway.

Certain features distinguish the carbohydrate metabolism of liver from that of muscle. Liver can and usually does synthesize glycogen from dietary glucose or by reversal of the Embden-Meyerhof pathway, using much of the lactic acid derived from muscle. Free glucose derived from stored glycogen or by synthesis from other compounds can be released into the circulation by liver after hydrolysis of glucose-6-phosphate by the enzyme glucose-6-phosphatase. Muscle, however, which does not have the enzyme glucose-6-phosphatase, cannot release glucose into the circulation; after glucose has been absorbed from the circulation, it can only be stored as glycogen, utilized with the concomitant production of lactic acid or, in the presence of sufficient oxygen, burned to carbon dioxide and water. Under anaerobic conditions, as during vigorous exercise, lactic acid accumulates and diffuses into the circulation. Part or all of the lactic acid can return to the liver and be utilized in the formation of glycogen, or it can be oxidized to carbon dioxide and water.

A large number of enzyme systems are involved in the synthesis and degradation of glycogen (Fig. 9-9). Deficiencies of activity of some of these have been implicated as causative factors for some of the clinical syndromes categorized as the glycogenoses.

Glucose enters into the synthesis of glycogen as uridine diphosphoglucose (UDPG). The enzyme uridine diphosphoglucose-glycogen-transglucosylase (UDPG-glycogen synthetase) adds glucose units derived from UDPG, one at a time, to the growing outer chains of glycogen. The attachment of these glucose units as 1-4 bonded groups is always such that it extends the chain linearly. For practical purposes the action of glycogen synthetase is not reversible. After a particular outer chain has grown to about 15 glucose units in length, another enzyme called amylo-1,4→1,6-transglucosidase (branching enzyme) dislodges a portion of this chain and transfers it intact onto a glucose residue of another chain, where it is attached at the 6 position, thus creating a branched structure. The glycogen molecule continues to grow by the combined action of these 2 enzymes. Yet another enzyme (amylo-1,4→1,4-transglucosidase) breaks off and transfers short linear chains from one part of the glycogen molecule to another point. These, however, are added onto existing chains in 1-4 linkages. In this phase the arrangement is entirely in a straight line, and there is no branching. This mechanism leads to elongation of the chain without branching.

The degradation of glycogen involves phosphorylase, an enzyme which exists in active and inactive forms; these differ by 2 molecules of phosphate. The active form is produced from the inactive form in the presence of another enzyme, phosphorylase kinase, and ATP; a phosphatase converts the active form back to the inactive one. Phosphorylase kinase is activated by adenosine-3', 5'-monophosphate (cyclic AMP), a compound whose formation is dependent upon the action of hormones such as epinephrine or glucagon. Phosphorylase removes glucose units, one at a time, from straight chains found at the outside of the glycogen molecule. From glycogen and inorganic phosphate this enzyme produces glucose-1-phosphate (G-1-P). The action of phosphorylase cannot proceed beyond a branch point in the glycogen formed by a glucose attached by a 1-6 bond and probably does not even reach to within 2 glucose residues from such branch points. Although phosphorylase can act in reverse to synthesize glycogen from glucose-1-phosphate in vitro, this is not its physiologic function, nor is it thought that much glycogen is synthesized by reversal of phosphorylase action in vivo. The few remaining glucose residues, other than the branch point itself, are removed by the action of amylo-1,4→1,4-transglucosidase. The enzyme which debranches glycogen at the 1-6 position, giving rise to free glucose, is called amylo-1,6-glucosidase. When the branch point is removed, phosphorylase may again proceed down the 1-4 linked chain, removing glucose units until it encounters the next branch point of this highly ramified molecule.

Another mechanism, entirely independent of the action of phosphorylase and amylo-1,6-glucosidase, exists within normal cells, capable of degrading glycogen to free glucose. Intracellular structures called lysosomes contain hydrolytic enzymes which act at acid pH to destroy virtually all the macromolecules normally found within the cytoplasm (glycogen, protein, nucleic acid). Among these enzymes is alpha-1,4-glucosidase (acid maltase), whose function is to hydrolyze glycogen. These lysosomal enzymes may hydrolyze the entire protoplasm of a cell and contribute to its destruction, but within viable functioning cells these enzymes destroy only portions of the protoplasm.

Thus the combined actions of the various enzyme systems are responsible for the degradation and resynthesis which maintain the protoplasm in a viable state.

Available evidence, based on pedigrees with affected siblings and in some instances consanguinity, indicates that most of the glycogenoses are probably inherited in an autosomal recessive manner. It has been suggested that type VI may be transmitted as a sex-linked characteristic, since virtually all examples occur in males. (See also comments above in respect to multiple disorders of glycogen metabolism in an individual and to different disorders in a kindred.)

TABLE 9-2.

PRINCIPAL ORGAN INVOLVED	EPONYM AND SYNONYM	TYPE	OTHER ORGANS INVOLVED	CLINICAL MANIFESTATIONS
Liver	von Gierke (hepato-renal)	Ia	Kidney, intestinal mucosa	Hepatomegaly, growth retardation, hypoglycemia, ketosis, hyperlipemia, hyperlactic acidemia; may have bleeding diathesis
		Ib	?	Same
	Forbes, Cori (limit dextrinosis)	IIIa	Muscle, heart not severely	Hepatomegaly, hypoglycemia with fasting, resembles type I; may have muscle weakness
		IIIb	None	Hepatomegaly, hypoglycemia with fasting, resembles type I
		IIId	Muscle	Hepatomegaly, hypoglycemia with fasting, resembles type I; may have muscle weakness
	Andersen (amylopectinosis)	IV	Kidney, heart, muscle, reticuloendothelial system, nervous system	Hepatosplenomegaly, portal cirrhosis of liver, no ketosis or acidosis; may be icteric; esophageal varices in 2 patients
	Hers (liver phosphorylase)	VIa	None	Hepatomegaly, hypoglycemia, acidosis. Range from mild to severe as in type I
		VIb	None	Same
	Lewis (aglycogenosis)	0	None	Severe hypoglycemia only after overnight fast. Mental retardation
Heart	Pompe (cardiac)	IIa	Muscle, liver, nervous system	Cardiomegaly hypotonia, death in first year of life
Muscle	Pompe	IIb	Liver, nervous system	Hypotonia; often survive more than 1 year
	Forbes, Cori (limit dextrinosis)	IIIc	None	Hypotonia
	McArdle (muscle phosphorylase)	V	None	Manifest as a rule in adulthood. Muscular fatigability and pain with exercise, especially after ischemic activity; myoglobinuria
	Tarui	VII	None	Same as V
	Thomson	VIII	None	Variable generalized muscular dysfunction; shortening of the gastrocnemius muscle

This table is an oversimplification of the categorization of the glycogenoses; many patients with disorders of glycogen metabolism do not fit within listed categories; however, patients have been observed and studied who qualify for each classification. Some patients have combined defects of the types noted.

THE GLYCOGENOSES

TESTS	GLYCOGEN STRUCTURE	CONTENT*	ENZYME DEFECTS
Poor hyperglycemic response to glucagon or epinephrine. Galactose or DHA increase blood lactic acid. Prediabetic type glucose tolerance curve	Normal	5-15 (L)	Glucose-6-phosphatase absent or very low
Same	Same	Same	Unknown
Hyperglycemia after glucagon only after feeding. Enzyme defect may be detected in WBC	Abnormal. Excessive branching, short outer chains	10-20 (L) 2-6 (M)	Amylo-1,6-glucosidase (debrancher) and amylo-1,4→1,4-trans-glucosidase absent or very low
Same	Same	10-20 (L)	Same
Same	Same	10-20 (L) 2-6 (M)	Amylo-1,4→1,4-trans-glucosidase absent or very low
Poor hyperglycemic response to glucagon; some response to epinephrine; abnormal glycogen can be measured in RBC. Enzyme defect may be detected in WBC	Abnormal. Very little branching, long outer chain	1-10 (L)	Low activity of amylo-1, 4→1,6-transglucosi-dase (brancher enzyme)
Poor hyperglycemic response to glucagon or epinephrine, good response to galactose. Enzyme defect may be detected in WBC	Normal	5-20 (L)	Liver posphorylase levels below 50% of normal
Same		Same	Phosphorylase kinase absent or very low
Poor hypoglycemic response to glucagon with fasting; normal response after feeding; no increase in urinary catecholamines after insulin	Normal	<0.5 (L)	UDPG-glycogen transglu-cosidase (glycogen synthetase) absent or very low
Normal tolerance tests (glucagon, epinephrine, glucose, galactose, etc.). Enzyme defect may be detected in WBC	Normal	5-15 (L) 5-10 (H) 5-15 (M) >Normal (N)	Lysosomal alpha-1,4-glucosidase (acid maltase) absent or very low
Normal tolerance tests (glucagon, epinephrine, glucose, galactose, etc.)	Normal	5-15 (L) 5-15 (M) >Normal (N)	Lysosomal alpha-1,4-glucosidase (acid Maltase) absent or very low
Normal liver function, but no increase in lactic acid after epinephrine in fasting	Abnormal. Excessive branching, short outer chains	2-6 (M)	Amylo-1,6-glucosidase (debrancher enzyme) absent or very low
No outpouring of lactic acid after epinephrine or ischemic muscular activity. Work capacity increased by glucose or fructose infusion	Normal	2-5 (M)	Muscle phosphorylase absent or very low
Same as V	Normal	2-5 (M)	Phosphofructokinase absent or very low
Very low outpouring of lactic acid after ischemic work, normal hyperglycemic response after epinephrine	Normal	3-13 (M)	Low activity of muscle phosphoglucomutase; also partial defects of other enzymes of glycolysis

*Contents in grams per 100 gm. of fresh tissue. Normal values and the symbols used are:
Liver (L), 1-5 gm./100 gm. fresh tissue.
Heart (H), 0.2-1.5 gm./100 gm. fresh tissue.
Muscle (M), 0.2-1.5 gm./100 gm. fresh tissue.
Nerve (N) by histochemical techniques only.

GLYCOGENOSES IN WHICH THE LIVER IS PRINCIPALLY INVOLVED

Hepatorenal Glycogenosis (Type I). In this disorder of glycogen metabolism, also known as von Gierke's disease, glucose-6-phosphatase activity is deficient in hepatic, renal and intestinal mucosal cells and results in accumulation of glycogen in these organs. The inability to release glucose from glucose-6-phosphate leads to hypoglycemia. This is accentuated after overnight fasting and during intercurrent illness. The excessive accumulation of lactic acid in the blood is evidence of impaired hepatic oxidation of carbohydrates and the glucogenic amino acids by the enzymes of the citric acid cycle. In the need for energy, fats (free fatty acids) are mobilized and are metabolized in the liver at an excessive rate to the 2-carbon level. As a consequence, glycogenolysis in liver proceeds only as far as pyruvic acid, which in turn is converted to lactic acid. These coeval events account for the ketosis, acidosis, hyperlipemia and fatty infiltration of the liver. The hyperlactic acidemia, ketosis and increased levels of free fatty acids in blood all disappear or ameliorate after administration of glucose. Since hypoglycemia is the normal state in these patients, increased mobilization of fat is almost constant, and explains the hypertriglyceridemia. Whereas the response to intramuscular injection of glucagon in the normal subject is hyperglycemia, in these patients it causes further elevation of lactic acid in the blood. The presence of normal or relatively increased fat depots and the deficient development of skeletal muscle may account for the doll-like appearance of many of these patients.

The enlarged, smooth liver may contain 5 to 15 per cent of glycogen in fresh tissue; the average normal content is 3 per cent (range 1 to 5 per cent). The hepatic cells are large, with small, centrally placed nuclei; the cytoplasm is filled with glycogen and in stained preparations appears as an empty space if the tissue is not properly fixed in 90 per cent ethanol. Intracellular fat is increased. The kidneys are enlarged, owing to accumulation of glycogen in the renal convoluted tubules. Histologic demonstration of apparent excess glycogen in liver cells is not sufficient evidence of hepatic glycogenosis; quantitative and qualitative chemical determinations of biopsied liver tissue are essential and should reveal more than 5 per cent of glycogen and a normal molecular structure.

The presence of excess glycogen in hepatic or renal cells is not necessarily evidence of a deficiency in glucose-6-phosphatase. In a few patients, who have otherwise conformed to the generally accepted criteria of this form of glycogenosis, no deficiency of glucose-6-phosphatase is demonstrable and the basic defect of the disorder is unknown. For the sake of categorization the disorder in these patients has been termed type Ib, and type Ia is applied to the form in which the enzyme deficiency is demonstrable.

CLINICAL MANIFESTATIONS. Both the severity and the prognosis of the illness vary. In the majority of instances the onset is insidious. Hepatomegaly is present at birth, but the abdominal enlargement may go unnoticed, since there are often no other symptoms during the first year of life. Gradually symptoms of hypoglycemia appear. Vomiting, more common at night, is frequent. Drowsiness, twitching and occasionally coma or convulsions may occur. Clinical manifestations of ketosis and acidosis are common complications of inanition accompanying intercurrent infections. Retardation of growth commonly results in dwarfism.

Occasionally the disorder is manifest within the neonatal period by dehydration and acidosis. Such infants are severely affected by the disorder and have fatty infiltration of the liver. Many die in early infancy.

Acetonuria is common and is increased during fasting. Ketoacidemia and elevated levels of lactic acid in the blood lower the plasma carbon dioxide content. The fasting level of blood glucose is low, though it is remarkable that hypoglycemic manifestations are often not evident even with blood glucose levels below 30 mg. per 100 ml. Hyperlipemia is common, and the serum inorganic phosphate levels may be low. A serious bleeding diathesis with thrombocytosis has been observed in a number of patients.

Several reports of adults with this disease suggest that the prognosis may not be as serious as was once suspected. In a few adults a defect in glucose-6-phosphatase activity has been associated with tophaceous gout. This was undoubtedly related to high levels of circulating uric acid, which are found in most examples of the type I defect, even in childhood, and appear to be secondary to hyperlacticacidemia; lactate competes with urate for renal excretion. Hepatic carcinomas have been observed in 3 adolescent patients with this disease.

DIAGNOSIS. Clinical studies are essential to determine whether a liver biopsy is indicated. Fasting hypoglycemia, hepatomegaly without evidence of parenchymal liver disease, and an abnormal response to intramuscular injection of glucagon (100 micrograms per kg.) suggest the diagnosis of hepatic glycogen disease. In the normal subject there is an increase in blood glucose of at least 70 mg. per 100 ml. within 30 minutes after injection of glucagon, whereas in patients with this disorder the increase will not be greater than 30 mg. per 100 ml. The glucose tolerance curve is characterized by a low fasting blood level of glucose, a high elevation following ingestion of glucose, which decreases slowly over several hours. A further increase in the usually elevated level of lactic acid follows ingestion of a test load of galactose, glucagon or dihydroxyacetone (DHA), a change not observed in normal persons.

Treatment. Though there is no corrective therapy for the biochemical defect in the liver, symptomatic measures can provide some relief by approximating physiologic levels of blood glucose. Four or more meals daily are advisable, the last being given at midnight. There is some rationale for limiting intake of lactose (milk), since galactose will augment the hyperlacticacidemia. A diet high in protein, though without effect upon levels of glucose in blood, may produce less postprandial hyperglycemia and thus may lessen release of insulin and in turn reduce the extent of the hypoglycemia. The administration of zinc glucagon immediately postprandially twice a day has been of value in some children.

Prolonged withholding of food for diagnostic procedures should be avoided. The ease with which acidosis and hypoglycemia develop in the course of an infection should be anticipated and prevented by provision of adequate amounts of fluid containing glucose and sodium lactate or bicarbonate.

Glycogenosis of Liver and Muscle (Type III; Limit Dextrinosis; Forbes's Disease). Debranching of glycogen involves 2 enzymes, amylo-1,6-glucosidase and amylo-1,4→1,4-transglucosidase. These enzymes are normally present in both liver and muscle. Deficiency of one or the other or of both enzymes can occur in liver or in muscle or in both tissues in varying combinations. Of the 15 possible combinations of defects, four have been described (see Table 9-2); two involve both liver and muscle, one involves only liver, and one involves only muscle. In all instances the glycogen which accumulates is abnormal not only in amount, but also in its molecular structure. Analysis reveals an excessive number of branch points, owing to deficiency of the debranching system.

The clinical manifestations are dependent on the tissues involved. The hepatic disturbances in types IIIa, IIIb and IIId are similar to those of type I glycogenosis, but are often milder. Muscular involvement is manifested by variable degrees of weakness.

Diagnosis. The responses to the various tolerance tests except that to glucagon are similar to those in patients with type I glycogenosis (see above). The response of the blood glucose to administration of glucagon is negligible in the fasting state, but after a meal high in carbohydrate there is a significant increase in the level of glucose. The administration of epinephrine, in the fasting state, will not result in an increase in blood lactic acid when there is involvement of the muscle. The amylo-1,6-glucosidase can be demonstrated in leukocytes; it is absent in some patients. Markedly increased amounts of abnormal glycogen have been demonstrated in erythrocytes in some patients and not in others. The significance of this discrepancy is not known; it is possible that it may be a distinguishing feature between subtypes, but in many of the earlier reported cases only 1 of the 2 enzymes was assayed.

Biopsy material should include muscle as well as liver. Glycogen from affected tissue has an excess of short outer branches. In some instances of type III glycogenosis the activity of hepatic glucose-6-phosphatase has also been low. This activity was brought to normal levels in at least one case by treatment with triamcinolone.

Glycogenosis Associated with Hepatic Cirrhosis (Type IV; Amylopectinosis; Andersen's Disease). In this very rare type of glycogenosis an abnormally structured glycogen accumulates in liver, kidney, spleen, muscle and nervous system. Clinically, there are growth retardation, hepatosplenomegaly, cirrhosis, and ascites, and, in some instances, icterus and esophageal varices. Hypoglycemic crises, ketosis and acidosis are absent, and the fasting blood sugar levels and the glucose tolerance curves are within normal ranges. The response to epinephrine and glucagon is poor. Impaired hepatic function is manifest by abnormal results in thymol turbidity and cephalin flocculation tests, by low serum albumin and elevated serum globulin levels, by Bromsulphalein retention, by increased serum bilirubin concentration, and increased levels of such serum enzymes as transaminases and aldolase.

The glycogen is characterized by an abnormal molecule with decreased branching resembling amylopectin. A deficiency of the enzyme amylo-1,4→1,6-transglucosidase has been demonstrated in hepatic tissue and in leukocytes of affected patients. The abnormal glycogen can be demonstrated in erythrocytes. The fibrosis which occurs in liver and on occasion in other tissues containing normal glycogen has been attributed to a foreign body reaction. Patients have all died in infancy or childhood. Treatment is entirely symptomatic. In one patient intravenous administration of α-glucosidase of fungal origin for 4 days resulted in a decrease of hepatic glycogen content from 11 to 1 per cent without altering the clinical course of the disease.

Glycogenosis Due to Deficiency of Liver Phosphorylase (Type VI; Hers's Disease). In this disorder an abnormal amount of normally structured glycogen accumulates in the liver (5 to 20 per cent of fresh tissue) and is associated with a decrease (50 per cent or more) in activity of liver phosphorylase. In some patients the defect is in the phosphorylase enzyme itself, whereas in others the defect is in the specific kinase which activates the phosphorylase. The clinical manifestations, which are mild, are similar to those of type I. The observed differences between the type I and type VI disorders include a lesser degree of fasting hypoglycemia and somewhat higher hepatic concentrations of glycogen in type VI, and a difference in the response to orally administered galactose. In type VI the administration of galactose results in a rise in glucose, but not in galactose levels in blood, and a significant increase in the lactic acid concentration, whereas in type I there is a significant increase in the already elevated blood level of lactic acid and no alteration in the level of glucose. A low activity of phosphorylase has also been demonstrated in leukocytes of patients with the type VI disorder. Analyses of several kindreds with this glycogenosis suggest a sex-linked mode of inheritance; however, the phosphorylase kinase variety may be inherited in an autosomal recessive manner.

Aglycogenosis (Defect in Synthesis of Glycogen). A form of glycogenosis in which the basic defect is inability to synthesize glycogen in adequate amounts has been described. A biopsy of the liver from one patient and autopsy material from another have revealed fatty metamorphosis, an abnormally low glycogen content (less than 0.5 gm. per 100 gm. of fresh tissue) and absence of activity of the enzyme UDPG-glycogen transglucosylase (glycogen synthetase). This enzyme is responsible for the glycogen synthesized in normal persons; a small amount of glycogen may possibly be produced by reversal of the phosphorylase action. Clinically, the outstanding manifestation is severe hypoglycemia after overnight fasting. Hypoglycemic convulsions, lethargy, vomiting and mental retardation have been observed. Response to the glucose tolerance test is characterized by a sharp rise in blood glucose from a low fasting level and a delayed return to hypoglycemic levels. There is essentially no response to the epinephrine test in the fasting state while the patient is hypoglycemic, and a normal response after feeding.

GLYCOGENOSES INVOLVING PRINCIPALLY CARDIAC MUSCLE

Type II; Generalized Glycogenosis (Pompe's Disease). In only one of the recognized glycogenoses (type IIa) is cardiac muscle sufficiently involved to be responsible for severe cardiac dysfunction. In types III and IV there is some deposition of abnormally structured glycogen in cardiac muscle, but no significant handicaps appear to be related to it. By contrast, in the classic form of Pompe's disease (type IIa), the significant clinical disorder is the cardiac involvement, though skeletal muscle and liver also have abnormal accumulations of glycogen (see Table 9-2).

Massive glycogen deposition in the cardiac muscle produces a "lacework" appearance of the fibers in microscopic sections and is responsible for massive enlargement of the heart. Accumulation of glycogen also increases the diameters of voluntary muscle fibers. In fact, the storage of glycogen in skeletal muscle in this illness is greater than that usually observed in other glycogenoses. The enzymatic defect in liver, cardiac and skeletal muscle is absence or deficient activity of lysosomal alpha-1,4-glucosidase (acid maltase). There are no detectable derangements of the Embden-Meyerhof pathway; the results of tolerance tests with glucagon, epinephrine, glucose or galactose are within the normal ranges. Serum

lipid concentrations are also within normal ranges.

Symptoms related to impaired cardiac function may be manifest at birth and in most instances become evident within the neonatal period. Cyanosis, dyspnea, tachypnea and restlessness are common. With advancing cardiac embarrassment, anorexia, listlessness and cough may appear. The heavy infiltration of glycogen in other tissues may produce clinical manifestations which are confusing. Mistaken diagnoses of Down's syndrome, cretinism and amyotonia congenita have been made on the basis of thickening of the tongue and extreme muscular hypotonicity. Neurologic abnormalities may be prominent when there is massive infiltration of the central nervous system with glycogen. The heart is greatly enlarged and has a circular appearance in roentgenograms. Murmurs are usually absent. Electrocardiographic tracings may show pronounced left axis deviation, inverted T waves and widened QRS complexes.

Though this disorder is rarely diagnosed before death, it should be considered a possibility in all infants under a year of age with cardiac enlargement and failure not otherwise readily explained. Demonstration of increased glycogen content in muscle and liver obtained at biopsy supports the diagnosis, but demonstration of lack of activity of alpha-1,4-glucosidase is necessary for definitive diagnosis. Leukocytes from patients with the disorder also have very low acid maltase activity, but some clinically normal persons also have deficiency of this enzyme.

Aberrant origin of a coronary artery from the pulmonary artery, transposition of the great vessels, cor pulmonale in cystic fibrosis, acute interstitial myocarditis and endocardial sclerosis, in particular, must be considered in the differential diagnosis.

Other than symptomatic therapy, no treatment is available. Alpha-glucosidase prepared from a mold has been used experimentally with only transient improvement. Death usually occurs within the first year of life.

GLYCOGENOSES WITH MUSCULAR MANIFESTATIONS

For some time after the identification of so-called von Gierke's glycogen storage disease of the liver and Pompe's glycogen storage disease of the heart, it was thought that these two represented the clinical variants of disordered glycogen metabolism. It has become evident, however, that there are other entities and that those involving the skeletal muscles or the nervous system are a relatively important segment of the glycogenoses (see Table 9-2).

Phosphorylase Deficiency (McArdle's Syndrome). The disorder in glycogen metabolism in type V glycogenosis, or McArdle's disease, is limited to the skeletal muscle. There is an abnormal accumulation of glycogen, owing to an absence or deficiency of phosphorylase in striated but not smooth muscle. Although the disease is usually manifest in childhood, most patients have not been detected until adulthood. The disorder is characterized by muscular weakness and pain following exercise which is out of proportion to the exertions; these symptoms may abate if exercise is continued. Exercise under ischemic conditions, with a cuff applied at greater than arterial pressure, can be carried out for only a short time. Under these conditions the usual increase in the lactic acid concentration of the venous blood returning from the ischemic muscle does not occur. Hyperlacticacidemia is not observed after the administration of epinephrine. Muscle biopsy reveals abnormal amounts of normally structured glycogen, and enzyme assays reveal absent or extremely low activity of muscle phosphorylase. Other enzymes involved in glycogenolysis are not altered. The heart is not involved, and patients tolerate the disorder well, provided they do not overexert. Myoglobinuria has been observed to follow prolonged exercise.

Phosphofructokinase Deficiency. Four patients, three of them siblings, of both sexes, have been studied who had all the clinical manifestations of McArdle's disease, including easy fatigability, cramps, myoglobinuria and inability to produce lactic acid after ischemic muscular exercise, but who differed biochemically in that they had a deficiency in their muscles of phosphofructokinase rather than of phosphorylase (type VII). In addition to elevated levels of glycogen, their muscles also accumulated abnormal amounts of glucose-6-phosphate and fructose-6-phosphate. Measurement of phosphofructokinase activity of blood cells revealed normal activity in leukocytes and about one-half normal activity in erythrocytes. In one of the studies both parents also had lower than normal levels in erythrocytes. The disorder appears to be inherited in an autosomal recessive manner.

Phosphoglucomutase Deficiency. Another form of glycogenosis with abnormal accumulation of normally structured glycogen in skeletal musculature has been described in one patient. The symptomatology was similar to that seen in McArdle's disease, but muscle phosphorylase activity was normal. In this patient a deficiency in the activity of muscle phosphoglucomutase and partial defects of other aspects of glycolysis were

demonstrated (type VIII). The patient was in good general health. His gastrocnemius muscles were bulky and were shortened to such an extent that he walked on the foreparts of his feet.

Amylo-1,4-Glucosidase Deficiency (Pompe's Disease). In type IIb of Pompe's disease there is little or no cardiac involvement, and the significant disturbance results from abnormal accumulations of glycogen in skeletal muscle and nervous tissue. The enzyme alpha-1,4-glucosidase is absent in liver and skeletal muscle. Clinically, the disturbance is characterized by hypotonia with muscular weakness and moderate hepatomegaly. Mental function is normal. It is one of the entities of the so-called amyotonia congenita syndrome. In contrast to type IIa with cardiac involvement, patients with type IIb live beyond the first few years of life.

Amylo-1,6-Glucosidase Deficiency (Limit Dextrinosis). In type III glycogenosis (limit dextrinosis, or Forbes's disease) there is muscular involvement in 3 of the 4 subtypes. In one type the disordered metabolism is limited to skeletal muscle and is manifest by hypotonia and weakness. The metabolic diagnosis is discussed above and outlined in Table 9-2.

DOUBLE ENZYMATIC DEFECTS

The simultaneous occurrence of 2 different enzymatic abnormalities such as those of phenylketonuria and cystathioninemia in the same person is very rare and is expected to happen by chance with a frequency which is the product of likelihoods of having each defect by itself. Among the glycogenoses, however, the occurrence of 2 enzymatic errors in the same person is not infrequent. This is particularly evident in type III. Other combinations of 2 enzymatic defects have been reported, and a number of sibships have been studied in which 2 children have different types of glycogenosis. The genetic mechanisms underlying these associations are poorly understood. One consequence of such observations is that biopsy material should in every instance be assayed for as many enzymes involved in carbohydrate metabolism as is technically feasible.

DEFECTS OF METABOLISM OF PYRIMIDINES AND PURINES

Purines and pyrimidines are heterocyclic nitrogen-containing compounds which, in conjunction with ribose or deoxyribose and phosphate, form the nucleotides. Ribonucleotides containing adenine and uracil are important energy-producing compounds or cofactors (ATP, UDPG, DPN,

TPN, and so on) involved in many metabolic reactions. The ribonucleotides make up ribonucleic acid, and the deoxyribonucleotides form deoxyribonucleic acid. Purines and pyrimidines are constantly being synthesized and degraded; genetic defects are recognized in each phase. The impor-

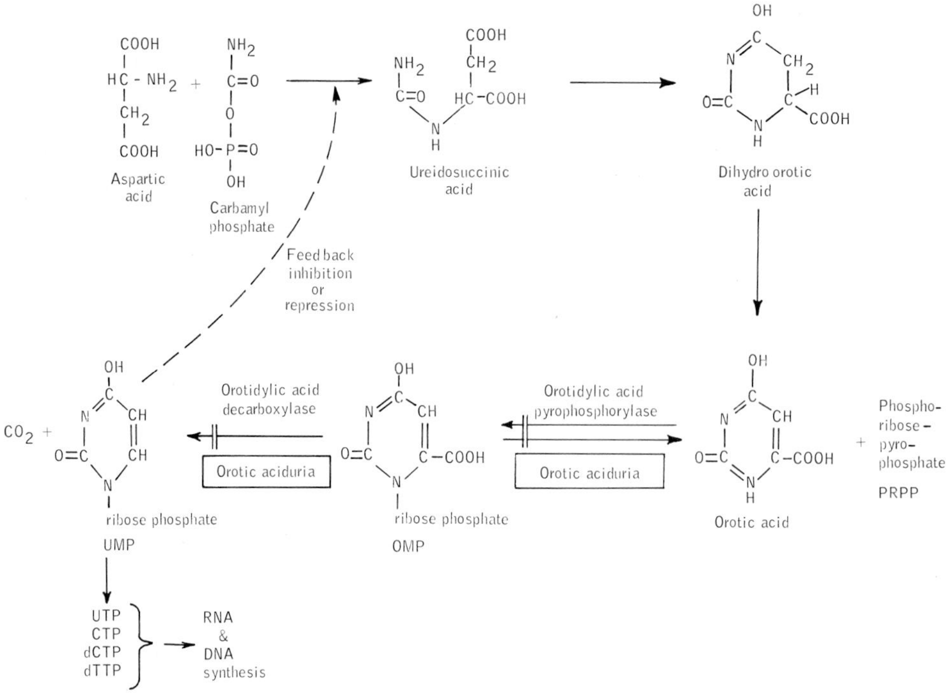

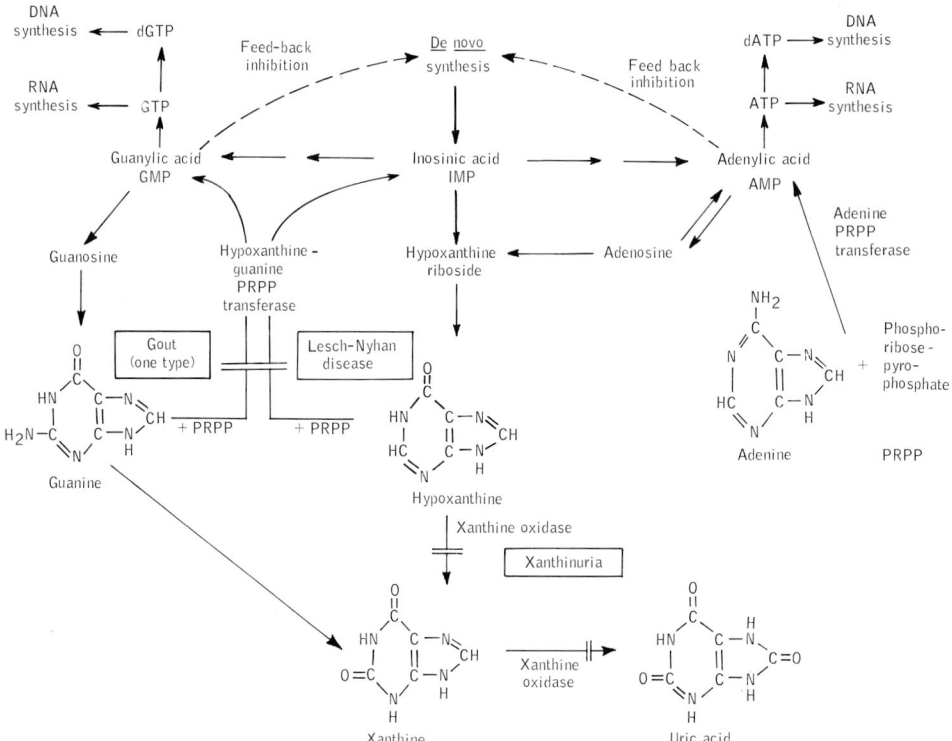

Figure 9-10. Pathways in pyrimidine biosynthesis. See legend for Fig. 9-1.

Figure 9-11. Pathways in purine metabolism and salvage. See legend for Fig. 9-1.

tant purines are adenine and guanine; the important pyrimidines are thymine, cytosine and uracil.

Orotic Aciduria. Orotic acid is an intermediate metabolite in the synthesis of pyrimidines. A block in the further metabolism of orotic acid, resulting in its excretion up to 1.5 gm. per day, has been observed in 5 persons. All had a megaloblastic anemia which did not respond to therapy with vitamin C, folic acid or vitamin B_{12}, and all formed orotic acid crystals in urine. In two of the patients therapy with a corticosteroid resulted in general improvement, but disappearance of abnormalities in the marrow and of excretion of orotic acid were noted only after administration of the pyrimidine nucleotides or nucleosides.

Two enzymes in the pathway distal to orotic acid, orotidylic acid pyrophosphorylase and orotidylic acid decarboxylase (see Fig. 9-10), were absent in liver, erythrocytes, leukocytes and fibroblasts grown in tissue culture. Heterozygotes have approximately half of both enzyme activities.

The effect of pyrimidine derivatives in lowering the excretion of orotic acid indicates that the enzymes in the pathway leading to orotic acid synthesis are under feed-back inhibition control. The hematologic response is directly due to the provision of essential material for DNA and RNA synthesis which cannot be made *de novo*. The fact that 2 enzymes in a sequence are missing indicates that the mutation probably involves a controller gene rather than a structural alteration of enzyme proteins. This view is further supported by the observation that fibroblasts from affected persons, grown in the usual tissue culture media, lack these enzyme activities, but exhibit near normal activities when grown in the presence of 6-azauridine, a compound which raises the activity of both enzymes in normal cells in tissue culture.

Xanthinuria. The catabolism of purines in man is completed at uric acid, which is then excreted in the urine. Xanthine is the immediate precursor of uric acid and is formed directly from certain purines, whereas hypoxanthine is formed from others. The oxidation of hypoxanthine to xanthine and of xanthine to uric acid is mediated by the enzyme xanthine oxidase, found in liver and intestinal mucosa (see Fig. 9-11).

Three patients with xanthinuria have been studied extensively. They have low levels of hypoxanthine and uric acid in the urine and plasma, and their excretion of uric acid decreases to zero on a purine-free diet. One of the patients, a 4½-year-old girl, had a xanthine stone; the other patients, both adults, did not have urinary stones. How many other persons with xanthine stones may have this defect is unknown. Jejunal biopsy of one of the affected adults revealed absence of activity of xanthine oxidase toward xanthine and only about 5 per cent of normal activity toward hypoxanthine. Increased renal clearances of xanthine and hypoxanthine are a natural consequence of their elevated blood levels.

Hyperuricemia (Gout). Hyperuricemia is transmitted by a dominant autosomal gene with different degrees of penetrance in the 2 sexes; it has been estimated to occur 6 to 7 times more frequently in males than in females. Among persons with hyperuricemia, gout occurs earlier and about 20 times more frequently in men than in women. Primarily a disorder of adults, gout rarely occurs in children. A notable exception is the child with type I glycogenosis in whom hyperuricemia is common and gouty tophi may develop.

Among adults with gout there are at least 2 genetic forms of the disease. In one, available evidence suggests that hyperuricemia is due to overproduction of uric acid; the disordered mechanisms are not understood. In the other group there is diminution to about 5 per cent of normal of the enzyme hypoxanthine guanine phosphoribosyltransferase (see Fig. 9-11). The enzyme has been measured in erythrocytes, leukocytes and fibroblasts, and its connection with purine metabolism is discussed below.

An association has also been described between gout and a variant erythrocyte glutathione reductase. This particular form of the polymorphic enzyme has higher activity than the usual form; both heterozygotes and homozygotes for increased glutathione reductase activity have a greater incidence of primary gout than the normal populations.

Lesch-Nyhan Disease. This disorder is characterized by mental retardation, choreoathetoid movements, scissoring position of the legs, self-mutilation and overproduction of uric acid. It is inherited by an X-linked gene; female carriers have been shown to have 2 populations of cells (Lyon hypothesis). The self-mutilation is not the result of an inability to feel pain, but of uncontrollable aggressive impulses which can be directed against others as well as self. Serum uric acid levels are in the same range (approximately 10 mg. per 100 ml.) as in patients with gout, and daily urinary excretion of uric acid approaches 1 gm. Gouty tophi appear in older patients and can be controlled with allopurinol; although it is effective in adults with gout, azathioprine does not lower serum uric acid levels in Lesch-Nyhan disease.

The enzymatic defect consists in the complete absence of hypoxanthine guanine phosphoribosyltransferase activity, and has been demonstrated in erythrocytes and fibroblasts. The role of this enzyme is of interest. Purines such as guanine and adenine, which are required for RNA, DNA and coenzyme synthesis, can be obtained from the diet or synthesized *de novo* from available metabolites. These same purine bases are normally catabolized via hypoxanthine and xanthine and excreted as uric acid. A reutilization mechanism conserves some of the hypoxanthine, which, with the addition of a ribose phosphate group, converts the base hypoxanthine to its nucleotide, inosinic acid. This is accomplished through the enzyme hypoxanthine guanine phosphoribosyltransferase. The same enzyme converts the base guanine to its nucleotide, guanylic acid (see Fig. 9-11). The concentrations of these 2 nucleotides and of adenylic acid (which is formed from the base adenine by a different enzyme) control by feed-back inhibition the rate of *de novo* synthesis of inosinic acid. In the absence of these salvage mechanisms for reutilization of hypoxanthine and guanine there is an inability to maintain the nucleotide levels required for feed-back inhibition of purine synthesis; excessive purines are synthesized and excess uric acid is excreted.

In Lesch-Nyhan disease, absence of the crucial enzyme for purine salvage and the clinical manifestations of the disorder appear to be referable to this occurrence. Only a few patients with gout have a significant deficiency (5 to 10 per cent of normal) of hypoxanthine guanine phosphoribosyltransferase activity. It is surprising that complete absence of activity produces the severe neurologic manifestation of Lesch-Nyhan disease, whereas 90 to 95 per cent loss of enzyme activity leads only to gout.

Miscellaneous Disorders Involving Purines. Pseudouridine is a nucleoside found in transfer RNA and microsomes and differs from uridine in that the ribose is attached to the uracil base at a carbon atom instead of a nitrogen atom. Some pseudouridine is normally excreted in urine, and increased amounts in persons with gout. Excretions of pseudouridine of 2 to 3 times the normal amount have been observed in 2 mentally retarded brothers. The cause is unknown.

Urinary stones consisting of uric acid have been found in 4 members in 3 generations of a family with normal serum uric acid levels and average daily excretion of uric acid. Uric acid crystals were found nevertheless in the distal urinary tract, leading to irritation. Studies suggested a specific disorder of tubular glutaminase as the causative factor responsible for a highly acid urine, precipitation of uric acid and formation of stones.

DEFECTS IN METABOLISM AND TRANSPORT OF LIPIDS

The hereditary defects in the metabolism and transport of lipids may be grouped in 4 categories: (1) excessive accumulations of lipids in the plasma, hypercholesterolemia and hyperglyceridemia; (2) deficiencies in plasma lipids, abeta-lipoproteinemia and analpha-lipoproteinemia; (3) accumulations of abnormal amounts of lipids within cells: Gaucher's disease, Niemann-Pick disease, Tay-Sachs disease and other syndromes; and (4) defective synthesis of adrenal steroid hormones (p. 1212.

In the lipidoses (p. 453) the accumulation of various lipids follows the genetic loss of an enzyme (usually lysosomal in location) which degrades the sphingolipids. Recently the first case of an enzyme deficiency in an anabolic pathway involving sphingolipids has been demonstrated. Krabbe's disease, or globoid leukodystrophy, is caused by the lack of an enzyme which transfers a sulfate molecule to hexose ceramide, forming a sulfatide. Patients with Krabbe's disease lack sulfatides. In metachromatic leukodystrophy these same sulfatides accumulate, owing to the absence of an enzyme which removes the sulfite group.

Generalized gangliosidosis (also known as G_M disease, Norman's disease or visceral Tay-Sachs disease) has recently been shown to be due to absence of the enzyme beta-galactosidase, which removes a galactose residue from glycolipid.

The disorder resulting from the absence of the serum enzyme lecithin-cholesterol acyltransferase is discussed on page 419.

Butyric and Hexanoic Acidemia. A syndrome characterized by weakness, lethargy, dehydration, convulsions and death by 1 month of age has been described in 5 infants in 2 families. The distinguishing feature of the syndrome was the odor of sweaty feet in breath, blood and urine. The compounds producing this odor were identified as butyric and hexanoic acids.

Long-chain fatty acids are degraded by a series of reactions removing 2 carbons at a time. Once a chain length of 6 carbon atoms is reached, a new specific enzyme, green acyldehydrogenase, is required to continue fatty acid catabolism through action upon hexanoyl-CoA and butyryl CoA. This enzyme is thought to be missing in this syndrome.

EPILOGUE

The number of *recognized* inborn errors of metabolism is constantly increasing. This is due in part to the clinical identification of new syndromes and to description of the biochemical nature of the metabolic block responsible for the condition. In addition, as new methods of diagnosis have become available, some disorders, such as phenylalaninemia and the glycogenoses, once thought to result from single enzymatic defects and manifesting a broad spectrum of clinical manifestations, are now being subdivided into several distinct clinical entities, each with a different enzymatic error.

The detection of many enzymopathies can now be made early in life; large-scale detection programs utilizing screening tests for blood or urine are currently carried out. Analysis of enzymes in readily available cells such as erythrocytes and leukocytes to confirm the diagnosis is becoming increasingly possible. For many conditions, particularly those associated with mental retardation, the earlier detection takes place and effective therapy is instituted, the better is the prognosis. A vigorous effort at early detection and treatment by dietary regulation of phenylketonuria has improved the mental development of these children significantly. Other inborn errors amenable to diet therapy include galactosemia, maple syrup urine disease, glycinemia and homocystinemia. The administration of massive amounts of certain vitamins can effectively overcome an enzymatic error when the mutant enzyme can no longer effectively bind the cofactor derived from the vitamin. This is exemplified by the beneficial effects of pyridoxine in one form of cystathioninemia and in hydroxykynureninuria (pyridoxine dependency) and by the beneficial effects of cobamide in some patients with methylmalonic acidemia and glycinemia.

Replacement of a missing enzyme has always seemed a logical and desirable goal of therapy, but has not been possible except in a very limited way. In cystic fibrosis the extracellular enzyme required for proper digestion can be administered conveniently, though the underlying defect is not ameliorated. When one is dealing with an intracellular enzyme, the problem is more complex. Nevertheless the experimental administration of hydrolytic enzymes such as α-glucosidase in the treatment of some forms of the glycogenoses is a step in this direction. The feasibility of injection of microencapsulated purified enzymes, avoiding the immunologic difficulties encountered by the repeated introduction of foreign proteins, has been demonstrated in animal studies.

Detection of some inborn errors of metabolism can now be made *in utero* by cultures of cells obtained by amniocentesis. These techniques permit prenatal diagnosis with the possibility of interruption of pregnancy, when a fetus has a disastrous disease for which there is no known effective treatment.

Finally, there is reason to anticipate that with increasing knowledge of genetic mechanisms it will be possible in the future to alter the genetic constitution of an individual and to overcome some of nature's more undesirable errors.

VICTOR H. AUERBACH
ANGELO M. DiGEORGE

REFERENCES

Only those references to new observations which are not contained in the four General References cited and which are considered pertinent are listed. Original reports are often listed in the more recent references given.

General

Harris, H.: *Garrod's Inborn Errors of Metabolism.* London, Oxford University Press, 1963.

Kalow, W.: *Pharmacogenetics, Heredity and the Response to Drugs.* Philadelphia, W. B. Saunders Company, 1962.

Nyhan, W. L. (Ed.): *Amino Acid Metabolism and Genetic Variation.* New York, McGraw-Hill Book Company, Inc., 1967.

Stanbury, J. B., Wyngaarden, J. B., and Fredrickson, D. S. (Eds.): *The Metabolic Basis of Inherited Disease.* 2nd ed. New York, McGraw Hill Book Company, Inc., 1966.

Defects of Protein Metabolism

Cleaver, J. E.: Defective Repair Replication of DNA in Xeroderma Pigmentation. *Nature,* 218:652, 1968.

Gottstein, U., Yoo, D. J., and Büttner, H.: C'I-Esterase und C'I-Esterase-Inhibitor in Serum von Kranken mit hereditärem genuinem Quincke-Ödem. *Klin. Wchnsch.,* 45:230, 1967.

Kontras, S. B., and Romshe, C.: Primary Family Erythrocytosis. *Am. J. Dis. Child.,* 113:473, 1967.

Lowe, C. U., and May, C. D.: Selective Pancreatic Deficiency. *Am. J. Dis. Child.,* 82:459, 1951.

Morris, M. D., and Fisher, D. A.: Trypsinogen Deficiency Disease. *Am. J. Dis. Child.,* 114:203, 1967.

Neitlich, H. W.: Increased Plasma Cholinesterase Activity and Succinylcholine Resistance: A Genetic Variant. *J. Clin. Invest.,* 45:380, 1966.

Norum, K. R., and Gjone, E.: Familial Plasma Lecithin-Cholesterol Acyltransferase Deficiency. *Scand. J. Clin. Lab. Invest.,* 20:231, 1967.

Sheldon, W.: Congenital Pancreatic Lipase Deficiency. *Arch. Dis. Childhood,* 39:268, 1964.

Defects of Erythrocyte Metabolism

Chang, T. M. S., and Poznansky, M. J.: Semipermeable Microcapsules Containing Catalase for Enzyme Replacement in Acatalasaemic Mice. *Nature,* 218:243, 1968.

Eng, L. L., and Tarail, R.: Carbonic Anhydrase Deficiency with Persistence of Foetal Haemoglobin. *Nature,* 211:47, 1966.

Ng, W. G., Donnell, G. N., and Bergren, W. R.: Deficiency of Erythrocyte Nicotinamide Adenine Dinucleotide Nucleosidase (NADase) Activity in the Negro. *Nature,* 217:64, 1968.

Defects of Amino Acid Metabolism

Alderman, M. H., and Frimpter, G. W.: Inherited Bone Disease with Glyclyproline Peptiduria. *Clin. Research,* 16:295, 1968.

Bejar, R. A., and others: Lactic and Pyruvic Acidemia with Hyperalaninemia. Society for Pediatric Research, April 1968, p. 158.

Brodehl, J., Gellissen, K., and Kowalewski, S.: Isolierte Cystinurie (ohne Lysin-, Ornithin- und Argininurie) in einer Familie mit hypocalcämischer Tetanie. *Monatsch. Kinderheilk.,* 115, 317, 1967.

Budd, M. A., and others: Isovaleric Acidemia. *New England J. Med.,* 277:321, 1967.

Carson, N. A. J., Scally, B. G., Neill, D. W., and Carré, I. J.: Saccharopinuria: A New Inborn Error of Lysine Metabolism. *Nature*, 218:679, 1968.

Carey, M. C., Fennelly, J. J., and FitzGerald, O.: Homocystinuria. II. Subnormal Serum Folate Levels, Increased Folate Clearance and Effects of Folic Acid Therapy. *Am. J. Med.*, 45:26, 1968.

Carey, M. C., Donovan, D. E., FitzGerald, O., and McAuley, F. D.: Homocystinuria. I. A Clinical and Pathological Study of Nine Subjects in Six Families. *Am. J. Med.*, 45:7, 1968.

Cohen, B. D., Stein, I. M., and Bonas, J. E.: Guanidinosuccinic Aciduria in Uremia. *Am. J. Med.*, 45:63, 1968.

Colombo, J. P., Bürgi, W., Richterich, R., and Rossi, E.: Congenital Lysine Intolerance with Periodic Ammonia Intoxication: A Defect in L-Lysine Degradation. *Metabolism*, 16: 910, 1967.

Crawhill, J. C., and others: Beta Mercaptolactate-Cysteine Disulfide: Analog of Cystine in the Urine of a Mentally Retarded Patient. *Science*, 160:419, 1968.

Dancis, J., and others: Hypervalinemia, A Defect in Valine Transamination. *Pediatrics*, 39:813, 1967.

Drummond, K. N., Michael, A. F., Ulstrom, R. A., and Good, R. A.: The Blue Diaper Syndrome: Familial Hypercalcemia with Nephrocalcinosis and Indicanuria. *Am. J. Med.*, 37: 928, 1964.

Gerritsen, T., and Waisman, H. A.: Hypersarcosinemia, an Inborn Error of Metabolism. *New England J. Med.*, 275:66, 1966.

Goodman, S. I., and O'Brien, D.: Transient Infantile Hypermethioninemia. *Pediatrics*, 42:528, 1968.

Goodman, S. I., and others: A Syndrome Resembling Lathyrism Associated with Iminodipeptiduria. *Am. J. Med.*, 45:152, 1968.

Guall, G. E., Rassin, D. K., and Sturman, J. A.: Significance of Hypermethionaemia in Acute Tyrosinosis. *Lancet*, 1:1318, 1968.

Jaiswal, R. B., Bhai, I., and Nath, N.: Tyrosine Crystals in Bone Marrow. *Lancet*, 1:1254, 1968.

Komrower, G. M., Wilson, V., Clamp, J. R., and Westall, R. G.: Hydroxykynureninuria. *Arch. Dis. Childhood*, 39:250, 1964.

Lieberman, E., Shaw, K. N. F., and Donnell, G. N.: Cystathioninuria in Galactosemia and Certain Types of Liver Disease. *Pediatrics*, 40:828, 1967.

Lonsdale, D.: Hyperalaninemia with Pyruvicemia. *New England J. Med.*, 278:1235, 1968.

Menkes, J. H.: Idiopathic Hyperglycinemia: Isolation and Identification of Three Previously Undescribed Urinary Ketones. *J. Pediat.*, 69:413, 1966.

Morrow, G., Barness, L. A., Auerbach, V. H., and DiGeorge, A. M.: Intermittent Glycinemia and Methylmalonic Aciduria. A New Syndrome? Society for Pediatric Research, April 1968, p. 20.

Morrow, G., III, and others: Metabolic Studies in Liver Homogenates from Patients with Methylmalonic Acidemia. *Fed. Proc.*, 28:628, 1969.

Mudd, S. H., Irreverre, F., and Laster, L.: Sulfite Oxidase Deficiency in Man: Demonstration of the Enzymatic Defect. *Science*, 156:1599, 1967.

Mundel, G., Fischl, J., and Israel, S.: Hydrindicuria: A Condition Due to Disturbed Indol Metabolism. *Am. J. M. Sc.*, 252:689, 1966.

Partington, M., Scriver, C. R., and Sass-Kortsak, A. (Eds.): Conference on Hereditary Tyrosinemia. *Canad. M.A.J.*, 97:1045, 1967.

Perry, T. L., and others: Carnosinemia. *New England J. Med.*, 277:1219, 1967.

Perry, T. L., and others: Cystathioninuria in Two Healthy Siblings. *New England J. Med.*, 278:590, 1968.

Price, J. M., Yess, N., Brown, R. R., and Johnson, A. M.: Tryptophan Metabolism. A Hitherto Unreported Abnormality Occurring in a Family. *Arch. Derm.*, 95:462, 1967.

Schneiderman, L. J.: Latent Cystathioninuria. *J. Med. Genet.*, 4:260, 1967.

Scriver, C. R., Pueschel, S., and Davies, E.: Hyper-β-alaninemia Associated with β-Aminoaciduria and γ-Aminobutyricaciduria, Somnolence and Seizures. *New England J. Med.*, 274:635, 1966.

Tada, K., Ito, H., Wada, Y., and Arakawa, T.: Congenital Tryptophanuria with Dwarfism. *Tohoku J. Exper. Med.*, 80:118, 1963.

Tada, K., Yokoyama, Y., Nakagawa, H., Yoshida, T., and

Arakawa, T.: Vitamin B_6 Dependent Xanthurenic Aciduria. *Tohoku J. Exper. Med.*, 93:115, 1967.

Whelan, D. T., and Scriver, M. D.: Cystathioninuria and Renal Iminoglycinuria in a Pedigree. *New England J. Med.*, 278: 924, 1968.

Defects of Carbohydrate Metabolism

Auerbach, V. H., and DiGeorge, A. M.: Genetic Mechanisms Producing Multiple Enzyme Defects. A Review of Unexplained Cases and a New Hypothesis. *Am. J. M. Sc.*, 249: 718, 1965.

Baker, L., Mellman, W. J., Tedesco, T. A., and Segal, S.: Galactosemia: Symptomatic and Asymptomatic Homozygotes in One Negro Sibship. *J. Pediat.*, 68:551, 1966.

Brown, B. I., and Brown, D. H.: Lack of an α-I, 4-Glucan: α-1,4-Glucan 6-Glycosyl Transferase in a Case of Type IV Glycogenosis. *Proc. Nat. Acad. Sc.*, 56:725, 1966.

Fernandes, J., and Huijing, F.: Branching Enzyme-Deficiency Glycogenosis: Studies in Therapy. *Arch. Dis. Childhood*, 43:347, 1968.

Fontaine, G., and others: La Sialuria: Un Trouble Metabolique Original. *Helv. Paediat. Acta*, 23: Suppl. 17, 1968.

Gitzelmann, R.: Hereditary Galactokinase Deficiency, a Newly Recognized Cause of Juvenile Cataracts. *Pediat. Res.*, 1:14, 1967.

Hommes, F. A., Polman, H. A., and Reerink, J. D.: Leigh's Encephalomylopathy: An Inborn Error of Gluconeogenesis. *Arch. Dis. Childhood*, 43:423, 1968.

Hug, G., Schubert, W. K., and Chuck, G.: Phosphorylase Kinase of the Liver: Deficiency in a Girl with Increased Hepatic Glycogen. *Science*, 153:1534, 1966.

Hug, G., Schubert, W. K., and Chuck, G.: Type II Glycogenosis: Treatment with Extract of *Aspergillus Niger*. *Clin. Res.*, 16:345, 1968.

Kobata, A., Grollman, E. F., and Ginsburg, V.: An Enzymic Basis for Blood Type A in Humans. *Arch. Biochem. Biophys.*, 124:609, 1968.

Layzer, R. B., Rowland, L. P., and Ranney, H. M.: Muscle Phosphofructokinase Deficiency. *Arch. Neurol.*, 17:512, 1967.

Montreuil, J., and others: Description d'un noveau type de melituria, la sialurie. *Compt. rend. Acad. d. ssc.*, Paris, 265: 97, 1967.

Moses, S. W., Levin, S., Chayoth, R., and Steinitz, K.: Enzyme Induction in a Case of Glycogen Storage Disease. *Pediatrics*, 38:111, 1966.

Oberholzer, V. G., Levin, B., Burgess, E. A., and Young, W. F.: Methylmalonic Aciduria. *Arch. Dis. Childhood*, 42:492, 1967.

Öckerman, P. A.: A Generalized Storage Disorder Resembling Hurler's Syndrome. *Lancet*, 2:239, 1967.

Parr, J., Teree, T. M., and Larner, J.: Symptomatic Hyperglycemia, Visceral Fatty Metamorphosis, and Aglycogenosis in an Infant Lacking Glycogen Synthetase and Phosphorylase. *Pediatrics*, 35:770, 1965.

Pollitt, R. J., Jenner, F. A., and Merskey, H.: Aspartylglycosaminuria, an Inborn Error of Metabolism Associated with Mental Defect. *Lancet*, 2:253, 1968.

Race, C., Zinderman, D., and Watkins, W. M.: An α-D-Galactosyltransferase Associated with the Blood Group B Character. *Biochem. J.*, 107:733, 1968.

Shen, L., Grollman, E. F., and Ginsberg, V.: An Enzymatic Basis for Secretor Status and Blood Group Substances Specificity in Humans. *Proc. Nat. Acad. Sc.*, 59:224, 1968.

Sparkes, R. S., Beutler, E., and Wright, S. W.: Galactosemia in 24 Year Old Man: Detection by Enzyme Studies. *Am. J. Ment. Def.*, 72:590, 1968.

Tarui, S., and others: Phosphofructokinase Deficiency in Skeletal Muscle. A New Type of Glycogenosis. *Biochem. Biophys. Res. Comm.*, 19:517, 1965.

Thomson, W. H. S., MacLaurin, J. C., and Prineas, J. W.: Skeletal Muscle Glycogenosis: An Investigation of Two Dissimilar Cases. *J. Neurol., Neurosurg. & Psychiat.*, 26:60, 1963.

Defects of Purine and Pyrimidine Metabolism

Haggard, M. E., and Lockhart, L. H.: Megaloblastic Anemia and Orotic Aciduria. *Am. J. Dis. Child.*, 113:733, 1967.

Kelley, W. N., Rosenbloom, F. M., Henderson, J. F., and Seegmiller, J. E.: A Specific Enzyme Defect in Gout Associated with Overproduction of Uric Acid. *Proc. Nat. Acad. Sc.*, 56: 1735, 1967.

Kihara, H.: Pseudouridinuria in Mentally Defective Siblings. *Am. J. Ment. Def.*, 71:593, 1967.

Krawczynski, J., Sagan, Z., Walajtys, E., and Ilowiecka, K.: Inborn Enzymatic Defect as the Probable Cause of the Formation of Renal Stones Consisting of Uric Acid. *J. Clin. Path.*, 18:219, 1965.

Long, W. K.: Glutathione Reductase in Red Blood Cells: Variant Associated with Gout. *Science*, 155:712, 1967.

Pinsky, L., and Krooth, R. S.: Studies on the Control of Pyrimidine Biosynthesis in Human Diploid Cell Strains. II. Effects of 5-Azaorotic Acid, Barbituric Acid, and Pyrimidine Precursors on Cellular Phenotype. *Proc. Nat. Acad. Sc.*, 57:1267, 1967.

Rogers, L. E., Warford, L. R., Patterson, R. B., and Porter, F. S.: Hereditary Orotic Aciduria. I. A New Case with Family Studies. *Pediatrics*, 42:415, 1968.

Seegmiller, J. E., Rosenbloom, F. M., and Kelley, W. N.: Enzyme Defect Associated with a Sex-Linked Human Neurological Disorder and Excessive Purine Synthesis. *Science*, 155:1682, 1967.

Defects of Lipid Metabolism

Bachhawat, B. K., Austin, J., and Armstrong, D.: A Cerebroside Sulphotransferase Deficiency in a Human Disorder of Myelin. *Biochem. J.*, 104:150, 1967.

Durand, P., Barrone, C., Della Cella, G., and Phillippart, M.: Fucosidosis. *Lancet*, 1:1198, 1968.

Okada, S., and O'Brien, J. S.: Generalized Gangliosidosis: Beta-Galactosidase Deficiency. *Science*, 160:1002, 1968.

Sidbury, J. B., Jr., Smith, E. K., and Harlan, W.: An Inborn Error of Short-Chain Fatty Acid Metabolism. The Odor of Sweaty Feet Syndrome. *J. Pediat.*, 70:8, 1967.

Van Hoof, F., and Hers, H. G.: Mucopolysaccharidosis by Absence of α-Fucosidase. *Lancet*, 1:1198, 1968.

Defects of Vitamin Metabolism

Arakawa, T., Fujii, M., and Hirono, H.: Tetrahydrofolate-Dependent Enzyme Activities of Erythrocytes in Formiminotransferase Deficiency Syndrome. *Tohoku J. Exper. Med.*, 88:305, 1966.

Arakawa, T., and others: Mental Retardation with Hyperfolicacidemia Not Associated with Formininoglutamicaciduria: Cyclohydrolase Deficiency Syndrome. *Tohoku J. Exper. Med.*, 88:341, 1966.

Arakawa, T., and others: Megaloblastic Anemia and Mental Retardation Associated with Hyperfolicacidemia: Probably Due to N⁵-Methyltetrahydrofolate Transferase Deficiency. *Tohoku J. Exper. Med.*, 93:1, 1967.

THE LIPIDOSES

A "lipidosis" is a syndrome resulting from an inborn constitutional defect which has as its demarcating expression an increase in the lipid content of tissues or serum. There is a large group of such diseases, some of which have rather superficial biologic relation to each other. The anatomic hallmark of the lipidosis process is the formation of the "foam cell"—a large, primitive histiocytic element in which increased cell volume is due to the intracytoplasmic accumulation of lipid materials (Fig. 9-13). Etiologic considerations are complicated by the observation that less specific foam cells may also develop in a wide variety of acquired disease conditions (e.g. granulomas, tumors, infections, toxic states) which may mimic the true lipidosis picture. Foam cell formation in an organ characteristically results in an increase in its size and weight, a paler color and a firmer texture, producing clinical "visceromegaly." Such an occurrence may lead to a variety of somatic problems, depending on the locus (e.g. liver, spleen, lungs, marrow cavity). A frequent accompanying handicap of more critical nature is alteration in neurologic function and development, perhaps produced by a separate though commonly associated defect.

For pedagogic purposes it is customary to make principal reference to the "type" lipid, accumulation of which is specific for any given syndrome (Fig. 9-12). This may be an unjustified oversimplification which obscures a wider consideration of the underlying pathogenesis. It is possible that the presently demonstrated lipid defects in the lipidoses are actually late or partial effects, and identification of each of these disorders may ultimately include the listing of other types of more basic biochemical handicaps. For example, it is probably more justifiable to describe Gaucher's disease as a syndrome *with*, rather than *of*, glyco-lipid accumulation. A large amount of investigative work remains to be done in this field.

The inborn nature of the biochemical defects in the lipidoses implies that the anomalies have hereditary aspects. For most of the syndromes the defect is passed by recessive transmission, only the homozygously involved person having identifiable handicaps. To date, no morphologic alterations have been found in the chromosomes of patients with lipidoses. No genetic cross relations are known among the various syndromes. All affected members of any one pedigree will have a reasonably uniform clinical picture (e.g. early or late onset, neurologic defect).

There are many theories designed to explain the pathogenesis of the tissue lipid accumulation. Leading hypotheses include increased rates of lipid synthesis, structural errors during biosynthesis, pernicious local tissue binding, and diminished activity of catabolic enzymes, the last having been emphasized in recent studies of several syndromes.

GAUCHER'S DISEASE

Gaucher's disease is an uncommon disorder, encompassing a group of syndromes in which "Gaucher cells" can be demonstrated in the viscera. This cell is highly characteristic, with intracytoplasmic accumulation of cerebroside-type glycolipids (Fig. 9-13). The most common form of the disease is a relatively benign disorder, with clinical manifestations usually first evident within the pediatric age period. An unusual type, with fatal outcome, is seen in infancy.

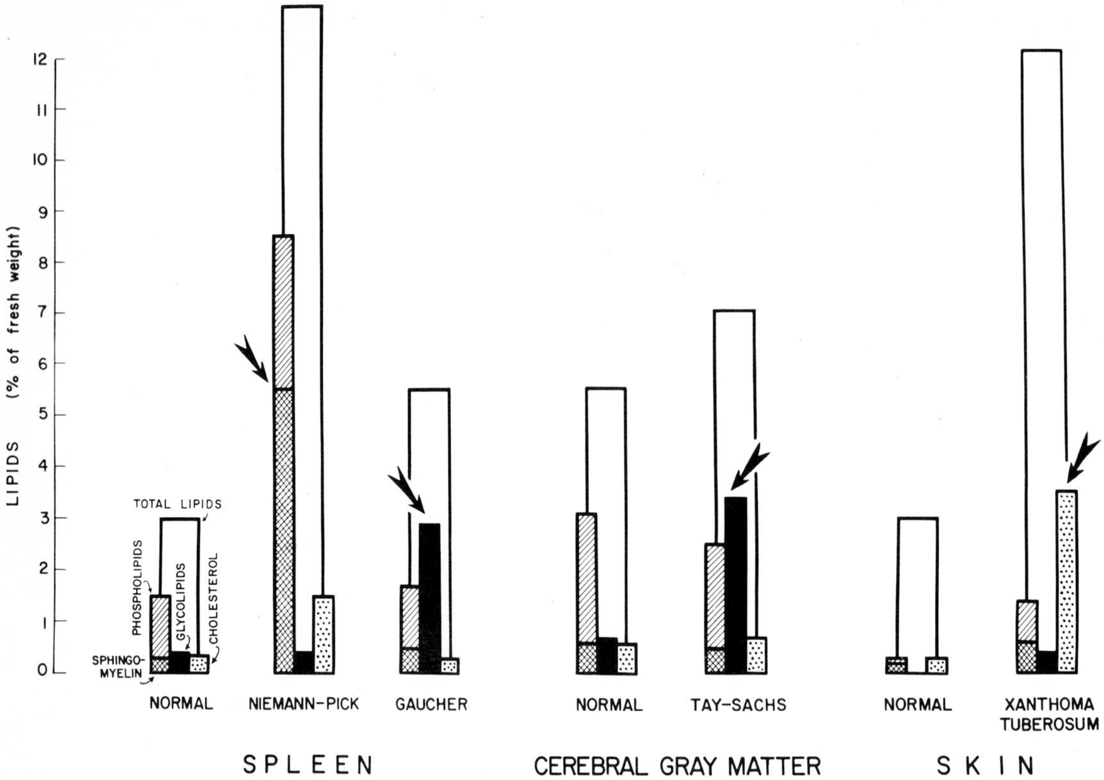

LIPIDS   (% of fresh weight)

12
11
10
9
8
7
6
5
4
3
2
1
0

TOTAL LIPIDS

PHOSPHOLIPIDS
GLYCOLIPIDS
CHOLESTEROL
SPHINGO-
MYELIN

NORMAL   NIEMANN-PICK   GAUCHER   NORMAL   TAY-SACHS   NORMAL   XANTHOMA
                                                                                                    TUBEROSUM

S P L E E N   CEREBRAL GRAY MATTER   S K I N

Figure 9-12. Typical results of analyses of tissue specimens from various lipidosis syndromes. Arrows indicate the most characteristic element of the lipid increase in each disease. (Note key to lipid components, on left.)

Etiology. In Gaucher's disease the majority of the glycolipid in the viscera is a glucocerebroside, instead of the usual form with galactose; there is a deficiency in glucocerebrosidase activity in these tissues and in the white blood cells and an elevation of acid phosphatase activity in the same tissues and in the serum. The majority of pedigrees demonstrate recessive transmission of the disease, with no abnormalities identifiable in the "carrier" heterozygotes; rare instances of undoubted dominant transmission for the chronic form have been described. About two thirds of all cases occur in Jewish pedigrees.

Pathology. The Gaucher cell is sufficiently unique in its appearance to allow tentative identification by common tissue techniques. It is a large, often multinucleated, cell with a fibrillar or wrinkled-appearing cytoplasm which is non-

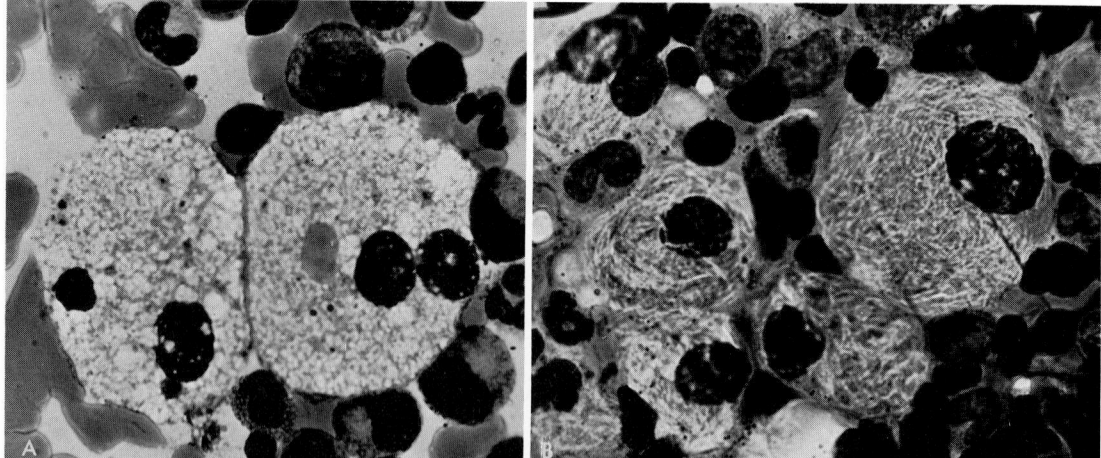

Figure 9-13. Smears from bone marrow aspirations (Giemsa stain) showing characteristic cells of Niemann-Pick disease *(A)* and Gaucher's disease *(B).* Note the bubbly, vacuolated appearance of the Niemann-Pick foam cells, as contrasted with fibrillar texture of the Gaucher cell cytoplasm.

vacuolated and pale-staining with most dyes. It is periodic-acid-Schiff positive and gives a strong acid phosphatase reaction. In chronic forms of the syndrome it is found in the bone marrow, the red and white pulp of the spleen, between liver cells and in lymphoid tissue. Splenomegaly is common; splenic weights are 5 to 18 times the normal for age.

In the infantile form, Gaucher cells are prominent in the lung, but are found in all areas of the body, even within the central nervous system. There are also some decrease in brain size, mild neuronal distention in the gray matter, neuronophagia, loss of nerve cells, gliosis and signs of poor myelination.

Clinical Manifestations. There is a wide spectrum of clinical involvement in Gaucher's disease, which can be classified in 2 general categories, each of which is constant within a given pedigree.

In the *acute* or *infantile* form there is an early onset of symptoms, which include slowed development, moderate enlargement of the liver and spleen, normal fundi, strabismus, retroflexion of the head, dysphagia and other signs of bulbar palsy, and increasing respiratory problems. Most of these infants do not survive beyond the first year of life, but occasional patients have lived until 2 to 6 years of age.

The *chronic* or *adult* form of the disease, 10 to 20 times more common than the infantile type, has a great variation in time of onset of symptoms. Abdominal enlargement is the most frequent first complaint, with splenic increase more notable than hepatomegaly. Owing to the sustained splenomegaly, the clinical signs of "hypersplenism," with suppression of the blood cell counts and even hemorrhagic manifestations, will appear. Symptoms related to the bones and joints, such as bone pain, rheumatic-like joint swelling and discomfort (often episodic and not dependent on trauma) and pathologic fractures, may also be early manifestations. The bone and joint symptoms occur only where overactivity in the medullary cavity has already produced radiologically identifiable changes. Less frequently, one finds a child who temporarily escapes the bone difficulties, but has poor growth and maturation and major enlargement of the liver with functional handicaps.

The usual time for onset of symptoms in the chronic form is middle childhood, but some patients go on to adult life before presenting medical problems. The development of scleral *pingueculae* and dermal pigmentation does not occur until after adolescence. For patients without neurologic involvement there should be no mortality from the disease itself, although the course may prove distressing because of the orthopedic difficulties. Bone pain may decrease in intensity after puberty.

Laboratory Data. Examination of bone marrow is the critical diagnostic procedure; the characteristic Gaucher cell is demonstrable in all forms of the disease. In addition, by the time the child has clinical manifestations it is usually possible to show bone changes by radiologic examination. These include signs of chronic marrow cavity overactivity with bone texture changes, extension of the usual limits of the medullary space, failure of tubulation, and occasional rarefactions in bone, seen best in the femora, but also found elsewhere as in the tibiae and humeri. In the severe situation there are fractures, "aseptic necrosis" and other deformities. Blood cell counts are normal, except with hypersplenism, when there is thrombocytopenia, anemia and leukopenia. The serum acid phosphatase level is elevated to some degree; the measurement should be made with a "Gutman-type" procedure (phenylphosphate substrate). In obscure situations, study of the removed spleen or a liver biopsy may be required for substantiation of the diagnosis.

Treatment. Clinical management of the patient with *chronic Gaucher's disease* involves (1) surveillance for signs of hypersplenism, for which splenectomy may be indicated, and (2) orthopedic supervision for the care of bone complications. Fractures are common, especially of the femoral neck, and may heal slowly. Collapse of vertebral bodies is less frequent. There may also be many disturbing periods of bone pain of less certain origin, which should be conservatively managed. The psychologic effects of the chronic and recurrent osseous problems may be severe and require much support. At present there is no effective chemotherapy, but under suitable circumstances trials of new drugs are justified. For the *infantile patient* the care program is similar to that for any severely brain-damaged baby (see p. 120).

NIEMANN-PICK DISEASE

Niemann-Pick disease includes a small, heterogeneous collection of conditions with a genetically determined abnormality. They have in common the occurrence, in such sites as bone marrow, spleen and liver, of vacuolated foam cells whose most striking chemical feature is the cytoplasmic accumulation of sphingomyelin (a phospholipid). Originally, Niemann-Pick disease was viewed as a syndrome with major neurologic handicaps, certain ethnic predilections and a uniformly fatal outcome in early life, but observations in recent years require a broader definition of the clinical picture.

Etiology. The principal hypothesis for the mechanism of Niemann-Pick disease suggests that the patient has synthesized (probably at a normal rate) a surfeit of phospholipid which he is not capable of catabolizing, either because he has formulated an abnormal tissue ingredient foreign to normal turnover systems, or because he congenitally lacks full enzymatic activity at the correct locus for phospholipid processing. Cholesterol and the monoaminophosphatides are also present in increased amounts (Fig. 9-12). The inconstant occurrence of simultaneous neurologic handicaps, and the otherwise wide variation in severity of the syndrome, require the postulation of several grades of dysfunction. To date, all pedigrees studied have demonstrated inheritance consistent with autosomal recessive transmission, and experience indicates that about one fourth of the patients in this country are of Jewish ancestry.

Pathology. The Niemann-Pick cell may be considered the prototype of foam cells. It has obviously vacuolated cytoplasm, a strongly positive reaction with fat stains (most specifically the Smith-Dietrich procedure), and is pale-appearing with other routine tissue stains (Fig. 9-13). It is widely distributed in the viscera, apparently reflecting the ubiquitous natural sites of its cell of origin. Niemann-Pick cells are most prominent in the bone marrow, spleen and lymphoid tissue of all types; they are commonly found in liver and lung, and may appear as a spurious element in the connective tissue or parenchyma of virtually any organ. Splenomegaly is important (the organ varies from 2 to 10 times normal weight for age); there is often a proportionate enlargement of the liver. When there is neurologic involvement, the brain is underweight, the gray matter is soft, with widespread neuronal distention, and there are mild deficiencies of white matter. Increased amounts of sphingomyelin can be demonstrated in cell cultures from Niemann-Pick tissues (marrow, skin and even amnion).

Clinical Manifestations. The clinical picture in Niemann-Pick disease has such broad variations, albeit relatively constant for any one pedigree, that generalizations do not pertain. At least 4 common clinical patterns are repeated, but even this list may need further extension or subdivision.

Group A. The originally described "classic" form of the syndrome has hepatosplenomegaly, early and severe handicaps, frequent occurrence of macular degeneration and blindness. Death occurs usually by 2 years of age.

Group B. A number of patients have been identified who have pathologic and biochemical abnormalities in most viscera, but no evidence (up to early adult life) of nervous system involvement. It is possible that survival potential may be normal in this interesting subgroup.

Group C. In the most common form, motor and intellectual handicaps appear in late infancy; the visceral abnormalities are quantitatively milder, and the fundi normal. The child survives to 3 to 6 years of age.

Group D. In this group affected persons have normal early development, but manifest neurologic disease in middle childhood which progresses to full dementia and paresis. Death occurs by 12 to 20 years of age.

The basic pathology for each of these groups is qualitatively similar (except for the normal brain in group B), and all must, by present definitions,

be described as having Niemann-Pick disease. Skin lesions are infrequent; occasional xanthomas are seen, but pigmentation of the skin is rarely observed.

Laboratory Data. Examination of the bone marrow is the most useful diagnostic procedure. Occasional aspirations, however, fail to yield an adequate number of abnormal cells, and in a few instances odd histiocytes with granular cytoplasm are seen. Similar foam cells may also be found in the bone marrow in other conditions, such as during cortisone therapy, in some liver tumors and in chronic hyperlipemia. Vacuolated lymphocytes and monocytes in the peripheral blood smear are a characteristic, but not invariable, sign of Niemann-Pick disease. These odd vacuoles, of uncertain origin, which occur in 1 to 10 per cent of otherwise normal agranulocytes, are seen elsewhere in comparable form only in the Swedish type of juvenile amaurotic idiocy, Wolman's disease and Norman-Landing disease (see Table 9-3). In Niemann-Pick disease there is suppression of white cells and platelets in the peripheral blood as occurs in any sustained splenomegalic syndrome; there is usually a moderate anemia. Roentgenographically, there may be diffuse pulmonary parenchymal abnormalities, especially in the first 2 clinical groups described, and the bones may show undermineralization or signs of marrow cavity overactivity. Increase of serum lipids, with moderate hypercholesteremia and even a turbid serum, is also characteristic of the patients in these 2 groups. When marrow examinations are unconvincing, or the clinical course is atypical, lipid analysis of tissues obtained by biopsy from the liver, spleen or lymph nodes may be required to establish the diagnosis.

Treatment. In contrast to Gaucher's disease, orthopedic problems are not a major issue in Niemann-Pick disease. Splenectomy may be indicated when there are significant evidences of hypersplenism. Special support for the patient with neurologic handicaps is of great importance in respect to feeding problems, mucus difficulties, seizures, and the like. To date no chemotherapeutic agent has been convincingly effective. Judicious trials of new drugs, however, are justified when adequate control can be maintained.

TAY-SACHS DISEASE

In this lipidosis one finds in the gray matter a large increase in the concentration of ganglioside, a water-soluble, neuraminic-acid-containing glycolipid (Fig. 9-12). It occurs in unique cytoplasmic organelles, masses of which distend the neuronal cell body. Many of the inborn-error syndromes have a slight increase in the content of brain ganglioside, but none to the magnitude of Tay-Sachs disease. Further, it has been shown that the increase is particularly in one special class of gan-

TABLE 9-3. PRINCIPAL FEATURES OF RECENTLY DESCRIBED LIPIDOSES

DESCRIPTIVE NAMES AND EPONYMS	AGE AT ONSET OF CLINICAL MANIFESTATIONS	PATHOLOGY	LIPID ACCUMULATED INTRACELLULARLY	INVOLVEMENT OF C.N.S.	COURSE
Primary familial xanthomatosis with involvement and calcification of the adrenals (*Wolman's disease*)	Early weeks of life	Diffuse foam cell formation in viscera, including small intestine Malnutrition	Cholesterol and triglycerides	Yes	Diarrhea, vomiting, nutritional failure Prominent calcification of the adrenals Familial involvement Death by 2-4 months of age
Angiokeratoma corporis diffusum universale (*Fabry's disease*)	Midchildhood to early adult life	Vacuolization of renal epithelial cells Changes in blood vessel walls and myocardium Neuronal distention	Ceramide trihexoside	Yes	X-linked transmission Cutaneous lesions (vascular rash) Corneal dystrophy Renal failure
Familial neurovisceral lipidosis; generalized gangliosidosis; pseudo-Hurler's disease (*Norman-Landing disease*)	Early months of life	Foam cells in viscera Glomerular epithelial cells swollen Distention of neurons	Ganglioside (G_{M1}), especially in brain Mucopolysaccharides in viscera	Yes	Spectrum of clinical expression (? includes several syndromes) Odd facies, varying visceromegaly, neurologic handicap, skeletal changes Death in 1-3 years
Tangier disease; familial high-density lipoprotein deficiency (*Fredrickson's disease*)	Childhood	Foam cells in tonsils and other reticuloendothelial tissues	Cholesterol esters (Low blood levels of cholesterol and phospholipid)	No	Large tonsils, with orange or gray color Occasional enlargement of spleen, lymph nodes or liver
Chronic reticuloendothelial cell storage disease (*Sawitsky's disease*)	All ages	Vacuolated or granular foam cells in marrow, lymph nodes, spleen and liver	? Glycolipid (not identified)	No	Asymptomatic hepatosplenomegaly May be anemic
Thrombocytopenic purpura with histiocytosis of the spleen	Middle childhood and later	Foam cells in red pulp of spleen; ? in bone marrow	Phospholipid (? especially sphingomyelin)	No	Clinical course similar to that of idiopathic thrombocytopenic purpura
Disseminated lipogranulomatosis (*Farber's disease*)	Usually early months of life Occasionally later in childhood	Granulomatous lesions of skin, synovia, viscera (some with foam cell formation); distention of neurons	Ceramide (also ganglioside and ? mucopolysaccharide)	Usual	Typically produces hoarse cry, subcutaneous nodules, arthropathy, irritability and nutritional failure Milder form also known
Pigmented lipid histiocytosis; chronic granulomatous disease of childhood (see p. 478)	Early childhood	Abscesses and reactive granulomas in lymph nodes and viscera Varying degrees of foam cell formation	Has chromolipoid (ceroid-like) Other materials not identified	No	Almost invariably males Increased susceptibility to infection, with debilitating course Phagocytic handicap in circulating granulocytes

glioside, so-called G_{M2} or "Tay-Sachs ganglioside." There are also minor electron microscopic and chemical changes in viscera other than the nervous system (e.g. liver). Of unknown pertinence is a deficiency in the serum of these patients of the enzyme, fructose 1,6-diphosphate aldolase, which is also partially reduced in relatives who are heterozygously involved (genetic carriers).

See page 1294 for the clinical description of the syndrome.

RECENTLY DESCRIBED SYNDROMES

In the past decade a large number of newly identified syndromes have been described as belonging in the lipidosis category. The principal features of 8 such diseases are given in Table 9-3. Most of these syndromes are rare, but it is likely that many more affected children will be found as familiarity is gained with the clinical and pathologic patterns. There are intriguing potentials for research in this special field. When tissue specimens are available from patients of this sort, it is advisable to retain portions in a frozen, unfixed state for study in one of the laboratories now doing investigative work in the lipids and mucopolysaccharides.

SYNDROMES WITH INCREASED BLOOD FAT

Secondary Hyperlipidemia. The content of fat in the blood of children may be increased in a variety of circumstances. The most common situations are *secondary*, dependent for degree upon the evolution of medical diseases in which lipid metabolism is altered as a byproduct of disturbances in the metabolism of carbohydrate or protein, as, for example, in diabetic acidosis, the von Gierke type of glycogenosis, and the nephrotic syndrome. During compensated phases of these illnesses the serum lipids return to normal or near-normal values. The hyperlipidemia provides an index of the progress of the disease, but it does not in itself require any special considerations in treatment beyond that directed at the primary metabolic disorder. The milky or lipemic appearance of the serum in the foregoing diseases is due principally to excess of triglycerides (neutral fat). One can expect a frank turbidity to appear whenever the triglyceride concentration exceeds 1000 mg. per 100 ml. (normal level 0 to 200 mg.). Characteristically, such patients also have moderate increases in the phospholipid and cholesterol values of the serum.

Significant increases in the blood lipids also occur, with a clear-appearing serum, in children with intrahepatic biliary atresia. In this instance the concentration of the triglycerides is not elevated, but there is a great increase in the phospholipid and cholesterol levels (up to 3000 to 5000 mg. per 100 ml.). The use of vegetable oil supplements in the diet lessens this hyperlipidemia considerably, as does also the use of bile-acid-absorbing resins. Other less frequent causes of increased blood lipid levels in children include hepatic tumors, hypothyroidism, severe anemia, and Niemann-Pick disease.

Primary Hyperlipoproteinemias. More critical elevations of blood fat occur in the *inborn-error syndromes*, identified collectively as the *familial hyperlipoproteinemias*. In these hereditary biochemical disturbances the basic defect appears to be in lipid metabolism. Fredrickson has brought order to this field by the identification of 5 major phenotypes, based on clinical features, enzymatic abnormalities and the serum lipoprotein electrophoretic patterns.

"Type I" hyperlipoproteinemia ("idiopathic familial hyperlipemia," Buerger-Grutz syndrome) is characterized by the presence of extremely lactescent serum (triglyceride levels of 2000 to 4000 mg. per 100 ml. or higher) in an otherwise well-appearing child who may have minor enlargement of the liver and spleen. On occasion there are bouts of abdominal pain and vomiting which may mimic an acute surgical crisis. Serum cholesterol levels are only mildly elevated; a deficiency of lipoprotein lipase ("clearing factor") can be demonstrated. The lipemia is responsive to a reduction in dietary intake of fat, but this is difficult to administer for long periods in children, and there seems little urgency to do so, since the prognosis for cardiovascular disease is not disturbing.

"Type II" familial hypercholesteremia is the most common of the constitutional hyperlipoproteinemias. The serum is clear, with the triglyceride level usually measuring near zero.

In *heterozygously involved* persons the serum cholesterol concentration characteristically is stable at about 350 to 450 mg. per 100 ml. Children with this disorder are asymptomatic and are identified only through family surveys. Adults, especially males, have a high incidence of coronary disease in the age range of 30 to 40 years. The hypercholesteremia is dominantly transmitted.

When both parents have the trait, the child may have the *homozygous abnormality*. Such a child will have a serum cholesterol concentration in the range of 700 to 1000 mg. per 100 ml. and will have skin and tendon xanthomas in the early years (see below). The homozygous state is incompatible with survival beyond early adult life, and deaths at 12 to 14 years of age are not infrequent from the complications of valvular and coronary atheromatosis. Lowering the hypercholesteremia by dietary therapy is of partial value only (use of vegetable oils, fish and poultry, instead of dairy and pork products) and should not be unduly pressed. Sitosterols, lecithin, lipotropic agents, heparin, estrogens and nicotinic acid have not been effective in children. Some newer agents appear to have more promise, particularly d-thyroxin and clofibrate.

"Types III, IV and V" familial hyperlipoprotein-emia are infrequently identified in childhood. Characteristically, there is a family history of diabetes mellitus and also often of heart disease. Affected persons may have a mildly abnormal glucose tolerance test result. The serum is often turbid (increase in triglycerides), sometimes markedly but inconstantly so; the cholesterol value is moderately elevated, and electrophoresis shows an important "pre-beta" factor in the lipoproteins. Xanthomas appear in adult life, and the cardiovascular prognosis is poor. The hyperlipoproteinemia often seems to be potentiated by a high intake of carbohydrates rather than of fat. Within the pediatric age range it is significant to realize that there are kinds of constitutional hyperlipemia which do not qualify for the more common types I and II and which will require more detailed study for full understanding. The child should be followed up with blood lipid measurements, for an extended period, the glucose tolerance examined in detail, and the other family members carefully investigated.

SKIN XANTHOMAS

Xanthomas of the skin have little direct importance in themselves, but serve as useful indicators for the detection of lipid disturbances, either in a localized, nonspecific fashion, or as part of a generalized metabolic dysfunction. These "yellow tumors" (also orange, brown or red) represent nodular collections of lipidized histiocytes and other related elements; their color is probably due to deposition of carotenoid material. The most pertinent cytoplasmic abnormality is the local accumulation of cholesterol. Only rarely is it necessary to substantiate the clinical impression of xanthoma by biopsy. The evaluation requires a general pediatric examination and careful measurement of the serum cholesterol level.

Xanthomas in Patients with Normal Serum Cholesterol Levels. These lesions are typically distributed in an axial fashion on the scalp, face, trunk and, occasionally, in the mouth. Such lesions are relatively common and are called "juvenile xanthogranulomas" (previously referred to as nevoxanthoendotheliomas). The lesions, which may range from one to a hundred or more, usually appear in the first months of life, increase for the next year or so, and then fade spontaneously by the time the child is 3 to 5 years of age (Fig. 9-14, *A*). The lesions are apparently benign new growths and require no specific therapy. The resulting scars are innocuous. In the characteristic situation there is no familial aspect, but some of the children

also have *café-au-lait* spots and may have a familial history of neurofibromatosis.

Clinical variants with more extensive involvement are also seen; these include minor degrees of hepatomegaly, light pulmonary infiltration, leukocytosis (monocytes and lymphocytes) and anemia. One of the rare forms is the so-called *leukemic xanthomatosis*, with a monocytic or monomyeloid leukemoid picture, in conjunction with manifestations of neurofibromatosis (Fig. 9-14, *B*). Such syndromes appear to be expressions of the overall histiocytosis reaction pattern, with an unknown type of provoking mechanism. There is similarity of the visceral lesions to those in true Letterer-Siwe disease. There may also be skin xanthomas and accumulation of cholesterol in foam cells in internal granulomatous lesions, especially in the dura, bone marrow and thymus in Letterer-Siwe disease. The differential diagnostic study of the child with normocholesteremic skin xanthomas requires consideration of the presence of leukocytic abnormalities and of Letterer-Siwe disease.

Another rare syndrome, termed "xanthoma disseminatum," also appears to be related. Clusters of brown xanthomas are found in the skin folds and on the oral mucosa, and at times in the larynx, on the meninges and on the cornea or sclera.

Xanthomas Associated with an Increase in the Serum Cholesterol Level. *Eruptive xanthomas* may appear on the skin in any syndrome in which there is a sustained elevation of blood lipids (see Syndromes with Increased Blood Fat). Diseases with which they are associated include von Gierke's disease, poorly controlled diabetes mellitus, chronic obstructive liver disease (Fig. 9-14, *C*) and "familial hyperlipemia" (Fredrickson type I hyperlipoproteinemia). Typically, the lesions occur in crops on the extensor surfaces of the extremities, where minor trauma is common, but occasionally they appear on the face, on the palate and on the sides of the toes. On the eyelids they are referred to as "xanthelasmata." When they first appear, there may be mild itching. Eruptive xanthomas tend to be transient and are dependent upon the course of the hyperlipidemia.

In the syndrome of familial hypercholesteremia (type II hyperlipoproteinemia) the xanthomatous lesions are more extensive. Heterozygously involved young adults may initially have xanthomas only on the eyelids and within the Achilles tendons, but with the passage of years more widespread lesions form, particularly in other tendons. Children are free of xanthomas in this syndrome unless they are homozygously involved (both parents have hypercholesteremia). In this circumstance, xanthomas begin to appear at 1 to 2 years of age, and progress steadily. Lumpy cutaneous lesions, referred to as "xanthoma tuberosum" (Fig. 9-14, *D*), form on the elbows and knees. Tendon lesions become large (heels, toes, knees, elbows, knuckles) and interfere with local comfort and function. On occasion their surgical removal may be justified as a temporary aid. In late child-

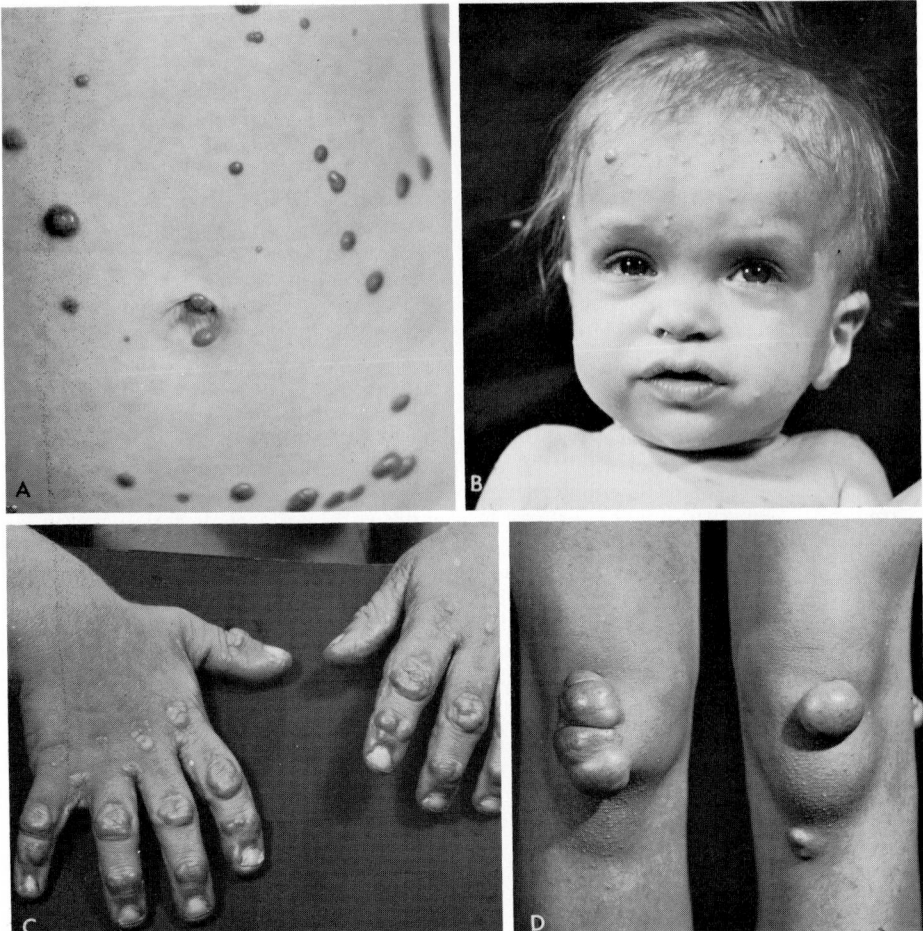

Figure 9-14. Skin xanthomas. *A,* Juvenile xanthogranuloma lesions on the abdomen of a 17-month-old girl. *B,* Xanthomas on the forehead and scalp of a 15-month-old boy with a histiocytic syndrome which included leukocytosis, hepatomegaly and *café-au-lait* spots. *C,* Eruptive xanthomas on the hands of a 4-year-old boy with intrahepatic biliary atresia. *D,* Xanthoma tuberosum lesions on the knees of a 12-year-old girl with homozygous involvement in "type II" hyperlipoproteinemia.

hood a corneal "arcus" may develop, and rarely xanthomatous lesions within the medullary cavity of bone. Cardiovascular lesions (atheromas) are of critical importance.

ALLEN C. CROCKER

REFERENCES

Lipidoses, General

Aronson, S. M., and Volk, B. W. (Eds.): *Inborn Disorders of Sphingolipid Metabolism.* Oxford, Pergamon Press, 1966.

Crocker, A. C.: The Cerebral Defect in Tay-Sachs Disease and Niemann-Pick Disease. *J. Neurochem.,* 7:69, 1961.

Crocker, A. C., and Farber, S.: Niemann-Pick Disease; A Review of 18 Patients. *Medicine,* 37:1, 1958.

Crocker, A. C., and Landing, B. H.: Phosphatase Studies in Gaucher's Disease. *Metabolism,* 9:341, 1960.

Pick, L.: A Classification of the Diseases of Lipoid Metabolism. *Am. J.M. Sc.,* 185:453, 601, 1933.

Thannhauser, S. J.: *Lipidoses; Diseases of the Intracellular Lipid Metabolism.* 3rd ed. New York, Grune & Stratton, Inc., 1958.

Recently Described Syndromes

Crocker, A. C., Cohen, J., and Farber, S.: The "Lipogranulomatosis" Syndrome—Review, with Report of Patient Showing Milder Involvement; in S. M. Aronson and B. W. Volk (Eds.): *Inborn Disorders of Sphingolipid Metabolism.* Oxford, Pergamon Press, 1966, p. 485.

Crocker, A. C., Vawter, G. F., Neuhauser, E. B. D., and Rosowsky, A.: Wolman's Disease: Three New Patients with a Recently Described Lipidosis. *Pediatrics,* 35:627, 1965.

Fredrickson, D. S.: Familial High-Density Lipoprotein Deficiency: Tangier Disease; in J. B. Stanbury, J. B. Wyngaarden and D. S. Fredrickson (Eds.): *The Metabolic Basis of Inherited Disease,* 2nd ed. New York, McGraw Hill Book Company, Inc., 1966, p. 486.

Holland, P., Hug, G., and Schubert, W. K.: Chronic Reticuloendothelial Cell Storage Disease. *Am. J. Dis. Child,* 110:117, 1965.

Landing, B. H., and Shirkey, H. S.: A Syndrome of Recurrent Infection and Infiltration of the Viscera by Pigmented Lipid Histiocytes. *Pediatrics,* 20:431, 1957.

Landing, B. H., and others: Familial Neurovisceral Lipidosis. *Am. J. Dis. Child,* 108:503, 1964.

Landing, B. H., Crocker, A. C., and others: Thrombocytopenic Purpura with Histiocytosis of the Spleen. *New England J. Med.,* 265:572, 1961.

Sweeley, C. C., and Klionsky, B.: Glycolipid Lipidosis: Fabry's Disease; in J. B. Stanbury, J. B. Wyngaarden and D. S.

Fredrickson (Eds.): *The Metabolic Basis of Inherited Disease.* 2nd ed. New York, McGraw-Hill Book Company, Inc., 1966, p. 618.

Syndromes with Increased Blood Fat and *Skin Xanthomas*

Crocker, A. C.: Skin Xanthomas in Childhood. *Pediatrics*, 3:573, 1951.
Fredrickson, D. S., and Lees, R. S.: Familial Hyperlipoprotein-

emia; in J. B. Stanbury, J. B. Wyngaarden, and D. S. Fredrickson (Eds.): *The Metabolic Basis of Inherited Disease.* 2nd ed. New York, McGraw-Hill Book Company, Inc., 1966, p. 429.
Liebman, S. D., Crocker, A. C., and Geiser, C. F.: Corneal Xanthomas in Childhood. *Arch. Ophthal.*, 76:221, 1966.
Rausen, A. R., and Adlersberg, D.: Idiopathic Hyperlipemia and Hypercholesteremia in Children. *Pediatrics*, 28:276, 1961.

DEFECTS IN PIGMENT METABOLISM

THE PORPHYRIAS

The porphyrias are a group of syndromes characterized biochemically by some error in pyrrole metabolism and clinically by photodermatitis and visceral and neuropsychiatric complaints. Incidence is estimated at 1:30,000 in the general population. These diseases are classified in Table 9-4 according to the organ system in which the error in pyrrole metabolism is localized: *erythropoietic* and *hepatic* forms are recognized. Most of the porphyrias have a dominant mode of inheritance. Family studies and close surveillance through adolescence are essential in order to identify cases in the latent stage; this is vital since most deaths occur during the late adolescent and early adult years and are attributable to delays in diagnosis which may lead to inappropriate and harmful therapy. Family studies entail determination of porphyrins in both urine and stool in all members; in cases of photosensitivity, measurements of erythrocyte protoporphyrin may also be necessary. With early diagnosis, proper fluid and dietary therapy and avoidance of contraindicated drugs, the prognosis for survival and symptomatic relief during acute visceral attacks is good.

TABLE 9-4. A CLASSIFICATION OF THE PORPHYRIAS

HEPATIC PORPHYRIAS

A. Acute intermittent porphyria (AIP, Swedish genetic porphyria)
B. Porphyria variegata (PV, South African genetic porphyria)
C. Hereditary coproporphyria
D. The cutaneous porphyrias (PCT, porphyria cutanea tarda)
   1. Hereditary types
   2. Acquired (but possible genetic predisposition associated with alcoholism, etc.)
   3. Toxic (hexachlorobenzene-induced)

ERYTHROPOIETIC PORPHYRIAS

A. Erythropoietic protoporphyria
B. Congenital erythropoietic porphyria

Relation of Abnormal Heme Biosynthesis to Disease States. Heme is the prosthetic group of hemoglobin, myoglobin, catalase, peroxidase and the cytochromes. It is formed from glycine, tricarboxylic acid cycle intermediates and iron via the metabolic pathway shown in Figure 9-15. This pathway is common to all mammalian cells, each cell synthesizing its own heme for the formation of its own particular hemoproteins. The initial step, formation of δ-aminolevulinic acid (ALA),* is mediated by ALA synthetase (Figure 9-15). This mitochondrial enzyme is inductible, and its availability is rate-limiting for the entire process.

Four basic porphyrin isomers are known and are designated as types I, II, III and IV. Types I and III are the only naturally occurring isomers. The isomeric forms of porphyrins are illustrated in Figure 9-16 using uroporphyrin (URO) as a model. Mammalian hemoproteins contain type III porphyrin isomers only. Protoporphyrin (PROTO) 9 is a type III isomer. Infinitesimal quantities of type I isomers are formed as byproducts of heme synthesis.

In *acute intermittent porphyria* excessive formation of ALA synthetase occurs in liver, and is responsible for the increased amounts of ALA and porphobilinogen (PBG) which characterize this disease. It seems likely that excessive ALA synthetase is common to all the hepatic porphyrias; this enzymatic abnormality has also been observed in red cells of patients with erythropoietic protoporphyria. Factors not yet elucidated account for differences in pattern of excretion of pyrroles in the various porphyrias.

The fundamental metabolic defect in *congenital erythropoietic porphyria* resides in the inability of approximately half of the developing erythroblasts to convert PBG to uroporphyrinogen (UROGEN) III (Fig. 9-15). Instead, URO I accumulates within the nuclei of these defective erythroblasts, diffuses into the circulation, is deposited in various tissues, including teeth and bone, and is excreted in the urine as a mixture of URO I and coproporphyrin (COPRO) I, with URO I predominant. In *erythropoietic protoporphyria* excessive amounts of PROTO 9 are produced in the

---

*The following abbreviations will be used in this chapter.
   ALA — δ-aminolevulinic acid.
   PBG — porphobilinogen.
   UROGEN — uroporphyrinogen.
   URO — uroporphyrin.
   COPROGEN — coproporphyrinogen.
   COPRO — coproporphyrin.
   PROTO — protoporphyrin.

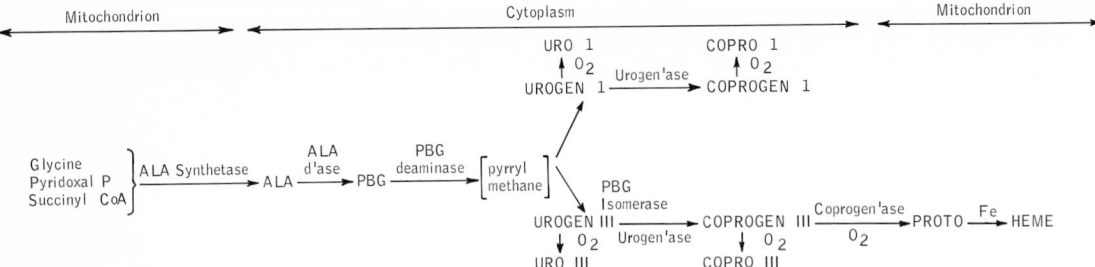

Figure 9-15. Intracellular organization of biosynthesis of heme. The initial and final steps in heme synthesis occur within the mitochondria. ALA is released in the cytoplasm. The metabolites formed in the cytoplasm are the ones found in the plasma and urine. ALA synthetase is the rate-limiting enzyme.

cytoplasm of erythrocytes both in marrow and in the circulation. The accumulated PROTO 9 is excreted in feces, but not in urine.

Only the fully reduced porphyrin intermediates, UROGEN III and coproporphyrinogen (CO-PROGEN) III can be utilized for heme formation (Fig. 9-15). These substances are colorless and unstable and do not exhibit fluorescence; hence they cannot be detected except by specialized techniques. Oxidation stabilizes porphyrin molecules and renders them fluorescent. Those portions of UROGEN and COPROGEN not utilized for heme synthesis are oxidized to UROs I and III and COPROs I and III (Fig. 9-15), and it is in this form that these porphyrins are usually detected in the tissues and excreta.

PBG and ALA are also colorless and do not fluoresce; they must be measured by chemical methods. Normally, the urinary excretion of PBG and ALA does not exceed 3 mg. a day. The qualitative Schwartz-Watson reaction for PBG (see p. 466) is positive only when a pathologic excess of PBG is present. Porphyrins normally appear in the excreta in very small amounts: fecal COPRO and PROTO should not exceed 100 μg. per gram of dry feces per day; COPRO is excreted in urine at a rate of 1 μg. per pound of body weight per day. Infections and accelerated erythropoiesis cause a two-fold to threefold increase in urinary COPRO; hepatitis (infectious and toxic) a tenfold to forty-fold increase in urinary COPRO; and lead intoxication a tenfold to fortyfold increase in both ALA and COPRO in urine. Porphyria may cause up to one thousandfold increases in pyrrole excretion. In acquired diseases COPRO always exceeds URO in urine, but in the heritable forms of porphyria the quantity of URO in urine always exceeds COPRO, if both are present. Increased fecal porphyrins virtually always indicate some heritable form of porphyria.

Relation of Metabolic Errors to Clinical Manifestations. *Photosensitizing effects of porphyrins.* Some but not all of the skin lesions of both erythropoietic and certain hepatic porphyrias are due to the photosensitizing effect of URO. Erythema, edema and vesiculation of the exposed skin result when persons with increased uroporphyrinemia are irradiated with a combination of near ultraviolet (4000 Å) and infrared (26,000 Å) monochromatic light sources. Urticaria and

eczematoid lesions may follow exposure to near ultraviolet light of subjects with greatly increased amounts of PROTO in their red blood cells and plasma. All the heme precursors (Fig. 9-15) have at one time or another been injected into both healthy and porphyric human subjects without demonstrable adverse effect other than photosensitization.

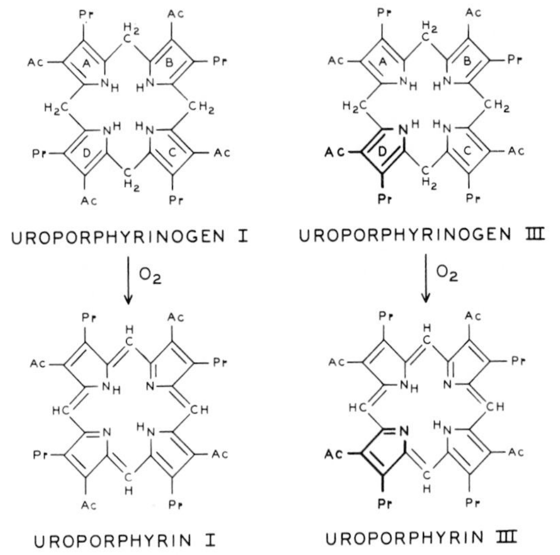

UROPORPHYRINOGEN I   UROPORPHYRINOGEN III

UROPORPHYRIN I   UROPORPHYRIN III

Figure 9-16. Isomers and oxidation states of uroporphyrin. The 4 pyrrolic nuclei of UROGENs I and III are derived from PBG and are labeled A, B, C and D in this figure. In UROGEN I all 4 nuclei have the same spatial orientation so that asymmetrical Ac and Pr side chains lie in alternating sequence around the periphery of the molecule. Type III isomers such as UROGEN III result when nucleus D (shown in bold face) is "flipped over" 180 degrees with respect to the others; now the Pr side chains of nuclei D and C are adjacent, which is crucial for attachment of heme to protein. UROs I and III represent the more stable oxidized state in which porphyrins are usually found in tissues and excreta. They are formed from UROGENs I and III by loss of 6 protons (two from the pyrrolic nitrogens and four from the methane bridges between each pyrrolic nucleus).

Abbreviations:

Porphyrin Side Chains	Bridges:	
	H_2	
Ac = CH_2COOH (acetic acid)	$-C-$	methane
Pr = CH_2CH_2COOH (proprionic acid)	H $=C-$	methene

Toxic and experimental hepatic porphyria. In patients with the hepatic forms of porphyria it is clear that the overproduction of ALA by the liver is responsible for the great accumulation of pyrroles in this organ and the excreta. What is not clear is how or whether this metabolic error is related to the visceral and neuropsychiatric disorders encountered in many such patients. Most cases of hepatic porphyria are clearly of genetic origin. When it is not possible to demonstrate this in family studies, such cases are usually designated as "acquired," but the possibility of genetic predisposition cannot be entirely excluded. New insight into these problems has been gained from studies of an outbreak of toxic cutaneous porphyria in Turkey.

Between 1956 and 1960 some 5000 cases of porphyria in southeastern Turkey were traced to the eating of seed wheat which had been treated with a fungicide, hexachlorobenzene. The resultant syndrome, seen predominantly in children, was characterized by cachexia, hepatomegaly, bullous skin lesions, photosensitivity, hyperpigmentation, hypertrichosis and increased porphyrin content of the excreta. "Rheumatoid" arthritic changes were noted ultimately in more than 50 per cent of the patients. A chronic porphyric state with all the features just enumerated persisted in most patients for at least 2 years after the cessation of hexachlorobenzene ingestion. Even 5 years later most still had hepatomegaly, arthritis, hypertrichosis and hyperpigmentation. Genetic factors were at first thought to be excluded, but recent work by Dogramaci suggests that those involved may have been genetically predisposed.

Acute intermittent porphyria is the first inborn error of metabolism in which the genetic defect causes an excess rather than a deficit of a specific

TABLE 9-5. Agents Used to Induce Chemical Hepatic Porphyria in Animals

"Chemicals"
Allylisopropylacetamide
Allylisoprophylacetylurea (Sedormid)
Hexachlorobenzene
3,5-dicarbethoxy-1,4-dihydrocollidine

"Drugs"
Sulfonal
Barbiturates
Sulfonamides
Griseofulvin
Chloroquine

"Endogenous Sex Steroids"
1. Potent porphyrin-inducing activity

C-19 Steroids	C-21 Steroids
(Etiocholanolone)	(Pregnanediol)
(Etiocholandiol)	(Pregnanolone)
(Etiocholandione)	(11-Ketopregnanolone)
(Etiocholanolone-17)	(17-OH Pregnanolone)

2. Weak porphyrin-inducing activity
   Testosterone
   Progesterone
   Estradiol
   Estrone
   Estriol

enzyme (hepatic ALA synthetase). Table 9-5 lists the drugs, chemical agents and endogenous metabolites which may induce hepatic porphyria in experimental animals. Granick has demonstrated that formation of ALA synthetase can be induced in vitro by hexachlorobenzene, griseofulvin, barbiturates, dihydrocollidines and steroids. The current hypothesis is that the level of ALA synthetase is controlled by operator and repressor genes. Granick proposes that hepatic porphyria is caused by a mutation in the operator gene which renders it poorly responsive to the repressor substance, which may consist of a protein aporepressor and heme as a corepressor. The inducing chemicals (Table 9-5) compete with heme, with the result that more ALA synthetase is formed in their presence. Granick has shown that certain C-19 and C-21 sex steroids are potent inducers of porphyrin synthesis. Included are etiocholanolone, pregnanediol and pregnanolone, which are produced in significant quantities daily and in the past were considered inert metabolites of hormone metabolism. In Granick's in-vitro system for studying induction of porphyrin formation the glucuronide conjugates of even the most potent steroid inducers are inert, whereas testosterone, progesterone, estradiol, estrone and estriol are weakly active. The fact that sex steroid metabolites are potent endogenous inducers may explain the delay in appearance of symptoms in hepatic porphyria until after puberty. These findings also emphasize a possible role of the liver in modifying hepatic porphyria, since the patient with porphyria may be protected from some potent inducers by the liver's ability to detoxify through conjugation.

Balance studies in patients with hepatic porphyria show that both severe caloric restriction and negative nitrogen balance are accompanied by a sharp increase in the excretion of pyrroles. This increase in pyrrole excretion can be suppressed if adequate caloric intake is restored by the administration of carbohydrates. Return to positive nitrogen balance is also accompanied by diminution in pyrrole excretion. The maintenance of a diet high in carbohydrate and adequate in protein is of considerable clinical importance.

Diagnosis and Management of the Porphyrias. *Clinical manifestations.* Although the porphyrias are generally genetically determined and associated with some metabolic error present from birth, clinical symptoms are rare before puberty in the hepatic forms. Three groups of clinical manifestations are recognized: cutaneous, visceral and neurologic. The onset of symptoms is insidious; once they occur, however, subtle cutaneous, visceral and neuropsychiatric complaints tend to run an undulating course throughout the remainder of the patient's life. The principal clinical syndromes and patterns of pyrrole excretion encountered in the porphyrias are summarized in Table 9-6.

Acute exacerbations of dermal lesions occur with exposure to sunlight. Visceral and neurologic

TABLE 9-6.   CLINICAL SYNDROMES AND PYRROLE EXCRETION PATTERNS IN HERITABLE FORMS OF PORPHYRIA

	HEPATIC PORPHYRIAS				ERYTHROPOIETIC PORPHYRIAS	
	ACUTE INTERMITTENT PORPHYRIA	PORPHYRIA VARIEGATA	"PORPHYRIA CUTANEA TARDA"	HEREDITARY COPROPORPHYRIA	ERYTHROPOIETIC PROTOPORPHYRIA*	CONGENITAL ERYTHROPOIETIC PORPHYRIA
Transmission	- Autosomal dominant -				- -	Recessive
Onset of clinical manifestations	- - - - - - - - - Puberty or later† - - - - - - - - -				- - - - Early childhood - - - -	Infancy
Acute visceral and neurologic attacks	Present	Present	Present	Present	Absent	Absent
Cutaneous lesions	Absent	Present	Present	?Absent	Present	Present
Pyrrole excretion‡ during acute visceral and neurologic attacks						
Urine						
ALA, PBG	+++	+++	±	+ to ++		
URO, COPRO	± to +++	± to +++	±	+ to ++		
Feces						
COPRO,	0	+++	+++	+++		
PROTO	0	+++	+++	±		
Pyrrole excretion‡ during remission of visceral and neurologic symptoms						
Urine						
ALA, PBG	±	0	±	0	0	0
URO, COPRO	±	0	0	±	0	+++
Feces						
COPRO,	0	+++	+++	+++	±	++
PROTO	0	+++	+++	0	+++	±

*Erythrocyte PROTO grossly increased in erythropoietic protoporphyria.
†In each group rare cases have been observed before puberty.
‡Increased URO in feces found in some cases of each group.
See page 461 for designations of abbreviations.

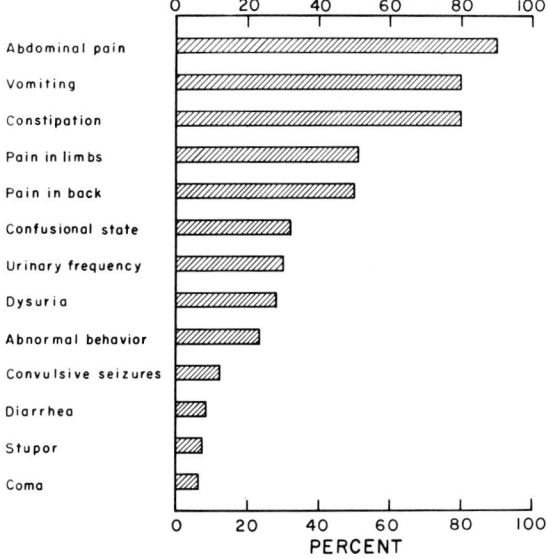

Figure 9-17. The acute attack of porphyria—relative frequency of symptoms. Based on an analysis of 107 acute attacks in 80 patients. (Adapted from L. Eales: Porphyria as Seen in Cape Town, a Survey of 250 Patients and Some Recent Studies. *S. Afr. J. Lab. & Clin. Med.,* 9:151, 1963.)

complaints, which almost invariably occur together, may be precipitated by infection, menstruation, pregnancy, alcohol, barbiturates and other agents listed in Table 9-5. Although the skin lesions are bothersome and may be disfiguring, it is the acute visceral and neurologic problems that threaten life. The relative frequency of various abnormal clinical findings encountered during the course of an acute attack are shown in Figures 9-17 and 9-18. None of these findings is pathog-

nomonic; early diagnosis depends upon recognition of the sequence in which the clinical manifestations appear, intensify and abate, and upon demonstration of excess pyrroles in the excreta. Colicky abdominal pain and varied neuropsychiatric symptoms are the usual presenting complaints.

Colicky abdominal pain is the initial symptom of an acute attack in most patients. The pain is felt most frequently in the epigastrium or right iliac fossa, but may be located anywhere in the abdomen or pelvis. There is considerable variation in the intensity of the pain. It tends to worsen in an undulating manner over a period of days. Severe colic may persist for hours and often cause the patient to writhe about or assume bizarre positions in bed. Vomiting and constipation shortly develop in all but the mildest attacks. Examination of the abdomen and pelvis reveals minimal signs which seem insignificant in comparison with the patient's pain. Diffuse tenderness of the abdomen is usually present, but does not localize, and rigidity and muscle spasm are rare. Leukocytosis and fever are often present. The acute visceral pain of porphyria has been confused with virtually every acute surgical condition of the abdomen, various painful gynecologic disorders and "hysteria." In the absence of other features and objective findings characteristic of these other conditions, the presence of tachycardia and hypertension makes porphyria a likely diagnosis.

Uncommonly, pain, weakness and paresthesia in back and limb muscles occur as presenting complaints in the absence of abdominal pain. *Personality changes* are observed in most patients suffering from visceral attacks, but they are rarely the predominating features. These patients are variously described as depressed, nervous, hy-

Figure 9-18. The acute attack of porphyria —relative frequency of signs and pertinent laboratory findings. Based on analysis of 107 acute attacks in 80 patients. (Adapted from L. Eales: Porphyria as Seen in Cape Town, a Survey of 250 Patients and Some Recent Studies. *S. Afr. J. Lab. & Clin. Med.,* 9:151, 1963.)

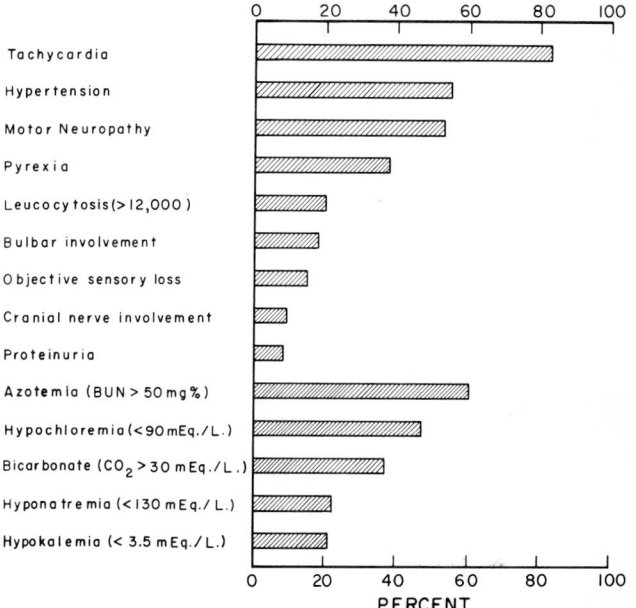

sterical, lachrymose or "peculiar." These traits wax and wane with the severity of the pain. In severe colic mental confusion, hallucinations and disorientation are often present.

After the patient with acute intermittent porphyria or porphyria variegata (Table 9-6) has had an exacerbation characterized by abdominal pain, vomiting, constipation, tachycardia and, in more severe cases, hypertension, the end of the attack may often be heralded by the resumption of normal pulse and blood pressure. The urine is apt to be colorless at first, although PBG is always present in high concentration and is diagnostic.

If the attack progresses, and especially if barbiturates are given, the urine usually becomes red, increasing motor restlessness is noted, and neurologic manifestations, rarely present initially, soon appear. These take the form of spotty weakness or paralysis, with diminished or absent tendon reflexes, and pain and tenderness in the involved muscle groups. Muscle paralysis is an ominous sign. There is patchy demyelination, and spotty paralysis which can spread unpredictably. Ill-advised abdominal or pelvic surgery may be quickly followed by catastrophic paralysis and coma. Weakness and paralysis may persist for months after the other features of an acute attack have subsided. Death, when it occurs, usually results from quadriparesis or respiratory failure.

There is a profound disturbance in water and electrolyte homeostasis in severe attacks of porphyria. The serum is hypotonic, with reduced concentrations of sodium and chloride (Fig. 9-18). The urine is hypertonic, owing in part to the excessive loss of sodium. This disturbance is attributed to inappropriate secretion of antidiuretic hormone. The severity of neurologic injury may be related to the degree of hyponatremia. Hypocalcemia and hypomagnesemia may occur, with and without tetany.

Burgundy red urine in the porphyric patient is due to the presence of URO. It is a constant finding in congenital erythropoietic porphyria and a frequent finding in patients with cutaneous manifestations of hepatic porphyria. In acute visceral attacks the urine is often colorless at first, and may or may not become red as the attack progresses.

A variety of *dermal lesions* may be observed in porphyria. Exposure to sunlight, particularly during the summer months, produces vesicles, bullae and edema on the exposed skin. These photosensitive lesions are prone to secondary infection and heal slowly, with chronic scars which become hyperpigmented. In some patients such lesions may also follow minor mechanical trauma and exposure to indoor sources of ultraviolet light. Macules, papules, eczematous plaques and urticaria are also seen. Nearly all patients with cutaneous forms of porphyria eventually have hypertrichosis and a violaceous hue to their skin. These changes develop insidiously over the years and are most prominent on the exposed parts of the body.

Differential diagnosis. Study of Figures 9-17 and 9-18 makes it clear that porphyria must be included in the differential diagnosis of essential hypertension, hyperthyroidism, painful gynecologic disorders, "hysteria," psychosis and all surgical conditions of the abdomen. Whenever diagnosis of such surgical conditions of the abdomen as ulcer, gallbladder disease or appendicitis cannot be made with confidence, a Schwartz-Watson test for PBG should be done prior to surgical exploration. A surprising number of porphyric patients are treated in error for hyperthyroidism. Serum protein-bound iodine is elevated in hepatic porphyria, but there are no evident disturbances in thyroxine metabolism. Cutaneous forms of porphyria should be included in the differential diagnosis of photosensitive dermatitides.

Laboratory diagnosis. Accurate diagnosis of porphyria requires examination of both urine and feces, and of blood in the case of erythropoietic protoporphyria (Table 9-6). The excreta of the patient and of his relatives must be examined to establish the type of pedigree and to identify latent cases. In the hepatic porphyrias, pyrrole excretion patterns may vary according to the presence or absence of visceral symptoms. Porphyrin excretion may be increased a thousandfold or more over the normal values. The red color imparted to urine by URO must be distinguished from that due to urates, bile, anthocyanin (from beets), melanin, eosin, hemoglobin or myoglobin.

The *Schwartz-Watson reaction for PBG* is almost always positive in acute visceral attacks. In *freshly voided* urine the test is simple, and diagnostic when performed as follows:

Five ml. of freshly voided urine (cooled to room temperature) is thoroughly shaken in a small separatory funnel for 30 seconds with 5 ml. of Ehrlich's aldehyde reagent [0.7 gm. of p-dimethylaminobenzaldehyde (A. C. S. reagent grade), 150 ml. of concentrated hydrochloric acid, and 100 ml. of distilled water]. The solution is then adjusted to pH 4 to 5 by mixing thoroughly with a saturated aqueous solution of sodium acetate (10 ml. usually required). The formation of a cherry-red or red-violet color at this point indicates the presence of porphobilinogen, urobilinogen or certain indolic compounds. The red pigments formed with Ehrlich's reagent by each of these substances can then be separated on the basis of differential solubility.

If red pigment is present, the solution is next extracted with 10 ml. of chloroform. Red color due to urobilinogen passes into the chloroform phase, which is discarded. Chloroform extraction is repeated until no more urobilinogen is obtained. If the remaining aqueous solution still contains red pigment, this aqueous solution is next extracted with 5 ml. of n-butanol. Red pigment due to indoles and other Ehrlich reactors passes into the n-butanol phase, while only red pigment formed from porphobilinogen remains in the aqueous phase. Butanol-extractable red pigment, as well as porphobilinogen, has been found in the urine of some patients with acute intermittent porphyria; so both the butanol and aqueous phases may contain red pigment after the final extraction.

If this test gives equivocal results, the urine should be treated with heat and acetic acid to convert all precursors to URO, which is then readily identified. The bibliography contains further references to analytical methods.

Treatment. Disturbances in water and electrolyte homeostasis are not usually seen in mild attacks; nevertheless they should be anticipated and the patient treated expectantly. When profound disturbances in water and electrolyte homeostasis are present, restriction of water and careful replacement of the sodium deficit may result in dramatic clinical improvement.

Because many chemical agents are capable of inducing porphyria, drug therapy must be approached with extreme caution. Pain and restlessness can be controlled with morphine and chloral hydrate. Cortisone and chlorpromazine have been beneficial in some cases, without obvious effect in others, and deleterious in a few. Adequate caloric and nitrogen intakes should be restored as rapidly as possible.

Successful long-term management requires careful control of infections, and the absolute avoidance of alcohol and of the drugs listed in Table 9-5. A diet adequate in nitrogen and high in carbohydrates is beneficial. Many patients are fearful of precipitating critical episodes and indulge in food fads. In some women, attacks are clearly related to the menstrual cycle; some have been treated with ovulatory suppressants, androgens and even oophorectomy, with apparent beneficial results. Oral contraceptives in the lowest effective dosage have been beneficial in some but not all cases of acute intermittent porphyria; they are apparently contraindicated in pedigrees with dermal symptoms. Persons with latent or manifest hepatic porphyria should wear "Medic Alert" bracelets.

The cutaneous lesions are usually satisfactorily managed by avoidance of excessive exposure to sunlight. When this is inadequate, the application of red veterinary petrolatum to the skin may be beneficial. Red veterinary petrolatum protects the skin from radiation in the near ultraviolet zone; the usual commercial sunscreens do not.

Infants of mothers with hepatic porphyria may have increased pyrrole excretion during the neonatal period; this *passive porphyria* is not associated with any symptoms. The excretion of pyrroles soon returns to normal.

ACQUIRED HEPATIC PORPHYRIA

The acquired forms of hepatic porphyria are clinically indistinguishable from the hereditary cutaneous syndromes (Table 9-6). Visceral manifestations are minimal or absent, and dermal features are usually less severe in the acquired disease, often being limited to hyperpigmentation and hypertrichosis. Acquired porphyria may occur as a rare complication of chronic alcoholism, cirrhosis, tumors involving the liver and such systemic diseases as Hodgkin's disease, disseminated lupus and leukemia. Red urine due to the presence of URO is usually the clue that leads to the diagnosis.

SPECIAL FEATURES OF GENETIC PORPHYRIA

One of the rarest of inborn errors of metabolism is *congenital erythropoietic porphyria.* Vastly increased amounts of URO I are found in bone marrow, circulating erythrocytes, plasma, urine and feces. Lesser amounts of COPRO I are also found in the excreta. The excretion of other pyrroles is normal. The accumulation of URO I in the tissues (including the teeth) and the associated hemolytic anemia account for all the clinical manifestations of this disease. The photodermatitis of this disease is devastating; severe disfigurement is the ultimate result. Splenomegaly results from the hemolytic anemia; splenectomy is beneficial in some cases. The excretion of urine which is burgundy red as passed, or becomes so upon exposure to light, begins at birth or shortly thereafter and continues for life.

Erythropoietic protoporphyria begins during childhood and continues through adult life. Two types of skin lesions follow exposure to sunlight: (1) an urticarial response which resolves without chronic dermal changes; and (2) erythema and edema followed by an eczematous eruption on the exposed parts. This eczematous eruption is chronic rather than recurrent and leaves considerable scarring. These patients also have dull, opaque fingernails without lunulae. Clinical manifestations are otherwise limited to the skin. Increased amounts of PROTO 9 are always found in erythrocytes, and usually in feces. Rigorous avoidance of sunlight is indicated.

Among the hepatic porphyrias the visceral, neurologic and dermal manifestations and the pattern of pyrrole excretion are usually constant within a given pedigree. There is, however, considerable variation from one pedigree to another. The features of 4 typical variants are shown in Table 9-6. Of these, *acute intermittent porphyria* and *porphyria variegata* are perhaps the most common. Although it is world-wide in distribution, acute intermittent porphyria is also referred to as "Swedish porphyria." In affected kindreds acute visceral and neurologic attacks are both most frequent and most severe in females of childbearing age. The disorder probably has an autosomal dominant mode of transmission, but the fact that the excreta may not contain excess pyrroles during the asymptomatic phase has impeded genetic studies. In such kindreds acute attacks often occur without obvious precipitating factors. The occurrence of visceral attacks before puberty has been reported.

Although it is frequently referred to as "South African genetic porphyria," *porphyria variegata* is also world-wide in distribution. Symptoms are most common between puberty and the fifth decade of life. Skin lesions are relatively more common in males, whereas acute visceral attacks are more frequent in females. A striking feature is the importance of administration of barbiturates in the precipitation of severe acute visceral attacks. In porphyria variegata there is clearly an autosomal dominant mode of transmission; 50 per cent of adult members of affected families have a constant increase in excretion of porphyrins in the feces whether symptoms are present or not.

In *"porphyria cutanea tarda"* visceral as well as dermal manifestations are present, but the visceral complaints tend to be mild in comparison with those seen in acute intermittent porphyria. The existence of a purely cutaneous, hereditary form of hepatic porphyria has been disputed, for it can be argued that these patients have never encountered an environmental agent which would precipitate a visceral attack.

It now appears that *hereditary coproporphyria* is transmitted by an autosomal dominant character and that it is not a symptomless trait, as previously thought to be. Clinically, it resembles acute intermittent porphyria, except that symptoms may begin during childhood. There may be chronic "nervousness" and other psychiatric complaints, with or without recurrent abdominal pain. The unique biochemical feature of this disease is increased excretion of COPRO III in the feces; urinary COPRO III may or may not be increased. In the majority of cases severe visceral attacks are provoked by barbiturates and possibly by other anticonvulsant and tranquilizing drugs; during such attacks urinary excretion of ALA, PBG and COPRO III is increased. Photosensitivity has been described in only 1 of 30 cases.

HEREDITARY METHEMOGLOBINEMIAS

Normally the iron of both oxygenated and deoxygenated hemoglobin is in the ferrous state (ferrohemoglobin); this is essential for its oxygen-transporting function. Oxidation of hemoglobin iron to the ferric state yields methemoglobin (ferrihemoglobin), which is nonfunctional and imparts a chocolate hue to the blood; in sufficient concentration it causes cyanosis. The blood of healthy persons contains methemoglobin, but the intraerythrocytic methemoglobin-reducing system maintains its concentration at less than 2 per cent of the total hemoglobin. "Normal" methemoglobin has a characteristic spectral absorption band at 632 millimicrons, which is abolished by treatment of the blood sample with cyanide (technique of Evelyn and Malloy). This technique is specific for assaying methemoglobin produced by exposure to certain chemicals such as aniline dyes, but yields erroneous results when hemoglobin M type pigments are present. In familial cases both recessive and dominant patterns of inheritance are recognized; each has a distinct metabolic error.

Hereditary Methemoglobinemia Associated with Defective Methemoglobin-Reducing System. Reduction of methemoglobin in normal erythrocytes can be effected by 4 known systems; ascorbic acid, glutathione, TPNH diaphorase and DPNH diaphorase. Among these, DPNH diaphorase (or DPNH methemoglobin reductase) is by far the most active.

In hereditary methemoglobinemia with a recessive pattern of inheritance there is complete absence of the DPNH-dependent methemoglobin reductase. In these patients the methemoglobin formed has the spectral and chemical properties of "normal" methemoglobin. Methylene blue is therapeutically effective because it is reduced to leucomethylene blue by both glutathione and TPNH diaphorase; leucomethylene blue in turn can reduce "normal" methemoglobin to hemoglobin.

Clinically, the disorder is characterized by cyanosis, the intensity of which varies with season and diet. The time at onset of the cyanosis also varies; in some patients it appears at birth, in others as late as adolescence. No associated abnormalities which might explain the cyanosis are found. Despite the fact that up to 50 per cent of the total circulating hemoglobin may be in the form of nonfunctional methemoglobin, there is little or no cardiorespiratory distress except on exertion.

The daily oral administration of ascorbic acid (200 to 500 mg. in divided doses) will gradually reduce the quantity of methemoglobin to about 10 per cent of the total pigment and will alleviate the cyanosis as long as therapy is continued. Methylene blue given intravenously (1 to 2 mg. per kg.) promptly eliminates both methemoglobin and cyanosis, and this effect can be maintained by the daily oral administration of methylene blue (3 to 5 mg. per kg.). Mental deficiency has been associated in a few cases, but not in most, and there is insufficient evidence to indicate that it is causally related to the methemoglobinemia.

Hereditary Methemoglobinemia Associated with Abnormal Methemoglobins (Hemoglobin M Diseases). The dominantly transmitted forms of methemoglobinemia are collectively known as the hemoglobin M diseases. When all the hemoglobin pigment in a blood sample is first oxidized to methemoglobin by treatment with potassium ferricyanide, the abnormal methemoglobin M type pigments can be separated from normal methemoglobin by means of starch gel electrophoresis. Amino acid "fingerprinting" of several hemoglobin M pigments reveals the substitution of an abnormal amino acid residue in the globin chain. Dissimilar substitutions have been found in different pedigrees. This situation is analogous to that of other hemoglobinopathies (hemoglobin S, hemoglobin C, and others). Theoretic considerations strongly suggest that the abnormal amino acid residue in each of the hemoglobin M pigments lies in a portion of the globin chain in close proximity to the prosthetic heme group where it can alter the properties of the heme moiety. Thus cyanosis is

TABLE 9-7. Some Spectral and Chemical Properties of the Hemoglobins M

Hb M TYPE*	ABNORMAL HEMOGLOBIN CHAIN	METHEMOGLOBIN SPECTRAL ABSORPTION MAXIMA IN VISIBLE RANGE† (mμ)	CYANOMETHEMOGLOBIN DERIVATIVE ABSORPTION SPECTRUM
Hb M$_{Boston}$	α	495 and 602	Abnormal
Hb M$_{Saskatoon}$	β	492 and 602	Normal
Hb M$_{Milwaukee-1}$	?	500 and 622	Normal
Hb M$_{Milwaukee-2}$	?β	490 and 588	Normal
Hb M$_{Iwate}$	α	485 and 590	Abnormal
Normal Hb A	—	502 and 632	Normal

*Geographic designation refers to residence of first pedigree studied; types are often abbreviated as follows: Hb M$_B$, Hb M$_S$, Hb M$_{M-1}$, Hb M$_{M-2}$, Hb M$_I$.

†In M/15 sodium phosphate buffer, pH 6.5.

Adapted from P. S. Gerald: *Pediatrics*, 31:780, 1963.

probably due to the unusual stability of the methemoglobin form of the M hemoglobins. Such a hypothesis would also explain the variable response of patients to ascorbic acid and methylene blue as well as the abnormal spectral properties and differing response to cyanide treatment of various hemoglobin M pigments. Among the several hemoglobin M pedigrees examined, 5 different hemoglobin M pigments have been identified. Some of their properties are summarized in Table 9-7. It is possible that the entity previously described as "congenital sulfhemoglobinemia" may fall within the hemoglobin M disease group.

Clinically, methemoglobinemia of the hemoglobin M type should be suspected when family studies suggest an autosomal dominant pattern of inheritance and when the blood of the cyanotic patient fails to show the absorption band at 632 millimicrons, characteristic of normal methemoglobin. The patient's methemoglobin may or may not react with cyanide (technique of Evelyn and Malloy) to yield a normal cyanomethemoglobin absorption curve. This varies with the pedigree (Table 9-7). In the hemoglobin M diseases the quantity of methemoglobin does not exceed 25 per cent of the total hemoglobin; the cyanosis, although persistent from early infancy, is not associated with any disability. There may be a compensatory polycythemia. Affected members of some pedigrees do not respond to ascorbic acid or methylene blue (hemoglobin M$_B$ and hemoglobin M$_{M-1}$). Fortunately, alleviation of cyanosis is not essential in the hemoglobin M diseases.

HEMOCHROMATOSIS

Hemochromatosis is one of several forms of iron storage disease. It is characterized by excessive deposition in many organs of hemosiderin, an iron hydroxide-protein complex which in liver, pancreas or heart eventually causes impaired structure and function. The familial form of the disease is called *primary hemochromatosis*, and is associated with increased gastrointestinal absorption of iron. The nature of the metabolic defect is unknown. It is not associated with any known cause of excessive iron absorption, such as increased erythroid activity or excessive dietary iron intake, which can cause *secondary hemochromatosis*. Untreated cases of primary hemochromatosis eventually exhibit the classic triad of hepatic cirrhosis, slate or bronze pigmentation of the skin and diabetes mellitus. These symptoms and signs do not appear before adulthood. Serum iron levels are increased in both latent and symptomatic adult members of affected families, but not in the children. The pattern of inheritance has not been established. Depletion of iron stores is the aim of treatment and will improve both symptoms and the function of affected organs. This is most conveniently achieved by repeated phlebotomy; in anemic patients with secondary hemochromatosis or hemosiderosis, chelation therapy with deferoxamine is preferred.

J. Julian Chisolm, Jr.

REFERENCES

Dean, G., and Barnes, H. D.: The Inheritance of Porphyria. *Brit. Med. J.*, 2:89, 1955.

Debre, R., and others: Genetics of Haemochromatosis. *Ann. Human. Genet.*, 23:16, 1958.

Dogramaci, I.: in S. Z. Levine (Ed.): *Advances in Pediatrics*. Chicago, Year Book Medical Publishers, Inc., 1964, Vol. 13, pp. 11-64.

Editorial: Diagnostic Tests in the Porphyrias. *Lancet*, 1:663, 1967.

Gerald, P. S., and Scott, E. M.: The Hereditary Methemoglobinemias; in J. B. Stanbury, J. B. Wyngaarden and D. S. Fredrickson (Eds.): *The Metabolic Basis of Inherited Disease*. 2nd ed. New York, McGraw-Hill Book Company, Inc., 1966, pp. 1090-99.

Goldberg, A.: Acute Intermittent Porphyria. *Quart. J. Med.*, 28: 183, 1959.

Goldberg, A., Rimington, C., and Lochhead, A. C.: Hereditary Coproporphyria. *Lancet*, 1:632, 1967.

Granick, S.: The Induction *in vitro* of the Synthesis of δ-Aminolevulinic Acid Synthetase in Chemical Porphyria: A Response to Certain Drugs, Sex Hormones and Foreign Chemicals. *J. Biol. Chem.*, 241:1359, 1966.

Granick, S., and Kappas, A.: Steroid Control of Porphyrin and Heme Biosynthesis: A New Biological Function of Steroid Hormone Metabolites. *Proc. Nat. Acad. Sci.*, 57:1463, 1967.

Hellman, E. S. Tschudy, D. P., and Bartter, F. C.: Abnormal Electrolyte and Water Metabolism in Acute Intermittent Porphyria. *Am. J. Med.,* 32:734, 1962.

Lamont, N. McE., Hathorn, M., and Joubert, S. M.: Porphyria in the African. *Quart. J. Med.,* 30:373, 1961.

Pollycove, M.: Hemochromatosis; in J. B. Stanbury, J. B. Wyngaarden and D. S. Fredrickson (Eds.): *The Metabolic Basis of Inherited Disease.* 2nd ed. New York, McGraw-Hill Book Company, Inc., 1966, pp. 780-810.

Rimington, C., Magnus, I. A., Ryan, E. A., and Cripps, D. J.: Porphyria and Photosensitivity. *Quart. J. Med.,* 36:29, 1967.

Runge, W., and Watson, C. J.: Experimental Production of Skin Lesions in Human Cutaneous Porphyria. *Proc. Soc. Exper. Biol. & Med.,* 119:809, 1962.

Schmid, R., Schwartz, S., and Sundberg, D.: Erythropoietic (Congenital) Porphyria: A Rare Abnormality of the Normoblasts. *Blood,* 10:416, 1955.

Schmid, R.: The Porphyrias: in J. B. Stanbury, J. B. Wyngaarden and D. S. Fredrickson (Eds.): *The Metabolic Basis of Inherited Disease.* 2nd ed. New York, McGraw-Hill Book Company, Inc., 1966, pp. 813-70.

Tschudy, D. P., and others: Acute Intermittent Porphyria: The First "Overproduction Disease" Localized to a Specific Enzyme. *Proc. Nat. Acad. Sci.,* 53:841, 1965.

Watson, C. J., Taddeini, L., and Bossenmaier, I.: Present Status of the Ehrlich Aldehyde Reaction for Urinary Porphobilinogen. *J.A.M.A.,* 190:501, 1964.

Welland, F. H., and others: Factors Affecting the Excretion of Porphyrin Precursors by Patients with Acute Intermittent Porphyria. I. The Effect of Diet. *Metabolism,* 13:232, 1964.

Welland, F. H., and others: Factors Affecting the Excretion of Porphyrin Precursors by Patients with Acute Intermittent Porphyria. II. The Effect of Ethinyl Estradiol. *Metabolism,* 13:251, 1964.

Zimmerman, T. S., McMillin, M., and Watson, C. J.: Onset of Manifestations of Hepatic Porphyria in Relation to the Influence of Female Sex Hormones. *Arch. Int. Med.,* 118:229, 1966.

10. Immunity, Allergy and Infectious Diseases

IMMUNITY AND ALLERGY

The prevention, diagnosis and treatment of infectious diseases and their complications occupy a large portion of the time of the pediatric physician. These functions require not only familiarity with available vaccines and the clinical pharmacology of antimicrobial drugs, but also knowledge of the epidemiology of the common viral, bacterial, fungal and parasitic infections and an appreciation of the variation of their clinical manifestations in children of different ages as a reflection of the anatomic, physiologic and immunologic development of the host. An attempt will be made to summarize the present state of knowledge of the host factors which affect response to infection and allergens in the following sections.

The immunologic system has two main functional divisions: the phagocytic cells and the cells of the lymphoid system with immunologic competence. The *phagocytic cells* are essential for the capture, killing and processing of antigens from invading microorganisms, a process which requires opsonins and is enhanced in its efficiency by specific antibody and complement. The cells of the lymphoid system have 2 functional subdivisions. First, there are the *lymphocytes*, which require the *thymus* in early life for establishment of their immunologic competence. They are found in the paracortical areas of the lymph nodes and in the periarterial sheaths of the splenic white pulp. They are essential for *cellular immunity*, as shown by (1) resistance to infection with many viruses, fungi and mycobacteria, (2) the capacity to develop delayed hypersensitivity, which influences the pathologic picture and clinical symptomatology of a wide variety of infections, and (3) recognition of cells from different individuals and, thus, rejection of allografts. The second functional subdivision includes cells which may have the morphology of lymphocytes at one stage of their development, but change into plasma cells when they carry out the protein synthetic function which makes them responsible for *humoral immunity*. These lymphoid cells are found in the lymphoid follicles of lymph nodes, spleen, and other tissues, and, when stimulated, change into plasma cells which may be found particularly in the medullary cords of the lymph nodes, red pulp of the spleen, lamina propria of the bowel mucosa and in other sites of inflammation in the tissues. There they synthesize and secrete specific immunoglobulins which protect against subsequent exposure to certain viruses (e.g. measles and poliomyelitis) and bacterial exotoxins, and which seem to be essential for immunity to most invasive bacterial infections. The immunologic "memory," upon which the accelerated tissue and antibody responses of the immune state depend, appears to be a property of "instructed" lymphoid cells. It appears likely that both subdivisions of lymphocytes have this functional capacity, inasmuch as the circulating as well as the tissue lymphocytes represent a mixed population of cells.

Development of the Immunologic System

COMPONENTS OF THE IMMUNOLOGIC SYSTEM

Although a great deal of new knowledge has been acquired in recent years about the various organs, cells and proteins comprising the immunologic system, the exact manner in which their functions are linked together in response to infection is far from clear.

Organs. The *thymus* plays a dominant role in the development of immunologic competence by the fetus and the young infant. Its epithelial portions develop as paired structures from endoderm of the third and fourth pharyngeal pouches and from ectoderm of the corresponding branchial clefts. By about 8 weeks of gestational age, Hassall's corpuscles begin to appear, and shortly thereafter the small lymphocytes (thymocytes) which pack the cortex of the normal thymus are formed from the epithelial portion of the gland under the inductive stimulus of the mesenchyme which makes up its stroma. Soon thereafter lymphocytes appear in succession in the developing lymph nodes, gut mucosa, spleen and bone marrow, coinciding with the development of immunologic responsiveness by the fetus of 12 to 14 weeks. In the absence of intrauterine infection the development of the clear-cut follicular architecture of the mature lymphoid tissues and the appearance of plasma cells do not take place until 4 to 6 weeks after birth. Although the *relative* size of the thymus is greatest in the first few years of life, it continues to grow until puberty, when involution normally begins.

The thymus plays a key role in the development of immunologic competence by the lymphocytes as manifested by the capacity to reject allografts and to develop the delayed type of hypersensitivity. These functions are markedly depressed in certain animal species if the thymus is removed at birth. The fact that they can be restored not only by reimplantation of the thymus, but also by its insertion in a millipore chamber, which prevents the ingress and egress of cells, suggests that the thymus may act in 2 ways: first, possibly, by supplying competent lymphocytes to the peripheral lymphoid tissues; and, second, by secreting a hormone which affects the function of these cells. In animals thymectomized neonatally there is a paucity of lymphocytes in the paracortical areas of the lymph nodes and in the periarterial sheaths of the white pulp of the spleen; lymphocytes of these "thymus-dependent" areas are thought to be derived from or controlled by the thymus.

In chickens a second central lymphoepithelial organ, the bursa of Fabricius, which arises from the cloaca, controls the development of antibody formation. This function is markedly depressed by early bursectomy and is restored by the injection of bursal lymphocytes. These cells, in contrast to the thymus-derived lymphocytes, localize around the germinal centers to form the cortical lymphoid follicles of the lymph nodes. Efforts to identify, in man or other mammals, a second lymphoepithelial organ analogous to the bursa of Fabricius and essential for development of the capacity to synthesize antibodies have failed thus far; tonsils, appendix and Peyer's patches have all been suggested. Nevertheless studies of patients with immunologic deficiency have revealed conditions in which the functional deficits and morphologic changes are those which would be predicted if there were 2 such lymphoid systems and if one were deficient while the other remained intact.

The *lymph nodes*, the most important immunologically active organs, are located at strategic sites along the peripheral lymphatic vessels and serve to collect macromolecules and particulate matter. Their structure, consisting of sinusoids lined by macrophages, provides for phagocytosis of foreign and particulate material; the sinusoids are closely related to a cortex consisting of lymphoid follicles, the number and size of which reflect the activity of the node. The paracortical, thymus-dependent area with its accumulation of lymphocytes lies below the cortex; the medullary cords, which lead toward the efferent lymphatic channel, have the greatest concentration of plasma cells in a stimulated node (Fig. 10-1).

The *spleen*, which bears a similar anatomic and functional relationship to the bloodstream as lymph nodes do to the lymphatic vessels, contains abundant sinusoids lined with macrophages, sheaths of lymphocytes around the arteries, lymphoid follicles in the white pulp, and plasma cells in the red pulp. Thus both lymph nodes and spleen have (1) phagocytic elements which clear the lymph or blood during passage through the respective organ, and (2) lymphoid follicles, lymphocytes and plasma cells, which mediate the specific immunologic responses to foreign antigens.

Cells. Three main groups of cells are involved in immunologic responses: phagocytes, lymphocytes and plasma cells. The *phagocytes* include the "fixed" macrophages of the reticuloendothelial system in lungs, liver, spleen, lymph nodes and bone marrow, as well as the "wandering" phagocytes—the polymorphonuclear leukocytes and monocytes of the blood and the macrophages of the connective tissues. Eosinophils seem to be involved in the phagocytosis of antigen-antibody complexes.

Lymphocytes play a key role in specific immunologic responses to histoincompatible cells, to many viruses and to foreign chemicals or antigenic configurations of microorganisms which evoke delayed hypersensitivity. The lymphocytes in the blood are almost certainly a heterogeneous population. Cells with similar morphology may be derived from thymus, bone marrow and peripheral

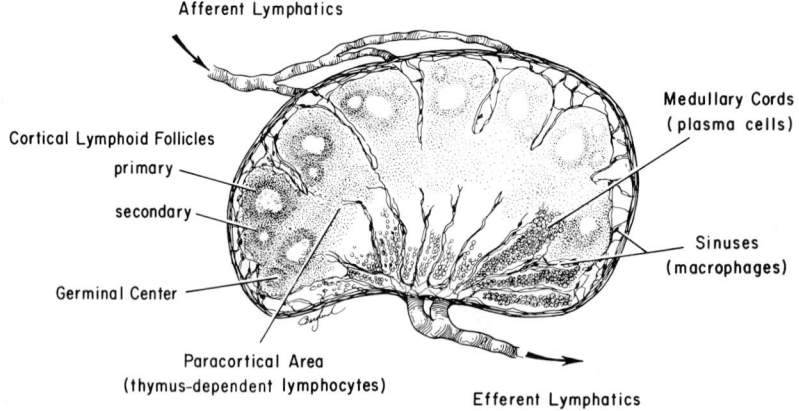

Figure 10-1. Diagram of a normal lymph node after antigenic stimulation.

TABLE 10-1. Human Plasma Immunoglobulins

CLASS OF IMMUNO-GLOBULINS	MOLECULAR FORMULA	MOLECULAR WEIGHT	CARBO-HYDRATE CONTENT	TURNOVER HALF-TIME (DAYS)	CONCENTRATION IN NORMAL ADULT SERUM (MG. %)	MATERNO-FETAL TRANSFER	FUNCTIONAL COMPONENTS
IgM	$(\mu_2\kappa_2)_5$	19S	10%	3-4	60-70	0	Antibodies formed in initial response
	$(\mu_2\lambda_2)_5$	900,000					Anti-O (bactericidal to gram-neg.) iso-hemagglutinins, Forssmann
IgA	$\alpha_2\kappa_2$	7-12S	7%	3-4	150-250	0	Serum IgA probably derived from locally formed "secretory IgA"
	$\alpha_2\lambda_2$	160,000-500,000					
IgG	$\gamma_2\kappa_2$	6.7S					Antibodies formed in later response
	$\gamma_2\lambda_2$	150,000	2%	20-30	700-1400	+	Antiviral Antitoxic Antibacterial Anti-H
IgD	$\delta_2\kappa_2$ $\delta_2\lambda_2$	160,000	—	—	3	0	—
IgE	$\epsilon_2\kappa_2$ $\epsilon_2\lambda_2$	180,000	—	—	0.03	0	Atopic reagins

lymphoid tissues (lymph nodes, spleen and Peyer's patches); some may have a life span of only a few days, whereas others have been reported to survive in the body for at least 1 or 2 years. Thymus-derived lymphocytes seem to move in the bloodstream only from the thymus to the thymus-dependent areas of the lymph nodes and spleen. Lymphocytes from the lymph nodes, on the other hand, undergo constant recirculation, passing first into the efferent lymphatics and the thoracic duct, thence into the bloodstream, and returning to the cortex of the lymph nodes from the blood by passing through the walls of the postcapillary venules. That this passage has a certain specificity is shown by the fact that when changes in the surface of the lymphocytes are produced by certain enzymes, passage of lymphocytes from the lumen of the venules into the cortex of the nodes is strikingly delayed.

Plasma cells are characterized by staining with methyl green-pyronin and by an abundant endoplasmic reticulum when examined under the electron microscope. They accumulate around small blood vessels in areas of inflammation, in the red pulp of the spleen and in the medulla of lymph nodes, as well as in such sites as the lamina propria of the gut mucosa. Their presence is associated with the formation of immunoglobulins, which can be demonstrated in their cytoplasm by specific immunofluorescence. It has not been settled whether plasma cells are derived solely from previously differentiated plasmablasts (preplasma cells) by mitosis after antigenic stimulation or also from the transformation of lymphocytes.

Immunologically Active Proteins. The *immunoglobulins* are synthesized by plasma cells and represent molecules specifically reactive with the antigens which stimulated their formation. Three main classes of immunoglobulins (IgM, IgA, IgG, or γ_M, γ_A, γ_G) are recognized when the plasma of normal adults is analyzed by immunoelectrophoresis; 2 additional classes, which are present in trace amounts in normal serum (IgD, IgE, or γ_D, γ_E) have been identified in recent years. The immunoglobulin molecules have a basic structure of 2 heavy (H) and 2 light (L) polypeptide chains joined by disulfide bonds. The L chains (κ or kappa and λ or lambda) are the same in all classes of immunoglobulins. Usually about two thirds of the molecules contain a pair of κ chains; one third of them, a pair of λ chains. On the other hand, the heavy or H chains of each class are different and account for the immunologic, structural and functional differences between the classes. Data concerning these differences are given in Table 10-1.

In addition, there are genetic differences between immunoglobulins from different persons. Thus far 4 different γ H chains have been identified from studies in myeloma patients (γ_a, γ_b, γ_c and γ_d). Therefore, one might write the formula for IgG globulins not just as $\gamma_2\kappa_2$ or $\gamma_2\lambda_2$, but as

$\gamma_{a2}\kappa_2$ or $\gamma_{a2}\lambda_2$, $\gamma_{b2}\kappa_2$ or $\gamma_{b2}\lambda_2$, $\gamma_{c2}\kappa_2$ or $\gamma_{c2}\lambda_2$, or $\gamma_{d2}\kappa_2$ or $\gamma_{d2}\lambda_2$. In those molecules containing γ_b or γ_c H chains, genetic variation is controlled by the G_M locus, and 20 variants have been identified. The Inv locus controls the structure of the κ form of L chains, with 3 determinants identified thus far. Because κ chains are present in all classes of immunoglobulins, this form of genetic variation affects them all and not just the IgG globulins, as in the case of the G_M locus.

Enzymatic and reductive cleavage of the immunoglobulin molecules has been used to investigate their structure and to alter them for therapeutic use. Three proteolytic enzymes — papain, pepsin and human plasmin — produce differing effects. Papain splits IgG globulin into 3 fragments, each with a sedimentation constant of approximately 3.5S, equivalent to a molecular weight of approximately 50,000; these fragments are known as the Fc fragment, which is without antibody activity, and 2 identical Fab fragments, each containing a single binding site for antigen. Pepsin digestion yields a single major 5S fragment ($F(ab')_2$) with a molecular weight of approximately 100,000, composed more or less of 2 Fab fragments, and with bivalent antibody activity. Properly controlled digestion of IgG globulin by human plasmin yields a major component with bivalent antibody activity and only slightly reduced molecular weight (6.5S), as well as smaller fragments. Purified and isotopically labelled fragments derived from pepsin and plasmin digestion of human IgG globulin have been shown to behave very differently after intravenous injection. The 5S $F(ab')_2$-like fragment of pepsin digestion has a very short half-life, while the 6.5S fragment obtained by plasmin digestion has a half-life close to that of normal IgG globulin (approximately 20 days). Both are much better tolerated on intravenous injection than are standard preparations of normal human serum gamma globulin, which contain small amounts of globulin complexes of higher molecular weight which produce severe reactions on intravenous injection, thus necessitating intramuscular administration. Gamma globulin fragments, some with molecular weights as low as 10,000, but still retaining bivalent antibody activity, are found in normal urine in very small amounts (5 to 10 mg. per liter).

IgM globulins are macroglobulins with a sedimentation constant of 19S and with a much higher valence and lower affinity for antigens than the IgG globulins, from which they may be distinguished by their susceptibility to reductive cleavage by mercaptoethanol, which destroys their activity as antibody. This type of antibody is the first to be detected after immunization or infection and is the "natural" bactericidal antibody in adult serum against the endotoxins of the gram-negative enteric bacilli. IgA globulins appear to be the antibody contained in body secretions, in which they appear as molecules with a weight of approximately 500,000 due to a combination of three 7S IgA molecules with an immunologically distinct "secretory" or "transport" piece which is not present in the circulating IgA globulins of the serum. Whether IgA globulins are synthesized by plasma cells in the sites of secretion or are simply transported from the blood into the secretions by combination with "transport piece" has not been definitely settled, but present evidence favors the former concept, the IgA globulins of the plasma representing overflow of locally synthesized IgA into the bloodstream.

Complement, originally described by Ehrlich as the heat-labile factor in serum essential for immunologically determined hemolysis, is a very complex system. For many years it was considered to have 4 components, but 9 separate proteins have now been identified. The complement system consists of a series of proteins (C′1 through C′9) that successively react with antigen-antibody complexes, with other macromolecular aggregates or with cells sensitized by antibody. In the course of this series of reactions, some of which require Ca^{++} or Mg^{++} ions, enzymes are activated which damage the bacterial or cell wall. Certain of the complement components themselves may be destroyed or altered by their participation in the reactions. In addition to the 9 known components of complement in serum, there are inhibitors which help to maintain an equilibrium in this system of interacting proteins, some of which are extremely labile. Thus C′1, the first component of complement, exists as a proesterase in serum, but is activated to an esterase (C′1 esterase) in the first step of the complement fixation reaction. Normal serum contains a C′1 esterase inhibitor, which can neutralize its activity; deficiency of this inhibitor in patients with hereditary angioneurotic edema results in recurrent attacks of localized swelling.

Research upon complement was handicapped in the past by the lability of many of its components and by the necessity for using immune hemolysis as the indicator system for measuring its activity. Recent advances in the purification of a number of the components of complement have made possible their measurement by immunochemical methods. C′3, or β_{1c} globulin, a relatively stable protein present in considerable amounts in normal serum, has turned out to be the limiting factor in immune hemolysis; its concentration is proportional to the hemolytic activity of fresh serum upon sensitized red cells. Thus immunochemical measurement of β_{1c} globulin concentration has been introduced as an easy method for measuring complement in clinical laboratories.

The components of complement appear to have a short half-life and rapid turnover in the body. Thus the level of C′2 or C′3 (β_{1c} globulin) is lowered only when there is a fairly massive fixation of C′ by antigen-antibody complexes (e.g. in acute glomerulonephritis, serum sickness or lupus erythematosus) or when synthesis is depressed.

Complement, or at least some of its components, probably plays an essential role in certain responses to infectious agents mediated by specific antibody – immune adherence, immune bacteriolysis, enhancement of phagocytosis and intracellular killing of virulent bacteria – as well as in certain aspects of the inflammatory reaction and the cellular damage produced by cytotoxic antibodies.

The *properdin system* is similar to the complement system in requiring specific and nonspecific proteins and Mg^{++} ions to produce immunologic injury. Lepow describes properdin as a "serum protein which is...distinct from the known immunoglobulins and which participates in a nonspecific manner in a variety of immunologic reactions of normal serum."

Interferon is a substance produced by cells infected with a virus. It inhibits viral multiplication in such cells. It is rapidly produced, nonspecific toward many viruses, but relatively species-specific in its action on cells. It probably plays an important role in recovery from certain viral infections. Interferon production may be stimulated by the injection of certain macromolecular substances such as double-stranded RNA, as well as by viral infection.

IMMUNOLOGIC RESPONSES

Inflammation. Most infections lead to inflammation, a nonspecific local response to injury characterized by migration first of polymorphonuclear leukocytes and later of mononuclear cells from dilated capillaries and venules, and by exudation of plasma proteins into the tissues at the site of infection. Small thrombi in blood vessels and lymphatics tend to localize the infection. The nature and intensity of the inflammatory response vary with the microbial agent as well as with the physiologic and immunologic status of the host. In general, the inflammatory reaction tends to be less intense in infants than in older persons. Study of the inflammatory response with a Rebuck chamber on the skin in newborn infants shows a greater than usual outpouring of eosinophils and a slower appearance of mononuclear cells.

Fever usually occurs in an infectious process, presumably as a result of the action upon hypothalamic nuclei of endogenous pyrogen released from leukocytes injured by bacterial endotoxins. Likewise, the *acute phase reaction*, which develops rapidly, is characterized by a series of changes in the plasma proteins which tend to parallel the intensity of the inflammation and to disappear when that subsides. These changes are (1) an increase in fibrinogen, producing a rapid sedimentation rate, (2) increases in α_1 antitrypsin, α_2 globulin and serum glycoprotein – principally haptoglobulins, and (3) the appearance of a β-globulin, the C-reactive protein.

Specific Immunologic Responses. While the local and systemic responses to infection are taking place, the immunologic response has already begun with phagocytosis of the infecting organisms by the leukocytes at the site of infection. This process requires *recognition* of the foreign nature of the infecting agent and the presence of "opsonins" in the plasma, and is greatly enhanced in the case of most virulent organisms by specific antibody and complement. If organisms invade the bloodstream, they are cleared through phagocytosis by the macrophages of the sinusoids of the liver and the spleen. The process of phagocytosis stimulates an increase in hexose monophosphate shunt activity and lipid turnover in the phagocytic cells, presumably to replenish the cell membrane pinched off to form the lining of the phagocytic vacuoles. Killing of the ingested bacteria is a complex process characterized by degranulation of the leukocytes and release of the lytic enzymes and bactericidal substances of the granules into the phagocytic vacuoles containing the ingested bacteria. The leukocytes may themselves be damaged or killed by the bacteria which they ingest, and release of their lytic enzymes as well as toxic products derived from the bacteria contributes to the intensity of the local inflammatory reaction.

Damaged cells, bacteria and the breakdown products derived from the action of the cellular enzymes on bacteria, tissues and plasma proteins are swept along in the lymph to the regional lymph nodes, where the macrophages ingest and digest these materials and somehow pass specific antigens along to the immunologically competent cells. Thus the process of phagocytosis results in the capture of infecting bacteria and their chemical processing to the actual antigens which initiate specific immunologic responses.

These responses may be divided into 2 groups: (1) those dependent upon the specific instruction of lymphocytes; and (2) those dependent upon the specific instruction of plasma cells. It is generally agreed that lymphocytes are responsible for the recognition of incompatible cells and hence for the rejection of allografts. They also are responsible for the delayed hypersensitivity which develops in varying degree in most infections. An intact thymus, at least in fetal and early neonatal life, appears essential for lymphocytes to develop their functional capacity to respond. Once "instructed" by an antigen, lymphocytes appear to carry "immunologic memory," so that subsequent encounter with the antigen evokes a rapid response. This memory may be due to gamma globulins, which have recently been separated from lymphocytes by chemical treatment and shown to be specifically reactive with antigens to which the donor had been immunized.

The cellular responses, which are the morphologic accompaniments to recognition of an antigen and to the antibody response, have been well described, but the biochemical events responsible for them are not clear. In vitro, when an antigen to which the host has been immunized is added to a culture of human peripheral blood lymphocytes, there is transformation of the cells to larger cells, and mitoses are induced in many

TABLE 10-2. CONTRAST BETWEEN PRIMARY AND SECONDARY
RESPONSES TO ANTIGENIC STIMULATION

	PRIMARY RESPONSE	SECONDARY RESPONSE
Basic process	*Instruction* of immunologically competent cells	*Immunologic memory* permits stimulation of previously instructed cells
Effect upon lymphocytes	Induction of state of delayed hypersensitivity (1-4 weeks)	Delayed hypersensitivity response (1-2 days)
Effect upon cells of plasma cell series	(1) Transformation to plasma cells (2) Synthesis of IgM globulin antibodies mainly	(1) Proliferation of plasma cells (2) Synthesis of IgG globulin antibodies
Antibody response	(1) Slow appearance (2) Low titer (3) Shorter duration of antibody	(1) Rapid appearance (2) High titer (3) Longer duration of antibody

of them. In vivo, the injected antigen is soon demonstrable in the lymph node draining the site of injection. The germinal centers of the primary follicles of the cortex enlarge, then secondary follicles develop at the periphery of the primary follicles, and, in a few days, plasma cells containing specific antibody appear in the margins of the follicles and, particularly, in the medullary cords.

Von Pirquet, in his studies of vaccinia, and von Pirquet and Schick, in their classic work on serum sickness, recognized that the difference between the initial response to an infectious agent or antigen and the response to a subsequent contact lay in a shortening of the interval between contact with the antigen and the manifestations of the immune response. These fundamental observations have been elaborated and applied in a practical way in recent years. A summary of the differences between the primary and secondary responses to an antigen or to an infectious agent is given in Table 10-2.

Another observation with important practical consequences, which has not been completely explained, is the action of adjuvants, originally described by Freund. By precipitation on aluminum salts of protein antigens, such as toxoids, or by adding oily substances or killed tubercle bacilli, the capacity of antigens to sensitize and to elicit antibody formation is greatly enhanced.

MATURATION OF IMMUNOLOGIC FUNCTION

By analogy with animal studies, immunologic competence is probably lacking during most of the first trimester of fetal life, so that *tolerance* to foreign cells and possibly to certain infectious agents may be established. This time corresponds to the period preceding population of the fetal lymphoid system with immunologically competent cells. During the subsequent 6 months of intrauterine life the fetus has the capacity to develop delayed hypersensitivity and to form plasma cells capable of synthesizing specific immunoglobulins. These are usually of the IgM and IgA classes; more than a trace of IgM globulin in cord blood provides suggestive evidence for prenatal infection. The human fetus probably does not synthesize IgG globulin, even though the level in the cord blood may be equal to or even slightly higher than that in the mother's blood at term; it manifests the same spectrum of antibody activity as the maternal IgG globulin and is almost certainly derived from transfer of maternal IgG globulin to the fetus through the placenta. This transfer is specifically related to the properties of the γH chains which are responsible for the immunologic specificity of the IgG globulins.

Postnatal development of the immunologic system is conditioned by the experience of the growing child. Animals raised in a germ-free environment, like human newborn infants, continue to have small lymph nodes, few plasma cells, and very low rates of immunoglobulin synthesis. Normally, soon after birth, the infant begins to respond to multiple antigenic stimuli from the bacterial flora which rapidly populate his skin, upper respiratory tract, and bowel, as well as from the microbial and parasitic infections (estimated roughly at one every 6 weeks until age 12) he acquires from his environment and from the vaccines he receives. If the immunologic system is normal, this immunologic experience is reflected in progressive hyperplasia of the follicles and gradual appearance of plasma cells in lymphoid tissues throughout the body, including enlargement of tonsils and lymph nodes from their relatively small size at birth. As the child's immunologic experience expands, there is an increase in immunoglobulin synthesis (Fig. 10-2).

An important aspect of immunologic development is that the maternally derived IgG antibodies are catabolized with a usual half-life of approxi-

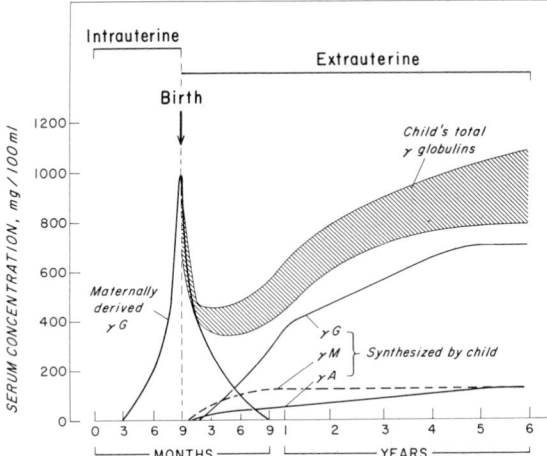

Figure 10-2. Average normal concentrations of the major immunoglobulins in the serum during fetal life and in the first few years of infancy and childhood. Considerable variations may occur as a result of infection or delay in the initiation of immunoglobulin synthesis after birth.

mately 30 days, so that passive immunity is gradually lost; the duration of immunity to a particular infection depends upon the level of the particular antibody in the mother's plasma during pregnancy and upon the amount of antibody required to protect the infant from that type of infection. Protection against pyogenic bacterial infections seldom lasts more than 1 or 2 months, whereas protection against measles or infectious hepatitis may last from 5 to 8 months. The striking frequency of sepsis or meningitis in newborn infants due to gram-negative enteric bacilli such as *E. coli*, probably depends, in part at least, upon the fact that bactericidal antibodies to this group of organisms are IgM globulins which are not transferred from mother to fetus.

The increasing immunologic experience of the child, derived from his contacts with various viruses, bacteria and fungi, is inscribed upon the memory of his specifically instructed lymphocytes which continue to circulate for several years and have the additional property of being able to transfer immunologic information to other lymphocytes through the "transfer factor" described by Lawrence. The induction of delayed hypersensitivity appears to have rather broad specificity for a whole species or group of organisms, whereas protective immunity is apt to be more strain- or type-specific. Thus the child who has already experienced a type XIV pneumococcal infection, for example, will react to infection with a type I pneumococcus with an accelerated and intensified inflammatory response, owing to the fact that certain lymphoid cells have become hypersensitive to antigens common to all pneumococci. The residual protective antibodies to the type XIV polysaccharide, however, will not protect against the type I infection. One concludes, therefore, that the formation of protective antibody to type I polysaccharide is in the nature of a primary response. It would appear that many of the relatively unique clinical pictures of infectious diseases during the first 3 years of life are due to the fact that these are primary infections occurring in the unsensitized host. By contrast in later childhood, delayed hypersensitivity to many of the common groups of organisms has already been established, even though protective immunity to the infecting strain is absent.

REFERENCES

Cooper, M. D., Peterson, R. D. A., South, M. A., and Good, R. A.: The Functions of the Thymus System and the Bursa System in the Chicken. *J. Exper. Med.,* 123:75, 1966.

Janeway, C. A., Rosen, F. S., Merler, E., and Alper, C. A.: *The Gamma Globulins.* Boston, Little, Brown & Co., 1967.

Lepow, I. H.: Serum Complement and Properdin; in M. Samter and others (Eds.): *Immunological Diseases.* Boston, Little, Brown & Co., 1965, p. 188.

Pirquet, C. F. H. von, and Schick, B.: *Serum Sickness.* Baltimore, Williams & Wilkins Company, 1951.

Smith, R. T., and Robbins, J. B.: General Physiology; The Specific Immune Response; Developmental Aspects of Immunity; in R. E. Cooke (Ed.): *The Biologic Basis of Pediatric Practice.* New York, McGraw-Hill Book Company, Inc., 1968, Section 6, pp. 495-507, 507-21, 521-36.

Immunologic Deficiency Diseases

The frequent complaint that a child has "poor resistance to infection" requires careful analysis. It may be due to unreasonable expectations of health, to environmental factors such as an overcrowded household into which older siblings bring multiple infections from their contacts at school or at play, or the child may truly have an unusual frequency or severity of infections. In the latter instance, *host factors* must be considered, but the physician should distinguish carefully between recurrent or persistent local infections, which suggest a local anatomic or physiologic defect, and the unusually severe, frequent infections which are suggestive of a generalized immunologic defect. The latter group of disorders will be described in this section on the basis of deficiencies of particular organs and cells, since this determines the type of functional impairment and the resultant clinical picture.

DEFICIENCIES OF THE PHAGOCYTES

THE WANDERING PHAGOCYTES

The polymorphonuclear leukocytes are the body's first line of defense against bacterial infections; wandering macrophages play an important supporting role. The polymorphonuclear leukocytes may be quantitatively or qualitatively deficient.

Neutropenia (see also p. 1072). Quantitative deficiency of the neutrophils may arise from a variety of causes. Failure to form them adequately in the bone marrow may occur as a rare congenital defect, either *reticular dysgenesis*, in which all white cells are absent and the infant survives only a few days, or *familial neutropenia*, a genetic defect (there may be more than one) which may result in death from infection within the first 1 or 2 years of life. *Acquired neutropenia* or *agranulocytosis* may develop at any age, either from direct suppression of the bone marrow or by the destructive action of autoantibodies. Thus it may be an expression of the toxic or sensitizing effects of various drugs, of invasion of the bone marrow by tumors or the action of the therapeutic agents used to suppress them, of damage by ionizing radiation, or of bone marrow injury from certain infections. It also may occur in recurrent cycles *(cyclic neutropenia)* of unknown cause.

The most common infection in patients with severe neutropenia is staphylococcal, usually arising from a local skin lesion, but other pyogenic infections, or invasion by gram-negative bacilli or anaerobic organisms from ulcerations in the oropharynx or gastrointestinal tract, may also occur. With the use of antimicrobial agents and the resultant distortion of the body's bacterial flora, invasive infections with drug-resistant gram-negative bacilli or fungi have become the principal causes of death.

Treatment of severe neutropenia consists in supportive therapy, the rational use of antimicrobial drugs, and protection of the hospitalized patient from infections by "reverse" precautions. Elimination of any drug thought to be responsible for the neutropenia, intensive antitumor therapy in cases of leukemia, good nutrition, and transfusion of fresh blood or concentrated white cells are all part of the relatively unsatisfactory treatment of neutropenia; the condition is best avoided by great care in the use of potentially toxic drugs and of those to which the patient is known to be sensitive.

Deficiency of Leukocyte Function. Two major disorders of leukocyte function have been identified thus far: chronic (fatal) granulomatous disease of children and the Chediak-Higashi syndrome.

Chronic granulomatous disease (p. 1074) is an X-linked recessive disease characterized by persistent and frequently fatal infections, often caused by organisms of low virulence which may be suppressed, but are not usually cured by antimicrobial therapy, and which result in lymphadenopathy, hepatosplenomegaly and hypergammaglobulinemia. The basic defect is an inability of both polymorphonuclear leukocytes and monocytes to kill ingested bacteria. There is a pronounced deficiency in the degranulation and stimulation of oxidative metabolism which nor-

mally accompanies phagocytosis, although the granules themselves contain a normal complement of enzymes and bactericidal substances. The metabolic abnormality of the leukocytes is the basis of the nitroblue tetrazolium (NBT) test, which is diagnostic for this disease and can be used to recognize heterozygous carriers (Fig. 10-3). Occasional heterozygous females may have trouble with persistent infections, and one female with the full-blown disease has been described. The exact enzymatic defect has not been identified, and specific immunologic responses (delayed hypersensitivity and antibody formation) are normal.

The *clinical picture* of the disease usually begins with infection of the skin, cervical lymph nodes or parenchyma of the lung; the middle ear or gut may be involved early. Lymphadenopathy, hepatosplenomegaly, and pulmonary consolidation with enlargement of the hilar nodes and hypergammaglobulinemia usually develop within weeks or months as infection recurs soon after antimicrobial therapy has been discontinued. Staphylococcal infection is most common, but gram-negative bacilli are often implicated as well. Locally, the pathologic reaction is a granulomatous one, with the formation of microabscesses which may give rise to draining sinuses. The peripheral blood picture varies; generally there is moderate anemia, mild neutropenia and a moderate increase in eosinophils and monocytes.

Antimicrobial *treatment* is often successful in

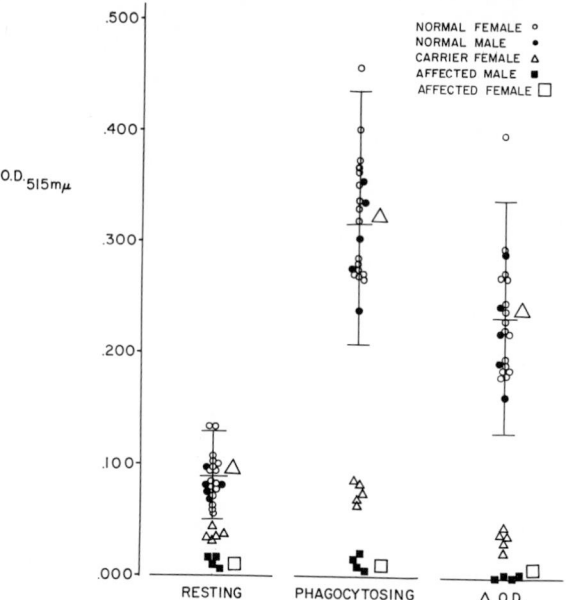

Figure 10-3. Chronic granulomatous disease. Quantitative NBT dye test on normal controls, mothers of affected males, affected males and 1 affected female and her parents (large symbols). Note that increased dye reduction during phagocytosis (as shown by change in optical density, △ O.D.) is nil for affected persons, marked in normals and slight but definite in carrier females. (Reproduced from *New England J. Med.*, 278:973, 1968, with permission of authors and publishers.)

suppressing the signs of invasive infection, but does little to eradicate the persistent low-grade infections or the immunologic responses which trouble these patients. The disease varies considerably in severity, but is generally fatal within the first 5 years in full-blown cases.

Familial opsonin deficiency, recently described in a mother and her daughter, is a condition somewhat analogous to chronic granulomatous disease. The defect is absence of a humoral factor necessary for the phagocytosis of particulate matter, including bacteria, by the polymorphonuclear leukocytes. Clinically, there are recurrent bacterial infections. The diagnosis is made by demonstrating the failure of leukocytes to ingest particulate matter (yeast particles) when incubated with the patient's plasma, but normal ingestion of the particles when the patient's leukocytes are incubated with the plasma of a normal person. Intravenous infusions of normal plasma result in temporary reversals of the defect.

The *Chediak-Higashi Syndrome* (see p. 1074) is a rare autosomal recessive disease characterized by the presence of giant granules in the leukocytes, undue susceptibility to bacterial infection, and diminution in the pigment of skin, hair and eyes. There are pyoderma, pneumonia, ulceration of the oral mucosa, and recurrent fever. Death usually occurs before adolescence with a terminal febrile illness characterized by enlargement of the reticuloendothelial organs, anemia, neutropenia and thrombocytopenia. Although the immunologic responses of these patients are normal, the giant granules found in the leukocytes represent a general phenomenon affecting many cells, apparently due to a failure of integrity of the membrane limiting subcellular particles; thus it appears to be a lysosomal disease, the connection of which with the abnormal susceptibility to infection remains unclear.

DEFICIENCY OF THE FIXED PHAGOCYTES OF THE SPLEEN

Bacteria that enter the bloodstream are usually rapidly cleared by the phagocytic action of the macrophages of the liver and the spleen. Smith demonstrated that when virulent pneumococci were injected intravenously into rabbits, the liver was responsible for removal of the majority of organisms in the immune animal, but that the spleen was principally responsible for this activity in the nonimmune animal. This experimental demonstration of the importance of the spleen has its counterpart in human disease, for clinical observation has shown that fulminating bacteremia and meningitis caused by the principal pyogenic invasive organisms—pneumococci, meningococci and *H. influenzae*—pose a very real threat to any child without a spleen. This has now been observed in 3 clinical situations: (1) *congenital absence of the spleen* (p. 1091), which occurs in association with certain cardiac malformations; (2) *familial*

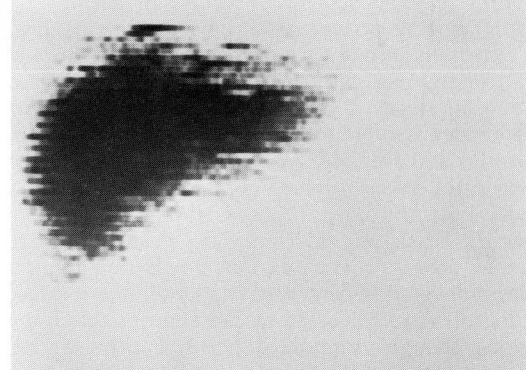

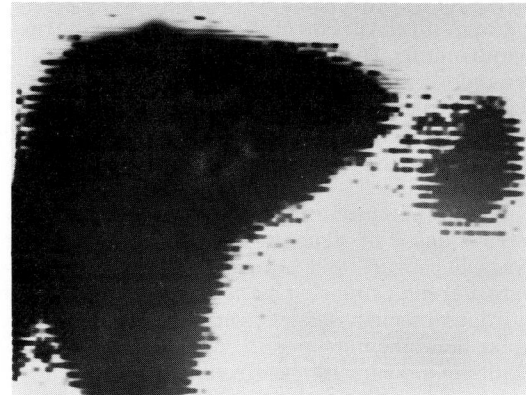

Figure 10-4. Hereditary splenic hypoplasia. Scintillation scan of the upper portion of the abdomen after injection of colloidal ^{198}Au. *Lower,* Normal scan of liver and spleen of unaffected sibling. *Upper,* Normal scan of liver, but no demonstrable spleen, in affected sibling. (Reproduced from *Pediatrics,* 42:755, 1968, with permission of the authors and publishers.)

splenic hypoplasia, observed in a family in which 3 siblings with severe fulminating bacteremia were shown to have structurally normal but minute spleens, whereas parents and siblings with no such infectious history had normal spleens (Fig. 10-4); and the (3) *postsplenectomy syndrome* (p. 1091), in which it has been statistically demonstrated that the younger the child in whom splenectomy is performed and the more serious the underlying disease, the greater the risk of subsequent fulminating bacteremia or meningitis. At present there is little one can do to prevent such infection except to be as conservative as possible in recommending splenectomy in young children, to warn the parents of a splenectomized child to be alert and to provide them with an effective broad-spectrum antimicrobial drug to be administered immediately at the onset of any febrile illness.

DISORDERS OF THE THYMUS

Because of the central role of the thymus in the development of immunologic competence, congenital thymic deficiency results in serious immunologic disturbances. Knowledge is too fragmentary to permit a rigid classification of diseases of the thymus, but certain clear-cut syndromes have emerged. In general, patients with thymic deficiency exhibit a severe defect in cellular immunity and are notably susceptible to certain viral (varicella, vaccinia) and fungal as well as bacterial infections, including those caused by acid-fast bacilli. In thymic deficiency the lymphocytes respond poorly to stimulation by phytohemagglutinin; delayed hypersensitivity cannot be induced, allografts are tolerated rather than rejected, and even though immunoglobulin synthesis and plasma cells may be found in some cases, antibody formation is seldom completely normal.

Congenital Aplasia of the Thymus (DiGeorge's Syndrome). This disease is characterized by congenital hypoparathyroidism with neonatal tetany, increased susceptibility to infections, particularly those due to viruses and fungi, failure to thrive, and anomalies of the mouth, neck and great vessels.

The grouping of anomalies suggests a developmental defect of structures arising from the pharyngeal pouches and branchial arches. Since the parathyroids and thymus are derived from the third and fourth pharyngeal pouches, combined aplasia of them is readily understood. The difficulty of inducing mitoses in cultured lymphocytes has hampered the search for chromosomal aberrations in this syndrome, and no genetic basis has been found for it.

Clinically, there are usually neonatal tetany and the low serum calcium and high serum phosphorus values seen in hypoparathyroidism. These manifestations respond to appropriate therapy, but within a few weeks or months a tendency to recurrent infections of the respiratory tract, diarrhea, moniliasis and failure to thrive becomes apparent. There are poor nutrition and growth, anomalies such as a fishmouth deformity of the lips and malformations of the ears, esophagus or great vessels (especially double aortic arch), and upper or lower respiratory tract infections.

The number of circulating lymphocytes is usually normal, but they respond poorly to stimulation with phytohemagglutinin. Efforts to elicit delayed skin reactions to antigens normally provoking them, such as *candida* antigen, or attempts to induce delayed skin hypersensitivity with potent sensitizers like dinitrofluorobenzene (DNFB), are unsuccessful. Usually the levels of immunoglobulins and of isohemagglutinins are normal for age, but specific antibody responses to injected antigens may be poor.

Pathologically, the stimulated lymph nodes display abundant follicles and plasma cells, but a depletion of lymphocytes in the paracortical ("thymus-dependent") areas (Fig. 10-6) and in the white pulp of the spleen. Thymic tissue usually cannot be found, and parathyroids are either absent or rudimentary.

Early diagnosis of these cases is essential and begins with suspicion of thymic deficiency in any young infant with a history of neonatal tetany or laboratory findings consistent with hypoparathyroidism. The increased susceptibility to infection is somewhat less severe than that observed in congenital thymic dysplasia, but sooner or later these patients succumb, generally before the age of 6 years, to some viral infection such as varicella or measles. *Transplantation of fetal thymic tissue*, resulting in establishment of immunologic competence and clinical improvement in the wasting and susceptibility to infection, has been carried out successfully in several infants and would appear to be the treatment of choice.

Hereditary Thymic Dysplasia (Thymic Alymphoplasia; Swiss Type Agammaglobulinemia). This disease gives rise to a severe form of immunologic deficiency characterized by persistent infections in early infancy, failure to thrive and death within the first 2 years. It is a genetic disease with both sex-linked recessive and autosomal recessive inheritance; no defect is demonstrable in the carrier of the trait.

Pathologically, the thymus is tiny, consisting only of a small, lobulated epithelial structure lacking corticomedullary differentiation, lymphocytes or Hassall's corpuscles (Fig. 10-5). The lymph nodes are tiny structures consisting mainly of stroma and sinusoids (Fig. 10-6), and the white pulp of the spleen and the lamina propria of the gut are devoid of lymphocytes and plasma cells; Peyer's patches are missing. The absence of lymphocytes in the tissues, except for a few in the bone marrow and blood, is striking.

The onset of persistent infection of the lungs, monilial infection of the oropharynx, esophagus and skin, chronic diarrhea and wasting and runting begins in the early months of life and progresses with monotonous regularity to a fatal termination despite all attempts at therapy. Examination usually reveals absence of tonsils, very small lymph nodes despite chronic infection, chronic pneumonitis evidenced by a pertussis-like cough, inspiratory retractions of the chest and rales, a somewhat distended abdomen with much wasting, and oral thrush.

Roentgenographic signs include pulmonary infiltration, and absence of a thymic shadow and of an adenoid shadow on lateral examination of the nasopharynx. There is usually an absolute decrease in the number of circulating lymphocytes, and occasionally neutropenia. In classic cases the immunoglobulins are markedly decreased, but variants have been described in which circulating immunoglobulins are normal or there is dysgammaglobulinemia. Plasma cells have been found in the tissues of such patients, but antibody formation is almost always somewhat impaired. Tests of delayed hypersensitivity give negative results: sensitization cannot be induced with dinitrofluorobenzene, cultured lymphocytes do not respond satisfactorily to phytohemagglutinin, and skin allografts are not rejected.

Treatment with grafts of immunologically com-

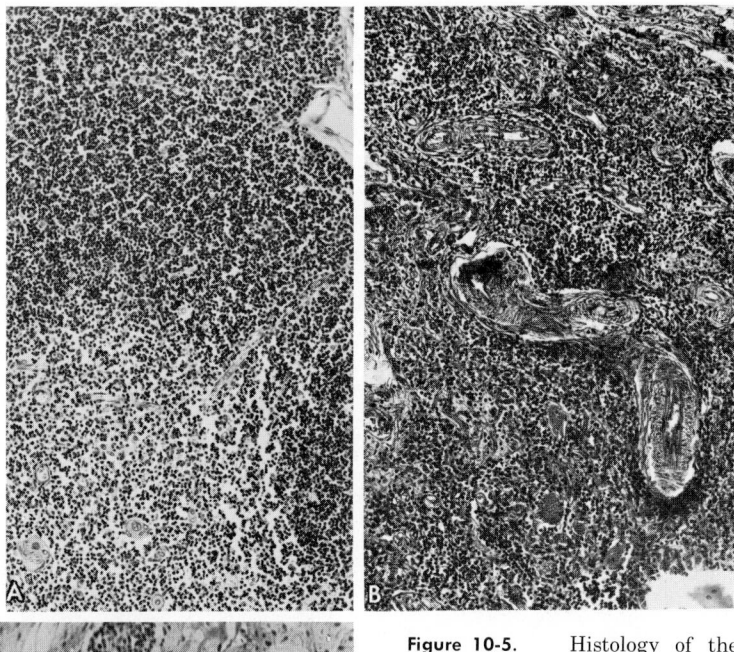

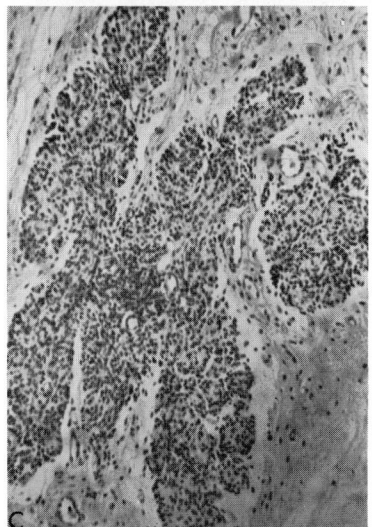

Figure 10-5.   Histology of the thymus. *A,* Portion of normal thymus. Note cortex *(top)* packed with lymphocytes and clearly differentiated medulla *(lower)* containing Hassall's corpuscles. *B,* Portion of thymus from patient with congenital agammaglobulinemia. The thymus is normal and contains Hassall's corpuscles, but there is involution as a result of fatal illness. *C,* Whole thymus from patient with hereditary thymic dysplasia (thymic alymphoplasia). Gland is minute and consists of lobulated epithelial structure without lymphocytes or corticomedullary differentiation of Hassall's corpuscles. (Reproduced from *New England J. Med.,* 275:775, 1966, and from *The Gamma Globulins,* Little, Brown & Co., 1967, with permission of the authors and publishers.)

petent cells derived from fetal or infant tissues or from adult bone marrow has thus far been unsuccessful in reversing the course of the disease, although a normal number of lymphocytes with ability to respond to phytohemagglutinin has been attained in several instances. The use of any but early fetal tissue may result in what appears to be a graft-versus-host reaction. Gamma globulin is ineffective in preventing infections, and antimicrobial therapy can provide only temporary relief. Immunization of these infants with BCG vaccine or with vaccinia or attenuated measles virus is strictly contraindicated, since this may lead to progressive fatal infections.

Other Types of Thymic Deficiency. Anatomic abnormalities of the thymus have been observed in other conditions. Interpretation of morphologic findings is difficult in view of the noted susceptibility of the thymus and other lymphoid structures

to depletion by wasting disease and by a number of therapeutic measures such as corticosteroid therapy.

Ataxia-telangiectasia (p. 1301) is an autosomal recessive disease in which abnormalities of the thymus have been found at postmortem examination. Progressive cerebellar ataxia begins in early childhood, associated with increasing telangiectasia. Gonadal dysgenesis and failure of sexual maturation may be present in those who survive beyond the first decade. In late childhood or subsequently many patients develop sinobronchial infections, including bronchiectasis, or malignant tumors, particularly of the lymphoid system.

The last 2 manifestations have suggested an immunologic disturbance affecting both cellular immunity and immunoglobulin metabolism. In many patients, blunting of delayed hypersensitivity reactions, failure to reject allografts nor-

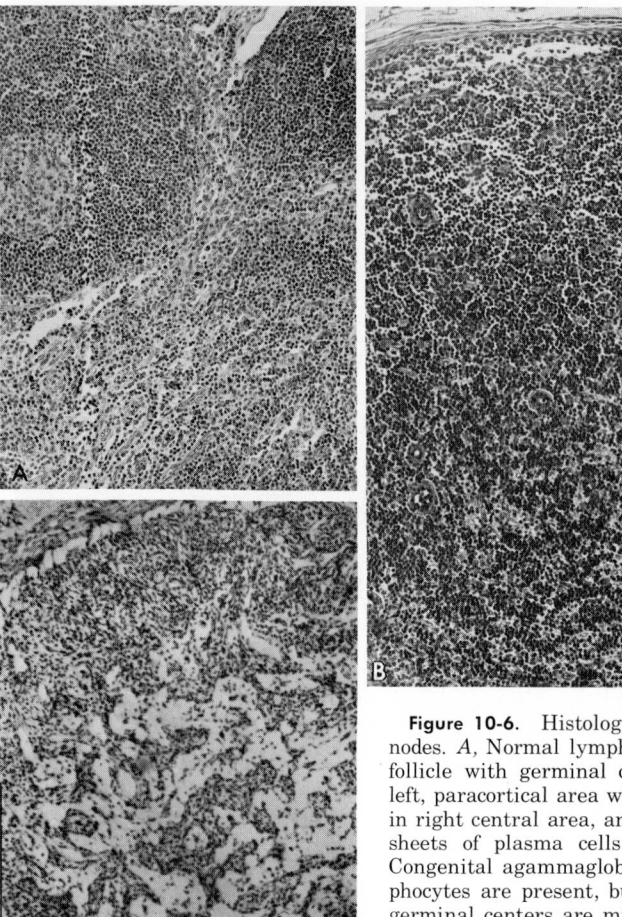

Figure 10-6. Histology of the lymph nodes. *A,* Normal lymph node. Cortical follicle with germinal center at upper left, paracortical area with lymphocytes in right central area, and medulla with sheets of plasma cells at bottom. *B,* Congenital agammaglobulinemia. Lymphocytes are present, but follicles with germinal centers are missing from cortex, and plasma cells are not present in medulla. *C,* Hereditary thymic dysplasia. The node consists only of sinuses and stroma. Lymphocytes and plasma cells are totally lacking. (Reproduced from *New England J. Med.,* 275:779, 1966, and from *The Gamma Globulins,* Little, Brown & Co., 1967, with permission of the authors and publishers.)

mally and reduced response of the lymphocytes to phytohemagglutinin suggest dysfunction of the thymic-dependent lymphocytes. At postmortem examination late in the disease the thymus is abnormally small and has a decreased number of lymphocytes, which have poor differentiation between cortex and medulla and decided diminution in Hassall's corpuscles. The number of circulating lymphocytes and the architecture of the lymph nodes vary considerably and do not always correlate well with the patient's history. The most consistent humoral defect is a low level or absence of IgA globulin in the serum, which occurs in about 70 per cent of affected persons and may precede clinical evidence of immunologic deficiency by a number of years. Thus, although ataxia-telangiectasia is a genetic disease in which many patients exhibit an immunologic disorder, it is not clear whether the thymic disturbance is primary or secondary.

Thymomas, consisting of spindle-shaped epi-

thelial cells, may also be associated with disturbances of immunity.

DEFICIENCIES OF LYMPHOCYTES

Quantitative or qualitative deficiency of some or all of the mixed population of cells which are morphologically lymphocytes may occur independently of primary disease of the thymus. The terms "lymphocytophthisis" and "alymphocytosis," originally used to describe clinical conditions subsequently recognized as *hereditary thymic dysplasia,* stress the importance of the deficiency of circulating lymphocytes and the absence of all types of lymphoid cells from lymph nodes and spleen which characterizes this syndrome (Fig. 10-6). Depletion of lymphocytes and depression of cellular immunity (delayed hypersensitivity and allograft rejection) have been described in instances of lymphangiectasia of the bowel, resulting in loss of lymph and lymphoid cells into the bowel lumen in a way somewhat analogous to chronic drainage of the thoracic duct which has been used to suppress homograft rejection in experimental animals.

Functional failure of the lymphocytes and even quantitative lymphocyte deficiency may develop late in the course of *ataxia-telangiectasia*, the *Wiskott-Aldrich syndrome* and in a few instances of *agammaglobulinemia*. A few cases of *"immunologic amnesia"* have been observed, in which recurrent infections have been associated with a reduction in circulating lymphocytes apparently due to the presence of a cytotoxic substance in the serum, resulting in a loss of immunologic memory. Though delayed hypersensitivity could be induced, it could not be retained. There was no "second-set" accelerated rejection of an allograft, and the antibody response to reinjection of an antigen was of the primary rather than of the secondary type. This state is somewhat analogous to that induced by the injection of antilymphocyte serum in order to prevent graft rejection. It is interesting that, after prolonged use of this agent in transplant patients, tumors, perhaps virus-induced, have occurred.

In *Hodgkin's disease* and also in *sarcoidosis*, both acquired diseases affecting the lymphoid system in a diffuse manner, many patients become "anergic." In Hodgkin's disease, antibody formation is usually not impaired, but the response to antigens normally eliciting delayed skin reactions is markedly reduced, allografts are tolerated by certain patients, and delayed hypersensitivity cannot be induced even by passive transfer of cells from sensitive donors. Thus there is a serious defect in cellular immunity to which the susceptibility of these patients to tuberculosis and fungal infections is probably related. Failure of cellular immunity due to destruction of normal lymphocytes in other lymphomatous diseases, such as acute leukemia, and by the antimetabolites used in therapy, undoubtedly plays a considerable role in the susceptibility of patients with these diseases to infections of all types, but notably to those caused by viruses and fungi.

DEFICIENCIES OF PLASMA CELLS

Deficiencies of the group of cells recognized by their characteristic morphology and staining with methyl green-pyronine as members of the plasma cell series result in inadequate synthesis of immunoglobulins and formation of antibodies, the so-called *antibody deficiency syndrome*. This syndrome is characterized by frequent, severe, recurrent infections caused primarily by the common pyogenic bacteria. If lymphocyte function is normal, as it is in the majority of instances, the patients tend to respond relatively normally to viral,

fungal and mycobacterial infections. The antibody deficiency syndrome encompasses a number of different clinical and pathogenetic entities.

Transient Hypogammaglobulinemia. Normally, the synthesis of immunoglobulins in response to infection and other antigenic stimuli begins after birth, with the result that the level of gamma globulins, which falls rapidly during the first month of life, levels off during the second month and soon begins to rise. Rarely, there is delay in the development of this important immunologic function; the level of IgG globulins received by passive transfer from the mother continues to fall and is not adequately replaced by immunoglobulins synthesized by the infant, so that within a few months the total gamma globulin level is much lower than usual for age. The infants have overt infections, unexplained episodes of fever and often bronchitis with wheezing. Regular injections of gamma globulin in full doses (see below) will protect them from severe, invasive infections. The injections may be discontinued when the IgG globulins begin to rise toward normal levels, usually before the age of 3 years. The cause and pathogenesis of this transient hypogammaglobulinemia are not known.

Congenital Agammaglobulinemia (Hypogammaglobulinemia; Bruton's Disease). This X-linked recessive disorder is the commonest form of the antibody deficiency syndrome. Though abnormalities of one or more immunoglobulins have been found among relatives of patients with the disease, no method has been found for detecting a carrier female, nor for diagnosing the disease in an affected male before several months of age.

Pathology. The thymus is normal (Fig. 10-5), but lymph nodes and spleen lack the usual follicular architecture. Germinal centers are absent, and there are few, if any, plasma cells in the medullary cords or red pulp (Fig. 10-6). Although the number of lymphocytes in the tissues appears diminished, they are present in the thymus-dependent areas, and normal numbers are found in the blood.

Clinical manifestations. The disease usually manifests itself in the second year of life, although the onset of the characteristically severe, recurrent infections may begin at any age from 8 months to 3 years. The infections are those caused by the common pyogenic organisms – *Staphylococcus aureus*, pneumococci, meningococci, *H. influenzae*, and less often beta hemolytic streptococci or salmonellae. They differ from infections in normal children only in their frequency, severity and the tendency for infection with the same organism to occur more than once. Pyoderma, purulent conjunctivitis, pharyngitis, otitis media, sinusitis, bronchitis, pneumonia, empyema, purulent arthritis, meningitis and sepsis occur with surprising frequency and may be associated with unusually high fever and unexpected elevation or depression of the leukocyte count. A rather indolent rheumatoid-like arthritis with sterile effusion into one

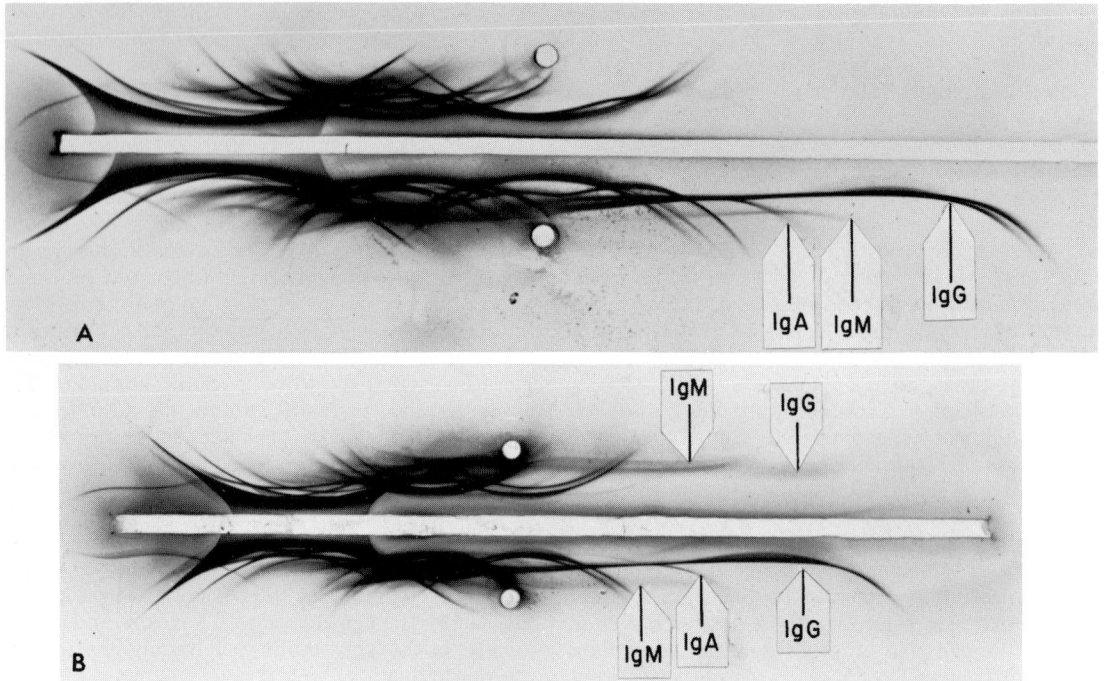

Figure 10-7. Immunoelectrophoresis of serum. *A, Top,* Congenital agammaglobulinemia. Complete absence of IgM, IgA and IgG bands. *Bottom.* Hypergammaglobulinemia, showing increased amounts of IgM, IgA and IgG. *B, Top,* Dysgammaglobulinemia. Marked increase in IgM, faint trace of IgG, absent IgA. *Bottom.* Normal serum.

of the large joints develops in about one third of patients and may be the presenting complaint. The children usually, but not always, handle most viral infections adequately, but progressive vaccinia, prolonged, severe varicella, and *Pneumocystis carinii* pneumonia have been seen in a few instances.

Diagnosis. There should be a high index of suspicion on the basis of the history of repeated severe bacterial infections. A careful family history may uncover instances of death from overwhelming infection or multiple severe infections in other male siblings, maternal uncles or male offspring of maternal aunts. Examination reveals little except the signs of infection, evidence of joint involvement if present, and unusually small, smooth tonsils. Lateral films of the pharynx fail to reveal an adenoid shadow. Lymph nodes are palpable, and regional nodes may become swollen and tender during episodes of infection. Proof of the diagnosis can be obtained by immunoelectrophoresis, which usually reveals a diminution of IgM, IgA and IgG globulins in the serum (Fig. 10-7). It is important to remember that, because of the individual variations and the low levels of IgM, IgA and IgG normally found in the early months of life, the diagnosis cannot be firmly established by immunoelectrophoresis until 6 to 8 months of age. Isohemagglutinins are usually absent or in very low titer. Injection of vaccines is not followed by an adequate antibody rise, and removal of a stimulated regional lymph node discloses absence of the expected germinal centers,

secondary follicles and plasma cells (Fig. 10-6).

Prognosis. Provided the diagnosis is made before infection has produced serious anatomic damage (e.g. bronchiectasis, middle ear deafness), the immediate prognosis for these children is excellent, and they gain and grow normally. In adolescence or early adult life, however, such complications may develop as hepatitis, dysgammaglobulinemia, and particularly a dermatomyositis-like picture with brawny edema, perivascular mononuclear infiltrates, and ultimately severe systemic symptoms and death (Fig. 10-8). The nature of this last complication is unknown, but neoplasia has been suggested; in our last case an enterovirus was repeatedly isolated from blood, stool and spinal fluid. Attempts to restore immunologic function with grafts of bone marrow or lymph nodes have not been successful, perhaps because cellular immunity and the capacity for graft rejection are intact.

Treatment. Vigorous antimicrobial therapy is indicated for individual infections, and regular injections of gamma globulin in doses adequate to maintain a plasma concentration of IgG globulin above 200 mg. per 100 ml. are essential. Maintenance therapy is initiated with a loading dose of 0.3 gm. (1.8 ml.) per kg. of IgG globulin. This may be given in divided doses over a period of a week in order to minimize discomfort. Thereafter an average dose of 0.1 gm. (0.6 ml.) per kg. per month (the volume of the injection may be scaled down if injections are given every 2 or 3 weeks) is required to maintain a protective

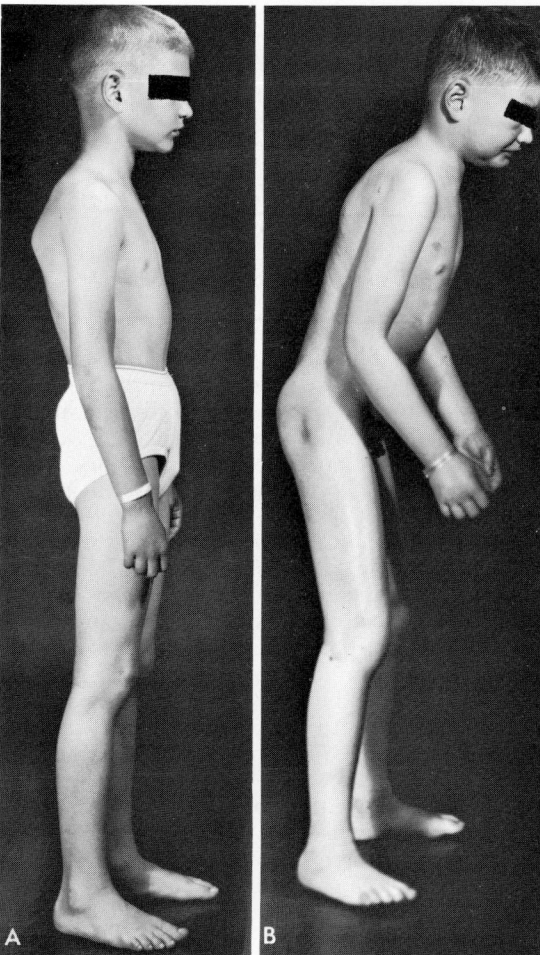

Figure 10-8. Congenital agammaglobulinemia. *A*, Age 11 years, in normal health. *B*, Age 12. Same patient 7 months after onset of dermatomyositis-like syndrome. Note brawny edema and contractures. Patient died 1 month later.

level of antibody. Intramuscular administration is necessary to avoid reactions with the standard preparation. A preparation satisfactory for intravenous administration is under study. Prophylaxis with gamma globulin is usually effective in preventing invasive bacterial infection and communicable disease, and its institution generally cures hydrarthrosis. It does not control localized superficial infection of skin or respiratory tract; in a few instances antimicrobial drugs may have to be given in addition.

Once a case of congenital agammaglobulinemia has been identified in a family, each subsequent male sibling or male offspring of a maternal aunt should be followed up carefully, with clinical examination and serial immunoelectrophoretic analyses of the serum at intervals of every 2 months from birth through the first year. Infants so detected and given prophylactic gamma globulin before severe infections have occurred, seem to thrive particularly well, but the physician must

be absolutely certain of the diagnosis before initiating such a program.

Acquired Agammaglobulinemia (Hypogammaglobulinemia). This antibody deficiency syndrome is similar to the congenital disease, except that it may develop at any age in patients of either sex. A predisposition may be inherited, since several instances of its development in siblings have been recorded; it has also been reported in only one of a pair of carefully studied monozygotic twins.

The main differences from congenital agammaglobulinemia are the lesser frequency of the rheumatoid arthritis-like picture, the greater frequency of a spruelike disorder, and the presence of somewhat higher levels of immunoglobulins, as well as low titers of serum antibodies. Pathologically, there may be necrobiotic change in the follicular architecture of the lymph nodes and spleen, and in some cases lymphadenopathy and splenomegaly result from reticulum cell hyperplasia. Many of these patients suffer bronchiectasis before the true cause of recurrent infections of the paranasal sinuses and lungs is recognized. Ultimately, malignant lymphoid tumors develop in an appreciable number of affected persons.

Management is the same as for congenital agammaglobulinemia.

Secondary Agammaglobulinemia (Hypogammaglobulinemia). In the 3 preceding forms of the antibody deficiency syndrome the deficiency of immunoglobulin synthesis is primary or idiopathic in the sense that it results from an unexplained inability to develop an adequate number of plasma cells in response to the stimulus of infection or immunization, so that there is failure of synthesis of adequate amounts of antibodies. Two types of antibody deficiency syndrome secondary to other disease processes may occur: (1) in diseases affecting the lymphoid system; and (2) in conditions responsible for hypercatabolic hypogammaglobulinemia.

Antibody deficiency syndrome due to known diseases of the lymphoid system. In extensive lymphomatous replacement of the normal lymphoid system, as well as in patients undergoing antimetabolite or radiation therapy for lymphoma or leukemia, many aspects of immunologic function, affecting both cellular and humoral immunity, are impaired. Hypogammaglobulinemia may develop, and, in chronic lymphatic leukemia in adults, becomes symptomatic in about one third of the cases. In multiple myeloma there may be a large increase in gamma globulin, which is monoclonal in type, from the neoplastic plasma cells, but there is often a severe antibody deficiency syndrome, which may be responsible for recurrent sepsis, frequently due to pneumococci.

Hypercatabolic hypogammaglobulinemia. The level of circulating immunoglobulins may be markedly reduced if there is extensive loss or rapid catabolism of plasma proteins, which results in a distinct shortening of their half-lives in the circulation. There may be loss of proteins through the skin in pemphigus, severe eczema or burns, into the lumen of the bowel in exudative enteropathy, or lymphangiectasis of the bowel, or into the urine in the nephrotic syndrome. There is usually a reduction of circulating albumin as well as of gamma globulin, but rarely, except in the nephrotic syndrome, is the deficiency of gamma globulin sufficient to produce undue susceptibility to invasive infection; plasma cells develop and immunoglobulin synthesis and antibody formation are normal even though the half-life of the immunoglobulin is greatly shortened. In the nephrotic syndrome several factors seem to be responsible for the increased susceptibility to infection: (1) age, since most of the patients are young children in whom recurrent infections are normally prevalent; (2) the nature of the edema fluid in the tissues and body cavities, with its low protein content, which makes it a good culture medium for certain organisms, notably pneumococci; and (3) the extremely low concentrations of gamma globulin in the edema fluid. The administration of prophylactic gamma globulin is of little use in instances of hypercatabolic hypogammaglobulinemia, since it is rapidly lost from the bloodstream.

Dysgammaglobulinemia. The term "dysgammaglobulinemia" is used for cases in which there are consistent deficiencies of one or 2 of the 3 major serum immunoglobulins. When such an abnormality is discovered, it must be considered in relation to the normally expected variation in concentration of these plasma proteins for the patient's age and condition at the time of the analysis. The significance of dysgammaglobulinemia lies in the fact that it is frequently associated with the antibody deficiency syndrome, whether congenital or acquired. Thus it is possible to have recurrent pyogenic infections with what appears to be a normal or only slightly low concentration of total gamma globulins.

Because there are 3 major classes of immunoglobulins, there are 6 possible types of dysgammaglobulinemia: three in which one and 3 in which two of the 3 immunoglobulins are missing. All 6 types have been observed, but only one has been reported in sufficient numbers to permit any sort of generalization. This type is one in which an elevation in the concentration of IgM globulin is associated with very low concentrations of IgG globulin and almost complete absence of IgA. The congenital form of this disease seems to occur almost entirely in males and has a suggestive X-linked pattern of inheritance. Except for a greater frequency of hematologic disorders (cyclic neutropenia, autoimmune hemolytic anemia, thrombocytopenia) the clinical course of these cases resembles that of congenital agammaglobulinemia. Histologically, there is disorganization of the follicular architecture in the lymphoid tissues similar to that of congenital agammaglobulinemia, except that PAS-positive plasmacytoid cells containing IgM globulin are present. In the acquired form of the disease, which may occur at any age in persons of either sex, the follicular architecture is better preserved, but similar plasmacytoid cells are found. In some infants with congenital rubella, hypogammaglobulinemia with very low IgG and IgA globulins, but persistently high IgM globulins, has been observed.

The most confusing situation arises in the case of an isolated deficiency of serum IgA globulin. In a few patients this may portend the later development of ataxia-telangiectasia, since it is present in about 70 per cent of such cases even before clinical symptoms begin. Yet an appreciable number of persons have been observed who remain completely healthy over many years despite deficiency of serum IgA globulin, so that such a finding is worth noting, but its clinical significance remains doubtful in any person.

Deficiency of Secretory IgA Globulin. Present evidence suggests that IgA globulin is synthesized in plasma cells closely related to the mucous membranes, but that it is secreted into colostrum, saliva, and respiratory and intestinal secretions as 3 molecules of IgA in combination with a "transport piece" which is separately synthesized in epithelial cells. IgA does not appear in secretions when it is not present in serum, but it can be secreted into the saliva in such patients in combination with "transport piece" if plasma containing IgA is infused intravenously. The total deficiency of serum and secretory IgA in certain patients with agammaglobulinemia and with ataxia-telangiectasia may be an important factor in their susceptibility to respiratory infections. It has been suggested that deficiency of IgA in the serum of some patients with steatorrhea or chronic diarrhea may be due to lack of IgA-producing cells in the bowel mucosa and that this is causally related to the diarrhea. The suggestion has further been made that recurrent otitis media in children with absence of IgA in the serum may represent the effects of deficiency of secretory IgA in the respiratory tract. These implications that a local antibody deficiency syndrome may be responsible for recurrent or persistent local infections are difficult to reconcile with the fact that some persons without IgA in the serum remain healthy all their lives; in some of these cases local secretion of IgM and IgG globulins has been demonstrated and may constitute a compensatory protective mechanism.

Unfortunately, standard preparations of gamma globulin contain very little IgM or IgA globulin, so that administration of such gamma globulin, which contains almost exclusively IgG globulin, cannot make up for their deficiency.

Wiskott-Aldrich Syndrome (p. 1086). The Wiskott-Aldrich syndrome is an X-linked recessive disorder which is usually manifested by eczema, thrombocytopenia, and a wide variety of infections beginning late in the first year, although it may present rarely as thrombocytopenia alone. Death may occur from hemorrhage, infection, or the development of a malignant process similar to the Letterer-Siwe type of reticuloendotheliosis.

TABLE 10-3. DIAGNOSTIC TESTS IN IMMUNOLOGIC DEFICIENCY DISEASES

FUNCTIONAL COMPONENT	DISEASE	SCREENING TESTS	DEFINITIVE TESTS
Phagocytes	Neutropenia	Low WBC, few neutrophils	Bone marrow examination
	Chronic granulomatous disease	Family history (X-linked recessive)	NBT dye test with WBC; phagocytic and bactericidal tests with WBC
	Congenital opsonin deficiency		No phagocytosis by WBC in patient's serum; satisfactory in normal serum
Spleen	Absence or hypoplasia	Absent splenic shadow by x-ray	Scan of upper abdomen after injection of radioactive colloid
	Thymic aplasia	Neonatal tetany (low Ca^{++}, high P) Skin tests negative	Failure of cultured lymphocytes to respond to: (1) Phytohemagglutinin (2) Monilia (3) Other antigens
Lymphocytes	Thymic dysplasia	Low lymphocyte count	(4) Allogenic lymphocytes Failure to reject skin graft Failure to become sensitized to DNFB
	Immunologic amnesia	Skin tests negative	Failure of anamnestic response Rejection first set graft; no second set rejection
Plasma cells	Antibody deficiency syndromes	Absent adenoid shadow (X-ray) Positive Schick test after DPT Low globulin (electrophoresis)	Immunoelectrophoresis—low to absent IgM, IgA, IgG Failure to form antibodies after immunization (primary or secondary)
	Agammaglobulinemia	Low to absent isohemagglutinins	Lack of plasma cells or germinal center in lymph node after stimulation
	Dysgammaglobulinemia	Moderate or no lowering of gamma globulin	Immunoelectrophoresis—deficiency of one or more immunoglobulins Failure to form antibodies Lymph node biopsy

The infections may be caused by a wide variety of microorganisms, including viruses, bacteria, fungi and *Pneumocystis carinii.* Transient episodes of arthritis have been observed.

Results of studies of the pathogenesis of the Wiskott-Aldrich syndrome are confusing. The lymphoid tissues appear normal early in the course of the disease, but as it progresses there may be a loss of lymphocytes from the thymus and paracortical areas of the lymph nodes. The peripheral lymphocyte count may decrease, and there is a variable loss of cellular immunity resulting in increased susceptibility to viral or fungal disease. Studies of immunoglobulin production in these patients suggest normal responses to a variety of antigens. IgM values are often low, and isohemagglutinins and Forssmann antibodies, normally present as "natural" antibodies, are usually lacking. The failure of these patients to respond to pneumococcal polysaccharides has led to the postulation that they have a general inability to respond to polysaccharide antigens, as opposed to normal responses to protein antigens. Whether this failure resides in the recognition system of the lymphocytes, in a deficit of the macrophages in processing such antigens or in a qualitative deficiency of plasma cell function is not clear. Since polysaccharides are widely distributed and important constituents of bacteria and fungi, it is reasonable that such a selective immunologic deficiency might have a serious impact upon resistance.

CHARLES A. JANEWAY

REFERENCES

Baehner, R. L., and Nathan, D. G.: Quantitative Nitroblue Tetrazolium Test in Chronic Granulomatous Disease. *New England J. Med.,* 278:971, 1968.

Bergsma, D., Good, R. A., Finstad, J., Miescher, P., and Smith, R. T. (Eds.): *Immunologic Deficiency Diseases in Man.* New York, The National Foundation, 1968, Birth Defects Original Article Series IV, No. 1.

Carson, M. J., Chadwick, D. L., Brubaker, C. A., Cleland, R. S., and Landing, B. H.: Thirteen Boys with Progressive Septic Granulomatosis. *Pediatrics,* 35:405, 1965.

Eraklis, A. J., Kevy, S. V., Diamond, L. K., and Gross, R. E.: Hazard of Overwhelming Infection After Splenectomy in Childhood. *New England J. Med.,* 276:1225, 1967.

Gitlin, D., Janeway, C. A., Apt, L., and Craig, J. M.: Agamma-globulinemia; in H. S. Lawrence (Ed.): *Cellular and Humoral Aspects of Hypersensitivity States: Symposium.* New York, Paul B. Hoeber, 1959, p. 375.

Hitzig, W. H., Barandun, S., and Cottier, H.: Die schweizerische

Form der Agammaglobulinämie. *Ergeb. inn. med. Kinder-heilk.*, 27:79, 1968.

Janeway, C. A., Rosen, F. S., Merler, E., and Alper, C. A.: *The Gamma Globulins.* Boston, Little, Brown & Co., 1967.

Kevy, S. V., Tefft, M., Vawter, G. F., and Rosen, F. S.: Hereditary Splenic Hypoplasia. *Pediatrics,* 42:752, 1968.

Kretschmer, R., Janeway, C. A., and Rosen, F. S.: Immunologic Amnesia. *Pediat. Res.,* 2:7, 1968.

Rosen, F. S., and Janeway, C. A.: The Gamma Globulins. III.

The Antibody Deficiency Syndrome. *New England J. Med.,* 275:709, 769, 1966.

Schulkind, M. L., Ellis, E. F., and Smith, R. T.: Effect of Antibody upon Clearance of I^{125} Labeled Pneumococci by the Spleen and Liver. *Pediat. Res.,* 1:178, 1967.

South, M. A., Cooper, M. D., Wollkeim, F. A., and Good, R. A.: The IgA System. II. The Clinical Significance of IgA Deficiency: Studies in Patients with Agammaglobulinemia and Ataxia-Telangiectasia. *Am. J. Med.,* 44:168, 1968.

Allergic Disorders

The allergic disorders of children comprise a relatively large and heterogeneous group of conditions which have in common immunologic hypersensitivity to molecular substances foreign to the individual. These foreign molecules serve as *antigens* which, when they produce symptoms, are designated as allergens.

Allergic disorders account for about one third of all chronic disease in children; asthma is the principal cause of chronic school absenteeism.

The term "allergic," often loosely used in reference to disorders of doubtful immunologic origin, has its clearest meaning when it refers to disorders which are generally given the name *atopy*, and of which the *immediate* reaction and the development of *reagins* are highly characteristic features. Certain more or less definite clinical patterns are recognized: urticaria, seasonal and perennial rhinitis, asthma, infantile and childhood eczema and certain drug reactions. Anaphylaxis, serum sickness, the Arthus phenomenon and certain other conditions, though not in a strict sense atopy, are closely related. Contact dermatitis, though it involves delayed rather than immediate reactivity, has been traditionally accepted as allergic. On the other hand, such disorders as lupus erythematosus, rheumatoid arthritis, scleroderma and dermatomyositis, and such autoimmune disorders as sympathetic ophthalmia and thyroiditis, in which the specificity of antibody is directed in whole or in part against the body's own tissues rather than against exogenous antigen, are not considered to be in the same general category as the allergic diseases.

The clinical heterogeneity of the allergic disorders requires that the clinician make every attempt to distinguish between allergic conditions and those disturbances which depend upon some other kind of idiosyncratic response to an exogenous agent. Examples of the latter are the intolerance of the child with galactosemia or lactase deficiency for milk, or the intolerance of the child with celiac disease for the gluten of wheat or other grains. In some conditions in which an evident intolerance for some environmental substance appears to exist, it will not be possible to determine whether the illness is an allergic one in the immunologic sense or an idiosyncrasy in some other sense. No useful purpose is served by designating as "allergic" vague or obscure conditions for which no adequate explanation can be found.

The *allergic* person is distinguished by the clinical features of an abnormal response of reactive cells to contact with antigen or allergen which does not occur when the nonallergic person is exposed to the same potential allergen. The heightened reactivity of the allergic person is often reflected in demonstrable alteration in local or general reactivity in tissues other than those exhibiting the principal symptom. For example, the skin may be reactive to the same allergens which produce nasal or bronchial symptoms upon inhalation. This feature is evidence that the reactivity of the allergic person is vested in wandering cells, rather than in the fixed cells of the involved tissue.

Adequate appraisal of the allergic child must take into account that the clinical manifestations are highly individual and highly variable and that a characteristic feature is the tendency to respond with allergic symptoms to a variety of situations. Among these situations may be distinguished (1) repeated exposure to foods, inhalants or contactants which have the potentiality of sensitizing; (2) infection, particularly of the upper and lower respiratory tracts; (3) acute or chronic emotional tension; and (4) sensory stimulation by certain nonallergenic irritants, such as heat, cold, trauma, dusts and the like.

No 2 children will have exactly the same allergic problem, so that the necessary insights for the optimal therapeutic program for any child will derive only from understanding him as completely as possible in the context of his own life situation. The emergence of symptoms in the allergic child is the result most often of not just a single allergenic stimulus. In many children, symptoms most likely depend upon the additive effects of genetic, dietary, inhalant, contactant, emotional, infectious and simple physical irritant factors.

It may be inferred that many different stimuli have the capacity to stimulate the effector tissue. In the case of immunologically active stimuli, the release of certain substances from reactive cells into tissues presumably produces symptoms. When allergic symptoms complicate otherwise undifferentiated respiratory infections, it is possible that in the atopic child the normal inflammatory response of involved tissues to infection is exaggerated by underlying allergic reactivity. The responsiveness of many allergic children to changes in ambient temperature or to irritating but nonantigenic dusts may also be an exaggeration of the response of an end-organ sensitized by allergic reactivity. It may be that the relative increase in parasympathetic tone during sleep explains in part the tendency of many allergic persons to have a worsening of their symptoms at night; and it may be through excitation of parasympathetic pathways, with vascular dilatation, smooth muscle spasm and increased secretion, that emotional stimuli produce symptoms in the allergic child.

Opinions differ as to whether emotional tensions act as primary initiators of the allergic state, but there can be no doubt of a relation between emotional tension and allergic symptoms in the reactive child. Not only will emotional turmoil precipitate allergic symptoms in some children, but also allergic symptoms may themselves provoke great anxiety in both child and parents. Management of eczema or asthma which fails to take into account emotional considerations is likely to fall short of optimal results.

Although hormones of the adrenal medulla and cortex are useful in management of allergic conditions, and possibly some allergic children may mobilize them less readily than other children, allergic reactivity of the atopic child has no well defined relation to his endocrine status.

Immunologically, there are 2 broad categories of allergic responses: the *immediate response*, mediated by chemicals released from sensitized cells on contact with an allergen and characteristic of *atopic reactivity*; and the *delayed response*, characteristic of bacterial and contact allergies.

The metabolic processes involved in the immunologic aspects of the allergic state are vested in the wandering cells of the lymphoid and reticuloendothelial systems; wherever a reaction occurs, these cells rather than the immobile cells of the involved organ are the ones which are primarily reactive. The reactive cells may, upon contact with allergenic particles, be stimulated to phagocytosis or incorporation of the particle, to the elaboration and release of chemical substances which may affect other cells in local or remote areas, or to increased production of antibody molecules specific for the antigen by which the cell is stimulated. Evidence suggests that these different responses are vested in morphologically different cells: phagocytosis in macrophages, the release of chemical mediators in basophils or mast cells, and the production of antibody in plasma cells. How these cells are related to the lymphocyte or histioblast or other reticuloendothelial cell which may be their common precursor remains uncertain.

The hallmarks of the *immediate allergic reaction* are the *wheal* and *flare* in the skin, edema, spasm of smooth muscle, and increased secretion by cells of involved membranes of the respiratory or gastrointestinal tract. A number of chemical mediators of the immediate reaction have been distinguished, the most important of which is histamine. Hista-

mine is found most abundantly in mast cells, and in lesser degree in eosinophils and neutrophils. Histamine is released from these cells in response to trauma, in states of shock, or upon contact with certain relatively simple chemical substances or with certain molecular complexes. The substances known as histamine-releasers include many antigen-antibody complexes, wasp and bee and snake venoms, and a number of drugs. These last include morphine, polymyxin, neomycin, tubocurarine and a variety of simple amines and diamines, among which are probably epinephrine and some antihistaminics.

Histamine released or injected into the tissues dilates the capillary bed, increases capillary permeability which leads to edema, contracts smooth muscle (including that of the arterioles) and stimulates glandular secretions. The glands of the stomach are exquisitely sensitive to histamine; this may be the prime normal stimulus for gastric secretion. Large doses of histamine in man produce hypovolemic shock rather than an increase in blood pressure. The body normally disposes of histamine partly through the action of the enzyme histaminase, partly through methylation of the ring portion of the molecule. It is possible that the eosinophil may have antihistaminic activity. This cell is likely to be associated with chronic allergic states or with the convalescent rather than the acute phase of acute allergic reactions.

The effects of histamine in the tissues may be in part blocked by drugs known as "antihistaminics." These generally act by blocking the effect of histamine upon the target cells. All effects of histamine are likely to be blocked in some degree by these agents except that upon gastric secretion. Other properties of antihistaminics include a general tendency to depress the central nervous system, antiemetic activity, some tendency to produce local anesthesia, and such atropine-like effects as drying of mucous membranes and possibly mild bronchodilatation. Some antihistaminics, like the closely related phenothiazines, may produce extrapyramidal central nervous system difficulties. Some are potent sensitizers when applied to the skin.

Other substances which play less clearly defined roles in the immediate allergic reaction include acetylcholine, serotonin (5-hydroxytryptamine), bradykinin, the "slow-reacting substance" and the Miles permeability factor. Bradykinin and the "slow-reacting substance" are polypeptides of unknown structure, and the Miles permeability factor is a proteose; the effects of these agents on capillary permeability or on smooth muscle are similar to those of histamine, but are not so rapid or intense.

Epinephrine and its analogues are the physiologic and pharmacologic antagonists of histamine. They promote capillary constriction, restoration of integrity of the capillary wall and relaxation of bronchial smooth muscle put into spasm by histamine. Active agents include, besides epinephrine, norepinephrine, ethylnorepinephrine, isopropylnorepinephrine, ephedrine, pseudoephedrine (an optical isomer of ephedrine), phenylpropanolamine and others. These agents differ as to their relative reactivities upon various tissues and in the degree to which they produce effects, such as the increases in heart rate or blood pressure, which may not be essential elements in controlling allergic symptoms. In asthma or allergic rhinitis, for example, in contrast to the circumstances in acute anaphylactic shock, these other effects of epinephrine may not be desired.

The differences among sympathomimetic drugs relate in considerable measure to whether they act upon α or β adrenergic receptors, or both. Alpha adrenergic activity stimulates smooth muscle of the blood vessels in skin and most viscera, stimulates the uterus, ureter, and the dilator of the pupil, and inhibits intestinal smooth muscle. Beta adrenergic activity inhibits the smooth muscle of blood vessels in muscle, in the coronary vasculature and in a few viscera; it stimulates the myocardium, and relaxes bronchial smooth muscle. Epinephrine, ephedrine and pseudoephedrine have both α and β adrenergic activity, whereas norepinephrine and methoxamine have predominantly alpha, and such drugs as isopropylnorepinephrine and isoetharine have predominantly beta activity.

It has been suggested that partial blockade or depressed reactivity of β adrenergic reactive sites may be a fundamental problem in the allergic diathesis. It is known, for example, that asthmatics are quite sensitive to bronchoconstrictive effects of such β adrenergic blocking agents as propanolol, which are therefore contraindicated or to be used with great caution in allergic persons. By contrast, it has been reported that asthma may be improved with the use of α adrenergic blocking agents, though they have no place in its current therapy.

Corticosteroids are capable of controlling many of the manifestations of atopic disease, but no clear relation with metabolism of histamine has been delineated. Ordinarily, the administration of corticosteroids does not modify the wheal and flare response to histamine or to skin testing. On the other hand, there is some evidence that the corticosteroids may impede the reaccumulation of histamine in tissue cells after its release, and that with prolonged administration the tissues may eventually be relatively depleted of histamine and so become unreactive. It is uncertain whether the anti-inflammatory action of the corticosteroids plays an important role in the control of symptoms due to the immediate type of allergic reactivity.

A highly characteristic feature of atopy is that the capacity to respond immediately to antigenic stimulation with the dermal wheal and flare reaction can be transferred by the intracutaneous injection of serum from an allergic person to a nonallergic one (Prausnitz-Küstner reaction). The recipient site becomes sensitized several hours after local injection of serum and may remain sensitized for a week or more. The transferred reactivity is highly specific for the antigens to which the donor of the serum is skin-sensitive.

The substances responsible for the transfer of reactivity from the allergic person to a nonallergic recipient have been given the name *reagins*. They are found among the immune globulins, predominantly if not exclusively in the fraction designated IgE, which is closely associated with IgA and, like IgA, does not cross the placenta.

Reagins can sensitize normal human leukocytes for release of histamine on exposure to specific allergens. It seems probable that cell-bound reagin is the essential ingredient in the *immediate* allergic response, which can be transferred passively with cells as well as with serum. Reagins do not normally induce passive cutaneous anaphylaxis (PCA) in the guinea pig, but IgE has induced it in the monkey. An exceptional capacity to produce reaginic IgE antibody *may be* a basic difficulty of the atopic person; it has been suggested that desensitization by means of allergenic vaccines may be through stimulation of increased production of IgG antibodies. Some of the IgG antibodies produced by desensitization in both atopic and normal persons have a high avidity for antigen and have the ability to "block" the union of antigen and reagin, with suppression of the immediate response. It has been postulated that the benefit derived from desensitization is the result of the production of these blocking substances. The titers of blocking activity, however, have not correlated well with clinical relief when studied with conventional skin test techniques. In contrast, recent work using the release of histamine from leukocytes as a sensitive indicator has shown that the appearance of blocking substances may bear a close relation to clinical relief from desensitization.

Delayed hypersensitivity is the form of allergic reactivity associated with a number of mycobacterial (tuberculosis), bacterial (brucellosis), viral (mumps), fungus (histoplasmosis) and parasitic (trichinella) diseases and with contact dermatitis. The presence of the delayed hypersensitive reaction is always good evidence of previous infection, and may indicate partial or complete immunity to the agent from which the antigen is derived.

Delayed hypersensitivity as elicited by skin testing is not manifest for 24 to 72 hours. The tuberculin reaction is typical of the delayed response. Delayed hypersensitivity is elicited by relatively complex antigens such as those of bacteria or viruses, and by such simple antigens as those of certain drugs or metals. It is thought that the antigenicity of the latter substances is related to their function as haptens.

Though the delayed form of hypersensitivity is not transferred from one person to another through the medium of serum, the transfer of sensitized lymphocytes or other reticuloendothelial cells or a soluble fraction of them does sensitize a local site in an appropriate recipient. Sensitization may be demonstrated immediately and may persist for many weeks.

The reaction of delayed hypersensitivity is essentially unmodified by epinephrine and its analogues, but may be completely abolished by the anti-inflammatory action of corticosteroids.

A principal difference between the immediate and delayed types of hypersensitivity is that nearly everyone appears capable of developing the delayed type, whereas the development of symptoms in association with the immediate type of hypersensitivity tends to occur in fewer people and to have strong familial tendencies. Not every person with reagins, however, actually suffers from atopic symptoms. The number of people with major allergic disorders has been estimated to be as much as 10 per cent of the population, whereas the number having minor intolerances to external antigens is estimated to be as high as 50 per cent.

METHODS OF STUDY OF THE ALLERGIC CHILD

History. Careful inquiry about the child's allergic difficulties is the most useful device leading to discovery of allergens or other factors which may be responsible for symptoms. The aim of history taking should be to relate allergic symptoms as accurately as possible with items in the diet, to places inside and outside the home, to the time of day, day of week or season of the year in which symptoms occur, to the presence or absence of concomitant signs of infection, and to emotional factors. The emotional response of parents and child to the child's illness should also be carefully and empathetically explored.

History taking is a continuous process, demanding detailed inquiry as to circumstances surrounding symptoms which have occurred since the last visit. This continuous history taking is both an essential diagnostic tool and the most useful medium for education of parents and child about continued therapy.

The focus of history taking will vary with the presenting symptoms. Gastrointestinal symptoms and eczema in the early months of life and allergic tension and allergic fatigue in the older child are particularly likely to be associated with foods. Respiratory symptoms may also be related to foods in infancy, but later are more often generated by infection or inhalant allergens. Accordingly, history taking in the older child should carefully review exposures inside and outside the home to such antigens as dust, feathers, animal danders, wool, pollens and molds.

In the search for inhalant allergens it is often appropriate to begin with the bedroom, and attempt to identify all potential allergens, especially the nature of pillows, blankets, mattress and box springs, and whether allergen-proof coverings are used on these items. The physician will need to determine how this room can be isolated from the remainder of the house, particularly if there is a hot air heating system. It will be helpful to know whether respiratory symptoms are manifest at times of housecleaning or in any particular area which may be characterized by a particular antigenic flora, such as in the basement, attic or barn.

The physician will need to know the many ways in which potential or known allergens may invade the diet or the environment of the allergic child without being readily detected. Some mothers, for example, who carefully avoid giving the child eggs may fail to take note of egg in custards. The infant highly reactive to milk may be given milk substitute as his feeding formula, but may have his cereal moistened with evaporated or whole milk. The child with an intolerance to chocolate sometimes has his characteristic difficulties when taking certain cola drinks.

Seventy-five per cent of allergic children have a positive family history of allergy on at least one side of the family, 35 per cent on both. Knowledge of the evolution of allergic symptoms in the parents or relatives may provide some evidence of the pattern or intensity of the genetic element. In the case of children with vague symptoms which *may* be allergic, the allergic symptoms of their parents may be equally vague. Some parents, for example, may deny allergic disease, but will readily acknowledge seasonal sinusitis or that as children they had symptoms similar to those manifested by the child, which were called bronchitis, recurrent pneumonia or an "unusual susceptibility to colds." The allergic history should always include details of previous studies and treatment, and should record the results of treatment, and for how long and in what season relief, if any, appeared to be obtained.

Avoidance of Suspected Allergens. When the history indicates possible offending allergens, their exclusion from the diet or environment may prove both diagnostic and therapeutic. The child who coughs only after going to bed at night and for a few minutes or hours in the morning may experience dramatic relief from the removal of a feather pillow from the bed. The infant who spits or vomits his cow's milk formula may eagerly accept a substitute for cow's milk with gratifying relief of his gastrointestinal difficulties. Unfortunately the control of allergic symptoms is not always so simple; most often symptoms do not depend upon a single allergen. There is also evidence that the reactive child may be tolerant of a single one of the substances to which he is reactive, but will react when exposed to two or more of them simultaneously. The management of seasonal respiratory symptoms, for example, is likely to require attention not only to pollens and molds, but also to house dust and to other inhalant or food allergens.

In control of inhalants, attention is focused primarily upon the bedroom, since the child spends more time in this room than in any other single area. As to foods, it is more helpful to reduce the diet to a nutritionally adequate selection of foods unlikely to be allergens than to eliminate single items serially from a diet which is otherwise uncontrolled and essentially unmonitored. Elimination diets (p. 1549) are helpful in this respect.

In the young infant the possibility of allergy to food can usually be determined relatively quickly by initially limiting the diet to a cow's milk formula for about 10 days. If symptoms are relieved, it can be inferred that some dietary item excluded from the diet was at fault. If symptoms continue, a hypoallergenic milk substitute should be used in place of cow's milk for an equal length of time.

In the older infant or child a diet of veal and lamb, rice and oat cereals, *root* vegetables such as potatoes, beets and carrots, *leaf* vegetables such as lettuce and other greens, cooked and canned fruits and fruit juices, gelatin desserts and synthetic vitamins is nutritionally adequate and does not contain foods of high sensitizing potential, such as wheat, egg, cow's milk, chocolate, fish, peas or beans, tomatoes, citrus fruit, spices or seafood. A period of trial on such a diet may quickly reveal whether cow's milk, wheat, egg, combinations of these, or other potent food allergens are likely to contribute in a large way to a child's difficulty. In the child with more or less continuous symptoms a trial of a week or two on such an elimination diet should be enough to disclose whether substantial relief has been attained. For the child with episodic symptoms the problem of identifying offending allergens is more difficult. It may be necessary to record scrupulously in a food diary everything eaten by the child so that an attempt may be made to relate symptoms to individual foods.

Skin Testing. When a carefully taken history and indicated trials of removal of possible or probable allergens from the diet or environment fail to bring adequate relief, or when uncertainties exist as to the nature or intensity of allergic reactivity in the patient, then skin testing may be useful. In the majority of allergic children some testing will usually be helpful. In a few a large number of tests will be necessary, but most often, with an adequate history, a dozen or so carefully chosen tests will be enough to provide a guide for therapy.

Techniques (see below) for testing include the scratch, intracutaneous, and patch tests, the passive transfer test, and direct application of a potential allergen to the conjunctiva or nasal mucous membrane. Each has advantages and disadvantages. The scratch test is the least sensitive, but many tests can be done relatively quickly, and systemic reactions are extremely rare. Many allergists feel that intracutaneous testing should be done only after negative reactions to scratch tests have been observed to the allergens which are to be given intracutaneously. Others feel that the increased sensitivity of the intracutaneous method warrants its initial use, and that there is

little danger of systemic reactions so long as the strengths of the extracts used are carefully selected.

The passive transfer technique (Prausnitz-Küstner reaction) (see below) will be necessary when the patient has little or no available normal skin for testing, or when other considerations make it unwise or difficult to use the patient's own skin.

Direct application of allergens to the mucous membranes is generally used only for pollens. The test is sensitive and specific for patients whose symptoms reside in the test area, but only a few tests can be performed at any one time.

Patch tests are used only for the detection of contactant allergens.

Skin testing will be most useful when the substances tested are carefully chosen after critical review of the patient's history. Testing may aim at (1) confirmation of suspicious clinical or historical findings, (2) the discovery of reactivities not otherwise suspected, or (3) determination of the dosage level at which desensitization can be undertaken without danger of systemic reaction.

Skin testing may also be helpful in determining whether a patient with vague symptoms, especially respiratory, has skin reactivity of the wheal and flare variety to common allergens. Dermal reactions to such agents as house dust, feathers or pollens will increase suspicion that vague symptoms may be generated at least in part by allergic reactivity, whereas absence of skin reactivity will suggest caution in making such an assumption.

Allergens responsible for positive skin reactivity may not be responsible for current symptoms; a direct relation between a positive reaction and the patient's symptoms may never occur, may have existed in the past, or may emerge in the future. By contrast, some patients with unquestioned clinical reactivity to a particular substance may have no dermal reaction to it. Such failure of skin reactivity may reflect the manner in which extracts are prepared, the use of a subthreshold dose in testing, a dissociation between reactivity in the superficial layers of skin and reactivity in the tissue where the clinical response is exhibited, or modification of reactivity by drugs taken during the 24 to 48 hours before testing. Antihistaminics are particularly active in suppressing skin reactivity, epinephrine analogues less so. Adrenocortical steroids do not generally suppress the wheal and flare response.

The interpretation of skin reactions, both positive and negative, must be made with caution. *No therapeutic program should be based solely on the results of skin tests.* When there are continuing unexplained symptoms, a positive reaction to a food or an inhalant with which the child comes in contact should not be ignored, unless it can be shown by repeated trials that the positive-reacting substance does not contribute to the clinical manifestations. On the other hand, a negative skin reaction does not exclude the possibility that the antigen may be responsible for clinical manifestations, and repeated clinical trials should be carried out to exclude such a possibility.

The allergens to be chosen for skin testing will generally be indicated by the patient's history. Attention should be focused upon those which are most difficult to remove from the diet or from the environment for a therapeutic trial. Most patients will be tested with house dust, certain pollens or molds, wheat, egg and cow's milk. It is often convenient to include other substances of relatively high sensitizing potential in the testing procedure, as well as substances rather unlikely to give clinical reactivity. With the inclusion of such different materials it will be easier to determine whether observed reactivity is likely to have real significance. When the patient has dermal sensitivity of such a high order that he reacts to most antigenic solutions, it may not be possible to correlate individual skin reactions with his clinical manifestations. Skin testing is most helpful when positive reactions can be clearly distinguished from negative ones and when some of the positive reactors are substances to which the patient is commonly exposed and which the clinical history indicates may be likely offenders.

In children with seasonal respiratory symptoms it may be sufficient to test for house dust and for the pollens and molds whose seasons correspond to the time of the patient's symptoms. For children who have no clear-cut seasonal distribution of their respiratory symptoms, tests will generally include house dust, regional trees and grasses, ragweed and certain molds, the most important being Alternaria and Hormodendrum. It may also be informative to test patients with respiratory symptoms for common food allergens, and to test older children with eczema for inhalant reactivity.

Skin testing is generally more reliable with inhalant allergens than with those of foods. Skin testing with bacterial antigens and drugs has little place in the management of the allergic child, except for patch testing with drugs which may have produced contact dermatitis. Although patients who have had anaphylactic or other generalized severe reactions to injected penicillin are apt to have a positive wheal and flare response to a skin test, the absence of such activity does not guarantee that a penicillin reaction will not occur again, nor is a positive skin reaction essential to a diagnosis of allergy to penicillin.

Particular care should be observed in performing intracutaneous tests with animal serums, extracts of animal danders, some animal proteins such as those of egg and fish, and with such strongly reactive substances as walnut, peanut, cottonseed or buckwheat. Preliminary scratch testing to these substances or intracutaneous testing with very dilute materials is essential to safety.

Scratch testing. Scratch tests are performed on the skin of the forearms or back. It is useful to identify the sites of the scratches to be made with dots made nearby with a ball-point pen. Scratches approximately ⅛ inch in length can be made with various instruments, a convenient one being an autoclaved 25-gauge hypodermic needle. The skin is held taut and the scratch made deep enough to disrupt the superficial cells of the skin, but not enough to draw blood. More uniform and deeper lesions can often be made with a spring-loaded device such as that used for tine tests; preliminary testing at sites so prepared should be with dilute extracts. Solutions of the appropriate allergens are gently rubbed into the scratches with dropper or toothpick. Tests should be observed continuously over a period of approximately ½ hour. Positive reactions generally reach their peak in about 20 minutes. As soon as a definitely positive reaction is seen, the allergen should be removed from the reactive site.

Reactions are graded in various ways, a convenient scale being as follows: 4+ reactions consist of wheal with flare with pseudopods; 3+ reactions, conspicuous wheal and flare without pseudopods; 2+ reactions, moderate wheal and flare; 1+ reactions exceed that of the control test with only diluent and have minimal wheal and flare formation; the reaction at the control site is designated as negative. It is important in grading skin reactions to take into account the overall reactivity of the patient's skin on a given day. When all test sites, including the control, are reactive 1+ or 2+, this is likely to be dermographia and not specific allergic reactivity. When the control site exhibits modest reactivity, those with clearly greater responses should be given a positive rating. In recording the results of skin tests, the sizes of the positive and of the control reactions should be indicated.

Intracutaneous tests. The intracutaneous test can be performed with a tuberculin-type syringe and a 27-gauge hypodermic needle. With the skin drawn taut the point of the needle is inserted into the skin almost tangent to it just to the point where the bevel of the needle is covered. Tension on the skin is relaxed and just enough extract is injected into the skin to blanch a small area around the tip of the needle. The amount need not exceed 0.01 ml.

Care should be taken to avoid injecting air into the test site; a drop or two of solution should be expressed from the needle just before the injection is made. If the needle is inserted into the deeper layers of the skin, a new test site should be chosen.

Intracutaneous tests are observed continuously for 20 to 30 minutes; the peak of reactivity is usually reached within 10 to 15 minutes. Positive reactions may be graded and recorded as described above for scratch tests.

Since systemic reactions are most commonly observed with intracutaneous testing, epinephrine must always be immediately at hand.

Patch tests. Patch testing is performed with potential allergens which act by contact. The suspected offending agent is placed on a ½-inch square of filter paper, centered on a larger square of cellophane (or waxed paper), and the cellophane covered with a larger patch of adhesive tape, unless the patient is sensitive to the adhesive. The test material is left in place for 24 hours, unless itching is severe at an earlier time, when it should be removed; at the end of another 24 hours the test site is examined for redness, papules and vesiculation. The interpretation of the reaction will need to take into consideration the primary irritant properties of some substances. In general, simple irritant reactions will be evident by 24 hours, and will subside within 24 hours after removal of the patch. By contrast, allergic reactivity emerging at 24 hours will tend to increase in intensity during the next day after the offending substance is removed.

Passive transfer. In passive transfer of immediate skin reactivity from the patient to a nonallergic person, a recipient must be found with no clinical or skin reactivity to those substances to which it is suspected the patient may react.

Serum is collected under sterile conditions from the patient, and 0.05 aliquots are injected at selected sites in the skin of the recipient. After 24 hours intracutaneous tests may be performed at these sites with antigens to which the patient would have been tested, similar injections being made into control sites. Conspicuous reaction at the transfer site and a negative control indicate the transfer of reactivity from donor to recipient. The same site can be used for several allergens, so long as positive reactions do not occur; an appropriate interval should be allowed between tests.

During a 24-hour period before transfer of serum and during testing, the recipient should not eat any foods to which the patient is known to be reactive, since such foods may evoke a positive reaction at all the injection sites, with consequent de-sensitization of them. Unless desensitized in this way or by testing, areas remain sensitized for 4 to 5 weeks.

Difficulties in the passive transfer technique include the need to identify an appropriate recipient, and the possibility of transfer of *homologous serum hepatitis*. The parent of the child may be used as recipient, but will sometimes be found to have a similar spectrum of reactivities. Use of a primate recipient (macaque) avoids these problems, but at such expense that it must remain a research tool.

Mucous membrane tests. The ophthalmic test may be used in testing clinical reactivity to pollens; a small amount of pollen is placed in the everted lower conjunctival sac with a toothpick. Alternatively, for nasal tests, the pollen can be sniffed from a toothpick placed at the nose. A positive reaction in the nasal mucous membrane consists of edema and serous exudate.

It is unwise to use the mucous membrane for pollen tests during the season in which the pollen is prevalent in the air. Disadvantages of the method include occasional severe local reactions.

Other Methods of Study. The following tests or measures of study are in the main only available in laboratories where they are used in research. In selected clinical problems, however, they may be helpful.

In the *hemagglutination test* an antigen is adsorbed to red blood cells; the addition of serum containing the antibody to this antigen in a medium containing the treated cells results in their agglutination. This test is considerably more sensitive than the usual antigen-antibody precipitation one. Hemagglutinins play a role in the Arthus phenomenon and in some other allergic and immunologic reactions, but not in atopy. High titers of hemagglutinating antibody against cow's milk or penicillin derivatives may correlate with specific clinical problems.

Monkey ileum may be used in the classic *Schultz-Dale technique* and appears to be a highly sensitive indicator of the presence of both reagins and hemagglutinins. The technique may be particularly useful as an indicator of reactivity to penicillin, and helpful in other clinical problems.

Leukocyte sensitivity or measurement of *histamine release from leukocytes* has added to an understanding of basic mechanisms in allergy. When the washed leukocytes of allergic persons are suspended in normal serum, the addition of the sensitizing allergen(s) will lead to release of an amount of histamine from the cells which correlates quantitatively with the amount of allergen added and with the clinical severity of symptoms associated with the allergen. Moreover, the leukocytes of about 20 per cent of normal persons can be passively sensitized by the serum of atopic persons and will release substantial amounts of histamine on exposure to appropriate allergens.

There are seasonal variations in leukocyte sensitivity; this sensitivity can also be shown to be modified by increasing titers of "blocking" substances in the patient undergoing desensitization.

The source of the histamine appears to be principally in the basophils (about 50 per cent) and eosinophils (about 35 per cent), and to a lesser extent in the neutrophils.

In the *passive cutaneous anaphylaxis test (PCA)*, serum suspected of containing antibodies is injected into the skin of the guinea pig or monkey. Subsequently antigen in a dye solution is injected intravenously. Extravasation of the dye at the site of the intracutaneous injection indicates a specific reaction of antigen with antibody. Human IgG induces PCA in the guinea pig; human IgE does not, but does in the monkey. The test is extremely sensitive, but has little current clinical applicability.

Lymphocyte transformation is a sensitive test that is likely to be most useful in identification of suspected *drug reactions*. In this test sensitized lymphocytes in tissue culture are stimulated to blast formation when the sensitizing antigen is added to the culture. Corticosteroids may inhibit lymphocyte transformation when given to the donor or when added to the cell culture.

GENERAL ASPECTS OF ALLERGIC MANAGEMENT

Fundamental to the adequate management of the allergic child is an awareness that the allergic state represents a pervasive tendency to react with allergic symptoms to a variety of factors. The parents, and ultimately the child himself, must learn to live within the limits imposed by this tendency. If physician, parents and child all understand this at the earliest possible moment, the possibility of devising an appropriate therapeutic program is greatly increased.

Prophylactic Measures. The child should be protected as completely as possible from contact with substances to which he is demonstrably reactive, and contacts should also be avoided with other substances of high sensitizing potential. Glaser fostered this viewpoint in recommending that some milk other than cow's milk or a milk substitute be used in early infancy for infants who have a family history of allergy and whose mother's supply of milk is inadequate.

Inhalant controls. Exposure of allergic children to house dust, feathers and other inhalants should be kept at a minimum, especially in the bedroom. Numerous programs have been suggested for rendering a bedroom relatively dust-free; one such is as follows.

PREPARATION AND MAINTENANCE OF AN ALLERGEN-FREE (DUST-FREE) ROOM. The most important dust is ordinary house dust, which is a mixture of many things, such as the wool fiber of rugs, feather dust from pillows, molds, insect scales, and the wool and cotton dust from upholstery, draperies, clothing, and the like. Practically anything which can wear out can produce dust. Though it is impossible to make a whole house or even a single room safe for a child who is allergic to dust by ordinary cleaning methods, special cleaning measures in the bedroom can be helpful.

Cleaning the room. Everything possible should be taken from the room, including pictures, rugs and curtains. If there is a closet, it should be emptied, or if it is used only for storage, it should be sealed off by wide Scotch tape. The room should be made as dust-tight as possible by closing all holes or cracks in the walls, ceiling or floor. If there is a hot-air outlet, it should be turned off in the basement and covered airtight in the room by plastic material or oilcloth. It is not necessary to supply heat for this room, since it is intended mainly for a bedroom and since any source of heat tends to collect dust and circulate it.

Once the room is tightly closed to the entry of dust, it should be cleaned thoroughly with soap and water. Remove every speck of dust from floors, walls and ceiling, including the dust on molding strips above doors and windows, in cracks in floors, on light fixtures, around pipes, and so on. A vacuum cleaner can be used to clean the room of large dust particles, but final cleaning should always be done with a damp cloth.

Furnishing the room. Furniture can be returned after it has been completely freed of dust by cleaning with soap and water. The bed should be taken apart to be cleaned carefully in every niche. Springs should be carefully wiped with a damp cloth. Only the following furniture is permitted: a bed, a small table, a simple wooden chair or two, and a chest of drawers (if the child's clothes cannot be kept in some other place). These things should all be carefully cleaned inside and out and should be of a material that is easily kept clean.

The mattress of the bed should be covered by plastic material specially made for allergic protection. Heavy plastic is necessary, such as is used in shower curtains. If there is a box spring, it should also be covered with plastic material. Foam rubber pillows should be used and should have plastic covers unless they are brand new. Foam rubber mattresses are desirable, and even they should be covered with plastic material.

Cotton blankets are preferable to wool. If wool must be used, it should be kept from the child by 1 or 2 sheets, so that the wool does not touch the child or have a chance to add dust to the room. Blankets should be washed frequently. Wool clothes are preferably not worn by the allergic child and in any event should be kept out of the bedroom.

The following should not be permitted in the room: rugs, upholstered furniture, curtains or draperies, bookcases, venetian blinds, or anything likely to make dust or to give it a resting place. Stuffed toys, such as animals, are not permitted. Toys should be as few as possible and be made of wood, metal or plastic.

If a floor covering is desired, linoleum should be used. If there are cracks in the floor which collect dust and cannot be filled, the floor should be covered with linoleum from wall to wall.

Pets are preferably excluded from the house and in any case should not enter the allergen-free room.

Maintenance. 1. Keep windows and doors closed except at night, when a window may be open. A screen door spring on the door will help to keep it closed.

2. Go over the room each day with a damp cloth, removing dust from all exposed surfaces.

3. Once a week clean room and furniture thoroughly with a damp cloth.

4. It is best if the child dresses and undresses in another room, using the bedroom only for sleeping.

5. The rest of the house should be kept as dust-free as possible by the measures outlined above and by frequent, careful damp cloth cleaning.

How far beyond the bedroom to extend the environmental modifications for the allergic child will depend upon the intensity of his reactivity and the circumstances under which his family lives. Drastic changes in family living should be avoided so far as possible.

Dietary controls. It is often wiser for psychologic reasons to eliminate certain substances of high sensitizing potential such as chocolate and nuts from the diet of the entire family than to limit such restrictions to the allergic child. Only rarely is it necessary to extend such dietary restrictions to wheat or cow's milk. Limitation of exposure to egg is easier and ought particularly to be urged for the child with eczema and his family. Many substances which act as allergens when ingested raw are less allergenic when

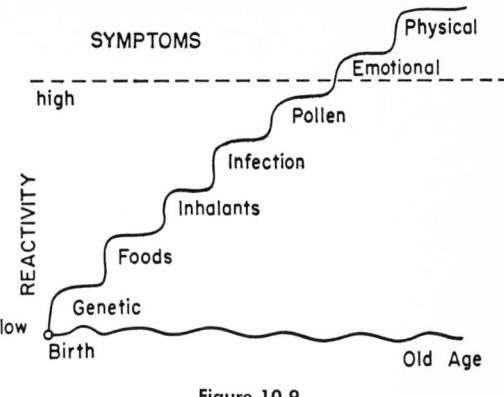

Figure 10-9.

cooked; and boiled, evaporated or powdered milk may be better tolerated than raw or pasteurized whole cow's milk.

Education. In educating parents and older children to the nature of the problem, the allergic state has been depicted in a number of ways. A convenient scheme, easily reproduced for parents in the course of a consultation, is embodied in Figures 10-9 through 10-12. These figures have the advantage over other schemes in that they include the important dimension of *time*. The level of allergic reactivity is plotted vertically and time horizontally. These diagrams can be easily drawn for the parents of the allergic child, or for the child himself, while the considerations depicted are discussed.

In Figure 10-9 the time-line begins at birth and ends at old age. The level of reactivity is depicted as reaching a threshold when symptoms appear. Various factors which may contribute to a level of reactivity above the zero level are indicated. Any or all of these factors might contribute to reactivity below the threshold level at which symptoms emerge.

Figure 10-10 charts the clinical reactivity of a hypothetical child with a relatively heavy genetic tendency to reactivity, in whom food reactivity gave rise to eczema in infancy, clearing so far as overt allergic symptoms are concerned, only to reappear in later childhood as asthma. At the time of this later clinical difficulty, one may imagine that genetic, food and inhalant reactivities are determining factors.

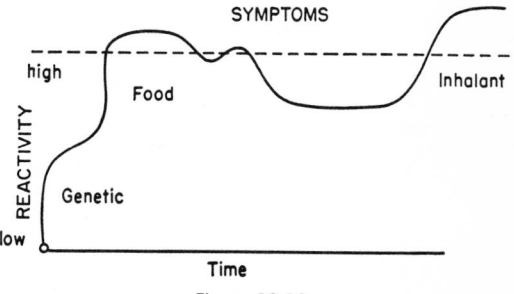

Figure 10-10.

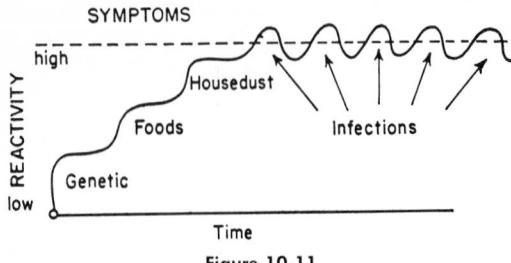

Figure 10-11.

Figure 10-11 will help to clarify the relation between infection and allergic symptoms. It is suggested that an allergic child whose degree of genetic, food and inhalant reactivity is below the threshold for symptoms may be in difficulty only when infection is superimposed. Clinical experience indicates that in many such children adequate prophylaxis against common food and inhalant factors will lower the general level of reactivity so that ordinary infections are tolerated without allergic symptoms.

Figure 10-12 introduces the important consideration that children who carry a fairly heavy allergic load may have a tendency to become more reactive, whereas if this load can be sufficiently lightened, the general level of reactivity abates. Attention given *only* to the symptoms representing reactivity above the threshold level will fail to meet the need for a more general abatement of reactivity. This extension of efforts at protection *beyond symptomatic control* has been labeled *prophylaxis* in the diagram. The aim of allergic management is to reduce the allergic load as far as possible below the threshold of reactivity, with the hope that a level can be reached at which the tendency to react in an allergic manner will ultimately disappear.

In making plans for the child, particularly in regard to prophylaxis, it is important to emphasize that the aim is to limit exposure to allergens to the extent that will permit the child to lead a normal life. Although everything necessary to relieve the child of symptoms should be done, the restrictions of his freedom or comfort should not be more rigid than are reasonable. Parents can be reassured that of the chronic diseases of children, the allergic disorders have the best prognosis for adequate control.

Specific desensitization. When adequate attempts at avoidance of inhalant or dietary allergens have not led to sufficient relief of allergic symptoms, immunologic desensitization (hyposensitization) may be considered. The manner in which desensitization accomplishes its effect is still largely unknown, though the weight of evidence now favors the development of "blocking" antibodies. Desensitization is limited mainly to inhalant allergens and ought to be restricted to allergens which cannot be easily avoided. It is undertaken only after adequate skin testing has been done to establish that the child is reactive to the agent to be used, and to determine the level of reactivity. Desensitization is not commonly carried out with allergens to which the child is not skin-reactive, unless clinical reactivity is clearly established.

There is lack of agreement as to use of bacterial vaccines for desensitization. Occasionally children seem to gain some relief from bacterial antigens of either stock or autogenous origin, when given intracutaneously, initially in low dilution and then in increasing doses. It may be reasonable to include a bacterial vaccine in the desensitization program when allergic symptoms are clearly augmented at the time of respiratory infection. The bacterial vaccines commonly used as "cold" shots should not, however, be expected to reduce the incidence of viral respiratory infections.

Desensitization is ordinarily carried out with extracts of appropriate antigens in buffered aqueous solutions, injections of increasing doses being given at regular intervals. The usual procedure in pollinosis is to initiate treatment 12 to 16 weeks before the onset of the pollen season, with the injection of increasing doses at weekly or more frequent intervals. For substances such as house dust and molds which have less evident seasons, desensitization may begin at any time.

We have generally found it satisfactory to initiate treatment with each antigenic substance in a concentration of 1:10,000 or 1:100,000, irrespective of differences of skin reactivity, choosing the more dilute solution when one or more allergens were highly reactive. Even more dilute solutions, to 1:10,000,000, may be necessary in the management of eczema. A typical desensitization program is outlined in Table 10-4 for a child with moderate reactivity to house dust, ragweed and molds. If the child is not improved at the end of 12 weeks, then a comprehensive re-evaluation is in order to ascertain what dietary, environmental, anatomic, infectious, emotional or immunologic stone was left unturned. The possibility that more or less antigen is indicated for desensitization should also be considered.

Although some children obtain satisfactory re-

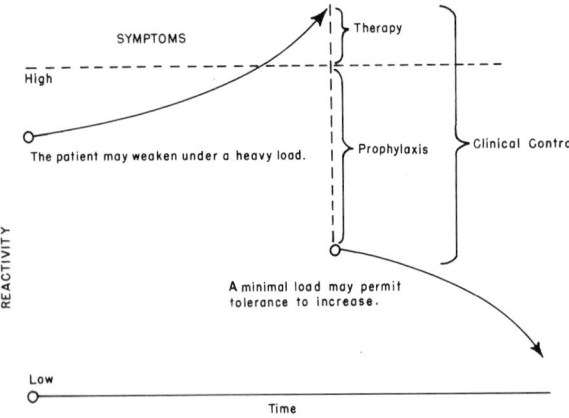

Figure 10-12.

TABLE 10-4. Sample Desensitization Program

Patient's Name_____

Extract Contains: House dust
Ragweed   ⎫ Vial #1 contains each antigen in a 1:10,000 dilution
Alternaria   ⎬ Vial #2 contains each antigen in a 1:1000 dilution
Hormodendrum ⎭

Desensitizing injections should be given at weekly intervals, according to the following program:

	AMOUNT	DILUTION	(DATE GIVEN)	(REACTION)
1st dose	0.05 ml.	1:10,000 (vial #1)		
2nd dose	0.075	"		
3rd dose	0.10	"		
4th dose	0.15	"		
5th dose	0.20	"		
6th dose	0.30	"		
7th dose	0.50	"		
8th dose	0.05	1:1000 (vial #2)	Note: After re-evaluation at 12 weeks a similar	
9th dose	0.075	"	stepwise increase in dose might be projected, using	
10th dose	0.10	"	extracts of greater strength. As the likelihood of	
11th dose	0.15	"	reaction increases, it becomes more prudent to	
12th dose	0.20	"	separate the individual allergens so that a reactor	
Maintenance dose	0.20 ml.	1:1000	can be more easily identified.	

INJECTIONS are given in the area of the triceps, subcutaneously, with precautions to prevent accidental intravenous administration. Reactions to these dosage levels are rare, but patients should remain under observation for 20 to 30 minutes after each injection so that any immediate reactions can be promptly managed with tourniquet, epinephrine, et cetera.

REACTIONS: An immediate general anaphylactic, asthmatic or urticarial reaction is alarming, and needs prompt treatment, as above. A *local* reaction of edema occurring within 20 to 30 minutes is generally benign and gone within 6 to 12 hours. A *delayed* general reaction consisting of nausea, vomiting and abdominal pain may occur 3 to 8 hours after injection and will generally need no therapy. *Other important types of delayed reactions* are (1) worsening of respiratory symptoms within 6 to 12 hours (usually more sneezing or coughing), (2) worsening of itching and redness of *eczema*, as late as 24 to 48 hours after injection, or (3) chronic worsening of an allergic condition during a course of treatment.

Any of the above-mentioned reactions indicates that *the optimum dose has been exceeded*. Delayed reactions are difficult to evaluate and may need to be confirmed by another dose given at the same level. In any event, if a reaction is suspected, the dose of extract *must not be increased*. Furthermore, *the dose should not be increased beyond any level at which a satisfactory clinical response has occurred*, since symptoms controlled at a low level may recur when that level is exceeded.

When satisfactory clinical improvement occurs, the interval between injections can be increased, first to every 2 weeks, then to every three, but injections *should generally not be given at intervals more widely spaced than every 4 weeks*, since reactions may occur. Injections should be continued usually until the patient has been symptom-free for a year.

lief with desensitization begun and maintained at low dosage levels, there is evidence indicating that relief (especially in pollen allergy) is best assured by gradual increases in dosage of allergen to the point at which the maximal physiologic tolerance for the injected allergen appears to be reached. The end-point is local edema and discomfort which lasts for a day or more, or a constitutional reaction. Those who wish to reach the maximal possible dosage in desensitization will sometimes aim toward 0.1 to 0.5 ml. of a 1:10 dilution of house dust extract, or of a 3 per cent pollen extract. If adequate relief of symptoms is obtained at lower levels, e.g. at 1:10,000 or 1:1000 dilution, there seems to be no reason to push beyond this level. Sometimes in the course of desensitization the child experiences initial relief only to have

symptoms recur as the dose is increased toward the projected goal. A return to the lower dosage level at which the child was free of symptoms may regain relief and maintain it for a long time.

Occasionally, when a patient is first seen with symptoms *during* a season in which a responsible pollen is prevalent, *coseasonal desensitization* may be helpful. This is best accomplished with intracutaneous injections of dilute extract (1:10,000) 3 or more times a week, increasing the dose (e.g. 0.025, 0.05, 0.075, 0.1, 0.15 ml.) to not over 0.2 ml. More concentrated extracts are not likely to be more helpful. Coseasonal therapy is suspended when relief occurs and reinstituted if symptoms recur; 1 or 2 doses are then often sufficient to re-establish control.

Desensitization in children is generally safe,

and severe reactions are uncommon. Scrupulous care should be taken to ensure that the dilution and dose of extract chosen are the ones intended, and that injections are not given intravenously. A careful inquiry should be made at each visit as to the possibility of evident or occult reactions to previous injections. A treatment sheet on which the projected program is outlined, which has space for recording dates of injections and reactions, and a description of the latter is shown in Table 10-4. Desensitization should be undertaken only when an anaphylactic reaction can be treated immediately in the event that the tolerated dosage level should be exceeded, either by accidental overdose or with the prescribed dose.

Several repository forms of allergic extracts are available; these include an alum-precipitate preparation (Allpyral). These products permit administration of relatively large amounts of antigen in each injection for release over a prolonged time. For children they probably have no substantial advantage over the traditional aqueous extracts.

Nonspecific controls of allergic reactivity. Many of the synthetic analogues of the hormones of the adrenal medulla and cortex are effective in the relief of allergic symptoms. The analogues of epinephrine are particularly useful since they generally bring prompt relief, and their use is not attended by prolonged, unwanted side effects. The area of usefulness of the corticosteroids is much more circumscribed, and they have side effects which are occasionally life-threatening. The use of corticosteroids or corticotropin should be reserved for allergic disorders which are immediately threatening to life or are normally sharply self-limited in duration. They should *not* be used as a substitute for other thorough conventional allergic management. Details of the use of these drugs will be given with the conditions for which they are prescribed.

The so-called antihistaminics include a large number of drugs which have some usefulness in allergic disorders, though less regularly so than epinephrine and its analogues. The various drugs differ in dosage and in frequency of such side reactions as drowsiness and personality changes. For the limited use which the physician should make of these agents, he will do well to acquaint himself thoroughly with one or two of them. Like the corticosteroids, they should not be used for prolonged symptomatic relief or as a substitute for adequate allergic investigation and management. The details of their use will be described with the conditions for which they may be prescribed.

Although there is evidence that allergic children generally have slightly lower levels of total serum gamma globulins than other children, and more variable levels of the component fractions of the gamma globulins, there is no indication how these differences may relate to the allergic state, nor any indication for administration of gamma globulins. On the contrary, administration of gamma globulins carries the risk of immunization to the various serotypes of the globulins and of post-poning the necessary development in the child of his own active immunity to prevalent viral agents.

Emotional tensions surrounding the child's allergic illness and contributing to his general level of reactivity are best handled by unhurried discussion with the parents of the child's difficulty, by avoidance of overdramatization of the child's illness, and by careful examination with the parents of those areas in which parent and child seem to be in conflict. The use of tranquilizers or sedatives as a substitute for an attempt to solve emotional problems through better understanding should be avoided.

ANAPHYLAXIS AND SERUM SICKNESS

Anaphylaxis and serum sickness are closely related and, in certain respects, are the prototypes of allergic illnesses. Anaphylaxis consists in a violent adverse physiologic response to an antigen to which the host has been sensitized. It is possible to produce anaphylaxis in a number of species of animals, in each of which the manifestations tend to be characteristic for the species. In man the development of the anaphylactic state bears no clearly defined relation to the capacity to develop allergic disorders of the atopic type.

The anaphylactic state is set up a varying period of time after exposure to a foreign antigen; in the case of horse serum in man, anaphylactic sensitization may be expected 10 to 14 days after initial exposure. At the end of this preliminary period and for an indeterminate time thereafter, a second injection of serum, which may be smaller in amount than the first, may produce violent symptoms. These symptoms are most likely the result of massive release of histamine from sensitized cells. The presence of antibodies in the blood of the sensitized person can usually be demonstrated. These antibodies are usually capable of transferring the anaphylactic state to another animal, if substantial amounts of serum are administered intravenously, and are usually capable of sensitizing human skin on passive transfer. In the person susceptible to anaphylactic reactions scratch, intracutaneous or conjunctival tests will usually yield specific positive reactions.

Serum sickness may be regarded as a subacute form of anaphylactic reaction. It characteristically appears 7 to 14 days after administration of heterologous serum, at the time when the level of foreign antigen has been rapidly falling and there begins to be an excess of homologous antibody. During the following days or weeks there may be continuing evidence of antigen-antibody reaction in the form of urticaria and angioneurotic edema, arthritis, sometimes polyarteritis, and rarely peripheral neuritis or encephalitis.

Etiology. In the past, anaphylactic reactions and serum sickness most commonly followed therapeutic use of animal serum in the treatment of diphtheria and tetanus. Penicillin and antibiotics derived from it are probably the most common cause of these reactions today. They are uncommon in children, but it may be that in childhood many persons are sensitized who will as adults manifest severe reactions. Anaphylactic reactions may also be caused by desensitizing injections and represent unusual sensitivity on the part of the patient.

Insect stings, particularly those of the bee, hornet, wasp and yellowjacket, are important causes of anaphylactic reactions. The reaction is due to the species-specificity of the protein injected by the insect, and not simply to the toxic agent. Anaphylactic reactions to insect stings commonly occur as the culmination of progressively severe reactions to repeated stings.

Toxic reactions resembling anaphylaxis may follow ingestion of foods, most commonly fish or other seafood, nuts, flaxseed or cottonseed, or buckwheat. These reactions are rarely seen in early infancy after ingestion of cow's milk.

Clinical Manifestations. The symptoms and signs of *the anaphylactic reaction* depend upon the tissues most intensely involved. When the cardiovascular system is primarily involved, syncope and shock may appear within a few seconds of injection of an antigen or of an insect sting; the blood pressure falls quickly to a very low level; the pulse is absent or rapid and feeble, and pallor gives way to cyanosis. Death may occur within a few minutes.

In less acute reactions respiratory and skin manifestations may be prominent. The patient may complain of tightness in the chest and of itching and may have rapidly progressive urticaria or angioneurotic edema. The edema may be most conspicuous around the eyes or may involve the oropharyngeal or laryngeal area, where it may impose an immediate threat to life. Dyspnea may become severe, with asthmatic wheezing, cough, cyanosis, and respiratory failure associated with bronchiolar obstruction. Peripheral vascular failure may supervene and prove fatal.

With the release of histamine in the anaphylactic reaction, there appears also to be a release of heparin, which may lead to postoperative hemorrhage when anaphylactic reaction is associated with surgery or the postoperative period.

The manifestations of *serum sickness* may occur a few minutes or hours to 7 to 14 days after exposure to the inciting agent; the earlier onset of symptoms presumably reflects past exposures which resulted in sensitization. The most prominent clinical features of serum sickness are urticaria and angioneurotic edema; the latter is particularly likely to involve the face, lips, tongue and oropharyngeal areas. Urticaria is likely to involve points of pressure on the skin, such as the belt line. Itching may be intense. Fever is commonly associated, and arthritis may occur which may be difficult to differentiate from rheumatic or rheumatoid involvement. Peripheral neuritis or headache, delirium, convulsions or coma may reflect edema or polyarteritis in the central nervous system.

Generalized lymphadenopathy is commonly present; the involved nodes may be tender, particularly in the area associated with the site of serum injection. The shorter the latent period between the administration of serum or drugs and the onset of the allergic reaction, the more likely is asthma to be manifest.

Laboratory Findings. Leukopenia is common. Protein and casts in the urine may be an indication of polyarteritis or some other renal lesion.

A wheal and flare reaction is usual in response to the intracutaneous injection of diluted antigen during serum sickness due to animal serums, but may not occur during that due to penicillin. Patients with acute severe anaphylactic reactions to penicillin are more likely to manifest skin reactivity than those in whom the reaction is delayed and milder. In the latter, hemagglutinating antibodies are more likely to be found to penicillin or its derivatives than are reagins. Skin testing of patients with serum sickness should be undertaken extremely cautiously, if at all.

Differential Diagnosis. The diagnosis of anaphylactic reaction is apparent when typical clinical manifestations follow quickly the exposure to a substance to which the patient may have been sensitized. In the child found in shock or with rapidly progressive symptoms, the examination should include inspection for the site of an insect sting.

Treatment. Treatment of an *anaphylactic reaction* should be prompt and vigorous. A tourniquet is placed proximal to the site of a sensitizing injection or sting in an extremity, and epinephrine is injected into another extremity in a dose varying from 0.2 to 0.5 ml. (1:1000 aqueous solution), which may be repeated after 10 to 20 minutes, if indicated. An antihistaminic agent should be given orally or intravenously as soon as possible in appropriate dosage for the drug used.

If the patient is in severe shock, other measures may be necessary, such as the intravenous administration of saline solution or plasma, and perhaps the administration of agents such as levarterenol to promote vascular tone. Oxygen should be given when there is dyspnea or cyanosis.

Since the corticosteroids require hours for therapeutic effect, they cannot be relied upon in the management of anaphylactic shock.

In the management of *serum sickness*, epinephrine and its analogues and the antihistaminics are the drugs of first choice. Epinephrine will often provide relief initially, which can then be sustained with ephedrine. Antihistaminic agents are usually helpful as adjuncts. Administration of one of them is continued for the 3 to 7 days of clinical activity. In patients in whom serum sickness is particularly severe with arthritic, nephritic or neuritic complications, the administration of a corticosteroid is indicated. Administration should be continued for 5 to 7 days.

Tracheotomy is occasionally necessary for relief of laryngeal obstruction.

Prevention. Since anaphylactic reactions and

serum sickness are commonly iatrogenic in origin, great care should be taken to prevent them. The occurrence of diphtheria or tetanus and the consequent need to use antiserum therapeutically represent a failure to provide adequate immunization at an earlier date. Therapeutic antiserum of human origin is now available for tetanus and should supplant animal serums. When human antiserum is not available and an animal serum must be used, careful testing for sensitivity should be carried out initially. If the patient proves to be sensitive, and the serum is *required* therapeutically, it should be given so as to permit rapid desensitization. Such desensitization can be facilitated by the concomitant administration of an antihistaminic agent.

Reactions of the anaphylactic or serum sickness type more commonly follow injection than oral administration of penicillin. Accordingly, the oral forms of penicillin should be used for systemic effect whenever possible in childhood. By contrast, surface administration of penicillin on the mucous membranes, e.g. through oral troches, has a high sensitizing potential and should be avoided. Of the injectable forms of penicillin, some, such as benzathine penicillin, may be more allergenic than crystalline sodium or potassium penicillin G.

Constitutional allergic reactions following wasp, bee, hornet or yellowjacket stings will need to be distinguished from acute toxic reactions which may be due to a large amount of toxic material from many simultaneous stings, usually ten or more. In the toxic reactions there is generally edema without urticaria; other manifestations include headache, fever, weakness, involuntary muscle spasms, and occasionally convulsions. Reactions to stings from these insects are also to be differentiated from nonallergic reactions to the potent toxins of such insects as the fire ant or black widow spider.

When a child has a history of increasingly severe reactions to insect stings, which extend beyond the local area, a program of desensitization should be undertaken. This should be carried out only after very cautious intracutaneous skin testing to establish the level of skin reactivity of the patient (scratch testing is not generally helpful). Testing for insect sensitivity cannot be done within 2 weeks of the sting, owing to a refractory period. Desensitization is usually initiated with a very dilute (1:1,000,000) solution of allergens, which should normally consist of whole body extracts of bee, wasp, hornet and yellowjacket. The polyvalent allergenic solution seems preferable, since identification of the stinging insect is not always possible. There is some cross reactivity. Desensitizing injections should be continued for at least 3 years. An attempt is made to attain a dose of 0.3 to 0.4 ml. of a 1:100 concentration of extract; injections may be given as infrequently as every 2 months during the second year of treatment, and every 3 months during the third year (Mueller).

Children extremely sensitive to insect stings should have a survival kit available whenever exposed to possible sting, and should know how to use it or to get help. An appropriate kit has a syringe containing epinephrine, a tourniquet, ephedrine and an antihistaminic.

URICARIA
(Hives)

Urticaria is relatively common in childhood. There are many causative factors, some of which are clearly not allergic or immunologic. Urticaria is seen as a manifestation of sensitivity to cold in association with cryoglobulinemia in Raynaud's disease and other conditions, with paroxysmal hemoglobinuria in congenital syphilis, with high titers of cold agglutinins and in the absence of protein or immunologic abnormality, e.g. in cold urticaria, in which histamine appears to be the mediating agent. Cold urticaria may follow serum sickness or viral illnesses, or may be related to helminthiasis. There is a form of *familial* cold urticaria which is inherited as an autosomal dominant.

Urticaria occurs as a response to heat in some persons, in whom it may be associated with hot foods, environmental temperature, exercise or emotional tensions. Heat urticaria seems to be mediated by acetylcholine in some persons. There is also a form of urticaria related to stimulation by light.

Urticaria is designated as allergic when a causative allergen can be demonstrated, and may be regarded as a mild equivalent of serum sickness or anaphylaxis. In children the exciting agents, when they can be found, are usually foods, and a careful search should be made for possible offenders. Cow's milk sometimes contains inhalant allergens, and may contain sufficient penicillin to cause urticaria in hypersensitive persons. The presence of other antibiotics in milk has not been clearly related to urticaria.

Angioneurotic edema, or *giant urticaria*, appears as a firm, nonpitting edema, most often of the eyelids, lips or cheeks and less commonly of the ears, tongue, larynx or extremities. Angioneurotic edema is commonly associated with urticaria, but may appear by itself; itching is less intense than with urticaria. The edema is usually limited in duration to a few hours, but may rarely become chronic and disfiguring.

Differential Diagnosis. The diagnosis presents no problem when hives appear in the course of a general or other localized typical allergic reaction, such as serum sickness or an asthmatic episode. When hives are the only manifestation of a possible allergic disorder, the establishment of the cause may be difficult. Allergic urticaria will need to be differentiated from other forms of urticaria, including the eruptions classified under the general term of erythema multiforme, which may represent transitions between allergic disease of the wheal and flare reaction type and more chronic collagen or connective tissue disorders.

Treatment. Treatment of urticaria is generally symptomatic. A careful search should be made for possible precipitating allergens; if one or more are identified, attempts should be made to avoid contact with them. If the cause remains obscure, and there are repeated attacks, a hypoallergenic diet may be tried.

Relief of urticaria and of itching is often obtained with epinephrine and may be sustained with ephedrine or antihistaminics.

Papular urticaria (see p. 1411) occurs as hard papules, commonly at the site of bites of insects such as fleas, mosquitoes or bedbugs. It tends to occur on exposed surfaces in crops, and often at night. Itching may be intense. Skin reactions with insect antigens may be positive. Measures directed at insect control constitute the most effective management.

ALLERGIC RHINITIS

Allergic rhinitis is the commonest clinical manifestation of the *atopic* disorders. There are many clinical patterns or variants, of which seasonal hay fever is the most typical; for some, differential diagnosis is difficult.

Etiology. As in other allergic conditions, the factors which may contribute to clinical reactivity are multiple. Foods are often the responsible agents in infancy, but after the first year or two of life, such inhalants as dust, pollens and molds become more important. In children with perennial allergic rhinitis, recurrent upper respiratory tract infections or a chronic *infectious* rhinitis may contribute to a high level of reactivity in the nasal mucous membrane.

Clinical Manifestations. The protean manifestations of allergic rhinitis warrant description of several of the clinical variants, but the illness in an individual child may include aspects of several of these patterns.

Allergic rhinitis during the first few months of life will most commonly result from food reactivity, cow's milk being the chief offender. The affected infant may seem to have a continuous "cold" and may have nasal obstruction severe enough to interfere with nursing or feeding.

Seasonal allergic rhinitis (hay fever or rose fever) is the most characteristic form and most often is due to sensitization to house dust, pollen or molds. Pollen allergy is rare during the first year of life and is uncommon before 4 or 5 years of age. In the season when a pollen or mold is prevalent, the affected child has attacks of sneezing, itching of the nasal mucous membrane and profuse watery rhinorrhea. Symptoms are likely to be most pronounced in the morning hours, with a tendency to improvement during the day. Onset of symptoms may be delayed beyond the beginning of the seasonal pollen and may continue for some weeks after its disappearance if other factors tend to keep the patient's reactive status at a symptomatic level.

House dust reactivity tends to be most evident in the winter months, especially when central heating units are in operation. Reactivity to ragweed pollen is most common from about the middle of August to the end of October. Rose fever is a misnomer, the reactivity ascribed to roses generally being the result of sensitization to grass pollen, and is coincident with the pollinating seasons of the various allergenic grasses. Sensitizations to tree pollens are usually clinically manifest only for a short time during the early spring. Clinical manifestations to molds are less clearly defined as to season and, even more than symptoms to pollens, may be dependent on weather.

Sporadic attacks of allergic rhinitis throughout the year may reflect repeated but intermittent exposures to a reactive agent, as, for example, in a cellar, attic or barn. In children who have bronchial asthma an attack of rhinitis may precede an asthmatic episode.

The nasal mucous membrane of the affected child is edematous, wet and usually pale; at times it may be almost gray or white. The uvula may also be pale and edematous. There is commonly an associated allergic conjunctivitis, with itching, edema, and redness of the conjunctivas.

In *perennial allergic rhinitis* there is no special seasonal pattern. Sensitization is usually to inhalants, such as house dust, feathers, wool and molds, and possibly to foods. The symptoms of perennial allergic rhinitis have a tendency to be less violent than those of hay fever, and in their least severe form may be manifest as mild nasal congestion with sniffling, a tendency to an itchy nose, postnasal drip and mouth-breathing. The "allergic salute," in which the child attempts to allay itching or to increase his nasal airway by pushing or rubbing upward against the cartilaginous septum, is a common manifestation, and may lead to a transverse crease across the nose just above the bulbous portion. Postnasal drip may lead to throat-clearing noises or to cough.

Allergic rhinitis may remain unsuspected for a long time, particularly in children who have frequent or prolonged respiratory infections. Such diagnoses as chronic rhinitis, chronic sinusitis, adenoiditis and chronic tonsillitis and "postnasal drip" are commonly made when the basic disturbance is allergic reactivity.

In perennial allergic rhinitis the appearance of the nasal mucous membrane may resemble that of seasonal rhinitis, but, when there is an associated purulent nasal discharge, as there often is, the characteristic pallor may be replaced by inflammatory response. Recurrent epistaxis is common. There may be some enlargement of adenoid and tonsillar tissues secondary to low-grade infection. Mouth-breathing is common. Particularly in young children, recurrent edema of the eyelids reflects congestion in the ethmoid area and tends to be most evident in the morning. In older children a characteristic discoloration of the lower eyelid occurs (allergic "shiners"). Otitis media is a common complication of perennial allergic rhinitis, and may be the presenting symptom on occasion. It often takes the form of recurrent or refractory serous otitis media.

Recurrent upper respiratory tract infections are often a manifestation of perennial allergic rhinitis.

Vasomotor rhinitis, presumably due to a labile vasomotor response to emotional or climatic change, is relatively uncommon in children. Some children with allergic rhinitis will sneeze upon entering air-conditioned rooms or upon leaving them, or with similar changes in ambient temperature. These responses may be more common in the atopic child than in the nonatopic one.

Diagnosis. The diagnosis of allergic rhinitis can usually be made with reasonable confidence on the basis of a detailed history, emphasis being placed upon seasonal occurrence of symptoms, and their relation to particular places or time of day, upon associated sensory phenomena, such as itchy nose or palate, allergic salute or other mannerisms, history of other past or current allergic reactivity, and family history. Parents of children with allergic rhinitis of the less typical varieties may not be aware of the allergic basis of their own symptoms, which they may think of as sinusitis.

Eosinophilia in the nasal discharge is suggestive of allergic origin for chronic rhinitis, more than 5 per cent of eosinophils being unusual in normal persons. When infection is present, however, eosinophilia may not be found; its absence therefore does not exclude the possibility of allergic rhinitis.

Skin reactions to potent allergens are an indication that the child with seasonal or persistent rhinitis has an allergic constitution. Failure to react creates doubt about the possibility of an allergic origin, but does not exclude it. Testing should not be done when the child is receiving antiallergic therapy.

Radiologic examination of the sinuses will often disclose some thickening of the maxillary sinus membranes and may demonstrate polypoid formations. Excess adenoid tissue can also be demonstrated roentgenographically or by direct vision.

Treatment. As with other allergic disorders, allergic rhinitis is best managed by a comprehensive program of allergic decontamination of the patient's environment, adequate control of infection, desensitization to allergens which cannot be adequately avoided, and limitation of exposure to potential sensitizers.

Symptomatic relief may be obtained from antihistaminics at the expense of side effects. Oral decongestants, such as pseudoephedrine, may be helpful. Nose drops are often difficult to administer and seldom helpful. They should not be given, in any case, for periods longer than 2 or 3 days. Nasal sprays, some with corticosteroids, may give temporary relief, but their use for more than a very short time is inappropriate; the recurrent use of preparations containing steroids may suppress adrenal function. None of these symptomatic measures should take the place of adequate allergic management.

Desensitization in allergic rhinitis is generally limited to house dust, pollens and molds, but occasionally includes other antigens, such as bacterial ones or other inhalants. Vaccines against windborne pollens are the ones most frequently used.

The role of infection in allergic rhinitis is often difficult to assess. Whenever feasible, the vicious cycle of infection and allergic reactivity should be interrupted. Occasionally in chronic infections it will be necessary to administer an antibiotic or a sulfonamide. Treatment with these drugs should usually be reserved for children who are carriers of susceptible pathogenic organisms, for which the in-vitro sensitivities have been determined. There is no justification for the use of gamma globulin except when a severe deficiency is demonstrated.

When there is polypoid formation in the nose or sinuses, surgical removal may be necessary. Polyps will occasionally shrink away after topical application of corticosteroids and may then be held in check by appropriate allergic management (see serous otitis media, p. 899).

The indications for tonsillectomy and adenoidectomy are the same in allergic children as in nonallergic ones (see p. 894). The operation at times appears to precipitate asthma as the next step in the evolution of the atopic diathesis.

ASTHMA

Asthma occurs when allergic reactivity is manifest by spasm of smooth muscle in bronchi and bronchioles. Edema and abnormal secretion of mucus are nearly always associated and, in conjunction with the spasm, are responsible for the symptoms and signs of generalized lower respiratory tract obstruction.

Etiology. Asthma in children is most often the result of allergic reactivity of the atopic variety. House dust is an important incitant at any age; foods are relatively important in the younger child, and pollen and molds in the older one. Asthma is commonly associated with undifferentiated respiratory infections in late infancy and early childhood. Vigorous physical activity may lead to episodes of asthma which tend to be relatively brief. Asthmatic children usually have more difficulty at night, often after sleep.

Psychiatric study of asthmatic children indicates that the onset of asthma may often follow closely upon a traumatic emotional experience, as, for example, the loss of or separation from a loved person, such as parent or grandparent. If the parent has unconscious feelings of rejection of the child, an impasse may develop which may need psychotherapeutic attention. In some children chronic or recurrent emotional tensions come to play a dominant role in occurrence of symptoms, even when these are determined at first predominantly by atopic reactivity. The dramatic symptoms and signs of severe asthma may become the focal point of parental anxiety or of a struggle between parent and child.

Pathology. The mucous membrane of the respiratory tract is pale and edematous, and there is increased secretion of mucus during an asthmatic episode. There is also narrowing of the lumen of the bronchi and bronchioles as a result of the spasm of smooth muscle. These changes are readily reversible in short-lived paroxysms or with specific medication.

If infection is associated with an acute asthmatic paroxysm, a mucopurulent exudate may be present, and there may be associated areas of bronchopneumonia. Obstruction of the larger bronchi with mucus plugs may give rise to atelectasis, especially of the right middle lobe. Occasionally, pneumothorax and pneumomediastinum are complications of severe asthma.

During the acute asthmatic episode the lungs are emphysematous, owing to the ball-valve type of obstruction of the smaller bronchi and bronchioles. In the child who has frequent occurrences of asthma over a long time the walls of the bronchioles may become thickened, and the persistent effort to aerate the lungs leads to chronic emphysema. The sternum becomes prominent, the back rounded, and the anteroposterior diameter of the chest increased.

Clinical Manifestations. The onset of asthma may be insidious or abrupt. Sudden onsets are often ushered in by a spell of coughing which may be associated with itching of the chin, anterior part of the neck or chest. The onset is apt to be gradual and resolution to be slower when the asthmatic attack complicates a respiratory infection; wheezing may appear a day or more after rhinorrhea and may resolve over a period of hours or days.

The asthmatic paroxysm is characterized by increasing dyspnea, with prolongation of the expiratory phase of respiration, by wheezing, and coarse and fine musical rales. A severe asthmatic paroxysm greatly limits pulmonary ventilation; the resulting air hunger is manifest by such signs as flaring of the alae nasi, the use of accessory muscles of respiration, and cyanosis and at times hypercapnia. The heart and respiratory rates are increased, and the child is restless and fatigued. Sweating may be prominent. There may be abdominal pain, particularly when coughing is severe, and the child may vomit. Vomiting may be followed by some relief of the dyspnea, but this is usually only temporary. The sputum of the child with acute asthma is tenacious and scanty until a response to treatment is seen, when it may become more abundant and loose. Then spirals of mucus which contain eosinophils are coughed up.

The chest is generally hyperresonant, with wheezing and musical and sibilant rales most prominent in the expiratory phase. Breath sounds may be suppressed, and occasionally the restriction of tidal air flow is so great that the breath sounds are barely audible. This is an ominous sign. The physical findings are those of generalized obstructive emphysema (see p. 934). If atelectasis, pneumothorax or pneumomediastinum occurs, then the chest findings will be altered, with a shift of the mediastinum to the side of atelectasis or to the side opposite the pneumothorax. When emphysema is severe, the liver and spleen may be felt below the costal margins.

Many attacks of asthma over a long time may lead to chronic emphysema. These changes may be largely or completely reversible with adequate therapy during childhood. Children with moderate to severe chronic asthma are likely to have fine lanugo hair over the shoulders and arms. Pulmonary osteoarthropathy is rare. Allergic rhinitis and sinusitis are common.

Laboratory Data. Eosinophilia can often be demonstrated in the peripheral blood, nasal secretions and sputum. There may be a polymorphonuclear leukocytosis in the presence of infection.

Pulmonary function studies will disclose diminished maximal breathing capacity, tidal volume, and timed vital capacity. The effective tidal volume, as determined from helium or nitrogen washout techniques, is low during the asthmatic attack and may improve in response to therapy with little change in the total vital capacity, presumably as unaerated components of lung become ventilated.

Early in an attack the patient with air hunger may move enough air to maintain a normal or even a low arterial pCO_2. When the pCO_2 begins to rise, ventilatory failure is occurring, and when the pCO_2 exceeds 50 or 60 mm. Hg, the patient is seriously ill and a candidate for assisted ventilation. He is likely now to have a rapidly falling pH and increasing respiratory acidosis.

Differential Diagnosis. Asthma of allergic origin must be differentiated from many other conditions which cause wheezing. An aspirated foreign body may produce typical asthmatic wheezing, and this may persist for weeks or months if the foreign body is retained. Chronic bronchopulmonary processes associated with bronchiectasis or cystic fibrosis may closely resemble asthma. True allergic asthma may be associated with cystic fibrosis, in which case allergic management added to other measures may be important to therapy.

In infancy, asthma of allergic origin is most often confused with acute bronchiolitis, from which it is sometimes distinguished with great difficulty. When bronchiolitis occurs for the first time in an infant and can be shown to be due to the respiratory syncytial virus or another viral agent or occurs as a part of an epidemic, there is little likelihood that the infant has asthma. On the other hand, when an infant responds to 2 or 3 respiratory infections or febrile illnesses with asthmatic paroxysms resembling bronchiolitis, then the possibility of allergic reactivity must be considered. Wheezing sometimes accompanies acute bronchitis and may lead to the designation of the illness as "asthmatic bronchitis." This term is vague in meaning and often constitutes an evasion of the diagnosis of bronchial asthma, with the latter's implied need for adequate allergic study and management.

Prognosis. With adequate treatment, asthma can be brought under satisfactory control in the majority of children. Some will continue to have periodic attacks over months or years, but most will be able to lead active normal lives within modest limitations imposed by their allergic condition. Results of long-term studies indicate that 20 years after the onset of asthma in childhood about 50 per cent of patients will be symptom-free, 35 to 40 per cent will have mild difficulties, and 10 per cent will continue to have severe asthma. The case fatality rate from asthma during this time is 1 per cent or less.

Treatment. *General management.* The basic treatment of the child with asthma consists in removal of the items from his diet or environment which can be shown to be productive of paroxysms, along with those general measures of allergic control which are apt to diminish the likelihood of the allergic state becoming more active or more broadly based. Desensitization is commonly utilized, but many children with infrequent, easily controlled attacks of asthma do very well without it.

When asthma complicates or is complicated by a bacterial infection, specific antibiotic therapy is indicated. Most respiratory infections associated with asthma, however, are viral in origin. In asthma, as in other diseases, the choice of an antibiotic should rest upon clear clinical indications, supported by adequate bacteriologic data. Occasionally, when uncontrolled chronic or recurrent asthma is associated with chronic sinusitis or persistent low-grade infections of the tonsillar or adenoid area, a course of therapy with antibiotic or chemotherapeutic agents for 2 to 3 weeks may be given a trial. Prophylactic administration of such drugs, however, is not recommended.

Tonsillectomy and adenoidectomy are often recommended and may be helpful when these tissues cause respiratory obstruction, or when they are chronically infected. Operation should not, however, be undertaken before the child has been shown not to respond to an adequate program of allergic management, including desensitization. It will commonly be observed that the tonsillar and adenoid tissues will become diminished after adequate allergic management.

A severe paroxysm of asthma may be anxiety-provoking to both child and parents. The immediate anxieties will be allayed by the understanding physician. Some parents, and even some physicians, may greatly overdramatize the occasion. The skillful physician will discern whether the manner in which parents respond to the asthmatic child reflects warmth and insight or whether a program of education as to the child's real needs is indicated.

When infants and small children need hospitalization, the continued presence of the mother or of some family member by the bedside may help allay anxiety. When it appears that conflicts or anxieties in the family initiate or perpetuate the child's asthmatic paroxysms and cannot be handled by simple supportive measures, psychiatric consultation should be sought. Rarely, the child's asthma is rooted in tensions and family situations which are not amenable to available psychotherapeutic help. In such circumstances the child may benefit from residence in an institution where adequate allergic, psychotherapeutic and other supportive treatments are available.

The asthmatic attack. Most asthmatic children need symptomatic therapy from time to time. Agents having some degree of effectiveness in relieving the dyspnea of an attack of asthma and in preventing the attack include epinephrine and its analogues, the antihistaminic drugs, aminophylline or theophylline, and the corticosteroids. Epinephrine and its analogues are the most generally useful. The variety of preparations is large, and includes analogues particularly compounded for long action or for freedom from unpleasant side effects. Some are preferentially given subcutaneously, others by inhalation.

Ephedrine has the advantages of prolonged action and oral administration. It should be given at the first sign of an attack. Dosage will vary from 8 mg. in the preschool child to 25 mg. in older children. In some children such doses produce tachycardia, central nervous stimulation, or vomiting. Pseudoephedrine, an isomer of ephedrine, is relatively free of some of these cardiovascular and central effects of ephedrine and may be a useful replacement. It can be given in about twice the dose of ephedrine. Either drug can be given prophylactically and may from time to time be particularly useful at bedtime in the avoidance of nocturnal paroxysms, or in anticipation of wheezing with exercise.

For the management of severe asthma, epinephrine is extremely useful. It is given subcutaneously in 1:1000 solution. It is preferable to use a small dose at approximately 20- to 30-minute intervals rather than to give an excessively large dose initially. Some patients become unresponsive to epinephrine; intravenous administration of diphenhydramine will at times re-establish responsiveness. For the infant 0.05 ml. is adequate as an initial dose of epinephrine; that for older children should not exceed 0.2 to 0.3 ml. Epinephrine is also given by inhalation in a 1:100 solution, *which must never be used for injection.*

Ethylnorepinephrine is free of some of the adrenergic effects of epinephrine; it may be given subcutaneously or intravenously.

Isopropylnorepinephrine is available for inhalation. Relief from aerosolized agents is often rapid. Control of the aerosols for children should be in the hands of a responsible adult, owing to the tendency of some children, especially in adolescence, to overmedication. Dosage will vary with the preparation used, 1 or 2 whiffs or sprays commonly bringing adequate relief. Administration at intervals more frequent than hourly or half-hourly is to be avoided. Prolonged use of aerosols may be a serious problem, owing to chronic alterations of bronchopulmonary physiology, with the result that other usual measures may be less effective and fatal status asthmaticus ensue.

Antihistaminic drugs have a limited place in the management of asthma; they are most useful when asthma follows or is associated with an acute allergic rhinitis, when early relief of obstruction in the upper respiratory tract may result in some relief of asthmatic distress. Otherwise, they are generally contraindicated, owing to their sedative and drying effects.

Aminophylline (theophylline ethylenediamine) and other preparations in which the active principle is theophylline may at times relieve a paroxysm when epinephrine has failed. They should be used with extreme caution. Severe reactions, occasionally fatal, may occur, especially when these drugs are administered in an excessive dose. *The physician must be familiar with the signs of toxicity.* The first signs are increasing restlessness, irritability and vomiting; if they appear, no more theophylline should be given. With increasing excitement or delirium, vomiting of blood or a convulsion, the level of intoxication has become life-threatening. Treatment consists of anticonvulsant medication, such as phenobarbital, and measures aimed at relieving cerebral edema.

Aminophylline is commonly given in rectal suppositories or instillations. *Doses should not exceed 3 to 4 mg. per kg. or be given more frequently than every 8 hours.* Its toxic effects may be potentiated by epinephrine or ephedrine, which should not be given concurrently unless the dose of aminophylline is reduced. Only whole suppositories of appropriate drug content should be used; the drug may be unevenly distributed between cut halves. Suppositories containing benzocaine are not recommended. Aminophylline may be given intravenously, but this route is dangerous; the injection must be given very slowly and with the *sure knowledge of what theophylline medication has been given within the past day.* Oral administration is less effective, owing to limited absorption and some gastric irritation.

Theophylline has been rendered more soluble in a number of preparations, such as choline theophyllinate and in elixir forms, some with added expectorants. Theophylline in these preparations should not be given in doses in excess of 3 to 4 mg. per kg., nor at intervals more frequent than every 8 hours. The total daily dose by all routes should not exceed 12 mg. per kg.

Expectorants are useful adjuncts to epinephrine and its analogues in the management of asthmatic paroxysms. Syrup of hydriodic acid may be mixed with equal parts of syrup of ephedrine or pseudo-ephedrine. The dose will be determined mainly by the child's need for ephedrine or pseudo-ephedrine. Potassium iodide and potassium guaiacholate may also be useful, often in combination with ephedrine or pseudoephedrine in syrups. Iodides may exceptionally be goitrogenic or may lead to increases in serum protein-bound iodine concentration. They should be used sparingly in adolescents, since they may aggravate acne. Inhalations of warm or cold vaporized water may add to the patient's comfort. There is no convincing evidence that the addition of wetting agents or volatile materials to such vapors is useful.

Sedatives should be used sparingly if at all in the management of the acute asthmatic attack. The effects of phenobarbital are unpredictable, particularly in small children; the mixture of somnolence, fatigue, anxiety and restlessness produced in some children may render other measures less effective than they might be otherwise. The use of opiates is contraindicated.

The child with asthma should be kept adequately hydrated and may need sodium bicarbonate intravenously for the correction of acidosis. The correction of acidosis may also re-establish responsiveness of the epinephrine-fast child to this drug.

Oxygen is indicated at the earliest appearance of cyanosis. The inhalation of 20 per cent oxygen with 80 per cent helium may be helpful in severe asthma, owing to the increased diffusion of oxygen in the presence of helium. The voice may be unexpectedly high-pitched after such inhalation.

If the drugs mentioned above and the other supportive measures have failed to bring adequate relief from an asthmatic paroxysm within several hours, a corticosteroid may be administered. At times 1 or 2 doses of cortisone orally in the amount of 25 mg., the second at an interval of 8 to 12 hours, will be sufficient. The place of these agents in the management of asthma, however, is limited. Their use for relatively mild attacks may lead to frequent administration with resultant suppression of adrenal activity. Prolonged use may lead to serious retardation of growth and to steroid dependency. It appears possible that a rising mortality rate of asthma in recent years has been contributed to by therapy with corticosteroids and aminophylline.

Respiratory failure in status asthmaticus. The child with severe asthma who fails to respond to epinephrine or aminophylline is said to be in status asthmaticus, the incidence of which appears to be increasing. Some feel that the recurrent use of corticosteroids, often for longer periods of time than are necessary, may be a factor; others suggest that the overuse of nebulized isopropylnorepinephrine may in some way make asthmatic attacks more refractory.

Respiratory failure is the most dangerous complication of the asthmatic paroxysm. It generally occurs during a prolonged or unusually severe attack in which inability to move sticky secretions has led to fatigue and diminishing pulmonary function. Breath sounds become diminished or absent, and cyanosis appears, even in 40 per cent oxygen atmosphere. Arterial pCO_2, which may have been normal, or even low during a period of relative hyperventilation, now rises, with the development of a mixed acidosis; the respiratory component is due to retention of carbon dioxide; the metabolic element, to anoxia. A pCO_2 above 60 mm. Hg may be an indication for assisted ventilation.

Children with status asthmaticus should be under intensive care with the participation of pediatrician, anesthesiologist, nurse, inhalation therapist, physical therapist and, at times, bronchoesophagologist. It is first necessary to ensure that hydration is adequately planned, including the correction of acidosis. Ineffectual overdoses of epinephrine or aminophylline should be avoided. Short-term therapy with a corticosteroid is indicated, and antibiotic therapy is justified on the possibility that infection may be a contributing factor or that considerable manipulation of the respiratory tract may be necessary.

Assisted ventilation may begin with intermittent positive-pressure breathing (IPPB), using a heavy aerosol of warm saline solution in an attempt to loosen secretions. The ultrasonic nebulizer is an effective way to administer water vapors, but, if overused, may overhydrate. It is doubtful whether wetting agents contribute to the effectiveness of aerosols; there is a possibility that acetyl cysteine may be helpful in depolymerizing thickened secretions, but some children find it irritating. The intravenous administration of sodium iodide (0.2 to 0.5 gm. per 500 ml. of fluids, up to 0.5 gm. per day) may help in liquefaction of secretions, or a bronchodilator such as isopropylnorepinephrine may be administered by IPPB every 4 hours, with care as to overuse.

Inflation of the chest should be slow, and the child should be encouraged to empty the chest with each expiration. Utilization of positive-pressure breathing may be intermittent or continuous. When its use by mask fails to bring relief, owing to inability of the child to cooperate, or if the child's condition deteriorates, then he should receive assisted ventilation through an endotracheal or nasotracheal tube, preferably using a volume-cycled respirator such as the Engstrom or Emerson machine. This can be accomplished only under sedation, and may also require the use of muscle relaxants.

The endotracheal tube will facilitate the aspiration of secretions from the bronchial passages, and may permit bronchial lavage with warm physiologic saline solution; bronchoscopic aspiration may be helpful in some instances. When necessary, a tracheostomy may permit more effective ventilation and easier bronchial lavage. Physiotherapy to the chest, with cupped hand percussion and postural drainage, may also make bronchial aspiration more effective.

Children receiving such heroic measures should be cared for only under conditions that permit continuous monitoring of body temperature, electrocardiogram, central venous pressure and peripheral arterial pressure. Frequent examinations of arterial blood for pH, pCO_2 and pO_2 are essential aids to adequate control of ventilation. Serum sodium, potassium and chloride values should also be determined at intervals.

Complications of such intensive manipulation include pneumomediastinum, pneumothorax, subcutaneous emphysema, cardiac arrest, and tracheal or glottic stenosis.

ECZEMA

The term "eczema" has had many meanings. In the relatively restricted sense in which it is used in pediatrics, it denotes a disorder of the skin generally held to be at least in part atopic. It is most common in infancy and is characterized by erythema, papules, vesiculation, oozing and crusting with intense itching. It is often, but not always, possible to demonstrate specific allergens which induce the eruption. There is a tendency to familial occurrence and for those who have eczema in infancy to have hay fever or asthma in later life.

Seborrheic dermatitis is commonly associated with eczema and on occasion may appear to be the initial feature. There is little evidence that uncomplicated seborrhea or seborrheic dermatitis has any strong allergic element, though some feel that allergic therapeutic measures are helpful in such severe seborrheic conditions as erythroderma desquamativa (Leiner's disease).

Etiology. Although it is usually easy to demonstrate allergic factors in eczema, it appears even more than other atopic disorders to be a complex problem in which nonimmunologic factors may determine the success or failure of therapy.

The onset of eczema in early infancy is commonly associated with the introduction of new foods to the diet. Eczema is uncommon in breast-fed babies and may appear shortly after cow's milk has been introduced into the diet, or when a relatively hypoallergenic form of cow's milk, such as evaporated milk, is replaced by whole pasteurized milk. Egg plays a conspicuous role, and sensitivity to egg on skin testing is so regularly found in afflicted children that intrauterine exposure to egg protein has been suggested as a causative factor. Skin reactivity can often be demonstrated to other potent allergens, such as wool and house dust, as well as to egg and milk.

Local factors in the skin unrelated to allergy, such as sweating and overhydration, tend to aggravate eczema, and dehydration of the skin tends to improve it.

The initial lesion in eczema may depend in large part for its evolution upon the scratching induced by the intense itching. Emotional tension and anger may lead to the skin becoming the focal point of a struggle between parent and child. When a mother feels that her child's eczema is unsightly, she may find it difficult to meet the child's needs for normal warm and affectionate handling, or may strive to erase the eruption with too energetic use of ointments and salves.

Infection of eczematous skin is common; it intensifies the itching and inflammation and results in the oozing of purulent material, which dries into crusts. Infection not only tends to make existing eczema more severe, but also may lead to involvement of new areas. Respiratory infections may also initiate exacerbations.

The importance of nonantigenic dietary factors in eczema is not clear. Hansen found that the level of unsaturated fatty acids in serum may be low and that the feeding of unsaturated fatty acids may at times be beneficial.

Clinical Manifestations. Eczema in the infant commonly appears first upon the cheeks as erythema, which may be quickly followed by papule and vesicle formation (see Fig. 10-12A, p. 628). The lesion may then spread to contiguous areas of the face or may develop independently in other parts of the body. It is particularly prone to occur on the flexural surfaces, in the antecubital and popliteal fossae, and on the volar surfaces of the wrist and forearms. The scalp is commonly involved, as may be the postauricular crease. Eczema may have its onset insidiously in lesions indistinguishable from seborrhea; cradle cap may be followed by generalized seborrhea of the scalp and extension to the forehead and cheeks. It may be difficult to separate seborrheic from eczematous factors.

Itching is characteristic of eczema rather than of seborrhea. The excoriation produced by scratching results in weeping and crusting, and the involved areas may be transformed into raw surfaces oozing serum, pus and blood. The infant with eczema is likely to be irritable and fretful. Infection of the involved skin is common, but, except for some degree of fever, systemic manifestations tend to be relatively mild. Generalized lymph node enlargement and splenomegaly are common.

With subsidence of the acute inflammatory process in eczema, erythema abates, edema disappears, and crusts dry and desquamate, leaving new and healthy epithelium. The lesion even in very severe eczema is usually completely reversible.

In chronic eczema the healing process associated with continued inflammation and the stimulation and irritation from scratching and rubbing cause the skin to become thickened and cracked. This lichenification is the hallmark of chronic eczema; it is particularly likely to be seen in flexural creases, at the volar surfaces of the wrist, occasionally on extensor surfaces of knees and elbows, and on exposed surfaces, such as face and neck, legs, and hands or arms below sleeve level. This distribution strongly suggests contactant factors, such as house dust, wool (felt) and the like. These changes of chronic eczema are more common in children than in infants.

The most common complication of eczema is infection of the eczematous skin by hemolytic streptococci or by staphylococci. Intractable itching may be a clue to such infections. The most severe infections are those in which eczema is complicated by vaccinia or by herpesvirus infection. Bacterial infections may extend beyond the eczematous lesion. Suppurative adenopathy is uncommon, and brain abscess is a rare complication. Other complications include undernutrition, at times with hypoproteinemia.

Differential Diagnosis. Seborrheic dermatitis and eczema are often difficult to differentiate. Either may have to be distinguished from eruptions on the scalp or body of nonlipid reticuloendotheliosis (Letterer-Siwe disease), in which the eruption may be hemorrhagic. The associated lesions of reticuloendothelial disease in lymph nodes or bone will aid in the differentiation; the histologic pattern of the dermal lesion is characteristic.

The Wiskott-Aldrich syndrome is a fatal sex-linked recessive condition characterized by hemorrhagic eczema, bloody diarrhea, periosteal hemorrhages, thrombocytopenia, chronic otitis media, and hypogammaglobulinemia (IgM deficiency). The familial occurrence in boys, the unusual clinical findings and the immunoelectrophoretic pattern should aid in diagnosis.

The possibility of phenylketonuria should be considered in infants with eczema, and appropriate tests obtained.

Laboratory Data. Eosinophilia is common. Atopic reactivity is generally found on skin testing, even in young infants, and may correlate well with clinical reactivity. Cultures of infected skin will commonly reveal streptococci or staphylococci. Staphylococci commonly overgrow and obscure streptococci unless special media are used, such as blood agar plates impregnated with gentian violet. When eczema vaccinatum or eczema herpeticum is present, viral inclusion bodies may be found in the exudate from lesions, or the infecting virus itself may be cultured.

Treatment. Few illnesses demand a more comprehensive approach than eczema. Attention should be focused upon avoidance of probable offending allergens, eradication of any complicating infection in the skin, control of itching and scratching and the instigation of local measures to improve the condition of the involved skin.

In addition to the avoidance of contact, so far as possible, with incriminated dietary and environmental allergens, other substances of high sensitizing potential should be avoided. For example, the exclusion of egg and chocolate from the diet of infants and children with eczema is recommended. The infant should be breast fed as long as possible.

Often infants seem to derive benefit from feeding of unsaturated fatty acids (see Etiology). Reduction of fat in the diet also at times seems to improve eczema; it may be that eczema is better tolerated by underfed or normally fed infants than by overfed ones.

Exposure to wool and house dust should be avoided so far as possible. Since both soap and water often seem to have adverse effects upon eczematous skin, skin cleansers containing mild detergents may be used in place of soap. Starch baths are often better tolerated than plain water.

The infant with eczema *must not* be vaccinated until his skin has been clear for a year or so, nor should he be exposed to other persons with fresh vaccinia lesions (see p. 646). The child with eczema should also be protected, as far as possible, from the virus of herpes simplex. He should be immunized in the usual way against diphtheria, pertussis, tetanus and poliomyelitis. Egg-grown vaccines should be avoided in egg-sensitive patients.

The ingenuity with which infants will find ways to rub the itching parts must be matched by the skill of the physician, nurse or parent in applying restraints, but these should be used for as short a period as possible. In infants the best restraints may be bulky wet dressings of cool Burow's solution, which will help alleviate the itching. Sedatives may also help allay itching; Hill recommends chloral hydrate. Antihistaminics such as diphenhydramine may be useful because of their joint sedative and antipruritic activity. The *local* use of antihistaminics and anesthetic agents *is contraindicated*, owing to their potential for skin sensitization. On mildly or moderately inflamed, uninfected skin in the older child *plain* calamine lotion may be soothing and antipruritic.

The local care of the infected skin is directed initially at removing debris and allaying the inflammatory reaction, which is practically always due in part to infection. Continuous applications (soaks) of Burow's solution are indicated until the skin has become relatively free of active inflammation and cleansed of debris. Then Lassar's paste or similar hydrophilic preparations may be used; a mild antiseptic such as hexachlorophene or benzalkonium chloride (1:10,000 aqueous solution) may be added. In severe infections of the eczematous lesion an antibiotic agent should be given systemically, the most useful being penicillin, owing to the frequency with which a beta hemolytic streptococcus is the pathogen or one of the pathogens. Even when staphylococcal organisms resistant to penicillin are found on the initial culture, unless there is a compelling need for some other agent, a trial of penicillin is warranted and will often be satisfactory. The oral route of administration is preferred; large doses are prescribed for at least 10 to 14 days. Sharply localized infections may sometimes be managed with the local use of antibiotic ointments; bacitracin and neomycin are the preferred agents for local use. Penicillin and the sulfonamides should not be used locally, owing to their high sensitizing potential.

When the skin has become dry and relatively free of active inflammation, a coal tar preparation will be effective in further clearing of the involved skin. It should be used in the mildest effective concentration. Many useful decolorized preparations are available, some of which contain small amounts of sulfur or salicylic acid, or both.

Topical therapy with a corticosteroid is helpful in abating the reactivity of acutely inflamed skin when the lesion is relatively limited in extent. When infection is present, it should be brought under adequate control before the steroid is applied. Systemic steroid therapy has a limited place in the management of eczema, since relapses usually follow its termination. It should be reserved for the most critical and troublesome situations and should be regarded solely as a temporary expedient.

When avoidance of allergens and local therapy have failed to control eczema, and when reactivity to inhalants is indicated by history or by skin testing, then desensitization may be helpful. This is applicable more commonly in older children than in infants.

Certain precautions are essential in skin testing children with eczema and in the administration of desensitizing materials. Some patients, usually children beyond infancy, have delayed systemic responses to skin testing or to desensitizing injections; these consist of malaise, nausea and vomiting, and intensification of the inflammation and of itching. This reaction occurs within a few hours or may be delayed as long as a day, and may last for 3 to 4 days. It may be easily overlooked or thought to be due to extrinsic factors in the diet or home. This reaction may occur with dilutions of desensitizing material as weak as 1:1,000,000 or weaker. This sensitivity will limit the dose of allergen which can be given in a desensitization program, but is not a contraindication to trial of desensitization at subreaction dosage levels.

The parents need to be reassured that the infant with eczema can be handled freely, and that he needs as much warm personal attention in the form of bodily contact as do other infants. He may need to be protected from contact with maternal clothing to which he is reactive or from contact with allergens which the parent may bring on clothing or hands. In older children, particularly when itching and scratching contribute to persistent unsightliness of the lesion, the physician will need to identify those situations in which scratching occurs in relation to feelings of frustration and in which attempts on the part of the parent to control scratching have made the skin the focal point of a struggle between parent and child. It may be helpful to make the care of the skin the child's responsibility as much as possible, as well as for the physician to explore other areas of parent-child conflicts.

Prognosis. Eczema usually undergoes a spontaneous and lasting remission in infants, after a variable course, by the second or third year of life. This termination more likely represents the result of developmental changes in the skin and in immune mechanisms than any fundamental change in the allergic diathesis, since many of these children will have other manifestations of atopy in later life. Asthma and hay fever are both common; asthma may appear for the first time before the eczema has remitted. A few children with infantile eczema will carry a continuing skin reactivity into the later years of childhood and into adult life, most often predominantly on the flexural surfaces of elbows and knees. In long-standing eczema (10 years or more) ocular cataracts are an occasional complication.

ATOPIC ERYTHRODERMA

This term was applied by Hill to a severe form of eczema observed in some infants in whom the seborrheic element is particularly strong. The eruption is generalized and may leave only the palms and soles free of involvement. During the acute phase and during exacerbations the skin and subcutaneous tissues may be edematous. Scaling and thickening of the skin may produce a pattern closely resembling that of Leiner's disease (p. 1403). The hands and feet may be cold and bluish. Generalized lymphadenopathy is commonly present. Itching is intense.

Children with atopic erythroderma give evidence of atopic sensitization, but respond poorly or not at all to therapy. Corticosteroid therapy may be necessary during periods of severe reaction. Spontaneous remissions occur after many months.

GASTROINTESTINAL ALLERGY

In allergic infants or children the gastrointestinal tract commonly serves as the *portal of entry* for allergens (food allergy) or as the *site of reaction* (gastrointestinal allergy). Although foods are the most common allergens causing symptoms in the gastrointestinal tract, food allergy and gastrointestinal allergy are not synonymous. Inhaled or injected material, as well as ingested, may produce in gastrointestinal tissues the characteristic allergic responses of edema, mucus exudation and smooth muscle spasm. Bleeding may also occur. Not all reactions to food necessarily represent histamine release, however. Other reactions to foods include cheilitis, aphthous stomatitis and perianal dermatitis. Foods may precipitate labial

herpes simplex in persons who harbor the virus. There may be an allergic element in some cases of peptic ulcer, regional ileitis or ulcerative colitis.

Clinical Manifestations. In early infancy the chief manifestations of gastrointestinal allergy include nausea, vomiting, diarrhea and abdominal pain, sometimes with refusal to take reactive foods. Rarely the onset is explosive and is accompanied by evidence of shock or a serious disturbance of fluid and electrolyte metabolism. Cow's milk is the chief offender; Bachman and Dees found evidence in 1 per cent of infants. The clinical pattern of intolerance to cow's milk is sometimes quite characteristic: a hungry infant, who appears otherwise well, is offered a bottle of cow's milk formula, takes a swallow or two eagerly, appears to find the formula distasteful and rejects the nipple, with further crying and evident hunger. With urging, after a minute or two the infant may accept the nipple and take an ounce or two of formula, which is then vomited. After this vomiting the remainder of the formula may be taken without incident, but the nursing period is followed by irritability, the appearance of colicky pain and the passage of frequent small, wet and gaseous stools.

Abdominal pain is common in infants, and there may be the typical picture of infantile colic. Aerophagia may contribute. Many infants with gastrointestinal symptoms of food allergy have an associated congestion of the upper respiratory tract or a skin eruption.

There is often an area of dermatitis in the intergluteal folds, more or less sharply delimited to the perianal region. The older child may also suffer from periodic irritation in this area, sometimes with pruritus, on exposure to reactive foods. Rubin described a number of infants in whom colic and diarrhea were associated with the appearance of mucus and bright red blood in the stool. Relief of symptoms following withdrawal of cow's milk from the diet was said to be prompt.

Gastrointestinal allergy in infants is often transient, presumably owing to the increasing impermeability of the gastrointestinal mucosa to large protein particles during the first 3 to 4 months of life. The condition is commonly terminated spontaneously by 6 months, though it will occasionally persist for many years.

A temporary intolerance to cow's milk may follow an acute diarrheal disorder in small infants; in the immediate postinfectious period the permeability of the intestinal mucosa to unsplit food protein may be increased. It may be wise to reinstitute oral feeding of cow's milk slowly or perhaps preferable to use a hypoallergenic cow's milk substitute for a brief time.

In older children the manifestations of gastrointestinal allergy may closely resemble the celiac syndrome. Heiner showed that in some infants with gluten-sensitive celiac disease there may be associated precipitins for wheat proteins, but the celiac syndrome induced by gluten is not generally regarded as allergic in nature (see p.

807). Gastrointestinal symptoms may be particularly striking in anaphylactoid purpura, in which they are the result of an immunologic injury to vascular endothelium. Only rarely, however, is anaphylactoid purpura clearly related to food allergy.

Diagnosis. Accurate diagnosis of gastrointestinal allergy may be difficult, owing to the frequency with which its symptoms may be associated with other conditions, to the possibility that food reactivities are multiple rather than single and to the nature of temporary food intolerance. A high index of suspicion is essential diagnostically, but confirmation requires a clear association of symptoms with an allergen and control of symptoms by its removal from the diet or environment.

The diagnosis of cow's milk intolerance is probably made more often than it is justified, but when the clinical manifestations subside promptly after substitution of a hypoallergenic milk, confirmation by further diagnostic testing scarcely seems necessary.

Skin testing is of limited help in food allergy, many clinical reactions being unaccompanied by skin responses. In infants with milk allergy, passive cutaneous anaphylaxis may be a useful technique of study (see p. 493).

Differential Diagnosis. In early infancy the vomiting of the allergic child may closely resemble that of hypertrophic pyloric stenosis and may even be associated with increased gastric peristalsis (see p. 785).

It is necessary to differentiate milk allergy from lactase deficiency and other enzyme deficiencies, which are probably more common than has been suspected (see p. 811).

Treatment. In gastrointestinal allergy a symptomatic response usually follows quickly the removal of the allergen from the diet or environment.

When cow's milk is the allergen, the substitution of a soybean "milk" may promptly control symptoms and re-establish nutrition. Supplemental vitamins and minerals are essential; the vitamins should preferably be of synthetic origin. When soy products are not tolerated, prepared formulas containing a protein hydrolysate or meat as the protein may be tried. When the symptoms have been clearly related to milk reactivity, it seems reasonable to continue a milk substitute for an extended period. When cow's milk is again given, evaporated milk will usually be better tolerated than whole milk, and its use should be continued as long as possible before pasteurized milk is resumed. The addition of other foods to the infant's diet should be undertaken cautiously, foods of high sensitizing potential being introduced last.

Prognosis. Gastrointestinal symptoms due to cow's milk or other allergens usually disappear in the latter part of the first year of life as the intestinal mucosa matures. Many children will have other evidences of allergy in later life, and cow's milk and other food allergens may continue to play an active role in the production of symptoms from reactivity in other tissues.

Prophylaxis. In families in whose members allergic manifestations have been particularly severe during infancy, it may be appropriate, if breast feeding is not possible, to initiate feeding with a cow's milk substitute, such as a soybean or other preparation (Glaser). In exceptional instances it may even be helpful to modify the diet of the mother during pregnancy in such a way that the exposure of the fetus to cow's milk or egg antigen is kept at a minimum. Needless to say, modifications of the diet for either infant or mother should ensure nutritional adequacy of the diet in every detail.

OTHER ALLERGIC DISORDERS

Pulmonary Hemosiderosis. See page 928.
Gastrointestinal Reactivity to Cow's Milk and Iron Deficiency Anemia. See page 1070.

VICTOR C. VAUGHAN, III

REFERENCES

Bachman, K. D., and Dees, S. C.: Milk Allergy. I. Observation of Symptoms and Incidence in "Well" Babies. II. Observations on Incidence and Symptoms of Allergy to Milk in Allergic Infants. *Pediatrics*, 20:393, 407, 1957.

Boisvert, P. L., and Powers, G. F.: Eczema and Hemolytic Streptococcal Disease in Children. *Yale J. Biol. & Med.*, 16:595, 1944.

Clein, N. W.: Cow's Milk Allergy in Infants. *Pediat. Clin. N. Amer.*, 1:949, 1954.

Dees, S.: Allergy to Cow's Milk. *Pediat. Clin. N. Amer.*, 6:881, 1959.

Kunz, M. L., Reisman, R. E., and Arkesman, C. E.: Evaluation of Penicillin Hypersensitivity by Two Newer Immunological Procedures. *J. Allergy*, 40:135, 1967.

Glaser, J.: The Prophylaxis of Allergic Disease in Infancy and Childhood. *Pediat. Clin. N. Amer.*, 6:901, 1959.

Gruskay, F. L., and Cooke, R. E.: The Gastrointestinal Absorption of Unaltered Protein in Normal Infants and in Infants Recovering from Diarrhea. *Pediatrics*, 16:763, 1955.

Heiner, D. C., Lahey, M. E., Wilson, J. F., and Peck, G. A.: Precipitins to Wheat in Steatorrhea. *Am. J. Dis. Child.*, 102:446, 1961.

Heiner, D. C., Sears, J. W., and Kniker, W. T.: Multiple Precipitins to Cow's Milk in Chronic Respiratory Disease: Syndrome Including Poor Growth, Gastrointestinal Symptoms, Evidence of Allergy, Iron Deficiency Anemia, and Pulmonary Hemosiderosis. *Am. J. Dis. Child.*, 103:634, 1962.

Hill, L. W.: The Treatment of Eczema in Infants and Children. *J. Pediat.*, 47:141, 357, 496, 648, 752, 1955. (Also as a monograph: St. Louis, C. V. Mosby Company, 1956.)

Hinkle, N. H., Hong, R., and West, C. D.: Identification of the Antigen and Symptomatology of Children with Precipitins to Milk. *Am. J. Dis. Child.*, 102:449, 1961.

McGovern, J. P., and Daeschner, C. W., Jr.: The Role of Fluid and Electrolytes in the Management of Severe Asthma. *South. M.J.*, 51:1197, 1958.

Miller, H., and Baruch, D.: Psychotherapy of Parents of Allergic Children. *Ann. Allergy*, 18:990, 1960.

Osler, A. G., Lichtenstein, L. M., and Levy, D. A.: *In Vitro* Studies of Human Reaginic Allergy. *Advances in Immunol.*, 8:183, 1968.

Richards, W., Siegel, S. C., Strauss, J., and Leigh, M. D.: Status Asthmaticus in Children. *J.A.M.A.*, 201:75, 1967.

Rubin, M. I.: Allergic Intestinal Bleeding in the Newborn; A Clinical Syndrome. *Am. J.M. Sc.*, 200:385, 1940.

Speer, F.: Allergic Tension-Fatigue in Children. *Ann. Allergy,* 12:168, 1954.

Tuft, L., and Ermilio, F.: Intracutaneous Asthma Vaccine Therapy in Asthmatic Children: Its Application and Clinical Value. *J. Pediat.,* 48:569, 1956.

Vaughan, V. C., III: Allergic Problems in the Upper Respiratory Tract, Including the Ear. *Pediat. Clin. N. Amer.,* 4:285, 1957.

Vaughan, V. C., III: The Allergic Child—A Philosophy of Management. *J. Med. Assoc. Georgia,* 49:171, 1960.

Wilson, J. F., and Lahey, M. C.: The syndrome of Milk-Induced Occult Gastrointestinal Bleeding. *J. Clin. Invest.,* 45:1086, 1966.

Diseases of Connective Tissue

("COLLAGEN DISEASES")

The disorders described in this section are grouped together because of similarities in symptomatology and pathology; in general, they are associated with inflammatory changes in various connective tissues throughout the body. Included are the following:

I. Juvenile rheumatoid arthritis
II. Ankylosing spondylitis
III. Systemic lupus erythematosus
IV. The vasculitis syndromes
   A. Henoch-Schönlein vasculitis
   B. Polyarteritis nodosa
      1. Infantile polyarteritis
      2. Wegener's granulomatosis
   C. Takayasu's arteritis
V. Dermatomyositis
VI. Scleroderma
   A. Morphea
   B. Progressive systemic sclerosis
VII. Miscellaneous
   A. Stevens-Johnson syndrome
   B. Erythema nodosum
   C. Goodpasture's syndrome
   D. Relapsing nodular nonsuppurative panniculitis

Certain diseases, discussed elsewhere, have points of similarity to these disorders, i.e. acute rheumatic fever, serum sickness, glomerulonephritis, the idiopathic nephrotic syndrome, ulcerative colitis, regional enteritis and thrombotic thrombocytopenic purpura.

The causes and pathogenesis of these disorders are unknown, and precise diagnostic criteria are lacking. They usually appear as clinically distinct entities, each generally presenting a characteristic picture. For example, rheumatoid arthritis is associated with chronic arthritis, dermatomyositis with inflammation of muscle, scleroderma with induration of skin, and the like. But each of these diseases can affect many organs throughout the body, as shown in Table 10-5, and overlapping symptoms and signs sometimes make precise diagnosis difficult. More critical techniques may show that one or more of these diseases represent a number of distinct entities, or that some are more closely related than we now know.

TABLE 10-5. CLINICAL MANIFESTATIONS OF SOME OF THE CONNECTIVE TISSUE DISEASES

TYPE OF INVOLVEMENT / DISEASE	ARTHRITIS	POLYSEROSITIS	CLINICAL NEPHRITIS	CHARACTERISTIC RASH	MYOSITIS	GASTROINTESTINAL MANIFESTATIONS	OCULAR MANIFESTATIONS	MYOCARDITIS OR ENDOCARDITIS	HEPATOSPLENOMEGALY LYMPHADENOPATHY	CNS MANIFESTATIONS	FEVER
Juvenile rheumatoid arthritis	⊕	+	−	⊕	+	±	⊕	−	+	±	⊕
Systemic lupus erythematosus	+	⊕	⊕	⊕	+	+	+	+	+	+	+
Henoch-Schönlein vasculitis	+	±	⊕	⊕	±	⊕	±	±	+	+	+
Dermatomyositis	±	±	±	⊕	⊕	+	±	±	+	±	+

⊕Disease characteristic when present.
+May be present, but not characteristic.
±Rare.
−Not associated.

JUVENILE RHEUMATOID ARTHRITIS
(STILL'S DISEASE)

Juvenile rheumatoid arthritis is a systemic disease with a broad spectrum of manifestations. Arthritis is characteristic, but patterns of joint involvement vary widely. Systemic manifestations may also be present, and be more conspicuous than the arthritis. Still believed in the 1890's that juvenile and adult rheumatoid arthritis were different diseases, but most observers now believe the two diseases are substantially the same, children having somewhat different reaction patterns.

Etiology and Epidemiology. The cause is unknown. Clinical onset often appears after an acute systemic infection or physical trauma to a joint, but no direct causative relation to such events has been shown. Two frequently mentioned hypotheses are that the disease represents a direct infection with an organism such as Mycoplasma, Bedsonia, or virus, or that it is a hypersensitivity or "autoimmune" reaction to unknown stimuli. There is no convincing evidence for either hypothesis at this time, however. The possible role of lysosomes in initiating or perpetuating joint damage by accelerated release of enzymes has been of recent interest. The disease may well represent a single form of response to a variety of stimuli.

There is no evidence that juvenile rheumatoid arthritis is a hereditary disease. The disease rarely occurs in siblings, although an increased frequency of rheumatoid arthritis and ankylosing spondylitis may be found in relatives of affected children. Exacerbations of activity often follow intercurrent illness or psychic stress.

The exact incidence of rheumatoid arthritis is not known, but it is not rare. About 5 per cent of all cases begin in childhood. It occurs more frequently in females than in males, different series showing ratios of female to male ranging from 3 to 1 to 1.5 to 1. The disease may begin at any time during childhood, but rarely before the second year. Two peak incidences of age at onset probably exist, the first between 1 and 4 years, and the second between 9 and 14 years.

Pathology. Rheumatoid arthritis is characterized by chronic nonsuppurative inflammation of the synovium; microscopically, edema, hyperemia, and infiltration with lymphocytes and plasma cells can be seen in the synovial tissues. Projections of thickened synovial membrane form villi which protrude into joint spaces, usually with increased amounts of joint fluid. As synovial invasion of the joint space continues, articular cartilages become eroded and progressively destroyed. Synovial tissue eventually fills the joint space, leading to narrowing, fibrous ankylosis and bony fusion.

Earliest changes consist of periarticular edema with little synovial reaction or joint effusion. Synovial inflammation soon becomes manifest. Osteoporosis and formation of periosteal new bone may occur adjacent to inflamed joints. Growth centers next to inflamed joints may undergo either premature epiphyseal closure or accelerated epiphyseal growth. Tendons and tendon sheaths are often involved with inflammation similar to that of synovial tissues. Inflammation of muscle may also occur.

Rheumatoid nodules, far less common in children than in adults, show fibrinoid material surrounded with chronic inflammatory cells; palisading of cells is said to be less prominent in children than in adults. Pleura, pericardium and peritoneum may show nonspecific fibrinous serositis; progression to such severe thickening as in chronic constrictive pericarditis occurs rarely, if ever. The rheumatoid rash histologically is characterized by a few inflammatory cells surrounding small vessels of subepithelial tissues without extravasation of red blood cells.

Clinical Manifestations. *Joints.* Joint involvement can occur with or without systemic symptoms. Onset of arthritis may be insidious with gradual development of joint stiffness, swelling, and loss of motion; or fulminant with sudden appearance of symptomatic arthritis. Initially any joint or combination of joints may be affected; knees, ankles, feet, wrists and fingers are frequently involved at onset. Up to half of children have arthritis confined to one (monoarticular) or a few (pauciarticular; also called oligoarticular) joints for three or more months after onset; this pattern of arthritis may persist for years or be superseded at unpredictable intervals by polyarticular disease. Joint involvement is usually symmetrical in children with polyarthritis.

Affected joints are generally swollen and warm without distinctive erythema. Swelling results

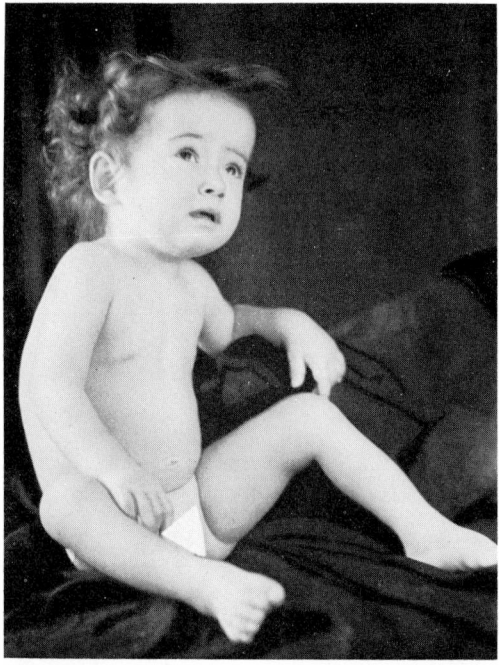

Figure 10-13. Characteristic posture of a child with rheumatoid arthritis, showing the anxious appearance and guarding of joints.

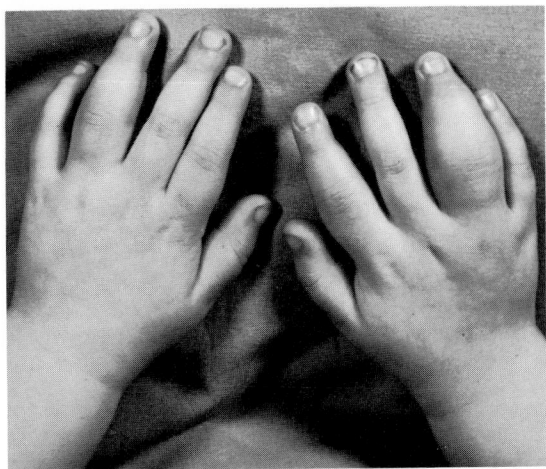

Figure 10-14. Fusiform changes (spindling) in juvenile rheumatoid arthritis involving the fourth finger of the left hand and the second and fourth fingers of the right hand.

from periarticular edema, joint effusion and synovial thickening. Some children initially have pain and stiffness of joints before development of objective changes. Affected joints may be tender to touch and painful on motion, although up to one third of children do not complain of pain in obviously inflamed joints. Inflamed joints usually have limitation of motion; this is related early to muscle spasm, later to actual joint destruction and fibrosis. Young children with polyarthritis often assume a characteristic posture, appearing irritable and anxious, and guarding their joints against movement (Fig. 10-13). Morning stiffness and "gelling" following inactivity (such as naps or car riding) occur in children, as in adults, with rheumatoid arthritis.

Tenosynovitis may be present, most often occurring in the hands and wrists. Weakness and atrophy of muscles about affected joints occur with great rapidity; myositis sometimes exists. Subcutaneous nodules are sometimes found over pressure points. Skin overlying inflamed joints may be altered by pigmentation or vitiligo. Chronically affected joints may become dislocated, deformed or fused.

Arthritis may ultimately affect any joint in the body. Knees, ankles, wrists, feet, fingers, toes, shoulders, elbows, neck, jaw, hips and sacroiliac joints are frequently involved. Inflammation of the proximal interphalangeal joints produces spindling, or fusiform changes, of the fingers (Figs. 10-14, 10-15) in about half of affected children; metacarpophalangeal involvement is equally common, and distal interphalangeal joints may also be affected. The cervical spine is involved, with neck stiffness and pain, in about half of patients, usually in those with polyarticular disease. Temporomandibular joint involvement with limited motion is common; the pain may be referred to as "earache" by young children. Hip involvement occurs in up to half of children, usually beginning

insidiously some time after the onset of polyarticular disease. Destruction of the femoral head may ensue; severe hip disease is a major cause of disability in late juvenile rheumatoid arthritis (Fig. 10-16). Radiographic sacroiliac joint changes are found in 25 per cent of cases; these are apparently unassociated with clinical symptoms, and are milder than in ankylosing spondylitis; the lumbodorsal spine is not involved. Rarely, the cricoarytenoid joint may be involved, causing hoarseness and laryngeal stridor. The involvement of sternoclavicular and costochondral junctions can cause chest pain.

Growth disturbances adjacent to inflamed joints may result in overgrowth or undergrowth of the affected part. Micrognathia following temporomandibular arthritis in young children is one of the hallmarks of juvenile rheumatoid arthritis. Small, deformed feet can result from foot involvement in early childhood.

Systemic. Systemic manifestations occur frequently. Irritability, anorexia and malaise are commonly present during active disease. Fever occurs in at least half of children; there may be daily spikes as high as 107°F. (41°C.), or it may be much lower and sustained. A characteristic fleeting rash of small, discrete pink macules with pale centers (Figs. 10-17, 10-18, p. 521) occurs in about

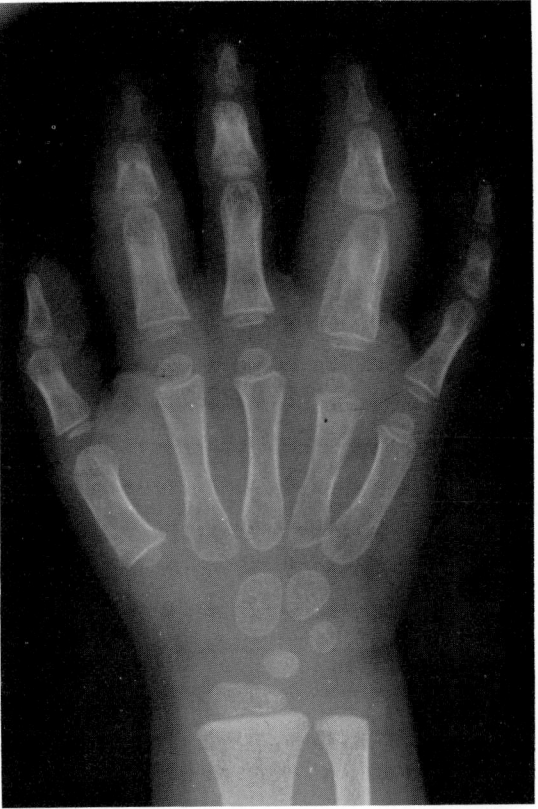

Figure 10-15. Radiograph of the right hand (Figure 10-14) showing soft tissue swelling and periosteal new bone formation adjacent to the second and fourth proximal interphalangeal joints.

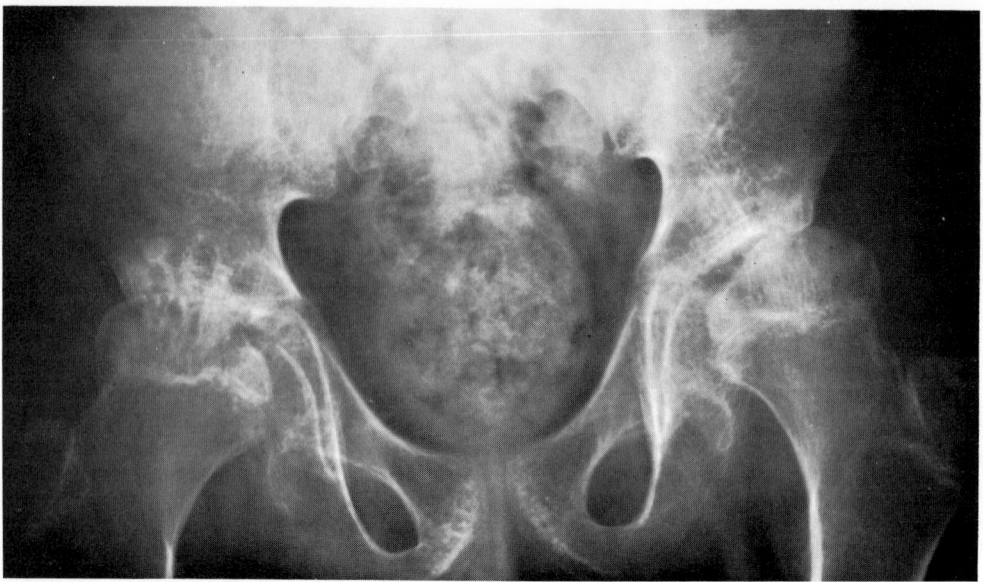

Figure 10-16. Severe hip disease in a 13-year-old boy with long-active juvenile rheumatoid arthritis, showing destruction of femoral heads and acetabula, joint space narrowing, and subluxation of the left hip. The patient had received corticosteroids systemically for 9 years.

one fifth of patients and is often overlooked. It occurs on the trunk and extremities and can be induced by fever, heat or psychic stress. Hepatosplenomegaly and generalized lymphadenopathy occur in about 20 per cent of patients; rarely there are disturbances of liver function. Anemia is common with active arthritis and may be profound; there may be evidence of decreased production or increased destruction of erythrocytes. Iron deficiency from anorexia can be a contributory factor. Pericarditis, with chest pain, cardiac enlargement and electrocardiographic abnormalities, is diagnosed

clinically in about 8 per cent of patients, but probably occurs more frequently. It may be recurrent, but is usually benign without development of cardiac failure or constrictive pericarditis. Myocarditis is rare, and endocarditis does not occur. Pleuritis with pleural thickening and small pleural effusions, visible radiographically, occurs occasionally. Chronic rheumatoid lung disease is extremely rare in children. Abdominal pain during active disease may be due to peritoneal inflammation or mesenteric adenitis. Rarely, tender cystic areas of inflammation resembling sterile abscesses occur in subcutaneous tissues and muscle.

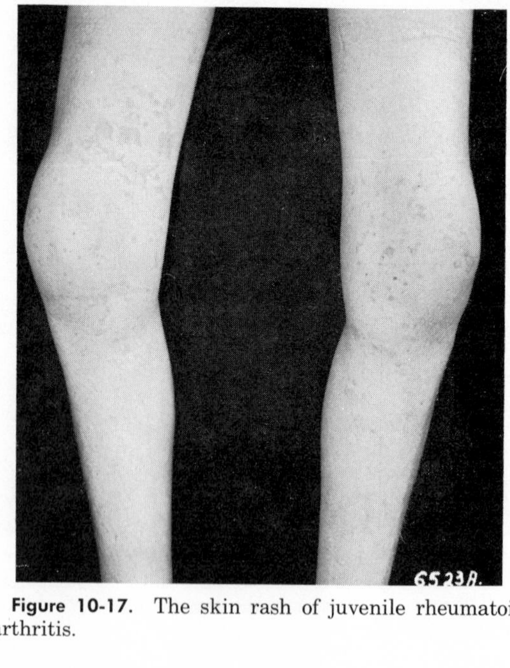

Systemic symptoms of profound toxicity, high spiking fever, hepatosplenomegaly, rash, anemia and polyserositis occur in 10 to 20 per cent of patients usually at the onset of disease. Such children usually develop significant polyarticular disease, sometimes severe. Most have joint manifestations within a few months of onset; a few have purely systemic manifestations for long periods of time before appearance of arthritis. Rarely, this constellation of systemic manifestations occurs without subsequent occurrence of significant arthritis, and definitive diagnosis cannot be made. Systemic manifestations may persist or recur, with or without joint exacerbations, for months or years, usually becoming less prominent as children grow older, even though active arthritis continues. Occasionally, however, severe systemic manifestations occur in older children and even in adults; the more common manifestations are anorexia and malaise, mild anemia and low-grade fever.

Inflammation of the eye, unilateral or bilateral, is the most serious extra-articular manifestation of juvenile rheumatoid arthritis; it occurs in 10 to

Figure 10-17. The skin rash of juvenile rheumatoid arthritis.

15 per cent of patients. Usually the iris and ciliary body are involved (iridocyclitis); rarely, the posterior uveal tract is affected as well (uveitis). The occurrence of eye involvement is not related to the severity of other systemic manifestations; it occurs most often in association with minimal joint disease and may occur when the arthritis is quiescent. Symptoms include redness and pain in the eye, photophobia, decreased visual acuity, and failure of the pupil to react to light. Often, however, there are no early symptoms, and the child presents late with irreversible eye damage, including scarring and adhesions about the iris, band keratopathy and cataracts. Prognosis for adequate vision in chronically affected eyes is poor.

Generalized retardation of growth is common in severely affected children; growth spurts often occur when the disease is controlled or goes into remission. Long-term corticosteroid treatment can contribute to growth retardation.

Course and Prognosis.   The outcome is unpredictable. Even with severe systemic involvement the disease is rarely life-threatening. There may be exacerbations and remissions, or symptoms may continue for years, with either mild arthritis causing little disability or severe arthritis with progression to joint destruction and permanent deformity. The disease does not always remit at puberty; some patients continue to have active arthritis into adulthood, and some have exacerbations after many years of apparently complete remission.

There appear to be no features which permit early prediction of outcome. The overall prognosis is good, however. At least 75 per cent of patients eventually go into remission without significant residual deformity or loss of function. Some patients end up with crippling joint deformities. Severe hip disease is particularly debilitating, as is loss of vision from iridocyclitis.

Laboratory Data.   There are no specific laboratory tests. The sedimentation rate is usually elevated during active disease; acute phase reactants such as C-reactive protein may appear in the serum. Anemia is common, usually with low reticulocyte counts and negative Coombs test results. The white blood cell count is often elevated; leukemoid reactions with peripheral white counts as high as 80,000 per mm.³ sometimes occur. Febrile proteinuria is common, but urinalyses are otherwise normal, except during salicylate therapy when a few erythrocytes and renal tubular cells may be seen. Serum proteins may be altered, with increase in the alpha$_2$ and gamma globulin fractions and decrease in albumin. Antinuclear factors are found in about 25 per cent of children with this disease, most frequently in young girls. There is no correlation with severity. Lupus erythematosus cells usually cannot be demonstrated.

Rheumatoid factor, detected by agglutination of gamma globulin-coated erythrocytes, or of latex or bentonite particles, is demonstrable in about 80 per cent of adults with rheumatoid arthritis, but is less frequently found in children, especially when disease begins in early childhood. Tests do not convert from negative to positive with long-active juvenile disease. The presence of rheumatoid factor correlates with rheumatoid nodules, but not with severity of disease. Rheumatoid factor is sometimes found in other connective tissue disorders in children, such as systemic lupus erythematosus and scleroderma.

Early radiographic joint changes consist of periarticular soft tissue swelling and osteoporosis, capsular swelling (from effusion), and juxta-articular periostitis. Regional epiphyseal closure may be accelerated, and local bone growth increased or decreased. In long-active joint disease subchondral erosions and narrowing of joint spaces may occur (Fig. 10-19). Changes in the cervical spine are characteristic, with narrowing and eventual fusion of apophyseal joints (most frequently seen at C2 to C3) (Fig. 10-20). Erosions of the odontoid process and atlantoaxial subluxation may occur. Vertebral joint spaces may be narrowed and vertebral bodies underdeveloped. Radiographic changes in the sacroiliac joints occur in 25 per cent of patients.

Diagnosis and Differential Diagnosis.   The diagnosis is clinical, and depends on the presence of persistent arthritis for three or more months and the exclusion of other diseases. Presence of typical systemic symptoms may aid in clinical diagnosis. In patients with only systemic symptoms, juvenile rheumatoid arthritis can be strongly suspected when recurrent high spiking fever and rheumatoid rash are present. Such patients usually develop arthritis within six months of onset. Rarely iridocyclitis is a presenting manifestation.

Early in the disease, pyogenic or tuberculous joint infection, sepsis, or arthritis associated with other acute infectious illnesses must be considered. Culture of joint fluid, tuberculin test and radiographs of involved joints are helpful. Acute leukemia can present with arthritis of one or more joints and should be considered when onset is recent, and particularly if there is severe anemia.

Acute rheumatic fever may be confused with rheumatoid arthritis; the migratory nature of the arthritis with lack of persistent changes in the joints and the presence of valvular carditis help in differentiation. Systemic lupus erythematosus may cause arthritis indistinguishable from rheumatoid arthritis, but the joint changes are usually less marked; L.E. cells and other systemic manifestations of lupus, including nephritis, should be sought. Ankylosing spondylitis may not be distinguishable before characteristic involvement of the lumbodorsal spine becomes manifest; the presence of early progressive sacroiliac changes associated with pain in the low back, hips and groin is suggestive. In other diseases, including the vasculitis syndromes, dermatomyositis, ulcerative colitis, regional enteritis, Whipple's disease, sarcoidosis, gonococcal infection, and psoriasis, there may be arthritis similar to that of rheumatoid arthritis.

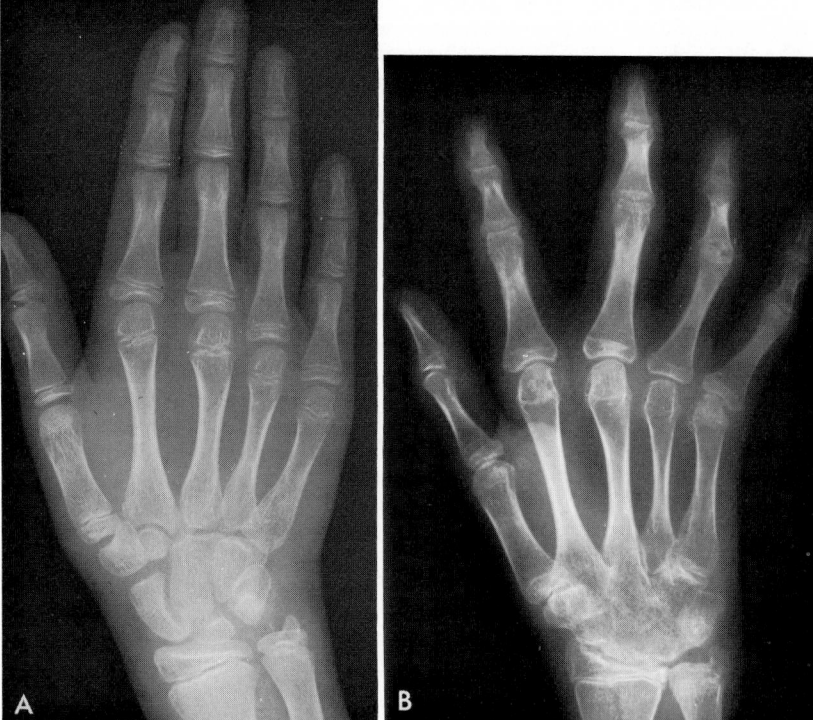

Figure 10-19. Progression of joint destruction in a girl with juvenile rheumatoid arthritis. *A,* Roentgenogram of hand at onset. *B,* Roentgenogram 4 years later, showing destructive changes and joint space narrowing in the distal and proximal interphalangeal, and metacarpophalangeal joints, and destruction and fusion of wrist bones.

Legg-Perthes disease and Osgood-Schlatter disease may initially mimic arthritis. Acute toxic synovitis of the hip, a self-limited condition of uncertain origin, does not progress to chronic arthritis. Reiter's syndrome (arthritis, urethritis and conjunctivitis) is rare in childhood. Pigmented

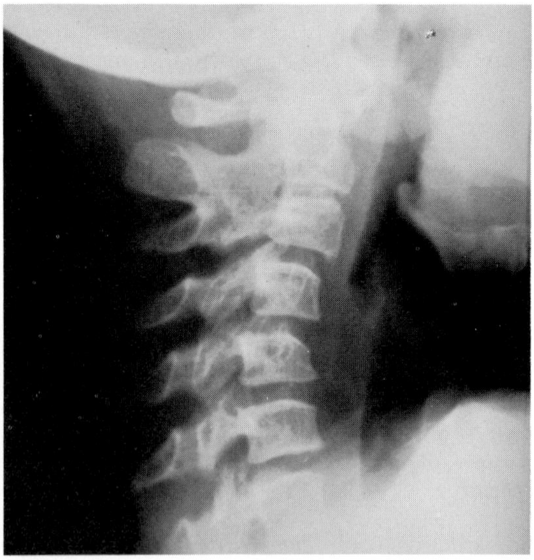

Figure 10-20. Cervical spine in long-active juvenile rheumatoid arthritis, showing fusion of apophyseal joints between C2 and C3, narrowing and erosions of the remaining apophyseal joints, and resulting abnormal curvature.

villonodular synovitis, an uncommon tumorous synovial overgrowth, usually affects only one joint.

Synovial biopsy may be useful, especially to exclude infection in monoarticular disease; however, it may not differentiate between the synovitis of rheumatoid arthritis, various other connective tissue disorders, and so-called postinfectious states.

Treatment. In planning therapy it is important to realize that, though this disease may be painful and of long and uncertain duration, and there is no specific cure, the overall outlook for remission is good, and life is rarely threatened. Management of these children and their families constitutes one of the severest tests of a physician's ability to treat the "whole child." Unpredictable exacerbations are discouraging and make evaluation of therapy difficult. There is a natural tendency to "shop" for medical help and to try fad cures. The eventual failure of any therapy to produce dramatic results may cause the family to give up, allowing unnecessary crippling deformity to occur.

The aims of immediate and long-term treatment are twofold: (1) to preserve good joint function and to provide adequate care of extra-articular manifestations without therapeutic harm; and (2) to support the outlook of the child and his family. Such care ideally requires the devoted attention of one coordinating physician, plus the consultation of numerous specialists, including a physiatrist or physical therapist, an orthopedist, an ophthalmologist, and sometimes an orthodontist, a psychiatrist or a social worker. This team approach is costly and is likely to be found only in group practice.

A number of drugs are effective in suppressing the inflammation in the joints; these include salicylates, corticosteroids and gold salts. Salicylates are the most satisfactory of the available drugs. In doses sufficient to maintain blood levels of 20 to 30 mg. per 100 ml., fever and inflammation, pain and stiffness of joints are usually alleviated. About 100 mg. of aspirin per kg. daily, divided into 4 or 6 doses, is needed to maintain such blood levels. There is considerable individual variation in required dosage; blood levels should be followed and the patient carefully watched for toxicity. A maximal therapeutic response may require weeks to months. When dosage and response are determined and stabilized, the medication can be given for years. The few patients who do not achieve adequate blood levels with regular aspirin may do so with other salicylate preparations, such as choline salicylate. Aspirin should probably be given with food. If gastrointestinal irritation occurs, antacids can be added, or buffered aspirin or choline salicylate substituted. Parents must be alerted to the early signs of salicylism: hyperventilation, drowsiness and gastrointestinal upset. Tinnitus, a common complaint of adults with salicylism, is not often noted in children.

There is no consensus about the therapeutic efficacy of corticosteroids. Although in sufficient dosage they dramatically suppress symptoms, they do not induce permanent remission or prevent joint damage, and with decreases in dosage symptoms reappear. Therapeutic doses cause adrenal suppression, and can suppress growth and produce other potentially dangerous side effects. The dose required for suppression of symptoms is unpredictable and may increase with prolonged therapy. Severe hip disease has occurred in association with long-term steroid therapy (Fig. 10-16), and it has been suspected that it may be a contributing factor. The risks of prolonged administration of corticosteroids do not seem warranted in a disease which is usually self-limited and not life-threatening.

Therapy with corticosteroids is indicated, however, when the disease threatens life, or when such therapy may possibly achieve an otherwise unobtainable goal. An initial dose of 1 to 2 mg. of prednisone per kg. per day will usually produce a therapeutic response. As soon as symptoms are suppressed, the dose should be decreased until a minimum suppressive dose is determined. When the desired result is achieved, the drug should be gradually discontinued. On withdrawal there is often a rebound of symptoms which can often be controlled by other medications, such as salicylates. Sometimes the rebound is so severe, however, that corticosteroids must be reinstituted and continued even for years.

Gold salts have not been widely used in juvenile rheumatoid arthritis, but have been considered an effective form of therapy in adults. Such therapy requires weekly injections and careful follow-up for possible toxicity (weekly physical examination, white blood cell count, and urinalysis). Gold does not appear to be more toxic in children than in adults. Several months are needed for therapeutic response.

Indomethacin may benefit some children with rheumatoid arthritis; it is still an experimental drug. Phenylbutazone is often not effective in rheumatoid arthritis, and has been associated with hematopoietic toxicity and gastric irritation. Chloroquine should not be used because of possible occurrence of irreversible retinal damage. Antimetabolites and alkylating agents such as 6-mercaptopurine and cyclophosphamide, respectively, have recently been used in adults; their use in children for symptomatic relief of a nonlife-threatening disease does not seem warranted until more is known of their long-term untoward effects.

Physical therapy is necessary to maintain and improve motion and muscular strength about affected joints. Parents should be instructed in supervision of these exercises so that they can be carried out at home on a regular daily basis. Night splints for knees and wrists may aid in preventing and correcting deformity. Cylindrical casts or prolonged immobilization of joints should be avoided.

Bed rest has little role in treatment of this disease. Children can usually determine their own activity; in general they should avoid only those activities which cause overtiring and joint pain. Orthopedic surgery is sometimes required to correct joint deformities. The value of synovectomy in children has not been established. Children with micrognathia may require orthodontic management.

Iridocyclitis is an emergency requiring prompt therapy. The eyes should be examined at each medical visit, and a slit-lamp examination should be made by an ophthalmologist twice a year. Parents should be cautioned to report any eye symptoms or decreased visual acuity at once. Therapy of iridocyclitis should be supervised by an ophthalmologist.

Affected children should be encouraged to lead as normal lives as possible. Parents and child need to know what to expect and to be treated optimistically. Children should not be led to believe that they are invalids, but should be taught to be as self-sufficient as possible. With encouragement most can lead active lives, attend school, and participate in usual activities except strenuous sports. Long hospitalizations should be avoided. Children with residual handicaps will need help in vocational planning for the future.

ANKYLOSING SPONDYLITIS

Ankylosing spondylitis is characterized by stiffness and pain in the back, with involvement of sacroiliac joints and variable progression to joints of the lumbodorsal and cervical spine. About half of patients also have arthritis of peripheral joints. Controversy exists over the relationship of ankylosing spondylitis to rheumatoid arthritis. Clinically, ankylosing spondylitis differs from rheumatoid arthritis in several respects: (1) characteristic involvement of sacroiliac joints and lumbodorsal spine, (2) predilection for males, (3) rarity of rheumatoid factor in affected adults, (4) extreme rarity of rheumatoid nodules, (5) high frequency of iritis in adults, (6) occurrence of a distinctive aortitis with resulting aortic insufficiency, and (7) significant familial incidence of the disease. Pathology of synovial tissue from affected synovial joints is similar in both disorders.

Ankylosing spondylitis is usually considered a disease of young and middle-aged adults. It may begin in childhood, however, usually in males over 6 years of age.

Clinical Manifestations. Peripheral arthritis may be the first manifestation; large joints (knees, ankles, shoulders and hips) are usually involved, although small joints of the hands and feet are occasionally affected. Distribution is often asymmetrical. Heel pain is common. Affected joints may be warm, swollen and painful. Peripheral arthritis is usually transient.

Characteristic involvement of sacroiliac joints and lumbodorsal spine may be present at the onset of disease or appear months to years later. Pain in the low back, hip girdles and thighs is characteristic. The pain is often transient, more severe at night, and relieved by moving about. Stiffness in the low back with loss of normal spinal mobility follows (Fig. 10-21). Spinal involvement of ankylosing spondylitis characteristically begins in the sacroiliac joints and proceeds in an ascending fashion, involving the lumbar, the dorsal and finally the cervical spine. By contrast, in juvenile rheumatoid arthritis the neck is involved and the lumbodorsal spine spared. Decreased expansion of the chest, related to involvement of costochondral junctions, may occur early in disease. Systemic manifestations of low-grade fever, anemia, anorexia, fatigability and growth retardation may occur.

Ankylosing spondylitis may arrest at any stage, or the entire spine may be involved over a number of years with loss of virtually all vertebral mobility. Prognosis for functional outcome, however, is usually good if good posture is maintained. Deformity of peripheral joints is uncommon, although some patients have destructive hip disease. Iritis and aortitis have not been described in children with ankylosing spondylitis, but occur in a significant number of adults with the disease.

Laboratory Data. There are no specific laboratory data. As in rheumatoid arthritis, sedimentation rates may be elevated or acute phase reactants appear in the serum. Anemia similar to that of rheumatoid arthritis occurs. Rheumatoid factor is absent in older children and adults. Involvement of the sacroiliac joints is demonstrable radiographically, usually within the first 3 or 4 years; destruction is progressive with eventual joint obliteration. Characteristic radiographic changes in the lumbodorsal vertebrae occur later in the disease.

Differential Diagnosis. Ankylosing spondylitis should be suspected in any child with persistent pain in hips, thighs or low back, with or without peripheral arthritis. Radiographic changes in the sacroiliac joints are necessary for diagnosis, but several years may be required for them to appear. In addition to juvenile rheumatoid arthritis, spinal cord tumors and anatomic defects of the vertebrae must be considered diagnostically in any child with persistent back pain, as must infections of the intervertebral disks and Scheuermann's disease. Legg-Perthes disease and slipped capital femoral epiphysis may cause persistent hip and thigh pain. Ulcerative colitis, regional enteritis, psoriasis and Reiter's syndrome may be associated with spondylitis.

Treatment. Aims of therapy are twofold: relief of pain and maintenance of good posture and function. For relief of pain, salicylates, as in rheumatoid arthritis, may suffice. Indomethacin and phenylbutazone may be helpful, but must be used with caution in children. (Indomethacin is still considered an experimental drug in children.) Gold is not usually effective, and corticosteroid therapy is rarely, if ever, indicated. Radiation therapy is contraindicated because of possible induction of leukemia.

To maintain good function, it is important to maintain good posture and to perform appropriate postural exercises. A firm mattress or bed board should be used for sleeping, and thick pillows avoided.

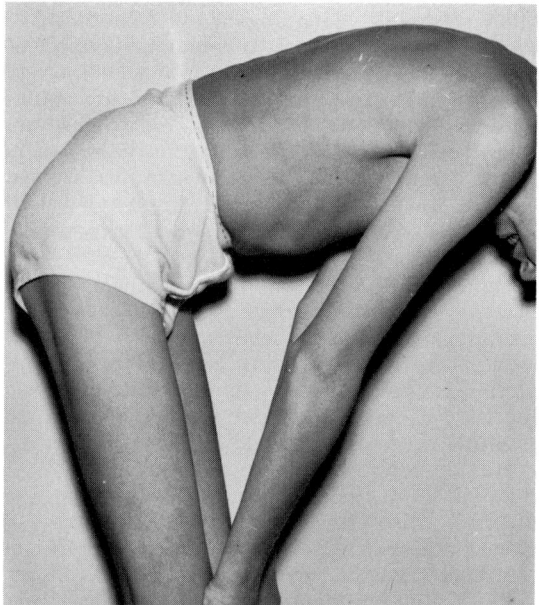

Figure 10-21. Loss of lumbodorsal spine mobility in a boy with ankylosing spondylitis: the lower spine remains straight when the patient bends forward.

SYSTEMIC LUPUS ERYTHEMATOSUS

Systemic lupus erythematosus (S.L.E.) is a connective tissue disorder which characteristically affects many organ systems. It was described clinically during the 1800 s; in 1948 the description of the lupus cell (L.E. cell) phenomenon by Hargraves provided a reasonably specific diagnostic test. The natural history of the disease is unpredictable; it is often progressive, terminating in death if untreated, but it may remit spontaneously or smolder for many years. It seems to be more acute and of greater severity in children than in adults.

Etiology and Epidemiology. The cause is unknown. There are a variety of immune phenomena, but it is not known whether they participate in the pathogenesis of the disease or they are secondary manifestations. Serum levels of gamma globulin are elevated and a number of abnormal antibodies are formed. These antibodies include the L.E. factor, antinuclear antibodies, antibodies against other cellular constituents (DNA, histones, cytoplasmic constituents) and against red blood cells, leukocytes, and platelets. There may be falsely positive tests for syphilis and circulating anticoagulants. Cutaneous hypersensitivity reactions to intradermal leukocyte injections have also been described.

The disease has been reported to follow exposure to a number of drugs, notably hydralazine, sulfonamides, penicillin, procainamide, and the anticonvulsants, hydantoins and trimethadione. Drug-induced disease may be indistinguishable clinically and pathologically from "spontaneous" S.L.E., but is often reversible when the offending agent is withdrawn. Cutaneous manifestations of S.L.E., and rarely systemic manifestations, may be exacerbated by sunlight. The onset of disease may appear related to infection, and exacerbations may occur after intercurrent infections. It is, moreover, suspected that there is an increased susceptibility to infections, perhaps on the basis of altered immune mechanisms. S.L.E. occurs frequently in some families and has occurred in identical twins; of interest in this respect is the observation of elevated values of serum gamma globulins, positive antinuclear factors, and other abnormal antibodies in apparently healthy relatives of patients with lupus. These phenomena suggest the possibility that S.L.E. may be a disease of altered immune reactivity in genetically predisposed persons.

The disease is not rare. The incidence is not known; it appears to have increased in recent years, but this may be related to more frequent recognition. S.L.E. begins in childhood in about 20 per cent of cases, usually in children over 8 years of age, but it has been reported in infants. Females are predominantly affected in all age groups (8 to 1). All races may be affected.

Pathology. Changes occur in connective tissue at multiple sites and may involve many of the organ systems. The presence of masses of amorphous, purple-staining extracellular material in hematoxylin-stained affected tissues is characteristic. These "hematoxylin bodies" probably represent degenerated cell nuclei and are considered similar to the inclusions of L.E. cells. Fibrinoid, an acellular, deeply eosinophilic material, is also found in loose connective tissue or in walls of blood vessels of affected tissues. This substance, of uncertain composition, is not specific for S.L.E. Fibrinoid deposition is usually accompanied by an inflammatory cellular reaction, predominantly with mononuclear cells. In the spleen perivascular fibrosis about affected vessels results in characteristic "onion-ring" lesions. Granulomas are sometimes found in affected tissues.

In the kidneys, lesions vary from mild glomerulitis, with small areas of glomerular hypercellularity and basement membrane thickening, to severe glomerulonephritis. Involvement may be confined to a part of the glomerulus, vary in severity between glomeruli, and spare some entirely. Changes in advanced lupus glomerulonephritis are characteristic and consist of local necrosis, fibrinoid deposition, cellular proliferation, and infiltration with inflammatory cells in the affected glomeruli. Hematoxylin-stained bodies may be found. The "wire-loop" lesions considered characteristic of lupus nephritis result from fibrinoid changes of glomerular capillary walls. Basement membrane thickening is often present. Adhesions and crescent formation may occur. Interstitial tissues may be infiltrated with inflammatory cells, and there may be tubular changes.

Clinical Manifestations. The disease may present insidiously with diverse symptoms, and time of onset may be difficult to determine. Symptoms may date back months or years before the diagnosis is suspected. In other instances the onset is fulminating with sudden appearance of involvement of many systems. The most frequent early symptoms in children are fever, malaise, arthritis or arthralgia, and rash. Fever occurs at some time in most affected children; it may be spiking or sustained in pattern. Malaise, anorexia, weight loss and debility are common.

Cutaneous manifestations are variable, but occur in most affected children at some time. The butterfly rash (Fig. 10-22, p. 521), which may consist only of an erythematous blush, or of scaly erythematous papules, involves the malar areas and usually spreads over the bridge of the nose. The rash may be photosensitive. Although involvement of the lower eyelids is common, upper lids are usually spared. The rash can spread to involve the entire face, scalp, neck, chest and upper arms in a patchy manner. Lesions may become bullous and secondarily infected. Discoid lupus with patches of erythematous scaling lesions on the face and other areas is rare in children in the absence of systemic disease. There are also other skin eruptions. Erythematous macules and punctate lesions on the palms, on the soles and on the fingertips are particularly distinctive; such lesions are secondary to vascular changes. Infarction with actual loss of tissue from involved areas may occur, as may Raynaud's phenomenon. Splinter hemorrhages and capillary tortuosity are seen at times in the nailbeds. Punctate lesions also occur on the palate and oral mucous membranes (Fig. 10-23, p. 521). Purpura, sometimes associated with thrombocytopenia, may appear on dependent or traumatized areas. Erythema nodosum or erythema multiforme is occasionally associated. Alopecia from inflammation about hair follicles may be patchy or generalized, and the hair coarse, dry and brittle.

Joint involvement is common. If it is an initial manifestation, the illness may be confused with rheumatic fever or rheumatoid arthritis. Any joints may be involved. Arthralgia and stiffness often occur without objective joint changes. Sometimes affected joints are warm and swollen, but persistent deforming arthritis is rare. Aseptic necrosis of femoral heads, presumably secondary to vasculitis, has been described. Tenosynovitis, myositis with myalgia, muscle tenderness and muscular weakness may occur.

Polyserositis with pleurisy, pericarditis and peritonitis is characteristic of the disease. Hepatomegaly, splenomegaly and generalized lymphadenopathy are common, as is some form of cardiac involvement evidenced by variable murmurs, friction rubs, cardiomegaly, electrocardiographic changes or congestive heart failure. Myocarditis, pericarditis or verrucous endocarditis (Libman-Sacks endocarditis) may be found at postmortem examination. Pulmonary symptoms may occur in association with parenchymal lung infiltrates; other infection must be excluded, however, before such changes can be ascribed to systemic lupus. Involvement of the nervous system may include personality changes, seizures, cerebral vascular accidents with resulting pareses, and peripheral neuritis. Gastrointestinal manifestations include abdominal pain, vomiting, diarrhea, melena, and even infarction of bowel secondary to vasculitis. Ocular changes may include episcleritis, iritis, or retinal vascular changes with hemorrhages or exudates (cytoid bodies).

Most children have clinical renal involvement, manifest by red cells, white cells, protein and casts in the urine, and occasionally by a nephrotic pattern. There is often progressive loss of renal function associated with azotemia and hypertension.

Laboratory Data. Demonstration of the L.E. cell is the most useful laboratory test. When the patient's serum is incubated in vitro with leukocytes (in practice by simply incubating the patient's whole blood), nucleoprotein of white cell nuclei becomes bound to the L.E. factor (a gamma globulin) from the patient's serum, forming homogeneous masses which are then phagocytized by polymorphonuclear leukocytes. The ingested particles form large cytoplasmic inclusion bodies, forcing the cell nucleus to the periphery (Fig. 10-24, p. 521). The L.E. cell phenomenon can be found in almost all patients with the disease. It is relatively specific, rarely being found in other illnesses in children.

Antibodies to other tissue components have been described in S.L.E. The antinuclear factors are a group of antibodies to components of cell nuclei; these are usually demonstrated by immunofluorescent staining procedures. Antinuclear factors are demonstrable in almost all patients with S.L.E., but are less specific than the L.E. phenomenon, since they appear also in a significant number of patients with other connective tissue disorders. Antibodies directed against other cellular constituents occur in S.L.E., but are less frequently identified diagnostically. Other abnormal antibodies which may be helpful if demonstrable are the biologic false-positive test for syphilis and the positive Coombs test. Serum gamma globulin levels are usually elevated in S.L.E.; alpha$_2$ globulin levels may be increased and albumin decreased.

Anemia, related to chronic inflammatory disease or hemolysis, is common. A positive Coombs test result may be present, and difficulties in typing and cross matching of blood arise, owing to presence of antibodies to isologous erythrocytes. Thrombocytopenia and leukopenia occur frequently; antibodies against these blood elements may be demonstrable. Idiopathic thrombocytopenic purpura may be the first manifestation of S.L.E. The serum complement titer is depressed with active disease. The urine may contain erythrocytes, white cells, protein and casts. Renal insufficiency is manifest by elevation of the blood urea nitrogen and abnormal renal function studies.

Prognosis. Sparing of the kidneys or mild, nonprogressive renal disease was in the past considered unusual in children, and S.L.E. has generally been considered a potentially or even a uniformly fatal disease. With increasing frequency of recognition, however, children with mild disease, and without progressive nephritis, are being found. It is now also recognized that some adults with S.L.E. have survived years of disease which started in childhood. Although spontaneous exacerbations and remissions of S.L.E. occur, prolonged spontaneous remission appears unusual in children. The advent of antibiotic and corticosteroid therapy has prolonged survival and perhaps improved the overall prognosis; however, the case fatality rate in published series of S.L.E. in children is still over 50 per cent.

Diagnosis and Differential Diagnosis. Diagnosis is based on the clinical pattern and is confirmed by the presence of L.E. cells. L.E. cells may not be demonstrable, but usually are at some time if persistently sought. The occurrence of antinuclear factors, elevated serum gamma globulin, positive Coombs test result, biologic false-positive test for syphilis, anemia, leukopenia, thrombocytopenia, and signs of nephritis may also be diagnostically helpful. Renal biopsy may confirm the diagnosis, but early histologic changes may not be specific for S.L.E., which may imitate many other diseases; any connective tissue disorder may be simulated. Thrombocytopenic purpura and hemolytic anemia may be presenting features, and the differential diagnosis of these manifesta-

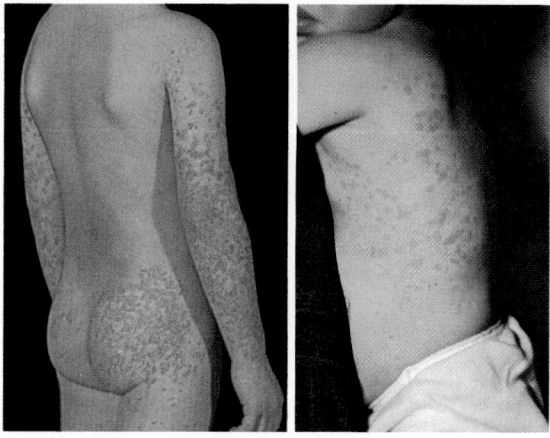

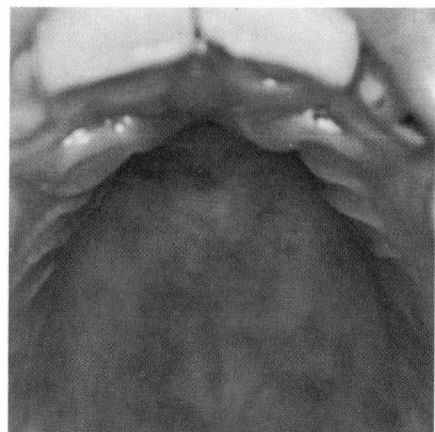

Figure 10-18. Rash of rheumatoid arthritis.
Figure 10-25. Henoch-Schönlein purpura (anaphylactoid purpura). (From G. W. Korting: *Hautkrankheiten bei Kindern und Jugendlichen.* Stuttgart, Germany, F. K. Schattauer Verlag, 1969.)

Figure 10-23. Palatal lesions of systemic lupus erythematosus.

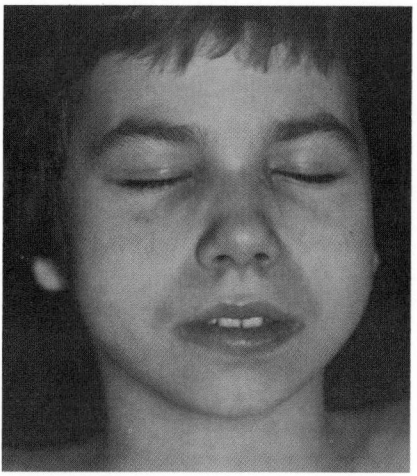

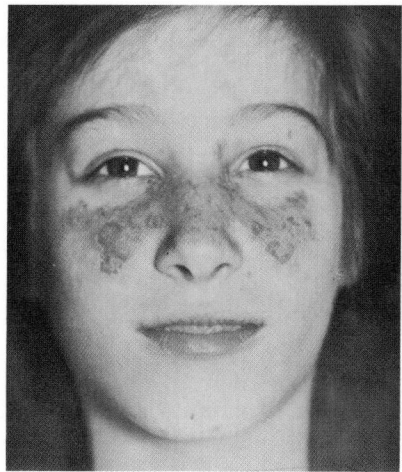

Figure 10-26. The facial rash of dermatomyositis. Note the faint erythema over the bridge of the nose and malar areas, and the heliotrope discoloration of the upper eyelids.

Figure 10-22. The butterfly rash of systemic lupus erythematosus.

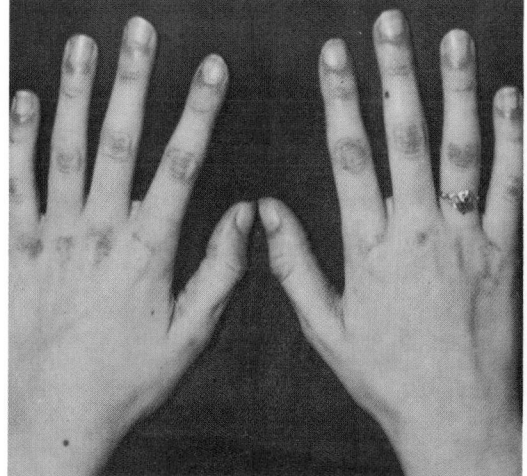

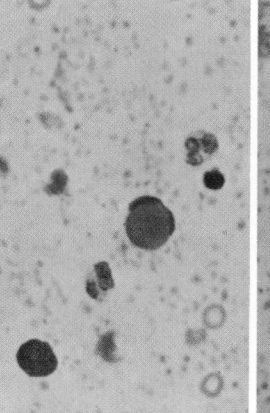

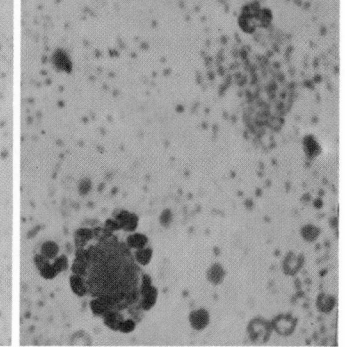

Figure 10-27. The skin changes over the knuckles in dermatomyositis.

Figure 10-24. An L.E. cell and "rosette" from incubated peripheral blood of a child with systemic lupus erythematosus.

521

tions should include S.L.E. Occasionally diagnostic manifestations of S.L.E. may not appear for years.

Treatment. Because of the possibility of drug-induced disease, inquiry should be made about possible offending agents; if identified, their administration should be discontinued. Corticosteroids are indicated to suppress symptoms, and hopefully to prevent progression when there is systemic disease with nephritis. Some observers think that the disease should be treated symptomatically and that the doses of steroids should be merely sufficient to suppress clinical symptoms. Others advocate large doses of steroids for prolonged periods of time in the hope of avoiding progressive nephritis. Such therapy is invariably associated with undesirable side effects. Whichever approach to corticosteroid therapy is chosen, it is well to begin with a high dose (1 to 2 mg. of prednisone per kg. per day, or 60 mg. of prednisone per square meter of body surface area per day) and then gradually reduce the dose to desired levels after acute manifestations have been controlled. There must be constant surveillance for dangerous side effects of corticosteroid therapy, particularly for adrenal insufficiency during intercurrent illness or stress, vertebral compression fractures secondary to osteoporosis, hypertension, masked infections, and peptic ulcer. Cushingoid appearance and growth suppression may be expected, but are reversible on withdrawal of the corticosteroids.

The renal status should be followed carefully by examinations of urinary sediment or 12-hour Addis counts, quantitative protein excretion, renal function studies, and perhaps renal biopsies. Low serum complement levels have been associated with active renal disease. If deterioration of renal status is evident, more vigorous therapy is indicated. Recent studies have shown possible effectiveness of such agents as cyclophosphamide, 6-mercaptopurine and azathioprine, but this therapy is still experimental.

Other agents have been used for symptomatic treatment in S.L.E. and may be useful in the absence of progressive renal disease. Salicylates may be effective in alleviating arthritis and other discomforts. Chloroquine has long been used in discoid and systemic lupus erythematosus, but should be used with extreme care because of retinal toxicity. Topical steroid preparations may be helpful in suppressing the facial rash.

VASCULITIS SYNDROMES

In these syndromes of primary nonspecific inflammation of blood vessels, the various patterns of disease depend on the size and location of affected vessels. When small nonmuscular vessels are involved, the disease takes the form of Henoch-Schönlein vasculitis, or anaphylactoid purpura. With involvement of larger muscular arteries the disease is called polyarteritis nodosa, many variants of which have been described, including infantile polyarteritis and Wegener's granulomatosis. Considerable overlap of these syndromes occurs, and it is reasonable to expect that in some instances vessels of various sizes may be involved in the same patient. In Takayasu's arteritis the aorta and other great vessels are the sites of inflammation.

Inflammation of vessels also occurs in other connective tissue disorders in children, notably lupus erythematosus, dermatomyositis and scleroderma; in hypertension; and in vessels exposed to local infection, trauma or thromboemboli.

The cause of these disorders is not known. Both Henoch-Schönlein vasculitis and polyarteritis nodosa have been reported to follow exposure to drugs or allergens. Serum sickness, a usually self-limited type of vasculitis occurring after exposure to foreign substances, is similar clinically and pathologically to Henoch-Schönlein vasculitis and to polyarteritis nodosa. Vasculitis has been produced in experimental animals by injection of antibodies against components of their own blood vessels, and by sensitization to foreign proteins. It is thus suspected that the vasculitis syndromes represent hypersensitivity reactions with blood vessels as target organs. In contrast to most other connective tissue disorders, Henoch-Schönlein vasculitis and polyarteritis nodosa affect predominantly males. In childhood, Henoch-Schönlein vasculitis is the most commonly encountered type of vasculitis.

HENOCH-SCHÖNLEIN VASCULITIS
(Anaphylactoid, Allergic or Rheumatic Purpura)

This distinctive clinical syndrome was described by William Heberden before 1800; Schönlein in the 1830's described the typical rash in association with joint manifestations, and Henoch in the 1870's recognized the association of gastrointestinal and renal manifestations. Osler pointed out the similarity between this disease and the hypersensitivity reactions, erythema multiforme and serum sickness. The skin lesion, which is not always purpuric, is the most obvious sign; the visceral lesions are less easily recognized, but are far more serious. The primary manifestations are due to vasculitis of small blood vessels; there are no hematologic changes which lead to spontaneous bleeding.

The cause is unknown. Allergy or drug sensitivity seems to play a role in some cases. The disease often follows an upper respiratory tract infection, sometimes with beta hemolytic streptococci, but this is of uncertain significance. The syndrome is not rare and may occur at any age; it is more common in children than in adults, most cases occurring in the age range from 2 to 8 years. Males are affected twice as often as females.

Pathology. In the skin small vessels of the corium are surrounded with an acute inflammatory exudate of polymorphonuclear and round cells; eosinophils and varying numbers of red blood cells may be present. Capillaries are most frequently involved, but small arterioles and venules may be affected. Scattered nuclear debris, edema, and swelling of collagen fibrils are found adjacent to affected vessels.

The renal lesion is characteristic. It usually begins as a focal glomerulitis with patchy areas of hypercellularity and accumulation of PAS-positive material in affected glomeruli. There is often variability in severity of lesions in adjacent glomeruli, and some may be spared. Lesions may heal with focal scarring, or progress to resemble those of subacute or chronic glomerulonephritis.

There is a paucity of data on histologic changes in other organs, but inflammation or hemorrhage may occur at other sites, notably in synovium, the gastrointestinal tract and the central nervous system.

Clinical Manifestations. Onset may be acute with simultaneous appearance of several manifestations, or gradual with sequential appearance of different manifestations over a period of weeks. Various combinations of symptoms and signs may occur. Malaise and low-grade fever are present in over half of cases.

Skin lesions are present in all identified patients; it is not known whether visceral manifestations occur in the absence of rash. The lesions usually appear on the buttocks and lower extremities, but may involve upper extremities, trunk and face as well. Dermatologic manifestations are extremely variable. The classic lesion begins as a small urticarial wheal with a central red punctum, or an erythematous maculopapular lesion. Lesions initially blanch on pressure, but lose this ability with progression. They may eventually become petechial or purpuric. Purpuric areas progress in the usual manner of ecchymoses, changing from red to purple, becoming rusty, and eventually fading. Skin lesions appear in crops, and at any time there may be a variety of lesions (Fig. 10-25, p. 521). Lesions are rarely pruritic. In addition to these characteristic lesions, the various patterns of erythema multiforme and erythema nodosum have been described. Angioneurotic edema involving the scalp, eyelids, lips, dorsa of the hands and feet, and perineum is common and may be striking; this occurs most frequently in young children.

Arthritis occurs in two thirds of affected children and may be a prominent complaint. Knees and ankles are most commonly involved; hips, wrists and elbows may also be affected. Small joints of the hands and feet are usually spared. The arthritis is mild. The joints may be swollen, tender, and painful on motion. Effusions may be present. Joint fluid is serous with leukocytosis, not hemorrhagic. Joint symptoms usually resolve after a few days without deformity or articular damage, but may recur during the period of active disease.

Gastrointestinal symptoms appear in two thirds of affected children. The most common complaint is colicky abdominal pain which may be severe and is often associated with vomiting. Stools show gross or occult blood in over half of patients, and hematemesis may occur. Failure to recognize this syndrome in children with sudden onset of acute abdominal pain may lead to unnecessary laparotomy. In such cases peritoneal exudate and enlarged mesenteric lymph nodes are usually found; segmental edema and hemorrhage into bowel wall may be present. Gastrointestinal radiographs may show decreased motility and segmental narrowing, presumably related to submucosal edema and hemorrhage. Rarely intussusception, obstruction, or infarction and perforation of bowel may occur.

Renal involvement is potentially the most serious manifestation, since it can result in chronic renal disease. It occurs in 25 to 50 per cent of children during the acute phase, the frequency depending in part on the adequacy of examination. It is usually manifest during the first few weeks of illness, but sometimes appears after other manifestations have become quiescent. Moderate azotemia and hypertension, and even oliguria and hypertensive encephalopathy, can occur. Presumably most children with acute renal involvement recover, although some continue to have abnormal urinary sediment, with or without abnormal renal function. A few children, usually over 6 years of age, suffer chronic renal disease within a few years of the acute phase.

A rare but potentially serious manifestation is central nervous system involvement, with seizures, pareses and coma. Hepatosplenomegaly and lymphadenopathy occur during acute phases of the disease. Rarely intramuscular hemorrhage, rheumatoid-like nodules, cardiac involvement, eye involvement and testicular swelling and hemorrhage have been reported.

Prognosis is excellent in the absence of significant renal disease. The course is variable. Often the disease is mild, lasting a few days and manifest only by transient arthritis and a few purpuric spots. In more seriously affected children the average duration is 4 to 6 weeks, and subsequently exacerbations and remissions may occur. Sometimes the illness may smolder for one or more years.

Laboratory Data. Laboratory tests are not diagnostic. Unless blood loss has been great, there is no anemia. The sedimentation rate may be elevated, and acute phase reactants appear in the serum. The white blood cell count is often increased, and eosinophilia may be present. Platelet counts, bleeding time, clotting time and clot retraction are normal. The tourniquet test is usually negative, although the trauma of the tourniquet may induce local purpuric lesions. With renal involvement red cells, white cells, casts and albumin are present in the urine. There may be gross or occult blood in the stools. Lupus erythematosus cells, rheumatoid factor and antinuclear factors are not usually found. Serum complement titers may be elevated, distinguishing this disease from acute glomerulonephritis, in which complement titers are low.

Diagnosis and Differential Diagnosis. The full-blown picture of Henoch-Schönlein vasculitis with rash, arthritis and gastrointestinal and renal manifestations is characteristic. Diagnostic confusion, however, may result when there is predominance of one symptom or failure to recognize the multiple system involvement. The rash may suggest a hemorrhagic diathesis or septicemia; platelet counts, blood clotting tests, and cultures will exclude these possibilities. In addition, the patient with septicemia usually appears more acutely ill. When gastrointestinal manifestations predominate, the syndrome may suggest a number of intra-abdominal emergencies. The possibility of Henoch-Schönlein vasculitis should be considered in any child with acute abdominal pain, and inquiry made for associated rash, nephritis and arthritis. With prominent renal findings, acute glomerulonephritis may be suggested; the presence of other manifestations of Henoch-Schönlein vasculitis should allow differentiation. In children with chronic renal disease a history of acute Henoch-Schönlein vasculitis in the past should be sought. Differentiation from other connective tissue diseases is rarely difficult. Acute rheumatic fever, juvenile rheumatoid arthritis, systemic lupus erythematosus, dermatomyositis, ulcerative colitis and regional enteritis may all be suggested clinically. In polyarteritis nodosa peripheral neurologic changes and cardiac manifestations are more common, but clinical distinction from Henoch-Schönlein vasculitis may be impossible to make.

Prognosis. During the acute phase, death may occur from gastrointestinal complications (massive hemorrhage, intussusception, bowel infarction), acute renal failure, hypertension or central nervous system involvement. The mortality rate in the acute phase, however, is probably less than 2 per cent. If death occurs later, it is usually from chronic renal disease, which may not become apparent for years after the initial phase of illness and may be indistinguishable from chronic glomerulonephritis. It is estimated that about 25 per cent of children with initial renal involvement have persistence of abnormal urinary findings for years; the eventual outcome for these patients is not known.

Treatment. There is no specific therapy. In the rare instance in which a specific allergen can be proved, the patient should be kept from contact with it. When the disease seems to follow a bacterial infection, particularly streptococcal, the patient should be vigorously treated to eliminate the organism; if the disease recurs, prophylaxis should be considered. Symptomatic treatment only is indicated for arthritis, rash, edema, fever and malaise. Salicylates will often alleviate these discomforts, which are all self-limited.

In the acute phase the patient's life may be endangered by intestinal hemorrhage, obstruction or perforation. These complications may perhaps be prevented by the early use of corticosteroids. Therapy with prednisone in dosage of 1 to 2 mg. per kg. per day is often associated with dramatic improvement, and at times seems lifesaving. Corticosteroid therapy is also indicated in the rare instances of central nervous system manifestations. Steroids do not, however, seem to affect renal involvement in the acute phase, nor prevent chronic disease, and may potentiate hypertension. Children with acute renal failure should be treated like those with acute glomerulonephritis. Intensive therapy with corticosteroids and antimetabolites (6-mercaptopurine, azathioprine) for persistent nephritis is still experimental. Should relapses occur, search for an offending allergen or related infection should be reinstituted.

POLYARTERITIS NODOSA

Medium-sized and small arteries are the sites of inflammation in polyarteritis nodosa. The disease can affect all age groups, but is rare in childhood. Males are affected more frequently than females. As with Henoch-Schönlein vasculitis, the cause is not known, but the disease has been reported to follow drug exposures. Pathologically, lesions are characteristically located in medium-sized vessels, often at bifurcations. Occasionally, smaller arterioles may be involved as well. Inflammation with polymorphonuclear leukocytes, eosinophils and round cells may involve the entire vessel wall. Necrosis, thrombosis or aneurysm formation may occur in affected vessels and result in infarction. Healed vessels become scarred or recanalized.

Clinical manifestations are diverse and depend on sites of vascular involvement. Signs of systemic illness, such as fever, anorexia, lethargy, weakness and loss of weight, are usually present. Arthralgia and arthritis are frequent, and myalgia and myositis may be present. Various cutaneous manifestations, including erythematous rashes, nodular lesions, petechiae and purpuric spots, cutaneous ulcers, and edema, are common. Rarely gangrene of extremities occurs. Peripheral neuropathy with pain, numbness, paresthesias and muscle weakness results from involvement of peripheral nerves adjacent to affected vessels. Abdominal pain, bleeding, ulcerations and infarction can follow involvement of gastrointestinal vessels. Renal involvement is a potentially serious manifestation; involvement of large renal vessels results in flank pain and gross hematuria, that of small vessels and glomeruli causes microscopic hematuria, proteinuria and cylindruria. Involvement of both types of vessels may result in renal failure and death. Hypertension is usually associated with renal involvement. Involvement of pulmonary vessels may cause cough, wheezing, pulmonary infiltrates and pleuritis. Central nervous system manifestations include seizures, encephalitic symptoms and stroke. Cranial nerve palsies may occur. Hepatosplenomegaly is common. Involvement of coronary vessels may produce tachycardia, congestive heart failure and myocardial infarction. Pericarditis may also be present. Orchitis and epididymitis are common. Iritis may occur.

There are no specific laboratory tests. The sedimentation rate may be elevated, and acute phase reactants present. Anemia is common. Eosinophilia is sometimes found. There may be gross or microscopic hematuria, and renal function studies may be deranged.

Polyarteritis nodosa is readily confused with many other diseases. Differentiation from other connective tissue disorders may be particularly difficult. The diagnosis is based primarily on clinical suspicion and on histologic changes in involved tissues on biopsy. Muscle biopsies may fail to identify vasculitis, even though the disease exists. Testicular biopsies are said to be helpful, but are seldom done. The diagnosis in children is probably most frequently made at autopsy.

The prognosis is poor; death occurs from renal failure, heart failure or severe gastrointestinal or central nervous system disease. Corticosteroids may suppress acute manifestations of the disease and effectively lengthen survival. Certainly a trial of steroid therapy in doses sufficient to suppress symptoms is indicated with severe disease. Long-term therapy may be required.

Infantile Polyarteritis

Polyarteritis occurs in infants less than 1 year of age; though rare, it presents a rather characteristic clinical pattern. Both sexes are affected. The cause is not known, but as in other forms of vasculitis, this disease has been reported in association with drug exposure (sulfonamides, penicillin). There is also a suggestive relation to viral and bacterial illnesses. Pathologic changes are similar to those of polyarteritis in older patients; fibrinoid necrosis of vessels is said to be less prominent.

The disease usually begins with a combination of fever, rhinitis, conjunctivitis and macular erythematous rash, suggesting an acute viral infection, but the illness persists. Involvement of the coronary arteries has been the predominant manifestation in most reported cases, resulting in tachycardia, cardiomegaly, congestive heart failure or pericarditis. The electrocardiogram may show right, left or combined ventricular hypertrophy, as well as evidence of myocardial ischemia or infarction. At autopsy, aneurysms of coronary arteries are frequently found, as well as myocardial infarcts and pericarditis. Aneurysms may perforate, causing hemopericardium.

Other reported manifestations include renal involvement (abnormal urinary sediment), hypertension, decreased blood pressure in or ischemia of an extremity, central nervous system manifestations (nuchal rigidity, pareses, cranial nerve palsies, seizures), hepatosplenomegaly, lymphadenopathy, gastrointestinal symptoms, and cough. Involvement of vessels in skeletal muscle is ap-

parently uncommon, and muscle biopsy is of little diagnostic usefulness. At autopsy widespread arteritis involving many organs has been found.

There are no specific laboratory tests. The white blood cell count is often elevated with eosinophilia. Sedimentation rates may be high. Diagnosis is usually made at autopsy, although awareness of this syndrome should permit presumptive clinical diagnosis.

The prognosis is very poor, all reported cases having terminated in death within an average of 1 month after onset. Death is usually sudden or related to progressive cardiac decompensation.

No satisfactory treatment has been found, but corticosteroid therapy appears worthy of trial.

Wegener's Granulomatosis
(Lethal Midline Granuloma)

Wegener's granulomatosis is a rare syndrome, considered a variant of polyarteritis nodosa by most observers, in which destructive granulomatous lesions of the upper respiratory tract and lungs are associated with a systemic necrotizing vasculitis, most prominent in lungs and kidneys. The upper respiratory and pulmonary granulomas may predominate in some cases, antedating recognition of systemic vasculitis by years. Indeed, it is postulated that limited forms of this syndrome, with only upper respiratory or pulmonary involvement, may occur. Males are predominantly affected (2 to 1). The syndrome is rare in children, occurring usually in late childhood. The cause is not known; as in other vasculitis syndromes, an association with drug sensitivity and allergy has been noted.

Symptoms referable to the respiratory tract are prominent. Persistent nasal discharge may be an early symptom, with crusted or pustular lesions in the nares. Lesions are progressively destructive and may result in perforation of the nasal septum, obliteration of nasal sinuses, and ulcerations of the palate, pharynx, larynx and trachea. Pulmonary symptoms of cough or hemoptysis may occur, and fever and prostration are common. Associated with respiratory symptoms in most instances are such manifestations of systemic vasculitis as arthritis, neuropathy, rash, splenomegaly, and severe progressive glomerulitis often terminating in renal failure. In cases with clinically inapparent systemic involvement, diffuse vasculitis may be found on postmortem examination.

There are no specific laboratory findings. Eosinophilia may be present. Roentgenograms may reveal bone destruction in the nose and sinuses and pulmonary infiltrates suggestive of tuberculosis or neoplasm. Urinalyses usually show evidence of nephritis, and renal function studies may be abnormal.

Diagnosis depends on demonstration of granulomatous lesions of the respiratory tract and systemic vasculitis, particularly nephritis. Biopsy of granulomatous lesions and kidney may be diagnostically helpful. The prognosis is poor, the disease having been described as uniformly fatal. Nevertheless some patients with more limited forms of disease survive for long periods of time. Involvement of the upper respiratory tract may be extremely disfiguring.

No curative therapy is known, but corticosteroids may suppress systemic vasculitis and prevent progression of destructive lesions in the upper respiratory tract. Recent experimental therapy with antimetabolites has been considered helpful in a few patients unresponsive to corticosteroids.

TAKAYASU'S ARTERITIS
("Pulseless Disease")

In this syndrome an inflammatory process involves the aorta and its major branches. The disease is rare and occurs predominantly in young adult females, with a significant number of cases occurring in late childhood. The disease has been described in infants. The majority of reported cases have been from Asia and Africa, but the disease has also been described in the United States and Europe. The cause is not known. Congenital defects of the great vessels have been associated in some cases. The disease is usually considered to represent a nonspecific inflammatory connective tissue disorder.

The basic pathologic alteration is an inflammatory panarteritis of the aorta and its major branches. Vasculitis of smaller vessels is not associated. Aneurysmal dilatation and rupture of affected vessels may occur; the aorta may be affected in any segment. Involvement of roots of the great vessels may cause weak or absent pulses and decreased blood pressure in the upper extremities, the so-called pulseless disease. Blood pressure in the legs may be higher than that in the arms, the reverse of the findings in coarctation. Occlusion of renal arterial orifices may cause renal ischemia with resulting hypertension. Decreased blood flow to the brain can result in central nervous system manifestations. Complaints of transient or permanent visual disturbances are common in older patients; cataracts, arteriovenous communications in retinal vessels, hyperemia of conjunctiva and sclerae, and retinal detachments may be present. Various rheumatic complaints, including arthralgia, myalgia, pleuritis, pericarditis, fever and rashes, have been described in some patients, these sometimes antedate the appearance of symptomatic aortitis by years.

In affected children the predominant finding has been hypertension, with hypertensive encephalopathy and congestive heart failure; hypertension is related to renal ischemia from occlusion of renal arteries. Fever is common. The pulseless manifestation and ocular disturbances seem to be uncommon during childhood. Rheumatic complaints have been reported, as has an association with chronic arthritis, similar to juvenile rheumatoid arthritis.

There are no specific laboratory data. The sedimentation rate is usually elevated, and serum gamma globulin values may be high. Positive lupus cell preparations have been reported. This disease should be considered in any child with hypertension of obscure cause, particularly if fever and increased sedimentation rate are associated. Angiography may demonstrate diagnostic changes in affected vessels.

The prognosis is variable. Some adult patients survive with few symptoms, but most reported children have succumbed with hypertension. In adult patients ruptured aneurysms have caused death.

No specific therapy is known. Corticosteroids have been considered helpful in some patients. Surgical intervention with endarterectomy or nephrectomy may be warranted.

DERMATOMYOSITIS

Dermatomyositis is a multisystem disease characterized principally by nonsuppurative inflammation of striated muscle. Affected children usually have associated characteristic cutaneous lesions. Adults may have polymyositis without skin manifestations.

Etiology and Epidemiology. The cause of dermatomyositis is unknown. The disease sometimes appears to begin after an acute infection, drug ingestion or exposure to sunlight. In adults, but rarely in children, there is a frequent association with malignancies (20 per cent of cases); the dermatomyositis often remits when the tumor is removed.

Dermatomyositis is less common than rheumatoid arthritis, systemic lupus erythematosus or Henoch-Schönlein vasculitis. It rarely begins before the second year of life; girls are affected more frequently than boys (3 to 2). There seems to be no familial clustering of the disease, but it has been reported in identical twins. There is no racial predilection.

Pathology. Tissue obtained by biopsy may provide supportive evidence for diagnosis. Lesions in skin, subcutaneous tissues, and muscles are irregularly distributed; care should be taken to choose an involved site for biopsy. The most prominent lesion in children appears to be a vasculitis involving arterioles, venules and capillaries in connective tissues of skin, subcutaneous tissue, muscle and gastrointestinal tract. Affected vessels are surrounded with inflammatory cells and may show intimal thickening and fibrin thrombi. In muscles the vasculitis is accompanied by patchy infarction, atrophy of muscle fibers, interstitial edema, and proliferation of connective tissue. In affected skin there is thinning of the epidermis, and edema and vasculitis in the dermis. In the gastrointestinal tract, vasculitis may result in mucosal ulcerations and tissue infarction. Glomerulitis has been found on renal biopsy. In the chronic phase, calcium deposits with surrounding inflammation may occur in skin, subcutaneous tissue and muscle.

Clinical Manifestations. Onset is usually insidious with slowly developing fatigability and weakness, often first apparent in the upper legs, shoulder girdle and neck. The child may develop an awkward gait and slowly lose capacity for functions such as climbing stairs, riding a bicycle and dressing. Infrequently the onset is more acute, and the affected muscles become stiff, sore and painful and are often brawny, indurated and tender. Skin and subcutaneous tissues may be thickened, and there may be nonpitting edema. The degree of muscle weakness varies from slight to extreme. All muscles of the body can be affected. Severe involvement of those of respiration and deglutition may lead to respiratory difficulty, aspiration and death. Arthralgia and transient arthritis sometimes occur. Raynaud's phenomenon may be present.

The skin lesions are characteristic. Erythema and induration occur over the malar areas and bridge of the nose in a butterfly distribution; this rash is rarely as severe as the similarly located one of systemic lupus erythematosus. The upper eyelids assume a pathognomonic violaceous discoloration (heliotrope eyelids) (Fig. 10-26, p. 521). Periorbital and facial edema may be associated. The skin over extensor surfaces of joints, particularly the knuckles, knees and elbows, becomes erythematous, atrophic and scaly (Fig. 10-27, p. 521). These areas later develop pigmentary changes with hyperpigmentation or vitiligo. A dusky erythema may cover the upper trunk and proximal arms. The skin over involved extremities often appears tight and glossy. In long-standing disease there may be cutaneous atrophy with binding of skin to underlying structures, and calcium may be deposited in affected subcutaneous tissues, muscles and fascia. These stony deposits sometimes break down and extrude in semisolid or solid form. Other rashes which may involve the trunk or extremities include maculopapular erythema, purpura, and pruritic lesions.

Low-grade fever is often present; other evidence of systemic involvement may be found, such as mucous membrane lesions, lymphadenopathy, hepatosplenomegaly, and renal, gastrointestinal or cardiac manifestations.

In untreated cases the fatality rate is about 40 per cent. Most deaths are related to palatorespiratory involvement or such gastrointestinal complications as hemorrhage and perforation and occur within 2 years of onset. Otherwise the disease slowly becomes inactive over a period of several years, after which subsequent exacerbations are uncommon. Infrequently, the disease may smolder for a long time. Most surviving patients are able to lead active lives, although they may have minor residual abnormalities. A few have severe contractures and crippling deformities. Evidence is

accumulating that the course of dermatomyositis can often be favorably modified by early vigorous treatment with corticosteroids.

Laboratory Data. Muscle inflammation is responsible for elevated serum levels of such enzymes as aldolase, transaminase and creatine kinase. The electromyogram of affected muscles is abnormal, with large numbers of brief, low-voltage action potentials and fibrillation potentials. The sedimentation rate may be elevated or normal. Rheumatoid factor and antinuclear factor are sometimes present. L.E. cells are not usually found. Infrequently there are proteinuria and a mild increase of blood cells in the urine. There may be gross or occult blood in the stool. Roentgenograms may reveal calcium deposits in soft tissues.

Diagnosis and Differential Diagnosis. In its typical form dermatomyositis should present little diagnostic difficulty. The combination of muscle weakness and characteristic rash, elevated serum levels of enzymes and abnormal electromyogram is diagnostic; muscle biopsy is usually not necessary. In the differential diagnosis various neuromuscular disorders such as poliomyelitis, Guillain-Barré syndrome, muscular dystrophy and myasthenia gravis should be considered, as should illnesses having predominantly muscular lesions, such as trichinosis. Such other connective tissue disorders as systemic lupus erythematosus, juvenile rheumatoid arthritis and scleroderma are distinguishable clinically and by laboratory tests. In the chronic phase, features of dermatomyositis and generalized scleroderma may overlap, making precise categorization difficult. When the onset is insidious, a period of observation may be needed to establish the diagnosis.

Treatment. During the acute phase, extreme care in evaluating palatorespiratory function may be lifesaving. If swallowing mechanisms are weak, soft or liquid diets should be provided under close observation. The patient should be closely watched for possible deterioration in respiratory function. Constant nursing care is mandatory for any child with palatorespiratory involvement, and equipment for nasopharyngeal suction, endotracheal intubation and tracheotomy should be available. A respirator may be required. The possibility of serious gastrointestinal manifestations during the acute phases of disease must also be kept in mind.

Functional recovery depends on preservation of adequate muscle strength and prevention of crippling contractures. Corticosteroids effectively suppress the inflammatory process in most patients. Serial analyses of serum levels of aldolase, transaminase or creatine kinase provide a helpful gauge of activity and therapeutic response. Prednisone in initial dosage of 1 to 2 mg. per kg. per day (or 60 mg. per square meter of body surface area per day) will usually reduce enzyme levels toward normal values within 1 to 2 weeks; clinical improvement with decreased pain and swelling in muscles and increasing muscle strength usually follows. When enzyme levels have declined significantly, the steroid dosage should be slowly decreased, with continued monitoring of the clinical course and serum enzyme levels. If the dose of steroids is reduced too rapidly, rebound in enzyme levels may occur; such rebounds are usually followed by deterioration in the clinical condition within a few weeks unless corticosteroid dosage is promptly increased. A low dose of steroids sufficient to suppress clinical symptoms and serum enzyme levels should be found and maintained for months; the small amount usually required is not apt to result in serious side effects. Sometimes low doses of steroids are required for years for suppression of the disease. The steroid preparations, triamcinolone and dexamethasone, associated with "steroid myopathy" and muscle weakness, should be avoided. Salicylates may occasionally be helpful as adjunctive drugs in relieving symptoms.

Physical therapy is essential to avoid contractures and rebuild muscle strength. During the acute phase when muscle weakness is pronounced, passive exercises can be used to maintain range of motion. With clinical improvement active strengthening exercises can be added. Appropriate splints to maintain good position of the limbs may be needed. Bed rest is not necessary, and immobilization without exercise is to be avoided at all times.

SCLERODERMA

Scleroderma ("hard skin") is a chronic inflammatory disturbance of connective tissue which classically involves skin, but may also affect the gastrointestinal tract, heart, lung, kidney and synovium. Cutaneous involvement, the hallmark of the disease, may occur either in focal, demarcated patches (morphea) or in a generalized, symmetric distribution. The latter is usually associated with systemic involvement (progressive systemic sclerosis) and is the usual form seen in adults, but is rare in children. Scleroderma in children usually has a patchy, focal distribution (morphea); systemic involvement is uncommon.

The disease is rare and of obscure origin. It affects females more frequently than males and may begin at any time during childhood. There does not seem to be any familial predisposition, although morphea has been reported in a mother and her child.

Histology of affected cutaneous tissues shows increased thickness and density of dermal collagen with perivascular infiltrates of mononuclear cells.

Clinical Manifestations. *Morphea.* The first signs are patchy asymmetric lesions of skin and subcutaneous tissues. These often have a linear pattern similar to the dermal distribution of peripheral nerves, and may occur primarily on one side of the body. During the early phases involved areas may be slightly erythematous and edematous, or may have an atrophic shiny appearance, and the child may complain of pain or a prickly sensation. As the disease progresses the skin lesions become indurated with violaceous, sometimes elevated borders and white or yellow waxy-appearing centers. Lesions enlarge peripherally and may coalesce to involve an entire extremity or a large portion of the body. Extensive scarring and fibrosis of the involved area may occur, with firm binding of cutaneous tissues to underlying structures ("hide-binding"), and be severe enough to limit growth of the affected part and produce crippling contractures (Fig. 10-28). Chronically involved areas may be hyperpigmented or depigmented. Active disease may arrest over a period of months to years, or may smolder for a long time. Prognosis for life is good in the absence of systemic involvement.

Progressive systemic sclerosis. Cutaneous involvement is symmetrical, involving hands, feet and distal extremities, and sometimes the trunk and face as well. Induration, pigmentary changes, and hide-binding of involved cutaneous tissues occur as with focal forms of the disease. Raynaud's phenomenon may be associated, and cutaneous ulcers occur. The disease may involve the gastrointestinal tract, heart, lungs, kidneys and joints. Systemic manifestations, particularly renal, cardiac and pulmonary, may be fatal. Esophageal dysfunction may result in chronic aspiration pneumonia.

Laboratory Data. There are no specific laboratory tests. The sedimentation rate is usually normal. Rheumatoid factor and antinuclear factors may be found in both focal and disseminated forms of the disease; L.E. tests usually give negative results. Radiographs may show dysfunction of esophageal and small bowel motility. Pulmonary function studies, electrocardiograms and chest radiographs may disclose cardiopulmonary involvement. Urinalyses and renal function studies are abnormal in the presence of renal involvement.

Diagnosis. The clinical picture is characteristic in both morphea and progressive systemic sclerosis. The disease may bear some superficial resemblance to dermatomyositis, but absence of myositis and the characteristic rash of dermatomyositis should allow differentiation. Subcutaneous fat necrosis and Weber-Christian nonsuppurative panniculitis may be suggested in morphea, but the course and histology are distinctive. *Scleredema adultorum* (of Bushke), a peculiar benign induration of subcutaneous tissues, may be confusing. This condition occurs acutely, usually following an intercurrent infection, particularly with beta hemolytic streptococci. Subcutaneous tissues of the neck, upper trunk, and arms become indurated; but skin is spared. This condition is self-limited and does not result in chronic scarring.

Treatment. No specific therapy is known. Many therapeutic agents, including corticosteroids, salicylates, chelating agents, chloroquine, radiation, dimethyl sulfoxide, para-aminobenzoic

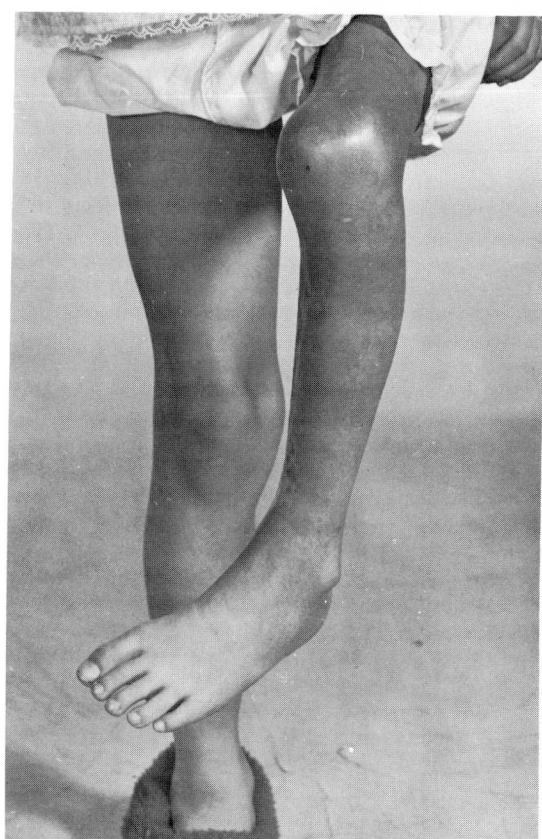

Figure 10-28. Extensive morphea involving the entire left leg, causing scarring, shortening and flexion contractures. Note the shiny appearance and patches of hyperpigmentation and vitiligo of affected skin.

acid and penicillamine, have been tried without clear-cut beneficial effects. Surgical excision of local patches of morphea does not seem to arrest the process. Systemic therapy with corticosteroids may be tried with severe systemic disease. Topical corticosteroids have been used for morphea. Vigorous physical therapy is important early in the course of morphea to prevent or minimize crippling contractures.

ERYTHEMA MULTIFORME EXUDATIVUM
(STEVENS-JOHNSON SYNDROME)

Erythema multiforme exudativum (bullosum) is characterized by lesions of skin and mucous membranes, with fever and systemic prostration. This syndrome was described by Hebra and Bazin over 100 years ago.

The disease occurs in children and young adults, and affects males more frequently than females. Onset often follows an upper respiratory tract infection. Evidence for a viral etiologic agent, especially herpes virus, has been inconclusive. The association of Stevens-Johnson syndrome with patchy pneumonia and increased titers of cold agglutinins has suggested an association with

primary atypical pneumonia and *Mycoplasma pneumoniae*. This organism has recently been isolated from patients with this syndrome, but the significance is not yet known. Association of the syndrome with ingestion of drugs, including sulfonamides, anticonvulsants, penicillin and barbiturates, has also been observed. The L.E. phenomenon has been demonstrated, and the possibility that the Stevens-Johnson syndrome represents a hypersensitivity state to a number of exogenous agents has been suggested.

The hallmark of the syndrome is an erythematous papular skin lesion which enlarges by peripheral expansion and usually develops a central vesicle. This eruption may involve most cutaneous surfaces, including the palms and soles, but spares the scalp. Lesions may be scattered or confluent. New lesions appear for 1 to 2 weeks after onset. Vesiculobullous lesions also occur on mucous membranes of the conjunctiva, nares, mouth, anorectal junction, vulvovaginal region and urethral meatus. Lesions have even been described in the larynx, trachea, bronchi, bladder and gastrointestinal tract.

The rash is often preceded by fever and general malaise. Severe prostration may occur at the height of the syndrome. About one third of affected patients have pulmonary involvement with a harsh, hacking cough and patchy changes on the chest radiograph. Periarticular swelling has been described. Involvement of cardiovascular, renal, hematopoietic and lymphatic systems does not usually occur. As the disease process reaches its peak, the patient presents a striking picture (Fig. 10-29). Stomatitis is particularly distressing;

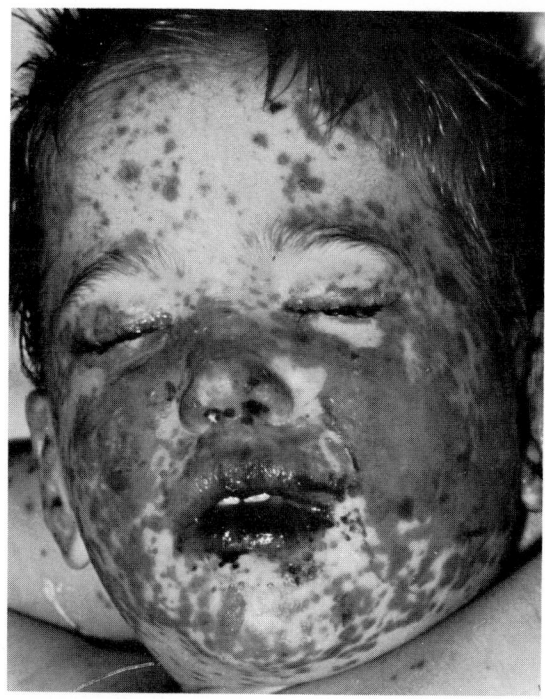

Figure 10-29. Cutaneous, oral, nasal and conjunctival involvement in severe Stevens-Johnson syndrome.

lesions erode, ulcerate, bleed and crust. Meatal involvement may make urination painful. Conjunctivitis results in photophobia, and purulent conjunctival discharge may be profuse. Corneal ulcerations may occur with resulting scarring and even blindness.

The case fatality rate may be as high as 10 per cent during the acute phase, particularly in patients with pulmonary involvement. After the acute phase the disease is self-limiting. Skin lesions gradually subside without scarring in 1 to 4 weeks. Mucous membrane lesions may persist for months. In about 20 per cent of cases the disease recurs, often in association with re-exposure to an offending drug.

During the acute phase symptomatic treatment is of great importance. Fluid requirements are high, and intravenous administration is often required. Cutaneous hygiene should be maintained to prevent secondary infection. Ophthalmologic consultation should be sought if serious conjunctivitis is present. Prednisone, 1 to 2 mg. per kg., is often used in children with serious disease. The efficacy of such therapy is not proved; it should be carefully supervised and is contraindicated whenever there is a possibility of herpetic infection of the eye. Appropriate antibiotic therapy is indicated if there is reasonable suspicion of infection with *Mycoplasma pneumoniae*.

and Europe streptococcal infections are now more frequently implicated as provocative stimuli. The eruption can also occur as a concomitant of sarcoidosis, histoplasmosis and coccidioidomycosis, and with underlying inflammatory disorders such as systemic lupus erythematosus, vasculitis, regional enteritis and ulcerative colitis.

Careful search for a precipitating infection or underlying disease should be instituted. The sedimentation rate is usually elevated, and other nonspecific evidences of inflammatory disease, such as acute phase reactants, are found. Suggestive etiologic evidence may include the demonstration of beta hemolytic streptococci in throat cultures or a rising antistreptolysin O titer; conversion of a previously negative tuberculin, histoplasmin or coccidioidin skin reaction; radiographic evidence of pulmonary tuberculosis or fungus disease; a positive Kveim test result; or evidence of an underlying disease such as systemic lupus erythematosus or inflammatory bowel disease.

Salicylates are usually adequate for symptomatic relief of erythema nodosum. The skin lesions and their constitutional manifestations may respond to corticosteroids, but such therapy is usually not warranted in a self-limited disease, and may be contraindicated because of the presence of underlying active infection.

ERYTHEMA NODOSUM

Erythema nodosum is characterized by the development of painful, indurated, shiny, red, hot, elevated, ovoid patches 1 to 3 cm. in diameter. They are most frequently distributed symmetrically over the shins, but may also occur on the calves, thighs, buttocks and upper extremities. Fever, malaise and arthralgia may precede or accompany the rash, and hilar adenopathy may be present on chest roentgenograms. The skin lesions have a characteristic progression: over a period of several days they become protuberant and present a brilliant display of violaceous colors. After 1 or 2 weeks as induration decreases, a dull purple discoloration predominates, and then fades, in the manner of a large bruise, leaving a brown residuum. Crops of lesions occur, usually over a period of 3 to 6 weeks. The disease then becomes quiescent and rarely recurs. The disease is uncommon in children under the age of 6 years, becoming progressively more frequent up to the third decade of life. Females are affected more frequently than males.

It is generally accepted that the skin lesions represent a hypersensitivity reaction to a variety of provocative stimuli. The eruption has been induced experimentally in patients with the disease by local injection of a single specific bacterial antigen. Epidemiologically, the disease was previously closely linked to tuberculosis, especially in Europe. In both the United States

GOODPASTURE'S SYNDROME

The combination of pulmonary alveolar hemorrhage and glomerulonephritis, called "Goodpasture's syndrome," appears to be a distinctive clinical entity, although there is some overlap with polyarteritis nodosa and with idiopathic pulmonary hemosiderosis. Young adult males are predominantly affected; the disease has been reported in children. The cause is not known. The disease often appears to begin after an acute illness, but no causative agent has been isolated. Recent evidence suggests that antibodies reactive with renal and lung tissue may be involved in pathogenesis.

The syndrome is characterized clinically by hemoptysis, anemia and nephritis. Dyspnea, cough, malaise and fever are often present; and rales and rhonchi may be heard on auscultation of the chest. Chest roentgenograms characteristically show bilateral flocculent infiltrates spreading from hilus to periphery in the lung fields. Hemosiderin-laden macrophages can be demonstrated in the sputum. Anemia, presumably related to pulmonary hemorrhage, is prominent. Urinalyses reveal varying degrees of proteinuria, hematuria, pyuria and cylindruria. Azotemia is frequent, and progressive renal failure often ensues. Histologically, focal glomerulitis or widespread glomerulonephritis may be demonstrated. Intra-alveolar hemorrhages, hemosiderin-laden macrophages, and thickening of alveolar septa are present in the lungs. Generalized vasculitis is not found; patients with concomitant vasculitis are usually considered to have polyarteritis nodosa, but this may prove to be an artificial separation.

The disease is usually rapidly fatal. Corticosteroid therapy has been considered helpful in a few cases, and recently alkylating agents and antimetabolites have been used on an experimental basis.

RELAPSING NODULAR NONSUPPURATIVE PANNICULITIS
(WEBER-CHRISTIAN SYNDROME)

Recurrent nodular nonsuppurative panniculitis is a rare disorder characterized by subcutaneous nodules of degenerating and inflamed fatty tissues. Its cause is not known; infection, drug reaction (especially to bromides and iodides), abnormal fat metabolism, hypersensitivity reaction and enzyme deficiency have all been suggested. It is probable that panniculitis results from a number of causative mechanisms, and does not represent a single disease. It has been reported in association with several connective tissue diseases (rheumatoid arthritis, acute rheumatic fever, systemic lupus erythematosus, glomerulonephritis, ulcerative colitis) and with corticosteroid withdrawal. Adults are predominantly affected, although the syndrome has been reported in all age groups. Females are affected more frequently than males.

Histologically, there are foci of degeneration and inflammation in subcutaneous fat. Mesenteric, perivisceral and periarticular adipose tissues may be affected; fatty metamorphosis of the liver and reticuloendothelial hyperplasia have been reported. Laboratory findings are not specific. Leukopenia and elevated sedimentation rates may be present, and rheumatoid factor, L.E. cells and cryoglobulins have been rarely observed.

Clinically the disease is characterized by the appearance of crops of subcutaneous nodules. Lesions may occur on any part of the body; thighs, abdomen, breasts and arms are most frequently involved. Nodules may vary in size from several millimeters to several centimeters, and may be painful with redness and warmth of the overlying skin. Nodules regress in days to weeks, usually leaving a pigmented depression. Fever is commonly associated with appearance of nodules, and at times with a variety of rheumatic complaints, including arthritis, arthralgia and myalgia. Hepatosplenomegaly and abdominal pain may be present. Uveitis and episcleritis have been reported. Recurrences of crops of nodules and systemic symptoms over a long period of time are the usual course of disease. Fatalities have occurred in association with Weber-Christian disease, but it is uncertain how many of these were caused by the panniculitis itself.

Diagnosis of Weber-Christian syndrome is made by the clinical picture and the histologic appearance of the lesions. Differential diagnosis includes erythema nodosum, vasculitis, morphea, erythema induratum, sarcoidosis, and postinjection subcutaneous fat necrosis. In subacute nodular migratory panniculitis, probably a related syndrome, plaques of inflamed subcutaneous fat which enlarge peripherally affect the lower extremities. Fat necrosis with subcutaneous nodules, arthritis and visceral involvement can occur as a manifestation of pancreatic disease, presumably from enzymatic action on fat cells.

No specific therapy is known. Symptomatic relief has been reported after therapy with corticosteroids, chloroquine and phenylbutazone. Recent experimental work suggests that heparin may abort attacks, perhaps by stimulating production of a deficient enzyme. Patients with underlying pancreatic involvement are benefited by appropriate therapy of the pancreatic disease.

RALPH J. WEDGWOOD
JANE SCHALLER

REFERENCES

General

Christian, C. L. (Ed.): Rheumatism and Arthritis. Seventeenth Rheumatism Review. *Arth. & Rheum.*, 9:93-266, 1966.
Decker, J. L. (Ed.): Primer on the Rheumatic Diseases. 6th ed. *J.A.M.A.*, 190:127, 425, 509, 741, 1964.
Hanson, V., and Kornreich, H.: Systemic Rheumatic Disorders ("Collagen Disease") in Childhood: Lupus Erythematosus, Anaphylactoid Purpura, Dermatomyositis, and Scleroderma. *Bull. Rheum. Dis.*, 17:435, 1967.
Hollander, J. L. (Ed.): *Arthritis and Allied Conditions*. 7th ed. Philadelphia, Lea & Febiger, 1966.
Wedgwood, R. J. (Ed.): Symposium on Collagen Diseases. *Pediat. Clin. N. Amer.*, 10:855-1093, 1963.

Juvenile Rheumatoid Arthritis

Ansell, B. M., and Bywaters, E. G.: Prognosis in Still's Disease. *Bull. Rheum. Dis.*, 9:189, 1959.
Ansell, B. M., and Bywaters, E. G.: Diagnosis of "Probable" Still's Disease and Its Outcome. *Ann. Rheum. Dis.*, 21:253, 1962.
Brewer, E. J., Blattner, R. J., and Wing, H.: Treatment of Rheumatoid Arthritis in Children. *Pediat. Clin. N. Amer.*, 10:207, 1963.
Bywaters, E. G.: Heberden Oration, 1966. Categorization in Medicine: A Survey of Still's Disease. *Ann. Rheum. Dis.*, 26:185, 1967.
Bywaters, E. G., and Ansell, B. M.: Monoarticular Arthritis in Children. *Ann. Rheum. Dis.*, 24:116, 1965.
Calabro, J. J., and Marchesano, J. M.: Fever Associated with Juvenile Rheumatoid Arthritis. *New Eng. J. Med.*, 276:11, 1967.
Cassidy, J. T., and Valkenburg, H. A.: A Five Year Prospective Study of Rheumatoid Factor Tests in Juvenile Rheumatoid Arthritis. *Arth. & Rheum.*, 10:83, 1967.
Grokoest, A. W., Snyder, A. I., and Schlaeger, R.: *Juvenile Rheumatoid Arthritis*. Boston, Little, Brown and Company, 1961.
Isdale, I. C., and Bywaters, E. G.: The Rash of Rheumatoid Arthritis and Still's Disease. *Quart. J. Med.*, 25:377, 1956.
Laaksonen, A. L.: A Prognostic Study of Juvenile Rheumatoid Arthritis. Analysis of 544 cases. *Acta paediat. Scand.*, Suppl. 166:1, 1966.
McMinn, F. J., and Bywaters, E. G.: Differences Between the Fever of Still's Disease and That of Rheumatic Fever. *Ann. Rheum. Dis.*, 18:293, 1959.
Smiley, W. K., May, E., and Bywaters, E. G.: Ocular Presentations of Still's Disease and Their Treatment: Iridocyclitis in

Still's Disease: Its Complications and Treatment. *Ann. Rheum. Dis.*, 16:371, 1957.

Still, G. F.: On a Form of Chronic Joint Disease in Children. *Med.-Chir.*, 80:47, 1897. (Reprinted in *Arch. Dis. Childhood*, 16:156, 1941.)

Sury, B.: *Rheumatoid Arthritis in Children*. Copenhagen, Munksgaard, 1952.

Ankylosing Spondylitis

Wilkinson, M., and Bywaters, E. G.: Clinical Features and Course of Ankylosing Spondylitis; As Seen in a Follow-up of 222 Hospital Referred Cases. *Ann. Rheum. Dis.*, 17:209, 1958.

Jacobs, P.: Ankylosing Spondylitis in Children and Adolescents. *Arch. Dis. Childhood*, 38:492, 1963.

Systemic Lupus Erythematosus

Cook, C. D., Wedgwood, R. J., Craig, J. M., Hartmann, J. R., and Janeway, C. A.: Systemic Lupus Erythematosus. Description of 37 Cases in Children and a Discussion of Endocrine Therapy in 32 of the Cases. *Pediatrics*, 26:570, 1960.

Dubois, E. L. (Ed.): *Systemic Lupus Erythematosus*. New York, McGraw-Hill, 1966.

Holman, H.: Systemic Lupus Erythematosus. A Review of Certain Recent Developments in the Study of This Disease. *J. Pediat.*, 56:109, 1960.

Jacobs, J. C.: Systemic Lupus Erythematosus in Childhood: Report of 35 Cases, with Discussion of Seven Apparently Induced by Anticonvulsant Medication, and of Prognosis and Treatment. *Pediatrics*, 32:257, 1963.

Peterson, R. D., Vernier, R. L., and Good, R. A.: Lupus Erythematosus. *Pediat. Clin. N. Amer.*, 10:941, 1963.

Pollak, V. E., Pirani, C. L., and Schwartz, F. D.: The Natural History of the Renal Manifestations of Systemic Lupus Erythematosus. *J. Lab. & Clin. Med.*, 63:537, 1964.

Robinson, M. J., and Williams, A. L.: Systemic Lupus Erythematosus in Childhood. *Aust. Paediat. J.*, 3:36, 1967.

Rothfield, N. F., McCluskey, R. T., and Baldwin, D. S.: Renal Disease in Systemic Lupus Erythematosus. *New England J. Med.*, 269:537, 1963.

Henoch-Schönlein Vasculitis

Ackroyd, J. F.: Allergic Purpura, Including Purpura Due to Foods, Drugs and Infections. *Am. J. Med.*, 14:605, 1953.

Allen, D. M., Diamond, L. K., and Howell, D. A.: Anaphylactoid Purpura in Children. (Schönlein-Henoch Syndrome): Review with a Follow-up of the Renal Complications. *Am. J. Dis. Child.*, 99:833, 1960.

Bywaters, E. G., Isdale, I., and Kempton, J. J.: Schönlein-Henoch Purpura; Evidence for a Group A β-Haemolytic Streptococci Aetiology. *Quart. J. Med.*, 26:161, 1957.

Gairdner, D.: The Schönlein-Henoch Syndrome. (Anaphylactoid Purpura). *Quart. J. Med.*, 17:95, 1948.

Osler, W.: The Visceral Lesions of Purpura and Allied Conditions. *Brit. Med. J.*, 1:517, 1914.

Vernier, R. L., Worthen, H. G., Peterson, R. D., Colle, E., and Good, R. A.: Anaphylactoid Purpura. Pathology of the Skin and Kidney and Frequency of Streptococcal Infection. *Pediatrics*, 27:181, 1961.

Wedgwood, R. J. P., and Klaus, M. H.: Anaphylactoid Purpura (Schönlein-Henoch Syndrome); Long Term Follow-up Study with Special Reference to Renal Involvement. *Pediatrics*, 16:196, 1955.

Polyarteritis Nodosa

Fager, D. B., Bigler, J. A., and Simonds, J. P.: Periarteritis Nodosa in Infancy and Childhood. *J. Pediat.*, 39:65, 1951.

Frohnert, P. P., and Sheps, S. G.: Long Term Follow-up Study of Periarteritis Nodosa. *Am. J. Med.*, 43:8, 1967.

Owano, L. R., and Sueper, R. H.: Polyarteritis Nodosa — A Syndrome. *Am. J. Clin. Path.*, 40:527, 1963.

Report to the Medical Research Council by the Collagen Disease and Hypersensitive Panel. Treatment of Periarteritis Nodosa with Cortisone: Results after 3 Years. *Brit. Med. J.*, 1:1399, 1960.

Rose, G. A., and Spencer, H.: Polyarteritis Nodosa. *Quart. J. Med.*, 26:43, 1957.

Infantile Polyarteritis Nodosa

Munro-Faure, H.: Necrotizing Arteritis of the Coronary Vessels in Infancy. Case Report and Review of the Literature. *Pediatrics*, 23:914, 1959.

Roberts, F. B., and Fetterman, G. H.: Polyarteritis Nodosa in Infancy. *J. Pediat.*, 63:519, 1963.

Wegener's Granulomatosis

Blatt, I. M., and others: Fatal Granulomatosis of the Respiratory Tract (Lethal Midline Granuloma — Wegener's Granulomatosis). *Arch. Otolaryng.*, 70:707, 1959.

Carrington, C. B., and Liebow, A. A.: Limited Forms of Angiitis and Granulomatosis of Wegener's Type. *Am. J. Med.*, 41:497, 1966.

Takayasu's Arteritis

Danaraj, T. J., Wong, H. O., and Thomas, M. A.: Primary Arteritis of the Aorta Causing Renal Artery Stenosis and Hypertension. *Brit. Heart J.*, 25:153, 1963.

Lee, K., and others: Primary Arteritis (Pulseless Disease) in Korean Children. *Acta paediat. Scand.*, 56:526, 1967.

Nakao, K., and others: Takayasu's Arteritis. Clinical Report of 84 Cases and Immunological Studies of 7 Cases. *Circulation*, 35:1141, 1967.

Strachan, R. W., Wigzell, F. W., and Anderson, J. R.: Locomotor Manifestations and Serum Studies in Takayasu's Arteriopathy. *Am. J. Med.*, 40:560, 1966.

Dermatomyositis

Adams, R. D., Denny-Brown, D., and Pearson, C. M.: *Diseases of Muscle.* 2nd ed. New York, Harper, 1962.

Banker, B. Q., and Victor, M.: Dermatomyositis (Systemic Angiopathy) of Childhood. *Medicine*, 45:261, 1966.

Bitnun, S., and others: Dermatomyositis. *J. Pediat.*, 64:101, 1964.

Carlisle, J. W., and Good, R. A.: Dermatomyositis in Childhood; Report of Studies on Seven Cases and a Review of the Literature. *J. Lancet*, 79:266, 1959.

Everett, M. A., and Curtis, A. C.: Dermatomyositis; A Review of Nineteen Cases in Adolescents and Children. *Arch. Int. Med.*, 100:70, 1957.

Pearson, C. M.: Patterns of Polymyositis and Their Response to Treatment. *Ann. Int. Med.*, 59:827, 1963.

Roberts, H. M., and Brunsting, L. A.: Dermatomyositis in Childhood; Summary of 40 Cases. *Postgrad. Med.*, 16:396, 1954.

Wedgwood, R. J., Cook, C. D., and Cohen, J.: Dermatomyositis; Report of 26 Cases in Children with Discussion of Endocrine Therapy with 13. *Pediatrics*, 12:447, 1953.

Scleroderma: Morphea and Progressive Systemic Sclerosis

Bradford, W. D., Cook, C. D., Vawter, G. F., and Berenberg, W.: Scleredema of Childhood. *J. Pediat.*, 68:391, 1966.

Chazen, E. M., Cook, C. D., and Cohen, J.: Focal Scleroderma. *J. Pediat.*, 60:385, 1962.

Christianson, H. B., Dorsey, C. S., O'Leary, P. A., and Kierland, R. R.: Localized Scleroderma: Clinical Study of 235 Cases. *Arch. Dermat.*, 74:629, 1956.

Jaffe, M. O., and Winkelmann, R. K.: Generalized Scleroderma in Children. *Arch. Derm.*, 83:402, 1961.

Kass, H., Hanson, V., and Patrick, J.: Scleroderma in Childhood. *J. Pediat.*, 68:243, 1966.

Rodnan, G. P.: A Review of Recent Observations and Current Theories on the Etiology and Pathogenesis of Progressive Systemic Sclerosis (Diffuse Scleroderma). *J. Chron. Dis.*, 16:929, 1963.

Erythema Multiforme Exudativum (Stevens-Johnson Syndrome)

Ashby, D. W., and Lazar, T.: Erythema Multiforme Exudativum Major. *Lancet*, 1:1091, 1951.

Foy, H. M., Kenny, G. E., and Koler, J.: *Mycoplasma Pneumoniae* in Stevens-Johnson Syndrome. *Lancet*, 2:550, 1966.

Rallison, M. L., Carlisle, R. E., Lee, R. E., Jr., Vernier, R. L., and Good, R. A.: Lupus Erythematosus and Stevens-Johnson Syndrome. *Am. J. Dis. Child.*, 101:725, 1961.

Stevens, A. M., and Johnson, F. C.: A New Eruptive Fever

Associated with Stomatitis and Ophthalmia. *Am. J. Dis. Child.*, 24:526, 1922.

Erythema Nodosum

"A Group of Pediatricians": Aetiology of Erythema Nodosum in Children. *Lancet*, 2:14, 1961.
Doxiadis, S. A.: Erythema Nodosum in Children. *Medicine*, 30:283, 1951.
James, D. G.: Erythema Nodosum. *Brit. Med. J.*, 1:853, 1961.

Goodpasture's Syndrome

Benoit, F. L., Rulon, D. B., Theil, G. B., Doolan, P. D., and

Watten, R. H.: Goodpasture's Syndrome. *Am. J. Med.*, 37: 424, 1964.

Relapsing Nodular Nonsuppurative Panniculitis

Perry, H. O., and Winkelmann, R. K.: Subacute Nodular Migratory Panniculitis. *Arch. Derm.*, 89:170, 1964.
Hallahan, J. D., and Klein, T.: Relapsing Febrile Nodular Nonsuppurative Panniculitis. Review of the Literature and Report of a Case. *Ann. Int. Med.*, 34:1179, 1951.
Sanford, H. N., Eubank, D. F., and Stenn, F.: Chronic Panniculitis with Leukopenia (Weber-Christian Syndrome). *Am. J. Dis. Child.*, 83:156, 1952.

Rheumatic Fever

Rheumatic fever is a multisystem disease, the acute manifestations of which may include arthritis and fever, carditis, emotional instability and choreiform movements and, less frequently, a characteristic rash (erythema marginatum) and subcutaneous nodules. The disease is naturally recurrent and derives its importance from the fact that it can result in chronic heart disease. Despite a gradual decline in severity and prevalence of acute rheumatic fever in recent years, rheumatic carditis is still the leading form of acquired heart disease in children.

Both acute and recurrent attacks are triggered by group A beta hemolytic streptococcal infections of the upper respiratory tract. Knowledge of this has led to practical approaches to control of rheumatic fever through the prevention and treatment of streptococcal pharyngitis.

Historical Aspects. Though acute rheumatic fever was apparently known to the ancient Greeks, it was many centuries before it became clearly separated from other forms of rheumatism. Sydenham, whose name is associated with chorea, also described the migratory arthritic pattern, but the association of the 2 manifestations was first recognized by Stoll a century later in 1780. Shortly thereafter Pitcairn, Jenner and Wells emphasized that rheumatic fever can damage the heart. Another century passed before the French pediatrician Roger recognized the relation of the various manifestations of the disease and before Cheadle pointed out the variations in the clinical patterns at different ages as well as the tendency of the disease to occur in families. Although earlier observers had described submiliary nodular reactions in the myocardium, Aschoff in 1904 is generally credited with stressing their specificity. The "criteria" introduced by Jones in 1944 brought order into the clinical classification.

The association of acute rheumatic fever with sore throat and the concept of a latent period were recognized during the nineteenth century, particularly by Haygarth, Fowler and Haig-Brown. The relation of scarlet fever and streptococcal tonsillitis to acute rheumatic fever was described by Schlesinger, Collis and Coburn in 1930 and 1931. The development of techniques for classifying streptococci by Lancefield and Griffith has led to firm documentation of the relation of group A streptococci to acute rheumatic fever. The description of the antistreptolysin O test by Todd in 1932 has permitted correlation of serologic with clinical, epidemiologic and bacteriologic findings.

MacLagon advocated salicylates for the treatment of acute rheumatism in 1876, and the era of steroid therapy was introduced in 1949 by Hench and co-workers. Control of recurrences by sulfonamide prophylaxis was demonstrated independently by Thomas and France and by Coburn and Moore in 1939. Treatment of acute streptococcal infections with penicillin was first shown to reduce recurrent attacks of rheumatic fever by Massell and colleagues and to prevent initial attacks by Rammelkamp and co-workers.

Pathogenesis. Rheumatic fever may properly be considered a *complication of streptococcal infection of the upper respiratory tract.* Although not all patients with acute rheumatic fever give a history of sore throat, evidence consistent with recent streptococcal infection can usually be obtained by careful laboratory examinations. Throat cultures taken at the time of the acute infection preceding an attack of rheumatic fever regularly yield beta hemolytic streptococci serologically identifiable as group A, but by the time of onset of rheumatic fever the numbers of group A streptococci may have diminished naturally or may have been suppressed by penicillin therapy to the point at which they are difficult to identify in throat cultures. Serologic evidence of a recent streptococcal infection (elevation of antistreptolysin O or other streptococcal antibodies) can usually be obtained. The demonstrated association of acute rheumatic fever with outbreaks of streptococcal sore throat or scarlet fever provides epidemiologic evidence of a relation between rheumatic fever and these streptococcal diseases. The striking reduction of first attacks of rheumatic fever when streptococcal infections are treated with penicillin and of secondary attacks in patients who are receiving continuous antimicrobial prophylaxis provides additional support for the role of streptococcal infections in the pathogenesis of both initial and recurrent attacks.

Despite the large number of *antigens and biologically toxic or active factors* associated with group A streptococci, none has been definitely identified in the development of rheumatic fever. The streptococcal factor(s) responsible for the appearance of rheumatic fever must be common to most strains, since clinical and epidemiologic evidence suggests that many if not all *serologic types* of group A streptococci frequently found in the throat can be associated with acute rheumatic fever. This is in contrast to acute nephritis, which is related to a limited number of serologic types. The further observation that acute rheumatic fever, again in contrast to acute nephritis, never seems to follow streptococcal infections of the skin indicates important pathogenetic differences with regard to the *location of infection*, reflecting either differences in host response or in the capacity of strains with different biologic capacities to infect different sites.

The importance of *host factors* is suggested by the fact that group A streptococcal infections are common, occurring about once every 3 to 5 years during childhood, and yet relatively few children acquire acute rheumatic fever. The tendency for rheumatic fever to occur in families points to the possible importance of genetic factors, but a clear-cut genetic pattern has not been found; in a study of monozygotic twins less than one fifth were concordant for rheumatic fever.

The resemblance of the clinical manifestations of acute rheumatic fever to those of serum sickness, including the presence of a latent period, has suggested the importance of *hypersensitivity* or *immunologic factors* in the pathogenesis of acute rheumatic fever. Although the delayed type of hypersensitivity of the skin can be demonstrated with a variety of streptococcal products in rheumatic patients, these reactions are also demonstrable in many healthy persons. A role for exaggerated antibody responses in the pathogenesis of acute rheumatic fever has been postulated on the basis that levels of antistreptolysin O and other streptococcal antibodies in patients with acute rheumatic fever are usually, but not always, higher than those in patients after uncomplicated streptococcal infections. The view that rheumatic fever may be an *autoimmune disease* is supported by the demonstration of antigenic cross-reactions between components of the streptococcus and human myocardium, but circulating cross-reacting antibodies are also found in persons who fail to acquire rheumatic fever as well as among those who do, and it is not known whether the cross-reactions are a cause or an effect of injury.

The possible significance of *living streptococci* in the pathogenesis of rheumatic fever is suggested by the demonstration that successful prevention of rheumatic fever by treatment of the preceding streptococcal infection depends upon eradication of the infecting organisms. Direct infection of heart valves is not supported by recent observations, and massive penicillin therapy during the course of acute rheumatic fever does not alter the course or prognosis of the disease. The possibility that wall-less forms of streptococci (*protoplasts or L-forms*), which would be resistant to penicillin, may survive or propagate in tissues has been entertained, but successful attempts to produce these aberrant streptococcal forms in the test tube and in experimental animals have not been matched by convincing success of efforts to recover them from patients.

No completely satisfactory *pathologic model* for acute rheumatic fever has been developed in experimental animals. This has hindered further exploration of the pathogenesis of this disease.

Epidemiology. The epidemiology of acute rheumatic fever is closely related to the epidemiology of streptococcal infections of the upper respiratory tract (pharyngitis, tonsillitis and scarlet fever).

Rheumatic fever, like streptococcal infections, occurs most commonly in children between 5 and 15 years of age, with a peak incidence of first attacks at 6 to 8 years of age. The rarity of rheumatic fever in infants under 3 years of age and in older adults is probably attributable to the rarity of streptococcal infections at these extremes. When adults have intimate and frequent exposures to streptococcal infections, as in military service or through close contact with school-age children, an increased risk of rheumatic fever may be expected.

The distinct *seasonal fluctuation* in onset of acute rheumatic fever coincides with the seasonal variation in streptococcal sore throat and scarlet fever. The incidence is highest in the winter and spring months. This may be related to the increased opportunity for spread of streptococcal infection by close contact during the colder and damper months.

Although traditionally considered to be a disease of temperate *climates*, rheumatic fever also occurs in the warmer ones. The high prevalence of rheumatic heart disease which may be found in some tropical or desert climates, as in India and Egypt, suggests that the pathologic process is common there, but may be clinically modified. This is in keeping with the observation in the United States that acute rheumatic fever appears to be more frequent in the North than in the South, but rheumatic heart disease is found at autopsy as often in Southern as in Northern clinics.

Crowding due to socioeconomic factors or to military exigencies seems to play an important role in the spread of streptococcal infections and in the incidence of acute rheumatic fever. When allowance is made for the effect of crowding, due to differences in housing, no significant *racial differences* have been established.

In contrast to acute nephritis, the *attack rate* of acute rheumatic fever following well documented streptococcal infections in epidemic situations is relatively constant; it is about 3 per cent. Lower attack rates, of the order of 3 per thousand, have been reported among children in nonepidemic situations, but it is not clear whether there is a true difference in attack rates or whether the apparent difference is due to the difficulties in identifying viral infections among streptococcal carriers. Although rheumatic fever appears to be more common in certain *families*, it is not known whether this is due to an increased group exposure to streptococcal infections or to differences in host or genetic factors.

There is no striking *sex difference* in the overall incidence of rheumatic fever, but chorea and mitral stenosis are more common in females, and aortic insufficiency is more common in males.

Morbidity and Mortality. There is evidence suggesting a decline in severity of first attacks of rheumatic fever, in prevalence of rheumatic heart disease and in mortality from it over the past several decades. The incidence of recurrent attacks of rheumatic fever has been gradually declining, but a definite decline in the frequency of first attacks is not so well established. Antibiotics have been generally held responsible for the *decline in the incidence of rheumatic fever*, but more credit is probably due to general improvement in social conditions leading to less crowded living conditions. Changes in the infecting organism or in the infected host may also be possible factors, but have not been documented.

The current *yearly incidence for first attacks* of rheumatic fever has been estimated to be about 50 per 100,000 children. In recent years *prevalence rates for rheumatic heart disease* among school children have been of the order of 0.7 to 1.6 per 1000. They are generally less than the current prevalence rates for congenital heart disease, but prevalence rates for college students and servicemen are about 6 to 9 per 1000, and rejection rates among military selectees are appreciably greater for rheumatic than for congenital heart disease.

In the United States in 1964 about 16,000 *deaths* were attributed to rheumatic fever or chronic rheumatic heart disease, an overall mortality rate of 8 per 100,000 population. Most of the deaths occur in adults, although the initial attack usually dates back to childhood.

Pathology. The pathologic response to acute rheumatic fever includes both exudative and proliferative reactions. The *exudative reactions* when manifest as arthritis subside spontaneously, but more rapidly with anti-inflammatory drugs, and leave no evidence of permanent damage; when manifest as pancarditis, they may be life-threatening. *Proliferative reactions* accompanied by permanent damage appear to be confined to the myocardium and endocardium.

The unique pathologic lesion of rheumatic fever, the *Aschoff body*, does not develop in brain tissue, and its occurrence in joints is doubtful. Although generally considered to be a granuloma, developing from injury to collagen fibers, some pathologists contend that the Aschoff body results from primary injury to the myocardium, and others believe that it may result from blockage of lymphatic channels in the heart. Biopsies of auricular appendages in patients with rheumatic heart disease may show Aschoff bodies many years after there has been any clinical evidence of rheumatic activity. Whether the *deposits of gamma globulin* which have been demonstrated in rheumatic heart tissue represent a primary cause or a secondary result of heart damage is not known. *Valvular damage* most frequently involves the mitral, less commonly the aortic, and rarely the tricuspid and pulmonary valves. Scarring sufficient to result in stenotic heart valves requires months or years to develop. There is little knowledge or understanding of the *pathology of Sydenham's chorea*, since patients do not often die with this form of rheumatic fever and the histopathologic changes can-

not be related to the clinical manifestations. Pathologic lesions similar to those of hyaline membrane disease of newborn infants have been reported in patients dying with rheumatic pneumonitis.

Clinical Manifestations. The first symptoms of rheumatic fever usually do not develop until the clinical manifestations of streptococcal infection have disappeared for some time. This *latent period* may last from 1 to 5 weeks and in chorea may be much longer (2 to 6 months).

The *presenting manifestation* of acute rheumatic fever is commonly arthritis or choreiform movements in school-age children and carditis in very young children. Abdominal pain which may be suggestive of appendicitis is occasionally the presenting complaint. The onset is usually abrupt when arthritis and fever are the initial manifestations, and may be with carditis, when chest pain or shortness of breath appears suddenly. The onset with carditis, however, is more apt to be insidious and unsuspected until an enlarged liver or a significant murmur is detected. A subtle onset is especially common in chorea and a perfunctory diagnosis of emotional disturbance is often made initially.

A *history of a recent sore throat* is obtained in about 50 per cent of instances. A *family history* of acute rheumatic fever or rheumatic heart disease can sometimes be elicited, but must be carefully differentiated from other arthritic and cardiac diseases. Patients presenting with well established rheumatic heart disease should be carefully questioned about the possibility of earlier attacks.

Fever is almost invariably present in the early stage, except in patients whose only manifestation is chorea or in those receiving salicylates or a corticosteroid. Prolonged fever without development of other manifestations is unusual. Without suppressive drugs the fever will often become low grade after the first week and may persist at this level for 2 to 4 weeks.

The *arthritis* of acute rheumatic fever characteristically involves the large joints and migrates from one joint to another for a few days to several weeks. Involvement of the most distal joints, such as the small joints of the fingers and toes, and the central ones, such as the hips and the spine, is unusual. Infrequently such joints as the temporomandibular joint may be involved. Pain on pressure or movement is characteristically intense and aggravated rather than alleviated by massage. The tenderness, though exquisite, is likely to be diffusely present over the entire joint. Swelling of the joint, increased heat and redness are commonly present. Pain without objective changes may occur in some joints and frank arthritis in others, or pain may be the only indication of joint involvement.

Carditis occurs in approximately 40 per cent of patients during the first attack of rheumatic fever and may be the only major manifestation, especially in infants and young children. It usually appears within the first week of illness. *Tachy-*

cardia, disproportionate to fever, present during sleep, and persisting after fever is under control, is highly suggestive of carditis. The first heart sound may be muffled, consistent with first-degree heart block, or both sounds may be distant in patients with pericardial effusion. *Significant murmurs* are almost always present with rheumatic carditis. Mitral valvulitis is manifested as an apical systolic murmur sometimes accompanied by an apical mid-diastolic murmur. The apical systolic murmur should be carefully differentiated from functional murmurs by its length (filling all of systole), by its blowing, high-pitched quality and by its persistence irrespective of position or phase of respiration. The low-pitched mid-diastolic murmur is more difficult to detect and must be differentiated from the third heart sound and the late-appearing murmur of mitral stenosis, with which there is presystolic accentuation. Involvement of the aortic valve, uncommon in children but relatively frequent in adult males, is manifest by the basal diastolic murmur of aortic regurgitation. Mitral stenosis and aortic stenosis are late manifestations of cardiac damage, which do not develop until months or years after the initial or repeated attacks. *Cardiomegaly, pericarditis*, with or without friction rub, and *congestive failure* may be present during the acute phase. In children with chronic rheumatic heart disease, changing murmurs or increasing heart size may be evidence of progressive or reactivated carditis.

Rheumatic pneumonia does occur, but is difficult to distinguish clinically from pneumonitis of other cause and from pulmonary congestion. It occurs especially in association with extensive heart damage. *Subcutaneous nodules* (Fig. 10-30) are also most often found in patients with well established rheumatic disease, often after multiple attacks of carditis. The nodules are firm and nontender, and range in size from 0.1 to 1 cm. in diameter. They are usually found over the extensor surfaces of both large and small joints, over the scalp, or near the superficial bony prominences of the spine and scapulae. The skin overlying the nodules is freely movable and is not inflamed. *Epistaxis*, occasionally an early sign, occurs in less than 10 per cent of patients with acute rheumatic fever; by itself it is not sufficient grounds for a rheumatic work-up. Patients with severe active heart disease may also have striking *pallor*, often accompanied by anemia.

The distinctive skin rash associated with rheumatic fever is *erythema marginatum* (Fig. 10-31). It occurs in about 10 per cent of patients with acute rheumatic fever and is rarely found in other diseases. The pink, often slightly raised, macules of the early stages fade centrally and coalesce to form a serpiginous pattern. The lesions are most common over the protected parts of the body and may be elicited or accentuated by the local application of heat. They may disappear after a few hours or days and may occur intermittently over a period of weeks or months. Although commonly occurring in association with other manifestations of rheu-

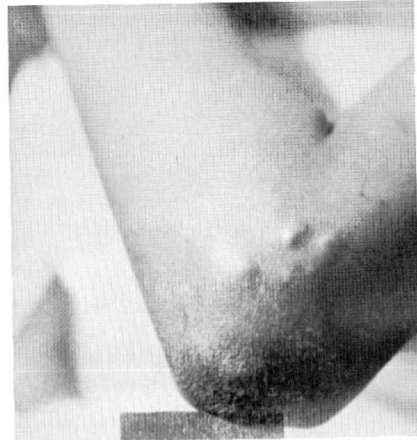

Figure 10-30. Rheumatic nodules at the elbow in a Negro girl 10 years of age. She had polyarthritis, endocarditis and pericarditis. She died 3 weeks after the picture was taken.

matic fever, erythema marginatum sometimes appears as an isolated physical finding.

Chorea, variously known as Sydenham's chorea, St. Vitus's dance or chorea minor, is one of the common and most peculiar manifestations of rheumatic fever. Not infrequently it is the only manifestation (pure chorea), but a significant number of patients have other manifestations or chronic heart disease following subsequent attacks of rheumatic fever. It occurs most often in prepubertal girls and is rare among adults of either sex. Its most striking feature is involuntary purposeless movements. These are usually bilateral, but sometimes unilateral. They develop gradually

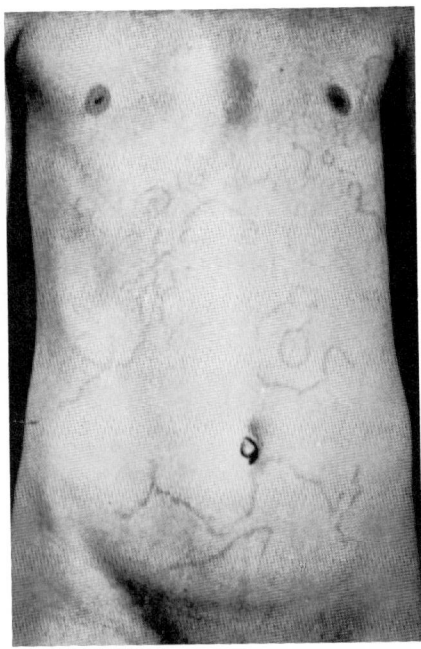

Figure 10-31. Erythema marginatum. Annular erythema on the chest and abdomen of a boy 8 years of age who also had rheumatic carditis.

over a period of weeks and vary in intensity from those which can be brought out only by excitement or conscious efforts to be still, to those which are so violent that they may result in self-injury. Deterioration in speech and in handwriting as well as general clumsiness may be noted. Serial samples of handwriting may be a useful manner of documenting the course of the affliction. The child may have difficulty in counting rapidly and in holding his protruded tongue still. He tends to hyperextend his fingers and wrists when holding his fingers outstretched and to turn his palms outward when he holds his arms above his head. He has a weak hand grip, and the examiner may detect intermittent muscular contractions or twitchings. Other evidence of muscular weakness is usually present. The patellar reflex is often manifest by a "hung-up" type of response. Emotional lability is characteristic and may be expressed by inappropriate outbursts of crying or laughter. Chorea is typically a delayed manifestation of rheumatic fever and may not develop until other signs of activity have subsided, or it may appear as the sole manifestation 2 to 6 months after a streptococcal infection.

Laboratory Data. Clinical impression of inflammatory activity can be confirmed by demonstration of a rapid *erythrocyte sedimentation rate* and of circulating *C-reactive protein*. These and other so-called acute phase reactants are not specific for rheumatic fever, but they are almost always demonstrable in the early stages of untreated acute rheumatic fever (except with pure chorea or with isolated erythema marginatum) and are useful in objectively documenting the presence or persistence of activity. Anemia and less certainly heart failure may influence the erythrocyte sedimentation rate, and low borderline rates may be difficult to interpret. The C-reactive protein test is not influenced by anemia and the problem of borderline tests does not exist, since the detection of even small amounts is significant.

Leukocytosis may occur in patients with acute rheumatic fever, but is not regularly present. A mild to moderate *anemia* is common during the active phase. Blood loss by epistaxis is usually not sufficient to account for the anemia, and the cause is often ill-defined.

Laboratory evidence of a preceding streptococcal infection can be obtained in most patients with acute rheumatic fever, except in those with chorea, in whom, because of the longer latent period, it is more difficult to document. The frequency with which *group A streptococci* can be isolated from the throat at the time rheumatic symptoms appear is related to the number of cultures taken and the care with which they are examined. The streptococci may be difficult to detect, owing to natural decline in numbers during the latent period or to suppression by antibiotics. *Streptococcal antibody tests* more regularly provide corroboration of recent streptococcal infection. They may be elevated even in the absence of clinical or bacteriologic evidence of streptococcal illness.

The antistreptolysin O (ASO) titer is the most widely used streptococcal antibody test. It measures the inhibition of hemolysis of rabbit red blood cells by specific antibody to streptolysin O, an extracellular product of beta hemolytic streptococci which in its reduced form is actively hemolytic for these cells. Normal levels of this and other streptococcal antibodies vary with the age of the population, the geographic location, the season of the year. Antistreptolysin O titers of 500 Todd units or greater are rarely found in normal school-age children and can be considered clear evidence of recent streptococcal infection (Fig. 10-32). About 20 per cent of normal school-age children will have titers of 250 or greater, and 10 per cent will have titers of 320 or greater. Therefore titers below 250 should be considered normal, and titers of 250 to 320 should be considered borderline elevated; about 80 per cent of patients with acute rheumatic fever will have ASO titers in this range and about 60 per cent will have titers of 500 or greater. In infants and older adults, who normally have lower levels of streptococcal antibodies, titers in the range of 200 to 250 may be significant. A demonstrated rise of 2 tubes or more on serially collected serums tested simultaneously is evidence of recent streptococcal infection regardless of the absolute level of the titers or the age of the patient.

In patients suspected of acute rheumatic fever who have normal or borderline elevated antistreptolysin O titers, the determination of antibody levels to another streptococcal antigen is often helpful. *Antistreptokinase* and *antihyaluronidase* titers have been used for this purpose, but have been somewhat difficult to standardize. More recently, antibody tests for streptococcal deoxyribonuclease B (DNAse B) and streptococcal diphosphopyridine-nucleotidase (DPNase) or nicotinamide-adenine-dinucleotidase (NADase) have been developed (Fig. 10-32). The *anti-DNAse B* and the *anti-DPNase (anti-NADase)* tests are dependent upon antibody neutralization of the activity of these specific enzymes produced by the streptococcus. Multiple antibody tests may be especially helpful in patients with pure chorea, who are less likely than other rheumatic patients to have distinct elevation of antistreptolysin O.

Patients whose disease is of several months' duration may have declining or normal titers of streptococcal antibodies. In patients receiving antistreptococcal prophylactic medication, serial streptococcal antibody titers may be useful in identifying new clinical or subclinical streptococcal infections which may result in recurrent attacks.

Roentgen examinations are useful in documenting cardiac enlargement and pericardial effusion. The presence of pericarditis may be suggested or supported by elevation of the ST segment on the *electrocardiogram*. Carditis should not be diagnosed on the basis of prolongation of the P-R interval alone, since this finding may occur in many infectious diseases. Although careful auscultation is usually sufficient for the differentia-

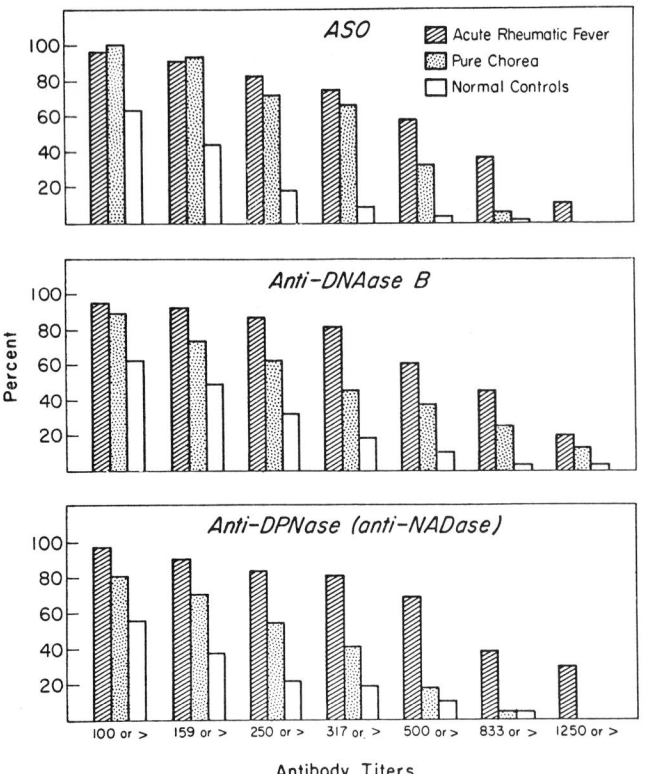

Figure 10-32. Distribution of various streptococcal antibody titers at certain levels or greater in patients with acute rheumatic fever, patients with pure chorea, and normal controls. (Adapted from data of Ayoub and Wannamaker: *Pediatrics*, 29:527, 1962; 38:946, 1966.)

tion of innocent from organic murmurs by physicians experienced with cardiac examinations in children, *phonocardiographic studies* may be helpful in substantiating or documenting the clinical impression.

Diagnosis and Differential Diagnosis. Since no single clinical or laboratory finding is pathognomonic for acute rheumatic fever, the diagnosis is based on a combination of manifestations characteristic for this disease and on the absence of evidence of other diseases which may mimic it. For this purpose the *Jones criteria*, as modified over the years, have proved useful (Table 10-6). The major manifestations are much more likely to be indicative of acute rheumatic fever than the minor ones, and for this reason a diagnosis based on 2 major manifestations is stronger than one based on 1 major and 2 minor manifestations. The possibility of other diseases should always be considered and, if possible, ruled out by appropriate tests, especially in patients with only 1 major manifestation, atypical findings, or no serologic evidence of recent streptococcal disease.

The combination of *fever, arthritis and positive acute phase reactants* is found in many different diseases, including rheumatoid and bacterial arthritis, serum sickness, penicillin hypersensitivity, systemic lupus erythematosus, subacute bacterial endocarditis, sickle cell anemia, Henoch-Schönlein purpura and acute leukemia. Some of these diseases, notably the latter three, may also present with *abdominal pain*, and some, as rheumatoid arthritis, serum sickness and penicillin

hypersensitivity, may also be accompanied by skin lesions which must be differentiated from erythema marginatum. *Skin reactions*, such as hives, erythema multiforme and erythema nodosum, should not be confused with the lesions of erythema marginatum, which do not itch, nor are they markedly elevated or painful.

The diagnosis of acute rheumatic fever in patients with nonmigrating or monoarticular arthritis unaccompanied by other major manifestations is particularly hazardous. *Osteomyelitis* and *local injuries* to the bones and joints may be confused with the early stages of acute rheumatic fever. *Growing pains*, vaguely localized and confined to the lower extremities, most often present at night and disappearing in the morning, are a common complaint in children. There is no pain on motion and no other objective findings, and, in contrast to rheumatic joints, there is often relief from massage.

Pericarditis or myocarditis, in the absence of other major manifestations, is often of viral origin, which should be considered in the absence of murmurs and streptococcal antibody responses typical of acute rheumatic fever.

The movements of chorea must be carefully differentiated from simple fidgeting, tics and athetosis. Healthy children in close association with patients with chorea may mimic the disease sufficiently well to cause problems in differential diagnosis.

Subcutaneous nodules occur in rheumatoid arthritis, particularly in older persons without evidence of heart involvement. Because they usually occur as a late manifestation in children with well established rheumatic heart disease, they are rarely helpful in differential diagnosis.

Except in patients with pure chorea, the *absence of serologic evidence of streptococcal infection* in 2 or more antibody tests should stimulate a search for other possible diseases. On the other hand, elevated streptococcal antibody tests should *never* be the basis for diagnosis of rheumatic fever in the absence of definitive clinical criteria.

Overdiagnosis of acute rheumatic fever on the basis of either clinical or laboratory findings should be assiduously avoided, since it may result in psychologic damage, a long-term commitment to unnecessary antimicrobial prophylaxis, and difficulties with regard to future insurability.

Treatment. Therapy with salicylates or corticosteroids should not be initiated until a firm diagnosis has been established, since it may leave the physician in unresolvable doubt as to the nature of the disease process (see above). Ordinarily the disease is full-blown by the end of the first or second week, but some patients may have low-grade symptoms for a longer time, leaving the diagnosis in doubt. Although a therapeutic trial of aspirin or a corticosteroid has sometimes been used in such patients, the response is not sufficiently specific to make a differential diagnosis.

Bed rest is recommended during the acute stages of the disease. Strict bed rest, including feeding by an attendant, should be insisted upon in patients with congestive failure or cardiac enlargement without evidence of stabilization. *Sedatives* may be required in such patients. *Digitalis*, perhaps in conjunction with diuretics, should be used when heart failure is present (see p. 1032). Although some patients may have unusual sensitivity to digitalis, requiring special caution in digitalization, there is consensus that rheumatic patients in congestive heart failure should be digitalized regardless of the presence or absence of active carditis.

The acute signs of rheumatic inflammation are quickly suppressed by *anti-inflammatory drugs.* Fever and joint manifestations disappear within a few days. The acute phase reactants, especially the sedimentation rate, may require several weeks to return to normal. *Corticosteroids* are more powerful suppressive agents than aspirin and may be somewhat more prompt in bringing the acute manifestations under control. They are the drug of choice for fulminating pancarditis. *Aspirin* may be the drug of choice for joint disease without evidence of carditis. Most physicians prescribe a corticosteroid when a firm diagnosis of carditis has been made in the acute stage. Opinions differ, however, and available evidence is conflicting as to the possible effect on residual heart disease.

The dosages of both aspirin and corticosteroids may have to be adjusted for individual patients to achieve suppression. For aspirin, a total daily dose of 60 mg. per pound, not to exceed 10 gm. per day, is usually adequate. Blood levels, occasionally helpful in patients who do not appear to respond to therapy or who show evidence of toxicity, should be maintained at about 25 to 35 mg. per 100 ml. Some patients tolerate aspirin poorly, owing to nausea and vomiting. Postprandial administration or enteric-coated pills may be helpful; sodium bicarbonate may reduce the effectiveness of sali-

TABLE 10-6. Clinical and Laboratory Manifestations of Acute Rheumatic Fever*
(Modified Jones Criteria)

MAJOR MANIFESTATIONS	MINOR MANIFESTATIONS	SUPPORTING EVIDENCE OF STREPTOCOCCAL INFECTION	OTHER FINDINGS
Carditis	Fever	Recent scarlet fever	History of recent sore throat
Polyarthritis	Arthralgia**	Throat culture positive for group A streptococci	Family history of rheumatic fever
Chorea	Previous rheumatic fever or rheumatic heart disease	Increased ASO or other streptococcal antibodies	Abdominal pain
Erythema marginatum .	Positive acute phase reactants Increased erythrocyte sedimentation rate C-reactive protein Leukocytosis		Epistaxis
Subcutaneous nodules...	Prolonged P-R interval††		Tachycardia Rheumatic pneumonia Pallor and anemia Precordial pain Weight loss Malaise

Adapted from the recommendations of the Committee of the American Heart Association (*Circulation*, 32:664, 1965).

*The presence of 2 major or of 1 major and 2 minor manifestations supported by evidence of recent streptococcal infection indicates a high probability of acute rheumatic fever.

**Should not be counted as a minor manifestation in patients in whom polyarthritis is counted as a major manifestation.

††Should not be counted as a minor manifestation in patients in whom carditis is counted as a major manifestation.

cylates. Tinnitus, decreased hearing acuity, and hyperpnea may occur and require temporary discontinuance or adjustment of the dose. Prednisone is usually favored over other steroids because the necessity for a low salt diet and added potassium is avoided. A dose of 50 to 75 mg. per day administered in divided doses is generally considered to be sufficient. High-dose, short-term (7-day) therapy has been used in some clinics. Moonface, abdominal fullness and other mild manifestations of Cushing's disease occur in patients after several weeks of steroid therapy, and severe reactions such as toxic psychoses, hypertension, overwhelming infection, growth retardation, gastric ulcers and compression fractures of the spine may occur, especially with prolonged administration. In patients with mild or moderate disease who respond promptly, especially those without evidence of carditis, aspirin can often be discontinued in about 10 days or the dose of the steroid can be tapered and then discontinued after a similar time. Steroid treatment for periods up to 4 to 6 weeks or even longer may be required for patients with severe carditis.

Rebounds occur after discontinuance of aspirin therapy and are even more common after steroid therapy. Arthralgia and fever are the usual manifestations; at times there is frank arthritis, and rarely severe carditis. Subclinical rebounds may be detectable only by laboratory tests (acute phase reactants). The most reasonable explanation for rebounds is that anti-inflammatory drugs have been discontinued before the disease has run its natural course, which may be 1 to 5 weeks in patients with arthritis and 2 to 6 months, sometimes longer, in patients with severe carditis. The clinical manifestations of rebounds usually respond to salicylate therapy.

There is no evidence that anti-inflammatory agents have any effect on erythema marginatum or Sydenham's chorea and only questionable evidence that they may influence the disappearance of subcutaneous nodules.

The *management of chorea* is supportive. The disease will subside spontaneously after a variable period of a few weeks or months; in unusual cases it may persist longer. Symptomatic care includes an environment free from noise and bright lights, patient and understanding attendants, and protection against tongue-biting and other self-injuries due to violent, uncontrollable movements. Phenobarbital and chlorpromazine are sometimes helpful. Some patients manifest increased agitation during therapy with sedatives.

Antimicrobial agents are important in the prevention of further streptococcal insults to lessen the possibility of new or additional cardiac damage and should be prescribed for all patients with acute rheumatic fever, including those with Sydenham's chorea. As soon as the diagnosis of rheumatic fever is established and cultures have been taken, therapeutic doses of penicillin should be prescribed to eradicate residual group A streptococci

and then should be followed by continuous prophylaxis (see below).

Gradual *ambulation* should be started when the clinical and laboratory signs of acute disease have subsided, as soon as 7 to 10 days in children with no evidence of heart disease. Bed rest for periods of 3 weeks to 3 months may be required for patients with carditis, depending on the severity and evidence of progression or stabilization. Prolonged bed rest should be avoided, if possible, and due attention should be given to the psychologic needs and school activities of the child. *After recovery no restriction of physical activity* is ordinarily required, except in patients with persistent cardiac enlargement, who will usually tolerate moderate exercise, but may not tolerate the vigorous exercise of active competitive sports.

Prevention. *Continuous antimicrobial prophylaxis* (Table 10-7) for patients with a well documented history of acute rheumatic fever or clear evidence of rheumatic heart disease is the most important feature in the control of this disease. Such prophylaxis has proved highly effective in preventing streptococcal infections and consequently recurrences of acute rheumatic fever with their added risk of serious heart disease. Intramuscular benzathine penicillin is preferable to oral preparations which depend heavily on patient cooperation and adequate absorption from the gastrointestinal tract. Prophylaxis by the oral route should be considered only in patients who are reliable, who have minimal or no heart disease, and who have not had repeated attacks of rheumatic fever. Penicillin prophylaxis should never be discontinued during childhood unless the original diagnosis is in doubt. Young adults should be urged to continue their prophylaxis, particularly while subjected to the hazards of exposure to streptococcal infections in the military service or by close contact with children as parents, baby-sitters, school teachers or in other occupations. Older adults, whose initial attack was many years previously, especially those without heart disease and with minimal exposure to streptococcal infection, may be in relatively little danger, but available information is insufficient to define their risk in discontinuing prophylaxis.

Prevention of first attacks of acute rheumatic fever (Table 10-7) is more difficult than prevention of recurrences because of problems in recognition and definition of streptococcal infection, assurance of adequate therapy, and uncertainty as to whether penicillin treatment will influence the ultimate development of permanent heart disease. A throat culture, carefully taken and processed, will help to determine those who are harboring beta hemolytic streptococci, but will not distinguish patients with current streptococcal infection from chronic carriers with non-streptococcal infection. This is a serious problem, since carrier rates among school-age children are often of the order of 20 to 25 per cent in the winter

TABLE 10-7. PREVENTION OF RHEUMATIC FEVER AND BACTERIAL ENDOCARDITIS

PREVENTIVE AIM	RISK	APPROACH	RECOMMENDED REGIMENS†	EFFECTIVENESS	LIMITATIONS AND PRECAUTIONS
First attacks of rheumatic fever in general population	0 to 5 cases per 100 cases of streptococcal respiratory infection	*Eradication of streptococcus by prolonged treatment of acute infection*	*Single intramuscular injection of benzathine penicillin:* < 10 yrs., 600,000 units; > 10 yrs., 900,000 units; adults, 1,200,000 units *Oral penicillin for 10 days:* 200,000 to 250,000 units 3 or 4 times daily *Erythromycin* in penicillin-sensitive patients (20 mg./lb./day, up to 1 gm. per day in older children and adults, for 10 days) Sulfadiazine and tetracyclines should not be used	90% effective with intramuscular benzathine penicillin. Oral regimens generally less effective, usually due to failure to take drug regularly for 10 days	Dependent upon *recognition* of streptococcal infection and *differentiation* from viral infections *Subclinical infections* (comprising about 50% of total) usually escape detection except in cultured family or school epidemic contacts Reculture at 2 weeks to confirm effectiveness of oral therapy
Recurrent attacks of rheumatic fever in patients with well documented history of rheumatic fever or definite evidence of rheumatic heart disease	10 to 50 cases per 100 cases of streptococcal respiratory infections	*Prevention of streptococcal parasitism by continuous administration of antimicrobial agents* (Acute streptococcal infections should receive vigorous and prolonged treatment, but complete reliance should not be placed on this approach)	*Intramuscular benzathine penicillin:* 1,200,000 units at monthly intervals. *Oral sulfadiazine:** < 60 lbs., 0.5 gm. once daily > 60 lbs., 1.0 gm. once daily *Oral penicillin:** 200,000 to 250,000 units once or preferably twice daily Erythromycin (100 mg. once daily) in penicillin-sensitive patients*	Recurrence rates are about 1 per 25,000 patient-years on intramuscular regimen and 1 per 2500 patient-years on oral regimens Oral sulfadiazine is at least as effective as oral penicillin	Faithful patient cooperation is essential in oral prophylaxis Monitor for possible reactions for first few months in patients receiving sulfadiazine. After this time reactions are extremely rare with either drug
Bacterial endocarditis in patients with rheumatic or congenital heart disease	Transitory bacteremia from *dental and other operative and diagnostic procedures* is frequent. Risk level of endocarditis not certain, but probably low.	*Prevent or minimize bacteremia; eradicate implanted bacteria before vegetation forms*	*Procaine penicillin:* 600,000 units plus crystalline penicillin 600,000 units intramuscularly 1 to 2 hrs. before procedure and daily for 2 days after procedure *or* *Large doses of oral penicillin* (at least 0.25 gm. penicillin V or phenethicillin or 500,000 units buffered penicillin G) q. 4 to 6 hrs. on day of procedure (with extra dose 1 hr. before procedure) and for 2 days thereafter. Add *streptomycin* (50 mg./kg., not to exceed 1 gm. per day in children) in procedures on lower gastrointestinal and genitourinary tracts (including childbirth) where bacteremia with penicillin-resistant enterococci may occur	Reduction in bacteremia has been demonstrated, but prevention of endocarditis is not documented	Do not give penicillin if any history of *sensitivity* is obtained. Use *erythromycin* in dose of 20 mg./lb./day (up to 1 gm./day in older children and adults) divided into 4 doses

†Adapted from American Heart Association recommendations (Circulation, 31:948, 1965).

*Before initiation of continuous prophylaxis, a full therapeutic course of penicillin or erythromycin should be given as outlined under treatment of acute infection (see above). This is to eradicate any possible residual streptococci which may or may not be demonstrable.

and spring months and may on occasion be much higher. This feature may explain why children appear to have a lower risk of acquiring acute rheumatic fever than do young adults with well documented epidemic streptococcal disease. The risk of development of rheumatic fever may be minimal in such children, unless they have clear physical signs of pharyngeal or tonsillar inflammation, such as exudate, or association with an epidemic in their family or school.

Eradication of the infecting streptococcus is essential for successful prevention of rheumatic fever. Patients who harbor group A streptococci after oral therapy should be retreated with injectable benzathine penicillin. Examination of *family contacts* will reveal evidence of streptococcal infection in about 1 out of 4 persons. Treatment may be beneficial in those who have clinical evidence of infection or large numbers of beta hemolytic streptococci in their throat culture. When there is a sequential pattern of infection within a family, treatment of all members should be considered.

Mass penicillin prophylaxis is rarely required in civilian populations and should be considered only when there is good evidence of epidemic streptococcal disease or multiple cases of acute rheumatic fever or acute nephritis. *Tonsillectomy* is ineffective in preventing initial or recurrent attacks of rheumatic fever and may increase the likelihood that streptococcal infections will go unrecognized clinically and therefore not be treated. Some *streptococcal vaccines* are currently being subjected to clinical trial, but the problem is a complex one because of the large number of serologic types, the question of whether primary immunization can be regularly achieved and the possible risks involved.

Prognosis. Prognosis is related chiefly to the development and persistence of *heart disease*. Fulminating carditis progressing to death during or after a single attack occurs in only a few patients. In approximately one fourth to one third of patients with carditis, the heart disease will regress during the acute episode or over a 10-year follow-up period. Arthritis is never permanently crippling. The neurologic manifestations of chorea subside completely with time, but a high percentage of *psychiatric disturbances* has been reported in long-term follow-up studies. Since psychologic disturbances may commonly exist prior to the onset of chorea, it is not clear whether this finding is a cause or a result of the disease. Patients with pure chorea may be somewhat less likely to develop carditis than patients with other rheumatic manifestations, but some reports indicate that a considerable proportion will develop rheumatic heart disease if not protected by prophylaxis.

Most chronic disability and deaths are related to *recurrent attacks*, which occur with high frequency in rheumatic children not protected by antistreptococcal prophylaxis. In one study more than two thirds of patients had one or more recur-

rences during a follow-up period averaging 8 years. The risk of rheumatic fever following streptococcal infection is about 10 times greater in persons who have had one attack than it is in the general population. Recurrences are most likely to occur in younger children, in the years immediately after an attack, in patients with heart disease, and in those who have had multiple attacks. Patients with rheumatic heart disease are susceptible to *subacute bacterial endocarditis* and should be protected against the possibility of this complication during dental and other surgical procedures which may result in bacteremia (Table 10-7).

LEWIS W. WANNAMAKER

REFERENCES

Albam, B., and others: Rheumatic Fever in Children and Adolescents: A Long-Term Epidemiologic Study of Subsequent Prophylaxis, Streptococcal Infections, and Clinical Sequelae. *Ann. Int. Med.,* 60: Supp. 5, No. 2, part II, 1964.

Aron, A. M., Freeman, J. M., and Carter, S.: The Natural History of Sydenham's Chorea. *Am. J. Med.,* 38:83, 1965.

Catanzaro, F. J., Rammelkamp, C. H., Jr., and Chamovitz, R.: Prevention of Rheumatic Fever by Treatment of Streptococcal Infections. II. Factors Responsible for Failures. *New England J. Med.,* 259:51, 1958.

Dorfman, A., Gross, J. I., and Lorincz, A. E.: The Treatment of Acute Rheumatic Fever. *Pediatrics,* 27:692, 1961.

Feinstein, A. R.: Standards, Stethoscopes, Steroids and Statistics. The Problem of Evaluating Treatment in Acute Rheumatic Fever. *Pediatrics,* 27:819, 1961.

Goldring, D., Behrer, M. R., Brown, G., and Elliot, G.: Rheumatic Pneumonitis. II. Report on the Clinical and Laboratory Findings in Twenty-Three Patients. *J. Pediat.,* 53:547, 1958.

Kuttner, A. G., and Mayer, F. E.: Carditis During Second Attacks of Rheumatic Fever. Its Incidence in Patients Without Clinical Evidence of Cardiac Involvement in Their Initial Rheumatic Episode. *New England J. Med.,* 268:1259, 1963.

Lendrum, B. L., Simon, A. J., and Mack, I.: Relation of Duration of Bed Rest in Acute Rheumatic Fever to Heart Disease Present 2 to 14 Years Later. *Pediatrics,* 24:389, 1959.

Marienfeld, C. J., Robins, M., Sandidge, R. P., and Findlan, C.: Rheumatic Fever and Rheumatic Heart Disease Among U.S. College Freshmen, 1956-60. *Pub. Health Rep.,* 79-789, 1964.

Markowitz, M., and Kuttner, A. G.: *Rheumatic Fever—Diagnosis, Management and Prevention.* Philadelphia, W. B. Saunders Company, 1965.

McCarty, M.: Missing Links in the Streptococcal Chain Leading to Rheumatic Fever. The T. Duckett Jones Memorial Lecture. *Circulation,* 24:488, 1964.

Stollerman, G. H.: Factors Determining the Attack Rate of Rheumatic Fever. *J.A.M.A.,* 177:823, 1961.

Taranta, A.: Relation of Isolated Recurrences of Sydenham's Chorea to Preceding Streptococcal Infections. *New England J. Med.,* 260:1204, 1959.

Uhr, J. W.: *The Streptococcus, Rheumatic Fever and Glomerulonephritis.* Baltimore, Williams & Wilkins Company, 1964.

United Kingdom and United States Joint Report: The Natural History of Rheumatic Fever and Rheumatic Heart Disease: Ten-Year Report of a Cooperative Clinical Trial of ACTH, Cortisone, and Aspirin. *Circulation,* 32:457, 1965.

Wood, H. F., and McCarty, M.: Laboratory Aids in the Diagnosis of Rheumatic Fever and in Evaluation of Disease Activity. *Am. J. Med.,* 17:768, 1954.

Zabriskie, J. B., and Freimer, E. H.: An Immunological Relationship Between the Group A Streptococcus and Mammalian Muscle. *J. Exp. Med.,* 124:661, 1966.

Clinical Use of the Microbiology Laboratory

Much of the responsibility for attaining satisfactory laboratory diagnosis of infectious diseases rests with the clinician. It is he, not the laboratory worker, who decides what specimens to collect, how to obtain them and which laboratory procedures to request. He must also see that the specimens are preserved properly until they can be delivered to the laboratory. Finally, he should be competent to make the correct interpretation of the results.

Choice of Specimens. The choice of specimens to be examined often makes the difference between diagnostic success and failure. The clinician, in many instances, will be guided by the patient's signs and symptoms as to the type of causative agent he should suspect. In other instances, however, the signs and symptoms may be so non-specific that he must ask the laboratory's help in ruling out a variety of agents. Material from the system of the body chiefly involved should be collected, e.g. cerebrospinal fluid from a patient with meningeal symptoms or blood from a patient with fever of undetermined origin. Consideration should also be given to possible portals of entry, such as the upper respiratory tract in patients with meningeal involvement.

In the choice of specimens the clinician must decide whether an attempt should be made to isolate the causative agent or to demonstrate the antibody response, or both. More than one culture is advisable when seeking a causative pathogen. In bacterial infections the method of choice is the demonstration of the offending organism by smear and culture, provided the disease is of short duration. As the infection progresses, however, isolation techniques may fail, and serologic tests should also be requested. Accurate diagnosis of viral diseases now depends largely on isolation of the infecting agent. Nevertheless a rise of specific antibody is required to prove that the isolate is causative rather than transient or nonpathogenic.

Collection and Preservation of Specimens for Isolation of Causative Agent. *Bacteria, fungi and protozoa.* A dry cotton or alginate swab is most efficient for the collection of specimens from the skin and mucous membrane. Contamination by insignificant organisms must be avoided through the removal of superficial organisms from skin lesions by the gentle application of alcohol-cotton before swabbing the deeper infected area. Despite the varied normal microbial flora on the mucous membranes, which cannot be removed, swabbing the infected area will often result in the isolation of an almost pure culture of the offending organism.

The proper preservation of swab specimens is important. Since drying is rapidly destructive to some pathogenic bacteria, swab specimens should be placed promptly in about 0.3 ml. of nutrient broth (Fig. 10-33). Swab specimens collected for

virus isolation also need careful attention (see below).

Specimens of body fluids should be collected aseptically. Culture of the blood is one of the most fruitful procedures in the diagnosis of bacterial disease. It should be done carefully before administration of antibiotics, using iodine-alcohol for skin cleansing. After the venipuncture a fresh needle should be used for inoculating the blood into at least 2 flasks of medium prewarmed to room temperature. If only 1 blood culture is possible before antibiotic therapy, then a sufficient sample should be obtained: e.g. 10 ml. from a newborn, 60 ml. from an adult, and proportional amounts between these ages. Not more than 10 ml. should be inoculated per flask. If penicillin therapy has been started, the bacteriologist must be notified so that he can add penicillinase immediately. Suprapubic puncture is the most satisfactory method of obtaining urine for culture. Cerebrospinal fluid from a patient with suspected bacterial meningitis should be incubated at 37°C. for 12 to 18 hours in addition to routine culture. Grossly turbid fluids may coagulate on standing, thus making the detection of organisms difficult and accurate cell counts impossible. In this situation a portion of the specimen should be collected in an oxalate tube for smear and cell count.

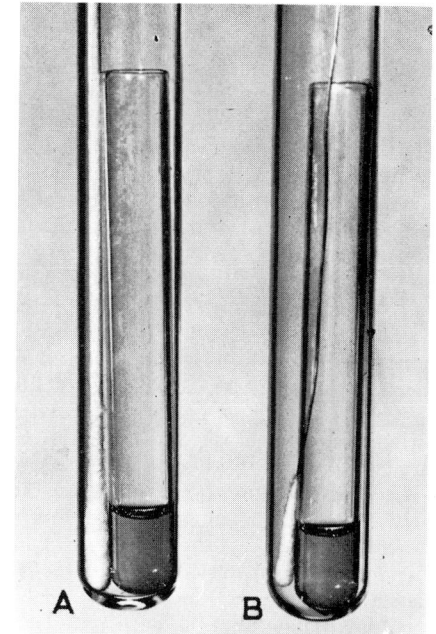

Figure 10-33. Throat and nasopharyngeal swab outfit. *A*, Wooden swab for collection of material from the throat and tonsils or for general use. *B*, Wire swab for collection of nasopharyngeal specimens. Both are contained in sterile cotton-plugged test tubes. After the test material has been obtained the swabs are immersed in the broth in the inner tube.

Immediate study of bacteriologic and parasite specimens is always desirable and in some instances essential. For example, darkfield examination for spirochetes is practically useless 30 minutes after the material has been collected. Whenever there is delay in transferring bacteriologic specimens to the laboratory, they should be stored in the refrigerator, but should not be permitted to freeze. Specimens of cerebrospinal fluid from patients with suspected bacterial meningitis should be stored at 37° C.

Viruses and rickettsiae. If viral disease is a diagnostic possibility when the patient is first seen, immediate steps should be taken to confirm the diagnosis, since delay usually nullifies attempts at isolation and makes serologic results more difficult to interpret. It is helpful to attempt isolation from several samples. Routinely, throat and stool or rectal swab specimens should be submitted. Throat specimens are best taken by means of vigorous throat swabbing which results in removing some superficial cells. For certain viruses, e.g. rubella, swabs should be taken from the nasal turbinates. The swab should be rinsed thoroughly in a fluid medium (nutrient broth or 0.5 per cent gelatin in Hanks' solution), squeezed against the glass and discarded. Discarding of the swab is important because the chlorine used for bleaching the stick is toxic for tissue culture cells in which virus isolation will be attempted. If the laboratory is reasonably close, storage of specimens at 4°C. for a few hours is permissible. For mailing, the specimen should be frozen and packed in sufficient dry ice for the journey. Isolation of virus from cerebrospinal fluid, owing to the low protein content, is ideally accomplished by immediate transfer to the virus laboratory.

Collection and Preservation of Specimens for Serologic Tests. Correct diagnosis from serologic tests requires at least 2 blood specimens. The first should be taken at the time of the first examination during the early acute phase of the disease ("acute serum"), the second ("convalescent") 14 to 21 days later. If this is taken earlier than 14 days, it is advisable to take a third blood specimen 4 to 6 weeks after the onset, since the rise of antibodies may be delayed, especially in infants. Great care must be taken to avoid contamination and hemolysis. An aseptic venous puncture, removal of the needle before emptying the syringe into the tube, avoidance of air bubbles and early separation of serum are all very important factors in obtaining the best results. Serum should be frozen for preservation, *but whole blood should never be.*

Laboratory Procedures. There are 2 principal types of diagnostic procedures in microbiology. The first is the direct method, whereby the infectious agent is identified in clinical material by direct microscopy, culture, injection into susceptible laboratory hosts or by a combination of these methods. The second is the indirect approach, through the detection of specific antibody either by skin tests or by serologic procedures. In general the direct method yields more reliable information for diagnosis, since the correct interpretation of immunologic tests is often difficult.

Direct visualization. It is sometimes possible to identify the agent by routine microscopy of clinical material at the time it is cultured. In order to do so the organism must have a characteristic physical appearance (spirochetes, amebae), unusual staining properties (tubercle bacillus) or be the only organism present in the specimen. By virtue of the larger size and more varied morphology of fungi, direct microscopy is an important diagnostic step for the mycoses; it is essentially the only one needed for the diagnosis of parasitic diseases. In certain viral infections, scrapings from the lesion reveal characteristically altered cells which are of immediate aid in differential diagnosis.

Fluorescent antibody (FA) technique has widened the diagnostic scope of direct microscopy (Table 10-8). A number of specific antiserums are now available commercially for several common pathogens. In these serums the antibody molecules have been conjugated with a fluorescent dye. The specific dye-labeled serum is added to the smear containing the suspected organism and the slide examined microscopically under ultraviolet light. If the organism is present, the antibody molecules are concentrated about it and the observer sees a bright fluorescence. The presence of only a few organisms in the smear can be detected in this manner. This is the *direct method*, which is the more useful if specific labeled serums are readily available. In the absence of such serums the *indirect method* is useful, although it leads to somewhat more nonspecific fluorescence than the direct. In this method there are 2 steps: (1) The slide is covered with the *unlabeled* specific serum; time is allowed for antibodies to fix, and then the excess of unfixed antibody is washed off. (2) The slide is then overlaid with a dye-labeled antispecies gamma globulin. The antigamma globulin antibodies are concentrated at the site of the specific microorganism-antibody complex and fluoresce.

Isolation of agent. Successful cultivation of the causative organism on artificial media is the mainstay of bacteriologic and mycologic diagnosis. Viruses and rickettsiae require living cells for propagation, namely, laboratory animals, embryonated hen's eggs or tissue cultures of human or animal cells.

Detection of antibodies. The host produces antibodies in response to infection even when it is subclinical. The amount of antibody varies with the nature of the infectious agent. Enteric gram-negative bacilli, exotoxin-producing agents, viruses and rickettsiae are good, whereas fungi and animal parasites are, as a rule, poor antigens.

Antibodies can be detected by a variety of specific serologic methods, one method being more appropriate than another for different agents.

Agglutination antibodies are primarily sought in the diagnosis of bacterial infections, the antigen being either the intact cell or a fraction of it adsorbed to a particulate carrier such as type O human erythrocytes or latex particles. A modification of the agglutination test, agglutination-lysis, is standard for the diagnosis of leptospiral infections. Rickettsial infections can also be diagnosed by identifying agglutinating antibodies using antigens prepared from infected yolk sacs. *Complement-fixing antibodies* are utilized in the diagnosis of syphilis and the majority of viral and rickettsial infections, and are being used with increasing frequency in the diagnosis of some fungal and protozoal diseases. *Hemagglutination-inhibiting antibodies:* Certain viruses, such as the myxoviruses, vaccinia and some enteroviruses, have the capacity to agglutinate erythrocytes. The presence of antibodies which prevent this can be detected by the extent to which a particular serum specifically inhibits hemagglutination. *Fluorescent antibodies* can be detected by the technique of indirect fluorescence (see above). *Precipitation antibodies:* These are useful in the serologic diagnosis of helminthic infections. They are detected by the appearance of a white precipitate when the antigen prepared from the suspected parasite is added to an antibody-containing serum. *Neutralizing antibodies* can be detected in all viral infections for which suitable laboratory hosts are available; this test has the advantage of a high degree of specificity, but is more complicated and expensive than those listed above.

Nonspecific methods. Certain infectious agents, including rickettsiae, PPLO organisms and certain viruses, lead to the development of antibodies to nonspecific antigens. For example, rickettsial infections can be suspected if the serum agglutinates one of the OX strains of proteus; mycoplasma-induced primary atypical pneumonia leads to the development of agglutinations for type O human erythrocytes in the cold; and infectious mononucleosis is associated with the presence of a certain type of heterophile antibody.

Skin tests. The presence of specific hypersensitivity to infectious agents can also be detected by immunologic procedures in which the suspected antigen is injected into the skin of the patient (see Table 10-8).

Interpretation of Results. Direct visualization of microorganisms in certain gram-stained clinical material is a rapid diagnostic aid which often permits initiation of rational therapy. It is of little help with specimens coming from mucous membranes, because few of the pathogenic bacteria are distinguishable microscopically from constituents of the normal flora. Even in the case of pathogens which have a distinctive morphologic feature, e.g. *M. tuberculosis* and *C. diphtheriae*, identification is still provisional unless specifically diagnosed by fluorescent antibody.

Culture methods are the principal diagnostic tools in bacteriology, and they are likely to remain so, since bacteria must be cultured to determine their chemotherapeutic susceptibility. Viral cultures also have diagnostic value.

It is important, however, to remember that the presence of a pathogen in a specimen does not in itself establish a causative relation, since the patient may only be carrying the organism. But, for practical purposes, the heavy growth of a particular pathogen, if consistent with the clinical picture, can be assumed to establish a causative relation. Proof of this requires the demonstration of a rising titer of specific antibody in the patient's serum.

Serologic tests, as noted above, are essential, when available, for establishing the etiology of a given pathogen. For diagnosis a fourfold rise of specific antibody against the isolated agent within the convalescent (3 to 6 weeks after onset of illness) serum, as compared with that in the acute one, is required. Without the isolation of a pathogen from the patient, the finding of a fourfold rise to a suspected agent, especially an enterovirus or enteric bacillus, may not be specific for that agent, but only represent a booster response to an antigen shared by a number of enteroviruses or enteric bacilli. For the clinician this may at least establish the causative agent as belonging to a group of pathogens, even if the individual agent cannot be categorized.

The finding of a positive titer against the suspected agent in a single specimen of serum, either late acute or convalescent, will not differentiate between a recent and a past infection, so that 2 serum specimens are usually mandatory for a definitive diagnosis. But under the following circumstances the study of a single serum can strongly support a clinically made diagnosis: (1) a high antibody level as compared with that of the population in general; (2) in neonates (up to 1 month) antibody in the IgM fraction; (3) antibody in the infant not present in the mother; (4) antibody in both infant and mother, but persisting at birth level in the infant; (5) in suspected mumps, the presence of antibody to the soluble ("S") fraction of the mumps virus in the acute serum. This antibody may be found as early as the second or third day of the disease when that to the viral ("V") antigen may be absent or very low; (6) in typhoid fever, the presence of Vi antibody.

The value of skin tests is limited by the inability to distinguish between recent and past infections and by the possibility of cross reactions.

T. F. McNair Scott
Stanley A. Plotkin

TABLE 10-8. SELECTION OF DIAGNOSTIC MICROBIOLOGIC SPECIMENS[1]

SUSPECTED AGENT	SPECIMENS	LABORATORY EXAMINATION
Systemic Infection		
Bacterial		
Meningococcus		Culture[2a, b, c, d, e]
Pneumococcus		Inoculate guinea pig for brucella and
Staphylococcus	Blood, whole, 10 ml.	glanders
Coliform bacilli	Lymph node or bone marrow	
Proteus		See also *Respiratory, Nervous System,*
Pseudomonas		and *Urinary Infections*
Glanders bacillus		
Listeria		
Streptobacillus		
Mima polymorpha		
Bacterioides		
Streptococcus	Blood, clotted, 5-10 ml.[3]	Comparative tube agglutination tests
Salmonella		Widal test for salmonella; antistrepto-
Brucella		lysin O, antihyaluronidase, and C-
Plague bacillus		reactive protein for streptococci
Tularemia bacillus		
Mycobacteria		See *Respiratory* and *Nervous System Infections*
Spirillum	Blood	Giemsa-stained thick smears
		Inoculate rat
Fungal		Giemsa- or silver-stained smears
Histoplasmosis†	Bone marrow; lymph node	Culture[2f]
Candida	Blood, heparinized, 10 ml.	See *Respiratory Infection*
Phycomyces	Blood, clotted 5-10 ml.[3]	Comparative CF[3] tests
Spirochetal		
Leptospira	Blood, whole	
	Cerebrospinal fluid and/or urine	Culture[2g]
Borrelia		Inoculate young guinea pig (lepto-spira) or young white rat (borrelia)
	Blood, heparinized, 5 ml.	Microscopic darkfield of blood from patient and inoculated animal (borrelia)
Protozoan		
Haemosporina (malaria)	Blood	Giemsa-stained thick smears
Toxoplasma†,[5]	Biopsy, lymph nodes, bone marrow	Giemsa-stained thick smears
Leishmania†		Inoculate mice or hamsters (toxoplasma)
Trypanosoma	Blood, whole	Culture[2h] (leishmania and trypanosoma)
	Blood, clotted, 5-10 ml.[3]	CF[3], HAI[3], slide agglutination
		Sabin-Feldman dye test (toxoplasma)
		indirect FA[3] (malaria)
Helminthic		
Trematodes		See *Gastrointestinal, urinary,* and *Respiratory Infections*
Cestodes		
Filariae†	Blood, usually taken at night	Giemsa-stained thick smears
Toxicara canis (cati)		
Echinococcus†	Biopsy of affected organ	Microscopic for larvae
Trichinella spiralis†		
All of above	Blood, clotted, 5-10 ml.[3]	CF[3], HA[3], latex slide agglutination, flocculation, precipitin reactions with appropriate worm antigens

MICROBIOLOGIC

TABLE 10-8. *Continued*

SUSPECTED AGENT	SPECIMENS	LABORATORY EXAMINATION
Viral[6]		
Mumps†	Saliva[4]	Inoculate appropriate tissue cultures (all); embryonated eggs (mumps, herpesviruses); suckling mice 48 hours old (enteroviruses, herpesviruses, ArBo viruses, LCM)
Cytomegalovirus	Urine (uncontaminated, at 4°C.)	
Enteroviruses[7]	Throat and rectal swabs[4]	
Measles / German measles	Nose and throat swabs[4]	
Herpesviruses[8]	Vesicle fluid, saliva[4] / Throat swabs	
ArBo viruses[9] / Lymphocytic chorio-meningitis virus (LCM)	Blood clot, emulsify / Keep frozen in dry ice	
EB virus (infectious mononucleosis)	Blood	Count and smear for atypical lymphocytes
For all above	Blood, clotted, 5-10 ml.[3]	CF[3] on acute serum for mumps viral and soluble antigens / Comparative CF[3], HAI[3], neutralization tests; indirect FA[3] (EB virus)
Rickettsial[5]		
Typhus fever group (epidemic; murine, scrub)	Blood clot, emulsified / Keep frozen in dry ice	Inoculate male guinea pigs and yolk sac of embryonated eggs
Rocky Mountain spotted fever		
Rickettsialpox	Blood, clotted, 5-10 ml.[3]	Comparative CF[3], ESS[3], Weil-Felix tests
Q fever		

Respiratory Infection (Including Mouth)

SUSPECTED AGENT	SPECIMENS	LABORATORY EXAMINATION
Bacterial		
Streptococcus, β-hemolytic	Throat or nasopharyngeal swabs[4]	Culture[2a, b, c]
Pneumococcus		Grouping for streptococcus and meningococcus
Meningococcus		
Influenza bacillus	Sputum[4]	"Quellung" reaction for pneumococci, meningococci and influenza bacillus
Staphylococcus		
Pseudomonas		
Proteus	Bronchial aspiration[4]	Coagulase for staphylococcus
Coliform bacilli		
Plague bacillus		See *Skin, Wound and Lymph Node Infections*
Diphtheria†	Pharyngeal, laryngeal or nasopharyngeal swabs[4]	Methylene blue-stained smears / Direct FA[3] / Culture[2a, 2i] / Toxigenicity test
Pertussis†	Nasopharyngeal swab[4]	Direct FA[3] / Culture[2j]
Mycobacteria†	Sputum, early morning specimen / Gastric aspiration × 3	Acid-fast-stained smears / Culture[2k] / Fluorescent-stained smears
Fusobacterium fusiforme	Scraping	Gram-stained smears / Culture[2a, 2l]

SUSPECTED AGENT	SPECIMENS	LABORATORY EXAMINATION
Mycoplasma		
M. pneumoniae (PPLO; Eaton's agent)	Throat swab, washings, sputum[4]	Culture[2m] at 36°C.
	Blood, clotted, 5-10 ml.[3]	Comparative CF[3]; cold agglutinins; indirect FA[3]
Protozoan		
Pneumocystis carinii	Lung puncture / Tracheal aspirate	Giemsa- or silver-stained smears

(Table continues)

TABLE 10-8. *Continued*

M
I
C
R
O
B
I
O
L
O
G
I
C

SUSPECTED AGENT	SPECIMENS	LABORATORY EXAMINATION
Fungal Actinomycetes Nocardia Coccidioides† Aspergillus Histoplasma† Cryptococcus Candida	Sputum[4] Pharyngeal swab[4] Pus and granules	Gram-stained smears for actinomycetes and nocardia; lactophenol-cotton blue, silver- or Giemsa-stained smears for others Culture[2f] Inoculate mice (coccidioides)
All of above	Blood, clotted, 5-10 ml.[3]	Comparative CF[3] and precipitin tests
Viral[6] Adenoviruses[10] Myxoviruses[11] Respiratory syncytial (RS) Rhinoviruses[12] IBV-like viruses[13] Enteroviruses[7] Reoviruses[14] Herpesviruses[8]	Nose, throat and rectal swabs[4]	Inoculate appropriate tissue culture (all); embryonated eggs (myxo- and herpesviruses); organ culture (IBV-like viruses)
All of above	Blood, clotted, 5-10 ml.[3]	Comparative CF[3], neutralization, HAI[3] tests
Rickettsial[5] Q fever	Blood clot, emulsified; Sputum – keep frozen in dry ice	Inoculate guinea pigs
	Blood, clotted, 5-10 ml.[3]	Comparative CF[3] and agglutination tests
Bedsonia[5] Psittacosis Ornithosis	Blood clot, emulsified; sputum; throat washings; vomitus; organ emulsions – keep frozen in dry ice.	Inoculate mice or embryonated eggs
	Blood, clotted, 5-10 ml.[3]	Comparative CF[3] tests
Gastrointestinal Infection *Bacterial* Salmonella Shigella Enteropathogenic E. coli Staphylococci	Rectal swab[4]	Direct FA[3] Culture[2a, 2c] Identification by serologic typing
Salmonella	Blood, clotted, 5-10 ml.[3]	Comparative slide and/or tube agglutinations Vi antibody, when indicated See also *Systemic Infection*
Vibrio cholera	Feces or rectal swab	Immediate culture[2n]
	Blood, clotted, 5-10 ml.[3]	Comparative agglutinations
Fungal Candida	Rectal swab[4]	Culture[2f]
Protozoan Entamoeba histolytica Giardia lamblia Balantidium coli Isospora belli and hominis	Fresh stool after purgation Keep warm Sigmoidoscopic specimen – same	Warm stage for trophozoites of E. histolytica, B. coli and G. lamblia
	Stool	Direct smears, concentration and flotation techniques for cysts

TABLE 10-8. *Continued*

SUSPECTED AGENT	SPECIMENS	LABORATORY EXAMINATION
Helminthic		
Trematodes (flukes)		
Fasciola buski and hepatica		
Clonorchis sinensis		
Schistosoma mansoni		
and japonicum		
Cestodes (tapeworms)	Stool	Direct smear, concentration and flota-
Taenia saginata and	Duodenal and/or proctoscopic	tion techniques for ova, larvae and
solium	aspirates	proglottids
Hymenolepis nana		
Diphyllobothrium latum		
Nematodes (roundworms)		
Ascaris lumbricoides		
(large roundworm)		
Necator americanus and		
Ancylostoma duodenale		
(hookworms)		
Trichuris trichiura		
(whipworm)		
Strongyloides stercoralis	NIH cellophane swab or Scotch	
Enterobius vermicularis	tape smear from perineum in	Microscopic of swab or tape for ova
(pinworm)	early morning	
Viral		See *Systemic and Respiratory Infec-* *tions*
Nervous System Infection		
Bacterial		
Pneumococcus		
Meningococcus	Cerebrospinal fluid; avoid delay	Cell count, sugar
Influenza bacillus		Gram-stained smears of sediment
Staphylococcus		
Streptococcus		
Coliform bacilli	Blood, whole, 10 ml.; add directly	Culture[2a, b, c]
Salmonella	to culture medium	Antibiotic susceptibility
Pseudomonas	Nasopharyngeal swabs[4]	Serologic typing when indicated
Proteus		Direct FA[3] (influenza bacillus, listeria)
Listeria monocytogenes		
Mima polymorpha		
For all (under special cir-	Blood, clotted, 5-10 ml.[3]	For comparative slide or tube aggluti-
cumstances, but not		nations
used as routine)		
Mycobacteria†	Cerebrospinal fluid	Cell count
		Direct fluorescent-stained and Ziehl-
		Neelsen acid-fast-stained smears of
		sediment or fibrin clot
		Culture[2k]
Spirochetal		
Leptospira		See *Systemic Infection*
Treponema pallidum		See *Genital Tract Infection*
Fungal		
Cryptococcus	Cerebrospinal fluid	Culture[2f]
		Inoculate mice
Candida		Gram-stained smears of sediment
Protozoan		
Toxoplasma†, [5]	Cerebrospinal fluid	Giemsa-stained smears of sediment
	Blood, clotted, 5-10 ml.[3]	Comparative HAI[3], Sabin-Feldman dye, CF[3] tests

(Table continues)

TABLE 10-8. *Continued*

SUSPECTED AGENT	SPECIMENS	LABORATORY EXAMINATION
Acanthamoeba (Hartmanella)	Cerebrospinal fluid Brain biopsy	Culture on HeLa cells or special medium[20]; Giemsa-stained smears of growth Warm-stage examination for motile forms Hematoxylin-eosin stained fixed sections
Trypanosoma rhodesiense (sleeping sickness)	CSF, lymph node aspiration	See *Systemic Infection*

Viral[6]

Rabies	Brain or spinal cord Take aseptically Store at −20°C. in glycerol or keep frozen in dry ice	Contact smears for Negri bodies and direct FA[3] Inoculate into mice
ArBo viruses[9] Mumps Lymphocytic chorio-meningitis (LCM) Enteroviruses[7] Herpesviruses[8] Cytomegalic inclusion viruses	Cerebrospinal fluid	Cell count, sugar Inoculate into suckling mice, eggs and tissue culture
	Throat and rectal swabs[4]	See *Systemic Infection*
For all of above	Blood, clotted, 5-10 ml.[3]	Comparative CF[3], neutralizing or HAI[3] tests

Genital Infection

Bacterial

Gonococcus Staphylococcus Streptococcus	Swabs from cervix, vagina and/or urethra	Direct FA[3]; Gram-stained smears Culture[2a, b]
Ducrey's bacillus	Aspirate from lesion	Gram-stained smear Culture[2p]
Mycobacteria		See *Skin, Wound and Lymph Node Infections*
Fusobacterium fusiforme	Scrapings from lesion	See *Respiratory Infection*

Spirochetal

Treponema pallidum	Scrapings from chancre in saline or buffer	Microscopic darkfield
	Blood, clotted, 5-10 ml.[3] Cerebrospinal fluid	Serologic tests[15]

Fungal

Candida	Swabs or saline washings from vagina	Microscopic of wet lactophenol-cotton blue mounts Culture[2f]

Protozoan

Trichomonas	Swab or saline washings from vagina	Microscopic of wet mounts

Helminthic

Filaria		See *Systemic Infection*

Viral

Herpesviruses[8]	Vesicle fluid, pus or cervical scraping[4]	Inoculate eggs, tissue culture, suckling mice
Bedsonia		
Lymphogranuloma venereum (LGV)†	Scraping of lesion	Giemsa-stained smears for giant cells (herpesviruses) and elementary bodies (LGV)
For both of above	Blood, clotted, 5-10 ml.[3]	Comparative CF[3], neutralization tests

M I C R O B I O L O G I C

TABLE 10-8. *Continued*

SUSPECTED AGENT	SPECIMENS	LABORATORY EXAMINATION

Urinary Infection
  Bacterial

Coliform bacilli Streptococcus Proteus Pseudomonas Staphylococcus Moraxella-Mima species	Aseptically collected urine by careful midstream or suprapubic puncture	Immediate colony count—uncentrifuged Culture[2q] centrifuged sediment Gram-stained smears of sediment
Mycobacteria†	As above (early morning specimen)	Decontaminate centrifuged sediment with NaOH 4% Digest with acetylcystine Culture[2k]

Helminthic
  Schistosoma hematobium ....As above ....Microscopic of sediment for ova

Skin, Wound and Lymph Node Infection
  Bacterial

Staphylococcus Streptococcus Enterococcus Anaerobic streptococcus Anthrax bacillus Pseudomonas Proteus Coliform bacilli Bacterioides Diphtheria	Swabs[4]	Direct FA[3] smears (diphtheria, streptococcus) Culture[2a, 2c] See also under *Respiratory Infection (Diphtheria)*
Tetanus Gas gangrene	Pieces of debrided tissue, ground up with broth	Gram-stained smears of tissue juice Culture[21] Toxigenicity test, if indicated
Tularemia bacillus Plague bacillus	Swab or aspirate from bubo Blood, whole, 10 ml.	Direct FA[3] and gram-stained smear Culture[2a, 2c]

Mycobacteria
  Tubercle bacillus†
  Atypical mycobacteria†
  Leprosy†
	Scraping
	
	Biopsy
		Culture[2k]
		Acid-fast and fluorescent-stained smears
		Microscopic for acid-fast organism in sections

For all	Blood, clotted, 5-10 ml.[3]	Comparative agglutination tests

Spirochetal

Treponema pallidum (syphilis) T. pertenue (yaws) T. carateum (pinta)	Scrapings from lesion Blood, clotted[3]	Microscopic darkfield Serologic tests with T. pallidum[15]

Protozoan
  Leishmania braziliensis ....See *Systemic Infection*

Fungal

Actinomycetes Blastomyces† Histoplasma† Coccidioides† Sporotrichum Allescheria Hormodendrum Dermatophytes	Pus with granules, crusts or scrapings	Microscopic of KOH 10% and/or lactophenol-cotton blue mounts; Giemsa- and Gram-stained smears Culture[2a, 2f]

MICROBIOLOGIC

(Table continues)

TABLE 10-8. *Continued*

SUSPECTED AGENT	SPECIMENS	LABORATORY EXAMINATION
Viral[6]		
Herpesviruses[8] Variola ············· [Vesicle fluid Vaccinia Scraping of lesion] ·············		Inoculate suckling mice, eggs, tissue culture Giemsa-stained smears for giant cells (herpesviruses) or elementary bodies (poxviruses)
For all ·················Blood, clotted, 5-10 ml.[3] ·················		Comparative CF[3], HAI[3] neutralization tests
Molluscum contagiosum··········Biopsy ·············		Microscopic for characteristic histology
Cat-scratch disease† ···········Pus from bubo ·················		Prepare heated skin test material

Eye Infection
  Bacterial

Staphylococcus Streptococcus Pneumococcus Gonococcus Influenza bacillus ···········Swabs[4]················· Proteus Pseudomonas Moraxella-Mima Kochs-Weeks bacillus		Gram-stained smears Culture[2a, b]

  Helminthic

Sparganum species·················Incision of eye lesion ···········Naked eye for larvae		
Onchocerca volvulus···············Aspiration anterior chamber ···············Microscopic of fluid for microfilariae		

  Bedsonia

Inclusion blennorrhea Lymphogranuloma ···········Scraping ············· venereum Trachoma		Giemsa-stained smears for inclusions and elementary bodies; direct FA[3] Inoculate embryonated eggs

  Viral[6]

Herpesviruses[8] Adenoviruses[10] ·········Swabs[4]·············		Inoculate suckling mice, eggs or tissue culture
Variola Vaccinia Newcastle disease ·········Scraping ············· Molluscum contagiosum		Giemsa-stained smear for inclusion and elementary bodies
Cat-scratch disease·················Not diagnostic ·················		Skin test with antigen prepared from infected lymph node

Both Bedsonia and Viral···········Blood, clotted, 5-10 ml.[3] ·················		Comparative CF[3], HAI[3], neutralization tests

† Skin test available.

[1] The help of Mr. John McKitrick (Bacteriologist to The Children's Hospital of Philadelphia) in the preparation of this table is gratefully acknowledged.

[2a] Blood plates and thioglycollate broth.

[2b] Neisseria; chocolate agar and incubate in 5-10% CO_2.

[2c] Enteric bacteria; blood, EMB, phenyl ethyl alcohol plates, S.S. agar plates and tetrathionate broth.

[2d] Brucella; special broth (Albimi Lab.) incubated in 25% CO_2.

[2e] Tularemia bacillus; blood dextrose cystine agar.

[2f] Blood agar at 36°C. and Sabouraud's glucose agar at 21°C. (room temperature).

[2g] Leptospira; 0.03 ml. into 15 ml. of tryptose-phosphate broth, enriched with 10% heat-inactivated rabbit serum; incubate at 28-30°C. for 28 days.

[2h] Inoculate 4 slants NNN medium; incubate in dark at 20°C.

[2i] Tellurite, Loefflers, K.L. virulence agar.

[2j] Bordet-Gengou medium.

[2k] Lowenstein-Jensen or Middlebrook media.

[2l] Anaerobic bacteria; blood plates in anaerobic jar, and thioglycollate.

[2m] Hayflick's Horse Serum medium.

[2n] Alkaline peptone broth, pH 8.4.

[20] Special Trypticase agar (⅕ the usual amount of trypticase soy medium ingredient in 1.5% agar); seed with a small inoculum of Aerobacter (singh) and incubate at room temperature (20-22°C.) for 24 hours. Inoculate with small droplets and leave at room temperature. Examine after 24 hours daily for clear areas of amebic growth.

[2p] Clotted rabbit blood in 5-10% CO_2.

[2q] Urine; blood plates, EMB plates, and thioglycollate broth.

[3] The bloods should be centrifuged to separate serums, which should then be preserved at −20°C. for subsequent testing. Serologic tests for circulating antibodies are most helpful when paired specimens are tested; the first obtained as early in the clinical course as possible, the second 1 to 3 weeks later. In some viral and fungal infections a third specimen, obtained at 6 weeks, should also be tested. Routine serologic tests include CF (complement fixation), FA (fluorescent antibody), HAI (hemagglutination inhibition), ESS (erythrocyte sensitizing substance) and neutralization.

[4] Saliva or swabs; if not inoculated immediately, place in 0.3 ml. of nutrient broth or Hanks' solution containing 0.5% gelatin.

[5] Dangerous to laboratory personnel, and isolation should not be undertaken without special precautions.

[6] Viruses listed under each system refer to the usual viruses isolated from that system.

[7] Enteroviruses consist of poliomyelitis viruses, Coxsackie groups A and B, and ECHO.

[8] Herpesviruses include H. hominis (simplex), H. varicellae (varicella and zoster), H. simii (B. virus).

[9] ArBo (arthropod-borne viruses). Many types exist; those of clinical importance include *group A* −Eastern, Western and Venezuelan equine encephalitis; Chikungunya; *group B* −dengue complex; yellow fever; St. Louis, Japanese B. and Murray Valley encephalitides; West Nile; tickborne encephalitis such as Omsk hemorrhagic fever, Kyasanur Forest disease; louping ill; *nongrouped* −California encephalitis type viruses, and a number of others.

[10] Adenoviruses; types 1, 2, 3, 4, 7, 8, 14, 21 are important causes of clinical illness. Pharyngoconjunctival fever, types 1, 3, 7. Epidemic keratoconjunctivitis, type 8.

[11] Myxoviruses include influenza A, B, C; parainfluenza 1, 2, 3, 4; respiratory syncytial virus; mumps; Newcastle disease; rubeola.

[12] Rhinoviruses require a low temperature (33°C.) and a neutral pH for propagation in rolled tissue culture. H. rhinoviruses only grown in human embryo kidney or human diploid fibroblasts. M. rhinoviruses grow also in several species of monkey kidney cells.

[13] I.B.V. stands for viruses morphologically similar to infectious bronchitis virus of chickens, detectable by their ability to interfere with ciliary action in tracheal organ culture.

[14] Reoviruses include types 1, 2, 3.

[15] Tests for syphilis include VDRL test, Kolmer (CF test for reagin), FTA (fluorescent treponemal antibody), T.P.I. (Treponema pallidum immobilization). The specificity of the last two has been increased by recent modifications.

REFERENCES

Bailey, W. R., and Scott, E. G.: *Diagnostic Microbiology*. 2nd ed. St. Louis, C. V. Mosby Company, 1966.

Culbertson, C. G.: Pathogenic Acanthamoeba (Hartmanella). *Am. J. Clin. Path.*, 35:195, 1961.

Dubos, R. J., and Hirsch, J. G.: *Bacterial and Mycotic Infections of Man*. 4th ed. Philadelphia, J. B. Lippincott Company, 1965.

Edwards, P. R., and Ewing, W. H.: *Identification of Enterobacteriaceae*. 2nd ed. Minneapolis, Burgess Publishing Co., 1962.

Faust, E. C., Beaver, P. C., and Jung, R. C.: *Animal Agents and Vectors of Human Disease*. 3rd ed. Philadelphia, Lea & Febiger, 1968.

Horsfall, F. L., Jr., and Tamm, I.: *Viral and Rickettsial Infections of Man*. 4th ed. Philadelphia, J. B. Lippincott Company, 1965.

Lennette, E. H., and Schmidt, N. J.: *Diagnostic Procedures for Viral and Rickettsial Diseases*. 3rd ed. New York, American Public Health Association, 1964.

Wilson, Sir Graham S., and Miles, A. A.: *Topley and Wilson's Principles of Bacteriology and Immunity*. 5th ed. Baltimore, Williams & Wilkins Company, 1964.

Isolation Measures for Infectious Diseases

The care of a patient with a communicable disease should include measures to prevent others from contracting it. Certain quarantine practices, which vary somewhat in different localities, have been set up for the protection of the community (Table 10-9). Quarantine regulations have at best a limited value in control of the spread of contagious diseases. In many places "placarding" is no longer practiced. Until effective vaccines for active immunization are widely available there are substantial arguments in favor of permitting children to contract German measles, chickenpox and mumps during the preadolescent years, provided they are in good health at the time. For the control of poliomyelitis, diphtheria, smallpox, pertussis and measles artificially induced immunity is of greatest importance.

The patient with a contagious disease should be isolated, not only to limit distribution of the disease, but also to protect him from secondary infection.

Isolation technique necessitates cooperation of physician, nurse and family, and, in hospitals, of all personnel, including orderlies and maids, who come in contact with the patient or his environment. An error in technique by any of these persons may defeat the efforts of the others.

The patient is regarded as a contaminated unit,

TABLE 10-9. SUGGESTIONS FOR QUARANTINE REGULATIONS

DISEASE	PATIENT IS RELEASED FROM ISOLATION AND MAY RETURN TO SCHOOL	SUSCEPTIBLE CONTACTS MAY RE-ENTER SCHOOL	IMMUNE CONTACTS MAY RE-ENTER SCHOOL
Diphtheria	On recovery, and after 2 or 3 successive negative cultures; each from nose and throat; taken after cessation of antimicrobial therapy and at intervals of not less than 24 hours.	When 2 or more successive cultures of nose and throat are negative, or not for at least 7 days after last exposure	If bacteriologically negative
Scarlet fever.....	Upon clinical recovery, but not less than 7 days from onset	No restriction	No restriction
Measles	On recovery; at least 8 or 9 days (5 days after appearance of rash)	Exclusion from school of no practical value; when practiced, at least 14 days must elapse after last exposure	No restriction
German measles	Quarantine is usually not imposed. Period of infectivity estimated from 7 days before and 4 to 5 days after appearance of rash	No restriction	No restriction
Smallpox	On recovery and after disappearance of scabs and crusts; usually 3 to 6 weeks	16 days after successful vaccination	If there is not continued exposure and if successfully vaccinated within 5 years. The person should be vaccinated whenever exposure occurs even if there has been a previous successful "take"
Chickenpox......	On recovery and when crusts have formed; not sooner than 7 days after onset	Exclusion from school of no practical value; when practiced, at least 21 days must elapse after exposure	No restriction
Pertussis	Not before 3 weeks after onset of typical paroxysms	14 days after exposure	No restriction
Poliomyelitis ...	One week after onset of symptoms or after defervescence, whichever is longer	No restriction	No restriction
Mumps............	When swelling has disappeared	No restriction	No restriction
Infectious hepatitis	After first week of illness	No restriction	No restriction

Adapted from several sources, principally from the Control of Communicable Diseases, The American Public Health Association, New York, 1960, and Report of the Committee on the Control of Infectious Diseases, American Academy of Pediatrics, 1966.

and the area in which he is—whether a room in home or hospital, a cubicle or space in a ward—as a contaminated unit area. The space between beds in an open ward should be at least 6 feet. Anything which comes in contact with the unit area must be considered contaminated. Isolation precautions for persons entering and leaving the unit area are based on "hand and gown technique"; all physicians and nurses should be familiar with an approved method. When the child is to be cared for by a nonprofessional attendant at home, e.g. the mother, adequate instruction should be given by the physician.

Infectious agents may also be transferred to another person by air conduction. The control of airborne infection is still not adequately solved for practical application. Oiling of floors and of bed blankets would appear to be as useful a method as any; air sterilization with ultraviolet irradiation or an aerosol has a limited effectiveness in reducing the spread of infection in institutions. Antibiotic treatment of bacterial infections is the most effective means for limiting their spread.

The unit area must be properly equipped to care for the patient, and nothing should be taken into it that is not necessary or cannot later be destroyed or sterilized. The trays and dishes—or the bottles for infants—should be sterilized after each use by boiling or autoclaving.

A bedpan should be provided for each patient. In the home a special bathroom reserved for the isolated area is a great convenience.

Bed linen and clothing, including diapers,

should be sterilized in an autoclave; in the home they should be boiled before being sent to the laundry.

Secretions from the eyes, nose, mouth and throat should be received on soft paper squares which are placed in a paper bag and burned.

All attendants should be in good health and free of infection of the respiratory tract.

The patient should be discharged from the unit area only after thorough bathing with soap and warm water, including a shampoo. He should not, of course, return to the contaminated area.

Other materials, as well as the floor and furniture of the room, should be thoroughly washed with soap and water, and the room aired for at least 24 hours before again being occupied.

Material in the unit area which cannot be burned is cleansed as follows: all clothing and linen, as already described; mattresses and pillows are aired for 6 to 8 hours, preferably on 2 successive days; all glass, rubber, china, enamelware and any instruments which permit it are boiled for 5 to 10 minutes, or autoclaved, or put into 2 per cent cresol solution or 1:5000 Zephiran for 18 hours.

When a patient is to be taken to an operating or x-ray room, or is transferred to another unit area, the accompanying attendant must wear a clean gown, and the patient should be wrapped in a clean sheet. Equipment in the operating or x-ray room which has been contaminated should be cleaned in the manner described for the unit area.

WALDO E. NELSON

Bacterial Infections

Streptococcal Infections

General Considerations

The streptococci collectively constitute a large group of microorganisms with varied biologic characteristics. They are gram-positive and tend to grow in chains. Strains which infect man are chiefly hemolytic, a property useful for cultural identification. Nonhemolytic streptococci are mostly saprophytes which inhabit the upper respiratory tract and the intestine. They are occasionally associated with infections of the heart valves, urinary tract and wounds.

Classification. Schottmüller (1903) grouped streptococci as hemolytic, green and indifferent, according to their action on red blood cells in culture. Brown (1919) described them as alpha, beta or gamma, according to whether they produce slight, distinct or no hemolysis of red blood cells. In this latter classification most pathogenic strains are in the beta group.

Studies of the antigenic structure of the streptococcus led to a useful serologic classification. Lancefield (1933) and others found that most strains can be arranged into 13 groups by means of precipitin reactions between the specific carbohydrate substance of a group A strain and an antiserum. These groups, designated by letter (Table 10-10), vary in source and pathogenicity. Practically all strains causing human infection belong to group A; a few to group B.

Within group A at least 40 types of streptococci have been identified upon the basis of the M substance, a protein fraction of the cell. Antibacterial immunity is related to the type specificity and usually is more or less permanent; subsequent beta streptococcal infections will be with a type new for the patient.

Group A strains produce a number of extracellular antigens of clinical importance. Among these are the erythrogenic toxin, produced by over 90 per cent of the strains; streptolysins O and S; streptokinase (fibrinolysin) and hyaluronidase.

The erythrogenic toxin is responsible for the rash and other toxic manifestations of scarlet fever. Streptolysin O induces an antibody, the demonstration of which in the blood indicates a recent streptococcal infection, an important diagnostic test. Antibody titers to streptolysin, streptokinase and hyaluronidase usually reach higher levels in the blood of rheumatic fever patients than in relation to streptococcal infections alone.

Epidemiology. The incidence of streptococcal infections in the United States varies geographically and seasonally. It is highest in northern regions and in late winter and spring. The low incidence in tropical areas may be more apparent than real; culture and antibody studies indicate that there may be more infections than are recognized clinically.

From a careful study of a representative pediatric practice in Rochester, New York, Breese estimated 1 case of streptococcal infection per 20 child patients. The carrier rate in this study was approximately 4 per cent. Crowding, e.g. under poor housing conditions and in military groups, is important in the spread of infection. Transmission is primarily by direct contact with an infected person; indirect routes of infection such as contaminated food, drink, fingers and objects are less commonly noted.

Age affects the nature of streptococcal infections. As described by Powers and Boisvert (1944), the initial infection in the infant may be of low grade, whereas a subsequent infection tends to be more severe, suggesting the development of a state of hypersensitivity (see p. 890).

In the past 3 decades the severity of streptococcal infections has diminished significantly, as illustrated by the morbidity and mortality rates of

TABLE 10-10. SUMMARY OF RECOGNIZED SEROLOGIC GROUPS OF STREPTOCOCCI

GROUP	USUAL HABITAT	USUAL PATHOGENICITY
A.....	Man	Many human diseases
B.....	Cattle	Mastitis
C.....	Many animals	Many animal diseases
	Man (human strains)	Mild respiratory infections
D.....	Dairy products Intestinal contents of man and animals (enterococci)	Genitourinary tract infections, endocarditis, wound infections
E.....	Normal milk	None known
	Swine	Pharyngeal abscesses of swine
F.....	Man	Questionable; found in respiratory tract
G.....	Man	Mild respiratory infections; rare
	Dogs	Genital tract infections in dogs
H.....	Man	Questionable; found in respiratory tract
K.....	Man	Questionable; found in respiratory tract
L.....	Dogs	Genital tract infections
M.....	Dogs	Genital tract infections
N.....	Dairy products	None
O.....	Man	Occur in upper respiratory tract, but not associated with disease. Endocarditis

Groups A to E were described by Lancefield (1933); groups F and G, by Lancefield and Hare (1935); groups H and K, by Hare (1935); and groups L and M, by Fry (unpublished). Group N was identified independently by several groups, and the letter "N" was assigned by Shattuck and Mattick (1943). Group O was described by Boissard and Wormald (1950).

From M. McCarty; in R. J. Dubos and J. G. Hirsch: *Bacterial and Mycotic Infections of Man.* 4th ed. Philadelphia, J. B. Lippincott Company, 1965, p. 360.

scarlet fever. Since this change began before the introduction of antibiotics, it seems likely that a decrease in virulence of the streptococcus or an increase in host resistance has occurred.

Immunity. Although antibodies to several of the antigens of group A streptococci can be demonstrated in the blood of patients recovering from infection, only two of them can readily be associated with resistance. One is antitoxic and is the specific antibody to the erythrogenic toxin; the other is antibacterial, a type-specific antibody to the M substance. The former is responsible for immunity to the rash and other toxic manifestations in scarlet fever. The type-specific antibody is responsible for long-lasting immunity, and reinfection by its streptococcus rarely occurs. There is evidence, however, that very early administration of penicillin may inhibit the establishment of complete immunity.

Diagnosis. With the exception of scarlet fever and erysipelas, few streptococcal infections can be accurately diagnosed without bacteriologic confirmation. A swab adequately charged with material from the suspected lesion should be properly spread upon the surface of a fresh, moist, sheep's blood agar plate. After 24 to 48 hours' incubation, characteristic hemolytic colonies may be identified. Secondary pure growths from suspected colonies may then be serologically grouped and typed.

A large number of colonies in the original culture combined with clinical symptoms is usually indicative of a streptococcal infection, whereas only an occasional colony in the culture from an asymptomatic subject is suggestive of the carrier state.

The demonstration of a significant antistreptolysin O titer, or an increasing titer, is indicative of a recent streptococcal infection and has diagnostic significance in glomerulonephritis and in rheumatic fever.

REFERENCES

Breese, B. B., Disney, F. A., and Talpey, W. B.: The Prevention of Type Specific Immunity to Streptococcal Infections Due to the Therapeutic Use of Penicillin. Occurrence of Second Attacks Due to the Same Type of Group A Hemolytic Streptococci. *Amer. J. Dis. Child.,* 100:353, 1960.

Breese, B. B., Disney, F. A., and Talpey, W. B.: The Nature of a Small Pediatric Group Practice. II. Incidence of Beta Hemolytic Streptococcal Illness in a Private Pediatric Practice. *Pediatrics,* 38:277, 1966.

Denny, F. A., Perry, W. D., and Wannamaker, L. W.: Type-Specific Streptococcal Antibody. *J. Clin. Invest.,* 36:1092, 1957.

Lancefield, R. C.: Specific Relationship of Cell Composition to Biological Activity of Hemolytic Streptococci. *Harvey Lect.,* 1940-1941, 36:251, 1941.

Lancefield, R. C.: Current Knowledge of Type-Specific M Antigens of Group A Streptococci. *J. Immun.,* 89:307, 1962.

McCarty, M.: The Hemolytic Streptococci; in R. J. Dubos and J. G. Hirsch (Eds.): *Bacterial and Mycotic Infections of Man.* 4th ed. Philadelphia, J. B. Lippincott Company, 1965, p. 365.

SCARLET FEVER

(SCARLATINA)

Definition. Scarlet fever, a streptococcal infection, is a combination of septic and toxic manifestations. From the usual primary site of infection in the pharynx, the organism may invade adjacent tissues and even the blood stream and cause a number of metastatic lesions. It also produces a potent soluble toxin which, absorbed into the blood, causes fever, headache, delirium, tachycardia, vomiting and the rash. Some of the clinical manifestations have been regarded as allergic.

Etiology. Any erythrogenic toxin-producing strain of beta hemolytic streptococcus can cause scarlet fever. In a given outbreak several types of group A organisms may be involved. In one outbreak 22 different types were found among 228 patients. Of these, types 14, 18, 28 and 3 were most frequently observed. Certain types, 12, 1, 4,

TABLE 10-11. RESUMÉ OF THE COMMON CONTAGIOUS DISEASES HAVING AN EXANTHEM OR ENANTHEM

	DIPHTHERIA	SCARLET FEVER	MEASLES	GERMAN MEASLES	SMALLPOX	CHICKENPOX
Etiology	*Corynebacterium diphtheriae*	Hemolytic streptococcus group A	Virus	Virus	Virus	Virus
Transmission	Usually direct contact with patient or carrier	Usually direct contact; occasionally indirect or by contaminated milk, etc.	Usually direct contact	Direct contact	Direct or indirect contact; probably airborne	Direct or indirect contact; probably airborne
Incubation	2-5 days	2-7 days	10-14 days	14-21 days	8-16 days	14-21 days
Mouth and throat	Pseudomembrane spreads beyond tonsillar area and is difficult to remove	Punctate scarlet enanthem, tonsillar exudate; strawberry tongue early; raspberry tongue later	Koplik's spots	Macular eruption on soft palate (Forcheimer's spots)	Lesions on mucous membranes	Vesicular enanthem
Eruption	None	Bright red, punctate; face little involved; first on neck and chest, then spreads downward; later (after a week), desquamation, especially of hands and feet	Reddish maculopapules, crescentically grouped; appear first on face; later (after a week), branny desquamation	Pale rose macules, variable in size, discrete; first on face, spreads rapidly (24 hours) over body. At times scarlatiniform rash	Macules, then papules, then vesiculation of papules, then (by sixth day) pustules. Attacks first face and wrists, then hands and arms, then trunk and legs (chiefly on exposed parts of body)	Macules, papules, then vesicles, then some become pustules; lesions superficial, and found simultaneously in all stages of development. Attacks first face and back, then spreads rapidly downward (chiefly on covered parts of body)
Important constitutional symptoms	Fever often not high; prostration; myocarditis	At onset: sore throat, fever, nausea or vomiting and headache	Photophobia: catarrhal symptoms. Fever may subside about third day of invasion, then rise sharply within 24 hours when the rash appears	Lymphadenopathy, especially postauricular nodes; slight fever or may be none	At onset: vomiting, headache, high fever. Improvement at onset of rash; fever again in pustular stage	Fever; usually slight
Blood	Polymorphonuclear leukocytosis usually not very marked	Leukocytosis	Absence of leukocytosis; neutropenia common	Absence of leukocytosis	May be leukopenia in prodromal stage; later leukocytosis, often with mononuclear increase	Slight leukocytosis
Important complications	Bronchopneumonia; cardiac failure; postdiphtheritic paralysis	Otitis; adenitis; arthritis; nephritis; carditis	Bronchopneumonia; otitis media; sinusitis; laryngitis; encephalomyelitis	Occasionally bronchopneumonia; encephalomyelitis	Laryngitis, bronchopneumonia; gangrene; encephalomyelitis	Pustular skin lesions; encephalomyelitis
Diagnosis: technical aids	By culture from membrane	Culture; Schultz-Charlton test				
Other features	May be nasal or laryngeal involvement, etc.	"Surgical" scarlet fever		Congenital rubella syndrome	May be modified by previous vaccination	

18, 25 and 49, appear to have a relation to acute glomerulonephritis.

Of the various soluble substances elaborated by the organism, the erythrogenic toxin is important, for it causes the rash. The toxin can be demonstrated in the serum early in the disease, and its disappearance coincides with the appearance of humoral antitoxin.

Epidemiology. Factors influencing the incidence and method of spread are essentially those of streptococcal infections in general (see preceding section).

About half of the cases of scarlet fever occur in children between 2 and 8 years of age; other streptococcal infections are also frequently encountered during the first 2 years of life. Certain families appear to be particularly susceptible, but in general the family communicability rate is only 5 to 10 per cent.

In the United States the reported combined incidence of scarlet fever and streptococcal pharyngitis for 1956 was 176,392, with 240 deaths. By 1964 the incidence had increased to 402,334 cases, with 94 deaths. No doubt better reporting supported by more frequently taken cultures accounted in part for the apparently increased incidence. Antimicrobial therapy may be responsible for the decreased mortality.

Scarlet fever, like other streptococcal infections, is more common during the winter and spring seasons and in the temperate and cold climates. In the United States it is more common in the North than in the South.

Immunity. Resistance to scarlet fever is both antibacterial and antitoxic. The latter is the more important, since it provides protection, usually permanent, against the erythrogenic toxin. Antibacterial immunity is type-specific. Though immunity to a given strain of streptococcus may be of long duration, repeated streptococcal infections such as tonsillitis, sinusitis and otitis media are the rule, each possibly being an infection with a different strain. The presence of antitoxic immunity (negative Dick reaction) would seem to account for the occurrence of "scarlet fever" without an eruption (*scarlatina sine exanthemata*).

Immunity to the erythrogenic toxin is measured by titrating the serum and is reflected within limits by the Dick test.

This skin test consists in injecting 0.1 ml. of standardized streptococcal toxin intradermally. The amount of toxin injected is the amount which will produce within 18 to 24 hours an area of erythema at least 1 cm. in diameter in the susceptible subject. This is known as one skin test dose (S.T.D.). The result is usually positive during the first few days of the disease and negative during convalescence. The test is more dependable with the heat-labile toxin than with the ordinary Dick toxin. The heat-labile toxin is obtained from ordinary toxin by precipitation with alcohol (Ando).

The relation of the incidence of positive Dick reactions to age is similar to that of the Schick test. During the first 3 to 6 months of life the Dick reaction is negative in the majority of infants, but this finding is not explained by the presence of demonstrable antitoxin in the blood. By 1 year of age about 80 per cent of infants have a positive Dick reaction. By 10 to 12 years only about 10 to 15 per cent have positive reactions, irrespective of whether they have a history of scarlet fever.

Effective antimicrobial therapy has diminished interest in passive immunization with immune serum in scarlet fever, especially since it concerns the antitoxic aspect of the disease. Interest is renewed in active immunity, however, with the hope that an effective antigen may be prepared to provide active immunity against all streptococcal infections.

Pathology. The local lesions result from bacterial invasion and consist of acute tonsillitis and pharyngitis. The tonsils are enlarged and hyperemic, and their crypts are filled with exudate. The mucous membrane of the pharynx is hyperemic and edematous. An infiltrate of polymorphonuclear leukocytes is present in the edematous submucosa as well as within the epithelium; the latter is covered by patches of mucopurulent or fibrinopurulent exudate. The regional lymph nodes reveal toxic hyperplasia or suppuration.

The exanthem and enanthem are the result of bacterial toxins. Hyperemia of the corium is responsible for the diffuse redness. In addition, there is edema of the skin with a lymphocytic and monocytic infiltrate around the hair follicles. The cellular and fluid exudate accumulates in the midzone of the epidermis, where an accelerated keratinization (pseudokeratosis) occurs. Separation of the outer layers of the epidermis from the intermediate keratinized zone is responsible for the desquamation. The "strawberry" appearance of the tongue results from erythematous papillae projecting from a gray-coated background; with desquamation a beefy red appearance ensues.

Visceral involvement consists of generalized hyperplasia of lymphoid tissue and perivascular and diffuse infiltration of lymphocytes and monocytes. These infiltrates are especially prominent in the heart, liver and kidney; in renal interstitial tissue they may rarely lead to uremia, which usually appears within a week after the eruption.

Clinical Manifestations. The incubation period is usually 2 to 4 days, with an upper limit of 6 to 7 days.

The primary infection, usually in the pharynx, is responsible for the toxic manifestations and the septicemia. The toxic manifestations include headache, fever, vomiting, rapid pulse, delirium, exanthem, enanthem, generalized lymphadenitis, myocarditis, nephritis and perhaps arthritis. The septic manifestations resulting from bacterial invasion of the tissues and bloodstream, in addition to cellulitis of the pharynx and neck, and cervical adenitis, may include otitis media, sinusitis, mastoiditis, pyelonephritis, endocarditis, meningitis and other metastatic lesions.

The typical case of scarlet fever begins with headache, fever, sore throat and vomiting, followed within 24 to 72 hours by the appearance of the rash.

The onset is sudden, with a temperature of 101 to 104°F., reaching its height about the second day and gradually subsiding to normal by the seventh to the tenth day. The pulse rate is increased out of proportion to the temperature. Nausea is common, and vomiting occurs in approximately 80 per cent of the cases in children. Headache is often severe, and prostration is common.

The throat is deeply injected, and petechiae are present on the uvula and soft palate. Edema of the soft tissues may be present. Mucopurulent exudate may be distributed over the surface of the tonsil resembling the early lesion of diphtheria. In severe cases a serosanguineous nasal discharge may be present. The cervical lymph nodes are usually palpable and are often enlarged and tender. There is also a generalized enlargement of the superficial lymph nodes.

The eruption is a diffuse, finely papular, bright red erythema which blanches on pressure. It begins 12 to 72 hours after the onset of symptoms about the base of the neck, in the axillae and groins, and later appears on the trunk and extremities. The cheeks are flushed, and a ring of pallor corresponding to the topical area of the orbicularis oris muscle encircles the mouth (circumoral pallor). Invasion of this area by a true exanthem does not occur, and frequently the remainder of the face is also spared. When there is a rash over the cheeks, it is less severe than elsewhere. In the creases on the flexor surface of the elbow are deeply injected transverse lines of hyperemia which do not fade on pressure (Pastia's sign). Petechiae are frequent in the more toxic cases and may occur in mild cases; the Rumpel-Leede test result is positive.

The rash may be locally blanched by the intradermal injection of 0.2 ml. of convalescent serum or diluted commercial antitoxin (Schultz-Charlton blanching phenomenon).

After 3 to 7 days the rash fades and is followed by a branny type of desquamation which is most noticeable in the axillae, groin, fingertips and at the base of the nails, but may occur anywhere on the body. The degree of desquamation is proportional to the intensity of the rash, and in mild cases it may be absent.

The so-called strawberry tongue is observed in more than half of the cases and is an important clinical sign. Early in the disease the tongue is coated and somewhat swollen, the borders and tip are deeply injected, and the papillae are prominent (white strawberry tongue). By the third or fourth day the coating desquamates, leaving a beefy red tongue with swollen papillae (red strawberry tongue). This type of tongue is frequently observed in streptococcal infections without eruptions.

The clinical patterns of scarlet fever vary in severity. The more toxic or septic the initial reaction, the more frequent and numerous are the complications and the more grave is the prognosis.

A secondary anemia, albuminuria and leukocytosis are usually present. The white blood cell count is 10,000 to 20,000, of which 75 to 90 per cent are polymorphonuclear cells. Eosinophilia (4 to 20 per cent) may be observed after the fourth day of the rash. It diminishes during the second week and often increases again during the third week.

Relapses occur in about 0.5 per cent of cases in the third to sixth week of the disease and are generally regarded as representing infection with a new strain of streptococcus. They are usually of shorter duration and less severe than the original attack.

Second attacks are rare and require clinical and bacteriologic proof. The few instances of suspected second attacks observed by the author usually occurred in allergic persons, and confirmatory evidence of one of the attacks was incomplete. Diagnosis of second attacks on clinical evidence alone is not reliable.

Differential Diagnosis. The typical case offers little difficulty in diagnosis. The characteristic onset with fever, sore throat and vomiting followed within 1 to 3 days by a diffuse erythematous rash constitutes a presumptive diagnosis of scarlet fever. In mild, atypical cases and in infants the diagnosis may be exceedingly difficult.

In *German measles*, which is perhaps most frequently confused with the mild type of scarlet fever, the intensity of the eruption is out of proportion to the symptoms. Enlargement of the occipital nodes and the rapidly changing and fading eruptions are characteristic. The throat symptoms are mild, and desquamation is rare.

Measles can usually be identified by the catarrhal symptoms, the morbilliform eruption with involvement of the face, the presence of Koplik's spots and leukopenia. The modified type of measles may offer considerable difficulty in diagnosis.

Exanthem subitum may on occasion present an eruption more scarlatiniform than morbilliform. The course of the disease and leukopenia are characteristic.

Infectious mononucleosis may be differentiated by serologic and hematologic data.

Drug rashes, particularly those caused by belladonna, the coal-tar derivatives, sulfonamides and irritants to which the patient is allergic, are common causes of error. Drug rashes are usually more intense on the extremities. The history of drug administration is helpful. The scarlatiniform type of eruption associated with serum disease is easily identified by its pruritic quality and its relation to an injection of serum.

Severe staphylococcal infections are sometimes associated with a scarlatiniform rash.

In general, the following evidence may assist in the positive diagnosis of a questionable case of scarlet fever: (1) history of exposure within a week; (2) concurrent streptococcal infections in siblings or close contacts; (3) subsequent desquamation or development of nephritis; (4) hemolytic streptococci in the throat culture or a rising ASO titer;

(5) positive rash-extinction test; (6) reversal of the Dick reaction during the illness.

Complications. The complications fall into 2 general groups: (1) those caused by septic infection by the hemolytic streptococcus or other secondary invading organism and (2) those caused by the toxin.

The incidence of the septic complications, suppurative cervical adenitis, sinusitis, otitis media, mastoiditis, lateral sinus thrombosis, epidural abscess, meningitis and endocarditis, has been greatly reduced by early treatment with effective antibacterial agents.

Sinusitis probably occurs in most cases, varying from a mild ethmoidal infection to severe pansinusitis. Retropharyngeal and peritonsillar abscesses are also complications.

The pain of acute *mesenteric adenitis* may resemble that of appendicitis.

Laryngitis is occasionally an early manifestation and may be obstructive. It may progress to diffuse laryngotracheobronchitis.

Bronchopneumonia is not common and is usually interstitial in type; empyema develops in about one third of untreated cases.

Cardiac disorders, which are of several types, occur in less than 1 per cent of cases. One of the most common is acute toxic myocarditis, which occurs early and is not unlike that of diphtheria. It is often transient. Bacterial endocarditis and pericarditis are septic in origin. If rheumatic carditis occurs, it usually does so during the second or third week.

Albuminuria with only an occasional cast or red blood cell occurs early in most severe cases. It usually disappears when the temperature subsides.

Clinically manifest acute *glomerulonephritis* occurs in about 1 per cent of cases in the second or third week of the disease. An increase of urinary protein and cellular components may be found in the majority of cases at this time, if studied by the Addis method (Lyttle).

Arthritis, usually involving the smaller joints, may occur in older children during the second or third week of the disease. It is probably caused by the toxin and subsides within a week or more. It resembles rheumatic fever, which may also occur at this time. Suppurative arthritis of pyemic origin is usually multiple and involves the large joints.

Paronychia is a common minor infection.

Prognosis. The mortality rate in the United States is now under 1 per cent. It is somewhat higher in infants, in whom septic features of the disease are more common. These complications should be controlled by early and adequate antimicrobial therapy. Late complications such as rheumatic fever and glomerulonephritis may occur regardless of the severity of the disease.

Prevention. Isolation measures have in general failed to control the spread of scarlet fever, owing to the many sources of group A beta hemolytic streptococci. The carrier rate appears to be little affected by quarantine.

Patients adequately treated with penicillin for 10 days rarely become carriers. If the mucous membranes of the nasopharynx appear normal and there are no purulent complications, isolation of the patient may be discontinued after 7 days.

Active or passive immunization is now seldom used. Among family contacts about 25 per cent of those exposed will acquire some form of streptococcal infection. They should be closely observed. If symptoms occur, and the throat culture reveals beta hemolytic streptococci, they should be treated with penicillin. If a contact has a history of rheumatic fever or chorea, he should receive continuous prophylaxis (p. 541).

Treatment. Rest in bed, adequate intake of fluids, and a liquid, soft or regular diet, as the child desires, are the general measures indicated in the acute stage. Codeine and aspirin may be required to relieve headache, sore throat and general discomfort.

Daily examinations of the patient and frequent urinalyses should be made during the febrile period. Inhalation of moist air is indicated when there is severe infection of the upper respiratory tract. Cold or hot local compresses may be applied to painful, swollen cervical lymph nodes; incision should be made only when fluctuation is obvious.

The pain of otitis media is relieved by codeine and aspirin and the local application of heat. Early myringotomy is indicated if the drum is bulging. The treatment of toxic myocarditis is identical with that described under Diphtheria (p. 567). The management of acute glomerulonephritis is discussed elsewhere. The secondary anemia quickly responds to administration of an adequate diet, iron and cobalt.

Adequate antibiotic treatment is important, for it may prevent complications such as rheumatic fever and glomerulonephritis.

Penicillin is the drug of choice, unless the patient is sensitive to it, when erythromycin may be substituted. Therapy should continue for 10 days. An intramuscular injection of 600,000 to 1,200,000 units of benzathine penicillin G according to the size of the patient is effective. The author prefers 2 injections of aqueous procaine penicillin (300,000 to 600,000 units) at 3-day intervals combined with the oral administration of 200,000 to 400,000 units of penicillin V every 6 hours for 10 days.

Surgical Scarlet Fever. In this type of the disease the focus of infection is somewhere other than the throat. It may be a traumatic or operative wound or a burn. It may follow any surgical operation, but particularly those of the ear, mouth or nose; the onset is usually within 2 to 4 days. The symptoms are usually mild, and complications are infrequent. The pharynx is not involved, and hemolytic streptococci can usually be cultured from the suspected focus.

REFERENCES

American Academy of Pediatrics: Report of the Committee on the Control of Infectious Diseases. Revised, 1966, p. 129.

Breese, B. B.: Beta Hemolytic Streptococcal Infections in Children. *Pediat. Clin. N. Amer.*, 7:843, 1960.

Dick, G. F., and Dick, G. H.: A Skin Test for Susceptibility to Scarlet Fever. *J.A.M.A.*, 82:265, 1924.

Dunnet, W. N., and Schallibaum, E. M.: Scarlet Fever-like Illness Due to Staphylococcal Infection. *Lancet*, 2:1227, 1960.

McCarty, M.: The Hemolytic Streptococci; in R. J. Dubos and J. G. Hirsch (Eds.): *Bacterial and Mycotic Infections of Man.* 4th ed. Philadelphia, J. B. Lippincott Company, 1965, p. 378.

Strom, J., and Turnevall, G.: Long-Acting (DBED) Penicillin and Procaine Penicillin in the Treatment of Scarlet Fever. A Clinical and Serobacteriological Follow-up Study. *Acta paediat.*, 44:571, 1955.

United States Department of Health, Education, and Welfare: Morbidity and Mortality. Annual Supplement Survey 1965, Vo. 14, #53.

ERYSIPELAS

(St. Anthony's Fire)

Erysipelas is an acute streptococcal infection of the skin and occasionally of the mucous membranes. It is characterized locally by a painful erythematous induration with sharply demarcated serpiginous borders and generally by constitutional symptoms.

Etiology.　A number of the subgroups of group A hemolytic streptococci may be the cause of erysipelas.

Epidemiology.　The disease exists endemically in all communities where streptococcal infections occur. Since the introduction of the sulfonamides and antibiotics it is relatively infrequent.

Immunity.　The newborn infant is highly susceptible. An attack of the disease confers no immunity against subsequent ones. Certain persons appear to be predisposed to the disease and have repeated attacks. In this respect erysipelas differs from scarlet fever, in which immunity to the erythrogenic toxin (rash) is conferred.

Pathology.　Streptococci are found in great numbers in and about the lymphatics of the skin near the border of the spreading infection. The surrounding area is hyperemic and edematous. Infiltration of mononuclear cells is appreciable, extending into the corium and subcutaneous fatty area. Suppuration is rare except in the subcutaneous region, where it may occur in infants. The regional lymph nodes are enlarged. In young infants septicemia is frequent and results in multiple metastatic purulent lesions which may include parenchymal lesions of the liver, kidneys, brain, heart and other organs.

Clinical Manifestations.　The local lesion is often the first evidence of infection, although at times fever, malaise, irritability, vomiting, loss of appetite or other general symptoms may precede it. The portal of entry is a wound of the skin which may be trivial or may be a surgical incision, or the lesions of such conditions as eczema, impetigo, varicella and vaccinia. The sites most frequently involved are the periumbilical area (newborn), the genitalia, face and extremities. When the face is involved, the infection may extend from one cheek across the nose to the other cheek (the familiar "butterfly" type). The inflamed area is red, hot and tender, and there may be vesiculation. The border is elevated and spreads in an irregular manner, avoiding areas of the skin where tension normally exists, such as bony prominences. The disease may be self-limited or may spread over a large portion of the body, fading in one area while extending in another. The fading area becomes branny and desquamates.

Erysipelas of the mucous membranes is relatively rare. It may occur as a hard, painful, swollen inflammation of the pharynx, nose, larynx or vulva. Extension into the larynx may lead to suffocation.

The temperature usually reaches a level of 104 or 105°F. Fever may be intermittent, but more often remains at a high level; it may last only a few days or may persist for one or more weeks. Occasionally it is of low grade; in overwhelming infections, especially in newborn infants, the temperature may be subnormal.

Leukocytosis is usually present, the white blood cell count ranging from 12,000 to 40,000 per mm.³ with a preponderance of polymorphonuclear cells. Except in infants, blood cultures are usually sterile.

Relapses are common, usually beginning in the areas of skin most recently infected. The course of a relapse is usually shorter and the symptoms are less severe than in the original attack.

Diagnosis.　The fully developed case of erysipelas offers little diagnostic difficulty.

Diffuse cellulitis, or infection of the subcutaneous tissue, especially staphylococcal infection in the newborn infant, is the condition most commonly confused with erysipelas. The characteristic elevated border of erysipelas is usually absent. Orbital cellulitis, secondary to ethmoidal sinus infection, is occasionally misdiagnosed as erysipelas. *H. influenzae* and other bacterial pathogens are occasional causes of orbital cellulitis and of erysipeloid lesions in other locations.

Dermatitis medicamentosa, particularly that due to mercurial ointment, may be differentiated by history and by lack of fever, as may eczema of the erythrodermic type.

Complications.　In infancy, septicemia, bronchopneumonia and peritonitis are the most important complications. Abscess formation occurs in 10 to 15 per cent of all cases. Sloughing with ulceration results most frequently in areas subject to pressure.

Suppurative lesions of the accessory nasal sinuses sometimes occur. More extensive forms of such infections may lead to thrombosis of the cavernous sinus or other dural sinuses, meningitis or brain abscess.

Prognosis.　The general mortality rate was formerly 5 to 10 per cent, and in infants as high as 80 per cent. When treatment is instituted early, recovery can be expected in practically all instances, even in infants.

Treatment.　The patient should be in strict isolation. Erysipelas responds dramatically to the systemic administration of penicillin or other antibiotics effective against the beta hemolytic streptococcus. Local treatment is not effective.

DIPHTHERIA

Definition. Diphtheria is a specific infectious disease caused by *Corynebacterium diphtheriae*. In its classic form it is characterized by a local pseudomembranous lesion, usually on the tonsils, pharynx and adjacent tissues, from which a powerful toxin is absorbed. This toxin produces the constitutional symptoms. The location of the lesion, its extent and the degree of toxemia vary greatly.

History. The modern concept of the disease began with the classic clinical description by Bretonneau in 1826, who called it *diphtherité*. Diphtheria, however, was known to the Hebrews before Christ. It is not known when the disease reached America; Samuel Bard (1771) probably described an epidemic in New York City and the Colony.

Klebs in 1883 demonstrated diphtheria bacilli in the pseudomembrane, and Loeffler in 1884 identified them in pure culture. In 1888 Roux and Yersin described the toxin, and in 1894 von Behring discovered its antitoxin. Theobald Smith suggested toxin-antitoxin for active immunization, and it was widely popularized by Park and Zingler (1913). Schick introduced the intracutaneous test for determining susceptibility in 1913, and in 1922 Ramon described the preparation of formalized toxin (toxoid). The introduction of tracheotomy (1825) by Bretonneau and of intubation (1895) by O'Dwyer were also important contributions.

Etiology. The diphtheria bacillus is polymorphous, but characteristically is a slender, slightly curved, sometimes clubbed organism. It is gram-positive, nonmotile and nonspore-forming. It is easily destroyed by heat (60°C. for 10 minutes) and is susceptible to weak antiseptics. It survives in ice for several weeks. In water, milk or dried mucus it may remain viable for several weeks.

Three types of the organism, gravis, mitis and intermediate, may be identified by the type of colony formed on a blood-agar medium containing potassium tellurite.

The diphtheria bacillus produces a powerful toxin. It is a heat-coagulable protein and accounts for practically all the clinical manifestations. It is a potent tissue poison which, within a few hours after absorption, produces characteristic cellular changes, especially in the cardiac, renal and nervous tissues. Freeman has shown that avirulent strains may become virulent when exposed to bacteriophages associated with virulent strains of the organism.

Epidemiology. Diphtheria is endemic and epidemic throughout the world, particularly in the temperate zones. It is more frequent during the winter. Negroes are said to have greater immunity than white persons.

Diphtheria has a characteristic age incidence, corresponding to the lack of humoral antitoxin. The disease is rare during the first 6 months of life; the incidence reaches its peak between the second and fifth years and declines rapidly beyond the age of 10. In the United States about 65 per

cent of cases have occurred in children under 5 years of age. There is, however, evidence of a rising age incidence, which may be the result of extensive active immunization among the younger age groups. Such evidence supports the continued use of "booster injections," at least throughout the school years (see p. 190).

The morbidity and mortality from diphtheria have declined rapidly in the United States since 1920. The number of reported cases decreased from 1568 in 1956 to 168 in 1965, and the number of deaths for these years from 103 to 16.

Diphtheria spreads in schools and other places where children of susceptible ages are grouped together. One or more chronic carriers may account for its persistence within a particular community. The discovery that, in the presence of a specific bacteriophage, certain avirulent strains can become permanently virulent adds importance to the role of the carrier.

Infection is due to contact with a person with the active disease or with a carrier of virulent organisms. Fomites and animals play an unimportant role in the transmission of the disease, as do water and milk. Chronic sinusitis and diseased tonsils and adenoids are important predisposing factors.

Immunity. Resistance to *C. diphtheriae* is of 2 types: passive and active.

Passive immunity may be obtained by the newborn infant transplacentally from an immune mother. It is almost absolute for the first 3 months of life and partial until about the sixth month. If the mother is susceptible to diphtheria, her baby is also susceptible. Passive immunity for about 3

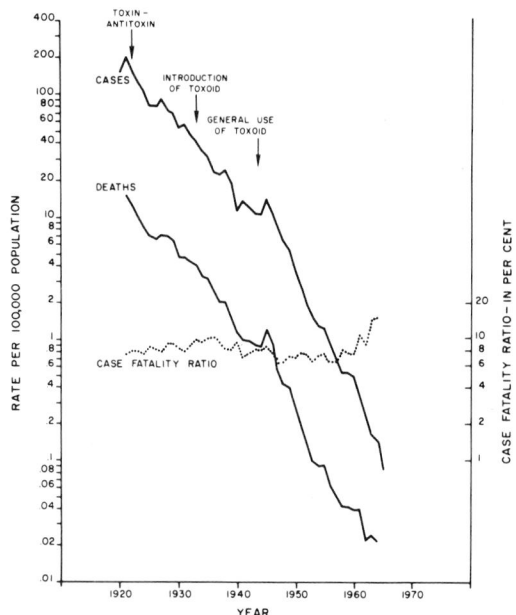

Figure 10-34. Diphtheria: reported annual case and death rates and case-fatality ratio, United States, 1920-1965. (From United States Department of Health, Education, and Welfare. Morbidity and Mortality, Vol. 14, No. 53, Oct. 14, 1966.)

weeks may be artificially obtained by subcutaneous injection of 1500 units of antitoxin.

Active immunity is acquired by having the disease or by receiving inoculations of one of several antigens. Not all persons recovering from the disease become immune; hence secondary attacks may occur. It is probable that the early injection of antitoxin, though curative, interferes with the patient's power to generate antibodies. Conversely, not all persons immune to diphtheria have had the classic disease; active immunity is presumably induced by inapparent diphtheritic infections. Occasionally a susceptible person lacking demonstrable humoral immunity as reflected by a positive Schick reaction fails to contract diphtheria in spite of repeated exposures to virulent organisms. This suggests that resistance may depend upon cellular as well as humoral immunity.

Schick test. The Schick test consists in intracutaneous injection of 1/50 M.L.D. of toxin contained in 0.1 ml. of a proper diluent. If the tested person is susceptible, an area of reddish-brown discoloration appears at the site of injection within 24 hours. In persons who have practically no antitoxin, vesication often occurs. After 5 to 7 days the reaction begins to fade, leaving a scaling, wrinkled area with brownish pigmentation which may last 4 to 6 weeks. If the tested person is immune, no local reaction occurs unless he is allergic to the autolyzed substance of the diphtheria bacillus or to other protein components of the culture medium or diluent solution. In this case a pseudoreaction manifested by a diffuse erythema with or without an urticarial wheal develops within a few minutes or hours. It usually disappears within 72 hours. A control test is performed with identical material except that the toxin has been destroyed by heat. In some clinics the control test is omitted, and the interpretation is made at the end of the fifth day, when pseudoreactions have usually disappeared.

Four types of Schick reactions are commonly observed: (1) positive reaction: patient susceptible to diphtheria and not allergic to protein material in test solution; (2) positive combined reaction: patient susceptible and also allergic to protein in test solution; (3) pseudoreaction: patient immune, but allergic to protein in test solution; (4) negative reaction: patient immune and nonallergic to protein material in test solution.

About 15 per cent of newborn infants have positive Schick reactions. In such instances the mother's reaction is almost always positive. The incidence of positive reactions gradually increases until the sixth month of age, when about 50 per cent are positive. At 1 year fully 90 per cent of nonimmunized infants have a positive reaction; after this age the incidence until recent years gradually diminished, until at 17 years only about 15 per cent remained positive. Surveys now indicate that 50 to 60 per cent of adolescents and adults have positive reactions.

Pathology. An exotoxin elaborated by the organisms tends to inhibit the local inflammatory response. As this response is overcome the bacteria multiply rapidly and produce more toxin, resulting in edema, hyperemia and necrosis of the epithelium. A pseudomembrane, consisting of fibrin, leukocytes, necrotic tissue, and bacteria, is formed and becomes adherent to the underlying tissue. Its removal exposes a raw, bleeding surface. Pseudomembranes may be absent in early or mild forms of the disease and may be present in diseases other than diphtheria.

Pharyngeal membranes may extend from the nasopharynx into the larynx, or the lesion may be localized to the larynx. Primary tracheal diphtheria is rare. The tracheal membrane may become loose and cause obstruction in the lower respiratory tract.

Lymph nodes draining the affected area, and at times more remote ones, reveal reactive hyperplasia. The malpighian corpuscles of the spleen and of the lymph nodes contain large toxic reaction centers.

In patients dying with toxic myocarditis the heart is soft and flabby, and the chambers, especially the left ventricle, are dilated. Scattered petechiae may be present. Histologically, there are interstitial edema and multiple areas of necrosis associated with an inflammatory infiltrate consisting predominantly of polymorphonuclear leukocytes.

Paralysis results from the effects of the toxin on the peripheral nerves. Degeneration and even destruction of myelin sheaths occur, and the axons may be swollen. Rarely is there irreparable axonal damage.

Cloudy swelling and occasionally focal necrosis may be present in the liver and kidneys; rarely is there acute interstitial nephritis.

Death may result from peripheral vascular collapse, respiratory obstruction, cardiac failure, respiratory paralysis or secondary bronchopneumonia.

Clinical Manifestations. The incubation period is from 2 to 7 days.

Faucial diphtheria. The disease may be overlooked or discovered only by bacteriologic examination, since catarrhal inflammation without membrane formation may occur, especially in partially immune persons.

In the moderately severe case there may or may not be soreness of the throat, but malaise and headache are usually present. Fever is usually of low grade, 101 to 103°F. During the first day there is congestion and slight swelling of the tonsillar and pharyngeal tissues, with slight enlargement of the cervical lymph nodes. Within 24 hours small yellowish-white spots appear upon the surface of the tonsils. They closely resemble those of follicular tonsillitis and are removed with difficulty. The spots coalesce and spread rapidly from the tonsillar surface to the pillars, uvula, soft palate and posterior pharyngeal wall (Fig. 10-35, p. 629). The membrane may extend upward into the nares and cause a bloody, serous nasal discharge. The odor is offensive, but not characteristic. Swelling of the soft tissues and cervical lymph nodes develops. Constitutional symptoms increase in severity, and the pulse becomes rapid and of less volume. The blood pressure falls, and prostration becomes pronounced. Difficulty in swallowing increases, and noisy breathing becomes evident even without laryngeal obstruction. A nasal voice or regurgitation of liquids through the nose during the act of swallowing suggests palatal paralysis. The patellar reflexes may be diminished or absent. In severe cases there is rapid reduction of erythrocytes and hemoglobin. Polymorphonuclear leukocytosis develops. The urine usually contains albumin, and often casts.

The more malignant type of the disease is usually a combined faucial and nasopharyngeal lesion. Toxemia in this form is extreme, and the sensorium is frequently disturbed. The local infection is extensive, and there may be secondary infection, frequently with the hemolytic streptococcus. Hemorrhages from the mouth and nose are common, and petechiae may appear in the skin and mucous membranes. The cervical lymph nodes may become greatly swollen and, with the firm, nonpitting edema in the surrounding skin and subcutaneous tissue, give a characteristic "bull-neck" appearance. The face becomes edematous and has a waxy pallor. Death usually occurs within a week from toxic myocarditis or bronchopneumonia.

Laryngotracheal diphtheria. In about one fourth of all cases the infection invades the larynx and trachea, the laryngeal lesion being an extension from a pharyngeal focus about 3 times as often as it is primary. It is more common in infants and has a high mortality rate. There is less toxemia in the primary form.

Hoarseness, a brassy cough and noisy breathing are the initial symptoms. Laryngeal obstruction is progressive with stridor that is mainly inspiratory. Anxiety and retractions of the episternal and subcostal regions increase; if the obstruction is not relieved, cyanosis develops, and death occurs from suffocation or cardiac failure. Laryngoscopic examination reveals edema, congestion and the pseudomembrane.

Nasal diphtheria. In about 2 per cent of all cases, more often in infants, diphtheria may occur primarily in the nose (Fig. 10-36, p. 629). The infection may remain localized or extend to the nasopharynx, throat and larynx. When the lesion is limited to the nose, constitutional symptoms are usually absent or slight, and the fever tends to be low. The only evidence may be a nasal discharge which characteristically is sanguineous and has a foul odor. Breathing may be obstructed. Nasal diphtheria, because of its chronicity, constitutes a continuous source of contagion if not treated.

Cutaneous diphtheria. Cutaneous infection is not unusual in the tropics, as was observed during World War II in Africa and in the Pacific area. In a series of 1423 cases of diphtheria (Los Angeles County Hospital, 1945-50) there were 6 instances of cutaneous infection and 10 of infection in the ear, conjunctiva, umbilicus or vagina.

The skin lesion may be primary or secondary. A common form consists of a gray membrane around the swollen edge of a wound. Other lesions may be eczematous, impetiginous, pustular or bullous. Constitutional reactions range from none to a fatal toxemia. The lesions usually respond promptly to specific treatment.

Other types of diphtheria. Primary infection may occur in unusual regions of the body, or these areas may become secondarily infected from a diphtheritic lesion in the upper respiratory tract. The vulva, vagina, umbilical cord, conjunctivas and cutaneous wounds are some of the unusual sites. Lesions on the lips and face may also occur. Wounds, especially those resulting from tonsillectomy, are at times infected. Tonsillectomies should be performed only on children known to be Schick-negative.

Diagnosis. There is nothing typical about the early tonsillar lesion, except the manner and rapidity of extension of the membrane. A throat swab should be obtained for culture and smear at the initial examination. If dependable bacteriologic facilities are not available, antitoxin should be administered immediately in each suspected case.

Bacteriologic diagnosis of diphtheria requires (1) good culture medium, (2) proper technique of taking the culture, and (3) expert interpretation of stained smears. The swab should be made from the base of the exudate or membrane. A fluorescent antitoxin test for immediate diagnosis has been proposed.

In doubtful cases, particularly in patients under observation in a hospital, the following routine may prove helpful: (1) an accurate history of previous active immunization and Schick reaction, (2) incubation of a culture from the lesion, (3) performance of a Schick test, (4) careful, regularly repeated examination of the throat lesion, and (5) immediate therapy with penicillin. If the membrane spreads, antitoxin should be administered even if the culture is negative. A rapid method of culturing the organism consists in the use of a swab impregnated with horse serum, the surface of which is coagulated by passing the swab through a flame. Charged swabs prepared in this manner, when incubated, often show growth of *C. diphtheriae* within 2 to 4 hours.

Differential Diagnosis. *Nasal diphtheria.* This lesion may be confused with any condition responsible for a persistent bloody nasal discharge. Ulcers produced by constant picking of the nose, a foreign body and congenital syphilis are the more common conditions that require consideration.

Faucial diphtheria. Faucial diphtheria is most likely to be confused with follicular *tonsillitis*, in which the temperature is usually high, swallowing is painful, and the follicular exudates, though they may coalesce, do not usually extend beyond the surface of the tonsils. In early *syphilis* primary or secondary ulcerative lesions may resemble those of diphtheria. They are more frequent in adults, and the specific serologic reaction is positive. Severe pharyngeal reactions to *herpes virus* occasionally suggest diphtheria; but characteristic herpetic lesions of the tongue, cheeks, lips and gums are usually present or soon develop. In severe or septic cases of *scarlet fever*, tissue swelling, ulceration and heavy mucoid exudate over the tonsil, soft palate and posterior pharyngeal wall may occur. The throat lesion of *infectious mononucleosis* may be confusing. *Thrush*, usually encountered during infancy, occurs in other areas of the oral cavity as a rule, and the exudates are whiter than that of diphtheria and are characteristically arranged as small linear (filaments) membranes. The membranes which characteristically form in *post-tonsillectomy wounds* have been mistaken for diphtheria. In certain *blood dyscrasias*, such as agranulocytosis and leukemia, necrotic lesions occur in the throat which may resemble those of diphtheria.

Laryngeal diphtheria (see also p. 907). This lesion is most frequently confused with *acute laryngitis* and *laryngotracheobronchitis*. Clinical differentiation of these conditions is often not possible. Direct laryngoscopic examination offers the best assistance both for direct visualization and for obtaining material for culture. *Spasmodic croup* produces an intermittent rather than progressive stridor. It often occurs in a child known to have had previous attacks and frequently responds to ipecac, sedatives, and a moist atmosphere. *Bronchopneumonia* in infants may be characterized by dyspnea, hoarseness and stridor with retraction; this is especially true of acute bronchiolitis (p. 922). The stridor of *bronchial asthma* is principally expiratory and usually responds to a test dose of epinephrine. Retropharyngeal or peritonsillar abscess, mediastinal tumor, edema of the glottis, papilloma of the larynx, and tetany are other conditions which at times must be considered.

Complications. Complications vary in epidemics and with the promptness with which specific antitoxin therapy is instituted.

Respiratory complications. *Bronchopneumonia* is common, particularly in infants and especially in conjunction with the laryngeal form of diphtheria. It occurs in over half of the fatal cases, and is usually caused by other organisms than *C. diphtheriae.*

Atelectasis is associated particularly with laryngeal and tracheal lesions.

Circulatory complications. *Circulatory failure* is one of the most important complications. Early circulatory failure is the result of toxemia. Late circulatory failure occurs during apparent convalescence and is due to changes in the peripheral vasomotor mechanism. *Cardiac failure* is due to acute toxic myocarditis with or without superimposed damage to the intrinsic conduction system. It may occur at any time during the disease, but most commonly between the fifth and twelfth days. The symptoms are fatigue, dyspnea and a weak, rapid pulse. At times the pulse rate is very slow, in some, but not all, instances caused by heart

block. The heart sounds, particularly the first, become feeble, and often there is an associated gallop rhythm. Enlargement of the liver, epigastric pain, vomiting, cardiac dilatation, pallor and diminished blood pressure are characteristic findings. The electrocardiogram reveals an increased P-R interval and inversion of the T wave in the first and second leads.

Renal complications. *Albuminuria* is common during the febrile stage of the disease. It is due to toxic degenerative changes in the renal epithelium. In the more' severe cases there is usually a mild generalized edema. The urine is diminished in volume and contains leukocytes, epithelial cells and hyaline casts, but seldom erythrocytes. Clinical evidence of *nephritis* exists in about 10 to 15 per cent of all cases; postmortem studies reveal renal changes in the majority of fatal cases.

Paralysis. Paralysis occurs in 10 to 15 per cent of all cases as the result of a toxic peripheral neuritis which is painless, usually persists for several days or weeks and may involve any muscle or group of muscles. The time of onset and the extent of the paralysis depend upon the severity of the disease and the time when antitoxin is given.

Palatal paralysis is the most frequent and usually the first type to appear, usually during the first or second week of the disease. The patient cannot elevate the palate, the voice becomes nasal, and regurgitation of fluids through the nares occurs upon attempts at swallowing. Palatal paralysis occasionally is recurrent.

Paralysis of the ocular muscles is the second most frequent type, usually involving the muscles of accommodation. Inability to read may be the first evidence. Strabismus, dilatation of the pupils and ptosis of the eyelid may occur. Ocular palsy occurs usually during the third week or later.

Progressive *general paralysis*, involving the face, neck, trunk and extremities, may follow the palatal or ocular type. It usually occurs after the fourth week of the disease. Inability to raise the head is characteristic. The deep tendon reflexes, especially the patellars, become diminished or absent, though at first they may be increased. The superficial reflexes are frequently obtainable. The Guillain-Barré syndrome has been observed in association with diphtheria.

Paralysis of the phrenic nerve usually occurs during the fourth to the eighth week. It is characterized by cough, dyspnea, thoracic breathing, and cyanosis. The forced respiratory efforts induced by the patient's fear of suffocation are impressive. It is often associated with pneumonia or myocarditis and may be fatal.

Paralysis of the pharyngeal and laryngeal muscles usually occurs during the third week and often results in accumulation of secretions and liquids in the lower respiratory tract. Aphonia obviously results.

Except for the unusual occurrence of monoplegia or hemiplegia resulting from thrombosis of a cerebral artery, there is complete recovery from diphtheritic paralysis. Though involvement usually lasts but 1 or 2 weeks, complete recovery may not occur for several months.

Unusual complications include pleurisy, arthritis, septicemia, empyema, thrombosis and embolism. Chronic laryngeal stenosis may follow tracheotomy, particularly when the incision is made too near the larynx (p. 686).

Occasionally there are relapses and recurrences of diphtheria, recurrences usually being less severe than the original attack.

Prognosis. The case fatality rate in diphtheria varied from 6.5 per cent in 1956 to 9.5 per cent in 1965. In general the prognosis depends on the stage of the disease when an adequate and properly administered amount of antitoxin is injected. When specific treatment is carried out on the first day of the disease, the mortality rate is about 0.3 per cent; on the third day, 4 per cent; on the fourth day, 12 per cent; and on subsequent days, 25 per cent. In young infants the fatality rate is higher, owing to the frequency of laryngeal involvement and of bronchopneumonia. Septic symptoms, cardiac involvement and hemorrhagic manifestations are unfavorable complications. The virulence of the organism and the location and extent of the membrane are important prognostic factors. Secondary infections obviously may influence the outcome.

Prevention. Immediate contacts should be subjected to Schick tests, nose and throat cultures and daily inspection. Penicillin should be given intramuscularly or orally.

Previously immunized contacts should receive a booster injection of fluid toxoid. Those with negative Schick reactions and positive cultures should be treated as carriers. Those with positive Schick reactions and positive cultures should be treated as active cases with antitoxin (2000 units) and with either penicillin or erythromycin. Contacts not previously immunized, but showing positive Schick reactions, should later be actively immunized.

When the foregoing regimen is not possible, it may be safer to provide passive immunity for the immediate contacts with a subcutaneous injection of 2000 units of antitoxin after proper testing for sensitivity. They should also receive penicillin.

The patient should be isolated until 2 negative cultures on consecutive days have been obtained from the nose and throat. The first culture should not be taken until a week after the onset of the disease. If the second culture is positive, 5 days should elapse before another culture is taken. The child should not return to school for at least 3 weeks after the onset of illness.

Active immunization (see p. 190). The most important preventive measure is active immunization during infancy. For this purpose the combined triple antigen is best. For older children and adults either the "adult type" of diphtheria-tetanus toxoid mixture or the fluid diphtheria toxoid is used. Booster injections are necessary during childhood to maintain adequate protection.

Early administration of antitoxin may interfere with production of immunity during an attack of diphtheria, a factor probably accounting for many of the second attacks. Hence it is advisable to Schick-test the patient convalescing from the disease after the antitoxin administered therapeutically has been eliminated (6 to 8 weeks). If the reaction is positive, he should receive active immunization.

Management of the carrier. Diphtheria is one of the classic "carrier diseases." In about three fourths of the cases the organisms disappear from the upper respiratory tract within 3 weeks after the acute phase. In the remaining fourth, organisms may be retained for months. The convalescent carrier and the carrier closely associated with an active case are epidemiologically important because they can be assumed to harbor virulent organisms. Only about 10 per cent of carriers discovered by surveys harbor virulent organisms.

The incidence of convalescent carriers is decreased when treatment during the acute stage includes antitoxin and penicillin.

The nonconvalescent carrier should be treated with penicillin or erythromycin. In persistent carriers foci of infection in tonsils, adenoids and sinuses should be eliminated. If the carrier is Schick-positive, the operation should be deferred until he has been actively immunized. Penicillin should be given immediately before and after the operation.

Carriers should be isolated until virulent organisms are no longer demonstrated by culture.

Treatment. **General care.** The patient should be kept absolutely quiet in bed for at least 2 weeks. If the membrane extends beyond the surface of the tonsils or if antitoxin was not given until late in the course of the disease, this period should be extended. Daily physical examinations are essential. If there is the slightest doubt about the status of the circulatory system, an electrocardiogram should be obtained. Intravenous injections of 10 per cent glucose solution (about 1 gm. per kg. per day) are indicated to counteract the tendency to hypoglycemia associated with toxemia. A fluid or soft diet ample in vitamin content should be given. Saline throat irrigations may be symptomatically helpful, and an ice collar is comforting when the cervical lymph nodes are swollen. Codeine and aspirin may relieve suffering from sore throat or headache.

Penicillin should be administered in addition to antitoxin, not as a substitute.

Specific treatment. This consists in the early injection of an adequate amount of antitoxin. From 10,000 to 20,000 units of antitoxin may be injected intramuscularly in cases of average severity. In the toxic, the complicated or the laryngeal case 20,000 to 40,000 units should be administered, one half intramuscularly and one half intravenously. If improvement in the local or general condition of the patient is not apparent within 24 hours, more antitoxin may be administered. Injected antitoxin neutralizes only the toxin free in the circulatory system and that which will be absorbed later; it has no effect upon that which is already bound by the body cells.

SENSITIVITY TEST. Preliminary testing of the patient for sensitivity to horse serum should always be made before antitoxin is administered. This is done by injecting 0.05 ml. of a 1:20 dilution of horse serum intracutaneously, or a similar amount of the antitoxin.

DESENSITIZATION. In the event of a local reaction (a wheal with an area of erythema appearing within 10 to 30 minutes) or general reaction to the preliminary test, careful desensitization of the patient should be carried out:

Serial injections of diluted antitoxin as indicated below may be made at intervals of 15 minutes, provided no reaction occurs. If a reaction occurs after an injection, one should wait an hour and then repeat the last dose which failed to cause a reaction.

1. 0.05 ml. of a 1:20 dilution of antitoxin, subcutaneously
2. 0.05 ml. of a 1:10 dilution of antitoxin, subcutaneously
3. 0.1 ml. of undiluted antitoxin, subcutaneously
4. 0.2 ml. of undiluted antitoxin, subcutaneously
5. 0.5 ml. of undiluted antitoxin, intramuscularly
6. 0.1 ml. of undiluted antitoxin, intravenously
7. The remainder of the therapeutic dose is slowly injected intravenously.

In a person known to be allergic to horse emanations extreme care should be used, or bovine antitoxin should be substituted. A syringe containing epinephrine chloride solution should always be available when antitoxin is being injected.

Complications. The management of complications, especially circulatory failure and paralysis involving the mechanisms of swallowing and respiration, is often difficult. The therapeutic principles for the management of diphtheritic myocarditis are the same as those in other types of acute myocarditis. Absolute rest is essential, and intravenous therapy is often necessary. Though once considered to be contraindicated, digitalis is now thought to be of value in diphtheritic myocarditis and should be given if possible before there is evidence of decompensation. Oxygen, sedatives, a salt-poor diet and diuretics are indicated in cardiac insufficiency.

For shock and peripheral circulatory collapse, measures, such as the use of plasma, blood and ephedrine, designed to raise the blood pressure and to restore blood volume should be instituted.

Paralysis or weakness of the extremities requires rest, splinting and appropriate physical therapy. A polyethylene tube is useful for gastric feeding when muscles concerned with swallowing are involved. The respirator (p. 686) should be used early for respiratory paralysis, and maintenance of an adequate airway should be ensured. The emotional problems of both child and parent must be taken into account.

Laryngeal diphtheria. In addition to the general and specific measures, relief of obstruction to breathing is necessary. If the patient can rest and sleep quietly in a moistened atmosphere, intervention may not be required. Increasing restlessness, anxiety, increasing retractions of the suprasternal and substernal structures, and significant decrease in the volume of air exchange as estimated by auscultation indicate obstruction which needs relief. Cyanosis indicates that relief is urgent. Sedatives should be withheld during this period of observation, for they may conceal important symptoms.

In certain instances aspiration of the membrane by direct laryngoscopy may provide an adequate airway, but has the disadvantage that more edema and further obstruction may result from the manipulation.

Tracheotomy is now regarded as the most effective and safest method. It can be performed under local anesthesia, with slight risk of pneumomediastinum if no dissecting is done during the procedure (p. 686). One of its greatest advantages is the ease with which suction may be carried out. The tube can usually be removed after 7 to 10 days. During this period antibiotic therapy should be maintained.

REFERENCES

Committee on the Control of Infectious Diseases, Evanston, Ill., American Academy of Pediatrics, 1966, p. 38.

Freeman, V. J.: Studies on the Virulence of Bacteriophage-Infected Strains of Corynebacterium Diphtheriae. *J. Bact.,* 61:675, 1951.

Funt, T. R.: Primary Cutaneous Diphtheria. *J.A.M.A.,* 176:273, 1961.

Murphy, W. J., Maley, V. H., and Dick, L.: Continued High Incidence of Diphtheria in a Well Immunized Community. *Pub. Health Rep.,* 71:481, 1956.

Pappenheimer, A. M., Jr.; in R. J. Dubos and J. G. Hirsch (Eds.): *Bacterial and Mycotic Infections of Man.* 4th ed. Philadelphia, J. B. Lippincott Company, 1965, p. 468.

Schick, B.: Die Diphtherietoxin-Hautreaktion des Menschen als Vorprobe der prophylaktischen Diphtherieheilseruminjektion. *Münch. med. Wchnschr.,* 60:2608, 1913.

United States Dept. of Health, Education and Welfare. Morbidity and Mortality. Annual Supplement Summary 1965, Vol. 14, 53, Oct. 14, 1966.

Whitaker, J. A., Nelson, J. D., and Fink, C. W.: The Fluorescent Antitoxin Test for the Immediate Diagnosis of Diphtheria. *Pediatrics,* 27:214, 1961.

PERTUSSIS
(WHOOPING COUGH)

Definition. Pertussis is an acute infection of the respiratory tract caused by *Bordetella pertussis.** In its typical form the disease is characterized by a series of repeated spasmodic coughs ending in a forced inspiration (the whoop) and at times followed by vomiting. In mild cases neither the whoop nor the vomiting may be present.

History. De Baillou in 1578 wrote the first classic description of the disease. Bordet and Gengou (1906) described a small coccoid bacillus which they found in the sputum of active cases.

---

*Because of their nutritional and antigenic relations, a separate genus (Bordetella) has been proposed to include *H. pertussis, H. parapertussis* and *Brucella bronchiseptica.*

Since then Shipley, Holt and others have experimentally reproduced the disease in the chimpanzee, and the MacDonalds, in susceptible children. Goodpasture and Gallavan, by an ingenious method of inoculating the chorioallantoic membrane of the developing chick embryo, produced a pathologic lesion of the bronchial epithelium which is essentially that found in the human disease. Leslie and Gardner (1931) demonstrated the differences between the antigenic properties of the smooth (phase I) and the rough (phase IV) types of organism.

Etiology. *Bordetella pertussis* is regularly present in the upper respiratory tract during the early stage of the disease. It is seldom found in persons without symptoms, but is occasionally recovered from immediate contacts of an active case.

Epidemiology. World-wide in distribution, pertussis exists in most of the thickly populated communities, where it prevails epidemically at intervals of 2 to 4 years. The communicability rate is high, approaching that of measles and of chickenpox. In family exposures it is 75 to 90 per cent.

Pertussis may occur at any age. The youngest patient observed by the author was 2 weeks of age, the oldest 77 years, but about 50 per cent of all cases occur under 4 years of age. The number of reported cases in the United States decreased from 31,732 in 1956, with 266 deaths, to 13,005 in 1964 with 93 deaths. The incidence varies in different regions of the country and is higher in the female, especially above the age of 10 years.

Immunity. Susceptibility to the disease is great. In contrast to the temporary immunity to measles and diphtheria, the newborn infant is usually highly susceptible to pertussis. Proved second attacks are rare, though they are often suspected clinically. Humoral antibodies, as demonstrated by the agglutinin titer, complement fixation and mouse protective test, appear during convalescence and after active immunization. The organism has more antigens in common with *B. bronchiseptica* than it does with *B. parapertussis*.

Pathology. The lesions are located principally in the bronchi and bronchioles, although changes are also present in the trachea, larynx and the nasopharyngeal mucosa. Numerous bacilli are entangled within the cilia of the columnar ciliated

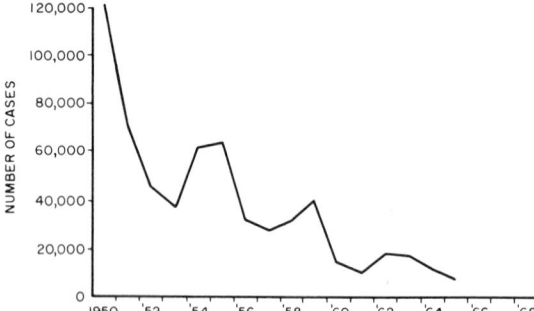

Figure 10-37. Pertussis: reported cases in the United States, 1950-1965. (From United States Department of Health, Education, and Welfare. Morbidity and Mortality, Annual Supplement Summary 1965, Vol. 14, No. 53, Oct. 14, 1966.)

epithelium, which may be covered by a muco-purulent exudate. The essential lesion consists in necrosis of the basilar and midzonal epithelium, with a focal infiltrate of neutrophils and macrophages. An infiltrate of lymphocytes and, to a smaller extent, of neutrophils is present in the walls of the respiratory passages and extends outward into the interalveolar septums to produce a peribronchial interstitial pneumonitis. Plugs of mucus are occasionally present in the small bronchi, with resultant obstructive emphysema and atelectasis. Little exudate is found in the alveoli unless secondary infection has occurred. Bronchiectasis may result from the pulmonary lesions. Small foci of hemorrhage may be found in the brain, but whether a true encephalitis occurs is not established.

Clinical Manifestations. The incubation period varies from 7 to 14 days. The course of the typical disease is about 6 weeks, representing 3 stages: catarrhal, spasmodic and convalescent, each lasting approximately 2 weeks.

The clinical course is extremely variable. The disease may exist in an extraordinarily mild form without vomiting, whooping or even spasmodic coughing. In 2 proved cases in nonimmunized persons the duration of cough was 1 week, and in a previously immunized patient only 4 days.

Catarrhal period. The onset is usually insidious with a mild cough, often nocturnal. During the next 10 days the cough becomes progressively intense, spasmodic and diurnal. Coryza, sneezing and anorexia are common, and hoarseness is occasionally present. In rare instances the disease resembles acute obstructive laryngitis.

Spasmodic period. Near the end of the second week the cough becomes aggravated. In the typical severe paroxysm a series of explosive efforts occurs, and the patient appears to strangle; the face becomes red and in some instances cyanotic; it temporarily appears swollen, and anxiety is apparent. The paroxysm ends with a sudden forceful inspiratory crow or whoop, often followed by vomiting or by the coughing up or swallowing of large amounts of thick, tenacious, mucoid sputum. Sweating, congestion of the neck and scalp veins, mental confusion, convulsions and exhaustion may follow the violent coughing. Infants may become so cyanotic that artificial respiration and oxygen inhalation are necessary. In small infants choking spells may replace the characteristic whoop. Activity, excitement, sudden changes in temperature or inhalation of irritating fumes tend to provoke paroxysms. Epistaxis often occurs, and subconjunctival hemorrhages and puffiness of the lower eyelids are common in severe cases.

Convalescent period. About the fourth week the number and severity of the paroxysms decrease, vomiting becomes less frequent, and the appetite returns. The hilar and basilar rhonchi disappear. An intercurrent infection, such as the common cold, may cause return of the major symptoms even to the point of resembling a new attack.

Diagnosis. Typical pertussis is readily recognized during the paroxysmal stage. In the early stage and in the atypical forms, however, it may be difficult to diagnose. The disease may be suspected when a progressive nocturnal cough becomes diurnal and continues in a spasmodic form, and when the physical examination reveals no obvious explanation of its cause. In such an instance the patient should be isolated and a culture taken.

The characteristic lymphocytosis appears during the late catarrhal or early paroxysmal stage. Average leukocyte counts range from 15,000 to 45,000 cells per mm.[3] of blood, with a progressive increase in the number of lymphocytes; infrequently the count may exceed 100,000. On occasion the lymphocytes may appear late, or the percentage of them may be equivocal.

The causative organism may be isolated from the upper respiratory tract by the cough-plate culture method or, preferably, by the nasopharyngeal swab method (see p. 543). Bacteriologic diagnosis is particularly helpful in the catarrhal stage and in the atypical case. A negative culture does not eliminate the possibility of pertussis.

Serologic tests for the presence of humoral antibodies include determination of the agglutinating titer, the complement-binding power or the mouse protective value. Since these all appear at the height or during the convalescent stage of the disease, they are of no value in early diagnosis.

Differential Diagnosis. A spasmodic cough similar to that of pertussis may be observed in tracheobronchitis, bronchiolitis and interstitial pneumonitis caused by a variety of agents. On occasion, epidemics of respiratory infection in infants and small children have so closely resembled pertussis clinically that it could be excluded only by failure to isolate *B. pertussis* and by absence of the usual changes in the white blood cells.

Other conditions which may resemble pertussis include sinusitis or adenoiditis with postnasal discharge, allergic rhinitis and bronchitis, endobronchial tuberculosis, foreign bodies in the larynx or trachea, the combination of tetany and upper respiratory tract infection and the respiratory infection associated with cystic fibrosis.

Parapertussis, caused by *B. parapertussis*, resembles mild pertussis so closely that it can be differentiated only by culture. An attack of one disease does not protect against the other.

Complications. *Respiratory tract.* The most frequent complications are in the respiratory tract. *Otitis media* is common, especially in infants, and is usually caused by secondary invading organisms. *Bronchitis* is so common that it may really be considered a part of the disease. *Bronchopneumonia* is by far the most important complication and is usually interstitial in type. Atelectasis is common, resulting from blocking of a bronchus with mucus. Vesicular or interstitial emphysema occurs in practically all severe cases. Air may reach the cellular tissues of the mediastinum and extend into the soft tissues of the neck. Cases in which there is widespread subcutaneous emphysema are often fatal. Pneumothorax and empyema are infrequent complications. *Bronchiectasis* is more frequent than is generally recognized. A pre-existing *primary tuberculous* infection may be disseminated. *Persistent pneumonia, atelectasis* and *pulmonary fibrosis* are not uncommon sequels. Cardiac dilatation involving chiefly the right side of the heart is most commonly associated with a diffuse pneumonic lesion.

Digestive tract. Severe and prolonged vomiting may result in emaciation. Prolapse of the rectum and hernia may be secondary to straining. Ulceration of the frenum may result from biting the tongue during the coughing spells; stomatitis may develop.

Nervous system. Convulsions are relatively common in infants. Tetany may occur when there is coexisting rickets and occasionally when there is alkalosis produced by loss of hydrochloric acid from excessive vomiting. Intracranial hemorrhages occur, but probably are infrequent as a cause of convulsions. Cerebral congestion and edema are common postmortem findings. Neurologic complications of pertussis include epilepsy, mental retardation, personality changes, spastic paralysis, myelitis, temporary or permanent visual disturbances, hemiplegia, monoplegia and aphasia. If caused by edema or congestion, they are temporary; if by hemorrhage or encephalitis, they may be permanent.

Hemorrhages. Hemorrhage is usually mechanical in origin, and occurs most often as epistaxis, hemoptysis and subconjunctival extravasations. The most serious type is intracranial.

Prognosis. From 1920 to 1963 the mortality rate from pertussis fell from 12.5 to 0.1 per 100,000 population. Although this decrease began before the introduction of effective active immunization and antibiotic therapy, there is little doubt that these factors now play important roles. Of the 269 deaths reported in the United States for 1959, 103 were in males and 166 in females. Pulmonary and cerebral sequels may constitute serious handicaps.

Prevention. (See also p. 190.) The infant should be carefully protected from exposure, but,

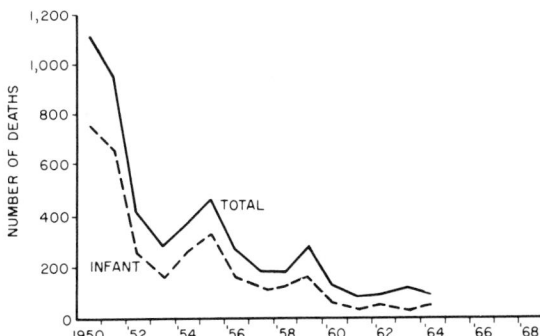

Figure 10-38. Pertussis: reported deaths in the United States, 1950-1964. (From United States Department of Health, Education, and Welfare. Morbidity and Mortality, Annual Supplement Summary 1965, Vol. 14, No. 53, Oct. 14, 1966.)

when exposed, should receive passive immunization. This may be accomplished by the intramuscular injection of 1.25 ml. of gamma globulin prepared from hyperimmune human serums (Hypertussis). Prophylactic doses of one of the broad-spectrum antibiotics may also be given.

The exposed subject should be isolated for 2 weeks, and active immunization should be started.

During the active phase the child should be isolated for 4 weeks to protect susceptibles and to protect him from possible secondary infections responsible for many of the serious complications.

Active immunization of all infants should be started by the third month of age or earlier. This can be accomplished by the intramuscular injection of a triple vaccine (D.P.T.) (see p. 190). Because *B. pertussis* has certain allergic attributes, and encephalopathy has occasionally followed injection of the vaccine, care should be observed in immunizing infants subject to seizures. In such instances small doses of vaccine should be given.

Treatment. Good nursing care is essential, especially for the seriously ill infant. When vomiting is persistent, feedings should be smaller and more frequent than usual. Sudden changes in temperature should be avoided.

Patients with convulsions or persistent dyspnea should be placed in an oxygen tent, even though acyanotic. Strangling from excessive mucus may be relieved by gentle suction and by placing the infant on his abdomen with the head lowered to facilitate drainage.

Infrequently, sedation with phenobarbital may be indicated, but excessive sedation should be avoided. Phenobarbital should be given intramuscularly for convulsions, and oxygen should be administered. Magnesium sulfate in doses of 0.05 ml. of a 50 per cent solution per pound (0.1 ml. per kg.) may be injected intramuscularly for its sedative effect, but not more often than twice a day.

Hyperimmune gamma globulin (1.25 to 2.5 ml.), injected intramuscularly, may be of benefit during the early stage of the disease.

The administration of pertussis vaccine or other antigens during the catarrhal period to a child previously immunized may have limited value.

Several drugs are effective in clearing the respiratory tract of the organism, though clinical symptoms often persist. The tetracyclines and chloramphenicol are about equally effective in doses of 10 mg. per pound per day (25 mg. per kg.) divided into 3 or 4 doses. Chloramphenicol is *not* recommended *for routine use* because of its potential toxic effect. Ampicillin (alpha-amino-benzyl penicillin) is effective in total daily doses of 75 to 100 mg. per kg. and currently is the drug of choice.

REFERENCES

Bradford, W. L.: The Bordetella Group; in R. J. Dubos and J. G. Hirsch (Eds.): *Bacterial and Mycotic Infections of Man.* 4th ed. Philadelphia, J. B. Lippincott Company, 1965, p. 742.

Byers, R. K., and Moll, F. E.: Encephalopathies Following Prophylactic Pertussis Vaccine. *Pediatrics*, 1:437, 1948.
Collier, A. M., Connor, J. B., and Irving, W. R., Jr.: Generalized Type 5 Adenovirus Infection Associated with the Pertussis Syndrome. *J. Pediat.*, 69:1073, 1966.
Nelson, J. D., Matteck, B. M., and McNabb, J.: Susceptibility of Bordetella Pertussis to Ampicillin. *J. Pediat.*, 68:222, 1966.
Olson, L. C., Miller, G., and Hanshaw, J. B.: Acute Infectious Lymphocytosis Presenting as a Pertussis-Like Illness: Its Association with Adenovirus Type 12. *Lancet*, 1:200, 1964.
United States Department of Health, Education, and Welfare: Morbidity and Mortality. Annual Supplement Summary, Vol. 14, #53, Oct. 14, 1966.
White, R., Finberg, L., and Tramer, A.: The Modern Morbidity of Pertussis in Infants. *Pediatrics*, 33:705, 1964.
Wiener, S. L., Tinker, M., and Bradford, W. L.: Experimental Meningo-encephalomyelitis Produced by Hemophilus Pertussis. *Arch. Path.*, 67:694, 1959.

PARAPERTUSSIS

Definition. Parapertussis is an acute infection of the respiratory tract caused by *Bordetella parapertussis*. The disease resembles mild pertussis, from which it can be distinguished only by bacteriologic methods.

History. Eldering and Kendrick, and Bradford and Slavin, independently isolated the causative organism in 1937 from patients clinically suspected of having pertussis. The organism was isolated in 1933 in Copenhagen, though its clinical relation was not recognized at the time.

Etiology. *Bordetella parapertussis* is a small, nonmotile, gram-negative coccobacillus, morphologically indistinguishable from *B. pertussis*. It has common antigenic fractions with both *B. pertussis* and *B. bronchiseptica*, but is identical with neither. *Bordetella parapertussis* is virulent for mice, producing pulmonary lesions after intranasal inoculation that resemble those of experimental murine pertussis. A similar, though less potent, toxin is produced.

Specific humoral antibodies develop during the course of the disease and may be demonstrable for at least 3 years. Second attacks have not been reported. An attack of either pertussis or parapertussis affords no immunity against the other disease. Active immunization against pertussis gives no protection against parapertussis.

Incidence. Bacteriologic and serologic evidence indicates that the disease is a common one which is usually overlooked clinically. From a random sample of routine hospital admissions in Rochester, New York, (1954) 7 per cent of the children had agglutinative titers of 1:320 or higher, compared to 34 per cent against *B. pertussis*.

Clinical Manifestations. The incubation period is not definitely known, but is probably 6 to 15 days. The onset is similar to that of pertussis, though it may be more abrupt. The cough is less severe, but is spasmodic and is sometimes followed by a whoop and less often by vomiting. The entire course of the disease is 1 to 3 weeks. The infection sometimes resembles tracheitis.

Complications are rare, though otitis media and

bronchitis have been observed. Two deaths have been reported in which the organism was isolated at autopsy.

Treatment. Active cases should be isolated. Therapy is usually only symptomatic. Experimentally, polymyxin B, Terramycin and chloramphenicol are effective, though treatment with them is rarely indicated because of the usually mild course of the disease.

REFERENCES

Bradford, W. L., and Slavin, B.: An Organism Resembling *Hemophilus Pertussis*, with Special Reference to Color Changes Produced by Its Growth upon Certain Media. *Am. J. Pub. Health*, 27:1277, 1937.

Eldering, G.: A Study of the Antigenic Properties of *H. Pertussis* and Related Organisms. II. Protection Tests in Mice. *Am. J. Hyg.*, 36:294, 1942.

Lautrop, H.: Parapertussis: *Bakterologiske, Epidemologiske og Kliniske under so gelser* (with an English summary). Kobenhavn, Ejnar Munksgaard, 1954.

Scherp, H. W., Bradford, W. L., Day, E., and Allen, R. M.: Humoral Antibodies and Intradermal Reactions to Chemical Fractions of Hemophilus Parapertussis. *Am. J. Dis. Child.*, 87:724, 1954.

Zuelzer, W. W., and Wheeler, W. E.: Parapertussis Pneumonia: Report of Two Fatal Cases. *J. Pediat.*, 29:493, 1946.

PURULENT MENINGITIS

For meningitis in the newborn infant, Tuberculous Meningitis, Lymphocytic Choriomeningitis, Cryptococcosis and the Acute Aseptic Meningitis Syndrome, see pages 404, 609, 693, 706 and 687.

General Considerations. Meningeal disturbances are caused by a variety of pathogenic agents. Nonsuppurative meningeal reactions include meningismus and serous meningitis; the latter (see p. 687) includes the meningitides produced by certain viruses, and syphilitic and tuberculous meningitis. Suppurative meningitis is characterized by a purulent exudate and is caused by the meningococcus, pneumococcus, streptococcus, *Hemophilus influenzae*, staphylococcus, colon bacillus and other pyogenic organisms. In the first 2 or 3 months of life gram-negative bacilli, especially *E. coli*, are the most frequent pathogens; from 3 months to 3 years or so of age, *H. influenzae is the most common one.* The typhoid bacillus and various types of the Salmonella group may cause meningitis in infancy and childhood, and nonhemolytic strains of streptococci and of staphylococci are occasionally encountered. Less frequently, organisms closely related to *Listeria monocytogenes* have been isolated from meningeal infections in human beings, as have the Friedländer bacillus, *Pseudomonas aeruginosa*, *Aerobacter aerogenes*, *Lactobacillus lactis*, the gonococcus and others.

Most bacteria, other than *M. tuberculosis*, usually cause a purulent reaction, although in the very early stage of infection, or as the result of inadequate (suppressive) antimicrobial therapy, the spinal fluid may not be purulent. In the majority of instances the meninges are infected hematogenously, but, on occasion, infection is by direct extension from a contiguous lesion, such as one in a mastoid, sphenoid sinus, dural sinus or meningocele. A fracture of the skull may provide a means of entrance.

Bacterial Diagnosis. Except in the young infant, the clinical picture is usually sufficiently characteristic to identify a meningeal infection. Etiologic diagnosis, however, depends upon identification of the bacterium in the spinal fluid. The presence of petechiae is suggestive of meningococcal infection.

Since the final outcome depends upon early diagnosis and adequate therapy, the spinal fluid should be examined whenever the diagnosis is suspected. The fluid should be collected in 3 separate tubes, when possible, and its appearance noted. From the fluid in the first tube a cell count and bacterial culture should be obtained, and a stained preparation of the centrifuged sediment should be made. The Gram stain often provides a clue to the proper culture media to be used; inoculation of a rabbit-blood-agar plate, an endo-agar plate and a tube of thioglycolate broth is usually indicated. Chocolate blood agar is an excellent medium for the growth of *H. influenzae*. The fluid in the second tube is used for chemical analysis of sugar, protein, chlorides, and the like; the third tube is frozen and saved for viral and other studies or is used for the culture, and a portion of the fluid in tube 1 is frozen and saved for the viral studies.

Therapy. Symptomatic and antimicrobial therapy should be started promptly. The appropriate drug for a known infecting bacterium is discussed under each of the several types of meningitis described in this section.

When no organism is found on a stained smear of the spinal fluid, or the identity of the one observed is uncertain, one of several therapeutic regimens should be initiated at once without waiting for the results of the bacterial culture: (1) a combination of penicillin and kanamycin, especially in the neonatal period, when the incidence of *E. coli* infection is high; (2) a combination of penicillin, sulfisoxazole (Gantrisin) and chloramphenicol, proved by experience to be effective (this combination should not be used for infants during the first 2 or 3 weeks of life); or (3) ampicillin, an antibiotic which has recently been shown to be as effective as the latter combination for *H. influenzae*, pneumococcal and meningococcal meningitides. Except in the neonatal period, ampicillin appears to be the selection of choice at the moment; it has the advantage of a single drug over multiple ones and avoids the use of the more toxic agent, chloramphenicol.

Changes in antimicrobial therapy should be made if a specific organism is identified which is not sensitive to in-vitro tests with the prescribed antibiotics or when the clinical response is not satisfactory.

The route of administration of antimicrobial agents should be the one most comfortable for the patient without sacrificing effectiveness. Kanamycin and streptomycin must be given intramuscularly. Chloramphenicol and sulfisoxazole should be given by mouth when possible, but the initial dose of chloramphenicol should be given intravenously. Sulfisoxazole may be given subcutaneously in a 5 per cent solution. Ampicillin and penicillin are best administered by periodic rapid drip or injection into the tube of a continuous intravenous infusion; the size and frequency of the doses result in undue pain and trauma to tissue when given intramuscularly for more than a few days. Intramuscular use of chloramphenicol or the tetracyclines is to be avoided whenever possible because of the frequency of local tissue necrosis.

Duration of therapy should be based upon clinical response and evidence that the causative agent has been eliminated. Treatment with antimicrobials should be given for a minimum of 7 days and should not be discontinued until the patient has been afebrile for at least 72 to 96 hours. The usual course is 10 to 14 days; among the variables are the promptness in initiating therapy and the infecting bacterium (see the following subsections). Subsequent examination of the spinal fluid 24 to 48 hours after institution of treatment is helpful in evaluating therapy, and examination before cessation of therapy is advisable.

Management of family contacts. Fortunately secondary cases are not common within family groups. When the meningococcus is the infecting agent, the members of the family and other close contacts may be given prophylactic therapy with a sulfonamide if the organism is sensitive to it. The recommended drug is sulfadiazine, the dose being 2 gm. every 12 hours for 4 doses for adults and 0.1 gm. per kg. every 12 hours for children under 20 kg. of body weight. Penicillin is not as effective in eliminating the carrier state unless used as in the treatment of meningitis.

If *H. influenzae* is the cause of the meningitis, there is a small but significant incidence of infection due to the same organism among family contacts under 3 years of age. Ampicillin in oral dosage of 50 mg. per kg. per day for 10 days is currently the drug of choice, but the adequacy of this regimen is in question.

Sequelae. The impressive decrease in mortality from bacterial meningitis has unfortunately been associated with a significant increase in numbers of patients with serious neurologic and mental sequelae. Among the more common complications is the subdural collection of fluid, especially in infants. Exploratory subdural taps should be performed in all instances when the clinical response is not optimal (see p. 1272).

MENINGOCOCCAL MENINGITIS AND MENINGOCOCCEMIA
(Cerebrospinal Fever; Epidemic Cerebrospinal Meningitis; Spotted Fever)

Etiology. The meningococcus (*Neisseria meningitidis*) is a gram-negative, biscuit-shaped diplococcus which in the body may be found extracellularly or intracellularly. It may be responsible for infection of the upper respiratory tract, septicemia, meningitis and other metastatic lesions, separately or collectively in a given patient.

The various immunologic types of meningococci are assigned to 4 groups: A, B, C and D. Strains belonging to groups A and C are encapsulated and definitely antigenic. Group B strains are less antigenic and do not have capsular swelling in antiserum. Group A strains cause the majority of outbreaks of the disease, whereas group B strains are usually responsible for sporadic cases. Very few group D strains have been isolated in the United States. A number of strains isolated from the pharynx do not fall into any of the major groups and probably do not have a significant pathogenic role.

Certain toxic properties of the organism are related to an endotoxin present in both living or dead forms. Group-specific exotoxins have not been established.

Epidemiology. The disease is endemic throughout the world; epidemics occur frequently. Since 1956 the annually reported number of meningococcal infections has varied between 2150 and 3040, and the number of deaths between 586 and 785.

Both endemic and epidemic infections occur most often in late winter and early spring months. Males are infected more often than females. About 45 per cent of all cases occur in children under 15 years of age, about 25 per cent in those under 5 years, and about 15 per cent in infants under 1 year. The case fatality rates are highest in infants and in adults over 50 years of age.

About 3 per cent of the population are carriers during interepidemic periods, and the rate may increase to 70 to 80 per cent during an epidemic. Upper respiratory tract infections may be caused by the meningococcus, and it may be that recovery from such an infection confers immunity against subsequent, more serious infections such as meningitis.

Immunity. One attack of the disease usually confers permanent immunity, but relapses and recurrences do occur. Probably the bactericidal power of the blood determines whether the organisms gain contact with the meninges. This mechanism of immunity, which would support the hematogenous theory of invasion, might also explain the low incidence of the disease during the first few weeks or months of life, when the infant may have protection from placentally transferred humoral antibodies.

Pathology. The mechanism of infection appears to be that of a bacteremia originating from a focus in the nasopharynx, the central nervous system being infected as a metastatic focus. The organisms multiply in the blood and elaborate toxin which aids in their dissemination and localization. Petechial and purpuric areas are characteristic of meningococcal septicemia and occur in the skin and in the mucous and serous membranes. Hemorrhagic and purulent metastatic lesions occur in the peritoneum, pericardium, pleura, joints, eyes and epididymis. Vegetative endocarditis may also occur.

The lesion of the central nervous system is a purulent inflammation of the arachnoid and pia mater, usually heaviest over the parietal and occipital lobes and over the cerebellum. The infection may extend to the ventricles and may obstruct the various openings, resulting in obstructive hydrocephalus. The intracranial portions of various cranial nerves, particularly the optic, facial and auditory, may be involved. Throughout the brain perivascular foci of leukocytes, round cells and red blood cells may be found, as well as hemorrhagic and necrotic areas. This aspect of the infection is often overlooked.

When there is an extensive purpuric eruption and death occurs suddenly in the initial stage, there is often a massive hemorrhage into the adrenal glands (the Waterhouse-Friderichsen syndrome, p. 1209).

Clinical Manifestations. Several clinical types of meningococcal infection are recognized, the most important being the meningitic and septicemic forms.

Meningitic form. Meningitis is the characteristic form of the disease. The onset is abrupt with general malaise, headache and irritability. Repeated and often projectile vomiting and prostration occur. Chills and convulsions, particularly in infants, are frequent. The temperature is high, the pulse is fast, and the respirations may be irregular. General muscular rigidity develops, especially in the muscles of the spine, producing the positive spine sign and even opisthotonos. Attempts to flex the neck produce pain and cause the patient to bend his knees and hips (Brudzinski's sign). If the leg is flexed at the hip, it cannot be straightened at the knee (Kernig's sign). *The rigidity of the neck and back is frequently absent in very young infants.*

Disturbances of the sensorium are frequent, causing delirium, stupor and even coma. Petechial or purpuric skin lesions are an early characteristic manifestation (Fig. 10-39). Herpes labialis is common. The *tache cérébrale*, a conspicuous linear mark produced by drawing the fingernail across the skin, indicates a disturbance of the vasomotor mechanism. A tense or bulging fontanel, choking of the optic disks and a positive Macewen sign are evidences of increased intracranial pressure. The last sign is a "cracked-pot sound" elicited by percussion over a distended lateral ventricle. Urinary retention, constipation, anorexia and rapid loss of weight may be clinical features.

The fulminating meningitic form is characterized by an explosive onset and rapid course, usually terminating in death. The entire course may last only 6 to 48 hours. The attack usually begins with violent headache, chills or convulsions, vomiting and high fever. Delirium or coma appears early, and the skin manifestations are pronounced; extensive involvement including massive hemorrhages in the adrenals is associated with profound shock and usually with sudden death (Waterhouse-Friderichsen syndrome, Fig. 10-40, p. 628).

Infrequently a meningitic infection may exist for days before suggestive signs lead to a lumbar puncture. This mild form usually occurs in infants as a sporadic case or near the end of an epidemic. Diarrhea and vomiting are common symptoms. Irritability is usually noted, but meningeal signs may be equivocal. Increased tension of the fontanel or weakness of an external ocular muscle may be the first clue. Relapses are common in this atypical form.

Chronic meningitic form. The clinical course may extend over a long time, usually characterized by emaciation, opisthotonos, hydrocephalus, cranial nerve palsies and by persistence of the meningococcus in the cerebrospinal fluid. The usual outcome is death, but the illness may last for months. Such clinical patterns are usually the result of delay in starting therapy or of *suppressive* rather than curative therapy.

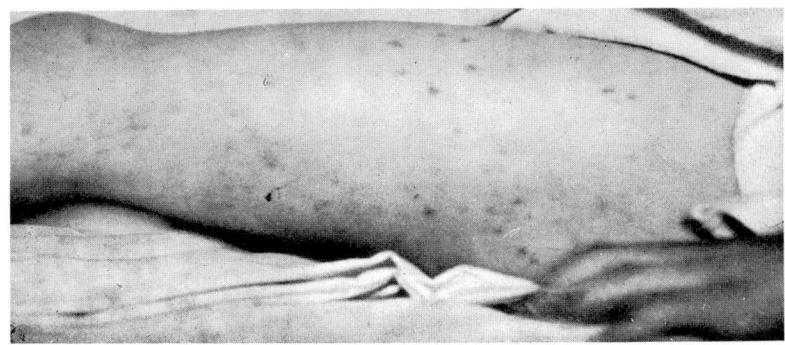

Figure 10-39. Purpuric eruption in meningococcal meningitis in a boy 6½ years of age.

Septicemic form. The onset is usually sudden, with fever, chills, vomiting and weakness. Skin lesions [Figs. 10-39 & 40 (p. 628)] develop rapidly If meningeal manifestations occur, they usually appear 1 to 3 days later. Most often if meningitis does not occur, the course of the septicemic form is rapid, ending either in death or, if therapy is effective, in recovery. In some instances low-grade fever with joint pains and muscular tenderness suggests a grippal infection or acute rheumatic fever, and the proof of meningococcemia by blood culture is unexpected.

Diagnosis. The meningitic form is diagnosed by examination of the cerebrospinal fluid, which is usually under increased pressure. The total cell count may range from only a few cells to several thousand per mm.[3] The majority of the cells are polymorphonuclear; rarely, at the outset, mononuclear cells may predominate. The protein content is elevated, the sugar content usually reduced, and the chloride content diminished. Though purulent cerebrospinal fluid containing intracellular and extracellular gram-negative diplococci is strong evidence in favor of meningococcal meningitis, a definite diagnosis is made only from culture. Samples of the cerebrospinal fluid should be taken in 3 sterile tubes: one for cell counting and direct smear, which is then placed in the incubator for future reference; the second for determinations of protein, chlorides and sugar; and the third for bacterial culture.

Cultures from the nasopharynx and from the blood are advisable before treatment is instituted. The white blood cell count is usually increased, sometimes as high as 20,000 to 30,000 per mm.[3] with a preponderance of polymorphonuclear cells.

Complications. *Hydrocephalus* and subdural collections of fluid (see pp. 1291, 1286) are frequent and important complications. Inability to obtain fluid by lumbar puncture when it is readily obtained by ventricular puncture may be the first indication of basilar obstruction. Unless the obstruction is relieved, either death occurs during the acute period, or hydrocephalus develops.

Other nervous system complications include headache which may persist for weeks or months, impairment of the intellectual faculties, chronic pachymeningitis, convulsions and various types of paralysis, spasticity and contractures.

Otitis media is common in the acute stage of the infection. Deafness is usually bilateral and permanent. It results from infection of the inner ear with or without associated middle ear infection.

Ophthalmia occurs in about 5 per cent of cases. There may be an optic neuritis, uveitis or purulent choroiditis which is usually embolic in origin and may lead to destruction of the eye. These lesions are usually unilateral. Optic atrophy may result, particularly in association with hydrocephalus. Conjunctivitis is common, and corneal ulcers may develop unless proper precautions are taken.

Arthritis of the large joints may occur, especially during the first week of the disease. *Endocarditis* is most frequently observed in meningococcemia without meningitis. *Pneumonia*, an occasional complication, is usually caused by secondary invading organisms.

Prognosis. The death rate from meningococcal meningitis varies considerably in different epidemics. Before the introduction of specific serum therapy the case fatality rate was about 75 per cent; in patients treated with serum it was about 20 to 30 per cent. The case fatality rate is now less than 10 per cent and is almost entirely limited to the group with adrenal inadequacy (Waterhouse-Friderichsen syndrome). As in other suppurative meningitides, there may be neurologic and psychotic sequelae.

Treatment. As in all types of bacterial meningitis, successful therapy depends upon early clinical recognition, proper identification of the organism, proper choice and administration of drugs, and adequate general care.

Until recently the sulfonamides were the drugs of choice. Recently there appears to be a significant increase, at least in certain geographic areas, of infections with type B meningococci, many of which are resistant to the sulfonamides. For this reason, penicillin, with or without a sulfonamide, is now considered to be the appropriate agent for therapy.

Penicillin G in aqueous solution should be given intravenously in doses approximating 400,000 units per kg. per day in 6 divided doses administered by rapid drip or push during a 1- to 10-minute period every 4 hours. Comparable results can probably be obtained by intramuscular administration of the same doses at the same time interval, but such doses cause pain and may cause local tissue damage, particularly in infants with a small muscle mass. It should be emphasized that very large doses of penicillin are necessary for reliable eradication of meningococci; many patients have arrived at the hospital with blood and spinal fluid cultures positive for meningococcus after several days of treatment of a respiratory infection with ordinarily adequate therapeutic doses of penicillin. Sulfisoxazole (Gantrisin) is equally effective as and less toxic than sulfadiazine. A total daily dose of 100 mg. per kg. is given intravenously in three 8-hourly doses. After the second day, or when possible, the same dose can be given orally and continued for 8 to 10 days. An adequate concentration of the sulfonamides in the cerebral spinal fluid is easily maintained. Blood cell counts and urine examinations should be made every other day. Certain reactions may occur, such as fever, rash or peripheral neuritis, at which time the drug should be discontinued.

The therapeutic role of the corticosteroids in circulatory collapse and shock (Waterhouse-Friderichsen syndrome) is controversial. The author favors the judicious use of them in severe cases. A single dose of hydrocortisone hemisuccinate sodium is given immediately, intravenously or intramuscularly (25 mg. to the infant, 50 mg.

to the preschool child, and 100 mg. to the older child). A similar dose is then given during each of the next 2 days, after which the dose is gradually diminished and discontinued after 5 days.

To correct hypotension, L-norepinephrine (Levarterenol) may be slowly introduced into the continuous infusion, guided by frequent checks of blood pressure. One milligram is dissolved in 500 mg. of fluid. Sloughing of the subcutaneous tissues may result from extravasation. The value of this drug in bacterial shock has recently been questioned. Stiehm and Damrosch suggest that dibenzyline, an adrenergic blocker and a vasodilator, may be more effective.

A second examination of the spinal fluid should be made 36 hours after treatment is begun if clinical response is not excellent, and a final examination should be made when therapy is discontinued.

General supportive treatment. Symptomatic care is often neglected. Adequate nutrition should be maintained; feeding by gavage is often necessary. Good nursing care serves to prevent the development of bedsores, stomatitis and the excessive drying of the conjunctivas in delirious patients. Distention of the bladder should be avoided, by catheterization if necessary. Excessive headache and restlessness may be relieved by administration of a suitable sedative, such as paraldehyde, and by spinal drainage. Excessive vomiting and fever quickly cause dehydration, which may be prevented or treated by the intravenous administration of 5 per cent glucose and saline. Solutions of amino acids are an efficient means of supplying nitrogen when parenteral feeding is required. Blood transfusions are indicated if the hemoglobin level is less than 9 gm. per 100 ml. The development of hyponatremia with water intoxication requires the use of a hypertonic solution of sodium chloride.

Before isolation precautions are discontinued it should be ascertained by culture of the nasopharynx that the child is not a carrier.

STREPTOCOCCAL MENINGITIS

The hemolytic streptococcus is a relatively infrequent cause of purulent meningitis. In the newborn infant the streptococcus may gain entry to the blood through a superficial infection, such as an umbilical one, or may reach the meninges directly through an infected meningocele. In older children otitis media, mastoiditis, sinus thrombosis, erysipelas or suppurative lesions of the head and scalp may constitute the portal of entry.

There is purulent exudate over the surface of the brain, resembling that of pneumococcal meningitis except that there is somewhat less fibrin in the exudate.

Streptococcal meningitis cannot be distinguished from other types of purulent meningitis except by bacteriologic examination of the cerebrospinal fluid, which should be made immediately if a meningeal infection is suspected.

Treatment. Treatment should be instituted at the earliest possible moment. Penicillin is the drug of choice and may be administered alone or in conjunction with a sulfonamide. Except in the extremely rare instance of penicillin-resistant beta hemolytic streptococci, penicillin is preferable to other antibiotics. In-vitro sensitivity tests of the infecting organism to the various antibiotics should always be obtained.

Whenever there is any question of a significant mastoid involvement, the mastoid should be opened and, if indicated at operation, the dura exposed. With early and adequate medical and surgical care the mortality rate should not be more than 10 per cent.

PNEUMOCOCCAL MENINGITIS

Pneumococcal meningitis is more prevalent among infants than among older children. The seasonal distribution is similar to that of pneumococcal pneumonia. There may be a history of pneumonia, upper respiratory tract infection or infection of the middle ear. Trauma, particularly fracture of the skull, may be a predisposing factor. Infection of the bloodstream is frequent.

Etiology. Any of the specific types of pneumococcus may be responsible for pneumococcal meningitis, but types III, V and XIV appear to be the more common ones.

Pathology. The lesions of the brain and meninges resemble those produced by the meningococcus. The heavy exudate of pus and fibrin may be more abundant over the anterior lobes and less over the basilar areas of the brain. For this reason spinal rigidity and opisthotonos may be slight or absent. The spinal meninges are usually only slightly involved.

Diagnosis. The clinical manifestations are similar to those of purulent meningitis caused by other pathogenic bacteria. The diagnosis depends upon the bacteriologic findings. The cerebrospinal fluid is purulent, containing many polymorphonuclear cells and gram-positive lancet-shaped diplococci which are usually easily recognized on direct smear and easily cultured on blood-agar medium. The sugar and chloride contents of the cerebrospinal fluid are decreased, and the protein is increased.

Complications. As with other purulent meningitides, the decreasing case fatality rate has been associated with a definite increase in serious complications, many of which are permanent and severely handicapping. There may be a variety of pneumococcal lesions outside the nervous system such as empyema, pericarditis, peritonitis and arthritis, but the more frequent and usually more important ones involve the central nervous system.

Prognosis. About 85 per cent of the patients

now survive. Both survival and the extent of residual damage are related to the promptness of instituting therapy and to its adequacy.

Treatment. Penicillin is the drug of choice, but many clinicians also use sulfadiazine in conjunction with it. Ampicillin is also effective.

Because the blood-brain barrier is high for penicillin, total doses of 2,000,000 to 12,000,000 units of the aqueous crystalline form are given daily by continuous intravenous drip for the first 3 days. After this, procaine aqueous penicillin is continued intramuscularly in doses of 1,000,000 units twice daily.

A sulfonamide, either sulfadiazine or sulfisoxazole (Gantrisin), may also be given (see p. 264).

All therapy is discontinued after 10 to 14 days, provided the clinical and cerebrospinal fluid findings are satisfactory. There is no indication for specific antiserum therapy.

Adequate fluid intake must be maintained. Sedation should be prescribed as indicated, but depression of the respiratory mechanism should be avoided. Early surgical drainage of foci, such as those of otitis media and mastoiditis, is indicated.

INFLUENZAL MENINGITIS

Etiology. *Hemophilus influenzae* is a common cause of bacterial meningitis in infants, the peak of incidence occurring between 6 and 12 months of age. It is rare during the first 2 months of life and infrequent after the fourth year. The strains causing meningitis are serologically related and are included in the group termed type b. In most instances the disease is preceded or accompanied by an infection of the upper respiratory tract which frequently includes involvement of the middle ear.

Clinical Manifestations. The clinical pattern of influenzal meningitis is essentially that of any other type of purulent meningitis. Though bacteremia is usually present, skin manifestations are rare. The cerebrospinal fluid rapidly becomes purulent, and in most instances the organism is readily identified. Infrequently in untreated cases for a short time and frequently when therapy has been suppressive rather than curative, the cerebrospinal fluid changes may be those of a lymphocytic type of response simulating tuberculous meningitis. The presence of gram-negative, pleomorphic, coccobacillary organisms in the direct smear of the sediment should suggest *H. influenzae*. Direct typing of the organisms from the cerebrospinal fluid may be made. The organism is easily cultured on a medium of chocolate agar.

Complications. Many complications of influenzal meningitis, but not all, seem to be related to delay in starting therapy, inappropriate selection of therapeutic agents or the use of appropriate agents in too small amounts for too short a time. Complications of the central nervous system include paralyses, mental retardation, nerve deafness and hydrocephalus. Subdural collections of fluid appear to be a factor in the production of some of these (see p. 1288).

Prognosis. Before the advent of effective antibacterial agents the mortality rate approximated 95 per cent; now the recovery rate should be about 95 per cent. But the incidence of serious and permanent complications has increased.

Treatment. A combination of chloramphenicol and sulfisoxazole (Gantrisin) has been the therapy of choice. Recent experience with ampicillin indicates that it is effective and safer than chloramphenicol. But with increasing use of ampicillin, reports of its failure to eradicate the infection are beginning to appear. Most of these failures have been among children who have received the drug by intramuscular injection after the first few days of treatment, or in whom the interval between administrations was longer than 4 hours, or both. On the basis of overall evidence, ampicillin remains the initial drug of choice, provided the physician is alert to the possibility of therapeutic failure and is prepared to substitute chloramphenicol when it is apparent that ampicillin is not adequate.

The recommended initial dose of ampicillin is 50 mg. per kg., followed by 25 mg. per kg. every 4

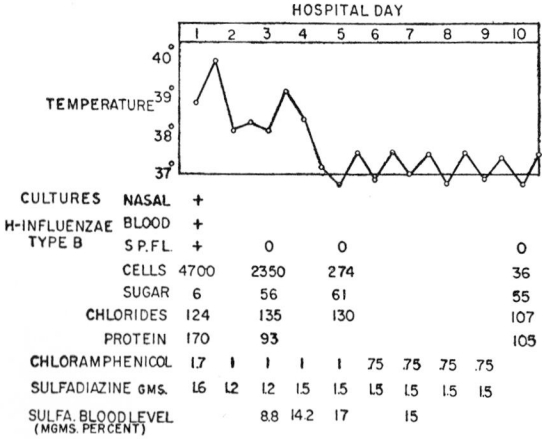

Figure 10-41. Chart of a female infant 6 months of age with *Hemophilus influenzae* meningitis. Onset 5 days before admission, with cold and diarrhea (2 siblings with "grippe"). One day before admission, fever, vomiting, irritability, stiff neck, full fontanel. No organisms seen in initial smear of cerebrospinal fluid; hence 3 million units of aqueous penicillin were injected daily for 2 days. Complete recovery.

hours (150 mg. per kg. per 24 hours). Because of its instability in solution, ampicillin should not be given by continuous intravenous drip. The drug is diluted with 5 ml. of isotonic saline and given over a period of 1 minute. Although the drug may be administered intramuscularly after 48 hours if the response to treatment is good, the most reliable regimen is one in which it is injected intravenously every 4 hours until the patient's temperature has been normal for 5 days. The average duration of treatment is 2 weeks.

If chloramphenicol is given, 50 mg. per kg. is given intravenously, followed by 25 mg. per kg. every 6 hours (100 mg. per kg. per 24 hours). The same dosage regimen may be followed by the oral route as soon as the patient can take and retain it. Sulfisoxazole (Gantrisin) is given in the manner prescribed for meningococcal meningitis (see p. 574).

STAPHYLOCOCCAL MENINGITIS

Staphylococcal meningitis is usually blood-borne from such primary foci as cutaneous lesions (especially in the newborn), otitis media, mastoiditis, sinusitis or sinus thrombosis. The infection may also be introduced at the site of a wound or from a surgical operation on the brain or meninges. There is widespread inflammation of the pia with a heavy accumulation of pus and frequently localized abscesses of the brain and meninges.

Diagnosis depends upon examination of the cerebrospinal fluid, in the sediment of which the organisms are usually numerous. The culture is confirmatory. Owing to the frequency of resistance of various strains of staphylococci to many of the antibiotics, especially penicillin, in-vitro testing to a number of them is mandatory at the time of the initial culture.

Before 1938 only nine recoveries had been reported; now the recovery rate is approximately 40 per cent.

Treatment. Initial therapy should provide coverage for both penicillin-sensitive and resistant organisms and should be continued until the results of the in-vitro sensitivity tests are available. Penicillin G in aqueous solution in combination with one of the semisynthetic penicillins, such as methicillin, nafcillin, oxacillin or cloxacillin, is recommended. Penicillin G should be given intravenously for the first 2 to 3 days and then intramuscularly; for the parenteral route of administration of the semisynthetic penicillins consult Table 5-16 (p. 251). When the results of the in-vitro sensitivity are known, the antibiotic therapy should be adjusted in relation to the demonstrated sensitivities of the organism and to the clinical response to the initial therapy. The prescribed drug(s) should be given in maximal dosage, based on age and size of the patient and continued for at least 8 to 10 days after *all* signs

of infection have disappeared. Careful search should be made for extrameningeal foci of infection; they should be treated surgically when this is possible. Currently there is interest in the cephalosporin antibiotics, which are effective against both penicillin-resistant and sensitive staphylococci. One or more of these agents should be included in the initial in-vitro testing of the pathogen.

REFERENCES

Barrett, F. F., Eardley, W. A., Yow, M. D., and Leverett, H. A.: Ampicillin in the Treatment of Acute Suppurative Meningitis. *J. Pediat.*, 69:343, 1966.

Eickhoff, T. C., Klein, J. O., Daly, A. K., Ingall, D., and Finland, M.: Neonatal Sepsis and Other Infections Due to Group B. Beta-Hemolytic Streptococci. *New England J. Med.*, 271: 1221, 1964.

Groover, R. V., Sutherland, J. M., and Landing, B. N.: Purulent Meningitis of Newborn Infants. *New England J. Med.*, 264: 1115, 1961.

Haggerty, R. J., and Ziai, M.: Acute Bacterial Meningitis in Children. A Controlled Study of Antimicrobial Therapy with Particular Reference to Combinations of Antibiotics. *Pediatrics*, 25:742, 1960.

Leedon, J. M., and others: Importance of Sulfadiazine Resistance in Meningococcal Disease in Civilians. *New England J. Med.*, 273:1395, 1965.

McCracken, G. H., Jr., and Eichenwald, H. F.: Antimicrobial Therapy in Infancy and Childhood. *Pediat. Clin. N. Amer.*, 13:231, 1966.

McKay, R. J., Jr., Ingraham, F. D., and Matson, D.: Subdural Fluid Complicating Bacterial Meningitis. *J.A.M.A.*, 152:387, 1953.

Mathies, A. W., Jr., and Wehrle, P. F.: Management of Bacterial Meningitis in Children. *Pediat. Clin. N. Amer.*, 15:185, 1968.

Morbidity and Mortality. Annual Supplement Summary 1965. Community Disease Center. United States Dept. of Health, Education, and Welfare, 14: No. 53, 1966.

Mortimer, E. A.: Rational Use of Prophylactic Antibiotics in Children. *Pediat. Clin. N. Amer.*, 15:261, 1968.

Pryles, C. V.: Antimicrobial Therapy in Staphylococcal Disease of Children. *Pediat. Clin. N. Amer.*, 15:167, 1968.

Stiehm, E. R., and Damrosch, D. S.: Factors in the Prognosis of Meningococcal Infection. *J. Pediat.*, 68:457, 1966.

TETANUS
(Lockjaw)

The systemic manifestations of tetanus are caused by the powerful exotoxin, liberated during the actively growing phase, of *Clostridium tetani,* a spore-forming organism. Like diphtheria, the infection remains localized. Infection is almost always acquired through an open wound.

History. Tetanus was produced experimentally before the organism was isolated in pure culture. In 1884 Carle and Rattone transmitted it to rabbits by inoculation of material from an acne pustule that represented the nidus of a fatal human case, and Nicolaier produced a tetanus-like disease in mice, guinea pigs and rabbits by inoculating them with suspensions of dirt. Nicolaier suggested that the disease was carried by organisms that multiplied locally and produced a strychnine-like poison. Kitasato (1889) isolated the organism in pure culture by heating pus to a temperature of 80°C. for 45 to 60 minutes. Von Behring and Kitasato (1890) demonstrated that tetanus toxin is antigenic, capable of producing antitoxin.

Etiology. *Clostridium tetani* is an anaerobic, spore-bearing organism, widely distributed in soil. The bacillus is frequently found in the intestinal tracts of herbivores and, at times, of man. Under suitable conditions the tetanus bacillus produces several poisons: a lysin for red blood cells, a substance injurious to leukocytes and a neurotropic toxin (tetanospasmin) which produces muscular rigidity and spasms. Unlike diphtheria toxin, tetanus toxin produces no skin reaction suitable for the assessment of immunity.

Epidemiology. Tetanus occurs most frequently in areas where soil contamination is heavy and standards of cleanliness and care of wounds are poor. It is rare in the newborn infant when aseptic obstetrics is practiced, but otherwise it is a relatively common and serious problem. During World War II active immunization of the military personnel with toxoid almost completely prevented its occurrence (8 cases with 3 deaths).

Pathogenesis. There is no typical wound that gives rise to tetanus. It may result from the most trivial scratch or insect bite, and the portal of entry is often not apparent. Injuries most likely to lead to tetanus are deep puncture wounds, because they afford ideal anaerobic conditions, and crushing wounds and burns, because they provide necrotic tissue. The site of infection has been reported in the tonsil, the alimentary tract and in ocular and aural lesions. Infection has resulted from contaminated catgut and serologic products. Though tetanus occasionally results from smallpox vaccination, it is practically always due to improper care of the secondarily infected lesion rather than to contaminated virus. Infection in the newborn infant is usually in the umbilical area.

The manner of absorption and the mode of action of the toxin have been the subject of considerable controversy. There are 2 main hypotheses: (1) that the toxin is absorbed at the motor nerve endings and reaches the anterior horn cells of the central nervous system by means of the axis cylinders; and (2) that the toxin is absorbed by the lymphatics and distributed to the central nervous system by arterial blood. After the toxin has become fixed to nerve tissue it apparently is not easily neutralized by specific antitoxin, but is in its free, circulating form.

Immunity. Immunity to tetanus may be natural or acquired. Mammals vary in susceptibility. The blood of naturally resistant animals contains practically no antitoxin; hence their immunity cannot be humoral. Persons of all ages are susceptible. The newborn has placentally transmitted antitoxin, but it is usually inadequate for protection.

The toxin is highly antigenic, and the prophylactic and therapeutic use of its specific antitoxin is of tremendous practical importance. It acts by neutralizing toxin, but does not prevent the germination of spores or multiplication of the bacilli in tissue. Modification of the toxin into toxoid by treatment with formalin affords a potent antigen for the production of active immunity.

Clinical Manifestations. The incubation period is usually 5 to 14 days, but may be prolonged to several weeks in mild infections or when the course has been modified by antiserum.

The clinical manifestations are usually generalized, but they may be localized to the area of injury when there is incomplete neutralization of toxin in the area of the injury, but complete neutralization of that in the blood. The action of the toxin in such instances is on the motor end-organs, resulting in localized spasm and rigidity.

The onset of the generalized form is usually insidious, with increasing degrees of muscle stiffness, especially in the jaw and neck. Within 48 hours the disease is well defined, and difficulty in opening the mouth (trismus) is evident. Difficulty in swallowing, restlessness, hyperirritability, headache, chilliness, and pain in the extremities are early symptoms. A clonic convulsion, caused by the effect of toxin on the anterior horn cells, is often the first symptom. Rigidity of the abdominal muscles may suggest an acute intra-abdominal lesion.

The spasm is characteristic. The body exhibits boardlike rigidity, while the head is drawn back in pronounced opisthotonos with legs and feet extended. The arms are stiff and the fists clenched. The spasm of the facial muscles results in a fixed expression (the sardonic grin, or *risus sardonicus*). The eyebrows are raised, and the mouth is distorted by the downward and outward drawing at the angles. The patient is apprehensive. The spasms at first are intermittent and often separated by apparently complete relaxation. Later the periods of relaxation are less obvious, and the seizures become painful. Intramuscular hemorrhage may result from violent contractions. Cyanosis and asphyxia may result from paroxysms affecting the respiratory or laryngeal muscles. Convulsions may be precipitated by the slightest stimulus, such as handling the patient, attempts to drink or even by visual or auditory stimulation. Profuse sweating is common. Retention of urine may be due to spasm of the urethral muscles. In rare instances spasms may be sufficiently severe to cause compression fractures of the spine; hence roentgenographic examination of the spine of a patient who has had unusually long and severe spasms should be obtained before he is permitted out of bed.

Fever is usually of a low grade, except that there is often an elevation during the terminal stage. Respirations are variable in rate and depth, and the pulse rate is increased. The cerebrospinal fluid is normal, except for some increase of pressure. There is usually a moderate leukocytosis.

Diagnosis. The diagnosis is usually not difficult. The history of a wound and the characteristic type of muscular spasticity, particularly of the jaw, are fairly conclusive. In infants other convulsive disorders may be confusing. Spasms due to strychnine rarely involve the jaw muscles and are interspersed by periods of more complete relaxation. Tetany may be recognized by chemical studies of the blood. Meningitis may be identified by examination of the cerebrospinal fluid. Tetanus is probably the only condition likely to be confused with rabies. The history of a bite, mental excitement, constant pharyngeal and laryngeal spasm, absence of trismus, and pleocytosis of the cerebrospinal fluid are distinguishing features of rabies. Local causes of stiffness of the jaw, such as enlarged cervical lymph nodes and retropharyngeal abscess, should be distinguished.

Prognosis. The case fatality rate is still high. In 1964, 289 cases were reported in the United States with 179 (62 per cent) deaths. Fatal cases usually terminate within a week or so and are more frequent after short incubation periods. Uncontrolled seizures, respiratory complications and grossly contaminated wounds contribute to an unfavorable outcome. Mortality rates are highest in newborn infants and the aged. Most deaths are precipitated by respiratory conditions such as obstruction by secretions, asphyxia from laryngeal spasm, prolonged anoxia, atelectasis and pneumonia. The judicious use of tracheotomy appears to have facilitated the management of these complications.

Prevention. The prevention of tetanus consists to a considerable degree in the prevention of injuries; it is, in part, an educational endeavor, which should include children. Most communities have legislation to control the sale of fireworks. Competent surgical care of wounds is essential.

The injection of antitoxin within a few hours of the occurrence of a wound produces *passive immunization* and prevents tetanus or lengthens the incubation period and results in a milder form of disease.

The generally recommended prophylactic dose of antitoxin is 1500 to 5000 units injected subcutaneously after a preliminary skin test to determine sensitivity to horse serum, but some give as much as 10,000 to 20,000 units. The difficulty of deciding when antitoxin should be used, the fear of anaphylaxis, the induction of serum sensitivity and the occurrence of tetanus even when passive immunization has been carried out are all practical objections to this form of prophylaxis. The use of tetanus immune globulin (human) U.S.P. obviates the danger of sensitization to horse serum. The recommended dose is 250 units. The administration of penicillin for 2 or 3 days after a severe injury may be an *additional* preventive factor because of its bactericidal effect.

When antitoxin is given to a child who has not had active immunization, it should be considered obligatory to give tetanus toxoid within the next few weeks.

Active immunization is effective in reducing the incidence of tetanus. Alum-precipitated, aluminum hydroxide-absorbed, and fluid toxins are available. Though each is definitely antigenic, alum-precipitated and aluminum hydroxide-absorbed toxoids produce more durable immunity than does fluid toxoid. On the other hand, fluid toxoid produces a more rapid secondary response

and therefore is the choice for a booster injection after a wound.

For basic immunization, 3 primary injections of toxoid at intervals of 1 to 3 months are advised, with subsequent booster injections (see p. 190). A severely wounded, immunized person, or one in whom the last injection of toxoid was made 4 or more years previously, is afforded maximal prophylaxis by the simultaneous injection of both antitoxin and fluid toxoid in different extremities. Recent evidence indicates that booster injections of tetanus toxoid are often given too frequently. If accurate dates of previous injections are available, an interval of one year appears to be a safe one for emergency injections.

Treatment. Constant attention to the general care and supportive measures are essential. The patient should be kept quiet, and external stimulation should be avoided. Oral and gastric feeding should be deferred until the dangers of vomiting and aspiration no longer exist. Immediate surgical care of the wound is important.

Sedatives. The ideal sedative would be one capable of controlling spasms and convulsions without respiratory depression. Unfortunately, this requirement is not easily met.

Chlorpromazine (Thorazine), especially in combination with a barbiturate, is considered by some to be the drug of choice. The dose of chlorpromazine is 2 mg. per kg. per 24 hours in 4 or 6 divided doses. An initial dose of 25 to 30 mg. may be given.

Paraldehyde given rectally is one of the safest and most effective sedatives. Avertin (tribromoethanol amylene hydrate) administered rectally in doses of 10 to 15 mg. per kg. (5 to 7 mg. per pound) is effective, but, since it is a respiratory depressant, its effect must be carefully watched. Phenobarbital in individual doses of 15 to 30 mg. by gavage is a satisfactory sedative in tetanus neonatorum.

Curare and related drugs should be used only when the spasms cannot be controlled by other measures, and then only by experienced personnel.

Since death is often related to respiratory obstruction, tracheotomy may be lifesaving and should be carried out when pulmonary ventilation is impaired. Oxygen and the use of the respirator may be required.

Penicillin should be given every 12 hours for its probable effect on *Cl. tetani* and to control secondary infection. Other antibiotics should be given when indicated to control specific secondary invaders.

Serum therapy. Antitoxin is the only specific agent. Fifty thousand units intramuscularly and 50,000 units intravenously should be given immediately. After the intravenous administration of antitoxin, 5000 to 10,000 units may be infiltrated around the wound in preparation for wide excision, if indicated. The patient should be tested intradermally for the possibility of sensitization to horse serum. If he is sensitive, rapid desensitization should be carried out (p. 567), or tetanus immune globulin (human) may be used in doses of

3000 to 40,000 units intramuscularly. The wound should be left open. Firor advises daily intramuscular injections of 5000 units to assure the maintenance of sufficient humoral antibody.

Active immunization should be started during convalescence.

REFERENCES

Brooks, V. B., Curtis, D. R., and Eccles, J. C.: Mode of Action of Tetanus Toxin. *Nature*, 175:120, 1955.

Edsall, G., Elliott, M. W., Peebles, T. C., Levine, L., et al.: Excessive Use of Tetanus Toxoid Boosters. *J.A.M.A.*, 202:111, 1967.

Report of the Council on Drugs: A New Agent for Prophylaxis of Tetanus, Tetanus Immune Globulin. *J.A.M.A.*, 192:471, 1965.

Smith, M. H. D.: Tetanus; in H. C. Shirkey (Ed.): *Pediatric Therapy*. 3rd ed. St. Louis, C. V. Mosby Company, 1968, p. 411.

Smolens, J., Vogt, A. B., Crawford, M. N., and Stokes, J., Jr.: The Persistence in the Human Circulation of Horse and Human Tetanus Antitoxins. *J. Pediat.*, 59:899, 1961.

Symposium on Tetanus: *Proc. Staff Meet., Mayo Clin.*, 32:141, 1957.

Volk, V. K., and others: Antigenic Response to Booster Dose of Diphtheria and Tetanus Toxoids. *Pub. Health Rep.* 77:185, 1962.

BRUCELLOSIS

(Undulant Fever; Malta Fever; Bang's Disease)

Brucellosis is an infectious disease which primarily affects domestic animals, but is transmissible to man, in whom it produces a variety of clinical patterns. Infection in children is less frequent than in adults.

Etiology. There are several strains of Brucella organisms, classified as follows: *B. melitensis* (goat), *B. abortus* (cattle) and *B. suis* (swine). These species may be differentiated by the dye-typing method of Huddleson and by their ability to produce hydrogen sulfide.

Though devoid of exotoxin, the bacillus has an endotoxin which plays a part in the pathogenesis of the disease. After invasion it enters and probably multiplies within the cells, thus creating a type of parasitism which accounts, in part, for the chronicity observed in both man and animal. Hypersensitivity is a feature of the disease which definitely contributes to the clinical manifestations.

Epidemiology. Human infection occurs principally by contact, ingestion, accidental inoculation and inhalation. The incidence is higher among farmers and slaughterhouse workers. Ingestion of raw milk accounts for about one fourth of the cases, the remainder originating from contact with infected animals or their environment. Infection in swine has served to a great degree in maintaining the disease. Skin and conjunctivas serve as important portals of entry, while inhalation of brucella-contaminated dust is a prob-able method of transmission. The laboratory is an occasional source of infection. The reported number of human infections, probably one fifth or less than the number of actual cases, has markedly decreased: 3510 in 1950; 1444 in 1955; 751 in 1960; 262 in 1965. States with a case rate of 0.50 per 100,000 population in 1965 were Idaho, South Dakota, Iowa and Arkansas.

The disease is relatively infrequent among infants and children. The apparent relative immunity of the young is not fully understood. McBride states that among 48 children who ingested contaminated milk, 9 developed agglutinins, and only 2 exhibited clinical manifestations of the disease. Obviously, children have less opportunity than adults for direct contact with infected animals. Intrauterine infection has been reported, and Brucella organisms have been demonstrated in the colostrum of an infected mother.

Pathology. The pathologic changes are nonspecific and appear to involve principally the reticuloendothelial system. Histologically, there are hyperplasia of the reticuloendothelial system, and granulomatous foci and focal necroses in the liver, spleen and lymph nodes.

Clinical Manifestations. The incubation period varies between 5 and 30 days, but is usually about 2 weeks.

Acute form. The onset of the acute form is often gradual, with fatigue, irritability, headache and malaise which may exist for several days or weeks before fever occurs. Pain in the chest with a nonproductive cough may be observed. In some instances the onset is sudden with fever, chills and nocturnal sweating. Frequently the patient feels well in the morning, but quite ill in the afternoon. This alternating daily cycle of well-being and extreme malaise eventually leads to weakness, loss of weight, and secondary anemia. Anorexia, constipation and abdominal pain are frequent complaints, and diarrhea and bloody stools occasional ones. The course may persist for several months. The febrile episodes are often intermittent, with fever lasting from 1 to 2 weeks, followed by afebrile periods.

The wide variety of localized manifestations of brucellosis and the relative infrequency of the infection in infants and children make it impossible to define a characteristic pattern except for the undulating fever. The liver and spleen may become enlarged and tender, and occasionally jaundice occurs. Lymph node involvement may be widespread, and there may be abscesses in them as well as in the subcutaneous tissue. Bone and joint involvement is relatively common, especially in the large joints and the spine. Ocular manifestations include keratitis, retinitis, uveitis, papilledema and optic neuritis. Purulent meningitis and infections of the urinary tract are occasional manifestations. At times skin lesions resembling rose spots occur.

There is usually a leukopenia with a relative

lymphocytosis, although the total leukocyte count may be normal and at times is even increased. An increase in the number of large mononuclear cells and eosinophils may also be observed. The clotting time may be prolonged, with imperfect clot retraction. Secondary anemia is common.

Chronic form. Chronic brucellosis presents a variety of symptoms. In young children there may be no characteristic symptoms, and in older children and adults they may be so vague as to suggest neurasthenia. Generalized weakness, prolonged malaise, low-grade fever, insomnia and vague aches and pains are common. The undulating fever frequently observed in the acute form is seldom seen in chronic brucellosis. Bursitis, periarthritis and spondylitis should suggest the chronic form of infection. Persistent lymphadenitis may be observed.

Diagnosis. A history of unexplained fever in a patient who has ingested raw milk products is suggestive of brucellosis. The disorders that may resemble brucellosis include typhoid fever and other salmonella infections, malaria, tuberculosis, Hodgkin's disease, rheumatic fever, influenza, tularemia, arthritis, appendicitis, cholecystitis, subacute bacterial endocarditis and even neurasthenia.

The diagnosis is established by identification of the organism in the blood, urine, bile, joint fluid, aspirates from abscesses, or bone marrow biopsy material. Cultures should be observed for 2 or 3 weeks.

Agglutinins may appear in the blood by the tenth day of the disease, or not until late in convalescence; in 5 to 10 per cent of active infections in man they may not be demonstrable at any time. On the other hand, agglutinins may be present in the blood serum of certain persons who have consumed raw milk, but are free from symptoms, and in those who have had intradermal tests with Brucella antigens. Though a titer of 1:80 to 1:160 is generally considered significant, the demonstration of a rising titer is of greater diagnostic significance. Falsely positive agglutinin titers may appear in tularemia and in persons immunized with cholera vaccine. Guinea pigs may be injected subcutaneously with suspected infectious material and their serum subsequently tested for agglutinins, and their tissues may be examined for lesions of brucellosis.

The *intradermal injection* of a suspension of heat-killed organisms or the nucleoprotein of the organism (brucellin) produces a dermal reaction in most infected persons. The reaction is an allergic one resulting from past or present infection; it is useful for epidemiologic surveys, but has limited value as a diagnostic aid.

Complications. In a disease whose natural course may be as prolonged as that of brucellosis and whose manifestations are as protean, it becomes somewhat arbitrary to designate particular lesions as chronic manifestations or as complications. In any event, arthritis with or without hydroarthrosis, osteomyelitis (especially spondylitis), pericarditis, peritonitis, pleurisy, meningitis, encephalitis, infection of the urinary tract, abscesses of the lymph nodes and subcutaneous tissues, and purpura have all been observed in cases of long standing. Endocarditis of the vegetative type may result from brucella infection superimposed on a previously damaged heart valve.

Prognosis. Death occurs in about 1 per cent of recognized cases. The prolonged disability, often lasting for months or years, is the important feature. In children the disease is less severe than in adults. Relapses are more frequent in persons in whom a definite increase of humoral antibodies (agglutinins) fails to develop, and in those with mild symptoms.

Prevention. Isolation of the patient is unnecessary, since human transmission seldom, if ever, occurs. Caution, however, should be exercised in handling infected tissues or exudates. The infection may possibly be transmitted by blood transfusions.

The prevention of brucellosis consists in (1) pasteurization of milk and its products; (2) eradication of the infection in domestic animals; (3) vaccination of persons intimately associated with diseased animals or who have laboratory contact with the organism; and (4) public education concerning the danger of consuming raw milk.

Treatment. Tetracycline is the drug of choice for the infection of average severity. It is given orally in a total daily dose of 40 to 50 mg. per kg. in 4 equal doses for 21 days. The course is repeated if there is a relapse. In severe infections or in those which do not respond to this treatment, streptomycin is given in conjunction with tetracycline. Streptomycin is given once or twice a day intramuscularly for 2 weeks in total daily doses of 0.5 to 1.0 gm. Corticosteroid therapy, though seldom necessary, may be beneficial in alleviating toxic manifestations.

Desensitization by injection of brucella antigen has been used with antibiotic therapy in chronic infections. Rest and, at times, psychotherapy are important adjuvants in the management of chronic infections.

REFERENCES

Bothwell, P. W.: Brucellosis in Children. *Arch. Dis. Childhood,* 37:628, 1962.

Bruce, D.: Note on Discovery of a Micrococcus in Malta Fever. *Practitioner,* 39:161, 1887.

Elberg, S. S.: The Brucellae; in R. J. Dubos and J. G. Hirsch (Eds.): *Bacterial and Mycotic Infections of Man.* 4th ed. Philadelphia, J. B. Lippincott Company, 1965, Chap. 28, p. 698.

Meyer, K. F.: Trends in Brucellosis Control. *Pub. Health Rep.,* 71:511, 1956.

Spink, W. W.: *The Nature of Brucellosis.* Minneapolis, University of Minnesota Press, 1956, p. 464.

Spink, W. W.: Current Status of the Therapy of Brucellosis in Human Beings. *J.A.M.A.,* 172:697, 1960.

Wallis, H. R. E.: Brucellosis in Children. *Brit. M. J.,* 1:617, 1957.

TULAREMIA
(Rabbit Fever)

Tularemia is an infectious disease of rodents which is transmissible to man.

History. Tularemia was identified in Tulare County, California, in 1910 by McCoy, who observed a "plaque-like disease" among ground squirrels. Wherry (1914) described the first case in a human being. Francis (1920) produced the disease in the guinea pig by inoculating it with the blood of a person who had died after the bite of a deerfly.

Etiology. *Francisella tularense* is a small, non-motile, gram-negative, coccoid bacillus. It is easily destroyed by the usual disinfectants and by heating at 56°C. for 10 minutes.

Epidemiology. In the United States important sources of infection are animals, insects and laboratory material. Although tularemia is commonly associated with wild rabbits, it also appears to be frequently transmitted by infected ticks (Assal). Birds (quails, chickens) and cold-blooded animals may also harbor the organism. Various insects serve as vectors; these include the wood-tick, dogtick, horsefly, bedbug, flea, louse; in Utah the deerfly plays an important role. In the southern United States Hopla demonstrated infestation in the lonestar tick. The seasonal incidence is influenced by the period of the year when ticks are prevalent or when rabbits or other game animals are being hunted or trapped.

Tularemia has been observed in the United States, Alaska and Canada, in Japan, where it is known as "Ohara's disease," and in Norway, Russia and other parts of Europe. In the United States the incidence is greatest in Arkansas, Kansas, Illinois, Missouri and Tennessee. The disease is more frequent among adults than among children.

Infection may be acquired by skinning or dressing of rabbits and such other animals as skunks, deer, foxes, rats and tree squirrels; it has followed the bites of such animals as dogs, cats, squirrels and raccoons. Contact with sheep may result in infection, especially among shearers, since the wool may contain infected ticks and contaminated fecal droplets. Infection may also be acquired by ingestion of inadequately cooked contaminated meat or the drinking of contaminated water; the organism has been demonstrated in the water of several streams. Transmission from man to man, though possible, is not probable. Laboratory infection is common; unless extreme care is exercised, practically everyone who handles fluid cultures or infected animals contracts the disease. One attack of the disease usually confers lasting immunity.

Pathology. In addition to the local lesion at the portal of entry and the lesions in the regional lymph nodes, there are focal necrotic areas in various stages of evolution throughout the body. Small yellow-white lesions are found in the spleen, liver, kidneys, lungs, lymph nodes and bone marrow. Histologically, the lesions may resemble miliary tubercles with or without central purulent exudate. In the central areas of these lesions polymorphonuclear cells are abundant, often associated with central necrosis and surrounded by an area of small round cell infiltration. In the more diffuse lesions, fibroblasts and mononuclear cells are abundant, particularly during the subacute stage of the infection.

Clinical Manifestations. The average incubation period is 3 to 5 days. Based somewhat upon the reaction at the portal of entry, 6 clinical types are generally recognized: (1) ulceroglandular, (2) oculoglandular, (3) glandular, (4) pulmonary, (5) typhoidal and gastrointestinal, and (6) oropharyngeal. Manifestations are both local and generalized.

The onset is abrupt, with fever, chills, headache and vomiting. Generalized pains, prostration and sweating are usually present. Sometimes the liver and spleen are enlarged. Various exanthems (macules, papules, pustules and petechiae) may be observed as well as jaundice. Fever lasts 1 to 2 weeks.

The local lesion, a papule, usually becomes ulcerated with enlargement and tenderness of the regional lymph nodes, which suppurate in about half of the cases.

When the portal of entry is the conjunctiva, photophobia, itching, lacrimation, hyperemia and swelling of the eyelid, usually the upper, occur. Preauricular and cervical lymph nodes enlarge and frequently suppurate. Though damage to the eye is rare, corneal ulcers may sometimes perforate and permanently impair vision.

The *pulmonary* type occurs from inhalation or by the hematogenous route. The pneumonia is patchy, confluent and often migratory. The mediastinal and peribronchial lymph nodes are enlarged.

The *oropharyngeal* type, resulting from ingestion of contaminated material, is characterized by ulcerated lesions of the oral cavity, throat and tonsils with cervical adenitis. The tonsils may be covered with exudate or a pseudomembrane, not unlike that of diphtheria. In children this type may be rapidly fatal.

Cryptogenic infection may occur, and the clinical course may resemble that of typhoid fever.

There is moderate leukocytosis and secondary anemia. Albuminuria is common.

Diagnosis. The disease may resemble atypical pneumonia, psittacosis, brucellosis, septicemia, influenza, tuberculosis and the typhoid-paratyphoid group of diseases. The typical case (ulceroglandular) in which the patient becomes ill after dressing or skinning a wild rabbit should offer little difficulty in diagnosis.

Confirmation may be obtained from agglutination and skin tests and from bacterial cultures and inoculation of laboratory animals. By the end of the second week of illness the patient's serum contains specific antibodies, and the agglutinin titer gradually increases, sometimes exceeding 1:1280. The skin test, described by Foshay, consists in the intracutaneous injection of a suspension of detoxified, formalin-killed *P. tularensis.* The tuberculin-like reaction is said to occur by the third day of illness.

Complications. Chronic bronchitis, bronchopneumonia and pleural effusions are probably more common than clinical symptoms suggest. Peritonitis, sometimes with persistent ascites, may develop. Pericarditis, thrombophlebitis, osteomyelitis, purulent meningitis and encephalitis have been described.

Prognosis. The case fatality rate is about 5 per cent. The pulmonary and the gastrointestinal types of the disease are extremely serious, often resulting in mortality rates as high as 60 per cent. The course of the disease is variable. Many patients are only mildly ill; in others there is extreme toxemia. The fever usually lasts 3 to 4 weeks, but the glandular enlargement may last 3 to 4 months, and convalescence may be prolonged even longer. Because *P. tularensis* is frequently an intracellular organism, it may remain viable in the tissues long after symptoms have disappeared.

Prevention. Prevention largely involves avoiding contact with infected rodents or other animals and with ticks and insect vectors. Face masks and rubber gloves should be worn by those handling infectious material in the laboratory. Proper cooking will eliminate rabbit meat as a source of ingestional infection. Prophylactic vaccination of animals or man has not proved entirely effective. Evidence suggests that a killed vaccine protects against or modifies the systemic infection in man resulting from intracutaneous transmission, but does not alter the local reaction. In Russia a viable attenuated vaccine is used.

Treatment. Streptomycin in doses of 50 mg. per kg. per day in divided doses every 6 hours is usually responsible for rapid recovery; treatment is usually continued for a week. Tetracycline (30 mg. per kg. per day) is also effective.

Symptomatic care is important. The discharges from open lesions should be handled so as to prevent spread of infection. Surgical incision of suppurative lesions is frequently followed by systemic reactions.

REFERENCES

Assal, N., Blenden, D. C., and Price, E. R.: Epidemiological Study of Human Tularemia Reported in Missouri 1949-1965. *Pub. Health Rep.,* 82:627, 1967.

Foshay, L.: Tularemia. *Ann. Rev. Microbiol.,* 4:313, 1950.

Francis, E.: Tularemia: A New Disease of Man. *J.A.M.A.,* 78: 1015, 1922.

Hopla, C. E.: The Transmission of Tularemia Organisms by Ticks in the Southern States. *South. M.J.,* 53:92, 1960.

Hughes, W. T.: Tularemia in Children. *J. Pediat.,* 62:495, 1963.

Meyer, K. F.: Pasteurella and Francisella; in R. J. Dubos and J. G. Hirsch (Eds.): *Bacterial and Mycotic Infections of Man.* 4th ed. Philadelphia, J. B. Lippincott Company, 1965, Chap. 27, p. 681.

Saslaw, S., Eigelsbach, H. T., Wilson, H. E., Prior, J. A., and Carhart, S.: Tularemia Vaccine Study. 1. Intracutaneous Challenge. *Arch. Int. Med.,* 107:689, 1961.

SALMONELLA INFECTIONS

Salmonella infection is currently of great concern because of its many sources in animals and man and the difficult problems of its control. From 200 to 500 weekly isolations of the organism from human sources are reported; these obviously are only a small portion of the actual incidence. In 1965, 17,161 cases of human infection (exclusive of typhoid fever) were reported, as compared to 6704 cases in 1956.

Etiology. Salmonella infections are caused by a great number of flagellated organisms which have a common relationship based upon antigenic structure. They are members of the Salmonella genus and have H (flagellar) and O (somatic) antigens. They are arranged in groups according to their O antigen characteristics. Within each subgroup they are further differentiated on the basis of their H components.

New species are continuously being added to the long list of several hundred already identified. Many of these species vary from others in a given group only by a minor antigenic factor or a biochemical reaction. Some of the more common ones are classified as follows:

Group A: *S. paratyphi* (paratyphoid A bacillus)
Group B: *S. schottmülleri* (paratyphoid B bacillus)
　　　　　S. typhimurium (Bacterium aertrycke)
Group C_1: *S. hirschfeldii (S. paratyphi C)*
　　　　　S. choleraesuis (Bacterium suipestifer)
　　　　　S. oranienburg
　　　　　S. montevideo
Group C_2: *S. newport*
Group D: *S. typhosa* (typhoid bacillus)
　　　　　S. enteritidis (Bacterium enteriditis)
　　　　　S. gallinarum
　　　　　S. pullorum
Group E: *S. anatis (Bacterium anatum)*

Those organisms which are primarily human pathogens and usually cause typhoid-like infections are *S. typhosa, S. paratyphi, S. schottmülleri* and *S. hirschfeldii.* Those which are primarily pathogenic for animals or birds, but occasionally cause human infection, chiefly through contaminated foods, are *S. typhimurium, S. choleraesuis, S. oranienburg, S. montevideo, S. newport, S. enteritidis* and *S. anatis. Salmonella gallinarum* and *S. pullorum* are also occasionally responsible for gastroenteritis through contamination of food. Certain species, notably *S. hirschfeldii* and *S. choleraesuis,* frequently invade the blood stream and produce localized purulent lesions such as osteomyelitis.

Epidemiology. In general, members of the Salmonella group of organisms have two common characteristics: (1) most of them (*S. paratyphi, S. schottmülleri* and *S. hirschfeldii* are exceptions) have a natural habitat in animals, and (2) they remain viable for considerable periods of time and multiply in contaminated food. Rats, mice, hogs, fowls, rabbits, cats, dogs, cows and horses may act as natural reservoirs. Meat, eggs, vegetables, milk and water are often contaminated, especially at warm temperatures, by food handlers, flies or the droppings of infected rodents. Packaged foods such as powdered egg can be responsible for wide dissemination. Man usually becomes infected by eating contaminated food, but also probably acquires infection by handling animals. Convalescent patients, especially infants, may be infectious for long periods of time. There are permanent carriers for *S. paratyphi* A and B, as well as for some of the other types.

Epidemics of paratyphoid and typhoid fever may coexist, and both infections may even occur simultaneously in the same patient. The incidence of typhoid fever in the United States (less than 500 cases reported annually) is continually declining. Whereas the value of typhoid vaccine is accepted, the inclusion of other members of the Salmonella group in the vaccine is not currently recommended.

Pathology. Tissue changes are similar to, though less severe than, those encountered in typhoid fever. Acute enteritis and superficial necrosis of the lymphoid tissue are the principal changes in the intestinal tract. Deep ulceration and frank hemorrhage are rare, and perforation of the bowel in children is practically unknown.

Clinical Manifestations. The clinical manifestations may be extremely variable, though the predominant symptoms are usually gastroenteric, pulmonic or septic. Two general clinical types may be recognized: (1) the typhoid-like type (paratyphoid fever) and (2) the food-poisoning type (gastroenteritis).

The incubation period may be as brief as a few hours in the food-poisoning type or as long as 12 days in typhoid-like infections. Headache, nausea and vomiting are initial symptoms. Abdominal pain and diarrhea are common in the typhoid-like type and invariably present in the food-poisoning type. The stools may be watery and at times contain mucus and blood suggestive of dysentery.

There may be considerable drowsiness, and in some instances the sensorium is disturbed. Meningismus is often striking, and in such instances the possibility of meningitis cannot be eliminated without a diagnostic lumbar puncture. In paratyphoid A, B and C infections, rose spots may be present. The spleen is not regularly enlarged, but abdominal distention is not uncommon. There may be either leukopenia or leukocytosis, the former occurring more often in paratyphoid B infections, the latter in *S. typhimurium* and *S. enteritidis* infections.

Suppurative lesions of the *joints, bones and soft tissues* are more common than in typhoid fever, and are particularly characteristic of infection with the members of group C, of which *S. hirschfeldii* and *S. choleraesuis* are the principal ones. An unusual predilection of patients with abnormal hemoglobins to develop salmonella osteomyelitis has been observed.

Meningitis may be the only manifestation or it may be associated with other lesions. It has a high fatality rate.

The duration of the disease, though variable, is shorter than that of typhoid fever. The temperature may remain moderately elevated or may be of the septic type. When death occurs, it usually follows a course of illness in which there have been extreme dehydration, toxemia and circulatory collapse.

Diagnosis. Typhoid fever, bacillary dysentery, acute appendicitis and staphylococcal and streptococcal food poisoning are among the more important conditions likely to be confused with salmonella infections.

The bacteriologic diagnosis consists in (1) isolation of the organism from the blood, stools, urine, spinal fluid or pus from a suppurative lesion; and (2) demonstration of a significant agglutinating titer of the patient's serum. Identification of an organism as a member of the Salmonella group is dependent upon serologic typing. Cross-agglutination reactions frequently occur because of the close antigenic relations among the Salmonella organisms. In instances in which contaminated food is suspected, it should be cultured.

Complications. The most common complications are those due to septic localization of the organism and include arthritis, osteomyelitis, meningitis and abscess of the soft tissues. Intestinal perforation is extremely rare. Bronchitis is frequently present in the early stage; bronchopneumonia may be a later complication.

Prognosis. The case fatality rate, though not accurately known, is less than that of typhoid fever. In 1964, in 17,144 cases of human infection reported, there were 67 deaths. The mortality rate appears to be higher in the paratyphoid type of infections than in cases of acute food poisoning.

Treatment. The patient should be isolated, and precautions similar to those recommended for typhoid patients should be practiced. When diarrhea and vomiting are excessive, it may be necessary temporarily to discontinue feeding by mouth. Adequate fluid administration is necessary. (See page 220 for treatment of diarrheal states.) Suppurative joints require surgical incision and drainage.

Drug therapy in salmonellosis is difficult to evaluate, since the course of the natural disease is extremely variable. Bacteriologically, some of the antibiotics appear to be effective in the acute phase; but upon cessation of treatment, positive cultures frequently recur. By then, however, the general condition of the patient is improved, and a certain degree of immunity established.

Specific drug therapy is generally not required for the food-poisoning type of infection, nor for infections of moderate severity with manifestations limited to the digestive tract, nor for the carrier state. In the more severe and protracted intestinal infections and for those in other locations, ampicillin appears to be the drug of choice over agents formerly used, such as chloramphenicol. The usual bacterial sensitivity tests should be made, since recent tests indicate increasing resistance of some strains to ampicillin.

REFERENCES

Abroms, I. F., and others: A Salmonella Newport Outbreak in a Premature Nursery with a One-Year Follow-up. Effect of Ampicillin. *Pediatrics*, 37:616, 1966.

Black, P. H., Kunz, L. J., and Swartz, M. N.: Salmonellosis—A Review of Some Unusual Aspects. *New England J. Med.*, 262:811, 864, 921, 1960.

Edwards, P. R.: Salmonella and Salmonellosis. *Ann. New York Acad. Sc.*, 66:3, 1956.

Newell, K. W.: Possibilities for Investigation and Control of Salmonellosis for This Decade. *Am. J. Pub. Health*, 57:472, 1967.

Rosenstein, B. J.: Salmonellosis in Infants and Children. *J. Pediat.*, 70:1, 1967.

Silver, H. K., Simon, J. L., and Clement, D. H.: Salmonella Osteomyelitis and Abnormal Hemoglobin Disease. *Pediatrics*, 20:439, 1957.

United States Department of Health, Education, and Welfare: Morbidity and Mortality. Annual Supplement Summary, Vol. 14, #53, Oct. 14, 1966.

TYPHOID FEVER
(Enteric Fever)

Although the causative agent of typhoid fever is antigenically a member of the Salmonella genus, the prototype features of the disease justify a separate discussion. The portal of entry of *Salmonella typhosa* is the gastrointestinal tract, and many of the essential features of the disease depend upon the occurrence of early bacteremia.

History. The intestinal lesions were described by Bretonneau in 1820; Louis described the disease and named it *fièvre typhoïde* in 1829. One of his pupils, Gerhard, observed an epidemic of typhoid and one of typhus fever in Philadelphia in 1837 and gave a clear clinical differentiation of the 2 diseases. Badel (1873), another pupil of Louis, emphasized the importance of feces as a source of the infecting agent and described the danger in the excretions of a convalescing patient, as well as the role of water and milk in the spread of the disease. In 1880 Eberth discovered the causative agent, and in 1896 Widal discovered the agglutination reaction. Russell (1909) used vaccine for the prevention of typhoid fever in the United States Army.

Etiology. *Salmonella typhosa* may be easily isolated from the blood during the early stage of the disease, and later from the urine and feces. During the bacteremia it may be found in the spleen, bone marrow, lymphatics and gallbladder. During the second week of the disease specific agglutinins appear in the blood serum.

The bacillus has at least 3 types of antigens, the H (flagellar), the O (somatic) and the Vi. Agglutinins against the H antigen result from a previous typhoid infection or vaccination. A high titer of agglutinins against the O antigen denotes active infection. The blood of chronic carriers usually contains Vi antibodies, but the antigen is not available for practical use. It has been suggested that H antibodies may have little protective value, whereas the O and the Vi are protective. In general, an agglutination titer of 1:160 or higher against a formalinized suspension of typhoid bacilli is significant. A progressively rising titer in subsequent tests is diagnostic. In most cases of typhoid the O agglutinins appear earlier than the H, and agglutination for them is therefore preferred in performing the Widal test. In the macroscopic method the O type produces a small, granular flaky reaction, the H type a large flaky one.

The rise in the agglutinin titer of the serum is usually associated with a decreasing bacteremia (Fig. 10-42). The maximum titer frequently coincides with clinical improvement.

Epidemiology. Typhoid fever is a preventable disease and does not exist to a significant degree where rigid rules of sanitation prevail. The most important source of infection is the human typhoid carrier.

Water- and milk-borne epidemics are characterized by explosive onsets. Foodstuffs such as milk, ice cream, butter, cheese and shellfish have been responsible for outbreaks.

The disease is found in practically all parts of the world; in the temperate zones it is more prevalent during the latter half of the year. It is typically a disease of childhood and early adult life, occurring most frequently between the ages of 15 and 30 years. It is rare in infancy, when the mortality rate is high. During the last decade in the United States the number of cases and of deaths reported decreased from 1700 cases and 54 deaths in 1956 to 501 cases and 14 deaths in 1964.

Immunity. Two of the immunologic aspects, the relapse and the so-called permanent immunity, are difficult to explain. The disease may continue or even relapse in the presence of an appreciable concentration of humoral antibodies. Organisms in such instances probably disappear from the blood and remain in the spleen, lymph nodes or other locations where they are protected from the action of antibodies in the serum, but where they liberate toxic factors.

In explanation of permanent immunity to typhoid infection, it is postulated that the tissues of a previously infected person probably remain highly sensitized even though the humoral anti-

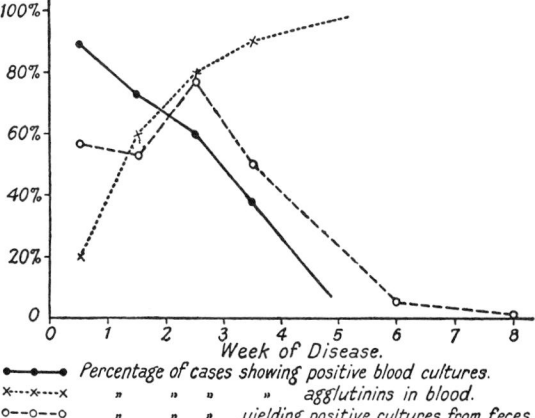

Figure 10-42. The time relations in typhoid fever of the occurrence of positive blood and stool cultures and agglutinins in the blood serum. (Topley and Wilson: *Principles of Bacteriology and Immunity.* Edward Arnold & Co.)

bodies have disappeared, and, when reinfected, respond to the antigenic stimulation with the immediate production of humoral antibodies sufficient to prevent another attack.

Pathogenesis. The bacillus enters the body tissues through the walls of the alimentary tract. In the bloodstream and particularly in the reticuloendothelial cells of the liver and spleen the organisms are destroyed by phagocytosis. In these organs the bacilli also multiply rapidly and secondarily reinfect the bloodstream. It has been suggested that the beginning of the second phase represents the clinical onset of the disease. Large numbers of organisms are eliminated from the liver, and heavy secondary infection of the intestinal tract occurs. In this manner the gallbladder is readily infected, and on occasion gallstones are formed.

The general symptoms of the disease, such as fever, malaise and headache, are caused by the action of toxins. Bacterial emboli in the capillaries of the skin produce the characteristic rose spots. The splenomegaly is caused by congestion of the splenic pulp, by the great accumulation of red blood cells and by endothelial hyperplasia. Ulceration of the bowel accounts to a great degree for the intestinal symptoms. The leukopenia results from the action of toxins on the bone marrow and from infiltration of it by phagocytic endothelial cells.

Pathology. The morphologic changes in infants are less striking than those in children; proliferation of cells of the reticuloendothelial system, as well as intestinal lesions, is apt to be mild or even not demonstrable. Peyer's patches become swollen, and necrosis of the mucosa occurs. The necrotic mucosa sloughs, leaving a round or oval ulcer with the long diameter in the long axis of the bowel; hemorrhage and perforation may occur.

The mesenteric lymph nodes become swollen, soft and hemorrhagic. In the intestinal lymphoid tissue, the lymph nodes and the bone marrow there is a nonsuppurative cellular reaction composed chiefly of large phagocytic cells from the reticuloendothelial system.

The spleen is enlarged, red and soft. The pulp contains great numbers of red blood cells and large phagocytes, and there are areas of focal necrosis. There may also be minute areas of necrosis in the liver and bone marrow and mild inflammation of the gallbladder. In typhoid meningitis, periostitis, osteomyelitis and arthritis, which are rare, the reaction is pyogenic. Bronchopneumonia is usually caused by a secondary infection.

Clinical Manifestations. *In children.* The clinical course of typhoid fever from the second year of life through childhood is similar to that in adults, except that it is usually less severe. The incubation period has been reported to vary from 3 to 40 days, but is usually between 10 and 20. It is said to be longest in water-borne, shorter in milk-borne and shortest in food-borne infections. The entire course of the infection is usually not more than 2 or 3 weeks; occasionally the febrile period lasts but 1 week. The temperature curve is more irregular than in adults, and the disproportion between the height of the fever and the pulse rate is not so constant. There is also a lesser degree of hypotension, and the dicrotic pulse is often not discernible. The onset may be either insidious or abrupt and often resembles that of an upper respiratory tract infection. Disturbances of the sensorium and prostration are less frequent and less pronounced. The intestinal symptoms are usually less severe than in adults. Tympanites tends to be moderate and is often associated with abdominal tenderness. Diarrhea occurs in about half of the cases. The stools are liquid and contain mucus. About the end of the first week the spleen becomes enlarged and tends to remain so until the temperature becomes normal, or longer in event of a relapse. The embolic skin reactions appear upon the trunk and extremities early in the disease. They are small erythematous macules about 2 to 5 mm. in diameter which may appear in successive crops and occur less frequently than in adults. A considerable degree of fatigue and emaciation often develops during the course of infection. The blood reveals evidence of a secondary anemia. There is a definite leukopenia, with disappearance of eosinophils and a relative increase in the number of mononuclear cells. Relapses occur in about 10 per cent of the infections, but are usually less severe than in the adult.

In infants. The infection may be present at birth, the organism having been transmitted through the placenta. In such instances the infant may be born prematurely and die soon after birth, though recovery is possible. The symptoms are variable and may include fever, convulsions, jaundice, diarrhea, and enlargement of the spleen. Diagnosis is established by isolating the organism from the blood or feces. A positive Widal reaction in the infant indicates infection of the mother and not necessarily of the infant.

When an infant acquires infection after birth, the clinical pattern may be far from typical. It may resemble that of sepsis or may suggest only a mild intestinal disturbance. Diarrhea, abdominal distention and vomiting are frequent, but there may be constipation. Distention may be related to low levels of potassium in the serum. The temperature is usually high and irregular, and rose spots are present in about half of the cases. The spleen is enlarged. An unexpected diagnosis is occasionally made from blood cultures in otherwise unexplained and atypical infections. The mortality rate of the disease among infants is about 10 per cent.

Diagnosis. Influenza, tuberculosis, malaria, brucellosis, atypical pneumonia, meningitis, rheumatic fever and other salmonella infections frequently must be considered in the differential diagnosis. In the infant the clinical manifestations may resemble those of bacillary dysentery or septicemia. Obviously typhus fever must be considered in localities where both diseases exist.

Bacterial cultures of the blood, feces and urine should be obtained in every suspected case. The organism can almost always be isolated from the bloodstream during the first week of the disease; the stool culture is usually positive, and in about one third of the cases the organism can be isolated from the urine. After the tenth day of illness the agglutination reaction (Widal) becomes positive in the majority of instances.

Complications. Complications, including hemorrhage and perforation of the bowel, are less frequent in children than in adults. Symptoms of *shock* accompany perforation of the intestine. Abdominal pain is great, and distention usually develops. The abdominal muscles are rigid. With beginning *peritonitis* the fever reappears and leukocytosis occurs. Peritonitis may occur without evidence of perforation. *Intestinal hemorrhage* seldom occurs in patients under 10 years of age. Extensive bleeding from the bowel is characterized by pallor, rapid pulse, fall in blood pressure and absence of abdominal pain. Epistaxis is the most common type of hemorrhage and may be severe. *Thrombosis* and *phlebitis* occur occasionally in children.

Hepatitis with icterus occurs occasionally. *Acute cholecystitis* and formation of gallstones are rare complications. *Infections of the respiratory tract,* particularly bronchitis, are frequent during the early stage of typhoid; bronchopneumonia may occur in the late stage. As in other salmonella infections, there may be localized *arthritic, periosteal* and *osseous* infections.

Infection of the urinary tract occurs in about one fourth of the cases. *Cutaneous* lesions include furuncles and bedsores which may be foci for staphylococcal or streptococcal septicemia. Sudamina, urticarial rashes, herpes, epilation, and grooving of the nails are other epidermal manifestations.

Nervous complications are relatively common, and such symptoms as delirium, stupor and mental depression are frequent. There are rarely residual defects from toxic encephalitis; aphasia, a rare late manifestation, is usually only temporary. Chorea, hemiplegia, optic neuritis and peripheral neuritis have been reported. Purulent meningitis and brain abscess are rare and often fatal.

The carrier. During convalescence the patient often continues to harbor the causative agent and excrete it in stools or urine. About two thirds of patients are free of organisms by 6 weeks; about 3 per cent continue to harbor organisms after a year and are considered chronic carriers. Adult chronic carriers are about 9 times as frequent as child carriers, and females apparently outnumber males.

The nidus of the organism in the permanent carrier is usually in the gallbladder; occasionally in the intestine, kidney or a fistula.

The bacteriophage technique of typing typhoid bacilli is useful for tracing the role of the carrier in the spread of the disease. In addition, a high titer of serum antibody against the Vi antigen is almost entirely confined to the carrier state.

Removal of the gallbladder is often effective in eliminating the chronic carrier state. The practical management of the carrier requires the closest cooperation of the carrier, his family and the health department.

Prevention. The establishment of good sanitation is the most important preventive measure. Routine immunization is not recommended in the United States, though selective vaccination is advised for (*a*) intimate continual exposure to a carrier, (*b*) in community or institutional outbreaks, and (*c*) for foreign travel to areas where the disease is endemic.

The following doses of typhoid vaccine are suggested: primary (for adults and children over 10 years), 0.5 ml. subcutaneously or 0.1 ml. intradermally; (for children 6 months to 10 years), 0.25 ml. subcutaneously on 2 occasions 4 to 5 weeks apart. Single booster injections of such dosages should be given under conditions of repeated exposure every 3 years or upon subsequent exposure.

Treatment. Good nursing care and the maintenance of proper nutrition are important. In uncomplicated cases a high caloric, smooth diet is desirable. The maintenance of fluid and electrolyte balance is especially important in infants and small children. There should be particular attention to the possibility of potassium deficiency when abdominal distention is associated with protracted vomiting or diarrhea. Opiates should not be used. Blood transfusions are indicated to correct anemia.

An antiserum, prepared according to the method of Felix, contains antibodies against Vi and O antigens; when injected early in the disease, it is said to be effective against the toxemia.

Chloramphenicol has been the drug of choice for the treatment of typhoid fever. It appears to be more effective than ampicillin, particularly in severe cases, but its potential toxicity must be carefully considered. The recommended dose is 50 to 100 mg. per kg. per day in 4 divided doses, injected intramuscularly, not to exceed a total dose of 2 gm. daily. For infants under 1 month of age, the dose should not exceed 25 mg. per kg. daily. Treatment should continue for 10 to 14 days.

The use of adrenal steroids should be limited to the acutely toxic patient during the first few days of illness.

The patient should be carefully isolated and screened against contact with flies. The urine, sputum and feces should be treated with Lysol before being discarded. Three negative urine and stool cultures should be obtained before the patient is released from isolation.

REFERENCES

Gerhard, W. W.: On the Typhus Fever Which Occurred at Philadelphia in the Spring and Summer of 1836; Illustrated by Clinical Observations at the Philadelphia Hospital; Showing the Distinction Between This Form of Disease and Dothienenteritis or the Typhoid Fever with Alteration of the Follicles of the Small Intestine: *Am. J. M. Sc.*, 19:289, 1837.

Salmonella Surveillance. Special Report on Typhoid Vaccine. Communicable Disease Center. United States Department of Health, Education, and Welfare, Report #51, Aug. 15, 1966, p. 7.

Sanders, W. L.: Treatment of Typhoid Fever: A Comparative Trial of Ampicillin and Chloramphenicol. *Brit. Med. J.*, 2: 1226, 1965.

Simon, H. J., and Miller, R. C.: Ampicillin in the Treatment of Chronic Typhoid Carriers: Report of Fifteen Treated Cases and a Review of the Literature. *New England J. Med.*, 274:807, 1966.

BACILLARY DYSENTERY

(Shigellosis)

Bacillary dysentery is caused by a variety of closely related organisms and involves chiefly the large bowel. It is characterized clinically by fever, general toxicity, abdominal pain, tenesmus and frequent loose stools containing mucus, pus and blood.

History. Hippocrates is said to have distinguished diarrhea from dysentery by associating diarrhea with the frequent passage of liquid stools and dysentery with the passage of bloody stools. In 1898 Shiga isolated a gram-negative bacillus from the feces and intestinal wall of dysenteric patients in Japan. In 1900 Flexner isolated several strains of dysentery-producing organisms in the Philippines, and in 1915 Sonne described *Shigella sonnei*, an organism which he isolated in Denmark.

Etiology. The Shigella organisms (*Enterobacteriaceae*) are nonmotile, gram-negative, non-encapsulated and nonspore-forming rods. All are easily killed by heat, sunlight and ordinary disinfectants. Although earlier methods of differentiation were based upon biochemical reactions, serologic methods are now more generally used.

The following is a practical classification of the important Shigellae:

Sh. dysenteriae:

Type 1.	(Shiga's bacillus); prevalent in tropical countries and in East Asia, occasionally encountered in the United States.
Type 2.	(Schmitz's bacillus); world-wide distribution, chiefly associated with institutional outbreaks in the United States.
Types 3-7.	(Large-Sachs bacillus); found chiefly in India, but reported from North Africa and the United States.

Sh. flexneri:

Type 1-6.	(Flexner's bacillus); also called *Sh. Panadysenteriae*, causes a significant proportion of dysentery in the United States.

Sh. sonnei:

	(Sonne-Dural bacillus); world-wide distribution, an important cause of diarrhea in the United States.

Sh. boydii:

Types 1-11.	(Boyd's bacillus); first isolated in India, 1930; isolated with increasing frequency in the United States.

Epidemiology. The prevalence of shigellosis varies with climate, living conditions and age. Studies of the presence of shigellae in the normal population reveal rates varying from 0.04 per cent in New York City to 20 per cent in certain southern areas of the United States. Unlike salmonellosis, the general incidence of shigellosis in the United States has remained fairly constant from 1959 (12,888 cases with 133 deaths) to 1964 (12,985 cases with 125 deaths).

Explosive epidemics are not common, but small outbreaks are frequent. Crowding in institutions and summer camps with poor sanitation offers favorable conditions for an outbreak. Inadequate refrigeration and food contaminated with soil or by flies that have access to human excrement are important factors. Unlike typhoid, bacillary dysentery is seldom water-borne. It appears that the disease is becoming more urban than rural and that the incidence among older children is increasing.

Shigellosis is almost entirely a disease of human beings. The mode of spread is from man to man. In untreated cases the carrier state may last for a month. Ordinarily carriers of the Shiga type are more persistent than those of the Flexner type. The organism may be excreted intermittently, a factor which adds to the difficulty of detecting it by culture.

Shigella infection varies with age. Its prevalence is low during the first 6 months of infancy, and increases during the next 6 months to a level which is maintained for several years. The disease is often severe, frequently fatal, in early infancy, but less severe and often mild after 3 years of age.

Pathology. Unlike typhoid fever, dysentery is a local infection which chiefly involves the colon; in about half or less of the cases the lower ileum is affected.

The mucosa of the intestine is thickened, hyperemic, inflamed and edematous; it may be covered by patches of fibrinopurulent exudate. Shallow ulcers are present which vary greatly in size; these seldom penetrate below the submucosa, and perforation is rare. Healing of the ulcers is usually complete. The mesenteric lymph nodes are somewhat enlarged, but the spleen is not involved.

Clinical Manifestations. The incubation period may vary from a few hours to 8 days, but is most frequently 2 to 4 days. The symptoms and signs are readily explained by the pathologic changes. The pain, tenesmus and diarrhea result from acute inflammation of the bowel; the mucus, pus and blood, from inflammation of the bowel epithelium. Since the disease is characteristically localized, septicemia and splenic enlargement are rare. Toxic encephalitis and peripheral neuritis occur occasionally.

The clinical severity of dysentery may vary from extreme mildness to such severity that death occurs on the first day. In the *mild* cases there may be practically no constitutional symptoms. Instances with little or no diarrhea have been recorded.

The onset is usually sudden with fever, vomiting and frequently abdominal pain. The temperature is usually high, 102 to 105°F. Meningeal signs are frequent. The passage of frequent, loose, thin stools within 6 to 24 hours of the onset which later contain mucus, pus and streaks of bright red blood suggests the diagnosis. The number of stools varies, but 10 to 20 a day is average. Abdominal cramps usually precede a passage, which is often accompanied by tenesmus. In some instances tenderness may be elicited by palpation along the course of the colon. There may be weakness, delirium and rapid loss of weight due to dehydration.

The acute symptoms usually last 5 to 10 days. The temperature tends to return to normal as the stools become formed. In some instances normal stools may not be noted for 2 to 3 weeks after the onset.

The onset of the *toxic*, or most severe, form is usually even more abrupt, and all the symptoms are exaggerated. The temperature is high, often septic in type, and diarrhea is severe. Tenesmus and often prolapse of the rectum are present. Sunken eyes, dryness of the mucous membranes, coating of the tongue and sordes of the lips and teeth indicate rapid loss of body fluids. Acidosis develops rapidly. Delirium, weakness and convulsions may occur. Abdominal distention in association with a decrease or cessation of bowel movements is an unfavorable situation.

In some instances the infection becomes *chronic*, persisting for weeks or months. The fever is low-grade, or the temperature may even be subnormal. The course is characterized by remissions of the diarrhea, the stools containing large amounts of mucus, but little or no blood. Continued poor nutrition, progressive loss in weight, and feeding difficulties are characteristic, and there may be abdominal distention, secondary anemia, nutritional edema and vitamin deficiencies. In such instances sigmoidoscopic examination may reveal a diffusely injected granular mucosa with follicular ulceration, cultures from which frequently reveal dysentery organisms.

Diagnosis. The majority of patients with an acute febrile disease associated with loose stools containing gross or microscopic blood, mucus and leukocytes have dysentery. Atypical cases, such as the chronic type, and acute cases in the prediarrheal stage, pose more difficult diagnostic problems. A mild diarrhea, without mucus, blood or pus, due to Shigella organisms is fairly common.

The diagnosis depends upon isolation of the organism from the stool or material obtained by rectal swab. The culture should be made immediately, since the organism dies rapidly upon drying. A highly selective medium such as SS agar (Shigella-Salmonella thiosulfate citrate bile) is used. Suspicious colonies are transferred to carbohydrate broths (lactose, glucose, mannitol, xylose, and the like) for detection of characteristic fermentation reactions. The organism is also tested for indole and hydrogen sulfide production and for motility. Finally, it is agglutinated with polyvalent and monovalent antiserums.

Differential Diagnosis. *Typhoid fever* and other types of Salmonella infection may closely resemble bacillary dysentery. *Amebic colitis* may be differentiated by identifying *Entamoeba histolytica*. In practice it is frequently difficult to differentiate *bacterial* from *viral diarrhea* until a bacteriologic report is obtained. Poh suggests that regardless of the total leukocyte count, if the differential count reveals more band neutrophils than segmented forms, shigellosis should be strongly considered.

Intussusception in its early stage may be mistaken for dysentery. The onset with spasmodic pain and recurrent vomiting, the appearance of an abdominal mass and the shocklike symptoms of intestinal obstruction should distinguish it.

Occasionally there is localization of abdominal pain over the cecum, with tenderness and a delay in the appearance of diarrhea. When there is a moderate leukocytosis, *acute appendicitis* must be considered, and removal of the appendix often is a justifiable, although not profitable, procedure.

Bleeding from focal lesions such as *Meckel's diverticulum*, *papilloma* or *duodenal ulcer* is usually not associated with the passage of frequent stools, nor with an acute febrile illness.

In the prediarrheal stage of dysentery, meningeal and encephalopathic symptoms are frequently present. *Meningitis* or the preparalytic stage of *poliomyelitis* may be suspected, and a lumbar puncture may be necessary for diagnostic purposes.

Complications. Pneumonia and otitis media are occasional complications, especially in infants. Invasion of the blood stream by the dysentery organism is rare; pyelonephritis is uncommon. Dural sinus thrombosis and venous thromboses have been observed, principally with severe dehydration; encephalitis and peripheral neuritis are rare and usually not permanent residuals. A late complication, more frequently encountered in adults, is nonsuppurative arthritis, particularly of the knee joints. Vaginitis may occur, but is not common. Dietary deficiencies are frequently observed in the chronic cases.

Prognosis. A certain degree of durable immunity appears to follow an attack of the disease. Whether this protection extends beyond group specificity is not established. Second attacks probably represent relapses occurring in a carrier. The disease usually lasts 1 to 6 weeks. The case fatality rate is high among infants. Death from toxemia occurs early in the disease; later in the disease it usually results from fluid imbalance and acidosis. Pre-existing malnutrition and concomitant infections are contributory factors to an unfavorable outcome. Infection caused by the Sonne organism is seldom fatal; that caused by the Shiga organism is most serious.

Prevention. The proper care and thorough washing of food which has been in contact with soil are important measures. The child with dysentery should be isolated and protected from flies. The carrier should be subjected to the same precautions as in typhoid fever, although chemotherapy appears to be more effective among dysentery carriers. There is no effective method of active immunization.

Treatment. The important aspects are correction of water and electrolyte imbalance, chemotherapy and diet.

The treatment of dehydration by maintaining the proper fluid and electrolyte balance is of the greatest importance, especially in infants. In the more severe cases an initial period (24 to 72 hours) of elimination of oral feeding during which parenteral fluids are administered is usually desirable (see p. 220). Only small amounts of glucose and saline solution are given orally during this phase. After this time other fluids can usually be given. Skimmed lactic acid milk containing scraped raw apple, apple powder, apple pectin-agar or pectin-kaolin mixtures is usually well taken, and banana powder may be added shortly, or fully ripe bananas may be given separately. High-protein, low-residue diets are, as a rule, well tolerated. Separate administration of all the vitamins in fairly large amounts is indicated. During the postdysentery period, feeding may be extremely difficult, and occasionally gavage may be necessary.

Shigella infections have responded to a number of antimicrobial drugs, but their relative effectiveness has not been clearly established. The readily absorbed sulfonamides and the tetracyclines cause early clearance of susceptible strains from the enteric tract with clinical improvement. Nevertheless so many strains of Shigella are now resistant to these drugs that sensitivity tests should precede selection of the therapeutic agent. This resistance may, in part, be transferable by the R-factor. Recently, ampicillin has been reported as the drug of choice when given in daily doses of 100 mg. per kg. for at least 5 days.

There is need of further studies concerning the effect of antimicrobial therapy on the duration of the carrier state. Length of treatment varies and should be dependent on control of symptoms and eradication of the dysentery organism, which can be expected in the acute cases within 4 to 7 days.

Paregoric is often indicated to relieve pain and tenesmus, and it may reduce the number of stools. Repeated colonic irrigations are harmful. In Shiga infections antitoxin is indicated if it can be injected early in the course of the disease.

WILLIAM L. BRADFORD

REFERENCES

Cooper, M. L., Keller, H. M., and Wallers, E. W.: Comparative Frequency of Detection of Enteropathogenic E. Coli, Salmonella and Shigella in Rectal Swab Cultures from Infants and Children. *Pediatrics*, 19:411, 1957.

Goodwin, M. H., Love, G. J., Mackel, D. C., and Wanner, R. G.: Observations of Familial Occurrence of Diarrhea and Enteric Pathogens. *Am. J. Epidem.*, 84:268, 1966.

Haltalin, K. C., and others: Double-Blind Treatment Study of Shigellosis Comparing Ampicillin, Sulfadiazine, and Placebo. *J. Pediat.*, 70:970, 1967.

Morgan, H. R.: The Enteric Bacteria; in R. J. Dubos and J. G. Hirsch (Eds.): *Bacterial and Mycotic Infections of Man.* 4th ed. Philadelphia, J. B. Lippincott Company, 1965, p. 634.

Poh, S.: Shigellosis: Clue to Early Diagnosis. *Pediatrics*, 39:119, 1967.

Salzman, T. C., Scher, C. D., and Moss, R.: Shigellae with Transferable Drug Resistance: Outbreak in a Nursery for Premature Infants. *J. Pediat.*, 71:21, 1967.

Winter, B. V., and Harding, H. B.: Shigella Sonnei Bacteremia, *J.A.M.A.*, 180:927, 1962.

CHOLERA

Cholera is a severe diarrheal disease which usually occurs in epidemics among crowded and poorly nourished populations; the case fatality rate is high among untreated patients.

Etiology. *Vibrio cholerae* is a small, highly motile, comma-shaped, polymorphic gram-negative organism. It occurs in 3 serotypes which share a common group antigen (A). The serotypes are Inaba (AC), Ogawa (AB) and Hikojima (ABC). The validity of the Hikojima serotype is questioned by some authorities. *Vibrio El Tor* is also widely accepted as a cause of cholera, but there is disagreement as to whether or not it is actually a vibrio separate from *V. cholerae*; the 2 strains are identical in many respects, including the serotypes. Other "noncholera vibrios" with different serotypes have been identified in association with diarrheal disease when searched for; their possible relation to common epidemic diarrheal disease of unknown origin is currently under investigation.

Epidemiology. The human bowel is the chief reservoir for *V. cholerae*. The organism is known to have been shed for as long as 4 years by an asymptomatic carrier, although the vibrio usually disappears from stools of patients about the third to fifth day of the disease. During epidemics the carrier rate may approach 10 per cent in the community and 20 per cent among family contacts. Contaminated food and water supplies have been responsible for household and community outbreaks; cholera tends to disappear in endemic areas as modern sewage disposal and water systems are installed. The vibrio may survive up to 2 weeks in food or water stored at room temperature, and longer in refrigerated or frozen foods. It is sensitive to drying and to an acid environment.

Bengal (India and East Pakistan) is the chief endemic center from which cholera is spread to cause recurrent epidemics, which have occurred as far away as Afghanistan, Egypt, Iran, Thailand, the Philippines, New Guinea, Hong Kong and Korea.

Secondary cases of cholera are rare among medical personnel who have close contact with patients and fomites, but are common among family contacts.

Immunity. It is rare for more than one attack of clinical cholera to occur in the same person. Coproantibody appears early in the disease, but recovery takes place before there is a demonstrable rise in serum antibody. Both serum and coproantibody appear in response to parenteral immunization, but immunized persons who contract the disease do not get a "booster type" response.

Pathology. The pathophysiology of the disease is unclear. The intestines contain an almost clear, whitish, watery fluid with a notable absence of bile. The intestinal mucosa is congested and studded with enlarged solitary lymph follicles, and Peyer's patches are enlarged and hypertrophied, but the mucosal surface remains intact. The liver and the spleen are congested, and the gallbladder is distended with bile. Tubular necrosis and other renal changes may be present in patients dying of postcholeric uremia.

Clinical Manifestations. Typically, after an incubation period of 6 hours to 3 days (rarely it may be as long as 7 days) there is sudden onset of profuse, watery diarrhea without griping, tenesmus or irritation of the skin around the anus. The stools are intermittent at first, then almost continuous; they resemble whitish, almost clear water, and contain flecks of mucus. The term "rice-water stool" is derived from the resemblance to water in which rice is being boiled. They have only a slight, inoffensive fishlike odor. Many children complain of crampy abdominal pains just before, during or after the onset of the diarrhea, at which times vomiting is also common. When the child is first seen, the rectal temperature is usually slightly elevated (about 38°C.), but may fall to levels below normal as shock deepens and death nears. Within a few hours the skin assumes a dusky hue, the eyes become sunken, with dark circles, the skin cold and clammy, and the facial expression anxious. The tips of the fingers may become shrivelled ("washer-woman's hands") as dehydration becomes severe. As the disease progresses, there are intense thirst, restlessness and cramps in the legs and abdomen. The blood pressure falls, the radial pulse becomes imperceptible, and urine volume decreases. Although lethargy, thick speech and a somnolent state occur usually within a few hours of onset, the patient rarely loses consciousness. Migration of ascaris out of the intestinal tract may be a striking feature; a Bengali word for cholera is translatable as "madness of the worms."

The usual duration of the acute symptoms is about 3 days, with a range of 1 to 10 days. The first sign of recovery is usually the reappearance of pigment in the stools; the cessation of diarrhea is usually rapid.

Complications. *Anuria* of 24 to 36 hours' duration or longer is not uncommon. If it is prolonged, it may be evidence of irreversible renal damage, which results in death from renal failure.

Dehydration, hypovolemic shock and circulatory failure in that sequence are the mechanisms to which anuria and renal damage were attributed in the past and are no doubt valid explanations among patients who are untreated or who first receive treatment late in the course of the disease. On the other hand, among children treated with the usual adult fluid regimens, anuria may be secondary to hypernatremia. Such patients, though their blood volume and plasma specific gravity have been restored to normal, remain extremely thirsty; relief of thirst and anuria follows the administration of "free water" by mouth or by vein. Fever, tachycardia, tachypnea, vomiting, twitching, delirium, coma, and convulsions occurring in children whose therapy included fluids with a high sodium content are likewise probably of hypernatremic origin.

Hypokalemia may be avoided by using solutions containing 15 to 20 mEq. of potassium per liter and by avoiding the unnecessarily heavy sodium loads contained in most solutions widely used in the treatment of adults with cholera. *Hypoglycemia* may be avoided by making sure that all intravenous solutions contain 3 per cent dextrose. *Pulmonary edema* is rarely, if ever, seen if fluid and electrolyte therapy is appropriate for the age, size and condition of the patient. Fever and shock may result from pyrogens contained in bacterially contaminated undistilled water used in the manufacture of homemade solutions for intravenous use, as well as from hypernatremia.

Prognosis. The case fatality rate is less than 0.5 per cent among adult patients who are treated early and adequately. With less than optimum treatment the mortality rate rises and is about 40 per cent in untreated cases. Reliable statistics are lacking for infants and small children, but the mortality rate among them is high for both treated and untreated patients.

Prevention. The avoidance of contact with patients and carriers and good personal and environmental hygiene, combined with good nutrition, are probably the best preventive measures against cholera. Patients with cholera should not be released from isolation until their stool cultures have been negative for 2 days; their contacts should be kept under surveillance. The effectiveness of immunization is variously estimated at 20 to 80 per cent. There is general agreement that single injections of cholera vaccine are not very effective and that protection lasts only a few months. Mass treatment with orally administered vibriocidal agents, particularly tetracycline, offers promise in epidemic situations and is currently under investigation.

Treatment. The treatment of cholera is fraught with problems related to the circumstances under which it must be carried out. Laboratory facilities tend to be inadequate or lacking, those responsible for management are rarely acquainted with the principles of intravenous therapy of children, and appropriate intravenous fluids and equipment are often not available. The children themselves often present the added complications of anemia and malnutrition.

Fluid therapy to combat dehydration, hypovolemia and circulatory failure is the essential element in the treatment of cholera. The results have been disappointing in children as compared to adults. This is probably related to differences in the electrolyte composition of pediatric as opposed to adult choleric stools (Table 10-12), to the use of intravenous solutions with electrolyte contents appropriate for adults, but not for children, and to the difficulty in getting children to drink adequate amounts of "free" water along with the intravenous administration of electrolyte solutions.

The few studies which have been done in children with cholera indicate that the sodium, chloride and bicarbonate contents of their stools are lower and the potassium content higher than in adults (Table 10-12). The concentrations of sodium, chloride and potassium in the serum are usually normal or slightly elevated at the time treatment is begun. Average fluid deficits at the start of treatment are approximately 100 ml. per kg., and continuing losses in the stools may be as high as 200 to 350 ml. per kg. per 24 hours.

Since peripheral vascular collapse with diminished or absent radial pulse is usually present when the patient is first seen, it is frequently necessary to surgically expose a vein for the initial rehydration. Ideally, the initial treatment of hypovolemic shock should probably be with Ringer's lactate or Dacca solution (see Table 10-12), with a change to a more hypotonic solution after the radial pulse has returned to normal volume and the patient is out of clinical hypovolemic shock. But the practicalities of treatment of cholera under epidemic circumstances dictate the use of a single solution, if possible. The N.A.M.R.U.-2 solution (Table 10-12) is recommended as a single solution which may be used. Even it may be too hypertonic if insensible fluid loss is high and the loss is not replaced through intake of additional "free" water.

The *rate of infusion* is usually limited by the size of the intravenous needle which can be introduced, but probably should not exceed 1 ml. per kg. per minute until a normal radial pulse volume has been restored; then the infusion should be slowed to a rate adequate to replace continuing gastrointestinal fluid losses milliliter for milliliter and to provide for the gradual recovery of normal skin turgor. Measurement of stool losses is accomplished by use of a "cholera cot," a canvas cot with a hole cut to accommodate the buttocks, under which a calibrated bucket is placed. Measurements of plasma specific gravity are helpful as a guide to treatment; a rule of thumb is rapid infusion of 5 ml. of fluid per kg. for each 0.001 over 1.025. Oral intake of water should be encouraged to replace insensible water loss, which is 500 to 1000 ml. per square meter of body surface per day in hot climates. If oral intake is impractical, this necessary "free" water should be supplied by vein.

Antibiotic therapy. The oral administration of 10 mg. of tetracycline per kg. every 6 hours for the first 72 hours of treatment reduces the duration of diarrhea from a mean of about 72 hours to a mean of about 24 hours, reduces the duration of need for intravenous therapy (an important practical consideration during an epidemic), and reduces the incidence of convalescent carriers.

R. James McKay

REFERENCES

Bushnell, O. A., and Brookhyser, C. S. (Eds.): *Proceedings of the Cholera Research Symposium*, January 24-29, 1965, Honolulu. Washington, D.C., Superintendent of Documents, U.S. Government Printing Office.

Griffith, L. S. C., Fresh, J. W., Watten, R. H., and Villaroman, M. P.: Electrolyte Replacement in Paediatric Cholera. *Lancet,* 1:1197, 1967.

PSEUDOMONAS INFECTIONS

Pseudomonas aeruginosa is representative of a large group of gram-negative bacilli whose natural habitat is soil and water. They are ubiquitous organisms only rarely pathogenic for man. Under appropriate circumstances, however, they can and do cause serious and even fatal disease. They are opportunists which exhibit their full pathogenic potentiality in debilitated persons whose resistance to infection is compromised by disease, malnutrition, trauma or foreign body, or by immunosuppressive drugs. Pseudomonads are not fastidious in their growth requirements and are somewhat more resistant to germicides than the gram-positive cocci. Pseudomonas strains can be differentiated one from another for epidemiologic purposes by serologic typing (O types), phage typing and pyocin typing. In contrast to the staphylococci, there is little evidence that "hot strains" of unusual epidemicity or pathogenicity exist. All strains are endowed with a highly sophisticated system for energy conversion which probably accounts for their resistance to most antibiotics.

Distribution. Since Pseudomonads are widely encountered in nature, it is to be expected that even small children will have frequent contact with them. They can be recovered occasionally from the skin of most people. Between 5 and 10 per cent of older children and adults carry these organisms in their stools, but they rarely become the predominating organism. It is not unusual to recover them from the throats of sick infants. Perhaps 20 per cent of children develop low titers of agglutinating antibodies to Pseudomonas in their serums by the first year, and practically 100 per cent do so by later childhood. The defenses of

TABLE 10-12. ELECTROLYTE CONTENT OF CHOLERIC STOOL AND OF SOLUTIONS RECOMMENDED FOR INTRAVENOUS TREATMENT OF CHILDREN

| | APPROXIMATE ELECTROLYTE CONCENTRATION (mEQ. PER LITER) | | | | | |
	Na	Cl	K	HCO₃	Ca	Mg
Adult's choleric stool.....................................	132	96	19	44	2	2
Child's choleric stool.....................................	97	74	23	32	2	2
Ringer's lactate solution...............................	130	109	4	28	—	—
SEATO 5:4:1/2 solution*...............................	133	92	7	48	—	—
Dacca solution**..	133	99	14	48	—	—
Recommended solution (N.A.M.R.U.-2 Pediatric Cholera Solution)***...............................	90	64	15	45	2	2

*5 gm. NaCl, 4 gm. NaHCO₃, 0.5 gm. KCl per liter.
**5 gm. NaCl, 4 gm. NaHCO₃, 1 gm. KCl per liter.
***2.6 gm., NaCl; 3.8 gm., NaHCO₃; 1.1 gm., KCl; 0.1 gm., CaCl₂; and 0.1 gm., MgCl₂ per liter.
All solutions should contain 30 gm. of dextrose (glucose) per liter.

Composition of N.A.M.R.U.-2 Pediatric Cholera Solution and review of manuscript courtesy of Dr. Lawrence S. C. Griffith.

the body against Pseudomonas seem to reside mainly in intact body surfaces and in such non-specific forces as phagocytosis and the natural bactericidal action of human serum against "non-pathogens." Because these defenses are not as well developed in the newborn infant as later on, serious and fatal infections are apt to occur during the first month of life (see p. 404).

Clinical Patterns. Pseudomonas produces 2 kinds of lesions: (1) in healthy persons introduction of these organisms into minor wounds may be followed by transient self-limited cellulitis or by frank pus formation, with the pus traditionally green or blue in the case of contamination of large surface wounds; (2) in debilitated persons Pseudomonas may overpower impaired local defenses and multiply in interstitial tissues so as to elaborate sufficient toxin (protease) to prevent a local neutrophilic reaction and pus formation. In this latter case unrestrained bacterial multiplication occurs, prodigious numbers of organisms propagating along paths of least resistance in and around blood vessel walls. Hemorrhagic necrosis results, producing lesions pathognomonic of Pseudomonas infections. In the skin these lesions may start as pink macules which progress to small subcutaneous hemorrhagic nodules, with or without vesiculation, and eventuate in coin-sized areas of necrosis with eschar formation surrounded by a bright red areola (ecthyma gangrenosum).

In hospitalized children, Pseudomonas causes serious systemic infections in several well recognized classes of patients. These are (1) newborn infants in the period following surgery of the gastrointestinal tract or repairs of meningoceles, (2) burned patients, (3) children under treatment for leukemia or aplastic anemia, (4) children with chronic obstruction of the urinary tract, and (5) children with cystic fibrosis. When several instances of Pseudomonas infection occur in a

hospital in rapid sequence, they can often be traced to contamination of inhalation apparatus, suction devices, antiseptic solutions or other items of hospital usage.

Secondary infections of wounds. Although the natural defenses of the body can eliminate a few bacilli of low virulence inoculated under the skin, such bacteria may easily colonize body surfaces compromised by trauma, obstruction or disease. The weeping proteinaceous surfaces of burns and the viscid bronchial mucus of children with cystic fibrosis are commonly populated by Pseudomonas and other gram-negative bacilli, which in such situations set up a low-grade inflammatory reaction. Since drainage is possible, however, deep and spreading invasion of the tissues usually does not occur. The mere presence of these bacteria in injured surfaces does not, therefore, necessarily require vigorous treatment with antibacterial agents.

Colonization, however, is the necessary fore-runner of invasion. Should circulation be impaired, a foreign body be present, or the leukocytic response of the patient deteriorate, or protein synthesis be compromised by drug or disease, colonization is likely to be followed by spread of the infection. Although often difficult to achieve, the most satisfactory management of these wound infections lies in adequate removal of bacterially contaminated secretion, débridement of devitalized tissue and foreign material, protection from colonization by additional bacteria, and in maintenance of a positive nitrogen balance in the patient. Frequent changes of moist bacteriostatic dressings, or alternating applications of bacteriostatic salves and their removal by washing, as in the *Sulfamylon* treatment of burns, is usually effective in keeping the concentration of surface bacteria sufficiently low to prevent tissue invasion and spreading infection. Systemic administration of toxic antibiotics should be reserved for treatment of spreading infection.

Leukemia. Leukemic patients in relapse are especially susceptible to invasion by Pseudomonas as a terminal event. Invasion is commonly by way of the intestine; it is insidious in onset, usually heralded by anxiety, anorexia, fever and diarrhea. Vasculitis of the intestinal and mesenteric vessels and hemorrhagic necrosis lead to septicemia. Metastatic lesions occur in many organs; in the skin they take the form of purplish nodules or ecchymotic areas which become gangrenous. Since leukemic patients often have a tendency to purpura, the infectious nature of these lesions is often not appreciated. Another frequent characteristic lesion in these patients is perirectal cellulitis, which also becomes hemorrhagic and gangrenous. Septicemia may lead to ileus, hypotension and shock. The severely burned patient has abundant neutrophils and may weather several attacks of septicemia, but few leukemic patients survive more than their first episode, despite antibiotic treatment and transfusions.

Cystic fibrosis (see p. 856). The majority of patients with cystic fibrosis who are maintained on antibiotic therapy acquire Pseudomonas in their sputum. Colonization of the bronchial secretions is not equivalent to tissue involvement. There seems little doubt that bacteria growing in profusion in mucus encourage the migration of pus cells into the sputum and promote an increase in its volume and viscosity. Frequently strains of Pseudomonas may be isolated which produce huge, watery mucoid colonies (slime producers). Slime production appears to be induced by infection of ordinary Pseudomonas organisms by lysogenic bacteriophage. Such strains may produce less pigment than rough strains and may appear in vitro to be more sensitive to antibiotics, even though they are isolated from patients receiving such antibiotics. They seem to produce a greater antibody response in the patient, indicating that they may be more pathogenic.

Pseudomonas may occasionally be suspected to be the cause of pneumonia in cystic fibrosis when appropriate antistaphylococcal therapy fails and sputum freshly obtained by "postural drainage" shows massive overgrowth of Pseudomonas. Such sputa, digested with N-acetyl cysteine and diluted 1:100,000 before culture, will reveal 10^6 or 10^7 organisms per cu. mm. Treatment of Pseudomonas pneumonia with systemic polymyxin is not very successful unless effective thinning and removal of bronchial secretions are possible through postural drainage and aerosol therapy. Probably the use of polymyxin B by aerosol inhalation, when it accompanies vigorous pulmonary physiotherapy, is superior to systemic administration. The large amount of nucleic acid in bronchial pus tends to inactivate neomycin and polymyxin.

Treatment. Mere colonization of infected body surfaces does not ordinarily demand antibiotic treatment. Abscesses demand drainage, and surface wounds demand cleansing and débridement.

Systemic infections with Pseudomonas are always serious, and usually yield only to systemic treatment with polymyxin B or colistin even though in-vitro antibiotic disk sensitivity tests may show larger areas of inhibition to some of the broad-spectrum antibiotics. Since polymyxin B (3 to 5 mg. per kg. per day) is neurotoxic and nephrotoxic, its use for longer than a week should be avoided if possible. Colistin may be equally effective if used in larger doses, but it is then equally toxic. Both must be used intramuscularly since neither drug is absorbed from the intestine. Meningitis must be treated intrathecally with polymyxin B (3 to 5 mg. [total dose, not per kg.] per day for 3 days) in addition to treatment by the intramuscular route. For aerosol inhalation 3 to 5 mg. of polymyxin B is diluted in 2 to 3 ml. of water or in 10 per cent propylene glycol solution and nebulized 2 to 5 times a day. Two experimental antibiotics, gentamycin and carbenicillin, show great promise in the treatment of serious pseudomonas infections.

Other Gram-Negative Bacilli. With the exception of the characteristic lesion of hemorrhagic necrosis with vasculitis caused by Pseudomonas, most of the considerations in the foregoing discussion apply also to infections with other gram-negative environmental bacteria. These organisms frequently include E. coli, Klebsiella-Enterobacter and Proteus, and less commonly Alkaligenes, Paracolon bacilli, Serratia, Mima, Flavobacteria and Achromobacter. Infection by these organisms is fostered by debility, the postoperative state, the leukemic state, obstructive uropathy, and the administration of steroids or immunosuppressive drugs. Prompt treatment even of septicemia is frequently successful if bactericidal drugs are used. Kanamycin is more frequently the drug of choice than any other, but antibiotic sensitivity to the individual strain involved should be determined, since some of these agents may have strange patterns of antibiotic resistance. Septicemia with any of them may lead to infectious shock due to gram-negative endotoxin. When shock occurs, antibacterial treatment is important, but the major part of management involves maintenance of blood volume, blood pressure, cardiac output and tissue perfusion, and the avoidance of intravascular clotting.

WARREN E. WHEELER

REFERENCES

Cooper, R. G.: Systemic Pseudomonas Infection in Childhood. *Med. J. Australia,* 1:527, 1967.
Teplitz, C.: Pathogenesis of Pseudomonas Vasculitis and Septic Lesions. *Arch. Path.,* 80:297, 1965.

TUBERCULOSIS

Tuberculosis has a uniquely important place in medical history. It has at all times been a main

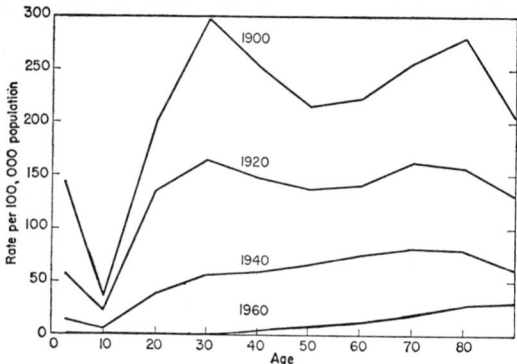

Figure 10-43. Tuberculosis death rates by age, United States, 1900-1960 (Expanding Death Registration States). (Department of Health, Education, and Welfare, Public Health Service, Communicable Disease Center, Tuberculosis Program, Atlanta, Georgia.)

cause of illness and of death in all climates. It was one of the first diseases to elicit widespread organized public health efforts, and the degree of control attained has proved the value of detection and isolation of infected persons. It stands as the prototype of infections which exist in man most often as a parasite without causing significant disease and yet capable of producing both acute and chronic disease patterns of sufficient seriousness to be one of the leading causes of death.

The steady decrease in death rates at all ages (Figs. 10-43, 10-44) is evidence of gain in the battle with the tubercle bacillus. Only in recent years

can credit for these gains be given to specific antimicrobial agents. It is essential to know by what means these gains have been made and to recognize that in our improving health situation, tuberculosis remains a serious problem, to be solved by the combined means of public health measures and medical therapy.

Etiology. Koch demonstrated in 1882 that tuberculosis is caused by the acid-fast bacillus *Mycobacterium tuberculosis*. Subsequently Smith showed that disease could be produced in man by bovine and human tubercle bacilli. (See also other mycobacterial infections, page 611.)

The tubercle bacillus does not contain or produce any chemical constituent which has measurable toxicity for tissues not sensitized to tuberculin; its tissue-necrotizing capacity exists in the protein fraction. The lipids of the tubercle bacillus give it the property of acid-fastness and appear to be a factor in the production of fibrosis as well as in the formation of epithelioid cells and tubercles.

Epidemiology. The exact incidence of tuberculosis is not known. Evidence of its frequency is limited to surveys using the tuberculin test, roentgenographic films, clinical recognition of the disease, and examination of autopsy material. Data indicate that the incidence of infection is declining throughout the world and in general is lowest in populations with high living standards. In all areas the incidence of tuberculous infection increases with age and is generally higher in urban than in rural areas.

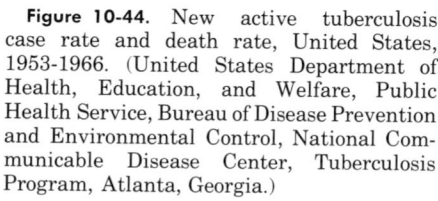

Figure 10-44. New active tuberculosis case rate and death rate, United States, 1953-1966. (United States Department of Health, Education, and Welfare, Public Health Service, Bureau of Disease Prevention and Environmental Control, National Communicable Disease Center, Tuberculosis Program, Atlanta, Georgia.)

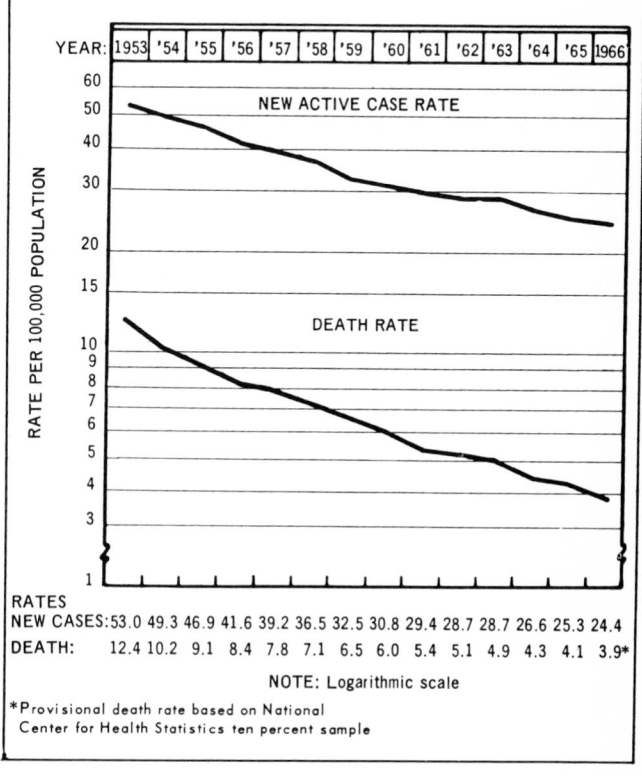

Predisposing Factors. The introduction of tubercle bacilli into the human body is not invariably followed by the development of significant disease. Pertinent to an understanding of this situation is why certain persons have greater rèsistance to infection than others, and why the resistance of a given person may vary from time to time.

Factors related to the tubercle bacillus which may affect the establishment of disease are principally of 2 orders: the relative virulence of the invading organisms and the number of organisms in the inoculum. Though there are distinct differences in the virulence of various strains of tubercle bacilli, strains of low virulence are rarely encountered in human infections.

Heredity. There is no evidence of an inherited tendency to tuberculous infection. Differences in constitutional patterns do, however, appear to influence resistance to disease. Animals of the same species vary in degree of resistance, and by selective breeding of those with a high degree the increased capacity for resistance can be transferred to the offspring. The question in man is not so simply answered.

Congenital or intrauterine infection occurs infrequently and is probably secondary to infection of the placenta.

Race. Differences in racial immunity are not well defined. There is a higher mortality rate from tuberculosis in the United States among the non-white population, especially among American Indians, than among the white, but it would seem that much of this difference can be attributed to hygienic and environmental factors, such as poor housing conditions and opportunities for frequent reinfection from ambulatory patients.

Age. Age is a factor in resistance to tuberculous infection, the fatality rate being higher during infancy and adolescence than in the intervening years of childhood. There are also differences in the nature of the lesion which is initiated at various age levels. These are described under Pathology.

Sex. Sex appears to be a factor only in the latter part of childhood and during adolescence, when the morbidity and mortality rates are higher in girls than in boys.

Temporary factors affecting resistance. Chronic illness and undernutrition may increase susceptibility to infection, as may chronic fatigue. Acute nontuberculous infections may activate a quiescent tuberculous lesion.

Allergy and Immunity. Two to 10 weeks after infection of a previously tuberculin-negative person with tubercle bacilli the presence of allergy can be demonstrated by a positive cutaneous reaction to tuberculin. With the development of allergy there is an alteration in the host response to tubercle bacilli, evidenced by exudation and a tendency to localize the infection. Certain other immune reactions also develop which are neither complete nor as adequately measured as in some other infections. Immunity is not complete; it may be sufficient to protect against moderate infections, but not against large numbers of invading bacilli or against those of exceptionally high virulence.

To what extent allergy and immunity are related phenomena is a controversial question. It is variously held (1) that they are related and perhaps identical, (2) that they are entirely separate phenomena, or (3) that they are opposing forces. It may be that the degree of hypersensitivity is the important factor. Thus moderate degrees of hypersensitivity appear to be effective in localizing the lesion and in bringing the phagocytic cells in contact with the bacteria more quickly; whereas greater hypersensitivity is responsible for such extensive destruction of tissue that spread of the infection may be increased by it.

Pathogenesis. Infection through the intact skin probably does not occur, but infections may be acquired in open wounds and through inapparent abrasions, and have been transmitted by a human bite. Direct bloodstream infection is a practical possibility only in placental transmission. Inhalation and, to a lesser extent, ingestion are the principal means by which tubercle bacilli gain entrance to the body and produce infection.

Pathology. The response of infants and small children to tuberculous infection differs in certain respects from that of older children and adults; there is, however, a good deal of overlapping. Thus lesions which have the characteristics of the "childhood type" are seen on occasion in adults, especially of the Negro race, and the "adult type" of infection may occur in children, especially in the latter part of childhood.

In general, the age differences are as follows: (1) The pulmonary lesion in infants and children may be in any part of the lung, but shows some tendency to be localized in the periphery. The site is more likely to be in the lower than in the upper part of the lungs. By contrast, in adolescents and adults there is a predilection for localization of the lesion either in the apical region or just below it in the infraclavicular area. (2) The regional lymph nodes are more often involved in infants and children than in adolescents and adults. Initial infections in adults usually show little or no evidence of extensive involvement of the lymph nodes. (3) Both the parenchymal and nodal lesions in children exhibit a strong tendency to heal by calcification, whereas in adults the tendency is to heal by fibrosis. (4) Hematogenous dissemination is much more likely to occur in infants than in older children. Miliary tuberculosis and tuberculous meningitis occur with much greater frequency in the first few years of life than subsequently.

At the site of the initial focus, e.g. in the parenchyma of the lung, there is at first an accumulation of polymorphonuclear leukocytes. This reaction is temporary and is followed by proliferation of epithelioid cells which surround the tubercle bacilli, creating the typical tubercle formation.

The tubercles are usually surrounded by an accumulation of lymphocytes, and giant cells are usually present. The tubercles may remain discrete or may become confluent; central caseous necrosis is commonly present. Foci of the primary infection vary considerably in size, but the majority apparently remain small (1 cm. or so in diameter). There is often only a single primary focus, but there may be more.

Lymph node involvement is almost a constant accompaniment of the initial parenchymal lesion in children. It has generally been considered that lymph node involvement is a characteristic of the initial lesion of tuberculosis and does not occur in association with the lesion of reinfection. This concept does not appear to be wholly correct. There is evidence suggesting that the extent of involvement of regional lymph nodes is determined in part by age factors, being less with increasing age. The nodes become enlarged, often matted together, and tend to adhere to adjacent structures. In the mediastinum they may exert pressure on the trachea, bronchi or blood vessels, and at times rupture into them.

The tendency of the primary lesions both in the parenchyma and in the lymph nodes is toward healing in the majority of instances. There are, however, 3 mechanisms by which the primary infection may be responsible for serious damage during its active phase: (1) progressive destruction at its initial site; (2) erosion of a bronchus with intrabronchial dissemination and the formation of other pulmonary lesions; and (3) hematogenous distribution resulting in one or more isolated foci in such parts of the body as the lungs, bones, kidneys, liver or brain, or in widespread miliary lesions involving some or all of the viscera.

The progressive primary tuberculous focus is a large, irregularly demarcated area of caseation with no definite capsule. The tissue surrounding this area tends to be pneumonic and the overlying pleura to be thickened. Softening and liquefaction may be generalized in the nodular mass or localized in one or more small areas. If the liquefied material is evacuated, there remains an irregular, shaggy excavation with a poorly defined capsule. Hematogenous distribution is more likely to occur during the stage of softening, but before the stage of liquefaction, whereas bronchogenic spread tends to result from the breakdown of an area of liquefaction.

Consolidated lesions in association with primary infections are usually atelectasis or tuberculous pneumonia, or a combination of the two. Bronchi may be occluded by external pressure from caseous lymph nodes, or there may be erosion of the bronchus and occlusion of the lumen by the resultant intrabronchial lesion. When the obstruction is incomplete, there may be greater hindrance to the exit of respired air than to its entrance, so that there is obstructive emphysema distal to the lesion; when the obstruction is complete, resorption atelectasis occurs.

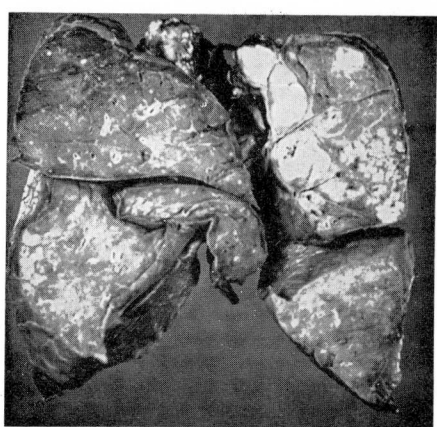

Figure 10-45. Tuberculous lesion (primary) in apex of left upper lobe (right upper corner) with associated massive involvement of regional lymph nodes (primary complex). Large wedge-shaped lesion in lower half (lateral portion) of left upper lobe. This last lesion (tuberculous pneumonitis) is secondary to bronchial erosion from a tuberculous node. (Courtesy of Drs. Charles Dunlap and James B. Arey.)

Massive hematogenous dissemination of tubercle bacilli from a tuberculous focus results in widespread formation of tubercles. Though the heaviest distribution is likely to be in the lungs, any or all of the viscera may be involved, especially the liver, spleen and kidneys. Tuberculous meningitis, as shown by Rich and McCordock, is more likely to result from breakdown of a tuberculoma in contiguity with the meninges. Isolated hematogenous lesions may be located in the brain, kidneys and bones and occasionally in other structures.

Clinical Forms. Tuberculosis may involve practically any organ or tissue of the body. Exogenous foci are naturally limited to structures which have an epithelial covering or lining, whereas tuberculosis of structures of the body which have no outside contact are of necessity blood- or lymph-borne from a pre-existing focus. Symptoms of any tuberculous lesion may be varied and may simulate many other disease entities. In the differential diagnosis of the majority of chronic infections and of many acute ones, the possibility of tuberculosis must be considered.

Intrathoracic tuberculous infection accounts for at least 90 per cent of recognized tuberculous disease in children. Although parenchymal and lymph node involvement always occurs, the foci are not always apparent by clinical or roentgenographic examination. The extent of the infection in the pulmonary parenchyma or in the lymph nodes is largely responsible for the various clinical patterns. Table 10-13 provides a classification of intrathoracic lesions based on clinical patterns rather than the more traditional one of primary and reinfection tuberculosis. Extrathoracic tuberculous lesions are tabulated in Table 10-15 (p. 607).

TABLE 10-13. CLASSIFICATION OF INTRATHORACIC TUBERCULOSIS

Hypersensitivity to tuberculin without clinically demonstrable disease
Apparently healed (calcified or fibrotic) pulmonary or tracheobronchial lymph node foci with hypersensitivity to tuberculin
Noncalcified pulmonary focus
Extensive pulmonary infiltration
Tuberculosis of the tracheobronchial lymph nodes
Intraluminal and extraluminal bronchial lesions
  Localized ulcerative or granulomatous endobronchial lesions
  Extraluminal bronchial compression
    Lesions distal to bronchial obstruction
      Emphysema
      Atelectasis
      Tuberculous pneumonitis
      Or any combination of above 3 lesions
Caseous bronchopneumonia
  Bronchogenic or hematogenous
Hematogenous tuberculosis
  Single or multiple pulmonary infiltrations (clinically indistinguishable from nonhematogenous lesions)
  Miliary tuberculosis
Apical and infraclavicular lesions
Pleurisy
(See page 607 for Classification of Extrathoracic Tuberculosis)

INTRATHORACIC TUBERCULOSIS

Clinical Manifestations. The initial lesion in the lung may be, and usually is, a localized one of 2 or 3 cm. From this lesion tubercle bacilli travel to and colonize in the regional lymph nodes. *The 2 lesions constitute the so-called primary complex.* The various possibilities are (1) healing, (2) persistence of indolent lesions, (3) extension at the local site with progressive destruction of tissue, (4) erosion of bronchial walls with partial or complete occlusion of the bronchial lumen (or such occlusions by external pressure of enlarged lymph nodes) with establishment of localized obstructive emphysema or atelectasis and at times with distribution of tubercle bacilli to other parts of the lung and establishment of a number of new lesions, (5) erosion of blood vessels with widespread distribution of tubercle bacilli (miliary tuberculosis) or with establishment of localized lesions at distant sites, (6) subsequent reactivity of the lesion, or (7) reinfection, endogenous or exogenous.

Detection of tuberculin sensitivity in any person requires careful study (1) to localize, if possible, the site of the lesion or lesions; (2) to determine whether the disease is active, quiescent or healed; and (3) to detect any existing tuberculous contacts.

When no lesion can be demonstrated in the child by physical examination or on a roentgenogram of the chest, and there is no evidence of active infection manifest by fever, increased sedimentation rate or blood cell counts, the child may be diagnosed as *hypersensitive to tuberculin without clinically demonstrable disease.* Specific treatment is recommended for such children under 4 years of age and for those of any age who are known to have become tuberculin-positive within recent months (see p. 605).

When there are one or more *calcified foci in the pulmonary parenchyma or calcified lesions in the tracheobronchial lymph nodes* (Fig. 10-46) in a child with a positive reaction to tuberculin and no reaction to histoplasmin or coccidioidin and no evidence of active disease, he may be considered to be in an inactive state of tuberculosis. Calcified foci, especially those close to the hilus, can usually be distinguished roentgenographically from blood vessels, which tend to have a smooth circular or elliptical homogeneous density, whereas calcified foci are usually irregular in outline and density. Such a situation suggests a healed state, but the child must be watched for the possibility of an exacerbation.

Demonstrable noncalcified lesions. The *noncalcified small pulmonary focus* appears on the roentgenogram as a more or less circumscribed area, usually not more than 1 or 2 cm. in diameter. There may or may not be evidence of associated hilar node involvement, but in infants and children there is likely to be. As a rule the child is not ill with this type of lesion. In the adolescent years such lesions are often located in the apex of the lung or the infraclavicular area, and in such circumstances initial tuberculous lesions may simulate the so-called reinfection lesions of adults.

On occasion the initial lesion in the lung is not confined to a small focal area, but extends into the surrounding lung tissue. Such an *extensive pulmonary infiltration* is often termed "progressive primary tuberculosis" (Fig. 10-47). Clinically, there are no certain methods for determining whether such a lesion is the initial one or is an exogenous reinfection or one resulting from hema-

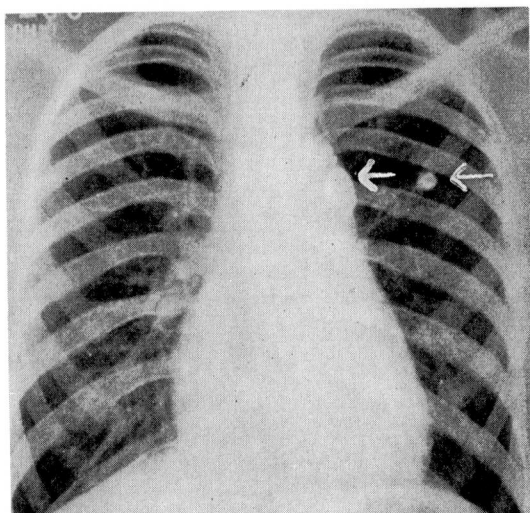

Figure 10-46. Calcified tuberculous focus (right arrow) and calcified tracheobronchial lymph node (left arrow) in a Negro girl 10 years of age.

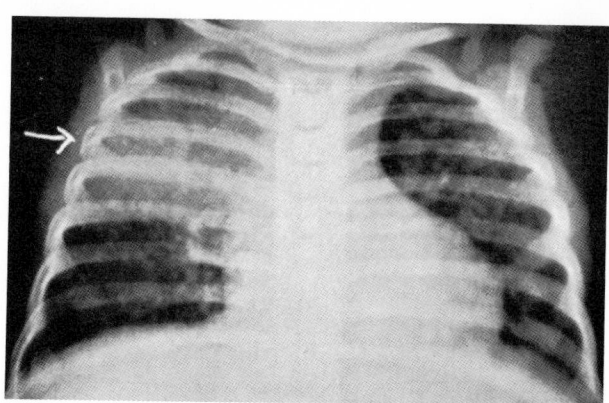

Figure 10-47. Extensive infiltrative lesion in the middle portion of the right lung in a white boy 20 months of age.

togenous or bronchogenic dissemination. Such lesions may involve several lobules or most of a lobe.

Though there may be symptoms, not infrequently extensive pulmonary lesions are detected roentgenographically in children who have no complaints and whose parents have not observed any unusual manifestations.

Physical findings vary considerably. There may or may not be impairment to percussion. Rales may or may not be present. Cavitation occasionally occurs, but, because it is likely to be farther away from the chest wall than in apical lesions, it may be missed on physical examination and even on roentgenograms. Bullous emphysematous lesions have also been infrequently observed, which appear after initiation of therapy and may persist for months, apparently without inhibiting recovery. Tubercle bacilli can frequently be found in the sputum or in lavaged gastric contents.

Infection of the hilar lymph nodes is an almost constant accompaniment of pulmonary tuberculosis in infants and children. The nodes on the side of the parenchymal lesion are the ones usually involved, but the contralateral ones may also be infected. Frequently the only manifestation of the primary infection is the involvement of the tracheobronchial nodes, the parenchymal lesion being so small that it is not demonstrable on the roentgenogram. The infection in the lymph nodes goes through the same stages as that of the parenchymal lesion and, until calcification is complete, is attended by the same danger of local extension and hematogenous dissemination.

There are frequently no symptoms (see p. 602). Though a brassy, paroxysmal cough is often attributed to enlarged nodes, it occurs so infrequently that it can scarcely be considered characteristic. Enlargement of the nodes is rarely demonstrable by physical signs. Cyanosis, edema of the face and dilatation of the superficial veins have been observed in association with extremely enlarged nodes, owing to compression of the larger blood vessels. Paravertebral dullness is rarely demonstrable. Roentgenographic demonstration of enlarged nodes in conjunction with a positive tuberculin reaction constitutes the best evidence for diagnosis.

Intraluminal and *extraluminal bronchial lesions* are of considerable importance in tuberculosis in children. Involvement of the bronchus is almost invariably from a contiguous lesion, rarely by direct infection from an outside source.

Intraluminal lesions are produced by extension from an adjacent tuberculous process, usually in a lymph node, through the bronchial wall with establishment of an ulcerative or granulomatous lesion. The lesion may partially or completely obstruct the lumen of the bronchus and may also result in dissemination of infected material to other portions of the tracheobronchial tree with establishment of tuberculous bronchopneumonia.

An *extraluminal lesion* is a partial or complete occlusion of a bronchus by enlarged adjacent and usually adherent tuberculous lymph nodes without erosion through the bronchial wall.

When a bronchus is partially obstructed by compression from without or by an intraluminal granulomatous lesion to a degree sufficient to interfere with the flow of air, the portion of the lung supplied by the bronchus becomes emphysematous (Fig. 10-48). When the obstruction is complete, absorption atelectasis occurs (Fig. 10-49). In each instance there may also be a tuberculous pneumonitis in all or part of the involved pulmonary area (Fig. 10-50).

Intrabronchial lesions may be responsible for cough, which may be brassy and may also be productive of variable amounts of sputum. Lesions in the major bronchi may be seen bronchoscopically. Biopsy material can often be obtained for histologic and cultural diagnostic purposes, and on occasion sufficient material can be removed to restore the bronchial airway.

Caseous bronchopneumonia may be localized in one area of the lung or widely disseminated. Material from a tuberculous focus in the parenchyma or in a lymph node discharged into a bronchus in a state of liquefaction is likely to be more widely distributed than when it is in a less fluid, caseous state. The lesions are particularly likely to be distal to the portion of the lung supplied by the eroded bronchus where conditions for localization are good, owing to interference with respiratory mechanics. In some instances all lobes are involved.

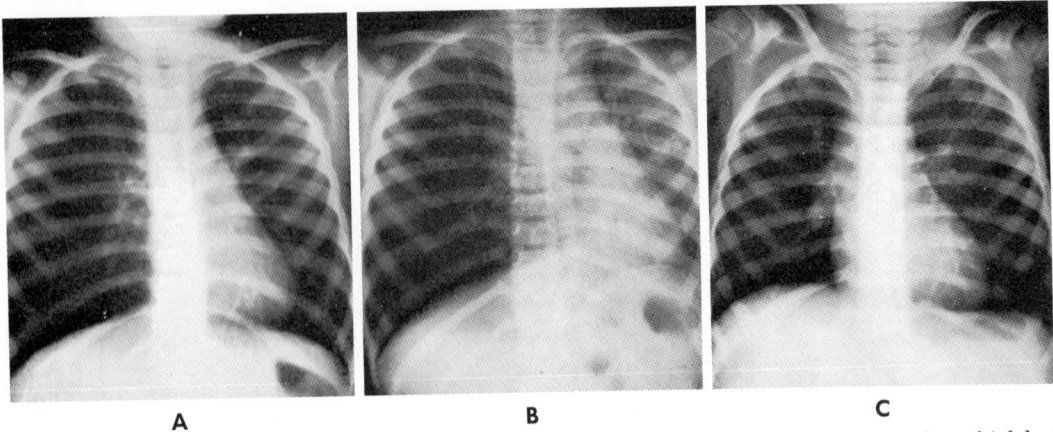

Figure 10-48. Obstructive emphysema of the right lung secondary to a granulomatous intrabronchial lesion. *A*, Inspiratory phase; *B*, expiratory phase, showing failure of right lung to contract, and shift of heart and mediastinal structures to left; *C*, film taken 24 hours after bronchoscopic removal of tuberculous tissue from right main stem bronchus, showing normal aeration of right lung.

Children with caseous bronchopneumonia tend to be quite sick. There is usually fever, malaise and, not infrequently, a loose, productive cough. The physical findings vary considerably. There may or may not be impairment to percussion, bronchial breathing or rales. If there is cavity formation, there may be pectoriloquy unless the lesion is too deeply situated. The extent of the involvement can be determined only from the roentgenogram. Tubercle bacilli can usually be discovered in the sputum or lavaged gastric contents.

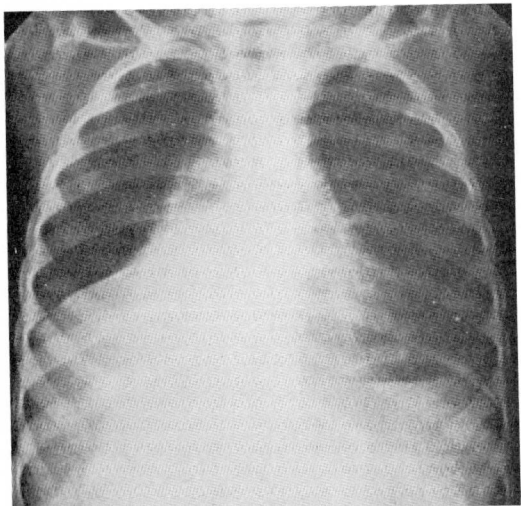

Figure 10-49. Atelectasis of right middle and lower lobes secondary to tracheobronchial tuberculous lymphadenitis and an endobronchial granulomatous lesion in a Negro child 4 years of age. Gastric washings were positive for tubercle bacilli. Two months before the exposure of this film the child suffered a partial bronchial occlusion which resulted in obstructive emphysema. Subsequently complete bronchial occlusion resulted in absorption atelectasis illustrated here. At this time a portion of the endobronchial granuloma was removed endoscopically. There was no immediate effect, but re-expansion occurred over the next 2 months.

Acute miliary tuberculosis is a blood-borne infection characterized by multiple tubercle formations. It is more frequent in infants than in older children. Practically all organs of the body may be involved, as may any serous membrane. Tubercle bacilli become lodged in the small capillaries; a lesion develops at each site, and necrosis tends to develop rapidly in each of the small foci. If the life of the child is sufficiently prolonged, there is an epithelioid response, and the lesions in the lungs become visible on the roentgenogram.

The symptoms are usually those of a general infection. The onset may be abrupt, although at times it is insidious. Fever soon develops and tends to run an irregular course, frequently with peaks as high as 104°F., and the patient appears extremely ill. Initially there may be no physical signs to indicate the extent of the involvement. Choroidal tubercles may be an early manifestation and may be detected by funduscopic examination. The spleen is often enlarged and the abdomen distended; these findings with the high fever and absence of other physical findings may suggest the possibility of typhoid fever. At times the early pulmonary manifestations may be those of generalized obstructive emphysema, and acute bronchiolitis may be suspected. Localized signs which disclose the true identity of the infection frequently do not appear until the last week or so of the illness in the untreated patient. Fine crepitant rales may be heard at this time over all portions of the chest, and the roentgenogram which previously failed to reveal pulmonary changes will show the characteristic, widely distributed miliary lesions, which create a mottled appearance and are frequently described as resembling snowflakes (Fig. 10-51). The white blood cell count is not distinctive; it may be increased, but leukopenia is the more frequent response.

Death usually occurs within 4 to 6 weeks in untreated cases, but recovery is possible in the majority of instances if treatment is instituted sufficiently early (see p. 606).

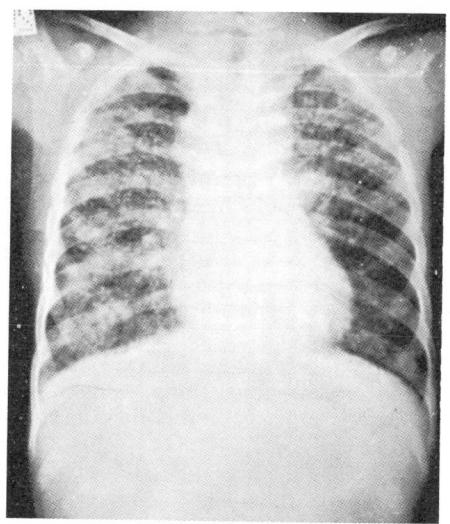 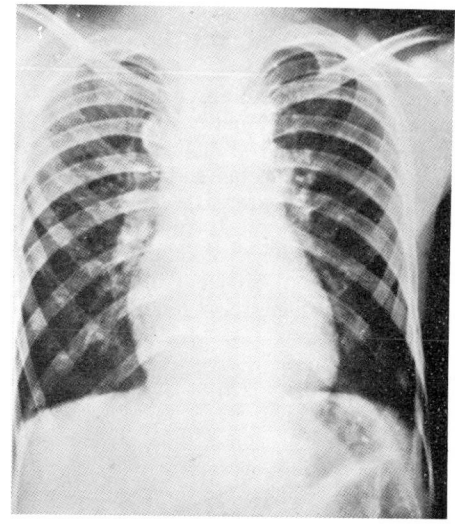

A   **B**

Figure 10-50. *A,* Extensive tuberculous bronchopneumonia in a child 5 years of age, more prominent on the right side. *B,* Appearance of lungs at 9 years of age, after recovery (prior to availability of specific antimicrobial therapy).

Apical and infraclavicular lesions are most commonly seen in adult life and are often termed "adult tuberculosis," "apical tuberculosis" or "reinfection tuberculosis." They are relatively uncommon before the adolescent period, when they become the most frequent type of tuberculous involvement, being more frequent in females than in males. These lesions have generally been considered to be the result of endogenous or exogenous reinfection; their tendency to remain localized and the absence of any extensive involvement of the regional lymph nodes are attributed to an altered response of the host because of a previous infection with the tubercle bacillus. Lesions will develop, however, in the upper portions of the lungs in previously tuberculin-negative as well as in tuberculin-positive adolescents and young adults which are clinically indistinguishable. For this reason these lesions are described simply on the basis of their location and roentgenographic appearance.

The clinical courses of these lesions can in general be grouped in 3 categories. In some there is retrogression toward healing almost from the time of recognition; in others the lesion is indolent and resists healing. In this latter type, activation of the lesion may be associated with any factor which lowers the host's general resistance. In the third type the lesion is persistently progressive, and there is destruction of lung tissue with cavitation.

The symptoms and physical findings are also variable. In some instances no symptoms are elicited. In others there may be the general symptoms of a chronic infection. Physical examination may or may not reveal fine rales; they are likely to be most consistently detected at the beginning of an inspiration which follows a slight cough after forced expiration. Cavity formation of any extent can usually be suspected on the basis of bronchophony and pectoriloquy. The diagnosis is established by roentgenographic examination, the detection of tubercle bacilli in the sputum or lavaged gastric contents, and upon the response to the tuberculin test. Similar lesions can be produced by coccidioidomycosis and histoplasmosis.

Tuberculous pleuritis may occur as a dry fibrinous pleurisy, as a serous effusion, and rarely as a necrotic involvement of the pleura stemming from

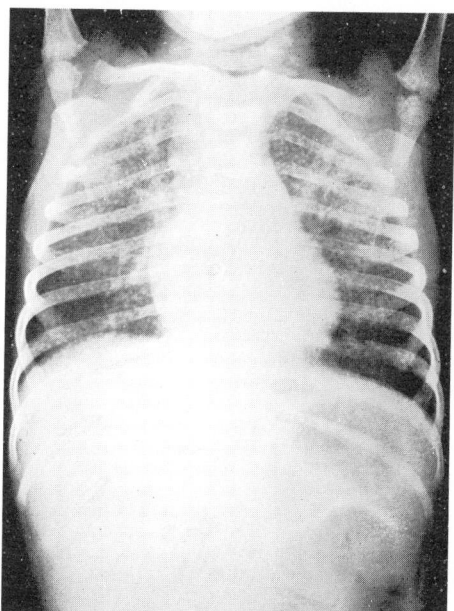

Figure 10-51. Miliary tuberculosis of the lungs in a white boy 3 years of age. His mother had pulmonary tuberculosis. The physical findings were fine, crackling rales throughout both lungs. Death occurred shortly after this roentgenogram was taken. The tuberculin reaction was positive.

a contiguous caseous focus in the lung. Most often the reaction is a serous one, and the process is nearly always unilateral.

Children rarely have complaints suggestive of pleural involvement. Occasionally during the dry stage there may be pleural pain with limitation of respirations on the affected side. Rarely an effusion may become so extensive that there is bulging of the intercostal spaces and respiratory embarrassment. The presence of pleural effusion is usually suspected from physical findings, and the diagnosis is confirmed roentgenographically and by pleural aspiration.

The prognosis is generally governed by the pulmonary lesion. Treatment is that of tuberculous infection; aspiration, other than for diagnostic purposes, is indicated only when there are severe symptoms of compression. Absorption of fluid is followed by pleural thickening and adhesions. There is no evidence that drainage will lessen such residuals or prevent reaccumulation of fluid.

Diagnosis of Pulmonary Tuberculosis. The diagnosis of pulmonary tuberculosis is established with certainty by the demonstration of tubercle bacilli in the sputum, aspirated bronchial secretions or gastric contents. In the absence of such information the diagnosis is based on the history of symptoms and of contact with tuberculous infection, on the physical examination, on the reaction to tuberculin and on roentgenographic examination of the lungs.

The evaluation of the child suspected or proved to have tuberculosis should include an estimate of whether the tuberculous lesion is in an active, quiescent or healed stage (see p. 604). In the absence of fever and other clinical evidences of disease such an evaluation is rarely clear-cut.

The appraisal is not complete without a careful search for the source of contact. Frequently open tuberculosis is present in some member of the family or other close associate without his being aware of it (Figs. 10-52, 10-53). For this reason tuberculin tests should be performed on the siblings; if the reaction is positive, roentgenograms of the chest should be obtained. All adult members should have a careful physical examination, tuberculin test and a roentgenogram of the chest. Grandparents and other older persons with whom there is contact should be included in this examination, since chronic, open tuberculosis is common among older people. It is a good policy to repeat the examination of the members who have no evidence of disease after an interval of about 6 months.

History. History of possible contact with open tuberculosis should be included in the appraisal of all children with or without symptoms of the disease (see above).

Symptoms of pulmonary tuberculosis vary considerably and to some extent are proportionate to the seriousness of the lesion. There are variations in this regard, however, and it is essential to know that pulmonary infections, even extensive ones, may not be productive of any recognizable symptoms. As a rule, symptoms in children are merely the general ones of chronic infection, such as fatigue, irritability and possibly some degree of undernutrition, and are usually not directly related to the respiratory system. When all or most symptoms such as cough with expectoration, hemoptysis, fever, fatigue, malaise, loss of weight, and night sweats are present, one may be certain that the lesion is extensive.

Physical examination. The examination

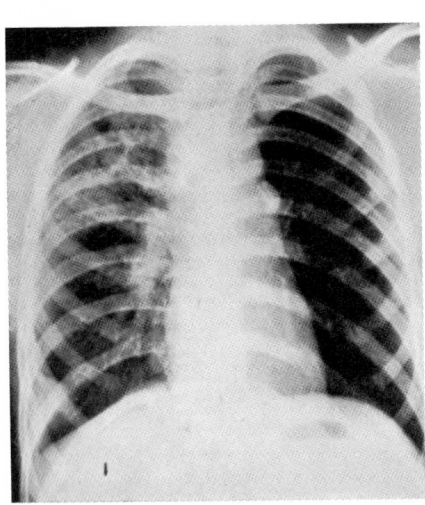
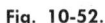
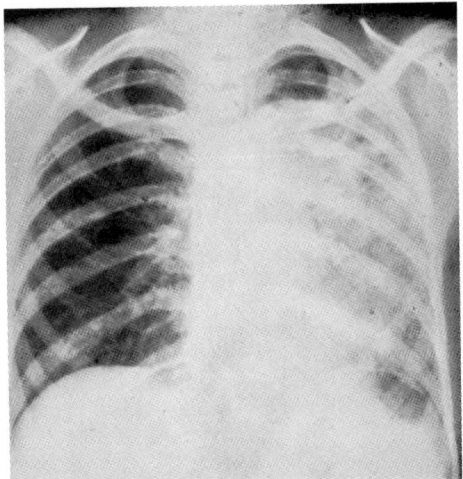

Fig. 10-52.   Fig. 10-53.

Figure 10-52. Calcified node in left hilar area and tuberculous lesions in upper part of right lung in a Negro child 12 years of age.

Figure 10-53. Extensive tuberculous lesion in the chest of the mother, who disclaimed any knowledge of illness or history of tuberculosis in any member of the family. Sputum was positive for tubercle bacilli. Roentgenogram of the mother was taken as part of a survey of the family because of detection of tuberculosis in the child.

should be complete, since tuberculous lesions may be present in other parts of the body and non-tuberculous conditions of the lungs or other parts of the body may be coexistent.

The physical findings of the lungs vary with the nature and extent of the lesion and have been described above. Not infrequently, extensive lesions are found by roentgenogram when no or only slight abnormal physical signs have been elicited. In general, physical signs of tuberculosis in children tend to be disproportionately few in relation to the extent of the pulmonary damage.

Roentgenographic examination. The common roentgenographic abnormalities have been described and illustrated in the descriptions of the various clinical types of intrathoracic tuberculosis. Chronic intrathoracic disease, such as histoplasmosis or coccidioidomycosis, cystic fibrosis, persistent bronchopneumonia, pulmonary changes following measles or pertussis, lymphoblastomas of the mediastinum, lung abscess, aspiration of foreign material, pulmonary infiltrations due to ascariasis, toxocariasis or *Pneumocystis carinii*, Löffler's pneumonia, Letterer-Siwe disease and others, are likely to simulate the lesions produced by pulmonary tuberculosis. Interpretation of roentgenograms without adequate knowledge of the history, physical findings and laboratory data will lead to many erroneous diagnoses.

The tuberculin test. SIGNIFICANCE OF A POSITIVE REACTION. A positive tuberculin reaction is evidence that the person has been infected with the tubercle bacillus or an unclassified acid-fast bacillus and is allergic or hypersensitive to its protein. The presence or absence of activity of the lesion cannot be deduced from the extent of the reaction. Properly used, the test constitutes the most reliable method for the detection of children who have had an infection with the tubercle bacillus or with one of the unclassified mycobacteria and who thus require further examination to determine whether the lesion is active or quiescent. Certain of the unclassified mycobacteria which are pathogenic for man have an antigenic relation with the tubercle bacillus, and their respective "tuberculins" will elicit cross-reactions. Reasonable probability of the infecting bacterium can be determined by comparative testing (see p. 612).

With certain exceptions, failure to elicit a positive reaction to tuberculin eliminates the possibility of the presence of tuberculous infection. For several weeks after the entrance of tubercle bacilli into the body there is no cutaneous reaction to tuberculin. During advanced or terminal stages of tuberculosis, allergy to tuberculin may occasionally disappear; at times it is temporarily inhibited by such nonspecific factors as severe inanition, dehydration, acute febrile illness and administration of corticosteroids. Tuberculin hypersensitivity may also be temporarily suppressed after immunization with live measles vaccine and possibly with smallpox vaccine. Duration of allergy to tuberculin after healing of the lesion, and the factors that govern it are not completely understood. In most instances cutaneous allergy persists for years in association with apparently healed lesions.

CHOICE AND DOSE OF TUBERCULIN. Since there is a common allergen for the human and bovine types of tubercle bacilli, the use of tuberculin from human tubercle bacilli is considered adequate to detect infection with either bacillus (See page 612 for use of "tuberculins" of unclassified mycobacteria.)

At present 2 tuberculins of the human tubercle bacillus are available: old tuberculin (OT) and purified protein derivative (PPD). The principal objection to OT has been the variation in potency of different batches of it. Purified protein derivative, now the most widely used tuberculin, contains no protein other than that of tubercle bacilli. Its antigenicity is reduced by heating. It is usually dispensed in the dried state in tablet form, and is dissolved in a measured amount of diluent before use.

The recommendations for dosages of tuberculin by the National Tuberculosis Association (Diagnostic Standards, 1957) are as follows:

For diagnostic and case-finding work and after BCG vaccination, the use of 5 international units (5 TU) of PPD is recommended as the best single dose, i.e. that amount of any standardized PPD prepared according to acceptable methods which is equal in potency to 0.0001 mg. of PPD-S, the international standard for human tuberculin. If there is no reaction, or a small one, and suspicion of tuberculous infection still exists, repetition of the test with the same dose is recommended. If there is reason to expect a severe reaction, 1:5 dilution of the foregoing dose may be used as a preliminary test. This dilution is made with sterile physiologic or buffered saline solution.

When OT must be used, it is recommended that the dosage be equivalent to the 5 TU dose of the international OT standard. If the OT used approximates the international standard in potency, the recommended dose would be 0.1 ml. of a 1:2000 dilution (0.05 mg.). Unfortunately, there is evidence that some commercial preparations of PPD and OT vary in potency which may lead to variations in results.

There is good evidence that doses greater than 5 TU produce some reactions which are not specific for tuberculous infection. For this reason, the larger doses are of doubtful diagnostic value.

In view of the similarity of certain fungus infections to tuberculosis, it may be wise to perform tests with their antigens simultaneously with the performance of the tuberculin test. This procedure is particularly applicable to histoplasmin in the central part of the United States and to coccidioidin in the far Western states.

TECHNIQUE. There are various methods of performing the tuberculin test, such as the scarification or cutaneous test of Pirquet, the intracutaneous test of Mantoux, the patch test of Vollmer and the multiple puncture tests (Heaf or tine). The percutaneous test of Moro is not used in this country, and the conjunctival test of Calmette is not a safe procedure. In clinical practice or when large numbers of tuberculin tests are to be performed, the intracutaneous or multiple puncture (tine) methods are recommended.

For the *intracutaneous test* a 1-ml. tuberculin type of syringe graduated to 0.1 ml. and a 27-

gauge, short-bevel needle should be used. Injections should be made intracutaneously and not subcutaneously. The tuberculin is so diluted that the testing dose is contained in 0.1 ml. of diluent.

Tuberculin is heat-stable, and it is practically impossible to remove traces of it from syringes or glassware by ordinary methods of cleaning. For this reason a syringe for tuberculin should be restricted to this testing material and should never be used for any other skin-testing solution. Thus, if a cutaneous reaction was obtained from Schick testing material injected from a syringe previously used for tuberculin, one could not be certain whether the reaction resulted from the Schick material or from the tuberculin.

Recommendations for interpretation of the tuberculin test according to the Diagnostic Standards (1961) of the National Tuberculosis Association are as follows:

The Mantoux intracutaneous test should be read 48 to 72 hours after injection. Readings should be made in a good light, with the forearm slightly flexed. Reactions are classified on the basis of induration (not erythema), which may be determined by inspection, palpation, and gentle stroking of the area with the fingers. Reactions should be measured and recorded in millimeters as the largest diameter of induration at right angles to the long axis of the arm.

Significance of reactions. Persons with good-sized reactions to the 5-TU test (10 mm. or more of induration) are at greater risk of having tuberculous disease than persons with smaller (5 to 9 mm.) reactions. Such reactors are also more likely to be household contacts of a person with tuberculosis. It is known that some small (5 to 9 mm.) reactions may be due to technical errors; they may represent recent infection with incompletely developed sensitivity; or they may be cross-reactions to other mycobacterial infections and not necessarily indicative of infection with *M. tuberculosis* or *M. bovis.* It is generally held that persons with these small reactions should be retested with the same dose of tuberculin.

It is recommended that reactions of 5 mm. or more be considered positive until further evidence is available, but also that the exact measurement of the reaction be recorded.

In extremely severe reactions to the intracutaneous test the inflammation may be decreased and sloughing of the necrotic center at times avoided by prompt application of an ice compress and a corticosteroid ointment.

In recent years the Heaf multiple puncture test or its modification, the tine test, has supplanted the Vollmer patch test for both diagnostic and screening testing.

The tine test, as developed by Rosenthal, consists of a stainless steel disk with 4 prongs each 2 mm. long, attached to a plastic handle. After the tines have been precoated with concentrated OT, the unit is packed and sterilized with ethylene oxide gas.

The test is performed on the volar surface of the forearm after the skin site has been cleansed, as with alcohol or acetone. The skin is stretched tightly with one hand while the other presses the disk smoothly and firmly against the skin for about 1 second so that the tines penetrate the skin, allowing the tuberculin to be deposited in the outer layer. The disk is then discarded.

The test area is carefully inspected 48 to 72 hours later under good lighting; careful palpation is performed to note the presence of induration. If the induration of one or more of the puncture sites is 2 mm. or more in diameter, the reaction is considered positive. The tine test is said to be standardized so that a positive reaction to it is equivalent to an intradermal reaction of 5 or more mm. to 5 T.U. or 0.0001 mg. of PPD.

If the results of the tine test are equivocal, an intradermal Mantoux test should be performed.

Bacteriologic examination. Tubercle bacilli can usually be isolated in children with active

lesions if a diligent search is made. It is the only basis for an absolute diagnosis of tuberculosis; *M. tuberculosis* must be distinguished from other acid-fast bacilli, including the unclassified strains of mycobacteria variously designated as anonymous or atypical strains. There are 3 principal means for detection of the tubercle bacillus: (1) by direct smear and staining of sputum, cerebrospinal fluid or discharges from such lesions as draining lymph nodes and sinuses of osseous lesions; (2) by guinea pig inoculation of any of these materials; and (3) by cultural methods on artificial media. The last is the most effective. In infants and children who are liable to swallow sputum the lavaged contents of the fasting stomach provide the best source of material for examination. The lavage should be performed early in the morning before the usual breakfast time.

Evaluation of clinical activity. The diagnosis of tuberculous infection is not complete without determining whether the lesion is active or quiescent. When there are such obvious signs of clinical activity as fever and malaise, no further evidence is required. When there are no apparent manifestations of active infection, however, other measures must be used. These include sedimentation rates, blood cell counts, serial roentgenograms, response to exercise and particularly continued observation of the child's apparent well-being and his growth pattern. Rectal temperature should not be taken for at least a half hour after active exercise, since it is normally elevated for a short time after physical activity. Failure to recognize this fact has often been responsible for unnecessarily confining a child to bed or reduced activity.

Prognosis. Most children recover from primary tuberculous infection, and the majority are unaware of its presence even during its active phase. The realization that recovery is frequent has resulted in the conclusion by some clinicians that the primary infection is a benign lesion. There is an apparent failure to recognize the relatively high fatality rate during the first 2 years of life, as well as the fact that hematogenous and bronchogenic lesions originate from the primary focus and, in such instances, are in reality a part of the primary infection.

Mortality rates have been relatively high in the first few years of life and during adolescence. The prognosis of pulmonary as well as of other forms of tuberculosis has been tremendously improved by the use of antimicrobial agents. Death, except in tuberculous meningitis, almost never occurs except in patients who are not treated or in whom the diagnosis is made in the terminal phase of the disease. Antimicrobial treatment of pulmonary tuberculosis has resulted in a striking decrease in hematogenous lesions. This observation has led to an extensive clinical trial (p. 605) with the prophylactic administration of isoniazid to young children with positive tuberculin reactions with or without roentgenographically demonstrable lesions and to older children who are known to have become tuberculin-positive within recent months. This study demonstrated that progression of the localized lesion is usually prevented, and the incidence of hematogenous dissemination is decreased.

Prevention. The only certain means for the prevention of tuberculosis is avoidance of contact with tubercle bacilli. Maintenance of an adequate nutritional status and avoidance of fatigue and of debilitating infections are factors in natural resistance, but none of them is sufficient to prevent infection.

As yet no method has been developed for production of a solid, artificially induced specific immunity.

Identification of tuberculous contacts. Perhaps the most important measure for the prevention of tuberculosis in children would be frequent examination of all adults for the presence of tuberculosis. In such a plan adults with positive tuberculin reactions would be examined roentgenographically at stated intervals. Unfortunately, this method of case-finding is not practical on a broad basis. It is desirable, however, that efforts be made to perform tuberculin tests on all children at intervals of 2 to 3 years.

In view of the high incidence of tuberculosis in crowded and urban areas where poor housing conditions prevail, it is obvious that correction of these conditions is an important public health measure.

Milk. If at all possible, only pasteurized milk from tuberculosis-free cattle should be used for the feeding of infants and children. Unpasteurized milk should not be used without boiling.

Artificial immunity. There have been numerous attempts to develop a satisfactory method for the stimulation of artificial immunity against tuberculosis. Of these, only BCG (Bacillus of Calmette and Guérin) vaccination merits continued use. The vaccine is composed of bovine tubercle bacilli whose virulence has been reduced by special cultural procedures. Administration of the vaccine to animals or man produces a limited immunity to reinfection with virulent tubercle bacilli. Intradermal injections seem to be somewhat more effective than subcutaneous ones and less likely to result in indolent ulcers. An occasional infant vaccinated during the first few months of life may acquire suppurative adenopathy, but such a complication almost never occurs in older infants or children. The usual intradermal dose is in the range of 0.1 to 0.15 mg. of freshly prepared vaccine. Positive tuberculin reactions develop in most instances after inoculation.

Controlled studies, chiefly in the Scandinavian countries and in the United States, have shown that BCG vaccination produces definite though incomplete protection against tuberculosis. The practice of administering BCG vaccine to children who live in areas with a high tuberculosis mortality rate or to those who are intimately exposed to adults with inactive or "arrested" tuberculosis is less frequently recommended than previously,

since equal or greater protection is afforded by the daily administration of isoniazid (see below).

At present BCG vaccine is prepared in only a few laboratories. Its distribution from these laboratories is usually controlled by local or state health departments.

Chemoprophylaxis. Extensive trials have demonstrated that the daily administration of isoniazid to children who have a high probability of exposure to tuberculosis significantly reduces the incidence of new tuberculous infections. The disadvantage of this form of prophylaxis is the need for continuous therapy. A significant advantage is the absence of any effect on the child's reaction to tuberculin, so that the test can continue to be useful in detecting infection, if it is acquired.

Treatment. It is generally agreed that all children with demonstrable active lesions of whatever order and in whatever location of the body should receive antimicrobial therapy. In addition, it is recommended that all tuberculin-positive children up to 4 years of age, all such older children who are known to have become tuberculin-positive within recent months and all who are or have been in recent contact with open tuberculosis, irrespective of the time of acquisition of their tuberculin sensitivity, should receive isoniazid in doses of 10 to 20 mg. per kg. per day for about a year whether or not they have demonstrable lesions. The reasons for this policy are the effectiveness of isoniazid in the control of progressive lesions, its apparently low degree of toxicity and, in particular, its effectiveness in the prevention of hematogenous dissemination.

The most useful drugs in the treatment of tuberculosis are isoniazid, streptomycin and aminosalicylic acid. Other agents include kanamycin, neomycin, viomycin, cycloserine and possibly pyrazinamide, ethionamide and ethambutol. Clinical experience with these drugs is limited in children. At the moment their usefulness is largely limited to patients infected with tubercle bacilli resistant to isoniazid and streptomycin.

Isoniazid is the most useful of the available agents. It can be administered orally or parenterally. Its toxicity is low, provided the daily dose does not exceed 10 to 20 mg. per kg. per day. The emergence of drug-resistant organisms is not rapid, and it can be used as a single agent in many patients with the less serious forms of tuberculosis. Patients with progressive, localized lesions, miliary tuberculosis and meningitis should receive an additional agent during the early part of their treatment (Table 10-14). Some adults who received isoniazid for a long time have had convulsive disorders. So far as known, such complications have not been observed in infants and small children. Such reactions have been minimized or averted by the continuous administration of pyridoxine.

Streptomycin is an active agent against *M. tuberculosis*, and its use is probably indicated in addition to isoniazid in all serious tuberculous infections. The drug must be administered by intramuscular injection. Long-term treatment is

TABLE 10-14.　Suggested Schedules for Antimicrobial Therapy of Pulmonary Tuberculosis in Infants and Children

TYPE OF DISEASE[3]	DRUG[1]	TOTAL DAILY DOSE PER KILOGRAM	DURATION
Positive tuberculin reaction in a child under 4 years of age or a positive tuberculin reaction recently acquired by a child of any age	Isoniazid	10 to 20 mg. (total daily dose should rarely exceed 500 mg.)[2]	One year
Asymptomatic pulmonary tuberculosis	Isoniazid	10 to 20 mg.[2]	One year or for a minimum of 6 months after lesion appears to be inactive
Progressive pulmonary lesions; progressive apical and infraclavicular lesions; pleurisy; miliary tuberculosis	Isoniazid and	10 to 20 mg. (total daily dose should rarely exceed 500 mg.)[2]	12 to 18 months or for a minimum of 6 months after lesion appears to be inactive
	Streptomycin or	20 to 40 mg. in 1 dose per day (dose not to exceed 1.0 gm./day)	Daily for 1 to 2 months, then 2 to 4 times weekly for 3 to 6 months (concurrently with isoniazid)
	Aminosalicylic acid (PASA)	200 to 300 mg. (dose not to exceed 12 gm./day)	For duration of isoniazid therapy. If streptomycin is given initially, then substitute PASA for it after its discontinuance. Some prescribe it only for an arbitrarily determined shorter time

1. See text for use of corticosteroids.
2. The smaller doses are used for large and overweight children. Pyridoxine is prescribed with isoniazid for adolescent children by some clinicians to lessen the likelihood of convulsive disorders.
3. See text for treatment of tuberculous adenitis and other forms of extrathoracic tuberculosis.

occasionally complicated by labyrinth disorders and less often by deafness, but these are uncommon if the drug is administered only once a day or less frequently. Streptomycin should not be used as the only antituberculous agent, owing to the rapid emergence of streptomycin-resistant organisms. This process can be retarded if another agent is administered concurrently. Dihydrostreptomycin is not recommended, since deafness is a common sequel.

Aminosalicylic acid (para-aminosalicylic acid) is tuberculostatic, but is not as effective as streptomycin or isoniazid. It rarely produces toxic reactions other than gastric irritation, which is occasionally sufficiently severe to prevent its administration. Drug-resistant tubercle bacilli have been infrequently observed. It inhibits the development of resistance by tubercle bacilli to both streptomycin and isoniazid and tends to increase serum levels of isoniazid by competing with it for acetylation.

Corticosteroid therapy in conjunction with antimicrobial drugs has not been clearly beneficial except in the treatment of endobronchial granulomas, in which improvement may be noted within a week or so and possibly in the prevention of hydrocephalus in patients with tuberculous meningitis. Pleural effusions may also resolve more rapidly with such treatment. In such circumstances corticosteroid treatment is continued for about 2 months.

Bronchial obstruction secondary to enlarged mediastinal lymph nodes is apparently not benefited by the administration of corticosteroids.

Suggested plans for antimicrobial treatment of the various clinical forms of tuberculosis are detailed in Table 10-14.

When patients with progressive pulmonary tuberculosis are treated by the suggested plan, symptomatic improvement is usually noted in 2 to 4 weeks. Improvement, as measured by changes in the roentgenograms of the chest, is slow, but extension of the lesion rarely occurs.

Patients with miliary tuberculosis tend to show somewhat more rapid improvement in response to treatment. There is apt to be regression or even disappearance of the miliary densities observed in the roentgenograms within 6 to 10 weeks from the start of treatment. Coexisting extensive pulmonary lesions follow the same pattern of slow improvement noted with other progressive pulmonary lesions. If meningitis develops, the patient should be treated as outlined on page 610.

The use of antibacterial agents in the treatment

of pulmonary tuberculosis does not eliminate the need for symptomatic and other general therapy.

Children with nonprogressive primary tuberculous lesions receiving isoniazid require no special care beyond that of assurance of adequate nutrition, avoidance of fatigue, prevention of exposure to open tuberculous infection and regular physical examinations, including roentgenograms of the chest. Active immunization against pertussis, measles and influenza is desirable for children with tuberculous lesions, as is the early treatment of all intercurrent infections in order to lessen the possibilities of activation of the tuberculous process.

Children who are sick with tuberculosis as evidenced by fever, malaise, loss of weight, anemia, abnormal white blood cell count, increased erythrocyte sedimentation rate or roentgenogaphic evidence of progression of the tuberculous lesion require general medical care.

Bed rest is indicated until there are substantial evidences of improvement. Other than maintenance of the necessary isolation procedures (p. 553), the management is that of any child with a chronic illness, whether in an institution or at home.

The *psychologic attitudes* of the child and his family are important. An atmosphere of cheerful optimism should prevail in which the child is provided some regularity of schedule and even some purposeful duties. Except in severe illness, there is no reason why the child should not be permitted to continue with his schoolwork.

Fresh air and *sunshine* are not important in treatment except as they add to the child's sense of well-being. Heliotherapy is not contraindicated except in excessive amounts in patients with pulmonary lesions. Burning of the skin should be scrupulously avoided. Tanning is permissible if it is acquired gradually.

The *nutritional intake* should be adequate, but forced feeding should be avoided. Special attention should be given to the protein, mineral and vitamin content of the diet. There is need for additional amounts of vitamin C; 100 to 200 mg. of ascorbic acid will meet the daily requirement in the average patient. There is no reason why this cannot be supplied by natural foodstuffs. Vitamins of the B complex should also be supplied in amounts somewhat in excess of average requirements. There is no need for extra amounts of vitamin D or for more than a quart of milk a day. Fresh fruits and vegetables should be given freely. Feeding of tuberculous infants is, with the exception of those with gastrointestinal disturbances, not different from that of other infants. Low-residue diets should be prescribed when there is chronic intestinal involvement.

Surgical procedures, other than bronchoscopy, are rarely indicated in the treatment of pulmonary tuberculosis in infants and children. Lobectomy is occasionally required for those with persistent atelectasis or bronchiectasis following endobronchial lesions.

EXTRATHORACIC TUBERCULOSIS

Tuberculous Infection of Tonsils and Cervical Lymph Nodes

Infection of the cervical lymph nodes is, in most instances, secondary to tuberculous infection of the tonsils, which may constitute the primary lesion or may be secondary to a pulmonary lesion. When the tonsillar infection is primary, it constitutes, in conjunction with the cervical lymph node involvement, a primary tuberculous complex. Such infections have become much less frequent with the decrease in incidence of bovine tuberculosis.

Clinical Manifestations. The local manifestations of tuberculosis of the cervical lymph nodes vary from slight enlargement of a single node to involvement of a number of them. The nodes of both sides are frequently affected, although usually more on one side than on the other. The initial inflammatory changes are responsible for the enlargement, and at this stage the node or nodes are discrete, firm and usually freely movable. When the lesions of the individual nodes become caseous, however, there is a tendency to erosion of the capsule, and the nodes in the immediate vicinity become matted together in a single, irregular nodular mass, often with variable degrees of firmness in different portions. The mass becomes attached to other adjacent structures and to the overlying skin and is no longer freely movable. The skin is often discolored and may be retracted in areas by the underlying adhesions, thus having an uneven contour.

If liquefaction of the caseous mass occurs, rupture into the adjacent tissues is likely. If the overlying skin is perforated, as it often is, one or more draining sinuses may be formed. When the nodes

TABLE 10-15. CLASSIFICATION OF EXTRATHORACIC TUBERCULOSIS

Tuberculosis of tonsils and cervical lymph nodes
Intra-abdominal tuberculosis
  Enteritis
  Mesenteric and retroperitoneal lymphadenopathy
  Peritonitis
  Liver
  Fistula in ano
Tuberculosis of central nervous system
  Tuberculoma
  Tuberculous meningitis
Tuberculosis of skin
Tuberculosis of bones and joints
Tuberculous pericarditis
Tuberculosis of genitourinary tract
  Kidney
  Bladder
  Female genital organs
  Male genital organs
Tuberculosis of eye
  Phlyctenular keratitis
  Chorioretinitis
Tuberculosis of middle ear

of the retropharyngeal area are involved or when the discharge from other nodes or from an osseous lesion in the cervical vertebrae finds its way into the retropharyngeal area, a chronic, burrowing retropharyngeal and retroesophageal abscess results. The draining sinuses on the surface of the neck persist until the involved lymphatic tissue is broken down and evacuated, the course without antimicrobial therapy being measured in months or, at times, in years. Indolent skin lesions frequently result, and healing leaves permanent scarring, discoloration and contractural deformities.

Not all tuberculous lymph nodes undergo such a course, and resolution may take place before extensive caseation occurs, or the caseous mass may become calcified and a number of nodes remain matted together and indurated without suppurating. Calcification may be visualized roentgenographically. During the period of active inflammation there may be a low-grade fever and other evidences of chronic infection.

Diagnosis. The tonsillar lesion can be identified only by microscopic examination of the enucleated tonsil.

The differential diagnosis is from other conditions which may cause chronic lymphadenitis, and should include the lymphoblastomas, Hodgkin's disease, carcinoma of the thyroid, actinomycosis, cat-scratch disease and toxoplasmosis. Particular difficulty is experienced in residual or low-grade cervical lymphadenitis associated with chronic upper respiratory tract infections. The likelihood of a tuberculous origin is increased in the presence of a positive tuberculin reaction, but the diagnosis is established only by isolation of tubercle bacilli from the excretions of a draining sinus or by microscopic examination of an excised lymph node.

Prognosis. This depends upon the stage at which diagnosis is established and treatment instituted. Most lesions eventually heal even when untreated. In such instances contractural deformities may be expected.

Treatment. Treatment varies with the stage of the lesion at the time of diagnosis. If the lymph nodes are still discrete, excision of the involved ones by careful surgical dissection is recommended. Streptomycin, 10 to 20 mg. per kg. per dose, should be administered 2 or 3 times at intervals of 12 hours before operation. After excision, streptomycin is continued for approximately 2 weeks, or longer if the operative site shows any drainage. Isoniazid is also administered postoperatively for 12 months in doses of 10 to 20 mg. per kg. per day.

If the lymph nodes have ruptured spontaneously, antibacterial therapy as recommended for progressive pulmonary tuberculosis in Table 10-14 should be instituted. If drainage persists after 2 weeks of treatment, secondary bacterial infection is probably present, and other antibiotic therapy should be given in addition to the antitubercu-lous therapy. In most instances the sinus tracts will close within several weeks. Surgical excision can then be performed; antimicrobial therapy should be carried out postoperatively as recommended above.

If the mass of lymph nodes is so extensive that surgical excision is not feasible, antimicrobial therapy as recommended for progressive pulmonary lesions is suggested.

Whether tonsillectomy should be performed several weeks after excision of the lymph nodes is not established.

Infection of Other Superficial Lymph Nodes

Tuberculosis of other superficial lymph nodes, such as those of the axilla, groin or occipital region, may occur, but is less frequent than infection of the cervical lymph nodes. Such infections are usually secondary to tuberculosis of the skin. The course of the infection is that described for cervical lymphadenitis.

Intra-abdominal Tuberculosis

Tuberculous enteritis may occur as a primary infection or may be secondary to a pulmonary lesion, the bacilli being transported in swallowed sputum. The stomach is rarely infected. Progressive ulcerative enteritis is more likely to be a secondary than a primary infection and is usually associated with advanced pulmonary disease. In both primary and secondary lesions the mesenteric and, at times, the retroperitoneal lymph nodes are involved. In primary infections the intestinal lesion is usually relatively unimportant and is overshadowed by the lymph node involvement, whereas the situation is essentially reversed in secondary infections. *Tuberculous peritonitis* may be part of a generalized hematogenous infection, but more frequently results from rupture of a caseous mesenteric lymph node or by extension from an ulcerative intestinal lesion. *Tuberculosis of the liver and spleen* is usually a part of generalized miliary tuberculosis. The incidence of intestinal tuberculosis in this country has decreased tremendously in recent years, owing in part to the almost complete eradication of bovine tuberculosis.

Fistula in ano may be secondary to tuberculosis, but is more frequently secondary to other gastrointestinal diseases such as granulomatous ileocolitis.

Tuberculous Enteritis

Small tuberculous ulcers frequently produce no symptoms and are discovered only at autopsy. With more extensive lesions the symptoms are those of ileocolitis with tenesmus and chronic diarrhea. There may be gross hemorrhage, but more often there is only slight bleeding. That the lesions are tuberculous may be suspected from the chronicity and also from the presence of tuberculous infection elsewhere in the body, especially in the lungs. Abdominal distention and tenderness may be present; there is irregular fever, wasting is often great, and anemia and debility are severe.

Treatment. The diet should be low in residue, but should have adequate caloric value and be high in vitamin content. In the more severe cases parenteral administration of vitamins may be indicated, as well as amino acids, blood and plasma. Antispasmodics such as paregoric and belladonna preparations may be given for the relief of tenesmus. Antimicrobial therapy for progressive pulmonary tuberculosis (Table 10-14) should be given.

Tuberculous Peritonitis

The incidence of tuberculous peritonitis has decreased markedly, and the lesion is now rare in the United States. Scattered miliary tubercles may be found upon the peritoneum in acute, generalized miliary tuberculosis. Tuberculous peritonitis usually originates from erosion of a caseous or liquefied lesion in a mesenteric lymph node; less often from an intestinal lesion which has penetrated through the outer coat, usually without perforation.

Clinical Manifestations. The onset is as a rule insidious and is characterized by gradually increasing abdominal distention, debilitation, vague abdominal pain or tenderness, and low-grade fever. The onset may, however, be more abrupt and severe and may be suggestive of appendicitis when the pain and tenderness are in the right lower quadrant. Vomiting may occur, but usually is not severe, and there are no characteristic changes in the stools except in the presence of an associated enteritis.

Clinically, tuberculous peritonitis has been divided into 3 general types: (1) the ascitic form, (2) the fibrinous or plastic form, and (3) the caseous or ulcerative form. All these processes are frequently present in a single case, and there may be no sharp distinction into a particular clinical pattern.

Prognosis. The natural course of tuberculous peritonitis is generally chronic. The outcome is determined not only by the type and extent of the local involvement, but also by the nature of the tuberculous lesions of other parts of the body. In general, the ascitic form has the most favorable prognosis, the caseous form the worst.

Treatment. The management of tuberculous peritonitis is essentially that of tuberculosis in general. If there is an associated enteritis, the diet should be low in residue; otherwise it may be adjusted to the patient's appetite. There should be adequate calories as well as a high vitamin and mineral content in the diet. Antimicrobial ther-

apy as recommended for progressive pulmonary tuberculosis is indicated (Table 10-14).

Tuberculosis of the Central Nervous System

Tuberculoma. Tuberculomas of the brain or spinal cord may be single or multiple, and may or may not be productive of neurologic symptoms. Though they are often recognized only at autopsy, they may be responsible for symptoms of increased intracranial pressure or localized peripheral manifestations and in such instances are indistinguishable clinically from intracranial neoplasms. Intracerebral calcification, demonstrable on the roentgenogram, may be tuberculous in origin, but more often is in the lesions of toxoplasmosis, cytomegalic inclusion disease, astrocytomas, Sturge-Weber syndrome or an organized hemorrhage. Tuberculomas at the surface of the brain constitute the principal means for infection of meninges.

Tuberculous Meningitis

Tuberculous meningitis is the principal cause of death from tuberculosis and is most frequent in the first few years of life. It is always associated with primary tuberculous infection, usually in the lung, and is most likely to occur within a few months after the initial manifestation of the primary lesion. The incidence is especially high in the Negro race. Frequently it is the initial and only clinical manifestation of tuberculous infection, although it is always a secondary lesion. Generalized miliary tuberculosis is observed in about 25 per cent of cases.

Pathogenesis and Pathology. The observations of Rich and McCordock indicate that the meninges are rarely directly infected by the hematogenous route, but rather are secondarily involved by the discharge of tubercle bacilli into the cerebrospinal fluid from contiguous older caseous foci such as a tuberculoma in the brain or spinal cord or osseous lesions of the vertebrae.

Tubercles are scattered over the pia and the surface of the brain. The dura is tense, the convolutions are flattened, and the arachnoid space and the ventricles contain serofibrinous exudate.

Clinical Manifestations. The clinical manifestations may vary, and at times meningeal symptoms are not present until the terminal stage. In general, however, there is a more or less typical pattern which in the untreated child may be divided into 3 stages: (1) a prodromal stage of irritation, (2) a transitional stage of increased intracranial pressure and meningeal symptoms, and (3) a terminal stage of paralysis and coma. These stages are not sharply demarcated, and not all may be present in a given case.

Prodromal stage. The onset is usually slow, with little or no fever, rarely acute with high fever. The initial manifestations are often vague.

Changes in disposition are frequent; a good-natured child becomes irritable. Periods of drowsiness are common, but sleep is frequently restless. Older children complain of headache. Anorexia, vomiting and constipation are common.

Transitional stage. Convulsions may occur during this stage, and the drowsiness becomes much deeper. Most frequent, however, are the evidences of meningeal irritation. There is nuchal rigidity, and stiffness of the back and extremities, at times sufficient to produce opisthotonos. The deep reflexes tend to be exaggerated. There may be bulging of the fontanel. Ocular paralyses are common, or there may be nystagmus or strabismus; the pupils are normal or contracted, and hippus may be present. Occasionally there is choking of the disk, and tubercles may be present along the vessels of the choroid. There is usually a well marked *tache cérébrale* and at times, because of vasomotor disturbances, irregular flushing of the trunk and face. The temperature is usually elevated, but is rarely high. The course is progressive, and the drowsiness tends to be replaced by stupor.

Terminal stage. The evidences of meningeal irritation are replaced by those of paralysis in the final phase. The child lapses into a comatose state with dilated and unresponsive pupils, insensitivity of the cornea, widespread paralyses, irregular pulse which may be slow or accelerated, and irregular respirations which are at times of the Cheyne-Stokes type. The temperature rises abruptly at the terminal stage, at times to as high as 107°F., and there may be hyperglycemia and glycosuria. Death occurs without recovery of consciousness.

Variations. The duration of untreated tuberculous meningitis is generally not more than 3 weeks after definite symptoms appear. In general, each of the 3 stages described averages about a week, although the initial one may be somewhat longer and the last stage shorter. In unusual instances, however, the terminal stage may be prolonged for several weeks. The course is also subject to other variations. The prodromal stage may be absent, with the onset sudden and the total course brief. Temporary improvement and even remissions have been recorded. As a rule, the onset in infancy is more abrupt than in childhood; generalized convulsions are more frequent, the symptoms are less characteristic, and the course is shorter. A clinical course unmodified by treatment is now rarely seen.

Diagnosis. A positive tuberculin reaction is only supportive evidence. In the terminal stage cutaneous sensitivity to tuberculin may be lost. The white blood cell count is not characteristic; in the early stages it may be decreased. In the late stage there is often a leukocytosis.

The *cerebrospinal fluid* provides the most important data, but an absolute diagnosis can be made from it only by isolation of tubercle bacilli. The fluid may be clear or only slightly turbid, the so-called ground-glass appearance. It is practically always increased in pressure and amount. The cell count ranges from 20 to about 500 per mm.[3] The cells are principally lymphocytes, though there is occasionally a predominance of polymorphonuclear cells in the early stage. The protein content of the cerebrospinal fluid is increased and is often more than 100 mg. per 100 ml.; the sugar content is usually decreased, and the chloride concentration is usually significantly reduced in the latter phase of the disease.

On standing, the cerebrospinal fluid usually forms a fibrinous web or pellicle in which tubercle bacilli may be enmeshed and in which they can be demonstrated on staining. The fluid should also be centrifuged and the sediment examined. When the organisms cannot be demonstrated by direct examination, they usually can be by culture.

The *differential diagnosis* is chiefly from other conditions responsible for an increase in lymphocytic cells in the cerebrospinal fluid (see Aseptic Meningitis Syndrome, p. 687). There is rarely any difficulty in the differential diagnosis of the various purulent meningitides, except as their course has been modified by suppressive but inadequate antimicrobial therapy. The demonstration of a tuberculous lesion in some other region of the body is strong supportive evidence in favor of a tuberculous cause for the meningitis.

Prognosis. Complete recovery from tuberculous meningitis is now possible. The mortality rate is still high, ranging from 10 to 50 per cent in different series of treated cases, and the incidence of permanent physical and mental residuals among the survivors is also high. The promptness with which specific therapy is instituted would seem to be a determining factor, although recovery has occurred in patients considered to be hopeless.

Treatment. The treatment of choice is a combination of streptomycin and isoniazid and adequate supportive measures.

The plan currently used in our clinic is as follows: streptomycin, 50 mg. per kg. intramuscularly every 12 hours (but not over 2 gm. per day) until there are signs of improvement, then 20 to 40 mg. per kg. every other day (but not over 1 gm. per dose) for a total of 3 to 6 months; and isoniazid in total daily oral doses of 20 to 40 mg. per kg. until there is improvement. Thereafter the dose is reduced to 10 to 20 mg. per kg. and is continued for at least 18 months. Intrathecal therapy with antimicrobial drugs is not used. In some clinics aminosalicylic acid is administered in conjunction with isoniazid after the streptomycin has been discontinued (see Table 10-14).

One of the main obstacles in the treatment of tuberculous meningitis is the development of obstruction to the flow of cerebrospinal fluid. Obstruction may apparently be prevented or at times relieved by systemic administration of a corticosteroid during the first months of therapy.

Supportive measures include adequate nutrition, which often necessitates gavage feeding, vitamin supplements, attention to fluid and electrolyte balance (see p. 226 for salt-losing syndrome), sedation, prophylaxis against bedsores, and early detection and treatment of intercurrent infections.

REFERENCES

General

Kendig, E. L.: *Disorders of the Respiratory Tract in Children.* Philadelphia, W. B. Saunders Company, 1967.
Lincoln, E. M., and Sewell, E. M.: Tuberculosis in Children. New York, McGraw-Hill Book Co., Inc., 1962.

Epidemiology

Trauger, D. A.: Editorial. A Note on Tuberculosis Epidemiology. *Am. Rev. Resp. Dis.,* 87:582, 1963.

Pathology

Auerbach, O.: Tuberculosis in Children. *Am. J. Dis. Child.,* 75: 555, 1948.
Terplan, K.: Morphologic Analysis of Fatal Tuberculosis in Children. *Am. Rev. Tuberc.,* 74:7, 1956.
Terplan, K.: Anatomical Studies of Human Tuberculosis. *Am. Rev. Tuberc.* (Supp.), 42:1, 1940.

Factors Influencing Development of Infection

Johnston, J. A.: *Nutritional Studies in Adolescent Girls, and Their Relation to Tuberculosis.* Springfield, Ill., Charles C Thomas, 1953.
Lurie, M. B.: Heredity, Constitution and Tuberculosis; Experimental Study. *Am. Rev. Tuberc.,* (Suppl), 44:1, 1941.
Pinner, M.: Pathogenesis of Tuberculosis. *J.A.M.A.,* 107:475, 1936.
Rich, A. R.: *The Pathogenesis of Tuberculosis.* Springfield, Ill., Charles C Thomas, 1944.

Age Factors in Tuberculous Infection

High, R. H., and Zwerling, H. B.: Variation with Age in the Frequency of Tuberculous Pulmonary Calcification. *Pub. Health Rep.,* 61:1769, 1946.
Israel, H. L., and Long, E. R.: Primary Tuberculosis in Adolescents and Young Adults. *Am. Rev. Tuberc.,* 43:42, 1941.

Lesions Simulating Tuberculosis

Christie, A., and Peterson, J. C.: Histoplasmin Sensitivity. *J. Pediat.,* 29:417, 1946.
Palmer, C. E.: Nontuberculous Pulmonary Calcification and Sensitivity to Histoplasmin. *Pub. Health Rep.,* 60:513, 1945.
Smith, C. E.: Coccidioidomycosis. *M. Clin. N. Amer.,* 27:790, 1943.

Tuberculin

Furcolow, M. L., Hewell, B., Nelson, W. E., and Palmer, C. E.: Quantitative Studies of Tuberculin Reaction. I. Titration of Tuberculin Sensitivity and Its Relation to Tuberculous Infection. *Pub. Health Rep.,* 56:1082, 1941.
Furcolow, M. L., Watson, K. A., Charron, T., and Lowe, J.: A Comparison of the Tine and Mono-vacc Tests with the Intradermal Tuberculin Test. *Am. Rev. Resp. Dis.,* 96:1009, 1968.
Nelson, W. E., Mitchell, A. G., and Brown, E. W.: Possibility of Sensitization to Tuberculin. *Am. Rev. Tuberc.,* 37:286, 1938.
Nelson, W. E., Seibert, F. B., and Long, E. R.: Technical Factors Affecting Tuberculin Test. *J.A.M.A.,* 108:2179, 1937.
Rosenthal, S. R.: The Disc-Tine Tuberculin Test (Dried Tuberculin—Disposable Unit). *J.A.M.A.,* 177:452, 1961.
Seibert, F. B., and Dufour, E.: A Study of Certain Problems in the Use of Standard Tuberculin. *Am. Rev. Tuberc.,* 58:363, 1948.
A Statement of the Committee on Diagnostic Skin Testing: Tuberculin Skin-Testing Techniques: Current Status. *Am. Rev. Resp. Dis.,* 87:607, 1963.

Prophylaxis

A United States Public Health Service Tuberculosis Prophylaxis Trial: Prophylactic Effects of Isoniazid on Primary Tuberculosis in Children. *Am. Rev. Tuberc.,* 76-6, 1957.

Palmer, C. E., Shaw, L. W., and Comstock, G. W.: Community Trials of BCG Vaccination. *Am. Rev. Tuberc.,* 77:6, 1958.
Report of AD HOC Advisory Committee on BCG to the Surgeon General of the United States Public Health Service. *Am. Rev. Tuberc.,* 76:5, 1957.

Treatment

A Statement by the Committee on Tuberculosis and Respiratory Disease in Children: Treatment of Tuberculosis in Children. *J. Pediat.,* 57:290, 1960.
Filler, J., and Porter, M.: Physiologic Studies of the Sequelae of Tuberculous Pleural Effusion in Children Treated with Antimicrobial Drugs and Prednisone. *Am. Rev. Resp. Dis.,* 88:181, 1963.
Matsaniotis, N., Kattamis, C., Economou-Mavrou, C., and Kyriazakou, M.: Bullous Emphysema in Childhood Tuberculosis. *J. Pediat.,* 71:703, 1967.
Nemir, R. L., Cardona, J., Lacoius, A., and David, M.: Prednisone Therapy as an Adjunct in the Treatment of Lymph Node-Bronchial Tuberculosis in Childhood. *Am. Rev. Resp. Dis.,* 88:189, 1963.
Smith, M. H. D.: Practical Management of Tuberculosis. *Pediat. Clin. N. Amer.,* 3:427, 1956.

INFECTIONS WITH UNCLASSIFIED MYCOBACTERIA (ATYPICAL OR ANONYMOUS MYCOBACTERIA)

The existence of acid-fast mycobacteria other than *Mycobacterium tuberculosis* has been known for many years, but until recently these organisms were only occasionally regarded as pathogenic for man. In the past few years an increasing amount of evidence has shown that infections with these organisms can produce lesions which closely simulate tuberculosis in human beings and can also induce cutaneous sensitivity to tuberculin derived from human strains of *M. tuberculosis* as well as to their own specific antigens.

Currently the term "unclassified mycobacteria" is used to designate species obtained from human sources. According to the 1961 Diagnostic Standards and Classification of Tuberculosis they are grouped as follows:

Photochromogens *(M. kansasii, M. luciflavum,* the yellow bacillus, Runyon group I): these strains become yellow-pigmented only after exposure to light
Scotochromogens (Runyon group II): the yellow-orange pigment of these strains is not completely light-conditioned
Nonchromogenic strains (the "Battey" type, Runyon group III): characteristics include variable pigmentation, late in appearance, not light-conditioned
Rapid growers (Runyon group IV): rapidly growing photochromogens.

Epidemiology. Human infections with unclassified mycobacteria have been reported from many areas of the world. In the United States the majority of the cases have been noted in the southeastern and southwestern or central states, where the most commonly isolated species are the "Battey" type and *M. kansasii,* respectively.

The unclassified mycobacteria have been isolated from a variety of sources, including soil, water, various animals and man. In man these organisms have most frequently been recovered from sputum, bronchial secretions, purulent discharges from infected lymph nodes, saliva and skin. In the rare instances of hematogenous dissemination they have been recovered from virtually every organ of the body.

Although the routes by which man acquires these infections are under intensive investigation, the epidemiologic pattern is not well understood. Outbreaks of cutaneous infections with *M. balnei* have been traced to infected water in swimming pools. Available data suggest that human contacts are relatively unimportant in the spread of these organisms.

Pathology. The macroscopic and microscopic lesions produced by infections with the unclassified mycobacteria simulate those produced by *M. tuberculosis*. Differentiation must be made by appropriate bacteriologic studies.

Clinical Manifestations. Human infections with the unclassified mycobacteria produce clinical manifestations which simulate those caused by *M. tuberculosis* and are therefore not described in detail. In adults the lungs are the most common site of infection, whereas in children most infections occur in the lymph nodes, especially in the anterior cervical and submandibular areas. Isolated hematogenous foci of infection, such as osteomyelitis, have been noted. A few cases of fatal generalized infections, simulating miliary tuberculosis and the Letterer-Siwe variety of reticuloendotheliosis, have been observed.

Cutaneous ulcers and chronic granulomas have been noted with infections caused by *M. ulcerans* and *M. balnei* (both unclassified).

Diagnosis. Infections with the unclassified mycobacteria can be diagnosed only by appropriate bacteriologic studies. Pathologic studies, including the demonstration of acid-fast bacilli in tissues, purulent discharges, sputum, and the like, do not permit differentiation from disease produced by *M. tuberculosis*.

Tuberculin tests. A number of antigens have been prepared from cultures of the unclassified mycobacteria by the method used for the production of PPD. These antigens are not commercially available, but may sometimes be obtained from state health departments or the United States Public Health Service. Intradermal tests with these antigens are applied and interpreted as described under the Mantoux test (p. 603).

The results of intradermal tests with PPD-like material from the unclassified mycobacteria have shown that many persons react to one or more of the antigens and that such reactors commonly also react to the standard PPD of *M. tuberculosis*. In general, persons who have a strong reaction to the standard PPD are likely to show a lesser reaction to PPD preparations of one or more of the unclassified mycobacteria. The reverse is also observed.

Available evidence suggests that in instances when there are dermal reactions to PPD of the human tubercle bacillus and to one or more PPD preparations from the unclassified mycobacteria, the largest reaction is apt to be produced by the antigen of the infecting organism.

Differential diagnosis includes those diseases described under Tuberculosis (pp. 598 and 607).

Prognosis. The outlook for spontaneous recovery from infections with the unclassified mycobacteria is generally good, probably more favorable than with infections caused by *M. tuberculosis*. Nevertheless fatalities from these infections occasionally occur.

Treatment of infections caused by the unclassified mycobacteria is largely symptomatic and supportive. Most species are moderately to strongly resistant to therapy with isoniazid and paraaminosalicylic acid. Some strains are moderately susceptible to streptomycin or cycloserine. The choice of antimicrobial therapy should be controlled by in-vitro sensitivity tests.

Infections of the lymph nodes or localized abscesses may be treated by excision or drainage.

ROBERT H. HIGH

REFERENCES

Bialkin, G., Pollak, A., and Weil, A. J.: Pulmonary Infection with Mycobacterium Kansasii. *Am. J. Dis. Child.,* 101:739, 1961.

Diagnostic Standards and Classifications of Tuberculosis. New York, National Tuberculosis Association, 1961.

Edwards, L. B., and Palmer, C. E.: Epidemiologic Studies of Tuberculin Sensitivity. *Am. J. Hyg.,* 68:312, 1958.

Hsu, K. H. K.: Nontuberculosis Mycobacterial Infections in Children. *J. Pediat.,* 60:705, 1962.

Kendig, E. L.: *Disorders of the Respiratory Tract in Children.* Philadelphia, W. B. Saunders Company, 1967, Chap. 54.

Mellman, W. J., and Barness, L.: Unclassified Mycobacteria. *Am. J. Dis. Child.,* 104:21, 1962.

Runyon, E. H.: Anonymous Mycobacterium in Pulmonary Disease. *M. Clin. N. Amer.,* 43:273, 1959.

Yakovac, W. C., Baker, R., Sweigert, C., and Hope, J. W.: Fatal Disseminated Osteomyelitis Due to an Anonymous Mycobacterium. *J. Pediat.,* 59:909, 1961.

LEPROSY

(HANSEN'S DISEASE)

Leprosy is a chronic infection caused by *Mycobacterium leprae*, which chiefly affects superficial neural and epithelial tissues.

It is estimated that there are approximately 3,000,000 leprous persons in the world, most of whom are to be found between the thirtieth parallels north and south of the equator. About 30,000 are in Central and South America and about 1000 in the United States, mainly in states bordering the Gulf of Mexico and in Hawaii. Until 400 to 500 years ago Europe, which is now virtually free of leprosy, had large numbers of cases originating from African and Mideastern trade routes.

There are no intermediate hosts involved in leprosy, transmission being dependent upon rather prolonged, intimate association with the disease. Children are more easily infected than adults, but

TABLE 10-16. Distinguishing Features in Tuberculoid and Lepromatous Leprosy

	TUBERCULOID	LEPROMATOUS
Usual lesions	Macules; plaques	Nodules
Distribution	Asymmetric; localized	Symmetric; general
Involvement	Skin; nerves	Skin; nerves; eyes; mucosa; viscera
Anesthesia; nerve damage	Early; in skin lesions	Late; not confined to skin
Fever	Rare	Frequent
Host resistance	Good	Poor
Lepromin test	Positive	Negative
Bacilli	Very sparse	Abundant

congenital infection does not occur. The basis for the variation in susceptibility among persons and races is probably genetic. In current times leprosy is infrequent among Caucasians.

Only since 1964-65 has it become possible to cultivate *M. leprae* in tissue culture and to study the disease by inoculating murine foot-pads. The use of these methods may uncover metabolic mysteries of *M. leprae* and result in improved treatment and control. Demonstration of organisms is otherwise dependent upon the use of scrapings and smears of tissues to reveal typical acid-fast rods in clusters and in oval aggregates. There is no other confirmatory method.

The lepromin skin test consists in the intradermal injection of autoclaved filtered human tissue containing *M. leprae*. A positive reaction in a leprous patient denotes host resistance and is most often seen in tuberculoid leprosy, which has a much better prognosis than lepromatous leprosy. The test, however, has limited value in establish-

ing a diagnosis; the result is positive in numerous persons living in areas where leprosy does not occur, owing to numerous cross-reactions with

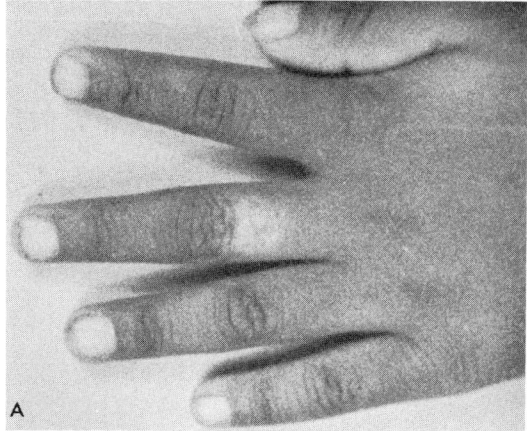

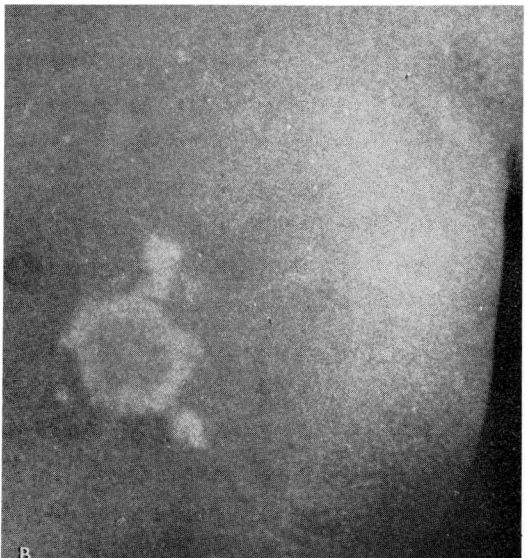

Figure 10-55. Tuberculoid leprosy. *A,* Early tuberculoid leprosy of finger: a hypopigmented anesthetic macule which had been present for 6 months. *B,* Tuberculoid leprosy on buttock. The well defined, anesthetic hypopigmented macule had been present for a year; the satellite lesions were of shorter duration. (Courtesy of Dr. A. B. A. Karat, India.)

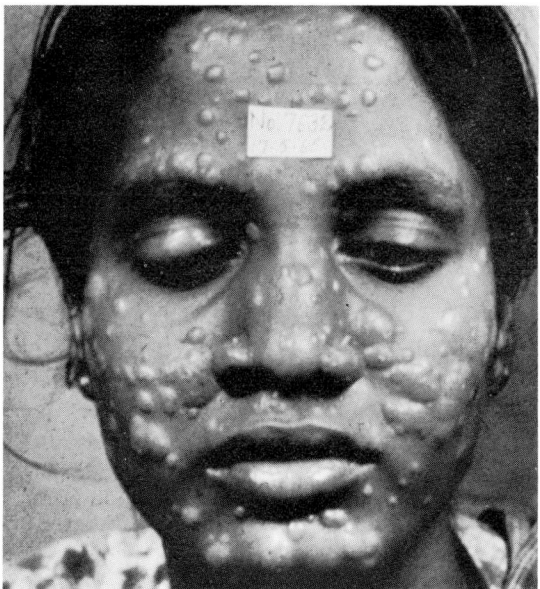

Figure 10-54. Lepromatous leprosy in an adolescent girl. Nodules are extensive, especially on exposed parts. The lepromin skin test result was negative.

other animal and human strains of mycobacteria, including wild and BCG strains of *M. tuberculosis.*

Clinical Manifestations. The diagnosis of leprosy is largely clinical and may be difficult, especially in the early stages of the disease and in nonendemic areas. Children may acquire either of the 2 main types of disease: *lepromatous* (nodular) and *tuberculoid* (neural). The 2 forms may coexist in the same child. Disfigurement and deformity result from the disease process itself and as a result of burns and other traumatic injuries in areas with diminished sensation. Trophic and motor changes in portions of the body supplied by involved nerves add to the problem.

There are numerous types of skin lesions. Slightly raised erythematous plaques, elevated thick plaques, flat, pale anesthetic areas, and nodular lesions are among the more common ones. Associated anesthetic changes are common. Involvement of the nasal, ocular, pharyngeal and laryngeal mucosal surfaces is less frequent in children than in adults.

The *lepromatous* (nodular) lesions are the most infectious; they yield many organisms when scraped for diagnosis. These lesions tend to be symmetrical, especially on the exposed parts such as face and hands. Patients regularly have a *negative lepromin skin reaction*, poor resistance and progression of disease. Moreover, the incidences of active tuberculosis and of falsely positive serologic test results for syphilis are much higher in such patients than in those with tuberculoid leprosy.

In *tuberculoid* leprosy, skin lesions consist chiefly of asymmetrical localized macules or of plaques associated with rapid neural changes. These may appear anywhere, including the clothed trunk of the body. Such lesions yield very few organisms, and the patients have good resistance, often with spontaneous arrest of the disease within a few years. They usually have a positive lepromin test result, seem to be less susceptible to tuberculosis

than those with lepromatous lesions, and seldom have falsely positive serologic test results for syphilis.

Control and Treatment. Bacteriologically negative patients need not be isolated. Young unaffected children should, however, be removed from infectious cases if possible. Isolation in leprosariums remains in vogue and is important for the *lepromatous* form of the disease. Recent trials in Uganda have created hope that BCG vaccine may reduce the incidence of childhood leprosy.

Until recently antimicrobial therapy was largely limited to chaulmoogra oil, the effects of which were at best slight. It is now apparent that diamino-diphylsulfone (Dapsone) administered over a period of several years is effective in arresting progression of the disease. Prolonged maintenance therapy is important except in patients whose natural resistance is indicated by a strongly positive lepromin reaction. Except for residual nerve destruction and tissue mutilation, recovery often ensues.

Surgical procedures are now available to restore usefulness of hands and feet affected by ulnar and peroneal nerve damage. Unfortunately, most patients reside in nonaffluent parts of the world where optimal surgical, occupational and social rehabilitation is not easily achieved. Children with tuberculoid leprosy who have little disfigurement or neurologic involvement should be able to lead fairly normal lives.

ALEX J. STEIGMAN

REFERENCES

Brown, J. A. K., Stone, M. M., and Sutherland, I.: BCG Vaccination of Children Against Leprosy: First Results of a Trial in Uganda. *Brit. Med. J.,* 1:7, 1966.
Bullock, W. E.: Studies of Immune Mechanisms in Leprosy. *New England J. Med.,* 278:298, 1968.
World Health Organization Bulletin, Vol. 34, No. 6, 1966.

Spirochetal Infections

Classification and Nomenclature. Spirochaetales is an order consisting of 2 families of motile spiral organisms: *(a)* Spirochaetaceae with its 3 genera (Spirochaeta, Saprospira, Cristispira) which do not cause human disease, and *(b)* Treponemataceae with its 3 genera (Treponema, Leptospira, Borrelia) which can cause human disease. These last 3 genera include species which are saprophytes, others which cause only animal disease, and still others, like certain leptospira, which may afflict man or animals.

The recognized spirochetal infections of man are listed in Table 10-17; they are major causes of human disease. There are numerous other species

of Spirochaetales which are saprophytic in man; for example, *T. microdentium* resides in the mouth and gums.

SYPHILIS

Syphilis is a systemic communicable infection characterized by periods of clinical activity and prolonged latency. The requirement of a premarital serologic test for syphilis (STS) and the widespread use of penicillin (not necessarily given for syphilis) have dramatically reduced the occur-

TABLE 10-17. MEMBERS OF TREPONEMATACEAE WHICH CAUSE HUMAN DISEASE

GENUS OF PATHOGENIC TREPONEMATACEAE	USUALLY TRANSMITTED BY	DISEASES
Treponema		
pallidum	Human contact	Syphilis
pertenue	Human contact	Yaws
carateum	Human contact	Pinta
Leptospira		
± 15 species	Direct or indirect contact with animals	Leptospiroses
Borrelia		
recurrentis	Lice; ticks	Relapsing fever
vincenti	Human (usually with B. fusiformis)	Vincent's angina, gingivitis, genital and topical ulcers, etc.

rence of infectious syphilis in the United States until lately, when a rising incidence has been noted, particularly in adolescents. In 1957, 6251 cases of primary and secondary syphilis were reported; in 1967 the figure was 21,091.

The organism responsible for syphilis, *Treponema pallidum,* is a fine, pale, spiral motile thread 5 to 15 microns long and about 0.15 micron thick, which cannot be cultured in vitro and which survives poorly outside of the body. It stains poorly even in tissue sections; its detection in fresh scrapings of lesions requires darkfield illumination and a competent observer. Life-long persistence of the organism despite successful treatment has been documented, especially in the eye.

Fetal syphilis is contracted from the mother, whose infection is usually latent. Acquired syphilis requires close contact between an infective lesion and a break in the skin or mucosa of the genitalia, anus, lips, mouth, face, fingers, or other parts of the recipient child or adult. Fomites, vectors, and the like, appear to have no role in transmission. Transmission by blood transfusion is now extremely rare.

CONGENITAL (FETAL) SYPHILIS

Epidemiology. The incidence of fetal syphilis is determined by the incidence of syphilis in pregnant women and by whether or not the disease is detected and treated early enough in pregnancy to protect the infant. The effectiveness of preventive measures would be increased if the STS required before marriage in many places would be repeated early in pregnancy, again in the third trimester, and in subsequent pregnancies, since fetal syphilis may be contracted from a mother whose syphilitic infection occurred during the current pregnancy or many years earlier and whose intervening pregnancies may have yielded infants without syphilis.

Congenital syphilis is often not recognized in early infancy; of all congenital syphilis officially reported in the United States in recent years, only about 10 per cent of cases were detected in the first year of life. Most cases reported were in patients beyond the age of 10 years, when late sequelae are noted. Prevention and control of congenital syphilis depend on high levels of clinical suspicion, supported by routine and diagnostic use of laboratory and radiologic aids.

Pathology. Since fetal infection prior to the fourth month of pregnancy is uncommon, anomalies of organ formation seldom occur. Syphilis only rarely causes abortion, but if the mother is untreated, stillbirths result in one fourth of cases. The other 75 per cent of untreated mothers deliver living offspring who may manifest no *clinical* abnormality for weeks or even months. The severity of disease depends upon the time in pregnancy when the fetus is infected, upon the dose of *T. pallidum* and its capacity to multiply in a given fetus, upon the state of maternal immunity and upon whether the pregnant mother received sufficient penicillin to cure or modify the infection. Penicillin might have been given to the mother inadvertently for some intercurrent infection or specifically for syphilis.

The fetal tissues most often extensively involved in stillborn infants or in those severely ill at or soon after birth are bone, bone marrow, lungs, liver and spleen. There may be considerable extramedullary hematopoiesis. Any organ system may be involved. Lesions of the skin and mucous membranes in early congenital syphilis, generally manifest a few weeks or months after birth, may occasionally be present at delivery.

Additional changes involving such tissues as cornea, teeth, bone, palate and nervous system become evident in later years when congenital syphilis is not treated in infancy.

Clinical Manifestations of Early Congenital Syphilis. The infant may seem normal for the first few weeks or months of life. General symptoms such as fever, anemia, failure to gain weight,

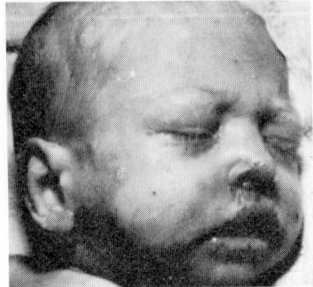 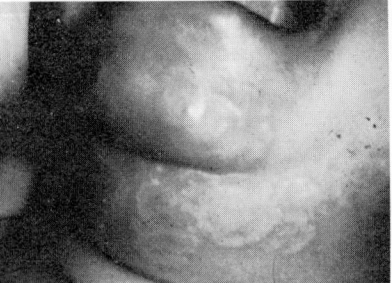 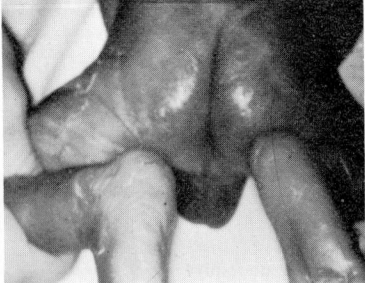

Figure 10-56.   **Figure 10-57.**   **Figure 10-58.**

Figure 10-56. Nasal snuffles, labial excoriation, macular eruption of forehead.

Figure 10-57. Circinate syphilide.

Figure 10-58. Desquamation with shiny, parchment-like appearance following bullous eruption.

restlessness, may first appear without any of the characteristic lesions of the skin or mucous membranes. On the other hand, local findings may erupt in an infant who appears quite well otherwise. This stage of congenital syphilis is roughly analogous to the systemic eruptive secondary stage of acquired syphilis. There is no lesion in congenital or in transfusion-acquired syphilis which corresponds to the primary or chancre stage of acquired syphilis.

The characteristic clinical changes of florid congenital syphilis include a variety of rashes, severe rhinitis ("snuffles"), moist lesions at the mucocutaneous junctions of the mouth, anus and genitalia, painful pseudoparalysis of limbs, and enlargement of liver, spleen and lymph nodes. Scrapings of the cutaneous and mucosal lesions reveal motile *T. pallidum* on darkfield examination.

The eruption in skin may be scant or diffuse. It is reddish and maculopapular, sometimes bullous or circinate, and involves palms and soles. The nails may be ridged, and syphilitic paronychia may occur from finger sucking. The rash may disappear spontaneously, only to recur a few weeks or months later. No permanent stigma remains from these eruptions in skin, whether or not specific therapy is given. But the nasal discharge of syphilitic rhinitis ("snuffles") commonly excoriates the upper lip, leaving fine scars, and the nasal structures may ulcerate, leaving a flat nasal bridge. Mucocutaneous lesions about the mouth, anus and genitalia are also moist and irritating, and produce fissures which heal with permanent scars ("rhagades"), especially around the corners of the mouth and on the chin. During the florid eruptive stage of early congenital syphilis raised plaques may be present in the perianal area, and even condylomata, which are more characteristic of later stages. The eruptions of early congenital syphilis do not itch.

A characteristic pseudoparalysis (Parrot's paralysis) may occur in one or more limbs, owing to the bone changes of syphilitic osteochondritis and periostitis. Lymph node enlargement is common, and involvement of the epitrochlear node is especially characteristic. Edema may be seen in severe cases, owing to hypoproteinemia and sometimes to renal involvement (syphilitic nephrosis). Anemia may stem from the syphilitic infection and from complicating secondary bacterial infection, especially of the respiratory tract.

Although the central nervous system is seldom clinically involved in early congenital syphilis, the spinal fluid should always be examined for cells, for abnormalities of protein content and for STS. Acute meningovascular syphilis in early infancy frequently has severe sequelae, which include mental retardation, low-grade hydrocephalus and convulsions. Other damage to the

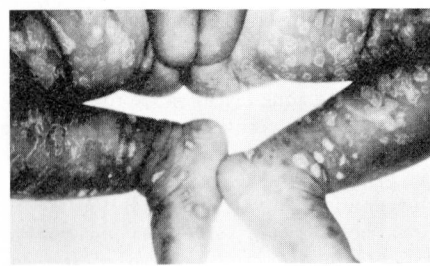 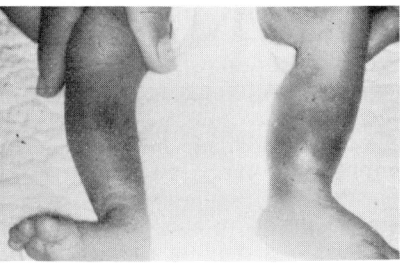

Figure 10-59. 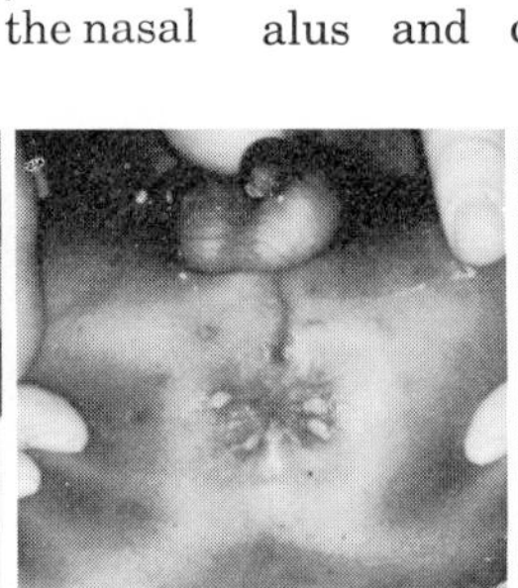   **Figure 10-60.**   **Figure 10-61.**

Figure 10-59. Generalized maculopapular syphilide.

Figure 10-60. Perianal condylomata.

Figure 10-61. Severe bilateral syphilitic osteomyelitis.

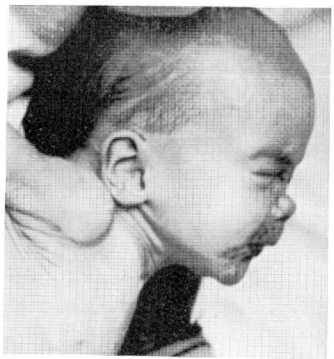 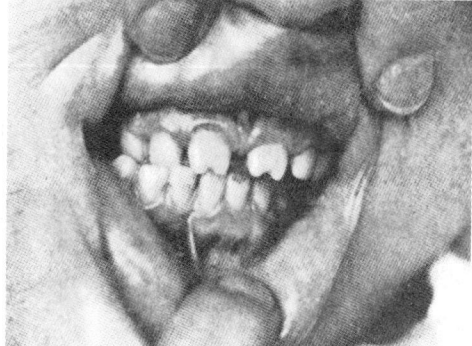 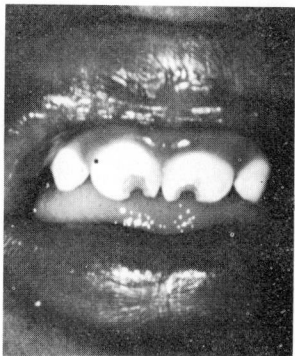

Figure 10-62.   **Figure 10-63.**   **Figure 10-64.**

Figure 10-62.   Saddle nose in early syphilis.

Figure 10-63.   Hutchinson's teeth in congenital syphilis in a boy 10 years of age.

Figure 10-64.   Dental dysplasia of deciduous incisors, nonsyphilitic, not to be confused with hutchinsonian incisors.

nervous system and organs of special sense may not become evident for years.

Radiologic changes in the skeleton are often diagnostic in early congenital syphilis and may be especially helpful when the serologic and clinical findings are ambiguous. Characteristic changes include multiple sites of osteochondritis at the elbows, wrists, ankles and knees, periostitis of several long bones and occasionally of the skull bones, widened and serrated epiphyseal lines and sometimes actual separation of epiphyses. Despite adequate therapy prenatally to the mother or to the infant after birth the periostitis may persist for many months.

Untreated, early congenital syphilis frequently subsides, but *T. pallidum* persists in the tissues. Recent evidence indicates that *T. pallidum* may persist in ocular tissues for 5 or 6 decades. The infant soon becomes noncontagious, however, and probably cannot be reinfected with acquired syphilis. Nor will the female child be able to give congenital syphilis to her offspring ("third-generation syphilis"). The child may bear *stigma of the early manifestations* such as a flat bridge of the nose, a square high forehead (cranial bossing), and fine scars around the puckered mouth and chin (rhagades). Other changes which were initiated early

take time to appear. For example, the buds of the permanent incisors and first permanent molars are being formed in the first weeks of extrauterine life, when the impact of early congenital syphilis may be great. Each permanent incisor may become rounded and peg-shaped with a central notch (Hutchinson's incisor) and the cusps of the molar surfaces may appear squeezed together (mulberry molar). The deciduous teeth do not appear deformed.

Clinical Manifestations of Late Congenital Syphilis. The term "late congenital syphilis" refers to those clinical manifestations which appear only after infancy. The most frequent and important of these involve the skeleton, the eye and the central nervous system. Much rarer are subcutaneous gummas, paroxysmal hemoglobinuria, and cardiovascular or other visceral changes more characteristic of late syphilis in adults.

The most frequent late ophthalmic change is *interstitial keratitis*, which may be unilateral or bilateral and appear at any age. Intense photophobia and lacrimation occur, and progressive corneal opacity may lead to blindness in a period of weeks or months. Less common late ocular manifestations include choroiditis, retinitis, vascular occlusions and optic atrophy.

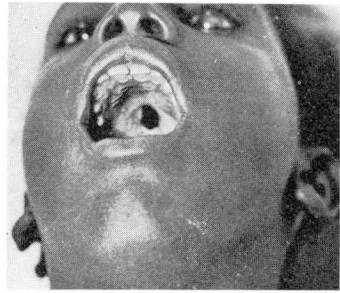 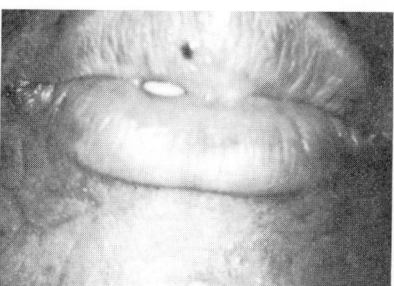 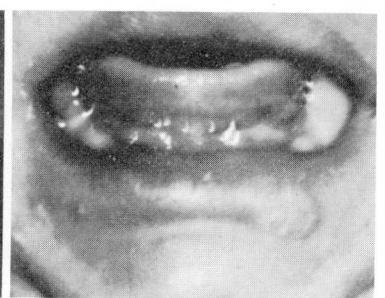

Figure 10-65.   **Figure 10-66.**   **Figure 10-67.**

Figure 10-65.   Syphilitic perforation of the palate in a girl 10 years of age.

Figure 10-66.   Rhagades as long-term residual from infantile snuffles and eruption.

Figure 10-67.   Chancre of lower lip, darkfield-positive.

The nervous system may harbor latent *meningovascular syphilitic infection* which may be abruptly manifest in prepubertal children by hemiplegia or convulsions. More often, however, the child with central nervous system syphilis is dull, retarded or irritable or exhibits antisocial behavior. *Juvenile paresis* is the counterpart of general paresis in the adult. *Juvenile tabes* with spinal cord involvement is rare. Involvement of the eighth cranial nerves may occur without other detectable central nervous system changes, and may produce rapidly progressive *deafness*. The classic *Hutchinson's triad* of late congenital syphilis consists of nerve deafness, interstitial keratitis and hutchinsonian incisors.

The skeletal changes include persistent or recurrent periostitis which causes chronic thickening of bone best exemplified in the tibia, where anterior curving produces the "saber shin." Dactylitis may occur as a late manifestation, and swollen joints may occur without evident cause from time to time, especially in adolescent boys and at the knee (Clutton's joints). Gummatous involvement of the bones of the nose or palate may lead to destruction of the nasal bridge or to perforation of the palate.

Table 10-18 lists most of the manifestations of late congenital syphilis.

Diagnosis. The diagnosis of congenital syphilis depends on clinical judgment and appropriate use and evaluation of microscopic, serologic, radiologic and sometimes epidemiologic data.

Darkfield examination of scrapings from moist cutaneous and mucocutaneous lesions in early congenital syphilis may reveal the *T. pallidum* to the experienced observer. The organism cannot be cultured in vitro.

Serologic tests for syphilis fall into two main groups: (1) a group using *nontreponemal* antigens (such as cardiolipin-synthetic lecithin reagents) to detect nonspecific *reagin* antibodies in complement-fixation tests (Wassermann, Kolmer) or in flocculation tests (VDRL, Kahn, Kline, Hinton, Eagle, Mazzini, and others); and (2) a group using *treponemal* antigens harvested from *T. pallidum* inoculated into rabbit testis to detect *specific* antibodies. The treponemal antigen tests are not widely available and are reserved for unravelling special problems, such as biologic falsely positive reagin reactions (BFP's).

Within both groups of tests there are numerous variations in procedures; the physician should familiarize himself with those used in his region. The reagin tests are highly satisfactory for screening, especially in *early* congenital syphilis, when the tests using treponemal antigen are not often needed to clarify an ambiguous situation. These tests are most helpful in dealing with questionable cases of *late* congenital syphilis and in adults who have been treated.

The original treponemal serologic test described in 1949 is the TPI (*T. pallidum* immobilization) procedure. This test is highly specific and sensitive, but its complexities restrict its use to a few highly specialized laboratories. Specific treponemal antibody, unlike the nonspecific reagin, is detectable for many years, often for life; it is little influenced by therapy unless this is given early in the course of infection. Other treponema-specific serologic tests have been developed since 1949, of which the FTA-ABS (fluorescent treponemal antibody-absorbed) is most favored at present. Commercially prepared slides containing dried *T. pallidum* (nonviable) are overlaid with the serum being tested. Syphilitic antibody globulin will attach to the *T. pallidum*, and can be revealed when fluorescein-tagged antibody to human gamma globulin is added and the treponemata viewed for fluorescence under ultraviolet light microscopy. Human serums may contain nonspecific treponemal antibodies; these can be absorbed out with a sonicate (the yield of organisms achieved by high intensity sonic vibration) of Reiter treponemes prior to the FTA-ABS test.

When there is doubt about the interpretation in an asymptomatic newborn infant of a positive STS, whether reagin or treponemal, repeated *quantitative* serial tests should be performed. The half-life of gamma globulin is such that a falling titer in the first 3 to 4 months of life is the usual finding associated with the passive transfer of maternal antisyphilitic antibody. The passively transferred reagin antibody usually declines in titer before the passively acquired FTA antibody disappears. The maternal history of intrapartum illnesses and antibiotic therapy, the maternal serology and the roentgenographic examination of the infant's skeleton must all be taken into consideration in deciding whether a positive STS reflects active disease requiring therapy in an asymptomatic infant.*

In response to various infections, including congenital syphilis, newborn and young infants have elevated serum levels of immunoglobin M (IgM). IgM is not passively transferred via the placenta; accordingly, elevated titers in the infant indicate *active* infection. The IgM fraction of umbilical cord or infant's serum can be tested by the indirect immunofluorescent technique against specific antigens, including *T. pallidum*. A positive reaction gives highly specific evidence of active syphilis.

Biologic falsely positive reagin reactions (BFP) occasionally create problems in the diagnosis of congenital syphilis. Tests using crude lipoidal antigen may give more BFP's than tests using purified cardiolipin. A positive STS which does not fit the clinical picture should be repeated by several techniques. BFP reactions may be found if the infant or his mother has a current or recent infection or recent immunization. BFP reactions are

---

*When there is reasonable doubt that a newborn infant with a positive STS who does not have any clinical manifestations of syphilis can be observed through the first few months of life, it would seem appropriate to treat him as if he had an active infection.

TABLE 10-18.   CLINICAL MANIFESTATIONS OF CONGENITAL SYPHILIS

	EARLY MANIFESTATIONS	STIGMAS	LATE MANIFESTATIONS
Skin	Maculopapular rash Diffuse inflammation of palms and soles Mucocutaneous lesions about nose, mouth and anus Condylomas *Café-au-lait* appearance Pemphigus Paronychia Deformities of nails Alopecia	Rhagades	Condylomas Syphilides Gummas
Mucous membrane	Rhinitis Mucous patches	Saddle nose	
Bones	Periostitis Osteochondritis (epiphysitis) Pseudoparalysis (Parrot's) Dactylitis	Bossing of head Hutchinson's teeth Mulberry molars	Osteoperiostitis Saber shin Gummas Hydrarthrosis Arthritis
Eye	Chorioretinitis Iritis	Keratotic scar Chorioretinitis Pupillary change Optic atrophy	Interstitial keratitis Chorioretinitis Optic atrophy
Nervous system	Meningitis Hydrocephalus	Deafness	Deafness Neurosyphilis
Other	Pneumonia alba Hepatitis Jaundice Splenomegaly Nephritis Lymphatic hyperplasia Orchitis Malnutrition Anemia Gastrointestinal disturbances Fever Hemorrhage	Syphilitic facies	Paroxysmal hemoglobinuria

common in some families, especially in those in which there have been so-called autoimmune diseases such as thyroiditis or lupus erythematosus. Apparently healthy pregnant women may occasionally have a BFP which appears in the newborn infant's cord blood. Such infants do not have elevated IgM levels, nor are specific treponemal test results positive.

Differential Diagnosis. The chief pitfall in diagnosis is not to think of syphilis. In *early congenital syphilis* the following diagnoses may be considered: diaper rash, scabies, epidermolysis bullosa, drug rashes, cutaneous moniliasis, pemphigus, Letterer-Siwe disease, the fetal rubella syndrome, cytomegalovirus infection, toxoplasmosis, acute poliomyelitis, scurvy, pyogenic osteomyelitis, Caffey's syndrome, the "battered-child syndrome," and others. The sometimes bloody nasal discharge, excoriating the upper lip, may suggest nasal diphtheria.

Late congenital syphilis may suggest phlyctenular conjunctivitis, undifferentiated mental retardation, osteomyelitis, epilepsy, idiopathic hemiplegia, acquired toxoplasmic chorioretinitis, and other conditions.

ACQUIRED SYPHILIS

Infants, children or adolescents may acquire syphilis from an infected adult. The older the patient, the more likely is the source of transmission through sexual play or exploration or participation in usual or unusual forms of intercourse. Transmission to a youngster by kissing or other innocent contact is not common, even from a parent or other adult in the rather highly infectious stage of secondary syphilis.

The primary sites of introduction of *T. pallidum* are chiefly on the genitalia, anus, face, neck, lips and mouth, but a detectable chancre is not common in children. It is often not until such manifestations of the secondary stage as rash, condylomata and mucous patches appear that the condition comes to medical attention.

When acquired syphilis is recognized and treated promptly, the infection is suppressed and seroconversion leads to negative reagin tests. Whether every *T. pallidum* is then entirely eradicated is doubtful. Recent evidence suggests long-term survival of *T. pallidum* even after seroconversion. The organism has been demonstrated in ocular fluids, spinal fluid, lymph nodes and liver by means of fluorescent antibody techniques. These organisms are relatively dormant, but may still be pathogenic, especially for ocular lesions. Penicillin acts most effectively on actively multiplying organisms; in these cases of dormancy the *T. pallida* are not reproducing regularly.

TREATMENT AND PROGNOSIS

In *early congenital syphilis* penicillin is the therapeutic drug of choice. Only in the most severe forms of penicillin allergy should the tetracyclines (60 mg. per kg. per day for 12 to 15 days) or erythromycin (15 mg. per kg. per day for 12 to 15 days) be substituted for penicillin, Injectable preparations are preferred to oral administration. Experience with semisynthetic penicillins and with cephalothin is too limited for any reliable recommendations to be made at this time. See Table 10-19 for treatment schedules.

When a full course of penicillin is given in early congenital syphilis, there is swift disappearance of lesions. Reversion to negative of the STS and of the reactivity of spinal fluid requires some months. Skeletal changes are more stubborn, especially those of the periosteum; these may not disappear radiographically for a long time, even when the mother received an adequate course of therapy during pregnancy.

Brief, febrile Herxheimer reactions occur in 15 to 20 per cent of patients, especially if excessive penicillin is given. These reactions are of little consequence and do not constitute an indication to change from penicillin to other drugs.

TABLE 10-19. Dose and Duration of Penicillin Therapy for Congenital Syphilis

AGE	CHOICE OF	DURATION
Under 2 years	15,000 units APP*/kg./day or	10 days
	50,000 units benzathine penicillin/kg.	Weekly for 3 doses
Over 2 years	20,000 units APP*/kg./day or	10 days
	100,000 units benzathine penicillin/kg.	Weekly for 3 doses

*APP = aqueous procaine penicillin.

The general and social management of these infants must not be neglected. Secondary bacterial infections, anemia, malnutrition and parental negligence in extreme degree sometimes coexist with syphilis in such infants.

In *late congenital syphilis* the antibiotic therapy is generally similar to that for early congenital syphilis. Interstitial keratitis requires additional treatment, which will include topical corticosteroids and topical cycloplegics. In interstitial keratitis, optic atrophy, chorioretinitis and iritis the cooperation of an ophthalmologic consultant in planning treatment is highly desirable. These lesions are generally considered to be manifestations of hypersensitivity to endogenous spirochetes and may result in painful and deep corneal scars and iritis.

YAWS

Yaws is an acute and chronically relapsing non-venereal treponematosis, primarily of children, caused by the introduction of *Treponema pertenue* into a break in the skin. *T. pertenue* cannot be distinguished microscopically from *T. pallidum*; patients with yaws have serologic reagin and treponemal antibody reactions identical to those of patients with syphilis. Because the biologic relation between the 2 treponemes results in considerable cross-immunity, syphilis, including congenital syphilis, has a lowered incidence in regions where yaws is endemic. Congenital yaws is unknown.

Yaws occurs chiefly in the wet tropical climate of Africa, Southeast Asia and some South Pacific Islands. It is also found in Central and South America, and was probably brought to the New World by West African slaves. Instances are reported of children infected in these endemic areas in whom lesions erupt after they arrive in areas where yaws is unknown.

One to 2 months after exposure to yaws a primary granuloma or papule appears at the inoculation site. An indolent papilloma usually persists some weeks to months, until the manifestations of the secondary stage appear.

The secondary stage is characterized by mild constitutional symptoms and by the eruption in crops of macules, papules and characteristic granulomas (yaws or frambesiomas), which are crusted granular lesions resembling raspberries. These lesions are infectious and may persist for months or years, after which they undergo spontaneous involution. Yaws may then become latent until the lesions of the tertiary stage appear.

The lesions of tertiary yaws may resemble cutaneous gummata, with some destruction of skin and subcutaneous tissues, and with painful thickening of the soles ("crab yaws") and sometimes of the palms. In a small percentage of patients, osteitis and periostitis of the extremities, and more rarely of skull, pelvis and spine, may occur, either in association with the infectious skin lesions or in later years after the skin lesions have regressed. In contrast to syphilis, yaws rarely if ever involves the nervous system, organs of special sense, or viscera.

Diagnosis requires alertness to the possibility of yaws and use of the same laboratory tests for confirmation as syphilis.

Penicillin therapy in the doses used for syphilis is remarkably effective. Eradication of yaws may be obtained with mass use of penicillin in endemic areas, together with improved conditions of general health.

PINTA

Thought before 1938 to be a fungus infection, pinta is caused by *Treponema carateum*, which is morphologically indistinguishable from *T. pallidum*. This nonvenereal trepanematosis is essentially confined to the skin. Visceral and osseous lesions do not occur. Congenital pinta is unknown. Patients with pinta have the same serologic reactions as do patients with syphilis or yaws.

Pinta is endemic in wide areas of Central and South America, and to a lesser extent in the West Indies, tropical Africa and some South Pacific Islands. Children and young persons are the chief victims, but marks of untreated pinta remain visible throughout life.

T. carateum enters a break in the skin. In several weeks the primary papular lesion occurs, which often looks like a patch of psoriasis or scaly eczema. The regional lymph nodes are slightly enlarged, and treponemata can be seen on darkfield microscopy of skin scrapings or in an aspirate of a lymph node. The primary lesion may spread slightly or seem to regress. After 6 to 8 months the secondary eruption occurs, which consists of small macules and papules, especially likely to appear on the face, scalp and other exposed parts. These are bluish to pink, nonpruritic, slightly scaly and darkfield-positive. Many lesions involute spontaneously; others coalesce, forming scaly pigmented patches resembling psoriasis. Their color ultimately changes to a violet-bluish tint. In time the skin becomes atrophic and depigmented, leaving areas of disfiguring vitiligo and mottled skin on the hands, wrists, ankles, feet, face and scalp. The chronic lesions of pinta may remain darkfield-positive for years.

Treatment with penicillin is as effective as for yaws.

LEPTOSPIROSIS

Many species of animals are carriers or victims of the 15 or more serotypes of Leptospira. The principal carriers throughout the world are wild rodents whose excreta—especially urine—may infect many species of domesticated and wild animals or contaminate water supplies. Cats, dogs, cattle, swine, deer, foxes, raccoons, skunks and opossums become infected with Leptospira through exposure to the excreta of rodents, and may become ill and die; but more often they become persistent urinary carriers. Human infection results from direct or indirect exposure to infected animals, their products or excreta. The diagnosis in man is considered frequently only in adults with occupational exposures, such as miners, veterinarians, herdsmen and farmers. The actual frequency of human infection is doubtless greater than reported (only 43 cases were reported in the United States in 1967).

Most human infections in the United States seem to be due to *L. icterohemorrhagica, L. canicola* and *L. pomona*, but all serotypes are potentially pathogenic for man. Unlike the treponemata causing human disease, Leptospira are fairly hardy and can be cultured in vitro and on chick-embryo membranes. Direct contact with animals is not necessary for transmission; indirect contact, such as bathing in contaminated waters, is sufficient. The incubation period is 1 to 2 weeks. Leptospirosis produces a wide range of clinical illnesses, from inapparent to fatal.

Because of its severity, *Weil's syndrome (icterohemorrhagic fever)* is the best known manifestation of leptospirosis, but it is relatively uncommon. The liver, kidneys, muscles and blood vessels are especially involved. Jaundice, proteinuria, azotemia, hematuria, anemia and thrombocytopenia occur, with hemorrhages into the skin and many viscera, including the nervous system. Macular and maculopapular rashes with no particularly distinctive features may appear. Although *L. icterohemorrhagica* is classically associated with Weil's syndrome, this organism may cause a very mild general illness not involving the liver, whereas Weil's syndrome may be caused by other Leptospira species.

Leptospirosis may run a biphasic febrile course, with the initial period ushered in abruptly with fever, headache, conjunctivitis, photophobia with scleral pain and hemorrhage, myalgia and chills. The clinical picture of aseptic meningitis is probably the most common expression of leptospirosis. Even in patients without nuchal or spinal rigidity, pleocytosis is frequently found on spinal fluid examination, especially 4 to 5 days after onset of symptoms (see p. 687).

A mild febrile illness with a macular or maculopapular eruption over the pretibial area *(pretibial fever, Fort Bragg fever)* has been ascribed to *L. autumnalis*, and has been reported in children.

The diagnosis of leptospirosis begins with suspicion of the disease. Children taken abruptly ill with a grippelike illness should be suspect, especially in summer or fall and if they have been swimming in questionably safe streams or otherwise exposed to animals. It is more usually epidemiologic data rather than clinical judgment that point toward the diagnosis of leptospirosis. Laboratory confirmation of the diagnosis is essential, and identification of the specific serotype of Leptospira involved is desirable as an aid in surveillance of disease in herds of domestic animals.

Blood, urine and spinal fluid may reveal Leptospira on culture. Serologic tests include agglutination, fluorescent antibody, and other techniques. Direct darkfield examination of blood, urine or spinal fluid is *not* recommended, owing to the frequency of confusing artifacts. A polymorphonuclear leukocytosis occurs, but is too variable to be useful in diagnosis.

Leptospirosis must be differentiated from aseptic meningitis, acute brucellosis, hemolytic-uremic syndrome, dengue fever, typhoid fever, nephritis, hepatitis, and the like.

Patients severely ill with leptospirosis require skillful management of fluids, electrolytes, and nutrition and the use of blood components as indicated. Penicillin does not have the same dramatic effect as in treponemal diseases; it does, however, reduce fever and somewhat shorten the period of illness. Penicillin should be given in preference to the tetracyclines.

REFERENCES

Syphilis

Goldman, J. N., and Girard, K. F.: Intraocular Treponemes in Treated Congenital Syphilis. *Arch. Ophth.,* 78:47, 1967.
Hunter, E. F., Deacon, W. E., and Meyer, P. E.: An Improved FTA Test for Syphilis: The Absorption Technique (FTA-ABS). *Pub. Health Rep.,* 79:408, 1964.
Proceedings of World Forum on Syphilis and other Treponematoses. Publication No. 997, U.S. Public Health Service, 1964.
Smith, J. L., and Israel, C. W.: The Presence of Spirochetes in Late Seronegative Syphilis. *J.A.M.A.,* 199:126, 1967.
Wells, J. A., and Smith, J. L.: The Fluorescent Antibody Tissue Stain in Experimental Ocular Syphilis. *Arch. Ophth.,* 77: 530, 1967.

Yaws

Hackett, C. J., and Lowenthal, L. J. A.: Differential Diagnosis of Yaws. World Health Organization Monograph Series, No. 45, Geneva, 1960.

Leptospirosis

Diesch, S. L., and McCulloch, W. F.: Isolation of Pathogenic Leptospires from Waters Used for Recreation. *Pub. Health Rep.,* 81:299, 1966.
Galton, M. M., and Heath, C. W., Jr.: Zoonoses Surveillance. Communicable Disease Center, Report No. 7, Leptospirosis. C.D.C., Atlanta, Ga., 1965.
Heath, C. W., Jr., Alexander, A. D., and Galton, M. M.: Leptospirosis in the United States. Analysis of 483 Cases in Man. *New England J. Med.,* 273:857, 1965.

RAT-BITE FEVER

Two forms of rat-bite fever may be distinguished clinically and bacteriologically. Despite the frequency of exposure to rats in depressed urban areas and in certain occupations, rat-bite fever is not common.

In both types of rat-bite fever it appears that the nature of the illness is determined both by infection and by an allergic response to the organism on the part of the host.

SPIRILLARY RAT-BITE FEVER
(SODOKU)

The spirillary form of rat-bite fever is caused by *Spirillum minus* and produces a clinical picture known as Sodoku, first described in Japan.

The initial bite heals promptly, to be followed within 10 to 30 days by a painful indurated ulcer at the site of the original bite, and by regional lymphadenopathy. In a few days the temperature may rise and a rash will appear, which consists of violaceous macules, more or less ovoid in shape and up to several centimeters in diameter. There is no pruritus. The eruption is in some ways analogous to that of secondary syphilis. Within a few days to a week the temperature will subside, but cycles of fever recur at irregular intervals.

Laboratory confirmation of the diagnosis may be difficult. Darkfield examination of scrapings from the lesion may show the relatively thick spirillary forms with 3 curls. The organism cannot be cultivated in vitro. Animal inoculation in expert hands may be confirmatory, but animals used must be free of morphologically related organisms. Falsely positive reagin serologic reactions for syphilis are common.

There is a prompt therapeutic response to either penicillin or streptomycin.

STREPTOBACILLARY RAT-BITE FEVER
AND
HAVERHILL FEVER

Streptobacillus moniliformis is carried by many rats, presumably as a saprophyte. The organism is an aerobic gram-negative bacillus; it may as-

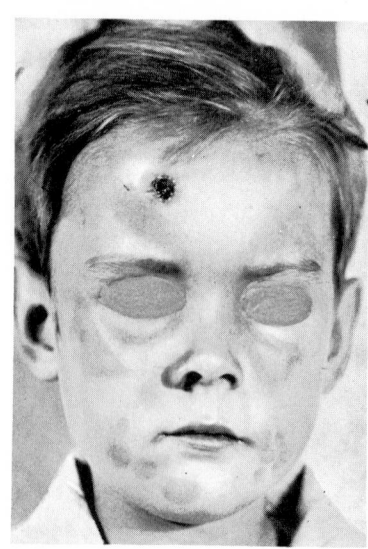

Figure 10-68. Chancre-like indurated ulcer at bite-site on forehead; secondary macular eruption of face.

sume a minute L form which is filterable and resistant to penicillin. In old cultures, especially in solid media, it forms chains with swellings resembling yeast buds; hence the designation moniliformis.

The incubation period following an infectious rat bite ranges from 2 to 7 days. The local lesion is not distinctive and may be overlooked even when fever erupts. In contrast to spirillary rat-bite fever, the streptobacillary form has a greater tendency to produce a maculopapular rash, arthralgia, arthritis, subcutaneous abscesses, endocarditis and erythema nodosum.

When *Streptobacillus moniliformis* infects man by the respiratory or alimentary tract instead of by rat bite, the resulting condition is referred to as *Haverhill fever*. The incubation period is short, often less than 5 days, with abrupt onset of fever, chills, vomiting, headache, muscle and joint pains and a maculopapular rash. Recurrent cycles of fever are characteristic, and at times large metastatic subcutaneous abscesses may appear. Arthritis is a prominent feature. Organisms may be recovered from any of the affected parts.

Laboratory tests are more readily confirmatory in streptobacillary rat-bite fever than in the spirillary form. The organism can be cultured in vitro or recovered by animal inoculation with patient's blood or material from an abscess or an affected joint. A rising titer of specific agglutinins is also helpful in diagnosis. The incidence of falsely positive reactions for syphilis is lower than in Sodoku.

Haverhill fever is more readily detectable in its epidemic form, such as may occur from ingestion of infected milk, than in individual sporadic cases, which are easily misdiagnosed. In epidemic form the fever, rash and intense muscle and joint pain may suggest dengue fever.

Penicillin therapy for 7 to 10 days is the treatment of choice.

ALEX J. STEIGMAN

Viral Infections and Those Presumed to Be Caused by Viruses

MEASLES
(RUBEOLA)

Definition. Measles is an acute communicable disease characterized by 3 stages: (1) an incubation stage of approximately 10 to 12 days with few, if any, signs or symptoms; (2) a prodromal stage with enanthem on the buccal (Koplik's spots) and pharyngeal mucosa, mild to moderate fever, slight conjunctivitis, coryza and an increasingly severe cough; and (3) a final stage with a maculopapular rash erupting successively over the neck and face, body, arms and legs and accompanied by high fever.

History. Sydenham described the disease as a separate entity in the seventeenth century.

In 1759 Home transmitted the disease by scarifying the arms of susceptibles and applying bandages soaked in blood from subjects during the early stages of measles. Hektoen in 1905 confirmed this observation by injecting blood from subjects in the early stage of measles into susceptible persons.

Anderson and Goldberger in 1911 first produced measles in *Macaca mulatta* (rhesus monkey) by injection of filtered material from acute cases and suggested a virus as the causative agent. The virus was later grown on the chorio-allantois of the chick embryo by Rake and Shaffer from filtered nasopharyngeal washings and blood of patients in an early phase of measles. Enders and his co-workers established the virus in successive tissue culture passages.

Etiology. The virus, classified tentatively as a member of the myxovirus group, is similar structurally to the mumps, Newcastle disease and parainfluenza viruses. It also shares biologic properties with the viruses of bovine rinderpest and canine distemper. The virus is present in the nasopharyngeal secretions and in the blood, at least during the prodromal period and for a short time after the appearance of the rash. It can remain active for at least 34 hours at room temperature, for at least 15 weeks after desiccation from the frozen state, for at least 4 weeks in storage at -72 to $-35°$C., and for several days at $0°$C. It is readily inactivated at a low pH.

The production of typical giant cells in successive passages in tissue cultures of human renal cells and in human amnion cells by Enders et al. has made possible the development of neutralization and complement fixation tests. Virus cultivated in the chorio-allantois has produced modified measles in *Macaca mulatta* and in man. After such modified disease the monkeys usually are immune when challenged with active virus. In man, after such modified disease, resistance to challenge inoculation has been variable.

Infectivity. Maximal virus dissemination by droplet spray from the respiratory tract occurs during the prodromal period (catarrhal stage). Transmission to susceptible contacts often occurs before the diagnosis of the original case has been established. An infected person becomes infective for others by the ninth or tenth day after exposure (beginning of the prodromal phase), in some instances as early as the seventh day. Isolation precautions to prevent spread, especially in hospitals or other institutions for children, should be maintained from the seventh day after exposure until at least 5 days after the rash has appeared.

Epidemiology. Except for isolated regions, including some areas of Greenland and certain islands of the Pacific, the endemicity of measles is world-wide. Epidemics occur irregularly, but in large urban centers they appear at 2- to 4-year intervals, probably resulting from the accumulation of large new groups of susceptible children. Approximately 90 per cent of susceptible children under 6 years of age with family exposure during an epidemic will contract the disease. Most of the remaining 10 per cent will contract it subsequently. There is no evidence that a carrier state exists, nor has any other mode of interepidemic transmission been established. During an epidemic the airborne route appears to be the commonest mode of spread, although direct contact and spread by droplet spray are important means of cross infection.

Rarely a person does not acquire immunity from an attack and has measles repeatedly. In most instances, however, so-called second or third attacks are not rubeola, but are rubella, exanthem subitum or Coxsackie or ECHO virus infections.

Infants acquire immunity transplacentally from mothers who have had measles. This immunity is usually complete for the first 4 to 6 months of life and disappears rapidly thereafter. Infants of susceptible mothers have no such immunity and may contract the disease with the mother before or after delivery.

It has been reported that permanent immunity follows in about 75 per cent of those children whose measles is attenuated by human immune globulin.

Pathology. The essential lesion of measles is found in the skin, in the mucous membranes of the nasopharynx and bronchi, and in the conjunctivas. It is a reaction of the capillary bed to the invading virus. Serous exudate and proliferation of mononuclear cells and a few polymorphonuclear cells occur around the capillaries. There is usually hyperplasia of the lymphoid tissue, where multinucleated giant cells up to 100 microns in diameter (Warthin-Finkeldey reticuloendothelial giant cells) may be found. In the skin the reaction is particularly notable about the sebaceous glands and hair follicles. Koplik's spots* consist of serous exudate and proliferation of endothelial cells similar to those in the skin rash. There is a general inflammatory reaction of the buccal and pharyngeal mucosa which extends into the lymphoid tissue and the tracheobronchial mucous membrane. Interstitial pneumonitis is occasionally associated with measles; in some instances it may be due to the measles virus. Hecht's giant cell pneumonia is an infrequent accompaniment (see p. 925). Bronchopneumonia due to secondary bacterial invasion is perhaps the most frequent pulmonary infection.

Clinical Manifestations. The incubation period is approximately 10 to 12 days if the first symptoms are selected as the time of onset, or approximately 14 days if the appearance of the rash is selected; rarely it may be as short as 6 to 10 days. A slight rise in temperature may occur 9 or 10 days from the date of infection and then subside for 24 hours or so.

The prodromal phase, which usually lasts 4 to 5 days, is characterized by low-grade to moderate fever, a slight hacking cough, coryza and conjunctivitis. These practically always precede Koplik's spots, the pathognomonic sign of measles, by 2 or 3 days. An enanthem or red mottling is usually present on the hard and soft palates. Koplik's spots are grayish-white dots, usually as small as grains of sand, with a slight reddish areola; occasionally they are hemorrhagic. They tend to occur opposite the lower molars, but may spread irregularly over the rest of the buccal mucosa. Rarely they are found within the midportion of the lower lip, on the palate and on the lacrimal caruncle. They appear and disappear rapidly, usually within 12 to 18 hours. As they fade there may remain red, spotty discolorations of the mucosa. Examination for Koplik's spots should be carried out, if possible, in bright daylight. Trauma from biting the cheeks may result in tiny ulcers with an areola which may simulate Koplik's spots. The conjunctival inflammation and photophobia lead one to suspect measles before Koplik's spots appear. In addition, a transverse line of conjunctival inflammation, as described by Stimson, sharply demarcated along the eyelid margin, may be of diagnostic assistance in the prodromal stage. As the entire conjunctiva becomes involved, the line disappears.

Occasionally the prodromal phase may be unusually severe, being ushered in by sudden high fever, at times with convulsions and even pneumonia. Usually the coryza, fever and cough are increasingly severe up to the time the rash has covered the body.

The temperature rises abruptly as the rash appears and often reaches 104 or 105°F. When the rash appears on the legs and feet, within about 2 days, the symptoms subside rapidly in uncomplicated cases. The patient up to this point may appear desperately ill, and yet within 24 hours after the drop in temperature, which is usually abrupt, he will appear to be essentially well.

The rash usually starts as faint macules on the upper lateral parts of the neck, along the hairline and on the posterior parts of the cheeks. The individual lesions become increasingly maculopapular as the rash spreads rapidly over the entire face, neck, upper arms and upper part of the chest within approximately the first 24 hours (Figs. 10-69, p. 629, 10-70). During the succeeding 24 hours it spreads over the back, abdomen, entire arms and thighs. As it finally reaches the feet on the second or third day it is beginning to fade on the face. The fading of the rash proceeds downward in the same sequence as that of its appearance. The severity of the disease is directly related to the extent and confluence of the rash. In mild measles the rash tends not to be confluent, and in very mild cases there are few, if any, lesions on the legs. In severe measles the rash is confluent, the skin being completely covered, including the

---

*So-called Koplik's spots were apparently first described by Dr. John Quier in his Fifth Letter written from the West Indies to London in 1774.

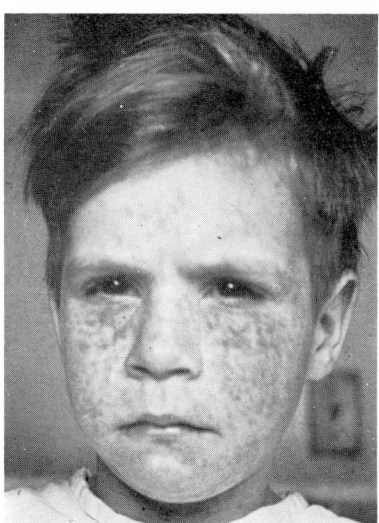

Figure 10-70. Purpuric rash of measles.

palms and soles, and the face is swollen and dis-figured.

The rash is often slightly hemorrhagic; in severe cases with a confluent rash, petechiae may be present in large numbers, and there may be extensive ecchymoses. Itching is generally slight, although on occasion it may be annoying. As the rash fades, there is a branny type of desquamation and a brownish discoloration, which disappear within 7 to 10 days.

Variations in types of rash may occur. Infrequently a slight urticarial, a faint macular or a scarlatiniform rash may appear during the early prodromal stage and disappear in advance of the typical rash. Complete absence of rash is rare except in patients who have received human antibodies during the incubation period. Occasionally death may occur before the rash has appeared. In the hemorrhagic type of measles ("black measles") bleeding may occur from the mouth, nose or bowel. In mild cases the rash may be less macular and more nearly pinpoint, somewhat resembling that of scarlet fever.

Lymph nodes at the angle of the jaw and in the posterior cervical region are usually enlarged, and slight splenomegaly may be noted. Gastrointestinal symptoms, such as diarrhea and vomiting, and otitis media and bronchopneumonia are more common in infants and small children than in older children.

The white blood cell count tends to be low with a relative lymphocytosis.

Differential Diagnosis. Diseases from which rubeola must be differentiated include exanthem subitum, rubella, infections due to ECHO viruses and Coxsackie viruses, meningococcemia, scarlet fever, rickettsial diseases, serum sickness and drug rashes, particularly those due to phenobarbital, Dilantin and sulfonamides.

Koplik's spots are pathognomonic for rubeola, and the diagnosis of unmodified measles should not be made in the absence of cough, a symptom rarely present in most of the illnesses from which it is to be differentiated.

Roseola infantum (exanthem subitum) is readily distinguished from measles because the rash appears as the fever disappears. The rashes of rubella and of enteroviral infections tend to be less striking than that of measles, as do the degree of fever and severity of illness. Although cough is present in many rickettsial infections, the rash usually spares the face, which characteristically is involved in measles. Headache is a more prominent feature of rickettsial infections. The absence of cough and the history of injection or ingestion of drug usually serve to identify serum sickness or drug rashes. Meningococcemia may be accompanied by a rash somewhat similar to that of measles; however, cough and conjunctivitis are usually absent. The diffuse, finely papular rash of scarlet fever, a confluent erythema with a "goose-flesh" texture most marked on the abdomen, is relatively easy to differentiate from that of measles.

The milder rash and the clinical picture of measles modified by immune globulin, or through partial immunity induced by measles vaccine, may be difficult or impossible to differentiate without virologic or serologic verification.

Complications. The chief complications of measles are otitis media, pneumonia and encephalitis. Noma of the cheeks and gangrene elsewhere are rare complications in severe cases.

Pneumonia may be caused by the measles virus itself; when this is the case, the lesion is interstitial. Bronchopneumonia is more frequent, however; it is due to secondarily invading bacteria, particularly the pneumococcus, streptococcus, staphylococcus and *Hemophilus influenzae*. Laryngitis, tracheitis and bronchitis are common and may be due to the virus alone.

One of the potential dangers of measles is exacerbation of an existing *tuberculous process*. There may also be a temporary loss of hypersensitivity to tuberculin.

Myocarditis is an infrequent serious complication; transient electrocardiographic changes are said to be relatively common.

Neurologic complications are more common in measles than in any of the other exanthems. The incidence of encephalomyelitis is estimated to be 1 to 2.0 per 1000 reported cases of measles. There appears to be no correlation between the severity of the measles and that of the neurologic involvement, nor between the severity of the initial encephalitic process and the prognosis. Rarely, encephalitis has been reported in association with measles modified by gamma globulin; it has not been reported in association with the use of live attenuated measles virus vaccine. Nevertheless the possibility of establishing a "slow virus infection" such as subacute sclerosing panencephalitis (Dawson's encephalitis) has been postulated. In a few instances encephalitic involvement is manifest in the pre-eruptive period, but more often the onset is 2 to 5 days after the appearance of the rash. The cause of measles encephalitis remains controversial. It is suggested that when encephalitis occurs early in the course of the disease, viral invasion plays a large role, whereas that which occurs later is predominantly demyelinating in nature. In this demyelinating type of reaction the symptoms and course do not differ from those of other parainfectious encephalitides (p. 689).

Prognosis. Case fatality rates in the United States have decreased in recent years to low levels for all age groups, in large part because of improved living conditions, but also because of effective antibacterial therapy for the treatment of secondary infections.

When measles is introduced into a highly susceptible population, the results may be disastrous. Such an occurrence in the Faroe Islands in 1846 resulted in the deaths of about one quarter, nearly 2000, of the total population regardless of age. At Ungava Bay, Canada, where 99 per cent of 900 persons had measles, the mortality rate was 7 per cent.

Prophylaxis. Quarantine is of little value, owing to the high communicability of the disease during its prodromal stage, when its presence is usually not suspected. Susceptibles known to have been exposed to the first case or group of cases may be permitted freedom for a week and then kept under strict isolation for 8 days. Under ordinary school or home conditions such attempts at isolation are ineffectual. The isolation of children with measles will decrease the opportunities for them to acquire secondary bacterial infections. Quarantine of the patient may be lifted 1 to 2 days after return of the temperature to normal.

Active immunization against measles has been achieved by vaccines which are still under evaluation: live attenuated virus vaccine and inactivated virus vaccine. Vaccines are being prepared chiefly from the Edmonston strain of Enders. The live attenuated virus vaccine is administered as a single subcutaneous injection of 0.2 to 0.25 ml. There is a short febrile illness of 2 to 3 days about a week after inoculation. The temperature range has been from 101 to 104°F. rectally. Koplik's spots and mild skin eruptions may be seen. The use of immune globulin, 0.02 to 0.04 ml. per kg. given intramuscularly from a separate syringe at a different site immediately after the inoculation of the vaccine, lessens the reaction to the vaccine. A more highly attenuated form of live virus vaccine (Schwarz) which produces less severe reactions is being evaluated.

Antibody levels induced by vaccines in serologically negative children are lower than those following the natural disease. Nevertheless vaccine-induced immunity is effective, and it is generally thought that this protection against measles will be as lasting as that following natural infection. Antibody level increases rapidly on subsequent exposure or challenge. During their febrile response vaccinated children do not appear to be an infection hazard for susceptible contacts.

As a rule, young infants who have received measles antibody from their immune mothers do not show a response to measles vaccine until about the eighth month of life, when the passively transferred maternal antibody has fallen to a low level.

Severe reactions, including neurologic involvement, following vaccination with live virus vaccine are rare. Regional lymphadenopathy, thrombocytopenic purpura and pneumonia have been recorded, as have febrile convulsions.

Allergic reactions have followed the use of chick embryo-cultured vaccine in persons sensitive to egg and the use of dog kidney-cultured vaccine in persons sensitive to canine antigens. Simultaneous administration of live virus measles vaccine and live attenuated poliovirus vaccine is not recommended; an interval of at least a month is suggested. The response to live measles vaccine is unpredictable if immune globulin has been administered in the 3 months preceding immunization. Anergy to tuberculin may develop and persist for a month or longer after administration of live attenuated measles vaccine. A child with active tuberculous infection should be receiving antituberculosis treatment when live measles vaccine is administered. A tuberculin test prior to active immunization against measles is desirable.

Use of live measles vaccine is not recommended for children with debilitating disease such as leukemia or in those receiving immunosuppressive drugs. When protection against measles is indicated, measles immune globulin (human) should be given intramuscularly in a dose of 0.25 ml. per kg. as soon as possible after exposure. This dose may need to be increased in children with acute leukemia.

The use of inactivated (killed) virus measles vaccine is not recommended. Unusual local or systemic reactions have occurred in recipients of killed virus measles vaccine who were later exposed to natural measles or were vaccinated with live attenuated measles virus. Such reactions to live virus vaccine have included severe local tenderness, swelling, erythema, heat and hemorrhagic or vesicular lesions, accompanied by malaise, fever and regional lymphadenopathy. Exposure to natural measles has resulted in a severe, atypical form of measles, with high fever, pneumonia and toxicity. The rash, which may be petechial, vesicular or urticarial, begins on the feet and extends upward, but is concentrated largely on the extremities. Such reactions do not seem to follow repeated inoculations of the attenuated live virus vaccine in children.

Passive immunization with pooled adult serum, pooled convalescent serum, placental globulin and gamma globulin of pooled plasma is effective for prevention and attenuation of measles. Measles can be prevented by the use of immune serum globulin (gamma globulin) in a dose of 0.25 ml. per kg. given intramuscularly within 5 days after exposure, but preferably as soon as possible after exposure. Complete protection is indicated for infants, for children with chronic illness and for contacts in hospital wards and children's institutions. Attenuation may be accomplished by the use of gamma globulin in a dosage of 0.05 ml. per kg. Gamma globulin, including that now prepared in the United States from placental blood, is approximately 25 times as potent in antibody titer as pooled adult serum. Attenuation is variable, and the modified clinical patterns may vary from those with few or no symptoms to those with little or no modification.

After the seventh or eighth day of incubation the amounts of immune bodies must be increased greatly for any degree of protection. If the injection is delayed until the ninth, tenth or eleventh day, slight fever may already have started, and only slight modification of the disease may be expected.

Treatment. Sedatives, antipyretics for high fever, skin lotions for itching or irritation, complete bed rest and an adequate fluid intake are the usual requirements. Humidification of the room may be necessary for laryngitis or an excessively irritating cough, and it is best to keep the room comfortably warm rather than cool. Because of conjunctival irritation, the patient should be protected from exposure to strong light. The complications of otitis media and pneumonia require appropriate antimicrobial therapy.

REFERENCES

Adams, J. M., Baird, C., and Filloy, L.: Inclusion Bodies in Measles Encephalitis. *J.A.M.A.,* 195:290, 1966.
American Academy of Pediatrics: Report of the Committee on the Control of Infectious Diseases. 15th ed. Evanston, Ill., 1966, p. 63.
Anderson, J. F.: Experimental Measles in the Monkey. *Pub. Health Rep.,* 26:847, 887, 1911.
Blattner, R. J.: Live Measles Vaccine and the Tuberculin Reaction. Comments on Current Literature. *J. Pediat.,* 63:174, 1963.
Blattner, R. J., and Heys, F. M.: Measles Encephalitis in Viral Encephalitis; in S. Z. Levine (Ed.): *Advances in Pediatrics.* Chicago, Year Book Publishers, Inc., 1962, Vol. 12, p. 77.
Christensen, P. E., and others: An Epidemic of Measles in Southern Greenland, 1951. II. The Epidemic Proper. III. Measles and Tuberculosis. *Acta med. scandinav.,* 144:430, 450, 1953.
Enders, J. F., and others: Studies on an Attenuated Measles Virus Vaccine: (Series of papers). *New England J. Med.,* 263:159, 1960.
Fulginiti, V. A., Eller, J. J., Downie, A. W., and Kempe, C. H.: Altered Reactivity to Measles Virus: Atypical Measles in Children Previously Immunized with Inactivated Measles Virus Vaccines. *J.A.M.A.,* 202:1075, 1967.
Goldberger, J., and Anderson, J. F.: An Experimental Demonstration of the Virus of Measles in Mixed Buccal and Nasal Secretions. *J.A.M.A.,* 57:476, 1911.
Goldfield, M., Boyer, N. H., and Weinstein, L.: Electrocardiographic Changes During the Course of Measles. *J. Pediat.,* 46:30, 1955.
Hektoen, L.: Experimental Measles. *J. Infect. Dis.,* 2:238, 1905.
Home, F.: *Medical Facts and Experiments.* London, A. Millar, 1759, p. 253.
Katz, S. L., and Enders, J. F.: Measles Virus; in F. L. Horsfall and I. Tamm (Eds.): *Viral and Rickettsial Infections of Man.* 4th ed., Philadelphia, J. B. Lippincott Company, 1965, p. 784.
Koplik, H.: The Diagnosis of the Invasion of Measles from a Study of the Exanthema as It Appears on the Buccal Mucous Membrane. *Arch. Pediat.,* 13:918, 1896.
Panum, P. L.: Observations Made During the Epidemic of Measles on the Faroe Islands in the Year 1846. Translated by A. S. Hatcher. New York, Delta Omega Society, American Public Health Association, 1940.
Scott, T. F., and Bonanno, D. F.: Reactions to Live Measles-Virus Vaccine in Children Previously Inoculated with Killed-Virus Vaccine. *New England J. Med.,* 277:248, 1967.
Shaffer, M. F., Rake, G., and Hodes, H. L.: Isolation of a Virus from a Patient with Fatal Encephalitis Complicating Measles. *Am. J. Dis. Child.,* 64:815, 1942.
Shaffer, M. F., Rake, G., Stokes, J., Jr., and O'Neil, G. C.: Studies on Measles. II. Experimental Disease in Man and Monkey. *J. Immunol.,* 41:241, 1941.
St. Geme, J. W., Jr., Wright, F. S., Jones, F., Halberg, F., and Anderson, J. A.: Failure to Detect Subtle Neurotropism of Live Attenuated Measles Virus Vaccine. *J. Pediat.,* 70:36, 1967.
Starr, S., and Berkovich, S.: The Effect of Measles, Gamma Globulin Modified Measles and Attenuated Measles Vaccine on the Course of Treated Tuberculosis in Children. *Pediatrics,* 35:97, 1965.

GERMAN MEASLES
(RUBELLA)

Definition. Rubella is a common communicable disease of childhood characterized ordinarily by mild constitutional symptoms, a rash similar to that of mild rubeola or scarlet fever, and enlargement and tenderness of the postoccipital, retroauricular and posterior cervical lymph nodes. In older children and adults the infection may occasionally be severe, with such manifestations as joint involvement and purpura.

Rubella in early pregnancy as a cause of severe congenital anomalies in the newborn infant was first recognized in 1941. Since the 1964 pandemic, other aspects of maternal rubella have received attention which have serious import for the newborn infant and significant epidemiologic implications. The congenital rubella syndrome is now recognized as an active contagious disease with multisystem involvement, a wide spectrum of clinical expression, and, as a rule, a long postnatal period of active infection with shedding of virus.

History. Designated as *Röteln* by German physicians in the eighteenth century, German measles was regarded as a variant of measles or scarlet fever. Maton described it as a separate entity in 1815; Wagner emphasized its distinction from rubeola and scarlet fever in 1829; and in 1866 Veale in Edinburgh called the disease rubella. Gregg (Australia) in 1941 observed severe congenital malformations in newborn infants whose mothers had rubella early in pregnancy. The pandemic of 1964 brought to light a new concept of congenital rubella as mentioned above.

Etiology. Rubella is caused by a viral agent, which in 1938 Hiro and Tasaka transferred successfully to children by filtered nasopharyngeal secretions from patients. Krugman in 1953 showed that the infectious agent was present in the blood 2 days before and on the first day of the rash.

Early attempts at tissue culture isolation were not successful because of the absence of cytopathic effect. Two methods are now available for virus assay and antibody study: use of cell lines in which rubella virus shows a visible effect, e.g. human amnion cells, and rabbit kidney cells; and by interference phenomena, i.e. the presence of rubella

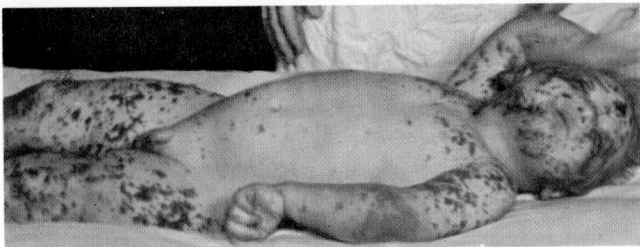

Figure 10-40. Fulminating meningococcemia in a child 2½ years of age. Onset 36 hours before admission, with vomiting and fever; 18 hours before admission, extensive purpuric eruption began; death 8 hours after admission. Blood culture positive, Meningococcus type II. Nasal and cerebrospinal fluid cultures negative. One sibling had meningitis; another was found to be a carrier.

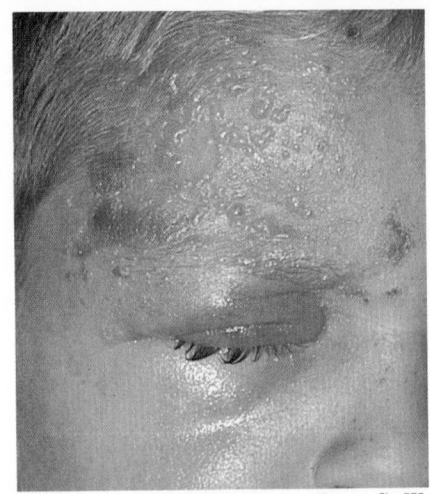

Figure 10-80. Herpes zoster ophthalmicus. (From G. W. Korting: *Hautkrankheiten bei Kindern und Jugendlichen.* Stuttgart, Germany, F. K. Schattauer Verlag, 1969.)

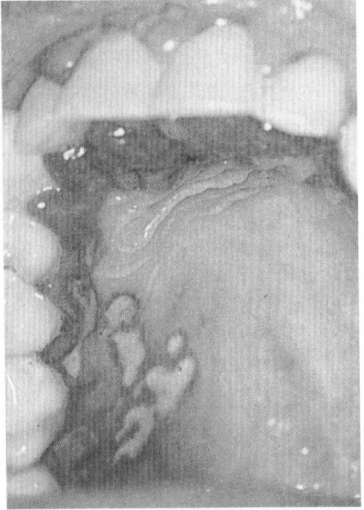

Figure 10-87. Herpangina. (From G. W. Korting: *Hautkrankheiten bei Kindern und Jugendlichen.* Stuttgart, Germany, F. K. Schattauer Verlag, 1969.)

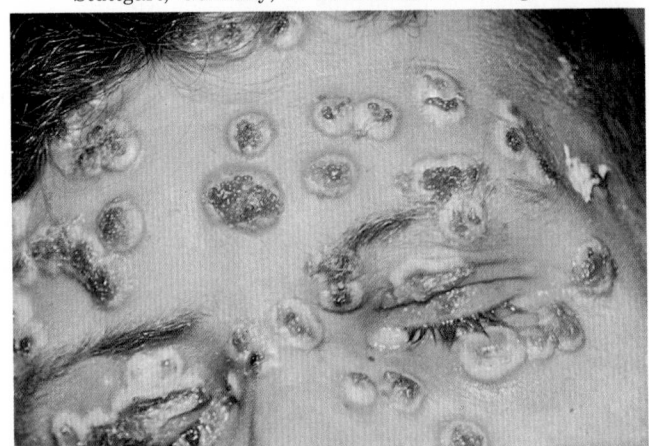

Figure 10-83. Eczema vaccinatum. (From G. W. Korting: *Hautkrankheiten bei Kindern und Jugendlichen.* Stuttgart, Germany, F. K. Schattauer Verlag, 1969.)

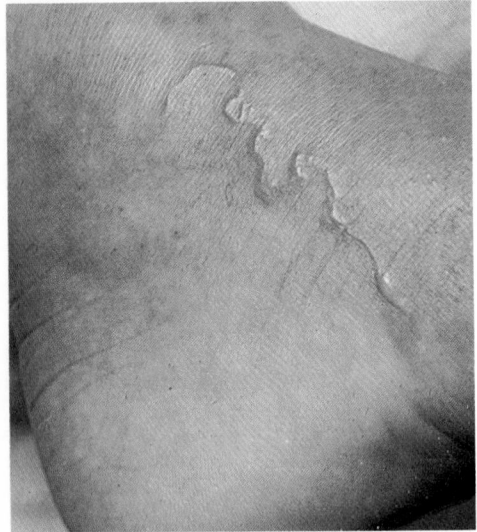

Figure 10-106. Creeping eruption of cutaneous larva migrans. (From G. W. Korting: *Hautkrankheiten bei Kindern und Jugendlichen.* Stuttgart, Germany, F. K. Schattauer Verlag, 1969.)

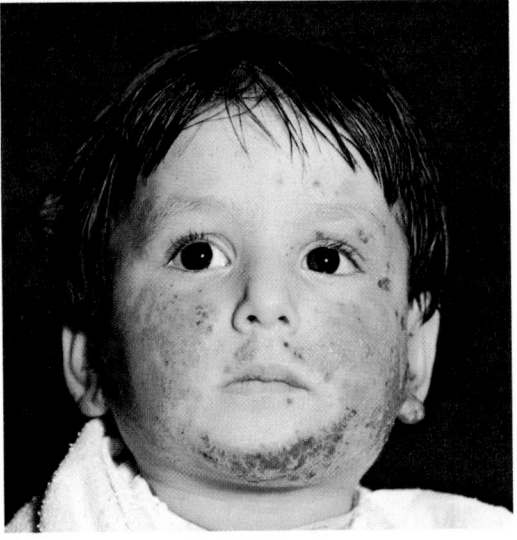

Figure 10-12A. Infantile eczema.

628

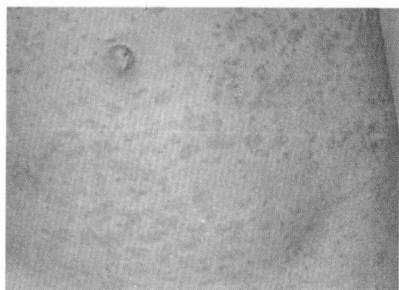

Figure 10-69. Maculopapular rash of measles. (From G. W. Korting: *Hautkrankheiten bei Kindern und Jugendlichen.* Stuttgart, Germany, F. K. Schattauer Verlag, 1969.)

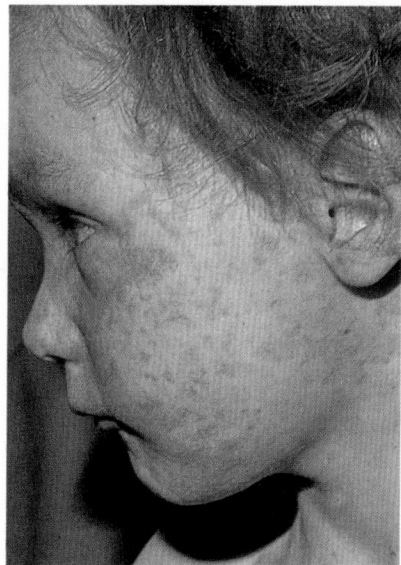

Figure 10-71. Rash of rubella (German measles). (From G. W. Korting: *Hautkrankheiten bei Kindern und Jugendlichen.* Stuttgart, Germany, F. K. Schattauer Verlag, 1969.)

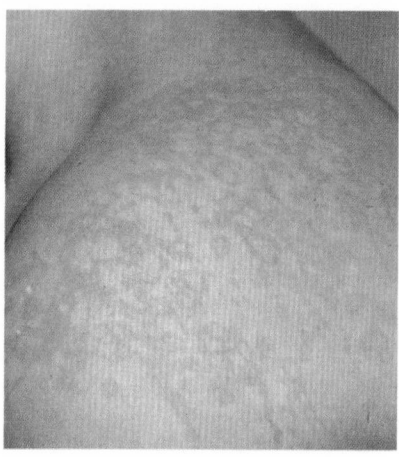

Figure 10-72. Erythema infectiosum. (From G. W. Korting: *Hautkrankheiten bei Kindern und Jugendlichen.* Stuttgart, Germany, F. K. Schattauer Verlag, 1969.)

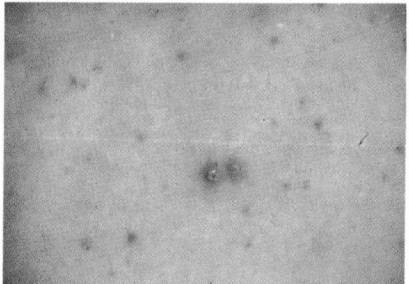

Figure 10-78. Skin lesions of chickenpox. Note the varying stages of development (macules, papules and vesicles) present at the same time. (Courtesy of Dr. P. F. Lucchesi.)

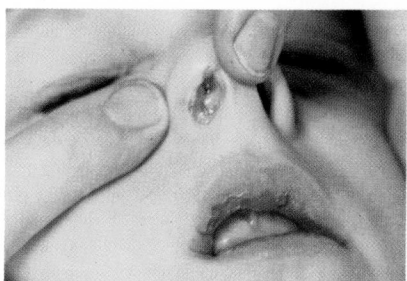

Figure 10-36. Nasal diphtheria. (Courtesy of Dr. Robert A. Lyon.)

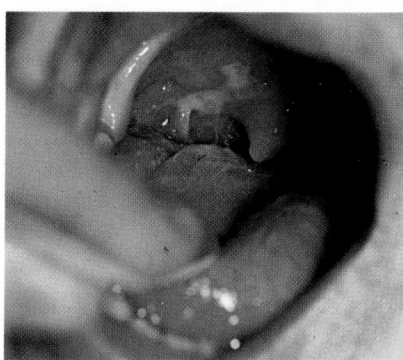

Figure 10-35. Pharyngotonsillar membrane of diphtheria. (Courtesy of Dr. Robert A. Lyon.)

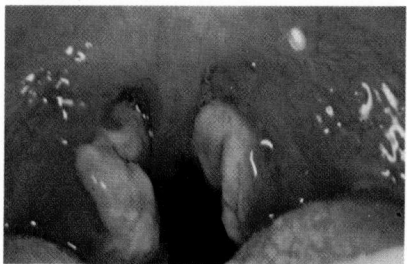

Figure 10-85. Pharyngitis with membrane formation in infectious mononucleosis. (Courtesy of Dr. Alex J. Steigman.)

virus interfering with the cytopathic effect of ECHO virus 11 and Coxsackie virus A_9 subsequently introduced into the culture. The virus appears to be of a single type with characteristics of the myxovirus group. During clinical illness it is present in nasopharyngeal secretions, blood, feces and urine. Virus has been recovered from the nasopharynx 7 days before the exanthem, and from 7 to 8 days after its disappearance. Subclinical infections are known to occur.

Epidemiology. Transplacental immunity is effective for the first 5 or 6 months of life. Epidemics occur approximately every 3 to 4 years. A single attack is thought to confer permanent immunity, and verified second attacks occur rarely. Most of the so-called second attacks are actually exanthematous manifestations associated with other virus infections such as with ECHO virus and Coxsackie virus. The incidence of rubella among adults is relatively high. Epidemiologic studies have confirmed the spread of rubella in families; as high as 60 per cent of the family was affected, and the ratio of inapparent to overt infection was 2:1.

In maternal rubella, the infection in the mother is primary and is transferred to her offspring by way of the placenta. In a considerable number of instances in which therapeutic abortion was performed because of clinical rubella in the first trimester, the rubella virus was recovered from the products of conception. In one particular case the mother was thought to be in the first week of pregnancy at the time of clinical rubella. Therapeutic abortion was performed at 18 weeks; the fetus had cataracts, and its development was impaired. Rubella virus was recovered from various fetal tissues.

In the congenital rubella syndrome, virus can be isolated from nasopharyngeal washings, stool, blood, urine and spinal fluid of the newborn infant. Virus shedding continues for periods as long as 12 to 18 months, making the infant a source of infection for contacts, such as older children who are not immune and nonimmume adults, including pregnant women and nursery personnel.

Clinical Manifestations. The incubation period for rubella is generally 14 to 21 days, but may be slightly shorter or longer. The prodromal phase of mild catarrhal symptoms is shorter than that of measles and may be so mild as to go entirely unnoticed. The most characteristic sign is retroauricular, posterior cervical and postoccipital adenitis. No other disease causes the tender enlargement of all these nodes to the same extent that German measles does. An enanthem often appears just before the onset of the skin rash. It consists of discrete rose spots on the soft palate which may coalesce into a red blush and may extend over the fauces.

Lymphadenopathy is evident at least 24 hours before the *rash* appears and may be present for a week or more. The exanthem is more variable than that of rubeola. It begins on the face (Fig. 10-71, p. 629) and spreads quickly. Its evolution is so rapid that the rash on the face may be fading by the time it appears on the trunk. Discrete maculopapules are present in large numbers, but in addition to this eruption, there are large areas of flushing which spread rapidly over the entire body, usually within 24 hours. The rash may be confluent, particularly on the face. During the second day the rash may assume a pinpoint appearance, especially over the trunk, resembling that of scarlet fever. The eruption usually clears by the third day. Any residual pigmentation disappears in a few days, and desquamation is minimal. Cases of rubella without a rash have been described.

The pharyngeal mucosa and the conjunctivas are inflamed slightly. Photophobia is not present, as in rubeola. Fever is slight, or not present at all. When present, it occurs at the height of the rash, and persists for 1, 2 or occasionally for 3 days. The temperature seldom exceeds 101°F. Anorexia, headache and malaise are not common in rubella. The spleen is often slightly enlarged. Mild itching may occur, but is not a problem. There are no characteristic changes in the white blood cells; the total count is normal or slightly reduced.

Infection in older children and adults can follow the usual course, be subclinical or be associated with severe manifestations, including joint involvement and purpura.

In the *congenital rubella syndrome* the most common permanent defects are cataracts, cardiac anomalies, especially patent ductus arteriosus, deafness and secondary mutism, microcephaly and mental deficiency. Less frequent conditions are microphthalmus, buphthalmus, retinal lesions, talipes equinovarus, syndactyly, hypospadias, generalized muscular weakness, cerebral diplegia, cleft palate and dental anomalies.

The degree of involvement of the infant at birth varies widely. In severe widespread infection, growth retardation, particularly in weight, is the most common finding at birth. Within the first few days of life the disease process may become more severe, and the infant may experience a stormy course for the first 6 months or so with such manifestations as thrombocytopenia, anemia, hepatitis, pneumonitis, encephalitis, rhinitis, otitis media, congestive heart failure and diarrhea. In the heart, the most common anomalies are patent ductus arteriosus and pulmonary artery branch stenosis. Skeletal abnormalities are common in infants with the rubella syndrome. In the skull, mineralization of the calvaria is poor, and sutures are prominent. The anterior fontanel is often large and may extend well into the frontal bone, involving the metopic suture. The long bones have an altered trabecular pattern characterized by longitudinal streaks of poor mineralization. Bone manifestations are most pronounced at the knees and bear some resemblance to rickets. These skeletal abnormalities are self-correcting if the infant thrives.

Central nervous system involvement is striking. The degree of involvement may be masked in the very ill infant, but surmised by a tense fontanel and hypotonia in the first few months of life. Overt neurologic disease may not be apparent until later in infancy. In one series in 1964 over half the deaths during the first year of life were in infants under 3 months of age. Persistence of virus infection is reflected by virus recovery from the cerebrospinal fluid. Virus can be isolated from inner layers of the lens of the eye for as long as 3 years.

Differential Diagnosis. Particularly in its more severe forms, rubella may be confused with the mild types of scarlet fever (p. 558) and rubeola (p. 632). *Roseola infantum* (exanthem subitum) is distinguished from rubella by the appearance of the rash at the end of the febrile episode rather than at the height of the signs and symptoms. *Drug rashes* may be extremely difficult to differentiate from rubella. The characteristic enlargement of the lymph nodes would support the diagnosis of rubella. In *infectious mononucleosis* a rash may occur which resembles that of rubella, and enlargement of the lymph nodes in both diseases may lead to confusion. Changes in the hematologic findings in infectious mononucleosis should be sufficient to distinguish the 2 diseases. ECHO virus infections, which may be accompanied by a rash, can be differentiated by their shorter incubation period and the absence of suboccipital adenopathy.

Prognosis and Complications. The prognosis is good, and complications are relatively uncommon in rubella in children. Neuritis and arthritis occur occasionally. Resistance to secondary bacterial infection is not altered significantly. Encephalitis similar to that seen with rubeola is not a common complication, but is serious when it occurs.

Prevention. Prophylactic measures in childhood are rarely indicated, but preventive measures are of the utmost importance to protect the fetus. It is important for girls to be exposed and to contract the disease before the childbearing age. Pregnant women, especially early in pregnancy, but also during the entire gestational period, should avoid exposure to rubella, *regardless of history of the disease during childhood.* Risk of damage to the fetus is considered to be reduced after the fourteenth week of gestation.

Should isolation for the exposed susceptible be indicated, strict isolation is recommended from about the tenth to the twenty-first day after exposure. In an exposed susceptible, protection from or attenuation of the disease may or may not be afforded by intramuscular injection of immune globulin, given in large dosage (0.12 to 0.20 ml. per pound) within the first 7 to 8 days after exposure. The effectiveness of immune globulin is not predictable, depending apparently upon the antibody content of the blood product used, or upon factors as yet undetermined. The value of immune serum globulin has been questioned also because in some instances rash was prevented, and clinical manifestations were absent or minimal, while at the same time viable virus was present in the blood. In general, however, the risk to the fetus appears to be reduced if the mother receives immune substance early and in adequate amount.

The current movement to liberalize abortion laws received its impetus in part from the epidemics of rubella in the early 1960's and from the episodes associated with the use of thalidomide. In most instances in which therapeutic abortion has been performed because of clinical rubella in the first trimester of pregnancy, the diagnosis of rubella and the indication for termination of the pregnancy have been reviewed, and the decision made on the advice of 3 or 4 qualified physicians. Recent developments in antibody detection, especially the hemagglutination and hemagglutination inhibition techniques, have facilitated verification of the diagnosis of rubella.

Although, at present, measures for active immunization against rubella are not perfected, prospects are good for a live attenuated vaccine prepared in tissue cultures. Pilot studies with several highly attenuated strains of virus grown in tissue culture have given encouraging results, with good immune response and a minimum of clinical manifestation. Nevertheless virus persists in the nasopharynx, and shedding may occur for as long as 3 weeks after vaccination. The serious risk is the possible spread of the virus to pregnant women, with potential damage to the fetus. Until this important problem is solved, universal use of rubella vaccine is not recommended.

Treatment. Unless bacterial complications occur, treatment is symptomatic. The patient should be kept at bed rest until the temperature is normal.

REFERENCES

Alford, C. A., Jr., Neva, F. A., and Weller, T. H.: Virologic and Serologic Studies on Human Products of Conception After Maternal Rubella. *New England J. Med.*, 271:1275, 1964.

Anderson, S. G.: Rubella in Volunteers. *J. Immunol.*, 62:29, 1949.

Baylor University College of Medicine: Rubella Study Group: Rubella: Epidemic in Retrospect. *Hospital Practice*, 2:27, 1967.

Desmond, M. M., and others: Congenital Rubella Encephalitis: Course and Early Sequelae. *J. Pediat.*, 71:311, 1967.

Gregg, N. M.: Congenital Cataract Following German Measles in the Mother. *Tr. Ophthal. Soc. Australia*, 3:35, 1941.

Gregg, N. M., and others: The Occurrence of Congenital Defects in Children Following Maternal Rubella During Pregnancy. *M.J. Australia*, 2:122, 1945.

Habel, K.: Transmission of Rubella to *Macacus Mulatta* Monkeys. *Pub. Health Rep.*, 57:1126, 1942.

Hiro, Y., and Tasaka, S.: Die Röteln sind eine Viruskrankheit. *Monat. f Kinderh.*, 76:328, 1938.

Ingalls, T. H., and others: Rubella: Epidemiology, Virology, and Immunology. *Am. J.M. Sc.*, 253:349, 1967.

Krugman, S., (Ed.): Rubella Symposium. *Am. J. Dis. Child.*, 110:345, 1965.

Krugman, S., and Ward, R.: Rubella: Demonstration of Neutralizing Antibody in Gamma Globulin and Re-evaluation of the Rubella Problem. *New England J. Med.*, 259:16, 1958.

Meyer, H. M., Jr.: Clinical Experience with Natural and Attenuated Rubella Virus Infection. Abst., Amer. Pediat. Soc., 77th Ann. Meet., Atlantic City, April 1967 (Program, p. 12).

Monif, G. R., Sever, J. L., Schiff, G. M., and Traub, R. G.: Isolation of Rubella Virus from Products of Conception. *Am. J. Obst. & Gynec.*, 91:1143, 1965.

Rawls, W. E., Desmyter, J., and Melnick, J. L.: Serologic Diagnosis and Fetal Involvement in Maternal Rubella. *J.A.M.A.*, 203:627, 1968.

Rawls, W. E., and others: Persistent Virus Infection in Congenital Rubella. *Arch. Ophthalmol.*, 77:430, 1967.

Rudolph, A. J., and others: Transplacental Rubella Infection in Newly Born Infants. *J.A.M.A.*, 191:843, 1965.

Schick, B.: Die Röteln. *Ergeb. d. inn. Med. u. Kinderh.*, 5:280, 1910.

EXANTHEM SUBITUM
(ROSEOLA INFANTUM)

Definition. Exanthem subitum is an acute viral disease of infants and young children, usually occurring sporadically, but occasionally in epidemics. It is unique in that the diagnostic rash and clinical improvement occur almost simultaneously. The disease is characterized by a period of high fever lasting 3 to 4 days, during which time there are insufficient clinical findings to explain the hyperpyrexia, and by an abrupt termination with a precipitous drop of the temperature to normal and the appearance of a generalized eruption, which fades quickly.

History. Zahorsky first described the disease in the United States in 1910 as roseola infantum; later Veeder and Hempelmann applied to it the more suitable term of "exanthem subitum."

Etiology. Available evidence supports viral origin. Blood serum, heparinized blood and throat washings obtained from patients on the third day of fever and also on the first day of the rash have been shown to be infective for susceptible infants, and for monkeys. Typical disease resulted in infants after an incubation period of 9 to 10 days, and in monkeys, 4 to 5 days.

Nothing is known of the pathologic changes of the disease.

Epidemiology. The degree of contagiousness is not known. There is a tendency for the disease to occur chiefly in the spring and fall. It attacks both sexes equally. In the rare epidemics described the incubation period was estimated to be from 7 to 17 days, usually about 10 days. The epidemiologic pattern is not clear. The occurrence of exanthem subitum sporadically in early life, with rare epidemics in older age groups, suggests the possibility of an endemic spread through most of the population in early infancy and childhood, with production of permanent immunity. Most of the cases occur between the ages of 6 months and 3 years, although the disease does occur infrequently in older children and even in adults. The peak incidence appears to be during the second year of life.

Clinical Manifestations. The onset is sudden, with fever which rises abruptly as high as 103 to 105°F.; convulsions may occur at this time. Although the pharyngeal mucosa is slightly inflamed at times and there may be slight coryza, there are no typical signs. The outstanding feature is the absence of physical findings sufficient to explain the height of the fever. The diagnosis is suspected chiefly by exclusion of other possible infections, particularly those which at this age are the most common causes of high fever and in which the diagnosis may not be evident, such as otitis media, acute pyelonephritis, pneumonia and meningitis.

Early in the febrile period, the first 24 to 36 hours, the blood cell count may be elevated, as high as 16,000 to 20,000 per cu. mm. with an increase in neutrophils. By the second day leukopenia becomes evident, with counts from 3000 to 5000 on the third to fourth day of fever. There is an absolute neutropenia with a relative lymphocytosis, which may be as high as 90 per cent. Occasionally a large number of monocytes is present.

The fever falls by crisis on the third or fourth day, and just before or shortly after the return of the temperature to normal a macular or maculopapular eruption appears over the body, starting on the trunk and spreading to the arms and neck, with slight involvement of the face and legs. The rash soon fades, rarely remaining as long as 24 hours. Desquamation is rare, and no pigmentation remains. In the rare epidemic outbreaks, cases without a rash may be suspected, but a definite diagnosis cannot be made. Clemens described an enanthem on the soft palate consisting of small erythematous spots and streaks. Slight periorbital edema has also been described. Occasionally the lymph nodes, especially in the cervical area, may be enlarged, but not to the extent that they are in rubella.

Differential Diagnosis. The principal difficulty in differential diagnosis is with *rubella*, from which exanthem subitum is distinguished chiefly by the prodromal period of high fever. *Rubeola* and *dengue* can be distinguished primarily by the time of appearance of their rash in relation to fever and other clinical findings. In measles, though there is usually a fever of variable degree for 3 or 4 days just before the rash, the temperature becomes abruptly elevated to 103 to 104°F. at the time of appearance of the rash and remains elevated for the next 2 days or so. The lack of Koplik's spots, severe coryza, conjunctivitis and cough also helps to distinguish exanthem subitum from rubeola. Certain allergic rashes, e.g. those resulting from sensitivity to drugs, may be difficult to distinguish from exanthem subitum, but the characteristic clinical pattern of the latter is usually sufficiently definite to establish the diagnosis.

Prognosis is good except in the rare patient who has encephalopathy or extreme hyperpyrexia.

Prophylaxis and Treatment. There are no known methods for shortening the course of the disease or for prophylaxis. In infants and young children who are prone to convulsions the administration of a sedative at the appearance of the sharp febrile onset of exanthem subitum may be effective as prophylaxis against such seizures. Aspirin may be of some help in partially reducing the fever and in allaying restlessness.

RUSSELL J. BLATTNER

REFERENCES

Berenberg, W., Wright, S., and Janeway, C. A.: Roseola Infantum (Exanthem Subitum). *New England J. Med.*, 241:253, 1949.

Burnstine, R. C., and Paine, R. S.: Residual Encephalopathy Following Roseola Infantum. *Am. J. Dis. Child.*, 98:144, 1959.

Clemens, H. H.: Exanthem Subitum (Roseola Infantum): A Report of Eighty Cases. *J. Pediat.*, 26:66, 1945.

Hellström, B., and Vahlquist, B.: Experimental Inoculation of Roseola Infantum. *Acta paediat.*, 40:189, 1951.

Kempe, C. H., Shaw, E. B., Jackson, J. R., and Silver, H. K.: Studies on the Etiology of Exanthem Subitum (Roseola Infantum). *J. Pediat.*, 37:561, 1950.

Letchner, A.: Roseola Infantum: A Review of Fifty Cases. *Lancet*, 2:1163, 1955.

Veeder, B. S., and Hempelmann, T. C.: A Febrile Exanthem Occurring in Childhood (Exanthem Subitum). *J.A.M.A.*, 77:1787, 1921.

Zahorsky, J.: Roseola Infantum. *J.A.M.A.*, 61:1446, 1913.

ERYTHEMA INFECTIOSUM

(Megalerythema Epidemicum; Fifth Disease)

History. The early reports on this disease came from Germany, where the first epidemic in 1886 was described as one of atypical rubella. In 1896 Escherich recognized the disease as a clinical entity, and the present name was accorded it by Stricker in 1899. In 1904 Plachte named it megalerythema epidemicum, and in 1905 the name "fifth disease" was introduced by Cheinesse of Paris.

Etiology. No proved agent has been identified.

Pathology. Biopsy of the skin lesions reveals nonspecific edema of the dermis and epidermis and lymphocytic perivascular infiltration.

Epidemiology. This mildly infectious disease tends to occur in family and small localized epidemics. The incubation period appears to be 6 to 14 days. The infection has a world-wide distribution; there is no sex predilection. The incidence is highest in children, but the disease can occur in infants and adults.

Clinical Features. Usually the first detectable evidence of illness is the appearance of a characteristic rash. In some patients, especially in adults, nonspecific symptoms of sore throat, coryza, mild myalgia or arthralgia may shortly precede the rash. The rash erupts in 2 stages; the first, often overlooked, appears on the malar prominences as an intensely erythematous, coalescent maculopapular rash ("slapped cheeks") which conspicuously spares the upper lip, nasolabial folds and often the chin. The affected area has a raised, defined edge, feels hot, but is not tender, and superficially resembles erysipelas. Faint macules can often be found at the hairline on the neck, forehead and chin. The rash remains on the face for 1 to 4 days as a rule. In the second stage, beginning about 24 hours after the first, an erythematous maculopapular rash appears on the extensor surfaces of the arms, backs of the hands and, within a few hours, on the thighs and buttocks (Fig. 10-72, p. 629). Occasionally there is an extensive rash over the trunk, but most often it is free of eruption or has only a few isolated faint macules. Within 24 to 48 hours the rash spreads to the flexor surfaces of the arms, and the lesions on the extensor surfaces begin to clear centrally. As this clearing of the rash proceeds, the faded areas coalesce, leaving the diagnostic lacework of bright, irregular red outlines. This stage lasts for several days to a week, and another week or more is required for the rash to fade completely. The entire course of the disease (rash) varies in the described epidemics from 2 to 24 days. One of the diagnostic features of the rash is its evanescent nature. Even during the height of the disease the rash may vary markedly in intensity from hour to hour. It is also characteristic for the rash to reappear for a few days when the skin is exposed to irritation such as sunlight or extremes of heat or cold, even weeks after the original rash has faded. Mild pruritus is occasionally present. There is no enanthem or lymphadenopathy.

As a rule the disease is afebrile, and the patients feel quite well. Temperatures up to 102°F. may occur early in the disease, occasionally in children and more commonly in adults.

Laboratory Data. There are no characteristic findings.

Diagnosis. This depends on interpretation of the rash. The butterfly distribution of the early rash on the face must be distinguished from erysipelas, certain enterovirus infections (e.g. ECHO-9), certain drug reactions (e.g. Aureomycin) and lupus erythematosus. The characteristic evolution of the rash and the benign course of the disease should easily clarify the diagnosis and thus avoid unnecessary isolation or treatment.

Complications. None has been reported.

Treatment. None is indicated. Isolation is not required.

REFERENCES

Bard, J. W., and Perry, H. O.: Erythema Infectiosum. *Arch. Derm.*, 93:49, 1966.

Greenwald, P., and Bashe, W. J., Jr.: An Epidemic of Erythema Infectiosum. *Am. J. Dis. Child.*, 107:30, 1964.

Lawton, A. L., and Smith, R. E.: Erythema Infectiosum. Clinical Study of an Epidemic in Branford, Connecticut. *Arch. Int. Med.*, 47:28, 1931.

HERPES SIMPLEX

Herpesvirus hominis is a common parasite of man that can produce a variety of clinical manifestations. These can be classified under diseases of the skin, the mucous membranes, the eye, the central nervous system and generalized systemic disease.

Two types of infection are recognized: (1) Primary: This is the susceptible host's first experience with the virus, which results in a subclinical infection in most instances. In the remainder, local superficial lesions usually occur (see below) accompanied by a varying degree of systemic reaction. In newborn infants and severely malnourished infants a fatal systemic infection, often without superficial lesions, may occur. Circulating antibodies develop in nonfatal cases. (2) Recurrent: These lesions are the result of reactivation of a latent infection in an immune host with circulating antibodies. Reactivation follows such nonspecific stimuli as changes in the external milieu, e.g. cold, ultraviolet light, or the internal milieu, e.g. menstruation, fever or emotional stress. The lesions are localized and, as a rule, unassociated with systemic reaction.

CLINICAL PATTERNS

Systemic Infection

In the Newborn Infant. Infection is acquired usually from passage through the birth canal of a mother with a primary herpetic vulvovaginitis. Infection of an infant, of a mother with a history of recurrent herpes labialis and circulating antibodies to type 1 virus, may occur during passage through a cervix infected with the type 2 virus, which differs antigenically from that causing her labial infection. Infants born of uninfected mothers can be infected from attendants with herpetic lesions. Rarely a transplacental infection has been postulated.

The infant with typical generalized infection appears well until the fifth to ninth day, when appetite fails and evidence of a widespread infection rapidly follows. The fully developed illness may simulate septicemia; the infant may have fever or hypothermia, dyspnea, increasing jaundice, vomiting, lethargy or convulsions. Myocarditis has been described, and circulatory collapse is often the terminal event. Hepatosplenomegaly is common. Purpura or other bleeding results from liver failure or thrombocytopenia. Vesicular lesions on the skin or mucous membranes or conjunctivitis may or may not be present; when the esophagus is affected, thick, yellow mucus accumulates. A terminal septicemia with *Pseudomonas aeruginosa* is not unusual. Some infants recover after a mild infection characterized only by a vesicular eruption and low-grade fever.

In Severely Malnourished Infants. The primary infection in infants who have severe protein malnutrition, often in their second year, may be generalized and fatal. The clinical and pathologic findings are similar to those in the newborn.

Lesions of the Skin and Mucous Membranes

Lesions of the Skin
(HERPES LABIALIS, FACIALIS, FEBRILIS)

Primary infection may, uncommonly, result in a generalized vesicular eruption in which the lesions are small and may continue to appear over a period of 2 to 3 weeks. If the systemic manifesta-

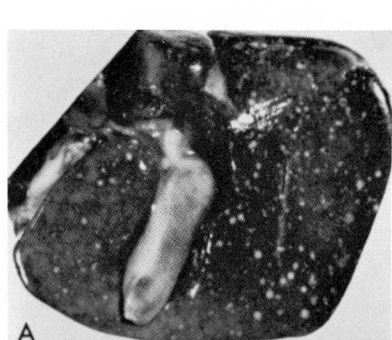
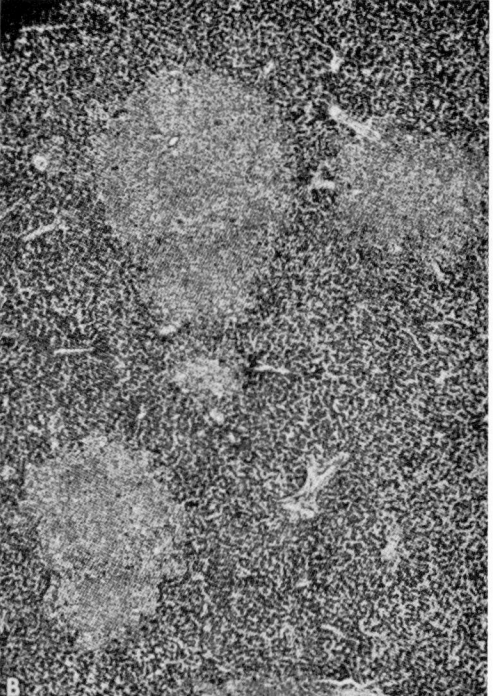

Figure 10-73. *A*, Right lobe of liver of an infant with generalized herpes simplex, who died at 10 days of age. The mother had vesicles on both labia; there were no lesions on the skin of the infant. Note the multiple discrete areas of necrosis. *B*, Photomicrograph of liver from an infant with generalized herpes simplex. There are multiple sharply demarcated areas of necrosis scattered throughout the parenchyma (× 38).

tions are mild, the infection must be differentiated from varicella; if severe, from variola.

Clinical lesions of recurrent herpes infection occur on the skin or mucous membranes. On the skin the lesion consists of aggregates of thin-walled vesicles on an erythematous base. These rupture, scab and heal within 7 to 10 days without leaving a scar except after repeated attacks or secondary bacterial infections; temporary depigmentation occurs in the Negro. The local lesions may be preceded by mild irritation or burning at the local site or by severe neuralgic pain in the region. In children the vesicles often become secondarily infected, introducing *impetigo contagiosa* into the differential diagnosis. The lesions tend to occur at mucocutaneous junctions, but may occur anywhere. They tend to recur at the same site.

Traumatic lesions of the skin can be readily infected by the ubiquitous herpesvirus. Primary lesions can also occur on apparently unbroken skin, as, for example, on the chin of drooling infants with herpetic stomatitis, in whom scattered isolated vesicles appear (contrast the grouped vesicles of recurrent attacks). When the skin of a limb is infected, vesicles appear in 2 to 3 days at the site of the trauma. There is often centripetal spread along lymph channels, causing enlargement of regional lymph nodes and scattered vesicles on the intervening undamaged skin. The final clinical picture may be mistaken for that of *herpes zoster*, especially if accompanied by neuralgic pain, unless the lesions are recognized as not being confined to a dermatome. The lesions heal slowly, often taking 3 weeks; recurrences at the site of the local trauma are common and may assume a bullous nature. Wrestlers and medical personnel are liable to herpetic infections of superficial abrasions (herpes gladiatorum and herpetic Whitlow). In the latter, infection of minor trauma about the nails leads to extremely painful, deep-seated spreading lesions with vesicles which resolve spontaneously in 2 to 3 weeks. Similar lesions occur on the fingers of "thumb suckers" who are suffering from herpetic gingivostomatitis. Treatment is symptomatic only; the lesions should not be incised.

Eczema Herpeticum
(KAPOSI'S VARICELLIFORM ERUPTION; JULIUSBERG'S PUSTULOSIS VACCINIFORMIS ACUTA)

This, the most serious manifestation of "traumatic herpes," results from a widespread and usually primary infection of the eczematous skin with herpesvirus. The severity of the complication varies; the attacks may be so mild as to be overlooked without a high index of suspicion and adequate laboratory facilities, or they may be fatal. In a typical severe primary attack, vesicles develop abruptly in large numbers over the area of eczematous skin. They continue to appear in crops for as long as 7 to 9 days. Isolated at first, they later

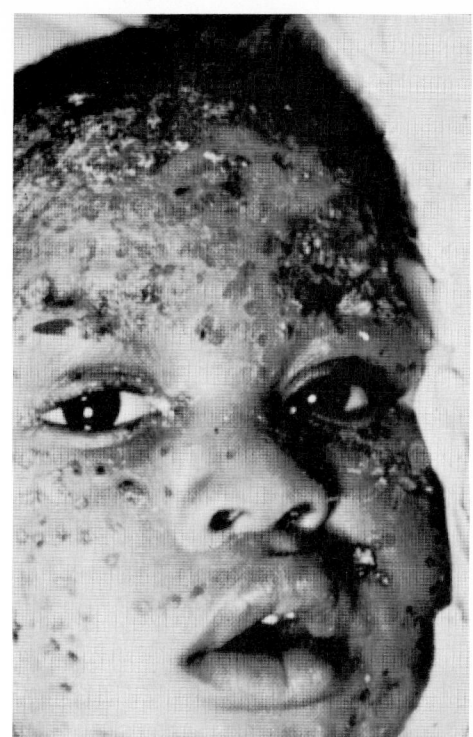

Figure 10-74. Eczema herpeticum. Note similarity of umbilicated vesicular lesions on face to those of eczema vaccinatum (p. 646).

become grouped and may occur on adjoining areas of normal skin. Wide denudation of the epidermis may occur. Scabs eventually form, and epithelization occurs. The systemic reaction varies, but temperatures of 103 to 105°F. for 7 to 10 days are not uncommon. Recurrent attacks can occur on chronic atopic skin lesions. The systemic, presumably hypersensitivity, reaction is usually less than in primary infection. Death may occur as the result of profound physiologic disturbances from loss of fluid, electrolytes and protein through the skin or from secondary bacterial invasion. A differentiation from *eczema vaccinatum* (p. 646) can usually be made clinically by determining with reasonable certainty that the child has not been exposed to vaccinia and by the occurrence of crops of vesicles in herpes. The diagnosis can be established by laboratory methods.

Acute Herpetic Gingivostomatitis
(ACUTE INFECTIOUS GINGIVOSTOMATITIS; APHTHOUS STOMATITIS; CATARRHAL STOMATITIS; ULCERATIVE STOMATITIS; VINCENT'S STOMATITIS)

This primary infection is probably the commonest cause of stomatitis in children between 1 and 3 years of age. It can occur in adults. The symptoms may appear abruptly with pain in the mouth, salivation, fetor oris, refusal to eat, and fever, often as high as 104 to 105°F. The onset may be

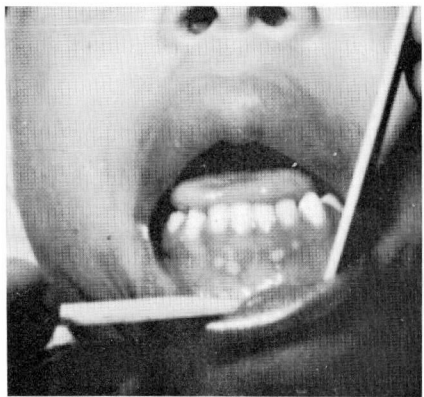

Figure 10-75. Herpetic stomatitis.

insidious, fever and irritability preceding the oral lesions by a day or two. The initial lesion is a vesicle, seldom seen because of its early rupture. The residual lesion is 2 to 10 mm. in diameter and is covered with a yellow-gray membrane. When this membrane sloughs, a true ulcer remains. Although the tongue and cheeks are most commonly involved, no part of the oral lining is exempt. Except in edentulous infants, acute gingivitis is characteristic of the disease and may precede the appearance of mucosal vesicles. Submaxillary lymphadenitis is common. The acute phase lasts 4 to 9 days and is self-limited. Pain tends to disappear 2 to 4 days before healing of the ulcers is complete. In some instances the tonsillar regions are involved early, and acute tonsillitis of bacterial origin or herpangina may be suspected. Failure of the lesion to respond to antibiotic therapy differentiates a bacterial infection, and the spread of the vesiculation to the buccal mucosa rules out herpangina.

Recurrent Stomatitis

Localized lesions may occur on the palate in association with a febrile illness or on the mucosa

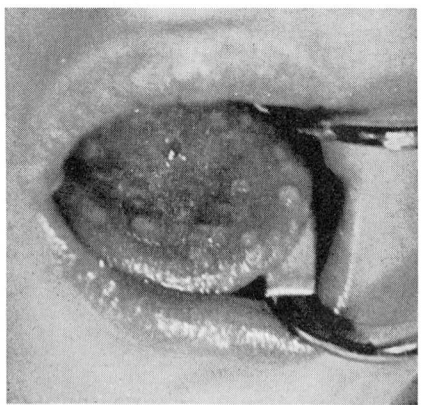

Figure 10-76. Lesions of herpetic stomatitis on the tongue.

adjacent to a lesion on the lip; recurrent aphthous ulcers, however, are not caused by herpesvirus. In some persons a generalized stomatitis recurs consistently 7 to 10 days after a recurrent herpetic lesion of the lip or elsewhere, and is often accompanied by skin lesions of erythema multiforme; this lesion is a hypersensitivity reaction to virus protein.

Herpes Progenitalis

Primary herpetic vulvovaginitis is not an uncommon lesion in childhood (due to either type 1 or type 2 virus). The patient complains of burning pain in the genitalia. The lesions resemble those in the mouth; they appear as vesicles which soon collapse and become covered with a yellow-gray membrane. These become eroded into superficial, painful ulcers (Fig. 10-77). There is associated enlargement of the inguinal nodes, and often a low-grade fever. The lesions heal spontaneously; sitz baths are advisable for cleanliness. In adult women herpetic ulcers of the cervix occur and recur; these are usually, but not always, caused by the genital (type 2) strain of virus.

Herpes progenitalis of males is rare in childhood. Primary infection, manifest by a cluster of tiny vesicles surrounding a reddened meatus, has been described. In recurrences, clusters of small erosions (eroded vesicles) appear on the glans or corona, sometimes associated with typical herpetic vesicles on the shaft.

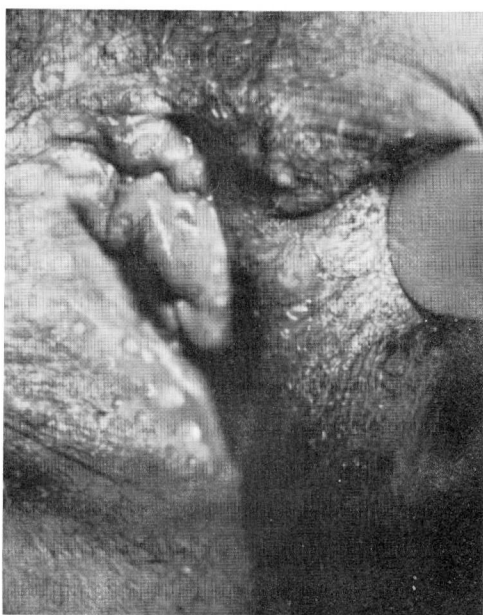

Figure 10-77. Primary herpetic vulvovaginitis. Note the similarity of the lesions to those of herpetic gingivostomatitis. (From Scott, Coriell, Blank and Burgoon: *J. Pediat.*, Vol. 41.)

Lesions of the Eye

Conjunctivitis and keratoconjunctivitis may occur as manifestations of either a primary or a recurrent infection. The conjunctiva appears congested and swollen with little, if any, purulent discharge. In the primary infection the preauricular node is enlarged and tender.

Corneal lesions may be superficial in the form of a dendritic ulcer, or deep, as a disciform keratitis. The diagnosis is suggested by the presence of herpetic vesicles of the lids and established by the isolation of the virus. The primary nature of the attack can be confirmed by demonstrating a rise in circulating antibodies after recovery. The highly contagious *epidemic keratoconjunctivitis* (shipyard conjunctivitis) due to adenovirus type 8 must be considered in the differential diagnosis.

Meningoencephalitis

See page 689.

GENERAL FEATURES OF HERPETIC INFECTIONS

Etiology.   *Herpesvirus hominis* is a DNA-containing virus. Each particle (virion) is 100 to 170 millimicrons in diameter and is made up of 162 capsomeres surrounded by an envelope derived from the host. The virus readily infects rabbits, guinea pigs, hamsters and mice; suckling mice are especially susceptible. It produces small superficial pocks on the chorio-allantoic membrane of the embryonated hen's egg and characteristic cytopathic changes in a variety of cells growing in monolayer tissue cultures. Two strains are recognized from biologic and antigenic characteristics: type 1 which commonly infects skin and mucous membranes, and type 2, which infects primarily the genitalia.

Epidemiology.   This virus is a parasite of man, which has developed an extremely compatible relationship with its host. In the majority of instances (approximately 85 per cent) the infection is subclinical; even when clinical manifestations are present, the host is only rarely disabled or killed. Under exceptional circumstances the primary infection may lead to institutional or family outbreaks of stomatitis. *The spread of infection appears to be determined in large measure by 2 factors: trauma and close bodily contact.* Prior to the onset of symptoms there is often a history or implication of trauma to the site such as teething, or a break in the skin. Since trauma decreases production of interferon in infected guinea pigs, the clinical manifestations may be the result of the combination of incidental seeding of the virus and depressed body defenses. Close bodily contact is common among young children. The overcrowding and lack of hygiene which exist among disadvantaged and primitive peoples results in extensive, up to 100 per cent, spread among children within the first 6 years or so of life. With improvement of living standards, the incidence of infection among children decreases with a consequent increase in the proportion of susceptible adults, among whom clinical manifestations of primary infection may be expected. The newborn infants of these adults will also be susceptible.

Once infected, the majority of people continue to carry the virus in an occult state and maintain an almost constant level of circulating antibodies. It has been shown that the level of antibodies may fall after a primary infection, and that several subclinical reinfections may occur before a stable antibody level is established. Carriers may distribute virus without the presence of a manifest lesion. The asymptomatic carrier is more common among children 7 months to 2 years of age than among adults.

Pathology.   The pathologic changes vary with the tissue infected. In general, a specific lesion is characterized by the presence of intranuclear inclusion bodies. These are homogeneous masses lying in the midst of a severely disorganized nucleus in which the basichromatin has marginated to the nuclear membrane. In the area of the specific lesion there is always evidence of an acute inflammatory reaction. In the skin and mucous membranes the typical lesion is a unilocular vesicle. This is formed by breakdown of epidermal cells which have undergone ballooning degeneration. In the skin the vesicle is tense; the roof is formed by the outer cells of the prickle layer and the keratinized cells beyond. Ballooned epithelial cells containing intranuclear inclusions can best be seen at the margins of the vesicle. The vesicular fluid contains infected epithelial cells, including multinucleated "virus" giant cells and leukocytes. In the corium there is no necrosis, but capillaries are dilated and there is infiltration with mononuclear and polymorphonuclear cells. In the mucous membrane, owing to maceration, there is early leakage of the vesicular fluid, resulting in a collapsed vesicle, mainly filled with fibrin. The edematous roof cells form a gray membrane over the lesion. In the brain there are petechial hemorrhages and some areas of necrosis in the cortex and subcortical white matter; in the meninges there are congestion and infiltration with mononuclear cells. There is vascular engorgement with perivascular cuffing by lymphocytes. In disseminated herpes, in addition to the changes in the central nervous system, interstitial pneumonitis, adrenal hemorrhage and focal necrosis of liver, spleen, kidneys and bone marrow occur. At the edges of the necrotic areas infected cells with intranuclear inclusions can be found; these are rare in brain lesions.

Clinical Laboratory Data.   No specific diagnostic aid is obtained from laboratory examinations, other than from viral tests (p. 543). There is a moderate polymorphonuclear leukocytosis in acute herpetic gingivostomatitis, eczema herpeticum and meningoencephalitis. In meningoencephalitis there is a cellular increase in the cerebrospinal fluid up to about 1000 cells per mm.[3], most of which are lymphocytes; the protein level is elevated, and the sugar is within the normal range. Characteristic giant cells may be found in scrapings from fresh lesions of the skin or mucous membrane.

Diagnosis. The diagnosis is based on any two of the following: (1) a typical clinical pattern; (2) isolation of the virus; (3) development of specific neutralizing antibodies; (4) demonstration of characteristic cells or histologic changes in scrapings or biopsy material.

Course and Prognosis. Primary infection with the herpes virus is a self-limited disease, usually lasting 1 to 2 weeks. Fatalities may occur in the newborn infant, in older infants with severe malnutrition and in patients with meningoencephalitis or severe eczema herpeticum; otherwise the prognosis is usually good. There may be frequent recurrent attacks, but they seldom cause more than a temporary inconvenience except in the eye, where they may eventually cause scarring of the cornea and blindness.

Treatment. The treatment of the ocular manifestations should be in the hands of a skilled ophthalmologist. The antiviral agent, thymidine analogue, 5-iodo-2'-deoxyuridine (IDU) is an effective local agent. It is applied as drops at hourly intervals during the day and at 2-hour intervals during the night. Approximately 80 per cent of the superficial infections respond favorably, but deep lesions usually do not. Other antiviral agents are becoming available for the treatment of strains resistant to IDU, such as cytosine arabinoside (CA), which is quite toxic, methylaminodeoxyuridine (MADU), which has low potency, and 5-trifluoromethyl-2'-deoxyuridine (F_3TDR), which appears to be nontoxic and potent. *Corticosteroids must not be used in the acute stage*, since corneal perforation may follow, but they may be valuable in patients with keratitis disciformis, probably a manifestation of hypersensitivity, if used in conjunction with one of the foregoing antiviral agents.

The thymidine analogue is useful in the treatment of cutaneous lesions only when injected by compressed air (e.g. Dermajet) or applied in dimethyl sulfoxide. It has also been used in therapy of herpetic encephalitis and neonatal infection.

Apart from this specific therapy, symptomatic and supportive therapy is of great importance. In infants especially, eczema herpeticum and stomatitis may lead to severe dehydration, shock and hypoproteinemia, requiring replacement of fluids, electrolytes and proteins.

Care of the mouth demands cleanliness by oral lavage; Ceepryn 1:4000 or Zephiran 1:1000 may be useful. Local analgesics, such as viscous Xylocaine or Benzocaine lozenges may allay pain and enable the older child to eat. A mouthwash with tetracycline (250 mg. in 30 to 60 ml. of water) is helpful in controlling pain. Analgesics should be used systemically as required. Antibiotics are useful only in the treatment of secondary bacterial infections.

The intake of food and fluid will be facilitated by acquiescing to the child's whims. Ice-cold fluids or semisolids are often accepted when other food is refused. Frequent recurrences are often due to emotional stress, which must be recognized and treated.

Neonatal infections may be treated by prophylactic cesarean section in presence of maternal genital infection. Otherwise, intravenous IDU (600 mg. per kg. per day) for five or more days is indicated despite its toxicity. Gammaglobulin (0.5 to 1.0 ml. per kg.) should also be given.

Prophylaxis. All newborn infants and infants and children with eczema should be kept from contact with manifest herpetic infection.

REFERENCES

Dowdle, W. R., Nahmias, A. J., Harwell, R. W., and Pauls, F. P.: Association of Antigenic Types of Herpesvirus Hominis with Site of Viral Recovery. *J. Immunol.*, 99:974, 1967.

Kaufman, H. E.: Chemotherapy of Herpesvirus Infections. 1st International Conference on Vaccines Against Viral and Rickettsial Diseases of Man. Pan American Health Organization, Pan American Sanitary Bureau, Regional Office of the World Health Organization, Washington, D.C., 1967, p. 604.

Nahamias, A. J., and Dowdle, W. R.: Antigenic and Biologic Differences in Herpesvirus Hominus. *Prog. Med. Vir.*, 10, 110, 1968.

Partridge, J. W., and Millis, Rosemary R.: Systemic Herpes Simplex Infection in a Newborn Treated with Intravenous Idoxuridine. *Arch. Dis. Childh.*, 43:377, 1968.

Scott, T. F., McNair, and Tokumaru, T.: The Herpesvirus Group; in F. L. Horsfall, Jr. and I. Tamm (Eds.): *Viral and Rickettsial Infections of Man.* 4th ed. Philadelphia, J. B. Lippincott Company, 1965, p. 892.

White, J. G.: Fulminating Infection with Herpes Simplex Virus in Premature and Newborn Infants. *New England J. Med.*, 269:455, 1963.

VARICELLA AND HERPES ZOSTER

Since the observations of Bokay (1888) there have been frequent reports that exposure of susceptible persons to a patient with herpes zoster could result in the acquisition of chickenpox. The work of Weller and his co-workers confirmed the impression that these 2 diseases are different clinical manifestations of the same causative agent.

Etiology. The common causative agent is now designated as *Herpesvirus varicellae*. The structure of viral particles as seen under the electron microscope is indistinguishable from that of *Herpesvirus hominis*. Each agent can be grown in a variety of primary cultures of human tissues, and each produces an identical focal area of cytologic changes. Either agent will produce chickenpox in human volunteers, and neither can be transmitted to lower animals or grown in the embryonated hen's egg. Serum antibodies in patients recovering from varicella react equally with the agents derived from varicella and herpes zoster vesicles.

The reasons for different clinical manifestations

of the 2 diseases are not understood. It seems probable that varicella is the primary response of a susceptible host, whereas herpes zoster may be the response of partial immunity when a latent infection is activated by some exogenous factor, e.g. stress, trauma, malignancy or x-radiation.

Pathology. The *skin lesions* of both diseases are identical and characteristic of the herpesvirus group and cannot be distinguished from those of *Herpesvirus hominis* (herpes simplex) (see p. 633). Although not usual in cases of average severity, necrosis with hemorrhage can be found in the mucous membranes of the mouth, trachea, esophagus and intestine.

Internally, the lesions vary somewhat in the 2 diseases. In fatal cases of *varicella* intranuclear inclusions can be found in the endothelium of the blood vessels; the vessel walls may undergo necrosis. Intranuclear inclusions have also been found in most organs of the body, including the salivary glands, the nervous system, and in the cells of the myenteric plexus of the stomach and intestine. In the brain perivenous demyelination is similar to that of other postinfectious encephalitides; necrosis of nerve cells and leptomeningitis have been described.

In *herpes zoster* the characteristic lesions are in the nervous system, particularly in the dorsal root ganglia. Early in the disease the cells of the dorsal ganglia of the affected dermatome contain intranuclear inclusions. Shortly thereafter the ganglia show only necrosis of cells, sometimes associated with hemorrhage. As the disease progresses evidence of inflammation and degeneration is found in the posterior roots and in the peripheral portions of the nerves. Unilateral and segmental necrosis of the nerve cells in the posterior horn may be found (*cf.* poliomyelitis, which involves the nerve cells of the anterior horn). Leptomeningitis occurs in the region of the involved nerves. Intranuclear inclusions have been found in the sympathetic ganglia, the neurilemma cells of the nerve twigs in the corium and in the myenteric plexus, and, in visceral herpes, in the walls of the bladder and other viscera.

VARICELLA
(Chickenpox)

Varicella is characterized by the appearance on the skin and mucous membranes of successive crops of typical vesicles generally accompanied by a mild constitutional reaction. Chickenpox, the term derived from *cicer* (chick-pea), was clearly distinguished from smallpox in 1767 by William Heberden.

Epidemiology. Varicella is extremely contagious, and therefore its incidence is mainly during childhood. It can occur at any age, including the neonatal period. The disease can be transmitted by direct contact or be airborne in the form of droplet nuclei. Air disinfection by ultraviolet light can materially decrease the spread of the disease. Epidemics of chickenpox have been initiated by exposure to herpes zoster. Patients are infectious from 24 hours before to 6 or 7 days after the eruption, at which time the vesicles have dried up. Scabs do not appear to be infectious. Second attacks are exceedingly rare.

Clinical Manifestations. The incubation period varies from 11 to 21 days, and is between 13 and 17 days in the majority of instances. At the end of the incubation period prodromal symptoms, except in the mildest cases, precede the characteristic rash by 24 hours. There may be slight fever, malaise or anorexia, accompanied at times by a scarlatiniform or morbilliform rash. It is characteristic of the specific rash to appear rapidly. Typically, it begins as crops of small, red papules which almost immediately develop into clear, often oval, "teardrop" vesicles on an erythematous base. These vesicles are usually not umbilicated. The contents become cloudy within about 24 hours. The vesicles are easily broken and become scabbed. Occasionally they dry before becoming cloudy. Except for the mildest cases in which few lesions occur, crops of widely scattered vesicles continue to erupt for 3 or 4 days, starting on the trunk and later spreading to the face and scalp, with minimal, if any, involvement of distal parts of the extremities. There is some tendency for the lesions to be concentrated in areas of skin pressure or irritation, but not to the same extent as in smallpox. Characteristically, at the height of the disease the eruption consists of papules, early and late vesicles, and crusts present at the same time (Fig. 10-78, p. 629). Rarely in severe disease the lesions appear as hard, pearly lumps mostly at the same stage of development and resemble those of smallpox. Pruritus is a constant and annoying characteristic of the rash. Vesicles may also be found on mucous surfaces and are common in the mouth, where they may resemble the lesions of herpetic stomatitis. Less commonly, lesions are found on the genital mucous membranes and on the conjunctiva and the cornea, where they are potentially dangerous to sight. Laryngeal involvement is rare. There may be generalized lymphadenopathy.

The severity of the disease varies from a few lesions with little evidence of systemic illness to many hundreds of lesions, and extreme toxicity with temperatures ranging from 103 to 105° F. Systemic manifestations occur only during the first 3 to 4 days, when the rash is erupting.

Infrequently the rash becomes hemorrhagic in association with a mild to severe thrombocytopenia. The more severe forms usually occur with other complications such as pneumonia or in patients receiving immunosuppressive therapy. Purpura fulminans, which occurs about the end of the first week associated with gangrene, probably represents a Shwartzman-like reaction.

Varicella bullosa is an uncommon variant in which many of the lesions appear as bullae instead of vesicles. The course of the disease is not changed.

Congenital varicella may be manifest at birth

or appear within a few days in infants whose mothers have an active infection. Such infections are usually fatal; in contrast, infections acquired postnatally by young infants are usually mild.

Laboratory Data. There may be a mild leukocytosis. Virus giant cells (see Herpes Simplex, p. 637) can be demonstrated in scrapings from the floors of fresh vesicles.

Diagnosis. This is not difficult in the average case. Most important is the distinction between chickenpox and smallpox, which may be exceedingly difficult in patients with mild smallpox or severe chickenpox. The following clinical points should be borne in mind: (1) The rash of chickenpox begins on the trunk and spreads toward the periphery, whereas that of smallpox tends to spread from the periphery toward the trunk. (2) The lesions of smallpox tend to be most frequent in areas of pressure or tightness of the skin, as over the bridge of the nose and the wrist or at the belt line, whereas those of chickenpox do not have this tendency to the same extent. (3) The lesions of chickenpox are more superficial and are not umbilicated, whereas the lesions of smallpox tend to be deeper and more "shotty" to the touch and are usually umbilicated. (4) The lesions of chickenpox are present in all stages of development at a given time, whereas those of smallpox are more or less in the same stage at each phase of the disease. (5) The prodromal symptoms of chickenpox are short (1 to 2 days) and usually mild; those of smallpox are longer (3 to 4 days) and may be severe with high fever which drops with the appearance of the rash.

Complications. These are rare, but infections such as erysipelas, ecthyma or furuncles may follow scratching. Hemorrhage into the skin may occur (see above); internal hemorrhage from ulcerations or into an adrenal may be fatal. Lesions in the larynx may lead to obstructive edema, and corneal infection can result in uveokeratitis. Interstitial pneumonitis, myocarditis, pericarditis, nephritis and acute myositis of the limb muscles have been described. Postinfectious encephalitis is the most common neurologic complication (see p. 695), acute cerebellar ataxia being a common manifestation; other lesions include the Guillain-Barré syndrome, transverse myelitis, facial nerve palsy, optic neuritis with transient loss of vision, and the hypothalamic syndrome with obesity and recurrent fever.

Patients who contract chickenpox during long-term therapy with corticosteroids may, but usually do not, have a prolonged and complicated course. Patients at particular risk are those with leukemia who are receiving a corticosteroid or one of the antimetabolites; in such instances the disease is often fatal.

Prognosis. The prognosis is usually good; fatalities occur from the complications.

Treatment. There is no specific treatment. Symptomatic treatment should be directed to alleviating itching by the use of systemic antipruritic agents and sedation as required. Scratch-

ing should be minimized by use of mittens and keeping the nails short. Daily changes of clothes and linen and antiseptic baths will reduce the incidence of secondary bacterial infection. If secondary infection occurs, systemic antibiotic therapy is indicated.

For patients acutely ill with pneumonitis, pharmacologic doses of a corticosteroid and oxygen are urgently indicated. In contrast, for those being treated for a chronic disease with steroid therapy, the dose should be decreased to little more than physiologic requirements if there is exposure to varicella or if the disease is contracted.

Prophylaxis. There is no proved and generally applicable method of prophylaxis. Pooled gamma globulin in a dose of 1.4 ml. per kg. is said to decrease the severity of the subsequent disease, if given within 3 days of exposure. An experimental varicella-zoster gamma globulin derived from serum drawn from donors at the height of antibody response (2 to 3 weeks after onset of herpes zoster) and injected intramuscularly in a dose of 0.1 ml. per kg. within 3 days of exposure appears to be effective in preventing chickenpox. Similarly obtained blood group compatible serum (2 to 4 ml. per kg.) may be used intravenously, but the risk of the disease must be balanced against the risk of hepatitis transmitted by the serum. These preparations should be reserved for use in *susceptible* patients who are at high risk, e.g. premature infants or patients with leukemia or nephrosis who are receiving immunosuppressive therapy or adrenal corticosteroids.

HERPES ZOSTER
(SHINGLES)

Herpes zoster is an acute infection characterized by crops of vesicles, usually confined to a dermatome and by neuralgic pain in the area of the affected dermatome.

Epidemiology. Herpes zoster is relatively uncommon under 10 years of age, after which its incidence increases steadily with each succeeding decade. Second attacks are rare, less than 1 per cent in one study of 206 patients. The patient with herpes zoster usually has a history of having had varicella. When this is not the case, the possibilities must be considered that a mild case of varicella may have been misdiagnosed or that there had been exposure in the neonatal period which resulted in clinically unrecognized disease. The severity of the disease increases with age. There is no sex or race predilection.

Clinical Manifestations. Herpes zoster has a pre-eruptive and a posteruptive phase. In the last days of the incubation period, which appears to be from 7 to 21 days, the patient usually has pain and tenderness along the involved dermatome. There is often generalized malaise and fever. Within a few days groups of red papules appear distributed along 1 or 2 adjacent dermatomes; the individual lesions quickly vesiculate (Fig.

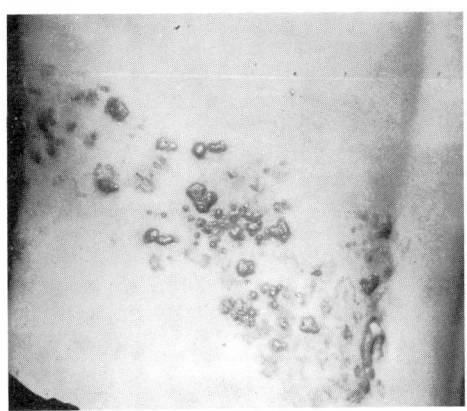

Figure 10-79. Herpes zoster. (Courtesy of Dr. Carroll S. Wright.)

10-79), become pustular, dry up and scab in the course of 5 to 10 days. The lesions tend to appear first at a point nearest the central nervous system. Successive crops of lesions continue to appear for 7 days, extending along the course of the nerve. The eruption clears in 7 to 14 days in most patients under 20 years of age, but when vesicles continue to appear for 7 days, healing may be delayed up to 5 weeks. The lesions, except in rare instances, are unilateral. Fever, pain and tenderness usually continue throughout the period of progression. The regional lymph nodes are invariably enlarged. Although the dermatomes of the second dorsal to the second lumbar nerves are the commonest sites under the age of 20 years, cephalic zoster and infection of the sacral nerves, producing lesions of the leg and genitalia, do occur in children. Transient paralysis of the affected part is a rare complication.

When there is infection of the fifth nerve, any or several of its branches may be affected; with involvement of the ophthalmic branch, lesions may appear over the forehead with local loss of hair, on the tip of the nose and on the cornea (herpes ophthalmicus, Fig. 10-80 [p. 628]), over the cheek and the homolateral palate, with infection of the maxillary branch, and over the homolateral mandible and tongue when the mandibular branch is affected. Infection of the seventh nerve or the geniculate ganglion results in the *Ramsay Hunt syndrome* of paralysis of the facial nerve and vesicles in the external ear canal.

A generalized rash may accompany herpes zoster; this tends to occur in elderly patients, but may occur in children who have had a mild attack of varicella in early infancy. Occasionally in children the first vesicles of varicella may be distributed along a dermatome.

Laboratory Data. Examination of the cerebrospinal fluid often reveals a mild lymphocytosis. Scrapings of the floors of vesicles in their initial stage contain virus giant cells (see Herpes Simplex, p. 637).

Diagnosis. Diagnosis may be difficult before development of the rash; the pain may resemble

that of pleural, cardiac or peritoneal origin, depending on the site of the lesion. Once the rash has appeared, its distribution and characteristics along with the pain make the diagnosis relatively simple. Occasionally, herpes simplex may simulate the distribution of zoster.

Course and Prognosis. In children the course is usually mild, and the ultimate prognosis is good.

Complications. Postherpetic pain does not occur in children. Keratitis and uveitis may follow fifth nerve involvement, and secondary bacterial infection is possible in any of the lesions.

Treatment. There is no specific therapy. Prednisone, approximately 1 mg. per kg. per day, has been reported to control pain and to shorten the course of the disease. In zoster ophthalmicus the treatment should be directed by an ophthalmologist. Otherwise treatment consists in preventing, as far as possible, secondary bacterial infection by cleanliness and prevention of scratching (see Varicella). If infection has occurred, suitable antimicrobial therapy should be considered. Pain, seldom a serious problem in children, can usually be controlled with aspirin and codeine.

Prophylaxis. The possibility that herpes zoster may follow exposure to chickenpox should be kept in mind. Conversely, since chickenpox can follow exposure to herpes zoster, it is unwise to admit to an open ward a child suffering from the latter disease.

REFERENCES

Burgoon, C. F., Burgoon, J. S., and Baldridge, G. D.: The Natural History of Herpes Zoster. *J.A.M.A.,* 164:265, 1957.

Charkes, N. D.: Purpuric Chickenpox. *Ann. Int. Med..* 54:745, 1961.

Elliot, F. A.: Treatment of Herpes Zoster with High Doses of Prednisone. *Lancet,* 2:610, 1964.

Weller, T. H.: Varicella-Herpes Zoster Virus; in Horsfall, F. L., Jr., and Tamm, I. (Eds.): *Viral & Rickettsial Infections of Man.* 4th ed. Philadelphia, J. B. Lippincott Company, 1965, p. 915.

SMALLPOX
(VARIOLA)

Smallpox is an acute communicable viral disease characterized by a papulovesicular, pustular rash and usually by severe systemic symptoms.

Etiology. There appear to be 2 stable types of virus, variola major and variola minor, which can usually be distinguished by the severity of the disease they cause. They can be dried under relatively unfavorable conditions and remain viable for months, e.g. in house dust. The virus particles, studied in the form of the identical-appearing vaccinia virus, are the prototypes of the poxvirus group. Under the electron microscope the particles are roughly rectangular, measuring 300 by 250 millimicrons. There is a dense central region 100 to 150 millimicrons across. On or near the surface is a complex network of filamentous structures, 6 to 8 millimicrons in diameter, resembling a loose ball of yarn; some particles have an envelope. The nucleic acid is DNA. The virus grows on a variety of mammalian cells in tissue culture; it grows readily on the chorio-allantoic membrane, where it produces small pocks similar to those of herpes simplex. In the rabbit it produces a keratoconjunctivitis after corneal inoculation (Paul's test).

Epidemiology. The disease is readily transmitted to susceptibles, probably by way of the respiratory tract. Fomites and letters can also spread the disease. The finding of elementary bodies in the crusts of lesions and on the bedclothes of a patient supports the airborne theory. No age or sex is immune, but the colored races appear to be more susceptible than the white. If the pregnant woman becomes infected, abortion commonly results, or, depending on the stage of pregnancy, the fetus may be infected in utero or the infection may be acquired during or after birth. Second attacks are extremely rare. Smallpox epizootics in monkeys have been reported in association with epidemics in man, and the virus can be transmitted to this host experimentally.

The great danger of dissemination is from mild sporadic cases which may go unrecognized or be misdiagnosed as chickenpox, or from patients with severe hemorrhagic disease who die before they exhibit the characteristic rash. Laboratory assistance should be sought whenever there is suspicion of smallpox.

Pathology. Specific changes are found in the skin, mucous membranes and many of the organs. The typical skin lesion starts with changes in the capillaries of the corium and is characterized by dilatation, endothelial proliferation and perivascular mononuclear infiltration. In the adjacent epidermis the cells of the middle and upper stratum spinosum swell, and the characteristic Guarnieri bodies make their appearance. These are spherical bodies lying close to the nucleus, consisting of collections of virus elementary bodies, and range in size from 2 to 8 microns; in rare instances intranuclear inclusions may be found. The swollen cells rupture, forming a vesicle divided into lobulations by thin septums of partially ruptured cellular membranes and thicker septums formed of the resistant ducts of sweat glands. The lower layer of the stratum spinosum and the basal layer beneath the growing vesicle also degenerate, and the vesicle eventually reaches the corium. The basal cells at the margin of the vesicle proliferate, leading to an increase in the thickness of the epidermis over that of the vesiculating portion. This gives rise to the early umbilication which is accentuated when the vesiculation surrounds a hair follicle. Umbilication disappears as the fluid increases, but reappears as desiccation and crusting begin. Healing occurs without scarring except on the face, where necrosis of sebaceous glands characteristically occurs, and in other areas where there has been secondary bacterial infection.

In the squamous epithelium of the upper diges-tive tract, changes occur coincidentally with those of the skin and consist initially in localized and then diffuse necrosis of the superficial cells and congestion and hemorrhage in the tunica propria. Grossly, these lead to the appearance of a diffuse pseudomembrane in the pharynx by the third or fourth day which disappears without scarring by the third week. The kidneys reveal the changes of interstitial nephritis. Orchitis occurs during the papulovesicular stage and consists in hyperplasia of the vascular endothelium followed in order by necrosis of the interstitial cells and of those of the seminiferous tubules; in boys the lesions resemble ischemic infarctions. There are hemorrhages in bone marrow in all types of smallpox; the megakaryocytes are profuse except in hemorrhagic smallpox, in which they are decreased. Small hemorrhages and mononuclear infiltrates may be found in other organs.

Clinical Manifestations. The incubation period is usually 12 to 14 days, but may be as long as 21 days in previously vaccinated persons and in variola minor.

Variola major. In a typical case the prodromal symptoms are severe and usually start abruptly. The initial clinical manifestations include headache, chills or chilliness, aching of the back and limbs, and fever, which mounts rapidly to 106 or 107°F. In children there may also be vomiting, drowsiness, convulsions or coma. Often delirium occurs, and the patient is prostrated.

During the first 2 days transient rashes are common, which may resemble scarlet fever or measles or may be petechial. They tend to be most prominent over the upper thighs and buttocks and disappear rapidly by the third or fourth day, when the raised macules of the typical cutaneous lesion begin to appear over the face. Widespread prodromal rashes and the early appearance of macules presage a severe attack.

There is usually diminution in severity of symptoms as the rash becomes papular, and the temperature may even become normal and remain so until the pustular stage. The individual lesions appear in a single crop and progress at the same rate, unlike the multiple crops in chickenpox. Initially the papules are 2 to 4 mm. in diameter and are firm and "shotty." Within about 24 hours the size of the papules increases, and vesicles appear. They tend to be umbilicated in the early and again in the late stages. Some of the vesicles are superficial, and others deeper and less readily recognized. A small red areola encircles each vesicle.

About the fifth or sixth day of the disease the vesicles become cloudy, and the pustular stage begins. The individual lesion is greenish or grayish-yellow and has an elevation slightly greater than its diameter. About the ninth day of the disease the lesions begin to dry, and the areolas disappear. They are usually crusted over by the end of the second week, and the scabs drop off about the end of the third or fourth week. The scabs persist longest on the palms and soles, where

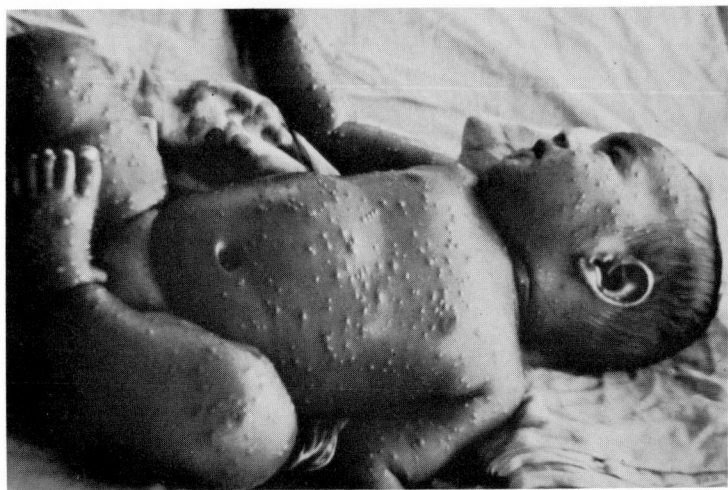

Figure 10-81. Variola in an unvaccinated infant. (Courtesy of Dr. Roger Feldman.)

they are known as "seeds," and may have to be enucleated with a needle.

The cutaneous areas chiefly involved in the early stages are those where the skin is tight, such as the wrists and the prominences of the face; the more exposed extensor surfaces of the forearms and upper arms are then involved, leaving the more protected flexor surfaces and the axilla relatively free. The rash then spreads to the chest. In severe cases the abdomen and the legs are heavily covered; in milder cases they may be only slightly involved. Concurrently with the skin lesions, the mucous membranes of the mouth, eyes and often the larynx become affected.

A striking feature of the disease, in contrast to chickenpox, is the profusion of lesions on the face, including the lips, and the presence of a relatively large number of lesions on the palms and soles. When the lesions become confluent, there is considerable edema of the face, so that there is difficulty in closing the eyes and mouth. The lesions on the mucous membranes also tend to be confluent. Scarring, greatest on the face, results from necrosis of sebaceous glands and is not greatly influenced by secondary infection. Intense pigmentation of the skin persists for a variable time after the scabs have fallen. In the fatal cases death usually occurs during the second week of the disease.

Hemorrhagic smallpox may occur in 2 forms: *vesicular hemorrhagic smallpox,* in which hemorrhages occur in the corium after the development of vesicles, and *"true hemorrhagic* or *black smallpox,"* in which a diffuse hemorrhagic rash begins on the second or third day of prodromal symptoms, followed by ecchymoses and hemorrhages into the mucous membranes. In the latter form the temperature may be subnormal, although the symptoms are severe. Death may occur before the characteristic rash of smallpox develops.

Variola minor (alastrim). This form differs from variola major chiefly in being less severe and rarely causing death. It apparently breeds true

and never develops into variola major; it is thought by some to be a distinct disease entity.

Varioloid. Smallpox modified by previous vaccination is usually termed "varioloid." Although varioloid lesions appear in a single crop and progress in a manner similar to those of more severe smallpox, they are entirely discrete, and the prodromal symptoms are mild. There is no secondary rise of temperature, and premature involution of many of the lesions occurs.

Abortive type. In persons who have been vaccinated shortly before exposure to smallpox a condition known as "variola sine eruptione" may occur. Macules or papules may involute with great rapidity, or there may be no eruption at all, and the patient has only a mild, febrile illness.

Laboratory Data. A neutropenia is characteristic of the early stages of the disease. In hemorrhagic smallpox this may be associated with a reduction of platelets. Large lymphocytes are characteristically present in small numbers. During the pustular stage a polymorphonuclear leukocytosis occurs. There is prolongation of the prothrombin time and a decrease in fibrinogen associated with the hemorrhagic type, probably dependent on extensive liver damage.

Diagnosis. The typical case of smallpox is readily diagnosed, but mild cases may be misdiagnosed as chickenpox, or missed altogether. In a doubtful case the patient should be isolated and viral studies obtained (see Diagnosis of varicella, p. 640).

Complications. Pyogenic infections of the skin and bacteremia, particularly with the streptococcus, were common before the availability of antibacterial agents. An enanthem of the larynx may lead to edema of the glottis and perichondritis of the laryngeal cartilages. Bronchopneumonia is relatively common. Viral osteomyelitis occurs occasionally in children and usually appears between the tenth and twentieth days of the disease. Multiple joints as well as bones are commonly infected, but severe systemic symptoms are not related to this involvement. Roentgenographic changes of bone destruction may be seen as early as the fourth day after onset of swelling and slight tenderness. Serious deformities such as flail joints, ankylosis, malformed bones and cessation of bone growth are common sequels. Central nervous system involvement is rare; symptoms usually begin 5 to 13 days after the appearance of the rash and resemble those of other postinfectious encephalomyelitides (see p. 695).

Prognosis. The case fatality rate varies with the type of the disease and the age of the patient. The rate during epidemics of variola minor is less than 1 per cent, whereas an overall rate of about 10 per cent may be expected in epidemics of variola major. The case fatality rate is considered to be about 5 to 6 per cent in discrete smallpox, 60 per cent in confluent smallpox and 80 per cent or over in hemorrhagic smallpox. The mortality rate is greatest in children under 5 and in persons over 45 years of age.

Treatment. No effective specific therapy is available once the disease has developed. Symptomatic treatment and nursing care are of extreme importance. The patient's room should be light and well ventilated; some odor-killing device is desirable. Severe cases of confluent and hemorrhagic smallpox should be treated for shock and dehydration by proper use of intravenous fluids, blood and plasma. Appropriate antibiotics in therapeutic doses should be used in severe disease when secondary bacterial infection is identified or suspected. Nutrition must be maintained, by tube feeding if necessary. Lesions of the eyes require frequent irrigation; this therapy should be supervised by an ophthalmologist. Crusts in the nose may be loosened with swabs moistened with oil. Sedation should be given as indicated. In the milder cases the general methods of treatment as outlined under Chickenpox are adequate (p. 640).

Prophylaxis. General prophylaxis of the population can be maintained only by adequate vaccination. If an inadequately vaccinated person is exposed to smallpox, vaccination alone may not prevent the disease. Hyperimmune vaccinia gamma globulin given at the time of vaccination raises the protection rate fourfold; Marboran (N-methylisatin beta-thiosemicarbazone) raises the protection rate sixteenfold. The drug is given orally as a 10 or 20 per cent suspension in syrup in doses of 3.0 gm. twice daily after meals for 4 days. There may be nausea and vomiting if the drug is not given after meals.

Patients should be strictly isolated until all the crusts have dropped off. Fomites, books, letters, and the like, must be sterilized, preferably by heat.

In the public health management of a smallpox epidemic the following steps, scrupulously enforced, can usually be relied on to control the spread of the disease, without mass vaccination: (1) listing of contacts; (2) surveillance of contacts for 3 weeks for any evidence of illness; (3) vaccination of contacts, preferably within 24 hours of exposure. Vaccination must produce reliable evidence of a take, and must be repeated if negative or doubtful.

REFERENCES

Bauer, D. J., St. Vincent, L., Kempe, C. H., and Downie, A. W.: Prophylactic Treatment of Smallpox Contacts with N-Methylisatin β-Thiosemicarbazone. *Lancet,* 2:494, 1963.

Bras, G.: The Morbid Anatomy of Smallpox. *Docum. Med. Geog. et Trop.,* 4:303, 1952.

Cockshott, P., and MacGregor, M.: The Natural History of Osteomyelitis Variolosa. *J. Fac. Radiologists,* 10:57, 1959.

Dixon, C. W.: *Smallpox.* London, J. & A. Churchill, 1962.

Downie, A. W.: Poxvirus Group; in F. L. Horsfall, Jr., and I. Tamm (Eds.): *Viral and Rickettsial Infections in Man.* 4th ed. Philadelphia, J. B. Lippincott Company, 1965, Chap. 44, p. 932.

Horne, R. W., and Wildy, P.: Virus Structures Revealed by Negative Staining. *Advances in Virus Research,* 10:101, 1963.

Kempe, C. H., and others: The Use of Vaccinia Hyperimmune Gamma Globulin in the Prophylaxis of Smallpox. *Bull. W.H.O.,* 25:41, 1961.

VACCINATION AGAINST SMALLPOX

The use of cowpox virus for vaccination against smallpox was the first successful development of a method for the protection of human beings against a serious epidemic disease. Although used by Benjamin Jesty, a Dorsetshire farmer, in 1774 to protect his own family, it was Dr. Edward Jenner in 1798 who conclusively proved that the inoculation of human beings with material from cowpox led to immunity to smallpox. Cowpox and variola belong to the "pox" group of viruses which affect many species of animals, each animal having its own specific pox infection which as a rule is not transmissible to another host. Cowpox, however, is sufficiently related to the human "pox" virus, variola, that it can and does affect man with a specific disease of the skin of the hands on close contact. The stable pox virus of vaccinia may have been derived from hybridization between variola and cowpox viruses. In the laboratory such hybrids resemble the virus of vaccinia and could have occurred from documented early accidental contamination of vaccine virus batches with variola virus. The great diversity of vaccine strains that exist at present may also be the result of the past practice of mixing different strains of vaccinia virus in order to produce an effective vaccine.

Age at Initial Vaccination. Although vaccination can be performed in the neonatal period, in nonendemic areas it is preferable to perform vaccination between the ages of 1 and 3 years. Statistical evidence indicates that the lowest incidence of complications is during these years. Vaccination should be considered a routine procedure in healthy children; most states in the United States require evidence of vaccination before entrance into school. The likelihood of exposure to smallpox, however, must be weighed against the risks of the procedure when there is any question about the child's health. Vaccination should be avoided, if possible, in young premature infants, in children with or recovering from an illness, and in those with eczema or other skin lesions, including "prickly heat." Contact between a recently vaccinated child and another with eczema must be prevented, or the eczematous contact should be protected by hyperimmune gamma globulin. Elective vaccination is contraindicated for children with known immunologic defects and in those receiving immunosuppressive drugs, and also for pregnant women.

Type of Vaccine. The usual type of vaccine is obtained from the pulp of vesicles of vaccinated calves, which is diluted 1:5 in 50 per cent glycerin-saline solution containing 1 per cent phenol. It is distributed in capillary glass tubes. The marketed vaccine is not completely free of bacteria; by law, it must contain less than 50 bacteria per dose and no pathogens. It is considered potent for 3 months if kept below 5°C.; it deteriorates rapidly at room temperature. Avianized vaccine prepared from vaccinia-infected chorio-allantoic membranes of embryonated hens' eggs is equally effective. Lyophilized dried vaccine which is stable at room temperature is advisable in the tropics or where refrigeration facilities are inadequate. A vaccine for subcutaneous administration, derived from a strain of virus attenuated by passage in chick embryo tissue culture, is now under study. It may prove to be the ideal vaccine for primary vaccination in smallpox-free areas. Revaccination, with its lower incidence of complications, should be with one of the standard vaccines.

Site of Vaccination. Vaccination should be performed on the skin over the insertion of the deltoid muscle or on the posterior axillary fold. The latter site is exposed to a minimum of trauma, and the scars are inconspicuous. Vaccination on the thigh is more exposed to contamination in the infant and proves more incapacitating during the height of the reaction in older persons.

Method of Vaccination. Although there is good evidence that there is direct correlation between protection against the disease and the number and extent of the vaccination scars, the present policy, in nonendemic areas, is to make only one inoculation. Where smallpox is endemic or after exposure, 2 to 4 sites of inoculation are advocated. The technique is as follows:

The skin should be cleansed with a volatile antiseptic, e.g. ether or acetone, care being taken to avoid making abrasions in which the virus could "take." The tube of lymph should be removed from the freezing section of the refrigerator only at the moment of use, the ends broken off after filing, and the contents expressed on the skin by means of a small rubber bulb. Introduction of the virus can be accomplished by one of 2 methods.

1. The *multiple pressure method* is most generally recommended in the United States. The needle is held almost parallel with the skin and the point pressed up and down against the skin through a drop of lymph in such a way that the surface cells are picked off, thus exposing the deeper-growing cells of the epidermis to the virus. Two or 3 pressures over an area of about 1/8 to 1/4 inch in diameter are usually sufficient for primary vaccination after the age of 6 months. In very young infants and for revaccination, 30 pressures are recommended. The area should become erythematous, but should not bleed.

2. The *scratch method* is generally recommended in the British

Isles and consists in making a scratch with a sterile needle through a drop of vaccine lymph. The scratch should be about 1/4 inch long and deep enough to get through the skin without drawing blood.

In each method the lymph is rubbed into the site with the shaft of the needle, the excess wiped off, and the remainder allowed to dry.

Type of Reaction. The reaction to smallpox vaccination is considered to be due to hypersensitivity as well as to the necrotic action of vaccinia virus on the infected cells. The usual reactions vary according to the degree of host sensitivity and are classified as primary, accelerated or vaccinoid, "early" reaction, or no visible reaction.

Primary reaction. This is the reaction of the nonimmune unsensitized person. There is little reaction at the site except a fading erythema until the third to fifth day, when a red, slightly itching papule appears. This rapidly vesiculates within about 24 hours and becomes surrounded by a red areola. The vesicle grows in size, becomes umbilicated and pearly-gray and is surrounded by an increasing area of erythema and induration. The reaction reaches its height about the ninth or tenth day, when the area is hot and tender, the regional lymph nodes are enlarged and painful, and the spleen may be enlarged. There is usually some systemic reaction, which may be mild with low-grade fever, malaise and headache or severe with temperatures of 104°F. or higher for 3 to 4 days. There is little change in the leukocyte count. After the peak of the reaction the vesicle undergoes desiccation, becomes covered with a dark scab which is shed about the twenty-first day. The pink, pitted scar, which slowly fades to white, remains as the only evidence that successful vaccination has been performed.

Vaccinoid or accelerated reaction. This is the reaction of the partially sensitized person. The lesion goes through the same general stages as does the primary take, but more rapidly. The greater the sensitization, the more rapid is the evolution. A papule may become vesiculated within 2 days and reach the peak of its reaction in less than a week. The size of the reaction is smaller than with the primary take, and there are few, if any, general signs or symptoms.

"Early" reaction. This reaction consists of a small area of redness and induration maximal at 8 to 72 hours; a vesicle may or may not be present. It occurs in highly sensitized persons and usually, but not always, indicates immunity. Nevertheless a similar lesion can be produced by inactivated vaccine in such persons, so that they should be revaccinated with a known potent vaccine, if exposed to smallpox.

No reaction. In some persons repeated vaccinations do not result in a local lesion. Poor technique or the use of inactivated virus may explain some of these failures. Obviously such persons should be vaccinated several times with potent vaccine and by an approved technique before it is assumed that they have been immunized. Laboratory tests for neutralizing antibodies will provide definite proof of immunization.

Revaccination. Revaccination is ordinarily indicated every 4 years, but must be performed whenever there is contact with a case of smallpox. In endemic areas revaccination is required at 6- to 12-month intervals. Under these circumstances a positive "take" is of such importance that at least 2 "insertions" should be made. Local skin immunity to vaccination can exist without systemic immunity; hence the site of revaccination should be at a location other than the original one; the forearm appears to be particularly sensitive.

WHO suggests "major" for any reaction present on seventh day and "minor" or "equivoid" for the earlier reactions.

Care of Site of Vaccination. Maintenance of dryness and free flow of air about the vesicle is essential. Shields should never be used. A relatively sterile surface may be maintained on the entire area surrounding the reaction by sponging gently with alcohol at least twice daily, being careful to leave the surface of the vesicle intact. If the vesicle ruptures because of excessive tension or trauma, the area should be sponged with alcohol 3 or 4 times daily and loosely covered with a piece of gauze attached to the skin above and below by adhesive tape placed well outside the indurated area. When the dressing is changed, it should be cut off and the fresh one taped over the original adhesive tapes. These should not be removed until the inflammation has subsided to avoid secondary lesions in the adhesive abraded areas.

COMPLICATIONS

Pyogenic Infections. As a result of scratching or neglect, the vaccination site can become contaminated with various bacterial pathogens, such as staphylococci and streptococci, giving rise to cellulitis, scarlet fever or septicemia. The size of the scar is always increased by such contamination. Vaccine lymph can be contaminated with tetanus spores; however, tetanus has occurred only in the presence of a tight shield or other occlusive dressing.

Abnormal Virus Distribution. *Local.* Transfer of infection to other parts of the body can result from scratching the primary lesion. Such infections may occur at any site, especially when the skin is traumatized, and they have occurred on the eye, tongue, lip, penis, vulva, and anus. In those autoinoculated, the secondary lesions heal, usually without scarring, at the same time as the primary lesion. When the lesion is at a potentially harmful site, as on the eye, specific treatment should be given (see below). Osteomyelitis from the viremia of a primary vaccination is a rare complication. A susceptible person can be infected by contact with the primary lesion of another person.

General. *Eczema vaccinatum* (Figs. 10-82, 10-83 [p. 628]), or vaccinia superimposed upon eczematous skin, can result from autoinoculation from infection of eczematous skin or from contact with a vaccinated person. There is probably spread of virus via bloodstream and lymphatics in addition to local inoculation. The eczematous skin is covered with umbilicated vesicles which involute like the primary ones. Infants are seriously ill; the mortality rate is in the range of 30 to 40 per cent. The condition must be distinguished from eczema herpeticum (p. 635), chiefly by history of exposure.

Abnormal Host Response. *Antibody formation.* Some persons have a delay in their sensitivity response to the protein of vaccine virus, but rapidly produce neutralizing antibodies (see No reaction), whereas others are slow in producing neutralizing antibodies and in responding by a delayed hypersensitivity reaction. The latter situation may result in various forms of *generalized vaccinia.* These include (1) *satellite or widespread vaccinal lesions,* which usually persist, along with the original lesion, for days or weeks beyond the normal time of healing until antibodies are eventually formed and all lesions heal together. Generalized vaccinia is sometimes mistakenly diagnosed when a coincidental skin eruption, e.g. varicella or impetigo, occurs in a child who has been vaccinated. Generalized vaccinia can be excluded if the original vaccination site is progressing normally without satellite lesions.

(2) *Prolonged progressive vaccinia or vaccinia gangrenosa.* There is spreading necrosis at the site of the primary inoculation which eventually destroys the area, and metastatic necrotic lesions occur throughout the body, including the bones. This complication is found in 2 types of patients: in those who cannot produce antibodies but have delayed hypersensitivity reactivity, and in those who are deficient in both functions. The condition may respond to hyperimmune serum therapy in the former, but is almost always fatal after a prolonged illness in the latter, despite treatment.

Hypersensitivity reactions. A variety of rashes, which can be included under the general term "erythema multiforme," occur at 7 to 11 days in about 1 of 5000 vaccinations. They are commonly mild and maculopapular ("roseola vaccinosa") (Fig. 10-84), papulovesicular or urticarial. Less frequently, there is a severe, generalized bullous

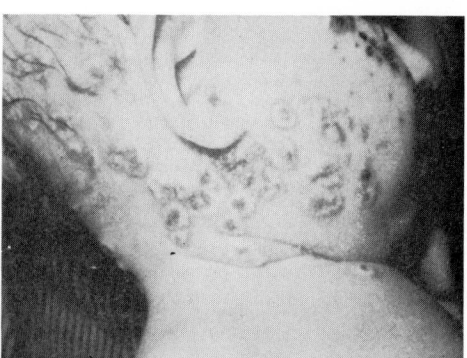

Figure 10-82. Eczema vaccinatum.

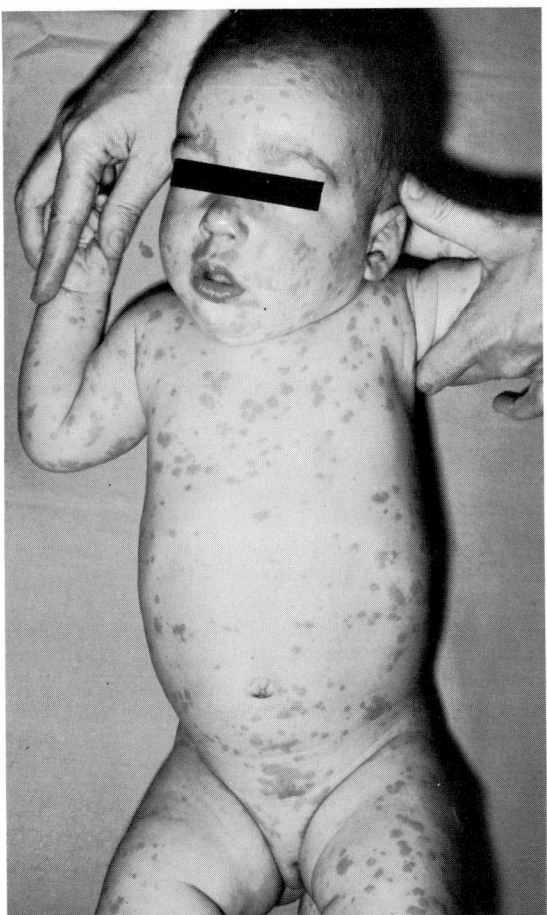

Figure 10-84. Erythema multiforme (roseola vaccinosa) complicating smallpox vaccination. Rash appeared 8 days after primary vaccination. Vaccination site is just visible in upper lateral aspect of left thigh.

rash which may also involve the mucous membranes of the mouth, anus and genitalia (erythema multiforme pluriorificialis).

CENTRAL NERVOUS SYSTEM. Postvaccinal encephalomyelitis is one of the allergic encephalitides (see p. 696). It usually appears 11 to 14 days after vaccination, but often earlier in infants. The clinical pattern varies and may be mainly encephalitic, encephalomyelitic, myelitic or meningitic. It occurs in approximately 1 of 100,000 vaccinations in the United States; in parts of Europe the incidence has been as high as 1 per 4000. The highest incidence is in children ranging in age from 5 to 15 years; 10 per cent of the cases and 20 per cent of the deaths have been in infants under 2 years of age. At this age the pathologic changes are those of anoxia, whereas in older patients the characteristic changes of demyelination are found. The case fatality rate is approximately 50 per cent; most of the deaths occur in patients with the encephalitic pattern. There is no evidence that a particular batch of vaccine is involved, and there appears to be no correlation with the size or severity of the local reaction or the number of inoculations. Encephalitis appears to be less common

and less severe after revaccination than after primary vaccination.

Treatment of Complications. Bacterial complications should be treated with appropriate antibiotic agents. Delay of antibody production leading to generalized vaccinia can be overcome by administration of hyperimmune vaccinal gamma globulin in a dose of 0.6 ml. per kg., which can be repeated as required. A single injection of the same amount of gamma globulin can be given prophylactically to contacts with eczema or to eczematous subjects at the time of a mandatory vaccination. Lesions due to autoinoculation or heteroinoculation in potentially dangerous sites should be treated with a similar dose of hyperimmune globulin except when the cornea is affected. Serotherapy aggravates this, and IUD drops should be used locally (see herpes). For *eczema vaccinatum*, 2 administrations may be required. For *progressive vaccinia* the administration must be repeated every week or two until healing is proceeding favorably, and until vaccinia virus can no longer be demonstrated in the lesions. N-methylisatin β-thiosemicarbazone, given orally as a 10 per cent suspension, has appeared to be effective in some patients in whom serotherapy has failed. The therapy for encephalitis is supportive (see p. 696), and there is no reason to give hyperimmune gamma globulin, because the normal development of antibodies is indicated by normal healing of the vaccinal lesion. Hyperimmune gamma globulin, given at the time of the primary vaccination, has been useful prophylactically in areas where the incidence of encephalitis is high.

REFERENCES

Bedson, H. S., and Dumbell, K. R.: Smallpox and Vaccinia. *Brit. Med. Bull.,* 23:119, 1967.

Cochran, W., Connolly, J. H., and Thompson, I. D.: Bone involvement After Vaccination Against Smallpox. *Brit. M.J.,* 2: 285, 1963.

Hansson, O., and Vahlquist, B.: Vaccinia Gangrenosa and Compound 33T57. *Lancet,* 2:687, 1963.

Kempe, C. H., Fulginiti, V., Minamitani, M., and Shinfield, H.: Smallpox Vaccination of Eczema Patients with a Strain of Attenuated, Live Vaccinia (CVI-78). *Pediatrics,* 42:980, 1968.

Kempe, C. H., Berg, T. O., and England, B.: Hyperimmune Vaccinal Gamma Globulin: Source, Evaluation and Use in Prophylaxis and Therapy. *Pediatrics,* 18:177, 1956.

Leahy, H. F.: Smallpox Vaccination and Its Complications. *Health News* (New York State Dept. of Health), 36:4, 1959.

Marsden, J. P.: Vaccination Against Smallpox; Critical Review of the Present Position. *Bull. Hyg.,* 21:555, 1946.

Ministry of Health Memorandum on Vaccination Against Smallpox. London, H. M. Stationery Office, 1956.

Pincus, W. B., and Flick, J. A.: The Role of Hypersensitivity in the Pathogenesis of Vaccine Virus Infection in Humans. *J. Pediat.,* 62:57, 1963.

Pincus, W. B., and Flick, J. A.: Successful Vaccinia Infection Without a Local Lesion. *Am. J. Pub. Health,* 53:898, 1963.

MUMPS
(EPIDEMIC PAROTITIS)

Mumps is an acute contagious generalized viral disease in which painful enlargement of the salivary glands, chiefly the parotids, is the usual presenting sign.

The disease was recognized as early as the fifth century B.C. by Hippocrates, who mentioned the complication of orchitis. In 1790 Hamilton also noted orchitis and the involvement of the central nervous system in certain patients. The frequency of the latter complication has been recognized increasingly during the present century, as has the fact that other organs, e.g. the pancreas, can also be infected.

Etiology. The viral origin was firmly established by Johnson and Goodpasture in 1934. The virus is classified as a myxovirus *(Myxovirus parotidis)*; it has a subtle relation to Newcastle disease and the parainfluenza viruses of man. The virus particle is roughly spherical, varying in size from 100 to 600 millimicrons in diameter. The heat stability varies with different strains, but the half-life of a number of strains at 35°C. has been reported as 8 hours. The virus can be preserved at −70°C. for several months. It produces interferon, hemolysin, hemagglutinin and CF antigens. The CF antigens are of 2 types: a smaller, noninfectious, soluble (S) antigen which is abundantly present in infected tissues, e.g. in egg membranes, and a larger viral (V) antigen which is the viral particle and is present in the extraembryonic fluids of the infected eggs. The virus can be transmitted to monkeys and dogs by the intraparotid route; domestic dogs are also reported to acquire mumps naturally. In other laboratory animals clinical disease is produced with difficulty and only after adaptation; guinea pigs, when infected, have a subclinical response with the production of antibodies and dermal hypersensitivity. The chick embryo was first described as a suitable host by Habel in 1945; the amniotic sac appears to be the most susceptible portion. The virus can also be grown in tissue culture cells. In HeLa cells cytopathic effects are produced in the form of giant cells; in monkey kidney cells cytoplasmic inclusion bodies are formed. The virus can also multiply without producing any visible change in the infected cells.

Epidemiology. Mumps is endemic in most urban populations; the virus is spread from a human reservoir by direct contact, airborne droplet nuclei, fomites contaminated by infectious saliva and possibly by urine. It has a world-wide distribution and affects both sexes equally; 85 per cent of the infections occur in children under the age of 15 years. Epidemics occur at all seasons of the year, although they are slightly more frequent in the late winter and spring. The source of infection may be difficult to trace, because 30 to 40 per cent of infections are subclinical.

It is uncertain how long a patient may be infectious, but virus has been isolated from saliva as long as 6 days before and up to 9 days after the appearance of salivary gland swelling. Under usual conditions, however, transmission does not seem to occur longer than 24 hours before the appearance of the swelling or later than 3 days after it has subsided. Virus has been isolated from the urine from the first to the fourteenth day after the onset of salivary gland swelling.

A lifelong immunity is produced by any type of clinical or subclinical infection; transplacental antibodies seem to be effective in protecting infants during the first 6 to 8 months of life. The presence of immunity and, therefore, of a previous infection (regardless of history) may be detected by 2 standard procedures: (1) the presence of CF antibodies to the V antigen of mumps, and (2) the development of a tuberculin-like skin reaction after intradermal injection of 0.1 ml. of inactivated infected allantoic fluid. The injection may produce an immediate wheal which disappears within 30 minutes and is nonspecific. Observation for the specific reaction should be made at 24 and 48 hours; only reactions with erythema and induration of 15 mm. or greater in diameter are considered positive. Sensitivity to egg should be checked by a parallel injection of uninfected fluid. A positive skin reaction usually indicates a previous infection, but it may be elicited during the incubation period of the disease.

Pathogenesis. The probable evolution of the disease is as follows: after entry and initial multiplication in the cells of the respiratory tract, the virus is blood-borne to many tissues, of which salivary and other glands seem to be the most susceptible. The swelling of the infected structures is probably the result of a hypersensitivity reaction to the locally multiplying virus, since the virus can be detected in the infected monkey parotid 4 to 5 days before clinical swelling occurs.

Pathology. Little information is available about the lesions caused by mumps in the human patient. In a parotid from which the virus was isolated 70 hours after onset of the disease the acini were well preserved, but there was periductal edema and lymphocytic infiltration extending slightly into the connective tissue. The main damage was to the ducts; the extent varied from slight epithelial swelling with a few polymorphonuclear cells in the lumen to complete desquamation of the epithelium and dilated lumens choked with debris. Some epithelial cells were observed with swelling of cytoplasm, but only rarely did one contain a large basophilic inclusion body. Other studies of parotid glands from patients with clinical mumps, without viral isolation, confirmed these general findings, although in some instances damage to the acini was observed. Changes in testes, biopsied within a day or two after onset of pain, have varied from mild interstitial edema and no disturbance of spermatogenesis in the majority of instances, to focal destruction of epithelium with extensive perivascular lymphocytic cuffing. The basic injury appeared to be vascular; irregular hemorrhages occurred in the more severe infections. Even in these, however, areas of normal germinal epithelium could be seen.

Clinical Manifestations. The incubation period ranges from 14 to 24 days, with a peak incidence at 17 to 18 days. In children prodromal symptoms and signs are rare, but may be manifest by fever, muscular pain, especially in the neck, headache and malaise. The onset of illness is usually characterized by pain and swelling in one or both parotid glands. The parotid swells in a characteristic way; it begins by filling the space between the posterior border of the mandible and the mastoid and then extends in a series of crescents downward and forward, being limited above by the zygoma. Edema of the skin and soft tissues usually extends further and obscures the limit of the glandular swelling, with the result that the swelling is more readily appreciated by sight than by palpation. The swelling may proceed extremely rapidly, reaching a maximum size within a few hours, although the peak is usually reached in 1 to 3 days. The swollen tissues push the ear lobe upward and outward. The swelling slowly subsides within 3 to 7 days; occasionally it lasts longer. Usually swelling of one parotid gland precedes that of the other by a day or two, but swelling limited to one gland is common. The swollen area is tender and painful, pain being especially elicited by tasting sour liquids such as lemon juice or vinegar, a useful diagnostic sign. Redness and swelling are commonly noted about the opening of Stensen's duct. Accompanying the parotid swelling there may be edema of the homolateral pharynx and soft palate displacing the tonsil medially; acute edema of the larynx has been described. Edema over the manubrium and upper chest wall may be found, probably owing to lymphatic obstruction. The parotid swelling is usually accompanied by moderate fever, but normal temperatures are common (20 per cent) and temperatures of 104°F. or over are rare; no correlation exists between extent of swelling and degree of fever.

Although the parotid glands alone are affected in the majority of patients, swelling of the submandibular glands occurs frequently and usually accompanies or closely follows that of the parotid glands. In 10 to 15 per cent of patients, however, only the submandibular gland(s) may be swollen. The swelling of the submandibular gland follows 2 patterns: the commoner is an ovoid enlargement extending forward and downward from the angle of the mandible; in the other the enlargement extends more directly downward in a half-egg shape. The deep portion of the gland is only rarely affected. Little pain is associated with the submandibular infection, but the swelling subsides more slowly than that of the parotids. Redness and swelling at the orifice of Wharton's duct frequently accompany swelling of the gland.

Least commonly the sublingual glands are infected, usually bilaterally; the swelling is evident in the submental region and in the floor of the mouth.

Complications. Viremia early in the infection probably accounts for the wide-spread complications which are mainly manifestations of mumps infection in organs other than the salivary glands.

Meningoencephalomyelitis. This is the most frequent complication in childhood. The true incidence is hard to estimate because subclinical infection of the central nervous system, as evidenced by a pleocytosis in the cerebrospinal fluid, has been reported in over 65 per cent of patients with parotitis. Clinical manifestations have been reported in over 25 per cent of patients. These occur more frequently in persons over the age of 15 years; in patients under 20 years of age there is a 3:1 higher incidence in males.

Meningoencephalitis begins typically with a sharp rise of temperature, headache, vomiting and sometimes a convulsion. There is moderate stiffness of the neck, but relatively little other change in the neurologic pattern. There is a polymorphonuclear leukocytosis in the peripheral blood. This clinical picture is indistinguishable from meningoencephalitis of other origin (see p. 689). The meningeal reaction, with its associated good prognosis, usually predominates, but in some patients the more serious "allergic" form of encephalitis occurs (see chapter on Encephalitis). Occasionally the presenting sign is muscular weakness, so that a diagnosis of poliomyelitis is considered. The neurologic complications as a rule appear 3 to 10 days after the onset of glandular swelling, but may precede it and, in an appreciable number of patients, occur in the absence of glandular swelling.

Orchitis, epididymitis. These lesions rarely occur in prepubescent boys, but are common (14 to 35 per cent) in adolescents and adults. The testis is most often infected with or without epididymitis, or epididymitis may occur alone. Rarely there is a hydrocele. The orchitis usually follows parotitis within 8 days, but sometimes is delayed, and it may occur without evidence of salivary gland infection. In about 30 per cent of patients with orchitis, both testes are affected. The onset is usually abrupt with a rise of temperature, chills, headache, nausea and lower abdominal pain; when the right testis is implicated, appendicitis may appear to be a diagnostic possibility. The affected testis becomes tender and swollen and the adjacent skin edematous and red. The average duration is 4 days. As the swelling subsides, the testis loses its normal turgor; approximately 30 to 40 per cent of affected testes atrophy. Impairment of fertility is estimated to be about 13 per cent, but absolute infertility is probably rare.

Oophoritis. Pelvic pain and tenderness are noted in about 7 per cent of female patients.

Pancreatitis. Severe involvement of the pancreas is rare, but mild or subclinical infection may be more common than is recognized. It may be unassociated with salivary gland manifestations and be misdiagnosed as gastroenteritis. Epigastric pain and tenderness are suggestive; these may be accompanied by fever, chills, vomiting and prostration. An elevated serum amylase value is characteristically present in any patient with mumps, with or without clinical manifestation of pancreatitis. The possibility that diabetes mellitus may be an infrequent sequel should be investigated.

Nephritis. Associated with viruria, severe and even fatal nephritis has been reported as an uncommon complication occurring 10 to 14 days after the parotitis.

Thyroiditis. Although uncommon in children, a diffuse, tender swelling of the thyroid may occur about a week after the onset of parotitis and has been followed by the development of antithyroid antibodies.

Myocarditis. Serious clinical manifestations are extremely rare, but mild infection of the myocardium is probably more common and overlooked. In one series of adults electrocardiographic tracings revealed changes, mostly depression of the S-T segment, in 13 per cent of them. Such involvement could explain the precordial pain, bradycardia and fatigue sometimes noted among adolescents and adults with mumps.

Mastitis. This is an uncommon occurrence in either male or female patients.

Deafness. Unilateral, or rarely bilateral, nerve deafness may occur after mumps; although the incidence is low, mumps is considered a leading cause of unilateral nerve deafness.

Ocular complications. These include *dacryoadenitis,* painful swelling of the lacrimal glands which is usually bilateral; *optic neuritis (papillitis)* with symptoms varying from loss of vision to mild blurring and with recovery in 10 to 20 days; *uveokeratitis,* usually unilateral, with photophobia, tearing, rapid loss of vision and recovery within 20 days; *scleritis; tenonitis* with resultant exophthalmos; and *central vein thrombosis.*

Arthritis. Arthralgia associated with swelling and redness of the joints is an infrequent complication which appears 12 to 14 days after the onset of parotitis; complete recovery is the rule.

Thrombocytopenic purpura follows mumps on occasion, as it does other infections.

Mumps embryopathy. There is no firm evidence that maternal infection with mumps leads to any damage to the developing fetus; a possible relation to endocardial fibroelastosis has been postulated, but is far from being established.

Diagnosis. The diagnosis of mumps parotitis is usually readily apparent from the symptoms and physical examination. When the clinical manifestations are limited to those of one of the less common lesions, the diagnosis is not as clear, but may be suspected especially during an epidemic. The routine laboratory tests are nonspecific; there is usually a leukopenia with a relative lymphocytosis, but complications often result in a polymorphonuclear leukocytosis of a moderate degree. An elevation of serum amylase is found in most patients with mumps; the rise, paralleling the parotid swelling, reaches its peak in a week and generally returns to normal over the course of the next 2 weeks. The etiologic diagnosis depends on the isolation of the virus from the saliva, urine, spinal fluid or blood or the demonstration of a significant rise in circulating CF antibodies during convalescence. Serum antibodies to the S antigen reach their peak early in about 75 per

cent of patients and are detectable at the time of the presenting symptoms. They gradually disappear within 6 to 12 months; antibodies against the V or viral antigen usually reach a peak titer in about a month, remain stationary for about 6 months and then slowly decline over the ensuing 2 years to a low level at which they persist. The presence of a high anti-S titer and a low anti-V titer during the acute stage of an otherwise undiagnosed meningoencephalitis, for example, would be strongly suggestive of a mumps infection which would be confirmed if a convalescent serum, taken 14 to 21 days later, revealed a fourfold rise of anti-V antibodies with little change in the titer of anti-S antibodies.

Differential Diagnosis. This includes *parotitis* of other origin, as in the rare instances of Coxsackie A and lymphocytic choriomeningitis infections which can be distinguished only by specific laboratory tests; *suppurative parotitis,* in which pus can often be expressed from the duct; *recurrent parotitis,* a condition of unknown origin, but possibly allergic in nature, which has frequent recurrences and a characteristic sialogram; *salivary calculus,* obstructing either a parotid or, more commonly, a submandibular duct, in which the swelling is intermittent; *preauricular* or *anterior cervical lymphadenitis* from any cause; *lymphosarcoma* or other rare *tumors* of the parotid; and *orchitis due to infections other than mumps,* e.g., the rare infections by Coxsackie A or lymphocytic choriomeningitis viruses.

Treatment. This is entirely symptomatic. Bed rest should be guided by the patient's needs; there is no statistical evidence that it prevents complications. The diet should be adjusted to the ability of the patient to chew. The headache of meningoencephalitis may be relieved by a lumbar puncture. Orchitis should be treated with local support and bed rest. Corticosteroids, preferably hydrocortisone in pharmacologic doses (10 mg. per kg. per day) for 2 to 4 days, relieve the pain, although evidence of any effect on length of illness or protection against atrophy is lacking.

Prophylaxis. *Passive.* Present evidence suggests that the use of hyperimmune mumps gamma globulin not only does not significantly reduce complications, but also in some instances actually increases their incidence.

Active. An attenuated live mumps virus vaccine has been developed (Mumpsvax [Merck, Sharp & Dohme]) which leads to the development of antibodies and has a protective effect on exposure. Although most useful for susceptibles in preadolescent and older ages, it may be included among the routine immunization procedures, but later revaccination may be required. There is no evidence that vaccination will protect any susceptible person exposed to mumps, but there is no contraindication to its use in exposed adolescents or adults who presumably have not had mumps.

T. F. McNair Scott

REFERENCES

American Academy of Pediatrics: Report of the Committee on the Control of Infectious Diseases, 1968.

Henle, W., and Enders, J. F.: Mumps Virus; in F. L. Horsfall and I. Tamm (Eds.): *Viral and Rickettsial Infections of Man.* 4th ed. Philadelphia, J. B. Lippincott Company, 1964, Chap. 32, p. 755.

Lindsey, J. R., Davey, R., and Ward, P. H.: Inner Ear Pathology in Deafness Due to Mumps. *Ann. Otology,* 69:918, 1960.

Reed, D., Brown, G., Merrick, R., Sever, J., and Feltz, E.: A Mumps Epidemic on St. Georges Island, Alaska. *J.A.M.A.,* 199:113, 1967.

Smith, R. E.: Mumps. *Guy's Hosp. Rep.,* 92:1, 1943.

Werner, C. A.: Mumps Orchitis and Testicular Atrophy. *Ann. Int. Med.,* 32:1066, 1950.

Young, M. L., and others: Experiences with Jeryl Lynn Strain Live Attenuated Mumps Virus Vaccine in a Pediatric Out-Patient Clinic. *Pediatrics,* 40:798, 1967.

EPIDEMIC INFLUENZA

Definition. Influenza is an acute communicable viral disease primarily affecting the respiratory tract. It occurs in pandemic waves usually separated by several decades, during which epidemics of less severity occur at 2- to 4-year intervals.

Etiology. Two viral agents appear to have been responsible for most of the outbreaks of respiratory infection resembling influenza since 1933: influenza A virus, identified by Smith, Andrewes and Laidlaw (1933); and influenza B virus, identified independently by Francis and by Magill in 1940. Subsequently 2 additional types of influenza virus have been isolated and identified. In 1949 Taylor isolated a virus which was designated as influenza C. Thus far it has been responsible for only mild epidemic disease. A viral agent isolated in 1953 in Japan (Sendai virus) was first identified as a possible influenza type D, but was later classified with the parainfluenza group of agents. It has been responsible for a severe form of pneumonitis in newborn infants in many parts of the world. Pandemic influenza, similar in worldwide prevalence, but not in severity, to that of 1918–19, occurred in 1957. The causative virus was a mutant strain—Asian strain—of type A influenza virus, to which immunity could not be produced by vaccines containing known strains of type A virus. Persons born before 1890 were usually found to have antibodies to the Asian strain, thus suggesting an antigenic relation of the new mutant to the virus responsible for the pandemic of 1889–90.

Influenza viruses A and B are distinct serologically with no cross immunity, and each type has a number of antigenic strains. In spite of antigenic differences the A and B viruses have common features. Both have an affinity for respiratory epithelium and produce the same type of lesion. A and B viruses multiply rapidly in embryonated eggs in contrast to type C, which multiplies slowly and requires amniotic transfer. They can be cultivated in tissue culture, and both are capable of producing hemagglutination of red cells.

After either experimental or natural infection with virus A or B, neutralizing and complement-fixing antibodies increase rapidly, reaching their peak within approximately 2 to 3 weeks, and then slowly diminish to their previous levels in approximately a year. A fourfold increase of antibodies in comparative tests of acute and convalescent serums is diagnostic.

The agglutination of chick red cells by both viruses and the inhibition of this phenomenon by previous addition to the viruses of an immune serum were developed independently by Hirst and Hare as a means of determining the presence and amounts of antibodies in unknown serums. This method of measuring antibody formation is more exact than the virus neutralization test, but not as accurate as the complement fixation test. The soluble antigen is the same for all type A strains (swine, A, A′, Asian); the soluble antigen of type B is quite different from that of type A.

In both pandemic and epidemic influenza the mortality is, to an extent, dependent on secondarily invading bacteria, of which *Hemophilus influenzae,* hemolytic streptococcus, pneumococcus and *Staphylococcus aureus* are the most frequent. In the 1957 epidemic, however, it became evident that rapidly fatal cases were not always due to superimposed bacterial infection, but could be caused by the virus itself.

Epidemiology. Influenza is probably the only remaining pandemic disease over which no effective control has been established. The pandemic of 1918 is estimated to have caused approximately 22,000,000 deaths throughout the world in about 3 months.

Serologic data relating to the pandemics of 1889, 1918 and 1957, together with identification of different strains of influenza A virus from various epidemics since 1930, suggest a pattern of recurrent outbreaks of influenza A infections which depends primarily upon mutant strains of virus and secondarily upon the accumulation of susceptible hosts, especially among the young and the middle-aged. Epidemics from the same strain may recur every 3 to 4 years, but a subsequent pandemic does not occur until a new mutant strain of virus again becomes widespread. Epidemics from strains of A virus tend to occur every year or two; while those of influenza B, less frequently. Epidemics usually occur in the late winter and early spring.

The viruses, which spread by the airborne route and by direct contact, are present in the upper respiratory tract of patients from the first to the fifth day of disease. Viremia has not been demonstrated.

Both sexes and all races appear equally susceptible. Young adults and children over 5 years of age appear to be more susceptible than infants and older persons. Experimental human infection has indicated a direct relation between the titer of serum antibodies and resistance to infection. A large number of inapparent infections occurs in any epidemic, as indicated by the rise of antibody titers in persons who have had no symptoms. No reservoir of the viruses for interepidemic survival has been found, nor have carriers been discovered.

Pathology. Uncomplicated influenza in man may be considered analogous to the disease in ferrets, in which there is severe inflammatory reaction in the mucous membrane of the upper respiratory tract with a loss of ciliated epithelium. Regeneration occurs by development of epithelium of a more squamous type over a period of several weeks, with slower regeneration of the columnar epithelium. During this transitional period the epithelium is resistant to further influenzal virus infections.

In severe cases hemorrhages with serosanguineous exudate often occur in the pharynx, larynx, bronchi and bronchioles, with edema of the entire respiratory tract. The alveolar ducts and bronchioles may be dilated and their walls frequently covered with hyaline material. There is necrosis of the mucous membrane, and emphysema is usually present in localized areas.

The pathologic picture may be altered by bacterial pathogens. When several different organisms are present, the pathologic changes are less uniform than when there is a single pathogen. With pneumococcus there is typically a lobular pneumonia tending to become confluent, with the influenzal bacillus, severe destructive changes in the bronchioles and interstitial pneumonia, often leading to bronchiectasis; with *Staphylococcus aureus*, an overwhelming infection characterized by hemorrhagic edema and multiple pulmonary abscesses; and with hemolytic streptococcus, an interstitial reaction with hemorrhagic edema and frequently with pleurisy and empyema.

Clinical Manifestations. The symptoms of pandemic and epidemic influenza are similar except for severity and extent of complications. Experimental infections of human susceptibles have simulated the milder cases of epidemics.

The incubation period is usually 36 to 48 hours. The onset is sudden with a chill or a chilly sensation, frequently in children with a convulsion; a sharp rise in temperature ranging from 102 to 106°F.; flushing of the face, neck and chest; headache; vertigo; a dry sore throat; and pains in the back and extremities. A short, dry, hacking cough is usually present soon after the onset and rapidly increases in frequency and severity. It often becomes paroxysmal and resembles the cough of pertussis. In young children vomiting and diarrhea may be the principal manifestations at the onset. The accompanying prostration may be extreme and is related not only to the severity of the disease, but also to the lack of complete bed rest from the onset of symptoms. The fever is often diphasic, with the 2 peaks separated by a period of 24 to 48 hours.

The mucous membranes of the throat appear dry and red with no exudate; those of the nose are red, but usually there is little or no discharge except when purulent sinusitis is a late complication. The conjunctivas are injected. Epistaxis is common. The pulse is usually rapid and often weak, as are the heart sounds when the cardiac muscle is seriously affected. Often the skeletal muscles are painful on pressure, and movements of the eyeballs cause considerable discomfort.

The usual increase in leukocytes during the early stages of the disease is soon replaced by a leukopenia with a relative lymphocytosis.

The milder uncomplicated cases rarely last more than 3 to 4 days.

In severe infections which extend into the lower respiratory tract fine moist rales may soon be detected bilaterally, and these may spread rapidly over the entire lung area with diminution of breath sounds, or a tendency to bronchial breathing if consolidation occurs. As the cough increases in frequency it becomes productive, often sanguineous at first and later mucopurulent. Diminution of breath sounds resulting from edema of the bronchial tree and alveoli is far more common than the localized consolidation of lobular pneumonia, and frequently the breath sounds almost disappear as patchy edematous and atelectatic areas are interspersed with areas of emphysema. In extremely severe infections the patient shows evidence of anoxia. Myocardial involvement results in distention of the right side of the heart, passive congestion of the liver, and, finally, extensive pulmonary edema and cardiac failure.

When secondary bacterial infections are present, the symptoms depend to a considerable extent upon the type of organism involved.

Diagnosis. During epidemics or pandemics the diagnosis is not difficult. The simplest diagnostic test is that of Hirst and Hare (p. 651); the complement fixation test, however, appears to be more reliable. The isolation of virus by intra-amniotic inoculation of throat washings is diagnostic.

Complications. In few other diseases are the complications such an integral part of the severe forms of the infection. Many of these have been mentioned under Clinical Manifestations and actually may be considered clinical variations.

Otitis media, mastoiditis, purulent sinusitis, pneumonia, bronchiectasis, pulmonary abscess and empyema are the more common respiratory variants of severe infections. Less common ones are pneumothorax and mediastinitis. Rare nonrespiratory complications include hematoma from rupture of the rectus muscles of the abdomen, epistaxis, intestinal hemorrhage, polyneuritis, postinfluenzal psychoses, nephritis, subcutaneous or intramuscular abscess, endocarditis, myocarditis, pericarditis, thrombophlebitis, meningitis and hemorrhagic encephalitis.

Prophylaxis. During epidemics, avoidance of fatigue and chilling, and of crowds is important. Specific resistance can be increased by the use of vaccines. Vaccination is preventive and not therapeutic. Febrile and local reactions to the vaccines are proportional to the amount of virus they contain. In rare instances persons sensitive to chick embryo proteins may have allergic reactions.

Recently isolated strains of influenza virus, such as A′ and Asian, have complicated the production of effective vaccines, since the older strains, such as PR8, do not protect against other prime strains. The present objective is the preparation of a vaccine containing multiple antigens which will induce broad immunity at all ages. The preparations now available contain strains representative of A_1, A_2, A_3, A_4 and of B_1 and B_2, and are considered to be 50 to 80 per cent effective. As a rule, persons who have some circulating antibodies respond promptly to this antigenic stimulus, and antibodies can be increased within 7 to 10 days. Serum antibody levels of 1:128 measured by the hemagglutination inhibition test appear to be associated with a high degree of immunity. Antibody levels tend to fall to half the attained level in 6 months to a year.

The recommended immunization schedule for adults is 1.0 ml. of vaccine subcutaneously, with the same dose repeated in 1 to 2 months. Children over 12 years of age tolerate the adult dose. For children 5 to 12 years of age a dose of 0.5 ml. is recommended, with a second dose in 10 to 14 days as part of the primary immunization. For children 3 months to 5 years of age intracutaneous or subcutaneous injection of 0.1 ml. has been proposed, to be repeated in 1 to 2 weeks. The antigenic effect of such a dose is small, however, and amounts up to 0.25 ml. have been recommended. In the event of epidemics prior vaccination against influenza appears to reduce complications.

Treatment.   No specific treatment is available. Complete bed rest from the earliest evidence of disease is absolutely essential and should be continued long into convalescence. Antimicrobial therapy is indicated for bacterial complications. The fluid intake should be ample. Acetylsalicylic acid and codeine may be used for discomfort and cough.

REFERENCES

Blattner, R. J.: Neurologic Complications of Asian Influenza. Comments on Current Literature. *J. Pediat.,* 53:751, 1958.
Blattner, R. J.: Virus Isolation in Fatal Human Cases of Asian Influenza. Comments on Current Literature. *J. Pediat.,* 55: 113, 1959.
Francis, T., Jr.: Influenza; in C. S. Keefer (Ed.): Symposium on Viral and Rickettsial Diseases. *M. Clin. N. Amer.,* 43:1309, 1959.
Hirst, G. K.: The Agglutination of Red Cells by Allantoic Fluid of Chick Embryos Infected with Influenza Virus. *Science,* 94:22, 1941.
Lief, F. S., and Henle, W.: Antigenic Analysis of Influenza Viruses by Complement Fixation. VI. Implications of Age Distribution of Antibodies to Heterologous Strains Following Infection and Vaccination. *J. Immunol.,* 85:494, 1960.
Magill, T. P.: A Virus from Cases of Influenza-Like Upper-Respiratory Infection. *Proc. Soc. Exper. Biol. & Med.,* 45:162, 1940.
McClelland, L., and Hare, R.: The Adsorption of Influenza Virus by Red Cells and a New in Vitro Method of Measuring Antibodies for Influenza Virus. *Canad. Pub. Health J.,* 32:530, 1941.
Mellman, W. J.: Influenza Encephalitis. *J. Pediat.,* 53:292, 1958.
Shope, R. E.: Swine Influenza. *J. Exper. Med.,* 54:349, 373, 1931.
Smith, W., Andrewes, C. H., and Laidlaw, P. P.: A Virus Obtained from Influenza Patients. *Lancet,* 2:66, 1933.
Taylor, R. M.: Studies on Survival of Influenza Virus Between Epidemics and Antigenic Variants of the Virus. *Am. J. Pub. Health,* 39:171, 1949.

RABIES
(HYDROPHOBIA)

Definition.   Rabies is an acute viral disease of the central nervous system which is transmitted by dogs, cats, bats and wild animals. In general, it is characterized by extreme excitation, severe and painful spasm of the muscles of the pharynx and larynx at the sight of food or liquids, which accounts for the name "hydrophobia," and finally by generalized paralysis and death within a few days.

History.   Rabies is one of the oldest recorded diseases in Europe and Asia. Democritus in 500 B.C. and Aristotle in 322 B.C. described rabies; Celsus in A.D. 100 advised cauterization of bites by rabid dogs, and Galen in A.D. 200 advised surgical excision of the bite. Apparently rabies had not occurred in North and South America before colonization.

In 1804 Zinke infected a normal dog with saliva from a rabid dog. Pasteur in 1881 to 1884 demonstrated the infective agent in the central nervous system of rabbits and named it a virus, from the Latin word for poison. There followed the development in his laboratories of the fixed virus and the study of vaccination with attenuated virus. Fermi in 1908 treated infected nervous tissue with phenol for use as a vaccine. In 1903 Negri demonstrated the inclusion bodies now known by his name. In 1921 Haupt found the vampire bat to be a symptomless carrier of the virus, a finding of great epidemiologic importance.

Etiology.   The rabies virus is neurotropic and travels by the injured peripheral nerves to the central nervous system. This natural virus is termed "street virus" and has a variable incubation period related to the distance of the injury from the head, the severity of the bite, and the amount of virus in the wound. The "street virus" invades the salivary glands and is usually transmitted in saliva. The "fixed virus" is the natural virus modified by repeated intracerebral passages in laboratory animals. This virus has a 4- to 6-day incubation period and does not invade the salivary glands. The "street virus" through multiple passage in the chick embryo loses its pathogenic properties and may be used without inactivation for vaccination.

Epidemiology.   Two categories of rabies have been suggested by Johnson: the sylvatic, existing in wild animals; and the urban, prevalent in domestic dogs. Sylvatic rabies is well recognized among wolves, foxes, coyotes, skunks, and more recently bats.

Symptom complexes in animals which in the past were not associated with rabies, such as "running fits" of dogs and paralytic syndromes in dogs and other animals, may be of rabid origin. In the United States and Canada deaths from rabies in human subjects have been estimated at less than 100 annually, although rabies appears to be increasing among dogs. In certain areas outside the United States the paralytic form of rabies has been more frequent. In Trinidad both man and cattle have been infected by vampire bats, which apparently are carriers and not victims of the disease.

Pathology. Fresh virus from a rabid animal will cause widespread degeneration and necrosis of neurons. Demyelination and degeneration of the axis cylinders are present in the white matter. The areas chiefly involved are the red nucleus, substantia nigra, pons and particularly the nuclei of the cranial nerves in the medulla. Here neuronophagia and infiltration with mononuclear cells are extensive. The pathognomonic sign in the neuronal cytoplasm and dendritic processes is the Negri body, which apparently is an inclusion body. It has eosinophilic cytoplasm with a basophilic granular corpuscle in the center. Since the neurons of the salivary glands at times show similar changes with Negri bodies, it is conceivable that the rabies virus enters the saliva by this route.

Clinical Manifestations. Since prophylaxis against the disease in man depends to a great extent upon an understanding of the early manifestations in the dog, they are described first.

In the dog, symptoms may be considered under 2 general types, although it is not possible to separate them completely.

1. The "furious" type results from increased excitation of the central nervous system, with fever, hyperesthesia and lack of appetite. The evidences of disease depend to a great extent upon the nature and training of the dog. The more aggressive dog will begin to snap and become excited and dangerous early in the course of the disease. The gentle dog in the early stages will more frequently seek seclusion and refuse food or will become excessively affectionate, after which it becomes agitated and restless. This is usually followed by irritability and snapping at strangers and a little later by snarling or snapping at imaginary objects and chasing and biting other animals. Finally, if free, it will run for miles, snapping at or biting all living things in its path until it falls paralyzed to the ground.

2. The "dumb" or paralytic type, despite its frequency (approximately 20 per cent), is rarely recognized by the dog's owners, primarily because no agitation or excitement is seen. The course is far more rapid, paralysis occurring in any group of muscles, but particularly in the lower jaw and in the muscles of deglutition. In such cases the tongue hangs out of the mouth, continuously dripping saliva; sympathetic persons, suspecting a foreign body in the dog's throat, may expose their hands to the infective saliva in an effort to relieve the dog. Rapidly extending paralysis soon results in death; occasionally dogs die suddenly without signs of illness, and encephalitis with Negri bodies is found at autopsy.

In man the incubation period is approximately 4 to 8 weeks, but may be months and, rarely, as long as a year. It may be shorter than 4 weeks when the lacerations are about the head or neck.

Clinical cases are usually characterized by 3 stages. In the *prodromal* phase, numbness, formication, tingling, burning or a sensation of cold may be felt about the wound and along the involved nerve trunks, followed by mild excitation with irritability, restlessness, dilatation of pupils, salivation, lacrimation, perspiration and insomnia or, at times, drowsiness and depression.

In the *second* phase, excitation increases rapidly, and there is apprehension and even terror. The neck is stiff, and there is delirium and twitching or mild convulsive movements. At this stage the sign appears which has characterized the disease, i.e. the strangulating and painful spasm of the throat at any attempt to swallow food or liquids and even at the sight of them (hydrophobia). Slight noises may initiate these spasms, as may tactile stimuli. At such times the patient is unable to breathe, and the body remains in a tonic convulsion during which death may occur. The temperature is usually elevated to 103 to 105°F., but may be lower. Blood-tinged vomitus or excessive saliva may give the impression of "frothing."

Within 1 to 3 days the patient passes rapidly into the *terminal* phase with increasing paralysis, cessation of spasms, coma and death within another day or two.

The paralytic form of the disease, which is far less common, begins with numbness or severe pains in the nerve trunks supplying the involved area, followed shortly by flaccid paralysis of the part, which extends first to the opposite side of the body, and then slowly ascends in a manner similar to Landry's paralysis, terminating with involvement of the respiratory and circulatory centers.

In each form there may be a polymorphonuclear leukocytosis, as great as 20,000 to 30,000 cells per mm.³ The cerebrospinal fluid usually has a slight increase of protein and occasionally of mononuclear cells, up to 30 to 100 per mm.³

Diagnosis. With classic symptoms and history of bite, the diagnosis is not difficult. History of bite may be lacking, however, and symptoms may be atypical. The paralytic form may be confused with poliomyelitis. In a few instances differentiation from tetanus has been a problem, since tetanus also may be transferred by animal bite. In rabies the incubation period is usually longer. In tetanus the cerebrospinal fluid shows no cellular response and no increase in protein level. Persistent muscle spasm, particularly trismus, is characteristic in tetanus, whereas the strangulating spasms of the muscles of deglutition characteristic of rabies are lacking.

Occasionally a person who has been bitten becomes hysterical and may present signs and symptoms which simulate rabies; however, differential diagnosis in this instance should not be difficult.

Prognosis. No recovery from rabies has been recorded.

Prevention. The most important prophylactic measure is control of dogs. In England, the Scandinavian countries and Canada, rabies has been nearly eliminated by precautions in the general handling of dogs. In some countries these include strict quarantine practices on entry of dogs into the country. Stray dogs should be eliminated, and all other dogs should be muzzled, confined or on leash. A dog bitten by a rabid animal should either be killed or isolated for at least 6 to 8 months. Vaccination of such a dog to be successful must include a sufficient number of injections; the customary single prophylactic injection is totally inadequate. The disappearance of a dog after biting an animal or man should be regarded with suspicion, since a dog frequently seeks seclusion

TABLE 10-20. INDICATIONS FOR SPECIFIC POSTEXPOSURE TREATMENT

| NATURE OF EXPOSURE | CONDITION OF ANIMAL | | RECOMMENDED TREATMENT |
	AT TIME OF EXPOSURE	DURING OBSERVATION PERIOD OF 10 DAYS	
I. No lesions Indirect contact only	Rabid	—	None†
II. Licks			
1. Unabraded skin	Rabid	—	None†
2. Abraded skin and abraded or un-abraded mucosa	(a) Healthy	Healthy	None
	(b) Healthy	Clinical signs of rabies or proved rabid	Start vaccine at first signs of rabies in animal
	(c) Signs suggestive of rabies	Healthy	Start vaccine immediately. Stop treatment if animal is normal on fifth day after exposure‡
	(d) Rabid, escaped, killed* or unknown	—	Start vaccine immediately
III. Bites			
1. Simple exposure	(a) Healthy	Healthy	None
	(b) Healthy	Clinical signs of rabies or proved rabid	Start vaccine at first signs of rabies in animal
	(c) Signs suggestive of rabies	Healthy	Start vaccine immediately. Stop treatment if animal is normal on fifth day after exposure‡
	(d) Rabid, escaped, killed* or unknown; or any bite by wolf, jackal, fox or other wild animal	—	Start vaccine immediately
2. Severe exposure (multiple; or face, head or neck bites)	(a) Healthy	Healthy	Hyperimmune serum immediately no vaccine as long as animal remains normal
	(b) Healthy	Clinical signs of rabies or proved rabid	As in III, 2, (a), but start vaccine at first sign of rabies
	(c) Signs suggestive of rabies	Healthy	Hyperimmune serum immediately, followed by vaccine. Vaccine may be stopped if animal is normal on fifth day after exposure
	(d) Rabid, escaped, killed* or unknown. Any bite by wild animal	—	Hyperimmune serum immediately, followed by vaccine

Hyperimmune serum to be effective must be given within 72 hours of exposure.
These indications apply equally well whether or not the biting animal has been previously vaccinated.
*The fluorescent antibody technique of examination of brain tissue may be used, if available, as a guide for vaccination.
†Start vaccine immediately when a reliable history cannot be obtained.
‡Alternative treatment would be to give hyperimmune serum and not start vaccine as long as animal remains normal.
Prepared by Expert Committee on Rabies of World Health Organization.

before death from rabies. Suspicion should also be attached to a previously gentle dog whose behavior suddenly changes. Any dog which has bitten a person, but which has no sign of rabies, should be kept under surveillance.

Infection from bats has often followed thoughtless disturbance of sleeping, injured or obviously sick bats. A few instances of unprovoked attacks have occurred.

Suggestions for prophylactic therapy are detailed in Table 10-20. Although no form of prophylaxis is 100 per cent effective, the regimens now recommended can be expected to prevent rabies from minor exposures and in at least 90 per cent of the more severe exposures. Modifications of these basic recommendations have been suggested. Cases must be individualized, as in the suspected exposure of young children who cannot give a reliable history. Very minor exposures may be covered by hyperimmune serum while the animal is being observed. In such instances longer observation of the dog in question is recommended: 12 to 14 days instead of a minimum of 5 days.

Rabies vaccine. Pasteur's method of active immunization consisted of daily injections of increasing quantities of attenuated ("fixed") virus in spinal cord suspensions from infected rabbits. This vaccine has now been replaced by some form of killed virus. Semple vaccine consists of infected rabbit brain sterilized by phenol. The multiple hen's egg-passive vaccine (HEP Flury) is used widely for the vaccination of dogs. In human subjects this Flury strain (HEP) has given variable results; however, recent modifications in preparation and administration promise more satisfactory response. The duck embryo vaccine appears to be the preparation of choice for ordinary exposures. In instances of a single bite, except on the head and neck, 1 ml. of this vaccine is administered subcutaneously once a day for 14 consecutive days. In the case of more severe exposure, as in multiple bites, or about the face, head or neck, this treatment is continued for 21 days.

Hyperimmune antirabies serum is prepared by the immunization of horses; it is standardized by mouse tests. Such hyperimmune serum is most effective when given within 24 hours after exposure, and is especially valuable in severe exposures. The usual single intramuscular dose is 0.5 ml. per kg. Sensitivity status of the patient to horse serum must be initially determined by skin or eye test. An additional 5.0 ml. of hyperimmune serum may be injected locally at the site of the wound. If 72 hours have elapsed since the bite, double the intramuscular dose is recommended.

The *wound* should be washed thoroughly with soap or detergent and water. Suturing should not be carried out immediately, since immediate closure is thought to contribute to virus spread. Cauterization of the wound with concentrated nitric acid has been a traditional procedure, and this acid does destroy the virus. The procedure is painful, however, and disfiguring. The use of a freshly prepared 1 per cent solution of Zephiran chloride has been recommended for final wound cleansing. The activity of such quaternary ammonium compounds is neutralized by soap, and the washed wound should be rinsed well with water before the application of Zephiran. Since tetanus spores as well as rabies virus may be introduced into the wound, tetanus toxoid or antitoxin is recommended if the patient has not been immunized within the past year.

Repeated exposure to rabies is not common; if it occurs within 3 months after vaccination, no retreatment is necessary beyond proper wound cleansing and prophylaxis for tetanus (see above). If re-exposure occurs within 3 to 6 months, 2 booster vaccine doses may be given a week apart. If the interval is longer than 6 months, antiserum and 7 daily injections of vaccine are recommended.

Reactions to antirabies vaccine. Minor reactions are those common in allergic conditions such as urticarial or erythematous rashes, and edema with occasional syncope. Of greater significance are such infrequent neurologic complications as polyneuritis of the Guillain-Barré type, ascending paralysis and meningoencephalitis. They are thought to be due to an antigen-antibody reaction in the perivascular tissues. Treatment of neurologic manifestations is chiefly symptomatic. In some cases antihistaminics or corticosteroids have been beneficial.

Treatment. Active treatment, once the disease has developed, is of little use. Sedatives should be used in large doses, and the patient's room kept darkened and quiet. Anesthesia may be required as the disease progresses. Attendants should be instructed carefully in the handling of the patient; human bite is possible, and contact with saliva from an infected person is hazardous.

REFERENCES

Anderson, G. R., Schnurrenberger, P. R., Masterson, R. A., and Wentworth, F. H.: Avian Embryo Rabies Immunization. I. Duck Embryo Vaccine Administered Intradermally in Man. *Am. J. Hyg.,* 71:158, 1960.

Blattner, R. J.: Rabies Infection Transmitted by Insectivorous Bats: Human Case with Virus Isolation from Spinal Fluid during Life. Comments on Current Literature. *J. Pediat.,* 58:433, 1961.

Blattner, R. J., and Heys, F. M.: Antirabies Treatment: in Viral Encephalitis, *Advances in Pediatrics.* Chicago, Year Book Publishers, Inc., 1962, Vol. 12, pp. 84-6.

Briggs, G. W., and Brown, W. M.: Neurological Complications of Antirabies Vaccine Treated with Corticosteroids. *J.A.M.A.,* 173:802, 1960.

Burns, K. F., Shelton, D. F., Lukeman, J. M., and Grogan, E. W.: Cortisone and ACTH Impairment of Response to Rabies Vaccine. *Pub. Health Rep.,* 75:441, 1960.

Johnson, H. N.: Rabies Virus; in F. L. Horsfall and I. Tamm (Eds.): *Viral and Rickettsial Infections of Man.* 4th ed. Philadelphia, J. B. Lippincott Company, 1965, p. 814.

Kent, J. R., and Finegold, S. M.: Human Rabies Transmitted by the Bite of a Bat: With Comments on the Duck Embryo Vaccine. *New England J. Med.,* 263:1058, 1960.

World Health Organization, Expert Committee on Rabies. Fifth Report, Geneva, 1966, Technical Report Series No. 321. See Also *Morbidity and Mortality, Weekly Report,* 16:152, Week ending May 13, 1967; United States Department of Health, Education and Welfare, Public Health Service.

Veeraraghavan, N., and Subrahmanyan, T. P.: Value of Antirabies Vaccine with and without Serum against Severe Challenge. *Bull. World Health Organization,* 22:381, 1960.

YELLOW FEVER

Definition. Yellow fever is an acute viral disease with severe constitutional symptoms accompanied by jaundice, hematemesis, and renal and cardiac involvement. Distribution is essentially tropical.

History. Carlos Finlay in 1881 first suggested the mosquito *Aedes aegypti* as the vector. The classic experiments of Reed, Carroll, Agramonte and Lazear in 1900 and 1901 verified its essential role, the need for mosquito control, and established the viral origin.

Etiology. The virus of yellow fever is small, averaging 20 to 23 millimicrons. Affinity of the virus for host cells is of 2 main types: neurotropism, an affinity for nervous tissue, and viscerotropism, an affinity for liver, kidney and heart. Under natural field conditions the virus is pantropic. Both viscerotropism and neurotropism of the virus can be greatly reduced by repeated passage in tissue cultures, whereas neutrotropism is increased and viscerotropism practically disappears after repeated intracerebral passage of the virus in mice.

In the laboratory the neurotropic strain developed from intracerebral mouse passage produces, when injected intracerebrally in the *Macaca mulatta,* fatal encephalitis with absence of hepatitis and other visceral lesions.

Immunologically, the strains of yellow fever virus may not differ, but clinically a differentiation appears necessary between *jungle yellow fever* and *urban yellow fever.* Jungle yellow fever occurs occasionally in man in close contact with the jungle in the absence of *Aedes aegypti,* its usual vector. In South America the virus has been found in mosquitoes of the genus Haemagogus and in *Aedes leucocelaenus,* while in Africa it has been found in *Aedes simpsoni* and *A. africanus.*

Epidemiology. In transmission of the more common form of the disease the aegypti mosquito bites an infected person during the first 3 days of the disease when the virus is circulating in the blood. After 9 to 12 days the mosquito becomes infective, and a susceptible host acquires the disease by bite, with clinical manifestations beginning within 3 to 6 days.

A possible mode of transmission in the laboratory without insect vector has been suggested. While the virus is circulating in the blood of monkeys it can apparently be transferred from one animal to another through minute cutaneous abrasions, or even through the intact skin. The passaged neurotropic virus may also be transmitted to mice and monkeys by intranasal instillation.

Outbreaks of urban yellow fever have occurred in areas adjacent to endemic areas of jungle yellow fever. In Central America jungle yellow fever has been spreading slowly northward from Panama since 1948. Urban yellow fever has not been present in the Western Hemisphere since 1934 and has not been reported in the Orient. Southeastern United States is considered a receptive area for yellow fever; constant vigilance against mosquitoes is essential.

Pathology. There is severe jaundice, combined with petechial hemorrhages or ecchymotic areas of the skin. Black bloody material may be present in the mouth, nasal passages, and stomach. The liver is normal in size or slightly enlarged and is stained a deep yellow. Hepatic cells undergo fatty degeneration, with a distinctive type of necrosis, which is typically midzonal, although in severe cases the entire lobule may be involved. The architecture of the liver is preserved, and in healing no cirrhosis occurs. Coalescent acidophilic areas of hyaline necrosis, widely scattered in the parenchymatous cells, are termed "Councilman bodies." Superficial hemorrhages are often seen in the mucous membranes of the stomach, particularly in the pyloric region, and in the intestines. Although the spleen is fairly normal in size, there is usually degeneration of the malpighian corpuscles. The tubular epithelium of the kidneys, and the cardiac muscle, show involvement similar to that in the liver. The brain at times shows perivascular hemorrhages.

Clinical Manifestations. The majority of infections are so mild that the diagnosis may not be suspected.

The onset is acute with severe headache, chills, backache, pain in the limbs, and flushing of the face. Photophobia and conjunctival injection are prominent features. At the onset, jaundice is absent or slight. Cough and evidence of upper respiratory tract infection are usually lacking. As a rule, during the first 2 or 3 days the temperature rises rapidly to 103 to 104°F. with an increasing pulse rate, and then diminishes relatively more slowly than the pulse rate in what is often termed a temporary remission. During this period, albuminuria develops, and there are epigastric pain and tenderness, and vomiting.

Subsequently the temperature is again elevated and prostration and depression are prominent features. The face is pale with a cyanotic appearance. Jaundice increases slowly. Hemorrhages into the skin and often into the gums appear at this time with epistaxis, a dry, brown tongue and a decreasing pulse rate to less than 50 per minute in spite of high fever (Faget's sign). Degenerative changes in the heart result in cardiac dilatation and low blood pressure. The urine contains large amounts of albumin and casts. There is usually vomiting of dark brown material. The leukocyte count is often as low as 3000 cells per mm.[3] In severe and fatal cases bile appears in the urine; at times there is anuria followed by convulsions or coma.

In nonfatal cases improvement starts about the sixth day, and the temperature often is normal by the eighth day. When convalescence begins, progress is continuous without complications. There is permanent immunity to the disease.

Diagnosis. Differential diagnosis may present a problem, especially in the milder cases. Early differentiation from leptospirosis is particularly difficult. In infectious and serum hepatitis the illness usually develops and subsides much more slowly. Cases of yellow fever with acute onset may be confused initially with influenza, malaria or dengue fever.

Diagnostic aids include animal inoculations and neutralization and complement fixation tests of acute phase and convalescent serums. Increasing titer of type-specific antibody during clinical recovery constitutes good presumptive evidence of the disease. Isolation of the virus from blood obtained during the first 3 to 4 days of illness has been accomplished with regularity by intracerebral inoculation of mice.

Prognosis. The overall case fatality rate is probably not over 5 per cent, but in any outbreak the fatality rate of recognized cases may be 50 per cent or more.

Prophylaxis. Two types of live virus vaccine are available: the neurotropic (French) vaccine, which is administered by scarification, and the 17-D strain vaccine, which is administered subcutaneously. The neurotropic virus is attenuated by mouse brain passage, and prepared in mouse brain. The 17-D virus is attenuated in tissue culture, and prepared in chick embryos. Experience indicates that the 17-D strain vaccine is preferable. Immunity is afforded within 8 days after inoculation and lasts for 8 years or longer.

About 5 per cent of all persons vaccinated have a mild reaction on the sixth to eighth day. Untoward reactions appear to be more prevalent in infants, and all recorded cases of encephalitis have been in this age group and have occurred within 1 to 2 weeks after administration of the vaccine. In most recorded cases recovery was spontaneous within 4 to 5 days with no apparent residual damage. In one instance, however, a 3-year-old child died of encephalitis following subcutaneous inoculation. Virus (17-D strain yellow fever virus) was recovered from the brain.

General experience with active immunization indicates that it is not advisable to give smallpox and yellow fever vaccine at the same time. An interval of 21 days is suggested.

In the event of suspected cases the patients should be protected from mosquitoes. Spraying of premises, house, room or ward with a satisfactory insecticide is recommended.

Treatment. Specific therapy is lacking; complete bed rest is essential to lessen the danger of cardiac failure and hepatic damage. Supportive treatment and good nursing care are important, with special attention to oral hygiene and control of fever. Vomiting should be kept under control; solid food should be limited. Maintenance of nutritional status and of fluid and electrolyte balance, and control of intercurrent infection are essential. Because of diminution in prothrombin and fibrinogen, vitamin K should be given, and, if possible, plasma concentrates which contain coagulation factors.

REFERENCES

Clarke, D. H., and Casals, J.: Yellow Fever; in F. L. Horsfall and I. Tamm (Eds.): *Viral and Rickettsial Infections of Man.* 4th ed. Philadelphia, J. B. Lippincott Company, 1965, p. 608.

Feitel, M., Watson, E. H., and Cochran, K. W.: Encephalitis after Yellow Fever Vaccination. *Pediatrics,* 25:956, 1960.

Langmuir, A. D., and others: Fatal Viral Encephalitis Following 17-D Yellow Fever Vaccine Inoculation: Report of a Case in a 3-Year-Old Child. A Joint Statement. *J.A.M.A.,* 198:671, 1966.

McLean, D. M.: Yellow Fever; in A. J. Rhodes and C. E. van Rooyen (Eds.): *Textbook of Virology for Students and Practitioners of Medicine.* 4th ed. Baltimore, Williams & Wilkins Company, 1962, Chap. 45, p. 333.

Reed, W., Carroll, J., Agramonte, A., and Lazear, J. W.: Yellow Fever: A Compilation of Various Publications. *United States 61st Congr., Third Session, Senate Doc. No. 822,* Washington, D.C., 1911.

LYMPHOGRANULOMA VENEREUM

(LYMPHOGRANULOMA INGUINALE)

The majority of children with lymphogranuloma venereum acquire the disease by direct transmission from an infected adult. The infectious agent is considered to be a virus closely related to those of the psittacosis-ornithosis group (Rickettsiales). The agent usually enters through a minor abrasion on the penis or vulva, or it may penetrate the urethra, resulting in a mild urethritis. Rarely, the primary lesion is at other sites, as the mouth or hand.

Clinical Manifestations. Enlargement of the inguinal lymph nodes is the most prominent manifestation of the disease and may be the first and only sign; the primary lesion is rarely discovered in children. Rectal and anal strictures are not common in children; when they do occur, obstruction from residual scarring may be the first indication. The site of the primary lesion determines the extent and location of the lymphadenitis. Cervical and axillary lymphadenopathy has been described following mouth and hand lesions, respectively.

The lymphadenopathy is chronic, and the involved nodes are tender and often painful. They suppurate frequently, draining sinuses form, and the nodes become matted together and to adjacent tissues. In some instances the nodes change little in consistency, remain firm and gradually become less tender. Although early stages of the condition may be characterized by fever and malaise, in general the systemic symptoms are mild. Joint involvement has been observed roentgenographically in children, with the joint space slightly increased. There may be diffuse, mild rarefaction of the bones. Scarlatiniform eruptions and erythema nodosum have been described, and in some instances splenic enlargement and generalized lymphadenopathy have occurred.

Parinaud's oculoglandular syndrome, a unilateral conjunctivitis followed by a chronic enlargement of the parotid gland and the anterior cervical nodes, may be caused by the virus of lymphogranuloma venereum, as well as by other infectious agents.

Central nervous system involvement has been reported in only a few instances, some of which, however, progressed to fatal outcome. Headache, nuchal rigidity and mental confusion were the presenting symptoms. The cerebrospinal fluid is under increased pressure with increased protein content and pleocytosis. The spinal fluid sugar content may be reduced moderately, and the colloidal gold curve may show a strong first-zone reaction. Encephalitis may develop in the absence of obvious lesions or enlarged nodes. The agent has been recovered from spinal fluid by chorio-allantoic or yolk-sac inoculation of embryonated eggs.

Diagnosis. Viremia may be demonstrated during most of the course. A fourfold increase or more in the titer of complement-fixing antibody during clinical recovery provides good presumptive evidence. A titer of 1:32 obtained on repeated tests is highly suggestive even without a further rise. The antigen usually used is derived from virus grown in chick embryo tissue culture.

The skin test (Frei) with heat-inactivated virus, usually material from a bubo, is performed by injecting 0.1 ml. of the antigen (Lygranum) intradermally into the flexor surface of the forearm, with a similar amount of control material injected into the other arm. A positive reaction consists of a firm papule 5 mm. or more in diameter which appears within 48 to 72 hours, with a negative or only a slight reaction at the site of the control inoculation. The reaction usually becomes positive within 3 to 8 weeks from the time infection has occurred, and may remain positive for years. Recently tissue-culture antigen has been used in the same manner. Transient positive skin reactions have been reported in patients with psittacosis, atypical pneumonias and syphilis.

Differential diagnosis includes distinction from other types of lymphadenopathy such as in chronic pyogenic bacterial infection, tuberculosis, tularemia, cat-scratch disease, and lymphoma or other neoplasm.

Treatment. Sulfonamide drugs, penicillin and the tetracyclines have been given, singly or in combination. The tetracyclines are generally considered the drug of choice, penicillin and chloramphenicol being less effective. Treatment must be continued for 10 to 14 days. Surgical excision of lymph nodes is rarely necessary.

REFERENCES

Banov, L., Jr.: Rectal Lesions of Lymphogranuloma Venereum in Childhood. *Am. J. Dis. Child.,* 83:660, 1952.

Beeson, P. B., Wall, M. J., and Heyman, A.: Isolation of Virus of Lymphogranuloma Venereum from Blood and Spinal Fluid of Human Being. *Proc. Soc. Exper. Biol. & Med.,* 62: 306, 1946.

Erskine, D.: Lymphogranuloma Venereum: A Review of Sixty-One Cases. *Brit. J. Ven. Dis.,* 34:163, 1958.

Greaves, A. B., Hilleman, M. R., Taggart, S. R., Bankhead, A. B., and Feld, M.: Chemotherapy in Bubonic Lymphogranuloma Venereum: A Clinical and Serological Evaluation. *Bull. WHO,* 16:277, 1957.

Levy, H.: Lymphogranuloma Venereum in Childhood. *J. Pediat.,* 11:812, 1937.

Roth, D., and Schulick, R.: Isolated Cervical Lymphogranuloma in a Child. *Pediatrics,* 8:480, 1951.

Sabin, A. B., and Aring, C. D.: Meningoencephalitis in Man Caused by the Virus of Lymphogranuloma Venereum. *J.A.M.A.,* 120:1376, 1942.

INFECTIOUS MONONUCLEOSIS

Infectious mononucleosis, which seems to occur most frequently in older children and young adults, is not uncommon in children between the ages of 2 and 10 years, and during epidemic periods it has been observed in infants. The variable manifestations and common occurrence of this disease make it a diagnostic possibility in throat infections, colds, influenza-like disease and generalized rashes. The essential feature of the disease is an increase in the mononuclear elements of the blood at some time during its course. The infectious agent is considered to be viral; blood from patients in the acute phase has produced similar disease when injected into monkeys and rabbits.

Recently the EB virus (Epstein and Barr), similar in structure to viruses of the herpes group, has been implicated in the causation of infectious mononucleosis. This virus, originally observed by electron microscopy in cultures of Burkitt-lymphoma cells, apparently replicates only in cells of the lymphatic series. Extensive seroepidemiologic studies by indirect immunofluorescence techniques strongly suggest a possible causative relation between the EB virus and infectious mononucleosis.

Clinical Manifestations. The incubation period is variable; it averages about 11 days. The onset may be insidious or acute. Common clinical manifestations are malaise, sore throat with pharyngitis, and prolonged fever characterized by morning remission. In children periorbital edema may be the initial sign. Enlargement of the lymph nodes may occur early or relatively late in the clinical course. The enlarged nodes are not tender, as a rule, and seldom suppurate. The salivary glands are rarely involved. The throat may be mildly or severely inflamed, at times with a membranous exudate which may simulate severe streptococcal disease or diphtheria (Fig. 10-85, p. 629). Splenomegaly is common and may persist for months. The spleen, not always tender, is palpable by about the seventh day of illness. A skin rash is present in 10 to 20 per cent of the cases, appearing between the fourth and tenth days of the disease, usually in the form of a discrete macular eruption (Fig. 10-86). Most prominent over the trunk, it is rarely seen on the hands, thighs, legs and feet. The rash may also assume a petechial, vesicular, morbilliform or scarlatiniform appearance.

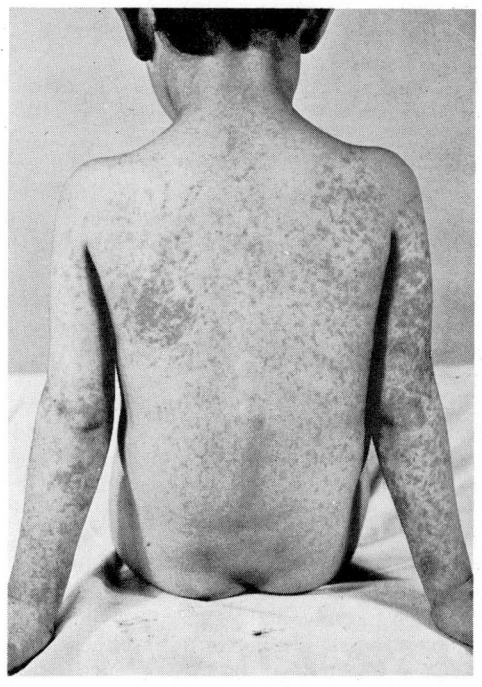

Figure 10-86. Morbilliform rash in mononucleosis.

Jaundice is an indication of hepatic involvement; there is good evidence, however, that the liver is frequently involved without discernible jaundice. Confusion of infectious mononucleosis with infectious hepatitis is possible in view of the lymphocytosis which may occur in hepatitis.

Neurologic manifestations occur occasionally and may precede, follow or occur simultaneously with the acute phase of the disease. The pattern may be that of an aseptic meningitis or a polyneuritis. Severe headache, nuchal rigidity, blurring of vision, mental confusion and occasionally convulsions have been noted. The cerebrospinal fluid may show an increase in mononuclear cells and in protein content. Concentration of sugar is normal.

Pericarditis with characteristic clinical manifestations and electrocardiographic changes may occur during the acute phase, prolonging the convalescence.

Diagnosis.   Essential laboratory data are the characteristic changes in the lymphocytes of the peripheral blood and a positive heterophil antibody test result.

The characteristic hematologic alteration is in the lymphocytes, which vary markedly in size and shape. Typically they are larger than mature lymphocytes, and have basophilic cytoplasm which is excessively vacuolated. The nucleus in these larger cells is frequently placed eccentrically, and is irregular or indented. Electron microscopic studies of the leukocytes in infectious mononucleosis have confirmed these characteristic features. Such atypical lymphocytes are also seen in smaller numbers (not more than 5 per cent) in other diseases such as infectious hepatitis, rubella and primary atypical pneumonia. In infectious mononucleosis, however, the increase in these atypical lymphocytes is characteristically greater, being 10 to 25 per cent of the leukocytes.

The leukocyte count is usually elevated, but may be normal or low. Although initially the polymorphonuclear cells are often increased in number, in a fully developed case the relative reduction in granulocytes is typical. The rise in lymphocytes usually begins on the fourth or fifth day, and by the seventh to the tenth day these cells constitute 60 to 90 per cent of the total leukocytes. In rare instances thrombocytopenia with purpura and prolonged bleeding time, agranulocytosis and anemia may occur.

The sheep-cell or heterophil agglutination test (Paul-Bunnell-Davidsohn) for the diagnosis of infectious mononucleosis is a nonspecific serologic reaction, the exact nature of which is not known. A characteristic antibody is present in the serum in infectious mononucleosis; it differs from other antibodies in human serums which agglutinate sheep cells, such as those usually found in low titer in normal human serum, or those which occur in relatively high titer after the administration of horse serum (serum sickness). These various antibodies can be differentiated through their selective absorption by certain cells. In infectious mononucleosis the sheep-cell agglutinins can be absorbed completely by ox erythrocytes, but not by guinea pig kidney tissue. The sheep-cell agglutinins of serum sickness can be absorbed completely by both ox erythrocytes and guinea pig tissue. Those sheep-cell agglutinins normally present in human serum cannot be absorbed by ox erythrocytes, but can be absorbed almost completely by guinea pig kidney tissue.

In each instance the antibody level can be titrated. In the case of infectious mononucleosis, titers of 1:10 to 1:40 are considered negative or borderline; titers of 1:80 to 1:160 are presumptive; and titers above 1:160 are considered diagnostic. The best criterion in the early stages of the disease is a rising titer. In 60 per cent of cases of infectious mononucleosis the heterophil antibody reaction becomes positive during the first week of the disease and remains so for varying periods of time; the titer may reach a peak quickly and subside rapidly. Falsely positive results may be obtained in patients who have received horse serum, as indicated above, and in rare instances in other infections.

Recent modifications of the differential tests are useful in confirmation. The capillary screening test is rapid and simple to perform. Slide tests with enzyme-treated cells, such as the ox-cell hemolysin test, are useful when the usual heterophil antibody titer is borderline. The Hoff-Bauer rapid slide test is a promising diagnostic tool, having a high degree of specificity, and being easy to perform.

Patients with infectious mononucleosis may have a falsely positive complement fixation (Wassermann or Kahn) reaction for syphilis which usually appears during the second week of the disease and becomes negative within 2 or 3 weeks. Patients in whom a rash develops appear more likely to have this falsely positive reaction than those who do not have an eruption.

Prognosis.   In general the prognosis is good, even in prolonged and the more serious cases. The convalescent period, however, is usually long, especially in older children; weakness and easy fatigability may persist. Fatalities have occurred as a result of rupture of the spleen. With the possible exception of chronic hepatitis, significant sequels do not occur.

Treatment.   Therapy is supportive and nonspecific. Bacterial complications are not common and may be treated as indicated. An initial period of bed rest is usually indicated. Increase in activity should be gradual, based on the patient's temperature and evidence of fatigue. Convalescent serum and gamma globulin have been used in some severe cases. In a few patients with liver involvement, azotemia and thrombocytopenia, good results with ACTH have been reported. The routine use of ACTH or corticosteroids in uncomplicated cases is not recommended.

REFERENCES

Bender, C. E.: The Value of Corticosteroids in the Treatment of Infectious Mononucleosis. *J.A.M.A.*, 199:529, 1967.

Davidsohn, I., and Lee, C. L.: The Laboratory in the Diagnosis of Infectious Mononucleosis: With Additional Notes on Epidemiology, Etiology, and Pathogenesis. *M. Clin. N. Amer.,* 46:225, 1962.

Davidsohn, I., and Lee, C. L.: Serologic Diagnosis of Infectious Mononucleosis: A Comparative Study of Five Tests. *Am. J. Clin. Path.,* 41:115, 1964.

Diehl, V., Henle, G., Henle, W., and Kohn, G.: Demonstration of Herpes Group Virus in Cultures of Peripheral Leukocytes from Patients with Infectious Mononucleosis. *J. Virol.,* 2:663, 1968.

Epstein, M. A., Barr, Y. M., and Achong, B. G.: Studies with Burkitt's Lymphomas. *Wistar Institute Symp. Monograph,* 4:69, 1965.

Evans, A. S., Niederman, J. C., and McCollum, R. W.: Seroepidemiologic Studies of Infectious Mononucleosis with EB Virus. *New England J. Med.,* 279:1121, 1968.

Henle, G., Henle, W., and Diehl, V.: Relation of Burkitt's Tumor-Associated Herpes-Type Virus to Infectious Mononucleosis. *Proc. Nat. Acad. Sci.,* USA, 59:94, 1968.

Hoff, G., and Bauer, S.: A New Rapid Slide Test for Infectious Mononucleosis. *J.A.M.A.,* 194:351, 1965.

Lee, C. L., Davidsohn, I., and Mih, N. L.: A Capillary Screening Test for Infectious Mononucleosis. *Am. J. Clin. Path.,* 44:162, 1965.

Mikkelsen, W., Tupper, C. J., and Murray, J.: The Ox Cell Hemolysin Test as a Diagnostic Procedure in Infectious Mononucleosis. *J. Lab. & Clin. Med.,* 52:648, 1958.

Schnell, R. G., Dyck, P. J., Bowie, E. J. W., Klass, D. W., and Taswell, H. F.: Infectious Mononucleosis: Neurologic and EEG Findings. *Medicine,* 45:51, 1966.

ACUTE INFECTIOUS LYMPHOCYTOSIS

This infection, originally thought to be a variant of infectious mononucleosis, was described and named by Carl Smith in 1941. The outstanding characteristic is the increase in the total number of lymphocytes in the peripheral blood and in the bone marrow, which persists over a relatively long time. Although the clinical course is usually mild, a variety of symptoms and signs has been recorded, such as fever, nasopharyngitis, abdominal complaints, skin rash and mild meningoencephalomyelitic manifestations.

Etiology and Epidemiology. No bacterial or viral agent has been isolated as the cause of this condition. Multiple cases have been reported in institutional epidemics and in families. The incubation period is estimated to be 12 to 21 days. Most of the cases described have been in children under the age of 10 years. The disease has been observed in the Western Hemisphere and in Europe. Nothing is known about the development of immunity.

Pathology. Microscopic examination of excised lymph nodes reveals degeneration of the lymph follicles and proliferation of the reticuloendothelium of the sinuses.

Clinical Manifestations. Many patients are asymptomatic, and there may be no abnormal physical findings. In some instances there may be fever at the onset and transient complaints. The manifestations may be those of an upper respiratory tract infection, sore throat predominating, or there may be gastrointestinal symptoms such as vomiting, diarrhea or abdominal pain. In a few instances symptoms simulating those of acute appendicitis have been present, suggesting a surgical emergency. The clinical pattern in a small number of recorded cases has been that of a meningoencephalitis with slight increase in the cerebrospinal fluid cell count. In one of these there was paralysis. A mild, generalized morbilliform rash similar to that in infectious mononucleosis may appear early in the course and last for several days. Slight enlargement of lymph nodes or the spleen has been observed, but is not common.

Laboratory Data. The only characteristic finding is the high white blood cell count, which ranges from 20,000 to 120,000 per mm.[3], the proportion of lymphocytes varying from 62 to 97 per cent. The lymphocytes are normal in appearance and chiefly of the small variety. A slight eosinophilia may be present. There is no abnormality in the erythrocytes or platelets.

The heterophil agglutination reaction is negative. The bone marrow contains an increased number of normal or postmature lymphocytes; otherwise it is not abnormal. These changes persist longer in the bone marrow than in the peripheral blood.

Diagnosis. From the hematologic point of view the condition must be differentiated from infectious mononucleosis, acute leukemia and infections associated with a lymphocytosis, principally pertussis. Less frequently the disease must be distinguished from acute abdominal conditions such as acute appendicitis, and from meningoencephalitis of other causes.

Infectious mononucleosis can be identified by the positive heterophil agglutination reaction and by demonstration in the peripheral blood of the abnormal lymphocytes typical of this disease. In addition, the clinical manifestations in infectious mononucleosis are more severe, including fever, malaise, sore throat, rash, jaundice and enlargement of lymph nodes and often of the spleen.

Differentiation from *acute leukemia* may on occasion be impossible without examination of the bone marrow.

Though in some of the more severe cases of *pertussis* extremely high lymphocyte counts are observed, the characteristic clinical manifestations in pertussis are usually sufficient for differential diagnosis.

When abdominal manifestations suggest a surgical condition, the high lymphocyte count supports a period of watchful waiting during which the diagnosis will usually become apparent in part because of the short duration of the abdominal complaints.

Course and Prognosis. Clinical manifestations, as a rule, are of short duration, and the prognosis is excellent. The lymphocytosis persists for weeks, however, and in one case was observed for 7 months. No sequels have been recognized and no deaths recorded.

Treatment is symptomatic.

REFERENCES

Barnes, G. R., Jr., Yannet, H., and Lieberman, R.: A Clinical Study of an Institutional Outbreak of Acute Infectious Lymphocytosis. *Am. J. Med. Sci.,* 218:646, 1949.

Lemon, B. K., and Kaump, D. H.: Infectious Lymphocytosis: A Report of an Epidemic in Children. *J. Pediat.,* 36:61, 1950.

Riley, H. D.: Acute Infectious Lymphocytosis. *New England J. Med.,* 248:92, 1953.

Ryder, R. J.: Acute Infectious Lymphocytosis. *Am. J. Dis. Child.,* 110:299, 1965.

Smith, C. H.: Acute Infectious Lymphocytosis; in *Advances in Pediatrics.* New York, Interscience Publishers, Inc., 1947, Vol. II, p. 64.

CAT-SCRATCH DISEASE

(BENIGN INOCULATION LYMPHORETICULOSIS; CAT-CLAW DISEASE; CAT-BITE FEVER)

The relation of cat-scratch disease in man to contact with the domestic cat seems to have been established.

Etiology. The causative agent, though not identified, has been thought to be a virus of the psittacosis-lymphogranuloma venereum group (Rickettsiales). Attempts to isolate the agent from suppurative lymph nodes have been unsuccessful, but transfer of the disease to monkeys and human volunteers has been accomplished. Stained sections of primary skin lesions and involved lymph nodes from both man and monkeys show large numbers of intracellular and extracellular granule-like bodies similar to those of psittacosis. On the basis of similarity in the type of elementary body, a possible relation between the causative agent of cat-scratch disease and that of feline pneumonitis has been suggested. This agent, which is related antigenically to the psittacosis-lymphogranuloma viruses, can be isolated readily and established in mice by intranasal passage. A similar transfer of material from infected nodes in cat-scratch disease has not produced disease in mice. Some complement fixation and hemagglutination studies have supported the concept of viral origin.

Epidemiology. Initially recognized about 1930 in France and the United States, the disease is world-wide.

Cats which transfer the agent to human subjects show no evidence of illness and have no reaction to the intradermal injection of the antigen.

Pathology. Examination of involved lymph nodes has revealed only nonspecific morphologic changes which can be classified into distinct phases: (1) an "elementary" phase of simple hyperplasia; (2) an "accentuated" phase in which, in addition to hyperplasia, areas of early cellular necrosis stain as acidophilic masses; and (3) the "ultimate" stage in which the lymph node architecture is displaced by multiple areas with central necrosis and by circumscribed foci of epithelioid cells and scattered giant cells of the Langhans type (pseudotubercles). The final phase corresponds to the clinical stage when the enlarged node becomes fluctuant.

Clinical Manifestations. Cat-scratch disease is a nonfatal systemic illness characterized by malaise, headache, low-grade fever and lymphadenitis. Although as a rule the patient does not appear acutely or chronically ill, the size of the involved lymph node, or nodes, is often striking. In most instances the history will reveal association with cats, with or without the recollection of a specific abrasion. The incubation period varies from 10 to 30 days. In a volunteer subject regional adenopathy began in 8 days and progressed to fluctuation in about 20 days. At the height of the lymph node response a skin papule appeared at the site of the primary intradermal inoculation and persisted for several days.

The foregoing sequence appears to be characteristic of the natural infection. At the time medical advice is sought there is usually an exacerbation of redness and swelling at the site where a primary lesion is in the process of healing. This lesion tends to heal slowly, and may resemble an insect bite, a small furuncle or a scab following simple trauma. The nodes involved are those which drain the area where the initial lesion occurred, commonly the epitrochlear, axillary, submandibular, cervical or inguinal nodes. The skin overlying enlarged nodes may show some redness, but more often is normal in appearance. Involved lymph nodes may be hard or soft, and vary in diameter from 1 to 5 cm.; on aspiration purulent fluid may be obtained.

Unusual clinical manifestations have included cervical adenitis, transient pulmonary infiltration and an oculoglandular form of the disease with conjunctivitis and enlargement of preauricular and cervical nodes. Purpura and skin rashes of the erythema multiforme and nodosum types have been observed. In one instance an osteolytic lesion which healed spontaneously was reported.

Central nervous system involvement, classified as encephalitis, encephalomyelitis, myelitis and radiculitis, may accompany or follow the acute phase. Onset of neurologic symptoms is usually abrupt with high fever. The spinal fluid shows a moderate increase in lymphocytes and in protein level.

Laboratory Data. There may be a moderate leukocytosis with a slight shift to the left. Otherwise there are no conclusive laboratory findings.

Skin Test. Patients with cat-scratch disease usually exhibit a skin reaction after the intradermal injection of an antigen prepared by the Frei procedure from an involved node of a known case. The skin test is performed by injecting intradermally 0.1 ml. of the antigen; the site should be observed at intervals of 48 and 72 hours. A typically positive reaction consists of an indurated, raised erythematous wheal 5 mm. or more in diameter, surrounded by a zone of erythema 30 to 40 mm. in diameter. The erythema may disappear in 1 to 2 days, but as a rule the wheal can be recognized for 4 or 5 days longer. A positive skin reaction may be obtained for years after cat-scratch infection. No regional adenopathy is associated with a positive reaction to the intradermal injection. Although the skin test is considered to have diagnostic significance, it must be recognized that the material used for preparation of antigen varies considerably from case to case.

Differential Diagnosis. Cat-scratch disease may be confused with simple pyogenic adenitis, but must be differentiated also from tuberculous adenitis, tularemia, bubonic plague, rat-bite fever, Hodgkin's disease, lymphoma, fungus infections and lymphogranuloma venereum.

Prognosis. The prognosis is uniformly good; the enlarged nodes regress spontaneously in 1 to 3 months. In some instances fibrosis may result in persistent enlargement.

Prevention. At present, detection of cats carrying the infective agent is not possible, since they are asymptomatic and do not have a positive skin reaction to the antigen. There are no control measures other than avoidance of contact with cats. Other possible means of transfer include abrasions by thorns and wood splinters, and by fragments of bone in meat handlers. The obvious question in such instances is whether the persons involved had subsequent contact with cats.

Treatment. No therapeutic measures are known to be of benefit. Occasionally drainage by aspiration will hasten resolution of fluctuant nodes; this procedure carries the risk of a draining sinus, which, however, usually heals with minimal scarring.

REFERENCES

Adams, W. C., and Hindman, S. N.: Cat-Scratch Disease Associated with an Osteolytic Lesion. *J. Pediat.,* 44:665, 1954.

Boyd, G. E., and Craig, G.: Etiology of Cat-Scratch Fever. *J. Pediat.,* 59:313, 1961.

Debré, R., and Job, J.-C.: La maladie des griffes du chat. *Acta paediat.,* 43 (Suppl. 96): 1, 386, 1954.

Margileth, A. M.: Cat Scratch Disease: Non-Bacterial Regional Lymphadenitis: The Study of 145 Patients and a Review of the Literature. *Pediatrics,* 42:803, 1968.

Mollaret, P., Reilly, J., Bastin, R., and Tournier, P.: Le virus de la lymphoréticulose bénigne d'inoculation. *Presse méd.,* 64:1177, 1956.

Naji, A. F., Carbonell, F., and Barker, H. J.: Cat Scratch Disease: A Report of Three New Cases: Review of the Literature, and Classification of the Pathologic Changes in the Lymph Nodes During Various Stages of the Disease. *Am. J. Clin. Path.,* 38:513, 1962.

Paxson, E. M., and McKay, R. J., Jr.: Neurologic Symptoms Associated with Cat Scratch Disease. *Pediatrics,* 20:13, 1957.

Small, W. T., and Sniffen, R. C.: Nonbacterial Regional Lymphadenitis (Cat Scratch Fever): Evaluation of Surgical Treatment. *New England J. Med.,* 255:1029, 1956.

Warwick, W. J., and Good, R. A.: Cat Scratch Disease in Minnesota. I. Epidemiology. II. Family Epidemics. III. Evaluation of Skin Test. *Am. J. Dis. Child.,* 100:228, 236, 241, 1960.

CYTOMEGALIC INCLUSION DISEASE

Cytomegalic inclusion disease is seen predominantly in young infants as a congenitally acquired infection, but it is encountered occasionally in older children and adults. It is a systemic disease characterized by the presence of intranuclear and intracytoplasmic inclusion bodies in enlarged cells of many viscera. Affected cells may be epithelial or mesenchymal. At necropsy inclusion-bearing cells have been demonstrated in almost all the organs of the body, including the respiratory system, kidneys, adrenals, liver, gastrointestinal system, hematopoietic tissues and the brain. Involvement of the central nervous system may be extensive. Although the tissue adjoining the involved cells may show no significant inflammatory response, in some instances there is an associated infiltration of lymphocytes, and on occasion focal areas of necrosis or fibrosis. Advanced periventricular cerebral necrosis has been observed in premature infants. Excessive extramedullary hematopoiesis may be present, especially in the spleen and liver of infants dying during the neonatal period. In premature and newborn infants who have acquired the infection in utero the inclusion bodies are prominent in the kidney. The intranuclear inclusion body occupies most of the enlarged nucleus of the infected cell, and characteristically is separated from the nuclear membrane by a clear halo. Small, multiple intracytoplasmic inclusion bodies occur less frequently.

Strains of the virus (DNA), which structurally resembles herpes simplex virus, are species-specific, affecting man, monkeys and other animals.

Serologic studies, still not adequate for diagnostic purposes, indicate that the virus is widespread. Antibodies have been demonstrated in a high proportion of human serums. After infection in the human subject the virus may be shed in the saliva for as long as 4 weeks, and in the urine for as long as 24 months. At necropsy it has been recovered from a variety of tissues, including salivary gland, kidney, brain and liver. It has also been recovered from adenoid and tonsillar tissue undergoing spontaneous degeneration in tissue culture, and from the urine of infants and children with no overt evidence of cytomegalic inclusion disease or other signs of clinical illness. Characteristic inclusion bodies have been observed as an incidental finding in the salivary glands of 8 to 32 per cent of fetuses and infants dying from a variety of causes. Such a finding does not warrant the diagnosis of cytomegalic inclusion disease. Similar inclusion bodies have also been observed in the tissues of infants, children and adults dying from pertussis and from debilitating diseases such as cystic fibrosis, leukemia, and lymphoma. The significance of these findings is not clear; it has been suggested that a latent viral infection may have been activated because of lowered host resistance.

Clinical manifestations of the congenitally acquired infection are apparent most often in the neonatal period or early infancy. Affected infants are often premature or below average birth weight for gestational age. Although any organ system may be involved, the manifestations are usually referable to the hematopoietic system, liver and the central nervous system. Hepatomegaly, splenomegaly, icterus, anemia, thrombocytopenia, purpura and cerebral calcifications are common findings. The cerebral calcifications are classically paraventricular, occurring mainly in the subependymal regions of the lateral ventricles; there may be poor development of the convolutions and dilatation of the ventricles with resultant microcephaly or hydrocephalus. Chorioretinitis, similar to that of congenital toxoplasmosis, may be a manifestation. Virus has been isolated from aqueous humor obtained from the anterior chamber.

In infants and children whose first manifestations of disease are apparent after the neonatal period the clinical pattern is more varied. The prominent signs and symptoms are apt to be those of interstitial pneumonitis or enterocolitis.

The **differential diagnosis** in the neonatal period includes erythroblastosis fetalis, sepsis, toxoplasmosis, congenital syphilis, generalized herpes simplex, congenital hemolytic anemia and congenital leukemia. The diagnosis is based on the demonstration of typical inclusion-bearing cells in the urinary sediment; and in fluid aspirated from the subdural space in one recorded case. For definite diagnosis, however, these observations must be correlated with other findings. The diagnosis has been verified by liver biopsy in a few instances.

The **prognosis** is grave. The fatality rate in recognized cases of the congenitally acquired infection is extremely high; accumulating evidence suggests, however, that there may be a relatively high incidence of clinically inapparent infections. Permanent cerebral damage, often present in infants who survive the clinically apparent disease, may vary in severity. Association of the disease with hypoparathyroidism and with residual adrenal or liver damage has been reported.

Prognosis for future pregnancies appears to be good. There is no conclusive evidence of a mother giving birth to a second infant with cytomegalic inclusion disease. Nevertheless in one recorded instance the clinical findings suggested possible infection of 2 infants of the same mother, born 15 months apart.

No satisfactory **therapy** is known; antibiotics, gamma globulin, corticosteroids and blood transfusions have been used without demonstrable benefit.

REFERENCES

Elliott, G. B., and Elliott, K. A.: Observations on Cerebral Cytomegalic Inclusion Disease of the Foetus and the Newborn. *Arch. Dis. Childhood,* 37:34, 1962.

Gear, J., Le Roux, A. F., Kessel, I., and Sichel, R.: Generalized Cytomegalic Inclusion Disease. *South African M.J.,* 36:8, 1962.

Hanshaw, J. B.: Congenital and Acquired Cytomegalovirus Infection. *Pediat. Clin. N. Amer.,* 13:279, 1966.

Medearis, D. N., Cytomegalic Inclusion Disease: An Analysis of the Clinical Features Based on Literature and Six Additional Cases. *Pediatrics,* 19:467, 1957.

Medearis, D. N., Observations Concerning Human Cytomegalovirus Infection and Disease. *Bull. Johns Hopkins Hosp.,* 114:181, 1964.

Smith, M. G.: The Salivary Gland Viruses of Man and Animals (Cytomegalic Inclusion Disease). *Progress in Med. Virology,* 2:171, 1959.

Weller, T. H.: Cytomegaloviruses; in F. L. Horsfall and I. Tamm, (Eds.): *Viral and Rickettsial Infections of Man.* 4th ed. Philadelphia, J. B. Lippincott Company, 1965, Chap. 43, p. 926.

INFECTIOUS NEURONITIS
(INFECTIOUS POLYNEURITIS; GUILLAIN-BARRÉ SYNDROME)

Infectious neuronitis is a disease of unknown origin involving the nervous system and manifested by varying degrees of motor and sensory disturbances. Characteristically, there is bilateral ascending paralysis. The existence of this disorder as a distinct entity has been questioned on the basis that it may represent a hypersensitivity phenomenon, and because it has been reported in association with diseases of divergent causes. The condition frequently follows an acute infection and is thought by many to be a toxic effect of the original infection. Others have suggested that the nervous system involvement may be due to an activated latent virus or to a concurrent viral infection. Experimental studies in animals have failed to demonstrate a specific causative agent. Diseases with which infectious neuronitis has been associated include diphtheria, scarlet fever, typhoid fever, mumps, influenza, respiratory infections, measles, infectious mononucleosis, tuberculous meningitis and infections with some of the enteric viruses. It has also been observed as a complication following the administration of tetanus antitoxin and various vaccines, including those for smallpox and poliomyelitis.

The incidence of the disease in children appears to be increasing. Although recorded cases suggest a higher susceptibility between the ages of 4 and 10 years, the condition can occur in infants under 1 year of age. The sexes appear to be equally susceptible.

The clinical picture is variable and may consist of acute ascending motor paralysis, of motor and sensory disturbances, or of a combination of signs and symptoms referable to the peripheral and cranial nerves. In most instances signs of peripheral neuritis develop symmetrically in the legs several days after an upper respiratory tract infection. The muscles become tender, and the deep tendon reflexes are abolished or greatly diminished; cutaneous reflexes are maintained, as a rule. Sensory loss is variable, but in children it is not often prominent. Cramping pains and paresthesias may occur. The paralysis tends to be symmetrical and ascending in its pattern of development, often involving the abdominal and thoracic muscles. Involvement of the cranial nerves is not common, except for the facial nerves, in which it may be bilateral. As a rule, muscular atrophy is not a feature of this disease, and recovery is usually complete, especially in children.

TABLE 10-21. VECTORS AND GEOGRAPHIC DISTRIBUTION OF DENGUE-LIKE DISEASES

ARBOVIRUS GROUP	VIRUS AND DISEASE	VECTOR	GEOGRAPHIC DISTRIBUTION
A................Chikungunya		*Aedes aegypti* *Aedes africanus*	Africa, India, Southeast Asia
A................O'nyong-nyong		*Anopheles funestus*	East Africa
B................West Nile Fever		*Culex molestus* *Culex univittatus*	Middle East, Africa, Southeast India

The course tends to be prolonged with a gradual return of function to the paralyzed muscles. Fatalities are uncommon, but may occur as a result of respiratory paralysis. Fever is an inconspicuous feature and may be absent.

When a cytoalbuminous dissociation coexists with polyneuritis, the condition has been designated as the Guillain-Barré syndrome. The characteristic increase in the protein level of the spinal fluid with little or no increase in cell count is an important diagnostic feature. The symmetry of the paralysis and the cerebrospinal fluid findings tend to distinguish the condition from acute anterior poliomyelitis.

Pathologic changes are found in the peripheral nerves and nerve roots; these consist chiefly in degeneration in the myelin and in the axis cylinders. There may or may not be evidence of inflammatory reaction. No characteristic central nervous system changes are found. Visceral lesions have been reported which consist in focal necroses with round cell infiltration in the liver, kidneys and adrenals.

Treatment is symptomatic; no specific therapy is available. Acceleration of recovery has been reported when therapy with a corticosteroid was initiated early in the course of the disease.

The **prognosis** in children is usually good, except in the most fulminating cases. Pneumonia is a common complication. The greatest danger is respiratory paralysis, in which early tracheotomy and mechanical respiratory aids may be lifesaving. Recovery is extremely slow and may require many months, but it is usually complete with no permanent residuals.

RUSSELL J. BLATTNER

REFERENCES

Berlacher, F. J., and Abington, R. B.: ACTH and Cortisone in Guillain-Barré Syndrome: Review of the Literature and Report of a Treated Case Following Primary Atypical Pneumonia. *Ann. Int. Med.*, 48:1106, 1958.

Eden, A. N.: Guillain-Barré Syndrome in a Six-Month-Old Infant. *Am. J. Dis. Child.*, 102:224, 1961.

Low, N. L., Schneider, J., and Carter, S.: Polyneuritis in Children. *Pediatrics*, 22:972, 1958.

Markland, L. D., and Riley, H. D., Jr.: The Guillain-Barré Syndrome in Childhood: A Comprehensive Review, Including Observations on Nineteen Additional Cases. *Clin. Pediatrics*, 6:162, 1967.

McFarland, H. R., and Heller, G. L.: Guillain-Barré Complex: A Statement of Diagnostic Criteria and Analysis of 100 Cases. *Arch. Neurol.*, 14:196, 1966.

Osler, L. D., and Sidell, A. D.: The Guillain-Barré Syndrome: The Need for Exact Diagnostic Criteria. *New England J. Med.*, 262:964, 1960.

DENGUE FEVER AND DENGUE-LIKE DISEASE

Definition. Dengue fever is a benign syndrome caused by several arthropod-borne viruses and characterized by biphasic fever, myalgia or arthralgia, rash, leukopenia and lymphadenopathy.

History. Epidemic dengue-like disease was first described by David Bylon in Java in 1779, and a year later in Philadelphia by Benjamin Rush. Large epidemics occurred frequently in temperate areas of the Americas, Europe, Australia and Asia until early in the twentieth century. Dengue fever and dengue-like disease are now endemic in tropical Africa and Asia. An unusually large dengue type 3 outbreak occurred in Caribbean countries in 1963.

Etiology. Dengue fever is caused by dengue viruses, of which there are at least 4 distinct antigenic types. In addition, 3 other arthropod-borne (arbo) viruses are frequently the cause of a similar or identical febrile disease with rash (Table 10-21).

Epidemiology. Dengue viruses are transmitted by mosquitoes of the Stegomyia family.

Aedes aegypti, a daytime biting mosquito, is the principal vector. All 4 virus types have been recovered from naturally infected *Aedes aegypti*. In most tropical areas *Aedes aegypti* is highly urbanized, breeding in water stored for drinking or bathing, or, alternatively in any container collecting rain water. Dengue viruses have also been recovered from naturally infected *Aedes albopictus*, and outbreaks in the Pacific area have been attributed to *Aedes scutellaris*. These species breed in water trapped in vegetation; *Aedes albopictus* frequently breeds in bamboo stumps. In Southeast Asia dengue may be maintained in a jungle cycle involving primates, since neutralizing antibody to dengue viruses is common in several species of Malaysian monkeys.

Dengue outbreaks in urban areas infected with

Aedes aegypti may be explosive; as many as 70 to 80 per cent of the population may be involved. Because *Aedes aegypti* has a limited flying range, spread of an epidemic is mainly through movement of viremic human beings. For this reason such outbreaks follow main lines of transportation. Sentinel cases may infect household mosquitoes and result in a large number of nearly simultaneous secondary infections, giving the appearance of a contagious disease. Where dengue viruses are endemic, children and susceptible foreigners may be the only persons to acquire overt disease, adults having become immune.

All dengue-like diseases may occur in epidemic outbreaks. Important epidemiologic features are determined by the vectors and their geographic distribution (Table 10-21). Chikungunya virus is widespread in the most populous areas of the world. In Asia, *Aedes aegypti* is the principal vector of infection to man; in Africa, *Aedes africanus*, which occupies the urban niche in place of *Aedes aegypti*, may be an important vector. In Southeast Asia, dengue and chikungunya outbreaks occur concurrently. Outbreaks of O'nyong-nyong and West Nile fever usually involve people living in villages or small towns, as opposed to the many urban outbreaks of dengue and chikungunya.

Pathology. Insufficient pathologic material has been obtained from virologically confirmed cases of dengue fever to present a comprehensive description. Fatalities are rare with chikungunya and West Nile infections; those recorded have been ascribed to viral encephalitis, hemorrhage or febrile convulsions (see p. 667) for description of Dengue Hemorrhagic Fever).

Clinical Manifestations. Biphasic fever and rashes are the most characteristic features of dengue. Manifestations vary with age and from patient to patient. In infants and young children the disease may be undifferentiated or characterized by a 1- to 5-day fever, pharyngeal inflammation, rhinitis and mild cough. In outbreaks a majority of patients have most of the findings described below.

After an incubation period of 2 to 7 days there is a sudden onset of fever which rapidly rises to 103 to 106°F., usually accompanied by frontal or retro-orbital headache. Occasionally back pain precedes the fever. A *transient*, macular, generalized rash which blanches under pressure may be seen during the first 24 to 48 hours of fever. The pulse rate may be slow in proportion to the degree of fever. Myalgia or arthralgia occurs soon after onset and increases in severity. Involvement of the knee may be particularly severe in patients with chikungunya or O'nyong-nyong infection. During the second to the sixth day of fever, nausea and vomiting are apt to occur, and during this phase generalized lymphadenopathy, cutaneous hyperesthesia or hyperalgesia, taste aberrations and pronounced anorexia may develop.

On the fifth to seventh day after onset of fever a generalized, morbilliform, maculopapular rash appears, which spares the palms and soles. It disappears in 1 to 5 days, and desquamation may occur. Rarely there is edema of the palms and soles. About the time of appearance of this second rash the body temperature, which has previously fallen to normal, may become slightly elevated and establish the biphasic temperature curve.

Epistaxis, petechiae and purpuric lesions, though uncommon, may occur at any stage of the disease. Swallowed blood from epistaxis passed by rectum or vomited may be interpreted by the unwary as bleeding of gastrointestinal origin. Convulsions may occur during extreme temperature elevations and are fairly common with chikungunya fever.

After the febrile stage prolonged asthenia, mental depression, bradycardia and ventricular extrasystoles, common in adults, occur infrequently in children.

Laboratory Data. Pancytopenia may be manifest on the third or fourth day of illness, and neutropenia may persist or reappear during the latter stage of the disease and may continue into convalescence. White blood cell counts as low as 2000 per cu. mm. have been recorded. Mild thrombocytopenia, rarely less than 100,000 cells per cu. mm., has been described in dengue and chikungunya infections confirmed by culture of the virus. Venous clotting, bleeding and prothrombin times and plasma fibrinogen values are within normal ranges. The tourniquet test infrequently gives positive results. Mild acidosis, hemoconcentration, increased transaminase values and hypoproteinemia have been described during primary dengue virus infections, particularly in infants. Sinus bradycardia, ectopic ventricular foci and prolongation of the P-R interval may be observed electrocardiographically.

Diagnosis and Differential Diagnosis. Clinical diagnosis derives from a high index of suspicion and a knowledge of the geographic distribution and of etiologic factors of causal viruses. Activities of the patient during the period preceding the onset of illness may give important clues to the possibility of infection.

Differential diagnosis includes a number of viral respiratory and influenza-like diseases and the early stages of malaria, scrub typhus, hepatitis and leptospirosis. Abortive forms of these latter diseases moderated by therapy or vaccine may never evolve beyond a dengue-like stage.

Three arbovirus diseases have dengue-like courses, but without rash: Colorado tick fever, sandfly fever and Rift Valley fever. Colorado tick fever occurs sporadically among campers and hunters in the western United States; sandfly fever, in the Mediterranean region, the Middle East, southern Russia and parts of the Indian subcontinent; and Rift Valley fever, in East, Central and South Africa.

Because of the variations in clinical findings and the multiplicity of possible causative agents, the descriptive term "dengue-like disease" should be used until a specific etiologic diagnosis is provided by the laboratory. Etiologic diagnosis can be made by serologic study or isolation of the virus. Blood for comparative and viral studies should be obtained during the febrile period, preferably before the fourth day of illness and during the convalescent phase, 14 to 21 days after the onset. The acute phase serum or plasma may be frozen, optimally at −65°C. or colder, to preserve the specimen if virus isolation is to be attempted. Serologic diagnosis is dependent on a fourfold or greater increase in antibody titer in the paired serums by hemagglutination inhibition, complement fixation or neutralization test. It may not be possible to distinguish the infecting virus by serologic methods alone, particularly when there has been prior infection with another member of the same arbovirus group, e.g. yellow fever immunization followed by dengue infection. For this reason, isolation of the virus should be attempted.

Prognosis. Primary infections with the viruses of dengue fever and dengue-like diseases are usually self-limited and benign. Fluid and electrolyte losses, hyperpyrexia and febrile convulsions are the most frequent complications in infants and young children, particularly in tropical countries. There is evidence that the prognosis may be adversely affected by previous infection with a closely related virus (see Dengue Hemorrhagic Fever).

Prophylaxis. Attenuated vaccines for dengue type 1 and chikungunya are efficacious, but are not available for general use. Prophylaxis consists in avoiding mosquito bite by use of insecticides, repellents, body-covering with clothing, and screening of houses. Destruction of *Aedes aegypti* breeding sites is also effective. If water storage is mandatory, a tight-fitting lid or a thin layer of oil may prevent egg laying or hatching. A larvicide, such as water-miscible DDT at a final concentration of 1 part per million, may be used. Only personal antimosquito measures are effective against mosquitoes in the field, forest or jungle.

Treatment. Treatment is supportive. Bed rest is advised during the febrile period. Salicylates or cold sponging should be used to keep body temperature below 104°F. Salicylates or mild sedation may be required to control pain. Fluid and electrolyte replacement therapy is required when there are deficits due to sweating, fasting, thirsting, vomiting or diarrhea.

REFERENCES

Casals, J., and Clarke, D. H.: Arboviruses; in F. L. Horsfall and I. Tamm (Eds.): *Viral and Rickettsial Infections of Man.* 4th ed. Philadelphia, J. B. Lippincott Company, 1965, pp. 583-684.

Sabin, A. B.: Research on Dengue During World War II. *Am. J. Trop. Med. & Hyg.,* 1:30, 1952.

Wisseman, C. L., and Sweet, B. H.: The Ecology of Dengue; in J. M. May (Ed.): *Studies in Disease Ecology.* New York, Hafner, 1961, pp. 15-40.

DENGUE HEMORRHAGIC FEVER

(Phillipine, Thai or Singapore
Hemorrhagic Fever; Hemorrhagic Dengue;
Acute Infectious Thrombocytopenic
Purpura)

Definition. Dengue hemorrhagic fever is a severe, often fatal, febrile disease caused by dengue viruses. It is characterized by shock, hemoconcentration, hypoproteinemia and abnormalities of hemostasis, and is currently thought to represent a hypersensitivity to a second or succeeding infection with dengue virus.

History. Hammon in 1956 established the causative relation of dengue infection to dengue hemorrhagic fever, which may have occurred in Australian children as early as 1897. Recent epidemics have involved most of Southeast Asia.

Etiology. At least 4 distinct types of dengue virus (types 1 through 4) have been isolated from patients with hemorrhagic fever.

Epidemiology. Dengue hemorrhagic fever occurs in areas where multiple types of dengue virus are simultaneously or sequentially transmitted. It is almost exclusively a disease of children. It is endemic in tropical Asia where warm temperatures and the practice of water storage in homes result in large, permanent populations of *Aedes aegypti*. Under these conditions, infections with dengue viruses of all types are frequent, and second infections with heterologous types are common. Nearly all patients with typical severe hemorrhagic fever have a secondary rise of antibody against dengue virus, indicative of a previous infection with a closely related virus.

Nonimmune foreigners, adults as well as children, exposed to dengue virus during an outbreak of hemorrhagic fever have classic dengue fever or even a milder disease. Since hemorrhagic fever has been described in a Caucasian child born in Thailand, the differences in clinical manifestations of dengue infections between natives and foreigners are probably related more to immunologic status than to racial susceptibility.

Pathology. Usually no gross or microscopic lesions are found which might account for death. In rare instances, death may be due to gastrointestinal or intracranial hemorrhages. Minimal to moderate hemorrhages are seen in the upper gastrointestinal tract, and petechial hemorrhages are frequent in the interventricular septum of the heart, on the pericardium and on the subserosal surfaces of major viscera. Focal hemorrhages are occasionally seen in the lungs, liver, adrenals and subarachnoid space. The liver is usually enlarged, often with fatty changes. Yellow, watery, at times blood-tinged, effusions are present in serous cavities in about three fourths of patients. Retroperitoneal tissues are markedly edematous.

Microscopically, there is perivascular edema in the soft tissues and widespread diapedesis of red blood cells. There may be maturational arrest of megakaryocytes in the bone marrow, and increased numbers of them are seen in the capillaries of the lungs, renal glomeruli and in sinusoids of the liver and spleen. Proliferation of lymphocytoid and plasmacytoid cells, lymphocytolysis and lymphophagocytosis occur in the spleen and lymph nodes. Granulomatous-appearing germinal centers are present in the spleen, and there is depletion of lymphocytes in the thymus. In the liver there are varying degrees of fatty metamorphosis, focal midzonal necrosis, hyperplasia of the Kupffer cells, and non-nucleated cells with vacuolated acidophilic cytoplasm, resembling Councilman bodies, in the sinusoids. Skin biopsies reveal minimal necrosis of endothelial cells during the acute stage of illness. Platelet or fibrin thrombosis or necrosis of vessel walls has not been described.

Dengue virus is almost invariably absent from tissues at the time of death; fluorescein-labeled antidengue gamma globulin has failed to reveal dengue antigen in tissues obtained either before or after death. These tissue suspensions, however, contain large quantities of dengue neutralizing substances.

Pathologic Physiology. Dengue hemorrhagic fever is characterized by 2 stages. Two to 5 days after the onset of a usual dengue illness the second phase, that of shock or hemorrhage, or both, occurs. At this time viremia is still present, and the patient has begun to produce large quantities of antidengue immunoglobulin (IgG). The association of hemorrhagic fever with sequential dengue virus infection and the high frequency of secondary antibody response suggests that the vascular damage is caused by a severe immunologic reaction. The capillary damage allows fluid, electrolytes, protein and, in some instances, red blood cells to leak into extravascular spaces. This internal redistribution of fluid, together with deficits due to fasting, thirsting and vomiting, results in hemoconcentration, hypovolemia, increased cardiac work, tissue hypoxia, metabolic acidosis and hyponatremia. The timing and sequence of dengue infections required to produce the aberrant host response are unknown, as is the mechanism of the immunologic reaction which produces the cellular damage.

Clinical Manifestations. The incubation period of dengue hemorrhagic fever is unknown, but is presumed to be that of dengue fever. The progression of the illness is characteristic in the severely ill child. A relatively mild first phase (see p. 666) with abrupt onset of fever, malaise, vomiting, headache, anorexia and cough is followed after 2 to 5 days by rapid clinical deterioration and physical collapse. In this second phase the patient usually manifests cold, clammy extremities, a warm trunk, flushed face and diaphoresis. He is restless and irritable. Frequently there are scattered petechiae on the forehead and extremities; spontaneous ecchymoses may appear, and easy bruisability and bleeding at sites of venipuncture are common. A macular or maculopapular rash may be present, and there may be circumoral and peripheral cyanosis. Respirations are rapid and often labored. The pulse is weak,

rapid and thready, and the heart sounds are faint. The pulse pressure is frequently narrow (20 mm. Hg or less); the systolic and diastolic pressures may be low or unobtainable. The liver may become palpable 2 to 3 fingerbreadths below the costal margin and is usually firm and nontender. Less than 10 per cent of patients manifest gross ecchymosis or gastrointestinal bleeding.

After a 24- to 36-hour period of crisis, convalescence is fairly rapid in the children who recover. The temperature may return to normal before or during the stage of shock. Bradycardia and ventricular extrasystoles are common during convalescence. Infrequently there is residual brain damage due either to prolonged shock or occasionally to intracranial hemorrhage. Death occurs in 10 to 40 per cent of patients with shock.

In contrast to the fairly characteristic pattern in the severely ill child, secondary dengue infections are relatively mild in the majority of instances, ranging from an inapparent infection through an undifferentiated, upper respiratory or dengue-like disease to an illness similar to that described above, but without apparent shock.

Laboratory Data. The most common hematologic abnormalities during clinical shock are a 20 per cent or greater increase in hematocrit over the recovery value, thrombocytopenia, mild leukocytosis (seldom exceeding 10,000 per mm.^{3}.) with 1 to 5 per cent of Türk's cells, prolonged bleeding time, and moderately prolonged prothrombin time (seldom less than 40 per cent of control) due to deficiencies in factors V, VII, IX and X. The tourniquet test gives a positive result early in the illness except in the moribund child.

Other abnormalities include moderate elevations of the serum transaminases, mild metabolic acidosis with hyponatremia and at times hypochloremia, slight elevation of serum urea nitrogen, and hypoproteinemia. Roentgenograms of the chest reveal bronchopneumonia and pleural effusions in somewhat less than 50 per cent of patients.

Diagnosis and Differential Diagnosis. In areas endemic for dengue, hemorrhagic fever should be suspected in children with a febrile illness who exhibit shock, hemoconcentration, hypoproteinemia and hemorrhagic manifestations with or without hepatic enlargement. Since many rickettsial diseases, meningococcemia and other severe illnesses caused by a variety of agents may produce a similar clinical picture, the diagnosis should be made only when epidemiologic or serologic evidence suggests the possibility of dengue fever. Hemorrhagic manifestations have been described in other diseases of viral or presumed viral origin; these include the hemorrhagic fevers observed in Argentina, Bolivia, Korea and the Soviet Union. These diseases differ clinically from dengue hemorrhagic fever. The bases for diagnosis of dengue fever are described on page 666.

Antibody response is of the secondary type, with rapid and pronounced rise of both hemagglutination-inhibiting (HI) and complement-fixing (CF) antibodies to dengue antigen. There are usually high and apparently fixed titers of HI antibody (1:640 or greater) and CF antibody (1:32 or greater) in both acute and convalescent serums. Such titers are regarded as presumptive evidence of recent dengue infection.

Prevention. Preventive measures are described on page 667. An attenuated, live dengue type 1 vaccine has been developed, but is not available commercially. The possibility exists that dengue vaccination may sensitize a recipient, so that ensuing dengue infection may result in hemorrhagic fever. Vaccination with yellow fever 17D strain has no effect on dengue illness.

Treatment. Management requires immediate evaluation of vital signs and degrees of hemoconcentration, dehydration and electrolyte imbalance. Close monitoring is essential for at least 48 hours, since shock may occur or recur precipitously early in the disease. Patients who are cyanotic or have labored breathing should be given oxygen. Intravenous replacement of fluids and electrolytes is frequently sufficient to sustain patients until spontaneous recovery occurs. When elevation of the hematocrit value persists after replacement of fluids, plasma or plasma protein preparations are indicated. Care must be taken to avoid overhydration, which may contribute to cardiac failure. Transfusion of fresh blood or of platelets suspended in plasma may be required to control bleeding, but should not be given during hemoconcentration, and should be given only after evaluation of hemoglobin or hematocrit value.

Paraldehyde or chloral hydrate may be required for children who are markedly agitated. Pressor amines, alpha adrenergic blocking agents, aldosterone and hydrocortisone have been widely utilized, but their use has not resulted in a significant reduction of mortality over that observed with simple supportive therapy.

SCOTT B. HALSTEAD

REFERENCES

Cohen, S. N., and Halstead, S. B.: Shock Associated with Dengue Infection. I. The Clinical and Physiological Manifestations of Dengue Hemorrhagic Fever in Thailand, 1964. *J. Pediat.,* 68:448, 1966.
Halstead, S. B., Nimmannitya, S., Yamarat, C., and Russell, P. K.: Hemorrhagic Fever in Thailand; Newer Knowledge Regarding Etiology. *Jap. J. Med. Sci. & Biol.,* 20:96, 1967.
Johnson, K. M., Halstead, S. B., and Cohen, S. N.: Hemorrhagic Fever of Southeast Asia and South America. A Comparative Appraisal. *Prog. Med. Virol.,* 9:105, 1967.
Mosquito-Borne Hemorrhagic Fevers of Southeast Asia and the Western Pacific. *Bull. World Health Org.,* 35:1-104, 1966.

Infections by Enteroviruses

The enteroviruses are members of a large family of picornaviruses, so called for their small size (pico) and ribonucleic acid (RNA) core. The picornaviruses are also represented by the rhinoviruses, as well as by a number of viruses derived from lower animals.

Enteroviruses, which primarily inhabit the alimentary tract of man, include the polioviruses, Coxsackie viruses and ECHO (enteric cytopathogenic human orphan) viruses. These agents have many properties in common. They are small (15 to 30 millimicrons in diameter), have a single-stranded ribonucleic acid core, that has been postulated to be surrounded by a small number, possibly 32, of protein subunits; they lack a lipid component, as reflected by their resistance to inactivation by ether. Infection has been induced by RNA extracted from representative polioviruses and Coxsackie and ECHO viruses. Viral activity is relatively stable at room temperature and well preserved at −20 to −70°C. Thermostability varies under different conditions, but inactivation is probably complete at 60 to 65°C. for 30 minutes. Viral activity persists at pH 3. Interference has been noted between different enteroviruses as well as between members of this group and other viruses. Enteroviruses have maximal prevalence in warm weather (summer season in temperate zones) and other similarities of epidemiologic pattern. Serologic surveys for detection of antibody in various populations have shown that human experience with these agents is ubiquitous and cumulative. Many of these viruses produce disease in man, and all induce recognizable infection in one or more of various experimental hosts, including primates, rodents and cells in tissue culture. The principal associations of enteroviruses with human diseases, as currently recognized, are indicated in Tables 10-22 and 10-23. Poliomyelitis is discussed on page 677.

COXSACKIE VIRUS INFECTIONS

Etiology. Coxsackie viruses, so named for the town in New York State where they were first encountered, have in common the capacity to induce fatal infection, frequently with paralysis, in suckling mice and hamsters. The route of inoculation, strain of virus and size of dose, as well as age of the host, influence the manifestations of infection. Dalldorf classified these agents into 2 groups based on the features of disease induced in newborn mice. Group A viruses characteristically cause flaccid paralysis attributable to extensive necrosis of skeletal muscle without lesions elsewhere, although massive excretion of myoglobin may result in renal damage similar to that observed in the crush syndrome. Group B viruses cause tremors, spasticity and paralysis with varying degrees of focal myositis as well as encephalomyelitis, myocarditis, hepatitis, pancreatitis, necrosis of brown fat and, less regularly, lesions in other organs. Group B viruses also in-

TABLE 10-22. ASSOCIATION OF ENTEROVIRUSES WITH HUMAN DISEASE

Enteroviruses
Poliomyelitis .... Paralytic poliomyelitis (mild to severe)
    Types 1, 2, 3   Polioencephalitis
                                         Ataxia (type 1)
                                         Nonparalytic poliomyelitis
                                         Abortive poliomyelitis, pharyngitis or undifferentiated febrile disorder

Coxsackie, group A .... Aseptic meningitis (epidemic, types 7, 9; sporadic, many
    Types 1-24   types)
    (type 23 same as ECHO   Paralysis (types 4, 7, 9)
       type 9)   Encephalitis (types 2, 5, 6, 7, 9)
                                           Ataxia (types 4, 9)
                                         Guillain-Barré syndrome (types 2, 5, 6, 9)
                                         Exanthem (see Table 10-23)
                                         Herpangina and other enanthems (see Table 10-23)
                                         Lymphonodular pharyngitis (type 10)
                                         Lymphadenitis (types 5, 6)
                                         Acute respiratory illness (types 9, 21, 24 in addition to herpanginal strains), pharyngitis or undifferentiated febrile disorder (many types)
                                         Hepatitis (types 4, 9, 10)

Coxsackie, group B .... Aseptic meningitis (types 1-6)
    Types 1-6   Paralysis (types 1-5)
                                         Encephalitis (types 1, 2, 3, 5)
                                         Epidemic myalgia (types 1-6)
                                         Encephalomyocarditis in early infancy (types 1-5)
                                         Myocarditis or pericarditis (types 1-5)
                                         Exanthem (see Table 10-23)
                                         Enanthem (see Table 10-23)
                                         Orchitis (types 1-5)
                                         Hepatitis (type 5)
                                         Acute respiratory illness, pharyngitis or undifferentiated febrile disorder (types 1-5)

ECHO .... Aseptic meningitis (types 1-7, 9, 11-23, 25, 30, 31)
    Types 1-33   Paralysis (types 1, 2, 4, 6, 7, 9, 11, 16, 18, 30)
    (types 10 and 28   Encephalitis (types 2, 3, 4, 6, 7, 9, 11, 14, 18, 19)
    deleted, type 8 same as   Guillain-Barré syndrome (types 6, 22)
    type 1, type 9 same as   Ataxia (type 9)
    Coxsackie A type 23)   Acute myocarditis (type 9)
                                             Exanthem (see Table 10-23)
                                         Enanthem (see Table 10-23)
                                         Diarrhea (types 11, 14, 18)
                                         Acute respiratory illnesses, pharyngitis or undifferentiated febrile disorder (types 1, 3, 6, 9, 11, 19, 20 and others)

From Committee on the Enteroviruses, National Foundation for Infantile Paralysis: The Enteroviruses. *Am. J. Pub. Health,* Vol. 47, with additions.

duce a form of pancreatitis in mature mice in which the islets of Langerhans are spared and the acinar tissue first becomes necrotic and then is replaced by fat. The greater susceptibility of newborn as compared to older mice may be attributable to the fact that only the latter produce interferon after infection by Coxsackie viruses. Moreover, cortisone, which increases susceptibility of mature mice, inhibits formation of interferon.

Twenty-four Coxsackie viruses of group A (designated A-1 to A-24) and 6 of group B (designated B-1 to B-6) have been recognized to date (A-23 is identical with ECHO virus type 9). Each of these agents is antigenically distinct and can be identified and differentiated by neutralization and complement fixation tests, and some strains (B-1, B-3, B-5, A-7, A-20, A-21, A-24) are identifiable by hemagglutination reactions with specific immune animal serums. A-9 and all the group B viruses share a common antigen which is detected by agar gel diffusion. Circulating antibodies can usually be found in the animal or human host within 2 weeks of infection or of the onset of symptoms and reach maximum titer in about 3 weeks. Neutralizing antibodies persist for years, apparently associated with resistance to homologous reinfection.

Animals other than mice have been infected with some strains of Coxsackie A and B viruses, but in general are less susceptible and have not

TABLE 10-23. ENTEROVIRAL EXANTHEMS AND ENANTHEMS

Exanthems
  Occurrence
    Epidemic...ECHO 16 (Boston exanthem)
                                                    ECHO 9
                                                    Coxsackie A-9
                                                    Coxsackie A-16 (hand, foot and mouth disease)
    Smaller outbreaks........................Coxsackie A-4, A-5, B-5
                                                    ECHO 2, 4, 11
    Sporadic......................................Coxsackie A-2, A-4, A-5, A-9, A-16
                                                    Coxsackie B, types 1-5
                                                    ECHO 1-7, 9, 11, 14, 16, 18, 19

  Type of rash
    Maculopapular
      ("rubelliform").........................Coxsackie A and B and ECHO viruses—all types
                                                    associated with rash
    Vesicular ....Coxsackie A, types 5, 16 (hand, foot and mouth disease);
                                                    Coxsackie A, types 4, 9; Coxsackie B, types 1, 4
    Petechial....................................ECHO 4, 9, 11'
                                                    Coxsackie A-9, B-3
    Urticarial...................................Coxsackie A-9, A-16, B-5
                                                    ECHO 11

Enanthems
  Herpangina...................................Coxsackie A, types 1-10, 16, 17, 22
                                                    Coxsackie B, types 1-5; ECHO 9, 17
  Lymphonodular pharyngitis ....Coxsackie A-10
  Gingivostomatitis............................Coxsackie A-3, A-5
  Miscellaneous................................Coxsackie A-5, A-9, A-16
                                                    Coxsackie B-2, B-3, B-5
                                                    ECHO 6, 9, 16

From D. M. Horstmann: Viral Exanthems and Enanthems. *Pediatrics*, 41:867, 1968, with additions.

been extensively used. A-7, A-14, A-16 and B-2 viruses induce poliomyelitis-like lesions in monkeys. All 6 group B and all but 6 group A viruses (types A-1, A-4, A-5, A-6, A-19 and A-22) produce characteristic cellular damage or cytopathic effect (CPE) in cultured normal or malignant primate cells. Cultivation in cells of other animals has been less successful. Plaques produced by Coxsackie viruses, when grown in susceptible cells under agar, are round and resemble those of polioviruses, but develop more slowly. Coxsackie B-3 virus has been observed to have an oncolytic effect after serial passage through HeLa tumors in rats.

Coxsackie viruses are small, approximately 28 millimicrons in diameter, and have a ribonucleic acid core which carries the hereditary determinants of infectivity and virulence. An A-10 strain has been purified and crystallized. By means of electron microscopy, crystalline arrays of B-5 virus have been observed within the cytoplasm of infected cells.

Coxsackie viruses are unusually stable. Viral activity is maintained at room temperature for many days and can be preserved for a long time if infected tissues are stored in glycerin or in a frozen state. In aqueous suspensions activity disappears after exposure to a temperature of 60°C. for 30 minutes. When these viruses are suspended in milk or ice cream, higher temperatures are required for their inactivation. Like polioviruses,

these agents retain their activity through a wide range of pH (2.3 to 9.4 for a day and 4.0 to 8.0 for a week). They are not inactivated by ether, 70 per cent ethyl alcohol, 5 per cent Lysol, 1 per cent Roccal, or antibiotics, but are inactivated rapidly by tenth-normal hydrochloric acid, 2 per cent tincture of iodine and 0.3 per cent formaldehyde.

Epidemiology. Coxsackie viruses have been encountered throughout the world in epidemic and sporadic distribution. Like other enteroviruses, they have been recovered most commonly from human feces and pharyngeal swabbings, and also from sewage and flies. Recently Coxsackie B-1, B-3 and B-5 viruses, as well as ECHO 6 virus, have been isolated repeatedly from nasal, pharyngeal and rectal swabbings of beagle dogs which presumably acquired infection from human sources. Strains of all the group B types and many different group A viruses have been recovered from the cerebrospinal fluid of patients with viral meningitis. Recovery of a Coxsackie virus during life from blood, urine or other human sources has been relatively uncommon. Virus in relatively high titer has been detected in the heart, brain and other organs of infants, and rarely of older persons, after death. No natural reservoir of infection other than man has been found, although flies, dogs and possibly cockroaches are able to transport these agents.

In temperate zones Coxsackie viruses have been

recovered mainly during the summer and fall, although in tropical areas and to a lesser extent elsewhere they may be encountered throughout the year. Infection is more common in children. Atypically, infection by Coxsackie A-21 virus and associated acute respiratory illnesses have been observed more frequently in young adults during the winter. The types of virus prevalent in a community vary from year to year. Transmission by fecal-oral or respiratory routes and strain differences may influence clinical manifestations. Spread is rapid through susceptible members of a household. Rates of infection may be higher in persons with poor living conditions. Some of these viruses cause epidemics of human disease, but at unpredictable intervals and locations. Successive infections with strains of a single type of Coxsackie virus have not been reported; immunity appears to be type-specific and relatively lasting. Communicability of infection by Coxsackie viruses is similar to that in poliomyelitis.

Pathology. Relatively few observations have been made of pathologic changes in man. Maculopapular and vesicular lesions of skin, papules, vesicles, ulcers and lymphonodular lesions of mucous membranes have been noted. Myocarditis, encephalitis, hepatitis, pancreatitis, pneumonia and inflammatory changes in the spinal cord have been observed in newborn infants with fatal disease attributed to a group B virus. On rare occasions fatal myocarditis has occurred in older persons. In a few instances myositis and degenerative changes have been observed in biopsies of skeletal muscle. In cases of sudden death among infants from whom group A and other enteroviruses have been isolated, the principal pathologic lesions were laryngitis, epiglottitis, pneumonia, bronchitis, myocarditis and erythroblastosis.

Clinical Disorders. Probably the commonest clinical expression of infection by an enterovirus is an acute, self-limited febrile illness without distinctive features occurring during the summer months and mainly affecting children. In some cases attention may be attracted to particular manifestations or lesions such as meningitis, myalgia, carditis, rash or enanthem. Two or more of these features may be encountered among different patients in a household, community outbreak, or even in the same patient; in other persons infection is clinically inapparent, recognized only by recovery of virus or demonstration of an antibody response. Usually, as shown in Tables 10-22 and 10-23, more than one but not every enterovirus can induce each of the various clinical syndromes which have been etiologically associated with these agents.

Aseptic meningitis. This syndrome (see p. 687) can be caused by any of a large number of viruses. Coxsackie viruses have frequently been found in association with sporadic cases and in epidemics during summer and fall. All the group B viruses and 16 different group A viruses have been re-

covered from patients with this disorder, the group B, A-7 and A-9 viruses in epidemic distribution. All the group B types and at least 12 of group A have been recovered from spinal fluid.

The clinical picture of aseptic meningitis caused by a Coxsackie virus is not distinctive. The onset may be sudden or gradual; in approximately half of the instances it is initiated by a prodromal phase. In 1 patient viremia with a B-2 strain was demonstrated 5 days before the appearance of meningeal signs. Anorexia, malaise, fever, nausea and abdominal pain are frequent early complaints. The temperature may be elevated to 104°F. Ultimately headache, drowsiness, vomiting and discomfort or stiffness of the neck or back may appear, occasionally associated with focal or generalized myalgia. Physical examination may reveal hyperemia of the pharynx, occasionally with discrete vesicles or ulcers and some degree of resistance to flexion of the neck and back. Persistent muscular stiffness or weakness is usually equivocal or absent. The tendon reflexes remain normal.

The white blood cell count is normal or only slightly elevated. The cells of the cerebrospinal fluid are increased, usually not in excess of 500 per mm.[3], but occasionally may exceed 2000. Initially 10 to 50 per cent are polymorphonuclear cells; later, lymphocytes predominate. Sugar values are usually normal; protein may be slightly elevated.

The course is characteristically uncomplicated and terminates in complete recovery; in older patients, however, fatigue and irritability may persist for several months.

Other neurologic disorders. Paralysis, encephalitis, ataxia and infectious neuronitis have infrequently been associated with Coxsackie viruses. Paralysis, in most instances mild and transitory, has been observed in patients infected with Coxsackie A viruses types 4, 7 and 9 and with B viruses types 1 to 5. Exclusive of newborn infants, encephalitis has been found in association with A types 2, 5, 6, 7 and 9 and B types 1, 2, 3 and 5. Coxsackie A viruses types 4 and 9 have been recovered from fecal specimens of patients with ataxia, and types 2, 5, 6 and 9 have been encountered in patients with the Guillain-Barré syndrome.

Pleurodynia (epidemic myalgia; devil's grippe; Bornholm disease). Pleurodynia, recognized in 1856 by Finsen in Iceland, has occurred in epidemics throughout the world, usually in summer or fall. The monograph by Sylvest in 1933 presents a classic description of an outbreak on the Danish island of Bornholm. Since 1948, Coxsackie viruses of group B have been shown to cause this disorder.

The incubation period is usually 2 to 4 days. The illness begins suddenly with fever, headache and pain in the muscles of the chest or abdomen on one or both sides. Characteristically sharp or stabbing, the pain may be extreme and is accentuated by respirations. Sometimes pain is localized in the lower part of the abdomen and may simulate an acute surgical condition. Superficial tenderness and palpable swelling of muscles in affected areas may be detected. The extremities are rarely involved. Although pleurisy may be suggested, auscultation and roentgenographic examination of the chest seldom reveal abnormalities. Splenomegaly is infrequent. The white blood cell count is not unusual.

Fever and pain subside within 2 or 3 days, but in about a fourth of the cases recur on one or more occasions after asymptomatic intervals of 2 or 3 days. Often several members of a family are affected with somewhat different manifestations and degrees of severity. Involvement of the central nervous system may be evidenced by convulsions, encephalitic manifestations or pleocytosis of the cerebrospinal fluid. Except for occasional meningeal involvement and orchitis in mature males, complications are unusual, and recovery is spontaneous.

Encephalomyocarditis in the newborn infant. Geer and his associates in South Africa first showed that group B Coxsackie viruses may cause generalized and sometimes fatal intrauterine or neonatal infection in human infants. Cases have occurred in relation to pleurodynia or meningitis, and to acute febrile illness in the mother about the time of delivery.

The infant usually becomes ill suddenly, most often within the first 10 days of life and sometimes shortly after a brief episode of diarrhea and anorexia. Tachycardia, dyspnea and cyanosis may appear early, and lethargy, grayish pallor and mild jaundice are typical manifestations. The temperature may be depressed or elevated. The heart, liver and sometimes the spleen are enlarged. Electrocardiographic changes are characteristic of myocarditis. The cerebrospinal fluid may be xanthochromic, and the leukocytes and protein may be increased.

The clinical course may be rapidly fatal or progress to complete recovery. In fatal cases virus has been recovered from the blood, brain and spinal cord as well as from the myocardium, and other organs. Postmortem examinations have revealed lesions in brain, heart, liver and other organs resembling those seen in experimentally infected newborn mice.

Acute myocarditis or pericarditis. Myocarditis or pericarditis may occur in older children or adults infected with a Coxsackie virus of group B or, less frequently, group A. In rare instances the virus has been recovered from pericardial fluid or, in fatal cases, from the myocardium. The etiologic role of enteroviruses recovered from the oropharynx or stools of surviving patients with acute cardiac disorders has been difficult to establish.

Herpangina. Herpangina, an acute, self-limited febrile disorder, is characterized by distinctive papular, vesicular and ulcerative lesions on the anterior tonsillar pillars, soft palate, tonsils, pharynx and posterior buccal mucosa. First described by Zahorsky in 1924, it was shown by Heubner and his associates in 1951 to be etiologically associated with 6 different group A Coxsackie viruses (types 2, 4, 5, 6, 8, 10). Since then additional group A viruses (types 1, 3, 7, 8, 9, 16, 17, 22) have been found in typical cases, and the characteristic enanthem has also been observed in patients infected with other Coxsackie (B types 1 through 5) and ECHO (types 9, 17) viruses, including some patients with additional manifestations of enteroviral infection, i.e. meningitis, pleurodynia or rash.

After an incubation period of 2 to 4 days the illness is usually initiated by an abrupt elevation of temperature to as high as 105°F. Anorexia and dysphagia are common, and patients over 2 years of age complain of sore throat. Headache and abdominal pain are encountered less often. Infrequently convulsions occur with the fever. The pharynx is usually hyperemic. Characteristic discrete lesions appear initially as white or grayish papules, or later as shallow ulcers 1 to 5 mm. in diameter, each surrounded by a red areola. They range from 1 to about 15 in number and are commonly located on the anterior pillars of the fauces, less frequently on the palate, tonsils, uvula or tongue (Fig. 10-87 [p. 628]). These lesions are not invariably present, however. Genital ulceration attributed to infection by A-10 virus has been described in a 7-year-old girl with herpangina. Acute parotitis complicating herpangina has also been reported. Rhinitis, cough, otitis media, sinusitis, diarrhea, generalized myalgia and meningeal irritation are not typical features of herpangina. The illness generally follows an uncomplicated course to recovery. Fever may last 1 to 4 days, and the ulcers heal within a week. The white blood cell count is usually normal or only slightly elevated.

Acute lymphonodular pharyngitis. Coxsackie A-10 virus was encountered in an outbreak of illness resembling herpangina. Patients complained of fever, headache and sore throat. Examination revealed small white or yellowish nodular lesions of the uvula, anterior pillars and posterior pharynx which subsided without vesiculation or ulceration. Histologic examination showed the papules to be heavily infiltrated with lymphocytes.

Fever with lymphadenitis. Coxsackie A viruses types 5 and 6 were associated in Africa with a febrile disorder resembling glandular fever which lasted 4 to 10 days. The illness was characterized by an abrupt onset and tender, swollen lymph nodes; stiffness of the neck and splenomegaly were noted in a few instances.

"Hand, foot and mouth disease." Coxsackie A viruses types 5 or 16 have been recovered mainly from infants and children with a syndrome called "hand, foot and mouth disease" characterized by vesicular and ulcerative lesions in the mouth, a maculopapular rash and vesicles on the hands and feet. In some cases a transient erythematous rash has been seen on the buttocks as well as the ex-

tremities. The course is acute and usually self-limited, although fatal cases in infants infected with Coxsackie A virus type 16 have been reported.

Exanthems. In addition to the maculopapular and vesicular skin lesions observed in some cases of infection with Coxsackie A viruses types 5 and 16, rashes have been reported in association with other types of Coxsackie A and B viruses. These are generally maculopapular, although vesicles and urticaria or petechiae have been seen in some cases of infection with Coxsackie A virus type 9, and B viruses types 3 and 5.

Hepatitis. Hepatic lesions occur in newborn infants with generalized infection by a Coxsackie virus of group B. Other Coxsackie viruses may affect the liver in older subjects. Coxsackie A virus type 10 and B virus type 5 have been encountered in outbreaks of mild hepatic disorder, and Coxsackie A viruses type 4 and 9 have been recovered, respectively, from the blood and from the liver, post mortem, in individual patients with signs of hepatitis.

Acute respiratory illness and other undifferentiated disorders. In addition to herpangina and other illnesses characterized by pharyngitis, Coxsackie A viruses have been found in association with acute respiratory illnesses, including both undifferentiated and typical forms. In an outbreak of illness among infants and children attributed to Coxsackie A-9 virus, 3 had pneumonia, and the virus was recovered from the liver and lung of one who died. A-21 virus (Coe) has been encountered repeatedly in outbreaks of acute respiratory infection, mainly among military recruits, and has been shown to cause "common colds" or mild febrile upper respiratory tract illness in human volunteers. A-24 virus (Pett) was recovered from the feces of children during an institutional outbreak of respiratory disease.

Infection with each of the Coxsackie B viruses has produced a varied spectrum of clinical manifestations within a community and often within a single family. Sore throat or other respiratory symptoms may occur during the prodromal stage in patients with aseptic meningitis or pleurodynia and may be the only features of illness in other members of the household. Coxsackie B viruses of several serotypes have been encountered in outbreaks of febrile respiratory illness in families, camps and institutions. Coxsackie B viruses types 3 and 5 were found in association with respiratory disease among infants and children during serial long-term studies in an orphanage. Coxsackie B viruses have also been recovered occasionally from patients with croup, bronchiolitis, vesicular pharyngitis, pneumonia and pleurisy, but are not considered to be principal causes of these clinical entities. On the other hand, mild respiratory illnesses are probably frequently attributable to Coxsackie B viruses, especially during the summer and fall.

Diagnosis and Differential Diagnosis. Diagnosis of infection by a Coxsackie virus is suggested by clinical and epidemiologic findings and confirmed by recovery of virus and demonstration of a related increase in titer of homologous neutralizing antibodies in serums obtained during the acute and convalescent phases of illness. Primary recovery of virus may be achieved by inoculation of newborn mice or, preferably, in the case of group B types 1 to 6, A-9 and A-23 viruses, by propagation in various tissue cultures. Coxsackie viruses which agglutinate human group O erythrocytes at 37°C. (in maximum titer with red blood cells from newborn infants) can be identified by hemagglutination-inhibition tests. Since infection by any one of these viruses may stimulate complement-fixing antibodies to heterologous strains, determinations by this technique are of limited diagnostic value. It should be emphasized that the establishment of a causative relation between a Coxsackie virus and associated disease requires careful correlation of pertinent clinical, epidemiologic and laboratory evidence.

Differentiation of aseptic meningitis caused by a Coxsackie virus from bacterial meningitis, leptospirosis, space-occupying lesions or infections of the central nervous system caused by other viruses such as poliomyelitis, mumps, lymphocytic choriomeningitis, equine encephalitis, and ECHO or herpes simplex virus is often indicated by clinical and epidemiologic evidence and can usually be verified in the laboratory. Recovery of a Coxsackie virus from cerebrospinal fluid collected during the acute stage of illness is positive diagnostic evidence. When both a Coxsackie virus and another viral agent, especially a poliovirus or ECHO virus, are isolated simultaneously from a patient, it may be difficult to determine the etiologic significance of each virus to the associated disease.

Paralysis caused by an enterovirus other than a poliovirus has been encountered occasionally in individual patients, but, with the possible exception of Coxsackie A virus type 7, not in epidemic distribution.

Pleurodynia attributable to a Coxsackie virus must be differentiated from other causes of thoracic pain, particularly pneumonia and pleurisy, and from other causes of abdominal pain, including acute gastroenteritis, appendicitis, volvulus, intussusception, peptic ulcer and disease of the gallbladder. Whether a group B Coxsackie virus can cause pancreatitis in man as in mice has not been determined. The superficial quality of the pain, the absence of deep abdominal or rectal tenderness, the relatively normal leukocyte count and the absence of abnormal roentgenologic findings should aid in the recognition of pleurodynia. Consideration of pleurodynia, particularly during the season of prevalence or in the presence of a local outbreak, may avert unnecessary surgery. Orchitis complicating pleurodynia or aseptic meningitis must be differentiated from that in mumps.

Generalized infection with myocarditis in the newborn caused by a group B Coxsackie virus is suggested by tachycardia, signs of myocarditis and circulatory collapse occurring during the neonatal period, particularly when epidemic myalgia is prevalent in the vicinity, or following an acute illness of the mother possibly attributable to infection by the same virus. This disorder must be differentiated from congenital heart disease and other neonatal infections.

In older patients carditis attributable to a Coxsackie virus may be difficult to distinguish from acute cardiac disease of different or undetermined origin.

Herpangina in the community is suggested by its occurrence in seasonal outbreaks and, in individual patients, by the presence of discrete vesicular or ulcerative lesions in characteristic distribution on the anterior pillars of the tonsils, the soft palate or uvula. In this respect the lesions differ from those attributable to herpes simplex virus. The latter may occur in the faucial areas, but commonly are distributed more diffusely in the gingival and buccal mucosa, on mucocutaneous borders and skin. Occasionally lesions typical of herpangina are seen in patients infected with Coxsackie B or ECHO viruses. Group A Coxsackie and herpes viruses are readily isolated from human sources by tests in suckling mice, but differ in their capacity to grow in various tissue cultures; each can be identified by appropriate procedures in the laboratory. The oral lesions of other bacterial and viral diseases, moniliasis, infectious mononucleosis, blood dyscrasias, deficiency diseases and heavy metal poisoning are unlikely to be confused.

Exanthems or enanthems occurring during the warm seasons, especially in epidemic distribution, should suggest enteroviral infection. The vesicular stomatitis and rash of the syndrome designated "hand, foot and mouth disease" should suggest infection with Coxsackie A-16 or A-5 virus. The rash associated with A-23 (ECHO 9) infection often appears with "violaceous" lesions on the cheeks spreading to the trunk and extremities and even to the palms and soles. The rashes associated with enteroviral infections are frequently described as maculopapular or "rubelliform," but may be vesicular, petechial or urticarial; they must be distinguished from those encountered in other exanthematous diseases of childhood and from those resulting from administration of drugs.

Enteroviruses are not generally regarded as important in the causation of respiratory diseases, and their role in these disorders may be overlooked or difficult to prove. The forms of enteroviral-related respiratory illnesses are multiple, not distinctive, and, probably in most instances, relatively mild. Enteroviral infection should be suspected in patients with respiratory disorders occurring during the seasonal prevalence of these viruses and especially in affected members of a household in which other members are experiencing enteroviral-related disease.

Prognosis. Complete recovery from disease caused by Coxsackie viruses can usually be expected except in newborn infants, in whom infection with a group B virus may prove fatal.

Treatment and Control Measures. No definitive therapy is known. Treatment is supportive and symptomatic. Specific measures to control infection by Coxsackie virus are not available.

ECHO VIRUS INFECTIONS

The introduction of tissue culture technique for recovery of virus from the alimentary tract led to the accidental discovery of a hitherto unrecognized group of enteroviruses, referred to initially as human cytopathogenic enteric or "orphan" viruses, and now called ECHO viruses. Many of these agents have since been shown to cause human disease.

Etiology. ECHO viruses, though less extensively studied, appear to have in common many of the biologic, chemical and physical properties of other enteroviruses, including comparable size and structure, RNA core, relative thermal stability and resistance to inactivation by ether, common antiseptics and antimicrobial agents. They are all cytopathogenic in variable degree for human or monkey cells in tissue culture and, when grown in appropriate cells under agar, produce distinctive plaques.

The ECHO viruses can be separated into 2 groups based on capacity for growth and kind of plaques found in cultures of cells from rhesus and patas monkeys. In general, ECHO viruses do not cause disease in suckling mice with the exception of type 9, which in this and other respects appears indistinguishable from Coxsackie virus A-23. Some of the ECHO viruses (types 1, 4, 6, 13) produce neuronal lesions in monkeys after experimental injection into the central nervous system or muscle; paralysis has been induced in these animals with virus types 7 and 14, and meningitis with types 6 and 16. Clinically inapparent infection associated with excretion of virus and homologous antibody response has been demonstrated in chimpanzees after oral administration of virus types 4 or 6. Interference has been observed between ECHO viruses and other enteroviruses, including active poliomyelitis vaccine strains, the latter in man as well as in the laboratory. Interference with the propagation in tissue culture of ECHO virus type 11 by rubella virus has been widely used as an indirect technique for detecting the presence of the latter.

Currently, ECHO viruses are identified by types, numbered 1 to 33, utilizing neutralization and complement fixation techniques, and, when possible tests for hemagglutination of human group O erythrocytes (types 3, 6, 7, 11-13, 19-21, 24, 29). Types 1 and 8 are now regarded as type 1, and type 9 is also recognized as Coxsackie virus A-23. Types 10 and 28 have been reclassified as type 1 rheovirus and rhinovirus, respectively. Considerable variation has been observed between individual strains of certain types, especially types 4 and 6. Although slight antigenic relations with other enteroviruses have been suggested, the ECHO viruses appear to be distinct entities, clearly distinguishable from other viruses which affect man. Similar viruses, however, have been encountered as natural parasites of other mammals.

Epidemiology. In general, ECHO viruses have exhibited the same epidemiologic characteristics as other enteroviruses. They have been detected in many parts of the world by both recovery of virus and demonstration of specific antibody in individual serums or gamma globulin. Infection has been more common among children in warm seasons, and among those in poor socioeconomic conditions, and virus has been recovered more readily from feces than from other sources. At different times and in widely separated localities, epidemics of meningitis have occurred which were caused by ECHO viruses of types 4, 6, 9, 11, 16 and 30. In sporadic distribution, meningitis has been attributed to 24 different types; strains of at least 17 types have been recovered from cerebrospinal fluid of patients with meningitis.

Exanthems have been noted in association with infection by 13 types of ECHO viruses, often in epidemics. Some patients infected with type 9 or type 4 virus had exanthems and meningitis. Patients infected with type 16 have shown either rash or enanthem. Whenever meningitis or rash attributable to an ECHO virus has been epidemic, instances of less distinctive and inapparent infections have also been prevalent in the same vicinity. The attack rate and rapid dissemination of infection by these viruses within families have indicated a high degree of communicability and a relatively short incubation period.

Pathology. Almost no information is available about the pathologic changes caused by ECHO viruses. A virus, identified as ECHO virus type 2, was recovered from the spinal cord of a child who died of a disease which clinically and pathologically resembled bulbospinal poliomyelitis. A type 9 virus was found in the medulla of another patient, and type 6 virus in the blood of other fatal cases with paralysis.

Clinical Disorders. Clinical disorders associated with ECHO viruses are indicated in Tables 10-22 and 10-23. The manifestations of illness resemble those seen with other enteroviruses, but, with the exception of meningitis and rash, they tend to occur in sporadic rather than epidemic distribution.

Aseptic meningitis. The clinical features and laboratory findings in meningitis caused by ECHO viruses generally correspond to those observed in patients infected with Coxsackie viruses. The illness is usually initiated abruptly with headache, often retrobulbar, and ensuing stiffness of the neck or back. Sore throat, nausea, vomiting and myalgia of the extremities may be present. In many patients with meningitis attributable to type 9 and less frequently in patients infected

with type 4 virus, a fine or blotchy, sometimes morbilliform, maculopapular erythematous rash may appear on the face and spread to the trunk and extremities. Occasionally, small ulcerations of the oral mucosa resembling the lesions of herpangina are also seen during infection with some ECHO viruses, particularly types 9 and 16. Cervical or generalized lymphadenopathy is not unusual. The illness in most patients is self-limited and relatively mild, although the duration and intensity of symptoms are extremely variable.

In most patients with ECHO virus meningitis the blood leukocyte count is normal. In the cerebrospinal fluid the leukocyte counts usually range up to 500 per cu. mm. and in cases of type 9 infection may exceed 1000. Polymorphonuclear leukocytes may be numerous (up to 90 per cent) early; eventually, lymphocytic cells predominate, and with type 4 infections may do so throughout the course of illness. The protein content is normal or slightly elevated; the sugar level is normal.

Other neurologic disorders. Individual cases of muscular weakness or paralysis with associated alterations of reflexes similar to poliomyelitis have been seen in association with at least 10 types of ECHO virus (types 1, 2, 4, 6, 7, 9, 11, 16, 18, 30), and fatal cases of infection with types 2, 6, 7, 9 and 11 are recorded. Thus clinical as well as experimental evidence indicates that some ECHO viruses induce poliomyelitis-like neuropathy.

Sporadic cases of encephalitis have been reported in association with 10 types of ECHO virus (types 2, 3, 4, 6, 7, 9, 11, 14, 18, 19), but the clinical pattern has been diverse and the evidence for a causative relationship inconsistent. Similarly, the role of ECHO viruses types 6 and 22 recovered from patients with the Guillain-Barré syndrome remains uncertain. Cerebellar ataxia has been seen in patients infected with type 9 virus.

Pleurodynia. Myalgia of the extremities is a common feature of ECHO virus infections, but typical pleurodynia has been reported infrequently in individual patients infected with types 1 or 9.

Myocarditis and pericarditis. ECHO viruses types 1, 9 and 19 have been detected in individual cases of pericarditis; myocardial involvement has been suggested by electrocardiographic changes observed in patients during infection with types 6 and 9, and type 9 virus has been isolated from the myocardium.

Exanthem. Maculopapular exanthems have been recognized as a characteristic feature of infection with types 4, 9 and 16 ECHO viruses. Rashes have been especially common in association with epidemics of type 9 infection both in patients with and in those without meningeal involvement. A rash *(Boston exanthem)* has also been a conspicuous feature in outbreaks of a mild febrile illness caused by strains of virus related to or identical with ECHO virus type 16. Rashes have also been observed in association with other ECHO viruses. The exanthems have most frequently been maculopapular, but vesicles, urticaria and petechiae have also been described.

These manifestations of infection appear to be more common in infants and children than in adults.

Diarrhea. The association of certain ECHO viruses, particularly types 11, 14 and 18, with diarrheal disease in infants and children has been observed, and a causative relationship suggested.

Acute respiratory illness. A number of ECHO viruses have been associated with acute respiratory illnesses. ECHO virus type 11 (U or Uppsala) virus was recovered in Sweden from children with nondiphtheritic croup. It was also found in children and adults with acute respiratory infections and with induced brief febrile illnesses in experimentally infected human subjects. ECHO virus type 6 has been recovered from patients with mild illnesses during epidemics of meningitis attributable to this agent and from cases of pharyngitis and conjunctivitis among children and adults in Japan. ECHO virus type 1 was reported, among infants in a Japanese institution, to be associated with upper respiratory tract infection, diarrhea and a rubella-like rash. A diagnosis of pneumonia was made in some cases during an epidemic of infection with ECHO virus type 9. ECHO virus type 19 has been encountered in infants and children with mild respiratory disease and was recovered from a fatal case during an outbreak of severe respiratory disease in premature infants. ECHO virus type 20 was found in infants with minor respiratory disorders and diarrhea. Volunteers experimentally infected with this agent had fever, pharyngitis and, in 2 instances, coryza. ECHO viruses, however, do not appear to be of great importance in the causation of respiratory disease.

Diagnosis. As with other enteroviruses, diagnosis of infection by an ECHO virus can be confirmed in the laboratory, but diagnosis of disease can be established only by careful correlation of associated clinical, epidemiologic and laboratory evidence. All the ECHO viruses are cytopathogenic and can be identified by neutralization tests with specific immune serum in cultures of renal cells from Rhesus monkeys. The presence of infection may be demonstrated by the detection of virus in the feces, oropharyngeal swabbings, blood, cerebrospinal fluid or other specimens from the patient and by the demonstration of a related antibody response in the patient's serum.

For discussion of differential diagnosis see under Coxsackie Virus Infections.

Prognosis. Disease caused by an ECHO virus is usually self-limited and uncomplicated and progresses rapidly to complete recovery. In cases with involvement of the central nervous system, muscular paralysis is an occasional complication. Fatal infection is rare.

Treatment and Control Measures. No definitive therapy is known. Treatment is supportive and symptomatic. Specific measures to control infection by Coxsackie virus are not available.

EDWARD C. CURNEN

REFERENCES

Andrewes, C. H.: Viruses and Noah's Ark. *Bacterial Rev.*, 29: 1, March 1965.

Curnen, E. C.: Immunology, Epidemiology and Clinical Aspects of Coxsackie Virus Infections; in *Poliomyelitis*, compiled and edited for the International Poliomyelitis Congress. Philadelphia, J. B. Lippincott Compnay, 1952.

Dalldorf, G., and Melnick, J. L.: Coxsackie Viruses; in F. L. Horsfall, Jr., and I. Tamm (Eds.): *Viral and Rickettsial Infections of Man.* 4th ed. Philadelphia, J. B. Lippincott Company, 1965.

Dalldorf, G., and Sickles, G. M.: An Unidentified Filtrable Agent Isolated from the Feces of Children with Paralysis. *Science,* 108:61, 1948.

Gear, J.: Coxsackie Virus Infections in Southern Africa. *Yale J. Biol. Med.,* 34:289, 1961-62.

Horstmann, D. M.: Viral Exanthems and Enanthems. *Pediatrics,* 41:867, 1968.

Huebner, R. J., and others: Herpangina; Etiological Studies of a Specific Infectious Disease. *J.A.M.A,* 145:628, 1951.

International Enterovirus Study Group: Picornavirus Group. *Virology,* 19:114, 1963.

Kibrick, S.: Current Status of Coxsackie and ECHO Viruses in Human Disease; in J. L. Melnick (Ed.): *Progress in Medical Virology.* Houston, Hafner Publishing Company, 1964, Vol. 6.

Kibrick, S., and Benirschke, K.: Severe Generalized Disease (Encephalohepatomyocarditis) Occurring in the Newborn Period and Due to Infection with Coxsackie Virus Group B: Evidence of Intrauterine Infection with This Agent. *Pediatrics,* 22:857, 1958.

Lerner, A. M., Klein, J. O., Cherry, J. D., and Finland, M.: New Viral Exanthems. *New England J. Med.,* 269:678, 736, 1963.

Melnick, J. L.: Echoviruses; in F. L. Horsfall and I. Tamm (Eds.): *Viral and Rickettsial Infections of Man.* 4th ed. Philadelphia, J. B. Lippincott Company, 1965.

Sylvest, E.: *Epidemic Myalgia: Bornholm Disease.* London, Oxford University Press, 1934.

Wenner, H. A.: The ECHO Viruses. *Ann. New York Acad. Sc.,* 101:398, 1962.

POLIOMYELITIS

Poliomyelitis is an acute viral infection occurring sporadically and in epidemics and characterized by varying degrees of neuronal injury with special localization in the anterior horns and the motor nuclei of the brain stem. There is a wide range in the clinical manifestations from inapparent infection to flaccid paralysis of many muscle groups with the possibility of death from asphyxia and involvement of vital centers in the brain stem.

Prior to the era of poliomyelitis vaccination it is estimated that 1 to 2 per cent of infected persons suffered neural disease ranging in severity from an aseptic meningitis syndrome to a fatal outcome. Another 4 to 5 per cent had a mild, undifferentiated abortive illness, while the rest had a clinically inapparent, permanently immunizing infection.

History. Epidemics of paralytic poliomyelitis have been described only in the past century, but there is some evidence that sporadic cases were recognized earlier. The first reference in the medical literature appeared in 1789 (Underwood in England). During the nineteenth century the disease was regarded as a rare affliction of infants, and a small group of isolated cases was accumulated by Heine in 1840 in Germany. The *epidemic* form was not clearly described until 1890 in Europe (Medin in

Stockholm) and 1894 in America (Caverly in Vermont). In 1908 Landsteiner produced paralysis in the monkey by intraperitoneal injection of human spinal cord tissue from fatal cases, and the filterability of the virus was established in 1910. A crucial observation was made in 1931 by Burnet and MacNamara that not all poliomyelitis virus strains are immunologically alike. The most significant contribution has been the cultivation of the virus in tissue cultures by Enders, Weller and Robbins. Their findings opened many conceptual and practical areas previously closed by the prevailing notion of the strict neurotropism of poliovirus. Vaccine production has been the most widely heralded of these, recently resulting in remarkable reduction of disease.

Etiology. Much more is known about poliovirus than about the predisposing factors which influence the clinical outcome.

The virus. Poliovirus is classified with the picornaviruses (*pico*, very small; RNA, ribonucleic acid), and is composed of a core of RNA and a protein coat whose total diameter is 28 mμ. It was the first animal virus to be crystallized (1955). The lack of lipid renders the virus resistant to ether, chloroform, bile and various detergents. Poliovirus is inactivated by strong oxidants, chlorine, formalin and ultraviolet irradiation. Unfortunately poliovirus deteriorates on desiccation; hence freeze-dried Sabin-type oral vaccine which would not require refrigeration is not feasible.

Fortunately there are only 3 serotypes (I, II, III); the above-mentioned characteristics apply to all. Within each type there may be different *strains*, some of which are more virulent than others, and some more immunogenic than others. To date, the largest epidemics of disease are ascribed to type I strains; some outbreaks have involved simultaneous occurrence of more than one type, and an occasional paralytic patient is found to have 2 serotypes of poliovirus. The occurrence of 2 separate paralytic illnesses each due to a different serotype is rare but documented.

Other viruses on rare occasion cause nonparalytic and paralytic disease distinguishable from poliomyelitis only by special virologic study; these are the enteroviruses (ECHO and Coxsackie) and mumps virus.

Predisposing factors. IMMUNE STATUS. Previous adequate exposure to a natural wild or a vaccine strain will protect against disease due to that serotype of virus, even though brief multiplication of that virus in the person's alimentary tract may occur.

NEUROVIRULENCE OR INVASIVENESS OF STRAIN. This characteristic affects the severity of epidemics as well as the neural response of infected persons.

OTHER HOST FACTORS. See Pathogenesis.

Epidemiology and General Control Measures. (See also *Immunity and Vaccines.*) Man is the sole natural reservoir for poliovirus and transmits infection by the oropharyngeal-fecal circuit. Casual unrecognized contact with alimentary content is probably the main source of virus transmission, with a much smaller role ascribable to oropharyngeal droplets. Human sewage becomes infected, but, together with flies and food vectors

(e.g. milk, water), appears to play a minimal role in transmission of poliovirus.

Most large outbreaks of poliomyelitis occur in the summer and early autumn months. Nevertheless poliovirus may be recovered from urban sewage in varying amounts through the entire year, and some outbreaks have occurred during periods of freezing weather.

Various control regulations are used to limit spread of wild virus strains. The greatest communicability from known cases occurs during the latter part of the incubation period and the first week of illness. A period of 7 to 10 days of isolation of patients is generally required, and a limited surveillance of household contacts. Indiscriminate closing of schools and other places of assembly is seldom recommended. During outbreaks it is wise to postpone elective surgery on susceptible persons, especially nasal, throat and dental operations.

Community outbreaks of poliomyelitis can now be brought under control by widespread oral immunization with attenuated monovalent oral poliomyelitis vaccine (Sabin) of the same wild virus serotype causing the outbreak.

Acutely ill paralytic patients should be managed in general or children's hospitals equipped to care for emergencies and to provide intensive aftercare. Isolation precautions to be observed are the same as those for typhoid fever.

Pathogenesis. Much of the knowledge of the pathogenesis of poliomyelitis has been obtained from experimental disease in other primates. When virus is *fed* to chimpanzees, they seldom become paralyzed. The usual response is the brief appearance of virus in the blood some days later, then in the stools, where it may remain for some weeks, and finally immunity as detected by the development of type-specific antibody. Chimpanzees which had no apparent disease may have scattered poliomyelitic lesions in their central nervous systems upon autopsy.

In man the virus generally enters the body through the oropharyngeal route and multiplies in the alimentary tract and in its related lymph nodes and other reticuloendothelial structures. Type-specific antibody is formed; if the response is of sufficient speed and magnitude, the virus particles are neutralized, no clinical disease occurs, and immunity to that type of poliovirus ensues. In this infectivity-antibody contest the virus may proliferate and become invasive before sufficient antibody is formed.

If virus gains direct access to nerve structures or to the blood-lymphatic system, direct infection of the central nervous system may occur. Thus bulbar poliomyelitis occurring soon after tonsillectomy may be due to virus gaining direct access to the medulla through severed cranial nerve filaments. Subcutaneously injected virus may follow nerve pathways and cause paralytic consequences initially in the injected limb, as it did in 1935 with the trial of incompletely inactivated vaccines and again in 1954. Although injected, the virus made its way centrifugally *from* the nervous system and appeared in the pharynx and feces, causing secondary cases in noninjected persons. There is no evidence that biting insects "inject" poliovirus into man.

Host factors are poorly understood; they operate at the cellular level, affecting the rate and perhaps the sites of virus multiplication. The influences of hormonal factors and of stress are evidenced by such observations as the following: (1) prepubertal boys have a paralytic rate of 2:1 as opposed to girls; (2) the incidence and severity of paralytic disease are higher in pregnant women than in the nonpregnant of similar age; (3) clinical severity of the disease increases with the age of the patient; (4) such stresses as muscular exhaustion, chilling and surgical procedures have deleterious effects once the virus has entered the body; concurrent or very recent tonsillectomy predisposes to bulbar poliomyelitis, and even remote tonsillectomy has a similar but less marked effect; excessive exertion and trauma may localize what might have been a nonclinical infection into a paralytic form, as may the injection of an arm with an irritating substance, such as alum-precipitated vaccine; and (5) cortisone increases the severity of certain forms of *experimental* poliomyelitis.

Pathology. *Neuropathology.* Unlike most viral infections of the central nervous system, the neuropathology of poliomyelitis is usually pathognomonic; only certain cells and areas of the neuraxis are susceptible to the virus. There is little histologic evidence of meningeal reaction.

Neuronal damage is due directly to virus multiplication. The clinical picture is dependent upon the number and location of involved neurons. The earliest changes consist in lysis of Nissl bodies in the cytoplasm, margination of the chromatin, acidophilic necrosis of the neuron followed by neuronal death, and finally neuronophagia, i.e. invasion by scavenger cells, including polymorphonuclears, plasma cells, lymphocytes and macrophages. There are also perivascular cuffing and some interstitial glial infiltration.

Not all affected neurons are killed. The injury may be reversible, and restoration of function may occur within 3 to 4 weeks after onset.

Histologic sections generally reveal more widespread lesions than would be estimated from the clinical findings. Considerable destruction of scattered neurons may occur without clinical disability.

The regions in which neuronal lesions occur are (1) spinal cord (anterior horn cells chiefly and to a lesser degree the intermediate and dorsal horn and dorsal root ganglia); (2) medulla (vestibular nuclei, cranial nerve nuclei and the reticular formation which contains the vital centers); (3) cerebellum (nuclei in the roof and vermis only); (4) midbrain (chiefly the gray matter, but also the substantia nigra and occasionally the red nucleus); (5) thalamus and hypothalamus; (6) the pallidum;

and (7) cerebral cortex (motor cortex). The virus *spares* the following areas, although they are invaded by the viruses of the arthropod-borne encephalitides: (1) the entire cerebral cortex *except* the motor area, (2) the cerebellum *except* the vermis and deep midline nuclei, and (3) the white matter of the spinal cord. It is the *distribution* of lesions which permits a histologic diagnosis of poliomyelitis.

Flaccid paralysis is the most obvious clinical expression of the neuronal changes. The ensuing muscular atrophy is due to denervation plus the atrophy of disuse. The pain, spasticity, nuchal and spinal rigidity and hypertonia of early illness are probably due to lesions of the brain stem, spinal ganglia and posterior columns. Respiratory arrhythmias, blood pressure and vasomotor fluctuations, cardiac arrhythmias, and the like, are reflections of damage to vital centers in the medulla.

Extraneural pathology. Although the virus seldom causes lesions outside the central nervous system, secondary lesions do occur elsewhere. When nervous control of ventilation is disturbed, secondary bronchopulmonary changes occur: viz., aspiration pneumonia, atelectasis and purulent bronchitis, owing to the inability to cough and to interference with thoracic movements. The cardiovascular changes may result in hypertension, cardiac failure and pulmonary edema. Long immobilization leads to negative nitrogen and calcium balances with urinary lithiasis, renal failure, hypertension with encephalopathy and convulsions; thrombophlebitis and pulmonary embolism are less common than might be expected. Treatment itself may cause untoward complications, such as urinary tract infection from improper catheterization, decubitus ulcers and psychotic disturbances. The virus does not affect the intellectual structures of the cerebral cortex. Ulcerations in the alimentary tract may result in serious bleeding and occasional perforation. Respiratory failure results in anoxic changes and respiratory acidosis.

Clinical Manifestations. The diagnosis of acute poliomyelitis rests upon clinical grounds; there is no generally available diagnostic laboratory test. Careful history, close examination of the unclothed patient, and recollection of conditions which may mimic poliomyelitis will obviate most diagnostic pitfalls.

When a susceptible person has had effective contact with poliovirus, one of the following responses may occur in this order of frequency: (1) *asymptomatic infection,* (2) *abortive poliomyelitis,* (3) *nonparalytic poliomyelitis,* (4) *paralytic poliomyelitis.* Any of these results in durable resistance to reinfection. One response may blend into a more severe form. This feature may result in a biphasic course ushered in by a minor febrile illness, a symptom-free interlude of a few days succeeded by a major episode (Fig. 10-88).

Abortive poliomyelitis. This presumptive clinical diagnosis is applicable only during obvious

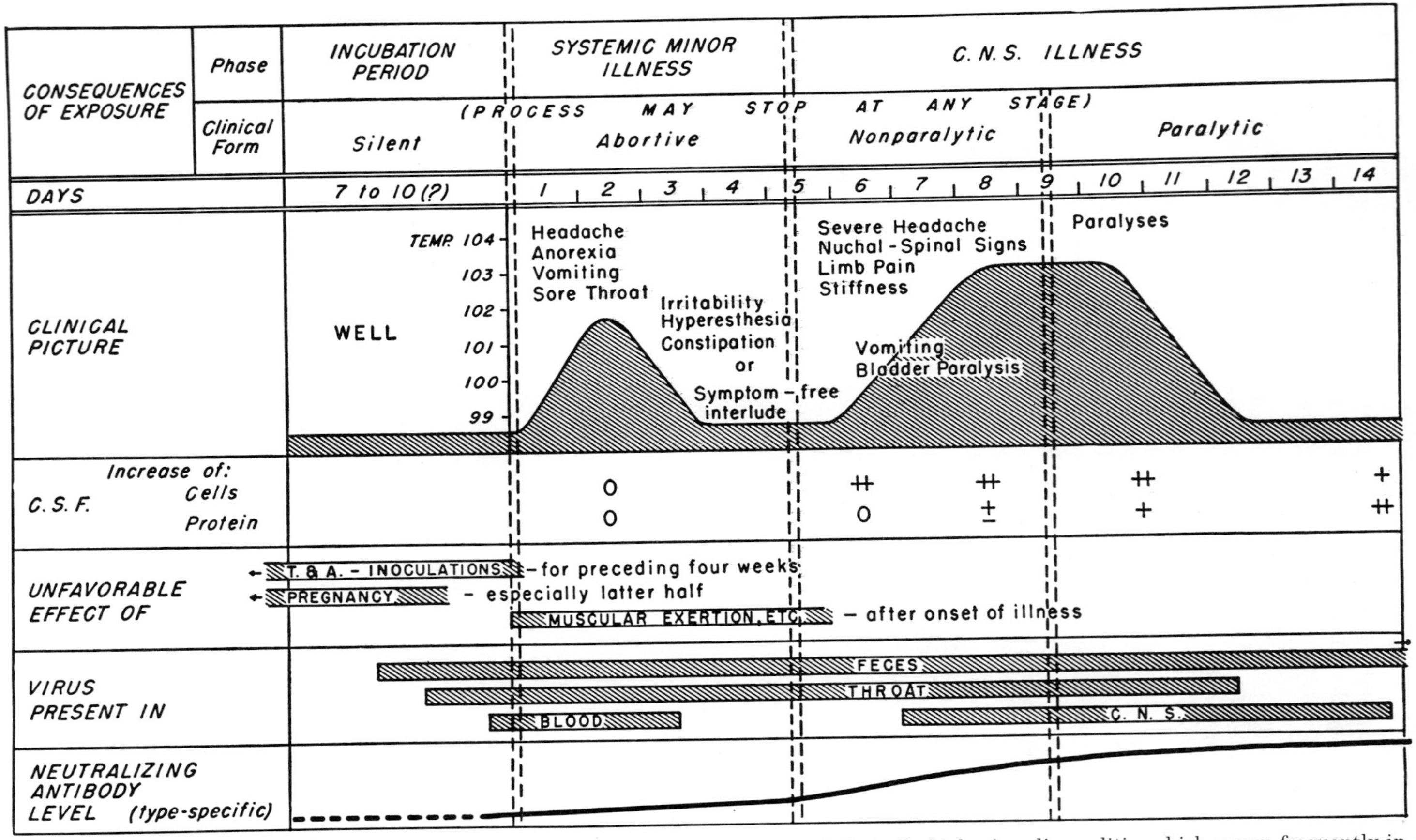

Figure 10-88. Schematic representation of major findings in the typical course of clinically biphasic poliomyelitis, which occurs frequently in children, but less so in adults, who tend to have an insidious monophasic course. *The evolution of the disease is often compressed into fewer days than shown diagrammatically.* Note that virus is present in feces and in throat swabs for relatively long periods, but the viremia period is short. Virus appears in the central nervous system prior to paralysis and tends to disappear in about 10 to 14 days, yet continues to be excreted in the feces. Muscular fatigue does not affect the course adversely unless continued. Antibody is present at the onset of symptoms and continues to rise. The influences of tonsillectomy, inoculations and pregnancy are exerted earlier. after onset of the minor illness phase, but the influences of tonsillectomy, inoculations and pregnancy are exerted earlier.

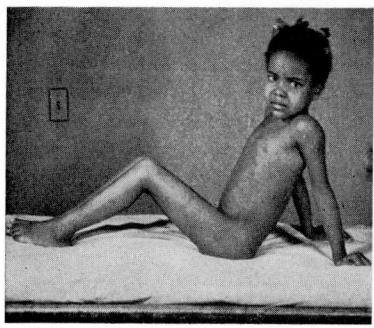 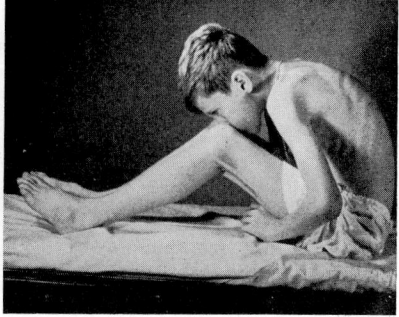

Fig. 10-89.   **Fig. 10-90.**

Figure 10-89. Tripod sign: characteristic position associated with stiffness of the spine. (From A. J. Steigman: Diagnosis and General Care of Acute Poliomyelitis. *Pediat. Clin. N. Amer.*, Vol. 1, No. 1A.)

Figure 10-90. Kiss-the-knee test: ability to complete the maneuver only by flexing the knee. Note tense appearance of the hamstrings. (From A. J. Steigman: Diagnosis and General Care of Acute Poliomyelitis. *Pediat. Clin. N. Amer.*, Vol. 1, No. 1A.)

poliomyelitis outbreaks, especially in patients known to have been exposed to a clearly recognizable form of the disease. A brief febrile illness occurs, with one or more of the following symptoms: malaise, anorexia, nausea, vomiting, headache, sore throat, constipation and unlocalized abdominal pain. The following are *uncommon* in abortive poliomyelitis: coryza, cough, pharyngeal exudate, diarrhea, localized abdominal tenderness and rigidity. A definitive diagnosis is impossible without viral identification. The fever seldom exceeds 103°F., and the pharynx shows little despite the frequent complaint of sore throat.

During poliomyelitis outbreaks patients presumed to have the abortive clinical form should have complete rest for about a week after defervescence and should be examined carefully about 2 months later to exclude muscular involvement previously undetected.

Nonparalytic poliomyelitis. The subjective symptoms are those enumerated for abortive poliomyelitis, except that headache, nausea and vomiting are more intense, and there is soreness and stiffness of the posterior muscles of the neck, trunk and limbs. Fleeting paralysis of the bladder is not uncommon, and constipation is frequent. Approximately two thirds of the children have a short symptom-free interlude between the first phase (minor illness) and the second phase (central nervous system or major illness) (Fig. 10-88). This 2-phase course is less common in adults, in whom the evolution of symptoms is more insidious. Nuchal and spinal rigidity is a necessity for the diagnosis of nonparalytic poliomyelitis during the second phase.

DETECTION OF NUCHAL-SPINAL SIGNS. The signs are first sought by *active tests*. The child is asked to sit up unassisted. If this causes undue effort, if the knees flex upward and he writhes a bit from side to side in sitting up and then places his hands on the bed behind him in the *tripod* supporting position, there is unmistakable spinal rigidity (Fig. 10-89). While he is still sitting, ask him to flex his chin to his chest and observe whether

nuchal rigidity is apparent. Then from the supine position, holding the knees down gently, ask him to sit up and *kiss his knees* (Fig. 10-90). If the knees draw up sharply or if the maneuver cannot be adequately completed, there is stiffness of the spine due to muscle spasm.

If still uncertain, the *passive tests* should be applied; these include the maneuvers which elicit Kernig's and Brudzinski's signs. Gentle forward flexion of the occiput and neck will elicit nuchal rigidity, which may antedate spinal rigidity.

Next one looks for *head drop* by placing the hands under the patient's shoulders and raising the trunk (Fig. 10-91). Normally the head follows the plane of the trunk, but in poliomyelitis it often falls backward limply. The frequency of the head-drop sign even in nonparalytic poliomyelitis with no subsequent residuals indicates that it is not due to true paresis of the neck flexors.

In struggling infants it may be difficult to distinguish voluntary resistance from clinically important involuntary nuchal rigidity. One may place the infant's shoulders flush with the edge of the table, support the weight of the occiput in the hand, and then flex the head anteriorly (Fig. 10-92). Nuchal rigidity that persists during this maneuver may be interpreted as involuntary. When not closed, the anterior fontanel may be tense or bulging as in meningitis.

In poliomyelitis the nuchal rigidity detected in the supine position (Fig. 10-93, *A*) often disappears when the patient is turned over. The nuchal rigidity associated with purulent meningitis generally persists in either position (Fig. 10-93, *B*). This paradoxical sign, though helpful, is not pathognomonic.

SUPERFICIAL AND DEEP REFLEXES. In the early stages the reflexes are normally active and remain so unless paralysis supervenes. Changes in reflexes, either increased or depressed, may *precede weakness* by 12 to 24 hours; hence it is important to detect them, especially in nonparalytic patients managed at home.

The *superficial* reflexes, i.e. cremasteric, ab-

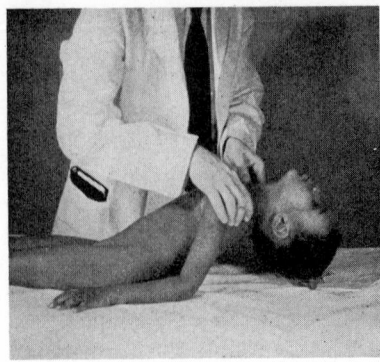
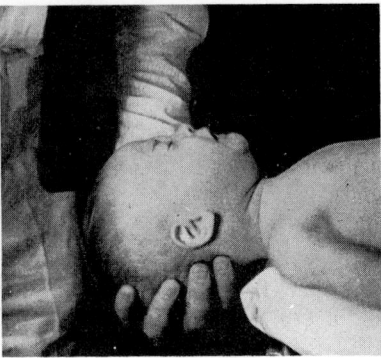

Fig. 10-91.   Fig. 10-92.

Figure 10-91. Head-drop sign: the head fails to continue in the plane of the body when the shoulders are elevated. This child had nonparalytic poliomyelitis. Tripod and head-drop signs appear in nonparalytic and paralytic poliomyelitis. (From A. J. Steigman: Diagnosis and General Care of Acute Poliomyelitis. *Pediat. Clin. N. Amer.*, Vol. 1, No. 1A.)

Figure 10-92. Testing nuchal rigidity in uncooperative, struggling infant: Place the shoulders at the edge of the table, supporting the occiput manually. Flex anteriorly. Only true involunatry rigidity persists. (From A. J. Steigman: Diagnosis and General Care of Acute Poliomyelitis. *Pediat. Clin. N. Amer.*, Vol. 1, No. 1A.)

dominal, and the reflexes of the spinal and gluteal muscles, are usually the first to be diminished. The spinal and gluteal reflexes are elicited by tapping segmentally downward on each side of the spine and buttocks. These reflexes may disappear before the abdominal and cremasteric ones.

Changes in the *deep* tendon reflexes, whether exaggerated or depressed, generally occur 8 to 24 hours after depression of superficial reflexes and indicate impending paresis of the extremities. There is absence of tendon reflexes with paralysis. Objective evidence of sensory defects does not occur in poliomyelitis.

DIFFERENTIAL DIAGNOSIS. A wide variety of diseases must be considered in an alert, febrile patient with meningeal signs whose muscular power and reflexes appear intact. In such a patient, when the cerebrospinal fluid reveals pleocytosis, no organisms and a normal sugar level, the differential diagnosis must include all causes of the acute *aseptic meningitis syndrome* (p. 687). Serologic procedures may be helpful in excluding many of these diseases. The clinical diagnosis of

nonparalytic poliomyelitis is made by exclusion of other conditions and the epidemiologic probability. Specific virus studies are now more feasible.

In their early stages *tuberculous* and *purulent meningitis* may simulate nonparalytic poliomyelitis. A lumbar puncture should be done; in addition to bacterial smears and cultures and a cell count, particular attention should be paid to the sugar content, since it is not depressed in the viral infections. Headache, fever and stiffness of the neck and back with tender extremities may occur in *acute rheumatic fever, rheumatoid arthritis* and *serum sickness*; the cerebrospinal fluid is normal, however, as it also is in the *meningismus* which may accompany the early stages of pneumonia, dysentery, typhoid, pyelitis and other infections. *Acute tonsillitis* and other conditions associated with cervical adenitis may cause a child to hold his head and neck immobile; this should not be confused with true nuchal rigidity.

Paralytic poliomyelitis. The manifestations are those enumerated for nonparalytic poliomyelitis plus weakness of one or more muscle groups,

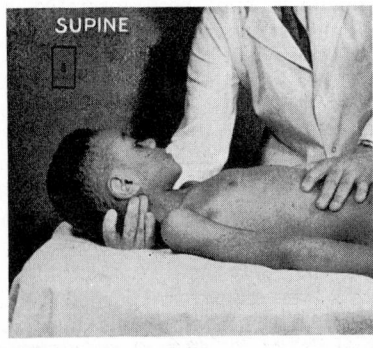
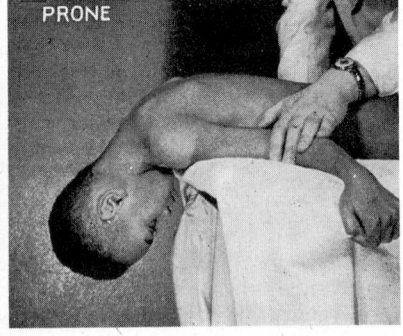

A   B

Figure 10-93. Supine versus prone postural test for nuchal rigidity in poliomyelitis. *A,* Nuchal rigidity elicited in conventional supine position. *B,* In prone position nuchal rigidity disappears in poliomyelitis, but generally persists in pyogenic meningitis. (From A. J. Steigman: Diagnosis and General Care of Acute Poliomyelitis. *Pediat. Clin. N. Amer.*, Vol. 1, No. 1A.)

either skeletal or cranial. These symptoms may be followed by a symptom-free interlude of several days and then a recurrence of symptoms, culminating in paralysis (Fig. 10-88). Bladder paralysis of 1 to 3 days' duration occurs in approximately 20 per cent of patients, and bowel atony is common, occasionally to the point of paralytic ileus. In infants muscular paralysis may be the first evidence noted.

CLINICAL CLASSIFICATION. The distribution of clinical paralysis is characteristically spotty and haphazard. To detect mild muscular weakness it is often necessary to apply gentle resistance in opposition to the muscle group being tested.

Spinal form. There is weakness of some of the muscles of the neck, abdomen, trunk, diaphragm, thorax or extremities.

Bulbar form. There is weakness in the motor distribution of one or more *cranial nerves* with or without dysfunction of the *vital centers of respiration and circulation.*

Bulbospinal form. Components of the preceding forms occur together.

Encephalitic form. There are irritability, disorientation, drowsiness and coarse tremors not explained by inadequate ventilation. Even during poliomyelitis epidemics this group can be recognized *only* if some peripheral or cranial nerve *paralysis* coexists or ensues. Hypoxia and hypercapnia due to inadequate ventilation from respiratory insufficiency may produce disorientation without true encephalitis.

DIFFERENTIAL DIAGNOSIS. *Conditions causing muscular weakness.* (1) *Infectious neuronitis* (Guillain-Barré syndrome) is the most common and difficult differential problem in this group. Generally the fever, headache and meningeal signs are less notable; characteristically there are few cells, but elevated globulin content in the cerebrospinal fluid. Paralysis is characteristically symmetrical in distribution. Sensory changes and pyramidal tract signs are common, but are absent in poliomyelitis. (2) *Peripheral neuritis*—postinjectional, toxic (lead, avitaminosis, and so forth), paralytic cranial herpes zoster, postdiphtheritic neuropathies—is excluded by history, sensory examination and related findings. (3) Arthropodborne viral *encephalitis, rabies* and *tetanus* have been confused with bulbar poliomyelitis. (4) *Botulism* may closely simulate bulbar poliomyelitis; nuchal-spinal rigidity and pleocytosis are absent. (5) *Demyelinizing types of encephalomyelitis* are associated with or follow the exanthems and other infections or occur as an untoward sequel of antirabies vaccination. (6) *Tick-bite* paralysis is uncommon; meningeal signs are absent, and removal of the tick is followed by swift recovery. (7) *Neoplasms* orginating in and around the spinal cord may rarely have a fairly abrupt onset. (8) *Familial periodic paralysis, myasthenia gravis* and *acute porphyria* are uncommon causes of weakness. (9) *Hysteria* and *malingering* are rare in children.

Conditions causing pseudoparalysis. In these, nuchal-spinal rigidity and pleocytosis are absent.

(1) *Unrecognized trauma* as from contusions, sprains, fractures and epiphyseal separation is a common cause of diagnostic confusion. (2) *Nonspecific (toxic) synovitis* produces a limp, usually unilaterally; the hip and the knee are the most common sites. There may be low-grade fever for several days. (3) *Acute osteomyelitis* has a more septic course; there is polymorpholeukocytosis, with localized signs, positive blood culture and later roentgenographic changes. (4) In *acute rheumatic fever* the clinical pattern is usually diagnostic. (5) *Scurvy* is revealed by history of inadequate intake of vitamin C and by roentgenographic changes in the bones. (6) *Congenital syphilitic osteomyelitis* of the acute painful type is found only in early infancy; serologic tests are indicated.

Bulbar and respiratory forms of poliomyelitis. A number of components acting together may produce insufficiency of ventilation (see Table 10-24). Adequate ventilation requires (1) intact neural mechanisms, including the rhythmic "drive" from the respiratory centers, and the neuromuscular integrity of the diaphragm and the intercostal muscles, (2) an open airway from the nostrils or lips to the alveoli, and (3) normal hemodynamics, especially of the pulmonary circulation.

The pathology of poliomyelitis is such that any or all 3 of these factors may become involved clinically. Although it may be convenient to consider the 3 factors separately, there is close interplay physiologically. Thus obstruction to airflow due to paralysis of pharyngeal muscles with accumulated secretions may result in hypercapnia sufficient to stimulate the respiratory center, but this particular vital center may be so diseased as to be unresponsive, or, if it is responsive, there

---

TABLE 10-24. COMMON SOURCES OF HYPOXIA AND HYPERCAPNIA IN POLIOMYELITIS

1. Cranial nerves IX to XII involved, with
   a. Pharyngeal paralysis and pooling of secretions
   b. Laryngeal involvement—either spasm of laryngeal muscles or paralysis of vocal cords
   c. Lingual paralysis
   d. Tracheal accumulation of secretions due to inability to cough
   e. Aspiration of vomitus
2. Vital center involvement with
   a. Inefficient, irregular respiration
   b. Cardiovascular disturbance
   c. Hyperpyrexia causing increased oxygen consumption
3. Cervical and spinal cord involvement causing paresis of the primary and accessory muscles of respiration
4. Pulmonary complications, viz., pneumonia, atelectasis, edema
5. Contributory factors
   a. Panic
   b. Gastric dilatation
   c. Sedation
   d. Inadequate equipment, viz., small-bore tracheostomy tubes, unsuitable respirator settings, and the like

may be incomplete response from the effector organs (the muscles of respiration) whose innervation may be involved.

The most serious biochemical changes are hypoxia and hypercapnia. These states produce effects on many other systems, such as the cardiovascular-renal one.

Respiratory insufficiency should be detected early in order to diminish its widespread effects. The objective is to maintain normal levels of oxygen and carbon dioxide in the blood; this requires proper assessment of the factors contributing to ventilatory failure. Since the situation may shift rapidly, continued clinical analysis is essential.

Despite weakness of the respiratory muscles, the patient may respond with so much respiratory effort that normal alveolar ventilation is maintained. In fact, the increased effort (associated with anxiety and fear) may actually produce overventilation at the outset, resulting in respiratory alkalosis. Such effort is fatiguing and soon leads to respiratory failure.

For clarity, certain terms will be defined: (1) *Pure spinal poliomyelitis with respiratory insufficiency* refers to tightness, weakness or paralysis of respiratory muscles (chiefly the diaphragm and intercostals) without discernible clinical involvement of cranial nerves or vital centers. The cervical and thoracic spinal cord segments are chiefly involved. (2) *Pure bulbar poliomyelitis* refers to paralysis of motor cranial nerve nuclei with or without involvement of the vital centers which control respiration, circulation and body temperature. Involvement of the ninth, tenth and twelfth cranial nerves is most important, since there is paralysis of the pharynx, tongue and larynx with resultant obstruction of the airway. (3) *Bulbospinal poliomyelitis with respiratory insufficiency* refers to involvement of the respiratory muscles with coexisting bulbar paralysis.

The clinical findings resulting from involvement of the *respiratory muscles* are (1) anxious expression; (2) inability to speak without frequent pauses, resulting in short, jerky, "breathless" sentences, which can be demonstrated by asking the child to count numbers serially; (3) increased respiratory rate; (4) movement of the alae nasi and of the accessory muscles of respiration; (5) inability to cough or sniff with full depth; (6) paradoxical abdominal movements due to diaphragmatic immobility from spasm or weakness of one or both leaves; (7) relative immobility of the intercostal spaces, which may be segmental, unilateral or bilateral. When the arms are weak, and especially when deltoid paralysis occurs, it is well to beware of impending respiratory paralysis, since the phrenic nerve nuclei are in adjacent areas of the spinal cord. In order to bring out minor degrees of paresis, splint the abdominal muscles manually and observe the patient's capacity for thoracic breathing. By lightly splinting the thoracic cage manually, the effectiveness of diaphragmatic movement may be assessed.

The clinical findings of *bulbar poliomyelitis* with respiratory difficulty (other than paralysis of extraocular, facial and masticatory muscles) include (1) nasal twang to the voice or cry, due to palatal and pharyngeal weakness — hard-consonant words such as "cookie" or "candy" bring this out best; (2) inability to swallow smoothly, resulting in accumulation of saliva in the pharynx and in partial immobility on holding the larynx lightly and asking the patient to swallow; (3) accumulated pharyngeal secretions which may cause irregular respiration, since each inspiration must be "planned" and cannot be "subconscious" in view of the risk of aspirating; the respirations may thus appear interrupted and abnormal even to the point of falsely simulating intercostal or diaphragmatic weakness; (4) the impossibility of effective coughing with resultant constant fatiguing efforts to clear the throat; (5) nasal regurgitation of saliva and fluids due to palatal paralysis with inability to separate the oropharynx from the nasopharynx during swallowing; (6) deviation of the palate, uvula or the tongue; (7) involvement of vital centers as reflected by irregularity in rate, depth and rhythm of respiration, by cardiovascular alterations which include blood pressure changes, especially upwards, alternate flushing and mottling of the skin, and cardiac arrhythmias; and by rapid changes in body temperature; (8) paralysis of one or both vocal cords causing hoarseness, aphonia and ultimately asphyxia unless recognized by laryngoscopy and managed by tracheotomy immediately; (9) the "rope sign," an acute angulation between the chin and larynx, due to weakness of the hyoid muscles. The hyoid bone is pulled posteriorly, narrowing the hypopharyngeal inlet.

Lumbar puncture in poliomyelitis. This procedure has diagnostic but not prognostic value. Although there are generally less than 500 leukocytes per mm.[3], the count may be higher, and rarely there may be no cellular increase. Early the cells are predominantly polymorphonuclear, but they soon become predominantly lymphocytic and decrease to normal numbers as early as 10 to 14 days after the onset. Absence of organisms on smear and culture and normal to elevated sugar content support the diagnosis of poliomyelitis. The protein content in the early stages is normal (up to 40 mg. per 100 ml.) or slightly elevated. Within 2 to 3 weeks after onset the pleocytosis diminishes, but the protein content frequently rises to as high as 300 mg. per 100 ml.

Complications. *Gastrointestinal tract.* Striking complications arise occasionally, including melena, which may be severe enough to require transfusion and is due to single or multiple superficial erosions. Gastrointestinal perforation is rare. Acute gastric dilatation may occur abruptly during the acute or convalescent stage, causing further embarrassment of respiration; immediate gastric aspiration and external application of ice bags are indicated.

Cardiovascular system. Mild hypertension of a few days' or weeks' duration is common in the acute stage, probably related to lesions of the vasoregulatory centers in the medulla, and especially to underventilation. In the later stages, owing to the protracted immobilization, hypertension may occur along with hypercalcemia, nephrocalcinosis and vascular lesions. Dimness of vision, headache and a lightheaded feeling in association with hypertension should be regarded as premonitory of a frank convulsion. Anticonvulsive therapy is indicated, and a program favoring increased mobilization should be instituted. Cardiac irregularities are uncommon; they vary from unexplained tachycardias which may yield to digitalization to cardiac arrest, for which measures to restore cardiac action are indicated. Electrocardiographic abnormalities indicative of myocarditis are not rare.

Acute pulmonary edema occurs occasionally, particularly in patients with arterial hypertension. Immediate management may be lifesaving. Pulmonary embolism is uncommon despite the immobilization.

Urinary tract. Transitory paralysis of the bladder in the acute stage has been mentioned. Skeletal decalcification begins soon after immobilization and results in hypercalciuria, which in turn predisposes to calculi, especially when urinary stasis and infection are present. A high fluid intake is the only effective prophylactic measure. The patient should be mobilized as much and as early as possible.

Prognosis. Overall mortality rates are influenced greatly by the percentage of bulborespiratory cases in an epidemic and by the completeness of reporting nonparalytic cases. Recorded case fatality rates in large urban epidemics in the United States have approximated 5 to 7 per cent. Most deaths occur within the first 2 weeks after onset. Fatality rates and the degree of disability appear to be greater after the age of puberty.

In general, the more extensive the paralysis in the first 10 days of illness, the more severe will be the ultimate disability. Unexpected improvement may appear soon after defervescence and again about 6 weeks after the onset, a time which corresponds to functional restoration of temporarily inactive neurons. The degree of functional recovery depends also upon the adequacy and promptness of therapy as related to proper body positioning, active motion, use of assistive devices and, of great importance, the psychologic motivation to return to as full and normal a life as possible.

Treatment. The broad principles of management are to allay fear, to minimize ensuing skeletal deformities, to anticipate and meet complications in addition to the neuromusculoskeletal ones, and to prepare the child and family for the prolonged treatment which may be required and for permanent disability, when this seems likely. A highly individualized approach with optimism blended with candor is essential.

Patients with the *nonparalytic* and mildly *paralytic* forms may be treated at home. No antibiotics are effective against poliovirus, and human immune globulin is ineffective after the onset of illness.

For the *abortive* form simple analgesics, sedatives, an attractive diet and bed rest until the child's temperature is normal for several days suffice. Avoidance of exertion for the ensuing 2 weeks is desirable, and there should be a careful neuromusculoskeletal examination 2 months later for any minor involvement.

Treatment for the *nonparalytic* form is similar to that for the abortive one, relief being indicated in particular for the discomfort of muscle tightness and spasm of the neck, trunk and extremities. Analgesics alone are not as effective as when combined with the application of hot packs for 15 to 30 minutes every 2 to 4 hours. Hot tub baths are sometimes useful. A firm bed is desirable and is improvised at home by placing table-leaves or a sheet of plywood beneath the mattress. A footboard should be used to keep the feet at a right angle with the legs. Muscular discomfort and spasm may continue for some weeks even in the nonparalytic form, necessitating hot packs and gentle physical therapy. Such patients should also be *carefully* examined 2 months after apparent recovery to detect minor residuals which might cause postural problems in later years.

Most patients with the *paralytic* form require hospitalization. A calm atmosphere is desired. Suitable body alignment is necessary to avoid excessive skeletal deformity. A neutral position with the feet at a right angle, knees slightly flexed, hips and spine straight, is achieved by use of boards, sandbags and occasionally light splint shells. Active and passive motions are indicated as soon as pain has disappeared. Opiates and sedatives are permissible only if no impairment of ventilation is present or impending. Constipation is common, and fecal impaction should be prevented.

When bladder paralysis occurs, a parasympathetic stimulant such as Urecholine (5 to 10 mg. orally, 2.5 to 5.0 mg. subcutaneously) may induce voiding in 15 to 30 minutes; some patients do not respond, and others have nausea, vomiting and palpitation. Bladder paresis rarely lasts more than a few days. If Urecholine fails, manual compression of the bladder and the psychologic effect of running water should be tried. If catheterization must be performed, the strictest asepsis is essential.

An interesting diet and a relatively high fluid intake should be started at once unless there is vomiting. Additional salt should be provided if the environmental temperature is high or if the application of hot packs induces sweating. Anorexia is common initially. An indwelling polyethylene gastric tube may be necessary to ensure adequate dietary and fluid intake.

The orthopedist and the physiatrist should see these patients as early in the illness as possible, and assume responsibility before fixed deformities develop.

The management of *pure bulbar poliomyelitis*

consists essentially in maintaining the airway and avoiding all risks of inhalation of saliva, food or vomitus. Gravity drainage of accumulated secretions is favored by the head-low (foot of bed elevated 20 to 25 degrees) *prone* position with the face to one side. Aspirators with rigid or semirigid tips are preferred for direct oral and pharyngeal use, and soft flexible catheters may be used for nasopharyngeal aspiration.

Fluid and electrolyte equilibrium is best maintained by intravenous clysis, since tube or oral feeding in the first few days may incite vomiting. After the first few days an indwelling polyethylene gastric tube may be used and sips of sterile water given from a spoon with increments as indicated by ability to swallow. In addition to close observation for respiratory insufficiency, the blood pressure should be taken at least twice daily. Hypertension is not uncommon and occasionally leads to hypertensive encephalopathy. Patients with pure bulbar poliomyelitis may require tracheotomy because of vocal cord paralysis or because of a "rope sign" with constriction of the hypopharynx.

The majority of patients with pure bulbar poliomyelitis who recover have little residual impairment; some patients exhibit mild dysphagia and occasional vocal fatigue with slurring of speech.

Management of respiratory failure due to inadequacy of respiratory muscles. This consists essentially in providing artificial mechanical respiration; familiarity in the use of the equipment selected is essential.

When placing a child in a respirator, it is essential to conceal any sense of haste or anxiety. The child and the parents should be told what is to take place; often the presence of the parents at the time of transfer reduces the child's terror and permits smoother synchronization to the machine. Suggestions for regulation of the respirator pressure and rate of respiration are given on page 878. Clinical evidence of improvement is detected by disappearance of restlessness, pallor or cyanosis, by adjustment to the machine's rhythm with cessation of extra efforts with the accessory muscles, and by an ability to doze.

Fever increases the oxygen requirement and should be controlled; in desperate instances the author has used induced therapeutic hypothermia. During the early febrile days it is better to err on the side of hyperventilation. If patients are hyperventilated too long, they may become "addicted," making the process of weaning from the respirator more difficult.

The amount of ventilation needed to maintain normal levels of oxygen and carbon dioxide in the arterial blood may vary widely within a short time. When blood gas determinations are not readily obtained, and since the oximeter gives no indication of carbon dioxide accumulation, close clinical supervision is required. Respiratory acidosis from accumulation of carbon dioxide may occur despite normal oxygenation achieved by oxygen therapy.

The only effective way to remove excess carbon dioxide is by augmented ventilation.

A combination of positive and negative pressures may be used with a cumulative net effect. A patient on occasion may require minus (−) 25 cm. of water pressure or more; this makes nursing care difficult because of the need to maintain a tight seal at the portholes. A combination of negative and positive pressures is then preferred, as for patients with hypotension and poor cardiac filling in whom "atmospheric" pressures, e.g. of minus (−) and plus (+) 10 cm. yielding a net pressure of 20 cm. The amount of ventilation prescribed must be "enough"; individualized judgment is required at *frequent* examinations. The thoracic cage of recumbent poliomyelitic patients acquires a lack of compliance or resistance to distensibility, so that pressures required to yield "enough" ventilation may be high.

Measurement of ventilation provides an index of the patient's requirement for artificial respiration and is especially useful in establishing the degrees of progress during the recovery stage (see p. 877).

TRACHEOTOMY. Tracheotomy is required for some patients with pure bulbar poliomyelitis, for some with pure spinal respiratory paralysis and for most patients with bulbospinal respiratory involvement. During epidemics it is generally possible for a busy nurse to maintain the airway more readily in respirator patients with a tracheostomy than by oropharyngeal aspiration alone. The operation is best done with a bronchoscope in situ to maintain ventilation, if necessary by attachment of the anesthetist's manual bag. An opening of the second tracheal ring is preferred, and the *largest* size tube admissible is inserted in order to reduce resistance to airflow. Respirator collar depressors are available for tracheotomized respirator patients. Standard tracheostomy tubes are often too long for these recumbent, head-low patients and may impinge upon the anterior tracheal wall, so that it may be advisable to cut 1 to 2 cm. from the distal end. The after-care requires extremely close attention to details. Strict asepsis is mandatory. Since the "prophylactic" administration of antibiotics may permit colonization of resistant bacteria, routine use of them is not advised. Nasopharyngeal wire swabs can be inserted down the tracheostomy tube to obtain material for bacterial culture. Frequent but swift endotracheal aspiration is required and is facilitated by instillation of a broncholavaging solution such as saline. Humidification of air or oxygen is important in preventing inspissation.

The tracheotomized patient with bulbospinal poliomyelitis differs from patients with tracheostomy for other acute airway problems in being unable to cough, frequently for many months. Tubes should not be removed too early, but may be corked and left in place until some tussive strength is restored.

Electronically activated mechanical devices

("exsufflators") are designed to produce sudden periodic high pressures on the chest wall of respirator patients during exhalation, thus forcing the bronchial secretions toward the glottis. Convalescent respirator patients whose cough is ordinarily feeble can also be trained to clear their bronchi several times daily by coughing while the chest is squeezed together by the attendant.

Weaning a patient from dependency on a respirator during convalescence is a part of the necessary rehabilitation. Much depends upon the initial psychologic and physical handling of the patient. The respirator should be opened periodically even if only for a few seconds, beginning on the first day of acute illness. *Strong verbal reassurance is given to the patient.* Gradually the pressure settings are lowered and the periods out of the respirator increased in duration and frequency. Cuirass respirators and the rocking bed are valuable devices in the weaning process, during which fatigue must be avoided. Speech therapists may be helpful in training these patients in glossopharyngeal ("frog") breathing. The weaning from respirators and the total rehabilitation of the severely involved ex-respirator patient may require several years of active work plus a supervised program for life. With adequate artificial devices and maintained motivation, patients with apparently overwhelming disabilities have been returned to productive lives.

Prevention. *Immunity and vaccines.* Newborn infants whose mothers' serum contains antibodies to all 3 serotypes of poliovirus are *passively immune* only for the duration of protective levels of transplacentally derived IgG. Pooled Human Immune Globulin contains poliomyelitis antibody, but this biologic preparation has no place in therapy and, in practical terms, no role in prophylaxis.

Prior to the advent of effective vaccines, life-long natural active immunity without illness came from adequate contacts with wild natural poliovirus strains. The increasing use of poliomyelitis vaccines will reduce the quantity of natural poliovirus in the general population. This situation underscores the importance of maintaining a high level of artificially acquired active immunity in the population by appropriate vaccination procedures.

Poliovirus vaccines. In the United States and in other countries in which large segments of the population have been vaccinated, reported cases of poliomyelitis are now infrequent. From 1950 through 1954 the number of cases reported in the United States totalled 190,000, i.e. approximately 25 per 100,000 population per year, mostly in children. The average of almost 40,000 cases reported per year has now dropped to approximately 100; these occur mostly in nests of unvaccinated children.

There are 2 kinds of vaccine: inactivated poliovirus vaccine (IPV-Salk) and an attenuated live oral poliovirus vaccine (OPV-Sabin). IPV-Salk is an injectable preparation containing all 3 poliovirus types, which were grown in tissue culture and inactivated by formalin. OPV-Sabin is available in a trivalent preparation containing all 3 types of virus and in monovalent (MOPV) preparations for each type of virus. OPV-Sabin is now used more widely than IPV-Salk. It is easier to administer and produces "natural immunity" (without extensive booster doses) of the alimentary tract as well as serum antibody. Except in direct control of an epidemic caused by a single type of virus, the trivalent OPV-Sabin is preferable to MOPV. No immunizing agent (including the superb tetanus toxoid) is 100 per cent effective and 100 per cent safe. Extensive experience with OPV-Sabin appears to justify the present confidence in it, and it has largely replaced IPV-Salk.

The recommended schedule for use of the available poliomyelitis vaccines is given on page 190.

ALEX J. STEIGMAN

REFERENCES

First International Conference on Vaccines Against Viral and Rickettsial Diseases of Man. Washington, D.C., Pan American Health Organization, Scientific Publication No. 147, May 1967.

Magoffin, R. L., Lennette, E. H., Hollister, A. C., Jr., and Schmidt, N. J.: An Etiologic Study of Clinical Paralytic Poliomyelitis. *J.A.M.A.*, 175:269, 1961.

Sabin, A. B.: Oral Poliovirus Vaccine. History of Its Development and Prospects for Eradication of Poliomyelitis. *J.A.M.A.*, 194:872, 1965.

Steigman, A. J.: The Control of Poliomyelitis. *J. Pediat.*, 59:163, 1961.

Steigman, A. J.: Clinical Paralytic Poliomyelitis Due to Enteroviruses Other than Poliovirus. *Arch. Gest. Virusforsch.*, 13:169, 1963.

ACUTE ASEPTIC MENINGITIS SYNDROME

The term "acute aseptic meningitis syndrome" includes a number of disorders which have in common an acute onset, usually a self-limited course with meningeal manifestations of varying degree, an increase in the cells of the spinal fluid and an absence of organisms on direct smear of it. The clinical significance is considerable, since over 3000 cases were reported in the United States during 1966.

The majority of these disorders are caused by viruses, especially enteroviruses with or without rashes, and by mumps virus with or without accompanying parotitis. There are numerous other causes, infectious and otherwise, as noted in Table 10-25, which often, or occasionally, present with this clinical picture.

The term "acute aseptic meningitis syndrome" is discarded in favor of a specific diagnostic one

TABLE 10-25.   Clinical Conditions Which May Induce the Acute Aseptic Meningitis Syndrome

DISEASE	AGENT
I. Infectious	
A. *Viral*	
Man to man	
Enteric, upper respiratory, neurologic infections	Enteroviruses (Coxsackie A and B and ECHO viruses, polioviruses); mumps virus
Common exanthems	Viruses of measles, rubella, herpes viruses (simplex, varicella-zoster)
Infectious mononucleosis	E B virus
Infectious hepatitis; influenza	Viruses of hepatitis, influenza
Rodent to man	
Lymphocytic choriomeningitis (LCM)	Lymphocytic choriomeningitis virus
Febrile meningeal reaction	Encephalomyocarditis viruses
Arthropod to man (Arbo)	
Meningeal and systemic illness	Arbo viruses A, B and nongroup; e.g. Eastern, Western, Venezuelan equine (group A); St. Louis, Japanese, Murray Valley, tick-borne encephalitis viruses (group B); California group of viruses (nongroup)
B. *Presumed viral*	
Infectious lymphocytosis; cat-scratch disease	Agents unknown
C. *Rickettsial*	
Rocky Mountain spotted fever	Rickettsia rickettsii
D. *Allergic*	
Postinfectious encephalitis	E.g. viruses of measles, rubella, mumps, varicella, variola
Postvaccinial encephalitis	E.g. vaccines against smallpox, rabies, influenza pertussis
E. *Bacterial*	
Incipient or partially treated meningitis	M. tuberculosis; atypical mycobacteria Common pathogens, especially H. influenzae
F. *Spirochetal*	
Leptospirosis	Leptospira icterohemorrhagica, canicola, pomona
Syphilis	Treponema pallidum
G. *Fungal*	
Disseminated coccidioidomycosis, moniliasis, cryptoccosis	Coccidioides immitis, Candida albicans, Cryptococcus neoformans
Nocardiosis	Nocardia (several species)
H. *Protozoal*	
Toxoplasmosis	Toxoplasma gondii
Acanthamoebiasis	Acanthamoebae (Hartmanella)
II. Noninfectious	
A. *Meningeal irritation from contiguous lesion*	E.g. abscesses, granulomas, hematomas, tumors, thromboses adjacent to or within CNS
B. *Tumor*	
Meningoencephalitis with increased intracranial pressure	Medulloblastoma
C. *Allergy*	
Meningeal reaction	
After vaccinations or infections	*See* I-D *above*
After other causes, e.g. serum sickness	Systemic foreign serum, antibiotics
D. *Miscellaneous*	
Leukemic meningitis	Leukemic infiltration
Meningeal reactions to	
Systemic poisoning	E.g. lead, toxins of gram-negative bacilli
Intrathecal injections	E.g. serum, antibiotics, contrast media
Implanted valves for treatment of hydrocephalus	Immediate postoperative or later bacterial infection

when clinical and laboratory data make this possible.

The epidemiology and the clinical patterns vary with the causative agent. The incidence tends to be higher in males in mumps and in certain enterovirus outbreaks. The section relevant for the individual agent should be consulted for details.

Immunity to a specific virus is long lasting. However, more than one attack of this syndrome may occur in view of the variety of etiologic agents, as, for example, the numerous serotypes of enteroviruses.

Clinical Manifestations. Although the onset may be insidious over a week or so, or even be preceded by a nonspecific acute febrile illness for a few days, it is generally fairly acute. The presenting manifestations in older children are headache and hyperesthesia; in infants, irritability and resentment at being handled. Fever, nausea and vomiting are frequent, but convulsions are rare. Preceding or accompanying exanthems may occur, especially with the ECHO viruses.

Examination reveals nuchal-spinal rigidity (see p. 681 for technique of the examination) without significant localizing neurologic changes.

Laboratory Data. The cerebrospinal fluid contains from 20 to several thousand cells; early in the disease these are often polymorphonuclear; later they are chiefly mononuclear. No organisms are seen on direct smears (bacteria, mycobacteria, protozoans, yeasts), and there are normal or slightly elevated levels of protein and of glucose. A decrease in glucose level can occur with medulloblastoma, leukemic infiltration and rarely in certain viral infections. In all instances the spinal fluid should be cultured for bacteria and mycobacteria, and in some instances special examinations are indicated for fungi, protozoa and other pathogens. Careful examination of the spinal fluid is most important, especially to assure that stains used for smears do not introduce artifacts and that the standard solutions used for glucose levels are accurate.

For special laboratory procedures to be used in the identification of viruses and other agents see page 543 and Table 10-8, p. 546.

Differential Diagnosis. Careful analysis of the history and epidemiologic circumstances may point toward one of the specific causes listed in Table 10-25. Especially during the summer and autumn, the presence of pleurodynia or of unexplained febrile eruptions in the community suggests the possibility of Coxsackie or ECHO viral infections; the coexistence of acute paralytic disorders in other patients suggests poliomyelitis; encephalitic infections in horses point to the possibilities of Eastern and Western equine encephalitis; swimming in waters contaminated by dead animals may suggest leptospiral infection. Knowledge of clear-cut exposure to or concurrent evidence of mumps or one of the common exanthems can be helpful in the differential diagnosis.

Most difficult from the diagnostic, therapeutic and prognostic points of view are instances of incipient or partially treated bacterial (especially *H. influenzae*) or mycobacterial meningitis. The clinical findings, the dosage of antibiotic previously used and the spinal fluid smear, culture and glucose level may be helpful in the former. When tuberculous meningitis is suspected, a careful evaluation of contacts and a positive tuberculin reaction may suggest the correct diagnosis. Medulloblastoma must be considered in the differential diagnosis, particularly if there is hypoglycorrachia and signs of increased intracranial pressure are prominent.

Finally, the possibility that the observed meningeal reaction is of neither viral nor bacterial origin must be recognized.

Treatment. Symptomatic measures, including aspirin, sponging and a cool room for relief of headache, hyperesthesia and fever, are useful. The withdrawal of spinal fluid for diagnosis often relieves headache. Codeine, morphine and the phenothiazine derivatives are best avoided, since they may induce misleading signs and symptoms. Assurance that recovery is likely may be considered part of therapy.

Several weeks after apparent recovery, careful neuromuscular assessment should be conducted to assure that muscular weakness has not been missed.

When the specific cause has been identified, the parents should be so informed. This is especially useful in the case of mumps in order to avoid anxiety following exposure to mumps in later life.

T. F. McNair Scott
Alex J. Steigman

Encephalitis

The manner in which the central nervous system may respond to abnormal influences is limited, so that similar signs and symptoms can result from a variety of noxious factors such as different infectious agents; toxins, e.g. lead or thallium; metabolic imbalances, e.g. uremia or hypertonic dehydration; circulatory disturbances, e.g. hypertension; and allergic reactions (see Aseptic Meningitis Syndrome, p. 687). Only encephalopathies of viral, suspected viral, and allergic origin will be discussed here.

Clinical Manifestations. Regardless of cause, the central nervous system responds by reactions which are predominantly meningeal, encephalitic, myelitic or radicular. When two or more of these reactions occur together, such terms as "meningoencephalitis" or "meningoencephalomyelitis" are used.

Meningeal manifestations. These are the most common; they are described elsewhere: aseptic meningitis syndrome (p. 687), poliomyelitis (p. 667), meningitis (p. 571) and meningitis in the newborn (p. 404).

Encephalitic manifestations. Characteristically, there is a history of sudden or insidious onset of headache, followed by drowsiness which may proceed to deep coma. Fever is usual. A convulsion may be the initial symptom, especially in infancy; the frequency decreases with age. Sometimes the onset is marked by hyperactivity, bizarre behavior or mental disturbance. Paralysis of one or more cranial nerves, a disorder of speech, ataxia, weakness of muscle groups, diplopia, alteration of reflexes and disturbances of the autonomic nervous system may be manifest singly or in combination. The cerebrospinal fluid is often within normal limits by routine tests; when a pleocytosis is found, it is moderate in extent, largely polymorphonuclear initially, but it becomes mononuclear after about the first 48 hours. The sugar content is usually normal, but on rare occasions it may be low; the protein content is either normal or moderately elevated. Recovery may be dramatically sudden within a few hours after the onset or may be delayed for weeks, months or even years. Permanent residual damage may result at all ages, although sequelae appear to be more frequent in very young infants. Persistent neurologic involvement is evidenced by such manifestations as seizures, hemiplegia or monoplegia, bizarre behavioral patterns and mental retardation. Residual damage may not be immediately obvious, but may manifest itself later as a deficiency in motor skills or learning ability. Apart from permanent residuals, transient neurologic changes and behavior disorders may be noted shortly after apparent recovery from the acute phase.

Myelitic manifestations. The onset is usually insidious. There is often paresthesia of the legs followed by weakness, which may be the initial symptom as in poliomyelitis. Sphincter and other autonomic nervous system disturbances are common early manifestations. There may be paralysis of various muscle groups, which may be symmetrical. Recovery is slow and often incomplete. There is usually an increase in cells in the spinal fluid and an increase in protein; the sugar content is usually normal.

Radicular manifestations. This may be monoradicular, as exemplified by the root pain in herpes zoster, or polyradicular as in the Guillain-Barré-Landry syndrome. The pathogenesis of the latter is considered to be an allergic swelling about the nerve roots. The onset may be associated with a known viral illness, an immunization procedure, or be unassociated with any recognized illness. Clinically and pathologically, it is usually only the peripheral nerve roots that are affected, but sometimes there are pathologic changes in the cord. In most patients, there is an elevation of the protein content of the cerebrospinal fluid at some time in the course of the disease, without a pleocytosis; a moderate increase in cells is seen occasionally. Both sensory and motor roots are involved in the characteristic Guillain-Barré syndrome, in which there is usually symmetrical weakness of muscle groups accompanied by loss of reflexes, by sensory loss which is most evident distally, and at times by exquisite muscle tenderness. If the disease predominantly affects the motor roots, paralysis often starts in the legs and, extending upward, may affect the diaphragm and the intercostal muscles. Death may result from respiratory failure, the sensorium remaining clear (Landry's paralysis).

Pathogenesis. Until recently it was customary to divide the encephalopathies, directly or indirectly associated with viral infections, into 2 groups: (1) viral and (2) allergic. Recent observations have suggested that these are not 2 qualitatively different entities, as their distinctive pathologic changes might indicate, but merely temporal or quantitative differences in host response to a viral infection.

After invasion by the virus the usual course of illness is as follows: Local multiplication occurs in the regional lymph tissue, until a concentration is reached sufficient for the virus to invade the bloodstream. This transient viremia results in seeding of susceptible cells. The systemic illness results from the seeded virus multiplying in various viscera, from which a second massive viremia is produced. By this time antibodies are forming, and the disease is finally brought to an end by a variety of host reactions.

Rarely the usually well protected nervous system is invaded, and a variety of neurologic signs and symptoms may result. These may be largely due to viral multiplication or to the host responses to the viral invasion.

Effects of viral multiplication. VIRAL MULTIPLICATION IN NEURONS AND SUPPORTING CELLS may follow one of several courses: (1) rapid multiplication in highly susceptible (usually young) cells leading to neuronal destruction with (e.g. herpes simplex) or without (e.g. Eastern equine encephalitis) intracellular inclusions; (2) slow multiplication leading to later destruction (e.g. rabies or kuru; (3) incorporation of the virus into the cell in such a way that it causes no detectable change in cellular morphology, its presence being revealed only by special techniques (e.g. fluorescent antibody). As the result of viral invasion the protein of the cell membranes is altered so that it becomes antigenic.

VIRAL MULTIPLICATION IN THE HIGHLY SUSCEPTIBLE ENDOTHELIUM OF BLOOD VESSELS may result in proliferation of the cells or necrosis; subsequent narrowing of vascular channels may result in tissue anoxia with consequent edema or frank necrosis. If necrosis supervenes, there is a breakdown of all tissue elements; when it occurs in the white matter, myelin sheaths are destroyed. At times, necrosis of vessel walls is associated with perivascular hemorrhage. Under these circumstances the clinical course of the disease is fulminating, and the cerebrospinal fluid contains both red cells and polymorphonuclear leukocytes. This combination of clinicopathologic events is referred to as *acute necrotizing hemorrhagic encephalitis.*

Effects of host reaction. ANTIVIRAL ANTIBODY PRODUCTION probably starts shortly after viral invasion, although it is not detectable in this early stage by present techniques. Two phases may be important in the pathogenesis of encephalitis: (1) Macroglobulins (IgM) may rarely leak into the cerebrospinal fluid. Their presence may actually increase viral multiplication, as has been shown experimentally with certain Arbo viruses. (2) The antigen-antibody complexes adhere to the walls of blood vessels, which may already be damaged by viral multiplication, fix complement and cause further cellular damage. When the meninges are involved, there are both pleocytosis and cellular infiltration within the subarachnoid and the Virchow-Robin spaces. In the gray matter the round cell infiltration may be associated with neuronal degeneration and neuronophagia. Serious consequences follow the cerebral swelling accompanying the inflammatory reaction. When the brain expands, the venous return is obstructed by pressure against the skull. The consequent stasis produces further swelling and anoxia, often resulting in widespread neuronal degeneration. Such secondary pathologic changes in the brain may on occasion dominate viral encephalitis.

ANTIHOST ANTIBODY PRODUCTION may be initiated by the elaboration of antigens from 2 sources: (1) Cellular protein, altered antigenically by the viral infection, stimulates antibody production by competent lymphocytes. These antibodies attack the infected cells. In addition, continued immunologic stimulation, as from the prolonged dissemination of the virus from cell to cell, broadens the spectrum of antibodies produced to include autoantibodies, which then react with uninfected nerve cells. The presence of such autoantibodies has been demonstrated in the cerebrospinal fluid. (2) The myelin, destroyed as the result of focal or perivascular necrosis, releases highly antigenic lipoproteins against which antibodies are formed locally. These in turn selectively destroy myelin sheaths, but have little effect on axis cylinders or adjacent neurons. This reaction is characteristic of so-called allergic encephalomyelitis. These events are illustrated diagramatically in Figure 10-94.

Although for clinicopathologic convenience the encephalitides are described under the headings of Viral, Probably Viral and Allergic, it must be emphasized that the events just described occur in a dynamic continuum. The pathologic differences found in individual patients merely represent various phases of this continuum and reflect the particular events which predominate at the time of death.

Pathology. The principal changes found at necropsy in encephalitis are (1) congestion and mononuclear infiltration of the meninges; (2) perivascular cuffing by lymphocytes and plasma cells which fill the Virchow-Robin spaces; (3) perivascular necrosis of tissue, including break-

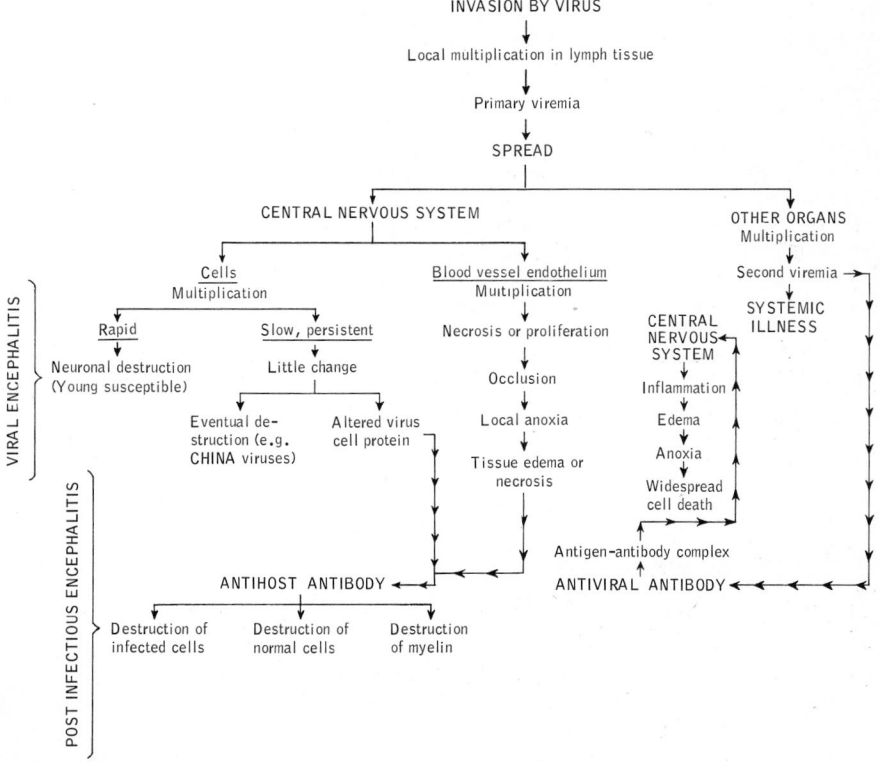

Figure 10-94.

down of myelin, and at times diapedesis of red cells so that the vessels are ringed with such cells (acute hemorrhagic leukoencephalitis); (4) selective demyelination with preservation of neurons and axis cylinders ("allergic" encephalitis); (5) neuronal degeneration with satellitosis and neuronophagia; (6) nonspecific ballooning of neurons; (7) inclusion bodies in neurons or glial cells, which may be *(a)* intranuclear, such as occur in infections with the herpesvirus group, cytomegalovirus, and measles, or *(b)* cytoplasmic, such as occur in rabies (Negri bodies), and also those that occur, in addition to the intranuclear inclusions, in infections with cytomegaloviruses and measles viruses; and (8) changes in the endothelial cells of blood vessels leading to proliferation or necrosis.

The extent and nature of the pathologic changes depend partly on the causative agent and partly on the rapidity and stage of the damage caused by the infecting agent and the host response. It seems probable that the peculiar susceptibility of some of the nerve cells to a given virus determines the areas of extensive damage characteristic of some encephalitogenic viruses. For example, the basal structures are most affected by rabies virus and the agent of von Economo's disease; the cortex, particularly that of the temporal lobe which is swollen, hemorrhagic and necrotic in parts, is characteristically involved by *Herpesvirus hominis* (herpes simplex); and the whole brain appears to be affected about equally by the arbo virus group. In allergic encephalitis the white matter is usually affected, and the gray matter most often is relatively unaffected. The findings of the neuropathologist can, only rarely, be diagnostic of the causative agent in themselves, but usually must be assessed in relation to the clinical and epidemiologic features.

Epidemiology. The epidemiologic pattern varies with the infecting agent. It is almost impossible to make an exact etiologic diagnosis clinically, but an epidemiologic evaluation may afford the basis for a well educated guess. For instance, an arthropod-borne viral infection might be suspected in a summer epidemic when suitable vectors are present in the environment, whereas a sporadic case of encephalitis might lead to a diagnosis of lymphocytic choriomeningitis if there is a history of exposure to mice. Epidemics of encephalitis due to one of the enteroviruses can be recognized only when the presence of such an agent in the community has been identified in the laboratory.

ENCEPHALITIS OF VIRAL ORIGIN

Arthropod-Borne (Arbo) Viruses. These viruses are transmitted by mosquitoes or ticks; many of them exist in nature by means of enzootic infections of lower animals, especially birds. Because of the epidemic nature of their spread, these viruses account for the majority of the documented viral encephalitides reported in the United States,

even though relatively few are known to be encephalitogenic for man. Categorically, these viruses are listed as *group A*, which includes the mosquito-borne Eastern, Western and Venezuelan equine encephalitis viruses and West Nile virus; *group B*, which includes the mosquito-borne St. Louis, Japanese and Murray Valley encephalitis viruses and the tick-borne encephalitis viruses, louping ill virus and Kyasnur Forest disease virus; and a *"nongroup"*, which includes the mosquito-borne California encephalitis viruses, 8 closely related but antigenically distinct agents.

The host-virus relation of the arbo viruses is complex and not fully worked out. In general, infection of man represents a tangential transmission of the agent from a natural cycle between blood-sucking vectors and reservoir animal hosts. The essential biologic requisites for maintenance of the virus in nature are *(a)* vertebrate hosts which support a high concentration and prolonged habitation of virus in their blood, *(b)* blood-sucking vectors with a preference for the virus-carrying hosts, so that the cycle in the reservoir host is continuous; *(c)* maintenance of the cycle through periods of time when the environment is unfavorable for the vector, e.g. winter. The mechanics of this last feature are not fully understood, but possibly, in certain hosts, viremia is prolonged and persists over such periods. Epidemics in man usually require an unusual concentration of the reservoir host and appropriate vector or vectors. The low level of viremia in man excludes him from the natural cycle, with the result that his infection is a terminal one for the parasite.

Nonarthropod-Borne Viruses. A relatively large number of viruses capable of causing encephalitis in man are transmitted directly by human contact or by contact with an animal host, which may or may not have clinical disease. In addition to those listed below, there are undoubtedly others, and it can be expected that many of these will be identified in the foreseeable future.

Enteroviruses (see p. 669). A great number of these exist in the human intestine; they are responsible for a variety of clinical disorders, but perhaps most often they are not associated with any clinical evidence of disease. They are divided into 4 groups: polioviruses, Coxsackie A viruses, Coxsackie B viruses and ECHO viruses. Neurologic disease has been identified with a number of them, including the 3 types of poliovirus; Coxsackie A viruses types 2, 4, 7, 9 and 10; Coxsackie B viruses types 1 through 6; and ECHO viruses types 1 through 7, 9, 11 through 23, 25 and 30 through 32.

Myxoviruses. MUMPS (see p. 647). Involvement of the central nervous system by this viral infection may be clinically manifest as meningitis or encephalitis. The *meningeal* form is relatively common and usually benign. Pleocytosis has been reported in as many as 50 per cent of patients with mumps parotitis, but symptoms and signs of meningitis are evident in only a small percentage of them and more often in boys than in girls. Mumps virus can be isolated from the spinal fluid of such patients.

Encephalitis is an uncommon but a serious complication. Permanent residuals are relatively common, and the case fatality rate is about 20 per cent. The pathologic changes are those of allergic encephalitis.

Other neurologic complications of mumps include the Guillain-Barré-Landry syndrome, transient or permanent weakness of muscle groups resembling that caused by poliomyelitis, and transient or permanent nerve deafness.

Aqueductal stenosis and subsequent hydrocephalus have been produced in suckling hamsters by intracerebral inoculation of mumps virus, but there is no evidence that mumps infection is related to hydrocephalus in man.

Influenza viruses. Although encephalitic symptoms do occur in some patients with influenza, there is little evidence that the symptoms are caused by direct invasion of the central nervous system by any of the influenza viruses. A neurotropic strain of influenza A virus has been recognized as causing encephalitis in mice.

Herpesvirus group. HERPES SIMPLEX (HERPESVIRUS HOMINIS) (see p. 633). Encephalitis may be a manifestation of a primary or of a reactivated latent infection. It may also be part of a generalized primary infection as in the newborn infant or in severely malnourished children, or it may occur as the sole manifestation, usually without superficial herpetic lesions. The clinical features may provide a diagnostic clue, since the herpesvirus tends to affect the brain locally, with a predilection for the temporal lobe, and may simulate a space-taking lesion. The course of the illness is often prolonged. There is a slight to moderate pleocytosis, usually mononuclear, and often many red cells in the spinal fluid. The diagnosis may be established by biopsy of the affected cerebral area; the virus can sometimes be isolated from brain tissue and the characteristic intranuclear inclusion bodies can be found in neurons or glial cells. Because a possibly specific anti-herpes virus agent is available for therapy, an etiologic diagnosis should be sought by any means (see Treatment below).

HERPES ZOSTER (HERPESVIRUS VARICELLAE) (see p. 640). As a rule this virus causes only radicular manifestations through infection of the posterior root ganglia. The presenting symptom is commonly pain, which precedes a vesicular eruption on the skin of one or two adjacent dermatomes. There is usually a lymphocytic pleocytosis, and, at times, clinical evidence of meningoencephalitis. Occasionally the virus spreads to the cord and affects the anterior horn cells with resultant paralysis of affected muscle groups.

B. VIRUS (HERPESVIRUS SIMIAE). This enzootic infection of monkeys causes stomatitis and skin lesions in its natural host. When man is infected by the bite of an animal with stomatitis or by contamination of his traumatized skin with infected saliva or even with infected monkey kidney cells

in tissue culture, a highly fatal encephalomyelitis occurs. The incubation period is 2 or 3 weeks; the central nervous system illness may be preceded by vesiculation at the site of the local trauma.

Lymphocytic choriomeningitis virus. The causative virus is enzootic in mice, and man may be incidentally infected. After an incubation period of 1 to 3 weeks there is a grippelike illness for 3 to 7 days which is followed, typically, by development of meningoencephalitis. Occasionally, only the systemic manifestations occur, and fatal pneumonitis without central nervous system involvement has been described in adults. The virus can be isolated from blood and cerebrospinal fluid. Recovery from the meningeal manifestations is the rule, although progressive fatal arachnoiditis has been recorded. Residual damage of some degree is usual after the encephalomyelitic forms.

Encephalomyocarditis viruses. These small RNA viruses cause a febrile disease of the central nervous system, sometimes with paralytic symptoms, accompanied by a pleocytosis. Myocarditis has not been described in the human disease, although the prototype virus causes encephalitis and myocarditis in the chimpanzee.

Rabies (see p. 653) is caused by an RNA virus resembling a myxovirus; it is transmitted through the bite of infected animals or by inhalation of airborne virus from the guano in bat-infested caves. After an incubation period of weeks to months a fatal encephalitis develops. The virus of rabies is included by some under the category, *Chronic Infectious Neuropathic Agents (CHINA),* as is the unidentified agent of Kuru (see below).

ENCEPHALITIS OF UNKNOWN ORIGIN, PROBABLY VIRAL

Kuru. This is a slowly progressive, afebrile disease of the central nervous system which is endemic among the Fore tribe of New Guinea. There is an insidious onset of ataxia, followed by tremors, increasing incoordination, dysarthria, progressive slowing of intellectual functions, emotional disturbances, and finally by complete incapacitation, loss of sphincter control, dysphagia and death. The incidence of kuru is declining, possibly as a result of diminished tribal eating of human flesh. The pathology is characterized by widespread neuronal degeneration: myelin loss, intense glial proliferation, scattered perivascular cuffing and "plaquelike" bodies, mainly in the cerebellum. An agent present in the brain of such patients is capable of producing the disease in chimpanzees after a long incubation period.

Von Economo's Disease (Encephalitis Lethargica). This clinical entity was observed in epidemic form for a period of about 10 years, beginning in 1917. The cause was not identified, although it was strongly suspected to be viral. In epidemics the clinical manifestations were of 2 main types: (1) somnolence and ophthalmoplegia and (2) hyperkinesia. Both types have been described successively in an individual patient. The striking feature of this infection was the insidious occurrence of severe sequels in apparently recovered patients. These might be manifested as parkinsonism, disturbance of sleep rhythm or behavior disorders. Especially typical were the so-called oculogyric crises, in which the child might stop all activity and often lie down, while spasms of the ocular muscles maintained the eyes in a fixed upward position for varying intervals of time.

Benign Myalgic Encephalitis (Iceland or Akrureyri Disease). This epidemic disease was first noted in Iceland, but has occurred subsequently in various parts of the world. Its cause is unknown. After an incubation period of a week the disease sometimes starts abruptly, but more often insidiously, with low-grade fever, accompanied by pain and tenderness in the nape of the neck, back and limbs, and sometimes paresis of various muscle groups. Relapses with paresis of other muscles may occur after intervals as long as 8 weeks. Paresthesia and hypalgesia are common. Deep tendon reflexes may be decreased. There is rarely evidence of nuchal rigidity, and the cerebrospinal fluid is not altered. Improvement may occur within a few days, but residual evidences of muscle and nerve involvement may persist for as long as 6 years after the acute episode, and delayed behavioral disturbances are not uncommon. Adolescents have been chiefly affected; the disease is rare under the age of 5 years.

Encephalohepatitis (Reye's Syndrome) (see also p. 847). This syndrome is usually preceded by an upper respiratory or other viral infection. Within 1 to 3 days there is severe and persistent vomiting, which is followed within hours to a day or so by convulsions and increasing coma. During the early stages there is often wild delirium with screaming and violent motion. Neurologic signs of progressive damage are usually present, such as changeable deep tendon and plantar reflexes, muscle tone and pupillary reactions. There is no pleocytosis. The prognosis is poor for life, but survival can occur; the survivors may or may not have serious brain damge. Pathologically there are edema and neuronal damage in the brain, and fatty degeneration in liver, kidneys and sometimes in the myocardium and pancreas. This syndrome has been related to a number of different viral agents, but most often the cause is not established. It is probable that it is a host reaction to a number of different agents.

Retino-meningoencephalitis. The clinical features are those of an acute meningoencephalitis, in which papilledema and retinal hemorrhages are prominent. The increased cellular content of the cerebrospinal fluid may be polymorphonuclear or mononuclear. The symptoms last 2 to 6 weeks, but recovery eventuates. The reported 3 patients had an associated rhinovirus infection; in a personal case arachnoiditis was demonstrated by pneumoencephalography.

Myoclonic Encephalopathy of Infants. This is a disease of unknown origin with a protracted, nonprogressive and ultimately self-limited course. The onset is sudden in otherwise healthy infants, although preceding respiratory or diarrheal diseases and immunization procedures have been reported. The clinical feature is one of shocklike contractions of voluntary muscles that completely disorganize voluntary movements. The eyeballs are notably affected with rapid, irregular conjugate movements of rotation and displacement; in addition there are irregular and variable incoordinate movements of the limbs and head, which are absent only during sleep. These may grossly resemble those of cerebellar ataxia. The symptoms rapidly reach a plateau, but may persist unchanged for months or even years. No changes have been observed in electroencephalograms, roentgenograms, pneumoencephalograms, brain biopsy or in the cerebrospinal fluid. Treatment with corticosteroids, especially ACTH, has been dramatically effective in some children. The suggested pathogenesis is that of an autoimmune process similar to that occurring in the allergic group of encephalitides.

Recurrent Encephalomyelitis. Occasionally a patient has repeated attacks of encephalitis. The first episode may, for example, follow measles, and recovery may appear to be complete. Subsequently, encephalitic episodes may follow other infections of known or unidentified causation, trauma or even occur without a recognized antecedent. Any one of the episodes may result in severe and irreversible damage or may end in apparent recovery. It is suggested that these attacks represent recurrent episodes of autoimmunization. It is also possible that, in some patients, these episodes represent early manifestations of multiple sclerosis.

Localized Encephalopathy. A clinical pattern suggestive of localized encephalitis has been described. The initial manifestation may be localized convulsions following an upper respiratory or diarrheal illness which may be characteristic of temporoparietal lobe seizures. Between convulsions, neurologic abnormalities are usually not noted, although there may be hemianopsia. Consciousness is not affected; there is no clinical evidence of increased intracranial pressure, and there are no associated systemic manifestations of illness. The cerebrospinal fluid is not affected, but there are abnormal electroencephalographic changes most prominent in the region of the brain corresponding to the origin of the convulsions. Arteriography may reveal local swelling of the brain, and a brain scan may be positive in the affected region. Treatment should be directed toward general support and the control of the seizures; anticonvulsant therapy should be continued until the electroencephalogram has returned to normal. The prognosis may be good with complete clinical recovery within days or weeks and with eventual return of the electroencephalographic pattern to normal. The process, however, may be prolonged with intractable convulsions over a long period of time. Pathologic changes in the brain, removed at therapeutic hemispherectomy, are those compatible with an encephalitis of viral origin. The recognition of this clinical entity and its differentiation from a space-taking lesion are of obvious importance in directing the course of therapy.

Acute Encephalopathies of Obscure Origin in Infants. Some neurologic syndromes, occurring mostly in infancy, have been categorized under this heading. The attacks are characterized by fever, convulsions, stupor or coma, decorticate or decerebrate postures, dystonic muscular movements and respiratory distress. Convulsions usually predominate initially, but may not occur when there is impaired consciousness. There is often a history of an ill-defined febrile illness at the onset. The cerebrospinal fluid is typically clear, without cells, but is usually under increased pressure. Respiratory difficulty may arise from involvement of the respiratory center or from paralytic obstruction of the airway, and the consequent hypoxia may cause additional damage. The pathologic changes are those of hypoxia. It seems probable that viruses, at present unidentified, may be the causative agents in some instances.

Other Encephalitides. Encephalopathy may on occasion be the predominant presenting feature in infections due to hepatitis viruses, in infectious mononucleosis and in adenovirus infections, although the causative relation of these agents to encephalitic phenomena is uncertain.

Progressive Multifocal Leukoencephalopathy (PMLE). Although this disorder has not yet been described in children, its existence should be mentioned. It occurs usually but not always in a patient with a chronic illness associated with immunologic unresponsiveness, e.g. Hodgkin's disease. The terminal fatal neurologic illness is relatively short, lasting 3 to 4 months. The clinical symptoms include ataxia, hemiparesis, cranial nerve palsies, visual and speech difficulties and mental deterioration. Pathologically, there are foci of demyelination, nuclear changes including the presence of eosinophilic inclusions in the oligodendrocytes and astrocytes, and hypertrophy of the cells in the granular layer of the cerebellum. Electron microscopic pictures reveal intranuclear structures with the characteristic structure of Papova viruses. No changes in the cerebrospinal fluid are noted by usual examinations.

Subacute Sclerosing Panencephalitis (SSPE). This clinicopathologic entity is now generally considered to include the encephalopathies originally reported as separate entities, as "inclusion encephalitis" by Dawson, "subacute sclerosing leukoencephalitis" by Van Bogaert and "panencephalitis" by Pette and Doering. The pathologic characteristics are the presence of type A intranuclear inclusion bodies, neuronophagia, perivenous mononuclear infiltration with demyelination and gliosis of the white matter. Any one of these features may predominate in an individual patient.

Three clinical stages are described. In the first there are insidious changes in personality, deterioration in behavior, impairment of intellectual function, and transient seizures resulting in frequent falls. In the second the child shows increasing impairment of mentality, easy fatigability, loss of memory and gradual loss of interest in the outside world, seizures of various types (especially myoclonic jerks), choreoathetoid or profound dystonic movements, including hemiballismus, and hyperkinesia. The third and final stage is one of increasing stupor and cachexia leading to death; the child may become blind, and frequently a decorticate spastic quadriplegia develops. There may be a terminal episode of hyperthermia. Diagnostic aids are (1) electroencephalographic changes, characterized in all leads by bursts of high voltage, stereotyped slow-wave complexes followed by suppression of activity occurring every 5 to 10 seconds at the time of myoclonic jerks; (2) a positive first zone in the colloidal gold test; and (3) an increase in gamma globulin at the expense of albumin and beta globulin in the spinal fluid. The diagnosis may be confirmed during life by cerebral biopsy; the procedure is justified for its prognostic value.

The pathologic findings in this clinical entity are in general similar to those found in the allergic encephalitides. Therefore it seems probable that this disease will be found to be the result of a host reaction to a number of different causative agents, most likely viruses. There is evidence that in some patients the disease has been associated with infection of the neurons and glial cells by measles virus. An unidentified agent, which is not a measles virus, has also been isolated from patients with this clinical disease which was passable to ferrets in series.

Multiple Sclerosis. This disease usually becomes clinically identifiable in late adolescence or early adult life. A transient attack of optic neuritis with or without associated encephalomyelitis in childhood should be considered a possible initial manifestation of this disease. There is increasing suggestion that multiple sclerosis is of exogenous origin and related to subacute sclerosing panencephalitis (see also Recurrent Encephalomyelitis).

ALLERGIC ENCEPHALITIS

The pathogenesis and pathology of this clinical entity have been discussed under their respective headings. The extensive and selective demyelination with perseveration of neurons and axis cylinders is characteristic. The pattern is indistinguishable from that of experimental allergic encephalitis (EAE) produced in animals by inoculation of brain tissue. The clinical reaction follows natural viral infections (postinfectious) and certain immunizing procedures (postvaccinal).

Postinfectious Encephalitis. After a number of exanthems and mumps, encephalitic manifestations may appear, usually after, but occasionally before, the characteristic systemic manifestations of the disease. The occurrence of this complication bears no relation to the severity of the original illness, and the incidence varies with different viruses and geographically. It is relatively common after measles in the United States (average 1:1000 cases), but apparently less common in continental Europe. It reportedly occurs in 1:2000 cases of smallpox and in 1:5000 cases of German measles. It is rare in association with varicella and mumps; the exact incidence is unknown, since mild varicella is often overlooked and there is a high incidence of subclinical infection in mumps. A similar encephalopathy has been described following upper respiratory tract infections which were probably viral in origin.

Postvaccinal Encephalitis. The incidence of encephalitis associated with active immunization varies with the procedure and also geographically. It is relatively high after rabies neural vaccine (1:3000 to 1:7000), but much less so after rabies non-neural vaccine (1:50,000). In the United States and Great Britain encephalitis is rare after smallpox vaccination (1:100,000 or more), but in parts of continental Europe the incidence is high (1:4000). It has been reported rarely after influenza, poliomyelitis (killed) and pertussis vaccines. In infants under 1 year of age encephalitis has followed yellow fever immunization. This may be the association of a neurotropic strain of virus and the highly susceptible cells of the infant's brain and so may not be appropriately placed in this classification.

DIAGNOSIS, PROGNOSIS AND TREATMENT

Diagnosis. Etiologic diagnosis is possible only by laboratory methods (see p. 543); either by isolation of the virus from the blood, cerebrospinal fluid, urine, throat, nose or rectal swabs or from the brain by biopsy or after death, or by demonstrating a rise of serum antibodies against a known virus.

Prognosis. This is extremely variable and may be surprisingly good despite severe neurologic manifestations. In general, however, the prognosis is better when the clinical manifestations are largely meningeal or localized, e.g. cerebellar, than when they are mainly encephalitic or encephalomyelitic. It is the clinical manifestation and *not* the causative agent that must guide the physician. Rapidly developing coma with increasing respiratory difficulty is usually associated with a fatal outcome. Prolonged coma, with preservation of intact vital signs, is often associated with subsequent brain damage, but, sometimes, apparently complete recovery may result.

Treatment. *Antimicrobial.* The antiviral drug 5-iodo 2′-deoxyuridine is currently under clinical trial in herpetic encephalitis. It has been given by intracarotid perfusion daily for 5 days at an average dose of 14 mg. per kg. per 24 hours and by continuous intravenous drip for 7 days at an average dose of 80 mg. per kg. per 24 hours. Suggestive improvement has been reported, and also drug toxicity. Because of the seriousness of this illness, further trials of this drug in documented herpetic infections seem justified.

General measures. The skillful application of supportive and symptomatic measures is of prime importance.

Careful *nursing care* is essential, with particular attention to care of the skin and mouth, frequent changes of position to avoid pressure sores and thoracic percussion to prevent lung collapse and hypostatic pneumonia.

Distention of the bladder must be anticipated and controlled by skillful Credé manipulation, suprapubic drainage through a Teflon tube or, as a last resort, catheterization. Cholinergic drugs, e.g. neostigmine, are usually not efficacious.

Constipation, and in particular fecal impactions, should be prevented by the use of mineral oil and enemas.

Water and nutrients usually must be administered intravenously in the early stage. Careful control of water intake is necessary to avoid water intoxication on the one hand, and dehydration on the other. Vitamins, including large amounts of vitamin C and the B vitamins, should be included in the daily intake. As soon as possible, feeding should be instituted through a nasogastric tube.

Obstruction of the airway may be anticipated when impairment of swallowing function results in pooling of secretions; it requires a head-low position and suction. Tracheotomy may be indicated. Failure of respiration may be due to paralysis of the respiratory muscles or to involvement of the respiratory center; it may require the use of an appropriate respirator.

Increased intracranial pressure may be manifest early by irregularities of respiration. Reduction of pressure is of prime importance, since avoidance of the consequent anoxia may preserve those cells that are not irreversibly damaged.* Various measures have theoretic potential for this purpose; trial with any one or all of them may be justified. (1) *Increase of serum osmolality.* If the encephalopathy is clearly due to water intoxication associated with inappropriate ADH secretion, the use of mannitol (1.5 to 2.0 gm. per kg. infused slowly over 1 to 1½ hours) may be justified. When capillary walls are damaged, such a maneuver would not be effective and might be harmful. The same probably applies to the use of glycerol by mouth (75 mg. of glycerol in an equal quantity of fruit juice is the adult dose). (2) *Hydrocortisone.* This steroid can be given in pharmacologic doses (10 to 15 mg. per kg. per 24 hours). Hydrocortisone is preferable to the synthetic steroids in an emergency, since, on occasion, the anti-inflammatory action is not produced by the latter. The

---

*The ability of some neurons to recover from a viral infection has been documented by Bodian in experimental poliomyelitis infection in the monkey.

effect should be observed over the course of 3 to 4 days, and continued administration should be determined on a clinical basis. (3) *Hypothermia.* Reduction of body temperature to levels of about 30° C. reduces cerebral edema and decreases the need of cells for oxygen. In whatever way the hypothermia is induced, shivering must be suppressed by slow intravenous infusion of chlorpromazine (0.25 to 0.5 mg. per kg.), sometimes accompanied by meperidine (0.5 mg. per kg.). During hypothermia accurate and frequent (hourly if possible) measurement of fluid intake and output is mandatory, since the decrease in reabsorption of water associated with the hypothermic state may rapidly lead to severe dehydration unless the intake is suitably increased. In a girl the use of a Foley catheter or a suprapubic Teflon tube is required for this purpose. (4) *Surgical decompression.* It is doubtful whether this procedure, even when the dura is left intact, is justifiable in children.

Control of convulsions. In the acute stage this can be accomplished by the intravenous use of anticonvulsants such as pentobarbital (1.0 mg. per kg.) or, in patients over 6 months of age, diazepam (Valium) (0.15 to 0.25 mg. per kg., repeated in 15 minutes). Other anticonvulsants (see p. 1256) may be indicated for several months during convalescence. Serial electroencephalograms may be helpful in evaluating the need for anticonvulsant therapy.

Antibiotic therapy. This is not indicated routinely in the types of encephalitis discussed. Antibiotics should be used in therapeutic doses when bacterial infection is superimposed. The use of antibiotics in patients receiving corticosteroid therapy or hypothermia measures is not routinely indicated. The use of bladder tubes for drainage introduces the risk of urinary tract infection. Meticulous catheter care should be observed, and the urine cultured frequently. If infection is found, appropriate antibiotics should be used. Prolonged therapy for at least 3 months, usually with sulfonamides, is indicated if infection becomes established. The high incidence of pseudomonas pneumonia in patients during hypothermia might warrant the use of therapeutic doses of polymixin B or other appropriate drug if artificial respiration is required.

Follow-up therapy. Physiotherapy, occupational therapy and corrective surgery should be utilized as necessary. Parents should be warned that transient, sometimes quite severe, emotional and behavioral aberrations are common and that children tend to return to normal more quickly when a permissive rather than a too restrictive attitude is adopted. They should also be encouraged with the prospect that there may be slow but continued improvement.

Prevention. Prophylactic vaccination is available against the viruses of poliomyelitis, but it seems unlikely that any of the other enteroviruses will soon be controllable by this means. Clinical rabies can often be prevented by vaccination sometimes accompanied by the use of rabies antiserum

(see under Rabies). The widespread use of live attenuated measles virus vaccine has dramatically lowered the incidence of measles in the United States and thus the incidence of postmeasles encephalitis. The judicious use of live attenuated mumps vaccine may reduce the incidence of serious mumps encephalitis. The availability of an effective vaccine for rubella within the near future seems probable. Killed vaccines developed for some of the arbo viruses have not been effective when tried on a large scale, e.g. vaccine against Japanese B encephalitis. More success may be expected from control of the arthropod vector by insecticide sprays and repellents. Extreme care and use of protective clothing are indicated when exposure to known animal reservoirs is necessary.

T. F. McNair Scott

REFERENCES

Aguilar, M. J., and Rasmussen, T.: Role of Encephalitis in Pathogenesis of Epilepsy. A.M.A. *Arch. Neurol.*, 2:663, 1960.

Brody, J. A., Henle, W., and Koprowski, H.: Chronic Infectious Neuropathic Agents (CHINA) and Other Slow Virus Infections. *Curr. Top. Microb. & Immun.*, 40:1, 1967.

Gajdusek, D. C., and Zigas, V.: Degenerative Disease of the Central Nervous System in New Guinea. The Epidemic Occurrence of "Kuru" in the Native Population. *New England J. Med.*, 257:974, 1957.

Gajdusek, D. C., Gibbs, C. J., and Alpers, M.: Transmission and Passage of Experimental "Kuru" to Chimpanzees. *Science*, 155:212, 1967.

Holzel, A., Smith, P. A., and Tobin, J. O'H.: A New Type of Meningo-encephalitis Associated with a Rhinovirus (Retinomeningoencephalitis). *Acta Pediat. Scand.*, 54:168, 1965.

Horsfall, F. L., and Tamm, I. (Eds.): *Viral and Rickettsial Infections of Man.* 4th ed. Philadelphia, J. B. Lippincott Company, 1965.

Katz, M., and others: Transmission of an Encephalitogenic Agent from Patients with Subacute Sclerosing Panencephalitis (SSPE) to Ferrets. *New England J. Med.*, 279:793, 1968.

Kennedy, C., and Scott, T. F. McN.: The Management of Acute Febrile Encephalopathies; in H. Eichenwald (Ed.): *The Prevention of Mental Retardation Through Control of Infectious Disease.* Bethesda, Md., Department of Health, Education, and Welfare, National Institutes of Health, 1966, p. 309.

Kennedy, C., and Wanglee, P.: Encephalitis: A Variable Syndrome in Response to Viral Infection. *Pediat. Clin. N. Amer.*, 14:809, 1967.

Kinsbourne, M.: Myoclonic Encephalopathy of Infants. *J. Neurol., Neuro. Surg. & Psychiat.*, 25:271, 1962.

Miller, H. G., Stanton, J. B., and Gibbons, J. L.: Para-infectious Encephalomyelitis and Related Syndromes. *Quart J. Med.*, 25:427, 1956.

Olson, L. C., Buescher, E. L., Artenstein, M. S., and Parkman, P. D.: Herpesvirus Infections of the Human Central Nervous System. *New England J. Med.*, 277:1271, 1967.

Reye, R. D. K., Morgan, G., and Baral, J.: Encephalopathy and Fatty Degeneration of the Viscera. A Disease Entity in Childhood. *Lancet*, 2:749, 1963.

Richardson, E. P.: Progressive Multifocal Leukoencephalopathy. *New England J. Med.*, 265:815, 1961.

Scott, T. F. McN.: Post Infectious and Vaccinal Encephalitis. *M. Clin. N. Amer.*, 51:701, 1967.

Sever, J. L. (Ed.): Conference on Measles Virus and Subacute Sclerosing Panencephalitis. *Neurology*, 18:192, 1968.

Webb, H. E., and Smith, C. E. G.: Relation of Immune Response to Development of Central Nervous System Lesions in Virus Infections of Man. *Brit. M.J.*, 2:1179, 1966.

Zu Rhein, G., and Chou, S. M.: Particles Resembling Papova Viruses in Human Cerebral Demyelinating Disease. *Science*, 148:1477, 1965.

Rickettsial Diseases

The rickettsiae are microorganisms which commonly inhabit the alimentary canal of certain insects and may be associated with disease in man. Stained preparations appear under the ordinary microscope as pleomorphic coccobacilli 0.3 to 0.5 micron in diameter. Most species are retained by bacterial filters, and all require the presence of living cells for multiplication. Biologically, the rickettsiae have some of the characteristics of bacteria and some of viruses and are classified in an intermediate position.

The rickettsial diseases of man, with the exception of Q fever, are febrile illnesses with rashes. They may be separated into 4 groups on the basis of clinical characteristics, insect vectors, etiologic agent and epidemiology (Table 10-26).

Epidemic typhus and endemic typhus are almost identical clinically and pathologically. The causative agents are so similar antigenically that cross reactions occur in Proteus or rickettsial agglutination tests. The 2 forms of the disease may be distinguished by specific complement fixation tests and by the inability of epidemic typhus to produce a scrotal reaction in guinea pigs. Brill's disease is a recrudescence of epidemic typhus.

There are many related strains of rickettsiae which cause spotted fever of variable severity in different parts of the world. The list includes boutonneuse fever of the Mediterranean regions, São Paulo, Tobia and pinta fevers of South America, Kenya or Nigeria fever of Africa, and many others. Rickettsialpox is included in the spotted fever group because of antigenic relations of *Rickettsia akari* to the causative agent of Rocky Mountain spotted fever.

Tsutsugamushi fever, or scrub typhus, was known in certain areas of Japan for many years, but not until the beginning of World War II was it learned that the disease was present also among the populations of India, Australia, Indonesia (Dutch East Indies) and Malaya. Effective vaccines are not available, and scrub typhus continues to be a hazard to those who enter endemic areas.

Q fever differs clinically, histologically and epidemiologically from the other diseases listed and is classified with them only because it is caused by a rickettsia.

The pathology, methods for making a laboratory diagnosis, and manner of treatment of each of the rickettsial diseases in man are so similar that it seems appropriate to discuss these topics as a whole before describing the individual diseases.

Pathology. The lesion of the arthropod-borne rickettsial diseases is sufficiently distinctive to be diagnostic in patients with a history of an exanthem. The main changes involve the small blood vessels, chiefly of the skin, subcutaneous tissue and central nervous system. The endothelial cells swell and occlude the small blood vessels, and thrombosis results. The occluded vessels are surrounded by cuffs of mononuclear cells, plasma

TABLE 10-26. RICKETTSIAL DISEASES OF MAN: SUMMARY OF PERTINENT INFORMATION

GROUP	DISEASE	CAUSATIVE AGENT	ARTHROPOD VECTOR	ANIMAL HOST	PROTEUS AGGLUTI-NATION*	GEOGRAPHIC DISTRIBUTION
Typhus...........	Epidemic typhus	*R. prowazeki*	Body louse	None	OX19	World-wide; rarely U.S.A.
	Brill's disease	*R. prowazeki*	None		OX19	Eastern coastal cities of U.S.A.; Israel
	Murine typhus	*R. mooseri*	Rat flea, louse	Rat	OX19	World-wide; southern states of U.S.A.
Spotted fever...	Rocky Mountain spotted fever	*R. rickettsii*	Tick	Rodents, mammals	Variable OX2 or OX19	North and South America; related diseases world-wide
	Rickettsial-pox	*R. akari*	Mite	House mice	None	Reported from eastern U.S.A.
Tsutsugamushi fever...........	Scrub typhus	*R. orientalis* (tsutsugamushi)	Mite	Rodents	OXK	Far East
Q fever...........	Q fever	*R. burneti* (*Coxiella burneti*)	Rarely ticks ?	Ticks, cattle, sheep, goats	None	World-wide; western U.S.A.

*Specific serologic procedures using rickettsial antigens in complement fixation, agglutination or neutralization tests are more reliable.

cells and macrophages. Rickettsiae localize in the endothelium of capillaries and extend via the intima into larger vessels. Rocky Mountain spotted fever may be distinguished histologically from other rickettsial diseases by the presence of rickettsiae in the smooth muscle cells of the media. This results in severe destruction of blood vessels and may explain the occurrence of necrosis of skin in sites such as the ear lobes, fingers, toes and scrotum.

The symptomatology of vector-transmitted rickettsial diseases correlates with the degree of involvement and the location of affected vessels. For example, the fall in blood pressure, an outstanding clinical feature of rickettsial disease, is generally conceded to be the result of changes in the peripheral vessels. Perivascular reactions in the lung may result in atelectasis and pneumonia. Vascular changes in the brain may produce central nervous system symptoms.

Q fever, which is not accompanied by a rash and does not require an insect vector, differs pathologically from the other rickettsial diseases. The principal, and usually the only, lesions occur in the lungs, where there is a patchy interstitial pneumonitis with copious exudate composed of fibrin and mononuclear cells. Alveolar walls, alveolar ducts and terminal bronchioles are infiltrated by large mononuclear cells.

Diagnosis. The diagnosis of a rickettsial infection in man usually requires laboratory confirmation, which is most readily established by demonstration of acquired specific antibodies. In unusual cases when serologic tests are unobtainable or equivocal it may be necessary to identify the causative agent.

Serologic diagnosis. During etiologic studies of typhus fever, Felix isolated a strain of *Proteus vulgaris* from the urine of a patient. This strain (OX19) was not the causative agent of typhus, but had sufficient antigenic similarity to *Rickettsia prowazeki* so that serum from patients convalescent from typhus fever contained high titers of OX19 agglutinin. Additional strains of Proteus related to the causative agents of tsutsugamushi (OXK) and Rocky Mountain spotted fever (OX2) were also discovered. These easily prepared antigens are used for agglutination tests in patients' serums (the Weil-Felix reaction).

In epidemic typhus fever the agglutination to OX19 usually reaches a titer greater than 1:160 during the second week of illness; the OX2 and OXK titers remain low. The agglutinin pattern observed with murine typhus is similar to that of epidemic typhus, and the 2 infections cannot be distinguished by this method. The Proteus agglutination test is of little value in the diagnosis of Rocky Mountain spotted fever, owing to the variations in the degree and types of response; classically, the patient should have a high titer of OX2 agglutinins and little, if any, antibody against OX19 and OXK. Proteus OXK agglutinin titers are high after tsutsugamushi disease. Convalescent serum from patients with Q fever or

rickettsialpox does not agglutinate to significant titer the Proteus strains used in the Weil-Felix reaction. Proteus titers do not persist and are usually below a significant level within 3 months after the illness.

Specific serologic procedures using rickettsial antigens in complement fixation, agglutination or neutralization tests are much more reliable than the Weil-Felix reaction and should be used to confirm the diagnosis of rickettsial infections. Two samples of serum, one obtained during the first week of illness and the other 2 or 3 weeks later, should be available to determine whether a significant increase in titer has occurred during the illness.

Culturing of rickettsiae. Rickettsiae may be propagated by inoculating susceptible experimental animals or the developing chick embryo. These techniques are seldom required to diagnose rickettsial infections, but may be used to study the effectiveness of various antibiotics or to detect the presence of rickettsiae in milk, dust or insects.

The culturing of rickettsiae in the laboratory is extremely hazardous and has been the source of infection for many investigators. This is a task for a special laboratory with proper facilities and immunized personnel. Serologic procedures, using killed antigen and heat-inactivated serums, involve little risk to the laboratory worker.

Treatment. Treatment of rickettsial infections is much more effective since the discovery of the broad-spectrum antibiotics. Mortality rates have fallen greatly, the morbidity rate has decreased, and complications have become infrequent. These drugs, however, are not immediately or invariably effective in influencing the course of the disease, and clinical relapses are not uncommon. Rickettsiae have been isolated from the blood of patients who received presumably adequate doses of an antibiotic. These difficulties are related to the fact that chloramphenicol and the tetracyclines suppress, but do not destroy, the rickettsiae. Final eradication of the microorganism depends upon the immune processes of the host.

The recommended dose of the tetracyclines or chloramphenicol for children is 50 to 100 mg. per kg. per day orally in 4 divided doses. The maximum or adult daily dose is 4 gm. When the intravenous route is used, 30 to 40 mg. per kg. per day of either drug should be administered in 3 equal doses. Drug therapy should be continued until the patient is afebrile for 48 hours; this is usually 5 to 9 days after initiation of treatment.

Early diagnosis and the proper use of antimicrobial agents are all that is necessary in the management of most rickettsial infections. Vigorous supportive therapy, parenteral fluids, transfusions, sedation and oxygen are necessary for the severely ill patient.

Corticosteroids have been used with an antibiotic in instances when the response to the antibiotic alone was not satisfactory. Although the results were described as good, sufficient information is not available to evaluate this therapy critically, and corticosteroids are not recommended for the average case.

TYPHUS FEVER

(Epidemic Typhus; Louse-Borne Typhus)

History. Typhus fever has been associated with misery since man donned clothing. Typhus was probably responsible for the plague of Athens, 430 B.C.; it existed during the Middle Ages and was associated with each of the serious famines in England before the discovery of America. Typhus was spread through Europe by louse-infected soldiers and was often the most important factor in determining the outcome of battles or the survival of nations.

In more recent years typhus has been an Old World disease with large outbreaks during time of war. In October 1943 the disease broke out in Naples as the Allied occupation troops arrived. Typhus was encountered in Nazi concentration camps and was spread through Europe by escaping inmates. Epidemics have occurred among immigrants in coastal cities in America, but typhus has not been common in the United States during recent years. The existence of endemic areas within a few hours of travel distance, however, makes epidemics of typhus in any country a possibility.

Etiology and Transmission. Man is the sole reservoir of *Rickettsia prowazeki*, the causative agent of epidemic typhus. The body or head louse may become infected by feeding upon the blood of a person with rickettsemia. The ingested organisms multiply within the cells lining the alimentary tract of the insect and are eliminated in the feces.

Contaminated feces may be introduced into a susceptible human host through abrasions or perforations in the skin, or by way of the conjunctival sac or upper respiratory tract. Inhalation of dried, infected louse excreta present in the clothing, bedding or furniture of a typhus patient is probably an important source of infection.

The infected louse dies soon after contracting typhus and seldom has more than a week to spread disease. The louse cannot fly or jump, but may crawl short distances to another human being, especially if his original host becomes uncomfortably hot or cold.

Pathology. See page 698.

Clinical Manifestations. Typhus fever was a much milder disease in children than in adults even before the availability of chemotherapeutic agents.

The clinical manifestations of typhus in children may include fever, transient rash and only few constitutional symptoms, which often make recognition of the disease difficult.

The incubation period is usually less than 14 days and is followed by an abrupt onset with severe frontal headache, weakness, malaise, generalized aches and pains, chills, and fever of 104°F. or more. Four to 7 days later the rash appears.

Faint, rose-colored spots of irregular outline 2 to 4 mm. in size which fade with pressure appear first over the chest and spread gradually over the abdomen, back and extremities. In 24 to 48 hours the lesions become dark red and no longer fade with pressure. The lesions may spread to include the palms and soles, but the face and scalp usually remain free. Petechial lesions occur in severe cases. The rash may be present for only a few hours or persist after the temperature has returned to normal. In general, the more profuse the rash, the more severe is the disease.

The appearance of the rash marks the beginning of the critical period. The fever remains high and unremitting, and periods of stupor are interrupted by bouts of violent delirium. The blood pressure is low, and renal output decreased. Oral intake is low and requires parenteral supplementation. In the absence of complications such as pneumonia, severe central nervous system involvement or renal insufficiency, which are frequently fatal, the patient begins to improve during the third week. The temperature gradually falls, the central nervous system symptoms disappear, and the headache ceases. Recovery from typhus is complete, and even in patients with evidence of diffuse involvement sequels are rare.

Laboratory Data. (See also page 699). Leukopenia with a relative lymphocytosis early in the disease is usually followed by a leukocytosis during the second and third weeks; a normocytic anemia is common. Urinary findings vary with the degree of renal involvement; albuminuria and microscopic hematuria are frequent.

Differential Diagnosis. Meningococcemia, typhoid, measles or smallpox may be confused with typhus, but the history, clinical course and laboratory data usually permit a proper diagnosis.

Control Measures. The immediate destruction of vectors with an insecticide with persisting effect such as DDT is an important measure in the control of an epidemic. Dust containing excreta from infected lice is also capable of transmitting typhus, and care must be taken to prevent its inhalation. This usually requires washing the patient's clothing, bedding and other possessions with hot water and a disinfectant after they have been dusted with DDT. Vaccination of persons likely to come in contact with typhus is recommended. The preferred vaccine is a killed preparation of a rickettsia grown in the yolk sac of the chick embryo. Insufficient data are available as to differences in sensitivity to broad-spectrum antibiotics by strains of rickettsiae, but if resistant forms do not occur, the administration of an antibiotic may be adequate prophylaxis for brief exposures to typhus.

Treatment. See page 699.

MURINE TYPHUS

(Endemic Typhus)

Etiology and Transmission. Unlike epidemic typhus, which is not seen among children in the United States, endemic typhus is fairly common, particularly in Texas and the southeastern states, and has been seen in most regions of this country.

It usually occurs in the summer and fall in contrast to typhus, which is characteristically a disease of winter and spring.

Murine typhus is a disease of rats caused by *Rickettsia mooseri*. It is usually transmitted from rat to rat by the rat louse or flea. In both the rat and the insect vectors murine typhus is a mild disease with no apparent effect on their life span. The eggs laid by infected fleas or lice do not transmit *R. mooseri* to the next generation. Man usually acquires murine typhus when bitten by an infected rat flea, but can also be infected by inhaling or possibly ingesting infected excreta of fleas.

Pathology. See page 698.

Clinical Manifestations. Murine typhus is a mild, seldom fatal illness that can be distinguished from epidemic typhus only by special laboratory procedures.

The incubation period is usually about 8 days. Prodromal symptoms such as headache, arthralgia and backache are followed by a gradually increasing temperature which may reach 106°F. in children and last 9 to 14 days. On the first to the eighth day of fever, most often by the fifth day, the rash appears. The eruption begins on the trunk and spreads to the periphery, rarely involving the face, palms or soles. Initially the skin lesion is a dull red macule with ill-defined margins which becomes slightly papular as it matures. It never becomes purpuric and persists for a much shorter period than the rash of epidemic typhus. Twenty per cent or more of children may have no rash or such a transient one that it is not noted. Central nervous system symptoms are uncommon, as is peripheral vascular collapse or other complications.

Diagnosis. See page 699.

Control Measures. Control of murine typhus requires elimination of the rat reservoir or the insect vector, or both. Immunization of personnel in contact with possibly infected rats is recommended. The vaccine is different from that used for epidemic typhus, although most persons who have recovered from one form of typhus are also immune to the other.

Treatment. See page 699.

BRILL'S DISEASE

Brill's disease is an unusual phenomenon in which a patient with a history of typhus suffers a recrudescence of his illness. It has been observed among immigrants from eastern Europe in the coastal cities of the United States and more recently in Israel. The strains of rickettsiae isolated from such patients are indistinguishable from those of epidemic typhus. It is presumed that organisms have persisted in the tissues of the host for years, and then, for reasons not understood, they increase in number and produce clinical symptoms. A patient with Brill's disease can infect lice and is a potential point of origin for a typhus epidemic when the vector is present. Brill's disease is not a problem in children.

SCRUB TYPHUS
(TSUTSUGAMUSHI FEVER; MITE TYPHUS)

Scrub typhus has been recognized in Japan and Formosa for centuries, but not until World War II was it realized that this disease could be found in localities stretching from India to the Philippines, including Burma, Malaysia, New Guinea, the Solomon Islands and Queensland. The incidence of scrub typhus among United States Army personnel in bases north of Australia during 1942 and 1943 was about 10 per 1000 troops per year with a case fatality rate of 3 to 10 per cent.

Etiology and Transmission. *Rickettsia tsutsugamushi*, also known as *R. orientalis*, is the causal agent of scrub typhus. The vectors which carry the agent are the larval forms of the "chigger" or trombiculid mites. The larvae feed on rats or other rodents and when not feeding are present on low-lying vegetation from where they can attack man. *Rickettsia tsutsugamushi* has been isolated from many species of rodents, and it seems likely that both mites and rodents can serve as reservoirs of rickettsiae.

Scrub typhus is mainly a disease of persons whose occupations bring them into contact with infected mites.

Pathology. See page 698.

Clinical Manifestations. The symptomatology of scrub typhus, although showing several distinctive features, is remarkably similar to that of other rickettsial infections. The disease may vary in severity, but characteristically has an abrupt onset 12 to 18 days after the bite by the infected mite. The initial symptoms are fever and headache, sometimes accompanied by anorexia and vomiting.

Some form of skin lesion is usually present at the site of the mite bite, which begins as an asymptomatic, pink papule, increases in size and becomes either an eschar, consisting of a central, black scab 4 to 8 mm. in diameter surrounded by a dull red areola, or, in moist areas (axilla, perineum), a pinched-out shallow ulcer. By the end of the first week of illness a maculopapular rash develops on the chest and abdomen and gradually spreads to involve the entire body, except usually the hands and face. Diffuse, tender adenopathy, greater in the region of the primary lesion, is a common part of the clinical syndrome.

Laboratory confirmation may be obtained by isolation of the causative agent in mice. The Weil-Felix reaction for Proteus OXK may become positive by the third week of the illness, but this is not invariable, especially in patients treated with antibiotics (see also p. 699).

In severe cases signs of pulmonary or cardiac involvement may develop during the second week of illness, and death results. In mild or treated cases improvement begins by the end of the second week, fever decreases, the rash fades, and the eschar heals. The mortality rate when antibiotics are used is less than 5 per cent.

Control Measures. The difficulties encountered in attempting to eliminate the widely prevalent mite vector of scrub typhus have led to investigations of control by vaccines. Unfortunately, the vaccines tested have not proved entirely satisfactory, owing to the many antigenically different strains of *R. tsutsugamushi* which are pathogenic for man. It is hoped that an effective polyvalent vaccine can be prepared. Until such time, protective clothing and early treatment with broad-spectrum antibiotics are the most useful aids to prevent death from scrub typhus.

Treatment. See page 699.

ROCKY MOUNTAIN SPOTTED FEVER

History. Rocky Mountain spotted fever is an exanthem of man first recognized in the Rocky Mountain region of the United States by Maxey in 1899. Ricketts inoculated monkeys and guinea pigs with infected human blood and was able to transmit the infection and demonstrate the causative agent. He later showed that the disease is spread by the wood tick and discovered infected ticks in the Bitter Root Valley of Montana. The name "Rocky Mountain spotted fever" gives a false impression of geographic limitation to a disease that has been observed throughout the United States. The attack rate in Virginia, Delaware and Maryland, for example, is as high as or higher than that in Nevada, Idaho and Montana.

Etiology and Transmission. The causative agent of Rocky Mountain spotted fever, *Rickettsia rickettsii*, is maintained in nature by many hosts, including the ground squirrel, jack rabbit, chipmunk, wood rat, meadow mouse and weasel; the animal hosts do not become ill. Transmission among animals and from animal to man is most commonly achieved through the wood tick, *Dermacentor andersoni*, or the dog tick, *Dermacentor variabilis.*

Sheepherders, hunters, woodsmen or others whose occupation or recreation brings them into the isolated tick-infested woods of Montana or Idaho are most likely to be bitten by an infected wood tick. In the eastern United States, however, more infections occur in children and women, who are probably bitten by infected dog ticks encountered during outings in the woods or while handling the family dog.

Infected female ticks may pass rickettsiae through eggs to the progeny and thus maintain a reservoir for a long time without infecting man.

Pathology. See page 698.

Clinical Manifestations. The incubation period in children varies from 1 to 8 days. The disease usually begins with such nonspecific symptoms as headache, fever, anorexia and restlessness. There is a history of tick bite in approximately half the reported cases, but local reaction at the site of the bite is uncommon. Discrete, pale, rose-red macules or maculopapules appear 1 to 5 days after the onset of illness; rarely there may be

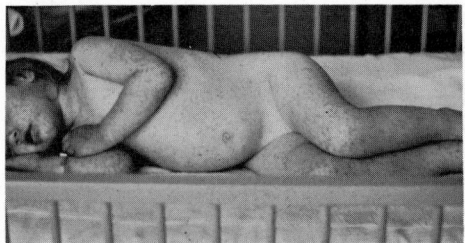

Figure 10-95. Patient with Rocky Mountain spotted fever. Note the greater concentration of skin lesions on the ankles, wrists and lower legs. (Courtesy of William H. Wood, M.D., Cleveland.)

little or no rash. The rash characteristically begins peripherally on the ankles, wrists or lower legs and then spreads, often rapidly, to involve the entire body, including the scalp, palms and soles. Early, the rash fades with pressure, but after 1 or 2 days it becomes more purple, papular and frequently petechial. Fever and headache persist; intense myalgia and malaise are frequent complaints. Bizarre central nervous system symptoms, edema of the face, electrocardiographic evidence of myocarditis, renal involvement, peripheral collapse and pneumonitis are the more severe manifestations. There have been reports of thrombocytopenia, hypofibrinogenemia and other clotting defects associated with Rocky Mountain spotted fever. Fatality rates among unvaccinated children before the availability of antibiotics varied from 10 to 40 per cent. It is generally accepted that rickettsial strains of high and low virulence exist throughout the United States. Recovery in uncomplicated cases occurs in the third week, initiated by a fall in temperature and gradual subsidence of symptoms.

The clinical **laboratory findings** are not specific. See page 699 for serologic tests.

Differential Diagnosis. Infectious mononucleosis, rubella, measles, ECHO exanthems, and meningococcemia are diseases frequently considered in patients with Rocky Mountain spotted fever. The spread of rash from distal portions of the extremities to the trunk and face, with involvement of palms and soles, is often the clue that leads to the diagnosis. Season of the year,

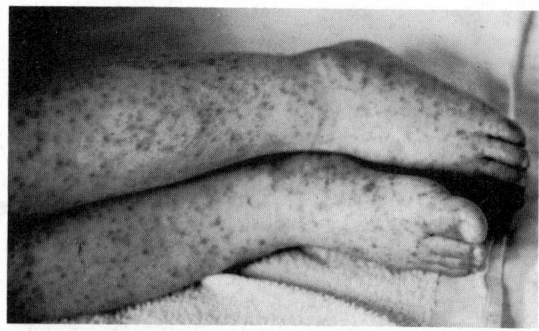

Figure 10-96. Ninth day of rash in Rocky Mountain spotted fever, showing hemorrhagic nature of rash and puffy edema of feet. (Courtesy of William H. Wood, M.D., Cleveland.)

negative blood cultures and normal spinal fluid are additional aids in reaching a correct diagnosis.

Control Measures. The reservoirs and vectors of spotted fever are so numerous and widespread that removal of the source of infection is not feasible. Protection from tick bite is best accomplished by the use of proper wearing apparel plus tick repellents or, optimally, the avoidance during the tick season of areas known to be infested.

Ticks rarely transmit infection until they have fed on the person for several hours; thus careful examination of children who have been playing in the woods and prompt removal of ticks may prevent disease. This is best accomplished by the use of gloves or forceps which will protect the operator from becoming infected by the crushed insect. The use of a hot match head or a coating of petrolatum to provoke the tick to remove his mouth parts is often recommended.

Vaccines are available and should be used by those whose pursuits require unusual exposure to virulent strains of rickettsiae.

Treatment. See page 699.

FIÈVRE BOUTONNEUSE

Fièvre boutonneuse is a relatively benign rickettsial disease, limited almost exclusively to Europeans in the countries surrounding the Mediterranean. The natives in this area are apparently infected early in life and develop long-lasting immunity. *Rickettsia conorii*, the causal agent, is transmitted by the dog tick, *Rhipicephalus sanguineus*. As in rickettsialpox or scrub typhus, a local lesion known as *tâche noire*, or primary eschar, develops, followed by a diffuse, maculopapular rash which later becomes petechial. Severe systemic manifestations are uncommon. The diagnosis is usually made on the basis of the clinical symptoms in an exposed person with a primary skin lesion. Agglutinins to both OX19 and OX2 occur during the second week of the disease and may be used to confirm the diagnosis if the more specific complement fixation test is not available. Treatment with broad-spectrum antibiotics is followed by rapid clinical improvement.

RICKETTSIALPOX

History. In 1946 an epidemic of an unusual febrile disease with varicelliform rash occurred in a New York housing development. The disease was recognized as a new entity caused by a previously unknown rickettsia, *Rickettsia akari*, and transmitted by the mouse mite, *Allodermanyssus sanguineus*. The illness, named rickettsialpox, has continued endemic in New York, and isolated cases have been reported from Boston, Philadelphia and Cleveland. The mite vector has been found in many cities of the United States.

Clinical Manifestations. Rickettsialpox is a mild illness characterized by an initial skin lesion followed by fever, chills, headache and a papulovesicular rash.

The initial lesion, presumed to be the site of the mite bite, has been observed in more than 90 per cent of cases. It may be located anywhere on the body, beginning as a nontender, nonitching, firm, red papule, 0.5 to 2.0 cm. in diameter. A deeply entrenched vesicle develops in the center of the papule and ruptures after several days, leaving a crusted, pigmented lesion or eschar which may persist 3 weeks or longer. Adjacent lymph nodes become enlarged and tender, but do not suppurate.

The initial lesion is followed in 2 to 7 days by fever, headache, chills and sweats. Temperature varies between 102 and 105°F., but the patient remains oriented and does not appear severely ill.

Within 24 to 72 hours after the onset of fever scattered erythematous maculopapules appear over the body, showing no preference for trunk, head or extremity. The lesions enlarge, become more papular and develop vesicles on the summit of each papule. The secondary lesions (rash) resemble the initial lesion except that they are smaller in size and heal, without leaving scars, in 4 to 7 days.

The duration seldom exceeds 7 to 10 days. Complications, sequels and fatalities are rare.

Except for leukopenia with relative lymphocytosis early in the disease, studies of blood, urine or stool show no characteristic changes.

Differential Diagnosis. The rash of rickettsialpox may be confused with that of chickenpox. In the latter the vesicles are superficial, thin, dewdrop lesions which appear in successive crops beginning on the chest. These differ from the deeply seated, randomly distributed firm vesicles of the rickettsial disease. The initial lesion and the presence of chills and fever before the rash may also help in differentiation. Other diseases to be considered include infectious mononucleosis, meningococcemia, Rocky Mountain spotted fever and typhus.

Control Measures. Preventive measures should include the eradication of rodent reservoirs as well as the mite vector. *Rickettsia akari* grows well in the yolk sac of the developing chick embryo, and a vaccine could be prepared if there were substantial need.

Treatment. See page 699.

Q FEVER

History. Q fever, a febrile disease without rash and often associated with an interstitial pneumonia, was originally observed among Australian abattoir workers in 1935. Initially the disease was infrequently diagnosed in this country except among laboratory workers. During World War II, epidemics of "pneumonia of unknown etiology" and "Balkan grippe" among military personnel in the Mediterranean theatre were shown to be Q fever. Since that time the disease has been reported from all parts of the world.

Etiology and Transmission. Q fever occurs naturally in cattle, sheep, goats and many wild animals. The causative agent of Q fever, *Coxiella burnetii*, has been found in many species of ticks, in which it may pass from the adult through ova to progeny.

Experimentally, Q fever has been transmitted by insect vectors through the skin and by inhalation. Careful studies of outbreaks of the disease in human beings have failed to incriminate insect vectors, although this mode of transmission may be important among animals. Person-to-person spread, if it occurs, is rare. Q fever epidemics in Italy during the war remained localized and involved only the inhabitants of specific quarters, a fact which led to the idea that Q fever was a "place infection." Later studies suggest that excreta from infected animals or insects may be a source of infection. In the endemic areas of California, human infections are related to contact with animals which show evidence of *Coxiella burnetii* infection. In northern California, sheep are the probable source of infection; in southern California, the dairy cow. The main route of infection appears to be inhalation of contaminated material from domestic animals or by direct exposure or by contact with wool, hides, hay or other contaminated materials.

Milk may be another source of infection for man. In a study of sporadic cases of Q fever in England, Marmion isolated *Coxiella burnetii* from 10 of the 20 (raw) milk sources used by the patients; *Coxiella burnetii* may survive pasteurization temperatures.

Pathology. See page 698.

Clinical Manifestations. Q fever may be a mild disease diagnosed only in retrospect by serologic survey, but, as commonly recognized, it is a disease of moderate severity with a duration in children of 2 to 3 weeks. The onset is characteristically sudden, but in some instances symptoms may increase slowly in intensity. Malaise, fever, chilliness and generalized weakness appear early, but the most prominent symptom is severe frontal headache, often associated with pain upon movement of the eyes. There is no rash. Complaints referable to the respiratory tract are mild and infrequent. Cough may occur late in the first week of illness with production of small amounts of blood-streaked sputum, and chest pain may be associated with pneumonitis or infrequently with pleural effusion.

Pneumonitis is common; rales may be audible, but the pulmonary involvement is usually established roentgenographically. Pulmonary consolidation is usually patchy and in the peripheries of the lower lobes; hilar involvement is rare. Resolution is slow and may require 3 to 6 weeks.

During the acute phase the temperature may reach 104 to 105°F., but may be remitting with wide daily swings. After 5 to 15 days the temperature gradually returns to normal, and most symptoms disappear. Convalescence may be prolonged for several weeks, but complications are rare. The mortality rate is less than 1 per cent.

Routine hematologic data are not significant. Serologic tests for syphilis may give falsely positive results during the illness.

Control Measures. Complete control of Q fever is not possible because of ignorance of the exact mode of spread. Recognition of the disease in livestock should alert communities to the risk of infection. Stockyard workers and others exposed to infected material might receive the formalinized vaccine, which at present is not generally available. Milk from infected herds must be pasteurized at temperatures sufficient to destroy the rickettsiae. Person-to-person spread of Q fever is not a problem, and special isolation measures are not necessary.

Treatment. See page 699.

ELI GOLD
FREDERICK C. ROBBINS

REFERENCES

Atkin, M. D., Strauss, H. S., and Fisher, G. U.: A Case Report of "Cape Cod" Rocky Mountain Spotted Fever with Multiple Coagulation Disturbances. *Pediatrics*, 36:627, 1965.

Commission on Acute Respiratory Diseases: Epidemics of Q Fever Among Troops Returning from Italy in the Spring of 1945. *Am. J. Hyg.*, 44:88, 1946.

Cooke, J. V.: Rocky Mountain Spotted Fever in Children. *Yale J. Biol. & Med.*, 16:495, 1944.

Greenberg, M., Pellitteri, O., Klein, I. F., and Huebner, R. J.: Rickettsialpox — Newly Recognized Rickettsial Disease; Clinical Observations. *J.A.M.A.*, 133:901, 1947.

Ley, H. L., Jr., and Smadel, J. E.: Antibiotic Therapy of Rickettsial Diseases. *Antibiotics & Chemother.*, 4:792, 1954.

Luoto, L., Casey, M. L., and Pickens, E. G.: Q Fever Studies in Montana. Detection of Asymptomatic Infection Among Residents of Infected Dairy Premises. *Am. J. Epidemiol.*, 81:356, 1965.

Marmion, B. P.: Q Fever; Natural History and Epidemiology of Q Fever in Man. *Tr. Roy. Soc. Trop. Med. & Hyg.*, 48:197, 1954.

Murray, E. S., and others: Brill's Disease; Clinical and Laboratory Diagnosis. *J.A.M.A.*, 142:1059, 1950.

Ormsbee, R. A., Parker, H., and Pickens, E. G.: The Comparative Effectiveness of Aureomycin, Terramycin, Chloramphenicol, Erythromycin and Thiocymetin in Suppressing Experimental Rickettsial Infections in Chick Embryos. *J. Infect. Dis.*, 96:162, 1955.

Pan American Health Organization: Vaccine Against Viral and Rickettsial Diseases of Man. *W.H.O.* No. 147, 1967.

Robbins, F. C., Ragan, C., and Rustigian, R.: Q Fever in Mediterranean Area; Report of Its Occurrence in Allied Troops; Laboratory Outbreak. *Am. J. Hyg.*, 44:64, 1946.

Smadel, J. E., Intracellular Infections. *Bull. New York Acad. Med.*, 39:158, 1963.

Mycotic Infections

ACTINOMYCOSIS

Definition and Etiology. Actinomycosis is a chronic infection, more suppurative than granulomatous, characterized by the formation of abscesses with multiple draining sinuses. The disease is more frequent in adults than in children, but must be considered in chronic infections of the lung and draining sinuses in the jaw, neck or thoracic or abdominal region.

The causative agent, the anaerobic *Actinomyces israeli*, appears in the lesion as small, hyaline-like to yellow "sulfur granules." On microscopic examination the crushed granule is a mass of branched mycelial filaments of approximately the same width as bacteria. The filaments in the periphery of the granule may be clubbed. The organisms must be cultured anaerobically, preferably in thioglycolate broth or brain-heart infusion agar. They can often be recovered from the mouth, tonsils and pyorrheal pus of patients without actinomycosis, suggesting an endogenous source of infection. The disease is not contagious.

Pathology. The lesions are those of a chronic granulomatous infection with a great tendency to suppuration with abscess formation, fibrosis, the formation of scars and multiple draining sinuses. The presence of typical "sulfur granules" is characteistic but not pathognomonic.

Clinical Forms. *Cervicofacial actinomycosis* (57 per cent of cases). The fungus enters through a carious tooth or the mucous membrane of the mouth or pharynx and produces a gradually enlarging hard or "woody" swelling in the jaw or neck. The tense overlying skin is often reddish or purple. The swelling later softens and drains to the outside through multiple sinuses, but can penetrate deeper to involve the bone and meninges. "Sulfur granules" may be found in the pus. Pain is minimal, and the general health is not greatly affected.

Abdominal actinomycosis (22 per cent of cases). Infection may appear several months after an appendectomy as a hard, irregular mass in the ileocecal region. This mass tends to soften and drain to the outside. Frequently, however, the infection extends through the diaphragm, after involving the liver and other abdominal organs, to produce thoracic lesions. With a severe infection there are chills, fever, night sweats and loss of weight.

Thoracic actinomycosis (15 per cent of cases). The clinical pattern is that of a chronic pulmonary infection with cough, sputum, fever, dyspnea, hemoptysis and loss of weight. Roentgenograms generally reveal bilateral involvement, usually in the lower lobes. Extension to the pleura causes accumulation of pleural fluid and involvement of the ribs and subcutaneous tissues with multiple sinus formation.

Diagnosis. The diagnosis requires finding the organisms in the pus or biopsy material from the sinus walls. A drop of pus is crushed under a coverglass and examined under the low power of the microscope for the typical "sulfur granules." The disease closely simulates tuberculosis, but other chronic bacterial and fungus diseases and amebic hepatic abscess must be considered.

Prognosis. This varies; widespread infection may be fatal.

Prevention and Treatment. Removal of chronically infected tonsils and treatment of pyorrhea may eliminate possible sources of infection. Penicillin is the drug of choice. Massive doses (1 to 20 million units per day intravenously for 6 to 8 weeks) may be necessary in severe infections. Penicillin can be used alone or preferably in combination with sulfadiazine. Potassium iodide may be useful in chronic actinomycosis and may be given with the more specific drugs for several months after the patient is apparently well. Surgical excision and drainage may be necessary. The broad-spectrum antibiotics (tetracyclines, chloramphenicol and erythromycin) may be used if the patient is sensitive to penicillin.

NORTH AMERICAN BLASTOMYCOSIS

Definition and Etiology. North American blastomycosis (Gilchrist's disease) is an infection with *Blastomyces dermatitidis* characterized by chronic granulomatous lesions and microabscess formation in any part of the body, but with a predilection for lungs, skin and bone. This disease is confined almost solely to the North American continent and especially to the southeastern and Mississippi Valley states. Evidence suggests that the usual portal of entry is the lungs and that both skin and bone lesions are metastatic.

The source of the infection is unknown. Blastomyces have been found in domestic animals (dog and horse), but not living free in nature (soil and wood). In tissues and in pus the fungus appears as a thick-walled, double-contoured, single-budding organism averaging 8 to 12 microns in diameter. On Sabouraud's medium at room temperature it grows slowly as a mold composed of branching filaments and small spores. The budding yeastlike forms are obtained on blood agar incubated at 37°C. Small forms of the organism must be distinguished by cultural means from Histoplasma and Monilia. The disease is not spread from man to man.

Pathology. The organism incites an inflammatory reaction which in the acute phase and in the advancing portions of the lesion is characterized by the formation of minute (micro-) abscesses. In the older portions of the lesion the reaction is essentially chronic and granulomatous, resem-

cosis, occurring in children otherwise in good health, has been reported from Indonesia and Africa. The disease begins as a painless subcutaneous nodule which gradually increases, sometimes to massive proportions. After several months to years of growth, spontaneous healing may occur. Histologically, the lesion resembles an eosinophilic granuloma containing the nonseptate hyphae of Basidiobolus species.

Diagnosis. The appearance of acute inflammation, infarction or necrosis in the lungs, gastrointestinal tract, nasopharynx, orbits or intracranial cavity in a patient debilitated by a chronic disease should suggest this serious complication. Bloody nasal discharge and a gray-black, ischemic necrotic lesion resembling dried blood are characteristic. The diagnosis depends upon recognition of the fungus in specimens of tissue or body fluid.

Prevention and Treatment. Prevention and treatment require scrupulous care of the underlying, predisposing debilitating illness. Amphotericin B is the drug of choice (see p. 709). Additional therapy includes surgical debridement or excision where possible, administration of large doses of iodides, desensitization with vaccine made from the fungus and antimicrobial treatment of any intercurrent bacterial infection.

NOCARDIOSIS

Definition and Etiology. Nocardiosis is a noncontagious, subacute or chronic suppurative disease primarily of the lungs, but with a tendency to hematogenous dissemination. The causative organisms belong to the same family as does Actinomyces. They are gram-positive with branching filaments, but, in contrast to Actinomyces, may be partially or strongly acid-fast, can be grown aerobically on simple media at room temperature and are found living free in nature (soil). Of the 9 recognized species, N. asteroides is the commonest cause of systemic infection.

Pathology. The basic histologic lesion is a focal area of necrosis surrounded by a variable cellular infiltrate. These abscesses are characteristically not encapsulated, but may show secondary fibrosis, or they may caseate and cavitate. Pulmonary infection (probably produced by inhalation of contaminated dust) begins as an acute pneumonitis which may become chronic. The lesions may extend locally and spread hematogenously to the subcutaneous tissues and to other organs, especially the brain. Differentiation from tuberculosis may be extremely difficult because of the histology, the acid-fastness of the organisms and their ready fragmentation into bacillary forms.

Clinical Forms. Aside from the localized primary cutaneous and subcutaneous infections which are uncommon in the United States, the clinical picture of nocardiosis is that of a chronic suppurative pulmonary disease, usually in persons with lowered resistance. Local and metastatic spread may occur. Twelve per cent of these cases have occurred in children—as early as 4 weeks of age. Common manifestations are cough, fever, anorexia, weight loss, malaise, night sweats, fatigue, dyspnea, chest pain and leukocytosis up to 50,000 cells per mm.[3] Local extension may result in empyema. A characteristic sequence is pulmonary disease followed by pustular eruption of the skin. There is a pronounced tendency to chronicity with remissions and exacerbations over many years. Secondary intracranial involvement results in cerebral abscess or meningitis. When the organisms, particularly Nocardia madurae, gain entrance through abrasions in the feet, they produce a burrowing infection of the subcutaneous tissues and bone, mycetoma pedis.

Diagnosis. Roentgenograms of the lungs usually reveal small infiltrative lesions or large lobular areas of consolidation, with the lower lobes of the lungs involved most often. Suppuration and cavitation may occur. The important features are chronicity with gradual progression, multiple lesions, refractoriness to antibiotic therapy and inability to establish the diagnosis by routine methods.

Differentiation must be made from actinomycosis by cultural means and by examination of the pus ("sulfur granules" are seldom present in N. asteroides infections). This is important, since therapy is different in the 2 conditions. Owing to the clinical resemblance to tuberculosis and the acid-fastness of the organisms, the differentiation is extremely difficult; it has been estimated that nocardiosis accounts for 1 to 5 per cent of patients in tuberculosis hospitals. When the lesion metastasizes to other organs, the resemblance to staphylococcal pyemia is striking. The chronic pulmonary disease has also been mistaken for cystic fibrosis. Cutaneous involvement may mimic tuberculosis, infections with atypical mycobacteria or cat-scratch disease.

Prognosis and Treatment. The overall mortality rate is probably over 50 per cent in untreated cases. Lesions respond well to symptomatic care and sulfonamide therapy in their early stage. Surgical excision may be necessary. The organisms are partially susceptible to the broad-spectrum antibiotics and streptomycin but resistant to penicillin.

SPOROTRICHOSIS

Etiology. Sporotrichosis is caused by Sporotrichum schenckii, a fungus which most frequently infects skin and subcutaneous tissues, producing a series of nodules and ulcerations. The fungus also may infect mucous membranes, lungs and other organs. It has been isolated from soil, plants and timber. Man is probably inoculated through abrasions in the skin.

Pathology. Section of a nodule usually shows

granulation tissue with epithelioid cells and giant cells surrounding a necrotic area, a lesion similar to that produced by tuberculosis or by other fungus infections.

Clinical Manifestations. The lesion begins usually in the skin or in the subcutaneous tissue as a small, hard nodule not attached to the skin. This nodule later adheres to the overlying skin, which becomes darker and finally ulcerates, discharging a small amount of purulent material. This primary "chancre" may persist for months and is usually followed by a chain of nodules along the course of the lymphatic drainage. These nodules may subsequently become attached to the skin and ulcerate. The patient is afebrile, and the general health is not affected. Sporotrichotic infections of the mucous membranes, lungs, bones and other organs occur, but are rare except for bone and joint infections, which comprise 17 per cent of total infections.

Diagnosis. The disease may resemble tuberculosis, syphilis or infections by other fungi. The local lesions suggest tularemia, but the general symptoms are not those of an acute bacterial infection. Diagnosis depends upon culturing the fungus from the chancre or subcutaneous nodule.

The fungi occur in the lesions as intracellular, small "cigar-shaped" bodies, 3 to 4 microns in length, and are demonstrated with difficulty. Direct smears cannot be depended upon as a diagnostic procedure. On Sabouraud's medium the fungus grows as a white or black mold identified as clusters of small, delicate, pear-shaped spores borne on short branches of narrow mycelial filaments.

Prognosis. Though the disease may persist for many months, the prognosis is good under adequate therapy.

Treatment. Oral administration of potassium iodide in increasing amounts up to tolerance is almost specific. The medication should be continued for at least a month after healing has occurred. Abscesses may be aspirated, but incision and curettage should be avoided. For patients who are sensitive to iodides or have systemic lesions, amphotericin B may be helpful.

ASPERGILLOSIS

Etiology. Aspergillosis is caused by various species (especially *Aspergillus fumigatus*) of the widely distributed, usually nonpathogenic genus Aspergillus. The organism most frequently causes granulomatous inflammatory lesions of the skin (external ear) and vagina, and may invade the nasal sinuses, orbit, bones, meninges and lungs. In the lungs the organism may grow in large masses ("fungus balls") in pulmonary cavities without eliciting much reaction or may invade the pulmonary parenchyma, causing necrosis and cavitation. Rarely dissemination occurs by the hematogenous route.

Pathology. Little reaction is seen to the "fungus ball." Invasion of the pulmonary parenchyma or blood vessels results in obstruction, thrombosis and extensive necrosis.

Clinical Manifestations. Infection with Aspergillus occurs only in persons with pulmonary lesions or in those who have an immunologic deficiency or are receiving prolonged treatment with corticosteroids, antibiotics or cancer chemotherapy. There are several clinical varieties.

Pulmonary aspergilloma. The fungus grows in a bronchiectatic, tuberculous or histoplasmosis cavity and forms masses of matted mycelia. The main symptoms relate to the underlying disease rather than to the fungus.

Pulmonary granulomatous aspergillosis. In patients debilitated by neoplasm, tuberculosis, systemic mycosis, or in whom immunity has been depressed by long corticosteroid therapy, intensive antibiotic, antineoplastic or anti-immune agents, infection may spread from the bronchus into the parenchyma, causing fever, cough, severe malaise, and hemoptysis.

Allergic type of migrating pneumonitis with or without eosinophilia. Acute invasive pulmonary aspergillosis. Massive inhalation of the spores has resulted in acute infections in children presumed to be immunologically deficient.

Differential Diagnosis. Aspergillosis, as well as other "opportunistic" fungus diseases, should be suspected in severely debilitated patients or in those whose immune responses have been suppressed for reasons mentioned above. The roentgenogram of the "fungus ball" in a pulmonary cavity is characteristic. Cultures may be misleading, since the organisms are widespread in nature and may be present as contaminants in routine cultures.

Treatment. Treatment must be directed against the underlying disease. Surgical therapy is necessary for localized aspergillomas. For patients with the invasive type of disease, amphotericin B (see below), sulfonamides and potassium iodide may be tried; none is particularly effective.

THERAPY WITH AMPHOTERICIN B*

Amphotericin B (Fungizone—Squibb) is a polyene antifungal antibiotic produced by a strain of

---

*X-5079C, a water-soluble polypeptide antibiotic derived from a streptomyces, is currently under investigation for the treatment of mycotic infections. Preliminary trials, in dosages of 3 to 5 mg. per kg. every 6 hours intramuscularly or subcutaneously for a week to 2 months, have shown it to be effective in the treatment of histoplasmosis, North American blastomycosis, and sporotrichosis. The drug is probably not fungicidal, and relapses are frequent in those initially responding to therapy (50 per cent). Little or no effect has been observed in the treatment of coccidioidomycosis, cryptococcosis or candidiasis. Except for hepatotoxicity, the drug has been well tolerated. All patients have shown delayed excretion of sulfobromophthalein and usually have increased serum concentrations of conjugated bilirubin. The changes have been reversible and have disappeared within 1 to 9 days after discontinuation of therapy. Caution is indicated in patients with liver disease.

streptomyces. It is insoluble in water, but may be dispersed in a colloidal suspension for intravenous use with desoxycholate and phosphate buffers. The colloidal suspension may be diluted with 5 per cent glucose, but not with salt solutions or any other diluents which may cause precipitation of the drug. The drug is poorly absorbed from the gastrointestinal tract, and subcutaneous or intramuscular injections are inefficient. The drug must be given intravenously. Little of it penetrates the cerebral spinal fluid. The renal threshold is high, and the drug is excreted very slowly. For this reason the drug is administered once daily or every other day. Solutions must be protected against prolonged exposure to light and should be discarded after 24 hours.

Method of Administration. The drug is used intravenously in a concentration of 0.1 mg. per ml. of 5 per cent dextrose solution. Therapy is usually started with a dose of 0.25 mg. per kg. and is increased *very gradually*, if tolerated, to a dose of approximately 1 mg. per kg. per day. The maximum dose should not exceed 1.5 mg. per kg. Depending upon tolerance, the drug is given on consecutive or alternate days. The infusion should take at least 6 hours in order to avoid serious toxic reactions. It is advisable to swirl the infusion bottle gently every 15 minutes in order to be certain that the drug is in proper colloidal suspension and that no precipitation whatsoever has occurred. Rapid administration or the use of high concentrations of the drug may lead to convulsions, ventricular fibrillations and cardiac arrest.

The duration of therapy for each infection depends upon its nature, severity and duration. Severe infections will require 1 to 3 months of therapy. The total dose ranges (for adults) from 2 to 4 gm. Relapses may occur and require additional courses of therapy.

In fungal meningitis amphotericin may be administered intrathecally on alternate days or twice weekly, beginning with 0.1 mg. dissolved in 2 to 3 cc. of spinal fluid or distilled water and increasing the dose to a maximum of 0.5 to 0.7 mg. if tolerated. Larger amounts may cause urinary retention, hyperpyrexia, arachnoiditis, and transverse myelitis which may be reversible, if the drug is discontinued. Transient paresthesias usually occur and are less extensive if the intraspinal administration is given while the patient is in the sitting position.

The drug may also be given topically as in the eye (1 to 5 mg.), intra-articularly (up to 25 mg.), intrathoracically (up to 3 mg.), into cutaneous lesions (up to 25 mg. with 1 to 2 per cent procaine every other day) or as an aerosol inhalant spray (5 mg. every 6 hours).

Toxicity. The reactions to intravenous administration of amphotericin are legion. Fortunately they seem to be less serious in children and tend to decrease during a prolonged course of therapy. Anxiety, anorexia, chills, fever and malaise are common and may be partly controlled by the prior administration (30 minutes) of aspirin, antihistaminics or chlorpromazine. Headaches, nausea, vomiting, abdominal pain and chest pains require a diminution in the total daily dose, particularly if these symptoms increase in severity or duration. With increasing doses, renal function is affected and the blood urea nitrogen level tends to rise. If the level is increased (over 20 mg. per 100 ml.; higher levels may be permissible if the patient is carefully watched), the drug should be discontinued until the level returns toward normal. The drug may then be given either in diminished doses or preferably every other day. Fortunately the effect on the kidneys seems to be temporary in most instances and disappears on discontinuation of the drug. Rarer toxic effects include albuminuria and other renal difficulties, anemia, thrombocytopenia, hypokalemia causing muscular weakness, duodenal ulcerations and hemorrhagic gastroenteritis. Observation should be made to detect these complications at an early stage, when they usually are reversible. Thrombophlebitis may occur, unfortunately probably more commonly in children, owing to their small veins, and cause technical difficulties in prolonged courses of therapy. Simultaneous administration of 20 to 100 mg. of soluble hydrocortisone in the intravenous infusion has been advocated to prevent toxicity, particularly from intrathecal injections.

Action and Uses. Amphotericin B is probably fungistatic rather than fungicidal, but has a broad spectrum of action, including *Coccidioides immitis, Histoplasma capsulatum, Cryptococcus neoformans,* Phycomyces species, Blastomyces species, Candida, Nocardia and Sporotrichum among others. There is no effect on bacteria or actinomyces.

In view of the many toxic effects of the drug and the difficulty of administration, amphotericin B should be reserved for the more serious infections and particularly for those which do not respond to other forms of therapy. It is the drug of choice in blastomycosis, cryptococcosis, disseminated coccidioidomycosis, chronic histoplasmosis and systemic moniliasis.

Treatment failures may be due to premature discontinuation of the drug, far advanced disease, insufficient amount of drug, death from associated diseases (e.g. leukemia), relapses (with steroid treatment, and metabolic disturbances), and disease due to resistant organisms.

JEROME S. HARRIS

REFERENCES

General

Conant, N. F., Smith, D. T., Baker, R. D., Callaway, J. L., and Martin, D. S.: *Manual of Clinical Mycology.* 2nd ed. Philadelphia, W. B. Saunders Company, 1954.

Fetter, B. F., Klintworth, G. K., and Hendry, W. S.: *Mycoses of the Central Nervous System.* Baltimore, Williams & Wilkins Company, 1967.

Haley, L. D.: *Diagnostic Medical Mycology.* New York, Appleton-Century-Crofts, 1964.

International Symposium on Opportunistic Fungus Infections. *Lab. Invest.,* 11:1017, 1962.

Wilson, J. W., and Plunkett, O. A.: *The Fungous Diseases of Man.* Berkeley and Los Angeles, University of California Press, 1965.

Actinomycosis

Peabody, J. W., Jr., and Seabury, J. H.: Actinomycosis and Nocardiosis–A Review of Basic Differences in Therapy. *Am. J. Med.,* 28:99, 1960.

Blastomycosis

Harrell, E. R., and Curtis, A. C.: North American Blastomycosis. *Am. J. Med.,* 27:750, 1959.

Smith, J. G., Jr., Harris, J. S., Conant, N. F., and Smith, D. T.: An Epidemic of North American Blastomycosis. *J.A.M.A.,* 158:641, 1955.

Cryptococcosis

Littman, M. L.: Cryptococcosis (Torulosis)–Current Concepts and Therapy. *Am. J. Med.,* 27:976, 1959.

Siewers, C. M. F., and Cramblett, H. G.: Cryptococcosis (Torulosis) in Children. *Pediatrics,* 34:393, 1964.

Phycomycosis (Mucormycosis)

Harris, J. S.: Mucormycosis. Report of Case. *Pediatrics,* 16:857, 1955.

Landau, J. W., and Newcomer, V. D.: Acute Cerebral Phycomycosis (Mucormycosis). *J. Pediat.,* 61:363, 1962.

Nocardiosis

Ballenger, C. N., Jr., and Goldring, D.: Nocardiosis in Childhood. *J. Pediat.,* 50:145, 1957.

Gundersen, G. A., and Nice, C. M., Jr.: Nocardiosis. A Case Report and Brief Review of the Literature. *Radiology,* 68:31, 1957.

Sporotrichosis

D'Alessio, D. J., and others: An Outbreak of Sporotrichosis in Vermont Associated with Sphagnum Moss as the Source of Infection. *New England J. Med.,* 272:1054, 1965.

Mikkelsen, W. M., Brandt, R. L., and Harrell, E. R.: Sporotrichosis. A Report of 12 Cases, Including Two with Skeletal Involvement. *Ann. Int. Med.,* 47:435, 1957.

Aspergillosis

Blattner, R. J.: Pulmonary Aspergillosis in Children. *J. Pediat.,* 70:139, 1967.

Heffernan, A. G., and Asper, S. P., Jr.: Insidious Fungal Disease. A Clinicopathological Study of Secondary Aspergillosis. *Bull. Johns Hopkins Hosp.,* 118:10, 1966.

Khoo, T. K., Sugair, K., and Leong, T. K.: Disseminated Aspergillosis. Case Report and Review of the World Literature. *Am. J. Clin. Path.,* 45:697, 1966.

Therapy

Butler, W. T.: Pharmacology, Toxicity, and Therapeutic Usefulness of Amphotericin B. *J.A.M.A.,* 195:371, 1966.

Utz, J. P.: Antimicrobial Therapy in Systemic Fungal Infections. *Am. J. Med.,* 39:826, 1965.

Utz, J. P., Andriole, V. T., and Emmons, C. W.: Chemotherapeutic Activity of X-5079C in Systemic Mycoses of Man. *Am. Rev. Resp. Dis.,* 84:514, 1961.

Witorsch, P., and others: The Polypeptide Antifungal Agent (X-5079C): Further Studies in Thirty-Nine Patients. *Am. Rev. Resp. Dis.,* 93:876, 1966.

HISTOPLASMOSIS

Histoplasmosis is an acute, subacute or chronic infectious disease caused by the fungus *Histoplasma capsulatum.* Once thought to be invariably fatal, it is now recognized as a relatively common benign (often clinically inapparent) or only moderately severe disease. At least 30 per cent of the observed cases of histoplasmosis have occurred in children.

Etiology. *Histoplasma capsulatum* has 2 distinct growth phases. When cultivated on artificial media at room temperature, it produces a white, cottony, aerial, mycelial growth and a brownish-yellow subsurface growth. In tissues and when first cultivated on enriched media at 37°C., it grows in a yeast cell phase, having a relatively thick, translucent capsule. It can be identified in the mycelial culture by the tuberculate chlamydospores. The fungus has been isolated from dogs, mice, rats and horses, and from soil, principally adjacent to chicken houses and pigeon lofts, but also in damp places, along streams and in caves. There is no evidence that the disease is transmitted from man to man or from animal to man.

Pathogenesis and Pathology. The fungus apparently enters the body through the skin or through the mucous membrane of the mouth, nasopharynx, respiratory tract or intestinal mucosa, producing an ulcerative lesion.

The granulomatous lesions of histoplasmosis may simulate those of tuberculosis, and the initial lesion, as, for example, in the pulmonary parenchyma with the subsequent involvement of the regional lymph nodes, simulates the primary complex of this disease. The yeast form of the fungus proliferates in the macrophages, initiating new cycles. In contradistinction to tuberculosis, this reaction produces relatively little inflammation in the adjacent tissues. Foci tend to become surrounded with giant cells and macrophages and to progress to central caseous necrosis. Calcium is often deposited in the healing lesion.

In infants and in debilitated older persons there is a tendency toward hematogenous dissemination, and the disease may manifest itself as a generalized process involving bone marrow, lung, liver, spleen and lymph nodes.

As in tuberculosis, the spread of the organism varies with the tissue resistance of the host, the size of the inoculum and the virulence of the strain. Hypersensitivity similar to that in tuberculosis occurs. Histoplasmin reactivity is established about 3 to 6 weeks after the primary inoculation.

Clinical Manifestations. Histoplasmosis may be manifest as a mild, moderately severe or severe infection, but most often it is clinically inapparent. In the severe form there is widespread infection, which may affect almost any of the tissues of the body. The mild and clinically inapparent infections are most often located in the thorax.

Severe form. The progressive form of the disease, which is more likely to occur in infants and young children or in debilitated adults, is generally recognized only after it has reached a moderately advanced stage, when the clinical pattern may be suggestive of leukemia. The temperature is irregularly elevated from 101 to 103°F. The signs and symptoms vary considerably; there may be a mild gastrointestinal disturbance

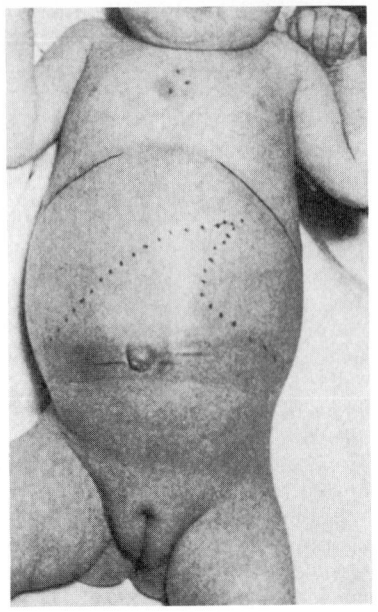

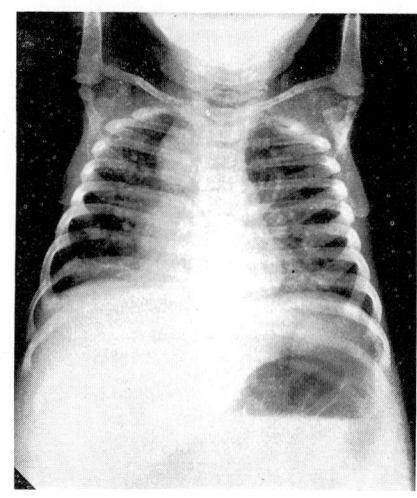

A   B

Figure 10-97. Histoplasmosis in an infant aged 5½ months, with pyrexia, anemia, hepatosplenomegaly and leukopenia. *A*, Note site of sternal puncture; yeast cells of *H. capsulatum* were found in smears and cultures of the sternal marrow. *B*, Chest roentgenogram shows diffuse pneumonitis and a mediastinal mass. Diagnosis confirmed by autopsy. (Hild: *Am. J. Dis. Child.*, Vol. 63.)

often with diarrhea, weight loss, malaise, irritability, pallor, indefinite joint and muscle pains or abdominal enlargement. Pneumonitis is common. The roentgenogram of the chest may reveal scattered parenchymal lesions or enlarged mediastinal nodes, which on occasion are responsible for localized obstructive emphysema. In most cases there is enlargement of spleen and liver. Purpura, ecchymoses and melena may be present in the terminal stages. Peripheral lymphadenopathy of a severe degree is uncommon in children. Meningitis with cerebrospinal fluid changes similar to those of tuberculous meningitis has been observed. In addition, there is a wide variety of manifestations which occur with variable frequency and depend on localization of the histoplasma infection as well as secondary ones; these include ulcerative lesions of the eyes, skin and mucous membranes, ulcerative colitis, adrenal insufficiency, pericarditis, myocarditis and endocarditis and lytic lesions of long bones.

Mild and moderately severe forms. Between 1930 and 1940 it became evident that a large number of persons living in the central and southern United States, especially in the Mississippi River Valley and along the western Appalachian slope, had what appeared to be calcified tuberculous lesions in the tracheobronchial lymph nodes and in the lungs, with a negative reaction to tuberculin. Subsequently it was discovered that most of these persons had a positive skin reaction to histoplasmin. It now seems apparent that they were infected with *H. capsulatum* and in most instances had not been aware of any acute illness.

Thus it appears that histoplasmosis, like tuberculosis and coccidioidomycosis, is a widespread infection with common benign and rare severe forms. It sensitizes the human host to its antigen, and its lesions in the benign form heal by calcification. Like coccidioidomycosis, it has a distinct geographic distribution. Noncalcified single and multiple focal lesions have been demonstrated in the lungs, with associated involvement of the hilar lymph nodes, which subsequently calcify. In neither stage are these lesions distinguishable from those of tuberculosis (Figs. 10-98, 10-99). When children with such lesions have positive skin reactions to histoplasmin and negative ones to tuberculin, it is assumed that they have active (noncalcified) or healed (calcified) histoplasmosis.

In a disease in which severe fatal forms and asymptomatic benign ones are recognized it would seem reasonable that there would be intermediate forms. *Histoplasma capsulatum* has been isolated from children with splenomegaly, ulcerations of the skin or mucous membranes and pulmonary infiltrations, who have recovered. These children have skin sensitivity to histoplasmin and complement-fixing antibodies.

Laboratory Diagnosis. Changes in the blood usually include a progressive hypochromic anemia and a leukopenia with a relative lymphocytosis. There may be pancytopenia, suggestive of an aleukemic phase of leukemia; the platelets, however, are usually not reduced until late in the course of the disease.

On occasion the parasites can be demonstrated in the white blood cells in the peripheral blood or in bone marrow. The yeast phase of the fungus as

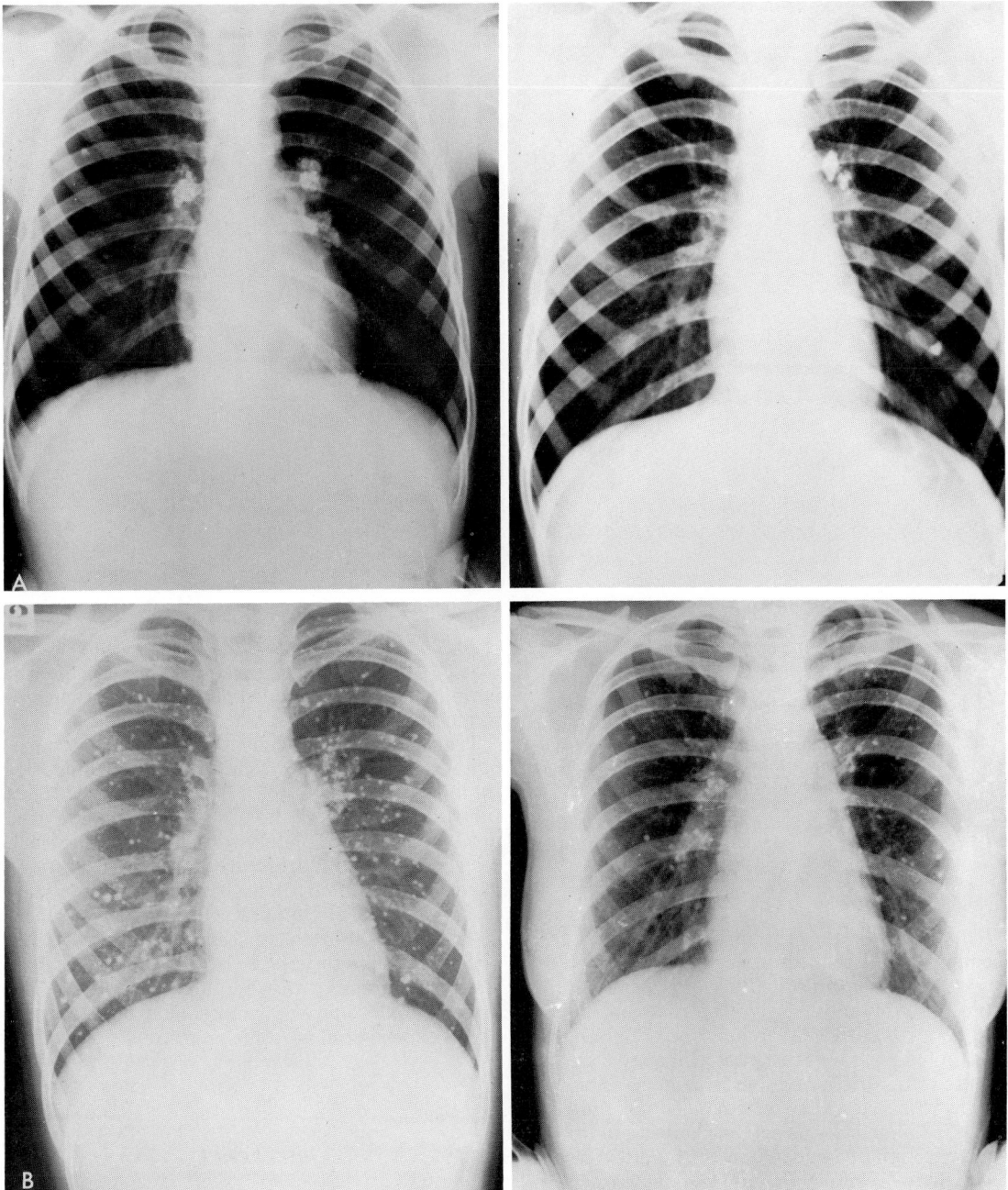

Figure 10-98. Examples of pulmonary and mediastinal calcifications in histoplasmin-positive and tuberculin-negative patients. *A,* Single pulmonary and mediastinal calcified masses strikingly similar to so-called healed pulmonary tuberculous complex. *B,* Multiple parenchymal calcifications suggestive of healed miliary tuberculosis.

it occurs in the cells of the body appears as a small (1 to 5 microns), encapsulated oval body in the large mononuclear cells. Thick-drop preparations or smears of the peripheral blood and bone marrow should be stained with Wright's or Giemsa's stain. Biopsy material from lymph nodes or from the liver or spleen, as well as bone marrow, sputum or material swabbed from an ulcerative lesion, can also be smeared and stained by one of these methods and cultured.

Technique of culture. The technique to be followed varies somewhat with the material. Biopsy specimens are ground to a thin paste, using a minimal amount of sterile saline solution. Swabs from infected areas are placed in test tubes containing 1 to 2 ml. of sterile saline solution. Blood is mixed with heparin, rather than citrate, as an anticoagulant, and is centrifuged at sufficiently high speed to allow separation of the white cells, which are pipetted off and placed in a test tube containing 1 to 2 ml. of sterile saline solution. After 1 hour, and again after 24 to 48 hours of incubation, the material is streaked heavily in each of 2 screw-cap bottles (25 by 50 mm.) containing slants of peptone or meat extract agar to which has been added 50 units per ml. of penicillin and 0.4 mg. per ml. of streptomycin and plasma or

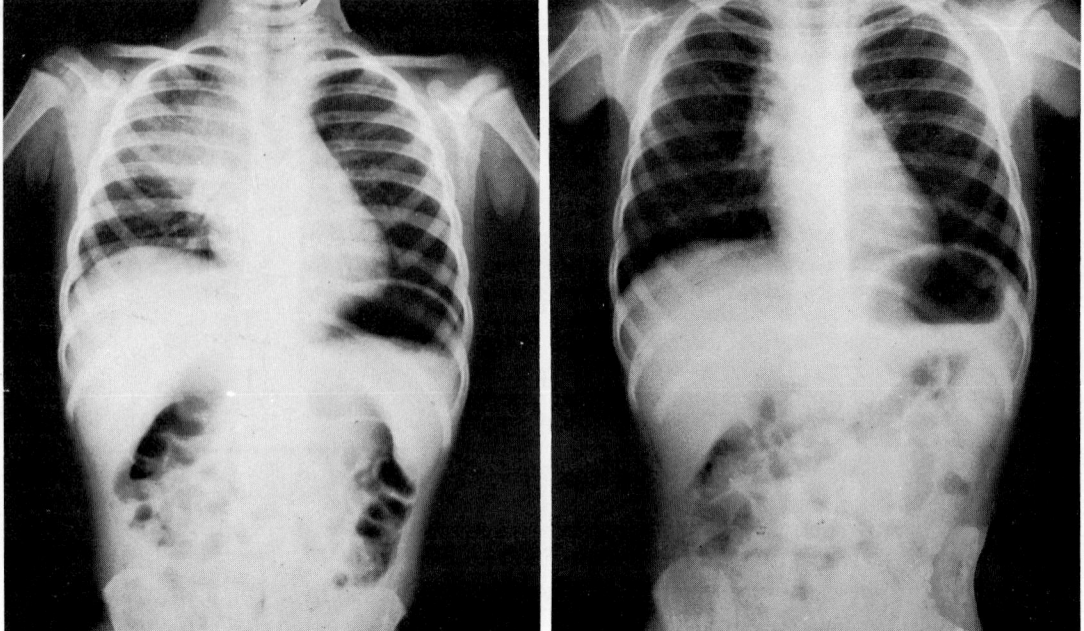

Figure 10-99. Primary histoplasmosis with resolution during sulfonamide therapy over a period of 7 months.

blood serum to a concentration of 5 per cent. The use of bottles instead of Petri dishes or plates decreases the chances of air contamination by fungi and permits small amounts of material to be studied. The bottles must be sealed; one bottle is incubated at 37°C., the other at room temperature. The cultures should be examined at intervals of 3 to 4 days and should not be considered negative until after an observation period of 4 weeks. Positive cultures which have been kept at 37°C. will frequently have colonies of yeast cells rather than of mycelium. At room temperature *H. capsulatum* grows only in the mycelial phase, producing the characteristic tuberculate chlamydospores. The older the mycelial culture, the more likely are chlamydospores apt to be present.

Histoplasmin test. The histoplasmin skin test resembles the tuberculin test. The testing material, a filtrate of a broth culture of *H. capsulatum*, is injected intracutaneously. The reaction is read at 48 hours; a positive reaction consists of an area of erythema with induration of at least 0.5 cm. in diameter. A positive reaction is evidence of sensitization to *H. capsulatum*, but does not indicate whether the infection is active. Conversion from a negative to a positive reaction within a few weeks or a positive reaction in infants is suggestive of an active infection. Persons with progressive disseminated histoplasmosis frequently fail to react to histoplasmin.

Serologic tests are useful to establish the presence of progressive infection.

Differential Diagnosis. Histoplasmosis may simulate a number of clinical conditions in addition to tuberculosis and coccidioidomycosis. The presence of progressive anemia, leukopenia and hepatosplenomegaly requires differentiation from leukemia, the lipid storage diseases, Banti's syndrome, malaria and brucellosis. Ulceration of the skin or mucous membranes must be differentiated from actinomycosis, leishmaniasis and toxoplasmosis; irrespective of lymph node enlarge-

ment, Hodgkin's disease and other malignant lymphomas must be ruled out, as must other systemic mycotic diseases.

Treatment. No chemotherapeutic or antibiotic agent has been found which satisfactorily inhibits the growth of *H. capsulatum* without injuring the tissue of the host. The commonly used antibiotics are completely without effect, and some may facilitate growth of the fungus. In the author's experience sulfonamides (triple sulfonamides) in doses sufficient to obtain blood levels of 15 to 20 mg. per 100 ml. have seemed to offer the most benefit. Amphotericin B may be used for the severe progressive disseminated infections. The drug is toxic, however, and should be used only by an experienced person (see p. 709).

Amos Christie

REFERENCE

Schwarz, J., and Baum, G. L.: The History of Histoplasmosis, 1906 to 1956. *New England J. Med.*, 256:253, 1957.

COCCIDIOIDOMYCOSIS
(San Joaquin Fever; Valley Fever; Desert Rheumatism; Coccidioidal Granuloma)

Etiology. Coccidioidomycosis is an infection caused by the fungus *Coccidioides immitis*. The minute spores of its so-called saprophytic phase are inhaled or, rarely, enter through an abrasion. They round up into spherules which develop endospores within doubly refractile walls, the characteristic sporangium of the so-called parasitic phase. These spherules do not spread from person to person or from animal to man; hence the infection is not contagious. The mycelial form frequently occurs in pulmonary cavities, but no cases of cross infection have been discovered. As they occur naturally, however, and on surface cultures, the arthrospores (chlamydospores) of the "saprophytic phase" are highly infectious. Although isolation is unnecessary, precautions should be taken with dressings and casts over open lesions lest the mycelial arthrospores develop as they do on surface cultures. Within the arid endemic areas of California's San Joaquin Valley, in scattered regions in southern California, in central and southern Arizona and even in western and southern Texas, from three quarters to nine tenths of long-time residents have been infected along with cattle, sheep, dogs and wild rodents. Infection apparently confers a permanent immunity. Therefore, where the population is stable, it is a childhood infection.

Clinical Forms. The human infection must be considered under two broad headings: (1) a benign, self-limited primary infection; and (2) a rare, disseminating, generally fatal disease.

Primary coccidioidomycosis. The incubation period varies from 1 to 3 weeks, with an average of 10 to 16 days. In 60 per cent of infected persons there are no clinical manifestations. Symptoms are influenzal in type, and the onset may be insidious, or abrupt with malaise, chills and fever. Night sweats and anorexia are common, and on occasion there is a persistent dry cough with which there may be a painful throat. There may be headache, backache and chest pain, which may vary from a mere sense of constriction to excruciating pleurisy.

There may be a generalized, fine, macular erythema within the first day or two. The most frequent dermatologic manifestation is erythema nodosum with or without erythema multiforme. These lesions develop at the time sensitivity to coccidioidin is maximal, 3 to 21 days after onset of symptoms. Skin lesions may occur, however, in persons otherwise asymptomatic. Other allergic manifestations, arthritis and phlyctenular conjunctivitis may occur concomitantly.

Physical examination of the chest rarely discloses positive findings, even though roentgenography reveals extensive consolidation. Infrequently dullness, a friction rub or fine rales may be detected. Pleural effusions occur at times and may be so massive as to embarrass respiration. Like tuberculous pleural effusions, they may develop without preceding respiratory symptoms. Infrequently a cavity may develop in an area of pulmonary consolidation; there are usually no symptoms related to it, and the diagnosis is made from the roentgenogram. Occasionally, however, there is hemoptysis which, although it may recur and be alarming, is seldom so severe as to impair health. Dissemination of the fungus from these cavities resulting in lesions in other areas is extremely rare. The infection appears to be localized as well in persons with cavities as in those without them. Pulmonary residuals sometimes persist, but are not harmful. They pose problems of differentiation from tuberculosis.

Disseminated or progressive coccidioidomycosis (coccidioidal granuloma). Certain persons seem to lack ability to localize the coccidioidal infection. Dissemination, which is rare and occurs mainly in males, especially in those of the dark-skinned races, usually follows the initial illness within 6 months, often without any interlude. The closest analogy is to progressive primary tuberculosis. Meningitis is the most serious of the disseminated lesions, being clinically similar to tuberculous meningitis. In white persons it is not unusual for meningitis to be the only extrapulmonary lesion. Papillomatous skin lesions and cold abscesses, both subcutaneous and osseous, occur most frequently in the dark-skinned races. Miliary dissemination and peritonitis are clinically and, except by demonstration of the causative agent, pathologically indistinguishable from tuberculosis. The case fatality rate of the untreated disseminated infection is at least 50 per cent, and of meningitis practically 100 per cent.

Diagnosis. Diagnosis of the disseminated infection may be established by biopsy or at autopsy. If histologic examination demonstrates the characteristic double-contoured spherules with endospores and without budding, the diagnosis is certain. In both primary and disseminated infections demonstration of the fungus by culture and animal inoculation is also diagnostic. Coverglass identification is not sufficient, since the diphasic nature of the fungus should be demonstrated. Sputum is generally scanty in the primary infection, so that gastric lavage may be advisable, especially in children. The fungus will not withstand the concentration procedures usually used for tubercle bacilli. The material should be cultured or, after treatment with penicillin and streptomycin or 0.05 per cent copper sulfate, injected intraperitoneally into a mouse or intratesticularly into a guinea pig. Any suspicious, white fluffy fungus should be injected into a mouse or guinea pig to demonstrate diagnostic spherules. Only especially qualified laboratories should undertake such procedures.

Coccidioidin test. The test is specific except for occasional cross reactions in histoplasmosis and blastomycosis. Like the tuberculin test, a positive reaction does not distinguish between a recent or old infection unless preceded within a reasonably short time by a negative test result. Obviously, its usefulness is restricted in residents of an endemic area. Coccidioidin is administered intradermally as 0.1 ml. of a 1:1000, 1:100 or even 1:10 dilution. The reaction generally reaches its peak at 36 hours and should be read at 24 and 48 hours. The criterion for a positive result is an area of induration more than 5 mm. in diameter. Patients with erythema nodosum suspected of being coccidioidal should have the weakest solution, since they are likely to be hypersensitive. Patients with disseminated infections are much less sensitive; on occasion even a 1:10 dilution may not elicit a reaction. Dermal sensitivity to coccidioidin does not appear to be as durable as is that to tuberculin. There is no danger of disseminating or activating a coccidioidal infection by a strong coccidioidin reaction, although there may be a systemic reaction as well as a local one. Coccidioidin does not evoke humoral antibodies, so that the skin test may precede serologic tests and provides information necessary for their interpretation.

Blood and cerebrospinal fluid. Serum precipitins and complement fixation appear after coccidioidin sensitivity has become demonstrable and persist during periods of anergy associated with overwhelming disseminated lesions. In general, the more severe the infection, the higher the titer of complement fixation. Humoral antibodies are generally not demonstrable in asymptomatic infections. The sedimentation rate is rapid in both primary and disseminated infections and is helpful in evaluating the clinical status. Eosinophilia is a common finding. The cerebrospinal fluid findings, other than a frequently encountered paretic type of colloidal gold curve, are similar to those of tuberculous meningitis. Fixation of complement by cerebrospinal fluid occurs in three fourths of patients with coccidioidal meningitis. This is usually diagnostic, though occasionally epidural coccidioidal lesions may also lead to complement fixation by the cerebrospinal fluid. Complement-fixing antibodies do not pass the blood-brain barrier, but are found in cord blood at the same titer as in the mother's blood. Passively transferred antibody in the infant disappears within 6 months. Congenital coccidioidal dissemination has been reported, but is rare.

Roentgenography. During the primary infection, roentgenograms of the chest may reveal no pulmonary changes, and those that occur are not diagnostic. Hilar adenopathy occurs frequently, and there may be single or multiple, sharply circumscribed or soft, feathery, small pulmonary densities or larger consolidated areas. Pulmonary cavities, when present, tend to be thin-walled. There may be pleural effusions of variable extent. The osseous lesions of the disseminated infection are usually multiple with a predilection for cancellous bone; the lesions often show considerable proliferation and are generally indistinguishable from those of tuberculosis.

Treatment. The treatment of primary coccidioidal infection consists in restriction of activity and in symptomatic measures. Treatment should be continued until the sedimentation rate is returning to normal, precipitins have vanished, the complement-fixing titer of serum is regressing, and radiographic improvement is noted. Pulmonary cavities frequently close spontaneously. When a cavity is located peripherally or when it persists or there is recurrent bleeding or secondary infection, excision should be considered. Infrequently, bronchopleural fistulas or recurrent cavitation may occur as surgical complications; rarely extensive dissemination may result. When extensive thoracic surgery is required, therapy with amphotericin B may be desirable.

Amphotericin B is the first antibiotic proved to be of value in the treatment of disseminated coccidioidomycosis. It is ineffective by oral administration. It is given intravenously in doses of 0.25 mg. per kg., increasing to 1.0 mg. per kg. daily in a 5 per cent dextrose solution containing 1 mg. of the drug per 10 ml. Immediate febrile reactions occur frequently, but may be reduced by pretreatment with thorazine or a similar drug. Its nephrotoxicity is reflected best by diminished creatinine clearance, but may also be detected by an elevation of the blood urea nitrogen level and at times by depletion of potassium. In such instances treatment may be reduced to 2 or 3 administrations a week. Thrombophlebitis is common even with scrupulous care in the intravenous administration. Anemia is constant during adequate administration of the drug, but is effectively controlled by transfusions and terminates when treatment is stopped. Agranulocytosis is rare, but hepatic insufficiency develops occasionally, mainly in those with pre-existing liver damage. The drug should not be used in primary infections except when dissemination seems imminent. Although the response is occasionally dramatic in the disseminated form of the disease, generally treatment must be continued for months and, if possible, until improvement is demonstrated by a significant reduction in complement-fixing antibodies. An increase in sensitivity to the coccidioidin is also favorable immunologic evidence. Cold abscesses should be drained, and if osseous lesions are accessible, excision should be considered.

Amphotericin B does not pass the blood-brain barrier in adequate amounts, but it may mask meningitis during intravenous treatment. Early treatment of coccidioidal meningitis is important. Intrathecal administration of the drug in doses of 0.5 mg. 2 or 3 times a week is usually necessary. Arachnoiditis is a hazard of intraspinal administration, and at least one instance of transverse myelitis has been reported. Only rarely is coccidioidal meningitis completely "cured," and intermittent intensive or continued "suppressive" treatment may be desirable even after complement-fixing antibodies are no longer demonstrable in the spinal fluid, and the chemical and cellular constituents have returned to normal. Continued close surveillance is imperative (see also p. 709).

CHARLES E. SMITH[*]
Revised by DEMOSTHENES PAPPAGIANIS

---

[*]Deceased.

REFERENCES

Ajello, L. (Ed.): *Symposium on Coccidioidomycosis.* Tucson, Ariz., University of Arizona Press, 1967. 2nd ed.

Fiese, M. J.: *Coccidioidomycosis.* Springfield, Ill., Charles C Thomas, 1958.

Smith, C. E.: Coccidioidomycosis. *Pediat. Clin. N. Amer.,* 2:109, 1955.

Idem: Human Coccidioidomycosis. *Bacteriological Rev.,* 25:310, 1961.

Winn, W. A.: Coccidioidomycosis and Amphotericin B. *Med. Clin. N. Amer.,* 47:1131, 1963.

Winn, W. A.: The Treatment of Coccidioidal Meningitis. The Use of Amphotericin B in a Group of 25 Patients. *California Medicine,* 101:78, 1964.

Parasitic Infections

Helminthic and Arthropod Diseases

Helminths and arthropods are Metazoa, i.e. many-celled animals, and both belong to the invertebrates. The parasitic helminths comprise 3 large groups: the Nematoda (roundworms), the Platyhelminthes (flatworms) and the Hirudinea (leeches). The arthropods constitute the largest group in the animal kingdom and include centipedes, scorpions, spiders, ticks, mites and insects.

Owing to the greater opportunities for exposure, diseases produced by most animal parasites occur most frequently in children. Furthermore, children are more likely to manifest acute evidences of these diseases, because in the early years of life there is no immunity or tolerance to many of the parasites. Later, as humoral and cellular resistance develops, the body tends to become more accustomed to the invader and may even develop a relatively solid immunity. Thus the morbidity and the mortality rates of animal parasitic diseases are higher in childhood than in later life, and as a general rule evoke more conspicuous and severe symptoms.

For information on the comparative epidemiology of these diseases see Table 10-27.

INFECTIONS PRODUCED BY ROUNDWORMS (NEMATODA)

All important roundworm infections are produced by species belonging to the phylum Nematoda, which includes the true roundworms. These are elongated, cylindroid, unsegmented animals covered with a tough, relatively impermeable cuticula secreted by the underlying tissue layer, the hypodermis. They have a complete digestive tract, consisting of a mouth which is frequently provided with lips, teeth or other organs designed for penetration and attachment, a muscular esophagus, a midgut in which digestion of food takes place, and a hindgut, or rectum. The nervous system is primitive and is elaborated only at the oral end. A conspicuous body cavity contains the organs of excretion and reproduction. With few exceptions the sexes are separate. The female reproductive opening (vulva) is midventral in position, near the equatorial plane or anterior to this level. The male reproductive system joins the rectum to form a cloaca, which opens externally at or near the posterior end of the body.

The most important roundworm infections (nematodiases) are ascariasis, enterobiasis (oxyuriasis), trichuriasis, the hookworm infections, strongyloidiasis, trichinosis, the filariases and dracontiasis, or dracunculosis.

ASCARIASIS

Etiology. Ascariasis is produced by the giant roundworm, *Ascaris lumbricoides*, which normally lives in the lumen of the host's small intestine. The mature female worm measures 20 to 35 cm. in length by 3 to 6 cm. in greatest diameter, and the male is about one fifth smaller. Both sexes have 3 fleshy lips surrounding the triangular mouth, and both taper to a sharp posterior end, although the male is curved ventrally at the posterior extremity. The female lays approximately 200,000 eggs each day. These are infertile if males are lacking, and some may be infertile if the female is just beginning to oviposit. The fertile eggs are passed in the patient's feces in the one-celled stage. They are broadly ovoidal, measure 35 to 50 microns in cross section by 65 to 75 microns in greatest diameter and are provided with a thin, resistant inner shell, a thick hyaline middle shell and a mammillated outer covering which is usually bile-stained. Within the shell covering is a densely granular, more or less spherical egg cell (Fig. 10-100).

Epidemiology. Ascariasis is widely distributed through the tropics and extends into the temperate zones as far north and south as latitude 40 degrees. The fertile eggs are able to survive practically all external conditions except heat and extreme desiccation. When the egg is deposited on the ground or on the floor of a house, it proceeds to embryonate and in warm weather within 9 days or more contains a motile first-stage larva. A week later, during which the larva molts once, the egg is infective. It does not hatch on the soil, but only after being swallowed. In favorable environments, as in the Gulf Coast area of the United States, the embryonated eggs may remain viable during the infective stage for months or even years. The worms are harbored principally by young children who find it more convenient to deposit their

TABLE 10-27. EPIDEMIOLOGY OF THE MORE IMPORTANT HELMINTHIC INFECTIONS ENCOUNTERED IN PEDIATRIC PRACTICE

PERORAL EXPOSURE	TRANSMISSION SOURCE	HELMINTH AND STAGE INVOLVED	DISEASE
1. From raw or inadequately processed foods	Fruits and vegetables	Ascaris and Trichuris (fully embryonated eggs)	Ascariasis, trichuriasis
	Water cress	Fasciola (encysted metacercariae)	Fascioliasis
	Water nuts	Fasciolopsis (encysted metacercariae)	Fasciolopsiasis
	Meat		
	Pork	Trichinella (encapsulated larvae)	Trichinosis
		Taenia solium (encapsulated cysticerci)	Teniasis
	Beef	*Taenia saginata* (encapsulated cysticerci)	Teniasis
	Porcupine, bear meat	Trichinella (encapsulated larvae)	Trichinosis
	Fish (fresh-water)	*Diphyllobothrium latum* (sparganum larvae)	Diphyllobothriasis
		Clonorchis, Opisthorchis, Metagonimus, Heterophyes (encapsulated metacercariae)	Clonorchiasis, etc.
	Crabs and crayfish	Paragonimus (encapsulated metacercariae)	Paragonimiasis
2. From fresh water	Cyclops and Diaptomus	Dracunculus (infective larvae); Sparganum (procercoid larvae)	Dracontiasis, sparganosis
3. From person-to-person contact	Anus→fingers→mouth or anus→clothing→fingers→mouth	Enterobius and *Hymenolepis nana* (fully embryonated eggs)	Oxyuriasis, hymenolepiasis
4. From contaminated soil	Dirty toys or candy; eating earth	Ascaris and Trichuris (fully embryonated eggs)	Ascariasis, trichuriasis
5. From contact with domestic mammals	Dog feces	Echinococcus (eggs)	Hydatid disease
		Toxocara canis (fully embryonated eggs)	Visceral larva migrans
	Cat feces	*Toxocara cati* (fully embryonated eggs)	Intestinal toxocariasis
	Dog and cat fleas	*Dipylidium caninum* (infective-stage larvae in fleas)	Dipylidiasis
	Rodent fleas	*Hymenolepis diminuta* (infective-stage larvae in fleas)	Hymenolepiasis

PERCUTANEOUS EXPOSURE	TRANSMISSION SOURCE	HELMINTH AND STAGE INVOLVED	DISEASE
1. From infested ground		Hookworms and Strongyloides (filariform larvae)	Hookworm disease, strongyloidiasis
2. From infested fresh water	Mollusca-intermediate hosts in water	Schistosoma species (cercarial larvae)	Schistosomiasis; schistosome dermatitis
3. From blood-sucking insects	Mosquitoes, coffee flies, mango flies, etc.	Filarial worms (filariform larvae)	Filariasis

excreta where they are playing than to use toilets. The eggs develop in the top soil, and children take some of them into the mouth on contaminated fingers or play objects, or as a result of eating dirt. Where these unsanitary conditions prevail, 60 to 100 per cent of children from 1 to 10 years of age are infected with Ascaris. Older children and adults are parasitized to a lesser degree and can usually trace their infections to sources provided by the younger groups.

Ascariasis is encountered occasionally among children in the northern United States, but the southern Appalachians and their extension into the Ozarks and the Gulf Coast states constitute the regions of high endemicity in the United States. Hard, permeable clay soils are most favorable for the development of Ascaris eggs, in contrast to moist, sandy humus for those of hookworms.

Hogs are infected with an Ascaris morphologically indistinguishable from that in man, but hog Ascaris is rarely infective for human beings under natural conditions.

Pathology. When infective-stage Ascaris eggs are swallowed and reach the duodenum, they hatch, and the escaping larvae enter the intestinal wall. The larvae penetrate into the mesenteric lymphatics or venules, commonly migrating through the liver, and are carried to the lungs through the right side of the heart. From the pulmonary capillaries the larvae invade the air sacs, causing the discharge of a minute pool of blood at each site of escape. An acute cellular infiltration typically occurs in the immediate vicinity, temporarily blocking the passage of the larvae up the respiratory tree (Fig. 10-101). If the number of larvae migrating through the lungs is appreciable, an atypical pneumonia results.

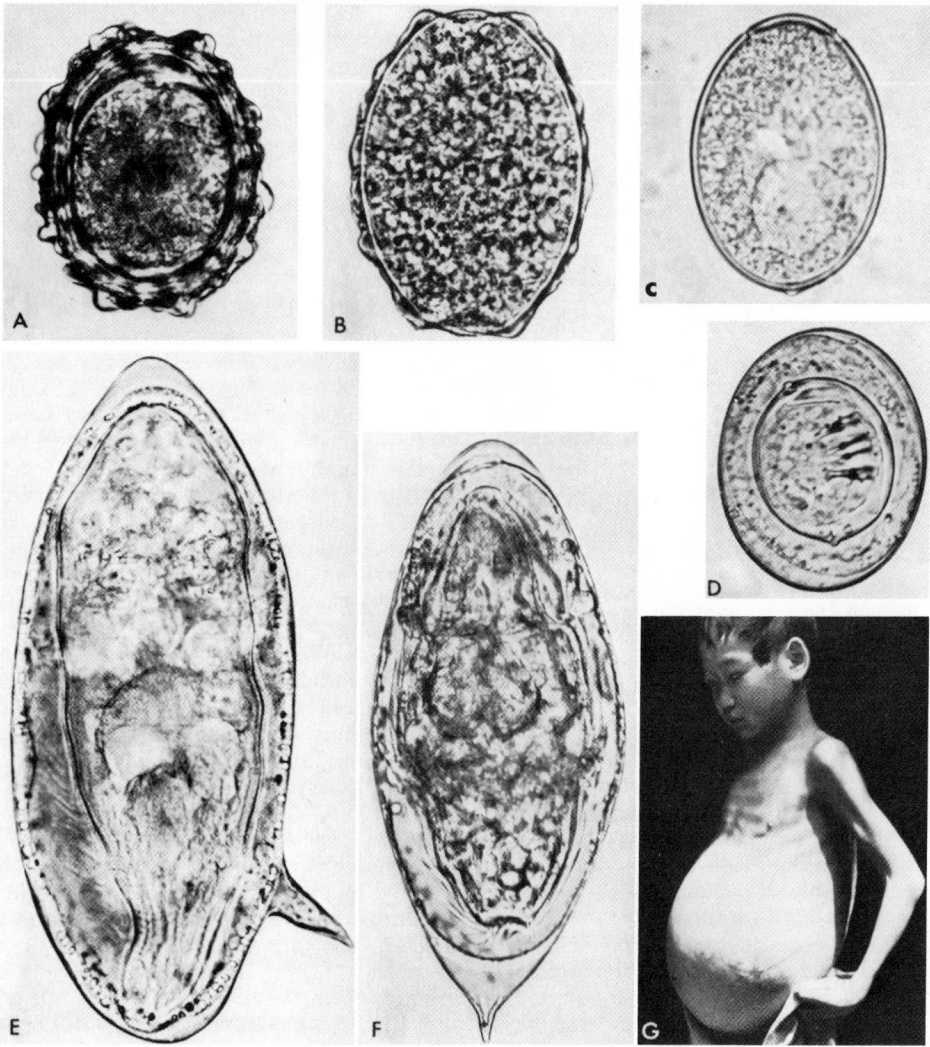

Figure 10-100. *A*, Fertilized egg of *Ascaris lumbricoides.* × 550. *B*, Unfertilized egg of *Ascaris lumbricoides.* × 550. *C*, Egg of *Diphyllobothrium latum.* × 550. *D*, Egg of *Hymenolepis nana.* × 550. *E*, Egg of *Schistosoma mansoni* from feces. *F*, Egg of *Schistosoma haematobium* from urine. × 550. *G*, Advanced stage of schistosomiasis japonica in a 13-year-old Chinese boy, with ascites resulting from hepatic cirrhosis, splenomegaly, fever, anemia and dysentery. (After E. G. Nauck: *Lehrbuch der Tropenkrankheiten.* Courtesy of Georg Thieme Verlag, Stuttgart.)

After a second larval molt in the lungs, the third-stage larvae reach the epiglottis, are swallowed and become established in the small intestine, where they grow into adult worms. Between the sixtieth and seventy-fifth days after the eggs have been swallowed, mature worms mate, and the females begin their egg-laying. If the worms become irritated by their environment, as, for example, owing to digestive disturbances or fever, they may pass down the bowel and be spontaneously evacuated; or they may enter the stomach to be vomited, or escape through the nares. They may block the appendiceal lumen, perforate the intestinal wall, block the common bile duct, migrate into the parenchyma of the liver or reach the pleural cavity. Extensive destruction of the hepatic parenchyma may occur as a result of their movements, their toxic metabolites and those of their eggs.

Clinical Manifestations. During their temporary stay in the lungs the immature worms may cause an atypical pneumonia. The sensitization produced by these migrating larvae is responsible for the manifestations of ascaris allergy frequently observed, including asthma, urticaria and eosinophilia.

Intestinal infection with Ascaris may be apparently symptomless, or there may be such manifestations as nausea and vomiting, anorexia, loss of weight, insomnia, slight fever, irritability, or physical and mental languor. The most common complaint of children is intestinal colic. Some patients are highly intoxicated by the by-products of the worms and may have a rapid rise in temperature. Acute symptoms accompany ectopic excursions of the worms. A mass of writhing worms knotted together frequently produces acute intestinal obstruction, at times resulting in per-

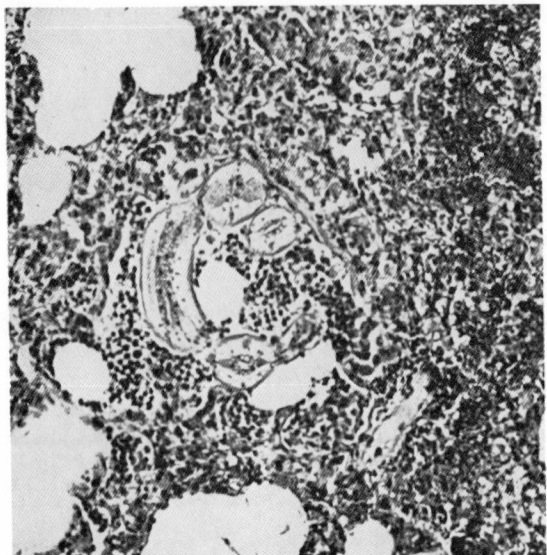

Figure 10-101. Larva of *Ascaris lumbricoides* in migration through the lung, in center of small pool of blood, with leukocytic infiltration. × ca. 200. (After Hunter, Frye and Swartzwelder: *A Manual of Tropical Medicine.*)

foration of the wall, in intussusception or in paralytic ileus.

Diagnosis. The diagnosis is commonly made by the recovery of fertile or infertile eggs in microscopic fecal films (Fig. 10-101). Direct unconcentrated films usually provide this evidence after the mature females have begun to oviposit. If only male worms occur (in less than 5 per cent of infections), clinical diagnosis may be confirmed by the therapeutic test. From time to time adult or immature worms passed in the stool or vomited or discharged from the nostril require diagnosis. Occasionally, during barium studies of the gastrointestinal tract for other purposes, ascarides are demonstrated.

Prognosis. Except when large numbers of Ascaris larvae in the lungs initiate lobular pneumonia or when adult worms produce intestinal obstruction or migrate into abnormal foci, the prognosis is good to excellent, provided a specific anthelmintic is administered.

Prevention. In highly endemic areas re-exposure is the rule, and reinfection takes place about every 3 months. Thus both the physician and the public health officer are concerned with problems of control. Children as well as adults should have comfortable, clean toilets and should be taught to use them habitually. Finally, all infected persons should receive specific medication.

Treatment. No chemotherapeutic agent has a lethal effect on Ascaris until the young worms arrive in the small intestine. The older ascaricidal drugs are not sufficiently effective or are too toxic in full therapeutic doses. *Piperazine citrate* (diethylene diamine) is an almost ideal drug for this infection. No pretreatment or post-treatment purgation or fasting is required, and the recom-

mended dosage produces no side effects. The syrup of piperazine citrate is given orally in a single dose of 3 or 4 gm. (30 to 40 ml. of syrup) and is repeated in 2 days. It may be introduced by intestinal catheter to children suspected of having intestinal or biliary obstruction resulting from ascariasis.

TOXOCARIASIS AND VISCERAL LARVA MIGRANS

See also Löffler's Syndrome (p. 928).

Etiology. Intestinal toxocariasis is produced by *Toxocara cati*, the cat ascarid, and visceral larva migrans by *Toxocara canis*, the dog ascarid. There are possibly 18 authentic records of intestinal infection with *T. cati* in children and only 1 questionable record of intestinal infection by *T. canis* in a child. By contrast, extraintestinal infection (visceral larva migrans) seems to be characteristic of *T. canis* in the human host. The life cycle of these worms in their normal hosts parallels that of human Ascaris, including a required migration through the lungs.

Epidemiology. Eggs of Toxocara embryonate on the ground. When they get into the mouths of children and reach the duodenum, they hatch, and the escaping larvae penetrate into the intestinal wall. Cumulative reports indicate that extraintestinal infection with the larval stage of *T. canis* is relatively common in children in the United States, especially in the deep South.

Pathology. Clinical investigations supplemented by experimental studies have shown that *T. canis* undertakes a migration through the viscera, but fails to develop. Usually it becomes trapped in a granulomatous tissue reaction, most frequently in the liver, at times in the lungs and eyeballs (Fig. 10-102), and rarely in the brain and other soft tissues. If thousands of infective-stage eggs are ingested, there may be a large number of granulomas, one surrounding each larva which has hatched and has attempted pulmonary migration. Once trapped, the larva may soon die and become fibrosed or calcified, or it may survive for months, but it does not proceed with normal growth in the human body and never completes its migration back to the intestinal tract to develop into an adult worm, as it would in the canine host.

Clinical Manifestations. The evidence may be solely a persistent eosinophilia, or there may be hepatomegaly, multiple pulmonary infiltrations (demonstrable roentgenographically), fever, cough, hyperglobulinemia or symptoms referable to the brain or eye.

Diagnosis. Diagnosis is made by demonstration of the larvae in granulomatous areas of the liver (biopsy), from enucleated eyes or at autopsy.

Prognosis. In limited invasions visceral larva migrans is a relatively benign disease, except when the larvae are trapped while migrating ectopically through the brain or eyeball. When multiple sites are involved, the prognosis is grave.

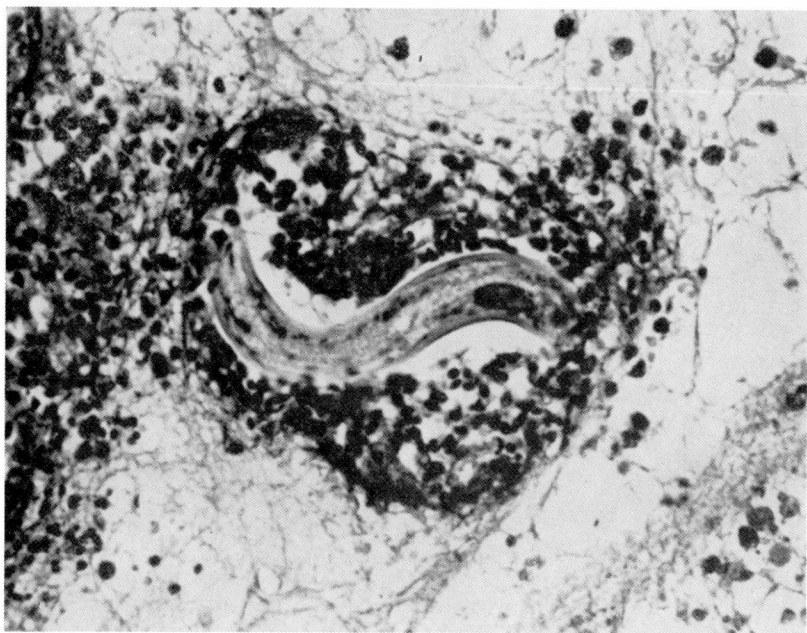

Figure 10-102. Visceral larva migrans. Second-stage larva of dog ascarid, *T. canis*, in center of granuloma in vitreous chamber of human eye. × 220. (After Wilder; courtesy of Armed Forces Institute of Pathology, and *Tr. Am. Acad. Ophth. & Otolaryng.*)

Prevention. Periodic deworming of household dogs is indicated.

Treatment. Thiabendazole is known to have been used in 1 successful trial to control visceral infection with *Toxocara canis* in man.

OXYURIASIS
(Enterobiasis)

Etiology. Oxyuriasis is produced by the pinworm, *Enterobius vermicularis* (seatworm, Oxyuris of older textbooks). The adult worms are small (males, 2 to 5 mm. in length, and curved ventrally at the posterior end; females, 8 to 13 mm. in length, robust in the middle and drawn out into a long sharp point posteriorly). The worms live attached by their lips to the mucous coat of the cecum and appendix. Gravid worms become detached, migrate down the bowel and characteristically crawl out the anus onto the perianal and perineal skin, where each female deposits several thousand eggs in a sinuous track. Eggs are laid within the bowel in only about 5 per cent of infections, and these are usually infertile or immature. The eggs laid outside the anus are elongated, ovoidal, somewhat flattened on one side, with a thick, slightly opalescent shell, and measure 50 to 60 by 20 to 30 microns. They contain a coiled larva at the time of oviposition (Fig. 10-103). At most they require only a few hours after deposition to become infective.

Epidemiology. This infection is world-wide in distribution. Children are particularly susceptible, and those in large families, schools in slum areas, and dormitory groups are more heavily parasitized than the population at large. They are exposed to infection by scratching the itching skin around the anus, where the eggs are lodged, or from soiled night garments or undergarments, bed linen or contaminated objects in the room, and in this way getting the eggs onto the tips of their fingers and then into their mouths, and from breathing airborne eggs. Fertile eggs remain in the average environment for at least 9 days.

Pathology. When viable eggs are swallowed and pass down the digestive tract, they hatch at the duodenal level, and the escaping larvae migrate to the cecum, become attached and develop into adults in 15 to 28 days. They usually produce no appreciable damage at the site of attachment, although they may cause hemorrhage from the appendiceal wall or provide an opening for pathogenic bacteria to initiate a submucous abscess. Gravid worms, crawling out the anus, usually at night, frequently cause a severe pruritus, and the inevitable scratching results in scarification and secondary infection of the skin. In the female patient the gravid worms may enter the genital tract, cause a salpingitis, become encapsulated in the tubules or enter the peritoneal cavity and provoke encapsulation.

Clinical Manifestations. The appendiceal lesions occasionally produce symptoms of acute or subacute appendicitis, with indications for excision of the organ. Pruritus ani is frequently complicated by bacterial invasion of the skin and the production of weeping, eczematous areas. Children, especially young girls, may exhibit irritability, loss of appetite and weight, and insomnia, resulting in chronic emotional disturbances. Vaginitis has been ascribed to direct invasion by

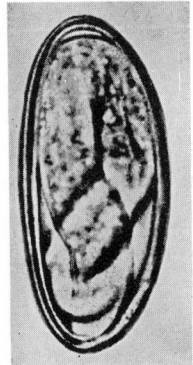

Figure 10-103. Fully embryonated egg of *Enterobius vermicularis* obtained by perianal swabbing. × 800. (From Cram: *Introduction to Nematology.* Bureau of Plant Industry, Washington, D.C.)

the worms. Eosinophilia may be produced, but is not present in all cases.

Diagnosis. Oxyuriasis is rarely diagnosed by fecal examination. The eggs (Fig. 10-103) can usually be recovered in one to several swabbings of the perianal and perineal skin, preferably in the morning before dressing, bathing or defecation.

A simple and probably the most efficient anal swabbing technique consists in the use of a 2-inch length of adhesive-cellulose tape, placed sticky side out on the end of a 3- by 1-inch clean microscope slide held in place with the thumb and index finger. As the tape is brought in contact with the anal sphincter and the perianal folds, it collects Enterobius eggs among the flecks of mucus and cellular debris. After swabbing, the tape is placed flat, sticky side down, on the slide. It may be examined microscopically at any convenient time by allowing a drop or two of toluene to filter between the slide and the tape.

Prognosis. This is usually good. When the adult worms spontaneously migrate out of the bowel or are removed by enema or catharsis, the infection may be permanently eliminated.

Prevention. Scrupulous personal and group hygiene is advised, but in itself will not eradicate oxyuriasis. Accurate diagnosis and treatment of all infected persons in a household, repeated several times if necessary, constitute an integral part of the control program.

Treatment. Pyrvinium pamoate, a cyanine dye, is used for single-dose treatment (5 mg. per kg.). Piperazine hexahydrate, as piperazine citrate syrup, is highly efficient and well tolerated. It is administered by mouth daily for 7 to 10 days in the amount of 1.5 gm. for adults, with correspondingly lesser amounts for children, depending on weight.

All infected persons in a family or dormitory *must* be treated simultaneously. Even if Enterobius is completely eradicated from a household, periodic reinfection may be anticipated from outside contacts, necessitating further chemotherapy.

TRICHURIASIS
(WHIPWORM INFECTION)

Etiology. This infection is produced by the whipworm, *Trichuris trichiura*, whose body is composed of a capillary anterior three fifths and a fleshy posterior two fifths. The males measure 30 to 45 mm. in length and are coiled ventrally at the posterior end. The females measure 35 to 50 mm. in length and have a club-shaped posterior end. These worms live with their anterior ends attached to or basted into the mucous coat of the cecum and appendix and, in heavy infections, in the adjacent parts of the ileum, ascending colon, and even in the sigmoid colon and rectum. The females daily lay a few thousand barrel-shaped eggs, which have mucus-like polar plugs and are commonly bile-stained (Fig. 10-104).

Epidemiology. Whipworm infection is widely distributed in warm, moist climates. It is most common in children over 5 years of age, but may be prevalent in younger patients. The eggs passed in feces and deposited on moist, shaded soil require 10 to 14 days to develop to the infective stage, at which time each contains a motile larva. When ripe eggs get into the mouth and are swallowed, they hatch at the level of the duodenum, and the escaping larvae slowly migrate to the cecum or appendix, become attached, and in about 3 months develop into adult worms.

Pathology. At each site of attachment there is a microscopic focus of inflammation. Toxic by-products at times provoke allergic manifestations, but usually the infection is well tolerated unless the worm burden is heavy (i.e. several hundred), as it frequently is in the tropics or the moist subtropics. In heavy infections the worms colonize the intestinal mucosa from the lower level of the ileum almost to the anal sphincter.

Clinical Manifestations. Many persons, especially in the southern United States, harbor a few worms without apparent symptoms, but a small proportion experience loss of appetite, loss of weight, insomnia, physical and mental apathy or nervous manifestations. Heavily infected patients typically have a secondary anemia, with pallor, shrunken skin, dull eyes, dry hair and, at times, edema of the abdomen and legs. In addition to the erythropenia there may be a neutropenia with monocytosis and a moderate eosinophilia. Children may fail to develop physically or sexually. In heavy infections there is profound irritation of the bowel wall, resulting in a bloody, mucous diarrhea, at times with an associated prolapse of the rectum.

Diagnosis. Diagnosis is made on the recovery of the characteristic eggs (Fig. 10-104) in direct or concentrated fecal films.

Prognosis. Prognosis is good in most patients, especially if a majority of the worms are removed by the use of anthelmintics.

Prevention. This consists in the habitual use of comfortable sanitary toilet facilities and the

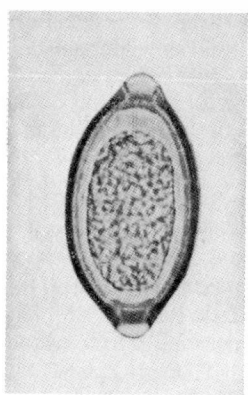

Figure 10-104. Egg of *Trichuris trichiura*, as seen in freshly passed feces. × 666. (After Faust, in Brennemann's *Practice of Pediatrics*. Courtesy of W. F. Prior Co.)

sanitary disposal of sewage. Children must be trained not to take contaminated objects and dirt into their mouths.

Treatment. For rapid treatment in hospitalized or clinic patients, high enemas of 0.2 per cent hexylresorcinol (Crystoids anthelmintic) are effective in removing a large proportion of the worms, and thus produce clinical cure. Before instilling the solution it is advisable to coat the buttocks, thighs and perineum with petroleum jelly to prevent burning of the skin from returned or spilled solution. For eradicative therapy, dithiazanine iodide was found to be efficacious, but its use has been discontinued, owing to its toxicity. Thiabendazole (see p. 245) is perhaps slightly less efficacious, but avoids the disturbing side effects produced by dithiazanine.

HOOKWORM INFECTIONS
(Uncinariasis; Ancylostomiasis)

Etiology. These infections are produced by certain species of hookworms which parasitize man: *Necator americanus*, the so-called American hookworm; *Ancylostoma duodenale*, the so-called Old World hookworm; *Ancylostoma ceylonicum* and *Ancylostoma braziliense*. The first two are exclusively parasites of man; *A. ceylonicum* and *A. braziliense* are typically parasites of dogs and cats. These worms are 7.5 to 13 mm. long and 0.3 to 0.4 mm. in greatest breadth. The males are slightly smaller than the females. The mouth of Necator is provided with a pair of upper and a pair of lower cutting plates; that of Ancylostoma, with 2 or 3 pairs of incurved upper teeth. The females have a bluntly pointed caudal extremity and a vulvar opening midventral in position near the equatorial plane. The caudal extremity of the male is drawn out into an umbrella-like expansion, the copulatory bursa, used to grasp the female during copulation. These worms are attached by their mouth capsule to the mucosa of the small bowel, typically at the level of the duodenum, jejunum and adjacent portion of the ileum.

After insemination each female hookworm lays several thousand eggs a day. These eggs (Fig. 10-105, *A*) are broadly ovoidal, thin-shelled and hyaline; they measure 60 to 76 by 36 to 40 microns. They are usually in an early stage of development when evacuated in the feces, but in constipated stools may be more advanced in development (Fig. 10-105, *B*).

Epidemiology. *Necator americanus* is the tropical hookworm of the Western Hemisphere; it is the only widely distributed hookworm in the Americas, including the southern United States. *Ancylostoma duodenale* is the hookworm of the Mediterranean basin and similar latitudes in Asia and is the more common species on the Pacific coast of South America. *Ancylostoma ceylonicum* is found in Southeast Asia and Brazil, while *Ancylostoma braziliense* has a spotted distribution in warm climates. Intestinal infection with this last species appears to be limited almost exclusively to canine and feline hosts.

Eggs of Necator and *A. duodenale* evacuated from the human bowel and deposited on a moist, sandy humus soil in a shaded site in warm climates embryonate rapidly and hatch in 24 to 48 hours. The escaping larvae feed ravenously on bacteria and organic debris, grow, molt, feed again and, between the fifth and tenth days, transform into infective-stage filariform larvae. Human exposure occurs when these third-stage larvae come in contact with the skin, as when persons walk barefooted on, or handle, infected soil. Infants and small children are seldom exposed to infection except in hyperendemic areas. Older children and adults, especially males, in highly endemic areas are subject to repeated infection. Thus man initiates the extrinsic phase of the life cycle by discharging hookworm eggs on the soil and, in turn, picks up the infection by direct contact with the soil.

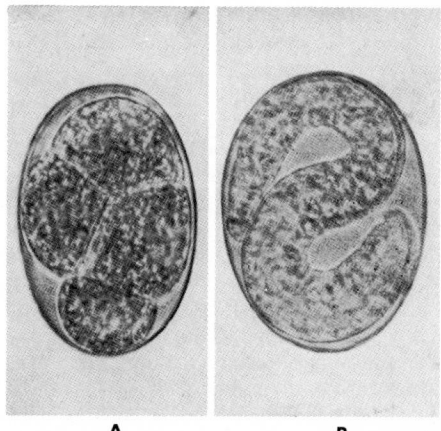

A   B

Figure 10-105. Eggs of human hookworm *Necator americanus*, as seen in freshly passed feces. *A*, 4-cell stage; *B*, maturing embryo. × 666. (After Faust, in Brennemann's *Practice of Pediatrics*. Courtesy of W. F. Prior Co.)

The canine and feline strains of *A. braziliense* are physiologically distinct. Man occasionally acquires intestinal infection with *A. ceylonicum* and incurs cutaneous larva migrans (creeping eruption) after exposure to *A. braziliense*.

Pathology. The infective-stage larvae of the human strains invade the human skin through hair follicles or under particles of desquamating epidermis. They migrate to the cutaneous blood vessels, enter the venules, are carried to the lungs through the right side of the heart and lodge in the pulmonary capillaries, where a third larval molt occurs. From the capillaries they penetrate the alveoli, migrate up the respiratory tract, pass over the epiglottis and are swallowed. On arrival in the small bowel, each develops a temporary mouth capsule, becomes attached to a villus and begins to digest tissues and suck blood, then develops a permanent mouth capsule under the earlier one, which is now shed, becomes sexually mature and copulates. In 5 to 10 weeks after invasion of the skin the females begin to lay eggs.

Temporary trauma and tissue reaction develop at the sites where the larvae invade the skin and where they pass from the pulmonary capillaries into the air sacs, but these manifestations are not serious unless the cutaneous lesions become secondarily infected or the number of invading larvae is large. After attachment to the villi in the small bowel, the adolescent worms secrete lytic juices which digest the epithelium and the walls of the capillaries. This partially predigested food of blood and epithelial cells is now sucked into and passes through the intestine of the worm. In part it is used as nourishment, but mainly as a source of oxygen, since hookworms are primarily anaerobic in their metabolism. Once this blood pumping is well under way, each worm may initially deprive the victim's body of as much as 0.67 ml. each day. The blood loss can be compensated if the number of worms is small, but frequently, when the number is more than 50 or the nutritional balance of the host is already precarious, decompensation occurs, with a resultant microcytic hypochromic anemia. This is the essential factor in hookworm disease.

Clinical Manifestations. As the intestinal infection develops, either rapidly as a result of a heavy single inoculation or cumulatively as a result of repeated exposure, digestion becomes disturbed and the stools are usually unformed, contain undigested food, and frequently are tarry with decomposed blood. Absorption of by-products of the worms results in systemic toxemia, but the more profound manifestations are the result of continued loss of blood. The skin has an ashen pallor or may have an icteric tinge. The eyes are dull, and the hair is lusterless. Owing to the anemia, there is a decreased oxygen-carrying capacity. The heart works at increased speed in an attempt to oxygenate the tissues and may become more or less permanently dilated. Mental apathy is pronounced. These conditions are more striking in children than in adults, and physical growth and sexual development are delayed.

In creeping eruption, *cutaneous larva migrans*, resulting from infection with canine or feline strains of *A. braziliense*, less commonly the cosmopolitan dog hookworm *A. caninum* and rarely the human hookworms *N. americanus* and *A. duodenale*, the larvae penetrate to the deeper layers of the skin, but, being unable to enter the peripheral blood vessels, continue to migrate for months (*larva migrans*) through serpiginous tunnels in the skin (Fig. 10-106, p. 628). This produces an inflamed appearance of the somewhat elevated channels, which usually become infected as a result of scratching the pruritic lesions.

At the end of the incubation period of human intestinal hookworm infection there is usually a moderate neutrophilic and eosinophilic leukocytosis. Later there is a neutropenia with monocytosis; there is also characteristically hypoproteinemia, which is often due to pre-existing malnutrition. In chronic infections the hypochromic anemia may be replaced by a hyperchromic macrocytic anemia.

Diagnosis. Diagnosis is based on identification of eggs (Fig. 10-105) in the stool.

Prognosis. Prognosis is usually good with specific treatment, provided reinfection is prevented, the hemoglobin content is returned to normal, and an adequate, balanced diet is provided.

Prevention. This consists in (1) detection and thorough treatment of all infected persons to reduce soil contamination; (2) provision and use of sanitary toilets; and (3) the habitual use of shoes in hookworm areas. Children on vacation in areas where hookworm infection exists should be warned about the danger of going barefooted, especially on the banks of streams and ponds.

Treatment. Several efficient anthelmintics are available, although not all are eminently safe. Before specific medication is undertaken it is desirable to provide the patient a well balanced, nutritious diet, reinforced with iron (ferrous sulfate). Infrequently a blood transfusion may be indicated. After a week or 10 days specific treatment may be safely undertaken. *Liver therapy is indicated only if there is a macrocytic type of anemia.*

The older anthelmintics previously used to treat hookworm disease are too toxic for general use. Tetrachloroethylene is well tolerated and has an efficiency of 90 per cent or more for worm removal, provided it is fresh and is kept in a cool place. It is most effective when given on an empty stomach, without pretreatment or post-treatment purgation. The dose is 0.2 ml. per year of developmental age; the adult dose is 3 ml. Treatment may be safely repeated in a week. When small children are in a poor physical state or when hookworm infection is complicated with ascariasis, hexylresorcinol crystoids (Crystoids anthelmintic) should first be administered. The single-dose plan is based on 0.1 gm. per year of developmental age up to 10 years. This drug is dispensed in 0.1- and 0.2-gm. capsules. It should be taken after overnight fasting and without pretreatment or post-treatment purgation and may be repeated safely in a week. It should remove about 90 per cent of the ascarids and 75 per cent of the hookworms. After 2 or 3 doses at weekly intervals the number of hookworms will usually be reduced below the level of clinical significance. In the event of an associated whipworm infection, this therapy should be followed by administration of thiabendazole by mouth (25 mg. per kg.).

The hydroxynaphthoate of bephenium has been effective in treating hookworm infection produced by *Ancylostoma duodenale*, even when administered in one fourth the recommended dose, but it appears to be less satisfactory for elimination of *Necator americanus*. The adult dose is 5 Gm. without preliminary purgation; it is administered after an overnight fast.

Creeping eruption of hookworm origin may be brought under control by freezing the infected area, especially the growing end, with ethyl chloride spray.

STRONGYLOIDIASIS

Etiology. This infection is produced by the threadworm, *Strongyloides stercoralis*. The delicate, threadlike parasitic females, which are barely visible to the naked eye, live primarily in the depths of the mucous coat of the intestine, from the pyloric wall of the stomach to the rectum, but for the most part at the duodenal level, where they lay eggs in the tissues. As the eggs filter out to the intestinal lumen, they mature and hatch, setting free the active larvae, which escape into the lumen of the bowel, feed and at times molt once in transit, and are evacuated in the feces. On deposition on the soil in a warm, moist, shaded site, the larvae grow and undergo one additional molt on or before the fifth day, becoming transformed into the third (infective) stage; or they may undergo one or more free-living cycles before they reach the infective stage.

Epidemiology. Strongyloidiasis is relatively common in warm, moist climates, but in the Western Hemisphere it is occasionally seen as far north as Canada. Exposure results from direct contact of the skin with infested soil, especially where there is a high ground-water level, as in the bayou regions of the Gulf coast of the United States, in tropical rainfall areas and in homes with dirt floors.

Pathology. The sites and methods of entry of Strongyloides into the skin and its migration to the intestine by way of the lungs are essentially the same as in hookworm infection (see p. 724). Occasionally, as these worms escape from the pulmonary capillaries, there is considerable cellular infiltration into the alveoli and bronchioles, but this does not destroy the worms, which continue to grow in the smaller respiratory passages and may even enter the bronchial or tracheal epithelium, where foci of infection are sometimes established. Nevertheless a majority of young worms reach the intestine; the females burrow into the mucosa and, about 26 days after exposure, begin to deposit eggs. The continued burrowing of the worms, together with the infiltration of their eggs, and the hatching and escape of the larvae contribute to the trauma and frequently to the sloughing of portions of the mucosa. There is a general irritation of the involved mucosa with secretion of excess mucus and impaired absorption of food.

Clinical Manifestations. There is only a temporary prickling pain at the site of entry of the infective-stage larvae into the skin. If the number of larvae migrating through the lungs is appreciable or if some become established in the bronchial epithelium, there may be symptoms of an atypical pneumonia. Owing to the changes in the bowel wall, normal tone and function are lost. There is usually dull or sharp pain in the epigastric region. There may be a debilitating, unchecked mucous diarrhea or diarrhea alternating with constipation. Dehydration and poor digestion may produce severe emaciation. During the chronic phase the larvae may transform to the infective filariform stage in transit down the bowel and produce internal autoinfection, or they may be responsible for perianal invasion. Cutaneous larva migrans due to perianal autoinfection was observed in Southeast Asia among white prisoners of war, but not in natives of the area. Patients with chronic infection are more likely to be constipated than to have diarrhea and frequently have neurotoxic manifestations.

The blood picture at the end of the incubation period is that of a leukocytosis with an eosinophilia of 25 per cent or more. In the chronic stage there is characteristically a neutropenia with a moderate eosinophilia and a monocytosis.

Diagnosis. This is based on the detection and identification of larvae in the stool (Fig. 10-107, *A*, *B*) or, more often, in material aspirated from the duodenum. A high eosinophilic count suggests the possibility of this infection.

Prognosis. The prognosis is fair to good in the recently acquired infection, provided specific treatment is adequately carried out. Absence of eosinophilia is a poor prognostic sign, indicating low cellular reaction and constitutional resistance.

Prevention. This requires sanitary disposal of human feces, treatment of infected persons and care not to expose the skin to polluted soil.

Treatment. For years the standard therapy was oral administration with meals of gentian violet medicinal in enteric-coated Seal-In tablets in 0.012- or 0.03-gm. (1/5 or 1/2 grain) sizes. This method of treatment was replaced by introduction of dithiazanine, which was more effective, but resulted in production of undesirable side effects. Thiabendazole has now been used as an effective, more acceptable preparation lacking the side ef-

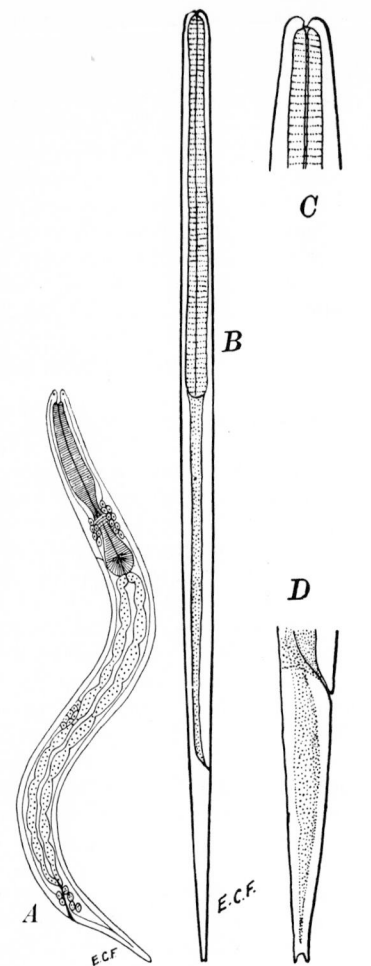

Figure 10-107. *Strongyloides stercoralis. A,* Rhabditoid larva, × 310; *B,* filariform larva, × 120; *C, D,* anterior and posterior ends of filariform larva, × 640. (Faust and Russell: *Clinical Parasitology.* Lea & Febiger.)

fects of dithiazanine. The oral adult dose is 25 mg. per kg. (see also p. 245).

TRICHINOSIS

Etiology. This infection is produced by *Trichinella spiralis.* The adult worms are microscopic and live in the mucous coat of the small bowel, especially at the duodenal level. The females produce living young (larvae) which gain access to the mesenteric venules and lymphatics, migrate through the bloodstream and usually filter out in skeletal muscle, where they become encapsulated in about 21 days.

Epidemiology. Trichinosis is common among pork-eating populations of the north temperate zone, in southern South America and in South Africa. Hogs (occasionally wild boars, other carnivorous mammals, and bears) are the source of infection, to which man is exposed by the consumption of infected meat in a raw or inadequately processed state. For this reason young children

are less commonly infected than older children and adults. Epidemic outbreaks of trichinosis still occur in the United States, frequently as a result of eating pork products from a single heavily infected hog, slaughtered on a farm.

Pathology. When meat containing viable trichina cysts is eaten, the cysts become separated in the stomach. In the duodenum the larvae break out of the cyst, burrow into the mucosa, mature in about 5 days, and mate. The females larviposit for about 6 weeks. There is inflammation as the excysted larvae enter the intestinal wall and mature. Inflammation continues as the larval progeny, having migrated through the bloodstream, become lodged in the muscular tissues.

Clinical Manifestations. Symptoms mimicking acute food poisoning begin within a few hours after ingestion of heavily infected meat and last 4 or 5 days, paralleling the entry of the excysted larvae into the bowel wall and their development into mature worms. During the larval migration there are typically intense muscular pains, stiffness and tenderness in the diaphragm, legs, and muscles of the throat, causing difficulties in breathing, walking, swallowing and talking. An increasingly toxic condition results in edema, especially around the eyes. During this stage or after encapsulation of the larvae there may be disturbances of the central nervous system (motor, sensory or of the higher centers), depending on the sites where migrating larvae have set up inflammatory reactions. There may also be clinical and electrocardiographic evidence of myocarditis from inflamed tracts in the heart muscle, through which the larvae have passed, but in which they do not encyst.

Beginning with the invasion of the duodenal mucosa and continuing through the weeks of larval migration, there is an elevation of temperature to 99 to 102°F. (37.2 to 38.8°C.) or even higher.

Early there is a leukocytosis with eosinophilia, later a leukopenia with eosinophilia and monocytosis.

When the infection is not heavy, there may be few or no apparent symptoms.

Diagnosis. During the incubation period and the early migration of the larvae diagnosis can be made only presumptively on clinical and epidemiologic evidence. After the larvae have become encapsulated (after the twenty-first day) the disease may be detected by biopsy of deltoid, biceps or gastrocnemius muscle strips, or by intradermal tests, using a 1:10,000 antigen, doing an immediate reading at 20 minutes and a final one at 24 hours. The positive intradermal test should be supplemented by the precipitin test to determine whether the infection is recent (ppt +) or of long standing (ppt−). Hemagglutination tests show considerable diagnostic promise. Many cases are diagnosed only at necropsy, and then merely as an incidental finding.

Prognosis. This varies from grave to excellent, depending on the severity of the infection.

Prevention. Thorough cooking, or freezing of all pork for at least 24 hours, will prevent human infection. Since this is not always done, the cooking of all garbage fed to hogs is a valuable preventive method.

Treatment. There is presently no specific therapy. However, in experimental mice and swine thiabendazole has been found effective in killing migrating larvae and those encapsulated in muscles of their host. Management includes administration of analgesics, abundance of citrus fruit juices and an ample fluid intake to maintain a good urinary output. If trichinosis is suspected during the first 2 or 3 days after exposure, daily saline purges with Glauber's salt (sodium sulfate) may serve to dislodge the young worms before they become embedded in the intestinal mucosa and the females start larvipositing.

FILARIASIS

Etiology. Filariasis is produced by one of several filarial worms, the most important being *Wuchereria bancrofti, Brugia malayi, Onchocerca volvulus* and *Loa loa.* The adult worms are threadlike objects characteristically living in certain body tissues. *Wuchereria bancrofti* and *B. malayi* inhabit lymphatic vessels and lymphoid tissues; Onchocerca adults are immured in fibrous subcutaneous nodules; *Loa loa* migrate through subcutaneous tissues. These worms all produce microscopic embryos called microfilariae, which eventually migrate through the superficial blood vessels or skin.

Epidemiology. *Wuchereria bancrofti* is widely distributed through the tropics in both hemispheres; *B. malayi* occurs in India, the Far East and the Southwest Pacific. Onchocerca is found in tropical Africa, in areas where Guatemala and Mexico are contiguous, in Venezuela and in one limited focus of Colombia, South America. The loa worm is found exclusively in tropical Africa.

Microfilariae are picked up by bloodsucking flies and develop to the infective-stage larvae in their thoracic muscles. *Wuchereria bancrofti* and *B. malayi* utilize mosquitoes; Onchocerca, species of black gnats (Simulium); *Loa loa*, the mango fly (Chrysops). After incubation in the appropriate insect host the larvae migrate to the tip of the fly's proboscis and enter the victim's skin in or near the puncture wound made by the fly. In endemic areas children are more commonly infected than older persons.

Pathology. The developmental period in Bancroft's filariasis may be as long as a year, but is not definitely known. Indirect evidence indicates that the larvae, on entering the skin, invade lymphatic vessels and may make long migrations through the lymphatic system before they reach the sites where they mature and mate, and the females begin to parturiate. During this period, if they lodge for any time in a lymph node and thus block lymph flow, they may produce an acute lymphangitis and associated lymphadenitis. At the end of the incubation period the microfilariae discharged by the female appear in the tissues around the parent worms, and within a short time those of Wuchereria, Brugia and *Loa loa* may be found in the blood. Tissue reaction may be temporary during the migration of larvae or adults, but in Bancroft's and Malayan filariasis there is usually a series of acute episodes of lymphangitis, often with fever, and subsequently there is fibrosis of the dead or dying parent worms, resulting at times in permanent blockage of lymphatic vessels. In onchocerciasis, fibrosis around the adult worms develops without acute local reaction, but almost invariably with systemic sensitization. In loa infection there is only temporary swelling in the subcutaneous tissues through which the worm is migrating.

Clinical Manifestations. In infection with Bancroft's and Malayan filariasis the incubation period may be marked by acute lymphangitis or allergic states. A second period, usually symptomless, begins when microfilariae are first recoverable, a year or more after exposure. Most patients have repeated attacks of lymphangitis, usually with fever. With fibrotic obstruction of lymph flow, elephantiasis gradually develops, and the skin becomes thickened and is deprived of practically all its blood supply. It cracks readily, providing easy entry for secondary pathogens. The subcutaneous tissues are remarkably thickened and consist of a matrix of fibrous tissue in which lymphatic fluid and adipose tissue are locked.

Onchocerca adults produce a painless swelling on any site of the body, but particularly at the junction of the long bones and on the temporal and occipital areas of the head. Their microfilariae, especially from parent nodules in the upper part of the trunk, neck and scalp, tend to migrate to the eyeball and optic nerve, causing diminished vision and, eventually, blindness. Loa usually produces only pruritus, but at times there is generalized edema or giant urticaria.

Diagnosis. This is suggested by the clinical manifestations, and is confirmed by recovery of the microfilariae in blood at night (*W. bancrofti, B. malayi*), in the daytime (*Loa loa*) or in biopsied skin (Onchocerca). When parent worms have died and during biologic incubation, microfilariae will be absent.

Prognosis. The prognosis depends on the degree of involvement and on the location of the lesions.

Prevention. This is difficult and requires control of the breeding of bloodsucking flies. DDT and other insect toxicants have provided a moderately effective means of control.

Treatment. There is no simple chemotherapy for any filarial infection, although Suramin (naphuride sodium) and Hetrazan (diethylcarbamazine citrate) are effective. Hetrazan has the advantage of oral administration. In Bancroft's filariasis, given in the amount for adults of 0.5 to 2.0 mg. per kg. for 2 to 3 weeks, it rapidly kills the microfilariae and acts more slowly on the adult worms. Allergic reactions to the drug are not uncommon. In onchocerciasis the drug is often not well tolerated. In onchocerciasis the subcutaneous tumors should be excised as soon as they appear, to lessen the possibility of grave ocular disease. In loaiasis the parent worm is readily removed when it crosses in front of the eye or over the bridge of the nose.

Immature filarial worms of species not adapted to complete maturity in man are occasionally found in subcutaneous nodules of the extremities, trunk and head in the southern United States, Latin America and Mediterranean countries.

DRACUNCULOSIS
(DRACONTIASIS)

Dracunculosis is produced by the dragon or Medina worm, *Dracunculus medinensis*, a distant relative of the filarial worms. It is prevalent in India, the Middle East, tropical Africa, Indonesia and Arabian countries and, to a less extent, in other areas. The meter-long adult female migrates from the viscera to the skin to deposit living young in fresh water when a small blistered area of the skin produced by the anterior tip of the worm breaks open in contact with the water, as, for example, during bathing or wading. Infection results from drinking or rinsing the mouth with water containing the infected intermediate host, Cyclops.

Treatment. In 1952 diethylcarbamazine (Hetrazan) was used in treating patients with incapacitating dracunculosis in an endemic village in French Sudan; the results were satisfactory. Subsequently (1965) a clinical test was carried out in heavily infected villages on the Ivory Coast of Africa with the drug CIBA 32644-Ba, also with favorable results.

No practical method of **prevention** has been developed.

INFECTIONS PRODUCED BY TAPEWORMS (CESTODA)

Tapeworms are flatworms (Platyhelminthes); they are invertebrate animals which have either a simplified digestive tract or none at all, a protonephridial excretory system, male and female genitalia usually in the same organism (hermaphroditism), no body cavity and, primitively, a ciliated ectodermal covering. Each tapeworm consists of a group of coordinated units: (1) a scolex or "head," provided with suckers and frequently with rostellar hooklets for attachment; (2) a "neck" or region of growth; (3) a series of proglottids or segments, beginning with immature ones arising from the distal part of the neck and becoming increasingly developed and finally gravid in the distal portion of the worm. The entire worm is called a strobila. Each mature proglottid contains a full set of male and female genitalia. The gravid proglottids are storehouses of eggs. Tapeworms have the following stages in their life cycle: egg, embryo, larva, adult.

The important tapeworm infections of man are teniasis (including the larval-stage infection cysticercosis), hymenolepiasis, diphyllobothriasis and hydatid disease. Dog tapeworm (*Dipylidium caninum*) infection occasionally occurs in children who fondle infected dogs or cats. The epidemiologic aspects of these infections are summarized in Table 10-27 (p. 718).

TENIASIS

Etiology. Teniasis is produced by the beef tapeworm, *Taenia saginata*, and the pork tapeworm, *Taenia solium*. The former has a length of 15 feet or more, contains about 1000 to 2000 proglottids or "segments" and has a head with 4 suckers, but no rostellar hooklets. *Taenia solium* seldom attains a length of more than 5 to 8 feet, has less than 1000 proglottids and has an apical ring of rostellar hooklets, as well as 4 head suckers. The most distal proglottids are gravid and contain fully embryonated eggs which may be passed in feces, but are more commonly excreted in proglottids (Fig. 10-108) which are detached from the parent worm.

Epidemiology. *Taenia saginata* infection is common in beef-eating peoples such as the Mohammedans and also occurs in the United States. *Taenia solium* infection occurs most often in eastern and southeastern Europe, is no longer

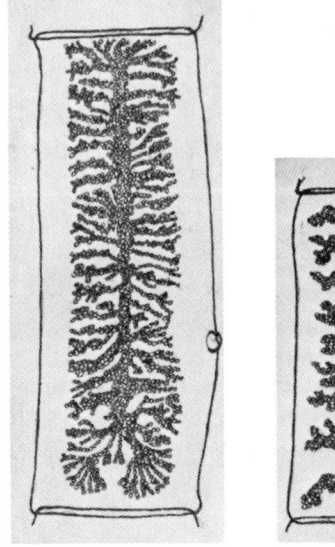

A   B

Figure 10-108. Gravid proglottids of *Taenia saginata* and *T. solium*, as passed in the feces or as they migrate from the anus, showing differential patterns of uteri. *A, T. saginata; B, T. solium*. (After Faust, in Brennemann's *Practice of Pediatrics*. Courtesy of W. F. Prior Co.)

indigenous in the United States, but is as common as *T. saginata* in Mexico and certain other Latin American countries. Gravid proglottids, discharged in human feces, disintegrate, and the contaminated soil is infective for cattle (*T. saginata*) or hogs (*T. solium*). The larval stage (cysticercus) develops in striated muscle of these animals, and the flesh becomes infective in about 3 months. Human beings who consume raw or rare beef or pork containing the cysticercus larvae are liable to infection.

Pathology. The larvae are digested out of the meat in the human stomach, become attached in the mucosa of the upper small intestine and, in about 3 months, develop into mature worms. Although there is slight inflammatory reaction at the site of attachment, the important pathogenic action is toxic and allergenic, with systemic reactions. Occasionally obstruction of the bowel may result from a tangled mass of worms or from detached proglottids which become lodged in the lumen of the appendix.

Clinical Manifestations. Toward the end of the incubation period there is considerable digestive disturbance, including mucous diarrhea due to the irritative action of the worm's by-products on the intestinal mucosa. There may be false hunger pains, especially at night. When the worm is mature, there may be no intestinal disturbance, but there may be other evidences, including (1) inconvenience from gravid proglottids which, having migrated from the anus, crawl down the leg; (2) nutritional drain on the patient; (3) appendiceal inflammation from detached proglottids; and (4) neurotoxic symptoms.

Man is also subject to infection with the cysticercus stage of *T. solium* by swallowing eggs in contaminations from his own or another person's intestinal infection. These cysticerci lodge in any soft tissue, including the brain, the meninges and the eyeball. Involvement of the brain usually results in a jacksonian type of epilepsy.

Initially there is a leukocytosis with moderate eosinophilia; later there is a slight neutropenia with monocytosis and, at times, a secondary anemia.

Diagnosis. Teniasis can be diagnosed by recovery of Taenia eggs in the stool or from anal swabs, but most patients do not pass eggs in appreciable numbers. Specific diagnosis can be made from a gross examination of gravid proglottids passed in the stool or migrating from the anus. When these are freed of debris and flattened in the fresh condition (not hardened in alcohol or formalin) between 2 glass slides, it is easy to count the number of main lateral arms of the uterus. In *Taenia saginata* the number is 15 to 21, in *T. solium,* 7 to 13 (Fig. 10-108).

Prognosis. This is good in intestinal teniasis if the worms are removed. Rarely, acute intestinal or appendiceal obstruction is a hazard. In cysticercosis the cerebral lesions may have serious consequences.

Prevention. Teniasis may be prevented by eating only previously frozen or well cooked beef and pork. More fundamental is the sanitary disposal of human feces.

Treatment. Oleoresin of male fern (aspidium filix-mas) and carbon tetrachloride are relatively toxic and require hospitalization of the patient. Quinacrine (Atabrine) is superior to either in effectiveness and ease of administration and is less toxic.

For treatment with Atabrine the patient should be on a light, nonconstipating diet for the preceding 48 hours and should have complete evacuation of the bowels the night before the drug is administered, preferably with castor oil purgation. In the morning on an empty stomach the adult patient takes five 0.1-gm. tablets of Atabrine by mouth preceded a half-hour earlier by administration of an antiemetic. For children the dose is reduced in proportion to developmental, not chronologic, age. One hour later castor oil purgation is advised to evacuate the worm, which is characteristically passed intact, deeply yellow-orange stained and contracted, but alive. Nausea and possibly vomiting may be anticipated. To reduce these side effects no food or carbonated drinks should be permitted until after a good bowel movement.

HYMENOLEPIASIS

Etiology. Hymenolepiasis is produced by the dwarf tapeworm, *Hymenolepis nana,* and the rat tapeworm, *H. diminuta.* The former is a small worm, only 1 to 2 cm. in length. Its head is provided with 4 suckers and a crown of rostellar hooklets. *Hymenolepis diminuta* is considerably larger (20 to 60 cm. in length) and has suckers but no hooklets on the head. The most distal gravid proglottids disintegrate as they become fully ripe, setting the characteristic eggs (Figs. 10-100, *D;* 10-109) free in the small bowel to be evacuated in the feces.

Epidemiology. The dwarf tapeworm, *Hymenolepis nana,* is cosmopolitan in distribution, except in cold climates. It is most commonly a parasite of children. Although this species is found in rats and mice, the strains are distinct and are not readily infective for man. Human infection with *H. diminuta* results primarily from contact with infected rat or mouse fleas. *Hy-*

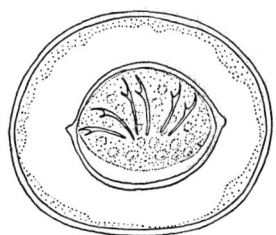

Figure 10-109. Egg of *Hymenolepis diminuta,* × 500. (Faust and Russell: *Clinical Parasitology.* Lea & Febiger.)

menolepis nana infections are common in children in the southern United States, in many countries of Latin America, India and in the Mediterranean area. Hymenolepis diminuta infections have been recorded from several countries, including the United States.

Eggs of H. nana passed in human feces are directly infective for man. They hatch soon after ingestion. On reaching the duodenum the escaping embryos bore into the villi, transform into larvae, return to the intestinal lumen, become attached, and grow into adults within a few weeks. Eggs of H. diminuta must undergo larval development in certain insects, usually rat fleas. Ingestion of these intermediate hosts is the source of infection for human beings.

Pathology. Except in heavy infections, the damage produced is largely toxic. There is suggestive evidence that in continued heavy infections with H. nana internal autoinfection occurs repeatedly.

Clinical Manifestations. There may or may not be clinical evidence of infection. A single H. nana in a child may at times evoke severe manifestations, with irritability, insomnia, loss of appetite and weight, and rarely convulsions. On the other hand, a moderate number in another child may evoke only mild symptoms. There is usually a moderate eosinophilia.

Diagnosis. This is made by demonstration of eggs (Figs. 10-100, D; 10-109) in the feces.

Prognosis. This is almost always good, provided specific medication is instituted promptly. In heavy infections with H. nana the prognosis may be poor, owing to repeated internal autoinfection.

Prevention. Dwarf tapeworm infection can be controlled only by the most careful personal and group hygiene and by treatment of all infected persons. Rat tapeworm infection may be eliminated as a human infection by campaigns against rats and mice and by use of DDT in rat runs or in nests to kill rodent fleas.

Treatment. See under Teniasis. Hexylresorcinol (Crystoids anthelmintic), as administered in ascariasis in association with hookworm infection (p. 724), is moderately efficient and should be tried first in small children because of its low toxicity. Atabrine (quinacrine) is probably more dependable in older children.

DIPHYLLOBOTHRIASIS

Etiology. Diphyllobothriasis is produced by the fish tapeworm, Diphyllobothrium latum, which measures 5 to 30 feet in length and has possibly as many as 3000 proglottids. The head is spatulate and is provided with a pair of longitudinal sucking grooves, one dorsal and one ventral in position. The proglottids never become strictly gravid, but discharge immature eggs.

Epidemiology. Fish tapeworm infection is prevalent in the lake districts of Minnesota and northern Michigan, adjacent territory in Canada and in the lake districts of Chile and Argentina, northern, eastern and southeastern Europe, U.S.S.R., including Siberia, Palestine, Syria, Japan and Australia. Elsewhere it is rarely endemic. Gefüllte fish may be a source of infection if it is eaten before it has been cooked. The immature eggs passed in feces are broadly ovoidal and operculate (Fig. 10-100, C). When discharged into cold fresh water, they must incubate for about 2 weeks, whereupon the shell opens to release a ciliated embryo. This swimming organism is eaten by little "water fleas" of the genera Diaptomus and Cyclops, in the bodies of which the embryos transform into procercoid (first-stage) larvae. Small fresh-water fish consume the infected water fleas and acquire infection in their flesh, the plerocercoid or sparganum (second-stage) larvae. Larger fish in turn consume the smaller ones and acquire the infection in their muscular tissues. Man, dogs or bears eat the fish in a raw or inadequately processed condition and become infected.

Pathology. Fish tapeworm infection frequently produces a toxic state, possibly due to absorption of unsaturated fatty acids, particularly if the worms are attached to the duodenal mucosa, where they prevent absorption of vitamin B_{12}.

Clinical Manifestations. In addition to the toxic symptoms, fish tapeworm may be associated with a primary anemia. It is believed that the tapeworm, when attached to the duodenal or jejunal mucosa, precipitates an anemic state in persons having an unstable equilibrium with respect to the antianemic intrinsic factor. There is usually a leukocytosis with eosinophilia, followed in the chronic period by a leukopenia with a monocytosis. At times there is a macrocytic or normocytic hyperchromic anemia.

Diagnosis. This is made on recovery of the eggs (Fig. 10-100, C) in the patient's feces.

Prognosis. This is good with specific treatment.

Prevention. Thorough cooking of all freshwater fish prevents infection. Prohibition of catching fish during the summer months when the fish are heavily parasitized would also reduce the hazard. Basic control consists in sanitary disposal of human excreta, since the reservoir hosts (dogs and bears) probably contribute little to human infection.

Treatment. See under Teniasis (p. 729).

HYDATID DISEASE
(ECHINOCOCCOSIS)

Etiology. Hydatid disease is produced by the larval stage (hydatid cyst) of Echinococcus granulosus and E. multilocularis, minute worms which live as adults in the small intestine of the dog and its wild relatives. A third species of Echinococcus, E. oligarthrus, has recently been reported to cause human infection in Panama; wild cats are the usual definitive hosts.

Epidemiology. *E. granulosus* is widely distributed wherever sheep, cattle and hogs are associated with dogs. It is particularly common in man in Australia, New Zealand, Palestine, Syria, Argentina, Uruguay, southern Brazil and Chile. Occasionally autochthonous cases occur in the United States. *Echinococcus multilocularis* is common in the highlands of Central Europe, where foxes replace dogs and wood mice replace sheep, cattle and hogs in the natural evolution of the infection (see below). This cycle also occurs in northern Alaska, Siberia and on a small adjacent island of Japan.

The eggs of *E. granulosus* passed in an infected dog's feces initiate the infection in practically any mammal, except a rodent, which ingests the eggs. These hatch in the duodenum; the escaping embryos bore into the intestinal wall, gain access to mesenteric venules or lymphatics and are carried to various parts of the body where they are filtered out. Dogs become infected from eating the carcasses of animals which have died of the disease. Man's association with infected sheep and cattle dogs and parasitized pet dogs provides the means for exposure to the disease.

Pathology. Unless the young larvae lodge in some vital location in the human body, they will usually develop to a considerable size before their presence is discovered. Thus infection acquired in childhood may not be detected until middle life. Although the little hydatid cyst provokes an acute inflammatory reaction at the site of implantation, it proceeds to vacuolate, to develop its germinative layer with many viable heads (scolices) and to accumulate fluid within the cavity. The cysts grow slowly, but in several years may reach the size of a grapefruit or larger. The outer layer is essentially a noncellular laminated structure which is friable; the entire cyst is surrounded by adventitia. The fluid of the *E. granulosus* cyst contains considerable foreign protein and is extremely toxic for the host if there is appreciable leakage. Rupture of a cyst may cause anaphylactic shock or may only set free a large number of viable scolices which become implanted elsewhere and develop secondary cysts. If the cyst reaches the shafts of long bones, it may proceed to grow as a syncytium (osseous hydatid). The most common sites of hydatid cysts in man are, in descending order, the liver, lungs, brain, peritoneal cavity and bone, but no tissues are exempt. The hydatid of *E. multilocularis* is alveolar and has no circumscribing membrane or adventitia. It almost invariably develops in the liver, and is essentially malignant in its growth.

Clinical Manifestations. If the larvae of *E. granulosus* lodge on a heart valve or in the brain or eye, the lesion causes grave symptoms relatively early in the infection. If it develops in the lungs, the first evidence may be a violent paroxysm of coughing with discharge of the contents of a ruptured cyst. If a unilocular cyst is hepatic in location, 20 or more years may pass before the weight of the mass causes sufficient discomfort to bring the patient to a physician. However, a blow on the abdomen may rupture the cyst and cause death from anaphylactic shock. The hydatid of *E. multilocularis* produces symptoms of hepatic disease.

Diagnosis. This is difficult before operation. Eosinophilia is suggestive, but depends on leakage from the cyst. Hydatid thrill is suggestive, but difficult to elicit. Serologic tests are the most reliable. These include complement fixation, bentonite flocculation, indirect hemagglutination and intradermal tests with antigen prepared from sterile hydatid fluid, which is usually obtained from infected sheep.

Prognosis. The prognosis of a unilocular cyst is fair if it is in an operable site. Recurrence resulting from the spilling of scolices from the parent cyst at the time of operation is difficult to avoid. Osseous hydatid disease is serious, and surgical intervention is rarely helpful. In alveolar hydatid disease the prognosis is always grave because the lesion is uncircumscribed.

Prevention. Control in endemic areas involves the deep burying of dead sheep, hogs and cattle. Periodic deworming of dogs with arecoline hydrochloride in endemic areas greatly reduces the amount of exposure to eggs. Man must be careful to keep dog feces from contaminating his food, drink or cooking utensils. Children should not be allowed to play with dogs which have access to sheep, cattle or pigs in endemic areas.

Treatment. No chemotherapy is available for treating the larval stage of the hydatid infections which occur in man. If the cyst is unilocular and in a favorable location for operation, an incision is made down to the outer cyst wall and the hydatid fluid is aspirated, with care not to spill a single drop in the operative area. Then the cyst wall is incised and enough 10 per cent formaldehyde is introduced into the cavity to sterilize the germinative layer. If possible, the entire cyst should be enucleated; if this is not feasible, the cyst should be collapsed and closed with sutures separately from closure of the operative wound. In inoperable cases desensitization with hydatid antigen, as in the treatment of bee allergy, offers some promise of relief.

INFECTIONS PRODUCED BY FLUKES (TREMATODES)

Flukes belong to a group of flatworms (Platyhelminthes) comparable to a single mature segment (proglottid) of a tapeworm. They have an incomplete digestive tract and are either unisexual or hermaphroditic. The flukes which parasitize man have a complicated life cycle, with a required development and multiplication in certain species of snails. Some flukes require a second intermediate host in which encystation occurs. The most important fluke infections are the schistosomiases and those due to the intestinal flukes, the liver flukes and the lung flukes (see Table 10-27, p. 718).

SCHISTOSOMIASIS

Etiology. This group of diseases is produced by the 2 intestinal blood flukes, *Schistosoma japonicum* and *S. mansoni*, and the vesical blood fluke, *S. haematobium*. These worms are unisexual and small enough to live as mated pairs in the smaller venules draining the intestine and the urinary bladder. The female, held in the ventral sex canal of the male (hence the name "schistosome," i.e. "split body"), deposits eggs which will completely fill the venule. Oviposition is repeated in adjacent venules into which the worms migrate, so that entire venous radicles may be crowded with eggs. These eggs are partially embryonated when deposited and soon secrete a lytic fluid which oozes through minute pores in the shell. By pressure on, and digestion of, the wall of the venule the eggs escape into the perivascular tissues and then through the mucous coat of the organ into its lumen, together with extravasated blood. Eggs of the intestinal types are passed in the stool; those of the vesical type, typically in the urine, but at times also in the feces (Figs. 10-100, *E,F*; 10-110).

Epidemiology. Blood fluke infections have an extensive distribution and involve millions of people in endemic territory. *Schistosoma japonicum* occurs in the Orient, especially in central, west and south China; in 5 foci in Japan, in one small focus in Thailand and in the Philippine Islands; *S. mansoni*, in Africa, Arabia, Puerto Rico, some of the Lesser Antilles, extensive areas of Brazil, coastal Surinam and foci in central north Venezuela; *S. haematobium*, in Africa, the Near East, Iran, Iraq, western India and the southern tip of Portugal. Children over 5 years of age are more frequently exposed than adults.

If eggs evacuated in feces or urine soon reach fresh water, they hatch, and the escaping ciliated larvae (miracidia) are enabled to attack and enter the soft tissues of appropriate species of snails. After development and 2 consecutive stages of multiplication in the snails, the parasite emerges in the fork-tailed larval stage (cercaria) and swims in the water, but eventually dies unless it infects man or certain other mammals.

Pathology. When man enters infested water, the blood fluke larvae attach themselves to the skin. They enter cutaneous blood vessels, producing slight injury, are carried to the lungs and gradually squeeze through the capillaries, and most are returned to the systemic circulation. Some larvae break out of the pulmonary capillaries with resultant petechial hemorrhage. The larvae which arrive by way of the mesenteric arteries in the portal blood stream feed on whole blood, grow and then migrate back into the mesenteric venules against the incoming portal blood. *Schistosoma japonicum* enters the drainage of the small bowel; *S. mansoni*, that of the large bowel; and *S. haematobium* typically migrates through the rectal and hemorrhoidal veins into the vesical venous plexus. There the worms mature and mate, and the females begin to lay eggs.

The approximate incubation periods are, for *S. japonicum*, 4 to 5 weeks; for *S. mansoni*, 6 to 7 weeks; and for *S. haematobium*, 10 to 12 weeks. During the incubation period, as the larval worms reach capillaries through which they cannot pass and where they perish, or as they rapidly increase in size in successful locations, an increasing amount of toxic metabolites is distributed throughout the patient's body, but especially among the tissues and organs in the vicinity of the worms. Then, as eggs are laid, there is initially extensive trauma as they escape from the blood vessels and filter through the tissues. Later, pseudoabscesses form around eggs which become lodged in the perivascular tissues. These lesions usually are transformed into pseudotubercles.

Clinical Manifestations. At each site of invasion of the skin by the cercariae there is a minute lesion with sharp needling pain which lasts only a few hours. As the larval worms pass through the lungs and later lodge elsewhere, there is considerable local and generalized reaction, particularly in the liver, which becomes greatly enlarged and tender, and on the skin, where giant urticaria typically develops. Toward the end of the incubation period there are late afternoon fever and night sweats. In the intestinal types there is a prodromal toxic diarrhea. Then, with the discharge of eggs, there is dysentery (*S. japonicum*, *S. mansoni*) or hematuria (*S. haematobium*). The patient usually becomes acutely ill

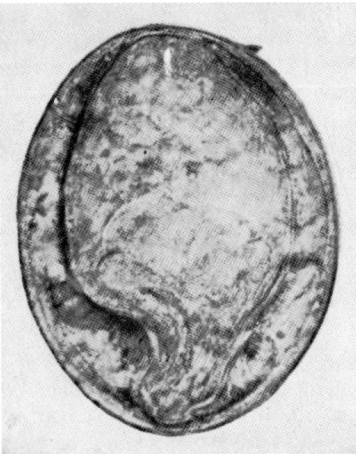

Figure 10-110. Egg of *Schistosoma japonicum* as seen in freshly passed feces, × 660. (After Faust, in Brennemann's *Practice of Pediatrics.* Courtesy of W. F. Prior Co.)

and, in the intestinal types, bedridden. After a few weeks of rest the dysentery is arrested, but on physical exertion is reactivated. Digestive disturbances are increased as fibrosis of the intestinal wall develops, and papillomas and cicatricial tissue prevent the normal passage of food or feces. There is periportal hepatic cirrhosis, the spleen becomes greatly enlarged, and the thoracic cavity is reduced in capacity by the increase in size of the abdominal viscera. In the vesical type the urinary bladder gradually becomes thickened, fibrosed and infiltrated with phosphatic salts. Renal colic is caused by bladder stones produced by deposition of uric acid crystals on the eggs as nuclei. In the intestinal types, ascites develops in the chronic stage, which occurs relatively early in the Oriental type. In the vesical type there is incontinence of urine. In both intestinal varieties of schistosomiasis, sepsis may be anticipated in the chronic stage, and carcinoma of the liver, intestinal wall or urinary bladder may develop as a result of constant irritation.

During the acute stage there is pronounced eosinophilia. Later there is a neutropenia with a moderate eosinophilia and monocytosis.

Diagnosis. This is made by recovery of the typical eggs in the stool (*S. japonicum*, Fig. 10-110; *S. mansoni*, Fig. 10-100, *E*) or in the urine (*S. haematobium*, Fig. 10-100, *F*, p. 719).

Prognosis. This is fair to excellent in the acute or early chronic stage with specific therapy, but is poor in long-standing or inadequately treated chronic infections. In highly endemic areas of China and the Philippines, children who are repeatedly subjected to heavy exposure die of the disease before reaching maturity.

Prevention. The use of the molluscicide, sodium pentachlorophenate (Santobrite), to kill the snails which are intermediate hosts and prohibition of wading or bathing in suspected water are temporary and relatively inadequate measures. Permanent control can be effected only by public health education, especially concerning sanitary disposal of human excreta. In endemic areas of *S. japonicum* infection the control problem is complicated by many mammalian reservoir hosts which can perpetuate the disease in the absence of human infection.

Treatment. Antimony salts are specific. Sodium antimony tartrate and potassium antimony tartrate (0.5 to 2 per cent solutions) are the drugs most likely to be effective in a single course of treatment, but their toxicity should be appreciated. The antimonials are introduced slowly into a vein, with care not to allow a single drop to escape into perivascular tissues and so cause painful necrosis. The patient must be recumbent during the period of administration and for at least a half-hour thereafter. The drug is administered 3 times a week for 4 to 12 weeks, beginning with 6 ml. and increasing to a tolerance of 20 ml. of the 0.5 per cent solution in adults with a weight of 50 kg., with proportional reductions for children.

Fuadin (stibophen), another antimony compound, is better tolerated and more easily administered than the antimony tartrates. It is injected intramuscularly and is more slowly absorbed, but its efficiency is considerably less, and treatment frequently must be repeated. The drug is administered as a 6 per cent solution 3 times a week. The first and second injections consist of 1.5 and 3.5 ml., respectively, and are followed by 9 injections of 5 ml. each. These dosages are for adults, but may be given to children 9 years of age or older. Fractional doses should be given to younger children.

The diaminoxanthone compound, Miracil D, which is administered orally, has been used with some success for *S. haematobium* infection, but is ineffective for intestinal schistosomiases.

In advanced chronic cases specific treatment is useless because of the irreparable visceral damage.

Cercarial (Schistosome) Dermatitis. The cercariae of human blood flukes do not produce "swimmer's itch." Swimmer's itch, or cercarial dermatitis, is caused by penetration of cercariae of blood flukes which are not able to complete their development in the human body. These are usually blood flukes of aquatic birds, occasionally of passerine birds or of domestic mammals. "Cercarial dermatitis" is widely distributed throughout the world, including the lake districts of northern United States and both fresh- and salt-water areas along the east and west coasts. These cercariae on entry into the epidermis are not able to get into the cutaneous blood vessels, and their presence causes a pruritic dermatitis (Fig. 10-111). Children are highly susceptible.

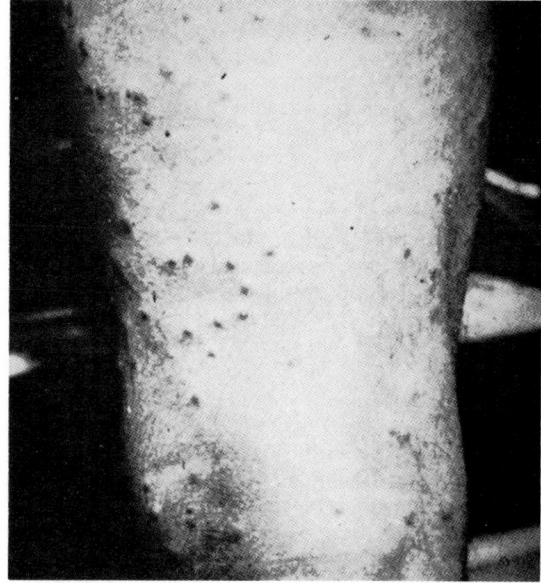

Figure 10-111. Papular eruption of leg in cercarial dermatitis (swimmer's itch) acquired in a Michigan lake. (After D. B. McMullen, Army Medical Graduate School, from Hunter, Frye and Swartzwelder: *Manual of Tropical Medicine.*)

INTESTINAL FLUKE INFECTIONS
(Intestinal Trematodiasis)

Etiology. Several groups of trematodes inhabit the intestine of man. These include *Fasciolopsis buski*, the giant intestinal fluke, which is fleshy and measures 20 to 75 mm. in length by 8 to 20 mm. in breadth; several species of echinostomes, which have a cervical collar of toothlike spines and vary in size from 0.5 to 20 mm. in length by 0.1 to 2.5 mm. in breadth; and the heterophyid species, which superficially resemble small seeds. These worms are most frequently attached to the duodenal and jejunal mucosae. Their eggs are operculate and vary in size from 140 by 85 microns (*F. buski*) to 28 by 16 microns (heterophyid species).

Epidemiology. *Fasciolopsis buski* has an extensive distribution in the Far East, southeast Asia and eastern India. It is contracted from the consumption of raw water plants such as the "water chestnut" and "buffalo nut," on which its larval stage is encysted. Echinostome species are found in the Far East, India and occasionally in the United States and the Balkans; infection with these species results from eating raw plant and animal tissues. Heterophyid species are present in the Orient, Egypt and the Balkans; they reach the human intestine in raw or inadequately cooked fresh-water and brackish-water fish. Some of the species occur commonly in reservoir hosts.

Pathology. The adult worms, especially the larger species, tend to erode the intestinal mucosa at the site of attachment. Moreover, their by-products are absorbed. Heterophyid flukes provide an additional grave hazard, since their minute eggs may get into the mesenteric lymphatics and venules and be carried to various vital organs such as the myocardium, where they cause small pseudotubercle formations.

Clinical Manifestations. When the adult worms of the larger species attach themselves to the intestinal mucosa, they provoke intestinal disturbances, including a mucous diarrhea. Their by-products, when absorbed, cause edema (especially around the eyes), ascites and even anasarca. These symptoms are frequent in children, the age group most commonly infected. When the minute eggs of the heterophyid flukes lodge in the heart muscle, they provoke a myocardial disturbance; in the central nervous system they embarrass motor and sensory functions.

Diagnosis. This is made by recovery of the particular type of egg from the feces.

Prognosis. This is good to excellent with specific anthelmintic medication, except in heterophyid infections in which eggs have infiltrated into critical centers.

Prevention. Control is particularly difficult, since the parasites exist in many hosts. Thorough cooking of all foods provides a safeguard, but is not likely in endemic areas.

Treatment. Tetrachloroethylene, as administered in hookworm infection, and hexylresorcinol crystoids (Crystoids anthelmintic) are efficient drugs.

LIVER FLUKE INFECTIONS
(Hepatic Trematodiasis)

Etiology. The important liver flukes which parasitize man are *Fasciola hepatica*, the sheep liver fluke; *Clonorchis sinensis*, the Chinese liver fluke; and *Opisthorchis felineus* and *O. viverrini*, the cat flukes. *Fasciola hepatica* is a moderately large species which lives in the proximal bile passages and the gallbladder. Clonorchis and Opisthorchis are delicate, lanceolate species which inhabit the bile ducts. Fasciola lays large eggs (140 by 75 microns) practically indistinguishable from those of *F. buski*. Eggs of Clonorchis measure 29 by 16 microns, and those of Opisthorchis 30 by 11 microns. These eggs are transported in bile and evacuated in feces.

Epidemiology. *Fasciola hepatica* exists wherever sheep are raised and is an important parasite in these and other herbivorous mammals. Human infections are uncommon, but there are several hundred autochthonous records from Latin America and southwestern France, and a few from Hawaii and California. Man frequently acquires fasciola infection from eating raw watercress. Clonorchiasis is common throughout the Orient, and is prevalent in eastern and southeastern Europe and U.S.S.R., including Siberia. Infection is acquired by man and other mammals that eat raw fresh-water fish.

Pathology. On consumption of food containing the encysted larvae and their passage into the duodenum, excystation occurs. The larvae of Fasciola migrate through the bowel wall, traverse the peritoneal cavity, penetrate Glisson's capsule and burrow through the hepatic parenchyma to the larger bile ducts. They produce extensive damage to the hepatic parenchyma. The larvae of Clonorchis and Opisthorchis migrate through the ampulla of Vater to the smaller bile ducts. Occasionally Fasciola larvae en route from the duodenum to the bile ducts via the peritoneal cavity lodge and develop in ectopic foci, as in the abdominal wall.

Clinical Manifestations. When the worms are established and mature, they provoke hyperplasia of the biliary epithelium, followed by fibrotic encapsulation of the duct and eventually by pressure necrosis of the parenchyma, occasionally terminating in periportal cirrhosis. The most frequent symptoms are those of cholecystitis and cholelithiasis.

Diagnosis. This is made by recovery of the eggs from feces or by biliary drainage. The latter method is more reliable in view of the close resemblance of the various eggs to those of intestinal trematodes.

Prognosis. This is fairly good if liver function is not seriously impaired.

Prevention. The only practical prophylactic

measure is thorough cooking of salad greens and fresh-water fish.

Treatment. Emetine hydrochloride (6 per cent solution), administered in the amount of 0.036 gm. (³⁄₅ grain) intramuscularly daily for 9 to 12 days, is fairly satisfactory for removing Fasciola, and in this dosage is relatively safe. There are no satisfactory drugs for treatment of clonorchis and opisthorchis infections, although Bithionol, as used in lung fluke infection (see below) has apparently been effective in some Japanese patients.

LUNG FLUKE INFECTION
(Pulmonary Trematodiasis; Paragonimiasis)

Etiology. The only fluke which produces pulmonary infection in man is *Paragonimus westermani*. This is a fleshy little worm somewhat resembling the kernel of a hazelnut. The eggs are broadly ovoidal, dark golden brown, have a relatively flat operculum, and measure about 90 by 55 microns.

Epidemiology. *Paragonimus westermani* is widely distributed through the Orient and the Southwest Pacific islands, and has been found in isolated regions of northwestern South America. Man, cats and dogs are exposed to infection when they eat raw or inadequately pickled crab and crayfish meat in infected areas.

Pathology. On arrival in the duodenum the larvae excyst and migrate through the intestinal wall, traverse the peritoneal cavity, bore through the diaphragm and reach the lungs by way of the pleural cavity. They migrate to sites near bronchioles and provoke tissue encapsulation. In addition, these worms may become lodged in nonpulmonary tissue, particularly the brain, abdomen, groin and neck.

In the lungs the worms become partly walled off, but invariably have an opening into an adjacent bronchiole. The eggs escape into the bronchiole and are coughed up, at times with blood.

Clinical Manifestations. In pulmonary infections there is excessive bronchial secretion which may have a rusty brown color, owing to the presence of eggs. Hemoptysis occurs periodically. In the abdomen the worms typically provoke abscess formation, and in the groin, a small hard tumor. Cerebral lesions may result in seizures, especially in infected children in Japan.

Diagnosis. Pulmonary infection requires differentiation from tuberculosis and other pulmonary diseases. The diagnosis is established by identifying the eggs in the sputum or, when swallowed, in the feces. Though this worm may be suspected as the cause of symptoms in other regions of the body, specific diagnosis depends on biopsy or on postmortem examination.

Prognosis. This is fair to good in pulmonary infection, fair in abdominal or groin involvement, and grave in cerebral infection.

Prevention. No effective control has been developed, but thorough cooking of crabs and crayfish would safeguard man.

Treatment. The Japanese synthetic drug, Bithionol (2.2-thiobis [4.6-dichlorophenol]), has helminthicidal effect on this worm in tolerated doses.

ARTHROPODS AS CAUSATIVE AGENTS AND TRANSMITTERS OF DISEASE

The role of arthropods (i.e. insects and their allies) in the production of disease is threefold: (1) certain arthropods elaborate venoms which they introduce into the human body; (2) other arthropods are tissue invaders; (3) many arthropods are mechanical transmitters of pathogenic microorganisms, and more are obligatory incubators and transmitters of disease-producing microorganisms.

VENENATING ARTHROPODS

This group of arthropods includes centipedes, scorpions, spiders, ticks, mites and several species of insects.

Centipedes. These animals have a pair of hollow jaws which serve as fangs to introduce into the skin toxic substances elaborated in their heads. The venom is relatively weak and at most, even in an infant, will produce an inflammatory reaction at the puncture site and mild lymphangitis. It may be treated with local compresses.

Scorpions. Many species of scorpions, including the dangerous ones in the southwestern United States, Latin America, many areas in Africa, southern Europe, Israel and India, have potent venom. This is elaborated in the swollen caudal segment and is introduced through the sharp, hollow caudal extremity into the skin of a person who accidentally steps on the animal or unconsciously brushes it with the arm.

The venom of some species produces only local tissue reaction, while that of other species is primarily neurotoxic in its action. The latter type of venom contains several fractions, including hemolysins, endotheliolysins and neurotoxins. In addition to an intense, aching pain, radiating from the site of the injury, and lymphadenitis, there is typically an ascending motor paralysis, with convulsions resembling those observed in strychnine poisoning, rapid weak pulse, extreme thirst, and dysuria; at times there is evidence of an acute pancreatitis. Deaths from scorpion stings occur particularly in children under 4 years of age. In most countries where the more dangerous species are common, standardized species-specific or group-specific antivenin is available for intramuscular administration.*

Supportive treatment consists initially in in-

---

*Antivenin for species of Centruroides in the southwestern United States is available from Laboratorias Myn, Avenida Coyoacán 1707, Mexico 12, D.F.

filtrating into the puncture wound a 2 per cent solution of procaine containing 1:1000 epinephrine to relieve pain, then parenteral administration of glucose and amino acid solutions. Shock should be treated with parenteral solutions, including blood plasma. Morphine is not indicated. Such patients can be controlled effectively by phenobarbital. Relatively large doses of sodium phenobarbital are necessary for irrational patients and those with convulsions. For example, 6 mg. per kg. of sodium phenobarbital may be injected subcutaneously initially in infants and children; subsequent doses of similar amounts are given at intervals of 20 or 30 minutes up to 4 or 5 administrations.

The application of residual sprays of the insecticides DDT or BHC in and around homes and outbuildings where scorpions hide will greatly reduce their numbers.

Spiders. All spiders produce venoms to stun or kill their prey, but relatively few species have powerful enough fangs or potent enough venom to endanger human beings as does the black widow spider of the United States, *Latrodectus mactans.* When her web is accidentally touched by the unprotected human body, this spider attacks. She strikes with her incurved fangs and inserts them deeply into tender skin. There is an immediate sharp pain at the site, with a burning, swollen, inflamed area around the puncture wound. The venom enters the bloodstream and produces dizziness, weakness, tremors, abdominal cramps and typically a spastic contraction of the muscles, particularly of the abdomen. There is rapid shallow respiration, tachycardia and high arterial blood pressure. Acute nephritis may develop as a result of the intoxication. Hemoglobinuria has been reported in small children. The double fang markings at the site of inoculation may provide a diagnostic clue, but diagnosis is usually from the clinical history.

Treatment consists in intramuscular injection of standardized species- or group-specific antivenin.* Pain can be reduced by the intravenous injection of 10 ml. of a 10 per cent solution of calcium gluconate. Barbiturates may be needed to allay muscle spasm and pain. Neostigmine bromide, U.S.P., may also be used to reduce spasms of smooth muscle. Most of the reported deaths have occurred because the patients were brought to the hospital too late for supportive or antivenin treatment.

Species of the hairy brown genus Loxosceles, which are domestic in their habitats, produce *necrotic arachnidism. Loxosceles laëta* and *L. rufipes* in South America cause topical necrosis and at times systemic hemolysis. In Missouri, Kansas and the southwestern United States the species *L. reclusa* is relatively common in closets, cellars and outbuildings. It is not aggressive, but when crushed or entangled in clothing, both the male and the female bite, causing severe local

pain, with rapid development of an indurated wheal which transforms into a violaceous sloughing ulcer, leaving a deep granulating base. Healing takes place slowly. Within 24 to 36 hours after the bite systemic reactions consisting of restlessness, fever and at times a scarlatiniform rash are observed. Experimentally, the venom has been found to contain a powerful necrotoxin. Parenteral administration of corticotropin to victims of Loxosceles bites will hasten healing of the wound.

Ten per cent DDT in kerosene sprayed on the spider's web is lethal to Latrodectus and to Loxosceles.

Ticks and Mites. Many species of ticks and several species of mites cause serious local irritation at the sites on the skin where they take blood meals. The most notorious mites are the chigger ("red bug") and the rat mite. These are particularly irritating for small children. The local lesion at the site of attachment can be effectively treated by application of phenolated camphor solution in pure mineral oil or Quotane ointment (containing 1[β-dimethylaminoethoxyl]-3-n-butylisoquinoline hydrochloride). Dusting of DDT into socks and pants, or rubbing of dimethyl phthalate on the ankles and legs, will usually prevent infestation with these mites.

Tick paralysis. Certain ticks, including the Rocky Mountain wood tick, introduce saliva which may produce a flaccid ascending motor paralysis which begins in the legs. Recovery is usually rapid and complete if the tick is removed quickly, but if it is allowed to remain, death may result from respiratory paralysis.

Insects. These include bees, wasps, ants, blister beetles, moth caterpillars and many bloodsucking insects. The honeybee worker releases her stinger along with venom; the bumblebee retains her stinger. Bees, wasps and ants have both acid and alkaline fractions as well as a histamine-like fraction in their venom. The stinger must be removed carefully after honeybee venenation. Hypersensitive persons who go into shock require prompt use of epinephrine, and then should be desensitized with whole bee extract made up in Coca's solution to minimize subsequent reactions.

Blister beetles produce a painful blister when their juices are brought in contact with the skin. Ammonia will partly neutralize the blister fluid, and a corticosteroid ointment will ease the pain. Certain caterpillars elaborate venom at the base of nettling hairs. When these hairs come in contact with the tender skin or mucous membranes, they produce a painful burn which heals slowly. The pain is partially eased by a corticosteroid ointment.

Many insects, such as mosquitoes, stable flies, fleas, lice and assassin bugs, introduce saliva into the skin before taking a blood meal. This foreign protein produces allergic manifestations in many persons. Since no method of treatment is eminently satisfactory, such hypersensitive persons must learn to protect themselves from these insects.

---

*Antivenin *Latrodectus mactans*, Merck, Sharp and Dohme, is specific.

TISSUE-INVADING ARTHROPODS

Among the arthropods which invade tissues the following are important: the itch mite (*Sarcoptes scabiei*), which produces scabies; the chigoe (*Tunga penetrans*); and the maggots or larval stage of many species of filth flies and their relatives, which cause myiasis.

Scabies. This disease, produced by *Sarcoptes scabiei*, is world-wide in distribution and is most frequent in lower economic groups whose personal hygiene is neglected. The adult mite is an 8-legged organism which burrows into the deeper layers of the skin and forms a tunnel nearly parallel to the surface. At the blind end of the tunnel the female lays about 10 eggs a week for 4 or 5 weeks. In 3 to 5 days the eggs hatch, and 6-legged larvae emerge. These young mites either make lateral tunnels or come out of the tunnel and form new ones. Since an entire life cycle may be completed in 11 to 15 days, an infestation, once established, develops rapidly. The tunnel appears superficially as a slightly raised, reddened, somewhat sinuous track. (See page 1412 for clinical discussion.)

Chigoe Infestation. *Tunga penetrans*, a flea, is a common skin parasite of dogs, pigs and bare-footed persons in the American tropics and tropical Africa. The most common sites of infestation are the spaces between the toes, into which the fleas burrow. The females swell to the size of a pea and produce painful, festering lesions. The gravid fleas should be removed with a sterile needle and the wounds painted with tincture of iodine to kill the remaining fleas and eggs. Since infestation is usually acquired from direct contact of the bare foot with dust or dirt harboring fleas from the feet of dogs or pigs, well shod feet practically guarantee safety from attack.

Myiasis. This results from penetration of animal tissues by the larval stage of several species of flies. It may be specific, semispecific or accidental, depending on the species of fly. Myiasis may affect the skin, eye, nasopharynx, ear, intestine or urethra.

Specific myiasis refers to a natural tendency of the gravid fly to deposit eggs or larvae on unbroken skin or uninjured mucous membranes. Certain species, such as the tropical warble fly (*Dermatobia hominis*), the sheep bot (*Oestrus ovis*), the cattle bots (Hypoderma species), the horse bots (Gasterophilus species) and the primary screwworm (*Callitroga hominivorax*), are myiasis-producing forms.

Semispecific myiasis-producing species are those which deposit their eggs or larvae either on or in clean or ulcerated tissues. These include the flesh flies (Sarcophaga species, Wohlfahrtia species) and the common American screwworm (*Callitroga macellaria*). Both groups produce mutilating wounds, which consist of long, serpiginous tunnels under the skin (larva migrans), deep wounds more or less perpendicular to the surface, or excavating lesions which become secondarily infected. Children are the most frequent victims. Death may be due to extensive deep penetration into the lungs, brain or abdominal viscera.

The third type of myiasis is purely accidental, and consists in the implantation of eggs or maggots in wounds, or their temporary lodgment in the intestine or urethra.

Maggots burrowing into tissues or breeding in wounds should be removed as soon as possible. The lesions should be irrigated, treated with a bactericidal ointment, and covered with a sterile dressing. In intestinal myiasis frequent saline purgation and enemas may be helpful. Young children, particularly those around stock farms, should be protected from flies by screening or mosquito netting, and any discharges from the eyes, nares or skin lesions should not be allowed to accumulate, since these attract myiasis-producing flies. Permanent control consists in eradication of breeding by these flies, especially around cattle, horses, hogs and domestic rabbits.

ARTHROPODS AS TRANSMITTING AGENTS OF DISEASE

Arthropods serve in 2 ways to transmit disease-producing microorganisms to man: (*a*) mechanically and (*b*) as essential biologic hosts or incubators of pathogens.

Mechanical Transmitters. The most important group of mechanical transmitters is that of the filth flies, including the common housefly, the lesser houseflies, stable flies, greenbottles, bluebottles, blowflies, the flesh flies, the hover flies, fruit flies and the cluster flies. During epidemics or when food and water are grossly polluted with human excreta, they are often responsible for the transmission of typhoid and other salmonella infections, shigellosis, cholera and amebiasis. Evidence is less conclusive that they play a conspicuous role in the spread of poliomyelitis and epidemic conjunctivitis.

Essential Transmitters. Arthropods which are biologic vectors of pathogens include (1) the ticks, which transmit tick spotted fever, Q fever, Colorado tick fever, hemorrhagic fever, relapsing fever and tularemia; (2) red mites, which transmit scrub typhus, and mouse mites, which transmit murine typhus and rickettsialpox; (3) lice, which transmit epidemic typhus fever, trench fever and relapsing fever; (4) fleas, which transmit plague, murine typhus and several other infections; (5) mosquitoes, which transmit malaria, yellow fever, dengue, a large number of other arboviruses causing viral encephalitis, filariasis and tularemia; (6) sand flies, which transmit kala-azar, cutaneous and mucocutaneous leishmaniasis, Oroya fever and pappataci fever; (7) Glossina flies, which transmit African trypanosomiasis; (8) black gnats, which transmit onchocerciasis; and (9) assassin bugs, which transmit Chagas' disease.

Children are particularly susceptible to all these diseases. In some instances protection can be afforded by vaccine, as in yellow fever, Rocky Mountain spotted fever and typhus fever. In some, individual prophylaxis consists in avoiding endemic territory. In certain diseases, the only practical safeguard consists in dusting the exposed person's clothing with DDT, as in louse-borne typhus fever, or using this insect toxicant as a residual spray, as in areas of rodent plague. One or both of these procedures have been effective in the control of epidemic typhus fever, malaria and filariasis. Another method of attack is the destruction of the reservoir host (i.e. rats in the case of plague and murine typhus). These arthropods are man's greatest enemy and today constitute one of his most serious challenges.

ERNEST CARROLL FAUST

REFERENCES

General

Faust, E. C.: *Human Helminthology.* 3rd ed. Philadelphia, Lea & Febiger, 1949.
Faust, E. C., Russell, P. F., and Jung, R. C.: *Craig and Faust's Clinical Parasitology.* 8th ed. Philadelphia, Lea & Febiger, 1969 (in press).
Faust, E. C., Beaver, P. C., and Jung, R. C.: *Animal Agents and Vectors of Human Disease.* 3rd ed. Philadelphia, Lea & Febiger, 1967.
Hunter, G. W., III, Frye, W. W., and Swartzwelder, J. C.: *A Manual of Tropical Medicine.* 4th ed. Philadelphia, W. B. Saunders Company, 1966.

Nematodes

Beaver, P. C.: The Detection and Identification of Some of the Common Nematode Parasites of Man. *Am. J. Clin. Path.,* 22:481, 1952.
Buckley, J. J. C.: On *Brugia* Gen. Nov. for *Wuchereria* spp. of the "Malayi" Group, etc. *Ann. Trop. Med. & Parasitol.,* 54:75, 1960.
Chaia, G., and Cunha, A. S. da: Terapêutica experimental com o Tiabendazol na estrongiloidíase. *Rev. Inst. Med. trop. S. Paulo,* 8:17, 1966.
Cuckler, A. C., Campbell, W. C., and Egerton, J. R.: The Effect of Thiabendazole on the Migratory Stages of Certain Tissue Invading Nematodes. *Proc. VII Int'l Congr. on Trop. Med. & Malaria,* 2:167, 1963.
Faust, E. C., and others: Unusual Findings of Filarial Infections in Man. *Am. J. Trop. Med. & Hyg.,* 1:239, 1952.
Hall, W. J., III, and McCabe, W. R.: Trichinosis. Report of a Small Outbreak with Observations of Thiabendazole Therapy. *Arch. Int. Med.,* 119:65, 1967.
Hawking, F.: The Chemotherapy of Filarial Infections. *Pharmacol. Rev.,* 7:279, 1955.
Jones, C. A.: Clinical Studies in Human Strongyloidiasis. I. Semeiology. *Gastroenterol.,* 16:743, 1950.
Jung, R. C.: The Predominance of Single-Brood Infections in Human Ascariasis. *J. Parasitol.,* 40:405, 1954.
Jung, R. C., and Beaver, P. C.: Clinical Observations on *Trichocephalus Trichiurus* (Whipworm) Infestation in Children. *Pediatrics,* 8:548, 1952.
Jung, R. C., and McCroan, J. E.: Efficacy of Bephenium and Tetrachlorethylene in Mass Treatment of Hookworm Infection. *Am. J. Trop. Med. & Hyg.,* 9:492, 1960.
March, H. N., Laigret, J., Kessel, J. F., and Bambridge, B.: Reduction in the Prevalence of Clinical Filariasis in Tahiti Following Adoption of a Control Program. *Am. J. Trop. Med. & Hyg.,* 9:180, 1960.
Marshall, C. L., and Yasukawa, K.: Control of Bancroftian Filariasis in the Ryukyu Islands: Preliminary Results of Mass Administration of Diethylcarbamazine. *Am. J. Trop. Med.,* 15:934, 1966.

Most, H., and others: The Treatment of *Strongyloides* and *Enterobius* Infections with Thiabendazole. *Am. J. Trop. Med.,* 14:379, 1965.
Nelson, J. D., McConnell, T. H., and Moore, D. V.: Thiabendazole Therapy of Visceral Larva Migrans: A Case Report. *Am. J. Trop. Med.,* 15:930, 1966.
Raffier, G.: Note préliminaire sur l'activité du CIBA 32644-Ba dans la dracunculose. *Acta Trop.,* 22:350, 1965.
Rodger, F. C.: *Blindness in West Africa.* London, H. K. Lewis & Co., Ltd., 1959.
Rousset, P.: Essai de prophylaxie et de traitement de la dracunculose par la notezine en Adrar. *Bull. Med. de l'Afrique-Occidentale Francaise,* 9:351, 1952.
Stone, O. J., and Mullins, J. F.: First Use of Thiabendazole in Creeping Eruption. *Texas Rep. Biol. & Med.,* 21:422, 1963.
Stone, O. J., Stone, C. T., Jr., and Mullins, J. F.: Thiabendazole— Probable Cure for Trichinosis: Report of First Case. *J.A.M.A.,* 187:536, 1964.
Swartzwelder, J. C., Miller, J. H., and Sappenfield, R. W.: The Treatment of Cases of Ascariasis with Piperazine Citrate. With Observations of the Effect of the Drug on Other Helminthiases. *Am. J. Trop. Med. & Hyg.,* 4:326, 1956.
Turner, L. H.: Studies on Filariasis in Malaya. Treatment of *Wuchereria Malayi* Filariasis with Diethylcarbamazine in Single Daily Doses. *Ann. Trop. Med. & Parasitol.,* 53:180, 1959.
Wilder, H. C.: Nematode Endophthalmitis. *Tr. Am. Acad. Ophthalm.,* 55:99, 1950.

Cestodes

Bonsdorff, B. von: *Diphyllobothrium Latum* as a Cause of Pernicious Anemia. *Exp. Parasitol.* (Rev. Sec.), 5:207, 1956.
Sodeman, W. A., and Jung, R. C.: Treatment of Teniasis with Quinacrine Hydrochloride. *J.A.M.A.,* 148:285, 1952.
Thatcher, V. E., and Souza, O. E.: *Echinococcus Oligarthrus* Diesing, 1863, in Panama and a Comparison with a Recent Human Hydatid. *Ann. Trop. Med. & Parasitol.,* 60:405, 1966.
Vogel, H.: Ueber den Entwicklungszyklus und die Artzuhörigkeit des europaischen Alveolarechinococcus. *Deutsch. med. Wchnschr.,* 80:931, 1955.
Vogel, H.: Ueber den Echinococcus Multilocularis Süddeutschlands. I. Das Bandwurm-stadium von Stämmen menschlicher und tierischer Herkunft. *Zeitsch. Tropenmed. u. Parasitol.,* 8:404, 1957.

Trematodes

Faust, E. C.: *Schistosomiasis Japonica:* Its Clinical Development and Recognition. *Ann. Int. Med.,* 25:585, 1946.
Faust, E. C., and Meleney, H. E.: Studies on *Schistosomiasis Japonica. Am. J. Hyg.,* Monogr. Ser., no. 3, 1924.
Most, H., and others: Schistosomiasis Japonica in American Military Personnel: Clinical Studies of 600 Cases during the First Year after Infection. *Am. J. Trop. Med.,* 30:239, 1950.
Olivier, L.: Schistosome Dermatitis, a Sensitization Reaction. *Am. J. Hyg.,* 49:209, 1949.
Sadun, E. H.: Studies on *Opisthorchis viverrini* in Thailand. *Am. J. Hyg.,* 62:81, 1955.
Sadun, E. H., and Maiphoon, C.: Studies on the Epidemiology of the Human Intestinal Fluke, *Fasciolopsii Buski* (Lankester) in Central Thailand. *Am. J. Trop. Med. & Hyg.,* 2:1070, 1953.
Wykoff, D. E., and others: *Opisthorchis Viverrini* in Thailand— The Life Cycle and Comparison with *O. Felineus. J. Parasit.,* 51:207, 1965.
Yokogawa, M., and others: Chemotherapy of Paragonimiasis with Bithionol. V. Studies on the Minimum Effective Dose and Changes in Abnormal X-ray Shadows in the Chest After Treatment. *Am. J. Trop. Med.,* 12:859, 1963.

Arthropods

Atkins, J. A., Wingo, C. W., Sodeman, W. A., and Flynn, J. E.: Necrotic Arachnidism. *Am. J. Trop. Med. & Hyg.,* 7:165, 1958.
Bogen, E.: The Treatment of Spider Bite Poisoning. In *Venoms,* Publ. 44, AAAS, Washington: 101, 1956.
Buxton, P. A.: *The Louse. An Account of the Lice Which Infest Man, Their Medical Importance and Control.* London, 1939.
Causey, O. R., Causey, C. E., Maroja, O. M., and Macedo, D. G.: The Isolation of Arthropod-Borne Viruses, Including Members of Two Hitherto Undescribed Serological Groups, in the Amazon Region of Brazil. *Am. J. Trop. Med.,* 10:227, 1961.

Cloudsley-Thompson, J. L.: *Spiders, Scorpions, Centipedes and Mites*. New York, Pergamon Press, 1958.

Hoogstraal, H.: Ticks and Tick-Borne Diseases—Some International Problems and Cooperation in this Study. *Int'l Rev. Trop. Med.*, 1:247, 1961.

Horsfall, W. R.: *Medical Entomology. Arthropods and Human Disease*. New York, Ronald Press Co., 1962.

James, M. T.: *The Flies That Cause Myiasis in Man*. U.S. Dept. Agr. Misc. Publ., No. 631. Washington, D.C., 1947.

Kirby-Smith, H. T.: Specific Treatment of Black Widow Spider Bite. *South. M.J.*, 38:696, 1945.

Kohls, G. M.: Vectors of Rickettsial Diseases. *Ann. Int. Med.*, 26:713, 1947.

Link, V. B., and Mohr, C. O.: Rodenticides in Bubonic-Plague Control. *Bull. WHO*, 9:585, 1953.

O'Rourke, F. J.: The Toxicity of Black Widow Spider Venom; in *Venoms*, Publ. 44, AAAS, Washington: 89, 1956.

Schenone, H., Semprevivo, L., and Schirmer, E.: Consideraciones propósito de dos casos Loxoscelismo cutáneo-visceral. *Bol. Chileno de Parasit.*, 14:17, 1959.

Schöttler, W. H. A.: On the Toxicity of Scorpion Venom. *Am. J. Trop. Med. & Hyg.*, 3:172, 1954.

Tropical Eosinophilia

Eosinophilia in the absence of an evident cause suggests occult helminthic infection. Trichinosis and larval toxocariasis (visceral larva migrans) are common forms of helminthic infection in which eosinophilia may be conspicuous while the causative worms are difficult to detect. Certain helminths, such as ascaris and hookworms, whose presence in the adult stage is easily detected by finding eggs in the feces, characteristically produce transient pulmonary infiltration and eosinophilia (Löffler's syndrome) during the period of larval migration through the lungs.

In tropical countries, particularly in India and other southeastern countries of Asia, there occurs, more frequently in adults than in children, a syndrome known as *tropical eosinophilia*. In addition to hypereosinophilia, the outstanding features are chronic or recurrent bronchial asthma and pulmonary infiltration (eosinophilic lung), both of which are relieved by diethylcarbamazine given orally in daily doses of 12 mg. per kg. in 3 divided doses for 4 days.

Tropical eosinophilia was recently shown to be a form of filariasis in which adult worms of an undetermined species, obscurely located, produce microfilariae that are filtered out of the bloodstream and destroyed in the lungs, causing small granulomas. The symptoms are those of bronchial asthma, and the lesions are demonstrable on roentgenograms of the lung. In visceral larva migrans, caused by larval Toxocara infection, the lungs are not usually affected, and in Löffler's syndrome, caused by larval ascariasis, the pulmonary phase and peripheral eosinophilia are notably transient, rarely persisting at remarkable levels for more than 3 weeks.

PAUL C. BEAVER

REFERENCES

Beaver, P. C.: Toxocariasis (Visceral Larva Migrans) in Relation to Tropical Eosinophilia. *Bull. Soc. Path. Exot.*, 55:555, 1962.

Beaver, P., and Danaraj, T. J.: Pulmonary Ascariasis Resembling Eosinophilic Lung. Autopsy Report with Description of Larvae in the Bronchioles. *Am. J. Trop. Med. & Hyg.*, 7:100, 1958.

Danaraj, T. J., Beaver, P. C., and others: The Etiology and Pathology of Eosinophilic Lung (Tropical Eosinophilia). *Am. J. Trop. Med.*, 15:183, 1966.

Gelpi, A. P., and Mustafa, A.: Seasonal Pneumonitis with Eosinophilia. A Study of Larval Ascariasis in Saudi Arabia. *Am. J. Trop. Med.*, 16:646, 1967.

Protozoan Diseases

MALARIA

Malaria results from the invasion of erythrocytes by one of 4 species of protozoan parasites of the genus *Plasmodium*. It is characterized by high fever, which is often intermittent, and by anemia and splenic enlargement. Despite world-wide campaigns aimed at eradication of malaria through interruption of its life cycle in the intermediate host (female mosquitoes of the genus Anopheles), the disease continues to be the principal health problem of warm climates; it is frequently imported to countries in the temperate zones where, in the summer months, it may be spread locally by mosquitoes.

For clinical and diagnostic purposes, malaria may be regarded as 2 disease entities: the more dangerous one, caused by *Plasmodium falciparum* and formerly termed "subtertian" or "malignant tertian malaria," can produce a great variety of acute clinical manifestations and may, if untreated, be fatal within a few days of its onset; the other, caused by *P. vivax* ("benign tertian malaria"), *P. ovale* (a rarity resembling *P. vivax*) or *P. malariae* ("quartan malaria"), is more typically paroxysmal and is almost never fatal. The latter may recur weeks after a primary attack has apparently been cured in contrast to falciparum infections, which, except in the case of drug-resistant strains, rarely recrudesce after standard treatment.

Etiology. Malaria is usually acquired from the bites of previously infected female anopheline mosquitoes. In other instances, malaria, particularly of the quartan type, has developed after the transfusion of infected blood, in which circumstances the pre-erythrocytic phase of the parasite's development in the liver is avoided. The usual evolution of the disease is as follows:

Pre-erythrocytic phase. The *sporozoites* injected by the biting mosquito reach the sinusoids of the liver through the blood stream and enter the cytoplasm of hepatic cells. Growth and nuclear division are rapid, and microscopic cysts (*schizonts*) are formed which contain *merozoites.*

At the end of approximately 6 days of development of falciparum cysts in the liver the cysts rupture, liberating some 40,000 merozoites from each cyst which penetrate red blood cells. In vivax infections as many as 10,000 merozoites develop in each cyst in 8 days, in ovale 15,000 in 9 days, and in quartan 15,000 in 15 days. Not all merozoites enter erythrocytes; some are believed to return to hepatic cells, paving the way for a relapse at a later date.

The prepatent or incubation period (the period between the infecting mosquito bite and the presence of parasites in the blood) varies with the species: *P. falciparum* is 10 to 13 days; *P. vivax* and *ovale*, 12 to 16; and *P. malariae*, 27 to 37, depending on the size of the inoculum. Malaria transmitted by the transfusion of infected blood becomes apparent in a much shorter time. Clinical manifestations of infection induced by any means may be suppressed for many months by subcurative doses of medications; this is particularly so in the cases of vivax and quartan malaria.

Erythrocytic phase. The merozoites which invade red blood cells appear first in stained smears as bluish rings or (*P. malariae*) bands of cytoplasm, with 1 or occasionally 2 red dots of nuclear chromatin. The growing parasites are named *trophozoites,* and appearing with them in the red cells are granules of yellow-brown pigment which consist of hematin derived from the hemoglobin consumed by the parasite to meet its protein requirements. The shape of the organism varies during growth until it becomes round and, with the scattered or clumped pigment, almost fills the red blood cell, which in the case of *P. vivax* is enlarged and stippled.

The nucleus of the parasite now divides asexually several times, its cytoplasm is arranged around the new nuclei, and the pigment aggregates into large clumps; this segmenter or mature *schizont* contains a varying number of merozoites depending on the species: 8 to 28 in *P. falciparum,* 12 to 24 in *P. vivax,* and 6 to 12 in *P. ovale* and *malariae.* The erythrocytes containing these merozoites rupture, and naked merozoites, pigment and erythrocytic debris are freed in the plasma. Those merozoites that escape phagocytosis enter fresh red blood cells. Thus an asexual cycle is begun each time a new crop of merozoites invades red cells, and this cycle, whose duration is of considerable clinical importance, lasts 48 hours in falciparum, vivax and ovale malaria and 72 hours in quartan malaria. The malarial paroxysm does not take place until enough cycles have occurred to produce the amount of parasitic material, pigment and red cell debris required to induce febrile or other reactions.

Certain of the growing parasites fail to divide, the nucleus remaining intact during the period of maturation. They are differentiated into male or female forms which continue to circulate within the host red cells for several weeks before degenerating, even after effective curative treatment. These forms, called *gametocytes,* are of no clinical importance, but are capable of infecting the mosquito.

Mixed infections and broods. Although mixed infections with 2 species may occur, almost invariably one species is responsible for the clinical pattern. Falciparum strains usually dominate vivax, and vivax dominate quartan; only when sufficient immunity is developed to the dominant strain does the other one begin to produce clinical manifestations.

In an infection with a single species distinct broods may develop. Since the merozoites in the liver are not released simultaneously and the erythrocytic schizonts do not all rupture at the same time, some groups of parasites begin their existence in red blood cells before or after the majority, often maturing in sufficient numbers to produce an independent clinical reaction. In vivax infections single broods will produce a febrile reaction every other day, whereas if 2 broods develop, there will be daily paroxysms; though this may also be the case initially in falciparum malaria, the classic picture of intermittent fever is soon disrupted. Two broods of *P. malariae* can be responsible for fever 2 days out of 3, and 3 broods for daily temperature rises.

Epidemiology. Only in regions where the people have gametocytes in their blood can anopheline mosquitoes become infected. Children may be especially important vectors. Transmission of malaria occurs in most tropical and some temperate zones; although North America is now free of indigenous malaria, focal outbreaks have occurred through infection of local mosquitoes by travelers and returning students and servicemen.

Congenital malaria, due to the transfer of the causative agent across the placental barrier, is believed to occur, but is extremely rare, particularly in endemic areas where mothers have acquired some immunity to the disease. Neonatal malaria, on the other hand, is less uncommon, and may result from mingling of infected maternal blood with that of the infant during the birth process.

Pathology. The extent of destruction of red blood cells characteristic of malaria depends upon the duration and severity of the infection. Hemolysis often leads to an increase in the serum bilirubin, and in falciparum malaria it may be sufficiently intense to result in hemoglobinuria (blackwater fever). In any malarial infection the degree of anemia is greater than that attributable solely to the destruction of cells by parasites. Hemolysis is probably contributed to by autoantigenic changes produced in the red cell by the parasite. Autoantigenic changes and increased osmotic fragility occur in all erythrocytes whether infected or not. Hemolysis may also be induced by quinine or primaquine in persons with hereditary glucose-6-phosphate dehydrogenase deficiency.

The pigment extruded into the circulation upon red cell disintegration accumulates in the reticuloendothelial cells of the spleen, the follicles of which become hyperplastic and sometimes necrotic, in the Kupffer cells of the liver, and in the bone marrow, brain and other organs. Deposition of sufficient pigment and of hemosiderin results in a slate-gray color of the organs.

The malignancy of falciparum malaria is peculiar to that species. The merozoites emerging from the liver are considerably more numerous than those of other species; there are as many in young children as in adults, so that children have a proportionately greater initial wave of infection. Young children are particularly prone to severe, often lethal, parasitemia.

Eight to 18 hours after the parasite has entered the red blood cells these cells become increasingly sticky and tend to adhere to the endothelial lining of blood sinuses and vessels, especially when the circulation is slow. A cross section of a small venule from a fatal case will usually reveal the remains of parasites or pigment in most of the red cells adjacent to the endothelium, and not in those lying in the lumen. The sticky cell is thus fixed and unable to return to the general circulation, although the parasite within it matures in the normal manner. As more cells adhere, flow within the vessel is progressively impeded, and occlusion or even rupture may occur.

The site and extent of this interference with vascular function, coupled with a selective localization of parasitized cells in various organs or systems, are responsible for the variety of symptoms from falciparum infections. Thus pneumonitis, encephalitis or enteritis may be manifest when the bulk of the infection is in the lungs, brain or intestinal tract, respectively. In the pregnant woman damage to the placenta may result in death of the fetus or in premature birth; infants born at full term to infected women have birth weights averaging one sixteenth less than those of infants born to uninfected mothers living under similar conditions.

The release of merozoites where the circulation is slowed facilitates the invasion of nearby red blood cells, so that falciparum parasitemia may be heavier than that of other species in which the rupture of schizonts takes place in the active circulation. Whereas *P. falciparum* invades all erythrocytes irrespective of age, *P. vivax* attacks primarily reticulocytes, and *P. malariae* invades mature red cells, features which tend to limit parasitemia of the latter 2 forms within 20,000 red cells per cu. mm. Falciparum infections in the nonimmune child may develop densities of as much as 500,000 parasites per cu. mm.; the prognosis is correspondingly grave.

Successful treatment stops the growth of parasites. Homologous immunity is vested in specific antibodies which may be associated with increased levels of 7S (IgG) gamma globulin in the serum of people repeatedly infected with a particular species. Antibody facilitates the phagocytosis of naked merozoites and of parasite-containing erythrocytes, which are ingested by reticuloendothelial cells and by large lymphocytes and neutrophils and particularly by monocytes. These antibodies do not, however, interfere with development of the parasite in the liver. A passive immunity, effective in restraining the severity of attacks of malaria for several weeks after birth, is conferred on infants born to mothers who have the disease. The beneficial effect of this transplacental acquisition of humoral immunity may be enhanced by persistence of fetal hemoglobin and by a diet limited to milk (low in PABA, hence inimical to growth of parasites). Certain hemoglobinopathies are also protective and tend to be genetically selective in endemic malarious regions. *P. falciparum* may fail to mature in children with the sickle-cell trait; *P. vivax*, in those with thalassemia and enzyme deficiencies; and *P. falciparum* is unable to attain high densities in children deficient in glucose-6-phosphate dehydrogenase.

Clinical Manifestations. Children who acquire malaria fall into 2 groups: those who have not had previous contact with the disease have little or no immunity and become severely ill unless treated; those who have been exposed to repeated infection since birth may survive early childhood to acquire a high degree of tolerance by about 10 years of age, though growth and development may be impaired. In the partially immune child heavy parasitemia may occur with few symptoms, or an intercurrent infection may initiate renewed activity of a quiescent malarial infection. Tolerance to malaria is most apparent among Africans and persons of African descent; it appears to be based on inherited factors that modify the severity of the disease.

In a nonimmune child clinical signs usually appear 8 to 15 days after infection, and may not be distinctive. Behavioral changes such as fretfulness, anorexia, unusual crying, drowsiness or disturbances of sleep may have been observed. Fever may be absent or increase gradually for 1 or 2 days, or the onset may be sudden with temperature up to 105 or 107°F., with or without prodromal chill. After varying periods of time the temperature falls to normal or below, and sweating occurs.

The febrile paroxysm may be extremely short or may last for 2 to 12 hours; its characteristic pattern is usually obscured in children less than 5 years of age. Complaints may be made of headache, nausea, generalized aching, particularly of the back, and occasionally of pain in the abdomen, when the spleen has swollen quickly and is tender. In vivax and quartan infections dominated by a single brood the fever is the characteristic manifestation, occurring at intervals of 48 hours in the former and 72 in the latter. If convulsions occur, they abate when the fever falls. Herpetic lesions of the mouth are not uncommon. The red blood cell count and hemoglobin level may decrease rapidly; leukopenia is variable, but monocytosis is common.

In falciparum infections the fever is less characteristic and may even be continuous; it may be overshadowed by severe manifestations related to the cerebral, pulmonary, intestinal or urinary systems. Cerebral complications are evidenced by convulsions or coma, with few localizing neurologic signs and (unless bacterial or viral infections of the central nervous system are superimposed) a normal cerebrospinal fluid. In cases of algid malaria, coma is preceded in the child by medical shock. Persistent nausea and vomiting, an enlarged and tender liver and progressive jaundice may evolve into hepatic failure; severe diarrhea may occur; or occasionally the signs of acute appendicitis may be imitated.

The spleen is more commonly enlarged in vivax than in falciparum infections; perisplenitis, infarction, even rupture may occur, and after repeated attacks the spleen may become very large and hard. "Idiopathic splenomegaly" (so-called big spleen disease of Africa) may constitute an abnormal immune response to *P. malariae* in malnourished children in underdeveloped countries. Enlargement of the spleen is accompanied by lymphocytic infiltration of liver sinusoids and an elevated fluorescent antibody titer for malaria, with or without scanty parasitemia.

Disturbances of renal function are shown by oliguria, and anuria may supervene. The *nephrotic syndrome* is associated with *P. malariae* in children inhabiting endemic malarious areas and is characterized by gross edema, massive proteinuria and severe hypoproteinemia; the prognosis is poor. *Blackwater fever,* now rarely seen, is associated with *P. falciparum.* Hemoglobinuria results from severe and sudden intravascular hemolysis, which may lead to anuria and to death from uremia.

Diagnosis. The diagnosis of malaria depends upon identification of parasites in the blood. In falciparum malaria, only ring forms are likely to be seen initially, crescents (gametocytes) joining them after 10 days; up to 20 per cent of the erythrocytes may be infected. All stages of the other species of parasites appear in the blood, but less than 2 per cent of red cells will contain them.

In the properly stained blood smear the parasites within the red cells have a red chromatin and bluish cytoplasm. In some leukocytes, particularly monocytes, remnants of phagocytized parasites and pigment may be seen. The parasites should first be looked for in thick blood films, since in light infections it may not be possible to find plasmodia in the thin film; the latter is best used for species differentiation. As parasites may not be seen at the height of the fever, examinations should be repeated preferably at intervals of 12 hours. Of the various stains available, the most suitable is Giemsa diluted 1:25 with distilled water preferably buffered to pH 7.0 to 7.2. Wright's stain may be used, 0.75 gm. of the powder being repeatedly shaken for 2 days with 65 ml. of pure methyl alcohol and 35 ml. of pure glycerin.

A falsely positive Wassermann reaction will be found in many cases.

Prevention. Infection of man does not occur where breeding of anopheline mosquitoes is prevented, where the adult mosquitoes are kept from contact with man by screens or bed nets, or where they are killed by natural enemies or insecticides before sporozoites have had time to mature. Children visiting endemic malarious areas should be protected by screens during the hours of mosquito activity, but as this is rarely entirely effective, they should also be given one of the chemoprophylactic drugs *regularly* throughout their stay and for 4 weeks thereafter. At least during this period, malaria should be suspected if febrile illness or chronic debility affects the child.

Chemoprophylactic drugs in common use are the following: the slightly bitter but extremely safe chlorguanide (proguanil), taken daily in amounts of 25 mg. (to 2 years), 50 mg. (2 to 6 years) or 100 mg. (older than 6); the tasteless but more toxic pyrimethamine (supplies of which should be particularly well guarded from inquisitive children), taken weekly in amounts of 6.25 mg. (to 2 years), 12.5 mg. (2 to 6 years) or 25 mg.; and chloroquine or amodiaquine taken weekly in amounts of 37.5 mg. of the base (to 1 year), 75 mg. (1 to 2 years), 112.5 mg. (2 to 6 years), 150 mg. (6 to 12 years) or 300 mg. The bitterness of chloroquine diphosphate and sulfate has been partially concealed in syrups which are available commercially, and a tasteless salt of chloroquine, the silicate, has been developed.

Proguanil and pyrimethamine not only suppress the development of parasites in the red blood cells, as do chloroquine and amodiaquine, but also interfere with the pre-erythrocytic stage in the liver. Unfortunately cross-resistance to the first 2 drugs is widely distributed, for which reason chloroquine and amodiaquine are generally preferred in prophylaxis. When resistance to the latter compounds also occurs, as in northern South America and southeast Asia, potentiating combinations of pyrimethamine with long-acting sulfonamides or sulfones may be taken by mouth, or an injectable repository preparation containing cycloguanil pamoate and diacetylaminodiphenylsulfone may prove effective.

Treatment. *Clinical treatment* falls into 4 categories: (1) specific chemotherapy of the attack, whether fresh infection, recrudescence or relapse; (2) supportive treatment and treatment of complications; (3) specific chemotherapy to prevent late relapse of vivax, ovale or quartan infections; (4) specific chemotherapy to destroy or sterilize gametocytes, and thus to protect the community should vector mosquitoes be present.

1. Any one of the drugs listed in Table 10-28 will effect a clinical cure of all types of malaria and provide a radical cure of falciparum malaria, unless drug-resistant parasites are present. Children who have inhabited malarious regions and acquired some immunity may be cured by one half of the quantities listed above, given in a single dose. Treatment must be repeated if vomiting occurs within an hour of ingestion of the drug; persistent vomiting is an indication for parenteral therapy.

Although specific treatment should not usually be undertaken until the diagnosis has been established, many experienced physicians, when confronted with a critically ill or comatose child whose history is suggestive of malaria or exposure thereto, would consider it advisable to administer quinine or chloroquine parenterally while awaiting the result of blood film examination.

Parenteral administration of chloroquine or quinine, although hazardous in children bordering on shock, is often essential for those who are vomiting persistently, who are in coma or who cannot be induced to swallow the drugs even if the bitterness is concealed. Parenteral therapy with antimalarial drugs should be replaced by oral administration as soon as possible. Chloroquine is given intravenously by slow drip in a glucose-saline solution, or intramuscularly; the dose by either route should not exceed 5 mg. base per kg. and should be repeated only once, 6 hours later, if treatment still cannot be given by mouth. Quinine dihydrochloride is administered intravenously in a dose of 10 mg. per kg. and may be repeated 12 hours later; it must be given only well diluted (not more than 1 mg. per ml.) and slowly, preferably by drip, but if by syringe, then no faster than 1 ml. per minute.

2. Supportive treatment includes that for hyperpyrexia; tepid sponging may add to the comfort when the temperature exceeds 104°F. The fluid and electrolyte needs should be maintained. Water, fruit juices and other fluids should be offered in small amounts at frequent intervals, and salt tablets may be used if sweating is excessive.

Metabolic requirements of the parasite rapidly

TABLE 10-28. TREATMENT OF UNCOMPLICATED MALARIA ATTACK

DRUG (U.S.P.)	SCHEDULE	DOSAGE IN MG. BASE (CHLOROQUINE AND AMODIAQUINE) OR MG. SALT (QUININE)*				
		Age under 1 year	Age 1-3 years	Age 3-6 years	Age 6-12 years	Older children
Chloroquine	Day 1-first dose	75	75	150	150	300
or	6 hours later	37.5	75	75	150	300
Amodiaquine	6 hours later	–	–	75	150	300
	Day 2-first dose	37.5	75	75	150	150
	6 hours later	–	–	–	–	150
	Day 3-first dose	37.5	75	75	150	150
	6 hours later	–	–	–	–	150
Quinine	Daily†	165	330	660	1000	2000

*Commercial tablets usually contain 250 mg. of chloroquine diphosphate or sulfate, of which 150 mg. is base: the quantity of base is stated on the label of the container, and should be prescribed as such.

†Given for 7 days in divided doses every 4 or 8 hours, as tolerated.

deplete the reserves of glucose, vitamins and co-enzymes, as well as of hemoglobin. Vitamin B₁ may be given, and, when the acute phase is passed, ferrous sulfate should be prescribed for a considerable time. Transfusion of packed red cells may be beneficial to children who have had long-standing infections and consequently severe anemia (hemoglobin 5 gm. per 100 ml. or less).

It is essential that children with severe falciparum infections receive fluids intravenously if dehydrated or in shock. Rapid expansion of the circulating blood volume with whole blood is more satisfactory than with dextran, plasma or glucose-saline solution. Although the full course of antimalarial therapy should not be instituted until the child is hydrated, out of shock and urinating, and quinine and primaquine are contraindicated in the presence of hemoglobinuria, nevertheless high parasitemia must be combated by the judicious use of chloroquine or amodiaquine. Should convulsions occur, they may be controlled with paraldehyde or barbiturates.

The nephrotic syndrome associated with quartan malaria is managed by the regimen described on page 1140, together with a course of chloroquine and primaquine.

3. Late relapse of vivax or ovale malaria rarely occurs more than 5 years after the primary attack, but much longer intervals have been recorded in the case of quartan malaria. Such relapses may be prevented by treatment of the child with primaquine (commencing on the second day of a concomitant clinical curative course of chloroquine, amodiaquine or quinine). The primaquine is given for 14 days in an age-adjusted dose equivalent to the adult one of 15 mg. base daily.

Children receiving primaquine should be watched for toxic manifestations such as methemoglobinemia, hemolytic anemia (sometimes accompanied by hemoglobinuria in children with G-6-PD deficiency), neutropenia and renal dysfunction. Quinacrine (mepacrine) should not be used simultaneously with primaquine, but since the former is obsolete as an antimalarial drug, the problem need not arise. Other synthetic antimalarial drugs are relatively nontoxic in therapeutic doses.

4. Gametocytes do not give rise to symptoms and disappear from the circulation soon after destruction of their asexual precursors by chloroquine, amodiaquine or quinine. Gametocytes may be destroyed by a single dose of primaquine, or their further development in the mosquito inhibited by single doses of chlorguanide or pyrimethamine, provided the parasite is not resistant to these drugs.

Drug resistance is of growing concern. Many strains of plasmodia are now resistant to chlorguanide and pyrimethamine, but a greater problem is posed by the spread in northern South America and in southeast Asia of *P. falciparum* resistant to chloroquine and amodiaquine; some strains are also tolerant to quinine. These strains are being introduced into countries such as the United States, where focal outbreaks may occur in the summer months, and children may become infected. Should the malarial attack not respond to chloroquine or amodiaquine, quinine should be used immediately. If this fails or, as is more usual, has only a temporary effect, a single dose of pyrimethamine in combination with a long-acting sulfonamide (dose-age or weight equivalent of 1.0 gm. adult dose) is effective: this combination may soon, however, be replaced by one containing a suitable sulfone or sulfonamide and trimethoprim, a dihydrofolate reductase inhibitor related to pyrimethamine, but less toxic.

DAVID F. CLYDE

REFERENCES

Chin, W., Contacos, P. G., Coatney, G. R., and King, H. K.: The Evaluation of Sulfonamides, Alone or in Combination with Pyrimethamine, in the Treatment of Multi-Resistant Falciparum Malaria. *Am. J. Trop. Med. & Hyg.,* 15:823, 1966.

Gilles, H. M.: Malaria in Children. *Brit. Med. J.,* 2:1375, 1966.

Russell, P. F., West, L. S., Manwell, R. D., and Macdonald, G.: *Practical Malariology.* 2nd ed. London, Oxford University Press, 1963.

Trowell, H. C., and Jelliffe, D. B.: *Diseases of Children in the Subtropics and Tropics.* London, E. Arnold, 1958.

Young, M. D.: Malaria; in G. W. Hunter, III, W. W. Frye, and J. C. Swartzwelder: *A Manual of Tropical Medicine.* 4th ed. Philadelphia and London, W. B. Saunders Company, 1966.

KALA-AZAR IN CHILDREN
(Leishmaniasis)

Three different clinical entities, kala-azar (visceral leishmaniasis), oriental sore (cutaneous leishmaniasis) and espundia (naso-oral leishmaniasis), are associated with what morphologically appears to be the same organism. Leishmania, a protozoal parasite which in the human body is a small ovoid or roundish organism measuring 2 to 4 microns in diameter, multiplies in the reticuloendothelial cells of the host. In the sandfly vectors (various species of *Phlebotomus*) and in cultures the Leishmania assume an elongated, motile, flagellated form.

There is some evidence that Leishmania responsible for the 3 above-mentioned clinical conditions represent different strains of the organism. This assumption is based in part on the distinctly different geographic distributions of the 3 diseases.

Epidemiology. Kala-azar is endemic in some parts of the eastern region of India (Assam, Bengal and Madras), in Ceylon and in areas of Africa, China and the U.S.S.R. It has also been reported in some areas of South America (Paraguay, Argentina and Brazil). In certain areas bordering the Mediterranean and on its islands (typically in Malta), kala-azar occurs mainly in infants and is termed "infantile kala-azar." The causative protozoan, *Leishmania donovani,* however, is the same as in the Indian, African and South American cases.

The disease is transmitted by the sandfly, which breeds in cracks and rubble. It flies low and only for short distances, so that multiple infections in the same household are common. The relation of human leishmaniasis to animal reservoirs of infection is intriguing. In the Mediterranean area, where infantile kala-azar is common, and in Morocco, Algiers and Iran, where human disease is rare, dogs commonly harbor leishmaniasis, whereas canine infection has not been found in endemic areas of India. Ground squirrels in Kenya, the striped hamster in China and the jackal in eastern Russia are naturally infected.

The incidence of kala-azar has been on the decline in recent years in the endemic areas of the world. The control of the sandfly and early diagnosis and specific treatment of the human host have presumably contributed to this decline.

Pathology. The parasites in visceral leishmaniasis are engulfed by the reticuloendothelial cells in the spleen, liver, bone marrow, and sometimes in the lymph nodes, and they multiply in them. The parasites often multiply until the cell ruptures, when the organisms are released into the bloodstream and may be transported to other viscera.

Clinical Manifestations. The onset in infants (*infantile kala-azar*) is acute with high fever and vomiting. Agranulocytosis, which is common, is responsible for the tendency to secondary infections and cancrum oris. Untreated infantile kala-azar is invariably fatal. In young children the onset is also often abrupt with typhoid-like fever and toxemia. The fever gradually rises to its peak in about a week and, after a couple of weeks of remittent or continuous fever, falls by lysis. If untreated, children are more liable than adults to such intercurrent infections as pneumonia and dysentery, which may be fatal. Slight generalized edema is common, as is enlargement of lymph nodes.

In the chronic form, common in older children and adults, low-grade remittent or intermittent fever, rarely over 102°F., is more or less persistent, often with 2 remissions in a 24-hour period. The fever for the initial 2 to 6 weeks is often continuous or remitting in type; this phase is often followed by one of apyrexia or low-grade fever, after which there may be long, irregular periods of fever. The spleen is usually enlarged early, being palpable a fortnight after the onset; it is rather soft in consistency and enlarges rapidly. The liver does not become appreciably enlarged for some months. Moderate enlargement of lymph nodes has been observed in the Mediterranean areas and China, but not in India. In the well established disease, emaciation with a protuberant abdomen due to gross enlargement of the spleen and a moderate anemia produce a typical appearance. In many long-standing cases the skin acquires a strange earthy-gray pigmentation, especially on the feet, hands and abdomen. Hence the name "kala-azar," which translated from the Indian dialect means "black sickness." The hair is likely to become sparse and brittle and may even fall out. A peculiar feature in adults and older children is that, in spite of systemic infection, the appetite is often good, the tongue clean, and the patient unaware that he has fever.

In the advanced stages secondary bacterial infections may supervene. Dysentery and pneumonia often cause death. Septic infection of the mouth may lead to cancrum oris and sloughing of the tissues in the cheek. Purpura, gingivitis and stomatitis are common. Pancytopenia may be evident and is probably due to displacement of the hematopoietic tissue of the bone marrow by parasitized reticuloendothelial cells. Progressive alteration of the plasma proteins occurs early; globulin is increased considerably, and albumin is decreased.

Hypopigmented macules or nodules on the face, chest and upper arms (postkala-azar dermal leishmaniasis; dermal leishmanoid) have been observed in India and the Sudan among patients who have had inadequate therapy.

Diagnosis. The early stage of kala-azar may be confused with malaria or typhoid fever. Prolonged or recurring fever may simulate tuberculosis, brucellosis and amebic abscess of the liver. The chronic stage may be confused with congestive splenomegaly (Banti's syndrome) or Indian childhood cirrhosis. The diagnosis depends mainly on the identification of the protozoa, which can usually be found in material aspirated from the bone marrow, spleen or liver and in the peripheral blood. Smears or cultures of the bone marrow are usually stained by the Leishman or Giemsa method. The parasites are usually sufficient in number for identification. Splenic puncture provides the highest percentage of positive results (95 per cent), but carries the risk of fatal hemorrhage, especially when there is anemia and a bleeding tendency. In smears of peripheral blood and in material obtained from lymph nodes the detection of organisms is less common; the percentage of identifications in blood is increased by culture of it in N.N.N. medium.

Among the available indirect diagnostic methods, the formol-gel test (aldehyde test) and Chopra's antimony test are useful for the diagnosis of chronic kala-azar. The complement fixation test (using an antigen from Kedrowsky's acid-fast bacillus) is useful for diagnosis during the early stage of the disease.

Prognosis. The introduction of specific therapy has greatly improved the prognosis; recovery can be expected if treatment is initiated in the early stage. Relapses are not uncommon, especially in Sudanese and African cases.

Treatment. The susceptibility of kala-azar to specific drug therapy appears to vary considerably in different parts of the world. The pentavalent antimonial drugs and the aromatic diamidines, such as pentamidine and stilbamidine, seem to have powerful antileishmanial properties. The disease in India is mostly cured by the pentavalent antimonials. These compounds are available for intramuscular or intravenous administration. Only an occasional patient is encountered who is resistant to antimony and for whom one of the diamidine drugs is required. These latter drugs, however, are not to be used in patients with hepatic or renal disease or a tendency to hemorrhage. Neuralgia is a side effect of the diamidines. Visceral leishmaniasis of the Sudan and East Africa is highly resistant to therapy; the Chinese and Mediterranean forms are intermediate in their response. In addition to specific treatment, it is important to combat malnutrition and to maintain strict oral hygiene to prevent stomatitis and cancrum oris.

The response of kala-azar to specific treatment is by and large good, but it may be slow even in the initial stage, and at times more than one course of therapy may be needed, and cure may not be achieved in less than at least a year or so.

Prevention. Sandfly control is not difficult to achieve with residual insecticides, such as DDT, and other measures. Early diagnosis and specific treatment of the human host have also contributed to the decline in incidence. The importance of treating postkala-azar dermal leishmaniasis cannot be overemphasized; such patients pose a serious public health problem. Destruction of infected dogs in Crete was followed by a decrease in incidence of kala-azar. A strain of leptomonad cultures of this protozoan obtained from ground squirrels is used for mass inoculation of those exposed to the infection in North Kenya. These animal strains of Leishmania are dermatropic and capable of producing artificial skin immunity without causing kala-azar. The use of repellant creams, insecticidal sprays and protective nets may help in personal prophylaxis against sandflies.

S. T. Achar[*]

TOXOPLASMOSIS

This disease results from infection with *Toxoplasma gondii*, an intracellular parasite first found in 1908 in animals in North Africa and Brazil. In 1939 Wolf, Cowen and Paige showed that Toxoplasma caused human illness; the organism was isolated from infants with congenital encephalomyelitis. It soon became apparent that there is a congenital form of infection, acquired in utero, and a postnatally acquired form. Sabin first pointed out that congenital toxoplasmosis is frequently manifest by a syndrome consisting of chorioretinitis, cerebral calcification, psychomotor retardation, hydrocephalus or microcephaly, and convulsions. By 1948 methods available for study of toxoplasmosis included the dye test, complement fixation, and a skin test.

Etiology. *Toxoplasma gondii* is generally considered a protozoan, but its precise classification remains in question. It is an oval or crescent-like organism measuring 2 to 4 by 4 to 7 microns and is best stained with Giemsa or Wright stain. It multiplies by endodyogeny only in the presence of living cells. The usual form is a trophozoite. Cysts are also produced early in the course of infection; these may contain hundreds of parasites, which seem to remain alive indefinitely. Toxoplasma is unique in that it invades all tissues of mammals and birds (with the exception of nonnucleated erythrocytes). Disease caused by Toxoplasma is expressed with remarkable similarity in different hosts, perhaps because the organism adapts to an unparalleled variety of cells. Only one species is known; all strains isolated have been serologically similar.

---

[*]Dr. Achar died during the final revision of this section. Dr. J. Viswanathan of Madras kindly completed the revision.

Epidemiology. The prevalence of Toxoplasma antibodies varies considerably among healthy persons in different parts of the world. Significant titers of dye test antibodies have been detected in 50 per cent or more of people in some localities and in less than 5 per cent in other areas. Similar variations in the evidence of frequency of infection are observed in wild and domesticated animals and birds. The interpretation of positive serologic findings in older children and adults is difficult unless changes in titer in serial samples suggest recent infection.

There is no evidence that Toxoplasma is communicated from person to person, except to the fetus from the mother. Given the high prevalence of subclinical infection in animals and man, it is difficult to relate with confidence infection in any human case to a specific animal. On the other hand, Desmonts has recently shown that young children may acquire antibodies for Toxoplasma by ingesting undercooked beef and mutton without exhibiting significant clinical symptoms. Jacobs has shown that freezing will usually render meat noninfectious. Infected meat may explain some instances of infection in man, but it cannot be the mechanism whereby vegetarians and herbivorous animals acquire parasites.

Hutchison has found that a nematode parasite of cats, *Toxocara cati*, can acquire toxoplasma. Subsequently the eggs of the worm may contain Toxoplasma and infect other cats. It is unlikely that the cat and its nematode represent a unique system, and on this basis similar relations are under investigation in other hosts.

Pathology. In both the congenital and acquired forms of toxoplasmosis histologic changes may be found in almost all tissues. In the congenital form changes are especially common in the central nervous system, the retina and the choroid; similar lesions have been noted in a few cases of acquired toxoplasmosis. Toxoplasma will usually be found encysted, especially in muscle; in severe acute infections individual organisms may also be found, often with surprisingly little tissue reaction. Gross or microscopic areas of necrosis may be found, however, in many tissues, especially in heart, lungs, skeletal muscle, liver and spleen. Areas of calcification may be present in necrotic areas of the brain in the congenital form; these have not been reported in acquired cases. The lesions of toxoplasmosis are not sufficiently characteristic to permit a specific diagnosis unless the parasite can be identified or other information supports the diagnosis. Parasites have been found in lymph nodes and tonsils, and their identity has been confirmed by animal inoculation. In congenital infection, tissue damage stabilizes early and tends not to progress, but live parasites may persist in the brain for years.

Clinical Manifestations. *Congenital toxoplasmosis.* Fetal infections appear to depend upon maternal acquisition of toxoplasma infection during the pregnancy. It is questionable whether congenital toxoplasmosis is ever inapparent; a few infants, however, suffer only minor damage.

The fetus infected with Toxoplasma may be stillborn, born prematurely or at full term. Illness may be apparent at birth or may not become evident for some days. Manifestations include malaise, fever, maculopapular rash, lymphadenopathy, hepatomegaly, splenomegaly, icterus, hydrocephalus, microcephaly, microphthalmia and convulsions, singly or in combination. Cerebral calcifications and chorioretinitis may be present at birth or appear subsequently.

Active congenital infection may terminate fatally in days or weeks, or the illness may become inactive, leaving as residuals varying degrees and combinations of hydrocephalus or microcephaly, chorioretinitis, psychomotor retardation, ocular palsies and convulsive disorders. The full impact of the infection upon development may not become evident until some weeks or months after its apparent cessation.

In a large series of cases of congenital toxoplasmosis (Feldman), premature birth was common (31 per cent) and carried a higher mortality rate (27 per cent) than if the infant was born at term (12 per cent). Chorioretinitis was noted in 99 per cent, cerebral calcification in 63 per cent, psychomotor retardation in 56 per cent and hydrocephalus or microcephaly in about half of the infants. Chorioretinitis was bilateral in 85 per cent of instances and almost equally distributed between the left and right eyes in the remainder. Residual damages in some cases were as slight as a minute peripheral patch of chorioretinitis or a single oculomotor palsy.

There is evidence that fetal infection occurs only after the placenta has been formed. All offspring in a multiple pregnancy are infected, but the degree of damage may be strikingly different in each fetus. Though toxoplasmosis may be responsible for premature birth, cerebral palsy, blindness and mental retardation, it does not appear to be a prominent cause of any of them. The disease occurs only in the offspring of one pregnancy of a given mother, so that subsequent pregnancies may be undertaken without fear of subsequent infection.

Acquired toxoplasmosis. Postnatally acquired toxoplasmosis is a relatively common inapparent infection and rarely a clinically apparent one. Parasitemia probably occurs in all cases and is the presumed means by which the fetus acquires infection from its mother. Except for occasional instances of lymphadenopathy, no clinical evidence of maternal infection has been noted.

When clinical manifestations are apparent in acquired toxoplasmosis, they may include almost any combination of the following: malaise, fever, myalgia, maculopapular rash, generalized lymphadenopathy, hepatomegaly, encephalitis, pneumonia and myocarditis. Chorioretinitis (usually unilateral) is uncommon. The rash, when present, persists for about 3 days. Symptoms may be evident for a few days or for some weeks; most patients recover spontaneously. The incubation period, source of infection and mortality rate are unknown.

Siim has reported generalized lymphadenopathy to be a frequent clinical sign of acquired toxoplasmosis in Denmark. Such cases may resemble infectious mononucleosis, Hodgkin's disease or other lymphadenopathies. The Paul-Bunnell test result is negative, and splenomegaly is rare. The involved lymph nodes are generally firm, nontender and nonsuppurative. Owing to the vagueness of this syndrome, the correct diagnosis is usually not considered until so late in its course that serologic confirmation is difficult, and in the author's experience such involvement has not been confirmed in many instances.

Laboratory Data. Congenital toxoplasmosis may be diagnosed in its active stage shortly after birth by demonstration of parasites in smears of sediment from cerebrospinal and ventricular fluids, which may be xanthochromic and contain cells (sometimes eosinophils) and increased protein. Otherwise identification depends upon isolation of the parasites in animals; mice are especially suitable. The inoculum should consist of suspensions of fresh tissue or of sediment from body fluids.

The dye test is the most sensitive and reliable indicator of toxoplasma antibody in human and animal serums. It is performed by incubating mixtures of various dilutions of inactivated serum of the patient with living parasites (mouse peritoneal exudate or tissue cultures), which have been suspended in fresh, antibody-negative human serum. The latter supplies a heat-labile serum component (activator) which is required for the action of the specific antibody. Methylene blue is added. In the absence of antibody, the parasite is stained blue. If antibody is present, the cytoplasm of the parasite will remain unstained. The end-point in titration occurs when 50 per cent of parasites are unstained. Toxoplasma antibodies identified by the dye test appear early in the course of infection and remain in high titer for months or years, when it diminishes gradually, but some antibody may persist for life. In the serums of infants or young children with congenital disease and of their mothers, titers of 1:1000 to 1:16,000 are usual for at least some months. If the infant's antibodies have been acquired only by passive transfer, there will be a sharp decline in titer by 3 months of age and almost total disappearance by 6 months.

The complement-fixation test is not as commonly done as the dye test, but it may offer additional aid. It becomes positive more slowly, so that early in the disease there may be a strongly positive dye, but a negative complement-fixation, reaction. On the other hand, the complement-fixation reaction tends to decrease relatively quickly, so that within months or years after the initial illness there may again be a negative complement-fixation and a positive dye reaction. An infant born with active disease and a positive dye reaction may have a negative complement-fixation reaction, although his mother has high titers by both procedures.

A skin test utilizing antigens from egg or from mouse peritoneal fluid is available, but it has little clinical diagnostic usefulness, since positive reactors are prevalent in many localities, and even negative reactors may have high titers of serum antibodies. The time required for the development of skin sensitivity which is of the delayed type is unknown; it appears to be about a year. Positive reactions are infrequently encountered in children under 4 years of age in general surveys.

Among more recently developed serologic methods the hemagglutination test is the most promising. The results generally parallel those obtained with the dye test, but there are sufficient differences so that they cannot, as yet, be substituted for one another. Remington has devised an ingenious procedure which may be of value in the early diagnosis of active toxoplasmosis: to slides containing Toxoplasma the patient's serum is added and then fluorescein-tagged anti-IgM serum. Fluorescence of the parasite then indicates that IgM toxoplasma antibodies are present and suggests a response to a recent infection. This method may prove to be useful in the diagnosis of infection in the newborn, since they will have had to make their own IgM antibodies.

Differential Diagnosis. Any manifestation of congenital toxoplasmosis may occur in other diseases. Neither the cerebral calcification (single or multiple) nor the chorioretinitis is pathognomonic. In our experience fewer than 50 per cent of children less than 5 years of age with chorioretinitis satisfy the serologic criteria for congenital toxoplasmosis. Others may have cytomegalic inclusion disease or chorioretinitis of unknown cause. The clinical picture in the newborn infant may suggest sepsis, syphilis or hemolytic disease.

Treatment. A combination of pyrimethamine (Daraprim) and sulfadiazine is superior to either drug alone in the treatment of experimental toxoplasma infections. The combination has also been used in human patients, and experience suggests it has been effective, but owing to the variable natural course of the disease, critical evaluation of any therapeutic regimen is difficult. In any case, this combination represents the best therapy currently available. Sulfadiazine should be administered in usual therapeutic dosage, and pyrimethamine, 1 mg. per kg. per day, in divided doses. The total daily dose of pyrimethamine should not exceed 25 mg., except that twice that dose is often prescribed for the initial 24 to 48 hours. Treatment should be continued for about 4 weeks. Both pyrimethamine, an antifolic agent, and the sulfonamide may produce severe leukopenia; accordingly, leukocyte counts should be obtained several times weekly. Thrombocytopenia induced by pyrimethamine may be alleviated by the administration of folinic acid, which will not interfere with the antiparasitic activity of the drug. Unfortunately, there is no evidence that this treatment affects intracellular or encysted organisms. In newborn infants with active disease the most that can be hoped for is that further damage will be prevented; regression of signs of tissue damage cannot be expected.

HARRY A. FELDMAN

REFERENCES

Feldman, H. A.: Toxoplasmosis (Medical Progress). *New England J. Med.,* 279:1370, 1431, 1968.
Jacobs, L.: Toxoplasmosis; in *Advances in Parasitology.* New York, Academic Press, 1967.
Maumenee, A. E.: Toxoplasmosis, with Special Reference to Uveitis. *Survey Ophthal.,* 6:700, 1961.
Siim, J. C.: Human Toxoplasmosis; in *Proceedings of the Conference on Clinical Aspects and Diagnostic Problems of Toxoplasma in Pediatrics.* Baltimore, Williams & Wilkins Company, 1960.

Intestinal Protozoa

The severity of disease produced by protozoa is not necessarily proportional to the size of the inoculum. Though protozoa are capable of developing colonies of limitless size, the ultimate population is limited by the area of suitable habitat and other factors. Once the colony is established, its reproductive potential is in part used for production of transfer-stages which infect other hosts.

The life cycle of an intestinal protozoan colony typically begins with a single cell, a *trophozoite* (vegetative stage), which has one or more nuclei and specialized structures for locomotion. The trophozoite grows and reproduces by binary fission (*Isospora* excepted). In some of the trophozoites the vegetative functions are interrupted, an enveloping membrane is secreted by the organism, and, thus immobilized, it is eliminated in the feces. In this stage it is infective and is referred to as a *cyst,* not to be confused with the eggs of higher animals or spores of other organisms. The protozoan cyst is fairly resistant to external conditions, but it rarely reaches a new host in a viable state except in relatively cool, moist media. When the cyst is ingested and reaches its normal habitat in the intestine, it ruptures its membrane, and the organism resumes its vegetative functions. Then by a succession of generations a new colony is formed, and the cycle is repeated.

Of the several species of protozoa found in the human intestine, 6 are amebae (*Entamoeba histolytica, E. hartmanni, E. coli, Endolimax nana, Iodamoeba buetschlii, Dientamoeba fragilis*), 3 are flagellates (*Giardia lamblia, Chilomastix mesnili, Trichomonas hominis*), 1 is a ciliate (*Balantidium coli*) and 2 are sporozoa (*Isospora* species). Only 2, *E. histolytica* and *Balantidium coli,* produce serious disease in man, although *Dientamoeba fragilis, E. hartmanni* and *Giardia lamblia* are frequently classified as pathogens. Isospora infection rarely occurs in man. It usually produces only mild symptoms and tends to be self-terminating.

AMEBIASIS

Etiology. Amebiasis is usually regarded as synonymous with *Entamoeba histolytica* infection.

If one of the other species is suspected of producing symptoms, the disease may be treated as infection with *E. histolytica.*

Entamoeba histolytica inhabits the colon. It is frequently found in symptomless carriers and is thought by some to be a harmless commensal in the majority of instances. Nevertheless it is capable of deep invasion of the bowel wall and of being transported to other organs, especially the liver, where it may cause serious damage.

Epidemiology. Amebiasis is found in all parts of the world, especially in the tropics, but, like other filth-borne diseases, its distribution and prevalence correlate more closely with standards of personal hygiene and sanitation than with climate. Infection rates may exceed 50 per cent in densely populated unsanitary areas and may be extremely low in well sanitated groups. In the United States amebiasis is probably most prevalent in the South Central States. In the Charity Hospital at New Orleans routine examinations reveal *E. histolytica* in approximately 2 per cent of stools. Possibly because amebiasis is more difficult to diagnose in children than in adults, surveys usually show a higher incidence in adults. Infrequently the disease appears in epidemic form. The mortality rate in the United States is less than 0.1 per 100,000 population.

Infection is passed from person to person by means of relatively nonresistant but extremely abundant cysts in feces which, in diverse but mostly unproved ways, contaminate food and water.

Infective cysts passed in stools vary from too few to be detected by ordinary means to many millions a day. Stools from 10 consecutive patients averaged 241 cysts per mg. of feces. A housefly or cockroach may ingest much more than a milligram of feces, the amebic cysts passing through its intestine unharmed.

Cysts are killed immediately by desiccation and by temperatures above 55°C., but may survive for months in water at temperatures below 20°C. They are killed by all commonly used disinfectants, but not by ordinary chlorination of water. There are no important animal reservoirs of amebic infection, although monkeys, apes and dogs may harbor natural infections, and other animals are readily infected in the laboratory. Amebic infection in dogs is relatively common, but as they rarely pass cysts they are not an important source of human infection.

Pathology. Some strains of *E. histolytica* are more pathogenic than others, and some which fail to produce symptoms in one person may readily produce disease in another. Infection may exist without evidence of disease, other than an abundance of cysts in the stools, and later develop into frank dysentery. Conversely, dysentery may be followed by a carrier state without evidence of disease.

Although massive colonization over its unbroken surface may deleteriously affect the mucosa, the only known means by which amebae produce disease is by tissue destruction in the colon or in other organs secondarily colonized by way of the bloodstream. The colon is most frequently invaded at the cecal and sigmoidorectal levels, but involvement varies greatly in area and in depth, the extreme being the full length of the organ and all layers even to, or through, the serosa. The older lesions are complicated by secondary bacterial invasion, and there are various degrees of inflammation and suppuration. Microscopically, the presence of amebae is diagnostic.

The hepatic lesion is more characteristic. Trophozoites diffusely distributed through the liver parenchyma produce multiple microscopic areas of necrosis which may coalesce to form a macroscopic lesion, the amebic liver abscess. It usually contains a characteristic pasty, brownish material. Occasionally this material is mixed with purulent exudate, and the demonstration of amebae, essential for positive diagnosis, is more difficult.

Clinical Manifestations. The signs and symptoms of intestinal amebiasis are largely those of nonspecific regional ulcerative colitis. Varying from mild irritation to extensive destruction of the bowel wall, from involvement of one or more local areas to that of the entire organ and from transient minor clinical disturbances to severe chronic disease, the manifestations of amebic infection are so diverse that intestinal amebiasis can never be ruled in or out without the aid of a microscope. Any abnormal bowel activity, unusual stools, abdominal complaints or physical findings suggestive of colonic disease should be an indication for microscopic examination of stools for amebae.

In severe amebic colitis, in contrast to bacillary dysentery, the onset is not likely to be sudden. Fever and leukocytosis are slight or absent, and the stools lack the odor and appearance of containing pus; i.e. the mucus is clear instead of being whitish or yellowish, and the odor is reminiscent of autolytic rather than suppurative processes. In this latter respect the diarrheas caused by *E. histolytica* and by whipworm (*Trichuris trichiura*) infections are identical.

The presence of an *amebic abscess of the liver* is suggested by chills, fever, leukocytosis and right upper quadrant tenderness or pain, especially if accompanied by physical signs or roentgenographic evidence of a bulging mass. The demonstration of colonic amebiasis would be supportive evidence, but other causes should be considered. In regions where *Ascaris lumbricoides* is endemic, abscess formation around adult worms in the liver, or enlargement and tenderness of the liver resulting from migrating larvae, is much more frequent in children than is hepatic amebiasis.

Diagnosis. The diagnosis of parasitic infections by stool examination presents 2 distinct problems: the detection of some stage of the organism and its identification.

Since all stages of amebae in feces or other material retain their normal appearance longer at room temperature than at body temperature and even longer under refrigeration (but not frozen), stools should be refrigerated promptly if examination is to be delayed more than 1 hour.

Abnormal elements in stools, such as mineral oil, fats, bismuth, kaolin, barium, certain foods such as bananas and milk and excessive amounts of undigestible pulpy fruits and vegetables, diminish the chances of finding amebae in the stools.

The specimen obtained by purgation, saline enema or proctoscopy has only the advantage of being delivered fresh and at a convenient time. A large specimen permits selection of favorable samples, but overemphasis of this factor may delay diagnosis, especially of waning dysentery. An ideal microscopic preparation contains only 1 to 2 mg. of feces, and most concentration methods require less than 1 gm. A fleck of feces obtained from the rectum on the gloved finger or from a saline enema may be sufficient.

If reliable diagnostic service is not locally available, fecal specimens and material aspirated from the colon or from liver abscesses may be satisfactorily preserved and mailed to distant laboratories by using one of the procedures described below. The material *must* be freshly collected and well mixed with the fixative-preservative.

Methods for preservation of stools. Full-strength commercial formaldehyde diluted 1 part with 9 parts of water is a good general fixative-preservative. An adequate specimen is 1 ml. of feces in 10 ml. of fixative. On reaching the laboratory the material is strained, mixed with ether and concentrated by centrifugal sedimentation. This is not satisfactory for dysenteric stools.

Preferred for dysenteric stools, and satisfactory for other types, is a fixative-preservative consisting of 2 solutions, stored separately and mixed immediately before use. Solution I is 40 parts of tincture of Merthiolate (Lilly), 5 parts of formaldehyde (U.S.P.) and 1 part of glycerin. Solution II is freshly prepared Lugol's solution (5 per cent iodine in 10 per cent aqueous potassium iodide solution). For use, combine 15 parts of solution I with 1 part of solution II. An adequate specimen is 1 ml. of feces in 8 to 10 ml. of preservative. Wet smears of the mixed specimen or the sediment are examined microscopically without further staining.

Cultures of fecal or aspirated material are generally not practical. Serologic tests are not used routinely.

Prognosis. Once a diagnosis of colonic amebiasis has been made, prompt eradication of the parasite is possible. Chronic refractory infections requiring long, varied treatments are exceptional. With proper corrective and supportive measures even severe dysentery can usually be controlled within a few days and cured within 2 or 3 weeks. Except for amebic abscess of the brain, which is rare even in adults, the prognosis is also good in extraintestinal infections diagnosed early.

Prevention. Contaminated water and food are probably the only important sources of amebic infection. In children the transfer of infection occasionally may be more direct. Water may be made safe by boiling. When this is impractical, hyperchlorination or halogenation with iodine by means of commercially available preparations is possible. Thoroughly dried foods may be regarded as safe. Rooty vegetables and fruits can be washed and peeled, and leafy vegetables can be safely eaten after immersion in aqueous iodine disinfectant or in full-strength vinegar (5 per cent acetic acid) for 15 to 20 minutes at room temperature. The prophylactic use of glycobiarsol or Diodoquin in doses of one sixth to one third of the therapeutic ones has been recommended.

Treatment. For children with acute dysentery or severe diarrhea due to *E. histolytica*, Milibis (glycobiarsol) is a relatively safe, inexpensive and effective drug. Tetracycline or emetine may be given for speedier control of symptoms, but, because of cost, toxicity and cure rates, they usually are not used as curative drugs. Milibis is administered orally in 250- or 500-mg. tablets 3 times daily with meals for 8 days, the single dose being 500 mg. for adults and for children over 6 years of age, and 250 mg. for younger children. Though the drug is generally nontoxic, treatment should be interrupted if such untoward symptoms as dizziness, severe headache, abdominal cramps or neuritis are noted. Tetracycline may be given alone or simultaneously with Milibis. The dosage for children is 5 to 10 mg. per pound 3 times daily for 2 to 4 days, or until acute symptoms subside. Emetine or dehydroemetine may be more effective and less expensive than the tetracyclines (see below for dosage). Although possibly less effective than Milibis, other drugs such as Diodoquin (diiodohydroxyquin) and chiniofon (Anayodin, Yatren) are often satisfactory.

Three or 4 stool examinations should be made at weekly intervals after completion of treatment. Because amebae may appear in the stools within a few days after reinfection, positive findings on treated outpatients should not be interpreted as necessarily indicating failure of treatment.

Hepatic amebiasis, in the presence of demonstrated colonic infection, is usually treated with chloroquine diphosphate. The drug is administered orally in 250-mg. tablets and may be given simultaneously with the treatment for colonic infection. The dose for children under 6 years of age is 250 mg. twice daily for 2 days followed by 125 mg. twice daily for 12 additional days; for older children and adults the dose is doubled. If treatment with chloroquine is not successful, emetine may be used. It is obtainable in 1-ml. ampules containing 65 mg. of emetine hydrochloride and is injected subcutaneously in doses of 0.5 mg. per pound per day for not more than 10 days, and never in excess of 65 mg. per day. Emetine may produce neuritis or irreversible myocarditis, so that its use should not be repeated in less than a month. Dehydroemetine apparently is less toxic and is comparable in action to emetine, and is administered in the same manner and dosage. Recently recommended for amebic dysentery or amebic liver abscess is metronidazole (Flagyl). It is administered orally in a dosage of 250 mg. twice daily for children 4 to 8 years of age, thrice daily for older children and adults, for 10 days.

ACANTHAMEBIASIS

Acute meningoencephalitis in children or older persons with a history of recent swimming in stagnant fresh water may be due to a type of amebic organism which, though ordinarily free-living, is capable of rapid invasion of the brain, apparently via the olfactory mucosa. Rapidly fatal cases were reported in Australia, eastern Europe, Florida, Texas and Virginia, there being altogether 34 cases reported since 1965. Although one was nonfatal, usually the infections were fatal within a few days after onset of symptoms. Amebae identified as Acanthamoeba (Hartmannella) or Naegleria were recovered from the spinal fluid or were seen in histopathologic sections of the brain. No specific treatment is known.

Ameboid organisms isolated during studies of respiratory and other diseases and assumed to be viruses have been shown to be Hartmannella species. Wang and Feldman detected 54 strains belonging to 3 species of Hartmannella in tissue cultures inoculated from throat swabs in the course of a search for agents of respiratory disease in a survey of "normal" families. The majority of these isolations were made from children under 5 years of age and most often from those less than a year of age. No relation between amebae and clinical illness was apparent.

The extent to which Hartmannella are responsible for human illnesses is unknown. Future studies may show these free-living amebae to be of greater clinical significance than is currently appreciated.

GIARDIASIS

Giardia lamblia is most frequently found in the tropics and subtropics, its distribution seeming to vary with economic, hygienic and sanitary conditions. Prevalence rates, generally highest in children 5 to 10 years of age, exceed 10 per cent in some communities. The parasite may be transmitted by food and water and by houseflies, or directly from person to person.

The flagellate usually lives in the duodenum and upper jejunum, where it may persist for years, or disappear spontaneously, especially in older children and adults. Trophozoites die within a few hours outside the body, but cysts may remain viable for several days.

The pathogenicity.of *Giardia lamblia* has not been satisfactorily demonstrated. It frequently occurs in stools of children with a variety of complaints referable to the intestinal tract, and conditions resembling sprue or celiac disease have been attributed to it.

Fortunately the infection is easily eradicated by drugs that are neither expensive nor very toxic. Quinacrine dihydrochloride (Atabrine) administered orally in 0.1-gm. tablets for 5 days in the following dosage rarely if ever fails to result in complete removal of Giardia: for adults and children over 8 years of age, 1 tablet 3 times daily; for children 4 to 8 years, ½ tablet on the same schedule; and for younger children, ½ tablet twice daily. Metronidazole (Flagyl) is also effective; it is given in doses of 250 mg. twice daily for children 4 to 8 years of age, or 3 times daily for older children and adults, for 5 days.

BALANTIDIASIS

Balantidium coli is a parasite which, like *E. histolytica*, colonizes the colon. More often than in man it is found in monkeys and pigs, both of which tolerate the infection without apparent damage. Although *Balantidium coli* is the only ciliate protozoon known to parasitize the human colon, numerous morphologically similar organisms are frequent in stools as contaminants and may lead to errors in diagnosis. Diagnosis is established by the presence of either the more or less uniformly ciliated, large, rapidly motile trophozoites or the large spherical cysts.

Balantidiasis is rare in the United States, but is relatively common in Puerto Rico, Mexico and various parts of South America. Most of the human infections apparently are derived from pigs. Under crowded or unsanitary conditions, person-to-person transfer of infective cysts commonly occurs. As a rule, however, cysts are formed only sparingly or not at all in the human intestine.

Typically, the infection is of short duration, producing in children a disease similar to amebic dysentery. The pathologic changes are similar in distribution and nature. The chief difference is the greater tendency of balantidiasis toward spontaneous cure. This factor has led to variable interpretations of the curative value of tested drugs. Satisfactory results appear to be obtained with tetracycline given orally in doses of 8 to 10 mg. per pound 3 times daily for 10 days, the total dose not to exceed 2 gm.

PAUL C. BEAVER

REFERENCES

General

Faust, E. C., Beaver, P. C., and Jung, R. C.: *Animal Agents and Vectors of Human Disease.* 3rd ed. Philadelphia, Lea & Febiger, 1968.
Harris, A. H., and Coleman, M. B. (Eds.): Intestinal Protozoa; in *Diagnostic Procedures and Reagents.* New York, American Public Health Association, Inc., 1963, pp. 808-20.

Amebiasis

Beaver, P., Jung, R., Sherman, H., Read, T., and Robinson, T.: Experimental Chemoprophylaxis of Amebiasis. *Am. J. Trop. Med. & Hyg.*, 5:1015, 1956.
Brooke, M. M.: Epidemiology of Amebiasis in the U.S. *J.A.M.A.*, 188:519, 1964.
Deschiens, R.: Chimiolprophylaxie par la thérapeutique anti-amibienne préventive. *Bull. Soc. Path. Exot.*, 58:67, 1965.
Powell, S. J., McLeod, I., Wilmot, A. J., and Elsdon-Dew, R.: Dehydroemetine in Amebic Dysentery and Amebic Liver Abscess. *Am. J. Trop. Med.*, 11:607, 1962.
Powell, S. J., McLeod, I., Wilmot, A. J., and Elsdon-Dew, R.: Metronidazole in Amoebic Dysentery and Amoebic Liver Abscess. *Lancet*, 2:1329, 1966.
Wilmot, A. J.: *Clinical Amoebiasis.* Philadelphia, F. A. Davis Company, 1962.

Acanthamebiasis

Blattner, R. J.: Primary Meningoencephalitis: Infection with *Hartmannella (Acanthamoeba). J. Pediat.*, 70:298, 1967.
Butt, C. G.: Primary Amebic Meningoencephalitis. *New England J. Med.*, 274:1473, 1966.
Callicott, J. H., and others: Meningoencephalitis Due to Pathogenic Free-Living Amoebae. *J.A.M.A.*, 206:579, 1968.
Culbertson, C. G.: Pathogenic Acanthamoeba (Hartmannella). *Am. J. Clin. Path.*, 35:195, 1961.
Fowler, M., and Carter, R. F.: Acute Pyogenic Meningitis Probably Due to *Acanthamoeba* Sp.: A Preliminary Report. *Brit. Med. J.*, 2:740, 1965.
Wang, S. S., and Feldman, H. A.: Isolation of *Hartmannella* Species from Human Throats. *New England J. Med.*, 277:1174, 1967.

Giardiasis

Cortner, J. A.: Giardiasis, a Cause of Celiac Syndrome. *Am. J. Dis. Child.*, 98:311, 1959.
Kuzmicki, R., Gajda, E., and Switalska-Kowalewska, E.: Wyniki leczenia lambliozy flagylem. *Wiad. Parazyt.*, 11:545, 1965.
Rubio, M., and Cuello, E.: Tratamiento de la giardiasis intestinal con un derivado del nitroimidazol. Estudio en Niños. *Bol. Chile de Parasit.*, 18:60, 1963.

Balantidiasis

Arean, V. M., and Koppisch, E.: Balantidiasis: A Review and Report of Cases. *Am. J. Path.*, 32:1089, 1956.
Shookhoff, H.: *Balantidium Coli* Infection, with Special Reference to Treatment. *Am. J. Trop. Med.*, 31:442, 1951.

11. The Digestive System

THE ORAL CAVITY

The condition of the oral cavity is important to physical and psychologic health and the sense of well-being. The recognition and treatment of oral abnormalities and diseases, particularly in infancy and early childhood, require cooperative effort between physicians and dentists. Initially the physician's role is predominant; later it is the dentist who has the most opportunity for periodic observation of the child as well as of his mouth. Many oral abnormalities are associated with systemic conditions and are best handled through coordinated efforts; the physician should identify and utilize the services of those dentists in his community, usually pedodontists or orthodontists, who share his concern for the psychologic and physical health of children.

The principal consideration in the oral health of children is the establishment of an intact, balanced, self-maintaining permanent dentition. Dental examination at 2½ to 3 years of age permits a careful evaluation of oral health, including the pattern of eruption and completeness of the dentition, tooth-to-tooth and arch-to-arch relations, facial growth, and condition of the enamel and dentin. Needed restorations may be made at this time, as well as plans for the treatment of other abnormalities. Regular, periodic surveillance is necessary throughout childhood to ensure that teeth are not lost through caries and that malocclusions receive timely correction; most periodontal disease of adults is often traceable to caries or malocclusion untreated during childhood.

ABNORMALITIES IN GROWTH AND DEVELOPMENT OF THE JAWS AND TEETH

DEVELOPMENT OF THE JAWS

The lower portions of the head mature much later than the cranium. The jaws and teeth continue to undergo change until late adolescence.

Maxilla. The maxillary bone is formed in utero from a fusion of the maxilla and premaxilla; the latter contains the upper incisors and anterior portion of the palate. Sutures are formed with the adjoining maxillary, zygomatic, frontal and palatine bones. The inclination of the sutures determines the direction of enlargement of the maxillary bone. Growth at these sutures results in forward and downward movement of the maxilla in relation to the base of the cranium. Remodeling and appositional bone growth result in the maxillary sinuses, alveolar ridges and mature facial contours. Transverse growth is by proliferation of bone at the median palatal suture and at the outer surface of the maxilla. As with other sutures, bony union occurs and growth terminates during adolescence.

Mandible. The mandible arises both from centers of ossification and from bony replacement of portions of Meckel's cartilage. Longitudinal growth is accomplished by interstitial bone growth at the condyles. The ramus maintains its configuration through resorption on the anterior border and deposition of bone on the posterior border. The body of the mandible also undergoes appositional growth at the alveolar ridges and inferior border. Although condylar growth normally stops during puberty, unlike a closed suture, the potential for further growth remains.

Abnormalities of Jaw Growth. Longitudinal growth of the upper and lower jaws occurs by dissimilar means. The maxillary bone moves forward and downward because of growth at the sutures, while the mandible enlarges in a similar direction through interstitial bone growth. Consequently disturbances which affect connective tissue alter maxillary growth; abnormalities in cartilaginous growth alter mandibular growth. For example, in cleidocranial dysostosis and craniofacial dysostosis sutural growth is retarded, and the maxillary complex is relatively smaller than the mandible. On the other hand, in acromegaly cartilage grows more rapidly than connective tissue, and the mandible becomes much larger than the maxilla, resulting in class III malocclusion (p. 758).

Facial Asymmetry. Molding of the head during birth is possible because the bones of the cranium are not fused and can override. No such mechanism of adjustment to the narrow birth canal is present in the face. The mandible is the only movable bone in the face and is attached to the cranium only at its condylar head by the muscles of mastication. Facial asymmetries resulting from excessive molding of the cranium or from displacement of the mandible during breech or face presentations are fairly common and are usually self-correcting. Facial asymmetry resulting from injury to the growing cartilage of the condylar head during birth, infancy or early childhood is also common, but the effects may be permanent. Traumatic injuries may occur during birth from the placing of obstetrical forceps over the area, or may result from blows on the chin during infancy and childhood.

Such injuries, acute infections or arthritis of the growing condylar cartilage may result in a partial (fibrous) or complete (bony) *ankylosis of the temporomandibular joint* and failure of that side of the mandible to grow. The normal side, meanwhile, continues to grow and pushes the midline toward the affected side. The midline deviation is exaggerated during mouth opening. Roentgenograms of the affected side reveal an increased preangular notch. Bilateral injuries to the growing cartilage result in failure of the mandible and chin to grow downward and forward, causing the entire mandible to be considerably smaller than normal and much retruded.

Hypoplasia of the Mandible. *Pierre Robin syndrome.* The Pierre Robin syndrome consists of micrognathia with associated pseudomacroglossia, glossoptosis, and high-arched or cleft palate. Posterior displacement of the attachment of the genioglossus muscle to the hypoplastic mandible prevents the normal anchorage of the tongue. Under the influence of gravity the tongue assumes a retruded position, obstructing the pharynx. A postalveolar cleft of the hard and soft palates is a common but not constant feature. In some instances the palate is high-arched.

Although the tongue is usually of normal size, the floor of the mouth is foreshortened and the buccal cavity reduced in size. The lack of space further contributes to the glossoptosis. The obstruction of the air passages, particularly on inspiration, usually requires treatment in order to avoid suffocation. The infant should be placed in the prone or partially prone position so that the tongue falls forward to relieve respiratory obstruction. In a number of instances further treatment, such as temporarily suturing the ventral surface of the tongue to the lower lip, or tracheotomy, is not necessary, since sufficient mandibular growth usually takes place within a few months to relieve the glossoptosis. A variety of splints and traction devices designed to pull the mandible forward have been unsuccessful. The feeding of infants with mandibular hypoplasia requires great care and patience, but can usually be accomplished without resort to gavage. Often the growth of the mandible will progress so that an essentially normal profile is achieved within 4 to 6 years. A variety of dental anomalies usually require individual treatment.

Mandibulofacial dysostosis. In mandibulofacial dysostosis (Treacher-Collins syndrome, Franceschetti-Klein syndrome) there is less severe micrognathia than in the Pierre Robin syndrome. The facial appearance is characterized by palpebral fissures sloping downward toward the outer canthi, coloboma of the lower eyelids, sunken cheekbones, blind fistulas opening between the angles of the mouth and the ears, deformed pinna, atypical hair growth extending toward the cheeks, receding chin and large mouth. Facial clefts, diseases of the ears and deafness are common. The disorder is transmitted as a dominant trait, but expression is often incomplete. The mandible is almost always hypoplastic; the under surface is often pronouncedly concave, the ramus may be deficient, and the coronoid and condyloid processes are flat or even aplastic. The palatal vault may be either high or cleft (about 40 per cent). Infrequently, unilateral or bilateral macrostomia, or failure of embryonic fusion of the maxillary and mandibular processes, may occur. Owing to poor maxillary development and palatal deformity, dental malocclusions are frequent. The teeth may be widely separated, hypoplastic, displaced, or have an open bite. Orthodontic and routine dental treatment is indicated.

Unilateral hypoplasia of the mandible is sometimes part of an anomaly complex that includes partial paralysis of the facial nerve, macrostomia, blind fistulas between the angles of the mouth and the ears, and deformed ear lobes. Because of the absence or hypoplasia of the mandibular condyle on the affected side, severe facial asymmetry and malocclusion develop. When there is early roentgenographic evidence of congenital condylar deformity, the deformity tends to increase with age. Plastic surgical procedures may be indicated early to minimize the deformity.

DISEASES OF THE JAWS

Caffey's Disease (Infantile Cortical Hyperostosis). See page 1359.

Osteomyelitis (see p. 1359). In the newborn infant, osteomyelitis tends to occur in the area of the premaxillary suture, but during childhood the mandible is the more common location. The infection is marked by swelling and redness of the oral mucosa or skin, associated with pain, fever and lymphadenopathy. Drainage should be established and the exudate cultured so that appropriate antibiotics may be administered. Large sequestra may require surgical removal.

Reticuloendotheliosis (Histiocytosis X) (see p. 1479). Oral lesions may occur in any of the syndromes and may be an early manifestation. Lesions of the jaws may produce pain, swelling, loosening of teeth, and fetid breath. Healing is often delayed after dental extraction. Dental roentgenograms may reveal spongelike patterns in bones with distinct "punched-out" areas.

Neoplasms (see p. 1471). *Benign tumors.* OSSIFYING FIBROMA is perhaps the most common tumor of the jaws. Prior to puberty its growth is rapid, after which it may slow or even cease. Cell-rich connective tissue invades bone and undergoes gradual ossification. Since the lesion is painless, a unilateral soft tissue swelling is usually the first sign. The roentgenographic features vary with the degree of mineralization; there is a transition from radiolucency to a mottled, "ground-glass" appearance. The tumor is benign; most patients can be treated by curettage. If the lesion is extensive, further surgical correction may be required.

CYSTS OF JAW. *Multiple basal cell nevoid syndromes.* See page 1386.

Malignant tumors. The malignant tumors of the jaws which occur in children include Burkitt's sarcoma, osteogenic sarcoma, lymphosarcoma, and more rarely fibrosarcoma.

DEVELOPMENT OF THE TEETH AND ASSOCIATED ABNORMALITIES

Initiation. The teeth form in dental crypts which arise from a band of epithelial cells incorporated into each developing jaw. Prior to the calcification of the maxilla and mandible a ribbon of epithelial cells grows inward from the oral epithelium into the underlying mesenchyme. By the eighth week of fetal life these epithelial bands, the *dental lamina*, each have 5 areas of rapid growth, which result in rounded, budlike enlargements. An accompanying organization of the mesenchyme adjacent to each area of epithelial growth takes place, and the 2 elements together constitute the beginning stages of a tooth. Five such areas on each side of the maxilla and of the mandible initiate the primary dentition.

The *permanent teeth* form in 2 groups. After the formation of the primary crypts a bandlike extension of the dental lamina proliferates lingually from each side to form another generation of tooth buds for the permanent incisors, cuspids and premolars, which erupt into sites previously occupied by primary teeth. This takes place from about the fifth gestational month for the central incisors to about 10 months of age for the second bicuspids. The permanent molars, on the other hand, arise from a backward extension of the dental lamina beyond the site of initiation of the second primary molars. Three budlike enlargements form sequentially at approximately 4 months of gestation, and 1 year and 4 to 5 years, respectively, for each of the 3 permanent molars.

Both failures and excesses of tooth initiation are observed. *Anodontia,* or absence of teeth, occurs when no tooth buds form. *Total anodontia* often occurs with ectodermal dysplasia. *Partial anodontia* results when a normal site of initiation is disturbed, as in the area of a palatal cleft, or from genetic failure, frequently familial, to code the formation of specific teeth. The third molars, maxillary lateral incisors and mandibular second premolars are the teeth which most commonly fail to form.

If the dental lamina produces more than the normal number of buds, *supernumerary teeth* occur. These are most often seen in the area of the maxillary central incisors. Since they tend to disrupt the position and eruption of the adjacent normal teeth, their identification as supernumer-

ary teeth by roentgenologic examination is important. *Natal teeth*, present at birth or erupting shortly thereafter, may be members of the normal primary dentition, but this should be verified roentgenologically, since they are often supernumerary teeth, which should be removed (see Natal Teeth, p. 756).

Histodifferentiation-Morphodifferentiation. As the epithelial bud proliferates, the deeper surface invaginates and a mass of mesenchyme becomes partially enclosed. Beginning with the crown, the epithelial cells assume the shape of the tooth they represent, lay down the organic matrix for calcification of the enamel, and induce the underlying mesenchymal cells to become columnar. These cells, in turn, lay down the organic matrix for calcification of dentin. The vascular, nerve and lymph structures (the *dental pulp* of the mature tooth) are confined in the mesenchyme of the hollow central portion of the tooth bud. Disturbances during histodifferentiation-morphodifferentiation may result in gross alterations in dental morphology. *Macrodontia* and *microdontia,* large and small teeth, respectively, are caused at this formative point. The maxillary lateral incisors may not only be absent owing to failure of initiation, but also may assume a slender, tapering shape (*"peg-shaped laterals"*).

Twinning, in which 2 teeth are joined together, is most often observed in the mandibular incisors of the primary dentition. It may result from 3 separate causative possibilities: germination, fusion or concrescence. *Germination* is the result of division of a single tooth germ to form a bifid or cloven crown on a single root with a common pulp canal. An extra tooth is then present in the dental arch. *Fusion* is the joining of incompletely developed teeth that under pressure of trauma or crowding continue to develop as a single tooth. Fused teeth are sometimes joined through their entire length; in other instances a single wide crown is supported on 2 roots. *Concrescence* is the attachment of the roots of closely approximated adjacent teeth by an excessive deposition of cementum. This type of twinning, unlike the others, is found most often in the maxillary molar region. *Dens in dente,* a "tooth in a tooth," is a roentgenologic finding in a tooth of normal appearance. It results from an invagination in the lingual surface, usually of a maxillary incisor, at the site of fusion between separate sites of calcification in the same tooth. Enamel continues to be formed, and an enamel-lined hollow space results. The dental roentgenogram shows the outline of a second dental structure within a tooth.

Congenital syphilis affects differentiation of permanent teeth, resulting in screwdriver-shaped incisors, often with central notches in their incisive edges *(Hutchinson's incisors),* and *mulberry molars* with lobular occlusal surfaces and narrow, pinched crowns (p. 617).

Calcification. Calcification, the deposition of the inorganic mineral crystals of mature enamel and dentin, takes place after the organic matrix has been laid down. Disturbances at this time affect the color, texture and thickness of the tooth surface. All teeth form from several sites of calcification which later coalesce. The characteristics of the inorganic portions of a tooth can be altered by (1) disturbances in formation of the matrix, (2) decreased availability of one or more of the minerals involved, and (3) the incorporation of foreign materials.

Amelogenesis imperfecta, a dominant genetic trait, results in faulty production of matrix. The teeth are covered by only a thin layer of abnormally formed enamel through which the yellow coloration of the underlying dentin is seen, giving a darkened appearance to the dentition. Usually all the teeth, both primary and permanent, are affected. Although susceptibility to caries is low, the enamel is subject to destruction from abrasion. Restorations offering complete coverage of the crowns are often placed for protection and improved appearance.

Dentinogenesis imperfecta, or hereditary opalescent dentin, is an analogous condition in which the odontoblasts fail to differentiate normally, and brown, poorly calcified dentin results. The junction between the enamel and dentin is altered, the enamel has a tendency to flake away, and the exposed dentin is then susceptible to abrasion. The teeth are opaque and pearly, and the pulp chambers are obliterated by calcification. Both primary and permanent teeth are usually involved. Unless the crowns of these teeth are covered early and completely, the abrasion of chewing often reduces them to the level and contour of the supporting alveolar bone.

Localized disturbances of calcification which correlate with periods of illness or malnutrition are frequent; they are analogous to the "growth disturbance lines" often seen in the long bones. An example is the *neonatal line* commonly observed on all the primary teeth and on the permanent central incisors and tips of cuspids at coronal levels consistent with the stage of calcification present at birth. Two general disturbances of the surface of the enamel are seen: Discoloration of the smooth surface, usually a more opaque white patch, is referred to as *hypocalcification*. A more severe disturbance, *hypoplasia*, may be manifest as pitting, or areas devoid of covering enamel. Hypoplasia is uncommon in the primary dentition because of the relative infrequency of intrauterine stress, as opposed to the frequent occurrence of illness or malnutrition during early infancy when the enamel of the outer third of the permanent incisors, cuspids and first molars is forming. Dental restoration of such areas is desirable to eliminate the sensitivity of exposed dentin, to prevent caries, and to improve the appearance.

Mottled enamel is found in persons whose early life is spent in areas where the fluoride content of the drinking water is greater than 2 parts per million; it is probably due to ameloblastic dysfunction. It varies from small, inconspicuous white patches to severe, brownish discoloration and hy-

poplasia; the latter changes are usually seen with fluoride concentrations over 5 parts per million.

Disturbances due to mineral deficiency are rare, but irregular dentin and enlarged pulp chambers have been observed with vitamin D-resistant rickets, and hypoplasia with vitamin D-deficient rickets.

Discolored teeth may result from incorporation of foreign substances into developing enamel. The hemolysis accompanying *erythroblastosis fetalis* may produce blue to black discoloration of the primary teeth, beginning at the neonatal line; the tips of the permanent first molars may also be affected. *Tetracyclines*, extensively incorporated into bones and teeth, may result in ugly, brownish-yellow discoloration and even hypoplasia of the enamel, if administered during the period of formation of enamel. This period extends from about the fourth month of gestation to the tenth month of life for the primary teeth and from about the fourth month to the sixteenth year of life for the permanent teeth. The enamel is completely formed on all but the third molars by about 8 years of age. Therefore, if possible, tetracyclines should not be prescribed for pregnant women or for children under 8 years of age. Discoloration of the teeth has been observed with *all* the tetracycline antibiotics. Fluorescence of the teeth under ultraviolet light is diagnostic.

Eruption. At the time of tooth bud formation each tooth begins a movement outward in relation to the bone; this movement is continuous. The full chronology of human dentition is given in Table 2-4 (p. 37); the relative times of eruption and shedding of the primary teeth and the times of eruption of the permanent teeth are listed in Tables 11-1 and 11-2.

The mandibular teeth usually erupt before their maxillary counterparts, as do those of girls before boys. As the teeth penetrate the gums, inflammation and sensitivity sometimes occur, a condition termed *difficult eruption*. The child may become irritable, and salivation markedly increase. Bacterial invasion through a break in the

TABLE 11-1. TIME OF ERUPTION AND SHEDDING OF THE PRIMARY TEETH

	ERUPTION		SHEDDING	
	Lower	Upper	Lower	Upper
	Age (Months)		Age (Years)	
Central incisor..	6	7½	6	7½
Lateral incisor..	7	9	7	8
Cuspid........	16	18	9½	11½
First molar....	12	14	10	10½
Second molar..	20	24	11	10½
Incisors......	Range ± 2 mos.		Range ± 6 mos.	
Molars........	Range ± 4 mos.			

From Massler and Schour: *Atlas of the Mouth.* American Dental Association, Chicago.

TABLE 11-2. Time of Eruption of the Permanent Teeth

	LOWER AGE (YEARS)	UPPER AGE (YEARS)
Central incisors	6– 7	7– 8
Lateral incisors	7– 8	8– 9
Cuspids	9–10	11–12
First bicuspids	10–12	10–11
Second bicuspids	11–12	10–12
First molars	6– 7	6– 7
Second molars	11–13	12–13
Third molars	17–21	17–21

From Massler and Schour: *Atlas of the Mouth.* American Dental Association, Chicago.

tissue or under a gingival flap covering the teeth may be responsible. A blunt, firm object for the infant to bite on is useful; incision of the gums is seldom indicated. There is no definite evidence to support claims of accompanying temporary systemic disturbances. Such disturbances, the most common of which are low-grade fever, facial rashes and mild diarrhea, are not attributable to eruption of teeth.

Delayed *eruption* of all teeth may indicate systemic or nutritional disturbances such as hypopituitarism, hypothyroidism, cleidocranial dysostosis and rickets. Local causes such as malpositioning of teeth, supernumerary teeth, cysts or retained primary teeth may be responsible for failure of eruption of single or small groups of teeth.

Early loss of primary predecessors is the most common cause of *premature eruption* of teeth. If the entire dentition is advanced for age and sex, an endocrine disorder such as hyperpituitarism must be considered.

Natal teeth. Erupted teeth are observed in approximately one of 2000 newborn infants. Usually there are two in the position of the mandibular central incisors. Their attachment is generally limited to the gingival margin, with little root formation or bony support; such teeth should not be considered supernumerary until a roentgenographic examination has proved them to be; a natal tooth may be a prematurely erupted primary tooth, an indication that generally early dental eruption may be expected.

The presence of teeth at birth may result in complications. Pain secondary to looseness and movement may interfere with nursing, as may maternal discomfort due to abrasion or biting of the nipple during feeding. There is danger of detachment with subsequent aspiration of the tooth. Since the tongue lies between the alveolar processes during birth, it may become lacerated, and occasionally the tip is amputated.

Supernumerary teeth should be extracted; the decision to extract prematurely erupted primary teeth must be made on an individual basis. Should extraction seem indicated, it should be performed by carefully dissecting away the gingival attachment to prevent tearing of the tissue and excessive hemorrhage.

Exfoliation failure occurs when a primary tooth fails to exfoliate prior to the eruption of its permanent successor; the primary tooth should be extracted.

DISORDERS OF THE TEETH ASSOCIATED WITH OTHER CONDITIONS

Osteogenesis imperfecta (p. 1342) is usually accompanied by *hereditary opalescent dentin*, also termed *dentinogenesis imperfecta*. Treatment is usually not indicated.

In *cleidocranial dysostosis* (p. 1345) there are a number of oral-facial variations. Frontal bossing, mandibular prognathism and a broadened base of the nose may be seen. Eruption of teeth is characteristically delayed. The primary teeth are abnormally retained, and the permanent teeth may remain unerupted. The presence of supernumerary teeth is common, especially in the premolar area. Erupted teeth are free of hypoplasia, but variations in size and shape are frequent. The primary dentition and those permanent teeth which do erupt should be restored if they become carious. Extraction of a primary tooth rarely results in the eruption of its permanent successor. The removal of the unerupted permanent teeth is also contraindicated. Their roots are usually crooked and curved, often leading to fracture during attempted removal.

In *ectodermal dysplasia* (p. 1387) the teeth are totally or partially absent. Since alveolar bone does not develop in the absence of teeth, the alveolar processes are usually either totally or partially absent, and the resulting overclosure of the mandible causes the lips to protrude. Cephalometric growth studies have shown, however, that facial development is otherwise not disturbed. Teeth, when present, are small and conical in form. Aplasia of the buccal and labial mucous glands, leading to dryness and irritation of the oral mucosa, has also been observed. Persons with ectodermal dysplasia need either partial or full dentures. The vertical height between the jaws is thus restored, improving the position of the lips and facial contours. Masticatory function is restored, and eating habits are thereby improved.

DISEASES OF THE TEETH

Dental Caries

Dental caries, or decay of the teeth, is a progressive, destructive lesion of the calcified dental tissues. Untreated, it eventually results in total destruction of involved teeth. Dental caries is the principal oral problem of children; by 2 years of age the average child has 2 carious lesions (Fig. 11-1).

Etiology. Dental caries is a bacterial disease, but many factors influence susceptibility to the

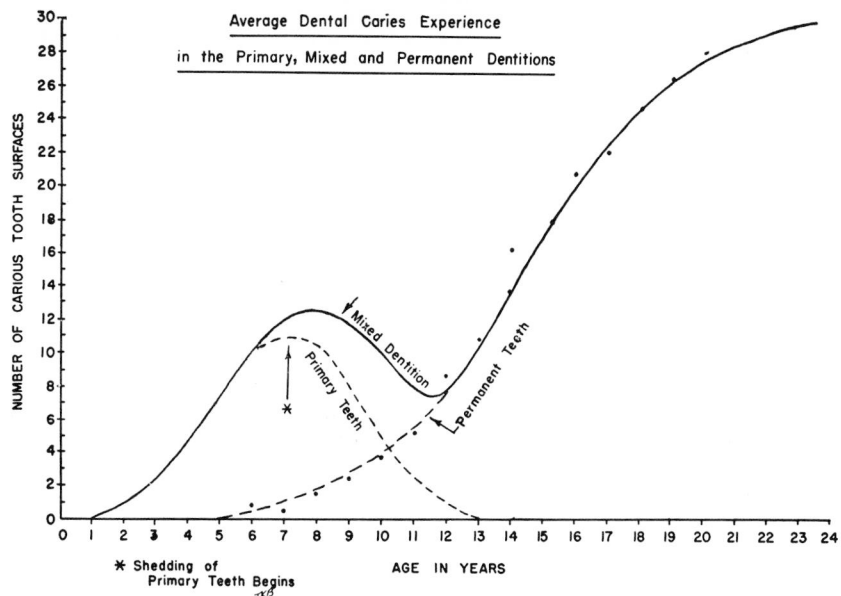

Figure 11-1. Average number of carious surfaces at different age periods. (J. C. Brauer et al.: *Dentistry for Children.* 4th Ed. New York, The Blakiston Division, McGraw-Hill Book Company, Inc., 1959.)

action of the causative organisms, which are principally streptococci. They produce extracellular polysaccharides that form a gelatinous plaque over the tooth to which the organisms adhere. Fermentable carbohydrates, chiefly sucrose, are the main substrate for the production of metabolic acids by the adherent bacteria (Fig. 11-2). The acids first decalcify the enamel, and then cause lysis of the protein of the organic matrix and destruction of the tooth.

Factors influencing caries. AGE. Caries is primarily a disease of childhood and adolescence. The periods of greatest carious activity are 4 to 8 years in the primary dentition and 12 to 18 years in the permanent dentition. Ninety per cent of rampant caries occurs during the latter period.

FLUORIDE. The incorporation of fluoride into mineral apatite crystals appears to increase their resistance to dissolution. Children living in communities where the drinking water contains more than 1.0 part per million (p.p.m.) of fluoride have 40 to 60 per cent less caries than those in areas where the fluoride content is under 0.5 p.p.m. The maximal reduction in dental caries appears to occur when the drinking water contains 1.0 to 1.5 p.p.m. of fluoride. If the fluoride content is over 2.0 to 2.5 p.p.m., mottling of the enamel becomes evident.

DIET. An important factor contributing to caries is the ingestion between meals of foods or fluids containing sucrose, particularly in forms which cling, such as taffy, or promote prolonged contact, such as lollipops and lozenges, with the teeth. Such ingestion provides the substrate for production of tooth-destroying acid by the bacteria adherent to the teeth. Sugars ingested at mealtime are less injurious, since the buffering capacity

of other foods and saliva tends to neutralize the acid.

The practice of putting small children to sleep with a bottle of milk results in pooling of the milk in the oral cavity. The acids produced by bacterial action on the milk substrate may also result in early, rampant caries.

ORAL HYGIENE. Lack of oral hygiene (rinsing and brushing, particularly after meals) permits the accumulation of food debris upon which the bacteria feed.

STATE OF HEALTH. In chronic debilitating dis-

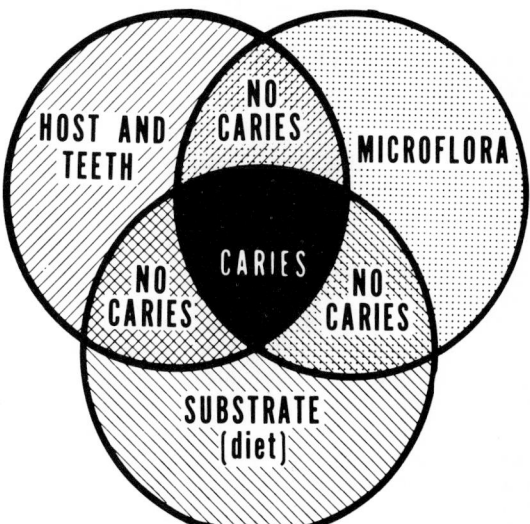

Figure 11-2. Factors involved in causation of dental caries. All factors must be operative before caries will develop. (Keyes: Etiologic Factors of Dental Caries. *Med. Ann. D.C.*, 34:463-7, 1968.)

eases both the quantity and the bacteriostatic quality of saliva may be reduced. Oral hygiene after each meal is even more important than for the healthy person.

Clinical Manifestations. Caries originates most often in areas where food may become impacted, as in the pits and fissures on the occlusal surfaces of the posterior teeth, between the teeth, or along the gum line at the neck of the tooth. The lesions may penetrate rapidly through the substance of the tooth, or their progress may be intermittent and slow. Rapidly burrowing caries is characteristic in children; the slow, intermittent type predominates in middle age.

Prevention. The most effective preventive measure against dental caries is *natural or artificial fluoridation of the water supply*, especially from birth until 8 years of age, by which time the enamel of most of the permanent teeth has been completely formed.

If an adequate amount of fluoride (1.0 p.p.m.) is not present in the water supply either naturally or by municipal fluoridation, 0.3 to 0.5 mg. of fluoride daily can be mixed with the water used to make the formula, or added directly to cow's milk. Although fluoride absorption from milk is delayed in comparison to that from water, it is essentially complete. Children over 1 year of age should receive 0.5 to 1.0 mg. of fluoride (1.1 to 2.2 mg. of sodium fluoride) per day. Recent studies have shown that a beneficial effect is obtained with oral fluoride preparations even after teeth have erupted. This is probably due to topical incorporation of fluoride into the surface dental enamel. Therefore, when liquid preparations containing fluoride are given, the dose should be deposited into the buccal area with the head turned slightly sideways, or the *chewable* tablet should be prescribed in order to encourage oral retention and give time for surface contact. Such fluoride preparations should not be used in areas where the water supply contains fluoride in excess of 0.7 part per million.

The prescription of *fluoride supplements* is not a substitute for fluoridation of community water supplies, since the latter ensures availability of adequate fluoride to *all* children in the area at a safe level and at a considerably lower cost. There is no definitive evidence that administration of fluoride to the pregnant woman reduces the incidence of caries in the child.

After dental eruption, biannual *topical application of fluoride* to the teeth increases the concentration of fluoride in the surface enamel where decay begins. Such applications are effective in areas with an adequate content of fluoride in the water supply, as well as in areas where the fluoride content of the water is inadequate.

Reduction of frequency of eating and *avoidance of sucrose-containing snacks, candies or drinks between meals* can markedly reduce the incidence of new carious lesions. The small child's "bedtime bottle" of milk should be avoided. If the habit has become established, replacement of the bottle with a cup of milk before brushing the teeth at bedtime is more effective than attempts at gradual withdrawal.

The *elimination of active lesions* by restoration of primary as well as permanent teeth reduces the bacterial population in the oral cavity and thereby the hazard to uninvolved teeth. Because of the rapid appearance and progression of new carious lesions, the usual 6-month interval between dental examinations may be inadequate; examination, particularly of the teenage child, should be at 3-month intervals.

Proper *oral hygiene* also is helpful in preventing caries. The mechanical removal of debris from tooth surfaces by brushing or at least rinsing the mouth soon after ingestion of food is important. Small children can be held in the lap. One hand can retract the lips while brushing is accomplished with the other. Brushing should be initiated on eruption of the first primary teeth. The child perceives the pattern and will eventually accomplish the procedure routinely without assistance. Electrically powered brushes are an advantage in facilitating the operation by the adult and in compensating for the child's poor manual dexterity.

Malocclusion

The oral cavity can be viewed as a masticatory machine. The cusps of the opposing posterior teeth interdigitate and slide around each other to reduce foodstuffs to a soft, moist bolus. The cheeks and tongue force the food into the areas of tooth contact. The incisal edges of the anterior teeth are apposed by mandibular manipulation for the purpose of biting off increments of larger food items.

The masseter and temporal muscles are the main forces of mandibular closure. Acting in conjunction with the interval pterygoid muscles, they produce very high pressures on contact of opposing teeth. If a number of teeth meet simultaneously, the force is distributed over a large area of bone to tooth attachment. In malocclusion, when only a few teeth touch, the same force is exerted over a much smaller area, and eventually in adulthood malocclusal deformities are a leading cause of loss of teeth. For this reason preventive measures in childhood should be directed at establishing proper relations of the upper and lower dental arches for physiologic as well as for cosmetic reasons. The Angle classification categorizes the variations in growth patterns into 3 main types of occlusion (Fig. 11-3).

Class I (Normal). The cusps of the posterior mandibular teeth interdigitate ahead of and inside the corresponding cusps of the opposing maxillary teeth.

Class II. The cusps of the posterior mandibular teeth are behind and inside the corresponding cusps of the maxillary teeth. This is the most common occlusal discrepancy; about 45 per cent of the population exhibits some form of it. There is an increased space between upper and lower anterior teeth which

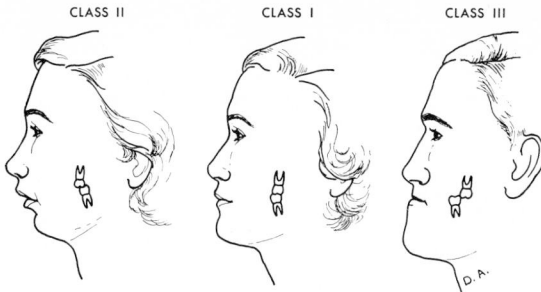

Figure 11-3. Angle classification of occlusion. The typical correspondence between the profile and molar relationship is shown. (R. E. Moyers: *Handbook of Orthodontics.* 2nd Ed. Chicago, Year Book Publishers, Inc., 1963.)

results in a receding chin and encourages sucking and tongue-thrust habits.

Class III. The cusps of the posterior mandibular teeth oppose cusps which are a cusp or more ahead of their maxillary counterpart. The anterior teeth are directly opposed, or the mandibular incisors are protruded beyond the maxillary incisors; the chin is prognathic.

Cross Bite. The mandibular teeth are normally in a position just inside the maxillary teeth, so that the outside mandibular cusps or incisal edges meet the central portion of the opposing maxillary teeth. A reversal of this relation is referred to as a cross bite.

Open and Closed Bites. If the posterior mandibular and maxillary teeth contact each other, but the anterior ones do not, the situation is termed an open bite. If the mandibular anterior teeth fit inside the maxillary anterior teeth in an overclosed position, the situation is referred to as a closed bite. If the overclosure is extreme, the mandibular incisors may strike the gingiva behind the maxillary incisors. The occlusal relation is determined by observing the positions of the teeth when the jaws are closed and the heads of the condyles are in the most posterior position within the glenoid fossa of the temporal bone.

Genetic factors are by far the most common cause of malocclusion. Nevertheless malocclusion may also result from abnormal growth; the mandibular protrusion seen with acromegaly is an example of abnormal growth leading to class III malocclusion. Habits such as thumb-sucking and tongue-thrusting are also important causative factors.

The severity of the malocclusion is the principal factor which determines the timing of treatment. Many cross bites, open bites and closed bites, and a few mild class II malocclusions can be corrected as early as they are diagnosed. Most class II and class III malocclusions are more easily correctable after the eruption of all the permanent dentition except the third molars.

The congenital absence of teeth also may cause occlusal discrepancies. These may be corrected either by prosthetic replacement of the missing tooth or teeth or by moving other teeth to close the vacant space. Early roentgenographic appraisal is important in establishing a plan for treatment.

Periodontal Disease

The roots of teeth are usually essentially conical in shape. Their retention and stability depend on the integrity of the surrounding alveolus and on a healthy periodontal membrane, with its fibers running from cementum to bone. In otherwise healthy adults, prolonged local insults may disturb one or both of these elements. This type of breakdown is relatively rare in childhood; apart from the normal sequence of eruption, either trauma or an underlying systemic condition is likely to be responsible for looseness or exfoliation. The differential diagnosis of noneruptive loss of teeth in children includes scurvy, osteomyelitis of the jaw, juvenile periodontitis, dysplasia of dentin, leukemia, acrodynia, vitamin D deficiency, vitamin D-refractory rickets, hypophosphatasia, Papillon-LeFevre syndrome (hyperkeratosis of palms and soles and disintegration of alveolar bone) and reticuloendotheliosis.

Periapical Infection (Alveolar Abscess). Teeth may become nonvital as a result of deep caries or trauma without an accompanying history of pain. Grayish discoloration, looseness and sensitivity on mastication are frequent symptoms. Localized alveolar swelling and redness are most commonly due to infection around the roots of nonvital teeth, which may also lead to chronic draining fistulas visible in the alveolus at the level of the apex of the root. Periapical infections of primary teeth may cause defects in the underlying permanent teeth. The roots of nonvital primary teeth may not follow the normal pattern of resorption, thus inducing abnormalities in eruption and decalcification of the enamel of the underlying teeth.

Periapical infections and nonvital teeth, which are potential foci for infection if not treated, should be referred promptly for dental treatment; surveillance for these conditions should be routine during pediatric physical examinations. After the reduction of acute symptoms the involved tooth may be extracted. Root canal therapy is usually contraindicated in primary teeth, but is valuable in the retention of permanent teeth.

Impacted Teeth. Though not actually a disease, impaction of teeth is a common dental problem in children. Previously erupted permanent teeth may prevent the subsequent eruption of another tooth which must occupy the same area of the alveolar ridge. The teeth most frequently involved are the maxillary canines and the mandibular third molars. The impacted tooth becomes lodged against the one impeding its eruption. Ectopic eruption, or resorption of the offending tooth, may result. Pain is common. Formation of a dentigerous cyst is the most serious consequence. Treatment consists in surgical removal of the impacted tooth. Unless otherwise contraindicated, impacted teeth should be extracted. If they are retained, periodic roentgenographic examinations should be made to be certain that complications do not arise.

Dentigerous Cysts. Impacted teeth retained in alveolar bone for long periods of time are the source of dentigerous cysts, or cystic degeneration of the enamel epithelium around the crown. The teeth most frequently involved are the mandibular third molars and the maxillary canines. Roentgenographically, the crown of the unerupted tooth is surrounded by a well demarcated radiolucent zone. A dentigerous cyst may dislodge the tooth with which it is associated, e.g. to the inferior border of the mandible or to the floor of the nasal cavity. The lesion requires complete enucleation or curettage; cysts arising from enamel epithelium have the potential of becoming ameloblastomas.

DENTAL INJURIES

The risk of accidental damage to the teeth is exaggerated with the protruding anterior teeth of class II malocclusions or protrusions of maxillary incisors due to finger-sucking or tongue-thrusting; protruding teeth should be brought into a less vulnerable position as soon as possible after the eruption of the permanent incisors. Sports are responsible for many dental injuries. Individually fitted protective mouthpieces are available and should be used. When injury does occur, prompt treatment of fracture or displacement improves the prognosis for subsequent alignment. Dental therapy usually should precede soft tissue treatment.

Fractured Incisors. Blows on the mouth usually strike the maxillary incisors, since they are the most anteriorly located hard structures. Fractures of the crowns and roots of these teeth are therefore frequent. If the cleavage of the crown does not include a portion of the pulpal cavity, treatment is limited to covering any exposed dentin, followed by placement of an esthetic restoration. If a small area of exposed pulp is covered very quickly, recovery may take place. With more extensive injury, the nerve must be removed. Treatment of the root canal, necessary to prevent possible periapical abscess, varies according to whether the root is fully developed or not.

Dislocated Teeth. When the force of a blow is not dissipated by fracture of a tooth, dislocation is common, usually accompanied by fracture of the cortical plate of the alveolar bone. The blood supply to the fractured portion of alveolar bone almost always remains intact, and healing is complete in 3 or 4 weeks. Nevertheless, because the alveolar ridge acts as a fulcrum, the apex of a tooth may be forced out of position, frequently severing the blood vessels and nerve which enter through the small apical foramen.

Dislocated teeth should be promptly repositioned and splinted. After a week, if the sensitivity of the tooth has not returned, root canal therapy will probably be required to prevent abscess formation.

Evulsed Teeth. Completely evulsed teeth should be placed in saline and taken immediately to a dentist for reimplanting. The devitalized tooth usually becomes firmly attached once again, but retention is limited, varying from 6 months to 12 years. Even so, reimplantation, by allowing adjacent dental structures to mature normally, increases the success of ultimate prosthetic replacement.

Habits Injurious to the Teeth.   The positions of the teeth significantly determine the contour of the alveolar bone and the shape of the face. The positions of the teeth, in turn, are dependent on a balance of forces. Normal pressure from the tongue is opposed by buccal and labial pressures; the force of eruption offsets the depression of mastication. Alteration in equilibrium between these forces can change the positions of teeth, disturb the interarch relations and, with time, change facial appearance.

Tongue Thrust.   Since swallowing occurs about once every 2 minutes during the waking hours, the common oral habit of thrusting the tongue forward during swallowing produces almost continuous lingual pressure on the teeth. Anterior inclination of the incisors, with frequent anterior open bite and a tight, protruding upper lip results. Pursing of the lips during swallowing identifies the habit. The placement on the palate of an appliance with a guard-reminder section is useful. Tongue exercises directed by a speech therapist may also be effective in treatment.

Finger-Sucking.   Sucking thumb, fingers or a pacifier between feedings is common in infants. Many children continue this habit well beyond infancy, frequently in response to stress. Weaning from a pacifier is usually less difficult than from a thumb or fingers. The outward pull, particularly of thumb-sucking, may produce a forward movement of the primary maxillary incisors and in turn may induce the associated alveolar bone to shift anteriorly. The permanent incisors then erupt in a more forward position. If the habit persists during eruption of these permanent teeth, they are frequently directed into a protruding inclination. Finger-sucking should be terminated by 5 years of age in order to prevent the displacement of permanent teeth when they erupt the following year.

After the age of 4 years finger-sucking is usually self-correcting in response to social pressures. Persuasion by the pediatrician or dentist may help furnish the motivation to stop. If the habit is very strong, an appliance with a guard in the region of the anterior palate may be successful. With the guard a palatal vacuum is unattainable, and interest in sucking is lost. An emotional problem usually underlies protracted cases.

ABNORMALITIES OF DEVELOPMENT OF THE PALATE AND SOFT TISSUES OF THE MOUTH

CLEFT LIP AND CLEFT PALATE

The incidence of cleft lip or cleft palate is from one in 600 to one in 1250 births according to

TABLE 11-3. APPROXIMATE RISK OF RECURRENCE OF CLEFT LIP AND CLEFT PALATE

AFFECTED	RISK FOR SUBSEQUENT OFFSPRING	
	Cleft Lip with or Without Cleft Palate	Cleft Palate Alone
Propositus	4-7%	2-5%
One parent	2%	7%
Propositus and one parent	11%	17%
Propositus and one sibling	10%	No data

From F. C. Fraser: Genetic Counselling in Some Common Paediatric Diseases. *Pediat. Clin. N. Amer.*, 5:475, 1958.

various studies. Twin studies indicate that genetic factors are of more importance in cleft lip with or without cleft palate than in cleft palate alone. The incidence of cleft lip with or without cleft palate is about one in 1000 births; the incidence of the cleft palate alone is about one in 2500 births. Cleft lip (harelip) with or without cleft palate is more frequent in males; cleft palate alone is more frequent in females. There appears to be an increased incidence of associated congenital malformations and of intellectual impairment among children with cleft defects; both are more common with cleft palate alone. These findings are partially explained by an increased incidence of impairment of hearing in children with cleft palate and by the frequency of cleft defects among children with numerical and structural abnormalities of the autosomes; many of the latter are stillborn or die in early infancy or childhood. The risks of recurrence of cleft defects within families are enumerated on page 345 and in Table 11-3.

Animal studies suggest that nongenetic influences may also be responsible for clefts if applied to a susceptible host at a critical period of organogenesis. Associated malformations are especially frequent in structures derived from the first branchial arch.

Cleft Lip. Cleft lip may vary from a small notch in the vermilion border to a complete separation extending into the floor of the nose. Clefts may be unilateral (more often on the left side) or bilateral, and usually involve the alveolar ridge. Deformed, supernumerary or absent teeth are additional anomalies. The nasal alar cartilage may also be displaced or deformed. Bilateral clefts of the lip are frequently associated with a deficiency of the columella and an elongation of the vomer producing a protrusion of the anterior aspect of the cleft premaxillary process (Fig. 11-4).

Cleft Palate. Clefts of the palate may occur alone or in association with cleft lip. Isolated cleft palate occurs in the midline and may involve only the uvula or extend into or through the soft and hard palates to the incisive foramen. When associated with cleft lip, the palatal defect may involve the midline of the soft palate and extend into the hard palate on one or both sides, exposing one or

both of the nasal cavities as a unilateral or bilateral cleft palate.

Management. The immediate problems of the infant with a cleft lip or palate are concerned with feeding and prevention of aspiration and infection. Most infants can be adequately managed by feeding in an upright position, using softened nipples with slightly enlarged openings. In some instances a medicine dropper or gavage feedings may be used to advantage. Special cleft palate nipples and plastic palatal coverings are usually not necessary.

Operation should be performed by a qualified plastic surgeon. Operation for *cleft lip* is usually at a month or two of age after the infant is gaining weight satisfactorily and is free of any oral, respiratory or systemic infection. The most common technique utilizes a staggered suture line to minimize notching of the lip from retraction of scar tissue. A Logan clamp (a wire bow attached by adhesive to the cheeks) is applied immediately after the operation to take tension off the suture line. The initial repair may be revised at 4 to 5 years of age. In most instances corrective surgery on the nose is better delayed until adolescence. Cosmetic results are dependent on the extent of the original deformity, absence of infection and the skill of the surgeon.

Since *clefts of the palate* vary considerably in size, shape, and degree of deformity, the timing for operation should be individualized. Criteria such as width of the cleft, adequacy of the palatal parts, the morphology of the surrounding areas (such as the width of the oropharynx) and the neuromuscular function of the soft palate and pharyngeal walls affect the decision. The goals of operation are union of the cleft parts, intelligible and pleasant speech, and avoidance of injury to the growing maxilla. The optimal time for palatal surgery varies from 6 months to 5 years of age, depending on the need to take advantage of the palatal changes which occur with growth. When operation is best delayed beyond the third year, a contoured speech bulb can be attached to the posterior of a denture so that contraction of the pharyngeal and

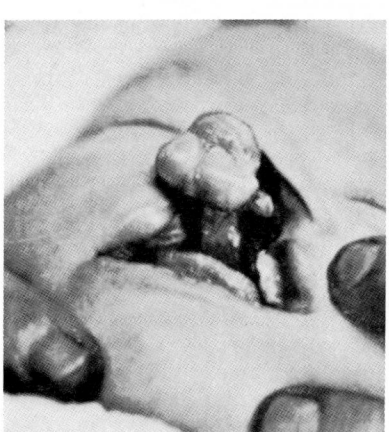

Figure 11-4. Double cleft lip and cleft palate in an infant 2 months of age. Note the intermaxillary process between the clefts.

villo-pharyngeal muscles can accomplish occlusion of the nasopharynx and help the child develop intelligible speech. Almost always the cleft crosses the alveolar ridge and interferes with the formation of teeth in the area. The missing elements of the dentition must be replaced by prosthetic devices; alterations in the positions of teeth may also be necessary.

PREOPERATIVE AND POSTOPERATIVE MANAGEMENT. Even the suspicion of infection is a contraindication to operation. If the child is in good nutritional state and in fluid and electrolyte balance, feeding may be permitted to within 6 hours of the operation. Fluid therapy is discussed on page 229.

During the immediate postoperative period *special nursing care is essential.* Gentle aspiration of the nasopharynx minimizes the hazards of the common complications of atelectasis or pneumonitis. The primary considerations in postoperative care are maintenance of a clean suture line and avoidance of strain on the sutures. For these reasons the infant is fed with a medicine dropper, and the arms are restrained with elbow cuffs. A fluid or semifluid diet is maintained for 3 weeks, and feeding is with a dropper or spoon. The patient's hands as well as toys and other foreign bodies must be kept away from the palate.

Complications. Recurrent otitis media and hearing loss are frequent complications. Excessive dental decay is not unusual and requires special care. Displacement of the maxillary arches and malpositions of the teeth usually require orthodontic correction.

Speech. Speech defects may be present even after good anatomic closure of the palate. Such speech is characterized by emission of air from the nose and by a hypernasal quality when certain sounds are made. The speech defect before and, at times, after palatal surgery is due to inadequacies in function of the palatal and pharyngeal muscles. The muscles of the soft palate and the lateral and posterior walls of the nasopharynx constitute a valve which functions to separate the nasopharynx from the oropharynx during swallowing and in the production of certain sounds. If the valve does not function adequately, it is difficult to build up enough pressure in the mouth to make such explosive sounds as p, b, d, t, h, g or the sibilants s, sh and ch, and such words as "cat," "boats" and "sisters" are not intelligible. After operation or the insertion of a speech appliance it may be necessary to institute speech therapy to lessen the persisting speech defect.

A *complete program of habilitation* for the child with a cleft lip or palate may require years of special medical, surgical, dental and speech treatment. Representatives of the specialties involved function more effectively on a team basis than individually. One of these, however, must be responsible for parental counseling and guidance. Ideally, this is the child's physician. A pediatrician, plastic surgeon, otolaryngologist, children's dentist, prosthetic dentist, orthodontist, speech pathologist, medical social worker, psychologist, child psychiatrist and public health nurse may make up such a *cleft palate team.* The child's physician may need to avail himself of such a group, usually located in the larger medical centers. Most states have programs for financial assistance for the medical care when the economic status of the family warrants.

PALATOPHARYNGEAL INCOMPETENCE

The speech disturbance characteristic of the child with a cleft palate can also be produced by other osseous or neuromuscular abnormalities in the oral and pharyngeal areas. The common denominator is the inability to form an effective muscular seal between oropharynx and nasopharynx during swallowing or phonation. The anomaly may be in the bony structures of the palate or pharynx or in the muscles attached to these structures. An adenoidectomy may precipitate the speech defect in a child who previously spoke normally, and the defect may be attributed to a previously unrecognized submucous cleft palate. In such instances it is assumed that the adenoid had a static function as a mass protruding into the epipharynx, allowing the soft palate to make contact with it when elevated. This became impossible after removal of the adenoid. If there is sufficient reserve neuromuscular function, compensation in palatopharyngeal movement may take place, and the speech defect disappears, although often some symptoms of palatopharyngeal incompetence may persist. In other instances slow involution of the adenoids may allow for gradual compensation in palatal and pharyngeal muscular function. This may explain why a speech defect does not become apparent in some children who have a submucous cleft palate or similar anomaly predisposing to palatopharyngeal incompetence.

Manifestations of Palatopharyngeal Incompetence

1. Hypernasal speech defect especially noted in the articulation of pressure consonants, such as p, b, d, t, h, v, f, s
2. Conspicuous constricting movement of the nares during speech
3. Inability to whistle, gargle, blow out a candle or inflate a balloon
4. Loss of liquid through the nose when drinking with the head down
5. Otitis media and hearing loss

Signs on Oral Inspection

1. Cleft palate or a relatively short palate with a large oropharynx
2. Absent, grossly asymmetric or minimal muscular activity of the soft palate and pharynx during phonation or gagging
3. A submucous cleft, as evidenced by the following pathognomonic signs
   (a) Bifid uvula
   (b) Translucent membrane in midline of soft palate revealing lack of continuity of muscles
   (c) Palpable notching in posterior border of hard palate instead of a posterior nasal spinous process
   (d) Forward or V-shaped displacement of grooving on the soft palate during phonation or gagging

The symptoms of palatopharyngeal disturbances are similar, although clinical signs will vary. The diagnosis can usually be made without difficulty if there is sufficient awareness of the entity.

Palatopharyngeal incompetence can be demonstrated roentgenographically. The head should be carefully positioned to obtain a true lateral view; one film is obtained with the patient at rest and another during continuous phonation of the vowel "u" as in "boom." The soft palate contacts the posterior pharyngeal wall in normal function, while in palatopharyngeal incompetence such contact is absent.

Treatment of palatopharyngeal incompetence is either surgical or prosthetic. In selected cases the palate may be retropositioned or a pharyngoplasty performed, utilizing a flap of tissue from the posterior pharyngeal wall. Dental speech appliances have also been used successfully. *Adenoidectomy should be avoided when there is a submucous cleft palate or a potential palatopharyngeal incompetence.*

DISEASES OF THE ORAL MUCOSA AND GUMS

Bednar's Aphthae (Pterygoid Ulcer). Abrasions of the palatal mucous membrane of the newborn infant, resulting from efforts to clear the mouth of debris, are termed Bednar's aphthae. Superficial trauma denudes a region of the posterior hard palate over which a grayish necrotic membrane forms typically on either side of the midline just anterior to the junction with the soft palate. The lesions heal spontaneously within 7 to 10 days.

Epstein's Pearls (Bohn's Pearls). See page 354.

Mucocele (Mucous Cysts). At any age from infancy to adulthood small mucus-containing cysts may occur in salivary gland-bearing areas of the oral cavity. They have a circumscribed, translucent, bluish appearance. Though usually elevated, they may be deep-seated and mobile on palpation. The cysts form after traumatic rupture of the excretory ducts of minor salivary glands. They are usually lined by granulation tissue, rarely by epithelium. Since recurrence is frequent if only drainage is accomplished, surgical removal of the cyst and the superficially located gland is recommended.

Fordyce Granules. Almost 80 per cent of adults have multiple, yellowish-white granules in clusters or plaquelike areas on the oral mucosa, most commonly on the buccal mucosa or lips. Histologically, normal sebaceous glands are seen in the lamina propria and submucosa. The glands are present at birth, but they hypertrophy and first appear as discrete yellowish papules during the preadolescent period in approximately 50 per cent of children. No treatment is necessary.

Epulis. See page 1440.

Oral Moniliasis (Thrush). Oral infection with the fungus *Candida albicans* is fairly common in the newborn infant (p. 392). The organisms are regular inhabitants of skin, and of oral, vaginal and intestinal mucosa and are spread to the infant during birth. The oral lesions in children are white, flaky plaques covering all or part of the tongue, lips, gingiva and buccal mucous membranes. They are removable, leaving a brightly inflamed base. Discomfort may interfere with food ingestion. The condition is likely to be acute in newborn infants and chronic in infants and young children with nutritional deficiencies and other debilitating conditions. Alterations in the oral flora due to antibiotic therapy also may be responsible. The diagnosis can usually be confirmed by direct microscopic examination and culture of scrapings from mucous membranes.

Though the infection in the newborn infant is usually self-limited, treatment is advisable to limit spread within the nursery and to avoid the occasional protracted infection. The simplest plan at the moment and as effective as any is the oral instillation of 1 ml. of a solution of nystatin (100,000 units per ml.) 4 times a day at intervals of 6 hours. The solution should be slowly and gently instilled so that there is an opportunity for it to be widely distributed throughout the oral cavity before it is swallowed.

Topical application of 1 per cent aqueous gentian violet is also effective, but it is temporarily disfiguring and stains clothing and bed linen (stains can be removed with a paste of sodium bicarbonate). Applications should be made on individual lesions, and care should be taken to avoid an excess of the solution, which may be irritating when swallowed. This can also be lessened if the infant is placed face downward after the application, so that saliva containing the drug will drain outward.

Of primary importance in the chronically ill or malnourished infant or child is the correction of the underlying disturbance. Topical treatment as described above is of course indicated.

Herpangina. See page 673.

Herpetic Stomatitis. See page 635.

Aphthous Ulcers (Canker Sores). The cause of aphthous ulcers is unknown. The lesions, which resemble somewhat those of herpetic stomatitis, but are more localized, occur singly and multiply on the oral mucosa, usually following situations of stress. Secondary infection by streptococci is the cause of much of the discomfort. Topical applications of tincture of benzoin are of value in the control of pain.

Necrotizing Ulcerative Gingivitis (Vincent's Infection; Vincent's Angina). Necrotizing ulcerative gingivitis is characterized by the formation of a gray necrotic membrane and small ulcers which are localized upon painful hyperemic gingivae. Fever, malaise and a prominent fetid odor are common. The infection is not a communicable disease as was once thought, but most often represents a decrease in resistance of gingival tissue to infection with the usual oral flora, and with an especially heavy overgrowth of fusiform bacilli and spirochetes. Such infections are largely limited to chronically ill, malnourished children. The acute stage of the infection responds dramatically, usually within 48 hours, to thorough cleansing of the mouth with oxidizing sprays or mouth rinses; hourly rinses with half-strength (3 per cent) hydrogen peroxide while awake are a useful regimen.

Since necrotizing ulcerative gingivitis is extremely rare in childhood, except in areas of extreme poverty, the diagnosis should be made with caution. Herpetic stomatitis and the oral manifestations of acute leukemia and the reticuloendothelioses may be similar and should be excluded.

Noma (Gangrenous Stomatitis; Cancrum Oris; Infective Gangrene of the Mouth). Noma is a rare progressive gangrene of the buccal mucosa which results in a perforating ulcer of the cheek (Fig. 11-5). It is caused by invasion of the buccal tissues by fusospirochetal organisms and other bacteria in children whose resistance has been lowered by concurrent disease or nutritional deficiency. The lesion usually begins as a small ulcer with few constitutional symptoms, but soon results in a gangrenous, greenish-black area on the gums, buccal mucosa or mucocutaneous borders. The gangrenous area spreads slowly but inexorably until the cheeks are perforated and the jaws denuded.

Intensive antibacterial therapy, based on susceptibility tests in vitro, should be instituted as soon as the diagnosis is made, and continued until all necrotic tissue, whether soft tissue or bone, has sloughed. Since malnutrition is frequent in these patients, an adequate diet should be introduced gradually with special emphasis on adequate amounts of protein and vitamins. Plastic surgical procedures may be indicated when healing is complete.

Chemical Burns. In addition to accidental ingestion of acids, alkalis or other caustic substances, incorrect self-medication may cause burns of the

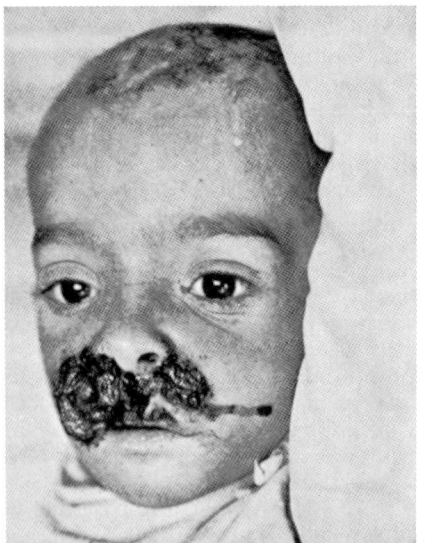

Figure 11-5. Gangrenous stomatitis, beginning in the lip.

oral mucosa which usually appear as white lesions. The most common example is the holding of an aspirin tablet locally against a painful tooth or gum, so that it dissolves slowly in the area. The result is a white, irregular patch of coagulated tissue. Camphor held in the mouth is another frequent cause of oral burns. The only treatment required is elimination of the practice; healing is spontaneous.

Dilantin Hyperplasia. A generalized enlargement of the gingiva occurs in about 10 to 30 per cent of patients who receive diphenylhydantoin sodium (Dilantin) for control of seizures. The gingiva is pale, firm, and granular and may hypertrophy to the point of covering the crowns of the teeth. Superimposed trauma or infection may cause inflammation and discomfort. Careful oral hygiene helps to avoid discomfort.

Fibromatosis Gingivae. Fibromatosis gingivae is a rare familial idiopathic gingival hyperplasia which resembles Dilantin hyperplasia. It may be associated with other developmental defects such as mental deficiency and hypertrichosis. The firm, smooth-surfaced, generalized enlargement of the gingiva consists of collagen covered by stratified squamous epithelium. The swelling may produce protrusion of the lips and migration of the teeth. The only effective treatment is surgical removal of the excess gingiva, but recurrence is common. Particular attention must be devoted to oral hygiene to prevent irritation and stimulation of further gingival overgrowth.

THE LIPS

Prominent Labial Frenum. In some instances the labial frenum appears prominent and thick. The fibers may pass between the maxillary central incisors, rather than attaching to the labial mucosa, and may appear to cause spacing, or diastema, of deciduous or permanent incisors.

A space between the primary maxillary incisors is common. If a wide band of the frenum with an attachment to the lingual side of the alveolar ridge persists after eruption of the permanent canines, the frenum may be suspected as being the cause of a diastema. In most cases the downward growth of the alveolar bone raises the attachment, and the lateral force of the erupting canines closes any existing space. When necessary, the attachment can be raised surgically, and a simple appliance can be used to bring the incisors together.

Cheilitis. Dryness of the lips followed by scaling and cracking and accompanied by a characteristic burning sensation is common in children. It is usually caused by sensitivity to contact substances (from toys and foods) plus photosensitivity to the sun's rays. It is aggravated by the habit of alternate wetting with the tongue and drying by the wind, especially in cold weather. Cheilitis also often occurs in association with fever. Frequent application of a bland ointment permits healing and is also preventive.

Angular Fissures. Maceration and fissuring at the angles of the mouth may be caused by an infection with *Candida albicans*. It usually causes no constitutional symptoms or pain. The infection usually extends inside the mouth. Treatment with a mild antiseptic is successful.

When fissuring is caused by a nutritional deficiency, it is termed *cheilosis*. Cheilosis is an early sign in riboflavin deficiency and is often accompanied by moniliasis. Fissuring also occurs in mentally deficient children who drool (rhagades in Down's syndrome).

Herpes Simplex (Herpes Labialis; Cold Sore; Fever Blister). Herpes simplex (see p. 634) is an aggregate of small transparent vesicles on an inflammatory base and is accompanied by itching or burning. It usually affects the mucocutaneous junction, but may affect the skin of the face or the mucous membrane of the mouth. It is self-limited, disappearing in 8 to 14 days.

Allergic Eruptions. Certain substances such as lipsticks and toothpastes may produce eruptions where they come in contact with the lips. The lesions may be vesicular or elevated reddish wheals (*urticaria*), and there may be a glossitis. There is usually a history of other allergic manifestations.

Angioneurotic edema (p. 500) is a variety of urticaria which may be responsible for a sudden diffuse swelling of short duration (1 to 2 days) in children with allergic tendencies. It often itches, but is seldom painful. There is no erythema, and the tissues appear to be normal in color, firm, and do not pit.

Mucous retention cysts are single teatlike projections covered by a thinned-out mucous membrane and filled with a clear fluid. They are caused by occlusion of the orifice of a labial or buccal mucous gland, resulting in retention of the secreted fluid.

THE TONGUE

The tongue in certain instances may assume an unusual appearance without undue clinical significance. The patient is often not aware of the unusual appearance.

Ankyloglossia (Tongue-tie). Occasionally the lingual frenum extends to near the tip of the tongue and interferes with its free protrusion; if the attachment reaches the anterior border, a notch may be visible. Owing to the possibility of bleeding or infection, and because it usually stretches with time, it is no longer thought advisable to clip the lingual frenum at birth. Should surgical correction be necessary (which it rarely is), the procedure can be carried out at any time after 8 to 10 months of age.

Fissured Tongue. The pattern may be foliaceous (leaflike) or cerebriform. The tongue may be somewhat enlarged and show imprints of the teeth at the sides. Fissured (scrotal) tongue is usually congenital, but may be acquired, especially in Down's syndrome. Occasionally fissuring may follow certain diseases such as scarlet fever, syphilis or typhoid fever.

Black Hairy Tongue (Lingua Nigra). This condition is characterized by an elongation of the filiform papillae into hairlike projections as long as $1/2$ to 1 inch. It is generally concentrated in a triangular area in front of the V-shaped line of circumvallate papillae. The patch may vary from brown to black. The condition is usually chronic, but often disappears spontaneously.

A similar condition also occurs in association with chronic intraoral hemorrhage, as in purpura and hemophilia. The filiform papillae become hypertrophied and are colored dark brown by the blood pigments. There is always a characteristic *fetor ex ore*, owing to the presence of blood in the mouth.

Hairy tongue may occur during prolonged antibiotic therapy, especially with oral troches.

Geographic Tongue (Wandering Rash). This benign lesion is characterized by one or more smooth, bright red patches often showing a yellowish, grayish or whitish membranous margin upon the dorsum of an otherwise normally roughened tongue. The patches are areas in which the filiform papillae have become completely desquamated, leaving a smooth, slick surface. The patches may be single or multiple, discrete or confluent (maplike). They travel by an extension of desquamation of the papillae at one edge and a regeneration of the normal papillae at the other. The condition is usually chronic, and a single cycle may last 2 to 7 days.

Temporary smooth red patches on the dorsum of the tongue simulating geographic tongue are frequent in children with low-grade fevers, particularly those accompanying the common cold and chronic systemic infections.

Macroglossia. The tongue in infants is often proportionately larger than the other oral structures because it grows at a relatively faster rate and is not confined by the teeth. In stocky infants the tongue is frequently so large and unconfined that it protrudes from the mouth, and occasionally has been mistaken for a manifestation of hypothyroidism. As the infant grows, the other oral structures gradually catch up and confine the tongue, so that its relative size is decreased.

A true hypertrophy of the tongue is rare. It may exist congenitally as a diffuse lymphangioma or as a muscular hypertrophy (rhabdomyoma). The tongue may reach such a size that it cannot be retained in the mouth, with the result that nursing and, later, speech are interfered with. In such cases the teeth are pushed into a malocclusion by the action of the tongue.

Treatment is surgical, although some relative adjustment usually occurs as the child grows older.

Hemangiomas and cysts may be responsible for diffuse or localized enlargement of the tongue. Enlargement is also present in cretinism, acromegaly and occasionally gargoylism.

White Coated Tongue. The accumulation of

food debris and bacteria among hypertrophied filiform papillae causes a *moist coated tongue*. The filiform papillae are present at birth, but are much shorter than even the fungiform papillae until about 5 years of age, so that the tongue appears smooth. Thus in the young child the cause should be sought for any coating of the tongue.

The condition of *dry furry tongue* (hypertrophied filiform papillae) is seen early in states of mild dehydration and low-grade fever.

A transitional stage from the white coated tongue to the raw red tongue is known as the *white strawberry tongue*. The appearance is that of an unripe strawberry. The engorged and enlarged fungiform papillae appear prominently above the level of the white, desquamating filiform papillae. It is seen early in scarlet fever and other acute febrile states.

Raw Red Tongue (Glossitis). When the filiform papillae of the white strawberry tongue or the coated tongue are shed, leaving the engorged fungiform papillae raised above the smooth, denuded surface of the tongue, the condition is known as red raspberry or red strawberry tongue. This is seen often in the later stages of febrile states and about the sixth or seventh day of scarlet fever.

When the papillae become flattened and edematous (mushroom-shaped), but not atrophied or shed, the *raw pebbly tongue* results. The color is a characteristic purplish-red (magenta) instead of pink. Edema of the tongue is common, and the indentations of the teeth can easily be seen. The edges of the tongue often become denuded and raw, resulting in a burning, painful sensation. Fissuring is common. Such lesions occur in *ariboflavinosis* in association with cheilosis, photophobia and lacrimation.

Complete atrophy of both the filiform and fungiform papillae results in a *smooth atrophic tongue*. The desquamated surface is usually dry and extremely sensitive (glazed tongue). *Atrophic glossitis* with a fiery red (scarlet) coloration of the tongue is characteristic of *niacin deficiency (pellagrous glossitis)*, especially when accompanied by infection. Atrophic glossitis with a pale salmon coloration of the tongue (*Hunter's glossitis*) occurs in *pernicious anemia*, and also in *sprue*, *achlorhydria* and *hypochromic anemia*.

Trauma. Accidental biting of the tongue, irritation by carious teeth, injuries by sharp objects placed in the mouth, and burns by hot foods occur frequently in children. Such injuries may result in a simple blister or ulcer which disappears in a few days, but even superficial ulcers are painful. In extreme cases the tongue may become swollen and edematous. Ice may be used to reduce the swelling. The food should be cool and in liquid form; it may be necessary to feed young infants through a nasal tube. A mild antiseptic mouthwash such as 1 per cent tincture of iodine in physiologic saline solution may be used.

Accidental injuries and burns resulting from ingestion of poisons are not uncommon in young children. Immediate care is determined by the poison ingested and the extent of the injury. In severe cases particular attention should be given to adequacy of the airway; occasionally tracheotomy is essential as a lifesaving measure.

Ulcerations of the frenum and the margins of the tongue are usually the result of herpetic infection; those limited to the frenum may be secondary to biting the tongue during paroxysms of coughing in pertussis. Such ulcers have also been observed in association with familial autonomic dysfunction.

SALIVARY GLANDS

Salivary secretions originate from 3 pairs of glands: the parotid, submaxillary and sublingual. The parotid fluid is serous and contains amylase and secretory immunoglobulin (IgA); that of the submaxillary glands is a mixed seromucoid fluid, and that of the sublinguals is a mucoid viscous fluid. The volume and composition of the mixed saliva are a function of the degree of secretory stimulation to each of the 3 pairs of glands, and are subject to many local and systemic influences.

With the exception of epidemic parotitis (p. 647), disease of the salivary gland is rare in children. Bilateral enlargement of the submaxillary glands may occur in cystic fibrosis, malnutrition and, transiently, during acute asthmatic attacks. Chronic vomiting and aspiration, as in achalasia, may also be accompanied by enlargement of the parotids.

Infants exhibit salivary discharge or drooling until muscular reflexes which initiate swallowing and lip closure are developed. Later, the irritation of teething in conjunction with the accompanying increase in oral activity may also lead to drooling. In some children with mental retardation, drooling is never overcome.

If salivary flow rates are decreased by medications, disease or irradiation, an increase in dental decay usually follows. In addition to the obvious washing action, saliva also appears to furnish the materials from which the cell-free film which covers dental enamel is formed. This film influences the surface equilibria between enamel and bathing fluids; its absence is accompanied by a pronounced increase in caries.

Excessive secretion of saliva occurs during teething, as a reflex to anticipated feeding or pain, from irritative lesions in the mouth, in conjunction with nausea, after administration of mercurial compounds, and in certain nervous affections such as encephalitis and chorea.

Xerostomia (Dry Mouth). Temporary dryness of the mouth occurs with fever, dehydration, and the ingestion of drugs such as the phenothiazine derivatives, atropine and other anticholinergic substances. In *congenital xerostomia* the mouth becomes glazed, dry and filled with debris. The condition responds to the administration of pilocarpine.

Recurrent Parotitis. Recurrent idiopathic swelling of the parotid gland may occur in otherwise healthy children. The swelling is usually unilateral, although both parotid glands may be involved simultaneously or alternately. As many as ten or more recurrences may be observed in an individual child. There is little pain associated with the swelling, which is limited to the gland and usually lasts 2 to 3 weeks. Subsidence is spontaneous and may be complete or partial. The incidence appears to be higher in the spring.

Suppurative parotitis, most often due to *Staphylococcus aureus,* may occur as a primary disease or as a complication of parotitis due to another cause. It is usually unilateral and may be accompanied by fever, and the gland becomes swollen, tender and painful.

Recurrent parotitis requires no treatment, but it may be confused with suppurative parotitis, which responds to appropriate antibacterial therapy based on culture of purulent discharge from Stensen's duct, or of pus obtained by infrequently required surgical drainage. Roentgen therapy appears to shorten the attacks of recurrent parotitis, and to decrease the number of recurrences. Owing to the potential hazards of irradiation of a growing child, it should be considered only in severe or prolonged cases.

Mikulicz's disease is a term applied to idiopathic bilateral, painless enlargements of the parotid and lacrimal glands, usually associated with dryness of the mouth and an absence of tears. The manifestations may also occur in diseases such as tuberculosis, leukemia and lymphosarcoma.

Ranula. Because of resemblance to the appearance of a frog's belly, a cyst associated with one of the major salivary glands in the sublingual area is termed a ranula. The large, soft, mucus-containing swelling occurs in the floor of the mouth and can be seen at any age, including infancy. The cyst should be excised and the severed duct exteriorized.

Frederick M. Parkins
Giulio J. Barbero

REFERENCES

Blayney, J. R., and Hill, I. N.: Fluorine and Dental Caries. *J. Am. Dent. A.,* 74:225, 1967.

Finn, S. B.: *Clinical Pedodontics.* 3rd ed. Philadelphia, W. B. Saunders Company, 1967.

Gorlin, R. J., and Pindborg, J. J.: *Syndromes of the Head and Neck.* New York, McGraw-Hill Book Company, Inc., 1964.

Keyes, P. H.: Research in Dental Caries. *J. Am. Dent. A.,* 76: 1357, 1968.

Kraus, B. S., and Jordan, R. E.: *The Human Dentition Before Birth.* Philadelphia, Lea & Febiger, 1965.

Lindahl, R. L., and Brauer, J. C.: *Dentistry for Children.* 5th ed. New York, McGraw-Hill Book Company, Inc., 1964.

Moyers, R. E.: *Handbook of Orthodontics.* 2nd ed. Chicago, Year Book Medical Publishers, 1963.

Richmond, J. B. (Ed.): Symposium on the Child's Mouth. *Pediat. Clin. N. Amer.,* 3:845-1137, 1956.

THE ESOPHAGUS

Symptoms suggestive of esophageal disease in infants and children are cough or choking on ingestion of fluids, dysphagia, complete inability to swallow, pain on swallowing, regurgitation of undigested food or fluids, and hematemesis. With any of these symptoms, swallowing function should be studied by cinefluoroscopy. Barium is the usual contrast medium used unless a tracheo-esophageal fistula or a complete esophageal obstruction is suspected, in which case an iodized oil should be used to avoid aspiration of barium into the trachea or bronchi. The esophagus may be examined directly with the esophagoscope, generally without anesthesia, in infants or children of any age. If a general anesthetic is preferred, airway patency must be maintained by an intratracheal tube to avoid compression of the soft tracheal walls by the esophagoscope.

CONGENITAL ANOMALIES

The esophagus is developed from the first part of the primitive gut, its upper part from the retropharyngeal segment, and the lower from the pregastric segment. As the neck differentiates and the heart and lungs push the stomach caudad, the esophagus elongates rapidly. Vacuoles appear in the epithelium to form a lumen by the eighth week. During the fourth week the laryngotracheal groove develops to become the larynx and trachea and the primordia of the lungs. Two furrows course longitudinally along the sides of this respiratory primordium and cut inward to separate it from the esophagus. This separation progresses in a cephalic direction. Congenital anomalies develop through a failure of one of these critical steps to be completed correctly, and vary from complete absence of the esophagus to duplication throughout its length (see p. 789).

TABLE 11-4. Average Measurements of the Esophagus at Various Ages

AGE	TEETH TO CRICOID	TEETH TO BIFURCATION	TEETH TO CARDIA
Birth	7 cm.	12 cm.	18 cm.
1 year	9 cm.	14 cm.	21 cm.
3 years	10 cm.	16 cm.	23 cm.
5 years	11 cm.	17 cm.	25 cm.
10 years	12 cm.	19 cm.	27 cm.
15 years	14 cm.	23 cm.	33 cm.
Adult	16 cm.	25 cm.	40 cm.

ATRESIA AND FISTULA
(Tracheo-esophageal Fistula)

Etiology. Atresia and fistula of the esophagus, the most common congenital anomalies, may be due to a deviation of the septum between trachea and esophagus, or to altered cellular growth along the septum. Absence of growth along the septum results in a fistula to the trachea; deficient growth of entodermal cells of the dorsal wall results in atresia.

Clinical Forms. Of the 5 types of atresia or fistula, the most common one (Fig. 11-6, *A*) consists of an upper segment which ends in a blind pouch at or slightly above the level of the bifurcation of the trachea, and a lower segment from the stomach which is connected to the trachea by a short fistulous tract. The *symptoms* are characteristic. The first swallow or two by the newborn infant is normal; then suddenly the fluids return through the nose and mouth; the child coughs, struggles, turns cyanotic and may stop breathing. The cycle is repeated with each attempt at nursing, and between feedings there is constant drooling from the dependent corner of the mouth. The stomach becomes distended with air, and bile and gastric secretion may be collected from the regurgitated material, owing to the fistula between the lower segment and the trachea. Pneumonia from aspiration of gastric secretions refluxed into the trachea is a serious problem prior to surgical correction.

In the second commonest type (Fig. 11-6, *B*) both segments are blind, neither being connected to the air passages. The *symptoms* are like those of the first type, but the roentgenogram shows an opaque abdomen devoid of gas in the stomach and intestines (Fig. 11-7). Since no gastric juice can enter the tracheobronchial tree, the pulmonary symptoms are produced entirely by overflow of milk and saliva from the esophagus, so that postural drainage and suction of the trachea are effective in clearing the obstruction. The lower segment is often rudimentary, and generally primary anastomosis is impossible.

Tracheo-esophageal fistula without atresia, the so-called H type (Figs. 11-6, *C*; 11-8), may be suspected in infants or children who show signs of

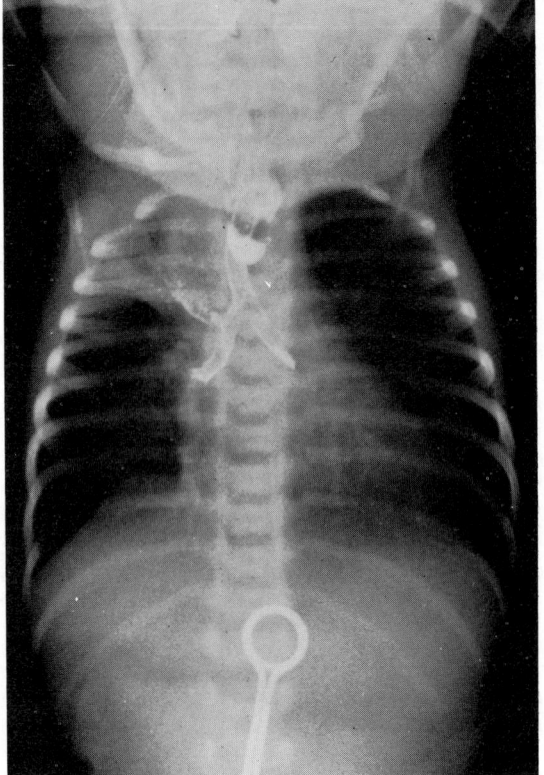

Figure 11-7. Roentgenogram of a newborn infant with esophageal atresia without tracheo-esophageal fistula (Fig. 11-6, *B*). Note absence of air in the gastrointestinal tract. Lipiodol was given by mouth, thereby demonstrating the upper blind pouch; some of the contrast material spilled over into the trachea and bronchi. The atelectasis of the right upper lobe is a common associated finding.

respiratory embarrassment and choking and coughing associated with fluid, as opposed to solid, feedings. There are usually gastric distention, and excessive amounts of mucus in the oropharynx. Repeated episodes of pneumonitis are common and may lead to the diagnosis only after the child is several months to a year or so of age. The fistula may be found at any point from the level of the cricoid cartilage to the midesophagus. The opening, which may be no more than pinpoint in

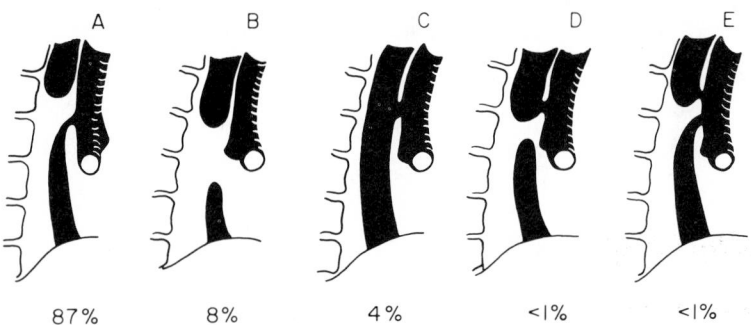

Figure 11-6. Diagrams of the 5 most commonly encountered forms of esophageal atresia and tracheo-esophageal fistula, in order of frequency.

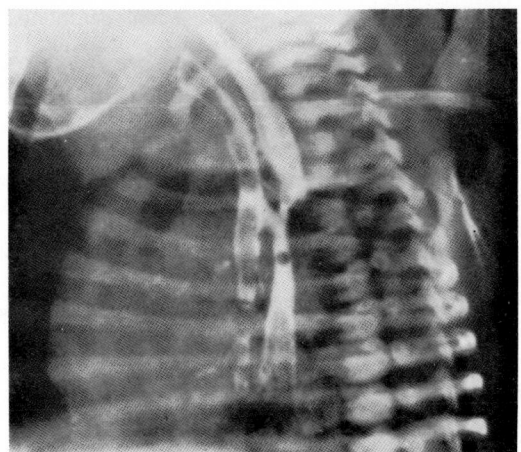

Figure 11-8. Tracheo-esophageal fistula (H type) without esophageal atresia. The infant was born prematurely; birth weight was 3 pounds 14 ounces. Respiratory distress appeared soon after birth and was progressive; it was accentuated when liquids were swallowed. The large fistula was demonstrated after the tip of the catheter had been positioned in the upper end of the esophagus and contrast material introduced through it. There is narrowing of the esophagus just above the site of the fistula.

size, is usually at a higher level in the trachea than in the esophagus.

In the least common types (Fig. 11-6, *D, E*) the upper segment of the esophagus opens into the trachea, and the infant may "drown" with the first feeding; coughing and cyanosis with feeding are prominent.

Diagnosis. Maternal polyhydramnios, commonly associated with atresia of the upper digestive tract, and excessive salivation or drooling in the newborn infant should arouse suspicion of esophageal atresia before the diagnosis is evident from choking, cyanosis or regurgitation on feeding. Roentgenologic confirmation may be obtained by demonstration that a radiopaque catheter will not pass into the stomach, or by use of contrast media. Iodized oil rather than barium should be used as the contrast medium for roentgenologic studies to avoid the danger of aspiration of barium. One-half cubic centimeter of the contrast material given by mouth with a medicine dropper or instilled in the esophageal pouch with a catheter is adequate for diagnostic purposes. The roentgenogram of the chest and abdomen taken in the upright position shows the round blind end of the esophagus at the level of the tracheal bifurcation, or it may demonstrate the fistulous tract into the trachea or the absence of air below the diaphragm, depending on the type of malformation.

The demonstration of an H type of fistula usually requires lateral or oblique cinefluoroscopy (Fig. 11-8) with contrast medium. Cinefluoroscopy is also helpful in distinguishing between a small fistula high in the trachea and pharyngeal overflow into the larynx in pharyngeal paralysis due to neurogenic abnormalities in the newborn infant.

Treatment. Most of the malformations can be corrected surgically. The success of operation is dependent on early diagnosis, before bronchopneumonia, dehydration and inanition have progressed to an irreversible degree.

The condition of the infant, particularly when the weight is less than 5 pounds, occasionally does not permit end-to-end anastomosis. In such instances a gastrostomy may be performed, the tracheal fistula to the lower segment ligated, and the upper segment exteriorized to avoid the otherwise inevitable pneumonia from aspiration. Later, when the infant's condition permits, the 2 ends are anastomosed to establish oral-gastric continuity.

Adequate preoperative and postoperative management is essential for the successful outcome of esophageal surgery. The following preoperative factors are considered important: (1) broad-spectrum antibiotic therapy for the treatment of pneumonia; (2) intermittent suction drainage of the upper esophageal pouch through an indwelling catheter, the tip of which should be maintained just above the lower end of the pouch; (3) maintenance of the infant in an upright position to avoid reflux of gastric juice into the trachea and lungs; (4) parenteral administration by slow, continuous intravenous drip of 5 to 10 per cent glucose in 0.2 per cent saline solution containing 1 to 2 mEq. of potassium per 100 ml. until the condition is deemed favorable for operation; (5) strict isolation technique, preferably in an enclosed incubator; (6) constant nursing supervision and care. Immediately before operation a cannula should be placed in a vein for administration of blood during the operation. Bronchoscopic aspiration may be required preoperatively or postoperatively if atelectasis persists; atelectasis of the right upper lobe is common.

Postoperatively, the infant should be placed in an oxygen tent or enclosed incubator. Feedings through the gastrostomy tube or through an esophageal-passed polyethylene tube may be started in 2 or 3 days. (Some surgeons are opposed to nasogastric intubation immediately postoperatively.) The first 2 or 3 feedings should consist of 0.5 per cent physiologic saline solution and then of 5 per cent glucose solution. If these are tolerated, a milk formula of gradually increasing strength may be given. Oral feedings are usually tolerated 8 to 10 days after the operation. There is a trend away from the use of prophylactic antibiotic therapy.

Stenosis at the operative site is not uncommon. A swallow of contrast material 10 days postoperatively observed fluoroscopically and recorded by spot films will determine the adequacy of the lumen. If there is stenosis, soft rubber mercury-filled bougies may be used to establish and maintain a satisfactory lumen. Too often the diagnosis of stenosis at the site of anastomosis is delayed because the diet is entirely liquid and the degree of obstruction is not apparent until semi-solids are added at 2 or 3 months of age. It must be stressed that early esophageal dilatations

TABLE 11-5. Survival of Patients with Type A Tracheo-Esophageal Fistula as Related to Some Associated Anomalies

ASSOCIATED ANOMALY	PATIENTS AFFECTED	SURVIVORS
None	478 (52%)	373 (78%)
Congenital heart disease	171 (19%)	37 (22%)
Genitourinary	98 (11%)	22 (22%)
Imperforate anus	88 (10%)	38 (43%)
Intestinal atresia	30 (3%)	4 (13%)
Other	51 (5%)	– – – –

Adapted from T. M. Holder, D. T. Cloud, J. E. Lewis, Jr., and G. P. Pilling, IV: Esophageal Atresia and Tracheo-esophageal Fistula. *Pediatrics,* 34:542, 1964.

of the soft stenosis at the point of anastomosis are more successful in maintaining a satisfactory lumen than later dilatations of fibrous scars.

The survival of patients with tracheo-esophageal fistula is influenced not only by prompt diagnosis and skilled surgical treatment, but also by the presence of other anomalies (see Table 11-5).

SHORT ESOPHAGUS

The esophagus may be abnormally short with a portion of the stomach displaced upward through the diaphragm into the thoracic cavity. Occasionally, temporary obstruction by a foreign body leads to a roentgenologic study which reveals a stricture in the midthorax at the esophagogastric junction with the short esophagus above it and true gastric mucosa with rugae below. These rugae can be followed through the diaphragm as a continuation of the rugae of the subdiaphragmatic stomach. The fact that the cardia becomes stenotic accounts for the symptoms. It has been suggested that the stricture may be the result of reflux of gastric contents due to an incompetence of the gastroesophageal mechanism as described under chalasia. The clinical picture is characterized by dysphagia, regurgitation, malnutrition and frequent attacks of complete obstruction of the esophagus.

Treatment. When there is no evidence of stricture, treatment consists in propping the infant in an erect position during and after feeding, as described for chalasia. When there is stenosis, repeated dilatations are indicated; the lesion is peculiarly resistant to therapy, and occasionally one must resort to gastrostomy and retrograde dilatation or, more rarely, to surgical reconstruction. Ulcers in the supradiaphragmatic stomach should be treated in a manner similar to other gastric ulcers.

STENOSIS

Congenital stenosis of the esophagus without a fistula can be found at any point, but usually in the distal third, as either a web or a long segment of esophagus with only a threadlike lumen. The symptoms are those of esophageal obstruction, usually first apparent when the infant begins to eat semisolid or solid food. The diagnosis is made by roentgenographic and esophagoscopic examinations. The treatment is esophagoscopic dilatation. These strictures respond more readily than does that of a congenitally short esophagus.

EXTERNAL COMPRESSION

Partial obstruction of the esophagus may be caused by compression from congenital cardiac or vascular anomalies and by mediastinal tumors such as tracheogenic or bronchogenic cysts, cystic duplications of the esophagus, teratomas or neurogenic tumors. Fluoroscopic studies of the esophagus with contrast material and recognition of both esophageal and tracheal compression by esophagoscopy and bronchoscopy assist in establishing the diagnosis. Angiocardiography is of value in questionable cases in which symptoms are severe. Treatment consists in surgical relief of the obstruction.

NEUROGENIC SWALLOWING DYSFUNCTION

Congenital anomalies of the medulla or cerebral birth injuries occasionally result in a lack of nervous stimulation of the muscles of deglutition. The infant is unable to swallow, and food and mucus constantly fill the pharynx and the trachea. Esophagoscopy, gavage and roentgenograms show the esophageal lumen to be entirely patent. Similar symptoms may occur in amyotonia congenita and bulbar poliomyelitis. Death may result from pneumonia.

Treatment. Postural drainage and suction of mucus are necessary to prevent pulmonary aspiration and pneumonia. Feedings must be entirely by gavage or gastrostomy.

CARDIO-ESOPHAGEAL RELAXATION
(CHALASIA)

This clinical syndrome is manifest by vomiting following feeding when the infant is in the horizontal position. The vomiting is the result of persistent relaxation of the lower end of the esophagus (chalasia). The cause in most instances is not demonstrable. The course tends to be self-limited, and for this reason chalasia has often been assumed to be the result of a temporary neuromuscular imbalance. Chalasia has been associated with cerebral defects, with obstruction at the pylorus or just below it and in one reported instance with a hemangioma at the cardia.

Vomiting begins a few days after birth, is more or less effortless, and can usually be avoided if the infant is maintained in the erect position. It may occur during feeding, but usually begins after the infant has been returned to the crib. In untreated cases the infant loses weight and becomes dehydrated. It may be that an occasional instance of rumination is the result of chalasia.

The diagnosis is established by observing the swallowing of barium under the fluoroscope. Persistent relaxation of the esophageal hiatus is observed with retrograde filling of the esophagus during inspiration or with increase of intra-abdominal pressure.

Therapy consists in feeding a relatively thick milk formula and in maintenance of the infant in an erect (propped sitting) position for several hours after feedings. Permanent relief is usually obtained after a month or two of such management.

ACQUIRED DISEASES

ESOPHAGITIS

Acute esophagitis may complicate practically any acute infectious disease; it may be associated with inflammation of other parts of the digestive tract or may follow lacerations produced by swallowing of foreign bodies or injuries caused by ingestion of hot liquids. The lesions generally last but a few days, and the prognosis is favorable. Symptoms may be substernal pain on swallowing, dysphagia and hematemesis, or may be entirely absent. Some benign esophageal strictures seen in later life originate from acute esophageal ulcers associated with infectious diseases in childhood.

The so-called *Rokitansky-Cushing ulcer*, which is an occasional accompaniment of severe lesions of the central nervous system, may be located in the lower third of the esophagus, in the fundus of the stomach or in the duodenum. Most often these lesions are identified at necropsy; occasionally they perforate before death.

Chronic esophagitis is not rare in early life. It may follow an acute process or be the result of venous congestion in chronic pulmonary or cardiac disease. Most commonly it is associated with congenital strictures or with a short esophagus.

Infrequent causes of esophagitis include diphtheria, thrush, variola, varicella, and perforation by a caseous lymph node.

Inflammatory strictures may follow any of the conditions mentioned as esophagitis. Symptoms and treatment are those of corrosive strictures. The diagnosis must be established from the history and from the roentgenographic and esophagoscopic appearances.

CORROSIVE STRICTURES

The most common cause of stricture of the esophagus (see also pp. 1494, 1499) is ingestion of caustic and corrosive agents such as lye, ammonia (readily available in the kitchen as cleansing agents and for flushing drains), acids – acetic, lactic, carbolic, nitric, sulfuric and hydrochloric – and bleaches (chlorates). Most accidents due to these agents occur because they are carelessly kept in a soft drink bottle, cup or jar similar to one the child uses for food or drink. The lesions vary from superficial pharyngitis and esophagitis to ulceration and necrosis of the esophageal or gastric wall with a chemical mediastinitis or peritonitis which may result in death in a few hours.

Clinical Manifestations. When a child swallows lye or an acid, the first mouthful causes intense burning and pain, and tends to inhibit further swallowing, but the damage has already been done. The lips, chin, tongue and pharynx become edematous and covered with exudate; similar changes occur in the esophagus and infrequently in the stomach (p. 796). In many cases the edema subsides after the first week, and the swallowing function returns to normal in 2 to 4 weeks.

The ensuing period may be symptomless, but if treatment is not carried out, difficulty in swallowing usually recurs insidiously over weeks or months as strictures develop in the burned areas. At first the child has difficulty in swallowing solid food. Eating becomes slow, food is frequently regurgitated, and, later, difficulty in taking liquids becomes apparent. Often the child is considered a "feeding problem" because the accident has been forgotten and the dysphagia is so gradual in its progress. Roentgenograms then reveal strictures of the esophagus, most pronounced in the areas of anatomic narrowing: the cervical region, the cardia, and the point at which the left bronchus crosses the esophagus. Children with long-standing esophageal strictures have numerous evidences of nutritional deficiencies.

Treatment. Emergency management for ingestion of alkalis consists in oral administration of large amounts of water, dilute vinegar or citrus fruit juices, and milk, egg whites, olive or mineral oil. For acid ingestion milk, lime water, soap solution or aluminum hydroxide gel, followed by egg whites, or olive or mineral oil, is appropriate. *Gastric lavage and emetics should not be used in either case.* For bleaches gastric lavage with warm water, emetics and saline cathartics are recommended. Patients with severe reactions following ingestion of any of these agents must be fed intravenously or by gastrostomy, and may require a tracheotomy because of pharyngeal or laryngeal edema.

After emergency treatment there is considerable variation in management, but it is imperative that an active regimen be initiated immediately. Hospitalization for observation is advisable. Broadspectrum antibiotics are usually prescribed for a week or so. Some use corticosteroids to lessen scar tissue formation, but the incidence of spontaneous hemorrhage or perforation of the esophagus or stomach associated with their use in acute esophageal burns is appreciable; furthermore, steroids alone do not prevent stricture formation.

Their use may be of some advantage, but should be limited to 10 to 14 days.

Early dilation of the esophagus after alkali and bleach burns is the *sine qua non* of their treatment. On the second or third day after ingestion, well lubricated rubber Hurst-type mercury-filled bougies are passed into the stomach. Beginning with bougies no. 14F and 16F, dilatations are done daily for the first week, every second day for the second week, then twice a week, weekly, twice monthly and then at monthly or bimonthly intervals. The size of the bougies is gradually increased to no. 24F for infants, 32F for children and 40F for adults. In mild acid burns this same routine may be followed. In severe acid burns early instrumentation is strictly avoided; a jejunostomy may be necessary for feeding purposes because of the severity of esophageal and gastric destruction.

With failure of early treatment, stricture formation or actual atresia may become apparent within 2 to 4 months; in some instances many years elapse before the stricture becomes severe enough to produce dysphagia. The generally accepted method of treatment of definitely formed strictures consists in esophageal dilatations which may be guided by a swallowed string, or visually through an esophagoscope. If the stricture is extremely tight, retrograde dilatation is preferred, the bougie being guided by a string advanced through a gastrostomy. When complete atresia of the esophagus follows ingestion of a caustic, endoscopic efforts at recannulization are generally successful, but occasionally external surgical procedures must be considered. Replacement of the esophagus by a section of colon or small bowel is preferred to resection of the stricture and gastroesophageal anastomosis.

SPASM OF THE ESOPHAGUS
(ACHALASIA; MEGA-ESOPHAGUS)

Esophagospasm, including cardiospasm, may be present even in newborn infants. Esophagospasm is usually characterized by severe sudden obstruction to swallowing and reverse peristalsis and, in older children, may be initiated by emotional stress. *Cardiospasm* (achalasia, preventriculosis) is the syndrome of nonorganic obstruction of the cardia associated with dilatation and hypertrophy of the esophagus (mega-esophagus). It is generally considered to be a failure of coordination of the mechanism at the cardia, preventing normal passage of food from the esophagus to the stomach. In long-standing cases there is fibrosis and disorganization of musculature of the lower end of the esophagus.

Clinical Manifestations. These are difficulty in swallowing, regurgitation of undigested food and fluid, cough from overflow of fluids into the larynx, especially at night, and failure to gain or loss of weight. The diagnosis is made by fluoroscopy or roentgenograms, which demonstrate the barium column in the dilated esophagus terminating in a fine point as it approaches the

diaphragm. Pulmonary infections, including bronchiectasis, may result from the constant overflow of food from the esophagus into the larynx.

Treatment. In uncomplicated cases treatment includes dilatations of the cardia by a pneumatic bag accurately placed under fluoroscopic guidance, by a Hurst mercury bougie, by an esophagoscope or by string-guided olive-tip bougies. Psychotherapy should be considered. In advanced cases retention of food and fluids produces esophagitis, periesophageal inflammation and fibrous strictures at the cardia. Surgical intervention may become necessary in extreme situations; such procedures as a Heller esophagocardial myotomy (similar to the Fredet-Ramstedt operation for pyloric stenosis) or an esophagogastrostomy may give permanent relief. Unfortunately, however, reflux esophagitis often leads to a recurrence of the symptoms and of the stricture itself, necessitating a return to dilatations or reoperation. Belladonna derivatives may be of some benefit if administered early, but are of no avail in advanced cases.

ESOPHAGEAL VARICES

Esophageal varices may occur in children with portal hypertension (Banti's disease, p. 1090) as one of the evidences of the attempt to return blood to the heart by circumventing the liver. The principal **symptoms** of the varices are recurrent, profuse hematemesis of bright red blood, tarry stools and systemic signs of severe hemorrhage. Careful roentgenographic studies with barium may outline the varices. Their presence may be confirmed by esophagoscopic examination.

Treatment. Treatment of portal hypertension is discussed elsewhere (p. 848). Acute hemorrhage may at times be controlled by some form of tamponade. The varices may be injected with sclerosing solutions, special long needles being used through the esophagoscope. These procedures are palliative in most instances, but prolong life, reducing the number and severity of the hemorrhages.

RETROESOPHAGEAL ABSCESS

The most frequent cause of retroesophageal abscess is extension of a retropharyngeal abscess downward to the retroesophageal component of this single, potential space; other causes are esophageal perforations, foreign bodies, spinal caries, pleuritis, pericarditis, ulceration from an intubation or tracheostomy tube, diphtheria of the pharynx or suppurating mediastinal lymph nodes. The abscess forms behind and around the esophagus and often displaces it to one side, while at the same time it compresses the more firmly seated trachea.

The **symptoms** are dyspnea, brassy cough, dysphagia and, as the trachea is pushed forward, swelling of the neck. Toxemia, pain, tenderness on palpation of the neck, and cervical emphysema may be present. The increased retrotracheal space can be demonstrated on lateral roentgenograms of the neck without the use of contrast medium; if the abscess is due to esophageal perforation, barium is contraindicated.

Prognosis. The abscess may rupture into the pleura, trachea or lung. Death may result from pressure of the abscess upon the vagus nerve or on the trachea with consequent asphyxia, or by an erosion into the great vessels of the neck with exsanguinating hemorrhage.

Treatment. Prompt surgical drainage is indicated. If the abscess is high, the retroesophageal space may be opened in the neck along the anterior border of the sternocleidomastoid muscle. Drainage here is effective to the level of the fourth dorsal vertebra. For retroesophageal abscesses occurring below this point a posterior mediastinotomy is generally indicated. Appropriate antibiotic therapy is indicated, but it should be recognized that such therapy could mask an advancing mediastinal infection, and that only repeated lateral roentgenograms of the neck and chest will indicate the situation in the post-tracheal area.

FOREIGN BODIES IN THE ESOPHAGUS

Infants and children swallow an unlimited variety and number of inedible objects which in most instances reach the stomach and pass through the gastrointestinal tract without complications. Occasionally they lodge in one of the 3 anatomically narrow points of the esophagus, from which they must be extracted.

The point of lodgment of most foreign bodies is the cervical esophagus, immediately below the cricopharyngeus muscle. Here the musculature is weak in comparison with the strong muscles immediately below. The narrowing at the hiatus of the diaphragm and the cardia constitutes the second most common site for the lodgment of foreign bodies, although few lodge there. The third and infrequent site for lodgment is the normal narrowing of the esophagus at the level of the arch of the aorta. Open safety pins are found most frequently in infants 7 to 15 months of age, and coins, small toys, buttons, marbles and jackstones in children from 3 to 6 years.

Strictures of the esophagus, congenital or acquired, are often responsible for the lodgment of foreign bodies which would pass through the normal esophagus. They are a constant problem in infants and children who have had a repair of a congenital esophageal atresia.

Clinical Manifestations. Initial symptoms of coughing, gagging, choking and dyspnea usually occur with ingestion of an object, no matter where it lodges. If it remains in the esophagus, pain localized in the region of the thyroid cartilage, dysphagia and drooling may follow. Once a foreign body becomes fixed, there is frequently a symptomless interval until edema around it produces evidence of obstruction, or until signs of infection resulting from esophageal perforation become evident.

Laryngeal symptoms may be produced by foreign bodies in the cervical esophagus. Dyspnea resulting from compression of the trachea may be severe enough to require a tracheotomy before the foreign body can be removed. This is especially true of marbles or jackstones. Cough and hoarseness follow obstruction of the cervical esophagus because of the irritation from secretions overflowing into the larynx. Similar symptoms occur if the foreign body erodes into the trachea.

Diagnosis. The diagnosis of a foreign body in the esophagus is most frequently made from the history. The child may state that he swallowed a button or coin, or the mother may state that the child placed some object in his mouth and choked on it. A history of difficulty in swallowing or the refusal of a child to take solid or liquid food suggests an esophageal foreign body.

A complete search of the gastrointestinal tract as well as of the respiratory system must be made to locate the object. Fluoroscopic examinations and roentgenograms of the cervical esophagus, with the introduction of radiopaque media, if necessary, and of the chest and the abdomen in the anteroposterior and lateral projections are indicated. On anteroposterior projection of the chest, the face of a flat foreign body, such as a coin or safety pin, is usually visible if it lies in the esophagus; if it lies in the larynx, the edge is visible.

Treatment. *Foreign bodies in the esophagus should be removed under direct vision through the esophagoscope.* The use of blind instrumentation in an attempt to force the foreign body into the stomach or attempted extraction by means other than by direct vision is liable to lead to esophageal perforation, mediastinitis and death. Attempts to force the foreign body into the stomach with dry bread, cabbage, cotton or roughage diets not infrequently necessitate the removal of this material as well as the foreign body. Such procedures may also wedge the foreign body more firmly into the esophageal mucosa.

PAUL H. HOLINGER

REFERENCES

Berenberg, W., and Neuhauser, E. B. D.: Cardioesophageal Relaxation (Chalasia). *Pediatrics*, 5:414, 1950.

Carré, I. J., Astley, R., and Smellie, J. M.: Minor Degrees of Partial Thoracic Stomach in Childhood. *Lancet*, 2:1150, 1952.

Chunn, V. D., and Geppert, L. J.: Spontaneous Rupture of the Esophagus in the Newborn. *J. Pediat.*, 60:404, 1962.

Cleveland, W. W., Chandler, J. R., and Lawson, R. B.: Treatment of Caustic Burns of Esophagus: Early Esophagoscopy and Adrenocortical Steroids. *J.A.M.A.*, 186:262, 1963. (See comment in Year Book of Pediatrics, 1964-65 Series, S. Gellis ed., Chicago, Ill., Year Book Medical Publishers.)

Herweg, J. C., and Ogura, J. H.: Congenital Tracheoesophageal Fistula with Esophageal Atresia. *J. Pediat.*, 47:293, 1955.

Holder, T. M., Cloud, T. C., Lewis, J. E., Jr., and Pilling, G. P., IV: Esophageal Atresia and Tracheoesophageal Fistula (A Survey). *Pediatrics*, 34:542, 1964.

Holinger, P. H., Johnston, K. C., and Potts, W. J.: Congenital Anomalies of the Esophagus. *Acta Oto-Lar.*, Suppl. 100 (1952).

Holinger, P. H., Johnston, K. C., Potts, W. J., and da Cunha, F.: The Conservative and Surgical Management of Benign Strictures of the Esophagus. *J. Thoracic Surg.*, 28:(Oct.) 1954.

THE GASTROINTESTINAL TRACT

Gastrointestinal Disturbances

Gastrointestinal symptoms may reflect disturbance of the gastrointestinal tract or of other systems, particularly of the central nervous system or of the psyche. Lack of appetite, vomiting, diarrhea, constipation, abdominal pain and rectal bleeding are common gastrointestinal manifestations which require diagnosis and management appropriate to the cause.

POOR APPETITE

Whenever the complaint is that of poor eating, the first step is to evaluate its significance in the light of the child's appearance and growth. Frequently the complaint arises from a misconception about normal food intake in early childhood, when physiologically diminished intake occurs as the rate of growth is decelerated significantly during the second and third years of life. Day-to-day variations in food intake also occur among children, as they do among adults. The dawdling of young children as they begin to explore self-feeding is likewise sometimes viewed as poor appetite. The finicky characteristic of liking a few foods and refusing to explore others, particularly of different texture, is noted among many children. The highly publicized value of "greens" or "a balanced diet" often leads to parental anxiety centered around food, forced feeding, and the development of a real dislike for eating. Children may pick up undesirable eating patterns of other members of their family; quarreling or chaotic conditions at mealtimes may also lead to dislike of eating. Complaints of poor appetite are made more frequently about only children, about children who are born many years after the last previous child, or about children whose parents are elderly. On occasion, lack of appetite may cause parental anxiety because of its association with illness experienced in previous offspring or during the parent's own childhood. Decreased appetite is common among children of families experiencing marital or other stresses and as a manifestation of either acute or chronic illness. It may be accompanied by temporary failure to grow, other causes of which must be carefully ruled out.

Neither a blunt statement that the child is well nor the prescription of a "tonic" will be successful in resolving the problem of poor appetite. A search in an atmosphere of patience and understanding for the factors responsible for the parental apprehension or stress, followed by sympathetic counseling, usually reduces the complaint and sometimes results in improvement of the child's appetite. The effort is worthwhile, since later psychosomatic or emotional difficulties may be rooted in early parent-child conflict over eating. Efforts to allay parental anxiety and improve the poor appetite of chronically ill children are rarely successful. Nevertheless the poor appetite of children with severe iron deficiency anemia often responds dramatically to iron therapy.

Anorexia Nervosa. Anorexia nervosa is an extreme form of poor appetite or self-starvation, usually observed in preadolescent and adolescent girls. It is accompanied by severe weight loss and in girls at times by amenorrhea or delayed puberty. Anorexia nervosa frequently starts as an attempt to lose weight by dieting. Normal physical activity may be maintained despite much loss of weight. Children with the disease often appear to have broken down in their ability to compete adequately in school and play; they manifest many patterns of emotional restriction, such as flat facial expressions and diminished verbal responses. *Treatment* includes appropriate nutritional surveillance and psychotherapy (p. 89).

Failure to Thrive. The term "failure to thrive" has come to be used for infants and children who, for relatively long periods of time and without superficially evident cause, fail to gain weight and to grow adequately, and often lose weight. This situation or syndrome is observed most often in infants and next most frequently in children just beyond infancy. Though in some instances the cause can be identified as dietary deprivation or as a not readily apparent organic lesion, in many there is no explanation beyond that of social neglect or abuse.

In general the clinical pattern is characterized by growth failure, developmental retardation and considerable psychosocial disruption, in conjunction with signs of physical and emotional deprivation such as apathy, poor hygiene, intense eye contact with people, withdrawing behavior, and disorders of food intake which may be manifest as anorexia, voracious appetite or pica. Such infants frequently improve in both weight gain and social response during hospitalization. Some may exhibit concurrent vomiting, regurgitation, diarrhea or general neuromuscular spasticity which may also improve or cease to exist during hospitalization without specific treatment. Failure to thrive may accompany or precede overt neglect or physical abuse. In many, but not all, instances the cause does not appear to be solely a defective intake of food, but rather some physical or emotional deprivation which may be secondary to family upheaval or illness.

Since failure to grow may be the presenting complaint for infants or children with nonovert but identifiable organic abnormalities, a thorough diagnostic workup is indicated. Renal insufficiency, urinary tract infection, congenital heart disease, neurologic lesions and the malabsorption syndrome are the more common conditions to be ruled out.

In the absence of identifiable organic disease a change of environment may be both diagnostic and therapeutic, particularly in children in adverse family circumstances. If the family situation is favorable, once progress is initiated in those without organic lesions, it usually continues. If not, temporary or permanent placement in a foster home may be necessary.

ABDOMINAL PAIN

Abdominal pain is a common symptom during childhood, arising in most instances from disturbances of the psyche or of the gastrointestinal or urinary tract. Except for *infantile colic* (p. 160), it is rare as a presenting complaint in early infancy, but may be associated with intestinal atresia or duplication, volvulus, visceral hernias, annular pancreas, Meckel's diverticulum, incarcerated hernia, intussusception and even appendicitis. Duodenal ulcer tends to present during infancy with vomiting rather than with abdominal pain. Urinary tract anomalies or infection may produce a complaint of abdominal pain at any age. During childhood, in addition to many of the conditions already enumerated, acute abdominal pain may be the presenting symptom or an interim manifestation of emotional crises, gastroenteritis, mesenteric adenitis, asthmatic attacks, diabetic acidosis, rheumatic fever, anaphylactoid purpura, right lower lobe pneumonia, pancreatitis, regional ileitis, primary peritonitis, infectious mononucleosis, the crises of sickle cell disease and torsion of the ovary, as well as of lead intoxication and porphyria. Patients with cystic fibrosis frequently have episodes of abdominal pain of uncertain origin, and *swallowed blood* may result in considerable epigastric pain. Abdominal pain is probably more frequently ascribed to roundworm infestation of the intestinal tract than is justified. Rarely, abdominal pain may be associated with cerebral dysrhythmia.

Recurrent Abdominal Pain. Recurrent abdominal pain without detectable disease of the urinary or gastrointestinal tract is a frequent complaint of children. It is often emotionally frustrating to the child and his parents, and diagnostically and therapeutically frustrating to the physician.

In many instances recurrent abdominal pain may represent a spastic form of the *irritable colon syndrome* (p. 799).

The frequent association of recurrent abdominal pain with signs of hyperactivity of the autonomic nervous system and with emotionally charged situations such as ambivalence about going to school gives support to the hypothesis that the syndrome of recurrent abdominal pain in children is often a psychosomatic illness. Further support for this hypothesis lies in the behavioral characteristics exhibited by children with the syndrome, such as generally strong sensitivity to other persons, varying degrees of fear for the health and happiness of parents and other persons close to them, and fears of being unacceptable to others in appearance or competence. Environmentally, the life of the family has frequently been punctuated by illness and acute situational crises, such as deaths, separations and accidents.

Treatment consists in reassurance and helping the child and his parents to gain insight into the nature of the problem. Implication that the abdominal pain is "in the head," "made up" or "put on" must be carefully avoided; the pain is real. Glib statements that the pain is psychologic or emotional are likewise hard for the parents to accept; they tend to have an unusual sensitivity to and sense of responsibility for pain of the body or spirit of their child. The physician must make a careful and unbiased exploration of possible organic causes for the pain, as well as a search for areas which may be recognized as emotionally stressful. Since anxiety over pain originally initiated by anxiety may result in a vicious circle, breaking the cycle may be helpful; a few patients respond to mild sedation or the symptomatic relief sometimes offered by antispasmodics. Such therapy should be intermittent and used only as seems necessary, in the early phase of psychosocial therapy. Continued drug dependence by the family or child should be avoided. The ritual of administration of an appropriate number of drops of tincture of belladonna in water 30 minutes before each meal may be more effective than the swallowing of a pill. If the abdominal pain is interfering with play or attendance at school, or if it has become an overwhelming focus of anxiety in the life of the family, hospitalization may be helpful in providing reassurance that every reasonable attempt has been made to rule out organic causes. The temporary removal from the home of the child who has become the source of parental anxiety may break the cycle of anxiety and in itself be therapeutic. The usual diminution of the complaint during hospitalization offers additional reassurance to the physician and family that the diagnosis is correct, and there is opportunity for calm and unhurried exploration of possible precipitating factors.

The measures outlined above are usually successful in temporarily or permanently alleviating the complaint of recurrent abdominal pain, but relapses are frequent. Fortunately, most children with recurrent abdominal pain eventually either recover or learn to accept the symptoms as a part of life, but a few may continue to have recurring episodes which are disruptive to their and their parents' lives. Even these children usually move on to eventual recovery. Psychiatric referral may be helpful for identified emotional problems with which the physician and parents are unable to cope on a more superficial basis.

Abdominal Epilepsy. Very rarely, recurrent abdominal pain may occur as an epileptic aura or equivalent. The diagnosis is based on the electro-encephalographic demonstration of cerebral dysrhythmia which coincides with the pain. The presence of minor electroencephalographic abnormalities in patients with recurrent abdominal pain, even if apparently relieved by anticonvulsant therapy, does not suffice to justify a diagnosis of epilepsy with its lifelong implications for the child.

GASTROINTESTINAL BLEEDING

Since many of the specific entities resulting in gastrointestinal bleeding are discussed elsewhere, only general comments will be made here. Gastrointestinal bleeding raises many questions of diagnosis and management, the resolution of which depends on the age of the child, severity and duration of bleeding, associated symptoms, and site of origin.

Below 1 year of age intussusception, Meckel's diverticulum, volvulus and gangrene of the small bowel are the chief causes of intestinal hemorrhage (Fig. 11-9), but *anal fissure, also more common under 1 year of age, is the most frequent cause of rectal bleeding in both infancy and childhood.* Polyps, esophageal varices and ulcerative colitis are more common beyond 1 year of age. Localized lesions are responsible for about 50 per cent of cases of gastrointestinal bleeding, and systemic disturbances (sepsis, hemorrhagic diseases, al-lergy) are responsible for 10 to 20 per cent. About one third of cases of gastrointestinal bleeding are not etiologically identifiable, even after exhaustive investigation. About half of the localized lesions causing bleeding from the intestinal tract are in the anus, rectum or colon; about one third are in the small intestine, and only about 10 per cent are above the ligament of Treitz.

Hematemesis. Hematemesis in childhood is most commonly due to blood swallowed during epistaxis or after a surgical or dental procedure. Such bleeding or accumulation of a large amount of blood in the gastrointestinal tract may be responsible for leukocytosis or fever. Blood-tinged vomitus and minor hematemesis are not infrequent after repeated vomiting of any cause. Otherwise hematemesis suggests upper gastrointestinal lesions such as esophageal varices, erosive esophagitis secondary to gastroesophageal hiatal hernia, peptic ulcer or, rarely, hemangioma or aberrant gastric mucosa in the esophagus.

Rectal Bleeding. Gross rectal bleeding may result from anal fissure, peptic ulcer, marginal ulcer associated with a Meckel's diverticulum or an intestinal duplication, gangrenous bowel secondary to volvulus, intussusception, gastrointestinal infection, ileitis, polyps, ulcerative colitis or amebic ulcer. Tarry stools may result from peptic ulcer, esophageal varices or bleeding diatheses. The association of vomiting, abdominal pain or shock with rectal bleeding suggests the possibility of a surgical emergency. Rectal bleeding with

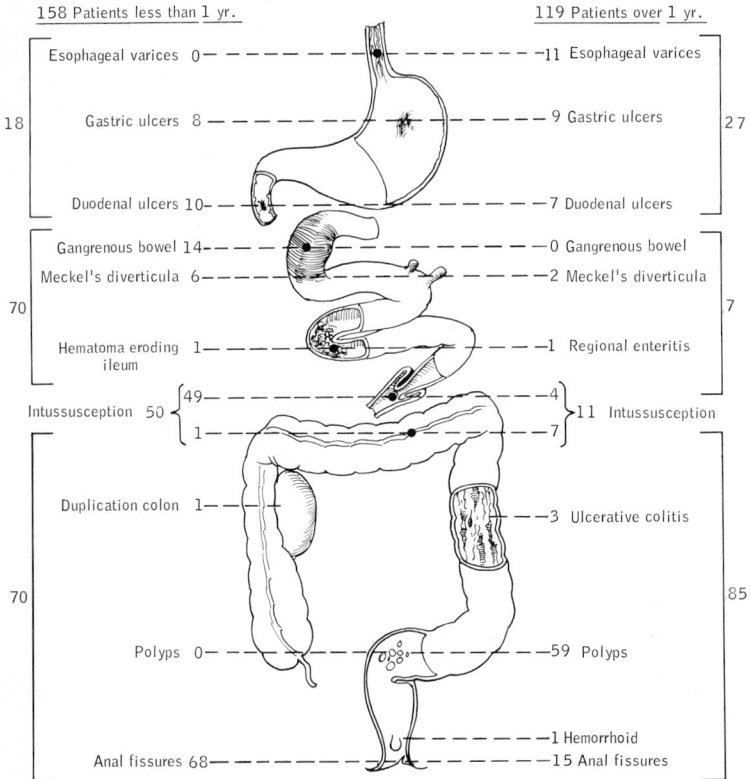

158 Patients less than 1 yr.   119 Patients over 1 yr.

Esophageal varices 0 — — — — — — — — — — —11 Esophageal varices

18   Gastric ulcers 8 — — — — — — — — — 9 Gastric ulcers   27

Duodenal ulcers 10 — — — — — — — 7 Duodenal ulcers

Gangrenous bowel 14 — — — — — — — 0 Gangrenous bowel

Meckel's diverticula 6 — — — — — — 2 Meckel's diverticula

70   Hematoma eroding 1 — — — — — — 1 Regional enteritis   7
ileum

Intussusception 50 {49 — — — — — — 4}   11 Intussusception
{ 1 — — — — — — 7}

Duplication colon 1 — — — — — — 3 Ulcerative colitis

70   85

Polyps 0 — — — — — — 59 Polyps

1 Hemorrhoid

Anal fissures 68 — — — — — — 15 Anal fissures

Figure 11-9. Lesions producing gastrointestinal hemorrhage in children under and over 1 year of age. (After Spencer: *Surgery*, 1963.)

diarrhea suggests infectious enterocolitis, ulcerative colitis, amebiasis or intussusception. Minimal or microscopic bleeding with recurrent or chronic anemia suggests Meckel's diverticulum, amebiasis, ulcerative colitis, infectious enterocolitis, hiatal hernia, or polyps; in infants, *milk allergy* is an occasional cause of such bleeding.

If the blood is bright red, diagnosis of the cause of rectal bleeding begins with careful examination of the anus for a crack, fissure or "sentinel tag." If any one of these is found, and the bleeding is minor or consists chiefly of blood-streaked stools or blood spots on the paper used to wipe the anus after defecation, particularly if there is a history of hard, large or painful bowel movements, the blood may be presumed to be from an *anal fissure.* Treatment consists in meticulous cleansing of the anus with soap and water after each defecation and of use of mineral oil or a stool softener to facilitate passage of stool until the lesion heals.

If an anal lesion is not found, thrombocytopenia, hypoprothrombinemia and other bleeding disorders should be ruled out; the rash associated with anaphylactoid purpura usually serves to identify it as a cause of intestinal bleeding. Sigmoidoscopic examination is useful to identify ulcerative colitis or polyps in the distal colon. Barium studies are useful to diagnose duodenal ulcer (because of the relative shortness and motility of the child's intestine, blood from a bleeding ulcer may be passed in virtually unaltered form), ileitis, ulcerative colitis, polyps, intussusception and volvulus; they are rarely informative for Meckel's diverticulum or duplication. Occasionally, air contrast study of the colon is useful in the diagnosis of polyps. Pigmented lesions on the lips suggest polyposis of the small bowel as part of the *Peutz-Jeghers syndrome* (see p. 1448). Although the passage of bright red blood does not rule out a lesion of the upper gastrointestinal tract, the passage of altered blood is almost pathognomonic for such lesions. In newborn infants hemorrhagic disease of the newborn (p. 396) and the "swallowed blood syndrome" (p. 397) may result in the passage of either bright red or altered blood.

Exploratory laparotomy may be indicated in selected cases of severe bleeding without historical, physical, laboratory or roentgenographic findings to explain the bleeding.

VOMITING

The causes of vomiting, one of the commonest symptoms of infancy and childhood, tend to vary according to age. In the absence of the frequent nonspecific association with almost any infection or emotional stress, vomiting is most frequently related to abnormalities of the central nervous, urinary and gastrointestinal systems.

Vomiting in the Neonatal Period. See pages 373 and 391.

Vomiting in Infancy After the Neonatal Period. Certain infants regurgitate or spit up small amounts of feeding at frequent intervals. They are usually well nourished, very active and responsive, and tend to regurgitate more when excited or exposed to an emotionally charged environment. Neither overfeeding nor other aberration in care seems to be a common causative factor. Formula changes rarely help. The vomiting tends to subside spontaneously in the second year of life, suggesting a maturational process. Treatment consists in reassuring the parents that organic disease is absent. Barium studies may be useful as much for parental reassurance as for ruling out abnormalities of the esophagus, stomach and duodenum. In some instances, provision of temporary or partial relief of an exasperated mother from the continual cleaning up of vomitus may be therapeutic.

Infants may respond with vomiting to the frustration of inhibition of free movement by body or leg casts applied for orthopedic treatment. The disturbance usually clears spontaneously within a few days.

Infants with neurologic disease or damage may have pharyngeal and esophageal dysfunction which results in vomiting and aspiration. Tracheostomy or gastrostomy may be required temporarily; in spite of progressive or persisting neurologic abnormality, the pharyngeal dysfunction usually improves sufficiently to permit oral feeding without complications by 2 years of age.

The validity of the popular assumption that vomiting is associated with *teething* is open to question. In some instances it is a manifestation of allergy to cow's milk (p. 509).

Rumination (Merycism). Rumination is a rare but serious form of chronic regurgitation, leading to severe growth failure in infancy. The onset is usually in the latter half of the first year of life. The condition appears to be of psychogenic origin and is often associated with maternal difficulty in establishing a warm, maternal relation with the baby. There may be general inability of the mother to develop a mature marital or parental role, or she may be unable to mother her infant because of a deep-seated fear that the baby will die; occasionally conception or birth has taken place near the time of the tragic death of a sibling. The possibility of an unconscious maternal death wish toward the baby has also been raised.

Chewing movements and mouthing of the regurgitated material and fingers often precede or accompany the regurgitation. Careful observation may disclose that the infant actively gags himself with his tongue or fingers. The large loss of nutrient may appear deceptively small; the infant lies continuously in a small pool of regurgitated liquid. In some cases such infants have been left for protracted intervals without appropriate emotional stimulation. A barium swallow and upper gastrointestinal series as well as urinalysis, blood urea nitrogen determination and a hemogram are valuable in ruling out chronic renal disease and upper gastrointestinal lesions such as hiatal hernia, esophageal stricture, chalasia, achalasia or duodenal ulcer.

Treatment involves an intensive relation with a warm, maternally inclined caretaker; rumination tends to stop while eye contact and verbal contact are established and maintained until the stomach empties. This usually leads to decreased regurgitation and to a gain in weight. Concomitant exploration of mother-child relations, together with warmth and support to combat the mother's feeling of inadequacy engendered by her malnourished infant, may allow her to regain her sense of adequacy, develop a warmer relation with the infant, and gradually take over the care of her child in the hospital. The prognosis is usually good for these infants if such a setting can be instituted. Otherwise death may result from malnutrition.

Vomiting in Childhood. Beyond infancy acute episodes of vomiting are usually due to readily ascertainable psychologic or infectious causes. Community epidemics of nausea, vomiting and diarrhea are common and presumably of viral origin. Appendicitis should always be considered when vomiting is coupled with abdominal pain and fever (p. 817). Ingestion of drugs or other toxic substances may lead to vomiting, which also may be an important symptom of chronic lead poisoning. Recurrent or prolonged vomiting should always arouse suspicion of an intracranial neoplasm.

Cyclic, Periodic or Recurrent Vomiting. Some children experience periodic attacks of unexplained vomiting. These episodes may be mild and accepted as a matter of course after intense activity or emotional stress. Other children, particularly preadolescent girls, have recurrent attacks of severe vomiting accompanied by intense parental anxiety. The bouts are characterized by violent retching, often of mildly bloodstained material, severe drooling and salivation, lethargy, withdrawn behavior and a striking facial flush. Intense thirst, headache and abdominal pain are frequent. The severity of the attacks often leads to suspicion of organic disease of the central nervous system or gastrointestinal tract, but physical, neurologic and roentgenographic examinations are normal. Occasionally electroencephalographic variations may arouse suspicion of an epileptic equivalent, but therapy with anticonvulsant drugs is usually disappointing.

Treatment of Vomiting. Vomiting should in all instances be viewed as a symptom, with principal attention directed toward determination and correction of its cause. Withholding oral intake for 4 to 6 hours, followed by frequent sips of clear fluids containing carbohydrate for the rest of the day, may be helpful. Phenothiazine derivatives are of limited value and may lead to disturbing central nervous system symptoms (p. 308). Severe or prolonged vomiting may lead to dehydration and hypochloremic alkalosis requiring parenteral fluid and electrolyte therapy, which should include glucose, most importantly, and potassium (p. 223). Attacks of *cyclic vomiting* may be aborted by hospitalization, administration of fluids intravenously, or both. In addition, a search should be made for sources of unrecognized or unadmitted frustration in the life of the child or the parents; environmental adjustment or the mere fact that the patient and parents gain insight into the existence of a problem may be sufficient to prevent recurrences. In any event, the attacks tend to subside as the child becomes older, though migraine may be a sequel during later life.

FECAL ELIMINATION

Normal Stools. The characteristics of the meconium stools of the first few days of life and of the transitional stools are described on page 21. When breast feeding is well established and the infant's intake is composed entirely of milk, the stools are yellow to golden, of salvelike consistency, faintly acid in reaction (pH 4.7 to 5.1), and may contain seedlike particles (*birdseed stools*). (See p. 159.)

When cow's milk is ingested, the stools vary from pale yellow to light brown, are firmer in consistency, less acid in reaction and may even be slightly alkaline (pH 6 to 8); there is a more decided odor, owing to decomposition of protein. Oral administration of acids or alkalis has little effect on the pH of the stools.

The number of stools per day varies considerably; the comfort and well-being of the infant are more important than the number and type of stools. Breast-fed infants average from 2 to 4 stools a day with a range of 1 to 7 during the first 3 or 4 months of life, whereas artificially fed infants average 1 or 2 stools. Occasionally the breast-fed infant may comfortably and normally have a bowel movement only once in 4 to 10 days, and yet the movements may remain of the usual consistency. By the end of the first year of life most infants have only 1 stool a day, although more or less than that is not abnormal.

Normal stools contain approximately 80 per cent water; the residue consists preponderantly of cellular elements, mucus and bacteria. Fat is present in the form of neutral fat, fatty acids and soaps. The fat is largely a residue from unabsorbed foods; some comes from bile, bacteria and cellular detritus, and some from lipids excreted from the blood. The fat content of infants' stools varies tremendously and may be as much as 35 per cent of the weight of the dried stool of artificially fed infants and 50 per cent of breast-fed infants. The sugar of the infant's diet is entirely absorbed. Starch is not completely digested and may be demonstrated in the stool by the iodine test. Only about 8 per cent of the protein ingested is lost in normal stools. From 8 to 10 per cent of the dried stool consists of mineral matter, chiefly calcium.

Curds may be found in the stools of both breast-fed and artifically fed infants and are of no particular significance. They are whitish, with an outer coating of yellow or brown; they are composed of a casein coagulum; those of breast milk stools are much smaller and less firm in consistency than those of cow's milk. The small white curds which appear in diarrheal stools represent undigested neutral fat.

Various enzymes are present in the stools, such as diastase, lactase, invertin, trypsin, rennin and a fat-splitting ferment.

Microscopically, the stools of an infant exhibit fat globules of various sizes, needles of fatty acids, innumerable bacteria, cholesterin plates, epithelial cells, small round cells, calcium salts in crystalline form, granular detritus, and occasionally bilirubin crystals, yeast fungi and protein matter.

As the infant grows older and the proportion of the diet contributed by milk becomes less, the stools acquire more of the characteristics of those of adults in both color and odor. By 2 years of age, stools become formed, although even young infants may pass fully formed stools, especially when their diet has a high protein content.

Mucous Stools. Mucus is often present in the stools of infants, and in small amounts may have no significance. During starvation the stools consist of thin mucoid secretions of the intestine which are stained a brownish tint (*starvation stool*). Mucus is generally present in considerable quantity after administration of a purgative such as castor oil. In older children it may represent a functional disturbance and be associated with emotional disturbances. It is present in large quantity in inflammatory conditions. Stools composed almost entirely of bloodstained mucus occur in dysenteric conditions, intussusception and ulcerative colitis. Undigested starch may resemble mucus in appearance, but can be distinguished by the iodine reaction.

Protein Stools. The odor of putrefaction may be present in the stools of infants who ingest large amounts of protein or whose digestion of protein is impaired. The color is brownish-yellow or sometimes greenish-black, and mucus may be present. Tough, yellowish, beanlike protein curds are often present after ingestion of unboiled milk.

Fat Stools. *Soap stool* depends upon an excess of fatty acids combined with calcium or magnesium to form a soap. The stool is white or gray, shiny, fairly firm, homogeneous, crumbly or salvelike, of acid reaction, and has a rancid or sour odor.

The fatty stool is yellow to gray and soft and bulky, has a greasy appearance, and will produce a grease spot when placed upon paper. If protein is also present in large amount, the odor is cheesy and offensive; when there is also undigested carbohydrate, the stool is frothy. Such stools are seen in the malabsorption syndromes.

Carbohydrate Stools. Stools from diets exceptionally high in carbohydrate are of normal consistency, smooth, brown or yellowish-brown, and have an acid reaction. Excess starch may be demonstrated by the iodine test. When there is indigestion of carbohydrate and decomposition of it in the intestinal tract, the stools become thin, frothy,

light yellow or often green, the odor is suggestive of acetic acid, and there is an acid reaction.

Green Stools. A faint pea-green color when the stool is passed or developing shortly thereafter is not abnormal; it results from oxidation of bilirubin (responsible for the yellow color) to biliverdin. Green watery stools are common in diarrhea.

Black Stools. Black or reddish-black stools may be seen after large amounts of blood have been swallowed or after extensive bleeding high in the gastrointestinal tract. Ingested iron causes the stools to become black, and bismuth causes them to be greenish-black.

DIFFICULTIES IN FECAL ELIMINATION

In many families the control and organization of the nature, timing and frequency of bowel movements arouse as much—or more—concern as do other aspects of the development of the child. There is little awareness among nonphysicians that the daily number of bowel evacuations may vary in normal persons from 3 or 4 a day to as few as one in 5 or 6 days; any variation from the family concept of what constitutes a normal pattern requires not only an adequate explanation, but often continued guidance for some time.

Although parents sometimes complain that their child has "diarrhea," by which they may mean increased frequency or any degree of decreased firmness of bowel movements, by far the most common complaint is of "constipation." This term may be applied by parents to painful or infrequent passage of bowel movements of normal consistency and size, or to hard or large bowel movements of normal or decreased frequency. In contrast, the significance of the soiling which frequently accompanies fecal withholding and impaction is seldom recognized. Likewise, chronic fecal impaction may present as a complaint of liquid stools (*paradoxical diarrhea*), which are probably due to irritation of the wall of the colon or to diminished capacity of the distended colon to absorb water.

Certain items of history should be explored in every child with a disorder of elimination. These are (1) whether the disorder has been continuous since birth or emerged subsequently, and, if so, when; (2) whether there is fecal retention; (3) whether the stools are bulky, scybalous or soft; (4) whether blood has ever accompanied bowel movements; (5) whether there is fecal soiling; and (6) whether behavior suggestive of voluntary withholding of stool is evident.

Acute Difficulties in Elimination (Constipation). In infancy acute difficulty in elimination may be manifested by straining and irritability at scattered times of the day. Quiescence follows an episode of explosive stool passage, sometimes accompanied by blood-streaking secondary to an anal fissure. The stools may vary from hard pellets to soft, pasty or loose, unformed feces. Such episodes may occur during acute infantile colic, an upper respiratory tract illness, travel, or a period of intensive emotional stimulation. Anal irritation due to diaper rash or fissure may result in discomfort and difficulty in passing feces. On occasion, particularly in infants between 1 and 2 years of age, the difficulty may arise in association with family upset caused by death, parental separation or strife, major illness, or a move to a new home.

Both infants and older children may withhold feces because of fear of pain on defecation. In such children there is often a history of an obviously painful, large, hard or blood-streaked bowel movement at the time of onset of the difficulty. Careful examination of the anus may reveal a small raw or bleeding fissure. Older children may withhold feces because of unavailability of a toilet at the time of colonic peristalsis. The unavailability may be actual or psychologic, owing to embarrassment in asking to use the toilet in school, or to aversion to using cold, unclean or malodorous facilities.

Most acute disorders of elimination are temporary, provided causative factors are eliminated and the disruption of parental or medical manipulation is not added. The physician should lend psychologic support in order to minimize parental inclination to intervene aggressively. Most disorders of elimination, including primary or secondary anal fissures, will subside spontaneously with reasonable hygienic measures. Gentle cleansing of the anus with soap and water after each bowel movement is more effective than the application of topical anesthetics, though they or a corticosteroid ointment to allay inflammation may be temporarily helpful. The use of suppositories and anal dilators may lead to undesirable alterations in the child's bowel habits and result in sensory disruption which may perpetuate a disorganized bowel habit rather than permit the establishment of one normal for the person. The inclination of both parent and physician to intervene inappropriately must be curbed. At times there may be justification for the temporary utilization of a mild laxative or stool softener, or a dietary change such as increased intake of fruit or fluid, or a change of formula.

In instances of sudden inability to defecate, the possibility of acute mechanical obstruction as by incarcerated hernia or volvulus must be considered.

Chronic Difficulties in Elimination. Failure to pass bowel movements is a symptom rather than a primary illness. Constipation dating from the neonatal period suggests hypothyroidism or aganglionic megacolon. The latter may present as acute intestinal obstruction in the first few weeks of life or as insidious difficulty in passage of stools, with chronic abdominal distention. Table 11-6 summarizes some of the characteristics which distin-

TABLE 11-6. DIFFERENTIATING FEATURES OF AGANGLIONIC MEGACOLON AND THE COMMON PATTERN OF FUNCTIONAL CONSTIPATION

	AGANGLIONIC MEGACOLON	FUNCTIONAL CONSTIPATION
Onset	Birth or neonatal period Symptoms of intestinal obstruction	About 60% in first year of life; most of remainder from 1 to 4 years
Course	Failure to pass formed bowel movements except by enema	Huge bowel movements at long intervals
Withholding efforts	Not present	Present
Soiling	None	At least two thirds of cases
Growth	Impaired	Usually normal
Abdominal findings	Distended; large fecal mass remains in same site	Variable distention and masses
Rectal examination	Rectum not dilated and usually empty of stool	Cavernous rectum, often filled with soft feces
Roentgenographic findings	Colon dilated proximal to an area of normal caliber; post-evacuation film shows poor evacuation of barium	Colon dilated to anus; post-evacuation film shows effective evacuation
Rectal biopsy	Absence of ganglion cells, large nerve bundles	Normal

guish aganglionic megacolon from functional constipation and to some extent from encopresis. Constipation is also a frequent accompaniment of mental retardation. If stool retention is protracted, there is a tendency for the colon to become dilated.

Chronic Constipation. The most common disorder of elimination is infrequency of bowel movements and difficulty in passage of stools. During the second and third years of life, as bowel control is being established in most children, bowel difficulty is often manifest by voluntary retention of feces while the body is held taut, by episodes of florid-faced straining, by holding the buttocks compressed together, and by crossing the legs, walking on the tips of the toes, or by jumping around without apparent reason. Fecal soiling may occur during some of these episodes. Some young children will be considerably distressed if placed on the toilet at this time. About two thirds of such children have a history, dating from the neonatal period, of straining at stool, of colic (p. 160), and of parental manipulations such as enemas, suppositories and formula changes. A few children have a history of chronic frequency of bowel movements during the second year, clinically misdiagnosed as a type of celiac disease. Boys are involved approximately 4 times as frequently as girls. The bowel movements are usually infrequent and bulky. Approximately two thirds of the children have fecal soiling as retention of stool becomes massive. Enuresis or occasional urinary retention is also reported in about two thirds of the cases. Such children usually have an emotional problem which is primary or contributory to the fecal retention.

Secondary behavioral or emotional problems are frequent as a result of interaction between parent and child over the stool difficulty. Many children shut out any reference to stools and give no outward sign of awareness of an urge to defecate, an urge that they may deny on questioning. They often prefer to be alone in a corner or lying on the floor during episodes of resistance to colonic peristalsis, and they may hide their soiled underclothing. Other children who withhold bowel movements are unable to tolerate even minor uncleanliness, such as dirty hands. Similarly, some parents of children who withhold bowel movements, particularly mothers, tend to be fetishly involved with housework and cleanliness as a compensation for feelings of inadequacy, which also lead to inability to tolerate any level of discomfort in their offspring. Adverse experiences during their own childhood may make it difficult for them to comfort a child over minor distress without intervening in some physical, manipulative fashion. Most such parents go through stages consisting in use of laxatives, cajoling, rewarding and punishing, all culminating in a feeling of desperation. They seem to interpret the whole process as a failure on their part and as defiance or "laziness" on the part of the child. They frequently describe the child as stubborn and "hard to understand." The children themselves tend to play poorly with peer groups and to be "loners," a problem which is contributed to by the malodor of their fecal soiling. In addition, feeding problems, overall restraint in expression of feeling, reading disability and infantile speech may be present in some cases.

Abdominal palpation in cases of chronic constipation usually reveals masses of retained feces of variable size, consistency and movability. On rectal examination one usually finds a markedly dilated rectal ampulla which is often filled with soft stool.

Treatment involves (1) attenuating parental fear of danger from retention of stool, and of physical defect beyond dilatation of the colon, and (2) assisting the child in interrupting the patterned withholding response to colonic peristalsis and in re-establishing a normal, regular bowel habit. This may be accomplished in many children by the oral administration of 1 or 2 teaspoonfuls (5 or 10 ml.) of mineral oil twice a day for a protracted period, usually 3 to 9 months. In cases of severe or longstanding retention of stool, particularly when accompanied by much parental anxiety, hospitalization may infrequently be justified to empty the dilated colon of retained feces and to break the adverse interaction between parent and child. Roentgenographic studies may be necessary to convince the parents of the absence of serious organic disease such as aganglionic megacolon. A series of warm saline enemas (a heaping teaspoonful of table salt per quart of water) given several hours apart 2 or 3 times a day until the returns are clear may be necessary to obtain complete emptying of the dilated colon. Subsequent administration of mineral oil with or without a stool softener such as dioctyl sodium sulfosuccinate will then usually suffice to maintain a regular pattern of bowel movements. The medication must be continued for at least 3 to 9 months in order to allow time for the colon to return to an undilated and more physiologically effective state, as well as for establishment of a regular bowel habit. In some instances a regular bowel habit may be established only through the addition as necessary of enemas when there has been no bowel movement by a predesignated time. Because of dislike of enemas on the part of mother or child, and the resulting psychologic conflict, a rectal suppository containing bisacodyl (marketed as Dulcolax) may be substituted for the enema.

In many instances of chronic constipation the precipitating factor has long since been removed, so that the condition itself has become a self-perpetuating source of conflict between parent and child. In such cases, relief of the symptoms of constipation and fecal soiling is sufficient to allow favorable psychologic readjustment, although exacerbations of the problem may recur under the stress of illness or emotional upset. In other cases, in which the underlying problem is a more deep-seated emotional one, psychiatric treatment is indicated. Psychiatric referral should be on the basis of the emotional disorder, however, rather than for the constipation itself, since the latter is frequently refractory to purely psychiatric therapy.

As improvement in the bowel problem takes place, the child may become more self-reliant, aggressive and outspoken, a situation in which parents frequently need the sympathetic support of the physician, as they do with the relapses and exacerbations which may characterize the problem.

Constipation with Rectal Scybala. In this type of constipation there tends to be more abdominal pain, more difficulty in passing feces, a less protracted history of retention, little abdominal distention, no bulky stool, some soiling with mucus or feces, less evidence of withholding and greater awareness of toilet and stool passage than in children with other types of chronic constipation. There may be vague abdominal tenderness, fecal masses or balls in the sigmoid, and minimal dilatation demonstrable by rectal examination or barium enema. These patients may be appropriately classified as having a variety of the irritable colon syndrome (p. 799). The condition is very responsive to help; infrequently hospitalization may be justified to provide a break with an unsatisfactory home routine. Small doses of mineral oil, with or without an antispasmodic drug, for short periods of time may be justified if the problem persists.

Encopresis. This term, which connotes the involuntary passage of feces unrelated to organic defect or illness, is used commonly to designate fecal soiling in association with voluntary withholding of bowel movements. The pattern may be continuous from infancy, during which it is normal, or it may arise after establishment of normal bowel control. Abdominal distention and dilatation of the rectal ampulla are variable. The anal sphincter usually has adequate tone. Recent experiments, however, with anal tonometry as a measure of the integrative reflexes of the rectum and anal sphincter show occasional failures of anal sphincter responses which may explain passage of feces at unpredictable times. Children with encopresis may also be hyperactive and have dyslexia or other learning disabilities, suggesting a degree of neural incoordination. Emotional instability is frequent, with a wide spectrum of manifestations ranging from intensive motor responses without facial expression to great sensitivity to criticism or a high level of basic anxiety, with easy crying. In most instances there is a disturbance in relations with both parents and peers. The condition is relatively rare in girls. Consultation with a physician is usually sought under the social impact of beginning school without bowel control. Older children seem to be able to hold back a bowel movement during school hours, only to drop their guard and to soil when they get home after school. They are usually exquisitely sensitive to the problem the soiling presents with respect to their relations with parents and peers and view themselves as failures because of it.

Since the natural history of encopresis is that it frequently, like enuresis, may become an organized habit if it is not resolved, careful neurologic examination, anal tonometry, psychologic evaluation and psychiatric consultation are indicated. Often a period of removal from their usual environment and associates helps these children. Pediatric and psychiatric counseling may be of considerable help.

DIARRHEA

Diarrhea, the passage of loose or watery stools, usually with increased frequency, is an important clinical manifestation of a large number of gastrointestinal disorders which collectively are one of the principal causes of illness and mortality among infants and children throughout the world. The problem is more serious during infancy than in later childhood, mainly because of the infant's greater susceptibility to infection and to water and electrolyte imbalances. The decrease in mortality from diarrheal disorders in countries with high standards of living and improved hygienic conditions has been largely responsible for the large overall decrease in infant mortality in these areas (Fig. 1-1). In countries with a high incidence of infectious diarrhea there is an increased number of cases during the warmer period of the year, whereas there is little seasonal variation in areas with a low incidence.

Etiology. The causes of the majority of acute diarrheal disturbances are unknown. Any of the known intestinal pathogens can infect a person of any age, but there are differences in the clinical and epidemiologic patterns at various ages; these will be discussed here. The clinical disturbances of the recognized enteric infections in which diarrhea is a significant manifestation are described elsewhere (see Bacillary Dysentery, Amebiasis, Salmonella Infections, Typhoid Fever, Cholera and Food Poisoning).

Diarrhea in the newborn (see also p. 407) is more serious when it occurs in epidemic form in a hospital nursery. Most of the intestinal pathogens, including enteropathogenic *Escherichia coli*, have been incriminated in individual epidemics. In addition, various bacteria not ordinarily considered pathogens, such as those of the paracolon, proteus, pseudomonas, staphylococcal and streptococcal groups, have been suspected in some epidemics in the neonatal period. Certain viruses also have been associated with diarrheal disease in the newborn infant.

The problem *in infancy after the neonatal period* varies greatly in different socioeconomic groups. In situations of poverty and poor sanitation, contamination of milk feedings and foods is probably the most important source of infection. Most infections in infants from higher socioeconomic groups are probably transmitted by infected persons or "carriers." Perhaps the most frequent causes at present are enteropathogenic *E. coli*, dysentery bacilli, salmonella and various viral agents. In addition to enteric viruses, it is possible that some respiratory viruses may be responsible for mild diarrheal disturbances in conjunction with respiratory infections; it is not uncommon to observe diarrhea in an infant of a family whose older members have an epidemic respiratory infection. Diarrhea may also arise by direct enteric infection by the staphylococcus in association with staphylococcal infections elsewhere in the body. Diarrhea associated with parenteral infections in the middle ear or in the urinary or respiratory tract is termed *parenteral diarrhea*. This form usually lasts only as long as the parenteral infection. Whether parenteral diarrhea represents a secondary intestinal infection with the agent causing the parenteral infection, or an intestinal reaction to the parenteral infection has not been defined.

In *childhood*, acute diarrheal disturbances become much less frequent and relatively less severe. Erratic eating, fatigue and nervous excitement may precipitate mild diarrheal disorders.

Diarrhea induced by therapy with antibacterial agents, especially when administered by mouth, is due in most instances to an upset in the normal balance among the flora of the intestinal tract. It may also be due in some cases to a direct irritative action of the drug on the intestine, or perhaps to stimulation by the drug of parts of the nervous system which influence intestinal motility. Ampicillin, chloramphenicol and the tetracyclines are the drugs most frequently involved, particularly when dosage is high or therapy is prolonged. Staphylococci, candida, proteus or pseudomonas are the organisms which most frequently become predominant and cause the diarrhea. *Treatment* is by cessation of oral administration of the offending drug so that the normal balance of intestinal flora can be re-established. Diarrhea usually ceases in 2 to 5 days. In some instances it may be necessary to stop *all* antibacterial therapy.

A number of *noninfectious conditions* may be responsible for diarrhea. These include allergy or intolerance to specific foods (p. 509); metabolic disorders such as hyperthyroidism, uremia and acidosis; emotional upset and fatigue; excessive ingestion of certain foods or unripe fruits; so-called starvation diarrhea, in which the stools contain an excessive amount of mucus and little fecal material; and malabsorption syndromes (p. 804). Diarrhea may be a prominent symptom of aganglionic megacolon; the cause may be enterocolitis, irritation of the wall of the colon by impacted feces, or disruption of the normal colonic mechanism for absorption of water from fecal material.

Chronic or persistent diarrhea may be a manifestation of genetic disorders in which there is an absence of intestinal sugar-splitting enzymes (p. 811). Temporary absence of such enzymes may be the reason for persistence of diarrhea after an acute diarrheal disorder; the diarrhea ceases if disaccharides are eliminated from the diet. Mild diarrhea may persist for months after an acute salmonella enteritis in infancy; it ceases after the organism has been finally eliminated. In areas in which amebiasis is endemic it may be responsible for chronic diarrhea. Two other forms of chronic diarrhea without demonstrable amebic infection may be benefited by the antiamebic agent, diiodohydroxyquin (Diodoquin): (1) *Acrodermatitis enteropathica (Danbolt-Closs syndrome)* is characterized by severe chronic diarrhea accompanied by areas of denuded skin around the mucocutaneous junctions, especially of the mouth and anus. This ill-defined condition was formerly considered universally fatal, but some cases have responded favorably to Diodoquin. (2) Cohlan has described a form of mild, chronic diarrhea in otherwise healthy infants and young children, usually from homes of good socioeconomic status and whose parents, especially the mother, are emotionally tense and insecure. Although amebic infection cannot be proved, some of these infants apparently respond well to Diodoquin, which usually must be continued for 6 to 12 months. (Also see p. 1394.)

Recurrent mild diarrhea (irritable colon syndrome, see also p. 799). Recurrent mild diarrhea is a common disturbance of childhood observed preponderantly between the ages of 1 and 3 years. It rarely leads to dehydration and almost never affects growth. It often begins or is exacerbated by a respiratory illness. There are usually 2 to 8 stools a day. The first stool of the day may be formed, the others progressively looser. Occasionally the diarrhea alternates with episodes of constipation. A bacterial or amebic basis for the diarrhea is rarely found, and clinical or laboratory signs of maldigestion or malabsorption are absent. The children are characteristically intense and hyperactive. First children are preponderantly involved. The fathers often work night and day; the young mothers are often lonely and find it hard to let their very active toddlers determine their own pattern of activity. If these children are hospitalized, they tend to improve promptly without medication. Diets and drugs are of little value; in some instances they seem actually deleterious. Clarification of the various diagnostic possibilities through reasoning rather than therapeutic action, together with understanding and sympathetic discussion with the parents about their questions and personal problems, usually provides the reassurance and support necessary to relieve the child of his emotionally reactive symptoms.

Clinical Manifestations. The descriptions here apply principally to infants and very young children; see also Diarrhea in the Newborn (p. 407) and the various specific infections responsible for diarrheal disturbances.

Mild diarrheal disturbances. Occasionally there are such prodromal symptoms as slight fever, irritability and a disinclination to eat. Severe vomiting is not a common symptom. The frequency of stools varies; there may be only 2 or 3 a day or as many as 10 or 12. Temporary reduction in oral feeding usually results in abatement of the diarrhea, and there is little or no evidence of dehydration.

Severe diarrheal disturbances can be placed in 2

groups: (1) cases in which the onset is only moderately severe and toxic manifestations are greatly accentuated when dehydration and electrolytic disturbances have become a factor; (2) cases in which the onset is abrupt with higher fever and extreme toxicity.

In the first group there may or may not be fever. There is often vomiting at the onset, but it is usually not persistent. It may return in the later stages. Diarrhea appears within 24 hours of onset; the stools are at first chiefly fecal, often contain small white curds, and are usually strongly acid. They quickly become liquid and greenish or greenish-yellow, contain increasing amounts of mucus, and at times are blood-tinged. Initially there are evidences of irritability and, at times, stupor and convulsions; these symptoms frequently disappear after the first day or so, but the irritability and restlessness return if dehydration and acidosis develop. The number of stools varies from a few to 20 or more a day. Evacuation is often preceded by pain, and the stools may be expelled with force.

The extent of dehydration and the rapidity of its development depend upon the amount of fluid lost in the stools, the presence or absence of vomiting, and the extent to which fluids are replaced parenterally. In untreated cases there is loss of subcutaneous tissues and elasticity of the skin. The pulse is rapid and weak, and there is increasing prostration. The output of urine is progressively decreased; the urine has a high specific gravity and often contains albumin and casts. Hemoconcentration varies with the severity of dehydration. Owing to the decrease in renal function and to the hemoconcentration, urea nitrogen levels of the blood are increased to as much as 50 mg. per 100 ml. or more. Acidosis is usually a prominent manifestation; in untreated cases plasma carbon dioxide levels may be less than 3 mEq. per liter, and the pH may approach 7. Hypertonic dehydration may be a problem, especially when skim milk feedings or oral electrolyte solutions are given (p. 222).

Cases which fall in the second category have been variously termed "acute toxic diarrhea" and food poisoning. They are characterized by an abrupt onset with high fever, often 104 to 106°F., and extreme prostration. Vomiting is frequently severe. An infant who otherwise has been well suddenly becomes prostrated. In some instances there is evidence of irritability, restlessness and even convulsions, but symptoms of collapse are more frequent. The infant in this latter instance is flaccid, and pallor is usually noticed. Respirations are rapid and may be hyperpneic. Diarrhea may be an early and severe manifestation or may not appear for some hours or even a day. Rarely, shock and death may occur without a diarrheal movement; at autopsy the bowel is filled with fluid of high electrolyte content. The fatality rate is extremely high, and death often occurs within the first 24 hours. Though acidosis and hemoconcentration are likely to be extreme, such peripheral manifestations of dehydration as loss of subcutaneous tissue and inelasticity of the skin are not prominent in the infants who die in the first day or two of the disease.

Diagnosis. There is no differential diagnosis beyond that of establishing the cause. Occasionally the history may indicate the source and nature of the infection or the possibility of food poisoning, but in most instances the cause can be determined, if at all, only by bacteriologic and virologic cultures of the stool. Samples of several stools in the first 24 hours of observation or, preferably, several rectal swabs at intervals of 8 to 12 hours should be planted immediately for culture.

Since the metabolic disturbances of diarrhea in infants are an important part of the clinical situation, no severe case can be adequately appraised without the assistance of laboratory data (see p. 219).

Prevention. Diarrheal disturbances are much more frequent in artificially fed infants than in breast-fed ones. With artificial feeding the mother should be instructed in the sterilization of formulas and in their proper storage until the time of feeding, so that contamination is prevented. During periods of unusually high environmental temperature and humidity or during any febrile disturbance, infants should be supplied with adequate amounts of fluid, and the intake of food should be temporarily reduced. Excessive clothing should be avoided.

Treatment is discussed under the various diarrheal entities. See Mild Diarrhea (p. 223), Acute Severe Diarrhea (p. 220), Diarrhea in the Newborn (p. 407), Bacillary Dysentery (p. 588), Amebiasis (p. 748), Salmonella Infections (p. 583), Botulism (p. 1485), Chronic Diarrhea (p. 783), Malabsorption Syndromes (p. 806), Gastrointestinal Allergy (p. 509) and Antibiotic and Sulfonamide Dosages (p. 245).

Congenital Anomalies of the Gastrointestinal Tract and Intestinal Obstruction

A variety of congenital anomalies of the gastrointestinal tract may be responsible for partial or complete obstruction. The majority of obstructions involve the rectum and the anus; the remainder are preponderantly in the small intestine. The important congenital anomalies may be listed as follows:

Pyloric stenosis
Atresia and stenosis
Anomalies of rotation (malrotation)
Duplications
Diverticula (Meckel's)
Anomalies of innervation (aganglionic megacolon)
Intra-abdominal hernias
Extra-abdominal hernias
Abnormalities of the pancreas

CONGENITAL HYPERTROPHIC PYLORIC STENOSIS

Pyloric stenosis is characterized by vomiting starting usually in the second or third week of life and becoming increasingly projectile. It affects approximately one in every 150 male and one in every 750 female infants and tends to occur in first-born children. Familial incidence has been observed; however, genetic study does not suggest any pattern of inheritance.

Etiology. The cause of pyloric stenosis is not known. In favor of a congenital origin is the high incidence in both of monovular twins, in contrast to the relative infrequency in both of binovular twins. There appears to be a probable, though undetermined, acquired factor involved in the pathogenesis of the lesion.

Pathology. The pylorus is elongated, thickened to as much as twice its usual size, and almost cartilaginous in consistency. There is severe narrowing of the lumen, due principally to the hypertrophy of the circular muscular layer. The stomach is usually dilated, and in long-standing cases there may be hypertrophy of its muscular coat.

Clinical Manifestations. Initially there is only regurgitation or occasional nonprojectile *vomiting*. The onset is rarely before 1 week of age, is usually in the second or third week, and is rarely delayed until the second or third month. The vomiting becomes projectile, usually within a week after onset, and generally occurs during or shortly after feeding, but at times as much as several hours later. In some instances there is vomiting after each feeding; in others it is intermittent. The infant is hungry and will take another feeding immediately. The vomitus consists only of gastric contents, but may be blood-tinged; it is not bile-stained. The stools may become very small and infrequent, depending on the amount of food that reaches the intestinal tract. Occasionally there is a starvation type of diarrhea.

Weight loss and *dehydration* may be extensive; weight may decrease to a level below that at birth. There is decreased elasticity of the skin and loss of subcutaneous tissue. The eyes may be sunken and the fat pads of the cheeks lost, so that the infant has a wrinkled, "old man" appearance.

Gastric peristaltic waves are visible as they progress from the left upper quadrant toward the pylorus in a manner suggesting the rolling of balls beneath the abdominal wall; they are most prominent immediately after feeding or just before vomiting (Fig. 11-10). At times the infant appears to be uncomfortable, although pain is not a prominent feature.

The pyloric tumor, which is usually the size and consistency of a medium-sized olive, can be palpated in the majority of instances midway between the umbilicus and the costal margin and just lateral to the right rectus muscle; its detection may require repeated examinations. Success in palpation depends on a relaxed, comfortable baby who is being fed by a relaxed, comfortable person while a relaxed, comfortable examiner sits with his hand gently lying across the upper portion of the infant's abdomen with the fingertips on the right upper quadrant. Kneading usually prevents the relaxation necessary to allow the fingers to sink and feel the tumor as it comes up during feeding. If the pyloric tumor cannot be felt, feeding should be continued until vomiting occurs, because this is followed by a momentary period of great relaxation during which the tumor can best be palpated.

Protracted jaundice, with hyperbilirubinemia of the indirect type, has been observed in a few infants with pyloric stenosis. A possible, but unexplained, relation is assumed.

Metabolic Alterations. Extensive and protracted vomiting in pyloric stenosis, as in other forms of high intestinal obstruction, may lead to critical deficits of potassium and sodium which,

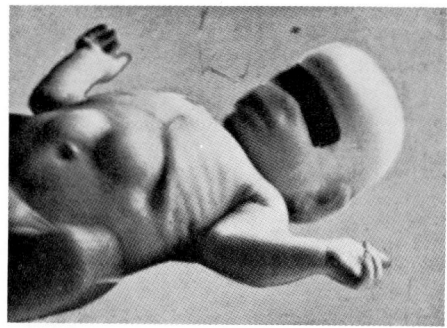

Figure 11-10. Gastric peristaltic waves of pyloric stenosis in an infant 3 weeks of age. (Courtesy of Dr. Carl Wagner, Cincinnati.)

owing to dehydration, may or may not be reflected by low values in the serum. Much more striking are the decrease in chloride concentration and increases in pH and in carbon dioxide content which constitute the characteristic serum chemical changes of *hypochloremic alkalosis* (p. 223). These chemical changes in the serum may lead the unwary to futile attempts at correction of hypochloremia and alkalosis through the intravenous administration of ammonium chloride solutions while ignoring the need for potassium and sodium. Intravenous administration of 5 per cent glucose in isotonic sodium chloride solution, to which 3 to 6 mEq. of potassium chloride per 100 ml. is added after the infant has been observed to urinate, will gradually and satisfactorily replace the calculated deficits (Table 5-9) of potassium, chloride and sodium and avoid the danger of hyponatremia which may ensue if hypotonic electrolyte solutions are used for replacement of fluid and electrolytes in dehydrated infants who have had protracted vomiting. The serum chloride level, which may vary from nearly normal to as low as 70 mEq. per liter, may be used as a rough index of potassium deficit; if the serum chloride is normal, the potassium deficit may be minimal, and care should be taken not to overload the infant with this ion.

Diagnosis. The usual case can be diagnosed by the characteristic clinical pattern and the identification of a pyloric mass. Congenital obstructions of the duodenum, if complete, are responsible for symptoms within a few hours after birth; if incomplete, as with stenosis, malrotation or constricting bands, vomiting may not become evident for days or even weeks after birth; however, there is no pyloric tumor, and the vomitus contains bile if the constriction is below the ampulla of Vater. Gastric waves are occasionally visible in small, emaciated infants who do not have pyloric stenosis. Chalasia of the esophagus and hiatal hernia usually result in vomiting in the first week of life and can be differentiated from pyloric stenosis by roentgenographic studies. Adrenal insufficiency may simulate pyloric stenosis; the absence of a palpable tumor, metabolic acidosis and elevated serum potassium and urinary sodium concentrations in adrenal insufficiency aid in differentiation. Allergy to cow's milk may be accompanied by projectile vomiting, but this vomiting is rarely so forceful as with pyloric stenosis. A family history of allergy and the presence of other signs of milk allergy (p. 509) usually indicate the diagnosis.

The principal diagnostic difficulty is with hyperkinetic infants who are exceptionally reactive to external stimuli and vomit frequently in the first few weeks after birth. Temperamentally, they bear a strong resemblance to infants with pyloric stenosis. The vomiting may be persistent and even projectile, but often diminishes or subsides completely when the feedings are given by a comfortable caretaker other than the mother, or if

phenobarbital or an atropine-like compound is prescribed. It is for this group of infants that the term *pylorospasm* has been used. Roentgenographic studies usually show delayed emptying of the stomach, but a normal pyloric lumen.

If the pyloric tumor can be palpated, roentgenographic studies are unnecessary, but they should be done if a pyloric tumor cannot be palpated. With pyloric stenosis there is not only delayed emptying and vigorous peristaltic activity of the stomach, but also delayed prepyloric opening time and, most importantly, a narrowed, elongated pyloric canal with a single streak of barium, the "string sign," or a double-track of barium outlining the canal, an antral "beak" at the beginning of the pylorus, and a curve of the pylorus upward and to the left.

Prognosis. When the diagnosis is made early in the course of the disease, and the infant is properly prepared for operation, the operative fatality rate is less than 1 per cent. Medical therapy has a higher mortality rate and, even when beneficial, must be continued for 3 to 8 months.

Treatment. Surgical relief of the pyloric obstruction as soon as the diagnosis is established and the metabolic imbalances are corrected is the treatment of choice. The correction of dehydration and electrolyte deficits with parenteral fluids has been described under Metabolic Alterations and in Section 5 (p. 223).

Surgical treatment. Well hydrated infants without evidence of electrolyte imbalance may be operated on without delay; delays of 24 to 36 hours for replacement therapy without oral intake are indicated in severely dehydrated infants. Gastric

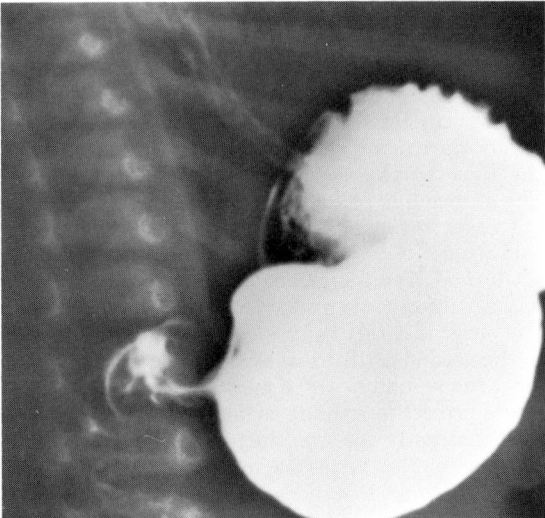

Figure 11-11. Hypertrophic pyloric stenosis. Note the elongated, narrow pyloric canal (string sign) as well as the blunt antrum. The base of the duodenal bulb is concave. Hyperperistalsis was noted fluoroscopically.

lavage with isotonic saline solution prior to operation is advised by some in the hope of diminishing gastric irritation which may cause postoperative vomiting; the tube may be left in the stomach during the operation in order to remove secretions and swallowed air. At operation the pyloric musculature is incised and separated longitudinally down to the mucosa (Fredet-Ramstedt pyloromyotomy). Eight to 12 hours postoperatively, oral feedings are begun in small amounts and increased gradually. An acceptable regimen is to give 4 ml. of 5 per cent glucose in saline solution hourly for 4 feedings. If no vomiting develops, 8 ml. are given hourly for the next 4 feedings, then 16 ml. hourly for 4 feedings. If these feedings are retained, 1 ounce of formula is given an hour after the last feeding of clear fluid and repeated 2 hours later. By stepwise increment the amount of feedings and the interval between them are increased until a full feeding program is in effect, usually within 48 hours. If vomiting occurs before formula feedings are begun, oral feedings are withheld for 4 hours, and the regimen is reinstituted from the beginning. Persistence of vomiting suggests an incomplete pyloromyotomy or possibly concomitant hiatal hernia or chalasia; occasional episodes of vomiting are not uncommon after operation, probably as the result of persisting gastritis. Feedings should ordinarily be maintained, but not increased, until a clear pattern of retention is sustained, at which time increases may be resumed. During the initial period of small feedings, intravenous administration of fluids is often required, depending on the fluid and electrolyte balance of the infant. A second pyloromyotomy is rarely required. Complete cessation of vomiting is the rule after operation, even though postoperative roentgenographic studies have shown that the pyloric canal may remain narrow for many months in the presence of complete well-being.

Nonsurgical treatment. The slowness of improvement (3 to 8 months), the higher case fatality rate, and the current high cost and probable adverse effect on emotional development of prolonged hospitalization have led to a virtual abandonment of nonsurgical treatment for pyloric stenosis, especially in the United States. Nevertheless, in cases of necessity, slow improvement will usually take place on a regimen of small, frequent feedings thickened with cereal, maintenance of a semi-upright position for an hour or so after feedings, sedation, administration of a cholinergic blocking agent, and parenteral administration of fluids as required. Emptying of the stomach by lavage when there is epigastric distention before a feeding may likewise decrease the chance of vomiting.

The foregoing measures are also useful in the treatment of infants with so-called pylorospasm. Phenobarbital is widely used for sedation in doses of 8 to 15 mg. half an hour before feeding 3 or 4 times a day; if drowsiness or apathy appears, the drug should be stopped until normal alertness is regained, at which time it may be resumed at a lower dose. The most widely used anticholinergic drugs for infants are atropine as a 1:1000 solution, tincture of belladonna, and a 0.6 per cent alcoholic solution of Eumydrin. Each is given by placing 1 drop on the infant's tongue about 20 minutes before each of 3 feedings a day. The dose may be increased first by giving it before more feedings, later by increasing the number of drops, until vomiting is controlled or flushing of the face or dilatation of the pupils appears, when the dose should be decreased. Care should be exercised that fresh solutions of these drugs are used.

CONGENITAL INTESTINAL OBSTRUCTION

General Considerations. Intestinal obstruction is observed in approximately one out of 1500 newborn infants. The cardinal signs of obstruction are (1) vomiting, (2) abdominal distention, and (3) failure to pass feces. Since a number of days may go by prior to full certainty that the infant has an obstructive lesion, early diagnosis depends on appreciation of the significance of vomiting and distention. *High intestinal obstruction* is characterized by vomiting, which tends to be persistent even when feedings have been stopped; distention may be absent. *Low obstruction* is characterized principally by distention, and vomiting may be only a late manifestation.

From an anatomic standpoint congenital obstructive lesions of the intestines can be divided on the basis of whether the obstructing factor is intrinsic, e.g. atresia, stenosis, meconium ileus and aganglionic megacolon, or extrinsic, e.g. malrotation, constricting bands, intra-abdominal hernias, duplications. Clinically, whether an intestinal obstruction is intrinsic or extrinsic is often not definable and is of secondary importance, since operation is always indicated. An attempt should be made, however, to locate the lesion preoperatively in order to guide the surgical approach.

When the obstruction is *complete*, there should be little difficulty in clinical recognition, but when incomplete, there may be considerable difficulty. Polyhydramnios is frequently an accompaniment of high intestinal obstruction, as it is of esophageal atresia. When polyhydramnios has been noted, an attempt to aspirate the infant's stomach immediately after birth may provide an important diagnostic clue. Failure to pass the tube into the stomach may disclose an esophageal atresia. Aspiration of 10 to 15 ml. or more of gastric fluid, especially if it is bile-stained, is suggestive of a high intestinal obstruction. When the obstruction is in the duodenum, symptoms may become manifest within a few hours; if it is in the large intestine, symptoms may be delayed for a day or so.

Meconium stools may be passed initially if the obstruction is in the upper part of the small intestine. The absence, on microscopic examination of the stool, of lanugo hairs and cornified epithelial cells, which are swallowed in amniotic fluid, is suggestive of complete obstruction (*Farber test*). This test has limited value, since a partially obstructive lesion may on occasion constitute as much of a surgical emergency as a completely obstructive one. In any event, the specimen to be examined should be taken from the center of the stool, since epithelial cells from the rectum and perianal area may adhere to the outside of the stool and be misinterpreted as swallowed epithelial cells.

Obstruction in the duodenal area is responsible for epigastric distention and, at times, for gastric waves similar to those of pyloric stenosis. The distention may not be persistent, however, since it may be relieved by vomiting. The vomiting may be projectile, and the vomitus will contain bile if the obstruction is below the ampulla of Vater, as it usually is.

Obstructions in the lower ileum, colon or rectum cause more generalized distention, often with bulging of the flanks. When the liver dullness is obliterated, there is a strong possibility that intestinal perforation has occurred. Vomiting with lower bowel obstruction may be delayed a day or so, but eventually may become fecal in type.

When the obstruction is *incomplete*, as, for example, with intestinal stenosis, constricting bands, including the so-called superior mesenteric artery syndrome, duplications and incomplete volvulus, symptoms (vomiting, abdominal distention, obstipation) may appear shortly after birth or may be delayed an indeterminate time. They may approach in severity those of a completely obstructive lesion, or they may be sufficiently mild and infrequent as to be overlooked until either an acute episode or diagnostic studies disclose the lesion.

Meconium ileus is described on page 860, meconium plug on page 392, aganglionic megacolon on page 791 and anal and rectal obstructions on page 814.

Valuable information on the location of congenital obstructive lesions in the intestine may often be obtained from roentgenograms of the abdomen without ingestion of contrast media, since with completely obstructive lesions there will be distention of the bowel above the obstruction and there may be a series of fluid levels with superimposed gas in the distended loops. An air-contrast study of the colon following an enema containing radiopaque material may provide additional localizing information, especially in respect to the possibility of a displaced cecum with malrotation of the intestine. Under usual circumstances, air is demonstrable roentgenographically in the stomach of the normal infant immediately after birth. Within an hour the proximal portion of the small intestine and segments of the colon are demonstrable. The distal parts of the colon may be visible as early as the third hour.

Prognosis. If a complete obstruction is not relieved promptly, the clinical course is rapid. Vomiting is persistent; dehydration, loss of weight, and prostration become severe, and the infant dies within a few days. When the obstruction is not complete, the infant may survive for weeks; minor obstructions may be compatible with life even without treatment. Recovery from both complete and incomplete obstructions can be expected in many instances with early diagnosis and appropriate management.

Treatment. Not every obstructive lesion is amenable to surgery, but infants can withstand massive resection of the small intestine when the lesion necessitates it. Preoperative preparation, including constant gastric aspiration, and postoperative care are of the greatest importance, especially in relation to the correction of dehydration and electrolyte deficits and to the maintenance of fluid balance and nutrition by parenteral means (p. 227).

ATRESIA AND STENOSIS

Atresia (complete occlusion) and stenosis (partial occlusion) of the gastrointestinal tract account for about one third of cases of intestinal obstruction. *Atresia* is the more common. The obstructive lesion is most frequently in the ileum (50 per cent) and duodenum (25 per cent), less frequently in the jejunum, rare in the colon and almost never in the stomach. There is an increased incidence of duodenal atresia, as well as of imperforate anus, in babies with Down's syndrome. About 15 per cent of intestinal atresias are multiple. The types of atresia are (1) a diaphragm-like occlusion of the lumen, (2) a blind end not in continuity with a distal segment, and (3) segments of bowel with cordlike connections.

The *diagnosis* of intestinal atresia should be suspected in the presence of maternal hydramnios, of Down's syndrome, and of vomiting or abdominal distention in the newborn infant. Upright roentgenograms of the abdomen show that the air in the intestinal tract has failed to progress beyond the level of the atresia. Intestinal stenosis results in signs of intestinal obstruction, the severity of which depends on the degree of the stenosis.

Treatment is surgical. In duodenal atresia or stenosis the surgical procedures of choice are duodenoduodenostomy or duodenojejunostomy to bypass the obstruction. Jejunal or ileal atresias are often associated with errors in rotation of the intestine, are subject to gangrene of the blind end of the bowel proximal to the atresia, and have a greater incidence of complications and of death.

ANOMALIES OF ROTATION
(MALROTATION)

Incomplete rotation, also incorrectly termed *malrotation of the intestine*, represents a failure of the bowel to rotate and become fixed normally. The normal embryologic sequence is as follows: the cecum rotates around the superior mesenteric artery, which acts as an axis, counterclockwise from a position in the middle of the abdomen just below the stomach. The colon, which lies on the left side of the abdomen, follows as the cecum rotates into the right upper quadrant and finally into the right lower quadrant. When rotation is completed, the ascending and descending mesocolon fuse to the back of the abdomen, anchoring the mesentery from the ligament of Treitz obliquely downward to the cecal area. In some instances rotation may be complete, but the mesentery is incomplete, so that there is abnormal mobility of the midgut and colon.

Most often in malrotation the cecum has failed to move into the right lower quadrant, and the bands fixing it to the posterior abdominal wall cross over and may obstruct the duodenum (Fig. 11-12). The narrow mesenteric stalk which suspends the small intestine in the area of the superior mesenteric vessels is liable to volvulus, resulting in intermittent or acute obstruction which may progress to strangulation. Obstruction occurs first at the upper portion of the duodenum, then at the lower end of the loop. Volvulus is present in more than half of the patients operated on for intestinal obstruction when the cecum is in the right upper portion of the abdomen. This problem usually presents with symptoms of acute or recurrent intestinal obstruction at birth or in the first year of life. Some children with malrotation present the clinical picture of celiac disease, which is relieved by surgical repair. Roentgenograms of the abdomen may show an abnormal colonic gas pattern, and barium enema confirms the abnormal position of the cecum. In acute obstruction, diagnosis is at

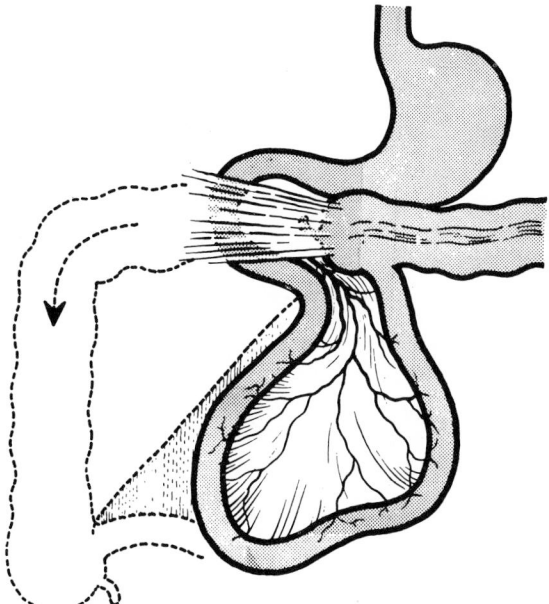

Figure 11-12. The mechanism of intestinal obstruction with incomplete rotation of the midgut ("malrotation"). The dotted lines show the course the cecum should have taken. Failure to rotate has left obstructing bands across the duodenum, and a narrow pedicle for the midgut loop, making it prone to volvulus. (Nixon and O'Donnell: *The Essentials of Pediatric Surgery,* 1961.)

laparotomy, and only an erect flat film of the abdomen is made to see the gas shadows.

Management includes fluid therapy to combat shock and disturbance of body fluids and electrolytes, followed by laparotomy at which the volvulus is unwound, transduodenal bands are divided, and the large intestine is straightened and placed in the left side of the abdomen with all the small bowel on the right.

DUPLICATION OF THE GASTROINTESTINAL TRACT

Duplications are congenital tubular or oval structures which have a smooth muscle wall and a mucous membrane similar to some part of the gastrointestinal tract, and which are intimately connected to the gastrointestinal tract. They vary widely in size and shape. Clinical manifestations usually arise during infancy and early childhood. They include symptoms of obstruction of adjoining intestine by compression, of intestinal bleeding from peptic ulceration secondary to gastric mucosa in the lining of a duplication which communicates with the intestine, of pain from secretory distention of a noncommunicating duplication, of gangrene of the bowel from obstruction of segmental vasculature or of a movable abdominal mass palpated on routine examination of the abdomen. Duplications are most frequent in the ileum, ileocecal region and esophagus, but may occur in any part of the gastrointestinal tract. In the abdomen a duplication may be the leading point of an intussusception. Duplications in the thorax are usually of the esophagus or the stomach, rarely communicate with either, but are evident through dysphagia and respiratory symptoms produced by esophageal and pulmonary compression, and are usually demonstrable roentgenographically. Associated anomalies of vertebrae are not uncommon, and often are at a higher level than the intrathoracic mass. Some intrathoracic duplications are of duodenal or jejunal origin.

Roentgenographic studies may show stenosis or compression of the intestinal lumen, but more frequently are normal. An intrathoracic duplication is usually visible as a mediastinal mass in roentgenograms of the chest. Very rarely barium studies may fill a communicating duplication.

Surgical removal is indicated, but is complex and usually involves removal of both duplication and adjoining intestine because of the common wall and blood supply, followed by primary anastomosis of the remaining ends of intestine.

DIVERTICULOSIS, DIVERTICULITIS AND ASSOCIATED DISORDERS

With the exception of Meckel's diverticulum, congenital and acquired single and multiple diverticula of the intestinal tract are extremely rare in

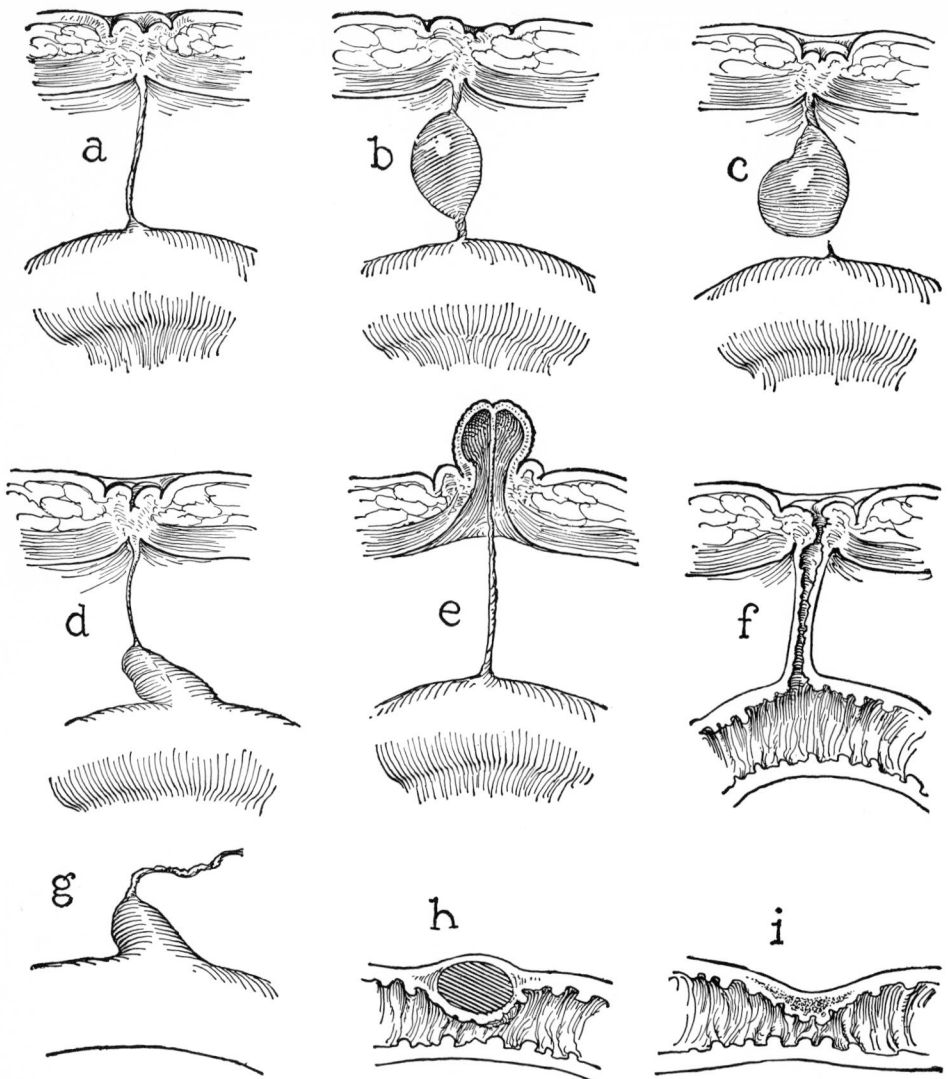

Figure 11-13. Diagrammatic representation of structures derived from remnants of the omphalomesenteric duct. *a*, Cord extending between umbilicus and ileum; *b*, cyst suspended between umbilicus and ileum; *c*, cyst suspended from umbilicus; *d*, Meckel's diverticulum with cord extending to umbilicus; *e*, everted mucocele attached by cord to ileum; *f*, fecal fistula between ileum and umbilicus; *g*, Meckel's diverticulum with free intraperitoneal cord; *h*, enterocystoma; *i*, stenosis from excessive evolution. (Brennemann: *Practice of Pediatrics.* W. F. Prior Co., Vol. 3.)

children. *Diverticulosis*, the presence of multiple outpouchings of the intestinal tract, usually in the colon, and *diverticulitis*, or inflammation of diverticula, are essentially diseases of adult life.

The omphalomesenteric duct, which connects the ileum with the yolk sac and disappears by the fifth or sixth week of fetal life, may persist in all or part of its course and be responsible for a variety of anomalies (Fig. 11-13). Of these, the most frequent is Meckel's diverticulum, which is estimated to occur in 2 to 3 per cent of all persons and is more frequently symptomatic in males than in females.

Pathology. Meckel's diverticulum is located on the antimesenteric side of the ileum within 18 to 36 inches of the ileocecal valve. Its mucosal lining may be gastric and ileal, or colonic and ileal in that order of frequency. Pancreatic cells, including

those of the islets of Langerhans, may also be present.

Clinical Manifestations. Symptoms from a Meckel's diverticulum can arise at any age, but occur more frequently in the first 2 years of life. *Hemorrhage* from a small peptic ulcer in or adjacent to aberrant gastric mucosa at the neck of the pouch is the most common symptom. The bleeding is unaccompanied by pain, a point which differentiates it from bleeding from an intussusception. Although the bleeding is usually acute, it may be intermittent and recurrent over an extended period of time. The blood may be dark red at first, but with massive bleeding it is bright red. *Abdominal pain* is the second most common symptom. It may be acute and due to diverticulitis with a clinical picture resembling that of acute appendicitis, or it may be vague and recurrent. Referral of the (ileal) pain to the umbilicus may suggest the true diagnosis. Perforation of an ulcer in the diverticulum may be responsible for peritoneal bleeding or inflammation. A Meckel's diverticulum may invert and become the leading point of an intussusception, or intestinal obstruction can result from herniation of a loop of bowel through a "ring" formed by the atrophied cord of the diverticulum. Volvulus may result from twisting of the intestine around or in association with persistence of an omphalomesenteric duct or cord. *Littre's hernia* is a rare condition in which a Meckel's diverticulum protrudes, along with the adjacent portion of the intestine, into the sac of an inguinal, femoral or umbilical hernia. The diverticulum is likely to become inflamed and adherent to the hernial sac with resultant incarceration.

Persistence of the omphalomesenteric duct may result in an umbilical sinus which discharges intestinal contents; if the ileal end is closed, there is only mucoid secretion. When both ends are closed, a cyst may form in the tract; the cyst may protrude through the umbilicus.

Roentgenographic studies are generally of little use in the diagnosis of Meckel's diverticulum. Very rarely abdominal films taken after the barium has cleared from the intestinal tract following gastrointestinal series or barium enema will show a residual blob of barium in the diverticulum. The blob is differentiated from barium in the appendix because it does not occupy a fixed position in the abdomen.

Treatment. If a Meckel's diverticulum or other anomaly of the omphalomesenteric duct is responsible for signs or symptoms, surgical extirpation is indicated. A diverticulum discovered during an abdominal operation for other conditions should be removed, if the situation otherwise permits.

MEGACOLON

The term "megacolon" denotes gross enlargement of the colon irrespective of cause; the principal responsible factors are chronic constipation from a variety of causes, chief of which are (1) voluntary withholding of feces because of physical discomfort or emotional conflict (chronic constipation, p. 780), congenital aganglionic megacolon, and anorectal stenosis (p. 814) or other anatomic obstruction to the passage of feces. *Dolichocolon* is a term used to describe enlargement and redundancy of the colon associated with chronic constipation. It is not clear whether the anatomic or physiologic abnormality is primary. The treatment is that of chronic constipation.

Congenital Aganglionic Megacolon
(Hirschsprung's Disease)

Congenital aganglionic megacolon is characterized clinically by obstinate and severe constipation dating from birth or soon thereafter, abdominal distention and, in severe cases, retardation of physical development. It is more common in males, and a familial pattern has been reported.

Pathology. The colon is greatly dilated and filled with feces and gas proximal to an area of narrowing, usually in the rectum or rectosigmoid. The muscular coat of the dilated bowel is hypertrophied, but in long-standing cases the wall of the dilated intestine may be extremely thin. Perforation is rare, but ulceration of the mucosa is not uncommon, particularly in infants.

Histologically, there is absence of the parasympathetic ganglion cells of the intramural plexus of the constricted portion of the bowel only. The *functional abnormality* is an increase in muscular tone and contractile activity of the aganglionic segment of bowel, without the reciprocal relaxation necessary to facilitate the onward movement of feces by the peristaltic activity of the colon proximal to the constricted aganglionic segment.

In 90 per cent of instances the aganglionic segment of bowel extends for 4 to 25 cm. proximally from the anus. Instances of involvement of the entire colon, of portions of the small bowel, and rarely of several aganglionic segments between normal areas have been reported.

Clinical Manifestations. In newborn infants the symptoms may be present at birth, with failure to pass meconium, or may appear during the first week and be those of partial or even complete intestinal obstruction with vomiting, abdominal distention and failure to pass stools. Temporary relief of symptoms may occur after a rectal examination, which is characteristically followed by an explosive discharge of feces and gas. Bile-stained and even fecal vomiting may occur, and the infant may lose weight and become dehydrated. Diarrhea of the "overflow" type may be the predominant symptom in the neonatal period and may occur in association with symptoms of intestinal obstruction. Hypoproteinemia and edema may develop in association with protein-losing enteropathy. Infants with aganglionic megacolon are prone to a severe, life-threatening enterocolitis.

When the symptoms are mild enough that the diagnosis is not made in early infancy, the clinical course is one of gradually increasing constipation and abdominal distention. Spontaneous bowel movements are rare, even in response to a laxative; enemas are usually necessary to produce evacuations. A large fecal mass is palpable in the left lower portion of the abdomen, but on rectal examination the rectum is not dilated and is almost invariably empty of feces, in contrast to the dilated, full rectum of children with chronic constipation due to withholding of feces. The stools, when passed, may consist of small pellets, be ribbon-like or have a fluid consistency; the large stools and fecal soiling of patients with functional constipation are absent. In mild cases the nutrition may not be greatly disturbed; in severe cases there is likely to be loss of subcutaneous tissue and failure to grow. The wasted extremities and large, protruding abdomen of such patients create a typical appearance, but one which may be confused with some of the *malabsorption syndromes* (p. 804), especially when "overflow" diarrhea is present. Hypochromic anemia is often present. Intermittent attacks of intestinal obstruction from impacted feces may be associated with pain and fever.

Diagnosis. Anorexia, obstipation, abdominal distention and vomiting in the absence of readily demonstrable anatomic obstruction are suggestive of aganglionic megacolon in early infancy. An "overflow" type of diarrhea may confuse the picture. Later the diagnosis is suggested by a history of obstipation and abdominal distention existing from early infancy.

Roentgenographic studies in the young infant with intestinal obstruction due to aganglionic megacolon show dilated loops of bowel throughout the abdomen on anteroposterior films taken in the erect position. In lateral erect films the rectal air, which is usually visible in the presacral area, is absent. The diagnostic findings on barium enema are (1) an abrupt change in caliber between the ganglionic and aganglionic sections of bowel, (2) irregular, "sawtooth" contractions of the aganglionic segment, (3) parallel transverse folds in the dilated proximal colon, (4) a thickened, nodular, edematous, proximal colon characteristic of protein-losing enteropathy (Fig. 11-14), and (5)

failure to evacuate the barium. In infants only a small amount of barium should be injected slowly through a small catheter whose tip is inserted barely beyond the anal sphincter, while the patient, in an oblique position, is being observed under the fluoroscope; the characteristic abrupt transition in caliber may be missed if the lower colon is flooded with too much barium. The possible existence of mechanical obstructions such as stenosis or stricture of the anus and membranous valvelike lesions in the rectum or rectosigmoid may be determined by sigmoidoscopic examination.

Rectal biopsy is useful when the clinical history is highly suggestive, but the roentgenographic studies are not diagnostic. This is particularly true in early infancy and in cases in which the thrust of the stool mass produces dilatation of a short aganglionic segment. The longitudinal biopsy of both layers of the muscularis reveals the absence of ganglion cells. *Anal tonometry* demonstrates absence of the normal reflex relaxation of the internal sphincter on rectal dilation with a balloon.

Roentgenographic examination of the urinary tract should also be obtained, since megaloureters have occasionally been demonstrated in conjunction with aganglionic megacolon.

Treatment. Retention enemas of 3 to 4 ounces of mineral or olive oil followed by repeated colonic

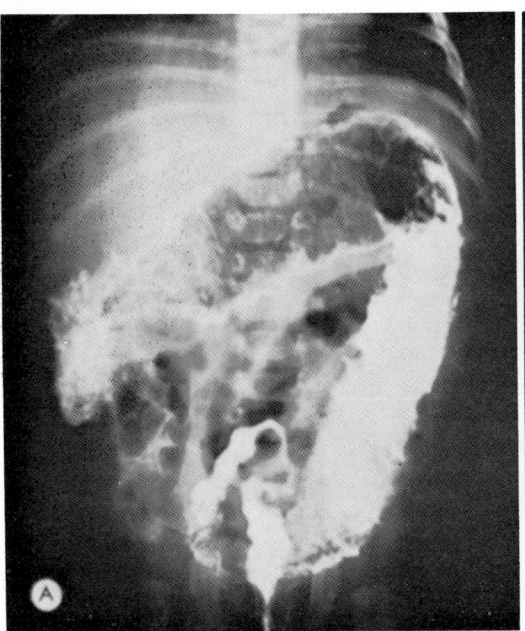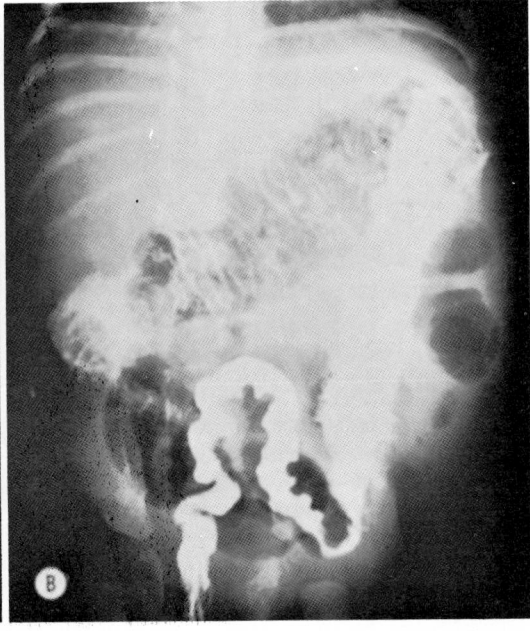

Figure 11-14. Roentgenographic findings in 8-week-old identical male twins with congenital aganglionic megacolon. Diarrhea gradually changed to constipation during the first 3 weeks of life in each. Both developed generalized edema and hypoproteinemia at 6 weeks of age. Plain roentgenograms of the abdomen of each twin showed a distended bowel with a relatively narrow rectum. *A,* Anteroposterior roentgenogram of the barium-filled colon of one of the twins shows irregular, bizarre, "sawtooth" contractions of the rectum and sigmoid. A zone of demarcation is noted at the junction of the sigmoid and descending colon, and parallel transverse folds are visible in the dilated proximal colon. Above this the colon is thick, nodular and edematous, producing a "shaggy" border suggestive of ulcerative colitis. This is the picture of exudative enteropathy. Histologic examination of the distal segment revealed the absence of ganglion cells. *B,* Anteroposterior roentgenogram of the barium-filled colon of the twin. (From J. W. Hope, P. F. Borns, and P. K. Berg: Roentgenologic Manifestations of Hirschsprung's Disease in Infancy. *Am. J. Roentgen.,* 95:217, 1965.)

irrigations with *isotonic saline solution* will usually remove most of the fecal accumulation. The rectal catheter should be inserted beyond the constricted segment. Attacks of syncope, shock and even death have been attributed to water intoxication following the use of tap water and soapsuds enemas. Magnesium poisoning has been reported following retention of enemas of magnesium sulfate in patients with congenital megacolon. Thus the use of solutions other than isotonic saline solution for rectal irrigation should be avoided.

Removal of the narrowed segment of bowel by the pull-through surgical technique devised by Swenson results in relief of symptoms and a return to normal bowel habits in the majority of instances. During operation it is essential to ascertain from biopsies of the bowel that ganglion cells are present in the proximal end of the resected bowel before the final anastomosis is made.

If an infant's condition prohibits the extensive surgery involved in a pull-through operation, a colostomy should be performed in the distal portion of the ganglionic part of the colon. Preoperative correction of anemia and of water and electrolyte deficits and adequate maintenance postoperatively are important. Later, when the infant is in good nutritional state and has been gaining weight, the pull-through form of resection of the bowel can be performed. Duhamel has utilized a longitudinal anastomosis between the descending colon and the rectum. Various modifications of this and other procedures are being evaluated.

INTRA-ABDOMINAL HERNIAS

An intra-abdominal hernia occurs when loops of intestine are trapped by an anomalous fold of peritoneum created by malrotation or malfixation of the duodenum or colon to the posterior abdominal wall. Loops of intestine also may herniate through congenital defects of the mesentery, particularly near the terminal ileum. The symptoms and signs are those of intermittent or acute intestinal obstruction. Gangrene of the intestine can occur if there is compression of the vasculature. Surgical reduction of the hernia and repair of the anomaly in order to prevent recurrence require great care and a knowledge of embryologic anatomy because of the danger of interference with intestinal blood supply.

EXTRA-ABDOMINAL HERNIAS

See Umbilical Hernia (p. 399), and page 821.

ABNORMALITIES OF THE PANCREAS

See Meconium Ileus (pp. 392, 860), Pseudomeconium Ileus (Meconium Plugs) (p. 392) and Annular Pancreas (p. 856).

ACQUIRED INTESTINAL OBSTRUCTION

Paralytic ileus, secondary to acute infections, especially pneumonia and peritonitis, and to uremia and electrolyte imbalance of any origin, is a frequent cause of intestinal obstruction. Pneumonia is probably the most frequent cause of paralytic ileus in infants; peritonitis, the most frequent in older children.

Incarcerated inguinal hernias and intussusception are the most frequent mechanical causes of intestinal obstruction in infants. Intestinal obstruction may also result from postoperative adhesions or those produced by acute peritonitis from which recovery occurred, or by chronic peritonitis, e.g. tuberculous peritonitis. Other causes are foreign bodies in the intestine, including fecal concretions and inspissated meconium in the newborn infant (p. 392), late obstruction by intraluminal contents in cystic fibrosis (pseudomeconium ileus), and by masses of roundworms; tumors of the bowel, including mesenteric cysts, may also be obstructive. Rectal stricture from lymphogranuloma venereum is rare in children.

Certain congenital anomalies responsible for intestinal obstruction may not manifest themselves until after birth. These include intra-abdominal herniations, volvulus resulting from malrotation of the intestine, and duplications of the bowel.

INTUSSUSCEPTION

Intussusception, an invagination of a portion of the intestine into a distal adjacent part, is a frequent cause of intestinal obstruction in infants and young children from 3 to 24 months of age, but is rare both earlier and later. It is more common in males and in all infants from 3 to 11 months of age. *Agonal intussusception* is relatively common and is presumably caused by loss of muscular tone preceding death.

Etiology. In most instances intussusception develops in healthy infants without demonstrable cause. Epidemiologic studies suggest that to some extent it may be correlated with viral infections of the gut affecting Peyer's patches. In about 5 per cent of the cases a specific lesion such as a Meckel's diverticulum, polyp, nodule of ectopic pancreas, duplication of the ileum, hypertrophied Peyer's patch, lymphoma of the bowel or intramural hemorrhage in anaphylactoid purpura (p. 522) serves as a lead point for the intussusception.

Pathology. Intussusceptions are most frequently ileocolic, ileo-ileocolic, and ileo-ileal in type with the upper portion (intussusceptum) invaginating into the lower (intussuscipiens), pulling the mesentery with it. Swelling begins promptly from edema and hemorrhage secondary to venous engorgement, with resultant intestinal incarceration and obstruction. Most intussusceptions do not strangulate the bowel in the first 24 hours, but may lead subsequently to intestinal gangrene and systemic shock. Agonal intussusception shows little evidence of swelling or inflammation and is without clinical significance.

Clinical Manifestations. In typical cases there is sudden onset of severe paroxysmal pain which recurs at frequent intervals and is accompanied by straining efforts and loud outcries. Initially, the infant may be comfortable and play normally between the paroxysms of pain, but if the intussusception is not reduced, he becomes progressively weaker and goes into a shocklike state in which the body temperature may rise as high as 106°F. The pulse becomes weak and thready, the respirations shallow and grunting, and the pain may be manifested only by moaning sounds. Vomiting occurs in most instances and is usually more frequent at the beginning. In the later phase the vomitus becomes bile-stained. Fecal matter of normal appearance may be evacuated during the first few hours of symptoms. After this time fecal excretions are small, or more often do not occur, and little or no flatus is passed. Blood generally appears in the first 12 hours, but at times not for 1 or 2 days and infrequently not at all. Stools consisting chiefly of blood and mucus are common and are termed *"currant jelly stools."*

Palpation of the abdomen usually reveals a sausage-shaped mass, sometimes ill-defined, which may increase in size and firmness during a paroxysm of pain and is most often in the right upper portion of the abdomen. It is most readily located by bimanual rectal and abdominal palpation between paroxysms of pain. The presence of bloody mucus on the finger as it is withdrawn after rectal examination supports the diagnosis of intussusception. Abdominal distention and tenderness develop as intestinal obstruction becomes more acute. On rare occasions the advancing intestine prolapses through the anus. This can be distinguished from prolapse of the rectum by the separation between the protruding intestine and the rectal wall, which does not exist in prolapse of the rectum.

Ileo-ileal intussusception may have a less typical clinical picture, the symptoms and signs being chiefly those of small intestinal obstruction. *Recurrent intussusception* is rare, with an incidence of no more than 2 per cent. *Chronic intussusception*, in which the symptoms exist in milder form for days or weeks, is more likely to occur with or following acute enteritis, or in older children.

Diagnosis. In intussusception the clinical history and physical findings are usually sufficiently typical for diagnosis. Roentgenographically, abdominal scout films may show a masslike density in the area of the intussusception. The film after a barium enema will show cupping in the head of barium as its advance is obstructed by the intussusceptum (Fig. 11-15). A central linear column of barium may be visible in the compressed lumen of the intussusceptum, and a thin layer of barium may be seen trapped around the invaginating intestine (coil-spring sign), especially after

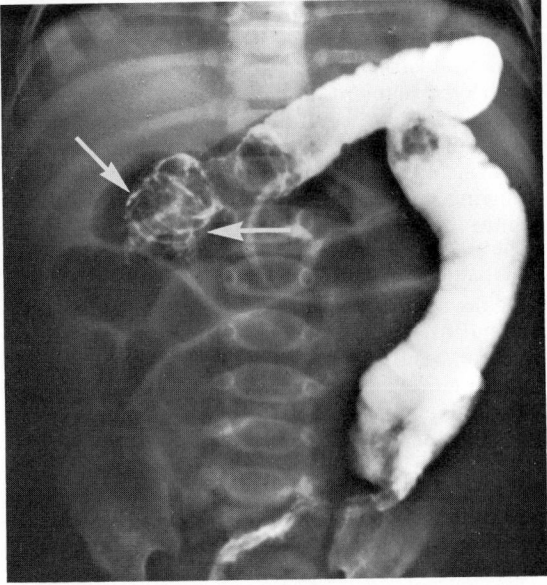

Figure 11-15. Intussusception in an infant. The obstruction is evident in the proximal transverse colon. Contrast material between the intussuseptum and the intussuscipiens is responsible for the coilspring appearance.

evacuation. Retrogression of the intussusceptum under the pressure of the enema, and gaseous distention of the small intestine from obstruction, are also useful roentgenographic signs. Ileo-ileal intussusception is usually not demonstrable by barium enema, but is suspected because of gaseous distention of the intestine above the intussusception.

Differential Diagnosis. Bloody bowel movements and abdominal cramps accompanying *enterocolitis* may usually be differentiated from intussusception because the pain is less severe and less regular and because the infant is recognizably ill between pains from the beginning. Bleeding from a *Meckel's diverticulum* is usually painless. The intestinal hemorrhage of *anaphylactoid purpura* is usually distinguishable by accompanying joint symptoms or purpura elsewhere. *It is important to keep in mind that intussusception may be a complication of any of the foregoing conditions,* none of which is accompanied by a palpable abdominal mass in the absence of intussusception. Since tenesmus and a discoverable tumor are usually absent in ileo-ileal intussusception, it may be confused with *ileal obstruction* from other causes. This is of little clinical importance, since surgical exploration is indicated in any case.

Prognosis. Untreated intussusception in infants is nearly always fatal; the chances of recovery are directly related to the duration of intussusception before reduction. The majority of infants will recover if the intussusception is reduced within the first 24 hours, but the mortality rate rises rapidly after this time, and recoveries are unusual when reduction is deferred to the third day. Spontaneous reduction during transport or preparation for operation is not uncommon.

Treatment.   Reduction of the intussusception is an emergency procedure to be carried out immediately after diagnosis and rapid preparation for operation with fluids and blood for shock and water and electrolyte repair. In many cases of short duration, when there are no signs of prostration, shock or peritoneal irritation, it may be possible to reduce the intussusception by hydrostatic pressure under fluoroscopic guidance and with the close consultation of a surgeon. The technique is described by Ravitch as follows:

The stomach is aspirated, intravenous administration of fluids is started, and a nonlubricated Foley bag catheter is placed in the rectum and inflated. The buttocks are compressed tightly and taped with adhesive plaster. A barium solution is then allowed to flow by gravity into the colon from a height of not more than 3 to 3½ feet above the fluoroscopic table. The abdomen is *not touched* during the procedure. Reduction of the intussusception is manifest by free filling of the small intestine, disappearance of the mass, passage of flatus or feces and improvement in the infant's condition. Charcoal is then administered by mouth, and its recovery in an enema 6 hours later is further evidence of intestinal patency. If there is any doubt about the completeness of the reduction, an exploratory operation is performed immediately.

Reduction by the hydrostatic technique is not effective in ileo-ileal intussusception and will resolve only the colonic component of ileo-ileocolic intussusception. With good surgical technique, operative reduction carries a very low mortality rate in early cases, and has the advantage of more certainty of reduction and of demonstration of any existing lead points, some of which may be removable. The recurrence rates for both operative and nonoperative methods are apparently about equal. When the intussusception is irreducible or the bowel gangrenous, the involved intestine must be resected promptly.

NEOPLASMS OF THE GASTROINTESTINAL TRACT

Neoplasms of the gastrointestinal tract are rare in childhood; primary carcinoma, sarcoma, lymphosarcoma, lipomas, polypoid adenomas and teratomas have been observed (p. 1448).

FOREIGN BODIES IN THE STOMACH AND INTESTINES

An object which reaches the stomach will in most instances pass through the gastrointestinal tract. Certain types of foreign bodies, however, are potentially dangerous. Needles, hairpins or bobby pins pass easily through the esophagus on their long axis, but may be unable to round the turns of the duodenum, where they become fixed and eventually perforate the intestine. Such potentially dangerous foreign bodies can usually be removed gastroscopically. Special attention should be paid to safety pins in the stomach. If they are small, they will probably pass without difficulty, whether

open or closed. If they are large, either closed or open, peroral removal is safe and is indicated.

If the foreign body has passed through the pylorus into the intestine, its progress should be observed by means of roentgenograms, and every stool should be examined for its presence. The stool can be placed in a fine-meshed sieve and disintegrated by allowing water to run through the sieve with some force. If serial roentgenograms show the foreign body to move progressively down the intestinal tract, perforation is not likely. If it remains stationary for a week, operation is indicated because of the dangers of ulceration and perforation of the bowel. If at any time such signs of perforation as tenderness, rigidity, pain, nausea or vomiting develop, surgery is indicated immediately. The diet should be normal, with no change from that to which the child has been accustomed. The bizarre roughage and wool or cotton diets sometimes recommended are valueless and may be dangerous. Laxatives are contraindicated, since the accelerated activity of the intestine increases the danger of perforation.

BEZOARS

Occasionally infants and children, particularly if emotionally disturbed or mentally retarded, acquire the habit of swallowing hair from their head or from dolls, brushes, or the like, or they may swallow fur, wool or cotton from wearing apparel

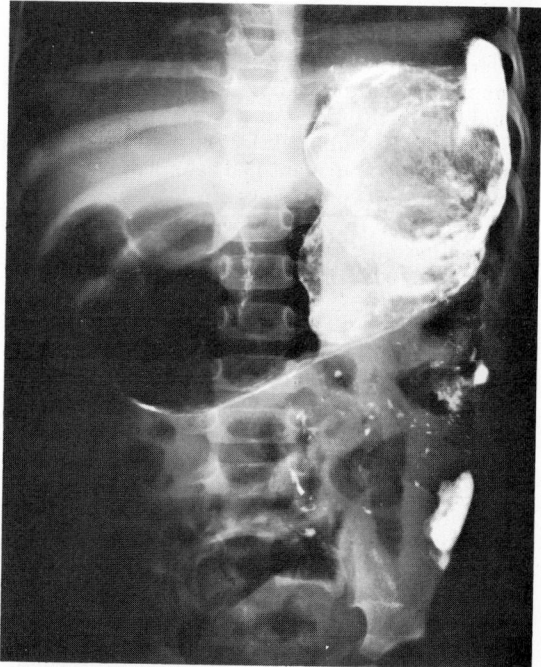

Figure 11-16.   Hairball (trichobezoar) in the fundus of the stomach of a girl 5 years of age; it is outlined by barium. The child was admitted to the hospital for intestinal obstruction resulting from a portion of the trichobezoar which had detached from the gastric mass and become impacted in the ileum.

or blankets. Some of this material may be passed through the intestines, but when the habit is persistent, there is an accumulation in the stomach with formation of the so-called *hairball* or *trichobezoar*. The symptoms are indefinite, but indigestion and gastric distress may be present. The tumor mass is often palpable, and may give a soft crackling sensation on palpation. A roentgenogram after administration of barium may disclose a mass outlined by barium (Fig. 11-16). A portion of the bezoar may be dislodged and subsequently become impacted in the intestine and cause obstruction. The diagnosis may be suspected from observation of the child in the act of swallowing these materials, and hair may occasionally be observed in the mouth or stools. The tumor should be removed surgically. The child's mental and psychologic status should be evaluated, and treatment provided as indicated.

Phytobezoars are accumulations of fibrous or mucilaginous materials such as that in persimmons and various tar products. The accumulation is usually rapid in comparison with that of the hairball.

Diseases of the Gastrointestinal Tract

Epidemic Gastroenteritis (Grippe-Like Infections). Community and family epidemics of highly contagious infections in which vomiting and diarrhea are prominent manifestations are common throughout the world. They are presumed to be due in large part to as yet unidentified pathogenic agent(s), probably viruses. Vomiting or diarrhea may occur among contacts without regard to the manifestations in the infecting person. The degree of illness may be mild or severe, but the duration is usually short, being only 1 to 3 days. Since the illness is likely to be much more severe in infants than in older children, every attempt should be made to protect infants from contact with affected persons. Treatment consists in limiting oral intake to frequent small amounts of clear fluids by mouth until the symptoms subside. If dehydration or electrolyte imbalance occurs, appropriate parenterally administered fluids should be substituted.

Specific Infections. Infections of the gastrointestinal tract due to identified agents are discussed elsewhere. See Typhoid Fever (p. 585), Escherichia Coli Infections (p. 405), Bacillary Dysentery (p. 588), Salmonella Infections (p. 583), Tuberculous Enteritis (p. 608), Enterovirus Infections (p. 669), Intestinal Protozoa (p. 748) and Intestinal Parasites (p. 717).

Acute Gastritis. Objective evidence of gastritis in children is infrequently available, and as an isolated lesion it must be rare. Gastric lesions are usually unsuspected during life since vomiting and anorexia are symptoms common to many infections. Bleeding may occur and be evident in the vomitus. Inflammatory lesions are occasionally observed at autopsy. Acute infections such as gastroenteritis, moniliasis, chickenpox, diphtheria, smallpox or scarlet fever may produce an inflammatory process in the stomach. *Drugs* such as acetylsalicylic acid, antibiotics and antileukemic agents may also cause acute or chronic gastritis in children, and an indwelling nasogastric tube may produce erosive lesions.

Corrosive gastritis is produced by strong acids or alkalis or by other irritants, such as calcium chloride, and may be accompanied by lesions of the mouth, pharynx and esophagus. Quantities of a swallowed irritant sufficient to produce an extensive gastritis frequently cause collapse and death. In most instances the esophageal lesion is the one of greatest importance.

Treatment. The general treatment of burns from acids and alkalis is discussed on page 1491, and of esophageal lesions on page 771. Administration of irritant drugs should be discontinued or they should be administered after a meal; protective demulcents such as aluminum hydroxide gel may be helpful. The only practical treatment of possible infectious gastritis is to diminish the oral intake until the primary infectious process subsides.

Gastric Dilatation. *Acute dilatation of the stomach,* and of the intestine (paralytic ileus) as well, may occur during the acute stages of pneumonia and other severe infections, after abdominal and thoracic operations or trauma, during peritonitis, with diabetic acidosis, hypokalemia and intestinal obstruction, and occasionally without discoverable cause. Gastric dilatation denotes a serious condition, especially when it occurs with pneumonia and peritonitis. Temporary relief can be provided by deflation through a stomach tube or, when there are accumulated gastric contents, by lavage. The use of the Wangensteen suction apparatus in postoperative conditions is helpful in avoiding and in treating paralytic ileus.

Chronic gastric dilatation may result from mechanical obstructions such as pyloric stenosis, external traction by adhesions, or pressure of a tumor in the pyloric area. It may also be a manifestation of chronic gastritis. During infancy a common cause is atony of the muscular wall in such conditions as rickets and extreme malnutrition.

The treatment depends upon the cause. A mechanical obstruction should be relieved. Chronic nutritional disturbances should be corrected.

Gastric Hemorrhage. Bleeding from the stomach may occur in association with purpura, hemophilia, hypoplastic anemias, leukemia, scurvy, peptic ulcer, cirrhosis of the liver, varices associated with other obstructions of the portal or splenic vein, and polypoid adenoma of the stomach.

Traumatic rupture of the stomach, injury from a swallowed foreign body, generalized infections, diabetic acidosis and persistent vomiting as in pyloric stenosis may also be responsible for gastric hemorrhage. Hemorrhagic disease of the newborn may result in gastric bleeding (p. 396).

Blood which is vomited (p. 776) may originate elsewhere than in the stomach; it may come from the nose, mouth, esophagus, lungs, or the fissured nipple of the nursing mother (p. 397). Blood expectorated from the lungs without swallowing is frothy. When hemorrhage from the stomach is copious, the blood is usually bright red, but if bleeding has taken place slowly and the blood has remained for some time in the stomach, the color will be dark brown or black (coffee-ground vomitus).

The *prognosis* depends upon the cause, but extensive gastric hemorrhage is usually serious.

Treatment. With extensive hemorrhage immediate steps should be directed toward its control, treatment of shock and replacement of lost blood. The child should be put at rest, an ice bag should be placed over the epigastrium, and morphine given hypodermically. When the hemorrhage is extensive, blood transfusions should be given as soon as possible to replace the lost blood. When the bleeding is continuous, gentle but constant aspiration through a Levin tube may aid in putting the stomach at rest, remove irritation from gastric secretions and provide an index of the extent of the bleeding.

Gastric Perforation. Perforation of the stomach or adjacent portions of the esophagus or duodenum is uncommon in infants and children; it is more often recognized at autopsy than during life. Rupture of the stomach in newborn infants has sometimes been recognized during life and repaired surgically with recovery of the infants.

The perforation of ulcers is the most readily explained; though infrequent, ulcers may be caused by an indwelling lavage tube, be associated with systemic diseases, usually acute ones, and especially with intracranial lesions (Rokitansky-Cushing ulcers) or be a sequel to corticosteroid therapy. Rupture of chronic gastric and duodenal ulcers is uncommon. Infrequently, spontaneous gastric perforation in otherwise apparently healthy newborn infants has been explained at autopsy; some have been associated with obstructive lesions, such as atresia of the pylorus, some with overdistention of the stomach from excessive ingestion (e.g. of partially cooked rice plus water), and some with defects of the gastric musculature.

Abdominal distention occurring suddenly in an infant should always suggest the possibility of perforation somewhere in the gastrointestinal tract, especially if there is obliteration of liver dullness. Vomiting, however, is usually the first symptom, and both the vomitus and the stool may contain blood. Cyanosis may appear if the distention is sufficient to interfere with respiration, and shock may be an early sign. The demonstration of air in the peritoneal cavity on a roentgenogram of the abdomen taken in the upright position is diagnostic.

Treatment consists in surgical repair as quickly as the infant can be prepared. Postoperatively, Wangensteen suction may be useful, and parenteral alimentation and hydration will be required.

PEPTIC ULCER

Gastric and duodenal ulcers are not common in childhood, but do occur at all ages, including the neonatal period. Nevertheless the high incidence of recurrent abdominal pain in children all too frequently leads to an erroneous diagnosis of ulcer. Gastric ulcers occur more frequently in early infancy; duodenal ulcers, more frequently in later infancy and childhood. Overall, the incidence of duodenal ulcer is at least 5 times that of gastric ulcer. Ulcerations of the upper gastrointestinal tract are more apt to be acute than chronic in the pediatric age range and are frequently secondary to conditions such as extensive burns (Curling's ulcer), neurologic lesions (Rokitansky-Cushing ulcer), intensive therapy with adrenocorticosteroids, severe infections (sepsis, gastroenteritis, meningitis, bronchiolitis) and marasmus.

The **symptoms** related to the ulcer may dominate the clinical picture, but often they are obscured by the primary disorder. Vomiting is the most common manifestation in infancy, but the ulcer may present with bleeding (hematemesis and melena) or with abdominal distention associated with perforation. In older children, as in adults, the chief symptom may be epigastric pain during the night or before meals; it is often relieved by eating. Frequently, however, in younger children the pain is periumbilical, erratic in timing, aggravated by eating, or the chief symptom is vomiting. Many children with ulcers are intense, driving youngsters who do well in school and are faced with emotional conflicts in their families. Peptic ulcer also appears to be somewhat more frequent in children with other chronic disorders of the gastrointestinal tract such as constipation or the irritable colon syndrome. In small children, ulcers sometimes appear to be related to "ulcerogenic" situations involving one or both parents.

The **diagnosis** of peptic ulcer should not be made without roentgenographic confirmation. In the very young infant free intraperitoneal air visible in abdominal films taken in the erect position should raise suspicion of a perforated gastric or duodenal ulcer. In such instances administration of contrast media is contraindicated; the nature of the perforation is determined at surgical exploration. The roentgenographic diagnosis of duodenal ulcer, most frequently located in the bulb, is based on a constant deformity of the bulb when it is well filled with barium: a persistent filling defect indicative of a crater, and a surrounding clear halo with convergent mucosal folds. Most duodenal ulcers are on the posterior wall; gastric ulcers are most frequently on the anterior wall and only rarely on the greater curvature. Postbulbar duodenal ulcers and ulcers of the pyloric canal (sometimes in conjunction with hypertrophic pyloric stenosis) are equally rare.

The roentgenographic identification of an ulcer in a child is difficult. A collection of barium caught between mucosal folds may resemble a crater, and it is difficult to obtain good compression films of the duodenum. Failure to fill the duodenal bulb with barium is not necessarily evidence of deformity or irritability, but may be solely the result of failure of filling secondary to pyloric spasm and increased duodenal reactivity in a frightened child; subsequent study usually shows that suspected "craters" or deformities are not present.

Gastric analysis, utilizing the augmented maximum histamine stimulation test, is of limited value in children; correlation with peptic ulcer has not yet been shown in children.

Prognosis. The case fatality rate is high among infants with perforated ulcers. Intractability and scarring of the duodenum is a rare sequel of peptic ulcer in childhood and the necessity for gastric or duodenal resection is rare. An estimated 50 per cent of children with ulcers have recurrent ulcers or ulcer-like pain as adults.

Treatment. Acute perforation requires immediate surgical closure. With acute hemorrhage the hematocrit should be followed closely and transfusions of blood given as indicated (see Gastric Hemorrhage, p. 797). Infants with hemorrhage but without perforation should be maintained on milk feedings; older children, on a bland diet. Hospitalization is usually warranted for initial therapy and a thorough investigation of the emotional interactions of the child and his family. After a few days on a bland diet a free diet is generally advocated, but any foods which are recognized as precipitating pain should be avoided. Gastric antacids or feedings between meals and at bedtime, as well as anticholinergic drugs shortly before meals, are therapeutically useful in children as in adults. Most ulcers of childhood heal rapidly, so that treatment need not be maintained beyond 3 or 4 weeks in most instances. If the pain does not improve with therapy, another origin of the pain is more likely than intractability of the ulcer. Follow-up roentgenographic studies should be carried out 1 or 2 months after treatment has been initiated.

MESENTERIC LYMPHADENITIS

Acute Mesenteric Lymphadenitis. Acute mesenteric lymphadenitis is frequently associated with an acute infection of the upper respiratory tract, especially of the pharynx. So much attention has been directed to this combination of inflammatory lesions, and the possibility that it may simulate acute appendicitis, that the physician may fail to recall that both acute and chronic involvement of the mesenteric lymph nodes may also be associated with infections of the appendix and the intestines.

Clinical manifestations. There is fever, abdominal pain, vomiting and at times constipation or diarrhea. The pain may be spasmodic, is often in the right lower quadrant, but may be in any part of the abdomen.

Differential diagnosis. When the pain is in the right lower quadrant and there is localized tenderness and muscular resistance, the possibility of appendicitis cannot be eliminated except by laparotomy. It has been suggested that in mesenteric adenitis there is a tendency for the area of tenderness to shift when the patient is rolled from side to side, whereas it remains fixed in appendicitis. Tenderness along the route of the mesentery on a line from McBurney's point upward to the left of the umbilicus is also said to favor a diagnosis of mesenteric adenitis. In the absence of physical signs of peritonitis or abscess, it is more common for the white blood cell count to be over 20,000 per mm.[3] with mesenteric adenitis than with appendicitis.

Complications. Suppuration of the lymph nodes is rare, but it may be responsible for localized or generalized peritonitis.

Treatment. Whenever appendicitis is a reasonable possibility, operation is indicated, since the danger of operation in mesenteric adenitis is much less than the danger of rupture of an inflamed appendix.

Chronic Mesenteric Lymphadenitis. Chronic infections of the lymph nodes may be sequels to an acute infection, or the involvement may be low-grade from the onset. In addition to conditions which may be responsible for acute adenitis, tuberculosis and histoplasmosis are causative possibilities. Involvement of lymph nodes is practically a constant accompaniment of chronic intestinal infections, but is usually overshadowed by the manifestations of the primary disease. Noninfectious lymph node involvement occurs with Hodgkin's disease, lymphosarcoma and neoplasms of the abdominal or pelvic organs.

NECROTIZING ENTEROCOLITIS

Necrotizing enterocolitis is a serious idiopathic disease of the newborn which occurs primarily in premature infants. It is characterized by gastric retention, abdominal distention, vomiting of bile, and blood-streaked and occasionally diarrheal stools. Earlier reports of "functional ileus," perforation of the ileum and colon, and colitis in the newborn infant probably represented forms of this condition.

The ileum and the colon are the most common sites of involvement; the duodenum is the least common. The condition usually complicates exchange transfusion or severe infections such as pneumonia, meningitis or omphalitis. *Patholog-*

ically, the intestine is dilated, necrotic and friable, with superficial ulcerations and submucosal hemorrhage. Perforation is common. Pneumatosis (intramural gas) of the intestinal wall is present and often is a premonitory sign of perforation. The *roentgenographic findings* are (1) multiple dilated loops of small intestine with air-fluid levels in the erect position and separation of loops suggesting mural edema or peritoneal fluid, (2) intramural gas, (3) free air in the peritoneum, and (4) gas in the portal vein. Therapy is mainly supportive; intravenous alimentation and hydration are usually necessary. Gastric suction, blood transfusions and antibiotic therapy are frequently indicated. Surgical treatment is required for intestinal perforation.

CHRONIC COLITIS

Chronic colitis, usually manifested clinically by chronic or recurrent diarrhea, may be divided into 4 categories: (1) infectious (amebic or bacillary dysentery, pp. 748, 588), (2) the irritable colon syndrome (spastic or mucous colitis), (3) chronic ulcerative colitis, and (4) granulomatous enterocolitis.

IRRITABLE COLON SYNDROME

The irritable colon syndrome is a frequent cause of recurrent abdominal pain in childhood. Its tendency to occur in emotionally sensitive children of overconcerned parents, together with accompanying signs and symptoms of autonomic hyperreactivity, suggests that it is a psychosomatic disease. See also sections on Abdominal Pain (p. 775) and Chronic Diarrhea (p. 783).

Clinical Manifestations. Characteristically, there is recurrent, intermittent, crampy abdominal pain which may be manifest in acute, sharp episodes. It may occur at any time of day or night; there is no consistent relation to eating or to bowel movements. Headache, facial pallor, dizziness, nausea and vomiting may on occasion lead the physician to suspect disease of the central nervous system. The stools are commonly described as hard pellets, suggesting spastic contractile activity of the colon, but diarrhea is also a frequent accompanying manifestation. Rarely, there may be blood in the stools. Poor appetite, low-grade fever and weight loss may lead to suspicion of granulomatous colitis, malignancy or other serious condition. There is abdominal tenderness over the colon, especially over the sigmoid and cecum.

Diagnosis. Granulomatous enterocolitis, ulcerative colitis, amebic and bacillary dysentery, and disorders of the urinary tract are ruled out by roentgenographic studies of the intestinal tract and colon using barium as the contrast medium, by intravenous urography, and by microscopic examination and culture of the stools. *Sigmoidoscopy* reveals pallor of the rectal and colonic mucosa, prominence of the blood vessels, some areas of erythematous flushing, increased mucus and prominent lymphoid follicles. The *family history* and relationships suggest the possibility of psychosomatic disease. The parents tend to be strikingly concerned about their children, and tend to set high standards of performance for themselves as well as their children. Illness during pregnancy has often led to both prenatal and postnatal anxiety about the child, and a history of death or severe illness in the family is frequent. Parental concerns have often led to an atmosphere of hovering anxiety over normal processes of behavioral development. As a result, the child often appears to be looking constantly for direction, reassurance and safety; relations with peers become restricted, and there is interference with normal childhood activities. School phobia is common.

Prognosis. Most children with the irritable colon syndrome gradually lose their symptoms with time, but a few retain them well into adulthood. As a group, their level of intellectual and material accomplishment tends to be high.

Treatment. Parent and child must learn that the child can cope with new environmental situations much better than either had believed possible. Ascertainment that no serious organic disease is present may help to relieve parental anxiety. Care should be taken not to imply to parent or child that the pain is "in the head." The physician's recognition of the reality of the pain should be stressed at the same time that an understanding and sympathetic explanation of its psychosomatic nature is made. Symptomatic therapy with an anticholinergic drug as needed is helpful in some instances. Older children with the irritable colon syndrome tolerate body contact sports poorly; prescribed relief from such compulsory activities may on occasion be helpful. Rarely, removal from the anxiety-laden environment is necessary, but on occasion a period with more relaxed relatives or rarely even in a hospital or convalescent home may break the cycle of anxiety.

CHRONIC ULCERATIVE COLITIS

Ulcerative colitis is a serious chronic inflammatory disease of the large intestine in which the mucous membrane becomes hyperemic and friable, bleeds easily, ulcerates, and tends to form pseudopolyps which are subject to malignant degeneration. The clinical course is marked by chronicity punctuated with acute exacerbations.

Etiology. Many theories based on infectious, allergic and psychogenic causes have been proposed for ulcerative colitis; none has been substantiated. The condition occurs more frequently among relatives of patients with the disease than would be expected from its incidence in the general population, and an inherited susceptibility to unidentified environmental factors has been suggested.

Pathology. The rectum and distal colon are principally affected, but all or any part of the colon may be involved, and the disease extends into the ileum in approximately one third of the cases. The mucosa becomes inflamed, edematous and friable, bleeds easily, and is covered with mucus and mucopurulent exudate. Histologically, the mucosa is infiltrated with polymorphonuclear leukocytes. "Crypt abscesses" are frequently located at the base of intestinal glands, and there is destruction of the mucous membrane to produce the ulceration which gives ulcerative colitis its name. As the disease progresses the ulcers enlarge and coalesce, and inflammatory tissue is piled up into pseudopolyps. With advanced disease the ulcers and inflammatory infiltrate penetrate more deeply into the bowel wall and ultimately result in fibrosis and in a decrease of both the internal diameter and length of the colon. Other tissue sites such as the skin, joints, liver and iris may have similar vascular and inflammatory changes during the course of the disease.

Clinical Manifestations. The onset may be insidious or acute and fulminating. Diarrhea is the most frequent presenting complaint, and careful questioning usually elicits a history of at least occasional loose bowel movements in the remainder. Rectal bleeding, weight loss, recurrent abdominal pain, arthritis, anemia, growth failure, erythema nodosum or even pyoderma gangrenosum may be the primary complaint that brings the child to the physician. The unformed stools usually contain mucus and blood. Abdominal cramps often precede the passage of stool, and explosive bowel movements, abdominal pain, tenesmus, hemorrhage of bright red blood, and even spastic constipation may occur. Other symptoms and signs are anorexia, fever, malaise, abdominal distention, nausea, vomiting and hepatosplenomegaly. Loss of bowel control is common and may accompany repeated urgent defecation during the night and on awakening in the morning. Growth and sexual maturation may be retarded. There may be severe headaches and abdominal cramps, particularly early in the course of the disease. Iron deficiency anemia may develop as the result of bleeding and poor dietary intake. In severe, chronic cases hypoproteinemia and edema may accompany emaciation. The serum albumin-globulin ratio may be reversed. The erythrocyte sedimentation rate is sometimes increased. There is usually mild to moderate tenderness on abdominal palpation, particularly in the left lower quadrant over the sigmoid.

Diagnosis. The diagnosis is suspected on the basis of the clinical pattern and by failure to isolate a specific agent. It is confirmed early in the disease by *sigmoidoscopy*; the mucosa is hyperemic and friable and bleeds easily. In more severe stages ulcers, mucus, exudate and polypoid changes may be seen. The demonstration of polymorphonuclear infiltration in a mucosal biopsy specimen is diagnostically helpful early in the disease. *Roentgenographic studies* with barium enema early in the disease may show only increased irritability of the involved segment at fluoroscopy and thickened mucosal markings on films taken after evacuation of barium. Later, ulcers appear as shaggy, barium-filled niches extending beyond the lumen of the colon. As the disease progresses, there is shortening and rigidity of the colon with loss of haustral markings ("pipestem colon"), particularly in the transverse and descending colon.

Children with ulcerative colitis tend to be dependent, passive and fearful, to expect the worst from every experience, and to be closely attached, yet with strong ambivalent feelings, to a parent, usually the mother. The parent, in turn, is closely, yet ambivalently, attached to the child. In some instances the child seems to be about the only reason for maintaining an incompatible marriage.

Course and Prognosis. The course is chronic and is usually marked by exacerbations and remissions over many years. Relapses may occur after remissions lasting up to 5 years. Ulcerative colitis may be complicated by arthritis and by such skin conditions as erythema nodosum, erythema multiforme and pyoderma gangrenosum. Death may occur from cachexia, during a fulminating episode with extreme dilatation of the colon, thrombosis of major blood vessels, or perforation of the colon. Some patients suffer carcinoma in pseudopolyps of the colon many years after the disease has appeared to be quiescent or nearly so. Overall, about 15 per cent of patients die of the disease, 30 per cent have prolonged remissions, and the remainder have symptoms persisting into adulthood.

Treatment. Hospitalization for initial evaluation and institution of therapy usually seems to produce better results than attempts at initial ambulatory management, perhaps because the child is removed from his usual psychologic stresses and the physician is able to develop a more effective relationship with patient and parents. Symptomatic treatment with tranquilizers, antidiarrheal and anticholinergic agents is of limited value. Initially, a low residue diet is helpful, but over the long term it may interfere with an adequate intake of food which is required. Supplements of vitamins and iron are indicated in children with severe diarrhea. Some patients benefit from the oral administration of salicylazosulfapyridine (Azulfidine) in a dosage of 150 mg. per kg. per 24 hours. If the process is limited to the distal part of the colon, nightly retention enemas of 50 to 150 ml. of tap water containing a soluble corticosteroid (50 to 100 mg. of hydrocortisone or 20 to 40 mg. of methylprednisolone) may provide some relief of symptoms, and may be continued according to clinical response. If the disease is more widespread, severe or resistant to other modes of medical therapy, trial with a corticosteroid or corticotropin (ACTH) is usually justified. Initial high dosage (8 mg. of hydrocortisone or 2.0 mg. of prednisone per kg. per 24 hours) may be necessary to achieve control. A maximum dose of 300 mg. of hydrocortisone or 75 mg. of prednisone is rarely exceeded. After one week the dose is reduced at weekly intervals by one fifth of the starting dose to the lowest maintenance dose which will keep the patient in remission, and is maintained at that level for at least 4 to 6 months. Administration of the total maintenance dose before breakfast every other day may help avoid undesirable side effects when the patient is in remission.

Surgical treatment by colectomy or ileostomy and partial colectomy is indicated for patients with fulminating ulcerative colitis not responding to corticosteroid therapy and for patients with chronic disease with an unsatisfactory response to other medical treatment.

Psychotherapy requires general psychologic support by the pediatrician or active treatment by a psychiatrist. In any event it is an important component of the overall program of management.

The proper care of children with ulcerative colitis requires a major, long-term commitment of interest on the part of the physician responsible for the patient. If this is not possible, he should consider referral to another physician who has a particular interest in the care of patients with the disease.

GRANULOMATOUS ENTEROCOLITIS
(REGIONAL ENTERITIS; CROHN'S DISEASE)

Granulomatous enterocolitis is a chronic, and occasionally an acute, inflammatory disease of the wall of the small or large bowel. Its cause is unknown.

Pathology. The lesion is usually limited to the terminal ileum (*regional ileitis*), but may extend into the jejunum and colon. Multiple involved areas may be separated by relatively intact bowel. The wall of the involved intestine is thickened, hyperemic and indurated, and extensions of mesenteric fat partially encircle the mucosa. The lumen is narrowed and may present a "cobble-stoned" appearance. Mucosal ulceration may lead to the formation of fistulas. Histologically, all layers of the intestinal wall are involved in the inflammatory process, but principally the sub-mucosa. The lymphoid tissue of the intestine is hyperplastic, as are the mesenteric lymph nodes, and there are noncaseating granulomas containing giant cells and epithelioid cells. Fibrosis may be present in the chronic stages.

Clinical Manifestations. In childhood, regional enterocolitis usually begins in the preadolescent period. The onset may be acute with a clinical pattern resembling that of acute appendicitis (*acute regional enteritis*). More often the onset is insidious, and the course is that of a low-grade chronic infection. There may be periodic bouts of fever without significant intestinal or abdominal symptoms or signs, or there may be recurrent abdominal pain, particularly after eating, mild diarrhea, intermittent constipation, low-grade fever, anorexia, and a sensation of rapid filling of the stomach at meals. The diarrhea may consist only of slightly loose stools which the patient considers to be unremarkable, or the stools may contain mucus, pus and, at times, blood. Loss of weight, delay of linear growth and delayed puberty in the absence of gastrointestinal symptoms other than anorexia may rarely lead to a mistaken diagnosis of anorexia nervosa. Iron deficiency anemia may occur. Pain is usually periumbilical or in the right lower quadrant; it is characteristically intermittent and cramping, but may be dull, aching or burning. External anal or abdominal fistulas should lead to suspicion of granulomatous enterocolitis. Erythema nodosum, clubbing of the digits, aphthous stomatitis and arthritis have been noted in a few patients. Complete or partial intestinal obstruction may be the presenting symptom.

Abdominal examination is uninformative unless there is a tender, fixed mass in the lower part of the abdomen, more often on the right than on the left or in the midline. Rarely, granulomatous pseudopolyps are palpable on rectal examination.

Children with granulomatous enterocolitis tend to be emotionally labile, to cry readily, to adapt poorly to new situations and to take a gloomy anticipatory view of any coming event. They often appear to be striving for high levels of performance in school and at home despite, or because of, lack of self-confidence or strong feelings of insecurity. Sometimes the disease accompanies or follows a series of major family stresses such as death and serious illness.

Laboratory data are of little aid in diagnosis. The erythrocyte sedimentation rate is elevated in about half the cases, and the normal ratio of albumin to globulin in the serum is reversed in an equal number.

Roentgenographic studies early in the disease may show thickening of the bowel wall manifested by an increase in the distance between gas or barium shadows in adjacent loops; later there are visible mucosal irregularities or rigidity of a segment of bowel wall, which in turn are followed by ulcerations, fissures, fistulas, pseudodiverticula, the cobblestone pattern of lymphoid granulomatous pseudopolyps or narrowing of a segment of bowel lumen. *Sigmoidoscopy* is useful only in the few patients with low colonic involvement which is manifested by an irregular, inflamed, cobblestoned appearance with little friability or bleeding.

Differential Diagnosis. When the onset has been abrupt, appendicitis may be suspected. Psychogenic abdominal pain, ulcerative colitis, tuberculosis, abdominal actinomycosis, anorexia nervosa, Hodgkin's disease or lymphosarcoma may be confused with the chronic form of granulomatous colitis.

Prognosis. The prognosis for life is usually good, but the course of the disease is persistent and chronic; spontaneous cures are infrequent, especially if fistulous tracts have developed. Rarely, an acute attack simulating appendicitis subsides spontaneously within a few weeks.

Treatment. No treatment is entirely satisfactory. Dietary restrictions have not been shown to be of benefit and may decrease food intake in a situation in which malnutrition is already a problem. Initially, corticosteroid therapy should be used, especially in patients with involvement of multiple or extensive segments of bowel and with disruption of a normal living pattern from weakness, loss of weight, anorexia, and absence from school. Hydrocortisone in a daily amount of about 8 to 10 mg. per kg., or preferably 2 mg. per kg. of prednisone, is recommended. A maximum dose of 300 mg. of hydrocortisone or 75 mg. of prednisone is rarely exceeded. The dose should be reduced by one fifth at 1- to 2- week intervals, depending on response, to a dose not much above the physiologic one (p. 295). This therapy may be maintained for 6 to 12 months. The dose should be sufficient to eliminate symptoms and perhaps to maintain a mildly "cushingoid" appearance of the patient; it has been suggested that those who do not have a "cushingoid" appearance often fail to benefit from such treatment.

Surgical resection of the involved area of bowel may be accompanied by a long remission or apparent cure. In acute cases resembling appendicitis, it is not indicated because of the possibility of spontaneous recovery. Because of a high rate of recurrence after surgery, an initial trial of medical therapy is indicated, particularly if the disease is extensive and would require resection of large segments of intestine. Nevertheless the majority of patients eventually require resection.

Anticholinergic drugs and antibacterial agents are of little benefit. The use of other chemotherapeutic agents, such as nitrogen mustard, has so far not been proved conclusively to be effective.

On occasion such symptoms as abdominal pain and diarrhea may diminish or disappear during hospitalization or other change of environment. Since the disease is a distressing one which frequently results in emotional depression in the child or parents, a strong supportive role by the physician is of considerable assistance to them.

PNEUMATOSIS CYSTOIDES INTESTINALIS

This is a rare condition characterized by multiple gas-filled cysts in the wall of the bowel. The cysts may be located in the small intestine, the colon, or both; in infants they are predominantly submucosal. The condition may occur at any age. In infants it is often associated with intrinsic disease of the gastrointestinal tract, e.g. enterocolitis, pyloric stenosis or congenital abnormalities. No symptoms directly related to pneumatosis in infancy are recognized. The diagnosis has been established roentgenographically (Fig. 11-17) and at laparotomy, but more frequently at autopsy. The pathogenesis of the cysts is not known, but may be related to mucosal defects with escape of intestinal gases into the lymphatics and wall of the bowel. Although pneumatosis intestinalis occurs in the

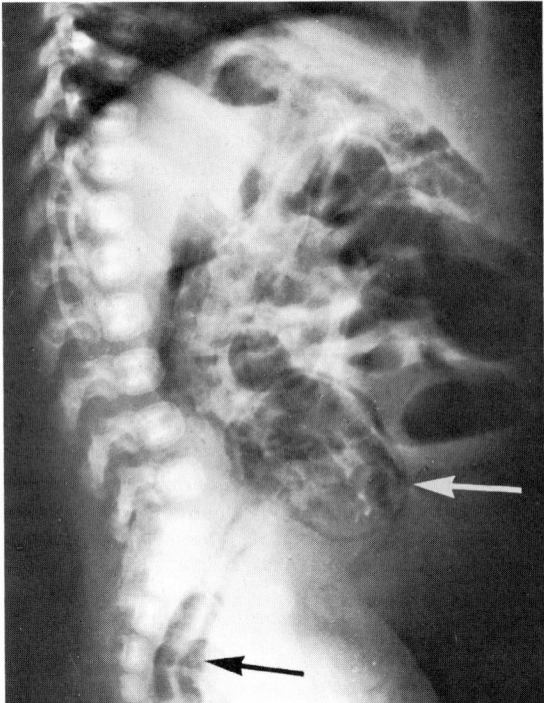

Figure 11-17. Lateral roentgenogram of the abdomen of an infant with aganglionic megacolon involving the entire colon. Pneumatosis of the colon was demonstrated before and after death in the walls of the rectum and sigmoid; note the apparent double contour of the intestinal walls (arrows).

course of other serious illnesses, it is not always a serious prognostic sign and will disappear if the primary disease improves. Death appears to result from some cause other than the pneumatosis.

GIULIO J. BARBERO

REFERENCES

Feeding Difficulties

Apley, J., and MacKeith, R.: Infant Feeding and Its Difficulties; in *The Child and His Symptoms: A Psychosomatic Approach.* Oxford, Blackwell Pub., 1962, Chaps. 12 and 13.
Barbero, G. J., and Shaheen, E.: Environmental Failure to Thrive: A Clinical View. *J. Pediat.,* 71:639, 1967.
Bliss, E. L., and Branch, C. H. H.: *Anorexia Nervosa.* New York, Paul B. Hoeber, 1960.
Patton, R. G., and Gardner, L. I.: *Growth Failure in Maternal Deprivation.* Springfield, Ill., Charles C Thomas, 1963.
Shaheen, E., Alexander, D., Truskowski, M., and Barbero, G. J.: Failure to Thrive—A Retrospective Profile. *Clin. Pediat.,* 7:255, 1968.

Abdominal Pain

Apley, J.: *The Child with Abdominal Pain.* Springfield, Ill., Charles C Thomas, 1959.
Kopel, E., Kim, I. C., and Barbero, G. J.: Comparison of Rectosigmoid Motility in Normal Children, Children with Recurrent Abdominal Pain and Children with Ulcerative Colitis. *Pediatrics,* 39:539, 1967.
Wood, J. L., Hardy, M. L., and White, H.: Chronic Vague Abdominal Pain in Children. *Pediat. Clin. N. Amer.,* 2:465, 1955.

Gastrointestinal Bleeding

Abrams, B., and Lynn, H. B.: Rectal Bleeding in Children. *Am. J. Surg.,* 104:831, 1962.

Baffes, T. G., and Potts, W. J.: Blood in the Stool of Infants and Children. *Pediat. Clin. N. Amer.,* 2:513, 1955.

Brayton, D.: Gastrointestinal Bleeding of "Unknown Origin." A Study of Cases in Infancy and Childhood. *Am. J. Dis. Child.,* 107:288, 1964.

Kiesewetter, W. B., Cancelmo, R., and Koop, C. E.: Rectal Bleeding in Infants and Children with a Hitherto Unreported Etiological Factor. *J. Pediat.,* 47:660, 1955.

Spencer, R.: Gastrointestinal Hemorrhage in Infancy and Childhood: 476 Cases. *Surgery,* 55:718, 1964.

Vomiting

Craig, W. S.: Vomiting in the Early Days of Life. *Arch. Dis. Childhood,* 36:451, 1961.

Hoyt, C. S., and Stickley, G. B.: Study of 44 Children with the Syndrome of Recurrent (Cyclic) Vomiting. *Pediatrics,* 25: 775, 1960.

Hughes, J. G.: The Etiology of Vomiting in Infancy and Childhood. *Pediat. Clin. N. Amer.,* 2:483, 1955.

Richmond, J. B., Eddy, E. J., and Green, M.: Rumination, a Psychosomatic Syndrome of Infancy. *Pediatrics,* 29:49, 1958.

Constipation

Anthony, E. J.: An Experimental Approach to the Psychopathology of Childhood; Encopresis. *Brit. J. Med. Psychol.,* 30:146, 1957.

Bellman, M.: Studies on Encopresis. *Acta Paediat. Scand.,* Suppl. 170, 1966.

Davidson, M., Kugler, M. M., and Bauer, C. H.: Diagnosis and Management in Children with Severe and Protracted Constipation. *J. Pediat.,* 62:261, 1963.

Pinkerton, P.: Psychogenic Megacolon in Children: The Implications of Bowel Negativism. *Arch. Dis. Childhood,* 33:371, 1958.

Prugh, D. G.: Childhood Experiences and Colonic Disorders. *Ann. New York Acad. Sc.,* 58:355, 1954.

Diarrhea

Barness, L. A. (Ed.): Symposium on Fluid and Electrolyte Problems. *Pediat. Clin. N. Amer.,* 11:789-1103, 1964.

Davidson, M., and Wasserman, R.: The Irritable Colon of Childhood (Chronic Non-Sepcific Diarrhea Syndrome). *J. Pediat.,* 69:1027, 1966.

Karelitz, S.: Diarrhea in Infants and Children. *Pediat. Clin. N. Amer.,* 3:137, 1956.

Congenital Hypertrophic Pyloric Stenosis

Bishop, H., and Hope, J. W.: Postoperative Roentgen Studies and Their Clinical Significance. *J. Pediat.,* 60:62, 1962.

Gross, R. E.: *The Surgery of Infancy and Childhood.* Philadelphia, W. B. Saunders Company, 1953.

Nixon, H. H., and O'Donnell, B.: *The Essentials of Paediatric Surgery.* Philadelphia, J. B. Lippincott Company, 1961.

Shuman, F. I., Darling, D. B., and Fisher, J. H.: The Radiographic Diagnosis of Congenital Hypertrophic Pyloric Stenosis. *J. Pediat.,* 71:70, 1967.

Intestinal Obstruction

Estrada, R. L.: *Anomalies of Intestinal Rotation and Fixation.* Springfield, Ill., Charles C Thomas, 1958.

Nixon, H. H.: Intestinal Obstruction in the Newborn. *Arch. Dis. Childhood,* 30:13, 1955.

Rickham, P. P.: *The Metabolic Response to Neonatal Surgery.* Cambridge, Harvard University Press, 1957.

Singleton, E. B.: *X-ray Diagnosis of the Alimentary Tract in Infants and Children.* Chicago, Year Book Publishers, Inc., 1959.

Swenson, O.: *Pediatric Surgery.* New York, Appleton-Century-Crofts, Inc., 1958.

Wasch, M. G., and Marck, A.: The Radiographic Appearance of the Gastrointestinal Tract During the First Day of Life. *J. Pediat.,* 32:479, 1948.

Intussusception

Gross, R. E., and Ware, P. F.: Intussusception in Childhood: Experiences from 610 Cases. *New England J. Med.,* 239:645, 1948.

Ravitch, M. M.: *Intussusception in Infants and Children.* Springfield, Ill., Charles C Thomas, 1959.

Aganglionic Megacolon

Bodian, M., Carter, C. O., and Ward, B. C. H.: Hirschsprung's Disease. *Lancet,* 1:302, 1951.

Duhamel, B.: A New Operation for the Treatment of Hirschsprung's Disease. *Arch. Dis. Childhood,* 35:38, 1960.

Hope, J. W., Borns, P. F., and Berg, P. K.: Roentgenologic Manifestations of Hirschsprung's Disease in Infancy. *Am. J. Roentgenol.* 95:217, 1965.

Madsen, C. M.: *Hirschsprung's Disease.* Springfield, Ill., Charles C Thomas, 1964.

Richards, M. R., and Hiatt, R. B.: Untoward Effects of Enemata in Congenital Megacolon. *Pediatrics,* 12:253, 1953.

Swenson, O., Fisher, J. H., and MacMahon, H. E.: Rectal Biopsy as an Aid in the Diagnosis of Hirschsprung's Disease. *New England J. Med.* 253:632, 1955.

Swenson, O., Neuhauser, E. B. D., and Pickett, L. K.: New Concepts of Congenital Megacolon. *Pediatrics,* 4:201, 1949.

Tobon, F., Nigel, C. R. W., Talbert, J. L., and Schuster, M. D.: Nonsurgical Test for the Diagnosis of Hirschsprung's Disease. *New England J. Med.,* 278:188, 1968.

Peptic Ulcer

Abramson, D. J.: Curling's Ulcer in Childhood: Review of the Literature and Report of 5 Cases. *Surgery,* 55:321, 1964.

Chenoweth, A. D., and Dimick, A. R.: Stress Ulcers in Infants and Children. *Ann. Surg.,* 161:977, 1965.

Judd, D. R., Heimburger, I. L., Vellios, F., and Waldhausen, J. A.: Zollinger-Ellison Syndrome in Adolescents. *Surgery,* 54:673, 1963.

Michener, W. M., Kennedy, R. L. J., and DuShane, J. W.: Duodenal Ulcer in Childhood. *Am. J. Dis. Child.,* 100:814, 1960.

Schuster, S. R., and Gross, R. E.: Peptic Ulcer in Childhood. *Am. J. Surg.,* 105:324, 1963.

Singleton, E. B., and Faykus, M. H.: Incidence of Peptic Ulcer as Determined by Radiologic Examinations in the Pediatric Age Group. *J. Pediat.,* 65:858, 1964.

Walker, E. E., and Grove, W. J.: Gastroduodenal Ulcers in Children with Brain Disease. *Arch. Surg.,* 89:559, 1964.

Gastric Perforation

Inouye, W. Y., and Evans, G.: Neonatal Gastric Perforation. *Arch. Surg.,* 88:741, 1964.

Pertsemlidis, D.: Neonatal Gastric Perforation. *J. Mt. Sinai Hosp.,* 31:97, 1964.

Granulomatous Enterocolitis

Lindner, A. E., Marshak, R. H., Wolf, B. S., and Janowitz, H. D.: Granulomatous Colitis. *New England J. Med.,* 269:379, 1963.

Marshak, R. H., and Lindner, A. E.: Ulcerative and Granulomatous Colitis, *J. Mt. Sinai Hosp.,* 33:444, 1966.

Rudhe, U., and Keats, T. E.: Granulomatous Colitis in Children. *Radiology,* 84:24, 1965.

Sobel, E. H., Silverman, F. N., and Lee, C. M.: Chronic Regional Enteritis and Growth Retardation. *Am. J. Dis. Child.,* 103:569, 1962.

Necrotizing Enterocolitis

Mizrahi, A., Barlow, O., Berdon, W., Blanc, W. A., and Silverman, W. A.: Necrotizing Enterocolitis in Premature Infants. *J. Pediat.,* 66:697, 1965.

Orme, R. L'E., and Eades, S. M.: Perforation of the Bowel in the Newborn as a Complication of Exchange Transfusion. *Brit. Med. J.,* 4:349, 1968.

Touloukian, R. J., Berdon, W. E., Amoury, R. A., and Santulli, T. V.: Surgical Experience with Necrotizing Enterocolitis in the Infant. *J. Ped. Surg.,* 2:389, 1967.

Ulcerative Colitis

Davidson, M., Bloom, A. A., and Kugler, M. M.: Chronic Ulcerative Colitis of Childhood; An Exhaustive Review. *J. Pediat.,* 67:471, 1965.

Kirsner, J. B., Raskin, H. F., and Palmer, W. L.: Ulcerative Colitis in Children. A.M.A. *J. Dis. Child.,* 90:141, 1955.

Lagercrantz, R.: Ulcerative Colitis in Children. *Acta Paediat.* (Stockholm), Supp., 75:89, 1949.

Michener, W. M., Brown, C. H., and Turnbull, R. B. J.: Ulcerative Colitis in Children. I. Diagnosis. II. Medical and Surgical Treatment. *Am. J. Dis. Child.,* 108:230, 236, 1964.

Pneumatosis Cystoides Intestinalis

Seaman, W. B., Fleming, R. J., and Baker, D. H.: Pneumatosis Intestinalis of the Small Bowel. *Seminars in Roentgenology,* 1:234, 1966.

INTESTINAL MALABSORPTION

The lumen of the small intestine is a large mixing pool in which exchange of fluids, electrolytes and nutrient compounds proceeds in both directions across the intestinal epithelial surface. The net balance of movement of materials from the intestinal lumen into the body is termed *absorption. Malabsorption* implies inefficient transfer of one or more nutrients across the intestinal mucosa, resulting in fecal losses which exceed normal values. In the majority of instances the most striking defect and the one that gives rise to symptoms is impairment of intestinal absorption of fat. There are many causes of steatorrhea and intestinal malabsorption in infants and children (see Table 11-7).

Physiology of Fat Absorption. The most important dietary lipid constituent is triglyceride (neutral fat), nearly all of which is normally absorbed when reasonable quantities are ingested. Separation of the dietary triglyceride into a coarse emulsion occurs principally in the stomach by mechanical churning and by admixture with phospholipids and other chyme components. The principal site of fat absorption is the upper jejunum; the process depends on many factors, but principally "digestion" or breakdown. The key to normal digestion is hydrolysis of triglycerides into diglycerides and monoglycerides and thence to their component fatty acids and glycerol. For this process pancreatic and perhaps other intestinal lipases are needed, while the various components of bile by activating this enzyme, by their emulsifying action and other processes greatly facilitate digestion. The mixture of monoglycerides, fatty acids and conjugated bile salts in the lumen of the small intestine forms water-soluble aggregates or complexes called micelles. These droplets progressively decrease in size as a result of further hydrolysis. The glycerol formed is water-soluble, is quickly absorbed by passive transport, and mostly enters the mesenteric venous blood, although a small fraction of it may be phosphorylated by enzymes in the intestinal cell cytoplasm. *Short-chain fatty acids* (fewer than 10 carbon atoms) are transported in the portal system, while *long-chain fatty acids* (more than 16 carbon atoms) are re-esterified in the mucosal cells and pass into the intestinal lymphatics.

Recent studies have shown that *medium-chain triglycerides* (MCT) (8 and 12 carbon atoms) are absorbed, transported and metabolized in an entirely different manner than are the longer chain ones which account for most of the fatty acids in the average American diet of both adults and children. After oral administration, MCT are rapidly hydrolized in the intestinal lumen by pancreatic lipase with the formation of fatty acids. Absence of bile does not affect their lipolysis, luminal solubility of the free fatty acid or the intestinal absorptive rate. Absence of pancreatic enzymes does not prevent limited intraluminal hydrolysis of the MCTs, which are then rapidly hydrolyzed intracellularly, which is not the case with the longer chain fatty acids. Under both normal and pathologic conditions MCTs are transported from the intestine into the portal vein as free fatty acids and not via the lymph to the thoracic duct as are the longer chain fatty acids.

Fat Absorption in Childhood. The absorption of fat from the intestine is less efficient at birth and in early infancy than it is later. Steatorrhea may be normal in a premature infant. Efficiency in handling dietary fat increases during the first few months of life. During the first 6 months infants have no overt signs of fat intolerance under normal circumstances. The maturation of their intestinal digestive processes, however, is not sufficient to enable them to cope with the stress imposed by serious illness. The result is impairment of fat absorption, steatorrhea and other symptoms of malabsorption.

TESTS FOR MALABSORPTION

Tests of Fat Absorption

Quantitative Determination of Fecal Fat by Balance Studies. The method recommended is described by van de Kamer. Steatorrhea may be defined as fecal loss of greater than 5 per cent of ingested fat. Often this balance is referred to in terms of the "coefficient of absorption" obtained from the formula:

$$\frac{(\text{Gm. ingested fat} - \text{gm. excreted fat}) \times 100}{\text{Gm. ingested fat}}$$

In children 1 year of age or older the coefficient of absorption is 95 per cent or above. Within reasonable limits the proportion of fat absorbed is not affected by the amount ingested. It is essential, however, for accurate results that the diet have a minimal fat content (30 to 50 gm.); excessive amounts of dietary fat (over 100 gm. per 24 hours) may lead to steatorrhea even in a normal child. Infants below 1 year of age normally may have a coefficient of absorption as low as 85 per cent.

Great variation in the fecal fat content may be encountered from day to day. Therefore *all* stools must be collected for a minimal period of 3 to 4 days and the total pool homogenized. Total fat content is then determined on aliquots and expressed in terms of grams of fecal fat per 24 hours or of the coefficient of absorption.

Only total fat need be determined; little additional information is gained by assessing the percentages of split fats and of neutral fats. This determination has been used to differentiate pancreatic from other types of steatorrhea; it has been shown to be unreliable, owing to lipolysis induced by bacterial activity and other factors. Likewise the expression of fecal fat as percentages of wet or dry weight of the total fecal material is no longer used because of the wide variation in water content of stools regardless of total fat content.

Fat Absorption Tests. *Absorption tests with neutral fats and fatty acids labeled with I^{131}.* A radio-iodine-labeled neutral fat, usually radiotriolein, is administered by mouth in a liquid "emulsified" breakfast. The diet otherwise does not have to be modified. Normal subjects excrete in their stools less than 5 per cent of the ingested radioactive material. Radioactivity of the serum at suitable intervals after ingestion of the test dose and of the urine in 48- to 72-hour collections also can be determined. The same procedure is followed if I^{131}-labeled fatty acids (e.g. radio-oleic acid) are administered.

Patients with all types of malabsorption will excrete larger amounts of labeled neutral fats than normal persons, but only those with pancreatic insufficiency will absorb fatty acids normally.

Drawbacks to this test are that it requires an elaborate laboratory set-up, that several factors may affect the results and that completely adequate base lines for normal children have not been established.

Vitamin A tolerance test. After ingestion of a test dose of the vitamin (7000 units per kg. in the form of a fish liver oil) the serum level of vitamin A in normal children rises at least 200 units above the fasting level in 4 to 6 hours. In patients with malabsorption the expected rise fails to reach this height, and the curve is flat. Most patients with intestinal malabsorption due to causes other than pancreatic achylia absorb vitamin A inadequately in either the ester or alcoholic form; children with pancreatic insufficiency (e.g. cystic fibrosis) absorb the alcoholic form satisfactorily, but not the esterified compound.

The results of this test are inconstant, since many factors, including the amount of dietary fat, influence the rate and degree of absorption.

Screening Tests for Steatorrhea

Serum Carotene Levels. This lipochrome is poorly absorbed in the presence of even moderate steatorrhea. In patients with malabsorption, serum carotene levels are frequently less than 10 to 20 gammas per 100 ml., whereas values in normal children are 40 to 150 gammas. This test is valid only when patients have been getting carotene-containing vegetables in their diets for some time.

If enough of the preformed vitamin has been regularly administered orally, serum vitamin A levels are apt to be normal even in the presence of steatorrhea and a low serum carotene (the precursor of vitamin A) concentration.

Lipiodol Tolerance Test. This test, which is a qualitative determination for iodine in urine collected 12 to 18 hours after the oral ingestion of iodized oil (Lipiodol), is useful and simple for estimating the fecal content (steatorrhea). For reliable results the correct technique must be carefully followed. A positive test for iodine in urine diluted 1:4 or more excludes steatorrhea.

Microscopic Examination of Stool for Fat. Microscopic examination of stool specimens is useful only in cases of severe steatorrhea (e.g. cystic fibrosis). If steatorrhea is only mild or moderate, the irregular distribution of fat in a stool specimen will often lead to erroneous conclusions.

In performing the test a drop of saline, a small amount of stool and a drop of saturated scarlet red in alcoholic solution are mixed well on a glass slide. A cover slip is placed over the mixture, which is then examined. The fat appears as globules of neutral fat or fatty acid crystals. If more than one fourth of the particulate matter takes the red stain, the reaction is rated as 3+ to 4+ and is considered significant.

Tests for Carbohydrate Absorption

Oral Glucose Tolerance Test. In most patients with severe malabsorption, oral glucose tolerance curves (p. 1170) are low; the blood sugar value rarely rises more than 40 mg. per 100 ml. of blood above the fasting level.

Xylose Absorption Test. Intestinal absorption of the pentose, D-xylose, is not influenced as much by renal and endocrine factors as is glucose; the xylose tolerance test result is abnormal principally in diseases with impaired absorption of both fat and carbohydrate from the upper small intestine. In normal children the recovery of xylose in urine over a 5-hour collection period after an orally administered dose is 20 per cent or more.

Microscopic Examination of Stools for Starch. Microscopic examination of the stools for extracellular starch granules has been advocated, but is not reliable and not recommended. Davidson demonstrated considerable amounts of extracellular starch granules in the feces of normal children, and starch granules are regularly present in diarrhea.

Tests for Gastrointestinal Loss of Protein

A wide variety of techniques have been proposed for the detection and quantitation of gastrointestinal plasma protein loss; these include metabolic balance studies, determination of plasma proteins in the gastrointestinal secretions by electrophoretic and immunologic methods, and the use of intravenously administered radioactively labeled macromolecules. Though each technique is of value, each has significant limitations; frequently a combination of two of them is required for an understanding of the protein metabolism. Waldmann has recently reviewed the results to be expected from the various studies.

Rapid disappearance of albumin and all globulin fractions from the serum can be demonstrated by degradation studies of albumin tagged with ^{131}I or ^{125}I, by the PVP test with ^{131}I polyvinylpyrrolidone or with ^{51}Cr-labeled albumin. Radio-iodinated PVP (polyvinylpyrrolidone), a plasma-protein substitute with a molecular weight approximating that of albumin, is injected intravenously; then urine and stools are collected for determination of radioactivity to assess the degree to which the injected material has passed into the intestinal lumen. Up to 1.5 per cent of the injected PVP has been collected in the stools of control subjects, whereas the recovery in patients with exudative enteropathy has ranged from 2.5 to 35 per cent. Somewhat similar technique is followed in the administration of ^{51}Cr-tagged albumin, which has some advantages over the PVP test, since the ^{51}Cr label is neither significantly absorbed from nor secreted into the gastrointestinal tract. Meaningful quantitation of enteric protein loss may be obtained if the fecal excretion is related to the serum radioactivity curves.

Peroral Intestinal Mucosal Biopsy

Peroral intestinal mucosal biopsy is a useful aid in the diagnosis of malabsorption, since characteristic changes may be present in gluten-induced enteropathy and intestinal lymphangiectasis. A variety of instruments designed to obtain mucosal peroral suction biopsy are available; each has advantages and drawbacks. The morphology of the small intestinal mucosa varies with the location from which biopsy is obtained; proper location of the source of the specimen and accurate histologic interpretation are essential. The range of normal variation in villous architecture varies considerably in various areas of the world. If maximal information is to be gained from the biopsy, the specimen must be prepared by highly specialized persons. Electron microscopic and enzymatic studies of intestinal mucosal specimens thus obtained can also be performed.

Complications are infrequent, but at least 3 cases of intestinal perforation and several of intestinal hemorrhage, at times severe, have been reported. Hydraulically operated tubes are slightly more risky than other types, but useful to obtain serial specimens for analysis.

Tests for Intestinal Disaccharidase Deficiencies

Stools can be screened for reducing substances with Clinitest tablets added to 15 drops of a mixture of 1 part of fluid stool to 2 parts of water. A color change indicating a concentration of 0.5 per cent or more of reducing substances in the mixture is considered abnormal. In all types of disaccharidase deficiency, lactic acid is increased; Weijers feels that a fecal level of this acid of 50 mg. per 100 ml. or higher is a reliable index except in breast-fed infants. Oral loads of different disaccharides and determination of the respective blood value of the component monosaccharides may also be helpful. Most effective is a direct study of the various disaccharidase activities in peroral biopsy specimens by quantitative, but not qualitative, methods, such as those described by Dahlquist.

Tests of Pancreatic Function

These are described on page 855.

Roentgenographic Pattern of Small Intestine in Malabsorption

In most patients with malabsorption there are roentgenographic changes associated with abnormal motility of the small intestine. These include dilatation of the loops of the small intestine, segmentation of the barium column, and coarsening and obliteration of mucosal folds. Clumping and coarsely granular flocculation of barium are also frequently present. Since all these patterns may be observed in normal infants and small children, roentgenographic studies in the younger age group may be misleading, and in older children they add little of diagnostic value for the individual patient.

MALABSORPTIVE DISORDERS
(THE CELIAC SYNDROME)

In 1889 Gee in London described a chronic disease of children and adults characterized by malnutrition, abnormal stools and a distended abdomen. He named it "celiac disease" from the Greek word for abdomen, κοιλία. In the subsequent 70 years it was realized that under this term there was included not one but a number of disorders distinct in causation, in clinical course and in ultimate outlook (see Table 11-7). These disorders have in common in varying degree the clinical manifestations of intestinal malabsorption: (1) malnutrition, (2) foul, bulky, greasy stools, (3) a distended abdomen due to accumulation of improperly digested and inadequately absorbed material and to abnormal accumulation of gas, and (4) secondary vitamin deficiencies. The symptom complex has also been called the "celiac syndrome."

History. The principal landmarks in the history of malabsorption in the pediatric age group have been (1) the recognition of cystic fibrosis as a separate disease entity by Fanconi, Andersen and others in the late 1930's, (2) the studies by Dicke, Weijers and van de Kamer in the early 1950's which identified gluten-induced enteropathy as one of the leading causes of severe malabsorption in children, (3) elaboration of the technique of peroral biopsy of intestinal mucosa by Shiner, Rubin and others, which

TABLE 11-7. Causes of Steatorrhea
and Malabsorption

A. **Impaired digestion of fat**
  1. *Inadequate lipolysis due to absence of pancreatic lipase:*
      Cystic fibrosis
      Congenital hypoplasia of exocrine pancreas
      Pancreatic insufficiency with bone marrow dysfunction
      Dietary protein deficiency

  2. *Inadequate emulsification of fat due to exclusion of bile from intestine:*
      Atresia of bile ducts
      Obstructive jaundice (e.g. viral hepatitis)

B. **Impaired absorption of fat**
  1. *Inadequate length of small bowel or increased transport time:*
      Extensive surgical resection
      Intestinal fistulas
      Increased intestinal motility due to diarrhea

  2. *Obstruction of intestinal lymphatics:*
      Exudative enteropathy due to lymphatic anomalies
      Tuberculosis
      Hodgkin's disease
      Lymphosarcoma

  3. *Inflammatory disease or involvement of intestinal mucosa in systemic diseases:*
      Intestinal infections and infestations
      Regional enteritis
      Ulcerative colitis
      Gaucher's disease
      Niemann-Pick disease
      Scleroderma

  4. *Biochemical dysfunction of mucosal cells:*
      Gluten-induced enteropathy
      Parenteral diarrhea (in infancy)
      Severe starvation

C. **Basic mechanism obscure**
      Incomplete obstruction of intestinal tract (malrotation, stenosis, blind-loop syndrome, etc.)
      Idiopathic steatorrhea
      Gastrointestinal allergy
      Acanthocytosis
      Hypoparathyroidism
      Sugar-splitting enzyme deficiencies
      Familial dysautonomia
      Catecholamine-secreting tumors
      Congenital defects in amino acid metabolism
      Acrodermatitis enteropathica
      Hypogammaglobulinemia and agammaglobulinemia

---

has made it possible to study and classify certain syndromes by their histologic patterns, and (4) the increasing number of specific causes for malabsorptive syndromes which have been uncovered in the last few years: intestinal disaccharidase deficiencies, gastrointestinal protein loss, acanthocytosis and others.

Classification. A classification of the many disorders responsible for steatorrhea and the symptoms of malabsorption is outlined above in Table 11-7.

Differential Diagnosis. In the differential diagnosis of the various disorders of the so-called celiac syndrome, it is important to demonstrate the presence of intestinal malabsorption and of steatorrhea and to determine the cause.

The tests for malabsorption are listed on page 804. The chemical determination of fecal fat by balance studies is unquestionably the most reliable test for steatorrhea, especially for estimating the milder degrees of it. It is time-consuming and technically involved. Adequate information may be obtained in many instances by such relatively simple screening tests as Lipiodol absorption and determination of the serum carotene concentration. The intestinal absorption of carbohydrates should also be evaluated.

These tests merely confirm the presence of steatorrhea and malabsorption and do not give an etiologic diagnosis. They should be complemented by appropriate investigations for the many separate disorders.

General Principles of Treatment. Similar dietary measures intended to counteract the effects of impaired intestinal absorption of fat are applicable in general in the management of almost all disorders giving rise to the celiac syndrome. The diet should be high in calories and protein and low in fat. Commercially available medium-chain triglyceride (MCT) preparations are useful. Simple sugars (monosaccharides and disaccharides) are usually not harmful and are needed to attain a high caloric intake; the traditional use of bananas in the treatment of these conditions is based on their high sugar content. Liberal amounts of fat-soluble vitamins should be given in water-miscible preparations to correct deficiencies and to compensate for fecal losses. The intake of starchy products and, at times, of disaccharides and other sugars will have to be restricted according to the disease under consideration.

Gluten-Induced Enteropathy
(Celiac Disease)

In gluten-induced enteropathy an unknown basic defect in enzymatic activity or metabolism is accentuated or precipitated by ingestion of wheat or rye gluten, which leads to impaired intestinal fat absorption. This disorder was formerly identified as idiopathic celiac disease, a term which has led to confusion and which should be discarded.

Etiology. The most acceptable theory is that this disorder is due to an inborn error of metabolism, which is triggered by a variety of mechanisms, including ingestion of wheat or rye gluten, dietary deficiencies, chronic infections and psychologic trauma, and is expressed somewhat differently in various age groups. It is thought that the disease in children and in adults (nontropical sprue) may be due to the same basic pathologic process. An increased familial incidence is in favor of this view. An inborn error of metabolism, however, is not the only possible explanation for gluten intolerance. An allergic reaction has been invoked as a contributory or sole factor, since cereal-grain proteins are antigenic.

Incidence.   Severe gluten-induced enteropathy has become increasingly rare in this country and in Western Europe, presumably owing to generally improved nutritional status and to the lowered incidence of chronic infections that may act as trigger mechanisms. Mild disturbances of intestinal absorption in children related to ingestion of wheat or rye gluten are not uncommon in pediatric practice. The predominant clinical symptom in such instances is intolerance to dietary starch; these cases have been categorized as "starch intolerant." Such patients respond satisfactorily to appropriate dietary treatment.

The disease has been seen in Caucasian children of almost all national origins; it is uncommon in Negroes and Mongolians. Both sexes are equally affected.

Pathology.   Gross and histologic changes were never consistently found at necropsy in children with "idiopathic celiac disease" or in adults with "nontropical sprue," presumably owing to autolytic changes in the intestinal tract soon after death. Peroral biopsy of the intestinal mucosa has made it possible to study the histologic changes during life. The mucosa is atrophic with blunting, fusion or absence of the villi, diminution of the surface goblet cells and an increase in plasma cells and eosinophilic and polymorphonuclear leukocytes in the lamina propria (Fig. 11-18, *A*, *B*). Rubin be-

lieves that these changes are specific for gluten-induced enteropathy, but others point out that the appearance of the intestinal mucosa in neomycin toxicity and in some other conditions leading to malabsorption may be similar.

There is also controversy as to the reversibility of the mucosal changes in gluten-induced enteropathy. Some patients, mostly children, have had a definite return to normal, whereas many, mostly adults, have not.

Pathogenesis.   *The role of gluten*.   The adverse effect of dietary wheat and rye products on clinical symptoms, volume of stools and degree of steatorrhea in many children with malabsorption (Fig. 11-19) was recognized in 1950 by Dicke and associates in Holland. The offending factor is not starch, but is the gluten or protein portion of wheat and rye flour which accounts for about 10 per cent of the weight of such flour.

Based on different solubilities in alcohol, 2 fractions can be distinguished in gluten: glutenin, which is relatively harmless, and gliadin, which is mainly responsible for malabsorption in patients with gluten-induced enteropathy. The amino acid glutamine accounts for 47 per cent of the weight of wheat gliadin; it has been implicated in the genesis of symptoms. When the glutamine is deaminated without breaking the peptide bonds, gliadin can be administered to sensitive patients without adverse effects. Administration of the amino acid itself to susceptible persons has not initiated or aggravated existing steatorrhea. Glutamine prob-

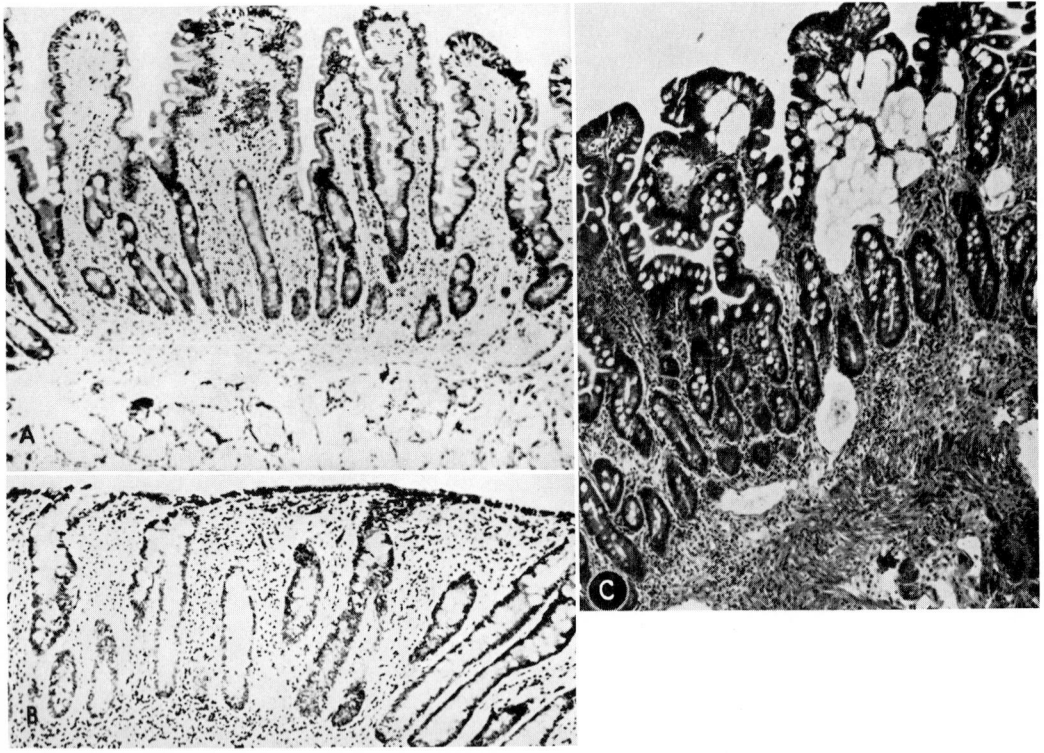

Figure 11-18.   Small intestinal mucosa; tissue obtained by peroral biopsy. *A*, Normal; *B*, gluten-induced enteropathy; *C*, exudative enteropathy. (*A* and *B*, Rubin et al.; *Gastroenter.*, Vol. 38; *C*, from Waldman et al.: *Gastroenter.*, Vol. 41.)

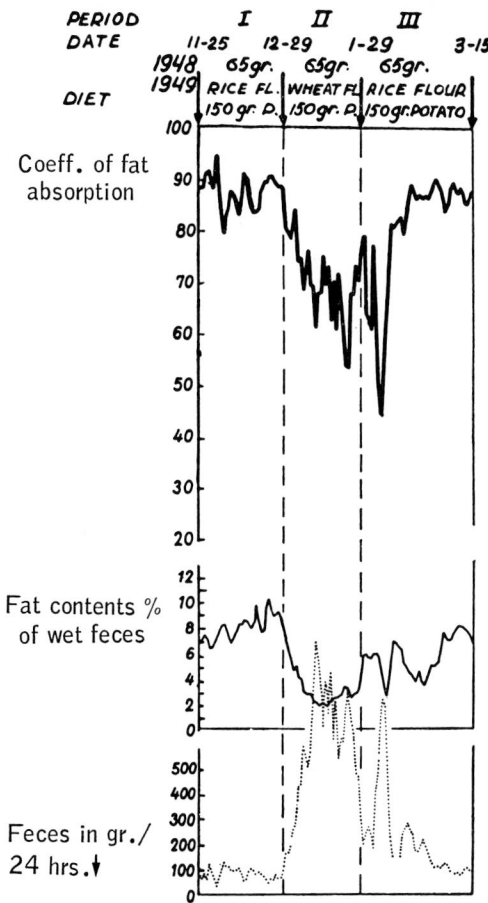

PERIOD

DATE

DIET

Coeff. of fat
absorption

Fat contents %
of wet feces

Feces in gr./
24 hrs.

Figure 11-19. The adverse effect of the introduction in the diet of wheat flour on the coefficient of fecal fat absorption and on the volume of stools in a patient with gluten-induced enteropathy. (From W. K. Dicke, H. A. Weijers and J. H. van de Kamer: *Acta paediat.,* Vol. 42.)

ably must be absorbed in a bound state, probably as a polypeptide, in order to manifest its adverse effect.

Clinical Manifestations. Chronic or recurrent diarrhea, progressive malnutrition and the effects of secondary deficiencies are the clinical hallmarks of severe gluten-induced enteropathy. The stools are characteristically foul, bulky and greasy, but during acute exacerbations there may be watery diarrhea. Anorexia may be prominent. The severe case presents a striking and unforgettable picture: a sad and fretful facies, a variably but usually greatly distended abdomen, and flattened buttocks with the skin hanging in folds, owing to the excessive loss of subcutaneous tissue. In contrast to the general malnutrition, the face may be full and plump. Commonly when the patient is first seen and is extremely anorectic, the abdomen is only moderately distended, but with improved appetite abdominal distention becomes greater.

The majority of patients presenting this symptomatology are between the ages of 6 and 18 months, but some symptoms may appear earlier. The ap-

parent earlier occurrence of this entity in recent years may be due in part to the early introduction of cereal into the diet.

The onset may be insidious. Over a period of weeks and months there are episodes of acute diarrhea frequently associated with respiratory infections, often accompanied by vomiting. Recovery is incomplete from these episodes. The stools, though numbering only one to three a day, tend to be abnormal. Hydrolability is common, with a gain or loss in a few hours of 5 or more per cent of body weight. If the condition persists, the full picture of intestinal malabsorption and chronic malnutrition becomes established. Growth and development are apt to be retarded. There may be profound changes in the behavior pattern. The ill humor and moodiness, the bursts of temper and hysterical behavior, alternating with periods of great timidity, make these children a trial to even the most patient and loving parent. With clinical improvement these symptoms disappear.

The characteristic chronic course may suddenly be interrupted by an episode of severe dehydration and acidosis, which has been termed the *celiac crisis.* It is often triggered by an upper respiratory tract infection. The child is prostrate, drowsy and dehydrated and has the characteristic clinical and laboratory manifestations of acidosis. There are large, watery stools and copious vomiting. The roentgenogram of the abdomen may reveal fluid levels in distended intestinal loops suggestive of mechanical intestinal obstruction. The "celiac crisis" is an acute medical emergency. It rarely occurs after 2 years of age, probably owing to the increasing stability of the water and electrolyte balance.

Laboratory and Roentgenographic Data. The percentage of ingested fat in the stools is rarely less than 75 to 85 per cent; it is usually in the form of soaps and fatty acids, since there is no difficulty in splitting neutral fats. Fecal nitrogen is within normal limits, a distinguishing feature from conditions with pancreatic involvement, notably cystic fibrosis.

The decreased rate of absorption of simple sugars is responsible for a low or flat oral glucose tolerance curve. Intravenous glucose and epinephrine tolerance curves are within normal limits and indicate that carbohydrates are handled normally after absorption from the intestinal tract. The impaired absorption of D-xylose is evidence of involvement of the upper portion of the small intestine.

Microscopic examination of the mucosa of the small intestine obtained by peroral biopsy reveals clubbing, fusion and atrophy of the villi (Fig. 11-18).

There may be iron deficiency anemia and hypoalbuminemia. Osteoporosis is commmon and may lead to spontaneous fractures. Formerly vitamin D deficiency rickets was common, owing to the large amounts of the liposoluble vitamin lost in the stools. For the same reason hypoprothrombinemia and bleeding consequent to vitamin K deficiency are occasionally seen.

The total serum protein level is an important indication of the severity of the disease. A level of less than 5 gm. per 100 ml. indicates a precarious situation, which can be easily upset by an intercurrent infection and lead to "celiac crises."

Diagnosis. At present the only way to establish the diagnosis unequivocally is to evaluate the patient's response to a gluten-free diet. Patients with gluten-induced enteropathy will show improvement in their well-being, gain in weight, improvement in the nature of the stools and disappearance of steatorrhea. In the milder cases no clear-cut improvement may take place within a few days, and it may be delayed as long as 6 to 8 weeks. There may also be a similar delay in the adverse response to reintroduction of dietary gluten.

Prognosis. The high mortality rate of former years (15 per cent in England before 1938) was in part but not wholly a reflection of the inclusion of cystic fibrosis in the category of what was then called "idiopathic celiac disease." With more precise diagnosis and improved management, death from gluten-induced enteropathy is unusual.

An excellent clinical response can be expected in most instances by excluding dietary wheat and rye gluten and by limiting the intake of fat (Fig. 11-20). For months or years relapses may occur during

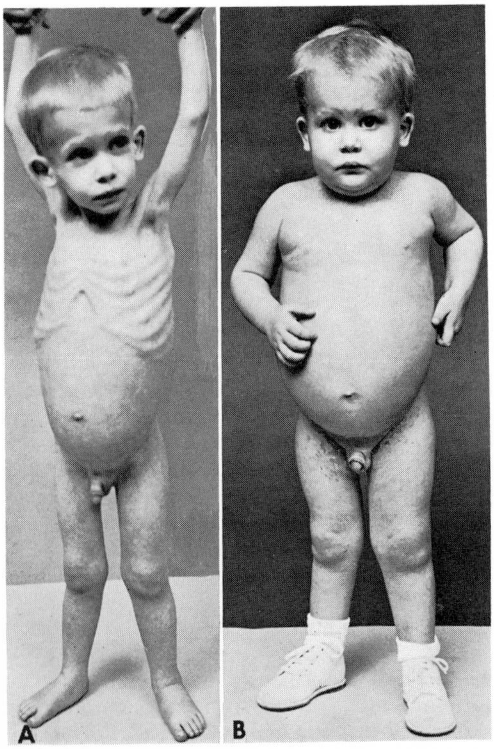

Figure 11-20. A 3-year-old boy with gluten-induced enteropathy proved on balance studies: *(A)* on admission and *(B)* after 52 days of treatment.

intercurrent upper respiratory tract infections or after dietary indiscretions. During such episodes watery diarrhea may be present.

Since gluten-induced enteropathy is a constitutional defect, it is doubtful whether actual cure takes place, at least in patients who once have had severe clinical manifestations. In some instances symptoms recur in adult life.

Treatment. Diet is of prime importance; wheat and rye products must be completely eliminated. Many commercially prepared foods which are usually not thought to contain wheat have wheat flour added; when this is the case, it will be indicated on the package. (See references at end of this chapter for permitted foods.)

Clinical management can be divided into 3 stages. In *stage I*, if the patient is in a so-called celiac crisis, intravenous therapy to replenish the depleted fluid and electrolyte stores must be undertaken promptly. When there is vomiting, as there frequently is during these episodes, all oral intake should be temporarily discontinued. If tetany occurs, calcium should be given intravenously; if parenteral infection is present, suitable antibiotic therapy should be prescribed. Corticosteroids are rarely needed by children. If given, relapse upon their withdrawal is not as constant in the pediatric age group as it is in adults with nontropical sprue.

When the acute situation has improved sufficiently to permit resumption of oral feedings (usually 1 to 3 days), *stage II* of the therapeutic program can be undertaken. A carefully prescribed high protein (6 to 8 gm. per kg.), relatively low fat, *starch-free* diet is offered to the infant. As the diagnosis of gluten-induced enteropathy is not usually clearly established at this time, it is essential to exclude all types of starch. Formulas with protein milk or skim milk, glucose, sucrose and banana powder are useful. Initially the feedings should be small; they can then be increased as the infant's appetite improves and there is no return of the vomiting or diarrhea. Liver extract, administered intramuscularly, may be beneficial at this time. Duration of this restricted dietary regimen will be 1 to 6 weeks.

In *stage III* the diet can be liberalized gradually, with individual foods added singly at intervals of several days to a week, and medium-chain triglycerides can be included. The diagnosis of gluten intolerance will have been made by this time, and wheat and rye products should not be allowed for a period up to several years. Gerrard has shown that even older children in the latent stage, who look well clinically, but still have tests showing abnormal fat absorption, may show further striking improvement in growth and development when dietary gluten is withheld. Water-miscible preparations of vitamins A and D should be prescribed in 2 to 3 times the usually suggested prophylactic dose. Oral preparations of vitamins of the B complex, vitamin C (50 to 100 mg. per day) and iron supplements (if anemia is present) should also be given. Administration of vitamin K is indicated if there is hypoprothrombinemia and bleeding.

Idiopathic Steatorrhea
(IDIOPATHIC CELIAC SYNDROME)

It was from this general category that gluten-induced enteropathy was separated as a specific clinical entity.

It is likely that the cases remaining in this *diagnostic* category include other relatively rare entities of varied but obscure origin. The clinical pattern, the diagnostic procedures and the principles of treatment are similar to those outlined for gluten-induced enteropathy. The main differences are the failure to respond to withdrawal of gluten from the diet and to reintroduction of it. Good results are obtained by following a diet similar to that prescribed for gluten-sensitive patients, except that *all* forms of starch should be withheld and the intake of fat should be limited. It is impossible to predict how long such restrictions will have to be continued—perhaps for several years; some restriction may be necessary throughout childhood. A retrial of any forbidden dietary item should be cautious.

Pancreatic Deficiency

Pancreatic achylia in cystic fibrosis (p. 856) is the commonest cause of severe malabsorption in the pediatric age group in this country. Several other rare disorders have been recognized recently in which pancreatic insufficiency is a part of the altered metabolism (p. 867).

Protein-Losing Enteropathy

Excessive loss of plasma proteins into the gastrointestinal tract may be a large factor in the pathogenesis of hypoproteinemia and edema. It can occur in association with a variety of generalized diseases such as nephrosis and hypogammaglobulinemia, in conjunction with a number of enteric disorders such as ulcerative colitis and regional enteritis, and as a transient complication in gluten-induced enteropathy. Study of excessive "leakage" of serum proteins through the gastrointestinal tract has also led to the recognition of some new syndromes affecting the gastrointestinal tract such as intestinal lymphangiectasis and so-called allergic gastroenteropathy.

Whatever the cause, there is a distinct reduction in the concentration of serum albumin and of all globulin fractions. The rapid disappearance of these proteins from the serum can be demonstrated by degradation studies of albumin-tagged with ^{131}I or ^{125}I or by the PVP test (radio-iodinated polyvinylpyrrolidone) of ^{51}Cr-labeled albumin studies (p. 805). Although the mechanism is not entirely clear, there is usually mild or moderate malabsorption with intermittent diarrhea and frequently with steatorrhea and moderate malnutrition.

Intestinal lymphangiectasis is one of the principal causes of protein-losing enteropathy in children. This congenital anomaly of intestinal lymphatics may or may not be associated with such other lymphatic anomalies as hemihypertrophy and chylous effusion. Waldmann has shown that dilatation of the intestinal villi can be recognized in many instances by peroral biopsy of the mucosa of the small intestine (Fig. 11-18, *C*). In most patients the defect is too extensive for surgical correction, though resection of a localized lesion within the gastrointestinal tract has been successful on occasion. A low fat diet and replacement of long-chain with medium-chain triglycerides in the diet has been helpful in a number of instances.

A syndrome characterized by edema, growth retardation, extreme hypoalbuminemia, anemia, eosinophilia and other allergic manifestations in which protein-losing enteropathy was a prominent part of the picture has been described by Waldmann and identified as *allergic gastroenteropathy.* Circulating antibodies to cow's milk and gastrointestinal blood loss were present in some patients, and, though removal of milk from the diet has appeared to be beneficial in some instances, a relation to gastrointestinal allergy is not established.

Disaccharidase Deficiency

The most important dietary carbohydrates are the polysaccharide, starch, and the disaccharides, sucrose and lactose. Hydrolysis of each of these to the monosaccharide form is necessary before significant absorption can occur.

Salivary and pancreatic amylases break starch down to maltose, in which 2 glucose units are joined by 1-4 α linkages, and isomaltose, in which 2 glucose units are joined by 1-6 α linkages. Intestinal maltase, of which several types have been recognized, then is needed to split them to the component monosaccharides. Sucrase hydrolyzes sucrose to glucose and fructose, and lactase liberates glucose and galactose from lactose.

Absence of one or more intestinal disaccharidases is often the basis of *disaccharide intolerance,* which may be "*primary*" and genetically determined or "*secondary*," often transient and present in many disorders affecting the intestine. As the intracellular localization of the disaccharidases is chiefly in the brush border, it is not surprising that these enzymes are vulnerable to any disease affecting the mucosal surface. Although information on distribution through the intestinal tract is inadequate, present evidence suggests that absolute levels tend to be higher in the jejunum and ileum than in the duodenum.

Primary deficiency of sucrase and isomaltase is the best established primary disaccharidase deficiency. The simultaneous absence of 2 enzymes in an "inborn error of metabolism" is of considerable genetic interest, and an altered polypeptide chain, common to sucrase and isomaltase, has been suggested as one possible explanation. The defect appears to be transmitted as a recessive trait, and enzyme levels tend to be low in heterozygotes. Diarrhea, at times profuse, with dehydration and severe malnutrition have been observed occasionally. Symptoms appear to improve with advancing age and may be absent or minimal despite lack of enzyme activity.

Primary lactase deficiency is not as well established an entity, and the mode of inheritance remains to be determined. Diarrhea is the predominant symptom and begins soon after ingestion of lactase. *Lactosuria* is a prominent feature in some infants with lactose intolerance; some investigators believe that it is a separate entity, and the term "hereditary alactasia" was suggested by Holzel. In infants with lactosuria other abnormalities have been noted, especially disturbed renal function, which has been postulated as a toxic effect of lactosemia.

Secondary disaccharidase deficiencies are not uncommon. The clinical manifestations are those of the underlying disorder plus the manifestation of intolerance to sugars. Usually there are low levels of all disaccharidases, though a disproportionate lowering of lactase is often found, suggesting that this enzyme may be more vulnerable than other disaccharidases. When mucosal damage is severe, frequently because of enteric infection, symptoms of intolerance to more than one disaccharide occur.

Clinical manifestations of both primary and secondary disaccharidase deficiencies are similar. Increased intestinal peristaltic activity, decreased transit time, and diarrhea which is probably due to 2 separate but concurrent mechanisms are common to all. The disaccharides by their osmotic power have considerable purgative effect. In addition, the unabsorbed carbohydrate is fermented by the bacterial flora in the ileocecal region and the proximal portion of the colon with an overgrowth of saccharolytic bacteria. The production of an excess of short-chain acids, especially lactic and acetic acids, is responsible for the acid, irritating quality of the stool, which in infants excoriates the buttocks. Symptoms tend to be more severe in infancy. Diarrhea, especially if watery, calls for investigation of disaccharidase deficiencies (p. 806).

The treatment is relatively simple. When the offending carbohydrates are removed from the diet, there is a prompt remission of symptoms. Secondary deficiencies of disaccharidase, especially of lactase, are in most cases temporary. Even in most primary deficiencies symptoms often diminish with advancing age.

Abeta-Lipoproteinemia
(Acanthocytosis)

(See also pages 418 and 1302.)

Bassen and Kornzweig in 1950 first reported this clinical entity in which some of the manifestations are similar to those of other disorders giving rise to malabsorption. Abeta-lipoproteinemia is a rare disease characterized by an absence of low-density lipoproteins from the plasma of patients who are probably homozygous for a single genetic defect. Another name for this condition is acanthocytosis because one of the striking features is an abnormal appearance of the red blood cells with thornlike projections. More than 20 cases have been reported so far, and although the first patients were Jewish, presently the majority of recorded cases are of different ethnic origin. At least 2 cases have been in Negroes.

Principal clinical manifestations are malabsorption with abnormal stools, steatorrhea and failure to thrive beginning in infancy or early childhood; progressive degeneration of the cerebellum and posterolateral columns causing weakness and ataxia and appearing in late childhood and adolescence; retinitis pigmentosa, also of late onset.

Laboratory findings are steatorrhea, an unusual crenation of many erythrocytes (acanthocytes) which is partially reversible in vitro, abnormally low plasma levels of cholesterol, phospholipids and triglycerides and absence of serum beta-lipoprotein. Peroral biopsy of the intestinal mucosa shows distinctive changes with gross engorgement of intestinal epithelial cells with triglycerides.

Abeta-lipoproteinemia should be suspected in any child with the celiac syndrome, especially if signs of ocular or spinocerebellar degeneration coexist. Conversely, examination of patients with any form of hereditary ataxia should exclude acanthocytosis.

Malabsorption improves to some extent during childhood, but the neurologic and ocular involvements are progressive and lead to severe disability. Though patients have not been followed up long enough to provide a reliable prognosis, several deaths have now been recorded in the third decade of life.

Gastrointestinal Allergy

(See also page 509.)

Gastrointestinal allergy has frequently been assigned a causative role in malabsorption. A recently described syndrome, "allergic gastroenteropathy," is mentioned in this section; a causative relation to allergy, however, is by no means proved. Most common is so-called allergy to cow's milk in infancy, a diagnosis frequently based on the finding of serum antibodies to cow's milk in the patients. But antibodies in the blood against different foodstuffs can often be demonstrated after their introduction in the diet in early infancy. Only in some instances do these antibodies give rise to clinical sensitivity through the antigen-antibody mechanism. Presumably this reaction occurs only in persons who have a so-called atopic constitution and are predisposed to the manifestations of allergy.

A recent study by Gryboski reaffirms that gastrointestinal allergy is an uncommon cause of severe intestinal malabsorption. In a 16-year period she was able to find only 21 infants with such a diagnosis in the records of a large medical center. All had severe symptoms: all had blood in their stools; in seven shock developed subsequent to "milk-challenge," and diarrhea was the predominant symptom. Far too often infants presenting with gastrointestinal symptoms of different degrees of severity and later proved to have gluten-induced enteropathy or cystic fibrosis are thought to have allergy to cow's milk. A variety of hypoallergenic formulas are then tried without success. Primary or more commonly secondary lactase deficiency should also be thought of and ruled out before gastrointestinal allergy is considered. Such patients are not hypersensitive *to*, but intolerant *of* unmodified cow's milk protein. Much valuable time would be saved if allergy were not the first etiologic explanation considered in such instances.

A trial of hypoallergenic formulas and other antiallergic measures is advocated under appropriate circumstances. The frequent use of the term "allergy" to cover one's failure to find the correct cause for a given disturbance, however, is deprecated.

Miscellaneous Causes of Malabsorption

There are many disorders in which malabsorption is occasionally or frequently a part of the clinical picture; in many steatorrhea also is present (Table 11-7). It is impossible to discuss all these conditions in detail; a few are mentioned for differential diagnostic purposes.

Chronic incomplete obstruction of the small intestine such as may be present in malrotation or stenosis or the so-called blind-loop syndrome may be responsible for malabsorption; the mechanism of this manifestation is not clearly understood. Some authors think that an altered bacterial flora is responsible for the impaired intestinal fat absorption.

Inadequate length of the small bowel, secondary to extensive surgical resection of the small intestine or rarely due to fistulous tracts between the stomach and the large intestine, may also result in malabsorption. In some instances surgical correction of the latter defects has resulted in disappearance of symptoms.

Transient steatorrhea may be encountered during periods of obstructive jaundice in *viral hepatitis* and *atresia of bile ducts*, and the subsequent biliary cirrhosis may also lead to impaired intestinal absorption of fat. In both instances inadequate emulsification of fat due to exclusion of bile salts from the intestine appears to be the cause. Although in biliary atresia dietary management may temporarily improve symptoms, permanent relief is obtained only in the small number of patients amenable to surgical repair.

Steatorrhea and malabsorption have been reported in association with a variety of defects in *amino acid metabolism* (cystine metabolism, Hartnup disease), with *catecholamine-secreting neural tumors* (p. 1220), with *acrodermatitis enteropathica* (p. 1394) and *familial dysautonomia* (p. 1308). The genesis of the altered intestinal physiology in these conditions is not understood.

Occasionally steatorrhea and malabsorption may be consequent to heavy parasitic infestation with Giardia, Trichurus and other parasites (p. 722); symptoms disappear when appropriate treatment is given.

Mild Idiopathic Malabsorption
(CHRONIC NONSPECIFIC DIARRHEA)

It is not uncommon in pediatric practice to encounter children usually between 1 and 3 years of age, who have episodes of recurrent loose stools. Mucus may be present in the feces, and in the more severe cases excoriation of the buttocks may be found. The patient otherwise appears healthy, and growth and development are not disturbed. There are none of the severe signs of malabsorption, and steatorrhea is not present.

At times the history is suggestive of sensitivity to wheat gluten, and it appears probable that some such patients represent mild cases of gluten-induced enteropathy which has not progressed to the more serious stage because of our better knowledge of nutritional requirements and the use of effective antibiotic agents. One of the disaccharidase deficiencies should also be considered, especially an absence of isomaltase, since isomaltose is produced in the digestion of starch and mild malabsorption may occur.

In many instances, however, infectious episodes, emotional disturbances, food allergies and anatomic defects appear to act as trigger mechanisms to a hyperirritable colon in initiating these diarrheal episodes. Occasionally there may be a family history of colon hypermotility.

After the known causes of malabsorption have been excluded the treatment is largely expectant, since symptoms rarely persist after 4 or 5 years of age. Reassurance and improvement in the social and psychologic environment are often of great therapeutic assistance. Unless there is a suggestive history of a specific food leading to symptoms, dietary restrictions are effective.

PAUL A. DI SANT'AGNESE

REFERENCES

General

Davenport, H. W.: *Physiology of the Digestive Tract.* 2nd ed. Chicago, Year Book Publishers, Inc., 1966.
di Sant' Agnese, P. A.: Malabsorption Syndrome; in S. S. Gellis and B. M. Kagan (Eds.): *Current Pediatric Theory* 3. Philadelphia, W. B. Saunders Company, 1968, p. 343.
Holt, P. R.: Medium Chain Triglycerides: Their Absorption,

Metabolism and Clinical Applications; in G.B.Y. Glass (Ed.): *Progress in Gastroenterology.* New York, Grune & Stratton, Inc., 1968, p. 277.

Laster, L., and Ingelfinger, F. J.: Intestinal Absorption — Aspects of Structure, Function and Disease of the Small Intestine Mucosa. *New England J. Med.,* 264:1138, 1192, 1246, 1961.

Morin, C., and Davidson, M.: Progress in Gastroenterology; Pediatric Gastroenterology. *Gastroenterology* 52:565, 713, 1967.

Senior, J. R.: Intestinal Absorption of Fats. *J. Lipid Research,* 5:495, 1964.

van de Kamer, J. H., ten Bokkel Huinink, H., and Weijers, H. A.: Rapid Method for the Determination of Fat in Feces. *J. Biol. Chem.,* 177:347, 1949.

Weser, E., Jeffries, G. H., and Sleisenger, M. H.: Progress in Gastroenterology: Malabsorption. *Gastroenterology,* 50:811, 1966.

Peroral Intestinal Mucosal Biopsy

Rubin, C. E., Brandborg, L. L., Phelps, P. C., Hawley, C., and Taylor, J.: Studies of Celiac Disease. I. The Apparent Identical and Specific Nature of the Duodenal and Proximal Jejunal Lesion in Celiac Disease and Idiopathic Sprue. *Gastroenterology,* 38:28, 1960.

Rubin, C. E., and Dobbins, W. O., 3rd: Progress in Gastroenterology: Peroral Biopsy of the Small Intestine. *Gastroenterology,* 49:676, 1965.

Gluten-Induced Enteropathy

Weijers, H. A., van de Kamer, J. H., and Dicke, W. K.: Celiac Disease; in *Advances in Pediatrics.* Chicago, Year Book Publishers, Inc., 1957, Vol. 9, p. 277.

Weijers, H. A., and van de Kamer, J. H.: Celiac Disease and Wheat Sensitivity. *Pediatrics,* 25:127, 1960.

Protein-Losing Enteropathy

Waldmann, T. A.: Progress in Gastroenterology: Protein-Losing Enteropathy. *Gastroenterology,* 50:422, 1966.

Waldmann, T. A., Steinfeld, J. L., Dutcher, T. F., Davidson, J. D., and Gordon, R. S. Jr.: The Role of the Gastro-intestinal System in "Idiopathic Hypoproteinemia." *Gastroenterology,* 41:197, 1961.

Disaccharidase Deficiency

Holzel, A.: Development of Intestinal Enzyme Systems and Its Relation to Diarrhea. *Pediat. Clin. N. Amer.,* 12:635, 1965.

Prader, A., and Auricchio, S.: Defects of Intestinal Disaccharide Absorption. *Ann. Rev. Med.,* 16:345, 1965.

Townley, R. R.: Disaccharidase Deficiency in Infancy and Childhood: Review Article. *Pediatrics,* 38:127, 1966.

Abeta-Lipoproteinemia

Farquhar, J. W., and Ways, P.: Abetalipoproteinemia; in J. B. Stanbury, J. B. Wyngaarden and D. S. Frederickson (Eds.): *The Metabolic Basis of Inherited Disease.* 2nd ed. New York, McGraw-Hill Book Company, Inc., 1966, p. 509.

Isselbacher, K. J., Scheig, R., Plotkin, G. R., and Caulfield, J. B.: Congenital Betalipoprotein Deficiency. *Medicine,* 43:347, 1964.

Gastrointestinal Allergy

Gryboski, J. D.: Gastrointestinal Milk Allergy in Infants. *Pediatrics,* 40:354, 1967.

Heiner, D. C., and others: Precipitins to Antigens of Wheat and Cow's Milk in Celiac Disease. *J. Pediat.,* 61:813, 1962.

Waldmann, T. A., Wochner, R. D., Laster, L., and Gordon, R. S.: Allergic Gastroenteropathy. *New England J. Med.,* 276:761, 1967.

Chronic Nonspecific Diarrhea

Davidson, M., and Wasserman, R.: The Irritable Colon of Childhood (Chronic Nonspecific Diarrhea Syndrome). *J. Pediat.,* 69:1027, 1966.

ANUS, RECTUM AND SIGMOID

Congenital anomalies of the anus and rectum are relatively common. The true incidence is not known, but it has been estimated that an anal or rectal anomaly of some extent can be expected in about one of each 400 births. Major anomalies which require surgical correction have been estimated to occur in about one of 1000 births.

MALFORMATIONS OF THE ANUS AND RECTUM

IMPERFORATE ANUS

There are several classifications of imperforate anus; in the one used here there are 2 main categories, identified as "low" and "high" lesions. The distinction is based on whether the bowel does or does not pass through the puborectalis muscle, which is a part of the pubococcygeus sling or levator mechanism. In the "low" lesions the bowel passes through the puborectalis muscle and ends abruptly at the skin or in a fistula to the median raphe of the perineum in both male and female patients. In the "high" lesions the muscle is not

traversed; if there is a fistula, it leads most often to the urinary tract in males or to the upper part of the vagina in females.

Embryology and Pathogenesis. In the normal embryology of the anus, after the cloacal stage there is a division of the cloacal cavity by a downgrowth of the mesoderm (the urorectal septum) into a ventral part, which will form the bladder and urethra, and a dorsal part, which forms the rectum. There is a small communication, the cloacal duct, between the 2 systems which is closed by the seventh week of gestation by a downgrowth of the urorectal septum. An ingrowth of mesoderm divides the cloacal membrane into the urogenital membrane ventrally and the anal membrane dorsally. During the seventh week the urogenital portion of the original cloaca has acquired an external opening, but the anal membrane does not rupture until later. The anus develops by an external invagination known as the proctodeum, which deepens toward the rectum, but is separated by the anal membrane. This membrane ruptures by the eighth week of gestation.

Interference with the development of anal-rectal structures at varying stages gives rise to a variety of anomalies which range from anal stenosis or incomplete rupture of the anal membrane (the

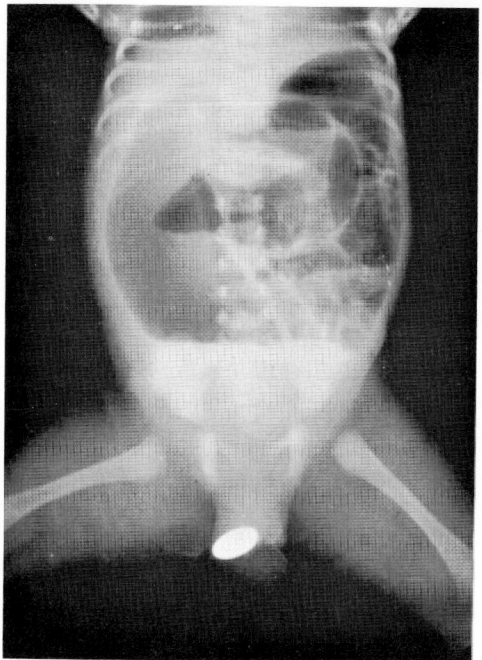
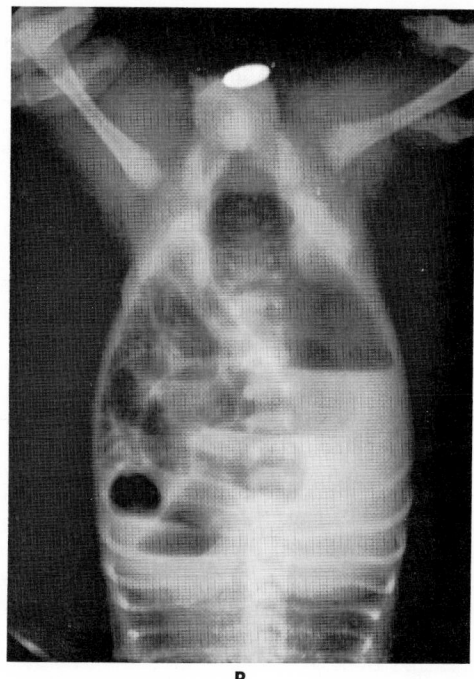

A   B

Figure 11-21. Wangensteen-Rice roentgenographic technique for demonstration of the position of the blind colonic pouch in the case of an imperforate or absent rectum. The infant is held head downward, causing the intestinal gas to rise to the blind end of the gut. *A*, Roentgenogram of child in upright position, showing transverse level of gas. The level of the obstruction is not demonstrated. *B*, The level of the obstruction is apparent when the roentgenogram is taken with the child in the inverted position. The site of the anus is marked by a lead disk.

"low" types) to complete failure of descent of the upper portion of the cloaca and failure of invagination of the proctodeum (the "high" types). The persistence of the communication between the urinary and rectal portions of the cloaca is responsible for the fistulas, which are more common in the male. In the female, rectal fistulas more commonly connect with the vagina than the urinary system.

Since the muscle of the anal sphincter is derived from exterior mesoderm, it is usually intact and not involved with the obstructive lesions of the anus and rectum.

Diagnosis. *Stenosis of the anorectal canal* may occur at any point or extend its entire length. The constriction may be crescentic or annular. Symptoms are dependent on the degree of obstruction; the common ones are straining at stool and obstipation. The constriction can be identified by digital and endoscopic examination.

In *true imperforate anus* the diagnosis can often be made by inspection. In "low" lesions the presence of a perineal fistula or bulging of the perineum is diagnostic. In the "high" lesions the perineum is more rounded, no bulge is noted, and the position of the external sphincter is difficult to define. When the fistula is not evident, the distance between the bowel and skin can be estimated by "upside-down" films or the Wangensteen-Rice view (Fig. 11-21) obtained after clinical distention is evident. A distance of more than 1.5 to 2 cm. from the bowel to the marker is indicative of a "high" lesion.

Most females have a rectovaginal or a rectoperineal fistula. Males with a "low" lesion may have a fistula to the median raphe of the perineum, and those with a "high" lesion to the urethra or bladder. The presence or absence of the fistula is not as important as the level of the lesion.

Associated urinary anomalies occur in nearly half the children with imperforate anus. Urinary investigation with excretory urography should precede definitive therapy in the "high" types and discharge in the "low" group. Particular attention should be paid to the anatomy of the bony pelvis; sacral anomalies may be important later in bowel and urinary functions.

Treatment. Anal stenosis can generally be treated by manual dilatations. All other forms of imperforate anus should be surgically corrected.

In the "low" types the bowel has the proper levator relationship, so that they can be repaired from below. A careful mucocutaneous reconstruction is essential.

The "high" types are best treated by a preliminary colostomy followed by a definitive repair in 3 to 6 months by an abdominoperineal, sacroperineal or sacroabdominoperineal approach, depending on the lesion and the preference of the surgeon. Careful positioning of the anus in the region of the external sphincter, and anatomic positioning of the bowel in the puborectalis sling are essential. Recognition of the fistula so that it can be eliminated is most apt to be accomplished when the reparative operation is delayed.

The surgical care of imperforate anus is not complete until the child has become bowel-trained and socially acceptable. The surgeon who knows the nature and degree of the disturbed anatomy and physiology must work closely with the child, the family and the pediatrician in order to achieve optimal results.

The higher the blind pouch and the more extensive the operation, the more difficulty one encounters in the postoperative period. With continuing care through the period of training a satisfactory functional solution can usually be expected. In a few instances there will be continuing problems due to stenosis, poor anal control or poor guidance. In the postoperative period constipation rather than, as one might expect, incontinence is the principal problem. The lack of sensation of fecal material in the rectum leads to fecal impactions with paradoxical or overflow diarrheal stools and gives rise to the acquired type of megacolon. Early attention to ensure regular evacuations will prevent massive fecal impactions and the social ostracism that results. As a rule the child should be taught to defecate at a given time of day rather than by the urge. In some instances a daily enema may be needed.

FISSURE IN ANO

Fissure in ano, a small slit or crack at the mucocutaneous line, is a common, acquired lesion in infancy and childhood. The cause is often not evident, but the lesion may be caused by trauma secondary to overzealous cleaning or to constipation, by scratching induced by irritation from *Oxyuris vermicularis* and by eczema and other perianal conditions.

Clinical Manifestations. Pain on defecation and often refusal to defecate are the principal manifestations. Bright red blood on the surface of the stool and sometimes bleeding following defecation may be observed. The diagnosis is made by inspection of the anal area while the child is straining.

Treatment. Most fissures will heal spontaneously if the local irritation is lessened or eliminated. This can usually be accomplished by the use of bland suppositories or instillations of mineral oil and by gentle dilatations of the anus. Oral medication to soften the stool may be indicated, and sitz baths may provide relief from the pain. A neglected, long-standing fissure in ano may result in serious constipation problems and eventually in acquired megacolon, with the associated psychologic disturbances from fecal soiling. Surgery is rarely necessary.

PRURITUS ANI

Anal itching in childhood is generally secondary to oxyuriasis, anal fissures and other local inflammatory lesions and to coarse or moist undergarments. Nocturnal itching is perhaps the most frequent evidence of pinworm infestation. Treatment consists in eradication of the underlying cause, and in cleansing the anal area with a mild soap and drying it with a soft cloth or tissue. Powders or solutions such as witch hazel may be used. In small infants exposure to sunlight or dry heat for as long as possible is helpful when the anal area is inflamed.

PROLAPSE AND PROCIDENTIA OF THE RECTUM AND SIGMOID

Prolapse is abnormal descent of the mucous membrane of the rectum with or without protrusion through the anal orifice; *procidentia* is abnormal descent of all the coats of the rectum or sigmoid with or without protrusion through the anus. These conditions are most common from 3 to 5 years of age. The infantile rectum lies on a lower plane than the other pelvic organs. This anatomic arrangement, combined with the effect of the nearly vertical infantile sacrum, predisposes to prolapse. Any factor causing suddenly increased intra-abdominal pressure may precipitate abnormal descent of the bowel wall. Malnutrition with absorption of ischiorectal fat is a contributory factor. Protrusion at stool initially recedes spontaneously, but later necessitates manual replacement. Bleeding and the passage of mucus may occur. The protruding mass varies from bright to dark red; it may be as much as 6 inches in length. In prolapse the striations or furrows radiate from the center of the anal aperture, in contrast to the concentrically arranged rosette of procidentia.

Treatment should be directed to dietary correction of constipation, to proper toilet training and to the elimination of any underlying disturbance, such as parasitic infection, diarrhea or polyps. Oral administration of mineral oil, rectal instillations of olive oil and strapping the buttocks together with adhesive tape, having first placed a cotton ball over the anal area, may be helpful.

Reduction of protrusion is aided by pressure with hot compresses. Cold packs are contraindicated. An easy method of reduction is to cover the finger with a piece of toilet paper, introduce it into the lumen of the mass, gently push it into the rectum and then immediately withdraw it. The toilet paper adheres to the mucous membrane, thus permitting release of the finger; the paper, when softened, is later expelled. For intractable cases perineal operation may be indicated. In procidentia of the rectum and sigmoid, abdominal sigmoidopexy is required.

ANORECTAL ABSCESS

An anorectal abscess is usually located in the ischiorectal fossa. Infection usually gains entrance through the anal crypts and the preformed spaces. The symptoms are pain and swelling. Defecation is painful, and the child is unable to sit comfortably. The temperature is not much elevated unless the perirectal space is invaded. A painful swelling overlies the ischiorectal fossa, with redness, heat, induration and fluctuation. Treatment consists in immediate incision and drainage under anesthesia. Hot sitz baths, 3 times daily, are helpful in the postoperative period.

FISTULA

Fistulas originating in the anus or rectum may be congenital or acquired and may extend to and communicate with the urinary bladder, urethra, vagina or perianal dermal area. Acquired fistulas are residuals of an abscess and usually open on the dermal surface. There is frequently a history of one or more incisions into the abscess.

The **symptoms** of an acquired fistula are those of a painful swelling which recurs intermittently, followed by a purulent discharge. Diagnosis is based on the presence of an opening into the skin beside the anal orifice into which a probe may be introduced (Fig. 11-22).

Treatment. Conservatism is indicated in the care of fistulas in infants. Many of the lesions will close spontaneously without resorting to surgery. If surgical extirpation is necessary, care must be taken to incise rather than excise the sphincter in order to prevent incontinence. Simple incision and removal of the fistulous tract with packing of the resultant defect is usually effective.

HEMORRHOIDS

Hemorrhoids are uncommon in infants and children. When they are encountered, one must

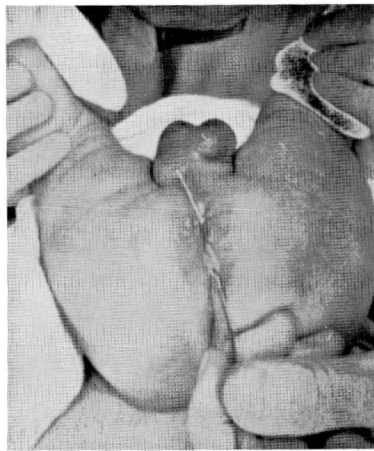

Figure 11-22. Complete anorectal fistula in a child 15 weeks of age; probe demonstrating external and internal openings. (Bacon: *Anus, Rectum and Sigmoid Colon.* J. B. Lippincott Company.)

look for the underlying cause, such as a venacaval or mesenteric obstruction, cirrhosis, portal hypertension, or other reasons for venous obstruction. Occasionally, chronic constipation, fecal impaction and straining at stool result in hemorrhoids as they do in adults. Operation is rarely indicated except for an acute external thrombus. The condition generally subsides when the primary condition is corrected.

NEOPLASMS

See page 1448.

CONGENITAL DEFECTS OF THE SACROCOCCYGEAL REGION

Pilonidal Sinus and Cyst. *Pilonidal sinus* is a congenital defect which probably results from faulty coalescence or invagination of the ectoderm in the midline over the sacrococcygeal region during early embryonic development. It is characterized by formation of a sinus tract in which are collected the products of dermal activity. Infection enters through the original site of invagination or through aberrant tracts which become manifest after puberty. A *pilonidal dimple* is commonly encountered, but is asymptomatic.

Pilonidal cysts and sinuses do not cause symptoms unless infection has occurred. The presence of swelling, heat, redness, tenderness, and fluctuation over the sacrococcygeal region is characteristic of an infected sinus. Purulent material may be discharged from one or more openings. If infection occurs, total excision should be performed. (See page 1307 for complications within the spinal canal.)

Tumors of the Sacrococcygeal Region. See page 1457.

REFERENCES

Kiesewetter, W. B., and Nixon, R. H.: Imperforate Anus. I. Its Surgical Anatomy. *J. Pediat. Surg.,* 2:60, 1967.
Rehbein, F.: Imperforate Anus: Experiences with Abdominoperineal and Abdominosacro-perineal Pull Through Procedures. *J. Pediat. Surg.,* 2:99, 1967.
Santulli, T. V., and others: Malformations of the Anus and Rectum. *S. Clin. N. Amer.,* 45:1253, 1965.

APPENDICITIS

Appendicitis, rare in the first year of life, has been noted in early infancy. The incidence increases after the first year of life; most cases occur in the first 3 decades. Males are slightly more prone to appendicitis than females. The mortality rate from this disease has progressively declined over a period of years. Nevertheless the percentage of children hospitalized with a ruptured appendix and localized or generalized peritonitis has not changed significantly. Further reduction in the morbidity from appendicitis can be accomplished only by more frequent recognition and treatment of the disease before the inflamed appendix ruptures.

Etiology. Obstruction is the primary factor in the pathogenesis of appendicitis. The obstruction may be secondary to inflammatory changes from blood-borne or enteric infections or may be mechanical as by pinworms, a fecalith, other foreign body, stenosis or kinking. Soft fecal material is commonly found in the lumen of the appendix, but has doubtful pathologic significance. In some instances appendicitis appears to be related to an infection of the upper respiratory tract, but a significant correlation is not established. Such systemic infections as rheumatic fever, measles, scarlet fever and other exanthems infrequently are responsible for appendicitis. Coliform organisms are most commonly found in the appendiceal abscess, though a mixed flora, including streptococci and staphylococci, may also be found.

Pathology. Inflammation begins in the mucosa, which may ulcerate; the wall is edematous and infiltrated with neutrophils; the lumen is distended, often enough to impair the blood supply and produce gangrene and perforation. In milder types there may be mucosal ulceration without obstruction. Bacteria may escape through a perforation or even the gangrenous wall to produce diffuse peritonitis or an abscess confined by adherence of adjacent omentum and intestines.

Clinical Manifestations. Epigastric pain shifting to the right lower quadrant and accompanied or followed by nausea, vomiting and low-grade fever is the classic pattern of acute appendicitis. It is the one observed commonly in older children, but relatively infrequently in infants and young children. About 70 per cent of children 5 years of age or younger who have acute appendicitis have a perforation of the appendix and peritonitis when first seen medically. The prodromal manifestations are usually not appreciated in the very young; perforation of the appendix takes place relatively quickly in the thin-walled appendix, and the omentum is not sufficiently developed to afford adequate protection against diffuse peritoneal spread.

Most children 4 years of age and under have difficulty in localizing pain; a finger pointed at the umbilicus or the mother's description of the positions of preference taken by the child, such as knees drawn up or reluctance to move the legs, is as much aid in localization as one may get. When perforation of the appendix has occurred in the very young child, he appears acutely ill with grunting respirations, a rigid abdomen, flaring of the alae nasi, an ashen color and an anxious expression. Extreme prostration may be preceded by an unaccustomed period of inactivity. Fever prior to rupture of the appendix may be absent or of low grade. After development of peritonitis the temperature is usually elevated to 103 to 105°F. Subnormal temperature in a prostrated child has serious implications. Active peristalsis may persist for some time with generalized peritonitis.

The initial symptom in the older child is usually persistent, rather than intermittent, pain, which increases progressively in severity. With localized ileus, secondary to appendiceal inflammation, the pain may be intermittent or crampy. The amount of vomiting appears to be somewhat related to the position of the appendix; if the organ is retrocecal or deep in the pelvis, no vomiting may occur. Peritoneal irritation and pain may also be masked by the position of the appendix. Constipation is more common than diarrhea, though a pelvic appendix irritating the bowel in the cul-de-sac may produce mucus and diarrhea. Frequency of urination may be produced by an inflamed appendix adjacent to the bladder.

Diagnosis. Persistent pain in the abdomen, insidious or abrupt in onset, accompanied by *persistent* localized tenderness in the right lower quadrant, muscular spasm and rigidity is evidence of localized intraperitoneal irritation. Nausea and vomiting are frequently present, and low-grade fever is more characteristic than chills and high fever at the onset of the disease.

Other signs of peritoneal irritation such as cough and rebound tenderness are helpful when elicited. A retrocecal inflamed appendix, however, may have deep tenderness as the only physical finding, and, when the appendix is in the pelvic area, there may be no abdominal findings. The rectal examination should be the final step in the physical examination, but must never be omitted, since it may provide valuable information.

Peristalsis is generally decreased or absent in the presence of intraperitoneal infection, but it may be hyperactive during the early stages. A positive psoas sign, or the tendency of the patient in bed to draw his legs up, is also suggestive of a right lower quadrant inflammatory lesion.

There is usually a mild leukocytosis of 14,000 to 16,000 cells per mm.^{3} with a preponderance of young polymorphonuclear cells. Excessively high total leukocyte counts are suggestive of an abscess or peritonitis. Leukopenia associated with prostration and a shocklike state may indicate overwhelming sepsis.

Differential Diagnosis. A history of antecedent or concomitant respiratory or enteric disease, poorly localized pain, fever out of proportion to the abdominal findings or variations in the intensity of pain may suggest *mesenteric adenitis*, but an exact differential diagnosis can be made only by laparotomy.

Prolonged, severe *constipation* may also simulate an acute surgical condition of the abdomen. When feces are easily palpated, and one has reason to suspect fecal obstruction of the bowel, a saline enema of moderate amount may be given. In contrast to the valid objections to catharsis under such a situation, an enema judiciously given may be valuable diagnostically.

Infection of the urinary tract may mimic appendicitis. Urinalysis is indispensable in evaluation of abdominal pain. The urinalysis may be within normal limits, however, in the presence of completely blocked hydronephrosis. On occasion an intravenous pyelogram may be required for differential diagnosis.

Pneumonia, especially of the right lower lobe, may simulate appendicitis. Abdominal tenderness and muscular tightness are apt to be somewhat higher with the pulmonary infection than with appendicitis. A roentgenogram of the chest will usually clarify the diagnostic situation.

The abdominal pain of *acute gastroenteritis* may on occasion suggest the possibility of appendicitis. Persistent *diarrhea* is rare as a symptom of appendicitis, though several loose stools may herald the onset of disease. If diarrhea persists after an acute abdominal episode, the possibility of a *pelvic abscess* should be considered. The differential diagnosis depends mainly on the physical findings. The 2 conditions may occur concomitantly.

Meckel's diverticulitis may simulate appendicitis. Blood, with or without mucus, in the stool favors diverticulitis. *Intussusception* must be considered particularly in children under 5 years of age. Intermittent sharp pain, the presence of an abdominal mass and blood by rectum are the differential features. A barium enema, which is contraindicated in appendicitis, may be useful in confirming and localizing the intussusception.

Ovarian lesions, such as cysts, ruptured follicles or a twisted pedicle, must be considered in girls, especially in the older ones.

Acute rheumatic fever, diabetes mellitus, regional enteritis, abdominal epilepsy, sickle cell crisis, infectious mononucleosis and nonicteric infectious hepatitis must also be considered diagnostic possibilities; these are described in their respective sections.

When one is confronted with evident peritonitis, the possibility of a primary infection as well as one secondary to a ruptured appendix must be considered. The former lesion is now encountered so infrequently, however, even in patients with nephrosis, and the consequences of continued drainage from a ruptured appendix are of such an order, that the differential diagnosis should be established by laparotomy.

Complications. Whether localized abscess formation (p. 821) and diffuse secondary peritonitis (p. 820) are to be considered complications or part of the natural course of acute appendicitis may be debatable, but they are the only common sequels. Perforation occurs earlier and more frequently in children than in adults, and there is less tendency for the infection to become localized. This failure to localize has been attributed to the relatively small size of the omentum in young children. A pelvic abscess occasionally occurs, but subphrenic abscess is rare. Less common complications are paralytic ileus and thrombophlebitis.

Postoperative complications of acute appendicitis include abscess of the operative wound, multiple intra-abdominal abscesses, intra-abdominal adhesions and intestinal obstruction.

Prognosis. There is great danger in postponing operation for appendicitis, since local or diffuse peritonitis consistently follows perforation, and almost negligible risk attends operation before perforation. Even when perforation has occurred, the mortality rate may be less than 1 per cent. This low rate is probably due to several factors, including improvements in preoperative preparation, operative technique, anesthesia, parenteral fluid therapy and antibacterial therapy.

Treatment. Once the diagnosis of appendicitis has been decided upon, the treatment is surgical. High fever, dehydration, overwhelming sepsis and a shocklike state are reasons for delay until appropriate preoperative correction can be attained. Convulsions during anesthesia are common in children with high fever. Induced hypothermia, hydration and antibiotic therapy are indicated. The temperature should be below 102° F., and the pulse below 120 before anesthesia is initiated.

Management of appendiceal abscess and of diffuse peritonitis is considered on page 820, and that of preoperative and postoperative fluid therapy on page 229. Reasonably early ambulation after removal of an unperforated appendix and dismissal from the hospital within a few days are usually possible.

REFERENCES

Fields, I. A., and Cole, N. M.: Acute Appendicitis in Infants Thirty Six Months of Age and Younger. *Am. J. Surg.,* 113: 269, 1967.
Holder, T. M., and Leape, L. L.: The Acute Surgical Abdomen in Children. *New England J. Med.,* 277:921, 1967.

PERITONEUM AND ALLIED STRUCTURES

MALFORMATIONS OF THE PERITONEUM

Congenital peritoneal bands may be responsible for intestinal obstruction (p. 787); numerous other anomalies may occur in the course of the development of the peritoneum, but are rarely of clinical importance. Intra-abdominal herniations infrequently occur through ringlike formations produced by anomalous peritoneal bands. Absence of the omentum or duplications of it are rare anomalies.

ASCITES

Etiology. The term "ascites" indicates an accumulation of fluid in the peritoneal cavity, but it is usually applied to accumulations of serous fluid. Renal, especially nephrotic, and cardiac conditions are most often responsible for ascites. It may represent an accumulation of fluid secondary to chronic adhesive pericarditis, or it may be part of a polyserositis in so-called Pick's syndrome. Other causes include obstruction of the portal circulation as in hepatic cirrhosis or by enlarged lymph nodes, tumors, thrombosis, chronic tuberculous peritonitis, rheumatic peritonitis or obstruction of the splenic vein.

Clinical Manifestations. The abdomen is distended; when distention is great, there is flattening or pouting of the umbilicus. Fluctuation can be detected on palpation; a wavelike impulse is obtained by sharp tapping on one side of the abdominal wall while the other hand is placed on the opposite side of the abdomen and an attendant's hand compresses it in the midline; shifting percussion dullness can often be demonstrated.

Ascites must be differentiated from other conditions which cause distention of the abdomen. These include gaseous distention of the intestines, fecal distention as in megacolon, tumor masses, including cysts of the mesentery, acute or chronic peritonitis, peritoneal hemorrhage, extreme distention of the bladder and simple obesity.

Prognosis and Treatment. The course, prognosis and treatment depend entirely upon the cause.

CHYLOUS ASCITES

The accumulation of chyle is an uncommon form of ascites which may occur at any age of childhood and is occasionally congenital in origin. True chylous ascites is caused by some anomaly, injury or obstruction of the thoracic duct within its abdominal portion. In the case of anomalies the condition is present at birth or shortly thereafter. At times in traumatic cases there is an associated chylothorax. Obstructions may be produced by enlarged lymph nodes or neoplasms. The fluid has the appearance of milk, owing to its high fat content. In chronic peritonitis, peritoneal fluid may have a somewhat similar color from degeneration of inflammatory products.

The prognosis of chylous ascites is unfavorable, but recovery may occur. The accumulation of chyle can apparently be reduced by decreasing the dietary intake of fat. Since there is a loss of considerable protein in this fluid, high protein diets should be prescribed. Abdominal exploration is justified to search for the site of the leak.

PERITONITIS

Acute infections of the peritoneum are arbitrarily designated as *primary* when the focus is outside the abdominal cavity and the infection is blood- or lymph-borne. The infection is termed *secondary* when it is disseminated by extension from or rupture of an intra-abdominal viscus or of an abscess of one of the solid organs.

Peritonitis in the neonatal period may arise from a transplacental infection in utero; more frequently it is the result of infection acquired during or shortly after birth. It may be a manifestation of septicemia, a direct extension from an umbilical infection, perforation of the intestine or, rarely, the sequel of a ruptured appendix. Meconium peritonitis is described on page 393. After the neonatal period, peritonitis is uncommon until later childhood, when appendicitis becomes relatively frequent.

ACUTE PRIMARY PERITONITIS

Etiology. Primary peritonitis has become a rare disorder in children. It is caused most often by the pneumococcus and the beta hemolytic streptococcus. It is more common in girls than in boys, and in some instances a preceding nongonorrheal vaginitis appears to be a portal of entry. Penumococcal peritonitis, at one time a relatively frequent complication of nephrosis, has become an uncommon one. Gonococcal peritonitis is a rare complication of gonorrheal vaginitis.

Clinical Manifestations. The onset is usually rapid with extreme prostration, some abdominal pain and vomiting. Intestinal peristalsis is usually continued until late in the disease, and diarrhea is common. The facial expression is likely to be anxious; there is often cyanosis, and the child appears toxic and weak. The temperature is usually septic in type, and may be as high as 104 to 105°F., although in very ill patients, and especially in young infants, it may be normal or subnormal. The pulse is rapid, small and compressible, and the respirations are rapid and shallow because of the pain which abdominal respiration produces. There is usually distention of the abdomen, moderate diffuse tenderness and a doughy resistance. Evidences of free fluid may be present. Rectal examination reveals tenderness. The white blood cell count is high, ranging from 20,000 to 35,000 cells per mm.[3]; 90 to 95 per cent are polymorphonuclear cells with an increase in immature forms.

Diagnosis and Treatment. When primary peritonitis is suspected, peritoneal aspiration, with smear and culture of any material obtained, may be in order. A pure culture of pneumococcus or streptococcus would exclude an enteric source of the infection, such as appendicitis, and would avoid a laparotomy. If mixed or enteric organisms are isolated, a laparotomy is indicated. Antibiotic therapy should be guided by bacterial culture and in-vitro sensitivity tests.

ACUTE SECONDARY DIFFUSE PERITONITIS

Etiology. This type of peritonitis usually results from perforation of an abdominal viscus, most often an inflamed appendix. Peritonitis secondary to intussusception, volvulus, incarcerated hernia, perforation of the intestine by a foreign body or rupture of a Meckel's diverticulum is infrequent. Perforation of the intestine in meconium ileus and spontaneous rupture of the stomach or intestines are infrequent causes in the neonatal period, and perforation of a peptic ulcer, though infrequent, is more common in early infancy than in later childhood. The invading bacteria are most often coliform bacilli with varying numbers of other organisms belonging mainly to the streptococcal and staphylococcal groups.

Clinical Manifestations. The manifestations of shock from a ruptured viscus or the early symptoms of acute appendicitis are followed by an increasing toxemia, as evidenced by greater restlessness and irritability, by a higher temperature, often 103 to 105°F., by an increase in the pulse rate and, at times, by chills or convulsions. In extreme situations and especially in early infancy, the temperature may be normal or subnormal. Vomiting, if previously present, is usually increased. The pain tends to be more diffuse over the abdomen, but may not be too notable if the patient remains quiet. Constipation is marked.

The child has an anxious expression, and there is progressive evidence of prostration. Dehydration and loss of electrolytes through vomiting are contributory factors. There are rapid pulse, splinting of the diaphragm, abdominal rigidity and diffuse tenderness, and rectal tenderness. Peristalsis may persist until late in the course of disease.

The white blood cell count is usually 16,000 to 25,000 per mm.[3], the polymorphonuclear elements usually being above 90 per cent.

Treatment. Adequate preoperative preparation is essential and may require 6 to 8 hours. These measures include rehydration, correction of electrolyte imbalance (p. 227), gastric suction and antimicrobial therapy. Relief of pain by Demerol, morphine or codeine contributes to improvement. The pulse rate should be reduced below 120 and the temperature below 102°F. if possible prior to operation. Severely ill patients may require mild hypothermia. Operative therapy consists in drainage and repair of the perforated viscus.

ACUTE SECONDARY LOCALIZED PERITONITIS
(Peritoneal Abscess)

Etiology. A single, localized pyogenic abscess, most often secondary to perforation of an inflamed appendix, is somewhat less common in children than in adults. The poor ability of young children to localize a peritoneal infection of appendiceal origin has been attributed to a lower order of resistance and to a relatively smaller omentum. Though localized peritoneal abscesses occur most often in the appendiceal region, they may be at any site, originating from various sources, or appendiceal infections may gravitate to other areas, notably the pelvic one. An abscess in the subdiaphragmatic area may originate from an appendiceal or other intra-abdominal infection or, rarely, from an empyema.

Clinical Manifestations. The general symptoms of *peritoneal abscess* are continued fever or recurrences of it, poor appetite, and vomiting following ingestion of food. The white blood cell count is increased, with a predominance of polymorphonuclear cells. In the appendiceal area, tenderness in the right lower quadrant is extended, and there is often a palpable mass.

A *pelvic abscess* is suggested by abdominal distention, rectal tenesmus with or without the passage of small stools containing mucus, or bladder irritability. Rectal examination may reveal a tender mass anteriorly.

A *subphrenic abscess* is evidenced by physical signs at the base of the lung, usually the right, due to elevation of the diaphragm, and frequently by the presence of pleural fluid. The diagnosis can often be established roentgenographically. The diaphragm is elevated and the liver depressed if the infection is on the right side, and there is frequently a pocket of air just below the diaphragm, owing to production of gas by bacteria.

Treatment. The abscess should be drained and appropriate antibiotic therapy provided. Initial broad-spectrum coverage should be modified, if indicated, by the results of sensitivity tests of the bacteria obtained from cultures. If the appendix cannot be removed at the initial operation, an appendectomy should be performed subsequently within 3 months.

TUBERCULOUS PERITONITIS

See page 609.

HERNIA AND HYDROCELE

Hernias of various types may be present at birth or develop subsequently, often because of congenital defects. The uncommon femoral hernia and the rare internal hernias other than that of the diaphragm will not be discussed. Congenital omphalocele and umbilical hernia are discussed on page 399.

INGUINAL HERNIA

Etiology and Pathology. Most inguinal hernias are of the indirect rather than the direct type and occur much more frequently in boys than in girls. These hernias may be present at birth or may appear at any age thereafter; they are situated more often on the right side than on the left, but frequently are bilateral.

During embryonic life, as the testis descends retroperitoneally from the genital ridge, a sac of peritoneum (the processus vaginalis) precedes it into the scrotum. The lower portion of this sac envelops the testis to form the tunica vaginalis, and the remainder normally atrophies by the time of birth. The indirect inguinal hernia results from a persistence of the processus vaginalis and becomes manifest as a mass in the inguinal region when an abdominal structure or peritoneal fluid is forced into it. The persistent sac may vary from a short one not extending beyond the external inguinal ring to one which extends into the scrotum and maintains its continuity with the tunica vaginalis. The hernial sac is thus present at birth, but it usually remains empty for a variable period of time. Later, commonly by 2 or 3 months of age, when the infant becomes more active and is able to increase his intra-abdominal pressure sufficiently to open the sac, peritoneal fluid or an abdominal organ is forced into it. The hernial sac then appears as a bulge in the inguinal region, extending into the scrotum or toward the labia.

Clinical Manifestations. There are no symptoms associated with an empty hernia sac. When abdominal contents are intermittently forced into it, symptoms of incomplete bowel obstruction with pain, fretfulness, difficult defecation, poor eating and local pressure may result. On the other hand, there may be few or no symptoms associated with a filled hernial sac. If a loop of intestine becomes incarcerated in the sac, there may be all the manifestations of intestinal obstruction ultimately leading to strangulation of the bowel and death. In female infants the ovary may prolapse into the hernial sac and appear as a 1- to 2-cm. movable, nontender, usually transient inguinal mass. Immediate surgical exploration and abdominal replacement of the ovary are indicated unless strangulation has destroyed the ovary, when excision is indicated. Occasionally the neck of the sac closes after peritoneal fluid has been forced into it and traps the fluid as an encysted, nontender irreducible hydrocele in the cord in the male or in the canal of Nuck in the female.

Diagnosis. A history of the intermittent appearance of a mass in the inguinal region of an infant or child is characteristic. If the hernial sac is full at the time of examination and can be emptied by gentle compression, or if it can be made to fill when the infant cries or strains or the older child stands or coughs, the diagnosis is established. Often, however, a suggestive history is the only criterion for diagnosis. Inspection may reveal a fullness on the affected side, especially after recent incarceration. Palpation for an enlarged internal ring by invaginating the scrotum is fruitless during the early developmental stage of the hernia, since the ring is not enlarged, nor are the muscles weakened. Gentle palpation by rolling a finger over the spermatic cord at the level of the pubic tubercle will reveal thickening of the cord on the involved side, and often the "silk glove" sensation may be elicited by rubbing together the 2 sides of the empty hernial sac. This maneuver should be performed as part of routine physical examinations in infants in order to discover the

presence of a hernial sac so that it can be removed before incarceration occurs.

The only difficulty in diagnosis is in distinguishing hernia from hydrocele. A hernial sac is often opaque to transmitted light, whereas the hydrocele is translucent. A hernia, however, may also be translucent if only distended and empty bowel is present in the sac. The inguinal hernia is usually reducible with gentle manipulation and tends to slip suddenly into the peritoneal cavity. By contrast, the encysted hydrocele is not reducible, and, although the communicating one is, reduction is usually accomplished with great difficulty and without sudden emptying of the sac. Characteristically it is reduced most readily after the patient has been in the horizontal position for a prolonged time, as during a night's sleep. The coexistence of a communicating hydrocele and an inguinal hernia is relatively common.

Treatment. The treatment of inguinal hernias in healthy infants and children is by surgical repair as soon as the defect is diagnosed. The operation consists essentially in removing the hernial sac and transfixing the neck at the internal ring. It is well tolerated by even small infants and obviates the possibilities of incarceration, testicular atrophy, secondary enlargement of the internal ring and weakening of the floor of the canal from prolonged pressure. Treatment by injection of sclerosing agents is contraindicated in infants and children.

Some surgeons recommend a bilateral operation in all children with a unilateral inguinal hernia on the basis that, in a significant number of instances, a hernia will subsequently appear on the apparently uninvolved side. We disagree with this policy and perform a bilateral operation in children with a unilateral hernia only when there is a history of hydrocele or thickening of the spermatic cord suggestive of a hernial sac.

Trusses are not recommended even for temporary use. They are difficult to apply correctly and impossible to keep clean. Every effort should be made to prepare the infant or child for surgical repair. When skilled pediatric anesthesiologists and surgeons are available, the operation can be performed with very little risk, even in the so-called high-risk patient, as, for example, the child with congenital heart disease.

Incarcerated Inguinal Hernia

Incarceration of inguinal hernias is common in children and occurs most often in the first 6 months of life. It is manifest by the appearance of a firm, tender, globular, irreducible swelling below the external inguinal ring. The infant is fretful and often vomits. Unless the condition is relieved, abdominal distention, cessation of bowel movements, persistent vomiting, fever and leukocytosis will develop as impairment of the blood supply progresses.

Manipulative reduction of an incarcerated hernia which has been present for less than 12 hours and has not been accompanied by a bloody stool is the treatment of choice. The infant is adequately sedated (with a barbiturate under 6 months of age or with morphine in an older patient). He is then placed in the Trendelenburg position with a roll of cloth under the buttocks, and an ice bag is placed on the affected side to decrease the edema. After an hour or more when the sedation has taken effect and the parents have quieted the infant to sleep, the mass is gently grasped with all fingers of the physician's warmed hand and squeezed with gentle equal pressure by all digits toward the inguinal canal. This maneuver frequently leads to reduction. The patient should then be observed closely for several hours for signs of peritoneal irritation to make certain that nonviable bowel has not been reduced. During the next several days the infant's metabolic disturbance is corrected, and the edema in the hernial sac is permitted to subside; elective herniorrhaphy can then be scheduled.

If the incarcerated hernia cannot be reduced or if it is inadvisable to attempt it because of its duration, emergency surgical correction must be undertaken.

HYDROCELE

A hydrocele is the presence of fluid anywhere within the course of the processus vaginalis.

Newborn male infants whose processus vaginalis has been obliterated often have residual peritoneal fluid in the tunica vaginalis of the testis. This common type of *noncommunicating hydrocele* forms an oval, fluctuant, tense, translucent sac, and the spermatic cord and ring can usually be felt above it. The fluid gradually absorbs during the first year of life, and surgical correction is rarely required.

If the processus vaginalis remains open, peritoneal fluid may be forced into it, forming a hydrocele of the spermatic cord or of the canal of Nuck in the female. An inguinal hernia is often associated. Frequently the parents note that the "testis seems larger" in the evening after an active day, and smaller the following morning. This history is highly suggestive of the *communicating hydrocele* (see Diagnosis under Inguinal Hernia). The length of the hydrocele is dependent upon the extent of the patency of the processus vaginalis. If it extends into the tunica vaginalis, then the elongated fluctuant mass extends to the lower part of the scrotum. When the occlusion is at a higher level, the hydrocele is a fluctuant swelling above the scrotum or extends only a short way into it. Occasionally the fluid becomes trapped in the sac and forms a firm globular mass which is irreducible and resembles an incarcerated inguinal hernia. If the fluid is at some distance below the external inguinal ring or has been present for several days and is neither tender nor symptomatic, the diagnosis of a hydrocele may safely be made. The sudden appearance of an irreducible hydrocele near the external ring is usually impossible to differentiate from an incarcerated hernia. Transillumination is of little value in such a case, since an incarcerated intestine may also transmit light before it becomes hemorrhagic. Emergency surgical exploration may be necessary for differentiation.

Since the appearance of a hydrocele some time after birth is evidence of a persistent processus vaginalis, the hydrocele should be extirpated by the inguinal route and the hernial sac removed. Aspiration of the tunica vaginalis or injection of sclerosing solutions is not warranted; either one may cause adhesions, which make the ultimate operation more difficult and may damage the testis.

EPIGASTRIC HERNIA

Epigastric hernias occur in the midline between the umbilicus and the lower end of the sternum. They are not common and, except for their location, are similar to umbilical hernias. They should be repaired surgically.

INCISIONAL HERNIA

Postoperative hernias should be repaired as soon as the local condition of the wound and the general condition of the child warrant it. There is no justification for permitting children to continue with the discomfort attendant on this type of hernia.

DIAPHRAGMATIC HERNIA

Diaphragmatic hernias may be congenital or acquired. Acquired hernias are usually traumatic in origin and are not considered here. Congenital herniation of abdominal contents into the thoracic cavity may be responsible for serious embarrassment of respiration and usually constitutes a medical-surgical emergency in the immediate neonatal period. Infrequently there is little or no respiratory embarrassment, and the hernia may not be detected until later in infancy or childhood. In addition to herniation through a defect in the diaphragm (see below), there may be partial herniation of the stomach through the esophageal hiatus (see p. 770), phrenic paralysis with displacement of abdominal contents upward, but not herniated (see p. 376), and eventration of the diaphragm. *Eventration is not a herniation*, but is also an upward displacement of abdominal contents into an outpouching or saclike structure of the diaphragm resulting from a weakness or absence of diaphragmatic musculature without an abnormal opening. The clinical manifestations of an eventration may simulate those of a diaphrag-

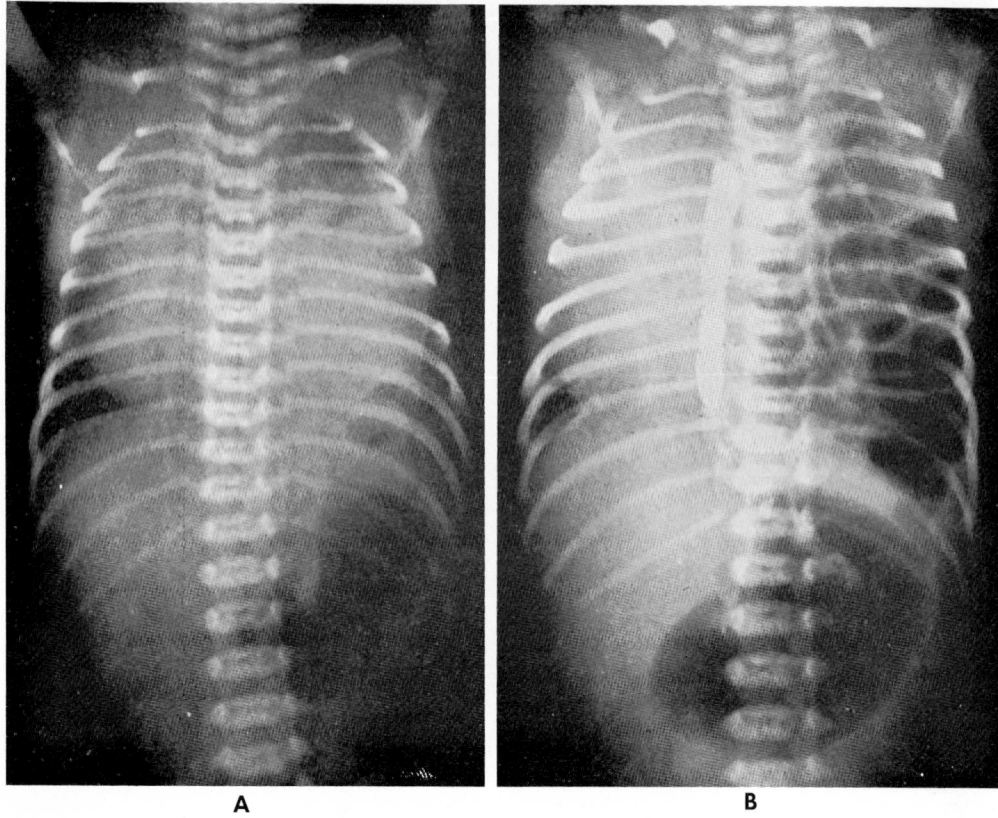

A   **B**

Figure 11-23. Congenital diaphragmatic hernia. *A*, Film exposed shortly after birth: distortion of shadow of left leaf of diaphragm, with huge, masslike density in left hemithorax displacing heart to right. *B*, Film exposed about 20 minutes after *A*. As the result of swallowed air, coils of air-filled small bowel are now demonstrated in the left hemithorax. The esophagus is outlined by swallowed contrast material. Operative correction was attempted because of extreme dyspnea. Infant died 5½ hours after birth.

matic hernia. Rarely there is complete absence of the diaphragm.

Etiology. Herniation occurs most often in the posterolateral segments of the diaphragm, and more often on the left than on the right side. The defect represents failure of the pleuroperitoneal canal to close completely during embryonic development (foramen of Bochdalek). Much less frequently the herniation is in the anterior portion of the diaphragm in the retrosternal area; this defect represents failure of midline fusion of the 2 anlagen of the diaphragm with elements of the pericardium (foramen of Morgagni). With this defect there may be herniation of intestine into the pericardial sac or, conversely, ectopia cordis with displacement of the heart into the peritoneal cavity. Umbilical defects are commonly associated with herniation through the foramen of Morgagni.

Pathology. There are various degrees of protrusion of the abdominal viscera through a diaphragmatic hernia into the thoracic cavity. In severe cases the stomach and a large part of the intestines and even, in rare instances, the spleen, liver and kidneys displace the lungs and heart. There may be associated incomplete rotation of the cecum, umbilical defects and duodenal constricting bands. The lung on the affected side is compressed and often hypoplastic. Hypoplasia of the opposite lung has also been observed.

Diagnosis. Severe respiratory distress, including dyspnea and cyanosis, is frequently present from birth. If symptoms are not present at birth, they may appear at any time during the neonatal period or later. These include vomiting, severe colicky pain, discomfort after eating and constipation as well as dyspnea. Symptoms and signs of acute intestinal obstruction may occur at any time. Infrequently there are no symptoms, and the condition may be discovered by chance roentgenographic examination.

The physical examination varies considerably, depending on the degree of displacement of abdominal contents into the thoracic cavity. When there is extensive displacement in the newborn infant, the abdomen is usually small and scaphoid in contour, and the infant is cyanotic and has obvious respiratory retractions. If the respiratory embarrassment is not relieved, shock and rapidly progressive hypoxia occur. In contrast, in mildly affected patients there may be no or only minimal respiratory distress and no digestive disturbance.

The percussion note over the part of the thorax containing the stomach and intestines may be more tympanic or duller than usual and the breath sounds absent, decreased or increased. Occasionally sounds of intestinal peristaltic movements can be heard over the chest.

The diagnosis can usually be established by

roentgenographic examination, often without the aid of contrast medium, or, if such is needed, air injected into the stomach may be sufficient. Characteristically, in the neonatal period there are fluid and air-filled loops of intestine in the chest which simulate cysts. The mediastinum is displaced toward the unaffected side, usually the right. Occasionally, in the case of cystic adenomatoid malformations in the chest, it may be necessary to use contrast material to demonstrate that the stomach and intestines are in the abdominal cavity.

Treatment. The newborn infant who is in respiratory distress should receive oxygen as required to relieve cyanosis. If positive-pressure ventilation is needed, caution must be used, since it may result in pneumothorax from the uneven distribution of intrapulmonary pressures established by the compression atelectasis and the associated pulmonary hypoplasia. The newborn infant in whom the diagnosis is suspected should immediately be positioned with his head and thorax higher than the abdomen and feet to facilitate the downward displacement of abdominal organs. Emergency definitive surgical correction is indicated in most instances. Elective operation may be justified later if there are no symptoms or if they are mild and intermittent, but the procedure should be performed as early in infancy as possible. The risks of both disease and surgery are high in the immediate neonatal period.

LAWRENCE K. PICKETT

REFERENCES

Baran, E. M., and others: Foramen of Morgagni Hernias in Children. *Surgery*, 62:1076, 1967.
Jackson, T. M.: Congenital Diaphragmatic Hernia. *Arch. Surg.*, 95:102, 1967.
McNamara, J. J., Eraklis, A. J., and Gross, R. E.: Congenital Posterolateral Diaphragmatic Hernia in the Newborn. *J. Thorac. & Cardiovasc. Surg.*, 55:55, 1968.
Swenson, O.: Diagnosis and Treatment of Inguinal Hernia. *Pediatrics*, 34:412, 1964.

THE LIVER

Anatomy. The liver of the full-term infant weighs 120 to 160 gm. at birth. The weight is doubled at 2 years and tripled at 3 years; at 9 years it has increased 6 times, and at puberty, 10 times. The liver of the adult is 12 to 13 times as large as that of the newborn infant. The relative sizes of the lobes of the liver change with age; at birth the right lobe is twice as large as the left lobe; in young children and adolescents it is about 3 times as large. The functional right and left lobes, drained by the right and left hepatic ducts and supplied with corresponding portal venous branches and hepatic veins, differ from the anatomic lobes. In the newborn infant the liver edge is usually less than 2 cm. below the costal margin in the right midclavicular line. The upper border of hepatic dullness is at the level of the fifth or sixth rib in the mammary line and extends nearly horizontally. In the axillary line it is usually in the seventh intercostal space and posteriorly in the ninth space. The lower border of the liver may be normally palpable about 1 cm. below the costal margin throughout childhood.

Extramedullary hematopoiesis, varying inversely in amount with the birth weight, may be found normally in the liver of infants for a few weeks after birth.

Congenital Anomalies and Malpositions. *Absence* of the liver has been reported in stillborn fetuses in association with other severe anomalies. The lobes of the liver may vary in size and shape; either one may be absent, or there may be more than two. Riedel's lobe is the tonguelike downward projection of the right lobe. A "floating liver" occurs when there is congenital elongation of the ligaments which support the organ. In situs inversus the liver is on the left side; rarely with diaphragmatic hernia it may be located in the thorax.

Downward displacement of the liver is produced by contractural deformities of the thorax (rickets), relaxation of the abdominal musculature (severe malnutrition, amyotonia congenita and other paralyses) or increased intrathoracic pressure (empyema, pneumothorax or pulmonary hyperaeration). Subphrenic abscess or a collection of air (perforation of the gastrointestinal tract) will also push the liver downward. The less common upward displacement may be caused by ascites, abdominal tumors or paralysis of the diaphragm.

Metabolic Functions. Owing to its important role in the metabolism of foodstuffs, the liver has been aptly termed the commissariat of the body.

The liver plays the leading role in maintenance of the normal blood sugar level. It forms and stores glycogen from glucose, levulose, galactose and dextrolactate. It converts the glycogenic amino acids and the glycerol fraction of fats into dextrose, which is deposited as glycogen (glycogenesis). Glycogen can be reconverted into glucose by the liver (glycogenolysis). Thus the liver serves as a storehouse of readily available glucose which can be delivered to the blood when required. The livers of infants contain proportionately less glycogen than those of children.

The liver is the site of both synthesis and oxidation of fat. Hepatic lipogenesis from acetate and pyruvate depends upon the normal functioning of both the anaerobic glycolytic (Embden-Meyerhof) and phosphogluconate pathways of carbohydrate metabolism. Most, if not all, of the fat mobilized in the liver is combined with lecithin and changed to phospholipid, a change which is apparently necessary for its transport and subsequent use. Dietary deficiency of lipotropic factors (e.g. choline, inositol or compounds which can contribute methyl groups for the formation of choline) prevents the formation of the more soluble phospholipid, so that fat accumulates in the liver. Cholesterol is formed in the liver from its esters or by synthesis from acetic acid. Cholesterol esters, i.e. compounds of cholesterol and fatty acids, which constitute 70 per cent of the plasma cholesterol, are also formed in the liver and are a means for the rapid transport of cholesterol. The plasma lipoproteins which transport triglycerides also appear to be, in part, formed in the liver.

The liver (and kidney) breaks down long-chain fatty acids into ketone bodies, which are burned by and supply energy to the muscles and other tissues which cannot form them. When fat is burned in excess (starvation and diabetes), large amounts of ketone bodies accumulate and are excreted in the urine.

Urea is formed exclusively in the liver by the deamination of amino acids. The liver is concerned with the formation of many fractions of the serum proteins. Fibrinogen, a globulin, is formed exclusively in the liver. Prothrombin and other coagulation factors and probably all the serum albumins are of hepatic origin. The liver also serves as a storage depot for protein. There is a large labile fraction of the hepatic proteins which increases with a high protein diet and decreases during starvation. In many disease states of the liver there is an increased concentration of serum globulins.

Vitamins A, C and D are stored in the liver, and considerable amounts of A and D remain for a long time after the administration of single large doses. The precursors of vitamin A are converted into vitamin A in the liver. The damaged liver has a reduced storage capacity for vitamin A and a lowered capacity for the conversion of its precursors. Riboflavin and vitamins E and K have important metabolic storage relations to the liver.

Influence of diet upon the liver. The vulnerability of the liver to toxic agents may be reduced or eliminated by various dietary constituents. A high carbohydrate diet has a protective action for the liver. This has been attributed to the resultant increased glycogen content of the liver, but may be due to other factors. An adequate protein intake also shields the liver from toxic injury; *methionine* and *cystine* are recognized as some of the protective elements in protein.

Dietary deficiencies lead to hepatic injury. A low protein diet results in massive hepatic necrosis, specifically as a result of cystine deficiency. Absence of tocopherol from the diet also predisposes to this type of liver damage. Protein deficiency of lesser degree or a high fat diet produces fatty infiltration of the liver which slowly progresses to diffuse hepatic fibrosis. This sequence of hepatic injury may be prevented by the inclusion of choline or methionine in the diet.

Blood Formation. The fetal liver is an active site of blood formation. Hematopoiesis is common in the livers of premature and occasionally of full-term infants as a remnant of this fetal function. In conditions such as hemolytic anemias in which excessive demands are placed on the blood-forming mechanisms the liver undergoes myeloid metaplasia and resumes its hematopoietic activity. The liver also serves as a storehouse for iron during the early months of infancy which is used when the infant's diet is chiefly milk and is low in iron. With depletion of this store by about the fifth month, hypochromic anemia develops if the diet does not contain a high iron content.

Detoxifying Functions. The liver can alter various exogenous toxic substances by conjugating them with sulfuric acid, glucuronic acid (an oxidation product of glucose) or amino acids. The conjugation mechanism is probably more concerned with increasing the solubility of the toxic substance so that it can be more easily transported through the body fluids and excreted than it is with a direct reduction in toxicity. Thus sulfanilamide is converted into the more soluble but more toxic compound, acetyl sulfanilamide. The liver also appears to be the principal site for removal of ammonia from the blood. The natural and synthetic estrogenic and androgenic substances are inactivated by the liver. Excess of these hormones in the body, when the damaged liver fails to dispose of them, results in abnormal physiologic effects.

Biochemistry of Liver Disease and Liver Function Tests

Knowledge of the wide variety of functions performed by the normal liver has led to the development of biochemical methods for their evaluation. Among these are tests useful in defining the ability of the liver to conjugate and excrete bilirubin, to synthesize serum proteins and coagulation factors, to contribute to carbohydrate homeostasis, to dispose of ammonia as urea, and to conjugate various drugs and hormones. Other indices of hepatic disturbance which are generally less specific reflect the immunologic response of the organ to injury. In this category are the flocculation and turbidity tests and electrophoretically determined alteration in gamma globulin concentration.

The acutely injured liver cell may permit spillage of intracellular enzymes into the blood, where their increased levels are measurable. Most widely studied of this group are the serum transaminases, glutamic-oxaloacetic (SGOT) and glutamic-pyruvic (SGPT).

Clinical evaluation of liver function may include examination of excretory capacity for certain dyes such as Bromsulphalein as well as physiologic substances normally excreted by this organ: cholesterol, bile acids, alkaline phosphatase and bilirubin. The quantity of bilirubin metabolites in the stool and urine gives valuable information relating to the adequacy of metabolic and anatomic excretory pathways.

Radiologic techniques are of great value in evaluating hepatic disorders. Cholangiography with introduction of contrast medium by oral, intravenous, transhepatic and direct injection into the gallbladder plays a part in the study of patients suspected of having disease of the gallbladder or of the extrahepatic biliary system. Contrast radiographic studies may disclose varices of the esophagus or, by distortion of the normal duodenal configuration, give suggestive evidence of the presence of obstructive dilatation of the common duct or mass lesions in the pancreas or its adnexa.

Transabdominal splenoportal venography with concomitant portal pressure measurements may confirm the presence of portal hypertension and document the presence of collateral circulation between portal and systemic venous systems. The same information may also be achieved by cannulation of the tiny lumen of the obliterated umbilical veins found in the falciform ligament as it passes extraperitoneally beneath the linea alba. The vessel is dilated to its entrance into the left portal vein, after which pressure measurements are made and venography is carried out. This procedure is more likely to show successfully the portal vein than is splenic venography, but more often it fails to show collaterals. It merits consideration also because it may be carried out under local rather than general anesthesia, avoids the occasional rupture of the spleen encountered in the usual venographic procedure, and also permits study of patients who have been subjected to splenectomy. Dye injected into the celiac axis through a catheter introduced into the femoral artery and threaded up the iliac to the aorta may give a good view of the intrahepatic arterial circulation, the portal vein and existent collaterals. Distortion of the intrahepatic circulation may disclose the presence of tumors or inflammatory masses. These lesions may also be seen by scintillation scanning techniques utilizing radioactive substances such as colloidal gold or ^{131}I-labeled Rose Bengal.

The hepatic circulation can also be evaluated by sampling hepatic venous and systemic arterial blood, utilizing dyes or radioactive substances extracted by the liver.

Bile Pigment Metabolism. The serum bilirubin concentration reflects a dynamic process of production and excretion. Bilirubin is derived from several sources. About 85 per cent of daily bilirubin production results from breakdown of senescent red cells, aged approximately 120 days. Studies with labeled precursors of bilirubin have shown the label to appear in the fecal bilirubin (stercobilin) within 10 days. This material, representing 10 to 20 per cent of the daily bilirubin production, is referred to as the "early labeled" fraction. It is derived from chromoproteins such as myoglobin, cytochrome C, catalase and tryptophan pyrrolase, and also from maturing red blood cells in the marrow. Each of these represents a potential source of overproduction.

Bilirubin is transported in the blood bound to serum albumin. It is carried to the liver cell, where it is freed of its albumin linkage. In its passage through the liver cell it is converted from a lipid-soluble pigment to one soluble in water. By utilizing the van den Bergh reaction, the pigment present in bile and in the serums of patients with obstructive jaundice gives an immediate red color with diazotized sulfanilic acid (conjugated, direct-reacting or one-minute bilirubin). Pigment in the serums of patients with hemolytic jaundice which has not passed through the liver cell requires the addition of alcohol before the diazo reaction can occur (unconjugated or indirect-reacting bilirubin). The biochemical process involved in this conversion has been clarified by Cole, Lathe and Billing. Using reverse-phase partition chromatography, they demonstrated 3 pigments in jaundiced serum. The first, free bilirubin, is the pigment responsible for the indirect van den Bergh reaction. The other two, pigment I and pigment II, give the direct reaction; they are the monoglucuronide and diglucuronide conjugates of bilirubin, respectively. It is probable that the monoglucuronide is a complex of unconjugated bilirubin and bilirubin diglucuronide. Conjugation with glucuronic acid converts bilirubin from a lipid-soluble, water-insoluble compound to one soluble in water. The conversion is enzymatic and requires uridine diphosphoglucuronic acid (UDPGA), which donates its glucuronic acid to the 2 propionic acid side chains of bilirubin. The reaction is catalyzed by the microsomal enzyme glucuronyl transferase according to the scheme below. It is of theoretic and perhaps practical importance that the transferase enzyme may be induced by large doses of barbiturate.

Bilirubin Excretion. Bilirubin in extravascular sites is in equilibrium with intravascular bilirubin. But salicylates or sulfonamides disrupt the linkage between albumin and bilirubin and lead to a rise in tissue concentrations and a fall in the serum value. This is particularly important in hemolytic disease in the newborn, since diffusible bilirubin is of critical importance in the development of bilirubin encephalopathy.

In the normal person the liver plays the primary role in the excretion of bile pigments. The bilirubin diglucuronide formed in the reaction outlined in Figure 11-24 is transported out of the liver cells via the bile canaliculi into the biliary duct system, from which it is delivered with other constituents of bile to the intestinal lumen. In adult mammals the secretion of conjugated bilirubin is limited more by the rate of hepatic clearance of bilirubin than by its uptake or conjugation. In neonatal mammals, conjugation and perhaps uptake are the rate-limiting factors.

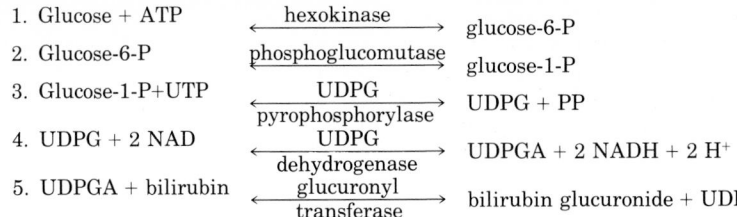

ATP = adenosine triphosphate
UTP = uridine triphosphate
UDPG = uridine diphosphoglucose
PP = pyrophosphate
NAD = nicotine adenine dinucleotide
UDPGA = uridine diphosphoglucuronic acid
NADH = reduced nicotine adenine dinucleotide

Figure 11-24.

The concentration of conjugated bilirubin in the serum is increased in hepatocellular and obstructive jaundice, and, because of its water solubility, the excess is excreted in the urine. After secretion into the bile and transport to the intestine, the bilirubin glucuronide is reconverted to free bilirubin by a beta-glucuronidase. The free bilirubin is readily reabsorbed into the circulation from the intestine, whereas conjugated bilirubin is not. In contrast to the adult, in whom the intestinal flora converts bilirubin into urobilinogen (stercobilinogen), the infant born with a sterile intestinal tract excretes unchanged bilirubin in the stool for weeks. The unconjugated bilirubin reabsorbed from the bowel enters an enterohepatic circulation. A small amount of stercobilinogen is also reabsorbed. That which is not re-excreted by the liver (about 4 mg. daily) is removed by the kidney as urobilinogen. This quantity is less than that detectable by the usual qualitative tests for urobilinogen.

Stercobilinogen which is not absorbed (about 100 to 200 mg. per day) gives the feces their brown color. Urobilinogen and stercobilinogen are oxidized readily to the chemically identical compounds, urobilin and stercobilin.

Bilirubin excretion in the newborn. Bilirubin formed by the fetus in utero can cross the placenta, where it is excreted by the maternal liver. After birth hepatic function for clearance of bilirubin is not adequate to prevent its accumulation in the blood during the first week of life. This phenomenon has been regarded as physiologic when it is limited to this age period and does not exceed a level of 12 mg. per 100 ml. in the absence of hemolytic disease.

Considerable emphasis has been placed on studies which explain neonatal jaundice in terms of reduced glucuronyl transferase activity noted in livers of fetal and newborn rats, guinea pigs, and monkeys and in recently expired premature infants. Recent observations, however, suggest that the transferase deficiency may have been overemphasized, since liver homogenates of newborn rats perform as well as those derived from

adult animals when sufficient UDPGA is added to the assay system.

Factors other than "hepatic immaturity" which may contribute to neonatal hyperbilirubinemia have been considered by Odell. Inhibitors of conjugation in serum and breast milk are important in some instances. Sterility of the intestinal tract in newborn infants prevents bacterial conversion of bilirubin to stercobilinogen, allowing reabsorption of bilirubin into the circulation with augmentation of the bilirubin pool. This process is dependent upon hydrolysis of bilirubin glucuronide in the intestine and may explain the hyperbilirubinemia which frequently accompanies intestinal obstruction in the newborn. The recent observation of lower bilirubin levels in the newborn infant fed "early" may be related to increased intestinal motility or to earlier introduction of intestinal bacteria, fostering reduction of bilirubin to stercobilinogen and its excretion in the stool. Persistent patency of the ductus venosus may also contribute to hyperbilirubinemia. In utero, the vessel permits oxygenated blood in the umbilical vein to bypass the liver and enter the inferior vena cava directly. At birth this bypass is normally functionally closed. Angiographic studies have shown that it may remain patent and permit portal vein blood, which constitutes about 80 per cent of the hepatic blood flow, to bypass the liver. Bypass of the liver has been documented in babies with the respiratory distress syndrome, in which hyperbilirubinemia is common. Increased bilirubin production in the absence of a hemolytic process may occur through operation of one or more of the "shunt" pathways from nonhemoglobin sources. In infants, 15N-labeled glycine appears in bile pigment in the stool within 48 hours in amounts greater than noted in adults.

Normal serum contains not more than 0.2 mg. per 100 ml. of conjugated bilirubin, and the total is less than 1.0 mg. per 100 ml. In jaundice due to hepatocellular injury and to obstruction the predominant pigment in the serum is conjugated bilirubin, and bile pigments are excreted in the urine. In jaundice secondary to hemolysis the indirect-reacting pigment predominates, and bile pigments do not appear in the urine unless the hemolysis is so intense that the serum concentration of conjugated bilirubin is also increased.

Stool color yields important clues to the origin of jaundice. Acholic stools are commonly seen during the early stages of hepatitis and are usual in complete obstruction of the extrahepatic biliary tree. Under these circumstances small amounts of bile pigment measured as urobilin may be found. Bilirubin may reach the intestine with intestinal secretions, where it is reduced by bacteria to stercobilinogen with later oxidation to urobilin. Quantitative estimations of fecal stercobilinogen are difficult, but have a place in obscure situations when increased hemolysis is suspected.

Bile Pigments in Urine. The Harrison spot and commercial tablet tests for bilirubin are useful and easily performed. In acute viral hepatitis, bilirubin appears in the urine before urobilinoginuria and jaundice are noted. Its presence in urine is an early sign of hepatotoxic effects in patients receiving chlorpromazine or iproniazid or who are exposed to carbon tetrachloride.

Qualitative tests for urobilinogen (Ehrlich's aldehyde reagent) and urobilin (Schlesinger) are easily done. An increase in urobilin is noted when hepatic function fails to re-excrete all bile pigment absorbed from the intestine. It is a highly sensitive test which may give a positive result when other routine test results are normal.

In viral hepatitis, urobilin in urine is increased early as a result of the depressed liver function. At the height of the illness the liver excretes little or no bilirubin, and urobilin disappears from the urine. It reappears with partial recovery and disappears again with complete restoration of hepatic function.

Urobilin is usually absent from the urine in complete obstructive processes and increases in association with the increased bile pigment production of hemolysis.

Serum Enzymes. The use of serum enzyme determinations in the study of liver disease is a consequence of their presence in large quantities in liver tissue and their loss to the circulation when the liver cell is injured or when egress of a particular enzyme is blocked by obstructive processes. Liver cells are particularly rich in enzymes exhibiting transaminase, dehydrogenase, peptidase, nucleotidase and alkaline phosphatase activities. Enzymes are rarely organ-specific, and changes in serum concentrations may indicate injury of more than one organ. Individual enzymes have been shown to be heterogeneous, composed of isoenzymes; with further delineation of these, organ specificity will no doubt be increased.

Phosphatases catalyze the hydrolysis of phosphoric acid esters. Serum alkaline phosphatase is normally at a level of 4 to 12 Bodansky units (3 to 13 King-Armstrong units) in childhood. With hepatocellular disease production of the enzyme is decreased, and with obstruction of the biliary tract its excretion is impaired; the enzyme

is normally secreted in bile. In starch gel electrophoresis bone and hepatic alkaline phosphatases have similar positioning. The serum of patients with intrahepatic or extrahepatic obstruction has 3 additional bands in the beta lipoprotein, alpha 2 and beta globulin regions. As this picture is also exhibited by normal bile, it appears that the changes in the serum are the result of regurgitation of bile from the biliary passages.

In obstructive jaundice, serum alkaline phosphatase concentrations usually exceed 30 King-Armstrong or 20 Bodansky units. In jaundice due to hepatocellular injury the levels, though raised, are usually below these. The levels in incomplete biliary obstruction as found in common duct stenosis or primary biliary cirrhosis are particularly high and out of proportion to the serum bilirubin concentration. It thus appears that the alkaline phosphatase level is a more sensitive indicator of bile stasis than is the serum concentration of bilirubin. Alkaline phosphatase levels are commonly elevated in the presence of hepatic tumors even in the absence of jaundice. The level is also raised with other space-occupying hepatic lesions such as amyloidosis, leukemia, abscess, tuberculosis or sarcoidosis. Elevation of alkaline phosphatase also accompanies disease of the bone, particularly rickets and hyperparathyroidism.

The serum transaminases are of particular value in indicating the presence of active hepatocellular injury. *Glutamic oxaloacetic transaminase (GOT)* is present in large amounts in the heart, liver, skeletal muscle and kidney and appears in increased amounts in the circulation when these tissues are involved in cellular destructive processes. Particularly high values accompany hepatocellular necrosis and myocardial infarction. *Glutamic pyruvic transaminase (GPT)* is present to a greater extent in liver cells than in cardiac or skeletal muscle. It is therefore a more specific index of hepatocellular injury. The differentiation of hepatic disease from myocardial infarction is not a significant clinical problem, and SGOT determinations alone are adequate. Except for the neonatal period, serum values for each of these 2 enzymes are usually 5 to 40 units. In the first weeks of life 90 to 120 units are in the physiologic range.

Transaminase determinations are of particular value in the early diagnosis of viral hepatitis, especially in anicteric patients. Values above 800 units for SGOT are strongly suggestive of viral hepatitis and may also be seen in infectious mononucleosis. The elevation may be transient with return to normal within a week of onset. Sustained elevations suggest continued activity of the disease process. Transaminase determinations are also helpful in detecting toxic hepatitis. Levels in cirrhosis are variable, with relatively higher concentrations in active juvenile cases. Moderate elevations, usually below 100 units, are found in obstructive jaundice; in biliary atresia, however, levels as high as 800 units have been encountered.

The *dehydrogenases* are catalysts in oxidation-reduction reactions. *Lactic dehydrogenase* (LD) is widely distributed in various tissues, including liver, heart, skeletal muscle and red cells. It is found in normal serum in concentrations up to 500 units. It is elevated in acute hepatitis, but not in cirrhosis or obstructive jaundice. A number of isoenzymes may be separated by starch gel electrophoresis. That from liver, LD_1, is easily distinguished from the isoenzyme derived from the heart, LD_5.

Isocitric dehydrogenase (ICD) is widely distributed throughout body tissues and occurs in normal serum in a concentration of 3 to 10 units. Its level is raised in any situation involving hepatocellular damage, including that of inflammatory, malignant or obstructive lesions. It is more specific for hepatic disease than SGOT, since it is not elevated in myocardial or skeletal muscle disease.

Serum cholinesterase which hydrolyzes acetylcholine and many other esters is present in normal serum at 2.2 to 5.6 micromoles per minute per ml. of serum. Low values occur with hepatocellular disease as well as with poor nutritional states.

Leucine amino peptidase is elevated in the serum in diseases of the pancreas or liver associated with biliary obstruction, hepatic infiltration or metastases. It is not affected by bone disease and may, therefore, aid in interpretation of elevated levels of alkaline phosphatase. Gellis has found it helpful in differentiating biliary atresia from other causes of obstructive jaundice in infancy. Normal levels of this enzyme are 150 to 250 units.

Serum 5-nucleotidase catalyzes the alkaline hydrolysis of phosphomonoesters only of the pentose-5′-phosphate nucleotides. It is therefore more specific than alkaline phosphatase. Its normal concentration is 0.3 to 3.2 Reis units. It is particularly elevated in obstructive in contrast to hepatocellular jaundice.

Dye Excretion Tests. The determination of the hepatic clearance of *Bromsulphalein sulfobromophthalein, (BSP)* is the most sensitive test of liver function. The injected dye is bound to albumin in the plasma and after clearance by the liver is excreted into the bile. BSP excretion by the liver involves selective uptake and concentration by the liver cell and the rate-limiting transport of both glutathione-conjugated and unconjugated dye into the bile canaliculi. In the standard test 5 mg. per kg. of the dye are injected intravenously. The normal person clears 90 and 96 per cent of the injected dye at 30 and 45 minutes, respectively. Additional information involving storage and excretory capacity for BSP may be obtained by measuring plasma clearance when the dye is infused intravenously. One or both of these values may be reduced when other usual tests of liver function give normal results. Changes in hepatic blood flow may reduce clearance of the dye in congestive heart failure or portal vein thrombosis. Clearance is also reduced with hepatocellular injury, metabolic abnormalities or obstructions to bile flow.

Proteins and Hepatic Function. *Albumin.*

When albumin synthesis is depressed as a result of hepatocellular disease, the serum albumin concentration and total body pool decrease. These changes are not rapid, owing to the slow rate of albumin degradation (half-life 12 to 18 days).

Globulins. In clinical laboratory evaluations, electrophoretic analysis of the serum globulin fractions is becoming routine. Alpha and beta globulin concentrations increase in a variety of infectious processes and in obstructive jaundice. They decrease when liver cell failure reduces their synthesis. Immunoglobulins increase in response to antibody formation stimulated by exogenous or tissue antigens. Although production of gamma globulin is not a function of the liver, its determination may be helpful in hepatic diagnosis. Extreme elevation may be found in children with postnecrotic or biliary cirrhosis as well as in lupoid hepatitis.

Serum haptoglobins. Haptoglobins are alpha$_2$-globulins which have the property of combining stoichiometrically with hemoglobin. It has been claimed that their level falls in cirrhosis and rises with obstructive jaundice. This has not been confirmed by Williams and colleagues. A decreasing concentration with increasing jaundice is characteristic of infectious hepatitis.

The flocculation and turbidity tests are not specific for liver disease. Flocculation or precipitation of the plasma proteins depends upon changes in various serum factors which tend to maintain the serum proteins in solution.

Coagulation Factors. Many of the active blood-clotting factors are synthesized by the liver. Among these are prothrombin, factors V, VII, IX and X and fibrinogen. A lowered concentration of these factors may result from impaired absorption of vitamin K, which is a requirement for the synthesis of prothrombin and of factors VII, IX and X. It may also reflect impaired hepatic synthesis of protein. Because of the rapid turnover (half-life 2 to 4 days) of a number of the coagulation factors, the one-stage prothrombin test serves as a sensitive indicator of changes in liver function in patients with acute liver disease. Persistence of abnormal values, after vitamin K has been given parenterally to correct the deficiency secondary to malabsorption, is indicative of severe liver damage.

Cholesterol. Variations in serum cholesterol concentrations reflect changes in serum lipoproteins. Cholestasis results in impaired excretion of cholesterol and bile acids, so that with normal synthesis of cholesterol serum concentrations of lipoproteins and cholesterol are increased. Impaired synthesis of hepatic lipoprotein with hepatocellular disease leads to decreased serum cholesterol levels.

Bile acids. Bile acids are the final products of cholesterol degradation; approximately 800 mg. are produced and excreted in the feces daily. Bile acids excreted in the bile are reabsorbed chiefly from the small intestine, forming an enterohepatic circulation; the rate of production is related to the quantity reabsorbed. In bile the quantity of trihydroxy acid (cholic acid) is approximately equal to the sum of the dihydroxy acids (chenodeoxycholic acid and deoxycholic acid). Estimation of bile acids in the serum is difficult; the total concentration is 1 to 2 mg. per 100 ml. The levels are increased in hepatocellular and in obstructive jaundice with little diagnostic discrimination; in obstructive jaundice the trihydroxy to dihydroxy ratio increases above the normal of 0.8.

The *bile salts* function in the emulsification of dietary fats and probably in their absorption. They have a cholagogue effect and assist in maintaining cholesterol in solution in the bile. They appear to be causally related to the pruritus of obstructive liver disease.

Needle Biopsy of the Liver. Percutaneous needle biopsy of the liver by an intercostal approach under local anesthesia is a relatively safe procedure. The Menghini needle (size 1 to 1.8 mm.), utilizing suction aspiration of the tissue, provides a more rapid and effective means of obtaining tissue than the Vim-Silverman needle.

In young infants in whom liver disease is almost invariably associated with hepatomegaly, a subcostal rather than a transthoracic approach is safer. Heavy sedation is necessary for all pediatric patents. The procedure is indicated in patients with otherwise unexplained jaundice, hepatomegaly and splenomegaly, as well as in evaluating progress in patients with subacute or chronic liver disease. It may also be useful in the diagnosis of unexplained fever, when biopsy may establish the presence of tuberculosis, sarcoidosis, brucellosis or neoplasia.

The procedure is contraindicated in patients with anemia, coagulation defects (prothrombin less than 60 per cent of control) and in infants in whom liver enlargement is not sufficient to permit a subcostal approach. The procedure should not be performed in patients suspected of having a vascular tumor of the liver. Hemorrhage from the biopsy site and leakage of bile from perforation of dilated intrahepatic ducts are unusual.

(See section on portal hypertension for discussion of venography and portal pressure measurements.)

Disorders Affecting Excretion of Bilirubin

Hyperbilirubinemia may be encountered with hepatic disease or with little or no evidence of it. The elevation in serum bilirubin which may be either of the conjugated or unconjugated type is the result of a failure of one or more steps involved in the normal pathway for excretion of bilirubin: uptake by the liver cell, glucuronide conjugation, transport from the conjugation site in the smooth endoplasmic reticulum, and excretion via the bile canaliculi.

These disturbances may be temporary or permanent and appear at birth or in later infancy and childhood. For purposes of diagnosis it is convenient to group hyperbilirubinemias on the basis of whether the increase is predominantly of unconjugated or conjugated bilirubin (Table 11-8).

UNCONJUGATED HYPERBILIRUBINEMIAS

Transient Neonatal Hyperbilirubinemia (Physiologic Jaundice of the Newborn, p. 394).
Delayed development of bilirubin conjugating system. Most full-term infants have mild unconjugated hyperbilirubinemia during the first 3 to 8 days of life. This is believed to be chiefly the result of delayed development of the bilirubin conjugating system, particularly involving glucuronyl transferase. Decreased activity of UDPG dehydrogenase has also been shown in guinea pig liver. Reabsorption of bilirubin which escapes conversion to stercobilinogen because of the rel-

ative sterility of the intestinal tract may be of greater importance. Production of increased quantities of bilirubin by "shunt" pathways and bypass of the liver through a patent ductus venosus as described above may also be contributing factors.

The serum unconjugated bilirubin usually does not exceed 10 mg. per 100 ml. in the full-term infant or 15 mg. per 100 ml. in the low-birth-weight infant (see also p. 393). Increased hemolysis does not play a significant role in this process, since it is usually not associated with declining hemoglobin or rising reticulocyte values. The risk of kernicterus in physiologic jaundice has not been clarified. It is generally believed to be less than in hemolytic disorders.

Inhibitors of conjugation. The *Lucey-Driscoll syndrome* is a form of intense, transient unconjugated hyperbilirubinemia which affects all newborn infants of certain mothers. The pathogenesis of this syndrome is not clear; the serums of the infants and their nonicteric mothers are several times more inhibitory to bilirubin conjugation by rat liver slices than the serums of unaffected infants and their mothers.

The breast-fed infant may exhibit a syndrome of severe and prolonged unconjugated hyperbilirubinemia. Rapid clearing of jaundice usually follows interruption of breast feeding. Pregnane-3 (alpha), 20 (beta)-diol isolated from inhibitory breast milk depresses glucuronyl transferase activity in vitro. Administration of this compound to infants is followed by unconjugated hyperbilirubinemia which clears after discontinuation of the compound.

Deficiency of red cell enzymes (see p. 1054).
Deficiency of red cell glucose-6-phosphate dehydrogenase is a common cause of neonatal hemolysis in the Mediterranean area. The incidence of especially severe cases in certain families suggests the presence of additional genetically determined hepatic factors. Other red cell enzyme deficiencies such as fructokinase have been similarly implicated.

Septicemia. Unconjugated hyperbilirubinemia may accompany septicemia and should be considered in patients with anemia and jaundice not resulting from blood group incompatibility (see neonatal sepsis, p. 404).

Drugs. Administration of certain drugs to pregnant women prior to delivery or to the newborn infant may accentuate unconjugated hyperbilirubinemia and increase the risk of kernicterus. Competition by the drug for bilirubin-binding sites on albumin may increase the quantity of bilirubin free to enter brain tissue. Long-acting sulfonamide drugs, especially sulfisoxazole (Gantrisin), have this effect and should not be administered to mothers before term or to newborn infants. Novobiocin appears to interfere with the

excretory phase of bilirubin transport through the liver. Synthetic vitamin K in doses larger than 1 mg. may act as an oxidizing agent producing hemolysis. The presence of glucose-6-phosphate dehydrogenase deficiency increases susceptibility to the potential toxic effects of excess administration of vitamin K.

Gastrointestinal obstruction in newborn infants. Unconjugated hyperbilirubinemia is relatively common in this situation, especially in pyloric stenosis. Increased shunting of blood through the ductus venosus and the consequent reduction in portal vein flow possibly related to increased intra-abdominal pressure may be an important factor in the increase in the unconjugated fraction of bilirubin. Reabsorption of bilirubin which escapes conversion to urobilinogen may also be a factor.

Hypothyroidism. Delayed development of the bilirubin conjugating system is thought to be the basis for the unconjugated hyperbilirubinemia which may accompany hypothyroidism in the young infant.

Persistent Jaundice with Defective Conjugation. *Crigler-Najjar syndrome (familial nonhemolytic jaundice with kernicterus).* This rare type of unconjugated hyperbilirubinemia is the result of hepatic deficiency of glucuronyl transferase activity. It is inherited as a mendelian recessive. The heterozygote may show decreased glucuronide conjugation of menthol in spite of a normal excretion pattern of injected bilirubin. Most affected patients have died in infancy with severe kernicterus. Occasional patients without severe central nervous system injury have survived. In this condition serum bilirubin levels may be reduced by administration of barbiturates. The mechanism appears to be induction of transferase activity.

Gilbert's syndrome (nonhemolytic jaundice). This syndrome has a varied origin. Klatskin suggests that if the term "Gilbert's syndrome" is to be used, it should encompass all instances of unconjugated hyperbilirubinemia which are not the result of overt hemolysis. Arias considers it desirable to abandon the term and use nomenclature based on the underlying defect. On this basis the following syndromes have been recognized: CHRONIC NONHEMOLYTIC ACHOLURIC JAUNDICE AS A RESULT OF DEFECTIVE GLUCURONIDE FORMATION IN VIVO AND VITRO. Serum bilirubin values from 8 to 20 mg. per 100 ml. were observed in one series and not above 6.2 mg. per 100 ml. in another and larger series. The syndrome appears to be hereditary in origin and may be related to the Crigler-Najjar syndrome. It differs from the latter in the lack of kernicterus, presence of bilirubin in bile and occasional late onset at puberty.

The disease occurs predominantly in males. The usual liver function test results are normal, as is the histologic pattern of the liver. The earliest onset in a large series was 10 years. About one third of the patients present with gastrointestinal complaints: nausea, abdominal pain, dyspepsia, constipation or diarrhea. A similar percentage of patients present with fatigue or malaise. In the remainder, jaundice is the presenting complaint. Treatment is symptomatic.

COMPENSATED HEMOLYTIC DISEASE WITHOUT OVERT SIGNS OF HEMOLYSIS, EXCEPT DURING CRISES. Affected persons have a decreased red cell survival time. They should be identified, since they are at risk of intermittent hemolytic crises.

MILD UNCONJUGATED HYPERBILIRUBINEMIA FOLLOWING VIRAL HEPATITIS. The serum bilirubin value is usually less than 5 mg. per 100 ml. Red cell survival and fecal urobilinogen excretion are normal. This syndrome may occur without evident antecedent viral hepatitis and with a variety of metabolic and infectious disorders. The cause is not known; reduced glucuronyl transferase activity and menthyl glucuronide excretion have been observed.

CHRONIC UNCONJUGATED HYPERBILIRUBINEMIA IN CIRRHOTIC PATIENTS WITH PORTOCAVAL SHUNTS.

CHRONIC HYPERBILIRUBINEMIA AT HIGH ALTITUDES, PRESUMABLY DUE TO ANOXIA.

Shunt Hyperbilirubinemia. *Israel's syndrome.* This disorder meets Klatskin's conditions for inclusion in the Gilbert syndrome. Because of common usage it is described here as a separate entity. Jaundice results from hemolysis and from increased production of bile pigment from sources other than mature, circulating red blood cells. Affected patients have exhibited splenomegaly, reticulocytosis and spherocytosis. Splenectomy corrects the shortened erythrocyte survival time, but jaundice persists. Increased destruction of erythrocytes within the bone marrow is the apparent main source of the unconjugated bilirubin.

Hemolysis Due to Maternal-Fetal Blood Group Incompatibilities. See page 1060.

Other Hemolytic Disorders. See page 1052.

CONJUGATED HYPERBILIRUBINEMIAS

Transient Neonatal Hyperbilirubinemia. Some infants with Rh hemolytic disease exhibit a sharp rise in serum conjugated bilirubin during the recovery phase when serum levels of unconjugated bilirubin are falling. Prolonged episodes of jaundice associated with evidence of hepatocellular obstruction have been called the *"inspissated bile syndrome";* they apparently are less frequent since the widespread use of exchange transfusions for the primary disorder. The syndrome reflects diffuse hepatic cellular injury rather than mechanical plugging of ducts with bile as the name implies.

Chronic Nonhemolytic Jaundice with Conjugated Bilirubin in Serum With and Without Pigment in Liver Cells. Dubin-Johnson's and Rotor's syndromes were distinguished initially by liver biopsy. In Rotor's syndrome the liver is histologically normal. The liver in the Dubin-

Johnson syndrome is macroscopically black, and microscopically dark brown pigment granules are seen in parenchymal cells, particularly in the centrilobular areas. In some families with the Dubin-Johnson syndrome, jaundiced patients without abnormal pigmentation of liver cells have been observed. Differences in the 2 syndromes in relation to the excretion of Bromsulphalein and cholecystographic agents do not appear to be clear-cut, and Scheuer and Williams recommend abandoning the effort to distinguish between the disorders. The main defect in both is excretory and results in regurgitation of conjugated bilirubin from the liver cell to the plasma. The excretory defect also involves cholecystographic agents, Bromsulphalein and other dyes. In 16 per cent of cases described by Dubin the onset was in the first 5 years of life. All patients exhibit jaundice, and approximately half have hepatomegaly and dark urine. The liver is frequently tender, and complaints of abdominal pain and weakness are common; nausea or vomiting, anorexia and diarrhea are also relatively common. Total bilirubin in the serum varies from 2 to 24 mg. per 100 ml. Bromsulphalein retention may be relatively normal or exceed 50 per cent of the injected dose. The gallbladder is usually not visible with cholecystographic agents, although visualization was achieved in the cases initially described by Rotor. Tests of hepatocellular function give essentially normal results.

The pigment accumulating in the liver cells in the Dubin-Johnson syndrome differs from lipofuscin histochemically and structurally. There is evidence that it is related to melanin and catecholamines. Mutant Corriedale sheep, which have a disorder apparently identical with the Dubin-Johnson syndrome, incorporate tritiated epinephrine or one of its metabolites into the pigment granules.

Recognition of these relatively benign syndromes permits their differentiation from other chronic liver diseases with jaundice.

Benign Familial Recurrent Cholestasis. This syndrome, initially described by Summerskill and Walshe, is characterized by recurrent episodes of jaundice accompanied by chemical and histologic evidence of cholestasis. Approximately half of the cases reported have been familial. The clinical pattern is characterized by recurrent attacks usually beginning with pruritus, anorexia and weight loss followed within an interval of 1 to 3 weeks by obstructive jaundice with clay-colored stools and dark urine. Serum alkaline phosphatase levels are elevated, and the elevated serum bilirubin level is predominantly of the conjugated form. Biopsy during symptomatic periods reveals bile stasis and cellular infiltration of the portal areas. Despite repeated episodes starting as early as 1 year of age and encompassing intervals as long as 38 years in one instance, there has not been persistent impairment of liver function. Cholestyramine may be helpful in relieving distressing pruritus.

Infections

NEONATAL HEPATITIS

The inflammatory processes which affect the liver in the early weeks or months of life have several features which distinguish them from those with onset in later childhood. Chief among these is a greater tendency to chronicity and progression to postnecrotic cirrhosis and death with hepatic failure. The liver of the infant so affected responds to injury with histologic changes, among which the formation of multinucleated giant cells is particularly prominent. This response, although not unique to the infant, is exaggerated beyond that usually seen in older subjects and may be so extensive as to involve what appears to be the entire hepatic parenchyma in a giant cell or syncytial transformation. This response has led to the use of the term "giant cell hepatitis" as a synonym for neonatal hepatitis.

Etiology. No single agent has been shown to be the cause of neonatal hepatitis. Most infections are probably viral in origin. Among the viruses incriminated by evidence derived from isolation and immunologic or transmission studies are those of serum hepatitis, cytomegalic inclusion disease, herpes simplex, rubella and Coxsackie infections. The virus of infectious hepatitis has also been considered but not proved to be a causative agent. Observations of newborn infants of women who had infectious hepatitis during pregnancy have not disclosed any evidence of fetal infection.

The protozoan parasite toxoplasma has also been found in newborn infants with hepatomegaly and jaundice, usually as a part of a generalized infection involving the central nervous system, the eye and the heart.

Hepatic involvement may also be associated with such bacterial infections as septicemia, pneumonia, pyelonephritis and listeriosis. Though syphilis may be responsible for neonatal hepatitis, significant clinical evidence of hepatic dysfunction is not common. Hepatocellular damage with jaundice and giant cell alteration occurs occasionally with Rh or other acquired hemolytic disease and commonly with uncontrolled galactosemia.

Pathology. The characteristic lesion of neonatal hepatitis is giant cell transformation of the hepatic cells. In severe involvement essentially the entire parenchyma may be so transformed, but even in the most severe examples the hepatic parenchyma may undergo repair. Unknown factors related to host resistance and the virulence of the infecting organism apparently influence the course toward recovery or chronicity, and on occasion to postnecrotic cirrhosis. In infants with apparent recovery, the liver tissue may appear normal on histologic examination, and biochemical evidence of residual damage may be limited to decreased excretory capacity for sulfobromophthalein.

Clinical Manifestations and Diagnosis. Commonly these infants present with persistent jaundice and the passage of acholic stools suggesting complete interruption of the flow of bile pigments from the liver to the intestinal tract. Approximately one third of these infants prove to have hepatitis, and most of the remainder have atresia of the extrahepatic biliary tree. The more or less characteristic clinical pattern of neonatal hepatitis consists of a history of late onset of jaundice in the second to third weeks of life, of initially normally colored stools which become acholic after several weeks, persistent conjugated hyperbilirubinemia, and positive qualitative test results for urobilinogen in urine and stool. Such a pattern suggests the presence of an acquired disease with partial obstruction; however, similar combinations of clinical findings have been noted in infants with proved extrahepatic biliary atresia (see p. 851).

The differentiation between obstructive jaundice on the basis of hepatocellular disease and that due to obstruction of the extrahepatic biliary tree is made difficult by a variety of factors. Among these are the frequency with which hepatitis leads to prolonged, essentially complete obstruction to the passage of bile into the intestinal tract, and the imperfect correlation of tests for hepatic parenchymal damage (flocculation, turbidity and transaminase) and the underlying disease process. Some clinicians have placed considerable reliance on serial determinations of serum bilirubin. Patients with hepatitis exhibit initially high levels (often above 10 mg. per 100 ml.) with a tendency toward an irregular decline with time. The infant with biliary atresia initially has lower values followed by a gradual increase in concentration.

In an occasional patient with biliary atresia esophageal varices, ascites and severe secondary biliary cirrhosis may develop as early as the third month of life. Awareness of this has led most workers to attempt to make a definite diagnosis by about 2 months of age, in order that the patient with operable biliary atresia may be spared the development of advanced biliary cirrhosis.

To this end operative liver biopsy and cholangiography have been generally relied on to accomplish the differentiation of biliary atresia from neonatal hepatitis. Though the risks of this procedure may not be as great as originally thought when surgical exploration of the extrahepatic ducts was commonly practiced, there is obvious reason to avoid subjecting patients with neonatal hepatitis to it. Additional considerations are the significant number of infants with neonatal hepatitis who have spontaneous resolution of their disease and the relatively small number (about 10 per cent) of infants with biliary atresia whose lesions are potentially correctable by surgery.

The clinical impression of hepatitis may be

supported by certain diagnostic procedures, and additional time may thus be allowed to determine whether there will be spontaneous clearing of the process, uncompromised by the hazards of anesthesia, open biopsy and cholangiography. Brent utilizes the radioactive rose bengal test for this purpose. After intravenous injection, if more than 5 per cent of the dye is excreted in the stool, complete obstruction is not considered to be present. If less than this amount is excreted, complete obstruction, on the basis of extrahepatic atresia or severe hepatocellular injury, is considered to be present. The author uses needle biopsy of the liver (technique described above) as an aid in the differential diagnosis of prolonged obstructive jaundice in infants.

The values for hemoglobin and bleeding, coagulation and prothrombin times must be adequate prior to the procedure. If the biopsy section is strongly suggestive of hepatitis, with giant cell transformation of the hepatic parenchyma and only minor evidence of portal fibrosis and bile duct proliferation, operation and cholangiography are delayed for 3 to 4 weeks to see whether the process will clear. If the histologic changes suggest biliary atresia, with relatively little alteration of the normal pattern of hepatic cell plates and definite evidence of portal fibrosis and proliferation of bile ducts, operative biopsy and cholangiography are undertaken. There is, however, considerable overlapping in the histologic changes observed in the 2 conditions. Some patients with biliary atresia have extensive giant cell transformation, and some patients with hepatitis have significant proliferation of bile ducts. Nor have cholangiographic studies proved to be infallible in distinguishing between neonatal hepatitis and biliary atresia. The reader is referred to the reported studies of Hays and colleagues for the variety of observations in a carefully studied series of patients with persistent jaundice.

Management. When a diagnosis of hepatitis is established and an additional period of a few weeks for observation shows no amelioration of jaundice, corticosteroid therapy should be tried. Prednisone in a dosage of 1 mg. per pound per day in divided doses is given initially for 2 to 4 weeks. The dose is then reduced by 25 per cent and continued for another 2 to 3 months. If no significant clearing of jaundice occurs during this time, there appears to be little likelihood of benefit from continued therapy. When a favorable effect is achieved clinically as well as in the lowering of serum bilirubin and transaminase values, an attempt should be made to maintain the dose at the lowest possible amount adequate to avoid exacerbation of jaundice. Though there is no reason to believe that steroids exert a curative effect, the anti-inflammatory action may lessen the obstructive process and foster excretion of bilirubin. The improvement in appetite induced by the steroid may also be beneficial.

Not uncommonly patients are seen at 4 to 6 weeks of age with clinical and laboratory findings suggesting neonatal hepatitis, in whom the process rapidly subsides without sequelae. It appears that prognosis for recovery varies inversely with the duration of disease. In our experience approximately one third of patients recover completely, and an equal number die or progress to postnecrotic cirrhosis. Only one infant has achieved complete recovery after remaining jaundiced for more than 6 months.

HEPATITIS IN THE OLDER INFANT AND CHILD

In a minority of families with more than one child affected by hepatitis, presumed to be transmitted transplacentally, the apparent onset of hepatic injury may be delayed for 6 to 8 months after birth. In these infants the course may be unremittent and progress to postnecrotic cirrhosis and death.

INFECTIOUS HEPATITIS
(Postnatal Viral Hepatitis)

Infectious hepatitis has its highest incidence, but lowest mortality, among children of school age. The disease remains, in the United States, the leading unconquered viral disease; most other viruses responsible for serious public health problems are being brought under control by the use of preventive vaccines. Although clinical hepatitis has been reproduced in human volunteers by feeding intestinal contents from patients in the acute phase of the disease, knowledge of the etiology and epidemiology of viral hepatitis is limited by the failure to find a suitable experimental animal or tissue culture system for the isolation and propagation of these viruses.

Etiology. Bacteria-free filtrates obtained from patients in the acute phase of the disease are capable of inducing viral hepatitis by serial passage in susceptible human subjects. The infectious agents are exceptionally stable; they resist heat at 56°C. for 30 minutes to an hour, chlorine at one part per million for 30 minutes and a number of chemicals which ordinarily inactivate bacteria and most other viruses.

Experimental and clinical observations of the naturally occurring disease or the experimental disorder in patients have shown that at least 2 viruses have etiologic roles. One, the "infectious hepatitis" virus or IH agent, produces clinical disease in susceptible persons after a relatively short incubation period of 14 to 40 days (mean 30 days). The second, the slow hepatitis, SH agent, homologous serum jaundice or transfusion hepatitis virus, has a much more prolonged incubation period of about 60 to 160 days. A further difference between the 2 viruses has appeared to reside in their means of transmission. It has been generally believed that the serum hepatitis virus is transmissible only by the parenteral route, whereas the infectious hepatitis virus may be transmitted by both oral and parenteral routes. Recent evidence (Krugman) suggests that the agent of serum hepatitis may also be transmitted from the patient to susceptible contacts by means other than parenteral inoculation. The virus of infectious hepatitis can be demonstrated in the stools of experimentally infected persons, whereas the serum hepatitis virus does not appear to be so excreted. Antigenic differences between the 2 viruses are evidenced by the development of immunity after infection with infectious hepatitis virus without immunity to the virus of serum hepatitis.

Gamma globulin obtained from pooled human plasma is capable of suppressing, but not preventing, clinical illness with both SH and IH agents. In each disease gamma globulin reduces the incidence of jaundice and the severity of the disease without reducing the incidence of the disease or interfering with active immune responses.

A number of different human viral pathogens have been isolated from patients with hepatitis. These include strains of ECHO and Coxsackie viruses, herpesvirus and adenoviruses. In most instances the presence of these viruses has been regarded as coincidental rather than etiologic; a number of "candidate viruses" are under study.

Of interest in the search for a suitable experimental animal host is the recent occurrence of more than 20 outbreaks of hepatitis in persons caring for immature primates, especially chimpanzees newly imported into the United States. In this animal there is a spontaneous disease clinically resembling human viral hepatitis. Studies with the South American marmoset are also relevant in this respect; histologic and biochemical evidence of hepatitis has been produced in this animal by serial passages of serum from a patient with typical viral hepatitis.

Pathology. Serial biopsy studies in adults reveal similar pathologic changes in the liver in both types of hepatitis. The hepatic lobules show varying degrees of cellular necrosis and autolysis, beginning in the center of the lobules and spreading radially as the disease advances. There is thickening of the reticular fibers. Evidences of cellular regeneration, i.e. increased mitotic figures, are prominent in the early stages of the disease. Accompanying the hepatocellular necrosis is widespread infiltration with inflammatory cells, polymorphonuclear leukocytes, lymphocytes, macrophages and plasma cells. In the later stages lymphocytes predominate. There is a diffuse reticuloendothelial reaction; the reticulum becomes thickened and assumes the staining properties of collagen. The periportal areas are widened because of infiltration with large numbers of inflammatory cells. Proliferating bile ducts appear in the perilobular portal areas, and bile stasis is visible. The clinical manifestations of viral hepatitis are expressions of the hepatocellular necrosis,

intrahepatic biliary obstruction, portal obstruction and diffuse inflammatory reaction in the liver. With recovery, complete regeneration of the liver cells occurs without scarring. In fulminating and fatal cases the hepatic changes are typical of yellow atrophy. About 15 per cent of the fatal cases studied by Lucké showed changes in the brain consisting in acute degeneration of ganglion cells and mild meningoencephalitis.

Clinical Manifestations. The incubation period of infectious hepatitis preceding the onset of jaundice is 14 to 40 days; if measured to the onset of initial symptoms, it may be 3 to 5 days less. The incubation period of serum hepatitis is 60 to 160 days. Clinical differentiation is more often suggestive than definitive. Infectious hepatitis is usually marked by an abrupt onset with fever, an autumn-winter incidence peak, and a predilection for children and young adults. Serum hepatitis, on the other hand, usually exhibits an insidious onset with little or no fever and a year-round incidence without an age preference.

Symptoms usually begin 4 to 5 days before the appearance of jaundice. Fever, malaise, mild headache and chilliness are present at the onset. Signs of a mild upper respiratory tract infection are common. Anorexia is invariably an early symptom, frequently followed by nausea and vomiting. The breath is often foul, and older children may complain of a sour or bitter taste. Upper abdominal distress and pain are frequent complaints. Constipation is more common than diarrhea. Bile usually is present in the urine 1 to 3 days before the appearance of jaundice.

On occasion jaundice appears without any preceding symptoms. Jaundice may vary from a slight discoloration of the scleras, where it is first seen, to a deep pigmentation involving the entire body. Fever usually disappears with the onset of icterus, but anorexia continues, and severe prostration and vomiting secondary to pylorospasm may occur, especially in deeply jaundiced patients. The stools are light or clay-colored at this stage. Pruritus is infrequent.

In more than half of the cases the liver is enlarged and tender; in a small number there is an enlarged, tender spleen. Ascites is rarely present. Bradycardia, common in the adult, is usually absent in children. Seborrheic dermatitis, morbilliform rashes and hemorrhagic phenomena are uncommon.

Diagnosis. The increase in the serum concentration of bilirubin is accounted for mainly by the conjugated (direct) form during the early days of jaundice. As recovery begins the unconjugated or indirect form increases, and in the late phase it may account for the total increase. Serum bilirubin values may be as high as 10 mg. per 100 ml. or more. With the onset of jaundice there is an increase in the urinary excretion of urobilinogen, owing to the inability of the damaged liver to excrete reabsorbed urobilinogen formed from bile which continues to enter the intestine, although in decreased amounts. Subsequently with complete failure of bile to reach the intestine and complete regurgitation of it into the circulation, urobilinogen disappears from the urine. With resumption of excretion of bile into the intestine, urobilinogen is again formed and appears in the urine in large quantities, the liver still being incapable of removing it completely from the blood.

The Bromsulphalein retention test result tends to parallel the retention of bilirubin in the blood, but often remains abnormal for a longer time. The serum glutamic oxaloacetic or glutamic pyruvic transaminases are elevated early in the course of the disease; their return to normal heralds the end of active disease and the beginning of recovery. The sedimentation rate is increased in most cases. There are no significant changes in the total serum protein concentration, but an increase in gamma globulin can be demonstrated by electrophoretic analysis.

There are no consistent changes in the leukocyte count, but a monocytosis as high as 25 per cent is occasionally observed. Serologic tests for syphilis may give falsely positive results.

Differential Diagnosis. The diagnosis of infectious hepatitis is dependent on the elimination of other causes of jaundice and of hepatitis with or without jaundice. The labial herpes, hemorrhagic exanthem, fever, leukocytosis, muscle pains and albuminuria occurring in *leptospirosis* should serve to distinguish it clinically. The specific agglutination test, the isolation of the spirochete from the blood or serum, or the successful inoculation of a guinea pig confirms the diagnosis of leptospirosis. Involvement of the liver, which clinically may mimic that in infectious hepatitis, is relatively common in *infectious mononucleosis*.

In the early preicteric phase, symptoms may be suggestive of influenza or gastroenteritis. Abdominal pain may resemble that of pneumonia or acute appendicitis. Drug-induced or toxic hepatitis must also be considered. Consideration should also be given to other types of conjugated hyperbilirubinemia discussed elsewhere in this section and to the possibility of an exacerbation of chronic liver disease.

Course and Prognosis. Compared with the clinical course in adults, the disease is characteristically milder and of shorter duration in children; the average duration is about 3 weeks, with a range of 4 to 80 days. Not infrequently a child feels improved by the time the jaundice appears; usually the other clinical manifestations are gone by the seventh day of jaundice. Complete recovery without relapse is usual. There is, however, a wide range in the clinical patterns of the disease, the principal examples of which are listed below.

Mild anicteric hepatitis is apparently more common among infants than the icteric form of the disease. The symptoms are those of a mild gastroenteritis or systemic infection, such as anorexia, diarrhea and vomiting. In an institutional epidemic of infectious hepatitis, which involved 36 infants, only one of them was jaundiced. The infants may excrete the virus in their stools for many months and constitute a potential source of infection to their attendants.

Hepatitis with predominant cholestasis is uncommon in children; it is also referred to as *cholestatic hepatitis* and *cholangiolitic hepatitis*. It is characterized principally by obstruction and dilatation of bile canaliculi with little evidence of hepatocellular necrosis. The clinical manifestations include jaundice with pruritus, bilirubinuria, pale stools with decreased fecal urobilinogen, and an enlarged, nontender liver. Laboratory examinations show increases in alkaline phosphatase, 5-nucleotidase and leucine aminopeptidase values in the serum with only slight increases in the serum transaminases.

Fulminant hepatitis. Fulminant hepatitis, or *acute massive necrosis*, is usually fatal within a few weeks after onset. Systemic manifestations during the preicteric phase are usually severe. Particularly prominent are high fever, abdominal pain and severe vomiting. Also indicative of an unfavorable outcome are rapid decrease in liver size, mental changes including lethargy, drowsiness, and confusion, electroencephalographic changes of encephalopathy, and an increase in prothrombin time not corrected by parenteral administration of vitamin K. Jaundice is usually intense, but death may precede its development. Transaminase levels may not be very high, perhaps reflecting failure of hepatic synthesis of the enzymes. Bleeding into skin and mucous membranes, ascites and deep coma are among the terminal manifestations.

Prolonged hepatitis, recurrent hepatitis and chronic hepatitis. Except in the very young infant, infectious hepatitis in childhood is usually a brief, self-limited illness. Only rarely do children with an apparently typical bout of hepatitis continue for months with hepatomegaly and biochemical evidence of continued hepatocellular injury. This type, of course, has been designated "prolonged hepatitis." Perhaps even more uncommon in children is recurrent hepatitis with exacerbation during the recovery phase. Patients with this course may be expected to recover ultimately unless subacute hepatic necrosis progresses to postnecrotic cirrhosis.

Treatment. Treatment is symptomatic and aimed at supporting the patient during the interval required for his own immunologic defenses to eradicate the invading virus. Maintenance of a reasonable state of nutrition during the illness appears to be beneficial; regeneration of damaged liver requires an adequate supply of protein and calories. An effort should be made to provide at least basal caloric requirements, utilizing the intravenous route if necessary.

After the initial anorexia has passed, a diet providing adequate calories and 1.5 to 2.5 gm. of protein per kg. per day should be provided. Restriction of fat intake is not necessary beyond the removal of gross fat from meats and avoiding fried foods and the use of oils in salad dressings. Milk, eggs and butter are usually well tolerated. Frequent feedings are helpful in achieving an adequate dietary intake. When vomiting or anorexia is prominent, intravenous infusion of a solution of 10 to 15 per cent glucose with maintenance levels of electrolytes should be given. Unusual gastrointestinal losses due to vomiting may require additional amounts of sodium and potassium chlorides.

Rest in bed is indicated until there is evidence of beginning clinical and biochemical recovery as manifest by disappearance of hepatic tenderness and decreases in serum bilirubin and transaminase values to 2 mg. and 40 units per 100 ml., respectively. Resumption of full activity should be allowed over a 2- to 4-week period, depending on the severity of the initial episode and the patient's own sense of well-being. In the more severely affected patients activity should be restricted until BSP excretion has fallen to normal.

Adrenocortical steroids are capable of inducing a prompt clinical remission in acute viral hepatitis, but this is not accompanied by an increased rate of resolution of the hepatic injury. Among the beneficial effects of steroid treatment are improved appetite and sense of well-being, increased extrahepatic clearance of bilirubin, lessening of intrahepatic obstruction by decreasing inflammation, and increased renal excretion of water. A more specific effect of these agents occurs in hepatic disease caused by allergy to drugs and by autoimmune processes.

Prednisone should be administered to patients with acute viral hepatitis only for the following indications: coma, persistent fever, severe bleeding and excessively abnormal chemical values, especially in serum bilirubin and in the prothrombin time. A dose of 1 mg. per pound per day is administered until the desired effects are noted; the drug is then discontinued gradually at a rate adequate to maintain clinical improvement.

Calamine lotion may alleviate itching to some extent. Cholestyramine, a bile-salt-sequestering resin, is useful when itching is a severe problem (1 to 3 gm. 4 times daily). Phenothiazines are contraindicated in acute hepatic injury. Sedation when needed is provided most safely by chloral hydrate or by short-acting barbiturates.

In the very severe cases of hepatitis additional problems which may require consideration are fluid retention, hepatic encephalopathy and severe bleeding.

Fluid retention and edema. Failure of renal excretion of sodium is the principal cause of edema. Treatment involves rigid restriction of sodium intake, which may necessitate the use of sodium-free milk in order to maintain adequate intake of protein. Combined use of hydrochlorothiazide (2 to 4 mg. per kg. per day) and an aldosterone-blocking agent, spironolactone (10 to 20 mg. per kg. per day), is usually required to promote adequate diuresis. Potassium deficiency may complicate therapy with these agents, and supplements may be necessary. Salt-poor albumin or mannitol may be helpful in treating edema if the serum albumin concentration is below 2.5 gm. per 100 ml. Hyponatremia is usually dilutional and is best treated by restriction of water intake. Abdominal paracentesis for ascites should be avoided unless abdominal and respiratory distress is severe.

Hepatic encephalopathy. Decreased liver function and shunting of portal blood to the systemic circulation are the chief factors responsible for the neurologic manifestations in hepatic disease. The effects of increased concentrations of blood ammonia are not clear, but levels above 100 micrograms per 100 ml. are commonly found in patients with hepatic coma. Blood ammonia values may rise with gastrointestinal hemorrhage, excessive protein intake or severe intestinal stasis. Potassium deficiency and anoxia may contribute to depressed functioning of the central nervous system and should be corrected.

To control intestinal production of ammonia, protein should be eliminated from the diet, and adequate calories as carbohydrate should be provided to limit endogenous breakdown of protein. Magnesium sulfate or mannitol should be administered orally to cleanse the intestinal tract of nitrogenous materials. Neomycin, 250 mg. 4 times daily, is used to reduce intestinal flora. In extreme situations consideration may be given to exchange transfusion. Perfusion of the patient's blood through the liver of a pig has been described by Watts.

Hemorrhage. This may be controlled by parenteral administration of vitamin K; it should be given to all jaundiced patients. Anemia is treated by blood transfusion. The treatment of bleeding varices is described in the section on portal hypertension.

Prevention. Isolation precautions appropriate for patients with intestinal infections are indicated during the period of hospitalization. The use of disposable needles and syringes is desirable in order to avoid the hazards resulting from their contamination. Other contaminated instruments should be autoclaved. Gamma globulin in a dose of 0.04 ml. per kg. should be used for the protection of susceptible contacts. Its use is of value up to 1 week before the appearance of the illness. It may be effective in preventing apparent disease in subjects exposed to the serum hepatitis virus when given in 2 doses of 10 ml. each at an interval of 1 month.

LIVER ABSCESS

SOLITARY ABSCESS

The single hepatic abscess is most often the result of a staphylococcal or streptococcal infection, but it may be due to a wide variety of infecting agents, including bacteria, fungi and protozoa.

Occasionally roundworms cause hepatic injury and permit secondary pyogenic infection. Amebic abscess, the commonest solitary abscess of adults, is relatively unknown in children.

Clinical Manifestations. Occasionally an abscess of the liver may be latent if it is well encapsulated, or it may be overshadowed by the symptoms of the disease from which it has its origin. Symptoms include fever, chills, sweating, prostration and nausea and vomiting. Pain is usually present over the liver and may be severe; at times it may be referred to the right shoulder or the epigastrium. Upward enlargement of the abscess may produce cough or dyspnea by irritation of the diaphragm. Mild icterus is present in many and ascites in a few cases. There is moderate enlargement of the liver.

The abscess may rupture spontaneously into the thorax, the peritoneum, the intestines or,

rarely, the pericardium. Metastatic abscesses of the lung or brain may occur.

The **diagnosis** is established by exploratory puncture, which is preferably performed when the liver is exposed by laparotomy.

Treatment. This consists of surgical drainage and appropriate antibiotic therapy determined, if possible, by culture and sensitivity tests.

MULTIPLE ABSCESSES

Multiple liver abscesses arise from septicemia or from ascending infection of the portal vein (pyelophlebitis). In the newborn infant, infection extending along the umbilical vein is a common cause of multiple hepatic abscesses. These abscesses are small and usually are not detected during life.

Chronic Liver Disease

In children chronic liver disease may present as a manifestation of a wide variety of disorders (see Table 11-9). In some it constitutes the principal clinical problem, e.g. the cirrhosis secondary to biliary atresia, whereas in others it is an associated disability of a systemic disturbance, e.g. cystic fibrosis.

The term "cirrhosis" indicates extensive destruction of hepatic parenchyma, with replacement by diffuse fibrosis. When hepatic cells are destroyed, new cells form from the cellular remnants. When death of cells is confined to individual lobules, orderly restoration of histologic and functional relations is possible. Destruction of many adjacent lobules with collapse of intervening stroma leads to regeneration of nodules which increase in size by growth at their periphery. New blood vessels surround the margins of the nodules and are compressed with continued growth. Compression decreases flow of blood more in the low-pressure veins than in the high-pressure arteries. This leads to dependence of the nodule on hepatic arterial blood for its nutrition, owing to shunting of portal blood past it and to impedance to outflow in the hepatic veins. Progress of the cirrhotic process is by further destruction of hepatic parenchyma, growth of regenerating nodules and contraction of scar tissue. Although fibrosis may be the most striking finding, the amount of functional parenchyma is of greater importance to the health and survival of the patient. Fibrosis may be largely reversible, as in hemochromatosis if excess iron is removed and in secondary biliary cirrhosis if the obstruction is removed. In conditions characterized chiefly by hepatic fibrosis, portal hypertension rather than parenchymal insufficiency may become the clinical problem, as, for example, in congenital hepatic fibrosis, multiple hemangiomas, scarring after abscess, and hepatic schistosomiasis.

In children it is convenient to consider chronic liver disease on the basis of whether it is acquired or results from hereditary defects. In some instances, as in neonatal hepatitis, a combination of factors, such as maternal viral infection and fetal genetic susceptibility, may be operative. Unidentified genetic factors may be important in apparently acquired liver disease, as in lupoid hepatitis and primary biliary cirrhosis.

ACQUIRED HEPATIC DISEASE

POSTNECROTIC CIRRHOSIS

Diffuse portal or Laennec's cirrhosis which involves all portal areas throughout the liver is rarely seen in children. Cirrhosis which commonly follows neonatal hepatitis is discussed on page 834. Infrequently cirrhosis is a sequel of infectious hepatitis in older infants and children. The resulting fibrosis is patchy and often extremely coarse. The inflammatory process may become quiescent, but more often there is a progressive process of inflammation and scarring. In children, in contrast to adults, most instances of postnecrotic cirrhosis are secondary to hepatitis. Children have fewer opportunities than adults for contact with such hepatic toxic agents as chloroform, carbon tetrachloride, chlorinated naphthalenes, arsenic and cinchophen.

Pathologically, postnecrotic cirrhosis differs from Laennec's cirrhosis in exhibiting larger nodules and wide bands of scar tissue. There is usually evidence of active inflammation, regeneration, and irregular vacuolated or multinucleated cells. Uninvolved lobules are also usually observed. These features are not always sufficiently de-

TABLE 11-9. Classification of Chronic Liver Disease in Childhood

I. **Acquired**
  A. Postnecrotic cirrhosis
  B. Chronic active hepatitis (lupoid hepatitis, juvenile cirrhosis)
  C. Primary biliary cirrhosis
    1. Idiopathic
    2. Post hepatitis
    3. Drugs
  D. Biliary cirrhosis secondary to extrahepatic biliary obstruction
    1. Atresia or stenosis of bile ducts
    2. Stone, sludge, tumor
    3. Recurrent pancreatitis
  E. Liver disturbances in ulcerative colitis
  F. Vascular congestion
    1. Cardiac
    2. Veno-occlusive disease

II. **Developmental abnormalities without cirrhosis**
  A. Polycystic liver disease
  B. Congenital hepatic fibrosis
  C. Hereditary hemorrhagic telangiectasis

III. **Hereditary disorders associated with cirrhosis**
  A. Hepatolenticular degeneration (Wilson's disease)
  B. Galactosemia
  C. Cystic fibrosis
  D. Fructose intolerance
  E. Sickle cell disease
  F. Porphyria, hepatic
  G. Hemochromatosis

IV. **Miscellaneous disorders**
  A. Idiopathic cirrhosis
  B. Indian childhood cirrhosis
  C. Sarcoidosis
  D. Progressive familial hepatic cholestasis of infants
  E. Tyrosinosis
  F. Cystinosis
  G. Glycogen storage disease
  H. Other storage diseases
    1. Hurler's disease
    2. Gaucher's disease
    3. Niemann-Pick disease
    4. Familial neurovisceral lipidosis
  I. Amyloidosis

From Iber and Maddrey.

veloped to permit a clear differentiation from portal cirrhosis.

In affected children the laboratory features include extreme elevation of gamma globulin values, persistent but fluctuating, predominantly direct hyperbilirubinemia and moderate elevation (200 to 400 units) of SGOT.

CHRONIC ACTIVE HEPATITIS

This condition has been described under a variety of designations, including plasma cell hepatitis, Kunkel's syndrome and lupoid hepatitis. Because none of these terms is completely satis-

factory, the term "active juvenile cirrhosis" has been proposed.

Clinical Features. Onset is commonly around puberty, with females predominantly affected. In approximately one fourth of the patients an ordinary episode of viral hepatitis progresses with continuation of jaundice and malaise or the development of edema. In others the disease becomes apparent during pregnancy, after operation or in the course of treatment of another disease. Patients usually appear quite well and are often taller than average. Fever is common, and direct hyperbilirubinemia (2 to 10 mg. per 100 ml.) is constant. The spleen is usually enlarged, the liver less commonly, and spider nevi are invariably present. Many patients have prominent cutaneous striae, and gynecomastia is frequent in males. Females usually have amenorrhea; jaundice and malaise are increased if menstruation occurs. Portal hypertension with bleeding and ascites occurs late in the course.

About 20 per cent of these patients have significant disease of other systems—nephritis, thyroiditis, myositis, arthralgia and hemolytic anemia. Serologic abnormalities, including antinuclear antibodies and typical lupus erythematosus cells, are common. The similarity to lupus erythematosus led to the characterization of this process as "lupoid hepatitis." This classification is probably not warranted, since typical systemic lupus is almost never associated with this form of hepatitis; the antinuclear antibodies in the 2 diseases can be shown to be different by ultracentrifugation, and the typical histologic picture of lupus is lacking. An autoimmune mechanism seems most likely to explain the features of the disease; "runt" disease and liver graft rejection exhibit histologic features similar to those noted in chronic active hepatitis.

Biochemical changes include hyperbilirubinemia and elevation of serum transaminase and gamma globulin values. Flocculation test results are positive; serum concentrations of albumin are variable. Lupus erythematosus cells are found in a minority of the patients, and the Wassermann reaction is usually anticomplementary. The portal zones examined histologically show a dense cellular infiltrate composed chiefly of lymphocytes and plasma cells. Hydropic degeneration and variation in size are seen in the liver cells, and there are many giant cells. Progressive necrosis and fibrosis result in a coarse postnecrotic cirrhosis.

Additional features which also resemble those of lupus erythematosus include skin rashes, pulmonary infiltrates, generalized lymphadenopathy and severe emotional disturbances. Ulcerative colitis may precede or follow the appearance of liver disease.

Treatment. The autoimmune mechanism apparently operative in this disease provides the rationale for corticosteroid therapy, which usually results in clinical and biochemical improvement. It is doubtful whether the basic process is altered, since progress to cirrhosis and duration of life are apparently not influenced by treatment. In some patients who have had unsatisfactory responses to steroid treatment, benefit has been observed with 6-mercaptopurine. Survival in this disease is of the order of 3 to 10 years. Some patients have survived beyond this period, suggesting a self-limited process.

PRIMARY BILIARY CIRRHOSIS

The clinical picture is characteristic, although histologic study late in the course of the disease may not permit a clear differentiation from other forms of cirrhosis. There is early onset of obstructive jaundice, with pruritus, dark urine and elevation in the serum levels of alkaline phosphatase, cholesterol and phospholipids. The liver is markedly enlarged, and xanthomas develop as the serum lipids increase. The course is benign for a number of years, but terminates with hepatic failure or bleeding from varices. The cause is unknown. Reactions to drugs such as chlorpromazine can produce a similar picture. The relation to hepatitis is unclear, but many patients have an early history and clinical course identical with that found in patients with postnecrotic cirrhosis.

The pathologic picture of intrahepatic or primary biliary cirrhosis is a progressive cholangiolitic hepatitis resembling that of drug hypersensitivity and infections with the hepatitis virus. Primary intrahepatic biliary cirrhosis has also been designated Hanot's hypertrophic as well as pericholangiolitic and nonobstructive cholangitic biliary cirrhosis.

In all forms of biliary cirrhosis, itching is a problem. Antihistamines, lotions and starch baths may be of some help. In severe conditions the administration of cholestyramine (1 to 3 gm. orally, 4 times daily), which binds bile salts in the bowel and thus prevents their reabsorption, may be of considerable benefit. In complete obstruction of biliary flow the drug can, of course, be of no help.

SECONDARY BILIARY CIRRHOSIS

Secondary biliary cirrhosis in childhood is the usual sequel to complete or partial obstruction of the extrahepatic biliary system. Less frequent causes in childhood are stone or sludge in the common bile duct, and tumor. It may also be the result of recurrent attacks of pancreatitis. In endemic areas the liver fluke, *Clonorchis sinensis,* may be responsible for a similar process.

THE LIVER IN ULCERATIVE COLITIS

Involvement of the liver may take various forms in ulcerative colitis. Fatty changes are the most frequent and appear in the periphery of the lobule and progress centrally. This alteration results from undernutrition secondary to anorexia, ane-

mia and intestinal loss of protein. *Postnecrotic cirrhosis* is common and probably is the result of serum hepatitis due to transfusion or other parenteral injections. *Pericholangitis* may result from portal toxemia and bacteremia arising from the inflamed colon. It may be benefited by prolonged treatment with a broad-spectrum antibiotic. *Chronic intrahepatic cholestasis* has also been described; the clinical picture resembles that of primary biliary cirrhosis.

CONGESTIVE DISTURBANCES

Cardiac failure is the principal cause of passive congestion of the liver. Though acute myocardial decompensation such as that associated with the crises of hemolytic anemias and with hypertensive acute glomerulonephritis will produce temporary passive hyperemia of the liver, more striking changes result from the prolonged passive congestion associated with chronic disease of the heart. Long-standing pulmonary disease with stasis in the right side of the heart will also engorge the liver. Occasionally a collection of pleural fluid or a thoracic tumor, by compressing the inferior vena cava, may retard the return of blood from the liver.

As the liver becomes congested, the central veins are distended, but the liver cords remain intact. With continuation of the hyperemia the liver cells surrounding the central vein undergo degenerative changes due to anoxemia and become atrophic, giving the liver the appearance described as the nutmeg liver.

The large, firm liver of either of these 2 stages may result in some pain or tenderness in the hepatic region. Subclinical or mild jaundice may be present.

With long-standing and particularly with recurrent episodes of congestive cardiac failure, cirrhosis may occur. Cirrhosis of this origin is rare in childhood.

Veno-occlusive disease of Jamaican children is associated with cirrhosis. It is believed to be due to prolonged ingestion of toxic substances in "bush teas" which contain Senecio alkaloids. This condition is discussed in relation to Indian childhood cirrhosis (p. 845).

FAMILIAL HEPATIC DISEASES

DEVELOPMENTAL ABNORMALITIES WITHOUT CIRRHOSIS

Polycystic Liver Disease. This relatively uncommon disease in which multiple cysts occur in the liver is usually associated with polycystic renal disease. The renal component more often leads to symptoms and has therefore been more fully studied. The form in which symptoms occur in adults is inherited as an autosomal dominant.

An autosomal recessive inheritance has been noted in subjects becoming symptomatic in infancy. The hepatic cysts are thought to represent dilated intralobular bile ducts which failed to undergo involution during embryonic development. They are invested with connective tissue which may become extensive enough to obstruct hepatic venous circulation and lead to portal hypertension. When documentation appears indicated, a biopsy specimen should be obtained. Portal hypertension may require treatment.

Congenital Hepatic Fibrosis. This is a developmental disorder marked by irregular broad bands of fibrous tissue located chiefly in the portal areas. Though hepatocellular function is usually well maintained, portal hypertension is often symptomatic and has been ascribed to defects in the terminal portions of the portal vein. Abdominal enlargement, hematemesis or hepatosplenomegaly usually leads to diagnosis by midadolescence. Portal pressure has been elevated in all instances in which it has been measured. Operative biopsy may be required to obtain sufficient tissue for diagnostic purposes. Portacaval shunts have been successful in reducing portal pressure. A relation to polycystic liver disease is suggested by the presence of polycystic kidneys in one of 3 siblings with hepatic fibrosis.

Hereditary Hemorrhagic Telangiectasia (Osler-Rendu-Weber Disease) (see p. 1384). This condition, inherited as an autosomal dominant, is rarely associated with clinically significant liver disease. Hepatic involvement may be of several types: *(a)* telangiectases, *(b)* telangiectases with fibrosis, *(c)* postnecrotic cirrhosis, and *(d)* discrete massive hemangiomas. Postnecrotic cirrhosis without hepatic telangiectases may be related to chronic active hepatitis, as these patients may also have immunologic defects.

HEREDITARY DISORDERS ASSOCIATED WITH CIRRHOSIS

Hepatolenticular Degeneration (Wilson's Disease) (see pp. 418, 1297). This disorder, inherited as an autosomal recessive, is predominantly a disease of young people. Clinical manifestations include cirrhosis; degenerative changes in the brain, predominantly in the basal ganglia; and the Kayser-Fleischer ring, a greenish-brown pigment most prominent at the inferior and superior margins of the cornea.

Two hypotheses have been proposed to explain the clinical manifestations. The first considers the disease a primary disturbance of copper metabolism. A second proposes a generalized disorder of tissue protein metabolism. Neither encompasses all the known facts of the disorder.

The normal adult ingests approximately 2.5 to 5.0 mg. of copper per day. High copper-containing foods include liver, shellfish, nuts and chocolate. Cow's milk contains only small amounts, but drinking water may contain significant quantities.

Approximately 95 per cent of serum copper is bound to a specific alpha-2 globulin called ceruloplasmin because of its blue color. Ceruloplasmin exhibits oxidase activity toward certain polyphenols and polyamines such as epinephrine and serotonin. Maximal oxidase activity is shown with paraphenylene-diamine as substrate. Markedly decreased ceruloplasmin concentration may be present in some healthy carriers of the abnormal gene of Wilson's disease. Serum ceruloplasmin can be measured, utilizing its oxidase activity. Normal values are 36.0 ± 5.6 and 40.9 ± 6.8 mg. per 100 ml. for males and females, respectively. In patients with Wilson's disease concentrations may vary from almost zero to 25 per cent of normal; occasionally, with severe liver involvement, ceruloplasmin values may be normal. Ceruloplasmin values may be increased in pregnancy, infections, thyrotoxicosis, cancer, hepatitis and cirrhosis. They are often decreased in the newborn infant and in anemic infants and in association with marasmus, sprue and nephrosis.

Approximately 5 per cent of the serum copper is bound to albumin and will react directly with diethyldithiocarbamate, a reaction used in determination of this fraction. The albumin-bound copper is responsible for transport of copper from the intestinal tract to the tissues and is the most metabolically active fraction. Copper is a normal component of red cells and exists in this site chiefly as erythrocuprein. In animals deficient in copper, an anemia morphologically similar to iron deficiency develops.

The body of a normal adult contains approximately 150 mg. of copper. Highest concentrations are present in the liver, central nervous system and kidney. Because of their mass, the muscles and bones contain more than half of the body's content of copper. Fetal liver contains about 10 times as much copper as does that of the adult; adult levels are attained by about 10 years of age. Copper is present in small quantities in most body fluids: saliva, sweat, tears, milk and bile. Urinary excretion is usually less than 0.1 mg. per day in the absence of significant proteinuria. Patients with Wilson's disease may excrete as much as 1.5 mg. of copper per day.

An increased copper content of the liver and the brain has been demonstrated in patients with Wilson's disease. In spite of the general decrease in ceruloplasmin in these patients, the serum copper value may be normal, although it is usually decreased. As urinary excretion of copper may be increased in many forms of cirrhosis, its determination may not be helpful in excluding Wilson's disease. The differentiation is best made by determination of serum ceruloplasmin and liver copper concentrations.

Copper within hepatic cells may be demonstrated histologically by rubianic acid, which forms a black precipitate with this metal. Copper deposition in the cytoplasm of the liver cells appears to precede the development of cirrhosis. In the brain, copper is deposited most extensively in the basal ganglia, although the cortex may also contain considerable quantities. The light-scattering properties of aggregates of copper in Descemet's membrane yield the characteristic brown or gray-green color of the Kayser-Fleischer ring.

Aminoaciduria occurs as a manifestation of a diffuse renal lesion. Renal plasma flow, glomerular filtration rate and tubular secretory capacity are all diminished. Glycosuria and increased excretion of bicarbonate and of uric acid are occasionally manifest. Phosphaturia may result in a decrease in serum phosphorus levels and contribute to osteomalacia.

Genetics. The disease is widespread, but most common in eastern European Jews, Italians from southern Italy, and Japanese. A high consanguinity rate supports inheritance as an autosomal recessive. The frequency of clinically normal heterozygous carriers of the abnormal gene has been estimated at approximately 1 in 500.

Clinical manifestations. The disease is apparently more common than has been realized. In addition to unrecognized asymptomatic subjects, some children thought to be suffering from chronic hepatitis and others dying of "subacute hepatitis" are so affected. Previously asymptomatic children may present with massive hematemesis. Uncommonly, the initial manifestations in young adults with Wilson's disease may reflect lenticular degeneration (see p. 1297). Although clinical evidence of hepatic disease may be absent, histologic evidence of cirrhosis is almost uniform. The pseudosclerosis of Westphal is a variant of Wilson's disease in which flapping tremor of wrists and shoulders overshadows signs of rigidity. The Kayser-Fleischer ring is the most important diagnostic sign of the disease. It is often difficult to see with the naked eye, and slit-lamp examination is necessary for its exclusion. The hepatic form of Wilson's disease in which frank clinical evidence of liver disease appears with little or no evidence of neurologic impairment is particularly common in childhood. Other clinical variants include severe behavior disturbances, seizures, hemiplegia and sudden coma.

Diagnosis. The disease should be suspected in siblings of affected patients and in children with manifestations of chronic liver disease not otherwise explainable, e.g. sudden hematemesis, cirrhosis or prolonged hepatitis. In late childhood unexplained tremor and rigidity should suggest Wilson's disease. Kayser-Fleisher rings are pathognomonic. Liver biopsy and determination of the copper content of the tissue are helpful in patients without clinical evidence of hepatic dysfunction. In Wilson's disease, copper content of the liver usually exceeds 100 micrograms per gm. dry weight. A decrease in serum ceruloplasmin below 20 mg. per 100 ml. is almost invariable.

Treatment. The goal of therapy is to decrease the total body store of copper. As a high protein intake increases urinary excretion of copper, a diet high in protein and low in copper is desirable. Potassium sulfide (10 to 40 mg. 3 times daily with meals) is given to decrease intestinal absorption of copper. D-penicillamine (β, β-dimethylcysteine) chelates with copper and increases its urinary excretion. It is given orally as Cuprimine (0.02 gm. per kg. per 24 hours) in divided doses. Toxic reactions are common; they include fever, maculopapular rash, nephrosis and leukopenia. Sensitivity may be transient. In patients unable to tolerate penicillamine, BAL (2,3 dimercaptopropanol), in doses of 2.5 mg. per kg., should be given twice daily in 5-day courses alternating with 2-day rest periods for as long as tolerated.

Asymptomatic siblings with persistently decreased ceruloplasmin values and increased hepatic copper concentrations should be treated as above. In newborn infants delay of therapy for 3 months or so will permit differentiation from the physiologic decrease in ceruloplasmin concentration characteristic of this age. Early prolonged treatment, however, yields excellent results. The untreated disease is progressive and invariably fatal.

Galactosemia (see p. 437). The liver is altered in nearly all patients with galactosemia, and frank cirrhosis is common. Fatty metamorphosis is present in the first weeks of life; later, liver plates are altered to pseudoglandular structures. The lesion progresses to cirrhosis with regenerative nodules.

Cystic Fibrosis (see p. 862). Focal cirrhosis has been found by Bodian in one fourth of 62 patients examined at necropsy, and in almost all patients living beyond 1 year. Cystic fibrosis, although a rather common cause of juvenile cirrhosis (16 per cent in the study of di Sant'Agnese and Blanc), is not often associated with symptomatic hepatic dysfunction. It should be considered, however, in all cases of portal hypertension in childhood and may antedate clinical evidence of pancreatic insufficiency.

Fructose Intolerance (see p. 436). Postnecrotic cirrhosis resembling that found in galactosemia may occur in patients with hereditary fructose intolerance.

Sickle Cell Disease. Sickle cell disease (SS) commonly is associated with significant hepatic injury, which may be of a variety of types: portal cirrhosis, ischemic necrosis and hemochromatosis. Hepatic damage appears to be secondary to ischemic infarcts produced by blockage of sinusoids with sickled erythrocytes, and by thromboses resulting from release of thromboplastin from sickle cells impacted in the sinusoids. Gallstones, which occur in approximately one third of patients, are usually asymptomatic. Viral hepatitis secondary to transfusion and hemosiderosis consequent to hemolysis often contribute to the hepatic damage.

Hepatic Porphyria. Cirrhosis has been observed in all forms of hepatic porphyrias except the acquired form. Fibrous changes, increased storage of hepatic iron and hepatomas may also occur.

Hemosiderosis and Hemochromatosis. The liver is the main storage depot for iron and plays an important role in conditions in which there is an iron overload. Intracellular storage of iron occurs in the form of 2 physically different compounds, ferritin and hemosiderin. These compounds function to bind excessive amounts of ionic iron and make iron available when needed. Ferritin consists of a protein shell, apoferritin, and micelles of a colloidal hydrated iron oxide-phosphate complex. Individual ferritin molecules are not visible under the light microscope and stain with Prussian blue only when present in large concentrations.

Hemosiderin is more complex and contains carbohydrate, protein, lipids and iron. In tissues it is seen as a golden yellow compound containing iron in a trivalent state and gives a positive Prussian blue reaction. It is the insoluble iron fraction of tissues separable by filtration, centrifugation and magnetic means. Hemosiderin granules have acid phosphatase activity and participate in the digestion of cellular material.

Pathogenesis of excess of iron. Increases in stores of iron are derived from administered blood or from increased absorption. The latter may occur with a normal dietary intake when abnormal conditions exist in the intestinal tract. Iron derived from blood transfusions is stored in the reticuloendothelial system. Parenchymal siderosis is not present without abnormal factors which lead to redistribution of iron. Increased absorption due to altered bowel conditions is operative in the siderosis of the Bantu and probably in alcoholics. In both, iron is deposited in the reticuloendothelial system and in the liver, but not in other tissues. In primary and secondary hemochromatosis increased absorption of iron occurs from a normal dietary intake. The mechanism in the former is unknown and appears to be genetically determined. In secondary hemochromatosis the principal disturbance is in the erythropoietic bone marrow. In both conditions there is heavy deposition of iron in many organs.

The following factors influence abnormal tissue deposition of iron: (1) manner of binding of circulating iron, (2) erythropoietic abnormalities, (3) disorders of hepatic cells, and (4) disorders of Kupffer cells.

Transferrin binding. Iron in the circulation is utilized in the marrow for synthesis of hemoglobin and in parenchymal cells for formation of catalase, cytochromes and other chromoproteins. The main utilization occurs in the marrow, and the unequal partitioning is accomplished through the unique attributes of the iron-binding protein, transferrin, and its relation to the red cell precursors of the marrow. Deposition in parenchymal cells may occur with disturbances of erythropoiesis, alterations in the binding capacity of the transport

system, or in increased affinity of the parenchymal cells. Transferrin bound to 2 atoms of trivalent iron adheres to the surface of young erythroblasts and yields its iron; it then returns to the plasma and acquires more iron. The mechanism permits transferrin to take up iron from the intestinal mucosa and reticuloendothelial system, bypass parenchymal cells, and deliver iron to the developing erythrocyte. Adequate operation of this mechanism requires a high degree of unsaturation of transferrin. Saturation of transferrin permits deposition in parenchymal cells before iron reaches the marrow. Unduly rapid absorption of iron, as in intestinal abnormalities, may overwhelm the binding capacity of transferrin and result in iron deposition in the liver.

Abnormal erythropoiesis. The key role of the young red cell in accepting iron leads to increased absorption of iron in erythroid hyperplasia and the opposite in hypoplasia. Defective erythropoiesis leads to failure of acceptance of iron in the marrow; the unused iron returns to plasma and increases the saturation of the transport protein and sets the stage for deposition in parenchymal cells.

The state of the hepatic cell may alter its affinity for iron, as in the siderosis following portacaval shunts. Of even greater importance may be the redirection of iron from the liver to other tissues in hepatocellular diseases.

The iron in the reticuloendothelial system arises from disintegrating red cells and is released to the circulation for incorporation into erythroblasts. In infections, iron is deposited excessively in these cells and is not available to the marrow. Changes in the balance of uptake and release of iron to Kupffer cells may play a role in parenchymal siderosis. All the foregoing factors, hemolysis, transfusion of blood, parenteral administration of iron, increased binding of transferrin, hepatocellular necrosis and altered Kupffer cell function, may contribute to siderosis. The mechanism by which iron overload produces hepatic and other tissue damage is not clear.

Clinical forms of iron overload. Siderosis or hemosiderosis (see also pp. 419, 1058) is used to describe an increase in iron storage without associated tissue damage. Distribution of iron deposits is further defined by the designation "reticuloendothelial and parenchymal siderosis." Hemochromatosis emphasizes parenchymal deposition in various organs and particularly associated tissue damage.

Of particular importance in the pediatric age group is the iron overload encountered with repeated transfusions in patients with chronic anemia. Prolonged iron therapy in patients with anemia not secondary to iron deficiency may also result in hemochromatosis.

Idiopathic hemochromatosis. See page 469.

Progressive Familial Hepatic Cholestasis of Infants. Siblings with a progressive disorder initially presenting with chemical and clinical evidence of obstructive jaundice have recently been recognized. Early histologic changes consist of bile staining of hepatic cells and variable degrees of bile plugging in canaliculi. The process progresses to fibrosis and finally to biliary cirrhosis. Clinical manifestations have included severe itching which may antedate jaundice by months or years. In some instances, however, jaundice may be apparent by 6 to 7 weeks of life. Hepatosplenomegaly, growth retardation, abdominal pain and facies marked by full cheeks and prominent eyes are common manifestations. A number of these children pass large, pale and foul stools. The skin is often greatly thickened as the result of scratching. Death has occurred from as early as the second year of life to the second decade.

Biochemical features include elevation of direct-reacting serum bilirubin, increased values of serum alkaline phosphatase, transaminases and cholesterol. Elevations of alpha$_1$, alpha$_2$ and beta globulins, retention of Bromsulphalein and an altered ratio of trihydroxy to dihydroxy bile acids are usually found.

The itching may be relieved by the bile salt-sequestering resin, cholestyramine.

The cause of the disease is not known, but may be an inborn error of bile acid metabolism, which permits overproduction of relatively insoluble acids, resulting in obstruction of excretory bile canaliculi.

Tyrosinosis (see p. 423). This condition, apparently an autosomal recessive disorder, may present as a fulminating neonatal disease with many of the characteristics of neonatal hepatitis. Evidence of renal tubular morphologic changes, as well as glycosuria and proteinuria, indicates the more widespread nature of the involvement in these cases. A number of cases of neonatal cirrhosis described in the past are probably examples of this disorder. The lesion in the liver may resemble biliary cirrhosis, hepatic cholestasis, portal fibrosis or a focal nodular cirrhosis. The disease has certain features resembling cystinosis and Wilson's disease.

Cystinosis (Fanconi Syndrome) (p. 1367). Cirrhosis may accompany this condition, though the renal tubular dysfunction and hypophosphatemic rickets are its paramount clinical manifestations.

Glycogenoses (Glycogen Storage Disease). See page 440.

Other Storage Diseases. In lipochondrodystrophy (Hurler's disease) impressive hepatosplenomegaly occurs along with other changes in the central nervous system, bone and eyes. Disturbance in metabolism of mucopolysaccharide leads to its accumulation in cells which is demonstrable by histochemical and chemical techniques (see p. 1337).

Hepatomegaly is also prominent in the familial lipidoses of Gaucher's disease, Niemann-Pick disease and familial neurovisceral lipidosis (p. 453).

Amyloidosis. See page 1478.

NUTRITIONAL LIVER DISEASES

Dietary protein deficiency produces 2 types of hepatic injury in experimental animals. One, acute massive hepatic necrosis with postnecrotic scarring, is caused by deficiency of sulfhydryl groups (cystine and methionine) and alpha tocopherol. Its analogue in human disease is the necrosis seen in fulminating viral hepatitis and various kinds of poisoning. The second type, fatty liver with fibrosis, results from the dietary deficit of lipotropic labile methyl groups (lecithin, choline and methionine) (see below). A number of clinical syndromes of human nutritional liver disease, collectively designated as *protein malnutrition* or *kwashiorkor* (see p. 166), occur among native populations of tropical and subtropical regions.

Other identified syndromes include the following: *Protein malnutrition complicated by Senecio (ragwort) poisoning* in South Africa. The Senecio alkaloids are hepatotoxic and are apparently ingested as a contaminant of wheat bread. Hepatomegaly and ascites are characteristic.

Protein malnutrition with siderotic cirrhosis of the liver in native South African children. The iron pigment in the cirrhotic liver appears to come from the iron cooking utensils in which carbohydrate foods are prepared.

Vomiting sickness of Jamaica, probably due to toxic substances in "bush teas" made from the bitter cassava or unripe ackee fruit which produce severe hepatic damage in malnourished children. Severe vomiting after meals, associated with *hypoglycemic manifestations,* characterizes this disorder, which is epidemic in the winter months. Death occurs in many instances in 2 to 3 days.

Veno-occlusive disease of West Indian children (see below).

ROBERT KAYE

INDIAN CHILDHOOD CIRRHOSIS

A greater prevalence of cirrhosis of the liver in children in the tropics and subtropics than in the temperate zones is generally recognized, but in 2 widely separated regions, Jamaica and India, it is sufficiently common to constitute a public health problem. There seem to be certain differences, however, between the types encountered in these 2 areas. The Jamaican cases, known also as *veno-occlusive disease,* have an abrupt onset with acute hepatomegaly and ascites followed by a subacute phase with persistent hepatomegaly, with or without ascites, and finally by chronic cirrhosis. By contrast, the onset of the cases in India is often insidious or subacute, and ascites is a later manifestation. Whereas neonatal hepatitis and biliary cirrhosis secondary to congenital atresia of the bile ducts occur in infants in India as in Europe and America, the frequent occurrence of cirrhosis of unknown origin in many areas of India among children, generally between 1 and 5 years of age, justifies the separate clinical designation, "Indian childhood cirrhosis."

Etiology. The cause or causes for this disorder in Indian children are not known. Congenital syphilis, malaria and kala-azar do not seem to be factors. Poor nutrition has been blamed, but does not seem to be directly responsible, since the condition is infrequent among the poorest classes, among whom kwashiorkor is endemic. Furthermore, progressive fibrosis of the liver is a rare sequel of kwashiorkor.

The similarity of histologic changes in the liver to those in the chronic phase of viral hepatitis and the frequency of jaundice at some stage of Indian childhood cirrhosis have given rise to speculation that some cases of the latter might represent the sequels of viral hepatitis. Unlike the situation in Jamaica, where a toxic alkaloid in the bush tea consumed by children is believed to be responsible for the hepatic changes, no hepatotoxic agent in the diets or medicaments commonly used in India has been incriminated. It is possible that there may be different causative factors in the Indian cases. The common occurrence of several cases in the same family has suggested the possibility of a genetic or an environmental factor.

Pathology. The most constant change in the early stage, as seen in liver biopsy specimens, is damage of the liver cells. Fatty vacuolation of the liver cells is absent at all stages. Cellular infiltrates are often present. In the stage of cirrhosis there is postnecrotic scarring with regenerating nodules. Occlusion of hepatic vein radicles, a common feature in the Jamaican cases, is apparently uncommon in the Indian ones.

Clinical Manifestations. The onset is usually insidious with vague symptoms of poor appetite and slight abdominal distention. The child lacks pep and is often peevish, and growth is retarded. Intermittent phosphaturia has been reported. Occasionally the onset is acute, comparable to that of viral hepatitis. Enlargement of the liver is invariably present from the beginning. Usually the liver extends to the umbilicus within a few months, contracting to some extent in the late stages, when it becomes increasingly firm. Jaundice is common in the late stages, and also often occurs for a short period in the early phase; occasionally there is a history of preceding jaundice.

Fever is inconstant, but never high. At times there is a discoverable cause such as an upper respiratory tract infection, but more often there is none, and the fever seems to be due to further hepatic parenchymal destruction. The child deteriorates during such febrile episodes. Portal hypertension with ascites, evidences of collateral circulation and hematemesis may be terminal manifestations. Splenomegaly and hypoproteinemic edema are also common in the late stages. The clinical manifestations can be attributed to hepatic dysfunction (peevishness, poor appetite, pale stools), to portal hypertension (ascites, tympanites, hematemesis) and to hypersplenism in

the late stages (anemia, leukopenia and purpura due to thrombocytopenia).

The course is from a few months to a year or two; even in the more severe and prolonged cases, recovery may rarely occur and be complete as shown by liver biopsies.

Treatment. Treatment is mainly symptomatic. Although a nutritious diet with moderate amounts of protein and vitamins, including vitamin B_{12}, can be expected to help these children, unusually large amounts of protein or lipotropic substances have not been beneficial. Cortisone has been used with the idea of suppressing fibroblastic reaction, but the results have not been uniformly encouraging. Surgery may be indicated for esophageal varices. Hematemesis may necessitate transfusion, and extensive ascites may require drainage.

S. T. ACHAR*

REFERENCES

Achar, S. T., Raju, V. B., and Sriramachari, S.: Indian Childhood Cirrhosis. *J. Pediat.*, 57:744, 1960.
Jelliffe, D. B., Gerrit Bras and Mukherjee, K. L.: Veno-occlusive Disease of the Liver and Indian Childhood Cirrhosis. *Arch. Dis. Childhood*, 32:369, 1957.

FATTY INFILTRATION

Fatty infiltration of the liver results from deposition of dietary or mobilized tissue fat in the hepatic cells. Various lipotropic factors prevent the accumulation or accelerate the removal of excessive hepatic fat in the experimental animal. Choline and a large number of its chemical analogues inhibit the deposition of neutral fats and cholesterol esters and cause more rapid removal of these lipids from the livers of animals fed excessive fat. Methionine has also been shown to be lipotropic.

Fat is deposited in normal liver cells and, in larger amounts, in damaged liver cells in a variety of clinical conditions. Fatty infiltration of the liver occurs in many metabolic disorders such as obesity, starvation, galactosemia, diabetes mellitus and familial hyperlipemia. It is encountered frequently in chronic tuberculosis and osteomyelitis and occasionally after pneumonia. It may occur rapidly during corticosteroid therapy. Large fatty livers occur in poisoning with phosphorus, phlorhizin, chloroform, alcohol, arsenic and mushrooms, and in severe anemic states in which it is assumed that the liver is damaged by anoxia. Fatty infiltration of the liver is also a common secondary condition in childhood.

Fatty infiltration of the liver should not be confused with *fatty degeneration* of hepatic cells, in

---

*Deceased.

which pre-existent invisible cell lipids are altered chemically and become visible as fat droplets. In fatty infiltration the normal lipid content of the liver (3 to 5 per cent) may increase to 40 per cent. In fatty degeneration there is a change in the cellular lipids with an alteration in the normal proportion between hepatic cholesterol and other hepatic lipids, but no absolute increase of liver fat. Occasionally, with hyperlipemia, the Kupffer cells of the liver will phagocytize fat droplets and become swollen.

Clinical Manifestations. Infiltration of the liver by fat is usually not directly responsible for symptoms or abnormalities in hepatic function. When hypoglycemia and ketosis are present, the hepatomegaly may be confused with glycogen storage disease. The usual clinical finding is hepatic enlargement, which may be extreme in some instances.

Treatment. Reduction of fat intake with a liberal allowance of protein is indicated. Beneficial effects have been described after administration of choline and its analogues (betaine), but are difficult to evaluate.

Acute Liver Disease

POISONING
(Acute Diffuse Hepatic Necrosis; Acute Yellow Atrophy)

Etiology. Acute atrophy of the liver is a rare disease, usually fatal, in which there is an acute, diffuse necrosis of the liver. Though the disease is commonly termed acute yellow atrophy, a red atrophy which is a later stage of yellow atrophy is also described. Different toxic agents are recognized as causative factors, such as phosphorus, arsenicals, chloroform, bismuth, trinitrotoluene, tetrachloroethane and mushrooms (*Amanita phalloides*). Syphilis has also been known to cause hepatic necrosis. Acute yellow atrophy is an infrequent sequel to infectious hepatitis, but the relation is not clear. It is possible that malnutrition, concurrent illness or individual hypersensitivity may be contributing factors.

Clinical Manifestations. The clinical picture is similar to, but more severe than, that of infectious hepatitis. Three stages of the disease are described, but, in some instances, fulminating hepatic necrosis without any prodromes leads to rapid death. The prodromal stage, consisting of constitutional disturbances (fever, headache, asthenia, articular pains) and gastrointestinal symptoms (anorexia, nausea and vomiting), is followed in 6 to 14 days by the icteric stage. In one sixth of the reported cases icterus was the initial symptom. The jaundice fluctuates in severity, but is usually extreme. In some cases death occurs so rapidly that icterus may not be apparent. Hemorrhagic phenomena are especially common during the terminal stage, which is characterized by the occurrence of grave nervous symptoms. Increased muscular irritability is followed by increasing drowsiness leading to coma. Convulsions are uncommon.

The breath often has a characteristic odor— "fetor hepaticus." The liver may be enlarged initially, but usually shrinks as the disease advances. The spleen is enlarged in almost all cases. All functions of the liver are depressed to low levels, and tyrosine is found in the urine.

Treatment. In most instances acute hepatic necrosis ends fatally. Fluids, electrolytes, glucose and protein (plasma and serum albumin) should be supplied by parenteral means to supplement the oral intake. Potassium-containing foods or 0.5 gm. of potassium chloride daily should be given to provide the needs of a high carbohydrate intake. Corticosteroids have had no measurable effect in children.

ACUTE ENCEPHALOPATHY AND HEPATOMEGALY WITH FATTY INFILTRATION
(Reye's Disease, p. 694)

Approximately 100 cases have been reported of a syndrome affecting chiefly infants and younger children which is characterized clinically by fever, vomiting, severe encephalopathic manifestations, including convulsions and coma, often with hepatomegaly and usually a fatal outcome. A nonspecific upper respiratory tract illness usually precedes the appearance of manifestations in the central nervous system, and at times a biphasic course is striking. A nonspecific erythematous rash occurs in about 10 per cent of patients; a varicella-like eruption has also been noted. Upper gastrointestinal bleeding is frequent.

Biochemical manifestations include high elevations of serum transaminase values with only a moderate increase of bilirubin. In about one third of the patients glucose concentrations in the blood and spinal fluid are decreased. Metabolic acidosis, elevation of blood urea nitrogen, ketosis and aminoaciduria have been found in the majority of instances.

The pathologic changes include cerebral edema and fatty infiltration of the liver. In some cases perilobular and focal necrosis with polymorphonuclear inflammatory response was noted, as well as infiltration of the portal triads, predominantly with lymphocytes and plasma cells. Fatty infiltration of renal tubular epithelium, erosion of the upper intestinal tract and small focal necroses within the adrenal cortex have also been observed.

A number of viruses, including reovirus, ECHO virus (types 8 and 11) and Coxsackie (A and B-4), have been isolated from brain, lung and feces in fatal cases. A viral origin seems most likely, but is not established. Some patients have recovered. Treatment is symptomatic.

PORTAL HYPERTENSION

(See Congestive Splenomegaly [Banti's Syndrome] p. 1090)

Etiology. In children, in contrast to adults, obstruction of the portal vein exceeds cirrhosis as a cause of symptomatic portal hypertension. Thrombosis may be secondary to omphalitis in the neonatal period or to cannulation of the umbilical vein for exchange transfusion or other purposes. The development of collaterals in the connective tissue around the thrombosed portal vein is a response to obstruction rather than a malformation.

The hepatic circulation at the time of birth is unique. The ductus venosus branches off the left portal vein and enters the inferior vena cava. The umbilical vein is in continuity with both the ductus venosus and the left branch of the portal vein. Sepsis in the umbilical region may, therefore, spread along the umbilical vein to the left branch of the portal vein and then to the main portal vein. Umbilical infection may spread to the hilus of the liver, where it may also result in portal vein obstruction. Rarely may the normal obliterative process involving the umbilical vein and ductus venosus extend to the portal vein. Anomalies of the portal venous system are rare; obstructive valves in the portal vein, however, have been demonstrated. Fistulas between the hepatic artery and portal vein and between the splenic artery and vein are also rare. Obstruction of the portal vein by neoplastic invasion is uncommon.

Portal hypertension is a common sequel to cirrhosis secondary to extrahepatic biliary obstruction or to postnecrotic hepatocellular disease. Because of the poor prognosis in these conditions, documentation of the presence of portal hypertension is often of only academic interest.

Acute thrombosis of the portal vein is usually followed by spread to the mesenteric veins with resultant diarrhea, peritonitis and intestinal gangrene.

Clinical Manifestations. In portal vein thrombosis, hepatic function is usually normal and the presenting signs are those resulting from portal hypertension. Hematemesis is common and is often accompanied by the passage of bright red blood per rectum.

Collateral circulation between the portal and systemic vessels may be noted on inspection of the abdominal wall; such vessels radiating from the umbilical region are referred to as *caput Medusae*. With development of extensive collateral circulation, venous hums may be audible over the xiphoid or umbilicus. The *Cruveilhier.Baumgarten syndrome* consists of cirrhosis with portal hypertension in association with a congenitally patent umbilical vein which permits development of a prominent caput Medusae.

The opportunities for communication between the portal and systemic circulations are many; these include: from vessels of the liver, esophagus and cardia of stomach to diaphragmatic and intercostal veins; from vessels in the falciform ligament to umbilical veins and from the surfaces of abdominal organs to contact vessels in the abdominal wall and in the retroperitoneal tissues; and also from portal and hemorrhoidal veins to pulmonary ones. Because most of the collateral vessels enter the azygos vein, a widened mediastinum may be demonstrated by tomography.

Of the varicosities accompanying portal hypertension, those arising in the esophagus and stomach are the most important because of their tendency to bleed massively (see below).

Pancytopenia (Banti's syndrome) related to the enlarged spleen is common (see Congestive Splenomegaly, p. 1090).

Ascites has generally not been considered to result from portal hypertension alone, though it has been recognized as a consequence of hemorrhage resulting in hypoproteinemia in association with extrahepatic portal obstruction without cirrhosis.

Diagnosis. Radiographic demonstration of esophageal varices is the simplest and safest means of establishing the presence of collateral circulation secondary to portal hypertension. The mucosa of the normal esophagus appears on contrast study to exhibit long, narrow, evenly spaced lines; these may be displaced by varices which appear as filling defects. Esophagoscopy entails some risk and is usually unnecessary for diagnosis. Under direct vision, varices appear as blue, rounded projections beneath the mucosa.

Measurement of intrasplenic pressure percutaneously yields a good approximation of the portal venous pressure. Portal venous pressure is normally about 7 mm. Hg, and the presinusoidal pressure determined in the spleen is slightly above this value. Determination of the elevated intrasplenic pressure also provides a baseline for evaluating the effectiveness of shunting procedures.

Splenic venography should be carried out, but demonstration of collaterals alone does not establish the presence of portal hypertension, since the collaterals may effectively decompress the portal system. Demonstration of normal wedged hepatic vein pressure with elevated intrasplenic pressure establishes the site of the vascular obstruction in the extrahepatic portion of the portal vein. This procedure is not often necessary in children, since the distinction between intrahepatic and extrahepatic portal vein obstruction is readily made on clinical and biochemical grounds.

In a normal splenoportogram the opaque medium reaches the liver in 2 to 3 seconds, and the only vessels seen are the splenic and portal veins. The procedure is useful in investigating the cause of intestinal bleeding and essential before carrying out anastomosis between portal and systemic circulations. It is also of value in the investigation of splenomegaly and in the delineation of liver masses.

Umbilical vein catheterization has been utilized as an alternate method for visualization of portal vein collaterals and determination of portal venous pressure. It can be carried out under local anesthesia and avoids the occasional occurrence of splenic rupture which may follow percutaneous splenoportography. The cordlike umbilical vein is located by extraperitoneal separation of the leaves of the falciform ligament midway between the umbilicus and xiphoid. The vessel is dilated and cannulated to its entrance into the left portal vein. A catheter is inserted, and radiologic and manometric studies are carried out. The procedure is of value in patients who have had a splenectomy.

Intrahepatic presinusoidal portal hypertension without elevation of wedged hepatic vein pressure has been encountered in schistosomiasis, congenital hepatic fibrosis and in infiltrations of the portal tracts with primitive hematopoietic tissue, as in myeloproliferative disease, myeloid leukemia, Hodgkin's disease and sarcoid.

In cirrhosis with portal hypertension, hepatic wedged pressure is also elevated, giving rise to the designation of "postsinusoidal intrahepatic portal hypertension." Connective tissue proliferation in the portal tracts may lead to anastomoses between portal and hepatic vein radicles (internal Eck-fistulas). In cirrhosis the main obstruction is to outflow from the hepatic vein which may remain elevated even after successful shunting procedures. In veno-occlusive disease, phlebitis of minute hepatic vein radicles also results in postsinusoidal intrahepatic portal hypertension.

Obstruction to the main hepatic veins by cardiac failure or constrictive pericarditis results in postsinusoidal extrahepatic portal hypertension.

Acute thrombosis of the hepatic vein may be followed by tender enlargement of the liver and in severe cases by shock, coma and death. In more chronic instances massive ascites, mild to moderate splenomegaly, slight jaundice and upper abdominal collateral veins are seen. Hematemesis from bleeding esophageal varices often occurs. This syndrome can be differentiated from one secondary to cardiac failure by normal venous pressure and circulation time. The enlargement of the liver serves to distinguish it from thrombosis of the portal vein. Laboratory findings are those of hepatic failure.

Primary portal hypertension has been described; it may be the result of excessive blood flow through an enlarged spleen.

Treatment. In infants and children with portal hypertension secondary to cirrhosis the prognosis of the underlying liver disease is often so poor as to contraindicate surgical treatment. In patients with Wilson's disease who have massive esophageal bleeding, amelioration of the portal hypertension by surgery may be indicated in view of the expected improvement in the hepatic disease with penicillamine treatment.

Extrahepatic portal obstruction leading to symptomatic portal hypertension requires careful consideration of operative intervention. There are a number of reasons for conservatism in relation to a surgical approach. The surgical problems are more difficult in young children because of the small size of vessels available for portal to systemic vein anastomosis. If bleeding is adequately controlled, the normal hepatic functions of these patients enable them to tolerate recurrent hemorrhages. A further basis for conservatism in respect to shunting procedures in children is the observation that variceal bleeding may cease spontaneously after repeated episodes. These considerations make the delay of surgical intervention until at least 4 to 6 years of age or older a reasonable course in most instances. Unfortunately, hemorrhage leading to peripheral circulatory failure with consequent cerebral hypoxia may result in brain damage.

In most instances of portal hypertension secondary to portal vein thrombosis the vessel is completely involved and thus unsuitable for anastomosis. Nevertheless patent proximal segments of the vessel may be seen by venography and used for anastomosis to the inferior vena cava. The portal vein branch most used for relief of portal hypertension in children is the splenic vein, which is anastomosed to the left renal vein, and the spleen is removed. Unfortunately, the splenic vein may be unsuitable because of size, extension of thrombosis, perisplenitis involving the vessels at the splenic pedicle, previous splenectomy or thrombosis of a previously attempted splenorenal shunt. It should be emphasized that splenectomy without a shunt procedure should not be done for obstruction of the portal vein, because it is ineffective in relieving portal hypertension and sacrifices the vessel most useful in definitive shunting procedures. Alternative approaches have been devised when the splenic vein is unsuitable for anastomosis.

ESOPHAGEAL AND GASTRIC VARICES

The clinical features are those of gastrointestinal bleeding with the added manifestations of portal hypertension. The bleeding may be slow and productive of melena, anemia and increased red cell production. It may also be heralded by massive hematemesis; bleeding may continue for days until controlled by treatment. In contrast to patients with portal hypertension caused by thrombosis of the portal vein with intact hepatic function, those with cirrhosis tolerate hemorrhage poorly.

When the source of bleeding is in doubt, a water-soluble barium solution may be used in the presence of bleeding to establish its site. The Sengs-taken tube, for compression of varices, may be used diagnostically as well as therapeutically. In obscure situations splenic venography may be used to detect varices.

In emergency treatment of bleeding varices, transfusion of whole blood, preferably guided by measurement of blood volume, is indicated. Esophageal tamponade with the Sengstaken tube, a three-lumen tube connected to balloons placed in the esophagus and upper part of the stomach and permitting aspiration of blood from the stomach, will usually control bleeding. The gastric balloon is filled with radiopaque material in order to verify by radiography its proper placement. The balloons are distended to a pressure of approximately 30 mm. Hg, and traction is applied over a pulley. The technique has the disadvantage of being uncomfortable and of giving rise to ulceration of the esophagus and pharynx.

Paracentesis to relieve tense ascites may be helpful in lowering portal pressure, and mannitol diuresis may also be useful. Failure of these measures is an indication for surgical ligation of varices prior to more definitive shunting procedures.

CYSTS

Conditions which may simulate hepatic cyst include hydrops of the gallbladder, choledochal cyst, hydronephrosis, mesenteric cyst, duplication of the intestine and tuberculous peritonitis.

Hepatic cysts are relatively uncommon in chil-dren. They have been classified by Jones as follows:

    A. Parasitic
        1. Echinococcal
    B. Nonparasitic
        1. Solitary — retention
        2. Multiple — polycystic disease
        3. Cystadenoma — proliferative
        4. Pseudocyst — degenerative
        5. Teratomas
        6. Lymphatic — lymphangiomatous
        7. Endothelial — ciliated epithelial

Large cysts may be manifest by abdominal enlargement and vague gastrointestinal symptoms. Displacement of adjacent structures may be apparent on contrast medium studies of the upper gastrointestinal tract. The echinococcal cysts are under relatively high tension, and the cyst wall characteristically exhibits circular calcification roentgenographically. Nonparasitic cysts have a predilection for the anteroinferior surface of the right lobe of the liver and may grow intrahepatically or extrahepatically. They are responsible for little or no impairment of liver function.

Treatment is by elective surgery, although bleeding into or rupture of the cyst may make surgical intervention an urgent matter. A plane for excision can usually be established between the fibrous layers of the cyst wall and the liver substance. When resection is not feasible, simple drainage or marsupialization is usually effective in causing regression of the cyst (see also echinococcal cyst, p. 730).

NEOPLASMS
See page 1450.

The Gallbladder

The gallbladder in the newborn infant is elongated, deeply embedded in the liver, and usually does not reach the liver edge. It gradually assumes its pear shape in later infancy. The volume is approximately 3.0 ml. in the young infant, 40 ml. in the adult.

Congenital Anomalies. Congenital anomalies of the gallbladder are rare. It may be bilobed or duplicated, or it may be absent with or without atresia of the extrahepatic ducts. Other anomalies include diverticulum, the so-called floating gallbladder, which is suspended from the liver by a mesentery and is freely movable, and various other malpositions, which may be left-sided, intrahepatic or retrodisplaced.

Cholecystitis. Acute inflammation of the gallbladder, though uncommon in childhood, is not as rare as it is generally thought to be. It may accompany a variety of acute infections, including bacterial pneumonia, meningitis, peritonitis and typhoid fever. The symptoms are nausea,

vomiting, fever, abdominal distention and pain in the right upper quadrant. In some instances the gallbladder may be palpable as a tense, excruciatingly tender mass in the right upper quadrant. The diagnosis is not easily made, since most pain in the right upper quadrant in children is not of gallbladder origin. In many instances a preoperative diagnosis of intestinal obstruction is made. With advancing symptoms, surgery is advisable, although with treatment of the associated infection, symptoms and signs often diminish rapidly.

Cholelithiasis. Biliary calculi are infrequent in early life, but are more common than infection of the gallbladder. Calculi have been reported in stillborn fetuses. In Ullen's series of 30 proved cases of cholecystitis in children, 43 per cent were jaundiced and 57 per cent exhibited stones. In 7 per cent of his cases the stone was in the common bile duct. Cholelithiasis in childhood occurs most frequently as a complication of the congenital hemolytic anemias in white children and sickle cell anemia in Negroes, though relatively few children with hemolytic diseases have gallstones. Though the stones are composed almost entirely of the excessive blood pigment liberated by hemolysis, calcium is deposited in some, yielding a shadow visible roentgenographically. Pure pigment stones cast no shadow and are demonstrable only by the use of contrast medium. Even gallstones associated with idiopathic cholecystitis in

children may fail to be visible by such means. Harris and Caffey have achieved good visualization in infants over 11 months of age with iopanoic acid (Telepaque) in a dose of 0.15 gm. per kg. In older children, 4 to 6 tablets are given in the evening with a fat-free meal, and films are taken the following morning. If the gallbladder is not visible, the dose is repeated and films are taken again in 6 to 8 hours. The treatment of symptomatic cholelithiasis is surgical.

The Bile Ducts

CYSTIC DILATATION AND PERFORATION
(CHOLEDOCHUS CYST)

Choledochus cyst, or cystic dilatation of the common bile duct, is generally considered to be an idiopathic congenital condition. In 80 per cent of recorded cases the patients are girls less than 10 years of age. Often there is no demonstrable mechanical obstruction. The dilatation is usually localized to the common duct, in contradistinction to the dilatation resulting from obstruction which involves the entire biliary tract and usually the gallbladder. Occasionally the dilatation may involve the cystic and hepatic ducts. Lee and Mitchell have described bile peritonitis in infants secondary to perforation of the common bile duct and have related the latter to the development of choledochal cysts. Exudate and fibrosis at the site of perforation may presumably result in formation of a bile-containing sac. A choledochus cyst may grow to large dimensions; cysts with a capacity of 2 liters are recorded.

The clinical manifestations of choledochus cyst are pain, jaundice and abdominal tumor. The liver may become enlarged and cirrhotic, and frequently there is cholangitis. Fever is indicative of infection. The pain is in the upper abdominal or umbilical region and is usually "dragging." Jaundice may be present.

Prolonged obstructive jaundice associated with high serum alkaline phosphatase values of 35 to 50 Bodansky units is suggestive of choledochal cyst or other incomplete obstruction to the common bile duct, as by stenosis or tumor. Direct radiographic visualization by oral or intravenous cholangiography may be diagnostic. Demonstration of distortion or impression on the duodenal loop by examination of the upper gastrointestinal tract with barium contrast material is suggestive of obstruction of the common duct and dilatation secondary to intrinsic disease or to infiltrative disease of the pancreas.

Treatment is surgical. The operation of choice is a primary anastomosis between the biliary system and the intestinal tract. The results following operation are usually good.

ATRESIA OF THE EXTRAHEPATIC BILE DUCTS

Etiology. Biliary atresia is generally thought to result from maldevelopment. In early fetal life the liver and its ductal system develop from a diverticulum from the ventral floor of the endodermal foregut.

The bile ducts and the gallbladder originate from the caudate portion; the liver proper arises from the cephalad portion. The ducts are initially patent, but become obliterated by epithelial proliferation and form solid cords. With further development the cords are recanalized. Failure of this last phase may involve all or part of the extrahepatic biliary tree and result in the clinical condition of biliary atresia.

It has also been suggested that biliary atresia may represent an acquired lesion related to neonatal hepatitis. This relationship is suggested because biliary atresia has rarely been found in stillborn infants and occurs only rarely in premature infants and also because some infants with histologic evidence of giant cell transformation have obstruction of the extrahepatic bile ducts.

Pathology. The tissues are deeply bile-stained, and the liver is enlarged and firm. During the first 4 to 6 months of life these changes become progressively more notable. Histologically, there is strikingly little distortion of the normal architecture of the hepatic plates. The outstanding feature is the extensive fibrosis within the portal triads, in which proliferating bile ducts are embedded. These changes have been noted in tissue obtained by needle biopsy during the first month of life. With progress in fibrosis and the development of cirrhosis there is interference with portal circulation and development of portal hypertension. The spleen becomes enlarged, and during the second half of the first year of life esophageal varices, ascites and the hematologic changes of hypersplenism make their appearance. In cases of long duration the bones may show osteomalacia as a result of the impaired absorption of calcium.

Effective surgical correction depends upon the presence of a patent portion of the extrahepatic ductal system in continuity with the intrahepatic biliary tree. This favorable circumstance has been reported to occur in 4 to 50 per cent of cases; its actual frequency is probably closer to the lower figure.

Clinical Manifestations. Jaundice and hepatomegaly are the most striking signs, but may not be detected for several weeks after birth. The hyperbilirubinemia is predominantly of the conjugated variety. The concentration of bilirubin in the serum is usually below 10 mg. per 100 ml. during the first 6 to 8 weeks of life, after which it steadily increases. Growth is impaired, especially in the latter part of the first year of life. The general appearance of well-being of these infants in the early phase is in striking contrast to their deep icterus. In the second half of the first year of life nutritional failure to the point of cachexia is common. Signs of portal hypertension and the manifestations of liver cell failure with hypoproteinemic edema, bleeding secondary to prothrombin deficiency and hyperammoniemia occur during this period. At this time the infants present a pathetic, irritable appearance with a skin color of greenish gray or bronze.

The stools are putty-like in consistency and white or clay-colored. Small amounts of bile pigments may be excreted on the surface of the stool. These are derived from intestinal secretions and epithelium and are responsible in the minority of patients for paradoxically positive reactions for urobilinogen (stercobilinogen) in the presence of complete obstruction of the extrahepatic biliary system.

The urine is always dark, resembling strong tea in color, and contains large amounts of direct-reacting bilirubin and bile salts. Urobilinogen is usually absent from the urine, as would be expected with exclusion of bilirubin from the intestinal tract, but occasionally may be present in small amounts if bilirubin enters the bowel with intestinal secretions and desquamated cells.

Laboratory Data. There is a moderate anemia, and a steady increase in the conjugated hyperbilirubinemia. Transaminase values in the serum are elevated, but in most instances remain below 400 units, and the serum leucine amino peptidase is usually elevated above 250 units. Serum alkaline phosphatase is also moderately elevated. Early in the course of the disease prothrombin concentrations are maintained in the normal range. When low values occur, correction is usually possible by parenteral administration of vitamin K until the late stage when hepatic cellular failure has developed.

Diagnosis. Congenital malformation of the bile ducts must be differentiated from other causes of obstructive jaundice in early infancy. The principal problem is differentiation from neonatal hepatitis (see p. 834 for suggested plan of study). Occasionally an infant with the early manifestations of biliary atresia will, during operative cholangiography, expel a mucous plug from the common duct, which is followed by complete clearing of symptoms.

Prior to the general use of exchange transfusion in the treatment of erythroblastosis fetalis, some affected infants had a prolonged episode of obstructive jaundice which was inappropriately labeled "the inspissated bile syndrome" on the assumption that the obstruction was related to excessive excretion of bilirubin. Now this syndrome, which results from hepatocellular injury associated with hemolysis rather than mechanical obstruction, has nearly disappeared.

Other relatively uncommon processes associated with prolonged obstructive jaundice in infancy include choledochal cyst, hepatic tumors (primary or metastatic), lymphomas, reticuloendothelioses, galactosemia, fructose intolerance and tyrosinosis. These are discussed elsewhere.

Management. When a portion of the extrahepatic biliary tree is demonstrated by cholangiography to be patent, surgical correction of the obstruction is mandatory. Interposition of a segment of small intestine between the biliary tree and small intestine will usually prevent pyogenic bacterial cholangitis due to ascending infection.

The demonstration at necropsy of potentially operable lesions not detected at laparotomy and the occasional necropsy evidence of impressive dilatation of portions of the intrahepatic biliary system suggest that in patients found to be inoperable initially, a second operative procedure should be considered after several months. Late dilatation of intrahepatic bile ducts may explain some of the reports of successful treatment of biliary atresia with implantation of tubes into the substance of the liver. Experience with liver transplantation is in the experimental stage.

For the infant with an inoperable lesion, symptomatic treatment should be provided. Vitamin K in a daily oral dose of 5 mg. may delay bleeding due to hypoprothrombinemia. The administration of vitamin D in a water-soluble medium in a dose of 1000 units per day will usually prevent manifest rickets. Antihistamines and starch baths should be given for itching, even though they may be of little help. Paracentesis for relief of ascites should be withheld in favor of diuretics, as discussed under the management of chronic liver disease.

Prognosis. Patients with inoperable lesions usually succumb in the second year of life. Adequate correction of operable biliary atresia by 3 to 4 months of age should be followed in most instances by satisfactory regression of biliary cirrhosis. Although early corrective operation increases the chances for a favorable outcome, good results are occasionally attained by surgery in older infants.

ATRESIA OF THE INTRAHEPATIC BILE DUCTS

Intrahepatic atresia of bile ducts has been observed most often in association with atresia of the extrahepatic biliary system and especially in infants with an unusually long survival time. It is likely that, in such instances, the intrahepatic atresia represents an atrophy of disuse of structures deprived of their normal function. Atresia of the intrahepatic biliary system coexisting with patency of the extrahepatic bile ducts is possible in view of the separate origin of the 2 portions of the biliary system from the cephalad and caudate portions of the foregut diverticulum, respectively. The outstanding clinical features of intrahepatic biliary atresia are prolonged survival, often to the end of the first decade, and hyperlipidemia with prominent cutaneous xanthomas. Treatment is symptomatic, including that for pruritus. Though cholestyramine should not be expected to be effective when the biliary obstruction is complete, it may be tried when other measures to allay itching are ineffective.

Robert Kaye

REFERENCES

General

Popper, H. P.: *Liver: Structure and Function.* New York, Blakiston Division, McGraw-Hill Book Company, Inc., 1957.
Schiff, L.: *Diseases of the Liver.* 2nd ed. Philadelphia, J. B. Lippincott Company, 1963.
Sherlock, S.: *Diseases of the Liver and Biliary System.* 3rd ed. Philadelphia, F. A. Davis Co., 1963.

Biochemistry and Function Tests

Hong, R., and Schubert, W. K.: Menghini Needle Biopsy of Liver. A.M.A. *J. Dis. Child.,* 100:42, 1960.
Kove, S.: Patterns of Serum Transaminase Activity—Diagnostic Aid in Neonatal Jaundice. *J. Pediat.,* 75:802, 1960.
Kowlessar, O. D., Haeffner, L. J., Riley, E. M., and Sleisenger, M. H.: Comparative Study of Serum Leucine Aminopeptidase, 5-Nucleotidase and Nonspecific Alkaline Phosphatase in Diseases Affecting the Pancreas, Hepatobiliary Tree and Bone. *Am. J. Med.,* 31:231, 1961.
MacLagan, N. F.: Liver Function Tests; in L. Schiff: op. cit.
Nagler, W., Bender, M. A., and Blau, M.: Radioisotope Photoscanning of the Liver. *Gastroenterology,* 44:36, 1963.
Seligson, D.: Biochemical Considerations of the Liver; in L. Schiff: op. cit.
Sharp, H. L., Krivit, W., and Lowman, J. T.: The Diagnosis of Complete Extrahepatic Obstruction by Rose Bengal I^{131}. *J. Pediat.,* 70:46, 1967.
Wheeler, H. O., Meltzer, J. I., and Bradley, S. E.: Biliary Transport and Hepatic Storage of Sulfobromophthalein Sodium in the Unanesthetized Dog, in Normal Man, and in Patients with Hepatic Disease. *J. Clin. Invest.,* 39:1131, 1960.
Wroblewski, F.: The Clinical Significance of Transaminase Activities in Serum. *Am. J. Med.,* 27:911, 1959.

Disorders of Bilirubin Excretion

Arias, I. M.: Hepatic Aspects of Bilirubin Metabolism. *Ann. Rev. Med.,* 17:257, 1966.
Crigler, J. F., and Najjar, V. A.: Congenital Familial Non-Hemolytic Jaundice with Kernicterus. *Pediatrics,* 10:169, 1952.
Dubin, I. N.: Chronic Idiopathic Jaundice: A Review of Fifty Cases. *Am. J. Med.,* 24:268, 1958.
Menken, M., Barrett, P. V. D., and Berlin, N. I.: Bilirubin Production and Excretion, Clinical Considerations. *J.A.M.A.,* 198:1273, 1966.
Odell, G. B.: "Physiologic" Hyperbilirubinemia in the Neonatal Period. *New England J. Med.,* 277:193, 1967.
Powell, L. W., Hemingway, E., Billing, B. H., and Sherlock, S.: Idiopathic Unconjugated Hyperbilirubinemia (Gilbert's Syndrome). A Study of 42 Families. *New England J. Med.,* 277:1108, 1967.

Schapiro, R. H., and Isselbacher, K. J.: Benign Recurrent Intrahepatic Cholestasis. *New England J. Med.,* 268:708, 1963.
Sherlock, S.: Biliary Secretory Failure in Man: Problem of Cholestasis. *Ann. Int. Med.,* 65:397, 1966.
Spiegel, E. L., Schubert, W., Perrin, E., and Schiff, L.: Benign Recurrent Intrahepatic Cholestasis with Response to Cholestyramine. *Am. J. Med.,* 39:682, 1965.

Neonatal Hepatitis

Brent, R. L.: Persistent Jaundice in Infancy. *J. Pediat.,* 61:111, 1962.
Danks, D. M., and Bodian, M.: A Genetic Study of Neonatal Obstructive Jaundice. *Arch. Dis. Childhood,* 38:378, 1963.
Gellis, S. S., Craig, J. M., and Hsia, D. Y-Y.: Prolonged Obstructive Jaundice in Infancy. IV. Neonatal Hepatitis. *Am. J. Dis. Child.,* 88:285, 1954.

Acute Liver Disease

Anspach, W. E.: Subphrenic Abscess in Children, with Special Reference to Roentgen Signs of Transphrenic Infection. *J. Pediat.,* 13:157, 1938.
Bradford, W. D., and Latham, W. C.: Acute Encephalopathy and Fatty Hepatomegaly. *Am. J. Dis. Child.,* 114:152, 1967.
Burnell, J. M., and others: Acute Hepatic Coma Treated by Cross-Circulation or Exchange Transfusion. *New England J. Med.,* 267:935, 1967.
Chalmers, T. C., and others: The Treatment of Acute Infectious Hepatitis. Controlled Studies of the Effects of Diet, Rest and Physical Reconditioning on the Acute Course of the Disease and on the Incidence of Relapses and Residual Abnormalities. *J. Clin. Invest.,* 34:1163, 1955.
Conrad, M. E., Schwartz, F. D., and Young, A. A.: Infectious Hepatitis—A Generalized Disease. A Study of Renal, Gastrointestinal and Hematologic Abnormalities. *Am. J. Med.,* 37:789, 1964.
Havens, W. P.: Viral Hepatitis. Clinical Patterns and Diagnosis. *Am. J. Med.,* 32:665, 1962.
Hillis, W. D.: Etiology of Viral Hepatitis. *Johns Hopkins Med. J.,* 120:176, 1967.
Klatskin, G.: Toxic and Drug-Induced Hepatitis; in L. Schiff: op. cit.
Krugman, S., Ward, R., Giles, J. P., and Jacobs, A. M.: Infectious Hepatitis: Studies on Effect of Gamma Globulin and on Incidence of Inapparent Infection. *J.A.M.A.,* 174:823, 1960.
Kutsunai, T.: Abscess of the Liver of Umbilical Origin in Infants; Report of Two Cases. *Am. J. Dis. Child.,* 51:3185, 1936.
Senior, J. R.: Post-Transfusion Hepatitis. *Gastroenterology,* 49:315, 1965.
Sun, N. C., and Smith, V. M.: Hepatitis Associated with Myocarditis: Unusual Manifestation of Infection with Coxsackie Virus Group B, Type 3. *New England J. Med.,* 274:190, 1966.
Ward, R., Krugman, S., Giles, J. P., Jacobs, A. M., and Bodansky, O.: Infectious Hepatitis: Studies of Its Natural History and Prevention. *New England J. Med.,* 258:407, 1958.

Chronic Liver Disease

Ahrens, E. H., Payne, M. A., Kunkel, H. G., Eisenmenger, W. J., and Blondheim, S. H.: Primary Biliary Cirrhosis. *Medicine,* 29:299, 1950.
Chalmers, T. C.: Pathogenesis and Treatment of Hepatic Failure. *New England J. Med.,* 263:23:77, 1960.
deLorimier, A. A., Simpson, E. B., Baum, R. S., and Carlsson, E.: Hepatic-Artery Ligation for Hepatic Hemangiomatosis. *New England J. Med.,* 277:333, 1967.
Klatskin, G.: Subacute Hepatic Necrosis and Postnecrotic Cirrhosis Due to Anicteric Infections with Hepatitis Virus. *Am. J. Med.,* 25:333, 1958.
Losowski, M. S., Jones, D. P., Lieber, C. S., and Davidson, C. S.: Local Factors in Ascites Formation During Sodium Retention in Cirrhosis. *New England J. Med.,* 268:651, 1963.
Page, A. R., and Good, R. A.: Plasma Cell Hepatitis. *Am. J. Dis. Child.,* 99:288, 1960.
Schiff, L.: The Use of Steroids in Liver Disease. *Medicine,* 45:565, 1966.
Shaldon, S., McLaren, J. R., and Sherlock, S.: Resistant Ascites Treated by Combined Diuretic Therapy. *Lancet,* 1:609, 1960.
Sherlock, S.: Primary Biliary Cirrhosis. *Gastroenterology,* 37:574, 1959.

Sherlock, S.: Hepatic Coma. *Gastroenterology,* 41:1, 1961.

Familial Liver Disease

Bearn, A. G.: Wilson's Disease; in J. B. Stanbury, J. B. Wyngaarden and D. S. Fredrickson (Eds.): *The Metabolic Basis of Inherited Disease.* 2nd ed. New York, McGraw-Hill Book Company, Inc., 1966.

Bensel, R. W., and Peters, E. R.: Congenital Hepatic Fibrosis Presenting as Hepatomegaly in Early Infancy. *J. Pediat.,* 72:96, 1968.

Gray, O. P. and Saunders, R. A.: Familial Intrahepatic Cholestatic Jaundice in Infancy. *Arch. Dis. Childhood,* 41:320, 1966.

Halvorsen, S., Pande, H., Loken, A. G. and Ghessing, L. R.: Tyrosinosis: A Study of 6 Cases. *Arch. Dis. Childhood,* 41: 238, 1966.

Iber, F. L., and Madrey, W. C.: Familial Hepatic Disease with Portal Hypertension with or Without Cirrhosis; in H. Popper and F. Schaffner (Eds.): *Progress in Liver Disease.* New York, Grune & Stratton, 1965, Vol. II.

Pollycove, M.: Hemachromatosis; in J. B. Stanbury, J. B. Wyngaarden, and D. S. Fredrickson, op. cit.

Scheinberg, I. H., and Sternlieb, I.: The Long Term Management of Hepatolenticular Degeneration (Wilson's Disease). *Am. J. Med.,* 29:316, 1960.

Scheuer, P. J., and Williams, R.: Genetic Disorders of the Liver; in H. Popper and F. Schaffner op. cit.

Portal Hypertension

Clatworthy, W. H., Jr., and de Lorimier, A. A.: Portal Decompression Procedures in Children. *Am. J. Surg.,* 107:447, 1964.

Kessler, R. E., and Zimmon, D. S.: Umbilical Vein Catherization in Man. *Surg., Gynec. & Obst.,* 124:594, 1967.

Koop, C. E., and Roddy, S. R.: Colonic Replacement of Distal Esophagus and Proximal Stomach in the Management of Bleeding Varices in Children. *Ann. Surg.,* 147:17, 1958.

Mikkelsen, W. P., Edmondson, H. A., Peters, R. L., Redeker, A. G., and Reynolds, T. B.: Extra- and Intrahepatic Portal Hypertension Without Cirrhosis (Hepatoportal Sclerosis). *Ann. Surg.,* 162:602, 1965.

Mikkelsen, W. P., Edmondson, H. A., Peters, R. L., Redeker, A. G., and Reynolds, T. B.: Extrahepatic Portal Hypertension in Children. *Am. J. Surg.,* 111:333, 1966.

Shaldon, S., and Sherlock, S.: Obstruction to the Extrahepatic Portal System in Children. *Lancet,* 1:63, 1962.

The Bile Ducts

Ahrens, E. H., Jr., Harris, R. C., and McMahon, H. E.: Atresia of the Intrahepatic Ducts. *Pediatrics,* 8:628, 1951.

Danks, D. M., and Campbell, P. E.: Extrahepatic Biliary Atresia: Comments on the Frequency of Potentially Operable Cases. *J. Pediat.,* 69:21, 1966.

Hays, D. M., and Others: Diagnosis of Biliary Atresia: Relative Accuracy of Percutaneous Liver Biopsy, Open Liver Biopsy, and Operative Cholangiography, *J. Pediat.,* 71:598, 1967.

Horne, L. M.: Congenital Choledochal Cysts. *J. Pediat.,* 50:30, 1957.

Kaye, R., Koop, C. E., Wagner, B. M., Picou, D., and Yakovac, W. C.: Needle Biopsy of the Liver. An Aid in the Differential Diagnosis of Prolonged Jaundice in Infancy. *Am. J. Dis. Child.,* 98:699, 1959.

Lees, W., and Mitchell, J. E.: Bile Peritonitis in Infancy. *Arch. Dis. Childhood.,* 41:188, 1966.

The Gallbladder

Flannery, M. G., and Coster, M. D.: Congenital Abnormalities of Gallbladder: 101 Cases. *Surg., Gynec & Obst.* (Internat. Abst. Surg.), 103:439, 1956.

Glenn, F., and Hill, M. R., Jr.: Primary Gallbladder Disease in Children. *Ann. Surg.,* 134:302, 1954.

Walker, C. H. M.: Aetiology of Cholelithiasis in Childhood. *Arch. Dis. Childhood,* 32:293, 1957.

THE PANCREAS

The pancreas contains 2 types of secreting glands: the acinar tissue is responsible for the exocrine secretion, and the islands of Langerhans for the endocrine secretion.

This section is concerned only with the disorders of the exocrine pancreas. Disturbances of the endocrine function (diabetes mellitus and hypoglycemia) are discussed on pages 1155 and 1164.

PHYSIOLOGY OF THE EXOCRINE GLANDS OF THE PANCREAS

Pancreatic juice is collected by a branching system of ducts and conveyed through the ducts of Wirsung and Santorini into the second portion of the duodenum. The principal ferments in pancreatic juice are trypsin, chymotrypsin, carboxypeptidase, amylase and lipase. Trypsin is secreted as a precursor, trypsinogen, which must be activated by the action of enterokinase, an intestinal hormone. Chymotrypsin is secreted as chymotrypsinogen and is activated by trypsin. Pro-carboxypeptidase is also activated by trypsin.

Trypsin and chymotrypsin, acting separately, digest proteins to peptides, which are then split to amino acids by pancreatic and intestinal carboxypeptidase (erepsin). Amylase is secreted in active form and digests starch to maltose, which later is hydrolyzed to glucose by intestinal maltase. Pancreatic lipase is activated by bile salts and splits the neutral fat molecule into its component fatty acid and glycerol. Whereas trypsin and to some extent lipase are present at birth, pancreatic amylase is absent from pancreatic juice during the first few weeks of life. Little provision has been made for the digestion at this time of any other food than the natural one: milk.

Pancreatic secretion is under both autonomic nervous (parasympathetic and sympathetic) control and hormonal regulation. Secretin, a hormone liberated by the mucosal cells of the upper intestinal tract in response to ingestion of food, is transported by the blood to the pancreas, where it stimulates the secretion of pancreatic juice, principally its water and inorganic constituents. Pancreozymin, a second pancreatic excitant, is also obtained from extracts of duodenal mucosa. Unlike secretin, it stimulates the secretion of trypsin, amylase and lipase, but exerts little or no effect on the volume of secretion.

TESTS OF PANCREATIC FUNCTION

Direct measurements of enzymatic activity of fluid obtained by duodenal drainage are the most reliable tests of pancreatic function. Good hydration and a reasonably good clinical condition of the patient are important prerequisites in order to ensure ample volume and enzyme content of the material obtained. An ordinary Levin tube can be used for the procedure, especially in infants and young children. It is important that no openings of the tube be in the stomach. A double-lumen tube can be used to advantage in older children.

Normally the duodenal fluid is clear, watery and of varying shades of yellow, depending on its bile content. Its pH is between 6.5 and 9; fluids of a lesser pH should not be accepted for testing. The volume obtained by drainage increases with advancing age: from an average of 3 to 5 ml. per hour in infants to as much as 6 to 30 ml. per hour in older children. Ordinarily assay for tryptic activity is sufficient for clinical purposes. In a simple screening method described by Andersen and Early the amount of proteolytic enzyme is estimated by the effects of duodenal fluid in varying dilution on a gelatin substrate. More precise measurements can be obtained by viscosimetric or enzymatic methods. Intravenous administration of secretin will stimulate pancreatic secretion, but is not needed in most instances.

Absorption Tests. Pancreatic function can be assessed indirectly by studies of fecal fat content or by fat absorption tests (p. 804). The rise of amino acid levels in blood after ingestion of a test meal of casein or gelatin has also been used as an indirect measure of pancreatic function.

The presence of tryptic activity in stools has been estimated by their capacity to digest the gelatinous coating of photographic film. The value of this test is limited, since proteolytic activity of bacterial origin may be present in stools. Ingestion of honeydew melon, pineapple or pancreatin may also give falsely positive results. Assessment of pancreatic enzymes from the tryptic and chymotryptic activity of fresh stool specimens on specific synthetic substrates as described by Barbero may be more satisfactory.

SWEAT TESTS FOR CYSTIC FIBROSIS

Determination of chloride and sodium levels in sweat is the principal diagnostic test for cystic fibrosis. The eccrine sweat glands number over 2 million in man. Their function is to help control body temperature through production of sweat. The sweat glands can be stimulated to secrete by environmental heat, by injection of cholinergic drugs or by iontophoresis.

Quantitative Sweat Test by Iontophoresis of Pilocarpine. Iontophoresis of pilocarpine, which utilizes a small electric current to carry this cholinergic drug into the skin and stimulate sweat glands locally, is safe, painless and reliable for diagnostic purposes.

The electric current source should supply direct current at a voltage between 0 and 22 volts. The current passing between electrodes is measured by a milliamperemeter which records accurately variations between 0 and 5 milliamperes. A simple wiring diagram for a battery-operated machine has been given by Gibson and Cooke.

The area to be iontophoresed is washed with distilled water and dried. The flexor surface of the forearm is used except in small infants, in whom the thigh may be substituted. Two milliliters of 0.2 per cent pilocarpine nitrate are pipetted on a 2- by 2-inch gauze square placed on a positive copper electrode (1.8 by 1.8 inches in size), which is then applied to the washed area. A negative copper electrode of similar size (permanently covered with gauze) is placed elsewhere on the same extremity, its gauze covering wet with 0.9 per cent sodium chloride solution. Both electrodes are firmly attached with rubber straps of the kind used for electrocardiography. The lead wires are then connected, and the current is gradually raised to 4 milliamperes in 15 to 20 seconds. Iontophoresis is continued for 5 minutes.

A current of 4 milliamperes passing through 4 square inches of skin is barely detectable. But if the positive electrode is not completely covered with gauze or the contact with the skin is poor, the current passes through a much smaller area and gives rise to a burning sensation. In this case momentary pressure should be applied to the offending electrode, or the strap should be tightened.

After completion of iontophoresis, the electrodes are removed, the gauze with pilocarpine solution is discarded, and the area of skin under the positive electrode is washed with distilled water and dried.

A thin pad of dry gauze, 2 inches square (a brand with low sodium content), or a low-ash filter paper of similar size is removed from a bottle, in which it was previously weighed, and placed over the area of skin in which the pilocarpine was iontophoresed. The gauze or filter paper is then covered with a plastic square ($2\frac{1}{2}$ by $2\frac{1}{2}$ inches) and sealed at the edges with waterproof adhesive tape to prevent evaporation.

The collecting gauze or filter paper is left in place for 30 to 45 minutes and then reweighed in the same flask. The difference between the second and the first weights represents the amount of sweat collected (usually 100 to 600 mg.*) In order to avoid contamination of the gauze or filter paper by fingers, a forceps should be used for all steps.

The sweat is then eluted from the gauze or filter paper with distilled water or other appropriate solution and analyzed for chloride by one of the titration methods and for sodium by flame photometry.

Quantitative Sweat Tests by Thermal Stimulation. In thermally induced sweating, secretion for analysis is collected on a sodium chloride-free dry gauze square covered with a plastic square and sealed at the edges with waterproof adhesive tape as described in the procedure using pilocarpine iontophoresis.

A constant-temperature room (90°F. and 50 per cent humidity) can be used to induce sweating. The patient lies on a bed and is covered with a blanket. An adequate amount of sweat for analysis will be obtained in 60 to 75 minutes. Plastic bags also have been widely used to induce sweating; however, several fatal accidents due to hyperthermia have been reported following their use. It is important as a precautionary measure not to use any source of external heat (e.g. electric pads) to increase sweating and not to prolong the period of collection beyond 45 to 60 minutes.

Quantitative sweat tests by thermal stimulation are used primarily for investigation, and the ion-

---

*Amounts of sweat less than 100 mg. do not give reliable analytic results if a flame photometer is used.

tophoresis of pilocarpine is recommended for diagnostic purposes.

Qualitative Screening Sweat Tests. Two general methods have been used to test sweat for screening purposes. In the first the reaction of chloride in palmar sweat on an agar plate impregnated with silver nitrate and potassium chromate is utilized. Patients with cystic fibrosis have a heavy palmar or finger imprint on the plate in contrast to the light imprint of normal subjects. Several simplified modifications of this test using filter paper or properly treated paper have been described. In the second group of screening procedures, the conductivity of sweat is measured; it is increased when the electrolyte concentration is elevated. Various modifications of the conventional Wheatstone conductivity bridge have been used for this purpose.

Each of these procedures has distinct limitations and should not be relied upon for a definitive diagnosis. If cystic fibrosis is suspected, a *quantitative* sweat test should be obtained.

ANOMALIES OF THE PANCREAS

Annular pancreas is often associated with obstruction of the descending duodenum, which it partially or completely surrounds. The condition may cause symptoms in the neonatal period or early childhood or may cause no disturbance until adult life. Duodenoduodenostomy or duodenojejunostomy has proved effective and safer than divisions of the pancreatic ring.

Ectopic pancreatic tissue (pancreatic heterotopia) is occasionally found in the wall of the duodenum or in other sites in the alimentary tract. In rare instances ectopic pancreatic tissue has served as the lead point of an intussusception. If present in Meckel's diverticulum or in a duplication, it may lead to ulceration and hemorrhage.

CYSTIC FIBROSIS*
(Fibrocystic Disease of the Pancreas; Pancreatic Fibrosis; Mucoviscidosis)

Cystic fibrosis is a hereditary disease of children, adolescents and young adults due to a generalized dysfunction of exocrine glands. In fully manifested cases there is chronic pulmonary disease, pancreatic deficiency, abnormally high sweat electrolyte levels and at times cirrhosis of the liver. Absence or only partial involvement of organs or glandular systems usually affected in cystic fibrosis is characteristic of the disorder and leads to many variations in the clinical pattern.

*The description of this disorder is given in this book under The Pancreas only as a matter of convenience and to avoid unnecessary repetition if some of the symptoms were described elsewhere.

History. Before the recognition of cystic fibrosis as a clinical entity, most patients died in infancy of bronchopneumonia; a small number in whom symptoms of malabsorption predominated were thought to have "celiac disease."

Cystic fibrosis was first noted as a separate entity by Fanconi in 1936; Andersen in 1938 gave the first complete pathologic and clinical description of the disorder. In recent years, owing to greater awareness of the entity, improved diagnostic techniques and the use of effective antibiotic agents to increase the life span of patients, the condition is recognized with increasing frequency.

Three distinct phases evolved in the study of cystic fibrosis: (1) The pathologic changes in the pancreas and the clinical effects of pancreatic deficiency attracted the attention of the early investigators and accounted for the name of the disease (Fanconi, Andersen, Blackfan and May). (2) In 1944 Farber pointed out that a widespread defect in mucous secretions could explain many symptoms of this disorder, and the name "mucoviscidosis" was suggested (Shwachman, Bodian). (3) With the demonstration in 1953 (di Sant' Agnese) of consistent involvement of sweat and salivary glands in this disorder, it became evident that cystic fibrosis is in reality a generalized disease affecting many and perhaps all exocrine glands, mucus-producing and others.

Cystic fibrosis, therefore, is not a disease limited to the pancreas, but one in which this organ is frequently, but not necessarily, involved. The name traditionally given this generalized disorder is a misnomer to be used only with the full realization of its limitations.

Etiology and Incidence. The basic defect in cystic fibrosis is unknown, but there is general agreement that it is genetically transmitted as an autosomal recessive trait. Most authors believe that a single mutant allele causes the disease. The overall incidence of the disorder among siblings is one in four, and both sexes are affected with approximately equal frequency, as would be expected from this hypothesis. Its occurrence in more than 25 per cent of siblings in small family groups is presumably due to chance distribution. The finding of the disease in first cousins and the rarity of affected offspring in remarriages of parents, as well as the recent observation that all 11 children of 10 mothers with cystic fibrosis were phenotypically normal, offer additional support for the thesis of a recessive transmission. Evidence is accumulating that homozygotes for the gene of cystic fibrosis have the full disease picture, whereas heterozygotes have no clinical manifestations.

From 2 to 4 per cent of autopsies in various children's hospitals in this country and abroad are in patients with cystic fibrosis. Several surveys indicate that the incidence of the fully manifested disease (homozygotes) is about 1 in 2000 live births in countries with populations predominantly of Caucasian descent. It follows that 5 per cent of the general population in the same areas presumably are carriers of the cystic fibrosis gene (heterozygotes). On this basis, cystic fibrosis appears to be the most frequent substantially lethal genetic disease among white children. All geneticists have been troubled by the unduly high mutation rate implied, especially because a heterozygote survival advantage cannot be demonstrated. Recent evidence from Switzerland and Australia that family size may be greater in cystic fibrosis families than in control ones, if substantiated, would point to greater reproduction fitness as a possible answer.

Cystic fibrosis has a striking racial distribution: it occurs equally in all groups of the Caucasian race, much less frequently in Negroes and principally among those in the United States. Only 4 patients have been reported so far in native African Negroes. A few possible cases have been described in children in Japan and two in children of Mongolian descent in Hawaii, but none from China or other areas with Mongolian population. It should be kept in mind, however, that in some underdeveloped countries with poor medical and public health facilities patients with cystic fibrosis may rarely survive long enough to be recognized.

In the United States cystic fibrosis is one of the most common serious chronic diseases of children. In this country cystic fibrosis accounts for almost all cases of pancreatic deficiency in the pediatric age group, for the majority of patients with chronic (nontuberculous) pulmonary disease and for some of the children with hepatic cirrhosis and portal hypertension.

In the past the disorder was confined to the pediatric age group by its high case fatality rate in infancy and early childhood, but cystic fibrosis is now seen with increasing frequency among adolescents and young adults. Among the most controversial of recent observations are those which suggest a possible relationship of cystic fibrosis to chronic pulmonary disorders in heterozygote adults.

Pathology. In the *mucus-producing glands* throughout the body abnormal secretions may accumulate and dilate them (Fig. 11-25). In some organs (e.g. pancreas and intrahepatic bile ducts) the secretions precipitate or coagulate to form eosinophilic concretions in the glands and ducts and obstruct the outflow of their secretions. Most of the pathologic changes and consequent clinical symptoms (e.g. pancreatic fibrosis and achylia) are thought to be secondary to this obstruction and not due directly to an abnormality of the secretions. The most striking changes are characteristically observed in the *pancreas*, which grossly is smaller, thinner and firmer than normal. Microscopically, the findings include obstruction of the pancreatic ducts by concretions, dilatation of the secretory acini and ducts and secondary degen-

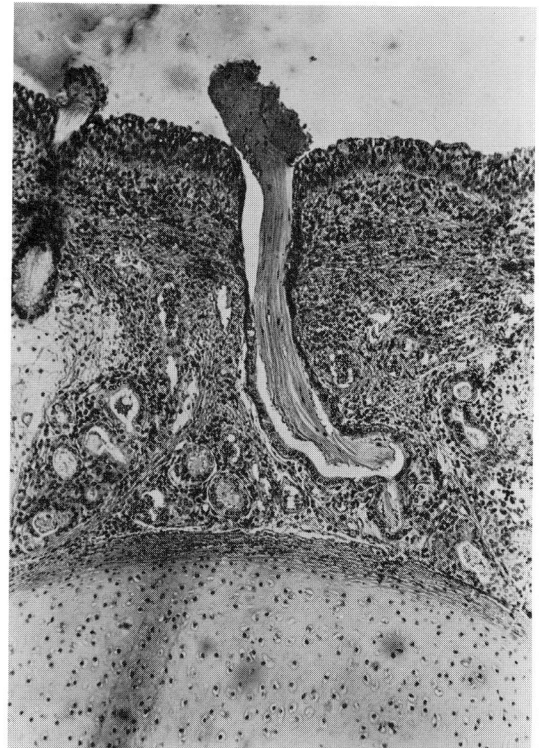

Fig. 11-25.

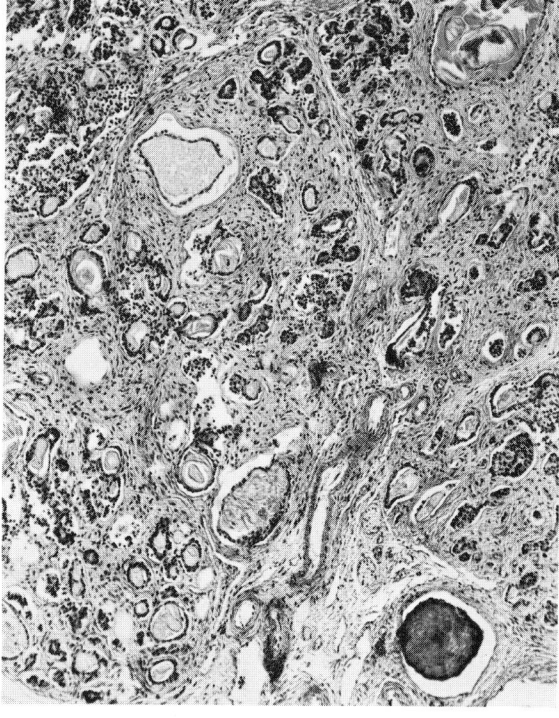

Fig. 11-26.

Figure 11-25. Microscopic section from trachea of patient who died at 6 months of age. Dense eosinophilic concretion obstructs a duct of the tracheal gland.

Figure 11-26. Microscopic section from pancreas of patient who died at 14 months of age. Note fibrosis, dilatation of ducts by eosinophilic inspissated secretion, calcified concretions and almost complete disappearance of acini.

eration of the exocrine parenchyma of this organ (Fig. 11-26). The pancreatic lesions are progressive. In the newborn infant most acinar cells appear normal, although the lumen contains concretions with initial fibrosis and inflammatory changes. After several years the picture is one of pancreatic atrophy with extensive fibrosis or replacement with fat. The entire process proceeds at variable speeds, and at a given age the pancreas of a patient may show different stages of evolution. The islands of Langerhans are usually normal, although they tend to decrease in number and exhibit increasing fibrosis with advancing age. Hyalinization or vascular changes in the islets are generally not present even when glucose intolerance and glucosuria are present.

Submaxillary, sublingual and labial *salivary glands* may be involved, with findings similar to those in the pancreas, although these changes are less widespread. In about one fifth of cases the *gallbladder* is small and contains a firm, gelatinous material which also fills the cystic duct.

Localized foci of biliary obstruction and fibrosis are common in the *liver* at necropsy, even in infants. These changes become progressively more extensive and may give rise to a distinctive type of multilobular biliary cirrhosis with large irregular nodules, at times with clefts. A trigger mechanism (e.g. nutritional injury or viral hepatitis) is postulated to account for the spreading of localized lesions. The onset of hepatic lesions before birth or in early infancy and the different growth rates of scar tissue and liver parenchyma may account for some of the bizarre morphologic findings. The fatty liver infiltration due to severe malnutrition described in earlier reports is uncommon nowadays, although occasionally present even though nutrition is adequate. Hepatic hemosiderosis may be seen in patients not treated with pancreatic replacement therapy. This is an expected finding, since pancreatic achylia of all causes is known to increase intestinal absorption of iron.

The *lungs* appear normal in most infants dying of complications other than chronic lung disease in the first few weeks of life. The initial lesion is a bronchiolar obstruction; later the main bronchi also are blocked by mucopurulent material. Acute and chronic bronchitis, peribronchitis, patchy atelectasis, bronchiolectasis and bronchiectasis are commonly found at autopsy in cases of long standing. Destructive emphysema as such is not commonly seen in patients with cystic fibrosis; rather a diffuse "obstructive overinflation" is usually prominent at necropsy.

Right ventricular hypertrophy is the dominant adaptive *cardiac change* and is probably directly related to the obstructive bronchial disease and pulmonary hypertension. Significant thickening of the arteriolar wall may be present in pulmonary vessels and has been considered a reversible change. It tends to increase with age and is probably secondary to contraction of the arteriolar muscle due to chronic hypoxia and acidosis. Occasional instances of perivascular myocardial fibrosis in scattered areas, predominantly of the left ventricle, have been reported.

Reproductive organs may be affected. Dilatation of cervical mucous glands is usually present in females. Extensive periurethral, glandular and prostatic concretions, as well as varying degrees of testicular fibrosis, have been found in most postpubertal males examined. In 2 recent studies it was found that spermatozoa were greatly reduced in number or that there was maturational arrest of them. Absence of the vas deferens in many instances explained the aspermia.

Considerable deposition of *ceroid pigment* as a consequence of vitamin E deficiency is present in the smooth muscle of the gastrointestinal tract of patients dying after the age of 3 years. Lesions in the striate muscle due to deficiency of vitamin E, however, have never been substantiated.

Nonmucus-producing glands (e.g. sweat glands or parotid glands) show no pathologic histologic changes, although the chemical composition of their secretions may be abnormal.

Pathogenesis. At present no one hypothesis satisfactorily places all the diverse and often conflicting observations into a single rational pattern. In particular, it is not possible to give a unified and reasonable explanation of the sweat defect and of the abnormal behavior of mucous secretions. Abnormal function of the autonomic nervous system leading to overstimulation of cholinergic glands throughout the body has been proposed as a common denominator and is a reasonable explanation for many of the features of cystic fibrosis, especially since this system innervates all exocrine glands. Nevertheless the supportive evidence to date is not substantial.

Glycoproteins. For many years cystic fibrosis has been considered an inborn error of glycoprotein metabolism. The evidence is far from conclusive, however, and further studies are needed to determine whether a structural change in glycoproteins indeed exists. At first attention was focused on the suggestion of Dische et al. that the primary alteration in glycoprotein fractions in cystic fibrosis might be in the carbohydrate moiety in the form of an increase in the methylpentose fucose and a consequent change in the fucose-sialic acid ratio, and some of the subsequent studies supported these results. But whenever detailed chemical analyses were performed (e.g. urinary macromolecules, Tamm-Horsfall urinary glycoprotein, salivary fractions, rectal mucus), no significant qualitative differences from normal values were found, though at times the quantity or relative content of some components was increased.

The recent observation of an interaction between calcium and glycoproteins in submaxillary saliva appears to be one of the best leads at the moment. The precipitation in various organs throughout the body of a relatively insoluble, calcium-glycoprotein complex might indeed explain most of the pathologic and clinical findings in cystic fibrosis, secondary as they are to obstruction.

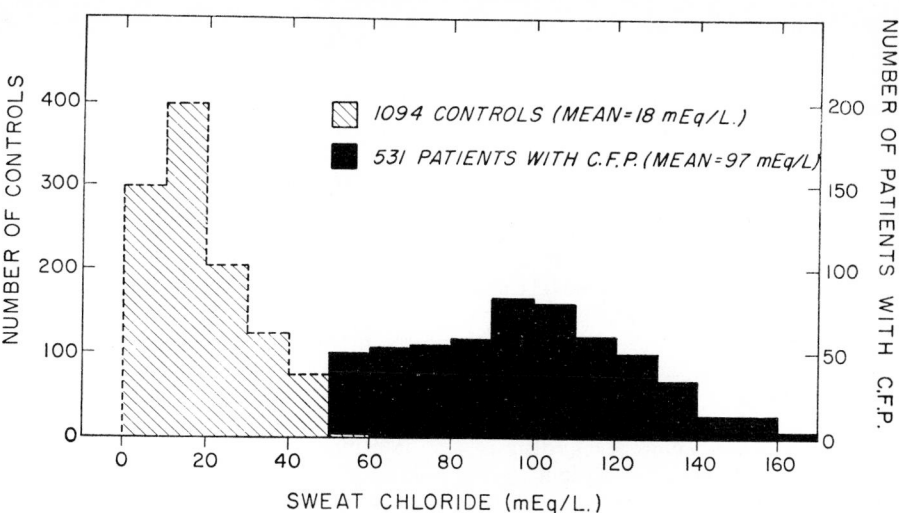

Figure 11-27. Sweat chloride levels. Patients with cystic fibrosis and control subjects. Age range up to 20 years. (From di Sant'Agnese and Powell: *Ann. New York Acad. Sc.*, Vol. 93.)

Sweat electrolyte defect. A striking increase above normal in the levels of sweat sodium, chloride and to a lesser extent potassium is present in virtually all patients with cystic fibrosis (Figs. 11-27, 11-28). The sweat electrolyte abnormality is present from birth and throughout life and is unrelated to either severity of the underlying disease or to involvement of other organs such as the pancreas and lungs; it is the most consistent and easily recognizable chemical abnormality in this disease.

In contrast to the elevated sweat concentration of sodium, chloride and potassium, the sweating rate and most other morphologic, physiologic and chemical parameters of the sweat gland studied so far are either normal or close to normal, including the calcium values and the composition of the precursor solution in the sweat gland coil. A defect in reabsorption of sodium and chloride in the sweat gland duct has been postulated. There is evidence, however, against its being a defect in active sodium transport, since this appears to be normally preserved in many sites throughout the body (e.g. kidney, erythrocytes).

In patients with cystic fibrosis adrenal function is normal, but sweat electrolyte levels remain abnormally high after such stimuli as heat, dietary restriction of salt or administration of salt-retaining steroids, which are effective in normal persons and in the case of the last in patients with adrenal insufficiency. Indeed, it is the dissociation between renal and sweat tubular functions which is a distinguishing feature of cystic fibrosis.

Salivary gland abnormalities. Salivary glands appear to be affected differently according to the glycoprotein content of their secretions.

Submaxillary saliva is rich in glycoproteins and shows striking abnormalities in patients with

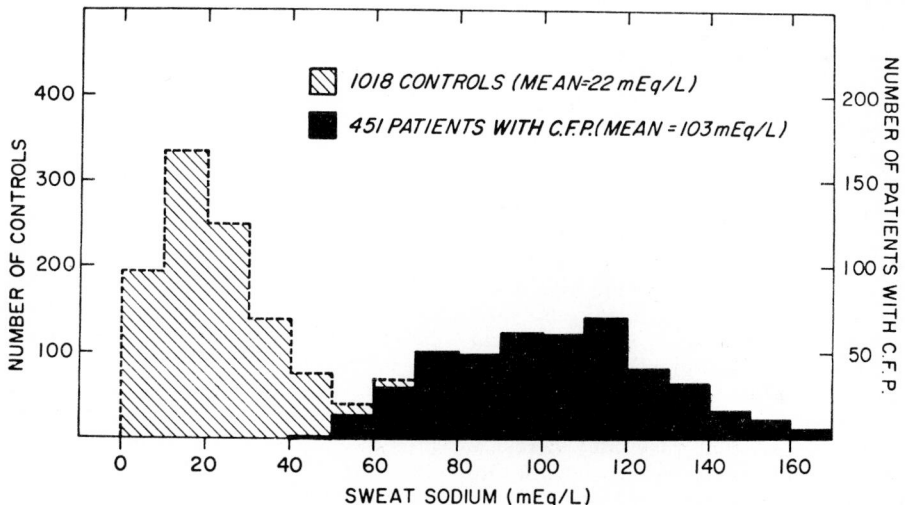

Figure 11-28. Sweat sodium levels. Patients with cystic fibrosis and control subjects. Age range up to 20 years. (From di Sant'Agnese and Powell: *Ann. New York Acad. Sc.*, Vol. 93.)

cystic fibrosis. Total protein, many of the enzymes and calcium and phosphorus values are elevated, while sodium, chloride and potassium concentrations as well as the secretory rate are within normal limits. An interaction between calcium and proteins has been shown to exist and results in an insoluble precipitate which gives a turbid appearance to submaxillary saliva in patients with cystic fibrosis, in contrast to the crystal-clear submaxillary saliva of normal persons.

Parotid saliva has low glycoprotein levels and is not very different from normal, except for some increase in secretory rate and a slight elevation in sodium and chloride concentrations.

Recent observations. At the time of this writing some preliminary observations have been made which may prove to be of great significance. Spock has found that serums from patients with cystic fibrosis and the euglobulin fraction of serum proteins from their parents disrupt the symmetrical ciliary beats of respiratory epithelium obtained from animals and grown in tissue culture. This factor is present in only 1 out of 25 control serums, the expected incidence of heterozygotes in the population.

Mangos has observed that when dilute saliva or sweat from patients with cystic fibrosis is introduced by retrograde injection into the parotid gland of rats, sodium reabsorption is inhibited, duplicating the effect of ouabain used in the same experimental fashion. If a substance inhibiting sodium reabsorption is present in some biologic fluids of patients with cystic fibrosis, it is not clear why it would exert a much greater action on the sweat glands than on the salivary glands.

Recently metachromasia has been observed in fibroblasts grown in tissue culture from skin biopsies of patients with cystic fibrosis. This and other evidence suggest that there is an increase in mucopolysaccharides in these cells; its significance at present is unknown.

Pathologic Physiology. *Cardio-pulmonary involvement.* Bronchial and bronchiolar obstruction by abnormally viscous and tenacious secretions is the primary and cardinal manifestation of the pulmonary involvement in cystic fibrosis. Ventilatory dysfunction is characteristic of the obstructive pulmonary disease, and the increase in airway obstruction parallels the advance in clinical severity. The changes include an increase in residual lung volume and its ratio to total lung capacity, a decrease in ventilatory flow rates and vital capacity, an increase in airway resistance, and uneven gas distribution throughout the lungs.

Compression of pulmonary blood vessels, variable degrees of atelectasis, acidosis, hypercapnia and hypoxia frequently lead to pulmonary hypertension and cor pulmonale. Catheterization studies show that intrapulmonary pressures are frequently increased and that they may decrease with administration of oxygen or bronchodilating agents. The fact that the effects of bronchiolar and bronchial obstruction may be reversible is a strong argument for the use of all methods for evacuating mucopurulent secretions by physical and inhalational therapy, as well as combating infection by the judicious use of antibiotics.

Pancreatic insufficiency. In more than 80 per cent of patients there is pancreatic achylia; trypsin, lipase and amylase are absent from duodenal contents. Steatorrhea and azotorrhea are excessive, reflecting the disturbances of alimentary absorption. In contrast to fats, proteins, though poorly absorbed, are well tolerated, making possible the attainment of positive nitrogen balance through increased dietary intake. Utilization of carbohydrates is less significantly impaired. Variable but large amounts of liposoluble vitamins are lost in the stools.

Recent observations indicate that even in patients in whom pancreatic function is preserved and intestinal absorption is normal there may be a decrease in water and electrolyte secretion by the pancreas, although production of enzymes is not measurably impaired.

Immunology. Except in the respiratory tract, fibrocystic patients do not have greater liability to infections than normal subjects of comparable ages; they are able to develop good levels of circulating antibodies to pathogenic bacteria and have adequate immunoglobulin responses to infection. The fact that the immune response of fibrocystic patients is normal makes their unusual susceptibility to respiratory infection difficult to understand; although bronchial obstruction precedes the pulmonary infection, it does not appear to be the whole answer.

Clinical Manifestations. *Meconium ileus* (see also p. 392). In about 5 to 10 per cent of patients with cystic fibrosis intestinal obstruction occurs with consequent symptoms within hours after birth (so-called meconium ileus); the lumen of the small intestine is plugged by putty-like, grayish meconium, usually near the ileocecal valve. Proximal to it the loops are distended by accumulation of viscid meconium, and volvulus occurs in about one third of patients. Perforation may occur. Occasionally the obstruction is higher in the small intestine, usually from antenatal volvulus. Meconium peritonitis and congenital peritoneal adhesions are not uncommon as a result of perforation in utero.

Chronic pulmonary disease. Chronic pulmonary disease is present in almost all patients, frequently severe and progressive. The time of onset is variable; clinical manifestations may appear weeks, months or years after birth. For some time the patient has a dry, nonproductive cough. Later, usually after an acute respiratory infection, the signs of generalized bronchial or bronchiolar obstruction and secondary infection appear. At this stage some degree of respiratory distress is present. At times it is severe, and the patient is quite ill. The infection may be brought under temporary control with antibiotic therapy, but some degree of bronchial obstruction usually persists. The cycle is repeated with subsequent respiratory infections and may result in a fatal episode.

According to Waring, so-called mucoid impaction of the bronchi occurs frequently. It consists of an accumulation of viscous mucus in one or more bronchi, resulting in their obstruction and dilatation. If the bronchi are irreversibly damaged, the pulmonary disease is progressive and eventually leads to pulmonary insufficiency, resulting in death through various complications within an average of 1 to 3 years. This sequence of events may be much shorter or persist for many years. If permanent damage has not been done to the bronchial wall, antibiotic and other therapy may be effective in keeping the disease in check.

As the pulmonary involvement progresses, compensatory emphysema or overaeration of the functioning alveoli tends to distend the chest, which becomes barrel-shaped. Except over large areas of atelectasis or other consolidations, the percussion note is tympanitic, and rales are commonly heard. Typically, there is roentgenographic evidence of generalized emphysema and bilateral parenchymal infiltrations (Fig. 11-29). Clubbing of fingers and toes is common in chronically ill patients.

Hemolytic *Staphylococcus aureus* is recovered from the nasopharynx, sputum and lungs of most patients. The nasopharyngeal flora has changed to some extent in recent times, probably owing to the common use of antibiotic agents. *Pseudomonas aeruginosa* has been found with increasing frequency, while *H. influenzae, E. coli,* Proteus and other organisms are isolated to a lesser extent. Most investigators agree that colonization with the pseudomonas has increased to a greater extent than with the staphylococcus, especially in the severer and more intensely treated patients. Recent studies suggest that the pseudomonas may not be of great significance in the pathogenesis of the pulmonary involvement in cystic fibrosis and that the staphylococcus is the main agent responsible for it.

Numerous complications arise in the course of severe pulmonary disease. In 5 to 10 per cent of patients *lobar atelectasis* (Fig. 11-30) with collapse of one or more lobes, usually on the right side, occurs early in the course of the illness. Small and multiple *lung abscesses* are common. Sudden death may occur from *asphyxia* due to flooding of the trachea with copious amounts of thick, tenacious bronchial secretions in a debilitated infant or small child. *Hemoptysis, spontaneous pneumothorax* and *mediastinal* and *subcutaneous emphysema* may be encountered, especially in the older age group. *Chronic cor pulmonale* with clinical and roentgenographic evidence of enlargement of the heart and cardiac failure may be seen with long-standing severe and progressive pulmonary disease. *Acute cor pulmonale* with dilatation of the heart may occur during attacks of sudden and severe bronchial obstruction. If the patient survives and responds to antibiotic treatment, the heart may return to its normal size.

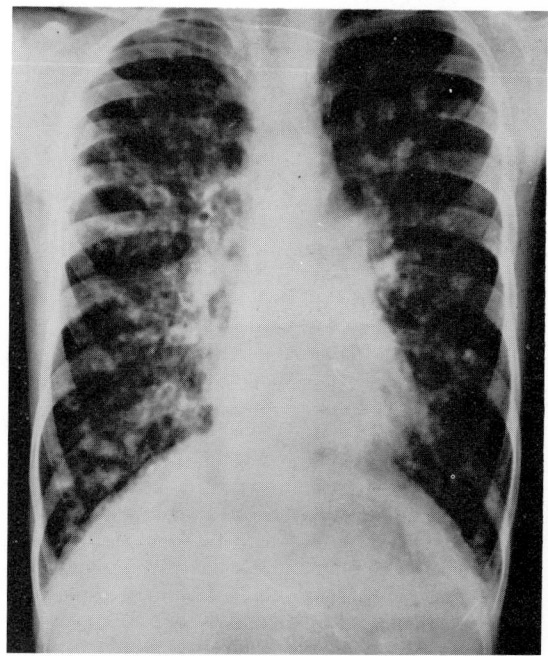

Figure 11-29. Advanced pulmonary disease in a 13-year-old boy with cystic fibrosis. There is a diffuse infiltrate with thickening of the walls of the bronchi and dilatation of bronchi. Note the evidence of overaeration.

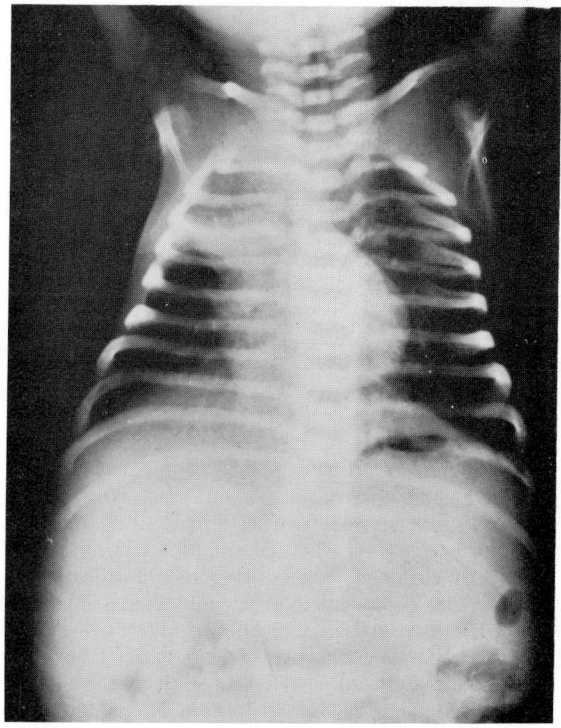

Figure 11-30. Cystic fibrosis in a 2-month-old infant. The lungs are overaerated, and there is evidence of generalized emphysema. The right upper lobe is atelectatic.

Involvement of the paranasal sinuses is usually demonstrable roentgenographically. A nasal voice, postnasal drip and polyps are common manifestations. Polyps often require surgical removal and tend to recur. Two cases of mucocele with complete nasal obstruction and extensive bony destruction are on record.

Pancreatic insufficiency is present in over 80 per cent of patients and gives rise to symptoms of intestinal malabsorption. Malnutrition may be striking despite excessive appetite and apparently adequate caloric intake. The abdomen is distended, and the stools are increased in number, bulky, greasy and foul. In most patients pancreatic achylia is present at birth, but in some children involvement of this gland may not be evident until later.

Because of the large amounts of preformed vitamin administered orally to most children, vitamin A deficiency is rarely a problem, although xerophthalmia was noted in the past. Vitamin D deficiency (rickets) has rarely been seen in patients with cystic fibrosis, a fact not clearly explained. Vitamin K deficiency leading to prolonged prothrombin time and subcutaneous bleeding is occasionally observed. Gordon and Nitowsky have shown that most children have a deficiency of vitamin E; one manifestation is creatinuria, which ceases on administration of the vitamin.

Cirrhosis of the liver. Focal biliary cirrhosis does not give rise to clinical manifestations, even if extensive. Only when there is progression to the diffuse type of multilobular biliary cirrhosis does the liver become hard and nodular. In about 2 per cent of patients there is portal hypertension with splenomegaly and at times hypersplenism, ascites and gastrointestinal bleeding. Owing to the focal nature of the process, the results of liver function tests are often within the normal range, and jaundice is absent or slight.

Other complications. Cystic fibrosis is by far the commonest cause of *prolapse of the rectum* in infancy and childhood. It is more frequent in the younger age group, but occurs at times in older children. Surgery is almost never needed, and relief follows pancreatic replacement therapy.

Regardless of age, all patients with cystic fibrosis are subject to intestinal obstruction due to inspissated or impacted feces because of the abnormality of their fecal contents. Small, hard *fecal masses* are frequently found in the large intestine, most often in the right lower quadrant. They are usually passed spontaneously, though fecal impaction has resulted from such masses. *Intussusception* is an occasional complication, even in children beyond the age of infancy. It appears to be precipitated by adherent intestinal content that cannot be propelled along the gut or through the ileocecal valve. *Adhesions* from previous surgery coupled with the abnormality of the intestinal content also increases the chances of obstructive complications.

Hypoalbuminemia is an occasional complication; there are 3 recognized causes for it: improper absorption and utilization of soybean protein in infancy; decreased synthesis of albumin with extensive hepatic cirrhosis; and hemodilution due to increased blood volume secondary to severe pulmonary disease and cor pulmonale. The last is the most common. In severely ill patients a combination of these factors may contribute to the hypoalbuminemia.

A progressively abnormal oral glucose tolerance curve and eventually *glycosuria* become manifest in some patients. Ketonuria, acidosis or vascular changes are not common as they are in classic diabetes mellitus. Dietary measures are usually sufficient for adequate control, although insulin may occasionally be needed. This inability to metabolize glucose adequately seems to be associated with increasing age and duration of the disease. When such patients are examined at autopsy, the islets seem to be disorganized by pancreatic fibrosis which presumably interferes with their function. This type of glucose intolerance is thus different from familial *diabetes mellitus*, which undoubtedly occurs coincidentally in some patients with cystic fibrosis.

High atmospheric temperatures, especially sudden heat, cause profuse sweating. Since the concentration of sodium and chloride in sweat of patients with cystic fibrosis is closely comparable to that in the serum, *massive salt loss* and hypoelectrolytemia may occur. The accompanying dehydration is made worse by vomiting, which occurs regularly when the loss of electrolytes is sufficiently great; reduction in extracellular fluid volume results and may lead to cardiovascular collapse. Hyperthermia, coma and death may then follow in fairly rapid succession.

Two types of *ocular lesions* are encountered; they may coexist in children with severe pulmonary involvement. Exudative retinopathy is present at times with severe pulmonary disease; the arteries and veins of the fundus are dilated, and hemorrhages and papilledema may be present. These changes parallel the extent of pulmonary involvement and do not appear to affect vision. Optic neuritis with diminution of visual acuity has been observed in patients receiving prolonged therapy with chloramphenicol. Discontinuance of the drug has resulted in variable degrees of visual improvement.

As in other types of chronic pulmonary disease, *pulmonary hypertrophic osteoarthropathy* develops occasionally and may give rise to arthritis and chronic periostitis. At times no symptoms are present, but periosteal new bone formation can be seen roentgenographically in the lower extremities.

Diagnosis. The 4 criteria required for diagnosis of cystic fibrosis are (1) increase in electrolyte concentration of sweat, (2) absence of pancreatic enzymes, (3) chronic pulmonary involvement, and (4) family history of the disorder. Frequently not all 4 criteria are present, but in addition to high concentration of sweat electrolytes, either chronic pulmonary disease or pancreatic insufficiency should be present. In the majority of instances the correlation of symptoms of chronic pulmonary disease and of intestinal insufficiency suggests the diagnosis. Recognition of cystic fibrosis may present difficulties in patients in whom only malabsorption or only chronic pulmonary disease is present. Such ancillary manifestations as malnutrition despite ravenous appetite, history of rectal prolapse, nasal polyps, hepatic cirrhosis, heat prostration in summer, meconium ileus or recurrent abdominal obstructive complications should suggest the diagnostic possibility of cystic fibrosis. The sweat test will be "positive" in all instances. All children and adolescents with recurrent respiratory infections or malabsorption should have a sweat test as part of their diagnostic work-up.

Diagnosis of cystic fibrosis also may be difficult in patients seen for the first time as adolescents or young adults, since they are not apt to present the classic textbook picture of the disease. The criteria for a definitive diagnosis should be more rigid than in children; this is especially so in view of the moderately higher concentrations of sweat electrolytes after the age of 18 or 20 years.

The "sweat test" (p. 855) is the simplest and most reliable laboratory method for the diagnosis of cystic fibrosis. Up to the age of 20 years a level of more than 60 mEq. per liter of sweat chloride is diagnostic of cystic fibrosis, and values between 50 and 60 mEq. are highly suggestive. Values for sweat sodium are about 10 mEq. per liter higher than those for chloride. Potassium concentration in sweat and sodium and chloride concentrations in saliva are not useful for diagnostic purposes. There are few conditions other than cystic fibrosis in which sweat electrolytes may be elevated. Untreated adrenal insufficiency is the most important one; occasionally elevations have been observed with glucose-6-phosphatase deficiency, glycogen storage disease, Pitressin-resistant diabetes insipidus, and, in one family group, with ectodermal dysplasia and sensorineural deafness.

Most children with pancreatic deficiency have cystic fibrosis; however, other causes of pancreatic achylia in this age group exist (see p. 868). All such patients have been found to have normal sweat test results and usually do not have chronic pulmonary disease.

Demonstration of characteristic pathologic changes in specimens of rectal mucosa and of labial salivary glands obtained by biopsy has been advocated as a diagnostic aid. We have not found it necessary so far to use these methods.

Roentgenography. Persistent, generalized emphysema, although not pathognomonic, is highly suggestive of cystic fibrosis. Children with chronic lung disease, but without the signs of generalized emphysema, usually have other disease entities. In moderately advanced and severe pulmonary lesions, there are a variety of additional roentgenographic changes which include disseminated infiltrative lesions of bronchopneumonia (Fig. 11-29), lobular and lobar atelectasis (Fig. 11-30) and widely disseminated miliary infiltrations

often indistinguishable from that of tuberculosis. At times mucoid impactions of the bronchi are demonstrated as grapelike nodular densities.

Changes in the roentgenographic patterns of the small intestine related to motility may be found in patients with pancreatic deficiency as in patients with other malabsorptive disorders. Since similar intestinal patterns are often seen in healthy infants and young children, roentgenographic studies of the intestinal tract are of little help diagnostically in the malabsorption syndromes. A moderate degree of osteoporosis is occasionally demonstrated on roentgenograms of the skeleton.

Cor pulmonale. Recognition of cor pulmonale may be difficult: cardiac signs are usually masked by the pulmonary manifestations; tachycardia may occur as the result of hypoxemia; the liver is frequently displaced downwards by the emphysema, and overt edema occurs rarely and usually as a terminal feature. Roentgenograms, electrocardiograms and vectorcardiograms are unreliable. According to Moss, clinical evidence of severe disease with a Shwachman score of less than 40, a vital capacity of less than 60 per cent of the predicted normal and inability to raise the oxygen tension above 300 mm. Hg after breathing 100 per cent oxygen for 10 minutes should suggest cor pulmonale. As hemodilution is by far the commonest cause of hypoalbuminemia in cystic fibrosis, a level of serum albumin of less than 3 gm. in the presence of severe pulmonary disease is suggestive of increased plasma volume due to incipient heart failure and may appear months or years before demise. In the later stages of the chronic lung disease other evidences of hemodilution also frequently appear, such as low serum electrolyte levels and a drop in hemoglobin values.

Pancreatic deficiency. Examination of duodenal contents for pancreatic enzyme activity as a confirmatory test and to evaluate pancreatic function may be performed when the diagnosis is uncertain (p. 855). For practical purposes *only* tryptic activity need be measured; it is absent in over 80 per cent of patients. The fluid obtained from patients with cystic fibrosis and pancreatic achylia is diminished in volume; its viscosity, although variable, is frequently much increased.

Intestinal malabsorption. Steatorrhea is present in more than 80 per cent of patients who have pancreatic achylia and can be demonstrated by tests described on page 804. Intestinal mucosa obtained by peroral biopsy is generally normal. The decrease or absence of lactase activity in oral biopsy specimens from many patients with cystic fibrosis is unexplained. Tests using polyvinylpyrrolidone and chromium-tagged albumin reveal slightly increased loss of serum protein through the gastrointestinal tract in some patients, not enough, however, to account for any decrease in serum albumin levels which may be present.

Blood chemical studies. Serum electrolytes are within the normal ranges in patients with cystic fibrosis when they are doing reasonably well clinically. When there is severe pulmonary disease, the serum electrolyte pattern is apt to be that of uncompensated or more frequently of compensated respiratory acidosis. There is hypoelectrolytemia in patients with heat prostration and shock resulting from the massive outpouring of electrolytes in sweat. Serum potassium levels may remain within apparently normal limits under these circumstances if the process is rapid, but will decrease if the loss occurs over a longer time. Hypoelectrolytemia has also been observed in infants with cystic fibrosis during cold weather, owing to moderate losses of salt through sweat combined with inadequate intake of salt. Such patients may be erroneously thought to have adrenal insufficiency.

Serum calcium and phosphorus levels are within normal limits. Serum protein values are usually normal in patients in reasonably good clinical condition. Hypoalbuminemia is discussed above. The globulin moiety may be increased by a rise in IgG and at times in IgA related to the respiratory involvement. IgM is generally within normal limits. Tests of liver function frequently do not reveal hepatic impairment.

Anemia is rarely a problem, and serum iron and iron-binding capacity are usually normal except as anemia due to chronic infection develops. Leukocytosis and elevation of the erythrocyte sedimentation rate reflect pulmonary or other infectious processes.

Prognosis. The pulmonary involvement usually dominates the clinical picture and determines the fate of the patient. The effects of pancreatic deficiency are less important to the ultimate outcome, although proper attention should be paid to maintenance of good nutrition, including avoidance of vitamin deficiencies. Infants who survive the operation for meconium ileus have essentially the same outlook as do other patients with cystic fibrosis. Uncontrollable bleeding due to portal hypertension and massive loss of salt in hot weather are occasional hazards in this disease.

Prognosis will improve further as diagnostic and treatment methods become more effective; at present about 50 per cent of affected children succumb before the age of 10 years, over 80 per cent before the age of 20 years, and almost all before 30 years of age. So-called cases of cystic fibrosis above the age of 30 years must be regarded with suspicion unless all or substantially all criteria are met.

Though early diagnosis, early treatment, and aggressive therapy during serious pulmonary complications are effective in prolonging the life of patients, the natural variation in the severity of cystic fibrosis is an important factor in determining the outcome.

As a group, patients over the age of 15 to 20 years are doing better than average, perhaps because their survival depended on the relatively mild degree of respiratory involvement. Males have a slightly better outlook than females, a fact which is unexplained. Despite the handicap of chronic pulmonary disease, many of the older patients have been able to carry on a full-time occupation.

Sinusitis and polyps, abdominal obstructive complications, hemoptysis and spontaneous pneumothorax, often recurring and sometimes bilateral, are common in young adult patients. On the other hand, digestion and absorption of food seem to become more efficient with increasing age, and less dietary restriction is necessary. Although retardation in growth has been considered an accompaniment of this disease, the eventual height as young adults generally approaches normal. Sexual maturation has been achieved, but at times is delayed. There is evidence that most males with cystic fibrosis may not be fertile (see Pathology).

At least 10 young women with cystic fibrosis have borne 11 normal children. Generally the course of the mother during pregnancy and delivery was roughly parallel to the preceding degree of pulmonary involvement. Two mothers died post partum as a result of their lung disease. Pregnancy in association with cystic fibrosis is a challenge in management and a potential hazard to the patient, especially in the presence of severe lung disease.

Treatment. The basic defect in cystic fibrosis is not known, and cure of this disease is not possible at present. Treatment has 4 main objectives: (1) general care of the patient, (2) control of the pulmonary infection, (3) maintenance of good nutrition, and (4) prevention or restoration of abnormal salt losses.

General care. Every effort should be made to permit the child to lead as nearly a normal life as possible. He should be encouraged to attend school if his condition permits, and physical activities should be restricted only as indicated by his tolerance. All routine immunizations should be performed at appropriate ages. Continued immunity against pertussis is desirable, and therefore booster injections are advised. Influenza vaccine and live virus measles vaccine are recommended and should be administered to all but the sickest patients, who may have untoward reactions.

A multidisciplinary approach to the manifold problems presented by the patient with cystic fibrosis and his family is needed. The role of the physician should be complemented by that of the social worker and the physical therapist.

The parents must clearly understand all the therapeutic measures to be carried out at home so that they can cooperate to the fullest extent, and the genetic aspects of this disease should be available to the family.

Cystic fibrosis is not only a medical problem, but a social one as well, owing to the devastating effects of the emotional and financial stresses on the family. Every effort must be made to prevent the fibrocystic patient from dominating the family emotionally and to allay the guilt feelings of the parents, which are apt to develop in relation to an inherited, severe disease. The support of a medical social worker familiar with the problems of this disorder is desirable to allay the family's emotional response as well as to help them to utilize to the fullest extent the resources of the community for patients with a chronic illness.

Control of the pulmonary infection. Active therapy of the pulmonary involvement deserves the principal emphasis. The use of antimicrobial agents and evacuation of mucopurulent secretions by physical methods and by use of aerosol solutions are essential to therapeutic success.

In *patients with severe pulmonary involvement* repeated courses of intensive antibiotic therapy in the hospital are usually indicated for periods of 2 to 4 weeks in an attempt to halt progressive deterioration. Patients with moderate pulmonary involvement should also be hospitalized for intensive treatment of acute pulmonary exacerbations. The choice of antibiotic agents should always be based upon in-vitro susceptibility tests of the bacterial pathogens isolated by culture from the respiratory tract. Large doses of single or multiple antibiotics are recommended during the period of hospitalization. The penicillinase-resistant penicillins and the cephalosporins are the most effective agents against penicillin-resistant staphylococci. Kanamycin and streptomycin are effective against most gram-negative bacteria, except Pseudomonas, but they should be used only when other agents have been proved ineffective because of their potential toxicity. Treatment of pseudomonas infections is, at best, unsatisfactory. Colistin alone or in combination with a tetracycline or chloramphenicol may be tried. Colistin should not be used for longer than 10 days because of its potential renal toxicity. The need for a nontoxic but effective antibiotic agent against infections with the Pseudomonas and other gram-negative organisms is obvious; the initial experience with gentamycin has been encouraging. Carbenicillin, a recently introduced semisynthetic penicillin, has also shown some promise in preliminary trials. Chloramphenicol is an effective agent, but because of the risks of depression of hematopoiesis and of optic neuritis, the latter especially after prolonged administration, its use should be avoided whenever equally effective antibiotics are available, and, if used, it should be only for a short time (1 to 4 weeks). Parents must be forewarned to seek immediate medical advice if diminution of visual acuity appears.

Antibiotic therapy by inhalation is to be regarded as a form of topical treatment and only as an adjunct to systemic therapy. In our experience neither neomycin nor polymyxin B has proved to be especially effective when administered in this manner.

Treatment should also include physical therapy measures to promote bronchial drainage if the patient's condition will permit, and continuous nebulization of aerosol solutions in an appropriate tent and by a suitable nebulizer. Compressed air can be used as a propellant. To penetrate to the smaller bronchial subdivisions aerosol particles must be 0.5 to 5.0 microns in size; hand-operated nebulizers do not deliver particles of adequate size. A small nebulizer such as those used in the treatment of asthma is sufficient for interrupted aerosol therapy, but for continuous nebulization in a "mist tent" a large-capacity nebulizer is needed. Ultrasonic nebulizers which produce a very thick mist are also commercially available. The aim of aerosol therapy is to increase the hydration of secretions in order to facilitate expectoration; among the various solutions used, one containing 10 per cent propylene glycol in distilled water has been as successful as any. In our experience the inclusion of detergents, enzyme preparations and mucolytic agents in the aerosol solution has not added to its effectiveness. As noted above, antibiotics (see Table 11-10) are frequently added for their potential topical effect, not as a substitute for systemic therapy.

When oxygen therapy is necessary, the child should be carefully observed, preferably with frequent monitoring of blood gas levels, in order to avoid excessive accumulation of carbon dioxide in the blood and so-called carbon dioxide narcosis. Intermittent administration of oxygen rather than continuous therapy may be useful in this regard. The use of intermittent positive-pressure machines (IPPB) should be limited to special circumstances and under close observation in the hospital. Digitalization is indicated for cardiac failure. Diuretics also may be helpful. Some cardiologists advocate long-term use of digitalis if cor pulmonale is thought to be present.

After completion of a course of therapy in the hospital, physical therapy to promote bronchial drainage and continuous nebulization of aerosol solutions in a tent at night are indicated in the home for an indefinite time. In addition, intermittent nebulization of propylene glycol and water solutions may be needed during the day (see Table 11-10). There is lack of agreement as to the advisability of continuous antibiotic therapy in relatively small doses when there is persistent clinical and roentgenographic evidence of pulmonary involvement. The principal argument against such therapy is the risk of increased resistance of strains of *Staphylococcus aureus* to antibiotics and the colonization of *Pseudomonas aeruginosa* and other resistant bacteria. In our experience, most severely ill patients cannot be controlled effectively without antibiotic therapy for long periods of time (months or even years). Several plans of continuous antibiotic therapy are currently used. Some clinicians prescribe intermittent therapy in which periods of 2 or 3 weeks of antibiotic administration are interrupted by a rest period of an equal time. Others prescribe antibiotics more or less continuously, but alternate the administration of several antibiotics, using a particular program for 2 or 3 weeks at a time. We favor continuation of oral therapy with the same antibiotic or combinations of antibiotics in the smallest effective doses as long as they appear to be helpful.

Pulmonary surgery is rarely indicated because

TABLE 11-10. TREATMENT OF PULMONARY INFECTION IN CYSTIC FIBROSIS
Therapeutic course (2 to 4 weeks)

A. ANTIBIOTIC THERAPY*

1. SYSTEMIC THERAPY

ANTIBIOTIC	DOSE	ROUTES OF ADMINISTRATION	INDICATIONS
Cephalothin.......... 50-100 mg./kg./24 hr.		I.M. or I.V.	Staphylococci resistant to pen-
Cephalotidine........30-60 mg./kg./24 hr.			icillins, Klebsiella, E. coli,
in 3 to 4 doses			P. mirabilis
Penicillins			
Penicillin G........1-4 million units/24 hr.		I.M. or I.V.	Nonresistant gram-positive cocci
			(infrequently used)
Ampicillin..........200 mg./kg./24 hr.		I.M. or I.V.	H. influenzae and other gram-
			negative bacilli, based on
			sensitivity tests
Methicillin......... 100 mg./kg./24 hr.		I.M. or I.V.	Penicillin-resistant staphylococci
Oxacillin............50-100 mg./kg./24 hr.		Oral	
Nafcillin........... 50-100 mg./kg./24 hr.		I.M. or I.V.	
Cloxacillin......... 50-100 mg./kg./24 hr.		Oral	
Erythromycin........ 40-100 mg./kg./24 hr.		Oral	Nonresistant staphylococci
Chloramphenicol....50-100 mg./kg./24 hr.		Oral or I.V.	Gram-negative bacilli
in 3 to 4 doses			
Kanamycin**.........15 mg./kg./24 hr. in 2 doses		I.M.	Most gram-negative bacteria
			except Pseudomonas
Colistin**............. 5 mg./kg./24 hr.		I.M.	Pseudomonas and coliform bac-
			teria
Streptomycin**......20-40 mg./kg./24 hr.		I.M.	Similar to kanamycin (rarely
(not more than 1 gm./24 hr.)			used)
Tetracyclines.........50 mg./kg./24 hr.		Oral	Broad-spectrum, bacteriostatic
			drug
Methacycline.........10-15 mg./kg./24 hr.		Oral	Similar to tetracyclines
Doxycycline...........2 mg./kg./24 hr.		Oral	Similar to tetracyclines
in 1 or 2 doses			

2. AEROSOL THERAPY†

ANTIBIOTIC	CONCENTRATION
Penicillin G	100,000 u./ml.
Methicillin	100-250 mg./ml.
Oxacillin	100-250 mg./ml.
Cephalotidine	100-250 mg./ml.
Colistin	5-10 mg./ml.
Polymyxin B	5-10 mg./ml.
Neomycin	50-100 mg./ml.

B. INHALATIONAL AND PHYSICAL THERAPY

Physical therapy
    Postural drainage, chest clapping, breathing exercises
Aerosol Therapy
    Solution recommended: 10% propylene glycol in distilled water (or isotonic saline)
    Equipment needed: Compressed air pump, appropriate nebulizer and tent
    Regimen advised:
        A. Continuous nebulization of propylene glycol 10% and distilled water during night and naps or for all 24
            hours
        B. Interrupted periods of nebulization
            Step 1: Nebulization of solution described for 10-15 minutes 3 or 4 times a day
            Step 2: Follow nebulization with postural drainage for 5 minutes
            Step 3: Nebulization of antibiotics as described (only if patient needs antibiotics by inhalation)

*Drug to be used should be selected whenever possible on basis of in-vitro sensitivity tests.
    N.B. Doses given here are for moderate and severe infections in infants beyond the neonatal period and in small
children. For doses for less severe infections, for maintenance therapy, and for all dosages for older children and
adolescents see Table 5-16, (p. 245). Also consult this table and the manufacturer's instructions (package insert)
for ranges of doses, routes of administration, as well as for cautions and contraindications applicable to each drug.
    **Not to be administered in a given course for longer than 10 days.
    †All antibiotics to be nebulized in solution of 2 cc. of isotonic saline solution. Whenever possible the same anti-
biotic is to be given by both systemic and aerosol routes.

of the generalized lung involvement. Bronchoscopy may be of assistance for drainage, especially in severely ill patients, when performed by a skilled operator; otherwise it should not be done. Bronchial lavage is indicated in selected cases; it is generally agreed that saline is less irritating than some of the mucolytic solutions. Corticosteroid therapy has not been helpful. Expectorants, antihistaminics and bronchodilators may be used and are occasionally effective, especially when there is an associated allergic component. A change of climate has not had strikingly beneficial effects on the course of the pulmonary involvement.

In *patients with a mild degree of pulmonary involvement* a full therapeutic course (Table 11-10) may be indicated during periods of acute relapse. Continuous nebulization of appropriate aerosol solutions at night in a tent* has helped to counteract the dry atmosphere, especially during the winter months. Physical therapy should also be used to promote bronchial drainage. Many patients will need continued antibiotic therapy by oral administration for long periods of time (Table 11-10). It may be possible to discontinue these drugs from time to time, especially during the summer months.

In *patients without pulmonary involvement* administration of antimicrobial agents prophylactically in order to avoid respiratory disease is ineffective. Matthews has advocated the use of physical and inhalational therapy as prophylactic measures as soon as the diagnosis of cystic fibrosis is made. It is not known whether this regimen will prove effective in preventing pulmonary involvement; it has not found universal acceptance.

Dietary therapy. The pancreatic achylia is readily compensated by a diet of high caloric, high protein and moderate fat content in conjunction with one of the pancreatic extracts. The patient's appetite should be a guide to the dietary intake. Commercially available powdered high-protein milk preparations can be used to advantage in the first few weeks of life; subsequently skim milk is advised until later childhood, when homogenized milk can be given if the patient tolerates it. Soybean milks do not provide adequate protein and should not be used for infants with cystic fibrosis. Hypoproteinemic edema has been a consequence of such feeding. Liposoluble vitamin supplements in water-miscible preparations should be provided every day in double the recommended dose. Pancreatic extract, which improves intestinal absorption and the nature of the stools, is needed with each meal. Many commercial products are available, and there is little evidence that any one has therapeutic advantage over the others. Dosage depends on the preparation selected and in particular on the patient's clinical response. Constipation and anorexia may result if the dose of the pancreatic extract is excessive. Medium-chain triglycerides (see p. 131) are absorbed better than other longer-chain fats, and dietary supplements of them have been advocated. At times anabolic steroids have been useful in increasing appetite and promoting weight gain, but to avoid side effects only short repeated courses are recommended. Claims that they have been effective in improving the respiratory disease do not seem to have been substantiated.

Dietary measures appear to become less necessary with advancing age, but individual variations are found in the need for dietary restrictions at all ages. The nutritional state is more closely correlated with the severity of the pulmonary infection than with pancreatic function.

Treatment of abnormal loss of salt. Massive salt depletion through sweating in hot weather may present a real medical emergency. The administration of saline solution intravenously is urgently needed in such instances to reconstitute the extracellular fluid volume and to avoid cardiovascular collapse; as much as 10 cc. of isotonic saline solution per kg. within 15 minutes may have to be given, followed by appropriate replacement therapy. Additional sodium chloride (2 to 4 gm. a day) should be taken orally by all patients in hot weather, regardless of their pancreatic status.

Other therapy. For that of meconium ileus, see page 392.

Beginning as early as 2 to 3 days postoperatively, 10 ml. of a 5 per cent solution of pancreatin powder is administered every 6 hours through a nasogastric tube. When feeding by mouth is deemed advisable, a dilute formula of one of the protein milk preparations and glucose can be started and increased in caloric value as rapidly as tolerated. Most infants with fibrocystic disease eventually will need as much as 150 calories per kg. per 24 hours in order to gain weight. Pancreatin powder should be put in each bottle (e.g. ½ teaspoonful in each of 6 bottles, equivalent to 3 teaspoonfuls when given with each of 3 meals).

Alternatively, preparations containing predigested amino acids and monosaccharides in a high-protein, low-fat milk (e.g. Probana [Mead-Johnson]) have been used to advantage for the first few weeks.

In patients with hepatic cirrhosis and portal hypertension severe gastrointestinal bleeding may require a surgical shunting procedure.

Treatment of rectal prolapse and of abdominal masses has been discussed. Repeated polypectomies may be indicated for nasal polyps if they recur. Associated allergy or diabetes mellitus should be treated as outlined in their respective sections.

PANCREATIC DEFICIENCIES NOT DUE TO CYSTIC FIBROSIS

Most patients with pancreatic achylia in the pediatric age group have cystic fibrosis, but sev-

---

*During summer months the temperature inside a tent may reach uncomfortable levels; a room air-conditioner is helpful in such instances.

eral other rare disease entities have been recognized in which pancreatic insufficiency is part of the clinical picture.

Congenital hypoplasia of the exocrine pancreas associated with pancreatic achylia and malnutrition was described in infants by Bodian (1952). At autopsy there was complete replacement of the parenchyma by fatty tissue, but notably there was no fibrosis and dilatation of pancreatic ducts. The islands of Langerhans appeared normal. Shwachman reported in 1964 six children ranging in age from 2 months to 10 years, 3 in one family, with shortness in stature and *pancreatic achylia and hematologic abnormalities,* including anemia, thrombocytopenia and neutropenia. In all these children the sweat test result was normal and there was no pulmonary involvement. Additional cases have since been recorded; in some there have also been other disorders which include metaphyseal dysostosis, Hirschsprung's disease, aplastic anemia, and hepatic cirrhosis with portal hypertension.

Trypsinogen deficiency has been identified in 2 unrelated infants with severe growth failure, hypoproteinemia and edema. The congenital absence of trypsinogen led to failure of activation of trypsin, chymotrypsin and carboxypeptidase and thus to impaired capacity to hydrolyze ingested protein. Pancreatic lipase and amylase were normal, as was the sweat test result; there was no pulmonary involvement. The importance of diagnosing this disorder is emphasized by the dramatic response to dietary management with protein hydrolysates. Both patients were anemic, and one had neutropenia.

Pancreatic deficiency has also been observed with the XXY Klinefelter's syndrome. This patient had pancreatic achylia, hypothyroidism, nerve deafness, chronic lung disease and dwarfism.

PANCREATITIS

Primary inflammatory disease of the pancreas is not common in childhood; acute pancreatitis is more common than chronic relapsing pancreatitis. About one third of patients reported with acute pancreatitis have signs suggestive of an acute surgical condition of the abdomen. The cause of acute pancreatitis is varied and often not identified. Presumed or proved causative factors have included trauma, blocking of the pancreatic duct by *Ascaris lumbricoides,* obstruction of the common bile duct and administration of corticosteroids. Malnutrition, especially protein deficiency, may lead to inflammatory changes in the pancreas and to eventual functional deficiency.

Pancreatitis may occur as a complication of mumps. Symptoms of severe epigastric pain, nausea and vomiting make an abrupt appearance 4 or 5 days after the onset of the parotid lesion. In rare instances there may be only pancreatic involvement. There frequently are fever, diarrhea

and leukocytosis. Transient hyperglycemia and glycosuria may occur occasionally during or after an acute attack. The prognosis is generally good, and complete recovery takes place in about a week. In mumps pancreatitis the finding of increased serum amylase concentration is not diagnostic, since it may be caused by inflammatory disease of the salivary glands.

Hereditary pancreatitis, or relapsing pancreatitis with lithiasis, has been described in 5 families as an autosomal dominant genetic disorder. Several members of each kindred have been involved. The diagnosis was established in most instances when the patients were adults, but the symptoms of severe recurrent abdominal pain lasting several days had started in childhood.

The absence of chronic pulmonary involvement, steatorrhea and malnutrition and normal electrolyte concentrations in sweat differentiate this entity from cystic fibrosis; pancreatic lithiasis has been seen only late in the disease. Aminoaciduria with loss of lysine and cystine occurs in some patients with hereditary pancreatitis.

CYSTS AND PSEUDOCYSTS OF THE PANCREAS

Congenital cysts of the pancreas are usually multiple. They are asymptomatic and are frequently associated with polycystic involvement of other organs.

Pseudocysts of the pancreas may occur as a complication of mumps or other acute pancreatitis or may follow trauma. Falls from bicycles and tricycles have been one of the most frequent causes. Pseudocysts should be considered in the differential diagnosis of abdominal masses in children, especially after blunt abdominal trauma. Surgical drainage and *marsupialization* followed some time later by excision may be needed. Pancreatic enzyme activity can be demonstrated in the contents of the pseudocysts, although the addition of enterokinase as an activator may be needed.

INVOLVEMENT OF THE PANCREAS IN SYSTEMIC DISEASE

Acute and chronic changes in the pancreas are often associated with a variety of systemic diseases without producing symptoms that would lead to clinical recognition of pancreatic involvement. Infiltration of the pancreas by leukemia, Hodgkin's disease and other lymphogranulomatous conditions is common. Severe congenital syphilis involving the pancreas causes widespread fibrosis. Fibrotic changes with extensive atrophy of acinar tissue result from chronic passive congestion of the pancreas produced by long-standing cardiac decompensation. Miliary abscesses occur in association with septicemia; tubercles, with miliary tuberculosis.

NEOPLASMS OF THE PANCREAS

Neoplasms of the pancreas in childhood are rare; they are discussed on page 1452.

PAUL A. DI SANT'AGNESE

REFERENCES

General

Davenport, H. W.: *Physiology of the Digestive Tract.* 2nd ed. Chicago, Year Book Publishers, Inc., 1966.

de Reuck, A. V. S., and Cameron, M. P. (Eds.): CIBA Foundation Symposium on the Exocrine Pancreas. Boston, Little, Brown and Co., 1962.

Tests

Andersen, D. H.: Pancreatic Enzymes in the Duodenal Juice in the Celiac Syndrome. *Am. J. Dis. Child.,* 63:643, 1942.

Barbero, G. J., Sibinga, M. S., Marino, J. M., and Seibel, R.: Stool Trypsin and Chymotrypsin. *Am. J. Dis. Child.,* 112: 536, 1966.

Gibson, L. E., and Cooke, R. E.: A Test for the Concentration of Electrolytes in Sweat in Cystic Fibrosis of the Pancreas Utilizing Pilocarpine by Iontophoresis. *Pediatrics,* 23:545, 1959.

Hadorn, B., and others: Quantitative Assessment of Exocrine Pancreatic Function in Infants and Children. *J. Pediat.,* 73:39, 1968.

Anomalies

Barbosa, J. J. de C., Dockerty, M. B., and Waugh, J. M.: Pancreatic Heterotopia – Review of the Literature and Report of 41 Authenticated Cases of Which 25 Were Clinically Significant. *Surg. Gynec. & Obst.,* 2:527, 1946.

Hays, D. M., Greaney, E. M., Jr., and Hill, J. T.: Annular Pancreas as a Cause of Acute Neonatal Duodenal Obstruction. *Ann. Surg.,* 153:103, 1961.

Cystic Fibrosis

Andersen, D. H.: Cystic Fibrosis of the Pancreas and Its Relation to Celiac Diseases; A Clinical and Pathologic Study. *Am. J. Dis. Child.,* 56:344, 1938.

Beier, F. R., Renzetti, A. D., Jr., Mitchell, M., and Watanabe, S.: Pulmonary Pathophysiology in Cystic Fibrosis. *Am. Rev. Resp. Dis.,* 94:430, 1966.

Bodian, M.: *Fibrocystic Disease of the Pancreas.* London, Heinemann, Ltd., 1952.

Bruce, G. M., Denning, C. R., and Spalter, H. F.: Ocular Findings in Cystic Fibrosis of the Pancreas. *Arch. Ophthal.,* 63:391, 1960.

Danes, B. S., and Bearn, A.: Cystic Fibrosis of the Pancreas: A Study of Cell Culture. *J. Exp. Med .:* April, 1969.

di Sant'Agnese, P. A., and Blanc, W. A.: A Distinctive Type of Biliary Cirrhosis of the Liver Associated with Cystic Fibrosis of Pancreas. *Pediatrics,* 18:387, 1956.

di Sant'Agnese, P. A., and Talamo, R. C.: Medical Progress: Pathogenesis and Physiopathology of Cystic Fibrosis of the Pancreas. *New England J. Med.,* 277:1287, 1344, 1399, 1967.

di Sant'Agnese, P. A., Darling, R. C., Perera, G. A., and Shea, E.: Abnormal Electrolyte Composition of Sweat in Cystic Fibrosis of the Pancreas. *Pediatrics,* 12:549, 1953.

Doershuk, C. F., Matthews, L. W., Tucker, A. S., and Spector, S.: Evaluation of a Prophylactic and Therapeutic Program for Patients with Cystic Fibrosis. *Pediatrics,* 36:675, 1965.

Farber, S.: The Relation of Pancreatic Achylia to Meconium Ileus. *J. Pediat.,* 24:387, 1944.

Grand, R. J., Talamo, R. C., di Sant'Agnese, P. A., and Schwartz, R. H.: Pregnancy in Cystic Fibrosis of the Pancreas. *J.A.M.A.,* 195:993, 1966.

Guide to Diagnosis and Treatment of Cystic Fibrosis of the Pancreas. National Cystic Fibrosis Research Foundation, 202 East 44th Street, New York, N.Y. 10017.

Kaplan, E., and others: Reproductive Failure in Males with Cystic Fibrosis. *New England J. Med.,* 279:65, 1968.

Lietman, P. S., di Sant'Agnese, P. A., and Wong, V.: Optic Neuritus in Cystic Fibrosis of the Pancreas. Role of Chloramphenicol Therapy. *J.A.M.A.,* 189:924, 1964.

Matalon, R., and Dorfman, A.: Acid Mucopolysaccharides in Cultured Fibroblasts of Cystic Fibrosis of the Pancreas. *Biochem. Biophysical Res. Communications* 33:954, 1968.

Matthews, L. W., and others: A Therapeutic Regimen for Patients with Cystic Fibrosis. *J. Pediat.,* 65:558, 1964.

Moss, A. J., Harper, W. H., Dooley, R. R., Murray, J. F., and Mack, J. F.: Cor Pulmonale in Cystic Fibrosis of the Pancreas. *J. Pediat.,* 67:797, 1965.

Mullins, F., Talamo, R. C., and di Sant'Agnese, P. A.: Late Intestinal Complications of Cystic Fibrosis. *J.A.M.A.,* 192: 741, 1965.

Shwachman, H., and Khaw, K-T: Cystic Fibrosis; in H. C. Shirkey (Ed.): *Pediatric Therapy.* St. Louis, C. V. Mosby Company, 1964, p. 499.

Shwachman, H., Kulczycki, L. L., and Khaw, K-T.: Studies in Cystic Fibrosis: 65 Patients over 17 Years of Age. *Pediatrics,* 36:689, 1965.

Schuster, S. R., Shwachman, H., Harris, G. B. C., and Khaw, K-T.: Pulmonary Surgery for Cystic Fibrosis. *J. Thor. & Cardiovasc. Surg.,* 48:750, 1964.

Waring, W. W., Brunt, C. H., and Hilman, B. C.: Mucoid Impaction of the Bronchi in Cystic Fibrosis. *Pediatrics,* 39:166, 1967.

Pancreatic Deficiencies Not Due to Cystic Fibrosis

Burke, V., Colebatch, J. H., Anderson, C. M., and Simons, M. J.: Association of Pancreatic Insufficiency and Chronic Neutropenia in Childhood. *Arch. Dis. Childhood,* 42:147, 1967.

Grand, R. J., Rosen, S. W., di Sant'Agnese, P. A., and Kirkham, W. R.: Unusual Case of XXY Klinefelter's Syndrome with Pancreatic Insufficiency, Hypothyroidism, Deafness, Chronic Lung Disease, Dwarfism and Microcephaly. *Am. J. Med.,* 41:478, 1966.

Shwachman, H., Diamond, L. K., Oski, F. A., and Khaw, K-T.: The Syndrome of Pancreatic Insufficiency and Bone Marrow Dysfunction. *J. Pediat.,* 65:645, 1964.

Townes, P. L., Bryson, M. F., and Miller, G.: Further Observations on Trypsinogen Deficiency Disease: Report of a Second Case. *J. Pediat.,* 71:220, 1967.

Pancreatitis

Frey, C., and Redo, S. F.: Inflammatory Lesions of the Pancreas in Infancy and Childhood. *Pediatrics,* 32:93, 1963.

Gross, J. B., Ulrich, J. A., and Maher, F. T.: Further Observations on the Hereditary Form of Pancreatitis; in A. V. S. de Reuck and M. P. Cameron (Eds.): *CIBA Foundation Symposium on the Exocrine Pancreas.* Boston, Little, Brown, and Co., 1962, p. 278.

Hendren, W. H., Greep, J. M., and Patton, A. S.: Pancreatitis in Childhood: Experience with 15 Cases. *Arch. Dis. Childhood,* 40:132, 1965.

Stein, D.: Pancreatitis – Acute and Relapsing – in Infancy and Childhood. *S. African Med. J.,* 37:1066, 1963.

Pseudocysts of the Pancreas

Kilman, J. W., Kaiser, G. C., King, R. D., and Shumacker, H. B.: Pancreatic Pseudocysts in Infancy and Childhood. *Surgery,* 55:455, 1964.

12. The Respiratory System

RESPIRATORY PHYSIOLOGY AND ITS APPLICATION TO PULMONARY DISEASE

Respiratory failure is the commonest cause of morbidity and death during the neonatal period, and respiratory diseases are the most frequent reasons for hospitalization of infants and children. Basic knowledge of the development and functions of the respiratory system is essential for understanding many of these respiratory illnesses. The respiratory system, whose function is to maintain adequate oxygen and carbon dioxide exchange between the body and the environment, is made up of (1) a control system which consists of respiratory centers in the brain stem, chemoreceptors in the midbrain and in the carotid and aortic bodies, and peripheral nerves, both motor (efferent) and sensory (afferent); (2) the respiratory muscles and "thorax" (including diaphragm, rib cage, abdominal wall and abdominal contents); (3) the lungs and air passages; and (4) the pulmonary vasculature. Any one or a combination of these parts may be involved in disease processes which may contribute to respiratory disability.

DEVELOPMENT OF THE RESPIRATORY SYSTEM AND INITIATION OF RESPIRATION

The respiratory centers in the midbrain are sufficiently developed early in gestation (at least by 20 or 22 weeks) to respond to sensory stimuli and changes in pH, P_{CO_2} and P_{O_2} by initiating gasps and even sustaining rhythmic, although frequently periodic, respiration. In the immature infant these centers are particularly sensitive to the depressant effects of severe hypoxia, severe hypercapnia, acidosis or drugs. Even with a normally functioning respiratory center, extrauterine survival is usually not possible until after 27 or 28 weeks' gestation because of limiting factors within the lungs themselves. Capillarization of the alveoli is not far enough advanced until 28 weeks to permit adequate gas exchange. In addition, until approximately the same stage of development, pulmonary vascular resistance is probably so high, even after lung expansion, that pulmonary blood flow is significantly reduced.

The *ability of the lungs to resist collapse* is dependent upon the appearance (also at approximately 28 weeks' gestation) of certain surface active phospholipids (surfactant) in the alveolar lining membrane. The important role of these phospholipids can best be appreciated when one considers the Laplace Equation, $P = \dfrac{2T}{r}$, representing the relation between the tension (T) of the wall of a sphere, its radius (r), and the pressure (P) within the sphere. If T were the same for all lung units (e.g. alveoli), then the smaller units would tend to collapse and the larger would expand. Actually, studies on extracts of lung lining layers suggest that, because of specific phospholipids, dipalmitoyl lecithin primarily and sphingomyelin in small part, the alveolar lining layer has a surface tension which varies with its degree of contraction (low surface tension) or expansion (high surface tension). This apparent adjustment of surface tension can explain the ability of air spaces of different sizes to coexist with equal pressures. Studies of experimental animals and of material obtained at autopsy from newborn infants indicate that the critical phospholipids are probably produced in type II (giant) alveolar cells in increasing amounts until enough is excreted into the alveolar spaces to allow formation of a continuous alveolar lining layer when the lungs are expanded for the first time with air. If only marginal amounts of the surface active compounds are present, production is apparently significantly decreased by various forms of stress (e.g. hypoxia or acidosis) and by hypothermia. Thus the atelectasis of the respiratory distress syndrome may be the result of immaturity of the phospholipid-producing cells of the alveoli alone or, in some cases, of immaturity combined with a variety of perinatal stresses.

The *onset of respiration* is the most critical adjustment required of the infant. During fetal life there is some inhibitory mechanism which ordinarily prevents anything more than occasional respiratory movements. At birth, if the infant is to survive, a series of important events must occur in the respiratory system. Sensory (tactile and thermal) and chemical (pH, P_{O_2} and P_{CO_2}) stimuli initiate respiration and, together with intrathoracic and intrapulmonary reflexes, sustain it. If the neuromuscular-thoracic structures are intact and adequately developed and the air passages are unobstructed, lung expansion will occur. For the initial inspiration, when air is introduced into the fluid-filled lung for the first time, large surface forces must be overcome. Transpulmonary pressures required for the first breath vary from 15 to 50 cm. of water. Although these high pressures are normally produced by the infant himself, alveolar rupture may occur either spontaneously or as a result of artificial respiration. If the surface active phospholipids are present in adequate quantities, air will tend to remain in the lung at the end of expiration, and subsequent respiration will require much smaller transpulmonary pressures, finally stabilizing at about 5 cm. of water for the quiet respiration of normal infants.

Concomitant with lung expansion in the normal infant is a striking reduction in pulmonary vascular resistance, an increase in pulmonary blood flow, and a rapid decrease in the shunting of blood from the right to the left side of the heart. This pulmonary vasodilatation is apparently the result of changes in blood gases and pH as well as lung expansion itself.

As part of the process of lung expansion, the fluid which fills the potential air spaces during fetal life must be rapidly removed. Some is removed through the nose and mouth, while much is apparently picked up by the capillaries and lymphatics. After the initiation of respiration the stiffness of the lungs gradually decreases, presumably as a result of removal of the fluid.

The respiratory mechanism at birth is most likely to fail as the result of (1) central nervous system depression or (2) abnormalities within the lungs. Drugs, intrauterine hypoxia and trauma may all depress the respiratory center. Unless morphine antagonists are indicated, little can be done to improve the responsiveness of the center except to supply it with oxygen and to remove excess carbon dioxide. Good obstetric and anesthetic procedures should greatly reduce the occurrence of respiratory center failure.

Expansion of the lungs may be limited because of airway obstruction, which can be removed if it is in the pharynx, trachea or main bronchi. If the obstruction is in the smaller air passages, as may occur with aspiration of meconium-containing amniotic fluid or with plugging of alveolar ducts with hyaline membrane material, the lungs may be resistant to expansion. The latter type of respiratory obstruction is the greatest single cause of death in the neonatal period.

Congenital malformations such as diaphragmatic hernias, lung cysts, intrathoracic tumors and tracheo-esophageal fistulas may also be the cause of respiratory difficulty in the neonatal period and may at times simulate conditions which have less specific therapy.

After the adjustments of the neonatal period, further development of the respiratory system is primarily a matter of growth. The surface area of the lungs is calculated to be approximately 2 to 3 square meters at birth and increases to approximately 70 square meters in the adult male. The larger air passages increase in radius by a factor of 3 from birth to adulthood. Alveoli continue to increase in number until the age of 8 years; after 8 years the increase in lung size is accomplished by expansion of the alveoli. The various lung volumes in the normal person can best be related to body size, particularly height, and these relations are approximately constant from shortly after birth through young adulthood.

CONTROL OF RESPIRATION

Regulation of alveolar ventilation and maintenance of normal arterial P_{O_2}, P_{CO_2} and pH are the principal functions of the medullary and peripheral chemoreceptors. The respiratory center in the brain stem is affected by reflexes from the lungs, the skeletal muscles and the carotid and aortic bodies and also by its chemical environment. Proprioceptive impulses from the lungs are carried in the vagi and diminish inspiratory activity when the lungs are inflated and increase this activity when the lungs are deflated (Hering-Breuer reflex). Impulses transmitted by sensory nerves from the muscles and joints also stimulate activity of the respiratory center and are probably responsible for much of the hyperventilation of exercise.

In the newborn infant, ventilation is initially adjusted to achieve a relatively low P_{CO_2} (28 mm. Hg versus 41 for the older child and the adult), presumably to compensate for metabolic acidosis. Periodic respiration occurs frequently in newborn and especially premature infants, and is usually diminished by the administration of oxygen.

Reduced arterial oxygen saturation stimulates chemoreceptors in the aortic and carotid bodies which, in turn, increase the activity of the respiratory center. Increases in arterial carbon dioxide stimulate the respiratory center directly without the mediation of a reflex arc. The actual stimulus to the center is probably due to the change in pH induced by the increase in P_{CO_2}. Although both hypoxia and hypercapnia stimulate the respiratory center at first, when they are prolonged and severe, they act as depressants. For this reason the primary aim in the management of central depression of respiration should be to increase the oxygen supply to the respiratory center. Drugs are useful as respiratory stimulants only as they improve the general circulation or specifically counteract a respiratory depressant (e.g. n-allylnormorphine).

Protective reflexes such as coughing and sneezing can alter the usual breathing patterns and act to eliminate foreign or obstructing matter from the respiratory tract. Respiration is also modified during swallowing and is altered reflexly by pain and variations of blood pressure.

MUSCLES OF RESPIRATION

In quiet, normal breathing only the inspiratory muscles are used; expiration occurs as a result of the elastic recoil of the lung as the inspiratory muscles are relaxed. The diaphragm is the most important muscle of inspiration, but with increasing inspiratory effort the intercostal, spinal extensor and neck muscles become active in that order. They increase the thoracic diameter and thus its volume; the intercostal muscles also serve to stabilize the rib cage so that the diaphragm can function more effectively.

The abdominal muscles are the ones primarily used for a forced expiration; they are assisted by the "spinal flexors," which increase intrapulmonary pressure for coughing. The intercostal muscles also assist expiration, but here, too, they function largely to stabilize the rib cage.

Patients with weakened abdominal muscles cannot cough well. Manual pressure over the abdomen after a maximal inspiration can produce a fair cough when the glottis is opened suddenly, but this technique is limited to cooperative patients. When muscular function is diminished, as with poliomyelitis or other neuromuscular disease, the forces developed may be so limited that artificial respiration is required.

The weak respiratory muscles and the pliable thoracic cage of the premature infant may seriously limit his abilities to achieve normal ventilation, particularly when his lungs are abnormally stiff as in the idiopathic respiratory distress syndrome. In addition, the premature infant's gag reflex is depressed and his ability to clear secretions markedly limited.

LUNG VOLUMES

The static or semistatic subdivisions of lung volume are shown in Figure 12-1, which represents a series of tidal volumes and a vital capacity.

The *vital capacity* is made up of the inspiratory capacity and the expiratory reserve volume, the proportion occupied by each varying with the position of the patient and with different respiratory conditions.

After each expiration a considerable volume of air, the *functional residual capacity,* remains in the lungs. This air serves as a buffer minimizing changes in the partial pressure of carbon dioxide and oxygen in the alveoli and arterial blood during the respiratory cycle. Since most air spaces remain open at end-expiration, surface forces are also reduced.

The volume of the functional residual capacity (the resting end-expiratory volume) is determined by the balance between the elastic recoil of the lungs and the tendency of the thorax to expand. The effective "thoracic" forces stem from the elastic characteristics of the rib cage, from the diaphragm and the abdominal wall, and from the hydrostatic force of the abdominal contents. The movement of the abdominal contents with shifts in position is largely responsible for the changes in the functional residual capacity; it is this movement on which the tilting method for artificial respiration is based. For example, in the supine position the diaphragm is pushed up and resting lung volume decreases, while in the upright position resting lung volume increases.

The *residual volume* is the amount of gas remaining in the lung at the end of a forced expiration; it is normally about 25 per cent of the total lung capacity. The functional residual capacity and especially the residual volume are increased when air is trapped beyond obstructed air passages as in bronchiolitis, asthma or cystic fibrosis. These lung volumes may be calculated by measuring the amount of nitrogen washed out of the lungs during the breathing of pure oxygen or by the dilution of known amounts of an inert gas such as helium in the lungs. In addition, plethysmographic methods allow rapid measurements of lung volumes.

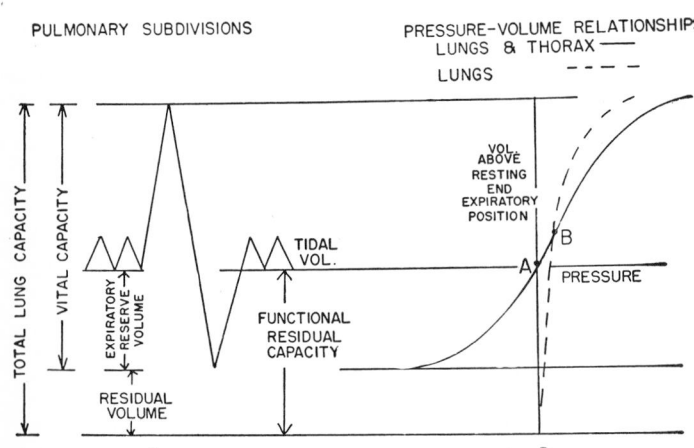

Figure 12-1. Static or semistatic subdivisions of lung volume.

TABLE 12-1. Normal Values for Pulmonary Studies (Ranges Include Approximately 95% of Normal Values; Volumes in Liters, BTPS)

AGE (YEARS)	NEWBORN	6	10	14	♂ 18	♀
LENGTH, HT. (CM.)	51	115	138	160	175	163
Vital capacity (L.)	0.100	1.0-1.8	1.7-2.9	2.6-4.5	3.4-6.3	2.7-4.8
Total lung capacity (L.)	0.140*	1.4-2.3	2.2-3.8	3.5-6.0	4.4-7.6	3.6-6.2
RV/TLC%	?	14-34	14-34	14-34	14-34	14-34
Vital capacity (2 sec.) % total–average	?	>90%	>90%	>90%	>90%	>90%
Maximal breathing capacity (L./min.)	?	30-60	42-106	65-140	90-175	62-147
Peak expiratory flow rate (L./min.)	7.1-10.1	130-236	217-391	294-534	370-770	295-535
Lung compliance (ml./cm. H_2O)	1-10	32-96	46-142	64-194	78-245	67-204
Flow resistance (cm. H_2O/L./sec.)	4-41†	3-14‡	2-9‡	2-6‡	1-5‡	2-6‡
Anatomic dead space (ml.)	5.6-12.8	40-78	59-120	84-170	105-205	82-162

Newborn values in supine position, all others in sitting position.
*Values represent extrapolation and need further verification.
BTPS–37° C. saturated with water vapor at ambient pressure.
†Nose-breathing.
‡Mouth-breathing.

MECHANICS OF RESPIRATION

The mechanical properties of the respiratory system may be divided into 2 components—one concerned with static or elastic forces and the other with the dynamic or flow-resistance forces. The resting end-expiratory position or functional residual capacity results from 2 forces—the tendency of the lungs to collapse and the tendency of the "thorax" to expand. This can be likened to the balance between 2 springs. Any deviation from the balance point requires work or an applied force; when the force is released, the springs return to their relaxation or balance point. In a comparable manner in normal breathing when the respiratory muscles contract, the "thorax" and lungs expand. When the muscles relax, the intrapleural pressure falls toward the resting end-expiratory pressure and expiration occurs.

The elastic or springlike characteristic is called *compliance* and is expressed as milliliters or liters per cm. of water pressure. In the case of the lungs it represents the change in pulmonary volume for a unit change of interpleural (i.e. transpulmonary) pressure and must be measured when there is no flow of air so that there is no flow-resistance component. The less the volume change produced by a given pressure change, the stiffer or less compliant are the lungs. Conversely, if the volume change for this same pressure difference is large, the lungs are highly distensible or compliant.

The lungs of infants are less compliant than those of older children and adults (Table 12-1), but when the difference in lung or body size is considered, they are found to be similar, and at all ages nearly the same transpulmonary pressure difference is required to produce the resting tidal volume. In order to measure the compliance of the lungs one must know the transpulmonary pressure changes. Pressure change in the thoracic esophagus may be used as an index of the trans-

pulmonary pressure change; this measurement and direct interpleural pressure measurements, although useful in understanding pathophysiologic changes, have little application to clinical pediatrics.

The volume-pressure relations of the lungs and "thorax" are shown in Figure 12-1. The resting end-expiratory volume has been continued as a horizontal line and also represents the pressure axis. Volume is represented by the vertical axis. Pressure changes to the right of the vertical axis are equivalent to positive airway or negative tank pressure, and pressures to the left represent negative airway or positive tank pressure. The volume-pressure characteristics of the lungs and "thorax" over the vital capacity range are represented by the solid curve. There is no scale because the values for subjects of different sizes are different; the shape of the curves, however, is similar. In the region of the tidal volume (between *A* and *B* on the curve) the relation of volume to pressure is essentially linear. With spontaneous respiration the effective strength of the respiratory muscles is an important factor in determining the magnitude of the maximum volume change. In addition, maximum inspiration is limited at large lung volumes by the decreased compliance of the lungs, the rib cage, and the abdominal wall and abdominal contents. Expiration, on the other hand, is limited by the compliance of the rib cage and the diaphragm.

Knowledge of the volume-pressure relation of the lungs and "thorax" is particularly useful during artificial respiration. In the older child and the adult, pressures required to produce suitable volume changes of the lungs plus "thorax" are approximately twice those required for the lungs alone. In the newborn infant, however, the "thorax" is so compliant that it requires little pressure for expansion.

A considerable part of the elastic characteristics of the lungs is the result of surface tension

TABLE 12-2. CHANGES IN PULMONARY FUNCTION IN 6 TYPES OF RESPIRATORY DIFFICULTY

	RESPIRATORY DISTRESS SYNDROME	CYSTIC FIBROSIS	ASTHMA	RESPIRATORY MUSCLE PARESIS	EMPHYSEMA	CONGESTIVE FAILURE
Total lung capacity	↓	↓	N or ↓	↓	↑	↓
Functional residual volume	↓	N or ↑	N or ↑	N	↑	N or ↑
Residual volume	?	↑	↑	↑	↑	↑
Vital capacity	↓	↓	N or ↓	↓	↓	↓
Timed vital capacity	?	↓	↓	N	↓	N or ↓
Lung compliance	↓	N or ↓	↓	↓	N or ↑	↓
Flow resistance	±	↑	↑	N	↑	N or ↑
Arterial blood P_{CO_2}	↑	Late ↑	N or ↑	N or ↑	↑	±
Arterial blood P_{O_2}	↓	Late ↓	N or ↓	N or ↓	↓	↓

forces created by the fluid-air interface within the air spaces. Particularly important is the surface-active material lining the lung (cf. above).

Thus far the force required to maintain the lungs under static conditions has been considered. During inflation and deflation dynamic factors are also present. These are the resistance of the airway to the flow of gases and the viscous resistance of the pulmonary tissues. They are combined in the measurement of pulmonary flow resistance, which is the force or pressure difference required to produce a specific flow of air and is expressed as centimeters of water per liter per second (Table 12-1). In diseases such as asthma or cystic fibrosis the pulmonary resistance may be increased to 10 to 15 times the normal value (Table 12-2). Since resistance to the flow of air through a tube is inversely related to the fourth power (to the fifth power when turbulence is present) of the radius of the tube, inflammation or mucus (e.g. croup, bronchiolitis) is most likely to produce serious obstruction and increases in flow resistance in infants and small children.

The respiratory muscles must have sufficient work capacity to overcome the elastic and flow resistance of the respiratory system. During normal resting respiration the amount of work is small, approximately 1 per cent of the resting metabolism. As ventilation is increased, the expenditure of energy for breathing increases more rapidly than the effective ventilation, especially at high ventilatory rates.

VENTILATION

Ventilation involves the exchange of gas in the alveoli with gas in the external environment and normally serves to maintain the body in oxygen and carbon dioxide equilibrium. When ventilation is adequate, alveolar oxygen tension (Pa_{CO_2}) and, secondarily, arterial oxygen tension (Pa_{O_2}) are approximately 100 mm. Hg, and carbon dioxide tension (Pa_{CO_2} and Pa_{CO_2}) is about 40 mm.

The partial pressures of gases at sea level in the normal person are presented in Figure 12-2.

These are not valid at altitudes much above sea level, since the lower barometric pressure reduces the partial pressure for all gases except that of water vapor. The latter is related to the temperature of the air and remains fixed at 47 mm. Hg at 37° C. If the patient is febrile, the vapor tension increases; an elevation of 2 to 3° C. adds about 10 mm. Hg to the partial pressure of water vapor, which then occupies more space and displaces other gases.

Owing to the differences in the P_{O_2} of alveolar gas and arterial blood, the sum of the partial pressures in the arterial blood does not equal the ambient barometric pressure. In normal persons virtually all this difference is due to a small venous admixture and ventilation-perfusion imbalance.

The volume of gas breathed into or out of the lungs with each breath is defined as the tidal

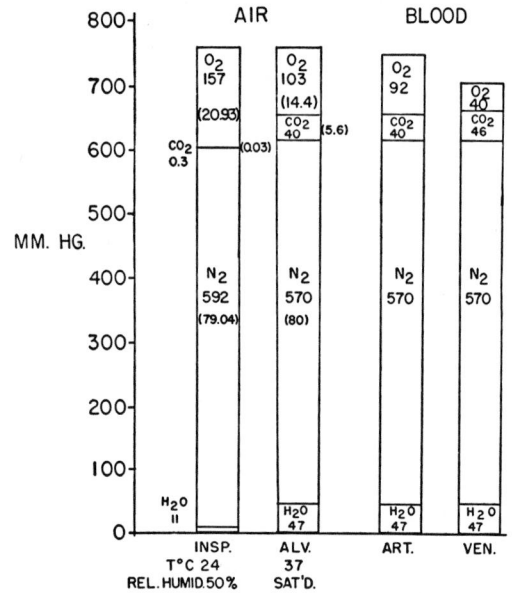

Figure 12-2. Partial pressures of gases in various physiologic media at sea level. (Barometric pressure, 760 mm. Hg.)

volume (V_T). This volume multiplied by the respiratory rate (f) gives the minute volume (V_E). Not all the tidal volume is effective in gas exchange; in the normal person about one third of each quiet respiration ventilates the nonfunctioning air passages or dead space (V_D), while the remaining portion (V_{Te}) enters the air sacs and alveoli and participates in gas exchange. Since alveolar ventilation (V_A) is a function of carbon dioxide production (V_{CO_2}) and the partial pressure of carbon dioxide in the arterial blood or alveoli, the following expressions are useful for defining the effective or alveolar ventilation:

$$V_T - V_D = V_{Te}$$

$$V_{Te} \times f = \dot{V}_A = k \frac{\dot{V}_{CO_2}}{Pa_{CO_2}}$$

As metabolism and carbon dioxide production increase, the alveolar ventilation must increase if the blood carbon dioxide tension is to remain at the usual level. Conversely, if $\dot{V}_A$ were doubled for a given $\dot{V}_{CO_2}$, then Pa_{CO_2} would be halved. It is also apparent that when the dead space increases secondary to disease or the use of anesthetic apparatus, V_T or f must increase to maintain a constant Pa_{CO_2}. The most effective way to increase alveolar ventilation is to increase the tidal volume. In this way alveolar ventilation is increased with a minimal increase in dead space ventilation.

In certain diseases such as emphysema or cystic fibrosis, parts of the lung which should participate in gas exchange are essentially functionless because of obliteration of their blood supply or large reduction in their ventilation due to local obstruction. Even in normal subjects, owing to varying degrees of resistance of the different air passages to the alveoli, there is a small degree of uneven ventilation and an imbalance in the ventilation-perfusion ratios. When parts of the lung are involved in diseases associated with either varying amounts of obstruction or regional differences in lung compliance, there will be a greater degree of uneven ventilation. Regions which, as a result, are underventilated will not fully saturate the blood which perfuses them; the overventilated regions cannot compensate, since they cannot supersaturate blood with oxygen. Therefore, even when the total amount of ventilation is normal, uneven ventilation causes an impairment in the uptake of oxygen. When ventilation is uneven with respect to pulmonary capillary blood flow, a fall in Pa_{O_2} occurs which is not accompanied by a rise in Pa_{CO_2} until the ventilation-perfusion imbalance is severe.

Alveolar ventilation may be impaired not only by intrapulmonary disease, but also by conditions interfering with control of respiration, e.g. depression of the respiratory center, paralysis of nerves supplying respiratory muscles, primary weakness of the muscles, and mechanical disorders of the lungs, chest or abdomen (including obesity as in the Pickwickian syndrome). When hypoventilation results from such extrapulmonary causes, a rise in Pa_{CO_2} is accompanied by an equal fall in Pa_{O_2}.

Normally there is a large reserve of ventilatory capacity. For example, a normal child may have a ventilation of 3 liters per minute at rest, but can increase this to 100 liters per minute for brief periods. When a disease is so severe that there is no longer any ventilatory reserve, the clearance of gas is impaired, and the composition of alveolar gas is changed, the Pa_{CO_2} increasing and the Pa_{O_2} decreasing. This affects the arterial tension of oxygen and carbon dioxide, but, because of the shape of the oxygen-hemoglobin dissociation curve, the ventilation has to be seriously impaired before there is much change in arterial oxygen saturation. On the other hand, Pa_{CO_2} and Pa_{O_2} change proportionately with changes in alveolar ventilation. Since arterial blood is a mixture from all the alveoli, its P_{CO_2} may be regarded as equal to the mean of all the different P_{CO_2}'s in various parts of the lung. Indeed, Pa_{CO_2} is particularly useful in measuring the level of alveolar ventilation because, unlike Pa_{O_2}, which may be affected by diffusion defects (cf. below) and the distribution of ventilation and blood flow in the lungs, carbon dioxide has a high solubility and the carbon dioxide-hemoglobin dissociation curve is almost linear. Its level, thus, is primarily a function of alveolar ventilation.

When the arterial P_{CO_2} rises, there is an accumulation of hydrogen ions, and pH decreases (uncompensated respiratory acidosis). In the course of a day or more the fall in pH is reversed by the retention of bicarbonate ions by the kidneys. When this occurs, the increased P_{CO_2} remains unchanged, but the pH will be near normal (compensated respiratory acidosis). In some respiratory disorders, when there is also an impairment in oxygen supply to the tissues, intermediate metabolites such as lactic acid accumulate in the blood, diminishing its buffering capacity (mixed respiratory and metabolic acidosis).

DIFFUSION

The uptake of oxygen by the lungs depends upon diffusion of the gas across the pulmonary membrane and chemical combination within the pulmonary capillary blood. Thus the total diffusing capacity of the lungs for oxygen, or for a test gas such as carbon monoxide, is the result of the diffusing capacity of the pulmonary membrane and the rate of uptake of the gas by the blood in the pulmonary capillaries. It is apparent that decreases in the diffusing capacity of the lungs may be the result of thickening of the alveolar membranes or a decrease in pulmonary capillary surface. Since carbon dioxide diffuses through living tissues approximately 20 times as rapidly as oxygen, its excretion is rarely limited by diffusion defects.

Although diffusion defects are rare in children, such conditions as pulmonary hemosiderosis, interstitial fibrosis, the Hamman-Rich syndrome, Niemann-Pick disease with pulmonary involvement and primary pulmonary artery hypertension with obliteration of many pulmonary capillaries are examples of pulmonary diseases associated with oxygen unsaturation secondary to abnormal diffusion. In adults, inhalation of a variety of toxic substances such as silica and beryllium leads to granulomatous lesions and fibrosis in the lungs and diffusion defects.

PULMONARY VASCULATURE

The interdependence of the pulmonary vasculature and pulmonary function is obvious, but frequently overlooked. For maintenance of normal oxygen and carbon dioxide equilibrium there must be a normal ventilation-perfusion relation throughout the greater part of the lung (cf. above).

In a number of pulmonary diseases, particularly those prolonged over months and years, pulmonary artery hypertension may develop. This may be due to actual compression of the pulmonary vascular system, as is apparently the case in scoliosis, or to vasoconstriction secondary to hypoxia, as in scoliosis or cystic fibrosis. In either case the chronic pulmonary hypertension tends to be progressive, and cor pulmonale finally ensues, so that many of the children with the most severe pulmonary disease terminally exhibit a combination of cardiac *and* pulmonary failure. In some cases the pulmonary vasoconstriction may be temporarily reversed by the administration of oxygen and the reduction of hypercapnia accomplished by assisted ventilation, but the course of the disease is rarely more than temporarily slowed.

When pulmonary vascular congestion occurs in infants as a result of left-to-right shunts associated with congenital heart disease, respiratory acidosis occurs. Respiratory function is further altered, since these infants are particularly apt to have serious difficulty with respiratory tract infections.

VENTILATION-PERFUSION RELATIONS

Ventilation ($\dot{V}_A$) and perfusion ($\dot{Q}$) relations vary from one part of the lungs to another, but the average $\dot{V}_A\dot{Q}$ ratio is 0.8. Although in the upright position both ventilation and perfusion are less at the apices than at the bases of the lungs, the difference is greater for blood flow, and hence $\dot{V}_A\dot{Q}$ is relatively higher at the top of the lungs and P_{O_2} is higher and P_{CO_2} lower than at the bases.

Congenital heart disease may affect ventilation-perfusion ratios. For example, the average value for $\dot{V}_A\dot{Q}$ is decreased when there is a left-to-right shunt and increased when there is decreased perfusion of the lungs as in pulmonic stenosis.

Ventilation-perfusion relations may be measured in several ways. When ventilated areas are not well perfused, the difference between the physiologic and anatomic dead space (the alveolar dead space) will be increased. The alveolar-arterial (A-a) gas tension gradient increases when there are uneven $\dot{V}_A\dot{Q}$ ratios in various parts of the lung, but an increased A-a P_{O_2} gradient may also be due to changes in diffusion or direct venous admixture. Yet if the A-a P_{O_2} gradient is measured at ambient *and* at high inspired oxygen tensions, uneven $\dot{V}_A\dot{Q}$ ratios will be associated with little change. If, on the other hand, the A-a P_{O_2} gradient increases at low inspired oxygen tensions, a diffusion abnormality is likely, whereas a large A-a P_{O_2} gradient at high oxygen tensions suggests a direct venous admixture.

Nonuniform $\dot{V}_A\dot{Q}$ ratios will also result in an increased A-a gradient for P_{N_2}, and this has been the basis for another technique for indirectly estimating such changes. Since the P_{N_2} of urine is a reflection of arterial P_{N_2}, the A-a P_{N_2} gradient can be measured in the steady state without drawing blood. In the newborn infant the normal value for A-a P_{N_2} gradient is about 20 mm. Hg or more, but within a few days of birth it approaches the adult value of 10 mm. or less.

CILIARY ACTIVITY

No discussion of the ventilatory system is complete without some consideration of the cilia and their activity. Normally, cilia line the air passages down to the level of the terminal bronchioles. The continuous activity of the cilia has been described as the natural defense mechanism against extraneous agents. In animal studies, at least, the cilia have been shown to beat approximately 1300 times a minute and to move mucus toward the upper part of the respiratory tract at about 1.5 cm. per minute.

Ciliary activity is directly related to the level of humidity in the inhaled gas, a fact which provides at least a partial scientific basis for the use of humidified air in infections of the upper respiratory tract. In addition, there is considerable evidence that any irritant, including inhaled cigarette smoke, may reduce the effectiveness of the cilia in keeping the air passages free of mucus and foreign material.

It has recently been shown that the ciliary activity of respiratory epithelial cells is adversely affected in vitro by perfusion with serums from patients with cystic fibrosis and their parents. The clinical significance of this finding remains to be determined.

Normally the lower respiratory tract is free of bacteria, but bacteria may be introduced by techniques for inhalation therapy or respiratory assistance. In addition, various conditions, such as cystic fibrosis, bronchiectasis, malignancy and chronic bronchitis, and broad-spectrum antibiotic therapy may predispose to lower respiratory tract infection. According to animal experiments, alveolar macrophages are effective in clearing these organisms from the lung, although the mucociliary "escalator" may also contribute.

METHODS OF ASSESSING VENTILATORY FUNCTION

Scrupulous history and physical examination combined with selected studies, including roentgenograms, bacterial and viral cultures and, on occasion, biopsy of the lung, are essential for the diagnosis of ventilatory abnormalities. Pulmonary function tests are rarely helpful in establishing specific diagnoses; rather they are useful in assessing the severity of disease, following the course of pulmonary conditions, evaluating the effect of therapy, or providing a better understanding of the disordered physiology.

Conditions affecting the function of the ventilatory system may be classified into 5 main groups: (1) restrictive disorders which limit the inflation and deflation of the lungs (e.g. respiratory muscle weakness), (2) obstructive diseases which lead to increased resistance to the flow of air within the lungs (e.g. asthma), (3) abnormalities in ventilatory control (e.g. central nervous system depression), (4) rarely, defects in the diffusion of gases, especially oxygen, across the alveolar membrane (e.g. idiopathic pulmonary hemosiderosis), and (5) abnormalities in the pulmonary circulation (e.g. primary pulmonary arterial hypertension). Fortunately the 3 most frequently encountered types of conditions, restrictive disorders, obstructive diseases, and abnormalities in control, are the most readily studied with pulmonary function tests (see Table 12-2). To quantitate ventilatory function, the appropriate test should be applied. Although many complex techniques are available, those mentioned below are either easily applicable or, in some cases, necessary for the quantitation of the type of condition suspected by the clinical examination. The fact that a high proportion of the tests require understanding and active participation on the part of the patient limits the use of many of the techniques to children 5 years of age or older.

Tests for Restrictive Disorders. In restrictive disorders the total excursion of the chest is limited and the vital capacity is thus reduced. Predicted values for vital capacity can be obtained from the following formulas:

5-15 YEARS	16+ YEARS
Males ....250 ml./yr. age	25 ml./cm. height
Females......200 ml./yr. age	20 ml./cm. height

These estimations are clinically useful, but not sufficiently accurate for research purposes. Normal values for children of various heights are given in Table 12-1.

Crying vital capacities have been measured in newborn infants by means of a face mask connected to a spirometer with low inertia. The average vital capacity for a full-term (3.0 kg.) infant is approximately 140 ml.

If the restrictive disorder is thought to be secondary to muscle weakness, effective muscle strength can be measured directly with an anaeroid manometer. In order for the results to be comparable to predicted values, it is necessary to measure expiratory strength starting at full inspiration and inspiratory strength starting at full expiration.

Tests for Obstructive Diseases. Obstruction to the flow of air is the primary physiologic derangement in many of the acute (e.g. bronchiolitis and croup) and chronic (e.g. asthma and cystic fibrosis) diseases of childhood. The direct measurement of airway resistance involves complex research techniques. Resistance (R) is related to pressure (P) and flow (F) in the following fashion:

$$R = \frac{P}{F}$$

If pressure or muscle strength is normal, measurement of flow provides a good index of airway obstruction. Air passages are compressed during forced expiration, and obstruction is more readily detectable during such a maneuver.

A number of different techniques are available for measuring flow rates. Recording a forced expiratory vital capacity on a rapidly revolving drum allows the measurement of the peak flow rate. In predicting normal values the effect of body size on lung volume can be disregarded when the proportion of the total vital capacity forcibly expired in the first 1, 2 or 3 seconds is calculated from a recording spirometer. It should be emphasized that the absolute values should also be recorded and will be influenced by body size and starting lung volume. The peak flow meter of Wright is also useful and is available in 2 sizes, one for small children and one for older children and adults. Predicted values for the Wright peak flow meter can be obtained from equation 1 (below).

In children 3 to 5 years of age a sensitive flow meter (a pneumotachygraph) has proved useful. In this age group, peak expiratory flow rates for children of both sexes may be obtained from the formula below (equation 2).

1. For boys: Peak flow rate (L./min.) = 5.70 × ht. (cm.) − 480
(S.D. = ±14.5%)
For girls: Peak flow rate (L./min.) = 4.65 × ht. (cm.) − 344
(S.D. = ±14.3%)
2. Peak flow rate (L./min.) = 11.62 × age (yr.) + 2.862 × ht. (in.)
− 60.12 (S.D. = ±24%)

Recently it has been demonstrated that measurement of maximal flow in relation to various lung volumes provides a sensitive method of demonstrating obstruction in patients with such conditions as asthma and cystic fibrosis. This technique allows for comparison of maximal expiratory flow rates at various lung volumes with normal values.

Tests for Regulation of Ventilation. Depression of the central nervous system secondary to asphyxia, trauma, infection, increased intracranial pressure or drugs is frequently associated with inadequate ventilation. There may be a decreased respiratory rate or disturbed rhythm (e.g. Cheyne-Stokes respiration). In addition, paralysis or muscle weakness may lead to hypoventilation.

The adequacy of ventilation can be estimated by measuring the minute volume ($\dot{V}_E$) by means of a recording spirometer or a ventilation meter. The measured tidal volumes are then compared with the predicted values obtained from a nomogram (Fig. 12-3) at the observed frequency of breathing. The use of the nomogram involves the assumption that the lungs themselves are relatively normal and that the body weight is a good index of the person's metabolism or carbon dioxide production. Knowing the weight and the frequency of breathing, one can then predict the required tidal volume.

This calculation is most applicable when regulating artificial respiration in respiratory muscle weakness or during apnea or anesthesia. Use of the nomogram is demonstrated by the following example:

A 40-pound male child requires artificial ventilation. His temperature is 40° C., he is breathing through a tracheostomy tube, he is not in coma, and he is at an altitude of 3000 feet. Respiratory frequency is set at 20 per minute. Corrections to be applied to basal tidal volume are listed on the nomogram (Fig. 12-3) and demonstrated below:

Basal tidal......................... 135 ml.
Awake + 10%..................... 14 ml.
Fever + 3 × 9 = 27%........... 36 ml.
Altitude + 1.5 × 5 = 7.5% ..... 10 ml.
                                    _____
                                    195 ml.
Tracheostomy − 40/2............. −20 ml.
                                    _____
                                    175 ml. predicted required V_T by tracheostomy tube

Predicted required minute volume ($\dot{V}_E$) is V_T times f; i.e. $\dot{V}_E$ is 175 × 20, or 3500 ml. per minute.

The adequacy of ventilation may be evaluated more accurately by measuring the alveolar or, more directly, arterial partial pressure of carbon dioxide. The determination of "alveolar" or end-

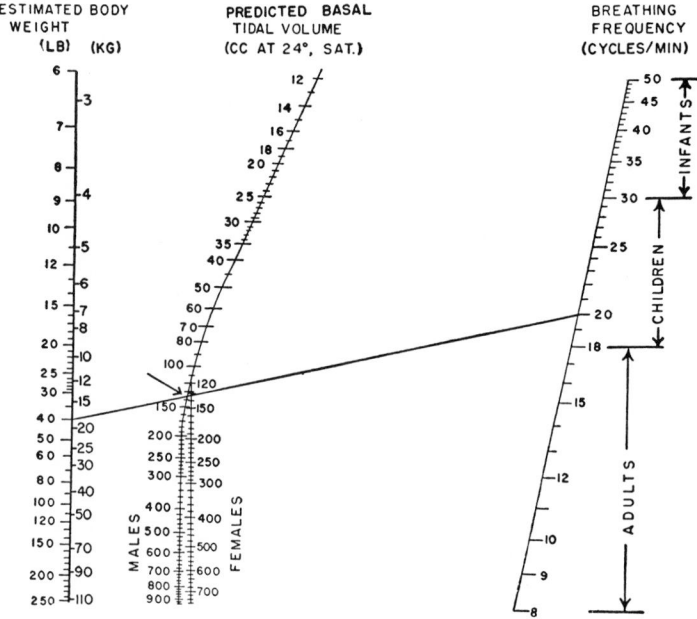

Figure 12-3. Nomogram for regulation of artificial respiration.

Corrections to be applied to basal tidal volume:

For metric system:

1. Add 10 per cent for daily activity (i.e. patient not in coma).
2. Add 9 per cent for each 1° C. above 37° C. rectal temperature.
3. Add 8 per cent for each 1000 M. altitude above sea level.
4. Subtract 1 cc./kg. weight if patient is breathing through a tracheostomy or endotracheal tube.

For English systems:

1. Add 10 per cent for daily activity (i.e. patient not in coma).
2. Add 5 per cent for each 1° F. above 99° F. rectal temperature.
3. Add 5 per cent for each 2000 ft. above sea level.
4. Subtract volume (cc.) equal to one-half body weight expressed as pounds if patient is breathing through a tracheostomy or endotracheal tube.

tidal P_{CO_2}, which can be continuously measured and recorded with an infrared carbon dioxide analyzer, is the most practical. End-tidal P_{CO_2}, however, will not reflect the alveolar gas tension unless the physiologic dead space is completely cleared.

Cyanosis is, of course, an indication of respiratory insufficiency except in patients with shock, cardiovascular disease or methemoglobinemia. If cyanosis occurs in spite of adequate ventilation as judged either by minute volume or, better still, by arterial P_{CO_2} measurements, then the need is for higher concentrations of oxygen and not for an increase in ventilation. Increased ventilation produces relatively little change in arterial oxygen saturation, but removes significant amounts of carbon dioxide from the body, lowers the P_{CO_2} and increases pH. A decreased P_{CO_2} even in the presence of a compensated pH is not a normal state and may cause temporary personality changes.

Tests for Diffusion Defects. Although rare in children, pulmonary diffusion defects may be suspected from roentgen findings consistent with generalized interstitial fibrosis or a clinical history consistent with pulmonary hemosiderosis. Since the oxygen diffusing rate is approximately one twentieth that of carbon dioxide, the principal failure of gas exchange in the presence of diffusing difficulties involves oxygen. Thus, with partial compensation resulting from hyperventilation, the typical blood gas findings are a low Pa_{O_2} and a normal or low Pa_{CO_2}. Further quantitation and definition (defective membrane diffusion or a decrease in pulmonary capillaries) of the diffusion defect require the actual measurement of lung diffusing capacity, most easily performed by using carbon monoxide as the indicator gas. This technique is difficult, however, especially in small children, and requires complex apparatus. Furthermore, when uneven ventilation is present, any interpretation of diffusion studies is of limited value.

Tests for Pulmonary Circulation. The pulmonary circulation, whether primarily involved in a disease process as in pulmonary artery hypertension or secondarily as in scoliosis, always requires for its investigation a fluoroscopic examination and usually necessitates cardiac catheterization (cf. section on heart disease). Measurement of pulmonary diffusing capacity at 2 oxygen tensions allows calculation of the pulmonary capillary blood volume, which tends to increase with left-to-right shunts and to decrease with various forms of interstitial fibrosis.

Differential Bronchospirometry. Localization of pulmonary dysfunction depends primarily on physical and roentgen examination. The insertion of a divided catheter is possible in children 12 years of age and older, and the ventilation, vital capacity and oxygen uptake of the right and left lungs may be compared.

Exercise Tolerance Tests. Provided the lungs alone are abnormal, their functional capacity may be measured indirectly by measuring exercise tolerance and comparing the results with standards established for children of comparable age and sex.

ARTIFICIAL RESPIRATION

Although obvious technical and quantitative differences exist, the basic principles of artificial respiration are the same for all ages and are as follows:

1. Maintenance of an adequate airway by
   a. Extension of neck with forward traction on mandible
   b. Gentle suction
   c. Intubation or tracheotomy
2. Institution of adequate ventilation as quickly as possible
3. Avoidance of injury to the patient

Severe hypoxia of only a few minutes may lead to irreversible damage, especially to the brain. Fortunately the newborn infant can tolerate hypoxia better than older persons, but, since the duration and severity of intrauterine hypoxia are impossible to gauge accurately, one should not delay resuscitative procedures even in the newborn. Oxygen administration is a useful adjunct, but is no substitute for adequate ventilation.

The methods of producing artificial respiration are (1) manual, (2) positive pressure applied to the airway, or negative pressure about the body, (3) rhythmic rocking of the patient, and (4) electrical stimulation of the phrenic nerve.

Newborn Infant. The normal newborn infant should not require resuscitation. If respiration has not started by 30 to 60 seconds after birth and is not fully established by 1 to 3 minutes, the central nervous system is probably depressed. Initially a free airway should be established. For this purpose an oral airway is usually adequate, although under special circumstances, and when an experienced person is available, tracheal intubation may be useful. Intubation by unskilled persons, however, may do more harm than good.

If not expanded, the lungs may most practically be inflated by positive pressure applied by a mask or through the endotracheal tube. The magnitude of the pressure necessary and its duration are variable for each infant. Available data suggest that transpulmonary pressures up to 20 cm. of water are usually safe, but in many instances pressures of 30 to 50 cm. may be necessary for adequate expansion. Certainly high pressures, if used at all, should be used with caution and for brief periods only, and only in infants with unexpanded or incompletely expanded lungs.

Pressures may be applied and controlled by a variety of machines and with practice and experience by mouth-to-mouth or mouth-to-tube resuscitation. The latter techniques have the disadvantage that there is a chance of cross infection between the patient and the physician, and pressure is difficult to gauge or control. Since hypoxia causes depression of the respiratory center

itself, supplemental oxygen should be supplied in
all instances until spontaneous respiration is
established. The apneic infant is already hyper-
capneic and acidotic, and the administration of
carbon dioxide may only lead to further depression.
In the newborn infant particularly, but in anyone
subjected to artificial respiration, the effectiveness
of the procedure should be checked not only by
observation of the excursion of chest and abdomen
and auscultation of the lungs, but also by measurements of the ventilation and alveolar P_{CO_2} and
blood gases.

For the infant whose lungs have never expanded, rocking will accomplish little; subsequently the effectiveness of rocking is in direct
proportion to the size of the infant. Hence rocking
is of little direct use in small infants as a ventilating maneuver. Central nervous system stimulants
(other than oxygen) are of little or no use and in
some instances may be harmful. Tubbing, spank-
ing, jackknifing and manual compression of the
thorax are all dangerous and ineffective. Phrenic
nerve stimulation produces a more natural type
of breathing, but has limited practical use because
of the need for special equipment and a trained
operator.

Infants and Older Children. Since the lungs
of older infants and children have already been
expanded, other techniques are applicable. Positive pressure (e.g. mouth-to-mouth) is useful once
a free airway has been established. In addition,
manual compression and expansion of the thorax
as in the back pressure-arm lift method or back
pressure-hip lift method can produce adequate
ventilation, provided there is no respiratory obstruction. Electrical stimulation of the phrenic
nerve is more practical than it is in the newborn
infant. For more prolonged artificial ventilation
the tank type of respirator, endotracheal positive
pressure, the rocking bed and special chest-type
or cuirass respirators can be used; the latter types
have limited usefulness in infants and small
children because the chest is compressed and
ventilation may be insufficient. When mechanical
artificial ventilation is required for a prolonged
period (hours or days), the patient should be given
deep breaths at regular intervals (2 or 3 times an
hour) in order to minimize the development of
atelectasis.

When apnea has been present for more than a
few minutes, the resulting acidosis should be
treated as soon as ventilation has been restored.

The effectiveness of various types of ventilating
devices is shown in Figure 12-4. The endotracheal
positive-pressure technique produces the greatest
tidal volume, owing to the compression of the gas
within the lungs. The effectiveness of the cuirass
respirators varies with the amount of the body
enclosed within them and the freedom of motion
allowed. The rocking beds are not included, since
there is great variation with the size of the patient.

There is no special pressure that should be used
for different age groups. The pressure or degree of
tilting should be set so that the required tidal

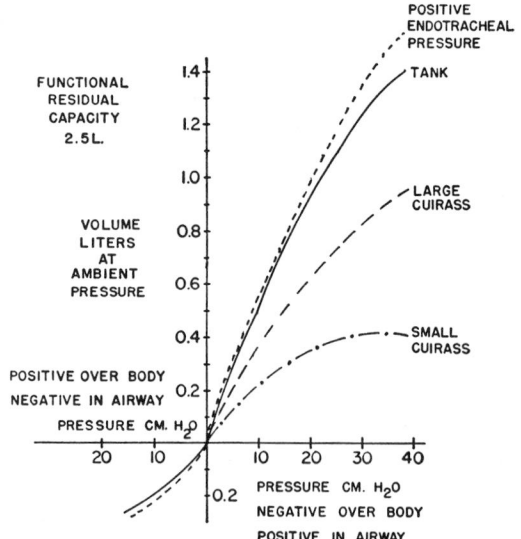

Figure 12-4. Effectiveness of breathing machines.

volume or an end-tidal P_{CO_2} of 40 mm. Hg is
obtained. This requires measuring the tidal
volume and comparing it with the predicted values
from the nomogram (Fig. 12-3) or measuring the
end-tidal P_{CO_2}. If the device is unable to produce
sufficient pressure at a given frequency, adequate
ventilation may be obtained by increasing the
frequency, which in turn usually increases the
pressure developed. A new calculation from the
nomogram will be necessary, since the predicted
tidal volume will be different. Optimally, blood
gas tensions should be checked in order to evaluate
the adequacy of ventilation.

INHALATION THERAPY

Besides oxygen, the most frequently used agents
for inhalation therapy are water, antibiotics and
bronchodilators, which are administered in compressed air or oxygen.

Oxygen. The therapeutic use of oxygen is not
without danger. In premature infants, concentrations of oxygen above that of room air increase the
incidence of retrolental fibroplasia. When 40 or
even 30 per cent oxygen is administered at sea
level, alveolar oxygen tensions may reach approximately 240 and 185 mm. Hg respectively. If a
mildly cyanotic infant is placed in such concentrations of oxygen, depending on the type of pathophysiologic change in the lungs, the possibility
of raising the arterial oxygen tension above the
safe (for retrolental fibroplasia) level is very real.
In addition to administering oxygen to premature
infants with primary pulmonary disease (e.g.
hyaline membrane syndrome), it is sometimes
necessary to give oxygen to those with episodes
of apnea. Often, however, the lungs are normal,
and under such circumstances arterial oxygen
tensions will approach the alveolar oxygen tension

as soon as regular respiration is reinstituted. Thus, if the risk of retrolental fibroplasia is to be minimized in the premature infant, it is imperative that the use of increased concentrations of oxygen be limited to those infants who are cyanotic. Furthermore, such therapy should be limited to the minimum concentration necessary to prevent cyanosis and should be discontinued as promptly as possible. There are, however, instances when oxygen therapy is necessary for the survival of a premature infant with severe hypoxemia; in such instances the potential benefit of the increased concentration of oxygen outweighs the potential risk of retrolental fibroplasia.

Oxygen therapy is also potentially dangerous in patients with chronic underventilation who are cyanotic. These patients may stop breathing and die, because the drive to breathe, which came from the low blood oxygen tension, is removed. Owing to chronic underventilation, blood carbon dioxide is high, and the respiratory center is no longer responsive to carbon dioxide. If the Pa_{CO_2} is initially about 80 mm. Hg, a further increase may reach narcotic levels, and the patient will become comatose. In such a situation artificial respiration may be necessary.

Environmental concentrations of oxygen greater than 60 per cent for a period of days are also toxic to the lungs themselves; hence the prolonged use of such high concentrations should be avoided if possible.

Water. The administration of air or oxygen supersaturated with water has long been used when there is evidence of increased or tenacious secretions and narrowing of the larger air passages (as with laryngitis or tracheobronchitis). Similarly, inhalation of water vapor is important in the management of patients breathing through a tracheostomy tube, when the normal humidifying action of the upper respiratory system is bypassed. Furthermore, in the premature infant, relatively high humidity (more than 60 per cent) helps to prevent heat loss and hence stabilizes the body temperature.

The use of vaporized water in peripheral pulmonary disease is less certainly effective. The air from the lower part of the trachea to the periphery of the lung is normally saturated with water at body temperature, whereas air saturated with water at room temperature (24° C.) is only 50 per cent saturated when raised to body temperature. Thus a saturated atmosphere does not necessarily supply saturated gas to the peripheral air passages.

Antibiotics. Inhalation of antibiotics in compressed air or oxygen (aerosols) is occasionally useful in the control of severe, diffuse pulmonary disease (e.g. cystic fibrosis). In most instances, however, the same agents may be as effective and more easily administered orally or parenterally. Furthermore, the distribution of ventilation, as well as the size of the droplets, the growth of the droplets, the polarization of the particles, and possibly other factors determine the penetration

of an aerosol into the smaller pulmonary units and thus impose limitations on aerosol therapy.

Bronchodilators. A number of bronchodilators can be effectively administered by inhalation. This route has the physical advantage that it is easy for the patient and the psychologic advantage that it is a means of treating directly the bronchoconstriction and thus the patient's symptoms. The disadvantage of this route is the difficulty in controlling dosage.

CHARLES DAVENPORT COOK

REFERENCES

Abramson, H. (Ed.): *Resuscitation of the Newborn Infant.* St. Louis, C. V. Mosby Company, 1960.

Avery, M. E.: *The Lung and Its Disorders in the Newborn Infant.* 2nd ed. Philadelphia, W. B. Saunders Company, 1968.

Barcroft, J.: *Researches on Pre-Natal Life.* Springfield, Ill., Charles C Thomas, 1947.

Bengtsson, E.: The Working Capacity in Normal Children, Evaluated by Submaximal Exercise on the Bicycle Ergometer and Compared with Adults. *Acta Med. Scand.,* 154:91, 1956.

Bucci, G., Cook, C. D., and Barrie, H.: Studies of Respiratory Physiology in Children. V. Total Lung Diffusion, Diffusing Capacity of Pulmonary Membrane and Pulmonary Capillary Blood Volume in Normal Subjects from 7 to 40 Years of Age. *J. Pediat.,* 58:820, 1961.

Colville, P., Shugg, C., and Ferris, B. G., Jr.: Effects of Body Tilting on Respiratory Mechanics. *J. Appl. Physiol.,* 9:19, 1956.

Comroe, J. H., Jr.: *Physiology of Respiration.* Chicago, Year Book Medical Publishers, Inc., 1965.

Cook, C. D., and Hamann, J. F.: Relation of Lung Volumes to Height in Healthy Persons Between the Ages of 5 and 38 Years. *J. Pediat.,* 59:710, 1961.

Cross, K. W., and Oppé, T. E.: The Effects of Inhalation of High and Low Concentrations of Oxygen in the Respiration of Premature Infants. *J. Physiol.,* 117:38, 1952.

Cross, K. W., Klaus, M., Tooley, W. H., and Weisser, K.: The Response of the Newborn Baby to Inflation of the Lungs. *J. Physiol.,* 151:551, 1960.

Dalhamn, T.: Mucous Flow and Ciliary Activity in the Trachea of Healthy Rats and Rats Exposed to Respiratory Irritant Gases (SO_2, H_3N, HCHO). *Acta Physiol. Scand.,* 36: Supplement, 123, 1956.

Ferris, B. G., Jr.: Studies of Pulmonary Function. *New England J. Med.,* 262:557, 610, 1960.

Ferris, B. G., Jr., and Smith, C. W.: Maximum Breathing Capacity in Female Children and Adolescents. *Pediatrics,* 12:341, 1953.

Ferris, B. G., Jr., Whittenberger, J. L., and Gallagher, J. R.: Maximum Breathing Capacity and Vital Capacity of Male Children and Adolescents. *Pediatrics,* 9:659, 1953.

Ferris, B. G., Jr., Mead, J., Whittenberger, J. L., and Saxton, G. A.: Pulmonary Function in Convalescent Poliomyelitis Patients. III. Compliance of Lungs and Thorax. *New England J. Med.,* 240:390, 1952.

Gaensler, E. A.: Analysis of the Ventilatory Defect by Timed Vital Capacity Measurements. *Am. Rev. Tuberc.,* 64:256, 1951.

Gluck, L., Motoyama, E. K., Smits, H. L., and Kulovich, M. V.: The Biochemical Development of Surface Activity in Mammalian Lung. I. The Surface Active Phospholipids; The Separation and Distribution of Surface Active Lecithin in the Lung of the Developing Rabbit Fetus. *Pediat. Res.,* 1:237, 1967.

Harned, H. S., Jr., Rowshan, G., Mac Kinney, L. G., and Sugioka, K.: Relationships of P_{O_2}, P_{CO_2}, and pH to Onset of Breathing of the Term Lamb as Studied by a Flow-Through Curvette Electrode Assembly. *Pediatrics,* 33:672, 1964.

Jackson, A. E., Southern, P. M., Pierce, A. K., Fallis, B. D., and

Sanford, J. P.: Pulmonary Clearance of Gram-Negative Bacilli. *J. Lab. & Clin. Med.,* 69:833, 1967.

Long, E. C., and Hull, W. E.: Respiratory Volume-Flow in the Crying Newborn Infant. *Pediatrics,* 27:373, 1961.

Mead, J.: Mechanical Properties of Lungs. *Physiol. Rev.,* 41:281, 1961.

Murray, A. B., and Cook, C. D.: Measurement of Peak Expiratory Flow Rates in 220 Normal Children from 4½ to 18½ years of Age. *J. Pediatrics,* 62:186, 1963.

Nelson, N. M.: Neonatal Pulmonary Function. *Pediat. Clin. N. Amer.,* 13:769, 1966.

Radford, E. P., Jr., Ferris, B. G., Jr., and Kriete, B. C.: Clinical Use of a Nomogram to Estimate Proper Ventilation During Artificial Respiration. *New England J. Med.,* 251:877, 1954.

Rivera, L. M., and Snider, G. L.: Ventilatory Studies in Preschool Children. I. Peak Expiratory Flow Rates in Normal and Abnormal Preschool Children. *Pediatrics,* 30:117, 1962.

Spock, A., Heick, H., Cress, H., and Logan, W.: In Vivo Study of Ciliary Motility: Asymmetrical Ciliary Beat Associated with Sera of Patients with Cystic Fibrosis. In 4th International Conference on Cystic Fibrosis, Berne, Switzerland, September 1966.

Sutherland, J. M., and Ratcliff, J. W.: Crying Vital Capacity. *Am. J. Dis. Child.,* 101:67, 1961.

RESPIRATORY DISTURBANCES

General Introduction. Disturbances in respiration are not necessarily related to lesions in or disease of the respiratory tract, because the process of breathing is influenced by the function of many organs other than lungs, and because the amount of respiratory exchange required depends on many factors extrinsic to the lung. Accordingly, in the differential diagnosis of respiratory disturbances, one must consider genetic (anatomic and metabolic) anomalies, traumatic, chemical (poisoning) or infectious factors. From an anatomic standpoint, the primary lesions may be in the respiratory system, or in the central nervous, cardiovascular, endocrine, urinary or gastrointestinal systems. The disturbed respiratory patterns found with disorders of other systems are discussed in their respective sections; here we will deal with primary diseases of the respiratory tract, excluding the conditions peculiar to the neonatal period.

Age as a Factor in Infectious Respiratory Disease. The clinical pattern of respiratory illness varies in considerable degree with the age of the patient. Differences in susceptibility to infection occur, the younger child being either more or less susceptible, according to the particular agent involved. Rates of infection among infants exposed to group A beta hemolytic streptococci are lower than among their older siblings, and a similar pattern has been demonstrated for influenza. Moreover, streptococcal disease in the young may differ strikingly from that in older children and adults. In the child under 2 years streptococcal infection rarely produces exudative pharyngotonsillitis, but is usually manifested as an insidious, subacute, protracted illness whose common manifestation is rhinorrhea. On the other hand, the infant may suffer severe disease from certain agents which produce relatively trivial illness in the older child. Whooping cough, a relatively harmless tracheobronchitis of childhood, is a serious and often fatal disease in the infant under a year of age. Tuberculosis is strikingly more severe in the infant, with a decided tendency toward hematogenous dissemination. The respiratory syncytial virus, the parainfluenza viruses and the adenoviruses produce generally mild illnesses in older children, but are often associated in infants with severe lower respiratory tract disease such as bronchiolitis, pneumonia, and croup. Why these differences should exist is not completely understood. They are believed to be due in part to anatomic differences between the 2 age groups (distances between corresponding points of the respiratory tract are shorter, orifices are smaller, and connective tissue is less dense, so that swelling can occur more readily). It is also possible that prior experience with some viral agents serves to protect the older child from serious disease when reinfection occurs.

Aside from considerations of severity of illness in infants as compared to older children, the manifestations themselves may be different, and organ systems may be involved in one age group which are not affected in another. For example, adenovirus type 3 infection in an older child is often associated with the syndrome of pharyngoconjunctival fever; in infants this same agent may cause diarrhea without associated respiratory tract disease. The changes in susceptibility and the different manifestations of infection that occur with age are the products of interaction of 3 basic factors: immunologic, environmental and metabolic. These are influenced in turn by a number of others such as anatomy, heredity and nutrition. The complexity of the situation is great, and little is known of the mechanisms through which these factors operate.

THE UPPER RESPIRATORY TRACT

THE NOSE

In man the primary functions of the nose are to adjust the humidity and temperature of inspired air and to remove foreign particles and bacteria from the air stream. Passage through the organ raises air temperature to nearly that of the body, and adjusts the relative humidity to approximately 80 per cent.

Bacteria and other foreign matter are impinged on the "mucous blanket" covering the ciliated pseudocolumnar epithelium of the nasal passages. This blanket is continuously propelled toward the pharynx by ciliary action, the movement being sufficiently rapid to require the replacement of the mucous layer approximately every 10 minutes.

The principal defense mechanisms of the nose appear to consist in the mechanical removal of bacteria and other noxious elements by means of this mucous blanket. Any intranasal medication which affects adversely the production of mucus, the integrity of the mucus or the behavior of the ciliary cells will reduce the efficiency of the protective barrier.

Nasal secretions contain specialized IgA antibodies, which presumably offer an immunologic barrier to infection and the enzyme lysozyme, whose action is capable of destroying bacteria, but whose exact protective function remains unknown.

Malformations. Structural nasal abnormalities of congenital origin are uncommon in contrast to acquired malformations. Occasionally, nasal bones are congenitally absent, and then the bridge of the nose will fail to develop, resulting in nasal hypoplasia. As part of a series of major malformations, congenital absence of the nose, complete or partial duplication, or a single centrally placed nostril will occasionally occur, but most of these are part of syndromes which are not compatible with life. Rarely, supernumerary teeth may be found in the nose, or teeth may grow into it from the maxilla and be absent from their usual site.

A more common defect is hypertelorism which results from overdevelopment of the lesser wings of the sphenoid. The most prominent physical manifestation is widening of the base of the nose, with the eyes widely separated. On occasion, nasal bones are sufficiently malformed to produce severe narrowing of the nasal passages. Often such narrowing is associated with a high and narrow hard palate. Patients with these defects may suffer from chronic or recurrent infections of the nasal and paranasal passages. Rarely, the alae nasi may be sufficiently thin and poorly supported to result in inspiratory obstruction.

The most common congenital abnormality of the nasal passages is *choanal atresia*. If only one side is affected, this does not give rise to severe symptoms at birth; however, if both nares are blocked by a membranous, cartilaginous or bony septum, the condition produces obvious symptoms in most but not all babies. Some infants are unable to breathe through their mouths when both nares are blocked, while others can mouth-breathe. Those infants unable to breathe through their mouths will make increasingly vigorous efforts at inspiration, with a sucking in of their lips, will become cyanotic quickly, and may soon die. Infants able to breathe through their mouths experience difficulty only in sucking and swallowing and will become cyanotic as they attempt to nurse. Bilateral choanal occlusion should be suspected in a newborn infant who persistently breathes through his mouth, or is cyanotic when at rest with his mouth closed, but returns to normal color when he cries. Unilateral choanal obstruction is usually asymptomatic until infection occurs, which results in profuse anterior nasal discharge, usually unilateral.

The obstruction can be demonstrated by the failure of a firm catheter or probe to pass into the nasopharynx. Other diagnostic possibilities can be eliminated with the instillation through a catheter of a radiopaque substance into each nostril while the infant is lying on his back. The nasal cavity will be outlined and the posterior block readily seen radiographically.

With bilateral choanal atresia, prompt establishment of an airway is urgent. In an emergency this is done most readily either by propping the jaws open with any suitable device or by making an airway from the mouth into the nasopharynx. The infant can then be fed by gavage until such time (usually 2 or 3 weeks) as he learns to breathe, as well as to eat, without the airway. Immediate surgery was formerly recommended, but operation can be delayed for weeks, months or even years. In those cases in which obstruction is unilateral, it is usually desirable to postpone operation until infection has been controlled and the infant is in otherwise satisfactory physical condition.

Deviation of the nasal septum is generally an acquired rather than a congenital condition and is rarely seen in young children. When this condition produces difficulty, operation is best deferred until the child is 14 or 15 years of age, since earlier operation often results in external deformities of the nose. *Perforation of the nasal septum* may rarely be a congenital defect, but is most likely caused by syphilis or tuberculosis. Other malformations of the septum, of the floor of the nose and of the external nose are frequently associated with harelip and cleft palate. An *encephalocele* protruding through a defect in the cribriform plate into the nasal cavity is a rare anomaly, but must be differentiated from polyps and tumors of extracranial origin.

Foreign Bodies in the Nose. Foreign bodies such as vegetables, nuts, erasers, paper wads, beads and stones are frequently introduced into the nose in early childhood. The object is usually situated well anteriorly at first, but through the unskillful efforts of the patient or others it may be forced deeper into the nose.

Initial symptoms are local obstruction, sneezing, relatively mild discomfort, and rarely pain. Irritation results in mucosal swelling, and, because some foreign bodies are hygroscopic and increase in size as water is absorbed, signs of local obstruction and discomfort may increase with time. Infection usually follows and gives rise to a purulent, malodorous or bloody discharge. Unilateral nasal discharge and obstruction should suggest the presence of a foreign body, which can usually be readily seen upon examination with a speculum or nasoscope. Removal should be promptly carried out in order to minimize the danger of aspiration of the object and to prevent local tissue necrosis. In most children, removal can be performed with topical anesthesia, using either forceps or nasal suction apparatus. Infection usually clears promptly upon removal of the object, and generally no further therapy is necessary.

The most frequent nasal growths are polyps, but rarely other tumors of the nose and nasopharynx occur (see p. 1438). Polyps are most often associated with allergic rhinitis and with cystic fibrosis; they usually produce obstructive symptoms as well as chronic nasal discharge. Treatment consists in their removal and attention to the underlying cause.

EPISTAXIS

Etiology. Nosebleeds are rare in infancy, common in childhood, and decrease in incidence after puberty. The condition is more common in males. The source of the bleeding generally is from the vascular plexus on the anterior septum and the mucosa of the anterior turbinates. By far the most common cause is trauma, including picking of the nose. Epistaxis is also encountered with adenoidal hypertrophy, with allergic rhinitis, sinusitis or polyps, and with a variety of acute infections such as rheumatic fever, scarlet fever, influenza, measles, varicella, typhoid fever, congenital syphilis, and diphtheria. In the last two conditions the discharge is generally both bloody and purulent. Especially severe bleeding may be encountered with such vascular abnormalities as telangiectasias or varicosities or if the child has such a generalized vascular condition as hypertension, venous congestion or a blood dyscrasia. Occasionally adolescent girls will have epistaxis at the time of menstruation.

Clinical Manifestations. Epistaxis usually occurs without warning, blood flowing slowly but freely from one nostril, occasionally from both. In children with nasal lesions, bleeding may follow physical exercise. When bleeding occurs at night, the blood is usually swallowed and may become apparent only when the child vomits or passes blood in his stools. Most nosebleeds stop spontaneously in a few minutes, but if bleeding continues, the child should be kept as quiet as possible in an erect position with the head tilted forward to eliminate blood trickling posteriorly into the pharynx. Local control of the hemorrhage can usually be achieved by compressing the nares. If these simple measures do not stop the bleeding, local application of a solution of epinephrine (1:1000) with or without topical thrombin may on occasion be useful. If bleeding persists, an anterior nasal pack should be inserted; if bleeding originates in the posterior nares, combined anterior and postchoanal packing is necessary. After bleeding has been controlled, and if a bleeding site can be identified, its obliteration by cautery with silver nitrate may prevent further difficulties. In patients with severe or repeated nasal hemorrhages, blood transfusions may be necessary, or special blood products and derivatives may be required for those patients who have an underlying hematologic disorder.

ELONGATED UVULA

Persistent enlargement of the uvula is rare; it may be congenital or may result from a chronic upper respiratory tract infection. The long uvula coming into contact with the base of the tongue produces an annoying cough and a constant desire to clear the throat. These symptoms tend to be exaggerated when the child is lying on his back. Enlargement associated with chronic infection may disappear with eradication of the infection. Otherwise, amputation of the tip of the uvula may be indicated.

Infections of the Upper Respiratory Tract

General Considerations. By a generally accepted definition, upper respiratory tract infections are those infectious processes primarily affecting the structures of the respiratory tract above the larynx. Some illnesses, however, affect the upper and lower portions of the tract simultaneously or sequentially; and others, more generalized, involve different portions of the respiratory tree at various times during the course of the illness. Diagnostic classification on an anatomic basis is, therefore, often arbitrary and depends largely upon which organ or area the physician or the patient concludes is most obviously involved.

Because large numbers of different microorganisms (chiefly viruses) are capable of causing primary upper respiratory tract disease, with few producing distinctive clinical syndromes, etiologic classification is of limited use. The same organism may cause clinical symptoms or syndromes of differing severity and extent in accordance with such host factors as age, sex, previous contact with the agent, allergy, nutritional status, and the like. For example, among different members of the same family a single virus may simultaneously produce typical colds in the parents, bronchiolitis in the infant, croup in a somewhat older child, pharyngitis in another, and a subclinical infection in another. Most of these agents, whether viral, bacterial or mycoplasma, can affect the respiratory tract in much the same way. There is, in a clinical sense, no true "cold" virus or "pharyngitis" agent; rather, any clinical syndrome involving the upper tract may be caused by a number of different organisms, not identifiable except by suitable laboratory investigations.

Etiologic Considerations of Nonbacterial Infections of the Respiratory Tract. It has become increasingly apparent that most acute respiratory tract infections are caused by viruses and mycoplasma. Exceptions are acute epiglottitis and the pneumonias of lobar distribution. Formerly, it was widely held that various bacteria, and especially *H. influenzae*, were responsible for significant proportions of these illnesses. With the advent of modern methods of virology it has been clearly established that the group A beta hemolytic streptococcus and the diphtheria organism are the only bacterial agents capable of causing primary nasal or pharyngeal disease; even in cases of acute tonsillopharyngitis, most illnesses are of nonbacterial origin.

Viruses and Mycoplasmas Which May Produce Acute Respiratory Disease. The viruses and mycoplasmas which can cause acute respiratory disease are listed in Table 12-3. Each of these organisms produces a spectrum of effects ranging from inapparent infection to severe respiratory tract illness. Though considerable overlapping exists, some microorganisms are more likely to produce a given respiratory syndrome than others. Certain agents have a greater tendency than others to produce severe disease.

The respiratory syncytial virus is the most important respiratory tract pathogen of the first years of childhood. It is the principal single cause of bronchiolitis, accounting for about one third of all cases. It is a common cause also of pneumonia, croup and bronchitis, as well as of undifferentiated febrile disease of the upper respiratory tract. Because of the severity of illnesses produced by infection with this agent, it accounts for a disproportionately large number of infants hospitalized with respiratory disease.

The parainfluenza viruses account for the majority of cases of the croup syndrome, but may also produce bronchitis, bronchiolitis and febrile upper respiratory tract disease. Type 1 is the agent most commonly associated with croup; type 3 is associated with croup as well as with other varieties of respiratory infection. Type 4 virus does not appear to be as pathogenic as the other three.

Except during epidemics, influenza viruses do not play much part in the various respiratory syndromes. In infants and children, influenza viruses account for more disease of the upper than the lower respiratory tract.

The adenoviruses account for less than 10 per cent of respiratory illnesses, many of which are

TABLE 12-3. Viruses and Mycoplasmas Which Cause Respiratory Disease in Infants and Children

	SEROTYPES		RELATIVE IMPORTANCE IN INDICATED SYNDROME*				
GROUP	TOTAL NUMBER	NUMBER ASSOCIATED WITH RESPIRATORY ILLNESS	BRON-CHIOLITIS	PNEU-MONIA	CROUP	BRON-CHITIS	URI
Myxovirus:							
Influenza	3	2 (A,B)	+	+	+	+	++
Parainfluenza	4	4 (1,2,3,4)	++	++	++++	+++	+++
Resp. syncytial	1	1	++++	++++	++	+++	+++
Adenovirus	30+	8 (1,2,3,4,5,7, 14,21)	++	+++	+	+++	+++
Picornavirus:							
Coxsackie A	24	8 (2,4,5,6,8, 10,21,22)					++
Coxsackie B	6	3 (2,3,5)					++
Rhinoviruses	60+	60+ (?)	++ (?)	++ (?)		++	++
Mycoplasmataceae	8	1 (M. pneumoniae)	+	++		++	+ (?)

*Relative importance graded on a scale of 0 to ++++.
Table modified from R. M. Chanock and R. H. Parrott: *Pediatrics, 36*:21, 1965.

TABLE 12-4. Ecology of Infection with Various Respiratory Tract Pathogens

GROUP	SEROTYPE	USUAL TIME OF PRIMARY INFECTION	PERSON-TO-PERSON SPREAD	PATTERN OF INFECTION	RISK OF INDICATED ILLNESS DURING PRIMARY INFECTION	REINFECTION
Myxovirus: Influenza	A,B	Infancy and childhood; any age for minor antigenic variants	Highly effective	Epidemic—every 2-4 years, usually winter	Influenza—75%	Common with new variants—less common with same variant
Parainfluenza	1,2,3,4	Infancy—type 3 Childhood—types 1,2,4	Highly effective—type 3; less effective—types 1,2,4	Endemic or sporadic—occasionally epidemic (types 1,3)	Febrile respiratory illness—50-75% (types 1,2,3)	Common—can be associated with URI
Resp. syncytial	—	Infancy	Highly effective	Epidemic, every year—fall, winter or spring	Febrile lower respiratory tract illness—45%	Common—often associated with URI
Adenovirus	1,2,3,5, 7	Infancy (1,2) Childhood (3,5,7)	Effective (1,2,5) or moderately effective (3,7)	Endemic (occasionally epidemic types 3,7)	Febrile respiratory disease—55-90%	Uncommon
Picornavirus: Coxsackie B		Infancy and childhood	Moderately effective	Epidemic—summer	Not known	Not known
Rhinovirus	60 or more	All ages	Ineffective	Endemic sporadic flurries of different types	URI 50%*	Occurs
M. pneumoniae	—	2nd and 3rd decades	Ineffective	Endemic or occasionally epidemic	Pneumonia 3—10%*	Uncommon

*Data for adult infection.
Table modified from R. M. Chanock and R. H. Parrott: *Pediatrics, 36*:21, 1965.

mild. A large proportion may be asymptomatic.

The activity of the rhinoviruses is limited almost entirely to the upper tract, most commonly the nose. They account for a significant proportion of the "common cold" syndrome. Rarely do they produce lower tract disease.

The Coxsackie A and B viruses produce primarily disease of the nasopharynx. This may be expressed as an undifferentiated febrile respiratory illness or, in the case of the group A organisms, as herpangina or exudative pharyngotonsillitis. Mycoplasma can produce both upper and lower respiratory tract illness, including bronchiolitis, pneumonia, bronchitis, and perhaps pharyngotonsillitis and otitis media. The frequency with which each of these organisms occurs in any age group varies from year to year, but in general mycoplasmas produce more disease in late childhood and early adult life than during infancy.

The ecology of infection, the seasonal pattern, the epidemiology, and the risk of reinfection are shown in Table 12-4. Several of these agents are encountered primarily during infancy, others at older ages, and some at all ages. They vary in contagiousness from very high to relatively low. With some, reinfection occurs readily, but a previous encounter may protect against subsequent serious disease.

Methods of Control. At present, vaccines exist only for influenza, and these are only moderately effective in preventing illness. Furthermore, the increased risk of febrile reactions to the vaccine with decreasing age has led to the recommendation that influenza vaccine not be given routinely to children, but only to those at special risk of complications, such as patients with cystic fibrosis, other types of chronic pulmonary conditions, or congenital heart disease.

No vaccines are available to protect children against infection from the other agents, nor is it likely that this situation will change in the near future. The multiplicity of viruses and strains alone would make the development of a "broad-spectrum" immunizing agent difficult; furthermore, even to the more important viruses potent vaccines are difficult to produce for a variety of technical reasons. The immunologic response is poor to vaccines against respiratory agents, and the protective effect of antibodies produced is relatively low. Even after the naturally acquired disease, reinfection occurs with many of these microorganisms. Some volunteers immunized against certain of these viruses and then challenged with the live agent have experienced severe illness.

It is not surprising that little protective effect can be expected from normal human gamma globulin. This substance is often administered to children with repeated respiratory infection, but its antibody content against the principal agents is low or undetectable, and even significant levels of antibody do not necessarily protect against disease.

Since bacteria do not play either a primary or secondary role in the undifferentiated upper respiratory tract diseases, the so-called bacterial cold vaccines can be expected to be ineffectual either in preventing illness or in changing the duration of disease.

ACUTE NASOPHARYNGITIS
("THE COMMON COLD")

The term "acute nasopharyngitis" designates that disease of children which corresponds to the common cold in adults. This difference in nomenclature is desirable because the disease in children differs clinically from that encountered among older persons. In children the infection is more extensive and involves the accessory paranasal sinuses, and usually the middle ear as well as the nasopharynx. It is usually accompanied by fever in children, whereas in adults the illness is usually afebrile as well as more limited in extent. Acute nasopharyngitis is the most common infectious condition of children, but its importance in pediatric practice depends primarily on the relative frequency with which complications occur.

Etiology. The illness is caused by a large number of different viruses; the principal agents appear to be the rhinoviruses. The period of infectivity is short, lasting from a few hours prior to the appearance of symptoms to a day or two after the illness has appeared. Since the activity of a virus in the respiratory tract impairs local host defense mechanisms, invasion of tissue by potentially pathogenic bacteria may occur during the course of the infection and be responsible for complications in the sinuses, ears, mastoids, lymph nodes and lungs. Bacteria most frequently involved in these complicating conditions are group A streptococci, pneumococci, *H. influenzae* and the staphylococci, the last two principally in the young child. Bacteria play no role in the course of the uncomplicated infection or in the pathogenesis of symptoms.

Contributory Factors. For reasons poorly understood, susceptibility to acute nasopharyngitis appears to vary in the same person from time to time. It is widely believed that various disturbances such as chilling, dampness, wet feet, and the like, greatly increase susceptibility to the infection, but there is no direct evidence to support this view. These "predisposing" events produce vasomotor effects and reduce the temperature of the nasal mucous membranes through vasoconstriction; this is later followed by vasodilatation, and on occasion by nasal irritation and discharge. These physiologic effects may exacer-

bate a chronic infection, but they do not cause a cold. The state of nutrition appears to have a moderate effect on susceptibility; frank malnutrition greatly increases the incidence of purulent complications.

Age does not appear to be a determining factor in susceptibility, but infection does result in a higher incidence of purulent complications in the young child. Infants under 6 months of age are susceptible, but do not commonly acquire colds because of the relative infrequency of exposure. In general, the frequency with which acute nasopharyngitis occurs in a child is directly proportional to the number of exposures to it.

Epidemiology. Susceptibility to the agents causing acute nasopharyngitis is universal. Infection can occur throughout the year, but in the north temperate zone there are usually 3 peaks: (1) in September about the time school opens; (2) in late January; and (3) toward the end of April. It has been estimated that the incidence in children ranges from 3 to 6 infections a year, but some children have a greater number. The illness is most common during the second and third years of life, and tends to be nearly endemic in nursery schools.

Pathology. The first changes are edema and vasodilatation in the submucosa. A mononuclear cellular infiltrate follows, which within a day or two becomes polymorphonuclear. The superficial epithelial cells separate and may slough, and there is profuse production of mucus, at first thin, later thicker and usually purulent.

Clinical Manifestations. Colds are more severe in the young child than in the older child and the adult. In general, children between the ages of 3 months and 3 years have fever early in the course of the infection, occasionally a few hours before localizing signs have appeared. Younger infants are usually afebrile; older children may have low-grade fevers. Purulent complications occur with increased frequency and severity in inverse relation to age. Persistent sinusitis, however, is more common in the older child, occurring rarely in infants.

The initial manifestations in infants more than 3 months of age are the sudden onset of fever, often in the range of 39 to 40° C. (102 to 104° F), and irritability, restlessness and sneezing. Nasal discharge begins within a few hours, quickly leading to nasal obstruction which interferes with nursing; in small infants with relatively great dependence on nose-breathing, signs of moderate respiratory distress may occur. During the first 2 to 3 days the eardrums are usually congested, and fluid may be noted behind the drum, whether or not purulent otitis media subsequently occurs. A few infants may vomit, and some have diarrhea. The febrile phase of the illness may last from a few hours to 3 days; the fever may recur with purulent complications.

In older children characteristically the initial symptoms are dryness and irritation in the nose and at times in the pharynx. This is followed within a few hours by sneezing, chilly sensations, muscular aches and a thin nasal discharge. Headache, malaise, anorexia and low-grade fever may be present. The secretions become thicker, usually within a day, and eventually purulent. The discharge is irritating, particularly during the purulent phase. Nasal obstruction leads to mouth-breathing, and this, through drying of the mucous membranes of the throat, increases the sensation of soreness. The acute phase lasts from 4 to 10 days.

Differential Diagnosis. Nasopharyngitis occurs early in the course of many contagious and acute infectious diseases of children. In the differential diagnosis one must also consider acute exacerbations of chronic upper respiratory tract infections, allergies, vasomotor responses to cold, diphtheria, and, in young infants, streptococcal infection and syphilis.

The initial manifestations of measles, pertussis, and to a lesser extent of poliomyelitis, hepatitis and mumps, are those of nasopharyngitis. A persistent nasal discharge, particularly if it is bloody, suggests nasal diphtheria or a foreign body and in the first weeks of life choanal atresia or congenital syphilis.

Allergic rhinitis differs from infectious rhinitis in that it is not accompanied by fever, the nasal discharge usually does not become purulent, and there is usually persistent sneezing, with itching of the eyes and the nose. The nasal mucous membranes in allergic rhinitis are usually pale, rather than inflamed, and nasal smears will often contain many eosinophils, rather than the polymorphonuclear leukocytes associated with infection. Antihistamines may produce rapid and relatively complete disappearance of signs and symptoms, whereas in infectious rhinitis their effect is slight. The proof of allergic rhinitis rests on the demonstration that removal of a specific allergen results in distinct improvement.

Complications. Complications of acute nasopharyngitis are primarily due to the invasion of paranasal sinuses and other portions of the respiratory tract by bacteria. The cervical lymph nodes may also become involved and occasionally suppurate. The commonest complication is otitis media, seen most frequently in the infant. Ear involvement may occur early in the course of infection, but usually appears after the initial acute phase of the nasopharyngitis is past and can therefore be suspected if fever recurs. Complications in the lower respiratory tract, such as laryngitis, bronchitis and pneumonia, occur much less frequently, but again are more common in the infant. Purulent sinusitis occurs more frequently in older children than in the infant; in the latter, however, acute ethmoiditis may occur.

Prevention. Since vaccines to the viruses causing acute nasopharyngitis do not exist, specific prevention is not possible. Gamma globulin does not reduce the frequency of infection; its use can-

not be recommended for frequent respiratory infections in children.

Because of the ubiquity of the common cold, it is not possible to isolate children from this condition. Since in the very young infant complications may be relatively serious, however, some attempt should be made to protect him from contact with potentially infected persons, particularly other children.

Therapy. There is no specific therapy. Antimicrobial therapy has no effect on the course of the illness, and when given during the acute phase not only does not reduce the incidence of bacterial complications, but also may even increase it. When bacterial complications do occur, they are usually obvious and can then be suitably treated.

Though rest in bed is generally recommended, there is no evidence that this shortens the course of the illness or has any effect on the outcome. Aspirin is usually helpful in reducing irritability, aching and malaise for the first day or two of the infection. Excessive use should be avoided.

Most of the distress of the child is related to nasal obstruction, and attempts should be directed at relieving this condition. Relief usually will permit the child to sleep, and to take fluids and food which he may previously have been unable to do.

The most consistently effective method for the relief of nasal obstruction is nasal instillation of suitable medications. Effective and relatively harmless are ephedrine or epinephrine in isotonic salt solutions, in concentrations approximately one half to one third of those used in adults. The more potent, longer-acting nose drops useful in adults tend to be too irritating for use in infants and occasionally are associated with the development of hyperexcitability or sedation (naphazoline). Nose drops in oily vehicles must be avoided because these are readily aspirated. Addition of antibiotics, corticosteroids or antihistamines to nose drops for children is expensive and adds nothing to their effectiveness.

Nose drops are best administered 15 to 20 minutes before feeding, and at bedtime. One to 2 drops are instilled in each nostril while the child is lying on his back with the neck extended. Since this will usually produce shrinkage only of the anterior mucous membranes, an additional 1 or 2 drops are instilled 5 to 10 minutes later. Introducing nasal decongestants by cotton-tipped applicators is not generally recommended in infants and small children, although this method is useful in the older child. Care must be taken that the cotton pledget extends beyond the anterior nares.

Bottles of nose drops should be used by only one person and for only one illness, since they usually become quickly contaminated with bacteria. Only older children should use inhalers producing a spray, and then only under adult supervision, since such applicators tend to be overused. In general, no medicament instilled into the nose should be used for periods in excess of 4 to 5 days; after this time any drug may become irritating and produce a chemically induced nasal congestion mimicking acute nasopharyngitis.

Nasal obstruction is most difficult to treat in infants. Various types of apparatus for suction of secretions from the nose have been used, but are relatively ineffective and occasionally dangerous. Best drainage can usually be obtained by placing the infant in the prone position, if this does not further embarrass respiration. A highly humidified environment such as provided by an efficient vaporizer usually provides substantial benefit.

Orally administered nasal decongestants are not particularly useful in young children, because of limited local activity and frequent increases in excitability. There is no advantage in combining these materials with other agents such as antihistamines, expectorants, and the like.

If the child is coughing, but has a profuse nasal discharge, potent antitussives should be avoided. Depressing the cough reflex may greatly increase the danger of aspiration of material from the nasopharynx.

Most children with acute nasopharyngitis will experience decreased appetite. There is no advantage in compelling them to take nourishment other than tolerated fluids. Fluids of the child's choice should be offered at frequent intervals. Transient constipation is common; this usually does not require treatment and will rapidly disappear when the child returns to his normal diet.

After the acute phase of the illness it is usually wise to limit the patient's contact with other children for a few days, because after such an infection the child appears to have increased susceptibility to the acquisition of potentially pathogenic bacteria and other viruses.

ACUTE PHARYNGITIS

The term "acute pharyngitis" refers to all acute infectious conditions of the pharynx, including tonsillitis and pharyngotonsillitis. The first term is preferred because the presence or absence of tonsils does not affect the frequency, the course or the complications of the illness or susceptibility to it. Pharyngeal involvement is part of most upper respiratory tract infections, and is also found with various acute generalized infections. When used in a strict sense, however, the term "acute pharyngitis" refers to conditions in which the principal involvement is in the throat. The disease is uncommon in children under 1 year of age, then increases in incidence, reaching its peak between the fourth and seventh years; it continues to occur throughout later childhood and adult life. In diphtheria, herpangina and infec-

tious mononucleosis pharyngeal involvement may be prominent; they are discussed elsewhere.

Etiology. Acute pharyngitis, whether febrile or not, is generally caused by viruses. The only common bacteria other than the diphtheria bacillus that cause this condition are group A beta hemolytic streptococci; except during epidemics this organism accounts for less than 20 per cent and probably less than 15 per cent of cases. *Mycoplasma hominis* may account for some cases. There are no epidemiologic data which suggest that pneumococci, *H. influenzae,* staphylococci or other bacteria are capable of producing acute pharyngitis; these organisms often proliferate during acute viral infections and may therefore be cultured in large numbers from the pharynx of the affected person.

Clinical Manifestations. These differ somewhat, depending on whether streptococci or viruses are the cause. There is, however, much overlapping of signs and symptoms, and it is often impossible to distinguish clinically one form of pharyngitis from another.

Viral pharyngitis is generally a disease of relatively gradual onset, which usually has as early signs fever, malaise and anorexia with moderate throat pain. Sore throat may be present initially, but more commonly begins a day or so after onset of symptoms and reaches its peak by the second or third day. Hoarseness, cough and rhinitis are also common. Even at its peak, pharyngeal inflammation may be relatively slight; but on occasion it is severe, and small ulcers may form on the soft palate and the posterior pharyngeal wall. Exudates may appear on lymphoid follicles of the palate and of the tonsils and be indistinguishable from those encountered with streptococcal disease. The cervical lymph nodes are usually moderately enlarged and firm, and may or may not be tender. Laryngeal involvement is common, but the trachea, bronchi and lungs are rarely involved. White blood cell counts may range from 6000 to above 30,000, an elevated count with predominance of polymorphonuclear cells being common in the early phase of illness. Leukocyte counts are therefore usually of little value in differentiating viral from bacterial disease. The entire illness may last less than 24 hours and usually does not persist more than 5 days. Significant complications are rare.

Streptococcal pharyngitis in the child over 2 years often begins with complaints of headache, abdominal pain, and vomiting. These symptoms may be associated with fever as high as 104°F., although occasionally a temperature elevation is not noted for 12 hours or so. Hours after the initial complaints, the throat may become sore, and in approximately one third of patients tonsillar enlargement, exudation and pharyngeal erythema are found. The degree of pharyngeal pain is inconstant and may vary from slight to sufficiently severe to make swallowing difficult. Two thirds of patients with acute streptococcal pharyngitis may have only mild erythema, with no particular enlargement of the tonsils and with no exudate. Anterior cervical lymphadenopathy usually occurs early, and the nodes are often tender. Fever may continue for 1 to 4 days; in very severe cases the child may remain ill for as long as 2 weeks. The physical findings most likely to be associated with streptococcal disease are diffuse redness of the tonsils and of the tonsillar pillars, with a petechial mottling of the soft palate, whether or not lymphadenitis or follicular exudation is found. These features, though common in streptococcal pharyngitis, are not diagnostic and occur with some frequency in nonstreptococcal infections.

Conjunctivitis, rhinitis, cough and hoarseness occur rarely with proved streptococcal pharyngitis, and the presence of two or more of these signs or symptoms suggests the diagnosis of viral infection.

The term *streptococcosis,* proposed by the Yale group in the 1940's, although not widely adopted as a diagnostic term, does imply descriptions of streptococcal disease in childhood which are worthy of perpetuation. In general it is suggested that infection with the beta hemolytic streptococcus has its pattern of clinical expression altered by an initial invasion of the host, in a manner somewhat analogous to tuberculous infection. Contact with the streptococcus is frequent, and it is postulated that the first infection is most likely to occur within the first few years of life. This first infection tends to be indolent and poorly localized, whereas subsequent infections tend to be localized, particularly in the throat, with acute manifestations of relatively short duration ("strep throat"). Scarlet fever, with its expression of the erythrogenic toxin, is included in this secondary infectional pattern, and glomerulonephritis and rheumatic fever are considered systemic manifestations of it. The presumption is that initial infection with one strain of beta hemolytic streptococcus group A will alter the reaction to subsequent infections with other strains.

The following is the description of the clinical patterns by Powers and Boisvert:

In the simplest form, the infant under 6 months shows irregular fever, under 102° F, a thin mucoserous nasal discharge causing some excoriation and crusting around the nostrils and some pharyngeal injection. There may be slight vomiting and diarrhea early in the course, and loss of appetite. The acute episode may last less than a week and except for persisting nasal discharge the patient may seem only somewhat peaked and slightly indisposed for . . . five or six weeks. Sometimes the disease . . . is almost asymptomatic with little or no complaint.

In the form most frequently demanding medical attention . . . the patients are children between 6 months and 3 years of age; they are more severely ill than those just described. The early symptoms and signs are those of coryza with postnasal discharge, a diffusely reddened pharynx, fever, vomiting, and loss of appetite. For a few days the temperature curve shows elevations of from 100° to 103° F and continues, in typical cases, to be irregular for . . . four to eight weeks gradually becoming normal. Within a few days of onset the cervical nodes begin to enlarge; they are usually modest in size and moderately resistant in consistency, there is some tenderness and pain when the mouth is opened. The course of the adenopathy follows roughly the fever with subsidence in about six weeks in the typical case.

This is one of the several "glandular fevers" and "catarrhal fevers." Swelling, reddening, softening, and suppuration may occur at any time in the six weeks' course; this complication is usually unilateral. Catarrhal otitis media, like persisting cervical adenopathy, is so frequently an accompaniment of streptococcal upper respiratory infections in infants that the conditions in some form may be regarded . . . as integral parts of the disease rather than as complications.

Diagnosis. It has been pointed out that it is difficult or impossible to differentiate viral from streptococcal disease on a clinical basis. The only reliable method is a throat culture. From 10 to 15 per cent of normal children carry group A streptococci in their throats, however, so that even a positive culture in a sick, febrile child is not necessarily conclusive evidence of streptococcal disease.

When a membranous exudate is present on the tonsils or pharynx, specific culture for diphtheria must be performed even though the clinical course of the patient may not suggest this diagnosis. The membranous exudate of infectious mononucleosis closely resembles that found in the partially immunized child with a diphtheritic infection. Herpangina, a specific viral infection, is not usually associated with tonsillar exudates, but rather with many vesiculoulcerative lesions on the anterior pillars, fauces and soft palate.

Agranulocytosis often is first manifested by symptoms of acute pharyngitis. The tonsils and the posterior pharyngeal wall may be covered by a yellowish or dirty white exudate, the mucous membranes under this exudate will usually become necrotic, and ulceration will extend into the mouth and tongue. The lesions are very painful, and dysphagia is severe. Enlargement of cervical lymph nodes commonly occurs, as do mucosal hemorrhages.

Pharyngoconjunctival fever is a form of epidemic sore throat described in both military and civilian populations. The condition is characterized by fever, sore throat, which is often rather mild, and conjunctivitis. The most striking feature is follicular injection of bulbar and palpebral conjunctivae, often affecting only one eye. There usually is scanty serous exudate which produces slight matting of the eyelids and increased lacrimation. Submandibular lymphadenopathy is common, as is involvement of the preauricular node on the side of the conjunctivitis.

Complications. With viral infections the complication rate is very low, although purulent otitis media may occur. In debilitated children both viral and streptococcal infections may lead to large, chronic ulcers in the pharynx associated with the presence of a variety of normal mouth flora. With streptococcal disease, peritonsillar abscess occasionally occurs, as do sinusitis, otitis media and rarely meningitis. Since acute glomerulonephritis and rheumatic fever may follow streptococcal infections, it is desirable to re-examine children with proved streptococcal disease within 2 to 3 weeks after illness.

Mesenteric adenitis is occasionally associated

with pharyngitis of either viral or bacterial origin. This may result in abdominal pain with or without vomiting which may closely simulate appendicitis.

Treatment. There is no specific therapy for viral pharyngitis. Streptococcal infection is best treated with penicillin, given orally if possible. This drug produces a prompt clinical response; if the patient is not afebrile within 24 hours after an appropriate dose of penicillin, the illness is not of streptococcal origin unless there is an existing complication. There is no reason, therefore, to continue administration of penicillin if the patient is not greatly improved within one day after start of therapy. In proved streptococcal disease it is generally recommended that the duration of therapy be 10 days. If penicillin cannot be used, owing to an allergy to the drug, erythromycin is a satisfactory alternative (p. 248).

Most children prefer to remain in bed during the acute phase of illness. When throat pain is severe, aspirin is often useful, as are hot or cold compresses to the neck, depending on the patient's preference. Gargles of warm saline solution offer some symptomatic relief for throat pain in children old enough to cooperate; in the younger patients the inhalation of steam occasionally produces similar effects. Because of pain on swallowing, cool bland liquids such as ginger ale are usually more acceptable to the child than solids or hot foods. No attempt should be made to force the child to eat.

The child with streptococcal infection is noninfectious to others within a few hours after penicillin therapy has begun. Children with viral disease remain infectious for several days. It is not possible to prevent viral pharyngitis. In children who require protection against streptococcal disease, such as those with a past history of rheumatic fever, penicillin or sulfonamide prophylaxis is usually satisfactory (see p. 540).

RETROPHARYNGEAL ABSCESS

During early childhood the potential space between the posterior pharyngeal wall and the prevertebral fascia contains several small lymph nodes, which usually disappear during the third or fourth year of life. The lymphatic channels which communicate with these nodes drain portions of the nasopharynx as well as the posterior nasal passages. With purulent infections of these areas, the nodes may become infected; this may, in turn, progress to breakdown of the nodes and to suppuration. The offending organism is usually a group A hemolytic streptococcus; staphylococci are occasionally involved. Occasionally a penetrating injury of the posterior pharyngeal wall, such as by a fishbone, can produce a retropharyngeal abscess.

Clinical Manifestations. The patient usually has a history of an acute nasopharyngitis or phar-

yngitis, and the clinical features of the earlier illness may still be present. There is generally an abrupt onset of high fever, with difficulty in swallowing and refusal of feeding, and with noisy, often gurgling respirations. The infant will usually lie with his head hyperextended. Respirations become increasingly labored, and secretions accumulate in the mouth, owing to the difficulty in swallowing.

A bulge in the posterior pharyngeal wall is usually readily apparent. Sometimes the abscess is located in an area of the nasopharynx where it may cause nasal obstruction and a bulging forward of the soft palate. A digital examination to determine whether the abscess is fluctuant or not must be performed with the patient in the Trendelenburg position and with provision for adequate suction in case the abscess ruptures. Retropharyngeal abscesses not detectable by simple inspection are uncommon, but occasionally roentgen examination of the neck may reveal abscesses bulging into the lower pharynx, too low to be visible or palpable through the mouth.

Differential Diagnosis. Nonfluctuant lymphadenitis in the retropharyngeal space may produce a bulge which, though tender, is not fluctuant. Caries of the cervical spine may on occasion produce a lateral retropharyngeal abscess; in this condition there is usually considerable rigidity of the neck and other signs of spinal involvement.

Course. If left untreated, the abscess may rupture into the pharynx spontaneously, resulting in aspiration of pus. The process may also dissect laterally and present externally on the side of the neck, or burrow into the esophagus, the mediastinum or auditory canal. Sudden death may occur if the abscess presses on the larynx, produces edema of the glottis, or erodes into major blood vessels.

If the abscess is incised as soon as it becomes fluctuant and proper antimicrobial therapy is given, the prognosis is good.

Treatment. As soon as retropharyngeal abscess is suspected, parenteral penicillin therapy should be given. Large doses of penicillin G are recommended. If the lymphadenitis is not fluctuant, the infection will often resolve with antibiotic therapy. As soon as the abscess is fluctuant, it should be drained; the operation is best performed under general anesthesia. Before incision is made, the mass should be aspirated to see whether retropharyngeal hemorrhage may not also be present from erosion of blood vessels. If no blood is obtained, an incision is made where the abscess is pointing, and the pus is carefully aspirated. If serious bleeding has occurred, ligation of the carotid artery is necessary.

LATERAL PHARYNGEAL ABSCESS

This condition occurs later in childhood than a retropharyngeal abscess. The process is usually so extensive that the entire pharyngeal wall is displaced medially, including the tonsil, the soft palate and the uvula.

Clinical Manifestations. The patient usually has high fever, appears acutely ill, and complains of severe pain and difficulty on swallowing. The bulge in the lateral pharyngeal wall is obvious. Cervical adenitis is usually present, and nuchal rigidity is common, owing to muscular spasm.

Treatment. Antibiotic therapy is identical to that of retropharyngeal abscess. As soon as the lesion is fluctuant, it should be incised.

PERITONSILLAR AND RETROTONSILLAR ABSCESSES

Both peritonsillar and retrotonsillar abscesses are uncommon in childhood and usually affect older children. Since these diseases rarely appear in patients who have had a tonsillectomy, the tonsil apparently represents the initial focus from which the process develops. The abscesses are almost always caused by group A beta hemolytic streptococci, rarely by *Staphylococcus aureus* and *H. influenzae.*

Clinical Manifestations. The abscesses are usually preceded by an attack of acute pharyngotonsillitis. There may be an afebrile interval of several days, or the fever of the primary infection may not subside. The patient complains of severe throat pain, has progressive difficulty in opening his mouth because of spasm of the pterygoid muscles, and often refuses to swallow or speak. Occasionally there is sufficient spasm of the homolateral muscles of the neck to produce torticollis. The fever may be septic and reach 40.5°C. (105°F.). The affected tonsillar area is markedly swollen and inflamed; the uvula is displaced to the opposite side. In untreated patients the abscess becomes fluctuant within a few days and usually points in the region of the anterior faucial pillar. If the abscess is not incised, spontaneous rupture will occur.

Treatment. If the condition is recognized prior to abscess formation, intensive antimicrobial therapy with penicillin G will sometimes prevent suppuration. Analgesic drugs may be needed for pain, such as aspirin for the younger child or meperidine for the older one. When the lesion becomes fluctuant, it should be promptly incised.

Subsequent attacks of peritonsillar abscess may be prevented by removal of the tonsils 3 to 4 weeks after inflammation has subsided.

SINUSITIS

The maxillary antrums and the anterior and posterior ethmoid cells are present at birth and are usually of sufficient size to harbor infection.

Each of the frontal sinuses develops from an anterior ethmoid cell. Though invasion of the frontal bone and pneumatization of the sinuses are demonstrable some time during the first 2 to 4 years of life, the frontal sinus is rarely a site of significant infection until the sixth to the tenth year. When there is severe ethmoidal disease in the first few years of life, the development and pneumatization of the frontal sinuses may be curtailed or even completely prevented. The sphenoidal sinus is present at birth; though there are variations in its development, it usually does not assume clinical significance until the third to the fifth year of life.

It can be assumed that the paranasal sinuses are involved in an exudative process in practically all acute nasal infections, but, as a rule, the sinus involvement does not persist after the nasal infection has subsided unless there has been a preexisting sinus infection. The incidence of both acute and chronic sinus infections increases in the latter part of childhood.

ACUTE PURULENT SINUSITIS

In addition to involvement of the sinuses during acute nasal infections, there may be acute empyema of one or more sinuses of sufficient severity to dominate the clinical picture.

Clinical Manifestations. The symptoms of acute sinusitis, in addition to those of rhinitis, are fever, localized pain, tenderness or a sense of fullness, headache and, at times, edema over the affected sinus. So-called sinus headaches, which tend to involve the region of the affected sinus, may assist in localization. In sphenoidal sinusitis the headache may be in the suboccipital region; in anterior ethmoidal sinusitis, in the region of the temples and over the eyes; and in posterior ethmoidal sinusitis, over the distribution of the trigeminal nerve, especially over the mastoid area. Unless the sinal ostia are obstructed, there is a purulent discharge which can be observed directly through a nasoscope. Pus in the middle meatus suggests involvement of the maxillary, frontal or anterior ethmoid sinuses; in the superior meatus, of the sphenoid or posterior ethmoid cells.

In acute ethmoiditis, especially in infants and small children, periorbital cellulitis with edema of the soft tissues and redness of the skin is a common manifestation.

Diagnosis. The roentgenogram will reveal an opaque shadow when a frontal or maxillary sinus is filled with pus, but a similar appearance may also be produced by thickening of the lining membrane. Transillumination may be helpful in older children, but not in young ones; it has greater limitations than the roentgenographic examination. It is rarely necessary in children to puncture a sinus simply to establish a diagnosis. Clouding of the ethmoid cells may be demonstrated on the roentgenogram in acute and chronic ethmoiditis.

Serious complications are otitis media, meningitis, cavernous sinus thrombosis, optic neuritis, orbital cellulitis and abscess, and nephritis.

Treatment. Treatment is essentially that of the rhinitis. Shrinkage of the nasal mucous membranes will often facilitate drainage from the sinus. Gentle suction or aspiration may be used, but may be more of an annoyance than a help, especially in infants. Drainage of a sinus is rarely necessary, but if there is persistence of local and systemic manifestations, it may be justified. Appropriate antimicrobial therapy should be used in full dosage.

CHRONIC SINUSITIS

Chronic infection of the paranasal sinuses should always suggest the possibility of a local or generalized disturbance which facilitates persistence of the infection. Search should be made for nasal deformities and infected and hypertrophied adenoids which might cause obstruction, for infected teeth as a source of maxillary sinusitis, and for such general disturbances as allergy and nutritional and thyroid deficiencies. The incidence of sinusitis is said to be greater in children who have had their tonsils and adenoids removed.

Clinical Manifestations. Symptoms of chronic sinusitis vary considerably. Fever, when present, is low-grade, and there is frequently malaise, easy fatigability, difficulty in mental concentration, anorexia and malnutrition. Nasal discharge, which may be bilateral or unilateral, varies from day to day, and may be greater during a certain portion of the day. Postnasal discharge or drip is common and, in the absence of infected adenoids, is practically diagnostic. Headaches are frequent, and pain or tenderness to palpation or percussion is helpful in localization. There are frequent attacks of sneezing; when there is an associated watery, nasal discharge, the possibility of allergic rhinitis must be considered.

Sinus disease should be suspected when there is persistent mouth-breathing, not otherwise explained, and constant pharyngeal irritation. Any of the complications of acute sinusitis may occur with chronic sinusitis, but probably the most frequent association is chronic bronchial infection. The term "sinobronchitis" is frequently used to designate the relationship.

Treatment. Attention should be given to the general health of the child, and the diet should be corrected as necessary. Locally obstructive nasal deformities should be corrected, if possible, and infected or hypertrophic adenoid tissue should be removed. Shrinkage of the mucous membranes by ephedrine or related compounds with the head in such a position as to facilitate entrance of the solution into the sinuses may be of some benefit. Either the so-called displacement method of Proetz or the lateral head-low posture of Parkinson may be used.

In the Parkinson method the child lies on his side with the shoulder elevated by a firm pad such as a folded blanket, and the head is bent down to a dependent position. The nasal solution which is then instilled can be expected to have contact with the various sinal ostia on both sides. The child should breathe through the mouth to prevent drawing the medication into the pharynx. The position is maintained for 5 to 6 minutes, and the face is then turned downward for a few moments to permit drainage of the nasal contents, or the child may sit up and place his head down between the knees.

Nasopharyngeal cultures and antibiotic susceptibility tests should be obtained as a guide in selection of antibiotic agents. Such therapy should be continued for about 2 weeks. Prolonged use of nasal solutions should be discouraged.

Every effort should be made to avoid operative procedures; but when there is persistence of chronic purulent sinusitis in spite of all nonoperative measures, surgery is indicated.

GENERAL CONSIDERATIONS OF CHRONIC INFECTIONS OF THE UPPER RESPIRATORY TRACT

THE PROBLEM OF CHRONIC COLDS

One of the disturbing problems of pediatric practice is that of the child with persistent or recurring upper respiratory tract infection with or without associated chronic bronchial involvement. Not all children with such chronic infections can be placed in any one category; but each must be studied to determine, if possible, the underlying factor or factors.

The age of greatest incidence of respiratory infections is from the latter part of the first year of life to 6 or 7 years. During this time it can be expected that the average child will have 3 to 6 "colds" a year. Recovery should occur after each attack, and the child should appear healthy between episodes. In the so-called chronic cases the child seems to recover from one acute attack, only to enter another, or there is more or less persistent rhinitis, cough and a general failure to do well. Such patterns may reflect what appears to be a familial or individual susceptibility or repeated exposure to respiratory infection within the home. Often there is some underlying disturbance in the child. Specifically included in the "chronic respiratory group" are chronic rhinitis, sinusitis, infected adenoids and tonsils, chronic otitis media, chronic bronchitis, bronchiectasis, tuberculosis, allergy and hypogammaglobulinemia.

CHRONIC RHINITIS

Chronic rhinitis as evidenced by a chronic nasal discharge, with or without a tendency to acute exacerbations, is usually a reflection of some particular underlying disturbance, such as infected adenoids, nasal polyps, chronic sinusitis, allergy, foreign bodies, deviated septum, various congenital malformations, nasal diphtheria or syphilis.

Chronic rhinitis should be considered merely a symptom, and the differential diagnosis should include the various disturbances enumerated. In addition, the possibility of a chronic debilitating infection or some nutritional or metabolic deficiency (as of the thyroid) must be considered.

Clinical Manifestations. Symptoms vary, but chronic nasal discharge is common to all cases. In the persistent cases the odor may be foul, and there may be excoriation of the anterior nares and upper lip. Bloody discharge is common in syphilitic and diphtheritic lesions and with foreign bodies, but may also occur in other conditions, especially if there is persistent picking of the nose. Disturbances of taste and smell are frequent. During exacerbations or superimposed infections, fever is common, but is otherwise usually absent. Chronic sinusitis, otitis media, pharyngitis and bronchitis are frequently associated.

Nasal polyps are commonly associated with allergy, sinusitis or cystic fibrosis; the symptoms are often predominantly unilateral. Their presence is determined by direct examination. They should be removed and the underlying disturbance treated (see *encephalocele*, p. 883).

Persistent *hypertrophic rhinitis* is also most often associated with chronic sinusitis or allergy. Especially in allergy the mucous membrane tends to be pale. The soft tissues are swollen and resistant to pressure. Nasal obstruction may occur in a cyclic pattern.

Atrophic rhinitis is uncommon; it is usually associated with some general debilitating condition, or it may be a sequel to long-continued nasal infection. The sense of smell is impaired. There may be little or no discharge, but considerable crusting and a sense of dryness in the nose and throat. In some instances there is a profuse, excessively foul nasal discharge *(ozena)*.

Treatment. Treatment must be directed toward the underlying disturbance. Particular emphasis must be placed upon eradicating foci of infection in sinuses, ears, adenoids or tonsils and upon the removal of or densensitization to known allergens. Attention should be given to such factors as nutritional status, rest and prevention of exposure to reinfection. In an attempt to provide symptomatic relief it is often difficult to avoid the use of such mucosal shrinking solutions as ephedrine and related compounds. It must be borne in mind, however, that their use is not without danger and that they may cause further damage. The use of antibiotics locally should be avoided, but systemic administration may be indicated in selected cases.

CHRONIC PHARYNGITIS

Chronic pharyngitis is essentially a secondary condition resulting from such chronic infections as those of the sinuses, adenoids and tonsils, although on occasion there is no other evidence of infection than that of the hypertrophied lymphoid tissue on the posterior pharyngeal wall and on the base of the tongue. The latter type of involvement occurs with frequency only in children whose faucial tonsils have been removed, some of whom have infected tonsillar tags.

Clinical Manifestations. There are likely to be repeated acute exacerbations; in the intervals there are complaints of discomfort in the throat such as dryness and raspy irritation. There are frequent efforts to clear the throat, and an irritative cough is common. The mucous membrane is usually inflamed, though on occasion it is pale, and the blood vessels are prominent. The pharyngeal wall is frequently covered with a mucopurulent secretion, and the lymphoid tissue is often hypertrophied and has a pebbled appearance.

Treatment. Treatment should be directed toward any disturbance in the sinuses, nose (deformities), adenoids or tonsils. Attention should also be given to the general nutrition and hygiene of the child.

TONSILS AND ADENOIDS

The term "tonsils" is used in its commonly accepted sense of indicating the 2 faucial tonsils; the term "adenoids," as synonymous with hypertrophy of the pharyngeal tonsil. The tonsils and adenoids are part of the lymphoid tissues which circle the pharynx and are known collectively as Waldeyer's ring. This consists of the lymphoid tissue on the base of the tongue (lingual tonsil), the 2 faucial tonsils, the adenoids (pharyngeal tonsil) and the lymphoid tissue on the posterior pharyngeal wall. This tissue naturally serves as a defense against infection; when its defense mechanism is overcome, it may become a site of acute or chronic infection.

The principal disturbances of the tonsils and adenoids are infection and hypertrophy. The latter is in most instances secondary to infection. The most important medical issue is the decision as to their removal. Though both tonsils and adenoids are usually removed at the same operation, there are good reasons for making the decisions for tonsillectomy and adenoidectomy separately, especially in children under 4 or 5 years of age.

Neoplasms of the Tonsils. Neoplasms of the tonsils are rare, although papilloma, lipoma, angioma, teratoma, fibroma, plasmocytoma and lymphosarcoma have been reported.

Acute Tonsillitis. Acute infections of the tonsils are considered in the same category as acute pharyngitis and are discussed on page 889; for peritonsillar abscess, see page 892.

CHRONIC TONSILLITIS
(Chronically Hypertrophic and Infected Tonsils)

The "tonsil problem" is of particular concern in pediatric practice, not only because of the frequency of chronic tonsillar involvement, but also because of its distortion by physicians and laity who have been too ready to attribute all sorts of complaints and ills to tonsillar involvement and have not been sufficiently critical in respect to tonsillectomy. A more critical attitude is developing. Tonsillar disturbances are not common during infancy.

Clinical Manifestations. These vary considerably; the more significant ones are recurrent attacks of sore throat or a persistent one, and obstruction to swallowing or breathing; the last is more often due to adenoids. There may be a sense of dryness and irritation in the throat, and the breath may be offensive, although neither of these is diagnostic. Constitutional symptoms are neither characteristic nor, as a rule, striking.

Indications for Tonsillectomy. Decision for removal of tonsils should be based so far as possible on symptoms and signs related to the tonsils; tonsillectomy should not be recommended as a possible panacea for unrelated disturbances. In general, the conditions for which tonsillectomy is considered are (1) factors directly related to the tonsils, (2) disturbances in closely related structures, and (3) systemic disturbances.

Local indications for removal are chronic infection and hypertrophy. True hypertrophy is usually the result of infection, acute or chronic, but may occur independently. *Many or even most tonsils considered to be hypertrophic actually are normal in size; the misinterpretation results from failure to appreciate that tonsils are normally relatively larger during childhood than in later years.* Tonsils may, however, virtually meet in the midline in some children who are quite asymptomatic. Tonsils of average size are projected toward the midline when the child is gagged and may be interpreted by the physician who is unaware of the relatively large size of the tonsil during childhood as being hypertrophic. On the other hand, infection does not always produce hypertrophy, and chronically infected tonsils may be small and embedded behind the faucial pillars. In the evaluation of chronic infection, history of repeated or essentially constant sore throat is of more value than examination. There is no certain way to demonstrate by direct observation whether tonsils are harboring chronic infection. The consistency or size of the tonsil and the presence of cheesy material within the crypts are not reliable guides. Persistent hyperemia of the anterior pillars is a more reliable sign, and enlargement of the cervical lymph nodes is supporting evidence. Persistent enlargement of the node just below and slightly in front of the angle of the jaw is especially significant. In contrast to the difficulty in determining the presence of chronic infection, hypertrophy sufficient to obstruct swallowing or breathing is readily detectable. Such tonsils practically meet in the midline when the throat is examined without gagging the patient. Before tonsillectomy is recommended it should be ascertained that the hypertrophy is chronic and not the result of a recent acute infec-

tion. Tonsils can increase in size greatly during an acute infection and recede after its subsidence.

Removal of tonsils and adenoids may be recommended for persistent carriers of diphtheria bacilli (p. 566).

Among the *disturbances in adjacent tonsillar structures,* peritonsillar (and retrotonsillar) abscess is the only definite indication for tonsillectomy. Other indications are less clear-cut. There are differences of opinion as to the value of tonsillectomy for sinusitis. When there are symptoms directly referable to the tonsils, there may be adequate justification for their removal. The physician who recommends removal before other treatment for the sinusitis will be wise if he does not promise relief from the sinusitis. In many instances removal of the adenoids is more likely to be indicated than is tonsillectomy. This is also true in cases of chronic otitis media and of middle ear deafness. Suppurative cervical adenitis, when the focus of infection is not traceable to structures other than the tonsils, may also be considered an indication for tonsillectomy. There is no evidence to indicate that the removal of tonsils is justified for infections in the lower respiratory tract, although such conditions are not a contraindication if there are other reasons for tonsillectomy.

No *systemic disturbance* in itself is an indication for tonsillectomy. The decision should be based on local indications. This applies to children with rheumatic fever or glomerulonephritis as well as to those with other infections in which the tonsils may be removed in a blind search for a focus of infection or as a remedy for undernutrition.

Tonsillectomy in relation to age of the child. Rarely it seems advisable to recommend tonsillectomy for children 2 or 3 years of age. Every attempt should be made, however, to postpone the operation. Frequently when the operation is postponed for reasons of age, the apparent need for tonsillectomy disappears within the next year or so. Actually, in the first few years of life the indications for adenoidectomy, though infrequent, are present more often than those for tonsillectomy. Neither procedure should be performed as a prophylaxis against the "common cold" at any age.

Tonsillectomy in relation to active infection. Tonsillectomy should be postponed until 2 or 3 weeks after subsidence of an infection. This, however, is not always possible; an occasional child seems never to be free of infection in and about the tonsils. In such a case it is justifiable to perform the operation if a sulfonamide or antibiotic is administered at therapeutic levels for a day or two before and 2 or 3 days after the operation.

Type of Operation. Though this is not the place to discuss operative procedures, certain generalizations are indicated. Careful removal by dissection should be carried out to ensure that all the tonsillar tissue is removed without destruction of adjacent tissues. Too frequently small amounts of tonsillar tissue are allowed to remain which later become infected and hypertrophied, or there is removal of adjacent tissue from the lateral pharyngeal wall, from the soft palate and even at times from the uvula. Aspiration of the throat during the operation will lessen the chances of pulmonary abscess or pneumonia. Bleeding should be completely controlled, and the child should not leave the operating room until he has dry tonsillar fossae.

Preoperative Preparation. This consists of a medical history which includes questions related to recent infection, to exposure to contagious diseases and to bleeding tendencies in the patient or his family. A thorough physical examination should include observation for loose or carious teeth, which should be removed or repaired before tonsillectomy. Bleeding and clotting times are usually obtained, but a careful history of bleeding tendencies is a more effective screening method than the commonly used poorly discriminating tests. The child should be told of the operation and the procedure explained, preferably by informed parents. There should be adequate preoperative preparation with one of the barbiturates and atropine. Though food is withheld for several hours before the operation, feeding should be adequate up to this time. In children who are undernourished or are readily susceptible to ketosis, preoperative intravenous administration of glucose is indicated.

Postoperative Care. This is usually not complicated. The child should be kept in bed for the remainder of the day and at rest for several more; it is wise to encourage eating and drinking as soon as the nausea from the anesthetic has disappeared. Rinsing the mouth with an alkaline solution has certain esthetic advantages. Aspirin may be prescribed for discomfort. Avoidance of contact with infection is of the greatest importance. The membrane which forms at the operative site is at times interpreted as being diphtheritic. Fusiform bacilli (Vincent's organisms) may be cultured from it with considerable regularity, but this by itself is not an indication for treatment.

Complications. Complications are not particularly frequent, but postoperative hemorrhage, lung abscess, pneumonia and septicemia do occur. Hemorrhage is, of course, the most frequent one, and should be controlled by packing or, in the case of severe bleeding, by ligation. Extensive bleeding will be responsible for severe anemia, leukocytosis, fever, and even dilatation of the heart. Transfusion is indicated in such cases.

Results to Be Expected from Tonsillectomy. No reduction in the incidence of epidemic respiratory infections is to be expected. The incidence of persistent throat infections may be decreased. Obstructive symptoms due to hypertrophied tonsils can be relieved. Otitis media and sinusitis are rarely benefited by tonsillectomy; the incidence of sinusitis may even be increased. Nasal allergy is not affected, nor is the incidence of laryngitis or of pulmonary infections. Neither the incidence of initial attacks of rheumatic fever nor that of recurrences appears to be affected by the operation.

Eradication of diphtheria bacilli from the throats of carriers after tonsillectomy is achieved sufficiently often to justify the operation in otherwise persistent carriers. The incidence of cervical lymphadenitis is decreased. In some instances nutrition is improved after tonsillectomy. In part this may be due to psychologic factors, but it is reasonable that general benefit should accrue when a focus of infection is removed. Care should be taken, however, in making predictions in this respect.

ADENOIDS
(HYPERTROPHY OF PHARYNGEAL TONSIL)

Disturbances of the lymphoid tissue of the nasopharynx (adenoids) tend to parallel those of the faucial tonsils. Hypertrophy and infection may occur separately, but usually occur together, infection, as a rule, being primary. The soft adenoid structure, which is normally widespread in the nasopharynx, especially on the posterior wall and the roof, undergoes hypertrophy, and masses of varying size up to 2 or 3 cm. are formed. These masses may almost fill the vault of the nasopharynx and interfere with the passage of air through the nose and obstruct the eustachian tubes.

Clinical Manifestations. Mouth-breathing and more or less persistent rhinitis are the most characteristic symptoms. Mouth-breathing may be present only during sleep, especially when the child is on his back, and in this position snoring is also likely to occur. In decided adenoid hypertrophy the mouth is kept open during the day as well, and the mucous membranes of the mouth and lips are dry. Chronic nasopharyngitis may be constantly present or recurs frequently. The voice is altered, developing a nasal, muffled quality. The breath is offensive, and taste and smell are impaired. A harassing cough may be present, especially at night, resulting from irritation of the larynx by inspired air which has not been warmed and moistened by passage through the nose. Impaired hearing is common. Chronic otitis media may be associated with infected, hypertrophied adenoids.

The **diagnosis** can be confirmed by direct digital palpation, examination of the vault of the pharynx by pharyngeal mirror, or roentgenographic examination. Otherwise the presence of adenoid hypertrophy can be suspected from such symptoms as mouth-breathing, snoring and persistent rhinitis with or without chronic otitis media.

An abscess in the adenoid tissue is uncommon, but may be a cause of protracted fever. Identification and drainage of the abscess have been achieved by digital expression. Appropriate antibiotic therapy followed by adenoidectomy is indicated.

Treatment. Adenoidectomy is indicated when there are symptoms such as persistent mouth-breathing, "nasal" speech, repeated attacks of otitis media, deafness and persistent or recurring nasopharyngitis which seem to be related to infected hypertrophied adenoid tissue. Although it is customary to remove the adenoids when tonsillectomy is performed, there are occasions, particularly in young children, when only adenoidectomy should be recommended. The same precautions for complete removal and control of bleeding points as recommended for tonsillectomy should be observed; for this reason, removal under direct vision is preferable to the use of the adenotome. If impaired hearing persists after adenoidectomy, radiation therapy may be considered.

HEINZ F. EICHENWALD
GEORGE H. McCRACKEN, JR.

REFERENCES

General Considerations

Chanock, R. M., and Parrott, R. H.: Acute Respiratory Disease in Infancy and Childhood: Present Understanding and Prospects for Prevention. *Pediatrics,* 36:21, 1965.
Chanock, R. M., Mufson, M. A., and Johnson, K. M.: Comparative Biology and Ecology of Human Virus and Mycoplasma Respiratory Pathogens. *Progr. Med. Virology,* 7:208, 1965.
Cramblett, H. G.: Viral Respiratory Illnesses of Infants and Children. *Bacteriol. Rev.,* 28:431, 1964.

Sterner, G., and Tunevall, G.: Acute Respiratory Illness in Children. A Combined Bacteriological and Virological Study. *Acta Pediat.,* 51:349, 1962.

Nasopharyngitis

Cate, T. R., Couch, R. B., and Johnson, K. M.: Studies with Rhinoviruses in Volunteers: Production of Illness, Effect of Naturally Acquired Antibody, and Demonstration of a Protective Effect Not Associated with Serum Antibody. *J. Clin. Invest.,* 43:56, 1964.
Freeman, G. L., and Todd, R. H.: The Role of Allergy in Viral Respiratory Tract Infections. *Am. J. Dis. Child.,* 104:330, 1962.
Gwaltney, J. M., Jr., and Jordan, W. S., Jr.: Rhinoviruses and Respiratory Disease. *Bact. Rev.,* 28:409, 1964.

Pharyngitis

Breese, B. B., and Disney, F. A.: The Accuracy of Diagnosis of Beta Streptococcal Infections on Clinical Grounds. *J. Pediat.,* 44:670, 1954.
Powers, G. F., and Boisvert, P. L.: Age as a Factor in Streptococcosis. *J. Pediat.,* 25:481, 1944.
Stillerman, M., and Bernstein, S. H.: Streptococcal Pharyngitis: Evaluation of Clinical Syndromes in Diagnosis. *Am. J. Dis. Child.,* 101:476, 1961.
Stillerman, M., Bernstein, S. H., Smith, M. L., Gittelson, S. B., and Karelitz, S.: Antibiotics in the Treatment of Beta-Hemolytic Streptococcal Pharyngitis: Factors Influencing the Results. *Pediatrics,* 25:27, 1960.

Retropharyngeal Abscess

Greenwald, H. M., and Messeloff, C. R.: Retropharyngeal Abscess in Infants and Children. *Am. J. Med. Sci.,* 177:767, 1929.

THE EAR

Malformations and Neoplasms. The complex embryology of the ear allows for the possibility of many developmental abnormalities. Minor malformations are common, but serious anomalies are rare. There are no precise definitions of normal size, configuration or position of the external ear; anything esthetically acceptable is considered normal. Occasionally the auricle is grotesquely small *(microtia)*, large *(macrotia)* or entirely absent *(anotia)*. Malformed, low-set ears may be associated with serious renal anomalies, mandibulofacial dysostoses and other congenital anomalies. Absence of the antihelix and superior crus results in "lop ear," which can be cosmetically improved by plastic surgery.

Hereditary cutaneous dimples or sinus tracts anterior to and above the tragus are common. They do not require surgical correction unless recurrently infected. Accessory auricular skin tags can be ligated; if there is cartilage or a broad base, they should be surgically removed.

Atresia of the external auditory canal is often associated with abnormalities of the external or middle ear. Roentgenographic examination is necessary to evaluate the bony canal, the ossicles and the middle ear cavity. If the conductive elements of hearing are present, reconstructive surgery can be attempted.

Chondromas and exostoses of the auditory canal are generally small and rarely require removal. Rare congenital tumors of the ear in childhood include hemangiomas, lymphangiomas and dermoid tumors.

Sebaceous cysts located in or near the lobule of the ear are common. They are prone to enlarge periodically with minimal tenderness, and to regress spontaneously.

Acquired malformations may result from trauma, frostbite or perichondritis. Frostbite is treated by moderately rapid warming to body temperature. Hematomas of the auricle should be evacuated promptly or the clot may organize and produce the deformity known as cauliflower ear.

Causes of the Painful Ear. Any acute inflammatory process in the external canal, middle ear or mastoid may cause pain. If suppurative material under pressure is allowed to drain, pain abates.

The sensory innervation of the ear involves branches of the fifth, ninth and tenth cranial nerves and the second and third cervical spinal nerves. Pain may be referred to the ear by disease in the parotid gland, temporomandibular joint, cervical spine, posterior ethmoid and sphenoid sinuses, third molars and the pharynx. Herpes zoster affecting the fifth cranial nerve may cause pain interpreted as earache in the pre-eruptive phase.

EXTERNAL AUDITORY CANAL

The outer, cartilaginous portion of the canal contains sebaceous glands and the specialized apocrine glands that secrete cerumen. These are not present in the inner, osseous portion. The normal extrusion of wax tends to cleanse the canal. Cerumen may be impacted against the tympanic membrane from attempts to clean the ear canal with a swab. Excessive cerumen is most easily removed by irrigation with water or isotonic saline, which should be at body temperature to avoid causing vertigo from labyrinthine stimulation. The syringe nozzle should be small enough that the auditory meatus is not occluded, or damage may be done by pressure. Hard wax is softened by instillation of mineral or lanolin oil twice daily for several days before irrigation. Cleaning the canal with a cerumen spoon or curet is a traumatic procedure and should be done only when there is urgency about examination of the ear and irrigation is unsuccessful.

The auditory canal of the newborn infant is filled with detritus of vernix caseosa which disappears after a few days.

Foreign Bodies. The curious child may insert an astonishing variety of vegetable and mineral matter into the auditory canal. Insects which find their way into the canal are particularly distressing because of their movement. They can be immobilized by alcohol or mineral oil before removal. Vegetable matter, such as paper, may absorb moisture and become more tightly impacted during irrigation and should instead be removed with small forceps. Most small objects can be removed by irrigation or with small forceps if the child is not hurt or anxious and can hold still during the procedure. General anesthesia is necessary if the child cannot cooperate and for removal of large objects or those deeply impacted.

Otitis Externa. Inflammatory conditions of the external auditory canal include furunculosis, acute bacterial and viral infections, and chronic disease related to bacteria, fungi or dermatoses. The normal bacterial flora of the canal consists of nonpathogenic corynebacteria ("diphtheroids") and *Staphylococcus epidermidis*. Acute external otitis is commonly caused by *Staphylococcus aureus* and streptococci. Subacute or chronic inflammations are likely to be associated with Proteus, Pseudomonas, Klebsiella-Aerobacter and fungi such as Candida and Aspergillus. Primary *Herpesvirus simplex* infection of the auricle and canal may be confused with impetigo.

With severe acute infections and furunculosis there is pain, fever and lymphadenitis. The pain is accentuated by movement of the tragus, a differential point from otitis media in which this manipulation does not increase pain. The preauricular, postauricular or cervical lymphadenitis is also helpful in differentiation from otitis media, because adenitis is not a feature of middle ear disease. The inflammatory process may obliterate the canal lumen; if the tympanic membrane can be seen, it may be normal or red.

Acute external otitis is treated with cleansing of the canal and frequent instillation of antibiotic drops (not ointment). A wick saturated with antibiotic solution is an effective means of local therapy. Local steroids are commonly used for anti-inflammatory effect. Systemic antibiotics are indicated for severe infections. Analgesics and local heat assuage pain.

Furunculosis due to *Staphylococcus aureus* occurs in the outer, cartilaginous portion of the canal. It is treated with incision and drainage and systemic antibiotics, usually penicillin G or a penicillinase-resistant penicillin.

In subacute or chronic infections there is discomfort or itching rather than pain, decreased hearing and foul-smelling discharge. Because of the itching, cleansing of the canal may be pleasurable rather than painful. The canal and tympanic membrane become insensitive to pain in chronic external otitis. Systemic antibiotic therapy is not helpful. Therapy consists in thorough cleansing of the canal and instillation of antibiotic ointments or drops.

The condition known as "swimmer's ear" is due to loss of protective cerumen and chronic irritation and maceration from moisture in the canal. Pseudomonas organisms are secondary invaders, not the basic cause. The distressing itching is temporarily alleviated by ointments, but the most effective therapy is cleansing and drying of the canal with alcohol after swimming and baths, and instillation of lanolin oil. Acute infection may supervene and necessitate antibiotic therapy.

THE TYMPANIC MEMBRANE

The tympanic membrane is situated obliquely in relation to the canal, with the superior and posterior portion most lateral. The major portion, or pars tensa, has a fibrous layer between the outer epithelial surface and the inner mucosal lining. At the periphery the fibrous layer forms a thick annulus attached to a groove in the temporal bone. The annulus is incomplete superiorly and traverses the membrane to the short process of the malleus forming the malleolar folds or ridges. Above these, the fibrous layer is absent in the pars flaccida, or Shrapnell's membrane.

The long handle of the malleus can be visualized through the normal tympanic membrane slanting downward and backward. From the umbo, or point of greatest concavity of the drum at the end of the handle of the malleus, a cone of light reflex fans out anteriorly and inferiorly (Fig. 12-5).

The tortuous S-shaped course of the auditory canal is protective to the tympanic membrane, but interferes with visualization. In the older child the canal can be straightened by pulling the auricle up, back and out; however, in young infants maximum exposure is obtained by pulling the auricle back and slightly downwards. Visualization of the tympanic membrane can be accomplished with a speculum and head mirror for reflected light, but most pediatricians prefer the illuminated otoscope with magnifying lens. The canal must be unobstructed, and a bright light is necessary. A dim light will make a normal tympanic membrane look red and dull. Familiarity with normal variations in anatomy and with the pink appearance of a normal membrane in a febrile, crying child is essential.

The tympanic membrane of the newborn infant is difficult to evaluate. The canal is filled with debris, and the drum appears dull. Lack of development of the osseous portion of the canal accentuates the normal obliquity of the tympanic membrane.

Perforation may occur secondary to foreign bodies, pressure, infection and surgical myringotomy. When myringotomy is performed, the canal and the drum should be cleaned with an antiseptic, and a semilunar incision made in the posterior inferior portion of the pars tensa. Perforations which fail to seal spontaneously predispose to chronic infection and require surgical correction.

Myringitis, or inflammation of the tympanic membrane, may accompany otitis externa or otitis media, but also occurs independently. Myringitis without bacterial infection is common in rubeola and exanthem subitum and must be differentiated from that secondary to bacterial otitis media. Bullous myringitis is a syndrome of pain and serous blebs on the membrane, with or without fever and adenopathy. Occasionally the blebs are hemorrhagic. The disease is thought to be due to unknown viruses and has been pro-duced experimentally by *Mycoplasma pneumoniae.* Pain is relieved by rupture of the bullae. Secondary bacterial infection is rare, and routine antibiotic therapy is not indicated.

THE MIDDLE EAR

Several factors contribute to the predisposition of infants to infection of the middle ear. The eustachian tube is short, the orifice patulous and easily compressed, and its horizontal position hinders drainage. Drainage is further impaired by the supine position in which the infant lies. Hypertrophy of the normally abundant nasopharyngeal lymphoid tissue from allergy or from upper respiratory tract infection may block the eustachian tube. The route of infection is presumed to be through the eustachian tube. Infection through the auditory canal probably occurs only with penetrating wounds. The importance of a hematogenous route is unknown.

For consideration of causative organisms and therapy, diseases of the middle ear are divided into 4 categories: serous (nonsuppurative), acute suppurative, recurrent, and chronic otitis media.

Serous Otitis Media. Serous effusions of the middle ear are believed to originate as a physical phenomenon secondary to blockage of the eustachian tube and to negative pressure in the middle ear cavity. The inciting cause of the obstructing edema or lymphoid hyperplasia may be nasopharyngeal inflammation or allergy. The increasing frequency of serous otitis in the antibiotic era suggests that some cases represent incompletely treated bacterial infections of the middle ear, but proof of this hypothesis is lacking. A viral origin has not been established.

The serous fluid produces a sensation of fullness in the ear, decreased hearing and a popping or clicking sound with swallowing or jaw movement. The tympanic membrane is bulging and dull with a few injected vessels, or a diffuse, dusky hue. Systemic symptoms are rare.

Initial management includes nasopharyngeal

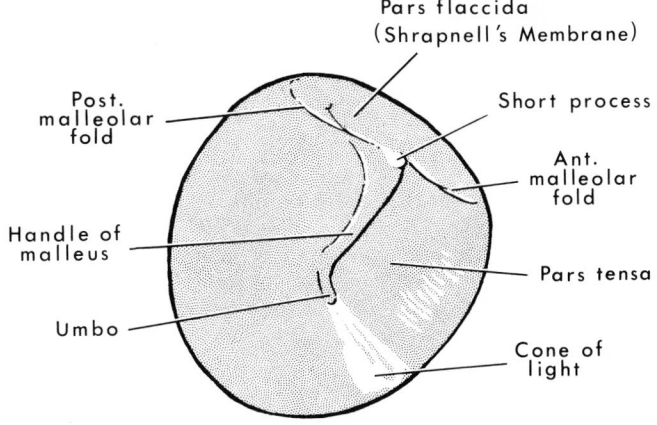

Post. malleolar fold

Pars flaccida (Shrapnell's Membrane)

Short process

Ant. malleolar fold

Handle of malleus

Pars tensa

Umbo

Cone of light

Figure 12-5.

decongestants. If the fluid persists without diminution after 3 weeks, myringotomy with removal by suction of the viscid material is done. If allowed to remain, the fluid eventually undergoes fibrinous changes, and permanent damage to the middle ear structures and deafness may result.

For recurrent or chronic serous effusions, adenoidectomy and repeated myringotomy may be indicated. Investigation for possible allergy should be made and appropriate treatment undertaken. Refractory cases may respond to implantation of a plastic tube into the middle ear cavity for continuous external drainage through the drum and for equalization of pressure.

Acute Suppurative Otitis Media. Acute bacterial infection of the middle ear is due to *Diplococcus pneumoniae* in over half of cases. Streptococci are less common invaders, and staphylococci are found in fewer than 5 per cent of cases. In infancy *Hemophilus influenzae* is an important causative agent, accounting for approximately one third of cases.

Pain, fever and constitutional signs occur early. At this time the tympanic membrane may show only redness, but as a purulent exudate accumulates there is bulging of the drum with loss of landmarks. The young infant may indicate pain by head-shaking or batting at the ears, but frequently there are only constitutional signs of fever and irritability, and at times vomiting and loose stools. If spontaneous perforation occurs, pain is relieved and fever decreases.

Therapy includes antibiotics, analgesics and nasal decongestants. The use of decongestants is based more on tradition than proof of efficacy. In children beyond infancy, penicillin is preferred in therapy. Adequate concentrations in the middle ear can be achieved with either parenteral or oral administration. In infancy, penicillin is frequently effective, but some strains of *Hemophilus influenzae* require high concentrations of penicillin for inhibition; ampicillin is effective therapy. Therapy is continued for 10 days or until signs of inflammation have been absent for several days.

Myringotomy is not always necessary. It should be performed if the patient fails to show any improvement after 48 to 72 hours of antibiotic therapy. Bacterial strains and culture of pus should be obtained. Discrepancy between the bacteriology of the middle ear and nasopharynx is so common that nasopharyngeal cultures are unreliable.

Serious complications of otitis media include mastoiditis and infection of the central nervous system.

Recurrent Otitis Media. Recurrence of infection within a few days or weeks of cessation of therapy is common in infancy. The spectrum of causative bacteria changes: pneumococci are much less common, but *Staphylococcus aureus, Hemophilus influenzae* and a variety of other bacteria may be involved. With recurrent infections, the tympanic membrane becomes thickened and may not show bulging or much inflammation, so that the physician fails to appreciate the presence of pus in the middle ear.

To establish drainage and to identify the causative organism, myringotomy is necessary in persistent or frequently recurring otitis media. Selection of antibiotics is based upon in-vitro sensitivity testing of cultured bacteria.

Investigation for predisposing causes such as abundant lymphoid tissue, mastoid infection or allergy should be undertaken and appropriate treatment given.

Chronic Otitis Media. The chronically infected ear often has associated mastoid infection. Characteristically there is decreased hearing and a painless discharge from the ear through a permanent defect of the tympanic membrane. A so-called cholesteatoma, or mass of desquamated epithelium with or without cholesterol crystals, may develop in the middle ear cavity with subsequent destruction of ossicles.

Cultures of the discharge generally reveal enteric gram-negative organisms, staphylococci or a mixed growth.

Acute exacerbation of infection may develop periodically and require antibiotic therapy, but, in general, systemic antibiotics are of little use in chronic otitis media. Local therapy consists in thorough cleansing of the ear and antibiotic ointments or drops. Predisposing causes should be investigated and treated. Ultimately the patient with chronic infection may require tympanoplasty with or without mastoidectomy and reconstruction of damaged ossicles.

Development of pain, vertigo or neurologic signs suggests complications such as meningitis, brain or epidural abscess, superior petrosal sinus thrombosis or labyrinthitis.

MASTOIDITIS

The mastoid antrum is present at birth, and pneumatization of the temporal bone starts in infancy. This is not an orderly, predictable process from individual to individual, nor in the 2 temporal bones of one person. Interpretation of roentgenographic changes before adolescence is therefore difficult, and normal variations in development may mimic pathologic changes of mastoid infection.

The mastoid process is not present at birth, so that the signs of redness, tenderness and swelling over the mastoid process seen in older children are not present in the infant with mastoiditis.

Acute inflammation of the mastoid air cells by direct extension from infection in the middle ear is treated with appropriate antibiotics. If destruction of bone, or osteomyelitis, occurs, there is risk of extension to the central nervous system. Intensive antibiotic therapy and simple mastoidectomy are required.

Infection of the petrous pyramid may produce sixth cranial nerve palsy. The constellation of pain, aural discharge and sixth nerve palsy is known as *Gradenigo's syndrome*.

The incidence of mastoiditis has been dramatically reduced since the availability of antibiotics; nevertheless it is still an important problem. Any child with recurrent or chronic middle ear infection should be suspected of having mastoiditis. Cholesteatoma formation in the mastoid may occur with chronic infection. Treatment of chronic mastoiditis is surgical.

JOHN D. NELSON

REFERENCES

Feingold, M., and others: Acute Otitis Media in Children. Bacteriological Findings in Middle Ear Fluid Obtained by Needle Aspiration. *Am. J. Dis. Child.*, 111:361, 1966.

Gorlin, J., and Pindborg, J. J.: *Syndromes of the Head and Neck.* New York, McGraw-Hill Book Company, 1964.

McGovern, J. P., Haywood, T. J., and Fernandez, A. A.: Allergy and Secretory Otitis Media. An Analysis of 512 Cases. *J.A.M.A..,* 200:124, 1967.

Mortimer, E. A., Jr., and Watterson, R. L.: A Bacteriologic Investigation of Otitis Media in Infancy. *Pediatrics,* 17:359, 1956.

Rifkind, D., Chanock, R., Kravetz, H., Johnson, K., and Knight, V.: Ear Involvement (Myringitis) and Primary Atypical Pneumonia Following Inoculation of Volunteers with Eaton Agent. *Am. Rev. Resp. Dis.,* 85:479, 1962.

Roddey, O. F., Jr., Earle, R., Jr., and Haggerty, R.: Myringotomy in Acute Otitis Media: A Controlled Study. *J.A.M.A.,* 197:849, 1966.

Silverstein, H., Bernstein, J. M., and Lerner, P. I.: Antibiotic Concentrations in Middle Ear Effusions. *Pediatrics,* 38:33, 1966.

van Dishoeck, H. A. E., Derks, A. C. W., and Voorhorst, R.: Bacteriology and Treatment of Acute Otitis Media in Children. *Acta Oto-laryng.,* 50:250, 1959.

THE LARYNX

Symptoms referable to the larynx are dyspnea, stridor, wheezing, hoarseness and aphonia. The dyspnea of laryngeal obstruction is characteristically associated with deep inspiratory indrawing at the suprasternal notch and supraclavicular spaces, as well as with stridor. Not all inspiratory indrawing at the suprasternal notch is the result of high obstruction; it occurs whenever the accessory muscles of respiration are brought into play as in generalized obstructive emphysema (see p. 934). In the latter situation the indrawing is more shallow. Stridor of laryngeal disease occurs in the inspiratory phase in contrast to the wheezing of asthma and other bronchiolitic disturbances, which is predominantly in the expiratory phase.

The only method of examining the larynx of a child under 6 or 7 years of age is by direct laryngoscopy. Direct laryngoscopic examination is indicated in the presence of the symptoms mentioned and may afford a means of treatment as well as diagnosis. Thorough physical examination, appropriate roentgenographic examination and bacteriologic studies may also be essential for the appraisal of laryngeal disease.

CONGENITAL MALFORMATIONS

CONGENITAL LARYNGEAL STRIDOR

Noisy, crowing respiratory sounds, usually associated with inspiration, are relatively common in the neonatal period and during the first year of life. Some infants merely have noisy breathing, whereas others have a laryngeal "crow," hoarseness or aphonia, dyspnea, and inspiratory retractions in the supraclavicular, intercostal and subcostal spaces. If inspiratory retractions are severe, deformity of the thorax may result. Infants with severe dyspnea frequently have difficulty in nursing, so that undernutrition is common. Cyanosis is rarely observed. Respiratory infections tend to exaggerate all the symptoms.

In the first few days of life it may be difficult to distinguish between congenital disturbances of the larynx and transient disturbances such as the laryngospasm of tetany of the newborn or laryngeal edema secondary to trauma or aspiration of irritant substances at birth. The history of aspiration at birth, hoarseness or aphonia and laryngoscopic examination establish the presence of postnatal laryngeal edema.

Stridor persisting or appearing after the first few days of life usually results from disturbances in or adjacent to the larynx. The most common of these is congenital deformity or flabbiness of the epiglottis and supraglottic aperture (laryngomalacia). Developmental malformations may be present, or there may be merely an exaggeration of the normal "omega" shape of the infantile epiglottis. Anomalies of the larynx include malformations of the laryngeal cartilages, intraluminal webs, and malformations or duplication of the vocal cords. At times generalized chondromalacia of the larynx and trachea may be observed. In such instances the larynx and the trachea tend to collapse with inspiration and to expand with expiration. Congenital tumors such as fibromas of the larynx are rare. Mucous retention cysts, branchial cleft cysts and thyroglossal duct remnants are other infrequent causes of stridor. Birth trauma must also be considered in the differential diagnosis.

Stridor may also be produced by extralaryngeal causes. Hypoplasia of the mandible permits the base of the tongue to displace the epiglottis posteriorly and cause laryngeal obstruction. Macroglossia from hypertrophy of the muscles, hemangioma, lymphangioma or cysts may have the same effect. Compression of the larynx by congenital goiters has been reported. Congenital vascular anomalies (p. 1010) may also cause stridor. Enlargement of the thymus is rarely, if ever, responsible for stridor.

Diagnosis. Most cases of congenital laryngeal stridor can be diagnosed only by direct laryngoscopy. Abnormalities of the epiglottis, the vocal cords and other parts of the larynx can be seen.

Extralaryngeal causes of stridor can often be established without the aid of direct laryngoscopy. Vascular anomalies which partially occlude the trachea and esophagus can often be detected by fluoroscopic observation during a "barium swallow" (p. 1011).

Treatment. The most common cause of laryngeal stridor, laryngomalacia, rarely requires treatment. The condition is seldom serious, and symptoms gradually become less severe, generally disappearing by about 1 year of age. Cysts, webs, tumors and malformations of the larynx require various specialized procedures, such as excision, dilatation, laryngoplasty or tracheotomy. The stridor associated with macroglossia or hypoplasia of the mandible can be relieved by pulling the tongue and mandible forward.

Particular attention must be given to the feeding of infants with stridor. Aspiration is an ever-present danger. Moreover, the respiratory efforts preclude normal sucking and swallowing in some infants. Slow, careful feedings from a small nipple or by dropper or glass are usually adequate. Feeding by gavage or even gastrostomy is occasionally necessary.

Infants with stridor must be protected from respiratory infections.

CONGENITAL WEB

This condition is not common, but its immediate diagnosis is essential. If the web is complete or almost complete, the newborn infant will quickly be asphyxiated. Laryngeal atresia has been associated with anophthalmia. In a few instances a web has been perforated or removed with sufficient promptness to save the infant's life. Often the obstruction is not complete, and there is only stridor and mild dyspnea.

Diagnosis and Treatment. Direct laryngoscopy affords the means for both diagnosis and treatment. In some instances it may be necessary to insert a tracheostomy tube while a series of dilatations is carried out. Direct laryngoscopic incision or excision of a congenital web is nearly always followed by prompt re-formation, and is thus rarely successful. An external operative approach may be helpful when the patient has reached 8 or 10 years of age.

TRAUMA OF THE LARYNX

Birth Trauma. Injury of the larynx during birth is not infrequent. It may result in *disloca-*

tion of the cricothyroid or *cricoarytenoid articulations.* Such an injury will result in hoarseness and at times in wheezing or fluttering respiratory sounds. The diagnosis is made by direct laryngoscopic examination. Treatment by direct laryngoscopic manipulations, using a laryngeal dilator, may be effectual, but tracheotomy should be done when there is evidence that the infant is not getting enough air.

Unilateral or *bilateral recurrent laryngeal paralysis* may also be produced by birth trauma, especially during instrumental delivery. When only one cord is paralyzed, there may be only hoarseness and slight stridor. There is usually no dyspnea. In bilateral paralysis there is dyspnea with stridor. Direct laryngoscopic examination will establish the diagnosis. Tracheotomy is usually necessary for bilateral paralysis. The older child may wear a valvular cannula, and a laryngoplasty may be done later to permit decannulation, unless breathing through the larynx has improved spontaneously.

Postnatal Trauma. Any trauma such as that brought about by a fall against a hard object may produce acute or chronic stenosis of the larynx, as may high tracheotomy and prolonged intubation. Immediate tracheotomy is required in the acute stage if there are signs of high obstruction.

LARYNGEAL STENOSIS

ACUTE LARYNGEAL STENOSIS

Acute stenosis may result from any acute infection, diphtheritic or nondiphtheritic, which is responsible for edema of the subglottic region, from inflammation secondary to the inspiration of a vegetal foreign body such as a peanut, and especially after instrumentation in the removal of such an object, from edema resulting from allergic factors or cardiorenal disease or from a foreign body lodged in the larynx.

Treatment. This consists in immediate provision of an airway by intubation or tracheotomy, after which appropriate medical treatment can be instituted.

CHRONIC LARYNGEAL STENOSIS

Chronic laryngeal stenosis is a frequent sequel of high tracheotomy, i.e. a tracheotomy in which the first tracheal ring or the cricoid cartilage has been damaged. It is rare when care is taken to keep these 2 structures intact. The laryngeal diseases which may be responsible for chronic stenosis include laryngeal diphtheria, acute laryngitis, syphilis, tuberculosis, burns by roentgen rays or radium, and external trauma.

Pathology. Scarring and stenosis most often develop in the subglottic region, and at times there is necrosis of cartilage.

Clinical Manifestations. These are generally limited to inability to decannulate the tracheotomized patient or to extubate the intubated patient. When neither intubation nor tracheotomy has been done, there will be dyspnea with audible stridor and indrawing at the suprasternal notch and at the supraclavicular and intercostal spaces.

Diagnosis. Diagnosis is by direct laryngoscopy, supplemented by palpation of the larynx and by roentgenographic examination.

The prognosis for eventual cure is good, though many patients require treatment for months or years.

Treatment. In the milder cases replacement of the tracheostomy cannula by a smaller one, and occlusion of this tube with a cork (at first a partial occlusion and then a complete one), will re-educate the patient to breathe through the mouth and permit removal of the cannula. If this is not successful, dilatation through a direct laryngoscope may accomplish the desired result. Such dilatation should not be done at too frequent intervals. When neither of these methods has sufficed to re-establish adequate breathing through the larynx, external surgery, with or without use of an indwelling mold, may be required.

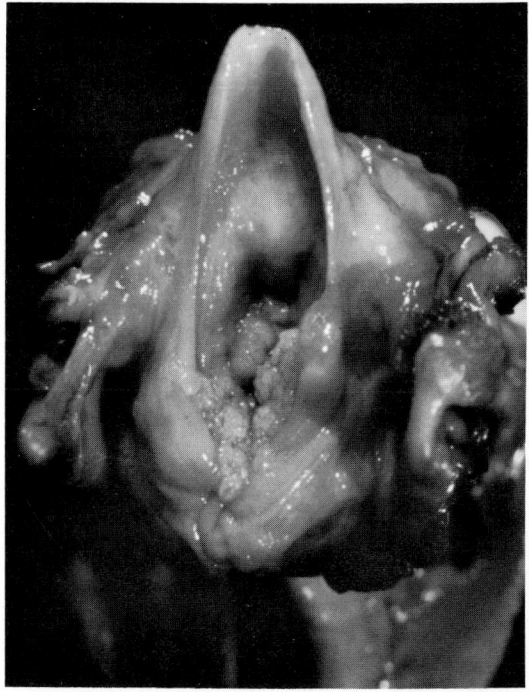

Figure 12-6. Obstructive glottic papilloma in a 5-year-old girl with a history of progressive dyspnea and aphonia (postmortem specimen). Although examined by a physician on several occasions, she was referred for treatment only when dyspnea became extreme; she died of asphyxia en route to hospital.

NEOPLASMS OF THE LARYNX
(See also p. 1445)

Papilloma is the most common benign tumor of the larynx in children. The lesions may grow profusely from any portion of the larynx, though usually from the vocal cords. The tumor rarely, if ever, becomes malignant, and often disappears after puberty. Initially, the only symptom is hoarseness; but if the condition is allowed to persist, there is likely to be dyspnea; asphyxia has occurred in unrecognized cases. The diagnosis may be made by direct laryngoscopy during the stage of hoarseness, even in an infant. The lesions are pinkish, warty tumors, which scalp off easily when grasped with forceps. The diagnosis should be confirmed histologically.

The best treatment is superficial removal of the tumors by forceps through the direct laryngoscope. Care should be taken not to damage normal tissues. Cure will ultimately be obtained, even though at first there is usually rapid recurrence. If recurrence is too rapid to be kept under control by this method, and asphyxia threatens, a tracheotomy should be done; a cannula should be left in place while the tendency to recurrence persists. More extreme therapeutic measures such as radical surgical excision or intensive irradiation are absolutely contraindicated. Recent evidence suggests that use of an autogenous vaccine prepared from freshly removed papilloma may retard regrowth.

Vocal nodules are small tumors which occur in children at the junction of the anterior and middle thirds of the vocal cords. They are generally bilateral. They have been called "screamer's nodes" or "singer's nodes." The only symptom is slight hoarseness. Regression may occur if strenuous use of the voice is avoided. Otherwise the nodules may be removed by small cupped forceps under direct laryngoscopic view.

FOREIGN BODIES IN THE LARYNX, TRACHEA AND BRONCHI

The air passages of children are frequent sites for the lodgment of foreign bodies; the carelessness of adults is the most important contributory factor.

Pathology. The changes produced by foreign bodies depend upon their nature and upon the degree of obstruction of the air passage. A sharp or irritating object lodged in the larynx will produce severe edema and later suppurative perichondritis. In the bronchus a nonobstructive foreign body may produce little pathologic change, whereas an obstructive object will produce atelectasis and later bronchiectasis, pulmonary abscess or empyema. A vegetal object, such as a peanut, may immediately produce a generalized inflammatory condition involving not only the portion of the tracheobronchial tree obstructed, but also the entire respiratory tract.

Clinical Manifestations. The initial symptoms of a foreign body in the air passages are choking, gagging, wheezing or cough. After the initial period there is often a symptomless interval which may last for hours, days or weeks. By the time symptoms reappear the initial ones may have been forgotten. The secondary symptoms usually give a clue to whether the foreign body is lodged in the air or food passages, and may indicate the level of lodgment. On occasion, however, dysphagia may occur from the swelling which results from lodgment of a foreign body in the region of the larynx, and foreign bodies in the upper esophagus may cause symptoms referable to the air passages by compression or by the overflow of food secretions into the larynx.

LARYNGEAL FOREIGN BODY

Clinical Manifestations. A foreign body in the larynx causes hoarseness, a cough which soon becomes croupy, and aphonia. Hemoptysis, dyspnea with wheezing, and cyanosis may occur. Obstruction resulting from the foreign body or the combination of it and the inflammatory reaction may prove fatal if the signs of high respiratory tract obstruction are not promptly recognized and appropriate treatment is not given.

Diagnosis. Roentgenographic and direct laryngoscopic examinations reveal the presence of a foreign body in the larynx (Fig. 12-7). An opaque foreign body in the neck will be clearly demonstrated on a lateral roentgenogram. When it is lodged anteriorly, it is obviously in the larynx; when it is behind the soft tissue shadows of the larynx, it is in the hypopharynx or the cervical esophagus. The plane in which the foreign body lies is another differential point in its localization. If it lies in the sagittal plane, it is in the larynx. If it is in the coronal plane, it is probably in the food passage. Even if the foreign body is not opaque, indirect evidence of its presence may be afforded by the roentgenographic examination. Films should always be taken from both the lateral and the anteroposterior projections. In some instances administration of a small amount of opaque material may be helpful. Direct laryngoscopy will confirm the diagnosis and provide access for instrumental removal of the foreign body. When there is a severe degree of dyspnea, it may be advisable to do a tracheotomy before the laryngoscopic examination.

TRACHEAL FOREIGN BODY

Though a foreign body in the trachea may be responsible for cough, hoarseness, dyspnea and cyanosis, the characteristic signs are the audible slap, the palpable thud and the asthmatoid wheeze. The diagnosis of tracheal foreign body may occasionally be made from the symptoms, physical signs and roentgenogram of the chest, but in most

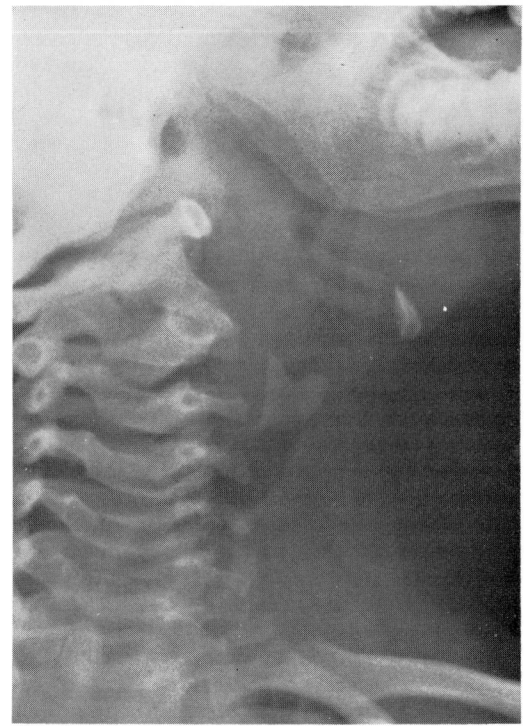

Figure 12-7. Foreign body (fragment of sea shell) in larynx of a 2-year-old child treated for "croup" 6 days before foreign body was suspected. Fortunately, tracheotomy was not required despite the presence of moderately severe laryngeal edema due to prolonged sojourn of the foreign body.

instances a definite diagnosis can be made only by bronchoscopy.

BRONCHIAL FOREIGN BODY

Clinical Manifestations. The initial symptoms are usually similar to those of foreign bodies in the larynx or trachea. Cough, blood-streaked sputum, and metallic taste in the case of metallic foreign bodies, are other symptoms which may be produced by bronchial foreign bodies. The degree of obstruction produced by a bronchial foreign body is a determining factor in the symptomology as well as in the pathologic changes. A *non-obstructive* foreign body may produce few symptoms even after prolonged sojourn. An *obstructive* foreign body quickly produces symptoms and signs and pathologic changes. When there is only a slight obstruction, a wheeze will be noted. When obstruction is of greater degree, obstructive emphysema or obstructive atelectasis will be produced; if either is allowed to persist, chronic bronchopulmonary disease may be a sequel. When both main bronchi are obstructed, there will be severe dyspnea and even asphyxia. If the foreign body is vegetal, e.g. a peanut, a severe condition known as *vegetal* or *arachidic bronchitis* will result. This is characterized by cough, a septic type of fever, and dyspnea. Chronic pulmonary sup-

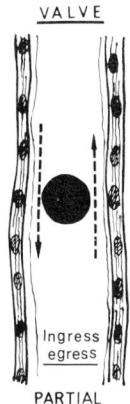
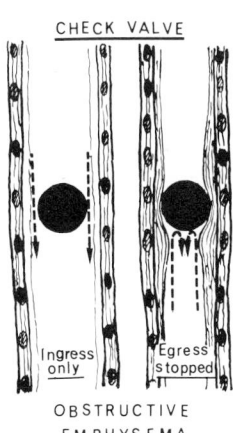
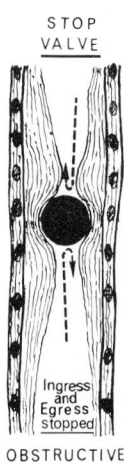

BY — PASS VALVE   CHECK VALVE   STOP VALVE

Figure 12-8. Valvular mechanisms in bronchial obstruction (see text).

Ingress egress

Ingress only   Egress stopped

Ingress and Egress stopped

PARTIAL OBSTRUCTION   OBSTRUCTIVE EMPHYSEMA   OBSTRUCTIVE ATELECTASIS

puration may be expected when a bronchial foreign body has been present for a long time.

Diagnosis. The symptoms of a bronchial foreign body depend upon the stage in which the patient is seen. The possibility of a foreign body must be considered in acute or chronic pulmonary lesions regardless of whether there is a history of a foreign body accident. The physical signs of bronchial obstruction from foreign bodies include limited expansion, decreased vocal fremitus, impaired (atelectasis) or hyperresonant (emphysema) percussion note and diminished breath sounds distal to the foreign body. When there is complete obstruction, with a so-called drowned lung or with atelectasis, there is absence of vocal resonance and vocal fremitus, which may lead to an erroneous diagnosis of empyema. Varying degrees

of tympany may be noted over areas of obstructive emphysema, which may persist for a time. Rales are more likely to be on the uninvaded side than on the invaded one.

Fluoroscopic examination is invaluable in detecting and localizing bronchial foreign bodies.

In order to understand the physical signs and the roentgenographic appearance of bronchial obstruction, it is helpful to recognize the analogies between the types of obstruction produced by foreign bodies and the different types of valves used to control the flow of fluids in pipes (Fig. 12-8).

A *first-degree* obstruction may be compared to a bypass valve, which allows passage of air or fluid in both directions, with only slight interference. In such cases a *wheeze* will be produced.

In a *second-degree* obstruction there is sufficient interference with the passage of air to permit it to go in one direction only. A "check-valve" action of this sort in the bronchial tree depends primarily upon the physiologic expansion of the bronchus on inspiration and its contraction on expiration. If the lumen is

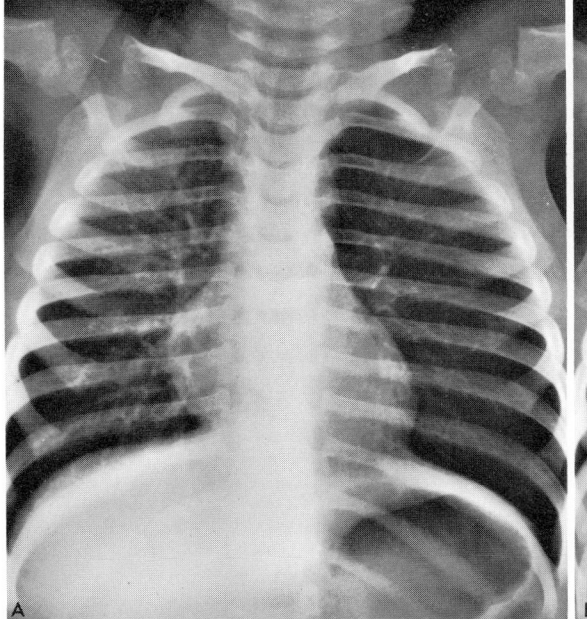
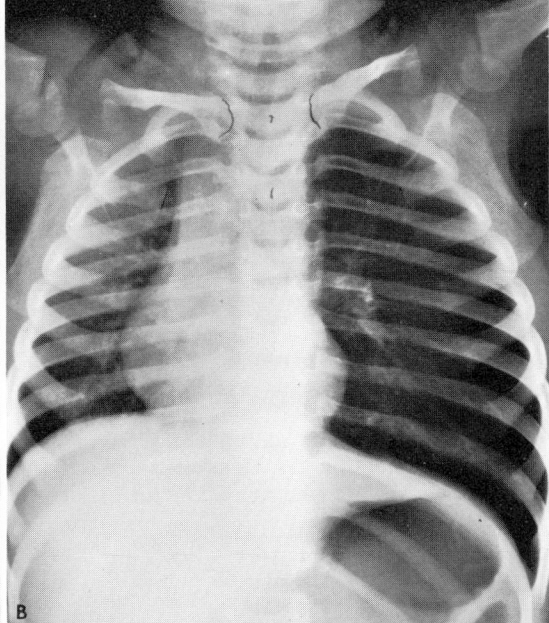

Figure 12-9. Obstructive emphysema due to peanut fragment in left main bronchus. Inspiratory film *(A)* appears relatively normal except for slight mediastinal shift to the right. In expiration *(B)* the left lung remains overaerated (check-valve mechanism), and the mediastinum moves far to the right.

obstructed by an object which is of just the right size to cause complete obstruction in the expiratory phase, but to allow air to pass in the inspiratory phase, air will enter the distal portion of the lung on inspiration, but little or none will escape during expiration. This type of obstruction produces *obstructive emphysema* (Fig. 12-9).

If blockage of the bronchus is complete, either by corking of the bronchus by the object itself or by an obstruction produced by the foreign body in combination with the inflammatory swelling of the bronchial mucosa, a stop-valve obstruction results, and the air in the distal portion of the lung is soon absorbed, leaving an area of *obstructive atelectasis* (Fig. 12-10).

These phenomena are most readily appreciated by observation under the fluoroscopic screen. In a bypass valve obstruction there is little or no roentgenographic evidence produced by a nonopaque foreign body.

When there is a check-valve type of obstruction, the *obstructive emphysema* makes it possible to localize a bronchial foreign body. The obstructed lung will remain expanded during expiration, while the heart and the mediastinum will shift to the opposite side as the unobstructed lung empties. The diaphragm is low, flattened and fixed on the obstructed side, while its excursion will be free and exaggerated on the unobstructed side. The differences between the lungs are much more evident on expiration than on inspiration. If a permanent record is desired, 2 films should be taken, one in full inspiration and one at the end of expiration.

When there is complete obstruction of the bronchus, producing *obstructive atelectasis,* the heart and the mediastinum are drawn toward the obstructed side and remain there during both phases of respiration. The diaphragm on the obstructed side remains high, while that on the unobstructed side moves normally. Films taken at the end of inspiration and of expiration will show only the slight difference resulting from the filling and emptying of the unobstructed lung. Observation of these phenomena under the fluoroscope and appreciation of the principles of the valvular mechanisms make it easier to understand the physical signs.

Opaque foreign bodies are clearly revealed on the roentgenogram. It is necessary to take films from both the anteroposterior and the lateral positions, with a sufficiently heavy exposure in the anteroposterior view to show a foreign body behind the heart.

Prognosis. Foreign bodies in the air passages which are not removed are sooner or later fatal in the majority of instances. Only 2 to 4 per cent of foreign bodies are coughed up spontaneously. About 99 per cent can be removed safely by the skilled bronchoscopist, and at least 98 per cent of patients so treated should recover completely.

Prevention. Much can be done to avoid foreign body accidents. If small objects are kept out of the reach of children, if children too young to masticate are not given candy containing nuts, and if toys which contain small parts loosely attached are not given to children, many serious cases of foreign body in the air passages will be prevented. Beads, the button box and coins should not be given to children as playthings. Safety pins should always be closed and not left near the baby's crib. The closed safety pin is not a dangerous foreign body, but the open one is among the most dangerous and the most difficult to remove safely.

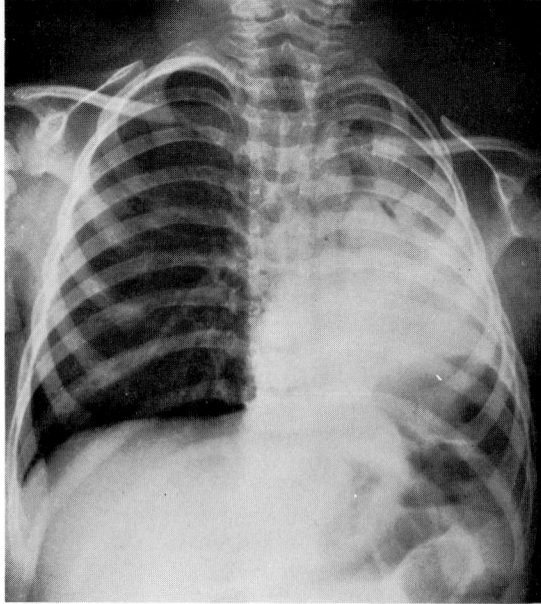

Figure 12-10. Foreign body lodged in left main bronchus, producing atelectasis of left lung. Note that the heart is drawn completely into the left side of the chest.

Adults should not set a bad example by holding pins or other objects in the mouth. The impulse to imitate is strong in a young child; frequently foreign body accidents occur because a baby or young child has imitated an adult by putting foreign objects in his mouth.

Treatment. The treatment of foreign body in the air passages consists in removal by direct laryngoscopy or bronchoscopy, with due consideration for the mechanical problem involved in the particular case. In some instances treatment of complicating conditions may be of equal importance. Removal of opaque foreign bodies lodged in the peripheral bronchi should be performed under the biplane fluoroscope. Any secondary infection should be treated with appropriate antimicrobial agents as indicated by laboratory sensitivity tests of the pathogenic organism.

CHARLES M. NORRIS

REFERENCES

Holinger, P. H., Johnson, K. C., and Schiller, F.: Congenital Anomalies of the Larynx. *Ann. Otol. Rhin. & Laryng.,* 63: 581, 1954.

Jackson, C., and Jackson, C. L.: *Bronchoesophagology.* Philadelphia, W. B. Saunders Company, 1950.

Acute Infections of the Larynx and the Trachea

General Considerations. Acute infections of the larynx are of relatively greater importance in infants and small children than in older children. This is true in part because of a somewhat greater incidence in the younger age group, but principally because the younger child has a relatively smaller airway which predisposes to greater respiratory distress.

The term "croup" is commonly applied to the heterogeneous group of infectious conditions characterized by inspiratory stridor, hoarseness, cough and signs of respiratory distress due to varying degrees of laryngeal obstruction. The infection in infants and small children is rarely limited to a single area of the respiratory tract, usually affecting in varying degrees the larynx, the trachea, bronchi and even the upper respiratory portion.

When there is sufficient involvement of the larynx to produce symptoms, the laryngeal part of the clinical picture is likely to overshadow other manifestations, owing to the severe effects upon vocalization and breathing.

Although an exact classification of acute laryngeal infection is not possible, there are several clinical varieties which seem to justify the following classification:

Acute diphtheritic laryngitis (p. 564)
Acute nondiphtheritic infections
  Epiglottitis
  Laryngitis
  Laryngotracheobronchitis
  Spasmodic laryngitis

ACUTE NONDIPHTHERITIC INFECTIONS
(INFECTIOUS CROUP)

Etiology. A large number of infectious agents, most often viruses, cause croup. Viral agents can now be identified for 60 to 75 per cent of patients studied, and it appears likely that they account for all or nearly all croup except that associated with diphtheria, pertussis and acute epiglottitis.

The agents most commonly isolated from patients with infectious croup are the parainfluenza viruses, which account for approximately two thirds of cases. The adenoviruses, the respiratory syncytial virus, influenza viruses and measles virus cause most of the remaining cases for which an agent can be identified.

Predisposing Factors. Regardless of cause, a number of factors predispose a child to this syndrome.

The majority of patients with viral croup are between the ages of 3 months and 3 years, whereas patients with croup due to bacterial agents such as *H. influenzae* and *C. diphtheriae* are more commonly between 3 and 7 years of age. For unknown reasons, the incidence of croup is higher in males than in females. The disease occurs most commonly during the cold season of the year.

In approximately 15 per cent of cases there is a strong family history of croup, and laryngitis does tend to recur in the same child.

Clinical Forms. *Acute epiglottitis.* This form of croup is a severe, rapidly progressive infection of the epiglottis and surrounding areas. Although *Hemophilus influenzae* type b is the organism classically associated with this severe illness, pneumococci and group A streptococci may produce an identical disease; a milder and superficially similar clinical picture due to moderate inflammation of the supraglottic area is commonly caused by viruses. The onset of illness is often abrupt, being preceded by a minor upper respiratory illness in about one fourth of the patients. The younger patient usually presents with sudden onset of high fever and difficulty in breathing. The older child often complains initially of severe sore throat and dysphagia. Within minutes or hours of the apparent onset of illness, the child will be in severe respiratory distress with inspiratory stridor, hoarseness, cough, dysphagia, irritability and restlessness. Fever ranges between 38 and 40.5° C. (100 to 105°F.) with an average of 39.5°C. (103°F.). Drooling, due to dysphagia, is commonly present.

The young child may assume a position of hyperextension of the neck, although other signs of meningeal irritation are absent. The older child may prefer a sitting position, leaning forward, with mouth open and tongue somewhat protruding. In some children the severity of illness may progress rapidly to a shocklike state characterized by pallor, cyanosis and impaired consciousness.

On physical examination the patient presents severe respiratory distress and characteristic inspiratory stridor. There is flaring of the alae nasi and inspiratory retractions of the suprasternal notch, the supraclavicular and intercostal spaces and the subcostal area. The pharynx is usually inflamed, and excessive mucus is present in the faucial regions. The diagnosis may be missed unless the tongue is depressed with a blade to show the large, edematous, cherry-red epiglottis, which is pathognomonic of epiglottitis. When the diagnosis is suspected in a seriously ill child, this procedure should be done only if tracheotomy can be performed at once. The maneuver may lead to sudden and complete obstruction. Mild to moderate cervical adenitis may be noted. The breath sounds are usually diminished bilaterally, indicating poor air exchange; there may be rhonchi due to mucus in the upper respiratory tract. When laryngoscopy is performed, intense inflammation is noted in the areas surrounding the epiglottis, as well as in the arytenoids and arytenoepiglottic folds, the vocal cords and subglottic regions. A pharyngeal or laryngeal membrane is rarely encountered.

REFERENCES

Berenberg, W., and Kevy, S.: Acute Epiglottitis in Childhood. A Serious Emergency, Readily Recognized at the Bedside. *New England J. Med.,* 268:870, 1958.

Cramblett, H. G.: Croup—Present Day Concept. *Pediatrics,* 25:1071, 1960.
Parrott, R. H.: Viral Respiratory Tract Illnesses in Children. *Bull. New York Acad. Med.,* 39:629, 1963.
Rabe, E. F.: Infectious Croup. I. Etiology. II. Virus Croup. III. Hemophilus Influenzae Type b Croup. *Pediatrics,* 2:255, 415, 559, 1948.

THE THORACIC CAVITY

For neoplasms of the lung, see page 1446.

MALFORMATIONS OF THE TRACHEA, BRONCHI AND LUNGS

Tracheo-esophageal fistula is the most important congenital anomaly of the trachea (p. 768). Rarely the trachea may be absent, or there may be tracheal stenosis of varying degrees. *Tracheal compression* may be produced by an anomalous aortic arch or other large vessel (p. 1010). *Tracheal diverticula* are blindly ending bronchus-like projections, which infrequently terminate in normal-appearing lung tissue (tracheal lobe). Other tracheal abnormalities are mentioned on pages 901 and 1337.

Bronchogenic cysts are usually located in the region of the bifurcation of the trachea. They rarely produce symptoms, and their clinical importance is based on the need to differentiate them from malignant tumors.

Anomalous fissures and lobes of the lungs are frequently observed roentgenographically and at autopsy, but are usually of no clinical significance. The so-called azygos lobe is actually a part of the right upper lobe. During fetal development the azygos vein normally shifts medially into the mediastinum and onto the vertebral column. If such a migration fails to occur, the vein cuts into the growing right upper lobe, leaving a deep azygos fissure, which separates the more medially placed azygos lobe from the remainder of the right upper lobe; there is no abnormality of the bronchial tree.

Congenital absence of both lungs is extremely rare. *Bilateral hypoplasia of the lungs* may occur in anencephalic monsters or may be associated with congenital diaphragmatic hernia; in the latter instance the lung on the side of the defect in the diaphragm shows greater reduction in size.

Unilateral pulmonary agenesis or hypoplasia is compatible with life. The heart and other mediastinal structures are shifted to the affected side, and the other lung is hyperexpanded and partially fills the thoracic cavity on the involved side. The stem bronchus on the affected side may be absent, rudimentary or of normal length and covered by a small rudimentary lung. Associated extrapulmonary anomalies may be present, especially hemivertebrae. Ipsilateral facial anomalies may occur with unilateral agenesis.

A *lower accessory lung* is a rare congenital anomaly. The accessory lung does not communicate with the tracheobronchial tree, and its blood supply is usually systemic rather than pulmonary in origin. It is almost always situated at the base of the left lung, rarely below the left diaphragm. Its structure varies from normal-appearing lung to that of a cystic space containing bronchial elements, but few or no alveoli.

Anomalous (nonpulmonary) circulation in a portion of a lower lobe (sequestered lobe) has been observed; there is a bronchial communication, but some maldevelopment of it. The blood supply is from the systemic circulation by way of an anomalous artery from the aorta. The lung tissue is usually replaced by multiple bronchial cysts or bronchiectatic cavities. Surgical removal of the involved lung is indicated.

Cysts of the lungs are occasionally present in infants early in the neonatal period and may be single or multiple, restricted to 1 lobe or distrib-

Figure 12-11. The lobar and segmental bronchi and the corresponding subdivisions of the lungs.

The subdivision of the lungs into parts smaller than the lobes aids in accurate localization of pathologic lesions and permits more economical resections in such diseases as bronchiectasis and tuberculosis. Although the lobes are classically identified by the interlobar fissures, the real basis of the division of the lungs into lobes is bronchial distribution. Each lobe is similarly subdivided by the branches coming from the lobar bronchus. For example, there are usually 3 branches of the right upper lobe bronchus, each of which supplies or branches out to form a definitive part of the lobe. The term "bronchopulmonary segment" is applied to that portion of a lobe supplied by a branch of the lobar bronchus. The smaller subdivisions identified on the basis of the distribution of the branches of the segmental bronchus are referred to as "subsegments." Each segment is named according to its position in the lobe of which it is a portion. For example, the 3 segments of the right upper lobe are termed anterior, apical and posterior. The bronchi are correspondingly named anterior, apical and posterior segmental branches of the right upper lobe bronchus.

At an intersegmental plane the alveoli at the periphery of one segment are separated from the alveoli of the adjacent segment by a small amount of fibrous connective tissue containing the tributaries of the pulmonary veins. The branches of the pulmonary arteries follow the bronchial branchings. (Prepared by Dr. John Franklin Huber, Professor of Anatomy, Temple University School of Medicine.)

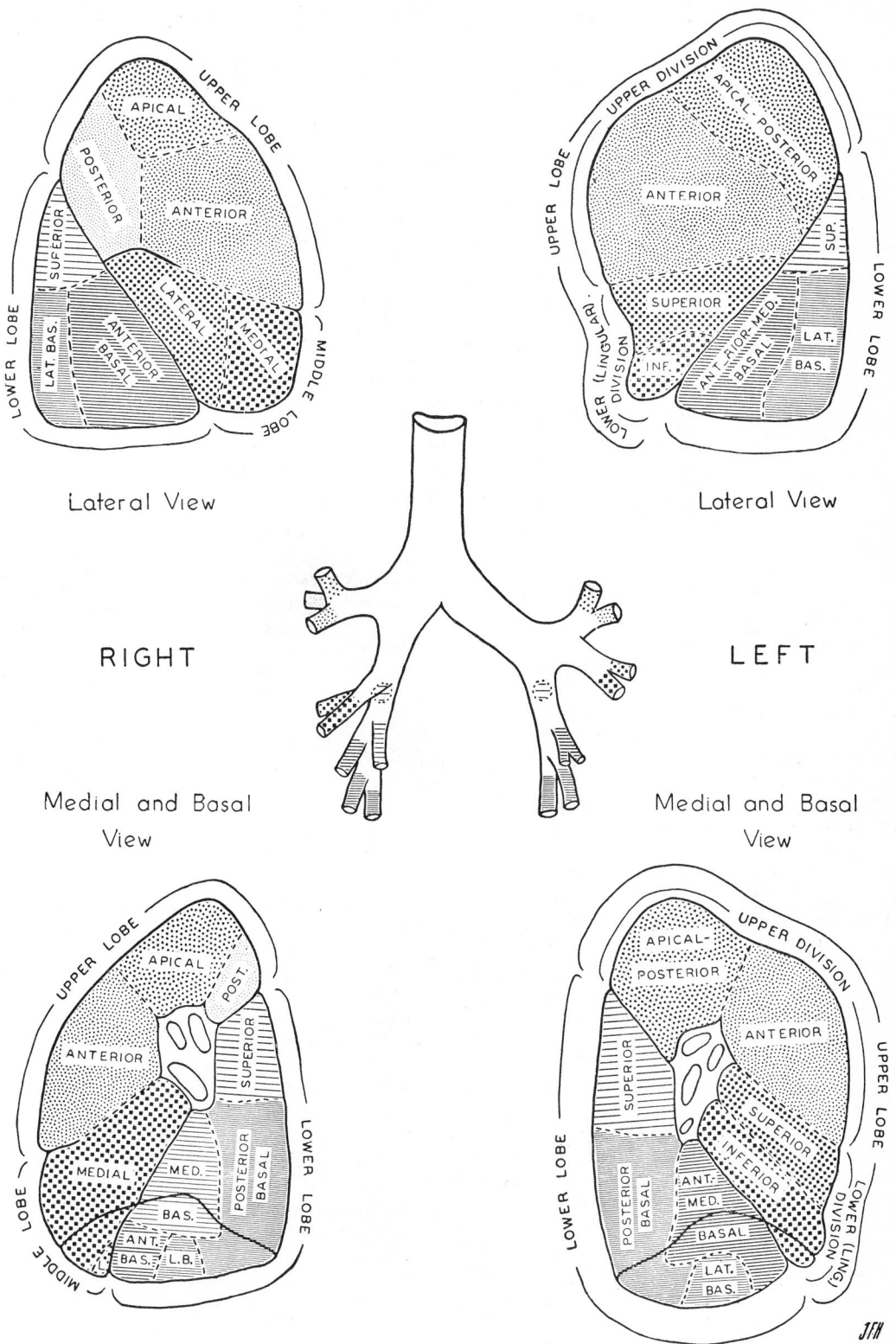

Lateral View

Lateral View

RIGHT

LEFT

Medial and Basal
View

Medial and Basal
View

Figure 12-11. *(Legend on opposite page)*

uted in 2 or more lobes. There is lack of agreement about the origin of many of them. It has been considered that those with an epithelial lining were congenital anomalies and that those without such a lining were the result of postnatal destructive processes. There is doubt whether this distinction is valid or whether the presence of cartilage in the wall of a cyst is in itself evidence of a congenital origin.

Cysts of congenital origin have been described in association with *adenomatoid malformations* of the lungs. The lesion, which apparently is most often limited to one lobe, may initially appear on the roentgenogram as a solid structure. The bronchi are malformed. As the lobe is irregularly aerated during the first few days of life, air accumulates in the potential cystic structures. These enlarge progressively and may cause severe respiratory distress. In the left lower lobe the condition may be confused with diaphragmatic hernia.

Most cystic structures in the neonatal period or later are acquired and result from destruction of the pulmonary architecture. This may occur during artificial respiration (see Pneumomediastinum, p. 389) and on occasion may be responsible for an accumulation of air (cyst) within one or more lobes (see Bullous Emphysema, p. 389). Partial blockage of a bronchus with creation of a ball-valve type of mechanism will permit retention of an increasing amount of air. Under such circumstances, whether the obstruction is inflammatory or purely mechanical and whether it is intrabronchial or extrabronchial, a so-called tension cyst is created. In other circumstances connection with the tracheobronchial tree is broken, alveolar sacs are ruptured, and the accumulation of air (bullous emphysema) remains for a long time before it is finally absorbed and the architecture of the lungs is realigned. Many factors can be responsible for such obstructions of the bronchi, some of which may be congenital in origin, but the majority are probably the result of postnatal disturbances, usually inflammatory. An unusual association with cytomegalic inclusion disease has been recorded. The cysts may be filled entirely with air or fluid or with a combination of them.

Most cysts eventually disappear without interference, but when a tension cyst continues to expand and compress the other lobes, it is usually necessary to remove the lobe containing it. Even such cysts, however, may establish an equilibrium with the uninvolved portions of the lung, become closed and eventually disappear. The decision for surgical removal must be based on the degree of respiratory embarrassment and whether it is progressive.

Lobar emphysema is discussed on pages 905 and 933.

REFERENCES

Boyden, E. A.: Developmental Anomalies of the Lungs. *Am. J. Surg.,* 89:79, 1955.

Caffey, J.: On the Natural Regression of Pulmonary Cysts During Early Infancy. *Pediatrics,* 11:48, 1953.

Craig, J. M., Kirkpatrick, J., and Neuhauser, E. B. D.: Congenital Cystic Adenomatoid Malformation of the Lung in Infants. *Am. J. Roentgenol.,* 76:516, 1956.

Ferencz, C.: Congenital Abnormalities of Pulmonary Vessels and Their Relation to Malformations of the Lung. *Pediatrics,* 28:993, 1961.

Gallager, H. S.: Cytomegalic Inclusion Disease of Infancy: Report of Case Associated with Cysts of Lung with Recovery Following Lobectomy. *Am. J. Clin. Path.,* 22:1147, 1952.

Gruenfeld, G. E., and Gray, S. H.: Malformations of the Lung. *Arch. Path.,* 31:392, 1941.

Huber, J. F.: Practical Correlative Anatomy of the Bronchial Tree and Lungs. *J. Nat. Med. A.,* 41:49, 1949.

Kergin, F. G.: Congenital Cystic Disease of Lung Tissue Associated with Anomalous Arteries. *J. Thoracic Surg.,* 23:55, 1952.

Laipply, T. C.: Cysts and Cystic Tumors of the Mediastinum. *Arch. Path.,* 39:153, 1945.

Potter, E. L., and Bohlender, G. P.: Intrauterine Respiration in Relation to Development of the Fetal Lung, with Report of Two Unusual Anomalies of the Respiratory System. *Am. J. Obst. & Gynec.,* 42:14, 1941.

BRONCHITIS

ACUTE BRONCHITIS

Though the diagnosis of "acute bronchitis" is frequently made, there is considerable doubt whether this condition exists in children as an isolated clinical entity. Rather, bronchitis occurs in association with a number of other conditions of the upper and lower respiratory tracts. The trachea is nearly always involved, and thus a more correct term would be "acute tracheobronchitis." The term "capillary bronchitis" (bronchiolitis) represents an entirely different illness, more closely related to the interstitial pneumonias.

Asthmatic bronchitis, a form of asthma with obscure pathogenesis, is often confused with acute bronchitis. Apparently, with a variety of upper respiratory tract infections, some children experience an exaggerated response of bronchi, with spasm and exudation similar to those encountered in older children with asthma.

Acute tracheobronchitis is most commonly found in association with an upper respiratory tract infection such as nasopharyngitis, but is also associated with such specific infections as influenza, pertussis, measles, typhoid fever (and other salmonelloses), diphtheria and scarlet fever. An acute, primary, undifferentiated tracheobronchitis also occurs, most commonly in older children and adolescents. It is likely that except for the bacterial diseases mentioned, acute tracheobronchitis is always of viral origin. Pneumococci, staphylococci, *H. influenzae* and various hemolytic streptococci may be isolated from the sputum of these patients, but their presence does not imply a bacterial origin, and intensive specific antimicrobial therapy does not appreciably alter the course of the illness.

Some children appear to be far more susceptible

to acute tracheobronchitis than others. The reasons are unknown, but it is thought that allergy, poor health, climate, air pollution and chronic infections of the upper respiratory tract, particularly sinusitis, are contributory factors.

Clinical Manifestations. Generally, the clinical manifestations of bronchitis are preceded by those of an upper respiratory tract infection. The illness is ushered in by a cough of relatively gradual onset, usually dry, hacking and unproductive. At this time the patient will often complain of low substernal discomfort, which is often aggravated by coughing. The child is frequently afebrile, but there may be fever to about 38.5°C. (102°F.). As the illness progresses, the patient will complain of soreness of the chest, occasionally of shortness of breath. Within 1 or 2 days the cough becomes productive, and the sputum, which may be clear initially, quickly becomes purulent. Vomiting is not uncommon, and is generally related to gagging on secretions or to the violence of the cough. Usually within 5 to 10 days the mucus thins and the cough gradually disappears. The considerable malaise often associated with the illness may continue for a week or more after acute symptoms have subsided.

Physical findings vary with the age of the patient and the stage of the disease. Early signs of nasopharyngitis and conjunctival injection are often noted. Later there may be some roughening of breath sounds, and rhonchi, coarse and fine moist rales and occasionally very fine bubbly rales may be heard over the entire chest.

In the otherwise healthy child, few if any complications occur. In undernourished children, or infants in poor health, such complications as otitis media, sinusitis or pneumonia are relatively common.

Treatment. There is no specific therapy. In small infants pulmonary drainage should be encouraged by frequent shifts in position. Older children are most comfortable in a highly humidified atmosphere, but there is no evidence that this shortens the duration of illness. Cough medicines are frequently given for symptomatic relief or for a supposed expectorant value, but none of the medications which can be safely given to children have been proved clearly beneficial. Potent cough remedies may suppress the cough reflex, but coughing is needed to clear the airway. If it is suppressed, obstruction of the bronchi by mucus may occur, which increases the possibility of suppuration. Antihistamines have an atropine-like action which tends to dry the secretions, and should be avoided. Antimicrobial therapy does not shorten the duration of the viral illness or decrease the low incidence of bacterial complications.

Children with repeated attacks of bronchitis should be carefully evaluated for the possibility of anomalies of the respiratory tract, foreign bodies, bronchiectasis, hypogammaglobulinemia, tuberculosis, allergy, and such chronic upper respiratory tract infections as sinusitis, tonsillitis or adenoiditis.

CHRONIC BRONCHITIS

There is considerable doubt whether chronic bronchitis as an isolated clinical entity exists in children. This condition is frequently diagnosed, but generally the child with a chronic cough and the chest signs of bronchitis either has an underlying allergy, so that wheezing is a common finding, or has a chronic infection of the sinuses or nasopharynx (adenoiditis) with postnasal discharge. Rarely, bronchial irritation may be secondary to the chronic inhalation of dust or noxious fumes. The condition is frequently confused with mild cases of bronchiectasis and cystic fibrosis.

Clinical Manifestations. The chief symptom is cough, with or without expectoration. The child will usually complain of soreness of the chest; characteristically, these signs and symptoms are worse at night. Physical findings are similar to those of acute bronchitis. The condition is usually associated with other respiratory or systemic disease.

Differential Diagnosis. Every attempt should be made to find the underlying condition which may be associated with chronic bronchitis. Roentgenograms of the chest and of the sinuses should be obtained, and bronchograms are essential for elimination of bronchiectasis. A nasal smear should be examined for eosinophils, and a search undertaken for inhalant allergens or other noxious factors in the child's environment.

Course and Prognosis. Both the course and the prognosis depend upon the possibility of appropriate management or eradication of any underlying illness. Complications will be those of the underlying illness.

Treatment. When an underlying cause for chronic bronchitis has been found, this should receive appropriate management. Allergic management may be helpful on occasion even when an underlying cause cannot be discovered. There is no evidence that autogenous vaccines or inhalation of antibiotics will serve a therapeutic purpose.

REFERENCES

Feingold, B. F.: Infection in Bronchial Allergic Disease: Bronchial Asthma, Allergic Bronchitis, Asthmatic Bronchitis. *Pediat. Clin. N. Amer.,* 6:709, 1959.

MacKeith, R.: Respiratory Disorders in Infants and Young Children, with Special Reference to Recurrent Stress Bronchitis. *Practitioner,* 175:692, 1955.

Williams, A.: Bronchitis, Asthma and Emphysema in Childhood. *Med. J. Australia,* 1:781, 1957.

PNEUMONIA

No clinical classification of pneumonia is entirely satisfactory. It has been common practice to separate the various clinical forms on the basis of their anatomic distribution, the principal designations being lobar pneumonia, lobular pneumonia or bronchopneumonia, and interstitial pneumonia or bronchiolitis. If separate categories are provided for the various aspiration pneumonias and for hypostatic pneumonia, most pneumonic infections can be grouped under these anatomic headings.

More or less characteristic lesions are produced by certain causative agents. For example, the pneumococcus produces an inflammatory lesion of the mucosa and an alveolar exudate, usually without destruction of the mucosal cells or extensive involvement of the interstitial tissues. The gross lesion is a consolidation of all or part of a lobe in the lobar variety, or of scattered lobules in the bronchopneumonic variety. In contrast, viral agents, *H. influenzae* and certain strains of the viridans group of streptococci invade or destroy the mucous membrane and produce principally bronchiolitis, peribronchiolitis and interstitial lesions. Secondary infections, especially in association with the primary viral infections, are often responsible for suppurative bronchiolitic, alveolar and interstitial lesions. Both the staphylococcus and Friedländer's bacillus tend to destroy tissue and to produce multiple small abscesses.

Most bacteriologic infections can be identified not only as to the causative agent, but also as to the specific type or strain of a given species. Such identification or the failure of it has both therapeutic and prognostic significance. Since, however, it is not possible to identify the etiologic agent in all instances, it is necessary to supplement etiologic classification with grouping on a pathologic basis. Most etiologically unclassified infections occur in infancy, and are probably of viral origin.

Within limits a clinical distinction can also be made on the basis of response to antimicrobial therapy. Most bacterial infections are susceptible to one or more of these agents, whereas viral infections usually are not.

The following classification is presented as a working basis:

I. BACTERIAL INFECTIONS
    Pneumococcus
    Streptococcus
    Staphylococcus
    H. influenzae
    Friedländer's bacillus
    Tubercle bacillus
    Treponema pallidum

II. VIRAL OR PROBABLE VIRAL INFECTIONS
    Bronchiolitis and interstitial pneumonitis
    Giant cell pneumonia
    Influenza

III. OTHER INFECTIONS
    Pneumocystis carinii pneumonia
    Q fever (p. 703)
    Mycoplasma pneumoniae pneumonia

IV. MYCOTIC INFECTIONS
    Coccidioidomycosis

    Histoplasmosis
    Blastomycosis
    Cryptococcosis
    Mucormycosis
    Nocardiosis
    Sporotrichosis
    Thrush

V. ASPIRATION OF
    Amniotic contents (fetal anoxia)
    Food
    Foreign bodies
    Zinc stearate
    Dust
    Kerosene
    Lipoid substances

VI. LÖFFLER'S SYNDROME

VII. HYPOSTATIC PNEUMONIA

BACTERIAL PNEUMONIA

General Considerations. In infants and young children with infection of the lower respiratory tract, signs and symptoms of pulmonary involvement are often nonspecific, and findings on physical examination may be sparse. Accordingly, roentgenographic evidence of pneumonia is frequently found in infants who clinically appear to have only upper respiratory tract infections, or only tachypnea and fever, without physical findings suggesting pulmonary involvement.

The defense mechanisms of the lower respiratory tract are extraordinarily efficient in preventing infection of the lungs. The defenses include (1) the epiglottal reflex, which prevents aspiration of infected secretions; (2) ciliary action of the intact respiratory epithelium, which serves to carry microorganisms away from the lung; (3) the cough reflex, which propels foreign material out of the lower tract; (4) the viscous secretions of the respiratory tract, to which airborne organisms adhere; (5) the lymphatics which drain the terminal bronchi and bronchioles; and (6) phagocytic cells which line the normal alveoli. In addition, the normal flora of the upper respiratory passage inhibits growth of nonindigenous microorganisms. When one or more of these defense barriers is altered, inhibited or destroyed, pulmonary infection may result from aspiration of infected secretions or the inhalation of droplets or particles containing bacteria.

The most common event disturbing the defense mechanisms is a viral infection, which alters the properties of normal secretions, inhibits phagocytosis, modifies the bacterial flora, and may temporarily disrupt the normal epithelial layer of the respiratory passages. A viral respiratory disease often precedes the development of bacterial pneumonia by a few days. Once pneumonia has occurred, a series of intricate mechanisms brings about resolution of infection and recovery. These include such systemic phenomena as fever, the mobilization of leukocytes, the stimulation of antibody production, and changes in the circulation surrounding the involved area. Local activities include an increase in acidity of the pulmonary exudate, the phagocytosis and digestion of pathogens and cellular debris by macrophages, the cytolytic action of substances released by disintegration of leukocytes, the local release of antibacterial (neutralizing antibody) from immunologically competent cells, and the formation of antiviral (interferon) substances.

Children with defects in defense mechanisms, or in the chain of events involved in recovery from infection, experience recurrent pneumonias or failure to resolve the disease completely. These defects occur with abnormalities of antibody production (agammaglobulinemia), cystic fibrosis, cleft palate, congenital bronchiectasis, tracheo-esophageal fistula, inability of mononuclear cells to phagocytize bacteria normally (granulomatous disease of childhood), neutropenia, increased pulmonary blood flow, deficient gag reflex, and so forth. Among iatrogenic factors promoting pulmonary infection are trauma, anesthesia, aspiration, and inappropriate antimicrobial therapy.

Pneumococcal Pneumonia

Though the incidence of pneumococcal pneumonia has declined over the last several decades, the disease remains the most common form of bacterial pneumonia encountered in childhood.

Epidemiology. Pneumococcal pneumonia most commonly occurs during the late winter and early spring when respiratory infections are at their peak. Pneumococci of serotypes 1 through 8 account for over 80 per cent of pneumonia in adults, but in children, types 14, 1, 6 and 19 are found most frequently.

Nontypable pneumococci and those with high type numbers are frequently encountered in the respiratory tracts of normal subjects. In contrast, the prevalence of carriers of the highly pathogenic serotypes is relatively low, except type 3, which is a common inhabitant of the normal pharynx. Asymptomatic carriers of pneumococci play a more important role in the dissemination of infective types than do patients ill with pneumonia. Upon recovery from pneumococcal pneumonia, the possession of type-specific antibody not only protects the person from reinfection, but also renders him less likely to become a carrier of that specific serotype of organism.

When high carrier rates of pathogenic types are encountered in a relatively closed community (e.g. orphanages, nurseries, schools), the occurrence of widespread viral disease of the respiratory tract may be followed by an epidemic of pneumococcal pneumonia. Except for these unusual instances, the disease occurs as a sporadic illness.

In childhood the highest attack rates are found during the first 4 years of life and then decline with increasing age.

Pathogenesis and Pathology. Pneumococci gain entrance to the lungs through the respiratory passages, usually by aspiration of infected secretions. Engorgement of interalveolar capillaries with outpouring of edema fluid supports proliferation of the organisms and aids in the spread of infection into adjacent portions of the lung. The involved lobe undergoes early consolidation, and polymorphonuclear leukocytes, fibrin, edema fluid, red blood cells and pneumococci fill the alveoli. This is the stage of *red hepatization*, which passes rapidly into that of *gray hepatization,* characterized by the deposition of fibrin over the pleural surfaces and the presence of fibrin and polymorphonuclear leukocytes in the alveolar spaces where phagocytosis of pneumococci now rapidly takes place. The interalveolar capillaries are no longer engorged. The final stage involves the *resolution* of infection. Increasing numbers of macrophages appear in the alveolar spaces, the neutrophils undergo fatty degeneration and necrosis, and the fibrin threads are digested and disappear. The clinical crisis in the untreated case occurs about the seventh day of illness; resolution and re-expansion require an additional 1 to 3 weeks. When antimicrobial therapy is instituted in the first several days of illness, the course is interrupted and the characteristic stages are not seen.

In older children and adults pneumococcal pneumonia characteristically involves one or more lobes, or parts of lobes, leaving the remaining bronchopulmonary system uninvolved. In infants the lesions may follow a bronchial distribution without the localization of lobar pneumonia.

Clinical Manifestations. The classic history of a shaking chill followed by high fever, cough and chest pain described for adults with pneumococcal pneumonia may be seen in older children, but is rarely observed in infants. The clinical pattern of pneumococcal pneumonia in infants and young children is considerably more variable than in older patients. In addition, the widespread use of antimicrobial therapy for upper respiratory tract infections has altered the symptoms, physical findings and characteristic course of pneumococcal pneumonia.

In infants. A mild upper respiratory tract infection characterized by stuffy nose, fretfulness and diminished appetite usually precedes the onset of pneumococcal pneumonia in infants. This mild illness of several days ends with the abrupt onset of fever to 39 to 40.5°C. (103 to 105°F.), restlessness, apprehension and respiratory distress. A generalized convulsion may accompany the high fever. Examination reveals an acutely ill infant with moderate to severe air hunger. The cheeks may be flushed, and circumoral cyanosis is often noted. The respiratory distress is manifest by flaring of the alae nasi, retractions of the supraclavicular, intercostal and subcostal areas, tachypnea and tachycardia. Cough is unusual at the onset of illness, but may be noted later.

Percussion of the chest is often unrevealing,

since the pathologic process is usually a patchy bronchopneumonia. Auscultation may reveal diminished breath sounds and fine, crackling rales on the affected side, but these findings are not noted as consistently as in older children and adults. On the opposite side the breath sounds may be exaggerated and almost tubular in nature. If dullness is found on percussion in young infants, the presence of pleural effusion or empyema should be suspected. Abdominal distention usually reflects gastric distention due to swallowed air or paralytic ileus. The liver may seem enlarged, owing to downward displacement of the right diaphragm or to superimposed congestive heart failure. Nuchal rigidity without meningeal infection (meningismus) is not uncommon, especially with involvement of the right upper lobe. Occasionally the infant may be slightly jaundiced.

The physical findings change little during the course of illness, although moist rales may become audible during resolution.

In children. The signs and symptoms of pneumococcal pneumonia in older children are similar to those of adults. After a brief upper respiratory tract infection the child usually experiences a shaking chill followed by high fever of 40 to 40.5°C. (104 to 105°F.). This is accompanied by drowsiness with intermittent periods of restlessness, rapid respirations, a hacking, unproductive cough, anxiety and occasionally delirium. Circumoral cyanosis may be present. The child is often noted to be splinting the affected side because of pleuritic chest pain and may lie on this side with the knees drawn up to the chest. Abnormal findings in the chest include dullness, diminished tactile and vocal fremitus, diminished breath sounds and fine and crackling rales on the affected side. On the first day of illness, dullness over the affected lobe is usually not evident, and the suppression of breath sounds on the affected side may lead to misinterpretation of the exaggerated breath sounds in the opposite lung as tubular breathing.

In older children, in contrast to young infants, the physical findings undergo greater change during the course of illness. Classic signs of consolidation are noted on the second or third day of illness and are characterized by dullness, increased fremitus, tubular breath sounds and the disappearance of rales. As resolution occurs, moist rales are heard and the signs of consolidation disappear. The initial dry, hacking cough gives way to one productive of large amounts of blood-tinged mucous material.

The development of a pleural effusion or empyema may cause a visible lag in respiration on the affected side, with exaggerated respiration on the opposite side. Examination usually reveals dullness over the area of the effusion with diminished fremitus and breath sounds. Tubular breathing is often noted immediately above the fluid level and on the unaffected side.

Laboratory Findings. The white blood cell count is usually elevated to 15,000 to 40,000 cells per mm.[3], with a preponderance of polymorphonuclear cells. White blood cell counts below 5000 per mm.[3] are often associated with a grave prognosis. The hemoglobin value is usually normal or only slightly diminished.

In most patients with pneumococcal pneumonia, pneumococci can be isolated from the nasopharyngeal secretions, but this finding cannot be considered proof of a causative relation; the isolation of pneumococci should be attempted from secretions obtained upon deep coughing, from gentle tracheal aspiration or from pleural fluid obtained at thoracentesis. Bacteremia is found in about 30 per cent of cases of pneumococcal pneumonia.

Roentgenographic Findings. The roentgenographic changes in pneumococcal pneumonia do not always correspond to the clinical observations. Consolidation may be demonstrated on x-ray film before it is detectable by physical examination, and resolution of the infiltrate may not be complete until several weeks after the child is clinically well. Lobar consolidation is unusual in infants and young children, but may be seen in the older child. The most common finding in infants is a patchy infiltration of one or several lobes. Pleural reaction with the presence of fluid is not uncommon; it may be seen early in the course of illness and, even in the untreated patient, is not necessarily indicative of developing empyema.

Differential Diagnosis. Pneumococcal pneumonia cannot be differentiated from other bacterial and viral pneumonias without suitable microbiological studies. Conditions which may be confused with pneumonia are bronchiolitis, congestive heart failure, acute exacerbations of bronchiectasis, aspiration of a foreign body, sequestered lobe, atelectasis, pulmonary abscess, and endotracheal tuberculosis with secondary bacterial pneumonia.

An older child with right lower lobe pneumonia may have pain referred to the right lower quadrant of the abdomen. Since ileus may accompany pneumonia, right-lower quadrant pain and absent bowel sounds may be misinterpreted as indicative of acute appendicitis.

When meningismus is severe and presents with opisthotonos or positive Kernig and Brudzinski signs, it can be differentiated from meningitis only by examination of the spinal fluid.

Complications. With the use of antimicrobial therapy bacterial complications of pneumonia have become unusual. The most common complication is empyema, resulting from extension of infection to the pleural surfaces. A thick, fibrinous exudate may develop with empyema and later compromise pulmonary function. This complication occurs most commonly in the young infant who has received medical attention late in the course of illness or has been inadequately treated. Purulent complications such as otitis media, meningitis, pericarditis, osteomyelitis and peritonitis are infrequent.

Prognosis. In the preantibiotic era the mortality rate from pneumococcal pneumonia in infants and small children ranged from 20 to 50 per cent and in older children from 3 to 5 per cent. Furthermore, the incidence of chronic empyema with altered pulmonary function was relatively high. With appropriate antimicrobial therapy instituted early in the course of the illness, the mortality rate during infancy and childhood is now less than 1 per cent, and long-term morbidity correspondingly low.

Treatment. The most important factor in therapy is the appropriate selection of an antimicrobial agent. The drug of choice is penicillin G, since all pneumococci are highly susceptible to this agent. In infants and young children a dose of 25,000 to 50,000 units per kg. per day is administered parenterally in 2 to 4 doses. In older children the total dose of penicillin should not exceed 1,000,000 units per day unless empyema or another suppurative complication is being treated concurrently. If allergy prevents the use of penicillin, erythromycin or cephalothin may be substituted.

The majority of older children with pneumonia can be treated at home, the decision to hospitalize depending on the degree of certainty of diagnosis and the severity of illness, the physical adequacy of the home and the ability of the mother or other members of the family to supply good nursing care. Pneumonia in the young infant is best treated in the hospital, since fluids may have to be administered intravenously. Furthermore, the course of illness in young infants is more variable and complications more common. Bed rest, liberal oral intake of fluids and the administration of aspirin for high fever are the principal adjuncts to therapy. The prompt administration of oxygen in patients with significant respiratory distress will greatly reduce the need for sedatives and analgesics, and it should be given long before the patient becomes cyanotic.

Streptococcal Pneumonia

Group A streptococci most commonly cause disease limited to the upper respiratory tract, but the organisms may spread to other areas of the body, including the lower respiratory tract. The frequency of streptococcal pneumonia and tracheobronchitis is unknown, but they are uncommon. Certain viral infections, particularly the exanthems and epidemic influenza, predispose the patient to these diseases, which are most frequently encountered in the child 3 to 5 years of age, and very rarely in the infant.

Pathology. Streptococcal infection of the lower respiratory tract may result in tracheitis, bronchitis or interstitial pneumonia. Lesions consist of necrosis of the tracheobronchial mucosa with formation of ragged ulcers and large amounts of exudate, edema and localized hemorrhage. The process may extend into the interalveolar septa and involve the lymphatic vessels. Infection may spread by way of the lymphatics to the mediastinal and hilar lymph nodes, or may proceed in a retrograde direction in occluded vessels and reach the pleural surfaces. Pleurisy is relatively common with streptococcal pneumonia; the effusion is often large and serous or thinly purulent, with a lower fibrin content than the exudate of pneumococcal pneumonia.

Clinical Course. The signs and symptoms of streptococcal pneumonia are similar to those of pneumococcal pneumonia. The onset may be sudden and characterized by high fever, chills, signs of respiratory distress and, at times, extreme prostration. On occasion the child appears only mildly ill, with cough and a low-grade fever. If an exanthem or influenza precedes the pneumonia, the onset may be seen only as an increasingly severe clinical course of the viral illness. Since streptococcal pneumonia is commonly an interstitial inflammatory process, the clinical findings on examination of the chest may be less impressive than the disseminated infiltration noted on x-ray examination. Serous or purulent pleurisy will be evidenced by the findings characteristic of pleural fluid.

Laboratory Data. The peripheral leukocyte count is elevated, with a predominance of polymorphonuclear cells. A rise in the serum antistreptolysin titer is supportive diagnostic evidence. Cultures should be taken from the nasopharynx, blood, and from pleural fluid when present. Isolation of group A streptococci from the nasopharynx alone does not establish the cause of the pneumonia; bacteremia occurs in approximately 10 per cent of cases.

Differential Diagnosis. The clinical course and radiographic findings of patients with streptococcal pneumonia with purulent pleurisy are often similar to those found with staphylococcal pneumonia. Pneumatoceles may be noted on x-ray examination in both conditions. The roentgenographic changes of uncomplicated streptococcal pneumonia may be indistinguishable from those of other interstitial pneumonitides, including those caused by *Mycoplasma pneumoniae* (primary atypical pneumonia). Chills and leukocytosis are more commonly observed in streptococcal pneumonia than in mycoplasma pneumonia.

Complications. Bacterial complications are common, and long-term morbidity is common in the untreated patient. Empyema occurs in about 20 per cent of children; the organizing exudate may inhibit expansion of the lung, requiring surgery for relief. Occasionally, septic foci develop in other organs such as the bones or joints, but otherwise, extension of the disease is uncommon.

Therapy. Treatment is similar to that described for pneumococcal pneumonia. Penicillin G is the drug of choice and should be given parenterally in a dose of 30,000 to 50,000 units per kg. per day in infants and from 500,000 to a million units per day in children. If empyema develops, a thoracentesis should be performed for diagnostic purposes and to remove the fluid. On occasion, closed drainage with indwelling chest tubes may be required if the fluid reaccumulates. The intrathoracic administration of antimicrobial agents or enzymes to liquefy pus or dissolve fibrin does not seem to contribute to the effectiveness of therapy.

Staphylococcal Pneumonia
(See also p. 388)

Pneumonia caused by *Staphylococcus aureus* is a serious and rapidly progressive infection which, unless recognized early and treated appropriately, is associated with prolonged morbidity and high mortality. Although it occurs less frequently than pneumococcal or viral pneumonias, its frequency has increased over the past decade, particularly in the infant.

Epidemiology. The incidence of staphylococcal pneumonia is highest during the winter months (October through May), corresponding to the season of greatest incidence of upper respiratory tract infections. As with other bacterial pneumonias, staphylococcal disease is usually preceded by a viral upper respiratory tract infection. Although it may occur at any age, staphylococcal pneumonia is found most commonly in the infant: 30 per cent of all cases occur under 3 months of age and 70 per cent before 1 year.

Although *Staphylococcus aureus* is commonly found on normal human skin and mucous membranes, serious disease is comparatively rare. Colonization of these surfaces begins early; nearly 90 per cent of normal infants become nasal carriers in the neonatal period. The carrier rate then gradually declines to approximately 20 per cent during the first 2 years of life, and by age 4 to 6 years the adult rate of 30 to 50 per cent is achieved.

The occurrence of epidemics of staphylococcal disease in nurseries is usually associated with certain specific pathogenic strains, identifiable by phage or serologic typing; they are commonly resistant to many antibiotics. Even during these outbreaks most of the colonized infants and hospital personnel or family contacts remain free from staphylococcal disease, but these healthy contacts may serve to spread the infection to others. The infant may exhibit disease within a few days after colonization or not until weeks later; most staphylococcal pneumonias of infancy are caused by organisms acquired in the nursery. Viral respiratory infections play a significant role in promoting dissemination of the staphylococcus among infants, and in converting colonization to disease.

Pathogenicity and Pathology. *Staphylococcus aureus* produces a variety of toxins and enzymes. Among the more important of these are the following: (1) hemolysin, which has been shown in certain animals to lyse red blood cells, to produce local necrosis after intradermal injection, and to be lethal if given intravenously; (2) leukocidin, which destroys human leukocytes by causing degranulation and membrane disruption; (3) staphylokinase, which causes clot dissolution by activation of plasma plasminogen; (4) coagulase, which interacts with a plasma factor to produce an active principle which converts fibrinogen to fibrin and thereby causes clot formation. A good correlation exists between coagulase production and virulence. Coagulase-negative staphylococci rarely produce serious disease.

Staphylococci cause confluent bronchopneumonia characterized by the presence of extensive areas of hemorrhagic necrosis and irregular areas of cavitation. The pleural surface is usually covered by a thick layer of fibrinopurulent exudate. Multiple abscesses occur, containing clusters of staphylococci, leukocytes, erythrocytes and necrotic debris. Rupture of a small subpleural abscess may result in a pyopneumothorax, which in turn may erode into a bronchus, producing a bronchopleural fistula. Septic thrombi may form in pulmonary veins in regions of extensive destruction and inflammation.

Clinical Manifestations. Most commonly the patient is an infant less than a year of age, often with a history of staphylococcal skin lesions and signs and symptoms of an upper or lower respiratory tract infection for several days to a week. Abruptly, the infant's condition changes with the onset of fever, cough and evidence of respiratory distress. Signs and symptoms include tachypnea, grunting respirations, sternal and subcostal retractions, cyanosis and anxiety. If left undisturbed, the infant appears lethargic, but upon arousing is irritable. Severe dyspnea and a shocklike state may be present. Some infants have associated gastrointestinal disturbances characterized by vomiting, anorexia, diarrhea, and occasionally abdominal distention. The rapid progression of symptoms is characteristic of staphylococcal pneumonia.

Physical findings depend on the stage of pneumonia. Early in the course of illness diminished breath sounds, scattered rales, and rhonchi are commonly heard over the affected lung. With the development of effusion or pyopneumothorax, dullness on percussion is noted, and breath sounds and vocal fremitus are markedly diminished. A lag in respiratory excursion often occurs on the affected side. Physical examination may, however, be misleading, particularly in the young infant with meager findings disproportionate to the degree of tachypnea.

Laboratory Findings. In the older infant and child a leukocytosis of 20,000 or more cells per mm.^{3} usually occurs, with the increase primarily among the polymorphonuclear cells; in the young infant the white blood cell count may remain within the normal range. As in other forms of bacterial infection, a count below 5000 cells is a poor prognostic sign. Mild to moderate anemia is common.

Material for diagnostic cultures should be obtained by tracheal aspiration or from a pleural tap. The finding of staphylococci in the nasopharynx is of no diagnostic value. Blood cultures are usually sterile.

Roentgenographic Findings. Most patients with staphylococcal pneumonia will have radiographic evidence of bronchopneumonia early in the illness. The infiltrate may be patchy and limited in extent or be dense and homogeneous and involve an entire lobe or hemithorax. The right lung alone is involved in about 65 per cent of cases; bilateral involvement occurs in fewer than 20 per cent of patients. A pleural effusion or empyema will be noted during the course in most patients; pyopneumothorax occurs in about one fourth. Pneumatoceles of varying size are common.

Though no roentgenographic change can be considered diagnostic, progression over a few hours from bronchopneumonia to effusion or pyopneumothorax with or without pneumatoceles is highly suggestive of staphylococcal pneumonia. Chest films should be obtained at frequent intervals if the diagnosis of early staphylococcal pneumonia is suspected. Clinical improvement usually precedes x-ray clearing by days or weeks, and pneumatoceles may persist as asymptomatic cysts for months.

Differential Diagnosis. The recognition of early staphylococcal pneumonia in the infant is often difficult. Abrupt onset and rapid progression of symptoms of pneumonia should be considered due to staphylococci until proved otherwise. A history of furunculosis, a preceding viral upper respiratory tract infection, a recent hospital admission or maternal breast abscess should also alert the physician to the possibility of this diagnosis in the infant.

Other bacterial pneumonias cause empyema or pneumatoceles and may thus be readily confused with staphylococcal disease. These include streptococcal, klebsiella, *H. influenzae* and pneumococcal pneumonias and primary tuberculous pneumonia with cavitation. Occasionally, the aspiration of a nonradiopaque foreign body followed by pulmonary abscesses may lead to a similar clinical and radiologic picture.

Complications. Since empyema, pyopneumothorax and pneumatoceles are so commonly seen with staphylococcal pneumonia, they are considered part of the natural course of the illness and not complications. Septic lesions outside the respiratory tract occur rarely except in the young infant, in whom staphylococcal pericarditis, meningitis, osteomyelitis and multiple metastatic abscesses in soft tissue have been recorded.

Prognosis. The case fatality rate ranges from 5 to 40 per cent and varies with the length of illness prior to hospitalization, the age of the patient, adequacy of therapy, and the presence of other illnesses and complications. Early recognition and immediate, adequate therapy are usually effective.

The course is usually prolonged, the hospital stay often being 6 to 10 weeks. The long-term morbidity is very low. Five-year follow-up examinations of recovered patients with staphylococcal pneumonia generally have revealed normal growth and development, with no increase in susceptibility to pulmonary infections, and with normal pulmonary function.

Therapy. Treatment of staphylococcal pneumonia consists in control of microorganisms with antimicrobial therapy and surgical drainage of collections of pus. The infant should be placed in oxygen in a semireclining position to relieve cyanosis and allay anxiety. The infant should not be fed orally during the acute phase of illness; caloric intake and hydration should be maintained intravenously. If the patient is severely anemic, blood transfusion may be beneficial.

Upon completion of diagnostic procedures, antimicrobial therapy must be initiated immediately when staphylococcal pneumonia is suspected. Methicillin in a dosage of 250 to 300 mg. per kg. per day should be administered parenterally. Since methicillin is potentially nephrotoxic, urinalysis should be performed daily to detect hematuria and increasing proteinuria. If the culture demonstrates that the responsible staphylococcus is susceptible to penicillin G, then this agent should be given in a dosage of approximately 100,000 to 400,000 units per kg. per day. There is no advantage to the concurrent use of several drugs; such use increases the frequency of adverse reactions. The duration of antimicrobial therapy should be in accordance with the clinical response of the patient; in the average patient 3 weeks is adequate.

When infection extends to the pleural surfaces, surgical intervention usually becomes necessary. With small amounts of effusion or empyema, repeated pleural taps may on occasion result in adequate removal of fluid, but generally pus reaccumulates so rapidly and is of such high viscosity that closed drainage is necessary, with a chest tube of the largest possible caliber. The appearance of pyopneumothorax is another indication for the immediate insertion of a catheter into the pleural space. It is often necessary to utilize several chest tubes when loculation occurs. Once the infant begins to improve and the lung has re-expanded, the tubes may be removed, even if they are still draining small amounts of pus. In general, tubes should not remain in the chest more than 5 to 7 days.

The instillation of antimicrobial agents or enzymes into the chest cavity does not help control the infection or promote drainage; in infants this procedure is associated with an increased incidence of pneumothorax and systemic toxic reactions.

Pneumonia Caused by Gram-Negative Organisms

Gram-negative organisms have accounted for fewer than 1 per cent of pneumonias in infants and children beyond the immediate postnatal period (see p. 405). The number, however, has increased in recent years, owing to the widespread use of antibiotics, to contamination of hospital equipment such as oxygen and humidification apparatus, and to the increasing use of immunosuppressive agents in the treatment of malignant disorders. The gram-negative organisms most commonly encountered are *Hemophilus influenzae* type b, *Klebsiella pneumoniae* and *Pseudomonas aeruginosa*; other organisms have been occasionally incriminated. The morbidity and mortality from these infections are rather high as a result of the pathogenicity of the bacteria and the altered host resistance in many of these patients.

Hemophilus Influenzae Pneumonia.   *Hemophilus influenzae* type b is one of the more frequent causes of serious bacterial infections in infants and young children. Nontypable *H. influenzae* are routinely found in the nasopharynx of normal persons; initial encounter with a typespecific encapsulated strain, however, especially with type b, usually results in a mild, febrile upper respiratory tract infection followed by lasting immunity. Nasopharyngeal infection precedes virtually all the clinical varieties of localized *H. influenzae* disease, such as otitis media, epiglottitis, pneumonia and meningitis. The factors that determine whether a child will have a mild upper respiratory tract infection or serious disease are not understood. A synergistic action has been demonstrated between *H. influenzae* and certain respiratory viruses, such as the influenza virus, or certain bacteria, such as the staphylococcus. This synergism in some way alters the dynamics of the bacterial population on respiratory epithelium and promotes the growth of bacteria which may result in pyogenic disease. An example of this phenomenon occurred in the viral influenza pandemic of 1918, when a high incidence of serious lower respiratory tract disease due to *H. influenzae* was noted.

H. influenzae pneumonia is usually lobar in distribution. Disseminated pulmonary disease and bronchopneumonia have also been described. Microscopic examination of lung tissue usually reveals extensive destruction of the bronchial and bronchiolar epithelium, interstitial inflammation and hemorrhagic edema. As with *H. influenzae* infection of the larynx, edema is often striking.

Clinically, *H. influenzae* pneumonia is difficult to differentiate from pneumococcal pneumonia; in contrast to pneumococcal infection, however, the onset of illness is often insidious, and the clinical course is usually subacute and prolonged over several weeks. In the young infant the disease is often associated with bacteremia and frequently with empyema.

The diagnosis may be difficult to establish. Predominant growth of *H. influenzae* type b in the nasopharynx is suggestive evidence of the cause, but only isolation of the organism from the blood or pleural fluid confirms the diagnosis. The usual radiographic findings are those of a lobar pneumonia. There is a moderate leukocytosis with a relative lymphopenia.

Complications are frequent, particularly in the young infant, and include bacteremia, pericarditis, cellulitis, empyema, meningitis and pyarthrosis. Empyema usually occurs early in the course of the pneumonia, while meningitis and pyarthrosis may occur late.

Treatment consists of the same symptomatic and supportive measures utilized in pneumococcal and staphylococcal pneumonias. When *H. influenzae* is suspected as the causative agent, ampicillin is the antimicrobial agent of choice and is given parenterally in a dose of 150 mg. per kg. per day. The development of empyema or pyarthrosis usually necessitates immediate surgical drainage.

Friedländer's Bacillus (Klebsiella Pneumoniae) Pneumonia.   *Klebsiella pneumoniae* is found in the respiratory and gastrointestinal tracts of approximately 5 per cent of normal persons. It is known to cause pneumonia in elderly patients and in those with diabetes mellitus, and frequently occurs as a secondary invader in the lungs of patients with chronic bronchiectasis, influenza and tuberculosis. Primary *Kl. pneumoniae* infection is unusual in infants and young children; it may occur, rarely, in nursery epidemics. During these epidemics many infants will carry the organism in their nasopharynges without signs of clinical illness; only an occasional baby will have severe disease. Contaminated fomites, including nursery equipment and humidification apparatus, are the primary source of nosocomial infection with the organism.

Pneumonia due to *Kl. pneumoniae* may be difficult to distinguish clinically from pneumonia due to other causes. In nursery epidemics, diarrhea and vomiting may be the presenting symptoms; the onset of respiratory difficulty is often abrupt. The disease may have a fulminant course characterized by copious, thick, purulent secretions and the formation of pulmonary abscesses and cavitation. A lobar infiltrate with bulging fissures on radiographic examination is suggestive of klebsiella pneumonia. Complications are common and include bacteremia, empyema and residual parenchymal damage. The case fatality rate in sporadic cases is about 50 per cent, but is lower during epidemics.

Isolation of the organism from purulent tracheal secretions, blood and pleural fluid establishes the diagnosis. Supportive treatment is similar to that given for other bacterial pneumonias; surgical intervention may be necessary to drain empyema or abscesses. The antimicrobial agent of choice is usually kanamycin, which is administered intramuscularly in a dosage of 7.5 mg. per kg. every 12 hours for 10 days to 2 weeks.

Pseudomonas Aeruginosa Pneumonia (see also p. 592). *Pseudomonas aeruginosa* produces a severe, progressive, usually fatal, necrotizing bronchopneumonia. It is rarely a primary infection of the lung, but occurs with chronic debilitat-

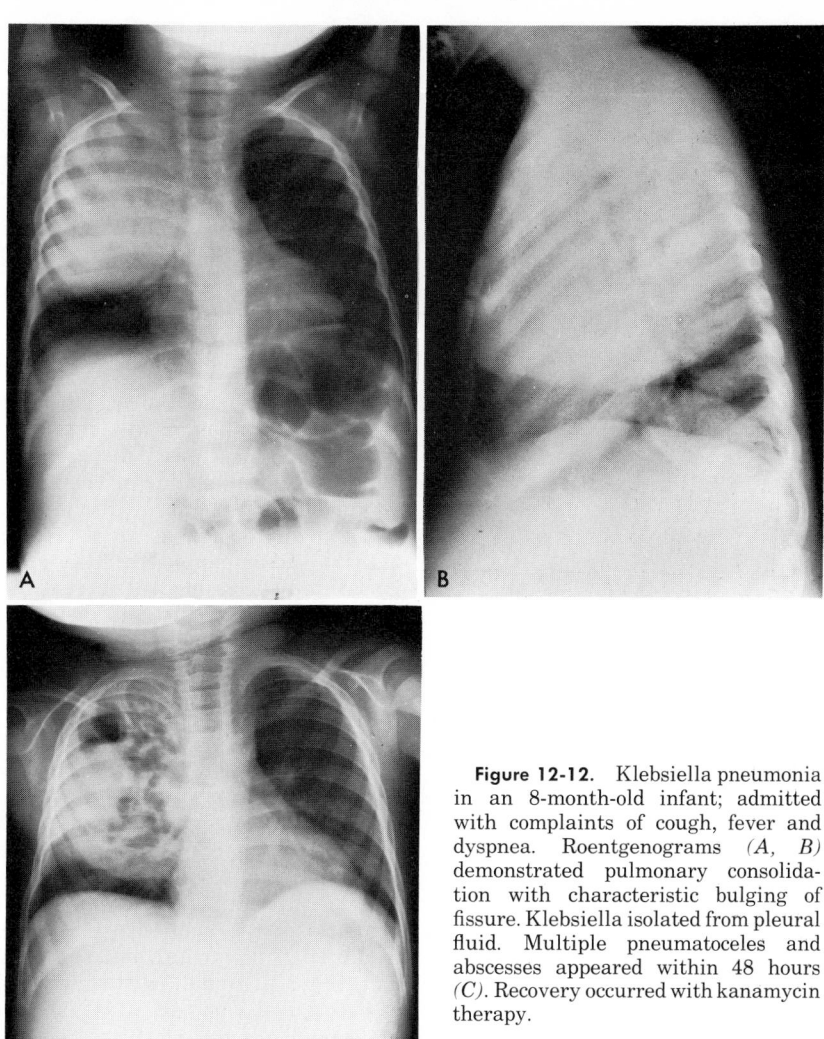

Figure 12-12. Klebsiella pneumonia in an 8-month-old infant; admitted with complaints of cough, fever and dyspnea. Roentgenograms *(A, B)* demonstrated pulmonary consolidation with characteristic bulging of fissure. Klebsiella isolated from pleural fluid. Multiple pneumatoceles and abscesses appeared within 48 hours *(C)*. Recovery occurred with kanamycin therapy.

ing illnesses such as cystic fibrosis and malignant disorders, with altered immunologic function, during prolonged antimicrobial therapy and in premature infants exposed to contaminated hospital equipment. The antimicrobial agent of choice is polymyxin B given intramuscularly, or intravenously initially if the infant is in shock, in a dose of 3.5 to 4.5 mg. per kg. per day for 10 days or so.

GEORGE H. MCCRACKEN, JR.
HEINZ F. EICHENWALD

REFERENCES

Pneumococcal Pneumonia

Hodges, R. G., and MacLeod, C. M.: Epidemic Pneumococcal Pneumonia. V. Final Considerations of Factors Underlying Epidemic. *Am. J. Hyg.,* 44:237, 1946.

MacLeod, C. M.: The Pneumococci; in R. Dubos and J. Hirsch (Eds.): *Bacterial and Mycotic Infections of Man.* 4th ed. Philadelphia, J. B. Lippincott Company, 1965, Chap. 16.
Smith, M. H. D.: Pneumococcal Pneumonia; in E. L. Kendig, Jr. (Ed.): *Disorders of the Respiratory Tract in Children.* Philadelphia, W. B. Saunders Company, 1967, pp. 283-8.
Wood, B. W.: Pneumococcal Pneumonia; in P. Beeson and W. McDermott (Eds.): *Cecil-Loeb Textbook of Medicine.* 12th ed. Philadelphia, W. B. Saunders Compnay, 1967, pp. 145-59.

Streptococcal Pneumonia

Keefer, C. S., Rantz, A., and Rammelkamp, C. H.: Hemolytic Streptococcal Pneumonia and Empyema: A Study of 55 Cases with Special Reference to Treatment. *Ann. Int. Med.,* 14:1533, 1941.
Kevy, S. V., and Lowe, B. A.: Streptococcal Pneumonia and Empyema in Childhood. *New England J. Med.,* 264:738, 1961.

Staphylococcal Pneumonia

Disney, M. E., Wolff, J., and Wood, B. S. B.: Staphylococcal Pneumonia of Infants. *Lancet,* 1:767, 1956.

Eichenwald, H. F., and Shinefield, H. R.: The Problem of Staphylococcal Infection in Newborn Infants. *J. Pediat.,* 56: 665, 1960.

Forbes, G. B., and Emerson, G. L.: Staphylococcal Pneumonia and Empyema. *Pediat. Clin. N. Amer.,* 4:215, 1957.

Huxtable, K. A., Tucket, A. S., and Wedgwood, R. J.: Staphylococcal Pneumonia in Childhood. A.M.A. *J. Dis. Child.,* 108: 262, 1964.

Williams, R. E. D.: Healthy Carriage of Staphylococcus Aureus: Its Prevalence and Importance. *Bact. Rev.,* 27:56, 1963.

Pneumonia Caused by Gram-Negative Organisms

Nyhan, W. L., Rectanus, D. R., and Fousek, M. D.: Hemophilus Influenzae Type b Pneumonia. *Pediatrics,* 16:31, 1955.

Riley, H. D., and Bracken, E. C.: Empyema Due to Hemophilus Influenzae in Infants and Children. *Am. J. Dis. Child.,* 110: 24, 1965.

Friedländer's Bacillus (Klebsiella Pneumoniae) Pneumonia

Morgan, H. R.: The Enteric Bacteria; in R. Dubos and J. Hirsch (Eds.): *Bacterial and Mycotic Infections of Man.* 4th ed. Philadelphia, J. B. Lippincott Company, 1965.

Thaler, M. M.: Klebsiella-Aerobacter Pneumonia in Infants. *Pediatrics,* 30:206, 1962.

PNEUMONIAS OF VIRAL ORIGIN

Acute Bronchiolitis

Acute bronchiolitis, a syndrome of respiratory tract obstruction at the bronchiolar level, is one of the more common diseases of the lower respiratory tract of infants. It occurs during the first 2 years of life, with a peak incidence at approximately 6 months of age, and, in many localities, is the most frequent cause of hospitalization of infants. The incidence is highest during the winter and early spring months. The illness occurs both sporadically and epidemically.

Etiology. Acute bronchiolitis is a viral illness. The respiratory syncytial virus has been incriminated as the causative agent in over 50 per cent of cases; the parainfluenza 3 virus, the Eaton agent (mycoplasma), some adenoviruses and occasionally other viruses, some probably not yet identified, produce the remaining cases. There is no firm evidence to support the view that bacteria cause this condition. Occasionally, bacterial bronchopneumonia may produce generalized obstructive emphysema and thus be confused clinically with bronchiolitis.

Pathophysiology. The most important pathologic lesion of acute bronchiolitis is bronchiolar obstruction due to edema and accumulation of mucus and cellular debris and invasion of the smaller radicles of the bronchial tree by virus. Since resistance to airflow in a tube is inversely related to the cube of the radius, even minor thickening of the bronchiolar wall in infants may produce a profound effect on airflow. Resistance to airflow in the small air passages is increased during both the inspiratory and expiratory phases, but is relatively greater during expiration. Partial (ball-valve) respiratory obstruction leads to air trapping and emphysema. Atelectasis occurs when obstruction becomes complete and trapped air is absorbed.

The pathologic process impairs the normal exchange of gases in the lung. Diminished ventilation of the alveoli results in hypoxemia. Carbon dioxide retention (hypercapnia) usually does not occur in mild cases of bronchiolitis, since adjacent functioning alveoli can compensate for the poor ventilation of their neighbors. But if a critical proportion of the alveoli are obstructed, such compensation becomes inadequate, and hypercapnia and respiratory acidosis occur. Generally, the higher the respiratory rate, the lower the arterial oxygen tension. Carbon dioxide retention is usually not found until respirations exceed 60 per minute; it then increases in proportion to the tachypnea.

Clinical Course. Most affected infants have a history of exposure to older children or adults with minor respiratory diseases within the week preceding onset of illness. The infant is first noted to have a serous nasal discharge and sneezing. These symptoms usually last several days, and may be accompanied by fever of 101 to 102°F. and diminished appetite. There is then gradual development of respiratory distress, characterized by paroxysmal cough, dyspnea and irritability. On occasion, in the more severely affected patients, these symptoms may develop more rapidly, within several hours. Other systemic manifestations such as vomiting and diarrhea are usually absent; the infant is commonly afebrile or has only a low-grade fever or may be hypothermic.

Examination reveals a tachypneic infant, often in extreme distress. Respirations range from 60 to 80 per minute; severe air hunger and cyanosis may be present. There is flaring of the alae nasi, and use of the accessory muscles of respiration results in intercostal and subcostal retractions, but these are shallow, owing to the persistent distention of the lungs by the trapped air (see p. 934). The liver and the spleen may be palpable several cm. below the costal margins as a result of the depression of the diaphragm due to emphysema.

Widespread fine rales may be heard at the end of inspiration and in early expiration. The expiratory phase of breathing may be prolonged, and wheezes are audible, particularly in the later course of illness. In the most severe cases, breath sounds are barely audible when bronchiolitic obstruction is nearly complete.

Roentgenographic examination reveals hyperinflation of the lungs, and an increased anteroposterior diameter on lateral view. Scattered areas of consolidation are found in about a third of patients, and are due either to atelectasis secondary to obstruction or to inflammation of the alveoli. Bacterial pneumonia cannot be excluded as a diagnostic possibility on radiographic grounds alone.

The white blood cell count is usually within normal limits. Lymphopenia, commonly associated with many viral illnesses, is usually not found. Nasopharyngeal cultures reveal normal flora except when the viral pathogen alters the ecology of the flora to allow growth of such microorganisms as *Hemophilus influenzae,* pneumococci or staphylococci. The presence of these bacteria does not imply that they are responsible for the illness.

Differential Diagnosis. The condition most commonly confused with acute bronchiolitis is bronchial asthma. Asthma occurs uncommonly in the first year of life, but frequently after this period. The presence of one or more of the following favors the diagnosis of asthma: a family history of asthma, repeated attacks in the same infant, sudden onset without preceding infection, markedly prolonged expiration, eosinophilia, and an immediate favorable response to the administration of a small dose of epinephrine. Repeated attacks represent an important differential point: fewer than 5 per cent of recurrent attacks of clinical bronchiolitis with obstructive emphysema have viral infections as a cause. Other entities which may be confused with acute bronchiolitis are congestive heart failure, foreign body in the trachea, pertussis, cystic fibrosis and bacterial bronchopneumonias associated with generalized obstructive emphysema.

Course and Prognosis. The most critical phase of illness occurs during the first 48 to 72 hours after the onset of cough and dyspnea. It is during this period that the infant appears desperately ill, when apneic spells occur in the very small infant and when respiratory acidosis is likely to be noted. After the critical period, improvement occurs rapidly and often dramatically. Recovery is complete in a few days. The case fatality rate is below 1 per cent; death may result from prolonged apneic spells, severe uncompensated respiratory acidosis, or profound dehydration secondary to loss of water vapor from tachypnea and the inability to drink fluids. Infants with such complications as congenital heart disease or cystic fibrosis have a higher mortality. Bacterial complications, such as bronchopneumonia or otitis media, are uncommon. Cardiac failure during bronchiolitis is rare. It has been reported that a significant proportion of infants with bronchiolitis have asthma during later childhood, but the interrelation of these 2 entities, if any, is not understood.

Treatment. Treatment is symptomatic. Infants should be placed in an atmosphere of high humidity, preferably produced by cold vapor rather than steam. Patients with dyspnea, whether cyanotic or not, should receive oxygen therapy. This serves not only to relieve the dyspnea and cyanosis, but also to allay anxiety and restlessness. Sedatives should be avoided whenever possible, owing to potential depression of respiration. When a sedative must be given, paraldehyde or chloral hydrate will be preferred. The infant is usually more comfortable if head and chest are slightly elevated in such a way that the neck is slightly extended. Tachypnea has a dehydrating effect, and oral intake of fluids must often be supplemented by parenteral fluids. In the event of respiratory acidosis, electrolyte and pH balance should be adjusted by suitable intravenous solutions. Mechanical assistance to ventilation is generally impractical in the young infant.

Since acute bronchiolitis is a viral illness, antimicrobial agents have no therapeutic value. Even in cases caused by the Eaton agent, no drug has been shown to have an effect on the course or outcome of the illness. The low incidence of bacterial complications is not made lower by antimicrobial therapy; thus no rationale for its use exists. Nor is there evidence that the use of corticosteroids is beneficial in bronchiolitis; these drugs may, under certain conditions, be harmful. Bronchodilating drugs are of no value; their use is, in fact, contraindicated, since they increase restlessness and oxygen requirements. Because the obstruction of bronchiolitis occurs at the bronchiolar level, tracheotomy cannot be expected to produce much benefit. The theoretical advantage which might be obtained by decreasing the dead air space of the respiratory passage is outweighed by the risk of performing this procedure in the acutely ill infant and the high rate of complications.

When bronchial asthma is considered a diagnostic possibility, a therapeutic trial of a single small dose of hypodermically administered epinephrine may be tried. If there is no response to this therapy within a short time, no additional epinephrine or other bronchodilators should be administered.

Primary Atypical Pneumonia
(EATON AGENT PNEUMONIA)

In the late 1930's the term "primary atypical pneumonia" was coined to describe a group of nonbacterial pneumonias presenting with an acute onset, moderate to severe constitutional symptoms, cough, and pulmonary infiltrates on radiographic examination with minimal or absent physical signs. Cold agglutinins were often found.

Etiology. It has become evident that atypical pneumonia represents a syndrome with multiple causes. The respiratory syncytial virus, influenza viruses A and B, parainfluenza type 3 and adenoviruses as well as certain of the rickettsiae are proved causative agents. These agents, however, are not regularly associated with those cases of atypical pneumonia characterized by elevated levels of cold agglutinins. In adults atypical pneumonia with cold agglutinins is a distinct epidemiologic and etiologic entity caused generally by *Mycoplasma pneumoniae* (Eaton agent), which is one of the Mycoplasmataceae, the smallest free-living organisms, similar in size to the myxoviruses.

Epidemiology. Unlike the influenza and respiratory syncytial viruses, *M. pneumoniae* does not produce sharply defined epidemics. Instead, infection occurs throughout the year, but most frequently during the early fall and winter months. The incidence and morbidity of mycoplasma pneumonia are higher in males than in females, particularly in the younger age groups. Though the organism causes lower respiratory tract illness in all ages, the majority of cases occur in childhood and through the third decade of life.

In an urban population the yearly incidence of mycoplasma pneumonia was found to be 1 to 1.5 cases per 1000 persons; in such closed populations as in military installations or institutions for the mentally retarded the annual incidence may be as high as 10 per 1000. These limited epidemics are caused by direct transmission by way of respiratory secretions, the degree of contact determining the contagiousness. The disease is not limited in its geographic distribution, and wide fluctuations in prevalence can occur in a given locality.

Pathology. The pathology of *M. pneumoniae* infection is not well known, since few patients die. The lungs usually have normal pleural surfaces, but occasionally there are patches of fibrinous pleural exudate. Areas of inflammation may be extensive or discrete, circumscribed and multiple. Nodular focal lesions resembling miliary granulomas may be present. Various stages of consolidation are seen, as well as areas of atelectasis and emphysema.

Microscopically, the principal pathologic process consists of an interstitial pneumonia with areas of necrotizing bronchitis and bronchiolitis. There is necrosis of the epithelial lining cells of the respiratory passage with desquamation and ulceration of the mucosa. The alveolar walls are hyperemic, and the septa are thickened with round cell infiltration and edema.

Clinical Manifestations. The effects of *M. pneumoniae* range from inapparent infection to pharyngitis, bullous myringitis, bronchitis, bronchiolitis and pneumonia. Most human infections do not become clinically apparent; it is estimated that only 3 to 10 per cent of infected persons undergo pneumonia.

The incubation period ranges from 1 to 3 weeks, averaging 12 to 14 days. The course of illness is extremely variable, particularly in the younger age groups. The onset is usually insidious; the initial complaints are often constitutional and nonspecific, such as headache, malaise, fever, chilliness, fatigue and anorexia. The principal respiratory symptoms include sore throat and cough. The cough is the most frequent and characteristic feature; it is usually dry in the initial stages, but may become productive of moderate amounts of blood-streaked sputum later in the illness. Headache is often a complaint, particularly in the older child. The duration and degree of fever vary widely; it is usually remittent and terminates by lysis in 4 to 14 days.

Generally, the older child and the adult do not appear to be as ill as the degree of fever might indicate. The pulse is slow in relation to the fever, and the respiratory rate is normal or slightly increased. Severe degrees of dyspnea are uncommon,

and cyanosis is rare. The paucity of abnormal physical findings is striking; often there are none at all. The throat may be mildly injected, and there may be slight enlargement of the cervical lymph nodes. The most characteristic finding late in the course of illness is the presence of fine, crepitant rales over the chest, with no signs of consolidation. A few patients have a maculopapular or urticarial rash, which usually disappears within 48 hours.

Roentgenographic examination often shows evidence of pneumonia before physical signs are apparent. Characteristically, the infiltrate appears to be most dense at the hilus and becomes progressively more feathery toward the periphery. The lesions may be confined to one lobe, more commonly a lower lobe, or may be present in several or all lobes. It is not uncommon for the infiltrate to spread, with resolution of early lesions as new infiltrates appear. Small pleural effusions are not uncommon. The roentgenographic changes are not distinctive or diagnostic.

Laboratory Data. The white blood cell count usually remains within normal limits. *Mycoplasma pneumoniae* may be recovered from pharyngeal swabs or sputum for as long as 4 weeks after infection. A specific serologic response can be demonstrated by immunofluorescent techniques or by complement-fixation and hemagglutination inhibition tests.

Some patients with atypical pneumonia have a variety of nonspecific immunologic reactions. Most adults with mycoplasma pneumonia develop cold hemagglutinins for group O human erythrocytes. Maximum titers are usually reached by the third or fourth week after onset of illness. Many of these patients also develop agglutinins for the MG strain of nonhemolytic streptococci. In children the development of cold agglutinins is erratic, and only a minority of patients have increases in titer. Cold agglutinins are also associated with lung infections due to other agents; the appearance of this antibody in children is related more to the degree of pulmonary involvement than to the specific cause.

Diagnosis. The clinical picture of atypical pneumonia associated with *Mycoplasma pneumoniae* is not sufficiently distinctive to allow differentiation from pneumonic processes caused by viral and rickettsial agents. In children a specific diagnosis can be made only if the causative agent is recovered or a rise in titer of specific antibody is demonstrated.

Course and Prognosis. The duration of the acute illness averages 8 to 10 days, with a convalescent period of an additional week. Complications are unusual, and the prognosis is excellent.

Treatment. Treatment is symptomatic, and hospitalization is rarely necessary. *Mycoplasma pneumoniae* is susceptible in vitro to the tetracyclines and to erythromycin. Although several studies have shown these agents to be useful in adults, the course of illness in children is not significantly altered by antibiotics.

Giant Cell Pneumonia
(HECHT'S PNEUMONIA)

Giant cell pneumonia is an uncommon interstitial pneumonitis of infancy and childhood. A definitive diagnosis depends on histologic demonstration of characteristic multinuclear giant cells with intranuclear and intracytoplasmic inclusion bodies in the lung. There are also a mononuclear infiltrate, squamous metaplasia of the bronchial and bronchiolar epithelium, proliferation of the alveolar lining cells and the occasional occurrence of giant cells in organs other than the lungs. There are some clinical and histologic similarities to distemper (a measles-like illness of animals); moreover, patients often develop giant cell pneumonia after measles. Rubeola virus has been recovered from the lung tissue of patients with giant cell pneumonia who had no clinical evidence of measles or had leukemia complicated by measles infection. The giant cell formation seen in Hecht's pneumonia and in cystic fibrosis is not, on the other hand, a histologic feature of the pneumonia commonly encountered with clinical measles. In the former group the process of giant cell formation originates in or near terminal bronchioles or alveoli, whereas in the latter it is of bronchial origin. Hecht's pneumonia may also follow immunization with attenuated measles vaccine in children who have leukemia or lymphomas.

Clinically, patients with giant cell pneumonia have moderate to severe respiratory distress manifest principally by tachypnea and dyspnea. Inspiratory and early expiratory rales and musical sounds are heard, but dullness is rarely present. Some patients will continue to excrete rubeola virus from the upper respiratory tract for weeks after the onset of illness. Roentgenographically, there are usually generalized, patchy infiltrates with areas of overinflation.

The course of illness may be prolonged over several weeks; clinical improvement may occur days to weeks prior to roentgenographic improvement. Occasionally, bacterial superinfection may occur. The mortality rate is high, particularly in patients with debilitating diseases such as leukemia and cystic fibrosis. Treatment is symptomatic; gamma globulin is of no value.

PNEUMONIAS OF MISCELLANEOUS CAUSES

Pneumocystis Carinii Pneumonia
(INTERSTITIAL PLASMA CELL PNEUMONIA)

Interstitial plasma cell pneumonia is an unusual infection of newborn infants and occasionally of children and adults with altered host resistance. The disease is caused by the protozoan *Pneumocystis carinii,* a ubiquitous organism whose exact affinities remain unknown, since it has not been grown in vitro.

Pathogenesis and Pathology. The majority of cases of *P. carinii* pneumonia occur among 3 different groups of patients: (1) premature and full-term infants, (2) patients under treatment for chronic debilitating illnesses, and (3) patients with primary immunologic deficiency syndromes.

In newborn infants an incompletely developed immunologic responsiveness and exposure to a humidified atmosphere contaminated with the parasite may interact synergistically to produce sporadic or epidemic disease in the nursery. In some infants intensive treatment of a respiratory tract infection with antibiotics may produce activation of a latent pneumocystic infection. Infants with cytomegalic inclusion disease or children with lymphoreticular malignancies treated with cytotoxic agents, corticosteroids or prolonged antimicrobial therapy are particularly susceptible to *P. carinii* pneumonia. Other susceptibles include patients with congenital or acquired immunologic deficiency diseases such as agammaglobulinemia and hypogammaglobulinemia.

Infection with *P. carinii* produces a characteristic intra-alveolar exudate of lacelike appearance which contains histiocytes, lymphocytes and plasma cells. The plasma cells are diminished or absent in agammaglobulinemia and hypogammaglobulinemia. Pneumocystic cysts are demonstrable in the exudate by a special staining technique. In the alveolar septa there are varying degrees of edema, inflammation and fibrosis.

Clinical Manifestations. The usual age at onset in infants is from the third to fifth week of life; in children with immunologic deficiency syndromes, onset ranges from 3 months to mid-childhood. The disease usually begins insidiously with cough and proceeds over a period of 1 to 4 weeks to severe respiratory distress. There is low-grade or no fever, and the absence or paucity of pulmonary findings to percussion and auscultation in a patient with severe distress is remarkable.

Roentgenographic findings are fairly characteristic. The lung fields are hyperexpanded and have a generalized granular pattern; bilateral pulmonary infiltrates, which originate at the hilus, extend peripherally, and eventually create a nearly solid appearance. The overaeration is most pronounced in the periphery. The white blood cell count is usually within normal limits or moderately elevated.

Diagnosis. The diagnosis of *P. carinii* pneumonia should be suspected in newborn infants and patients with altered host resistance who have severe respiratory distress with minimal physical findings and suggestive radiologic changes. The definitive diagnosis rests on the demonstration of the organism. At present a lung biopsy is the most satisfactory means of demonstrating the presence of *P. carinii;* silver stains of tracheal aspirates or of tonsillar smears may occasionally be satisfactory. A complement fixation test has been developed.

Course and Prognosis. *P. carinii* pneumonia usually lasts from 3 to 6 weeks, but may continue over many months. The death rate is variable; in infants with no complicating illness the most recent European case fatality rate is about 15 per cent.

Therapy. Pentamidine isothionate has been used in a number of patients with moderate success. Gamma globulin may be useful in those children with immunologic deficiency diseases. If the disease develops in a patient on immunosuppressant or corticosteroid therapy, it is usually necessary to reduce dosage or discontinue these drugs.

REFERENCES

Acute Bronchiolitis

Heycock, J. B., and Noble, T. C.: 1230 Cases of Acute Bronchiolitis in Infancy. *Brit. Med. J.,* 2:879, 1962.

Reynolds, E. O. R.: Bronchiolitis; in E. L. Kendig, Jr. (Ed.): *Disorders of the Respiratory Tract in Children.* Philadelphia, W. B. Saunders Compnay, 1967, Chap. 20.

Wright, F. H., and Beem, M. O.: Diagnosis and Treatment: Management of Acute Viral Bronchiolitis in Infancy. *Pediatrics,* 35:334, 1965.

Primary Atypical Pneumonia (Eaton Agent Pneumonia)

Sussman, S. J., and others: Cold Agglutinins, Eaton Agent and Respiratory Infections of Children. *Pediatrics,* 38:571, 1966.

Pneumocystis Carinii Pneumonia (Interstitial Plasma Cell Pneumonia)

Patterson, J. H., Lindsey, I. L., Edwards, E. S., and Logan, W. D.: Pneumocystis Carinii Pneumonia and Altered Host Resistance. *Pediatrics,* 38:388, 1966.

Robbins, J. B.: Pneumocystis Carinii Pneumonitis. A Review. *Pediat. Res.,* 1:131, 1967.

MYCOTIC PULMONARY INFECTIONS

See also Coccidioidomycosis, Histoplasmosis, Blastomycosis, Cryptococcosis, Mucormycosis, Nocardiosis and Sporotrichosis in their respective sections.

Thrush Pneumonia
(PULMONARY CANDIDIASIS)

Pulmonary infections with *Candida albicans* are rare in the pediatric age group in spite of the relatively high incidence of oral thrush (p. 763) in early infancy. This fact has been attributed to a natural resistance of columnar epithelium to invasion by the fungus. Emanuel summarized data on 17 cases (15 from the literature) in infants; the oldest was 8 weeks. All had respiratory distress; about half had oral thrush, but there was no clinical or roentgen characteristic to suggest the cause of the pulmonary infection. Cystic fibrosis may dispose to pulmonary candidiasis in infancy.

REFERENCE

Emanuel, B., Lieberman, A. D., Goldin, M., and Samson, J.: Pulmonary Candidiasis in the Neonatal Period. *J. Pediat.,* 61:44, 1962.

BRONCHIAL AND PULMONARY LESIONS SECONDARY TO ASPIRATION OF FOREIGN MATERIALS

Aspiration Pneumonia

For Fetal Anoxia with Aspiration of Excessive Amniotic Debris, see page 378.

Aspiration of Food. Infants with obstructive lesions, such as tracheo-esophageal fistula and duodenal obstruction, and weak and debilitated infants who have no obstructive lesions may aspirate, or regurgitate and then aspirate, an amount of food sufficient to cause significant pulmonary damage. Aspiration may rarely be an immediate cause of death by asphyxiation. More frequently the irritated mucous membrane becomes a site for bacterial invasion. Prophylaxis is of the greatest importance. Care should be taken to avoid amounts of feedings that will overdistend the stomach; this is especially true for infants whose feeding is by gavage. After the infant has been fed he should be placed on his abdomen or on his right side. When he is in the supine position, his head should not be lower than the rest of his body. While the infant is lying on his abdomen, however, drainage from the lungs may be materially aided by lowering the head of the bed.

Aspiration of Zinc Stearate. Aspiration pneumonia resulting from inhalation of zinc stearate powder, once relatively common, has become rare because of efforts discouraging the use of this powder for infants. Containers have also been equipped with an automatic closing device, but this is not infallible. Severe respiratory distress follows inhalation almost immediately. There is a generalized obstructive emphysema with an expiratory type of dyspnea. The embarrassment to respiration appears to be the result of an inflammatory reaction caused by the irritation of the zinc stearate. Owing to the extreme lightness of the powder, it is almost immediately drawn into the finer bronchioles, and for this reason bronchoscopic aspiration is of little avail except to remove the secretions which subsequently accumulate.

Immediate treatment is by oxygen therapy in an atmosphere of high humidity. Bronchoscopic aspiration is indicated when there is an excessive accumulation of secretions in the larger air passages.

Kerosene Pneumonia

Pulmonary disturbances are frequently associated with the ingestion of kerosene. (See Hydrocarbons [p. 498] for other manifestations of kerosene poisoning.)

There are conflicting interpretations of the **pathogenesis** of the pulmonary lesions. Some investigators contend that most of the kerosene reaches the lungs after absorption from the gastrointestinal tract, whereas others believe that aspiration during swallowing, vomiting or gastric lavage is the principal means of pulmonary contamination. Consequently there are divergent views as to the advisability of gastric lavage after the ingestion of kerosene or other hydrocarbons. The pulmonary changes observed in animals are edema, inflammation and hemorrhage.

Coughing and vomiting follow ingestion almost immediately. There is an elevation of temperature (100 to 104°F.), and the child may be drowsy or comatose. The pulmonary findings may be diminished resonance on percussion, suppressed or tubular breath sounds and rales. Pneumonic involvement is disclosed more frequently by roentgenographic examination than by physical findings. Pneumothorax, subcutaneous emphysema of the chest wall and pleural effusion, including empyema, have occurred as **complications.** In spite of the stormy clinical course, which averages 2 to 5 days, recovery occurs in most instances.

Treatment. When only small amounts of kerosene have been ingested, and especially if several hours have elapsed, gastric lavage probably should be omitted. When large quantities of kerosene or other hydrocarbons have been ingested, lavage should be performed with great care to avoid aspiration. In either instance a saline cathartic should be administered. The administration of an oil apparently decreases absorption from the gastrointestinal tract. There are conflicting data, however, in respect to different oils. Ashkenazi found reduced absorption after administration of paraffin oil. Gerarde's data, however, seem to indicate that mineral oil promotes absorption, whereas olive oil retards it. If there is dyspnea or cyanosis, the child should be placed in an oxygen tent. An antibiotic should be administered prophylactically, or therapeutically if a secondary infection has occurred.

Lipoid Pneumonia

Lipoid pneumonia is a chronic, interstitial proliferative inflammation resulting from aspiration of lipoid material; it occurs principally in debilitated infants.

The factors which may be responsible for aspiration of oil include (1) intranasal instillation of medicated oils, (2) any condition which interferes with the swallowing act, such as cleft palate, debilitation, and a horizontal position during feeding, and (3) forced feeding and especially the administration of cod liver oil, castor oil or mineral oil to crying children.

The severity of the pulmonary reaction depends upon the kind of oil inhaled. Vegetable oils are generally the least irritating, such oils as olive, cottonseed and sesame producing no inflammation; chaulmoogra, a vegetable oil, on the other hand, is responsible for extensive damage. Animal oils, owing to their high fatty acid content, are the most damaging. Cod liver oil belongs in this category. Liquid petrolatum is chemically inert and not so irritative as some of the other oils, but does act as a foreign body.

The reaction within the lung begins as an interstitial proliferative inflammation with which there may be an exudative pneumonia. In the second stage there is diffuse, chronic, proliferative fibrosis. Acute bronchopneumonia is not infrequently superimposed in this stage. In the third stage there are multiple localized nodules, the so-called tumor-like paraffinomas. Microscopically, there are numerous macrophages in the involved areas, with giant cell formation of the foreign body type. The lipoid substance is both intracellular and extracellular. The oil-laden cells may be carried through lymphatic channels to the hilar lymph nodes.

Clinical Manifestations. There are no characteristic signs or symptoms. The most common symptom is cough, and in severe cases there may be dyspnea. Unless there is a superimposed infection, there is usually no fever or physical sign. With extensive involvement there may be some impairment to percussion and increased or decreased voice and breath sounds. Secondary bronchopneumonic infections are common.

The only characteristic finding is the roentgenographic appearance. When there is only a mild involvement, there is an increase in both the density and the extent of the hilar shadows. With increasing involvement there is greater density of the perihilar shadows with widening in all directions (Fig. 12-13). In a few instances the pulmonary changes have been limited to the right lung, and in the infant who is recumbent most of the time the changes may be mainly in the right upper lobe.

Prognosis. The prognosis is guarded. It depends upon the extent of pulmonary damage, the discontinuance of oil inhalation, the general condition of the infant, and the avoidance of intercurrent infections.

Prevention. Intranasal medication in an oily vehicle should never be used. Concentrated preparations of vitamins A and D in water-miscible vehicles should be substituted for cod liver oil. Administration of mineral oil and castor oil should

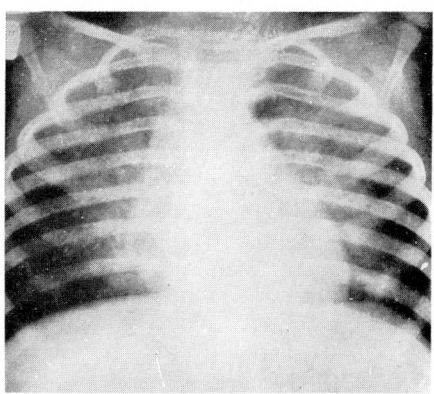

Figure 12-13. Roentgenogram showing increased density radiating from the hilus of each lung in an infant 13 months of age after intranasal application of liquid petrolatum 3 times a day for 5 months.

be avoided. Infants who regurgitate or vomit frequently should be placed on their abdomens to lessen the likelihood of aspiration.

Treatment. There is no specific treatment. The infant's position should be changed frequently to lessen the chances of hypostatic pneumonia.

REFERENCES

Zinc Stearate

Heiman, H., and Aschner, P. W.: Aspirations of Stearate of Zinc in Infancy. *Am. J. Dis. Child.*, 23:503, 1922.

Kerosene Pneumonia

Ashkenazi, A. E., and Berman, S. E.: Experimental Kerosene Poisoning in Rats. *Pediatrics*, 28:642, 1961.
Gerarde, H. W.: Toxicological Studies on Hydrocarbons. V. Kerosene. *Toxicol. Appl. Pharmacol.*, 1:462, 1959.

Lipoid Pneumonia

Bromer, R. S., and Wolman, I. J.: Lipoid Pneumonia in Infants and Children. *Radiology*, 32:1, 1939.
Nathanson, L., Frenkel, D., and Jacobi, M.: Diagnosis of Lipoid Pneumonia by Aspiration Biopsy. *Arch. Int. Med.*, 72:627, 1943.

LÖFFLER'S SYNDROME
(EOSINOPHILIC PNEUMONIA)

This syndrome is characterized by widespread, transitory pulmonary infiltrations which roentgenographically vary in size, but may resemble those of miliary tuberculosis, and by a blood eosinophilia which may be as high as 70 per cent. The clinical course is, as a rule, not particularly severe and varies from a few days to several months. Features more or less common to the reported cases are paroxysmal attacks of coughing, dyspnea, pleurisy and little or no fever. Zuelzer and others called attention to the association of hepatomegaly in this syndrome, especially in infants and young children. Biopsy sections of the livers reveal multiple focal areas of necrosis, granuloma formation and eosinophilic infiltration. These children have hyperglobulinemia, presumably as the result of hepatic dysfunction. Autopsy studies have revealed evidences of eosinophilic infiltrations in the lungs and in other organs. Instances have been recorded of localized pneumonic consolidation with an associated eosinophilia.

Löffler's syndrome is not a clinical entity. It has been considered by some to be an unusual allergic manifestation to a variety of antigens. In children it would appear to be most often a manifestation of helminthic infections. The term *visceral larva migrans* is used for extraintestinal invasion by the larvae of a variety of roundworms. Perhaps the most common pathogen in this country is the larva of the dog ascarid, *Toxocara canis,* and less often of the cat ascarid, *Toxocara cati* (see Toxocariasis, p. 720). Other roundworms may also be responsible for the syndrome; these include the hookworms, *Ascaris lumbricoides* (usually responsible for transient pulmonary lesions), and *Strongyloides*

stercoralis. So-called tropical eosinophilia (p. 739) may be manifest as Löffler's syndrome, and is probably caused by a number of different helminths. Paragonimiasis caused by a lung fluke (p. 735) may produce the syndrome, as well as extrapulmonary manifestations.

REFERENCES

Beaver, P.: Wandering Nematodes as a Cause of Disability and Disease. *Am. J. Trop. Med. & Hyg.*, 6:433, 1957.
Yun, D. J.: Paragonimiasis in Children in Korea. *J. Pediat.*, 56:736, 1960.
Zuelzer, W. W., and Apt, L.: Disseminated Visceral Lesions Associated with Extreme Eosinophilia: Pathologic and Clinical Observations on a Syndrome of Young Children. *Am. J. Dis. Child.*, 78:153, 1949.

HYPOSTATIC PNEUMONIA

Hypostatic pneumonia occurs after prolonged passive pulmonary congestion and may occur in any marantic state. Lying for a long time in one position favors its development. Pathologically, there is dependent congestion, edema and pneumonia.

Clinical Manifestations. The symptoms are not characteristic. There is neither dyspnea nor fever, unless these symptoms are dependent upon some other factor. The physical signs are principally slight dullness on percussion, feeble respiratory sounds and the presence of moist rales. Hypostatic congestion is usually a terminal event.

Treatment. Treatment is that of the primary affection. Prophylaxis is of the greatest importance; the position of the patient should be changed frequently when there is a possibility of development of passive pulmonary congestion.

PULMONARY HEMOSIDEROSIS

The term "pulmonary hemosiderosis" is used to describe a number of rare conditions characterized by an abnormal accumulation of hemosiderin in the lungs. Hemosiderin deposits follow diffuse alveolar hemorrhage and may occur either as a primary disease of the lungs or secondary to cardiac or systemic vascular disease. In children primary hemosiderosis occurs more frequently than the secondary varieties. There appear to be 3 types of primary pulmonary hemosiderosis: *(a)* an idiopathic form, *(b)* a form occurring in association with myocarditis, and *(c)* a form associated with progressive glomerulonephritis (Goodpasture's syndrome). Two types of secondary pulmonary hemosiderosis are recognized; one occurs with mitral stenosis and chronic left ventricular failure of any cause, and the other is associated with collagen diseases and anaphylactoid purpura.

Idiopathic Primary Pulmonary Hemosiderosis. The cause of this illness is unknown. Onset is usually in childhood, rarely later than early adult life. Symptoms are those of recurrent or chronic pulmonary disease, and include cough, hemoptysis, dyspnea, wheezing and occasional cyanosis, associated with fatigue and pallor. The cough may be productive of bloody sputum or the infant or child may simply vomit large quantities of blood. During acute attacks, which usually last 2 to 4 days, the child may be febrile.

The usual clinical features of fever, tachycardia, tachypnea, leukocytosis, respiratory distress and abnormal radiologic findings may suggest a bacterial pneumonia, and only prolonged follow-up will reveal the correct diagnosis. In some children, however, the early manifestations of the illness are related to chronic iron deficiency anemia, often refractory to therapy, and the characteristic pulmonary symptoms do not appear until much later. Paradoxically, the child may have severe pulmonary manifestations without roentgenographic abnormalities, or the roentgenographic picture may be abnormal before pulmonary symptoms have occurred.

The anemia is typically microcytic and hypochromic; serum iron concentrations are low. The stool usually contains occult blood, presumably swallowed. Hemosiderin can usually be demonstrated in macrophages of the sputum and in material obtained by gastric lavage. Roentgenographic changes range from minimal infiltrates to massive pulmonary involvement with secondary atelectasis, emphysema and hilar lymphadenopathy; significant changes may be seen from day to day. A biopsy may be necessary to establish the diagnosis. Histologic features are alveolar epithelial hyperplasia, large numbers of macrophages containing hemosiderin, varying amounts of interstitial fibrosis, and sclerosis of small blood vessels. Approximately 50 per cent of patients die within 1 to 5 years of the onset, usually from acute pulmonary hemorrhage and respiratory failure.

In some patients, corticosteroids may have produced remissions; in others these drugs have not been beneficial. Maintenance corticosteroid therapy has been used between attacks, with variable results. Immunosuppressant drugs and deferoxamine have also been advocated, but there are inadequate data to evaluate them.

Primary Pulmonary Hemosiderosis with Myocarditis. Some patients with idiopathic pulmonary hemosiderosis have inflammation of the myocardium, varying from minimal lesions to extensive disease. If significant myocardial disease is present when pulmonary symptoms are first noted, it may be impossible to determine whether the pulmonary hemosiderosis is a primary or secondary phenomenon. The clinical picture does not differ from that of idiopathic disease except that the heart may be enlarged, owing to the myocarditis, and electrocardiographic signs compatible with this cardiac lesion may be present.

Primary Pulmonary Hemosiderosis with Glomerulonephritis (Goodpasture's Syndrome) (see p. 530). This is a disease primarily of young adults and is rarely observed in children. The clinical picture is initiated by pulmonary involvement with hemoptysis and iron deficiency anemia. At this stage the disease may be virtually identical to idiopathic pulmonary hemosiderosis, but careful study will disclose a proliferative or membranous glomerulonephritis at the time of the first pulmonary attack. Patients with this syndrome usually have progressive renal disease which leads to renal failure and death.

Primary Pulmonary Hemosiderosis with Precipitins to Cow's Milk. A small number of patients with signs and symptoms of primary pulmonary hemosiderosis have had unusually high titers in serum of precipitins to multiple constituents of cow's milk. These patients may also have chronic rhinitis, otitis media and growth retardation. On a cow's-milk-free diet some patients with these serologic findings of milk reactivity appear to improve, others do not. The causative relation of milk reactivity to pulmonary hemosiderosis remains unknown; in any event, the majority of children with this condition do not have unusual amounts of precipitins to milk proteins.

Pulmonary Hemosiderosis Secondary to Heart Disease. Any form of heart disease producing chronic increase in pulmonary capillary pressure can lead to secondary pulmonary hemosiderosis. The most common primary lesion is mitral stenosis.

Pulmonary Hemosiderosis as a Manifestation of Diffuse Collagen Disease or Anaphylactoid Purpura. The vascular changes of polyarteritis nodosa occasionally are initially limited to the lungs, and may cause pulmonary hemosiderosis. In most instances, polyarteritis progresses to involve other organs. Other collagen diseases such as rheumatoid arthritis, lupus erythematosus and rheumatic fever have occasionally produced pulmonary hemosiderosis as an effect of a generalized, diffuse vasculitis.

A few patients have had pulmonary hemosiderosis in association with anaphylactoid purpura or thrombocytopenic purpura.

REFERENCES

Heiner, D. C., Sears, J. W., Kniker, W. T.: Multiple Precipitins to Cow's Milk in Chronic Respiratory Disease. A syndrome including poor growth, gastrointestinal symptoms, evidence of allergy, iron deficiency anemia, and pulmonary hemosiderosis. Am. J. Dis. Child., 103:634, 1962.

Irvin, J. M., and Snowden, P. W.: Idiopathic Pulmonary Hemosiderosis: Report of a Case with Apparent Remission from Cortisone. Am. J. Dis. Child., 93:182, 1957.

Launay, C., Bach C., Thiriez, H., et al.: Idiopathic Pulmonary Hemosiderosis. Ann. Pediat. (Paris), 10:379, 1963.

Soergel, K. H., and Sommers, S. C.: Idiopathic Pulmonary Hemosiderosis and Related Syndromes. Am. J. Med., 32:499, 1962.

PULMONARY ALVEOLAR PROTEINOSIS

Pulmonary alveolar proteinosis is a syndrome of unknown origin characterized by progressive dyspnea and cough. The onset of the illness may or may not be marked by a febrile episode. The patient may complain of increased fatigability and loss of weight. Cough may or may not be productive. The physical findings are relatively few, but roentgenologic changes are characteristic. These consist of a fine, diffuse, feathery-soft density radiating from the hilus to the periphery and are due to eosinophilic material rich in protein and lipid in the alveoli.

Death may result from anoxemia produced by the progressive filling of alveoli by this material, or from superimposed fungal or bacterial infection.

REFERENCES

Fraimow, W., Cathcart, R. T., and Taylor, R. C.: Physiologic and Clinical Aspects of Pulmonary Alveolar Proteinosis. *Ann. Intern. Med.,* 52:1177, 1960.

Hall, G. F.: Pulmonary Alveolar Proteinosis. *Lancet,* 1:1383, 1960.

IDIOPATHIC DIFFUSE INTERSTITIAL FIBROSIS OF THE LUNG
(HAMMAN-RICH SYNDROME)

Idiopathic diffuse interstitial fibrosis of the lung is a rare chronic, usually progressive and fatal, disorder of unknown origin, usually observed in adults, but occasionally in infants and children. The clinical pattern is characterized by progressive pulmonary insufficiency resulting from interstitial fibrosis and alveolar-capillary block. Onset is usually insidious, with dyspnea generally the first symptom, initially occurring only with exercise, but later present even at rest. Cough is frequent and may be productive of blood. The patient is usually afebrile. As the disease progresses, anorexia, weight loss and fatigability occur, and finally cyanosis, clubbing of the fingers and evidences of right-sided cardiac failure. Serial roentgenograms show progressive, widespread granular or reticular mottling or small nodular densities. Intercurrent infections are frequent and often serious.

The pulmonary pathology is variable. During the early stage of the disease, fibrosis is usually not present, but there is cellular infiltration of the walls of the alveoli, alveolar ducts and peribronchial tissue by lymphocytes, plasma cells and occasionally eosinophils. This usually progresses to extensive and diffuse proliferation of fibrous tissue throughout all the lobes of the lung, associated with organization of intra-alveolar exudate.

The cause is unknown; some cases may be familial in origin.

Corticosteroids appear to give some symptomatic relief, but do not alter the progression of the disease or improve the degree of pulmonary function. Other therapy is also symptomatic.

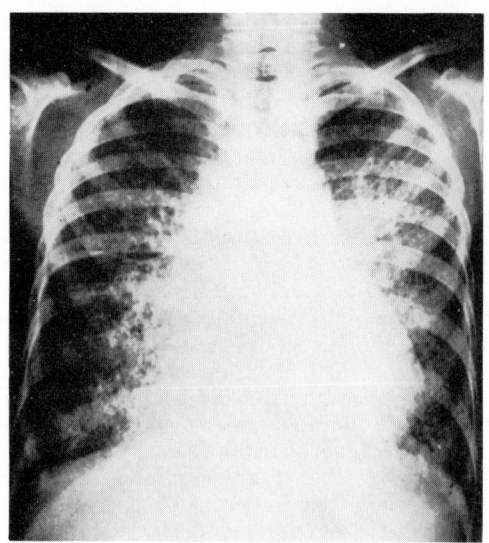

Figure 12-14.   Roentgenogram of chest of a 7-year-old boy with pulmonary alveolar microlithiasis. (From R. B. Clark, III, and F. C. Johnson: *Pediatrics,* Vol. 28.)

REFERENCES

Ivemark, B. I., and Wallgren, C. G.: Diffuse Interstitial Pulmonary Fibrosis (Hamman-Rich Syndrome) in an Infant. Report of a case with histologic and respiratory studies. *Acta Paediat.,* 51:97 (Supp. 135), 1962.

Rubin, E. H., and Lubliner, R.: The Hamman-Rich Syndrome: Review of the Literature and Analysis of 15 Cases. *Medicine,* 36:397, 1957.

Sheridan, L. A., Harrison, E. G., Jr., and Divertie, M. B.: The Current Status of Idiopathic Pulmonary Fibrosis (Hamman-Rich Syndrome). *Med. Clin. N. Amer.,* 48:993, 1964.

PULMONARY ALVEOLAR MICROLITHIASIS

This rare disease appears often to have its onset during childhood, but the clinical manifestations tend to be delayed to later years. It is characterized by widely disseminated intra-alveolar calculi, which create a rather characteristic pattern on the roentgenogram (Fig. 12-14). The appearance has been likened to that of an overfilled normal bronchogram. If the disease is identified in childhood, it is apt to be by roentgenographic examination before symptoms have appeared or when they are still minimal. The disease usually progresses slowly and terminates in cardiopulmonary failure during the middle years of adulthood.

The cause is unknown; there are no known metabolic abnormalities, including those of calcium and phosphorus. Some cases have shown a familial pattern; there is no sex predilection.

There is no known effective treatment.

REFERENCE

Clark, R. B., III, and Johnson, F. C.: Idiopathic Pulmonary Alveolar Microlithiasis. *Pediatrics,* 28:650, 1961.

ATELECTASIS

Congenital atelectasis is discussed on page 381.

ACQUIRED ATELECTASIS

Etiology. Atelectasis, the imperfect expansion or the collapse of air-bearing tissue of the lung, is relatively common in infants and children. Collapse may be produced by any factor which completely obstructs the intake of air into the alveolar sacs and persists sufficiently long to permit absorption of alveolar air into the bloodstream. In general, the causes may be divided into 2 groups: (1) external pressure directly upon the pulmonary parenchyma or a bronchus or bronchiole, and (2) intrabronchial or intrabronchiolar obstruction. Any factor responsible for a continuously decreased amplitude of respiratory excursion or for respiratory paralysis may be contributory. Reflex stimuli have also been considered initiating factors. De Takats demonstrated that at least 3 distinct stimuli, namely, pulmonary embolism, intra-abdominal manipulation and trauma to the chest wall, are capable of initiating bronchoconstriction and increased bronchosecretion. Allergy may be responsible for atelectasis through spasm of the bronchial or bronchiolar musculature and production of an exudate which occludes the lumen. This latter may also be responsible for atelectasis in patients with cystic fibrosis.

Atelectasis from external pressure. External factors may be operative in one of 4 ways: (1) interference with the movements of the thoracic cage (neuromuscular abnormalities as in cerebral palsy, poliomyelitis, spinal muscular atrophy, myasthenia gravis; osseous deformities as in rickets, scoliosis, kyphosis; scleroderma; splinting of the chest by casts and surgical dressings); (2) defective movement of the diaphragm (paralysis of phrenic nerve, increased abdominal pressure); (3) direct interference with expansion of lungs (pleural effusion, pneumothorax, intrathoracic tumors, diaphragmatic hernia), and (4) external compression of a bronchus completely obstructing ingress of air (enlarged lymph node, tumors, cardiac enlargement).

Atelectasis from intrabronchial or intrabronchiolar obstruction (see also p. 905). Complete intraluminal obstruction of a bronchus may be produced by a foreign body, by a neoplasm, by granulomatous tissue as in tuberculosis or by secretions as with cystic fibrosis, bronchiectasis, pulmonary abscess, allergy, chronic bronchitis or acute laryngotracheobronchitis.

Obstruction of one or more bronchioles in a given area may be produced by any of the conditions mentioned, but widespread bronchiolar obstruction is most often produced by bronchiolitis or interstitial pneumonitis and by asthma. Generalized obstructive emphysema is the initial result of such bronchiolar obstructions; but as the pathologic changes progress, some of the bronchioles may become completely obstructed, and there are then interspersed small areas of atelectasis and emphysema. Patchy atelectasis is relatively common in acute bronchiolitis or asthma, and is probably always present in advanced chronic diffuse infections such as the pulmonary infection associated with cystic fibrosis.

Pathology. The atelectatic areas are airless, congested, deep red, of a firm consistency, and depressed below the neighboring healthy or emphysematous lung. When there is extensive atelectasis of one or more lobes, there is usually compensatory emphysema of the air-bearing lung.

Clinical Manifestations. Symptoms vary with the cause and extent of the atelectasis. When only a small area is atelectatic, there are likely to be no symptoms referable to it. When a large area of the lung becomes atelectatic, and especially when it does so suddenly, there is dyspnea with rapid shallow respirations, tachycardia, and often cyanosis. If the obstruction is removed, the symptoms disappear rapidly. Even atelectasis of an entire lobe may not be responsible for changes in the percussion note, owing to the compensatory emphysema of the adjacent lung tissue. Breath and voice sounds are decreased or absent over extensive atelectatic areas.

Diagnosis. The diagnosis can usually be established by roentgenographic examination (Fig. 12-15). Small areas may be indistinguishable from pneumonic consolidations, but those that involve as much as several lobules of a lobe can usually be identified by the contraction of the area. When one or more lobes are atelectatic, the roentgenographic findings are those of massive collapse. Bronchoscopic examination will reveal a collapsed main bronchus when the obstruction is at the tracheobronchial junction and may also disclose the nature of the obstruction.

Prognosis. This depends upon the underlying cause. If the obstruction disappears spontaneously or is removed, the atelectasis usually disappears unless there is secondary infection. In persistent cases bronchiectasis is a frequent complication and pulmonary abscess an occasional one.

Treatment. Bronchoscopic examination is indicated when an isolated area of atelectasis persists for several days, and immediately if it is the result of a foreign body or if there is reason to believe that it is due to any bronchial obstruction which may be relieved. Frequent changes in the child's position and deep breathing may be beneficial. Oxygen therapy is indicated when there is dyspnea. Morphine and atropine are contraindicated.

MASSIVE PULMONARY ATELECTASIS

Massive collapse of one or both lungs is most often a postoperative complication, but occasionally results from other causes such as trauma,

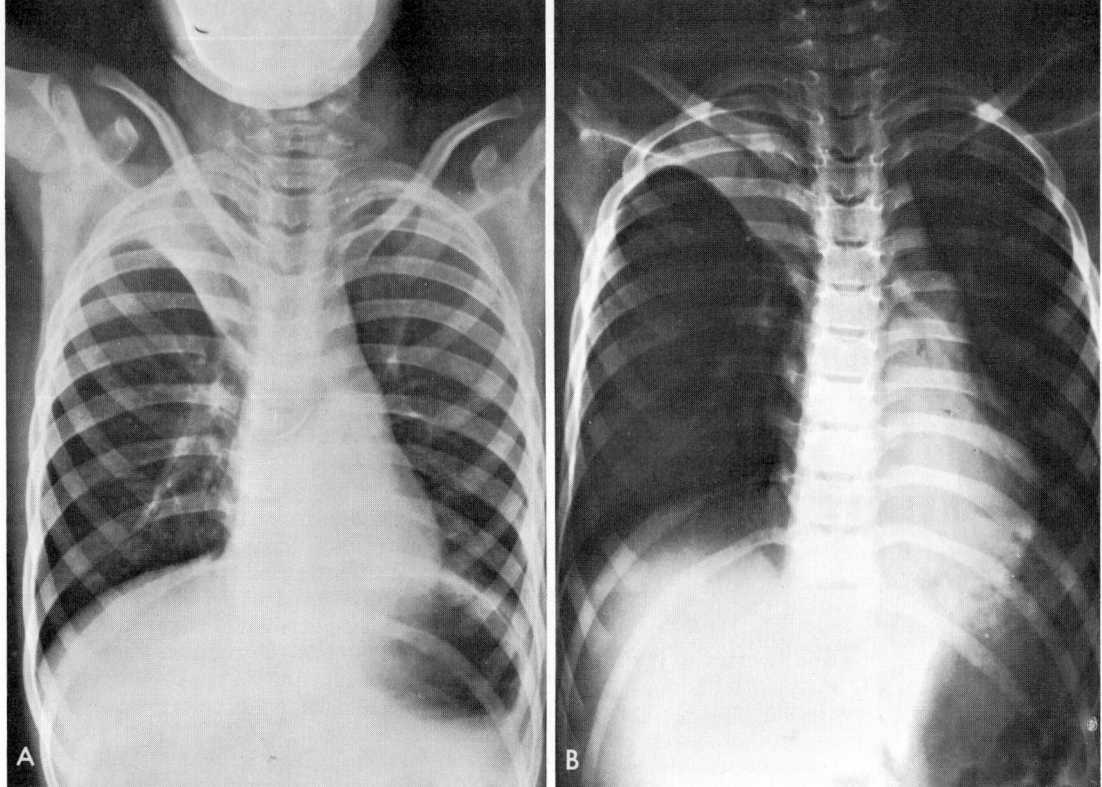

Figure 12-15. Atelectasis. The right upper lobe and the left lower lobe are collapsed. The atelectasis of the left lower lobe is demonstrated on the overpenetrated film (B). The atelectasis occurred postoperatively and disappeared spontaneously.

asthma, pneumonia, tension pneumothorax, the aspiration of foreign material (either a solid object large enough to obstruct a main stem bronchus or liquids such as water or blood) or paralysis such as that in diphtheria or poliomyelitis. Massive atelectasis is usually produced by a combination of factors: immobilization or decreased use of the diaphragm and the respiratory muscles, obstruction of the bronchial tree and abolition of the cough reflex.

Clinical Manifestations. The onset in postoperative cases is usually within 24 hours after operation, but may not occur for several days. There is dyspnea, cyanosis and tachycardia. The child is extremely anxious, there is likely to be prostration, and, if he is old enough, he usually complains of pain in the chest. The temperature may be as high as 103 or 104°F.

The physical signs are characteristic. The chest on the affected side appears flat, and there is decreased respiratory excursion on that side. There is dullness to percussion. Breath and voice sounds are feeble or absent. Lower lobes are more frequently involved than upper ones. The heart and the mediastinum are displaced toward the affected side. Roentgenograms show the collapsed lung, elevation of the diaphragm, narrowing of the intercostal spaces and displacement of the mediastinal structures and heart toward the affected side.

Prognosis. Bilateral massive collapse is usually rapidly fatal, although prompt bronchoscopic aspiration and artificial respiration may be lifesaving. In the unilateral cases the prognosis is usually good.

Prevention. Prophylaxis is of the greatest importance. The incidence of postoperative atelectasis can be reduced by adequate ventilation during anesthesia. After operation the child's position in bed should be changed frequently, collections of secretions in the oropharynx should be aspirated, and when consciousness returns, the child should be encouraged to breathe deeply. Tight thoracic or abdominal binders should be avoided.

Treatment. When there is bilateral atelectasis, bronchoscopic aspiration should be performed immediately. When there is only unilateral atelectasis, the child should be placed on the unaffected side. Forced coughing or crying while the child is lying on the unaffected side may also be helpful. When these measures are not successful, bronchoscopic aspiration should be performed.

Relapses are not infrequent, and the child should be kept under constant observation.

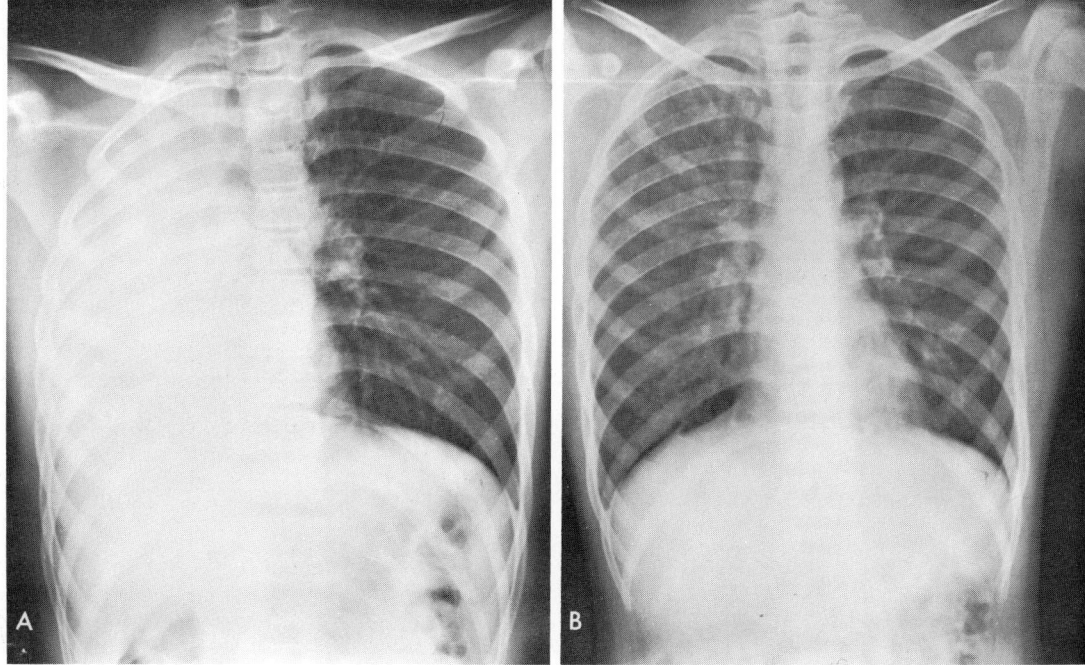

Figure 12-16. *A,* Massive atelectasis of the right lung, with *(B)* comparison study after reaeration following bronchoscopic removal of a mucous plug from the right stem bronchus. The patient is asthmatic. The heart and the other mediastinal structures are shifted to the right during the atelectatic phase.

EMPHYSEMA

Pulmonary emphysema is a distention or rupture of the alveoli. It may be generalized or localized and involve part or all of one lung. From a causative standpoint it may be compensatory or obstructive.

Compensatory Emphysema. This may be either acute or chronic. It occurs in normally functioning pulmonary tissue when for any reason a sizable portion of the lung is partially or completely airless, as may occur with pneumonia, atelectasis, empyema and pneumothorax.

OBSTRUCTIVE EMPHYSEMA

Obstructive emphysema results from partial obstruction of a bronchus or bronchiole when the difficulty of getting air out of the alveoli becomes greater than getting it in, so that there is a gradually increasing accumulation of air distal to the obstruction. This is the so-called bypass or check-valve type of obstruction. Such obstructions may be intrabronchial or extrabronchial (see p. 905).

Localized Obstructive Emphysema

When a bypass type of obstruction partially occludes the main stem bronchus, the entire lobe is emphysematous; only individual lobules are affected when the obstruction is that of a secondary bronchus. Localized obstructions which may be responsible for emphysema include foreign bodies and the inflammatory reaction to them, intrabronchial tuberculosis or tuberculosis of the tracheobronchial lymph nodes and intrabronchial and mediastinal tumors. When most or all of a lobe is involved, the percussion note will be hyperresonant over the area and the breath sounds decreased in intensity. The distended lung may extend across the mediastinum into the opposite hemithorax. Fluoroscopically, during expiration the emphysematous area does not decrease in size, and the heart and the mediastinum shift to the opposite side.

Congenital obstructive lobar emphysema may account for severe respiratory distress in early infancy. Symptoms may become apparent in the neonatal period or may be delayed for as much as 5 or 6 months. A part or usually all of a lobe may be involved, the left upper lobe being most often affected. In some instances the obstruction is not demonstrable, but it is assumed to be produced by a check-valve type of mechanism. Such obstructions have been attributed to defective cartilage in the bronchi, mucosal folds which create a valve-like obstruction, bronchial stenosis and external compression by aberrant vessels, tumors, and the like. When the distention is considerable, the emphysematous lung compresses the unaffected lung below or above it and the opposite lung by

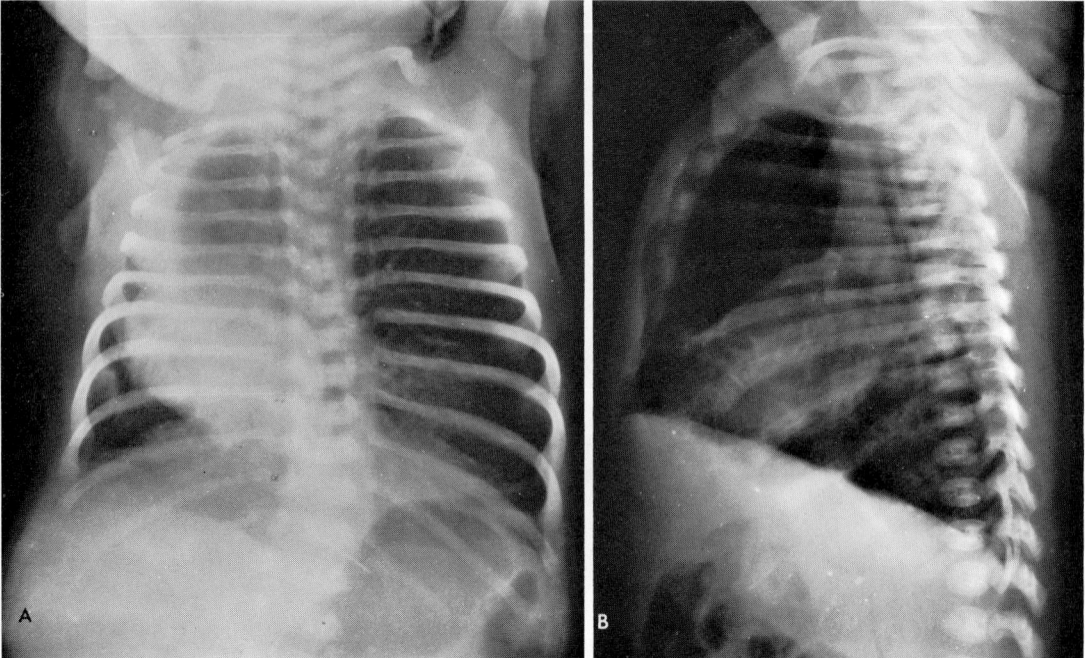

Figure 12-17. Congenital lobar emphysema in an infant 4 weeks of age. Severe dyspnea and wheezing of 4 days' duration. The left upper lobe is emphysematous and protrudes across the midline anteriorly (note lateral projection). The mediastinal structures are displaced to the right. Relief of symptoms followed removal of the left upper lobe.

extending across the mediastinum (Fig. 12-17). In most instances lobectomy is indicated.

Emphysema of all 3 lobes of the right lung has been produced by anomalous location of the left pulmonary artery, which partially constricts the right main bronchus.

Generalized Obstructive Emphysema

This depends upon widespread involvement of the bronchioles. It occurs more commonly in infants than in children and may be secondary to a number of clinical conditions, including respiratory infections associated with cystic fibrosis of the pancreas, acute bronchiolitis, interstitial pneumonitis, atypical forms of acute laryngotracheobronchitis, aspiration of zinc stearate powder, chronic passive congestion secondary to a congenital cardiac lesion, and miliary tuberculosis. Asthma is a relatively frequent cause in older children, but an uncommon one in infants.

The emphysematous portion of the lung is paler than usual, usually a light pink, and is distended and does not readily collapse. In chronic emphysema there is permanent loss of elasticity; many of the alveoli are ruptured and communicate with one another, producing distended saccules. As a result of the rupture of the alveoli, air may enter the interstitial tissue *(interstitial emphysema)* and result in pneumomediastinum and pneumothorax (see p. 389).

Clinical Manifestations. Generalized obstructive emphysema is characterized by an expiratory type of dyspnea. Owing to the relatively greater difficulty in expiration than in inspiration, air is trapped in the alveoli, the lungs become increasingly overdistended, and the chest remains expanded during expiration. Just the reverse happens in laryngeal obstruction, in which interference with exchange of air is relatively greater during inspiration and the lungs do not become fully inflated. There are an increased respiratory rate and decreased respiratory excursions in emphysema, owing to the overdistention of the pulmonary alveoli and their inability to be normally emptied through the narrowed bronchioles. Air hunger is responsible for forced respiratory movements, and the accessory muscles of respiration become overactive. The action of these muscles results in indrawing at the suprasternal notch, the supraclavicular spaces, the lower margin of the thorax and the intercostal spaces. This indrawing is not nearly so great, however, as it is in laryngeal or tracheal obstruction, since the overinflated lungs will not permit it. There is scarcely any reduction in size of the overdistended emphysematous chest during expiration, in contrast to the flattened chest during both inspiration and expiration when there is laryngeal obstruction. There is no hoarseness or stridor as there is in laryngeal obstruction; there is usually audible wheezing in asthma. Cyanosis is common in the severe cases. The percussion note is hyperresonant, and on auscultation the inspiratory phase is usually less prominent than the expiratory phase, which is prolonged and roughened. Fine or medium rales may be present.

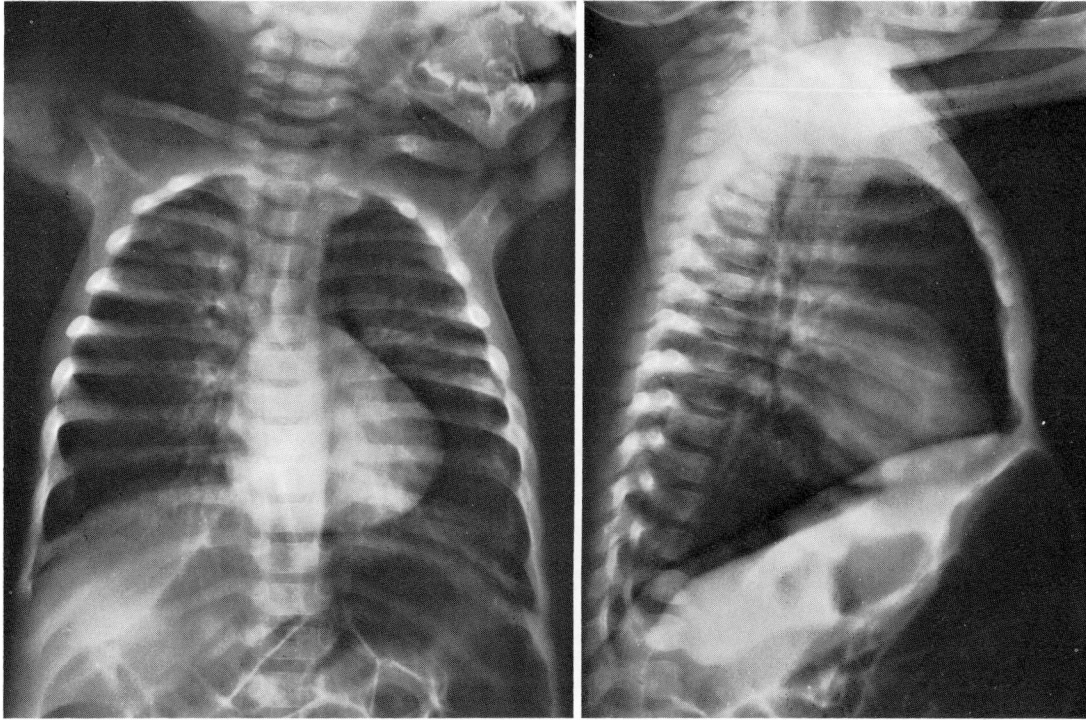

Figure 12-18. Generalized obstructive emphysema: dorsal projections of thorax in inspiratory and expiratory phases of respiration. Notice the relative failure of the lungs to empty in the expiratory phase. The left lung is less obstructed than the right (empties to a greater degree in the expiratory phase). This difference between the lungs is not apparent from a study of the diaphragm, which moves very little during respiration; it is evident, however, in the upper portions of the left lung space. (From Nelson and Smith: *J. Pediat.,* Vol. 26.)

Roentgenographic and fluoroscopic examinations of the chest are of the greatest help in establishing the diagnosis. Both leaves of the diaphragm are low and flattened, the ribs are farther apart than usual, and the lung fields are less dense (Fig. 12-18). There is a decided restriction in the movement of the diaphragm, which is demonstrated best by fluoroscopic examination. The normal "doming" of the diaphragm during expiration is decreased, and the excursion of the low, flattened diaphragm in the severe cases is barely discernible. Another evidence of retention of air in the lungs during expiration is a paradoxical increase in the horizontal diameters of the chest during this phase, suggesting that the emphysematous lungs are merely being forced into a different position by the diaphragmatic activity (the abdominal respiratory effort is relatively stronger than that of the intercostals) rather than emptied of any significant amount of trapped air.

Bullous Emphysema

Bullous emphysematous blebs or cysts (pneumatocele) result from overdistention and rupture of alveoli during birth or shortly thereafter (p. 391), or they may be sequels of pneumonia and of other infections. They have been observed in tuberculous lesions while the patient was being treated with specific antibacterial therapy. These emphysematous areas presumably result from rupture of distended alveoli so that a single or multiloculated cavity is formed. At times the cysts may assume large proportions (Fig. 12-12). They may contain some fluid, and an air-fluid level may be demonstrated on the roentgenogram. The differential diagnosis must be made from pulmonary abscess. In most instances the cysts disappear spontaneously within a few months, although they may persist for a year or so.

There is almost never any indication for treatment; aspiration or surgery should be avoided unless there is severe respiratory and cardiac embarrassment.

Subcutaneous Emphysema

Subcutaneous emphysema occurs whenever free air finds its way into the subcutaneous tissue. It may be a complication of a fracture of the orbit permitting air to escape from the nasal sinuses. In the neck and over the thorax, emphysema may follow tracheotomy, deep ulcerations in the pharyngeal region, esophageal wounds or any perforating lesion of the larynx or trachea. It is an occasional complication of thoracentesis. Air may also be formed in the subcutaneous tissues by gas-producing bacteria.

REFERENCES

Caffey, J.: *Pediatric X-ray Diagnosis.* 4th ed. Chicago, Year Book Publishers, Inc., 1961.

Currarino, G., and Silverman, F. N.: Roentgen Diagnosis of Pulmonary Disease of the Newborn Infant. *Pediat. Clin. N. Amer.,* 4:27, 1957.

Kress, M. B., and Finklestein, A. H.: Giant Bullous Emphysema Occurring in Tuberculosis in Childhood. *Pediatrics,* 30:269, 1962.

Landing, B. H.: Anomalies of the Respiratory Tract. *Pediat. Clin. N. Amer.,* 4:73, 1957.

Nelson, W. E., and Smith, L. W.: Generalized Obstructive Emphysema in Infants. *J. Pediat.,* 26:36, 1945.

PULMONARY EDEMA

Etiology. Pulmonary edema results from the escape of serous fluid from the pulmonary capillaries into the alveolar spaces and the bronchioles. It is usually associated with circulatory or neuro-circulatory collapse and consequently is often a terminal event in a variety of diseases. Though pulmonary edema may vary in severity, even in its mildest stages it is an ominous finding. It is a common manifestation of myocardial failure in acute or chronic rheumatic carditis and in congenital heart disease, or it may be due to hypervolemia from a rapid transfusion of blood or, more rarely, of plasma; it may be a manifestation of acute or chronic nephritis or, rarely, of pneumonic and other infections with substantial degrees of toxicity. Poisoning by such substances as barbiturates, morphine, epinephrine and alcohol may be responsible for the development of pulmonary edema, as may the inhalation of toxic gases, such as illuminating gas, ammonia and nitrogen dioxide, or the ingestion and consequent aspiration of highly volatile hydrocarbons such as lighter fluid.

Clinical Manifestations. The onset is variable, but rapid in most instances. The child often complains of a sense of oppression or pain in the chest. Cough is usually present and often produces a frothy, pink-tinged sputum. Pulse is rapid and feeble. The child is usually very pale and may be cyanotic. On physical examination, dullness to percussion and moist, bubbly rales are heard in the lower portions of the chest.

Treatment is directed at the primary disease causing the pulmonary edema. Management of myocardial failure, nephritis and the various poisonings is discussed elsewhere. The administration of oxygen is often useful in relieving some of the chest pain, and when possible is best accomplished by intermittent positive pressure. Dyspnea can often be relieved by morphine sulfate in a dosage of 0.15 mg. per kg. Antifoaming agents are not useful, and though atropine has been recommended, it is of doubtful value. If pulmonary edema is secondary to excessive parenteral administration of fluids or blood or to cardiac failure, the application of tourniquets or inflated blood pressure cuffs to the extremities or the withdrawal of blood may be lifesaving.

PULMONARY EMBOLISM AND INFARCTION

Pulmonary embolism as a recognized cause of disturbance in infants and children is rare. Emboli most often arise from thrombi in the femoral and pelvic veins and are usually postoperative complications. Fat emboli are most likely to be derived from fractured bones; on occasion they stem from necrotic tissue in the bone marrow of patients with sickle cell disease. Multiple pulmonary infarcts resulting from small emboli may be associated with severe dehydration in diarrheal disease, cyanotic heart disease, bacterial endocarditis and long-standing nutritional deficiencies. The clinical pattern is apt to be interpreted as a pneumonic process, and the diagnosis is usually made at autopsy. Emboli carrying bacteria may be responsible for multiple pulmonary abscesses.

Embolism of the pulmonary artery or its larger branches has a characteristic clinical picture. There is sudden pulmonary pain which is usually substernal, but may be pleural and radiate to the shoulder. There are dyspnea, tachycardia and signs of collapse. Though there are often no physical signs, if the infarct is sufficiently large (the base at the periphery and the apex toward the midline at the point of infarction), there may be impaired resonance and a pleural friction rub. Breath sounds may be distant or absent, and there may be moist rales. Expectorated material, which may be profuse, often contains blood. The case fatality rate is high, but recovery may occur even when the area of infarction is relatively large. Secondary infection may result in abscess formation.

Prevention. The prevention of pulmonary infarction depends essentially upon (1) prevention of vascular stasis and (2) maintenance of a good nutritional status. The latter is especially important in bedridden children. Substances which decrease the coagulability of the blood such as heparin have a limited usefulness in pediatric practice.

Treatment. Embolism of the larger branches of the pulmonary artery is a medical emergency. The child should be given morphine sufficiently often to induce quietness and allay fears, and should be placed in an oxygen tent for the relief of dyspnea and cyanosis.

REFERENCE

Robbins, S. L.: *Pathology.* 3rd ed. Philadelphia, W. B. Saunders Company, 1967.

PULMONARY SUPPURATION

BRONCHIECTASIS

The term "bronchiectasis," as commonly used, is somewhat misleading. In the strict sense the connotation is simply dilatation of bronchi, whereas the process identified consists in inflammatory destruction of bronchial and peribronchial tissue which permits accumulation of exudative material in dependent bronchi and hence distention of them in some instances. The classification of bronchiectasis based on such anatomic terms as cylindrical, fusiform, saccular or cystic has little clinical value.

Bronchiectasis is frequently misdiagnosed as chronic bronchitis, asthma or recurrent pneumonia; on the other hand, it may be present for some time without producing respiratory symptoms or may produce only minor ones. The possibility that a nonopaque foreign body may be the cause of bronchiectasis is often overlooked.

Etiology. Some cases probably represent *congenital bronchiectasis.* Though its pathogenesis is obscure, it has been postulated that an arrest in bronchial development has occurred which leads to formation of cysts; if these become infected, there is apt to be destruction of the bronchial wall. *Kartagener's syndrome* consists of dextrocardia, sinusitis and bronchiectasis, and has been reported to be manifest as early as infancy. Approximately 5 per cent of children with dextrocardia eventually have bronchiectasis; the bronchial defect is unknown, but has been thought to include defective cartilage rings. Rarely, extreme forms of pectus excavatum or scoliosis may be associated with bronchiectasis, probably as a result of inadequate pulmonary drainage. There is evidence that some cases of bronchiectasis may be familial.

In the majority of instances bronchiectasis is probably acquired after birth without relation to congenital factors, but the mechanisms involved are poorly understood. Obstruction of the bronchial tree followed by infection is one possible inciting cause. For example, it is likely that atelectasis or aspiration followed by pulmonary infection during early infancy may be a contributing factor. Measles, pertussis and pneumonia in general, once regarded as frequent antecedent infections, are rare causes of bronchiectasis. At present cystic fibrosis is the single most common underlying factor in children. Here the bronchial involvement is generalized rather than localized. Other predisposing factors include aspiration of a foreign body, often a nonopaque one, enlarged bronchopulmonary nodes due to tuberculosis, recurrent and chronic lung infections, sarcoidosis, neoplasm, lung abscess, localized cysts and emphysema with compression of other lung parenchyma, allergy, asthma and chronic sinusitis. Patients with agammaglobulinemia and dysgammaglobulinemia may have bronchiectasis, usually after repeated attacks of bacterial pneumonia and bronchitis.

It has recently been postulated that the most common cause of bronchiectasis is gastroesophageal reflux leading to chronic aspiration of gastric contents; this view is not generally accepted.

The *"middle lobe syndrome"* consists of subacute or chronic pneumonitis, bronchial obstruction and atelectasis, and is generally caused by extrinsic compression of the middle lobe bronchus by hilar nodes, followed by peribronchitis and chronic infection. On occasion this syndrome is related to congenital anomalies of the bronchi.

Reversible bronchiectasis, or "pseudobronchiectasis," occurs relatively commonly after pertussis as well as with lobar and interstitial pneumonias. Shortly after or during these illnesses the bronchi will appear cylindrically dilated on bronchography, but if these studies are repeated some months later, the changes have disappeared.

Tracheobronchomegaly is a rare congenital condition in which the distal trachea and the main bronchi are grossly dilated. A similar condition may be associated with recurrent pneumonia.

Pathology. The exact mechanism producing dilatation of peripheral bronchi is unknown, but the first destructive change is a loss of ciliated epithelium, which is regenerated as cuboidal and squamous epithelium. Concurrently, the elastic tissue within the bronchial walls disappears and thickening occurs, owing to interstitial edema, fibrosis and round cell infiltration, together with involvement of adjacent parenchymal and peribronchial tissue. In these peribronchial areas multiple abscesses may develop, and there usually is characteristic obstructive endarteritis of the small pulmonary vessels. Generally, bronchiectasis follows a segmental distribution, except in cystic fibrosis. The areas most frequently involved depend somewhat on the basic cause; most frequently affected are the right middle lobe segments, the basal segments of the lower lobes, and the lingular segments of the left upper lobe. The right lower lobe is commonly involved by aspiration of a foreign body, whereas the right middle lobe is most frequently affected by hilar lymphadenopathy.

Clinical Manifestations. In symptomatic cases, cough is invariably present and produces copious mucopurulent sputum during acute respiratory infections. The sputum is generally swallowed by young children. Physical activity of the patient or change in position, particularly while reclining, will often initiate a bout of coughing.

Recurring infections of the lower respiratory tract are common; they tend to persist and are difficult to control. The patient may be afebrile, or fever may be the only symptom. Later in the course of bronchiectasis, and particularly during acute exacerbations, hemoptysis may occur, varying in severity from streaking of the sputum to exsanguinating hemorrhage. Bronchiectasis characteristically follows a remitting and relapsing course; new pulmonary areas may or may not become involved.

Physical findings are often few, and may be absent. Moist rales may be heard; during acute exacerbations physical signs of atelectasis or diffuse pneumonitis are often present. The usual roentgen examination is never pathognomonic, although such predisposing factors as mediastinal lymph nodes or radiopaque foreign bodies may be demonstrated, as well as suggestive increased bronchovascular markings near the hilus of the lung. Atelectasis is relatively common.

With extensive bronchiectasis there is persistent dyspnea, and physical development is retarded. Ventilatory and diffusion studies may reveal more widespread or severe pulmonary involvement than suspected otherwise. Pulmonary osteoarthropathy occurs relatively late, and probably represents a systemic reaction to arteriovenous shunting.

Bronchography is essential for diagnosis, as well as to delineate the extent of disease and the segments involved. To exclude the possibility of foreign bodies, strictures or tumors, bronchoscopy is essential. When the procedure is performed, secretions of the bronchi should be obtained for culture.

Every patient with suspected or proved bronchiectasis should be examined for the presence of such possible causative factors as sinusitis, agammaglobulinemia, tuberculosis, asthma or other respiratory allergy, and cystic fibrosis.

Therapy.   Therapy of bronchiectasis in children is primarily medical. Surgery should be contemplated only in patients with localized, severe disease who fail to respond to adequate medical management. Conservative treatment includes elimination of all foci of infection in the respiratory tract, effective postural drainage and, when indicated, antimicrobial therapy. Postural drainage must be carried out intensively as long as secretions are being formed and is one of the most important aspects of medical management. Its effectiveness may be enhanced by such physiotherapeutic measures as cupped-hand percussion.

Systemic antimicrobial therapy is usually administered only during acute exacerbations in short courses of 5 to 7 days or rarely up to 2 weeks. The appropriate drug is selected on the basis of the tested antimicrobial susceptibility of bacteria isolated from sputum, obtained preferably by bronchoscopy. If cultures contain only normal flora, antibiotic therapy should not be used. The administration of antimicrobial agents by aerosol inhalation immediately following appropriate postural drainage may also be helpful, but should not be continued for excessively long periods of time, since this will encourage the establishment of a drug-resistant bacterial flora, pseudomonas being particularly likely and troublesome.

In the infrequent instances when localized disease progresses despite adequate medical management, segmental or lobar resection should be considered, even though the long-term results are often discouraging. Surgery may also be indicated when an extrinsic anatomic obstruction of the bronchus is found or when suppurative lesions exist due to aspiration of fragmented foreign bodies, especially such vegetable objects as grass fibers or fragments of peanut which elude bronchoscopic removal.

PULMONARY ABSCESS

Abscesses of the lung occur when pulmonary parenchyma becomes obstructed, infected, and then suppurative and necrotic. Abscesses may be single or multiple, and be caused by a single organism, usually aerobic, or by anaerobic flora, usually mixed. Klebsiella and staphylococcal pneumonias often result in multiple abscesses, which occur infrequently in pneumococcal, streptococcal and *H. influenzae* pneumonias. Multiple abscesses may also be associated with tuberculous or mycotic infections. More often, multiple abscesses occur in patients with such chronic pulmonary disease as cystic fibrosis or bronchiectasis, or with illnesses associated with diminished host resistance (agammaglobulinemia, agranulocytosis, the sex-linked chronic granulomatous disease of childhood, and so forth).

Solitary lung abscesses may be tuberculous or follow pneumococcal or staphylococcal pneumonia, or may stem from infected congenital cysts or be found in sequestered pulmonary tissue. Most commonly, however, a solitary lung abscess follows aspiration of a foreign body or other infected material or such surgical manipulations as tonsillectomy, adenoidectomy and tooth extractions. Abscesses associated with aspiration of tissue or foreign bodies are usually infected by bacteria normally found in the nasopharynx, such as anaerobic bacteroides, spirochetes, and various streptococci, generally not group A.

Whatever the cause, the pathologic evolution of abscess formation is similar. Initial inflammatory changes are followed by suppuration and thrombosis of the local blood vessels, which result in necrosis and liquefaction. Granulation tissue forms around the periphery of the abscess and may succeed in walling off the area, but more commonly the abscess will rupture into a bronchus and be evacuated. Contents of the abscess may be coughed up, or aspirated into other parts of the pulmonary tree, with additional abscess formation. Sputum is usually fetid, may separate into layers, and usually contains elastic fibers.

Peripheral abscesses may involve the adjacent pleura, with development of a plastic or occasionally a serofibrinous pleurisy. Abscesses may rupture into the pleural cavity and produce empyema.

On occasion, pulmonary abscesses may occur within interlobar fissures, where they are usually well encapsulated and respond poorly to antimicrobial therapy.

Clinical Manifestations.   The onset of lung abscess is occasionally insidious, but more commonly there is the sudden appearance of fever, cough and chest pain, often associated with dyspnea and tachypnea. The fever curve is often septic in type, and leukocytosis is usually marked. Physical examination may or may not reveal an area of pulmonary consolidation, depending on the location of the abscess and its size. At an early stage roentgenographic examination will usually show a wedge-shaped area of consolidation.

In untreated patients the abscess will often rupture into a bronchus within a week to 10 days after onset, with production of purulent or putrid sputum; hemoptysis is common in older children. At this time roentgenographic examination will usually reveal a cavity, with or without a fluid level, surrounded by an area of consolidation. Spontaneous drainage of the abscess may result in disappearance of symptoms within about a month. During this interval, clubbing of the fingers may appear and recurrent hemoptysis may be seen.

Treatment. Adequate treatment of pneumococcal pneumonia with penicillin will usually prevent pulmonary cavitation. With staphylococcal and klebsiella pneumonias, cavitation often occurs despite treatment, but rarely requires special therapy. It is generally enough if the underlying pneumonia is treated vigorously with suitable antimicrobial therapy. When a foreign body is suspected, bronchoscopic examination should be performed promptly for verification and removal, if possible. Bronchoscopy should be done also as soon as an abscess ruptures into a bronchus, to aspirate the purulent material and to secure bacteriologic cultures, by aerobic and anaerobic techniques. Repeated bronchoscopic aspirations will be needed for the patient who continues to cough up large quantities of purulent material. Intensive and appropriate antimicrobial therapy should be continued for at least 2 weeks. The instillation of proteolytic enzymes or antibiotics into the abscess cavity has not contributed significantly to therapy. For as long as the patient continues to bring up sputum, he should receive postural drainage and physical therapy to the chest.

When patients do not respond to initial bronchoscopic aspiration and intensive antimicrobial therapy, repeated aspirations of the abscess may lead to eventual closure of the cavity. If conservative management has not given satisfactory results in 1 month, surgical removal of the affected segment or lobe is usually carried out.

PULMONARY GANGRENE

Gangrene of the lung is extremely rare in children. It occasionally follows measles, and is seen in persons with severe immunologic deficits. The onset is usually sudden and is associated with early pulmonary hemorrhage; there is rapid development of pneumothorax and putrid empyema, death occurring quickly. Treatment consists of adequate pleural drainage and intensive antimicrobial therapy.

PULMONARY SEQUESTRATION

Pulmonary sequestration is a congenital condition in which nonfunctioning embryonic and cystic lung tissue supplied by systemic arteries is contained within otherwise normal lung parenchyma, or, less commonly, is found at an extralobar location.

This condition apparently results from maldevelopment of the primitive vascular and respiratory tissue during the time when the lungs bud from the main tracheobronchial apparatus. Histologically, the tissue is of fetal appearance and is cystic and disorganized. Most commonly, sequestered lung tissue is found in the region of the lower lobes.

Pulmonary sequestration becomes symptomatic if the tissue is infected; this may occur either by way of a fistula to normal lung tissue or through a similar connection to the digestive tract. Sequestered lung may also become infected by extension of pneumonia from neighboring lung. The primary manifestations of the condition become those of a recurrent, progressive, persistent pulmonary infection, often with suppuration and abscess formation. The patient is febrile and has cough, hemoptysis and weight loss; the signs and symptoms are indistinguishable from those found with other types of lung abscess. Roentgenographic findings do not differentiate the process from pneumonia and other lung abscesses, except that the process is generally limited to the basal segments of the lower lobes. The diagnosis of pulmonary sequestration is suggested by repeated episodes of injection involving the same basal area of the lung. Definitive diagnosis can be accomplished by bronchography or aortography. On bronchography the area of sequestration will not fill with dye, but its borders can be outlined by bronchi which are filled. Aortography will demonstrate anomalous arterial supply and give proof of the nature of the pulmonary density.

When the diagnosis has been established, resection of the sequestered area should be performed. Antimicrobial therapy is indicated prior to surgery.

REFERENCES

Bronchiectasis

Biering, A.: Childhood Pneumonia, Including Pertussis Pneumonia and Bronchiectasis: A Follow-up Study of 151 Patients. *Acta paediat.,* 45:348, 1956.

Clark, N. S.: Bronchiectasis in Childhood. *Brit. Med. J.,* 1:80, 1963.

Field, C. E.: Bronchiectasis in Childhood. I. Clinical Survey of 160 Cases. II. Aetiology and Pathogenesis, Including a Survey of 272 Cases of Doubtful Irreversible Bronchiectasis. *Pediatrics,* 4:21, 231, 1949.

Field, C. E.: Bronchiectasis: A Long-Term Follow-up of Medical and Surgical Cases from Childhood. *Arch. Dis. Childh.,* 36:587, 1961.

Visconti, R. J.: Agammaglobulinemia with Bronchopulmonary Manifestations. Report of a case. *Dis. Chest,* 48:530, 1965.

Williams, H., and O'Reilly, R. N.: Bronchiectasis in Children: Its Multiple Clinical and Pathological Aspects. *Arch. Dis. Childh.,* 34:192, 1959.

Pulmonary Abscess

Bernhard, W. F., Malcolm, J. A., and Wylie, R. H.: Lung Abscess: A Study of 148 Cases Due to Aspiration. *Dis. Chest,* 43:620, 1963.

Collins, H. A., and Daniel, R. A., Jr.: Primary Lung Abscess. *J. Thorac. & Cardiov. Surg.*, 47:383, 1964.

Pickar, D. N., and Ruoff, W. F.: Pulmonary Abscess: A Study of 70 Cases. *J. Thorac. Surg.*, 37:452, 1959.

Pulmonary Gangrene

Lewis, J. M., and Barenberg, L. H.: Pulmonary Gangrene Due to Spirochetes and Fusiform Bacilli. *Am. J. Dis. Child.*, 37:351, 1929.

Pulmonary Sequestration

Asp, K., Heikel, P. E., and Pasila, M.: Pulmonary Sequestrations in Children. *Ann. Paediat. Fenn.*, 9:270, 1963.

Simopoulos, A. P., Rosenblum, D. J., Mazumdar, H., and Kiely, B.: Intralobar Bronchopulmonary Sequestration in Children: Diagnosis by Intrathoracic Aortography. *Am. J. Dis. Child.*, 97:796, 1959.

Talalak, P.: Pulmonary Sequestration. *Arch. Dis. Childh.*, 35:57, 1960.

Diseases of the Pleura

PLEURISY

Inflammatory processes in the pleura are usually divided into 3 general types: (1) dry or plastic, (2) serofibrinous or serosanguineous, and (3) purulent pleurisy or empyema.

DRY OR PLASTIC PLEURISY

Dry or plastic pleurisy may be associated with pneumococcal pneumonia, or other acute bacterial pulmonary infections. Occasionally there is no obvious pulmonary involvement; in such instances the signs and symptoms usually develop during the course of an acute upper respiratory tract illness. The condition also is associated with tuberculosis and with mesenchymal diseases such as rheumatic fever.

The pathologic process is usually limited to the visceral pleura, which is roughened in appearance and covered with thick, yellowish-green fibrin. There are usually small amounts of yellow serous fluid, which clots rapidly upon removal. Adhesions between the pleural surfaces develop rapidly, particularly in tuberculosis, in which thickening of the pleura often occurs. Occasionally, fibrin deposition and adhesions may be sufficiently severe to produce a fibrothorax, which markedly inhibits the excursions of the lung.

Clinical Manifestations. Signs and symptoms are often overshadowed by the primary disease. The principal symptom of dry pleurisy is pain, which is exaggerated by deep breathing, coughing and straining. Often the pain is not only localized over the chest wall, but also may be referred to the shoulder or the back. Pain with breathing is responsible for grunting and guarding of respirations, the child often lying on the affected side in an attempt to decrease respiratory excursions. Early in the illness a leathery, rough, to-and-fro friction rub may be audible, but this usually disappears rapidly. Occasionally, increased dullness on percussion and suppressed breath sounds are heard when the layer of exudate is thick. On occasion, pleurisy is asymptomatic and is detected only on roentgenography. Two different radiologic pictures may be found; one consists of a diffuse haziness at the pleural surface, the other of a dense shadow which may be sharply demarcated. The latter finding may be indistinguishable from small amounts of pleural exudate. Chronic pleurisy is occasionally encountered with such conditions as atelectasis, pulmonary abscess, mesenchymal diseases and tuberculosis.

Differential Diagnosis. Plastic pleurisy must be distinguished from other diseases such as epidemic pleurodynia or trauma to the rib cage, particularly fracture of a rib, and from lesions of the dorsal root ganglia, tumors of the spinal cord, herpes zoster, gallbladder disease and trichinosis. Even if evidence of pleural fluid is not found on physical or x-ray examination, a pleural tap in suspected cases will often result in the recovery of small amounts of exudate, which, when cultured, will usually reveal the underlying bacterial cause in cases associated with an acute pneumonia. When pleurisy and pneumonia continue for more than a week, tuberculosis must be considered a causative possibility.

Treatment. Treatment should be aimed at the underlying disease. In the presence of pneumonia neither immobilization of the chest with adhesive plaster nor therapy with drugs capable of suppressing the cough reflex should be undertaken. If pneumonia is not present, or is under good therapeutic control, strapping of the chest to restrict expansion may afford relief from pain.

SEROFIBRINOUS PLEURISY

Serofibrinous pleurisy is most commonly associated with infections of the lung or with inflammatory conditions of the abdomen or mediastinum. Less commonly it is found with such mesenchymal diseases as lupus erythematosus, periarteritis or rheumatic fever. On occasion this type of effusion is seen with neoplasms of the lung, pleura or mediastinum, which may be primary or metastatic; tumors are, however, more commonly associated with a hemorrhagic pleurisy. Of infectious diseases, tuberculosis has been the most frequent cause of serofibrinous effusion, but in population groups where mycobacterial disease occurs infrequently, pneumococci have become the most common infectious agents.

Clinical Manifestations. Since serofibrinous

pleurisy is often preceded by the plastic type, the early signs and symptoms may be those of the latter illness. As fluid accumulates, pleuritic pain may disappear and the patient become asymptomatic so long as the effusion remains small, or there may be only the signs and symptoms of the underlying disease. If a large amount of fluid collects, there may be cough, dyspnea, tachypnea, orthopnea or cyanosis. Physical findings depend to some degree on the amount of effusion. Dullness to flatness may be found on percussion. There is a decrease or absence of breath sounds, a diminution in tactile fremitus, a shift of the mediastinum away from the affected side, and, on occasion, fullness of the intercostal spaces. If the fluid is not loculated, these signs may shift with changes in position. In infants, physical signs are less definite; sometimes, instead of decreased or absent breath sounds, bronchial breathing will be heard. If extensive pneumonia is present, rales and rhonchi may also be audible. Friction rubs are usually present only during the early or late plastic stage. The process is usually unilateral.

Roentgenographic examination shows a more or less homogeneous density obliterating the normal markings of the underlying lung. Small effusions may cause only obliteration of the costophrenic or cardiophrenic angles or a widening of the interlobar septa. Examination should be performed both in the supine and in the upright positions to demonstrate a shift of the effusion with change in position. The decubitus position may also be helpful.

Differential Diagnosis. Thoracentesis should always be done when pleural fluid is known to be present or is suspected. Examination of the fluid is essential to identify acute bacterial infections and may disclose tubercle bacilli. Furthermore, thoracentesis can differentiate between serofibrinous pleurisy, empyema, hydrothorax, hemothorax and chylothorax. In hydrothorax the fluid has a low specific gravity, below 1.015, and only a few mesothelial cells rather than leukocytes. Chylothorax and hemothorax usually have fluid distinctive in appearance. It is not possible to differentiate serofibrinous from purulent pleurisy without bacterial examination of the fluid. The fluid of serofibrinous pleurisy is clear or slightly cloudy and contains relatively few white cells and, occasionally, some red cells. Serofibrinous fluid may rapidly become purulent; its nature may depend on the time during the course of illness when thoracentesis is performed.

Course. Unless the fluid becomes purulent, it usually disappears relatively rapidly, particularly with bacterial pneumonias. It persists somewhat longer with mesenchymal diseases and tuberculosis and may remain or recur for a long time with neoplasms. As the effusion is absorbed, adhesions usually develop between the 2 layers of the pleura, but no functional impairment results. Pleural thickening may develop and is occasionally mistaken for small quantities of fluid or for

pulmonary infiltrates. Residual pleural thickening may persist for a long time. In general, however, the process disappears, leaving no residua.

Treatment. The treatment is that of the underlying disease. When a diagnostic thoracentesis is done, as much fluid as possible should be removed. If the underlying disease is adequately treated, there is usually no necessity for further drainage, but if sufficient fluid reaccumulates to embarrass the patient's respiration, repeated drainage should be performed.

PURULENT PLEURISY

Purulent pleurisy, or empyema, is an accumulation of pus in the pleural spaces. At present the condition is most often associated with pneumonia due to staphylococci, less frequently with pneumococci, *H. influenzae* and klebsiella. In pediatric practice, empyema is most frequently encountered during infancy.

The disease may be produced also when a lung abscess ruptures into the pleural space, by contamination introduced from trauma or thoracic surgery, or rarely by mediastinitis or by the extension of intra-abdominal abscesses.

Pathology. Most commonly, purulent pleurisy is an extensive process, consisting of a series of loculated areas involving a large portion of one or both pleural cavities. Thickening of the parietal pleura occurs. If the pus is not drained, it may dissect through the chest wall *(empyema necessitatis)*, into lung parenchyma, producing bronchopleural fistulas and pyopneumothorax, or into the abdominal cavity. Pockets of loculated pus may eventually develop into thick-walled abscess cavities, or, as the exudate organizes, the lung may collapse and be surrounded by a thick, inelastic envelope.

Clinical Manifestations. Since most purulent pleurisy occurs early in the course of bacterial pneumonia, the initial signs and symptoms are primarily those of the underlying disease. Patients treated inadequately or with inappropriate antimicrobial agents may have an interval of a few days between the clinical phase of pneumonia and the evidence of empyema. In infants, manifestations of the disease may consist only of moderate exacerbation of respiratory distress. The older child is apt to appear more toxic and in greater respiratory difficulty. Physical and radiologic findings are identical to those described for serofibrinous pleurisy; the 2 conditions can be differentiated only by thoracentesis, which should always be performed when empyema is suspected. The maximum amount of pus obtainable should be withdrawn. The physical appearance of pus produced by different organisms is not particularly distinctive; cultures must always be obtained and Gram-stained smears examined for the presence of microorganisms. Staphylococci and klebsiella are usually numerous and thus easily identified;

pneumococci and *H. influenzae* occasionally are present only in small numbers, particularly if antimicrobial therapy has been given previously.

Complications. With staphylococcal and klebsiella infections, bronchopleural fistulas and pyopneumothorax commonly develop. Other local complications encountered with any bacterial agent include purulent pericarditis, pulmonary abscesses, peritonitis secondary to rupture through the diaphragm, osteomyelitis of the ribs, and such septic complications as meningitis, arthritis and osteomyelitis. With staphylococcal empyema, septicemia occurs infrequently; it is often encountered in klebsiella, *H. influenzae* and pneumococcal infections.

Treatment. If pus is obtained by thoracentesis, closed drainage should be instituted immediately, and controlled either by an underwater seal or by continuous suction. A catheter with the largest possible internal diameter should be inserted into the site where accumulation of pus is suspected; sometimes several tubes are required to drain loculated areas. Closed drainage is usually necessary only for a week or so, even though small amounts of material will continue to drain after this time; this material is usually formed in response to the presence of the tube in the pleural cavity. There is no need to withdraw the tube gradually; rather, it should be removed all at once.

The introduction of fibrinolytic agents or proteolytic enzymes commonly produces severe systemic reactions in small children, and they do not appear to promote drainage substantially. If the chest tube is of sufficient caliber and is kept clear, a free flow of pus is obtained. The instillation of antibiotics into the pleural cavity does not improve results obtained with systemic antimicrobial therapy alone and is associated with local reactions. No attempt should be made to control empyema by multiple aspirations of the pleural cavity rather than by closed continuous drainage.

Systemic antimicrobial therapy is required; the selection of the antibiotic should be based on the in-vitro sensitivities of the responsible organism. Staphylococcal empyema in infancy is best treated by parenteral routes with penicillin G or, when applicable, with one of the penicillinase-resistant penicillins. Pneumococcal infection responds to penicillin, klebsiella to kanamycin, and *H. influenzae* to ampicillin. There is no advantage in the use of multiple antimicrobial agents. With staphylococcal or klebsiella infections, resolution of the process is slow, and systemic antimicrobial therapy is required for 3 or 4 weeks. In patients with inadequately treated empyema, extensive fibrinous changes may take place over the surface of the collapsed lungs; these may require decortication at a future date. If pneumatoceles form, no attempt should be made to treat them surgically, or by aspiration, unless they reach sufficient size to embarrass respiration or become secondarily infected.

REFERENCES

Middlekamp, J. N., Purterson, M. L., and Burford, T. H.: The Changing Pattern of Empyema Thoracis in Pediatrics. *J. Thorac. & Cardiov. Surg.,* 47:165, 1964.

Ravitch, M. M., and Fein, R.: The Changing Picture of Pneumonia and Empyema in Infants and Children. A Review of the Experience at the Harriet Lane Home from 1934 through 1958. *J.A.M.A.,* 175:1039, 1961.

Riley, H. D., Jr., and Bracken, E. C.: Empyema Due to Hemophilus Influenzae in Infants and Children. *Amer. J. Dis. Child.,* 110:24, 1965.

PNEUMOTHORAX

Pneumothorax in the neonatal period may be related to factors incident to birth and be associated with interstitial emphysema and pneumomediastinum (p. 389). In staphylococcal pneumonia in infancy the incidence of pneumothorax is relatively high (p. 918). Aside from the accidental introduction of air into the pleural cavity during thoracentesis, pneumothorax is uncommon during childhood. Pneumothorax may occur in pneumonia, usually in connection with empyema; it may also be secondary to pulmonary abscess, gangrene, infarct, rupture of a cyst or an emphysematous bleb, foreign bodies in the lung and external thoracic trauma or surgical procedures. In association with mediastinal emphysema it is an occasional complication of tracheotomy.

Pneumothorax may be associated with a serous effusion *(hydropneumothorax)* or a purulent effusion *(pyopneumothorax).* In pneumothorax the lung collapses toward the hilus, unless prevented by adhesions. Rarely is there a bilateral pneumothorax.

Clinical Manifestations. The onset is usually abrupt. When the pneumothorax is extensive, there may be pain, dyspnea and cyanosis. In infancy both symptoms and physical signs may be difficult to recognize. If the pneumothorax is only moderate in extent, there may be little displacement of intrathoracic organs and few or no symptoms.

The percussion note over the involved area is tympanitic; on auscultation respiratory sounds are feeble or absent. Larynx, trachea and heart may be shifted toward the unaffected side. The breath sounds may have an amphoric quality if there is an open fistula from air-bearing tissues into the pleural cavity. When fluid is present, there is usually a sharply delimited area of tympany above a level of flatness to percussion. It is important to determine whether the pneumothorax is an open *(tension pneumothorax)* or a closed one. The presence of amphoric breathing or of gurgling sounds synchronous with respirations when fluid is present in the pleural cavity is suggestive of an open fistula. Confirmatory evidence is provided when the pneumothorax fills rapidly after aspiration of it. Another means for determining whether a fistula is open is examina-

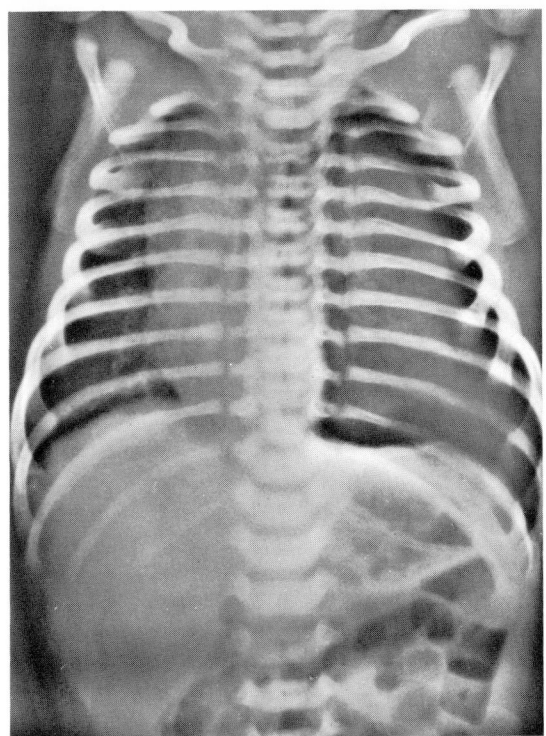

Figure 12-19. Pneumothorax in a newborn infant. The air in the left pleural cavity has resulted in partial collapse of the left lung and shift of the heart and mediastinal structures to the right.

tion of the aspirated air for its oxygen content. If a fistula is present, the oxygen content of the air in pneumothorax remains constant. If there is no connection with the bronchial tree, the oxygen content is low, since it is rapidly absorbed. The diagnosis can usually be established by roentgenographic examination (Fig. 12-19).

Differential Diagnosis. Pneumothorax must be differentiated from localized or generalized emphysema, from an extensive emphysematous bleb, from large pulmonary cavities or other cystic formations, from diaphragmatic hernia and from gaseous distention of the stomach. In most instances a simple roentgenogram will be all that is necessary for the differentiation. In the case of diaphragmatic hernia, however, a small amount of barium may be necessary to demonstrate that a portion of the gastrointestinal tract is in the thoracic cavity.

Prognosis and Treatment. The prognosis depends upon the cause. When there is no fistula connecting the air-bearing tissue and the pneumothorax, the air is usually absorbed within a week or so, and no treatment is necessary unless there are symptoms of excessive pressure, when the air should be aspirated.

Tension pneumothorax with a communicating fistula is usually best managed with a closed thoracotomy and drainage of the trapped air through a catheter whose external opening is kept in a dependent position under water. If the broncho-

pleural fistula is large, negative pressure in the drainage tube may be necessary. If the tension pneumothorax is not relieved by this means, surgical closure of the fistula should be considered. Treatment of a coexisting empyema is of course essential (p. 942).

HYDROTHORAX

In hydrothorax the fluid is noninflammatory in origin and has a lower specific gravity (less than 1.015) than that of a serofibrinous exudate. It contains less protein and fewer cells, which are mesothelial rather than leukocytic, and is usually associated with an accumulation of fluid in other parts of the body such as the peritoneal cavity and the subcutaneous tissues. Hydrothorax is most often associated with cardiac or renal disease, although on occasion it may be a manifestation of severe nutritional edema, and rarely it results from venous obstruction by neoplasms, enlarged lymph nodes or adhesions. Hydrothorax is usually bilateral in renal disease and in nutritional edema and may be in myocardial disease, although in this instance it may be limited to the right side or greater on the right than on the left side. The physical signs are those described under Serofibrinous Pleurisy (p. 940), but there is more rapid shifting of the level of dullness with changes of position. The treatment is that of the primary disorder; aspiration may be necessary when pressure symptoms are notable.

HEMOTHORAX

Extensive bleeding into the pleural cavity may result from erosion of a blood vessel in association with such inflammatory processes as tuberculosis and empyema, but is not common. It is also an occasional manifestation of intrathoracic neoplasms and blood dyscrasias, and may be the result of thoracic trauma. Rupture of an aneurysm is not likely during childhood. When a pleural hemorrhage occurs in association with a pneumothorax, it is termed *hemopneumothorax*. The diagnosis of a hemothorax can be made only by thoracentesis. In every instance an effort must be made to determine the cause, the treatment obviously depending upon it. Surgical intervention may be required to control active bleeding, and transfusion is necessary when loss of blood is excessive.

CHYLOTHORAX

Chylothorax is a rare condition at any age, but especially in childhood, though it has been observed even during the neonatal period. It depends upon the escape of chyle from the thoracic duct into the thoracic cavity. In most instances thoracic trauma has produced rupture of the duct, but the escape of chyle apparently can occur without rupture as a result of the pressure of enlarged lymph nodes or neoplasms. Thrombosis of the duct or the subclavian vein and congenital anomalies of the duct system have also been reported as causes. Chylothorax is rarely bilateral, usually being on the left side.

The symptoms and physical signs are those related to the presence of fluid in the thoracic cavity. The diagnosis is established when thoracentesis demonstrates a chylous effusion, a milky fluid containing fat, protein and other constituents of chyle. A pseudochylous milky fluid has been reported in cases of serous effusion in which the fatty material was assumed to be due to the degenerative changes within the fluid and not the presence of lymph. It has been suggested that this type of fluid can be distinguished from one containing chyle by shaking it with alkalis or ether; the fluid containing chyle tends to become clear.

Spontaneous recovery has occurred in over half of the reported cases in infants under a year of age. Repeated aspiration may be required to relieve the symptoms of pressure. The aspirated chyle has been reinjected intravenously without untoward reactions, although there is some doubt whether it has any particular benefit. The diet should be low in fat content and high in protein. The lowered intake of fat is thought to be associated with a decreased production of chyle. The high protein intake is required because of loss of protein in the chyle. The total caloric intake must be above the average requirement, and several times the daily requirements of the various vitamins, especially the fat-soluble vitamins A and D, should be added.

HEINZ F. EICHENWALD
GEORGE H. McCRACKEN, JR.

REFERENCES

Decancq, H. G., Jr.: Treatment of Chylothorax in Children. *Surg., Gynec. & Obst.,* 121:509, 1965.

Riker, W. L.: Lung Cysts and Pneumothorax in Infants and Children. *S. Clin. N. Amer.,* 36:1613, 1956.

Watson, E. H., and Foster, L. F.: Spontaneous Chylothorax in Infancy: Prognosis and Management. *Am. J. Dis. Child.,* 72:89, 1946.

13. The Cardiovascular System

THE HEART AND CIRCULATION IN HEALTH AND DISEASE

Inspection and Palpation. In early life the heart is situated somewhat higher in the chest in a more nearly horizontal position than in later years. The apex beat in the newborn infant may be palpated in the fourth left interspace in or just lateral to the left midclavicular line. After the age of 2 years the apical impulse is usually in the fifth intercostal space in or just medial to the midclavicular line. The flexibility of the mediastinum permits the heart to shift toward the side on which the patient lies. Although the relation of the apical thrust to the position of the midclavicular line is not an accurate index of cardiac size, it is helpful in making an estimate.

A hyperdynamic thrust, often extending over one or more interspaces, may accompany hypertrophy and dilatation of the ventricles. When the left ventricle is enlarged, the apex is likely to be 1 or 2 interspaces lower and farther to the left than normally. Enlargement of either ventricle, but especially of the right, tends to push the left side of the chest wall forward if the cardiac disease develops in early life when the ribs are soft and pliable. Displacement of the apex beat to the right or left without cardiac enlargement may be caused by pulmonary conditions such as empyema, atelectasis or the collapse of one lung, and sometimes by scoliosis of the spine or defects of the diaphragm.

A clinical evaluation of ventricular hypertrophy can be made by palpation of the apical impulse. In the presence of right ventricular hypertrophy the sensation of a *tap* is transmitted to the hand, whereas in left ventricular hypertrophy the apical impulse is *heaving*. Right ventricular hypertrophy is usually associated with clockwise rotation of the heart, so that the right ventricle accounts for nearly all the anterior surface of the heart. This can be appreciated by palpation of a sternal and a parasternal lift. Epigastric pulsations are commonly seen and felt in the presence of right ventricular hypertrophy, owing to the proximity of that chamber to the diaphragm. Biventricular hypertrophy can be suspected by a combination of the foregoing signs, namely, a sternal and parasternal lift associated with a left ventricular apical thrust.

Thrills may be detected during palpation; they should be timed in relation to the cardiac impulse. If the child is able to cooperate with the examiner, thrills should be felt during full expiratory apnea. Apical thrills are felt more easily in the left lateral position, and basal thrills with the patient sitting and leaning forward. Abnormal pulsations may also be detected, such as those produced by aneurysms or collateral vessels.

Percussion. Percussion of the cardiac borders in infants is difficult, owing to the thick layers of subcutaneous fat on the chest wall and the barrel shape of the thorax. The value of percussion in the diagnosis of heart disease is frequently overstressed. This method can be helpful in the evaluation of pericardial effusion, dextrocardia and movement of the mediastinum secondary to pulmonary or pleural space disease. Accurate assessments of cardiac size, shape and position can usually be made only by radiography.

Auscultation. It is generally agreed that the principal components of normal heart sounds are due to the closure of valves. The composition of these sounds is influenced by the fact that there is a normal asynchronous contraction of the ventricles whereby the onset of left ventricular systole precedes that of the right ventricle. Thus the first heart sound consists of 2 components: the first is due to mitral valve closure, and the second, to tricuspid valve closure. Similarly, the normal second sound consists of 2 components: the first is due to aortic and the second to pulmonic valve closure. This physiologic splitting of the second sound is best heard in the pulmonary area and can be detected in most normal children (Fig. 13-1). Furthermore, the split widens in inspiration and narrows in expiration, owing to the respiratory variation of pulmonary valve closure. The inspiratory delay of closure of the pulmonary valve is probably due to an increase in right ventricular stroke volume during this phase of respiration.

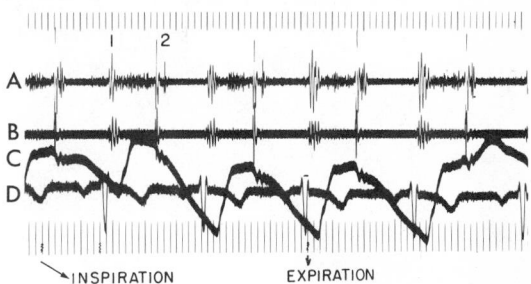

Figure 13-1. Physiologic splitting of second heart sound in a 5-year-old child with an innocent systolic murmur. Tracings from above are *(A)* phonocardiogram at pulmonary area, *(B)* phonocardiogram at apex, *(C)* carotid pulse, *(D)* electrocardiogram. Time lines 0.04 second. *1*, First heart sound; *2*, second heart sound.

Recognition of the variations in the normal splitting of the second heart sound is of considerable diagnostic importance. Wide splitting of this sound is often associated with conditions causing left-to-right shunting of blood such as may occur in atrial septal defect. In the presence of severe pulmonary stenosis the intensity of the systolic murmur frequently obscures the aortic element of the second heart sound. This produces a single soft second sound which arises from late closure of the pulmonary valve. In tetralogy of Fallot the pulmonary element of the second sound may not be audible, resulting in a single second sound due to aortic valve closure.

Ejection sounds. Aortic or pulmonic ejection sounds occurring early in systole are related to dilatation of or hypertension in the aorta and pulmonary artery. They may be mistaken for a split first heart sound. The aortic variety is more widely transmitted and may be heard at the apex, whereas pulmonary ejection sounds are heard best along the left sternal border, especially during expiration.

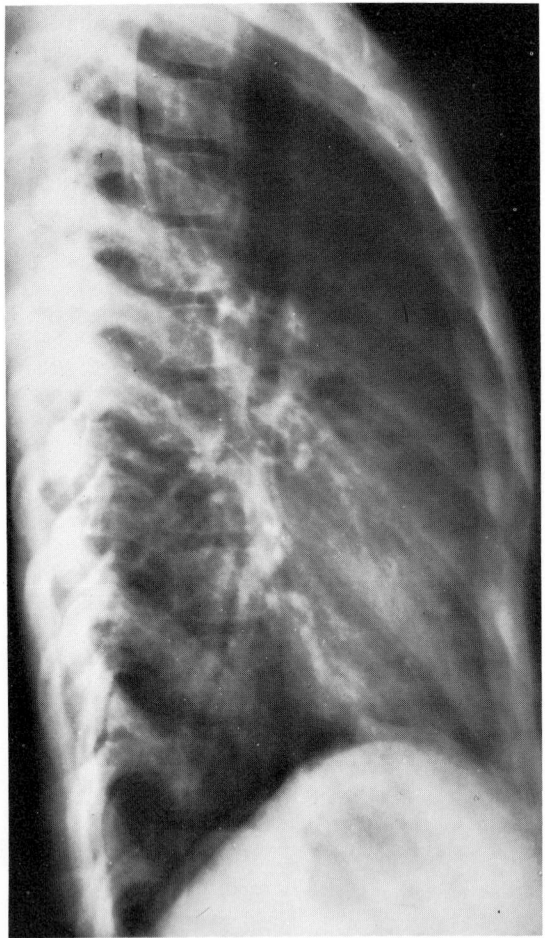

Figure 13-2. Straight-back syndrome which was associated with an innocent systolic murmur. Lateral teleroentgenogram shows absence of normal kyphosis of upper thoracic spine and narrow anteroposterior diameter of the chest.

Systolic clicks. Early systolic clicks are synonymous with ejection sounds described above. The mechanism of midsystolic and late systolic clicks and multiple systolic clicks is unknown. They are heard best at the left sternal border and apex, and their intensity and timing are affected by respiration and position of the body. In the majority of instances the clicks are innocuous and are not indicative of heart disease. It is important to recognize their benign nature and to differentiate them from pathologic sounds such as a diastolic gallop rhythm, widely split second sound and an opening snap. A functional systolic murmur may be initiated by a click. In rare instances a systolic click may initiate a late systolic murmur of mitral incompetence.

Systolic murmurs. A practical and clinically applicable classification of systolic murmurs based on abnormal hemodynamics has been described by Leatham. These murmurs have been divided into ejection and pansystolic types based on the timing of the murmur in relation to the first and second heart sounds.

EJECTION SYSTOLIC MURMURS. These are produced by (1) stenosis of the pulmonary or aortic valves or infundibular stenosis, (2) dilatation of the aorta or pulmonary artery, (3) increased blood flow through a semilunar valve, and (4) combinations of these factors. These murmurs are found clinically in aortic and pulmonary stenosis and in conditions associated with a large left-to-right shunt. Their nature is related to the timing of valve closure on the side of the heart from which it originates. Ejection murmurs start after the first heart sound because blood flow, and consequently the murmur, only begins when the ventricle raises its pressure sufficiently to open its respective semilunar valve. The murmur increases in intensity in early, mid or late systole and ends before the normal or delayed semilunar valve closure of the affected side of the heart.

PANSYSTOLIC (REGURGITANT) MURMURS. These are caused by the flow of blood from a ventricle or artery that retains a higher pressure throughout systole than the receiving chamber or vessel. They are heard most frequently in patients with mitral or tricuspid insufficiency and in ventricular septal defect. Blood flow, and consequently the murmur, begins soon after the first heart sound and continues up to the second heart sound.

Diastolic murmurs. Diastolic murmurs may be divided into the following: (1) rumbling mid-diastolic mitral or tricuspid murmurs due to increased atrioventricular flow (as in left-to-right shunts) or atrioventricular valve disease with or without stenosis, (2) early, high-pitched diastolic murmurs due to incompetence of the aortic or pulmonary valves, and (3) atrial systolic murmurs (presystolic) due to active atrial contraction in the presence of stenosis of the atrioventricular valve or to increased atrial stroke volume.

Sounds and murmurs produced by valves are not always heard at the positions of the chest wall to which these sounds might be expected to be transmitted. For example, the ejection systolic murmur of aortic stenosis may be heard best at the apex. Therefore care should be taken to auscultate the whole precordium and not to localize the examination to certain predetermined points on the left side of the chest. Murmurs of congenital heart disease in children may be widely transmitted, so that it is necessary also to auscultate both sides of the neck and the back. On the other hand, the friction of a pericardial rub may be localized fairly accurately over the area from which it emanates.

In older, cooperative children, sounds and murmurs may be more easily heard by varying the child's position, listening in various phases of respiration and noting the effects of exercise. Thus mitral systolic and diastolic murmurs are more easily heard with the child in the left lateral position, especially after exercise, and basal murmurs may be more obvious in the forward sitting position with the patient in full expiratory apnea.

Innocent murmurs. The terms "functional," "accidental" and "insignificant" have been used synonymously to designate murmurs unrelated to any demonstrable cardiac disturbance or anatomic abnormality. Though common usage has been responsible for their continuation, the term "innocent" is preferred because it stresses the innocuousness of the murmur. At a single, random auscultation approximately 30 per cent of children may be found to have an innocent murmur; the number is higher with repeated auscultations of the same children over a period of years.

In the newborn infant it is not unusual for soft midsystolic murmurs to be heard, usually to the left of the sternum in the third and fourth interspaces, but they generally disappear after a few days or weeks. In older children soft, sometimes musical or squeaky midsystolic murmurs may be heard in the area to the left of the sternum or at the base of the heart (Fig. 13-3). They may become less audible or disappear completely when the patient changes from a supine to an upright position, after mild exercise or during various phases of respiration. The loudness and even the presence of the murmur may be variable from examination to examination. Occasionally they remain constant under all conditions and persist until adolescence. Soft murmurs often develop during an acute illness or severe anemia and disappear during convalescence. The intensity of innocent systolic murmurs is usually increased during an intercurrent acute infection. The quality, location and variability of these murmurs usually indicate their innocuousness, and these patients have normal electrocardiograms and x-ray films.

The mechanism of these murmurs is not understood clearly. They may represent an increase in intensity of normal vibrations in the pulmonary artery, or a series of systolic clicks may simulate a murmur.

It is important to reassure the parents of the innocence of the murmur and to avoid unnecessary limitations of the child's activities.

A *venous hum* is produced by turbulence of blood in the jugular venous system. The hum has no pathologic significance and may be heard in the neck or anterior portion of the upper chest. It consists of a soft humming sound heard in both systole and diastole, which can be exaggerated or made to disappear by varying the position of the head or by light compression over the jugular venous system in the neck. These simple maneuvers are sufficient to differentiate a venous hum from the murmurs produced by organic cardiovascular disease, particularly patent ductus arteriosus, from which the sound is frequently indistinguishable.

Innocent cardiac murmurs may also be produced by the *straight-back syndrome.* This consists of loss of the concavity of the upper thoracic spine with resultant decrease of the anteroposterior diameter of the chest. This syndrome results in innocent systolic ejection murmurs; at times the murmur is accentuated in late systole. Lateral chest x-rays are diagnostic, since they demonstrate the straight dorsal spine (Fig. 13-2).

Arterial Pulse. The *cardiac rate* of newborn infants is rapid and subject to wide fluctuations. The average rate, ranging from 120 to 140 beats per minute, may increase to 170 or more during crying and activity and drop to between 70 and 90 during sleep. As the child grows older the average pulse rate becomes slower. Table 13-1 lists rates compiled from several sources.

Throughout childhood the pulse rate is labile and increases rapidly in response to muscular activity or emotional stimuli. The average rate is

TABLE 13-1. AVERAGE PULSE RATES AT REST

AGE	LOWER LIMITS OF NORMAL	AVERAGE	UPPER LIMITS OF NORMAL
Newborn	70	120	170
1-11 months	80	120	160
2 years	80	110	130
4 years	80	100	120
6 years	75	100	115
8 years	70	90	110
10 years	70	90	110

	GIRLS	BOYS	GIRLS	BOYS	GIRLS	BOYS
12 years	70	65	90	85	110	105
14 years	65	60	85	80	105	100
16 years	60	55	80	75	100	95
18 years	55	50	75	70	95	90

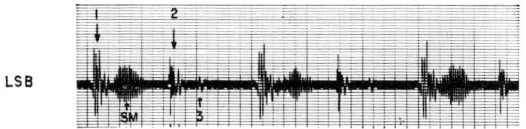

Figure 13-3. Phonocardiogram of innocent systolic murmur. *LSB,* Left sternal border; *1,* first heart sound; *2,* second heart sound; *3,* third heart sound; *SM,* short musical systolic murmur. Time lines 0.04 second.

generally higher in the afternoon than in the morning and more rapid after than before eating.

Tachycardia persisting for weeks or months has been observed in adolescents, especially girls, without any discernible cause. Persistent tachycardia (over 200 in newborns, 150 in infants or 120 in older children) should be investigated to exclude pathologic arrhythmias. The apprehension induced by a visit to the physician will often cause a fast rate at the time of examination. In order to determine the cardiac rate when it is not influenced by external stimuli, the pulse rate should be recorded several times throughout the day or night when the child is quiet or asleep.

Slow pulse rates are rare in children until the adolescent period, when rates as low as 50 to 60 per minute may be encountered, particularly in athletic boys.

The *rhythm of the cardiac beat* in the newborn infant is often irregular and seems to be closely related to respiration. When the infant is asleep, there may be periods of apnea and a slow cardiac rate, but when respiratory movements are resumed, the pulse rate speeds up again. This arrhythmia is exaggerated in premature infants and in those who have suffered from shock or intracranial hemorrhage.

Diagnostic information may also be obtained by analysis of the *quality* and *amplitude* of the peripheral pulse. A water-hammer pulse in the forearm or a Corrigan pulsation in the carotid arteries signifies a large pulse pressure commonly found in patent ductus arteriosus, aortic insufficiency or general vasodilatation. Capillary pulsation often accompanies such a finding. An anacrotic or plateau pulse of small volume signifies aortic stenosis, and pulsus bisferiens suggests combined aortic insufficiency and stenosis. Examination of the peripheral pulse should not be localized to the radial artery, but should include inspection and palpation of all major accessible arteries. Comparison of the amplitude of pulsation of the arteries on both sides of the body may help to localize a point of proximal compression. Routine examination of all infants and children should include palpation of the femoral vessels. Characteristically, the femoral pulsation is diminished or delayed in nearly all cases of coarctation of the aorta.

Arterial Blood Pressure. It is often difficult to determine arterial blood pressure with accuracy in infants and young children. The patient must be quiet, and the arm cuff should be wide enough to cover about two thirds of the upper arm. Erroneously high readings are obtained with narrower cuffs, and the converse with wider cuffs. When the thigh is used as the site for measuring blood pressure, the cuff should likewise cover two thirds of its surface area, especially when the pressure in this location is to be compared with that in the arm. Ordinarily the pressure in the legs with the cuff technique is about 20 mm. Hg higher than in the arms.

The *flush method* for estimating blood pressure is frequently used in infants because of the diffi-

TABLE 13-2. AVERAGE BLOOD PRESSURES OF CHILDREN

AGE	SYSTOLIC	DIASTOLIC
4	85	60
5	87	60
6	90	60
7	92	62
8	95	62
9	98	64
10	100	65
11	105	65
12	108	67
13	110	67
14	112	70
15	115	72
16	118	75

culties of the auscultatory method in these small patients. The infant must be quiet and in the supine position. A blood pressure cuff is applied to the wrist or ankle. The part of the extremity distal to the cuff is compressed by firm wrapping. The cuff is inflated to about 200 mm. Hg and the wrapping removed. The pressure in the cuff is released slowly until the blanched part of the extremity flushes. This point is an approximate index of mean arterial pressure.

The *oscillometric method* is also applicable to infants. As the pressure in the inflated cuff is lowered, an abrupt increase in oscillations indicates the systolic pressure; subsequent diminution indicates the diastolic pressure.

The blood pressure varies with the age of the child and is closely related to his height and weight. Significant increases occur during adolescence, with many temporary variations before the more stable levels of adult life are attained. Exercise, excitement, coughing and straining may raise the systolic pressure of children as much as 40 to 50 mm. above their usual levels. Variability of blood pressure among children of approximately the same age and body build must be expected. Table 13-2 was prepared by averaging data of the blood pressures of normal children from several studies.

In infancy and early childhood the blood pressure readings are approximately the same as those of the 4-year-old child listed in the table.

Persistent elevation of the systolic and diastolic pressures, and especially of the latter, requires investigation. The renal causes of persistent hypertension include acute and chronic glomerulonephritis, pyelonephritis, hydronephrosis, hypoplastic kidneys, Wilms's tumor, stenosis of the renal artery, and renal trauma. Coarctation of the aorta (thoracic or abdominal) or aortic arteritis may result in persistent hypertension. Adrenal causes include pheochromocytoma, adrenogenital syndrome, neuroblastoma, Cushing's disease and primary hyperaldosteronism; hypertension may also complicate steroid therapy.

Venous Pulse. Inspection of the cervical veins may yield considerable diagnostic information.

The patient should be propped in bed at an angle of about 45 degrees with his neck muscles relaxed. Distention of the external jugular veins, owing to constriction of their passage through the deep cervical fascia, occurs in many normal children. Distention and pulsation of veins situated above the sternal angle are otherwise abnormal. Increased venous pressure transmitted to the internal jugular vein may appear as venous pulsations without visible distention. Such pulsation does not occur in normal children reclining at an angle of 45 degrees. The height of venous pressure can be measured by observing the vertical height to which the distended and pulsating portion of the vein rises above the sternal angle. This clinical observation is of great help, since the difficulties of measuring the resting venous pressure by venipuncture in small patients often preclude the determination of exact pressure.

Venous pulsations may be distinguished from those of arteries in the following ways (Wood): (1) Venous pulsations undulate, yield readily to pressure, vary with the position of the patient, and usually have multiple components, whereas those of the carotid artery are single, abrupt, only compressible with moderate pressure and do not vary with the patient's position. (2) Abdominal pressure, especially over the right hypochondrium, increases the height of the venous pulse, but has no effect on the arterial pulsation. (3) Mild compression of the external jugular vein in the supraclavicular fossa will abolish venous pulsations and distend the vein, but will not affect the carotid pulsation. (4) The height of venous pulsation will increase with expiration and decrease with inspiration. Arterial pulsations are not affected by respiration.

The normal jugular phlebogram or direct tracings from the superior vena cava show 3 positive components corresponding to each cardiac cycle. They are termed "a," "c" and "v," respectively (Fig. 13-4). The "a" wave is synchronous with atrial systole, the "c" wave with early ventricular systole, and the "v" wave with atrial diastole. Since the great veins are in direct communication with the right atrium, changes of pressure and volume of this chamber are transmitted to the veins.

For example: (1) In congestive cardiac failure the increased right atrial pressure is transmitted to the cervical veins. The main pulsation at the upper part of distribution of these veins appears to be in late diastole. (2) Cardiac compression due to pericardial effusion or constriction increases the jugular pressure, but the amplitude of venous pulsation is small. (3) In relatively severe pulmonic stenosis the right ventricular diastolic pressure may be elevated. Emptying of the right atrium is dependent upon a systolic pressure in excess of the right ventricular diastolic pressure. A conspicuous presystolic "a" wave is present under these conditions. Similar "a" waves may be detected in patients with pulmonary stenosis and right ventricular hypertrophy with a normal right ventricular end-diastolic pressure. In these instances the

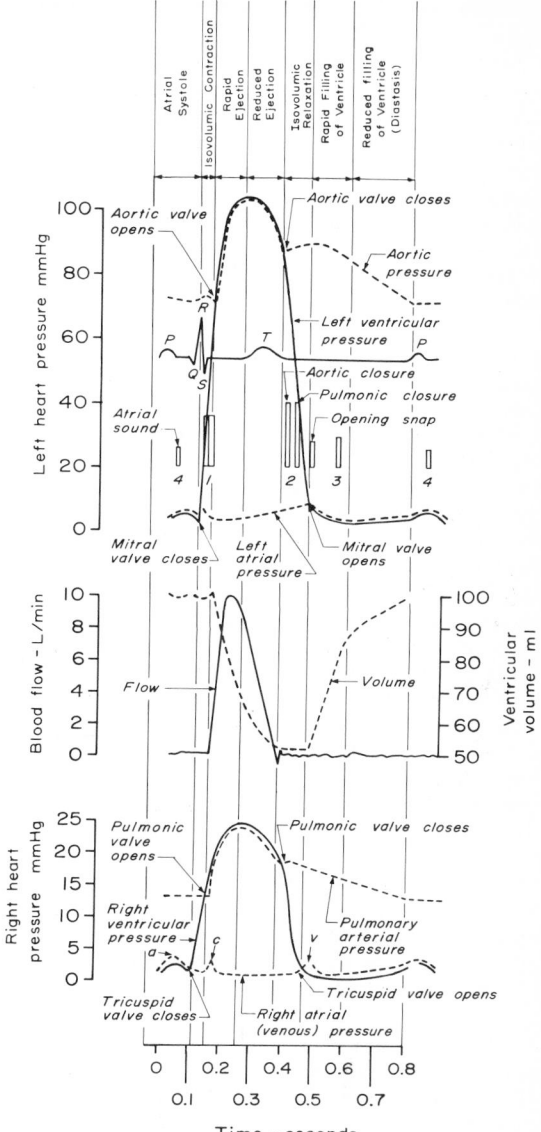

Figure 13-4. Idealized diagram of temporal events of a cardiac cycle.

mechanism of the "a" wave is due to a decreased distensibility of the right ventricle during diastole. (4) A presystolic "a" wave may be present in tricuspid stenosis or atresia, and the transmission of this wave to the inferior vena cava and hepatic veins produces presystolic hepatic pulsations. (5) In tricuspid insufficiency some of the right ventricular systolic pressure is transmitted to the right atrium, resulting in large conspicuous venous pulsations, which correspond to ventricular systole and produce a fusion of the "c" and "v" waves. (6) In complete heart block the occurrence of cervical venous pulsations will depend on the position of the tricuspid valve at the time of atrial systole. If the right atrium contracts when the tricuspid valve is closed, a large venous pulsation will occur. (7) In superior vena caval obstruction the jugular venous pressure is increased, but the veins do not pulsate.

Direct determinations may be made by inserting a needle in a peripheral vein. The venous pressure may be read on a water manometer, using the sternal angle as the reference point. By this method the average venous pressure of children over the age of 3 years is about 50 mm. of water.

Roentgenographic Examinations. Roentgenographic examinations furnish the most accurate information about cardiac size and shape. Many variations occur, owing to differences in body build, the phase of respiration or cardiac cycle, abnormalities of the thoracic cage, subdiaphragmatic pressure or pulmonary disease which may displace the heart to one side or the other.

Fluoroscopy. Fluoroscopic examination, utilizing image intensification to reduce exposure to harmful rays, provides important information about the size, configuration and pulsation of specific cardiac chambers and great blood vessels. Recording on video tape allows review of the findings after the study is completed; recording on motion pictures increases the amount of irradiation. Not only the heart, but also the great vessels, lungs, thoracic cage and diaphragm must be observed.

In infants the thymic shadow may overlap the shadow cast by the base of the heart. In the posteroanterior view the left border of the cardiac shadow consists of 3 convex shadows produced from above downwards by the aortic knob, the pulmonary arc and the left ventricle, respectively (Fig. 13-5). In cases of moderate to gross left atrial enlargement the atrium may project between the opposing movements of the pulmonary artery and of the left ventricle. Angiocardiographic and cardiac catheterization studies have conclusively proved that the outflow tract of the right ventricle or the pulmonary conus does not contribute to the shadows formed by the left border of the heart (Fig. 13-5). The aortic knob is not as easily seen in infants and children as in adults. Three structures also contribute to the right border of the cardiac silhouette; from above downward they are the superior vena cava, the ascending aorta and the right atrium. It is of fundamental importance also to assess the degree of pulmonary vascularity as represented by the intrapulmonary shadows. Angiocardiographic studies have shown that the hilar shadows are mainly vascular. Pulmonary overcirculation is usually associated with left-to-right shunts, and undercirculation with stenosis of the outflow tract of the right ventricle or pulmonary valve.

Fluoroscopic examination is not complete until the cardiac shadows have been studied in both oblique and lateral views (Fig. 13-5). The right anterior oblique view is optimal for the study of the left atrium and main pulmonary artery, whereas the left anterior oblique view is used for evaluation of the left and right ventricles, the aorta and the left atrium.

The esophagus is closely related to some of the cardiac chambers and great blood vessels, and its visualization with a barium emulsion helps further to delineate these structures, especially in the right anterior oblique view. The esophagus is

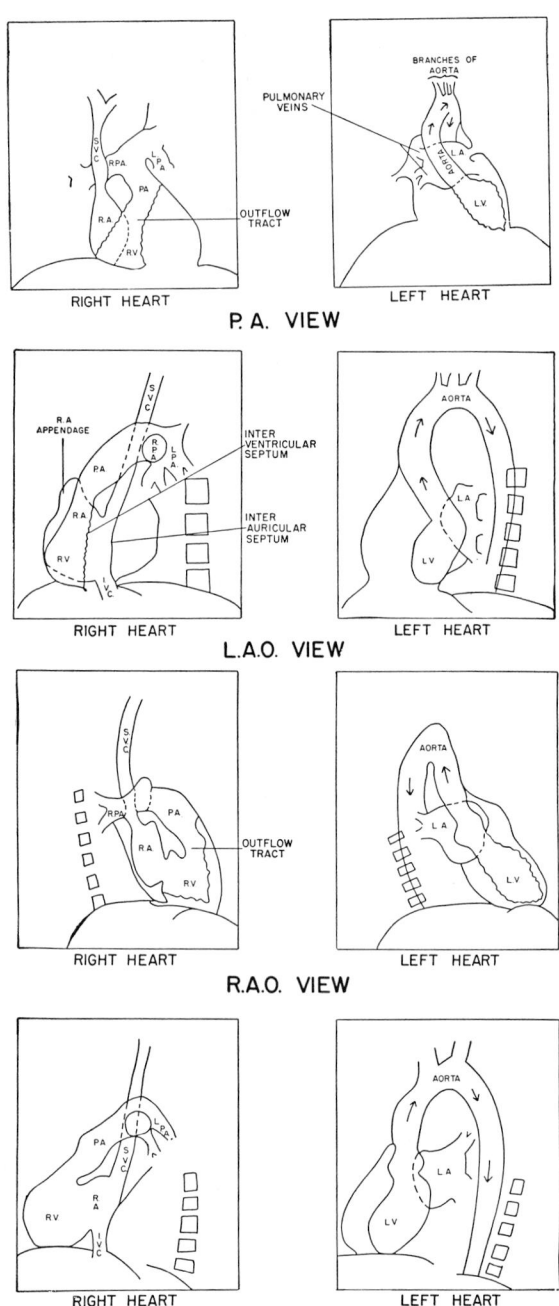

Figure 13-5. Idealized diagrams showing the normal position of the cardiac chambers and great blood vessels. Abbreviations are as follows: *P.A.*, posteroanterior; *L.A.O.*, left anterior oblique; *R.A.O.*, right anterior oblique; *S.V.C.*, superior vena cava; *R.A.*, right atrium; *R.V.*, right ventricle; *P.A.*, pulmonary artery; *R.P.A.*, right pulmonary artery; *L.P.A.*, left pulmonary artery; *L.A.*, left atrium; *L.V.*, left ventricle; *I.V.C.*, inferior vena cava. (Adapted and redrawn from Dotter and Steinberg: Angiocardiographic Interpretation. *Radiology,* Vol. 53.)

indented in turn by the aorta, pulmonary artery and left atrium from above down.

Interpretation of atrial or ventricular enlargement in infants and children by radiographic means is difficult. A hypertrophied ventricle may displace a normal chamber, giving a false impression of ventricular enlargement. Thus posterior displacement of a normal left ventricle by a hypertrophied right ventricle may cause the radiographic picture to resemble that of biventricular enlargement. The roentgenograms of patients with tetralogy of Fallot may not indicate the presence of right ventricular hypertrophy; conversely, the cardiac silhouette of patients with tricuspid atresia and an underdeveloped right ventricle may give the false impression of right ventricular hypertrophy. It is therefore apparent that the radiographic findings should be complemented by an electrocardiogram, which is a more sensitive and accurate index of ventricular enlargement.

Teleroentgenograms. Taken with the roentgen tube approximately 6 feet from the patient, teleroentgenograms represent fairly accurately the size of the heart and chest. For a complete assessment of cardiac configuration, posteroanterior, oblique and lateral views are essential. The positions of the various cardiac chambers and great vessels are shown in Figure 13-5.

The most frequently used measurement of cardiac size is the maximum width of the cardiac shadow in posteroanterior teleroentgenograms. When the cardiac width is more than half of the maximal chest width,* the heart is usually enlarged. The cardiothoracic ratio is a less accurate index of cardiac enlargement in infancy than in subsequent years, because the horizontal position of the heart may increase the ratio to more than half in the absence of true enlargement. In children with vertical hearts the cardiothoracic ratio will tend to give an erroneously low impression of the true heart size.

The width of the heart also bears a fairly definite relation to other body measurements. The transverse diameter is approximately 7 or 8 per cent of the body height and is more closely related to this factor than to age or weight.

The Electrocardiogram. The electrocardiogram in pediatric practice is not only of diagnostic aid in congenital and rheumatic heart diseases, but also is frequently helpful in the detection and management of disturbances of electrolyte metabolism, endocrine and metabolic diseases and acute infections. Electrocardiographic examination is not complete unless the standard leads are supplemented by the unipolar limb leads and multiple chest leads. It is beyond the scope of this text to discuss the physiologic concepts of unipolar

electrocardiography. A study of standard leads is valuable in the diagnosis of arrhythmias and for measurements of the duration of various parts of the cardiac cycle.

A wide electrocardiographic exploration of the chest is advised in children and especially in infants. In addition to the conventional leads of V_1 through V_6, leads over the right chest (V_{4R} or V_{3R}) are essential for adequate assessment of right ventricular activity.

The normal electrocardiogram.[†] In the majority of children the electrical position of the heart is vertical with varying degrees of clockwise rotation[‡] (Fig. 13-6). In a minority of cases the heart may assume a horizontal position. The unipolar chest leads have a different pattern from that observed in the normal adult. In infants the right ventricular surface leads show an Rs pattern which usually persists for the first 2 years of life and may be found up to the age of 4 years (Fig. 13-7). The T waves are inverted in V_{4R}, V_{3R}, V_1, V_2 and V_3 in almost all infants and may remain inverted in V_{4R}, V_{3R} and V_1 up to the middle of the second decade of life. In the first 24 to 48 hours of life the T wave is usually upright in V_{4R}, V_{3R} and V_1, and may be inverted in V_5 and V_6. Because of these normal patterns of the QRS-T in infants and children, the changes produced by right ventricular hypertrophy are different from those in adults. The diagnosis of ventricular hypertrophy is sometimes based on the increased voltage of the R and S waves in the unipolar chest leads. Nevertheless, since the height of these waves is mainly governed by the proximity of the exploring electrode to the surface of the heart, and since the chest wall of infants and children is relatively thin, the diagnosis of ventricular hypertrophy should not be

---

[†]In this text capitalized letters refer to waves of high voltage (tall or deep waves), and small letters are used to designate waves of low voltage.

[‡]In clockwise rotation the right ventricle moves to occupy more of the anterior surface of the heart.

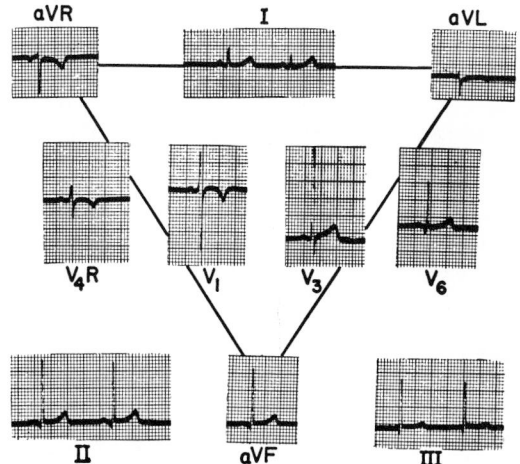

Figure 13-6. Electrocardiogram of a normal child. Note the relatively tall R waves and inversion of the T waves in V_{4R} and V_1.

---

*To obtain the maximal cardiac width in a posteroanterior midinspiration teleroentgenogram, a vertical line is drawn down the middle of the sternal shadow, and perpendicular lines are then drawn from the sternal line to the extreme right and left borders of the heart. The sum of the lengths of these lines is the maximal cardiac width. The maximal chest width is obtained by drawing a horizontal line between the right and left inner borders of the rib cage at the level of the top of the right diaphragm.

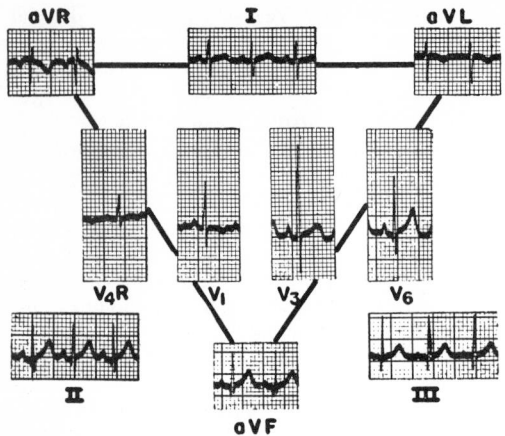

Figure 13-7. Normal infant's electrocardiogram. Note the tall R and small s waves in V_{4R} and V_1 and the inverted T wave in these leads.

based on voltage changes alone. The normal electrocardiographic pattern of infants and children has been described by Ziegler and others.

Electrocardiographic abnormalities. See abnormalities of cardiac rhythm (p. 1017).

The P wave. Tall, narrow and spiked P waves are seen in congenital pulmonary stenosis (Fig. 13-8), Ebstein's anomaly of the tricuspid valve (p. 980), tricuspid atresia and sometimes in cor pulmonale. These abnormal waves are probably due to right atrial hypertrophy, are usually taller than 2.5 mm. and are most obvious in standard lead II and leads V_{4R}, V_{3R} and V_1. Similar waves are sometimes seen in thyrotoxicosis. Flat and widened P waves, commonly bifid, are seen in chronic mitral stenosis and are probably due to left atrial hypertrophy. Flat P waves may be found in hyperkalemia. Inversion of the P wave occurs in all leads in nodal rhythm, in standard lead I in dextrocardia and occasionally in standard leads II and III without obvious cause.

Prolongation of the P-R interval. This abnormality is a form of heart block. Permanent prolongation of the P-R interval may be congenital or due to scarring from rheumatic carditis. Any active carditis, including acute rheumatic fever, may produce transient prolongation of the P-R interval. Other causes of temporary prolongation include digitalis therapy and carotid sinus pressure. No treatment is required specifically for this abnormality.

Right ventricular hypertrophy. *Right ventricular surface leads* of infants and children differ from those of adults, and tracings of the right side of the chest (V_{4R} or V_{3R}) are essential in young children. Review of electrocardiographic tracings in infants with known *right ventricular hypertrophy* has shown that the following changes may occur singly or in combination (Fig. 13-9): (1) a qR pattern in the right ventricular surface leads; (2) a positive T wave in leads V_{4R} through V_3 after the first 24 to 48 hours of life; (3) a monophasic R wave in V_{4R}, V_{3R} or V_1; (4) prolongation of the ventricular

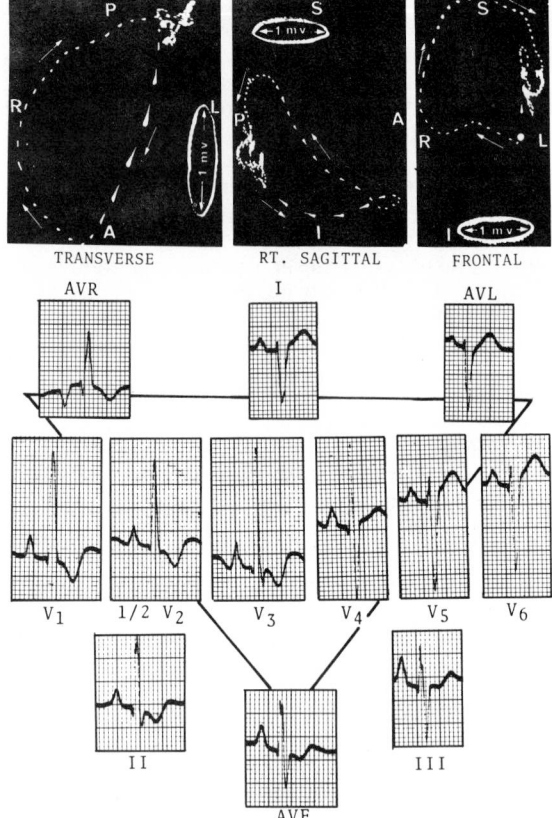

Figure 13-8. Electrocardiogram and vectorcardiogram of a 10-year-old girl with severe pulmonary hypertension. Prominent right atrial and ventricular hypertrophy is evident. Note prominent P waves and qR in right precordial leads. The QRS loop is of large voltage and is displaced anteriorly and to the right.

activation time in right ventricular surface leads to greater than 0.03 second; (5) the R wave in the right chest leads is usually taller than 7 mm., but this sign alone is not sufficient for the diagnosis; (6) aVR may show a QR pattern; (7) in the presence of incomplete right bundle branch block, right ventricular hypertrophy is indicated by a tall secondary R wave.

Older children and adolescents who have right ventricular hypertrophy show the same changes, but in addition may have the following abnormalities of the R and S waves of the unipolar leads: (1) the sum of RV_1 or RV_{3R} and SV_5 or SV_6 totals 11 mm. or more; (2) the depth of the S wave in V_1, V_{3R} or V_{4R} is less than 2 mm. It cannot be overstressed that the evaluation of ventricular hypertrophy should not be based on voltage changes alone.

Cabrera and Sodi-Pallares have correlated abnormal hemodynamics with electrocardiographic patterns. They have shown that obstruction to right ventricular and pulmonary flow (e.g. with pulmonary stenosis and primary pulmonary hypertension) is associated with a *systolic overload pattern.* This is characterized by an increasingly tall and late R wave in the right precordial leads.

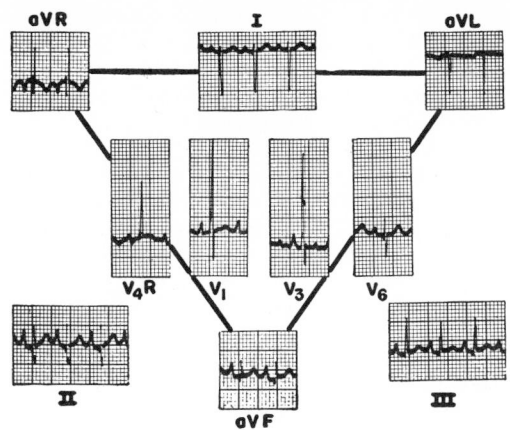

Figure 13-9. Electrocardiogram showing right ventricular hypertrophy in an infant with tetralogy of Fallot. Note the spiked P waves in lead II, monophasic wave in V_{4R}, delay in the ventricular activation time in V_{4R} and V_1 and the positive T waves in V_{4R} and V_1.

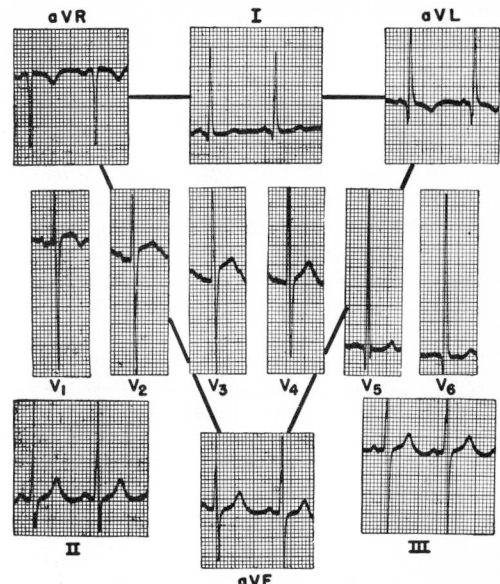

Figure 13-10. Electrocardiogram showing left ventricular hypertrophy in a 12-year-old boy with chronic rheumatic heart disease. Note the tall R in V_6, deep S in V_1, deep, wide Q and inverted T in a V_L.

In these leads the T wave is initially upright and later becomes inverted (Figs. 13-8, 13-9). In contradistinction, *diastolic overload* of the right ventricle (e.g. with atrial septal defect) is characterized by the pattern of incomplete or occasionally complete right bundle branch block (Fig. 13-11). Although this concept appears to be true in extreme examples, there are many instances in which the dynamics of systolic overload may be associated with right ventricular hypertrophy showing a pattern of incomplete right bundle branch block.

Left ventricular hypertrophy. The following features, alone or in combination, suggest dominance of the left ventricle (Fig. 13-10): (1) depression of the S-T segment and inversion of the T waves in left ventricular surface leads (i.e. V_5, V_6 or V_7; aVF if the heart is vertical and aVL if the heart is horizontal); (2) delayed onset of the ventricular activation time in V_5 or V_6 (greater than 0.04 second); (3) increased voltage of the QRS complex; and (4) a significant Q wave in left ventricular surface leads. In older children or adolescents the sum of the left ventricular potentials (i.e. RV_6 and SV_1) is greater than 35 mm. Also RV_5 or RV_6 exceeds 26 mm. If the heart is vertical, RaVF exceeds 20 mm., and in a horizontal heart RaVL exceeds 11 mm. It is again stressed that the evaluation of ventricular dominance should not be based on voltage changes alone.

Cabrera and Sodi-Pallares applied their concept of overload of the ventricles to the left side of the heart. They suggest that *systolic overload of the left ventricle* is characterized by depression of the S-T segment and inverted T waves in the left precordial leads. *Diastolic overload of the left ventricle* is suggested by tall R waves with a late activation time and tall upright and symmetrically peaked T waves in the left precordial leads. The foregoing electrocardiographic diagnoses, especially diastolic overload of the left ventricle, are frequently difficult to establish (Nadas).

Bundle branch block. Complete right or *left bundle branch block* is not frequently encountered in pediatric practice, except in patients who have undergone ventriculotomy during open-heart surgery. The electrocardiographic pattern does not differ from that in adults. *Incomplete right bundle branch block* with or without right ventricular hypertrophy is not uncommon. Incomplete right bundle branch block is suggested by an early r wave and a late R′ in the right precordial leads and a relatively broad SV_6. This can be a normal variant. Right ventricular hypertrophy, however, especially of the outflow, may produce the same pattern. In these patients the secondary R wave may be taller (Fig. 13-11). If there is associated right ventricular hypertrophy, the secondary R wave in the right precordial leads is tall and

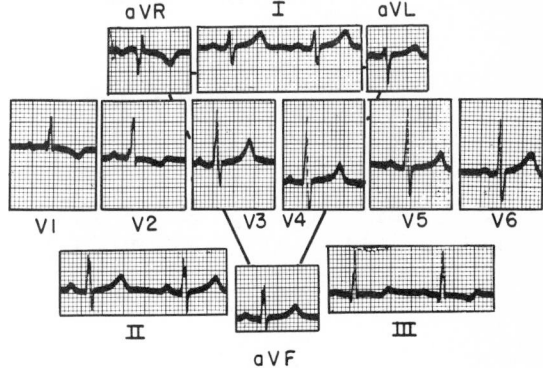

Figure 13-11. Electrocardiogram showing right ventricular outflow hypertrophy in a patient with an ostium secundum atrial septal defect. Note rsR′ in V_1 and deep, stumpy S in V_6.

usually exceeds 10 mm. It is often difficult to differentiate incomplete right bundle branch block from right ventricular hypertrophy, and it has been suggested that the pattern of incomplete right bundle branch block may in fact be due to right ventricular outflow hypertrophy.

Duration of electrical systole (Q-T interval). The duration of the Q-T interval (electrical systole) varies with the cardiac rate, and many formulas have been devised in an attempt to adjust this differential. Taran and Szilagyi's modification of Bazett's formula states that the corrected Q-T interval (Q-TC) equals the measured Q-T interval divided by the square root of the cycle length (R-R interval). The normal Q-TC is variously given as 0.38 ± 0.04. It is often lengthened in children with hypokalemia, hypocalcemia and in some patients with myocarditis (Figs. 13-12, 13-13). In

hypokalemia and hypocalcemia prolonged electrical systole is due to a lengthened Q-U interval. A shortened Q-TC may be found after administration of digitalis and with pericarditis or hyperkalemia.

S-T segment and T wave abnormalities. In generalized pericarditis superficial epicardial involvement may cause elevation of the S-T segment, followed by abnormal T wave inversion as healing progresses. Administration of digitalis is associated with sagging of the S-T segment and abnormal inversion of the T wave. Depression of the S-T segment may also occur in conditions producing myocardial hypoxia, e.g. anemia and carbon monoxide poisoning.

A group of abnormalities of special interest which produce S-T segment depression and sharp inversion of the T waves and which usually cannot be differentiated by the electrocardiogram alone includes endocardial sclerosis, aberrant origin of the left coronary artery from the pulmonary artery, glycogen storage disease of the heart, myocardial tumors and gargoylism. Aberrant origin of the left coronary artery from the pulmonary artery may lead to changes indistinguishable from those seen in acute myocardial infarction in adults. Similar changes may occur in progeria with degenerative coronary artery lesions and calcinosis of the coronary arteries.

In any form of carditis, especially diphtheritic, simple inversion of the T wave may occur. Hypothyroidism may produce flat or inverted T waves in association with generalized low voltage. In hyperkalemia the T waves are commonly of high voltage and are tent-shaped (Fig. 13-14).

Vectorcardiography. Vectorcardiography (VCG) is a study of the whole electrical activation of the heart. The spread of depolarization and repo-

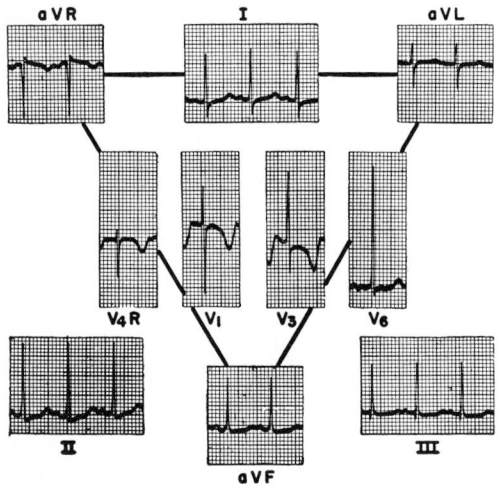

Figure 13-12. Electrocardiogram in hypocalcemia and hypokalemia (serum calcium 1.8 mEq./L.; serum potassium 2.2 mEq./L. at time of tracing). Note prolongation of electrical systole due to long S-TU segment. This graph also shows left ventricular hypertrophy.

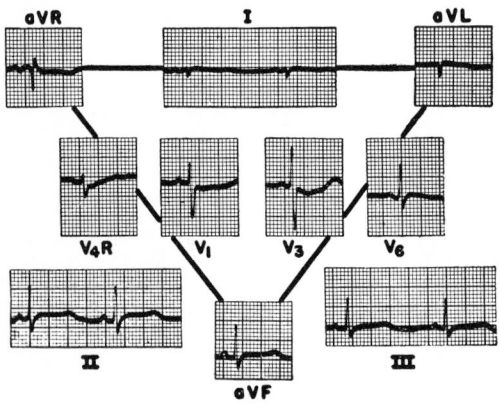

Figure 13-13. Electrocardiogram in hypokalemia (serum potassium 2.7 mEq./L.; serum calcium 4.8 mEq./L. at time of tracing). Note the prolongation of electrical systole due to a widened TU wave, especially in leads II, III and aV$_F$; also depression of the S-T segment in V$_{4R}$, V$_1$ and V$_3$.

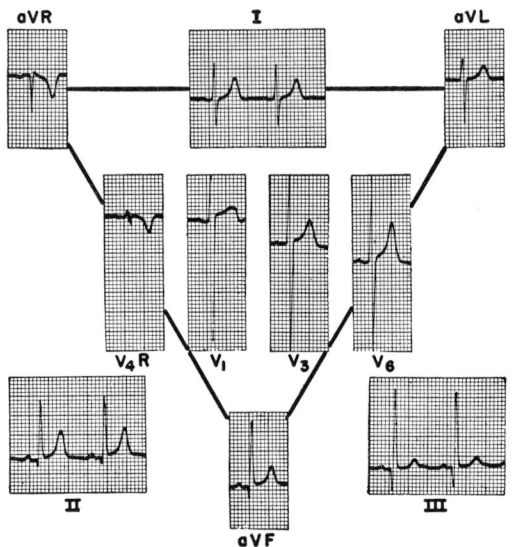

Figure 13-14. Electrocardiogram in hyperkalemia. (Serum potassium 6.5 mEq./L.; serum calcium 5.1 mEq./L.) Note the tall, tent-shaped T waves, especially in leads I, II and V$_6$.

larization through the heart muscle is a succession of innumerable instantaneous electrical forces or vectors. The recording of the direction, magnitude and orientation of these vectors in a single curve constitutes the vectorcardiographic loop (VCGsE). It is considered that these electrical forces arise from a common site, the so-called electromotive (E) point or zero (0) point. Three loops are recorded with each cardiac cycle: P loop (PsE), QRS loop (QRSsE) and T loop (TsE). Reference lead systems have been devised to record the vectorcardiogram in 3 planes: transverse or horizontal, sagittal and frontal. Analysis of vectorcardiographic loops includes evaluation of spatial position, direction of rotation (clockwise or counterclockwise), speed of inscription and spatial relation of QRS and T loops. Normal loops end at their point of origin (E point), resulting in a closed loop.*

The normal P loop is small, is inscribed slowly, rotates counterclockwise in the horizontal or frontal plane and is usually oriented to the left, forward and downward. The normal QRS loop has a great amplitude, is inscribed rapidly, rotates counterclockwise in the horizontal plane and clockwise in the sagittal plane. In the frontal plane the rotation is either clockwise or counterclockwise. QRSsE is oriented to the left downward and backward. The intermediate portion of the loop is inscribed most rapidly. The normal T loop is inscribed slowly, is small and is enclosed in QRSsE in at least 2 planes. In the child it is directed backwards.

Right ventricular hypertrophy or overload is associated with QRSsE located to the right and forward. In the horizontal plane the loop is oriented clockwise and counterclockwise in the sagittal plane (i.e. opposite to normal). *Left ventricular hypertrophy or overload* is associated with an exaggeration of the normal physiologic dominance of the left ventricle. QRSsE shows a predominance of the electrical forces directed to the left and backward.

Although the vectorcardiogram is a useful tool for the better understanding of the electrical phenomena of the heart, its place in the clinical management of children with heart disease is difficult to evaluate. The many different reference lead systems in use make vectorcardiograms difficult to analyze uniformly and to correlate with physiologic and pathologic findings.

Hematologic Data. The normal variations of the blood picture in infancy should be borne in mind in evaluation of cardiovascular disease. These include the normal polycythemia of the neonatal period and the relative anemia and leukocytosis of infancy. Persistent polycythemia after the first month of life is frequently associated with right-to-left shunts and cyanosis. Anemia and polymorphonuclear leukocytosis may be encountered in active rheumatic fever and in subacute bacterial endocarditis.

Intensely cyanotic patients may have abnormalities of coagulation which may cause difficulty during surgery. Generally 2 groups are recognized: *(1) consumption coagulopathy*, in which intravascular coagulation utilizes clotting factors to an extent that they are decreased in the circulating plasma, and *(2) circulating fibrinolysins*, which prevent normal clot formation. Coagulation abnormalities apparently unrelated to their heart disease have also been recognized in acyanotic patients, e.g. plasma thromboplastin antecedent (factor XI) inhibitor. Thus all patients with congenital heart disease who are to undergo elective surgery should be evaluated and treated for abnormalities of coagulation. The role of repeated small venesections in the preoperative management of the cyanotic polycythemic patient is not clear.

Cardiac Catheterization. All the chambers of the heart and the great vessels entering or leaving them are accessible for measurements of pressure, sampling of blood, injection of contrast and indicator materials and introduction of intravascular electrodes and phonocardiographic pickups. The majority of congenital cardiac lesions can be diagnosed after a careful clinical history and examination, and cardiac catheterization should not be used indiscriminately in young patients, owing to the hazards of injury and even death. Abnormal findings which may be encountered in patients with congenital heart disease are shown in Tables 13-3 and 13-4.

Cardiac catheterization in infants and children presents problems not encountered in adults. In many instances it is necessary to sedate or even anesthetize the patient. Volatile gas mixtures such as ether should not be used, because manometric blood analyses done in the presence of these substances are inaccurate. The calculations of cardiac output, shunts, resistances and valve areas should be interpreted cautiously if the study is made during anesthesia because their validity depends upon the patient's being in a "steady state," which is difficult to obtain during deep narcosis.

Right cardiac catheterization. The technique consists in passing a radiopaque catheter under sterile conditions into a peripheral vein and guiding it with the aid of fluoroscopy into the great veins, the right heart chambers and pulmonary artery (Fig. 13-15). In some congenital cardiovascular abnormalities the catheter may pass through intracardiac defects or into abnormally placed vessels (Fig. 13-16). Samples of arterial blood may be obtained simultaneously from an indwelling needle in the brachial or femoral arteries. Oxygen consumption and carbon dioxide production may be calculated from samples of expired air. These studies are of value in determining the presence of intracardiac shunts and pressures, as well as for measurements of cardiac outputs and indices (Table 13-5). Calculations may also be made of the

---

*All vectorcardiograms in this text were obtained with the Frank lead system. In all instances the loop is interrupted at 2.5 milliseconds so that every 4 teardrops represent 1/100 second. The stout part of the teardrop represents the front end. Sensitivity mark indicates 1 millivolt. Abbreviations in all vectorcardiograms are as follows: *A*, anterior; *P*, posterior; *L*, left; *S*, superior; *I*, inferior.

TABLE 13-3. Analysis of Oxygen Content in Blood (Cardiac Catheterization)

	VENAE CAVAE	RIGHT ATRIUM	RIGHT VENTRICLE	PULMONARY ARTERY	ARTERIAL OXYGEN SATURATION	REMARKS
Patent ductus arteriosus	Comparable →			Higher than R.V., R.A. and V.C.	Normal	(a) Rarely, with right-to-left shunt, arterial unsaturation present (b) If associated pulmonary valve insufficiency, high R.V. samples comparable to P.A.
Atrial septal defect	Lower than R.A., R.V. and P.A.	Comparable →			Normal	
Ventricular septal defect	Comparable →		Higher than R.A. and V.C. →		Normal	Rarely, direct shunt into P.A. without mixing in R.V. when P.A. higher than R.V., R.A. and V.C.
Anomalous pulmonary veins	(a) If empty into S.V.C., I.V.C. lower than S.V.C., R.A., R.V. and P.A. (b) If empty into I.V.C., S.V.C. lower than I.V.C., R.A., R.V. and P.A.	If empty into R.A., V.C. lower than R.A., R.V. and P.A.	Comparable →		Normal	Arterial saturation may be decreased with total anomalous pulmonary venous return
Isolated pulmonary stenosis	Comparable →				Normal	If right-to-left shunt, e.g. through foramen ovale, arterial unsaturation
Aorticopulmonary septal defect	Comparable →			Higher than R.V., R.A. and V.C.	Normal	
Tetralogy of Fallot	Comparable →				Usually gross unsaturation	In many instances R.V. and P.A. samples higher than R.A. and V.C. Venous blood grossly unsaturated
Tricuspid atresia	Comparable →		→		Usually gross unsaturation	
Transposition of great vessels	Depends on presence of associated defects such as atrial defect, ventricular septal defect and patent ductus arteriosus				Gross unsaturation	Contents vary in same chamber because shunt is in both directions
Eisenmenger "physiology," i.e. pulmonary hypertension with bidirectional shunt	Depends on site of defect. Commonest is ventricular septal defect when R.V. and P.A. higher than R.A. and V.C.				Unsaturation	In atrial defect, V.C. lower than R.A., R.V. and P.A. In patent ductus P.A. higher than R.V., and brachial artery higher than femoral artery

Normally the difference in oxygen content between the venae cavae and right atrium is less than 1.9 volumes per cent, between the right atrium and right ventricle less than 0.9 volume per cent, and between the right ventricle and pulmonary artery, less than 0.5 volume per cent.

P. A. = pulmonary artery, R. V. = right ventricle, R. A. = right atrium, V. C. = venae cavae, S. V. C. = superior vena cava, I. V. C. = inferior vena cava.

TABLE 13-4. PRESSURES DURING CARDIAC CATHETERIZATION (mm. Hg)

	VENAE CAVAE	RIGHT ATRIUM	RIGHT VENTRICLE	PULMONARY ARTERY	PULMONARY CAPILLARY	REMARKS
Normal	0–5	0–5	18–30/0–5	18–30/6–12 Mean 13–17	6–12	Normal left atrial pressure 4–8
Patent ductus arteriosus	Normal	Normal	Normal to increased	Normal to increased	Normal to increased	Right atrial and caval pressures increased in congestive failure
Atrial septal defect	Normal	Normal	Normal to increased	Normal to increased	Normal	
Ventricular septal defect	Normal	Normal	Normal to increased	Normal to increased	Normal to increased	Right atrial and caval pressures increased in congestive failure
Anomalous pulmonary veins (partial)	Normal	Normal	Normal to increased	Normal to increased	Normal	
Isolated pulmonary stenosis	Normal to increased	Normal to increased	Increased	Normal to decreased	Normal	Left atrial pressure normal, and right atrial pressure curve may show prominent "a" wave
Aorticopulmonary septal defect	Normal	Normal	Increased	Increased	Normal to increased	
Tetralogy of Fallot	Normal	Normal	Increased	Normal to decreased	Normal	Pressure differentials may be noted in continuous tracing as catheter passes from pulmonary artery to infundibular chamber and to right ventricle
Tricuspid stenosis	Increased	Increased	———	———	———	Left atrial pressure normal Right atrial pressure curve shows prominent "a" wave
Transposition of great vessels	Normal	Normal	Increased	Increased	Increased	Right atrial and caval pressures increased in congestive failure
Eisenmenger physiology	Normal to increased	Normal to increased	Increased	Increased	Normal	

pulmonary and peripheral arteriolar resistances, the work of the heart, the volume of various shunts and the areas of intracardiac defects and valves.

Left cardiac catheterization. The technique consists in passing a catheter under sterile conditions into a peripheral artery (brachial or femoral) and guiding it with the aid of fluoroscopy into the ascending aorta and left ventricle. In some instances the catheter may enter the left atrium from the left ventricle. If the atrial septum is intact, the left atrium may be entered by puncturing the atrial septum through a catheter which has been advanced from the saphenous vein into the right atrium. In pediatric practice, left cardiac catheterization is used primarily for the assessment of the nature and severity of aortic stenosis and for the injection of contrast material to evaluate the ventricular septum and mitral valve. Catheterization of the posterior ventricle and pulmonary artery is of great value to assess the presence of pulmonary vascular obstruction or pulmonic stenosis in transposition of the great arteries.

Combined right and left cardiac catheterization. The techniques described above are frequently used simultaneously. It is again stressed that these methods of study are not without hazard, and they should be undertaken only with the specific ob-

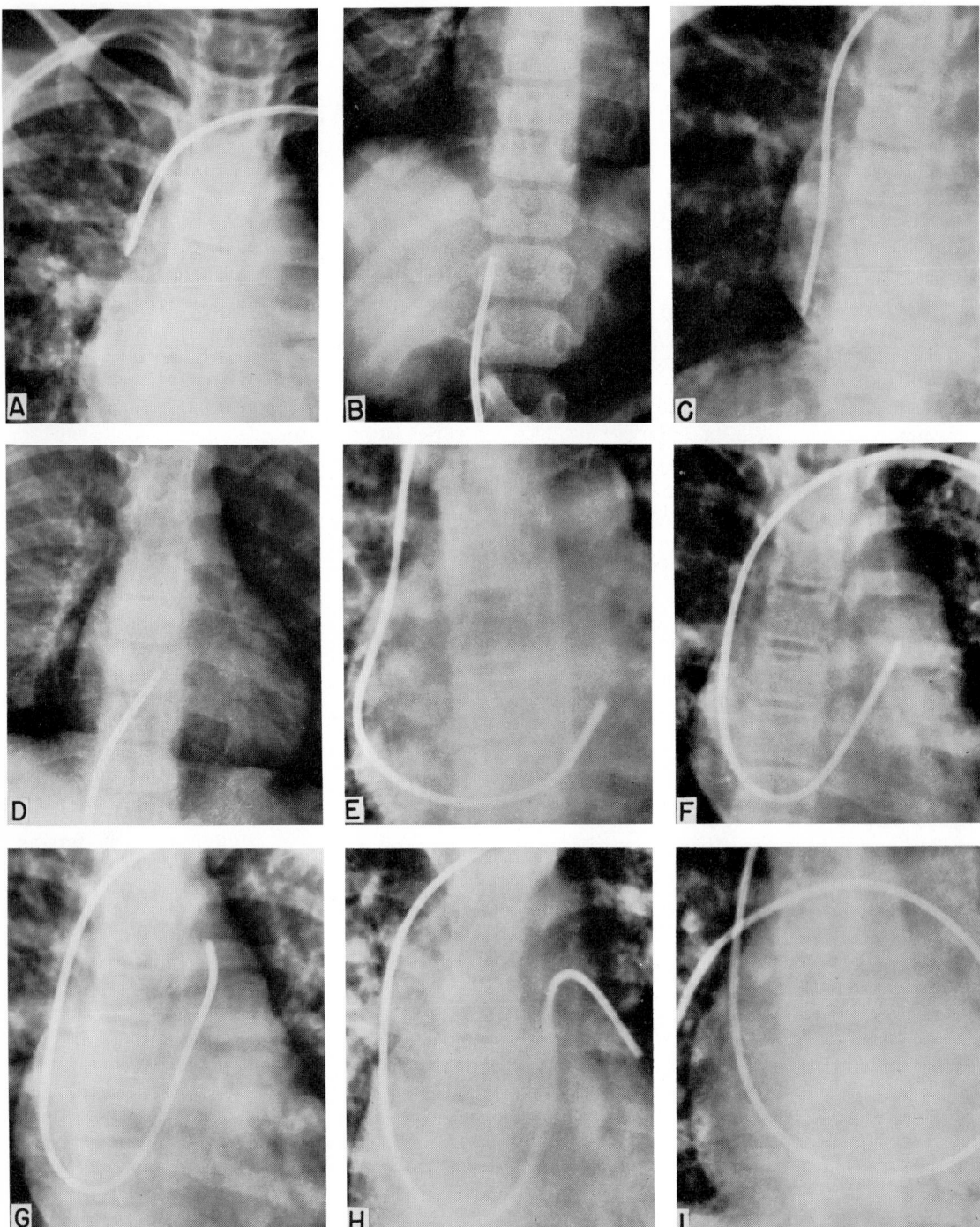

Figure 13-15. Roentgenograms showing the positions of the cardiac catheter from which pressures and blood samples may be obtained. *A*, Superior vena cava. Catheter inserted from antecubital vein. *B*, Inferior vena cava. Catheter inserted from saphenous vein. *C*, Low right atrium. *D*, Right atrium in region of tricuspid valve. *E*, Low right ventricle. *F*, High right ventricle in region of outflow tract. *G*, Main pulmonary artery. *H*, Left pulmonary artery. *I*, Right pulmonary artery.

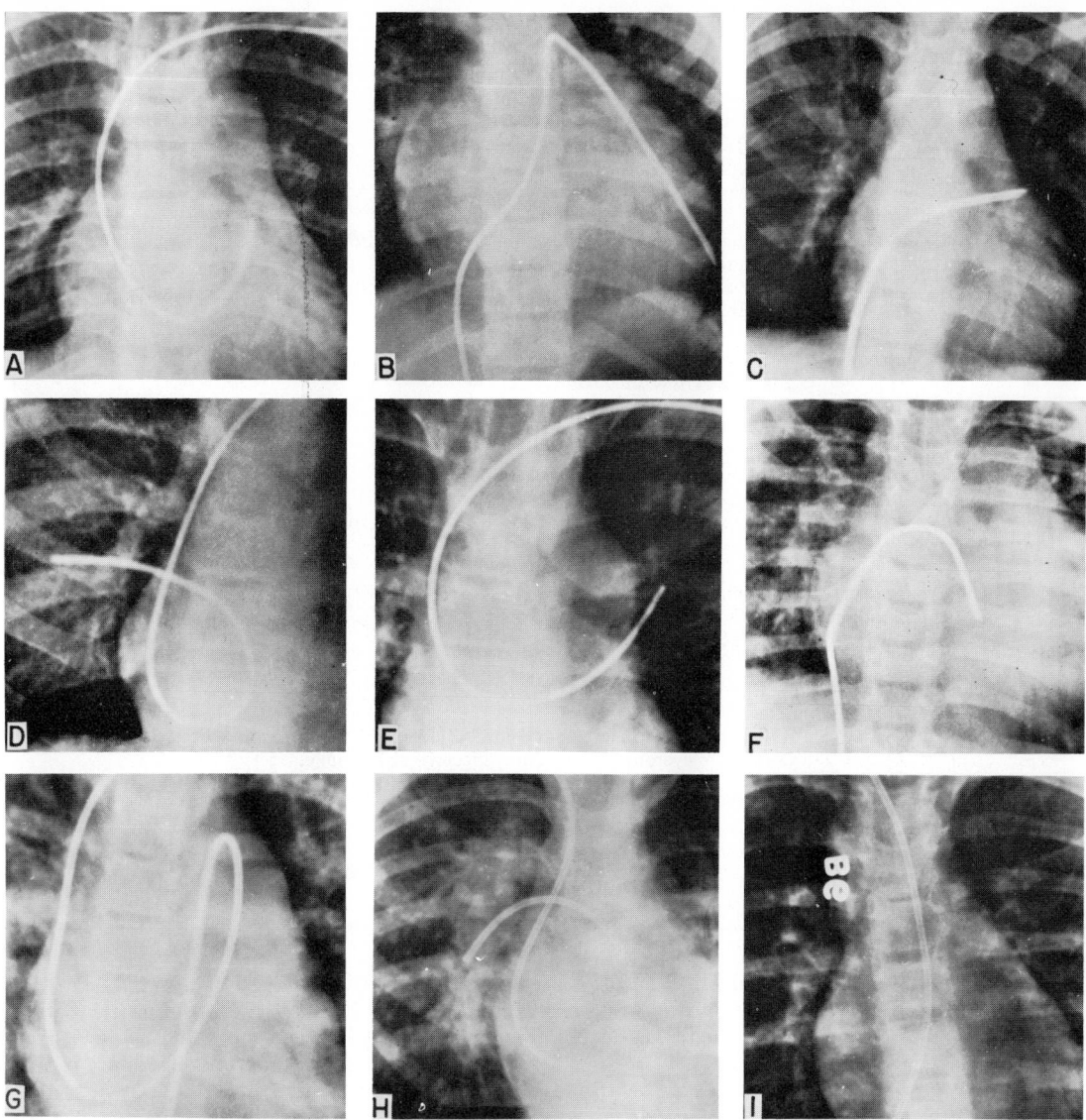

Figure 13-16. Roentgenograms showing positions of the cardiac catheter. *A*, Coronary sinus: compare with Figure 13-15, *F*. *B*, Pulmonary wedge or "capillary" via left pulmonary artery. *C*, Catheter has passed from the right to left atrium across an atrial septal defect. *D*, Catheter has passed across an atrial septal defect and entered a right pulmonary vein. This picture is frequently confused with an anomalous pulmonary vein entering the right atrium. *E*, Catheter tip in a left pulmonary vein after passing from the right to left atrium across an atrial septal defect. *F*, Catheter has passed from the inferior vena cava into the right atrium, across an atrial septal defect into the left atrium, and then through the mitral valve into the left ventricle. *G*, Catheter has passed from the superior vena cava to the right atrium, right ventricle and pulmonary artery, through a patent ductus arteriosus and down the descending aorta. *H*, Catheter tip in right pulmonary artery in a patient with corrected transposition of great vessels. Compare with Figure 13-15, *G* and *I*. *I*, Catheter advanced from inferior vena cava to the right atrium and right ventricle and then through a ventricular septal defect into the aorta.

jective of gaining information to help in the management of children with heart disease. These sophisticated methods of study do not supersede careful clinical evaluation and routine laboratory techniques.

Indicator Dilution and Appearance Techniques. If a bolus of indicator material is injected intravenously or into the right side of the heart, it traverses the pulmonary circulation and enters the left side of the heart and then the arterial circu-

lation. This indicator material may then be detected in the arterial blood. A continuous record of the circulation of indicator in normal subjects shows 2 peaks (Fig. 13-17). The time between the instant of injection and the detection of the indicator in arterial blood is known as the appearance time and is a measure of circulation time. The first peak of the indicator curve is due to the passage of indicator past the arterial detector, and the second to recirculation through the systemic arterial and

TABLE 13-5. Normals and Formulas for Determination of Hemodynamics in Cardiac Catheterization

1. Cardiac index 3.1 ± 0.4 liter/min./square meter
2. Arteriovenous oxygen difference 4.5 ± 0.7 ml./100 ml.
3. Oxygen consumption 140-160 ml./square meter/min.
4. Arterial oxygen saturation 94-100%
5. Difference in oxygen content between venae cavae and right atrium < 1.9 vol. %
6. Difference in oxygen content between right atrium and right ventricle < 0.9 vol. %
7. Difference in oxygen content between right ventricle and pulmonary artery < 0.5 vol. %
8. Normal mean left atrial pressure 4 to 8 mm. Hg
9. Pulmonary arteriolar resistance 50-150 dyne sec. cm. $^{-5}$(1 unit $= 80$ dynes)
10. Cardiac output ml./min. $=$
$$\frac{O_2 \text{ intake (ml./min.)}}{\begin{cases} O_2 \text{ content arterial blood (vols. \%)} \\ \text{minus } O_2 \text{ content of mixed venous blood} \end{cases}} \times 100$$
11. Cardiac index $=$ cardiac output (L./min.) per square meter of body surface area
12. Pulmonary artery flow $=$
$$\frac{O_2 \text{ intake (ml./min.)}}{\begin{cases} O_2 \text{ content of pulmonary venous blood (vols. \%)} \\ \text{minus } O_2 \text{ content of pulmonary arterial blood (vols. \%)} \end{cases}} \times 100$$
If a pulmonary venous sample is not obtained, it is assumed to be saturated 95% of capacity
13. Systemic flow $=$
$$\frac{O_2 \text{ intake (ml./min.)}}{\begin{cases} \text{systemic arterial } O_2 \text{ content (vols. \%)} \\ \text{minus mixed venous } O_2 \text{ content (vols. \%)} \end{cases}} \times 100$$
14. Effective pulmonary artery flow $=$
$$\frac{O_2 \text{ intake (ml./min.)}}{\begin{cases} \text{pulmonary venous } O_2 \text{ content (vols. \%)} \\ \text{minus mixed venous } O_2 \text{ content (vols. \%)} \end{cases}} \times 100$$
15. Total left-to-right shunt $=$ pulmonary artery flow minus effective pulmonary artery flow
16. Total right-to-left shunt $=$ systemic flow minus effective pulmonary artery flow
17. Pulmonary arteriolar resistance $R = \dfrac{PA - PC}{PF} \times 1332$

Where $\quad$ R $=$ pulmonary arteriolar resistance in dyne seconds cm.$^{-5}$
$\qquad$ PA $=$ mean pulmonary artery pressure in mm. Hg
$\qquad$ PC $=$ mean pulmonary "capillary" pressure in mm. Hg
$\qquad$ PF $=$ pulmonary flow in ml./sec.

---

venous systems, pulmonary circulation and reappearance in the arterial tree. If the concentration of circulating indicator is known, cardiac output can be computed (Fig. 13-17).

Localization of intracardiac and extracardiac shunts may be facilitated by the use of these methods. *Right-to-left shunts* are characterized by an abnormally short transit time for some of the indicator from the site of injection to the point of intra-arterial detection. Curves obtained after the injection of indicator at or upstream from the site of a right-to-left shunt show a short appearance time because of the escape of indicator across the defect (Fig. 13-17). This initial curve is followed by a second peak produced by the indicator which has traversed the longer normal pathway through the lungs. In contradistinction, curves obtained from injection of indicator downstream from the site of a right-to-left shunt show a normal appearance time.

In the presence of *left-to-right shunts* some of the indicator has a normal transit time to the detection site, whereas the remaining indicator recirculates through the lungs, resulting in a prolonged transit time. Curves recorded from systemic arterial blood have normal appearance times, reduced peak concentration and prolonged disappearance times (Fig. 13-17). Similar curves may be obtained in the presence of valvular regurgitation. Left-to-right shunts may be *localized* by the following methods: (a) Indicator is injected upstream or downstream from the site of the shunt, and curves are recorded from a systemic arterial detector. Downstream injections result in normal curves. If indicator is injected at or upstream to the site of shunt, the curve is as described above (Fig. 13-17). (b) The second method requires the use of 2 cardiac catheters. The first is placed in the distal pulmonary artery or left side of the heart for injection of indicator. The second is placed in the lesser circulation for sampling of blood containing indicator from the vena cava, right atrium, right ventricle or pulmonary artery. After injection of indicator into the distal pulmonary artery, it traverses the pulmonary circulation and appears in the left side of the heart and systemic circulation. If a left-to-right shunt is present, detectable indicator re-enters the right side of the heart and pulmonary circulation (Fig. 13-17), and comparison of curves localizes the site of left-to-right shunt. (c) A third method uses the same principle as (b), but the indicator detector is incorporated in the cardiac catheter, avoiding the necessity of inserting a second catheter and the sampling of blood (see Ascorbic Acid Polarography).

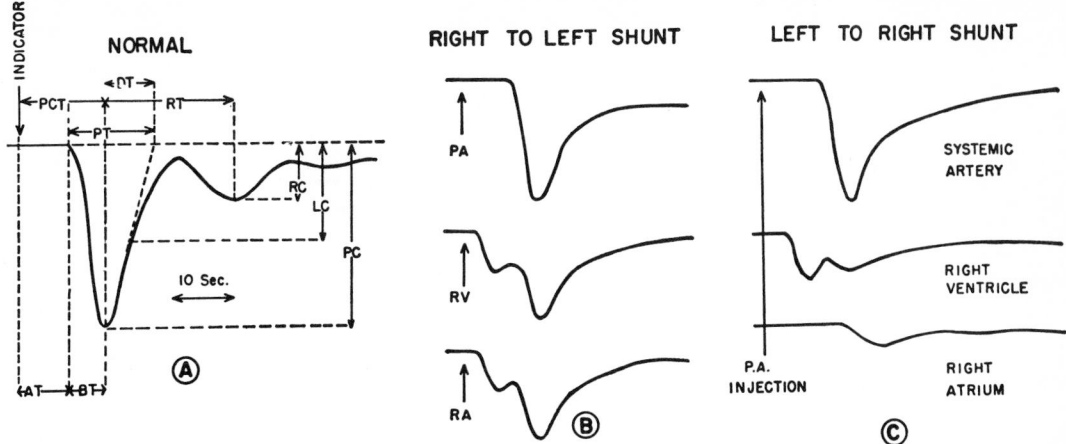

Figure 13-17. Idealized diagrams of the application of indicator dilution curves. *A*, Normal curve showing time and concentration components. Instant of indicator injection in right side of heart shown by arrow at top left. Curve obtained from detector in a systemic artery. Abbreviations: *AT*, appearance time; *BT*, build-up time; *PCT*, peak concentration time; *RT*, recirculation time; *PT*, passage time; *DT*, disappearance time; *PC*, peak concentration; *RC*, maximal recirculation concentration; *LC*, least concentration. Extrapolation of declining slope of concentration is easier if the curve is plotted on a logarithmic scale. Cardiac output may be computed by the formula $\dfrac{60I}{c\,(PT)}$, where I = amount of indicator, c = mean concentration of indicator, PT = passage time.

B, Localization of *right-to-left shunt*. Instant of injection of indicator shown by arrows. Example illustrates shunt at ventricular level. Site of injection: *PA*, pulmonary artery; *RV*, right ventricle; *RA*, right atrium. Indicator detector in systemic artery in all instances. PA injection (i.e. downstream from shunt level) shows normal appearance time. RV and RA injections (i.e. at and upstream from shunt level) show early appearance times.

C, Localization of *left-to-right shunt*. Example illustrates shunt at ventricular level. Indicator injected into distal pulmonary artery *(PA)* in all instances. In upper tracing indicator detector is in a systemic artery, and curve shows prolonged disappearance time. Middle curve is from indicator detected in right ventricle and shows an early appearance time because of ventricular septal defect. Right atrial curve shows normal appearance time.

Generally, indicator dilution methods are more sensitive than blood oxygen analyses for the detection of intravascular shunts. Available techniques for indicator curves include the following:

1. *Dyes.* The most frequently used material is indocyanine green. The detector is either an oximeter or densitometer. Accurate application of this method usually requires the continuous withdrawal of blood for the inscription of the dye dilution curve.

2. *Ascorbic Acid Polarography.* Anodically polarized platinum electrodes are depolarized and hence allow current to flow by certain readily oxidizable substances such as ascorbic acid. This technique has a particular advantage in infants and children because the platinum detector is placed intravascularly, avoiding the necessity for withdrawal of blood for the inscription of the ascorbate dilution curve. The platinum electrode may be inserted intra-arterially for localization of right-to-left shunts and incorporated in the wall of the cardiac catheter for detection of left-to-right shunts.

3. *Physiologic saline solution* is used as the indicator and is detected by the continuous withdrawal of blood through a conductivity cell.

4. *Radioactive materials,* including iodinated human serum albumin and radiophosphorus. Radioactive gases such as krypton-85 or ethyl iodide containing ^{131}I have also been used for the localization of left-to-right shunts by principles similar to those under The Hydrogen Electrode.

The hydrogen electrode. A platinized platinum electrode capable of sensing hydrogen is incorporated in a cardiac catheter which is inserted intravascularly or in the cardiac chambers (usually right). The detection and localization of *left-to-right shunts* depend on the fact that the electrode develops a potential in the presence of blood which has been exposed to hydrogen in the lungs; this is accomplished by having the patient take a breath of hydrogen. The instant the hydrogen appears in the nasal passages may be timed with another hydrogen electrode mounted in a flexible tube which has been brought into contact with the mucosa of the nose (airway signal). Some prefer to use an arterial hydrogen electrode for timing. Thus it is possible to time accurately the inhalation of hydrogen and its subsequent appearance in any part of the circulatory system. For example, in patients with ventricular septal defect and left-to-right shunt, the hydrogen appearance time will be normal in the venae cavae and right atrium (Fig. 13-18, *B*). Curves obtained from the right ventricle and pulmonary artery will show an early appearance time because left heart blood containing hydrogen has been shunted across the ventricular defect (Fig. 13-18, *B*).

The detection and localization of *right-to-left shunts* depend on the fact that saline solution saturated with hydrogen is completely cleared of hydrogen after passing through the normal lung. After the hydrogen electrode has been inserted into the aorta, hydrogenated saline is injected via a

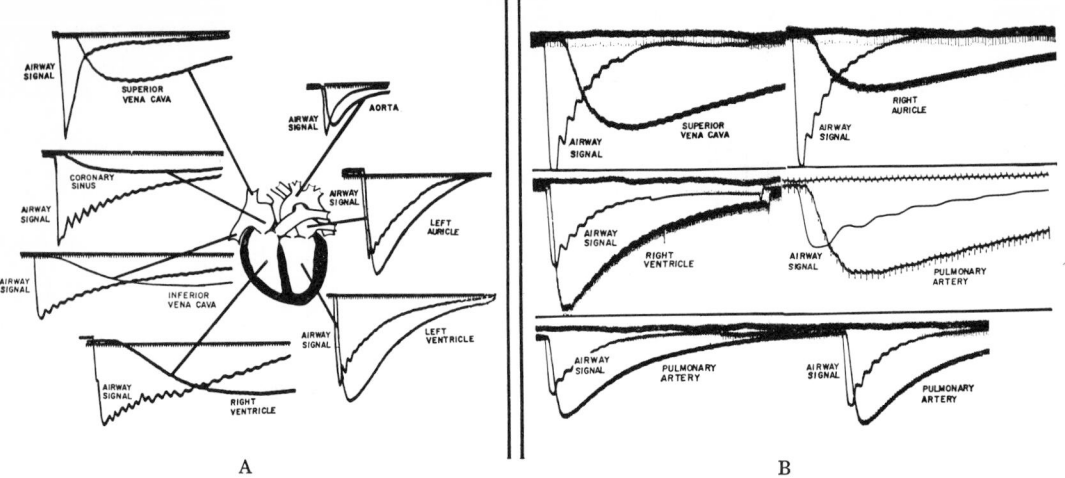

Figure 13-18. Hydrogen electrode curves. Airway signal curves from electrode in nasal passage, and these serve to time entrance of hydrogen into respiratory passages. *A,* Normal curves from various chambers of the heart. Note normal early appearance time in left as compared to right side of heart. *B,* Ventricular septal defect. Early appearance of hydrogen in right ventricle as compared to right atrium demonstrates left-to-right shunt at ventricular level. Right middle curve (pulmonary artery), at faster paper speed, demonstrates intracardiac electrocardiogram superimposed on hydrogen curve. (Courtesy of Dr. Leland C. Clark, Jr.)

cardiac catheter into the various right heart chambers. If the injection is made upstream from the site of right-to-left shunt, the arterial electrode will instantly detect the dissolved hydrogen. For example, in a patient with tetralogy of Fallot and right-to-left shunt across the ventricular defect, hydrogenated saline solution injected into the right atrium or right ventricle will be immediately detected by the aortic electrode. But if the injection is made downstream (i.e. in the pulmonary artery), the hydrogen is cleared by the lung and is not detected by the electrode.

The hydrogen electrode technique is particularly useful in infants and children because of its simplicity, extreme sensitivity, and elimination of repeated sampling of blood. The principal disadvantages are that the method is not quantitable, and hydrogen gas is explosive.

Arterial Oxygen Saturation. The arterial oxygen saturation or tension may be determined by analysis of blood obtained by direct puncture of the brachial or femoral artery, or by oximetry. Normal arterial blood has an oxygen saturation between 94 and 98 per cent. These levels are reduced in veno-arterial shunts and in disease of the pulmonary epithelium or vasculature which results in failure of proper oxygenation of the blood. The response of arterial oxygen saturation to exercise is a measurable index of the incapacity of the patient. In cyanotic congenital heart disease (e.g. tetralogy of Fallot) the resting arterial oxygen saturation is low; it is further reduced on exercise and the time taken for recovery to the control level is prolonged.

Angiocardiography. The great blood vessels and individual cardiac chambers may be seen by selective angiocardiography, i.e. injection of contrast material into specific cardiac chambers or

great vessels. This method allows identification of specific abnormalities without the superimposition of the shadows of normal chambers. Serial roentgenograms may be obtained in 2 planes at a rate of 6 to 14 per second.

Photofluorography with image intensification has made possible cardiac catheterization and selective angiocardiography simultaneously. The method has been combined with closed-circuit television to monitor the fluoroscopic screen and allow visualization of the cardiac silhouette and the cardiac catheter. After the cardiac catheter has been introduced into the specific chamber to be studied, a small amount of contrast medium is rapidly injected, and moving pictures are exposed at 30 to 60 frames per second. Biplane cine-angiocardiography allows detailed evaluation of specific cardiac chambers and blood vessels in 2 planes with the injection of a single bolus of contrast material. Angiocardiograms may also be monitored with video-tape systems, but at present the detail is not as precise as with cine techniques.

The injection of contrast medium into the circulation is not without hazard and should be used with discrimination. Deaths have been reported from iodine sensitivity, cardiac arrhythmia, cerebrovascular complications and pulmonary edema. The risk has been reduced, however, by the introduction of better contrast agents.

"Idealized" diagrams of the normal angiocardiogram are shown in Figure 13-5. The indications for this study are outlined under the individual congenital lesions.

Arteriography. In infants the arterial circulation may be visualized after retrograde injection of dye through a cannula placed in the brachial artery (Keith and Forsyth). This study may be of value in the diagnosis of patent ductus arteriosus, peripheral arterial aneurysms, some instances of coarctation of the aorta and arterial malformations (e.g. the study of the renal vessels in patients with suspected renal hypertension). The indications for arteriography have decreased with the introduction of combined cardiac catheterization and selective angiocardiography. The latter techniques allow the diagnosis of these anomalies and also may identify unsuspected associated malformations.

Roentgenokymograms. Roentgenokymograms are produced by interposing a slotted cassette between the film and the patient. During continuous roentgen exposure for about 2 seconds the film moves downward and records in 1 picture the variations of the cardiac size during systole and diastole. The excursion of pulsation of the heart and great vessels may also be measured with a photoelectric cell and recorded as a continuous tracing on a moving film.

Circulation Time. Many of the tests of circulation time depend on subjective sensations which are commonly difficult to evaluate in young patients. A sharp end-point may be obtained with injection into an arm vein of a sodium cyanide solution which makes the child gasp when it reaches the aortic body, or of fluorescein, which produces a green fluorescence of the lips when viewed under an ultraviolet lamp. The average time required for circulation of blood (as measured by the fluorescein method) from a peripheral arm vein to the heart through the lungs and finally to peripheral capillaries is about 7 seconds in infants and 11 seconds in older children.

Phonocardiography. Graphic records of heart sounds and murmurs are recorded simultaneously with electrocardiograms and intravascular pressure pulses. The function of phonocardiography is not to replace, but to corroborate the findings of clinical auscultation. In many instances hemodynamic abnormalities may be evaluated fairly accurately. For example, the severity of isolated valvular pulmonary stenosis may be assessed by clinical auscultation supplemented with phonocardiography.

Sound pickups incorporated in cardiac catheters may be introduced intravascularly for recording sounds and murmurs (intracardiac phonocardiography). This method localizes the cardiac chamber or blood vessel from which murmurs or abnormal sounds originate.

Arteriogram and Phlebogram. Recordings of the arterial pulsations from a peripheral vessel may be obtained directly from an indwelling needle or indirectly by recording the movement of an expansile capsule over the surface of the artery. The former method is more accurate and is preferable. Most abnormal contours can be discerned by the palpating finger, but records of the peripheral arterial wave are also helpful. Details of the peripheral venous pulsations (phlebogram) have already been described.

Ballistocardiography. Recoil of the body in the opposite direction to the ejection of blood from the heart may be recorded graphically if the subject is placed on a suitable table. Small tables for children have been constructed to record body movements in "head-to-foot" and "side-to-side" directions. Coarctation of the aorta is associated with an absent or small K wave.

REFERENCES

General

Cassels, D. E., and Morse, M.: *Cardiopulmonary Data for Children and Young Adults.* Springfield, Ill., Charles C Thomas, 1962.
Gasul, B. M., Arcilla, R. A., and Lev, M.: *Heart Disease in Children.* Philadelphia, J. B. Lippincott Company, 1966.
Keith, J. D., Rowe, R. D., and Vlad, P.: *Heart Disease in Infancy and Childhood.* 2nd ed. New York, Macmillan Company, 1966.
Moss, A. J., and Adams, F. H.: *Heart Disease in Infants, Children and Adolescents.* Baltimore, Williams & Wilkins Company, 1968.
Nadas, A. S.: *Pediatric Cardiology.* 2nd ed. Philadelphia, W. B. Saunders Company, 1963.
Rowe, R. D., and Mehrizi, A.: *The Neonate with Congenital Heart Disease.* Philadelphia, W. B. Saunders Company, 1968.
Taussig, H. B.: *Congenital Malformations of the Heart.* 2nd ed. Cambridge, Harvard University Press, 1960.
Watson, H.: *Paediatric Cardiology.* St. Louis, C. V. Mosby Company, 1968.

Cardiac Sounds and Phonocardiography

Caceres, C. A., and Perry, L. W.: *The Innocent Murmur: A Problem in Clinical Practice.* Boston, Little, Brown and Company, 1966.
Leatham, A.: Systolic Murmurs. *Circulation,* 17:601, 1958.
McKusick, V. A.: Symposium on Cardiovascular Sound. *Circulation,* 16:270, 414, 1957.
Rushmer, R. F., and Morgan, C.: Meaning of Murmurs, *Am. J. Cardiol.,* 2:722, 1968.

Roentgen Examination

Caffey, J.: *Pediatric X-Ray Diagnosis.* 5th ed. Chicago, Year Book Medical Publishers, Inc., 1967.
Edwards, J. E., Carey, L. S., Neufeld, H. N., and Lester, R. G.: *Congenital Heart Disease: Correlation of Pathologic Anatomy and Angiocardiography.* Philadelphia, W. B. Saunders Company, 1965.

Electrocardiogram and Vectorcardiogram

Cabrera, E., and Monroy, J. R.: Systolic and Diastolic Loading of the Heart. I. Physiologic and Clinical Data. II. Electrocardiographic Data. *Am. Heart J.* 43:661, 669, 1952.
Guntheroth, W. G.: *Pediatric Electrocardiography.* Philadelphia, W. B. Saunders Company, 1965.
Hoffman, I., and Taymor, R. C.: *Vectorcardiography.* Philadelphia, J. B. Lippincott Company, 1967.
Sodi-Pallares, D., and Calder, R. M.: *New Bases of Electrocardiography.* St. Louis, C. V. Mosby Company, 1956.
Ziegler, R. F.: *Electrocardiographic Studies in Normal Infants and Children.* Springfield, Ill., Charles C Thomas, 1951.

Cardiac Catheterization

Braunwald, E., and Swan, H. J. C.: Cooperative Study on Cardiac Catheterization. *Circulation,* 37: Supplement 3, 1968.
Clark, L. C., and Bargeron, L. M.: Detection and Direct Recording of Left to Right Shunts with the Hydrogen Electrode Catheter. *Surgery,* 46:797, 1959.
Wood, E. H.: Diagnostic Applications of Indicator Dilution Technics in Congenital Heart Disease. *Circulation Res.,* 10:531, 1962.
Zimmerman, H. A.: *Intravascular Catheterization.* 2nd ed. Springfield, Ill., Charles C Thomas, 1966.

Angiocardiography and Arteriography

Abrams, H. L.: Cinefluorographic Equipment in Cardiovascular Studies. *Prog. Cardiovasc. Dis.,* 5:440, 1963.
Rowe, R. D., Vlad, P., and Keith, J. D.: Selective Angiocardiography in Infants and Children. *Radiology,* 66:344, 1956.
Sones, F. M., Jr.: Cinecardioangiography; in American College of Chest Physicians: *Clinical Cardiopulmonary Physiology.* 2nd ed. New York, Grune & Stratton, Inc., 1960.

CONGENITAL HEART DISEASE

Fetal Circulation.   Blood flows from the fetus by way of the umbilical artery to the placenta, where it exchanges carbon dioxide and other waste products for oxygen and nutritive material. The oxygenated blood returns to the fetus through the umbilical vein; part of it goes directly into the inferior vena cava by way of the ductus venosus, and the remainder passes through the liver on its way to the heart. The blood entering the heart from the inferior vena cava is therefore a mixture of oxygenated and deoxygenated blood. The blood from the superior vena cava passes directly to the right ventricle through the tricuspid orifice, while the blood from the inferior vena cava divides into 2 streams, one directed into the right ventricle and the other through the open foramen ovale into the left atrium. In this way a part of the blood entering the right atrium is shunted directly to the left atrium and ventricle and out through the aorta without passing through the lungs. The blood which enters the right ventricle is directed toward the lungs, but, since the lungs are not expanded and the pulmonary vascular resistance is high, most of it is shunted into the aorta by way of the ductus arteriosus. Thus the blood in the aorta which circulates to all parts of the body is a mix-

ture of partly oxygenated and deoxygenated blood. A portion flows by way of the hypogastric arteries to the umbilical arteries and then to the placenta (Fig. 13-19).

Circulation in the Newborn Infant.   Changes in circulation occur rapidly after birth. When the cord is clamped and the lungs expand, the pulmonary circulation increases greatly in volume. The low resistance of the placental circulation is eliminated, with resultant increase in systemic vascular resistance. The foramen ovale, the ductus arteriosus and ductus venosus are no longer needed, but their closure proceeds gradually. The foramen ovale is functionally closed by the third month of life, though it is possible to pass a probe through the overlapping flaps in 25 per cent of adults (Patton). In the studies of Christie the ductus was closed in 88 per cent of infants by the end of the eighth week, and the foramen ovale in 87 per cent by the end of the twelfth week. During this period of adjustment there are rarely physical signs of patency of these structures. Nevertheless in some premature and occasional normal newborn infants an evanescent systolic murmur with late accentuation may be audible and is attributed to ductal flow. On rare occasions emboli to the ab-

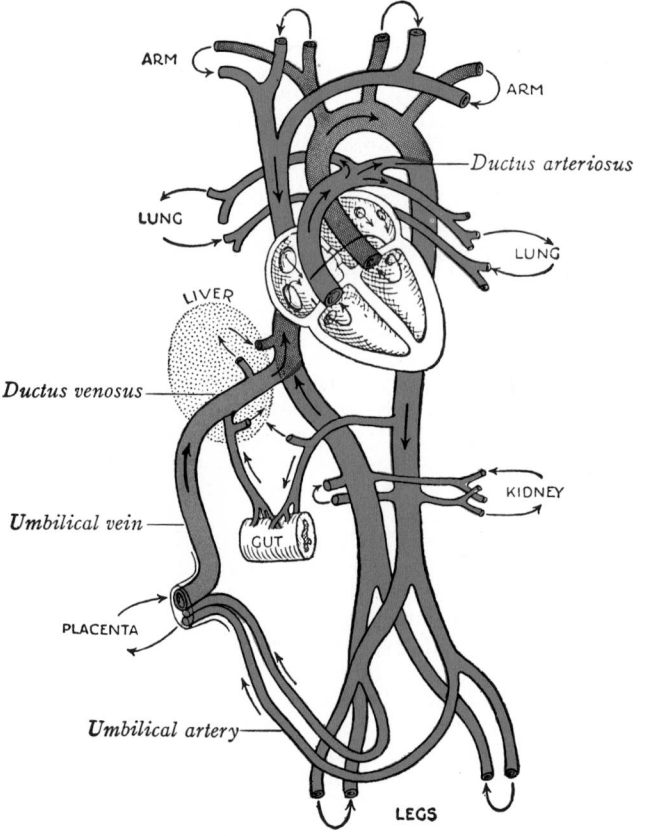

Figure 13-19.   Plan of the human circulation before birth (partly after Dodds). Colors show the quality of the blood, and arrows indicate its direction of flow (Arey).

dominal aorta and its branches (especially mesenteric) may arise from thrombosis in the ductus arteriosus. The pulmonary hypertension and high vascular resistance which are present in the normal fetus regress to normal levels generally within 10 to 14 days after birth.

Incidence of Congenital Heart Disease. The 2 important conditions which produce cardiovascular disease in children are congenital heart disease and rheumatic fever. The introduction of antimicrobial agents for the treatment and prophylaxis of streptococcal infections has resulted in a large decrease in the incidence of rheumatic fever. Simultaneously, great advances have been made in the diagnosis and surgical treatment of congenital cardiovascular diseases. In centers where diagnostic and surgical facilities are available new patients with congenital heart disease are almost 10 times more frequent than those with acute rheumatic fever.

The incidence of cardiovascular malformations at birth is about 6 per 1000, and they account for about 50 per cent of the deaths caused by congenital defects in the first year of life.

Table 13-6 provides a reasonable estimate of the incidence of selected malformations in different age groups; there is, however, considerable variation in different clinics. The development of palliative and corrective procedures has changed the frequency with which various malformations, especially transposition of the great vessels, are seen in older children. Patent ductus arteriosus is now seldom seen in adults, since surgical treatment is undertaken even in asymptomatic young children. Although small ventricular septal defects are common in children, they are uncommon in adults.

Etiology. *Maternal infection* may result in congenital heart disease. Congenital rubella is associated particularly with patent ductus arteriosus and pulmonary arterial branch stenosis. Coxsackie virus B has been implicated in the causation of endocardial fibroelastosis and has been demonstrated as a cause of acute myocarditis in neonates. Although a positive skin reaction to mumps antigen may be present in patients with endocardial fibroelastosis, the role of mumps virus as a teratogen is not clear. The protozoa of toxoplasmosis may be found in the heart, but functional cardiac disturbance seldom occurs. Late manifestations of congenital syphilis only rarely include aortitis and aneurysm. Cytomegalovirus and adenovirus have been isolated from cultures of cells (especially from the kidney) obtained from infants who have succumbed with congenital heart disease, but the mechanism and time of infection are not clear.

The teratogenic effect of *drugs and radiation* is well recognized. To date the highest incidence (about 10 per cent) of congenital heart disease has been associated with the thalidomide syndrome.

The incidence of patent ductus arteriosus appears to be higher among populations living at high altitudes, and cardiac malformations, especially arterial transposition and ventricular septal defect, appear to be more common among the offspring of prediabetic mothers.

Familial studies indicate that whereas the incidence of congenital heart disease in the population as a whole is about 6 per 1000, the incidence in liveborn siblings of probands is between 14 and 22 per 1000. The reported concordance of the lesions in siblings varies from 35 to 56 per cent. Information concerning the incidence of congenital heart disease in parents, other relatives and offspring of probands is scanty, but this incidence appears to be low. Generally only one of a pair of twins is affected by congenital heart disease.

The incidence of *atrial or ventricular septal defects* among siblings with these anomalies is about 1 per cent. Isolated instances of atrial septal defect have also been reported in several generations. *Patent ductus arteriosus* may aggregate in families and has been reported in 3 successive generations. *Truncus arteriosus* has been reported in siblings, as has *primary pulmonary hypertension.* Patients with *aortic stenosis* have occasionally had similarly afflicted siblings. The incidence of *coarctation of the aorta* in siblings is low, but that of *pulmonary stenosis* is probably highest of any form of

TABLE 13-6. PERCENTAGE INCIDENCE OF CONGENITAL CARDIOVASCULAR MALFORMATIONS AMONG AFFECTED PERSONS IN 3 DIFFERENT AGE GROUPS

	INFANTS	CHILDREN	OLDER CHILDREN AND ADULTS
Ventricular septal defect	28.3	24	15
Patent ductus arteriosus	12.5	15	15.5
Atrial septal defect	9.7	12	16
Coarctation	8.8	4.5	8
Transposition	8	4.5	2
Fallot's tetralogy	7	11	15.5
Pulmonary stenosis	6	11	15
Aortic stenosis	3.5	6.5	5
Truncus	2.7	0.5	—
Tricuspid atresia	1	1.5	1
All others	12.5	9.5	7
Total	100.0	100.0	100.0

Adapted from M. Campbell; in H. Watson (Ed.): *Paediatric Cardiology.* London, Lloyd-Luke, Ltd., 1968, Chap. 5.

congenital heart disease (almost 3 per cent). A relatively high incidence of consanguinity of the parents has been reported with situs inversus. Primary endocardial fibroelastosis has been reported in siblings.

Associated noncardiac malformations are common, especially with ventricular septal defects and double outlet right ventricle, whereas they are relatively uncommon with arterial transposition and aortic atresia; renal anomalies and cleft pal-ate are the commoner ones. Scoliosis occurs more frequently with cyanotic congenital heart disease. The common cardiovascular diseases associated with specific syndromes are listed in Table 13-7.

Genetic counseling concerning recurrence risk is of great practical importance. Generally parents can be supported in a decision to have additional children when one child has congenital heart disease, since the recurrence rate is about 2 per cent.

TABLE 13-7. CARDIOVASCULAR INVOLVEMENT IN SYNDROMES

SYNDROME	COMMON CARDIOVASCULAR INVOLVEMENT
HERITABLE AND POSSIBLE HERITABLE SYNDROMES AND DISORDERS	
Ellis-van Creveld	Single atrium (other defects in 30%)
Holt-Oram	Atrial septal defect (other defects common)
Kartagener's	Dextrocardia
Laurence-Moon-Biedl	Variable, including tetralogy of Fallot
Neurologic and muscular diseases:	
Friedreich's ataxia	Cardiomyopathy
Muscular dystrophy	Cardiomyopathy
Riley-Day	Episodic hypertension, postural hypotension
Refsum's	Arrhythmia, sudden death
Tuberous sclerosis	Rhabdomyoma, cardiomyopathy
Rendu-Osler-Weber	Arteriovenous fistula (lung, liver, mucous membranes)
Familial deafness	Occasionally arrhythmia, sudden death
Familial dwarfism and nevi	Cardiomyopathy
Congenital hypertrophic subaortic stenosis	Obstructive cardiomyopathy
Familial elfin facies, mental retardation, infantile hypercalcemia	Supravalvular aortic stenosis, pulmonary arterial branch stenosis
Scimitar syndrome	Hypoplasia of right lung, anomalous pulmonary venous return to inferior vena cava
Rubenstein-Taybi	Patent ductus arteriosus
CHROMOSOMAL ABNORMALITIES	
Down's	Endocardial cushion defect, atrial septal defect, ventricular septal defect, patent ductus arteriosus
Trisomy E	Ventricular septal defect, patent ductus arteriosus, pulmonic stenosis
Trisomy D	Ventricular septal defect, double outlet right ventricle, patent ductus arteriosus, atrial septal defect
Cri du chat	Ventricular septal defect in a minority
Turner's syndrome:	
Phenotypic female	Coarctation of aorta, pulmonic stenosis, aortic stenosis
Phenotypic male	Pulmonic stenosis, aortic stenosis
INBORN ERRORS OF METABOLISM	
Pompe's disease	Glycogen storage disease of heart
Homocystinuria	Pulmonary arterial and aortic dilatation, intravascular thrombosis, flushing of skin
CONNECTIVE TISSUE DISORDERS	
Marfan's	Aortic dilatation with aortic incompetence, mitral incompetence, dilatation of pulmonary artery
Hurler's	Multivalvular and coronary artery disease
Morquio-Ulrich	Aortic incompetence
Scheie	Aortic incompetence
Pseudoxanthoma elasticum	Peripheral arterial disease
Ehlers-Danlos	Arterial dilatation
Osteogenesis imperfecta	Aortic incompetence
Arterial calcification of infancy	Calcinosis of coronary arteries

Adapted from C. A. Neill; in A. J. Moss and F. A. Adams (Eds.): *Heart Disease in Infants, Children and Adolescents.* Baltimore, Williams & Wilkins Company, 1968, Chap. 3.

But if 2 siblings are affected, it is probable that the recurrence rate is higher. The incidence of cardiovascular malformation in the offspring of patients who have been treated for congenital heart disease is less than 3 per cent. Cyanotic women who become pregnant have an increased risk of spontaneous abortion, and, if they go to term, the infant is usually small.

Diagnosis of Congenital Heart Disease. The development of surgical procedures effective for certain congenital cardiovascular defects has made accurate diagnosis essential. Most often the diagnosis can be established from the history, physical findings and customary roentgenographic and electrocardiographic examinations. When doubt exists, cardiac catheterization, selective angiocardiography and aortography often supply the necessary confirmatory information. Because early surgical intervention may save many of them from death, severely ill newborn and young infants with cardiovascular malformations should be subjected to any necessary diagnostic procedures.

Classification of Congenital Heart Disease. Abbott established the custom of dividing congenital heart diseases into 2 groups: (1) those with cyanosis at rest, and (2) those without cyanosis or manifesting it only under certain adverse conditions, e.g. high pulmonary resistance. Taussig makes a similar division on the basis of malformations which do or do not permit an adequate supply of oxygen to the body. This classification has been criticized, and other, more complicated ones have been suggested; they depend on hemodynamic and anatomic factors, including the direction of shunt. In congenital heart disease persistent cyanosis is usually caused by the shunting of venous blood from the right to the left side of the heart, so that it passes into the systemic circulation without being oxygenated in the lungs. In this text the following classification of the more common anomalies will be used: (1) right-to-left shunts (i.e. with cyanosis), (2) left-to-right shunts (i.e. without cyanosis), (3) no shunt at all. It is appreciated that there is overlapping in these groups.

Congenital Cardiac Disease with Cyanosis (Dominant Right-to-Left Shunt)

TETRALOGY OF FALLOT

The combination of (1) obstruction to right ventricular outflow (pulmonary stenosis), (2) ventricular septal defect, (3) dextroposition of the aorta and (4) right ventricular hypertrophy constitutes the tetralogy of Fallot. It is the most common condition accompanied by persistent cyanosis and accounts for more than 75 per cent of cyanotic congenital heart disease in patients over the age of 1 year. Obstruction to pulmonary arterial flow is usually at the right ventricular infundibulum and pulmonary valve, though the pulmonary arterial trunk is generally smaller than usual. The pulmonic valve may have a small ring, be bicuspid, and occasionally be the only site of stenosis. Hypertrophy of the crista supraventricularis contributes to the infundibular stenosis and results in the formation of an infundibular chamber of variable size and contour. The ventricular septal defect is generally large, anterior, just below the aortic valve, involves part of the membranous septum and is separated from the infundibular chamber by the crista supraventricularis. The normal continuity of the mitral and aortic valves is maintained. The aorta arches to the right in 20 per cent of these patients, is large and straddles the ventricular septal defect. The aorta is considered to be dextroposed because a varying proportion of its origin is from the right ventricle.

Hemodynamics. Systemic venous return to the right atrium and right ventricle is normal. When the right ventricle contracts, the outflow of blood is resisted by the pulmonary stenosis and blood is shunted across the ventricular septal defect into the aorta. This results in persistent arterial unsaturation and cyanosis. The pulmonary blood flow is restricted by the obstruction to right ventricular outflow, but may be supplemented by bronchial collateral circulation and occasionally by a patent ductus arteriosus. The systolic and diastolic pressures in each ventricle are usually similar, as are the mean pressures in the atria. A measurable gradient of pressure is always detected across the outflow of the right ventricle, owing to the pulmonary stenosis.

The major defects in the tetralogy of Fallot are the obstruction to right ventricular outflow and the ventricular septal defect. When these conditions exist without right-to-left shunt, the anomaly is termed *acyanotic Fallot* (see Pulmonary Stenosis and Ventricular Septal Defect, p. 1001).

Clinical Manifestations. *Cyanosis,* one of the outstanding manifestations, may not be present at birth. Apparently, as long as the ductus arteriosus remains open, sufficient blood passes through the lungs to prevent cyanosis. As it closes during the first months of life, cyanosis may become apparent gradually or develop suddenly when the infant has an infection. The cyanosis is most prominent in the mucous membranes of the lips and mouth and in the fingernails and toenails, but the entire skin surface has a dusky, bluish color. The sclerae are gray, and the blood vessels at the periphery are likely to be engorged, giving the appearance of mild conjunctivitis. The blood vessels of the retina are large and dark. The mucous membranes of the pharynx are purple, and the tongue is deep blue and often large and fissured, with prominent papillae. The gums are frequently inflamed and bleed easily from light pressure. The eruption of the teeth may be delayed; histologic examination reveals dilatation and engorgement of the capillaries in the dental pulp and poor calcification of the dentin. *Clubbing* of the fingers and toes is a conspicuous sign generally presented by the age of 1 or 2 years. *Hemoptyses* may be recurrent, but are rare.

Dyspnea occurs on exertion. Infants and toddlers will play actively for a short time and then sit or lie down. Older children may be able to walk a block or so before stopping to rest. The capacity for exercise depends on the severity of the cardiac lesion, which is often reflected by the intensity of the cyanosis. Characteristically, children assume a *squatting* position for the relief of dyspnea due to physical effort. This results in an increase in arterial oxygen saturation so that the child is able to resume physical activity within a few minutes. Assumption of the squatting position may result in decreased venous return and increased systemic arterial resistance, each of which would tend to decrease the right-to-left shunt and increase pulmonary blood flow.

Paroxysmal dyspneic attacks (anoxic "blue" spells) are a particular problem during the first 2 years of life. The infant becomes dyspneic and restless, cyanosis increases, and gasping respirations ensue. During the spell the cry is usually weak, but may be loud. Occasionally some infants clutch or scratch over the anterior portion of the chest as if they had precordial pain. Temporary disappearance or decrease in intensity of the systolic murmur is usual. The spells may last from a few minutes to a few hours and are occasionally fatal. Shorter episodes are followed by generalized weakness and sleep. Severe spells may progress to unconsciousness and occasionally convulsions or hemiparesis. Their onset is spontaneous and unpredictable, though they may follow feeding (especially breakfast), crying or a bowel movement, or may be precipitated by infection or iron deficiency anemia. The spells are associated with a reduction of an already compromised pulmonary blood flow, which results in hypoxia and metabolic acidosis. The disappearance or attenuation of the systolic murmur and reduction of arterial oxygen saturation and pulmonary arterial pressure suggest that blue spells are associated with spasm of the right ventricular outflow tract. Guntheroth et al. postulate that hyperpnea precipitates an attack by increasing systemic venous return. In the presence of fixed or decreased pulmonary blood flow, the right-to-left shunt is increased. The resultant arterial hypoxia, metabolic acidosis and increased pCO_2 further stimulate the respiratory mechanism

to maintain continuing hyperpnea. Depending on the frequency and severity of the attacks, one or all of the following procedures should be tried in sequence: (1) placement of the infant on his abdomen in the knee-chest position, making certain that there is no constricting clothing; (2) administration of oxygen; (3) injection of morphine in doses of 0.5 to 1 mg. per 10 pounds of body weight; this is especially effective. Since metabolic acidosis develops when the arterial pO_2 is below 40 mm. Hg, rapid correction (within several minutes) is necessary if the spell is severe and there is lack of response to the foregoing therapy. This may be accomplished with intravenous administration of sodium bicarbonate or tris-hydroxyaminomethane (THAM). Recovery from the spell is rapid once the pH is returned to normal. Repeated blood pH measurements are necessary because rapid recurrence of acidosis is common. Beta-adrenergic inhibition by intravenous administration of propranolol may be considered in patients with uncontrollable recurrent severe spells.

Growth and development may be delayed. The stature and nutritional status are usually below the average for the age, and the muscles and subcutaneous tissues are flabby and soft. Puberty is delayed.

The *pulse* is usually normal, as are the venous and arterial pressures. The left anterior hemithorax may bulge forward. The heart is usually normal in size, and the apical impulse is tapping. A *systolic thrill* is felt in 50 per cent of cases along the left sternal border in the third and fourth parasternal spaces.

The *systolic murmur* is frequently loud and harsh; it may be transmitted widely, but is most intense at the left sternal border. The murmur may be either ejection or pansystolic (Fig. 13-20), and it may be preceded by a click. In many instances the second heart sound is single and is produced by closure of the aortic valve. When closure of the pulmonary valve is audible, it is delayed and diminished. In a small number of instances the systolic murmur is followed by a diastolic murmur. This continuous murmur may be audible in any part of the chest, anteriorly or posteriorly; it is produced by enlarged bronchial collateral vessels or rarely by persistence of a patent ductus arteriosus and occurs frequently in pulmonary atresia.

Polycythemia and an elevated *hematocrit* are usual. The defects in coagulation have been described (p. 955).

Roentgen Examination. The typical configuration in the anteroposterior position shows a narrow base, concavity of the left border in the area usually occupied by the pulmonary artery and a normal heart size. The rounded apical shadow situated rather high above the diaphragm is produced chiefly by the hypertrophied right ventricle and has been likened to the shape of a sheep's nose; the entire cardiac silhouette, to that of a wooden shoe (*coeur en sabot*) (Fig. 13-21). In the lateral projection the anterior clear space may or may not be encroached upon by the hypertrophied right

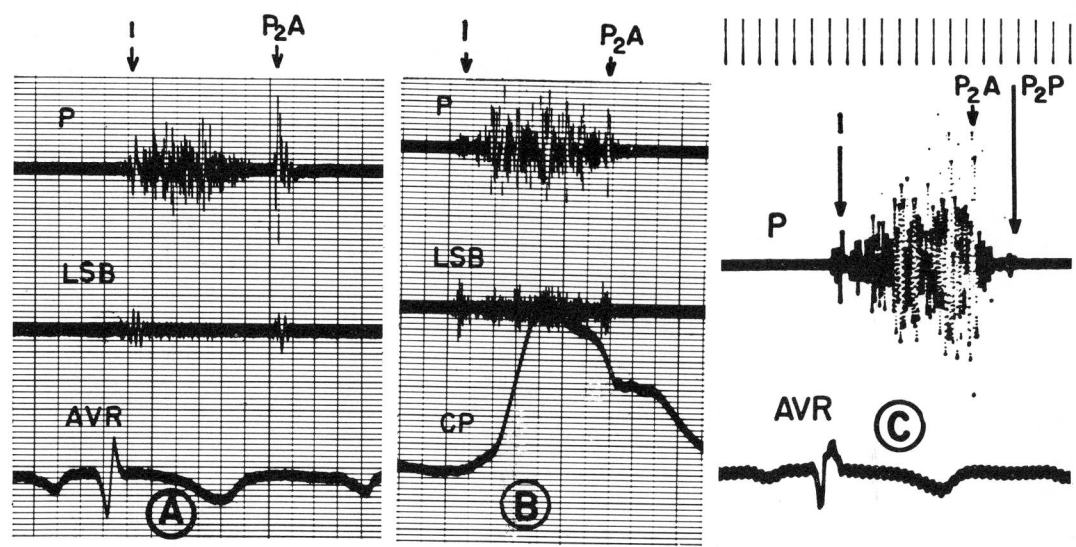

Figure 13-20. Phonocardiograms illustrating the variability of auscultatory findings in cyanotic tetralogy of Fallot. Abbreviations: *P*, pulmonary area; *LSB*, left sternal border; *AVR*, electrocardiogram; *CP*, carotid pulse; *1*, first heart sound; *P₂A*, aortic component of second heart sound, *P₂P*, pulmonic component of second heart sound. The systolic murmur may be early *(A)*, or when long *(B)* or accentuated in late systole *(C)*, it ends at P₂A. The second heart sound is single, owing to aortic valve closure *(A and B)* or split with a delayed soft pulmonic component *(C)*. Time lines 0.04 second.

ventricle. In many patients the right ventricle displaces the normal left ventricle posteriorly so that the posterior border of the heart may overlap the spine in the left anterior oblique view. Although all these features suggest right ventricular enlargement, the electrocardiogram is a more sensitive index of right ventricular hypertrophy.

The aorta is usually large, and its position is important. In about 20 per cent of instances the aorta arches to the right instead of the left; this may be clearly visible in the anteroposterior view

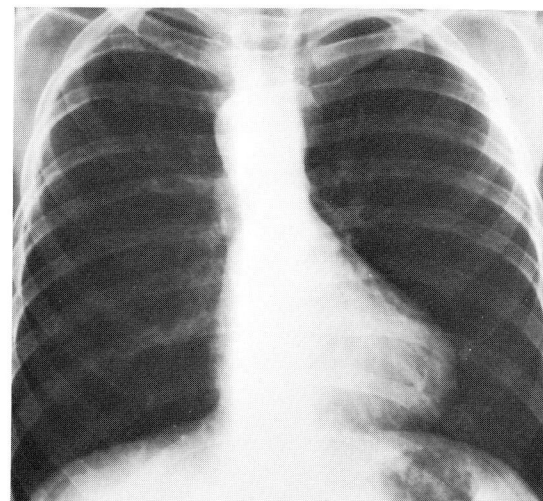

Figure 13-21. Teleroentgenogram of an 8-year-old boy with tetralogy of Fallot. Note the normal heart size, some elevation of the cardiac apex, concavity in the region of the main pulmonary artery, pulmonary vascularity and right aortic arch.

or may be confirmed by displacement of the barium-filled esophagus to the left. In the left oblique view a right aortic arch may indent the esophagus.

The hilar areas of the lungs are relatively clear and usually pulsate little or not at all, owing to the diminished pulmonary blood flow. The lung fields are remarkably clear for the same reason; this constitutes an important diagnostic sign.

Variations from the typical radiographic picture include poststenotic dilatation of the pulmonary artery, which is usually associated with valvular pulmonic stenosis. Occasionally pulmonary vascularity is made prominent by a reticular pattern of collateral bronchial circulation which radiates from the hilus of the lungs. Localized proximal infundibular stenosis with an infundibular chamber may produce a bulge at the upper left cardiac border in the frontal projection, which is distinguished from that of the pulmonary artery because it remains prominent in the right anterior oblique view.

Electrocardiography. The electrocardiogram reveals evidence of right axis deviation and right ventricular hypertrophy. Evidence of right ventricular dominance, without which the diagnosis of tetralogy of Fallot is unlikely, is found in the right precordial chest leads where the configuration of the QRS complex is Rs, R, qR, qRs, rsR′ or RS. In these leads the T wave may be positive, which is further evidence of right ventricular hypertrophy. The P wave is tall and peaked or sometimes bifid in about one third of patients (Figs. 13-8, 13-9).

Other Tests. In the majority of instances the diagnosis of tetralogy of Fallot can be made with the aid of the foregoing studies. Preoperative

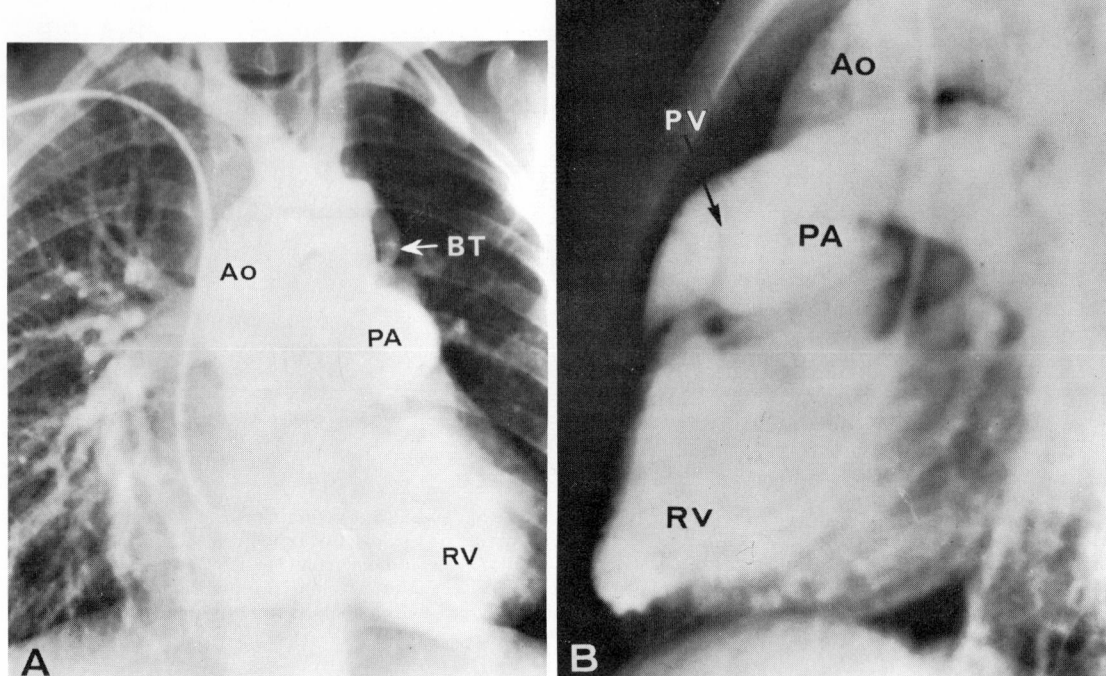

Figure 13-22. Selective right ventriculogram in 9-year-old boy with tetralogy of Fallot who had undergone a Blalock-Taussig operation at the age of 2 years. *A*, Anteroposterior view; *B*, lateral view. Simultaneous opacification of aorta and pulmonary artery from the right ventricle. Aortic root is dextroposed, and the pulmonary artery is anterior to the aorta. Abbreviations: *RV*, right ventricle; *PA*, pulmonary artery; *Ao*, aorta; *PV*, pulmonic valve; *BT*, subclavian-pulmonary artery anastomosis of previous Blalock-Taussig operation.

cardiac catheterization and angiocardiography are essential, however, in order to elucidate the anatomic abnormalities and to exclude other defects which may mimic the tetralogy of Fallot, especially double outlet right ventricle with pulmonic stenosis and arterial transposition with pulmonic stenosis.

Cardiac catheterization reveals systolic hypertension in the right ventricle and a sudden fall of pressure as the catheter enters the infundibular chamber or pulmonary artery. Serial pressure determinations taken from the region of stenosis of the right ventricular outflow tract may in some instances differentiate between valvular and subvalvular stenosis. In valvular stenosis the change in pressure from the pulmonary artery to the right ventricle is abrupt, whereas in infundibular stenosis 3 pressure differentials are recorded as the catheter tip is withdrawn from the pulmonary artery to the infundibular chamber and right ventricle (Fig. 13-23). The systolic pressure in the right ventricle is at the systemic level, usually between 80 and 110 mm. Hg.

The mean pulmonary arterial pressure is commonly between 5 and 10 mm. Hg; the right atrial pressure is usually normal. The aorta may be entered from the right ventricle through the ventricular septal defect (Fig. 13-16, *I*). The degree of arterial unsaturation depends on the magnitude of the right-to-left shunt and at rest is usually 75 to 85 per cent. Samples of blood from the venae cavae,

right atrium, right ventricle and pulmonary artery are frequently similar in oxygen content, indicating absence of a left-to-right shunt. In many patients, however, a left-to-right shunt is demonstrated at the ventricular level (Table 13-3). Indicator dilution curves localize the site of right-to-left or bidirectional shunt at the ventricular level.

Selective right ventriculography is of great diagnostic value. The contrast medium outlines the heavily trabeculated right ventricle. The infundibular stenosis varies in length, width, contour and distensibility. An infundibular chamber may also be demonstrated. The pulmonary valve may be normal, but frequently the leaflets are thickened and domed and the valve ring is small. Nearly simultaneous opacification of the aorta and pulmonary artery is usual. The size of the pulmonary trunk varies considerably. In severe cases it is small or hypoplastic. The ventricular septal defect is usually large and is situated below the hypertrophied crista supraventricularis. The large aorta is usually well opacified.

Prognosis. Without operation the prognosis varies with the severity of the pulmonary stenosis and the amount of collateral circulation. Deeply cyanotic children who have dyspnea on slight exertion rarely live until late childhood. Others may succumb during the adolescent period, and a few may live beyond the third decade.

Complications. The principal complications are as follows: *(a) Cerebral thromboses*, venous or

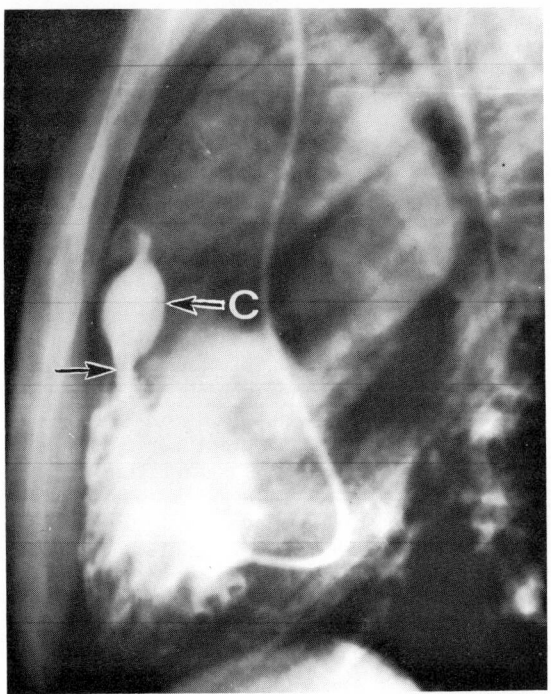

Figure 13-23. Lateral view of selective right ventriculogram in patient with Fallot's tetralogy. Arrow points to infundibular stenosis which is below the infundibular chamber (C).

arterial, are more common in the presence of extreme polycythemia and may be precipitated by dehydration. They occur more frequently in patients under the age of 2 years. Therapy includes adequate hydration, especially in the comatose patient. Intravenous heparin is useful if begun within 12 hours after onset. Physical therapy to the affected extremities should be instituted as early as possible. (b) *Brain abscess* is rarer than cerebral thrombosis, but in some instances the differential diagnosis is difficult. Patients with brain abscess are usually over the age of 2 years; the onset of the illness is often insidious; fever is usually of low grade; localized skull tenderness may be present; and the erythrocyte sedimentation rate and white cell count may be elevated. Massive antibiotic therapy may help to localize the infection, but surgical drainage of the abscess is frequently necessary. (c) *Bacterial endocarditis* is rare in patients unoperated on; nevertheless the usual preventive therapy should be given in all patients during intercurrent infections and prophylactically to cover surgical procedures in the mouth, throat and ear (see pp. 988 and 1023). (d) *Bleeding tendencies* (see p. 955). (e) *Congestive heart failure* is rare, but in infancy may be precipitated by iron deficiency anemia.

Associated cardiovascular anomalies are common and are difficult to recognize clinically. *Patent foramen ovale* and *patent ductus arteriosus* are frequent during infancy. Recognition of the drainage of a persistent left superior vena cava into the coronary sinus is important prior to surgical correction, since temporary occlusion of systemic venous return is essential prior to cardiotomy. *Atrial septal defects* of the secundum type are recognized during cardiac catheterization. Closure of defects in the atrial septum, including patent foramen ovale, is advised during radical surgery, since high venous pressure in the immediate postoperative period may result in cyanosis from a right-to-left shunt. *Absence of the pulmonic valve* produces a distinct syndrome; cyanosis is mild or absent, the heart is large and hyperdynamic, and loud to-and-fro murmurs are present. Aneurysmal dilatation of the pulmonary artery often produces wheezing respiration and recurrent pneumonitis from bronchial compression. The incidence of *stenosis of a branch of the pulmonary artery* has been estimated to be as high as 25 per cent. The diagnosis depends on visualization of the areas of obstruction by selective pulmonary arterial or right ventricular angiocardiography. Significant stenosis of major pulmonary arteries must be relieved during radical surgical correction. *Absence of a pulmonary artery* can be suspected if the roentgenographic appearance of the pulmonary vasculature differs on the 2 sides. Generally the left pulmonary artery is absent, so that the right lung appears more vascularized. This may be associated with hypoplasia of the left lung. Sometimes it is difficult to differentiate absence of the left pulmonary artery from severe stenosis with occlusion. It is of utmost importance to recognize absence of a pulmonary artery prior to the creation of an anastomosis between the systemic circulation and the single remaining pulmonary artery since occlusion of the latter during operation seriously compromises the already reduced pulmonary blood flow. Other associated anomalies include *relative hypoplasia of the left heart, aortic or subaortic stenosis, bicuspid aortic valve, aberrant coronary artery* and *anomalies of the aortic arch.*

Treatment. *General management.* Although the majority of patients require surgical treatment, astute management is necessary before operation. The prevention or prompt treatment of dehydration is important to avoid hemoconcentration and possible thrombotic episodes. The treatment of paroxysmal dyspneic attacks has been described (p. 968). In infancy these attacks may be precipitated by a relative iron deficiency. Iron therapy may decrease their frequency and also improve exercise tolerance and general well-being. In some infants the frequency of the dyspneic episodes may be decreased with mild sedation as by promethazine (Phenergan). Intercurrent infections should be vigorously treated with suitable antibiotics. It appears that the safest level of the hematocrit is between 55 and 65 per cent. Venesection is seldom indicated even if the hematocrit value is high. Even if undertaken cautiously and the blood volume is maintained with plasma, phlebotomy may result in peripheral vascular collapse.

Surgical ANASTOMOTIC PROCEDURES. Taussig observed that the prognosis was better when the ductus arteriosus was patent. She and Blalock devised the operation whereby an artificial ductus is created by anastomosis of a branch of the aorta to the homolateral branch of the pulmonary artery. The most common procedure is anastomosis of the end of the left subclavian artery to the side of the pulmonary artery. Potts and his associates achieved the same objective by side-to-side anastomosis of the upper descending thoracic aorta to the pulmonary artery. Pulmonary blood flow may also be increased by side-to-side anastomosis of the ascending aorta to the right pulmonary artery (Waterston). Palliative therapy with shunt procedures carries an operative mortality of about 7 per cent and is advised in severely handicapped patients under 4 to 5 years of age; total correction is generally undertaken only in older children.

The *postoperative course* of patients with a successful anastomosis is generally smooth. In addition to the usual postoperative complications following a thoracotomy, chylothorax, Horner's syndrome and postoperative cardiac failure may occur. Chylothorax is due to trauma to the thoracic duct or its tributaries and is treated with repeated thoracenteses. Suture of the duct is undertaken if chylothorax persists. Horner's syndrome is usually temporary and does not require treatment. Postoperative cardiac failure may be due to the large size of the anastomosis; its treatment is described on page 1032. Vascular problems in the upper extremity supplied by the subclavian artery which has been used for anastomosis are rare.

After a successful anastomosis there is a striking improvement in symptoms. Exercise tolerance is increased, and the habit of squatting is discontinued. The degree of cyanosis and clubbing diminishes. A machinery-type murmur, sometimes accompanied by a thrill, is detected after operation, and is indicative of a functioning anastomosis.

The duration of symptomatic relief tends to be short-lived after the Blalock-Taussig operation, especially if it is done during infancy. Therefore this operation is generally reserved for children over 2 years of age. Relief of symptoms of hypoxia is maintained well after the Potts operation, but late complications are frequent; they include cardiac failure, bacterial endocarditis and pulmonary hypertension. At present the Waterston operation is advised in infants because palliation is prolonged, and during later corrective surgery the shunt is closed with greater ease than after a Potts anastomosis. Late complications following the Waterston shunt are similar to those following the Potts anastomosis.

BROCK PROCEDURE. Brock suggested a direct surgical attack on the right ventricular outflow obstruction with infundibular resection or pulmonary valvotomy. With these procedures about two thirds of patients are greatly improved, and one sixth are benefited. It is possible that this approach steadily improves the size of the right ventricular outflow tract so that eventual surgical correction can be undertaken without the frequent need to use outflow patches.

DIRECT-VISION INTRACARDIAC SURGERY (WITH A PUMP OXYGENATOR) (p. 1014). The ideal surgical therapy is relief of obstruction to right ventricular outflow, together with closure of the ventricular septal defect. Although total correction is sometimes undertaken in a 3- or 4-year-old child previously unoperated upon, it is usually deferred until beyond the age of 4 or 5 years. While the patient's circulation is temporarily maintained by an artificial heart-lung machine, the right ventricle is opened extensively, the infundibular stenotic area resected, coexistent pulmonary stenosis relieved, and the ventricular septal defect is closed. The outflow tract of the right ventricle is enlarged with a pericardial patch if a significant gradient of pressure persists between the right ventricle and the pulmonary artery. If the pulmonary valvular ring and pulmonary trunk are small, it may be necessary to enlarge this area with a pericardial patch, even though it produces pulmonary valvular in-

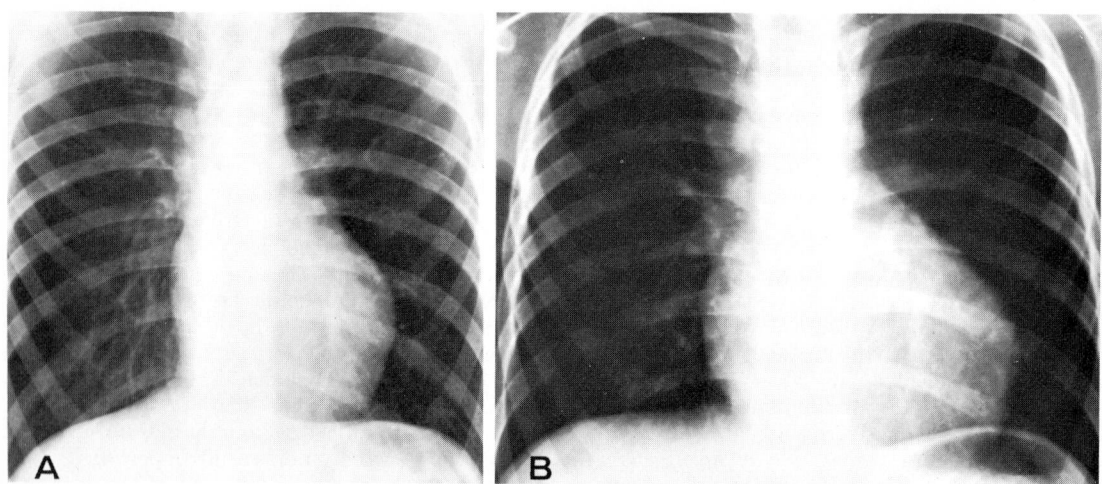

Figure 13-24. Teleroentgenogram of a 6-year-old boy with tetralogy of Fallot. *A,* Preoperative. *B,* Postoperative, after resection of right ventricular outflow obstruction and closure of ventricular septal defect. Some increase in heart size is not infrequent after operation.

competence. A previously established systemic-pulmonary shunt must be closed prior to cardiotomy. The Blalock-Taussig anastomosis is dissected and ligated immediately after establishing a cardiopulmonary bypass. The Potts anastomosis is closed from within the pulmonary artery after the induction of deep hypothermia and temporary total circulatory arrest. The Waterston shunt is closed from within the aorta after total cardiopulmonary bypass has been established, and after temporary occlusion of the ascending aorta just below the level of the innominate artery.

The surgical risk of total correction has currently fallen to less than 10 per cent. Factors that have contributed to this increasing success include optimal total body perfusion, adequate myocardial protection during bypass, relief of right ventricular outflow obstruction and prevention of air embolism. The presence of a previous anastomosis does not increase the operative risk significantly. Increased bleeding in the immediate postoperative period is common in markedly polycythemic patients, but should not seriously affect the outcome. The operative risk is higher if there is marked deformity of the right ventricular outflow tract, and in older adolescents and adults.

After successful total correction, the patients are asymptomatic and able to lead unrestricted lives. The shunt at the ventricular level is abolished and the resistance to right ventricular outflow is reduced greatly. The long-term effects of right ventricular outflow prostheses are unknown. They appear to be well tolerated if the ventricular septum is intact and the right ventricular pressure is near normal. The long-term effects of isolated pulmonary valvular incompetence are likewise unknown. Patients who have a significant left-to-right shunt postoperatively, or obstruction to right ventricular outflow, exhibit moderate to marked cardiac enlargement. A right ventricular outflow aneurysm may also be present at the site of ventriculotomy or outflow patch. Reoperation is generally necessary in such patients. The incidence of permanent complete heart block has decreased, but artificial pacing may be necessary for a few days or weeks because of temporary heart block.

ORIGIN OF BOTH GREAT VESSELS FROM THE RIGHT VENTRICLE WITH PULMONARY STENOSIS

The importance of this anomaly is due to the fact that in many instances it cannot be distinguished from tetralogy of Fallot. In this condition both the aorta and pulmonary artery arise from the right ventricle, and the only outlet for the left ventricle is through the ventricular septal defect. The aortic and mitral valves lose their normal continuity, and the ventricular defect is inferior to the crista supraventricularis. The history, physical examination, electrocardiogram and roentgenograms are similar to those described under Tetralogy of Fallot. The possible clue to the diagnosis is the demonstration by selective angiocardiography that the aortic and pulmonary valves lie in the same horizontal body plane. This study also demonstrates the abnormal anterior position of the aorta, which arises exclusively from the right ventricle. The angiocardiographic distinction between Fallot's tetralogy and the anomaly under discussion may be difficult because of the anterior position of the aorta in some patients with Fallot's tetralogy. Corrective surgical treatment is difficult, since a tunnel must be produced which allows an adequate outlet from the left ventricle to the aorta and at the same time closes the ventricular defect. The pulmonary obstruction also is removed. Palliative anastomotic procedures to increase pulmonary blood flow result in significant symptomatic improvement.

PULMONARY ATRESIA

With Ventricular Septal Defect. Sometimes called *pseudotruncus arteriosus*, this condition is an extreme form of Fallot's tetralogy. There is no direct communication between the right ventricle and pulmonary artery, since the pulmonary valve is atretic, rudimentary or absent. The pulmonary trunk is also atretic or hypoplastic. The entire ventricular output is ejected into the aorta. Pulmonary blood flow is dependent on bronchial collaterals or a patent ductus arteriosus.

The clinical manifestations are much the same as those of the tetralogy with the following exceptions: Cyanosis usually appears within a few days after birth in contrast to later in the first year in the tetralogy. The systolic murmur is absent or soft. The first heart sound is frequently followed by an ejection click. The second sound at the base is moderately loud and single. Continuous murmurs due to a patent ductus arteriosus or bronchial collateral flow may be heard anywhere in the chest, anteriorly or posteriorly, but are usually heard best under the clavicles. The heart may be enlarged roentgenographically, with a striking concavity of the pulmonary arterial segment. The reticular pattern of the bronchial collateral flow may be present.

The best diagnostic study is *right ventriculography*, which demonstrates immediate opacification of a large aorta from the ventricular septal defect and also the pathway of pulmonary blood flow from the aorta.

Since hypercyanotic spells and increasing hematocrit are frequent during infancy, a surgical systemic-pulmonary arterial anastomosis is indicated. The ideal patient has 2 reasonably sized pulmonary arteries available for anastomosis. In later years corrective surgery can be undertaken by closure of the ventricular septal defect and insertion of a homograft to act as the pulmonic valve and main pulmonary artery (Ross and Somerville).

Unfortunately, many patients have malformations of the primary divisions of the pulmonary arteries in the form of hypoplasia, multiple branch stenosis or absence of a pulmonary artery, with large bronchial collaterals. These are difficult to treat surgically even with anastomotic procedures.

Acquired total obstruction of right ventricular outflow may occur after a systemic-pulmonary anastomosis for Fallot's tetralogy (Sabiston et al.). In these patients the right ventricular outflow tract is stenotic but patent before the anastomotic procedure. Some time after operation there may be a return of symptoms in association with total obstruction at the infundibulum or pulmonic valve. The systolic murmur due to pulmonic stenosis is attenuated or disappears, and the completeness of outflow obstruction is confirmed by right ventriculography. Corrective surgery is similar to that for Fallot's tetralogy.

With Intact Ventricular Septum. In the majority of instances this anomaly is associated with a hypoplastic but thick-walled right ventricle lined by thick endocardium; the orifice of the tricuspid valve is small. In 15 to 20 per cent of cases the right ventricle is normal or large and the tricuspid valve functionally incompetent. Intermediate forms between the 2 extremes are common. Since there is no egress from the right ventricle, right atrial blood is shunted into the left atrium via the foramen ovale or an atrial septal defect, mixes with pulmonary venous blood, and is pumped by the left ventricle into the aorta. Pulmonary flow is via a patent ductus arteriosus and bronchial vessels.

Cyanosis occurs in early infancy, but may not be intense if the ductus is widely patent. Cardiac failure occurs early, especially in the presence of tricuspid incompetence. Cardiomegaly is usual. The second heart sound is single and continuous murmurs are common, especially in older infants and children. In others only systolic murmurs are audible. If the right ventricle is small, electrocardiographic signs of left ventricular hypertrophy are usual and the frontal QRS axis is either normal or to the right. This helps to exclude tricuspid atresia, in which left axis deviation is common. If the right ventricle is normal or large, right ventricular hypertrophy is noted. *Roentgenographically*, there is extreme variability in size of the heart. Generally it is normal in neonates with a small right ventricle, but enlarges progressively during the first few weeks of life. Marked cardiomegaly occurs when the right ventricle is normal or large. Pulmonary undercirculation is usual.

Cardiac catheterization demonstrates right atrial and ventricular hypertension if the right ventricle is small. Right ventriculography outlines a small cavity. Right ventricular outflow is absent, and flow of contrast medium is successively from a large right atrium to the left atrium, left ventricle and aorta. These findings are indistinguishable from those of tricuspid atresia if the right ventricle is not catheterized. Varying degrees of right ventricular hypertension are present if the ventricle is normal or large. Tricuspid incompetence is recognized by regurgitation of contrast medium from the large right ventricle to the right atrium.

Pulmonary valvotomy will relieve obstruction if the tricuspid valve, right ventricle, pulmonary valvular ring and pulmonary artery are nearly normal in size. If the right ventricle is hypoplastic, as in the majority of cases, the surgical treatment is a systemic-pulmonary arterial anastomosis and the creation of a large atrial septal defect. If there is doubt about the size of the right ventricle, a pulmonary valvotomy may be attempted first. Since there is no blood flow through the main pulmonary artery, it can be clamped temporarily during operation.

TRICUSPID ATRESIA

In tricuspid atresia the tricuspid orifice is absent and the right ventricle hypoplastic. The presence and size of a ventricular septal defect determine the size of the pulmonary valve and trunk. Generally the ventricular defect is small and pulmonary arterial hypoplasia is present. Pulmonary atresia is usual if the ventricular septum is intact. In a minority of instances the pulmonary artery is nearly normal in size, especially if the ventricular septal defect is large. Tricuspid atresia with transposition of the great arteries is discussed elsewhere. When pulmonic stenosis is present with tricuspid atresia and arterial transposition, the hemodynamics and clinical picture simulate those of tricuspid atresia with normal relations of the great arteries.

Since there is no inflow into the right ventricle, right atrial blood escapes into the left atrium via the foramen ovale or an atrial septal defect. Here the blood mixes with pulmonary venous blood and enters the left ventricle. The larger portion of the mixed blood passes into the aorta, but some is shunted through the ventricular septal defect and passes from the hypoplastic right ventricle into the pulmonary artery. A patent ductus arteriosus provides pulmonary blood flow if the pulmonary trunk is hypoplastic.

Clinical Manifestations. Cyanosis, polycythemia, easy fatigability, exertional dyspnea and anoxic hypercyanotic (paroxysmal dyspneic) attacks develop early, especially if pulmonary blood flow is seriously compromised. After infancy, clubbing is usual, but squatting is not as common as in tetralogy of Fallot. If the interatrial communication is small, right atrial hypertension results in a prominent jugular "a" wave and presystolic pulsations of an enlarged liver. These signs are easy to elicit but uncommon in infants. The heart may or may not be enlarged with a heaving left ventricular apical impulse. In very ill small infants, murmurs may not be prominent, but in the majority a pansystolic or ejection systolic murmur

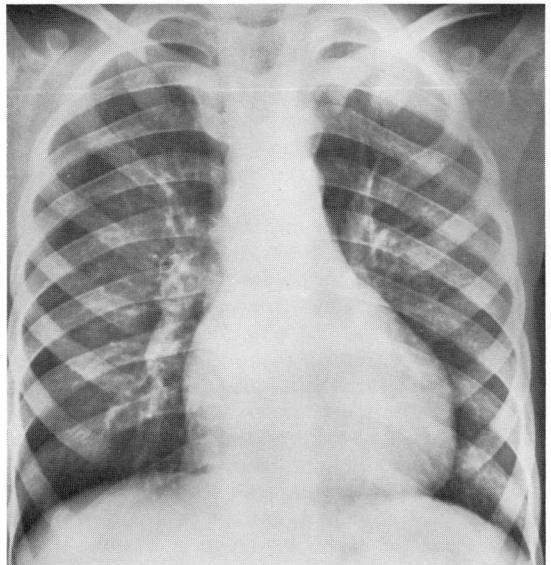

Figure 13-25. Teleroentgenogram in tricuspid atresia with underdeveloped right ventricle (see text).

is audible maximally down the left sternal border. The second heart sound is single, owing to absence of the pulmonary element.

Roentgenographic studies show pulmonary undercirculation and deficiency of shadows of the pulmonary artery (Fig. 13-25). The heart is normal in size or slightly enlarged. The cardiac contour is variable. In the posteroanterior view the right border may be straight or rounded by the large right atrium; the apex is high. In the left anterior oblique view the posterior border of the heart

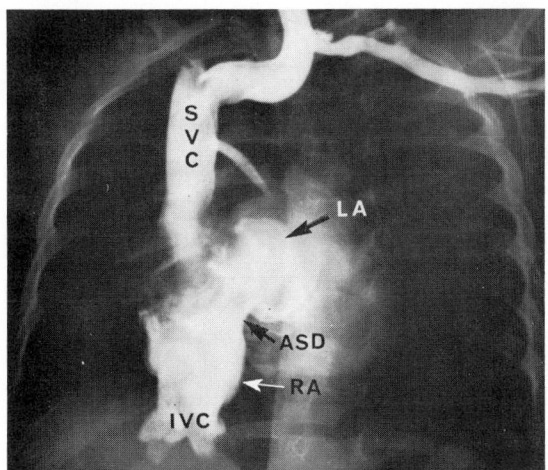

Figure 13-26. Angiocardiogram to demonstrate the course of the circulation in tricuspid atresia with underdeveloped right ventricle. Systemic venous blood flows from the right to the left atrium. Absence of right ventricular opacification due to tricuspid atresia. Abbreviations: *SVC*, superior vena cava; *IVC*, inferior vena cava; *RA*, right atrium; *LA*, left atrium; *ASD*, interatrial communication through atrial septal defect.

overlaps the spine because of the large left ventricle. The anterior border may be normal, recede from the sternum or be displaced forward by the large left ventricle. In many patients the cardiac silhouette is indistinguishable from that seen in Fallot's tetralogy, or is nonspecific in contour.

The *electrocardiogram* is a much more sensitive index of the state of the ventricles. Left axis deviation, left ventricular hypertrophy and abnormal P waves are the usual findings. In the right precordial leads the normally prominent R wave is replaced by an rS complex. The left precordial leads show a qR complex followed by a normal, flat, diphasic or inverted T wave. R_{V6} is normal or tall and S_{V1} generally deep. Although the P waves may be normal, they are usually tall and spiked, but sometimes diphasic or bifid.

Cardiac catheterization shows normal or elevated right atrial pressure with a prominent "a" wave. If the catheter is introduced from the saphenous vein into the inferior vena cava and right atrium, it usually passes with ease across the foramen ovale or atrial septal defect into the left side of the heart (Fig. 13-16, *C*, *E*).

With *selective angiocardiography* there is immediate opacification of the left atrium from the right atrium followed by left ventricular filling and visibility of the aorta (Fig. 13-26). Absence of flow to the right ventricle results in a filling defect between the right atrium and left ventricle in early films in frontal projection. The tiny right ventricle is opacified if a ventricular septal defect is present. Otherwise, pulmonary arteries are filled via a patent ductus arteriosus. The presence of associated transposition of the great vessels and pulmonic stenosis may be demonstrated by selective left ventriculography.

Prognosis and Treatment. The prognosis is poor, and many infants fail to survive the first few months of life unless pulmonary flow is adequate and the interatrial communication large. Surgical treatment is designed to increase pulmonary blood flow. This may be accomplished by a systemic-pulmonary arterial anastomosis, preferably of the Waterston type. If the interatrial defect is small, it may be enlarged by the Blalock-Hanlon operation. Although improvement after surgery may be striking, generally it is not as gratifying as with treatment of Fallot's tetralogy. Disappointing results are due to left ventricular failure or failure to recognize and enlarge a small interatrial communication (p. 978). Good results may also be obtained from end-to-end anastomosis of the superior vena cava to the right pulmonary artery.

EISENMENGER SYNDROME

The term "Eisenmenger syndrome" is used here for the combination of pulmonary hypertension with reversed or bidirectional shunt through either a ventricular septal defect, atrial septal

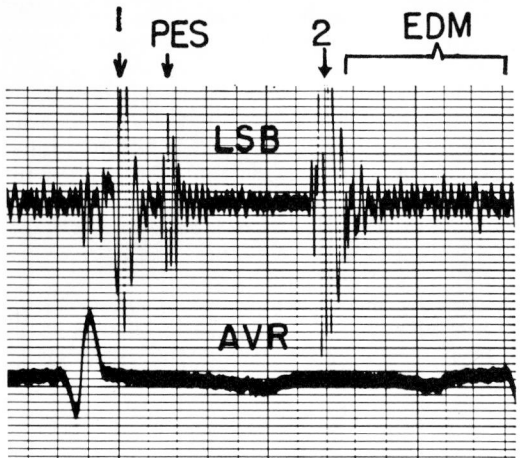

Figure 13-27. Phonocardiogram which illustrates auscultatory findings of patient with Eisenmenger syndrome associated with a ventricular septal defect. Abbreviations: *LSB*, left sternal border; *AVR*, electrocardiogram; *1*, first heart sound; *2*, second heart sound; *PES*, pulmonic ejection sound; *EDM*, early diastolic murmur due to pulmonary valve incompetence. Time lines 0.04 second.

defect or patent ductus arteriosus (or other communications between the aorta and lesser circulation). This concept implies that the principal physiologic abnormality is elevation of the pulmonary vascular resistance. In normal infants at, or soon after, birth the pulmonary vascular resistance is high. Within a few weeks the structure of the pulmonary arterioles changes to that of the adult with a thin wall and a large lumen, and the pulmonary vascular resistance falls to normal adult levels. In the Eisenmenger syndrome the pulmonary vascular resistance remains high. This abnormal resistance is probably present from birth, although in a minority of patients with large ventricular septal defects pulmonary resistance falls somewhat, only to rise again in later childhood or adult life.

Clinical Manifestations. Symptoms are usually present in the first year of life, especially in patients with ventricular septal defect. These include dyspnea, feeding difficulties, fatigue, failure to gain weight and recurrent pneumonia. As the child gets older dyspnea on effort is obvious, especially when there are ventricular and atrial septal defects. Squatting, angina pectoris, hemoptysis and episodes of syncope occur occasionally. Cyanosis, which may be present early, increases in intensity as the child approaches puberty, and is associated with clubbing and polycythemia. If there is a patent ductus arteriosus, venous blood from the pulmonary artery is shunted down the descending aorta and results in differential cyanosis (blue lower extremities and pink upper extremities).

Venous pressure is increased when congestive heart failure or functional tricuspid insufficiency is superimposed. Heart size is extremely variable, being normal in many cases with ventricular

defect, but usually enlarged with atrial defect. A conspicuous left parasternal, right ventricular heave with palpable pulmonary arterial pulsations is frequent. A systolic murmur of varying intensity is usual and is frequently preceded by a pulmonic ejection click. The second heart sound is loud and booming. It is closely split or single in many cases of ventricular defect, but widely split with atrial defect. Functional incompetence of the pulmonary valve resulting in a blowing diastolic murmur down the left sternal border (Graham Steell murmur) is common and is associated with a normal peripheral arterial pulse.

Roentgenographically, the heart varies in size from normal to greatly enlarged. The larger hearts are seen with atrial defects and the smaller ones with ventricular defects, but there is a large overlap. The pulmonary artery is usually enlarged. The pulmonary vessels are enlarged in the hilar areas and diminish in caliber in the peripheral branches. The right ventricle and atrium are prominent.

The *electrocardiogram* frequently shows right ventricular hypertrophy, occasionally associated with incomplete right bundle branch block. The P wave may be tall and spiked. Sometimes the electrocardiogram is balanced and does not reveal the ventricular hypertrophy.

Cardiac catheterization usually shows a bidirectional shunt at the site of the defect; e.g. in patients with a ventricular septal defect a left-to-right shunt is demonstrated at the ventricular level and is associated with a decrease in the arterial oxygen saturation due to the right-to-left shunt. There is, of course, a definite decrease in arterial oxygen saturation when there is only a right-to-left shunt. The catheter frequently tra-

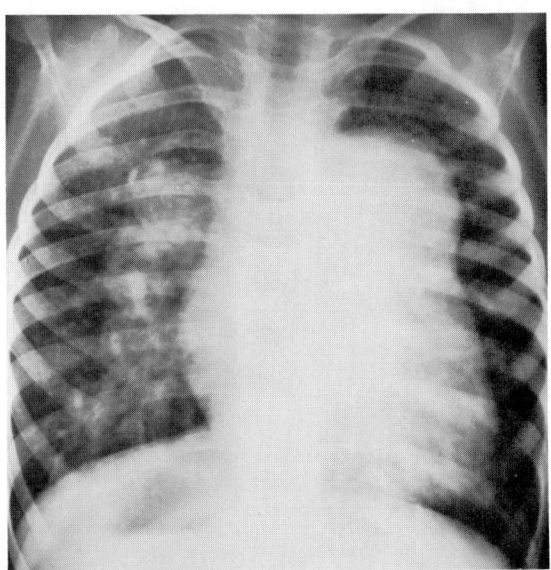

Figure 13-28. Teleroentgenogram in Eisenmenger syndrome due to a ventricular septal defect. Note the dilatation of the pulmonary artery and gross pulmonary overvascularity.

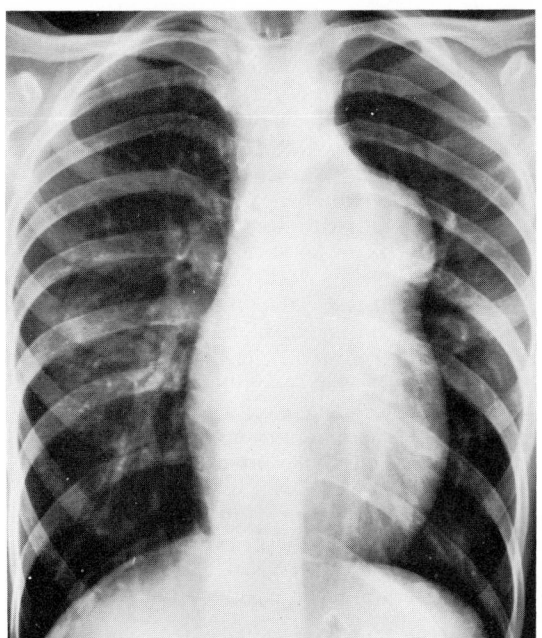

Figure 13-29. Teleroentgenogram in Eisenmenger syndrome due to a patent ductus arteriosus. The heart size is normal, the pulmonary artery segment is dilated, and the pulmonary vascularity is normal or slightly increased.

verses the defect, especially with a patent ductus arteriosus or atrial septal defect. The systolic pressures are usually equal in the systemic and pulmonary circulations. The pulmonary vascular resistance is elevated. *Indicator dilution curves* demonstrate the bidirectional shunts or the unidirectional right-to-left one. *Selective angiocardiography* is helpful in locating the site of the shunt. With patent ductus arteriosus contrast medium enters the descending aorta from the pulmonary artery.

Treatment. The presence of the Eisenmenger syndrome contraindicates surgical closure of the defect. But pulmonary hypertension with increased pulmonary blood flow, but without a right-to-left shunt, is not the Eisenmenger syndrome and surgery may be lifesaving. Medical treatment of the Eisenmenger syndrome is entirely symptomatic. Older children and adolescents with significant polycythemia may be improved by cautious, repeated small venesections.

TRANSPOSITION OF THE GREAT VESSELS (ARTERIES)

In this condition the aorta arises from the right ventricle and the pulmonary artery from the left ventricle. The systemic veins return to the right atrium, and the pulmonary venous return is to the left atrium. Thus the blood from the right side of the heart passes to the aorta. The pulmonary venous blood is returned to the lungs. The 2 in-

dependent circuits do not support life unless the foramen ovale or the ductus arteriosus remains open or unless there is a defect in the atrial or ventricular septum to permit some mixture of blood. This condition accounts for the majority of deaths in infants under the age of 1 year with cyanotic congenital heart disease. It is of interest that this condition occurs predominantly in males and that a significant number have a family history of diabetes mellitus.

Generally the aorta is anterior and to the right of the pulmonary trunk. Less commonly the aorta is directly in front of the pulmonary artery, or anterior and to the left of it, or the vessels are side by side. The pulmonary valve is continuous with the mitral valve (in the normal the mitral and aortic valves are continuous). Defects of the ventricular septum occur in about 50 per cent and are situated anywhere in the septum. Generally the right coronary artery arises above the posterior sinus of Valsalva and the left above the left sinus (in the normal the right coronary artery arises above the right sinus and the left above the left sinus).

The pulmonary circulation determines the hemodynamics, clinical course and prognosis. Infants generally have an increased pulmonary blood flow with a moderate or marked increase of pulmonary arterial pressure. In these patients the ventricular septum is intact or there can be a ventricular septal defect of varying size. Marked increase of pulmonary vascular resistance may be present early, but is generally found in older children, and usually with a large ventricular septal defect.

Clinical Manifestations. Cyanosis, congestive cardiac failure, dyspnea, tachypnea and retardation of growth dominate the clinical picture. Cyanosis appears shortly after birth or in the first few weeks of life. It is present at rest and progressive in intensity. Polycythemia and arterial unsaturation are usual in older infants. Occasionally cyanosis of moderate intensity appears late in patients who have a heavy pulmonary flow. In some patients the legs are less cyanotic than the rest of the body because of the flow of arterialized blood across a patent ductus arteriosus from pulmonary artery to descending aorta. Differential cyanosis is usually seen only if there is associated preductal aortic coarctation. Hypercyanotic blue spells are rare. Congestive cardiac failure occurs early, frequently in the neonatal period, and generally before the age of 4 months. Cardiomegaly with a hyperactive precordium and a right ventricular lift is usual, especially after the first month of life, but the heart size may be normal in the neonate. The first heart sound is sharp, and the second sound is single or narrowly split. Appreciation of splitting of the second sound is helpful in differentiating arterial transposition from hypoplastic left heart syndrome. Systolic murmurs are inconstant and frequently absent in the sick infant with an intact ventricular septum. When a ventricular defect is present, a systolic ejection murmur is generally audible, and often soft in quality.

With pulmonary vascular obstruction and reduced pulmonary blood flow, cyanosis is intense, but heart failure is minimal. Clubbing is marked in older children. Signs of pulmonary hypertension are obvious on auscultation and include a systolic ejection click, a booming second heart sound, a short systolic ejection murmur and sometimes an early diastolic murmur of pulmonary incompetence.

The typical *roentgenogram* reveals progressive cardiomegaly, increased pulmonary vasculature and a narrow cardiac base in frontal projection. During the first week of life these signs are not obvious. Progressive generalized cardiomegaly develops rapidly, however, and is much more striking if pulmonary blood flow is excessive. There is increased pulmonary vasculature bilaterally, which may be more striking in the right upper lobe. The narrow cardiac base in frontal projection is due to superimposition of the shadows of the aorta and pulmonary trunk; it may be obscured by a large thymic shadow. When pulmonary vascular obstruction is present, cardiomegaly is only mild to moderate, and the pulmonary vessels are prominent in the hilar areas, but appear narrow peripherally.

The *electrocardiogram* shows right axis deviation, right ventricular hypertrophy and frequently P pulmonale. In patients with a large pulmonary flow the axis is usually either to the right or normal, but occasionally it is to the left; there may be biventricular hypertrophy or occasionally dominance of the left ventricle. Right ventricular hypertrophy is usual when pulmonary vascular obstruction supervenes. In the newborn the electrocardiogram may be normal or show right ventricular hypertrophy.

Cardiac catheterization shows right ventricular hypertension. The catheter enters the aorta directly from the right ventricle; it may pass across the foramen ovale or an atrial septal defect into the left heart chambers, or across a ventricular septal defect into the pulmonary artery. The blood in the pulmonary artery has a higher oxygen content than that in the aorta; this finding is diagnostic. The direction of the shunt across the atrial and ventricular septa and the ductus arteriosus varies considerably. Marked systemic venous unsaturation is usual. The degree of arterial unsaturation is variable, but can be extreme in the hypoxic infant. If the ventricular septum is intact, the left ventricular peak systolic pressure may be lower than that in the right ventricle.

Selective right ventriculography is diagnostic. It demonstrates the origin of the anteriorly placed aorta from the right ventricle. The aortic valve is at a higher level than the pulmonic valve (reverse of normal). *Selective left ventriculography* demonstrates that the pulmonary artery arises from the posterior ventricle. Associated anomalies such as ventricular septal defect and patent ductus arteriosus may be demonstrated by selective injection of contrast medium into either ventricle. The origin of the coronary arteries is determined from an injection of contrast medium at the aortic root.

Prognosis. The majority of patients succumb during the first year of life. The onset of congestive heart failure, especially in the first few months of life, is an ominous sign. The few patients who survive beyond the age of 3 years usually have a ventricular septal defect with an increased pulmonary vascular resistance. The poorest prognosis is in infants who have an intact ventricular septum with a small foramen ovale and ductus arteriosus; most succumb during the first month of life.

Treatment. Confirmation of the diagnosis is an emergency in hypoxic neonates and infants. Recognition and early correction of metabolic and respiratory acidosis and hypoglycemia are also essential. After the diagnosis of arterial transposition has been confirmed by angiocardiography, particularly if the ventricular septum is intact, a large interatrial communication may be created at the time of cardiac catheterization by the balloon atrial septostomy technique of Rashkind. This method usually results in temporary but rapid improvement of hypoxia and acidosis so that future palliative surgical therapy can be undertaken electively. Surgical treatment depends on the nature of associated defects and the reaction of the pulmonary circulation. It is carried out preferably between the ages of 2 and 5 years. Relief of hypoxia and heart failure by balloon septostomy may be temporary, so that it may have to be repeated, or excision of the interatrial septum (Blalock-Hanlon) may be necessary. If a ventricular septal defect of significant size is present, the pulmonary vascular tree should be protected by banding of the pulmonary artery. A simultaneous Blalock-Hanlon operation is undertaken if intracardiac mixing is inadequate as indicated by severe hypoxia. These patients may also be relieved by atrial septostomy at the time of cardiac catheterization.

Good results may be obtained by the corrective operation described by Mustard. An intra-atrial

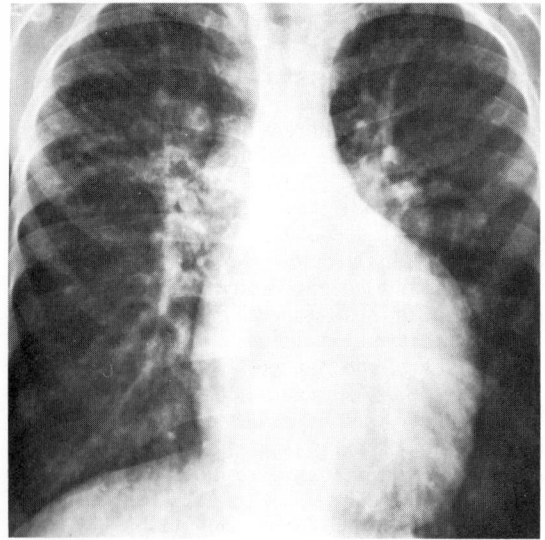

Figure 13-30. Teleroentgenogram in complete transposition of the great vessels (arteries) with intact ventricular septum, showing cardiomegaly, gross pulmonary overcirculation and a narrow cardiac base.

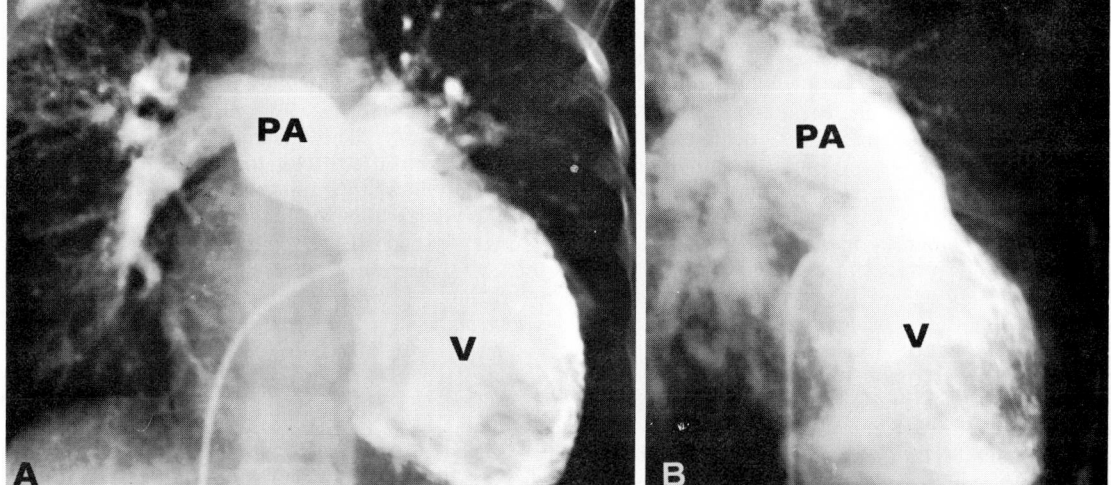

Figure 13-31. Transposition of great vessels. Injection of contrast medium into a smooth-walled posterior (left) ventricle. Pulmonary artery arises exclusively from the posterior ventricle, and the interventricular septum is intact. A, Anteroposterior view; B, lateral view. Abbreviations: PA, pulmonary artery; V, posterior (left) ventricle.

baffle of pericardium is developed which directs systemic venous blood to the mitral valve and posterior (left) ventricle and pulmonary venous blood to the tricuspid valve and anterior (right) ventricle. Thus systemic venous blood is pumped by the left ventricle to the lungs, and pulmonary venous blood is ejected by the right ventricle to the aorta. The ideal candidate for this operation is the 2- or 3-year-old child whose ventricular septum is intact or who has a small ventricular defect and does not have pulmonary vascular obstruction. Generally these patients have had a palliative operation during the first few months of life. Pulmonary vascular obstruction contraindicates surgery. During surgery the pulmonary artery is debanded and the ventricular septal defect closed; subsequently, persistent atrial dysrhythmias are common.

Although of limited value, medical treatment with digitalis and diuretics should be used vigorously.

TRANSPOSITION OF THE GREAT VESSELS (ARTERIES) IN ASSOCIATION WITH OTHER DEFECTS

With Pulmonary Stenosis. This condition assumes importance because it may mimic tetralogy of Fallot. In the majority of instances a ventricular defect is present. The onset of symptoms varies from soon after birth to late infancy and is manifest by cyanosis, hypercyanotic (paroxysmal dyspneic) episodes, decreased exercise tolerance and poor physical development. Congestive heart failure is not common in infancy, but may occur in later years. On examination the findings are similar to those described under tetralogy of Fallot. The cyanosis is usually more intense, however, and the heart may be slightly enlarged. The pulmonary vasculature as seen on roentgenogram is somewhat diminished or normal and in some in-

stances may be increased, especially if the pulmonic stenosis is not severe. The electrocardiogram usually shows right axis deviation, right ventricular hypertrophy and sometimes tall, spiked P waves. Acquired pulmonary stenosis may develop after the creation of an atrial septal defect for the relief of hypoxia due to arterial transposition.

During cardiac catheterization the pulmonary artery may be entered after the catheter has traversed the ventricular defect. The pulmonary arterial pressure is low, and its oxygen saturation exceeds that of the aorta. Selective right and left ventriculography demonstrates the origin of the aorta from the right ventricle, the origin of the pulmonary artery from the left ventricle, the ventricular defect and the pulmonary stenosis.

Treatment is difficult. Systemic-pulmonary arterial anastomosis is generally undertaken in cyanotic patients with severe pulmonic stenosis and ventricular septal defect who are not in congestive cardiac failure. At the same time an atrial septal defect may be created surgically (Blalock-Hanlon), especially if left atrial hypertension is present or if there is an insignificant rise in systemic arterial oxygen saturation from the shunt alone. Although anastomosis of the superior vena cava to the right pulmonary artery (Glenn) may result in palliation, later surgical correction may be compromised. Surgical correction by the Mustard operation with simultaneous closure of the ventricular septal defect and pulmonary valvotomy is possible. Another form of treatment consists of: (1) repair of the ventricular septal defect with a patch to connect the left ventricle and aorta, (2) division of the pulmonary artery, (3) reconstruction of the pulmonary artery with an aortic homograft, including the aortic valve, which is anastomosed between the right ventricle and the distal stump of the pulmonary artery (Rastelli et al.).

With Tricuspid Atresia. If arterial transposition is associated with tricuspid atresia and pulmonic stenosis, the syndrome is similar to that described under Tricuspid Atresia. If pulmonic stenosis is absent, however, and pulmonary flow excessive, cyanosis is mild and seldom conspicuous. Tachypnea, feeding difficulties, poor weight gain, recurrent respiratory infections and heart failure are usual. Increased venous pressure may result in presystolic pulsations of a large liver and a prominent "a" wave in the jugular venous pulse. Cardiac enlargement is moderate or marked. Systolic ejection murmurs of varying intensity are usual, and the second heart sound is loud and single. Although the electrocardiogram may show prominent P waves, left axis deviation and left ventricular hypertrophy, many patients have right axis deviation. Cardiac enlargement is confirmed roentgenographically; increased pulmonary vascularity is usual. The diagnosis is confirmed by selective left ventriculography, which delineates a large left ventricle, small right ventricle, arterial transposition and the relative size of the pulmonary artery and aorta. Generally the prognosis is poor, especially when the aorta is hypoplastic and pulmonary flow torrential. Surgical palliation is achieved with pulmonary arterial banding, which is most effective when the aortic root is near normal in size.

Transposition of Aorta and Overriding Pulmonary Artery
(TAUSSIG-BING SYNDROME)

In this malformation the aorta arises from the right ventricle, and the pulmonary artery, which is large, overrides the ventricular septum. A ventricular septal defect is always present. The clinical picture is dominated by the presence of severe pulmonary hypertension. Cyanosis of varying intensity is usually present from birth. Tachypnea, frequent respiratory infections, decreased exercise tolerance and poor physical development are usual. Cardiac enlargement may be present during infancy, but in older children the heart is near normal in size because pulmonary vascular disease restricts pulmonary blood flow. Auscultatory findings are produced by pulmonary hypertension and include an early ejection systolic click, a midsystolic ejection murmur, a booming second heart sound and sometimes an early diastolic murmur of pulmonary valvular incompetence. The systolic murmur is longer and louder if pulmonary blood flow is torrential. Pulmonic stenosis is rarely present.

The electrocardiogram shows right ventricular hypertrophy with prominent P waves. Left ventricular hypertrophy is seen in infancy when a large pulmonary flow is present. The chest x-ray shows cardiomegaly and increased pulmonary vasculature during infancy. As pulmonary vascular obstruction develops, the heart size decreases, the major branches of the pulmonary artery become prominent, and there is attenuation of the vascular pattern in the outer lung fields. Cardiac

catheterization reveals right ventricular and pulmonary hypertension, and the pulmonary arterial oxygen saturation exceeds that of the aorta. Selective right ventriculography demonstrates the abnormal anatomic positions of the aorta and pulmonary artery. The prognosis is variable, but many patients survive to adult life. Surgical correction now appears to be feasible by closure of the ventricular septal defect and interatrial venous transposition (Mustard operation). Pulmonary vascular obstruction contraindicates operation.

EBSTEIN'S DISEASE

This abnormality consists in downward displacement of an abnormal tricuspid valve into the right ventricle. The anterior cusp of the valve retains some attachment to the valve ring, but the other leaflets are attached to the wall of the right ventricle. The latter chamber is divided into 2 parts by the abnormal valve; the first is continuous with the cavity of the right atrium, and the second consists of a thin-walled ventricle. The right atrium is huge, and the tricuspid valve may or may not be competent. The effective output from the right side of the heart is decreased because of the small size of the functioning right ventricle and possible obstruction produced by the large, saillike, anterior tricuspid leaflet. Similar hemodynamics are produced by thinning of the right ventricular wall due to hypoplasia of the myocardium (*Uhl's anomaly*).

The severity of symptoms appears to depend on the degree of displacement of the tricuspid valve. In many patients, symptoms are mild and the only complaint is fatigue. Cardiac dysrhythmias are frequent, the commonest being numerous extrasystoles or attacks of paroxysmal tachycardia, usually supraventricular. The presence of cyanosis depends on the integrity of the atrial septum. If the foramen ovale is open or an interatrial defect is present, a right-to-left shunt at this level produces cyanosis and polycythemia. This symptom can appear at any age and in some patients is intense. The venous pressure is normal or, if there is associated tricuspid insufficiency, increased. On palpation the precordium is quiet. A systolic murmur, sometimes accompanied by a thrill, is audible over most of the anterior left side of the chest. Gallop rhythm is common, as is a diastolic murmur at the left sternal border. This murmur is superficial and may mimic a pericardial friction rub. A series of systolic ejection clicks and an opening snap of the tricuspid valve may also be audible.

The *electrocardiogram* shows incomplete or complete right bundle branch block, normal or tall and broad P waves and normal or prolonged P-R interval. Sometimes the pattern of the Wolff-Parkinson-White syndrome is present.

On x-ray examination the heart size varies greatly. In some instances it is normal, and in others there is cardiomegaly because of great enlargement of the right atrium and ventricle. In patients with large hearts the amplitude of cardiac pulsations is decreased; the intrapulmonary vasculature is normal or decreased, and the aorta is small.

Cardiac catheterization and selective angiocardiography confirm the presence of a large right atrium and demonstrate the right-to-left shunt at the atrial level, if this exists. The right atrial pressure may be normal, but it is frequently elevated, as is the right ventricular diastolic pressure. Simultaneous intracardiac electrocardiograms and pressures are of great value when they reveal the following 3 patterns: (1) right ventricular pressure with a right ventricular intracavity electrocardiogram, (2) from the atrialized portion of the right ventricle – atrial pressure curve with a right ventricular intracavity electrocardiogram, and (3) from the right atrium – atrial pressure curves and atrial intracavity electrocardiogram. These studies should not be undertaken lightly because of the hazard of precipitating cardiac arrhythmias or even rupture of the right atrium.

The prognosis is extremely variable, many patients living well into adult life. Medical treatment is directed toward control of cardiac failure and supraventricular dysrhythmias. In deeply cyanotic patients, anastomosis of the superior vena cava to the right pulmonary artery (Glenn) has resulted in symptomatic improvement. Replacement of the abnormal tricuspid valve with a prosthesis has been performed successfully.

TRUNCUS ARTERIOSUS

This condition is characterized by a single arterial trunk leaving the ventricular portion of the heart and supplying the systemic, pulmonary and coronary circulations. A ventricular septal defect is always present, and the number of semilunar valve cusps varies from 2 to 6. In the majority of instances the pulmonary arteries arise from the ascending portion of the truncus proximal to the origin of the innominate artery. The pulmonary arteries may arise as a single vessel from the truncus or as 2 separate arteries. In some instances the pulmonary arteries and ductus are absent so that the pulmonary blood flow is derived from collateral vessels, usually bronchial. If there is a remnant of a pulmonary artery leaving the right ventricle and pulmonary blood flow is supplied from the aorta via a ductus arteriosus, the condition is considered to be pulmonary atresia (see p. 973).

Hemodynamics. Both ventricles empty their blood at systemic pressure into the truncus. In the presence of a normal pulmonary vascular resistance, the blood flow to the lungs is greatly increased, the arteriovenous oxygen difference small, and cyanosis is minimal or absent. When the pulmonary resistance is high, the pulmonary circulation is inadequate, and cyanosis is intense. If pulmonary arteries are absent and collateral bronchial vessels supply the lungs, pulmonary blood flow is usually inadequate and cyanosis appears in early life.

Clinical Manifestations. Owing to the extremely variable hemodynamics, the clinical picture varies. In the majority of infants pulmonary blood flow is torrential, and the flow picture is dominated by dyspnea, fatigue, heart failure, recurrent respiratory infections and poor physical development. Cyanosis is minimal or absent. The runoff of blood from the truncus to the pulmonary circulation may result in a wide pulse pressure. The heart is usually enlarged, and the precordium is hyperdynamic. A systolic ejection murmur, sometimes accompanied by a thrill, is usual down the left sternal border. The murmur is frequently preceded by an ejection click. The second heart sound is loud and generally single, though it may be closely but clearly split. A mid-diastolic apical rumbling murmur is frequent, and occasionally an early diastolic murmur is audible. In older children with restricted pulmonary blood flow, progressive cyanosis, polycythemia and clubbing develop. When pulmonary arteries are hypoplastic, cyanosis and dyspnea are present from infancy; cardiomegaly is moderate, and continuous murmurs may be produced by the bronchial collateral flow.

The electrocardiogram is variable and shows pure right, pure left or combined ventricular hypertrophy. There is considerable variation of the appearance of the chest on roentgen examination. Cardiac enlargement is due to prominence of both ventricles. The truncus may produce a prominent shadow which follows the normal course of the ascending aorta and aortic knob; it arches to the right in one third to one half of the patients. The shadow of the main pulmonary artery is not clearly discerned. Sometimes a high bulge, seen to the left of the aortic knob, is produced by the main or left pulmonary artery. The pulmonary vascularity is increased in the presence of normal pulmonary resistance; it decreases as the resistance rises. A diffuse reticular pattern in the lung fields with retroesophageal vessels demonstrated by barium esophagogram may be seen in patients with bronchial collateral blood flow to the lungs.

The **diagnosis** is confirmed by cardiac catheterization and by selective right ventriculography. The catheter may enter the pulmonary arteries from the truncus. A left-to-right shunt is demonstrated at the ventricular level, and the systolic pressures in both ventricles and the truncus are similar. Selective angiocardiography reveals the large truncus arteriosus and the origin of the pulmonary arteries.

The **prognosis** is variable, but the majority of patients succumb during the first 2 years of life. Nevertheless, if pulmonary blood flow is via adequate collateral vessels, the patient may survive well into adult life with little incapacity.

Treatment is not standardized. Infants with

large pulmonary blood flow have been treated with banding of both pulmonary arteries. Corrective surgery is possible with closure of the ventricular septal defect and insertion of a homograft to act as a pulmonic valve and main pulmonary artery. Severe pulmonary vascular obstruction or hypoplastic pulmonary arteries preclude surgical treatment.

SINGLE VENTRICLE

With a single ventricle both atria empty through 2 separate atrioventricular valves into a single ventricular chamber from which the aorta and pulmonary artery arise. Associated cardiac anomalies are usual and consist of one or any combination of the following: (1) a rudimentary outlet chamber in the region usually occupied by the right ventricular outflow and separated from the single ventricle by a muscular ridge, (2) transposition of the aorta and pulmonary artery, (3) pulmonic stenosis, (4) dextrocardia or other cardiac malposition, (5) aortic outflow obstruction with or without coarctation, (6) defects of the atrial septum, (7) common atrioventricular canal. The more frequent associations are (1) single ventricle, arterial transposition and rudimentary outlet chamber from which the aorta arises; and (2) single ventricle with pulmonic stenosis.

The hemodynamics and clinical picture are extremely variable because they depend on the associated intracardiac anomalies and the degree of pulmonary blood flow. If a single ventricle is associated with pulmonic stenosis, cyanosis is present in infancy and increases in intensity during childhood when clubbing and polycythemia also appear. Dyspnea and fatigue are frequent, and paroxysmal dyspneic spells may occur. Cardiomegaly is mild or moderate; a left parasternal lift is palpable, and a systolic thrill common. The systolic ejection murmur is usually loud; an ejection click may be audible, and the second heart sound is single and loud. When a single ventricle is associated with a rudimentary systemic outflow tract, pulmonary blood flow is torrential. These patients have tachypnea, dyspnea, poor physical development, recurrent pulmonary infections and congestive heart failure. Cyanosis is only mild or moderate. Cardiomegaly is generally marked, and a left parasternal lift is palpable. The systolic ejection murmur is generally not intense, and the second heart sound is loud and closely split. A third heart sound is frequent and may be followed by a short mid-diastolic murmur. The development of pulmonary vascular disease may restrict pulmonary blood flow so that cyanosis increases in intensity, heart size decreases, and signs of cardiac failure appear to improve.

The electrocardiogram is nonspecific. P waves are normal, spiked or bifid. Usually right axis deviation is present, but occasionally left axis deviation is observed. The precordial lead pattern suggests right ventricular hypertrophy, combined ventricular hypertrophy or sometimes left ventricular dominance. The initial QRS forces are usually to the left and anterior. Roentgenographic examination confirms the degree of cardiomegaly. The rudimentary systemic outflow chamber may produce a bulge on the upper left border of the cardiac silhouette in the posteroanterior projection. In the absence of pulmonic stenosis, pulmonary vasculature is increased with prominence of the major branches of the pulmonary artery. Attenuation of the size of the peripheral pulmonary arteries occurs with the development of obstructive pulmonary hypertension. If pulmonic stenosis is present, pulmonary vasculature is decreased to varying degrees.

Cardiac catheterization reveals a left-to-right shunt at the ventricular level. Varying degrees of arterial unsaturation are present. The arterial oxygen saturation is markedly decreased in the presence of severe pulmonic stenosis or obstructive pulmonary hypertension, but is near normal when pulmonary blood flow is increased. The pressure in the single ventricle is high, and a gradient may be demonstrated between it and the rudimentary outflow tract or the pulmonary artery in the presence of pulmonary stenosis. Severe pulmonary hypertension is present when pulmonary stenosis is absent. Selective ventriculography is diagnostic and demonstrates the single ventricle and the position and relation of the pulmonary artery and aorta. Also the presence or absence of pulmonic stenosis or a rudimentary outflow chamber is identified.

A number of these patients succumb during infancy from congestive heart failure and superimposed pulmonary infection. Others may survive to adolescence and early adult life, but finally succumb to the effects of pulmonary hypertension. The prognosis appears to be better if there is associated pulmonary stenosis. If pulmonary stenosis is present, a systemic-pulmonary arterial anastomosis can result in improvement, but some patients suffer heart failure some months after operation. Anastomosis of the superior vena cava to the right pulmonary artery may be beneficial in patients with pulmonary stenosis. Pulmonary artery banding is advised for patients with a large pulmonary flow.

HYPOPLASTIC LEFT HEART SYNDROME
(Aortic Atresia)

The term "hypoplastic left heart syndrome" is used to describe varying degrees of underdevelopment of the left side of the heart. The anomalies include underdevelopment of the left atrium and ventricle, stenosis or atresia of the aortic or mitral orifices, and hypoplasia of the ascending aorta. Associated defects include endocardial fibroelastosis of the left ventricle, and atrial and ventricular septal defects. The left ventricular cavity is small, but the wall may be thick if obstruction to left ventricular outflow is associated with mitral stenosis. If aortic atresia and mitral atresia co-exist, the left ventricular cavity is minute.

Since the left ventricle is virtually nonfunctional, the right ventricle maintains both pulmonary and systemic circulations. Pulmonary venous blood passes through an atrial or ventricular septal defect from the left to the right side of the heart, where it mixes with systemic venous blood. If the ventricular septum is intact, all the right ventricular blood is ejected to the pulmonary arteries; the systemic circulation is supplied via the ductus arteriosus. With a ventricular septal defect and a patent but small aortic orifice, right ventricular blood is ejected to the small left ventricle and ascending aorta as well as to the pulmonary artery. The major hemodynamic abnormalities are inadequate maintenance of the systemic circulation and pulmonary venous hypertension.

Signs of heart failure appear within the first few weeks of life and include dyspnea and hepatomegaly. All peripheral pulses are weak or impalpable. Although cyanosis may not be obvious in the first 48 hours of life, a grayish-blue color of the skin is soon apparent. Differential cyanosis may be striking if the aortic valve has a small opening. In these patients oxygenated blood from the left ventricle enters the ascending aorta and innominate artery, resulting in a normal color in the right arm and right side of the head and neck with a contrasting cyanosis in the rest of the body. Cardiac enlargement is usual with a palpable right ventricular parasternal lift. In many cases, murmurs are not audible and, if present, are short and midsystolic. Roentgenographically, the heart is variable in size in the first few days of life, but moderate or gross cardiomegaly develops rapidly and is associated with increased pulmonary vascularity.

The electrocardiogram generally shows prominent P waves, right axis deviation and right ventricular hypertrophy. The diagnosis can be confirmed by angiocardiography and aortography. Most of the contrast medium flows from the right ventricle to the pulmonary artery, through a patent ductus arteriosus and into the descending aorta. The hypoplastic ascending aorta is best demonstrated by aortography, which may also show the coronary arterial system.

Most patients succumb during the first month of life, usually during the first week. Treatment is symptomatic.

ABNORMAL POSITIONS OF THE HEART: DEXTROCARDIA AND LEVOCARDIA

An approach to the classification and diagnosis of abnormal cardiac position has been suggested by Van Praagh et al. *Atrial localization* is facilitated by radiologic demonstration of the position of the abdominal organs, since atrial situs is the same as visceral situs; if the abdominal organs are in normal position, the atria have a normal position. Abdominal situs inversus is associated with the left atrium to the right and right atrium to the left. If the abdominal situs cannot be determined, as with a centrally located liver, atrial localization is difficult and asplenia or rudimentary spleen is common. *Localization of the ventricles and great arteries* depends on the direction of development of the embryonic cardiac loop. Initial protrusion to the right (d-loop) carries the future right ventricle to the right, and the left ventricle remains on the left. Protrusion to the left (l-loop) carries the future right ventricle to the left, and the left ventricle is on the right. In both types of loop the relations of the great arteries may be normal or transposed. Angiographic demonstration of the relations of the aorta and pulmonary artery indicates the type of cardiac loop and the relative location of the ventricle. The clinical picture of abnormal cardiac position is dominated by the associated cardiovascular anomalies.

Dextrocardia with or without situs inversus is frequently complicated by severe malformations, including combinations of single ventricle, arterial transposition, pulmonic stenosis, ventricular and atrial septal defects, complete atrioventricular canal, anomalous pulmonary venous return, tricuspid atresia, and pulmonary arterial hypoplasia or atresia. The patient with dextrocardia, cyanosis and signs of pulmonic stenosis generally has arterial transposition, pulmonic stenosis and ventricular septal defect. Generally dextrocardia with situs inversus is associated with other severe cardiovascular anomalies; a few of those who survive have functionally normal hearts. Some of the older patients have *Kartagener's syndrome* (complete situs inversus, paranasal sinusitis and bronchiectasis).

Abnormalities of the lung, diaphragm and thoracic cage may result in displacement of the heart to the right, mimicking dextrocardia. Hypoplasia of a lung may be accompanied by anomalous pulmonary venous return from that lung. The electrocardiogram is helpful in diagnosis, but frequently difficult to interpret. Inversion of the P wave in lead I is indicative of atrial inversion. Q waves produced by right ventricular hypertrophy may make interpretation of ventricular dominance difficult. Deep Q waves or QS in V_1, V_2 and a V_L are seen in patients with dextrocardia and normally related great arteries.

Levocardia with situs inversus is usually associated with severe cardiovascular defects, frequently of the cyanotic type. These include combinations of abnormal systemic venous return (bilateral superior vena cava; absence of inferior vena cava with venous drainage of the lower part of the body into the azygous system), anomalous pulmonary venous return, arterial transposition, pulmonary stenosis or atresia, atrial or ventricular septal defect, common atrioventricular canal,

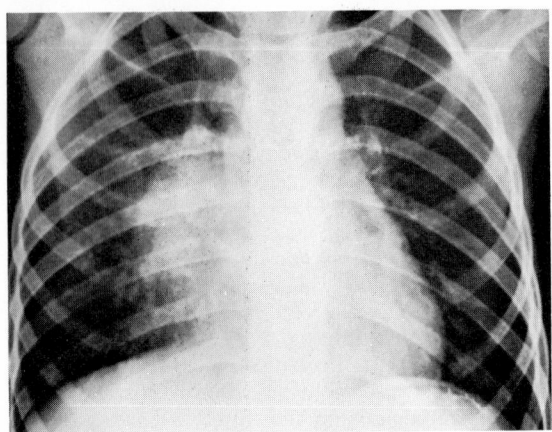

Figure 13-32. Teleroentgenogram in pulmonary arteriovenous fistula, showing a localized increase in pulmonary vascularity in the right lung.

single ventricle and patent ductus arteriosus. These patients have a high incidence of asplenia or rudimentary spleen, which may be suspected when Howell-Jolly bodies (nuclear remnants) or Heinz bodies (precipitated hemoglobin) are seen in the red cells.

Treatment of abnormal cardiac position is determined by the underlying defect. Cyanotic infants with pulmonic stenosis and ventricular septal defect as a part of the malformation improve after anastomosis of the systemic and pulmonary blood supplies. Lesions such as atrial or ventricular septal defect and Fallot's tetralogy have been repaired successfully.

PULMONARY ARTERIOVENOUS FISTULA

Fistulous vascular communications in the lungs may be large and localized or multiple, scattered and small. They may be a manifestation of the Rendu-Osler-Weber syndrome (hereditary hemorrhagic telangiectasia) with angiomas of the nasal and buccal mucous membranes, gastrointestinal tract or liver. A rare variant is a direct communication between the pulmonary artery and left atrium.

Venous blood in the pulmonary artery is shunted through the fistula into the pulmonary vein without exposure to alveolar air, enters the left heart and results in systemic arterial unsaturation. The shunt across the fistula is at low pressure and resistance, so that pulmonary arterial pressure is normal, cardiomegaly unusual, and heart failure rare.

The clinical picture depends on the magnitude of shunt. Dyspnea, cyanosis, clubbing and polycythemia occur with large fistulas. Hemoptysis is rare, but may be massive. Features of the Rendu-Osler-Weber syndrome occur in about half of the patients (or other members of their family) and

include recurrent epistaxis and gastrointestinal bleeding. Transitory dizziness, diplopia, aphasia, motor weakness or convulsions may result from cerebral thrombosis, abscess or paradoxical emboli. The heart is normal on examination, but soft systolic or continuous murmurs may be audible over the site of the fistula.

The electrocardiogram is normal. Roentgenographic examination of the chest may show opacities produced by large fistulas; multiple small fistulas may be visualized by fluoroscopy (abnormal pulsations) or tomography. Selective pulmonary arteriography demonstrates the site, extent and distribution of the fistulas (Figs. 13-32, 13-33).

Excision of solitary or localized lesions by lobectomy or wedge resection results in complete disappearance of symptoms. If the fistulas are widely distributed, extensive pulmonary resection may be followed by postoperative growth of smaller fistulas and recurrence of symptoms. Direct communications between the pulmonary artery and left atrium are obliterated by division and suture.

ECTOPIA CORDIS

This is a rare malformation in which the heart is in an abnormal location. In the commonest form, thoracic in type, the sternum is split, and the heart protrudes outside the chest. In others the heart protrudes through the diaphragm into the abdominal cavity, or may be situated in the neck. Associated intracardiac anomalies are common. Death occurs in the first few days of life in the majority of instances. Occasional patients with the abdominal type have survived to adulthood, but surgical attempts to replace the heart in the chest have failed.

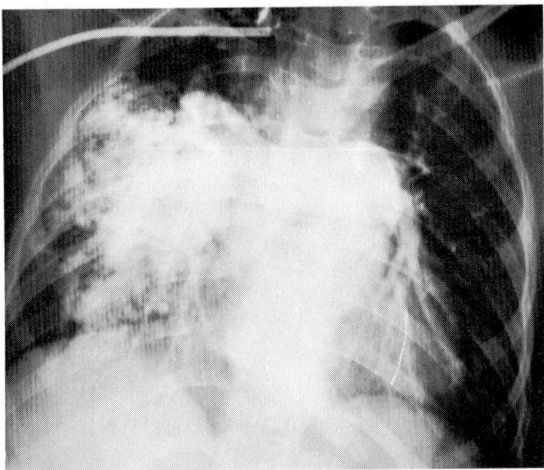

Figure 13-33. Angiocardiogram in pulmonary arteriovenous fistula. (Same patient as Figure 13-32.) The contrast medium has delineated the extent of the fistula in the right lung.

DIVERTICULUM OF THE LEFT VENTRICLE

In this rare anomaly a diverticulum of the left ventricle protrudes into the epigastrium. The lesion may be isolated, or associated with complex cardiovascular anomalies. A pulsating mass is visible and palpable in the epigastrium. Systolic or systolic-diastolic murmurs produced by blood flow in and out of the diverticulum may be audible over the lower sternum and the mass. The electrocardiogram shows a pattern of complete or incomplete left bundle branch block. Roentgenograms of the chest may or may not show the mass. Surgical resection should be attempted because the diverticulum may rupture.

Congenital Heart Disease with Little or No Cyanosis (Dominant Left-to-Right Shunt or No Shunt)

VENTRICULAR SEPTAL DEFECT

Isolated defects of the ventricular septum are among the commonest cardiac malformations. The majority lie inferior to the crista supraventricularis in close relation to the aortic valve and septal leaflet of the tricuspid valve; they may be between the crista supraventricularis and the papillary muscle of the conus or posteroinferior to this area to include the membranous portion of the septum. Defects superior to the crista supraventricularis are uncommon; they lie just below the pulmonic and aortic valves. Defects involving the inflow portion of the ventricular septum are muscular in type and may be isolated or multiple.

Effects on the cardiac chambers and pulmonary vascular tree depend to a large extent on the size of the defect and the response of the pulmonary vasculature. If the defect is small, the cardiac chambers and pulmonary vascular bed are normal. The significant left-to-right shunt and pulmonary hypertension produced by large defects result in varying degrees of right and left ventricular hypertrophy and dilatation, as well as in enlargement of the left atrium. The pulmonary arterial trunk is large. During infancy the media of the small muscular pulmonary arteries and arterioles are thick; this may represent retention of the normal fetal pulmonary vasculature, or a response to pulmonary hypertension. Intimal changes are variable; nonspecific intimal fibrosis may be the only lesion. In other instances there may be a plexiform lesion consisting of a papillary mass of endothelial cells in the lumen of the small vessel, with peripheral dilatation and thinning of the wall. Necrotizing arteritis may occur, but is uncommon.

Hemodynamics. Because of the normally nearly equal systemic and pulmonary arterial pressures and resistances during fetal life, the presence of a ventricular septal defect probably does not alter blood flow in the heart and lungs. After birth, blood flow across the defect is determined to a large extent by the magnitude of the normal fall in pulmonary vascular resistance as well as by the size of the defect. Defects up to 6 mm. in diameter ordinarily do not permit large left-to-right shunts, and right ventricular and pulmonary arterial pressures are normal. Larger defects allow enough communication between the left and right ventricles that the magnitude of the shunt is inversely related to the pulmonary vascular resistance; a marked increase in pulmonary vascular resistance may not only limit the magnitude of a left-to-right shunt, but also may result in a bidirectional shunt or a predominantly right-to-left shunt (see Eisenmenger Syndrome).

Levin and his co-workers have demonstrated that shunting of blood from left ventricle to right ventricle through a septal defect occurs throughout the cardiac cycle as long as right ventricular pressure is normal or moderately elevated. When ventricular pressures are nearly equal, right-to-left shunting occurs during isovolumic relaxation. In all patients a left-to-right shunt into the body of the right ventricle is present during diastole. Also, a left-to-right shunt is augmented during isovolumic contraction immediately preceding opening of the aortic valve.

In the presence of a left-to-right shunt the right ventricular output is supplemented by blood shunted across the defect; pulmonary arterial flow is increased, as is the return of pulmonary venous blood to the left atrium and ventricle. The factors which determine pulmonary hypertension are not clear; although increased pulmonary flow contributes to increased pressure (hyperkinetic pulmonary hypertension), closure of the shunt is not always followed by immediate reduction of pulmonary arterial pressure.

Clinical Manifestations. The manifestations of ventricular septal defects are determined by the hemodynamics; they vary according to the size of the defect and the reaction of the pulmonary circulation. *Small defects* with trivial left-to-right shunts and normal pulmonary arterial pressures are the most frequent. The patients are asymptomatic and the cardiac lesion is found accidentally during routine physical examination. Characteristically, there is a loud, harsh or blowing left parasternal pansystolic murmur, heard best over the lower left sternal border and frequently accom-

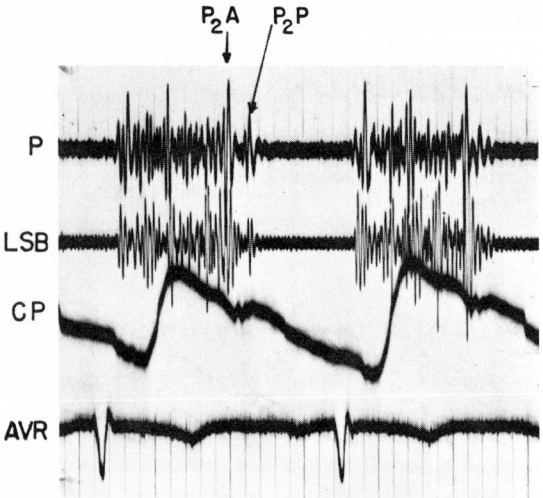

Figure 13-34. Phonocardiograms (*P,* pulmonary area; *LSB,* left sternal border) to illustrate auscultatory findings in moderate-sized ventricular septal defect with normal pulmonary arterial pressure. Long pansystolic murmur is evident. Abbreviations: *CP,* carotid pulse; *AVR,* electrocardiogram; P_2A, aortic components of second sound; P_2P, pulmonary component of second sound.

panied by a thrill. In a few instances the murmur ends well before the second sound, presumably because of closure of the defect during late systole; this atypical murmur becomes pansystolic after the administration of phenylephrine.

Roentgenograms are usually normal, although minimal cardiomegaly and a debatable increase in pulmonary vasculature may be observed. The electrocardiogram is usually normal, but may suggest isolated left or combined ventricular hypertrophy.

Ventricular defects of moderate size may result in large left-to-right shunts and mild to moderate increases in pulmonary arterial pressures and resistances. During infancy the symptoms are chiefly tachypnea, dyspnea, feeding difficulties, slow physical development and recurrent pulmonary infections with or without congestive cardiac failure. Improvement after the first year or two of life is usual, presumably due to relative or absolute decrease in size of the defect. Some prominence of the left precordium and sternum may be observed. A systolic thrill is usual. The characteristic pansystolic murmur is loud and harsh, has a wide distribution over the whole precordium, and is sometimes audible in the back, but is loudest at the lower left sternal border. The second heart sound at the apex is normal or moderately split and is normal or somewhat accentuated at the upper left sternal border. The increased pulmonary blood flow produces a systolic ejection murmur heard best at the upper left sternal border. The increased pulmonary venous return results in a large flow across the mitral valve, which, in turn, generates a rumbling mid-diastolic murmur best heard at the apex. This murmur may be preceded by a third heart sound.

Roentgenograms of the chest show mild to moderate cardiomegaly with some prominence of both ventricles and the left atrium. The shadow of the main pulmonary artery may be normal or prominent, and pulmonary overcirculation is usual. The electrocardiogram generally shows biventricular hypertrophy. Prominence of Q and R waves over the left precordium indicates left ventricular dominance; mild right ventricular overload is suggested by RS or rSr' in the right precordial leads.

Large defects with excessive pulmonary blood flow and pulmonary hypertension produce symptoms in infancy. These babies are dyspneic, have feeding difficulties, grow poorly, perspire profusely and suffer from recurrent pulmonary infections and episodes of heart failure. Cyanosis is absent, but a dusky plethora is sometimes noted during infections or crying. In the absence of heart failure, arterial and venous pulses are normal. Protrusion of the anterior portion of the chest is common, especially of the left precordium and sternum. Cardiomegaly is usual, with a palpable parasternal lift and apical thrust. Systolic thrills are common. The characteristic systolic murmur is similar to that of moderate-sized defects, but the sound of pulmonary valvular closure is louder and the second sound is narrowly split. The presence of an apical diastolic murmur indicates an appreciable left-to-right shunt.

Roentgenographically, gross cardiomegaly is usual, with prominence of both ventricles, the left atrium and pulmonary artery. The ascending aorta and aortic knob are relatively small, and intrinsic pulmonary arterial pulsations are common. The electrocardiogram shows biventricular hypertrophy or dominance of either the left or right ventricle. P waves may be notched or peaked.

If the shunt across the defect is limited by a significant elevation of pulmonary arterial resistance, the symptoms may appear to be less severe. Nevertheless physical underdevelopment and easy fatigability are usual. Mild cyanosis due to concomitant right-to-left shunt may be observed during intercurrent pulmonary infections. A precordial bulge is usual. Cardiomegaly is moderate, with a prominent left parasternal lift. A pulmonic ejection click is frequent and initiates a systolic ejection murmur. The second sound is narrowly split, with a booming pulmonary component. An early diastolic murmur of pulmonary valvular incompetence is sometimes heard. Roentgenographic examination confirms the moderate cardiomegaly; there is some prominence of both right and left ventricular shadows. Minimal left atrial enlargement may also be present. Prominence and increased pulsation of the pulmonary arterial trunk and its primary divisions may contrast with the relatively narrow peripheral branches of the pulmonary arterial tree. The electrocardiogram shows dominance of the right ventricle, but associated signs of left ventricular hypertrophy may also be seen. The P waves are either peaked or notched.

Special Studies. The effects of a ventricular septal defect on the pulmonary and systemic circu-

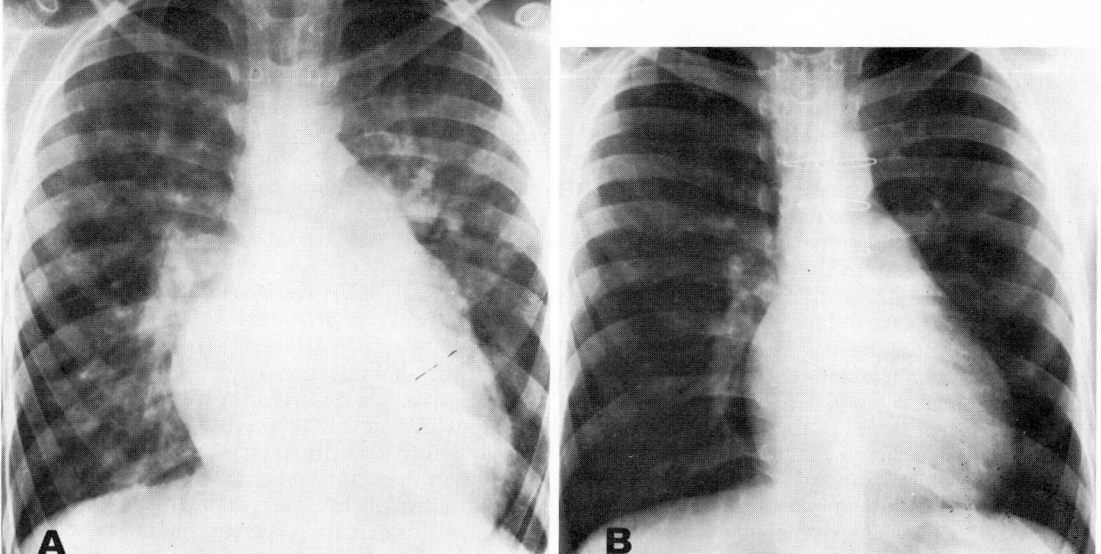

Figure 13-35. *A*, Preoperative teleroentgenogram in ventricular septal defect with large left-to-right shunt and pulmonary hypertension. Significant cardiomegaly, prominence of the pulmonary arterial trunk and pulmonary overcirculation are evident. *B*, Three years after surgical closure of defect. There is marked decrease in heart size, and the pulmonary vasculature is normal.

lations may be quantitated by cardiac catheterization, which also serves to determine if there are any clinically undetected anomalies. Since oxygenated blood passes across the defect from the left ventricle, blood from the right ventricle is significantly higher in oxygen than that from the right atrium. Occasionally mixing of blood in the right ventricle is inadequate, so that a definite rise in oxygen content is apparent only in the pulmonary arterial blood. If the right ventricular blood sample is obtained close to the defect, a falsely high oxygen content may be obtained. Conversely, small shunts may not result in a detectable increase in oxygen content of blood from the right ventricle, but may be demonstrated by indicator dilution tests (preferably hydrogen [Fig. 13-18] or indocyanine green [Fig. 13-17]), intracardiac phonocardiography or left ventriculography.

The nature of hemodynamic changes may be quantitated by pressure and flow measurements. Small defects are associated with normal right heart pressures and pulmonary vascular resistance. Pulmonary and systemic blood flow in patients with large defects with nearly equal pulmonary and systemic pressures is determined primarily by the resistance of the pulmonary and systemic circuits.

The location and number of ventricular defects may then be demonstrated by injection of contrast medium, which passes across the defect to opacify the right ventricle and pulmonary artery. Passage of the cardiac catheter across the defect into the left ventricle furnishes indisputable evidence for the presence of a ventricular septal defect. Intracardiac phonocardiography may show that the murmur is localized to the right ventricle and pulmonary artery and is inaudible in the right atrium.

Prognosis and Complications. The spectrum of the natural course of ventricular septal defects is illustrated by observations of the author in 400 patients. (1) A large number of children remained asymptomatic without evidence of increase in heart size, pulmonary arterial pressure or resistance. (2) Subacute bacterial endocarditis occurred in less than 1 per cent. (3) A small but significant number of infants had repeated episodes of respiratory infection and congestive heart failure; the case fatality rate was high. (4) Some had pulmonary hypertension. The majority of reports indicate lack of progression of pulmonary hypertension during childhood, but pulmonary resistance probably does increase in some children, and especially in adolescents and adults. (5) A small number acquired pulmonary stenosis, which served as a protection to the pulmonary circulation (in these patients the clinical picture changes from that of ventricular septal defect with large left-to-right shunt to that of ventricular septal defect with pulmonic stenosis [p. 1001]). (6) In some the ventricular septal defect closed spontaneously.

Treatment. With open-heart surgery ventricular septal defects can be repaired. The left-to-right shunt is obliterated, the hyperdynamic heart becomes quiet, thrills and murmurs are abolished, and the pressures in the lesser circulation return toward normal. In some instances after successful operation systolic ejection murmurs of low intensity persist for some months.

The most clear-cut candidate for surgical treatment is the symptomatic patient over the age of 2 years who has moderate pulmonary hypertension and a large left-to-right shunt. In these patients the surgical mortality rate is 3 per cent or less. Patients who have pulmonic systolic pressures at or approaching the systemic level, but without demonstrable right-to-left shunt and with large left-to-right shunts, are still good candidates for surgery, but the surgical mortality rate is higher. It appears that patients with significant right-to-left shunts and small left-to-right shunts are inoperable (see Eisenmenger Syndrome). Infants with symptomatic ventricular defects present a difficult problem in management, since open-heart surgery has a high mortality rate during the first 6 months of life. In this age group it is often possible to avoid episodes of heart failure and pulmonary infection with diligent and careful medical treatment. If these measures fail, surgical production of pulmonary stenosis by banding of the pulmonary artery should be considered; this relieves congestive heart failure, and the number of intercurrent infections is reduced. In later years surgical closure of the ventricular defect and removal of the pulmonary arterial band may be undertaken. Surgical treatment is not recommended for patients who are asymptomatic, and have a normal-sized heart, normal electrocardiogram and normal pressures in the lesser circulation.

Medical management in the years before operation is important. Therapy for the symptomatic infant has been mentioned. As a protection against subacute bacterial endocarditis, the integrity of the primary as well as the permanent teeth should be carefully maintained, and the child should receive large doses of penicillin for 48 hours before and 72 hours after dental extractions, tonsillectomy and adenoidectomy. Similarly, intercurrent infections should be treated diligently with suitable antibiotics.

VENTRICULAR SEPTAL DEFECT WITH AORTIC INSUFFICIENCY

In rare instances ventricular septal defect is complicated by prolapse of the aortic valve and aortic insufficiency. The physical signs of aortic insufficiency (diastolic murmur and wide pulse pressure) are added to those of ventricular septal defect and may be confused with patent ductus arteriosus or other defects associated with aortic runoff. Treatment is difficult because it is frequently necessary to replace the aortic valve after the ventricular defect has been closed.

VENTRICULAR SEPTAL DEFECT WITH LEFT VENTRICULAR, RIGHT ATRIAL SHUNT

Ventricular defects may be closely associated with an abnormal septal leaflet of the tricuspid valve. During left ventricular systole arterialized blood is ejected through the defect into the right atrium. The physical signs are those of ventricular septal defect or ostium primum defect. High right atrial pressure is manifest as a large systolic venous pulsation in the neck. Cardiac catheteriza-

tion reveals a left-to-right shunt at the atrial level and may result in a misdiagnosis of atrial septal defect. The diagnosis may be confirmed by left ventriculography; the right atrium opacifies immediately after delivery of contrast medium to the left ventricle. Also, the pansystolic murmur is recorded in the right atrium with intracardiac phonocardiography. These patients are treated surgically by closure of the ventricular defect.

ORIGIN OF BOTH GREAT VESSELS FROM THE RIGHT VENTRICLE

In this anomaly both the aorta and the pulmonary artery arise from the right ventricle. The only outlet from the left ventricle is a ventricular septal defect. The clinical picture closely simulates that of an uncomplicated ventricular septal defect with a large left-to-right shunt. In the majority of instances pulmonary hypertension is present. The electrocardiogram simulates that seen in ostium primum defects. The condition may be recognized by right ventriculography, which demonstrates the site of origin of the aorta and the fact that the aortic and pulmonary valves are at the same level. Although this anomaly has been treated successfully, surgical therapy is more complicated than for simple ventricular septal defect. Therefore it is important to differentiate these conditions before operation.

CORRECTED TRANSPOSITION OF THE GREAT VESSELS

In this malformation the systemic venous blood returns normally through the venae cavae into a normal right atrium. Venous blood then passes through a bicuspid atrioventricular valve into a right-sided ventricle and is ejected to the pulmonary artery. Pulmonary venous blood returns to a normal left atrium, passes through a tricuspid atrioventricular valve into a left-sided ventricle and is then ejected into the aorta. The right-sided ventricle has the internal appearance of a normal left ventricle, and the internal structure of the left-sided ventricle is that of a normal right ventricle. The pulmonary artery and ascending aorta are parallel, and the former is medial. Thus the course of the blood is normal in patients with uncomplicated corrected transposition. In the majority of instances, however, associated anomalies coexist, the common ones being ventricular septal defect, abnormalities of the left atrioventricular valve with or without incompetence, pulmonary valvular stenosis and atrioventricular conduction disturbances, frequently with complete atrioventricular dissociation.

Symptoms and signs are dominated by the associated lesions, since patients with uncomplicated corrected transposition have normal hemodynamics. Posteroanterior chest teleroentgenograms may suggest the abnormal position of the great arteries, since the ascending aorta occupies the upper left border of the cardiac silhouette. In addition to atrioventricular conduction disturbances, electrocardiograms may show abnormal P waves, absent QV_6, initial Q waves in leads III, aVR, aVF and V_1 and upright T waves across the precordium. The position of the great vessels is confirmed by cardiac catheterization (Fig. 13-16) or ventriculography.

Surgical treatment of the associated anomalies, especially of ventricular septal defects, has been difficult because of the unusual course of the coronary arteries, associated preoperative heart block and unrecognized disease of the left atrioventricular valve.

OTHER DEFECTS ASSOCIATED WITH VENTRICULAR SEPTAL DEFECT

The availability of surgical treatment for ventricular septal defects makes the diagnosis of associated cardiovascular malformations of paramount importance.

Patent Ductus Arteriosus. During cardiopulmonary bypass for the repair of ventricular defects arterialized blood from the heart-lung apparatus is returned to a branch of the aorta. If there is an associated patent ductus arteriosus, blood leaks into the pulmonary artery, flooding the surgical field with blood and contributing to postoperative pulmonary complications. In some instances the signs of the ventricular septal defect dominate, so that the murmur of the patent ductus is inaudible. In such cases the passage of the cardiac catheter from the pulmonary artery through the ductus and into the descending aorta is diagnostic.

In other instances the signs of patent ductus arteriosus predominate, although a systolic murmur and thrill are often present along the lower left sternal border. In these cases cardiac catheterization, hydrogen electrode and indicator dilution studies and angiocardiography reveal the left-to-right shunt at the ventricular level, as well as the patent ductus arteriosus.

The ventricular defect and the patent ductus are closed at the same operation. If the presence of the ductus is appreciated, the surgical risk is the same as that for the ventricular defect.

Multiple Ventricular Septal Defects. In rare instances there are multiple defects involving the ventricular septum. Generally these patients present with signs of a large left-to-right shunt and pulmonary hypertension. Usually, multiple defects cannot be appreciated clinically or by cardiac catheterization, but can be recognized by left ventriculography. Exploration of the entire ventricular septum is indicated during open cardiotomy to ensure that all defects have been treated. Nevertheless, even with careful exploration some defects may be missed. The postoperative period can be hazardous in these patients, especially if significant left-to-right shunts and pulmonary hypertension persist.

Atrial Septal Defect. In patients with a ventricular defect and an ostium secundum the physical signs are usually dominated by the ventricular defect. The clinical picture is similar to that of moderate-sized or large ventricular septal defects. This combination of defects may be suspected during cardiac catheterization if left-to-right shunts are demonstrated at both the atrial and ventricular levels. During right ventriculotomy or atriotomy for closure of ventricular defects the atrial septum is easily explored; if both defects are present, they can be repaired during the same procedure.

Coarctation of the Aorta. The signs of coarctation of the aorta are clear, but those of the ventricular defect may be confused with the signs produced by the collateral circulation secondary to the coarctation. It may be necessary to repair these lesions at separate surgical procedures.

Persistent Left Superior Vena Cava. This condition is not clinically diagnosable. It is proved by cardiac catheterization when the catheter enters the persistent left superior vena cava from the coronary sinus. Surgical treatment of ventricular defects with cardiopulmonary bypass requires occlusion of the venous inflow; if the left superior vena cava is not occluded, large volumes of venous blood enter the heart during cardiotomy. The persistent left superior vena cava in itself does not require treatment.

Endocardial Sclerosis. Thickened white areas are frequently found in the endocardium of the right ventricle in patients with ventricular septal defect. These areas are presumably produced by the jet of blood shunting across the defect to the opposite right ventricular wall. Endocardial sclerosis involving the left atrium and ventricle is infrequent with ventricular defects.

Complete Heart Block. This arrhythmia is rare in patients with ventricular septal defect, although systolic murmurs of varying intensity are not unusual in patients with complete heart block. They are produced by the turbulence associated with the large stroke volume. Patients with ventricular septal defect and complete heart block should be suspected of having corrected transposition of the great vessels. These abnormalities do not contraindicate closure of the ventricular defect, but surgical treatment is more difficult.

ATRIAL SEPTAL DEFECT

PATENT FORAMEN OVALE

At or soon after birth the foramen ovale closes. In about 80 per cent of normal hearts the closure is permanent; in the remainder a small slitlike opening persists.

An isolated patent foramen ovale is of no clinical significance. If the right atrial pressure is increased (e.g. secondary to pulmonary stenosis or pulmonary hypertension), venous blood may be shunted across the patent foramen ovale into the left atrium and result in cyanosis. A cardiac catheter introduced from the saphenous vein into the inferior vena cava and right atrium may pass easily across a patent foramen ovale into the left atrium.

Because of the anatomic structure at the valve of a patent foramen ovale, blood cannot be shunted from the left atrium to the right atrium.

An isolated patent foramen ovale does not require treatment.

OSTIUM SECUNDUM DEFECT

This is a defect in the region of the fossa ovalis and is associated with normal atrioventricular valves. The defects may be multiple, and in symptomatic older children openings of 2 cm. diameter or more are not unusual. Large defects may extend inferiorly toward the inferior vena cava and ostium of the coronary sinus, superiorly toward the superior vena cava, or posteriorly to the fossa ovalis.

Hemodynamics. A considerable shunt of oxygenated blood flows from the left to the right atrium. This blood is added to the normal venous return to the right atrium and is pumped by the right ventricle to the lungs. Pulmonary blood flow is usually 2 to 4 times systemic flow. Since the defect is closely related to the orifices of the right pulmonary veins, a greater volume of blood passes through it from the right lung than from the left. Although the left atrial pressure exceeds that of the right atrium by a few millimeters of mercury, the principal factor which determines the direction of shunt is the compliance of the chambers of the right side of the heart. The greater distensibility of the right atrium and ventricle allows a torrential left-to-right shunt. The paucity of symptoms in infants with atrial septal defects has been related to the structure of the right ventricle in early life when the ventricle is thick and less compliant, thus limiting the left-to-right shunt. As the infant gets older the right ventricular wall becomes thinner and the left-to-right shunt across the atrial defect increases. The large blood flow through the right side of the heart results in enlargement of the right atrium and ventricle and dilatation of the pulmonary artery. In spite of the large pulmonary blood flow, the pulmonary arterial pressure is usually normal or only moderately elevated. The left ventricle and aorta are smaller than usual, owing to the decreased amount of blood they carry. Progressive dilatation of the right ventricle may lead to heart failure. Cyanosis is extremely rare; it is seen occasionally with congestive heart failure or with the complicating features of the Eisenmenger syndrome.

Clinical Manifestations. An ostium secundum defect may be asymptomatic in many instances; it is often discovered during routine physical examination. Ostium secundum defects rarely produce heart failure in infancy. The history in older children usually includes recurrent episodes of pneumonitis, frequently complicated by segmental pulmonary collapse, and varying degrees of exercise intolerance. Although physical development may be significantly retarded (gracile habitus), it is normal in the majority of patients.

The pulse is normal or small and the venous pressure normal unless there is associated tricuspid insufficiency or heart failure. The heart may be normal in size or moderately or greatly enlarged. A hyperdynamic right ventricular systolic lift is usually palpable and extends from the left sternal border to the midclavicular line. The systolic murmur is ejection in type, soft, and seldom accompanied by a thrill. It is best heard at the upper left sternal border and is produced by turbulence of the torrential flow in the dilated pulmonary artery. In some patients with thin chests the murmur may be loud and accompanied by a thrill. The murmur is preceded by a loud first heart sound and sometimes by a pulmonic ejection sound. In 95 per cent of patients the second heart sound at the upper left sternal edge is widely split and fixed in all phases of respiration. This auscultatory finding is so characteristic that the diagnosis of uncomplicated atrial septal defect is questionable in its absence. The widely split second sound is probably due to prolongation of right ventricular systole because of large stroke volume which cannot be reduced (as in the normal) on expiration. A mid-diastolic murmur produced by the torrential flow across the tricuspid valve may be audible at the apex or at the lower left sternal edge. The diastolic murmur of pulmonary incompetence may be heard, but is rare.

Associated abnormalities which may be found on physical examination include pigeon chest, kyphoscoliosis and high-arched palate. Congenital or rheumatic mitral stenosis with atrial septal defect (*Lutembacher syndrome*) is rare.

Roentgenograms show varying degrees of

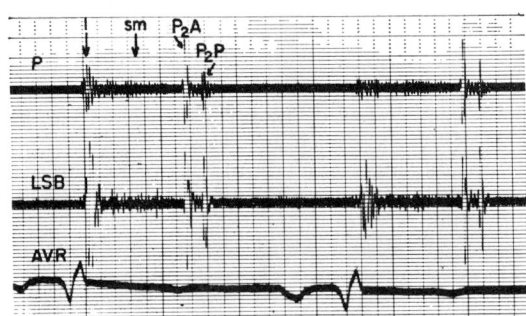

Figure 13-36. Phonocardiograms (*P*, pulmonary area; *LSB*, left sternal border) to illustrate auscultatory findings in ostium secundum atrial septal defect. Abbreviations: *AV$_R$*, Electrocardiogram; *1*, first heart sound; *sm*, systolic murmur; *P$_2$A*, aortic component of second sound; *P$_2$P*, pulmonary component of second sound. Note wide splitting of second sound. This splitting persisted in all phases of respiration. Time lines 0.04 second.

cardiac enlargement due to prominence of the right ventricle and atrium. The pulmonary artery is large, the pulmonary vascularity greatly increased, and hilar dance is not unusual. The left ventricle and the aorta are small. These signs vary and may not be conspicuous in less advanced cases.

The *electrocardiogram* shows right axis deviation and right ventricular hypertrophy (the so-called incomplete right bundle branch block); the diagnosis of an uncomplicated secundum atrial septal defect is in doubt if they are absent. Infrequent electrocardiographic abnormalities include tall P waves, prolonged P-R interval, dysrhythmias (e.g. atrial fibrillation and complete heart block), Wolff-Parkinson-White syndrome, complete right bundle branch block and left axis deviation. Occasionally the electrocardiogram is normal.

The diagnosis may be confirmed by *cardiac catheterization*, which demonstrates a significantly higher oxygen content of the blood from the right atrium as compared to samples from the superior vena cava. This finding is not diagnostic, since it may be evident with anomalous pulmonary venous return to the right atrium, with ventricular septal defect with tricuspid insufficiency, with ventricular septal defects associated with left ventricular-right atrial shunts, and with aortic-right atrial communications (e.g. ruptured sinus of Valsalva). The physical signs produced by these anomalies generally differ greatly from those of atrial septal defects, and their presence can usually be confirmed by selective angiocardiography. In a minority of patients, mixing of blood is incomplete in the right atrium, so that the principal site of shunt appears to be at the ventricular level.

The catheter frequently enters the left atrium from the right atrium, especially if it is introduced into the heart from the inferior vena cava. Indicator dilution curves may be used to demonstrate the site of the left-to-right shunt and the presence of anomalous pulmonary veins. Streaming of inferior vena caval blood across the defect to the left

atrium occurs in some patients with uncomplicated atrial septal defects. This minute right-to-left shunt may be demonstrated by indicator dilution curves, but does not result in arterial unsaturation or cyanosis. The pressures in the right side of the heart are frequently normal, but may show moderate right ventricular and pulmonary hypertension. Pressure gradients may be measured across the right ventricular outflow in the absence of organic pulmonic stenosis and are probably produced by functional pulmonic stenosis due to the large pulmonary flow. The pulmonary arteriolar resistance is usually normal, but occasionally may be increased. The shunt is also variable, but is usually considerable (as high as 20 liters per minute per square meter of body surface).

Intracardiac phonocardiography demonstrates an ejection systolic murmur in the pulmonary artery, sometimes preceded by a click. A mid-diastolic murmur may be recorded in the inflow of the right ventricle, owing to the large flow across the tricuspid valve.

Complications and Prognosis.   Secundum atrial septal defects are well tolerated during childhood, so that symptoms usually appear only in the third decade or later. Pulmonary hypertension, atrial dysrhythmias, tricuspid incompetence and heart failure are uncommon in childhood, although these complications are seen occasionally in infants. Bacterial endocarditis is rare; if it occurs, it suggests the presence of an associated cardiovascular anomaly. The principal guides to prognosis appear to be the presence or absence of symptoms and of continuing cardiac enlargement.

Secundum atrial septal defects are usually isolated, although they may be associated with partial anomalous pulmonary venous return, pulmonary valvular stenosis, ventricular septal defect, pulmonary arterial branch stenosis and persistent left superior vena cava.

Treatment.   Direct-vision, open-heart surgery

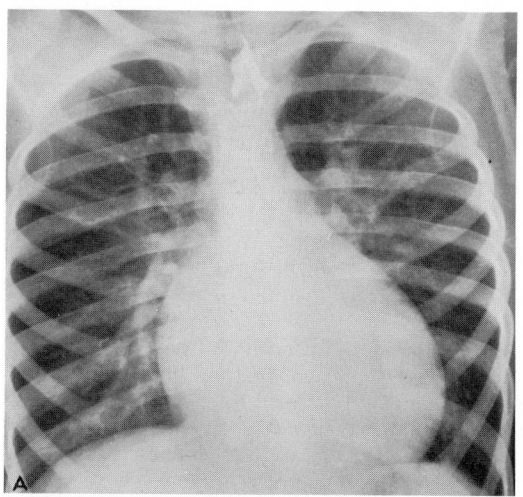 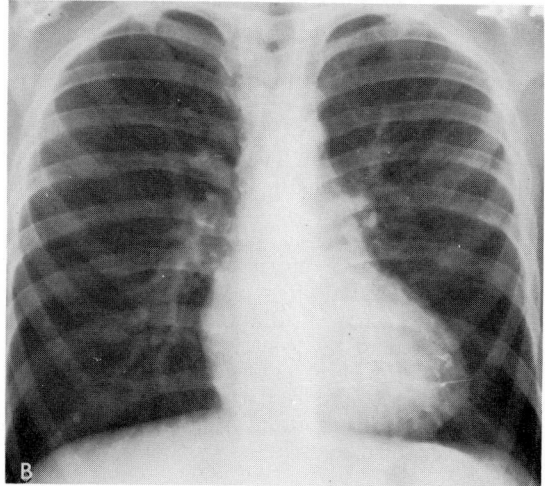

Figure 13-37.   Preoperative *(A)* and 1 year postoperative *(B)* teleroentgenograms in atrial septal defect (ostium secundum). Preoperative x-ray film shows cardiomegaly, prominent pulmonary artery segment and pulmonary overcirculation. Postoperative x-ray film shows decrease in heart size and normal pulmonary circulation.

allows accurate closure. It may be accomplished by hypothermia or with the use of a pump oxygenator and cardiopulmonary bypass. We prefer the latter because the defect may be closed leisurely and because associated defects may be treated during the same procedure. The mortality rate from surgery is less than 2 per cent.

SINUS VENOSUS DEFECT

These defects are situated in the upper part of the atrial septum in close relation to the entry of the superior vena cava. One or more pulmonary veins (usually from the right lung) drain anomalously into the superior vena cava. Sometimes the superior vena cava straddles the defect, so that some systemic venous blood enters the left atrium. The abnormal hemodynamics are similar to those of secundum atrial septal defect, consisting primarily of a volume overload of the right ventricle. The clinical picture, electrocardiogram and chest x-ray are similar to those of secundum atrial defect. Generally the anomalous pulmonary veins are not recognized on routine chest x-ray, although a bulge of the superior vena caval shadow may suggest the diagnosis. During cardiac catheterization the catheter may enter the pulmonary veins from the superior vena cava. Anatomic correction usually requires the insertion of a patch to ensure the entry of anomalous veins into the left atrium; surgical results are good.

OSTIUM PRIMUM DEFECT AND COMMON ATRIOVENTRICULAR CANAL
(ENDOCARDIAL CUSHION DEFECTS)

These abnormalities are grouped together because they have a common embryologic relation, and the clinical pattern may be similar.

An *ostium primum defect* is situated in the lower portion of the atrial septum and overlies the mitral and tricuspid valves. In the majority of instances there is a cleft in the anterior leaflet of the mitral valve. The tricuspid valve is usually normal, although some thickening of the septal leaflet may be present. The ventricular septum is usually intact functionally, but its proximal part is anatomically deficient.

Common atrioventricular canal consists of an interatrial and interventricular defect with an atrioventricular valve which is common to both ventricles and consists of an anterior and a posterior leaflet related to the ventricular septum with a lateral leaflet in each ventricle. The lesion is more common among children with Down's syndrome than among other children; other congenital heart defects may also occur in association with Down's syndrome.

Transitional varieties of these defects also occur. These include ostium primum defects with clefts in the anterior mitral and septal tricuspid valve leaflets, and, less commonly, ostium primum defects with normal atrioventricular valves. In others the atrial septum is intact, but the ventricular septal defect simulates that found in common atrioventricular canal. These defects are also associated with deformities of the atrioventricular valves.

Hemodynamics. In *ostium primum defects* the basic abnormality is a left-to-right shunt across the atrial defect, with associated mitral incompetence. The shunt is usually moderate or large. The degree of mitral incompetence is ordinarily mild or moderate. Pulmonary arterial pressures are usually normal or only moderately increased.

In *common atrioventricular canal* the left-to-right shunt is transatrial as well as transventricular. Pulmonary hypertension and increased pulmonary vascular resistance are common. Atrioventricular valvular incompetence results in regurgitation of blood from the ventricles to the atria. Some right-to-left shunting occurs at both atrial and ventricular levels, but is usually small in volume and seldom results in significant arterial unsaturation. Established or progressive pulmonary vascular disease increases the right-to-left shunt, however, so that clinical cyanosis may develop.

Clinical Manifestations. Many children with *ostium primum defect* are asymptomatic, and the anomaly is discovered during routine physical examination. In these patients with moderate shunts and trivial mitral incompetence the physical signs are similar to those of atrial defect of the secundum type. Clues to the correct diagnosis include an apical systolic murmur and a classic electrocardiogram (see below).

A history of effort intolerance, easy fatigability and recurrent pneumonitis may be obtained, especially in patients with large left-to-right shunts and significant mitral incompetence. In these patients cardiac enlargement is moderate or marked, a precordial bulge is common, a hyperdynamic parasternal right ventricular lift is palpable, and a left ventricular apical heave suggests significant mitral incompetence. The auscultatory signs produced by the left-to-right shunt include a normal or accentuated first sound, wide, fixed splitting of the second sound, a pulmonary ejection systolic murmur sometimes preceded by a click, and a rumbling mid-diastolic murmur at the lower left sternal edge. Signs of mitral incompetence are superimposed and usually consist of an apical pansystolic murmur which radiates to the left axilla; this murmur is variable in nature and may be short or musical.

In the majority of patients with common *atrioventricular canal*, congestive heart failure and intercurrent pulmonary infection appear in infancy. During these episodes minimal cyanosis may be evident. The jugular venous pressure may be increased because of pulmonary hypertension, congestive heart failure or incompetence of the atrioventricular valve. Cardiac enlargement is

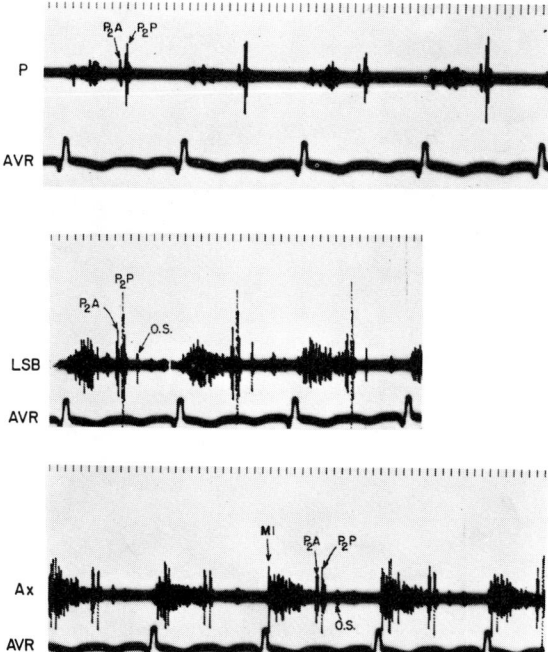

Figure 13-38. Phonocardiograms to illustrate auscultatory findings in ostium primum atrial septal defect. Abbreviations: *P,* Pulmonary area; *LSB,* left sternal border; *Ax,* apex; *AVR,* electrocardiogram; P_2A, aortic component of the second sound; P_2P, pulmonary component of second sound; *MI,* mitral component of first sound; *OS,* opening snap. The systolic murmur is ejection in type at the pulmonary area and pansystolic at the left sternal border and apex. Splitting of the second sound is fixed. The opening snap is either tricuspid or mitral in origin. Time lines 0.04 second.

moderate or marked, and a systolic thrill is frequently palpable. The first heart sound is normal or accentuated and is followed by a widely distributed, harsh systolic murmur. The second heart sound is widely split if pulmonary flow is torrential; if severe pulmonary hypertension develops, the width of splitting may not be striking, but pulmonary valve closure is loud. A low-pitched mid-diastolic murmur is audible at the lower left sternal edge, and a pulmonic systolic ejection murmur is produced by the large pulmonary flow.

Roentgenograms in endocardial cushion defects confirm the cardiac enlargement, which is due to prominence of both ventricles. The pulmonary artery is large; pulmonary vascularity is increased, and hilar dance is not unusual. The aorta is small or normal in size. (See Fig. 13-39.)

The *electrocardiogram* in endocardial cushion defects is unusual and diagnostic. The principal abnormalities are (1) superior orientation of the mean frontal QRS axis, with left axis deviation or occasionally extreme right axis deviation, (2) counterclockwise inscription of the superiorly oriented QRS vector loop, (3) signs of biventricular hypertrophy or sometimes isolated right or left ventricular hypertrophy, (4) normal or tall P waves, and (5) prolongation of the P-R interval.

Cardiac catheterization and angiocardiography confirm the diagnosis. These studies demonstrate the magnitude of the left-to-right shunt, the severity of pulmonary hypertension and increased pulmonary vascular resistance, and the degree of atrioventricular valve incompetence. The shunt is usually demonstrable at the atrial level; in some patients with inadequate mixing of blood it appears to be primarily at the ventricular level. The arterial oxygen saturation is normal except when severe pulmonary hypertension is present. In these patients a small right-to-left shunt may be demonstrable. Patients with ostium primum defects usually have normal or only moderate elevation of the pulmonary arterial pressure and resistance. Nevertheless common atrioventricular canal is usually associated with right ventricular and pulmonary hypertension as well as a moderate increase in pulmonary vascular resistance. The cardiac catheter enters the chambers of the left side of the heart with ease from the right side, especially if there is a common atrioventricular canal.

Selective left ventriculography is extremely helpful in the diagnosis of endocardial cushion defects. This study demonstrates the deformity of the mitral or common atrioventricular valve and the distortion of the outflow of the left ventricle. The latter has been described as a "gooseneck" deformity. The abnormal anterior leaflet of the mitral valve is serrated, and mitral incompetence may be demonstrable.

The **prognosis** of endocardial cushion defects depends on the magnitude of the left-to-right shunt, the degree of pulmonary vascular resistance and the severity of mitral incompetence. Death from congestive cardiac failure during infancy is not uncommon with common atrioventricular canal, but many patients with ostium primum defects are asymptomatic or have only minor, nonprogressive symptoms until they reach the third or fourth decade of life.

Treatment. Direct-vision intracardiac surgery with an artificial heart-lung machine and cardiopulmonary bypass is now a feasible form of treatment for endocardial cushion defects. Ostium primum defects are approached from an incision in the right atrium. The cleft in the mitral valve is located through the atrial defect and is repaired by direct suture. A cleft in the tricuspid valve is also treated by direct suture. The defects in the atrial and ventricular septa are usually closed by insertion of a prosthesis. The surgical mortality rate for primum defects is low, but that for complete atrioventricular canal is high.

PATENT DUCTUS ARTERIOSUS

During fetal life a large percentage of pulmonary arterial blood is shunted through the ductus arteriosus into the aorta. Functional closure of the ductus normally occurs soon after

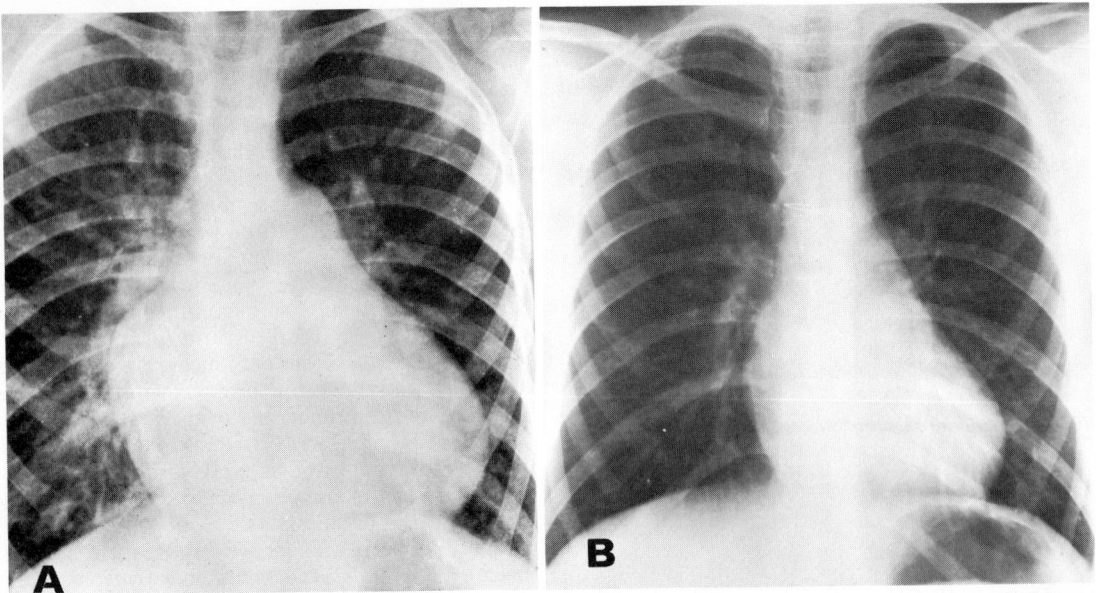

Figure 13-39. Ostium primum atrial septal defect with torrential pulmonary flow and normal pulmonary arterial pressure. *A,* Preoperative. Cardiomegaly is associated with prominence of the main pulmonary trunk, pulmonary overcirculation and an inconspicuous aorta. *B,* Postoperative. The cardiac silhouette and pulmonary circulation are within normal limits.

birth, but if the ductus remains patent, aortic blood is shunted into the pulmonary artery. The aortic end of the ductus is opposite and usually distal to the origin of the left subclavian artery, and it enters the pulmonary artery at its bifurcation. Patent ductus arteriosus is peculiar among congenital cardiac defects in that it occurs frequently as an isolated anomaly. It occurs about twice as frequently in females as in males and is one of the commonest congenital cardiovascular anomalies associated with maternal rubella during early pregnancy.

Hemodynamics. As a result of the higher aortic pressure the blood flow through the ductus is from the aorta to the pulmonary artery. The degree of shunt depends on the size of the ductus and the pressure gradient between the aorta and the pulmonary artery. In extreme cases one half to two thirds of the left ventricular output may be shunted through the ductus, and the oxygenated blood recirculates through the pulmonary circulation. In the majority of instances the pressures within the pulmonary artery, the right ventricle and right atrium are normal, but the pulmonary arterial and right ventricular systolic pressures may be elevated moderately or even to systemic levels (see Eisenmenger Syndrome). There is a wide pulse pressure. The total blood volume is increased; it returns to normal limits after surgical closure of the ductus.

Clinical Manifestations. There are usually no symptoms, but symptoms may develop at any age and include slowly progressive exertional dyspnea, followed by left ventricular failure or frank congestive cardiac failure. Retardation of physical growth may be the main manifestation. Rarer symptoms include precordial pain, probably due

to complicating neurocirculatory asthenia, and hoarseness from involvement of the adjacent recurrent laryngeal nerve.

The paucity of symptoms contrasts with the striking physical signs. Dynamically, a patent ductus arteriosus is an arteriovenous shunt of considerable extent; signs of a large pulse pressure are produced, including water-hammer radial pulsations and conspicuous arterial Corrigan pulsations in the neck. The low diastolic blood pressure may fall further after exertion. The heart is usually normal in size, but may be moderately or grossly enlarged. The apical impulse is normal or left ventricular and, with cardiac enlargement, is heaving. A thrill, maximal in the second left interspace, is present in many instances and may radiate toward the left clavicle, down the left sternal border, or toward the apex. The thrill is usually systolic in time, often extends into diastole and in some instances may be palpated throughout the cardiac cycle. The classic murmur has been variously described as machinery, humming top, millwheel or rolling thunder in quality. It begins soon after the onset of the first sound, reaches maximum intensity at the end of systole and wanes in late diastole. It may be localized to the second left intercostal space or radiate down the left sternal border or to the left clavicle. The murmur is harsh and does not have the blowing quality common in acquired lesions. A few patients have atypical murmurs, especially if there is pulmonary hypertension, when there is only a systolic murmur. Rarely the murmur is confined to diastole; this is probably due to pulmonary valvular insufficiency. In patients with a large left-to-right shunt a low-pitched mitral diastolic murmur may be audible and is probably due to the large blood flow

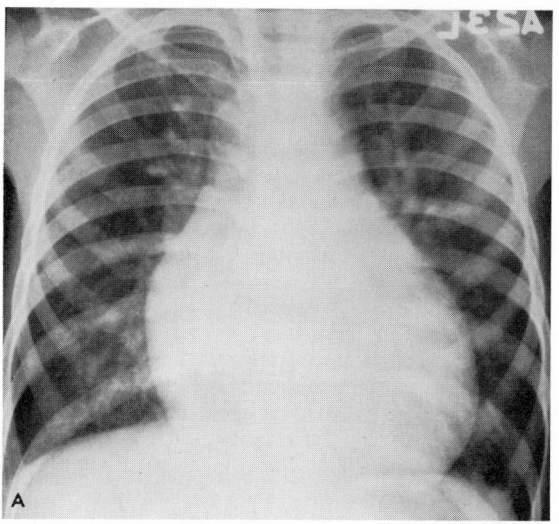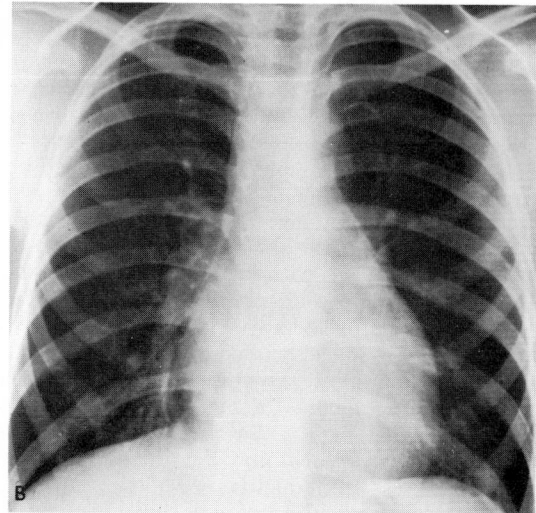

Figure 13-40. Preoperative *(A)* and 3 years postoperative *(B)* teleroentgenograms in patent ductus arteriosus. Preoperative x-ray film shows cardiac enlargement, prominent aorta and pulmonary artery and increased pulmonary vascularity. The decrease in heart size and degree of pulmonary vasculature is evident in the postoperative x-ray film.

across the mitral valve. The second heart sound may be split paradoxically.

The *electrocardiogram* is normal in the majority of instances. If the ductus is large, left ventricular hypertrophy may be present. The diagnosis of uncomplicated patent ductus arteriosus is untenable in the presence of electrocardiographic evidence of isolated right ventricular hypertrophy.

Roentgenographic studies commonly show a prominent and vigorously pulsating pulmonary artery. The intrapulmonary vascular markings are increased and sometimes exhibit an intrinsic pulsation or hilar dance. The cardiac size depends on the degree of left-to-right shunt; it may be normal, or moderately or grossly enlarged (Fig. 13-40). The chambers involved are the left atrium and ventricle. The aortic knob is normal or prominent and pulsates vigorously. Rarely, there may be calcification in the wall of the ductus.

The clinical pattern is sufficiently distinctive to allow an accurate diagnosis in the majority of patients. In patients with atypical murmurs further confirmatory studies are indicated.

Cardiac catheterization reveals a normal or increased pressure in the right ventricle and pulmonary artery. The presence of oxygenated blood in the pulmonary artery confirms a left-to-right shunt, as do hydrogen and indicator dilution curves. Samples of blood from the venae cavae, right atrium and right ventricle have a comparable oxygen content. With pulmonary valvular insufficiency some oxygenation of right ventricular blood may be present. The catheter may pass through the ductus into the descending aorta (Fig. 13-16, *G*). Injection of contrast material into the outflow tract of the right ventricle may show a washing away of the dye in the pulmonary artery by the shunt of blood from the aorta. Aortography by injection of contrast medium into the ascending aorta shows opacification of the pulmonary artery from the aorta.

Patent Ductus Arteriosus in Infancy. Aside from the symptoms described above, an uncomplicated patent ductus arteriosus may on occasion produce symptoms of left-sided heart failure or severe congestive failure during the first 2 years of life. These symptoms are frequently precipitated by respiratory infections.

As in older children, the presence or absence of the diastolic component of the murmur depends on the pressure relations between the aorta and the pulmonary artery. If secondary pulmonary hypertension has developed, there is little or no flow of blood during diastole, and only a systolic murmur is present. If the pulmonary arterial pressure is normal or only moderately elevated, the typical machinery murmur may be present early, even in infants a few weeks of age. In addition, the pulse pressure is wide, and the heart is moderately to grossly enlarged, the main chambers involved being the left ventricle and atrium.

Roentgenographic studies confirm the enlargement of the chambers and also reveal prominent pulmonary arteries and increased aortic pulsations. The *electrocardiogram* may be normal or show evidence of left ventricular dominance or biventricular hypertrophy.

The diagnosis of symptomatic uncomplicated patent ductus arteriosus in infancy is important because surgical treatment of the lesion produces dramatic relief of symptoms. Surgical therapy is indicated in all symptomatic patients irrespective of age and has been successfully performed in very young infants.

Differential Diagnosis. The diagnosis of uncomplicated patent ductus arteriosus is usually not difficult at any age. There are other conditions, however, which, in the absence of cyanosis, produce systolic and diastolic murmurs in the pulmonic area which may be misinterpreted.

The characteristics of a *venous hum* have been described elsewhere. *Aorticopulmonary septal defect* may be clinically indistinguishable from a patent ductus. Similarly, difficulty in diagnosis may occur in patients with a *ruptured sinus of Valsalva into the right side of the heart or pulmonary artery* and in patients with *coronary arteriovenous fistulas.* In these 3 conditions the dynamics are those of an arteriovenous fistula with a machinery murmur and a wide pulse pressure. Sometimes the murmur is not maximal in the pulmonic area, but is heard along the lower left sternal border. *Truncus arteriosus* with torrential pulmonary flow may be extremely difficult to differentiate from patent ductus, especially in infancy. *Pulmonary branch stenosis* is associated with systolic and diastolic murmurs, but the pulse pressure is normal. *Arteriovenous fistulas* of medium-sized intrathoracic vessels, e.g. the internal mammary, also produce signs which may be indistinguishable from those of patent ductus.

Ventricular septal defect with aortic insufficiency and *combined rheumatic aortic and mitral insufficiency* may be confused with patent ductus arteriosus because the combination of murmurs produced by these lesions superficially resembles those of patent ductus arteriosus. Careful auscultation and the absence of pulmonary overcirculation usually resolve the diagnostic problem.

Symptomatic infants with a large patent ductus arteriosus and pulmonary hypertension may have a clinical picture resembling a large ventricular septal defect. In others a widely patent ductus is associated with a ventricular septal defect; a wide pulse pressure may suggest the presence of the ductus, and confirmatory cardiac catheterization is indicated.

Prognosis and Complications. Because many patients with patent ductus arteriosus are asymptomatic, the impression may be gained that this lesion is benign. Keys and Shapiro estimated that a patent ductus was responsible for an average reduction of life expectancy of about 23 years in men and 28 in women. There are occasional instances of patients living a normal span with little or no cardiac embarrassment. Children and young adults who have this anomaly are subject to complications, however (see below), the frequency of which is great enough to make it clear that the lesion is not an innocuous one. Spontaneous closure of the ductus after infancy is extremely rare.

It has been mentioned that infants may succumb to congestive cardiac failure. This complication, which is not infrequently preceded by attacks of left ventricular failure, may occur at any age, but is most common in the third decade of life. Cardiac failure is treated along the usual medical lines, but it is an urgent indication for operation when the patient's condition permits.

Subacute bacterial endarteritis, the most frequent complication in late childhood, may occur at any age. Pulmonary emboli are common, and when the ductus is involved, systemic emboli may occur. This complication should be vigorously treated with suitable antibiotics and surgical closure of the ductus. The optimum time for surgical treatment is about 3 months after cure of the infective process.

Rarer complications include aneurysmal dilatation of the pulmonary artery or the ductus, calcification of the ductus, noninfective thrombosis of the ductus with embolization, paradoxical emboli and acquired rheumatic heart disease. Patent ductus arteriosus with pulmonary hypertension (Eisenmenger syndrome) has been described (p. 975).

Treatment. Irrespective of age, patients with a patent ductus arteriosus or similar shunt will derive great benefit from surgical closure of the abnormality (see above). If congestive cardiac failure develops, surgical treatment should not be postponed too long after adequate digitalis, diuretic and low-salt diet therapy, even if some signs of failure persist.

Because the mortality rate with surgical treatment is less than 1 per cent, and the risk otherwise is greater, ligation or division of the ductus is indicated in the asymptomatic patient, preferably between the ages of 3 and 10 years. Operation in this age group is performed with relative facility, whereas in older persons the regional vessels are more rigid or associated with degenerative changes, and the cardiac reserve is reduced (Gross). The upper age limit for surgical repair in the asymptomatic patient is about 35 years. If serious symptoms develop at any age, there should be no hesitation to operate. Pulmonary hypertension is not a contraindication to operation if it can be demonstrated that the shunt is from aorta to pulmonary artery and not reversed.

Surgical closure is by ligation or by division and suture of the ductus; the latter is preferred if technically feasible.

After closure, symptoms of frank or incipient cardiac failure rapidly disappear. If the patient was physically stunted, there is usually an improvement in physical development within a year or two. The pulse and blood pressure return to normal, and the machinery murmur is replaced by 2 normal heart sounds. In a small number of patients a systolic murmur over the pulmonary area may persist; the murmur may be due to turbulence in a persistently dilated pulmonary artery or rarely to an unsuspected associated ventricular or atrial septal defect. The roentgenographic signs of cardiac enlargement and pulmonary overcirculation also disappear (Fig. 13-40), and the electrocardiogram becomes normal. Pulmonary hypertension, if present preoperatively, also recedes.

AORTICOPULMONARY SEPTAL DEFECT

This defect is a communication between the ascending aorta and main pulmonary artery. The presence of pulmonary and aortic valves and an intact ventricular septum distinguishes this anomaly from truncus arteriosus. Symptoms resembling those of a large ventricular septal defect may appear at any age and include recurrent pulmonary infections, congestive heart failure and occasionally minimal cyanosis. In the absence of severe pulmonary hypertension, physical signs are a wide pulse pressure, cardiac enlargement and a variety of cardiac murmurs. The murmurs may be only systolic, systolic and diastolic or continuous. The electrocardiogram shows either left, right or biventricular hypertrophy. Roentgenographic studies confirm the cardiac enlargement and demonstrate prominence of the pulmonary artery and intrapulmonary vasculature.

This condition may simulate a patent ductus arteriosus. Cardiac catheterization reveals a left-to-right shunt at the level of the pulmonary artery with varying degrees of pulmonary hypertension. The course of the catheter may be diagnostic. In patent ductus arteriosus the catheter enters the pulmonary artery and passes across the ductus into the descending aorta (Fig. 13-16, G). In aorticopulmonary septal defect the catheter enters the ascending aorta from the pulmonary artery. Selective aortography with injection of contrast medium into the ascending aorta can demonstrate the lesion accurately.

Aorticopulmonary defects can be cured by surgical treatment. In the majority of instances the defect is in the intracardiac portion of the aorta, and cardiopulmonary bypass is necessary for the surgical repair.

FISTULA OF A CORONARY ARTERY

A congenital fistula may exist between a coronary artery and vein, or a coronary artery may empty directly into the heart, usually the right ventricle. In both instances the signs are similar to those of patent ductus arteriosus, but the machinery murmur may be more diffuse. In patients with *coronary arteriovenous fistula* arterialized blood enters the coronary veins, which in turn empty into the coronary sinus. In such cases the right atrial blood has a higher oxygen content than samples from the cavae. When a *coronary artery empties directly into the right ventricle*, there is a left-to-right shunt at the ventricular level. The anatomic abnormality is demonstrable by injection of contrast medium into the ascending aorta. Treatment consists in surgical abolition of the fistula.

RUPTURED SINUS OF VALSALVA

One of the sinuses of Valsalva of the aorta may be weakened by congenital or acquired disease and result in aneurysmal formation and rupture, usually into the right atrium or ventricle. The clinical manifestations are similar to those of patent ductus arteriosus, except that the machinery murmur may be in an unusual site. Cardiac catheterization demonstrates the left-to-right shunt at the atrial or ventricular level. Aortography with injection of contrast medium into the ascending aorta demonstrates the site of aneurysm and rupture. Surgical obliteration of the shunt during cardiopulmonary bypass is usually necessary.

PULMONIC STENOSIS (WITH NORMAL AORTIC ROOT)

Pulmonic stenosis may exist as an isolated abnormality or with defects in the atrial or ventricular septa. In all instances, however, the origin of the aorta is normal. This distinction aids in separating the malformatiom under discussion from tetralogy of Fallot, in which the aorta is dextroposed. Experience from direct-vision open-heart surgery indicates that in many instances dextroposition of the aorta (even in tetralogy of Fallot) may be more apparent than real.

The following is a modification of the classification of pulmonic stenosis with normal aortic root as suggested by Abrahams and Wood:

1. Simple pulmonic stenosis
   a. Valvular
   b. Infundibular
   c. Combined valvular and infundibular
2. Pulmonic stenosis (valvular or infundibular or both) with arteriovenous shunt
   a. Pulmonic stenosis with atrial septal defect
   b. Pulmonic stenosis with ventricular septal defect (acyanotic Fallot)
   c. Pulmonic stenosis with patent ductus arteriosus
3. Pulmonic stenosis (valvular or infundibular or both) with veno-arterial shunt
   a. Pulmonic stenosis with ventricular septal defect (hemodynamically similar to tetralogy of Fallot)
   b. Pulmonic stenosis with reversed interatrial shunt (through patent foramen ovale or atrial septal defect)

SIMPLE VALVULAR PULMONIC STENOSIS

In this, the commonest type of isolated pulmonic stenosis, the valve cusps exist as a dome-shaped membrane of varying thickness with a small central or eccentric opening. The ventricular and atrial septa are intact.

Hemodynamics. The obstruction to passage of blood from the right ventricle to the pulmonary artery results in increased systolic pressure and hypertrophy of the right ventricle. The degree of these changes depends on the degree of pulmonic stenosis. In severe cases right ventricular pressure may be much higher than systemic systolic pressure. Pulmonary artery pressure is low or normal. Arterial oxygen saturation is normal, and in severe cases the cardiac output is low and fixed.

Clinical Manifestations. With mild or moderate pulmonic stenosis there are usually no symptoms. If the stenosis is severe, there is usually

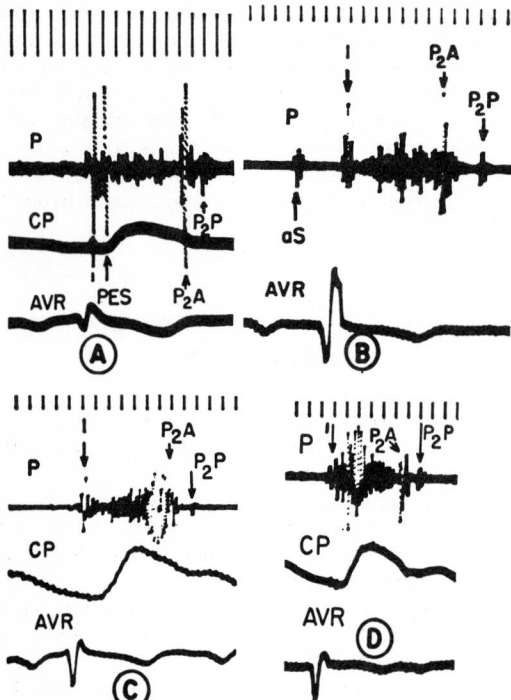

Figure 13-41. Phonocardiograms to illustrate auscultatory findings in valvular pulmonic stenosis of varying severity. Abbreviations: *P,* Pulmonary area; *CP,* carotid pulse; *AVR,* electrocardiogram; *PES,* pulmonic ejection sound; *P₂A,* aortic component of second sound; *P₂P,* pulmonary component of second sound; *aS,* atrial sound. Time lines 0.04 second.

A, *Mild pulmonic stenosis.* Ejection sound followed by midsystolic murmur. Second sound split with delayed, diminished pulmonic component. B, *Severe pulmonic stenosis.* Systolic murmur accentuated in late systole and extends beyond P₂A. P₂P delayed and diminished. C, *Severe pulmonic stenosis (preoperative).* Compare with B. D, Same patient as in *C,* 1 week postoperative. Murmur is now in early systole and midsystole. P₂P more accentuated and closer to P₂A. Compare with *A.*

some degree of effort dyspnea, and exercise tolerance may be reduced to walking a few yards. Squatting may occur, but is not as common as with tetralogy of Fallot. Substernal pain and effort syncope are rare manifestations in severe cases.

The physique is frequently normal. The facies of patients with a severe type of pulmonic stenosis have been described as being round, bloated or moon-shaped.

With *stenosis of a mild degree* the venous pressure and pulse are normal. The heart is not enlarged; the apical impulse is normal and the right ventricle is not palpable. A loud pulmonary systolic ejection murmur, frequently accompanied by a thrill, is audible maximally over the pulmonic area. The murmur is usually preceded by a pulmonic ejection sound. The second heart sound is split with a delayed pulmonary element of normal intensity. The electrocardiogram is normal, or reveals minimal right ventricular hypertrophy. The only abnormality on roentgenographic examina-

tion is poststenotic dilatation of the pulmonary artery. The heart size, the right ventricle and the pulmonary vascularity are within normal limits.

In *stenosis of a moderate degree* the physical signs are those described above with variable exaggeration. The venous pressure may be slightly elevated with an intrinsic "a" wave. A right ventricular sternal lift may be palpable. The systolic ejection murmur is accentuated in later systole, and a pulmonic ejection sound may or may not be present. The second heart sound is split with a delayed and diminished pulmonary component. The electrocardiogram reveals varying degrees of right ventricular hypertrophy (systolic overload), sometimes with a prominent spiked P wave. Roentgenographic examination reveals the heart to be normal in size or mildly enlarged, owing to prominence of the right ventricle; intrapulmonary vascularity may be decreased.

In *stenosis of a severe degree* peripheral cyanosis is sometimes present, owing to a small cardiac output, to compensatory vasoconstriction and to sluggish blood flow through the skin. The arterial oxygen saturation is normal. The venous pressure is usually elevated, owing to a large presystolic jugular "a" wave, which is sometimes transmitted to the liver as a presystolic pulsation. Occasionally a large jugular "c" wave is evident and is due to functional tricuspid incompetence. The heart is moderately or greatly enlarged with a conspicuous sternal and parasternal right ventricular lift which frequently extends to the midclavicular line. A loud systolic ejection murmur, frequently accompanied by a thrill, is audible maximally in the pulmonic area and may radiate widely over the whole precordium, into the neck and to the back. The murmur has late systolic accentuation, frequently encompasses the aortic component of the second

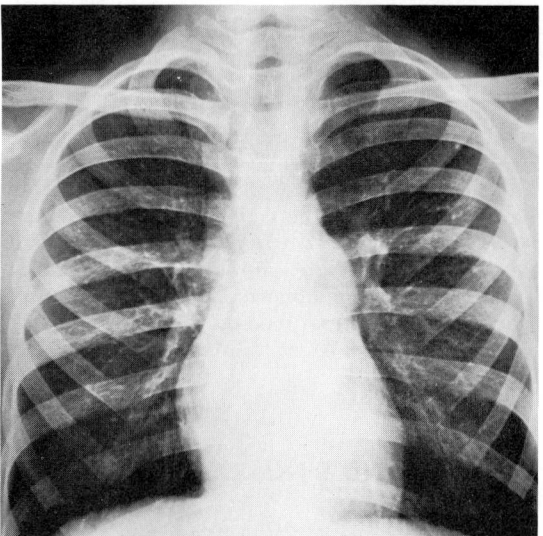

Figure 13-42. Teleroentgenogram in valvular pulmonic stenosis with normal aortic root. The heart size is within normal limits, but there is poststenotic pulmonary artery dilatation.

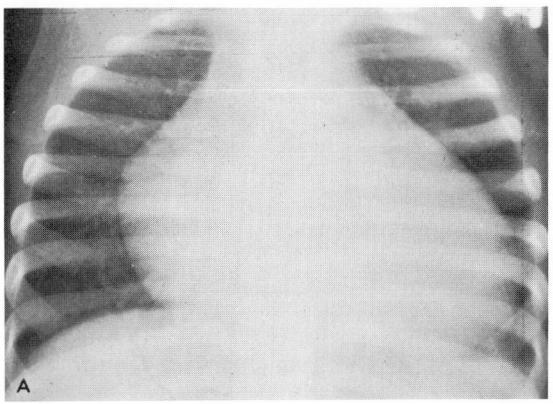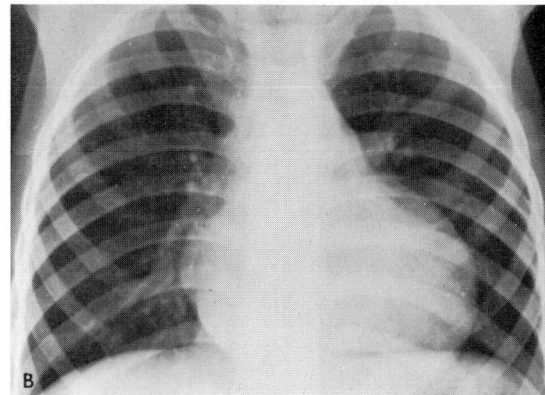

Figure 13-43. Teleroentgenograms in an infant with valvular pulmonic stenosis. *A,* Preoperative, showing massive cardiomegaly; *B,* 2 years after operation, showing decrease in heart size.

sound, and is sometimes preceded by an ejection sound. The pulmonary element of the second sound is either inaudible or very late and soft. A right atrial presystolic gallop is usually heard in the presence of a large venous "a" wave (Wood). The electrocardiogram shows gross right ventricular hypertrophy frequently accompanied by a tall spiked P wave (P pulmonale). Roentgenographic studies confirm the moderate or gross cardiac enlargement with prominence of the right ventricle and atrium. The pulmonary artery segment is prominent, owing to poststenotic dilatation. The intrapulmonary vascularity is decreased.

Cardiac catheterization demonstrates an abrupt gradient of pressure across the pulmonary valve, the magnitude of which depends on the severity of obstruction. The pulmonary arterial pressure is normal or low. The right ventricular systolic pressure is about 30 to 50 mm. Hg in mild cases, about 50 to 100 mm. in moderate cases, and in severe cases is frequently higher than the systemic systolic pressure. In severe and in some moderate cases the right atrial pressure shows a prominent, frequently giant, "a" wave. *Selective right ventriculography* clearly demonstrates the obstruction. The flow of contrast medium through the stenotic valve in ventricular systole produces a jet of dye which fills the dilated pulmonary artery. The abnormal pulmonary valve is frequently visible. This study also indicates that the ventricular septum is intact.

Complications. Congestive cardiac failure, the most common complication, occurs only in severe cases and at any age, even during the first month of life. The development of cyanosis from a right-to-left shunt across a foramen ovale is described on p. 1001. Subacute bacterial endocarditis is not common.

Course and Prognosis. Children with mild stenosis can lead a normal life without specific treatment, as may many with moderate stenosis, although their progress should be evaluated at regular intervals. Progression of obstruction to right ventricular outflow is indicated by change in the systolic murmur with the development of late

systolic accentuation. Generally, there is good correlation between the width of splitting of the second heart sound and peak right ventricular pressure, so that the duration of split (in milliseconds) approximates the peak pressure (mm. Hg); e.g. right ventricular systolic pressure is about 80 mm. Hg when the duration of split of the second sound is 80 milliseconds. Progressive electrocardio-

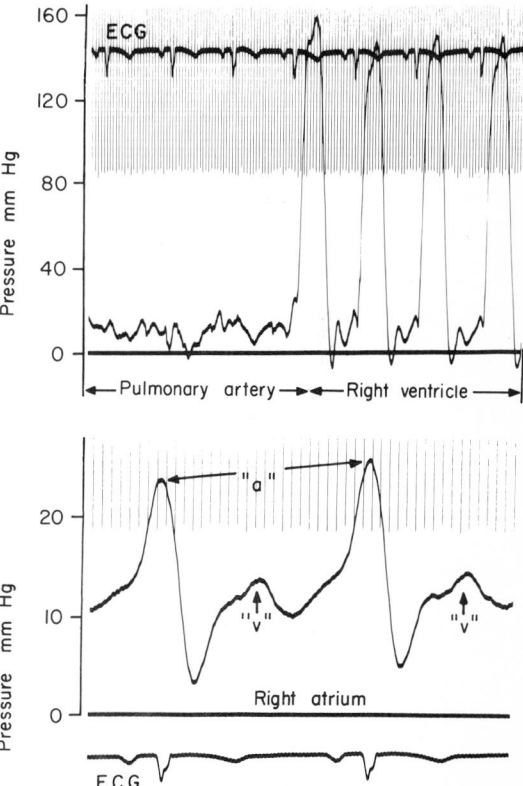

Figure 13-44. Pressure curves in severe valvular pulmonic stenosis. *Top,* Pressure record as catheter is withdrawn from pulmonary artery to right ventricle demonstrates a high peak systolic pressure gradient. *Bottom,* Right atrial pressure curve shows prominence of "a" wave.

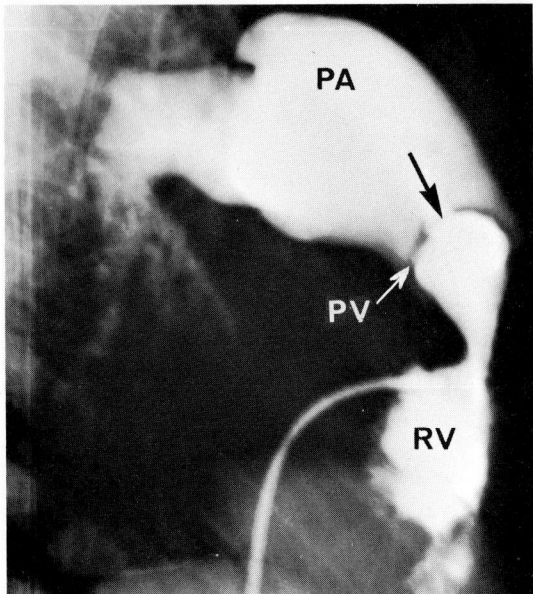

Figure 13-45. Lateral projection of selective right ventriculogram in severe valvular pulmonic stenosis. Arrow points to jet of contrast medium through minute opening of pulmonary valve. Subvalvular infundibular hypertrophy is also present. Abbreviations: *PV,* thickened pulmonary valve; *PA,* poststenotic dilatation of pulmonary artery; *RV,* right ventricle.

graphic signs of right ventricular hypertrophy also indicate increasing obstruction to right ventricular outflow. With severe stenosis the course is rapidly downhill with the development of congestive cardiac failure. Even newborn infants with severe stenosis require surgical treatment as promptly as possible.

Treatment. As indicated above, mild cases and many of moderate severity do not require specific treatment, and such patients should be encouraged to lead normal lives. Dental, ear, nose and throat surgery must be covered with prophylactic penicillin as described on p. 988.

All patients with severe isolated pulmonic stenosis require surgical therapy (*pulmonary valvotomy*). The valve can be cut and dilated blindly through a transventricular approach (Brock procedure); it can be approached through the pulmonary artery with inflow and outflow occlusion of the heart with or without hypothermia, or the valvotomy can be performed under direct vision during cardiopulmonary bypass.

Good results should be obtained in the majority of instances. The gradient across the pulmonary valve is reduced or abolished. A pulmonary diastolic murmur due to surgically created pulmonary valvular incompetence is not unusual, but appears to have little clinical significance.

INFUNDIBULAR STENOSIS

This condition is due to failure of involution of the bulbus cordis, resulting in a muscular or fi-

brous obstruction in the outflow tract of the right ventricle. The site of obstruction may be close to the pulmonary valve or well below it; an infundibular chamber is present between the right ventricular cavity and the pulmonary valve. When the pulmonary valve is abnormal (*combined valvular and infundibular stenosis*), the infundibular stenosis is frequently due to hypertrophy of the right ventricular outflow tract secondary to pulmonary valvular stenosis.

The *hemodynamics* and *clinical manifestations* are similar to those described under Simple Valvular Pulmonic Stenosis with the following exceptions: (1) The systolic thrill and murmur are frequently maximal in the third and fourth left parasternal spaces, but radiate widely. The murmur is long and seldom preceded by an ejection sound, and pulmonary valvular closure is soft and delayed. (2) Poststenotic dilatation of the pulmonary artery may be present, but is not usual. (3) With an infundibular chamber and valvular pulmonic stenosis, 2 pressure gradients may be noted during cardiac catheterization: between the right ventricle and the infundibular chamber and between it and the pulmonary artery. (4) Selective angiocardiography can be diagnostic in the majority of instances. When contrast material is injected into the right ventricle, the site of the infundibular stenosis is demonstrated, the presence of an infundibular chamber is evident, and associated abnormalities of the pulmonary valve are shown. It is important to prove that the ventricular septum is intact because the clinical picture of isolated infundibular stenosis closely mimics that of acyanotic tetralogy of Fallot.

The complications, course and prognosis are similar to those described under Simple Valvular Pulmonic Stenosis.

In severe cases surgical treatment is indicated. The infundibular stenosis is relieved under direct vision, and a pulmonary valvuloplasty performed if there is associated pulmonic stenosis. After operation the pressure gradients are reduced or abolished.

PULMONIC STENOSIS WITH ARTERIOVENOUS SHUNT

Valvular or infundibular pulmonic stenosis, or both, may be associated with a left-to-right shunt across an atrial septal defect, a ventricular septal defect or a patent ductus arteriosus. The clinical features depend on the degree of stenosis and the magnitude of the left-to-right shunt.

Pulmonic Stenosis and Atrial Septal Defect. In patients with dominant valvular pulmonic stenosis and a small left-to-right shunt across an atrial septal defect, the clinical picture is indistinguishable from that described under Simple Valvular Pulmonic Stenosis. If the shunt across the atrial defect is large and the pulmonic stenosis slight, the clinical manifestations are similar to those described under Atrial Septal Defect, but the systolic murmur is harsh and frequently accompanied by a thrill. The diagnosis can be made during cardiac catheterization when a left-to-right shunt is demonstrated at the atrial level, and the pulmonic stenosis is shown by the presence of a pressure gradient across the valve. Selective angiocardiography also shows the presence of pulmonic stenosis, and indicator dilution curves confirm the left-to-right shunt across the atrial defect.

Pulmonic Stenosis and Ventricular Septal Defect. When the ventricular septal defect is dominant and the pulmonic stenosis is slight, the clinical picture is that of ventricular septal defect, and the presence of pulmonic stenosis is not recognizable. During cardiac catheterization, however, a gradient is demonstrated across the pulmonary valve, and the left-to-right shunt is demonstrated at the ventricular level. The recognition of a small ventricular septal defect with dominant valvular or infundibular pulmonic stenosis is also difficult. Rarely, in patients with ventricular septal defects progressive ventricular hypertrophy may result in the development of infundibular pulmonic stenosis which obscures the presence of the septal defect. Even during cardiac catheterization the small shunt across the ventricular defect may not be demonstrated, and the diagnosis of isolated pulmonic stenosis may be made erroneously. Selective left ventriculography proves whether or not the ventricular septum is intact.

Pulmonic Stenosis and Patent Ductus Arteriosus. In addition to the signs of pulmonic stenosis, a machinery murmur is audible over the pulmonic area. This combination of anomalies is suspected in patients with the signs of patent ductus arteriosus and right ventricular hypertrophy. Pulmonary atresia is excluded by the absence of cyanosis and the presence of poststenotic dilatation of the pulmonary artery.

Treatment. These anomalies are treated by direct-vision surgery. Defects in the atrial or ventricular septa are closed and the pulmonic stenosis is relieved by infundibular resection or pulmonary valvuloplasty. If the ductus is patent, it is divided during the same procedure. Surgery is recommended only for severe or progressive cases. If operation is successful, the left-to-right shunt is obliterated, and the gradient across the valve is reduced or abolished.

PULMONIC STENOSIS WITH VENO-ARTERIAL SHUNT

With Atrial Septal Defect or Patent Foramen Ovale (Trilogy of Fallot). As indicated above, patients with moderate or severe valvular or infundibular stenosis have right ventricular systolic hypertension. If, in addition, the right atrium has difficulty in emptying during right ventricular diastole (which occurs during right atrial systole), the right atrial pressure rises. This results in reversal of the shunt to a right-to-left one across the

atrial septal defect and in cyanosis. A similar sequence of events occurs if the foramen ovale is patent.

Cyanosis may be present at birth or appear later, frequently during adolescence, and is accompanied by clubbing of the digits and polycythemia. The jugular venous pressure is increased in many instances with an intrinsic "a" wave. Other physical signs and technical data are similar to those described under severe valvular pulmonic stenosis. The right-to-left shunt produces arterial oxygen unsaturation.

Surgical therapy is required in all cases and consists in valvotomy and closure of the atrial septal defect.

With Ventricular Septal Defect. This condition is similar to tetralogy of Fallot (see p. 967).

PULMONARY ARTERIAL BRANCH STENOSIS

Single or multiple constrictions may occur anywhere along the major branches of the pulmonary artery. The type and degree of stenosis vary from mild and localized to extensive and multiple. This condition may occur as an isolated anomaly, but frequently is associated with other types of congenital heart disease, especially pulmonary valvular stenosis, tetralogy of Fallot, patent ductus arteriosus, ventricular septal defect, atrial septal defect and supravalvular aortic stenosis. A familial tendency has been recognized in some patients with peripheral stenosis. A high incidence has been found in infants with the congenital rubella syndrome. Supravalvular aortic stenosis with pulmonary arterial branch stenosis has been observed with idiopathic hypercalcemia of infancy.

If the constriction is mild, there is little effect on the pulmonary circulation. In patients with multiple severe constrictions there is an increase in pressure in the right ventricle and pulmonary artery proximal to the site of obstruction. When the anomaly is isolated, the diagnosis is suspected by the presence of murmurs in unusual locations over the chest, anteriorly or posteriorly. These murmurs are usually midsystolic, but may be continuous or systolic and diastolic. Frequently the physical signs are dominated by the associated anomaly, e.g. tetralogy of Fallot. If the stenosis is severe, there is electrocardiographic evidence of right ventricular and right atrial hypertrophy.

Cardiomegaly and prominence of the main pulmonary artery are present in severe lesions. Generally, the pulmonary vasculature is normal; in some cases small intrapulmonary vascular shadows are seen which may be shown by pulmonary arteriography to be areas of poststenotic dilatation. Pressure gradients across the areas of obstruction are demonstrable by cardiac catheterization. These gradients may not be easily identified if right ventricular outflow obstruction coexists, since the pressure in the main pulmonary artery is normal or low in such patients. In severe bilateral pulmonary arterial branch stenosis without other malformations the pulse pressure curve from the pulmonary artery shows a deep dicrotic notch and a flattened diastolic descent. Severe obstructions of the main pulmonary artery and its primary branches should be resected. This is especially important during corrective surgery for Fallot's tetralogy or valvular pulmonic stenosis.

PULMONARY VALVULAR INSUFFICIENCY

Pulmonary valvular insufficiency usually accompanies other cardiovascular diseases, especially those which result in severe pulmonary hypertension. Isolated congenital incompetence of the pulmonary valve is rare and usually is asymptomatic, since the incompetence is mild. The prominent abnormal sign is a diastolic murmur at the upper left sternal border which simulates in quality the murmur of aortic incompetence. In pulmonary incompetence, however, the murmur may start later, has a lower pitch and may increase in intensity during inspiration. Roentgenograms of the chest show prominence of the main pulmonary artery. The electrocardiogram is normal or shows minimal right ventricular hypertrophy. The diagnosis is confirmed by cardiac catheterization, which demonstrates a low pulmonary arterial diastolic pressure. Selective pulmonary arteriography shows the incompetent valve, and intracardiac phonocardiography identifies systolic and diastolic murmurs in the region of the pulmonic valve and outflow tract of the right ventricle. Aortography excludes the presence of aortic incompetence. Generally, isolated pulmonary valvular incompetence is well tolerated and does not require treatment other than prophylactic measures against bacterial endocarditis.

Absence of the pulmonic valve is usually associated with other defects, especially tetralogy of Fallot and ventricular septal defect. The pulmonary arteries become markedly dilated, and compress the bronchi, resulting in recurrent episodes of wheezing, pulmonary collapse and pneumonitis. Florid pulmonary valvular incompetence is not well tolerated, and death may occur in infancy from bronchial compression and heart failure. Though a homograft valve may be inserted at the time of correction of the ventricular defect and infundibular stenosis, gross dilatation of the pulmonary arteries remains.

COARCTATION OF THE AORTA

Constrictions of varying length may occur at any point between the arch and the bifurcation of the aorta, but 98 per cent of them occur as a localized stricture just below the origin of the left subclavian artery. They are about twice as frequent in males as in females.

Hemodynamics. Owing to the obstruction of the aorta, extensive collateral circulation usually develops, chiefly from the branches of the subclavian artery, the superior intercostal artery and the internal mammary with its intercostal, superior epigastric and musculophrenic branches. The thoracic and subscapular branches of the axillary artery may also enlarge as collateral channels. These vessels unite with the intercostal branches of the descending aorta and inferior epigastric branches of the femoral artery to create a channel for arterial blood to bypass the area of coarctation. The vessels contributing to the collateral circulation become enormously enlarged and tortuous by early adulthood.

The blood pressure is elevated in the vessels arising proximal to the coarctation; below it the amplitude of pulsation is diminished, and the pressure below the constriction is lower than that above it. The basis for the hypertension is not clear. It does not appear to be due to the mechanical obstruction alone, nor does renal ischemia play a large role.

Clinical Manifestations. Although incapacitating symptoms are not usual during the first decade of life, they may develop at any age and are the result of the hypertensive state, decreased myocardial performance or a deficient circulation in the legs. Hypertension may result in epistaxes and throbbing headaches, and the symptoms of left ventricular or frank congestive cardiac failure may occur secondary to the hypertensive state. Cerebral hemorrhages are not uncommon. Deficient circulation to the legs may be evidenced by cold feet and occasionally by intermittent claudication.

The classic sign of coarctation of the aorta is the disparity in pulsations and blood pressures between the arms and legs. The femoral, popliteal, posterior tibial and dorsalis pedis pulsations are weak and delayed or absent, in contrast with the bounding pulses of the arms and carotid vessels. In normal persons the systolic blood pressure in the legs as obtained by the cuff method is about 20 to 40 mm. Hg higher than that in the arms. In coarctation of the aorta the blood pressure in the legs is much lower than that obtained in the arms; frequently it cannot be obtained. Elevation of blood pressure in the arms may appear at any age from infancy, but hypertension of some degree is the rule in older patients. There is also a rise of blood pressure in response to exercise. It is essential to determine the blood pressure in both arms; a difference of more than 30 mm. between the right and left arms suggests involvement of the left subclavian artery in the area of coarctation.

The collateral arterial circulation may give rise to visible and palpable pulsations and to systolic murmurs, especially in the back between the scapulae and at their angles. These signs are usually more striking after the first decade of life, as is cardiac enlargement with a left ventricular apical impulse. Murmurs are variable in location, intensity and quality and are not diagnostic. The common murmur is systolic in time, ejection in nature, maximal over the base of the heart; it radiates down the sternum to the apex and to the interscapular area and frequently is loudest in the back. The murmur may be produced by the coarctation, by tortuous collateral vessels, by abnormalities of the aortic valve or by associated structural anomalies of the heart such as septal defects. Occasionally there is also a diastolic element, which may be due to associated congenital or rheumatic aortic insufficiency; it is heard best over the base of the heart and down the left sternal border. A continuous murmur over the pulmonic area radiating to the left clavicle suggests an associated patent ductus arteriosus. Rarely a diastolic murmur is heard in the back. A rumbling, apical diastolic murmur of uncertain origin may also be present.

The findings on *roentgenographic examination* depend on the age of the patient and on the effects of hypertension and collateral circulation. In infancy there are usually no changes except cardiac enlargement if congestive cardiac failure develops. During childhood the findings are not striking except when the left ventricle is prominent. After the first decade the heart tends to be mildly or moderately enlarged, owing to left ventricular prominence. The enlarged left subclavian artery commonly produces a prominent shadow in the left superior mediastinum. Notching of the inferior border of the ribs due to pressure erosion from enlarged collateral vessels is common by late childhood, except in the upper or lower 2 or 3 ribs. Rarely erosion is unilateral and is due to one of the subclavian arteries arising below the area of coarctation. In the majority of instances there is an area of poststenotic dilatation of the descending aorta. This may be manifest by displacement of the barium-filled esophagus and by discontinuity of the lateral margin of the aorta below the arch (Fig. 13-46). Prominent serrations on the posterior aspect of the barium-filled esophagus suggest the presence of large intercostal arteries entering the aorta below the coarctation. Occasionally scalloping in the soft tissues may be seen retrosternally; it is due to dilated internal mammary arteries.

The *electrocardiogram* is usually normal in children, but may reveal evidences of left ventricular hypertrophy and occasionally of left bundle branch block. Other cardiovascular anomalies should be suspected if right ventricular hypertrophy is present. The pattern of incomplete right bundle branch block may be present without associated anomalies. The ballistocardiogram is usually abnormal, showing a shortened J-K stroke due to a small or absent K wave.

Most often the diagnosis can be made by physical examination. Routine examination of all hypertensive subjects and of all infants in whom cardiovascular defects are suspected should include palpation of all the major accessible peripheral

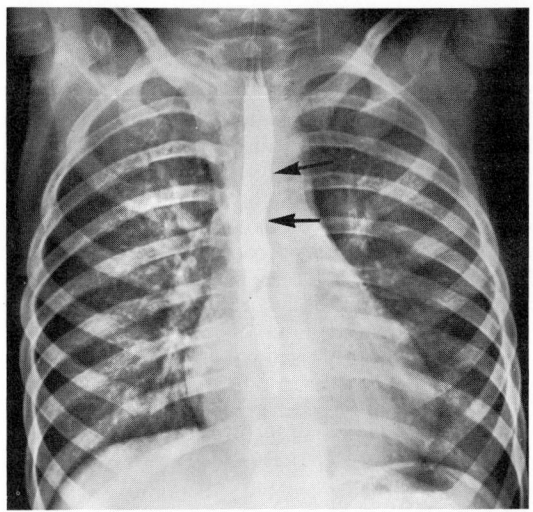

Figure 13-46. Teleroentgenogram of a 6-year-old boy with coarctation of the aorta. The barium-filled esophagus shows indentations produced by the aortic knob and left subclavian artery *(upper arrow)* and poststenotic dilatation *(lower arrow)*. These 2 indentations produce the E sign. The left ventricle is prominent, but there is no evidence of rib notching.

arteries. This simple maneuver should make the correct diagnosis obvious. The segment of coarctation can be demonstrated by aortography or angiocardiography, but these are seldom indicated except when the site of coarctation is considered to be unusual, e.g. involvement of the abdominal aorta.

Associated Abnormalities. Associated defects may produce gross physical signs which allow a correct diagnosis. Bicuspid aortic valves are rela-

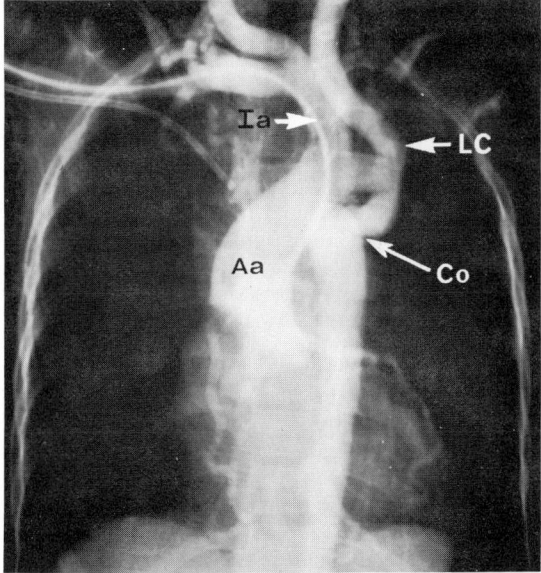

Figure 13-47. Aortogram in coarctation of the aorta. The left subclavian artery was hypoplastic and at operation was found to arise at the site of coarctation. Abbreviations: *Aa*, ascending aorta; *Ia*, innominate artery; *LC*, left carotid artery; *Co*, site of coarctation.

tively common, but usually do not produce signs unless aortic incompetence or stenosis develops. Rheumatic mitral stenosis and aortic insufficiency are rare complications. The association of patent ductus arteriosus and coarctation of the aorta is discussed later. Ventricular and atrial septal defects may be suspected by the additional signs of left-to-right shunt.

Severe neurologic damage or even death may occur from associated cerebral vascular disease. Subarachnoid or intracerebral hemorrhage may result from rupture of congenital aneurysms in the circle of Willis, of other vessels with defective elastic and medial tissue or of normal vessels; these accidents are secondary to the hypertensive state. Abnormalities of the subclavian arteries may also occur and include involvement of the left subclavian artery in the area of coarctation, stenosis of the orifice of the left subclavian artery and anomalous origin of the right subclavian artery.

Prognosis and Complications. The majority of untreated patients with coarctation of the aorta succumb between the ages of 20 and 40 years, though some may live well into middle life without serious handicap. Symptoms may appear in infancy and are nearly always present by the age of 25 years. The common serious complications are related to the hypertensive state, which may result in congestive cardiac failure or intracranial hemorrhage. Heart failure is frequently related to complicating anomalies, e.g. bicuspid aortic valve with aortic stenosis or insufficiency. Subacute bacterial endocarditis or endarteritis is also a frequent complication and most commonly involves abnormal aortic valves. Rupture of the aorta may occur and is due to defective elastic and medial tissue. Aneurysms of the descending aorta or of the enlarged collateral vessels are not unusual. The natural course in the individual case is unpredictable.

Treatment. In view of the natural course of coarctation of the aorta, most patients should be treated surgically. The optimum age for operation is between 8 and 15 years, because at this time the aorta has good elasticity, few if any degenerative changes, and the lumen after anastomosis is adequate to carry the patient through adult life (Gross), and the mortality rate at this age is less than 2 per cent. After the second decade the operation is more hazardous, owing to decreased cardiac reserve and degenerative changes or even aneurysms around the area of coarctation. Nevertheless, if the cardiac reserve is sufficient, the condition may be satisfactorily repaired well into midadult life. The mortality rate in this age group is about 5 per cent. Associated valvular lesions producing severe hemodynamic changes greatly increase the hazards of surgery.

The operation of choice is excision of the area of coarctation, and primary anastomosis. If the length of aortic constriction does not allow primary anastomosis, grafts may be used (Gross). Sympathectomy is of no value in the treatment of hypertension due to coarctation.

After operation there is a striking improvement in the amplitude of pulsations in the femoral artery. Patients may note a definite increase in the temperature of their legs. Headaches and epistaxes disappear, and symptoms of cardiac failure are improved. The relief of hypertension may be delayed for 3 or 4 weeks. Murmurs may not disappear after operation; they are probably due to persistent enlargement of the collateral vessels or to aortic valvular disease.

Postoperative mesenteric arteritis may cause hypertension with abdominal pain in the immediate postoperative period. The pain varies in severity and may subside without treatment. In other instances it is associated with anorexia, nausea, vomiting, leukocytosis and even signs of small bowel obstruction. These patients usually respond to therapy with antihypertensive drugs and intestinal decompression; corticosteroids may help to alleviate the symptoms and avoid surgical exploration for bowel obstruction.

Coarctation of the Aorta in Infancy. Severe congestive cardiac failure may rarely complicate coarctation of the aorta during infancy, possibly owing to closure of the ductus arteriosus in the absence of a well developed collateral circulation, to a particularly severe degree of coarctation at birth, or to associated endocardial sclerosis. Other associated anomalies which may contribute to heart failure are patent ductus arteriosus, ventricular septal defect and aortic valvular disease.

Symptoms of cardiac failure usually appear within the first 3 months of life. The infant is irritable and severely ill and has tachypnea. There are hepatomegaly, rales in the chest, and increased venous pressure. Absent or weak femoral arterial pulsations contrast with normal or bounding radial pulses. The heart is greatly enlarged, and a systolic murmur over the whole precordium and gallop rhythm are frequent. Roentgenograms confirm the cardiac enlargement; the heart shape is globular. The electrocardiogram reveals left ventricular hypertrophy, frequently with T wave inversion over the left precordium. Right ventricular hypertrophy may be associated.

Vigorous therapy for congestive heart failure is indicated. This includes digitalis, mercurial diuretics, low-salt diet and oxygen. In the majority of instances there is a slow but definite response over a period of weeks. These patients tend to do well after infancy, and surgery is undertaken between the optimal ages of 8 and 15 years. Surgery is indicated during infancy only when there is failure to respond to anticongestive therapy. If symptoms develop in the first month of life, the mortality rate is high with medical or surgical therapy.

COARCTATION OF THE AORTA AND PATENT DUCTUS ARTERIOSUS

Many anatomic and physiologic classifications have been devised in an attempt to describe the nature of these coexisting abnormalities. The anatomic classifications depend on the site and length of coarctation, the site of the aortic opening of the ductus and the size of the aorta proximal to the coarctation. The direction of blood flow across the ductus depends primarily on the pulmonary vascular resistance. In the majority of instances the pulmonary vascular resistance is lower than the systemic resistance, so that the shunt is from aorta to pulmonary artery. This occurs irrespective of the site of aortic opening of the ductus in relation to the coarctation. The signs of patent ductus arteriosus are superimposed on those of coarctation of the aorta; both lesions may be treated surgically simultaneously.

In infancy a large patent ductus arteriosus entering below a coarctation may be associated with high pulmonary vascular resistance. This results in a reversal of blood flow across the ductus, so that the aorta below the coarctation is supplied with venous blood from the pulmonary artery. In infants these lesions are also frequently associated with other cardiac malformations such as endocardial sclerosis with or without mitral and aortic valvular disease, transposition of the aorta and pulmonary artery and ventricular septal defect. Symptoms occur early and include dyspnea, cyanosis, superimposed pulmonary infections and feeding difficulties. Congestive cardiac failure also occurs early. Because the descending aorta is supplied with venous blood, differential cyanosis may be expected below the pelvic brim and a normal color of the upper half of the body. Unfortunately this sign is not always conspicuous, even if carefully looked for. The femoral pulses are present, but are sometimes weak. The heart is enlarged. The murmur is systolic, is heard over the whole precordium and is usually followed by a loud second sound. The electrocardiogram shows right ventricular hypertrophy. Roentgen examination confirms the cardiac enlargement and also reveals increased pulmonary vascularity. The prognosis is usually poor. Generally, the response to anticongestive measures is inadequate. Surgical therapy consists in resection of the coarctation, division of the patent ductus arteriosus and banding of the pulmonary artery if a large ventricular septal defect coexists. This therapy is associated with a high risk, especially during the first few months of life.

ANOMALOUS PULMONARY VENOUS RETURN

Abnormal development of the pulmonary veins may result in their anomalous drainage into the systemic venous circulation. The abnormal entry may be into the right atrium, into the superior or inferior vena cava or one of their major tributaries or into a persistent left superior vena cava which opens into the coronary sinus. Rarely, the pulmonary veins may enter the portal vein. An associated atrial septal defect is frequently present. All or only part of the pulmonary venous return may empty into the systemic venous circulation.

Partial Anomalous Pulmonary Venous Return. A varying number of pulmonary veins may enter the systemic venous circulation or right atrium. This results in a left-to-right shunt of oxygenated blood, which is increased if there is an associated atrial septal defect. Partial anomalous pulmonary venous return usually involves some or all of the veins of only one lung, more frequently the right (see Sinus Venosus Defect). The history, physical signs, electrocardiogram and roentgenographic findings are indistinguishable from those of atrial septal defect (ostium secundum). Occasionally an anomalous vein draining into the inferior vena cava is visible radiologically as a crescentic shadow of vascular density along the right border of the cardiac silhouette.

During *cardiac catheterization* the catheter may enter the anomalous pulmonary vein from the superior vena cava or right atrium or may traverse the associated atrial septal defect. The site of left-to-right shunt depends on the point of entry of the pulmonary veins and may be in the superior vena cava or right atrium. Frequently the oxygen content and saturation of the caval and right atrial blood are indistinguishable from those of atrial septal defect. Indicator dilution curves are valuable to demonstrate the presence of anomalous pulmonary veins. They may also be demonstrated by *selective pulmonary arteriography.*

The prognosis is similar to that for atrial septal defect (ostium secundum).

In symptomatic patients surgical therapy is indicated, usually during cardiopulmonary bypass. An associated atrial septal defect should be closed in such a way as to direct the pulmonary venous return to the left atrium.

Total Anomalous Pulmonary Venous Return. There is no venous connection with the left atrium, and all the blood returning to the heart (the systemic and pulmonary venous blood) enters and mixes in the right atrium. Some of the blood passes into the right ventricle and pulmonary artery, and the remainder passes through an atrial septal defect or patent foramen ovale to the left atrium.

Usually the pulmonary veins form a single trunk before entering the systemic venous circulation at one of the following sites: left superior vena cava (43 per cent), coronary sinus (19 per cent), right atrium (14 per cent) and right superior vena cava (12 per cent) (Keith et al.). The remainder enter the portal vein or ductus venosus.

Most often symptoms occur during the first 2 years of life and include tachypnea, poor weight gain and congestive heart failure. Cyanosis may not be definite, especially in early life, but in some infants with undue elevation of pulmonary vascular resistance it may be striking. The left side of the chest is frequently protuberant, and the heart enlarged. Gallop rhythm is usual. In early life, murmurs may not be audible, but in the majority

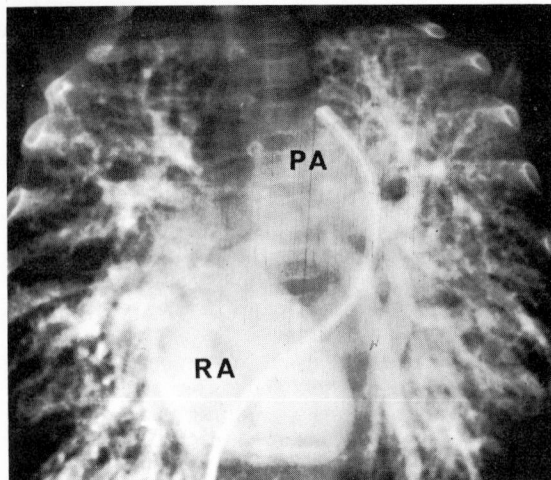

Figure 13-48. Total anomalous pulmonary venous return to the coronary sinus. Injection of contrast medium into the pulmonary artery *(PA)* opacifies the pulmonary arterial tree. The contrast medium returns to the coronary sinus, which drains into the densely opacified right atrium *(RA)*.

persistent left superior vena cava (Fig. 13-49). There is a large supracardiac shadow with a "figure-of-eight" or "snowman" appearance. The supracardiac shadow is produced by the dilated left superior vena cava, left innominate vein and right superior vena cava. If the pulmonary veins drain elsewhere, the heart is enlarged, the pulmonary artery and right ventricle are prominent, and the pulmonary vascularity is increased.

Cardiac catheterization shows that the oxygen saturation of blood in both atria, both ventricles and the aorta is more or less similar and higher than that of peripheral systemic venous blood. In older patients the pulmonary arterial and right ventricular pressures may be only moderately elevated, but in infancy pulmonary hypertension is usual. *Selective pulmonary arteriography* shows the anatomy of the pulmonary veins and their point of entry into the systemic venous circulation.

The prognosis is usually poor, and survival beyond infancy is unusual; death is due to congestive heart failure. Patients who survive beyond 2 years of age may have surprisingly few symptoms. Surgical treatment is now possible and is undertaken preferably during cardiopulmonary bypass. The common pulmonary venous trunk is anastomosed to the left atrium, the atrial septal defect is closed, and the connection to the systemic venous circuit is obliterated. Although the surgical results are good in older children, the risk is high in infancy.

The clinical picture of *infradiaphragmatic total anomalous pulmonary venous return* differs somewhat from that described above. Symptoms are usually present within the first few months of life and are dominated by grayish cyanosis and signs of increased pulmonary venous pressure (pul-

of instances a systolic murmur is heard maximally down the left sternal border and may be followed by a diastolic murmur. A continuous murmur with the quality of a venous hum may be audible over the pulmonary area and sometimes under the right clavicle.

The *electrocardiogram* demonstrates right ventricular hypertrophy (usually a qR pattern in V_{4R} and V_1), and the P waves are frequently tall and spiked. Roentgenograms are pathognomonic if the pulmonary veins enter the innominate vein and

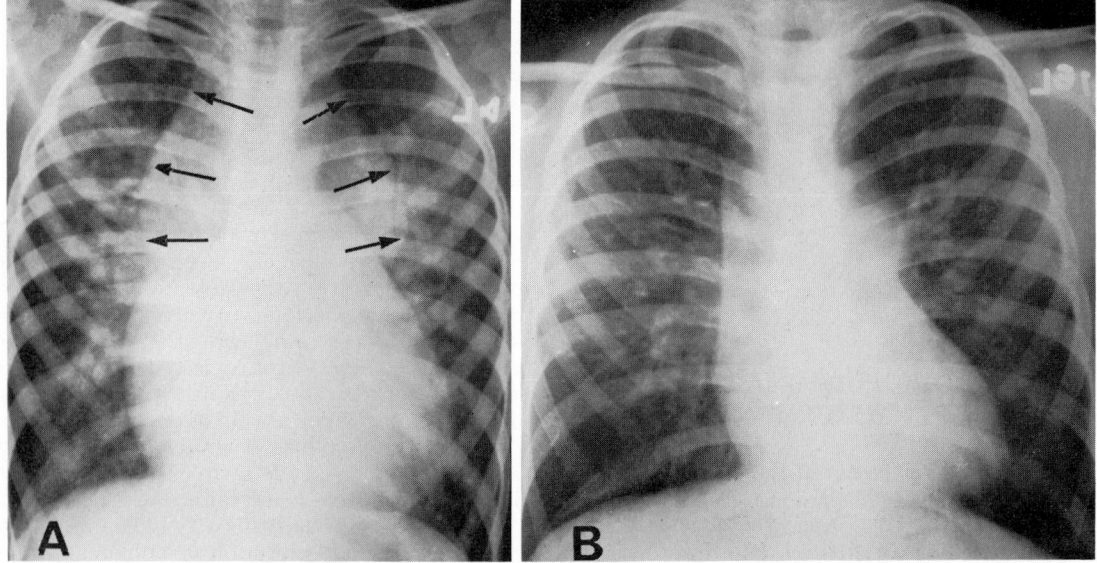

Figure 13-49. Teleroentgenogram in total anomalous pulmonary venous return to the left superior vena cava. *A*, Preoperative. Arrows point to the supracardiac shadow, which produces the "snowman" or figure-of-8 configuration. Cardiomegaly and increased pulmonary vascularity are evident. *B*, Postoperative, showing decrease in heart size and the supracardiac shadow.

monary edema). Radiographically, the heart may be normal in size, but the intrapulmonary vasculature is stippled because of prominent pulmonary veins and pulmonary edema; the chest films may superficially resemble those of newborn infants with hyaline membrane disease. The prognosis is extremely poor. This condition is potentially treatable by surgical anastomosis of the common pulmonary vein to the left atrium.

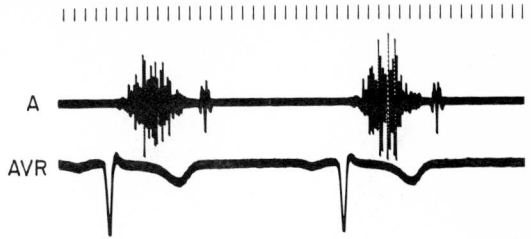

CONGENITAL AORTIC STENOSIS

Congenital aortic stenosis accounts for about 3 per cent of all cardiac malformations; it is more common in males (3:1). In the majority of instances the stenosis is valvular, the leaflets are thickened and the commissures fused in varying degrees. In others the stenosis is subvalvular (subaortic) with a discrete fibrous or muscular obstruction to the left ventricular outflow below the aortic valves. In rare instances the stenosis is supravalvular. Supravalvular aortic stenosis is sometimes associated with pulmonary arterial branch stenosis, and it may be sporadic, familial or associated with a syndrome of mental retardation and a typical facies (full face, broad forehead, flattened bridge of nose, long upper lip and rounded cheeks). Idiopathic hypercalcemia of infancy has been associated with this syndrome (p. 1369), and a causative relation to deranged metabolism of vitamin D in fetal life, possibly associated with excessive maternal intake of vitamin D, has been suggested.

Most often the child with aortic stenosis is asymptomatic, the physical development is good, and the abnormality is discovered during routine physical examination. But with severe obstruction to left ventricular outflow, fatigue and effort intolerance may be present. In these patients, angina pectoris, dizziness, syncope or episodes of pulmonary edema due to left ventricular failure indicate the presence of critical aortic stenosis. The pulse is usually normal; it sometimes has a small volume and infrequently is anacrotic. The heart size and apical impulses are usually normal. In severe cases the heart may be enlarged with a left ventricular apical thrust. A coarse, rasping systolic ejection murmur, usually accompanied by a thrill, is audible maximally in the aortic area and radiates to the neck and down the left sternal border and toward the apex. In some patients the systolic murmur may be maximal down the left sternal border or even at the apex, but retains its ejection nature. In valvular aortic stenosis the murmur is usually preceded by an aortic ejection click best heard at the apex and left sternal edge (Fig. 13-50). Clicks are unusual in discrete subaortic stenosis. Diastolic murmurs are not infrequent. Concomitant aortic insufficiency, which in some instances may dominate the picture, produces an aortic blowing diastolic murmur. Rarely an apical mid-diastolic rumbling murmur is audi-

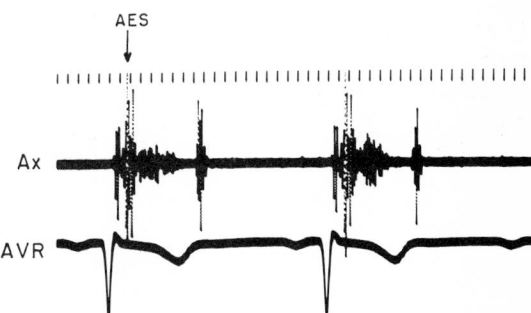

Figure 13-50. Phonocardiogram to illustrate auscultatory findings in congenital aortic valvular stenosis. At the aortic area the systolic murmur is ejection in type. At the apex the systolic murmur is initiated by an aortic ejection sound. Abbreviations: *A*, aortic area; *Ax*, apex; *AVR*, electrocardiogram; *AES*, aortic ejection sound.

ble in the presence of a normal mitral valve. The normal splitting of the second heart sound is present in mild cases. In patients with severe obstruction aortic valve closure is diminished, or the second sound may be split paradoxically. A prominent fourth heart sound is audible, especially when the obstruction is severe.

If the gradient of pressure across the aortic valve is small, the *electrocardiogram* is normal. It may also be normal in some children with severe obstruction, but evidence of left ventricular hypertrophy and strain is frequent in these patients. Children with severe obstruction and a normal electrocardiogram may have an abnormal vectorcardiogram. Roentgenograms may show signs of left ventricular enlargement. The ascending aorta is frequently prominent, but the aortic knob is normal. Valvular calcification has been noted even in children. Left cardiac catheterization demonstrates the magnitude and site of pressure gradient from the left ventricle to the aorta. The site of obstruction can also be identified by selective left ventriculography. The aortic pressure curve is abnormal if obstruction is severe; there are an early-appearing anacrotic notch, a slow, prolonged and delayed systolic upstroke, a narrow pulse pressure and a delayed dicrotic notch. In patients with severe obstruction the left atrial pressure is increased. Since a patient with severe aortic stenosis may be asymptomatic and have a normal electrocardiogram, vectorcardiogram and roentgenogram, whenever there is doubt otherwise

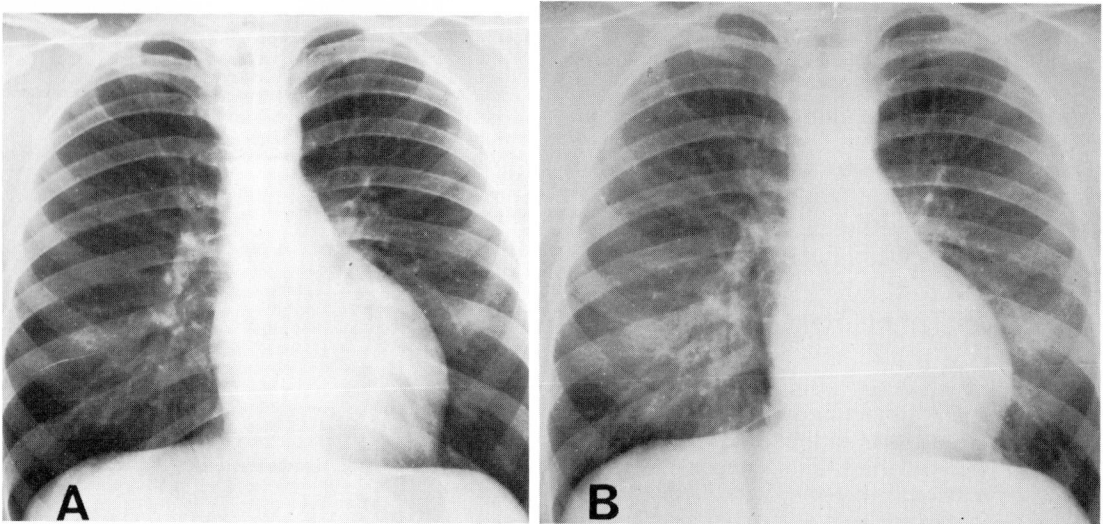

Figure 13-51. Teleroentgenograms in congenital discrete subaortic stenosis with a resting systolic gradient of 120 mm. Hg across the left ventricular outflow. *A*, Preoperative. Some prominence of the left ventricle is present, but in spite of the severity of the lesion, cardiomegaly is not prominent. The aorta is normal in size. *B*, Postoperative, after adequate resection of obstruction.

about the severity of the lesion, left cardiac catheterization should be undertaken.

The prognosis is good in the majority of children; however, in a small number sudden death, frequently precipitated by severe physical exertion, has been reported. In these patients there is usually, but not always, evidence of gross left ventricular hypertrophy. The prognosis is also affected by associated malformations, including ventricular and atrial septal defects, coarctation of the aorta and pulmonary stenosis. Infants with aortic stenosis who die from congestive heart failure frequently have endocardial sclerosis of the left ventricle and atrium and of the mitral valve.

Surgical treatment is indicated in symptomatic patients and in those with electrocardiographic

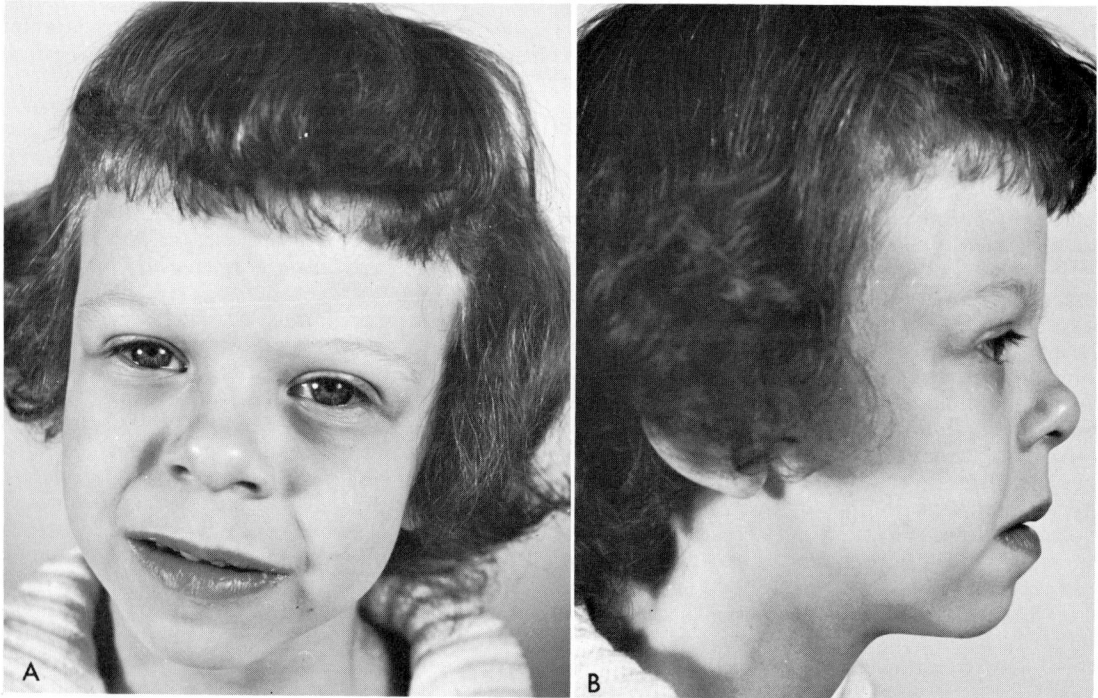

Figure 13-52. Patient with documented hypercalcemia during infancy who had supravalvular aortic stenosis relieved surgically at age 8 years. The upper lip is prominent, the bridge of the nose is flat, the nose is short and upturned, and hypertelorism is present.

evidence of gross left ventricular hypertrophy. Obstructions to left ventricular outflow are treated during cardiopulmonary bypass. After the ascending aorta has been occluded just below the innominate artery, the aorta is incised and the site of obstruction identified.

Aortic valvular stenosis is usually treated by valvotomy, but a minority of patients may require valve replacement. Discrete subaortic stenosis can usually be resected without damage to the aortic valve, anterior leaflet of the mitral valve or the conduction system. Relief of supravalvular stenosis can be achieved if the area of obstruction is discrete and is not associated with a hypoplastic aorta. Postoperative evaluation is difficult, especially when aortic insufficiency is produced or aggravated by surgery. Nevertheless the electrocardiographic improvement with alleviation of the signs of left ventricular hypertrophy indicates that the gradient across the aortic valve has been abolished or improved. Surgery is not indicated in the absence of definite evidence of left ventricular hypertrophy or of a significant gradient across the aortic valve. The definition of a "significant gradient" is difficult because the gradient depends on the degree of left ventricular obstruction as well as on cardiac output. The latter is difficult to measure in many small children, and a low cardiac output in the presence of severe aortic stenosis can result in the measurement of a relatively small gradient. It is generally agreed that surgery should be considered when the peak systolic gradient between the left ventricle and aorta exceeds 50 mm. Hg at rest or when the calculated aortic valve orifice is less than 0.7 square centimeter per square meter of body surface.

There is probably some danger in allowing patients with aortic stenosis to participate in active competitive sport, but otherwise they should lead normal lives. The status of each patient should be reviewed annually and surgery advised if progression of signs is definite. Since subacute bacterial endocarditis may develop in these patients, penicillin prophylaxis is indicated at the time of tonsillectomy, dental extractions or oral surgery.

CONGENITAL MITRAL STENOSIS

This relatively rare anomaly can be isolated or associated with other defects, the commonest ones being patent ductus arteriosus, aortic stenosis and coarctation of the aorta. The role of endocardial sclerosis in its origin is not clear. The mitral valve is funnel-shaped, its leaflets are thickened, and the chordae tendineae are shortened and deformed.

Symptoms usually appear within the first 2 years of life. The infants are underdeveloped and usually have obvious dyspnea; cyanosis or pallor is not infrequent. Episodes of pulmonary edema and congestive heart failure are common. The heart is usually enlarged, owing to dilatation and hyper-

trophy of the right ventricle and left atrium. Although a variety of murmurs have been described (mainly systolic in time), our cases had rumbling diastolic murmurs followed by a loud first sound. The second sound is loud and split. An opening snap of the mitral valve may be present. The electrocardiogram reveals right ventricular hypertrophy, with normal, bifid or spiked P waves. Roentgenograms usually show left atrial and right ventricular enlargement and pulmonary congestion. At cardiac catheterization there is an increase in right ventricular, pulmonary arterial and wedge pressures, and associated anomalies such as patent ductus arteriosus may be demonstrated. Angiocardiography may show delayed emptying of the left atrium.

The prognosis is usually poor; the majority of children succumb during the first 2 years of life. The results of surgical treatment have been poor, but occasional patients have been salvaged.

CONGENITAL MITRAL INSUFFICIENCY

This anomaly can be isolated or associated with patent ductus arteriosus, coarctation of the aorta, ventricular septal defect, corrected transposition of the great vessels, anomalous origin of the left coronary artery from the pulmonary artery, endocardial fibroelastosis and Marfan's syndrome. It is frequently associated with congestive cardiomyopathy. Mitral incompetence is an integral part of many endocardial cushion defects.

The mitral valve annulus is usually dilated; the chordae tendineae are short and may insert anomalously; the valve leaflets are deformed; and endocardial sclerosis of varying degree is usual. In significant mitral incompetence the left atrium enlarges to accommodate the regurgitant flow. The left ventricle hypertrophies and dilates, further increasing the degree of mitral incompetence. Increased pulmonary venous pressure results, with ultimate right ventricular and atrial hypertrophy and dilatation. Mild lesions produce no symptoms; the only abnormal sign is the murmur of mitral incompetence. In the majority of patients, however, significant regurgitation results in symptoms which can appear at any age. These include poor physical development, frequent respiratory infections, fatigue on exertion and episodes of pulmonary edema or congestive heart failure. Some degree of cardiac enlargement is usual, as is the typical apical pansystolic murmur of mitral insufficiency. An associated apical mid-diastolic or late diastolic rumbling murmur is frequent. The pulmonary component of the second heart sound is accentuated in the presence of pulmonary hypertension. The electrocardiogram usually shows bifid P waves, signs of left ventricular hypertrophy and sometimes signs of right ventricular hypertrophy. X-ray examination shows enlargement of the left atrium, which at times is aneurysmal. The left ventricle is prominent, the aorta small, and the pulmonary vascularity normal or increased.

Selective left ventricular angiocardiography outlines the left atrium by contrast medium which has regurgitated across the mitral valve. Cardiac catheterization shows an elevated left atrial pressure and at times pulmonary hypertension. Mitral valvuloplasty has resulted in striking improvement in symptoms and heart size. Before consideration for surgery, associated anomalies must be identified. In children beyond 3 or 4 years it may be difficult to exclude rheumatic fever as the cause of the mitral insufficiency.

PULMONARY VENOUS HYPERTENSION

A variety of lesions may result in pulmonary venous hypertension followed by pulmonary arterial hypertension and congestive heart failure. These include congenital mitral stenosis, mitral insufficiency, some varieties of total anomalous pulmonary venous return and left atrial myxomas, as well as less frequent ones, such as *cor triatriatum* (stenosis of the common pulmonary vein), *individual pulmonary venous stenosis* and *supravalvular stenosing ring of the left atrium*. In these conditions the symptoms are irritability, episodes of pulmonary edema, recurrent pulmonary infections and congestive heart failure. Physical signs are dominated by the presence of pulmonary hypertension. The electrocardiogram shows right ventricular hypertrophy with spiked P waves. X-ray studies show cardiac enlargement, and prominence of pulmonary veins, the right ventricle and atrium and the main pulmonary artery; the left atrium is normal in size or only slightly enlarged. Cardiac catheterization excludes the presence of a shunt and demonstrates pulmonary

hypertension with an elevated pulmonary arterial wedge pressure. The left atrial pressure is normal. Selective pulmonary arterial angiocardiography may delineate the anatomic lesion. It is important to recognize this clinical pattern, since cor triatriatum and some cases of supravalvular stenosing ring can be cured surgically.

ANOMALIES OF THE AORTIC ARCH

Right Aortic Arch. In this abnormality the aorta curves to the right and descends on the right side of the vertebral column; it is usually associated with other cardiac malformations. It is found in 20 per cent of cases of tetralogy of Fallot and is common in truncus arteriosus. A right aortic arch without other anomaly is asymptomatic. It can be demonstrated roentgenographically, to the right of the sternum. The barium-filled esophagus is indented on its right border at the level of the aortic arch.

Vascular Rings. Congenital abnormalities of the aortic arch and its major branches result in the formation of vascular rings around the trachea and esophagus with varying degrees of compression on them. The following are the more common anomalies: (1) double aortic arch (Figs. 13-53, 13-54), (2) right aortic arch with left ligamentum arteriosum, (3) anomalous right subclavian artery arising as the last major thoracic branch of a normally placed aorta (Fig. 13-55), (4) anomalous innominate artery arising further to the left on the arch than usual, (5) anomalous left carotid artery arising further to the right than usual and passing anterior to the trachea, (6) anomalous left pulmonary artery (vascular sling). The abnormal vessel arises from an elongated main pulmonary artery or from the right pulmonary artery. It courses between and compresses the trachea and esophagus.

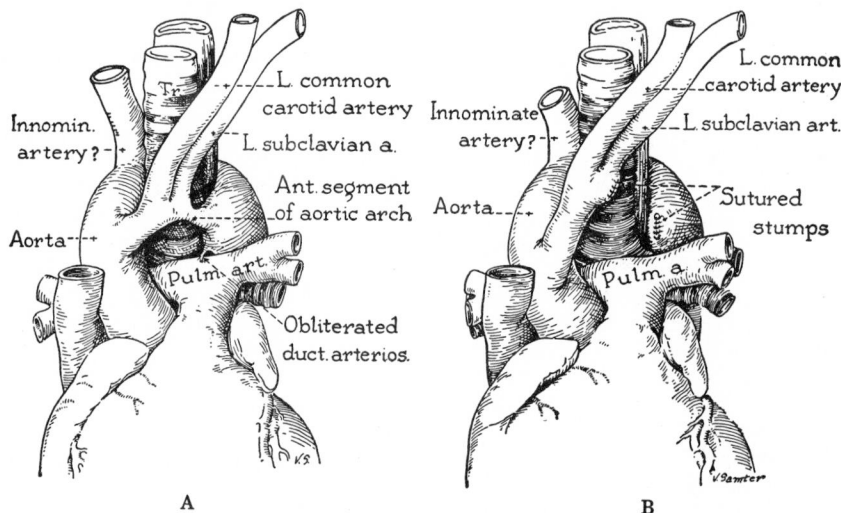

A   B

Figure 13-53.   Double aortic arch. *A*, Small anterior segment of double aortic arch (most common type). *B*, Operative procedure for release of vascular ring. (Courtesy of Dr. Willis J. Potts.)

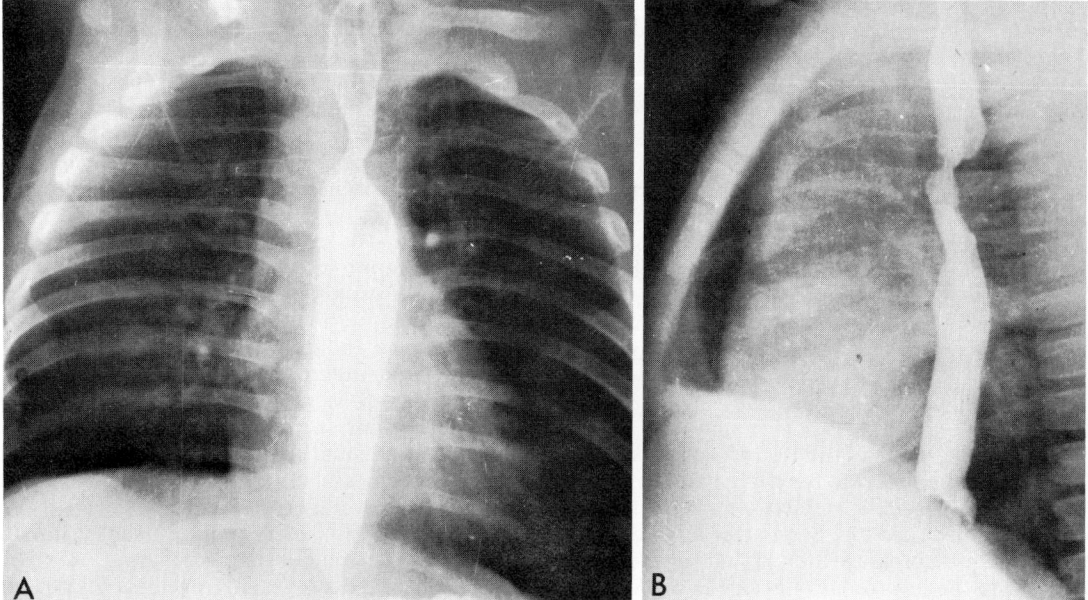

Figure 13-54. Double aortic arch in an infant aged 5 months. *A,* Anteroposterior view. The barium-filled esophagus is constricted on both sides. *B,* Lateral view. The esophagus is displaced forward. The anterior arch was the smaller and was divided at operation. (Courtesy of Drs. Eugene Saenger, Frederick Silverman and Edward McGrath.)

The clinical patterns are extremely variable. In some instances, especially with anomalous right subclavian artery, the condition is asymptomatic. If the vascular ring produces compression of the trachea and esophagus, symptoms are frequently present during infancy. Respirations are wheezing and are aggravated by crying, feeding and flexion of the neck. Extension of the neck tends to relieve the noisy respiration. Vomiting is frequent. There may be a brassy cough, and pneumonia is common. Examination of the barium-filled esophagus and of the air- or Lipiodol-filled trachea, during fluoroscopy and on roentgenograms (Figs. 13-54, 13-55), discloses the anomaly.

Surgery is advised in symptomatic patients with radiographic evidence of tracheal or esophageal compression. The appropriate vessel is divided in patients with double aortic arch (Fig. 13-53).

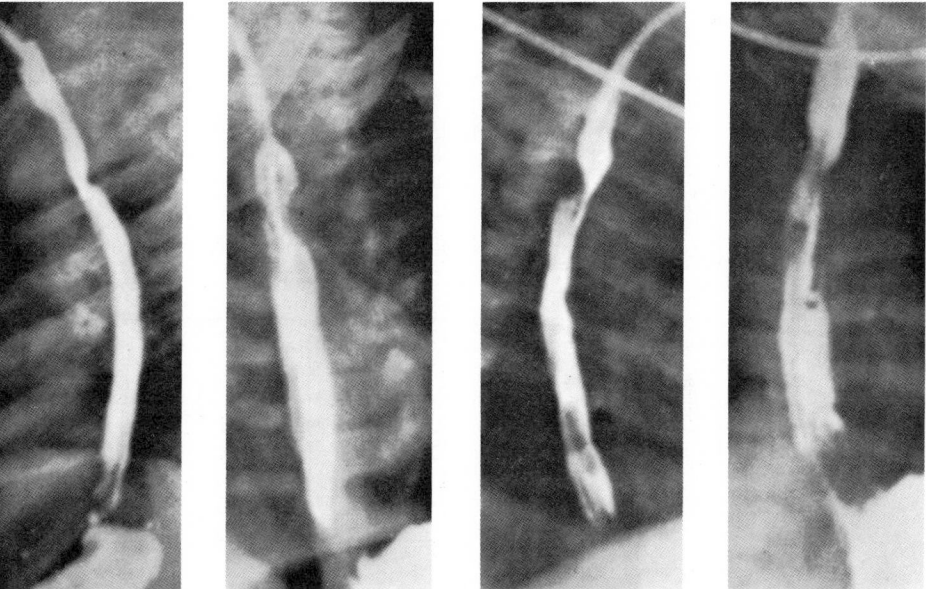

Figure 13-55. Esophagram of a child with aberrant origin of the right subclavian artery as a last branch from the arch of the aorta. The positions from left to right are lateral, left anterior oblique, right anterior oblique, anteroposterior. A constant defect is visualized on the posterior aspect of the esophagus.

Compression produced by a right aortic arch and left ligamentum arteriosum is relieved by division of the latter. An anomalous right subclavian artery is divided at its origin from the aorta. Anomalous innominate or carotid arteries cannot be divided; the tracheal compression is relieved by attaching the adventitia of these vessels to the sternum. Anomalous left pulmonary artery is treated by division at its origin and reanastomosis to the main pulmonary artery after the anomalous vessel has been brought in front of the trachea.

ANOMALOUS ORIGIN OF CORONARY ARTERIES

Anomalous Origin of the Left Coronary Artery from the Pulmonary Artery. In this condition there is a compromise of blood supply to the left ventricular myocardium. Soon after birth the pulmonary arterial pressure falls so that the perfusion pressure to the left coronary artery is inadequate. Interarterial anastomoses may develop between the right and left coronary arteries. This results in reversal of flow so that blood flows from the left coronary artery to the pulmonary artery. The left ventricle becomes dilated and somewhat hypertrophied with patchy fibrosis and microscopic deposition of calcium. Localized aneurysms may develop in the left ventricle.

In the majority of instances, symptoms occur during the first few months of life, and are those of congestive heart failure, frequently associated with or precipitated by respiratory infections. Recurrent attacks of discomfort, restlessness, irritability, sweating, dyspnea and pallor with or without mild cyanosis could be interpreted as being produced by angina pectoris. Cardiac en-largement is moderate to marked. Gallop rhythm is common. Generally in infants there are no murmurs, but short, nonspecific apical systolic murmurs may be audible. Older patients with abundant intercoronary anastomoses may have continuous murmurs. Roentgen examination confirms the cardiomegaly, but the contour and pulsations are not specific unless there is a complicating ventricular aneurysm. The electrocardiogram resembles the pattern described in anterior myocardial infarction in adults. A QR pattern followed by inverted T waves is seen in leads I and aVL. The left ventricular surface leads (V_5 and V_6) show deep wide Q waves and may also exhibit elevated S-T segments and inverted T waves. Aortography is diagnostic; there is immediate opacification of only the right coronary artery. Generally this vessel is large and tortuous. After filling of the intercoronary anastomoses, the left coronary artery and the pulmonary artery are in turn opacified. Selective pulmonary arteriography usually fails to opacify the anomalous left coronary artery. Selective left ventriculography reveals a dilated left ventricle which empties poorly.

In the majority of instances death from heart failure occurs within the first 6 months of life. The exceptional patients who survive have unusually abundant intercoronary anastomoses. Symptomatic infants should have surgical exploration with the object of ligation of the left coronary artery at its origin from the pulmonary artery. This increases the perfusion pressure of the left ventricular myocardium. Success of this procedure depends on adequate intercoronary anastomoses.

Anomalous origin of both coronary arteries from the pulmonary artery is extremely rare and may be associated with other severe cardiac malformations. After birth, blood flow to the myocardium is severely compromised because the coro-

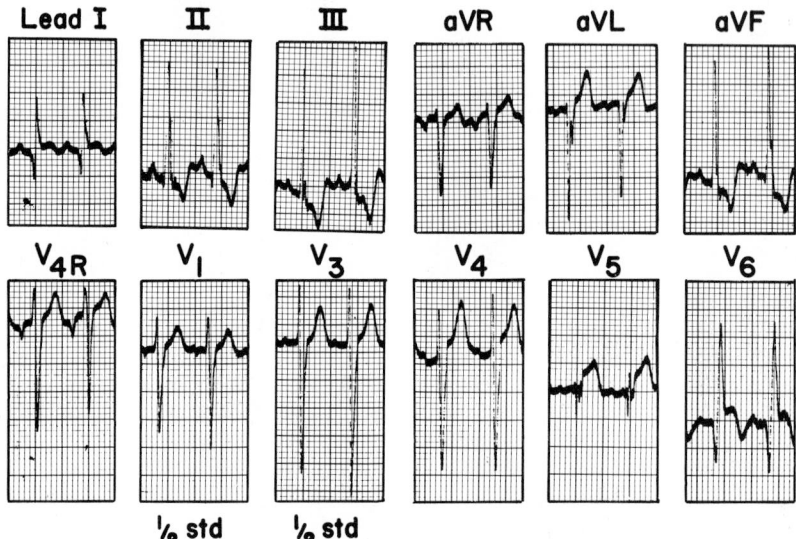

Figure 13-56. Electrocardiogram of a 3-month-old child with anomalous origin of the left coronary artery from the pulmonary artery. Anterolateral myocardial infarction is present because of abnormally large and wide Q waves in leads I, V_5 and V_6, elevated S-T segment in V_5 and V_6 and inversion of TV_6.

nary arteries are perfused with venous blood at a low pressure. The prognosis is usually poor.

Anomalous origin of the right coronary artery from the pulmonary artery is also rare; it does not produce signs or symptoms. The prognosis is good.

PRIMARY PULMONARY HYPERTENSION

Primary pulmonary hypertension is a disease of unknown origin characterized by hypertension of the lesser circulation and right-sided heart failure. The disease may occur at any age and may be clinically recognizable during childhood and adolescence. The pulmonary hypertension is associated with precapillary obstruction of the pulmonary vascular bed, owing to hyperplasia of the muscular and elastic tissues and the thickened intima of the small pulmonary arteries and arterioles. Atherosclerotic changes may be found in the larger pulmonary arteries. Other causes of pulmonary heart disease (chronic cor pulmonale) are absent, and there is no evidence of emphysema, pancreatic fibrosis or kyphoscoliosis. Recurrent pulmonary emboli may produce the same clinical picture, but this disease is rare in childhood. Severe pulmonary hypertension may result from myriads of minute microemboli from the cardiac end of a ventriculo-jugular shunt tube inserted for the treatment of hydrocephalus. Significant pulmonary hypertension may also result from persistent obstruction of the upper airway, e.g. by gross enlargement of the tonsils and adenoids; it may also be an accompaniment of extreme obesity, as in the Prader-Willi syndrome.

Hemodynamics. The pulmonary hypertension places a mechanical burden on the right ventricle and pulmonary artery with resultant right ventricular hypertrophy and dilatation of the pulmonary artery. Frequently the cardiac output is decreased. Sooner or later right-sided heart failure develops, at times with tricuspid insufficiency.

Clinical Manifestations. The predominant symptoms include effort intolerance and fatigability; occasional patients complain of precordial chest pain, dizziness or syncope. Peripheral cyanosis may be present and is associated with cold extremities and a nearly normal arterial oxygen saturation. If right-sided heart failure has supervened, the jugular venous pressure is elevated, and hepatomegaly and edema are present. Jugular venous "a" waves are present, and if functional tricuspid insufficiency has supervened, a conspicuous jugular "c" wave develops with systolic hepatic pulsations. The heart is slightly to moderately enlarged with a right ventricular apical tap. Thrills are absent, and murmurs may be insignificant. The first heart sound is frequently followed by a pulmonic ejection click. The systolic murmur is soft and short and is sometimes followed by a blowing diastolic murmur due to pulmonary incompetence. The second heart sound is closely split, loud, sometimes booming, and frequently palpable. A presystolic gallop rhythm may be audible down the left sternal border.

Roentgenograms reveal a prominent pulmonary artery and right ventricle (Fig. 13-57). The pulmonary vascularity in the hilar areas may be prominent and contrast with the peripheral lung fields, which are clear. The *electrocardiogram* shows right ventricular hypertrophy with spiked P waves.

The **diagnosis** is confirmed by *cardiac catheterization*, which reveals right ventricular and pulmonary hypertension with a normal pulmonary arterial wedge pressure. The cardiac output is usually low, and the arterial oxygen saturation is nearly normal.

Difficulty may arise in differentiating this condition from the Eisenmenger syndrome. Generally these may be differentiated by cardiac catheterization, which demonstrates the site, direction and magnitude of the shunt which has resulted in pulmonary hypertension. This study also excludes left-sided lesions which result in pulmonary venous hypertension; in these conditions the pulmonary arterial wedge pressure is elevated significantly. If primary pulmonary hypertension is associated with a reversed intra-atrial shunt through a foramen ovale, the clinical picture may simulate that of the Eisenmenger syndrome.

Rarely, *congenital intracranial arteriovenous fistulas* (p. 1037, 1281) in newborn infants may simulate primary pulmonary hypertension or heart failure due to other causes. Tachypnea and intermittent cyanosis are the presenting symptoms; congestive heart failure may follow. Roentgenographic, electrocardiographic and cardiac cathe-

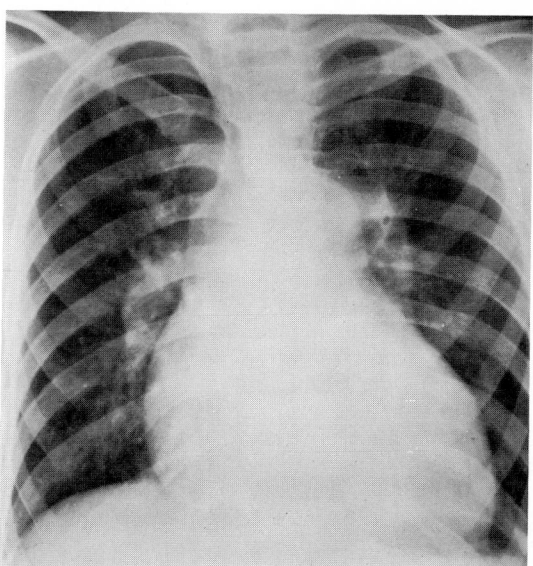

Figure 13-57. Teleroentgenogram in primary pulmonary hypertension, showing moderate cardiac enlargement, dilatation of the pulmonary artery and relative pulmonary undervascularity in the outer two thirds of the lung fields. This roentgen picture may simulate that found in valvular pulmonic stenosis with normal aortic root.

terization findings are superficially similar to those of primary pulmonary hypertension. The diagnosis is suspected on the basis of increased oxygen saturation of blood from the superior vena cava and of rapid, visible return of the contrast medium through the superior vena cava to opacify the right side of the heart after selective left atriography. Cerebral angiography is diagnostic. An analogous pattern may be seen with a large hepatic arteriovenous fistula.

Primary pulmonary hypertension is progressive, and the results of **treatment** are disappointing. Some relief may be obtained by the usual measures adopted for congestive cardiac failure.

MARFAN'S SYNDROME: CARDIOVASCULAR MANIFESTATIONS

The frequency of congenital malformations of the heart in Marfan's syndrome (p. 1345) has probably been overstressed. The common lesion is di-

latation of the aorta, beginning at the aortic valve and usually confined to the ascending portion. The valve ring is stretched, and the resultant aortic insufficiency may be pronounced. Progressive left ventricular failure occurs with or without angina pectoris. Dissecting aneurysm of the aorta is a common terminal event or may result in the development of aortic valvular incompetence. Cardiac symptoms may occur as early as the fifth year of life, but frequently do not appear until adult life.

The pulmonary artery and valve may be involved in a similar way to that of the aorta, resulting in dilatation of the pulmonary artery. This syndrome may explain some cases of *idiopathic pulmonary arterial dilatation.* Mitral insufficiency may result from redundant cusps and chordae tendineae. Subacute bacterial endocarditis may be a complication. Congenital cardiac malformations have been reported in occasional patients. These include atrial and ventricular septal defects, Fallot's tetralogy, patent ductus arteriosus, coarctation of the aorta, pulmonary arterial stenosis and anomalous pulmonary venous return.

Principles of Treatment in Congenital Heart Disease

The following principles of treatment apply to all patients with congenital heart disease. Owing to rapid advances in diagnosis and surgical treatment, an attitude of guarded optimism should be adopted. A level of life as nearly normal as possible should be encouraged because untold psychologic trauma is imposed by unnecessary restriction. The parents' attitude toward the child can be more relaxed if it is pointed out that sudden death is rare in congenital heart anomalies in contradistinction to some degenerative diseases in adults. Rigorous restriction of physical activities is usually not indicated, since children soon learn their own capacity for exercise. If cardiac enlargement is present or if there is a history of congestive heart failure, competitive sports should be discouraged.

General management includes a well balanced diet, the supplementation of iron and vitamins during the first few years of life and the usual immunization program.

The prevention or prompt treatment of dehydration in cyanotic patients is important so that hemoconcentration and possible thrombotic episodes will be averted. Infections should be vigorously treated with suitable antibiotics to prevent the onset of subacute bacterial endocarditis or congestive heart failure. Ear, nose and throat surgery and dental extractions must also be covered with antibiotics, preferably penicillin. Treatment with iron of a "relative hypochromic anemia" in cyanotic patients may improve their exercise tolerance and general well-being. The treatment of congestive heart failure and of paroxysmal dysp-

neic attacks is described on pages 1032 and 968 respectively.

Surgical Treatment. The standardized surgical therapy of patent ductus arteriosus, coarctation of the aorta and vascular rings has been described.

Open-heart surgery. This technique is used when surgical treatment of intracardiac defects under direct vision is indicated. The systemic venous return to the heart is diverted to an artificial heart-lung machine, and arterialized blood is returned to the systemic arterial system (*cardiopulmonary bypass*). Thus the principal source of blood flow through the heart and lungs is diverted, and the chambers of the "bloodless" heart may be opened widely. The systemic venous return to the heart is picked up by cannulae in the superior and inferior venae cavae, usually inserted through the right atrium. The arterialized blood is returned from the heart-lung machine to either the femoral artery or ascending aorta. In the former instance the body is perfused in a retrograde direction. With this system of cannulation coronary and bronchial flows are not disturbed, and the heart continues to beat. Mild or moderate hypothermia can be induced by controlling the temperature of the extracorporeal blood. Prolonged, deep hypothermia without perfusion has resulted in postoperative cerebral complications in children. If it is desired to abolish coronary flow, this is accomplished by intermittent occlusion of the ascending aorta or by selective hypothermia of the heart.

The postoperative period. With successful total body perfusion and direct-vision open-heart surgery, the postoperative course is frequently benign. Nevertheless many of these patients may be in a delicate or precarious state. The following complications are listed as a guide to management.

PLEURAL SPACE COMPLICATIONS. Pneumothorax and hemothorax are treated along usual lines.

PULMONARY COMPLICATIONS. Patchy areas of pulmonary atelectasis with or without edema and hemorrhage occur more frequently in patients with pulmonary hypertension and elevated pulmonary resistance. Decompression of the pulmonary vascular tree by cannulation of the left atrium or ventricle during cardiopulmonary bypass probably decreases the severity.

PULMONARY VENTILATION. Respiratory exchange may be increased by the use of respirators. Temporary artificial ventilation can be accomplished via a nasotracheal tube, but tracheostomy may be necessary if artificial ventilation is prolonged for more than a few days. Care must be exercised to avoid pulmonary damage from excessive concentrations of oxygen.

SHOCK. This complication is encountered within the first few hours or days after operation and may be seen after prolonged perfusion, in the presence of hypovolemia or cardiac tamponade, or when surgical correction is incomplete (e.g. inadequate relief of obstruction to right ventricular outflow). The clinical picture is dominated by hypotension, increased venous pressure (except in some patients with hypovolemia), peripheral vasoconstriction and cyanosis, oliguria and acidosis. In patients in whom hypovolemia and cardiac tamponade have been excluded artificial ventilation and correction of acidosis are usually required. The effects of small transfusions should be assessed by measurement of venous and arterial pressures, cardiac output and urinary volume. Although the use of corticosteroids with or without epinephrine or isoproterenol is debatable, these agents have had a salutary effect in some critically ill patients.

CARDIAC FAILURE. If heart failure was present before operation, many days or weeks may elapse before compensation is restored; anticongestive therapy is continued during this time. The appearance of heart failure for the first time after operation suggests volume overload of the ventricle (e.g. the development of aortic incompetence after aortic valvotomy) or inadequate relief of an obstructive lesion (e.g. persistent right ventricular outflow tract obstruction in pulmonic stenosis). Temporary increase of venous pressure is common after correction of Fallot's tetralogy and is probably related to the high pressure necessary to fill the recently incised right ventricle.

HEMORRHAGE. Although operation is conducted with the patient heparinized, postoperative bleeding should not be a problem. If it occurs, it may be an expression of inadequate perfusion. Deeply cyanotic patients may have an abnormal clotting mechanism preoperatively (p. 955).

COMPLETE HEART BLOCK. Trauma to the bundle of His during an intracardiac procedure may be produced by a suture or may result from local edema and myocardial anoxia. Fortunately, permanent heart block is becoming less frequent, but temporary episodes lasting from a few hours up to 3 or 4 weeks are seen. This complication is usually recognized at operation, but may develop during the first few postoperative days. If the slow heart rate results in inadequate cardiac output, treatment is required and consists of artificial pacing with an external pacemaker delivering the stimulus to an internal electrode sutured into the wall of the ventricle at the time of operation. This myocardial wire electrode is removed when sinus rhythm is restored. If heart block is permanent, an implanted pacemaker with a transvenous catheter is indicated. Generally the pacing electrode is advanced from the external jugular vein to the apex of the right ventricle and is attached to the permanent pacemaker, which is buried under the tissue below the right clavicle. Intravenous administration of isoproterenol (Isuprel) is useful in emergency situations. Although we have observed a number of children with surgically induced permanent heart block who have not required artificial pacing, the implantation of a pacemaker is advisable because of unpredictable Stokes-Adams attacks.

OTHER DYSRHYTHMIAS. The common causes of ventricular dysrhythmias after open-heart surgery are digitalis intoxication and hypokalemia; atrial dysrhythmias are common after extensive incision of the right atrium for correction of atrial septal defect or especially after interatrial correction of transposition of the great vessels. The dysrhythmia may take the form of ectopic atrial rhythms, atrial flutter or fibrillation, intra-atrial block, atrioventricular dissociation or sinus bradycardia. Generally these disturbances of rhythm are transient, but they may be recurrent or permanent, especially after treatment of arterial transposition.

ACIDOSIS. Minor degrees of respiratory acidosis are common and do not require therapy. Severe metabolic acidosis may occur and is usually an indication of inadequate blood flow during cardiopulmonary bypass or inadequate cardiac output after operation (see p. 225).

POSTCARDIOTOMY SYNDROME. Toward the end of the first postoperative week, or sometimes weeks or months after operation, a febrile illness due to pericarditis and pleurisy with or without fluid may develop. In most patients the condition is benign. In others, fever, chest pain and pleurisy may be complicated by collections of pericardial fluid and the resulting danger of cardiac tamponade. Symptomatic patients usually respond to salicylates and bed rest. If there is no response, corticosteroids may be used. In some patients there is a tendency for the condition to recur.

POSTPERFUSION SYNDROME. Within 3 to 12 weeks after cardiopulmonary bypass, fever, malaise and splenomegaly may develop, with or without hepatomegaly and a maculopapular rash. The total leukocyte count varies from 3000 to

15,000 per mm.[3], of which 40 to 80 per cent are atypical lymphocytes. The heterophil antibody test result may be positive. The mechanism of this complication is unknown, but its recognition and differentiation from bacterial endocarditis are important. The course is usually benign; salicylates may relieve the general discomfort.

HEMOLYTIC ANEMIA. Hemolysis of probable mechanical origin may be seen after treatment of endocardial cushion defects or the insertion of an artificial prosthetic valve. It may be due to unusual turbulence associated with jets of blood at high pressure, since it tends to occur if there is residual mitral incompetence after treatment of an ostium primum defect when jets of blood impinge on the plastic prosthesis used to close the defect. Intravascular hemolysis may also be seen after insertion of an artificial valve, especially if the valve is incompetent. The anemia may be controlled with iron therapy, although reoperation may be necessary in patients with severe and progressive hemolysis who require frequent blood transfusions.

INFECTION. Sepsis with bacterial endocarditis is a serious complication, especially when prosthetic patches or valves are used. Common infecting organisms are *Staphylococcus aureus*, *Staphylococcus albus* and *Pseudomonas aeruginosa*. Less often, unusual bacteria and fungi, including some that are generally considered noninvasive, have also been the offending organisms. Treatment is difficult, but prolonged and diligent therapy with combinations of antimicrobial drugs have occasionally been successful. Infected prostheses may require replacement before the infection can be eliminated.

REFERENCES

General

See page 963.

Incidence and Etiology

Campbell, M.: The Incidence and Later Distribution of Malformations of the Heart; in H. Watson (Ed.): *Paediatric Cardiology*. St. Louis, C. V. Mosby Company, 1968, pp. 71-83.

Neill, C. A.: Genetic Aspects of Congenital Heart Disease; in A. J. Moss and F. H. Adams (Eds.): *Heart Disease in Infants, Children and Adolescents*. Baltimore, Williams & Wilkins Company, 1968, pp. 36-46.

Tetralogy of Fallot and Pulmonary Atresia

Guntheroth, W. G., and Morgan, B. C.: Physiologic Studies of Paroxysmal Hyperpnea in Cyanotic Congenital Heart Disease. *Circulation*, 31:70, 1965.

Kaplan, S., and others: Results of Palliative Procedures for Tetralogy of Fallot in Infants and Young Children. *Ann. Thoracic Surg.*, 5:489, 1968.

Kirklin, J. W., Wallace, R. B., McGoon, D. C., and DuShane, J. W.: Early and Late Results After Intracardiac Repair of Tetralogy of Fallot. *Ann. Surg.*, 162:578, 1965.

Lillehei, C. W., Levy, M. J., Adams, P., and Anderson, R. C.: Corrective Surgery for Tetralogy of Fallot: Long Term Follow-up by Postoperative Recatheterization in 69 Cases and Certain Surgical Considerations. *J. Thoracic & Cardiovasc. Surg.*, 48:556, 1964.

Malm, J. R., and others: Factors That Modify Hemodynamic Results in Total Correction of Tetralogy of Fallot. *J. Thoracic & Cardiovasc. Surg.*, 52:502, 1966.

Nagao, G. I., Daoud, G. I., McAdams, J., Schwartz, D. C., and Kaplan, S.: Cardiovascular Anomalies Associated with Tetralogy of Fallot. *Am. J. Cardiol.*, 20:206, 1967.

Paul, M. H., Miller, R. A., and Potts, W. J.: Long Term Results of Aortic-Pulmonary Anastomosis for Tetralogy of Fallot. *Circulation*, 23:525, 1961.

Ross, D., and Somerville, J.: Correction of Pulmonary Atresia with a Homograft Aortic Valve. *Lancet*, 2:1446, 1966.

Sabiston, D. C., and others: The Diagnosis and Surgical Correction of Total Obstruction of the Right Ventricle. *J. Thoracic & Cardiovasc. Surg.*, 48:577, 1964.

Taussig, H. B., Crawford, H., Pelargonio, S., and Zacharioudakis, S.: Ten to Thirteen Year Follow-up on Patients After a Blalock-Taussig Operation. *Circulation*, 25:630, 1962.

Eisenmenger Syndrome

Wood, P.: Pulmonary Hypertension. *Mod. Con. Cardiovas. Dis.*, 28:513, 1959.

Transposition of the Great Vessels

Aberdeen, E., and others: Successful "Correction" of Transposed Great Arteries by Mustard's Operation. *Lancet*, 1:1233, 1965.

Miller, R. A., Baffes, T. G., and Wilkinson, A. A.: Transposition of Great Vessels. *Pediat. Clin. N. Amer.*, 5:1109, 1958.

Mustard, W. T., Keith, J. D., Trusler, G. A., Fowler, R., and Kidd, L.: The Surgical Management of Transposition of the Great Vessels. *J. Thoracic & Cardiovasc. Surg.*, 48:953, 1964.

Noonan, J. A., Nadas, A. S., Rudolph, A. M., and Harris, G. B. C.: Transposition of the Great Arteries. *New England J. Med.*, 263:592, 1960.

Rashkind, W. J., and Miller, W. W.: Creation of an Atrial Septal Defect Without Thoracotomy: A Palliative Approach to Complete Transposition of the Great Vessels. *J.A.M.A.*, 196:991, 1966.

Taussig-Bing Syndrome

Daicoff, G. R., and Kirklin, J. W.: Surgical Correction of a Taussig-Bing Malformation: Report of Three Cases. *Am J. Cardiol*, 19:125, 1967.

Ebstein's Disease

Genton, E., and Blount, S. G.: The Spectrum of Ebstein's Anomaly. *Am. Heart J.*, 73:395, 1967.

Watson, H.: Electrode Catheters in the Diagnosis of Ebstein's Anomaly of the Tricuspid Valve. *Brit. Heart J.*, 28:161, 1966.

Atrial Septal Defect

Evans, J. R., Rowe, R. D., and Keith, J. D.: Clinical Diagnosis of Atrial Septal Defect in Children. *Am. J. Med.*, 30:345, 1961.

Kaplan, S.: Atrial Septal Defect; in H. Watson (Editor): *Paediatric Cardiology*. St. Louis, C. V. Mosby Company, 1968, p. 376.

Leatham, A., and Gray, L.: Auscultatory and Phonocardiographic Signs of Atrial Septal Defect. *Brit. Heart J.*, 18:193, 1956.

Rastelli, G. C., Kirklin, J. W., and Titus, J. L.: Anatomic Observations on Complete Form of Persistent Common Atrioventricular Canal, with Special Reference to Atrioventricular Valves. *Proc. Mayo Clin.*, 41:296, 1966.

Weyn, A. S., Bartle, S. H., Nolan, T. B., and Dammann, J. F., Jr.: Atrial Septal Defect, Primum Types. *Circulation*, 32 (Supp. 3):13, 1965.

Zaver, A. G., and Nadas, A. S.: Atrial Septal Defect, Secundum Type. *Circulation*, 32 (Supp. 3):24, 1965.

Ventricular Septal Defect

Edwards, J. E.: The Pathology of Ventricular Septal Defect. *Seminars in Radiol.*, 1:2, 1966.

Hoffman, J. I. E.: Natural History of Congenital Heart Disease: Problems in Its Assessment, with Special Reference to Ventricular Septal Defects. *Circulation*, 37:97, 1968.

Kaplan, S., and others: Natural History of Ventricular Septal Defect. *Am. J. Dis. Child,*, 105:581, 1963.

Kirklin, J. W., and DuShane, J. W.: Indication for Repair of Ventricular Septal Defects. *Am. J. Cardiol.*, 12:75, 1963.

Levin, A. R., and others: Intracardiac Pressure-Flow Dynamics in Isolated Ventricular Septal Defects. *Circulation*, 35:430, 1967.

Ritter, D. G., Feldt, R. H., Weidman, W. H., and DuShane, J. W.: Ventricular Septal Defect. *Circulation*, 32 (Supp. 3):42, 1965.

Smith, G. W., Dammann, J. F., Littlefield, J. B., and Muller, W. H., Jr.: Banding of the Pulmonary Artery: Indications and Results; in D. E. Cassels (Editor): *The Heart and Circulation in the Newborn and Infant.* New York, Grune & Stratton, Inc., 1966, p. 389.

Weidman, W. H., DuShane, J. W., and Kirklin, J. W.: Observations Concerning Progressive Pulmonary Vascular Obstruction in Children with Ventricular Septal Defects. *Am. Heart J.*, 65:148, 1963.

Pulmonary Stenosis with Normal Aortic Root

Abrahams, D. G., and Wood, P. H.: Pulmonary Stenosis with Normal Aortic Root. *Brit. Heart J.*, 13:519, 1951.

Brock, R. C.: The Surgical Treatment of Pulmonary Stenosis. *Brit. Heart J.*, 23:337, 1961.

Leatham, A., and Weitzman, D.: Auscultatory and Phonocardiographic Signs of Pulmonary Stenosis. *Brit. Heart J.*, 19:303, 1957.

Levine, O. R., and Blumenthal, S.: Pulmonic Stenosis. *Circulation*, 32 (Supp. 3):33, 1965.

Anomalous Pulmonary Venous Return

Burroughs, J. T., and Edwards, J. E.: Total Anomalous Pulmonary Venous Connection. *Am. Heart J.*, 59:913, 1960.

Cooley, D. A., Hallman, G. L., and Leachman, R. D.: Total Anomalous Pulmonary Venous Drainage. Correction with the Use of Cardiopulmonary Bypass in 62 Cases. *J. Thoracic & Cardiovasc. Surg.*, 51:88, 1966.

Hastreiter, A. R., Paul, M. H., Molthan, M. E., and Miller, R. H.: Total Anomalous Pulmonary Venous Connection with Severe Pulmonary Venous Obstruction. *Circulation*, 25:916, 1962.

Snellen, H. A., and Dekker, A.: Anomalous Pulmonary Venous Drainage in Relation to Left Superior Vena Cava and Coronary Sinus. *Am. Heart J.*, 66:184, 1963.

Aortic Stenosis

Hohn, A. R., VanPraagh, S., Moore, A. D., Vlad, P., and Lambert, E. C.: Aortic Stenosis. *Circulation*, 32 (Supp. 3):4, 1965.

Lees, M. H., Hauck, A. J., Starkey, G. W. B., Nadas, A. S., and Gross, R. E.: Congenital Aortic Stenosis. *Brit. Heart J.*, 24:31, 1962.

Mitral Stenosis

Daoud, G., Kaplan, S., Perrin, E. V., Dorst, J. P., and Edwards, F. K.: Congenital Mitral Stenosis. *Circulation*, 27:185, 1963.

Dextrocardia and Levocardia

VanPraagh, R.: Malposition of the Heart; in A. J. Moss and F. H. Adams (Editors): *Heart Disease in Infants, Children and Adolescents.* Baltimore, Williams & Wilkins Company, 1968, p. 602.

Principles of Treatment

Anderson, R., and Larson, O.: Fever, Splenomegaly and Atypical Lymphocytes After Open Heart Surgery. *Lancet*, 2:947, 1963.

Drusin, L. M., Engle, M. A., Hagstrom, J. W. C., and Schwartz, M. S.: The Postpericardiotomy Syndrome, A Six Year Epidemiologic Study. *New England J. Med.*, 272:597, 1965.

Pirofsky, B., Sutherland, D. W., Starr, A., and Griswold, H. E.: Hemolytic Anemia Complicating Aortic Valve Surgery. *New England J. Med.*, 272:235, 1965.

Williams, J. F., Morrow, A. G., and Braunwald, E.: The Incidence and Management of "Medical" Complications Following Cardiac Operations. *Circulation*, 32:608, 1965.

DISTURBANCES OF RATE AND RHYTHM OF THE HEART

SINUS ARRHYTHMIA

(Respiratory Arrhythmia)

This rhythm, an acceleration of the heart rate during inspiration and a decrease during expiration, is physiologic in childhood. It is usually associated with cardiac rates under 90 to 100 per minute. It is exaggerated during convalescence from febrile illness and by drugs which increase vagal tone, such as digitalis, and is usually abolished by exercise or atropine. Some children have such great degrees of sinus arrhythmia that the presence of other arrhythmias such as extrasystoles is suspected, and an electrocardiogram is necessary for diagnosis.

EXTRASYSTOLES

(Premature Contractions)

Extrasystoles are produced by the discharge of an ectopic focus situated anywhere in atrial, nodal or ventricular tissue. They occur less frequently in children than in adults. In the majority of instances extrasystoles are of no clinical or prognostic significance. Under certain circumstances premature beats may be due to organic heart disease, e.g. in acute rheumatic or diphtheritic car-

ditis. Drugs, especially digitalis and epinephrine, may also produce extrasystoles. Atrial premature contractions may precede atrial fibrillation in rheumatic mitral stenosis.

The clinical signs of extrasystoles include the prematurity of the beat followed by a compensatory pause, especially if the ectopic beat arises in the ventricles. In the majority of instances, extrasystoles disappear during the tachycardia of exercise. If they remain or become exaggerated during exercise, associated organic heart disease is suggested. Ectopic beats produce a smaller stroke and pulse volume than normal and, if very premature, may not be audible with a stethoscope or palpable at the radial pulse. Extrasystoles may assume a definite rhythm, e.g. alternating with normal beats (*pulsus bigeminus*) or occurring after 2 normal beats (*pulsus trigeminus*). This rhythmicity is frequent in digitalis intoxication. The site of origin of the extrasystoles is determined by the electrocardiogram.

Most patients are unaware of premature contractions. The basis of therapy is convincing reassurance that the arrhythmia is not due to structural heart disease. If extrasystoles are produced by digitalis, the drug should be discontinued or its dose reduced. If relief is sought for palpitations, sedatives, quinidine sulfate or procainamide may be used.

PAROXYSMAL TACHYCARDIA

Paroxysmal tachycardia is produced by ectopic beats arising from the same focus in rapid succession. The ectopic focus may be anywhere in the atrial, nodal or ventricular tissue. Paroxysmal tachycardia may occur at any age and has been reported in the last month of fetal life. In the majority of instances the ectopic focus is situated in an atrium (paroxysmal atrial tachycardia or flutter). Paroxysmal ventricular tachycardia is rare in infants and children.

In older children, attacks of *paroxysmal atrial tachycardia* are characterized by abrupt onset and cessation. If an attack is not witnessed, its occurrence may be elicited by an accurate history. It may be precipitated by an acute infection. Attacks may last from a few seconds to several weeks, but usually persist for a few hours and seldom exceed 2 or 3 days. The cardiac rate usually exceeds 180 and occasionally may be as rapid as 300 per minute. The only complaint may be awareness of the rapid cardiac rate. If it is exceptionally rapid or if the attack is prolonged, precordial discomfort and congestive cardiac failure may supervene.

In young infants the diagnosis may be more obscure. Since the normal cardiac rate at this age is rapid and increases greatly with crying, a persistent tachycardia during quiet periods or sleep suggests the diagnosis. The cardiac rate during paroxysms is frequently in the range of 300 per minute, and signs of congestive cardiac failure rapidly supervene if the attack lasts a few hours or more. The infant is acutely ill, has an ashen and slightly cyanotic color and is restless and irritable. Tachypnea and hepatomegaly are the prominent signs of cardiac failure. Paroxysms may be associated with fever and leukocytosis. The diagnosis is confirmed by the electrocardiogram (Fig. 13-58), which also identifies the site of the ectopic focus.

Treatment. In supraventricular paroxysmal tachycardia (atrial or nodal) simple procedures of vagal stimulation such as pressure over the eyeballs or over the carotid sinus may abort the attack. Older children may have discovered some maneuver to abolish the paroxysm, such as self-induced vomiting, breath-holding, drinking ice water or the adoption of a particular posture. In infants and many older patients these measures fail, and digitalis should be given in full therapeutic doses. This drug abolishes the tachycardia in more than 95 per cent of patients. In infants, digitalis should be used even if the paroxysm was abolished by vagal stimulation, since the recurrence rate is high; therapy should be maintained for about one year after the paroxysm. In rare instances when paroxysms persist and congestive heart failure progresses, electrical cardioversion or beta adrenergic antagonists (propranolol) are used. Other agents which have been used to abolish paroxysmal supraventricular tachycardia include infusions of phenylephrine (Neo-Synephrine)

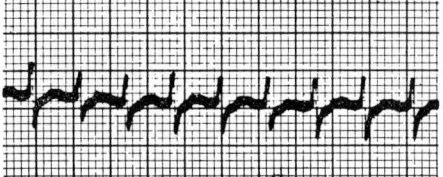

LEAD I

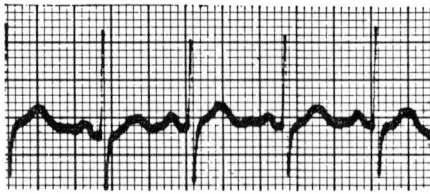

LEAD I

Figure 13-58. Electrocardiogram in paroxysmal atrial tachycardia. Upper tracing taken during paroxysm with heart rate of 240 per minute. Lower tracing, taken during recovery, is within normal limits.

diphenylhydantoin (Dilantin) and oral quinidine sulfate. It is important to relieve the apprehension associated with a prolonged paroxysm by sedation, preferably with morphine.

In most instances of paroxysmal atrial tachycardia there is no underlying structural cardiac disease. If cardiac failure supervenes during the paroxysms, cardiac function rapidly returns to normal after cessation of the attack. Between attacks some children may exhibit the electrocardiographic signs of the *Wolff-Parkinson-White syndrome*, which is probably due to an anomalous connection by special conducting fibers between the right atrium and the ventricles. Electrocardiography shows a widened QRS complex at the expense of a shortened P-R interval so that the P-S interval as measured from the beginning of the P to the end of the S is normal (Fig. 13-59). In the majority of instances there is no associated cardiac disease. Paroxysmal atrial tachycardia occurs in about 50 to 60 per cent of patients with the Wolff-Parkinson-White syndrome, and about 5 per cent of patients with paroxysmal tachycardia exhibit this syndrome between attacks of tachycardia.

Spontaneous *ventricular tachycardia* is rare in children. It may be seen in the immediate postoperative period after cardiac surgery or occasionally during severe myocarditis. Patients with ventricular tachycardia usually appear critically ill, with restlessness, pallor and hypotension. The diagnosis is confirmed by electrocardiography. Abolition of the paroxysm is urgently indicated and is best accomplished by electrical cardioversion. Drugs of choice are xylocaine, procainamide and quinidine sulfate.

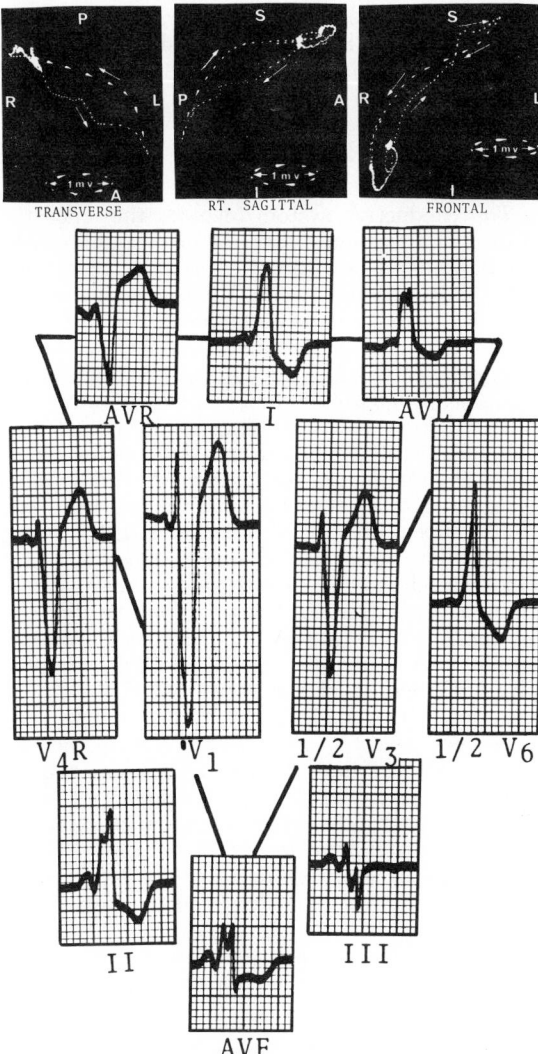

Figure 13-59. Electrocardiogram and vectorcardiogram in Wolff-Parkinson-White syndrome. Short P-R interval and wide QRS are present. The vectorcardiogram shows a slow inscription of the initial QRS.

ATRIAL FLUTTER

This arrhythmia is due to rapid and regular but abnormal atrial contractions. Lewis attributed these contractions to a circus movement in the atria; Prinzmetal suggested that they are due to an irritable focus in the atrial muscle similar to that of paroxysmal atrial tachycardia and atrial extrasystoles. The rate of atrial beats ranges from 250 to 400 per minute. Because the atrioventricular node cannot transmit such rapid impulses, the ventricles respond to every second, or even to every third or fourth, atrial beat.

Atrial flutter is not frequent in children, but may sometimes complicate myocarditis of any cause and occasionally acute infectious diseases. It should be suspected in patients with a regular tachycardia which is not influenced by effort,

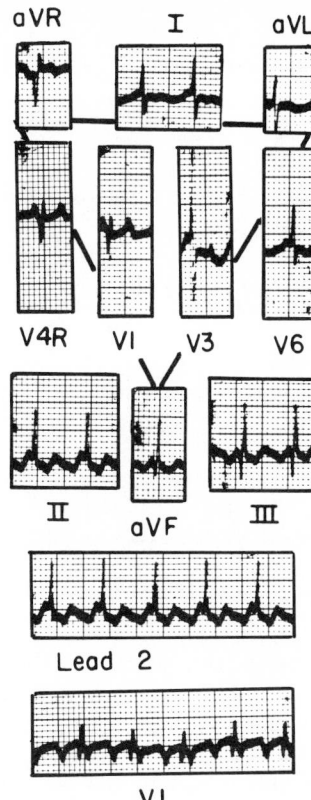

Figure 13-60. Atrial flutter in newborn. F waves present in leads II and V_1.

emotion or posture. Atrial flutter may precipitate congestive cardiac failure. Carotid sinus pressure frequently produces a temporary slowing of the cardiac rate. The diagnosis is confirmed by electrocardiography, which demonstrates the rapid and regular atrial flutter or "f" waves.

Treatment is by digitalization to convert the arrhythmia into atrial fibrillation. Normal sinus rhythm may then be restored when the digitalis is discontinued. If atrial fibrillation persists, quinidine sulfate is used. If atrial flutter still continues, the administration of digitalis is resumed. Uncontrollable atrial flutter may also be treated with electrical cardioversion.

ATRIAL FIBRILLATION

The mechanism of this abnormality is similar to that of atrial flutter; the atrial excitation is irregular and more rapid (300 to 500 per minute). The arrhythmia occurs most frequently in older children with rheumatic mitral valve disease. It has been reported as a complication of atrial septal defect and patent ductus arteriosus.

The rhythm is grossly irregular (Fig. 13-61) and associated with a pulse deficit. Atrial fibrillation may complicate or precipitate congestive cardiac failure.

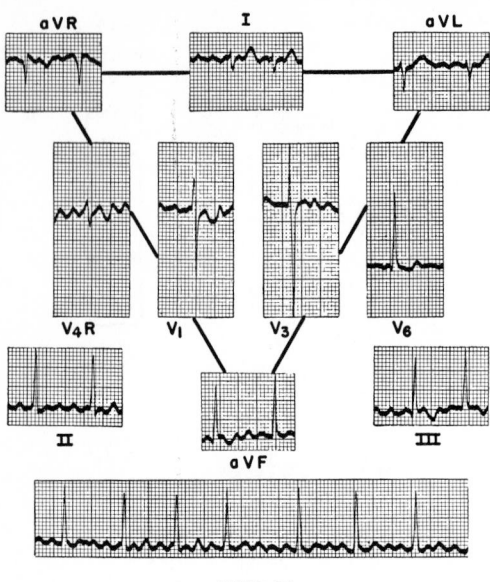

LEAD II

Figure 13-61. Electrocardiogram of an 11-year-old girl with rheumatic heart disease and mitral stenosis. The tracing reveals the presence of atrial fibrillation.

Treatment is by digitalization, which restores the ventricular rate to normal, although the rhythm remains irregular. Normal sinus rhythm may then be restored with quinidine sulfate. Electrical cardioversion also restores sinus rhythm. Maintenance of sinus rhythm is not usual in the patient whose atrial fibrillation was associated with florid mitral valve disease and cardiomegaly. Continuation of prophylactic therapy with digitalis and quinidine is usually required in these patients.

VENTRICULAR FIBRILLATION

This irregular ventricular action (Fig. 13-62) results in death unless an effective ventricular beat is restored. Occasionally this arrhythmia occurs during or shortly after cardiac surgery and explains some of the deaths due to intravenous drug therapy. The only effective therapy is cardiac massage (preferably external) and electrical defibrillation.

BRADYCARDIA

A slow pulse rate may occur during convalescence from acute infections such as rheumatic fever, typhoid fever or infectious hepatitis and in association with lesions of the brain which cause increased intracranial pressure. Older children and young adults who lead active lives frequently have pulse rates of about 60 per minute at rest. Bradycardia of this degree may occur as a family

trait. Rates of less than 80 per minute in the first 2 years of life and less than 50 in older children may be due to heart block.

HEART BLOCK

The conductive system includes the sinoatrial node, the atrial muscle, the atrioventricular node, the bundle of His with its left and right branches, and the Purkinje network. The conductive system may be blocked at any site along this pathway. When the block occurs at the sinoatrial node so that occasional beats are delayed or dropped, it is designated *sinoatrial block*. When the impulse is blocked in its pathway from the sinoatrial node through the atrioventricular node, it is termed *atrioventricular block*. Partial atrioventricular block may have only a prolonged P-R interval (*first-degree block*) or may be associated with dropped ventricular beats (*second-degree block*). Second-degree block may occur at regular intervals so that there are 2 or 3 atrial beats to 1 ventricular beat (2:1 or 3:1 partial atrioventricular block). Another type of partial atrioventricular block is a progressive lengthening of the P-R interval from cycle to cycle until a ventricular beat is dropped (*Wenckebach phenomenon*, Fig. 13-62). When no impulses pass through the atrioventricular node so that the atria and ventricles contract independently of each other, the condition is known as *complete atrioventricular block*. Finally, the impulse may be blocked in either the left or right branch of the bundle of His, and the condition is designated as *left* or *right bundle branch block*.

Complete heart block and first-degree partial block are the common types encountered in children.

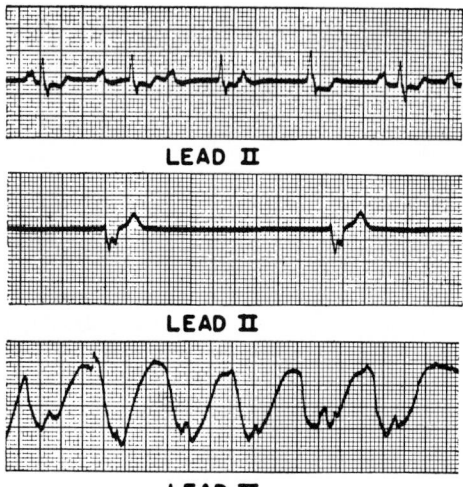

LEAD II

LEAD II

LEAD II

Figure 13-62. Electrocardiogram tracings showing various types of arrhythmias. Upper tracing shows the Wenckebach phenomenon. Note progressive prolongation of the P-R interval. Middle tracing shows idioventricular rhythm with a heart rate of 30 per minute. Lower tracing shows ventricular fibrillation.

Congenital Complete Heart Block. In children complete block is probably the result of a congenital defect in the main stem of the bundle of His. Although atrial or ventricular septal defects may be associated lesions, it is doubtful whether they are directly responsible. The majority of patients with atrial or ventricular septal defects have normal cardiac rhythms, and heart block usually occurs in patients with intact septa.

The condition is commonly asymptomatic, although attacks of syncope may occur. Congenital heart block is suspected if the cardiac rate is less than 80 in infants or less than 50 in older children. On this basis the condition has been occasionally suspected in the fetus. The peripheral pulse is of the water-hammer type, owing to the large ventricular stroke volume and peripheral vasodilatation, and the systolic blood pressure is elevated. Jugular venous pulsations occur irregularly and may be large when the atrium contracts against a closed tricuspid valve. Inconspicuous venous pulsations may occur independently of ventricular contractions. The first cardiac sound has a changing intensity, and isolated atrial contractions may be audible down the left sternal border or at the apex. Taussig observed that exercise and atropine, which have no effect in increasing the cardiac rate of adults with complete heart block, may produce an acceleration of 10 to 20 beats per minute in the child. Heart block in itself produces cardiac enlargement. Systolic murmurs along the left sternal border are frequent and do not indicate the presence of a ventricular septal defect. Apical mid-diastolic murmurs are not unusual.

The diagnosis is confirmed by electrocardiograms; the P waves and QRS complexes have no constant relation (Fig. 13-63). The shape and amplitude of the individual waves are generally normal.

The prognosis is usually favorable; patients who have been observed to the age of 30 to 40 years have lived normally active lives. In some patients,

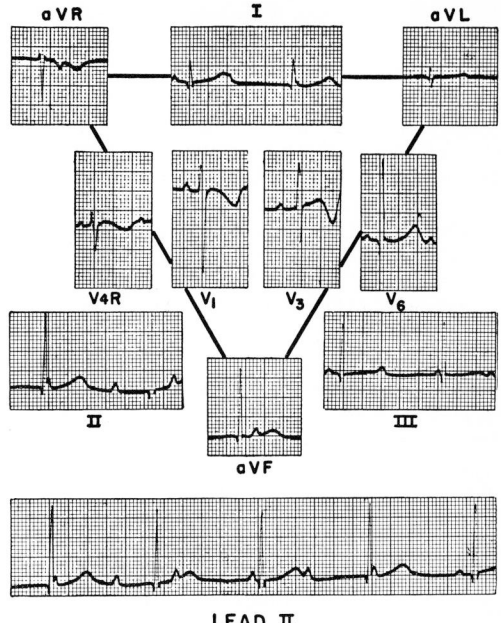

Figure 13-63. Electrocardiogram of 5-year-old boy showing complete heart block (see text).

however, episodes of dizziness with or without syncope (Stokes-Adams attacks) may occur. This complication requires the implantation of a permanent pacemaker.

REFERENCES

Campbell, M., and Thorne, M. G.: Congenital Heart Block. *Brit. Heart J.,* 18:90, 1956.

Nadas, A. S., Daeschner, C. W., Roth, A., and Blumenthal, S. L.: Paroxysmal Tachycardia in Infants and Children: Study of 41 Cases. *Pediatrics,* 9:167, 1952.

Paul, M. H.: Cardiac Arrhythmias in Infants and Children. *Prog. Cardiovas. Dis.,* 9:136, 1966.

DISEASES OF THE ENDOCARDIUM

ACUTE OR MALIGNANT ENDOCARDITIS

Acute endocarditis has been observed at all ages, including the neonatal period, when it may have been acquired during fetal life. The infection may occur suddenly in a previously well child or may complicate congenital or rheumatic heart disease. The commonest infecting agent is *Staphylococcus aureus.* Less frequently encountered organisms are gram-negative bacilli, enterococci, pneumococci and fungi. Vegetations develop on the endocardium of the valves and cardiac chambers, more frequently on the left side than on the right. They consist of bacteria in an exudate of fibrin and blood. Ulceration and the formation of friable granulation tissue occur early. Destruction of valvular tissue progresses rapidly, resulting in acute incompetence of valves, usually the mitral or aortic. Cardiac performance is further impaired by extension of the infection into the myocardium. Parts of the vegetations or necrotic tissue may embolize to any part of the body, obstructing blood flow and establishing secondary foci of infection.

Clinical Manifestations. The onset of acute endocarditis is explosive, with high fever and prostration. Abdominal pain, hematuria, diarrhea or paralysis of parts of the body may be produced by septic emboli. Cardiomegaly may or may not be present. Cardiac murmurs are either absent or produced by previously underlying heart disease.

Retinal hemorrhages, splenomegaly or the loss of pulsation of a major artery may be detected. In many patients the cause of the infection is not clear, but in some there is a history of recent furunculosis, osteomyelitis or infected pilonidal cyst. Polymorphonuclear leukocytosis is usual. Albuminuria, microscopic hematuria and pyuria are common. Blood cultures are usually positive.

Prognosis. The prognosis is generally grave, and death usually occurs within a few days unless treatment is started early. The cause of death is either toxicity from infection or relentless progression of cardiac failure. The latter complication may occur weeks or months after the infection is cured, owing to rupture or the development of defects in the valves (usually mitral or aortic).

Treatment. Since the prognosis is so poor if therapy is delayed, 3 blood cultures should be drawn within 1 to 2 hours and treatment started on the presumption that the causal organism is *Staphylococcus aureus*. Large intravenous doses of methicillin should be used until the results of the cultures and the antibiotic sensitivity of the organism are available. The duration of therapy should never be less than 4 weeks. Penicillin G (20 to 40 million units daily) may be used if the organism is sensitive to this antibiotic; the blood level may be increased with probenecid. Supportive therapy, including blood transfusion and intravenous fluid, is the same as for other acute infections. The complication of heart failure is treated with the usual anticongestive measures. Emboli to major vessels, especially in the lower extremities, should be removed surgically as an emergency.

SUBACUTE BACTERIAL ENDOCARDITIS

This disease resembles the acute form in many ways, but its course is more insidious and protracted. The infection usually develops at the site of congenital or acquired defects of the heart. It rarely occurs in infancy, but has been noted occasionally in children 3 or 4 years of age; the incidence increases with advancing age.

The commonest causative organism is *Streptococcus viridans*. Other infecting agents include enterococci (group D streptococci), *Staphylococcus albus* or *aureus* and fungi. Although predisposing factors are not clear in all patients, infection with *Streptococcus viridans* may follow oral or pharyngeal surgery, especially dental extractions. Enterococci may enter the bloodstream after instrumentation of the genitourinary or gastrointestinal tract. Organisms which are generally considered to be nonpathogenic may result in subacute (or acute) bacterial endocarditis after open-heart surgery.

The vegetations are usually smaller than those in the acute type. They may destroy the endocardial lining and underlying muscle and even perforate valves or septa. When superimposed upon acquired cardiac disease, the subacute form usually attacks the left rather than the right side of the heart. In congenitally malformed hearts the bacterial invasion begins at or near the site of the defect.

Clinical Manifestations. Initially, symptoms are obscure and ill-defined, including pyrexia, malaise, lassitude, pallor, anorexia, weight loss and arthralgia. Chills and night sweats may occur. Signs of pre-existing heart disease are present, and new murmurs may appear during the course of the disease, e.g. from mitral or aortic incompetence. Unexplained heart failure in a previously well compensated patient may be an early sign. Petechiae are common and are usually located in oral mucous membranes, conjunctivae and around the ankles and wrists. Splinter hemorrhages may be seen under the fingernails and toenails; occasionally retinal hemorrhages are present. The older literature stressed other classic signs of subacute bacterial endocarditis such as Osler's nodes (small, tender, palpable erythematous lesions in the pads of fingers or toes), Janeway's lesions (painless, hemorrhagic nodules in the palms and soles), Roth spots (hemorrhagic areas with a white center seen in the retina) and clubbing of the fingers. These signs are late manifestations of the disease and are now rarely seen. Splenomegaly may be present, but is not constant. Left upper quadrant pain may be produced by splenic infarction. A normochromic, normocytic anemia is usual. Albuminuria is common, and microscopic hematuria may be present. The emphasis of the clinical picture may be altered by systemic embolization, which may result in infarction, hemorrhage, abscess formation or gangrene. When the underlying cardiac disease is associated with a left-to-right shunt, pulmonary infarction may occur. Occasionally, bacterial endocarditis presents with meningitis, convulsions, hemiparesis or subarachnoid hemorrhage.

Diagnosis. Anemia and leukocytosis are common and the sedimentation rate is increased. Identification of the causative organism by blood culture is the most important laboratory finding. Six blood cultures (aerobic and anaerobic) taken over a period of 2 to 4 days usually suffice; if these are negative, subsequent cultures are rarely positive.

Prognosis. With early adequate treatment most children recover completely. The disease may run a mild course during its first weeks or even months so that the diagnosis may not be suspected until severe valvular disease has resulted. If therapy is inadequate, recurrences are usual.

Treatment. Identification of the infecting organisms is essential to successful therapy, but antibiotic treatment may be initiated, pending the results of in vitro sensitivity tests after the organism has been isolated. It is important that the blood level of antibiotics exceed the minimal inhibiting concentration of antibiotic in broth. Bactericidal agents should be used whenever possible, since bacteriostatic drugs are seldom successful in eradicating bacteria from cardiac vegetations.

Streptococcus viridans is almost always exquisitely sensitive to penicillin; i.e. growth is inhibited by 0.005 to 0.2 μg. of penicillin per ml. of serum. Infection with this organism is treated with a combination of penicillin and streptomycin, since the latter is synergistic with penicillin. The route of administration of penicillin and the duration of therapy are controversial. In many institutions penicillin G is given intravenously or intramuscularly in doses varying from 600,000 to 3,000,000 units every 4 hours for 2 to 6 weeks. We have had great success with oral phenoxymethyl penicillin (penicillin V) in a dose of 600 to 750 mg. every 4 hours for 2 weeks. We have not encountered instances in which the antibiotic had to be abandoned because of inadequate absorption or gastrointestinal symptoms (nausea, vomiting, diarrhea). Streptomycin is given intramuscularly every 12 hours, and the dose should not exceed 1 gm. per day even in adolescents. It is advisable to measure the antistreptococcal activity of the patient's serum against his own organism. Treatment is progressing satisfactorily if a serum dilution of 1:8, 1:16 or more inhibits growth of the organism.

Enterococci (group D streptococci) are usually more resistant to penicillin; these patients require intravenous therapy with penicillin G (15 to 25 million units daily) for 4 to 6 weeks. Streptomycin is used concomitantly; the dose should not exceed 1 gm. daily.

Endocarditis due to *gram-negative bacteria* is difficult to manage and in children is generally seen as a complication of open-heart surgery. The choice of antibiotic depends on the in vitro sensitivity of the causal organism. The antibiotics generally considered for use are kanamycin, the polymyxins, streptomycin and ampicillin. Toxic effects of these drugs are described elsewhere.

Penicillin sensitivity should be carefully confirmed by history. Barring a history of serious reaction, it is the drug of choice, and the following regimen may be used: (1) oral prednisone; (2) a gradual buildup in penicillin dosage (given at half-hourly intervals) as follows: (*a*) 10 units intradermally, (*b*) 100 units subcutaneously, (*c*) 1000 units subcutaneously, (*d*) 10,000 units intramuscularly, (*e*) 100,000 units intramuscularly. If no reaction occurs, the usual schedule of penicillin therapy may be followed even if urticaria is observed during the course of treatment.

Clinically acceptable but *bacteriologically unproved* endocarditis is a difficult therapeutic problem. Generally it is assumed that the organism is sensitive to penicillin, and so it is infused intravenously in a dose of at least 10 million units daily for not less than 4 weeks, frequently supplemented with intramuscular streptomycin. The adequacy of therapy is gauged by the clinical course. When there is lack of response to therapy, the dose of penicillin is increased or other bactericidal agents are added. Probenecid may be used to increase the blood level of penicillin.

A condition clinically indistinguishable from subacute bacterial endocarditis or endarteritis may be seen in children with *ventriculocardiovascular shunts* for the treatment of hydrocephalus. The colonization of bacteria is usually in the valve of the artificial shunt. Management is similar to that for subacute bacterial endocarditis, except that it is rarely successful without removal of the shunt and replacement with an uncontaminated substitute.

Prophylaxis. All children with rheumatic heart disease and congenital cardiovascular anomalies are exposed to the hazard of subacute bacterial endocarditis. Therefore these patients should be protected with large doses of penicillin for 48 hours before and after operations on the ears, nose or throat, and dental extractions. Acute bacterial infections should be vigorously treated with suitable antibiotics.

RHEUMATIC ENDOCARDITIS

Rheumatic infections (p. 533) are not limited to the endocardium, but involve other parts of the heart and other organs of the body; only the endocardial changes will be mentioned here.

Rheumatic involvement of the valves and endocardium is by far the most common type of endocarditis in children. The lesions begin as small verrucae composed of fibrin and blood cells along the borders of the valves. The mitral valve is affected most often, the aortic next most frequently, and the tricuspid and pulmonary valves less commonly. As the infection subsides, the verrucae tend to disappear and leave scar tissue. With each repeated infection more small lesions of this type form near the previous ones, and the mural endocardium and chordae tendineae also become involved.

Clinical Patterns of Valvular Disease. *Mitral insufficiency.* Mitral insufficiency which prevents normal closure of the mitral valve is most frequently rheumatic in origin. There is usually some loss of substance of the valve, and the chordae tendineae may be shortened and thickened. There is often associated mitral stenosis due to sclerosis of the base of the mitral ring and cusps.

During ventricular systole, blood regurgitates from the left ventricle to the left atrium. This may result in left atrial enlargement, which is sometimes aneurysmal. Owing to the greater work load and filling pressure of the left ventricle, this chamber may also enlarge. The increased left atrial pressure may be reflected through the pulmonary bed to the right side of the heart, producing enlargement of the right ventricle and atrium, with subsequent congestive cardiac failure. In the majority of children the lesion is of mild or moderate severity, is well tolerated, and is asymptomatic. The principal physical sign is the apical systolic murmur of mitral incompetence (see below). In moderately severe or florid lesions the dominant symptoms are fatigue, poor weight gain, weakness, dyspnea on effort, and palpitations. The heart is enlarged, and an apical systolic thrill may be palpable. The first heart sound is normal; the second sound may show wide expiratory splitting because of the shortened duration of left ventricular systole. Pulmonary valvular closure is loud in the presence of complicating pulmonary hypertension. A third heart sound is prominent and is due to the large early diastolic filling of the left ventricle. The usual murmur is pansystolic and radiates to the left axilla and to the left sternal edge; in a minority of instances it is short and on rare occasions may be absent. A diastolic murmur due to increased blood flow from the left atrium across the mitral valve may be audible even in the absence of mitral stenosis.

The electrocardiogram and roentgenograms are normal if the lesion is mild. With more severe lesions the electrocardiogram shows prominent bifid P waves, signs of left ventricular hypertrophy and sometimes associated right ventricular hypertrophy. Roentgenographically, there is prominence of the left atrium and ventricle. When pulmonary hypertension or congestive heart failure supervenes, the pulmonary artery segment and right heart chambers are prominent. Signs of pulmonary venous hypertension are also seen sometimes. Calcification of the mitral valve is rare in children.

Cardiac catheterization and left ventriculography are undertaken only if there is rapid progression of the disease and surgical treatment is contemplated. The cardiac output is normal or decreased in florid lesions. The left atrial pressure is frequently but not always increased. The pulse curve of the left atrium shows a steep rise in early systole to the peak of the "v" wave and is followed by a rapid "y" descent. A diastolic gradient may be measured across the mitral valve even in the absence of mitral stenosis. The left ventricular end-diastolic pressure rises during exercise or in the presence of left ventricular failure. Left ventriculography results in opacification of the left atrium. The degree of opacification is used as a qualitative assessment of the severity of incompetence.

A frequent problem is evaluation of an apical systolic murmur without other signs in patients who have had a mild attack of rheumatic fever or a history of recurrent upper respiratory tract infections. Though many of these patients are considered to have organic mitral insufficiency, the diagnosis is often incorrect. In some the murmur is extracardiac, and sometimes an innocent murmur is transmitted to the apex. Many children with murmurs suggestive of mitral insufficiency lose all evidence of cardiac disease after some years. Patients may require careful follow-up studies for many years before the cause of the murmur becomes apparent. Untold harm may be done if the patient's activities are reduced on the basis of the presence of a murmur alone.

During convalescence children with mild cardiac disease often make great improvement, while those with far advanced cardiac disease suffer from the effects of rapid growth. If rheumatic infections recur, the valvular condition may become progressively worse. For prophylactic therapy, see page 541.

Complications. Severe mitral incompetence may result in cardiac failure. This may be precipitated by progression of the rheumatic process, the onset of atrial fibrillation with rapid ventricular response or subacute bacterial endocarditis. Pulmonary congestion is common, but frank left ventricular failure is unusual. Right-sided heart failure may be accompanied by tricuspid or pulmonary incompetence. Bacterial endocarditis may complicate rheumatic mitral valvular disease, especially when dominant incompetence is associated with moderate stenosis. Occasional atrial or ventricular extrasystoles are well tolerated. First-degree heart block may persist for years after the original rheumatic infection or be due to digitalis therapy. Atrial fibrillation is more common when mitral incompetence is associated with a large hypertensive left atrium.

Treatment. In the majority of patients with mitral insufficiency, prophylaxis against recurrences of rheumatic fever is all that is required, since the lesions are mild and well tolerated. The treatment of complicating heart failure, dysrhythmias and bacterial endocarditis is described elsewhere. Surgical treatment is indicated in a minority who, in spite of adequate medical therapy, suffer from recurrent episodes of heart failure, extreme dyspnea with moderate activity and progressive cardiomegaly with pulmonary hypertension. Although annuloplasty gives good results in some children and adolescents, the majority require valve replacement.

Mitral stenosis. Congenital mitral stenosis is described on page 1009.

Organic mitral stenosis is nearly always rheumatic in origin and results from fibrosis of the mitral ring, commissural adhesions and contracture of the valve leaflets, chordae and papillary muscles. It may take 2 years or more for the lesion to become fully established, although the process may be accelerated in some children. Mitral stenosis is often associated with mitral insufficiency.

Mitral stenosis of critical degree is considered to exist if the valve orifice is reduced to 25 per cent or less of the expected normal. In established lesions the left atrium has difficulty in emptying, which results in hypertrophy and increased pressure in this chamber. The increased pressure results in pulmonary venous hypertension, increased pulmonary vascular resistance and pulmonary hypertension. Right ventricular and atrial dilatation and hypertrophy ensue and are followed by right-sided heart failure.

Generally there is a good correlation between symptoms and severity of obstruction. Patients with mild lesions are asymptomatic. More severe degrees of obstruction are associated with effort intolerance and dyspnea. Critical lesions can result in orthopnea, paroxysmal nocturnal dyspnea and overt pulmonary edema. These symptoms may be precipitated by uncontrolled tachycardia, atrial fibrillation or pulmonary infections. Congestive heart failure is usually associated with moderate or severe pulmonary hypertension. Right ventricular dilatation may result in functional tricuspid incompetence, hepatomegaly, ascites and edema. Hemoptysis may occur, owing to ruptured bronchial or pleurohilar veins and occasionally pulmonary infarction. Blood-streaked sputum occurs during episodes of pulmonary edema. Bacterial endocarditis and systemic emboli are uncommon in children.

With severe lesions, cyanosis and a malar flush are seen. The jugular venous pressure is increased in the presence of congestive heart failure, tricuspid valve disease or severe pulmonary hypertension. The heart size is normal with minimal disease. Moderate cardiomegaly is usual with severe mitral stenosis and sinus rhythm, but cardiac enlargement can be great, especially when atrial fibrillation and heart failure supervene. The apical impulse is brief and tapping, and a parasternal right ventricular lift is palpable when pulmonary vascular resistance is high. The principal auscultatory findings are a loud first heart sound, an opening snap of the mitral valve and a long, low-pitched, rumbling mitral diastolic murmur with presystolic accentuation. Severe obstruction is present when (1) the diastolic murmur is long (in the absence of mitral incompetence), (2) the Q-1 interval is long (i.e. time between the Q wave of the electrocardiogram and the first heart sound), and (3) the 2-OS interval is short (i.e. time between aortic valve closure and the opening snap). The mitral diastolic murmur may be absent in congestive heart failure. Presystolic accentuation of the diastolic murmur disappears during atrial fibrillation. An apical systolic murmur may be audible even in the absence of mitral incompetence and in some is due to complicating tricuspid incom-

petence. In the presence of pulmonary hypertension, pulmonary valvular closure is accentuated. An early diastolic murmur is usually due to associated aortic incompetence, since pulmonary valvular incompetence is not as common.

Electrocardiograms and roentgenograms are normal if the lesion is mild. More severe obstruction is associated with prominent and notched P waves and varying degrees of right ventricular hypertrophy. Moderate or critical lesions are associated with roentgenographic signs of varying degrees of left atrial enlargement, prominence of the pulmonary artery and right heart chambers and a normal or small aorta and left ventricle. Severe obstruction is associated with a redistribution of pulmonary blood flow so that the apices of the lung show a greater perfusion (i.e. reverse of normal). Serial films of patients with progressive stenosis will show more pulmonary vascular markings at the apices with prominence of the pulmonary veins. Septal lines at the costophrenic angles may also be present. Cardiac catheterization quantitates the diastolic gradient across the mitral valve, the degree of pulmonary hypertension and the severity of increase of pulmonary vascular resistance.

Treatment. Prophylaxis against recurrences of rheumatic fever and the treatment of cardiac failure and dysrhythmias are similar to those described under Mitral Insufficiency. Surgical treatment is undertaken when there are signs of recurrent pulmonary edema, high pulmonary vascular resistance or systemic emboli. Since extreme valvular distortion and calcification are rare in children, closed mitral valvotomy generally yields good results.

Aortic insufficiency. In the majority of instances aortic insufficiency results from rheumatic heart disease, but sometimes is associated with congenital cardiovascular lesions (see Coarctation of the Aorta, Aortic Stenosis and Ventricular

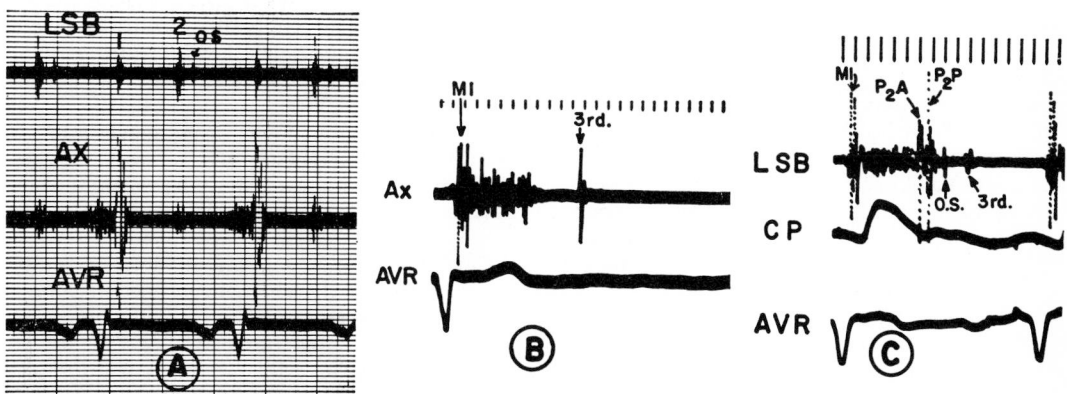

Figure 13-64. Phonocardiograms to illustrate auscultatory findings in proved cases of mitral valve disease. Abbreviations: *LSB,* Left sternal border; *AX,* apex; *AVR,* electrocardiogram; *CP,* carotid pulse; *1,* first heart sound; *2,* second heart sound; *P₂A,* aortic component, second sound; *P₂P,* pulmonary component, second sound; *OS,* mitral opening snap; *3,* third heart sound. A, Pure mitral stenosis. Note presystolic murmur, loud first sound, opening snap, prolonged Q-1 interval and 2-OS interval of 0.06 second. B, Pure mitral insufficiency. Note pansystolic murmur and loud third sound. C, Combined mitral insufficiency and stenosis. Note pansystolic murmur, opening snap and third heart sound.

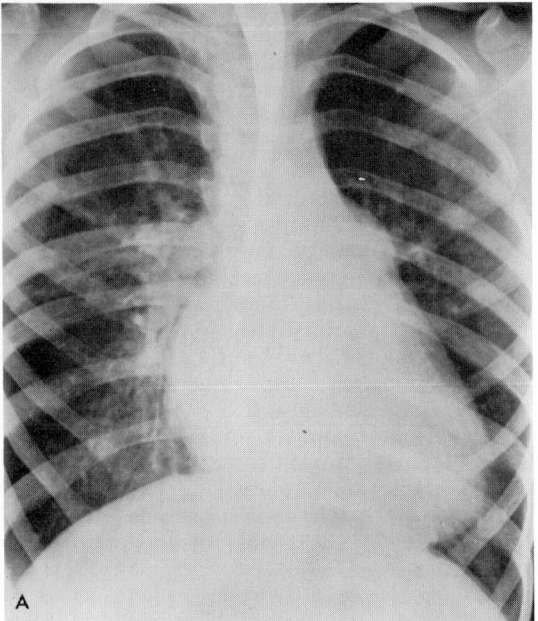
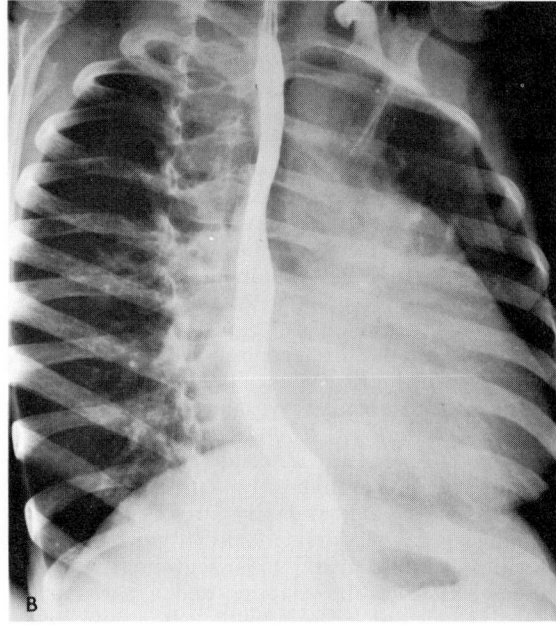

Figure 13-65. Teleroentgenograms in isolated rheumatic mitral stenosis. *A,* Posteroanterior view showing cardiomegaly and prominent main pulmonary artery. Vascular shadows in lungs due to prominent pulmonary arteries and veins. *B,* Right anterior oblique view showing indentation of esophagus by large left atrium. This patient required mitral valvotomy at age 8 years.

Septal Defect). In chronic rheumatic aortic insufficiency, sclerosis of the aortic valves results in distortion and retraction of the cusps. Regurgitation of blood results in a volume overload with dilatation and hypertrophy of the left ventricle. Secondary mitral incompetence may follow progressive left ventricular dilatation. Left ventricular failure results in left atrial hypertension. Congestive cardiac failure may occur insidiously or be preceded by bouts of pulmonary edema.

Symptoms are unusual except in gross aortic incompetence. The large stroke volume and forceful left ventricular contractions may result in palpitations. Excessive sweating and heat intolerance are related to vasodilatation. Dyspnea on effort progresses to orthopnea and pulmonary edema. Angina pectoris may occur during heavy exertion. In adolescents with florid incompetence, nocturnal attacks with nightmares, sweating, tachycardia, chest pain and hypertension may occur.

Owing to the reflux of blood through the aortic valve during diastole and to associated vasodilatation, the radial pulses are water-hammer in type, and the carotid arteries show bounding Corrigan pulsations. Associated signs of severe aortic insufficiency include capillary pulsations in the lips or fingernails, an audible systolic shock over the peripheral arteries (pistol shot) and systolic and diastolic murmurs over the femoral arteries if pressure is applied to the artery just distal to the stethoscope *(Duroziez's sign).* The systolic blood pressure is elevated, the diastolic lowered.

In severe aortic insufficiency the heart is enlarged with a left ventricular apical heave. Thrills

are absent unless there is an associated aortic stenosis. The typical murmur is early in diastole and is heard over the upper and middle left sternal border with radiation to the apex and to the aortic area. Characteristically, it has the hollow, fading quality of a whispered "ping." Generally the murmur is more easily audible in full expiration with the patient leaning forward, or it may be louder in the recumbent position. A systolic ejection murmur sometimes preceded by a click is frequent and is produced by the large stroke volume. An apical presystolic murmur (Austin-Flint) resembling that of mitral stenosis is heard sometimes. It is probably due to interference with valvular function by the large regurgitant blood flow which deflects the aortic cusp of the mitral valve.

Roentgenograms show prominence and exaggerated pulsations of the left ventricle and aorta. The electrocardiogram may be normal, but in severe cases reveals signs of left ventricular hypertrophy with prominent P waves.

Cardiac catheterization is seldom necessary and is undertaken only when surgery is contemplated because of a progressive lesion. The degree of elevation of left ventricular end diastolic, left atrial and pulmonary arterial pressures is quantitated, and ascending aortography demonstrates the regurgitant flow across the aortic valve into the left ventricle.

Mild and moderate lesions are well tolerated. Many adolescents with severe regurgitation are symptom-free and tolerate advanced lesions well into the third and fourth decades. Unfavorable signs are the onset of congestive heart failure, recurrent episodes of pulmonary edema or angina pectoris.

Treatment consists in prophylaxis against the recurrence of acute rheumatic fever and occurrence of subacute bacterial endocarditis, as well as encouragement to lead as active and normal a life as possible. Surgical treatment (usually valve replacement) is undertaken only when there is progressive deterioration from heart failure, pulmonary edema or angina pectoris.

Aortic stenosis. Aortic stenosis in children is usually the result of a congenital lesion. Rheumatic aortic stenosis is rare, although some degree of it may be associated with aortic insufficiency. The signs of pure aortic stenosis are described on page 1007.

Tricuspid valvular disease. Tricuspid involvement is rare. *Tricuspid insufficiency* is usually functional, secondary to right ventricular dilatation resulting from severe left-sided lesions. The signs produced by tricuspid insufficiency include prominent pulsations of the jugular veins with a "c-v" wave, systolic pulsations of the liver and a blowing systolic murmur in the fourth and fifth left parasternal spaces which increases in intensity during inspiration. Concomitant signs of mitral or aortic valvular disease with or without atrial fibrillation are frequent. Signs of tricuspid incompetence improve or disappear when heart failure produced by the left-sided lesions is treated.

Acquired tricuspid stenosis is rare. It is usually associated with rheumatic mitral or aortic valvular disease. The signs are increased jugular venous pressure with prominence of the "a" wave, presystolic hepatic pulsation and a rumbling diastolic murmur in the fourth and fifth left parasternal spaces. Hepatomegaly, edema and ascites are present with severe lesions. Cardiac catheterization shows a gradient of pressure across the tricuspid valve.

Pulmonary valvular disease. Pulmonary insufficiency is rarely due to organic disease and is usually functional, secondary to pulmonary hypertension or dilatation of the pulmonary artery. Occasionally it complicates severe mitral stenosis (Graham Steell murmur). The murmurs are similar to those of aortic insufficiency, but the peripheral arterial signs are absent in pulmonary insufficiency. Pulmonic stenosis is usually congenital in origin (see p. 997).

REFERENCES

Endocarditis

Blount, J. G.: Bacterial Endocarditis. *Am. J. Med.*, 38:909, 1965.

Blumenthal, S., Griffith, S. P., and Morgan, B. C.: Bacterial Endocarditis in Children with Heart Disease. *Pediatrics*, 26:993, 1960.

Geraci, J. E.: Antibiotic Therapy of Bacterial Endocarditis. *Heart Bull.*, 12:90, 1963.

Hamburger, M., Kaplan, S., and Walker, W. F.: Subacute Bacterial Endocarditis Caused by Penicillin-Sensitive Streptococci. *J.A.M.A.*, 175:554, 1961.

Lerner, P. I., and Weinstein, L.: Infective Endocarditis in the Antibiotic Era. *New England J. Med.*, 274:199, 1966.

DISEASES OF THE MYOCARDIUM

CONDITIONS CAUSING MYOCARDIAL DAMAGE

The status of the myocardium is the factor which most influences the prognosis of cardiac disease. If, in spite of congenital cardiac malformations, acquired valvular disease or arrhythmias, the myocardium is able to provide satisfactory circulation of blood, the child will be able to maintain adequate nutrition, growth and activity. The myocardium may be affected by infections, mesenchymal diseases, endocrine disorders, metabolic and nutritional diseases, neuromuscular diseases, blood diseases, tumors, hypertension and congenital anomalies.

Bacterial Infections. *Diphtheria.* The toxin of diphtheria bacilli may produce peripheral circulatory failure or toxic myocarditis. These complications occur from all types of diphtheria, including the cutaneous form. Peripheral circulatory failure occurs within the first 2 weeks of the disease and is associated with a rapid, thready pulse, cold, pale and clammy skin, and hypotension. In addition to therapy for diphtheria (p. 566), these patients are treated for cardiogenic shock.

Toxic myocarditis is characterized by the development of arrhythmia in the form of partial or complete heart block, bundle branch block or extrasystoles. Congestive cardiac failure occurs later and is associated with cardiac enlargement and gallop rhythm. In addition to the arrhythmia, the electrocardiogram shows S-T segment depression and T wave inversion in most leads. The immediate prognosis is grave (about 50 per cent mortality). Treatment (see also p. 566) includes strict bed rest until all signs of myocarditis have disappeared. Digitalis is reserved for patients with frank congestive heart failure.

Typhoid fever. Toxic myocarditis may be inferred if there is electrocardiographic evidence of T wave inversion in most leads. This sign may be transient, however, and by itself is of no clinical significance. Cardiac failure is rare, and peripheral circulatory failure is no longer common.

Acute glomerulonephritis (p. 1124). Myocardial involvement is evidenced by congestive cardiac failure, cardiac enlargement, gallop rhythm, an apical systolic murmur and electrocardiographic abnormalities. Cardiac failure is evidenced by dyspnea and pulmonary congestion, which are soon followed by increased venous pressure and hepatomegaly. It is usually difficult to determine whether cardiac failure contributes to edema in acute nephritis or whether hypervolemia contributes to cardiac failure. In these patients roentgenographic evidence of pulmonary edema is common. The electrocardiogram is frequently normal, but there may be T wave inversion, prolonged electrical systole or signs of left ventricular hypertrophy.

In addition to antihypertensive drugs, digitalization is indicated for cardiac failure. The response is good, and digitalis may be discontinued after a week or two.

Other bacterial infections. Circulatory involvement in bacterial infections is manifest as peripheral circulatory collapse or toxic myocarditis. The incidence of toxic myocarditis is difficult to gauge because it frequently depends on minor pathologic evidence such as cloudy swelling or fatty degeneration. Toxic myocarditis as evidenced by tachycardia, gallop rhythm and cardiac enlargement may complicate pneumonia, bacterial endocarditis and septicemia. The prognosis depends on the control of the primary infection.

Viral Infections. Myocarditis complicating such viral infections as measles, chickenpox and mumps is exceedingly rare. It is difficult to gauge the incidence of myocarditis in *poliomyelitis*; hypertension is not uncommon, but cardiac failure is rare. Terminal pulmonary edema may occur. Electrocardiographic abnormalities are not common. Severe myocarditis has been identified with *Coxsackie B virus* (p. 673).

Parasitic and Fungal Infections. Lesions in the myocardium have been described in association with *histoplasmosis*, *coccidioidomycosis*, *toxoplasmosis* and *trichiniasis*. In these conditions the cardiac lesion seldom produces clinical signs of myocarditis. *Actinomycosis* may involve the pericardium and myocardium by direct contiguity as, for example, from a pulmonary abscess. *Hydatid cysts* of the pericardium may be found on routine roentgenograms of the chest and usually produce symptoms only when they rupture. *Schistosomiasis* may produce pulmonary hypertension and cor pulmonale. *Cruz trypanosomiasis* (Chagas' disease) seldom occurs in North America. It may produce acute or subacute myocarditis and sudden death.

Mesenchymal Diseases. *Rheumatic carditis* is described on pages 535 and 1023.

The cardiovascular manifestations of *rheumatoid arthritis, disseminated lupus erythematosus, periarteritis nodosa, dermatomyositis* and *scleroderma* are described elsewhere. In *rheumatoid arthritis*, pericarditis is not uncommon. In patients with rheumatoid arthritis and mitral or aortic valvular disease the latter may be due to coincidental or past rheumatic carditis.

Endocrine Disorders. *Hyperthyroidism* produces tachycardia, vasodilatation, wide pulse pressure, cardiac enlargement and, rarely, atrial fibrillation. *Cretinism* seldom produces gross cardiac involvement, but the electrocardiogram discloses bradycardia, low voltage of all complexes, but especially of the P and T waves, left axis deviation and prolonged electrical systole. These signs may disappear within a month of adequate thyroid therapy.

Metabolic and Nutritional Diseases. Among vitamin deficiency diseases, *beriberi* (p. 171) causes the most conspicuous cardiac damage. In patients with malnutrition the deficiencies are often multiple, and it is difficult to separate the cardiac lesion of one nutritional disease from that of another.

Neuromuscular Diseases. In the original description of *Friedreich's ataxia*, heart disease was noted in 5 of the 6 cases. In most instances, however, there are few cardiac symptoms, the most common evidence of cardiac involvement being an abnormal electrocardiogram with T wave inversion in the left ventricular surface leads. Arrhythmias may also occur and consist of atrial tachycardia or fibrillation or extrasystoles. Cardiac failure has been reported.

In *progressive muscular dystrophy* (p. 1325) 50 per cent of children have postmortem evidence of myocardial involvement similar to that of the striated muscle. Cardiac symptoms, however, are not common, but the electrocardiogram is frequently abnormal and may reveal tachycardia, abnormalities of the P waves, short P-R interval and abnormal Q and T waves. Minimal evidence of right or left ventricular hypertrophy may also occur, and some patients have congestive heart failure.

Blood Diseases. In infants and children, anemia is the most common blood disease associated with cardiac involvement, as, for example, in leukemia, hemolytic anemias, severe iron deficiency and hemorrhage. Although cardiac output increases when the hemoglobin is below about 7 gm. per 100 ml., cardiac enlargement with or without congestive heart failure occurs only with an extreme reduction in hemoglobin to 3 or 4 gm. or less. The heart rate is rapid, the pulse pressure is widened, and the venous pressure is increased. An apical or left sternal border systolic murmur is usual, diastolic murmurs may occur in the same areas, and gallop rhythm is common. The electrocardiographic changes include depressed S-T segments and flat T waves. Occasionally minimal signs and symptoms are present when extreme states of anemia have developed gradually.

Treatment is directed toward the cause of the anemia. If blood transfusions are indicated in the presence of cardiomegaly or cardiac failure, small volumes (4 to 5 ml. per kg.) of packed cells are preferred. Venous pressure measurements during transfusion may be used as a guide for the rate and volume of transfusion.

Tumors of the Heart. See page 1444.

Carcinoid (p. 1449) of the small intestine may be accompanied by pulmonic and tricuspid valvular disease.

CONGENITAL ANOMALIES

ENDOCARDIAL SCLEROSIS
(ENDOCARDIAL FIBROELASTOSIS)

This condition has been described under a variety of other terms, including fetal endocarditis, endocardial fibrosis, prenatal fibroelastosis and elastic tissue hyperplasia. The term "endocardial sclerosis" is used in this text because it describes the gross appearance of the heart at autopsy and implies no age predilection or causative factor.

No cause has been definitely established. Proposed possibilities include inflammation or infection before or after birth, maldevelopment and inadequate blood supply to the endocardium. Black-Schaffer suggested that the endocardial changes are secondary to myocardial disease which results in cardiac dilatation and subjects the endocardium to a great stretch which initiates fibroelastic proliferation. Frühling suggested that intrauterine or early extrauterine infection with Coxsackie B virus may be the causal factor. Noren found a high incidence of positive mumps skin reactions in infants with endocardial sclerosis. The relation between mumps virus infection and endocardial sclerosis is not clear, since the positive skin reaction is seldom associated with a rise in mumps antibody titer and has been negative in patients proved to have the disease. The disease may occur in siblings.

Pathologically, there is a white, opaque fibroelastic thickening of the endocardium, especially of the left side of the heart, which frequently obscures the trabeculation of the inner surfaces of the cardiac chamber. The lesion may spread to involve the valves, especially the aortic and mitral ones. There may be coexisting congenital cardiovascular lesions. Microscopically, the lesion consists of a fibroelastic thickening of the endocardium which follows the course of the trabecular sinusoids and may result in subendocardial degeneration or necrosis of muscle with vacuolation of muscle fibers. The involved valve leaflets show a myxomatous proliferation with an increase in collagenous elements.

The clinical picture is variable. Most patients are in one of 3 groups:

1. Young infants, usually less than 6 months of age, who apparently have been in good health until the sudden onset of congestive cardiac failure, which is frequently precipitated by a respiratory infection. Death occurs early.

2. Infants with similar symptoms, but of milder degree and with periods of remission. At some time during the first 2 years of life they may manifest some dyspnea, refusal of feeding, failure to gain weight adequately and recurrent pulmonary infections. There are repeated episodes of congestive cardiac failure, finally ending in death.

3. A miscellaneous group in whom valvular lesions or associated congenital cardiovascular defects are predominant.

The majority of patients fall into groups 1 and 2. During episodes of congestive cardiac failure the infant is acutely ill with dyspnea, cough and anorexia. Cyanosis is infrequent, but is sometimes found in the terminal phase or as a sign of associated congenital cardiovascular defects. The jugular venous pressure is elevated, the liver greatly enlarged, and edema of the extremities, sacral area or face may be present. Rales and rhonchi in the lung fields are due to intercurrent pulmonary infection and congestion. The heart is moderately or greatly enlarged with a normal or left ventricular apical impulse. Thrills are not common, and murmurs are insignificant. About 25 per cent of patients have a grade I or II blowing systolic murmur down the left sternal border.

Roentgenograms confirm the cardiac enlargement (Fig. 13-66). There may be signs of intercurrent pulmonary infection. The electrocardiogram is usually abnormal, but not pathognomonic (Fig. 13-67). In the majority of cases tall R waves and inversion of the T waves over the left ventricular surface indicate dominance of the left ventricle. These signs are associated with inversion of the T waves in the standard leads and sometimes with a deep S in the right precordial leads. These electrocardiographic changes may also be seen in primary myocardial disease, gargoylism, glycogen storage disease of the heart, aberrant origin of the left coronary artery from the pulmonary artery, and medial necrosis or calcinosis of the coronary arteries.

More than 90 per cent of patients succumb during the first 2 years of life; occasional patients survive to adult life. In rare instances symptoms may appear for the first time at 5 or 6 years of age.

Treatment is directed toward alleviation of congestive cardiac failure and prevention of intercurrent infections.

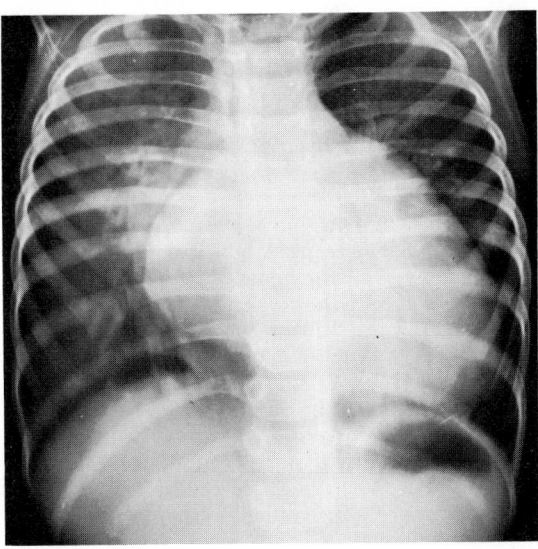

Figure 13-66. Teleroentgenogram of a 7-month-old girl with endocardial sclerosis. The enlarged heart is of an undistinctive contour.

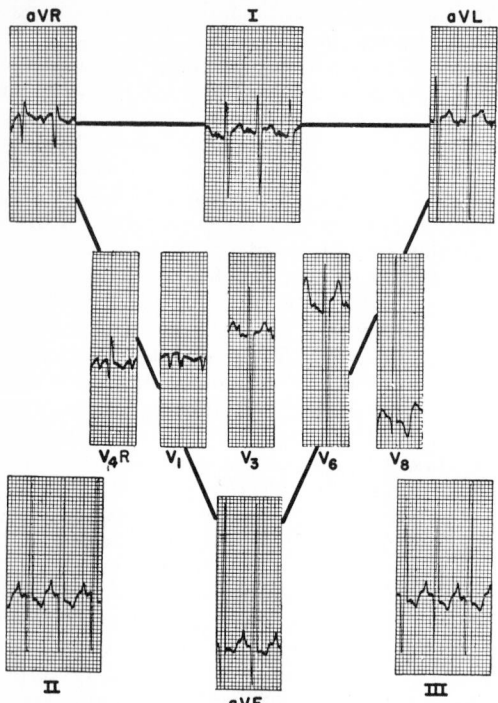

Figure 13-67. Electrocardiogram of 3-month-old girl with endocardial sclerosis. Note the abnormal T waves in leads II, aVF and V_8 and the deep Q and tall R waves in aVF and V_8.

CARDIOMYOPATHY

Hypertrophy of either ventricle of unknown origin has been recognized with increasing frequency. The disease may be familial, and the hypertrophy may be massive. The left ventricle is more frequently involved than the right. There are 2 principal clinical patterns:

Obstructive. Outflow of blood from the left ventricle is obstructed by muscular hypertrophy, producing symptoms and signs which may closely simulate aortic stenosis. In the less frequent right ventricular type the signs may simulate pulmonary stenosis. In other instances the signs mimic those of mitral insufficiency. With left ventricular outflow obstruction a systolic pressure gradient is demonstrable between the left ventricle and aorta. There is great lability of the gradient, however, even from moment to moment. Rapid ejection from the left ventricle occurs in early systole, but with further contraction, obstruction develops to outflow of blood. The severity of obstruction depends on the force of left ventricular contraction and on the volume of the left ventricular cavity. Thus a postextrasystolic beat does not result in the normally expected increase of arterial pressure. Also, factors which reduce left ventricular systolic volume intensify the gradient, e.g. Valsalva maneuver and inotropic agents, including digitalis. Administration of nitroglycerin or isoproterenol also intensifies the gradient. The compliance of the hypertrophied ventricles is poor.

Many children are asymptomatic and are evaluated because of a heart murmur. In others the clinical picture is dominated by weakness, fatigue, dyspnea on effort, palpitations, angina pectoris, dizziness and syncope. The pulse is brisk because of the early systolic ejection of blood from the ventricle. The heart is enlarged with a prominent left ventricular lift and double apical impulse. The first and second heart sounds are normal, although paradoxical splitting of the second sound is associated with a large gradient. The rarity of systolic ejection clicks helps to differentiate this condition from valvular aortic stenosis. A third sound is not common, but a fourth sound may be audible. The systolic murmur is ejection in type, of medium intensity and heard maximally at the left sternal edge and apex. The electrocardiogram shows left ventricular hypertrophy with or without S-T segment depression and T wave inversion (Fig. 13-68). The Wolff-Parkinson-White syndrome or other intraventricular conduction defects may be seen. Roentgenograms show cardiomegaly with prominence of the left ventricle and sometimes the right ventricle. The ascending aorta and aortic knob are usually normal.

The diagnosis is confirmed by cardiac catheterization, which demonstrates the unusual gradient described above. Left ventriculography shows encroachment on the left ventricular cavity by the hypertrophied muscle, especially the interventricular septum. The prognosis is unpredictable, especially in the asymptomatic patient; sudden death may occur, presumably from dysrhythmia or

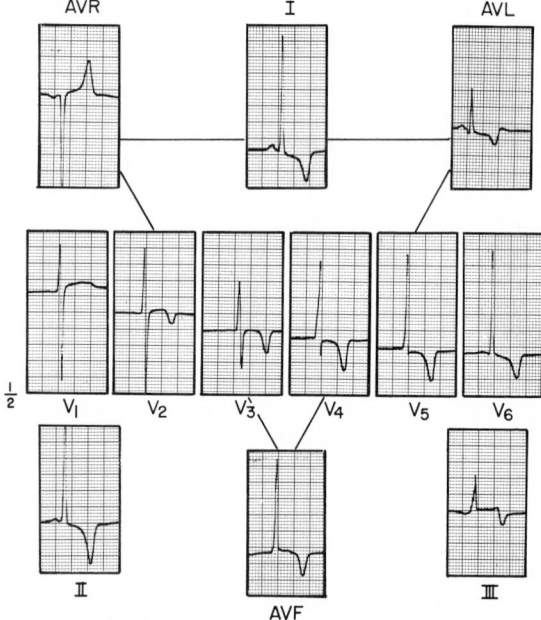

Figure 13-68. Electrocardiogram from 12-year-old boy with cardiomyopathy. All chest leads are at half-sensitivity. Although an intraventricular conduction defect is not excluded, the large voltage of R waves in V_5 and V_6, the deep SV_1 and widespread T wave inversion indicate severe left ventricular hypertrophy.

sudden intensification of the gradient. Treatment is not standardized. Digitalis and nitroglycerin should be used with extreme caution, since they intensify the obstruction. Beta adrenergic blocking agents (propranolol) have been used successfully. Some prefer surgical incision or resection of the left ventricular outflow tract.

Nonobstructive. In children the nonobstructive type of cardiomyopathy is more common. The enlarged hearts show diffuse hypertrophy, especially of the ventricular septum, and disorganization of the arrangement of muscle bundles. The symptoms are those of chronic congestive heart failure, sometimes with angina pectoris and palpitation. Physical examination reveals cardiac enlargement, nonspecific systolic murmurs and gallop rhythm, but apical murmurs of gross mitral incompetence may be present. Chronic congestive heart failure may result in tricuspid incompetence from right ventricular dilatation. The electrocardiogram usually indicates left ventricular hypertrophy. X-ray films confirm the generalized cardiomegaly with left ventricular prominence and pulmonary congestion. The prognosis is poor, and treatment is directed toward relief of heart failure.

Restrictive cardiomyopathy occurs occasionally. The mechanisms producing symptoms are probably related to poor ventricular compliance, so that diastolic filling of the heart is compromised. This results in a clinical picture which closely simulates that of constrictive pericarditis. In its overt form restrictive cardiomyopathy results in dyspnea, edema, ascites, hepatomegaly, increased venous pressure and pulmonary congestion. The heart is mildly or moderately enlarged, and murmurs are nonspecific. The electrocardiogram shows prominent P waves, frequently normal QRS voltage, S-T segment depression and T wave inversion. Roentgenographic examination shows slight or moderate cardiomegaly with poor cardiac pulsations. The prognosis is generally poor. Treatment is directed toward relief of edema with diuretics.

OTHER MYOCARDIAL DISEASES

The principal type of **glycogen storage disease** which affects the heart is the generalized form, also known as Pompe's disease or type II (p. 446). The clinical picture may be dominated by skeletal muscle weakness, macroglossia and hepatomegaly. Cardiomegaly is massive, but murmurs are insignificant. Pulmonary collapse with secondary infection is common and is related to compression from the large heart. The electrocardiogram shows prominent P waves, signs of left ventricular hypertrophy or intraventricular conduction defects. Roentgenograms confirm the striking cardiomegaly with prominence of the left ventricle. The prognosis is poor, and the majority of infants succumb before the age of 2 years. Effective therapy is not available.

In **gargoylism** (see p. 1338) the lesion in the heart and great vessels is the same as that in the connective tissue elsewhere in the body. The most pronounced lesions are found in the valves and coronary arteries, but abnormalities in the pericardium and aorta are not uncommon. The heart may be moderately enlarged with electrocardiographic signs of left ventricular hypertrophy. Cardiac murmurs may result from incompetence and stenosis of the mitral and aortic valves. Sometimes the pulmonary and tricuspid valves are also involved. Coronary arterial disease may result in angina and perhaps explain the not infrequent occurrence of sudden death. The prognosis is poor, and many children succumb before the age of 10 years with heart failure and pulmonary infection (Figs. 22-14, 22-15).

Calcinosis of the coronary arteries is a rare disease of infancy. Familial incidence has been recorded. The coronary arteries are tortuous and calcareous, and the ventricles, especially the left, are hypertrophied. Other blood vessels may be similarly involved. The onset of cardiac failure is sudden; death usually occurs in infancy.

CONGESTIVE HEART FAILURE

In older children the signs and symptoms of congestive heart failure are similar to those in adults. Fatigue, effort intolerance, anorexia, abdominal pain and cough are frequent. In addition to breathlessness at rest, the systemic venous pressure is elevated as gauged by clinical assessment of the jugular venous pressure, the liver is enlarged and tender, and edema may be present. Orthopnea and basal rales are commonly present, and edema usually occurs in dependent portions of the body. Older children may occasionally prefer to lie in the flat position, which causes generalized anasarca. Cardiomegaly is invariably present. Auscultatory findings are those produced by the basic lesion; gallop rhythm is common.

During infancy the presence of congestive heart failure may be more difficult to determine. Symptoms are dominated by tachypnea, feeding difficulties, poor weight gain, excessive perspiration, irritability, weak cry and noisy, labored respiration with costal and subcostal retractions. Flaring of the alae nasi and sternal retractions are frequent. Signs of pulmonary congestion are difficult to interpret, since they may be indistinguishable from those produced by bronchospasm. Pneumonitis with or without collapse of part of the lung is common. Dyspnea and hepatomegaly are nearly always manifest, and cardiomegaly is invariably present. In spite of pronounced tachycardia, gallop rhythm can be recognized frequently. The other auscultatory signs are those produced by the cardiac lesion which resulted in heart failure. A sudden increase in weight which decreases after diuretic therapy is common. A clinical assessment of the jugular venous pressure in infants may be difficult, owing to the shortness of the neck and the difficulty of securing a relaxed state, although it should always be attempted. Edema in infants with cardiac failure is frequently not detectable clinically. When present, the edema may be generalized, involving the eyelids as well as the sacrum, legs and feet.

TREATMENT

The underlying cause of cardiac failure must be removed or alleviated if possible. If the cause is a congenital cardiovascular anomaly amenable to surgery, medical treatment is indicated before the surgical procedure and is continued in the immediate postoperative period. For some diseases, such as hyperthyroidism, hypothyroidism, anemia and beriberi, specific therapy is available, but in the majority of instances only general measures are adaptable.

Bed rest in a comfortable position is essential. Some patients prefer to lie flat, but for most of them breathing is easier in a semireclining position. Initially sedatives or analgesics may be necessary to produce complete relaxation; the most frequently used drugs are morphine, codeine and the barbiturates.

A *low sodium diet* is efficacious in the treatment of cardiac edema and paroxysmal cardiac dyspnea. The oral intake of sodium should be reduced to 0.5 gm. daily; the diet may be made more palatable with a salt substitute. Formulas with a low sodium content are available for infants.

Oxygen administered by any method which is effective and comfortable for the patient will help to relieve dyspnea and cyanosis.

Diuretics relieve the edema and pulmonary congestion of heart failure. Currently available diuretics have a wide range of potency; the most frequently used agents are mercurials and thiazides. *Mercurial diuretics* in the form of mercaptomerin sodium and meralluride sodium (p. 290) are most effective, but should not be used if there is associated nephritis. The dose of mercurial diuretics varies according to the age of the patient and the severity of cardiac failure. In the newborn 0.125 ml. may be given intramuscularly daily or on alternate days in the early stage of treatment. In older children the dose is 0.5 to 1 ml. The easiest method of gauging the efficacy of the drug is by comparison of daily body weights. When a constant level is reached, it should be maintained. When the acute stage of cardiac failure is over, the injection of a mercurial diuretic is necessary in a few patients once or twice weekly. Mercurials act primarily by depressing renal tubular mechanisms responsible for the transport of sodium and fixed anion. Water excretion occurs because of decreased electrolyte reabsorption. Inhibition of reabsorption of sodium and chloride is associated with excretion of potassium in the urine. A decrease in venous pressure parallels the diuresis. In adults the action of mercurial diuretics is supplemented with orally administered ammonium chloride, but this is seldom necessary in children. *Thiazides* are moderately potent diuretic agents. Since they can be given orally (chlorothiazide syrup), they are useful in the long-term management of cardiac failure in infants and children. They act by increasing renal excretion of sodium and chloride with an accompanying volume of water. The usual dose of oral chlorothiazide (Diuril) is 1 to 1.5 gm. per square meter of body surface per day. Patients maintained on chlorothiazide should also be given potassium to supplement the usual dietary intake. Other diuretics used in conjunction with mercurials include the xanthine derivatives, theobromine and theophylline. *Spironolactone* (Aldactone), the aldosterone antagonist, and *Triamterene* are seldom used alone in the management of heart failure, although they are used occasionally to supplement mercurial or thiazide therapy. *Ethacrynic acid* and *furosemide* are extremely potent diuretics and are effective when given orally or parenterally. They act by markedly inhibiting salt transport in the renal tubules. The induction of diuresis is rapid (within 30 minutes), the action short-lived (about 4 hours), and indiscriminate use is not advised, since they may produce a massive diuresis. The principal indication is in the management of acute cardiac failure or pulmonary edema. They may be used cautiously when mercurials or thiazides fail to produce the desired diuresis. *Corticosteroids* generally produce water retention, but are sometimes used in patients whose diuretic-resistant cardiac failure is due to inflammatory disease, e.g. rheumatic carditis. *Carbonic anhydrase inhibitors* have little effect on cardiac edema, although they are sometimes used in heart failure due to cor pulmonale.

Cardiac failure which is resistant to therapy or breakdown of response to previously successful management may be due to (1) infection such as reactivation of rheumatic fever, superimposed subacute bacterial endocarditis or intercurrent pulmonary or urinary tract infection, (2) electrolyte imbalance, especially hypokalemia, hypochloremic alkalosis or hyponatremia, (3) development of arrhythmia such as atrial fibrillation with rapid ventricular response, or (4) pulmonary embolism, a rare complication in children. If ascites or pleural effusions produce discomfort, fluid should be removed by paracentesis.

Digitalis should be used in all forms of cardiac failure. The most satisfactory response is obtained in failure due to rheumatic heart disease, paroxysmal tachycardia and myocardial diseases. In general, patients with primary left ventricular failure respond better than those with primary right-sided failure. The response of patients with congestive cardiac failure due to cyanotic congenital cardiovascular disease is unpredictable because hypoxia, acidosis and hypoglycemia may complicate the picture.

Many preparations of digitalis are available, but familiarity with only a few is necessary. The ones most frequently used are digoxin and digitoxin for slow digitalization and maintenance, and lanatoside C (Cedilanid) for rapid digitalization. The dose of digitalis (p. 284) and the rapidity of administration depend on the weight of the patient, the severity of congestive cardiac failure, the type of preparation, and subsequently on the response of the patient.

Digoxin is the form of digitalis used most frequently in pediatric practice because of availability in liquid form and the relative ease of control when inadequate or toxic doses have been given. The maximal effect of digoxin occurs about 4 hours after administration; it is excreted within 48 to 72 hours. The recommended dosage schedule is as follows: For *newborn and premature infants,* the digitalizing dose is 0.03 to 0.05 mg. per kg., with a daily maintenance of one tenth to one fifth of the digitalizing dose. For *infants beyond the neonatal period, but under 2 years of age,* the oral digitalizing dose is 0.06 to 0.08 mg. per kg., with a daily maintenance dose of one fifth to one third of the digitalizing one. In this age group the parenteral digitalizing dose is 0.04 to 0.06 mg. per kg., with a daily parenteral maintenance dose of one tenth to one fifth of the digitalizing dose. For *children over 2 years of age* the oral digitalizing dose is 0.04 to 0.06 mg. per kg., with a daily oral maintenance dose of one fifth to one third of the digitalizing one. In this age group the parenteral digitalizing dose is 0.02 to 0.04 mg. per kg. The author prefers to use a digitalizing dose of 1.5 mg. of digoxin per square meter of body surface (see nomogram, p. 236) in patients beyond the neonatal period, with the total digitalizing dose not exceeding 2.5 mg. The daily maintenance dose is one fifth to one third of the digitalizing dose. In newborn and premature infants the digitalizing dose is 0.75 mg. per square meter of body surface, with a daily maintenance dose of one tenth to one fifth of the digitalizing dose. The *timing of administration* has considerable individual variation. Frequently half of the digitalizing dose is given initially, followed by one fourth of the total dose in 6 to 8 hours, and the remaining fourth is given in another 6 to 8 hours. The daily maintenance dose may be started 12 hours later and is given preferably in 2 equally divided doses.

The average adequate digitalizing dose of *digitoxin* (oral or intramuscular) for children varies from 0.02 to 0.04 mg. per kg. Infants require 0.04 to 0.06 mg. per kg., and full-term and premature newborn infants are given 0.015 to 0.03 mg. per kg. Owing to the wide variations of these dosage schedules, it may be preferable to calculate the digitalizing dose of digitoxin in older age groups on the basis of 0.75 mg. per square meter of body surface (see nomogram, p. 236). Full-term and premature newborn infants usually require 0.375 mg. per square meter of body surface. The daily maintenance dose of digitoxin is one tenth of the digitalizing dose. The full digitalizing dose is given in divided doses within 12, 24 or 48 hours, depending on the severity of congestive failure. If digitalization is required within 12 hours, half of the digitalizing dose may be given immediately and the remaining half in divided doses over 12 hours. The total dose may be more evenly distributed if 24 or 48 hours are taken for digitalization. The optimal effect of digitoxin occurs 4 to 8 hours after administration, and its excretion is slow (10 to 14 days).

Lanatoside C (Cedilanid) is used for rapid intravenous digitalization; it should be reserved for emergency situations. It begins to act within 3 to 15 minutes after administration, and maximal effects are achieved in about 1 hour; it is excreted within 24 to 36 hours. The digitalizing dose is 0.325 to 0.75 mg. per square meter of surface area (see nomogram, p. 236). This preparation is seldom used in full-term or premature newborn infants. Cautious redigitalization with digoxin or digitoxin is started about 24 to 36 hours later.

It cannot be overemphasized that *any dosage schedule of any digitalis preparation is only a guide,* since there are individual differences among patients. The dose may need to be modified after part or all of the calculated digitalizing dose has been given. Full-term and premature newborn infants have a distinct intolerance for digitalis preparations. In these patients, digitalization should be controlled by careful and repeated physical examination supplemented by electrocardiography. In some infants the only reliable guide to digitalis intoxication is electrocardiographic evidence of arrhythmia.

The digitalizing dose is effective if the cardiac rate is reduced, the venous pressure and liver size are decreased, dyspnea is relieved and diuresis occurs. Electrocardiographic evidences of digitalis effect include shortening of electrical systole, depression of the S-T segment with T wave inversion and lengthening of the P-R interval. In many patients the difference between an adequate and toxic dose of digitalis is small.

The signs of digitalis toxicity include anorexia, nausea, vomiting, diarrhea, visual symptoms, dizziness, headache and arrhythmias. The arrhythmias include atrial and ventricular extrasystoles, paroxysmal atrial tachycardia with block, atrial flutter or fibrillation, bundle branch block, ventricular tachycardia and intra-atrial block. If signs of digitalis toxicity occur, the drug must be discontinued temporarily, and potassium chloride may be given orally or by intravenous drip, if the arrhythmia warrants therapy.

The convalescent care of children who have suffered from congestive cardiac failure is important. As the child improves, greater freedom of activity may be permitted, and schoolwork may be resumed.

REFERENCES

Black-Schaffer, B.: Infantile Endocardial Fibroelastosis: A Suggested Etiology. *Arch. Path.,* 63:281, 1957.

Braunwald, E., Lambrew, C. T., Rockoff, S. D., Ross, J., Jr., and Morrow, A. G.: Idiopathic Hypertrophic Subaortic Stenosis. *Circulation,* 30 (Supp. 4):3, 1964.

Frühling, L., Korn, R., Lavillaureix, J., Surjus, A., and Foussereau, S.: La myo-endocardite chronique fibro-élastique du nouveau-né et du nourrisson (fibro-elastose). *Ann. Anat. Path.,* 7:227, 1962.

Gersony, W. M., Katz, S. L., and Nadas, A. S.: Endocardial Fibroelastosis and Mumps Virus. *Pediatrics,* 37:430, 1966.

Goodwin, J. F.: Disorders of Outflow Tract of the Left Ventricle. *Brit. Med. J.,* 2:461, 1967.

Levine, O. R., and Blumenthal, S.: Digoxin Dosage in Premature Infants. *Pediatrics,* 29:1, 1962.

Noren, G. R., Adams, P., Jr., and Anderson, R. C.: Positive Skin Reactivity to Mumps Virus Antigen in Endocardial Fibroelastosis. *J. Pediat.,* 62:604, 1963.

Robinson, S. J.: Digitalis Therapy in Infants and Children. *J. Pediat.,* 56:536, 1960.

DISEASES OF THE PERICARDIUM

Congenital malformations of the pericardium are rare. They are chiefly defects of the parietal pericardium and are of little clinical significance. Roentgenographically and electrocardiographically, they may simulate pulmonic stenosis.

Pericardial cysts are usually asymptomatic and discovered on roentgenograms of the chest. The cardiopericardial shadow is increased and distorted, depending on the location and size of the cyst. The electrocardiogram is normal. The cysts, which are usually benign, may be removed surgically.

PERICARDITIS

Etiology. Pericarditis may be primary (rheumatic, viral, postcardiotomy, purulent, traumatic or tuberculous) or an intercurrent manifestation of systemic disease (effusion due to congestive cardiac failure, or associated with uremia, rheumatoid arthritis, disseminated lupus, periarteritis nodosa, primary or secondary neoplastic disease, and hematologic diseases such as leukemia, Cooley's anemia and congenital hypoplastic anemia). Pericarditis may also occur in parasitic and mycotic infections, ulcerative colitis, hypothyroidism, Friedreich's ataxia and glycogen storage disease.

Hemodynamics. The effects on the circulation depend largely on the amount of pericardial fluid, the speed of its accumulation and the myocardial efficiency. Thus a small amount of fluid in the pericardium with a normal myocardium is compatible with normal cardiovascular dynamics, whereas the rapid accumulation of large amounts of fluid in the pericardium with a normal myocardium may result in cardiac compression or *cardiac tamponade.* Smaller amounts of pericardial fluid with a diseased myocardium may also result in cardiac tamponade as in acute rheumatic fever. Cardiac compression also occurs in long-standing chronic constrictive pericarditis.

The physiologic abnormality in cardiac compression is inadequate diastolic filling of the ventricles, which results in increased pressure in both atria and in the venous systems. The stroke volume is small and more or less fixed. Cardiac output is maintained by tachycardia, and reflex vasoconstriction maintains the blood pressure.

Clinical Manifestations. Pain may or may not be present and varies in intensity, location and distribution. Since the lower third of the pericardium is innervated by the phrenic nerve, pain may be referred to the neck or shoulder. The pain may be precordial and pleural when it is aggravated by inspiration and coughing and may be referred to the back. Or it may be precordial, constant and uninfluenced by respiration, but aggravated by rotating the trunk or by swallowing. The pain is either sharp or a dull, oppressive, poorly localized ache.

The venous pressure varies with the intrapericardial pressure. If the latter is raised, the venous pressure is elevated, especially during inspiration. Hepatomegaly, ascites and edema may also be present. The pulse is normal and small in volume or paradoxical; it depends on the degree of cardiac compression. A small, rapid pulse is found in patients with a tense pericardium and a low cardiac output. *Pulsus paradoxus* indicates that the pulse becomes smaller or disappears during inspiration; this sign may be confirmed by measuring the blood pressure during the phases of respiration. In the presence of cardiac compression the precordium is quiet to palpation. A large amount of fluid may be detected by percussion, shifting dullness and by recognizing that the apical impulse is well within the border of cardiac dullness. The heart sounds may be normal or distant. A pericardial friction rub may be audible even in the presence of large amounts of fluid. The rub is heard anywhere over the heart, but frequently over the lower left sternal border. It is superficial, of varying intensity and does not have any definite relation to the heart sounds.

Pericardial effusion may result in pressure on the left main stem bronchus with collapse of the left lung resulting in percussion dullness and bronchial breathing at the left base (*Ewart's sign*). Similar signs may occur from secondary pleural effusion.

The findings on *roentgen examination* vary according to the amount of pericardial fluid. In dry pericarditis there are no abnormal findings. If the accumulation is large, the cardiopericardial shadow is enlarged, the normal contours are obscured, and the amplitude of cardiac pulsation is decreased. Other nondiagnostic signs include changes in the shape of the cardiac silhouette with changes in posture, divergent vascular shadows at the base, an acute right cardiophrenic angle and rapid changes in the size of the cardiopericardial shadow. The roentgenographic findings are not pathognomonic and may be simulated closely by acute cardiac dilatation. Pericardial calcification due to chronic constrictive pericarditis is rare in children.

The *electrocardiographic* abnormalities are widespread and involve most of the leads. In the acute phase the S-T segment is elevated, and the QRS voltage may be low. As healing progresses the S-T segment becomes isoelectric or depressed, and the T waves are flattened, diphasic or inverted. The graph returns to normal when the pericarditis heals, although T wave inversion may persist for many months after clinical recovery. This electrocardiographic pattern may be transient and localized and may be recognized only with serial tracings.

In the presence of cardiac compression *cardiac catheterization* reveals an increased pulmonary "capillary" and right atrial pressure. The pulmonary artery and right ventricular pressures are normal or moderately elevated, and there is a conspicuous dip in the right ventricular pressure curve during early diastole. If the catheter is coiled in the right atrium, the width of the pericardial shadow can be detected. The diagnosis may be confirmed also by angiocardiography, which delineates the cardiac chambers and separates that part of the cardiac silhouette which is produced by pericardial effusion. Reflection of ultrasound may also be used in diagnosis; in pericardial effusion 2 echoes are recorded from the posterior part of the heart. The first is produced by the posterior wall of the heart and the second from the posterior wall of the pericardium. Radioisotope scanning after injection of iodinated human serum albumin may outline the intracardiac pool and indicate that it is significantly smaller than the roentgenographic cardiac silhouette.

Cardiac tamponade, whatever the cause, is a medical emergency. If the cardiac output is not maintained during cardiac compression, the patient goes into shock. The intrapericardial pressure must be reduced immediately, usually by pericardiocentesis.

Rheumatic Pericarditis. Rheumatic pericarditis is usually fibrinous or serofibrinous; a large accumulation of fluid is unusual. The child is usually acutely ill with fever, dyspnea and pericardial pain. The heart is frequently enlarged, and a pericardial friction rub is common. The electrocardiographic changes are as described above. Treatment is directed toward the rheumatic illness as a whole and the relief of pain, and pericardiocentesis is done in the rare instances of cardiac tamponade. Rheumatic pericarditis does not produce serious after-effects and does not lead to constrictive pericarditis, but there is usually extensive carditis and therefore a potentially poor long-term prognosis.

The differential diagnosis of rheumatic pericardial effusion from acute cardiac dilatation may be difficult. In some patients it may be necessary to resort to pericardiocentesis to establish the presence or absence of significant amounts of pericardial fluid. The essential difference between dry rheumatic pericarditis and other forms of dry pericarditis, such as acute benign pericarditis, is the presence in the former of significant systolic or diastolic murmurs as well as other evidence of acute rheumatic fever.

Septic Pericarditis. Septic pericarditis is produced by a variety of bacteria, including *Hemophilus influenzae*, *Staphylococcus aureus*, streptococci and pneumococci. Foci of infection, usually pneumonia, are frequently present at other sites. The purulent exudate in the pericardium is of varying consistency, and coagulated masses of fibrin and pus are common.

The patients are acutely ill with fever, pericardial pain and tachypnea. The heart is enlarged, murmurs are insignificant, and a friction rub may or may not be present. The electrocardiographic and radiologic pictures are described above. The diagnosis is confirmed by pericardiocentesis. This procedure may yield only small amounts of pus, owing to the consistency of the exudate and the multiple loculations. Surgical drainage is usually necessary and should be instituted early. This therapy with the use of appropriate antibiotics gives excellent results, and the long-term prognosis is usually good.

Acute Viral or Idiopathic Pericarditis. This disease frequently follows an upper respiratory tract infection with an average latent period of 12 days. The onset is usually acute with fever, and pericardial pain and a friction rub are common. Varying amounts of straw-colored pericardial fluid are present, but cardiac compression is rare. The electrocardiogram usually shows the typical pattern of pericarditis.

Although the disease is usually benign without any after-effects, recurrences, sometimes multiple, have been noted in up to 20 per cent of patients. Symptomatic treatment with aspirin is all that is usually necessary. Corticosteroid therapy may be considered in the severe forms of the disease or in patients with multiple recurrences.

Pericarditis in Rheumatoid Arthritis. Pericarditis may occur at any stage of rheumatoid arthritis and may precede the typical joint manifestations. Pericardial effusion is rare, and a pericardial friction rub common. Therapy is directed toward the primary disease, since pericarditis improves when the rheumatoid disease is stabilized.

Pericarditis in Uremia. In the terminal stages of uremia a pericardial friction rub may be heard. The pericarditis seldom produces symptoms, and the electrocardiographic changes are minimal.

Tuberculous Pericarditis. Tuberculous pericarditis is usually secondary to a lesion in the hilar nodes or in the lung. Pericardial effusion is common and is followed by a fibrotic reaction which may result in constrictive pericarditis. The onset may be insidious or associated with cough, dyspnea, fever, weight loss and night sweats. The

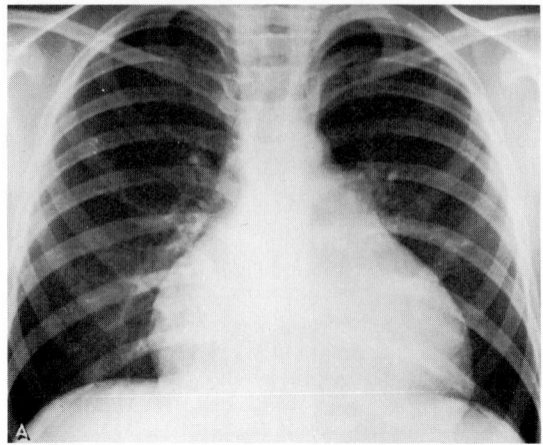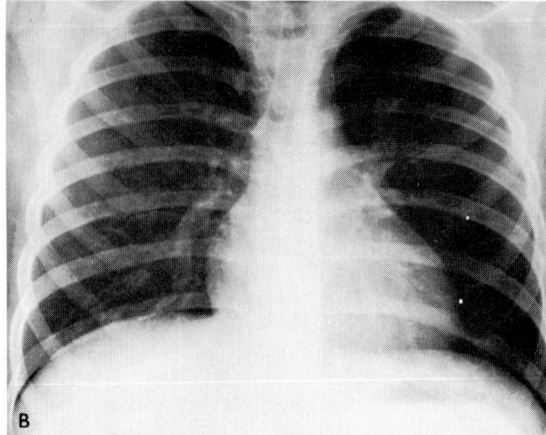

Figure 13-69. Teleroentgenograms in acute nonspecific pericarditis. *A,* Increase in cardiopericardial shadow due to pericardial effusion. *B,* One month later after complete recovery.

diagnosis depends on signs of tuberculosis elsewhere in the body and on recovery of the organism from the sputum, gastric washings or the pericardial fluid. Treatment is that of the tuberculous infection (p. 606). The effusion is cleared more rapidly with added corticosteroid therapy.

Chronic Constrictive Pericarditis. This disease is rare in children. In the majority of instances the cause is unknown, or the disease may follow tuberculosis. Occasionally septic or acute nonspecific pericarditis may be followed by constrictive pericarditis. The hemodynamics and clinical picture are those of chronic cardiac compression and must be distinguished from chronic congestive heart failure and restrictive cardiomyopathy. Atrial fibrillation may occur. If the constriction is severe, pericardiectomy is advised.

Postoperative Pericarditis. Postoperative pericarditis may follow any direct surgical procedure in the heart. Friction rubs are common during the first 2 weeks after operation. Some patients, however, may have the postcardiotomy syndrome (see p. 1015).

REFERENCES

Benzing, G., III, and Kaplan, S.: Purulent Pericarditis. *Am. J. Dis. Child.*, 106:289, 1963.

Cayler, G. G., Taybi, H., Riley, H. D., and Simon, J. L.: Pericarditis with Effusion in Infants and Children. *J. Pediat.*, 63:264, 1963.

Nadas, A. S., and Levy, J. M.: Pericarditis in Children. *Am. J. Cardiol.*, 7:109, 1961.

DISEASES OF THE BLOOD VESSELS

ANEURYSMS AND FISTULAS

Aneurysms are not common in children and occur most frequently in the aorta in association with coarctation of the aorta, patent ductus arteriosus and Marfan's syndrome and in intracranial vessels (p. 1281). They may also occur secondary to an infected embolus, infection contiguous to a blood vessel, trauma, congenital abnormalities of structure, especially of the medial coat, and arteritis, e.g. periarteritis nodosa.

Arteriovenous fistulas may be limited to small cavernous hemangiomas or may be extensive (pp. 1382, 1463). The commonest sites for arteriovenous fistulas in infants and children are intracranial, hepatic or in the extremities. They have also been described in other parts of the body, however, especially in vessels in or near the thoracic wall. The fistulas, though usually congenital, may follow trauma or be a manifestation of hereditary hemorrhagic telangiectasia (Rendu-Osler-Weber syndrome).

Cardiovascular manifestations occur only in association with large communications. In these patients arterial blood flows into a low pressure venous system, increasing local venous pressure and decreasing arterial flow below the fistula. Systemic arterial resistance falls because of the runoff of blood through the fistula. Compensatory mechanisms include tachycardia and increased stroke volume, so that cardiac output rises. Plasma volume is also increased. Cardiac failure may develop with large arteriovenous fistulas.

The clinical manifestations of arteriovenous fistulas appear to depend primarily on the size of the shunt across the fistula and the associated vasodilatation. Discoloration of the skin, prominence of the superficial vessels and local edema may occur at the site of the fistula or involve a whole extremity. Prominent arterial pulsations and a continuous machinery bruit may be heard over the site of the lesion, especially in the traumatic types. The venous pressure is elevated in an affected extremity, the temperature of the skin may be higher at the site of the lesion, and the venous oxygen saturation distal to the fistula is higher than that of venous blood taken from a similar site on the unaffected side. In extensive fistulas there is left ventricular hypertrophy and dilatation, a widened pulse pressure and congestive heart failure. Arteriograms with the injection of contrast material into an artery proximal to the fistula confirm the diagnosis.

Intracranial arteriovenous fistulas are usually congenital, although they may follow trauma. Congenital fistulas usually involve the Galenic venous system. Neonates with large fistulas suffer heart failure early (p. 1013). In later infancy progressive hydrocephalus or convulsions may occur (p. 1281). Older children suffer from headaches or subarachnoid hemorrhage. Clues to the correct diagnosis include venous engorgement over the scalp and neck as well as cranial bruits. The latter sign is not diagnostic, since bruits may be heard in normal infants, especially over the anterior fontanel.

Hepatic arteriovenous fistulas may be localized or generalized in the liver. In others the fistula is between hepatic artery and ductus venosus or portal vein. Congenital hemorrhagic telangiectasia may be associated with hepatic fistula. Large arteriovenous fistulas are associated with a large cardiac output and heart failure. Hepatomegaly is usual, and systolic or continuous murmurs may be audible over the liver.

Peripheral arteriovenous fistulas normally involve the extremities. These lesions are associated with disfigurement, swelling of the extremity and visible hemangiomas. Only a small minority result in large arterial runoff, so that cardiac failure is not common.

Treatment. Surgical extirpation of the fistula is indicated when cardiac enlargement or heart failure occurs. Surgical treatment is difficult in many patients because of the diffuseness of the lesion.

FROSTBITE

Frostbite may occur in the face or extremities from prolonged exposure to cold. The mechanism of cellular injury is related to intravascular thrombosis or ice crystal formation in the tissues. The skin first becomes red and then pale or rarely cyanotic, as the arterioles remain in spasm in an effort to preserve body heat. During thawing, hyperemia occurs, and blisters may form on the skin. Gangrene may occur if early relief is not obtained.

Treatment consists in rapidly rewarming the skin of the affected area which is still white. Analgesics are usually necessary. Massage of the damaged area or rubbing with snow or ice is contraindicated. Other therapeutic measures which have yielded equivocal results include anticoagulants (especially heparin), low-molecular-weight dextran, and sympathectomy. Meticulous local care to the injured area is essential. Recovery of an extremity from apparent severe frostbite can be striking and in the absence of infection, amputation or excision of tissue should be postponed for as long as possible.

EMBOLISM

Emboli, consisting of bacteria and fibrinous material, usually arise from mural thrombi or vegetations in the heart or large blood vessels, as for example in subacute bacterial endocarditis. Within weeks after bacteriologic cure of bacterial endocarditis, sterile embolization to major vessels may occur; this does not necessarily indicate reactivation of infection. Other, rarer causes of emboli include fat (secondary to trauma) and foreign material, such as air, introduced accidentally into the vascular system during therapeutic procedures. In patients with atrial or ventricular septal defects, emboli arising in the systemic venous system may pass across the defect and enter the systemic arterial system (*paradoxical embolus*).

When emboli lodge in an artery, the blood flow through the vessel is compromised. If the collateral circulation is inadequate, necrosis or gangrene supervenes; if the collateral circulation is adequate, the emboli may be silent. Thus an embolus to the arteries of the forearm may not give rise to symptoms and is detected only when the radial or ulnar pulse disappears.

The symptoms and signs produced by arterial emboli depend on their location: e.g. an embolus to the middle cerebral artery may result in hemiparesis; an embolus to the femoral artery may result in ischemia with or without gangrene in the leg. If the emboli are infected, an abscess forms locally.

Treatment consists in eradication of the source of the emboli, e.g. subacute bacterial endocarditis, and in increasing the collateral circulation to the affected area. Surgical therapy such as embolectomy, sympathectomy and amputation may be indicated in specific instances.

Pulmonary embolism is not as frequent in children as in adults. Thrombosis of the calf veins with secondary pulmonary embolism is rare in children. Pulmonary emboli may arise secondary to subacute bacterial endocarditis in patients with a left-to-right shunt and have also occurred in association with ventriculo-cardiovascular shunts for hydrocephalus. Occasionally pulmonary embolism is seen in older children with chronic rheumatic heart disease and atrial fibrillation. Multiple, small pulmonary emboli have been described elsewhere (see Primary Pulmonary Hypertension, p. 1013).

THROMBOSIS

Frequently *arterial thrombosis* in children is associated with polycythemia secondary to severe cyanotic congenital heart disease. A frequent site for such thrombi is the brain, but they may occur anywhere in the body. They may be precipitated by dehydration.

Venous thrombosis may occur in veins used for prolonged intravenous therapy or in an area surrounding an infective process. The inflammation in the vein (*phlebitis*) is usually local, and the thrombi seldom give rise to emboli.

Any severe illness associated with intense dehydration may be complicated by venous thrombosis. This complication is relatively frequent in infants with severe diarrhea or septicemia and in children with cyanotic congenital heart disease and polycythemia who become dehydrated. The common site for thrombosis is in the sagittal sinus of the brain and in the renal vein with extension into the inferior vena cava. (See Vascular Disorders of the Central Nervous System [p. 1281] and Hemorrhagic Infarction of the Kidney [p. 1149].

SAMUEL KAPLAN

14. Diseases of the Blood

DEVELOPMENT OF THE HEMATOPOIETIC SYSTEM

As long as animals remained small and the cells of their bodies had direct access to the surrounding sea water, exchange of gas and nutrients was easily effected by simple diffusion. With the evolution of multicellular and terrestrial organisms came development of a vascular system and hemic fluid. Blood probably originated as a simple saline solution similar to sea water; cellular components with specialized functions must have appeared soon thereafter. Among the principal functions of blood cells are transport of respiratory gases, hemostasis, and phagocytosis and other defense mechanisms. Most advanced organisms have separate lines of blood cells, each concerned with a specialized function.

Blood formation in the human embryo can be recognized as early as the third week after conception. Large, primitive hematopoietic elements are then widely scattered through mesodermal tissues, intimately associated with developing vascular channels. By 2 months active hematopoiesis is established in the liver, which is the main site of blood formation during the middle portion of fetal life. After about 6 months hematopoiesis shifts gradually to the medullary spaces,

and by birth most blood formation normally takes place in bone marrow.

Active hematopoietic tissue (red marrow) fills the medullary spaces of the bones of infants. During childhood fatty tissue (yellow marrow) gradually replaces hematopoietic tissue in the long bones, so that in the older child and the adult active blood formation is concentrated in ribs, sternum, vertebrae, pelvis, skull, clavicles and scapulae. The yellow marrow of the extremities has the potential for reconversion to active hematopoiesis in response to certain severe hematologic stresses.

Study of the bone marrow provides valuable information in the evaluation of many hematologic diseases. Marrow aspiration is a safe and technically simple procedure. In the infant the preferred sites for aspiration are the proximal tibia and posterior iliac crest. In older children the posterior iliac crest provides a large marrow-bearing space which is not adjacent to major blood vessels or vital organs. Table 14-1 lists the types and proportions of cells which occur in marrow of normal infants and children.

TABLE 14-1. DIFFERENTIAL COUNTS OF BONE MARROW DURING INFANCY AND CHILDHOOD

AGE	BLASTS	PRO-MYELO-CYTES	MYELO-CYTES AND META-MYELO-CYTES	BANDS AND POLY-MORPHO-NUCLEARS	EOSINO-PHILS	LYMPHO-CYTES	NUCLE-ATED RED BLOOD CELLS	MYELOID/ERY-THROID (M:E) RATIO
Birth 1	2	5	40	1	10	40	1.2/1
7 days...............1	2	10	40	1	20	25	2.1/1
6 months to								
2 years...........0.5	0.5	8	30	1	40	20	2.0/1
6 years..............1	2	15	35	1	25	20	2.7/1
12 years............1	2	20	40	1	15	20	3.2/1
Adult................2	2	22	44	2	10	20	3.5/1

The Red Cells

Synthesis of red cells requires a constant supply of amino acids, iron, certain vitamins and other trace nutrients. Production of red cells is regulated by a specific erythroid-stimulating hormone—erythropoietin. This hormone is largely produced in the kidney and is responsive to changes in tissue

oxygenation. The principal action of erythropoietin is to induce the differentiation of primitive stem cells into an erythrocytic sequence. The early erythrocyte precursors then undergo several successive cellular divisions. The processes of cellular differentiation which occur as the red cell attains

1039

maturity include condensation and extrusion of the nucleus and production of a complement of hemoglobin. Ninety per cent of the dry weight of the mature red cell is hemoglobin.

Hemoglobin. The combustion which is essential to life requires a constant supply of oxygen to the tissues of the body. The capacity of sea water and its internal equivalent, the plasma, to transport dissolved oxygen is limited. The evolutionary development of oxygen-carrying proteins, the hemoglobins, has increased the ability of blood to transport this gas. Further, because of the remarkable way in which hemoglobin combines with and dissociates from oxygen, the entire transport process is accomplished without expenditure of metabolic energy.

Hemoglobin is a complex protein consisting of the iron-containing heme groups and the protein moiety, globin. A dynamic interaction between heme and globin is responsible for the unique physiologic properties of hemoglobin in the reversible transport of oxygen. The hemoglobin molecule is a tetramer; i.e. it is made up of 2 pairs of protein polypeptide chains. The polypeptide chains of each kind of hemoglobin are of chemically different types. For example, the hemoglobin of the normal adult (Hgb. A) is made up of 2 pairs of chains called the alpha (α) and beta (β) polypeptide chains. Hemoglobin A can therefore be represented as $\alpha_2\beta_2$. Alpha and beta chains are markedly different in their chemical structure, and their synthesis is directed by separate genes.

The human hemoglobins are not homogeneous. Within the red cells of the embryo, fetus, child and adult, 5 different hemoglobins may be detected. They can be classified as the embryonic hemoglobins, Gower 1 and Gower 2; the fetal hemoglobin, Hgb. F; and the adult hemoglobins, Hgb. A and A$_2$. These variants have different electrophoretic mobilities, which reflect their different chemical structures. The compositions of the polypeptide chains of human hemoglobins

TABLE 14-2. THE NORMAL HUMAN HEMOGLOBINS

HEMOGLOBIN NAME	FORMULA	COMMENT
Gower 1	ϵ_4	Major embryonic hemoglobins
Gower 2	$\alpha_2\epsilon_2$	Not present after third month of gestation
Fetal (Hgb. F)	$\alpha_2\gamma_2$	Predominant hemoglobin throughout fetal life Alkali-resistant
Adult (Hgb. A)	$\alpha_2\beta_2$	Major adult hemoglobin
A$_2$	$\alpha_2\delta_2$	Minor adult hemoglobin Detectable postnatally

are listed in Table 14-2. The the time of appearance and quantitative relations between these hemoglobins are determined by complex developmental processes. The relations are depicted in Figure 14-1.

The embryonic hemoglobins. The blood of early human embryos contains 2 slowly migrating hemoglobins called Gower 1 and Gower 2. The Gower hemoglobins contain a unique type of polypeptide chain called the epsilon chain. Hemoglobin Gower 1 has the structure ϵ_4, and Gower 2, $\alpha_2\epsilon_2$. In embryos of 4 to 8 weeks' gestation the Gower hemoglobins predominate, but by the third month they have disappeared.

Fetal hemoglobin. Hemoglobin F contains gamma polypeptide chains which are different from the beta chains of Hgb. A. Hemoglobin F can be represented as $\alpha_2\gamma_2$. It resists denaturation by strong alkali, and the technique of alkali denaturation is usually used for quantitation. After the eighth gestational week it is the predominant hemoglobin, and in the 6-month-old fetus constitutes 90 per cent of the total hemoglobin. After this a gradual decline occurs, so that at birth Hgb. F averages 70 per cent of the total. Synthesis

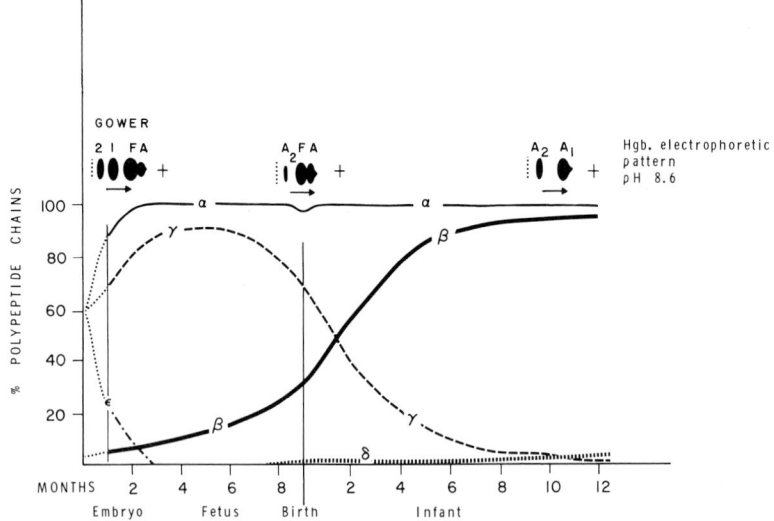

Figure 14-1. Proportions of the various human hemoglobin polypeptide chains through early life. The hemoglobin electrophoretic pattern typical for each period is also shown. (From H. A. Pearson: *J. Pediat.,* 69:466, 1966.)

of Hgb. F decreases rapidly postnatally, and by 6 to 12 months of age only a trace is present. Less than 2.0 per cent can be detected by alkali denaturation in older children and adults.

The adult hemoglobins. Some Hgb. A ($\alpha_2\beta_2$) can be detected even in the smallest embryos, and by the sixth month of gestation Hgb. A is present to about 5 to 10 per cent. A steady increase follows, so that at term Hgb. A averages 30 per cent. By 6 to 12 months of age the normal adult hemoglobin pattern appears. The minor adult hemoglobin component Hgb. A_2 contains delta (δ) chains and has the structure of $\alpha_2\delta_2$. It is seen only when significant amounts of Hgb. A are also present. At birth less than 1.0 per cent of Hgb. A_2 is seen, but by 12 months of age the normal level of 2.0 to 3.4 per cent is attained. Throughout life the proportion of Hgb. A to A_2 is about 30 to 1.

Normal relations of the various hemoglobins. During fetal life and early childhood there is an inverse relation between the rates of synthesis of gamma and beta chains and hence between the amounts of Hgb. A and Hgb. F. How this reciprocal relation is regulated is uncertain. By borrowing heavily upon the models of microbiologic biochemical genetics, a "switch mechanism" involving regulator genes has been postulated. During fetal life this mechanism facilitates gamma chain synthesis, while beta and delta chain production is repressed. After birth the "switch" is reversed, so that fetal hemoglobin synthesis is inhibited and the adult hemoglobins accumulate. Crucial factors influencing these regulatory mechanisms have not been clearly defined.

Alterations of the hemoglobins by disease. The relative proportions of the various hemoglobins are not usually altered by hematologic disease.

Since hemoglobins containing epsilon chains are normally present only very early in intrauterine life, they are largely of theoretic interest. Small amounts of the Gower hemoglobins have been detectable in a few newborn infants with the syndrome of D, (13-15) trisomy.

Levels of fetal hemoglobin may be influenced by a variety of factors. In patients heterozygous for β thalassemia (β-thalassemia trait), the postpartum decrease of Hgb. F is retarded, and about half of these patients have elevated levels of Hgb. F (more than 2.0 per cent) in later life. In homozygous thalassemia (Cooley's anemia) and in hereditary persistence of fetal hemoglobin large amounts of Hgb. F are characteristically seen. In patients with major beta chain hemoglobinopathies (Hgb. SS, SC, and so on) Hgb. F is usually elevated, particularly during childhood. Finally, moderate elevations of Hgb. F may be seen in many diseases accompanied by hematologic stress, such as hemolytic anemias, leukemia and aplastic anemia. This is often due to the presence of a small population of red cells which contain increased amounts of Hgb. F.

The normal adult level of Hgb. A_2 (2.4 to 3.4 per cent) is seldom altered. A level of Hgb. A_2 exceeding 3.4 per cent is found in most persons with the β-thalassemia trait, and moderate increases have been documented in those with megaloblastic anemias secondary to vitamin B_{12} and folic acid deficiency.

Metabolism of the Red Cell. The nucleated red cell in the bone marrow is able to perform a variety of metabolic functions, including active protein synthesis. After extrusion of the nucleus much of this metabolic capacity is lost, and the mature red cell is unable to synthesize proteins. Although loss of the nucleus makes the red cell a more perfect vessel for oxygen transport, it does impose upon the red cell a finite life span, for the cell cannot replace or repair its vital enzymatic proteins. The mature red cell contains more than 40 enzymes. Many of these are essential for cellular viability, but genetically determined deficiencies of others, such as catalase, do not interfere with normal survival.

The mature red cell is not metabolically inert. Glucose is utilized and lactic acid produced mostly by anaerobic glycolysis (Embden-Meyerhof pathway); about 10 per cent of glucose is metabolized oxidatively through the pentose phosphate pathway. Figure 14-2 depicts these pathways and shows the enzymes essential to metabolism of glucose by the mature red cell. Three uses for the energy generated by glucose metabolism have been identified as essential for normal cell viability: (1) Maintenance of electrolyte gradients. The principal intracellular cation of the red cell is potassium, while that in the plasma is sodium. There is a constant tendency for sodium to enter the red cell and concomitantly for potassium to leak out. Reversal of these flows and preservation of normal ionic gradients are accomplished by an energy (ATP)-dependent membrane mechanism, the cation pump. When the cation pump fails, sodium and water accumulate within the red cell, causing it to swell and ultimately to hemolyze. (2) Maintenance of the red cell membrane and shape. The red cell membrane is a complex phospholipid structure, and maintenance of these phospholipids consumes energy. Maintenance of the biconcave shape is probably also energy-dependent. (3) Maintenance of heme iron in the reduced (ferrous) form. Oxidative potentials within the red cell may cause oxidation of the iron of hemoglobin. Hemoglobin containing ferric (methemoglobin) is ineffective in oxygen transport. If peroxides and other oxidant substances are not inactivated, hemoglobin may be denatured and precipitated. Cells containing such denatured hemoglobin are rapidly removed from the circulation. Protection of the red cell from the detrimental effects of oxidation ultimately depends upon TPNH and DPNH. These compounds are constantly regenerated by activities of the glycolytic pathway and pentose shunt. Genetically determined deficiencies of a number of the glycolytic and pentose pathway enzymes have been identified, many of which produce hemolytic states because the energy necessary to perform these vital functions cannot be generated.

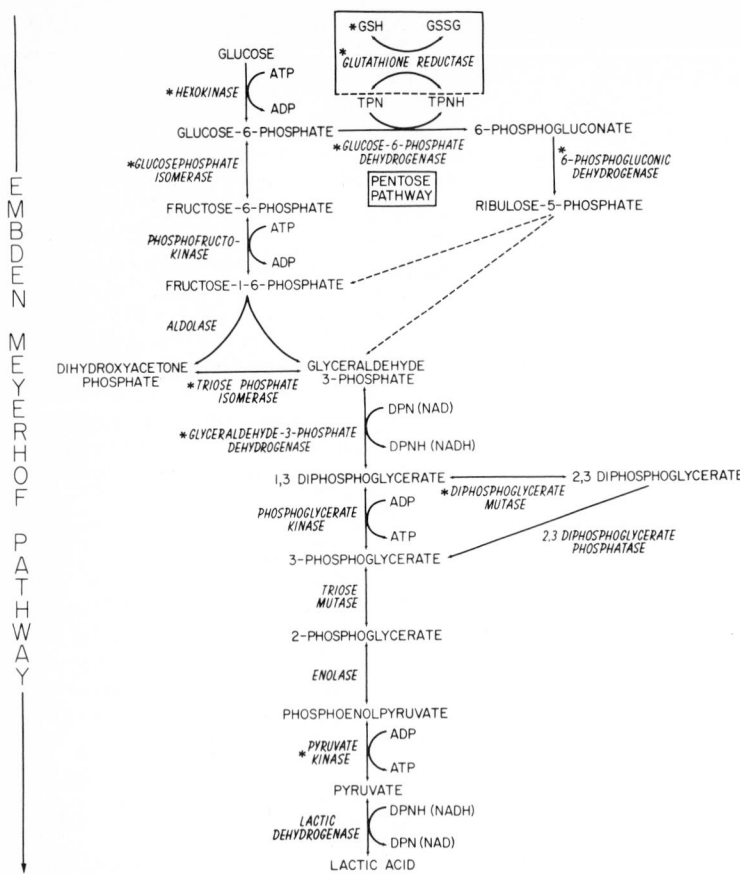

Figure 14-2. Metabolic pathways of glucose metabolism in the mature red blood cell. Congenital deficiency states have been described for the enzymes indicated by an asterisk (*).

THE ANEMIAS

Anemia is defined as a reduction of the red cell volume or hemoglobin concentration below the range of values occurring in healthy persons. Because these ranges vary with age and sex, the child's blood values should not be reported as "per cent" of an arbitrary standard (usually that of the adult male). Table 14-3 lists the means and ranges for hemoglobin and hematocrit values by age groups of well nourished children.

Although reduction in amount of circulating hemoglobin decreases the oxygen-carrying capacity of the blood, few physiologic disturbances occur until the hemoglobin level falls below 7 to 8 gm. per 100 ml. Below this level, pallor becomes evident in skin and mucous membranes. Physiologic adjustments to anemia include tachycardia, increased cardiac output, a shift in the dissociation curve which makes oxygen more readily available to the tissues, and a deviation of blood flow toward vital organs and tissues. When moderately severe anemia develops slowly, surprisingly few

symptoms or objective findings may be evident, but weakness, tachypnea, shortness of breath on exertion, tachycardia, cardiac dilatation and congestive heart failure ultimately result from increasingly severe anemia, regardless of its cause.

Anemia is not a specific entity, but is an indication or manifestation of an underlying pathologic process or disease. A useful physiologic classification of the anemias of childhood divides them into 2 large groups: (1) those resulting primarily from decreased production of red cells or hemoglobin; and (2) those in which increased destruction or loss of red cells is the predominant mechanism. In Table 14-4 the important anemias of childhood are classified by these criteria. In every case of significant anemia it is essential to describe the morphologic characteristics of the red cells, to determine the relative importance of defective red cell production and of cell destruction in the genesis of the anemia, and, when possible, to identify the basic etiologic process.

TABLE 14-3. HEMATOLOGIC VALUES DURING INFANCY AND CHILDHOOD

AGE	HEMOGLOBIN GM./100 ML. %		HEMATOCRIT %		RETICULOCYTES %	WBC/MM.³ %		NEUTROPHILS %		LYMPHOCYTES % (RELATIVELY WIDE RANGE)	EOSINOPHILS %	MONOCYTES %	NUCLEATED RED CELLS /100 WBC
	MEAN	RANGE	MEAN	RANGE	MEAN	MEAN	RANGE	MEAN	RANGE	MEAN	MEAN	MEAN	
Cord blood	16.8	13.7-20.1	55	45-65	5.0	18,000	(9-30,000)	61	(40-80)	31	2	6	7.0 (3-10)
2 weeks	16.5	13.0-20.0	50	42-66	1.0	12,000	(5-21,000)	40		48	3	9	0
3 months	12.0	9.5-14.5	36	31-41	1.0	12,000	(6-18,000)	30		63	2	5	0
6 mos.-6 yrs.	12.0	10.5-14.0	37	33-42	1.0	10,000	(6-15,000)	45		48	2	5	0
7-12 yrs.	13.0	11.0-16.0	38	34-40	1.0	8,000	(4500-13,500)	55		38	2	5	0
Adult Female Male	14 16	12.0-16.0 14.0-18.0	42 47	37-47 42-52	1.6	7,500	(5-10,000)	55	(35-70)	35	3	7	0

All values represent compromises between a number of standard sources and published reports. Greatest variations in "normal" are seen in infancy and early childhood.

The decreases in hemoglobin and hematocrit values and in the red blood cell count which occur in all infants during the first 2 or 3 months of life have been designated **"physiologic anemia"** of infancy. The erythrocytes are normocytic and normochromic, and there is no unusual reticulocytosis. These decreases are apparently related to the relatively short life span of the fetal red cell and to the dilutional effects of the infant's expanding blood volume. The pattern is not altered by the administration of iron or other "hematinic" substances. Low birth weight accentuates this "anemia" of early infancy; in such infants hemoglobin values may fall as low as 6.0 to 7.0 gm./100 ml. Usually there are no symptoms, even with this degree of anemia, but, if the infant is failing to grow or thrive, a small (5 ml. per kg.) transfusion of sedimented compatible red blood cells may be beneficial.

Although iron medication does not prevent this "physiologic anemia" the iron stores of infants of low birth weight and of infants who have had significant perinatal blood loss should be replenished by administration of medicinal iron or by feeding of an iron-fortified milk formula.

TABLE 14-4. CLASSIFICATION OF THE ANEMIAS

I. Anemias resulting primarily from inadequate produc-
tion of red cells or hemoglobin
  A. Decreased numbers of red cell precursors in the
     marrow
     1. "Pure red cell" anemias
        a. Congenital pure red cell anemia
        b. Acquired pure red cell anemias
  B. Inadequate production despite normal numbers of
     red cell precursors
     1. Anemia of infection, inflammation and cancer
     2. Anemia of chronic renal disease
  C. Deficiency of specific factors
     1. Megaloblastic anemias
        a. Folic acid deficiency
        b. Vitamin B_{12} deficiency
        c. Orotic aciduria
     2. Microcytic anemias
        a. Iron deficiency
        b. Pyridoxine-responsive and X-linked hypo-
           chromic anemias
        c. Lead poisoning
II. Hemolytic anemias
  A. Intrinsic abnormalities of the red cell
     1. "Structural" defects
        a. Hereditary spherocytosis
        b. Hemolytic elliptocytosis
        c. Paroxysmal nocturnal hemoglobinuria

     2. Enzymatic defects (nonspherocytic hemolytic
        anemias)
        a. Enzymes of glycolytic pathway; pyruvate
           kinase, hexokinase and others
        b. Enzymes of the pentose phosphate pathway
           and glutathione complex
     3. Defects in synthesis of hemoglobin
        a. Hgb. S, C, D, E, etc., alone and in combina-
           tion
        b. Thalassemia
  B. Extrinsic (extracellular) abnormalities
     1. Immunologic disorders
        a. Passively acquired antibodies (hemolytic
           disease of the newborn)
           (1) Rh isoimmunization
           (2) A or B isoimmunization
           (3) Other blood group families
        b. Active antibody formation
           (1) Idiopathic autoimmune hemolytic ane-
               mia
           (2) Symptomatic—lupus, lymphoma
           (3) Drug-induced
     2. Nonimmunologic disorders
        a. Toxic from drugs, chemicals
        b. Infections—malaria, clostridium
     3. Infantile pyknocytosis

See also anemia in pancytopenias (p. 1067) and leukemia (p. 1075).

Anemias Resulting from Inadequate Production of Red Cells

These anemias result when the bone marrow is unable to produce sufficient numbers of new red cells to replace those removed from the circulation. A slight reduction in the red cell life span may be present, but generally this is insufficient to cause anemia if hematopoiesis is adequate. Low reticulocyte counts are observed in most anemias of this group.

CONGENITAL PURE RED CELL ANEMIA
(CONGENITAL HYPOPLASTIC ANEMIA; DIAMOND-BLACKFAN SYNDROME)

This rare condition usually becomes symptomatic in early infancy. The most characteristic diagnostic feature is a deficiency of red cell precursors in an otherwise normally cellular bone marrow. Other congenital anomalies are not usually associated.

Etiology. A genetic basis is suggested by several instances of familial occurrence. Males and females are affected in equal numbers. Although an ill-defined abnormality of tryptophan metabolism has been reported in some children, the biochemical basis for the disease is still uncertain. High levels of erythropoietin are present in serum and urine.

Clinical Manifestations. Although some of these infants appear pale even in the first few days of life, hematopoiesis must have been generally adequate during intrauterine life. Profound anemia usually becomes evident by 2 to 6 months of age, occasionally somewhat later. Unless blood transfusions are given, the anemia progresses to such severity that heart failure and death occur. The liver and spleen are not enlarged initially.

Laboratory Data. The red blood cells are normochromic and normocytic; there are no morphologic or biochemical abnormalities. The most important feature is the lack of evidence of erythropoietic activity in blood and bone marrow. Reticulocytes are diminished even when the anemia is severe. Red cell precursors are markedly reduced in the marrow, resulting in myeloid-erythroid ratios of 10:1 to 200:1. In some cases a few pronormoblasts may be present, but not more mature forms. A normal complement of white cells, platelets and megakaryocytes is present. Serum iron is elevated, with a decrease in the iron-binding capacity. Red cell survival is normal.

Differential Diagnosis. Congenital hypoplastic anemia must be differentiated from other anemias in which there are low peripheral reticulocyte counts. The anemia of the convalescent phase of hemolytic disease of the newborn may, on occasion, be associated with markedly reduced erythropoiesis. This terminates spontaneously at 5 to 8 weeks of age, whereas congenital hypoplastic anemia is not usually recognized before this time. Aplastic crises, characterized by reticulocytopenia and decreased numbers of red cell precursors, may complicate various types of hemolytic disease. These episodes are transient, and evidence of antecedent hemolytic disease is usually present.

Course. Unless corticosteroid therapy produces remission of hypoplastic anemia, survival depends upon blood transfusions given as needed, usually at intervals of 4 to 8 weeks. By late childhood these children may have had a hundred or more transfusions, and hemosiderosis is an inevitable consequence. The liver and spleen enlarge, and secondary hypersplenism with leukopenia and thrombocytopenia may occur. Growth retardation is usual, and puberty may not occur.

Death usually occurs in the second decade. Chronic congestive heart failure due to ischemic and siderotic myocardial disease is a common terminal event. Despite this grave prognosis, spontaneous remissions occasionally occur, some after very extended periods of dependency upon transfusion.

Treatment. When anemia becomes severe, blood transfusions must be given. Corticosteroid therapy is frequently beneficial if begun early; the mechanism of its effect is unknown. Relatively large doses, 2 to 4 mg. per kg., of prednisone or its equivalent are administered initially. One to 3 weeks after therapy is begun red cell precursors appear in bone marrow, and then a brisk peripheral reticulocytosis occurs. The hemoglobin may reach normal level in 4 to 6 weeks. The dose of corticosteroid may then be reduced gradually until the lowest effective dose is found. This is often a very small amount, such as 2.5 mg. per day of prednisone or less, which may produce no adverse side effects or growth suppression. Intermittent administration every other day or for 3 or 4 consecutive days each week may also be effective. Therapy should be discontinued periodically to determine whether the child is still dependent upon steroids.

About 25 per cent of cases do not respond to corticosteroid therapy, and transfusions are necessary to sustain life. A large number of other therapies, including all known hematinics, cobalt and testosterone, have had no beneficial effect. Splenectomy is usually of no value, but may decrease the need for transfusion if hypersplenism or isoimmunization has developed. Because of the possibility of spontaneous remission, children refractory to corticosteroid therapy should be maintained as long as possible by transfusions, preferably of freshly drawn, packed red cells.

ACQUIRED PURE RED CELL ANEMIAS

A number of forms of acquired anemia with reticulocytopenia and reduced red cell precursors in the marrow have been described. The cause of most of the acquired instances is uncertain. In some cases a tumor of the thymus has been present, and remissions have followed its removal. In some other cases an erythropoietin-inhibiting antibody has been demonstrated in the plasma. The acquired pure red cell anemias may respond to therapy with corticosteroids, and a trial is indicated in any chronic case.

Administration of large doses of chloramphenicol inhibits erythropoiesis. Reticulocytopenia, erythroid hypoplasia and vacuolated pronormoblasts in the marrow are reversible pharmacologic effects of this drug (see also Pancytopenias, p. 1067).

ANEMIAS OF CHRONIC INFECTION, INFLAMMATION AND RENAL DISEASE

Anemia complicates a number of chronic systemic diseases associated with infection, inflammation or tissue breakdown. Examples of such conditions include chronic pyogenic infections such as bronchiectasis and osteomyelitis; chronic inflammatory processes such as rheumatic fever, rheumatoid arthritis and ulcerative colitis; and advanced renal disease. Despite diverse underlying causes, the erythrokinetic abnormalities are similar. The red cell life span is moderately decreased, but the principal factor determining the degree of anemia is a relative inability of the bone marrow to fabricate red cells. How these systemic diseases inhibit the marrow activity is not clear, but inadequate production of erythropoietin is not the primary mechanism.

Clinical Manifestations. Few symptoms are attributable to the moderate degree of anemia usually present; the important symptoms and signs are those of the underlying disease.

Laboratory Data. Hemoglobin concentrations usually range from 6 to 9 gm. per 100 ml. The red blood cell count and hemoglobin and hematocrit levels are proportionately decreased, resulting in a normochromic and normocytic anemia. Occasionally a modest degree of hypochromia and microcytosis is observed. Reticulocyte counts are normal or low. Leukocytosis is often present. Serum iron is low; however, there is no increase in total iron-binding capacity as in iron deficiency anemia. Rather, a decrease may result in a fairly normal saturation percentage. This pattern of serum iron and iron-binding protein is a regular and valuable diagnostic feature. The bone marrow has normal cellularity. The red cell precursors are adequate, and granulocytic hyperplasia may be present. Increased hemosiderin can often be demonstrated in marrow.

Treatment and Prognosis. Since these anemias are secondary to another disease process, they do not respond to iron or hematinics. Transfusions raise the hemoglobin concentration only temporarily and are rarely indicated. If the underlying systemic disease can be controlled, the anemia corrects spontaneously.

MEGALOBLASTIC ANEMIAS

The megaloblastic anemias all have in common certain abnormalities of red cell morphology and maturation which are diagnostic. The red cells at every stage of development are larger than normal and have a peculiar open, finely dispersed arrangement of nuclear chromatin and an asynchrony between the maturation of nucleus and cytoplasm. Almost all cases of megaloblastic anemia result from a deficiency of either folic acid or vitamin B_{12} or from a combined deficiency of them. Both substances are necessary cofactors in the synthesis of nucleoproteins.

FOLIC ACID DEFICIENCY
(Megaloblastic Anemia of Infancy)

This disease is caused by a decreased intake or absorption of folic acid. The dietary deficiency is usually compounded by rapid growth or infection, which may increase folic acid requirements. The normal daily requirement is small, having been estimated at 20 to 50 micrograms per day. Human and cow's milks provide adequate amounts of folic acid. Goat's milk is clearly deficient, and folic acid supplementation must be given when it is the main food. Unless supplemented, powdered milk may also be a poor source of this vitamin. Ascorbic acid deficiency probably impairs the availability of dietary folic acid conjugates.

Clinical Features. Megaloblastic anemia has a peak incidence at 4 to 7 months of age, somewhat earlier than iron deficiency anemia. In addition to the usual features of severe anemia, these infants are irritable, fail to gain weight adequately, and have chronic diarrhea. Thrombocytopenic hemorrhages occur in advanced cases. Concomitant signs and symptoms of scurvy may be present. Prematurity may be a predisposing factor.

Laboratory Data. The anemia varies in degree, but is progressive. Because the red blood cell count is disproportionately lower than the hematocrit levels, the anemia is macrocytic. Nevertheless considerable variations in red cell shape and size are common (Fig. 14-3, C). The reticulocyte count is low, but nucleated red cells demonstrating megaloblastic morphology are often seen in the peripheral blood. Neutropenia and thrombocytopenia may be present. The neutrophils are large, with hypersegmented nuclei; more than 5 per cent of the neutrophils will have 5 or more nuclear segments. Serum folic acid activity, as measured by microbiologic assay, is less than 3 millimicrograms per ml. Levels of iron and vitamin B_{12} in serum are normal or elevated. Formiminoglutamic acid is excreted in the urine, especially after an oral dose of l-histidine. The bone marrow is hypercellular because of erythroid hyperplasia. Megaloblastic changes are prominent,

though some normal red cell precursors may also be present. Large, abnormal neutrophilic forms (giant metamyelocytes) with cytoplasmic vacuolization are seen, as well as hypersegmentation of the nuclei of megakaryocytes.

Treatment. Initially folic acid may be administered parenterally in a dose of 2 to 5 mg. per day. Since a hematologic response can be expected within 72 hours, transfusions are indicated only when the anemia is severe or the child very ill. Folic acid therapy should be continued for 3 to 4 weeks. Satisfactory responses have been obtained with doses of folic acid as low as 50 micrograms per day. These "physiologic" doses have no effect on primary vitamin B_{12} deficiencies; a therapeutic test using such low amounts may be used, therefore, to differentiate between primary folic acid and vitamin B_{12} deficiencies. If there is a likelihood that juvenile pernicious anemia may be present, or if the anemia recurs after therapy, the prolonged use of folic acid should be avoided, since in pernicious anemia folic acid may produce a partial response of anemia without benefiting the neurologic abnormalities. If signs of scurvy are present, therapeutic doses of ascorbic acid should be given. Antibiotic therapy should be used for superimposed bacterial infection.

Folic Acid Deficiency of Malabsorption Syndromes (see also p. 804). Folic acid is absorbed throughout the small intestine, and diffuse inflammatory or degenerative disease of the intestine may markedly impair absorption. Celiac disease, chronic infectious enteritis and enteroenteric fistulas may lead to folic acid deficiency and megaloblastic anemia.

Folic Acid Deficiency Complicating Hemolytic Anemias. Folic acid is necessary for normal hematopoiesis, and it is possible that chronic hemolytic processes may increase the requirement for this vitamin. Frank megaloblastic erythropoiesis may complicate hemolytic anemia, leading to more severe anemia and increased need for transfusion. The bone marrow should be examined for megaloblastic changes if there is an unexplained worsening of chronic anemia or increased transfusion requirements in chronic hemolytic states. Folic acid supplementation is not ordinarily necessary in the management of such patients.

Folic Acid Deficiency Associated with Anticonvulsants and Other Drugs. Many patients have low serum levels of folic acid during therapy with certain anticonvulsant drugs (e.g. Dilantin, Mysoline), but they usually have no anemia or symptoms. Rarely such patients do have a frank megaloblastic anemia, which responds to folic acid therapy, even if administration of the offending drug is continued. Malabsorption of folic acid induced by diphenylhydantoin is the probable mechanism for folate deficiency.

A number of drugs have antifolic acid activity as their primary pharmacologic effect and will regularly produce megaloblastic anemia. Methotrexate and aminopterin prevent the utilization of folic acid by inhibiting its enzymatic reduction

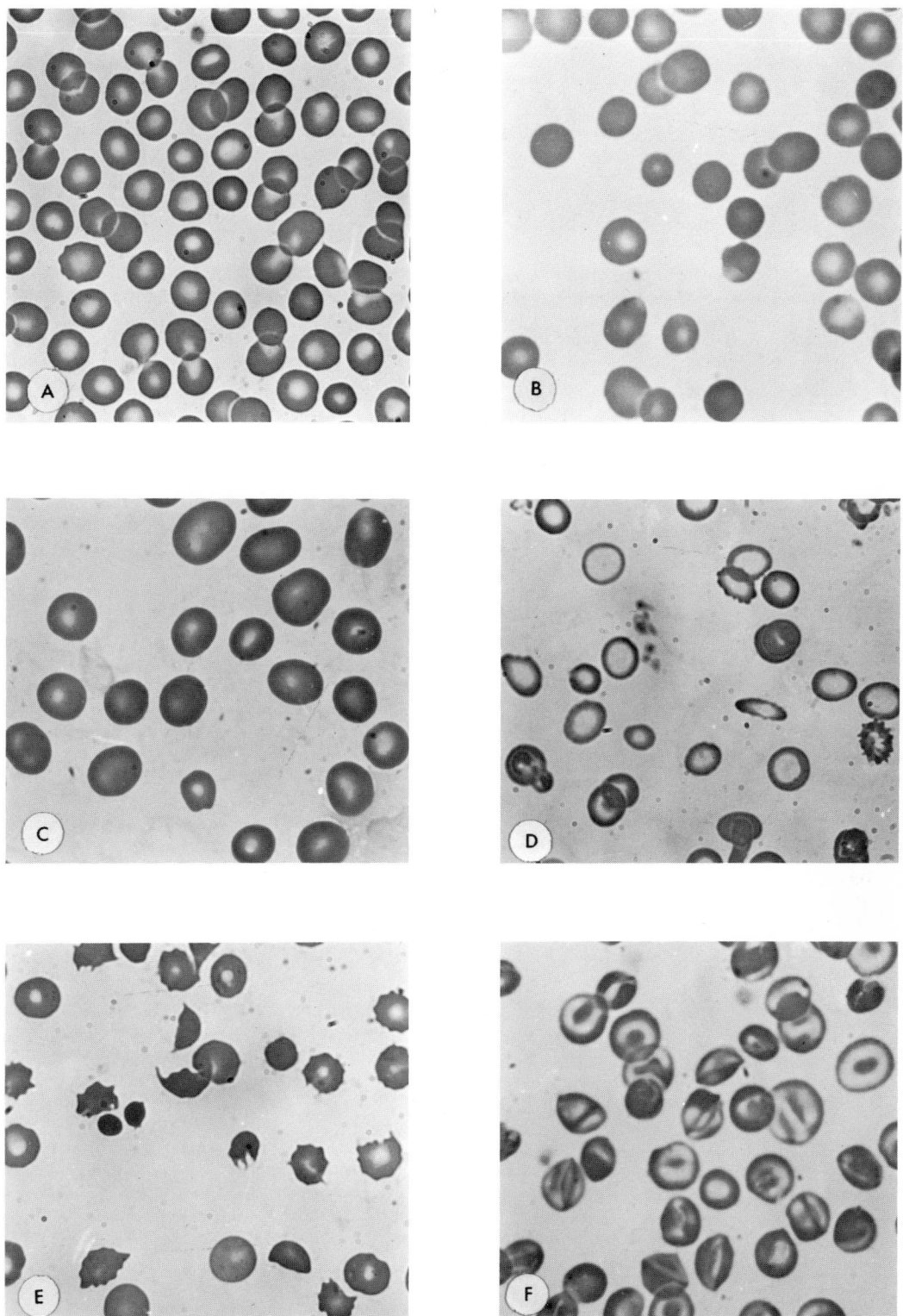

Figure 14-3. Morphologic abnormalities of the red cell. *A,* Normal. *B,* Spherocytes (hereditary spherocytosis). *C,* Macrocytes (folic acid deficiency). *D,* Hypochromic microcytes (iron deficiency). *E,* Schizocytes (hemolytic uremic syndrome). *F,* Target cells (Hgb. CC disease).

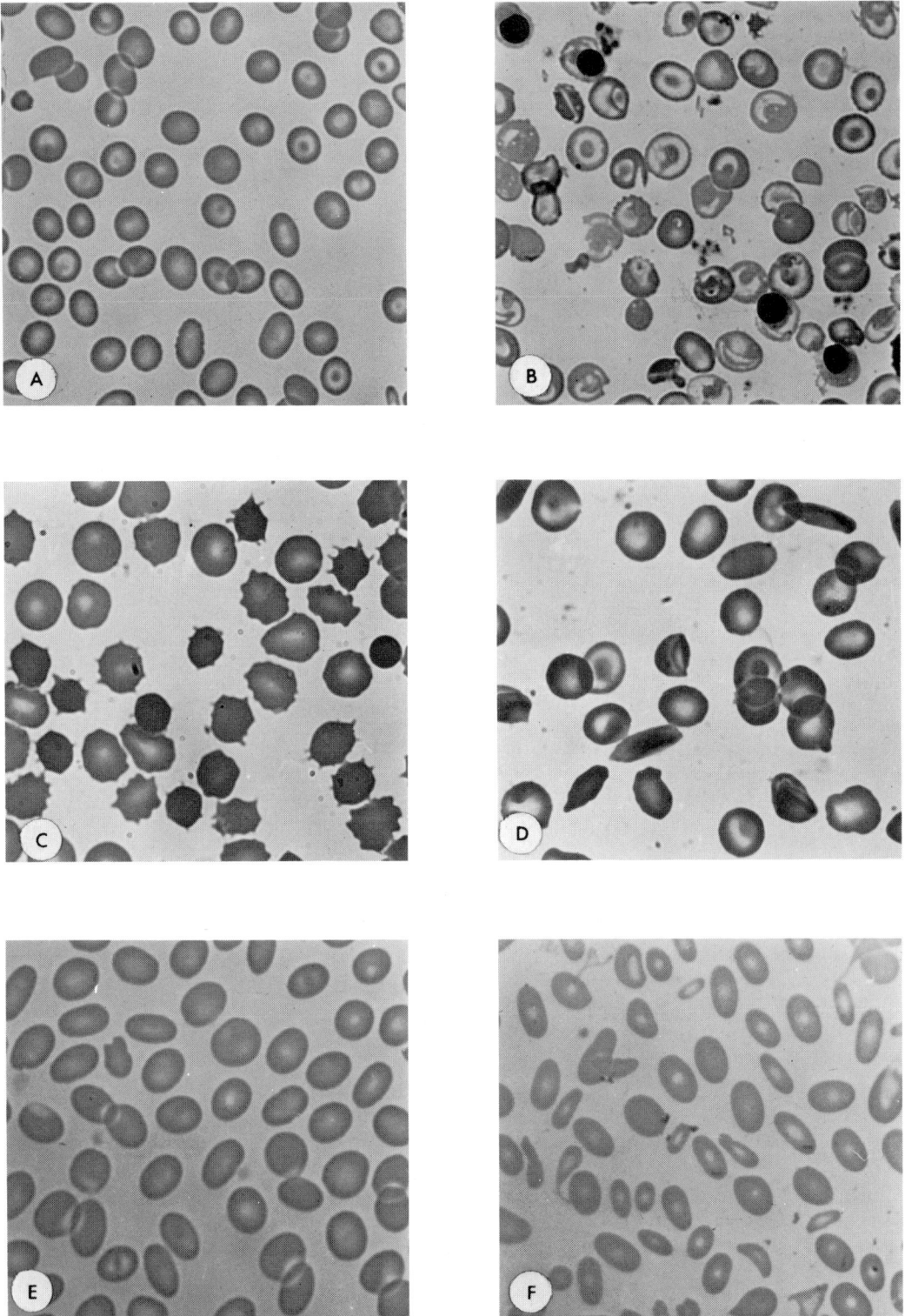

Figure 14-4. Morphologic abnormalities of the red cell. *A*, Thalassemia trait. *B*, Thalassemia major. *C*, Acantho-cytes (a-beta-lipoproteinemia). *D*, Sickle cells (Hgb. SS disease). *E*, Elliptocytes (hereditary elliptocytosis). *F*, Bizarre elliptocytes (hemolytic elliptocytosis).

to active coenzymatic forms. Daraprim and pentamidine isethionate, which are used in the therapy of toxoplasmosis and *Pneumocystis carinii* pneumonia, respectively, may induce folic acid deficiency and megaloblastic anemia.

VITAMIN B₁₂ DEFICIENCY

In order to be absorbed, dietary vitamin B_{12} must combine with a glycoprotein (intrinsic factor) secreted by the parietal cells of the gastric fundus. The B_{12}-intrinsic factor complex passes to the terminal ileum, where specific absorptive sites exist. In the presence of intrinsic factor and ionic calcium, vitamin B_{12} traverses the intestinal mucosa and enters the blood. Vitamin B_{12} deficiency may therefore result from (1) inadequate intake, (2) lack of secretion of intrinsic factor by the stomach, (3) consumption or inhibition of the B_{12}-intrinsic factor complex, or (4) abnormalities involving the receptor sites in the terminal ileum.

Because vitamin B_{12} is present in many foods, dietary deficiency is rare. An instance has been reported in a breast-fed infant whose mother was also markedly deficient. Vitamin B_{12} deficiency in childhood usually relates to inadequate intrinsic factor.

Juvenile Pernicious Anemia

This rare disease is due to inability to secrete gastric intrinsic factor. It differs from the typical disease in adults in that the stomach normally secretes acid and is histologically normal. Consanguinity is common in parents of affected children, and a mendelian recessive inheritance pattern is suggested.

Clinical Features. The symptoms of juvenile pernicious anemia become prominent at 9 months to 4 years of age. This interval is consistent with exhaustion of the stores of vitamin B_{12} acquired in utero. As the anemia becomes severe, irritability, anorexia and listlessness occur. The tongue is smooth, red and painful. Neurologic involvement is manifested by ataxia, paresthesias, hyporeflexia, Babinski responses, clonus and coma.

Laboratory Data. The anemia is macrocytic with prominent macro-ovalocytosis of the red cells. The neutrophils are large and hypersegmented. In advanced cases neutropenia and thrombocytopenia are seen. Serum vitamin B_{12}, as measured by radioactive techniques or microbiological assay, is below 100 micromicrograms per ml. Concentrations of serum iron and serum folic acid are normal or elevated. Serum antibodies directed against parietal cells or intrinsic factor cannot be detected. Gastric acidity may be reduced initially, but returns to normal when vitamin B_{12} therapy is instituted. Biopsy reveals a normal gastric mucosa, but intrinsic factor activity is absent in the gastric secretion.

Absorption of vitamin B_{12} is usually assessed by the Schilling test, using radioactive vitamin B_{12}. When a normal person ingests a small amount of vitamin B_{12} containing ^{57}Co or ^{60}Co, the radioactive vitamin combines with the intrinsic factor in the stomach secretions and passes to the terminal ileum, where absorption occurs. As the absorbed vitamin is bound to blood proteins and tissues, none is normally excreted in the urine. If a large (1000 micrograms) dose of nonradioactive vitamin B_{12} is then injected parenterally ("flushing dose"), from 10 to 30 per cent of the previously absorbed radioactive vitamin will appear in the urine. Patients with pernicious anemia excrete 2 per cent or less under these conditions. That malabsorption of vitamin B_{12} is due to lack of intrinsic factor can be confirmed through a modification of the standard Schilling test: 30 mg. of intrinsic factor is administered along with the radioactive vitamin; if absence of intrinsic factor is the basis of the B_{12} malabsorption, normal amounts of radioactive vitamin should now be absorbed and flushed out. On the other hand, when vitamin B_{12} malabsorption is due to disease of the ileal receptor sites or other intestinal causes, no improvement in absorption will be seen with intrinsic factor. The Schilling test result will remain abnormal in pernicious anemia, even when therapy has completely reversed the hematologic and neurologic manifestations of the disease.

Treatment. A prompt hematologic response follows parenteral administration of vitamin B_{12}. The physiologic requirement for vitamin B_{12} is 1 to 5 micrograms per day, and hematologic responses have been observed with these small doses. If there is evidence of neurologic involvement, 1 mg. should be injected intramuscularly daily for at least 2 weeks. Maintenance therapy will be necessary throughout the patient's life; monthly intramuscular administration of 1 mg. of vitamin B_{12} is sufficient. Attempts at oral therapy are contraindicated.

Vitamin B₁₂ Deficiency in Older Children

Vitamin B_{12} malabsorption has been described in late childhood associated with atrophy of the gastric mucosa and achlorhydria, and in some instances in combination with a familial syndrome of cutaneous moniliasis, hypoparathyroidism and other endocrine deficiencies. The serum contains antibodies against parietal cells and intrinsic factor. The Schilling test result is abnormal, but is corrected by addition of exogenous intrinsic factor. Parenteral vitamin B_{12} should be administered regularly to these patients to prevent the development of megaloblastic anemia.

Vitamin B₁₂ Malabsorption Due to Intestinal Causes

A few cases have been reported of familial occurrence of a specific intestinal defect in the absorption of vitamin B_{12}, in some instances associated with proteinuria. Surgical resection of the terminal ileum or such inflammatory diseases as regional enteritis or tuberculosis may also impair absorption of vitamin B_{12}. An overgrowth of intestinal bacteria within diverticula or duplications of the small intestine may cause vitamin B_{12} deficiency through consumption of the vitamin or the splitting of its complex with intrinsic factor. Similar mechanisms may operate when the fish tapeworm *Diphyllobothrium latum* infests the upper small intestine. When megaloblastic anemia occurs in these situations, the serum vitamin B_{12} level is low, the gastric juice contains intrinsic factor, and the abnormal Schilling test result is not corrected by the addition of exogenous intrinsic factor.

OROTIC ACIDURIA

Orotic aciduria is a genetically determined defect in nucleoprotein synthesis associated with a severe megaloblastic anemia and crystalluria due to excretion of orotic acid. Physical and mental retardation is frequently present. The anemia is refractory to vitamin B_{12} or folic acid, but responds promptly to administration of the nucleic acid precursor, uridine. Inheritance is autosomal recessive.

MICROCYTIC ANEMIAS

IRON DEFICIENCY ANEMIA

Anemia resulting from insufficient iron for synthesis of hemoglobin is by far the most frequent hematologic disease of infancy and childhood. The prevalence of this deficiency is related to certain basic aspects of iron metabolism and nutrition. The body of the newborn infant contains about 0.5 gm. of iron in contrast to the iron content of the adult, which is estimated at 5.0 gm. In order to make up this 4.5 gm. discrepancy, an average of 0.8 mg. of iron must be absorbed each day during the first 15 years of life. To this growth requirement an additional small amount is necessary to balance normal losses through excretion of iron. Accordingly, to maintain a normal positive iron balance in childhood, 0.8 to 1.5 mg. of iron must be absorbed each day. As only about 10 per cent of dietary iron is absorbed, a diet containing 8 to 15 mg. of iron is necessary for optimal nutrition. During the first years of life, because relatively small quantities of iron-rich foods are taken, it is often difficult to attain these amounts. At best, the infant is in a precarious situation with respect to iron. Should the diet become inadequate or should abnormal external blood loss occur, anemia ensues rapidly.

Etiology. A preponderance of the iron of the newborn is contained in the circulating hemoglobin. Low birth weight and significant perinatal hemorrhage are associated with a decreased neonatal hemoglobin mass and store of iron. As the high hemoglobin concentration of the newborn decreases during the first 2 to 3 months of life, considerable iron is reclaimed and stored. These reclaimed stores are usually sufficient for blood formation for the first 6 to 9 months of life; but in low-birth-weight infants or with perinatal blood loss, stored iron may be depleted earlier, and dietary sources become of paramount importance. Anemia due solely to inadequate dietary iron is unusual during the first 4 to 6 months, but becomes common from 9 to 24 months of age. Thereafter it is relatively infrequent. The usual dietary pattern observed in infants with iron deficiency anemia is the consumption of large amounts of milk and of carbohydrates, unsupplemented with iron.

Blood loss must be considered a possible cause in every case of iron deficiency anemia, particularly in the older child. Chronic iron deficiency anemia from occult bleeding is usually due to a lesion of the gastrointestinal tract such as peptic ulcer, Meckel's diverticulum, polyp or hemangioma. In some geographic areas hookworm infestation is an important cause.

Histologic abnormalities of the mucosa of the gastrointestinal tract are present in advanced iron deficiency anemia, as are significant decreases in intracellular iron-containing enzymes in the mucosal cells. The morphologic changes may be a direct manifestation of tissue deficiency of iron. A syndrome of gastrointestinal intolerance to whole cow's milk has also been described, which includes histologic abnormalities of the mucosa, chronic gastrointestinal bleeding and secondary iron deficiency anemia.

Clinical Manifestations. Pallor is the most important clue to iron deficiency. When the hemoglobin level falls below 5.0 gm. per 100 ml., irritability and anorexia are prominent. Tachycardia and cardiac dilatation occur, and systolic murmurs are often present.

The spleen is palpably enlarged in 10 to 15 per cent of cases, and in long-standing ones widening of the diploë of the skull similar to that seen in congenital hemolytic anemias may occur. These changes disappear after adequate therapy. The child with iron deficiency anemia may be obese or underweight with other evidences of undernutrition. Pica is sometimes prominent. The irritability and anorexia characteristic of advanced cases may reflect deficiency in tissue iron, for with iron therapy striking improvement in behavior frequently occurs before significant hematologic improvement.

Laboratory Data. In progressive iron deficiency a fairly definite sequence of biochemical and hematologic events occurs. First, the tissue iron stores represented by liver and bone marrow hemosiderin disappear. Next there is a decrease in serum iron to less than 50 μg. per 100 ml. Concomitantly, the iron-binding capacity of the serum increases to more than 350 μg. per 100 ml. and the per cent saturation falls below 15 per cent. As the deficiency progresses, hematologic changes ensue. The red cells become smaller than normal, their hemoglobin content decreases, and with increasing severity the red cells become deformed and misshapen. These changes result in the characteristic morphologic findings of microcytosis, hypochromia and poikilocytosis (Fig. 14-3, *D*), without which a diagnosis of significant iron deficiency anemia is untenable. The reticulocyte count is normal or minimally elevated; nucleated red cells may occasionally be seen in the peripheral blood. White blood cell counts are normal. Thrombocytosis, sometimes of a striking degree (600,000 to 1,000,000 per cu. mm.) may occur. On the other hand, in some cases significant thrombocytopenia is present. The mechanism of these platelet abnormalities is not clear; they return to normal with iron therapy. The bone marrow is hypercellular with erythroid hyperplasia. The normoblasts have scanty, fragmented cytoplasm with poor hemoglobinization. Leukocytes and megakaryocytes are normal.

Differential Diagnosis. Iron deficiency must be differentiated from other hypochromic microcytic anemias. The red cells in lead poisoning are morphologically similar, but coarse basophilic stippling of the red cells is prominent, and elevations of blood and urinary content of lead and of urinary coproporphyrins are seen in plumbism. The blood changes of thalassemia trait resemble those of iron deficiency, but characteristic alterations in the levels of Hgb. A_2 and Hgb. F are present, whereas they are not in iron deficiency. Thalassemia major with its pronounced erythroblastosis and hemolytic component should present no diagnostic confusion.

Treatment. Oral administration of simple ferrous salts (sulfate, gluconate, fumarate) provides inexpensive and satisfactory therapy. There is no evidence that addition of any trace metal, vitamin or other hematinic substance significantly increases the response to simple ferrous salts. On the other hand, absorption of some iron chelates may be suboptimal. For routine clinical use the physician should familiarize himself with an inexpensive preparation of one of the simple ferrous compounds. The therapeutic dose must be calculated in terms of elemental iron; ferrous sulfate is 20 per cent, and ferrous gluconate is 10 to 12 per cent elemental iron by weight. A daily total of 6 mg. per kg. of elemental iron in 3 divided doses provides an optimal amount of iron for the stimulated bone marrow to utilize. Doses of elemental iron in excess of 6 mg. per kg. per day do not result in a more rapid hematologic response. Better absorption may result when medicinal iron is given between meals. Ingestion of large amounts of milk may significantly decrease absorption of iron. Intolerance to oral iron is extremely rare; malabsorption of oral iron is more frequently invoked than documented. A parenteral iron preparation (iron-dextran) is currently available for pediatric use. This is an effective, reasonably safe form of iron when given in a properly calculated dose, but the response to parenteral iron is no more rapid or more complete than that obtained with proper administration of iron orally.

While adequate iron medication is given, the family must be educated about the patient's diet, and the consumption of milk should be limited to a reasonable quantity. When the re-education of child and parent is not successful, parenteral iron medication may be indicated. Within 72 to 96 hours after administration of iron to the anemic child, peripheral reticulocytosis is seen. The height of this response is inversely proportional to the severity of the anemia. Reticulocytosis is followed by a rise in the hemoglobin level, which may increase as much as 0.5 gm. per 100 ml. per day. Iron medication should be continued for 4 to 6 weeks after blood values are normal. Failures of iron therapy occur when the child does not receive the prescribed medication, when it is given in a form which is poorly absorbed, or when there is continuing unrecognized blood loss. An incorrect original diagnosis of iron deficiency anemia may be revealed by therapeutic failure of iron medication.

Since a rapid hematologic response can be confidently predicted in typical iron deficiency, blood transfusion is indicated only when the anemia is very severe or when superimposed infection may interfere with the response. It is not necessary and may be dangerous to attempt rapid correction of severe anemia by transfusion, owing to associated hypervolemia and cardiac dilatation. Slow administration of 5 ml. per kg. of packed or sedimented red cells is usually sufficient to raise the hemoglobin to a safe level, at which the response to iron therapy can be awaited.

INHERITED MICROCYTIC ANEMIAS

Although dietary deficiency of pyridoxine (vitamin B_6) does not ordinarily result in anemia, there is a rare form of severe hypochromic microcytic anemia with iron overload which is responsive to large amounts of pyridoxine. In most cases the abnormalities of tryptophan metabolism and other findings of B_6 deficiency are not seen. Familial incidence has been observed; males are more frequently involved.

Another variety of hereditary hypochromic microcytic anemia is transmitted as an X-linked recessive trait, but the biochemical defect is not known.

LEAD POISONING

(See also page 1486.)

Lead interferes with iron utilization and hemoglobin synthesis, so that a hypochromic microcytic anemia is a prominent finding in chronic lead poisoning. The red cells are hypochromic and microcytic, with coarse basophilic stippling. Examination of the red cells with the ultraviolet microscope reveals intense fluorescence due to markedly increased levels of protoporphyrin.

Hemolytic Anemias

The fundamental basis of the hemolytic anemias is a shortened survival time of the red blood cells. Red blood cells normally spend 100 to 120 days in the circulation; about 1 per cent of red cells (senescent ones) are removed from the blood each day and are replaced by an equal number of new cells released from the bone marrow.

In response to a shortened peripheral survival of red cells, the activity of bone marrow increases. The peripheral reticulocyte count exceeds 2.0 per cent. The sustained reticulocytosis in conjunction with a steady hemoglobin level is presumptive evidence of a hemolytic disorder. Hyperplasia of the erythropoietic marrow elements occurs, with lowering of the myeloid-erythroid ratio. In the chronic hemolytic processes of childhood, hypertrophy of the marrow may expand the medullary spaces and result in striking roentgenographic changes, particularly in the skull.

Products of red cell breakdown increase with hemolysis. Elevations of unconjugated (indirect) bilirubin accompany many hemolytic states, but if hepatic function is not impaired, readily distinguishable jaundice is unusual, and bilirubin levels may even be normal. Accelerated destruction of red cells increases the quantity of heme pigments excreted in the bile. These products of hemoglobin catabolism can be quantitated by the tedious and unesthetic measurement of fecal urobilinogen. Pigmented gallstones composed of calcium bilirubinate may be formed as early as 4 years of age, and a chronic hemolytic process should be considered likely in any case of cholelithiasis in childhood. Plasma concentrations of hemoglobin increase in hemolytic anemias, and the free hemoglobin combines irreversibly with specific binding proteins called haptoglobins. The large haptoglobin-hemoglobin complex is cleared from the circulation by reticuloendothelial activity. In severe hemolytic states the loss of haptoglobin exceeds the synthetic capacity of the liver, and serum haptoglobin is decreased or absent.

In addition to these indirect indicators of hemolysis, red cell survival can be directly estimated by isotopic techniques. Sodium chromate ($Na_2{}^{51}CrO_4$) and diisofluorophosphate ($DF^{32}P$) are the radioactive compounds most often used as red cell "tags." The ^{51}Cr technique is the most frequently used because of its simplicity. After injection of ^{51}Cr-tagged red cells, blood radioactivity normally decreases to 50 per cent of its initial level in 25 to 35 days (^{51}Cr T$^{1/2}$ or half-life). A shortened red cell survival is likely when the ^{51}Cr T$^{1/2}$ is reduced below 20 days. $DF^{32}P$ is expensive and more difficult to count, but permits an actual measurement of red cell survival. In practice, it is rarely necessary to use these specialized isotopic techniques.

The stimulated normal bone marrow can ordinarily increase its output sixfold to eightfold. By such compensation red cell survival can theoretically be reduced to 15 to 20 days without producing anemia, but most often in childhood chronic hemolysis results in some degree of anemia. Patients with hemolytic anemias of whatever type may have transient episodes of bone marrow failure. These *aplastic crises* are characterized by reticulocytopenia and markedly decreased numbers of red cell precursors in the marrow. Profound and life-threatening anemia may develop quickly because the shortened red cell survival is no longer even partially compensated. These episodes of acute marrow failure are self-limited and last 10 to 14 days. Aplastic crises are usually associated with infection, and may occur within a few days in several affected members of a family.

The hemolytic anemias may be divided into 2 large classes: (1) those due to premature destruction by intrinsic abnormalities of the red cell and (2) those due to noxious extraerythrocytic factors. Table 14-4 lists the important hemolytic anemias of childhood. In hemolytic states associated with intrinsic defects, red cell survival is short in normal persons receiving a transfusion of the patient's red cells, as well as in patients themselves. In contrast, red cells from patients with anemias due to extrinsic factors have an adequate life span when transfused to a normal recipient.

Hemolytic Anemias Due to Intrinsic Abnormalities of the Red Cell

HEREDITARY SPHEROCYTOSIS
(Congenital Hemolytic Anemia; Congenital Acholuric Jaundice)

This is the most common of the hereditary hemolytic states in which there is no abnormality of hemoglobin. The classic features are a congenital and familial hemolytic process associated with splenomegaly and with red cells which are spherical in shape. Typical cases have been reported in most ethnic groups, but the disease is particularly prevalent among persons of northern European origin.

Etiology. Hereditary spherocytosis is transmitted as an autosomal dominant trait. About 20 per cent of cases are sporadic and presumably represent new mutations. Although he basic defect has not been precisely delineated, its expression is an abnormality of the red cell membrane, which renders these cells unduly permeable to sodium. An increased concentration of intracellular sodium leads to an increased utilization of ATP to drive the so-called cation pump. Premature senescence and destruction of red cells are thought to result from metabolic overwork. Spherocytosis is the morphologic expression of these biochemical abnormalities.

The spleen is intimately involved in the hemolytic process. The splenic circulation imposes a metabolic environment which is particularly stressful to the spherocytic cell, and damage from repeated passages through this unfavorable environment results in their sequestration and destruction. The hemolytic process abates after splenectomy, even though the biochemical and morphologic abnormalities persist.

Clinical Manifestations. The disease has its onset in infancy and may present in the neonatal period with anemia and hyperbilirubinemia severe enough to require exchange transfusions. The anemia varies considerably in severity during infancy and childhood, but tends to be similar within families. Slight jaundice is usually present. Moderate expansion of the marrow cavity of the skull may occur, but not so extreme as in thalassemia or the hemoglobinopathies. After infancy the spleen is almost always palpably enlarged. Although pigmentary gallstones have been reported as early as 4 to 5 years of age, they usually do not develop until late childhood or adolescence. Approximately 85 per cent of untreated patients will ultimately form gallstones. Aplastic crises are the most serious complications which occur during childhood.

Laboratory Data. The usual evidences of hemolysis, including reticulocytosis, anemia and hyperbilirubinemia, are present. The characteristic spherocytic red cell is smaller than the normal erythrocyte and lacks the central pallor of the biconcave disk (Fig. 14-3, *B*). This morphologic change may be subtle, and only a relatively small proportion of the cells may be spherocytic. Though there is erythroid hyperplasia in the bone, the red cell precursors are not spherocytic. There are no abnormal hemoglobins.

The basic abnormality of the red cell can be demonstrated by osmotic fragility studies. When red cells are placed in hypotonic saline solutions, water enters the cells, causing them to swell. The normal red cell of biconcave shape can increase its volume, but the spherical cell already contains the maximum volume for its surface area. Imbi-

bition of small amounts of water causes the spherocyte to rupture. In 10 to 20 per cent of cases of hereditary spherocytosis the abnormality may be demonstrated only if the blood is incubated at 37°C. for 24 hours before determining osmotic fragility. The autohemolysis test is also useful in hereditary spherocytosis. When normal blood is incubated under sterile conditions for 48 hours at 37°C., less than 5 per cent of the red cells hemolyze. Red cells of patients with hereditary spherocytosis have markedly increased rates of autohemolysis (15 to 45 per cent). Abnormal autohemolysis can be corrected by the addition of small amounts of glucose to the blood before incubation.

Differential Diagnosis. Hereditary spherocytosis must be differentiated from other congenital hemolytic states. The family history, blood smear, and studies of osmotic fragility and autohemolysis are of most diagnostic value. Acquired spherocytosis of the red cells is seen in autoimmune hemolytic anemias; here the spherocytosis is more noticeable than in hereditary spherocytosis, and the Coombs test result is usually positive. It may be difficult to differentiate hereditary spherocytosis in the newborn infant from hemolytic disease due to A or B incompatibility when an appropriate blood group incompatibility is coincidentally present. A period of observation may be necessary to clarify the diagnosis.

Treatment. Splenectomy invariably produces a clinical cure. Elective splenectomy should be planned for the patient at 4 to 6 years of age. If anemia is severe enough to impair growth or if aplastic crises are frequent, the operation may be performed earlier. Splenectomy prevents gallstones and eliminates the threat of aplastic crises. After splenectomy, jaundice and reticulocytosis rapidly disappear, and the hemoglobin attains the normal range. Thrombocytosis may occur in the immediate postoperative period, but anticoagulation therapy is not routinely indicated. The syndrome of overwhelming sepsis after splenectomy is not a significant threat to patients with hereditary spherocytosis.

HEREDITARY ELLIPTOCYTOSIS

Oval or elliptical shape of red cells occurs as a benign, dominantly inherited morphologic curiosity in about 1 in 2000 persons (Fig. 14-4, *E*). Hemolysis is not usually present; however, in about 10 per cent of cases there may be a significant hemolytic anemia.

Etiology. The cause is uncertain. Family studies of affected children usually reveal one parent with elliptocytosis without hemolysis, while the other parent is normal. A few cases may have represented homozygous inheritance. The gene for elliptocytosis is sometimes linked with the Rh locus. No biochemical abnormality of the red cell has been defined.

Clinical Manifestations. Hemolytic elliptocytosis may manifest as jaundice in the neonatal period even though characteristic morphologic abnormalities may not be evident at that time. The usual features of a chronic hemolytic process are seen later, manifest by anemia, jaundice, splenomegaly and osseous changes. Cholelithiasis may occur in late childhood, and aplastic rises have been reported.

Laboratory Data. The morphology of the red blood cells is the most important diagnostic feature (Fig. 14-4, *F*). Elliptical cells are prominent, but many bizarre poikilocytes, microcytes and spherocytes are also present. The reticulocyte count is greatly increased. Erythroid hyperplasia is present in the bone marrow, but red cell precursors are not elliptical. There is no abnormal hemoglobin.

Treatment. Splenectomy decreases the hemolytic component of this disease and should be performed if there is significant chronic hemolysis. The red cell morphology is not corrected by the operation and may be considerably more abnormal in the postoperative period.

OTHER STRUCTURAL DEFECTS

Paroxysmal Nocturnal Hemoglobinuria. Paroxysmal nocturnal hemoglobinuria is a rare chronic anemia with prominent intravascular hemolysis. The hemolysis is characteristically worse during sleep, and morning hemoglobinuria is a classic finding. The disease is not congenital. It results from an ill-defined intrinsic defect of the red cell, which renders it susceptible to hemolysis in an acid medium. In addition to chronic hemolysis, there may be pancytopenia. Pyogenic infection and thrombosis are serious complications. Since a number of cases have followed aplastic anemia, it has been suggested that the same agent causing aplastic anemia may predispose to paroxysmal nocturnal hemoglobinuria. The diagnosis is established by a positive result in the acid hemolysin test. Splenectomy is not indicated. Prolonged anticoagulation therapy may be of benefit when thromboses occur.

Hereditary Stomatocytosis. Hereditary stomatocytosis is a rare morphologic abnormality of the red cells, characterized by a mouthlike slit in place of the usual circular area of central pallor. There may be hemolytic anemia. Extreme permeability of the red cell membrane to cations has been observed in one patient. Splenectomy has not been consistently effective, but may be indicated in patients with severe hemolysis.

Acanthocytosis. In this rare defect of lipid metabolism the distorted red cells have sharp projections (Fig. 14-4, *C*), but there is no hemolytic anemia. The striking morphologic changes presumably result from decreased levels of cholesterol and beta-lipoprotein in the serum. (See A-beta-lipoproteinemia, page 812.)

ENZYMATIC DEFECTS OF THE RED CELLS

Development of techniques for quantitating various red cell enzymes has permitted the identification of a number of specific entities within a group of diseases which have been collectively identified as congenital nonspherocytic hemolytic anemias because of the lack of spherocytes and normal osmotic fragility. Abnormalities of enzymes may involve the major pathways of glucose catabolism, the anaerobic Embden-Meyerhof pathway or the oxidative pentose phosphate shunt (Fig. 14-2).

PYRUVATE KINASE DEFICIENCY

This congenital hemolytic anemia is due to the homozygous occurrence of an autosomal gene which carries a decided reduction of red cell pyruvate kinase activity. Generation of ATP is impaired, and the life span of the red cell is reduced because of a deficient source of energy.

Clinical Manifestations and Laboratory Data. Jaundice and anemia may be manifest in the neonatal period. During later life the severity of the hemolytic component varies considerably. Spherocytes are not found in the peripheral blood, and osmotic fragility is normal. Autohemolysis is moderately or markedly increased, but glucose does not regularly correct this abnormality, as it does in hereditary spherocytosis. Diagnosis is based upon demonstration of reduced pyruvate kinase activity of the red cells. Heterozygous parents of patients have moderately reduced activity of this enzyme. Other red cell enzymes are normal or elevated. There are no abnormalities of hemoglobin, and the white blood cells have normal pyruvate kinase activity.

Treatment. Transfusions are indicated for profound anemia or aplastic crises. Splenectomy is not curative, but may be beneficial when there is a severe hemolytic component.

DEFICIENCIES OF OTHER GLYCOLYTIC ENZYMES

Inherited deficiencies of red cell hexokinase, triphosphate isomerase, 2-3 diphosphoglycerate mutase and possibly adenosine triphosphatase have been responsible for congenital nonspherocytic hemolytic anemia. The red cell morphology and osmotic fragility are normal. Splenectomy has not been beneficial. It is likely that other inborn errors of red cell metabolism will be described as enzymatic studies are extended.

DEFICIENCIES OF ENZYMES OF THE PENTOSE PHOSPHATE PATHWAY AND RELATED COMPOUNDS

The most important function of the pentose pathway, through which about 10 per cent of the glucose utilized by the red cell passes, is to provide reduced triphosphopyridine nucleotide (TPNH, NaDPH$_2$) for the red cell. TPNH, in turn, is necessary for conversion of oxidized to reduced glutathione, which is essential for the physiologic inactivation of oxidant compounds such as hydrogen peroxide which accumulate within the red cell. If glutathione or any of the compounds or enzymes necessary for maintaining it in the reduced state are decreased, hemoglobin may become denatured and precipitated into red cell inclusions called *Heinz bodies*. Once Heinz bodies have formed, the red cell is rapidly removed from the circulation.

GLUCOSE 6-PHOSPHATE DEHYDROGENASE DEFICIENCY (G-6-PD)

G-6-PD deficiency, the most important disease in this group, is responsible for 2 clinical syndromes: an episodic hemolytic anemia induced by certain drugs, and a spontaneous chronic nonspherocytic hemolytic anemia.

Drug-Induced Hemolytic Anemia Associated with G-6-PD Deficiency
(PRIMAQUINE SENSITIVITY)

Synthesis of red cell G-6-PD is determined by genes borne on the X chromosome. Diseases involving this enzyme occur, therefore, more frequently in males than in females. About 10 per cent of American Negro males and 2 per cent of Negro females have a defect which results in a deficiency of red cell G-6-PD. Italians, Greeks and other Mediterranean, Middle Eastern, African and Oriental ethnic groups also have high frequencies ranging from 5 to 40 per cent. The G-6-PD activity of the homozygous female or the hemizygous male is one tenth to one twentieth of normal. The heterozygous female has an intermediate enzymatic activity, and, as an example of random X chromosome inactivation (Lyon hypothesis), has 2 populations of red cells; one is normal, the other deficient in G-6-PD activity. The heterozygous female does not, however, have clinical hemolysis after exposure to oxidant drugs. There appears to be considerable variation in the defect among various racial groups; the defect in Negroes is less severe than in affected Caucasians. The basic defect appears to be production of an unstable enzyme which becomes inactive much more rapidly than normal.

In the usual pattern of G-6-PD deficiency no evidence of hemolysis is apparent until 48 to 96 hours after the patient has ingested a substance which has oxidant properties. Drugs which have these properties include antipyretics, sulfonamides, antimalarials and naphthaquinolones. The fava bean, a Mideastern dietary staple, is also particularly potent. The degree of hemolysis varies with the agent and the amount ingested. In severe cases, hemoglobinuria and jaundice are seen and the hemoglobin concentration may decrease 60 to 70 per cent. Even if administration of the responsible drug is continued, recovery is the rule, with evidence of a compensated hemolytic process. Occasionally infection may result in a moderate degree of hemolysis. This defect may be a cause of neonatal hyperbilirubinemia and kernicterus in Greek and Chinese newborn infants.

Laboratory Data. Hemoglobinemia and hemoglobinuria are manifest in severe acute cases. Unstained or supravital preparations of the red cell reveal the multiple small round inclusions called Heinz bodies, which are not visible on Wright-stained blood smears. Because cells containing these inclusions are rapidly removed from the circulation, they are not seen after the first 3 to 4 days of illness. Recovery is heralded by reticulocytosis and increase in hemoglobin concentration.

Diagnosis is dependent upon direct or indirect demonstration of reduced G-6-PD activity in red cells. By direct measurement, enzyme activity in affected persons is one tenth of normal or less. Satisfactory screening tests are based upon decoloration of methylene blue and upon reduction of methemoglobin. Immediately after a hemolytic episode reticulocytes and young red cells predominate. These young cells have significantly higher enzyme activity than older cells; therefore testing may have to be deferred for a few weeks before a diagnostically low level of enzyme can be shown.

Treatment. Prevention of hemolysis constitutes the most important therapeutic measure. When possible, males belonging to ethnic groups in which there is a significant incidence of G-6-PD deficiency should be tested for the defect before drugs are given which are known to be oxidant. When hemolysis has occurred, supportive therapy may include blood transfusions. Spontaneous recovery is the rule.

Other Hemolytic Anemias Associated with Deficiencies of G-6-PD and Related Substances

A rare form of chronic nonspherocytic hemolytic anemia has been associated with profound deficiency or absence of G-6-PD. The anemia is inherited as an X-linked recessive, and most reported cases have been in males of northern European origin. Chronic hemolytic anemia is maintained, and worsening of the hemolytic process may follow ingestion of oxidant drugs. Splenectomy is of no value. A mild, chronic nonspherocytic anemia has also been reported in association with a genetically determined deficiency of red cell glutathione.

6-Phosphogluconic dehydrogenase deficiency has been associated with drug hemolysis. Hyperbilirubinemia has been related to a deficiency of glutathione peroxidase in several newborn infants.

HEMOGLOBINOPATHIES

The clinically important abnormal hemoglobin syndromes result from single amino acid substitutions in the alpha or beta chains of adult hemoglobin. Although a large number of hemoglobin variants have been described, only a few of these are relatively prevalent.

Tremendous advances have been made in the biochemical characterization of the hemoglobins. Alpha and beta chains consist of about 150 amino acids, and the precise sequence of these amino acids in the polypeptide chains has been defined by a sophisticated analytic technique called "fingerprinting." By means of this technique it is possible to localize precisely and identify single amino acid substitutions which result in the abnormal hemoglobins (see also pp. 413 and 1041).

SICKLE CELL HEMOGLOBINOPATHIES

The sickle cell hemoglobinopathies serve as superb models for demonstrating the mechanism of molecular disease, from the levels of gene structure and action to the ultimate clinical syndrome in the patient. The basic defect is a mutant, autosomal gene which causes a valine residue to be substituted for a glutamic acid one in the no. 6 position of a beta polypeptide chain ($\alpha_2\beta_2^{6\ val.}$). This minor substitution has profound physiochemical consequences: deoxygenation results in a surface change which facilitates stacking of sickle hemoglobin molecules into monofilaments, which aggregate into elongated crystals, distorting the red cell membrane and forming the sickle cell.

Sickle Cell Trait. Heterozygous occurrence of the sickle gene is associated with a benign clinical course. About 10 per cent of American Negroes have the trait; there is a much greater prevalence in parts of Africa. Typical cases also occur in other ethnic groups from Mediterranean and Mid- and Near-Eastern areas. Possession of a sickle gene is believed to confer a degree of resistance to falciparum malaria. The individual red cells of persons with the trait contain a mixture of normal and sickle hemoglobins (Hgb. A and Hgb. S). The Hgb. S proportion varies from 25 to 45 per cent. With these low proportions of Hgb. S, sickling does not occur under physiologic conditions. On rare occasions severe hypoxia resulting from shock or flying at high altitudes in unpressurized aircraft may be associated with vaso-occlusive phenomena. Spontaneous hematuria, usually from the left kidney, and hyposthenuria may also occur; but anemia, hemolysis or other clinical abnormalities are not generally attributable to the uncomplicated sickle trait.

Sickle Cell Anemia

Sickle cell anemia is a severe, chronic hemolytic anemia occurring in persons homozygous for the sickle gene. The clinical course is marked by episodes of pain due to occlusion of small blood vessels by spontaneously sickled red cells.

Clinical Manifestations. Manifestations of sickle cell disease do not usually appear until the latter part of the first year of life. Coincidentally with the postnatal decrease in Hgb. F, the concentration of Hgb. S rises. Intravascular sickling and evidences of a hemolytic process then occur. Patients with sickle cell anemia experience episodes which traditionally have been called "crises." These are of several varieties, however, and the "crisis" is not a specific diagnostic entity.

Most frequent are the painful or *thrombotic crises.* These result from occlusion of small blood vessels with distal ischemia and infarction. They may be precipitated by infections or develop spontaneously in any or in many parts of the body. Symmetrical, painful swelling of the hands and feet (hand-foot syndrome) caused by infarction in the small bones of the extremities may be the initial manifestation of sickle cell anemia in infancy. Striking bony destruction with periosteal reaction may be observed radiographically. In older patients the large joints and surrounding parts may become painful and swollen. Severe abdominal pains, resembling those of an acute surgical condition of the abdomen, are often due to splenic infarction. Strokes due to cerebral occlusion are serious and, if not immediately fatal, may leave hemiplegias. Extensive pulmonary infarction is difficult to differentiate from pneumonia. Thrombotic crises are not associated with pronounced changes in the hematologic picture.

A second type of crisis, seen only in the young patient, is the so-called *sequestration crisis.* For unknown reasons large amounts of blood become acutely pooled in the liver and the spleen. The spleen becomes massively enlarged, and signs of circulatory collapse develop rapidly. If the patient is supported by hydration and by blood transfusion, much of the sequestered blood is remobilized. This sort of episode is a frequent cause of death in the infant with sickle cell disease and occurs in older patients with sickle cell variants in whom splenomegaly persists into later life.

The third well characterized type of crisis is the *aplastic crisis* previously described (p. 1052).

Hyperhemolytic crises are unusual, but may result when a person with homozygous sickle cell disease, who coincidentally has G-6-PD deficiency, ingests an oxidant drug.

In addition to the acute crises, a wide variety of clinical signs and symptoms result from severe hemolytic anemia and chronic vaso-occlusive disease. Progressive impairment of liver function contributes to the visible jaundice these patients regularly demonstrate. Gallstones have been seen in patients as young as 3 years of age. Renal function is progressively impaired by diffuse glomerular and tubular fibrosis. The spleen is initially considerably enlarged, but, because of repeated infarctions, soon becomes small and fibrotic, and is rarely palpable after childhood. Persons with sickle cell disease appear to have an unusual susceptibility to salmonella osteomyelitis and pneumococcal septicemia. Although growth may be initially normal, by later childhood most of these patients are underweight, and puberty is delayed. As a consequence of the varied and severe problems, many of these patients die during the first 2 decades of life.

Laboratory Data. Hemoglobin concentrations range from 6 to 8 gm. per 100 ml. A peripheral blood smear usually contains sickled cells (Fig. 14-4, *D*). Observation of spontaneous sickling almost always indicates classic homozygous sickle cell disease; it is not observed in the trait and is infrequently present in the sickle cell variants. Target cells, poikilocytes and hypochromia are frequently seen. The reticulocyte count ranges from 5 to 15 per cent, and nucleated red cells and Howell-Jolly bodies are often present. The total white blood cell count is elevated to 15,000 to 25,000 per cu. mm. with a predominance of neutrophils. The platelet count may be increased; the sedimentation rate is slow. Other changes include abnormal liver function test results, hyperbilirubinemia and diffuse hypergammaglobulinemia. The bone marrow is markedly hyperplastic.

Study of the red cells and hemoglobin is essential to establish the diagnosis. The most rapid and simple test to determine the presence of Hgb. S is the sickle cell preparation, in which red cells are deoxygenated or exposed to reducing agents such as sodium metabisulfite. Virtually 100 per cent of the red cells can be induced to sickle in both sickle disease and sickle trait; but sickling is more rapid and extreme in the disease state than in the trait. A decreased percentage of sickling occurs only after transfusion or during early infancy. Electrophoretic examination of hemoglobin is important for precise diagnosis. After infancy the red cells of patients with sickle cell anemia contain approximately 90 per cent Hgb. S, 2 to 10 per cent Hgb. F, and a normal amount of Hgb. A_2. No Hgb. A is present. Each parent has either the sickle cell trait or one of the sickle variants.

Differential Diagnosis. Sickle cell disease may be associated with a wide variety of clinical signs and symptoms. The presence of painful joints plus the heart murmurs of anemia may suggest acute rheumatic fever or rheumatoid arthritis. Osteomyelitis and leukemia are occasionally difficult to differentiate. Because of the varied signs and symptoms of sickle cell anemia, it is important to perform electrophoretic studies on Negro patients whose red cells sickle, particularly if they are anemic.

Treatment. No therapy is necessary, except during acute episodes. Administration of extra quantities of vitamins and of hematinics is of no value; iron therapy is contraindicated. There is no treatment of the painful crisis which has proved of consistent value. Analgesics are usually sufficient for the discomfort and pain. Dehydration and acidosis should be vigorously corrected. Complicating bacterial infections require appropriate antibiotic therapy. Blood transfusions are of little benefit during the painful crises, but are essential in sequestration and aplastic episodes. Splenectomy is not indicated unless recurrent sequestration crises have occurred or hypersplenism can be shown to be present.

OTHER HEMOGLOBINOPATHIES

Hemoglobin C ($\alpha_2\beta_2^{6\ \text{lys.}}$). Hemoglobin C, an abnormal hemoglobin with slow electrophoretic mobility, occurs in about 2 per cent of American Negroes. In the heterozygous state (Hgb. AC) no anemia or disease is present, although increased numbers of target cells are seen in the peripheral blood. In the homozygous person (Hgb. CC disease) a moderately severe hemolytic anemia and splenomegaly are observed. The peripheral blood contains a striking number of target cells (Fig. 14-3, *F*).

Hemoglobin D. Hemoglobin D represents several varieties of abnormal hemoglobin with electrophoretic mobilities similar to that of Hgb. S, but with different biochemical and physical properties. Sickling does not occur in Hgb. D syndromes. The homozygous state (Hgb. DD) is characterized by a mild hemolytic anemia with splenomegaly.

Hemoglobin E ($\alpha_2\beta_2^{26\ \text{lys.}}$). Hemoglobin E is prevalent in persons from Southeast Asia, particularly Thailand. The clinical and hematologic findings are similar to those associated with Hgb. C.

Hemoglobin S-C Disease. When the genes for both Hgb. S and Hgb. C are present in the same person, a moderately severe anemia with splenomegaly results. Although there are thrombotic episodes, they are usually less frequent and milder than those of sickle cell disease. Aseptic necrosis of the femoral head is an occasional complication. The hemoglobin concentration averages 9 to 10 gm. per 100 ml. Target cells are numerous, but sickled cells are usually not present. Hemoglobin electrophoresis reveals a nearly equal mixture of Hgb. S and Hgb. C with slight elevation of Hgb. F. Aplastic and sequestration crises are potential threats to life. Hgb. S-C disease does not usually affect growth and is compatible with survival into adult life.

Miscellaneous Hemoglobins. A group of recently described hemoglobins are associated with molecular instability, resulting in spontaneous denaturation and precipitation of the hemoglobin within the red cells. Among these unstable variants is *hemoglobin Zurich*, with which hemolysis occurs only when sulfonamides are ingested. *Hemoglobin Köln* and other similar heat-precipitable variants are associated with chronic hemolysis and with the presence of Heinz bodies in the circulating red cells, especially after splenectomy.

The *hemoglobin M diseases* are dominantly inherited methemoglobinemias associated with the presence of abnormal hemoglobin variants. The amino acid substitutions are strategically located in respect to a heme group so that a stable complex is formed with the iron moiety. This combination converts iron to the trivalent or oxidized form characteristic of methemoglobin. With the hemoglobin M variants resulting from beta chain substitutions, cyanosis is not present in the first few months of life, whereas in alpha chain variants cyanosis is congenital.

THALASSEMIA
(Mediterranean Anemia)

The thalassemias are a group of heritable hypochromic microcytic anemias of varying degrees of severity. The genetic defect results in deficient synthesis of adult hemoglobin (Hgb. A). There may be a severe hemolytic process. Unlike other hemoglobinopathies, no abnormal hemoglobin can be demonstrated, but characteristic alterations in the proportions of Hgb. A_2 and Hgb. F are seen. The most common genetic variety of thalassemia is associated with impaired production of beta-polypeptide chains and is called β-thalassemia. Although the gene is relatively prevalent among so-called Mediterranean peoples, typical cases occur in most racial groups. Like the sickle gene, that of thalassemia appears to be associated with resistance to malaria, which may account for its geographic distribution. Most cases can be clinically classified as thalassemia minor or major, corresponding in general to a heterozygous or homozygous genotype.

Thalassemia Minor (Thalassemia Trait). Heterozygous thalassemia is associated with mild anemia. The hemoglobin concentration averages 2 to 3 gm. per 100 ml. lower than normal. The red cells are hypochromic and microcytic and manifest poikilocytosis, ovalocytosis and sometimes basophilic stippling (Fig. 14-4, *A*). Target cells are present, but usually are not prominent and should not be considered specific for thalassemia. Although a mild decrease in red cell survival can be documented, no overt signs of hemolysis are present. The serum iron level is normal or elevated. More than 90 per cent of persons with the β-thalassemia trait have diagnostic elevations of Hgb. A_2 to 3.4 to 7.0 per cent. About 50 per cent of affected persons have slight elevations of Hgb. F, from 2 to 6 per cent. A small proportion of them have normal levels of Hgb. A_2, with Hgb. F levels ranging from 7 to 15 per cent.

Thalassemia Major
(Cooley's Anemia)

Homozygous thalassemia becomes symptomatic as a severe, progressive hemolytic anemia during

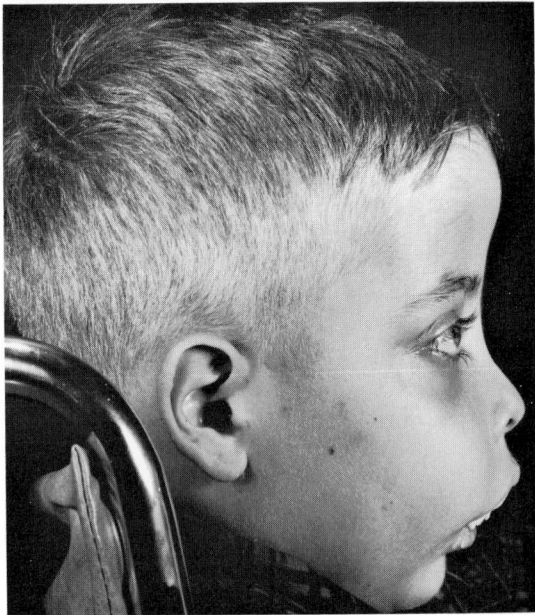

Figure 14-5. Appearance of patient with thalassemia major (Cooley's anemia). Note the maxillary hyperplasia and resulting dental abnormality.

the second 6 months of life. Regularly spaced blood transfusions are necessary to prevent profound weakness and cardiac decompensation due to anemia. In response to severe anemia and hemolysis, hypertrophy of erythropoietic tissue occurs in medullary and extramedullary locations. The bones become thin, and pathologic fractures may occur. Massive expansion of the marrow of the face and skull (Figs. 14-5, 14-6) produces a typical facies. Pallor, hemosiderosis and jaundice combine to produce a greenish-brown complexion. The spleen and liver are enlarged because of extra-

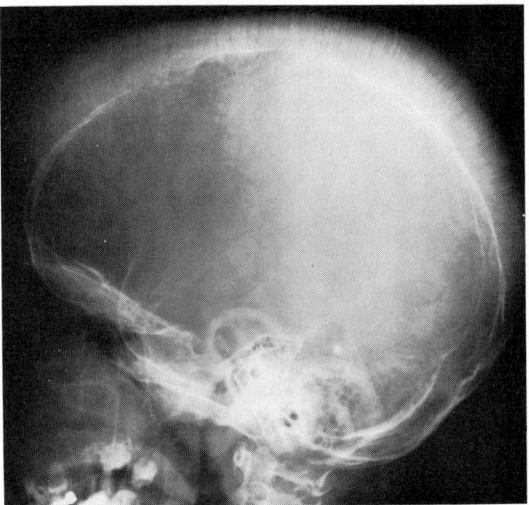

Figure 14-6. Roentgenogram of skull, showing overgrowth of the maxilla with opacification of the sinuses. The diploic spaces are widened with prominent vertical trabeculae (hair on end).

medullary hematopoiesis and hemosiderosis. In older patients the spleen may reach such proportions that it causes mechanical discomfort and secondary hypersplenism. Growth is impaired in older children, and puberty rarely occurs. Cardiac complications such as pericarditis and chronic congestive heart failure are frequent terminal events; death usually occurs during the second decade.

Laboratory Data. The red cell changes of thalassemia major are extreme. In addition to severe hypochromia and microcytosis (Fig. 14-4, *B*), many bizarre, fragmented poikilocytes and target cells are present. Large numbers of nucleated red cells circulate, especially after splenectomy. Intraerythrocytic precipitations thought to represent excess alpha chains are also seen after splenectomy. In the usual case the hemoglobin level falls progressively to less than 5 gm. per 100 ml. unless transfusions are given, but about 10 per cent of patients with homozygous thalassemia can maintain hemoglobin levels of 6 to 8 gm. per 100 ml. without transfusions. The unconjugated serum bilirubin level is elevated. The concentration of serum iron is high, with saturation of the iron-binding capacity. Progressive dysfunction of the liver and occasionally of the pancreas may occur as a result of hemosiderosis.

A striking biochemical characteristic is the presence of large amounts of fetal hemoglobin in the red cells. The level of Hgb. F is greater than 50 per cent during the early years of life, but has a tendency to decline with increasing age. Quantitation of fetal hemoglobin is imprecise because of frequent transfusions. Hemoglobin A_2 level is usually less than 3 per cent, but the ratio of Hgb. A_2 to Hgb. A is markedly increased.

Treatment. Transfusion is the only therapy available for these children. Hematinics are of no regular value, and iron is contraindicated. Transfusions should be given to maintain the hemoglobin above a level which permits activity with comfort. This is usually about 6 gm. per 100 ml. Careful cross matching should be performed to forestall isoimmunization, and the use of packed, fresh red cells is desirable. Experimental programs are currently evaluating the possible benefit of maintaining the hemoglobin at nearly normal levels by a more vigorous transfusion regimen, but long-term advantages of such a program have not been proved. Increases in hemoglobin levels are beneficial when cardiac complications develop. Hemosiderosis is an inevitable consequence of prolonged transfusion therapy; removal of iron by various chelating agents has not been sufficiently effective to warrant routine use. Splenectomy is often necessary because of the massive size of the organ or because of secondary hypersplenism, but has no effect on the basic hematologic disease. In a large number of patients who have had splenectomy severe, overwhelming sepsis may develop, and for this reason the operation should be performed only for significant indications and should be deferred if possible until after infancy or early childhood.

Other Thalassemic Syndromes

Hemoglobin S-Thalassemia. Combination of a thalassemia gene with that of an abnormal beta-chain hemoglobin results in clinical disease more severe than either trait alone. Hemoglobin S-thalassemia is a moderately severe hemolytic anemia with mild to moderate vaso-occlusive symptoms and significant splenomegaly. The hemoglobin electrophoretic pattern shows a predominance of Hgb. S, ranging from 60 to 80 per cent, the remainder being Hgb. F and Hgb. A. In some instances no Hgb. A can be detected, and the electrophoretic pattern is indistinguishable from that of sickle cell disease. In such instances family studies will usually reveal one parent to have thalassemia trait and the other, the sickle cell trait.

Hemoglobin C-Thalassemia and D-Thalassemia. Hemoglobin C-thalassemia and D-thalassemia are mild hemolytic anemias with significant splenomegaly. Hemoglobin electrophoresis reveals that the abnormal hemoglobin, C or D, constitutes more than 60 per cent of the total.

Alpha-Thalassemia. A group of diseases resulting from genetically determined blocks in alpha-chain synthesis are called α-thalassemia. No specific alterations in the proportions of the minor hemoglobins A_2 or F are seen in the heterozygous state. Special techniques may reveal traces of hemoglobin tetramers lacking alpha chains (Hgb. H and Barts) within the red cells. In the homozygous state, α-thalassemia produces the clinical picture of hydrops fetalis. In these cases the predominant hemoglobin is Hgb. Barts, γ_4. This variant has abnormal oxygen dissociation properties which make oxygen unavailable to the tissues under physiologic conditions.

Alpha-thalassemia is also involved in the Hgb. H syndromes. These are moderately severe anemias resembling Cooley's anemia. They are characterized, however, by the presence of a fast-moving, unstable hemoglobin component called Hgb. H or β_4. The combination of α-thalassemia with genes for beta-chain hemoglobin abnormalities or β-thalassemia results in hematologic diseases which are no more severe than with either trait alone.

Hereditary Persistence of High Fetal Hemoglobin. This interesting condition is associated with very high levels of normal fetal hemoglobin, but with no other abnormalities. It is thought to result from a genetically determined inability to convert from gamma- to beta-chain synthesis at the time of birth. The trait occurs most frequently in Negroes, Italians and Greeks. In the heterozygous person the level of Hgb. F is 20 to 30 per cent. There is an even distribution of fetal hemoglobin through the red cell population, in contrast to the thalassemias, in which Hgb. F content shows variation from cell to cell. A single instance of homozygosity for the high fetal gene has been observed. This patient's hemoglobin was completely Hgb. F, but he had no significant hematologic disease. When both the high fetal gene and the sickle gene are present in the same person, hematologic manifestations are very mild. The large amount of Hgb. F prevents the sickling process under physiologic conditions.

Hemolytic Anemias Due to Extrinsic (Extracellular) Abnormalities of the Red Cell

A number of agents with capacity to damage red blood cells may lead to their premature destruction. Among the most clearly defined of these are antibodies associated with immune hemolytic anemias. These antibodies, directed against specific intrinsic antigens, so damage the red cell that viability is compromised and rapid destruction ensues. The hallmark of this group of diseases is the positive result of the Coombs test, which detects a coating of immunoglobulin on the red cell surface. The most important immune hemolytic disorder encountered in pediatric practice is hemolytic disease of the newborn (erythroblastosis fetalis), caused by passive transplacental transfer of a maternal antibody active against the red cells of the fetus.

HEMOLYTIC DISEASES OF THE NEWBORN DUE TO Rh INCOMPATIBILITY

Human red cells contain a complex system of genetically related antigens designated the Rh system. The genetics of Rh is complex and is becoming increasingly more difficult to comprehend as new factors and interrelations are described. More than 25 blood factors are currently known to belong to the Rh system. From a practical point of view, the important Rh antigens may be divided into 3 sets: D (Rho) and its allele d (hr$_o$); C (rh') and c (hr'); and E (rh'') and e (hr''). These antigens are inherited as linked groups, and each individual possesses 3 sets, e.g. $\frac{CDE}{cde}$, of the 6 basic antigens. Of the large number of possible combinations, only about a half dozen reach appreciable frequency. The antigen D (Rho) is responsible for most cases of severe hemolytic disease of the newborn.

Pathogenesis. Approximately 15 per cent of Caucasian women and men are Rh-negative (d/d). Their red cells do not have the D antigen; when Rh-positive blood is infused into such women, they usually become immunized. Modern procedures have virtually eliminated mismatched blood transfusions as a basis for sensitization, and almost all cases now result from pregnancy. Minute quantities of fetal blood enter the maternal circulation during pregnancy and especially at delivery. If this transfused fetal blood contains the D antigen inherited from an Rh-positive father, primary maternal sensitization may occur.

Fortunately, only about 5 per cent of Rh-negative women ever have babies with hemolytic disease. This lower than expected incidence is due to several factors: most importantly, sensitization rarely occurs during the first pregnancy, and small family size reduces the chances of sensitization. The genotype of the father is also important, for about 55 per cent of Rh-positive men are heterozygous (D/d) and may have Rh-negative offspring. Finally, the capacity of Rh-negative women to form antibodies appears to be variable, some producing very low titers even after adequate challenge. When primary sensitization of a woman has occurred, her subsequent Rh-positive infants are at risk. If maternal antibodies reach a sufficiently high level, they may cross the placenta and become fixed to the fetal red cells, leading to hemolytic anemia.

Clinical Manifestations. A wide spectrum of disease may be observed in Rh-positive infants born of a sensitized woman. The chief clinical findings are due to the hemolytic anemia and to the processes marshalled by the infant to compensate for it. In about 15 per cent of cases the disease is so mild that no clinical manifestations are present, and the diagnosis is essentially a serologic one. As the severity of the disease increases, so does the anemia. Compensatory hyperplasia of erythropoietic tissue develops, especially in extramedullary sites, and the liver and spleen become massively enlarged. When the compensatory capacity of the hematopoietic system is exceeded, anemia becomes profound. Cardiac decompensation may then result in massive anasarca and the clinical picture of *hydrops fetalis*. Hydrops fetalis almost invariably results in death in utero or shortly after birth.

In severe cases, bilirubin pigments stain the amniotic fluid and the vernix caseosa yellow. Jaundice, however, is not usually present at birth because of clearance of bilirubin through the placenta to the mother. In the affected infant, jaundice is usually evident within the first day of life. Unconjugated bilirubin accumulates rapidly postnatally and may reach extremely high levels (20 to 50 mg. per 100 ml.). At these high levels the bilirubin pigments may penetrate cells of the nuclear masses of the brain and brain stem, staining them a yellow color (kernicterus), and produce cellular dysfunction and profound damage in these vital centers. This damage is clinically manifested by lethargy, poor feeding and loss of the Moro reflex. Characteristic spasms occur: the infant stiffly extends his arms with inward rotation and clenching of the fists, assumes a position of opisthotonos and emits sharp, high-pitched cries. Clinical signs of kernicterus are of grave prognostic import; 75 per cent or more of such infants die, and survivors often have mental retardation, deafness, spastic quadriplegia and choreoathetosis.

Laboratory Data. The most important laboratory finding is a positive direct Coombs or antiglobulin test result. The Coombs test utilizes an antihuman gamma globulin serum to detect the presence of a coating of immune globulin (antibody) on the red cell. A diagnosis of hemolytic disease due to Rh incompatibility cannot be made in the absence of a positive Coombs test result. Anemia is usually present. The hemoglobin concentration in cord blood may be less than 13.5 gm. per 100 ml., and with hydrops fetalis may be as low as 3 to 4 gm. The red cells are macrocytic. Nucleated red cells, most having their origin in the extramedullary hematopoietic sites, are present in markedly increased numbers. Reticulocytes are also increased. When correction is made for the nucleated red cells, the white blood cell count is normal, although immature forms are present. Thrombocytopenia may be present in severe cases. The level of bilirubin in cord blood is often elevated above 3.0 mg. per 100 ml. The level of serum bilirubin rises rapidly postnatally and may reach extremely high levels in the first 96 hours of life. Hepatic dysfunction may be present and is reflected by an elevated conjugated bilirubin level, hypoalbuminemia and hypoprothrombinemia.

Serologic Findings. Maternal antibodies to the Rh factor D are of 2 types. Antibodies of the 19-S or γ-M class, which agglutinate red cells in saline media, do not cross the placenta. The titer of antibody in a saline medium is not, therefore, of clinical or diagnostic importance. 7-S or γ-G antibodies, on the other hand, agglutinate Rh-positive red cells only in albumin or other colloidal media; they may also be detected by the Coombs technique. These antibodies readily cross the placenta. Significant fetal disease is usually associated with a maternal titer of albumin-active

antibodies of 1:8 or greater. Titers of more than 1:64 are associated with a relatively high frequency of stillbirth and hydrops fetalis. The height of the maternal titer is, however, imperfectly correlated with the severity of fetal disease. The information derived from examination of amniotic fluid may provide a more precise prognosis and guide to therapy.

Amniocentesis. Amniotic fluid obtained by direct transuterine aspiration is normally clear and colorless, but when the fetus has severe hemolytic disease, the fluid has a yellow color. This results from bilirubin and related pigments excreted by the affected fetus. The quantity of the bilirubin pigment is proportional to the severity of the hemolytic process.

The pigments are quantitated by spectrophotometric analysis. When the optical densities of normal amniotic fluid are measured at wavelengths from 350 to 700 millimicrons and plotted on semilogarithmic paper, a straight line is obtained (Fig. 14-7). Bilirubin pigments in the amniotic fluid produce a peak of density in the region of 450 millimicrons; the magnitude of this increase correlates closely with the severity of the hemolytic process in the fetus.

Accumulation of data from amniotic fluid analyses of a large number of affected pregnancies has permitted the definition of 3 zones into which the magnitude of the 450 density peak at various gestational ages may be assigned. Amniotic fluid with a 450 peak in zone 3 is associated with a high probability of fetal death and may indicate the necessity for induction of labor or intrauterine transfusion. A 450 peak in zone 1 generally means that the infant is mildly affected or has no hemolytic disease. Amniocentesis has proved to be a safe and generally reliable technique in the management of Rh hemolytic disease of the newborn.

Treatment. Treatment is directed to 2 main

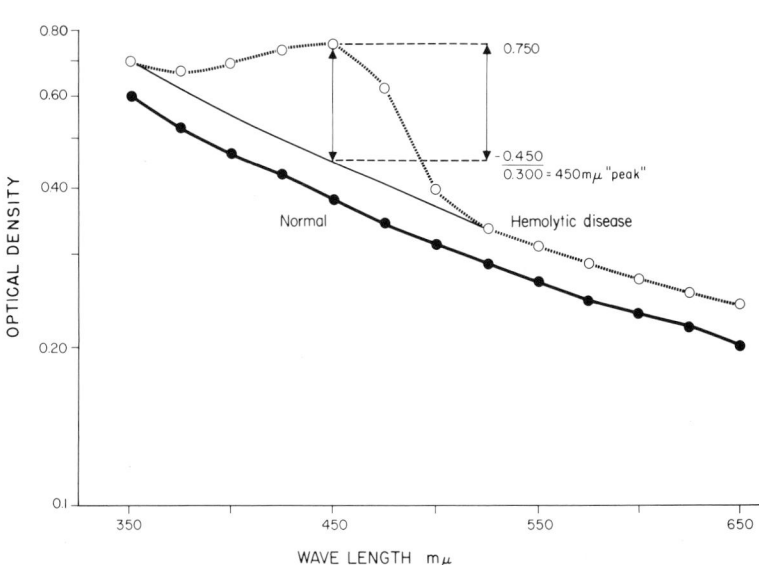

Figure 14-7. Spectrophotometric analysis of amniotic fluid. The method for measuring the 450 mμ peak is indicated.

goals: first, to detect and treat severe disease in utero in order to prevent hydrops fetalis and still-birth; and second, to prevent kernicterus in the liveborn infant. Rh typing of maternal red cells should be performed in the first 3 months of every pregnancy. If a woman is found to be Rh-negative, her serum should be screened for antibodies. If antibodies are found, or if there is a history of a previously affected infant, amniocentesis should be performed at 20 to 24 weeks' gestation. If anti-bodies are not present at the beginning of the preg-nancy, the antibody screening test should be re-peated at 20 to 24 weeks; if the result is positive, amniocentesis is indicated. Results of amniocen-tesis repeated at weekly intervals may be more reliable than a single determination. Maternal antibody detection and amniotic fluid examina-tion, alone or in combination, permit identification of most infants who are likely to die of hydrops fetalis before 36 weeks of gestation. Some medical centers use amniocentesis exclusively when sensi-tization has been established.

Intrauterine transfusion. The presence of a large 450-millimicron peak in the amniotic fluid (zone 3) is frequently associated with severe hemo-lytic disease and a significant possibility of intra-uterine fetal death before 34 weeks. The technique of intrauterine transfusion has permitted salvage of some of these babies. One or more transfusions of Rh-negative red cells can be administered by transuterine cannulation of the fetal peritoneum. Because this is a difficult technique which is poten-tially hazardous to both mother and infant, it is indicated only when fetal death is likely, and should be performed by a skillful, experienced operator. Intrauterine transfusion is not, in gen-eral, indicated after the thirty-fourth week of gestation, when delivery is usually preferable. Intrauterine transfusions are probably not indi-cated if roentgenographic signs of hydrops fetalis are already present.

Treatment of the liveborn infant. Infants iden-tified by maternal titer or amniocentesis as se-verely affected, who are at least 34 weeks of gestational age, should be delivered by early in-duction of labor. Elective induction of any sensi-tized woman at 36 weeks of gestation may help assure optimal management of the affected infant.

The physician who will care for the infant should attend the birth. Fresh group O Rh-negative blood, carefully cross-matched against the mater-nal serum, should be immediately available. If clinical signs of a severe hemolytic anemia such as pallor, hepatosplenomegaly or edema are evi-dent at birth, exchange transfusion should be performed immediately. With immediate therapy it is possible to save some very severely affected infants, though hydropic babies rarely survive. Care of such severely ill infants need not await laboratory studies. Otherwise cord blood should be examined in all infants born of Rh-negative women, without regard for signs of illness. If the direct Coombs test result is positive, hemolytic disease is presumed to be present, and its severity

can then be related to concentrations of hemo-globin and serum bilirubin.

The aim of therapy of the liveborn infant with hemolytic disease is to prevent kernicterus by avoiding dangerous degrees of hyperbilirubinemia during the first days of life. This is done by ex-change transfusion. Anemia and hypervolemia can be corrected concomitantly. Cord hemoglobin levels less than 13.0 gm. per 100 ml. or cord bili-rubin levels exceeding 3.5 mg. per 100 ml. are indicative of severe disease and warrant immedi-ate exchange transfusion. If immediate exchange transfusion is not necessary, the level of serum bilirubin should be followed carefully. If the rate of rise of the serum bilirubin exceeds 0.5 mg. per hour, if the unconjugated fraction exceeds 10 mg. per 100 ml. during the first 12 hours of life, or if the unconjugated bilirubin level exceeds 20 mg. per 100 ml. in the first 5 days of life, exchange transfusion should be carried out. Kernicterus can be essentially eliminated by keeping the serum bilirubin concentration below 20 mg. per 100 ml. by use of exchange transfusions.

Blood for exchange transfusion should be fresh. Heparin or acid-citrate-dextrose (ACD) may be used as anticoagulants. Heparinized blood makes the procedure technically easy and eliminates the need for calcium replacement, but should not be used if thrombocytopenia is present. The blood should be Rh-negative. Use of group O blood per-mits selection of a donor before delivery. The donor red cells should be tested against the maternal serum by the Coombs technique to assure com-patibility. Shortly before the transfusion is begun, the blood should be carefully warmed to room temperature. The infant should be prepared for transfusion by aspiration of the stomach, and the procedure should be performed in a bassinet or other device which permits maintenance of body temperature. A competent medical or nursing assistant should attend the infant in order to provide suction, monitor respirations and pulse, and tally the volumes of blood exchanged.

The umbilical vein is cannulated with a poly-ethylene catheter with strict aseptic technique. When free blood flow is obtained, the tip of the catheter is usually located in a large hepatic vein or the inferior vena cava. The venous pressure should be measured immediately. Twenty to 30 mm. of the infant's blood are aspirated and replaced with 10 to 20 ml. of donor blood. Alter-nating withdrawals and infusions of 10- or 20-ml. increments are done until a volume approximately twice the infant's estimated blood volume (2 × 85 ml. per kg.) has been exchanged. The exchange transfusion should be performed expeditiously and not take longer than an hour. If citrated blood has been used, 2.0 ml. of 10 per cent calcium glu-conate should be cautiously injected after each 100 ml. exchanged. When heparinized blood is used, 10 mg. of protamine sulfate may be injected intravenously at the conclusion of the transfusion.

Infants with severe hemolytic disease and hy-drops fetalis may have elevated venous pressure (higher than 10 cm. of water). This has been interpreted as indicating hypervolemic congestive heart failure, and initial withdrawal of larger amounts of blood (40 to 50 ml.) to lower the venous pressure has been advocated. Recent studies of blood volume and arterial blood pressures have demonstrated that the traditional concept of an expanded blood volume may not always be valid. Some babies may, in fact, be hypovolemic. Measurement of arterial blood pressure through the umbilical artery may be of value. Infants severely affected by hemolytic disease may also have the superimposed metabolic abnormalities of hypoglycemia and acidosis, which require appropriate therapy.

The efficiency of an exchange transfusion performed for removal of bilirubin can be increased by the intravenous injection of 1 gm. per kg. of human albumin in a 25 per cent salt-free solution 1 hour before the exchange. Alternatively, 50 ml. of the plasma of the donor blood may be replaced by an equal volume of 25 per cent albumin. Albumin should be used cautiously if there is elevated venous pressure or other evidence of congestive failure. After exchange transfusion the bilirubin level must be determined at frequent intervals (every 4 to 8 hours). If the level of the indirect fraction significantly exceeds 20 mg. per 100 ml., or if the infant exhibits neurologic symptoms suggestive of kernicterus, second or repeated exchange transfusions are mandatory. Prophylactic antibiotics are not necessary as a routine precaution, and sulfonamide drugs are contraindicated, owing to competitive attachment to albumin.

Exposure of jaundiced infants to blue light may reduce the level of serum bilirubin. This form of therapy is being evaluated and may prove of value, especially in jaundice not associated with hemolytic disease.

The infant with hemolytic disease must be observed carefully during the first 6 to 8 weeks of life, because the convalescent phase is sometimes marked by development of profound anemia. If the hemoglobin level falls below 5 to 6 gm. per 100 ml., simple transfusions with small amounts of Rh-negative blood will sustain the infant until hematologic recovery is indicated by reticulocytosis and a rise in the hemoglobin level. Iron and other hematinics are not necessary.

Prevention of Rh Sensitization. The initial sensitization of Rh-negative mothers is preventable by eliminating potentially antigenic fetal cells from the mother's circulation through intramuscular injection of 300 to 400 mcg. of human anti-D gamma globulin within 72 hours after delivery. Because of a limited supply of the antibody, it is currently recommended only for previously unsensitized Rh-negative women who deliver Rh-positive infants or who abort or miscarry infants of unidentified Rh type. Though there is evidence that 2 to 3 per cent of women at risk may be sensitized antenatally and though sensitization to other blood group factors will still result in sporadic cases, this procedure seems certain to reduce the incidence of hemolytic disease.

HEMOLYTIC DISEASE OF THE NEWBORN DUE TO A OR B INCOMPATIBILITY

Incompatibility in respect to the major blood groups results in a form of hemolytic disease which is generally mild. Usually the mother is type O and the infant type A or B. Although type O mothers regularly have anti-A and anti-B isoagglutinins in their serums, only a small proportion of A or B infants are affected. This is because most of the naturally occurring isohemagglutinins are 19-S, γ-M globulins which do not cross the placenta. Only the few type O mothers who have high levels of 7-S, γ-G antibodies which can cross the placenta are likely to have severely affected infants.

Clinical Manifestations. The disease is usually manifest by visible jaundice beginning in the first 24 hours of life. The infant is not usually severely affected at birth, pallor is not present, and hydrops fetalis is extremely rare. The liver and spleen are not greatly enlarged. The jaundice may become severe, and kernicterus can occur if the serum bilirubin concentration rises rapidly to high values and exchange transfusion is not done (see above). Hereditary spherocytosis is occasionally difficult to differentiate, especially if coincidental blood group incompatibility is also present.

Laboratory Data. The most important laboratory finding is incompatibility between mother and infant. The infant's hemoglobin level is usually normal, but occasionally may be as low as 10 to 12 gm. per 100 ml. Reticulocytes are increased to 10 to 15 per cent, and there are extensive spherocytosis, polychromasia and increased numbers of nucleated red cells. Although the direct Coombs test result may be negative, modern antiglobulin reagents with greater potency and sensitivity may give weakly positive results in 60 to 70 per cent of cases. Free anti-A or anti-B antibody may be present in the serum of the infant. The unconjugated serum bilirubin value is elevated and in 10 to 20 per cent of cases may increase to 20 mg. per 100 ml. or greater.

Treatment. Therapy is directed at preventing dangerous postnatal hyperbilirubinemia by exchange transfusion. Group O Rh-compatible blood cross-matched against the maternal serum should be used, as previously described; albumin increases the efficiency of bilirubin removal, and may be safely given in this disease when there is excessive hyperbilirubinemia.

HEMOLYTIC DISEASE FROM OTHER FACTORS

Less than 5 per cent of cases of hemolytic disease of the newborn are due to maternal-fetal incompatibilities involving factors other than A, B and

D. Among the most important antigens involved in these unusual cases are the Rh factors c (hr') and E (rh'') and antigens from other blood groups, especially Kell (K). These sensitizations may all be associated with severe hemolytic disease and sometimes hydrops fetalis. The direct Coombs test result is invariably positive. Exchange transfusion is indicated for severe anemia and hyperbilirubinemia. The blood chosen for transfusion should lack the antigen responsible for maternal sensitization, and should always be carefully cross-matched against the maternal serum.

AUTOIMMUNE HEMOLYTIC ANEMIAS

In the autoimmune hemolytic anemias abnormal antibodies directed against red cells are produced by the patient himself. The pathogenic mechanism of these disorders is uncertain. One theory postulates the basic cause to be an autonomous proliferation of a forbidden clone of immunologically competent cells which do not have the capacity of recognizing self-antigens. An alternative explanation suggests that drugs or infectious agents in some way alter the red cell membrane so that it becomes "foreign" or antigenic to the host.

Autoimmune hemolytic anemias associated with an underlying disease process such as lymphoma or lupus erythematosus are said to be secondary or symptomatic. In other instances the disease is termed idiopathic because no underlying cause can be found. A number of drugs may act as haptens which combine with proteins of the red cell membrane to form antigenic complexes. Penicillin and certain related drugs and methyldopa are occasionally involved in these drug-induced hemolytic processes. Readministration of the drug may result in a Coombs-positive hemolytic anemia.

Clinical Manifestations. Anemia may develop acutely with prostration, pallor and jaundice. The spleen is usually palpably enlarged, and lymphadenopathy is often present. In secondary cases, manifestations of an underlying disease may be prominent.

Laboratory Data. In many cases the anemia is profound, with hemoglobin levels less than 6 gm. per 100 ml. Considerable spherocytosis and polychromasia are present on the peripheral smear. More than 50 per cent of the circulating red cells may be reticulocytes, a large number of them nucleated. Leukocytosis is common. The platelet count is usually normal, but occasionally a concomitant immune thrombocytopenic purpura is present (Evans syndrome).

The direct Coombs test result is strongly positive, and free antibody can often be demonstrated in the serum. These antibodies are active at 37°C. Antibodies from the serum, and those eluted from the red cells, react with many different red cells, including those of the patient. Although they have often been regarded as nonspecific panagglutinins, careful studies have revealed many to have specificity for certain red cell antigens. A number of such antibodies have had anti-e (hr'') specificity. Since more than 95 per cent of the red cell population have the e antigen, the antibody might be considered a panagglutinin unless careful tests were performed. Sometimes spontaneous agglutination of the patient's own red cells occurs in all testing serums, so that the patient may be mistakenly blood-typed as group AB Rh-positive.

Treatment. Transfusions are usually of only transient benefit, but may be necessary. It may be extremely difficult to find compatible blood; in selecting blood the red cells giving the least positive in-vitro reaction by the Coombs technique should be chosen. The mainstays of therapy are the corticosteroids. Prednisone or its equivalent should be administered in a dose of 2.5 mg. per kg. per day. This should be continued until the evidence of hemolysis disappears, and then the dose is gradually reduced. If relapse occurs, resumption of full dosage may be necessary. The disease tends to remit spontaneously within a few weeks or months. The Coombs test result may remain positive even after hemolysis has subsided. When hemolytic anemia remains severe despite corticosteroid therapy, or if very large doses are necessary to maintain a reasonable hemoglobin level, splenectomy may be beneficial. Recently immunosuppressive agents have been of some benefit in chronic cases refractory to conventional therapy.

Course and Prognosis. Idiopathic autoimmune hemolytic disease in childhood is usually acute and may be severe, but is self-limited. Corticosteroid therapy has permitted most of these patients to be sustained until recovery has occurred; deaths are unusual. In immune hemolytic anemia secondary to lymphoma or lupus erythematosus the status of the basic disease determines the ultimate prognosis.

HEMOLYTIC ANEMIAS OF INTOXICATIONS AND INFECTIONS

Arsenic and phenylhydrazine are obligate hemolytic agents in any person when administered in a sufficient dose.

Hemolytic anemias may complicate a variety of infections. Direct red cell damage by microorganisms or their toxins may be the basis of hemolysis observed in septicemia. Actual parasitism of the red cell occurs in malaria.

Very high levels of the so-called cold antibodies which develop after certain viral pneumonias may coincidentally damage the red cell and produce a severe hemolytic process. The antibody is usually a macroglobulin. Specificity for red cell antigens, especially the i antigen, is present in some cases.

INFANTILE PYKNOCYTOSIS

Infantile pyknocytosis is an acute, self-limited hemolytic anemia occurring during the first 3 months of life. The peripheral blood contains large numbers of characteristically malformed red cells called pyknocytes. These are contracted, densely stained cells with irregular contours and several sharp spinelike projections. A small number of pyknocytes (0.5 to 2.0 per cent) may be present in the blood of normal newborn infants, and premature infants may have as many as 5 per cent. Pyknocytosis must be differentiated from crenation, which is a technical artifact of fixation and staining of blood smears. The cause is uncertain, but the condition does not result from an intrinsic defect; abnormalities of the red cell's environment may be important. Low levels of serum vitamin E have been found in premature infants with a hematologic syndrome resembling infantile pyknocytosis. Some of these infants had G-6-PD deficiency, but this may have been coincidental.

Clinical and Laboratory Data. Affected infants frequently become jaundiced during the neonatal period. Pallor and signs of anemia are evident after the second or third week. The spleen and liver are usually enlarged.

The anemia may be severe, with hemoglobin levels as low as 4 to 5 gm. per 100 ml., and reticulocytosis is also present. Twenty to 50 per cent of the circulating red cells are pyknocytes. Survival studies reveal that life spans of both transfused red cells and those of the patients are shortened.

Treatment. Exchange transfusion may be required in the neonatal period for hyperbilirubinemia. If the anemia becomes severe, transfusions with packed or sedimented red cells may be given. Oral vitamin E (alpha tocopherol) in a dose of 200 mg. per day has been of apparent benefit in some cases. Even without therapy the hemolysis abates, and by 4 months or so of age the patients are hematologically normal.

REFERENCES

The Red Cells: General

Harris, J. W.: *The Red Cell.* Cambridge, Harvard University Press, 1963.
Oski, F. A., and Naiman, J. L.: *Hematologic Problems in the Newborn.* Philadelphia, W. B. Saunders Company, 1966.
Smith, C. H.: *Blood Disease of Infancy and Childhood.* 2nd ed. St. Louis, C. V. Mosby Company, 1966.
Wintrobe, M. M.: *Clinical Hematology.* 6th ed. Philadelphia, Lea & Febiger, 1967.

Congenital Pure Red Cell Anemia

Allen, D. M., and Diamond, L. K.: Congenital (Erythroid) Hypoplastic Anemia – Cortisone Treated. *Am. J. Dis. Child.,* 102:416, 1961.
Diamond, L. K., Allen, D. M., and Magill, F. B.: Congenital (Erythroid) Hypoplastic Anemia. *Am. J. Dis. Child.,* 102:403, 1961.

Anemias of Chronic Infections, Inflammation and Renal Disease

Cartwright, G. E., and Wintrobe, M. M.: The Anemias of Infection. XVII. A Review; in W. Dock and I. Snapper (Eds.):

Advances in Internal Medicine. Chicago, Year Book Publishers, Inc., 1952, Vol. V, p. 165.
Desforges, J. F., and Dawson, J. P.: The Anemia of Renal Failure. *Arch. Int. Med.,* 101:326, 1958.
Reinhold, J.: The Survival of Transfused Red Cells in Acute Rheumatic Fever, with Reference to a Latent Haemolytic Mechanism. *Arch. Dis. Childhood,* 29:201, 1954.

Megaloblastic Anemias

Dahlke, M. B., and Mertens-Roesler, E.: Malabsorption of Folic Acid Due to Diphenylhydantoin. *Blood,* 30:341, 1967.
Herbert, V.: *The Megaloblastic Anemias.* New York, Grune & Stratton, Inc., 1959.
Huguley, C. M., Jr., Bain, J. A., Rivers, S. L., and Scoggins, R. B.: Refractory Megaloblastic Anemia Associated with Excretion of Orotic Acid. *Blood,* 14:615, 1959.
Klipstein, F. A.: Subnormal Serum Folate and Macrocytosis Associated with Anticonvulsant Drug Therapy. *Blood,* 23:68, 1964.
Luhby, A. L: Megaloblastic Anemia in Infancy. III. Clinical Considerations and Analysis. *J. Pediat.,* 54:617, 1959.
McIntyre, O. R., Sullivan, L. W., Jeffries, G. H., and Silver, R. H.: Pernicious Anemia in Childhood. *New England J. Med.,* 272:981, 1965.

Microcytic Anemia

Dallman, P. R., and Schwartz, H. C.: Distribution of Cytochrome C and Myoglobin in Rats with Iron Deficiency. *Pediatrics,* 35:677, 1965.
Erlandson, M. E.: Iron Metabolism and Iron Deficiency Anemia. *Pediat. Clin. N. Amer.,* 9:673, 1962.
Horrigan, D. L., and Harris, J. W.: Pyridoxine-Responsive Anemia: Analysis of 62 Cases. *Advances Int. Med.,* 12:103, 1964.
Moe, P. J.: Iron Requirements in Infancy. Longitudinal Studies of Iron Requirements During the First Year of Life. *Acta paediat.* (Suppl. 150), 52:54, 1963.
Naiman, J. L., Oski, F. A., Diamond, L. K., Vawter, G. F., and Shwachman, H.: The Gastrointestinal Effects of Iron-Deficiency Anemia. *Pediatrics,* 33:83, 1964.
Rundles, R. W., and Falls, H. F.: Hereditary (? Sex-Linked) Anemia. *Am. J.M. Sc.,* 211:641, 1946.
Schulman, I.: Iron Requirements in Infancy. *J.A.M.A.,* 175:118, 1961.
Wilson, J. F., Heiner, D. C., and Lahey, M. E.: Milk-Induced Gastrointestinal Bleeding in Infants with Hypochromic Microcytic Anemia. *J.A.M.A.,* 189:568, 1964.

The Hemolytic Anemias: General

Dacie, J. V.: *The Haemolytic Anemias.* 2nd ed. New York, Grune & Stratton, Inc., 1962.

Hereditary Spherocytosis

Jacob, H. S.: Hereditary Spherocytosis; A Disease of the Red Cell Membrane. *Seminars in Hematology,* 2:139, 1965.

Hereditary Elliptocytosis

Baker, S. J., Jacob, E., Rajan, K. T., and Gault, E. W.: Hereditary Haemolytic Anaemia Associated with Elliptocytosis. A Study of Three Families. *Brit. J. Haemat.,* 7:210, 1961.
Jensson, O., Jönasson, T., and Olafsson, Ö.: Hereditary Elliptocytosis in Iceland. *Brit. J. Haemat.,* 13:844, 1967.
Josephs, H. W., and Avery, M. E.: Hereditary Elliptocytosis Associated with Increased Hemolysis. *Pediatrics,* 16:741, 1955.

Paroxysmal Nocturnal Hemoglobinuria

Miller, D. R., Baehner, R. L., and Diamond, L. K.: Paroxysmal Nocturnal Hemoglobinuria in Childhood and Adolescence. *Pediatrics,* 39:675, 1967.
Damshek, W.: Riddle: What Do Aplastic Anemia, Paroxysmal Nocturnal Hemoglobinuria (PNH) & "Hypoplastic" Leukemia Have in Common? *Blood,* 30:251, 1967.

Hereditary Stomatocytosis

Zarkowsky, H. S., Oski, F. A., Sha'Afti, R., Shohet, S. B., and Nathan, D. G.: Congenital Hemolytic Anemia with High Sodium, Low Potassium Red Cell. *New England J. Med.,* 278:573, 1968.

Enzymatic Defects of the Red Cells

Beutler, E.: Glucose-6-Phosphate Dehydrogenase Deficiency and Nonspherocytic Congenital Hemolytic Anemia. *Seminars in Hematology,* 2:91, 1965.

Tanaka, K. R., Valentine, W. N., and Miwa, S.: Pyruvate Kinase (PK) Deficiency Hereditary Nonspherocytic Hemolytic Anemia. *Blood,* 19:267, 1962.

Zinkham, W. H., and Lenhard, R. E., Jr.: Metabolic Abnormalities of Erythrocytes from Patients with Congenital Nonspherocytic Hemolytic Anemia. *J. Pediat.,* 55:319, 1959.

Autoimmune Hemolytic Anemia

Hitzig, W. H., and Massino, L.: Treatment of Autoimmune Hemolytic Anemia in Children with Azathroprine (Imuran). *Blood,* 28:840, 1966.

O'Connor, W. J., Vakiener, J. M., and Watson, R. J.: Idiopathic Acquired Hemolytic Anemia in Young Children. *Pediatrics,* 17:732, 1956.

Hemoglobinopathies

Diggs, L. W.: Sickle Cell Crises. *Am. J. Clin. Path.,* 44:1, 1965.

Porter, F. S., and Thurman, W. G.: Studies of Sickle Cell Disease: Diagnosis in Infancy. *Am. J. Dis. Child.,* 106:35, 1963.

Rucknagel, D. L., and Neil, J. V.: The Hemoglobinopathies; in A. G. Steinberg (Ed.): *Progress in Medical Genetics,* New York, Grune & Stratton, Inc., 1961, Vol. 1.

Scott, R. B.: Sickle Cell Anemia. *Pediat. Clin. N. Amer.,* 9:649, 1962.

Thalassemia

Fink, H. (Ed.): Problems of Cooley's Anemia. *Ann. New York Acad. Sci.,* 119:369, 1964.

Weatherall, D.: *The Thalassemia Syndromes.* Blackwell Scientific, Oxford, 1965.

Hemolytic Disease of the Newborn

Allen, F. H., Jr., and Diamond, L. K.: *Erythroblastosis Fetalis.* Boston, Little Brown & Co., 1958.

Bowman, J. M., and Pollock, J. M.: Amniotic Fluid Spectrophotometry and Early Delivery in the Management of Erythroblastosis Fetalis. *Pediatrics,* 35:815, 1965.

Diamond, L. K.: Prevention of Erythroblastosis. *Pediatrics,* 41:1, 1968.

Lucey, J. F.: Diagnosis and Treatment. Current Indications and Results of Fetal Transfusions. *Pediatrics,* 41:139, 1968.

Mollison, P. L., and Cutbush, M.: Haemolytic Disease of the Newborn Due to Fetal-Maternal ABO Incompatibility; in L. M. Tocantins (Ed.): *Progress in Hematology.* New York, Grune & Stratton, Inc., 1959, Vol. II, p. 153.

Odell, G. B., Bryan, W. B., and Richmond, M. D.: Exchange Transfusion. *Pediat. Clin. N. Amer.,* 9:605, 1962.

Queenan, J. T.: Modern Management of the Rh Problem. New York, Paul B. Hoeber, 1967.

Van Praagh, R.: Diagnosis of Kernicterus in the Neonatal Period. *Pediatrics,* 28:870, 1961.

Infantile Pyknocytosis

Oski, F. A., and Barness, L. A.: Vitamin E Deficiency: A Previously Unrecognized Cause of Hemolytic Anemia in the Premature Infant. *J. Pediat.,* 70:211, 1967.

Tuffy, P., Brown, A. K., and Zuelzer, W. W.: Infantile Pyknocytosis. *Am. J. Dis. Child.,* 98:227, 1959.

POLYCYTHEMIA

(Erythrocytosis)

Polycythemia may be diagnosed when the red cell count, the hemoglobin and hematocrit levels, and the total red cell volume significantly exceed the upper limits of normal. In the older child the levels of hemoglobin and hematocrit which can be considered to represent polycythemia are 16 gm. per 100 ml. and 55 per cent, respectively, corresponding to a total red cell mass exceeding 35 ml. per kg. A decrease in plasma volume, such as occurs in acute dehydration and burns, may result in disproportionately high levels of hemoglobin and hematocrit. In these situations, more accurately designated hemoconcentration rather than relative polycythemia, the actual red cell volume is not increased. Expansion of the plasma volume or rehydration restores the hematocrit to normal levels.

Measurement of the red cell volume by dye dilution or radioisotopic techniques is essential in the differential diagnosis of polycythemia. True polycythemia is characterized by increases of both the red cell and total blood volumes.

Secondary Polycythemia. Polycythemia may be present in any clinical situation associated with arterial oxygen desaturation. Hypoxia of the kidney results in increased production of erythropoietin. This in turn stimulates increased production of red cells which ultimately results in greatly expanded red cell mass. Cardiovascular defects involving right-to-left shunts and pulmonary diseases interfering with proper oxygenation are the most common causes of secondary polycythemia. Examples of such conditions are cyanotic congenital heart disease, cystic fibrosis, asthma, emphysema and bronchiectasis. Clinical findings usually include cyanosis, hyperemia of sclerae and mucous membranes and clubbing of the fingers. The red blood cell count and hemoglobin and hematocrit values are all increased. The oxygen saturation of arterial blood is decreased. Living at high altitudes also causes a secondary polycythemia.

More subtle forms of hypoxia may also cause polycythemia. Congenital methemoglobinemia due to a deficiency of DPNH-reactive diaphorase may cause familial cyanosis and polycythemia. This condition is transmitted as an autosomal recessive. Dominantly transmitted cyanosis and polycythemia may be associated with the hemoglobin M syndromes, in which oxygen is not transported effectively. An abnormal hemoglobin named Hgb. Rainier has also been found to cause a benign familial polycythemia; it too is transmitted as an autosomal dominant trait. Hemoglobin Rainier has abnormal oxygen dissociation properties which make oxygen relatively unavailable to tissues, even at normal oxygen content of the blood. Transient benign polycythemia is said to occur in otherwise healthy adolescents; this syndrome has not been studied sufficiently to determine its nature and cause.

Polycythemia has also been reported in association with renal tumors and cysts and with vascular tumors of the cerebellum. Excessive red cell production occurs because these tumors secrete erythropoietin.

Polycythemia Rubra Vera (Erythremia). This severe disorder is characterized by polycythemia, leukocytosis, thrombocytosis, and hyperplasia of the bone marrow. Only a few children thought to have this syndrome have been described. Most of these were not studied with modern diagnostic tests; it is uncertain, therefore, whether this disease has occurred in childhood.

Plethora of the Newborn. High levels of hemoglobin and hematocrit are characteristic of the newborn infant. The range of normal hemoglobin at birth is 13 to 20 gm. per 100 ml., and the hematocrit 45 to 65 per cent. The blood volume of normal term newborns is 70 to 100 ml. per kg., and the red cell volume, 40 to 60 ml. per kg. Occasionally the blood values of newborn infants significantly exceed these ranges. Some of these plethoric infants have respiratory distress, tachycardia, congestive heart failure and hyperbilirubinemia. Monozygotic twins with placental vascular anastomosis may have unequal distribution of the circulation, so that one twin is born with anemia and hypovolemia, while the other twin is plethoric. On rare occasions maternofetal transfusion and congenital adrenal hyperplasia may be associated with neonatal polycythemia. In most instances no cause can be discovered. When these infants have symptomatic difficulties, phlebotomy may be indicated to reduce hypervolemia (see p. 396).

THE PANCYTOPENIAS

Aplasia of bone marrow, or replacement of its hematopoietic elements by other tissue, results in profound depression of all the formed elements of the blood. The clinical manifestations which result are anemia, thrombocytopenic hemorrhage, and decreased resistance to infection, because of neutropenia. The pancytopenias have traditionally been classified with the anemias, but the consequences of the thrombocytopenia and the neutropenia are much more striking and serious than the anemia. The pancytopenias may be constitutional, often due to ill-defined genetic factors, may be acquired as a result of damage to the marrow by a variety of chemical or other agents, or may result from invasion by abnormal tissue. In these conditions underproduction of blood cells is due to hypocellularity or replacement of marrow. Examination of an adequate sample of marrow is essential to diagnosis.

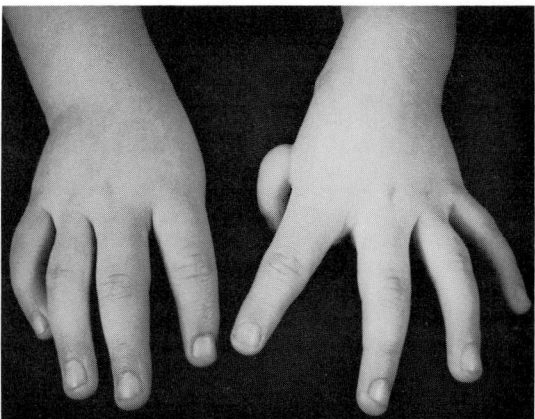

Figure 14-8. Hands of a child with constitutional aplastic pancytopenia. The thumb is absent on the right and rudimentary on the left.

CONSTITUTIONAL APLASTIC PANCYTOPENIA

The constitutional aplastic anemias are familial disorders inherited on an autosomal recessive basis. About half of affected children have evident congenital anomalies; especially common are microcephaly and absence of the radii and thumbs (Fig. 14-8); abnormalities of eye, heart and kidney are also relatively common (Fanconi syndrome). Some affected children have no serious anatomic defects, but are short in stature and have a peculiar dark pigmentation of the skin, as do many of those with structural anomalies.

Pancytopenia is not usually present at birth or during early infancy. Bruising, the first indication of hematologic disease, is usually observed by 3 to 12 years of age. The consequences of a progressively severe anemia and leukopenia are noted shortly thereafter.

Laboratory Data. Severe pancytopenia is evident in peripheral blood. The bone marrow is strikingly hypocellular with depression of all the cell types and an increase in fatty tissue. Reticulum, plasma and mast cells are prominent. A surgical or needle biopsy of the bone marrow is useful as an adjunct to aspiration, for it provides a large specimen in which to judge cellularity. Analysis of the hemoglobin reveals an increase in the percentage of Hgb. F of 5 to 15 per cent. This abnormality may antedate development of marrow aplasia and pancytopenia. Chromosomal studies reveal an abnormally high percentage of chromatid breaks and unusual chromosomal alignments; these also may precede frank pancytopenia.

Treatment. In addition to symptomatic treatment with blood transfusions and antibiotics, therapy with androgenic steroids is beneficial.

Testosterone propionate is given as sublingual tablets in a dose of 1 to 2 mg. per kg. per day to a maximum of 60 mg. per day. Alternatively, 400 to 600 mg. may be given as an intramuscular injection every 4 weeks. Relatively small doses of corticosteroids, such as 5 to 10 mg. of prednisone or equivalent, are also given. In a majority of instances a hematologic response becomes evident within 2 to 4 months. The marrow develops greater cellularity, and the hemoglobin rises to normal levels. The response of the neutrophils is usually less complete, and platelets may show only a moderate increase in numbers. When the hemoglobin has reached normal levels, it is often possible to reduce the dose of androgen. But if the drug is too rapidly or drastically decreased, relapse occurs. These effective doses of androgen regularly produce signs and symptoms of masculinization, including acne, hirsutism, deepening of the voice, and enlargement of the penis or clitoris. Synthetic androgen derivatives (oxymethalone, stanazol) have fewer of these side effects, but some degree of masculinization is probably inevitable. Prior to the advent of testosterone therapy these patients usually died during late childhood of hemorrhage, infection or the complications of multiple transfusions. An increased incidence of leukemia has been reported in children with this disease. Experience with androgen therapy is still too recent to know what the ultimate prognosis may now be.

ACQUIRED APLASTIC PANCYTOPENIAS

A number of physical, chemical and infectious agents may severely damage the bone marrow and lead to severe pancytopenia. Some of these agents have the capacity to produce marrow aplasia in any person who is exposed to them in a sufficient dose. Such obligate marrow depressants include ionizing radiation, chemotherapeutic drugs such as nitrogen mustard, 6-mercaptopurine and methotrexate, and certain organic solvents, especially benzene. A second group of agents produce aplastic pancytopenia only in a small, often a remarkably small, number of persons exposed to them. In these latter persons the adverse hematologic reactions must reflect idiosyncrasies. The drug most frequently associated with aplastic pancytopenia is chloramphenicol. It has been estimated that only one in 24,000 to 60,000 patients taking chloramphenicol suffers marrow aplasia; nevertheless the drug is involved in more than half of the drug-related aplastic pancytopenias. Other drugs associated with an appreciable incidence of marrow aplasia are sulfonamides, phenylbutazone and certain anticonvulsants. Severe infections may also produce severe marrow damage, but it is often difficult to decide whether the infection represents cause or effect. A number of cases of marrow aplasia have been described following typical infectious hepatitis. In about half of cases of aplastic pancytopenia no history of exposure to toxins or other agents can be elicited. These cases are usually designated as idiopathic, although the possibility of an environmental factor or toxin cannot be excluded with certainty.

Clinical and Laboratory Data. Hemorrhage secondary to thrombocytopenia is usually the first clinical manifestation. The signs and symptoms of anemia and neutropenia become apparent subsequently. The spleen and lymph nodes are not enlarged. Profound depression of red cells, platelets and neutrophils is present. The level of fetal hemoglobin may be increased. The marrow aspirate is scanty; the particles are fatty, and lymphocytes, plasma cells and reticulum cells predominate.

Treatment. The patient must immediately be removed from contact with any potentially toxic drugs or agents. When the onset of the disease is acute, with massive hemorrhage and serious sepsis, aggressive therapy with platelet concentrates and antibiotics is necessary; choice of antibiotic should be based upon bacterial culture and sensitivity tests. In any fully developed case, therapy with testosterone and corticosteroids should be given, as described for constitutional pancytopenia. Because response to these medications may not be evident for 2 to 4 months, an early start is advisable. Other forms of therapy are not of regular value. Hematinics are worthless, and splenectomy is hazardous. Bone marrow transfusions are of no help unless an identical twin is available as a donor.

Course. Approximately a third of patients die very quickly as a result of uncontrollable hemorrhage and infection. Pseudomonas and staphylococcal septicemias are frequent causes of death. The remaining two thirds of children have a subacute clinical course. In these patients androgen therapy often has a beneficial effect. Half of this group ultimately recover completely; the other half have a chronic course, many succumbing to sepsis and hemorrhage months or years after onset. Leukemia and paroxysmal nocturnal hemoglobinuria have developed in some children after recovery from aplastic anemia.

PANCYTOPENIA DUE TO MARROW REPLACEMENT

Diffuse replacement of marrow space by nonhematopoietic tissue results in peripheral pancytopenia. *Neuroblastoma* is the childhood tumor which most frequently metastasizes to the bone marrow. *Osteopetrosis,* or marble bone disease, is frequently associated with anemia and thrombocytopenia, owing to marrow obliteration; an element of hypersplenism may also be present. *Acute leukemia* occasionally presents with pancytopenia and a reticular appearance of the initially aspirated marrow. Adequate sampling or biopsy of the marrow from other sites will usually provide the proper diagnosis.

TRANSFUSIONS*

The most important indications for transfusions are to restore blood volume and treat shock following acute blood loss and to provide red cells for maintenance of the blood hemoglobin level. An individual component of blood, such as red cells, platelets, plasma or specific plasma proteins, may often be effectively used in place of whole blood.

INDICATIONS FOR TRANSFUSION

Acute Hemorrhage. The signs and symptoms accompanying hemorrhage vary with the magnitude and rapidity of the blood loss. When 15 to 20 per cent or more of the circulating blood volume is acutely lost, tachycardia, hypotension and shock may develop, accompanied by weakness, restlessness and syncope. Immediately after acute hemorrhage the hemoglobin or hematocrit level may be deceptively high, but hemodilution soon reduces this to a value reflecting the magnitude of the blood loss. Thrombocytosis and neutrophilia occur within a few hours and reticulocytosis within a few days of an acute bleeding episode. The most common causes of severe acute hemorrhage are trauma and gastrointestinal bleeding from peptic ulcers, Meckel's diverticulum and esophageal varices. In patients with defects of the hemostatic mechanism exsanguinating hemorrhage may occur from nosebleeds or gastritis.

Severe bleeding in the perinatal period may result in the clinical picture of asphyxia pallida. Pallor, shock, tachycardia and low venous pressures are seen. External hemorrhage may occur from the umbilicus or the gastrointestinal tract. The fetus may bleed before and during birth into the maternal circulation, and fetofetal transfusions between identical twins are not infrequent.

Laboratory data. The anemia of acute blood loss is usually normochromic and normocytic. Depending upon the duration of the hemorrhage and timing of the tests, compensatory reticulocytosis and normoblastemia may be seen. In the newborn infant with hemorrhage, the Coombs test result is generally negative and the level of serum bilirubin low.

Treatment. When possible, local measures to control the hemorrhage should be taken. Whole blood transfusions should be given to restore blood volume and treat shock; 20 ml. per kg. of blood should be administered initially. The need for additional blood will be guided by the clinical response and by physical and laboratory findings. Plasma or plasma expanders may be used to sustain the patient in shock until blood can be made available, but if the blood loss has been great, red cell replacement will be necessary.

Chronic Anemias. In anemias which develop slowly and which stabilize at a level of 6 to 9 gm. per 100 ml. remarkably few symptoms may be experienced by the patient. Transfusions are usually not routinely indicated in management. When such anemias result from deficiency of a specific factor such as folic acid or iron, a rapid response will follow replacement therapy. Transfusion is indicated only if the anemia is profound or if infections or other complications are present. No hard and fast rule can be made about the hemoglobin level at which transfusion is recommended. Some children with iron deficiency anemia may have hemoglobin levels of 4 to 5 gm. per 100 ml. with few signs of clinical or cardiorespiratory distress.

In progressive refractory anemias such as thalassemia major and pure red cell anemias, transfusions are necessary to sustain life. Packed or sedimented red cells are preferred for the correction of such chronic anemias. The maximum dose of packed red cells to be given in one transfusion is 15 ml. per kg.; if signs of congestive heart failure are present, considerably smaller amounts should be used. In extreme anemia with secondary heart failure, multiple small transfusions of 2 to 4 ml. per kg. of packed red cells may be helpful, or even exchange transfusion. Digitalis and oxygen are of limited value.

Platelet Transfusions. Platelets may be transfused to attain temporary hemostasis in some patients with thrombocytopenic hemorrhage. Although administration of fresh whole blood produces inconsequential rises in the recipient's platelet count, clinical hemorrhage is often controlled. Use of platelet-rich plasma or platelet concentrates prepared from fresh blood drawn in plastic equipment permits attainment of more nearly normal platelet counts. Platelet transfusions are beneficial in thrombocytopenias due to inadequate production such as hypoplastic pancytopenia and leukemia, but are useless or of only transient value in states characterized by peripheral hyperdestruction of platelets such as idiopathic thrombocytopenic purpura.

White Blood Cells. Because of the brief intravascular life span and low concentration of leukocytes in normal blood, transfusions of normal blood have no practical value for the supply of white blood cells. Transient clinical and hematologic benefit in neutropenias has been reported from use of donor blood from patients with chronic granulocytic leukemia who have very high total white blood cell counts.

Plasma and Plasma Concentrates. In acute dehydration when the plasma volume is decreased, but the red cell mass is adequate, plasma can be used effectively to expand the blood volume, and to restore circulation and renal blood flow. The usual dose of plasma is 10 ml. per kg. The use of fresh plasma and of concentrates of plasma such as factor VIII and fibrinogen preparations for bleeding disorders is described elsewhere. The usual gamma globulin preparations cannot be administered intravenously because they form large reactive aggregates which may produce hypotension and shock.

---

*See page 1062 for Exchange Transfusion.

SPECIAL CONSIDERATIONS

Choice of Blood for Transfusion. Storage of blood at 4°C. results in a decrease in red cell viability which is proportional to the length of storage time. When blood is given for acute hemorrhage, this is of no consequence, but in children who must receive transfusions repeatedly the blood selected should be as fresh as possible.

Blood for transfusion should be of the same blood group (O, A, B or AB) as the recipient's. The donor red cells should always be tested for compatibility with the recipient's plasma (major cross match) by the Coombs technique. Compatibility for the Rh antigens between donor and recipient is desirable. Rh-negative (d/d) persons should never receive Rh-positive blood; the reverse is permissible. Though considerable battlefield experience indicates that the use of so-called universal donor blood (group O Rh-negative blood with a low titer of anti-A and anti-B isohemagglutinins) is safe, with adequate modern blood banking facilities this is rarely necessary except in an emergency.

Risks of Blood Transfusion. Although modern technology has made blood transfusion a generally safe procedure, a definite risk is involved. Transfusions should be given, therefore, only when the benefit to the patient exceeds the inherent danger of the procedure. It has been estimated that of every 2000 persons receiving a blood transfusion, one dies as a result of the immediate procedure or its consequences. Problems may arise from (1) *Clerical errors.* The mislabeling or faulty identification of containers may lead to a patient's receiving the wrong blood. If a type O patient receives type A or B blood, fatal intravascular hemolysis may occur. (2) *Red cell isoimmunization.* In almost every blood transfusion the donor red cells have some antigenic factor which the recipient does not possess. Many such factors are poor antigens, but some evoke intense antibody formation, the immunized person being at increased risk if another transfusion is given. (3) *Hepatitis.* A small proportion of the normal population are asymptomatic carriers of the agent for homologous serum hepatitis. There is no way to detect carriers with certainty, nor to inactivate the agent in blood, the risk in pooled plasma being proportional to the number of donors to the pool. (4) *White cell, platelet and plasma protein immunization.* White cells, platelets and some of the serum proteins have polymorphic antigens; multiple transfusions may be associated with development of antibodies against these components. (5) *Circulatory overload.* Patients with chronic anemia have expanded plasma volume and increased cardiac output; infusion of blood or plasma may precipitate congestive heart failure; rapid administration of large volumes of blood should be avoided. (6) *Depletion of labile substances.* Storage of blood is associated with loss of platelets and decreasing activities of the labile coagulation factors, such as factor VIII. When massive or exchange transfusions of stored blood are given, a complex disturbance of hemostasis may ensue. Use of fresh blood will avoid these complications. Acute citrate toxicity may also occur. (7) *Iron overload.* Each 500 ml. of blood contains about 250 mg. of iron. Patients with refractory anemias who require frequent transfusion ultimately have hemosiderosis. Iron is deposited in skin, liver, spleen and other organs, and may interfere with normal function.

Reactions to Blood Transfusion. (1) *Allergic reactions* occur in association with 1 to 2 per cent of transfusions. The most common clinical manifestation is urticaria; occasionally wheezing and arthralgia occur. The mechanism of these reactions is not certain, but they may be due to allergenic substances or to antibodies in the donor plasma. The development of urticaria alone does not necessitate discontinuing the transfusion; therapy with antihistamines or corticosteroids is effective in treating or preventing this type of reaction. (2) *Febrile reactions.* The use of disposable plastic equipment has eliminated most external pyrogenic substances. Sensitization to white cell antigens may produce febrile reactions to transfusions. The use of packed cells, excluding the buffy coat, and liberal use of salicylates may modify these reactions. Rarely a unit of blood may be contaminated with bacteria. Severe febrile reactions, shock and death may occur if infected blood is transfused. (3) *Hemolytic transfusion reactions.* Hemolytic reactions result in massive intravascular destruction of red cells, manifest clinically by fever, chills, headache and back pain. These symptoms do not appear when the patient is anesthetized. In severe reactions, shock and acute renal failure may ensue. Hemoglobinemia and hemoglobinuria are usually observed. When a hemolytic reaction is suspected, the transfusion should be *terminated immediately.* Diagnosis is proved by re-examining the blood types of donor cells and the recipient, repeating the crossmatch, and examining plasma and urine for free hemoglobin. The patient generally survives the initial acute episode; if he can be sustained through a period of renal failure, recovery is the rule.

REFERENCES

Polycythemia

Brines, J. K., Gibson, J. G., Jr., and Kunkel, P.: The Blood Volume in Normal Infants and Children. *J. Pediat.,* 18:447, 1941.

Michael, A. F., Jr., and Mauer, A. M.: Maternal-Fetal Transfusion as a Cause of Plethora in the Neonatal Period. *Pediatrics,* 28:458, 1961.

Naeye, R. L.: Human Intrauterine Parabiotic Syndrome and Its Complications. *New England J. Med.,* 268:804, 1963.

The Pancytopenias

Bloom, G. E., Warner, S., Gerald, P. S., and Diamond, L. K.: Chromosome Abnormalities in Constitutional Aplastic Anemia. *New England J. Med.,* 274:8, 1966.

Deller, J. J., Cirksena, W. J., and Marcarelli, J.: Fatal Pancytopenia Associated with Viral Hepatitis. *New England J. Med.,* 266:297, 1962.

Huguley, C. M., Jr., Lea, J. W., and Butts, J. A.: Adverse Hematologic Reactions to Drugs; in E. B. Brown and C. V. Moore (Eds.): *Progress in Hematology.* New York, Grune & Stratton, Inc., 1966, Vol. V, p. 105.

Shahidi, N. T., and Diamond, L. K.: Testosterone-Induced Remission in Aplastic Anemia of both Acquired and Congenital Types. *New England J. Med.,* 264:953, 1961.

Shahidi, N. T., Gerald, P. S., and Diamond, L. K.: Alkali-Resistant Hemoglobin in Aplastic Anemia of both Acquired and Congenital Types. *New England J. Med.,* 266:117, 1962.

Transfusions

Chown, B.: The Fetus Can Bleed. *Am. J. Obst. & Gynec.,* 70:1298, 1955.

Grove-Rasmussen, M., Lesses, M. F., and Anstall, H. B.: Transfusion Therapy. *New England J. Med.,* 264:1034, 1088, 1961.

Purugganan, H. B., and Naiman, J. L.: Exchange Transfusion in Severe Iron Deficiency Anemia Prior to Emergency Surgery. *J. Pediat.,* 69:804, 1966.

DISORDERS OF THE LEUKOCYTES

The leukocytes of the blood and their precursors in the bone marrow are easily studied, enumerated and classified. Leukocyte functions are concerned with resistance to infection and disposal of products of cellular breakdown. Because characteristic changes occur in many diseases, the white blood cell and differential counts are important as general screening tests. Normal values are listed in Table 14-3 (p. 1043).

The leukocytes are divided into 2 major classes: the granulocytes, consisting of neutrophils, eosinophils and basophils; and the nongranulated lymphocytes and monocytes. White cells have cellular antigens different from those of the erythrocyte. Some of these may be related to histocompatibility antigens of the host.

TYPES OF LEUKOCYTES

Neutrophils. Neutrophils are the predominating type of granulocyte. The nuclei of these cells have 1 to 5 segments which account for their designation as polymorphonuclear leukocytes. They have ameboid motility, chemotaxis and the capacity for active phagocytosis. Their fine cytoplasmic granules have a light purple (neutrophilic) color when stained with Wright's stain. These granules are lysosomes and contain digestive enzymes of several sorts, including proteases, cathepsins and lysozymes. When bacteria or other particles are ingested by neutrophils, degranulation occurs as the enzymes of the granules are discharged into a vacuole formed about the ingested material. Degranulation requires TPNH (NADPH$_2$) and involves activation of the pentose phosphate pathway. Subtle aberrations of the biochemistry of phagocytosis and intracellular digestion may result in markedly impaired resistance to disease.

The neutrophils occupy definable compartments or pools within the body. The *mitotic compartment* consists of myeloblasts, promyelocytes and myelocytes of the bone marrow. The *maturation compartment* consists of metamyelocytes and band forms, which are relatively completely differentiated, but have lost the capacity to divide, but still reside within the marrow. The *marrow storage compartment* consists of a rapidly mobilizable reserve of mature neutrophils. It has been estimated that it takes 6 to 11 days for a cell to pass through the stages of differentiation from a myeloblast to a mature neutrophil emerging into the peripheral blood.

The neutrophils of the peripheral blood exist in 2 exchangeable pools of approximately equal size. The *circulating granulocytic compartment* is in equilibrium with a *marginal compartment* consisting of neutrophils sequestered in small blood vessels. Vigorous exercise or injection of epinephrine causes the marginal pool to be mobilized into the circulation. The half-time of granulocytes within the circulation is 6 to 9 hours, after which they enter the *tissue pool,* where they carry out their primary function of phagocytosis. Little is known of their survival in the tissues.

Techniques are available for studying the various neutrophil compartments. The intramedullary mitotic and maturation compartments are generally estimated by examining bone marrow tissue. Hypertrophy of the neutrophilic series is reflected in alterations of the ratio between myeloid and erythroid elements (M/E, or myeloid-erythroid, ratio). The usual M/E ratio of between 2 and 4 to 1 may be markedly increased to between 5 and 10 to 1 in the presence of chronic inflammatory processes. Adequacy of the marrow storage compartment can be estimated from changes in the peripheral leukocyte count after intravenous injection of extracts of bacterial endotoxin. Normally, a twofold to fourfold increase in the numbers of circulating neutrophils results from such stimulated release of cells from the marrow storage compartment. In states of marrow hypoplasia or failure, no increase occurs. Radioisotopic techniques have been devised for estimating the time required for maturation and release of neutrophils from the marrow, as well as rate of turnover of neutrophils.

Eosinophils. The eosinophils are characterized by large coarse granules of a prominent red color with Romanowsky stains and by a nucleus with 1 or 2 segments. They normally account for less than 5 per cent of the circulating leukocytes. Eosinophil counts are depressed by high levels of adrenocortical hormones and increased in parasitic and allergic disorders. The most pronounced eosinophilia encountered in this country accompanies such diseases as visceral larva migrans and trichinosis, in which actual invasion of the tissue by parasitic helminths occurs.

Basophils. These leukocytes are distinguished by coarse, deep blue granules which fill the cytoplasm and obscure the nucleus. They contain large amounts of heparin and histamine. They normally account for less than 1 per cent of the circulating leukocytes. Increases occur in chronic myelogenous leukemia and in generalized mast cell disease.

Lymphocytes. Lymphocytes constitute 30 to 60 per cent of the blood leukocytes. Most are small cells measuring 10 microns in diameter, with a round, dark, blue-black nucleus and scanty blue cytoplasm. Other lymphocytes, probably younger forms, have more abundant blue cytoplasm. Lymphocytes are actively motile, but not phagocytic. The lymphocytes appear to be of 2 types. One of these has a brief life span, whereas the other is exceedingly long-lived. Small lymphocytes have the capacity to undergo blastic transformation and mitosis when stimulated by phytohemagglutinin. The lymphocytes are intimately involved in various aspects of the immune mechanism, especially in transmission of delayed immunity, and in immunoglobulin synthesis. A pronounced lymphocytosis is characteristic of pertussis and the syndrome of infectious lymphocytosis. In infectious mononucleosis characteristically atypical lymphocytes appear in large numbers. Thymic alymphoplasia is associated with profound lymphopenia and immunoglobulin deficiency.

Monocytes. These large phagocytic cells are characterized by a large lobulated nucleus and an abundant gray cytoplasm containing fine azurophilic granules. They normally account for 1 to 5 per cent of the circulating leukocytes, but are increased in such diseases as tuberculosis, systemic mycosis, bacterial endocarditis and certain protozoan infections.

Quantitative Disorders of the Neutrophils

Absolute neutrophil counts vary widely in normal subjects. The relative proportion of neutrophils and lymphocytes in the blood varies with age. Neutrophils predominate at birth, but decrease rapidly in the first few days of life. During infancy they constitute 30 to 40 per cent of the circulating leukocytes. Parity between neutrophils and lymphocytes occurs by about 5 years of age, but the approximately 70 per cent predominance of neutrophils characteristic of the adult is not attained until puberty. In normal healthy children, therefore, from 30 to 70 per cent of the total circulating white blood cells may be neutrophils. In absolute terms they number 2500 to 6000 per cu. mm. Levels exceeding this range are designated neutrophilia.

NEUTROPHILIA

Neutrophilia accompanies a wide variety of localized and generalized pyogenic infections as well as some noninfectious inflammatory processes. Both the total white blood cell count and the proportion of neutrophils increase. In addition, larger numbers of nonsegmented (band) neutrophils and even more immature cells (metamyelocytes and myelocytes) may be seen ("shift to the left"). In general, younger children demonstrate more pronounced responses to infections than adults and manifest higher white cell counts with greater numbers of immature forms. When the total white cell count exceeds 40,000 per cu. mm., a "leukemoid" blood picture is said to be present. A presumptive cause is usually evident for leukemoid reactions, such as infection, intoxication, and the like, but occasionally the blood picture may be difficult to differentiate from chronic myelogenous leukemia. The neutrophilia of infection or inflammation is accompanied by increased activity and hypertrophy of the entire neutrophilic series. On the other hand, the transient neutrophilia accompanying acute stress reflects shifts of previously formed neutrophils between circulating and marginal pools rather than actual increased production, and is not accompanied by changes in marrow.

NEUTROPENIA

Neutropenia is a reduction below normal of the numbers of circulating neutrophils. This occurs in a substantial number of congenital and acquired diseases and results from either underproduction or peripheral hyperdestruction of neutrophils. When the absolute neutrophil count is less than 1500 per cu. mm., the patient becomes unusually susceptible to bacterial infections, especially to those of the skin and respiratory tract. Buccal and rectal ulcerations are also frequently associated.

Infantile Lethal Agranulocytosis. This familial disease is characterized by the onset in early infancy of recurrent, severe pyogenic infections, especially of the skin and the lung. Neutrophils are totally absent in the blood or present in reduced numbers; there are absolute monocytosis and eosinophilia. The platelets are normal, and primary anemia is absent. The bone marrow contains markedly decreased numbers of neutrophilic precursors. The neutrophilic series is represented by a few promyelocytes and myelocytes. Lymphocytes and plasmacytes are prominent. The erythrocytic and megakaryocytic elements are normal.

There is no specific or effective therapy. Hematinics, corticosteroids and splenectomy produce no beneficial effect. Although antibiotics may be of temporary value, death frequently occurs during infancy or the first few years of life as a result of overwhelming sepsis. The disease appears to be genetically determined; most pedigrees suggest an autosomal recessive transmission. The basic enzymatic or metabolic defect is unknown.

Chronic Benign Neutropenia. This disease usually produces relatively mild clinical manifestations and is differentiated from the preceding disorder by its mildness and sporadic occurrence. The child experiences recurrent pneumonia, pyoderma and mouth ulcerations. The peripheral white blood cell count is decreased, and there is a striking paucity of neutrophils. There is no anemia, and the platelets are normal. Monocytosis and eosinophilia are usually present. Serum protein studies demonstrate diffuse hypergammaglobulinemia. In the bone marrow there is maturation arrest at the myelocyte or metamyelocyte stage and plasmacytosis, but no alteration of the erythrocytic and megakaryocytic elements. Some of these patients appear to be able to mobilize a neutrophilic response when challenged by significant pyogenic infections.

Infections can be controlled by appropriate antibiotic therapy. Attempts to stimulate granulopoiesis with corticosteroids or other therapy are usually ineffectual. Affected children tend to improve with age and may undergo total remissions in late childhood. Although most cases are sporadic, at least 2 pedigrees suggesting autosomal dominant inheritance have been described.

Acquired Neutropenia. Decrease in the total white blood cell count and concomitant neutropenia occur in many viral infections, particularly roseola infantum, rubella, rubeola and influenza. Neutropenia is also characteristic of typhoid and paratyphoid infections and brucellosis. In severe pyogenic infections the observation of neutropenia is an ominous prognostic sign, often indicating the overwhelming nature of the disease. In some cases of rheumatoid arthritis and lupus erythematosus neutropenia also occurs. The pathogenesis of the leukopenia in these diseases is uncertain, but may represent peripheral sequestration or hyperutilization.

Neutropenia results from marrow insufficiency in leukemia, aplastic pancytopenia and disseminated neoplasms such as neuroblastoma. In advanced megaloblastic anemia due to deficiency of vitamin B_{12} or folic acid, neutropenia regularly occurs, possibly owing to ineffective leukopoiesis. On the other hand, an enlarged spleen may filter large numbers of neutrophils from the circulation. Ionizing radiation and such drugs or chemicals as nitrogen mustard, methotrexate and benzene regularly cause marrow depression and neutropenia in any person receiving them in sufficient amounts.

DRUG-INDUCED NEUTROPENIAS
(MALIGNANT AGRANULOCYTOSIS)

This syndrome is characterized by a profound reduction of neutrophils in the blood and of their precursors in the bone marrow, accompanied by severe systemic infection. It is usually self-limited, but occasionally lethal.

Etiology. The drugs or agents which produce this situation do so in a relatively small number of patients so that an idiosyncrasy would seem to be partly responsible. In some instances, such as in neutropenia associated with aminopyrine, an immunologic basis is probable. This drug acts as a hapten in combination with a protein of the neutrophil, forming an antigenic complex which stimulates formation of a leukocidal antibody. Currently, the drug most frequently producing neutropenia is the aminopyrine derivative, dipyrone (Pyralgin). The use of this potentially dangerous drug for its symptomatic effect on fever is inappropriate. Other drugs associated with a significant incidence of neutropenia include thiourea derivatives, phenothiazines and sulfonamides. In many cases of neutropenia no cause can be discovered.

Clinical Manifestations. An abrupt onset with a racking rigor occurs in aminopyrine-induced neutropenia. In other cases the onset may be insidious. Ulcerations of the mouth and rectum, cutaneous infections, and pneumonia are frequent. Despite the absence of neutrophils, the temperature curve is septic, with frequent high spikes. Purulent exudates are not formed, so that the usual physical findings of pyogenic infections may not occur. Death results from overwhelming sepsis in the first week of the disease in about 20 per cent of cases. Intestinal perforations may occur.

Laboratory Data. The total white blood cell count is reduced. Circulating neutrophils are low, but a compensatory monocytosis and eosinophilia are frequently present. There is no anemia or thrombocytopenia. Bone marrow changes depend upon the stage of illness. At the height of the disease the marrow is cellular, with normal numbers of erythroid precursors and megakaryocytes, but neutrophilic precursors are reduced. Five to 20 per cent of the nucleated cells may be plasma cells. Recovery is presaged by a return of granulopoiesis in the marrow, which proceeds as a surge of maturation through the several stages of development. Bone marrow examination in this early recovery stage may be misinterpreted as showing a maturation arrest. Four to 5 days after the return of precursors to the marrow, mature neutrophils reappear in the blood. Coincident with their reappearance, prompt defervescence and clinical improvement usually ensue.

Treatment. The most important therapeutic measure is immediate discontinuation of any medications which may be causative. Infection should be treated with therapeutic doses of antibiotics, the choice of which should be determined by culture and sensitivity studies; when feasible, bactericidal antibiotics should be used. Prophylactic antibiotics are not indicated, and there is no practical way to transfuse effective numbers of neutrophils. Corticosteroid therapy is not of significant value. Once a patient has acquired neutropenia after administration of a specific drug, that drug or closely related agents should not be administered again.

CYCLIC NEUTROPENIA

This ill-defined disease is characterized by periodic episodes of fever and oral ulcerations accompanied by profound neutropenia. Neutropenia persists from 5 to 10 days, after which the white blood cell count returns to normal and the symptoms abate. Such episodes occur at cycles of 14 to 45 days. The bone marrow during the period of neutropenia shows diminished numbers of neutrophilic precursors or maturation arrest. Between episodes the blood and marrow are normal. Therapy is symptomatic.

TRANSITORY NEUTROPENIA OF THE NEWBORN

Neutrophilia is characteristic of the immediate postnatal period, but with severe infections such as cytomegalic inclusion disease, toxoplasmosis or bacterial sepsis striking neutropenia may occur. Newborn infants have been described with familial neutropenia and superimposed bacterial infections. In some of these cases the mother has also been neutropenic, suggesting transmission of a humoral inhibitor or antibody from mother to infant. Isoimmunization to neutrophil antigens analogous to Rh sensitization has been suggested as causative in some instances. Bacterial infections usually respond to vigorous antibiotic therapy. The duration of the neutropenia is 4 to 7 weeks.

Inherited Abnormalities of the Leukocytes

Ninety per cent of the neutrophils in the peripheral blood of normal persons have 2 to 4 segments. Only about 5 per cent are unsegmented (bands), and less than 5 per cent have 5 segments. An increase in unsegmented forms, or "shift to the left," usually indicates infection or inflammation, whereas hypersegmentation, or "shift to the right," most commonly occurs in megaloblastic anemias due to folic acid or vitamin B_{12} deficiency.

Hereditary Hyposegmentation (Pelger-Huet Anomaly). This defect of neutrophilic segmentation is inherited as an autosomal dominant trait. In heterozygous persons more than 90 per cent of circulating neutrophils and eosinophils are either unsegmented or have only 2 lobes. Despite this abnormal nuclear configuration, their phagocytic capacity is normal, and no predisposition to infection is associated with the trait. The homozygous state may be lethal.

Hereditary Hypersegmentation (Undritz Anomaly). This rare condition is characterized by predominance of neutrophils with 4 and 5, or even more, segments. The anomaly is inherited as an autosomal trait. No adverse clinical effects are associated with its presence.

May-Hegglin anomaly. This rare, dominantly transmitted anomaly involves the neutrophils and platelets. A majority of the neutrophils contain irregular blue cytoplasmic inclusions similar to Döhle bodies. Döhle bodies consist of precipitated nucleoprotein material and are usually observed in patients with severe systemic infections. In patients with the May-Hegglin anomaly no infection need be present. There may be abnormally large platelets, and at times thrombocytopenia. The thrombocytopenia responds to splenectomy.

Alder anomaly. In this condition, which is probably transmitted as an autosomal recessive trait, the neutrophilic granulations are larger and stain much more prominently than normal. The granules are distinctly lavender or blue, a circumstance which permits their differentiation from eosinophils. A very small proportion of patients with the Hunter-Hurler syndrome may show somewhat similar granulations in their neutrophils (Reilly bodies).

Chediak-Higashi disease. This recessively transmitted syndrome has striking clinical features, including albinism, photophobia and markedly impaired resistance to infection. The neutrophils contain large, greenish-brown cytoplasmic inclusions which represent giant, abnormal lysosomes. The granulations of the eosinophils and basophils are also very large. Patients with this disease usually die in childhood of sepsis. A high incidence of lymphoreticular malignancy is seen.

Chronic granulomatous disease (See pp. 457, 478 and 487). This is the first disease in which a specific metabolic abnormality of the granulocytes has been recognized as a basis for increased susceptibility to infection. The disease is inherited as an X-linked recessive trait. Affected males suffer from severe repeated infections and large infectious granulomas. Their neutrophils do not undergo normal degranulation with ingestion of bacteria, and the latter are not killed and digested. The basic defect appears to be an inability to activate the pentose phosphate pathway, which results in a relative deficiency of TPNH.

The Leukemias

Leukemia is a uniformly fatal malignant disease due to uncontrolled neoplastic proliferation of leukocyte precursors in blood, bone marrow and reticuloendothelial tissues.

Etiology. The cause of leukemia has thus far eluded definition, but there are a number of clues. A genetic predisposition is suggested by a high concordance rate (25 per cent) in identical twins, whereas the disease has not been observed in both of fraternal twins. Except in identical twins, familial occurrence is rare. Certain hereditary conditions which demonstrate chromosomal instability are associated with an increased rate of leukemia, such as Fanconi's aplastic anemia and Bloom's syndrome. Diseases associated with disorders of the immune mechanism, such as agammaglobulinemia and ataxia-telangiectasia, have an increased incidence of leukemia and other lymphoreticular malignancy, and in Down's syndrome the rate of leukemia is increased to 10 to 20 times normal. There is an increased incidence in children of high socioeconomic backgrounds.

A great deal of interest has been centered on a possible infectious origin; certain animal leukemias are of proved viral origin. Epidemiologic evidence possibly supporting an infectious factor in human leukemia includes the observation of geographic and temporal "clusters" of cases markedly in excess of expected frequency. In addition, virus-like bodies can be demonstrated by electron microscopy in the blood and bone marrow of many leukemic patients. Circumstantial evidence indicates a virus origin for the Burkitt lymphoma, which sometimes terminates in leukemia. A simple infectious viral cause seems unlikely for childhood leukemia, since despite more than 250 instances of maternal leukemia during pregnancy, in only 2 instances has the infant been known subsequently to have the disease.

Leukemia has a striking peak of age of onset in children at 3 to 4 years of age, a phenomenon which was not seen prior to about 1940. There is a slightly increased incidence in males. In Negroes the disease seems to be somewhat less frequent, and the peak of onset at 4 years not so striking.

Types of Leukemia. The leukemias of childhood are classified according to the morphologic characteristics of the abnormal leukemic cells rather than the symptoms or length of survival. During childhood acute leukemias predominate. The abnormal cells of acute leukemia are primitive, undifferentiated forms called "blast" or stem cells. About 80 per cent of cases of childhood leukemia are the acute lymphoblastic type (ALL). In about 15 per cent of cases the disease may be classified as acute granulocytic or myelogenous (AGL), and chronic granulocytic leukemia (CGL) accounts for 3 to 5 per cent. Erythroleukemic, eosinophilic, monocytic and plasmacytic varieties are rare. Chronic lymphatic leukemia has not been convincingly documented in childhood. Although it is not always possible to classify precisely the type of a given case of acute leukemia, attempts should be made for prognostic purposes. Acute lymphoblastic leukemia frequently responds to chemotherapy, whereas in other acute varieties a response is far less predictable.

Clinical Manifestations. The presenting signs and symptoms of leukemia result from anemia, neutropenia and thrombopenia, and from diffuse infiltration of organs and tissues.

Anemia of a profound degree is frequently present, with its attendant symptoms of weakness, lassitude and dyspnea. The skin has a peculiar lemon-yellow hue. Cardiac dilatation, tachycardia and systolic-flow murmurs are often present. Petechiae and purpura are often the first recognized signs of the disease. Extensive bruising of the legs and large ecchymoses after minor trauma, as well as cutaneous petechiae, are frequently present. Epistaxis and oral and scleral hemorrhages may be prominent. Occasionally hematuria and melena occur. Blood loss may significantly increase the severity of anemia.

Bone and joint pain may be prominent, and leukemia should be considered in the differential diagnosis of children with unexplained bone pain or limp. This pain results from infarction and bone destruction, from subperiosteal hemorrhage and possibly from pressure exerted by hyperplastic neoplastic tissue within the medullary space. Areas of bone destruction and periosteal elevation are seen roentgenographically. A transverse line of radiolucency is frequently seen at the metaphysis of the long bones.

Although leukemia represents an uncontrolled proliferation of abnormal white cells, leukemic cells do not have effective phagocytic function, and pyogenic infections of skin and lung are common. Fever may reflect a hypermetabolic state due to rapid growth and destruction of leukemic tissue; substantial pyrexia usually indicates infection, however, and antibiotic therapy should be instituted upon this premise.

Another prominent group of signs and symptoms of leukemia is due to proliferation of leukemic cells in abdominal viscera and lymph nodes. The testes and kidneys are sometimes diffusely enlarged. The liver and spleen are usually significantly enlarged, and nodular infiltrates of skin occasionally occur, particularly in cases of granulocytic leukemia. The lymph nodes are enlarged and firm, but not painful or tender. Enlargement of mediastinal lymph nodes may produce respiratory distress due to pressure on the bronchial tree. In about 5 per cent of patients the liver, spleen and lymph nodes are not significantly enlarged.

Laboratory Data. The diagnosis of acute leukemia is established on demonstration of leukemic blast cells in blood, bone marrow and other tissues.

It cannot be overemphasized that leukemic infiltration of the marrow or other tissues must be shown unequivocally before a diagnosis of this fatal disease can be made.

The accompanying anemia is normochromic and normocytic. The reticulocyte count is low, but a few nucleated red cells may be observed on the peripheral smear. Severe thrombocytopenia is usually present, with platelet counts of less than 40,000 per cu. mm. The total leukocyte count is variable. In about half the cases the leukocyte count is within the normal range (7000 to 12,000 per cu. mm.). Five to 10 per cent of cases demonstrate severe leukopenia (white blood cells less than 3000 per cu. mm.). In the remaining cases varying degrees of leukocytosis are seen, and markedly elevated white cell counts occur occasionally. The predominant circulating cell is the blast cell. In acute lymphoblastic leukemia this is a large cell with scanty blue cytoplasm which contains no granulations. The nuclear chromatin is dispersed in a finely stippled pattern. One or more nucleoli may be seen. Occasionally, prominent, sharp punched-out vacuoles may be seen within the blast cells; these represent degenerative changes. In addition to the blast cells, more mature cells of the lymphocytic series are present. In the 15 per cent of cases of childhood leukemia classified as granulocytic, the leukemic cells correspond to myeloblasts and promyelocytes and many contain primitive granulations. Occasionally red, needle-like, cytoplasmic crystals called Auer rods are present.

In the stained aspirate of bone marrow the varied, colorful appearance of normal marrow is replaced by monotonous sheets of blast cells. Fat spaces are reduced, and megakaryocytes and erythroid precursors are markedly diminished; the marrow may be so hypercellular that aspiration is unsuccessful. A "dry tap" almost always indicates an abnormal marrow. A specimen suitable for diagnosis can be obtained from the iliac crest with a Silverman or Westerman-Jensen needle or by surgical biopsy. In a small proportion of cases the initial sampling of marrow does not reveal typical findings, but hypoplasia or fibrillar reticulum tissue may be observed. Although aspiration from another site may reveal typical morphology, on rare occasions it may initially be impossible to differentiate between leukemia and aplastic anemia. Since therapy with most antileukemic drugs is disastrous in aplastic anemia, these chemotherapeutic measures should be withheld until an unequivocal histologic diagnosis is made. In these cases of so-called aleukemic leukemia, conventional findings usually become apparent in a short time. Other laboratory findings are relatively unimportant and inconstant. Hyperuricemia may occur, particularly when high white blood cell counts are present. There are no specific or regular chromosomal changes observed in acute leukemia, but peripheral blood and bone marrow cultures frequently reveal aneuploidy.

Differential Diagnosis. Leukemia should be included in the differential diagnosis of any child with unexplained depression of any of the formed elements of blood, and complete hematologic investigation, including examination of the bone marrow, is mandatory. Diseases sometimes confused with leukemia include idiopathic thrombocytopenic purpura and other forms of thrombocytopenia, scurvy, acute rheumatic fever, rheumatoid arthritis, aplastic anemia, sickle cell disease, osteomyelitis, and infectious mononucleosis and lymphocytosis.

Other malignant processes mimic acute leukemia. About 25 per cent of patients with lymphoma exhibit hematologic changes of acute leukemia during the course of their disease. In disseminated neuroblastoma the marrow may be sufficiently replaced by metastatic disease that morphologic differentiation from leukemia may be difficult. In metastatic neuroblastoma there is a tendency to form syncytia, with a mosaic appearance and occasional pseudorosettes. In addition, most patients with neuroblastoma excrete large amounts of urinary catecholamines.

Course and Prognosis. The course of untreated acute lymphoblastic leukemia of childhood is short. Death from infection or hemorrhage occurs within 6 months in most instances. Symptomatic therapy with blood transfusion and antibiotics is of only transient benefit. Before the chemotherapeutic era a few children had spontaneous remissions, with temporary return of blood and bone marrow to normal status. These remissions usually followed severe infections and were of short duration, survivals for more than 9 to 10 months being remarkable. The development of specific chemotherapeutic agents for acute leukemia has changed the survival time significantly. In most instances of acute lymphatic leukemia it is possible to induce remissions which may be maintained for a relatively long time. Recent reports describe median survivals of 18 to 24 months. An appreciable number of children now survive from 2 to 3 years after diagnosis; some children with acute leukemia are alive 5 years or longer after initial diagnosis. The possibility that some of these may represent cures has been entertained.

Treatment. Treatment of acute leukemia may be divided into supportive and specific types. General supportive therapy includes transfusions and antibiotics. Fresh whole blood and platelet concentrates can be given to control hemorrhage and to correct anemia. Infections must be vigorously treated. Antibiotic therapy should be used when bacterial infection is likely, and based upon appropriate cultures and sensitivity tests whenever possible. Pseudomonas and staphylococcal septicemia are common. Because of their debilitated state and altered resistance, affected children may also become infected by saprophytes, such as fungi, *Pneumocystis carinii* and the cytomegalic inclusion virus.

Chemotherapeutic agents. The drugs used in the therapy of leukemia are listed in Table 14-5. These drugs belong to several classes; in general, there is no cross resistance among them. All have the capacity to induce remissions. A remission is defined as eradication of morphologic evidence of leukemia from blood and bone marrow with restoration of normal health. During remissions a histologic diagnosis of leukemia cannot be made. Two agents, corticosteroid and vincristine, act rapidly and induce remission in a high percentage of cases of acute lymphoblastic leukemia. Because the remissions are usually of short duration, these 2 drugs may be used in conjunction with other agents which prolong remissions. The latter drugs include 6-mercaptopurine (6-MP), a substituted purine base; methotrexate, a folic acid antagonist; cyclophosphamide, a polyfunctional alkylating agent; and Daunomycin, an antibiotic. Newer drugs are continuously being developed and tested. All are potent agents with significant adverse side effects and should be used only when careful observation by an experienced physician is available.

Several therapeutic programs utilizing the foregoing drugs have been developed. In the regimen most frequently used, initial remission is rapidly induced with a corticosteroid or vincristine. Hyperuricemia and precipitates of uric acid in the kidneys may accompany the rapid lysis of cells; adequate hydration and alkalinization of the urine will usually avoid this complication. Allopurinol in a dose of 10 mg. per kg. per day is also effective. When remission is attained, corticosteroids and vincristine are discontinued, and therapy with 6-MP, methotrexate or cytoxan is begun. Maintenance therapy definitely prolongs the remission. When relapse occurs, as indicated by reappearance

of clinical and hematologic manifestations of the disease, a new attempt at control is begun with a different drug. It is often possible to attain 3 or more successive remissions before the patient becomes refractory to all therapy.

In an attempt to forestall development of resistance to the drugs, cyclic regimens have been used in which drugs were changed every 4 to 8 weeks, but recent studies have shown no increased survival with such therapeutic programs. More recently, more aggressive programs involving simultaneous administration of 4 or more drugs have been used in an attempt to eliminate all residual leukemia cells, in hope of producing longer remissions or even cures. These programs entail considerable morbidity and even mortality and require vigorous supportive treatment during a prolonged induction phase. Ten to 15 per cent of children with leukemia respond poorly to all therapeutic attempts. Even in those children who respond favorably, after one or more remissions and varying times, the leukemic process becomes refractory to all available therapy.

It is important to attempt to identify cases of acute granulocytic leukemia, for the response to therapy is less predictable and survival is generally not as long as in the lymphoblastic variety. Despite frequent unresponsiveness, a chemotherapeutic approach similar to that described for lymphoblastic leukemia should be attempted, and good results are obtained occasionally. A new agent, cytosine arabinoside, may be effective. In some instances a dramatic worsening of the clinical and hematologic manifestations of acute granulocytic leukemia has occurred coincidentally with corticosteroid therapy, which should on that account be used cautiously.

All therapy should be directed toward quickly

TABLE 14-5. DRUGS USEFUL IN THE TREATMENT OF LEUKEMIA

GENERIC NAME	TRADE NAME AND MANUFACTURER	ROUTE OF ADMINISTRATION	USUAL DOSAGE	PREDOMINANT TOXICITY
Amethopterin.........................	Methotrexate (Lederle)	(a) Oral (b) Intermittent— intravenous or oral (c) Intrathecal	(a) 1.25 to 5 mg./day (b) 20 to 30 mg./m.² twice a week (c) 0.5 mg./kg. up to 10 mg. every 2 to 4 days until CSF clears	Myelotoxicity Affects gastrointestinal mucous membrane
Corticosteroids: e.g. prednisone (other preparations available for parenteral use)	Meticorten (Shering)	Oral	2 mg./kg./day	Cushing's syndrome
6-Mercaptopurine...................	Purinethol (Burroughs-Wellcome)	Oral	2.5 mg./kg./day	Myelotoxicity
Vincristine...........................	Oncovin (Lilly)	Intravenous	0.075 mg./kg./week for 4 to 6 doses	Peripheral neuropathy, alopecia
Cyclophosphamide...................	Cytoxan (Mead Johnson)	(a) Oral (b) Intravenous	(a) 2.5 mg./kg./day (b) 5 mg./kg./day for 10 days	Myelotoxicity, alopecia Chemical cystitis
Busulfan.............................	Myleran (Burroughs-Wellcome)	Oral	1 to 4 mg./day	Myelotoxicity

restoring the child to normal health, and maintaining this for as long as possible. Relapses and other complications should be detected as early as possible so that drug changes can be made before the child becomes so ill that hospitalization is necessary. With skillful management, hospitalizations can be kept to a minimum.

Central Nervous System Leukemia. About 25 per cent of children with leukemia suffer leukemic infiltration of the meninges. The symptoms and signs are those of increased intracranial pressure, with headache and morning vomiting as frequent initial manifestations. Papilledema and increased head circumference are seen, and spreading of the sutures is evident roentgenographically. This complication of acute leukemia usually occurs after a period of successful chemotherapy, but may rarely be present at the onset of the disease. Lumbar puncture reveals increased pressure, increased protein and a mononuclear pleocytosis of 50 to 5000 per cu. mm. of leukemic blast cells. It has been postulated that leukemic cells may be protected from the effects of systemic chemotherapy by the blood-brain barrier, since the levels of these drugs in the spinal fluid are less than one tenth those in the serum.

The complication can be treated effectively by 3 or 4 injections of 5 to 10 mg. of methotrexate into the subarachnoid space by lumbar puncture. This therapy is effective even when the systemic disease has become refractory to methotrexate. Roentgen therapy in a dose of 400 to 600 r directed to lateral skull ports may also be effective. In some medical centers the spinal cord is also irradiated. If this complication is not recognized and prompt therapy initiated, ocular palsies and even blindness may ensue.

Counseling the Family of the Child with Leukemia. There are few situations in pediatric practice in which wise and sympathetic support and counseling are of greater value.

The possibility of leukemia should not be discussed unless the diagnosis is unequivocal, and consultation or referral should be considered in any questionable case. If leukemia is present, the parents must be told the diagnosis. The skillful management of the initial interview profoundly affects subsequent relations between family and physician.

The physician must state the diagnosis without equivocation and without using euphemisms. A less positive approach, or expressed doubts of the diagnosis, may raise false hopes in the parents' minds. A number of questions, fears and feelings of guilt are so common in parents that they should be anticipated by the physician. The parents should be told that leukemia is not hereditary or contagious, so that there is no significantly increased risk to siblings or playmates. The parents can be told that acts of omission and commission do not cause leukemia, and that there is no known way that the disease could have been prevented. Reassurance can be given that delays in diagnosis do not in general affect the long-term results.

A brief explanation of the nature of the disease and its clinical manifestations should be given. The remission should be described and the probability that remissions can be attained in a majority of cases should be emphasized. A definite prediction of survival should not be given, but it can be stated that remissions often last for many months or even years. The family can be advised that the treatment of leukemia is fairly standardized; scientific communications are well developed so that as definitive therapies are discovered, information is rapidly disseminated throughout the medical community. Parents can, therefore, be assured that there is in general little to be gained by taking the child to distant centers in search of novel therapy or cures. Finally, the parents can be told that leukemia is not usually associated with pain, and in most instances it is possible to prevent undue suffering.

During the early days of the disease, frequent reassurance and discussions help the family make the necessary adjustments to the diagnosis and the realization that their child will ultimately die. Management and support of the older child or adolescent with leukemia present particular challenges. These children will often themselves learn of their diagnosis from friends or neighbors, and it may be better that they be told by their parents or physician if questions arise.

Acute Leukemia in the Newborn. Leukemia in newborn infants is generally of the acute granulocytic type. They have profound anemia and thrombocytopenia, and markedly elevated white cell counts with large numbers of circulating blast cells are common. There may be nodular leukemic infiltrations of the skin and massive hepatosplenomegaly. Response to chemotherapy has been poor. Leukemia must be differentiated from various neonatal diseases such as syphilis, cytomegalic inclusion disease, toxoplasmosis, rubella and hemolytic disease of the newborn (erythroblastosis fetalis). A few newborn infants with Down's syndrome have had a hematologic syndrome indistinguishable from acute granulocytic leukemia and have had remissions of very long duration. It is impossible to say whether this represents a variant of leukemia or an unusual leukemoid reaction. In any case, caution is indicated in diagnosing leukemia in newborns with trisomy 21.

Chronic Granulocytic Leukemia. About 5 per cent of leukemias in children are of the chronic granulocytic variety (CGL). The spleen usually becomes gigantic in size, often descending into the left pelvis. White blood cell counts may exceed 70,000 per cu. mm., and blast cells, promyelocytes, myelocytes and metamyelocytes, as well as more mature granulocytes, are present in the blood. Nucleated red blood cells and an absolute eosinophilia and basophilia are also observed. The more mature granulocytes in this disease have very low alkaline phosphatase activity, in contradistinction to the high activity of granulocytes in leukemoid reactions. Serum levels of vitamin B_{12} are also very high in this form of leukemia.

Chronic granulocytic leukemia is the only human malignancy in which a characteristic cytogenetic abnormality occurs and has been regularly observed. Peripheral blood and bone marrow culture reveals an abnormal G group or 21 chromosome which has lost material from both long arms; a minute fragment results, called the Philadelphia or Ph chromosome. Although most typical cases of chronic granulocytic leukemia have the Ph chromosome, a number of infants with otherwise typical hematologic findings have not had it. An elevated level of fetal hemoglobin is characteristic of this latter variety, and affected infants pursue an acute fulminating clinical course; they do not respond well to therapy.

Chronic granuloctyic leukemia may be treated with busulfan (Myleran), a nitrogen mustard derivative. This is given orally in a dose of 1 to 4 mg. per day until the white blood cell count drops below 20,000 per cu. mm. Maintenance therapy at a lower dose may then be begun, or the drug discontinued until relapse occurs. Mercaptopurine (6-MP) is also effective. The disease may be controlled for many months or even years, but ultimately large numbers of blast cells appear in the circulation. At this point the disease may be indistinguishable from acute granulocytic leukemia, and death usually occurs in a short time.

REFERENCES

General

Cartwright, G. E., Athens, J. W., Boggs, D. R., and Wintrobe, M. M.: The Kinetics of Granulopoiesis in Normal Man. *Series Hematologica*, 1:1, 1965.

Davidson, W. M.: Inherited Variations in Leucocytes. *Brit. Med. Bull.*, 17:190, 1961.

Neutropenia

Kauder, E., and Mauer, A. M.: Neutropenias of Childhood. *J. Pediat.*, 69:147, 1966.

Leukemia

Dameshek, W., Necheles, T. F., Finkel, H. E., and Allen, D. M.: Therapy of Acute Leukemia. *Blood*, 26:220, 1965.

Evans, A. E., D'Angio, G. J., and Mitus, A.: Central Nervous System Complication of Children with Acute Leukemia: An Evaluation of Treatment Methods. *J. Pediat.*, 64:94, 1964.

Evans, A. E.: If a Child Must Die. *New England J. Med.*, 278:138, 1968.

Freireich, E. J., and Frei, E., III: Recent Advances in Acute Leukemia; in C. V. Moore and E. B. Brown (Eds.): *Progress in Hematology.* New York, Grune & Stratton, Inc., 1964, Vol. IV, p. 187.

James, K. J., and Kay, H. E. M.: Some Aspects of Current Therapy in Acute Leukemia. *Lancet*, 1:206, 1967.

Reisman, L. E., and Trujillo, J. M.: Chronic Granulocytic Leukemia of Childhood. Clinical and Cytogenetic Studies. *J. Pediat.*, 62:710, 1963.

HEMORRHAGIC DISEASES

The blood is in dynamic equilibrium between fluidity and coagulation. This balance must be precisely maintained to assure that exsanguination does not result from trivial trauma or that spontaneous thrombosis does not occur. The hemostatic mechanism is complex and involves local reactions of the blood vessels, the several activities of the platelet, and finally the interactions of a number of specific coagulation factors which circulate in the blood. The vascular endothelium is the primary barrier against hemorrhage. When small blood vessels are transected, active vasoconstriction and local tissue pressure control minute areas of bleeding even without mobilization of the coagulation process, but the platelet is essential for maintenance of small blood vessels and of their endothelial stability. Hemostatic defects due to abnormalities of the vessels are manifest by small intracutaneous hemorrhages and petechiae. Hemorrhagic states related to the platelets and the soluble coagulation proteins are more dramatic and urgent.

Schema of Coagulation. The classic schema of coagulation, formulated at the turn of the century, pictured coagulation as proceeding in 3 phases. In phase I a hypothetical substance called thromboplastin was formed by interaction of plasma, platelets and tissue juice. In phase II, prothrombin was converted to thrombin in the presence of thromboplastin and calcium. Finally, in phase III, thrombin converted soluble fibrinogen into the visible fibrin clot. Although this simple scheme, involving only 6 substances, has been expanded so that a dozen factors have now been defined, retention of the concept of a basic 3-phase reaction has considerable merit. Table 14-6 lists the currently recognized coagulation factors and their common synonyms. The modern view of coagulation is depicted in Figure 14-9.

In phase I, in addition to an increased number of factors, intrinsic and extrinsic systems have been recognized. The intrinsic mechanism involves the successive enzymatic conversion of the inactive forms of factors XII, XI, IX, VIII to their active forms. Active factors VIII and a phospholipid substance (partial thromboplastin) derived from platelets catalyze the successive conversion of inactive factors X and V to active counterparts. The extrinsic mechanism involves the conversion of inactive factor VII to its active state by a substance derived from tissue fluid. In the extrinsic system active factor VII does not require the platelet phospholipid to activate factors X and V. A specific substance which has been identified as thromboplastin probably does not exist.

Phase II of coagulation is concerned with the enzymatic cleavage of inactive prothrombin into active thrombin. This step requires factor II as substrate, as well as active factors X and V and calcium.

Finally, in phase III, thrombin splits 2 small

TABLE 14-6. THE COAGULATION FACTORS

INTERNATIONAL NUMBERS	SYNONYMS	COMMENT
I..........	Fibrinogen	Number rarely used—congenital deficiency known (afibrinogenemia)
II..........	Prothrombin	Number rarely used—congenital deficiency known
III..........	Thromboplastin	No specific factor identified
IV..........	Calcium	Number rarely used
V..........	Labile factor proaccelerin	Congenital deficiency known (parahemophilia, Owren's disease)
VI..........	Activated labile factor, accelerin	No longer differentiated from V
VII..........	Stable factor, SPCA, proconvertin	Congenital deficiency known
VIII..........	Antihemophilic factor (AHF) or globulin (AHG)	Hemophilia A (classic hemophilia) results from congenital deficiency
IX..........	Christmas factor, plasma thromboplastin component (PTC)	Hemophilia B results from congenital deficiency
X..........	Stuart-Prower factor	Congenital deficiency known
XI..........	Plasma thromboplastin antecedent, PTA	Congenital deficiency known
XII..........	Hageman factor	No clinical symptoms associated with congenital deficiency
XIII..........	Fibrin stabilizing factor	Congenital deficiency known

peptides from the fibrinogen molecule, uncovering reactive sites in the fibrin monomer. These monomers then spontaneously polymerize to form long chains of fibrin. Factor XIII facilitates lateral bonding between fibrin strands to form a stable 3-dimensional clot.

Tests for Evaluation of the Hemostatic Mechanism. Laboratory tests are of considerable value in the diagnosis of hemorrhagic disorders, but the importance of the history, including the family history, and of the physical examination cannot be overemphasized. Significant congenital defects are almost invariably associated with histories of easy bruising or prolonged bleeding after minor injury.

The platelet count, tourniquet test and bleeding time are used to assess the integrity of the small blood vessels. The *tourniquet test* is performed by inflating a blood pressure cuff to a point midway between the systolic and diastolic pressures for 5 minutes. Normally this stress results in fewer than 5 petechiae on an area of skin on the forearm 2.5 cm. square. A greater number of petechiae indicates thrombocytopenia, increased fragility, or dysfunction of the small blood vessels. The *Ivy bleeding time* also assesses the vascular and platelet phases of hemostasis. A blood pressure cuff is applied to the arm and inflated to 40 mm. Hg, and a stab incision 2 mm. long and deep is made with a scalpel blade. At 30-second intervals drops of blood are blotted from the margin of the incision. Normally blood flow stops within 4 to 8 minutes. A *platelet count* or estimation is essential in the evaluation of any patient suspected of having a hemostatic disorder. When the platelet count is less than 40,000 per cu. mm., those tests which rely upon platelet function, such as the bleeding

time and tourniquet test, usually give abnormal results.

The *whole blood clotting time* tests the entire coagulation mechanism. The interval for a firm blood clot to form in a glass test tube is normally 8 to 12 minutes; if a careful 3-tube technique is used, the upper limit of normal is 15 to 19 minutes. The clotting time is a very gross assessment of the hemostatic mechanism, since fairly severe defects may be present in spite of a normal clotting time. The capillary tube clotting time is unreliable.

The 3 phases of coagulation can be individually assessed by simple, accurate tests. In any hemorrhagic state the adequacy of phase III should be ascertained first. Unless adequate fibrinogen is present, the blood is incoagulable, and the other laboratory tests in which the formation of a visible clot is the end-point give, perforce, abnormal results. Phase III can be evaluated by the thrombin time, the time required for plasma to clot after the addition of bovine thrombin. The normal thrombin time is 15 to 20 seconds. Prolongation indicates hypofibrinogenemia or a circulating anticoagulant.

Phase II in its entirety is assessed by the prothrombin time, the time taken for plasma to clot after the addition of thromboplastin and calcium. Normal prothrombin time is 12 to 14 seconds. If phase III is intact, a prolonged prothrombin time indicates a deficiency involving factors II, V, VII or X, alone or in combination. Specific assays for all these factors are available. The level of ionized calcium must be less than 2.5 mg. per 100 ml. in order to interfere with blood coagulation.

Phase I, the most complex part of the coagulation mechanism, can be evaluated by several tests. The partial thromboplastin time (PTT) is the time

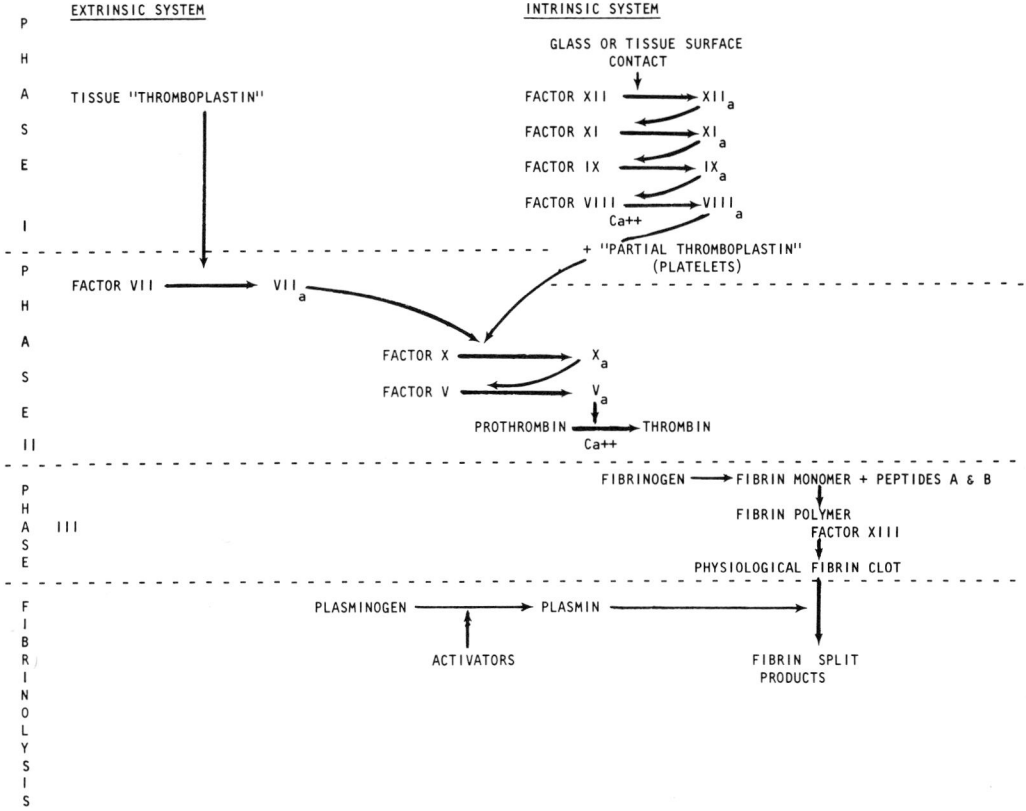

Figure 14-9. The coagulation mechanism.

required for plasma to clot when calcium and platelets, or a lipid substitute for platelets (partial thromboplastin), are added to plasma. The normal time is 60 to 90 seconds. The PTT is a simple, inexpensive and reliable way to assess the adequacy of factors XII, XI, IX and VIII. The *prothrombin consumption time* is a standard prothrombin determination performed on serum instead of plasma. Because prothrombin is used up during coagulation, the serum normally contains little prothrombin, and the serum prothrombin time is prolonged to 35 seconds or greater. Deficiencies of the phase I factors are associated with poor utilization of prothrombin. If the serum prothrombin time does not differ significantly from that obtained with plasma, deficiency of one of the phase I factors is likely.

The *thromboplastin generation* test is the most sensitive of all the tests of phase I. The thromboplastic activity of an incubated mixture of plasma, serum and platelet substrate is estimated at regular intervals. A deficiency of any of the phase I factors will be reflected in an abnormal generation test result. This test can be modified so as to quantitate precisely factors VIII and IX.

There is considerable difference in sensitivity among these tests. For example, a plasma level of factor VIII which is only 1 or 2 per cent of normal is sufficient for a normal clotting time. A level of factor VIII at 3 to 5 per cent of normal produces a normal prothrombin consumption test. The PTT and thromboplastin generation test results become abnormal when the factor VIII level is 15 to 20 per cent of normal or less.

If the PTT, prothrombin consumption or thromboplastin generation test results are abnormal, the way in which they can be corrected identifies the specific deficiency. Normal plasma adsorbed with barium sulfate retains factors VIII and XI. Normal serum contains factors IX and XI. Therefore, if an abnormal test result can be rectified by adsorbed plasma, but not by serum, factor VIII deficiency is proved. If an abnormal result is corrected by serum, but not by adsorbed plasma, factor IX deficiency is present. If both serum and plasma are corrective, factor XI deficiency may be present.

Coagulation Disorders

PHASE I DISORDERS— THE HEMOPHILIAS

The hemophilias are the most common and serious of the congenital coagulation disorders. They are associated with genetically determined deficiencies of factors VIII, IX or XI.

FACTOR VIII DEFICIENCY
(Classic Hemophilia; Hemophilia A)

About 80 per cent of cases of hemophilia are caused by a gene carried on the X chromosome which results in a profound depression of the level of factor VIII in the plasma. The disease is transmitted by asymptomatic female carriers to affected sons. In most instances it is impossible to detect the carrier state by laboratory tests. In 80 per cent of cases the family history is positive. Sporadic cases may represent new mutations. The clinical severity depends upon the level of factor VIII in the plasma, severe cases having less than 3 per cent of the normal level; the degree of severity tends to be constant within a given family.

Clinical Manifestations. Since factor VIII does not cross the placenta, a bleeding tendency may be evident in the neonatal period. Hematomas after injections and bleeding from circumcision are common, but many affected newborns exhibit no clinical abnormalities. As ambulation begins, excessive bruising is observed. Large intramuscular hematomas result from minor trauma. A relatively minor traumatic laceration, as of the tongue or lip, which bleeds persistently for hours or days is frequently the event that leads to diagnosis. The hallmark of hemophilia is hemarthrosis. Hemorrhages into the elbows, knees and ankles cause pain and swelling and limit movement of the joint. Repeated hemorrhages may produce degenerative changes, with osteoporosis, muscle atrophy and ultimately a fixed, unusable joint. Spontaneous hematuria is a troublesome, but not usually serious, complication. Intracranial hemorrhage and bleeding into the neck constitute life-threatening emergencies.

Patients with levels of factor VIII greater than 5 per cent may not have severe spontaneous symptoms. These patients with "mild hemophilia" may experience only prolonged bleeding following tooth extractions or surgery.

Laboratory Data. The only significant laboratory abnormalities occur in coagulation tests and are due to serious deficiency of factor VIII. The partial thromboplastin time (PTT) is prolonged to greater than 120 seconds. Prothrombin consumption is so markedly impaired that the serum and plasma prothrombin times may be similar. The thromboplastin generation test result is grossly abnormal. The abnormal tests can be corrected by normal plasma adsorbed with barium sulfate, but not by serum. In less severe cases only the PTT and thromboplastin generation test result may be abnormal.

Treatment. Prevention of trauma constitutes a most important aspect of care for the hemophilic child. During early life the crib and the playpen should be padded, and the child should be carefully supervised while he is learning to walk. As he becomes older, physical activities which do not entail a risk of trauma should be encouraged. It is important that a course somewhere between over-protection and permissiveness be followed in the supervision of these patients.

When bleeding episodes occur, replacement therapy is essential to prevent pain, disability or life-threatening hemorrhage. The aim of therapy is to increase the level of factor VIII in the plasma to assure hemostasis. Presently this can be done only by the intravenous infusion of fresh plasma or plasma concentrates. The factor VIII level can be effectively increased by infusion of fresh or fresh-frozen plasma in a dose of 10 to 15 ml. per kg. every 12 hours. This regimen maintains a plasma level between 10 and 25 per cent of normal. Because of danger of circulatory overload, no more than 30 ml. per kg. of plasma should be administered in a 24-hour period.

Several factor VIII concentrates are currently available. The most inexpensive of these is cryoprecipitate, which may be easily prepared from fresh plasma. One unit of cryoprecipitate can be harvested from 250 ml. of plasma. After a priming dose of 1 unit per 5 kg., a dose of 1 unit per 10 kg. every 12 hours results in an average plasma factor VIII level of 25 to 50 per cent of normal. Factor VIII-rich fibrinogen and glycine-precipitated factor VIII are commercially available and are excellent, but expensive, sources of factor VIII.

When the hemophilic child has significant bleeding, local measures should include application of cold and pressure. For ordinary hemarthroses, therapy with plasma or cryoprecipitate should be administered for 72 to 96 hours. Immobilization is indicated initially, but passive exercises should be begun within 48 hours to prevent joint stiffness and fibrosis. The necessity of aspiration of blood from the joint is somewhat controversial. When the skin overlying the joint is very tense, aspiration of blood, when adequate factor VIII has been given, may provide relief of pain. Replacement therapy is probably the most important part of management of hemarthrosis, since equally good results have been obtained by groups who routinely practice aspiration and by others who do not. Aggressive replacement therapy with factor VIII and careful orthopedic management of hemarthroses can prevent much severe deformity and crippling. When hemorrhage occurs in vital areas such as the brain or neck, or when surgery or dental extractions are contemplated, intensive therapy using factor VIII concentrates is indicated to maintain the plasma level above 25 per cent. Venipunctures should be performed only from superficial veins; aspiration from femoral or internal jugular veins is hazardous.

Factor VIII Inhibitors. A small number of patients with hemophilia become refractory to factor VIII therapy, owing to development of a circulating inhibitor or antibody. The development of inhibitors is not related to the number of plasma transfusions. These inhibitors are IgG globulins and are specifically active against factor VIII. It is virtually impossible to overpower an inhibitor, but when hemorrhage occurs, massive doses of factor VIII concentrates or exchange transfusions with fresh blood should be given and may be of temporary benefit.

FACTOR IX DEFICIENCY
(CHRISTMAS DISEASE; HEMOPHILIA B)

About 15 per cent of cases of hemophilia are due to a genetically determined deficiency of factor IX. This disease is clinically indistinguishable from factor VIII deficiency, and is also transmitted as an X-linked recessive trait. The disease has a wide range of clinical severity, which in general corresponds to the level of factor IX in the serum.

Laboratory Data. The partial thromboplastin time (PTT), prothrombin consumption and thromboplastin generation test results are usually abnormal. These in-vitro abnormalities can be corrected by normal serum, but not by adsorbed plasma.

Treatment. Since there is no factor IX concentrate yet available commercially, replacement therapy is accomplished by infusions of plasma. Ten to 15 ml. per kg. should be given every 12 to 24 hours during bleeding episodes. The response to fresh or fresh-frozen plasma is superior to that obtained with stored plasma.

FACTOR XI DEFICIENCY
(PTA DEFICIENCY; HEMOPHILIA C)

This usually mild bleeding disorder is inherited as an autosomal dominant trait, and typical cases are seen in both sexes. The usual clinical manifestations are nosebleeds, and excessive hemorrhage and hemarthroses are rare. The PTT, prothrombin consumption and thromboplastin generation test results are abnormal in the more severe cases. Both normal plasma and serum correct the deficiency. Plasma therapy in a dose of 10 to 15 ml. per kg. every 12 to 24 hours should be given for significant clinical hemorrhage.

FACTOR XII DEFICIENCY
(HAGEMAN FACTOR DEFICIENCY)

This fascinating condition is due to homozygous occurrence of an autosomal gene which results in a profound deficiency of factor XII. Despite abnormal test results of the first phase of coagulation, these patients have no clinical abnormalities.

VON WILLEBRAND'S DISEASE
(VASCULAR HEMOPHILIA)

This dominantly inherited disease is complex. It is characterized by a capillary defect manifest by prolonged bleeding time, a deficiency of factor VIII in many cases, and decreased platelet adhesiveness. The clinical manifestations are nosebleeds and increased bleeding after trauma or surgery. The tourniquet test result and bleeding time are usually abnormal. Although fresh plasma infusions result in increases in the factor VIII level which are sustained for several days, owing to *de novo* synthesis, they have an inconsistent effect on the bleeding time. Cryoprecipitate has recently been shown to correct the prolonged bleeding time. It is of interest that the synthesis of factor VIII is controlled by both autosomal (von Willebrand) and X-linked (hemophilia A) genes.

PHASE II DISORDERS

Factors II, V, VII and X are involved in the second phase of coagulation and are designated the *prothrombin complex*. The factors are produced in the liver, and all except factor V require vitamin K for normal synthesis. The laboratory diagnosis of these deficiencies depends upon a prolonged prothrombin time. Significant bleeding does not usually occur until the prothrombin time exceeds 30 to 35 seconds, corresponding to a level of 10 to 15 per cent of normal.

Genetically determined congenital deficiencies of factors II, V and VII have been described, the most common of which is factor V deficiency (parahemophilia, Owren's disease). The clinical manifestations of these deficiencies are mucocutaneous hemorrhages, bleeding into tissues, and hemorrhages after injury. Hemarthroses occur frequently. These deficiencies are refractory to vitamin K therapy, and fresh plasma should be administered for active hemorrhage.

HEMORRHAGIC DISEASE OF THE NEWBORN

Hemorrhagic disease of the newborn is a self-limited bleeding disorder usually occurring on the second or third day of life, and resulting from a deficiency of the coagulation factors dependent upon vitamin K.

The levels of factors II, VII, IX and X are nearly normal in umbilical cord blood, but decline rapidly to reach a nadir at 48 to 72 hours of life. In 0.25 to 0.5 per cent of infants the decline is so extreme that severe hemorrhage may result.

Clinical Manifestations. In most instances hemorrhagic manifestations become evident on the second or third day of life. Melena, bleeding from the navel and hematuria are frequent signs of the disorder. The most serious complications are intracranial hemorrhage and anemic shock.

Treatment. Prophylactic administration of vitamin K_1 to the newborn prevents the postnatal decline of the factors of the prothrombin complex and virtually eliminates hemorrhagic disease of the newborn. Preparations of vitamin K_1 are indicated, for they do not have a hemolytic effect as do large doses of synthetic vitamin K analogues. Although vitamin K given to the mother may be beneficial, a therapeutic effect is more certain if the drug is administered to the newborn infant. As little as 25 micrograms of vitamin K prevents the postnatal decline of the prothrombin complex; the currently recommended dose of 1.0 mg. of vitamin K_1 is safe and effective. Larger doses do not increase the therapeutic effect.

In overt hemorrhagic disease 1.0 mg. of vitamin K_1 should be given by intravenous or intramuscular injection. Clinical hemorrhage usually stops within 2 hours. If intracranial or other serious hemorrhage has occurred, an infusion of 10 to 15 ml. per kg. of fresh plasma will immediately correct the hemostatic defects. Profound anemia and shock may be corrected by infusions of fresh blood.

Premature infants may experience a complex hemorrhagic state involving multiple coagulation factors as well as a platelet deficiency. Vitamin K therapy is ineffective in correcting the abnormalities, owing to hepatic immaturity. Fresh plasma infusions are indicated if significant hemorrhage occurs.

Vitamin K deficiency rarely occurs after the neonatal period. Intestinal malabsorption of fats and prolonged administration of broad-spectrum antibiotics may, however, result in vitamin K deficiency, and cystic fibrosis and biliary atresia may be complicated by disorders of the prothrombin complex. Prophylactic administration of water-soluble vitamin K is indicated in these situations. In advanced liver disease, synthesis of the factors of the prothrombin complex may be compromised, owing to hepatocellular damage. Vitamin K therapy is not fully effective in correcting the disorders if advanced liver disease is present. The anticoagulant properties of Dicumarol and other coumadin derivatives depend on interference with synthesis of factors II, VII and X. Vitamin K_1 is a specific antidote.

PHASE III DISORDERS

Congenital afibrinogenemia is a rare hemorrhagic disorder due to homozygous occurrence of an autosomal recessive gene. Despite totally incoagulable blood, these patients usually do not have severe spontaneous hemorrhages or hemarthrosis, but trauma or surgery may be followed by severe bleeding. Therapy with 100 mg. per kg. of concentrated fibrinogen provides a hemostatic plasma level. Since the plasma half-life of fibrinogen is 5 days, frequent infusions are not necessary. A very high risk of homologous serum hepatitis is attendant upon use of fibrinogen concentrates.

Factor XIII Deficiency (Fibrin Stabilizing Factor). A deficiency of factor XIII is the most recently recognized inherited hemorrhagic disease. Onset is most often in infancy with bleeding after separation of the umbilical cord stump. Gastrointestinal, intracranial and intra-articular hemorrhages have been the most common clinical manifestations. Routine coagulation studies are normal. Factor XIII deficiency is diagnosed by finding an abnormal solubility of the clot in 5M urea and a short euglobulin lysis time.

REFERENCES

Aballi, A.: The Actions of Vitamin K in the Neonatal Period. *South. Med. J.*, 58:48, 1965.

Aballi, A. J., and de Lamerens, S.: Coagulation Changes in the Neonatal Period and in Early Infancy. *Pediat. Clin. N. Amer.*, 9:785, 1962.

Biggs, R., and Macfarlane, R. G.: *Human Blood Coagulation and Its Disorders.* 3rd ed. Philadelphia, F. A. Davis Company, 1962.

Dallman, P. R., and Pool, J. G.: Treatment of Hemophilia with Factor VIII Concentrates. *New England J. Med.*, 278:199, 1968.

McMillan, C. W., Diamond, L. K., and Surgenor, P. M.: Treatment of Classic Hemophilia: The Use of Fibrinogen Rich in Factor VIII for Hemorrhage and for Surgery. *New England J. Med.*, 265:224, 1961.

Perkins, H. A.: Correction of the Hemostatic Defects of von Willebrand's Disease. *Blood*, 30:375, 1967.

Pool, J. G., and Shannon, A. E.: Production of High Potency Concentrates of Antihemophilic Globulin in a Closed-Bag System. *New England J. Med.*, 273:1443, 1965.

Stefanini, M., and Dameshek, W.: *The Hemorrhagic Disorders.* 2nd ed. New York, Grune & Stratton, Inc., 1962.

The Purpuras

The purpuras are a group of diseases in which small hemorrhages occur into the superficial layers of the skin, producing areas of purple discoloration. Minute extravasations of blood about the small vessels are recognized as petechiae; more extensive hemorrhages cause ecchymoses. Bleeding may also occur from the mucous membranes and into other organs and tissues. The purpuras may be classified into 2 general groups according to platelet count. In *thrombocytopenic purpuras* the platelet count is reduced below 40,000 per cu. mm., and hemorrhages are due to this quantitative deficiency. In *nonthrombocytopenic purpuras*, bleeding results from defects in the small blood vessels or from defective platelet function despite their adequate numbers.

NONTHROMBOCYTOPENIC PURPURAS

Platelets are non-nucleated, cellular fragments produced by the megakaryocytes of the bone marrow. The large size of the megakaryocyte reflects its polyploidy. As the megakaryocyte reaches maturity, extreme fragmentation of the cytoplasm occurs, and large numbers of platelets are liberated. They have a life span in the circulation of 7 to 10 days. The platelet has a number of intrinsic antigens, which are distinct from those of the red blood cell, but some are shared by the leukocytes.

The platelets are intimately involved in both the vascular and the clotting aspects of hemostasis. They are necessary for integrity of the vascular endothelium; when small blood vessels are transected, platelets accumulate at the site of injury, forming a hemostatic plug. Platelet aggregation and degranulation are initiated by contact with extravascular components and perhaps by ADP. Serotonin and histamine are liberated during these processes, and increase local vasoconstriction. Platelets have a phospholipid with partial thromboplastin activity, which makes an important contribution to coagulation. They also transport other blood coagulation factors through adsorption to the platelet surface. Finally, the platelet is necessary for normal clot retraction.

The *normal platelet count* is 150,000 to 400,000 per cu. mm. Counts below this range indicate thrombocytopenia, owing either to inadequate production or to excessive destruction or removal of platelets. Inadequate production is almost always due to marrow dysfunction which decreases the number of megakaryocytes. By contrast, in the thrombocytopenias due to increased destruction, the megakaryocytes are quantitatively normal or increased. The hypomegakaryocytic thrombocytopenias result from aplasia of the marrow or from

its infiltration by abnormal or neoplastic tissue. Because of the grave prognosis of such disorders, bone marrow aspiration is indicated in every case of significant thrombocytopenia. Bone marrow aspiration can usually be performed without serious bleeding even in the presence of severe thrombocytopenia, since thromboplastins in marrow juice will usually effect hemostasis.

Purpura Associated with Normal Numbers of Platelets. The most common nonthrombocytopenic purpura is *anaphylactoid purpura*, or *Henoch-Schönlein syndrome* (see p. 522), an acute inflammatory process of unknown origin involving the small blood vessels of the skin, joints, gut and kidney. The striking centrifugal distribution of the rash and involvement of the legs and buttocks are characteristic, particularly when combined with arthritis, nephritis or gastrointestinal bleeding. The petechiae must be differentiated from those of early meningococcemia or septicemia due to other microorganisms. Demonstration of bacteria in blood expressed from the cutaneous lesions of septicemia is a valuable method for early diagnosis. Septic emboli cause the petechiae observed in bacterial endocarditis. Toxic vasculitis may produce a hemorrhagic rash as a reaction to drugs such as arsenicals and iodides. Similar findings may occur during viral or rickettsial infections.

The *thrombasthenias,* or thrombocytopathic purpuras, are associated with quantitatively normal platelets with defective function. Abnormal function is reflected in petechiae and excessive bleeding. The abnormality of platelet function may also be revealed by defective clot retraction or by failure of the patient's platelets to support normal thromboplastin generation.

THROMBOCYTOPENIC PURPURAS

IDIOPATHIC THROMBOCYTOPENIC PURPURA

Idiopathic thrombocytopenic purpura (ITP), the most common of the thrombocytopenic purpuras of childhood, is associated with mucocutaneous bleeding and hemorrhages into tissues. There is a profound deficiency of circulating platelets despite adequate numbers of megakaryocytes in the marrow.

Etiology. The disease often appears to be related to sensitization by viral infections, for in about 50 per cent of cases there is an antecedent disease such as rubella, rubeola or viral respiratory infection. It seems likely that an immune mechanism is the basis for the thrombocytopenia. Platelet antibodies can rarely be detected in acute cases, probably owing to limitations of current methods. During the early stages of the disease the hemorrhagic manifestations are so acute and generalized that a vasculitis or defect of the capillary endothelium has been postulated.

Clinical Manifestations. The onset is frequently acute. One to 4 weeks after a viral infection, or without antecedent illness, bruising and a generalized petechial rash occur. Hemorrhages in mucous membranes may be prominent, with hemorrhagic bullae of the gums and lips. Nosebleeds are often severe and difficult to control. The most serious complication is intracranial hemorrhage, which occurs in less than 1 per cent of cases. The liver, spleen and lymph nodes are not enlarged. Except for the signs of bleeding, the patient appears clinically well. The acute phase of the disease associated with spontaneous hemorrhages lasts for only a week or two. Even though thrombocytopenia persists, spontaneous mucocutaneous hemorrhages then subside. In some instances the onset is insidious with moderate bruising and few petechiae.

Laboratory Data. The platelet count is reduced below 40,000 per cu. mm., and those tests which depend upon platelet function such as the tourniquet test and bleeding time and clot retraction give abnormal results. The white blood cell count is normal, and anemia is not present unless significant external blood loss has occurred.

Bone marrow aspiration reveals normal granulocytic and erythrocytic series, and numerous megakaryocytes. Some of the latter are immature, with deep basophilic cytoplasm; platelet budding may be scanty, but there is no pathognomonic or diagnostic morphology of the megakaryocytes.

Differential Diagnosis. Idiopathic thrombocytopenic purpura may be differentiated from aplastic or infiltrative processes of the bone marrow by marrow examination. Significant enlargement of the spleen will suggest primary liver disease with congestive splenomegaly, lipidosis or reticuloendotheliosis. Thrombocytopenic purpura may be an initial manifestation of systemic lupus erythematosus, but this sequence is unusual in children.

Treatment. Idiopathic thrombocytopenic purpura has an excellent prognosis even when no specific therapy is given. Seventy-five per cent of patients recover completely within 3 months, most within 8 weeks. Severe spontaneous hemorrhages and intracranial bleeding are usually confined to the initial phase of the disease. After the initial acute phase, spontaneous manifestations tend to subside. Nine to 12 months after the onset, 90 per cent of affected children have regained normal platelet counts, and relapses are unusual.

Fresh blood or platelet concentrates are of only transient benefit, owing to the very short survival of transfused platelets, but they may be useful when life-threatening hemorrhage occurs. Corticosteroid therapy is of great value; though it has not decreased the number of chronic cases, it does reduce the severity and shorten the duration of the initial phase.

When the disease is mild and hemorrhages of the retina or mucous membranes are not present, no specific therapy may be indicated. The affected child should be protected from falls or trauma. Bacterial infections should be treated with appropriate antibiotics. Vitamins K and C have no therapeutic effect. Although infusions of plasma are occasionally followed by sustained rises of platelet count, the value of plasma therapy in ITP remains undetermined. For the severe cases, therapy with a corticosteroid, such as prednisone in a dose of 1 or 2 mg. per kg. or its equivalent, is indicated. This therapy is continued until the platelet count is normal or for 3 weeks, whichever comes first. Prolonged corticosteroid therapy is not indicated and may, in itself, depress the bone marrow. If thrombocytopenia persists for 4 to 6 months, a second short course of corticosteroid therapy may be given. Splenectomy should be reserved for chronic cases and for the severe ones which do not respond to corticosteroids, in which considerable improvement can be expected in most instances. Only about 2 per cent of cases of ITP in children tend to be chronic and refractory to all therapy.

OTHER THROMBOCYTOPENIC PURPURAS

Drug-Induced Thrombocytopenias. A number of drugs may be associated with immune thrombocytopenia. It has been clearly shown that quinidine and Sedormid function as haptens which combine with proteins on the platelet surface and stimulate antibody formation. Administration of these drugs to sensitized persons is followed by severe thrombocytopenia. This syndrome is unusual in pediatric practice because the responsible drugs are rarely prescribed. In any case of thrombocytopenia, however, a careful search for any drug exposure should be made, and the patient removed from contact with potential offenders.

Wiskott-Aldrich Syndrome and Other Inherited Thrombocytopenias. The Wiskott-Aldrich syndrome consists of cutaneous eczema, thrombocytopenic hemorrhage, and increased susceptibility to infection due to an immunologic defect. The disease is transmitted as an X-linked recessive trait. Bloody diarrhea or hemorrhage during the first months of life is usually the initial clinical manifestation. The bone marrow contains a normal number of megakaryocytes, but many have bizarre nuclear morphology. Homologous platelets survive normally when transfused into these patients. Wiskott-Aldrich syndrome may represent a unique circumstance in which thrombocytopenia results from abnormal platelet formation or release despite quantitatively adequate numbers of megakaryocytes. The immunologic defect involves macroglobulin (IgM) synthesis, as indicated by absence of isohemagglutinins. Splenectomy is contraindicated; it has been followed most often by overwhelming sepsis and death when it has been performed. A significant number of patients have had lymphoreticular malignancies.

A number of other types of inherited thrombocytopenias have been described. Some are X-linked, and some have autosomal transmission. Responses to therapy, including splenectomy, have usually been disappointing.

Thrombopoietin Deficiency. A single child has been described (Schulman) with chronic thrombocytopenia presumably resulting from a deficiency of a megakaryocyte maturation factor contained in normal plasma. Plasma infusions repeatedly produced a sustained peripheral rise in the platelet count.

Thrombocytopenia with Cavernous Hemangioma. Some infants with large cavernous hemangiomas of the trunk or extremities have severe thrombocytopenia. Histologic and isotopic studies indicate that platelets are trapped and destroyed within the extensive vascular bed of the tumor. The peripheral blood is normal except for thrombocytopenia, and the bone marrow contains adequate numbers of megakaryocytes. Spontaneous thrombosis within the tumor may lead to obliteration of the vascular channels and spontaneous recovery; radiation therapy in a single dose of 600 to 800 r may accelerate this process, but repeated courses may be necessary. When anatomically feasible, external compression or total excision may be attempted, but surgery may be associated with uncontrollable hemorrhage. Other forms of therapy are without effect, including corticosteroids. Splenectomy is contraindicated.

NEONATAL THROMBOCYTOPENIA

Thrombocytopenia of the newborn has unique aspects which merit special consideration. Thrombocytopenia may reflect primary systemic diseases of the infant's hematopoietic system or be due to transfer of abnormal factors from the mother.

Septic Thrombocytopenias. A variety of fetal and neonatal infections may result in significant thrombocytopenic bleeding. These include virus infections (especially rubella and cytomegalic inclusion disease), protozoal infections such as toxoplasmosis, syphilis, and bacterial infections, especially those caused by gram-negative bacilli. Hemolysis is usually also present in infants with prominent anemia and jaundice. The liver and spleen are considerably enlarged. The bone marrow changes are variable, but reduced numbers of megakaryocytes may be seen.

Immune Neonatal Thrombocytopenia. About 50 per cent of infants born of mothers with idiopathic thrombocytopenic purpura (ITP) have thrombocytopenia in the neonatal period, owing to transplacental transfer of antiplatelet antibodies. Petechiae are not present initially, but appear in a generalized distribution within a few minutes after birth. Bleeding from bowel and kidney and intracranial hemorrhage may occur. In mild cases there may be few abnormal findings.

Hepatosplenomegaly is not present. The duration of the thrombocytopenia is 2 to 4 months. Although therapy is not strikingly successful, fresh blood, exchange transfusions or platelet transfusions may be of temporary value. Corticosteroid therapy has not been convincingly beneficial. Because of the self-limited nature of the disease, splenectomy is contraindicated.

When the fetus has platelet antigens which the mother does not have, isoimmunization may occur. If maternal antibodies to fetal platelet antigens reach a sufficiently high titer, they may cross the placenta and produce thrombocytopenia in the fetus. The disease may be familial, and first-born infants are frequently affected. The clinical signs include petechiae and other hemorrhagic manifestations. By use of sensitive tests involving complement fixation, antiplatelet antibodies can be demonstrated in about 50 per cent of cases.

When the mother has drug-induced thrombocytopenia, both antibody and drug may cross the placenta and cause neonatal thrombocytopenia. Corticosteroid therapy and especially exchange transfusions should be considered when bleeding manifestations are severe.

Congenital Hypoplastic Thrombocytopenia with Associated Malformations. Severe thrombocytopenia has been described as a familial condition associated with aplasia of radius and thumbs, and cardiac and renal anomalies. Severe hemorrhagic manifestations are evident in the first days of life. Hemoglobin levels are normal; leukocytosis has been documented in some cases. The only recognized abnormality of the bone marrow is absence of megakaryocytes.

The combination of anomalies in this disease is identical with that observed in Fanconi's pancytopenia, in which the hematologic abnormalities are not usually observed until the third and fourth years of life. No infants with congenital hypoplastic thrombocytopenia have been followed up to see whether the Fanconi syndrome developed, nor have cases of both conditions been observed in the same family.

THROMBOCYTOSIS
(THROMBOCYTHEMIA)

Platelet counts in excess of 750,000 per cu. mm. may be designated as thrombocytosis. Markedly elevated counts may accompany hemorrhage, iron deficiency anemia, hemolytic anemias and primary myeloproliferative disorders. After splenectomy for ITP or hemolytic anemia the platelet count often rises precipitously and may exceed 1,000,000 per cu. mm. 5 to 10 days postoperatively. In general, no specific therapy such as anticoagulation is necessary, for thrombosis is extremely rare.

A case of primary thrombocytosis associated with thrombotic episodes and myocardial infarction has been described.

REFERENCES

Canales, M. L., and Mauer, A. M.: Sex-Linked Hereditary Thrombocytopenia as a Variant of Wiskott-Aldrich Syndrome. *New England J. Med.,* 277:899, 1967.

Lusher, J. M., and Zuelzer, W. W.: Idiopathic Thrombocytopenic Purpura in Childhood. *J. Pediat.,* 68:971, 1966.

Pearson, H. A., Shulman, N. R., Marder, V. J., and Cone, T. E., Jr.: Isoimmune Neonatal Thrombocytopenic Purpura. Clinical and Therapeutic Considerations. *Blood,* 23:154, 1964.

Schulman, I.: Diagnosis and Treatment: Management of Idiopathic Thrombocytopenic Purpura. *Pediatrics,* 33:979, 1964.

Schulman, I., Pierce, M., Lukens, A., and Currimbhoy, Z.: Studies on Thrombopoiesis. I. A Factor in Normal Human Plasma Required for Platelet Production, Chronic Thrombocytopenia Due to Its Deficiency. *Blood,* 16:943, 1960.

Spach, M. A., Howell, D. A., and Harris, J. S.: Myocardial Infarction with Multiple Thrombosis in a Child with Primary Thrombocytosis. *Pediatrics,* 31:268, 1963.

Wolff, J. A.: Wiskott-Aldrich Syndrome: Clinical, Immunologic and Pathologic Observations. *J. Pediat.,* 70:221, 1967.

Zinkham, W. H., Osborn, J. E., and Medearis, D. N., Jr.: Blood and Bone Marrow Findings in Congenital Rubella. *J. Pediat.,* 67:985, 1965.

CONSUMPTION COAGULOPATHIES AND FIBRINOLYTIC STATES

Consumption coagulopathy is a relatively new unifying concept for a group of conditions associated with disseminated intravascular coagulation. Disseminated intravascular coagulation has been described in a large number of clinical states, including incompatible blood transfusions, cyanotic congenital heart disease, hemangioma with thrombocytopenia, fulminating meningococcemia with Waterhouse-Friderichsen syndrome, purpura fulminans and acute promyelocytic leukemia. In some of these states intravascular hemolysis appears to initiate thrombosis. In others diffuse vasculitis may be the primary abnormality, and an endotoxin may be of primary importance in some. Depletion of the consumable coagulation factors (I, II, V and VIII) may be a consequence of this process. Clinical and pathologic features of some of these syndromes have been compared to those of the generalized Shwartzman reaction. Thrombocytopenia and hemolytic anemia with bizarre red cell changes are often prominent.

The Fibrinolytic Mechanism. Fibrinolysis, the process of dissolution of the clot, is an essential physiologic mechanism. This mechanism is complex and involves a number of fairly well defined factors, the most important of which is a fibrinolytic enzyme called plasmin and its inactive precursor plasminogen. Thrombin and a urokinase found in urine are particularly potent in the conversion of inactive plasminogen to its active enzymatic form. The fibrinolytic system is activated at the same time that coagulation occurs, with the result that in diseases associated with diffuse intravascular coagulation, increased fibrinolytic activity of the plasma can often also be found. Increased fibrinolytic activity is demonstrated in the test tube by spontaneous dissolution of the clot on incubation of clotted blood, or by a shortened euglobulin lysis time. Spontaneous fibrinolytic states may on rare occasions be associated with hemorrhagic symptoms. It may be difficult to differentiate these primary fibrinolytic states from consumption coagulopathies, in which

fibrinolysis is a secondary phenomenon. In consumption coagulopathies, factors I, II, V and VIII and platelets are usually decreased, whereas in fibrinolytic states platelets are usually normal and the other factors inconstantly affected. Treatment with epsilon aminocaproic acid (EACA) may be of value in fibrinolytic states, but is not indicated in consumption coagulopathies.

Hemolytic-Uremic Syndrome (see also p. 1133). This acute disease of infancy and early childhood usually follows an episode of acute gastroenteritis. Shortly thereafter signs and symptoms of hemolytic anemia, thrombocytopenia and glomerulonephritis develop. Bilateral renal cortical necrosis may occur, and case fatality rates as high as 30 per cent have been reported. Its sometimes epidemic occurrence suggests that an infectious agent may be involved.

Laboratory data. The hemolytic anemia is associated with characteristically bizarre red cell morphology. Many of the red cells are contracted and distorted, with prominence of spherocytes, burr cells and helmet-shaped forms (Fig. 14-3, *E*). A depressed platelet count despite normal numbers of megakaryocytes in marrow indicates excessive peripheral destruction. Tests of the coagulation mechanism may give abnormal results. Protein, red cells and casts are present in the urinary sediment, and grave renal damage is reflected in oliguria and azotemia. Renal biopsy reveals fibrinoid deposits in small blood vessels and glomeruli, which may represent deposition of fibrin on a diffusely damaged endothelium.

Treatment. For management of uremia and anuria, see page 1143. Transfusions are indicated for severe anemia. Corticosteroid therapy has not been convincingly beneficial. Heparin, in doses of 50 to 100 units per kg. given intravenously every 4 to 6 hours, may halt intravascular coagulation.

Thrombotic Thrombocytopenic Purpura. This rare and serious disease has many similarities to the hemolytic-uremic syndrome. Diffuse embolism and thrombosis of the small blood vessels of the brain are evidenced by shifting neurologic signs such as aphasias, blindness and convulsions. The prognosis is grave. Laboratory findings include thrombocytopenia and a hemolytic anemia associated with distorted and fragmented red cells. Treatment has been of dubious success, but large doses of ACTH or corticosteroids and emergency splenectomy have been advocated. Anticoagulant therapy may also be of value.

Purpura Fulminans. Purpura fulminans is an unusual disease which usually occurs in the convalescent phase of a bacterial or viral infection. Diffuse symmetrical hemorrhages occur, with prominent inflammatory vasculitis and necrosis of skin and subcutaneous tissues, particularly involving the buttocks and lower extremities. Systemic toxicity may be extreme, and mortality is high. In nonfatal cases large areas of gangrenous skin and muscle may slough, leaving areas requiring plastic surgical repair. The platelet count is normal or low. Fragmented red cells may be seen on blood smear. The levels of consumable coagulation factors, especially of fibrinogen, are decreased. Replacement therapy with fibrinogen and fresh plasma transfusions, as well as high doses of corticosteroids, have appeared to be helpful on occasion. Intravenous administration of heparin, 50 to 100 units per kg. (0.5 to 1 mg. per kg.) every 4 to 6 hours, or the use of dextran infusions may arrest the progression of the cutaneous lesions and correct the coagulation defects.

REFERENCES

Abildgaard, C. F., Corrigan, J. J., Seeler, R. A., Simone, J. V., and Schulman, I.: Meningococcemia Associated with Intravascular Coagulation. *Pediatrics,* 40:78, 1967.

Allen, D. M.: Heparin Therapy of Purpura Fulminans. *Pediatrics,* 32:211, 1966.

Edson, J. R., Krivit, W., White, J. G., and Sharp, H. L: Intravascular Coagulation in Acute Stem Cell Leukemia Successfully Treated with Heparin. *J. Pediat.,* 71:342, 1967.

Gianantonio, C. A., Vitacco, M., Mendilaharzu, F., Rutty, A., and Mendilaharzu, J.: The Hemolytic-Uremic Syndrome. *J. Pediat.,* 64:478, 1964.

Good, R. A., and Thomas, L.: Studies on the Generalized Shwartzman Reaction: IV. Prevention of the Local and Generalized Shwartzman Reactions with Heparin. *J. Exp. Med.,* 97:871, 1953.

Hardaway, R. M., III: *Syndromes of Disseminated Intravascular Coagulation.* Springfield, Ill., Charles C Thomas, 1966.

Lanzkowsky, P., and McCrory, W.: Disseminated Intravascular Coagulation as a Possible Factor in the Pathogenesis of Thrombotic Microangiopathy. *J. Pediat.,* 70:460, 1967.

Rodriguez-Erdmann, F.: Bleeding Due to Increased Intravascular Blood Coagulation. *New England J. Med.,* 273:1370, 1965.

MacWhinney, J. B., Jr., Packer, J. T., Miller, G., and Greendyke, R. M.: Thrombotic Thrombocytopenic Purpura in Childhood. *Blood,* 19:181, 1962.

THE SPLEEN

The spleen has excited speculations of man since antiquity. Pliny believed it to be the seat of mirth and laughter; Galen pronounced it an organ full of mystery. Although no unique cells or tissues occur within the spleen, their particular arrangements and the anatomic relations are responsible for unique functions. The spleen is a large mass of lymphoid and phagocytic reticuloendothelial cells with a complex network of tortuous capillaries and fenestrated sinusoids. These impart the important properties of a biologic filter to the spleen.

A number of functions can be assigned to the spleen, and some of these are germane to hematologic processes and diseases: (1) *Reservoir function.* In lower animals the spleen is a contractile organ, owing to the presence of considerable smooth muscle in the capsule and trabeculae. In man little muscle is present, and the reservoir function is normally not very great. The normal spleen contains only about 25 ml. of blood, but when the spleen enlarges for any reason, its content of blood increases. The sequestration crisis of sickle cell states is an exaggeration of reservoir function. (2) *Hematopoiesis.* The spleen is a site of active blood formation during fetal life, but by about 6 months of gestation hematopoiesis disappears unless a condition such as hemolytic disease of the newborn is present. In a few exceptional diseases such as thalassemia and osteopetrosis, hematopoiesis persists or is resumed postnatally. The stimulus for this is not known. (3) *"Culling."* This term has been used to describe the ability of the spleen by virtue of its unique circulation and structure to remove damaged or abnormal blood cells from the circulation. This function is clearly demonstrated by the fact that red cells and platelets lightly coated by antibodies are selectively sequestered and destroyed by the spleen. The spleen's activity in destroying spherocytes is another example of culling. (4) *"Pitting."* The spleen has the ability to remove structures such as Howell-Jolly bodies or siderotic granules from within the red cell without destroying the cell. The peripheral blood of a person with no spleen contains relatively large numbers of these intracellular inclusions. (5) *Destruction of old red cells.* The spleen is probably the principal site of destruction of senescent red cells. This function is easily assumed by other portions of the reticuloendothelial system, however, and red cell life span is not significantly increased in the absence of spleen. (6) *Membrane effect.* The normal spleen is postulated to have an ill-defined effect on the red cell membrane. When the spleen is absent, red cells are flatter and thinner than normal, increased numbers of target cells are seen, and osmotic fragility is decreased. (7) *Filtering and immunologic functions.* Because of the intimate relation of the circulating blood with lymphoid and reticuloendothelial elements within the spleen, this organ plays an important role in primary defense against bacteria which gain access to the circulation. The spleen is especially vital in the immature and nonimmune person, for it constitutes the primary site of clearance of organisms such as pneumococci in the absence of specific antibody. (8) *Hormonal function.* It has been postulated that the spleen produces a hormonal substance ("splenin") which exerts an effect on bone marrow activity. There is little evidence for such a hormone, and "hypersplenism" is better explained on the basis of excessive filtering or culling activities.

Clinical Examination of the Spleen. Careful and gentle palpation of the relaxed abdomen provides reliable information about the size of the spleen. The tip can be felt at the left costal margin in 5 to 10 per cent of normal children and in a higher proportion of children with viral infections. The spleen must be increased to 2 or 3 times average size before it can be regularly felt on physical examination. Lesser degrees of enlargement can be detected radiographically. An enlarged spleen must be differentiated from other masses in the left upper quadrant. Useful physical characteristics which aid in identifying the spleen include concealment of its upper margin by the rib cage,

the presence of a palpable notch, and the absence of overlying bowel. When it is impossible to be certain of the identity of a mass, angiographic or isotopic scanning studies may be helpful, but laparotomy is more definitive.

The spleen has vascular, lymphatic and reticuloendothelial components; pathologic processes involving any of these systems may be manifested as splenomegaly. Table 14-7 lists important causes of splenic enlargement.

CONGESTIVE SPLENOMEGALY
(Banti's Syndrome)

The venous outflow from the spleen may be obstructed within the liver or in the portal or splenic veins. This vascular obstruction produces congestion and ultimately splenomegaly. Liver diseases associated with parenchymal inflammation, fibrosis and vascular constriction include postnecrotic cirrhosis, galactosemia, Wilson's disease, cystic fibrosis and biliary atresia. Septic omphalitis, either primary or following umbilical vein cannulation, may progress to portal vein thrombophlebitis and thrombosis. Rarely, congenital or acquired anomalies of the splenic or portal veins may cause obstruction and secondary splenomegaly. In some areas of the world schistosomiasis and malaria are important causes of splenomegaly.

Clinical Manifestations. Observation or palpation of an enlarged spleen may be the initial indication of the disease. The enlarged spleen may filter out and destroy increased numbers of blood cells and platelets, resulting in thrombocytopenic hemorrhage and anemia. As a response to portal vein obstruction, collateral circulation develops through the short gastric, esophageal, superficial abdominal and hemorrhoidal veins. In a significant proportion of cases, massive gastrointestinal hemorrhage from ruptured esophageal varices may be the first clinical manifestation of congestive splenomegaly.

Laboratory Findings. Pancytopenia of varying degrees of severity is seen. The bone marrow shows active hematopoiesis with abundant megakaryocytes. Liver function tests may indicate hepatocellular disease. It is possible to measure portal venous pressure, and injection of radiopaque dyes into the spleen will permit radiologic visualization of the splenic and portal veins. This should usually be done under direct vision, for percutaneous needling may lead to laceration of the splenic capsule.

Treatment. The site of obstruction must be determined. If only the splenic vein is involved, splenectomy is curative. In cases in which the portal vein is extensively involved or in which intrahepatic obstruction is present, splenectomy will correct pancytopenia, but will not relieve portal hypertension. Portacaval anastomosis, which in general is preferred to splenorenal shunting in

TABLE 14-7. Some Causes of Splenomegaly in Children

I. *Hematologic diseases*
   Hemolytic anemias—due to extramedullary hematopoiesis and reticuloendothelial hyperplasia
   A. Congenital hemolytic anemias
   B. Hemoglobinopathies and thalassemia

II. *Infections*
   A. Bacterial: septicemias; typhoid; endocarditis
   B. Viral: infectious mononucleosis
   C. Protozoal: malaria, toxoplasmosis

III. *Congestive splenomegaly*
   A. Secondary to portal or splenic vein obstruction
   B. Secondary to intrahepatic disease—cirrhosis
   C. Chronic congestive heart failure

IV. *Infiltrations*
   A. Lipidoses—Niemann-Pick, Gaucher's diseases
   B. Nonlipid reticuloendothelioses

V. *Cysts*
   A. Congenital
   B. Acquired

VI. *Neoplasms*
   A. Leukemia and lymphosarcoma
   B. Hodgkin's disease
   C. Hemangioma and lymphangioma

VII. *Miscellaneous*
   A. Rheumatoid arthritis (Still's disease)
   B. Lupus erythematosus
   C. Cysts

the young child, is indicated when portal hypertension is clearly shown or when bleeding from esophageal varices has occurred. Successful relief of portal hypertension may result in decrease in splenic size and improvement of pancytopenia.

ANOMALIES AND TRAUMA

Congenital Absence of the Spleen. Absence of the spleen occurs as part of an unusual group of anomalies, including complex abnormalities of the heart and great vessels with severe cyanotic congenital heart disease. Apparent dextrocardia and varying degrees of heterotopia of the abdominal viscera are seen. The condition can be suspected from examination of the blood: target cells, increased numbers of spherocytes, intraerythrocytic inclusions such as Howell-Jolly and Heinz bodies and hemosiderin granules are easily demonstrated. The incidence of overwhelming sepsis appears to be increased in congenital asplenia.

Hypersplenism. Hypersplenism is not a specific diagnosis, but rather a descriptive term for a clinical complex which includes (1) depression of one or more of the cellular elements of the blood; (2) active formation of that element in the bone marrow; (3) an enlarged spleen, which may be due to a large number of causes (Table 14-7); and (4) correction of the hematologic abnormalities by splenectomy. A diagnosis of primary hypersplenism is difficult to establish; other causes of splenomegaly with secondary pancytopenia must be excluded.

Rupture of the Spleen. Traumatic injury of the spleen may result from a hard, direct blow to the left flank or left side of the abdomen, such as may occur during automobile accidents or contact sports. If the tear in the splenic capsule is small, the symptoms may be moderate and include left upper quadrant or left shoulder pain and signs of peritoneal irritation due to blood. In more extreme cases, shock may develop rapidly. When the spleen is pathologically enlarged, rupture may occur after relatively minor trauma. This occurs in the newborn infant with hemolytic disease, and in the older child with infectious mononucleosis. Laparotomy and splenectomy are indicated when rupture is suspected or diagnosed.

SPLENECTOMY

Removal of the spleen is a common operation which is performed for a variety of indications. Primary surgical indications include (1) rupture of the spleen; (2) removal of tumors, cysts or vascular anomalies involving the spleen; (3) when

necessary for adequate surgical exposure of the left upper portion of the abdomen; (4) as part of certain shunting procedures; (5) for relief of mechanical distress due to massive enlargement in thalassemia major or Gaucher's disease.

Hematologic indications include (1) congenital hemolytic states such as hereditary spherocytosis and elliptocytosis, and some cases of nonspherocytic anemias such as pyruvate kinase deficiency; (2) autoimmune hemolytic anemia when chronic and refractory to corticosteroid therapy; (3) chronic idiopathic thrombocytopenic purpura (ITP) and (4) hypersplenism. The results derived from the operation vary considerably with the basic disease process.

Overwhelming Sepsis Following Splenectomy. There is general agreement that removal of the spleen alters host resistance and that overwhelming and often fatal meningitis and septicemia are seen with increased frequency in asplenic persons. The consequences and risks vary considerably, depending primarily upon the disease for which splenectomy is performed and to a less extent upon the age of the patient.

The risk of overwhelming sepsis is low when splenectomy is done for traumatic rupture, hereditary spherocytosis and ITP. A high incidence of infection is seen when the indication is thalassemia major, Wiskott-Aldrich syndrome, histiocytosis and lipidosis. The risk is somewhat increased in all categories for younger infants and children. Severe infections after splenectomy, usually meningitis and septicemia, are characterized by an acute and fulminating course, death frequently occurring within 12 to 24 hours after onset of symptoms. In more than 60 per cent of cases, pneumococci are the responsible agents; *Hemophilus influenzae* and meningococci are responsible for a smaller number of infections. Because of this risk, splenectomy should be performed only for pressing indications, and when possible the operation should be deferred until after 3 to 4 years of age. Prophylactic penicillin has been advocated for the young child during the first year or two after splenectomy, but there are no data on the effectiveness of such management.

REFERENCES

Crosby, W. H.: Normal Functions of the Spleen Relative to Red Blood Cells; A Review. *Blood*, 14:399, 1959.
Ellis, E. F., and Smith, R. T.: The Role of the Spleen in Immunity. *Pediatrics*, 37:111, 1966.
Eraklis, A. J., Kevy, S. V., Diamond, L. K., and Gross, R. E.: Hazard of Overwhelming Infection after Splenectomy in Childhood. *New England J. Med.*, 276:1225, 1967.
Schulkind, M. L., Ellis, E. F., and Smith, R. T.: Effect of Antibody upon Clearance of I^{125}-Labelled Pneumococci by the Spleen and Liver. *Pediat. Res.*, 1:178, 1967.

THE LYMPHATIC SYSTEM

The lymphatic system includes the free lymphocytes of the blood and lymph as well as the organized lymphatic structures such as lymph nodes, spleen, Peyer's patches, appendix and tonsils. The origin of lymphocytes is uncertain; some are believed to originate in the embryonic thymus, from which their progenitors migrate to populate other lymphatic tissues. Others, or all, may arise from other tissues such as the lymphoid areas of the gastrointestinal tonsillar tract area, or the appendix.

The lymph vessels start as small capillaries between the cells of all organs except the brain and the heart. Small lymphatic capillaries join to form progressively larger channels which drain the extremities, trunk and head. The largest of the lymphatic vessels is the thoracic duct, which discharges most of the central return of body lymph into the left subclavian vein.

The lymph channels are characteristically interrupted by lymph nodes. These well defined structures are networks of dilated sinusoids lined by reticuloendothelial elements and surrounded by masses of actively proliferating lymphocytes. The lymph nodes are located in groups, through which the lymphatic drainage of well defined anatomic areas passes. Because of their locations and structure, the lymph nodes function as protective barriers to the spread of infections. They also filter particulate antigens, and the lymphocytes and plasma cells within lymph nodes actively participate in antibody formation.

The superficial lymph nodes are evaluated by palpation. Small nodes can normally be felt in the neck, axillae and groin. Roentgenograms of the chest assess enlargement of the mediastinal lymph nodes. Lymphangiography permits evaluation of the size and structure of the pelvic and retroperitoneal lymph nodes.

The lymph is a clear fluid. It has a protein content intermediate between that of interstitial fluid and plasma and contains a substantial number of small lymphocytes.

DISEASES OF THE LYMPH VESSELS

Acute Lymphangitis. This is an inflammation of the lymphatics draining an area of acute infection, usually bacterial. It is manifested as red painful streaks radiating proximally from the infected site. Painful swelling of the regional nodes is also usually present.

Lymphedema. Lymphedema is a diffuse, permanent pitting edema due to obstruction of the lymph drainage of an area, usually an extremity. Congenital lymphedema occurs in so-called Milroy's disease and as part of the syndrome of gonadal dysgenesis. Acquired lymphedema may result from inflammatory processes or from surgical or radiologic obliteration of lymph nodes or lymph channels.

DISEASES OF THE LYMPH NODES

Enlargement of the lymph nodes occurs in response to a wide variety of infectious, inflammatory and neoplastic processes. Enlargement of a single node or group of nodes is most frequently due to an infection in the area it drains. Generalized lymphadenopathy occurs in many acute infections, especially rubella, rubeola, typhoid, tularemia and infectious mononucleosis. Leukemia, lymphoma and reticuloendotheliosis are sometimes accompanied by striking degrees of lymph node enlargement. Malignant tumors such as neuroblastoma sometimes metastasize to lymph nodes, and large numbers of lipid-bearing histiocytes may be present in the lymph nodes of Gaucher's disease and other lipidoses.

ACUTE LYMPHADENITIS

As a result of cellulitis or other infections, bacteria and toxins and other by-products of acute inflammation are carried in the lymph to regional lymph nodes where an acute inflammatory process occurs. Bacteria may cause abscess formation. Acute cervical adenitis secondary to acute pharyngitis and inguinal lymphadenopathy resulting from infections of the lower extremity are common. The involved nodes become swollen and painful, and the overlying skin is hot and red. Although the primary infectious process is usually obvious, the site of inoculation may not be apparent, as in cat-scratch disease. Mediastinal lymphadenitis secondary to pulmonary infections may produce obstructive symptoms and cough. Mesenteric lymphadenopathy may, on occasion, be associated with crampy abdominal pain simulating appendicitis.

Treatment. Antibiotic therapy which is appropriate for the primary infection will benefit the lymphadenitis. When suppuration occurs, needle aspiration or surgical drainage is necessary.

CHRONIC LYMPHADENITIS

Chronic infection or inflammation is frequently associated with hyperplasia of the lymph nodes. Tuberculous infections regularly result in regional lymphadenopathy. Scrofula, or chronic cervical lymphadenopathy, may be secondary to infection of the nasopharynx with bovine tuberculosis. This organism is uncommon in the United States, where chronic lymphadenopathy is more often due to infection by atypical acid-fast organisms.

The organisms are trapped in the nodes, where granuloma and caseous necrosis occur. Affected nodes are hard, nontender and frequently matted to adjacent tissues. Biopsy may be necessary to differentiate chronic infections from malignant processes.

LYMPHORETICULAR MALIGNANCIES

The lymphoreticular malignancies are lymphosarcoma, including reticulum cell sarcoma, and Hodgkin's disease. In so-called reticulum cell sarcoma large undifferentiated cells thought to represent the most primitive form of the lymphocyte series predominate. In the lymphoblastic varieties of lymphosarcoma, slightly more differentiated cells corresponding to lymphoblasts are seen. Reticulum cell sarcoma usually has more aggressive clinical characteristics than other lymphosarcomas.

In Hodgkin's disease a varied histologic picture is seen. The predominating cell type is a large, primitive reticulum-like malignant cell. In addition, multinucleated giant cells (Reed-Sternberg cells) constitute a diagnostic feature. Varying degrees of eosinophilia, lymphocytosis and fibrosis are also present. In general, tumors containing substantial numbers of lymphocytes and eosinophils are associated with less malignant clinical behavior.

Etiology. The cause of the lymphoreticular malignancies is unknown. They occur with markedly increased frequency in diseases involving defects of the immune mechanism, such as Wiskott-Aldrich syndrome and ataxia-telangiectasia. One particular form, the *Burkitt lymphoma of African children,* is the first human malignancy in which evidence for a viral origin or relation is considered convincing. This tumor has a clinical predilection for the jaws. The histologic picture is characteristic. Sheets of primitive lymphoblasts are interspersed with large, pale, lipid-filled histiocytes. This tumor is prevalent in areas of Africa where climactic conditions are favorable for virus-bearing arthropod vectors; viruses can be demonstrated and grown in tissue cultures from these tumors. It is not clear, however, whether or how viruses are related to the more usual cases of lymphoreticular malignancy.

Clinical Manifestations. The main clinical features of the lymphoreticular malignancies are similar. Lymph node involvement is the most common initial manifestation. The area most commonly affected is the posterior cervical triangle; next, the axillary and inguinal regions. Mediastinal and retroperitoneal areas may be affected in the absence of superficial involvement. Rarely, the primary affected site may be extranodal. Involvement of nodes of a given area may be single or multiple. Involved nodes are firm and nontender; the overlying skin is not red or hot. Mediastinal lymphadenopathy may produce respiratory symptoms or cough by compressing the airway. In addition to mechanical symptoms due to the enlarged nodes, systemic manifestations are frequent. Fever, sweating and weight loss are common constitutional symptoms.

The degree of dissemination of lymphoreticular malignancy has considerable prognostic significance. In stage I, the disease is restricted to a single anatomic site or localized group of lymph nodes, and no constitutional symptoms are present. In stage IIa, 2 or 3 adjacent lymph node areas on the same side of the diaphragm are involved without systemic illness. In stage IIb constitutional symptoms are present. Finally, in stage III the disease is widely disseminated, involving multiple lymph node areas and other organs. Precise assessment of the degree of involvement depends upon complete physical examination, chest x-ray, intravenous pyelography, and newer techniques such as lymphangiography and inferior venacavography.

In about 20 per cent of cases of lymphosarcoma the blood and bone marrow may be invaded, with a clinical and hematologic picture indistinguishable from that of acute lymphoblastic leukemia.

Treatment. Surgical biopsy is essential to obtain adequate tissue for histologic diagnosis. If complete excision of the affected node is feasible at the time of biopsy, this is advisable, but extensive surgical procedures are not usually indicated.

The lymphoreticular malignancies are sensitive to radiation, which constitutes the mainstay of therapy. In stages I and IIa, cure is possible. Aggressive radiotherapy should involve tumoricidal doses to the primary lesion and to the adjacent lymph node regions. When respiratory symptoms are present, this therapy should be administered cautiously, for edema may occur, temporarily aggravating the degree of obstruction. Chemotherapy may be particularly useful in this situation.

In stages IIb and III smaller amounts of radiation delivered to the most significant tumor masses are of considerable palliative value.

Chemotherapy is useful in these diseases, and the alkylating agents, nitrogen mustard and cyclophosphamide, are most frequently used. Nitrogen mustard in a total dose of 0.4 mg. per kg. is administered in 1 or 2 intravenous injections. Care should be exercised, for the drug is vesicant when extravasation occurs. Cyclophosphamide may be given either orally in a daily dose of 2.5 mg. per kg. or intravenously in a weekly dose of 10 to 15 mg. per kg. Nitrogen mustard therapy usually results in prompt relief of constitutional symptoms and reduction in size of the lymph nodes. The clinical improvement following chemotherapy may last for many months. When relapse occurs, another course is indicated. The response is usually shorter with successive treatments, and ultimately the disease becomes refractory.

The periwinkle alkaloids, vincristine and vinblastine, may also be beneficial. Corticosteroids may be of some value in ameliorating constitutional symptoms and are especially valuable in treating the autoimmune hemolytic anemias which occasionally develop. In those cases of lymphosarcoma in which leukemic dissemination has occurred, therapy with folic acid antagonists and 6-mercaptopurine may be helpful.

Course and Prognosis. The prognosis in general is very grave. Only about 10 to 20 per cent of unselected patients are still alive 5 years after diagnosis, with a mean survival of 3 to 4 years. If the illness presents in stage I or stage IIa, the outlook is much better; 5-year survival rates of 50 to 80 per cent have been reported. In general, the more histologically differentiated tumors have a somewhat better prognosis. In disseminated disease palliative therapy is often effective in extending comfortable life for many months. Ultimately, however, the disease becomes refractory to all therapy, death resulting from general inanition and associated complications.

Howard A. Pearson

REFERENCES

Aisenberg, A. C.: Primary Management of Hodgkin's Disease. *New England J. Med.*, 278:93, 1968.

Burkitt, D.: Determining the Climactic Limitations of Children's Cancer Common in Africa. *Brit. Med. J.,* 2:1019, 1962.

Jones, B., and Klingberg, W. G.: Lymphosarcoma in Children—A Report of 43 Cases and a Review of the Recent Literature. *J. Pediat.,* 63:11, 1963.

Lee, B. J., Nelson, J. H., and Schwarz, G.: Evaluation of Lymphangiography, Inferior Venacavography and Intravenous Pyelography in the Clinical Staging and Management of Hodgkin's Disease. *New England J. Med.,* 271:327, 1964.

Peters, M. V.: Hodgkin's Disease: Radiation Therapy. *J.A.M.A.,* 191:28, 1965.

Rosenberg, S. A., Diamond, H. D., Dargeon, H. W., and Craver, L. F.: Lymphosarcoma in Childhood. *New England J. Med.,* 259:505, 1958.

15. The Urinary System

ANATOMY

The intimate integration of structure and function is nowhere better illustrated than in the kidney. The nephron is the anatomic and functional unit of the kidney; there are approximately 1,000,000 nephrons in each kidney, each composed of a glomerulus and an unbranched tubule which joins a collecting duct to drain into the renal pelvis. The spatial arrangement of the tubule and glomerulus is such that the distal tubule is adjacent to the glomerular stalk; at this point a portion of the tubular surface becomes the macula densa and is in intimate contact with the afferent and efferent arterioles. Together, these structures form the juxtaglomerular apparatus at the hilus of the glomerulus.

The juxtaglomerular apparatus is involved in renal sodium regulation and the production of renin. This intimate relation of the distal tubule to the renin-producing cells has, along with variations in the granulation of the cells of the juxtaglomerular apparatus, physiologic relevance to absorption and excretion of sodium, changes in the appearance of the adrenal cortex (zona glomerulosa), the production of aldosterone, and hypertensive states.

Filtration is the only known function of the glomerulus (capillary tuft). Figure 15-1 diagrammatically demonstrates the 3 layers constituting the capillary wall: the inner layer of endothelial cells, the middle layer or basement membrane with its layers of varying density, and the outer layer of epithelial cells. The normal separation of the individual foot processes of the epithelial cells is lost (smudged) during excessive proteinuria such as occurs in the nephrotic syndrome, and gaps or pores are seen in the endothelial lining. Pathologic processes in the kidney particularly involve the appearance of the epithelial cells, the numbers of endothelial cells, and the structure of the basement membrane. The third type of cell of interest is the so-called intercapillary or mesangial cell, which resides in the amorphous substance, or mesangium, of the stalk of the glomerulus. In many pathologic states there are decided increases in amount of this amorphous substance and in the number of mesangial cells. The function of the mesangial cell is not clearly understood.

The tubule has an elongated, hairpin shape, and can be anatomically divided into the proximal convolution, the descending limb, the loop (of Henle), the ascending limb and the distal convolution; these segments have been shown to localize various functions. The length of the tubule varies. In the premature and the young infant there is a relatively large number of short limbs. This may be an important factor in the decreased concentrating ability in early infancy (see Renal Function in Infancy, p. 1102).

The interlobular arteries originate from the arcuate arteries and are arranged anatomically parallel to the medullary rays. The afferent artery to each glomerulus takes its origin from the interlobular artery. At its exit from the glomerulus the vessel becomes the efferent arteriole. There is little evidence that there is in man any significant bypassing of the glomerulus directly from afferent to efferent arteriole. The efferent arteriole splits up into a capillary network between the tubules which is their only blood supply (postglomerular); these capillaries become the vasa recta which follow the general hairpin shape of the renal tubules and in their intimate relation with the tubules form the basis of the countercurrent mechanism for renal regulation of water balance. These capillaries finally return to the arcuate veins, which enter the renal veins.

There are striking functional differences between the kidney of the early months of life and that of the adult, not all of which are presently explicable. Some differences do not depend just on obvious anatomic variation, but may reflect enzymatic and biophysical factors.

From a study of human fetuses Vernier and Birch-Andersen observed that the process of glomerulogenesis in the fetus appears to proceed by growth of the cortex toward the capsule in such a way that the more mature glomeruli are near the corticomedullary junction. The glomeruli considered to be most immature consist of spherical masses of cells in which the clearly recognizable glomerular anlage is surrounded by a cup-shaped layer of epithelial cells, with or without an evident Bowman's space. Slightly more developed glomeruli demonstrate a well defined Bowman's space, early evidence of flattening of the capsular (parietal) epithelial cells and a less densely packed glomerular structure, which contains 6 to 8 well defined capillaries. More mature glomeruli resemble those of the adult and are composed of a tuft of capillaries enclosed by a thin, single layer of parietal epithelium, a crescent-shaped Bowman's space, and a single layer of visceral epithelial cells. The capillary tuft is less complex than in the adult and contains fewer capillary loops.

About 20 per cent of glomeruli are mature at 9 weeks of gestation; at 19 weeks about 30 per cent. It appears that the number of glomeruli also increases in proportion to fetal development.

Electron micrographs show that somewhat flattened, parietal epithelial cells form the capsular layer. The visceral epithelial cell layer is 2 to 3 cells in thickness, and these cells, as well as their nuclei, are typically rounded or rectangular. Differentiation of subcapsular glomeruli has been shown (Potter and Thierstein) to continue until about 35 weeks of gestation. The majority of glomeruli in the kidney of the newborn infant have well differentiated epithelial cell foot processes, as well as normal morphology by light microscopy. The mean diameter of glomeruli increases gradually after birth (diameter about 100 microns) to reach the adult diameter (about 200 microns) by about 20 years of age.

1095

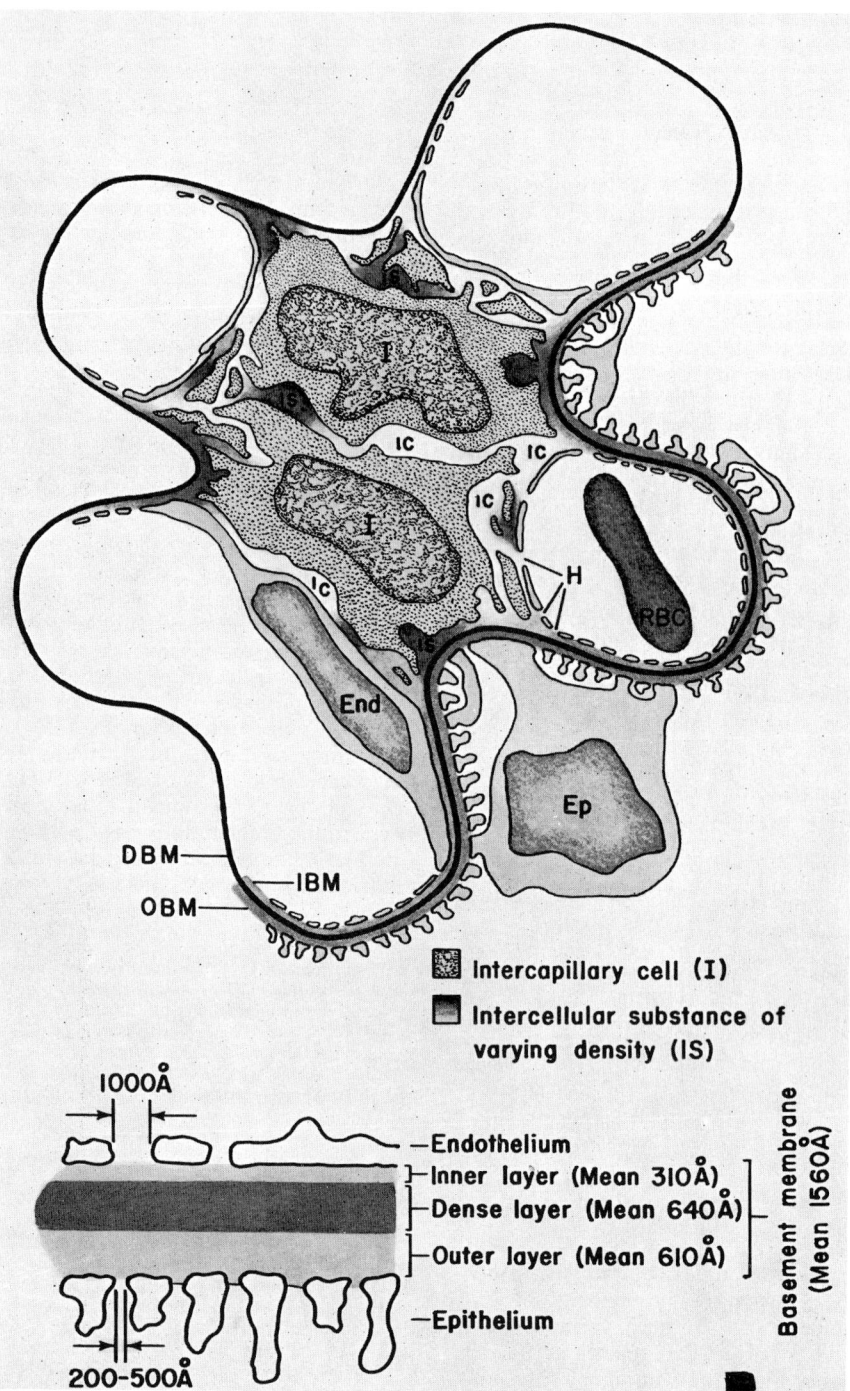

Figure 15-1. Glomerular lobule with its centrolobular region (mesangium). Measurements of the peripheral basement membranes based on a study of rats. Abbreviations: *DBM,* dense layer of basement membrane (lamina densa); *OBM* and *IBM,* outer and inner layers, respectively, of basement membrane; *Ep,* epithelium; *End,* endothelium; *IC,* intercapillary channel; *H,* holes or gaps in endothelium; *RBC,* red blood cell. (From H. Latta, A. B. Maunsbach and S. C. Madden: *J. Ultrastruct. Res.,* 4;455, 1960.)

Grunewald and Popper have proposed that the improvement of renal function which occurs in the early months of life results from sloughing of the epithelial cells during neonatal glomerular development. Vernier and Birch-Andersen demonstrate, though, that many glomeruli from fetuses of 5 months of gestation appear structurally fully capable of function. They believe that the low glomerular filtration rate of infants is related to other factors such as (1) the decreased capillary bed available for filtration in the small glomeruli of fetuses and infants and (2) the low blood pressure characteristic of infants.

Sclerosis of a few glomeruli (usually less than 1 per cent) is common in the newborn. Rarely, a much higher percentage of glomeruli may be so involved, as in the rubella syndrome. It is thought that in rare cases there may be sufficient numbers of glomeruli involved to result in renal failure.

Section of the kidney of the newborn infant often reveals reddish-yellow streaks in the apices of the papillae. These are deposits of urates (uric acid infarcts), chiefly in the straight portions of the tubules in the medulla. Sodium, calcium and phosphorus salts and oxalic acid may also be found.

The bladder of the infant is practically an abdominal organ, since the small pelvis is not capable of containing it.

PHYSIOLOGY

RENAL CIRCULATION AND METABOLISM

The kidneys represent less than 1 per cent of body weight, but normally receive about 20 per cent of the cardiac output. This large blood flow ensures a high perfusion rate despite fluctuations in systemic blood pressure, and allows the kidneys to receive the entire blood volume about every 5 minutes. Such a blood flow is an important homeostatic advantage in regulating volume and composition of body fluid. In moderate to severe systemic hypotension, renal blood flow is reduced directly in proportion to blood pressure, and renal filtration and urine volume fall in proportion.

Although blood flow cannot be measured directly, a reliable estimation can be made by means of the Fick equation. The substance used, paraaminohippurate (PAH), is not destroyed or synthesized in the body and can be measured accurately. At low plasma concentrations (less than 5 mg. per 100 ml.) normal adult kidneys remove 90 per cent of PAH in 1 passage through them. If the amount of PAH eliminated through the kidneys in a given unit of time and the arterial and venous plasma concentrations of PAH during this interval are known, an estimate of effective renal plasma flow is obtained. Effective flow excludes the blood perfusing the renal capsule, fat and other nonexcretory tissues. This method has proved useful in relating renal blood flow to other measures of renal function.

Ninety per cent of renal blood flow perfuses the cortex through glomeruli and their postglomerular capillary beds; about 10 per cent perfuses the medulla. Medullary blood has a higher packed cell volume and a slower rate of flow; perfusion of the vasa recta is essential to the concentrating process.

The renal circulation depends upon adequate systemic blood pressure. Under normal conditions renal filtration and local blood perfusion are controlled from within the kidney, probably by local changes in the tone of the smooth muscle in the walls of the vessels. This autonomous control by the kidneys is remarkably effective in maintaining renal filtration and perfusion despite moderate variations of systemic pressure. Sympathetic stimulation may depress renal blood flow profoundly, diverting large volumes of blood to perfuse the more vital organs, brain and heart. The kidneys have no systemic vasodilator nerves.

The kidneys have a high consumption of oxygen in proportion to their weight. Unlike that in other organs, renal oxygen consumption varies with blood flow, correlating directly with filtration rate. When a given filtration rate is sustained, consumption of oxygen varies directly with sodium reabsorption.

For reasons not yet clear, the renal medulla appears to have a high rate of anaerobic metabolism. This is in accord with the lower blood flow through the medulla, and may relate to the concentrating function.

GLOMERULAR FILTRATION

The initial step in formation of urine is in the glomeruli, where a cell-free, essentially protein-free ultrafiltrate of blood passes into the tubule. It seems clear that substances from the blood passing through the glomerulus traverse 3 distinct histologic structures. Nevertheless the chemical composition of the ultrafiltrate is very like that which would be formed by filtration through an inert membrane having pores of limited size. The hydrostatic pressure in the glomerular vessels (about 60 mm. Hg) is of the right magnitude to produce such an ultrafiltrate against the opposing forces of plasma oncotic pressure (about 25 to 30 mm. Hg) and glomerular intracapsular pressure.

Because of its importance in determining renal function, measurement of the rate of formation of glomerular filtrate in patients is often desirable. The glomerular filtration rate may be less than 50 per cent of normal in asymptomatic renal disease, and it drops to below 10 per cent of normal in terminal renal failure. This measurement can be estimated only indirectly, and requires the presence of an inert substance free in the plasma (not bound to protein or cells), which is completely filtered through the glomeruli, and neither reabsorbed nor secreted by the renal tubules. The inert polysaccharide inulin is ideal for this purpose.

Because it is excreted solely by filtration, the clearance of inulin serves as a standard of reference for the renal excretion of other substances. Substances with clearances lower than inulin must undergo some reabsorption beyond the glomeruli.

Substances whose clearance exceeds that of inulin must undergo some secretion or synthesis beyond the glomeruli. Since both reabsorption and secretion of the same substance may occur, only the net result can be judged by comparison with inulin clearance. This method of comparison treats the functions of the entire renal tubule as a single process, which of course is a simplifying assumption.

Expressed in terms of the surface area of a "standard man," the normal value for rate of glomerular filtration in the male is approximately 120 ml. per minute. Variation is great, owing to fluctuations within the individual and between different persons. The control of glomerular filtration is predominantly renal and autonomous under usual circumstances; how this occurs is not certain. Systemic blood pressure and blood volume may affect the glomerular filtration rate, and under conditions of hypervolemia or generalized sympathetic stimulation, glomerular filtration rises or falls appropriately. A large change in the rate of glomerular filtration generally is reflected in urine volume, but tubular function primarily determines urine volume, nine tenths of glomerular filtrate being reabsorbed under all conditions.

Because of the considerable independence of glomerular filtration and tubular function, as well as the autonomy of renal circulation, it is useful to know the fraction of renal blood flow which is filtered. This may vary independently of total renal blood flow because of the autonomous regulation of filtration rate. This "filtration fraction" is calculated from the separately estimated rate of glomerular filtration (clearance of inulin) and "effective renal blood flow" (clearance of para-aminohippurate at low plasma concentration). The determinations should be made simultaneously because of constantly changing filtration and perfusion. Determined in this manner, filtration fraction is normally about 0.22.

TUBULAR FUNCTION

Tubular function determines the ultimate volume and composition of glomerular filtrate as urine and involves transport of substances from and to urine. Two main types of transtubular movement for substances occur: (1) active and (2) passive. Passive transport implies movement down a gradient of concentration for the substance being considered from an area of higher concentration to one of lower concentration. In the case of an ionized substance (electrolyte) passive transport may also occur down an electrochemical gradient from an area of higher potential to one of lower potential. If both gradients are present, the resultant of the 2 forces determines the direction of passive transport of the ion. When these gradients are measured experimentally, the direction of the passive transport can be predicted. If the substance moves in the direction opposite to that predicted, active transport is present. Both types of transport occur across the renal tubules, but active transport accounts for the major expenditure of energy of the kidney. By this means over 400 gm. of sodium per day are reabsorbed in the adult.

Substances which are actively transported across the tubule may behave in one of 2 ways when the transport system is saturated. Saturation never occurs physiologically, but does in certain disease states. An absolute maximal rate of transport may be demonstrated for nonelectrolytes and weakly ionized substances. This maximal rate of transport is called tubular maximum (TM).

The behavior of substances which have a reabsorptive TM can be illustrated by the titration curve for glucose transport. If glucose is infused to elevate progressively plasma glucose concentration and the glomerular filtration rate (C_{inulin}) is measured, the filtered load of glucose is indicated by the product of inulin clearance (GFR) and the plasma glucose concentration in milligrams per ml. The amount filtered minus that excreted equals the amount of glucose reabsorbed per minute. At low plasma levels, reabsorption is complete. The glucose *threshold* is the highest concentration at which reabsorption is complete. Above the threshold some glucose appears in urine while reabsorption continues to rise. A higher plasma level is then reached at which reabsorption is maximal (the TM).

For a defined physiologic state the TM is a reproducible value for any substance and does not depend on the rate of glomerular filtration. The major electrolytes (except bicarbonate) exhibit no TM and are called gradient-time limited substances. The maximal rate of transport appears to be governed by the chemical gradient across the tubular cell membrane for the ion in question. The maximal rate of transport is affected by the rate of glomerular filtration. Specific examples of these types of transport are given below.

The volume of water reabsorbed by the kidneys is enormous; even severe diabetes insipidus produces only a slight proportionate fall, as can be seen from the total amount of glomerular filtrate formed in a day (over 170 liters in an adult, 14 liters in a newborn infant). Water reabsorption throughout the renal tubules is secondary to the osmotic gradients created. Current concepts indicate that the renal tubules are freely permeable to water everywhere except in the ascending limb of Henle's loop. Two types of water reabsorption can be distinguished: (1) isosmotic reabsorption and (2) hyperosmotic reabsorption, according to the presence or absence of a measurable osmotic gradient across the renal tubule. Isosmotic reabsorption accounts for four fifths of all water reabsorbed and occurs secondary to sodium reabsorption in the proximal tubule. This water reabsorption takes place independently of body water content. It has, therefore, been called obligatory and has no role independent of sodium in body homeostasis. Hyperosmotic reabsorption of water takes place in the distal tubule and collecting ducts where the concentrating mechanism resides. Like proximal reabsorption of water, distal reabsorption is passive, occurring secondary to an osmotic gradient.

The anatomy of the medulla is the clue to the current concept of medullary concentration, for which there is now much evidence. Two anatomic features essential to the concentrating process are the loops of Henle of the juxtamedullary glomeruli and the vasa recta, both of which dip deep into the renal medulla (Fig. 15-2).

As noted, urine is isosmotic throughout the proximal tubule. When it reaches the early distal tubule, it is hyposmotic, regardless of whether the final urine is to be dilute or concentrated. Renal medullary tissue and blood are, accordingly, consistently hyperosmotic to plasma and cortex. This increase in medullary osmolality is due primarily to sodium (with matching anions) and urea. The unifying concept is that of a sodium pump in the ascending loop of Henle, which creates the hyperosmotic medulla and renders the urine hyponatremic at the beginning of the distal tubule. The ascending loop is presumed to be poorly permeable to water; the permeability of the distal tubule is controlled by antidiuretic hormone (ADH). The hyperosmotic medullary interstitium effects distal reabsorption of water when ADH is secreted, which increases tubular permeability to water. When ADH is not secreted, distal water reabsorption is precluded by low tubular permeability, and diuresis occurs.

Both glomerular filtration rate and degree of

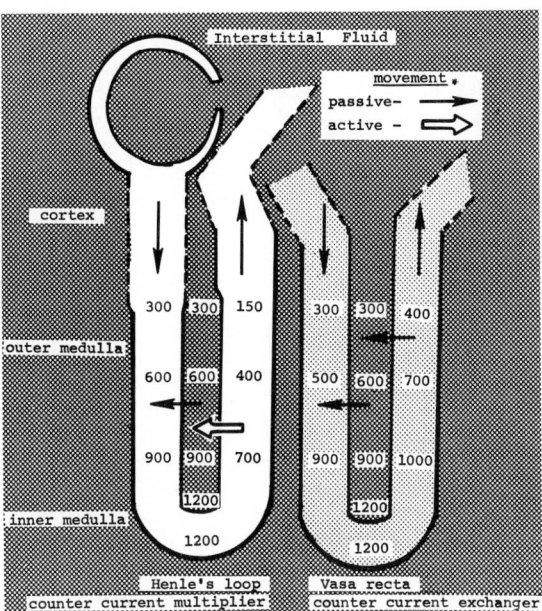

Figure 15-2. Schematic diagram of osmotic events in renal medulla. Numbers represent values of osmolality in mOsm. per liter. Water diffuses freely everywhere except in the ascending loop of Henle, which must be impermeable to water. (Adapted from R. W. Berliner et al.: *Am. J. Med.,* 24:730, 1958; and R. F. Pitts: *Physiology of Kidney and Body Fluids.* Chicago, Year Book Medical Publishers, Inc., 1963, p. 113.)

proximal reabsorption participate in renal regulation of water balance through alteration of the volume of fluid presented for concentration or dilution. In dehydration, reduced glomerular filtration and slowed tubular flow increase the concentrating operation. In overhydration the higher volume of filtrate per unit of time and higher rate of tubular flow increase water excretion.

Sodium is the principal cation of extracellular water. Although it actually comprises but 45 per cent of the osmolality of extracellular water, effectively it accounts for 90 per cent of extracellular osmolality. This is because the kidney appears to regulate sodium balance primarily, the matching (Cl^- and HCO^-_3) being controlled indirectly. Sodium controls the volume of body water through the limits of osmolality tolerated by osmoreceptors of the hypothalamus, which normally maintain the osmolality of body fluids between 280 and 300 mOsm. per liter. The total volume of extracellular fluid is determined primarily by the amount of sodium in this compartment.

The kidneys regulate sodium homeostasis in 4 important ways: (1) through changes in the rate of glomerular filtration; (2) through the adjustment of proximal tubular sodium reabsorption to the rate of glomerular filtration; (3) through their response to aldosterone; and (4) through adjustment of proximal tubular sodium reabsorption independently of glomerular filtration rate. Sodium retention raises plasma volume and the glomerular filtration rate. Since the proximal tubule reabsorbs a relatively constant fraction of glomerular filtrate, a rise in filtration rate leads to a rise both in the amount of sodium reabsorbed and in the amount excreted. Some of the excess sodium in the body is thereby excreted. The increment in sodium excretion tends to continue until glomerular filtration rate falls to normal. In sodium depletion, on the other hand, the reduced plasma volume which generally exists causes a lower rate of glomerular filtration. If the *fraction* of glomerular filtrate reabsorbed proximally stays constant, a reduction in the amounts of sodium reabsorbed and excreted will occur. The reduced excretion helps to correct sodium depletion and tends to continue until the glomerular filtration rate rises to normal. In sodium depletion, aldosterone activity also increases tubular reabsorption of sodium. Other homeostatic alterations in proximal tubular reabsorption of sodium independent of filtration rate have been shown to occur, but the mechanisms are not known.

Reabsorption of most of the *chloride* in the glomerular filtrate takes place passively in the proximal tubule in conjunction with active reabsorption of sodium. Since the concentration of chloride in plasma is limited by the concentration of sodium, the filtered load of chloride which can be presented to the tubules is limited. Within this limitation no restriction on the rate or amount of chloride which can be reabsorbed or excreted is known. The concentrations of chloride and bicarbonate anions vary inversely in disease; an elevation of plasma bicarbonate promotes a chloruresis with a fall in plasma chloride, and a reduction in plasma bicarbonate increases chloride reabsorption. Since, in chloride depletion, the tubules can remove virtually all chloride from urine, some active reabsorption of chloride must be possible in the distal nephron. The latter is a minute fraction of proximal reabsorption.

Potassium is both reabsorbed and secreted by the renal tubules. It is probable that all filtered potassium is reabsorbed, primarily in the proximal tubule, and that potassium in urine accrues from tubular secretion. Secretion is dependent upon the body stores of potassium, upon the reabsorption of sodium, and upon acid-base equilibria. The renal tubules conserve potassium when the body stores are reduced and secrete potassium when the body stores are plentiful. Urinary excretion of potassium can be raised a hundredfold, but cannot be reduced below about 10 mEq. a day, even during potassium deficiency.

Since potassium and hydrogen ion secretion apparently occurs in part by an ion exchange for sodium or hydrogen, an increase in sodium reabsorption tends to promote secretion of potassium. Whether potassium or hydrogen is selected preferentially depends on the relative stores of each available. Acidosis promotes H^+ secretion over K^+, whereas alkalosis promotes secretion of K^+ instead of H^+. These considerations are the basis for the relation between renal potassium excretion and acid-base equilibrium, and explain why a patient with alkalosis and potassium deficiency (e.g. in pyloric stenosis or Cushing's syndrome) may excrete an acid urine.

The *bicarbonate* in plasma appears in glomerular filtrate and then undergoes either reabsorption or excretion. Reabsorption is thought to take place with the active transport of sodium, in both the proximal and the distal tubules. At both sites, reabsorption is intimately related to the simultaneous reabsorption of sodium and secretion of hydrogen ion (Fig. 15-3). During reabsorption of bicarbonate 1 mEq. of sodium bicarbonate is added to peritubular blood for each milliequivalent which has been removed from tubular urine. This process produces no net change in plasma bicarbonate or acid-base equilibrium, since it serves only to return filtered bicarbonate to blood. The steps in this process involve intracellular decomposition of carbonic acid to hydrogen ion and bicarbonate ion. The latter combines with reabsorbed sodium to return to blood. The hydrogen ion remaining is secreted into urine and combines with bicarbonate in the urine to form carbonic acid. Either carbonic acid or carbon dioxide resulting from its decomposition diffuses back into tubular cells. Urine contains very small amounts of carbonic acid and carbon dioxide. The continuous production of carbon dioxide from metabolic activity and the large content of water in the body ensure an endless supply of these substances. Carbonic anhydrase accelerates the formation and decomposition

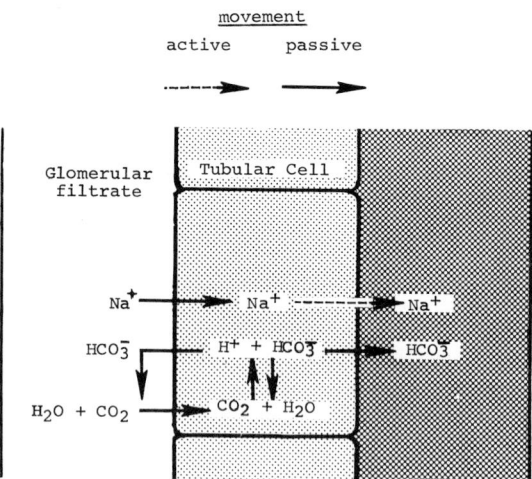

Figure 15-3. Bicarbonate reabsorption in the proximal tubule.

of carbonic acid in tubular cells. It appears to be important only in the distal reabsorption of bicarbonate. The partial pressure of carbon dioxide in blood (pCO_2) affects the magnitude of bicarbonate reabsorption, an elevated pCO_2 providing more bicarbonate and hydrogen ions in the tubular cell.

Although the proximal tubule accounts for the greater volume of bicarbonate reabsorption, final reabsorption of filtered bicarbonate is accomplished in the collecting duct. Here urine can be made free of bicarbonate. An acid urine (lower than pH 6.0) requires both complete reabsorption of bicarbonate and excretion of titrable acid and ammonium ions.

Renal excretory mechanisms for *hydrogen ion* help the body deal with the excess of acid in the usual human diet. In discussing hydrogen ion transport a distinction must be made between the final result accomplished, net excretion or net retention, and the separate chemical steps leading to this result. Only net excretion can be determined. This depends on the excretion of bicarbonate and of ammonium, as well as of hydrogen ion. Net excretion is determined by the algebraic sum of these 3 ions in urine. No tubular reabsorption of hydrogen ion occurs, but hydrogen ion is secreted into the tubules, where it combines with phosphate (or other buffer) or ammonia. This process takes place almost entirely in the distal nephron and depends on the availability of hydrogen ions from the cells, as well as upon ammonia and buffer anions in urine.

The availability of hydrogen ions in cells depends on the pCO_2 as well as on the free hydrogen ion concentration. Ammonia originates within tubular cells, whereas phosphate anions are supplied from filtered plasma. As mentioned previously, hydrogen secretion is probably by ion exchange, which depends upon reabsorption of sodium. Potassium may be substituted for hydrogen. Consequently, potassium stores influence the availability of hydrogen ion for secretion. Under conditions favoring maximal acidification urinary pH cannot be reduced below 4, a limit probably representing the maximal hydrogen ion gradient attainable between tubular cells and urine.

Phosphorus in plasma exists as univalent and bivalent *phosphate* anions. Because these chemical forms cannot be measured accurately, measurements of total inorganic phosphorus are used to estimate phosphates in plasma. This custom should not obscure the fact that phosphate anions are the chemical forms present in vivo. A small fraction of plasma phosphate may be bound to proteins and not filterable through the glomeruli. Filtered phosphate is actively reabsorbed in the proximal tubules. Phosphate reabsorption exhibits a tubular maximum which is close to the normal load of filtered phosphate. In consequence, a rise in plasma phosphate may deliver to the proximal tubules more phosphate than they can reabsorb, whereas a reduction in plasma phosphate will lead to complete reabsorption of filtered phosphate. In this manner the level of plasma phosphate regulates renal phosphate excretion.

Renal excretion of phosphate is also influenced by acid-base equilibrium, parathormone, osseous metabolism and vitamin D. Acute acidosis causes both release of phosphate from tissues into plasma and reduced tubular reabsorption of phosphate; these effects provide more urinary phosphate buffer for the excretion of hydrogen ions. Parathormone inhibits tubular reabsorption of phosphate, causing phosphaturia. For a person in phosphorus balance, the renal excretion of phosphorus equals the absorption from the gut. Excretion varies, then, according to intestinal absorption.

Urinary *ammonium* arises from ammonia synthesized by proximal and distal tubular cells. Synthesis and excretion are determined primarily by acid-base equilibrium. Ammonia produced within tubular cells appears to diffuse passively into tubular fluid, where it combines with secreted hydrogen ion to form ammonium. The latter ion does not diffuse freely across cell membranes and is trapped within tubular fluid and excreted along with available anions (chloride). Under physiologic conditions about two thirds of renal excretion of hydrogen ion is by combination with ammonia. Renal ammonium excretion rises severalfold in persistent acidosis.

Sulfate concentration in plasma is normally 2 to 3 mEq. per liter. It is filtered freely at the glomeruli and actively reabsorbed by the tubules. Maximal rate of tubular reabsorption is low, so that any appreciable rise in filtered sulfate leads to quantitative sulfaturia. Plasma sulfate level rises in renal failure.

Unlike the univalent cations of plasma, bivalent *calcium* is partially bound to plasma proteins. Only the fraction not bound is filterable through the glomeruli. In normal plasma about 50 per cent of the calcium is filterable. Calcium is actively reabsorbed throughout the length of the nephrons. Under many conditions reabsorption and excretion of calcium parallel those of sodium.

Magnesium resembles calcium in being bivalent and partly bound to plasma proteins. Normally about 60 per cent of plasma magnesium is not filterable. Filtered magnesium is reabsorbed by the distal tubules. The questions of proximal reabsorption and tubular secretion have not been settled. Magnesium excretion parallels calcium excretion under many circumstances. A circadian rhythm of urinary calcium and magnesium excretion has been shown in normal subjects.

Urea is the chief end-product of nitrogen metabolism. It diffuses freely into plasma and is completely filtered in the glomerulus. Variable degrees of tubular reabsorption occur in both proximal and distal nephrons, depending upon reabsorption of water at these sites. In the proximal tubule probably a third of filtered urea is reabsorbed passively under physiologic conditions. Distally, reabsorption of urea appears to accompany reabsorption of water and is therefore affected by changes in tubular permeability with antidiuretic hormone activity. Medullary recirculation of reabsorbed urea apparently occurs in antidiuresis and increases the maximal osmolality attainable in urine by further raising the medullary osmolality; this effect is augmented during ingestion of a high protein diet.

Creatinine is a low-molecular-weight endproduct of nitrogen metabolism. It is freely filtered at the glomerulus and may also undergo tubular secretion in the proximal tubule at higher plasma levels. Daily excretion in urine correlates well with the body muscle mass and, unlike urinary urea, is unaffected by changes in dietary protein. In normal man, endogenous creatinine clearance approximates the clearance of inulin. In renal disease, however, the ratio of creatinine to inulin clearance varies from 1 to 4.

Uric acid is an end-product of purine metabolism. In man it is completely filterable from plasma and is actively reabsorbed. The tubular maximum for reabsorption is above the values attainable under natural conditions, but urate is present in urine because of wide differences in the completeness of reabsorption among different nephrons. A small amount of tubular secretion may occur in man. Uricosuric agents act by interfering with the reabsorptive process.

Glucose is filtered and actively reabsorbed in the proximal tubules. The renal threshold for glucose reabsorption normally lies above 150 mg. per 100 ml. of plasma. Above this threshold, glucose begins to appear in urine. At higher plasma levels tubular reabsorption continues to rise, however, until glucose TM is reached, normally between 300 and 400 mg. per minute per 1.73 square meters. Despite this wide range of normal, glucose TM is remarkably constant for each person.

The small amounts of amino acids circulating in plasma (only 2.5 to 3.5 mM. per liter) are freely filtered; 98 per cent of the amount filtered is actively reabsorbed in the proximal tubule.

Numerous other *organic substances,* both endogenous and exogenous, are transported by the renal tubules during renal excretion. Small amounts of citrate, lactate, malate, acetoacetate and β-OH butyrate present in plasma are filtered and then reabsorbed. Since the tubular maxima for reabsorption of acetoacetate and butyrate are low, they appear in urine when high levels occur in plasma, as in diabetic ketoaciduria.

Several exogenous organic substances, such as phenolsulphonphthalein, penicillin, salicylate and weak organic bases, are both filtered and secreted by the tubules, sometimes competitively. In addition, salicylate can be passively reabsorbed in the distal nephron from acid urine.

Radiopaque substances containing 2 or 3 iodine atoms in an organic molecule are cleared by filtration and tubular secretion.

Two unrelated *hormones* appear to originate from the kidneys. Renin is found in the cortex; it is concentrated in the area of the juxtaglomerular apparatus. This substance has not been purified, but can be detected in normal renal venous blood through its ability to release angiotensin from plasma. Angiotensin produces a rise in systemic blood pressure. The second hormone, erythropoietin, probably arises in the kidneys to a large extent. It stimulates maturation of the erythroid elements in the bone marrow.

Diuretic substances increase the rate of renal excretion of water. Some act extrarenally; only those which act on the renal tubules will be considered here. Useful agents are limited to those which increase renal excretion of sodium, because without loss of sodium too little water can be lost to benefit the patient. Each diuretic has a characteristic action upon the tubules which ultimately limits its efficacy, and combinations of diuretics frequently are effective, when one agent is not. To prescribe effectively, therefore, familiarity with the mode of action of each diuretic is necessary.

Organic mercurial diuretics partially block reabsorption of sodium and chloride, which results in a concomitant loss of water. Potassium loss may occur, but is not excessive. Hyperchloremic acidemia potentiates the diuretic effect of mercurials, for reasons unknown. These agents are ineffective during hypochloremia. Recent micropuncture studies indicate that organic mercurial diuretics, previously thought to act on the proximal tubule, have their locus of action in the distal nephron.

Osmotic diuretics are chemically inert substances which exert their effect solely by osmotic force. This osmotic force results from their restriction to one side of a semipermeable membrane (within the renal tubular lumen). To exert a significant effect they must be of low molecular weight and be present in high concentration; they are freely filtered, but not reabsorbed. Examples are mannitol and urea. Because they are held in the tubular lumen they limit water absorption and carry water with sodium and anions into the urine. Under certain unnatural conditions sodium (in addisonian crisis) or glucose (in hyperglycemia) may act as osmotic diuretics.

Carbonic anhydrase inhibitors may be useful diuretics. In appropriate dosage an increased volume of alkaline urine results, which may lead to metabolic acidemia. Their effectiveness is assumed but not proved to be due to inhibition of intratubular carbonic anhydrase, which reduces coupled sodium-hydrogen ion exchange. This would favor either no reabsorption of sodium or exchange of sodium for potassium; either result would lead to a loss of sodium or potassium bicarbonate in urine.

The potent benzothiadiazides inhibit tubular reabsorption of sodium and chloride independent of the acid-base equilibrium of blood. With optimal doses a moderate kaliuresis usually occurs, and hypokalemia may occur with prolonged usage. Ethacrynic acid is a newer diuretic similar in action to the benzothiadiazides, but more potent in doses clinically used. Its diuretic effect occurs within a few hours after oral administration; in massive diuresis a secondary metabolic alkalosis may occur. Furosemide has recently been shown to be as potent as ethacrynic acid, but with a shorter duration of action. Loss of potassium in urine occurs, but not to the extent produced by the thiazide drugs. The mechanisms of diuretic action of furosemide, ethacrynic acid and benzothiadiazides are currently thought to be the inhibition of sodium transport from the ascending limb of Henle. All three may cause retention of uric acid, apparently by competing with uric acid secretion in the proximal tubule.

RENAL FUNCTION IN INFANCY

In the absence of an absolute standard of reference or any single appropriate physiologic basis of reference for the expression of renal function at different ages, measurements of function are most often referred to the unit 1.73 M^2, which represents the body surface of a standard adult. Choice of such a unit of reference permits one to compare directly the values for renal functions at different ages. Such relative values will vary, of course, with the unit of reference chosen, whether it is body surface area, body weight, renal weight or some other unit.

Glomerular filtration rate adjusted for body surface area is low in infancy, reaching the adult norm of 120 ml. per minute per 1.73 $M^2 \pm 20$ in early childhood. At birth the corrected clearance of inulin varies between 10 and 50 per cent of the norm for older children. Infants of low birth weight have filtration rates comparable to normal term infants. The huge individual variability, which approaches 50 per cent of the filtration rate, produces a wide range of values in normal infants. This variability is not due to differences in body size or age, and diminishes with maturity. Though only a few longitudinal studies have been reported, a progressive rise in filtration rate occurs from birth to the age of 6 to 18 months, when the childhood norm is attained. The greatest increment in the filtration rate takes place in the first month of life. During this period an increase of 100 to 200 per cent in filtration rate is common.

PAH clearance at low plasma levels is low in relation to body surface in infancy and reaches the childhood and adult norm at about 2 years of age. This indicates a relatively low effective renal perfusion during infancy. The variation in persons of the same age is about 300 per cent after birth and lessens with age. Filtration fraction, $\frac{C_{inulin}}{C_{PAH}}$, in the first few months of life appears to be similar to values in older subjects when both clearances are adjusted to body surface area.

Infants can not concentrate urine as well as older subjects after dehydration. Many factors affect maximal urine osmolality. Edelman and co-workers have shown that the lower excretion of urea by infants accounts for some of the lower "maximal" urine osmolalities reported in infants. Normal infants can concentrate urine to about $2\frac{1}{2}$ times plasma osmolality, or 750 mOsm. per liter, after a 24-hour thirst and fast. Urine osmolalities exceeding 1000 mOsm. per liter have been attained in young infants after 5 days of normal solute and reduced water intake. By the age of 6 months the infant can concentrate urine as well as the adult. The infant's response to antidiuretic hormone appears equal to that of older subjects.

Infants excrete less acid in the first week of life than children or adults; the difference may be due solely to differences in nitrogen metabolism and previous intake of protein. By 1 week of age infants excrete as much titratable acid and ammonium per volume of glomerular filtrate as do adults.

Edelman and co-workers have reported that plasma values for renal bicarbonate threshold in infants (20 to 23 mEq. per liter) are lower than those in normal adults (26 to 28 mEq. per liter). This may explain why the normal level of plasma bicarbonate is significantly lower in infants than in older subjects.

DIAGNOSTIC TESTS FOR RENAL DISEASE

Examination of the Urine. *Urinalysis* is the single most reliable test for the evaluation of renal disease. A variety of simple and accurate tests using dip sticks are available. It is important to differentiate those tests specific for glucose from those which measure reducing substances in general.

When the specimen is not to be examined soon after being voided, it must be refrigerated or a chemical preservative must be added if reliable information is to be obtained. No urinalysis is complete without a careful microscopic examination. Formed elements disintegrate rapidly in dilute or alkaline urine. Centrifugation of 5 to 10 ml. of urine for 3 to 5 minutes in a conical tube concentrates the formed elements. The sediment so obtained normally has fewer than 3 erythrocytes, 5 leukocytes and 1 cast per high-power microscopic field (about 430×). The normal range varies

slightly with the method of preparation and the size of the microscopic field. In addition to cells, one may see unexpected crystals, microorganisms or oval fat bodies of diagnostic importance. An unusual color of urine may have significance. Urine which turns blue on standing suggests indicanuria, associated with nephrocalcinosis. Red urine may be due to hemoglobin and its derivatives, urates, anthocyanins (from ingestion of beets) or other benign ingested pigments.

Quantitative estimation of formed elements, of specific gravity and of protein can be obtained by the Addis count. Fluids are withheld after lunch, and the patient receives a dry supper. He voids completely about 8 p.m. All urine is collected for the next 12 hours. This specimen normally has a specific gravity greater than 1.021, a pH less than 6.0, and a protein content below 50 mg. Leukocytes, erythrocytes and casts are counted in a hemocytometer. There are normally less than 500,000 leukocytes, epithelial cells and erythrocytes and less than 10^4 casts per ml. Unless stained, leukocytes may not be distinguishable from epithelial cells. Cells may originate anywhere within the genitourinary tract; except in casts, which derive only from the renal tubules.

Diurnal variations are common in proteinuria; its severity is best determined in a 24-hour collection; the normal 24-hour protein excretion is below 150 mg. in adults.

Bacteriologic culture of urine requires careful preparative cleansing of the genital area and collection in a sterile container. Since the urethra frequently contains organisms of no apparent significance, a midstream collection is the most reliable. Immediate inoculation of media should be done, or refrigeration provided. Reliable interpretation requires that bacteriuria be quantitated for each organism present. Except in established or recurrent infection, counts below 1000 colonies per ml. are considered harmless, and those between 1000 and 100,000 per ml. equivocal. Counts above 100,000 per ml. indicate pathologic bacteriuria in urine collected under appropriate conditions. Catheterization for culture should be resorted to only after equivocal results have been obtained on 2 or more "clean catch" specimens. Sterile technique is essential for reliable results and to minimize the hazard of introducing bacteria into the urinary tract.

Suprapubic puncture of the bladder is a safe and reliable technique for obtaining urine cultures in experienced hands. This method requires that the patient have a distended, palpable bladder. The urethra is compressed manually (by rectal finger in the female), and the suprapubic area sterilized with iodine and alcohol. A perpendicular midline puncture is made just above the symphysis. Bacterial counts in urine obtained by this technique are lower than those in "clean catch" specimens. The recovery of gram-negative organisms indicates significant bacteriuria, whereas gram-positive bacteria in small numbers may represent failure of aseptic technique. The technique is especially valuable in neonates, owing to the difficulty in obtaining reliable voided specimens. In neonates, however, the bladder may be more difficult to distend by hydration, because of frequent voiding.

Renal concentrating ability can be determined most reliably by determining maximal urinary osmolality after a 12- to 24-hour thirst and fast. Normal values after early infancy are above 800 mOsm. per liter (specific gravity 1.024) and depend on the duration of dehydration and on the dietary intake of protein and sodium; high intakes of either raise the osmolal value. Specific gravity may be distorted by severe proteinuria or glycosuria. One gram per cent of protein raises the urine specific gravity about 0.003; one gram per cent of glucose raises it about 0.004. Determination of urine concentration by refractometry is simple and requires only a drop of urine. It is accurate in the absence of moderate proteinuria or glycosuria.

The measurement of excretion of phenolsulfonphthalein provides a simple index of proximal tubular function; more accurate values are obtained by measuring the excretion of para-aminohippurate. These tests are less reliable in the azotemic patient.

Renal acidification may be measured by determining the net hydrogen ion excretion after administration of an acidifying salt. Ammonium chloride, in an oral dose of 120 to 160 mEq. per 1.73 square meters of body surface area, is given for 3 to 5 days in divided doses. A mild fall in plasma carbon dioxide content often occurs by the third day, and after 3 to 5 days there is normally a twofold to threefold increase in total urinary acid excretion. The latter is measured as the algebraic sum of titratable acid (titrated to the patient's plasma pH) and ammonium excretion, minus bicarbonate. Most of the rise in hydrogen ion excretion results from increased urinary excretion of ammonium. Neonates of low weight excrete less ammonium and total hydrogen ion in relation to body surface than do normal neonates. At all ages individual variability is large.

Measurement of *residual urine* by catheterization of the bladder after complete voluntary voiding demonstrates the adequacy of vesical evacuation. Aseptic technique must be observed. If ureteral reflux is suspected, "triple voiding" should precede the catheterization. Three successive attempts to void over a 5-minute period will ensure emptying of the ureters prior to catheterization. Children should have less than 15 ml. of urine after voiding.

Examination of Blood. The serum levels of nonprotein nitrogenous catabolites (serum urea nitrogen [SUN] and total nonprotein nitrogen [NPN]) are useful indices of renal function. The levels are influenced by protein metabolism and the state of hydration as well as by renal function. Serum creatinine level is less affected by daily fluctuations in protein metabolism, but is more difficult to determine accurately. Severe renal failure causes a rise in the serum level of nonprotein nitrogenous catabolites (urea, creatinine, uric acid and NPN), as well as of phosphorus and potassium. Metabolic acidemia occurs and is reflected in a reduced carbon dioxide content (or bicarbonate concentration) of serum. The concentration of undetermined anions rises, as estimated from the difference between the serum sodium concentration and the sum of the concentrations of chloride and bicarbonate. Normally this value is between 5 and 18 mEq. per liter. In renal failure undetermined anions are made up principally of phosphate and sulfate. Blood pH tends to fall, depending partly on the degree of respiratory compensation.

Tubular dysfunction may produce derangements of serum electrolytes in patients without glomerular failure or azotemia. An example of this is the hypokalemia of renal potassium wasting. Serum protein fractions may show characteristic alterations in various renal diseases. The erythrocyte sedimentation rate often gives an indication of the activity of a disease process, as in acute glomerulonephritis and in the nephrotic syndrome.

Clearance Studies. Reasonably accurate information on renal filtration requires clearance studies. Techniques for determination of clearances of endogenous urea and creatinine do not require the infusion of a test substance. A timed collection of urine and a blood sample are needed. Urine flow must be at least 2 ml. per minute for reliable data (1.0 ml. per minute may be sufficient under 2 years of age). A blood sample is taken at the midpoint of urine collection. Clearance of creatinine can be determined from 24-hour collections in outpatients. Because the serum creatinine concentration is relatively constant, the serum specimen may be taken just before, during or after the urine collection. The clearance of urea ranges from 48 to 75 ml. per minute per 1.73 square meters. The clearance of endogenous creatinine approximates inulin clearance (130 ± 20 ml. per minute per 1.73 square meters), except in azotemia, in which creatinine-inulin clearances vary from 1.0 to 4.0. The convenience of these methods and their reproducibility make them useful for serial measurements.

Radiography. Although radiographic methods give no precise quantitative estimate of renal function, they are of great value in revealing structural abnormalities of the kidneys and in following the course of certain renal diseases. *Intravenous urography* outlines the position, size and shape of the kidneys, in addition to demonstrating promptness of excretion of opaque media. Urography may be made satisfactory in the presence of the azotemia of mild or moderate renal failure by varying the amount of dye injected or the speed and mode of injection. If there is urinary tract obstruction, intravenous urography may fail to demonstrate one or both kidneys or ureters, and *retrograde pyelography* may be required. Functioning renal tissue can be demonstrated by a *renal scan* after injection of a radioactively tagged substance which is excreted by the tubules, such as isotopic mercury or technetium. *Renal angiography* demonstrates the main renal vascular branches arising from the aorta or returning to the vena cava.

Radiologic study of the lower urinary tract should be performed (1) if the clinical picture suggests lower urinary tract disease, (2) in recurrent urinary tract infection, and (3) whenever there is unexplained evidence of urinary tract disease. The value of *cystography* is enhanced when radiography is carried out during voiding, when visualization of any ureteral reflux and of urethral caliber may be achieved. Only rapid-sequence films permit such study. Cinefluoroscopy entails more radiation exposure, but may be required to demonstrate dysfunction in a few patients. An estimate of adequate vesical evacuation can be obtained by instillation into the bladder of 5 to 10 ml. of Lipiodol, which floats on urine and normally is eliminated promptly. The demonstration of residual Lipiodol in a film of the bladder 48 hours after instillation indicates urinary retention.

Renal Biopsy. Renal biopsy is a valuable tool in the evaluation and management of selected renal patients. Percutaneous puncture is usually done after intravenous urography has established the presence and position of both kidneys. Coagulation studies to assure adequate hemostasis should also be done prior to the biopsy. Severe hypertension, a bleeding diathesis, solitary kidney, tumor, infection or serious illness of the patient contraindicate percutaneous renal biopsy. It is most often needed in patients whose renal disease is atypical or chronic. In these situations information obtained by biopsy may help to indicate the future course of the disease and influence decisions regarding drug therapy.

W. JOSEPH RAHILL

REFERENCES

General

Campbell, M. F.: *Urology.* 2nd ed. Philadelphia, W. B. Saunders Company, 1963.

Heptinstall, R. H.: *Pathology of the Kidney.* Boston, Little, Brown and Co., 1966.

Smith, H. W.: *The Kidney.* New York, Oxford University Press, 1951.

Strauss, M. B., and Welt, L. G.: *Diseases of the Kidney.* Boston, Little, Brown and Co., 1963.

Third International Congress of Nephrology, Washington, 1966. New York, S. Karger, 1967, Vol. 2.

Vernier, R. L., and Birch-Andersen, A.: Studies of the Human Fetal Kidney. 1. Development of the Glomerulus. *J. Pediat.,* 60:754, 1962.

Renal Physiology

Barnett, H. L., Hare, K., McNamara, H., and Hare, R.: Measurement of Glomerular Filtration Rate in Premature Infants. *J. Clin. Invest.,* 27:691, 1948.

Calcagno, P. L., and Rubin, M. I.: Renal Extraction of Para-Aminohippurate in Infants and Children. *J. Clin. Invest.,* 42:1632, 1963.

Edelman, C. M., Jr., Barnett, H. L., and Troupkou, V.: Renal Concentrating Mechanisms in Newborn Infants. *J. Clin. Invest.,* 39:1062, 1960.

Edelman, C. M., Jr., Soriano, J. R., Biochis, H., Gruskin, A. B., and Acosta, M. I.: Renal Bicarbonate Reabsorption and Hydrogen Ion Excretion in Normal Infants. *J. Clin. Invest.,* 46:1309, 1967.

Pitts, R. F.: *Physiology of the Kidney and Body Fluids.* Chicago, Year Book Medical Publishers, Inc., 1963.

Rubin, M. I., Bruck, E., and Rapoport, M.: Maturation of Renal Function in Childhood: Clearance Studies. *J. Clin. Invest.,* 28:1144, 1949.

Starkiewiczowa, J., Bajorek, J., and Sliwinska, H.: Renal Clearance Studies in Premature and Newborn Infants. *Pediat. Pol.,* 38:467, 1963.

Strauss, M. B., and Welt, L. G.: *Diseases of the Kidney.* Boston, Little, Brown & Company, 1963.

Renal Function Tests

Dodge, W. F., and others: Percutaneous Renal Biopsy in Children. *Pediatrics,* 30:287, 1962.

Lyttle, J. D.: The Addis Sediment Count in Normal Children. *J. Clin. Invest.,* 12:87, 1933.

Peonides, A., Levin, B., and Young, W.: The Renal Excretion of Hydrogen Ions in Infants and Children. *Arch. Dis. Childhood,* 40:33, 1965.

Pryles, C. V., Atkin, M.D., Morse, T. S., and Welch, K. J.: Comparative Bacteriologic Study of Urine Obtained from Children by Percutaneous Suprapubic Aspiration of the Bladder and by Catheter. *Pediatrics,* 24:983, 1959.

Winberg, J.: Determination of Renal Concentration Capacity in Infants and Children Without Renal Disease. *Acta Pediat.,* 48:318, 1959.

URINE AND URINATION

NORMAL URINE AND URINATION

Urine formation in the human kidney begins about the ninth week of fetal life, and urea has been detected in the amniotic fluid as early as $2\frac{1}{2}$ months of gestation. Urine has been found in the bladder of the 4-month fetus. In bladder urine of 2 of 12 fetuses aged 12 to 19 weeks Vernier and Birch-Andersen found a small amount of protein. At 7 months' gestation uric acid has been found in the kidney.

Amount. Urine is usually present in the bladder at birth, but little is secreted during the first 2 or 3 days of life. Occasionally infants have considerable edema at birth, and much of this fluid may be excreted in the urine during the next 48 hours. As soon as the child begins to take fluid, the urinary secretion is increased and is proportionately greater throughout childhood than in adult life. The amount is variable and influenced by many factors, such as the amount of liquid ingested, the environmental temperature and the states of the digestive and nervous systems. Oliguria or polyuria may be a reflection of altered

TABLE 15-1. AVERAGE DAILY EXCRETION
OF URINE

AGE	MILLIMETERS
First and second days	30-60
Third to tenth day......................	100-300
Tenth day to 2 months................	250-450
2 months to 1 year	400-500
1-3 years.................................	500-600
3-5 years.................................	600-700
5-8 years.................................	650-1000
8-14 years	800-1400

renal function. In prolonged anuria an obstructive lesion should be suspected.

Frequency of Micturition. The frequency varies from 2 to 6 times in the first and second days of life. Commonly the infant does not void until more than 12 hours after birth, and may not void until the second or even the third day of life. Subsequently excretion is frequent during infancy, varying from 5 to 30 or 40 times in 24 hours; the urine is often retained for several hours during sleep. After control of the bladder has been attained the frequency of urination varies from 6 to 8 times in 24 hours.

Physical and Chemical Characteristics of Urine. The specific gravity during the first few days of life is relatively high (1.012), but after the ingestion of milk has begun it falls rapidly to 1.002 to 1.006. The infant's kidneys, however, are capable of concentrating during restriction of water; in the premature infant this capacity is limited. The full-term infant attains the ability of the adult to concentrate urine by about 3 months of age. The loss of concentrating capacity is evidence of renal disturbance. When solid food is added to the diet, the specific gravity of the urine gradually increases.

The urine is at first highly colored and slightly turbid, owing to its concentration and to the presence of urates and mucus. Later, even during childhood, it is generally paler yellow than in adult life. Sometimes in infancy, particularly in the newborn, it stains the diaper faintly red through the decomposition of urates. The reaction of the

TABLE 15-2. ELEVATION OF SPECIFIC GRAVITY
OF URINE

QUANTITIES OF SUBSTANCES NEEDED TO ELEVATE SPECIFIC
GRAVITY OF URINE 0.001 AT 15° C.

Urea.................................	3.595 gm./liter
Glucose............................	2.700 gm./liter
Sodium phosphate	3.792 gm./liter
Disodium phosphate	0.979 gm./liter
Sodium chloride	1.473 gm./liter
Sodium sulfate....................	1.405 gm./liter
Albumin............................	3.892 gm./liter

From Albarran, in A. M. Fishberg: *Hypertension and Nephritis.*
4th ed. Philadelphia, Lea & Febiger.

initial urine of the newborn is decidedly acid, but after a few days approaches neutrality; that of the morning urine is less acid than that of the afternoon. The pH varies between 5 and 7. Odor is almost absent in freshly voided urine in infancy and even in childhood unless the urine is highly colored. The ammoniacal odor often noted in the nursery is due to delay in changing diapers, the urine decomposing after it has been passed.

There is little *urea* in the urine at birth. The proportion is increased by the third day, but remains relatively low during infancy and varies with the protein content of the diet. Phosphates, chlorides and sulfates are present. The concentrations of these are increased when a mixed diet is started, but are less than in adults. McCance showed that infants after the first few days of life reabsorb a greater percentage of their filtered sodium and chloride than do adults. The amount of urea is greater in childhood than in adult life on the basis of body weight, but forms a smaller percentage of the total nitrogen excreted than in adults. Approximately 80 per cent of the urinary nitrogen is excreted as urea, 5 to 15 per cent as ammonia, and the rest as uric acid, creatine and creatinine. (Approximately 2 per cent of the total urinary nitrogen is excreted as alpha amino nitrogen, and approximately 2 per cent of the milliequivalents of organic acids in the urine consist of amino acids.) The percentage of uric acid is especially high in the neonatal period, after which it falls, but remains higher in childhood than in adult life. The relation of uric acid to urea is 1:14 in the newborn and about 1:70 in the adult.

About 7 to 10 mg. of *creatinine* per kg. are excreted daily by the newborn, about 20 mg. at 2 years of age, and 30 to 40 mg. in adult life.

Creatine is excreted in variable and large amounts by infants and to a less degree by children up to puberty; in the male its excretion ceases a few years before this time. For some unexplained reason premature infants excrete almost no creatine. Creatinuria has an important relation to

TABLE 15-3. CHEMICAL COMPOSITION OF URINE

SUBSTANCE	24-HOUR EXCRETION RATES
Urea..........................	Approximately 300 mg./gm. protein in diet
Amino acids................	1-5 mg./kg.
Ammonia	1-3 mEq./kg.
Titratable acid	1-2 mEq./kg.
Calcium	1-5 mg./kg.
Phosphorus................	15-20 mg./kg.
Citrate.....................	About 6-12 mg./kg.
Bicarbonate	0 when the pH is below 6.8
Sodium*	
Chloride*	
Potassium*	
Na/K ratio approximately 2.0	

From P. Royer, R. Habib and H. Mathieu: *Problèmes actuels
de néphrologie infantile.* Paris, Editions Médicales Flammarion.
*Varies considerably, depending on the diet.

thyroid activity, being low in the cretin and rising to normal levels with thyroid administration.

Indican is not usually found in the urine of healthy breast-fed infants, but traces are generally present in those fed artificially. Older children on mixed diets excrete indican to the same extent as do adults. Excessive excretion of indican and other indole derivatives has been reported in some metabolic disorders. It is thought to result from excessive bacterial degradation of tryptophan. This in turn leads to excessive indole production and to indicanuria, which on oxidation to indigo blue causes a peculiar bluish discoloration of the diaper which has been given the term "the blue diaper syndrome."

Protein in small amounts may often be found in the urine of healthy newborn infants during the first 10 days of life. Some of the apparently positive test results, however, may result from the excretion of mucin and urates. Throughout childhood, with very sensitive tests, small amounts can usually be discovered (average, 35 mg. per 12 hours).

Sugar detectable by ordinary clinical methods is frequently found in the urine of the newborn and in early infancy, when relatively large amounts of sugar have been ingested. With tests more sensitive than the usual copper reduction one, both fermentable and unfermentable carbohydrates may be discovered in the urine of children (between 0.3 and 0.9 gm. per 24 hours).

Casts, red blood cells and white cells are present in small numbers in normal urine (see Addis count, p. 1103).

Disorders of Urinary Excretion

Decreased urinary output may result from decreased formation of urine or retention of it in the bladder.

Urine may be secreted in small amount (*oliguria*) or, temporarily, not at all (*anuria*). This situation may be normal in the first 24 hours of life. Pathologic causes in the newborn infant include renal agenesis, anomalies such as polycystic formations and obstructions resulting in hydronephrosis, acquired lesions such as thrombosis of the renal vein or artery and renal infarction and, most often, dehydration. After the neonatal period any of these factors may be causative, anhydremia, as in diarrheal disease, being the most frequent one. Suppression of urine is characteristic of acute glomerulonephritis, of poisonings by various metals and drugs and of conditions productive of shock and tubular necrosis. Obstruction of the renal tubules by crystallization of sulfonamide drugs is an example of mechanical blockage.

When there is *retention of urine*, formation of urine is not necessarily impaired, but there is failure of the bladder to expel it. In the newborn this may be due to phimosis, atresia of the labia or urethral obstruction by abnormal folds of mucous membrane, uric acid crystals or a calculus. Balanoposthitis, vulvovaginitis, or inflammation of the meatus may cause retention, owing to the pain (*dysuria*) which urination produces. Disturbances in the innervation of the bladder and various reflex or direct inhibitions are factors, as in myelomeningocele, meningitis, myelitis, rectal irritation, spasm of the vesical sphincter, hysteria, mental depression, and the debility associated with severe febrile diseases.

Polyuria is a large increase in the amount of urine. It occurs in a variety of conditions, including diabetes mellitus, diabetes insipidus, chronic renal disease and the recovery phase of so-called lower nephron nephrosis (tubular necrosis). It also occurs when a large amount of fluid is imbibed and during the reduction of edema. Nervous excitement and chilling of the body surface may temporarily increase urinary secretion.

Frequent urination (pollakiuria) is normal in the first 2 years of life. It also occurs with polyuria, cystitis and nervous excitement and from reflex stimulation by renal calculi. A highly concentrated acid urine causes it by irritation of the urethra.

Incontinence depends upon a variety of causes. It is observed with phimosis, cystitis, impaction of a calculus in the urethra, paralytic conditions of the bladder resulting from disease of the brain or spinal cord, including spina bifida, and in profound exhaustion or coma. The bladder becomes overdistended until there is persistent overflow, or sometimes an intermittent expulsion of urine without the patient's intent. Malformations such as exstrophy of the bladder, abnormal openings of the ureters into the vagina, persistent urachus and absence of the vesical sphincter allow the urine to flow constantly. With partial obstruction, as from a malformation in the posterior urethra, the overdistended bladder often produces a constant dribble of urine. Incontinence is common among the severely mentally retarded.

Enuresis (see also p. 87) is "involuntary discharge of urine," but in clinical practice the problem in children is largely limited to involuntarily wetting the bed at night. Bladder control at night is usually gained by 3 years of age; however, many children do not develop control until they are 5, 6 or 7 years of age. An occasional wetting of the bed may be seen in 10 to 20 per cent of children even as late as 9 or 10 years of age. The incidence tends to be higher in the institutionalized and children in the lower socioeconomic groups. In most instances, enuresis is a continuation of bed wetting from birth. It may commence, however, after a period in which bladder control had been gained.

It is now generally believed that enuresis is in most children related to psychologic disturbances.

In children who have complete control of their bladder during the day and irregularly wet the bed at night, a defect of the sphincter mechanism would seem unlikely. Abnormalities of the sphincter mechanism are usually associated with other localized neurologic defects, such as loss of sensation over the perineal area and thighs, deficient anal sphincter tone or alteration in neuromuscular control of the legs. A gross anomaly of the lower part of the spine may or may not be associated with a neurologic defect.

Owing to the variability in age at which bladder control is finally established, it is difficult to state when enuresis requires urologic study. If there are symptoms referable to the urinary tract, episodes of unexplained fever or neurologic findings and spine defects as described above, then certainly the urine and voiding function must be evaluated. At any rate, if bed wetting continues after 3 or 4 years or beyond the period when bladder control is usually obtained within a family pattern, careful study should be made of renal concentrating capacity, with examination for abnormalities of composition and for significant bacteriuria. Observation of the urinary stream is helpful in determining excretory function of the bladder; diminished force of the stream, constant dribbling, the need for several efforts to empty the bladder completely or an enlarged bladder bespeak the need for urologic investigation.

Alterations in Composition of Urine

PROTEINURIA

PHYSIOLOGIC OR BENIGN PROTEINURIA

Delicate tests will demonstrate protein in the urine of most persons; the average normal excretion in 12 hours is between 30 and 50 mg. Proteinuria of greater degree may occur transiently during the neonatal period, and subsequently is common during acute infections, states of dehydration, diarrheal diseases, cardiac failure, and, in older children, after violent exercise, overeating and cold bathing.

ORTHOSTATIC (POSTURAL) PROTEINURIA

In this entity, protein appears in the urine after the child has been standing and disappears in the recumbent position, provided the urine secreted during the period of standing has cleared the urinary tract. The pattern of composition is similar to that of the serum proteins. This condition should be suspected when proteinuria is found irregularly in a series of urinalyses. Its demonstration may require putting the patient in an exaggerated lordotic posture. The normal person increases his proteinuria in the erect position, but to a much less degree. Most of the protein excreted in a 24-hour period by the normal person may occur during the time spent in an upright posture.

Vigorous exercise in the normal person may also result in hematuria, hemoglobinuria, proteinuria and even red cell casts, which may persist for a day or two after strenuous exercise, such as competitive sports in adolescence.

Exaggeration of proteinuria may also occur in the upright position in patients with active renal disease; in the recovery phase of acute renal disease, proteinuria may be elicited only as postural proteinuria. It is necessary, therefore, in postural proteinuria to exclude nephritis and pyelonephritis through careful urinalysis. Addis counts may be helpful in such evaluation.

The cause is by no means clear. It has been shown that the erect posture produces renal vasoconstriction; this is thought to be the critical factor by some investigators. Mechanical interference with renal circulation in the erect position is also widely believed to be a factor; but faulty posture is not present in many of these patients, nor do all children with lumbar lordosis exhibit proteinuria. In a small group of children with orthostatic proteinuria and normal renal biopsies, proteinuria was found to disappear with the administration of adrenal corticosteroids, and to return when the steroids were withdrawn. Whatever the basis for the disorder, steroid therapy appears to decrease the glomerular leak of protein in a manner similar to that in which it alters protein leakage in nephrosis.

Orthostatic proteinuria may be found in the preschool child; its frequency increases with age, reaching a peak incidence at 13 to 15 years of age. It occurs with equal frequency in males and females.

The child's health is generally good. He is often lordotic, and tends to be tall and asthenic. There may be periods when the proteinuria disappears for days or months. There is no evidence that the protein stores of the body are depleted. In most patients the disorder seems to disappear after adolescence, but may persist into adult life.

The quantity of protein in the urine varies from a trace (less than 150 mg.) to 3 to 4 gm. a day. Electrophoretic studies show a pattern similar to that of normal serum proteins. In some cases, casts may also be found. Proteinuria may be demonstrated only when the patient has been in the hyperlordotic position for 15 to 20 minutes.

The benign nature of orthostatic proteinuria is now being questioned through follow-up studies; some adults who had such a diagnosis in childhood have become constantly proteinuric, some with microscopic hematuria and cylindruria suggesting latent glomerular nephritis. In addition, renal biopsy in apparently healthy young men with orthostatic proteinuria has shown varying degrees of glomerular alterations, and in some the lesions have resembled those of membranous nephritis.

Treatment. There is no specific treatment. Protein intake should not be restricted. Attention should be paid to improvement of muscle tone and correction of any faulty posture, and the child should be allowed a normally active life.

FEBRILE PROTEINURIA

Proteinuria occurs commonly in association with high, continued fever from any cause, but disappears on cessation of the fever. The urine is highly colored and concentrated, and contains a small amount of protein and occasionally a few hyaline or epithelial casts.

ADVENTITIOUS PROTEINURIA

The presence in the urine of blood or purulent material in sufficient quantity will produce proteinuria. Bence-Jones type of protein is found in the urine of patients with multiple myeloma.

LITHURIA

Some uric acid is always excreted in the urine, even during complete starvation. The amount rises with increased destruction of tissue, as in leukemia, anemia, lead poisoning, and pneumonia; and with increased ingestion of purine bases. In the urine of the newborn infant precipitated urates may form a whitish or reddish deposit upon the diaper. Uric acid may be precipitated in the bladder when the urine is highly acid, and give rise to pain on micturition. In the newborn infant uric acid infarctions of the kidney may produce attacks of abdominal pain, but are otherwise without importance. When treatment is deemed necessary, water should be given freely and the urine alkalinized.

LIPURIA

Fat in the urine is frequently found in small amounts during uncontrolled diabetes mellitus, in nephrosis and in the nephrotic stage of chronic nephritis.

In *chyluria* there is sufficient fat to give the urine a milky appearance, and there may be proteinuria and red blood cells as well. Chyluria results from blockage of the lymphatic system, with leakage of chyle into the urinary system; some cases are due to filariasis.

HEMATURIA

Hematuria may produce a blood-red urine or may be so slight that it is detected only on microscopic examination. Since blood cells disintegrate in an alkaline and dilute medium, urine should be examined soon after voiding. Hematuria must be distinguished from hemoglobinuria, in which only blood pigment is present, and from the bright red anthocyaninuria sometimes seen after ingestion of beets. In the newborn, hematuria must be distinguished from the brick-red staining caused by urates.

Etiology. Large hemorrhages are most often renal in origin, whereas blood appearing only at the onset or termination of micturition is likely to be from the lower urinary tract. The 2-glass test may help determine whether hematuria occurs only during a phase of micturition or throughout the voiding. Cystoscopic examination and ureteral catheterization may be necessary to determine the source. Red cell casts indicate hematuria of renal origin.

Among the causes are acute and chronic glomerulonephritis; neoplasms, usually of the kidney; renal tuberculosis; calculus; trauma and foreign bodies; renal angioma; hemorrhagic cystitis; acute and chronic urinary tract infection; and chemical and toxic irritants, such as urotropin, turpentine, carbolic acid and some sulfonamides. Thrombosis of the renal and intrarenal veins and bilateral cortical necrosis may produce hematuria, often in association with renal failure. In the newborn uric acid infarction in the kidney can be a cause. A common cause for slight bleeding is ulceration at the meatal opening of the penis produced by irritation of ammoniacal urine; the blood is bright red and appears only in the first few drops of urine passed. There are numerous systemic causes for hematuria: sepsis, leukemia, purpura, aplastic anemia, sickle cell anemia, hemophilia and other blood dyscrasias. Scurvy is often manifested early by the presence of a few red blood cells in the urine. Vitamin K deficiency may result in hematuria. Congestive cardiac failure may be a cause. Strenuous physical exercise may cause transitory hematuria. In some cases, varicosities of the renal vessels have been found. Allergic hematuria has been described in association with certain foods. Bleeding also occurs in Schönlein-Henoch purpura (anaphylactoid purpura).

AMMONIACAL URINE

In most instances, ammonia appears in the urine only after exposure to the air. In some instances, however, the conversion of urea to ammonia occurs almost immediately on passage of the urine. In many infants the ammonia is highly irritating to the skin and often results in varying degrees of dermatitis as well as meatal ulcers.

In long-standing urinary tract infections, including cystitis, the breakdown of urea to ammonia may occur in the bladder.

ABNORMAL PIGMENTS

For porphyrinuria and tyrosinuria, see pages 461 and 422.

Red urine may be due to blood, hemoglobin, porphyrinuria or ingestion of beets (anthocyaninuria) or certain dyes. Urates produce a reddish precipitate. Bile may produce a reddish-yellow color. A green or blue urine may be caused by ingestion of methylene blue; purple by fuchsin; magenta by phenolphthalein; red with a greenish fluorescence by eosin; black by ingestion of carbolic acid, in alcaptonuria, or by the presence of melanin; bright yellow by ingestion of carotene-containing foods. Some of these colorations may follow ingestion of certain artificially colored candies.

HEMOGLOBINURIA

Hemoglobin appears in the urine when blood destruction is too rapid for the reticuloendothelial cells to dispose of it. A positive benzidine reaction in the absence of red blood cells indicates hemoglobinuria, but spectroscopic examination offers the most conclusive evidence. The experimental injection of hemoglobin in normal man or animals seems to produce no adverse effects on the kidney; however, if it is given when the animal is dehydrated, tubular necrosis may occur. With tubular necrosis there is rapidly developing renal failure. The urine is light or dark red or reddish-brown, at times almost black. Hemoglobinuria may be caused by hemolytic blood dyscrasias; severe infections; burns; parasitic diseases, such as malaria; poisoning, as with carbolic acid, potassium chlorate, oxalic acid, arsenic, phosphorus, carbon monoxide, chloroform, quinine, naphthol, aspidium, snake venom and mushrooms; G-6-PD deficiency (p. 1055); and by transfusion with incompatible blood. Sulfonamides may also cause hemoglobinuria.

Besides removal of the primary cause of the hemoglobinuria, immediate therapy consists in hydration and alkalinization. (See Treatment of Acute Renal Failure, p. 1143.)

MELANURIA

Excretion of melanogen is rare, occurring in some cases of melanotic neoplasms, and has been reported, perhaps incorrectly, in other conditions such as cachexia, pneumonia, intestinal obstruction, and after exposure to roentgen and solar rays.

REFERENCES

Herdman, R. C., Michael, A. F., and Good, R. A.: Postural Proteinuria: Response to Cortical Steroid Therapy. *Ann. Int. Med.*, 65:286, 1966.

Lecocq, F. R., McPhaul, J. J., and Robinson, R. R.: Fixed and Reproducible Orthostatic Proteinuria. *Ann. Int. Med.*, 64: 557, 1966.

Maxson, W. T.: Benign Proteinuria of Childhood and Adolescence: A Survey. *Clin. Pediat.*, 2:662, 1963.

Rennie, I.D.B., and Keen, H.: Evaluation of Clinical Methods for Detecting Proteinuria. *Lancet*, 2:489, 1967.

MALFORMATIONS OF THE URINARY TRACT

Malformations of the urinary tract are found in 5 to 12 per cent of autopsies. Many produce no symptoms or disturbances of function.

The kidneys may be absent, dysplastic, hypoplastic, hypertrophic, duplicated, ectopic, polycystic or fused (*horseshoe*). There may be absence of one or both ureters; they may be hypoplastic, duplicated, dilated or ectopic; or they may be obstructed by strictures, valves, kinks or abnormally placed blood vessels. The bladder may be absent or hypoplastic, or there may be hemiatrophy of the trigone, exstrophy, a ureterocele or diverticulum. The urachus may remain patent or persist as a cystic structure. Fistulas may extend from the bladder to the rectum or the vagina. The urethra may be absent, hypoplastic or obstructed by a stricture, or there may be a hypospadias or epispadias. The urethra may be connected with the rectum by a fistula.

Anomalies of the external genitalia are often associated with anomalies of the urinary tract, most commonly obstructive in nature. There is also an association between renal anomalies and malformations of the external ear. Absence of abdominal musculature is often associated with obstructive uropathy. Megaloureters, by permitting stasis of urine, may be responsible for partial obstruction; they may occur with or without anatomic obstruction at a lower site; infrequently they are associated with Hirschsprung's disease. Spinal cord lesions may produce the so-called neurogenic bladder and obstructive uropathy.

RENAL AGENESIS

Bilateral renal agenesis is a rare condition, more frequent in males than in females. The affected infant is usually stillborn or lives only a few hours or days. There may be other malformations, such as fusion of the legs. The diagnosis may be suggested by the peculiar facies, first described by Potter: the distance between the eyes is increased; the palpebral fissures are flattened or even mongoloid in their configuration; there are prominent epicanthi; the nose is "parrot-beaked"; the ears are large and low-set; and the chin is receding. There is a high incidence of anomalies of other organs: the bladder, urethra and gonads may be absent.

Unilateral renal agenesis is not uncommon. It occurs more frequently in males, and is usually associated with complete absence of the ureter on the affected side; rarely, a patent ureter may be present with a normal orifice. When a mass unrecognizable as normal renal tissue is found in the expected location, it is termed "renal dysgenesis." The opposite kidney is usually hypertrophied, but otherwise normal. The single kidney may be pelvic in location and its ureteral orifice open into the midline of the bladder. Malformations of the genital tract are present in over half of the patients; defects of the heart and spine occur, and esophageal atresia may coexist. Diagnosis can be established by urography or arteriography.

RENAL HYPOPLASIA AND DYSPLASIA

Renal hypoplasia may involve one or both kidneys. When the condition is bilateral, as is usually the case, renal insufficiency is present. This anomaly must be differentiated from secondary contraction of kidneys from ischemia, pyelonephritis or other fibrosing renal diseases. Enumeration of renal lobules is of more diagnostic importance than renal mass; a truly hypoplastic kidney has 5 or fewer reniculi and calices, in contrast to the normal 10 or more. Hypoplasia and dysplasia are often present in the same kidney. The severity of renal insufficiency parallels the reduction in volume of functional renal parenchyma.

Renal dysplasia is relatively common and varies considerably in the extent of maldevelopment. It may be bilateral, unilateral or segmental within a kidney, and, as noted above, the involved kidney(s) is often hypoplastic. In many instances there are cystic formations. The basic or underlying anatomic pattern consists of epithelial-lined tubular structures, surrounded by concentric bands of undifferentiated mesenchymal tissue, in which there may be strands of smooth muscle. Small plaques of cartilage may also be present. The pelvis is usually absent, and the ureter is almost always abnormal. Anomalies of other organ systems frequently coexist and are similar to those associated with renal agenesis. With unilateral lesions there may be no apparent loss of renal function. Hypertension, however, may be a manifestation; it has been eliminated by removal of a unilateral dysplastic kidney.

Extensive cystic formation, at least as recognized clinically, is usually unilateral and is generally designated as *multicystic kidney disease*. It is a more common cause of a unilateral, abnormal abdominal mass in the newborn infant than either Wilms's tumor or neuroblastoma, but is probably less common than hydronephrosis.

POLYCYSTIC DISEASE OF THE KIDNEYS

In line with what appears to be current usage, the term "polycystic disease of the kidneys" is used here to designate the 2 forms of genetically transmitted, bilateral malformations of the kidney: the so-called *infantile* and *adult forms*. These 2 forms are distinguishable on genetic and usually on morphologic and clinical bases.

In each type the kidneys are enlarged, but retain their usual shape; in the infantile type the enlargement has rarely been sufficient to interfere with delivery. Myriads of minute cysts give the cortex and medulla a spongy appearance; the cysts may be so minute, however, as to be overlooked on superficial examination of the renal surfaces. In the infantile type, however, minute, white to yellowish elevations may be visible. The reader is referred to pathologic texts for histologic descriptions; the important difference would appear to be in the relative quantity of functioning renal tissue, which is minimal in the infantile form and most often greater in the adult form. The pelves and calices are present, but distorted by the increased bulk of the surrounding tissue. (See Figure 15-4.)

The *infantile form* is transmitted on an autosomal recessive basis. Clinically, there is evidence of renal dysfunction within the neonatal period, and death occurs in infancy. There is associated involvement of the liver, usually as cystic malformations. Cysts of other organs, e.g. the lungs, spleen and pancreas, are not common, and other malformations are infrequent, in contrast to the frequency of their occurrence with renal dysplasia.

Urinary tract infection or nephritis may complicate the clinical course. Severe hypertension may be present even in the first few months of life and may be associated with cardiomegaly and signs of congestive cardiac failure. Secondary infection may occur in both the renal and the hepatic cysts.

The *adult form* is transmitted on an autosomal dominant basis. It is infrequently manifest in infancy or childhood and usually does not become clinically evident until after the fourth decade of life; about 10 per cent of affected persons do die, however, in the first decade. It is estimated that in about 20 to 30 per cent of instances there are cystic lesions in the liver and distinctly less frequently in the lungs. Cerebral aneurysms are reported as occurring in about 10 per cent of affected persons. There is suggestive but inconclusive evidence that there is an unusual frequency of other vascular malformations.

Pyelography characteristically reveals elongation of the renal pelves and major calices ("spider pelvis") with flattening of the minor calices; a variety of patterns may be produced, however, and the roentgenographic findings are not pathognomonic. (See Figure 15-4C.)

A hereditary form of hepatic fibrosis, resulting in portal hypertension, has been described in association with polycystic kidneys in older children. Renal function is usually not grossly impaired.

MEDULLARY CYSTIC DISORDERS

There appear to be one or more distinct clinicopathologic entities in which the underlying structural abnormalities include medullary cystic formations or tubular dilatations which have been designated as medullary sponge kidney, medullary sponge kidney with uremia, familial nephronophthisis, and renal tubular ectasia.

In the so-called *medullary sponge kidney* there are multiple, small cysts in the medulla which usually connect with the collecting ducts. It is the accumulation of contrast material in these dilated areas which is responsible for the characteristic spongy roentgenographic picture, which has also been described as renal tubular ectasia. The cases which have been included in this category have not had evidence of primary renal dysfunction, and the disorder is compatible with average longevity. Most instances have been identified by roentgenographic examinations initiated because of evidence of urinary tract infection or lithiasis. These seem to be the most common complications. Both kidneys are usually affected. Treatment is limited to that of the complications.

Medullary cystic disease with uremia may be a variant of the medullary sponge kidney; some clinicians, however, think that it is an entity. In contrast to the latter, as described above, there is also cortical involvement with sclerosis of glomeruli, tubular atrophy, interstitial fibrosis and cystic formation. Affected persons are usually detected in childhood or as young adults because of renal failure with azotemia. The possibility of genetic transmission has been suggested.

Familial nephronophthisis as described by Fanconi has much in common with medullary cystic disease with uremia, both pathologically and clini-

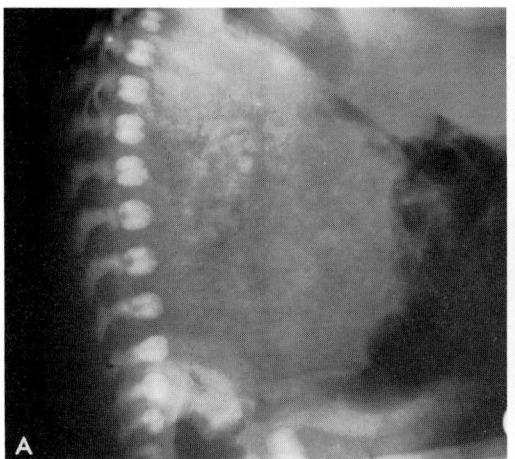
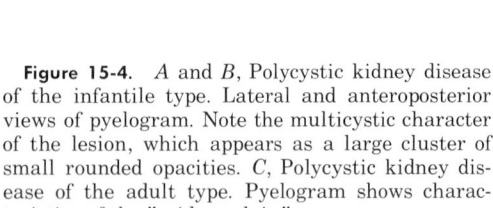
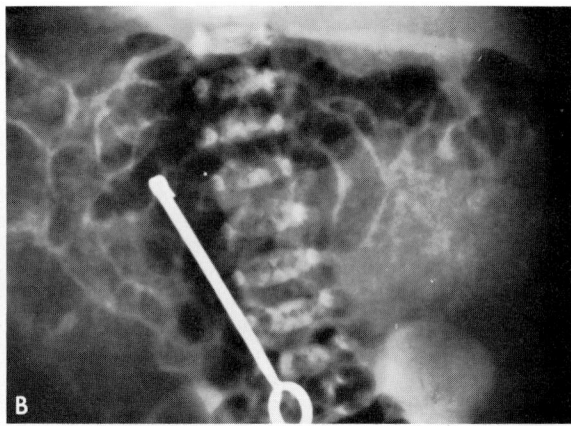
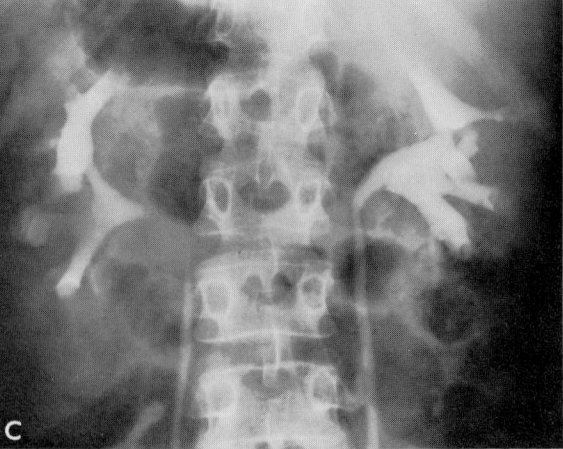

Figure 15-4. *A* and *B*, Polycystic kidney disease of the infantile type. Lateral and anteroposterior views of pyelogram. Note the multicystic character of the lesion, which appears as a large cluster of small rounded opacities. *C*, Polycystic kidney disease of the adult type. Pyelogram shows characteristics of the "spider pelvis."

cally. Death usually occurs before puberty. The condition is also thought to be genetic, but the mode of transmission is not clear. Until more information is available, it cannot be decided whether these 2 conditions are separate entities.

Renal tubular ectasia, or dilatation of the collecting tubules, is essentially a roentgen diagnosis (see medullary sponge kidney, above) and can be demonstrated in excretory urograms when renal function is adequate, or by retrograde urograms when it is not. Renal tubular ectasia has also been described with the combination of renal and hepatic cystic formations as a familial disorder. In some instances there have been no clinical manifestations; in some the hepatic involvement has dominated the clinical pattern with evidences of cirrhosis and portal hypertension. Whether this condition is a clinical entity or a variant of the medullary cystic kidney is unclear. In addition, it has been suggested that the roentgen pattern of the infantile form of polycystic disease of the kidney may simulate that of renal tubular ectasia.

SOLITARY RENAL CYST

Simple renal cysts are usually solitary and unilateral, but several cysts involving one kidney or bilateral solitary cysts may occur. They usually present as an abdominal mass. The cysts are normally unilocular and do not as a rule communicate with the renal pelvis. They should be differentiated from polycystic disease of the kidneys, multicystic kidneys, hydronephrosis and Wilms's tumor.

MALFORMATIONS PRODUCING OBSTRUCTION TO THE URINARY FLOW

Though urinary obstruction leading to the production of hydronephrosis is usually caused by a congenital defect within the urinary tract, it may also be caused by external pressure as by an aberrant blood vessel on the kidney pelvis or ureter or by a neoplasm (usually of the kidney). Urinary calculi, kinking of a ureter secondary to a prolapsed kidney, inflammatory strictures, neuromuscular lesions of the bladder or ureter and extreme phimosis are other causes of obstructions.

Care must be exercised in deciding whether a kidney pelvis is slightly enlarged because of back pressure or is simply within the upper range of normal in size. The absence of evident obstruction below the pelvis and of blunting of the calices would favor the latter probability. But when the obstruction is at the pelvic-ureteral junction, there will be no ureteral dilatation below this level. In some instances the pelvis is extrarenal and therefore appears enlarged; or there may be congenital absence of a major calyx, or one calyx may be larger or smaller than the others without having any special significance.

It is advisable to divide obstructive lesions into 2 groups: (1) those at the bladder neck and below it and (2) those above the bladder and involving one or both ureters or ureteral orifices. Since there is dilatation of the structures proximal to the obstruction, the bladder will become dilated and its walls hypertrophied when the obstruction is distal to it, but will not be involved when the obstruction is above it.

When the obstruction is at or below the bladder neck, the ureters and renal pelvis as well as the bladder become dilated; when the obstruction is proximal to the bladder, only the portion of the ureter above the obstruction and the renal pelvis are distended. In both instances, if the obstruction is not removed, hydronephrosis develops, with progressive atrophy of renal tissue, and often with recurrent or persistent infection.

Owing to the seriousness of delay in recognition of urethral obstruction, the newborn infant should be observed for frequency of voiding and force of the urinary stream before he is dismissed from the newborn nursery. Urographic studies are indicated whenever infection occurs. Efforts must be made to relieve an obstruction at the earliest possible moment.

OBSTRUCTIVE LESIONS INVOLVING THE BLADDER NECK OR URETHRA

Although a tight phimosis may partially obstruct the urinary flow, it is rarely a cause of serious trouble. When obstructive uropathy and phimosis coexist, a careful search for another obstruction should always be made. Meatal strictures, inflammatory and otherwise, may rarely cause obstruction.

Congenital obstructions in the urethra are found in both boys and girls. Congenital narrowing or partial absence of the urethra rarely occurs. In males the common anomaly consists of 1 or 2 membranous folds with 1 end attached to the verumontanum and the other usually to the lateral urethral walls. As the urine flows from the bladder, these folds acting as *valves* are ballooned out, causing a diminution in the urethral caliber. At times an obstruction resembling an iris diaphragm may partially or completely encircle the posterior urethra below the verumontanum. Since often there is no obstruction to the passage of a urethral catheter into the bladder, there may be some difficulty in establishing the presence of urethral valves. They can usually be demonstrated, however, by cystourethrography.

Of children with recurrent or persistent infection in the urinary tract, about one quarter have urethral stenosis, most of whom are girls. Most of these have residual urine in the bladder, as demonstrated by retention of Lipiodol instilled in the bladder 48 hours previously, and a third or more have associated ureteral reflux. It is thought by some that the urethral stenosis is secondary to infection, by others that there is a congenital basis. In any case the rate of recurrence of infection is significantly reduced after urethral dilation.

Campbell states that stricture in the female urethra is frequently overlooked, that many female children have congenitally tight external meatuses, and that in a lesser number there is comparable narrowing of the vesical outlet. Urethrotrigonitis is frequent in girls and may be associated with periurethritis or congenital or acquired stricture. Congenital contracture of the vesical outlet and congenital stenosis of the external meatus, the commonest lesions producing lower tract obstructions in girls, frequently coexist in the same patient. It is generally believed that contracture of the vesical outlet is due to muscular hypertrophy of the internal sphincter, which may be analogous to the lesion in pylorospasm. Others feel that this muscular hypertrophy is secondary to more distal urethral stricture or stenosis, the dilated proximal urethra producing a false image of bladder neck obstruction, more often in girls than boys. Congenital stricture of the ureterovesical junction, with dilation of the upper urinary tract, may be associated. Less commonly obstruction of the neck of the bladder results from a shelf or bar of hypertrophied muscle on the floor of the bladder at its junction with the posterior urethra. There is some evidence that this lesion is progressive and may not produce serious obstruction during infancy.

Bodian has demonstrated fibroelastosis of the posterior urethra in the male; it results in resistance to normal distention of this area during voiding, and thus to obstructed urine flow. These changes are believed to represent an abnormality in the developing prostatic tissue. It is conjectured that hypertrophy of the detrusor and of the bladder neck musculature is secondary to the obstruction to urine flow. *Prostatic hypertrophy* is an infrequent cause of urinary obstruction; transient prostatic hypertrophy causing urinary obstruction has been noted after hormonal therapy for cryptorchidism.

Obstruction of the bladder neck occurs most often in females and apparently more commonly in white than in nonwhite children. The lesion usually involves concentric hypertrophy of the bladder neck; mucosal folds may also be present. In the early stages the upper urinary tract often appears normal on urography, but hydronephrosis eventually develops. The presenting symptoms may be those of infection or obstruction. The bladder wall is usually trabeculated, and even though the bladder is often not palpable, the voiding cystourethrogram invariably reveals urinary retention. Floating Lipiodol can be used to detect residual urine in children too young to void on request. Normally the Lipiodol is excreted within 24 hours.

In some instances of vesical and ureteral dilatation with hydronephrosis *no obstructive lesion can be found*. In a few cases neuromuscular dysfunctions may be due to demonstrable lesions of the spinal cord, with or without spina bifida or other malformations of the lower spine. Swenson and Fisher observed a diminution in ganglion cells in the bladder walls of children of both sexes with megaloureter and megalobladder unassociated with an obstructive lesion of the urinary tract. They termed the condition aparasympathetic bladder. These patients seem to have a loss of sensation in the bladder, but are not incontinent. Megaloureters and megalobladder have on occasion been noted in conjunction with aganglionic megacolon.

The term "megaureter-megacystis" has been applied to a condition in which great dilatation of a smooth and thin-walled bladder is accompanied by vesicoureteral reflux and dilated ureters. Involved children have an enlarged urinary tract, but may go for years without evidence of bladder retention, which would be unlikely in obstruction at the bladder neck. Transient obstruction may occur with urinary tract infections, and renal failure may appear in late childhood in patients in whom infection has not been controlled.

Elevated intravesical pressure on voiding has been reported in children with recurrent urinary infection in whom no anatomic obstructive lesion could be demonstrated. It has been postulated that distal obstruction to urine flow must exist in these children, at least on a functional basis.

Slight enlargement, blunting and distortion of the calices and widening of the ureters may occur in pyelonephritis without evident anatomic obstruction. If the infection is of short duration, and treatment is effective, these changes may be reversible. In prolonged infection with destruction and scarring of the renal mass, distortion of the pelvis and calices may be progressive and permanent.

Hydroperitoneum has been associated with congenital obstructive lesions of the urinary tract in the newborn, most often with obstruction of the urethra.

OBSTRUCTIVE LESIONS INVOLVING THE URETEROVESICAL JUNCTION, URETER, PELVIS OR KIDNEY

Anomalies involving the ureters are common. Complete or partial absence of one or both ureters may occur. Duplication, complete or partial, of one or both ureters is fairly common; the duplication may be limited to the renal pelvis. Partial obstruction of the ureter, usually due to a narrowing of the lumen, occurs most often at the pelvic-ureteral or the vesicoureteral region; it may occur where the ureter crosses the iliac vessels. In any of these locations the narrowing of the lumen may be due to an inflammatory stricture, a congenital anomaly or compression of the ureter from without, as, for example, by an aberrant blood vessel near the pelvic-ureteral junction.

Ureteral reflux is commonly associated with recurrent and persistent urinary tract infection. There is reason to believe that deficiency in the vesicoureteral "valve" mechanism, secondary to infection involving the intravesical portion of the ureter, may prevent adequate closure when intravesical pressure rises during voiding. Alternatively, in some patients a congenital defect in the valve seems to be the basis for reflux, as suggested by the common association of reflux with double ureters and anomalies of the bladder neck. Reflux may lead to dilatation of the upper tract.

When ureteral obstruction is due to a fold in the mucosa at the vesical orifice or an extreme narrowing at the orifice, there may be a ballooning of the ureteral wall into the bladder, producing a *ureterocele*, or intravesical cyst. This anomaly, which is really a prolapse of the ureter, may be unilateral or bilateral. When the intravesical portion is large, it may result in complete blockage of ureteral urine flow and hydronephrosis. In the early stages, correction can often be obtained by endoscopic incision or amputation; when there is significant renal damage, partial or complete nephrectomy and ureterectomy are indicated for unilateral lesions.

Diverticula of the ureters are rare; they may be responsible for obstruction and may be difficult to demonstrate. Retrograde urography offers the best chance of detection.

Hydronephrosis

Dilatation of the renal pelvis and calices is due to obstruction in their drainage. Rarely, obstruction of the renal pelvis results from displacement of a movable kidney. If the obstruction is infravesicular, the hydronephrosis is bilateral (Fig. 15-5) and develops somewhat more slowly than when the obstruction is supravesicular; in either instance, however, hydronephrosis may be well advanced at birth. Several years may elapse before maximal dilatation is obtained, or hydronephrosis may progress rapidly over a period of a few months, especially in unilateral lesions. If there are obstructive lesions in both ureters, the hydronephrosis is also bilateral. If only one side is obstructed, then the hydronephrosis is unilateral (Fig. 15-6). If the obstruction produces back pressure in the ureters, they become dilated, at times thickened, and often increased in length with great tortuosities. In long-standing lesions the renal substance is greatly atrophied as a result of the pressure on the tissues and their blood supply, and the kidney may ultimately consist of a thin-walled cystic mass with little functioning renal tissue. The calices appear on the urogram as large balls, and there may be little or no renal tissue separating them. At times the combined mass of a unilateral hydronephrotic kidney and

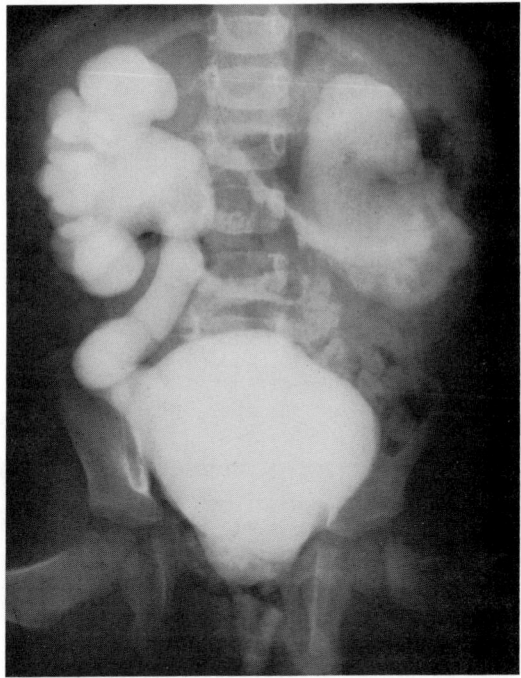

Figure 15-5. Hydronephrosis. Reflux pyelogram showing bilateral hydronephrosis and hydroureters and enlargement of the bladder secondary to obstruction produced by a congenital "valve anomaly" in the posterior urethra.

dilated ureter will produce a large cystic tumor filling half or more of the abdominal cavity. A history of an abdominal mass fluctuating in size and associated with changes in urinary volume is suggestive of hydronephrosis secondary to obstructive uropathy.

Clinical Manifestations. The symptoms resulting from obstructive uropathy can, in general, be divided into 3 categories: (1) interference with the flow of urine, (2) infection, and (3) renal insufficiency.

Manifestations resulting from interference with the flow of urine. In *infravesicular obstruction* or with *primary bladder dysfunction* these symptoms are more striking than when the obstruction is above the bladder. The presenting symptom is often an abdominal tumor (distended bladder) noted by the mother. There may be some hesitation or difficulty in initiating the urinary stream and even periodic inability to void at all. It is important to question the mother about the voiding habits of the child and especially to watch the child void. A thin, weak or dribbling urinary stream is the most important physical sign in the detection of bladder obstruction. Residual urine in the bladder can be demonstrated by catheterization immediately after a voluntary voiding or by the instillation of floating Lipiodol. Dilatation of the bladder, trabeculation of its wall and ureteral reflux can be revealed by urography (cystourethrogram).

In the so-called *cord bladder* there may be complete paralysis with overflow incontinence. Reflex

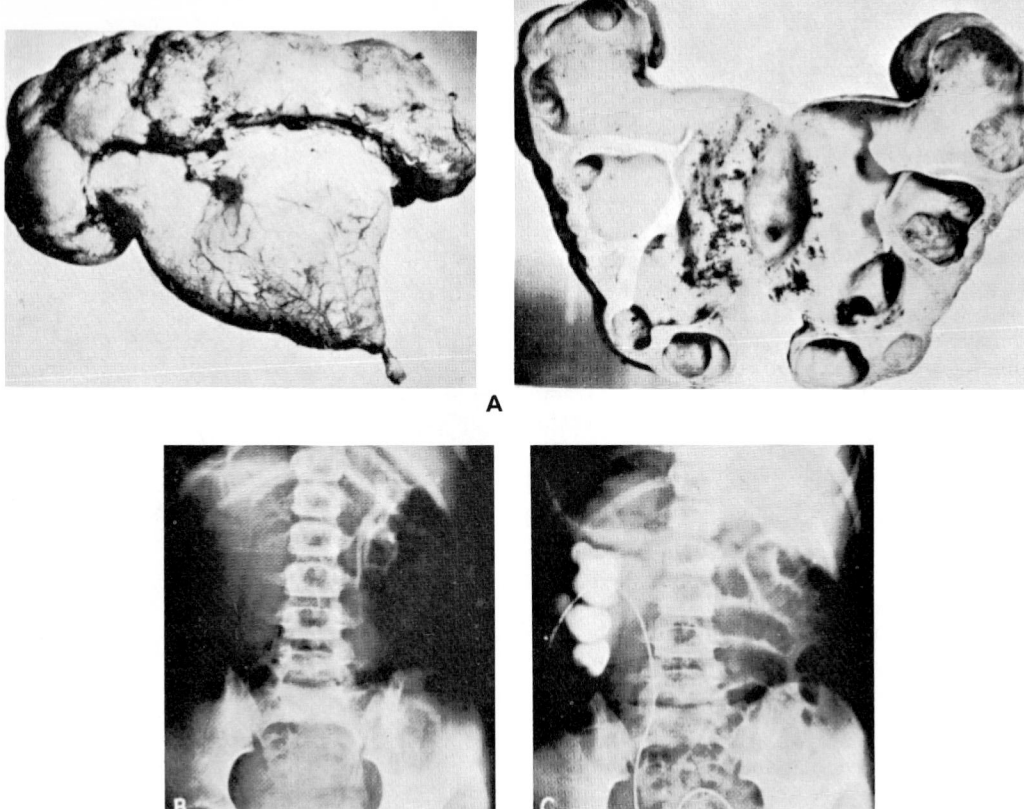

Figure 15-6. Congenital obstruction at the ureteropelvic junction due to fibrosis of the ureteral wall. An anomalous renal artery crossed the ureter at this point and may have precipitated these fibrotic changes. *A*, Kidney removed at operation. Note the stricture at the ureteropelvic junction and the greatly dilated renal pelvis and calices. *B*, Intravenous urogram showing normal right renal pelvis. The left renal pelvis is not visible, probably because of poor renal function and great dilution of the Diodrast. *C*, Retrograde pyelogram showing greatly dilated calices on the left side which were not visualized at all in the intravenous urogram (*B*).

automatic voidings usually develop with associated dribbling, but residual urine usually remains in the bladder. Relaxation of the rectal sphincter is most often an associated lesion. In so-called aparasympathetic megalobladders the defect in function is said to be less pronounced than with cord bladders, and incontinence does not occur.

In *supravesicular obstruction*, symptoms referable to the urinary tract may be lacking. In some instances there may be intermittent periods in which large quantities of urine are voided, owing to the release of an obstructed and greatly distended ureter or hydronephrosis. Many of these children complain of vague or even severe colicky abdominal pains variously referred to the renal region or midanterior area of the abdomen. The pain may also radiate to the groin or thigh and resemble a Dietl's crisis. Large masses which may give the impression of being cystic are often palpated in either or both flanks.

In infants with relaxed abdominal walls the kidneys can normally be palpated. This examination is best conducted bimanually with one hand pressing upward in the flank and the other downward over the anterior abdominal wall. When the kidneys are too easily palpable or appear at all enlarged, a thorough urologic study is indicated.

Manifestations resulting from infection. Obstruction of the urinary tract above the bladder is more commonly asymptomatic than is obstruction below it and is less likely to lead to infection. Irregular bouts of fever, with or without chills or convulsions in the young infant, are commonly present. Intermittent or persistent bacteriuria, pyuria, microscopic hematuria and rarely gross hematuria occur. In some long-standing cases, even though the renal substance is infiltrated with small round cells, the urine finally becomes free of leukocytes and bacteria. There may be malaise and eventually cachexia. Children whose malnutrition is not readily explainable on other grounds should have a thorough examination of their urinary system.

Manifestations of renal insufficiency. If the obstruction is not relieved, there is progressive renal dysfunction and death. Pyuria may or may not persist, casts and red cells are often present, and the urine, which is increased in volume, has a fixed, low specific gravity. The blood nonprotein nitrogen is increased, the blood pressure is often elevated, and there is a state of acidosis with which the urine may be relatively alkaline (pH above 6). All phases of renal function are reduced. The blood inorganic phosphorus level may be elevated and that of calcium reduced, resulting in tetany, renal hyperparathyroidism, and dwarfism with bony deformities somewhat similar to those of rickets. At this stage it may be difficult to differentiate obstructive disease from chronic glomerulonephritis.

Diagnosis. Suspicion of a congenital malformation of the urinary tract should lead to immediate urologic study. This includes observation of the urinary stream, urinalysis, measurement of the blood urea nitrogen level and intravenous urography; a postvoiding roentgenogram should be made to detect any residual urine. Voiding cystography with the instillation of floating Lipiodol will often demonstrate an infravesicular obstruction with retention and reflux into the dilated ureters during voiding, even when bladder residual is not disclosed following the intravenous pyelogram.

The child should be tested for sensitivity to the contrast material to be used for intravenous urography before it is injected. In some instances, usually with high concentrations of blood urea nitrogen, intravenous urography will fail to demonstrate the congenital defect, because of poor glomerular filtration or loss of concentrating capacity; retrograde urography is then required. Differences in function between kidneys can be detected by examination of urine obtained from each by ureteral catheterization. Owing to leakage around ureteral catheters, estimation of concentrations rather than clearance measurements of excreted substances (e.g. creatinine) may be preferable. Cystometric studies and studies of ureteral peristaltic activity may be helpful in evaluating the lesion and gauging prognosis.

Neurologic examination is essential in instances of disordered urinary flow, and should include examination of perineal sensation and rectal examination to determine sphincter tone, which may be spastic or atonic. Roentgenograms of the lower spine may detect skeletal abnormalities associated with neurologic defects.

Treatment. The treatment of obstructive uropathy involves surgical relief of the obstruction and management of infection and renal insufficiency when they exist.

Since the sudden release of urine from a greatly distended bladder may result in shock and even fatal anuria, the bladder should be emptied by gradual decompression through an indwelling catheter. A rapid improvement in renal function often follows this drainage, even in cases of longstanding obstruction. Reduction in the hydronephrosis may not be apparent for several months.

After prolonged dilatation, sclerosis and atony of the bladder wall may prevent adequate evacuation of urine, even after removal of the obstruction. But improvement almost regularly follows relief of obstruction, control of infection and treatment of renal insufficiency. Preliminary drainage by indwelling catheter or cystostomy should not delay surgical removal of the obstructive lesion for a very long time. Infection is likely with an indwelling catheter and usually is not prevented by the use of antibiotics, except that irrigation of the bladder with an antibacterial agent such as neomycin may help reduce the likelihood of infection. When the ureters are elongated and tortuous, drainage of the ureters and renal pelvis from below is often not effective, and ureterostomy or nephrostomy may be necessary, even in the newborn.

When infection is present, antibacterial therapy is mandatory (see p. 1123). Attention must be given to fluid balance (loss of concentration capacity), to the biochemical disorders due to renal dysfunction, and to the anorexia and vomiting commonly encountered.

Obstruction due to urethral stenosis or stricture may be relieved by dilatation. When the obstruction is not relieved by dilatation, revision of the bladder neck may be required to correct bladder retention.

The construction of an ileal conduit may be necessary in the patient with a "neurogenic bladder" if bladder neck revision does not relieve the obstruction to urine flow. In patients with ureteral reflux, transplantation of ureters to form more competent ureterovesical valves is often necessary, but may be successful only if bladder neck revision is also done.

Patients with so-called aparasympathetic bladders must be taught to make sustained efforts to empty the bladder completely; manual suprapubic pressure is often necessary. Three separate efforts to empty the bladder at each voiding are often helpful in reducing residual urine. A schedule of 4 or 5 voidings a day and 1 or 2 at night can be recommended. Resection of the bladder neck may be necessary to relieve urinary retention.

Even when considerable renal function has been lost, surgical relief should be attempted. A prolonged useful life is possible, even with a considerably lowered renal function, and it is often surprising to what extent renal function will improve after an obstruction is relieved. In mild cases there may be almost complete restoration of the urinary tract to normal size and complete recovery of renal function; hence the *urgency for early diagnosis.*

DUPLICATION OF THE URETER

Duplication of the ureter is found in approximately 1 in every 160 autopsies and is often associated with duplication of the pelvis. It is often bilateral. The upper pelvi-caliceal system is usually the smaller and drains the upper major calyx. The lower element drains the remainder of the kidney. The condition is more common in girls than in boys. When the function of a portion of the kidney drained by the smaller of the 2 segments is depressed, the duplication may not be detected by the intravenous pyelogram, and the diagnosis will be established only by retrograde urography. Sometimes the upper, smaller segment may not drain well, and the radiopaque substance may persist in the pelvic area. The duplication is not always complete; when it is, the ureter from the upper pole of the kidney usually enters the bladder caudally and medially to the ureter from the lower segment. The ureter may also open into the urethra, or into the vagina or vulva. If reflux occurs, it is most commonly into the ureter draining the lower segment of the kidney.

Frequently there are no clinical disturbances associated with duplication of a ureter. When there are, the major one is obstruction to urine flow in one or more of the ureters, either at its lower end or where they join. The lesion is commonly discovered when urography is done for recurrent infection. Constant wetting will occur when the aberrant ureter inserts below the bladder sphincter.

Recurrent infection should be treated as described on page 1123. Surgery is indicated when there is obstruction to urinary flow, when the aberrant ureter produces constant wetting, or when reflux contributes to recurrent infection. When hydronephrosis and renal infection are apparently limited to the upper, smaller segment, heminephrectomy may be indicated.

DISPLACEMENT OF THE KIDNEY

Dystopia. Accompanying or independent of some of the malformations mentioned, one or both kidneys may be displaced. For example, both may be on the same side or one or both may be above or below the usual positions. Most often, the left kidney is displaced downward. Palpation of the displaced kidney may suggest such conditions as intussusception, fecal accumulation and appendiceal abscess. Displacement may be associated with ureteral obstruction and hydronephrosis, or the displaced kidney may obstruct the ureter of the other kidney. There may be no symptoms, or the kinking of the ureter may cause pain and dysuria. Pyelography and arteriography will reveal the location of the kidney and the nature of its blood supply. As a rule the shortness of its blood vessels prevents its replacement. Nephrectomy is indicated if the kidney is nonfunctioning, constantly or recurrently infected as a result of hydronephrosis, or when by its location it also interferes with function of the other kidney.

Movable Kidney. This relatively uncommon condition may be congenital or acquired. The acquired form is seen oftener in girls than in boys during late childhood and may result from poor posture and asthenia. Symptoms, if present, are a sensation of pressure or dragging in the abdomen or lumbar region, attacks of renal colic (Dietl's crisis) and perhaps chronic urinary tract infection. General splanchnoptosis may also be present. Hydronephrosis may develop from kinking or twisting of the ureter. In establishing a diagnosis it should be remembered that it is often possible to palpate the lower pole of the kidney in normal children. Intravenous pyelography in the supine and upright positions will usually establish the diagnosis. It should be recognized, however, that the normal kidney is mobile, and one must be cautious in concluding what extent of movement is abnormal. Treatment consists in efforts to strengthen the musculature and to correct abnormal posture. Surgical measures are seldom required.

Horseshoe kidney is about 4 times as common in boys as in girls. Fusion usually occurs between the lower poles of the kidney; the isthmus is most commonly anterior to the great vessels, rarely behind them. The pelves are directed more anteriorly than normal, and on pyelography the ureters appear to come straight down from the lower pole of each kidney. The isthmus is sometimes palpated as a prevertebral mass, where it is susceptible to trauma. Obstruction of the ureters as they pass over the isthmus may lead to hydronephrosis. When there are symptoms referable to the kidney, they may include abdominal pain due to obstruction, urinary stasis with infection, formation of calculi, hypertension and hematuria.

REFERENCES

Bodian, M.: Some Observations on the Pathology of Congenital Idiopathic Bladder Neck Obstruction. *Brit. J. Urol.*, 29:393, 1957.

Eagle, J. F., and Barrett, G. S.: Congenital Deficiency of Abdominal Musculature with Associated Genitourinary Abnormalities. *Pediatrics*, 6:721, 1950.

Herdman, R. C., Good, R. A., and Vernier, R. L.: Medullary Cystic Disease in Two Siblings. *Am. J. Med.*, 43:335, 1967.

Hinman, F., and Hutch, J. A.: Atrophic Pyelonephritis from Ureteral Reflux Without Obstructive Signs ("Reflux Pyelonephritis"). *J. Urol.*, 87:230, 1962.

Immergut, M., Culp, D., and Flocks, R. H.: The Urethral Caliber in Normal Female Children. *J. Urol.*, 97:693, 1967.

Kissane, J. M.: Congenital Malformations; in R. H. Heptinstall (Ed.): *Pathology of the Kidney.* Boston, Little, Brown and Co., 1966.

Lattimer, J. K., Uson, A. C., and Melicow, M. M.: Urologic Emergencies in Newborn Infants. *Pediatrics*, 29:310, 1962.

Mongeau, J. G., and Worthen, H. G.: Nephronophthisis and Medullary Cystic Disease. *Am. J. Med.*, 43:345, 1967.

Reilly, B. J., and Neuhauser, E. B. D.: Renal Tubular Ectasia in Cystic Disease of the Kidneys and Liver. *Am. J. Roent.*, 84:546, 1960.

Waterhouse, K.: The Dilated Posterior Urethra. I. Male. *J. Urol.*, 91:72, 1964.

Williams, D. I.: Congenital Bladder Neck Obstruction and the Megaureter. *Brit. J. Urol.*, 29:389, 1957.

INFECTIONS OF THE URINARY TRACT

Infection of the urinary tract is relatively common in children; its true incidence is not known. Among presumably healthy school children Kunin found significant bacteriuria in 1.2 per cent of the girls and 0.03 per cent of the boys. The incidence was 3.5 per cent among adolescent Negro girls. In the author's clinic significant bacteriuria was found in 1.5 per cent of presumably well infants. Bacteriuria in itself is not diagnostic of pyelonephritis; clear evidence of kidney involvement is required. It is difficult to differentiate upper from lower urinary tract infection.

Anatomic or functional obstructions in the urinary tract dispose to infection of the kidney. When *E. coli* are injected intravenously into the normal rat or rabbit, pyelonephritis does not occur in the normal kidney. When one ureter is tied, however, infection occurs in the kidney on the obstructed side. Obstruction is said to be a common basis for urinary tract infections during pregnancy, and urinary infection is common in paraplegia: e.g. in the child with spina bifida and neurogenic bladder.

Infection of the urinary tract is thought to be second in frequency only to infections of the respiratory tract. It accounts for approximately 5 to 6 per cent of pediatric hospital admissions in some areas. The reported incidence at autopsy in children varies from 2 to 4.5 per cent. Autopsy data may be misleading, however, because of the variable criteria used in the histologic diagnosis of pyelonephritis. Moreover, autopsy data in children do not reflect the seriousness of the disease, since renal failure may be slow and inapparent until adult life. In spite of the lack of precise data, it is evident that infection of the urinary tract is common in childhood, frequently overlooked, and deserving of intensive medical care.

Infection of the kidney by way of the bloodstream may be the common mode in the newborn, but beyond this age period infection is generally believed to be due to upward spread from the bladder, by way of the lumen of the ureter into the renal tubules or directly into the interstices of the kidney. On the other hand, when infection complicates obstruction limited to the upper urinary tract, the infecting agent may have entered the kidney from the bloodstream.

Infection is 10 to 30 times more common in girls than in boys, except in the neonatal period, when the incidence is essentially equal; this has been ascribed to the short female urethra, the orifice of which is readily contaminated with feces. Michie observed that water readily entered the bladders of girls who stood and sat 10 times in a tub of water. It is presumed that the antibacterial capacity of the bladder mucosa and the mechanical washing out with free urine flow keep the incidence of urinary infection relatively low. With anatomic obstruction, infection is facilitated.

Normally the pressure on the wall of the full bladder closes off the vesicoureteral valve. Vesicoureteral reflux occurs rarely if at all in the normal urinary tract, but is frequently found in children with congenital anomalies of the lower urinary tract and residual urine in the bladder, and with acute and recurrent urinary tract infection, even where there is no demonstrable obstructive lesion. Murphy found that some infected children with no obstruction demonstrable by the usual means raised their intravesical pressures to very high levels during voiding, suggesting some kind of functional obstruction.

The length of the intravesical portion of the ureter is considerably smaller in the infant than in the adult and may therefore more readily decompensate. Some congenital defect has been postulated as a cause for reflux during voiding. In support of this possibility is the fact that in patients with double ureters, reflux is more common in the lower ureter. Pyelonephritis has been demonstrated more frequently in the portion of the kidney drained by the refluxing ureter. Infection itself may be the primary event leading to reflux; reflux disappears on occasion after control of the infection. Presumably, infection produces a stiffness of the intravesical portion of the ureter and a failure of the valvelike mechanism. Whether bladder neck and urethral obstruction lead to reflux without anatomic defect in the ureterovesical valve is not clear. There is a high incidence of reflux with neurogenic bladder, with the megaureter-megacystis syndrome associated with congenital bladder neck obstruction, and with atonic ureters. The demonstration of reflux may on occasion be fortuitous: it may appear and disappear during an examination; and it may be seen in the cystourethrogram during voluntary voiding when it is not demonstrable during anesthesia.

PYELONEPHRITIS; PYELITIS

Acute infection of the urinary tract may be suspected from the clinical symptoms (though in many cases there are none related directly to the urinary tract). The diagnosis is established only by demonstration of increased numbers of white blood cells or bacteria in the urine, whose origin is not from a contaminating extraurinary source such as vaginitis.

Etiology. The incidence of *acute pyelonephritis* is highest during the diaper age, being somewhat less during the first few weeks of life than during the remainder of infancy. Pyelonephritis is the most common renal disease of childhood, and in its chronic forms is not an uncommon cause of chronic renal failure, particularly in the presence of obstructive uropathy.

Many different bacteria may infect the urinary tract. Organisms of the colon bacillus group are responsible for about 80 per cent of acute infections. Recurrent episodes of infection are also commonly caused by *E. coli*, and not infrequently by different strains. Certain *E. coli* serotypes tend to predominate, in both acute and recurrent episodes. There is evidence that the serotype of *E. coli* isolated from the urinary tract tends to be identical to that in the intestinal tract at the time, suggesting that the intestinal tract is the source of organisms infecting the urinary tract by way of the urethra. Enteropathogenic *E. coli* which cause diarrhea in newborn and young infants rarely infect the urinary tract.

Acute infection may also be caused by staphylococci, hemolytic streptococci, *Streptococcus faecalis*, and less commonly such organisms as typhoid, salmonella or dysentery bacilli and *M. tuberculosis*. In long-standing cases and in patients who have had prolonged treatment with antibacterial agents and especially in those with obstruction and who have had instrumentation, Proteus, *Pseudomonas aeruginosa* and staphylococci are common infecting agents. It is not unusual to find mixed organisms in patients with chronic infection.

It has been suggested that protoplasts or L forms (forms of bacteria with altered cell walls) may play a role in the persistence of infectious organisms within the kidney. Under ordinary cultural methods these protoplasts are not detected. Since cell walls are the site of action of some antimicrobial agents, these protoplasts devoid of cell wall may not be adversely affected by them; other antibiotics, however, which affect both the cytoplasmic membrane and intermediary metabolism, such as erythromycin, tetracycline, and others may be effective against these forms.

Pathology. In the early stages of pyelonephritis the kidney is usually enlarged because of the associated inflammation, with scattered minute wedge-shaped abscesses, the apices of which point toward the pelvis. There are congestion and leukocytic infiltration in the renal pelvis and widening of the calices with some blunting of the papillae. In the areas of abscess there is destruction of the proximal tubules, with an intense cellular infiltration of leukocytes and round cells. Heptinstall has shown that in experimental pyelonephritis there is a rapid change in a few days from polymorphonuclear to round cells. These inflammatory cells are found within the tubule as well. The glomeruli stand out as islands of uninvolved normal tissue, and the blood vessels show little change. Uninvolved tissue appears normal. The early changes are severest in the medullary portions of the kidney, as the infection spreads from the pelvis.

In chronic pyelonephritis there is characteristic irregular scarring and atrophy, with reduction of the total kidney mass. In the areas of atrophy the renal calices are considerably distorted, and the distance is reduced between the papillae and the kidney surface. The distortion of the pelvis and the narrowing of the adjacent cortical tissue are diagnostic in the intravenous pyelogram. Acute lesions may coexist with chronic ones. The chronic microscopic lesion is characterized in the areas of scar tissue by interstitial fibrosis, round cell infiltration, and glomeruli in varying stages of hyalinization. Some glomeruli show intense periglomerular fibrosis, and others may show the proliferative and necrotic changes characteristic of ischemia. Changes may even resemble those of chronic glomerulonephritis. Subcapsular deposits of collagen are said to be common, crowding the glomerular tuft. The tubules are dilated, and there is atrophy of the cells. Characteristically, they are filled with eosinophilic, homogeneous material. The arteries and arterioles in these areas often show intimal thickening and perivascular fibrosis, arteriolosclerosis and necrotizing arteriolitis. The vascular changes are more striking when hypertension is present. As the disease progresses, the intervening normal tissue becomes more and more involved, and the total mass of the kidney greatly shrunken.

In most instances some inflammatory reaction is seen in the submucosa of the ureters and bladder. In long-standing infection secondary to infravesicular obstruction, the bladder and ureters may be dilated and their walls greatly thickened. Infection itself is said to produce some dilatation of the kidney pelvis and ureter. Occasionally inflammatory thickening of the ureter is responsible for its obstruction and for proximal dilatation of the ureter and pelvis. With subsidence of infection in such cases, the ureter and pelvis may return to their normal size. With long-standing obstruction of the urinary tract the renal tissue may be compressed into a thin shell surrounding the greatly dilated calices (Fig. 15-6). With increasing destruction of renal tissue, renal function progressively fails.

Owing to the spotty distribution of the renal lesions, renal tissue obtained by percutaneous needle biopsy may not be diagnostic.

Clinical Manifestations. Typically, in *acute pyelonephritis* the onset is abrupt, and the child appears acutely ill. The temperature frequently reaches 104°F., but is rarely sustained at such a level for over a day or two; characteristically, there are wide fluctuations. On occasion there may be little or no fever.

In the infant there are usually no localizing signs to indicate that the infection is in the urinary tract, except perhaps urinary frequency, which is difficult to evaluate at this age. During the period of high temperature the infant is likely to be irritable, and other central nervous symptoms such as convulsions and meningismus may be manifest. In the newborn infant there may be no fever. Gastrointestinal manifestations are common, vomiting often being a striking symptom. It may be projectile, associated with exaggerated gastric peristaltic waves and persistent enough to simulate pyloric stenosis. Diarrhea occurs occasionally and may result in dehydration. Anorexia is usually severe. Clinical signs of sepsis, including jaundice, may dominate the picture, especially in the newborn infant.

In older children there may be localizing symptoms. When there is an associated cystitis, frequency of urination, urgency and dysuria may be present. There may also be pain, sharp or dull, over the renal area with muscular spasm and tenderness on palpation. It cannot be overemphasized that at any age *all symptoms may be lacking or none may be related to the urinary system*, and the diagnosis is established, if at all, by urinalysis and culture. This is particularly true in recurrent infection. Enuresis in a child with previous bladder control may be the presenting symptom of infection, or in approximately 10 per cent of cases there may be hematuria, which may persist for only a day or two.

In most untreated cases the fever, if any, lasts 7 to 10 days, and the urinary changes about 3 weeks. The acute clinical manifestations usually last for only the first few days of the disease. If the kidney lesion remains active, however, mild anemia, anorexia and failure to thrive may persist for weeks after the urine has returned to normal. In the unusual, severe form when large areas of the kidney are abscessed, there is great intoxication; in such infections death may occur within a week or two after the onset of the illness. The fatality rate, however, is low among the ordinary acute cases. In both treated and untreated infections there is a tendency to recurrence. Nosocomial infections play a part in reinfection of the urinary tract, probably through the use of the catheter and similar instruments.

Chronic and recurrent infections present serious problems; they are often, but not invariably, associated with obstructive lesions of the urinary tract. Instead of subsiding after 2 or 3 weeks, the infection may persist for months or years in a latent, clinically unexpressed phase, or there may be intermittent fever, pyuria, bacteriuria and progressive involvement of the renal parenchyma leading to interference with renal function and to hypertension. The principal symptoms, inanition, anemia and failure to grow, are often unexplained unless the urinary tract is investigated. In most children, growth failure correlates with renal functional loss; when normal renal function is maintained, growth tends to proceed at normal rates.

Acute exacerbations are common. During early childhood greatly reduced renal function may not restrict activity to a great extent. The ultimate renal failure often comes during periods of rapid growth, as in puberty. In many instances, although the infection after some years becomes quiescent or is "burnt out," and pus and bacteria no longer appear in the urine, the kidney is irreparably damaged.

Loss of renal function is reflected in loss of concentrating capacity, which is reversible in the acute phase; in chronic infection the loss may resemble that in nephrogenic diabetes insipidus. Whereas in glomerulonephritis there is reduction of the glomerular filtration rate with loss of concentration, in pyelonephritis the filtration rate is maintained. Renal salt-wasting, as reflected in an increase in urinary sodium concentration, is not uncommon in chronic pyelonephritis.

Progressive renal failure with pyelonephritis is most commonly associated with obstruction to urine flow and in childhood is seen most frequently in the first year or two of life. In the older children with recurrent bacteriuria in the absence of "detectable" obstruction to urine flow and other primary renal disease, overall renal function may be surprisingly well maintained. Death from renal failure in this latter group of patients is uncommon during childhood. Since the manifestations of the renal insufficiency are not unlike those of chronic nephritis, the true cause of the renal lesion may be overlooked unless a history of past infection is obtained or a congenital malformation of the urinary tract is demonstrated. Differential diagnosis may be made by needle biopsy.

Secondary hyperparathyroidism may be a complication. Hypertension may be severe and may be responsible for cardiac failure or cerebral hemorrhage. A hereditary form of chronic pyelonephritis with renal insufficiency in the male has been described. Deafness is associated in some instances (see p. 1133).

In unilateral chronic pyelonephritis renal function may not be significantly reduced, owing to hypertrophy of the nonaffected nephrons in the diseased kidney and in the uninfected kidney.

Diagnosis. The most essential aspect of diagnosis is demonstration of bacterial infection by quantitative cultures of urine. Bladder urine is normally sterile, but readily contaminated during and after voiding. Pyuria reflects the degree of acute renal inflammatory response and may be absent in as many as 50 per cent of patients with persistent or recurrent episodes of infection. In late, burnt-out infections, with advanced renal scarring and functional failure, both bacteriuria and pyuria may be absent. White blood cell casts are of particular diagnostic importance, since they are indicative of acute intrarenal infection.

In assessment of pyuria the examination of a freshly voided, clean specimen is of prime importance. Formed elements, particularly cellular casts, disintegrate rapidly after a half hour, and especially in alkaline urine. The early morning specimen is best for examination, since it is likely to be a concentrated and acid specimen; both factors tend to preserve the formed elements. Urine contains a small number of white blood cells under normal circumstances. Addis counts of healthy children (voided in boys, catheterized in girls) demonstrate less than one-half million white blood cells in the urine excreted in a 12-hour period. In a fresh, uncentrifuged specimen obtained by similar means there should not be more than 1 or 2 white blood cells per low-power microscopic field; a freshly shaken specimen should not contain more than 1 cell per 10 high-power fields. Stansfeld and Webb found 10 or fewer white blood cells per mm.³ of uncentrifuged urine in 98 per cent of boys free of urinary infection; the majority had either zero counts or but one cell per mm.³ Similar counts were obtained in catheterized urine of a comparable percentage of infant girls and in 84 per cent of older girls.

Vaginal secretions are the most common source of pus in the urine. Many girls are treated for months for so-called pyelitis when the origin of the pus cells is in the vagina. When pus cells are found in the urine, a "clean" specimen must be obtained.

The external vaginal orifice and the surrounding perineum must be thoroughly cleansed before collecting urine for slide examination or culture; pHisoHex and Zephiran 1:1000 are used for this purpose. In boys the foreskin should be retracted and the glans cleansed. If possible, only the latter portion of the voiding should be collected. Urine collected under these conditions shows a close correlation in white cell counts and bacterial counts with that obtained by catheterization. In older girls in whom cleansing may be more difficult, catheterization, after cleansing, may be necessary to obtain reliable cultures. Catheterization should be deferred until the results of a noncatheterized specimen are known.

The quantitative estimation of bacteriuria has been a great advance in the study of urinary tract infection. Isolation of a few bacteria in catheterized specimens from girls or in voided specimens collected in midstream from boys is not diagnostic of urinary infection. Infected urine usually contains more than 100,000 bacteria per ml. in a specimen cultured within 1 hour of voiding. Counts approximating 10,000 should be considered suspicious, and further examinations should be made. We have found that counts above 10,000 usually indicate infection. Lower counts usually represent contamination. On the other hand, counts as low as 1000 per ml. have been associated with rises in specific antibodies in serum, particularly in recurrent infections, in which they often represent infection with a new organism. It may be particularly difficult to obtain "clean-catch" cultures with low counts from female newborn infants. In these young infants or even in older children, when clean specimens cannot be obtained and the diagnosis of infection remains in doubt, suprapubic aspiration of the bladder will recover uncontaminated urine. Urine aspirated from the bladder by needle puncture should be sterile or essentially so, and we accept a single positive culture obtained by this method as diagnostic of infection. Otherwise, diagnosis is established by 2 successive cultures from which the same strain of organism is obtained. Urine obtained from the upper urinary tract is sterile if the bladder is sterile. Bacterial counts from ureteral urine may be low even in the presence of infection; multiplication of bacteria occurs as urine remains in the bladder.

Low bacterial counts in urine of patients with infection may result from suppressive therapy, rapid excretion (not permitting sufficient time for bacterial multiplication in the bladder), acid urine with pH below 5.5 or an alkaline urine above 8.5. Organisms such as group A streptococci, some strains of staphylococci and enterococci may grow poorly in urine and thus produce few bacteria. Low bacterial counts may also be found in chronic and in healed pyelonephritis.

Though less reliable than cultural methods, the direct examination of a *cleanly* voided specimen of urine, even in girls, gives a reasonable indication of urinary infection. The absence of bacteria in a fresh uncentrifuged drop of urine stained with Gram's stain is suggestive evidence against the existence of urinary infection. The presence of bacteria in such preparations is usually associated with bacterial counts of 100,000 per ml. or more.

During the first 2 or 3 days of pyelonephritis, while the fever and associated symptoms are most severe, the urine may be normal. Pyuria may be intermittent, especially in chronic infections. The initial absence of pyuria may be due to failure of interstitial pyogenic collections to rupture into the renal tubules; subsequently temporary absence of pyuria may be due to ureteral obstruction in a unilateral infection. If the child's dietary intake has been restricted or if there has been persistent vomiting, there may be acetonuria. Proteinuria is usually minimal unless the pyelonephritis is a complication of some other primary renal disease. The urine most often contains a few red blood cells; red cell and hemoglobin casts will help in the differentiation from acute glomerulonephritis.

There is a mild anemia, more severe in the graver cases, and a varying degree of polymorphonuclear leukocytosis.

In every instance of persistent or recurring pyuria of urinary tract origin the child should be examined by intravenous and, if necessary, retrograde urography in search of structural or neurologic abnormalities which might be responsible for stasis and thus for persistence of an infection. The possibility of ureteral reflux or residual urine after voiding should be investigated by voiding cystourethrography with floating Lipiodol.

Percutaneous renal biopsy is not generally used as a diagnostic procedure in pyelonephritis because of the spotty nature of the renal pathology, but if other diseases are to be excluded, such biopsies may be helpful diagnostically.

Treatment. The aims in therapy of urinary tract infection are the eradication of infective organisms, the elimination of any obstruction to urine flow, and the correction of any renal functional impairment. Neither symptomatic response nor the disappearance of pyuria can be taken as evidence that bacteriuria has been eliminated. Symptoms in acute urinary tract infection often subside within a few days regardless of therapy. Treatment should therefore be preceded by careful bacteriologic diagnosis, to make certain that the urinary tract is indeed infected and to identify the infecting agent.

In the acutely ill child with appreciable pyuria it is advisable to obtain a "clean-catch" or a catheterized or aspirated specimen of urine for culture and begin therapy immediately. If the illness is not severe or the diagnosis not obvious, it is well to wait for a definitive diagnosis supported by at least 2 urine cultures.

The acutely ill and febrile patient will be best treated at bed rest with symptomatic therapy for fever, restlessness or convulsions. Fluids should be given freely, since there is evidence that a high osmolality of the medullary interstitium of the kidney may decrease phagocytosis and increase bacterial growth.

Since *E. coli* is the commonest agent in acute infections, the sulfonamides are widely used in treatment. Bacterial resistance to these drugs is not rapidly established. Sulfisoxasole (Gantrisin) is more soluble than many other sulfonamides and is thus less likely to produce crystalluria. Effective doses of sulfonamides range from 0.1 to 0.2 gm. per kg. per day, in 3 divided doses. An effective drug level is established by making the first dose of the drug one third to one half of the calculated total daily dose. In a few instances the daily dose may need to be increased. In the case of sulfonamide-resistant bacteria, the sulfonamide may be combined with an antibiotic chosen on the basis of in-vitro sensitivity tests, or the selected antibiotic may be given alone. Sterilization of the urine by sulfonamides occurs in a high percentage of patients infected with *E. coli*. With infections due to aerobacter, Proteus and Pseudomonas clinical responses may not be good, and a sterile urine is often not obtained. It is wise to obtain blood levels of sulfonamides periodically as a check on drug ingestion, and when impaired renal function creates a danger of overdosage. A high fluid intake and large urine output help prevent precipitation of crystals in ureters or bladder.

Nitrofurantoin (Furadantin) is the second most commonly used drug in our clinic. It is both bacteriostatic and bactericidal against most of the pathogens of the urinary tract except pseudomonas, which is highly resistant. Various strains of Proteus differ widely in their sensitivity. Use of the drug should be based on in-vitro sensitivity tests (see p. 262 for dosages and for contraindications in respect to use of this drug). Recurrences of infection following the discontinuance of nitrofurantoin therapy may occur more quickly than recurrences following sulfonamide therapy.

Antibiotic therapy should always be based on carefully controlled in-vitro sensitivity tests of the infecting bacterium; doses and contraindications of the antibiotics in current use are listed in Table 5-16, p. 237.

Methenamine mandelate has been of limited usefulness in the control of chronic urinary infection because it is effective only if the urine is acid (less than pH 5). At this pH methenamine may be a relatively effective antibacterial agent for such organisms as Proteus, Pseudomonas, the coliform group and staphylococci. Methionine and ascorbic acid have been used successfully as acidi-

fying agents (see Table 5-16). Bacterial counts of less than 10,000 colonies per ml. in voided urine are used as an indication of the effectiveness of methenamine and the amount of it to be prescribed. The principal use of methenamine is for prolonged therapy after the primary urinary infection has apparently been cleared by appropriate antibacterial drugs.

Although it is still to be proved, there is some agreement among investigators that the recurrence rate after apparently successfully treated urinary tract infections is reduced by prolonged therapy. Some think that long-term therapy is essentially prophylaxis and that the infecting organisms are usually eliminated by 2 weeks of therapy. Schedules for prolonged therapy vary considerably in length, ranging from several months to a year. If the patient has no adverse reaction to the drugs, bacterial suppression can often be maintained over many months by their use. Discontinuation of treatment may be followed, however, by prompt return of bacteriuria. At least 2 negative cultures at an interval of 4 to 6 weeks should be obtained after cessation of therapy before it is considered that the infection has been eradicated. Even then the patient should be kept under continued surveillance for the possibility of recurrence.

Though antibacterial therapy is of prime importance in the treatment of urinary tract infection, correction of any interference with urine flow is also essential. An intravenous pyelogram and a voiding cystourethrogram should be obtained as soon as the acute infection is under control. If an obstructive lesion is found, it should be relieved as promptly as possible to avoid renal damage or to preserve remaining function when irreversible damage has already occurred.

Since a large percentage of children with infections of the urinary tract require long-term treatment, their parents should be educated as to the nature of this disease, which with so few symptoms may lead to serious disability. Appropriate insight should also be given to older children by a sympathetic and understanding physician. Unless parents and children appreciate the nature of the problem, there is apt to be unadvised stoppage of prolonged drug therapy by the child or parents when symptoms have abated.

PERINEPHRITIS
(Perinephric Abscess)

Perinephritis is an inflammatory reaction in the soft tissues surrounding the kidney. The infection is ordinarily unilateral and usually proceeds to suppuration unless checked by therapy. Pus accumulates below the kidney and may extend in any direction, usually along the lumbar muscles toward the pelvis. It may rupture into the iliocostal space, above Poupart's ligament, or into the peritoneum, intestines, kidney, bladder or pleura.

Etiology. Perinephritis may follow trauma over the renal area, it may be blood-borne from suppurative infections elsewhere, or it may be a direct extension from a neighboring focus. Staphylococcal infections of the skin frequently antedate the renal infection. In the majority of instances, infection of the perinephric space results from rupture of an embolic renal cortical abscess.

Clinical Manifestations. The symptoms come on abruptly with fever, chills and other signs of acute infection. The fever is usually remittent. Signs localizing the disease to the renal region appear early with pain in the lumbar region of the affected side which may be referred to the groin, hip, thigh or knee. Movement of the spine causes discomfort, so that the patient walks with difficulty or prefers to lie on his back and, because of the spasm of the iliopsoas muscle, keeps his thigh flexed. Extension of the flexed leg is resisted, owing to the induced pain, but movement of the hip and knee joint in other directions is unhampered. Locally, there is tenderness with muscle spasm over the renal area and eventually an indefinite swelling, at times with demonstrable fluctuation. The overlying skin and subcutaneous tissues may become reddened and edematous.

Urinary symptoms are usually lacking, though in about half the cases there is pyuria during the course. On the roentgenogram the shadow of the abscess may obliterate that of the psoas muscle; elevation and decreased excursion of the diaphragm are evident during fluoroscopy. Acute cases may terminate within several weeks with gradual subsidence of all symptoms and signs; or the infection may become chronic and persist for months before rupture of the pus into one of the areas mentioned.

Prognosis and Treatment. The prognosis is influenced by the primary disease. Treatment includes rest in bed, local application of heat during the early stages, administration of an appropriate antibiotic, and, if suppuration occurs, surgical drainage. Blood and urine cultures may aid in establishing an etiologic diagnosis and thus permit a more effective selection of the antibacterial agent.

REFERENCES

Ambrose, S. S., and Nicolson, W. P.: Ureteral Reflux in Duplicated Ureters. *J. Urol.,* 92:439, 1964.

Andersen, H. J., Lincoln, K., Ørskov, F., Ørskov, I., and Winberg, J.: Studies of Urinary Tract Infections in Infancy and Childhood. V. A Comparison of the E. Coli Antibody Titer in Pyelonephritis Measured by Means of Homologous Urinary and Fecal E. Coli Antigens. *J. Pediat.,* 67:1073, 1965.

DeLuca, F. G., Fisher, J. H., and Swenson, O.: Review of Recurrent Urinary-Tract Infections in Infancy and Early Childhood. *New England J. Med.,* 268:75, 1963.

Fairley, K. F., Bond, A. G., Brown, R. B., and Habersberger, P.: Simple Test to Determine the Site of Urinary Tract Infection. *Lancet,* 2:427, 1967.

Gutman, L. T., Schaller, J., and Wedgewood, R. J.: Bacterial L-Forms in Relapsing Urinary Tract Infection. *Lancet,* 1:464, 1967.

Hinman, F., and Hutch, J. A.: Atrophic Pyelonephritis from Ureteral Reflux Without Obstructive Signs ("Reflux Pyelonephritis"). *J. Urol.,* 87:230, 1962.

Holland, N. H., and West, C. D.: Prevention of Recurrent Urinary Tract Infections in Girls. *Am. J. Dis. Child.,* 105:560, 1963.

Hutch, J. A., Miller, E. R., and Hinman, F., Jr.: Vesicoureteral Reflux. *Am. J. Med.,* 34:338, 1963.

Kass, E. H., and Ziai, M.: Methionine as a Urinary Tract Antiseptic. *Antibiotics Annual,* 1957-1958. New York, Medical Encyclopedia, Inc., 1958, p. 80.

Kunin, C. M.: A Guide to the Use of Antibiotics in Patients with Renal Disease. *Ann. Int. Med.,* 67:151, 1967.

Kunin, C. M., Southall, I., and Paquin, A. J.: Epidemiology of Urinary Tract Infections. *New England J. Med.,* 263:817, 1960.

Little, P. J., and de Wardener, J. E.: Acute Pyelonephritis — Incidence of Reinfection in One Hundred Patients. *Lancet,* 2:1277, 1966.

MacDonald, R. A., Levitin, H., Mallory, K., and Kass, E. H.: Relation Between Pyelonephritis and Bacterial Counts in the Urine. *New England J. Med.,* 256:915, 1957.

Murphy, J. J., Schöenberg, H. W., and Tristan, T. A.: Diagnoses and Management of Lower Urinary Tract Dysfunction in Children. *J. Urol.,* 89:192, 1963.

Neter, E., Steinhart, J., Calcagno, P. L., and Rubin, M. I.: Urinary Tract Infection in Children. I. Studies on Antibody Response; in E. H. Kass (Ed.): *International Symposium on Pyelonephritis: Progress in Pyelonephritis.* Philadelphia, F. A. Davis Company, 1965.

Neumann, C. G., and Pryles, C. V.: Pyelonephritis in Infants and Children. *Am. J. Dis. Child.,* 104:215, 1962.

North, A. F., Jr.: Bacteriuria in Children with Acute Febrile Illness. *J. Pediat.,* 63:408, 1963.

Pryles, C. V., and Eliot, C. R.: Pyuria and Bacteriuria in Infants and Children. *Am. J. Dis. Child.,* 110:628, 1965.

Rubin, M. I.: Pyelonephritis: Certain Aspects. *Pediat. Clin. N. Amer.,* 11:649, 1964.

Stamey, T. A., and Pfau, A.: Some Functional, Pathologic, Bacteriologic, and Chemotherapeutic Characteristics of Unilateral Pyelonephritis in Man. II. Bacteriologic and Chemotherapeutic Characteristics. *Invest. Urol.,* 1:162, 1963.

Steele, R. E., Leadbetter, G. W., and Crawford, J. D.: Prognosis of Childhood Urinary Tract Infection. *New England J. Med.,* 269:883, 1963.

Still, J. L., and Cottom, D.: Severe Hypertension in Childhood. *Arch. Dis.,* 42:34, 1967.

Turck, M.: Broad Spectrum Penicillin and Other Antibiotics in the Treatment of Urinary Tract Infections. *Ann. New York Acad. Sc.,* 145:344, 1967.

Waterhouse, K., and Hamm, F. C.: The Importance of Urethral Valves as a Cause of Vesical Neck Obstruction in Children. *Tr. Am. A. Genito-Urinary Surgeons,* 53:138, 1961.

Winberg, J.: Renal Function Studies in Infants and Children with Acute Nonobstructive Urinary Tract Infections. *Acta Paediat.,* 44:577, 1959.

DISTURBANCES OF THE KIDNEY

NEPHRITIS

ACUTE GLOMERULONEPHRITIS

Acute glomerulonephritis is a disease largely of childhood and is the most common form of nephritis in children. Its true incidence is not known, since many of the milder cases are unrecognized; it accounts for about 0.5 per cent of hospital admissions. It is uncommon under 3 years of age, but it has been observed in the neonatal period and as a congenital lesion. It seems to be more common in boys than in girls.

Etiology.   Acute glomerulonephritis appears to be an antigen-antibody reaction secondary to an infection elsewhere in the body. The typical reduction in serum complement level and the precipitation of antibody globulins and components of complement on the glomerular basement membrane support this assumption. As in rheumatic fever, the initiating infection is most often in the upper respiratory tract and most often caused by a group A beta hemolytic streptococcus. Streptococcal skin infections are also common precipitants. Beta hemolytic streptococci can be cultured from the nose and throat or the skin in most patients with acute glomerulonephritis who have not been treated with an antibacterial agent effective against this organism. The rise in ASO antibody titer, which is sometimes not more than 100 units, is found in over 80 per cent of cases. When examination is made for two or more of the antistreptococcal antibodies, the percentage of cases showing evidence of recent streptococcal infection approaches 95 per cent. For example, the antistreptokinase titer may be elevated without a rise in ASO titer. Elevation of the ASO titer may persist for several months. Type-specific antibody to the cellular antigen develops more slowly and persists for years. Early penicillin therapy inhibits the development of ASO titer and of type-specific antibody; inhibition of the latter might theoretically increase the risk of a subsequent infection with the same nephritogenic strain. It may be this latter antibody which determines the rarity of second attacks of acute glomerulonephritis.

Not all strains of streptococci are nephritogenic; type 12 appears to be the most common of the nephritogenic strains; types 4, 25, and 45 are somewhat less common. Moreover, the rate of renal involvement in infections with the so-called nephritogenic strains appears to vary in different epidemics. Nephritis occurs in about 1 per cent of cases of scarlet fever, the incidence varying widely in different epidemics, up to 18 per cent. Other organisms such as the pneumococcus, staphylococcus and viridans strains of the streptococcus have also been thought to be infrequent causative agents; a viral origin has also been suggested.

The serum complement level is almost always low in acute glomerulonephritis (now usually measured as β_{1C} globulin) and is presumably bound to antigen-antibody complexes. The complement level usually returns to normal by the end of the third week of illness. Persistence of lowered complement levels is associated with continued renal disease (hypocomplementemic persistent glomerulonephritis).

Focal nonsuppurative glomerulonephritis may occur at the height of a variety of infections. The proteinuria and hematuria in these conditions are usually transient. Transient mild hematuria has also been observed on the second or third day in 5 to 10 per cent of patients with acute streptococcal infections and occasionally with nonstreptococcal infections.

See also nephritis in anaphylactoid purpura (p. 522) and Focal Glomerulonephritis (p. 1133).

Pathology.   In acute glomerulonephritis the kidneys are slightly enlarged, pale, and dotted with small, punctate hemorrhages on the cortical and cut surfaces. The histologic changes vary considerably in degree and may be minimal.

The essential lesion is a proliferation and swelling of the endothelial cells of the glomerular capillary wall. All glomeruli are involved, but the intensity of proliferation varies among them. It is not always possible to correlate the clinical picture with the severity of renal changes. The glomerular tuft is swollen and fills Bowman's space. Erythrocytes may be found in large numbers in Bowman's space. Polymorphonuclear leukocytes appear in the glomeruli in varying numbers; within 2 or 3 weeks after the onset, however, while proliferation is still extensive, biopsy may show only an occasional polymorphonuclear leukocyte. The epithelial cells may be somewhat swollen, but appear otherwise normal. The glomerular capillaries appear compressed and devoid of blood. The intercapillary space is swollen, and there is an increase in the size and numbers of the mesangial cells in this space, which accounts for much of the cellularity of the glomerulus in this disease. There is an increase also in PAS-positive amorphous material in the intercapillary space, especially at the stalk. The basement membrane is usually normal. Occasionally epithelial crescents and adhesions between the tuft and Bowman's capsule may be seen as early as 2 to 3 weeks after the onset of the disease; they have been noted to disappear on serial biopsies, and therefore do not necessarily represent early chronic glomerulonephritis.

By immunofluorescent staining, deposits of β_{1C} and IgG globulin are found on the basement membrane in a characteristic granular or lumpy pattern. They correspond to the subepithelial electron-dense deposits observed in electron micrographs and are suggestive of the presence of antigen-antibody complexes on the glomerular capillaries. By immunofluorescent staining, fibrinogen deposits have also been demonstrated within the glomerulus. With regression of the proliferation in the glomerulus, these substances are no longer detectable.

The cells of the tubules are swollen and granular and contain hyalin and fatty droplets. Both red and white blood cells and casts are found in the tubular lumen. The interstitial tissues tend to be edematous and congested with a minimal amount of inflammatory cellular reaction.

By electron microscopy the predominant lesion is proliferation and swelling of the endothelial cells and hypercellularity of the glomeruli. The basement membrane of the glomerular capillary loops of unhyalinized glomeruli is not altered in early primary proliferative glomerular disease in adults (Jennings and Earle). Focal thickenings (deposits) are seen on the subepithelial side of the membrane (humps). The foot processes of the epithelial cells appear to be normal even in advanced lesions. In some instances leukocytic exudation in the glomerulus may be the predominant feature; this kind of reaction is more common in adults whose disease progresses toward chronicity.

When acute glomerulonephritis heals, there may be no residual evidence of the disease. Hypercellularity may persist for several months in some glomeruli, however, even when all evidences of clinical disease have disappeared.

In persistent glomerulonephritis the kidney is large and pale. Histologically, there is disappearance of some nephrons, whereas others have undergone a compensatory hypertrophy. The remaining glomeruli reveal changes similar to those described in acute glomerulonephritis, but often with more numerous capsular adhesions and with proliferation of the epithelial cells of the capsule which leads to the formation of epithelial crescents. Focal areas of lymphocytic infiltrate are present in the areas of atrophic renal parenchyma.

Though it is postulated that capillary damage in glomerulonephritis is not limited to the kidney, there is little anatomic or other evidence of it. In some organs other than the kidney small extravascular collections of red cells appear. Cerebral edema is present in some instances; its exact cause is not clear. It may depend on vascular injury, and it has been associated with a high venous pressure.

Clinical Manifestations. The onset of symptoms of glomerulonephritis occurs 1 to 3 weeks after the onset of streptococcal infection. There is great variability in the clinical patterns. The attack may be so mild as to be unnoticed, or may be detected only by repeated urinalyses after a streptococcal infection such as scarlet fever. At the other extreme the onset may be abrupt and severe, and there may be some or all of the following: high fever, severe headache, malaise, gross hematuria, oliguria or anuria, hypertension with encephalopathy, and severe circulatory congestion. Death may occur during such acute episodes. The clinical pattern of the average case is sufficiently characteristic to permit its description.

As a rule the child is not very ill. The most frequent presenting symptom is hematuria. The parents have usually forgotten the preceding acute respiratory infection, and its history is elicited only by questioning. At times the respiratory infection is still present when the hematuria appears. Puffiness about the eyes may antedate the onset of hematuria or appear with it. For the first few days the urine is grossly bloody, but usually not bright red (at times there is only microscopic hematuria). It then acquires a smoky, dirty, brownish hue. Edema may be generalized and influenced by posture. Severe edema is usually not seen in acute glomerulonephritis unless excess fluids have been given in the presence of oliguria or when there are associated manifestations of nephrosis. The temperature varies considerably; it may be as high as 103 to 104°F. for 3 to 5 days, then gradually falls to about 100°, fluctuating at this level for some days. At times there are such gastrointestinal symptoms as loss of appetite and

vomiting; less often, diarrhea. Some patients complain of headache.

On examination little may be found other than a residual upper respiratory tract infection or slight puffiness about the eyes. Varying degrees of hypertension may be present. When the blood pressure is elevated, the pulse rate is slow if the cardiac action is good. The urine is usually decreased in amount, of a high specific gravity, and contains protein, varying amounts of red blood cells, some white blood cells, and hyaline, granular and cellular casts (principally red cells). The levels of blood urea nitrogen and of all other waste products excreted by way of the kidney are usually elevated, in inverse relation to the urinary volume. There is acidosis, the severity of which is directly related to the degree of oliguria.

There is often a slight decrease in the levels of serum albumin, probably largely the result of expanded extracellular fluids. In some cases a large urinary loss of protein can be an additive factor. Anemia tends to develop quickly, also related to the expended plasma volume; urinary blood loss is probably not a significant factor. The anemia differs from that seen in chronic glomerulonephritis, in which hemolysis and inadequate red cell production are major factors. The erythrocyte sedimentation rate is usually elevated. In some patients the serum cholesterol level is slightly elevated, most often in patients with greater than usual falls in levels of serum protein, in which case there may be rather extensive edema, and the clinical pattern resembles that of nephrosis. The clinical course in these latter patients, however, may be otherwise that of uncomplicated, acute glomerulonephritis.

Some abnormality can often be detected on serial electrocardiograms. The cause is not clear. Frequently the heart is enlarged, with roentgen evidences of pulmonary vascular congestion.

Improvement, manifest by abatement of the constitutional symptoms, usually begins within 1 to 2 weeks, and grossly visible blood disappears from the urine about this time. Diuresis usually commences after 3 or 4 days, and the patient may lose 5 to 7 pounds even though edema had not been clinically evident. There is a correlation between the onset of diuresis and the abatement of circulatory congestion. As a rule the blood pressure returns to normal after about a week, and the blood chemical findings during the second week.

Microscopically, the urine returns to normal in an average of about 6 weeks. Several urinalyses are needed to establish the cessation of active disease, since red blood cells may be absent and reappear subsequently. Occasionally, gross hematuria returns after having subsided for a few days. The Addis count usually shows abnormal numbers of red blood cells in the urine for about 4 to 8 months. Abnormal proteinuria often disappears before red cells. The urine may not be completely normal for a year or more.

The erythrocyte sedimentation rate can usually be used as an indicator of activity of the disease. It remains rapid in the average case for about 3 months. The prognostic value of the sedimentation rate depends on the fact that it remains rapid in patients whose disease persists, even though the Addis count may temporarily be normal. Occasionally the sedimentation rate returns to normal at the usual time and the Addis count remains abnormal; we have observed this sequence when renal biopsy revealed persistent glomerulonephritis.

Urinary findings. Urinary abnormalities (proteinuria, hematuria and casts) may be the only manifestation of acute disease in about 10 per cent of patients. The smoky brown discoloration is due to conversion of the hemoglobin to acid hematin. The specific gravity of the urine during the acute phase is usually high. Rarely, even early in the disease, if there is severe renal damage, the specific gravity of the urine may be low. In most instances the volume of urine is reduced, and in about 5 per cent of cases there is oliguria approximating anuria. There is no correlation between generalized vasospasm or arterial hypertension and the volume of urine or its specific gravity.

Though a definite diagnosis of glomerulonephritis cannot be made in the absence of hematuria, infrequently only a few red blood cells can be detected microscopically at any time in the course of the disease. In rare cases a normal urine is found in the presence of clinical manifestations and typical biopsy findings. Gross hematuria occurs in about half the cases. Freshly passed urine should be examined for both red blood cells and casts, since both may disappear when alkaline or dilute urine is allowed to stand. Red cell casts are a common and important diagnostic feature. White blood cells are increased in number; occasionally so many are present as to suggest pyelonephritis.

The amount of protein in the urine varies greatly (usually below 3 gm. per day) and is not correlated with the severity of the disease. The amount decreases as the renal process heals, and usually parallels the decrease in red blood cells (see above). Postural proteinuria may be present during recovery or in the chronic phase.

Hypertension. Hypertension of some degree is present in about 60 to 70 per cent of patients. The existence of a slight elevation may be appreciated only when the child is well and the pressure has returned to its normal level. Hypertension may appear at any time during the acute phase; systolic pressures may be as high as 200 mm. Hg, with diastolic pressures of 100 to 120. The rise may be sudden: e.g. from a normal level in the morning to high levels by afternoon. The drop may be just as precipitous. In most instances the hypertension is present during the first 4 or 5 days of the illness, slowly returning to normal levels by the end of the first week. In some cases, usually those with more extensive renal damage, the hypertension may persist for weeks; in progressive cases it may be permanent.

The mechanism of hypertension in acute glomerulonephritis is considered to be generalized vasospasm, possibly resulting from the production of hypertensive agents by the kidney. Expansion of plasma volume may also be causative.

Hypertension is directly correlated with cerebral symptoms (hypertensive encephalopathy), and it most often coexists with cardiovascular symptoms.

Cerebral symptoms. Cerebral symptoms appear after an acute rise in blood pressure in 2 to 10 per cent of patients and are probably due to cerebral ischemia resulting from vasospasm. Symptoms persist during hypertension and are chiefly headache, drowsiness, convulsions and vomiting. Restlessness, dimness of vision and diplopia may be associated. The pulse is slow. When the blood pressure is reduced (relaxation of the vasospasm), the cerebral symptoms disappear. There is no correlation between these episodes and the degree of renal impairment or water retention.

Cerebral edema may occur, but certainly is not the total or usual explanation for hypertensive encephalopathy, since measures which reduce the vasospasm result in disappearance of the cerebral symptoms, whereas diuretics which induce cerebral dehydration usually do not. The cerebrospinal fluid pressure is usually within normal limits, and there is no papilledema except in some cases with cerebral edema. Constriction of the retinal arteries is usually the only fundal finding in the acute phase; retinal hemorrhages and exudation are observed in chronic nephritis.

Episodes of hypertensive encephalopathy usually last a day or two and spontaneously end with the fall in blood pressure. Death may occur during the cerebral attack. Recovery under appropriate treatment is usually rapid and complete. Residual disturbances may occasionally result from prolonged anoxia.

Cardiovascular manifestations. Evidence of cardiovascular disturbance is present in many patients. In the early phase of the illness the clinical picture closely resembles that of congestive heart failure, with cardiac enlargement, systolic apical murmur, gallop rhythm, tachycardia, dyspnea, hepatic enlargement and pulmonary edema. These symptoms may appear suddenly, usually in the presence of hypertension, and may be the presenting symptoms of glomerulonephritis. Hypertension is not the sole cause of the cardiovascular symptoms, though it may contribute to the symptom complex.

These clinical manifestations have been considered to represent myocardial failure, but there is no clear evidence of severe myocardial damage in glomerulonephritis. The circulation time and oxygen extraction (arteriovenous oxygen difference) are not abnormal. Plasma volume is frequently increased, presumably as the result of retention of water and sodium. The symptoms of this hypervolemia are indistinguishable from those ascribed to noncardiac circulatory congestion. Evidence also suggests that peripheral venoconstriction is an added factor in the production of vascular congestion.

The pulse rate during the acute hypertensive

phase of glomerulonephritis tends to be relatively slow; a rapid rate is suggestive of cardiovascular decompensation.

The changes commonly seen in the electrocardiogram may be secondary to biochemical alterations. The most striking changes are observed in the T wave and consist chiefly in flattening or inversion in one or more leads, although a transient increased amplitude of the T wave occurs late in the acute phase and is often preceded, especially in leads I and II, by a slightly depressed, upward bowed segment. Transient inversion of the T wave occurs as frequently in lead III as in lead I.

In the acute phase of acute glomerulonephritis, and even without symptoms of cardiac decompensation, roentgenograms of the chest may show prominent pulmonary vasculature, pulmonary edema and pleural fluid, which reflect the vascular congestion of this disease.

The "cardiac" manifestations usually subside rapidly with the onset of diuresis and the fall in blood pressure.

Renal dysfunction. Renal function is impaired in most patients early in the disease; infrequently there is anuria. The glomerular filtration rate is generally somewhat reduced, and may be greatly reduced. The extent of reduction correlates poorly with the chances of ultimate recovery. The fall in urine volume is at least in part related to reduced filtration; evidence suggests that increased tubular reabsorption of filtered water may also contribute to oliguria and edema, glomerular function being disproportionately reduced in relation to tubular function. The greater impairment of glomerular function is consistent with the predominantly glomerular pathologic lesion. Circulatory and humoral factors may also be important in water and salt retention. In most instances the urinary volume may be used as a guide to overall renal function. The volume of urine cannot be used alone as a guide, however, for when concentrating capacity is lost, even early in nephritis, there may be a large volume of dilute urine. If the volume is not sharply reduced (with an adequate intake) and the specific gravity of the urine is within normal limits, there is no serious functional loss. Persistent oliguria not due to severe dehydration is an ominous sign and an indication of renal failure. Retention and elevation of the serum levels of nonprotein nitrogenous substances, phosphates, sulfates and potassium correlate with the degree of fall in glomerular filtration rate. Acidosis may result from a combination of factors: ketosis due to starvation, retention of metabolically produced H ions and loss of base. Dilutional hyponatremia (hypervolemia) may develop if fluids are not appropriately restricted in the presence of true oliguria (not due to dehydration).

Renal plasma flow as measured by para-aminohippurate may be normal, or even high. Thus the filtration fraction is almost always reduced. Tubular excretory capacity as measured by maximal excretion of para-aminohippurate is reduced in about 50 per cent of patients during the acute phase.

Recovery of renal function is gradual and usually occurs with clinical recovery, but may be somewhat delayed and return to normal only after several months. Rarely, progressive renal insufficiency may lead to death in the acute stage of the disease. Severe oliguria persists infrequently beyond 5 to 7 days, but may last 2 or 3 weeks or more, with complete recovery.

Diagnosis. In the usual case of acute glomerulonephritis there are no diagnostic difficulties; the coexistence of hematuria, proteinuria and slight edema, in the absence of circulatory congestion, establishes the diagnosis. In cases in which symptoms of vascular congestion occur early, they may dominate the picture so that initially the nephritis may not be suspected.

"Embolic" nephritis, which may strongly resemble acute glomerulonephritis may occur during bacteremia such as that of subacute bacterial endocarditis; it is transient and often disappears when the bloodstream becomes free of bacteria.

Transient hematuria during *acute pyelonephritis* may be a diagnostic problem; about 10 per cent of patients with acute urinary infections have gross hematuria. Large numbers of pus cells in the urine in comparison with red blood cells and bacteriuria aid in differentiation from glomerulonephritis.

It may be impossible initially to differentiate the hematuria, decreased urinary output and occasional azotemia resulting from *sulfonamide crystals*. The disappearance of the hematuria and other urinary symptoms within a day or two after withdrawal of the drug is strong evidence against glomerulonephritis. A clinical picture indistinguishable from glomerulonephritis is also occasionally seen in *sulfonamide "intoxication."* Other causes of hematuria such as *cystitis* (p. 1153), *scurvy, blood dyscrasias, calculi, diseases involving the renal vasculature, tumors and tuberculosis* of the urinary tract may also require differentiation. The urinary findings associated with the nephritis commonly seen in *anaphylactoid purpura* also require differentiation (p. 522). The *nephrotic syndrome* may have an onset with gross hematuria. In young adults benign and transitory hematuria, proteinuria and occasionally cylindruria may follow *vigorous exercise*.

An entity called *benign hematuria* is sometimes seen in children. There are usually no acute manifestations. The hematuria is usually microscopic, but at times may be gross. There are no evidences of renal dysfunction or of a hematologic disorder. Some renal biopsies have been reported as being normal, others to have glomerular changes consistent with acute glomerulonephritis or focal nephritis. It may be difficult to separate these 2 conditions except through prolonged observation.

If hematuria is sufficiently great (hematocrit of the urine greater than 2 per cent), the supernatant urine will contain an increased amount of protein. Trauma, foreign bodies, neoplasms and renal infarction must be excluded as causes for hematuria. These latter conditions do not produce casts.

At times acute *exacerbations of chronic glomerulonephritis* suggest acute glomerulonephritis. The history of illness, the evidences of advanced renal dysfunction, presence of severe anemia or growth failure, and renal biopsy will clarify the picture. *Acute tubular necrosis* may at times be difficult to distinguish from acute glomerulonephritis; it often follows prolonged hypotension, a transfusion reaction, sepsis, trauma, or exposure to nephrotoxic agents. Hematuria may be less striking, and there tend to be more casts than in acute glomerulonephritis. The specific gravity of the urine is usually high in acute glomerulonephritis and low in tubular necrosis; the sodium excretion is the reverse, high in tubular necrosis.

The *hemolytic uremic syndrome* may also be confused with acute glomerulonephritis. It is more commonly seen, however, in a younger age group (see p. 1133). *Hereditary nephritis, renal infarction, Zeeks angiitis* (diffuse), *lupus and focal nephritis* (see Index) must also be considered in differential diagnosis of acute glomerulonephritis.

In severe states of *dehydration* the concentrated urine often contains protein and hyaline casts, which tend to disappear quickly when the child is hydrated. *Febrile and other benign proteinurias* at times create diagnostic problems. Febrile proteinuria is usually recognized by its transitoriness. Since the erect posture may occasionally increase proteinuria in subacute or chronic glomerulonephritis and since the urine in *orthostatic proteinuria* may rarely contain a slightly increased number of red blood cells and casts, differential diagnosis may be difficult.

Course and Prognosis. In mild cases the entire course may extend for only 10 to 14 days. In general, the abnormalities of the urine as demonstrated by routine examination usually disappear within 6 or 8 weeks, and the erythrocyte sedimentation rate becomes normal in about 3 months, the Addis count in about 4 to 8 months. In protracted cases urinary changes may continue for a year, and rarely for a longer time, and still terminate in complete recovery.

Although the prognosis of acute glomerulonephritis is generally good, it is unpredictable in the individual case. Thus the mild case may progress to a subacute stage (see Chronic Glomerulonephritis, p. 1131), whereas a patient with fulminating symptoms at the onset with hypertensive encephalopathy, "cardiac failure" or renal shutdown may recover completely. There is, however, a positive correlation between the severity of the onset and the fatality rate during the acute stage. Death is usually the result of renal failure or cardiovascular congestion. Mortality rates during the acute phase have varied from 1 to 5 per cent. Since antibacterial therapy has been available the rates in most clinics have approached the lower figure. The incidence of progression to chronic nephritis is of about the same order, though rates as high as 5 to 10 per cent have been reported. Progression toward chronicity is char-

acterized by episodes of gross hematuria, often associated with acute respiratory infection.

Second attacks of glomerulonephritis are extremely rare. Recrudescence of the disease before healing is complete, however, is not uncommon in association with fresh respiratory infections, which need not be of streptococcal origin.

Treatment. *General measures*. No therapeutic measures have been shown to modify the inflammatory process in the glomeruli. The treatment is largely symptomatic, but should be based on recognized physiologic principles. The child should be confined to bed during the acute phase and until gross urinary changes subside. Ordinary activity after the first 2 or 3 weeks of the disease does not seem to affect the course adversely. Subsequently the child's urine should be closely watched, and he should be guarded against respiratory infection and overexertion.

Since positive nasopharyngeal cultures for streptococci are often found at the onset of clinical nephritis, full therapeutic doses of penicillin should be given for 10 days. Subsequently it may be desirable to maintain prophylaxis with penicillin, 250,000 units orally 3 times daily for 2 or 3 months, to lessen the chances of bacterial upper respiratory tract infections which might initiate an exacerbation of the nephritis.

During the oliguric phase, or with acute renal failure, the diet should be free of protein and potassium. Salt-free diets are not generally prescribed unless edema or vascular congestion is excessive, but during the acute phase, salt should not be added to the food. There is little evidence that the protein in the diet needs restriction, except during the height of the acute stage. There is no clear indication that adrenocortical steroids or ACTH is beneficial.

Surgical procedures should be restricted to those absolutely essential. Abscesses of the middle ear or in other locations should be drained, but tonsillectomy should not be performed during the first 2 or 3 months of the disease. If the operation is performed later, antibiotic therapy should precede and follow it by 2 or 3 days in an attempt to prevent bacterial spread. Nephritis of itself is not an indication for tonsillectomy.

Specific measures. FLUID BALANCE. The most critical stage of the disease is in the first few days. The immediate threats to life are the development of uremia, of vascular congestion with pulmonary edema or of hypertensive encephalopathy. Treatment is guided by urinary output, blood pressure determination, extent of edema, the status of the cardiovascular system, and by blood chemical values which indicate the severity of renal functional loss, such as blood urea nitrogen or creatinine levels, acidosis, hyperkalemia, hyponatremia, hyperphosphatemia and lowered blood hematocrit.

It is important to know the patient's urinary outputs at 8-hour intervals. This period is usually long enough to determine whether the patient has a sustained adequate output, and yet not so long as to endanger his condition from either severe fluid restriction or excessive intake of fluids. After the patient is weighed his need for water for the first 8 hours will be the estimated insensible water loss during this period; for an average 7-year-old child this will be about 400 to 500 ml. per day, or 130 to 165 ml. per 8 hours. At the end of this 8-hour period and for every 8 hours until it is clear that urine output is adequate, the fluid intake should be the estimated insensible water loss plus the urine output of the previous 8 hours. Even with this cautious regimen there is a greater danger of *overhydration*, with vascular congestion and pulmonary edema, than there is of dehydration. The child should be weighed daily. During the oliguric phase of illness a daily weight loss of about 100 to 150 gm. is desirable. A rising body weight represents water retention and the threat of intravascular expansion.

When severe vascular congestion leads to pulmonary edema, tachycardia, respiratory distress and hepatomegaly, peritoneal dialysis with a hypertonic concentration of glucose in the dializing fluid can rapidly remove water, potassium and urea, and aid in correcting hyponatremia, acidosis and hyperphosphatemia. Hypertension is also often reduced by dialysis.

When glomerular filtration is greatly reduced, diuretics are of little benefit in promoting the excretion of edema fluid. When severe pulmonary congestion exists, however, chlorothiazide or ethacrynic acid may be tried. These are potent natriuretic agents with low nephrotoxicity. Digitalization is ineffective in circulatory congestion unless there is myocardial insufficiency. When myocardial insufficiency is suspected, the possible beneficial effects of digitalis justify its use with an opiate.

HYPERTENSION. The blood pressure should be carefully determined at frequent intervals. A diastolic pressure of 100 mm. Hg or more is an indication for the administration of antihypertensive drugs. For patients with mild hypertension, reserpine in doses of 0.01 to 0.04 mg. per kg., up to 1.2 mg., may help reduce the pressure to normal levels. Hydralazine hydrochloride (Apresoline) in increasing doses may be added if needed. For patients severely hypertensive on admission a combination of reserpine and Apresoline has been found to be most effective. Reserpine may be given up to a dose of 0.07 mg. per kg. simultaneously with Apresoline, 0.1 mg. per kg. intramuscularly. This combined therapy has an effect within ½ hour which may persist for 12 or more hours; it may need to be repeated after 12 hours, but a single administration is adequate in the majority of instances. When hypertension has been relieved, the 2 drugs may be administered orally to forestall recurrence. At the prescribed dosage levels it is rarely necessary to give vasopressor drugs. Magnesium sulfate was widely used in the past to reduce hypertension in acute glomerulonephritis, but with these newer drugs available its use has been largely abandoned.

With reduction in blood pressure either spontaneously or through the use of antihypertensive drugs, cerebral symptoms of hypertensive encephalopathy usually abate quickly. Convulsions, however, may require administration of barbiturates or Dilantin, and oxygen therapy may also be indicated.

RENAL FAILURE. In correction of the biochemical imbalance resulting from renal insufficiency, the most urgent concern is hyperkalemia. Fluids and diet should be free of potassium, and release of potassium from cells should be minimized by provision of 100 to 150 gm. of glucose each day as hard candy, keeping in mind the need for fluid restriction. The electrocardiogram offers a rapid method for detection of hyperkalemic effects on the heart. Should the serum potassium concentration rise to levels above 6 mEq. per liter, a cation exchange resin, such as Kayexalate, is effective in binding potassium; it is given orally or by high retention enemas. The use of an osmotic cathartic such as sorbitol in conjunction with the resin is sometimes recommended, but this is rarely needed in children. Since the sodium exchange resin may in large quantities result in the administration of a large amount of sodium, use of a calcium exchange resin may at times be preferred. When there are conspicuous changes in the electrocardiogram with the risk of cardiac arrest, the rapid infusion of hypertonic glucose with insulin or of sodium bicarbonate solution may promote transfer of potassium into the cells. If the foregoing measures fail to control the level of blood potassium, then peritoneal dialysis should be utilized.

Because administration of alkali may aggravate water retention, it is well to disregard minor degrees of acidosis. Severe acidosis is best corrected by dialysis, which also corrects the hyperphosphatemia. If the blood calcium level is low, calcium should be given intravenously.

LUPUS NEPHRITIS

See Systemic Lupus Erythematosus (p. 519).

NEPHRITIS IN ANAPHYLACTOID PURPURA

See Schönlein-Henoch syndrome (p. 522).

PULMONARY HEMORRHAGE AND GLOMERULONEPHRITIS

See Goodpasture's syndrome (p. 530).

IRRADIATION NEPHRITIS

Acute and progressive glomerulonephritis may follow roentgen therapy of the abdominal area. The interval between irradiation and the manifestations of nephritis varies from a few weeks to several months. The prognosis is generally poor.

CHRONIC GLOMERULONEPHRITIS

The cause of chronic glomerulonephritis is much debated, but certain concepts seem to be reasonably well established. Whereas acute glomerulonephritis is much more common in children than in adults, the reverse is true for chronic nephritis. In children, progression of acute poststreptococcal glomerulonephritis to a chronic phase only rarely occurs; on the other hand, acute glomerulonephritis is more frequently followed by chronic nephritis in adults than it is in children. About 15 per cent of adult patients with chronic glomerulonephritis have a history indicative of acute glomerulonephritis (Relman). A latent period of varying duration is common between the acute disease and the chronic phase. In both children and adults chronic glomerulonephritis may be ushered in by a nephrotic syndrome without any antecedent acute episode. The majority of such patients have neither a past history nor immunologic evidence of acute glomerulonephritis. Chronic nephritis more commonly follows the nephritis of anaphylactoid purpura than that of the poststreptococcal disease. Hereditary nephritis is another important cause of chronic glomerulonephritis in children. Chronic nephritis may be a late manifestation of the nephrotic syndrome (see p. 1136).

Chronic glomerulonephritis may also occur as a complication of such diseases as the hemolytic-uremic syndrome, lupus erythematosus, periarteritis nodosa and amyloidosis.

Pathology. The pathology varies with the cause. The kidneys are usually reduced in size, with narrowing of the cortex, except in children with the nephrotic syndrome. In most of the glomeruli there are pathologic changes, varying from slight abnormalities to complete scarring. A reduction in total number of glomeruli suggests that some have disappeared completely. Endothelial proliferation with fibrosis and hyalinization of the glomerulus is common, as is epithelial proliferation with crescents and scars. There are mesangial thickening and cellularity, and localized thickenings of the basement membrane. Many tubules are atrophic or have disappeared; the remaining ones are often enlarged. Scar tissue replaces the areas from which nephrons have disappeared. The arterioles may be narrow, and the reduction in blood supply probably contributes to renal destruction.

Clinical Manifestations. The clinical expression of chronic glomerulonephritis varies from no obvious symptoms to those associated with severe renal failure and hypertension. When renal function is well maintained, the health status of the child may appear to be good, the only manifestations of the disease being reflected in the urinalysis and in the renal biopsy.

The disease is often accidentally discovered by routine urinalysis. In some patients fatigability and pallor may be the only manifestations.

Hypertension may be the presenting symptom. The symptoms of progressive renal failure may become more apparent during adolescence. In some patients the disease may be rapidly progressive, or there may be intervals of relative freedom from symptoms interrupted by acute exacerbations, the latter often closely following respiratory infections, streptococcal or viral. These exacerbations may result in transient or progressive functional deterioration. The child may look and act well when renal function has been reduced almost to the vanishing point, and the disease may not be recognized until renal failure is well advanced.

In the so-called dry type of chronic nephritis edema is not a striking feature, although it may be present more or less constantly about the eyes and ankles. In the nephrotic phase of chronic glomerulonephritis, edema may be severe, with reversal of the albumin-globulin ratio in the serum and elevation of the serum cholesterol level. Not infrequently during this phase of chronic glomerulonephritis there is a decrease in retention of nonprotein nitrogen and in the hypertension; hematuria may be inconstant. When chronic glomerulonephritis follows the nephrotic syndrome, the pattern of edema and proteinuria usually becomes less intense. When renal function is notably impaired, polyuria and low, fixed specific gravity of the urine become evident, and edema often is minimal. The patient may even become dehydrated and salt-depleted; when cardiac failure is associated with hypertension, the edema may return.

The urinary changes are extremely variable. Proteinuria is constant, but varies in amount. In the final stages, owing to the dilution of the urine, there may be only traces of protein. Hematuria also varies in degree, blood being present usually in only microscopic amounts and at times entirely absent. There may be gross hematuria during an acute exacerbation. Casts are found irregularly in the ordinary examination, but by the Addis technique they are consistently increased in number. Glycosuria and aminoaciduria are also occasionally present in the late phase. The creatinine and other clearances show gradual but progressive loss of function, which is also evidenced by the low, fixed specific gravity of the urine. As a consequence of the reduction in glomerular filtration, the blood urea nitrogen level is elevated, and there is usually an associated elevation of plasma phosphate, sulfate and often potassium. The plasma sodium and chloride are usually reduced, as is the pH, and acidosis may be severe.

Moderate hyperglycemia and a diabetic glucose tolerance curve are occasionally seen in azotemic renal failure, sometimes with low values for total exchangeable body potassium. When the total exchangeable body potassium is raised by oral potassium supplementation over a period of 10 to 14 days, the glucose tolerance test may return toward normal. With repletion of potassium the blood urea nitrogen level may fall, without a concomitant fall in the blood creatinine concentration; this suggests that there is no improvement in glomerular function.

Temporary improvement in chronic glomerulonephritis may seem to occur, but the course is progressively downward. Hypertension is usually present, with sudden elevations. Anemia is progressive and may be severe. Headache, lassitude and anorexia are common. There may be episodes of encephalopathy and cardiac failure; death may occur at such times. As the terminal stage is reached the child loses his appetite, complains of headaches and muscular cramps and may have convulsions, diarrhea and vomiting. Ulceration of the gastrointestinal tract may occur late in the disease. Arteriolar changes appear in the retinal vessels at this stage, resulting in hemorrhages and exudation, and edema of the optic disks. A tendency to skin and visceral hemorrhages is not uncommon in the uremic phase. These patients are highly susceptible to infection, which may precipitate uremic coma and death.

The anemia has both hemolytic and aregenerative elements. It is usually normocytic and normochromic and has been shown to result primarily from depression of erythropoiesis. Blood loss is usually not a significant factor unless there are gastrointestinal hemorrhages. The bleeding tendency is usually associated with normal or slightly reduced numbers of platelets, which are said to be functionally defective. Marked decrease in platelet factor III has been found in some patients. With sepsis other clotting defects may occur.

So-called renal rickets with osseous changes is less likely to occur in this form of chronic renal disease, but vitamin D resistance, stunting of growth, retention of phosphate and low blood calcium levels may be observed, in association with tetany.

Complement Levels in Chronic Glomerulonephritis. Under the terms "hypocomplementemic" and "normocomplementemic persistent (chronic) glomerulonephritis," West has suggested that chronic glomerulonephritis as generally seen in children can be divided into 2 categories, according to persistently low or persistently normal levels of serum β_{1C} globulin. There are relatively minor clinical differences in these 2 groups, but renal biopsies show distinctive differences. Most patients studied in both groups were thought initially to have acute glomerulonephritis, and in several there was elevation of the serum ASO titer. The patients with low β_{1C} levels had an onset more typical of acute nephritis. Those with normal β_{1C} levels were more frequently labeled as having the nephrotic syndrome at onset.

Pathologic findings were extensive proliferative changes in the glomerulus, often with lobulation of the glomerular tuft, with adhesions of the capillary tuft to Bowman's membrane, and at times with crescent formation. Sometimes the lesions resembled the chronic membranous glomerulonephritis more commonly found in adults. In the hypocomplementemic form a unique alteration is reported in the degree of argyrophilia of the capillary wall, resulting apparently from splitting of the basement membrane by nonargyrophilic

material. The glomerular tuft tended to be markedly lobulated, as in chronic lobular glomerulonephritis. In normocomplementemic patients, lobulation was not prominent, and the basement membrane, though thickened, remained argyrophilic. There were no other distinct clinical or laboratory differences between the 2 groups.

West suggests that hypocomplementemic disease is a progression from acute poststreptococcal glomerulonephritis, whereas a variety of separate disease entities may be represented in the normocomplementemic group. Biopsies in the latter group showed lesions in all stages of chronicity, as well as specific lesions of allergic angiitis, chronic focal nephritis and membranous glomerulonephritis.

Differential Diagnosis. The differential diagnosis from *congenital polycystic* and *hypoplastic kidneys* or *obstructive uropathy* may be difficult without urographic studies. Periarteritis nodosa, lupus erythematosus and other connective tissue diseases which involve the kidney may resemble chronic glomerulonephritis, as may the terminal phase of pyelonephritis. Postural proteinuria (see p. 1108) must be differentiated, even though there may be postural exaggeration of the proteinuria in glomerulonephritis.

Prognosis. The decrease in renal function may be slow, but the downward course is inevitable; in an occasional case progression downward is rapid, and death occurs from uremia within a few months. More often death takes place within 5 to 10 years.

Treatment. Though the downward course of the disease cannot be significantly altered by therapy, many children can have their lives prolonged and made happier by appropriate management. The child should be permitted to lead as normal a life as possible. Vigorous activity is known to produce renal ischemia and hematuria, proteinuria and cylindruria; it is therefore wise to restrict such activity. A healthy mental attitude toward his limitations should be established in the child; it is also important that the parents maintain as hopeful an attitude as possible in the face of the impending catastrophe.

Nutritional needs should be met. Reduction in protein intake to 0.5 gm. per kg. per day (proteins of high biologic value) may help to increase the intervals between required dialyses. An adequate caloric intake should be maintained. Salt restriction is indicated during a nephrotic phase, in the presence of edema due to congestive cardiac failure or when hypertension is severe. But hypochloremia and hyponatremia during nephritis may further depress renal function. During episodes of acute hypertension with impending cardiac failure and hypertensive encephalopathy, reserpine, alone or in appropriate combinations with hydralazine, may be tried. In persistent hypertension the combined use of antihypertensive and natriuretic drugs should be given a trial.

In the late stages of the disease, control of the hypertension is difficult; a variety of antihypertensive agents may be tried, such as guanethidine, methyldopa or ganglionic blocking agents such as hexamethonium or pentolinium, but the use of these drugs is limited by their adverse effects.

Digitalization is indicated when there is heart failure. In renal failure there is reduced renal excretion of digoxin, and the half-life of labeled digoxin is about doubled. Accordingly, smaller than usual doses will maintain digitalization during renal failure. Peritoneal dialysis recovers only small amounts of digitalis or its analogues.

Severe anemia requires transfusions for its correction. Hyperphosphatemia and hypocalcemia are treated with aluminum hydroxide gel and calcium lactate orally in amounts needed to correct the plasma values. Sedatives and anticonvulsant drugs may be needed in the late stages. Peritoneal dialysis, which can be repeated, may clear the uremic state and improve the biochemical aberration for a few days or weeks after its use. Periodic dialysis over prolonged periods is now used in preparation for renal transplantation. The interval between dialyses should not be prolonged until there are severe biochemical changes and a decompensated clinical status. Renal transplantation using appropriate donors is being increasingly used in advanced disease.

All drugs which are primarily excreted by the kidney should be given in reduced amounts in order to avoid toxic blood levels. For example, the serum half-life of penicillin G may be 15 to 20 times longer than normal in the oliguric patient. The half-life of erythromycin is 3 to 4 times normal, of tetracycline 10 or more times normal, and of kanamycin up to 20 to 25 times normal.

FOCAL GLOMERULONEPHRITIS

Periodic episodes of gross hematuria may be precipitated by an acute infection in children who have persistent microscopic hematuria, and varying amounts of proteinuria and cylindruria in the intervals between gross hematuria. They may for long periods have no evidences of renal functional impairment, appearing physically well, and may ultimately recover. In other instances a single episode of hematuria may be associated with infection and bacteriuria, as in bacterial endocarditis. The pathologic lesions found at biopsy in these patients, who are felt to have focal nephritis, vary from all normal glomeruli to mixtures of normal and pathologic glomeruli. The characteristic glomerular change is proliferation localized to a single lobule, usually at its periphery. Less commonly there is generalized proliferation of the entire glomerulus while other glomeruli still appear normal. This is unlike poststreptococcal glomerulonephritis, in which this irregularity in glomerular involvement is uncommon.

The prognosis is said to be good, few patients going on to chronic renal failure. On the other hand, the renal lesion is characteristically focal in Schönlein-Henoch purpura, in systemic lupus erythematosus and polyarteritis nodosa, at least in their early stages, and in angiitis and in Goodpasture's syndrome. In these conditions the renal lesion commonly progresses to chronic glomerulonephritis and renal failure.

HEREDITARY NEPHRITIS

Several syndromes have been described which are characterized by hematuria, proteinuria and casts, including red cell casts, and a renal lesion which is essentially that of glomerulonephritis. Hematuria varies from microscopic to gross, remissions are common, and exacerbations may be associated with infections.

The most common of these syndromes is designated as *Alport's syndrome*; this syndrome includes deafness and is transmitted as a sex-linked dominant. It is more severe and progressive in the male than in the female; in females it is often compatible with a normal life span. Most patients are discovered only when routine urinalysis discloses microscopic hematuria. Proteinuria may occur without hematuria. Many patients are first given a diagnosis of acute glomerulonephritis. In hereditary nephritis, however, the β_{1C} levels are normal.

Clues to the diagnosis are the demonstration of similar urinary findings in other members of the family, the history of similar illnesses in several generations, and the finding of high-tone nerve deafness in the patient or other family members. Deafness occurs especially in the male, but it is not always present and may exist without apparent renal involvement. Its detection may require audiometric studies. The nephritic lesion is slowly progressive; in the male renal failure and death often occur before the fourth decade of life.

In a second type of hereditary nephritis, very similar to Alport's syndrome, nerve deafness does not occur. In a third type there are congenital abnormalities of the eyes, including cataracts. In a fourth type there are congenital renal malformations, mental retardation, nerve deafness and hyperprolinemia (see p. 428).

In these conditions the microscopic pathology varies from essentially normal glomeruli and tubules to the classic lesions of chronic glomerulonephritis. Collections of "foam cells" in the interstitium are common.

THE HEMOLYTIC-UREMIC SYNDROME

This syndrome combines acute renal failure, severe hemolytic anemia, thrombocytopenia and changes in shape of red cells, which are often described as "burr cells." The disease affects primarily infants, but occurs in children and adults as well. The essential lesion involves the walls of the arterioles and glomerular capillaries, with secondary thrombosis, almost always fibrinoid in nature. The elementary lesion involves the endothelium, which is swollen and often layered, resembling an onion on cross section. There may also be subintimal fibrinoid necrosis, which may occupy only a portion of the vessel wall. The glomerular lesion is variable, with swelling of the capillary endothelium, dilated capillaries, fibrinoid thrombi, epithelial hypertrophy of the capillary tuft and Bowman's capsule, and sometimes complete hyalinization of the capillary tuft. Tubular cells are flattened or swollen and contain hyalin granules. There is no tubular necrosis. Interstitial edema occurs, and sometimes interstitial fibrosis. The vascular lesions and the fibrin thrombi strongly resemble the pathology of the Shwartzman phenomenon, now widely accepted to result from intravascular clotting.

The hemolytic-uremic syndrome has been described in association with renal cortical necrosis and with extrarenal vascular lesions. It is not clear whether cortical necrosis simply represents a more severe form of the disease.

Gianantonio has found that cases seem to appear in small "epidemics" in Argentina, with the lowest incidence during the South American summer months (January to March). He and his associates have isolated viral agents which may have some etiologic significance.

The onset of the disease resembles that of an infection of the respiratory tract in combination with gastrointestinal symptoms. There are coryza, slight fever, anorexia, vomiting and diarrhea, the stool often being watery and bloodstained. Abdominal pain, intense pallor, prostration and severe oliguria or anuria develop rapidly. The patient is restless, often stuporous, and may have convulsions. There may be cutaneous hemorrhages. The clinical manifestations of severe renal failure become apparent within the first days after onset of the illness, resulting in metabolic acidosis, severe azotemia, hyperkalemia and often hypertension. Anuria occurs in about half of the patients. The mortality rate is high, but can be considerably reduced by proper treatment. After a few days or weeks in surviving patients the diuretic phase gradually begins. Some of the surviving patients may have persistently abnormal urinary sediment and hypertension; serial biopsies reveal evidences of slowly progressive, chronic renal disease.

The hemolytic anemia develops rapidly, and the reticulocyte count and serum bilirubin level rise concomitantly. Anemia rapidly recurs after tranfusion, and hemolytic crises may occur for several days. Distorted and fragmented red cells are a striking feature of the blood smear. They may persist for some months in patients who have survived the acute disease. Thrombocytopenia is striking in most patients; in some the bleeding from the bowel may be severe. Purpura is not usually pronounced. Subdural and retinal hemorrhages may occur. There is usually a moderate leukocytosis; the Coombs test result is negative.

The urine contains protein and casts and is often grossly bloody, but the hematuria may be only microscopic. Hemoglobinuria may be present. Evidence of renal failure includes elevations of blood urea nitrogen, hyperkalemia, hyperphosphatemia and metabolic acidosis. With heavy proteinuria and markedly reduced serum protein levels the patients may show some manifestations of the nephrotic syndrome.

Cardiomegaly and circulatory congestion are common, and may be secondary to excessive administration of fluids and blood. Hypertension may be severe, and the picture may strongly suggest cardiac failure; as in acute glomerulonephritis, it is difficult to differentiate circulatory congestion due to hypervolemia from that due to myocardial failure. An occasional patient may have transient or even permanent evidence of central nervous system damage.

Treatment is symptomatic and includes that described for acute renal failure. Transfusions with packed red cells are needed to maintain a reasonable hemoglobin level; care should be taken not to overexpand the plasma volume. The transfusions may be given as small exchange transfusions. There is no clear evidence of benefit from the administration of adrenal corticosteroids. The use of heparin has been thought to be efficacious in some patients when a consumption coagulopathy has been demonstrated.

Thrombotic thrombocytopenic purpura resembles the hemolytic-uremic syndrome in some of its clinical and pathologic manifestations. There are hemolytic anemia, purpura, nausea and vomiting, muscular pains, and neurologic manifestations, including paresthesias, cranial nerve paralysis, hemiplegia and convulsions. The red cells have bizarre shapes, and there is a decrease in platelets. The fundamental morphologic lesion is the occlusion of arterioles by eosinophilic masses, previously thought to be platelet thrombi, but now shown by fluorescent antibody studies to be derived from fibrinogen or fibrin. The vascular changes are found in numerous organs besides the kidneys. Hematuria, proteinuria, cylindruria and nitrogen retention reflect the renal involvement. In most patients the disease is rapidly progressive to death within weeks of the onset. Treatment is as for the hemolytic-uremic syndrome.

VASCULAR NEPHRITIS
(ARTERIOLAR NEPHROSCLEROSIS)

This condition, common in adults, is rare in children, but may occur even in infants. There is arteriolosclerosis of the entire vascular system. Localized vascular involvement may also occur, resulting in focal scarring. The media of small arterioles are at first thickened and then become hyalinized, decreasing the diameter of the lumen. The renal vascular changes are similar to those in chronic pyelonephritis associated with longstanding hypertension. In the latter instance there may also be changes in the arterioles of other organs, but they are minimal. The differential diagnosis between so-called essential arteriosclerosis and severe hypertension secondary to pyelonephritis may be difficult and, at times, impossible except at autopsy or by renal biopsy. Glomerular sclerosis develops with advancing disease.

Renal impairment and hypertension are regularly present. Death usually results from cardiac failure, cerebral hemorrhage or uremia. There is slight to moderate proteinuria. Rarely, massive hematuria occurs, but hemorrhages from other organs, as from the gastrointestinal tract, may occur.

Cerebral symptoms often dominate the picture with headache, drowsiness and episodes of hypertensive encephalopathy, or signs of cerebral hemorrhage. Retinal changes are common and consist in constriction of the arterioles, hemorrhages, exudation, and choking of the disks. Vomiting and abdominal pain may be prominent features. The course of the disease is usually rapidly downward.

UNILATERAL RENAL DISEASE WITH HYPERTENSION

Goldblatt and others demonstrated that hypertension would result when the blood flow to one kidney was reduced by constriction of the renal artery. Butler demonstrated the reduction of hypertension in a child with unilateral pyelonephritis following nephrectomy.

The onset of this type of hypertension is characteristically abrupt in the adult, and the progression is rapid. In children, information concerning the onset is less well known, since blood pressures are not often recorded prior to the time when symptoms bring the patient for study. Headache is a common complaint and is usually associated with papilledema; in long-standing cases retinal exudate and hemorrhages may appear in children without any previous history of chronic renal disease. The frequency with which unilateral chronic pyelonephritis is the basis for the unilateral contracted kidney and hypertension is controversial. Habib feels that in most instances in which hypertension is associated with a unilateral small kidney, this kidney is a congenitally dysplastic one. Unilateral renal thrombosis with infarction, renal tumors and cysts may also be a basis for hypertension.

Hypertension may also be associated with abnormalities of the renal artery. Among the arterial lesions may be stenosis of the renal artery, aneurysm of it, or compression of it by a ganglioneuroma.

The mechanism of renal hypertension is related to the renin-angiotensin system. It is thought that a decrease in renal blood flow stimulates the juxtaglomerular apparatus to the elaboration of renin, which causes angiotensin I to be split from an alpha-2 globulin (a plasma substrate). In the presence of a "converting enzyme," angiotensin I is converted to angiotensin II, a powerful pressor substance which is thought also to be responsible for the release of aldosterone from the adrenal gland. Aldosterone increases the tubular reabsorption of sodium.

Several methods have been recommended for the detection of unilateral renal disease. Initially, one must exclude primary aldosteronism, pheochromocytoma, chronic nephritis and pyelonephritis with urinary obstruction. An intravenous pyelogram may demonstrate differences in function of both kidneys or a decrease in size of the affected kidney. The Howard test may be helpful if it reveals a decrease of approximately 50 per cent in water excretion and of 15 per cent in sodium concentration on the affected side. Stamey and others have recommended the inulin or creatinine U/P ratio as a means for estimating the increased tubular reabsorption of water in the involved kidney. They used infusions of urea and other substances to amplify the differences in total water reabsorption between the ischemic and the normal or less ischemic kidney. The radioactive renogram described by Winter is also a useful diagnostic tool. Most observers, however, consider the aortogram, showing the renal arteries and their branches, to be the most helpful single test. Renin values may be determined in peripheral venous blood and in the blood of each renal vein. A differential elevation of values may have diagnostic significance.

Emphasis has been placed on surgical correction of the renal artery anomalies, when possible, rather than on nephrectomy; this has been accomplished by grafts, endarterectomy or splenorenal arterial anastomosis. Nephrectomy is obviously contraindicated if there is advanced functional damage of the opposite kidney; minimal impairment of it is not a contraindication to removal of an ischemic kidney when repair of the arterial supply is not possible. With mild hypertension due to unilateral renal vascular disease it may be reasonable to attempt management with an antihypertensive agent, owing to the risks of surgery; if the blood pressure cannot be controlled, surgery may then be indicated. Even after several years of persistent hypertension, relief may be obtained by operation. In most instances, blood pressure falls rapidly to normal within a few hours after operation, but the fall may be delayed for several months.

REFERENCES

Ammuann, P., and Rossi, E.: Allergic Hematuria. *Arch. Dis. Childhood*, 41:539, 1966.

Barry, K. G., Schwartz, F. D., Hano, J. E., Schrier, R. W., and Canfield, C.: Peritoneal Dialysis: Current Applications and Recent Developments; in *Proceedings of 3rd International Congress of Nephrology*, Washington, D.C. New York, S. Karger, 1967, p. 288.

Bernstein, S. H., and Stillerman, M.: A Study of the Association of Group A. Streptococci with Acute Glomerulonephritis. *Ann. Int. Med.*, 52:1026, 1960.

Doherty, J. E., Perkins, W. H., and Wilson, M. C.: Studies with Tritiated Digoxin in Renal Failure. *Am. J. Med.*, 37:536, 1964.

Earle, D. P., and Jennings, R. B.: Glomerulonephritis; in *Proceedings of Third International Congress of Nephrology*, Washington, 1966. 3:51, New York, S. Karger, 1967, p. 51.

Eichna, L. W.: Circulatory Congestion and Heart Failure. *Circulation*, 22:864, 1960.

Eisenberg, S.: Blood Volume in Patients with Acute Glomerulonephritis as Determined by Radioactive Chromium Tagged Red Cells. *Am. J. Med.*, 27:241, 1959.

Etteldorf, J. N., Smith, J. D., and Johnson, C.: The Effect of Reserpine and Its Combination with Hydralazine on Blood Pressure and Renal Hemodynamics During the Hypertensive Phase of Acute Nephritis in Children. *J. Pediat.*, 48:129, 1956.

Fleisher, D. S., and others: Hemodynamic Findings in Glomerulonephritis. *J. Pediat.*, 69:1054, 1966.

Goldman, R., and Haberfelde, G. C.: Hereditary Nephritis; Report of a Kindred. *New England J. Med.*, 261:734, 1959.

Hume, D. M., and others: Experiences with 108 Consecutive Non-Twin Renal Homotransplants in Man; in *Proceedings of 3rd International Congress of Nephrology*, Washington, 1966. New York, S. Karger, 1967, p. 351.

Jennings, R. B., and Earle, D. P.: Post-Streptococcal Glomerulonephritis: Histopathologic and Clinical Studies of the Acute, Subsiding Acute and Early Chronic Latent Phases. *J. Clin. Invest.*, 40:1525, 1961.

Kark, R. M.: Renal Biopsy and Prognosis. *Ann. Rev. Med.*, 18:269, 1967.

Kirkpatrick, J. A., and Fleisher, D. S.: The Roentgen Appearance of the Chest in Acute Glomerulonephritis in Children. *J. Pediat.*, 64:492, 1964.

Kolff, W. J., and Nakamoto, S.: Progress in Dialysis; in *Proceedings of 3rd International Congress of Nephrology*, Washington, 1966. New York, S. Karger, 1967, p. 274.

Large, J. P., Lange, R. D., and Moore, C. V.: Characterization of the Anemia Associated with Chronic Renal Insufficiency. *Am. J. Med.*, 24:4, 1958.

Lerner, R. A., Glassock, R. J., and Dixon, F. J.: The Role of Anti-Glomerular Basement Membrane Antibody in the Pathogenesis of Human Glomerulonephritis. *J. Exper. Med.*, 126:989, 1967.

McCluskey, R. T., and Baldwin, D. S.: Natural History of Acute Glomerulonephritis. *Am. J. Med.*, 35:213, 1963.

McCrory, W. W., Fleisher, D. S., and Sohn, W. B.: Effects of Early Ambulation on the Course of Nephritis in Children. *Pediatrics*, 24:395, 1959.

Metcoff, J. (Ed.): *Acute Glomerulonephritis.* Proceedings of 17th Annual Conference on the Kidney. National Kidney Foundation. Boston, Little, Brown and Co., 1967.

Michael, A. F., Drummond, K. N., Good, R. A., and Vernier, R. L.: Acute Poststreptococcal Glomerulonephritis: Immune Deposit Disease. *J. Clin. Invest.*, 45:237, 1966.

Spergel, G., and others: The Effect of Potassium in the Impaired Glucose Tolerance in Chronic Uremia. *Metabolism*, 16:581, 1967.

Stetson, C. A., Rammelkamp, C. H., Jr., Krauss, R. M., Kohen, R. J., and Perry, W. D.: Epidemic Acute Nephritis: Studies on Etiology, Natural History and Prevention. *Medicine*, 34:431, 1955.

Thomson, G. E., Waterhouse, K., McDonald, H. P., Jr., and Friedman, E. A.: Hemodialysis for Chronic Renal Failure. *Arch. Int. Med.*, 20:153, 1967.

West, C. D., Northway, J. D., and Davis, N. C.: Serum Levels of Beta 1_C Globulin, a Complement Component in the Nephritides. *J. Clin. Invest.*, 43:1507, 1964.

West, C. D., Holland, N. H., McConville, J. M., and McAdams, A. J.: Immunosuppressive Therapy in Persistent Hypocomplementemic Glomerulonephritis. *J. Pediat.*, 67:1113, 1965.

West, C. D., McAdams, A. G., McConville, J. M., Davis, N. C., and Holland, N. H.: Hypocomplementemic and Normocomplementemic Persistent (Chronic) Glomerulonephritis. *J. Pediat.*, 67:1089, 1965.

Wilson, S. G., and Heymann, W.: Acute Glomerulonephritis with the Nephrotic Syndrome. *Pediatrics*, 23:874, 1959.

Focal Nephritis

Ayoub, E. M., and Vernier, R. L.: Benign Recurrent Hematuria. *Am. J. Dis. Child.*, 109:217, 1965.

Bodian, M., Black, J. A., Kobayashi, N., Lake, B. D., and Shuler, S. E.: Recurrent Haematuria in Childhood. *Quart. J. Med.*, 34:359, 1965.

Ferris, T. F., Gorden, P., Kashgarian, M., and Epstein, F. H.: Recurrent Hematuria and Focal Nephritis. *New England J. Med.*, 276:770, 1967.

Familial Nephritis

Alport, A. C.: Hereditary Familial Congenital Nephritis. *Brit. Med. J.*, 1:504, 1927.

Schafer, I. A., Scriver, C. R., and Efron, M. L.: Familial Hyperprolinemia, Cerebral Dysfunction and Renal Anomalies Occurring in a Family with Hereditary Nephropathy and Deafness. *New England J. Med.*, 267:51, 1962.

Williamson, D. A. J.: Alport's Syndrome of Hereditary Nephritis with Deafness. *Lancet*, 2:1321, 1961.

Hemolytic Uremic Syndrome

Gianantonio, C. A., Vitacco, M., and Mendilaharzu, F.: The Hemolytic-Uremic Syndrome; in *Proceedings of 3rd International Congress of Nephrology*, Washington, 1966. New York, S. Karger, 1967, pp. 24-36.

Gianantonio, C., Vitacco, M., Mendilaharzu, F., Rutty, A., and Mendilaharzu, J.: The Hemolytic-Uremic Syndrome. *J. Pediat.*, 64:478, 1964.

Habib, R., Mathieu, H., and Royer, P.: Le syndrome hémolytique et urémique de l'enfant. *Nephron*, 4:139, 1967.

Shumway, C. N., and Miller, G.: An Unusual Syndrome of Hemolytic Anemia, Thrombocytopenic Purpura and Renal Disease. *Blood*, 12:1045, 1957.

Unilateral Kidney Disease

Duffie, E. R., Jr., and Holliday, M. A.: Hypertension and Renal Disease. *Pediat. Clin. N. Amer.*, 11:723, 1964.

Goldblatt, H., Lynch, G., Hauzal, R. F., and Summerville, W. W.: Studies on Experimental Hypertension. 1. The Production of Persistent Elevation of Systolic Blood Pressure by Means of Renal Ischemia. *J. Exper. Med.*, 59:347, 1934.

Maxwell, M. H.: Renal Arterial Hypertension, Clinical Features, Diagnostic Tests, Results of Surgery; in *Proceedings of 3rd International Congress of Nephrology*, Washington, 1966. New York, S. Karger, 1967, p. 131.

Peart, W. S.: Pressor Assays in the Evaluation of Renal Hypertension; in *Proceedings of 3rd International Congress of Nephrology*, Washington, 1966. New York, S. Karger, 1967, p. 140.

Stamey, T. A., Nudelman, I. J., Good, P. H., Schwentker, F. N., and Hendricks, F.: Functional Characteristics of Renovascular Hypertension. *Medicine*, 40:347, 1961.

Still, J. L., and Cottom, D.: Severe Hypertension in Childhood. *Arch. Dis.*, 42:34, 1967.

NEPHROTIC SYNDROME
(NEPHROSIS)

The term "nephrotic syndrome" has been used for a symptom complex with varied clinical and pathologic manifestations, variable prognosis and variable responses to therapeutic agents, particularly to the adrenocortical steroids. From data obtained from renal biopsies and from immunologic studies a number of different entities responsible for the nephrotic syndrome have been defined. Unfortunately, such separation cannot often be made on clinical grounds early in the disease. Each of the various types of nephrosis is characterized early by edema, heavy proteinuria, striking hypoalbuminemia and hypercholesterolemia. All types may have hematuria, hypertension and azotemia. In so-called lipoid nephrosis (minimal disease) hematuria, hypertension and azotemia are often absent or, if present, usually minimal and transient. In the other forms of nephrosis, hematuria is usually more striking and persistent, and azotemia and hypertension may or may not appear early. In lipoid nephrosis, light microscopy generally reveals essentially normal glomeruli, whereas distinct pathologic lesions of the glomeruli occur early in the second group, and often resemble focal or chronic glomerulonephritis.

The nephrotic syndrome is said to afflict each year about 7 children per 100,000 population under the age of 9 years. It is estimated that there are 14 active cases per 100,000 children in this age group. The so-called minimal disease is primarily a disease of early childhood: the average age at onset is about 2½ years; it is uncommon in the first year. This form of the disease is also seen in adults. A nephrotic syndrome occasionally seen in the neonatal period may be a different disease, as may be the nephrotic syndromes associated with acute glomerulonephritis in older children and with Schönlein-Henoch purpura, focal nephritis, lupus nephritis and various forms of chronic glomerulonephritis, including membranous nephritis.

Etiology. The cause of nephrosis as commonly seen in childhood is not known. Relatively rare instances of the nephrotic syndrome are associated with specific diseases such as syphilis, amyloid disease, diffuse angiitis, thrombosis of the renal vein, disseminated lupus erythematosus, diabetes mellitus and chronic glomerulonephritis and with poison oak dermatitis, bee sting and nephrotoxic agents such as trimethadione, paradione, penicillamine, gold salts and mercury.

In most instances it is not possible to relate the onset of nephrosis to another disturbance. Sometimes an upper respiratory tract infection precedes it. Recurrences and exacerbations, however, are often associated with acute respiratory infections.

It is now generally held that lipoid nephrosis is not a stage of acute glomerulonephritis. Its pathology is strikingly different from the proliferative glomerular lesions of acute glomerulonephritis. Occasionally, however, patients with urinary and blood chemical findings of acute glomerulonephritis will have excessive edema, heavier than usual proteinuria, greater than usual reduction in serum albumin and moderate elevation of serum cholesterol. Such children generally follow the expected course of acute glomerulonephritis, with complete recovery.

Because lipoid nephrosis resembles a syndrome produced in rats by antikidney serum, it has been thought that nephrosis may be an autoimmune disease. Circulating antikidney antibodies have not been unequivocally demonstrated in patients. Improvement or induction of remission by the use of adrenocortical steroids and other immunosuppressive agents does not itself indicate that nephrosis has an immunologic origin.

Pathology. Renal biopsy studies in the nephrotic syndrome have demonstrated variations in the renal lesion which are not expressed clinically.

In the so-called lipoid nephrosis, which has also been called by some "foot-process" disease, by others "minimal change," the kidneys are large, edematous and pale, with a smooth, external surface and often flecks of lipid on the cut surface. With light microscopy and various staining techniques the glomeruli appear essentially normal. In an occasional patient mild endothelial and mesangial proliferation is seen. As the disease persists, with recurrent edema and proteinuria, the glomeruli may continue to appear normal for many years, possibly in part because steroid therapy may alter the pathologic process. Vernier, Worthen and Good suggest that in some patients, however, glomeruli are damaged progressively with increasing duration of the nephrotic syndrome, even in those who apparently recover. The progressive lesion with diffuse glomerular scarring and proliferation is more likely to occur in patients who fail to respond to therapy.

By electron microscopy there is fusion and swelling of the foot processes of the epithelial cells lining the basement membrane, in some but not all of the lobules of the capillary tuft, even in active disease. Since the epithelial changes are reversible when the proteinuria disappears, it is uncertain whether they are primary or secondary to the proteinuria; most investigators believe the latter. Minimal focal modeling and splitting of the basement membrane have been described by several investigators.

In "minimal" disease Drummond et al. found neither IgG or β_{1c} immunofluorescent globulin on the capillary wall by immunofluorescent technique.

In the early stage there are fine vacuolations in the tubular cells from fatty deposits and hyalin droplets, presumably reabsorbed protein. There is no atrophy, and casts are found in the collecting ducts. Tubular atrophy, interstitial edema with fibrosis, and collections of small round cells may be found in the progressive cases.

The second major category of patients with the nephrotic syndrome have been classified under the general term of chronic glomerulonephritis and further subdivided into (1) proliferative; (2) membranous; (3) membranoproliferative; (4) lobular; (5) chronic; and (6) focal.

The *proliferative* group may or may not represent a stage of poststreptococcal acute glomerulonephritis. It is in patients of this group, in whom the pathology differs little from that of chronic glomerulonephritis, that Drummond found globulin precipitates on the basement membrane. Proliferation, however, may be minimal and without globulin precipitates.

The *membranous* type is more common in adults than in children. In the early stages it may not be possible to distinguish the membranous type from lipoid nephrosis. With advancing disease, thickening of the basement membrane produces thickening of the capillary wall. There may be some focal thickening of the mesangium. As seen by electron microscopy, the foot processes are fused. Cellular proliferation of the glomerulus is characteristically absent. Immunofluorescent studies show that there is gamma globulin in the thickened capillary basement membranes.

In the *membranoproliferative* type, thickening of the membrane is associated with proliferative glomerulonephritis. This is the form of membranous disease we have seen more commonly in children. Whether this represents a different disease from the so-called membranous (adult) form is not clear. There is a patchy, tubular loss with vacuolization and hyalin deposits in the remaining tubules. With and without proliferation, large numbers of lipid-containing macrophages may be present in the interstitium. Such cells are actually present in many patients with the nephrotic syndrome, and resemble the foam cells seen in hereditary nephritis.

A *lobular* form has also been described by Habib; it is characterized by endocapillary and intercapillary proliferation, occasionally with the presence of polymorphonuclear cells. PAS-positive hyalin is precipitated within the lobule, giving the glomerular tuft a rather stiff, segmented appearance. It is generally believed, without convincing proof, that this condition begins as a poststreptococcal proliferative nephritis and is not a stage of membranous glomerulonephritis.

The pathologic lesion may be that of a *focal* glomerulonephritis, with proliferative changes occurring segmentally within an individual glomerulus. Some glomeruli appear to be entirely normal.

No extrarenal lesions have been discovered in childhood nephrosis except as complications, or when the nephrosis is a complication of some generalized disease.

The pathogenesis of edema in nephrosis is not entirely clear. The low intravascular osmotic pressure secondary to hypoproteinemia is an important factor. The loss of edema fluid when the serum albumin is still at a low level, however, suggests that some additional factor must operate in control of the edema. Luetscher demonstrated an increase in aldosterone in the urine of nephrotic patients during the edema phase and its return to normal levels after diuresis. The primary stimulus for the increased aldosterone secretion is thought to be a reduction in the plasma volume brought about by the lowered serum albumin (leakage of plasma water into the interstitial spaces). It is also postulated that hyponatremia, also a stimulus for aldosterone secretion, may result from increased production of antidiuretic hormone secondary to the reduction in plasma volume (increased water reabsorption by the tubules). During diuresis the excretion of sodium and chloride in the urine increases and may continue for some time after weight loss has ceased.

It is generally believed that the principal reduction in serum albumin is due primarily to urinary loss. Studies of Gitlin, however, suggest that there may be an associated increase in catabolism of serum albumin.

Clinical Manifestations. Edema is the usual presenting symptom, most often appearing between 2 and 4 years of age. At the onset the child rarely appears ill, except when an acute infection precipitates the attack. The development of severe generalized edema may be abrupt, but more often the edema initially is slight and inconstant, appearing only about the eyes and ankles. Finally, edema fluid accumulates in great quantity; in some instances the patient almost doubles his true weight. This phase may last several weeks to months. Characteristically, the course of nephrosis is one of recurrent accumulations of edema fluid after partial or complete remissions resulting from spontaneous or induced diuresis.

The urinary output in the early stages varies inversely with the edema. As the disease becomes well established, pallor develops, but may not be related to any significant degree of anemia. The appetite fails, lassitude and irritability generally develop, and malnutrition may become severe. During edematous phases the loss in body tissue is masked, only to become glaringly apparent when the edema is lost. The edema may become so extensive that it seems as if the skin would rupture; at such times, ascites is usually striking, and there may be bilateral hydrothorax. Intense edema of the scrotum is characteristic. The edema in the peripheral tissues is dependent and shifts with change in posture. In well established cases the peripheral edema may be minimal, with large accumulations of ascitic fluid. Diarrhea and vomiting are not uncommon during the periods of generalized edema; edema of the intestinal wall may be the factor in the intestinal disturbance. Under such circumstances there may be faulty intestinal absorption.

Most of the physical characteristics of the disease (respiratory distress, abdominal distention, dilatation of veins of the anterior abdominal wall and lower portion of the thorax, umbilical and inguinal hernias, rectal prolapse and decreased ambulation) are related to the extent of the edema. The liver is often moderately enlarged. In the absence of infection there is no fever; in fact, there may be no fever even with a severe infection.

Children with nephrosis are unusually susceptible to infection. Repeated acute upper respiratory tract infections with a variety of infectious agents, both bacterial and viral, often antedate a recurrence by a day or two. Clouding of the paranasal sinuses on roentgenography is probably more dependent on the edema of the mucous membrane than on the existence of bacterial infection. On rare occasions there has been complete recovery from nephrosis after an acute bacterial infection. Remissions following measles are common. Primary peritonitis, usually due to the pneumococcus, was formerly a common complication. With use of antibiotics this has become rare, but must be considered in patients with unexplained fever. Unsuspected sepsis may occur without fever in children receiving corticosteroid therapy, whose infection may be expressed only by a shocklike state.

Erysipeloid lesions occasionally occur on various

parts of the body, and consist of red, blotchy, tender patches, accompanied by fever and other signs of acute illness and often bacteremia. The urinary volume may sharply decrease at this time, and the edema becomes more extensive; on occasion, diuresis ensues.

Hematuria, azotemia and hypertension may be present in minimal degrees for a few weeks. Occasionally, gross hematuria occurs at the onset and suggests acute glomerulonephritis. At present there is little basis on which to separate the patients with such findings from those without them, since the clinical courses, the renal findings and the responses to therapy are often similar.

When the nephrotic syndrome is associated with the various forms of glomerulonephritis, it is usually in older children (5 years and above). Hematuria is usually more striking and persistent, but rarely gross, except in those with focal glomerular lesions. Hypertension and evidences of glomerular failure with azotemia and acidosis tend to occur late and are progressive. In the early stages, however, the clinical picture most often cannot be differentiated from that of lipoid nephrosis. The differentiation of these various categories of disease early in their course can often be made only by renal biopsy.

Xanthomatous lesions may be associated with high (total) blood lipid and cholesterol levels. The basal metabolic rate is usually within the normal range if correction is made for the overweight due to the edema fluid.

Laboratory Data. The most important laboratory finding is proteinuria, which usually consists mainly of albumin. Heymann noted that the excretion of globulin exceeded that of albumin in patients whose disease was progressive. The total daily urinary output of protein commonly ranges from 2 to 10 gm.; it may be higher. During the accumulation of edema fluid the urinary volume is reduced, and the specific gravity of the urine is high. Diuresis of large amounts of urine accompanies disappearance of the edema. Hyaline, granular and cellular casts are found in large numbers, and many contain doubly refractile lipoid bodies. These lipoid bodies are also found free in the urine. There may be some increase in leukocytes. Neither the presence nor the absence of a small number of red blood cells early in the course of the disease seems to have prognostic significance. The development of persistent hematuria, however, is a more serious prognostic omen. There may also be transient and moderate nitrogen retention; it does not necessarily indicate progressive renal failure. There is little tendency toward acidosis in the early stage of the disease. In the "non-nephritic" phase renal function tests, such as measurements of the glomerular filtration rate and renal plasma flow, often reveal normal and even elevated capacities; maximal concentrating ability and acidification of the urine are maintained. With progressive glomerular involvement in the "nephritic" phase there is progressively decreasing function.

The characteristic changes in the blood are a lowering of the serum albumin sufficient to produce a reversal of the albumin-globulin ratio and an increase in the blood lipids, particularly in the cholesterol fraction, with levels of 300 to 1800 mg. per 100 ml. The ratio of free to esterified cholesterol is unaffected. There is an increase in the ratio of total cholesterol to phospholipids, the greatest increase occurring in the fraction of cholesterol bound to beta-lipoprotein.

The hyperlipemia is thought to result essentially from an endogenous metabolic error. It is not affected by a diet low in exogenous lipids. Hypoproteinemia was long thought the basis for the hyperlipemia, but in the experimental animal hyperlipemia precedes hypoproteinemia. It has been suggested that the urinary loss of albumin and of a heparin-like clearing substance (for lipids) could be causative, and further that the low concentration of plasma albumin causes an increased synthesis of low-density or lipid-rich beta lipoproteins and a decreased rate of conversion to high-density beta lipoproteins. The relation of plasma albumin levels to the lipid level, however, is not clear. Hyperlipemia may persist long after the albumin concentration has returned to normal.

The major reduction in serum protein is in the albumin fraction; edema develops at levels of about 2.5 gm. per 100 ml. In most cases the albumin is reduced below 1 gm. per 100 ml. These low levels may persist even after edema has entirely disappeared, and then slowly rise as the disease process subsides. The total globulin fraction may be normal or slightly elevated; the gamma globulin fraction is reduced and the alpha-2 fraction increased. The fibrinogen is often increased. The plasma volume is reduced in most cases, but rises during diuresis.

The level of serum complement activity is usually normal and that of β_{1C}–β_{1A} is normal in lipoid nephrosis (minimal glomerular change); these levels may remain normal in this type even when there are progressive glomerular changes, focal or diffuse. On the other hand, West found a persistent reduction in serum β_{1C} in a small group of patients with clinical manifestations of the nephrotic syndrome with persistent glomerulonephritis.

Low levels of protein-bound iodine have been found in some patients without clinical signs of hypothyroidism, presumably owing to proteinuria; other factors may be operative.

A deficiency of coagulation factor IX was found in about 10 per cent of children with the nephrotic syndrome, in whom the abnormality was reversed by steroid therapy. In two of our patients this finding led to deferment of renal biopsy.

Slight or even severe secondary anemia may be present. The erythrocyte sedimentation rate is rapid. The serum calcium level is frequently reduced, primarily in the protein-bound fraction. Tetany is not common, but in chronic glomerular disease is an occasional complication. In advanced disease, glycosuria occasionally occurs without a coexisting hyperglycemia. Woolf and Giles found 2 patterns of aminoaciduria: one suggestive of a defect in renal tubular reabsorption and the other of a disturbance primarily in amino acid metabolism.

Severe skeletal changes, including rickets, seem to be restricted to patients with nephrotic syndrome who have severe glomerular or tubular insufficiency. Short-period balance studies suggest a resistance to vitamin D therapy similar to that seen in renal failure.

The ascitic fluid is nearly always opalescent, appearing like slightly soapy water. The protein content averages about 0.2 per cent.

Prognosis. The course of nephrosis is variable, but in general is characterized by recurrent episodes of edema of varying length. Though the untreated child is seldom completely free of edema during the active phase of the disease, he may appear to be so after rapid loss of large quantities of edema fluid. Even in cases which go on to recovery, proteinuria may persist for weeks or months, and the return of the other chemical changes to normal may be slow. The cholesterol level is usually the last blood abnormality to return to normal; it may remain elevated for months, and is an important index of persistent disease. The erythrocyte sedimentation rate usually remains rapid as long as the disease exists.

Mild hematuria and azotemia in the early stage of the disease do not in themselves indicate a grave prognosis. They may disappear, and the patient may eventually recover, or they may be an indication of progressive glomerulonephritis. Excessive or persistent hematuria is strongly suggestive of extensive or progressive glomerular damage and carries a more serious prognosis. Renal biopsies may aid in gauging prognosis.

Antibacterial therapy has greatly reduced the death rate from infection, but seems to have had little effect on the progression to glomerulonephritis.

Corticosteroid therapy has greatly influenced the course of the disease. Remissions in the clinical and biochemical aspects of the disease are induced in over 80 per cent of instances, and recurrences are considerably reduced. The renal lesion often fails to progress, and eventually, even after several years, clinical recovery may occur.

When the proteinuria is predominantly albumin ("selective"), the response to corticosteroids is usually good; it is less when the proteinuria is less "selective" and consists of increasing proportions of proteins of higher molecular weight, globulins.

There is increasing evidence that such immunosuppressive agents as the alkylating agent cyclophosphamide and the purine antagonist azathioprine may be effective in patients who are corticosteroid-resistant or corticosteroid-dependent. These drugs have been reported to reduce the frequency of recurrences and to improve the renal lesion. They are particularly helpful when the nephrotic syndrome is associated with various forms of glomerulonephritis in which corticosteroids have been ineffectual. Whether the ulti-

mate course of the disease is altered with these new agents cannot as yet be stated.

After effective antibacterial agents became available, and before the availability of corticosteroid therapy, recovery rates were estimated at 30 to 50 per cent. A collaborative study (Riley et al.) of approximately 800 patients over a period of 5 years indicated that the survival rate of patients with intensive steroid therapy was 75 per cent, whereas that of a control group was 60 per cent. Other studies have provided similar results. Owing to the long intervals between recurrences, up to 9 years in our experience, and with recovery occurring after many years of illness, final evaluation of these data must be deferred.

Treatment. Treatment aims at prevention and control of acute infections, establishment of good nutrition, readjustment of the disturbed metabolic processes, control of edema, control of progression of the renal lesion, and establishment of good mental hygiene. In view of the chronic and recurrent features of the disease, which cause great discouragement to both child and parents, time must be spent in acquainting the parents with the nature of the illness and the rationale of the therapy. The child should be kept in bed only during periods of severe edema or when other constitutional symptoms are present. Otherwise he should be out of bed and active, but should have adequate rest and be reasonably guarded against exposure to infection. On exposure to or in the presence of acute bacterial infections the patient should be treated promptly with appropriate therapy. Careful nursing attention is needed to protect the edematous skin from injury and subsequent secondary infection. The flagging appetite should be tempted with attractively prepared food which is easily handled by the disturbed gastrointestinal tract. The diet should be well balanced and contain an adequate amount of protein. In the presence of edema, salt should not be added to food during or after cooking. After diuresis, when hyponatremia may develop, administration of salt may be necessary.

Although edema is usually the symptom which calls attention to the disease and the outward expression which causes the greatest concern to parents, primary emphasis should not be placed on it, but rather on attempts to control the renal disease process.

Many regimens of corticosteroid therapy have been described, and several are currently used. Owing to a number of variables, it is not possible to evaluate them adequately from a comparative standpoint. The following represents the current practice in the author's clinic. Prednisone is the steroid most commonly used; it is prescribed in daily doses of 60 mg. per square meter of body surface per day up to 80 mg. per day, in 4 divided doses. This dose is given for 3 to 4 weeks, by which time there is usually a clinical remission with diuresis, disappearance of proteinuria and a restoration of the serum protein values to normal, with the serum cholesterol concentration approaching normal. Diuresis and reduction of proteinuria usually occur within 7 to 14 days; if a biochemical remission has not occurred by the end of 4 weeks, the dosage of prednisone may be increased to 70 or 80 mg. per square meter. It has been recommended that side effects of steroid therapy may be lessened when the steroids are administered on alternate days, double the above recommended dosage being given each alternate day as a single dose. Occasionally a remission is induced by daily treatment, when it is not by the alternate day program. Once an initial remission has occurred, various programs of steroid therapy may be used to maintain the remission. For maintenance therapy the daily dose of the steroid may be given on the first 3 days of each week, with none on the remaining 4 days, or may be given on alternate days as a single dose. If the patient remains in remission, this maintenance therapy is continued for a period of 2 months by some, for 6 months by others and for 12 months by still others. We prefer a 12-month maintenance period. If recurrence develops during this period of intermittent therapy or after its completion, a full course of continuous therapy is again instituted to produce a remission, after which the intermittent therapy is again given. The tendency to relapse is decreased with prolonged therapy. Rarely, corticotropin therapy, 2 units per kg. per day, appears to have been effective when corticosteroid therapy has failed.

Patients with the so-called minimal glomerular changes appear to have the best prospects for successful therapy. Those in whom the nephrotic syndrome is an aspect of glomerulonephritis tend to be less responsive to therapy and are more likely to become dependent upon prolonged steroid therapy to maintain remission. After numerous complete clinical and biochemical remissions, even those patients with minimal glomerular changes may ultimately become resistant, or may have only a partial remission, with persistent proteinuria as evidence of continuing disease.

Steroid therapy should be delayed until any existing infection is brought under control and any serious electrolyte imbalance is corrected. Severe hypertension is also a contraindication and should be controlled before steroid therapy is initiated. Hematuria, minimal azotemia and minimal hypertension are not contraindications. Complete clinical and biochemical remissions are less likely and complications of steroid therapy more likely in patients with evidences of advanced glomerular damage (thickening of basement membrane, endothelial changes and glomerular sclerosis). After months or years of persistent albuminuria, however, clinical recovery may result, either from treatment or spontaneously.

West first reported the greater frequency of induction of remission when hormone therapy was combined with mechlorethamine (HN-2), an immunosuppressive agent. Since then other immunosuppressive agents have been used, alone or in combination with steroids, to induce remission in patients who have not responded to steroid therapy alone or to prolong the interval between recurrences. Both the alkylating agent cyclophosphamide (Cytoxan) and the purine antagonist azathioprine (Immuran) have been used (Ettledorf et al.; Grupe and Heymann; Michael et al.; West et al.). These agents have also been used in patients for whom further steroid therapy was contraindicated because of hypercorticism as manifest by growth failure, hypertension, severe osteoporosis or glycosuria.

Heymann and Grupe recently observed that proteinuria which had appeared to be resistant to steroid therapy decreased or disappeared in a number of nephrotic children when the steroid therapy was discontinued. The drug had been discontinued with the intent of substituting immunosuppressive therapy. It would appear essential to defer immunosuppressive therapy in children whose proteinuria is apparently steroid-resistant until the effects of discontinuing the latter therapy have been ascertained.

The ultimate benefit from these immunosuppressive agents must await more prolonged observations. Nevertheless they have already added considerable benefit to immediate care. The development of leukopenia (bone marrow depression), though reversible, must be carefully observed when using these agents. The continued use of corticosteroids helps to maintain the level of circulating granulocytes against the dangerous complication of sepsis. Hemorrhagic cystitis and alopecia are complications of cyclophosphamide therapy.

Diuretics are useful adjuncts to therapy, especially early in the course of treatment, when steroids may actually aggravate the edema. The thiazide diuretics have been effective in inducing diuresis in most of these patients. Chlorothiazide is usually given orally in a dosage of 20 mg. per kg. per day in 2 divided doses. The associated loss of potassium, which may be further aggravated by the corticosteroid therapy, may result in potassium depletion. The simultaneous administration of an aldosterone antagonist, spironolactone (Aldactone), is often more effective than the thiazides alone. We have given spironolactone orally in a dosage of 60 mg. per square meter per day in 4 divided doses. When diuresis is not produced by these agents, ethacrynic acid may be effective. Its action may also be enhanced by the simultaneous use of spironolactone. Ethacrynic acid is first administered in a dosage of 25 mg., and the dose increased by 25 mg. twice a day; the maximal total daily dose for adults is said to be 200 mg. It may be effective given every other day. When these potent saluretic agents are used, it is important that the blood electrolytes be carefully observed so that severe depletion may be avoided. When the serum potassium concentration is greatly reduced, 2 to 4 gm. daily of potassium chloride may be given orally so long as there is an adequate urinary output (see p. 1144).

It is strongly recommended that mercurial diuretics not be given intravenously to patients with nephrosis; fatalities from such are reported.

Prior to the advent of steroids the intravenous administration of 20 to 50 gm. of concentrated salt-poor albumin per day was often used to induce diuresis. At best the effect was only temporary, owing to the rapidity with which it filtered through the kidney and was lost in the urine. In addition, the preparation is expensive. At present it is infrequently used; on occasion use may be justified as a temporary adjunctive agent to induce immediate diuresis.

Water restriction is of little value in limiting the accumulation of edema, and may actually be harmful. In the so-called steady state of edema, water restriction is often paralleled by decreased urinary output. Hypovolemia and its concomitant shocklike syndrome may exist in the presence of peripheral edema.

Significant elevation of the blood pressure is an indication for withdrawal of steroid therapy, if the hypertension cannot be controlled with antihypertensive drugs. Prophylactic administration of antibacterial agents is not recommended during steroid therapy, but the patient should be observed for evidences of masked infection. With combined steroid and immunosuppressive therapy the usual clinical indications of existing infection may be absent and often discovered only by bacterial cultures, and particularly by blood cultures. If a generalized infection is suspected, it is well first to obtain appropriate material for culture, then to treat vigorously with antibiotics appropriate for both gram-negative and gram-positive organisms until the laboratory report is available.

Signs of Cushing's disease usually do not appear during short courses of therapy. Any tendency to "moon facies" disappears after reduction or withdrawal of therapy. In patients on prolonged steroid therapy there may be growth failure and severe osteoporosis, with fractures of the vertebral bodies. This process is usually reversed with the cessation of steroid therapy. Transient glycosuria may occur. Other untoward features of steroid therapy include azotemia before the onset of diuresis, hypokalemic alkalosis with convulsions, atherosclerosis with central nervous system symptoms, pseudotumor cerebri with papilledema, headache, diplopia and other neurologic signs and convulsions even in the absence of hypertension.

In patients with large ascitic collections, peritoneal drainage may be necessary to relieve respiratory and cardiac distress or disturbances from pressure on the gastrointestinal tract. Such drainage is rarely required for patients receiving corticosteroid and diuretic therapy.

If urinary tract infection is suspected, appropriate cultures of the urine should be obtained. The diagnosis should not be based entirely on the finding in renal biopsy of focal interstitial cellular infiltration, since such findings occur in renal diseases in which infection does not exist.

For the treatment of advanced renal failure see therapy of chronic glomerulonephritis (p. 1132) and of renal failure (p. 1145).

INFANTILE NEPHROSIS

Two forms of nephrosis which occur in early infancy have been described, each of them characterized by resistance to corticosteroid therapy and an almost invariably fatal outcome.

The type described by Oliver as "infantile microcystic renal disease" has been found mostly in infants of Finnish extraction as a congenital nephrotic syndrome with an autosomal recessive mode of inheritance. Prematurity is said to be common. The renal lesion is characterized by dilatation of the proximal tubule, segmental atresia of the tubules, and increase in the size of the glomeruli, with distention of Bowman's space. There may be minimal proliferative changes, sometimes focal, sometimes resembling glomerulonephritis. In some cases the glomeruli are essentially normal. On electron microscopy the epithelial foot processes are characteristically fused as in other forms of the nephrotic syndrome, but the basement membrane is not thickened. A genetic abnormality in the permeability of the glomerular basement membrane has been postulated as a possible cause of this disorder.

Edema is usually evident in the neonatal period and may be present at birth. In the early stages the laboratory findings are similar to those of nephrosis in older children. The serum cholesterol level is usually not so high, and susceptibility to water and electrolyte imbalance and to infection is exaggerated. The disease proceeds rapidly to renal failure and death within the first year or two.

The second form of infantile nephrosis may also be manifest in the neonatal period; the clinical manifestations, biochemical alterations and renal lesions are similar to those in the nephrotic syndrome in older children. Microcysts are not seen. The clinical course is rapidly progressive, death from renal failure usually occurring within the first 2 years. Like microcystic disease, the process is unresponsive to corticosteroid therapy.

Renal vein thrombosis is not rare in the neonatal period, but rarely causes the nephrotic syndrome at this age. These conditions are more frequently associated in the adult.

Hereditary proteinuria and hypercholesterolemia without hypoproteinemia and edema have also been described; the fundamental defect in this disorder is not known.

REFERENCES

Arneil, G. C., and Lam, C. M.: Long-Term Assessment of Steroid Therapy in Childhood Nephrosis. *Lancet*, 2:819, 1966.

Calcagno, P. L., and Rubin, M. I.: Physiologic Considerations Concerning Corticosteroid Therapy and Complications in the Nephrotic Syndrome. *J. Pediat.*, 58:585, 1961.

Cameron, J. S., and White, R. H. R.: Selectivity of Proteinuria in Children with the Nephrotic Syndrome. *Lancet*, 1:463, 1965.

Cornfeld, D., and Schwartz, M. W.: Nephrosis. *J. Pediat.*, 68:507, 1966.

Churg, J., Grishman, M. D., Goldstein, M. H., Yunis, S. L., and

Porush, J. G.: Idiopathic Nephrotic Syndrome in Adults. *New England J. Med.*, 272:165, 1965.

Dixon, F. J.: The Pathogenesis of Immunologically Induced Nephritis; in *Proceedings of 3rd International Congress of Nephrology*, Washington, 1966. New York, S. Karger, 1967, Vol. 2, p. 97.

Dodge, W. F., and others: Percutaneous Renal Biopsy in Children. III. The Nephrotic Syndrome. *Pediatrics*, 30:459, 1962.

Drummond, K. N., Michael, A. F., Good, R. A., and Vernier, R. L.: The Nephrotic Syndrome of Childhood: Immunologic, Clinical and Pathologic Correlations. *J. Clin. Invest.*, 45:620, 1966.

Ettledorf, J. N., and others: Cyclophosphamide in the Treatment of Idiopathic Lipoid Nephrosis. *J. Pediat.*, 70:758, 1967.

Grupe, W. E., and Heymann, W.: Cytotoxic Drugs in Steroid Resistant Renal Disease. *Am. J. Dis. Child.*, 112:448, 1966.

Hallman, N., and Hjelt, L.: Congenital Nephrotic Syndrome. *Pediat.*, 55:152, 1959.

Handley, D. A., and Lawrence, J. R.: Factor-IX Deficiency in the Nephrotic Syndrome. *Lancet*, 1:1079, 1967.

Heyman, W., and Grupe, W. E.: Increase in Proteinuria Due to Steroid Medication in Chronic Renal Disease. *J. Pediat.*, 74: to be published.

Hoyer, J. R., Michael, A. F., Good, R. A., and Vernier, R. L.: The Nephrotic Syndrome of Infancy: Clinical, Morphologic and Immunologic Studies of Four Infants. *Pediatrics*, 40:233, 1967.

Jones, J. H., Peters, D. K., Morgan, D. B., Coles, G. A., and Mallick, N. P.: Observations on Calcium Metabolism in the Nephrotic Syndrome. *Quart. J. Med.*, 36:301, 1967.

Lerner, R. A., Glassock, R. J., and Dixon, F. J.: The Role of Antiglomerular Basement Membrane Antibody in the Pathogenesis of Human Glomerulonephritis. *J. Exper. Med.*, 126:989, 1967.

McCrory, W. W., Rapoport, M., and Fleisher, D. S.: Estimation of Severity of the Nephrotic Syndrome in Children as a Guide to Therapy and Prognosis. *Pediatrics*, 23:861, 1959.

Michael, A. F., Drummond, K. N., Vernier, R. L., and Good, R. A.: Immunologic Bases of Renal Disease. *Pediat. Clin. N. Amer.*, 11:685, 1964.

Michael, A. F., and others: Immunosuppressive Therapy of Chronic Renal Disease. *New England J. Med.*, 276:817, 1967.

Rennie, I. D. B., and Keen, H.: Evaluation of Clinical Methods for Detecting Proteinuria. *Lancet*, 2:489, 1967.

Shearn, M. A.: Normocholesterolemic Nephrotic Syndrome of Systemic Lupus Erythematosus. *Am. J. Med.*, 36:250, 1964.

Vernier, R. L., Farquhar, M. G., Brunson, J. G., and Good, R. A.: Electron Microscopic Pathology of the Various Forms of the Nephrotic Syndrome. *Am. J. Dis. Child.*, 94:514, 1957.

West, C. D., McAdams, A. G., McConville, J. M., Davis, N. C., and Holland, N. H.: Hypocomplementemic and Normocomplementemic Persistent Glomerulonephritis. *J. Pediat.*, 67:1089, 1965.

West, C. D., Northway, J. D., and Davis, N. C.: Serum Levels of Beta 1c Globulin, a Complement Component in the Nephritides. *J. Clin. Invest.*, 43:1507, 1964.

Wilson, S. G. F., and Heymann, W.: Acute Glomerulonephritis with the Nephrotic Syndrome. *Pediatrics.*, 23:874, 1959.

IDIOPATHIC HYPERCALCIURIA

Idiopathic hypercalciuria connotes excessive loss of calcium in urine, with normal serum levels of calcium. It has been described mainly in adults. In children it is accompanied by growth failure, vitamin D-resistant rickets, renal lithiasis, proteinuria (said to be of tubular type) and Pitressin-resistant hyposthenuria. Mental retardation may occur. On microscopic examination the kidneys may present a normal picture or that of interstitial nephritis, with nephrocalcinosis. The tubular regulation of acid-base balance is reported to be normal, but the renal excretion of calcium is more than 6 mg. per kg. per 24 hours, reaching 10 mg.

per kg. The serum concentration of calcium is not increased.

Idiopathic hypercalciuria must be differentiated from hypercalciuria secondary to idiopathic hypercalcemia, osteolytic bone lesions, chronic renal tubular acidosis, vitamin D intoxication, and various disorders of the parathyroids, adrenals or ovaries. Secondary hypercalciuria is also seen with prolonged immobilization and administration of corticosteroids.

Reduction of the calcium intake to less than 0.5 gm. or less per day may be helpful in reducing the tendency toward renal calcification. Vitamin D may aid in the healing of rickets. Royer has suggested the use of thiazide diuretics.

REFERENCES

Albright, F., Henneman, P., Benedict, P. H., and Forbes, A. P.: Idiopathic Hypercalciuria. *J. Clin. Endocrinol.*, 13:860, 1953.

Royer, P., Habib, R., and Mathieu, H.: *Problèmes actuels de nephrologie infantile.* Paris, Editions Medicales Flammarion, 1963.

ACUTE RENAL FAILURE

This term is used for severe renal dysfunction resulting in pronounced oliguria or anuria of whatever cause. It may be completely reversible, revert to a pre-existing state of chronic renal insufficiency, or occasionally be irreversible. It is convenient clinically to divide acute renal failure into 3 categories: prerenal failure secondary to decreased renal plasma flow, intrarenal failure associated with parenchymal damage, and postrenal failure due to obstruction of the urinary tract.

Prerenal Failure. Mild or moderate decreases in renal blood flow may result in acute renal failure which is usually completely reversible when normal renal plasma flow is restored. Diarrhea with dehydration, diabetic acidosis, hemorrhage, burns, trauma with shock, and heart failure are examples of conditions in which this type of renal failure can be expected. Severe impairment of renal blood flow may lead to ischemia of the kidney, resulting in parenchymal damage.

Intrarenal Failure. The pathogenesis of acute renal failure secondary to parenchymal damage has been divided into 2 categories by Oliver: nephrotoxicity and ischemia.

Nephrotoxicity. Microdissection of individual nephrons has shown that the lesion produced by nephrotoxins involves uniform necrosis of tubular epithelium, without essential damage to the basement membrane except in the most severe cases. The lesions occur primarily in the proximal convolutions, but may involve other portions of the tubule as well.

Ischemia. This type of renal tubular lesion is designated a tubulorrhexis by Oliver and is used synonymously with the term, "lower nephron nephrosis." The latter term is inappropriate, since any segment of the tubule may be involved.

In addition to disruption and necrosis of the epithelial lining, there are fraying or disintegration and breaks in the basement membrane. There is dissolution of the continuity of the tubule, which may involve the entire tubule or may be fragmentary with normal sections interspersed with areas of complete disruption. Casts may be found in the tubular lumens. Peritubular reaction and interstitial edema may be prominent. Re-epithelialization does not occur in areas where the basement membrane has been disrupted, but since not all the nephrons are affected even in severely damaged kidneys, restitution of function is possible. The glomeruli are uninvolved except in the more severe ischemic lesions wherein large numbers of nephrons are totally destroyed, and infarction leads to cortical necrosis. Unless there is extensive cortical necrosis, which is not common, survival and recovery may occur, owing to the patchiness of the lesion.

Views concerning the mechanism of tubular necrosis and of the consequent uremia are controversial. In one theory it is assumed that toxins or ischemia damages the tubules, permitting leakage of tubular fluid into the interstitium, with a resultant rise in intrarenal pressure, which mechanically obstructs renal blood flow. But data with regard to increased intrarenal pressure or reduction in renal blood flow are contradictory. Some question whether damaging hypoxia occurs despite the fall in renal blood flow.

A variety of conditions may result in an ischemic lesion: blood loss, surgical shock, shock associated with sepsis, crush injuries to muscle, and burns, hypovolemia secondary to severe dehydration (as with vomiting, diarrhea, intestinal obstruction, hypoadrenalism and diabetic acidosis), hemolytic disorders, incompatible blood transfusion, the intravenous injection of distilled water, and drug sensitivities.

Acute glomerulonephritis is the commonest cause of acute renal failure in childhood. It is usually associated with moderate oliguria; however, there may be severe oliguria or anuria. In the majority of instances this is transitory, and the patient usually recovers completely. Acute renal failure may occur during chronic uremia with rapid deterioration of the clinical condition. It may represent an acceleration of the underlying disease process or may be secondary to water and electrolyte depletion. The hemolytic-uremic syndrome exemplifies acute intrarenal failure.

Vascular thromboses with infarction may occur in association with dehydration or sepsis, especially in young infants.

Postrenal Failure. In children the commonest cause of urinary tract obstruction leading to acute renal failure is a congenital malformation of the urinary tract. Acute renal failure commonly ensues when pyelonephritis complicates an obstructive lesion or bilateral renal hypoplasia. Other obstructions which may result in renal failure include tumors, edema and inflammation of the ureterovesical orifices secondary to ureteral catheterization, and trauma to the urethra. Obstruction by crystals such as sulfonamide, uric acid, or renal calculi is an uncommon cause of renal failure in children.

Acute renal failure may be divided into 3 phases: (1) oliguric, (2) diuretic, and (3) recovery.

Oliguric Phase. In young infants this phase may be overlooked, especially in the presence of severe disease, such as sepsis, in which the nonrenal manifestations may overshadow those of the kidney. There may be a profound reduction in urine flow within a few hours of the precipitating cause; the urine volume may be 10 to 30 ml. per day. Anuria is usually not present; however, recovery of urine on catheterization may provide the only evidence of urine formation.

In acute prerenal failure resulting from severe dehydration, the glomerular filtration rate may be reduced to 5 to 10 per cent of normal and be responsible for oliguria. Loss of tubular function may also be present and result in decreased concentrating capacity (low specific gravity) even when the supply of antidiuretic hormone is adequate. Osmotic diuresis in the residual functioning nephrons must also be a factor in the excretion of the dilute urine. The decreased excretion of sodium which occurs may result from increased tubular reabsorption, the reduction in glomerular filtration, and a low dietary intake. Back-diffusion of urea from the tubular fluid and protein catabolism may be additional factors in the elevation of the blood urea nitrogen level. Urinary acidity is usually maintained. Minimal glycosuria and aminoaciduria may occur.

In nephrotoxic renal damage the onset of oliguria may be delayed for several days. The duration of oliguria may vary considerably, up to 5 to 10 days, or longer. During this phase there is a fall in renal plasma flow, and blood may be shunted from the cortex through the juxtamedullary glomeruli. Experimental studies with nephrotoxic agents have demonstrated that active, though reduced, glomerular filtration occurs in spite of the absence of urine formation. Thus it must be assumed that reabsorption of the plasma filtrate is complete under such circumstances.

With hydrogen ion retention cellular potassium may shift to the plasma, and the resultant hyperkalemia is often severe enough to endanger life. The plasma bicarbonate level falls, and severe acidosis develops. The serum sodium and chloride levels are commonly reduced, most probably reflecting an increase in total body water due to inappropriate intake or administration of fluids, and in part to "metabolic water" from fat catabolism. Vomiting may increase the loss of electrolytes, especially chloride. The urine usually contains red cells and casts; when intravascular hemolysis occurs, hemoglobinuria may be present.

During the early phase of oliguria, unless the causative disease is overwhelming, the child may be surprisingly well. In late oliguria all the signs of uremia with its concomitant evidences of potassium intoxication and acidosis may exist to produce symptoms referable to the cardiovascular, gastrointestinal, neuromuscular and respiratory systems. Hypertension may be severe.

Diuretic Phase. Diuresis may begin abruptly or may slowly increase to reach polyuric proportions. With large volumes of urine, dehydration and weight loss may ensue. During this phase the urine is hypotonic or isotonic to plasma and may remain so for months; it may contain large numbers of casts and white blood cells, a few red cells and a moderate amount of protein. As diuresis increases, so does the excretion of sodium, chloride and potassium (salt-wasting). Renal blood flow and the filtration rate return toward normal; the blood urea nitrogen level may actually rise above previous levels as a result of dehydration, glomerulotubular imbalance, and urea back-diffusion. The clinical signs of uremia may become intense and be associated with hypertension and convulsions; death may occur even though urine flow is re-established.

Recovery Phase. There is finally a decrease in the high urinary output with a decline in the symptoms of uremia and return of the biochemical status toward normal. The deficiency in the ability to concentrate urine is often the last of the functions to return to normal. Renal function may be permanently impaired, and proteinuria may be present for a long time.

Prognosis. The majority of patients in acute renal failure, when properly managed, recover renal function spontaneously. Even after weeks of severe oliguria, recovery is possible if the biochemical status of the patient is maintained with reasonable adequacy and if treatment is guided by physiologic principles.

Treatment. It is of prime importance to determine whether oliguria or anuria is of renal or extrarenal origin. Initially this may not be readily apparent. When clinical dehydration is apparent or blood loss has occurred, the need for fluids or restoration of blood volume is obvious. In uncertain situations the intravenous administration of one-third isotonic solution of sodium chloride in 5 per cent glucose solution (350 ml. per square meter), given within 1 hour, will usually expand plasma volume sufficiently to induce urine flow (before correction of dehydration) when oliguria is caused by dehydration. Further fluids may be necessary to induce urine flow if dehydration is severe. When there is evidence of impending or existing vascular congestion or cardiac insufficiency, fluid should be administered slowly and the volume reduced. The danger of administration of hypotonic solutions is that the further expansion of body water or plasma volume may induce or aggravate pulmonary edema, cardiac failure or water intoxication. In the presence of vascular congestion with pulmonary edema it may be necessary to *remove water* by peritoneal dialysis using hypertonic glucose. Potassium-containing solutions should not be administered until adequate urinary

TABLE 15-4. POTASSIUM CONTENT OF COMMONLY USED BEVERAGES, FRUIT JUICES AND MILK

	mEq. OF POTASSIUM/LITER
Ginger ale	0
Pineapple juice	36
Orange juice	44
Whole milk (cow's)	36

flow is established, and hyperkalemia is not present (Table 15-4).

If the administration of fluids as described above does not produce urine flow, diuresis with mannitol or a diuretic such as ethacrynic acid may be attempted. This therapy is most effective when begun as soon as oliguria is confirmed. If using mannitol, it is well to start with a test dose in order not to overexpand plasma volume. A dose of 0.2 gm. per kg. should be given in 3 to 5 minutes as a 20 per cent solution. If there is adequate urine formation within a 2- or 3-hour period, then the full dose (100 gm. per 24 hours in adults) may be given.

Experimentally, the induction of osmotic diuresis with mannitol and hypertonic urea solutions during or immediately after burns decreases the incidence of renal failure, and intravenous administration of mannitol has been used clinically in the early stages of acute renal shutdown with some success. In the presence of hypertension the possibility of overexpansion of the plasma volume must be considered.

Decapsulation of the kidney and the administration of corticotropin have not been clinically successful in the induction of diuresis.

If urine flow is not established by the above-mentioned maneuvers, then fluid intake must be restricted. In the presence of oliguria, fluid intake should equal urinary output plus insensible water loss only. Insensible loss is usually about 300 to 400 ml. per square meter per day. The value will vary somewhat with the activity and temperature of the child and the temperature and humidity of the environment. Fluid requirements should be recalculated frequently; a weight loss of 100 to 200 gm. per day should occur.

During oliguria, carbohydrate, in the form of ginger ale, candy, syrups, and the like, can be given if the patient is able to take oral feedings. If not, glucose should be given intravenously. About 100 to 150 gm. of sugar per day will prevent ketosis and excessive protein catabolism.

Potassium intoxication can be corrected by several methods. The administration of sodium as the bicarbonate or chloride will counteract hyperkalemia most rapidly, but the duration of effect is only 1 to 2 hours, and there are dangers of overexpanding the extracellular fluid volume and of pulmonary edema. The effect of the administration of 25 to 30 per cent glucose and insulin may last several hours. Insulin should be given in a ratio of 1 unit to 3 gm. of glucose. The serum concentration of potassium may also be reduced by oral or rectal administration of a cation exchange resin which may be combined with sorbitol, a laxative, though this may not be necessary in children. The resin (Kay-Exelate, Winthrop) exchanges sodium for potassium.

Acidosis can be corrected, if necessary, by the administration of sodium bicarbonate or lactate; in the recovery phase, Shohl's solution* may be used to counteract excessive loss of base.

Hypocalcemia may occur and require the administration of calcium.

Replacement of electrolytes in the oliguric phase is rarely indicated. Rarely, when acute water intoxication occurs, sodium may be given cautiously as a hypertonic solution. The possibility of pulmonary edema with such treatment must be recognized. Unless the serum sodium concentration is extremely low, or there is obvious loss from the gastrointestinal tract, replacement is not indicated.

Peritoneal dialysis can be used to correct acidosis, electrolyte disturbances, uremia, and water imbalance in the oliguric phase. It is efficient in children, well tolerated by them, and does not require special equipment or the insertion of an arteriovenous shunt, as is necessary with hemodialysis.

Prophylactic antibiotic therapy is not indicated in acute renal failure. If used to combat infections during renal failure, the doses should be reduced appropriately.

Hypertension may complicate renal failure and lead to cardiac failure. Reserpine may be given in doses of 0.01 to 0.04 mg. per kg. per dose. If this is not effective, the dose may be increased to 0.07 mg. per kg., and hydralazine (Apresoline) added when reserpine alone fails (see p. 1130).

Congestive cardiac failure is treated with fractional doses of digoxin (see p. 1032). The maintenance dose of digitalis should be decreased in patients with renal failure. Morphine and oxygen are also helpful in the management of pulmonary edema and of cardiac failure. If there is severe anemia, cardiac function may be improved by the cautious administration of small amounts of sedimented erythrocytes.

MITCHELL I. RUBIN

REFERENCES

Calcagno, P. L., and Rubin, M. I.: Effect of Dehydration Produced by Water Deprivation, Diarrhea and Vomiting on Renal Function in Infants. *Pediatrics*, 7:328, 1951.

Franklin, S. S., and Merrill, J. P.: Acute Renal Failure. *New England J. Med.*, 262:711, 761, 1960.

Kunin, C. M.: Problems of Antimicrobial Drug Therapy in Renal Failure; in *Proceedings of 3rd International Congress of Nephrology*, Washington, 1966. New York, S. Karger, 1967, Vol. 3, p. 193.

Oliver, J., MacDowell, M., and Tracy, A.: The Pathogenesis of Acute Renal Failure Associated with Traumatic and Toxic Injury. Renal Ischemia, Nephrotoxic Damage and Ischemuric Episode. *J. Clin. Invest.*, 30:1307, 1951.

Rubin, M. I., and Calcagno, P. L.: Acute Renal Failure: Pathogenesis and Management. *Pediat. Clin. N. Amer.*, 9:155, 1962.

Shigeto, A., and Kolff, W. J.: Treatment of Renal Failure with the Disposable Artificial Kidney. *Am. J. Med.*, 23:565, 1956.

TUBULAR DYSFUNCTIONS ASSOCIATED WITH GENERALIZED RENAL OR URINARY TRACT DISEASE

Concentrating Defects. In renal failure defective urinary concentration is the rule, and is due in part to the elevated solute excretion per nephron imposed on the remaining functional nephrons. A reduced medullary osmolality may also play a role. Pitressin-resistant isosthenuria may occur in chronic pyelonephritis, obstructive uropathy and medullary cystic disease. This may result from the destructive changes which take place in the medulla. Defective concentration can occur also in hypercalcemia or in the hypercalciuria of immobilization. The latter may be secondary to reduced tubular permeability to water and reduced medullary osmolality. With relief of urinary tract obstruction or recession of hypercalciuria (or hypercalcemia) normal renal concentrating ability may return. In other instances a liberal dietary intake of water must be ensured, and unnecessary ingestion of salt should be eliminated.

Renal Electrolyte Wasting. Renal wastage of sodium, potassium or calcium singly or in combination may occur in diffuse renal disease. The symptoms reflect the specific (sodium, potassium or calcium) depletion; reduced serum concentrations suggest the disorders. Calcium depletion may present as rickets or osteomalacia. These disorders arise more often in chronic pyelonephritis and other diseases which alter renal tubular architecture than in chronic glomerulonephritis. Provision of increased amounts of sodium, potassium or calcium orally is indicated. The amounts needed must be determined by trial and error unless balance studies are possible. One and a half to 4 times the usual intakes of these salts may be needed.

Defects in Acid-Base Regulation. In renal failure renal acidification is impaired, primarily from a reduced excretion of ammonium. Quantitatively, this dysfunction appears to be the major one, but defective hydrogen ion excretion also occurs and urinary pH may not fall below 6.0 despite metabolic acidemia. Bicarbonate wasting may occur, but can rarely be distinguished from ammonium or hydrogen ion excretion without special study. Any of these 3 functional defects may occur in renal disease without glomerular insufficiency. Therapy is limited to administration of alkali, orally or parenterally. Sodium

---

*Shohl's solution:
Citric acid	98 gm.
Sodium citrate	140 gm.
Water, q.s.	1000 ml.

TABLE 15-5. DISORDERS OF RENAL
TUBULAR FUNCTION

Disorders associated with extrarenal disease
Acquired
    Potassium deficiency
    Vitamin C or D deficiency (pp. 175, 178)

Heritable
    Galactosemia (p. 437)
    Wilson's disease (pp. 418, 842, 1297)
    Vitamin D-refractory rickets (p. 1363)
    Cystinosis (p. 1367)
    Pseudohypoparathyroidism (p. 1203)
    Hartnup disease (p. 426)
    Oculo-cerebro-renal (Lowe's) syndrome (p. 1368)

Disorders limited to the tubules
Acquired
    Renal tubular acidosis (p. 1367)
    Fanconi's syndrome (p. 1366)

Heritable
    Renal glycosuria (p. 1147)
    Cystinuria (p. 426)
    Nephrogenic diabetes insipidus (p. 1148)
    Glycinuria (p. 429)

**Disorders associated with generalized renal
or urinary tract disease**
    Concentration defects
    Renal electrolyte wasting
    Defects in acid-base regulation
    Proximal tubular dysfunction

---

bicarbonate or a modified Shohl's solution (10 gm. of sodium citrate and 6 gm. of citric acid in 100 ml. of water) is recommended in a dose of 2 to 8 mEq. of citrate per kg. (3 to 12 ml. per kg.) daily. If edema or hypertension is present, administration of alkaline salts of sodium may have to be restricted. Dialysis (peritoneal or extracorporeal) ameliorates the metabolic acidosis temporarily.

Proximal Tubular Dysfunctions. Glycosuria, generalized aminoaciduria or renal electrolyte wasting occur infrequently in diffuse renal disease. The presence of diffuse renal disease is indicated when there is a combination of both glomerular and tubular dysfunctions.

Potassium deficiency may lead to disturbances in tubular function; vasopressin-resistant hyposthenuria is a common sequel of potassium depletion. Polydipsia and polyuria not attributable to a renal tubular defect also occur in some instances, suggesting a primary hypothalamic defect in the release of antidiuretic hormone or an inappropriate thirst. Vacuolation of the proximal convoluted tubules is seen in potassium depletion. The renal abnormality is confined to a defect in ability to concentrate urine. The mechanism appears to be a reduced medullary osmolality or reduced permeability of the collecting ducts to reabsorption of water. Potassium depletion may occur in chronic diarrhea or vomiting, prolonged use of thiazide diuretics, hyperaldosteronism, ureterosigmoidostomy and primary renal potassium wasting. Depletion occurs only if dietary potassium is too low to replace excessive losses.

Symptoms include anorexia and nausea, generalized weakness and hypotonia. Cardiac arrythmias, mental confusion or paralytic ileus may also occur. These findings in conjunction with polydipsia and polyuria should suggest potassium depletion. Urinary acid excretion is high in spite of alkalemia ("paradoxical aciduria"), owing to conservation of renal potassium. Potassium deficits of 2 to 9 mEq. per kg. may occur. Unless life-threatening consequences of potassium depletion occur, such as serious cardiac arrythmias or muscular paralysis, oral potassium therapy of 1 to 3 mEq. per kg. daily should be given. Repletion of severe deficits of intracellular potassium requires weeks of therapy, during which time subsidence of the clinical signs and symptoms occurs. The renal functional defect is nearly always reversible.

Renal tubular acidosis represents a defect in renal acid-base control without glomerular insufficiency or generalized tubular dysfunction. Although the cause is unknown, the disorder has been termed primary renal tubular acidosis to distinguish it from a similar defect associated with generalized tubular dysfunction. Most patients present either with transient metabolic acidemia in infancy or with persistent metabolic acidemia which has its onset after infancy. Affected infants exhibit anorexia, vomiting, irritability and growth retardation. The persistent form in older children is often manifest by hypercalciuria, nephrolithiasis, renal potassium wasting and defective urinary concentration. All patients have elevations in serum chloride values proportional to the reduction of the carbon dioxide content. Most cannot acidify the urine below pH 6.0 in spite of acidemia. In most instances the tubular defect is an inability to establish a maximal hydrogen ion gradient in the distal nephron. Titratable acidity and ammonium excretion are reduced, but can be raised by infusion of phosphate. The limitation in ammonium excretion results from the reduced hydrogen ion gradient between tubular cell and urine. Edelman has observed 2 infants with renal tubular acidosis in whom urinary acidification was normal, but who had lowered threshold for bicarbonate reabsorption. His patients had no defect in distal acidification or ability to lower urine pH, but they wasted bicarbonate. Since most bicarbonate reabsorption occurs in the proximal tubule, Edelman's patients apparently had a different functional defect, which he termed "proximal RTA." Oral therapy with sodium citrate or bicarbonate improves the acidemia and ameliorates the signs and symptoms. The transient form remits after several months, with no sequelae, whereas persistent renal tubular acidosis usually terminates in uremia after a number of years. Most cases are sporadic, but a familial incidence has been reported.

Renal glycosuria is a benign heritable disorder in the proximal tubular reabsorption of glucose. Its importance rests in distinguishing it from diabetes mellitus by the absence of hyperglycemia. The plasma level at which glycosuria occurs varies among patients, occurring in some only after meals, but in others during fasting. Tubular threshold for reabsorption of glucose is reduced in all patients. Some have a normal, others an increased reabsorptive threshold in the tubules. Inheritance appears to occur by autosomal dominant transmission; the disorder may not become manifest until adulthood. No treatment is indicated. Glucose TM is apparently normal in these patients in contrast to those with renal glycosuria associated with other tubular dysfunctions.

Cystinuria (p. 426) is a group of recessive hereditary defects in the renal tubular reabsorption of 4 amino acids: cystine, lysine, arginine and ornithine. Defective intestinal absorption of these amino acids has also been shown in cystinuric persons and has been further confirmed by in-vitro studies of their jejunal biopsies. Aside from recurrent urolithiasis, there are no abnormal symptoms or signs. Formation of urinary calculi is directly due to the high concentration of cystine in urine. The other 3 amino acids are completely soluble in human urine in the concentrations excreted. Calculi may lodge anywhere in the genitourinary tract. About 3 per cent of cystinurics form calculi, which may become manifest in infancy or not until adult life. Hexagonal cystine crystals can be seen microscopically in acid urine. Most calculi are radiopaque and composed essentially of only cystine. The solubility of cystine in urine increases 100 per cent from pH 5.5 to 7.5. Excretion of continuously alkaline urine, however, is virtually impossible to achieve. Hydration and the oral administration of acetazolamide or alkali at bedtime definitely retard the formation of cystine stones. Recently d-penicillamine, a chelating agent which can form a mixed disulfide with cystine in vivo, has improved the management of patients with cystine stones. Although the drug has toxic side effects, these are usually mild in doses that reduce free urinary cystine below levels at which stones are formed.

Nephrogenic diabetes insipidus is a congenital insensitivity of the renal tubules to antidiuretic hormone. Antidiuretic activity has been found in the blood and urine of affected persons. The disease appears to be inherited as an X chromosome-linked characteristic, affected females having a milder disorder. It becomes manifest in infancy with polyuria, dehydration, fever and growth failure. Vomiting, constipation and convulsions may occur. Deaths have occurred before the condition was recognized. In older children mental retardation is frequent. The typical triad of polydipsia, polyuria and persistent hyposthenuria occurs only when hydration is adequate. Polyuria unresponsive to Pitressin may also occur in potassium deficiency, hypercalcemia, cystinosis, medullary cystic disease, obstructive uropathy and uremia. The defect is not as severe in these conditions. All renal functions except concentration are normal in subjects with nephrogenic diabetes insipidus.

Diagnosis is made by the finding of a low urine osmolality (less than 400 mOsm. per liter) or specific gravity (less than 1.012) upon administration of Pitressin to a patient with an isolated defect in concentrating urine. Pitressin sensitivity is determined by collection of urine for specific gravity or osmolality at 30-minute intervals after an oral water load of 20 ml. per kg. and Pitressin. Beginning with 0.2 ml. of aqueous Pitressin, the dose should be raised at hourly intervals until an increase in urine concentration occurs or side effects (blanching, abdominal cramps) occur. Water voided should be replaced by oral ingestion. Partial response to vasopressin occurs in some females. Treatment consists in restriction of solute intake and free access to water. In infancy extra water must be offered frequently. A low protein diet (1 to 2 gm. per kg. per day) and low salt (0.5 to 1.0 gm. of NaCl per day) intake reduce the water requirement and urine volume. This diminishes the continual need to drink and void which has hindered food intake and caused megabladder and hydronephrosis in some patients. Growth may be subnormal because of repeated bouts of dehydration and hyperosmolality, or secondary to low protein intake. Chlorothiazide may be useful in controlling the symptoms by producing salt depletion. Older children able to drink freely may be managed on a more liberal diet (see also p. 1179).

Renal hyperglycinuria (see p. 429) has been found in 5 rare familial disorders, in which it does not appear to cause any symptoms. In one type it was associated with oxalate urolithiasis in females of 3 successive generations. It has been found without urolithiasis in a father and son of another family. In familial glucoglycinuria, hyperglycinuria is accompanied by renal glycosuria. Renal hyperglycinuria has also been found in familial hypophosphatemic rickets and in familial hyperprolinemia.

W. Joseph Rahill

REFERENCES

Milne, M. D.: Renal Tubular Dysfunction; in M. B. Straus and L. B. Welt (Eds.): *Diseases of the Kidney.* Boston, Little, Brown and Company, 1963.
Stanbury, J. B., Wyngaarden, J. B., and Frederickson, D. S.: *The Metabolic Basis of Inherited Disease.* 2nd ed. New York, McGraw-Hill Book Company, Inc., 1966.

SUPPURATIVE NEPHRITIS
(Abscess of the Kidney)

Suppurative nephritis occurs most often in adults, but it may occur in the neonatal period and at any age thereafter.

Etiology. The infection may be hematogenous in origin, or it may reach the kidney by contiguity from another suppurating lesion; or it may result from the presence of a calculus, from trauma or from urinary obstruction secondary to a congenital anomaly. Many microorganisms may be causative, but the more common ones are the streptococcus, staphylococcus and colon bacillus. Pathologically, the lesions vary somewhat with the origin. In those of hematogenous origin both kidneys are usually involved, with numerous abscesses of varying size. At times there may be a localized abscess (*renal carbuncle*), the remainder of the renal structure being normal.

Clinical Manifestations. The symptoms of suppurative nephritis, when it is a manifestation of another severe infection, are overshadowed by those of the primary infection. When, in conjunction with a generalized septic infection, a kidney is enlarged and tender or there is tenderness over the renal area in conjunction with pus and blood in the urine, the possibility of a renal abscess should be considered. In cases of abscess secondary to pyelonephritis the urinary findings are inconclusive. If the abscess is walled off, the urine may be normal.

Prognosis. The prognosis is unfavorable in the metastatic cases. In other forms the outlook is grave, being best when there is free communication with the urinary tubules to afford drainage. A perinephric abscess may develop, or the pus may burrow beyond the perinephric region.

Treatment. The treatment for abscess of the kidney which is part of a septicemia is primarily that of the general infection. Removal of an abscessed kidney may be indicated when it is reasonably certain that the other kidney is healthy. Appropriate antibiotic therapy is indicated in all instances.

TUBERCULOSIS OF THE KIDNEY

Tuberculosis of the kidney is uncommon in early life except as a manifestation of generalized miliary tuberculosis. Pathologically, it is manifest by the presence of small tubercles on the surface and in the parenchyma of the kidney. There are rarely any symptoms related to the kidney.

Localized tuberculous lesions of the kidney are rare in infants and children. At autopsy the lesions are usually bilateral, even though the clinical manifestations have been unilateral.

There may be no symptoms, but most often there are general symptoms of fever and emaciation, and localized ones of pain, tenderness and enlargement in the renal region. There is frequent and painful urination, the urine being acid and usually containing blood, pus and tubercle bacilli. A persistently sterile pyuria is suggestive of tuberculous infection. The duration of caseous renal tuberculosis depends upon the local lesion and upon the course of tuberculous lesions elsewhere in the body.

Renal tuberculosis may be differentiated from pyelonephritis by identification of tubercle bacilli in the urine; care must be taken to differentiate them from smegma bacilli. Occasionally, urographic studies aid in the diagnosis by showing deformity of the renal pelvis. The tuberculous process may spread to the renal pelvis and ureter, leading to obstruction. The first lesions in the bladder appear around the ureteric orifice of the affected side; the lesion spreads and may produce small ulcerations. Fibrosis and infiltration produce a rigid, contracted bladder wall.

Treatment. All possible means must be used to sustain the general health. Operative removal is indicated in extensive unilateral lesions, if the other kidney is shown to be functioning normally and is not infected. Streptomycin and isoniazid should be used with or without para-aminosalicylic acid (see p. 606).

HEMORRHAGIC INFARCTION OF THE KIDNEY
(Thrombosis of the Renal Vein)

This condition usually occurs in the early weeks of life; most of the reported patients are under 1 year of age, but it may occur in any age group. An increased incidence in infants of diabetic and prediabetic mothers has been reported. It is usually associated with thrombosis of the renal veins, although it may occur in the absence of demonstrable thrombosis. Conversely, thrombosis of the renal vein may occur without hemorrhagic infarction of the kidney.

Thrombosis of the renal veins is rarely primary. It is usually secondary to an infectious process in some other part of the body, or to severe dehydration, especially that associated with diarrhea and vomiting. The symptoms may be masked by the primary disturbance, but the sudden appearance of protein and blood in the urine of an infant with severe dehydration secondary to diarrhea is sufficient reason to consider renal thrombosis in the differential diagnosis of the renal lesion. In a tabulation of 27 cases with survival the prominent manifestations were flank mass 81 per cent, microscopic hematuria 67 per cent, gross hematuria 30 per cent, proteinuria 56 per cent, oliguria 15 per cent, elevated nonprotein nitrogen 44 per cent, and "shock" 3 per cent. In about half the cases the thrombosis is unilateral; the intravenous pyelogram may show a nonfunctioning kidney, and retrograde pyelography may demonstrate a normal or distorted renal pelvis. The thrombus may progress from one side to the other; such progression has been described even following unilateral nephrectomy.

Thrombosis of the renal veins may lead to the nephrotic syndrome, but usually does not in infancy.

Treatment of the unilateral lesion is prompt surgical removal of the infarcted kidney and of the thrombus.

It is often not possible to tell whether the thrombus has extended to involve the opposite kidney. In the absence of infection of the suspected infarcted kidney, anticoagulant therapy may lessen the tendency for the thrombus to spread. In bilateral renal vein involvement anticoagulant therapy is of primary importance.

REFERENCES

Miller, H. C., and Benjamin, J. A.: Acute Idiopathic Renal Vein Thrombosis in Infant. *Pediatrics*, 30:247, 1962.

Sandblom, P. H.: Renal Thrombosis with Infarction in the Newborn: Two Different Forms. *Acta Paediat.*, 35:160, 1948.

Zuelzer, W. M., Seymour, C., Kurnetz, R., Newton, W. A., Jr., and Fallon, R.: Circulatory Diseases of the Kidneys in Infancy and Childhood. *Am. J. Dis. Child.*, 81:1, 1951.

RENAL CALCULUS

Etiology. Benign uric acid infarcts of the kidney occur in the newborn infant (p. 1109). Renal calculi may occur in infants and children of all ages. Calculi are found more frequently in some geographic regions than in others. It has been suggested that this geographic distribution may be dependent upon such factors as poor nutrition, alkaline-ash diets and vitamin A deficiency. In most instances the basis for calculus formation is not known. Deficiency of some substance in the urine which normally prevents calcium precipitation (citrate, hyaluronic acid and others) or an increase of an agent which tends to promote calcium precipitation (a mucopolysaccharide) has been postulated as a basis for stone formation. An inherited tendency has also been suggested. Suppuration of bone, prolonged immobilization, and obstruction with stasis and infection of the urinary tract may be contributing factors (see also, nephrocalcinosis below). Precipitation of the acetyl forms of sulfonamides in the kidney may produce obstruction. Urinary calculi are common in parathyroid disease, in cystinuria and in renal tubular acidosis. *Oxalosis* is associated with the widespread deposit in the tissues of calcium oxalate crystals.

Pathology. The chemical composition of the calculi varies. In a large series of children the largest number were composed of uric acid or its salts. In other series, stones consisting of oxalates, phosphates or carbonates have been relatively more common. Cystine and xanthine calculi occur less frequently. The stones vary in number and in size from that of gravel to calculi which fill the entire pelvis of the kidney. In about 20 per cent of cases both kidneys are involved. There may be inflammation of the tissue surrounding stones in the renal parenchyma and in the urinary tract, and secondary hydronephrosis may develop.

Clinical Manifestations. In many instances there are no symptoms. The more common ones are tenderness in the renal region, pyuria, hematuria, attacks of renal colic, with pain radiating to the lower part of the abdomen, the external genitalia and thigh, and a frequent desire to urinate.

Vomiting may occur with the renal colic. The attack lasts for a few hours or sometimes, with remissions, for several days. A calculus which has descended into the ureter may return to the pelvis of the kidney, or advance and be passed into the bladder and later voided as a single stone or as gravel. In infancy, symptoms may be absent or indefinite, and the pain of renal colic may be misinterpreted as intestinal in origin. In some instances there is hematuria without colic, particularly when the calculi are in the substance of the kidney. Infection of the urinary tract is often present and may dominate the clinical picture, with fever the prominent symptom. Roentgenograms and pyelograms are of value, although uric acid stones do not cast a shadow. Intravenous pyelography may demonstrate a stone as a filling defect. Calculi may be seen on cystoscopy. The appearance of uric acid crystals in the urine does not necessarily mean that they have been passed from the kidney, since they may have been precipitated after the urine was voided.

Nephrocalcinosis is a disseminated form of nephrolithiasis in which calcium salts, usually oxalate or phosphate, are deposited within the renal interstitial tissues and nephrons, in the majority of cases without clinical expression. There may be renal calculi, recurring hematuria, urinary infection and renal dysfunction, especially tubular but also glomerular. Hypertension may be present. The causative factors are varied, there being no evidence that nephrocalcinosis is a primary disorder. Nephrocalcinosis in infancy may be associated with idiopathic hypercalcemia and possibly with excessive vitamin D intake, and may be reversible. Nephrocalcinosis occurs in connection with widespread damage to renal tissues such as that by infection secondary to urinary stasis and is probably dependent on secondary disturbances of calcium and phosphate metabolism. It also occurs in association with hyperparathyroidism and other conditions responsible for hypercalcemia with hypercalciuria, such as hypervitaminosis D or increased responsiveness to it, metastatic bone disease, cortisone administration, Cushing's disease, and prolonged immobilization (p. 1370). Nephrocalcinosis may also be a manifestation of certain renal tubular disorders which are apparently dependent on metabolic disorders. These include cystinuria and primary hypercalciuria without hypercalcemia. Nephrocalcinosis may aggravate the primary renal dysfunction and often contributes to persistence of infection in the kidney. The roentgenogram will at times reveal the multiple deposits of calcium salts widely distributed throughout the renal parenchyma.

Prognosis. The prognosis of calculi is usually good in children when there is no systemic disease (see p. 1148). There is a tendency for new calculi to form. If the stone is impacted, pyonephritis or hydronephrosis may develop. In long-standing cases renal function may be permanently impaired.

Treatment. During attacks of colic, morphine and atropine can be administered. Ureteral catheterization may be necessary to dislodge an impacted stone. Persistent renal stones should be removed surgically. After an attack any infection of the urinary tract should be treated, and an attempt made to discover whether other stones are present and to detect the existence of obstructive uropathy. To aid in preventing recurrence, water should be taken freely. If the stone passed is composed of uric acid, it may be advisable to keep the reaction of the urine alkaline and to avoid excessive ingestion of meat. In the case of phosphate calculi the urine should not be alkalinized. When calculi result from tubular dysfunction with loss of base producing an acidosis, alkali therapy may be helpful (see p. 1146). When a basic disease is causative, as in nephrocalcinosis, it should be treated. Early ambulation and passive exercise for the bedridden patient are important considerations for the prevention of nephrocalcinosis. Reduction of the calcium intake to 0.5 gm. or less per day may be helpful in reducing the tendency toward renal calcification. In the presence of hypercalcemia, cortisone therapy may be of use in reducing the intestinal absorption of calcium; the vitamin D intake should be at a minimum. Such foods as rhubarb, eggplant, spinach and asparagus increase the urinary excretion of oxalates.

REFERENCES

Combes, M. A.: Calcium Excretion During Orthopedic Immobilization in Children. *Am. J. Dis. Child.,* 96:612, 1958.

Daeschner, C. W., Singleton, E. B., and Curtis, J. C.: Urinary Tract Calculi and Nephrosclerosis in Infants and Children. *J. Pediat.,* 57:721, 1960.

Drummond, K. N., Michael, A. F., Ulstrom, R. A., and Good, R. A.: The Blue Diaper Syndrome: Familial Hypercalcemia with Nephrocalcinosis and Indicanuria. *Am. J. Med.,* 37:928, 1964.

Fellers, F. X., and Schwartz, R.: Etiology of Severe Form of Idiopathic Hypercalcemia of Infancy: A Defect in Vitamin D. Metabolism. *New England J. Med.,* 259:1050, 1958.

Lightwood, R., and Stapleton, T.: Idiopathic Hypercalcemia in Infants. *Lancet,* 2:255, 1953.

Shanks, R. A., and MacDonald, A. M.: Nephrocalcinosis Infantum. *Arch. Dis. Childhood,* 34:115, 1959.

DISTURBANCES OF THE URINARY BLADDER

EXSTROPHY OF THE BLADDER

Exstrophy of the bladder occurs chiefly in boys. When the defect is complete, the entire lower urinary tract from the apex of the bladder to the external urethral meatus is exposed and everted on the abdominal wall. The trigone and the ureteral orifices can be seen in the center of the mass. There is an associated complete epispadias of a short penis; in girls the clitoris may be fissured and the labia separated. In some instances the exstrophy is not complete, and only a part of the bladder is exposed. The exposed bladder mucosa is bright red, has numerous folds, and is extremely sensitive to touch. With advancing years this sensitivity decreases, and portions of the bladder mucosa are replaced by squamous epithelium. There is a wide diastasis of the rectus muscles below the umbilicus; the pubic rami are widely separated, causing the child to walk with a waddling gait. The testes are usually in the abdomen, and bilateral inguinal hernias may be present. In girls the vagina may be absent or replaced by a cloaca including vagina and rectum. At times there are defects of the lower bowel. These patients are quite uncomfortable. The surrounding skin is often badly excoriated, and ulcerations of the bladder mucosa are common. Rarely there are malignant lesions. Exstrophy of the bladder is not incompatible with a full life span.

When the exstrophy is not complete, a satisfactory plastic closure of the abdominal and bladder walls may be obtained. For a complete exstrophy, successful functional and cosmetic results are relatively uncommon (5 to 20 per cent of cases). The principal danger is progressive renal damage due to hydronephrosis and infection. Transplantation of the ureters into the sigmoid is now less commonly performed than previously, owing to the frequency with which urinary infection led to progressive renal damage. If diversion of the urinary stream is necessary, an ileal loop poses less threat to the kidney. Poor rectal sphincteral tone commonly leads to leakage from the bowel when sigmoid implantation is performed.

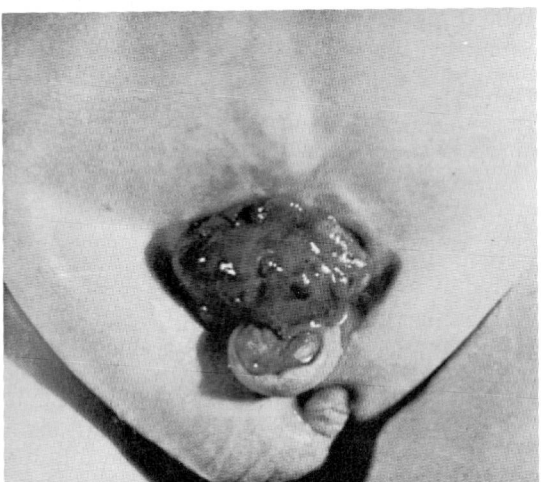

Figure 15-7. Exstrophy of the bladder in a boy 10 years of age. Below the bladder is the atrophic penis and, below it, the empty scrotum. There is also a right inguinal hernia.

Closure of the bladder is usually attempted between 6 months and 2 years of age. Renal decompensation often determines the immediacy of the operation. Lattimer and his associates, on the other hand, recommend early operation, when the infant can withstand a 6- to 7-hour operation, preferably before 3 to 4 months of age. They report a procedure in which the bladder is rolled into a sac and replaced within the abdomen, with good functional and cosmetic results. The pubic bones are approximated at the time of operation, and a stable symphysis is constructed. Before surgical repair the surrounding skin will need protection; this may be achieved with silicone preparations.

Mild degrees of hydroureter and hydronephrosis are common; occasionally there is a severe degree of hydronephrosis. Pyelonephritis is not infrequent, but can usually be controlled by antimicrobial therapy. The colon bacillus is the most common infecting organism. Adequate renal function can usually be maintained for many years. The ultimate prognosis depends in great measure on the extent of renal damage from back pressure and infection.

PATENT URACHUS AND URACHAL CYST

In early embryonic life the bladder extends to the umbilical region, subsequently descending along the anterior abdominal wall. During this descent the upper portion becomes attenuated to form the narrow tubelike urachus, which later is obliterated. On rare occasions an open lumen persists, permitting discharge of urine into the umbilicus in postnatal life. This type of urachal defect is usually associated with obstruction of the urinary tract at the bladder neck. Deficiency of abdominal musculature is also commonly present. In some instances there is only an external communication at the umbilicus, and the rest of the urachal tract is closed off; in others there is only an internal communication to the bladder. The most common urachal lesion is a blind cyst occurring usually at the upper end of the tract just under the umbilicus and extraperitoneally.

When the entire urachus is patent, there is a constant flow of urine from the umbilical region. The diagnosis can be established by means of dyes excreted through the urine, by chemical analysis of the discharge, and by roentgenography after injection of contrast material into the bladder or into the umbilical opening. The urachal cyst exists as a deep midline swelling below the umbilicus attached to the internal part of the abdominal wall.

Urachal cysts may become infected, and at such times the symptoms are those of a midline abscess. The abscess may rupture internally into the bladder with infection extending to the kidneys, or into the peritoneum, or externally through the umbilicus.

Urachal cysts should be removed when diagnosed and before infection has occurred. If infection has already occurred, surgical drainage is indicated with subsequent removal of the cyst. If there is an obstructive lesion of the bladder neck, repair is imperative.

Less common malformations of the bladder include agenesis, complete duplication, incomplete duplication, hourglass bladder, congenital vesicovaginal fistula, and vesical diverticula.

NEUROGENIC BLADDER

Traumatic lesions, tumors and inflammatory diseases of the spinal cord may result in the neurogenic bladder, but by far the commonest causes are congenital spinal cord lesions, such as spina bifida. There is poor correlation between the severity of bony deformity and the nerve lesion. Spina bifida occulta is common in children and usually produces no bladder difficulties. The typical neurogenic bladder is usually enlarged, flaccid, and thin-walled, without trabeculation, and lacking a sensation of fullness. The lack of bladder wall hypertrophy in congenital lesions is in contrast to the pattern in the autonomous bladder resulting from later traumatic injuries. Urethral resistance is low, and there is dribbling of urine. In the absence of obstruction the upper urinary tract is normal. Infection in the bladder may result in acute retention of urine. Some patients with neurogenic bladder due to congenital spinal cord lesions have evidence of bladder outflow obstruction (spastic external sphincters), with a dilated posterior urethra, trabeculation, ureteral reflux and varying degrees of upper urinary tract dilatation. Expression of urine from such bladders is less adequate than from the more common type. In a third type (Williams) there may be some bladder sensation. There are residual urine, bladder trabeculation and funnel-neck dilatation of the urethra. If urethral resistance is low, treatment is primarily by training. Incontinence in the girl may necessitate the construction of a diversional ileal loop. When there is resistance to emptying and residual urine remains in the bladder, surgery of the bladder neck should be considered.

VESICAL CALCULUS

About two thirds of urinary calculi are found in the bladder. Vesical calculi during childhood are most common from the age of 2 to 7 years, and occur oftener in boys, since the short, wide female urethra permits stones to be passed while they are still small. The calculus is usually formed in the kidney, but increases in size in the bladder. Occasionally a foreign body introduced into the bladder or long-standing catheter drainage forms the nucleus for a stone. Obstructive lesions at the bladder outlet and neurogenic bladder dysfunction with urinary retention and infection may also be contributory.

The symptoms are vesical irritability, enuresis and often attacks of pain, especially at the close of micturition. Pain is felt in the neck of the bladder or at the end of the penis, or in the vagina, rectum or perineum. Tenesmus is frequent both on urination and on defecation, and may produce prolapse of the rectum. There may be a sudden arrest of micturition, accompanied by severe pain and straining. Pain may be relieved by having the child void while lying down if the stone is not lodged in the urethra. Priapism is common, and incontinence may occur. If cystitis develops, the symptoms are accentuated, and the urine contains mucus, pus and red blood cells. The only positive diagnosis is by cystoscopic or roentgenographic examination. The prognosis depends upon the size of the stone and upon treatment. Medical treatment is similar to that for renal calculi. Large stones must be removed surgically, smaller stones by crushing. Any urinary obstruction will need surgical relief.

FOREIGN BODIES IN THE BLADDER

Occasionally boys and girls, especially at puberty, introduce foreign bodies into the urethra, and these may pass into the bladder. The nature of the bodies is varied, among them being hairpins, pencils, shot, beads, and the like. They may give rise to inflammation, form the basis of a calculus or contribute to the development of infection. Treatment usually consists in removal through the operating cystoscope, or surgical removal if necessary. There may also be a need for psychotherapy.

CYSTITIS

Cystitis as an isolated infection is uncommon; it is usually associated with pyelonephritis or an obstruction at the neck of the bladder or in the urethra. Other causes include vesical calculi, foreign bodies, tumors, rupture of an abscess into the bladder or extension of a gonococcal infection. Actually, the bladder is relatively resistant to infection; if an associated infection is controlled or an obstructing or irritating lesion removed, the cystitis tends to disappear spontaneously except when there are extensive changes in the vesical wall in long-standing infections. A rare form is *cystitis emphysematosa*, in which there are gas-containing vesicles in the wall of the bladder. Chronic infections of the upper urinary tract may be associated with the appearance of small, cystlike masses in the region of the bladder neck known as *cystitis cystica*.

The constitutional **symptoms** include fever, restlessness and anorexia. The local disturbance varies in intensity, being greater in older children, in whom there is pain and tenderness in the region of the bladder and painful and frequent urination. The straining may produce prolapse of the rectum, and there may be constant dribbling of urine. In infants the painful urination may be evidenced only by crying. The urine is cloudy and contains white and red blood cells, mucus, vesical epithelium and bacteria. The **diagnosis** is established by cystoscopic examination.

An acute, apparently infectious, *hemorrhagic cystitis* is occasionally seen in infants and children as well as in adults. Low-grade fever, urinary frequency and dysuria are common manifestations. Bacteria are not usually isolated from the urine, and the possibility of a viral origin has been considered. Recently adenovirus type II has been isolated from the urine of several patients with hemorrhagic cystitis. Gross bleeding may last for several days, and acute glomerulonephritis must be differentiated. The lesion tends to be self-limited.

Treatment. The only effective treatment for secondary infections of the bladder is removal of the cause. In acute cases, bed rest is required, and the child should be encouraged to drink large amounts of water. Bacterial infections should be treated with a sulfonamide or an appropriate antibiotic in full therapeutic doses. Pain and straining may be relieved by hot or cold applications over the bladder or by administration of opiates or other analgesics. In severe and obstinate cases, lavage may be indicated. Instillation into the bladder of a 0.1 per cent solution of neomycin, containing Elase (bovine fibrinolysin and deoxyribonuclease), and allowing it to remain for 30 minutes, then washing it out with several instillations of sterile water, has been suggested as adjunctive treatment.

TUBERCULOSIS OF THE BLADDER

This infection, infrequent during childhood, may exist with tuberculosis of other parts of the genitourinary system, especially the kidney, or it may be the only tuberculous lesion in the urinary tract. The lesion may consist of scattered, grayish, caseous nodules, or of ulcers in the mucous membrane. The clinical manifestations are those of chronic cystitis with hematuria. The diagnosis can be made by the discovery of tubercle bacilli in the urine and by cystoscopic examination (see Treatment, p. 606).

SPASM OF THE BLADDER

This symptom is more frequent in early childhood than later. Among causes are sudden chilling of the body, vesical calculus and secretion of highly concentrated urine. It may also be a reflex symptom of renal calculus or disorders of the rectum, vulva, urethra, hip joint, appendix or other neighboring structures. There may be a spasm of the sphincter, and the child is unable to void; more commonly there is irritation of the detrusor apparatus, resulting in frequent emptying of the bladder. In the former instance there is pain and straining without passage of urine. In the latter the urine is passed frequently, sometimes only in drops, and there may or may not be pain.

Treatment consists in elimination of the cause if possible. When the urine is highly acid, alkali may be given, water should be ingested freely, and atropine with or without a sedative may be administered. During spasm of the sphincter hot compresses may be applied over the bladder, or the child may be placed in a warm bath. Catheterization is rarely required.

MITCHELL I. RUBIN

REFERENCES

Darwish, M. E., Staubitz, W. J., Scheuller, E. F., Rubin, M. I., and Neter, E.: Antibody Response of Dogs to Experimental Infection of the Bladder Pouch. *Invest. Urol.*, 6:66, 1968.

Fairley, K. F., Bond, A. G., Brown, R. B., and Habersberger, P.: Simple Test to Determine the Site of Urinary Tract Infection. *Lancet*, 2:427, 1967.

Kjellberg, S. R., Ericsson, N. O., and Rudhe, U.: *The Lower Urinary Tract in Childhood.* Chicago, Year Book Medical Publishers, Inc., 1957.

Lattimer, J. K., Uson, A. C., and Melicow, M. M.: Urologic Emergencies in Newborn Infants. *Pediatrics*, 29:310, 1962.

Williams, D. I.: Congenital Bladder Neck Obstruction and the Megaureter. *Brit. J. Urol.*, 29:389, 1957.

16. Metabolic Disorders

DIABETES MELLITUS

Diabetes mellitus is a complex disorder of metabolism characterized clinically by hyperglycemia and glycosuria and, in the untreated child, progressively by ketonemia, ketonuria, undernutrition and loss of weight, and finally by acidosis and coma. The metabolism of fat and protein, as well as that of carbohydrate, is deranged.

Incidence. It is estimated that there are more than 3,000,000 diabetics (known and unknown) in the United States, and that perhaps 4 per cent of them are less than 15 years of age.

Etiology. Diabetes mellitus is a hereditary disease and in most instances appears to be transmitted as a recessive character. Evaluation of the genetic pattern is complicated by the variability in the clinical expression of the disease. This situation is reflected by such factors as (1) the wide age range (infancy to old age) in which the disease may become manifest, (2) the variability in clinical severity, some cases being clinically inapparent, perhaps at times indefinitely, and (3) the similarity of clinical patterns in newborn infants of diabetic mothers and prediabetic mothers. Diabetes occurs more frequently in both members of identical twins than in those who are not identical. When only one of identical twins has overt diabetes, the other member frequently manifests some evidence of the prediabetic state.

Doubt has been expressed that diabetes is transmitted by a single mutant gene or that it represents a single defect; rather it is postulated that 2 or more defects exist in the person who becomes overtly diabetic (multifactorial inheritance). The basic question, of course, is what is inherited. The possibilities currently under consideration include (1) impaired response of beta cells of the pancreas to hyperglycemia, (2) an abnormal insulin, (3) an increase of a normal insulin antagonist (Vallance-Owen "synalbumin") or (4) an abnormal insulin antagonist. Another important and unanswered question is the relation, if any, of the vascular changes (microangiopathy) and of the retinopathy to the metabolic defect(s) in carbohydrate metabolism.

Whether certain factors or stresses may precipitate manifest disease in the potentially diabetic person is of some importance. Obesity may be a factor in the adult, but there is no evidence that either overindulgence in eating or obesity is related to the onset of diabetes in childhood.

The relation of endocrine glands other than the pancreas to the metabolism of carbohydrates is recognized, but incompletely understood. Diabetes can be produced in the experimental animal by the appropriate injection of anterior pituitary extract. Hyperglycemia is occasionally associated with such endocrine disturbances as acromegaly, Cushing's syndrome, hyperthyroidism and pheochromocytomas. These disturbances of carbohydrate metabolism usually disappear if the endocrine disturbance is controlled.

Infection has been suggested as a cause of diabetes. The evidence does not support such a relation; it does, however, indicate that acute infection may frequently be the stress activating a latent state of diabetes mellitus in children.

A progressive loss of glucose tolerance has been observed in some children with cystic fibrosis. In some instances this glucose intolerance may represent the coincidental occurrence of 2 diseases: diabetes mellitus and cystic fibrosis. In the majority of instances, however, the disturbance in glucose metabolism appears to result from direct interference with the function of the islets of Langerhans by the fibrotic changes in the pancreas (see p. 862).

Pathologic Physiology. When there is insufficient insulin activity, a sequence of events is set up which terminates in diabetic acidosis, coma and death. The metabolic pattern which evolves is far more complicated than simple interference in the utilization of sugar, and many aspects of the disrupted metabolic pattern are not understood. What follows is merely an attempt to enumerate some of the metabolic derangements which contribute to the clinical expressions of this disease. These include (1) impaired transport of glucose across cellular membranes and impaired utilization of it within the cell, (2) impaired glycogen formation in the liver and in the muscles, and (3) increased glycogenolysis. As a result there is hyperglycemia, which, when it exceeds the renal threshold, is responsible for glycosuria. The diuresis initiated by the hyperglycemia accounts not only for the excretion of excess glucose, but also for excessive losses of electrolytes and water.

The breakdown of tissue and the consequent freeing of potassium and phosphates result in abnormally high levels of these electrolytes in the blood at a time when total body stores of them are being significantly depleted. The loss of body water results in hemoconcentration and dehydration, which in turn are responsible for decreased renal function. The shift of electrolytes from the intracellular to the extracellular spaces, the hemoconcentration and the renal dysfunction create a relative

1155

hyperelectrolytemia which, except as it is interpreted in the light of the altered physiology, may create a false impression of the body stores.

The tissue breakdown results in part from osmotic forces, in part from tissue catabolism secondary to the inability to use glucose for fuel. Both protein and fat are oxidized at abnormally rapid rates. The increased rate of breakdown of fat in the liver results in overproduction of ketones and in discharge of them into the blood at a rate exceeding the capacity of the peripheral tissues to oxidize them and of the kidneys to excrete them. Ketonuria may occur at blood levels which do not disturb the acid-base equilibrium, but the accumulation of ketone bodies in the blood of the uncontrolled diabetic does become sufficient to be a substantial factor in the development of acidosis. The other factors in the development of acidosis are dehydration, renal dysfunction secondary to anhydremia and loss of fixed base. Late contributory factors are loss of water through the hyperpnea caused by the acidosis and accumulation of lactic acid during cardiac failure.

The specific causes of coma are not apparent, but cerebral cellular activity is probably adversely affected by the various metabolic derangements. Whether hypoxia is a cause or merely an accompaniment is not known, but Kety's observation of diminished cerebral oxygen uptake during coma with acidosis is an argument in favor of the correction of excessively low pH levels early in the course of therapy of diabetic acidosis. Acidosis also inhibits restoration of the disrupted metabolism in the uncontrolled diabetic state in other ways. Guest and his co-workers showed that lowering of the pH and alkali reserve of the body fluids leads to hyperglycemia, hemoconcentration, losses of intracellular labile phosphates and potassium and inhibition of insulin action.

In summary, in the uncontrolled diabetic patient there are hyperglycemia, severe losses of body water and electrolytes, depletion of fixed base, lowering of the plasma carbon dioxide content, a shift of the pH of the blood to the acid side and depletion of glycogen stores in the liver and muscles. Therapy, to be rational, must be directed toward restoration of metabolic equilibrium.

Pathology. There is a decrease in the number of beta cells in the islands of Langerhans; it has been estimated that the number is usually less than 10 per cent of normal. Existing beta cells are said to show evidence of hyperactivity. Lymphocytic infiltration, believed to be a response to a pre-existing injury rather than a primary change or cause, is common. Hydropic degeneration may be present, but hyalinization, a common finding in adults with diabetes of long duration, is rare in children. Hepatomegaly is not uncommon; chemical studies reveal a depletion of glycogen. Histologic studies reveal little or no glycogen in the cytoplasm, but deposition of it in the nuclei. Arteriosclerosis and other degenerative changes occur with increasing frequency in young adults after 15 years or so of clinical diabetes.

Preclinical Phases of Diabetes Mellitus. Considerable interest is being manifest in the detection of diabetes before it is clinically overt. The importance of such information, beyond adding to a better understanding of the pathophysiology of the disease, would appear to be relatively greater for adults than for children. This is the case in several respects: for example, the development of the active clinical state is in general much more rapid in the child than in the adult, so that early detection is much less likely and perhaps less important; pregnancy is one of the more common stress situations which may temporarily and even permanently activate the diabetic state; and reduction of weight by the obese adult with an abnormal glucose tolerance curve may postpone, perhaps avoid, overt diabetes. Obesity is rarely a problem in the preclinical or early stages of diabetes in the child.

In order to provide a means for categorizing the preclinical phases, to identify factors which may activate the prediabetic state, and to establish a common terminology, the Committee on Professional Education of the American Diabetes Association has proposed the following classification:

Overt diabetes mellitus. Frank disease in which there is fasting hyperglycemia, and a glucose tolerance test is not required for diagnosis.

Chemical or latent diabetes. The patient has no symptoms of diabetes; the fasting blood glucose level is usually normal, but the postprandial level is frequently elevated. Oral or intravenous glucose tolerance curves, in the absence of stress, are in the diabetic range.

Suspected diabetes mellitus (including "stress" hyperglycemia). Temporary carbohydrate intolerance during certain physiologic or pathologic situations is considered a reason to suspect diabetes mellitus, particularly when there is a family history of diabetes. Impaired carbohydrate tolerance during periods of "stress" requires that the patient be re-evaluated frequently in respect to his diabetic status. These stressful situations include pregnancy, obesity, infections, trauma, vascular accidents, burns, impaired nutrition, severe emotional disturbances, treatment with such pharmacologic agents as corticosteroids or thiazides, and endocrinopathies such as acromegaly, Cushing's syndrome, thyrotoxicosis and pheochromocytoma.

Prediabetes. This term is applied to the time prior to the onset of identifiable diabetes mellitus (overt, chemical or latent). This state cannot be assumed with reasonable certainty, except in the nondiabetic identical twin of a diabetic patient and possibly in the offspring of 2 diabetic parents.

Clinical Manifestations of Overt Diabetes. In general the symptoms of diabetes mellitus in children are similar to those in adults. The principal differences are that the onset is likely to be more rapid in children, the diabetic child at the time of onset is more likely to be underweight in contrast to the frequency of obesity in adults, and diabetic hyperglycemia in the child does not respond favorably to oral hypoglycemic agents. A few diabetic children have had idiopathic hypoglycemia during infancy.

The common clinical manifestations in the early stage of diabetes are loss of weight, increased thirst and appetite and polyuria. The symptoms are somewhat more variable than in adults, and not infrequently the onset is so rapid that none of them has been noticed, or their existence is brought out only by leading questions. The child may be brought for medical attention because he has failed to gain weight in spite of a voracious appetite. One of the more frequent evidences of polyuria is bedwetting in a previously trained child. In untreated and long-standing cases dryness of the skin and pruritus are not uncommon, and there may be hypertrichosis. Skin infections are common, but the converse—a high incidence of diabetes in association with chronic infections of the skin—is not the case. Intertrigo and secondary skin infections are particularly common about the genital region in small children.

The presenting symptoms are often those of coma or stupor (diabetic acidosis), particularly when there is an existing acute infection or if there has been a recent one. In the precomatose state there are drowsiness, dryness of the skin, flushed cheeks, cherry-red lips, acetone breath, hyperpnea, nausea and vomiting, abdominal pain and often general body pains. In complete coma the hyperpnea becomes greater (*Kussmaul breathing*), the eyeballs are soft and sunken, the abdomen is rigid, the pulse is rapid and weak, and the temperature and blood pressure may be subnormal.

Chemical Changes. The characteristic alterations in the nonacidotic state include glycosuria, with or without ketonuria, and hyperglycemia. The absence of a fasting hyperglycemia does not rule out the possibility of diabetes mellitus. In rare instances the fasting blood sugar of an infant or young child who has only recently manifested diabetes may not be above the normal level, and a glucose tolerance test will be required to establish the diagnosis. Ketonuria may exist without measurable disturbance of the acid-base equilibrium, and there is no consistent relation between the degree of hyperglycemia and the absence or presence of ketonuria or its degree. Blood sugar levels as high as 800 to 1000 mg. per 100 ml. have been observed without an associated ketonuria in children who have eaten large amounts of carbohydrate. The blood cholesterol and lipid levels may be elevated in untreated diabetics.

With the development of acidosis there is a lowering of the carbon dioxide content of the blood, and a shift of the pH to the acid side. There is often an elevation of the nonprotein nitrogen. Protein and casts are frequently present in the urine at such times, but disappear when the acidosis is corrected.

Diagnosis. Children in whom the diagnosis of diabetes mellitus must be considered may be divided into 3 general categories: (1) those who have a history suggestive of diabetes; (2) those who have a transient or persistent glycosuria; and (3) those who have clinical manifestations of acidosis with or without stupor or coma. In all instances the diagnosis depends upon laboratory data. Glycosuria associated with a fasting hyperglycemia is for practical purposes diagnostic of diabetes mellitus. It is necessary, however, to eliminate the rare possibilities of Cushing's syndrome, hyperthyroidism and pheochromocytoma. Transitory glycosuria may be the result of emotional disturbances, of overeating (alimentary glycosuria), of acute infections, of cerebral injuries, of lead poisoning and of the ingestion of certain drugs. Salicylates may be responsible for a reduction of Benedict's solution which may simulate that by sugar.

Renal glycosuria is the result of a lowered renal threshold for glucose, but there is no hyperglycemia, and the glucose tolerance curve is within or below the usual range. The level of the renal threshold for sugar can be established by the sugar clearance test. It is important to bear in mind that not all urinary sugar is glucose, and steps should be taken to ensure that the unusual instances of *pentosuria* and *galactosemia* are not diagnosed as diabetes mellitus.

Whenever glucose is detected in the urine, fasting and postprandial blood glucose determinations should be obtained. If acetone is also present, a blood glucose determination should be obtained immediately. If the blood sugar is more than 200 mg. per 100 ml., a tentative diagnosis of diabetes mellitus is justified; if it is under this level, a fasting specimen of blood should be obtained the following morning; if the level is then within the normal range, a glucose tolerance test should be performed. The glucose tolerance test should be reserved for questionable cases; fasting and postprandial blood sugars will usually serve both for diagnosis and for evaluation of treatment.

Diabetic acidosis with or without coma must be differentiated from acidosis or coma from other causes, e.g. hypoglycemia, uremia, gastroenteritis, lead poisoning, salicylate poisoning, encephalitis, cerebral hemorrhage and other intracranial lesions. The symptoms previously described aid in differentiation, but the diagnosis must be based on laboratory analyses. Abdominal pain, tenderness, muscular rigidity, vomiting and leukocytosis are commonly present in diabetic acidosis. Though it is possible that acute appendicitis or other intra-abdominal infection may be the inciting cause of diabetic acidosis, the differential diagnosis cannot be made until the symptoms of acidosis have been relieved. High white blood cell counts may exist in association with diabetic acidosis, and do not in themselves indicate an infection.

Complications. Except in cases of long duration or in inadequately treated ones, complications are uncommon. Gangrene is a rare complication, but has been observed even in newborn infants. Stunting of growth, lack of development, failure to develop secondary sexual characteristics, and amenorrhea are seen in children whose diabetes has been uncontrolled over long periods of time. Hepatomegaly, though not a frequent complication, apparently occurs more often in inadequately treated children than in adults. Cataracts may occur at any age, but their incidence increases with duration of the disease. Arteriosclerosis, including renal lesions (see below), is seen with frequency only after the disease has existed for 10 to 15 years. Xanthomatous deposits in the skin occur occasionally in uncontrolled diabetes in association with hyperlipemia. *Necrobiosis lipoidica diabeticorum* is an uncommon cutaneous lesion characterized by elevated red papules 1 to 3 mm. in diameter, which eventually develop a yellowish tint. Carotenemia with resultant discoloration of the skin is more frequent in diabetics than in nondiabetics, and apparently is a reflection of hepatic dysfunction in the conversion of the provitamin A, carotene, to vitamin A. In poorly treated diabetic children, infections not only are common, but also show less tendency to heal.

Complications associated with the injection of insulin are lipodystrophy (atrophy of the subcutaneous fat), lipomatosis (a lipoma-like swelling) and allergy to insulin. Lipomatosis and possibly also lipodystrophy are the results of repeated injections of insulin into the same area, and perhaps of too superficial an injection.

Course and Prognosis. Before the introduction of insulin in 1922 the life expectancy of diabetic children was only about 2 years after the onset of the disease. What the expectancy is for the insulin-treated patient is not known, but the outlook has become less bright than it seemed in the earlier years of the "insulin era." The reason for this apparent change is based primarily upon the relative frequency with which serious degenerative lesions are appearing in young adults who have had diabetes for 10 to 20 years. These complications include principally arteriosclerosis with hypertension, retinal and lenticular changes and nephropathy, the characteristic lesion being intercapillary glomerulosclerosis (Kimmelstiel-Wilson syndrome). The incidence of complications in persons who have had diabetes for 20 years or more is as high as 85 per cent in a large series (White). The high incidence of vascular degenerative disease constitutes the most important problem in juvenile diabetes. There are those who view these complications as manifestations of a phase of diabetes which is not affected by presently available therapy. Some attach causal significance to deviations in clinical control sufficient to result in high blood cholesterol levels and frequent episodes of ketosis and acidosis. There is no clear evidence that the development of degenerative vascular changes or length of life after the onset of clinically manifest diabetes is related to degree of control as measured by variations in hyperglycemia and glycosuria or by strict adherence to a prescribed diet. There is limited evidence to suggest that the newborn infant of an adolescent diabetic girl is more apt to survive if the mother's diabetic control during gestation is good.

Physical growth and development are related to control of the diabetes. To what extent they are related to a degree of control which approximates normoglycemia is not known. Beal's data on a group of children whose diabetic control was probably well above average show a slight delay in growth in stature, but a tendency to approximate average adult heights after a somewhat prolonged growth period.

The so-called *Mauriac syndrome*, the underlying problems of which are not understood, consists of dwarfism, hepatomegaly and obesity in association with diabetes mellitus.

Comparatively little difficulty is encountered in management of the average preadolescent diabetic child, provided both the child and his family are properly instructed in the technique of diabetic care and assisted in making the necessary psychologic adjustments. The adolescent, however, has a natural inclination to rebel against authority and restraint, which is often reflected in breaks in diabetic control. At such times both the physician and the parents must take care that they do not lose the confidence and cooperation of the patient.

Treatment. The aims of treatment are restoration of the diabetic child to average physicial status and health, and subsequent maintenance of them. Control of the metabolic aspects of diabetes is merely a means to an end. The child who is not physically, mentally and socially able to compete with his colleagues cannot be considered an adequately treated diabetic child.

The essentials of treatment are (1) insulin in an amount adequate to approximate glycemic equilibrium; (2) a diet adequate for normal growth and activity and sufficient to satisfy the child's appetite; (3) instruction of the child and his parents in the ordinary routine care of diabetes so that it may be satisfactorily managed in the home; and (4) acceptance on the part of the child and his family that he is a "normal" healthy person able to compete with children of his own age.

Treatment may be divided into 4 phases: (1) acidosis; (2) postacidotic stage; (3) establishment of glycemic equilibrium; and (4) supervision of the controlled diabetic child.

Diabetic acidosis. Diabetic acidosis is a medical emergency requiring constant attention and teamwork among physician, nurse and laboratory. Recovery is directly related to the duration and degree of the acidosis and the state of consciousness of the patient and to the quantitative aspects of treatment. When it is not known that the patient is diabetic, the diagnosis can be established only by laboratory means. A sample of blood should be taken immediately for determinations of the blood sugar level, pH and the carbon dioxide content, and a specimen of urine should be obtained, by catheterization if necessary, for examination for sugar and acetone.

A plan for fluid and insulin therapy is detailed on page 224. The plan of therapy in our clinic differs in only one feature. For the patient who is in a severe state of acidosis (pH less than 7.1, carbon dioxide less than 6 to 8 mEq. per liter) we administer sodium bicarbonate after the initial expansion of the vascular volume with saline solution. This policy is based on clinical experience and on the physiologic considerations stated previously. In comparative observations in children and in animals, recovery as based on return of consciousness and ability to take and retain oral feedings has been more rapid when bicarbonate was administered early in therapy. Further, we have not observed any untoward results from such therapy. It should be clearly understood that only enough bicarbonate is given to raise the carbon dioxide level to 12 to 15 mEq. per liter (p. 225). Continuous clinical observation and frequent monitoring of blood sugar concentrations are essential in the management of the acidotic child.

Potassium is administered relatively early, as indicated on page 219. Potassium chloride can be added to the glucose-saline solution being administered intravenously in an amount so that its concentration does not exceed 0.15 per cent or 20 mEq. per liter, or it can be administered as a separate solution subcutaneously.

Gastric lavage is invariably beneficial in the acidotic patient. It will not only avert vomiting as the child regains consciousness, but it will also shorten the time until fluids can be taken by mouth. After the stomach has been thoroughly emptied of its contents, which often contain digested blood, several grams of sodium bicarbonate in solution may be introduced as an emollient. The lavage may be delayed until after the parenteral fluid therapy has been started.

Hyperosmolar diabetic coma, which has been described principally in adults, has also been observed in children. Four of 6 children with this syndrome observed in one clinic (Rubin et al.) had pre-existing neurologic lesions. Their blood chemical data revealed hyperglycemia, hyperosmolality, metabolic acidosis and little or no ketosis. Four of the children died; only those who received very small amounts of glucose in the initial parenteral fluid therapy survived.

Postacidotic stage. Parenteral fluid therapy can usually be terminated in less than 24 hours. For the next 24 to 48 hours the child will require special attention. As soon as he is ready to take fluids by mouth, sips of water or chilled ginger ale (for some reason carbonated drinks seem to be retained at this stage more often than orange juice) may be given for a few hours or until it is evident that vomiting or gastric distention is not likely to occur. A soft or liquid diet consisting chiefly of carbohydrate may then be started and given to the child at approximately 3-hour intervals during the day. Such foods as fruits, fruit juices, skimmed milk, fat-free ice cream, and gelatin desserts are taken well. The insulin dosage during this time is entirely empiric and is based on urine analyses for sugar. It is best to give small doses of regular insulin at frequent intervals rather than large doses at infrequent intervals. Careful check should be maintained to avoid insulin shock or the return to hyperglycemia. After a day or two on this regimen the child should be ready for an average diet.

Establishment of glycemic equilibrium. The suggestions made here are also applicable to the child who has not been in acidosis, but is not in satisfactory diabetic control. There are no hard and fast rules; each child is an individual problem for whom a satisfactory diet must be arranged and the insulin dosage determined. No attempt should be made to avoid the use of insulin.

Diet. There has been a gradual transition in types of diets prescribed for diabetic children. The prescription of low carbohydrate diets has for practical purposes ceased, and the tendency now is to provide a diet which approximates that of the average child and conforms to the family's dietary pattern. Principal differences are now in whether the diet is measured or is unrestricted ("free diet"). The so-called free diet is usually restricted to the extent that the child is advised to avoid dietary excesses, especially of "sweets" and foodstuffs of high carbohydrate content. There is no doubt that one of the essentials in the management of the diabetic child is complete acceptance of the disease and its management without the sense of undue restriction or of being different from other children. Such an ideal situation is usually not attained; if the free diet could be the determining factor in attaining it, its use would be justified. In our experience, however, we have felt that most often both child and parents profit initially from some guidance in the dietary program.

It is our practice to prescribe the initial diet for the child while he is in the hospital. After the first week or so of the insulin adjustment period, the child is consulted about his satisfaction with his diet and requested to participate in planning his home diet both qualitatively and quantitatively. The method devised by Stare (p. 1547) is used, and the child and his mother are given a copy of the Exchange Lists. They should know that the diet is not a rigid one, that gross household measures are adequate, and that occasional quantitative deviations are of no great consequence. Though the diet is not an entirely unrestricted one, it can be a self-determined one and can vary markedly from child to child to conform to individual desires and to family dietary patterns. Certainly dietary instruction can be given on a very general basis and without a precise prescription. The goals of any plan are (1) to ensure a qualitatively satisfactory intake; (2) to secure an adequate distribution of caloric intake at the various meals; and (3) to teach the child by experience the self-serving of meals at a later age. The essentials of an adequate diet are (1) sufficient caloric value for activity and growth; (2) a protein intake not less than 1.5 gm. per pound for children under 3 years of age, and 1 gm. per pound for older children; (3) 40 to 50 per cent of the calories as carbohydrate; (4) optimal intake of vitamins and minerals; and (5) participation in the diet by the entire family.

A reasonable distribution of calories can be obtained by the use of one of the following formulas:

Carbo-hydrate		Protein		Fat		Calories	
Gm. per		Gm. per		Gm. per		per	
Kg.	Lb.	Kg.	Lb.	Kg.	Lb.	Kg.	Lb.
9	4	3	1.5	2.5	1.5	= 70	35
9	4	2	1.0	2.5	1.5	= 66	33
7	3.5	3	1.5	2.0	1.0	= 58	29
7	3	2	1.0	2.0	1.0	= 54	25

See page 129 for average caloric requirements at different age levels.

Stabilization should be carried out, if at all possible, while the patient is normally active. Even in the hospital the child may be permitted considerable activity. The initial diet should subsequently be adjusted on the basis of the appetite and the growth response (as indicated by the weight curve). If growth is normal and appetite is satisfied, the diet remains as planned; if growth is not proceeding and appetite is not satisfied, the diet is increased; if there is no gain in weight, but the appetite is satisfied, more food is prescribed and more concentrated foods are substituted for relatively bulky ones; or, if the patient is gaining, but the appetite is not satisfied, the bulk of the diet is increased without increasing the caloric value. There is no need to use commercial diabetic foods.

Insulin. Insulin is the *sine qua non* of diabetic therapy. No juvenile diabetic can be treated without it. The principal question is the degree of control of hyperglycemia which is attempted. A few clinicians believe that, except as hyperglycemia is sufficient to cause excess diuresis, it is not harmful; otherwise their only concern is ketosis. Others hold that a reasonable attempt should be made to achieve a normoglycemic status; we subscribe to this goal, but only so far as it can be attained without hypoglycemic attacks, other than as rare occurrences, and without too great dietary rigidity. Practically all children excrete small amounts of sugar daily on this plan.

The sulfonylureas, as orally administered hypoglycemic agents, are widely used in the treatment of adults with mild diabetes. These agents stimulate the production of insulin. Since the capacity to produce insulin is usually rapidly and largely lost in diabetic children, the sulfonylurea drugs are rarely able to evoke any significant increase in the production of insulin in them. In the infrequent instances in children when there is a slow onset and the chemical pattern of diabetes is not severe, the sulfonylurea agents may be as effective as they are in mild diabetes in the adult.

The biguanides (Phenformin–DBI) are another class of drugs used in the oral treatment of diabetes. These agents lower blood glucose levels by altering carbohydrate metabolism. In our experience, Phenformin has not been useful in the management of children with diabetes. The incidence of side reactions is high, and, even when satisfactory chemical control of the diabetes was achieved, growth was significantly retarded.

There are now available at least 7 different forms of insulin. These are listed in Table 16-1 and are grouped according to the rapidity and duration of their hypoglycemic effect.

The physician will be well advised to become thoroughly familiar with the use of 2 or 3 insulins and to limit his prescribing of insulins to them. As a rule, working familiarity with one of the "inter-mediate action" insulins and one of the rapidly acting ones is sufficient. In maintenance therapy, if one of the "intermediate" (NPH or Lente) insulins is given as the basic product, most children will require a supplementary dose of a rapidly acting insulin (see below). Our experience has been largely with Lente and NPH insulin among the intermediate-acting ones and with unmodified or regular insulin among the rapidly acting ones.

If sufficient Lente or NPH insulin is administered as the prebreakfast dose, an effect can be secured for 24 hours or so. Occasionally they will provide sufficient insulin action to avoid significant glycosuria during the day and still maintain nocturnal control without hypoglycemia. More often, however, unmodified insulin will have to be administered along with Lente or NPH insulin to avoid significant diurnal glycosuria, if diurnal control without insulin shock is desired. The majority of our diabetic children receive a combination of Lente and unmodified insulin. One of the advantages of Lente and NPH insulin over protamine zinc insulin is that the unmodified insulin can be included in the same syringe without being altered; it thus behaves as if it were a separate injection. Lente insulin contains no protamine, so that the slight possibility of induced allergy to it is eliminated. For infants and children up to 4 or 5 years of age unmodified insulin for the prebreakfast and prelunch injections and Lente insulin for the evening injection often provide an effective plan of insulin therapy.

The daily requirements of insulin are estimated from qualitative tests of the urine for sugar. Specimens of urine should be collected 4 times a day: (1) before breakfast (7 to 8 a.m.), (2) before the noon meal (11:30 a.m. to 12 noon), (3) before the evening meal (5 to 6 p.m.), and (4) before retiring (7 to 9 p.m.). The results of analyses of these specimens will be of greater aid in estimating insulin dosage if the child voids (discarding the specimen) from $1/2$ to 1 hour before each of the 3 specimens to be tested is obtained.

After the first day or two of the postacidotic stage as described above, unmodified (regular) insulin is given before each meal. Individual doses are usually in the range of 10 to 15 units; estimates can be made from the experience of the preceding days, and adjustments made daily on the basis of the qualitative urine test for sugar in specimens voided about 3 hours after each meal, as noted above. After 2 days or so a reasonable estimate of the total daily dose of insulin which is sufficient to effect a reduction in the urinary sugar without causing insulin shock can be made.

At this time one may initiate the permanent plan for insulin therapy. It is our practice to give about 75 per cent of the previous day's total dose of insulin as Lente insulin and the remainder as unmodified insulin before breakfast. Subsequent adjustments of the dose of each insulin are made on the basis of the presence or absence of sugar in the urine or by the occurrence of insulin shock. The dose of Lente insulin is adjusted so that the urine

TABLE 16-1. FORMS OF INSULIN COMMERCIALLY AVAILABLE

| | APPROXIMATE HYPOGLYCEMIC EFFECT IN HOURS | | |
	ONSET	PEAK	DURATION
Rapid Action—Short Duration			
Insulin product			
Regular (unmodified, zinc crystalline)..........	$1/2$	2-4	6-8
Semi-Lente..	$1/2$	2-4	10-12
Intermediate in Rapidity of Action—Relatively Long Duration			
NPH (isophane)	2	8-10	28-30
Lente (70% Ultra-Lente and			
30% Semi-Lente).....................................	2	8-10	20-26
Globin	2	8-16	Up to 24 hours
Delayed Action—Long Duration			
Protamine zinc (PZI)	4-8	14-20	24-36
Ultra-Lente...	4-8	14-24	36 or more

of the following morning contains little or no sugar and so that the child does not have insulin shock during the night or prebreakfast hours. The dose of the unmodified insulin is estimated on the basis of the urinalyses preceding the noon and evening meals or the occurrence of insulin shocks during this portion of the day. Under such a plan an attempt is made to secure an average blood sugar level the following morning and urine tests at noon and in the afternoon which indicate only small amounts of glycosuria. Occasionally, satisfactory glycemic equilibrium is obtained with only Lente insulin, but most often unmodified insulin will also have to be continued in the prebreakfast injection. Rarely is an additional dose of unmodified insulin given before the evening meal to avoid glycosuria during the evening hours. If there is only a transitory spilling of sugar after the evening meal and if, on the following morning, the blood sugar level approximates the normal range or the urine contains little or no sugar, there is no need for injection of insulin before the evening meal.

The urine can be made essentially sugar-free within about a week by this regimen. The dose of insulin at this stage, however, does not represent the child's maintenance dose. During the next 2 to 3 months it will usually have to be decreased progressively. The need for decreasing it is determined on the basis of aglycosuria, or of blood sugar levels below the normal range or by hypoglycemic shock.

This period of improvement in carbohydrate tolerance occurs early in the initial treatment of practically all diabetic children, provided their insulin dosage has been reasonably appropriate. The period has been termed restoration of metabolic equilibrium and diabetic remission; neither is appropriate. A general metabolic adjustment takes place gradually and there is no known way to shorten this period. The low level of insulin dosage is attained about 12 to 16 weeks after initiation of therapy. Infrequently the need for

exogenous insulin may then disappear for a short time, and injections can be temporarily discontinued. Daily urinalyses, however, must be continued, since glycosuria will become evident again within a few weeks, and the administration of insulin will have to be resumed. *It is obviously essential that the parents and the older child should understand this phase and its management.*

There are distinct advantages in keeping the child hospitalized, but not inactive, for the first 2 weeks or so of the initial adjustment period. The latter part of this period can then be managed in the child's home, provided instruction of the patient and his family has been adequate and careful records of urinalyses for sugar will be kept.

Insulin should be administered subcutaneously, care being taken that it is not injected too near the skin. Definite instruction should be given for changing the site of injection: e.g. successively into the right upper arm, the left upper arm, the left thigh, the right thigh. Each extremity may be used for several weeks without making 2 injections into the same site, provided a systematic plan is followed. Thus, starting at the inner and upper corner of an area to be used, each succeeding injection is made $1/2$ inch below the preceding one, and when each vertical line is complete, the site selected is moved outward $1/2$ inch at the upper level, and injections then proceed downward in a similar vertical manner. Other sites which may be used are the upper part of the buttocks, the back and the abdomen. If signs of induration appear at the sites of injection, these areas should be carefully avoided for several weeks after all evidences of local irritation have disappeared. Patients receiving insulin should bathe at least every other day, and sterile technique should be practiced in preparing the needle, syringes, bottle caps and the skin at the site of the injection.

Antibody production to the exogenous insulin being used is common, and perhaps occurs to some extent in all insulin-treated patients. Infrequently, the diabetic child may manifest evidences of allergy to insulin or of insulin resistance. In either instance, discontinuance of the insulin being used and substitution of a sulfated insulin or one from a different species of animal is advisable.

Among the factors which vary the need for, or utilization of, insulin are diet, physical activity, infection and, to a less extent, growth. No definite rule can be stated about the possible need for increased insulin with increase in diet or body weight. Many children require gradual increases in insulin dosage up to puberty, and then often further but temporary increases during early adolescence, whereas others do not. Increased dietary intake usually does not require proportionate increase of insulin dosage, often none at all.

Exercise tends to lower the blood sugar level of children receiving otherwise adequate amounts of insulin and may thus initiate insulin shock. Diabetic children should, however, be encouraged to be normally active; so far as possible, exercise should be regulated in quantity and time so that allowance may be made for it in the adjustment of insulin dosage. The child should be instructed to carry sugar with him at all times and to take it whenever the first symptoms of shock are noted. When it is known that there is to be an increase in physical activity, the caloric intake for that day can be increased or the dose of insulin can be reduced by an amount determined by experience to be satisfactory.

Infection increases the requirement for insulin and is the most potent factor in initiating acidosis. During mild infections, such as those of the upper respiratory tract, the only treatment required for the diabetic condition is sufficient extra insulin to prevent excessive glycosuria. In severe infections fat should be decreased in the diet, extra carbohydrate should be administered if the child's appetite requires it, and additional insulin should be injected as needed. An adequate plan for adjustment of insulin dosage during infection in children receiving a combination of Lente and unmodified insulins is to maintain the quantity of Lente insulin at the previous dose and to add extra unmodified insulin at breakfast, lunch and dinner in amounts estimated from the results of the urinary test for sugar. It is important to bear in mind that the dose of insulin must be reduced again during convalescence.

Insulin shock may result from an overdose of insulin, from reduction in diet or from increase in exercise without a corresponding reduction in insulin. Early symptoms are sudden hunger, weakness, restlessness, pallor, sweating and dilated pupils; if carbohydrate is not administered, tremor, vertigo, unconsciousness, convulsions and in rare instances even death will occur. In shock from overdose of protamine insulin and to a less extent of Lente and NPH the onset may be less abrupt, and the reactions usually, but not always, less severe. Vomiting during and after shock from the long-acting insulins may occur, but practically never from unmodified insulin. The slower onset of shock from the long-acting insulins, together with the vomiting, may lead to an incorrect diagnosis of diabetic acidosis.

The time of occurrence of hypoglycemic shock after injection of insulin may aid in the differential diagnosis of shock from coma. Shock from unmodified insulin usually occurs 3 to 8 hours after injection, that from Lente, NPH and protamine insulins usually 8 to 24 hours after injection. If, however, it is not clear whether unconsciousness is the result of hypoglycemia or diabetic acidosis, 20 to 10 ml. of 20 or 50 per cent glucose should be injected intravenously. If unconsciousness is the result of hypoglycemia, consciousness will be quickly restored; no harm will be done by the injection of glucose if the child is in diabetic acidosis.

The emotional response of the diabetic child to insulin shock tends to follow a stereotyped pattern characteristic of him. The variations in response are somewhat similar to those of different persons to alcoholic intoxication. Thus one child may become despondent and cry readily, whereas another one is exuberant and even hilarious, and an occasional child becomes belligerent.

Insulin shock is, under ordinary circumstances, such a transient affair, and the disappearance of symptoms is so complete, that there is often failure to recognize that it may have serious consequences. When shock of an extreme degree is allowed to persist, there may be cerebral damage responsible for permanent motor defects, mental deficiency and even death.

The treatment of shock usually requires nothing more than the ingestion of sugar or some food such as orange juice which contains readily available simple sugars. If the child is unable to take food by mouth, it may be necessary to give glucose intravenously (see above) or epinephrine or glucagon subcutaneously.

Glucagon is packaged for emergency and can be used within the home by a parent or other caretaker who has been appropriately instructed. When the shock from insulin overdosage is so profound that the child cannot take sugar orally, an injection of glucagon (0.5 to 1.0 mg.) will usually elevate the blood glucose level within a few minutes and restore the child to consciousness. Sugar can then be given by mouth. In such instances transportation to the hospital for intravenous administration of glucose may be avoided. It would seem wise to keep an emergency kit containing glucagon in the home of the diabetic child.

Supervision of the Diabetic Child. Diabetic children can be normally healthy and active, and it is the physician's responsibility to assist the child and his family in making an adequate psychologic adjustment. Instruction in daily care should be given to the patient and his family so that they can be essentially independent of the physician for the ordinary care of diabetes. These instructions should include (1) dietary planning; (2) administration of insulin and minor adjustments in dosage which are required by changes in activity and even minor infections; (3) examination of the urine for sugar; (4) the keeping of daily records; (5) the need for personal cleanliness; (6) recognition of early signs of shock and method of treatment; and (7) recognition of early signs of acidosis and of the need for immediate medical assistance. The diabetic child should assume his share of family responsibilities and compete on an equal basis with his schoolmates. He should not look upon his diabetes as a handicap or as a reason for asking for quarter.

Unfortunately a truly adequate psychologic adjustment by the child and his family is frequently not attained. In some instances this is largely due to the physician's failure to provide early guidance and particularly to his failure to permit the child and his parents to achieve a sense of sufficiency for the ordinary management of the diabetes. The daily management can become as routine as other features of personal hygiene. No attempt should be made to hide the fact that the child has diabetes; on the other hand, it should not be used as a "crutch" or defense mechanism. The child should be permitted and encouraged to develop his natural talents, but the *sense of direction* should exist in him. The differences in the attitudes and adjustments of diabetic children in various clinics attest to the importance of guidance by medical and ancillary personnel — or in certain respects, perhaps, to lack of it.

During adolescence the problems of the diabetic child are likely to be accentuated. Rebellion at the regularity of insulin injections may result in lapses of medication and hence acidosis, or rebellion may be expressed in other ways, such as aggressiveness or withdrawal and even delinquency. Parents and physicians require a fine understanding; above all, they must have the confidence of the child if he is to be brought to maturity adequately adjusted to compete on an equal basis with his peers.

THE DIABETES MELLITUS SYNDROME IN THE NEWBORN INFANT

A few instances of a transient state of diabetes mellitus developing in the neonatal period, persisting for weeks or months and terminating apparently in complete recovery, have been reported. Clinically, the syndrome fulfills the diagnostic requirements: viz., hyperglycemia, glycosuria and clinical control with exogenous insulin. It is most likely to occur in infants less than 6 weeks of age whose birth weight was low for gestational age. The onset may be sudden with severe dehydration, polyuria, fever and metabolic acidosis; if the condition is not treated with insulin and supportive therapy, brain damage or death may result. Ketonuria may not occur; if present, it is usually mild. Ketonemia may exist in the absence of ketonuria in the neonatal period. Occasionally, transient hypoglycemia in the newborn may precede the development of transient diabetes mellitus. Infection has not seemed to be an important instigating factor. The management is that of diabetes mellitus, but extreme care must be taken to avoid hypoglycemia and to determine when administration of insulin is no longer required. By contrast with the true disease, complete recovery occurs and, so far as is known, is permanent.

True diabetes mellitus is also rare in newborn infants, but it does occur. Differentiation from the transient state can be made only after sufficient time has elapsed to determine whether the diabetic state is permanent.

WALDO E. NELSON

See page 1171 for References to Diabetes Mellitus.

HYPOGLYCEMIA

Hypoglycemia is a state in which there is an abnormally low level of blood glucose, the principal circulating hexose and physiologically the most important one. Enzymatic assay (glucose oxidase) is required for the specific quantitation of blood glucose concentration; methods which depend on the reducing properties of sugar such as the Nelson-Somogyi and ferricyanide ones also identify other sugars (e.g. galactose) as well as glucose.

The fasting blood glucose level varies with age; it is lower in infants than in adults. In normal infants during the first few days of life, values as low as 20 mg. per 100 ml. are not uncommon. Low-birth-weight infants may continue to have such low values for a longer time. Thereafter the normal values range from 50 to about 100 mg. per 100 ml. Although values below 50 mg. per 100 ml. (below 30 mg. in the newborn) are generally accepted to represent chemical hypoglycemia, a low blood glucose level may be considered clinically significant only when it is associated with characteristic clinical manifestations.

Physiologic Considerations. Glucose may be derived directly from dietary intake by intestinal absorption, by conversion of other hexoses after absorption (galactose, fructose), by hydrolysis of polyglucose units (maltose, starch, glycogen) or by combinations of these processes (lactose, sucrose). Glucose can also be derived from dietary or endogenous amino acids, but there is no *net* synthesis of glucose from exogenous or endogenous lipids.

Figure 16-1 depicts in simplified form some of the pathways of glucose metabolism. Although free glucose may passively diffuse through most cell membranes, it is usually taken up from the lumen of the intestinal tract by the mucosal cells, from the lumen of the renal tubules by their epithelial cells, or from the bloodstream by various parenchymal cells against a concentration gradient. Such an active process requires energy and

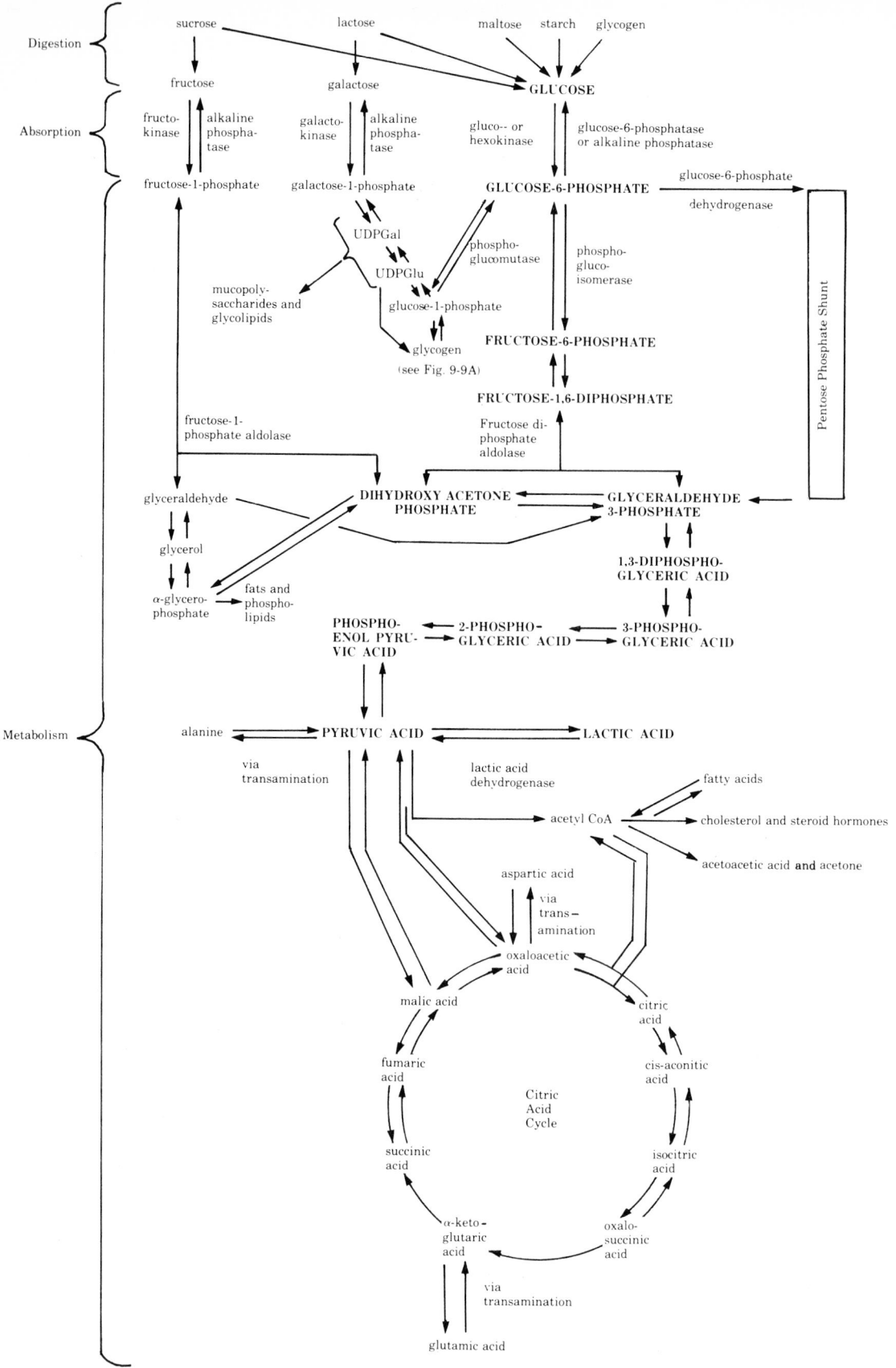

Figure 16-1. The metabolism of glucose. The compounds of the Embden-Meyerhof pathway are indicated in bold face type.

is brought about by the phosphorylation of glucose, using ATP and either hexokinase or glucokinase. Once within the cells, the glucose-6-phosphate may be metabolized or may be hydrolyzed to glucose, which is then free to diffuse out of the cell again. The main routes of metabolism are as follows: (1) The Embden-Meyerhof pathway of anaerobic glycolysis converts the 6-carbon glucose to 3-carbon acids (pyruvic and lactic) with a small release of energy. (2) The pentose-phosphate shunt, which is initiated by the enzyme glucose-6-phosphate dehydrogenase, yields ribose among other sugars or joins the Embden-Meyerhof scheme at the level of glyceraldehyde-3-phosphate. The reduction of TPN along this pathway is important for lipid synthesis and for the maintenance of glutathione in the reduced form. (3) Glucose is also converted to glucose-1-phosphate, which is in equilibrium with galactose-1-phosphate through a combined form involving uridine diphosphate. In this form, glucose is used for the synthesis of the 1,4 chains of glycogen (p. 440).

The ultimate product of glycolysis is pyruvic acid. After the addition of carbon dioxide or after oxidization to acetyl coenzyme A, it enters the citric acid cycle (tricarboxylic acid or Krebs cycle). Acetyl coenzyme A can also be used in the synthesis of fatty acids, cholesterol and steroid hormones or to form the ketone bodies (acetone, acetoacetic acid and beta-hydroxybutyric acid). The enzymes of the citric acid cycle are found in the mitochondria within the cells where most of the energy resident in glucose is released and captured in the form of ATP. It is in the citric acid cycle that many amino acids are in equilibrium with glucose. By transamination or oxidation, glutamic acid is converted to alpha-ketoglutaric acid, aspartic acid to oxaloacetic acid, and alanine to pyruvic acid.

Many of the enzyme systems involved in the metabolism of glucose are under hormonal control. The mechanisms and exact sites of action of the various hormones are poorly defined. Insulin is known to increase the activity of glucokinase, to increase permeability of the cell membrane for glucose and to facilitate removal of glucose from the circulation and to increase its utilization. Glucagon stimulates hepatic phosphorylase, resulting in increased glycogen breakdown and hyperglycemia. Epinephrine acts in the same manner as glucagon and also reduces peripheral utilization of glucose. Many of these hormones stimulate the enzymatic formation of cyclic $3',5'$ AMP, a compound which has many physiologic and pharmacologic effects. The enzymatic sites of action of growth hormone, corticotropin and glucocorticoids on glucose metabolism are unknown; they produce hyperglycemia. Glucocorticoids promote gluconeogenesis from protein.

Pathologic alterations of endocrine systems, toxins and inherited enzymatic defects can be responsible for hypoglycemia.

Although muscle, liver, kidney and other non-neural tissues can utilize sugars other than glucose as a source of energy, the normal brain usually utilizes only glucose for its metabolic requirements. Hence hypoglycemia is manifest principally by evidences of central nervous system dysfunction.

Etiology. Since hypoglycemia may result from a wide variety of factors, and rational treatment and prognosis depend upon the nature of the disorder, it is essential to make every reasonable effort to determine its cause.

Hypoglycemia due to impaired intestinal absorption of glucose. Unlike most adults, children and especially infants may exhibit lowering of the blood glucose level when carbohydrate is withheld for 24 to 48 hours. Fasting, however, by itself is rarely, if ever, a cause of clinical hypoglycemia, but may be a precipitating factor when other defects that may cause hypoglycemia are present. This may be the case when the blood glucose value is lowered by impaired intestinal absorption accompanying chronic diarrhea, celiac disease or the edematous phase of the nephrotic syndrome. There are several specific defects in the intestinal absorption of sugars (p. 811) such as of glucose and galactose, of sucrose and isomaltose, and of lactose, which are characterized by diarrhea, but they do not lead to significant hypoglycemia. Delayed absorption of glucose occurs in hypothyroidism, but rarely is of sufficient magnitude to lead to hypoglycemia.

Hypoglycemia due to renal glycosuria. Glycosuria due to defective tubular reabsorption of glucose occurs in a variety of clinical entities. It occurs as an isolated hereditary condition, in combination with glycinuria, in the de Toni-Fanconi syndrome, and in some patients with lead poisoning. It is rare that any of these conditions leads to hypoglycemia.

Hypoglycemia due to decreased delivery of glucose into the blood by the liver. HEPATIC DAMAGE. Severe hepatic damage may disturb the metabolism of carbohydrates sufficiently to produce hypoglycemia. Hepatotoxic agents, such as phosphorus, halogenated hydrocarbon (carbon tetrachloride) and hydrazine, may be responsible for hypoglycemia. Extensive infiltration of the liver by neoplastic cells, fibrous tissue, granulomas or fat may also lead to hypoglycemia, as may acute and chronic infectious hepatitis in the terminal stages. The mechanism is not completely understood, but the hypoglycemia probably results from failure to store glycogen, impaired release of glucose into the bloodstream and decreased net synthesis of glucose from amino acids.

Ingestion of ethyl alcohol precipitates hypoglycemia in normal adults after a fast of 2 to 3 days, but in persons in whom the gluconeogenic reserve is decreased the hypoglycemic potential of alcohol is revealed after only 12 hours or so of fasting. The hypoglycemia is not mediated by an increase in insulin secretion and is not responsive to glucagon administration. It has been shown that pure ethanol, and not congeners or denaturants, is responsible for the hypoglycemia; the effect appears to result from interference with intrahepatic mechanisms for gluconeogenesis.

Addiction to alcohol or chronic alcoholism is not necessary for the hypoglycemic effect; the accidental ingestion of alcohol by children has produced hypoglycemia sufficient to cause seizures, coma and even death.

In the syndrome of *encephalopathy and fatty degeneration of viscera (Reye's syndrome)* (p. 847), blood glucose levels below 25 to 30 mg. per 100 ml. are relatively common. The hypoglycemia is believed to be the result of the severe fatty degeneration of the liver.

GLYCOGENOSES. Hypoglycemia occurs only in those glycogenoses (glycogen storage diseases) which primarily affect the *liver* (p. 440), whereas those which primarily affect *muscle* are not associated with hypoglycemia. In type I glycogenosis (von Gierke's), glucose-6-phosphatase activity is absent or markedly diminished in the liver as well as in the kidney, and release of glucose from the liver is decreased. Severe hypoglycemia may occur in the fasting state and 4 to 6 hours postprandially. Levels of glucose as low as 0 mg. per 100 ml. have been reported; it has been assumed that the brain of such a person does not depend solely on glucose as a source of energy. It is believed that amino acids and fatty acids are metabolized by the brain, since affected patients are not as a rule mentally retarded or excessively prone to convulsions. In type III glycogenosis the debrancher enzyme is absent, and in type VI glycogenosis there is decreased activity of hepatic phosphorylase. Both types III and VI result in limited ability to degrade glycogen and are also associated with hypoglycemia, although it is not as severe as in von Gierke's disease (type I). In aglycogenosis, the condition in which there is deficiency of glycogen synthetase, only small amounts of glycogen can be synthesized in the liver. In this disorder severe hypoglycemia occurs after an overnight fast. These observations emphasize the cardinal role of the liver in glucose metabolism. In type IV glycogenosis the brancher enzyme is deficient and an abnormal amylopectin-like glycogen is synthesized, but hypoglycemia has not been found in the few patients observed.

GALACTOSEMIA. Hypoglycemia may be one of the clinical manifestations of galactosemia (p. 437). The total blood sugar level (Nelson-Somogyi method) is normal or elevated, but the glucose level may be low; the difference is accounted for by galactose. This situation accounts for hypoglycemic manifestations in infants with normal concentrations of total blood sugar. Hypoglycemia may occur after ingestion of milk, and, during the course of a galactose tolerance test, blood glucose may fall to as low as 10 mg. per 100 ml. The mechanism responsible for the hypoglycemia is not completely understood; it has been suggested that an elevated blood level of galactose stimulates release of insulin. On the other hand, it has also been suggested that the toxic amounts of galactose-1-phosphate and dulcitol found in this disorder not only cause renal damage, cataracts and cerebral damage, but also interfere with glucose release from the liver by inhibition of phosphogluco-mutase and glucose-6-phosphatase.

FRUCTOSEMIA (HEREDITARY FRUCTOSE INTOLERANCE). The ingestion of fructose leads to abnormally elevated blood levels of fructose (fructosemia) in 2 conditions. One of these, essential or benign fructosemia, is an asymptomatic disorder (p. 436) resulting from a deficiency of fructokinase. The other disorder, known as hereditary fructose intolerance or as fructosemia, is a serious disorder of infancy, and one of the easily treated causes of hypoglycemia.

The clinical symptoms of hypoglycemia are associated with other systemic manifestations. Affected infants do not exhibit symptoms until fructose is added to the diet. The infant then becomes anorexic, vomits and fails to thrive. Hypoglycemic manifestations include drowsiness during feeding, excessive sweating, pallor, rolling of the eyes, twitching and convulsions. Jaundice and hepatosplenomegaly develop and may be the presenting manifestations. Renal tubular involvement may result in glycosuria, aminoaciduria, proteinuria and acidosis. A low blood glucose concentration may be masked by fructosemia, unless the measurement is made by the glucose oxidase method. The disorder may ultimately lead to death, if it is not recognized and treated. The development of an aversion to fruits and other fructose-containing foods (sucrose) results in the spontaneous amelioration of symptoms and may account for survival into childhood before recognition of the disorder.

Fructosemia is a genetic disorder transmitted in an autosomal recessive manner. The primary defect is a structural mutation of one of the 2 isozymes of aldolase known as liver type. This enzyme normally reacts with both fructose-1-phosphate and fructose-1,6-diphosphate. The muscle type aldolase which remains in the liver reacts more readily with the diphosphate than the monophosphate, resulting in accumulation primarily of fructose-1-phosphate.

The mechanism of the hypoglycemia is not known; it is not associated with increased levels of insulin. It has been suggested that accumulation of fructose-1-phosphate may inhibit hepatic enzymes involved in the release of glucose.

Ketotic hypoglycemia. Ketotic hypoglycemia accounts for approximately half of the cases of hypoglycemia in childhood. The onset is usually after 1 year of age. Boys are affected more often than girls, and the number of affected children who are born at low birth weight is disproportionately high. The attacks are episodic and occur after a period of food deprivation; acetonuria is associated with the hypoglycemia. There is rapid response to administration of glucose, but not to administration of glucagon. The child is in apparent good health between attacks, which decrease in frequency with advancing age.

Between attacks carbohydrate tolerance tests

most often give normal results, but hypoglycemia can be precipitated by prolonged fasting or by administration of a ketogenic diet. Neither the ketogenic diet nor administration of tolbutamide is associated with increased release of insulin. The precise mechanism of the disorder is unsettled, but there appears to be a defect in gluconeogenesis, and this may be secondary to an inability to secrete sufficient insulin to accumulate hepatic stores of glycogen.

Hypoglycemia due to pituitary and adrenal cortical insufficiency. Corticotropin and growth hormone are the principal anterior pituitary hormones with carbohydrate-regulating properties.

The manner in which growth hormone affects glucose metabolism is not known; it is known, however, that in normal children plasma levels of growth hormone rise in response to hypoglycemia and after prolonged fasting. By contrast, about half of the children with isolated deficiency of growth hormone do not respond in this manner to hypoglycemia, and some of them do have symptomatic hypoglycemia. When other pituitary tropic hormones (ACTH and TSH) are also deficient, the incidence of hypoglycemia and the unresponsiveness of growth hormone to it are even higher.

The effect of corticotropin on carbohydrate metabolism is an indirect one through its control of adrenal secretion of glucocorticosteroids. The principal actions of glucocorticosteroids on carbohydrate metabolism are an increase in gluconeogenesis and a decrease in utilization of glucose by the tissues. A deficiency of corticotropin or of adrenal cortical secretion may thus lead to hypoglycemia by a combination of these effects. Patients with congenital virilizing adrenal hyperplasia occasionally have hypoglycemia due to inability of the adrenal cortex to produce adequate amounts of hydrocortisone (p. 1214).

Hypoglycemia associated with adrenal medullary unresponsiveness. In normal persons the secretion of epinephrine is stimulated by hypoglycemia; the urinary excretion of epinephrine during hypoglycemia increases 5- to 20-fold above that of euglycemic periods. The increased circulating epinephrine tends to restore the level of blood glucose to normal. Children have been observed in whom the normal increase in epinephrine does not occur in response to spontaneous hypoglycemia or to that provoked by insulin administration. Most children so affected have had a low birth weight for gestational age, but did not appear immature. Symptoms of hypoglycemia may begin in the neonatal period or may be delayed for many months.

Although there is defective release of epinephrine, it is not known whether the disturbance is in the adrenal medulla, the hypothalamus or the autonomic nervous system. Nor is it known whether the adrenal medullary unresponsiveness is a primary defect or a consequence of the hypoglycemia; hypoglycemia is rare in adrenalectomized patients receiving adequate corticosteroid

therapy. A 2-year-old child with hypoglycemia and adrenal medullary unresponsiveness has been reported who also had an isolated deficiency of ACTH. It was speculated that in this instance the deficiency of glucocorticoids resulted in failure of activation of the adrenal medullary enzyme system which converts norepinephrine to epinephrine.

Extrapancreatic neoplasms. Hypoglycemia has been observed repeatedly in association with some extrapancreatic tumors. The tumors are usually large mesodermal neoplasms (sarcomas) arising in the abdominal or thoracic cavity. Although the majority of reported patients have been adults, this phenomenon has been observed in a 5-year-old child with Wilms's tumor and in an infant with a congenital neuroblastoma. Tumor hypoglycemia is probably underdiagnosed, since fasting blood glucose levels are not determined routinely in children with extensive tumors. Although the mechanism by which hypoglycemia develops is still unsettled, evidence suggests that an insulin-like compound or an insulin potentiator is produced by the tumor.

Hypoglycemia due to pancreatic dysfunction. ORGANIC HYPERINSULINISM. A functioning *islet cell adenoma* of the pancreas is a rare lesion in the pediatric age range; it has been reported in about 30 children. In most instances the onset of symptoms has been after 4 years of age, but in a few instances hypoglycemia has occurred during the first days of life. Although hypoglycemia is presumably the result of secretion of excessive amounts of insulin, it has not always been demonstrable even when serum levels of insulin were measured. The symptoms may be severe and unremitting or may be mild and intermittent. The adenoma is usually solitary, but may be multiple, and rarely there is diffuse *adenomatosis* of the pancreatic islets.

Hyperplasia of the beta cells of the islets of Langerhans is common in newborn infants of diabetic and prediabetic mothers. Increased insulin content of the pancreas and increased plasma insulin levels have been found in such infants; hypoglycemia is common and often symptomatic. The disorder is believed to be caused by the maternal hyperglycemia to which the fetus is exposed.

In newborn infants with moderate or severe hemolytic disease, clinical manifestations of hypoglycemia and blood glucose levels under 30 mg. per 100 ml. have been observed with some frequency. Hyperplasia of the pancreatic islets has been observed in many infants dying with this disorder, and elevated pancreatic insulin content has been demonstrated recently. The pathogenesis of the islet hyperplasia is unknown.

Hyperplasia of the pancreatic islets has also been observed in the recently described *syndrome of macroglossia, omphalocele and visceromegaly (Beckwith syndrome).* Large kidneys, hyperplasia of the pancreas, and cytomegaly of the adrenal fetal cortex are common features of the disorder.

Hypoglycemia occurs in the first days of life and usually disappears spontaneously after a few weeks or months.

Hyperplasia of the islets has also been found in infants with *leucine-sensitive hypoglycemia* (see below).

Deficiency of pancreatic alpha cells and presumably deficiency of glucagon as a cause of hypoglycemia in siblings was first reported 2 decades ago. The observation has been questioned, but recently several additional instances of hypoglycemia associated with deficiency of pancreatic alpha cells have been reported. The disorder has not been established unequivocally by immunoassay of glucagon in plasma in the pancreas.

FUNCTIONAL HYPERINSULINISM. Hypoglycemia secondary to increased insulin levels without discernible pathologic changes of the islets of Langerhans has been termed functional hyperinsulinism.

Increased secretion of insulin occurs in the condition known as *leucine-induced hypoglycemia*. When leucine is administered to normal children, there is only a small decrease in blood glucose levels (5 to 10 mg. per 100 ml.), whereas, in children with this disorder, the blood glucose level falls to about half of the fasting level. The increased responsiveness of the islet cells to the administration of leucine is thought to be due to a deranged homeostatic mechanism. Approximately 30 per cent of patients with "idiopathic" hypoglycemia are leucine-sensitive. This phenomenon is sometimes familial; it has been observed in siblings and in a child and one parent, but the pattern of inheritance is not clear.

A similar defect occurs in some functioning *islet cell adenomas* as demonstrated by the hypoglycemia-provoking effect of leucine while the patient is harboring the tumor and its disappearance when the tumor is removed.

Abnormally increased secretion of insulin has also been observed 2 to 4 hours after a meal and after administration of glucose. Nervous impulses through the right vagus originating in the hypothalamic parasympathetic center can stimulate insulin secretion; a functional type of true hyperinsulinism based on abnormal nervous stimulation in this center has been postulated. Affected patients are emotionally unstable persons who are tense and anxious. This form of hypoglycemia is frequent in adults, but relatively uncommon in children.

Early in the course of *diabetes mellitus*, hypoglycemia is relatively common 3 to 5 hours after meals, especially in adults. The glucose tolerance test in such persons is characterized by a normal or slightly elevated fasting blood level of glucose, hyperglycemia for the first 2 to 3 hours, and a sudden fall to hypoglycemic levels between the third and fifth hours.

Miscellaneous causes of hypoglycemia. Salicylates and related compounds such as acetaminophen may on occasion produce hypoglycemia in some infants and children. This effect does not appear to be mediated through increased release of insulin, but it is possible that these drugs interfere with enzyme systems involved in glucose homeostasis.

Hypoglycemia has been observed in untreated patients with *maple syrup urine disease*. It has been postulated that the elevated leucine levels which occur in this disorder may provoke increased insulin secretion. In one treated patient, however, this has not been the case, and the mechanism of the hypoglycemia is unknown.

Maternal chloropropamide therapy during pregnancy has resulted in therapeutic concentrations in the serum of the fetus, and the newly born infant has prolonged symptomatic hypoglycemia. Exchange transfusion has been effective in treatment.

The ingestion of "bush tea," made from unripe ackee fruit, is responsible for the *vomiting sickness of Jamaica*. This disorder is characterized by severe prostration, vomiting, drowsiness, convulsions, coma and hypoglycemia with blood glucose levels below 20 mg. per 100 ml. The mortality rate is high, death occurring on the first day. There are severe hepatic changes, including fatty degeneration. A hypoglycemic amino acid, hypoglycin A, has been found in the seeds and fruit of the ackee nut, but the mechanism of its action is uncertain. It is noteworthy that hypoglycin A is an analogue of leucine and inhibits the oxidation of fatty acids and leucine.

Mild hypoglycemia is a complication of *kwashiorkor*, in which it may be secondary to impaired gluconeogenesis.

Hypoglycemia has occurred in *phenylketonuric* children during the course of treatment when dietary restriction of phenylalanine has been too severe. In these instances general malnutrition has been thought to be the principal factor causing the hypoglycemia.

Idiopathic hypoglycemia of infancy. In many instances of hypoglycemia in the pediatric age group no pathologic or metabolic lesion can be identified. The symptoms usually begin in early infancy, and there is a tendency to spontaneous improvement in subsequent years. In the absence of an understanding of the pathogenesis such cases of hypoglycemia have been termed idiopathic hypoglycemia of infancy. This group is undoubtedly a heterogeneous one consisting of several different defects.

Transitory hypoglycemia is occasionally observed in the neonatal period, especially in low-birth-weight infants (see p. 403).

Clinical Manifestations. There is no constant relationship between blood glucose levels and the development or severity of symptoms of hypoglycemia in different patients or even in the same patient at different times. The rate of fall of blood glucose seems to be an important determining factor for the appearance of symptoms; a rapid fall, irrespective of the actual level reached, is especially likely to produce symptoms. Even at extremely low blood levels of glucose, children manifest great variability in their responses. Many become conditioned to repeated hypoglycemic episodes or to hypoglycemia of long duration, so that they have few or no symptoms. This is evidenced by children with type I glycogenosis (von Gierke's disease). The symptoms of hypoglycemia are derived chiefly from disturbances of the central nervous system. Neural tissue has little stored carbohydrate and, unlike other tissues, cannot utilize sugars other than glucose, so that it is dependent upon a continuous and adequate supply of blood glucose to maintain its normal functions. There is evidence that neural tissue can utilize free fatty acids or amino acid as sources of energy; this is thought to be the case in children with prolonged hypoglycemia who are asymptomatic.

Hypoglycemic symptoms are protean, but often produce more or less characteristic patterns in individual patients. Some of the more frequent symptoms are fatigue, headache, pallor, sweating, speech and visual disturbances and motor disturbances, such as tremulousness, incoordination, paralyses, syncope and convulsions. Hunger is prominent; vomiting is inconstant. The temperature is often subnormal. Tachycardia and extrasystoles occur as a result of stimulation of the sympathetic nervous system. Psychic disturbances such as irritability, negativism, drowsiness and alterations in behavior are common in older children. In the ranks of emotionally disturbed children there are certainly some unhappy, ill-behaved or maladjusted children requiring sugar as well as guidance.

In newborn and young infants, recognition and evaluation of symptoms may be difficult except as the possibility of hypoglycemia is considered. Convulsions are often the first recognized manifestation, but irritability, poor feeding, lethargy, excessive drowsiness, eye-rolling, sweating and twitching are more common symptoms.

Diagnosis. Two distinct diagnostic problems are posed: (1) the detection of hypoglycemia and (2) the determination of its cause. Many children exhibit clinical manifestations on one or more occasions which suggest hypoglycemia, but hypoglycemia can be demonstrated in them only under specific conditions or it may never be demonstrated. In others, hypoglycemia is readily demonstrated by blood glucose determinations. Even when the diagnosis is established, it is often difficult to establish the cause. There is no routine approach for the study of patients with manifestations of hypoglycemia; individualization in the choice of diagnostic procedures is essential.

Measurement of fasting levels of blood glucose and a 6-hour glucose tolerance test are indicated as the initial procedures for the establishment of the hypoglycemic state. If the fasting blood glucose level and the glucose tolerance test are normal, then a more prolonged period of fasting, as long as 24 hours, may be necessary to provoke symptoms and to demonstrate hypoglycemia.

If these procedures fail to induce hypoglycemia, further measures are usually not indicated. But if hypoglycemia is established, one must then evaluate the information garnered from the history and physical examination before undertaking exhaustive tests of carbohydrate function. Since many of the causes for hypoglycemia are genetically determined, a family history of other affected persons or of consanguinity may be pertinent information. The initial episode of hypoglycemia caused by ingestion of alcohol or other toxins can usually be identified by the history. The infant with galactosemia usually has other clinical manifestations to suggest the diagnosis before hypoglycemia is suspected. A history of aversion to fruits and sweets, and the occurrence of gastrointestinal manifestations as well as those of hypoglycemia following ingestion of foods containing fructose should suggest hereditary fructose intolerance. Aggravation of hypoglycemic symptoms by meals rich in protein suggests leucine-induced hypoglycemia. Hypoglycemic episodes following periods of undereating or of vomiting or diarrhea are suggestive of ketotic hypoglycemia.

Hepatomegaly should alert one to the hepatic causes of hypoglycemia. Growth failure directs attention to pituitary hypofunction, whereas manifestations of Addison's disease lead to consideration of adrenal hypofunction. The association of large tumors in the thoracic or abdominal cavity with hypoglycemia should suggest a causative relation. Tolerance tests utilizing fructose, galactose, leucine, glucagon or epinephrine are indicated when these disorders are under consideration.

Other possibilities are a functioning islet cell adenoma and the idiopathic type of hypoglycemia. The former is rare in the pediatric age range. It is more likely to be manifest in childhood than in infancy, whereas the latter is more apt to occur in infancy. There is no test which clearly separates these 2 conditions. Both disorders have been associated with elevated and normal insulin levels, and administration of tolbutamide may result in a prolonged hypoglycemic response in each one. Furthermore, the leucine-induced form of hypoglycemia cannot be differentiated easily from functioning islet cell adenomas, which are themselves leucine-sensitive. In such instances laparotomy may be necessary to establish the diagnosis.

Laboratory Data. Tests for the evaluation of carbohydrate metabolism (Table 16-2) are usually performed after an overnight fast except in young infants, for whom a 6-hour period is adequate. Occasionally, owing to the severity of the hypoglycemia, shorter periods of fasting are indicated. When the expected response of a given test is a lowering of the blood glucose level, the fasting glucose level should be 50 mg. per 100 ml. or higher to permit a sufficient differential in glucose levels for comparative purposes. The patient should be in reasonably good nutritional state and free of fever when a test is performed.

The *glucagon tolerance test* is a useful pro-

TABLE 16-2. Tolerance Tests for the Evaluation of Carbohydrate Metabolism

COMPOUND	ROUTE	DOSE	TIME TO OBTAIN SAMPLES IN MINUTES	METHODS AND COMMENTS
Glucose	Oral	1.75 gm./kg.	0, 30, 60, 120, 180, 240, 300, 360	Nelson-Somogyi (N-S) or glucose oxidase (G.O.)
	I.V.	0.4 gm./kg. as 10-20% solution over 4-min. period	0, 5, 10, 20, 30, 40, 50, 60	N-S or G.O.; determine slope of line
Galactose	Oral	1.75 gm./kg.	0, 30, 60, 90, 120	Glucose by G.O.; galactose by galactose dehydrogenase or by difference between N-S and G.O.
Fructose	Oral I.V.	0.5 gm./kg. 0.25 gm./kg. as 10% solution over 4-min. period	0, 30, 45, 60, 90	Glucose by G.O., fructose by resorcinol or by difference between N-S and G.O. Also measure serum phosphorus levels
L-Leucine	Oral I.V.	150 mg./kg. as 2% solution or slurry 75 mg./kg. as 2% solution in 0.45% NaCl	0, 15, 30, 45, 60, 75, 90, 120	N-S or G.O.; also measure insulin by immunochemical method
Epinephrine	I.M.	0.03 mg./kg. (0.3 mg. maximum)	0, 10, 20, 30, 45, 60, 90, 120	N-S or G.O.; also measure nonesterified fatty acids (NEFA)
Glucagon	I.M.	30 μg./kg. (1 mg. maximum)	0, 10, 20, 30, 45, 60, 90, 120	N-S or G.O.
Insulin	I.V.	0.1 unit/kg. of crystalline insulin (0.05 units/kg. for sensitive patients, such as hypopituitarism)	0, 15, 30, 45, 60, 90, 120	N-S or G.O.; also measure growth hormone by immunochemical method
Tolbutamide	I.V.	20 mg./kg. (1 gm. maximum)	0, 20, 30, 40, 60, 90, 120	N-S or G.O.; also measure insulin by immunochemical method

cedure to study the ability of the liver to release glucose into the circulation from stored glycogen. The *epinephrine tolerance test* has been replaced by the safer glucagon test. Normally a rise of blood glucose of at least 50 mg. per 100 ml. should occur within 60 minutes. Failure of an adequate response may be due to depletion of liver glycogen by starvation or hepatic disease. In all the glycogenoses in which the liver is the principal organ involved, there is also a poor hyperglycemic response to glucagon. Children with ketotic hypoglycemia exhibit an inadequate response to glucagon during the hypoglycemic episode or after a 24-hour fast, but respond normally between attacks.

The *galactose tolerance test* should not be used for the diagnosis of galactosemia, since it may induce severe hypoglycemia; direct assay of uridyl transferase activity is the appropriate diagnostic method. The galactose tolerance test is informative in the differentiation of the hepatic forms of glycogenoses when lactic acid levels are also measured.

The *fructose tolerance test* is primarily of use in the detection of hereditary fructose intolerance. Administration of fructose to patients results in a decrease of blood glucose to hypoglycemic levels and a rise in the level of blood fructose. In addi-

tion, the level of serum inorganic phosphorus is decreased, the concentration of lactic acid is increased, and the insulin level remains unchanged. For this test the blood glucose level must be measured by the glucose oxidase method, since the total concentration of reducing sugar (Nelson-Somogyi) remains relatively constant.

The *leucine tolerance test* is used to determine whether this amino acid provokes hypoglycemia. In sensitive persons the concentration of blood sugar is decreased about 50 per cent within 30 to 60 minutes after intravenous or oral administration of leucine. The concentration of insulin in the blood increases as the concentration of glucose decreases.

The *insulin tolerance test* provides a direct method of determining the ability of the patient to recover from hypoglycemia. Normally the level of blood glucose drops to about 50 per cent of the fasting level in 15 to 30 minutes and returns to normal within 60 to 90 minutes. The glucose level fails to return to normal within this time in patients with hypofunction of the adrenal or pituitary gland, because insulin is unopposed by hyperglycemic hormones from these glands. This test may be dangerous in the hypoglycemic child and should never be performed without constant surveillance during the procedure and without provision to terminate the hypoglycemia promptly if alarming symptoms develop.

The *tolbutamide tolerance test* measures the ability of the pancreas to release insulin as determined by the degree and duration of the hypoglycemic response. In normal children the blood glucose level falls about 40 per cent within 20 to 30 minutes and returns to normal within 2 hours. In the diabetic child there is a markedly decreased response, and in hypoglycemic patients there is an exaggerated response. Failure of blood glucose to return to the normal range 2 to 3 hours after administration of tolbutamide is strong presumptive evidence for the presence of a functioning islet cell adenoma in the adult. Infants with functional as well as organic hyperinsulinism, however, may exhibit a profound and prolonged response to tolbutamide. Thus the test is of limited usefulness in the detection of functioning islet cell adenomas in infants and young children.

Abnormal *electroencephalographic patterns* resulting from hypoglycemia are difficult, if not impossible, to differentiate from those occurring in epileptic patients. In patients with infrequent hypoglycemic attacks, abnormalities in the electroencephalogram are usually not present between attacks. They may be present on a continuing basis in children who have permanent cerebral damage from severe and prolonged hypoglycemia, as, for example, in the infrequent instances of inappropriate administration of insulin to diabetic patients in hypoglycemic shock whose manifestations were misinterpreted as representing hyperglycemic diabetic acidosis without measuring the blood sugar concentration. In the case of neurologically damaged children who were hypoglycemic in the neonatal period (see p. 403), it is possible that in the majority of instances both their neurologic damage and their neonatal hypoglycemia were the result of the same noxious influence, possibly severe hypoxia. There is no clear evidence that the residual neurologic damage and any persistent electroencephalographic abnormalities were caused by the hypoglycemia, though it may in some instances have been an additive factor.

Treatment. During a hypoglycemic attack the child should under no circumstances be left unattended. The immediate symptoms may be relieved by the administration of glucose, but it should be kept in mind that hypoglycemia of either the organic or functional type may be only temporarily abated by the administration of glucose and may rebound to hypoglycemic levels as the release of additional insulin is evoked. In such situations frequent feedings of small amounts of carbohydrates are advisable until the patient is stabilized.

Glucagon in a dose of 1.0 mg. intramuscularly is usually effective in terminating a hypoglycemic episode. This form of therapy is a useful emergency measure which parents can be trained to utilize in the home. It is *not* effective in the glycogenoses, in other hepatic disease or in ketotic hypoglycemia. Even when it is effective, it should be followed by the oral administration of sugar in some readily absorbable and acceptable (to the child) form.

When the cause of the hypoglycemia is established, treatment should be related to it. Patients with galactosemia or fructosemia must be maintained on diets free of the offending sugar: galactose or fructose. Those with leucine-induced hypoglycemia should be given diets low in protein and particularly low in leucine, but not free of this essential amino acid; administration of glucose solution orally, 20 to 30 minutes after feedings, is also advisable.

Children with functional hypoglycemia other than the leucine-induced form or with organic or idiopathic hypoglycemia should have the protein content of the diet increased. This rationale is based on the steady conversion of amino acids to glucose (gluconeogenesis) at a rate to avoid hyperglycemia and hence to avoid undue stimulation of insulin secretion.

Ephedrine may be useful in the treatment of hypoglycemia resulting from decreased responsiveness of the adrenal medulla, but is otherwise of little value.

Hydrocortisone tends to restore normal carbohydrate metabolism in patients with corticotropin or adrenal cortical insufficiency. Corticotropin has been effective in maintaining normal glycemic levels in infants with idiopathic hypoglycemia, and hydrocortisone and other glucocorticosteroids administered orally appear to be equally effective. The dose must be adjusted to the lowest effective amount. Every 6 months or so attempts should be made to discontinue the drug gradually.

Diazoxide, a nondiuretic benzothiadiazine, is an effective agent in controlling hypoglycemia when other forms of therapy have failed. This drug is currently available only to qualified investigators. The most consistent undesirable side effect is hypertrichosis. The drug acts primarily by suppressing insulin release and appears to be particularly effective in conditions in which glucose and leucine stimulate excessive release of insulin.

For the patient with protracted hypoglycemia which is unresponsive to dietary measures, corticotropin or corticosteroids, and is also unresponsive to diazoxide, an exploratory laparotomy is indicated. If a pancreatic adenoma is not found on surgical exploration, partial pancreatectomy is frequently helpful in reducing the frequency and severity of hypoglycemic attacks.

Psychologic guidance of the hypoglycemic child and his family is of paramount importance.

Angelo M. DiGeorge
Victor H. Auerbach

REFERENCES FOR DIABETES MELLITUS

Beal, C. K.: Body Size and Growth Rate of Children with Diabetes Mellitus. *J. Pediat.*, 32:170, 1948.
Bell, E. T.: Renal Vascular Disease in Diabetes Mellitus. *Diabetes*, 2:376, 1953.
Colwell, J. A.: Diminished Insulin Response to Hyperglycemia in Prediabetes and Diabetes. *Diabetes*, 16:560, 1967.

Committee on Professional Education, American Diabetes Association: Classification of Genetic Diabetes Mellitus. *Diabetes*, 16:540, 1967.

Elliott, R. R., O'Brien, D., and Roy, C. C.: An Abnormal Insulin in Juvenile Diabetes Mellitus. *Diabetes*, 14:780, 1965.

Gentz, J. D. H., and Cornblath, M.: Transient Diabetes of the Newborn. *Advances in Pediatrics*, Vol. XVI, 1969.

Gepts, W.: Pathologic Anatomy of the Pancreas in Juvenile Diabetes Mellitus. *Diabetes*, 14:619, 1965.

Gerrard, D. M., and Chin, W.: The Syndrome of Transient Diabetes. *J. Pediat.*, 61:89, 1962.

Guest, G. M.: The Mauriac Syndrome. *Diabetes*, 2:415, 1953.

Guest, G. M., Mackler, B., and Knowles, H. C., Jr.: Effects of Acidosis on Insulin Action and on Carbohydrate and Mineral Metabolism. *Diabetes*, 1:276, 1952.

Jackson, R. L., and others: Degenerative Changes in Young Diabetic Patients in Relation to Level of Control. *Pediatrics*, 5:959, 1950.

Kety, S. S., Polis, B. D., Nadler, C. S., and Schmidt, C. F.: The Blood Flow and Oxygen Consumption of the Human Brain in Diabetic Acidosis and Coma. *J. Clin. Invest.*, 27:500, 1948.

Klein, R., Marks, J. F., Roldan, E., Sherman, F. E., and Fetterman, G. H.: The Occurrence of Peripheral Edema and Subcutaneous Glycogen Deposition Following the Initial Treatment of Diabetes Mellitus in Children. *J. Pediat.*, 60:807, 1962.

Knowles, H. C., Jr., Guest, G. M., Lampe, J., Kessler, M., and Skillman, T. G.: The Course of Juvenile Diabetes Treated with Unmeasured Diet. *Diabetes*, 14:239, 1965.

Larsson, Y. A., Sterky, G. C., and Christiansson, G.: Long-Term Prognosis in Juvenile Diabetes Mellitus. *Acta Paediat.*, 51:1, 1962 (Suppl. 135).

Little, J. A., and Arnott, J. H.: Sulfated Insulin in Mild, Moderate, Severe and Insulin-Resistant Diabetes Mellitus. *Diabetes*, 15:457, 1966.

Mirsky, I. A.: The Etiology of Diabetic Acidosis. *J.A.M.A.*, 118:690, 1942.

O'Sullivan, J. B., and Mahan, C. M.: Prospective Study of 352 Young Patients with Chemical Diabetes. *New England J. Med.*, 278:1038, 1968.

Parker, M. L., Pildes, R. S., Kuen-Lan, C., Cornblath, M., and Kipnis, D. M.: Juvenile Diabetes, a Deficiency in Insulin. *Diabetes*, 17:27, 1968.

Post, R. H.: An Approach to the Question, Does All Diabetes Depend upon a Single Genetic Locus? *Diabetes*, 11:56, 1962.

Rimoin, D. L.: Genetics of Diabetes Mellitus. *Diabetes*, 16:346, 1967.

Rubin, H. M., Kramer, R., and Drash, A.: Hyperosmolality Complicating Diabetes Mellitus in Childhood. *J. Pediat.*, 74:177, 1969.

Sherman, L.: The Vallance-Owen ("Synalbumin") Insulin Antagonist. *Diabetes*, 15:149, 1966.

Shwachman, H., and Kulczycki, L. L.: Diabetes and Cystic Fibrosis of the Pancreas. *Am. J. Dis. Child.*, 104:625, 1962.

REFERENCES FOR HYPOGLYCEMIA

Antony, G. J., Underwood, L. E., and Van Wyk, J. J.: Studies in Hypoglycemia of Infancy and Childhood. Diagnosis and Treatment. *Am. J. Dis. Child.*, 114:345, 1967.

Baker, L., Kaye, R., Root, A. W., and Prasad, A. L. N.: Diazoxide Treatment of Idiopathic Hypoglycemia of Infancy. *J. Pediat.*, 71:494, 1967.

Brunjes, E., Hodgman, J., Nowack, J., and Johns, V. J., Jr.: Adrenal Medullary Function in Idiopathic Spontaneous Hypoglycemia of Infancy and Childhood. *Am. J. Med.*, 34:168, 1963.

Colle, E., and Ulstrom, R. A.: Ketotic Hypoglycemia. *J. Pediat.*, 64:632, 1964.

Combs, J. T., Grunt, J. A., and Brandt, I. K.: New Syndrome of Neonatal Hypoglycemia: Association with Visceromegaly, Macroglossia, Microcephaly and Abnormal Umbilicus. *New England J. Med.*, 275:236, 1966.

Cornblath, M., and Schwartz, R.: *Disorders of Carbohydrate Metabolism in Infancy.* Philadelphia, W. B. Saunders Company, 1966.

Cummins, L. H.: Hypoglycemia and Convulsions in Children Following Alcohol Ingestion. *J. Pediat.*, 58:23, 1961.

DiGeorge, A. M., Auerbach, V. H., and Mabry, C. C.: Leucine-Induced Hypoglycemia. III. The Blood Glucose Depressant

Action of Leucine in Normal Individuals. *J. Pediat.*, 63:295, 1963.

Dodge, P. R., Mancall, E. L., Crawford, J. D., Knapp, J., and Paine, R. S.: Hypoglycemia Complicating Treatment of Phenylketonuria with a Phenylalanine-Deficient Diet. *New England J. Med.*, 260:1104, 1959.

Donnell, G. N., Leiberman, E., Shaw, K. N. F., and Koch, R.: Hypoglycemia in Maple Syrup Urine Disease. *Am. J. Dis. Child.*, 113:60, 1967.

Drash, A., and Schultz, R.: Islet Cell Adenoma in Childhood: Report of a Case. *Pediatrics*, 39:59, 1967.

Driscoll, S. G., and Steinke, J.: Pancreatic Insulin in Severe Erythroblastosis. *Pediatrics*, 39:448, 1967.

Ehrlich, R. M., and Martin, J. M.: Tolbutamide Tolerance Test and Plasma-Insulin Response in Children with Idiopathic Hypoglycemia. *J. Pediat.*, 71:485, 1967.

Freinkel, N., and others: Alcohol Hypoglycemia. I. Carbohydrate Metabolism of Patients with Clinical Alcohol Hypoglycemia and the Experimental Reproduction of the Syndrome with Pure Ethanol. *J. Clin. Invest.*, 42:1112, 1963.

Garces, L. Y., Drash, A., and Kenny, F. M.: Islet Cell Tumor in the Neonate. Studies in Carbohydrate Metabolism and Therapeutic Response. *Pediatrics*, 41:789, 1968.

Grollman, A., McCaleb, W. E., and White, F. N.: Glucagon Deficiency as a Cause of Hypoglycemia. *Metabolism*, 13:686, 1964.

Haworth, J. C., and Coodin, F. J.: Idiopathic Spontaneous Hypoglycemia in Children. Report of Seven Cases and Review of the Literature. *Pediatrics*, 25:748, 1960.

Hung, W., and Migeon, C. J.: Hypoglycemia in a Two-Year-Old Boy with Adrenocorticotropic Hormone (ACTH) Deficiency (Probably Isolated) and Adrenal Medullary Unresponsiveness to Insulin-Induced Hypoglycemia. *J. Clin. Endocrin. & Metab.*, 28:146, 1968.

Jelliffe, D. B., and Stuart, K. L.: Acute Toxic Hypoglycaemia in the Vomiting Sickness of Jamaica. *Brit. M.J.*, 1:75, 1954.

Joassin, G., Parker, M. L., Pildes, R. S., and Cornblath, M.: Infants of Diabetic Mothers. *Diabetes*, 16:306, 1967.

Levin, B., Snodgrass, G. J. A. I., Oberholzer, V. G., Burgess, E. A., and Dobbs, R. H.: Fructosaemia. Observations on Seven Cases. *Am. J. Med.*, 45:826, 1948.

Limbeck, G. A., Ruvalcaba, R. H. A., Samols, E., and Kelley, V. C.: Salicylates and Hypoglycemia. *Am. J. Dis. Child.*, 109:165, 1965.

Loutfi, A. H., Mehrez, I., Shahbender, S., and Abdine, F. H.: Hypoglycaemia with Wilms' Tumour. *Arch. Dis. Childhood*, 39:197, 1964.

Lucey, J. F., Randall, J. L., and Murray, J. J.: Is Hypoglycemia an Important Complication in Erythroblastosis Fetalis? *Am. J. Dis. Child.*, 114:88, 1967.

Nadler, H. L., Newman, L. L., and Gershberg, H.: Hypoglycemia, Growth Retardation, and Probable Isolated Growth Hormone Deficiency in a One-Year Old Child. *J. Pediat.*, 63:977, 1963.

Nordmann, Y., Schapira, F., and Dreyfus, J. C.: A Structurally Modified Liver Aldolase in Fructose Intolerance: Immunologic and Kinetic Evidence. *Biochem. & Biophys. Res. Commun.*, 31:884, 1968.

Ruvalcaba, R. H. A., Limbeck, G. A., and Kelley, V. C.: Acetaminophen and Hypoglycemia. *Am. J. Dis. Child.*, 112:558, 1966.

Salinas, E. D., and others: Functioning Islet Cell Adenoma in the Newborn. *Pediatrics*, 41:646, 1968.

Shapiro, M., Sincha, A., Rosenmann, E., and Shafrir, E.: Hypoglycemia Associated with Neonatal Neuroblastoma and Abnormal Responses of Serum Glucose and Free Fatty Acids to Epinephrine Injection. *Israel J. Med. Sci.*, 2:705, 1966.

Slone, D., Taitz, L. S., and Gilchrist, G. S.: Aspects of Carbohydrate Metabolism in Kwashiorkor; with Special Reference to Spontaneous Hypoglycaemia. *Brit. M.J.*, 1:32, 1961.

Snyder, R. D., and Robinson, A.: Leucine-Induced Hypoglycemia. *Am. J. Dis. Child.*, 113:566, 1967.

Steinke, J., and Driscoll, S. G.: The Extractable Insulin Content of Pancreas from Fetuses and Infants of Diabetic and Control Mothers. *Diabetes*, 14:573, 1965.

Unger, R. H.: The Riddle of Tumor Hypoglycemia. Editorial. *Am. J. Med.*, 40:325, 1966.

Woolf, L. I.: Inherited Metabolic Disorders: Galactosemia. *Advances Clin. Chem.*, 5:1, 1962.

Zucker, P., and Simon, G.: Prolonged Symptomatic Neonatal Hypoglycemia Associated with Maternal Chlorpropamide Therapy. *Pediatrics*, 42:824, 1968.

17. The Endocrine System

DISORDERS OF THE PITUITARY GLAND

The pituitary gland consists of an anterior lobe and a posterior lobe. The anterior lobe develops from the ectoderm of the stomodeum (Rathke's pouch); fetal rests of the original connection of Rathke's pouch with the primitive oral cavity may persist in postnatal life as a craniopharyngeal duct. Sometimes tumors develop from the remnants of this duct (craniopharyngiomas) and give rise to symptoms of pituitary and hypothalamic dysfunction. The posterior lobe is derived from the infundibulum of the diencephalon and is histologically and functionally distinct from the anterior lobe.

Function. *Anterior lobe.* Seven well defined hormones and possibly other hormonal peptides are produced by the anterior pituitary. Three cell types can be distinguished in the anterior lobe by the use of hemotoxylin-eosin stain: eosinophilic, basophilic and chromophobe cells. With special staining techniques, however, other specific types of cells have been identified; these include 4 types of basophils, each of which synthesizes a different hormone. The eosinophilic cells produce growth hormone and prolactin. The basophilic cells are the source of thyrotropin (TSH), corticotropin (ACTH), melanocyte-stimulating hormone (MSH), follicle-stimulating hormone (FSH) and luteinizing or interstitial cell-stimulating hormone (LH or ICSH). Chromophobe cells are regarded as undifferentiated precursors of the secretory cells, though secretory potential is suggested by chromophobe tumors which produce corticotropin. The pituitary hormones act either directly on the body cells or on other endocrine glands to affect almost every organ, and are reciprocally affected by the hormones produced by the target endocrine glands.

The pituitary gland itself is under the control of the hypothalamus. A number of hypothalamic secretions (hypophysiotropic hormones) have been identified, and each independently regulates specific pituitary target cells. These neurosecretions are transferred to nerve endings of the median eminence and thence to the blood supply through the hypothalamic-hypophyseal portal system. Known secretions include corticotropin-releasing hormone (CRH), growth hormone-releasing hormone or somatotropin-releasing hormone (GRH or SRH), follicle-stimulating hormone-releasing hormone (FSH-RH or FRH), and luteinizing hormone-releasing hormone (LH-RH or LRH). Gonadal steroids, thyroxine and cortisol appear to have feed-back control directly on hypothalamic

centers ("long" negative feedback). Certain pituitary hormones, such as LH and possibly FSH and ACTH, also have a direct feedback on hypothalamic centers ("short" feed-back loop). Some of these hypothalamic hormones have been prepared in highly purified form and appear to be polypeptides. They are found in very small amounts; e.g. only 2.8 mg. of thyrotropin-releasing hormone (TRH) could be derived from 100,000 porcine hypothalami.

Growth hormone is a protein with a molecular weight of 27,100; it is effective only when administered parenterally. It acts directly on all tissues, promoting growth without affecting maturation or sexual development. Decreased production of growth hormone occurs in the absence of thyroid hormone. The secretion of growth hormone is also responsive to the level of blood glucose; administration of glucose suppresses, and hypoglycemia acts as a potent stimulus to, secretion. Sensitive immunoassays for circulating growth hormone are now in clinical use. Measurement of the concentration of growth hormone in the plasma during induced hypoglycemia is a direct test of pituitary somatotropin function. There is species specificity for growth hormones; only growth hormone from monkey and human pituitaries is effective in man. Deficiency of somatotropin results in dwarfism, and an excess in gigantism or acromegaly.

Gonadotropic hormones include 2 specific substances. The follicle-stimulating hormone (FSH) is gametokinetic and stimulates growth of the ova in the female and of the sperm cells in the male. The luteinizing hormone (LH), sometimes called the interstitial cell-stimulating hormone (ICSH), regulates formation of the corpus luteum in the female and growth of the Leydig cells of the testes in the male. Both hormones are probably of minor significance under normal conditions in girls before the age of 10 years or in boys before the age of 12 years. In castrates or in patients with primary hypogonadism there are overproduction of gonadotropins and increased urinary excretion of them; their secretion is inhibited by estrogens or androgens.

Specific bio-assays indicate that FSH is present in urine before puberty and increases 2.5-fold in adolescence, whereas LH is barely detectable in urine prior to puberty, but increases tenfold afterwards. The initiation of adolescent changes may be related not only to the increases in FSH and LH which occur, but also to the change in the FSH-LH ratio. Immunoassay techniques for the measurement of FSH and LH in plasma have been developed and should contribute to further understanding of physiologic and pathologic processes.

Thyrotropic hormone (TSH) stimulates the thyroid; an excess may result in hypertrophy and hyperplasia, whereas a deficiency results in inactivity and atrophy of the thyroid gland. A reciprocal relation exists between the anterior pituitary and the thyroid. Thyroid hormone inhibits production of pituitary thyrotropin, and a low level of circulating thyroid hormone results in accelerated production of thyrotropin. Thyrotropin prepared from the pituitary glands of cattle is commercially available and is useful in differentiating pituitary hypothyroidism from primary thyroid deficiency. Recently a very sensitive radio-immunoassay for TSH content of plasma has been applied to the study of clinical problems.

Corticotropin (adrenocorticotropic hormone, ACTH) is the hormone which stimulates the synthesis and release of steroids from the adrenal cortex. The principal hormone liberated by the human adrenal cortex when stimulated by corticotropin is hydrocortisone; corticosterone is second in importance. There is evidence that androgens, estrogens and progesterone, or precursors of these compounds, are also liberated.

The principal actions of corticotropin are mediated by adrenocortical steroids. A reciprocal relation exists between corticotropin and production of adrenocortical hormones. When an exogenous corticosteroid is administered, there is a reduction in corticotropin production. If this administration is prolonged and then suddenly stopped, adrenocortical insufficiency is induced as a result of the pituitary inhibition. The increased corticoid secretion induced by exogenous corticotropin also depresses corticotropin output by the pituitary in a manner similar to that of exogenous cortisone. Therefore adrenocortical insufficiency follows sudden withdrawal of corticotropin therapy. The severity of the adrenal insufficiency depends upon the duration of therapy, the dose used and the rapidity of withdrawal. This adrenal insufficiency is usually temporary and can be prevented by slowly tapering the dosage and increasing the interval between doses of either corticotropin or cortisone.

Posterior lobe. The posterior lobe of the pituitary is part of a functional unit known as the neurohypophysis, which consists of (1) the neurons of the supraoptic and paraventricular nuclei of the hypothalamus; (2) their axons, which form the pituitary stalk; and (3) the posterior lobe of the pituitary. The neurohypophysis is the source of vasopressin (antidiuretic hormone) and oxytocin, which are 2 very similar octapeptides. These hormones, produced by a process of neurosecretion in the hypothalamic nuclei, are transported along the axons down the pituitary stalk and stored in the posterior pituitary until they are secreted into the blood.

The most clear-cut example of neurohypophyseal deficiency is diabetes insipidus. The closer a lesion is to the hypothalamic nuclei, the more complete is the deficiency of antidiuretic hormone. More than 85 per cent of the hypothalamic-hypophyseal tracts must be severed before clinical diabetes insipidus becomes manifest. Removal of only the posterior lobe of the pituitary rarely results in diabetes insipidus.

NEOPLASMS

Primary tumors of the anterior pituitary may arise from any of the 3 principal types of cells. Chromophobe adenomas are the most common type, but rarely occur in children. They may cause pituitary insufficiency by compression of functioning pituitary tissue. Other symptoms are caused by pressure on adjacent structures. Basophilic adenomas are rare in children; they may occur with untreated Cushing's syndrome. The tumors which occur months or years after bilateral adrenalectomy for Cushing's syndrome due to adrenal hyperplasia are usually chromophobe in nature rather than basophilic (p. 1217). They may cause enlargement of the sella and ocular manifestations, but rarely cause other neurologic symptoms. Eosinophilic adenomas produce abnormal growth through overproduction of growth hormone (p. 1177).

HYPOPITUITARISM

PITUITARY DWARFISM

Etiology. Any lesion which destroys the anterior pituitary causes cessation of growth. Destructive lesions are not selective, and evidence of multiple pituitary hormonal deficiencies will be present. The most common lesion responsible for this type of dwarfism in childhood is the craniopharyngioma (p. 1285). The growth failure almost always antedates the neurologic signs and symptoms. In some instances, pituitary function is relatively normal initially, but the operative procedure itself causes hypopituitarism. In rare instances, tuberculosis, syphilis, sarcoidosis, xanthomatous lesions (Hand-Schüller-Christian disease), toxoplasmosis, intracranial aneurysms, chromophobe adenomas of the pituitary or hypothalamic tumors are the cause of pituitary destruction. These lesions are frequently associated with detectable roentgenographic changes. Enlargement of the sella or deformation or destruction of the clinoid processes usually indicates a tumor. Intrasellar or suprasellar calcifications are usually indicative of a craniopharyngioma.

In more than half of patients with pituitary dwarfism there is no demonstrable lesion of the pituitary (idiopathic hypopituitarism). About half of these children have *isolated deficiency of growth hormone*. The insidious loss of growth hormone may lead to gradual deceleration of the growth rate. The cause is not known in most instances; deficiency might result from a defect in the hypothalamic growth-hormone-releasing hormone or from a deficiency of or a defect in the acidophilic cells of the pituitary. Isolated deficiency of growth hormone may occur as a sporadic disorder, but is often familial and transmitted as an autosomal recessive disorder. Since it has been observed in one of identical twins, environmental factors may be responsible in some instances.

Siblings with dwarfism have been observed who have high levels of growth hormone, but exhibit a normal response to the administration of exogenous human growth hormone. It appears that such children synthesize a *biologically inactive growth hormone*, owing to a recessive genetic defect. On the other hand, the African pygmy has normal levels of growth hormone, but fails to respond normally to exogenous human growth hormone; this suggests that growth failure is due to an inherited *defect in end-organ response* to endogenous growth hormone.

Approximately half of the children with growth hormone deficiency also have deficiencies in other pituitary tropic hormones. It is unsettled whether the primary defect is in the hypothalamus or the pituitary. The multiple deficiency of tropic hormones may be present in infancy, or there may be progressive development of the various deficiencies. For example, a child with only growth hormone deficiency initially may eventually exhibit TSH and corticotropin (ACTH) deficiencies.

Clinical Manifestations. *In patients without demonstrable lesion of the pituitary.* Pituitary dwarfs are usually of normal size and weight at birth. The retardation of growth has a variable onset; in about half of the affected children the retardation of growth is noticed by 1 year of age. In others there may be a regular but slow growth in height with the increments always below those of coevals, or periods of lack of growth may alternate with short spurts of growth. Delayed closure of the epiphyses permits growth beyond the time when normal persons cease to grow.

The head is round, and the face short and broad. The frontal bone is prominent, and the bridge of the nose depressed and saddle-shaped. The nose is small, and the nasolabial folds are well developed. The eyes are somewhat bulging. The mandible and the chin are underdeveloped and infantile, and the teeth, which erupt late, are frequently crowded. The neck is short and the larynx small. The voice is high-pitched and remains high after puberty. The genitalia are usually undeveloped. The extremities are well proportioned, the hands and feet being small (acromicria). The skin is often wrinkled and lies in folds, particularly in the face *(geroderma)*. Facial, axillary and pubic hair is usually absent; the hair of the scalp is fine. Sexual maturation may be delayed or absent. Hypoglycemic attacks may occur, and there may be failure of the usual glycemic response following insulin-induced hypoglycemia.

The intelligence of pituitary dwarfs is usually normal. Their physical peculiarities influence their emotions and behavior as they grow older, and they may become shy and retiring.

In patients with demonstrable lesion of the pituitary. The child is normal initially, and manifestations similar to those seen in the idiopathic pituitary dwarf gradually appear and progress. When complete or almost complete destruction of the pituitary gland occurs, severe manifestations of pituitary insufficiency are present, and the disorder is known as *Simmonds's disease*. Atrophy of the adrenal cortex, thyroid and gonads results in loss of weight, asthenia, sensitivity to cold, mental torpor and absence of sweating. Sexual maturation fails to take place, or regresses if already present. Thus there may be atrophy of the gonads and genital tract with amenorrhea and loss of pubic and axillary hair. There is a tendency to hypoglycemia and coma. Growth ceases. Diabetes insipidus may be present early, but tends to improve spontaneously with progressive destruction of the anterior pituitary.

If the lesion is an expanding tumor, symptoms such as impaired vision, ocular disturbances, pathologic sleep, mental retardation and other neurologic signs may be present. In some patients the neurologic manifestations antedate the endocrine symptoms; the evidence of pituitary insufficiency often follows surgical intervention.

Laboratory Studies. A technique for the measurement of the serum level of growth hormone is now available and should simplify the diagnosis of growth failure due to deficient production of this hormone. Under basal conditions, however, the amount of growth hormone in serum is very small, even in the normal child. Therefore, to secure significant measurement of it, it is necessary to provoke temporarily increased secretion of the hormone. This may be accomplished by inducing hypoglycemia with insulin or by the intravenous infusion of L-arginine. These agents induce a distinct increase in the level of circulating growth hormone in normal persons, but not in patients with growth hormone deficiency. Great care must be taken in the administration of insulin to patients with hypopituitarism because of their decreased ability to overcome hypoglycemia. Failure of sexual maturation beyond the appropriate age in association with growth failure is strong presumptive evidence for gonadotropin deficiency.

The protein-bound iodine level is low, and the uptake of radioactive iodine by the thyroid is decreased when there is deficiency of thyrotropin. Differentiation from primary hypothyroidism is possible on demonstration of normal thyroid reserve after stimulation with exogenous thyrotropin. Corticosteroid excretion may be decreased when corticotropin is deficient. Direct measurement of corticotropin levels is possible, but is not a clinical procedure; an indirect method for measuring pituitary corticotropin reserve is available. Administration of metyrapone results in increased urinary corticoid levels in the presence of normal pituitary corticotropin reserve. This agent (an 11-hydroxylase inhibitor) interferes with hydrocortisone synthesis, which in turn leads to increased corticotropin production. Increased production and excretion of compound S (a precursor of hydrocortisone) ensue. Since compound S is also measured as a corticosteroid by the usual test procedure, increased levels are noted. In the absence of corticotropin, metyrapone has no effect on corticosteroid production. In such instances it is necessary to establish that the adrenals are normally responsive to exogenously administered corticotropin.

Roentgenographic Examination. The fontanels remain open beyond the second year; in the occipital suture wormian bones may be found. The bones of the vault are thin, and osteoporosis may be noticed. The long bones are slender and poor in minerals. The centers of ossification appear late, and the epiphyseal clefts remain open. The sella turcica is often small, but there is great variation in the size of the sella in normal persons, and the evaluation of a small sella is difficult.

Differential Diagnosis. When the diagnosis of pituitary dwarfism is established, every effort must be made to determine whether there is a destructive intracranial lesion. A history of nausea, vomiting, loss of vision, headache or increase in circumference of the head suggests increased intracranial pressure. The eyegrounds must be carefully examined, and roentgenograms may be helpful in localization of a tumor.

Children with constitutional delay in growth and sexual maturation rarely are as dwarfed as children with deficiency of growth hormone, and they have no other evidence of pituitary deficiency. Dwarfism resulting from the chondrodystrophies, osteogenesis imperfecta, pseudohypoparathyroidism or the various types of rickets can be recognized by features characteristic of each of them. When retardation in growth is due to cardiac, renal, hepatic or intestinal disease, the cause can be identified by the diagnosis of the underlying disorder.

In girls gonadal dysgenesis must always be considered. When this is associated with the usual characteristic congenital deformities, the diagnosis is not difficult; such patients are chromatin-negative and have an XO chromosomal karyotype. The girl with an XO/XX karyotype has few characteristic abnormalities other than shortness of stature; chromosomal analysis is necessary to establish the diagnosis (p. 1231). After puberty, gonadotropin secretion is elevated in the patient with gonadal dysgenesis, whereas it is absent in the pituitary dwarf. The osseous development of pituitary dwarfs is greatly retarded, whereas girls with gonadal dysgenesis have only a slight delay in epiphyseal development.

Emotional deprivation may lead to severe retardation of growth and mimic hypopituitarism. Although the mechanisms whereby sensory and emotional deprivation interfere with growth are not fully understood, some degree of functional hypopituitarism may be indicated by decreased pituitary response to metyrapone administration and by inadequate rise of growth hormone levels in response to provocative stimuli. Appropriate history and careful observations reveal disturbed mother-child or family relations which provide clues to diagnosis. Emotionally deprived children frequently have perverted or voracious appetites, are excessively passive or aggressive, and are borderline or dull-normal in intelligence. Improved growth rates are noted when child-rearing practices are altered or when the child is placed in a more stimulating environment.

In *primordial dwarfism* the growth retardation begins during intrauterine life, is present at birth, and is frequently associated with other minor or major defects. This is a heterogeneous group with diverse causative factors. Growth hormone levels are normal.

Prognosis. Prognosis for life depends upon the causative factor, and whether it can be eradicated. In the absence of an anatomic lesion the affected person may reach old age.

Prognosis of ultimate height is difficult, since continued growth is possible long after the usual age of adolescence, owing to the persistence of open epiphyses. Sexual maturation may also take place 10 or 20 years later than in normal persons. Catch-up growth is frequently observed in children who have had surgical treatment of a craniopharyngioma, even in some patients in whom deficient growth hormone responses persist.

Treatment. In patients with demonstrable organic lesions, treatment should be directed to the underlying disease process.

In contrast to the failure of growth hormone prepared from bovine and porcine pituitary glands to stimulate growth in the human dwarf, growth hormone prepared from human and monkey pituitary glands is effective. The hormone is not generally available, owing to the inadequate supply of human pituitary glands obtained at autopsy from which to extract the hormone. One pituitary yields about 5 mg. of growth hormone. Although optimum dosage schedules have not evolved, it appears that 1 to 2 mg. by intramuscular injection 2 or 3 times a week is effective in establishing growth in children with pituitary dwarfism.

Protein anabolic agents such as methyltestosterone and analogues of testosterone have been used to induce growth. These compounds increase the rate of growth of the dwarf. Yet even with the least androgenic of the available agents, the ultimate height attained is almost always compromised, apparently owing to accelerated osseous maturation with early closure of epiphyses. These agents should not be used in the young child with pituitary dwarfism and should be used with great caution in the older child only when human growth hormone is not available or when growth hormone is no longer effective, owing to the development of antibodies.

Replacement therapy with thyroid hormone or hydrocortisone, or both, is indicated when deficiency of either or both is present. If sexual maturation does not occur, administration of gonadal hormones may be necessary.

PITUITARY GIGANTISM AND ACROMEGALY

Tumors of the anterior pituitary gland may produce excessive amounts of growth hormone. In young persons with open epiphyses, overproduction of growth hormone results in gigantism; in persons with closed epiphyses, acromegaly results. When onset occurs during adolescence, both patterns are manifest.

Pituitary gigantism is rare. The cause is most often an eosinophilic adenoma; occasionally gigantism results from a chromophobe adenoma. In most of the recorded cases the abnormal growth became evident at puberty, and the abnormal height was attained within the next few years. Such giants may grow to a height of 8 feet and more. After closure of the epiphyses, acromegaly may be superimposed upon gigantism; often some acromegalic features are seen with gigantism even in children and adolescents.

Acromegaly consists chiefly in an enlargement of the distal parts of the body, but the manifestations of abnormal growth actually involve all portions. The circumference of the skull increases, the nose becomes broad, and the tongue is often so enlarged that it protrudes between the thick lips. The mandible grows excessively, and the teeth become separated. The fingers and toes grow chiefly in thickness. There may be a dorsal kyphosis. Fatigue and lassitude are early symptoms; signs of increased intracranial pressure appear later. Visual loss may be demonstrable only by careful determinations of visual fields.

The adenoma may compromise anterior pituitary function through growth or cystic degeneration. Decreased secretion of gonadotropins may result in delayed sexual maturation or in hypogonadism. Secretion of TSH and ACTH may also be impaired. Serum levels of growth hormone and of phosphorus are elevated. Carbohydrate tolerance is decreased, and mild diabetes may result.

Roentgenograms of the skull reveal enlargement of the sella turcica and of the paranasal sinuses; those of the hands reveal tufting of the phalanges. Osseous maturation is normal.

Differential Diagnosis. In the differential diagnosis hereditary tall stature must be considered. In this condition there is usually abnormal height in one or both parents or in close relatives. Such tall persons are well proportioned and free of signs of increased intracranial pressure. Abnormal growth during preadolescence in obese children is a temporary state; though such children may become tall, they do not attain the height of giants. Children with precocious puberty are often unusually tall, but do not develop into giants, since their epiphyses close early and growth ceases prematurely. Cerebral gigantism, a condition which is far more common than pituitary gigantism, can usually be differentiated on clinical grounds (see below).

Treatment. If there is evidence of increased intracranial pressure, surgical intervention is indicated. In the absence of such ocular symptoms as choked disks and constricted visual fields, irradiation may be an effective form of therapy; its effectiveness should be estimated by serial measurements of levels of growth hormone. Replacement therapy for hormone deficiencies may be necessary.

CEREBRAL GIGANTISM

This disorder, like pituitary gigantism, is characterized by rapid growth; however, growth hormone levels in the serum are not elevated, and evidence suggests a cerebral defect for the pathogenetic mechanism. Birth weight and length are above the ninetieth percentile in most affected infants, and macrocrania may be noted. Growth is rapid, and by 1 year of age all affected infants are over the ninety-seventh percentile in height. Accelerated growth continues for the first 4 to 5 years, and then a normal rate is observed. Puberty usually occurs at the normal time, but may occur slightly early. The hands and feet are large, with thickened subcutaneous tissue. The head is large and dolichocephalic, and the jaw is prominent; there is hypertelorism, and the eyes have an anti-mongoloid slant. Clumsiness and awkward gait are characteristic, and affected children have great difficulty in sports, in learning to ride a bicycle and in other tasks requiring coordination. Mental retardation is almost always present; though it may vary considerably in degree, it is not progressive.

Radiographs reveal a large skull, a high orbital roof, a sella of normal size but slightly posterior inclination, and an increased intraorbital distance. Osseous maturation is consistently advanced and compatible with the patient's height. Growth hormone levels are normal, and 17-ketosteroids are only slightly increased. Abnormal electro-

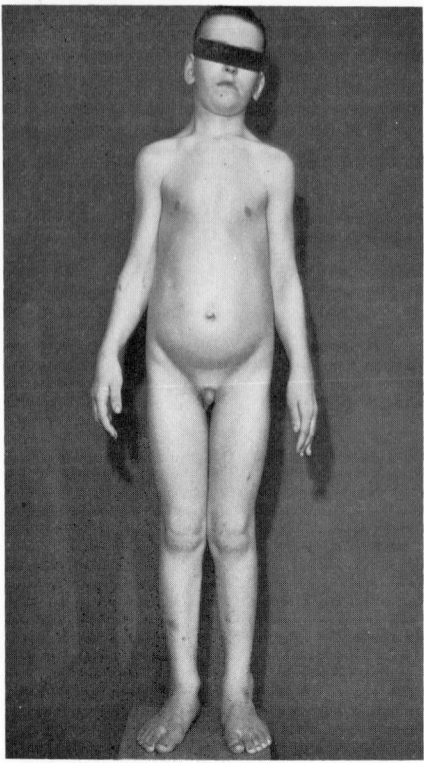

Figure 17-1. Cerebral gigantism in an 8-year-old boy. Height age was 12 years; bone-age, 12 years; I.Q. 60; abnormal electroencephalogram. Note prominence of forehead and jaw and the large hands and feet. Sexual development was consistent with chronologic age. Hormone studies were normal except for slightly elevated 17-ketosteroids. Adult height was 6 feet 10 inches; normal sexual development. He wears size 18 shoes.

encephalograms are common, and pneumoencephalography frequently reveals a dilated ventricular system.

The cause of the disorder is unknown, and it is not clear whether all patients with this syndrome have the same defect. It may be that this syndrome represents a disturbance in the production of the hypothalamic growth hormone-releasing hormone in the fetus and in the young infant.

DIABETES INSIPIDUS

Diabetes insipidus may result from pathologic changes in any part of the close functional unit made up of the posterior lobe of the pituitary, the supraoptic and paraventricular nuclei of the hypothalamus and the hypothalamico-hypophyseal fibers. Such changes result in deficiency of antidiuretic hormone (vasopressin), which acts directly on the distal tubules and collecting ducts to facilitate reabsorption of water. This disorder is characterized by inability of the kidney to produce a concentrated urine. When antidiuretic hormone is administered, there is a remarkable decrease in the amount of urine excreted and an increase in its specific gravity.

Etiology. Any acquired lesion which damages the neurohypophysis or hypothalamus may result in diabetes insipidus. Tumors, particularly craniopharyngiomas, are the most common cause, and in such instances, symptoms of increased intracranial pressure may accompany those of diabetes insipidus or may follow years later. Diabetes insipidus may result from operative procedures in the region of the pituitary and the hypothalamus and may be transitory or permanent. Injuries of the head, such as basal skull fractures, may lead to diabetes insipidus immediately, or symptoms may appear after several months. In the Hand-Schüller-Christian syndrome the disturbance of water metabolism may be accompanied by exophthalmos and defective areas in the skull. Encephalitis, tuberculosis, leukemia, actinomycosis and syphilis may occasionally cause diabetes insipidus. In a small percentage of instances, diabetes insipidus may occur as a hereditary disorder; transmission is usually in an autosomal dominant manner, but is occasionally sex-linked recessive. In such patients there is a primary degeneration of the nerve cells of the supraoptic and paraventricular nuclei of the hypothalamus.

In many instances no specific cause can be determined. The search for a lesion should be continued indefinitely, since diabetes insipidus may be the first recognizable sign of an intracranial tumor and antedate neurologic signs by years.

Clinical Manifestations. Polydipsia and polyuria are the outstanding symptoms of diabetes insipidus. In families with the hereditary disorder the polyuria is noted in early infancy. The infant cries excessively and will be dissatisfied when additional milk is offered, but is quieted when given water. Hyperthermia, rapid loss of weight and collapse are common in infancy. Vomiting, constipation and growth failure may be observed. Dehydration in early infancy may result in brain damage and mental deficiency.

In a child who has acquired bladder control, enuresis may be the first symptom. The excessive thirst is a disturbing symptom and interferes with play, learning and sleep. Children with diabetes insipidus do not perspire, and their skin is dry and pale. Anorexia is a common symptom; there is a preference for carbohydrates.

Other signs and symptoms depend on the primary lesion; thus patients with tumors in the region of the hypothalamus may have disturbance of growth, progressive cachexia or obesity, hyperpyrexia, sleep disturbance, sexual precocity or emotional disorders. Lesions initially causing diabetes insipidus may progress and eventually destroy the anterior pituitary. In such instances the symptoms of diabetes insipidus tend to ameliorate or disappear completely.

Laboratory Data. The daily volume of urine may be 4 to 10 liters or more. The urine is pale or colorless, and the specific gravity varies from 1.001 to 1.005 and does not exceed 1.007 except during extreme dehydration; the urine is hypotonic to the blood. Renal function studies other than the inability to concentrate urine are within normal limits.

Roentgenograms of the skull may reveal such evidence of an intracranial tumor as calcifications, enlargement of the sella turcica, erosion of the clinoid processes or increased width of the suture lines. Roentgenograms of the skull or other bones in patients with the Hand-Schüller-Christian syndrome may reveal areas of rarefaction.

The neurohypophysis can be stimulated to determine whether there is any reserve of antidiuretic hormone by the intravenous administration of hypertonic saline solution or of nicotine under controlled conditions.

Differential Diagnosis. Polydipsia may occur in psychopathic patients and is easily confused with diabetes insipidus. Such persons are usually able to produce a concentrated urine when fluids are withheld. Occasionally, however, the ability of such patients to secrete antidiuretic hormone becomes impaired, and they cannot concentrate urine normally. Antidiuretic hormone activity returns to normal when the compulsive drinking of water is discontinued.

Polydipsia, polyuria and impaired concentration of urine are common manifestations in patients with chronic renal disease. In nephrogenic diabetes insipidus the renal disorder is restricted to the tubular deficiency in the reabsorption of water. Hypercalcemia and potassium deficiency also are responsible for polydipsia and polyuria.

After the diagnosis of diabetes insipidus has been established, the underlying process must be determined.

Prognosis. The prognosis depends upon the underlying condition. It is favorable in the hereditary and idiopathic types, when treatment is adequate. If the disorder follows trauma, spontaneous cure may occur. The prognosis of patients with a brain tumor depends upon the site of the lesion and upon the type of neoplastic cell.

Treatment. The causative factor deserves first consideration in the treatment. Tumors will require surgical intervention in the majority of instances. Appropriate treatment is indicated for other specific lesions.

Symptomatic treatment with vasopressin (Pitressin) is indicated regardless of the cause. The treatment of choice is intramuscular injection of Pitressin tannate in oil, 0.5 to 1 ml. every 1 to 3 days, as determined for the individual patient. Careful attention must be given to adequate resuspension of the Pitressin tannate in the viscous oil. Polyuria and polydipsia are diminished in the majority of instances. Pitressin may also be administered intranasally as snuff or nose drops, or synthetic lysine-8-vasopressin may be administered as a liquid nasal spray; but these forms of therapy are less satisfactory.

Nephrogenic Diabetes Insipidus (Vasopressin-Insensitive Diabetes Insipidus). This is a renal tubular disorder occurring nearly always in boys. These patients have normal production of antidiuretic hormone, but failure of end-organ response in the renal tubule. Despite considerable controversy, most of the evidence favors an X-linked mode of inheritance; heterozygous females are usually asymptomatic, but may exhibit a variable defect in concentration which is probably explained by Lyon's hypothesis of sex-chromosome inactivation.

The onset is shortly after birth, the symptoms

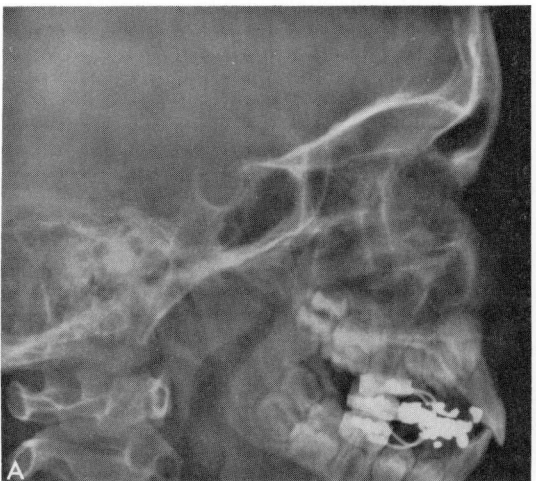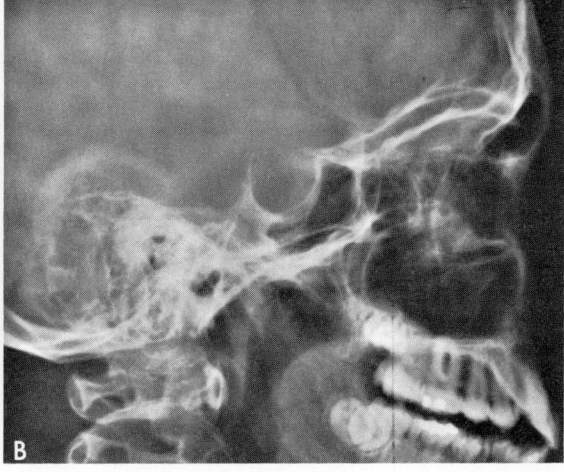

Figure 17-2. *A,* Radiograph of skull of 9-year-old boy with polydipsia, polyuria, nocturia and enuresis. Urine specific gravity was 1.016 after water deprivation. Growth was normal, and the sella turcica was considered to be at upper limit of normal, but was probably enlarged. Over the ensuing 6 months the symptoms of diabetes insipidus abated. *B,* The patient returned at 14 years of age because of growth failure and delay in sexual maturation. Studies revealed a deficiency of growth hormone, gonadotropins, corticotropin and a partial deficiency of thyrotropin. Note enlargement and thinning of the sella turcica, but absence of intrasellar or suprasellar calcification. Neurologic and ophthalmologic examinations were normal. There was exacerbation of diabetes insipidus with administration of hydrocortisone and thyroxine. Surgery revealed a large craniopharyngioma.

being those of diabetes insipidus. In addition to polyuria and polydipsia, unexplained fever, irritability, vomiting, constipation and failure to thrive are common. Fluid restriction or elevated environmental temperature may result in hyperpyrexia, rapid loss of weight and peripheral collapse. Growth is retarded, and mental development may be impaired.

Hyperelectrolytemia and azotemia are almost constant findings in early infancy, but tend to subside later in life. The urine has a low specific gravity, which may rise to about 1.010 during severe dehydration. Administration of vasopressin fails to induce antidiuresis and has no effect on the volume or specific gravity of urine.

Treatment consists in administration of water at frequent intervals in amounts sufficient to prevent dehydration and fever. It is almost impossible to maintain normal serum electrolyte levels without giving a low solute diet, which is justifiable in early life, even if growth is retarded.

Diuretics, particularly the thiazides, paradoxically reduce the polyuria. The precise mechanism of action is still unsettled, but the beneficial effect of these drugs appears to be to decrease free water clearance. Chlorothiazide or hydrochlorothiazide, in 3 divided doses totalling 0.1 gm. per square meter per day, has been used successfully when coupled with low solute diets. Since refractoriness to therapy and bone marrow toxicity have been observed, these drugs should be used with caution and administered only to patients with severe manifestations of the disorder (see also p. 1148).

PRECOCIOUS PUBERTY

The average age of children at the onset of puberty in the United States is 11 to 12 years in girls and 12 to 13 years in boys; there is, however, a wide range of normal variation. Puberty may be delayed to 18 to 20 years of age or may take place much earlier than usual. The following physical changes are accepted as evidence of abnormally early sexual development: (1) breast enlargement before 8 years of age; (2) menarche before 10 years; (3) pubic or axillary hair before 9 years, especially if dark and coarse; (4) enlargement of the clitoris or penis disproportionate to the age of the child; or (5) other associated phenomena at a disproportionate age such as facial hair, acne, change in voice, pigmented areolas of the nipples and pigmentation of the sexual organs.

The physiologic mechanism which initiates the onset of puberty is not known; evidence suggests that it may originate in the hypothalamus as a neurohumoral stimulus to the pituitary. Release of gonadotropic hormones from the pituitary then stimulates the Leydig cells of the testes to secrete testosterone and the follicles of the ovary to secrete estradiol. At the same time, androgen production by the adrenal cortex increases, and these steroid hormones act on the various end-organs to produce the secondary sex characteristics.

TABLE 17-1. Conditions Causing Precocious Puberty

A. **True precocious puberty**
   1. Cerebral lesions
      Brain tumors, pineal tumors, postencephalitic scars, tuberous sclerosis, hydrocephalus, hypothalamic hamartomas
   2. McCune-Albright syndrome
   3. Syndrome of precocious puberty and hypothyroidism
   4. Syndrome of short stature and elevated gonadotropins (Silver's syndrome)
   5. Gonadotropin-producing hepatoblastoma
   6. Secreting choriocarcinoma
   7. Therapeutic administration of gonadotropin
   8. Complication of corticosteroid therapy for virilizing adrenal hyperplasia
   9. Idiopathic (constitutional; functional; no demonstrable lesion)
      a. Sporadic
      b. Familial

B. **Precocious pseudopuberty**
   Females
      Isosexual (feminization)
         1. Ovarian tumors
            a. Granulosa cell tumor
            b. Theca cell tumor
            c. Teratoma
         2. Autonomous functional cyst of ovary
         3. Adrenal cortical tumor
         4. Medications (estrogens)
      Heterosexual (virilization)
         1. Congenital adrenal hyperplasia
         2. Adrenal cortical tumor
         3. Adrenal rest tumor in ovary
         4. Medications (androgens)
   Males
      Isosexual (masculinization)
         1. Congenital adrenal hyperplasia
         2. Adrenal cortical tumor
         3. Leydig cell tumor
         4. Teratoma (containing adrenal cortical tissue)
         5. Medications (androgens)
      Heterosexual (feminization)
         1. Adrenal cortical tumor
         2. Medications (estrogens)

C. **Partial precocious puberty**
      Premature pubarche (adrenarche)
      Premature thelarche

Precocious pubertal development may be divided into true puberty, pseudopuberty, and partial (p. 1185) precocious puberty. True precocious puberty is always isosexual and indicates not only precocity of the secondary sexual characteristics, but also an increase in the size of the gonads with premature production of mature sperm or ova. In precocious pseudopuberty only the secondary sex characteristics appear; the gonads do not mature, and there is no spermatogenesis or ovulation. In pseudopuberty the precociously appearing sex characteristics may be isosexual or heterosexual. This latter group will be discussed in the sections on Adrenocortical Hyperfunction (p. 1211) and on the Primary Le-

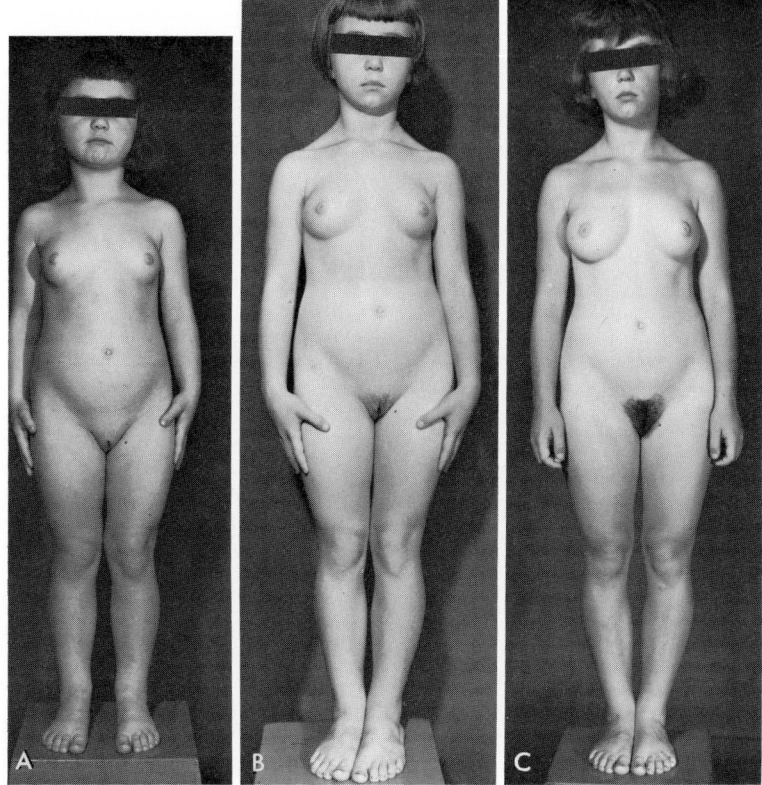

Figure 17-3. Constitutional precocious puberty. Patient at *(A)* $3^{11}/_{12}$, *(B)* at $5^{8}/_{12}$ and *(C)* at $8^{1}/_{2}$ years of age. Breast development and vaginal bleeding began at $2^{1}/_{2}$ years of age. Osseous age was $7^{1}/_{2}$ years at $3^{11}/_{12}$, and 14 years at 8 years of age. Repeated estrogen assays have varied between 12 and 132 mouse units. Urinary gonadotropins were not demonstrable until the child was 5 years of age. 17-Ketosteroids varied between 1.6 ,and 2.1 mg. per 24 hours during the first 5 years of life. Intelligence and dental age are normal for chronologic age. Growth was completed at 10 years; ultimate height was 56 inches.

sions of the Ovary (p. 1233) and of the Testis (p. 1230).

TRUE PRECOCIOUS PUBERTY

Precocious Puberty Without Other Pathologic Findings (Constitutional)

When no causative factor can be found, the early onset of puberty is considered a physiologic process which begins at an unusually early age. Most instances of true sexual precocity are of this type, and most of these physiologic variants occur in girls. Presumably the hypothalamic mechanism which initiates puberty is precociously activated. Sexual precocity has been observed as a familial disorder in 11 kindreds; in these instances only males were involved.

Clinical Manifestations. Sexual development may begin at any age. In girls the first sign is development of the breasts; pubic hair may appear simultaneously, but more often appears later. Development of the external genitalia, the appearance of axillary hair and the onset of menstruation follow. The early menstrual cycles may be more irregular than with normal puberty. Men-

arche has been observed within the first year of life. Although the initial cycles are usually anovulatory, pregnancy has been reported as early as $5^{1}/_{2}$ years of age.

In boys there are enlargement of the penis and testes, appearance of pubic hair, acne, and frequent erections. The voice deepens, and linear growth is accelerated. Spermatogenesis has been observed as early as 5 or 6 years of age, and nocturnal emissions may occur. Testicular biopsies have shown all elements of the testes to be stimulated. If the precocity is complete, various degrees of spermatogenesis are present; even if it is incomplete, the interstitial cells are present.

In both girls and boys there is advancement of growth in height and weight and of osseous maturation. The increased rate of ossification results in early closure of epiphyses, so that ultimate stature is less than it would have been otherwise. Approximately one third of patients do not achieve a height of 152 cm. (5 feet) as adults. Dental age and mental development, however, are usually compatible with chronologic age.

Laboratory Data. Urinary excretion of 17-ketosteroids and estrogens may correspond to that in normal mature men and women. Gonadotropins, on the other hand, are frequently not

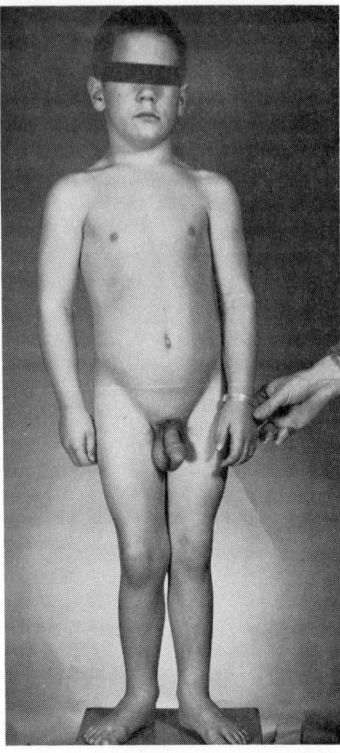

Figure 17-4. Precocious puberty without a demonstrable lesion in a 3½-year-old boy. Height age was 5 years and bone-age 8 years. Urinary gonadotropins were demonstrable; 17-ketosteroids, 1.9 mg. per 24 hours. Note well developed testes; testicular biopsy revealed Leydig cells and well developed tubules with adult spermatogonia. At 5 years of age the boy had a height age of 10 years and osseous maturation of 14 years. Growth ceased at 9 years; ultimate stature was 58½ inches. He had no neurologic abnormalities, and was bright-normal in intelligence and well adjusted emotionally.

demonstrable in the urine of children with true precocious puberty, although early release of gonadotropins is believed to be essential to the development of the disorder. This apparent inconsistency sometimes reflects the low sensitivity of analytic techniques routinely used in clinical laboratories. With more sensitive techniques and testing of multiple specimens, increased gonadotropin excretion is more often demonstrated. Stained vaginal smears reveal cornification and other estrogenic effects. In many children there are electroencephalographic abnormalities, suggesting a primary cerebral abnormality as the cause of the disorder.

Differential Diagnosis. In girls, lesions of the central nervous system, tumors of the ovaries, feminizing adrenal cortical tumors, McCune-Albright syndrome and accidental ingestion of estrogens must be considered in the differential diagnosis. A carefully obtained history, a complete physical examination and appropriate laboratory studies usually resolve the diagnosis. A pelvic examination under anesthesia may be necessary to determine whether there is an ovarian tumor.

In boys cerebral lesions, the adrenogenital syndrome, a Leydig cell tumor and a gonadotropin-producing hepatoma must be considered diagnostic possibilities. In the *adrenogenital syndrome* the testes are small relative to the degree of sexual maturation. A *Leydig cell tumor* can usually be detected on physical examination, and a *hepatoma* usually causes hepatomegaly.

When there is no evidence of a cerebral lesion from the initial examination, the child must be carefully and repeatedly observed for several years before the possibility of an intracranial lesion can be excluded.

Treatment. Treatment consists essentially in psychologic management of patient and family. A detailed explanation to the parents with the reassurance of the harmlessness of the condition is imperative. They should also be told that the precocious manifestations will persist, but that by the age of 10 to 14 years the child will not be different from other children. Such children should also be guarded against abuses that could result in pregnancy. The few data available indicate that these patients have a normal reproductive span and that menopause takes place within the usual time.

Medroxyprogesterone acetate, a progestational compound which inhibits gonadotropin production, appears useful in slowing sexual development in both boys and girls with true precocious puberty. If therapy is instituted early enough, osseous maturation may be decelerated; the prognosis for ultimate stature should be improved, but this remains to be established. The value of this agent is yet to be convincingly demonstrated.

Precocious Puberty with Polyostotic Fibrous Dysplasia and Abnormal Pigmentation
(McCune-Albright Syndrome)

When fibrous dysplasia of the skeletal system is associated with patchy cutaneous pigmentation and endocrine dysfunction, the clinical combination is frequently referred to as the McCune-Albright syndrome. The most common endocrine disturbance is sexual precocity; the syndrome occurs principally in the female. The pathogenesis is not known, but the disease is thought to be the result of a congenital disorder of development involving the skeleton, the skin and the hypothalamus.

Vaginal bleeding has occurred as early as 4 months of age and secondary sex characteristics at 6 months, but the average age at menarche is 3 years. Thyroid enlargement with or without hyperthyroidism, gynecomastia and acromegalic features have occasionally been observed. In one instance of the McCune-Albright syndrome bilateral adrenal cortical hyperplasia produced Cush-

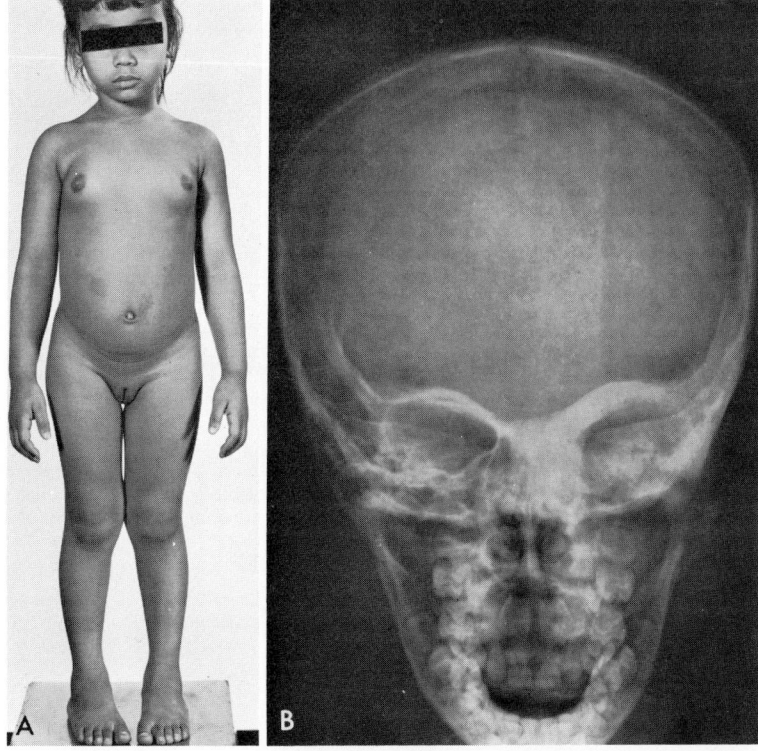

Figure 17-5. Precocious puberty associated with polyostotic fibrous dysplasia (McCune-Albright syndrome) in a girl 4½ years of age; at this time her height age and osseous age were normal. Menarche at 4 years. *A,* Note bilateral breast development, hyperpigmented spots on abdomen and prominence of left side of face. *B,* Roentgenograms revealed fibrous dysplasia in the distal end of the left ulna and thickening of the bones about the left orbit and the maxillary portion of the frontal bones.

ing's syndrome in early infancy, prior to the onset of pubertal changes.

The symptoms of precocity, the demonstrable hormonal deviations and the treatment are the same as those of constitutional precocious puberty. Serum calcium and phosphorus levels are normal; that of alkaline phosphatase is normal or increased. Prognosis is favorable for longevity, but deformities may result from the bony lesions and repeated pathologic fractures. The disease becomes static in adult life.

Precocious Puberty Resulting from Organic Brain Lesions

A wide variety of lesions of the central nervous system such as tumors, postencephalitic scars, tuberculous meningoencephalitis, tuberous sclerosis, neurofibromatosis and hydrocephalus have been associated with sexual precocity. Such lesions may involve the hypothalamus by invasion or pressure. Sexual precocity may be the initial manifestation of a hypothalamic hamartoma. This lesion is a benign nodule composed of nerve cells and is attached to both the mammillary bodies and tuber cinereum.

About one third of prepubertal boys who have tumors of the pineal body undergo precocious puberty by involvement of the posterior hypothalamus or by pressure on the aqueduct of Sylvius and posterior hypothalamus (see choriocarcinoma below).

Precocious puberty secondary to a lesion of the central nervous system is always isosexual; precocity of this origin is more common in boys than in girls. The endocrine pattern of affected patients is identical with that observed in children with true precocious puberty without demonstrable organic lesions. Since some of the intracranial lesions, such as hamartomas, may grow slowly and produce no signs other than precocious puberty, a child who is considered initially to have precocious puberty without a lesion may eventually exhibit signs of increased intracranial pressure and be found to have a hypothalamic tumor. Other hypothalamic signs or symptoms such as diabetes insipidus, hyperthermia, obesity, cachexia, unnatural crying or laughing may suggest the possibility of an intracranial lesion. A history of convulsions, retarded mental development or other neurologic signs should also make one suspect a lesion of the central nervous system.

Roentgenographic examination of the skull and electroencephalographic studies, although rarely of value, are essential parts of the examination, and on occasion pneumoencephalography, ventriculography or cerebral angiography is indicated.

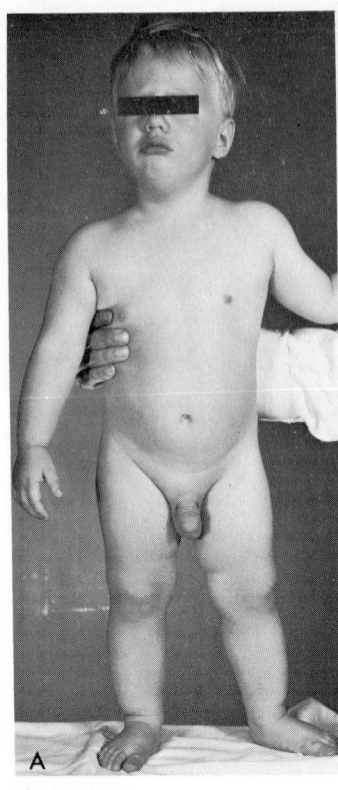
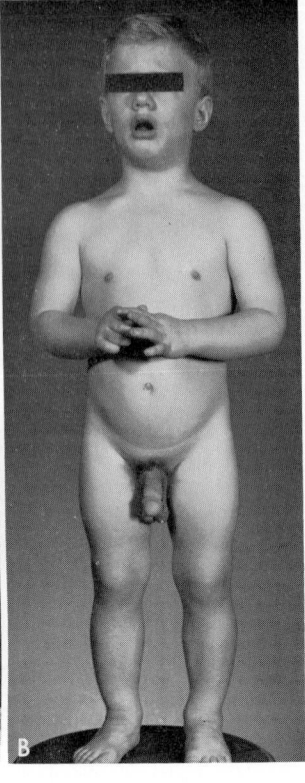

Figure 17-6. Precocious puberty with central nervous system lesion. Photographs at *(A)* 1½ and *(B)* 2½ years of age. Accelerated growth, muscular development, osseous maturation and testicular development were consistent with the degree of secondary sexual maturation. Urinary gonadotropins were repeatedly negative, 17-ketosteroids usually 2 to 3 mg. per 24 hours. In early infancy he began having frequent episodes of rapid, purposeless spells; later in life he had episodes of uncontrollable laughing with ocular movements. At 7 years he exhibits emotional lability, aggressive behavior and destructive tendencies. Although a hypothalamic disorder has been suspected, repeated studies have failed to reveal a space-taking lesion.

Treatment depends on the lesion. Surgical decompression followed by roentgen therapy is usually indicated when removal of a tumor is not possible.

Gonadotropin-Producing Hepatoblastoma

Six instances of precocious puberty in boys with malignant hepatomas have been recorded. In all instances, gonadotropins were detected in the urine or blood, and hyperplasia of the interstitial cells of the testes were demonstrated. The tumor produces a gonadotropin-like hormone which stimulates precocious maturation of the testes and which has been detected in one instance in tumor extracts. The age at onset varied from 1 to 7 years, and all patients have had an enlarged liver or mass in the right upper quadrant. Treatment for these tumors is the same as that for other carcinomas of the liver (p. 1451).

Syndrome of Precocious Puberty and Hypothyroidism

Puberty is usually delayed in children with untreated hypothyroidism. Therefore precocious maturation in a child with untreated congenital or acquired hypothyroidism presents a striking appearance. Fifteen of the 18 reported instances involved girls; 5 patients also had Down's syndrome. The high incidence of females may reflect the greater frequency of hypothyroidism in females; the high incidence of Down s syndrome may be related to the known association of this disorder to thyroid autoimmunity. Sexual development has most often appeared at 7 to 9 years of age. In spite of advanced development, pubic and axillary hair is absent or sparse. The usual manifestations of hypothyroidism were present, including retardation of growth and of osseous maturation. Ten of the children had enlargement of the sella turcica. Galactorrhea, excessive pigmentation and papilledema were present in some. In all instances, treatment with thyroid hormone resulted in regression of the sexual precocity.

It has been suggested that in these cases of sexual precocity an oversecretion of gonadotropins accompanies the excessive secretion of thyrotropic hormone which occurs in primary hypothyroidism. Urinary gonadotropins have not usually been found in these children. Sensitive and specific immunoassays for TSH, LH, FSH, and other pituitary hormones may clarify relations and mechanisms in the future.

Syndrome of Congenital Asymmetry, Short Stature and Elevated Gonadotropins
(SILVER'S SYNDROME)

Silver's syndrome consists of short stature, congenital hemihypertrophy, normal genitalia and slightly to moderately increased excretion of gonadotropins. Affected children have low birth weight, even though born at term, a small mandible and shortened and incurved fifth fingers. Osseous maturation is delayed and is consistent with the height-age. Urinary and serum levels of gonadotropins may be increased despite lack of sexual development; other laboratory studies give normal results. The cause of the disorder is unknown.

In spite of the short stature and retarded osseous development, a few of these children have undergone precocious sexual maturation, presumably as a result of early production of gonadotropins.

Heterogeneity of this disorder is suggested by reports of Silver's syndrome with a variety of chromosomal aberrations.

Precocious Puberty Due to Secreting Choriocarcinoma

Choriocarcinomas secrete excessive amounts of chorionic gonadotropins which may stimulate the gonads to initiate precocious sexual maturation. In the prepubertal male these tumors are most apt to arise *in the pineal body*. The precocity is produced by the tumor itself and is not to be confused with the situation which occurs with most pineal tumors in which involvement of the hypothalamus is the cause of the sexual precocity (p. 1183). In the prepubertal female, choriocarcinomas have occurred principally *in the ovary*. Sexual precocity is produced by stimulation of the opposite ovary. These tumors are usually highly malignant, and the child may be cachectic in association with the sexual precocity.

In boys there is hyperplasia of the Leydig cells and tubular maturation. In one boy only spermatocytic precursors were found; in other instances, spermatogenesis has been observed. The ovary may contain numerous follicular cysts, but there may be no mature follicles or corpus luteum. Although choriocarcinomas may not always produce mature sperm or ova, they are considered a cause of true precocious puberty.

The diagnosis is readily established if the urine contains large amounts of chorionic gonadotropin and there is a positive pregnancy test result. Other hormone assays are consistent with the degree of sexual maturation.

INCOMPLETE (PARTIAL) PRECOCIOUS DEVELOPMENT

Isolated manifestations of precocity without development of other signs of puberty are not unusual. Development of the breasts and growth of sexual hair are the 2 most common ones.

Simple Hypertrophy of the Breasts (Premature Thelarche). Precocious enlargement of the breasts may occur without any other secondary sex change. In such instances, enlargement of the breasts is usually manifest between the first and third years of life. There may be enlargement of only one breast. Enlargement of the breasts may be the first sign of true or pseudoprecocious puberty, but more often is a benign abnormality. Thorough diagnostic study and a prolonged period of observation are indicated in all instances. The hypertrophy of the breasts may disappear spontaneously. It has been suggested that the mammary gland may be unusually sensitive to small amounts of estrogens secreted by the ovaries, whereas other structures, being normally responsive, do not react until greater amounts are produced at puberty. The usual tests for urinary estrogens are not sensitive enough to detect their presence. There is no cornification of the vaginal epithelium, and urinary excretion of gonadotropins and 17-ketosteroids is not increased. Other aspects of growth and osseous maturation are within normal limits; menarche occurs at the normal time.

Premature Development of Sexual Hair (Premature Pubarche). The appearance of sexual hair at an early age without any other evidence of maturation has been termed "premature pubarche" and "premature adrenarche." It occurs much more frequently in girls than in boys. Hair appears first on the labia majora, then in the pubic region, and finally in the axilla. Affected children

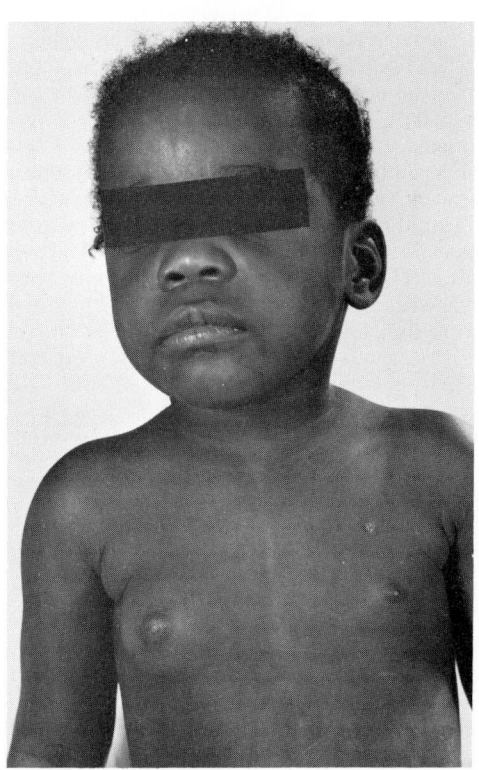

Figure 17-7. Premature thelarche. Simple hypertrophy of the breasts in a 23-month-old girl. No demonstrable urinary estrogens or gonadotropin. Normal genitalia and growth. Note the disparity in size of the breasts. This is a common finding in this condition as well as in normal puberty.

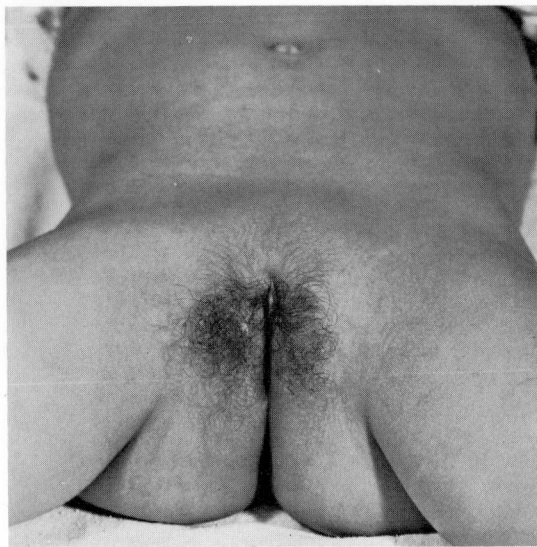

Figure 17-8. Premature pubarche. Isolated development of sexual hair in a 6-year-old girl with cerebral palsy. Urinary 17-ketosteroids varied between 1.5 and 3.4 mg. in 24 hours.

are taller than average, and their osseous age is generally 1 to 4 years in advance of their chronologic age. Urinary 17-ketosteroids may be slightly increased beyond values normal for the age, but there is no evidence of true virilization. When this disorder occurs in children with cerebral damage, as it often does, the child is usually small for his chronologic age, and osseous maturation is not advanced.

This condition appears to result from premature activation of the adrenal cortex, with secretion of adrenal androgens before the pituitary gonadotropic mechanism becomes activated. The reason for the relatively frequent association of the disorder with cerebral damage is not known. Premature pubarche must be differentiated from early true precocious puberty, adrenal cortical tumors and adrenal hyperplasia. Parents should then be assured that this condition is a harmless variation of development.

MEDICATIONAL PRECOCITY

Although this is a type of pseudopuberty, it is included here to emphasize that a variety of medicaments can induce the appearance of secondary sexual characteristics which may be confused with precocious puberty. A careful history to exclude accidental exposure to or ingestion of sex hormones is of paramount importance. Precocious pseudopuberty in both boys and girls accidentally ingesting stilbestrol has been reported. Exogenous estrogens may induce an intense, dark brown color to the areola of the breasts which is not usually seen in endogenous types of precocity. The precocious changes disappear after cessation of administration of the exogenous hormones.

REFERENCES

General

Wilkins, L.: *The Diagnosis and Treatment of Endocrine Disorders in Childhood and Adolescence.* 3rd ed. Springfield, Ill., Charles C Thomas, 1965.
Williams, R. H.: *Textbook of Endocrinology.* 4th ed. Philadelphia, W. B. Saunders Company, 1968.

Pituitary Dwarfism

Farquharson, R. F.: *Simmonds' Disease: Extreme Insufficiency of the Adenohypophysis.* Springfield, Ill., Charles C Thomas, 1950.
Goodman, H. G., Grumbach, M. B., and Kaplan, S. L.: Growth and Growth Hormone. II. A Comparison of Isolated Growth-Hormone Deficiency and Multiple Pituitary-Hormone Deficiencies in 35 Patients with Idiopathic Hypopituitary Dwarfism. *New England J. Med.,* 278:57, 1968.
Greenwood, F. C., Hunter, W. M., and Marrian, V. J.: Growth Hormone Levels in Children and Adolescents. *Brit. Med. J.,* 1:25, 1964.
Henneman, P. H.: The Effect of Human Growth Hormone on Growth of Patients with Hypopituitarism. A Combined Study. *J.A.M.A.,* 205:828, 1968.
Holmes, L. B., Frantz, A., Rabkin, M. T., Soeldner, J. S., and Crawford, J. D.: Normal Growth with Subnormal Growth-Hormone Levels. *New England J. Med.,* 279:559, 1968.
Laron, Z., Pertzelan, A., and Mannheimer, S.: Genetic Pituitary Dwarfism with High Serum Concentration of Growth Hormone. A New Inborn Error of Metabolism? *Israel J. Med. Sci.,* 2:152, 1966.
Martin, M. M., and Wilkins, L.: Pituitary Dwarfism: Diagnosis and Treatment. *J. Clin. Endocrinol. & Metab.,* 18:679, 1958.
Merimee, T. J., Rimoin, D. L., Cavalli-Sforza, L. C., Rabinowitz, D., and McKusick, V. A.: Metabolic Effects of Human Growth Hormone in the African Pygmy. *Lancet,* 2:194, 1968.
Raben, M. S.: Growth Hormone. 1. Physiologic Aspects. 2. Clinical Use of Human Growth Hormone. *New England J. Med.,* 266:31, 82, 1962.
Roth, J., Glick, S. M., Yalow, R. S., and Berson, S. A.: Secretion of Human Growth Hormone: Physiologic and Experimental Modification. *Metabolism,* 12:577, 1963.
Seip, M., van der Hagen, C. B., and Trygstad, O.: Hereditary Pituitary Dwarfism with Spontaneous Puberty. *Arch. Dis. Childhood,* 43:47, 1968.
Silver, H. K., and Rinkelstein, M.: Deprivation Dwarfism. *J. Pediat.,* 70:317, 1967.
Steiker, D. D., Bongiovanni, A. M., Eberlein, W. R., and Leboeuf, G.: Adrenocortical and Adrenocorticotropic Function in Children. *J. Pediat.,* 59:885, 1961.

Pituitary Gigantism

Frasier, S. D., and Kogut, M. D.: Adolescent Acromegaly: Studies of Growth-Hormone and Insulin Metabolism. *J. Pediat.,* 71:832, 1967.
Hook, E. B., and Reynolds, J. W.: Cerebral Gigantism: Endocrinological and Clinical Observations of Six Patients, Including a Congenital Giant, Concordant Monozygotic Twins and a Child Who Achieved Adult Gigantic Size. *J. Pediat.,* 70:900, 1967.
Milunsky, A., Cowie, V. A., and Donoghue, E. C.: Cerebral Gigantism in Childhood. A Report of Two Cases and a Review of the Literature. *Pediatrics,* 40:395, 1967.
Poznanski, A. K., and Stephenson, J. M.: Radiographic Findings in Hypothalamic Acceleration of Growth Associated with Cerebral Atrophy and Mental Retardation (Cerebral Gigantism). *Radiology,* 88:446, 1967.
Saxena, K. M., and Crawford, J. D.: Acromegalic Gigantism in an Adolescent Girl. *J. Pediat.,* 62:660, 1963.
Sotos, J. F., Dodge, P. R., Muirhead, D., Crawford, J. D., and Talbot, N. B.: Cerebral Gigantism in Childhood. *New England J. Med.,* 27:109, 1964.

Diabetes Insipidus

Barlow, E. D., and DeWardener, H. E.: Compulsive Water Drinking. *Quart. J. Med.,* 52:235, 1959.
Blotner, H.: Primary or Idiopathic Diabetes Insipidus: A System Disease. *Metabolism,* 7:191, 1958.

Braverman, L. E., Mancini, J. P., and McGoldrick, D. M.: Hereditary Idiopathic Diabetes Insipidus. A Case Report with Autopsy Findings. *Ann. Int. Med.*, 63:503, 1965.

Crawford, J. D., Kennedy, G. C., and Hill, L. E.: Clinical Results of Treatment of Diabetes Insipidus with Drugs of the Chlorothiazide Series. *New England J. Med.*, 262:737, 1960.

Dingman, J. F., Benirschke, K., and Thorn, G. W.: Studies of Neurohypophyseal Function in Man. *Am. J. Med.*, 23:226, 1957.

Gautier, E., and Simpkiss, M.: The Management of Nephrogenic Diabetes Insipidus in Early Life. *Acta paediat.*, 46:354, 1957.

Holliday, M. A., Burstin, C., and Hurrak, J.: Evidence That the Antidiuretic Substance in the Plasma of Children with Nephrogenic Diabetes Insipidus Is ADH. *Pediatrics*, 32:384, 1963.

Martin, F. I. R.: Familial Diabetes Insipidus. *Quart. J. Med.*, 52:573, 1959.

Rallison, M. L., and Tyler, F. H.: Treatment of Diabetes Insipidus in Children with Lysine-8-Vasopressin. *J. Pediat.*, 70:122, 1967.

Robinson, M. G., and Kaplan, S. A.: Inheritance of Vasopressin-Resistant ("Nephrogenic") Diabetes Insipidus. *A.M.A. J. Dis. Child.*, 99:164, 1960.

Ruess, A. L., and Rosenthal, I. M.: Intelligence in Nephrogenic Diabetes Insipidus. *A.M.A. J. Dis. Child.*, 105:358, 1963.

Schotland, M. G., Grumbach, M. M., and Strauss, J.: The Effect of Chlorothiazides in Nephrogenic Diabetes Insipidus. *Pediatrics*, 31:741, 1963.

Precocious Puberty

Aarskog, D., and Tveteraas, E.: McCune-Albright's Syndrome Following Adrenalectomy for Cushing's Syndrome in Infancy. *J. Pediat.*, 73:89, 1968.

Bauer, H. G.: Endocrine and Other Clinical Manifestations of Hypothalamic Disease; A Survey of 60 Cases with Autopsies. *J. Clin. Endocrinol. & Metab.*, 14:13, 1954.

Beas, F., Zurbrügg, R. P., Leibow, S. G., Patton, R. G., and Gardner, L. I.: Familial Male Sexual Precocity: Report of the Eleventh Kindred Found, with Observations on Blood Group Linkage and Urinary C_{19}-Steroid Excretion. *J. Clin. Endocrinol. & Metab.*, 22:1095, 1962.

Bruton, O. C., Martz, D. C., and Gerard, E. S.: Precocious Puberty Due to Secreting Chorionepithelioma (Teratoma) of the Brain. *J. Pediat.*, 59:719, 1961.

Bulbrook, R. D., Greenwood, F. C., and Snaith, A. H.: Hormone Excretion in Precocious Puberty in Girls. *Arch. Dis. Childhood*, 33:295, 1958.

Cook, C. D., McArthur, J. W., and Berenberg, W.: Pseudoprecocious Puberty in Girls as a Result of Estrogen Ingestion. *New England J. Med.*, 248:671, 1953.

Curi, J. F. J., Vanucci, R. C., Grossman, H., and New, M.: Elevated Serum Gonadotropins in Silver's Syndrome. *Am. J. Dis. Child.*, 114:658, 1967.

Ferrier, P., Shepard, T. H., II, and Smith, E. K.: Growth Disturbances and Values for Hormone Excretion in Various Forms of Precocious Sexual Development. *Pediatrics*, 28:258, 1961.

Ferrier, P. E., and Ferrier, S. A.: Silver's Syndrome: Report of a Case with Chromosomal and Dermatoglyphic Study. *J. Pediat.*, 70:438, 1967.

Fine, G., Smith, R. W., Jr., and Pachter, M. R.: Primary Extragenital Choriocarcinoma in the Male Subject. *Am. J. Med.*, 32:776, 1962.

Hertz, R.: Accidental Ingestion of Estrogens by Children. *Pediatrics*, 21:203, 1958.

Kaplan, S. A., Ling, S. M., and Irani, N. G.: Idiopathic Isosexual Precocity Therapy with Medroxyprogesterone. *Am. J. Dis. Child.*, 116:591, 1968.

Kulin, H. E., Rifkind, A. B., Ross, G. T., and Odell, W. D.: Total Gonadotropin Activity in the Urine of Prepubertal Children. *J. Clin. Endocr.*, 27:1123, 1967.

List, C. F., Dowman, C. E., Bagchi, B. K., and Bebin, J.: Posterior Hypothalamic Hamartomas and Gangliogliomas Causing Precocious Puberty. *Neurology*, 8:164, 1958.

Pabst, H. F., Pueschal, S., and Hillman, D. A.: Etiologic Interrelationship in Down's Syndrome, Hypothyroidism, and Precocious Sexual Development. *Pediatrics*, 40:590, 1967.

Rifkind, A. B., Kulin, H. E., and Ross, G. T.: Follicle-Stimulating Hormone (FSH) and Luteinizing Hormone (LH) in the Urine of Prepubertal Children. *J. Clin. Invest.*, 46:1925, 1967.

Root, A. W., Bongiovanni, A. M., and Eberlein, W. R.: A Testicular-Interstitial-Cell-Stimulating Gonadotropin in a Child with Hepatoblastoma and Sexual Precocity. *J. Clin. Endocr.*, 28:1317, 1968.

Schoen, E. J.: Treatment of Idiopathic Precocious Puberty in Boys. *J. Clin. Endocr.*, 26:363, 1966.

Sigurjonsdottir, T. J., and Hayles, A. B.: Precocious Puberty. A Report of 96 Cases. *Am. J. Dis. Child.*, 115:309, 1968.

Silverman, S. H., Migeon, C., Rosemberg, E., and Wilkins, L.: Precocious Growth of Sexual Hair Without Other Secondary Sexual Development: "Premature Pubarche," a Constitutional Variation of Adolescence. *Pediatrics*, 10:426, 1952.

Stool, S., and Cohen, P.: Silver's Syndrome. Syndrome of Congenital Asymmetry, Short Stature, and Altered Patterns of Sexual Development. *Am. J. Dis. Child.*, 105:199, 1963.

Thamdrup, E.: *Precocious Sexual Development. A Clinical Study of 100 Children.* Springfield, Ill., Charles C Thomas, 1961.

Visser, H. K. A., and Degenhart, H. J.: Excretion of Six Individual 17-Ketosteroids and Testosterone in Four Girls with Precocious Sexual Hair (Premature Adrenarche). *Helv. paediat. Acta*, 21:409, 1966.

Wolman, L., and Balmforth, G. V.: Precocious Puberty Due to a Hypothalamic Hamartoma in a Patient Surviving to Late Middle Age. *J. Neurol., Neurosurg. & Psychiat.*, 26:275, 1963.

DISORDERS OF THE THYROID GLAND

GENERAL CONSIDERATIONS

The main function of the thyroid gland is to synthesize thyroxine (T_4) and triiodothyronine (T_3). Triiodothyronine differs from thyroxine in having 3 rather than 4 atoms of iodine. It is physiologically 4 to 5 times as active as thyroxine and has a much shorter latent period. Iodine is essential for the production of these hormones; the daily requirement has been estimated to be about 40 to 100 micrograms. Regardless of the chemical form upon ingestion, iodine eventually reaches the thyroid gland as iodide. Thyroid tissue has a special avidity for this element and is able to trap, transport and concentrate it for synthesis of thyroid hormone.

Before trapped iodide can react with tyrosine it must be oxidized; this reaction is catalyzed by thyroidal peroxidase. The thyroid cells also elaborate a specific thyroprotein, a globulin with approximately 120 tyrosine units. After iodination of tyrosine to form monoiodotyrosine and diiodotyrosine, 2 molecules of diiodotyrosine couple to form 1 molecule of thyroxine, or 1 molecule of diiodotyrosine and 1 of monoiodotyrosine combine to form triiodothyronine. It is uncertain whether a coupling enzyme exists. Once formed, hormones are stored as thyroglobulin in the lumen of the follicle (colloid) until ready to be delivered to the body cells. Thyroglobulin has a molecular weight of about 660,000 and under normal conditions does not enter the circulation except perhaps in very small amounts. T_4 and T_3 are liberated from thyroglobulin by activation of proteases and peptidases.

The thyroid gland is regulated by hypothalamic-pituitary mechanisms as well as by intrinsic mechanisms. Certain basophilic cells of the anterior pituitary produce the thyroid-stimulating hormone (TSH), a glycoprotein with a molecular weight of about 25,000. This hormone activates proteolytic enzymes in the thyroid gland to effect release of thyroid hormones. An excess of TSH results in hypertrophy and hyperplasia of the thyroid cells, increased trapping of iodine and increased synthesis of thyroid hormones. TSH secretion is increased in states of decreased production of thyroid hormone, and is inhibited by the thyroid hormones released. Exogenous thyroid hormone also inhibits TSH production, leading to decreased synthesis of endogenous thyroid hormone. Pituitary TSH is under control of a hypothalamic neurohumor known as thyrotropin-releasing hormone (TRH). This hormone is active in doses less than a nanogram, but its chemical nature is uncertain. Thyroid hormones inhibit this factor as well as TSH.

Approximately 90 per cent of circulating thyroid hormone is T_4 and is firmly bound to thyroxine-binding globulin (TBG) and thyroxine-binding prealbumin (TBPA). Measurement of this protein-bound iodine (PBI) usually furnishes an accurate index of the circulating thyroid hormone.

The serum level of PBI for euthyroid children or adults is 4 to 8 micrograms per 100 ml. At birth the PBI of the infant approximates that of the mother, with a mean value of 8.3 micrograms per 100 ml. This value increases during the first week of life to reach a mean value of 12 micrograms per 100 ml. The TSH level in cord plasma usually exceeds that in maternal plasma and increases during the first few hours of life; it probably accounts for the changes in PBI in the first week. The PBI gradually decreases, reaching a mean value as low as that of older children by about 1 year of age. In hypothyroidism the PBI is usually below 3 micrograms per 100 ml.; in hyperthyroidism it is above 9 micrograms.

There are many medications, diagnostic agents, and disorders other than hypothyroidism and hyperthyroidism which result in abnormal PBI levels. Ingestion of inorganic iodide in Lugol's solution or in cough medication, or application of tincture of iodine to the skin may elevate levels of PBI for as long as a month. The amount of iodide in iodized salt or in radioactive iodine used for uptake studies does not interfere with the level of PBI. Contrast media used for urography, cholecystography, bronchography and myelography result in elevated levels of PBI which last from a few weeks to a year, depending on the agent used. Iophenoxic acid (Teridax), an agent formerly used for cholecystography, has been estimated to elevate the PBI for more than 30 years. This agent can cross the placenta, and even many years after ingestion by the mother will produce in her offspring elevated PBI levels which persist for many years.

The physiologic elevation of thyroxine-binding globulin (TBG) in pregnancy or in newborn infants results in elevated PBI levels. Estrogens, including oral contraceptive agents, increase PBI levels by increasing TBG.

An increase of TBG also occurs as a hereditary defect. An otherwise unexplained elevation of the serum PBI level should lead to measurement of the level of TBG. The PBI levels range between 9 and 16 micrograms per 100 ml., and thyroxine-binding globulin is proportionally increased. Patients are clinically euthyroid, and other tests of thyroid function are usually within normal range. The defect appears to be X-linked, genetically.

Abnormally low levels of PBI in euthyroid persons are caused by several mechanisms. Patients with nephrosis and severe hypoproteinemia have low PBI levels as a result of loss of TBG in the urine. Inherited diminution or absence of TBG occurs as an X-linked trait; affected males have PBI levels below 3 micrograms per 100 ml., but are clinically euthyroid. Certain medications, such as diphenylhydantoin sodium (Dilantin), depress the serum level of PBI by displacing thyroxine from thyroxine-binding globulin, without causing hypothyroidism. Testosterone and other androgens decrease PBI by decreasing TBG levels, whereas salicylates decrease PBI levels by inhibiting the binding of T_4 to TBPA.

The butanol-extractable iodine (BEI) measures almost exclusively thyroxine. This test has been largely replaced by the thyroxine-by-column method, which is a more reliable index of thyroid hormone concentration in the presence of excess iodides, with some contrast media, and with biologically inactive thyroproteins (p. 1192).

The iodine-trapping or concentrating mechanism of the thyroid can be evaluated by radioactive iodine. ^{131}I, with a half-life of 8 days, or ^{132}I, with a half-life of 3.2 hours, is given to the patient orally (usually by gavage to infants). The radioiodine is concentrated in the thyroid gland, where the gamma rays emitted can be measured (usually 24 hours later) by placing a "counter" over the patient's thyroid. Normal values vary, depending upon the equipment and technique used. An uptake of less than 10 per cent usually indicates hypothyroidism. Falsely low values may be due to vomiting of the radio-iodine, ingestion of large amounts of iodine as either food or medicine, or administration of exogenous thyroid. Patients with hypothyroidism due to a defect in thyroid hormone synthesis have normal or elevated uptakes of radio-iodine (p. 1192).

The thyroid hormones increase the metabolic processes of the body by increasing basal consumption of oxygen, but the mechanism of this calorigenic effect is uncertain. There are other widespread biochemical effects, such as stimulation of protein synthesis and effects on carbohydrate, lipid and vitamin metabolism. The thyroid hormones are needed for the conversion of carotene to vitamin A; patients with hypothyroidism often have low serum vitamin A and high carotene levels (carotenemia).

Congenital athyreosis results in stunting of mental, physical and sexual development. Thyroid hormones are not capable of stimulating growth in the absence of growth hormone. Recent studies have shown that in children with hypothyroidism diminished growth hormone secretion accounts in part for the growth retardation; treatment with thyroid hormone restores normal secretion of the growth hormone.

The synthesis of hormone by the thyroid is disturbed by certain "antithyroid drugs." The thiocyanate ion prevents concentration of iodide in the gland and causes a discharge of stored iodide. Propylthiouracil and related compounds do not interfere with collection of iodide by the gland, but in some way prevent its fixation in organic combination. The interference with formation of thyroid hormone results in increased production of thyrotropic hormone and in enlargement of the thyroid. Thus these compounds are termed goitrogens.

HYPOTHYROIDISM

Hypothyroidism results from deficient production of thyroid hormones. The disorder may be manifest very early in life as a congenital defect, or it may be acquired after a period of apparently normal thyroid function.

CONGENITAL HYPOTHYROIDISM
(SPORADIC CRETINISM)

Many infants with congenital hypothyroidism have rudiments of thyroid gland which are hypoactive and may be found in ectopic locations between the base of the tongue and the normal position in the neck; some have no thyroid tissue. Little is known of the factors which interfere with embryologic development of the thyroid. The disorder rarely appears in more than 1 member of a family. In the rare instances in which two or more siblings have congenital hypothyroidism, the possibility of genetic origin should be suspected. The occurrence of congenital hypothyroidism in only one of monozygotic twins, on the other hand, points to a deleterious factor operating during intrauterine life. It has been demonstrated that thyroid antibodies are present more frequently in mothers of athyreotic cretins than in mothers of normal infants, but the role of autoimmunity in the pathogenesis of congenital thyroid defects is unsettled. The administration of therapeutic doses of radio-iodine to women during

TABLE 17-2. CLASSIFICATION OF HYPOTHYROIDISM

I. **Congenital (cretinism)**
  A. Aplasia, hypoplasia or maldescent of thyroid
    1. Maternal radio-iodine
    2. Autoimmune disease (?)
    3. Embryonic defect of development
  B. Defective synthesis of thyroid hormone (nonendemic goitrous cretinism)
    1. Iodide-trapping defect
    2. Iodide-organification defect
    3. Coupling defect
    4. Deiodinase defect
    5. Abnormal secretion of iodoproteins
  C. Maternal ingestion of medications during pregnancy
    1. Goitrogens (propylthiouracil, methimazole)
    2. Iodides
  D. Iodide deficiency (endemic cretinism)

II. **Juvenile hypothyroidism (acquired)**
  A. Thyrotropin deficiency
    1. Isolated
    2. Associated with other tropic hormone deficiencies
  B. Hypoplasia or maldescent of thyroid
    1. Autoimmune disease (?)
    2. Embryonic defect of development
  C. Partial defect of thyroid hormone synthesis
  D. Autoimmune disease
    1. Goitrous (Hashimoto's thyroiditis)
    2. Nongoitrous
  E. Thyroidectomy — partial or complete
    1. Thyrotoxicosis
    2. Cancer
    3. Lingual or other ectopic thyroid
  F. Medications
    1. Iodides
    2. Cobalt
    3. Propylthiouracil and methimazole
    4. Para-aminosalicylic acid
  G. Iodine deficiency

pregnancy for treatment of cancer of the thyroid or of hyperthyroidism is an infrequent cause of fetal thyroid damage. Before radio-iodine is administered to women, it should always be ascertained that they are not pregnant. The administration of radioactive iodine to lactating women is also contraindicated, since it is readily excreted in human milk.

Congenital hypothyroidism with a goiter may be due to a defect in the synthesis of thyroid hormone (goitrous cretinism), or it may be caused by the ingestion of medications during pregnancy (congenital goiter). Except for enlargement of the thyroid gland, the clinical manifestations are the same as in patients with athyreosis.

Clinical Manifestations. Congenital hypothyroidism is about 3 times as common in girls as in boys. It is recognized only rarely at birth, since the signs and symptoms are usually not sufficiently developed. It can be suspected and the diagnosis established during the early weeks of life if the initial but less characteristic manifestations are recognized. Cretins may be significantly heavier at birth than normal newborn infants, but, owing to the great variation in birth weights, there is little diagnostic value to this observation. Unusual prolongation of physiologic icterus, owing to delayed maturation of glucuronide conjugation, may be the earliest sign. Feeding difficulties, especially sluggishness, lack of interest, somnolence, and choking spells during nursing are often present during the first month of life. Respiratory difficulties, owing in part to the large tongue, include apneic episodes, noisy respirations and nasal obstruction. These infants cry little, sleep much, have poor appetites and are generally sluggish. There is obstinate constipation which usually does not respond to laxatives. The abdomen is large, and an umbilical hernia is usually present. The temperature is subnormal, and the skin, particularly of the extremities, may be cold and mottled. The pulse is slow; heart murmurs and cardiomegaly are common. Anemia is often present and is refractory to treatment with hematinics.

These manifestations progress; retardation of physical and mental development becomes greater during the following months, and by 3 to 6 months of age the clinical picture is fully developed. When there is only a partial deficiency of thyroid hormone, the symptoms may be milder, the syndrome incomplete and the onset delayed.

The child is stunted in growth, the extremities being short, and the head seems large. The anterior fontanel is widely open, the eyes appear far apart, and the bridge of the broad nose is depressed. The palpebral fissures are narrow and the eyelids swollen. The mouth is kept open, and the thick and broad tongue protrudes from it.

Dentition is delayed, and the erupted teeth have a tendency to decay rapidly. The neck is short and thick, and there may be deposits of fat above the clavicles and between the neck and shoulders. The hands are broad and the fingers short. The skin is dry and scaly, and there is little perspiration. Myxedema manifests itself particularly in the skin of the eyelids, of the back of the hands and of the external genitalia. Carotenemia may cause a yellow discoloration of the skin, but the scleras remain white. The scalp is thickened, and the hair is coarse, brittle and scanty. The hairline reaches far down on the forehead, which usually appears wrinkled.

The muscles are usually hypotonic. In rare instances generalized muscular hypertonia has been observed (*Debré-Sémélaigne syndrome*); its pathogenesis is unknown, but a genetic origin of the syndrome is suspected. Such children may have an athletic appearance due to pseudohypertrophy of the muscles.

The mental development of cretins is usually retarded. They appear lethargic and are late in sitting and standing. The voice is hoarse, and they do not learn to talk. The degree of physical and mental retardation increases as they become older. Sexual maturation is delayed or does not take place at all. Precocious sexual maturation is an occasional complication (p. 1184).

Laboratory Data. Retardation of osseous development can be shown roentgenographically at birth in a high percentage of cretins and indicates some deprivation of thyroid hormone during intrauterine life. In untreated patients there is an increasing discrepancy between chronologic

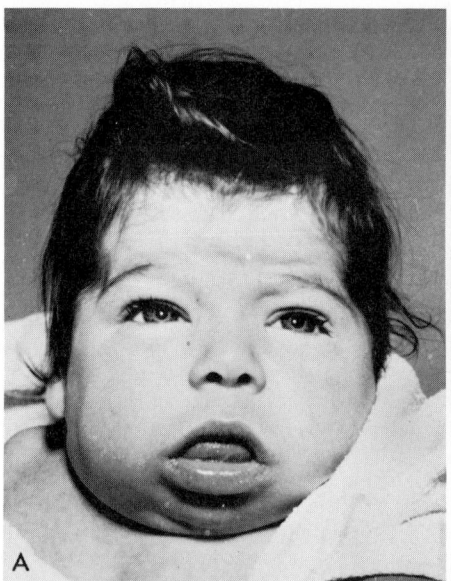 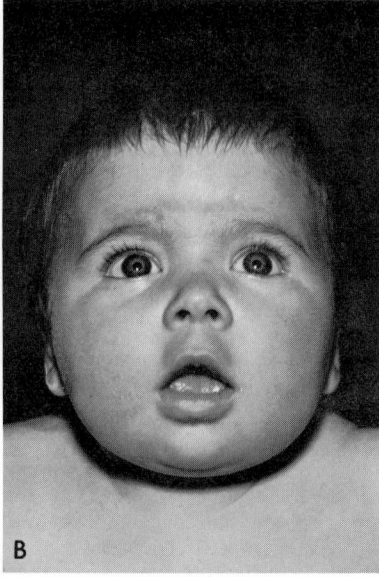

Figure 17-9. Congenital hypothyroidism in an infant 6 months of age. The infant fed poorly in the neonatal period and was constipated. She had a persistent nasal discharge and a large tongue, was very lethargic, and had no social smile and no head control. *A,* Note puffy face, dull expression, hirsute forehead. Serum cholesterol, 172 mg. per 100 ml.; alkaline phosphatase, 4.8 Bodansky units; negligible uptake of radio-iodine. Osseous development was that of newborn. *B,* Four months after treatment with U.S.P. thyroid. Note decreased puffiness of face, decreased hirsutism of forehead and alert appearance.

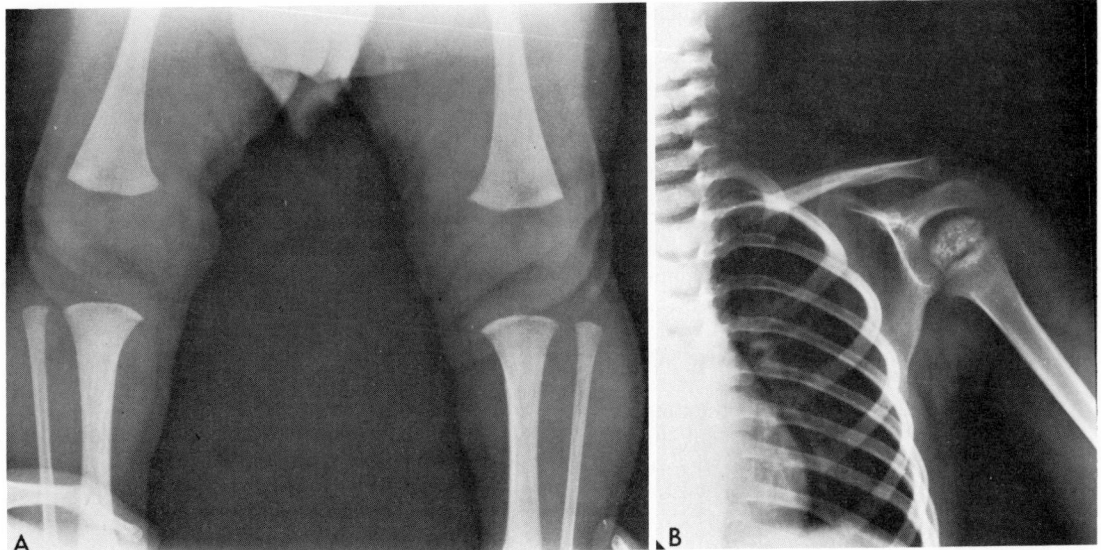

Figure 17-10. Congenital hypothyroidism. *A*, Absence of distal femoral epiphysis in a 3-month-old cretin who was born at term. This is evidence for the onset of the hypothyroid state during fetal life. *B*, Epiphyseal dysgenesis in the head of the humerus in a 9-year-old girl who had been inadequately treated with thyroid.

age and roentgenographically demonstrable osseous development. The epiphyses often have multiple foci of ossification (epiphyseal dysgenesis); deformity ("beaking") of the twelfth thoracic or first or second lumbar vertebra is common.

The protein-bound iodine (PBI) or thyroxine level of the serum is the most reliable measurement of thyroid function and is usually under 2 micrograms per 100 ml. In mild instances of hypothyroidism the PBI level may be in the range of 2 to 3.5 micrograms per 100 ml. Uptake of radioactive iodine by the thyroid gland is decreased. Plasma levels of TSH are characteristically elevated.

In older children with hypothyroidism, the serum level of cholesterol is usually increased; the extent varies markedly. Values up to 500 mg. per 100 ml. are not unusual. In infants with hypothyroidism the serum level of cholesterol is rarely sufficiently elevated to be of any diagnostic help. Elevated cholesterol levels rapidly return to normal after institution of treatment and increase again 6 to 8 weeks after treatment has been discontinued.

The serum level of phosphatase is decreased, and the carotene level is often increased. Responses of serum levels of growth hormone to arginine and to hypoglycemia are usually impaired and return to normal after treatment with thyroid. The electrocardiogram of infants with hypothyroidism may show low voltage P and T waves with diminished amplitude of QRS complexes. The electroencephalogram frequently shows low voltage.

Differential Diagnosis. Since the symptoms appear gradually, the early diagnosis of hypothyroidism may be difficult, but one should think of it in any instance of retarded physical or mental

development. Roentgenographic evidence of retardation of ossification is a helpful diagnostic aid only when the discrepancy with the chronologic age is great. A low PBI or serum thyroxine level is the most useful single diagnostic test.

Down's syndrome, gargoylism and chondrodystrophy may be mistaken for cretinism, but can be readily differentiated by clinical manifestations and by appropriate laboratory studies. Pituitary dwarfism is frequently accompanied by some degree of hypothyroidism and presents a greater diagnostic problem (p. 1174).

Prognosis. Without treatment, cretins may die of respiratory obstruction or intercurrent infections. Those who live become mentally deficient dwarfs. Treatment with thyroid hormone results in normal linear growth, osseous maturation and sexual development. Mental development, however, is much less predictable. Thyroid hormone is critical for normal cerebral development both in the late months of fetal life and in early months of postnatal life. Hence the diagnosis must be made early in life and effective treatment initiated promptly in order to minimize irreversible brain damage. Only about half of infants with hypothyroidism who are treated adequately before 6 months of age will achieve an intelligence quotient of 90 or more. In general, the more profound the deprivation of the thyroid hormone in the early months of life, the poorer is the prognosis for mental development. In fact, there is evidence that impairment of cerebral development often begins in utero in completely athyreotic infants. There is no conclusive evidence that treatment of the pregnant woman with huge doses of thyroid hormone to enhance transplacental transfer of protective levels of hormone to the hypothyroid fetus is effective. When clinical evidence of hypothyroidism is delayed in onset, the outlook for normal mental development is much better; children who acquire hypothyroidism after 2 years of age and are treated appropriately have a good prognosis for mental development.

Treatment. Desiccated thyroid in tablet form is given orally as substitution therapy. It must be given continuously, and the dose may need to be altered from time to time. Increased doses may be required for the periods of rapid growth, puberty and reproduction. It requires some time to saturate the tissues of the body with the hormone, which then has a cumulative effect. Thus an immediate effect of therapy cannot be expected, and the dose should not be judged by the results after a few days of administration. The total daily requirement is given as a single dose. As soon as the diagnosis of cretinism is made an initial dose of 30 mg. of desiccated thyroid (U.S.P.) should be given daily. Further increases should be made at intervals of 2 weeks, but the increment should not exceed 15 to 30 mg. In the first year of life adequate daily doses are in the range of 60 to 90 mg., and in older children doses of 120 to 200 mg. will usually prove satisfactory. The dose must be adjusted to the demands of the individual child. Determination of the protein-bound iodine or thyroxine level is the best laboratory procedure to evaluate the adequacy of therapy. One should attempt to maintain levels between 6 and 8 micrograms per 100 ml.

Sodium L-thyroxine given orally is also effective and has the advantage over desiccated thyroid of being a stable preparation with a long shelf life and constant biologic activity. Each 0.1 mg. is equivalent to approximately 60 mg. of desiccated thyroid. When thyroxine is used, the levels of PBI must be maintained between 9 and 12 micrograms per 100 ml. to provide a euthyroid state.

Triiodothyronine also affords adequate replacement therapy, but seems to have no advantages for maintenance therapy. Because of its rapidity of action, it may be useful in the initial period of treatment in an attempt to achieve a euthyroid state quickly. Protein-bound iodine levels are of no value in determining adequacy of therapy when this compound is used.

SPORADIC GOITROUS CRETINISM

An enlarged thyroid gland (goiter) associated with hypothyroidism may result from a defect in synthesis of thyroid hormone. The gland becomes goitrous as a result of stimulation by excessive thyrotropin secretion in response to the low level of circulating thyroid hormone. At least 5 separate defects in the synthesis of thyroid hormone have been delineated. The available evidence indicates that each defect is genetically determined and is transmitted in an autosomal recessive manner.

The defects are the following:

1. *Iodide-trapping defect.* There is failure of accumulation of iodide by the thyroid gland; hence the uptake of radio-iodine by the thyroid is low. In the other 4 defects the ^{131}I uptake is usually elevated.

2. *Iodide organification defect.* Iodine is avidly accumulated by the thyroid gland as demonstrated radioactively, but administration of thiocyanate or perchlorate rapidly eliminates it. The iodide is discharged because it is not bound to tyrosine residues. It has been suggested that there is lack of an iodine peroxidase which normally oxidizes iodide. A partial form of this defect seen in patients with nerve deafness is known as Pendred's syndrome (p. 1196).

3. *Coupling defect.* There is failure of coupling of monoiodotyrosine and diiodotyrosine in the thyroid gland, resulting in inadequate synthesis of thyroxine and triiodothyronine. Deficiency of a coupling enzyme has been proposed.

4. *Deiodinase defect.* Free monoiodotyrosine and diiodotyrosine in the thyroid gland are deiodinated by a deiodinase. This enzyme is also found in liver, kidney and other tissues. The iodine liberated is reutilized in synthesis of hormone. Patients with deiodinase deficiency have large amounts of monoiodotyrosine and diiodotyrosine in the blood and urine; neither of them is normally found outside of the thyroid gland.

5. *Abnormal serum iodoprotein.* Patients with this disorder release iodinated proteins or polypeptides which are calorigenically inactive. The iodide is included in determinations of PBI, but it is not included in measurements of thyroxine. Goiter results because these hormonally inactive compounds comprise the major output of the thyroid.

The **clinical manifestations** of goitrous cretinism are those of hypothyroidism; they vary in severity and time of onset, depending upon the completeness and type of defect. The goiter may be present at birth or may not make its appearance until later in childhood. Except in patients with the iodide-trapping defect, the thyroid gland accumulates iodide normally, often avidly. The serum protein-bound iodine level may be low, normal or elevated, depending upon which defect is present.

The **diagnosis** of type 1 defect is suspected when hypothyroidism and goiter are associated with a low radio-iodine uptake. The second type of defect is identified by demonstration of rapid discharge of radio-iodine from the thyroid gland within a few hours after the oral administration of thiocyanate. The fourth type of defect requires chromatographic techniques for demonstration of iodotyrosines in blood or urine. The fifth type may be suspected when there is a significant disparity between the serum levels of PBI and thyroxine.

Treatment for goitrous cretinism is the same as for athyreotic cretinism. It is of interest that defects 1 and 4 have been successfully treated by large doses of iodides, but, as for all patients with hypothyroidism, treatment with thyroid hormone is preferable.

JUVENILE HYPOTHYROIDISM
(ACQUIRED HYPOTHYROIDISM)

The development of hypothyroidism in a child who previously was euthyroid may be due to a wide variety of factors. A congenitally hypoplastic thyroid gland may furnish amounts of hormone sufficient for the first few years, but the deficiency may become manifest when demands on the gland are increased by rapid growth of the body. Such hypoplastic glands are frequently ectopic. Although the defect is congenital, clinical manifestations may present as in patients with acquired lesions of the thyroid.

Complete or subtotal thyroidectomy for thyrotoxicosis or cancer may result in hypothyroidism, as may removal of an anomalous thyroid, when it constitutes the sole source of thyroid hormone. For example, when the thyroid is ectopically placed at the base of the tongue (lingual thyroid), it is often the only thyroid tissue. Likewise the entire thyroid gland may consist of a midline nodule mistaken for a thyroglossal duct cyst and excised. Such nodules may be split and each half with its vascular pedicle be transplanted beneath the sternocleidomastoid muscle on each side of the neck.

Deficiency of pituitary thyrotropin, either as an isolated defect or in association with deficiency of other pituitary hormones, may also result in hypothyroidism. Hypothyroidism in association with a goiter may be caused occasionally by chronic infectious processes or by the protracted ingestion of medications such as iodides or cobalt. Acquired hypothyroidism, however, most often results from Hashimoto's thyroiditis, which may or may not be associated with a goiter (p. 1196).

The clinical manifestations depend upon the age of the child at onset and upon the extent of dysfunction. The later in life hypothyroidism is acquired, the less will be the impairment of growth and development. Nevertheless myxedematous changes of the skin, constipation, sleepiness and a mental decline may be manifest at any age. Cessation or retardation of growth in a child whose growth has previously been normal should always alert one to the possibility of hypothyroidism (Fig. 17-11). Obese children are frequently, but usually erroneously, considered to have hypothyroidism. Most obese children have warm moist skin, a ruddy complexion and normal thyroid function.

Deficiency of pituitary thyrotropin may be suspected when there are signs of deficiency of other anterior pituitary hormones, such as gonadotropins, corticotropin and growth hormone. It is possible to differentiate primary and secondary hypothyroidism by studying the response of the thyroid to parenterally administered thyrotropin. After an initial study to determine the radioiodine uptake or serum PBI level, TSH is administered intramuscularly for several days, and the study is repeated; the results are then compared

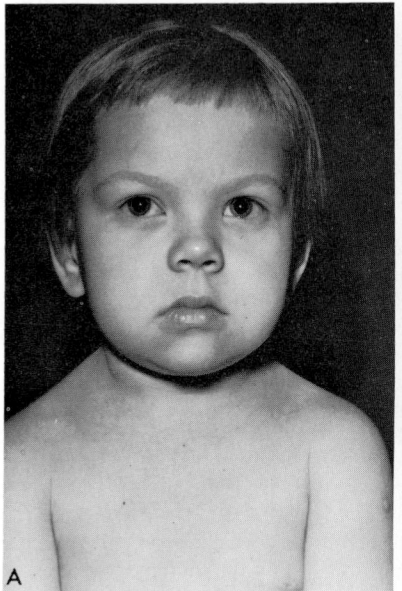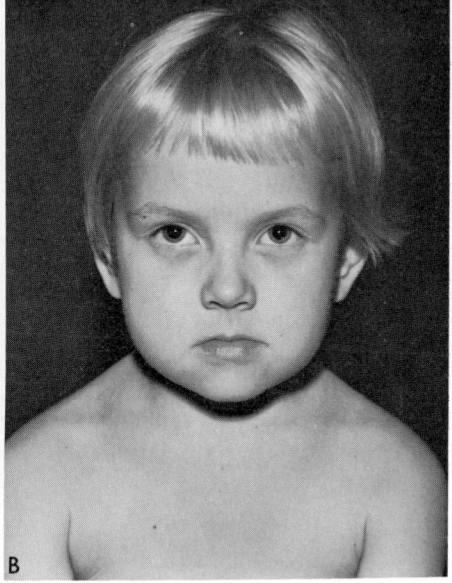

Figure 17-11. Acquired hypothyroidism in a girl 6 years of age. She was treated with a wide variety of hematinics for refractory anemia for 3 years. She had almost complete cessation of growth, constipation, and sluggishness of 3 years' duration. Height age was 3 years; bone age, 4 years. She had a sallow complexion, and immature facies with a poorly developed nasal bridge. *A,* Serum cholesterol, 501 mg. per 100 ml.; alkaline phosphatase, 1.8 Bodansky units; radio-iodine uptake, 7 per cent at 24 hours; PBI, 2.8 micrograms per 100 ml. *B,* After therapy for 18 months. Note nasal development, increased luster and decreased pigmentation of hair and maturation of face. Height age was 5½ years; bone age, 7 years. There was decided improvement in her general condition. Menarche occurred at 14 years; ultimate height was 61 inches. She graduated from high school. She was well controlled with 0.2 mg. of sodium-L-thyroxine daily.

with the original data. In primary thyroid failure there is little or no change, whereas in hypothyroidism associated with deficiency of thyrotropin there is a significant increase in thyroid uptake of radio-iodine and of the PBI level. Although the optimal dose of TSH for this diagnostic test has not been definitely determined, it appears that 5 to 10 units given intramuscularly once daily for 3 days is effective.

Treatment consists in administration of thyroxine or desiccated thyroid. The dose must be adjusted to the demands of the individual child (see p. 1192). The prognosis with adequate replacement therapy is good.

GOITER

A goiter is an enlargement of the thyroid gland. Persons with enlarged thyroids may have normal function of the gland (*euthyroidism*), thyroid deficiency (*hypothyroidism*) or overproduction of the hormone (*hyperthyroidism*). Goiter may be congenital or acquired, endemic or sporadic.

The goiter most often results from increased secretion of pituitary thyrotropic hormone in response to decreased circulating levels of thyroid hormone. Thyroid enlargement may also result from infiltrative processes which may be inflammatory or neoplastic. Goiter in patients with thyrotoxicosis is caused by the long-acting thyroid stimulator (LATS).

CONGENITAL GOITER

Congenital goiters due to iodine deficiency are common in endemic goitrous areas. Sporadic congenital goiter is frequently the result of the administration of antithyroid drugs or of iodides during pregnancy for the treatment of thyrotoxicosis, or of iodides for asthma. Goitrogenic drugs and iodides cross the placenta and interfere with synthesis of thyroid hormone in the fetus. Some congenital goiters are the result of a defect in synthesis of thyroid hormone (p. 1192); in a few no causative factor is identifiable.

The enlargement of the thyroid at birth may be sufficient to cause respiratory distress which interferes with nursing and may even cause death. The head may be maintained in extreme hyperextension. When respiratory obstruction is severe, partial thyroidectomy rather than tracheotomy is indicated. Administration of thyroid hormone generally hastens the disappearance of the goiter. Most of the infants are euthyroid, but a few have evidence of hypothyroidism, which is rarely permanent.

ENDEMIC GOITER

Iodine is deficient in the water and natively grown foods in certain areas, such as the north-western states and the states surrounding the Great Lakes in the United States. The dietary iodine deficiency is even greater in certain mountainous districts in Switzerland, Austria and France, in the Carpathian, Himalayan and Andean mountains, and in many other regions. In such areas, except as iodine is provided in foods from other areas, in iodized salt or in a prophylactic medication, goiter is endemic. Seawater is rich in iodine, and the iodine content of fish and shellfish is also high. Endemic goiter is therefore rare in populations living along the sea. In persons who have only a mild deficiency of iodine the enlargement of the thyroid does not become noticeable except when there is an increased demand for the hormone. This is true during periods of rapid growth as in adolescence and during pregnancy. In regions of moderate iodine deficiency, goiter may be observed in school children. It may disappear when maturity is reached and reappear in pregnancy and during the period of lactation. Many more girls than boys have goiters.

Pathogenesis. The thyroid produces and stores thyroid hormones. If there is a deficiency of iodine, the demand can be satisfied by increased efficiency in synthesis of thyroid hormone. Iodine liberated in the tissues is returned quickly to the gland, which resynthesizes the hormone at a higher rate than normal. This increased activity is achieved by compensatory hypertrophy and hyperplasia. The cells become enlarged and change from a flat-cuboidal to a columnar shape. As soon as the hormone is formed it must be transported to the tissues, and storage of colloid does not occur. The radio-iodine uptake is frequently elevated and may be 70 per cent or more of the administered dose. Usually during childhood the thyroid continues to function even when there is a scarcity of iodine; thus the demand of the tissues for thyroid hormone is satisfied.

Decompensation and hypothyroidism as a result of iodine deficiency in children result in *endemic cretinism*, which is nonexistent in the United States. In other parts of the world where endemic goiter occurs in mountainous regions, endemic cretinism may also be found. Although a correlation exists between the iodine deficiency in the soil, food and water of these regions and endemic goiter and cretinism, there are other causes as yet unknown. Iodine deficiency is believed to lead to goiter in the mother and, if the deficiency persists during pregnancy, to cretinism in some of her children. Endemic goiter and cretinism may occur without iodine deficiency. A hyperendemic area of goiter has been found in the highlands of New Guinea. Nearly half of the population have goiters, most have damage of the nervous system, and many are deaf. The cause of congenital goitrous cretinism in this locality has yet to be determined.

The endemic cretin is usually born with an enlarged thyroid gland. Such a congenital goiter is poor in colloid; the cells appear large and crowded, and the blood vessels distended and filled with blood. Compression of the trachea may interfere

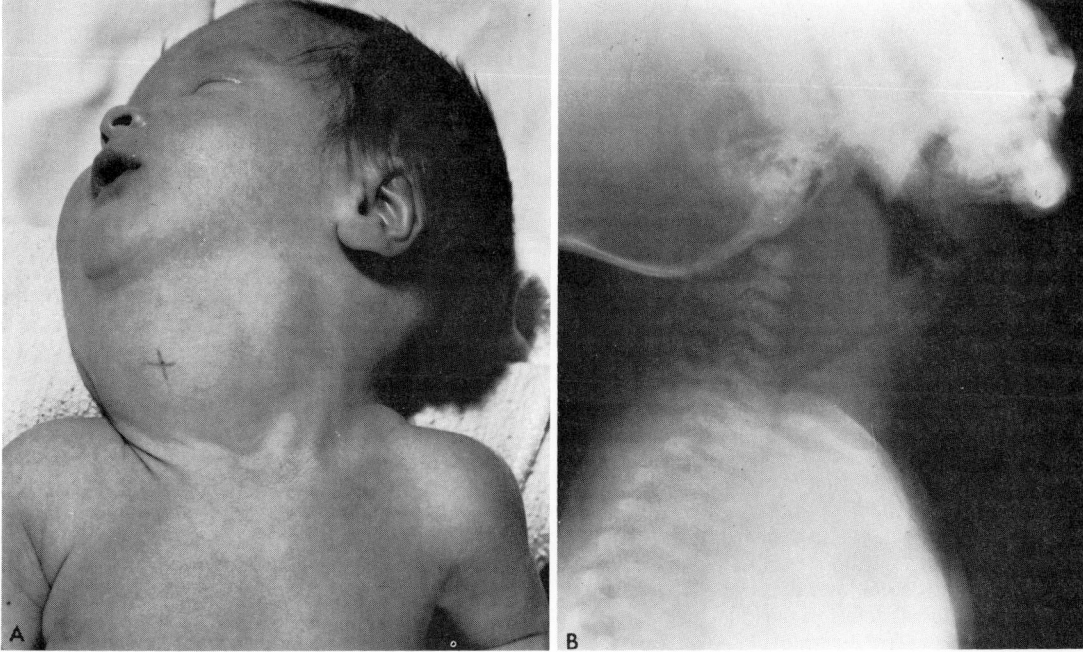

Figure 17-12. Congenital goiter in infancy. *A*, Large congenital goiter in an infant born to a mother with thyrotoxicosis who had been treated with iodides and methimazole during pregnancy. *B*, A 6-week-old infant with increasing respiratory distress and cervical mass since birth. Operation revealed a large goiter which almost completely encircled the trachea. Note anterior deviation and posterior compression of the trachea. Partial thyroidectomy completely relieved the symptoms. No cause for goiter was found. It is apparent why a tracheotomy is not adequate treatment for these infants.

with respiration in early infancy and be a lethal factor. In children who survive, degenerative processes in the thyroid result in atrophy of the glandular tissue and in hypothyroidism. At such times, goiter may be absent.

Clinical Manifestations. The thyroid gland is palpable and visible; its surface is smooth and its consistency soft. The enlargement is usually moderate, and pressure symptoms are rare. Bruits may be heard on auscultation of the gland. Signs of endocrine disturbance usually do not develop, but when present are the same as for hypothyroidism of any origin, with the exception that deafness is an additional frequent finding.

Treatment. Endemic goiter and congenital goiter, as well as endemic cretinism, are disappearing in goitrous areas where iodized salt is used by most of the population. Iodized salt in the United States contains 0.01 per cent of potassium iodide, and provides excellent prophylaxis. For the child with endemic cretinism substitution therapy is required. If desiccated thyroid is administered soon after birth, some symptoms of hypothyroidism can be avoided, but mental retardation cannot be prevented by treatment after birth.

SPORADIC GOITER

This type of goiter is seen most frequently in pubertal girls. It occurs sporadically in areas where the food and water are not deficient in iodine. Though the cause is not apparent in some instances, it is now clear that the majority of such goiters are a manifestation of Hashimoto's thyroiditis (see below).

Some instances of sporadic goiter may be the result of an intrinsic biochemical defect in the synthesis of thyroid hormone. When this derangement is slight, compensatory hypertrophy of the thyroid gland is sufficient to maintain the patient in a euthyroid state. Severe defects of thyroid synthesis result in goitrous cretinism (see p. 1192).

Sporadic goiter may also be iatrogenic. Prolonged administration of para-aminosalicylic acid or cobalt and externally applied resorcinol may apparently cause goiter. In allergic children treated for a long time with iodide preparations, goiter has occasionally developed. In such instances, hypothyroidism eventually develops if the goitrogen is not discontinued.

The enlargement of the thyroid is usually only moderate. Constitutional symptoms are infrequently present; occasionally there is evidence of hypothyroidism. Only rarely are there local pressure symptoms. Many patients have an elevated 24-hour radio-iodine accumulation. Other thyroid functions are usually within normal limits.

Small goiters require no treatment; the larger ones are treated primarily for cosmetic reasons. The treatment of choice is sodium-L-thyroxine, 0.2 to 0.3 mg. a day, which may be continued for a year or longer as needed. Desiccated thyroid, 120 to 180 mg. a day, may also be used.

If permanent remission does not occur within a year, it is unlikely that it will occur thereafter, and continued treatment may be necessary to suppress the goiter.

GOITER AND CONGENITAL DEAFNESS
(PENDRED'S SYNDROME)

A syndrome of deafness and goiter is transmitted in a simple recessive fashion. The relation of the thyroid and auditory defects is not known. This disorder is not to be confused with the deaf-mutism seen in goitrous persons in areas of endemic goiter, nor with the minor impairment of hearing which may be found in severely hypothyroid persons. Affected persons are euthyroid or only mildly hypothyroid. The thyroid enlargement may be barely detectable or may be pronounced; it makes its appearance during childhood, and the gland tends to become nodular in adult life. The deafness is congenital and is most severe for high tones. Affected persons are otherwise normal in mental and physical development.

Administration of thiocyanate or perchlorate causes a significant discharge of iodide from the thyroid gland, indicating a defect in organification of iodide. The discharge of iodide is similar to, but slower and less complete than, that seen in patients with type 2 defect of thyroid hormone synthesis (p. 1192). The enzymatic defect appears to be the same in both disorders except for quantitative differences.

Administration of thyroid preparations is effective in decreasing the goiter.

INTRATRACHEAL GOITER

One of the many ectopic locations of thyroid tissue is within the trachea. The intraluminal thyroid is beneath the tracheal mucosa and is frequently continuous with the normally situated extratracheal thyroid. The thyroid tissue has an unusual susceptibility to goitrous enlargement, which involves the normally situated as well as the ectopic thyroid. The reason for goiter formation is not known, but a defect in thyroid hormone synthesis has been suggested. When there is obstruction of the airway associated with a goiter, it must be ascertained whether the obstruction is extratracheal or endotracheal. If obstructive manifestations are mild, administration of thyroid hormone (120 to 180 mg. per day) will usually cause the goiter to decrease in size. When symptoms are severe, surgical removal of the endotracheal goiter is indicated.

THYROIDITIS

Lymphocytic Thyroiditis
(STRUMA LYMPHOMATOSA; HASHIMOTO'S THYROIDITIS)

This condition is characterized histologically by lymphocytic infiltration of the thyroid. Early in the course of the disease there may be only hyperplasia; this is followed by infiltration of lymphocytes and plasma cells between the follicles, and by atrophy of follicle. Germinal follicles are frequently present. Epithelial degeneration is variable, and fibrosis is absent or minimal. An autoimmune mechanism appears to be responsible for the disorder. Although circulating thyroid antibodies are usually demonstrable, these do not appear to be directly responsible for the disorder. The factors initiating the autoimmune mechanism are not known; viral infections have been suspected.

A high incidence of lymphocytic thyroiditis has been found in some families, in which about half of the siblings of affected patients have circulating antibodies. This type of thyroid disorder occurs frequently in patients with Turner's syndrome; circulating thyroid antibodies are also frequently found in infants with Down's syndrome and in their mothers. The pathogenetic mechanism for these associations is not known.

Clinical Manifestations. The disorder, formerly thought to be rare, is now known to be a common cause of goiter and accounts for many lesions incorrectly designated as sporadic goiter or adolescent goiter. It occurs most frequently in girls (90 per cent) between the sixth and fifteenth years of life. The goiter may appear insidiously; the thyroid is diffusely enlarged, firm and nontender. In about a third of the patients the gland is lobular and may seem to be nodular.

Most affected children are euthyroid and asymptomatic, but some have clinical and laboratory signs of hypothyroidism; a few have manifestations suggestive of hyperthyroidism. The clinical course is variable. The goiter may become smaller or disappear spontaneously, or it may persist unchanged for years and the patient remains euthyroid. A significant percentage of patients who are euthyroid initially gradually exhibit hypothyroidism over the course of months or years. It is now clear that many patients with nongoitrous juvenile hypothyroidism also have lymphocytic thyroiditis as the destructive thyroid lesion (p. 1193).

Laboratory Data. The PBI level may be normal, elevated or low. In most instances the serum levels of PBI exceed that of thyroxine by more than 2 micrograms per 100 ml.; the normal difference is only 0.5 to 1.0 microgram per 100 ml. This finding reflects the presence of calorigenically inactive iodinated thyroproteins in the serum of patients with lymphocytic thyroiditis. The level of PBI may suggest thyrotoxicosis in a patient with normal thyroxine level, or the PBI may be in the euthyroid range when the patient is actually hypothyroid and has a low serum thyroxine level. The difference between PBI and thyroxine levels is sufficiently diagnostic so that both studies should be performed in all goitrous children.

The radioactive iodine uptake may be normal, elevated or low; a subnormal response to TSH administration is common, indicating loss of the thyroid's reserve capacity. If only one method of assay (hemagglutination; complement fixing; cytotoxic) is utilized, circulating antibodies will be found in only about one half of patients, but if examination is made by more than one technique, they will be found in most patients. The definitive diagnosis can be established by needle or open biopsy of the thyroid.

Treatment. Corticosteroids effectively suppress the autoimmune process and produce a decrease in the antibody level; however, when therapy is discontinued, clinical and laboratory manifestations usually return. The preferred treatment is administration of desiccated thyroid in doses sufficient to suppress thyrotropin (120 to 180 mg. per day). The goiter slowly decreases in size, but antibody levels may remain unchanged. Treatment should be continued for several years. In some of the patients, hypothyroidism eventually develops, and therapy must continue indefinitely.

Other Causes of Thyroiditis. Other types of thyroiditis in children are rare. Specific agents such as those of cat-scratch disease, tuberculosis and mumps virus have been incriminated, but in most instances the cause is not known.

Acute suppurative thyroiditis is usually preceded by a respiratory tract infection or is secondary to trauma. When suppuration occurs, incision and drainage and administration of antibiotics are indicated.

HYPERTHYROIDISM

(Thyrotoxicosis; Toxic Goiter; Graves's Disease; Exophthalmic Goiter)

Etiology. Excessive secretion of thyroid hormone results in hyperthyroidism. In most instances the thyroid is diffusely enlarged, and often exophthalmos is present. The pituitary appears to play no part in the origin of hyperthyroidism, and secretion of TSH is suppressed. Although it is still not known what initiates Graves's disease, it is maintained by the long-acting thyroid stimulator (LATS), which is an IgG globulin. This antibody presumably represents the response to a thyroid antigen; it may be one of a spectrum of antibodies against thyroid produced by an autoimmune reaction. Graves's disease, Hashimoto's thyroiditis and idiopathic hypothyroidism are frequently seen at different times in the same patient or in different members of a sibship. An autoimmune mechanism with production of a variety of antibodies could explain these findings. There appears to be a genetic predisposition to the development of thyroid autoimmunity, but the basic stimulus or immunologic defect is not known. The pathogenesis of the ocular manifestations is unknown; LATS does not appear to be a causative factor. Other causes of hyperthyroidism in children such as autonomously functioning thyroid adenomas or hyperfunctioning thyroid carcinoma are extremely rare.

Approximately 1 per cent of all patients with hyperthyroidism are less than 15 years of age, and, of these, 80 per cent are between the ages of 10 and 15 years. The disease has been observed in infants as young as 1 year. The incidence is about 6 times higher in girls than in boys. Infectious diseases or psychic trauma may precipitate the disease. Hyperthyroidism occurs occasionally with polyostotic fibrous dysplasia and sexual precocity (p. 1182).

Pathologically, there are hypertrophy, hyperplasia and striking vascularity. The epithelial cells are high and columnar, and the colloid is reduced. There may be areas of adenomatous tissue which may contain colloid.

Clinical Manifestations. The earliest signs in children may be emotional disturbances accompanied by motor hyperactivity. They become irritable and excitable and cry easily. Their schoolwork suffers, and their restlessness, which may resemble that of chorea, causes conflicts. Tremor of the fingers can be noticed if the arm is extended. There may be a voracious appetite combined with loss of or no increase in weight. The thyroid is enlarged, visible and palpable, and bruits may be audible over it. Exophthalmos is noticeable in the majority of patients, but is rarely severe. *Graefe's sign* (lagging of the upper eyelid as the eye looks downward), *Moebius' sign* (inability of convergence) and *Stellwag's sign* (retraction of the upper eyelid and infrequent blinking) may be present. The skin is smooth and flushed, and there is excessive sweating. Muscular weakness progresses as the disease continues. Tachycardia, palpitation, dyspnea and cardiac enlargement and insufficiency cause discomfort and may endanger the patient's life. The systolic blood pressure and the pulse pressure are increased. Children with hyperthyroidism are usually tall; their osseous development is advanced for their age, but sexual maturation is delayed.

Thyroid "crisis" or "storm" is a form of hyperthyroidism manifested by an acute onset, hyperthermia, and severe tachycardia and restlessness. There may be rapid progression to delirium, coma and death. "Apathetic" or "masked" hyperthyroidism is another variety of hyperthyroidism characterized by extreme listlessness, apathy and cachexia. A combination of both forms may also occur. These symptom complexes are rare in children.

Laboratory Data. The basal metabolic rate is increased, glucose tolerance is decreased, and there may be glycosuria. Lymphocytosis is found in the blood; the cholesterol level tends to be low. The protein-bound iodine in the serum is high, most levels being in the range of 12 to 20 micrograms per 100 ml. Uptake of radioactive iodine is rapid, the majority of patients having an uptake of over 50 per cent.

Differential Diagnosis. Simple goiter may be as large as or larger than the goiter of hyperthyroidism, and a bruit may be heard on auscultation of the gland, but the absence of toxic symptoms and a normal serum level of PBI differentiate the two. The cardiac symptoms may simulate organic heart disease, but the presence of goiter and exophthalmos favors hyperthyroidism. The restlessness and agitation may suggest chorea. The clinical pattern of pheochromocytoma may resemble that of hyperthyroidism in many respects, but the elevation of blood pressure is greater, the level of serum PBI is within normal limits, and that of catecholamines is elevated. Lymphocytic thyroiditis may on occasion present manifestations of hyperthyroidism and must be differentiated on the basis of appropriate laboratory studies.

Treatment. There is general agreement that most children with thyrotoxicosis should be given a trial of medical therapy before surgery is considered. During adolescence in particular an attempt should be made to tide the child over this period of rapid growth with antithyroid drugs in the hope of inducing a permanent remission.

Excitement should be avoided, and an adequate and liberal diet with supplementary vitamins is indicated. A sympathetic understanding by the family of the physical and emotional problems is essential.

The recommended antithyroid drugs are propylthiouracil and methimazole (Tapazole). These compounds inhibit incorporation of trapped inorganic iodide into organic compounds and thus produce a progressive decrease in the synthesis of thyroid hormone. Toxic reactions occur with about equal frequency with both drugs. The initial dose of propylthiouracil is 100 to 150 mg., 3 times daily, and that of methimazole is 10 to 15 mg., 3 times daily. Subsequently the dose is increased or decreased as indicated. Smaller initial doses should be used in early childhood. Because these drugs are excreted rapidly, an attempt should be made to space doses at fairly regular intervals. Overdosage can lead to a hypothyroid state. Clinical response becomes apparent in 2 to 3 weeks, and adequate control in 1 to 3 months. The dose of the medication is then reduced to the minimal level that will maintain the child in a euthyroid state.

The thyroid frequently becomes larger after initiation of treatment, but eventually it usually decreases in size. The drug should be continued for 1 to 2 years, when it should be discontinued slowly. Approximately 75 per cent of children will have a permanent remission; if a relapse occurs, it will usually appear within 3 months and almost always within 6 months after therapy has been discontinued. Therapy may be resumed in case of a relapse. In pubertal children it is advisable to continue treatment throughout early adolescence.

Less than 2 per cent of patients treated in this manner have minor toxic reactions such as fever, pruritic or urticarial skin rash, nausea, diarrhea, abdominal cramps and headache. More serious reactions such as agranulocytosis are rare.

Operation is indicated when adequate cooperation for medical management is not possible or when adequate trial of medical management has failed to result in permanent remission. Subtotal thyroidectomy, a rather safe procedure, is performed only after the patient has been brought to a euthyroid state. This may be accomplished with propylthiouracil or methimazole over a 2- to 3-month period. After a euthyroid state has been attained 5 drops of a saturated solution of potassium iodide per day are given in addition for 2 weeks before operation in order to decrease the vascularity of the gland. Complications of surgical treatment include recurrence of thyrotoxicosis, hypothyroidism, hypoparathyroidism (transient or permanent) and paralysis of the vocal cords.

Radioactive iodine should not be used for treatment in children because, theoretically, permanent harmful irradiation effects might occur either in the thyroid or in other tissues. A period of observation of many years will be needed to exclude this possibility. In the exceptional patient in whom medical treatment is not feasible and operation is contraindicated or refused, radioiodine may have to be resorted to.

CONGENITAL HYPERTHYROIDISM

Hyperthyroidism in the newborn infant is rare and occurs only in infants of thyrotoxic mothers. It is caused by the transplacental passage of the long-acting thyroid-stimulating hormone (LATS); the clinical course is consistent with its estimated half-life of 3 weeks. Treatment of thyrotoxicosis during pregnancy does not necessarily prevent this complication. The infant is extremely restless, irritable and hyperactive and appears anxious and unusually alert. The eyes are widely opened and appear exophthalmic. There is extreme tachycardia (200 per minute or more) and tachypnea (100 per minute or more). The temperature is elevated. Without treatment, there is progression of symptoms; weight loss occurs despite a ravenous appetite, hepatomegaly increases, and jaundice may become manifest. Cardiac decompensation is common. The illness is transient and resolves in 6 to 12 weeks, but the infant may die if therapy is not instituted promptly. The serum level of protein-bound iodine is markedly elevated.

Treatment consists in administration of Lugol's solution (1 drop, 3 to 6 times daily) or propylthiouracil or methimazole. Parenteral fluid therapy, sedation and digitalization may be indicated.

CARCINOMA OF THE THYROID

Carcinoma of the thyroid is a rare lesion in children. The cause is unknown, but about 80 per cent of 227 patients in whom an attempt was made to obtain a history were found to have had irradiation during infancy to the neck and adjacent areas for such benign conditions as "enlarged" thymus, hypertrophied tonsils and adenoids, hemangiomas, nevi, acne, eczema and "cervical adenitis." Irradiation for thymic enlargement in infancy has been found to carry a 4 per cent risk of thyroid carcinoma and an approximately 30 per cent risk of thyroid nodularity.

Girls are affected twice as often as boys. The average age at diagnosis is 9 years, but the onset may be as early as the first year of life. A painless nodule in the thyroid is the first evidence of disease in about one fourth of the children. Cervical lymph node involvement is usually present at the time of the initial diagnosis and is often bilateral. The lungs are the most common site of metastases beyond the neck. There may not be any clinical manifestations referable to them; roentgenographically, they appear as diffuse miliary or nodular infiltrations, principally in the basal portions. They may be mistaken for tuberculosis, histoplasmosis or sarcoidosis. Other sites of metastases include the mediastinum, long bones, skull and axilla. On rare occasions the carcinoma may be functional and produce symptoms of hyperthyroidism.

Every identified thyroid nodule in a child should be removed and examined; the incidence of carcinoma in nodular lesions is estimated to be about 70 per cent. The neoplasm frequently grows slowly and may even remain dormant for years; undifferentiated neoplasms, however, may have a rapidly fatal course. The case fatality rate is approximately 20 per cent; death usually occurs in the first postoperative year.

The treatment of proved carcinoma of the thyroid is controversial. Some recommend thyroidectomy (hemithyroidectomy with removal of the isthmus if the disease is unilateral), dissection of any enlarged cervical nodes and postoperative roentgen therapy. Others recommend total thyroidectomy and regional dissection of lymph nodes, even though there is no evidence of involvement of them. Inoperable tumors should be removed as completely as possible along with any normal thyroid tissue, in preparation for the possible use of radio-iodine. Radio-iodine should be used only when the lesion cannot be completely removed surgically and when the cancerous tissue is capable of concentrating cancericidal doses of the drug. Regression of extensive pulmonary metastases has been observed to follow the use of radio-iodine.

All patients with a differentiated carcinoma should also be treated with thyroid hormone in doses sufficient to suppress thyrotropin on the possibility that tumor remnants which are thyrotropin-dependent may regress.

Medullary carcinoma of the thyroid may account for 5 to 10 per cent of all thyroid carcinomas. The tumor is characterized by sheets of cells with eosinophilic granular cytoplasm. There is deposition of amyloid in the stroma, and calcification is common. The most frequent symptom is goiter or a palpable thyroid nodule. Regional lymph node metastases are common; distant metastases also occur. Death may result, but 5-year survivals are known, and year-long survivals are not uncommon. Though this tumor is rare in childhood, it has special interest because it secretes calcitonin

and because it is frequently associated with other disorders such as pheochromocytoma (p. 1220). Medullary carcinomas of the thyroid probably arise from the parafollicular cells of the thyroid. Hypocalcemia occurs only rarely; perhaps increased parathyroid hormone secretion compensates for the hypercalcitonemia.

REFERENCES

General

Williams, R. H. (Ed.): *Textbook of Endocrinology.* 4th ed. Philadelphia, W. B. Saunders Company, 1968.

Hypothyroidism

Andersen, H. J.: Studies of Hypothyroidism in Children. *Acta paediat.*, 50 (Suppl. 125), 1961.

Carr, E. A., Jr., and others: The Various Types of Thyroid Malfunction in Cretinism and Their Relative Frequency. *Pediatrics*, 38:1, 1961.

Cross, H. E., Hollander, C. S., Rimoin, D. L., and McKusick, V. A.: Familial Agoitrous Cretinism Accompanied by Muscular Hypertrophy. *Pediatrics*, 41:413, 1968.

Fisher, W. D., Voorhess, M. L., and Gardner, L. I.: Congenital Hypothyroidism in Infant Following Maternal I[131] Therapy. *J. Pediat.*, 62:132, 1963.

French, F. S., and Van Wyk, J. J.: Fetal Hypothyroidism. *J. Pediat.*, 64:589, 1964.

Little, G., Meador, C. K., Cunningham, R., and Pittman, J. A.: "Cryptothyroidism," The Major Cause of Sporadic "Athyreotic" Cretinism. *J. Clin. Endocr.*, 25:1529, 1965.

Lowrey, G. H., and others: Early Diagnostic Criteria of Congenital Hypothyroidism. A Comprehensive Study of Forty-Nine Cretins. *A.M.A. J. Dis. Child.*, 96:131, 1958.

MacGillivray, M. H., Aceto, T., Jr., and Frohman, L. A.: Plasma Growth Hormone Responses and Growth Retardation in Hypothyroidism. *Am. J. Dis. Child.*, 115:273, 1968.

Moncrief, M. W., and McArthur, R. G.: Hypothyroidism in One of Monozygotic Twins. *Postgrad. Med. J.*, 44:423, 1968.

Neel, J. V., Carr, E. A., Beierwaltes, W. H., and Davidson, R. T.: Genetic Studies on the Congenitally Hypothyroid. *Pediatrics*, 27:269, 1961.

Smith, D. W., Blizzard, R. M., and Wilkins, L.: The Mental Prognosis in Hypothyroidism of Infancy and Childhood. A Review of 128 Cases. *Pediatrics*, 19:1011, 1957.

Goitrous Cretinism

Stanbury, J. B.: Familial Goiter; in J. B. Stanbury, J. B. Wyngaarden, and D. S. Fredrickson (Eds.): *The Metabolic Basis of Inherited Disease.* 2nd ed. New York, McGraw-Hill Book Company, Inc., 1966.

Goiter

Chamberlain, J. L., III: Thyroid Enlargement Probably Induced by Cobalt. *J. Pediat.*, 59:81, 1961.

Choufoer, J. C., Van Rhijn, M., and Querido, A.: Endemic Goiter in Western New Guinea. II. Clinical Picture, Incidence and Pathogenesis of Endemic Cretinism. *J. Clin. Endocrinol.*, 25:385, 1965.

Costa, A., and Cottino, F.: Research on Iodine Metabolism in Endemic Goiter in Piedmont. *Metabolism*, 12:35, 1963.

Gajdusek, D. C.: Congenital Defects of the Central Nervous System Associated with Hyperendemic Goiter in a Neolithic Highland Society of Netherlands New Guinea. I. Epidemiology. *Pediatrics*, 29:345, 1962.

Galina, M. P., Avnet, N. L., and Einhorn, A.: Iodides During Pregnancy. An Apparent Cause of Neonatal Death. *New England J. Med.*, 267:1124, 1962.

Greer, M. A., and Astwood, E. B.: Treatment of Simple Goiter with Thyroid. *J. Clin. Endocrinol.*, 13:1312, 1953.

Kimball, O. P.: Prevention of Endemic Goiter in Man. *Arch. Int. Med.*, 107:290, 1961.

Marine, D.: Endemic Goiter: A Problem in Preventive Medicine. *Ann. Int. Med.*, 41:875, 1954.

Martin, M. M., and Rento, R. D.: Iodide Goiter with Hypothyroidism in Two Newborn Infants. *J. Pediat.*, 61:94, 1962.

Paris, J., McConahey, W. M., Owen, C. A., Jr., Woolner, L. B., and Bahn, R. C.: Iodide Goiter. *J. Clin. Endocr.*, 20:57, 1960.

Randolph, J., Grunt, J. A., and Vawter, G. F.: The Medical and Surgical Aspects of Intratracheal Goiter. *New England J. Med.*, 268:457, 1963.

Srinivasan, S., Subramanyan, T. A. V., Sinha, A., Deo, M. G., and Ramalingaswami, V.: Himalayan Endemic Deafmutism. *Lancet*, 1:176, 1964.

Studer, H., and Greer, M. A.: A Study of the Mechanism Involved in the Production of Iodine-Deficiency Goiter. *Acta Endocrin.*, 49:610, 1965.

Pendred's Syndrome

Bax, G. M.: Typical and Atypical Cases of Pendred's Syndrome in One Family. *Acta Endocrinol.*, 53:264, 1966.

Fraser, G. R.: Association of Congenital Deafness with Goiter (Pendred's Syndrome). A Study of 207 Families. *Ann. Hum. Genet.*, 28:201, 1965.

Nilsson, L. R., Borgfors, N., Gamstorp, I., Holst, H., and Lidén, G.: Nonendemic Goitre and Deafness. *Acta Paediat.*, 53:117, 1964.

Thould, A. K., and Scowen, E. F.: Genetic Studies of the Syndrome of Congenital Deafness and Simple Goitre. *Ann. Hum. Genet.*, 27:283, 1964.

Thyrotoxicosis

Darby, C. P.: Three Episodes of Spontaneous Thyroid Storm Occurring in a Nine-Year-Old Child. *Pediatrics*, 30:927, 1962.

Hayles, A. B., Kennedy, R. L. J., Beahrs, O. H., and Woolner, L. B.: Exophthalmic Goiter in Children. *J. Clin. Endocrinol. & Metab.*, 19:138, 1959.

Hung, W., Wilkins, L., and Blizzard, R.: Medical Therapy of Thyrotoxicosis in Children. *Pediatrics*, 30:17, 1962.

Kogut, M. D., Kaplan, S. A., Collipp, P. J., Tiamsic, T., and Boyle, D.: Treatment of Hyperthyroidism in Children. *New England J. Med.*, 272:217, 1965.

McKendrick, T., and Newns, G. H.: Thyrotoxicosis in Children: A Follow-up Study. *Arch. Dis. Childhood*, 40:71, 1965.

McKenzie, J. M.: Humoral Factors in the Pathogenesis of Graves' Disease. *Physiol. Rev.*, 48:252, 1968.

Root, A. W., Bongiovanni, A. M., Harvie, F. H., and Eberlein,

W. R.: Treatment of Juvenile Thyrotoxicosis. *J. Pediat.*, 63:402, 1963.

Congenital Hyperthyroidism

Farrehi, C., Mitchell, M., and Fawcett, D. M.: Heart Failure in Congenital Thyrotoxicosis. *Pediatrics*, 37:460, 1966.

Martin, M. M., and Matus, R. N.: Neonatal Exophthalmos with Maternal Thyrotoxicosis. *Am. J. Dis. Child.*, 111:545, 1966.

McKenzie, J. M.: Neonatal Graves' Disease. *J. Clin. Endocr.*, 24:660, 1964.

Lymphocytic Thyroiditis

Clayton, G. W., and Johnson, C. M.: Struma Lymphomatosa in Children. *J. Pediat.*, 57:410, 1960.

Doniach, D., Nilsson, L. R., and Roitt, I. M.: Autoimmune Thyroiditis in Children and Adolescents. *Acta Paediat.*, 54:260, 1965.

Fialkow, P. J.: Autoimmunity and Chromosomal Aberrations. *Am. J. Hum. Genet.*, 18:93, 1966.

Humbert, J. R., Gotlin, R. W., Hostetter, G., Sherrill, J. G., and Silver, H. K.: Lymphocytic (Auto-immune, Hashimoto's) Thyroiditis. *Arch. Dis. Childhood*, 43:80, 1968.

Leboeuf, G., and Bongiovanni, A. M.: Thyroiditis in Childhood. *Advances in Pediat.*, 13:183, 1964.

Saxena, K. M., and Crawford, J. D.: Juvenile Lymphocytic Thyroiditis. *Pediatrics*, 30:917, 1962.

Solomon, I. L., and Blizzard, R. M.: Autoimmune Disorders of Endocrine Glands. *J. Pediat.*, 63:1021, 1963.

Winter, J., Eberlein, W. R., and Bongiovanni, A. M.: The Relationship of Juvenile Hypothyroidism to Chronic Lymphocytic Thyroiditis. *J. Pediat.*, 69:709, 1966.

Carcinoma of the Thyroid

Pincus, R. A., Reichlin, S., and Hempel-Mann, L. H.: Thyroid Abnormalities After Radiation Exposure in Infancy. *Ann. Int. Med.*, 66:1154, 1967.

Sussman, L., Librik, L., and Clayton, G. W.: Hyperthyroidism Attributable to a Hyperfunctioning Thyroid Carcinoma. *J. Pediat.*, 72:208, 1968.

Williams, E. D., Brown, C. L., and Doniach, I.: Pathological and Clinical Findings in a Series of 67 Cases of Medullary Carcinoma of the Thyroid. *J. Clin. Path.*, 19:103, 1966.

Winship, T., and Rosvoll, R. V.: Childhood Thyroid Carcinoma. *Cancer*, 14:734, 1961.

DISORDERS OF THE PARATHYROID GLANDS

The 2 hormones principally involved with maintainence of calcium homeostasis are *parathyroid hormone* (PTH), synthesized by the parathyroid glands, and *calcitonin*, synthesized in the thyroid gland. Disturbances of production of these hormones result in a variety of clinical disorders.

Parathyroid Hormone. The principal known function of parathyroid hormone is the maintenance of calcium balance, though it is indirectly, through its effect on calcium metabolism, a controlling factor (1) in the structure of bone, (2) in the regulation of neuromuscular activity, (3) in the conduction of cardiac impulses, (4) in the coagulation of blood, (5) in the permeability of cellular membranes, and (6) perhaps in the regulation of other functions of the body. Secretion of parathyroid hormone is regulated by the plasma level of calcium: hypocalcemia stimulates and hypercalcemia inhibits secretion. Hyperphosphatemia stimulates secretion of the hormone only indirectly by inducing hypocalcemia. PTH is a small polypeptide with both calcium-mobilizing and phosphaturic activity. Its effects appear to be mediated through the formation of cyclic 3',5'-adenosine monophosphate (AMP) at the cell membrane.

If administration of parathyroid extract is discontinued in a parathyroidectomized person, there is a decrease in the urinary excretion of phosphorus and a rise in serum phosphorus which is quickly followed by a fall in serum calcium and a decrease in urinary excretion of calcium. When parathormone therapy is resumed, these metabolic alterations are reversed. The calcium in the blood is principally in 2 forms: calcium ions and calcium proteinate. Since the total serum calcium concentration may be reduced by a decrease in the serum protein level, the ionized or active serum calcium cannot be evaluated adequately without knowledge of the concentration of serum protein (see Nomogram, p. 1541).

Parathormone has a direct action on the renal tubular mechanism, causing a phosphate diuresis by the kidney. It also causes resorption of bone, possibly through direct action on the matrix. A direct action of the hormone on mitochondria where it stimulates respiration and uptake of phosphate as well as the release of calcium has been demonstrated.

Calcitonin. Calcitonin, discovered in 1961, has hormonal effects antagonistic to parathyroid hormone. In birds, amphibians and teleost fish, calcitonin is synthesized in a discrete structure known as the ultimobranchial body, derived from the fifth pharyngeal pouch. In mammals this structure is incorporated into the thyroid gland as the parafollicular cells of the thyroid follicle. The hormone is a polypeptide consisting of 32 amino acids and has been synthesized; a sensitive radio-immunoassay has been developed. Calcitonin is secreted in response to hypercalcemia. Its main function is believed to be to restore normocalcemia during periods of hypercalcemia; another function appears to be regulation of bone remodeling. Its physiologic role has not been completely assessed.

Calcitonin deficiency, e.g. following thyroidectomy, does not appear to result in gross disturbance of calcium homeostasis, perhaps because some calcitonin is also found in the thymus. A syndrome of calcitonin excess occurs in patients with medullary carcinoma of the thyroid (p. 1199).

HYPOPARATHYROIDISM

Etiology. Temporary dysfunction of calcium homeostasis is observed in so-called *tetany of the newborn* (p. 401). Hypocalcemia has its onset during the first few days of life and rarely persists longer than a week. The role played by the parathyroids in this condition remains to be resolved by direct measurements of parathyroid hormone.

Occasionally hypocalcemia may be manifest later and may persist for several months; this is thought to result from *congenital transient hypoparathyroidism*. Although the cause is usually not known, in some instances the condition is due to maternal hyperparathyroidism. In such instances it is presumed that exposure to elevated levels of maternal serum calcium results in suppression of parathyroid function in the fetus; tetany may be manifest in the infant until normal functional activity is established.

Congenital permanent hypoparathyroidism usually results from aplasia or hypoplasia of the parathyroid glands; frequently there are other developmental defects, such as aplasia of the thymus (p. 480), right-sided aortic arch with or without other cardiovascular abnormalities, and absence of the isthmus of the thyroid. Micrognathia and abnormalities of the ears are occasional external clues. The disorder occurs sporadically, and the cause is unknown.

Familial congenital hypoparathyroidism also occurs; since all affected infants have been males, it appears to be transmitted by a sex-linked recessive gene. The nature of the defect is not known, and it does not appear to be associated with other congenital defects.

Removal or damage of the parathyroid glands may occur as a complication of thyroidectomy *(surgical hypoparathyroidism).* Hypoparathyroidism has developed even when the parathyroid glands had been identified and left undisturbed at the time of operation. This, presumably, is the result of interference with the blood supply or of postoperative edema and fibrosis. Symptoms of tetany may occur abruptly postoperatively and be permanent or temporary. In some instances symptoms develop insidiously and go undetected until months after thyroidectomy. Occasionally the first evidence of surgical hypoparathyroidism may be the development of cataracts. All patients subjected to thyroidectomy should be carefully studied to determine the status of parathyroid function.

Idiopathic hypoparathyroidism may be acquired at any age. In many of the reported patients who were adults when the diagnosis was established clinical manifestations had begun in childhood. The cause is unknown, but an autoimmune mechanism is suggested by the demonstration that over a third of such patients have parathyroid antibodies. This assumption is further supported by the frequent association of hypoparathyroidism with other disorders believed to have a similar origin, such as Addison's disease, lymphocytic thyroiditis and pernicious anemia. Addison's disease and hypoparathyroidism may occur in the same patient or may alternate in members of the same family. Mucocutaneous moniliasis occurs frequently in patients with idiopathic hypoparathyroidism or Addison's disease; there is abundant evidence that it is not the cause of the endocrinopathy. An inherited abnormality of the immunologic mechanism probably accounts for all these findings. At autopsy no parathyroid tissue is demonstrable.

Clinical Manifestations. Neurologic manifestations usually dominate the clinical picture. Convulsions with loss of consciousness may occur at intervals of days, weeks or months. They may begin with abdominal pain, followed by general tonic rigidity, retraction of the head and cyanosis. Hypoparathyroidism is frequently mistaken for epilepsy. Headache, vomiting, increased intracranial pressure and papilledema may be associated with convulsions, and the differentiation from a brain tumor may be difficult. Muscular pain and cramps are early manifestations which progress to numbness, stiffness and tingling of the hands and feet. Manifestations of tetany are usually present. There may be only positive Chvostek and Trousseau signs or there may be laryngeal and carpopedal spasms.

The teeth erupt late and irregularly. Enamel formation is irregular, and the teeth may be unusually soft. The skin may be dry and scaly, and the nails of the fingers and toes may have horizontal lines. Manifestations of a wide variety

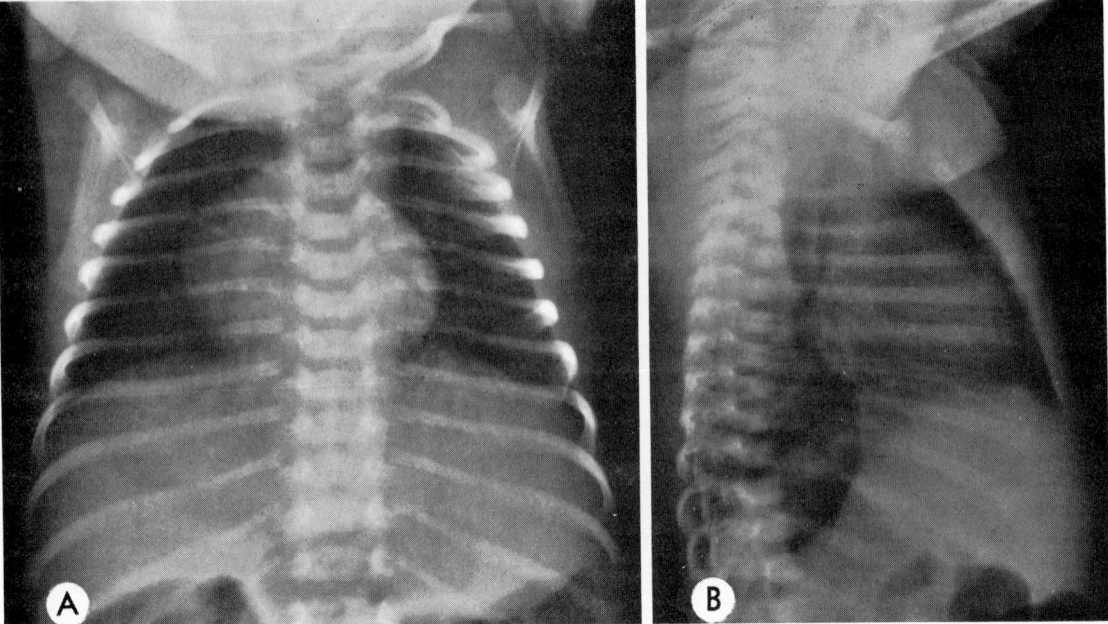

Figure 17-13. Congenital absence of parathyroid glands; roentgenograms of chest exposed at 6 days of age reveal no evidence of thymus. *A,* The mediastinum is narrow; *B,* the substernal area is radiolucent. (From Kirkpatrick and DiGeorge: *Am. J. Roentgenol.,* 103:32, 1968.)

of other disorders which are not a direct consequence of parathyroid hormone deficiency may also be seen. Mucocutaneous candidiasis often antedates the development of hypoparathyroidism; the monilia infection most often involves the nails, the oral mucosa, the angles of the mouth and less often the skin. Patients with hypoparathyroidism may also have abnormal loss of hair, manifested as thinning or patchy loss or as complete alopecia.

Cataracts in patients with long-standing untreated disease are a direct consequence of hypoparathyroidism; other ocular disorders such as keratoconjunctivitis may also be associated. Manifestations of Addison's disease, Hashimoto's thyroiditis, pernicious anemia, hepatitis and primary gonadal insufficiency may also occur in association with those of hypoparathyroidism.

Permanent physical and mental deterioration occurs if initiation of treatment is delayed for a long time.

Laboratory Data. The serum calcium level is low (5 to 7 mg. per 100 ml.) and the phosphorus elevated (7 to 12 mg. per 100 ml.) The serum phosphatase level is normal or low. The Sulkowitch test gives a negative result, and renal function is normal. Even a moderate amount of calcium in the urine is strong evidence against hypocalcemia. Parathyroid hormone in serum is detectable only in small amounts or not at all even in the presence of hypocalcemia. Roentgenograms of the bones rarely reveal an increased density limited to the metaphyses, suggestive of heavy metal poisoning, or an increased density of the lamina dura. Roentgenograms of the skull may reveal calcifications in the basal ganglia.

There is a prolongation of the Q-T interval on the electrocardiogram, which disappears when the hypocalcemia is corrected. Electroencephalographic tracings usually reveal widespread slow activity; the tracings return to normal after the serum calcium has been within the normal range for a few weeks unless irreversible brain damage has occurred or unless the parathyroid insufficiency is associated with epilepsy. When hypoparathyroidism occurs concurrently with Addison's disease, the serum level of calcium may be normal, but hypocalcemia appears after effective treatment of the adrenal insufficiency.

Treatment. Emergency treatment for tetany consists in intravenous injections of 5 to 10 ml. of a 10 per cent solution of calcium gluconate at the rate of 0.5 to 1 ml. per minute. Initially either vitamin D or dihydrotachysterol should also be administered. Since dihydrotachysterol acts more rapidly, it is preferable in the early stages of treatment and may be given in doses of 1 to 4 ml. daily. Foods with a high phosphorus content, such as milk, eggs and cheese, should be eliminated from the diet.

Maintenance therapy consists in oral administration of vitamin D in daily doses of 50,000 to 250,000 I.U. During the period of stabilization some patients require supplemental calcium, which can be given orally in the form of calcium gluconate or calcium lactate (3 to 9 gm. per day).

Clinical evaluation of the patient and frequent determinations of the serum calcium level are indicated in the early stages of treatment in order to determine the dosage requirements of vitamin D and of calcium. Maintenance treatment must be continued indefinitely. If vitamin D therapy is discontinued, the serum calcium level may remain normal for 6 to 18 months; hence a permanent remission cannot be assumed until there has been an adequate period of observation. If hypercalcemia occurs, vitamin D should be discontinued and resumed at a lower dose after the serum calcium level has returned to normal. In cases of long standing, repair of cerebral and dental changes is not likely. Pigmentation, lowering of the blood pressure or weight loss may indicate adrenal insufficiency, which requires specific treatment (p. 1208).

PSEUDOHYPOPARATHYROIDISM

In this syndrome, in contrast to the situation in idiopathic hypoparathyroidism, the parathyroid glands are normal or hyperplastic histologically, and they can synthesize and secrete parathyroid hormone. Serum levels of parathyroid hormone are increased when the patient is hypocalcemic. It is believed that the primary defect is a failure of the end-organs, particularly of the kidney and skeleton, to respond to parathormone. Administration of parathormone fails to raise the serum level of calcium or to lower the serum level of phosphorus.

In addition to clinical and chemical findings similar to those of idiopathic hypoparathyroidism, patients have a short, stocky build and a round face. Growth failure may be striking. There is brachydactylia; the first, fourth and fifth metacarpals are most often involved, and the first and fifth metatarsals are also often affected. As a result, the index finger may be longer than the middle finger. There may be other skeletal abnormalities, such as short and wide phalanges, bowing, exostoses, thickening of the calvaria and general demineralization of the bones. These patients frequently have calcium deposits and metaplastic bone formation subcutaneously. Mental retardation is common, as are calcifications of the basal ganglia and lenticular cataracts.

Resorption of subperiosteal bone and elevated levels of serum alkaline phosphatase in some patients indicate that the osseous system may not be as resistant as the renal tubules to endogenous parathormone.

The hypocalcemia characteristically does not respond to parathyroid extract, but does to vitamin D. Therefore treatment is the same as for idiopathic hypoparathyroidism.

Pseudo-pseudohypoparathyroidism is a term that has been used to describe patients with the usual anatomic stigmata of pseudohypoparathyroidism, but in whom the serum calcium and phosphorus levels are normal. Evidence indicates that this syndrome is a variant of pseudohypoparathyroidism; transition from one form to another has been observed. Furthermore, there are pedigrees with both variants in more than one generation. Transmission would appear to be by a sex-linked dominant form of inheritance. Turner's syndrome has been observed in some of these patients.

HYPERPARATHYROIDISM

Excessive production of parathyroid hormone may result from a primary defect of the parathyroid glands such as an adenoma or idiopathic hyperplasia *(primary hyperparathyroidism)*. A wide variety of neoplasms in adults, particularly carcinomas of the lung and kidney, have been reported to produce sufficient parathyroid hormone to result in hyperparathyroidism. Presumed fetal hyperparathyroidism has been observed in infants of mothers with inadequately treated hypoparathyroidism. The manifestations involved primarily the bones and were transitory.

More often the increased production of parathyroid hormone is a compensatory phenomenon, usually aimed at correcting hypocalcemic states of diverse origins *(secondary hyperparathyroidism)*. In vitamin D-deficient rickets (p. 1363) and in the malabsorption syndromes (p. 804) intestinal absorption of calcium is deficient, but hypocalcemia and tetany are averted by increased activity of the parathyroid glands. In chronic renal disease, hyperphosphatemia and the consequent hypocalcemia result in compensatory hyperparathyroidism with increases in serum levels of parathyroid hormone. If stimulation of the parathyroids is sufficiently intense and protracted, the glands become autonomous in their secretion of parathyroid hormone. This situation is known as *tertiary hyperparathyroidism* and is manifest in patients with chronic renal disease by the development of normocalcemia or hypercalcemia in the presence of hyperphosphatemia. They have the extensive osseous lesions of hyperparathyroidism and frequently are benefited by parathyroidectomy. The autonomous nature of parathyroid function in such patients is being increasingly revealed after restitution of normal renal function by renal transplantation.

PRIMARY HYPERPARATHYROIDISM

Primary hyperparathyroidism is uncommon in children and is usually due to a single adenoma. Less frequently it may be due to hyperplasia of all the parathyroid glands. When the disorder is caused by an adenoma, symptoms generally begin after 10 years of age, whereas symptoms are present in infancy when the disorder is caused by diffuse primary hyperplasia of the parathyroids. In some instances, adenoma of the parathyroid glands, with or without adenomas of other endocrine glands, is inherited as an autosomal dominant disorder. In such cases the adenomas are apt to be multiple. In affected families the parathyroids may vary histologically, some patients having adenomas and others hyperplasia. The occurrence of hyperplasia of the parathyroid glands in infant siblings from a consanguineous mating suggests an autosomal recessive mode of inheritance.

Clinical Manifestations. In older children the manifestations tend to resemble those in adults. At all ages the clinical manifestations of hypercalcemia of any cause include muscular weakness, anorexia, nausea, vomiting, constipation, polydipsia, polyuria, loss of weight, and fever. Calcium may be deposited in the renal parenchyma, resulting in nephrocalcinosis, and progressively diminishes renal function. Renal calculi may be formed and be manifest by renal colic and hematuria. Osseous changes may be responsible for pain in the back or extremities, disturbance of gait, deformities, fractures and tumors. There may be decrease in height from compression of vertebrae, and the patient may become bedridden.

Less common findings are abdominal pain, alopecia areata, denting and thickening of the fingernails and toenails and clubbing of the fingers. Duodenal ulcers are common in adults with hyperparathyroidism, but not in children. The so-called parathyroid crisis is manifest by progressive oliguria, azotemia, stupor and coma.

In infants, failure to thrive may be the earliest manifestation. Mental retardation, convulsions and even blindness may be expected. Enlargement and tenderness of the epiphyseal regions have been observed, and the anterior fontanel may be large and bulging.

Laboratory Data. The serum calcium level is elevated, often above 15 mg. per 100 ml. The serum phosphorus level is reduced to about 3 mg. per 100 ml. or less. When there is skeletal involvement, serum phosphatase is increased. The level of serum magnesium is low, and that of nonprotein nitrogen may be elevated. The urine may have a low fixed specific gravity. Urinary excretion of calcium and phosphorus may be increased.

Roentgenograms of the bones may reveal generalized rarefaction, cysts, tumors, fractures and deformities. The most consistent and characteristic findings are resorption of subperiosteal bone and disappearance of the lamina dura. Resorption of bone is seen best along the margins of the phalanges of the hands. In the skull there may be gross trabeculation or a granular appearance resulting from focal rarefaction. In infants, cupping and fraying are seen at the ends of the long bones, and the distance between the calcified diaphysis and epiphysis is increased. These changes, as well as flaring of the ends of the ribs, are suggestive of rickets. Radiographs of the abdomen may reveal renal calculi or nephrocalcinosis.

Differential Diagnosis. *Hypercalcemia* of any origin results in a similar clinical pattern and must be differentiated from hyperparathyroidism. A low serum phosphorus level in association with hypercalcemia is usually diagnostic of primary hyperparathyroidism. Pharmacologic doses of corticosteroids lower the serum calcium level to normal in patients with hypercalcemia from other causes, but generally do not affect the calcium level in patients with hyperparathyroidism. This may be a useful test in differential diagnosis. *Vitamin D intoxication* can be excluded by history, by a normal level of serum phosphorus and by roentgenographic evidence of increased bone density. *Idiopathic hypercalcemia* of infancy may be easily confused with hyperparathyroidism; however, the serum phosphorus level is normal or slightly elevated and, roentgenographically, the increased bone density of idiopathic hypercalcemia contrasts strikingly with the rarefaction of primary hyperparathyroidism. *Hypophosphatasia*, especially when severe, is frequently associated with mild to moderate hypercalcemia. The serum phosphorus level is normal, and that of alkaline phosphatase is depressed. Roentgenograms of the bones may reveal complete disappearance of the zone of provisional calcification and lack of calcification of the metaphyseal bone. Elevated serum calcium levels may also be observed in patients with sarcoidosis, thyrotoxicosis, malignant disease with osseous metastases, and during periods of prolonged immobilization. Hypercalcemia has also been observed in association with subcutaneous fat necrosis. In rickets and in renal tubular disorders the serum phosphorus level is low, but that of serum calcium is normal or low.

When renal disease and evidence of hyperparathyroidism coexist, it is frequently difficult to decide whether the hyperparathyroidism is primary, secondary or tertiary.

Treatment. Surgical exploration is indicated in all instances. All glands should be carefully inspected; if an adenoma is discovered, it should be removed. If there is only generalized hyperplasia, a subtotal parathyroidectomy should be performed. The patient should be carefully observed postoperatively for the development of hypocalcemia and tetany; intravenous administration of calcium gluconate may be required for a few days. The serum calcium level then gradually returns to normal, and, under ordinary circumstances, a diet high in calcium and phosphorus need be maintained for only several months after operation.

The **prognosis** is good if the disease is recognized early and there is appropriate surgical treatment. When extensive osseous lesions are present, permanent deformities may persist; when renal disease has occurred, the prognosis is less hopeful. A search for other affected family members is indicated.

REFERENCES

Blizzard, R. M., Chee, D., and Davis, W.: The Incidence of Parathyroid and Other Antibodies in the Sera of Patients with Idiopathic Hypoparathyroidism. *Clin. Exp. Immunol.,* 1:119, 1966.

Bronsky, D., Kushner, D. S., Dubin, A., and Snapper, I.: Idiopathic Hypoparathyroidism and Pseudohypoparathyroidism: Case Reports and Review of the Literature. *Medicine*, 37: 317, 1959.

Bronsky, D., Kiamko, R. T., Moncada, R., and Rosenthal, I. M.: Intrauterine Hyperparathyroidism Secondary to Maternal Hypoparathyroidism. *Pediatrics*, 42:606, 1968.

DiGeorge, A. M.: Congenital Absence of the Thymus and Its Immunologic Consequences: Concurrence with Congenital Hypoparathyroidism; in D. Bergsma and R. A. Good (Eds.): Birth Defects Original Article Series, No. 1. New York, The National Foundation, 1968, Vol. IV.

Fanconi, A., and Prader, A.: Transient Congenital Idiopathic Hypoparathyroidism. *Helv. Paed. Acta*, 22:342, 1967.

Hartenstein, H., and Gardner, L. I.: Tetany of the Newborn Associated with Maternal Parathyroid Adenoma: Report of the Seventh Affected Family. *New England J. Med.*, 274: 266, 1966.

Hillman, D. A., Scriver, C. R., Pedvis, S., and Shragovitch, I.: Neonatal Familial Primary Hyperparathyroidism. *New England J. Med.*, 270:483, 1964.

Jackson, C. E., and Boonstra, C. E.: The Relationship of Hereditary Hyperparathyroidism to Endocrine Adenomatosis. *Am. J. Med.*, 43:727, 1967.

Kunstadter, R. H., Oh, W., Tanman, F., and Cornblath, M.: Idiopathic Hypoparathyroidism in the Newborn. *Am. J. Dis. Child.*, 105:499, 1963.

Lee, J. B., Tashjian, A. H., Streeto, J. M., and Frantz, A. G.: Familial Pseudohypoparathyroidism. Role of Parathyroid Hormone and Thyrocalcitonin. *New England J. Med.*, 279: 1179, 1968.

Lobdell, D. H.: Congenital Absence of the Parathyroid Glands. *A.M.A. Arch. Path.*, 67:412, 1959.

Mann, J. B., Alterman, S., and Hills, A. G.: Albright's Hereditary Osteodystrophy Comprising Pseudohypoparathyroidism and Pseudopseudohypoparathyroidism. With a Report of Two Cases Representing the Complete Syndrome Occurring in Successive Generations. *Ann. Int. Med.*, 56:315, 1962.

Melvin, K. E. W., and Tashjian, A. H., Jr.: The Syndrome of Excessive Thyrocalcitonin Produced by Medullary Carcinoma of the Thyroid. *Proc. Nat. Acad. Sci.*, 59:1216, 1968.

Nolan, R. B., Hayles, A. B., and Woolner, L. B.: Adenoma of the Parathyroid Gland in Children. Report of Case and Brief Review of the Literature. *A.M.A. J. Dis. Child.*, 99: 622, 1960.

Peden, V. H.: True Idiopathic Hypoparathyroidism as a Sex-Linked Recessive Trait. *Am. J. Hum. Genet.*, 12:323, 1960.

Sherwood, L. M.: Parathyroid Hormone and Thyrocalcitonin in Calcium Homeostasis. *New England J. Med.*, 278:663, 1968.

Tashjian, A. H., and Melvin, K. E. W.: Medullary Carcinoma of the Thyroid Gland. Studies of Thyrocalcitonin in Plasma and Tumor Extracts. *New England J. Med.*, 279:279, 1968.

DISORDERS OF THE ADRENAL GLANDS

GENERAL CONSIDERATIONS

The adrenal gland is composed of 2 endocrine systems: the chromaffin system contained in the medulla, and the interrenal system of the cortex. The medulla is of ectodermal origin, and its cells are derived from sympathetic ganglia. The cortex is of mesodermal origin and is formed in the embryo by about 6 weeks' gestation from perineal mesothelium.

In a fetus of 2 months the adrenals are larger than the kidneys, but from the fourth month the kidneys grow rapidly, becoming about twice as large as the adrenals by the end of the sixth month. At birth the adrenal gland is one third the size of the kidney, and the combined weight of both glands is 7 to 9 gm. in the full-term infant.

The adrenal cortex in the fetus and the newborn infant is composed of 2 histologically distinct components: an outer portion, the true cortex, and a more central portion, known as the "fetal cortex." At birth this fetal cortex makes up about 80 per cent of the gland. Within a few days after birth it involutes, undergoing a 50 per cent reduction in total mass by 2 weeks of age. Fetal cortex has steroidogenic activity, but its specific function in the fetus is unknown.

The true cortex consists of 3 zones. In the zona glomerulosa, situated beneath the capsule, there is an alveolar arrangement of the cells; in the broader zona fasciculata the columns of cells are radially arranged; in the zona reticularis the cells form a network next to the medulla.

Function. Removal of both adrenal glands results in death, which is preceded by vomiting, thirst, anuria, muscular weakness, tachycardia, fall in blood pressure, and coma.

The *adrenal cortex* secretes various steroid compounds essential to life. The known compounds can be divided into several general categories:

1. *Glucocorticoids.* These steroids have a 21-carbon structure and are also referred to as 17-hydroxycorticosteroids or simply as corticosteroids. The principal one is hydrocortisone, which is also known as cortisol or compound F. Cortisone (compound E) is another member of this group.

These substances have carbohydrate-regulating and antiphlogistic properties. The fall of the blood sugar level in fasting, adrenalectomized animals is attributed to a lack of these hormones; in their absence, formation of new sugar (gluconeogenesis) from endogenous protein is impaired. The influence of these adrenocortical hormones on fat metabolism is illustrated by the obesity in children with Cushing's syndrome. Excessive amounts of these substances lead to protein catabolism, osteoporosis and growth failure. They also result in sodium and water retention and loss of potassium.

The corticosteroids and their metabolites are excreted in urine; the amounts excreted can be measured chemically. Methods are also available for measurement of their blood levels; "normal values" differ somewhat according to the method used. In patients with Addison's disease or pituitary insufficiency the levels of corticosteroids are reduced, and in those with Cushing's disease increased.

The rate of corticosteroid production is under control of pituitary adrenocorticotropin (ACTH). Measurement of blood or urinary levels of the corticosteroids before and after the administration of corticotropin is used to assess adrenocortical reserve. Pituitary reserve is tested by the administration of Metopirone (metyrapone), a compound which selectively inhibits 11-hydroxylation and the formation of cortisol. Normally the impairment of cortisol synthesis leads to increased pituitary secretion of corticotropin, which in turn stimulates the adrenal to increased secretion of the precursors of cortisol. Appropriate measurements of urinary steroids after metyrapone provides indirect evidence as to whether corticotropin has been produced.

Many synthetic analogues of cortisone and hydrocortisone are available. Derivatives with an additional double bond in ring A are known as prednisone and prednisolone. They are 3 to 4 times as potent in anti-inflammatory and carbohydrate activity as the natural steroids, but have less effect on salt and water retention. Halogenated derivatives are also available. Thus 9-alpha-fluorohydrocortisone is approximately 15 times as active as hydrocortisone in anti-inflammatory activity, but is more than 20 times as active in salt and water retention. Triamcinolone (delta-1, 9-alpha-fluoro, 16 alpha-hydroxy-hydrocortisone) is approximately 5 times as potent as hydrocortisone, and beta-methasone and dexamethasone are approximately 25 times as potent; none of them is thought to affect the retention of water and electrolytes. These analogues are usually used in pharmacologic doses for their anti-inflammatory or immunosuppressive properties.

2. *Aldosterone.* Aldosterone is the 18-aldehyde of corticosterone and is produced primarily in the zona glomerulosa of the adrenal cortex. It is the most potent mineralocorticoid, and unlike the glucocorticoids its secretion is regulated by the state of activation of the renin-angiotensin system and only to a minor degree by corticotropin. Renin is a proteolytic enzyme which acts upon angiotensinogen to convert it to the inactive decapeptide, angiotensin I. A converting enzyme then immediately changes angiotensin I to the biologically active octapeptide, angiotensin II. Angiotensin II is a potent pressor agent, but its principal known physiologic role is to act directly on the adrenal cortex to stimulate the secretion of aldosterone. The adrenal also secretes 2 other mineralocorticoids, desoxycorticosterone (DOC) and corticosterone (compound B); their effects on electrolyte metabolism vary, but excessive secretion leads to hypokalemic alkalosis and hypertension.

Sodium deprivation is a potent stimulus to secretion of aldosterone. Changes in intake of sodium result in small changes in blood volume, arterial pressure and renal blood flow. These changes are sensitively monitored by the juxtaglomerular cells on the renal afferent arterioles, which form the receptor site or volume receptor.

Activation of the juxtaglomerular apparatus results in increased output of angiotensin II followed by increased secretion of aldosterone.

The principal action of aldosterone is the maintenance of electrolyte equilibrium, which in turn contributes to the stabilization of blood volume and blood pressure. Aldosterone controls sodium reabsorption (and hence water reabsorption) in the distal tubule of the kidney.

3. *Androgens.* Dehydroepiandrosterone, androstenedione and testosterone are representative of this group. These hormones are capable of increasing retention of nitrogen, potassium, phosphorus and sulfate. They promote growth and have an androgenic effect, properties which are most conspicuous under pathologic conditions when adrenal hyperplasia or adrenal tumors induce precocious growth and development of secondary male sex characteristics. There is evidence that the adrenal androgens are partly responsible for the development of axillary and pubic hair in the female.

Metabolized adrenal androgens are excreted in the urine as 17-ketosteroids. Their measurement can be accepted as an index of the production of adrenal androgens in the female. In the male approximately one third of the urinary 17-ketosteroids can be attributed to testicular and two thirds to adrenal androgens. In children prior to 8 to 10 years of age the urinary excretion of these substances is small (p. 1224), but there is a constant increase throughout adolescence until adult levels are reached. Under pathologic conditions increased production of adrenal androgens is reflected in increased secretion of urinary 17-ketosteroids.

4. *Estrogens.* Adrenal cortical production of estrogens is most strikingly illustrated in patients with feminizing adrenal cortical tumors (p. 1220).

The *adrenal medulla* consists of irregularly shaped cells and of blood sinuses located between the strands of cells.

The principal hormones of the adrenal medulla are the physiologically active catecholamines: dopamine, norepinephrine and epinephrine. The sequence of reactions representing the biosynthetic route is depicted in Figure 17-14. Catecholamine synthesis also occurs in brain, in sympathetic nerve endings, and in chromaffin tissue other than in the adrenal medulla. The principal metabolites of the catecholamines excreted in the urine are vanilmandelic acid, or VMA, metanephrine and normetanephrine. The relatively large amount of VMA excreted in urine and its relative ease of chemical estimation have made its determination the method of choice for the detection of functioning tumors of the adrenal medulla.

The proportions of epinephrine and norepinephrine in the adrenal vary at different ages. In early fetal stages there is practically no epinephrine, and even at birth norepinephrine is predominant. In adults, norepinephrine makes up only 10 to 30 per cent of the total pressor amines in the medulla.

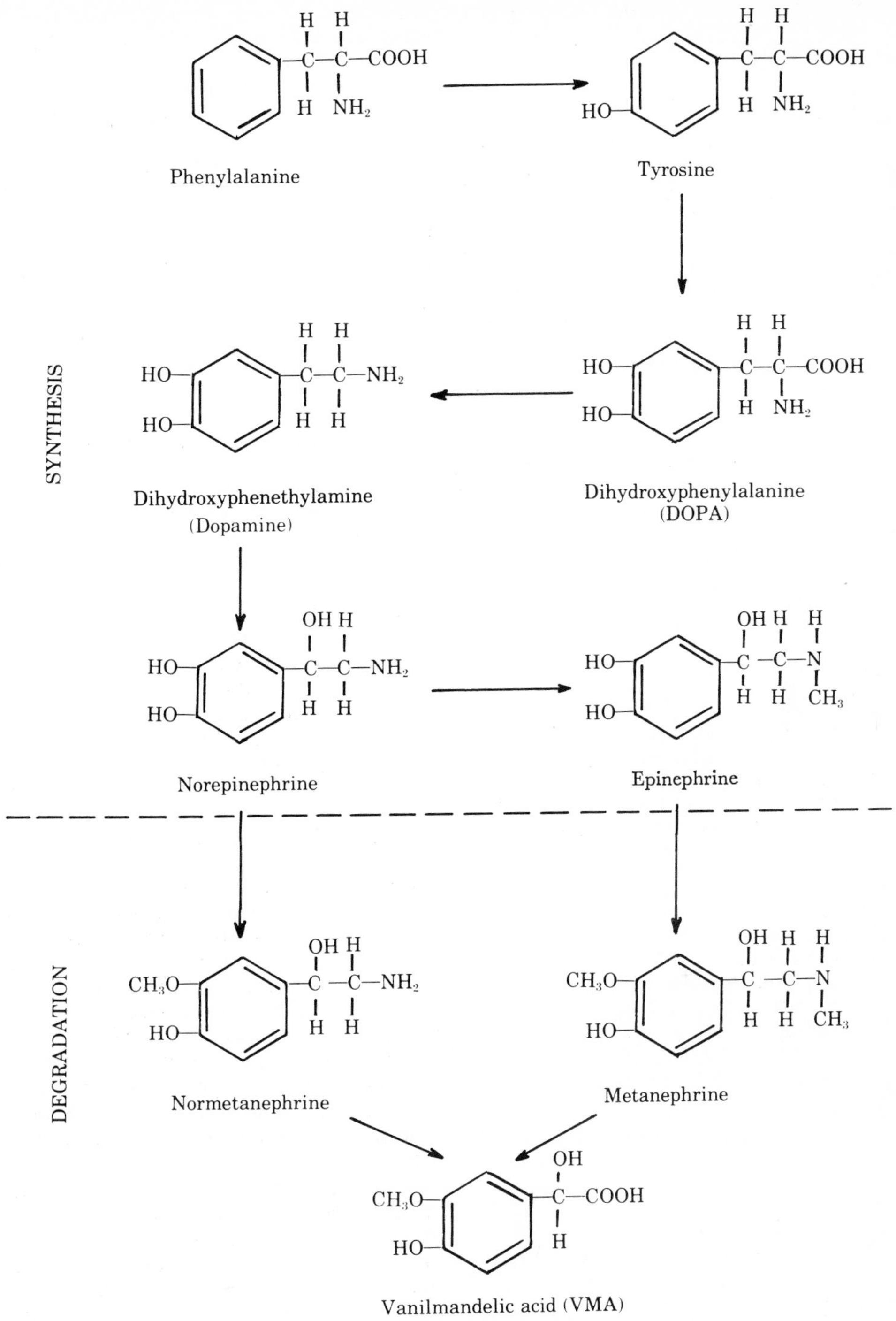

Figure 17-14. Biosynthesis and inactivation of the catecholamines: norepinephrine and epinephrine.

Both epinephrine and norepinephrine increase the mean arterial blood pressure. Norepinephrine accomplishes this without changing the cardiac output. By increasing peripheral vascular resistance, it increases systolic and diastolic blood pressures with only a slight reduction in the pulse rate. Epinephrine increases the pulse rate and, by decreasing the peripheral vascular resistance, decreases the diastolic pressure. The hyperglycemic and calorigenic effects of norepinephrine are much less pronounced than those of epinephrine. Both hormones are believed to be excreted into the bloodstream in approximately the same proportion as elaborated in the adrenal.

ADRENAL CORTICAL INSUFFICIENCY

Deficient production of corticosteroids and aldosterone may result from a wide variety of congenital or acquired lesions of the pituitary or adrenal cortex (Table 17-3). Depending upon the pathologic lesion, the symptoms may be severe or mild; the deficiency may be temporary or permanent, and symptoms may be manifest abruptly or insidiously.

Etiology. *Onset in infancy.* ABSENCE OR HYPOPLASIA OF THE PITUITARY. The adrenal gland may be markedly hypoplastic because of absence or deficiency of corticotropin. This situation is common in anencephaly and in holoprosencephaly, since the pituitary is absent or hypoplastic in these conditions. Failure of normal pituitary development is rare in infants with an intact cranium. A congenital defect of the hypothalamus with deficiency of corticotropin-releasing hormone could also result in corticotropin deficiency, but no patient with such a lesion has yet been described.

PRIMARY ADRENAL APLASIA OR HYPOPLASIA. This condition occurs most often in males and has been reported in brothers and in half-brothers with different fathers, strongly suggesting an X-linked gene as the causative factor. It is not yet clear whether the few instances of affected females depend upon an autosomal gene or are not genetically transmitted. Histologic examination of the hypoplastic adrenal cortex in males with this disorder reveals disorganization and cytomegaly, a finding not present in the adrenals from corticotropin-deficient infants.

Congenital adrenal cortical insufficiency occurs most frequently in infants with *defective synthesis of adrenal cortical hormones.* Approximately 30 per cent of infants with the 21-hydroxylase type of *congenital adrenal hyperplasia* have a deficiency of cortisol and of aldosterone, and manifest salt-losing symptoms in the neonatal period (p. 1215). Such symptoms are also consistently present in infants with lipoid adrenal hyperplasia and in those with the 3β-dehydrogenase defect. More recently a salt-losing syndrome in infancy has been described resulting from isolated *defects in synthesis of aldosterone.* Two defects are known: in one there is failure of the 18-hydroxylation of corticosterone; in the other, failure of dehydrogenation of 18-hydroxy-corticosterone (see Fig. 17-17). Evidence suggests that both defects are inherited in an autosomal recessive manner.

Adrenal hemorrhage may occur in the neonatal period as a consequence of difficult labor or of asphyxia. The hemorrhage may be sufficiently extensive to result in death from exsanguination or from hypoadrenalism. Often the hemorrhage is asymptomatic initially and is identified by calcification of the adrenal later in life. On rare occasions gradual impairment in function resulting from progressive fibrosis or cystic changes may culminate in adrenocortical insufficiency in infancy or childhood.

Onset after infancy. *Deficiency of corticotropin* as an isolated finding is rare at all ages; it is an infrequent cause of hypoglycemia (p. 1167). It occurs frequently in association with other pituitary tropic hormone defects resulting from a variety of factors (p. 1174). Patients with defects in steroidogenesis occasionally are asymptomatic in infancy and present with hypoadrenalism during childhood (p. 1214). Likewise, an occasional patient with congenital *adrenal hypoplasia* may have sufficient functioning adrenal tissue to pass asymptomatically through infancy. The precise defect causing *isolated corticosteroid deficiency* is unknown, but it may be related to defective adrenal cortical development; evidence suggests that the defect is inherited in an autosomal recessive manner.

TABLE 17-3. CLASSIFICATION OF ADRENAL HYPOFUNCTION

A. **Onset in infancy**
1. Corticotropin deficiency
    a. Pituitary hypoplasia or aplasia
    b. Hypothalamic defect?
2. Primary adrenal hypoplasia or aplasia
    a. Sex-linked type
    b. Autosomal recessive type?
    c. Sporadic
3. Defective steroidogenesis
    a. Lipoid adrenal hyperplasia
    b. 3-beta-hydroxysteroid dehydrogenase
    c. 21-hydroxylase defect (30% of patients)
    d. Defect of 18-hydroxylation of corticosterone
    e. Defect of dehydrogenation of 18-hydroxycorticosterone
4. Adrenal hemorrhage

B. **Onset after infancy**
1. Corticotropin deficiency
    a. Isolated deficiency
    b. Multiple pituitary deficiency
        1. Sporadic
        2. Familial
2. Defect in steroidogenesis
    a. 21-hydroxylase defect
    b. 11-hydroxylase defect
    c. 17-hydroxylase defect
3. Primary adrenal hypoplasia
    a. Sex-linked type
    b. Autosomal recessive type?
    c. Sporadic
4. Isolated corticosteroid deficiency
5. Destructive lesions of adrenal (Addison's disease)
    a. Granulomatous lesions, e.g. tuberculosis
6. Autoimmune adrenalitis (Addison's disease)
    a. Isolated
    b. Associated with other autoimmune endocrinopathies or candidiasis
7. Addison's disease with cerebral sclerosis
8. Addison's disease with spastic paraplegia
9. Neonatal hemorrhage
10. Acute infection (Waterhouse-Friderichsen syndrome)
11. Iatrogenic
    a. Abrupt cessation of exogenous corticosteroids or corticotropin
    b. Removal of functioning adrenal tumor

Bilateral adrenalectomy or the removal of one adrenal in the absence of the other will result in death unless replacement therapy is maintained.

Another cause of adrenal insufficiency is the *abrupt cessation* of administration of corticotropin or a corticosteroid. Symptoms are most likely to occur after these substances have been given in large doses for a long time to patients who are subsequently subjected to stressful situations such as severe infections or surgical procedures. Administration of these substances results in impaired pituitary or adrenal cortical function, and these effects may sometimes outlast treatment for a long time.

Bacterial infection associated with hemorrhage into the adrenal glands and a characteristic state of shock has been termed the *Waterhouse-Friderichsen syndrome*. Although the syndrome has been most often recognized in patients with fulminating meningococcemia, it also occurs with septicemia caused by other organisms. The circulatory collapse in patients with this syndrome has been attributed to impaired adrenal cortical function; in most patients, however, blood levels of corticoids are elevated. In some children, on the other hand, hemorrhagic adrenals at autopsy were associated with undetectable levels of serum corticoids. The circulatory collapse is in most instances probably the result of the severe toxemia, but may be aggravated by hypoadrenocorticism. The various lesions, including the adrenal hemorrhage, have been attributed to a generalized Shwartzman reaction.

A more common cause of adrenal insufficiency is a destructive lesion of the adrenal gland; this is referred to as *Addison's disease*. Tuberculosis, once the most frequent cause of Addison's disease, is no longer a large factor. Histoplasmosis, coccidioidomycosis, torulosis, mycosis fungoides, amyloidosis and metastatic malignancies have been identified as causative agents in adults, but not in children. A *"cytotoxic"* degeneration or idiopathic atrophy is noted in most instances. The adrenal glands may be so small that they are not visible at autopsy, and only remnants of tissue are found in microscopic sections. The medulla, however, is usually not destroyed, and there is lymphocytic infiltration in the area of the former cortex and in the medulla. Antibodies against adrenal tissue have been found in many patients and suggest an autoimmune basis for Addison's disease. In some instances adrenal antibodies have been demonstrated before the development of Addison's disease; there is no evidence, however, that the antibodies are themselves responsible for the disorder.

Addison's disease may occur as an isolated disorder; when it does, it is more apt to affect males. Often it occurs in association with other endocrinopathies, particularly hypoparathyroidism; lymphocytic thyroiditis, diabetes mellitus and gonadal abnormalities are less frequently associated. Hypoparathyroidism usually precedes development of Addison's disease; the reverse is less frequent. Other nonendocrine disorders such as partial or complete alopecia, pernicious anemia, juvenile cirrhosis and ocular abnormalities also occur in association with Addison's disease or hypoparathyroidism.

Another disorder commonly associated with Addison's disease is chronic mucocutaneous candidiasis. Although the candidiasis antedates the other disorders, there is no evidence to suggest that it causes any of them. The primary defect responsible for the concurrence of this varied assortment of disorders is probably a disturbed immune mechanism. Some patients have a defect in acquisition of delayed hypersensitivity.

The fundamental defect is thought to be inherited through an autosomal recessive gene, but affected siblings may exhibit heterogeneity of manifestations; e.g. one sibling may have adrenal insufficiency, and another hypoparathyroidism.

A few children with Addison's disease in association with *diffuse cerebral sclerosis* of the sudanophilic type have been reported. The age at onset of Addison's disease varied, but occurred as early as 3 years and usually antedated the neurologic manifestations by ½ to 2 years. That all the patients were males suggests that the syndrome is caused by an X-linked gene. Cutaneous pigmentation has been a striking feature in some cases; this indicates that corticotropin secretion is increased and that the adrenocortical atrophy is not secondary to a central nervous system defect.

Addison's disease has been described in association with *spastic paraplegia* in a few adult patients of both sexes.

Clinical Manifestations. *Acute adrenal cortical insufficiency* may be manifest abruptly and, if untreated, runs a rapidly fatal course. The patient suddenly becomes cyanotic; his skin is cold and clammy and his pulse rapid and weak. The blood

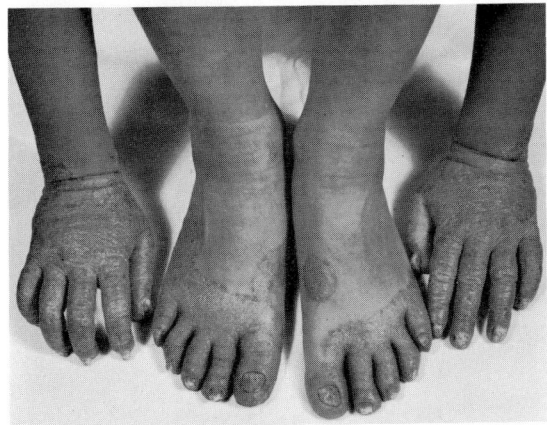

Figure 17-15. Chronic mucocutaneous candidiasis in a boy with Addison's disease. Candida infection was first noted on the tongue and buccal mucosa at 9 months; fingernails were first involved at 2 years of age. The lesions have resisted treatment and progressed to involve hands, feet and other cutaneous areas. Addison's disease developed at 8 years of age; no other endocrinopathies have developed by 10 years of age.

pressure falls, respirations are rapid and labored, and he becomes comatose. This symptom complex is known as *adrenal crisis;* it may occur in connection with any of the conditions listed in Table 17-3 in which a severe deficiency of cortisol and aldosterone occurs. Crises can also be precipitated in patients with inadequately treated chronic adrenal insufficiency by infection, trauma, excessive fatigue, or drugs such as morphine, barbiturates, laxatives, thyroid hormone or insulin.

In the *chronic form* the onset is more gradual and is characterized by weakness, lassitude, anorexia, loss of weight, vomiting and diarrhea. Abdominal pain may simulate an acute abdominal process. There may be an intense craving for salt. If water and salt are withheld, dehydration rapidly ensues and is followed by circulatory collapse and death. Other physical findings are muscular weakness, general wasting, low blood pressure and microcardia (Fig. 17-16). The presenting manifestations may be those of hypoglycemia. Increased pigmentation about the genitalia, umbilicus, axillae, nipples and joints may be seen in children with severe cortisol deficiency due to primary adrenal disease. It may be first apparent on the face and hands or, rarely, may be generalized. At times vitiligo-like pale spots may be interspersed with the dark areas. In the buccal mucosa the pigmentation is usually bluish-brown.

Laboratory Data. In adrenal cortical insufficiency the sodium and chloride concentrations in the serum are low, and that of potassium is elevated. Hypoglycemia may be striking, or it may not become manifest until after prolonged fasting. The oral glucose tolerance curve is relatively flat

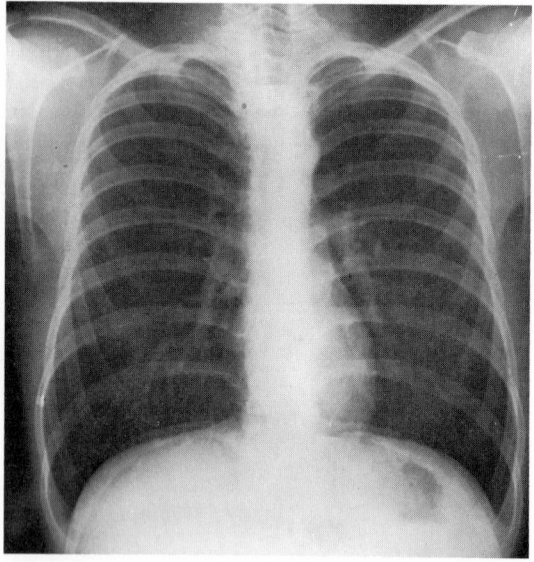

Figure 17-16. Addison's disease in a 10-year-old boy. On admission he was dehydrated; there was bronzing of the skin and hypotension. Note the microcardia characteristic of untreated Addison's disease. Hypoparathyroidism developed subsequently. One sibling had hypoparathyroidism and superficial moniliasis, and another died of Addison's disease.

for the first 2 hours, after which hypoglycemia may develop and be prolonged, leading to clinical symptoms. The nonprotein nitrogen and protein concentrations of the plasma are normal unless the patient is dehydrated. The urine may contain small amounts of protein and a few casts; the specific gravity tends to be low. There is an increase in the urinary excretion of sodium and chloride and a decrease in that of potassium.

The circulating eosinophils are usually increased in number, but may not be and may even be absent during crises. Since pronounced eosinopenia is usually present during acute infections when the function of the adrenal glands is adequate, a normal eosinophil count in the sick child is suggestive of impaired adrenal function. Roentgenograms of the abdomen occasionally reveal calcified areas in the region of the adrenals, especially when tuberculosis or hemorrhage has been the causative factor. A small and narrow roentgenographic shadow of the heart reflects the hypovolemia. Electrocardiographic changes are related to potassium levels, and abnormalities in the electroencephalogram include absence or a greatly decreased number of low-voltage, fast-frequency waves.

Tests of adrenal function permit confirmation of the diagnosis. The most definitive test is the measurement of urinary or plasma levels of corticosteroids before and after the administration of corticotropin. Resting levels of corticosteroids are low in the urine and plasma, and there is no increase after administration of corticotropin. In occasional instances the resting levels of corticosteroids are normal, but there is no increase after administration of corticotropin, indicating the absence of adrenocortical reserve. A low initial level followed by a significant increase in urinary or blood levels of corticosteroids may indicate adrenal insufficiency secondary to pituitary corticotropin insufficiency. When corticotropin deficiency is suspected, residual reserve of pituitary corticotropin can be evaluated by using an 11-beta hydroxylase inhibitor (p. 1206). The urinary 17-ketosteroids are decreased in men and absent in women with Addison's disease. These changes are not apparent in children until the immediate prepubertal years, when the 17-ketosteroids are normally excreted in significant amounts.

Prognosis. The mortality rate is high in infants and children with acute adrenal insufficiency unless the diagnosis is suspected and adequate replacement therapy is instituted. The prognosis in chronic adrenal insufficiency must be guarded despite the advances in therapy. Patients with this disorder are like those with diabetes in their need for constant supervision; acute crises may develop suddenly and on slight provocation. The patient may become dehydrated quickly during minor infections or periods of salt restriction, and death may ensue if therapy is not prompt or adequate.

Treatment. Treatment for *acute adrenal insufficiency* or for *crises* must be instituted immediately and must be vigorous. Five per cent glucose in saline solution is given intravenously at a rate permitting the administration of about 75 to 100 ml. per kg. per day. This may be modified, depending on the deficits of the patient. Administration of plasma or, in case of a low hemoglobin level or adrenal hemorrhage, whole blood is indicated. Concomitantly a water-soluble form of hydrocortisone, such as the sodium salt of the hemisuccinate, should be given intravenously. High levels may be achieved instantaneously in this manner; large doses can be used safely. As much as 25 mg. for infants and 50 mg. for young children may be given immediately and then continued by intravenous drip on the basis of the foregoing doses for each 6-hour period. Intramuscular administration of the steroid should be instituted when intravenous therapy is discontinued. Desoxycorticosterone acetate in oil should be added in doses of 1 to 5 mg. intramuscularly to maintain electrolyte balance.

Norepinephrine can be given intravenously in instances of shock and circulatory collapse. Four milligrams per liter may be added to the intravenous solution; the blood pressure should be measured at frequent intervals. Oxygen administration is indicated. In newborn infants with adrenal hemorrhage, vitamins K and C should also be given. In acute adrenal insufficiency associated with infection appropriate antibiotic therapy is essential.

Patients with *chronic adrenal insufficiency* (Addison's disease) require replacement therapy for their deficiencies of electrolyte-controlling hormones and of glucocorticosteroids. Desoxycorticosterone acetate (DOCA) is the salt-retaining hormone of choice in the initial regulation of the patient, though fluorohydrocortisone may be used for maintenance therapy. DOCA in sesame oil is administered intramuscularly in single daily injections; maintenance doses usually range from 1 to 3 mg. The dose depends upon the intake of sodium chloride, which must be kept constant while the maintenance dose is determined. The daily requirements of sodium chloride are usually 4 to 8 gm. in addition to that contained in the food; sodium chloride can be administered in 1-gm. enteric-coated tablets. During the first few months of treatment there is a gradual decrease in requirements for DOCA. After the maintenance dose has been determined, daily intramuscular administration can be replaced by use of the long-acting preparation, desoxycorticosterone trimethylacetate, a single intramuscular injection of which can provide a constant supply of the hormone for about a month. In lieu of intramuscular administration, subcutaneous implantation of pellets may be used. A pellet containing 125 mg. of DOCA is equivalent to daily injections of about 0.5 mg. of this drug for about 12 months.

When the salt-retaining hormone fluorohydrocortisone is administered in the place of DOCA, oral doses of 0.1 to 0.2 mg. daily are usually adequate.

Overdosage with DOCA or salt results in retention of sodium chloride and water and in excretion of excessive amounts of potassium; edema, hypertension, cardiac enlargement and muscular weakness or paralysis are clinical manifestations.

Hydrocortisone should also be administered to all patients with adrenocortical insufficiency in order to maintain normal carbohydrate metabolism and normal vigor. It may be given orally in doses of 5 to 20 mg. twice daily. During situations of stress, such as periods of infection or operative procedures, the dose of hydrocortisone should be increased. Antibiotic therapy is indicated for all infections, even minor ones, since they are poorly tolerated.

Hypoaldosteronism. When a selective deficiency of aldosterone is due to a defect either in the 18-hydroxylation of corticosterone or in the dehydrogenation of 18-hydroxycorticosterone (Fig. 17-17 and p. 1213), initial manifestations include poor feeding, occasional vomiting, and failure to gain weight; they progress to dehydration, shock and death. There is no unusual pigmentation. In mild cases, failure to thrive and poor growth may be the only manifestations, and serum electrolytes may be normal. Some adaptation or compensation appears to occur, since amelioration of the salt-losing manifestations is evident with increasing age. Some instances of transient adrenal insufficiency may be examples of a mild defect or of delayed maturation of the 18-hydroxylation enzyme system. Hyponatremia and hyperkalemia are usually present. Urinary 17-ketosteroids, cortisol and pregnanetriol are normal. Aldosterone secretion rate is decreased, especially considering the state of sodium depletion. Renin activity is elevated. In the defect involving dehydrogenation of 18-hydroxycorticosterone this latter substance accumulates in the urine and gives a positive Porter-Silber reaction. Porter-Silber chromagens are elevated in this condition; they are not suppressed by dexamethasone, but are decreased by administration of DOCA and salt. This provides a method for detection of the syndrome. Treatment is by DOCA and salt. The disorder must be differentiated from all the other causes of salt-losing syndromes.

ADRENAL CORTICAL HYPERFUNCTION

Four syndromes are attributable to hyperadrenocorticism: the *adrenogenital syndrome, Cushing's syndrome, hyperaldosteronism* and *feminization* (Table 17-4). The adrenogenital syndrome results from hypersecretion of androgenic hormones; it may be due to a congenital defect in steroidogenesis or may be acquired, caused by a tumor of the adrenal cortex. Cushing's syndrome resulting from hypersecretion of hydrocortisone and primary hyperaldosteronism resulting from excessive secretion of aldosterone may also be due either to adrenal hyperplasia or to a tumor.

(see text).

TABLE 17-4. CLASSIFICATION OF ADRENAL CORTICAL HYPERFUNCTION

I. **Excess androgen secretion (adrenogenital syndrome)**
   A. Congenital adrenal hyperplasia
      1. 21-hydroxylase defect
      2. 11-hydroxylase defect
      3. 3-beta-hydroxysteroid dehydrogenase defect
   B. Tumor
      1. Carcinoma
      2. Benign adenoma

II. **Excess cortisol secretion (Cushing's syndrome)**
   A. Bilateral adrenal hyperplasia
      1. Origin unknown (hypothalamic origin?)
      2. Pituitary corticotropin-producing tumor?
      3. Extra-adrenal corticotropin-producing tumor
      4. Exogenous corticotropin
   B. Tumor
      1. Carcinoma
      2. Benign adenoma

III. **Excess mineralocorticoid secretion (hypertensive hypokalemic syndrome)**
   A. Primary hyperaldosteronism*
      1. Adrenal hyperplasia
         a. Congenital aldosteronism
         b. Partial 17-hydroxylase defect
      2. Tumor
         a. Carcinoma
         b. Benign adenoma
   B. Desoxycorticosterone excess
      1. Adrenal hyperplasia
         a. 11-hydroxylase defect
         b. 17-hydroxylase defect
      2. Tumor
         a. Carcinoma

IV. **Excess estrogen secretion (adrenal feminization syndrome)**
   A. Tumor
      1. Carcinoma
      2. Adenoma

V. **Mixed hypercorticism**
   A. Tumor

*Excess aldosterone secretion also occurs secondarily to a variety of other disorders (see text).

Feminization resulting from excessive adrenal production of estrogen has been observed only with adrenal tumors.

ADRENOGENITAL SYNDROME

Congenital Adrenal Hyperplasia

Pathogenesis. This disorder is caused by an inborn defect of biosynthesis of certain steroids of the adrenal cortex, the primary disturbance being an inability to synthesize hydrocortisone from its precursors. The deficiency of hydrocortisone, a potent inhibitor of pituitary activity, results in increased secretion of corticotropin, which in turn leads to adrenocortical hyperplasia and overproduction of intermediary metabolites and of androgens. Administration of hydrocortisone or one of its analogues inhibits the production of corticotropin, which in turn results in reduced production of androgens.

Four distinct enzymatic defects of adrenal steroid biogenesis are known to result in the adrenogenital syndrome.

1. The most common form of the disorder is due to a deficiency of *21-hydroxylase*. Excess production of adrenal androgens results in pseudohermaphroditism in the female and in premature virilization in the male. Urinary metabolites consist predominantly of C-21 methylsteroids; large amounts of pregnanetriol are also constantly present. Most affected persons produce small amounts of hydrocortisone, but sufficient to maintain electrolyte balance. When salt-losing manifestations are present, the defect is complete, and there is no synthesis of hydrocortisone. Complete deficiency of 21-hydroxylase also results in failure of synthesis of aldosterone.

2. A much less common defect is deficiency of *11-hydroxylase*. Large amounts of the immediate precursor of hydrocortisone, compound S, are characteristically present in the urine. Hypertension is an almost constant clinical manifestation and is attributed to the sodium retention caused by the excessive formation of desoxycorticosterone. Only moderate amounts of pregnanetriol are found in the urine. These patients are virilized to the same degree as those with the 21-hydroxylase defect. The hypertension as well as the virilization is relieved by treatment with hydrocortisone.

3. A rare defect is lack of *3-beta-hydroxysteroid dehydrogenase*. Affected persons are salt-losers, and the males are usually incompletely virilized. This enzyme is required for the biosynthesis of testicular hormones, and its absence in fetal testes probably explains the incomplete virilization of affected newborn males.

4. Another rare defect is the failure of conversion of cholesterol into pregnenolone, presumably due to the absence of one of the 3 enzymes needed for this conversion (Fig. 17-17). A large accumulation of lipids and cholesterol in the adrenal cortex results in the condition known as congenital *lipoid adrenal hyperplasia*. Total failure of synthesis of any adrenal steroids results in salt-losing manifestations, and urinary 17-ketosteroids are not elevated. The enzymatic defect also prevents synthesis of testicular hormones, and males with this condition are completely feminized, whereas females exhibit no genital abnormalities. All infants with the complete defect have died in early infancy, but an incompletely masculinized male with partial defect did not exhibit symptoms of hypoadrenalism until 7 months of age and survived until 10 months of age.

Congenital adrenal hyperplasia is inherited as an autosomal recessive trait. Each defect is

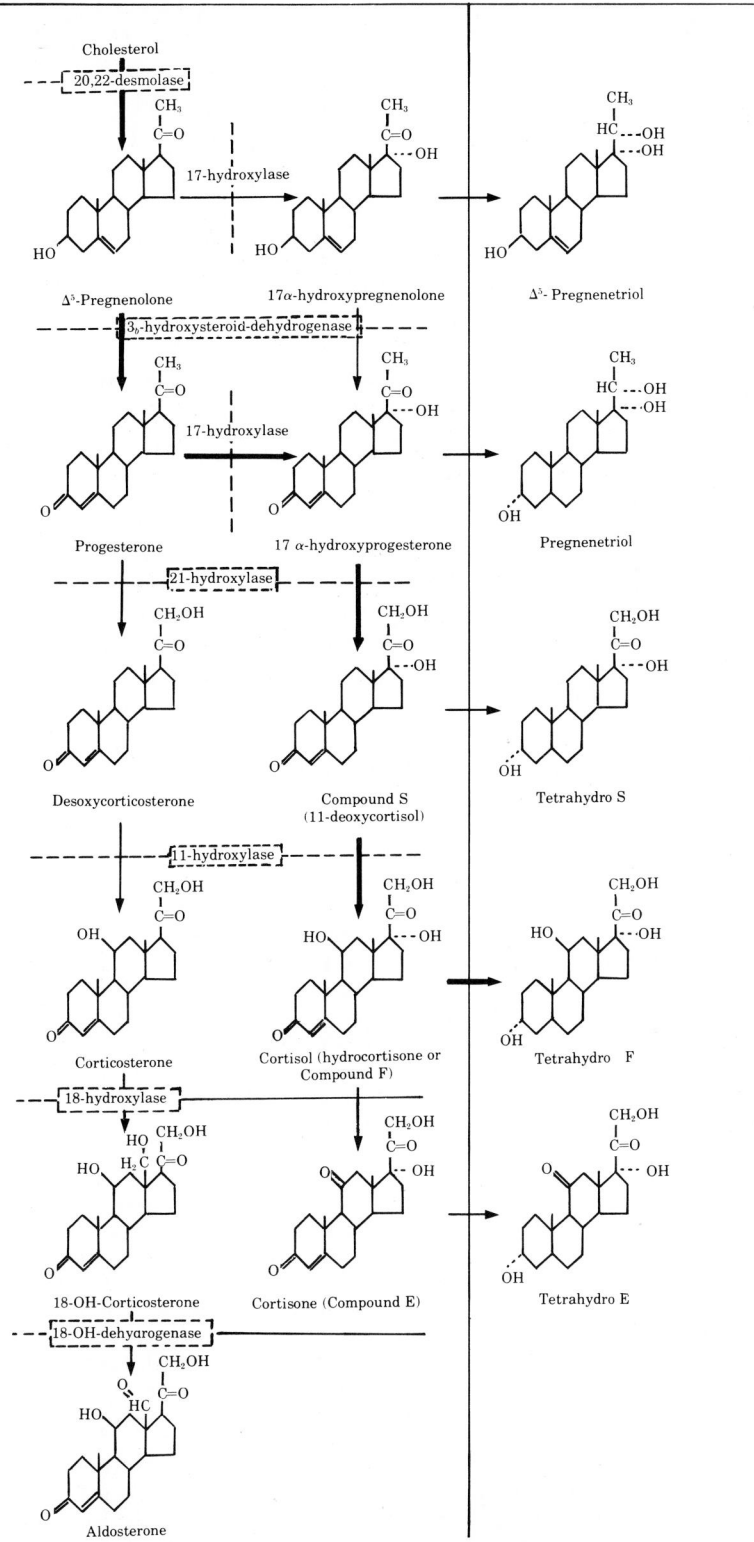

Figure 17-17. The synthesis of hydrocortisone is shown to the left of the vertical line. The heavy arrows indicate the principal pathway, and the light arrows show alternate pathways of steroid genesis. The enzymatic defects which cause virilizing adrenal hyperplasia and the defects in aldosterone synthesis are shown by horizontal dotted lines. Vertical dotted lines show the defect in 17-hydroxylation. To the right of the vertical line are each of the predominant urinary metabolites found in patients with one of these enzymatic defects, as well as the normal urinary metabolites.

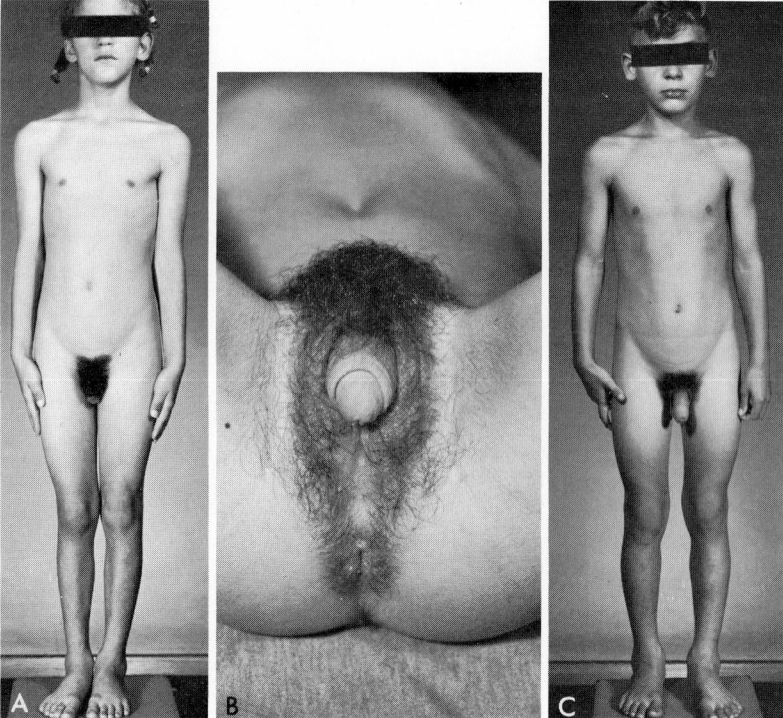

Figure 17-18. *A*, A 6-year-old girl with congenital virilizing adrenal hyperplasia. Height age, 8½ years; bone-age, 13 years; urinary 17-ketosteroids, 50 mg. in 24 hours. *B*, Note clitoral enlargement and labial fusion. *C*, Five-year-old brother of girl in *A* was not considered abnormal by parents. Height age 8 years, bone-age, 12½ years, urinary 17-ketosteroids, 36 mg. in 24 hours.

genetically specific; if one form occurs in a family, subsequently affected infants will have the same defect.

Clinical Manifestations in the Most Common Form of Congenital Virilizing Adrenal Hyperplasia. Approximately 90 per cent of patients with virilizing adrenal hyperplasia have the defect in 21-hydroxylation.

In the *male* the main clinical manifestations are those of premature isosexual development. The infant usually appears normal at birth, but signs of sexual and somatic precocity may appear within the first half-year of life or develop more gradually and not become evident until 4 or 5 years of age or later (Fig. 17-18). Enlargement of the penis, scrotum and prostate, appearance of pubic hair, and development of acne and of a deep voice are noted. The muscles are well developed, and the bone age is advanced for the chronologic age (infant Hercules; macrogenitosomia praecox). Owing to premature closure of the epiphyses, growth stops relatively early, and the adult stature is stunted.

The testes are normal in size, so that they appear relatively small in contrast to the enlarged penis. Occasionally, ectopic adrenocortical cells are present in the testes of patients with adrenal hyperplasia; these cells may become hyperplastic just as the adrenal glands do and produce enlargement of the testes. Spermatogenesis does not take place. Mental development is usually normal, but

the abnormal physical development may result in behavioral problems.

In the *female*, congenital adrenal hyperplasia results in female pseudohermaphroditism. Since the disorder of steroidogenesis begins early in fetal life, there are almost always evidences of some degree of masculinization of the female fetus. It is manifest at birth by enlargement of the clitoris and variable degrees of labial fusion. The vagina has a common opening with the urethra (urogenital sinus). The clitoris may be so enlarged that it resembles a penis, and, since the urethra opens below this organ, a mistaken diagnosis of hypospadias and cryptorchidism is often made. Occasionally the urogenital sinus extends to the tip of the phallus, and the genitalia resemble those of a cryptorchid male. The severity of the virilization is in general greater in infants who are salt-losers than in those who are not. The internal genital organs are those of a normal female.

After birth the masculinization progresses. Pubic and axillary hair develops prematurely, acne appears, and the voice assumes a masculine quality. These girls are tall for their age, ossification is advanced for their age, and they show good muscular development and, in general, have the body build of a boy. Although the internal genitalia are female, breast development and menstruation do not occur unless the excessive production of androgens is suppressed by adequate treatment.

Hypoglycemia occurs only rarely in patients

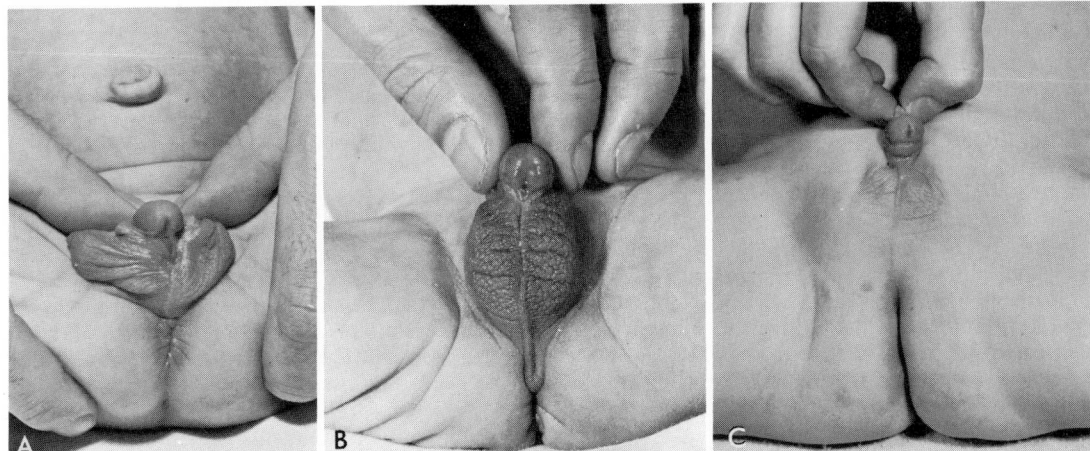

Figure 17-19. Three female pseudohermaphrodites with untreated congenital adrenal hyperplasia. All were erroneously assigned male sex at birth, and each had normal female sex-chromosome complement. Infants A and B were salt-losers and were diagnosed in early infancy. Infant C was referred at 1 year of age because of bilateral cryptorchidism. Note completely penile urethra; such complete degrees of masculinization in females with adrenal hyperplasia are not extremely rare, but most such infants are salt-losers.

with virilizing adrenal hyperplasia. Another rare manifestation in these patients is periodic fever, which has been attributed to excessive circulating levels of unconjugated etiocholanolone, a steroid known to provoke fever in man.

Manifestations Specific for Each Enzymatic Defect. *21-Hydroxylase defect.* Symptoms characteristic of adrenal cortical insufficiency are seen in approximately one third of the infants with the 21-hydroxylase defect; they are referred to as *"salt-losers."* The symptoms begin during the first month of life in more than 90 per cent of infants so affected. Anorexia, vomiting, diarrhea, loss of weight and extreme dehydration are the outstanding manifestations. Restriction of fluid and salt intake results in sudden collapse and death.

The salt-losing defect is a genetically specific form of the disorder. Since the defect is transmitted as a recessive autosomal trait, boys and girls are affected with equal frequency. The diagnosis is established more frequently, however, in females than in males, because the hermaphroditic external genitalia direct attention to the correct diagnosis. In the male the clinical manifestations are more apt to lead to the incorrect diagnosis of pyloric stenosis, intestinal obstruction or a diarrheal disorder. Disturbances in cardiac rate and rhythm, with cyanosis and dyspnea, may erroneously suggest heart disease; electrocardiograms, however, reveal the changes of hyperkalemia.

The mechanism for salt wasting is unknown. Patients with the salt-losing form of the disorder have a more complete enzymatic block of 21-hydroxylation, and their rate of aldosterone secretion is decreased. In the simple virilizing form of the disorder the enzymatic defect is incomplete and aldosterone secretion is normal. Intermediate cases are also known in which the

salt-losing tendency is noted only under conditions of stress or sodium deprivation. Since renin levels are elevated in these infants, it has been suggested that in the salt-loser natriuresis may be aggravated by high levels of angiotensin. The familial homogeneity of each type suggests 2 different genetic defects of the 21-hydroxylating enzyme.

11-Hydroxylase defect. The association of clinical manifestations of virilizing adrenal hyperplasia with hypertension is strong presumptive evidence for a defect in 11-hydroxylation. Salt-losing manifestations are rarely, if ever, seen with this defect.

3-Beta-hydroxysteroid dehydrogenase defect. Males with this defect are incompletely virilized and have hypospadias with or without cryptorchidism. Severe salt-losing manifestations are almost always present, and most of the recognized patients have succumbed in infancy.

Laboratory Data. The 3 forms of virilizing adrenal hyperplasia are characterized by higher than normal levels of urinary 17-ketosteroids for the age of the patient. Young infants may excrete as much as 10 mg. in a 24-hour period, and older patients as much as 80 mg. or more. Owing to the somewhat normally elevated 17-ketosteroid levels during the first few days of life (2 to 3 mg. per day), there may be difficulty in diagnosis at this time, and repeated determinations may be indicated. The urinary concentration of pregnanetriol, the metabolite for 17-hydroxyprogesterone, is elevated to diagnostic levels in patients with the usual form of the disorder (21-hydroxylase defect). Urinary gonadotropins may be at adult levels; presumably the compensatory pituitary hyperactivity involves not only corticotropin, but also gonadotropin secretion. The plasma level of testosterone, derived from adrenal androgens, is markedly elevated and accounts in large measure for the virilization.

In the hypertensive form of the disorder (11-hydroxylase defect), urinary concentration of pregnanetriol is only moderately increased, but increased urinary concentration of tetrahydro S is characteristic.

The 3-hydroxysteroid dehydrogenase defect is characterized by the presence of compounds with the Δ^5-3β-OH configuration.

Female pseudohermaphrodites with virilizing adrenal hyperplasia are chromatin-positive and have normal chromosomes for a female. Roentgenograms taken after injection of contrast medium into the urogenital sinus may demonstrate the vagina and the uterus. Osseous maturation is advanced; the degree depends on the severity of the disorder and the age of the patient before treatment.

"Salt-losers" have low serum concentrations of sodium and chloride and elevated levels of potassium and nonprotein nitrogen. Elevation of the serum potassium level may be responsible for electrocardiographic abnormalities.

Diagnosis. A history of congenital adrenal hyperplasia in siblings should always alert one to the diagnosis. The salt-losing form of the disorder must be suspected in any infant who fails to thrive and especially in female infants with ambiguous external genitalia. When virilization occurs postnatally, in either the male or female, a virilizing adrenocortical tumor must be considered in the differential diagnosis.

An adrenal tumor may be palpable or suggested by displacement of the adjacent kidney as demonstrated by pyelography. Urinary 17-ketosteroid excretion is elevated with congenital hyperplasia and with cortical tumors, but very high values favor the diagnosis of a neoplasm. Large amounts of urinary pregnanetriol are highly suggestive of adrenal hyperplasia. A therapeutic test with a corticosteroid is a reliable differential procedure; administration of cortisone or one of its analogues quickly reduces excretion of urinary 17-ketosteroids to normal levels in patients with congenital adrenal hyperplasia, but does not do so in those with a virilizing tumor. Cortisone, by inhibiting secretion of corticotropin, reduces the excessive stimulation of the adrenals in patients with hyperplasia, whereas adrenal cortical tumors are not subject to pituitary regulation.

In males with virilization an interstitial cell tumor of the testis and true precocious puberty must also be considered in differential diagnosis. In true precocious puberty, gonadotropins may be present in the urine; the urinary 17-ketosteroid level is never above normal adult values; pregnanetriol is not found in the urine; the testes are usually well developed, and interstitial cells may be seen in biopsy specimens.

Females with this condition must be differentiated from those with other causes for ambiguity of the external genitalia. Only in this condition, however, are urinary 17-ketosteroids elevated. Males with the 3-beta-hydroxysteroid dehydrogenase defect may be confused with female pseudohermaphrodites, owing to lack of normal virilization of the external genitalia. These male patients are chromatin-negative and do not have elevated urinary pregnanetriol levels; they are thus easily differentiated from the chromatin-positive female pseudohermaphrodite.

Treatment. Hydrocortisone is effective in inhibiting excessive production of adrenal androgens and in stemming the progressive virilization. The maintenance dose may be administered orally as follows: 10 to 20 mg. per day to children under 5 years of age; 20 to 30 mg. per day to children between 5 and 12; 30 to 50 mg. per day after 12 years of age. These doses should be divided into 2 or 3 daily administrations. Such amounts suppress excessive secretion of androgens without producing undesirable effects. Analogues of hydrocortisone or cortisone are effective in suppressing adrenal androgens, but do not provide complete physiologic replacement; they are therefore contraindicated in the treatment of adrenal hyperplasia. Repeated determinations of the urinary excretion of 17-ketosteroids and pregnanetriol and careful measurements of growth are important guides in determining the adequacy of dosage.

Patients who have a disturbance of electrolyte regulation ("salt-losers") must have a high salt intake and receive desoxycorticosterone acetate in addition to hydrocortisone. Dehydrated infants may require 4 to 8 gm. of sodium chloride for adequate replacement therapy during the first 24 hours. For maintenance, 2 to 6 gm. of salt per day should be added to the diet, and 2 to 5 mg. of DOCA should be given daily by intramuscular injection. After the maintenance dose of DOCA has been determined, we prefer the subcutaneous implantation of pellets of DOCA for long-term maintenance. When the pellets are exhausted, usually in a year, oral therapy is instituted with fluorohydrocortisone, in once daily doses of 0.1 to 0.2 mg. This medication is continued indefinitely in salt-losers.

The administration of hydrocortisone must be continued indefinitely in *all* patients. Increased doses are indicated during periods of stress such as infection or surgery, or during periods of decreased salt intake; this is true not only of "salt-losers," but also of all patients, including those with the 11-hydroxylase defect, since they all have defective adrenal reserve. Surgical correction of the abnormal genitalia of females is best performed before 2 years of age. When treatment is instituted early in life, normal sexual maturation occurs at the usual time. If the osseous age is in the pubertal age range when treatment is begun, true precocious puberty develops.

Virilizing Adrenocortical Tumor

Tumors of the adrenal cortex may result in masculinization in girls and pseudoprecocious puberty in boys. Hypertension is common in both sexes. *In males* the symptoms are usually the same as those occurring with congenital adrenal hyperplasia. It is virtually impossible to differentiate the 2 conditions on clinical grounds. *In females* virilizing tumors of the adrenal cause masculinization of a previously normal female, whereas congenital adrenal hyperplasia is almost always associated with genital abnormalities at birth (p. 1212). There have been a few instances of adrenal hyperplasia in which virilization had its onset postnatally, and an adrenal adenoma is known to have caused intrauterine virilization manifest by clitoral enlargement and mild labial fusion.

These tumors are frequently associated with other congenital defects, particularly hemihypertrophy, genitourinary tract and central nervous system abnormalities, and hamartomatous defects. Patients also appear to have a proclivity to other malignancies such as astrocytomas. Urinary 17-ketosteroids are usually markedly increased and may exceed 100 mg. per day; on occasion, however, only modest elevations are found. The differential diagnosis of virilizing adrenal hyperplasia and adrenal cortical tumor is discussed on page 1216.

The treatment is surgical; a transperitoneal approach is usually recommended. Some of these neoplasms are highly malignant and metastasize widely, but cure with regression of the masculinizing features may follow removal of less malignant encapsulated tumors.

A neoplasm of one adrenal may be responsible for atrophy of the other one, owing to excessive production of cortical hormones by the tumor and suppression of the normal gland. Consequently adrenal insufficiency may follow surgical removal of the tumor. This situation can be avoided by giving 100 mg. of cortisone daily, starting on the day of operation and continuing for 3 or 4 days postoperatively. It may also be necessary to give corticotropin concurrently with cortisone to reactivate the atrophied gland. Adequate quantities of water, sodium chloride and glucose must also be provided. On rare occasions the tumors are bilateral and in at least 5 instances the contralateral adrenal was absent; in such instances, replacement therapy must be continued indefinitely.

The recurrence rate of these tumors is high. Urinary excretion of 17-ketosteroids returns to normal postoperatively if removal of the tumor is complete. The 17-ketosteroid level should be measured at monthly intervals to detect recurrences early. Intensive therapy with o,p′ DDD, an isomer of DDD, is indicated for inoperable tumors and for recurrences. This agent can induce regression of metastases and of abnormal steroid excretion, but no cures have been recorded.

CUSHING'S SYNDROME

Cushing's syndrome, a characteristic pattern of obesity in association with hypertension, is the result of maintenance of abnormally high blood levels of hydrocortisone caused by hyperfunction of the adrenal cortex.

The adrenal lesion in infants is often a *functioning tumor*, which is usually a malignant cortical carcinoma; only rarely is it a benign cortical adenoma or bilateral nodular cortical hyperplasia. Patients with cortical tumors often exhibit a mixed form of hypercorticism, owing to overproduction of such other steroids as androgens, estrogens and aldosterone.

Bilateral hyperplasia of the adrenal glands is found more frequently than a tumor in children over 10 years of age. In only a small percentage of such cases is a pituitary tumor demonstrable at the time of initial diagnosis of Cushing's syndrome.

Although the initiating factor for the adrenal hyperplasia is not known, a hypothalamic disturbance is suspected. When Harvey Cushing described the entity in 1932 he attributed it to a basophilic adenoma of the pituitary. Such tumors are rarely demonstrable before treatment, but a number of patients have had pituitary tumors months or years after total adrenalectomy. In this form of adrenal hyperplasia there is increased secretion of corticotropin, loss of normal circadian rhythm in its concentrations in serum, and relative resistance to suppression of its secretion by glucocorticoids. This and other evidence suggest that the primary defect may be in the hypothalamus and that pituitary tumors result from overstimulation of the pituitary by the cerebral defect.

Cushing's syndrome with bilateral adrenal hyperplasia has been found occasionally in association with pheochromocytoma or other functioning neural tumors. It has been suggested that excessive secretion of catecholamines may cause the adrenal hyperplasia in these instances.

Cushing's syndrome may be associated with *extra-adrenal tumors*, such as malignant tumors of the thymus or pancreas, and particularly of the respiratory tract; such an association has been reported in a 2-year-old boy with an islet cell tumor of the pancreas. These tumors produce substances with ACTH-like activity which stimulate the adrenal cortex to produce excessive hydrocortisone.

Prolonged exogenous administration of corticotropin or hydrocortisone or its analogues results in a clinical pattern identical to the spontaneous disorder and is frequently referred to as "cushingoid syndrome."

Clinical Manifestations. Symptoms may begin in the neonatal period or at any time thereafter. In this form of adrenocortical hyperfunction, the "buffalo" type of obesity is a characteristic pattern, though generalized obesity is more frequent. The characteristic appearance of patients is determined by the accumulation of fat on the cheeks, chin and upper parts of the trunk; sometimes there is a relative lack of fat on the extremities. In spite of their monstrous appearance, such patients are not much above average weight, and they are frequently stunted in growth.

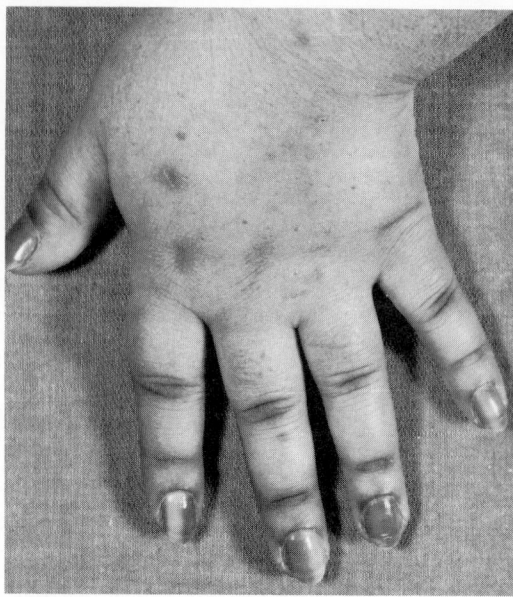

Figure 17-20. Pigmentation of skin in a 12-year-old girl with postadrenalectomy pituitary tumor. Note pigmentation of nails and skin folds. Adrenalectomy was performed for Cushing's syndrome due to bilateral adrenal hyperplasia when the girl was 10 years of age. Pigmentation, headaches and enlargement of the sella turcica developed 1 year after adrenalectomy.

The skin appears plethoric, and the cheeks, in particular, are intensely red; acne is a frequent manifestation even in very young children. Purplish striae on the hips, abdomen and thighs are seen mainly in older children. There is hypertrichosis on the face, trunk and in the pubic region. The voice becomes deep and coarse. In girls the clitoris is frequently enlarged. Sometimes breast development and menstruation begin precociously. Thus signs of abnormal masculinization and feminization may be seen simultaneously in such girls. Cessation of the menses is a common manifestation in postpubertal girls. In boys the external genitalia are usually normal, but evidence of virilization may be present. The blood pressure is elevated, the heart often enlarged, and cerebral hemorrhage may occur. Patients with pituitary tumors may have oculomotor or optic involvement or may exhibit hyperpigmentation, whereas patients with adrenal tumors may have a palpable abdominal mass. The mentality is initially normal, but as the disease progresses the children frequently become listless, apathetic and dull. Cushing's disease in childhood may have a gradual onset with obesity and deceleration or cessation of growth as the only manifestations.

Laboratory Data. The red blood cell count and hemoglobin level are usually in the range of high normal values, and there is usually an eosinopenia. The blood glucose level may be high, and there may be glycosuria. On occasion there may be high serum concentrations of sodium and bicarbonate and a decrease in that of potassium. Patients with Cushing's syndrome have elevated levels of corticosteroids in blood and urine; elevation of free cortisol in urine is particularly characteristic. These levels may fluctuate from day to day, and repeated determinations may be required to establish the diagnosis. The urinary output of 17-ketosteroids may also be increased. Ossification may be normal or advanced for the patient's age, and there may be osteoporosis with spontaneous fractures. The pituitary sella is enlarged in 10 to 15 per cent of patients with adrenal hyperplasia; an unusually small pituitary fossa is occasionally seen in patients with adrenal tumors.

Special studies are usually necessary to establish the diagnosis and to differentiate the various causes of the syndrome, and multiple tests may be necessary, particularly in those children with adrenal hyperplasia who have only moderate symptomatology. Evaluation of diurnal variation of serum corticoid levels is a useful test. In approximately 90 per cent of patients with Cushing's syndrome the normal diurnal rhythm is abolished; false-positive results are frequently noted, however, particularly in patients with central nervous system disorders.

One of the most valuable and simple screening tests is based on the lack of the usual suppressive effect of dexamethasone on the blood cortisol level in patients with Cushing's syndrome. One microgram of the drug is administered at 11 p.m. and the blood cortisol level is determined at 8 a.m. the next morning. Blood cortisol levels over 10 micrograms per 100 ml. are found in over 95 per cent of patients with Cushing's syndrome, and only rarely in other patients. A positive response is an indication for additional tests of pituitary suppression of adrenal function. For example, administration of 0.5 mg. of dexamethasone every 6 hours for 2 days results in reduction of urinary excretion of corticosteroids to less than 2.5 mg. per 24 hours on the second day of the test in normal persons, but not in patients with Cushing's syndrome. The same test with a larger dose, 2 mg. every 6 hours for 2 days, results in a 50 per cent or greater decrease in excretion of corticosteroids on the second day of the test in 80 per cent of patients with Cushing's syndrome due to bilateral adrenal hyperplasia, but only rarely in those with adrenal cortical tumors.

Cushing's syndrome is frequently suspected in children with obesity, particularly when there are striae and hypertension. Differential diagnosis is complicated by the frequent occurrence of elevated urinary concentrations of corticosteroids in obese persons. The increased cortisol production is thought to be secondary to the obesity and not a cause of it. Rapid suppression of excretion of corticosteroids is induced by oral administration of dexamethasone in persons with simple obesity.

Treatment. Since an adrenal tumor accounts for many instances of Cushing's syndrome in children, treatment is primarily surgical. If the lesion is a benign cortical adenoma, unilateral adrenalectomy is indicated. Benign cortical adenomas causing Cushing's syndrome are occasionally bilateral; in such instances the treatment of choice is subtotal adrenalectomy. In either instance an excellent therapeutic result is achieved by removal of the tumor. Adrenal cortical carcinomas, on the other hand, frequently metastasize, especially to the liver and lungs, and the prognosis may be unfavorable, in spite of the removal of the primary lesion. Treatment with o,p′ DDD or aminoglutethimide is warranted in such instances.

There is lack of consensus as to the optimal treatment of bilateral adrenal hyperplasia. Some recommend subtotal adrenalectomy, others prefer bilateral adrenalectomy. After subtotal adrenalectomy the remaining segment of the adrenal frequently undergoes hyperplasia, and symptoms recur. After complete adrenalectomy a significant number of patients subsequently exhibit a tumor of the pituitary. The appearance of increasing pigmentation of the skin despite adequate replacement therapy with cortisone after total adrenalectomy is usually the first evidence of a pituitary tumor. Increased synthesis of melanocyte-stimulating hormone by the tumor accounts for the pigmentation.

In order to avoid these complications of adrenalectomy, therapy of adrenal hyperplasia by external irradiation of the pituitary or by implantation of radioactive substances into the pituitary is under investigation. Treatment of adrenal hyperplasia with aminoglutethimide has been attempted, but this agent appears to have limited usefulness.

Management of adrenalectomy requires adequate preoperative and postoperative replacement therapy with a corticosteroid. Tumors which produce corticosteroids usually cause atrophy of the opposite adrenal, and replacement therapy with both cortisone and corticotropin is required. Patients with adrenal hyperplasia must be carefully watched after adrenalectomy for the development of a pituitary tumor, most likely to be a chromophobe adenoma. Periodic examinations of the pituitary fossa and of the ocular system are essential.

EXCESS MINERALOCORTICOID SECRETION

The principal mineralocorticoid secreted by the adrenal is aldosterone. Increased secretion may result from a primary defect of the adrenal (primary hyperaldosteronism) or from factors which activate the renin-angiotensin system (secondary hyperaldosteronism). When excess mineralocorticoid secretion occurs, hypertension or hypokalemia is usually present, except in those patients who have secondary hyperaldosteronism.

Desoxycorticosterone is a precursor of aldosterone with only about one thirtieth the sodium-retaining potency of aldosterone (see Fig. 17-17), and overproduction of desoxycorticosterone occurs in 2 different defects of adrenal steroidogenesis. The first of these is a defect in 11-hydroxylation, which also leads to androgen excess and presents clinically as the hypertensive form of the adrenogenital syndrome (p. 1215). The second defect involves 17-hydroxylation, and presents as hypogonadism since the defect impairs the synthesis of androgens and estrogens as well as of adrenal steroids.

Desoxycorticosterone excess (17-hydroxylase deficiency) has recently been described in several young adult women with hypertension, hypokalemia and lack of sexual maturation. A deficiency of 17-hydroxylation in adrenal and ovary was deduced from study of steroids in blood and urine; corticotropin, desoxycorticosterone and corticosterone were present in excess, whereas cortisol, estrogens and androgens were deficient. Low levels of aldosterone and of renin in these patients may reflect inhibition of the renin-angiotensin system by the high level of mineralocorticoid synthesis. In 2 children with almost identical findings, aldosterone secretion was increased. A partial 17-hydroxylase defect has been proposed to explain these findings. The father of one child and the mother of the other were similarly affected. In both the adult and the juvenile cases the hypertension responded dramatically to administration of adrenal suppressive therapy such as with prednisone or dexamethasone.

Primary hyperaldosteronism occurs most often in the third and fourth decades of life and is rare in childhood. The most common cause in affected adults is a functioning adrenal cortical tumor (aldosteronoma). Such tumors have been found in 5 children, the youngest being a 3-year-old child. In another 10 children, hyperaldosteronism has been associated with adrenal hyperplasia of unknown origin; the term *congenital aldosteronism* has been used to describe this condition. Demonstration of low renin levels provides strong supportive evidence for a primary adrenal defect; this was the case in the 2 instances in which it was measured. Since most patients improved after resection of the adrenal, it is presumed that the adrenal disorder is primary in these children. Clinical manifestations always include hypertension; it is usually severe and leads to retinopathy and cardiomegaly.

Secondary hyperaldosteronism. Aldosterone secretion is increased in conditions in which there are low body sodium, excessive accumulation of potassium, and dehydration; it is a normal homeostatic response. Hyperaldosteronism also occurs in many common disorders such as the nephrotic syndrome, congestive cardiac failure and cirrhosis of the liver. Since the extracellular fluid volume is increased in these conditions, the mechanism for the increased aldosterone excretion is paradoxical and unknown. Increased secretion of aldosterone may also occur in conditions in which renin is increased, such as in stenoses of the renal artery and in malignant or essential hypertension.

BARTTER'S SYNDROME is characterized by hypochloremia, hypokalemic alkalosis, normal blood pressure, growth failure and increased secretion of renin and aldosterone. Renal biopsy reveals hyperplasia of the juxtaglomerular apparatus. Since infusion of angiotensin II fails to raise the blood pressure of affected patients, it is postulated that the primary defect is an inherited hypo-responsiveness of the blood vessels to angiotensin II. This results in increased production of renin, which in turn results in increased production of angiotensin and stimulation of aldosterone secretion.

PSEUDOHYPOALDOSTERONISM has been described in 5 male infants with a salt-losing syndrome despite hyperaldosteronism. Evidence suggests that these infants have a renal tubular insensi-tivity to salt-retaining hormones and that the increased aldosterone secretion is a compensatory mechanism. Administration of salt suppresses secretion of aldosterone and alleviates the symp-toms. In most instances the salt supplementation could be discontinued during the second year of age.

Clinical Manifestations. Besides hyperten-sion, excess production of mineralocorticoids may produce polydipsia, polyuria, nocturia, pares-thesias, visual disturbance, intermittent paralysis, tetany, fatigue and muscle weakness and dis-comfort. The severe growth retardation and mus-cular weakness which may occur are probably caused by potassium depletion.

The urine is neutral or alkaline, and the kid-neys lose their ability to concentrate urine normally. The serum pH, carbon dioxide content and sodium concentrations are elevated, and the serum potassium, chloride and magnesium levels are decreased. Tetany occurs in spite of normal serum levels of calcium. Urinary excretion of 17-ketosteroids and 17-hydroxycorticosteroids is within normal limits, but urinary excretion of aldosterone is increased. The abnormalities of renal function are attributed to "clear-cell ne-phrosis," a lesion characteristic of chronic hypo-kalemia.

Diagnosis. In patients with hypertension and increased excretion of aldosterone it may be difficult to separate primary from secondary hyper-aldosteronism. Urinary aldosterone levels are only moderately increased in any case, and it is essential to the diagnosis of primary aldosteronism to demonstrate relative unresponsiveness to sodium restriction and administration of sodium. The most important diagnostic finding is the low level of serum renin during sodium restriction. In secondary hyperaldosteronism, serum renin is high or rises during a low salt diet, whereas in primary adrenal hypersecretion of aldosterone the renin-angiotensin system is suppressed.

Treatment. Differentiation of children with functioning adrenal adenomas from those with adrenal hyperplasia can be established only by exploratory laparotomy. A course of therapy with prednisone is indicated preoperatively in all patients in order to eliminate the possibility of a partial 17-hydroxylase defect.

Removal of an aldosteronoma results in cure. The electrolyte abnormality is usually corrected within 10 days, but the blood pressure may not return to normal for several months after opera-tion. In instances of congenital aldosteronism bilateral adrenalectomy is indicated; the results are excellent. Adrenal replacement therapy is, of course, required.

FEMINIZING ADRENAL TUMORS

Adrenocortical tumors associated with excessive production of estrogens with feminization have been recorded in 56 males, but only 4 of these patients were children. Gynecomastia, the initial clinical manifestation, developed between 2 and 7 years of age. Growth and development may be normal, or virilization may be present as evidenced by acne, deep voice, phallic enlargement and advanced osseous maturation. Hypertension is common in adults, but has not been observed in children. The demonstration of abnormally high concentration of urinary estrogens and, in some instances, of 17-ketosteroids supports the diag-nosis. The tumor may be a benign adenoma or a carcinoma. Gynecomastia regresses after removal of the tumor, and hormone values return to nor-mal.

An instance of an adrenal tumor causing femini-zation (isosexual precocity) in a 5½-year-old girl has also been recorded. In this child there was no clinical evidence of Cushing's syndrome or of virilism, and 17-ketosteroids as well as estrogens were in the adult range.

EXCESSIVE SECRETION OF CATECHOLAMINES

PHEOCHROMOCYTOMA

The pheochromocytoma, a catecholamine-se-creting tumor, arises from the chromaffin cells. The most common site of origin is the adrenal medulla; they may develop, however, anywhere along the abdominal sympathetic chain, and are particularly apt to be located near the aorta at the level of the inferior mesenteric artery or at its bifurcation. They also appear in the peri-adrenal area, the urinary bladder or ureteral walls, the thoracic cavity and the cervical region. Less than 5 per cent of reported instances have been in children. Tumors vary in size from about 1 to 10 cm. in diameter; they are found more often on the right side than on the left. In 20 per cent of affected children the adrenal tumors are bilateral, and in 30 per cent tumors are found both in the adrenal and in extra-adrenal areas or only in an extra-adrenal area.

Pheochromocytoma is frequently inherited as an autosomal dominant trait. In affected families the age of patients at the time of diagnosis has varied from the first to the fifth decade of life, and more than half the patients have had multiple tumors.

Pheochromocytoma is frequently associated with other syndromes or tumors. Approximately 5 per cent of patients with pheochromocytoma have neurofibromatosis. Sporadic as well as familial instances of pheochromocytoma have been noted in patients with von Hippel-Lindau disease. Kinships have been reported in which some affected members also have asymptomatic islet cell adenomas, and some in which members with pheochromocytoma are asymptomatic, although urinary concentration of catecholamines is elevated.

Coexistence of pheochromocytoma with thyroid cancer has long been recognized; it is now known that the thyroid tumor is almost invariably of the medullary type (p. 1199). Some patients with these 2 tumors may also have multiple mucosal neuromas. The neuromas appear early in life and affect primarily the tongue and lips; they may also affect the gingival, buccal or conjunctival mucosa (p. 1440). Parathyroid hyperplasia also occurs in some patients with this syndrome.

These syndromes are all inherited in a dominant fashion; in a single kindred there may be individuals with only a limited number of the manifestations and some with complete expression of the syndrome.

Clinical Manifestations. These are due to excessive secretion of epinephrine and norepinephrine; the variability of the clinical picture is related to the quantitative variations in their secretion. All patients have hypertension at some time. Although the hypertension is usually sustained, it is often *paroxysmal*. The latter, in particular, should suggest the possibility of pheochromocytoma as a diagnostic possibility. When there are paroxysms of hypertension, the attacks are usually infrequent at first, but become more frequent and eventually are replaced by a continuous hypertensive state. Between attacks of hypertension the patient may be free of symptoms. During attacks the patient complains of headache and palpitation, and pallor, vomiting and sweating are noticed. Convulsions and other manifestations of hypertensive encephalopathy may occur. In severe cases precordial pains radiate into the arms, and pulmonary edema and cardiac and hepatic enlargement may develop. The child has a good appetite, but does not gain weight, and severe cachexia may develop. Polyuria and polydipsia can be sufficiently severe to suggest diabetes insipidus. Growth failure may be striking. The blood pressure may range from 180 to 260 systolic and 120 to 210 diastolic, and the heart may be enlarged. Ophthalmoscopic examination may reveal papilledema, hemorrhages, exudate and arterial constriction.

Laboratory Data. The urine contains protein, a few casts and occasionally glucose. Gross hematuria suggests that the tumor is in the bladder wall. In many instances the basal metabolic rate may be as high as +50 or +60. Polycythemia is occasionally noted.

The most direct and specific test is the demonstration of increased urinary excretion of catecholamines or of VMA (3-methoxy-4-hydroxymandelic acid), a major metabolite of epinephrine and norepinephrine (Fig. 17-14). The daily urinary excretion of catecholamines and VMA by normal children increases with age, but when adjusted to surface area, they are equivalent to those of adults. There is a direct relation between the concentrations of catecholamines in the tumor and in the urine. Norepinephrine is increased in the urine in all patients; when epinephrine is also increased, it strongly suggests that the tumor is adrenal in location. Pharmacologic tests using adrenergic blocking agents or histamine were utilized for diagnosis; they are not as reliable as determinations of VMA and are rarely indicated.

Differential Diagnosis. The various causes of hypertension in children must be considered, such as renal disease, coarctation of the aorta, acrodynia, thallium intoxication, hyperthyroidism, Cushing's syndrome, congenital adrenal hyperplasia and essential hypertension. A nonfunctioning kidney may result from compression of a ureter or of a renal artery by a pheochromocytoma. If the hypertension is paroxysmal, the diagnosis of familial dysautonomia must also be considered. Urinary excretion of VMA is low in familial dysautonomia, owing to a defect in release rather than in synthesis of catecholamines. Cerebral disorders, diabetes insipidus, diabetes mellitus and hyperthyroidism must also be considered in the differential diagnosis.

Neuroblastoma, ganglioneuroblastoma and ganglioneuroma frequently produce catecholamines. Secreting neurogenic tumors commonly produce hypertension, excessive sweating, flushing, pallor, rash, polyuria and polydipsia. Diarrhea may also be associated with these tumors, particularly with ganglioneuroma, and may at times be sufficiently persistent to suggest the "celiac syndrome."

Treatment. Localization of the tumor is often difficult; only rarely can it be discovered by palpation. Pyelography may reveal the location of the tumor, but often it is demonstrated only by surgical exploration. Retroperitoneal gas insufflation, aortography or venous catheterization and sampling of blood at different levels for catecholamine determinations are only rarely necessary to localize the tumor. Since these tumors are often multiple, especially in children, a thorough transabdominal exploration of all the usual sites of localization offers the best insurance for locating all of them. Removal of the tumor(s) results in cure. Although these tumors often appear malignant histologically, only rarely has malignancy been unequivocally established, as demonstrated by metastases to lymph nodes of hormonally active chromaffin cells. The operation is not without danger, because an extreme rise of blood pressure may result from massive discharge of hormone during the operative manipulation. Shock from a precipitous drop of blood pressure during operation or within the first 48 postoperative hours is also a danger. These risks can be lessened by the proper preoperative preparation of the patient, by careful monitoring during surgery, and by continuous postoperative surveillance. The urinary excretion of VMA should be determined after operation as a measure of the completeness of the surgical removal. Prolonged follow-up is indicated, since functioning tumors at another site may become manifest many years after the initial operation. Examination of relatives of affected patients may reveal other persons harboring unsuspected tumors. In one family with 10 affected individuals the highest blood pressures and urinary concentrations of catecholamines were found in the children, whereas some of the affected adults were normotensive and had only moderately elevated urinary concentrations of catecholamines and VMA.

OTHER CATECHOLAMINE-SECRETING NEURAL TUMORS

Elaboration of excessive catecholamines is not exclusive to pheochromocytomas, but frequently occurs with other neurogenic tumors (neuroblastoma, ganglioneuroblastoma and less frequently ganglioneuroma). As a consequence, many of the systemic manifestations characteristic of pheochromocytoma may be seen in patients with other tumors of neural origin. Hypertension, excessive sweating, flushing, pallor, rash, polyuria and polydipsia are the most common findings. Chronic diarrhea may be the only symptom, or it may occur in association with other manifestations. Diarrhea is rarely a prominent manifestation in patients with pheochromocytoma, and the biochemical basis for this symptom in patients with neural tumors is not known. Diarrhea is more apt to occur in association with ganglioneuromas, but it may occur with ganglioneuroblastoma or neuroblastoma. Benign adrenal cortical hyperplasia with Cushing's disease has been observed in children with these neural tumors; the relationship between them is not clear.

A high percentage of patients with these tumors have increased excretion of dopa, dopamine, norepinephrine, normetanephrine, homovanillic acid and vanilmandelic acid (VMA). Patients with pheochromocytoma excrete only epinephrine, norepinephrine, their methoxy analogues and VMA (Fig. 17-14). Differentiation on a biochemical basis between neuroblastomas, ganglioneuroblastomas and benign ganglioneuromas is not possible. Repeated determinations of VMA and catecholamines, and particularly of norepinephrine and dopamine, are helpful in detecting recurrences and in assessing the effectiveness of therapy. Excretion of these compounds returns to normal if the tumor is completely removed.

A few catecholamine-secreting glomic tumors (chemodectomas) arising in the carotid or jugular bodies have been observed. Whether the cells comprising these tumors are neural in origin is unsettled.

CALCIFICATION WITHIN THE ADRENAL

Calcification within the adrenal glands may occur in a wide variety of situations, some serious and others of no obvious consequence. Adrenal calcifications are often detected as an incidental finding in radiographic studies of the abdomen in infants and children. One may elicit a history of anoxia or trauma at birth. Hemorrhage into the adrenal at or immediately after birth is probably the common factor which leads to subsequent calcification. Although it is advisable to assess the adrenal cortical reserve of such patients, there is rarely any functional disorder.

Neuroblastomas, ganglioneuromas, cortical carcinomas, pheochromocytomas and cysts of the adrenal gland may each be responsible for calcifications, particularly if hemorrhage has occurred within the tumor. Calcification in such lesions is almost always unilateral.

The most common infection associated with calcifications within the adrenal is tuberculosis, and the patient usually has the clinical manifestations of Addison's disease. Calcifications may also develop in the adrenal glands of children who recover from the Waterhouse-Friderichsen syndrome; such patients are usually asymptomatic.

Infants with the *Wolman syndrome*, a rare lipid storage disease, have extensive bilateral calcifications of the adrenal glands. The clinical manifestations and pathologic changes mimic those of Niemann-Pick disease; rapid clinical deterioration and death by 3 to 4 months of age are the usual course. The lipid stored in the affected tissues is a cholesterol-triglyceride mixture and not phospholipids as in Niemann-Pick disease. Deposition of this lipid is especially heavy in the adrenal, but the cause of the calcifications is not known. The disorder is recessively transmitted. It is probable that the patients who have been reported to have had adrenal calcifications in association with Niemann-Pick disease have had this form of xanthomatosis.

REFERENCES

General

Johannisson, E.: The Foetal Adrenal Cortex in the Human. Its Ultrastructure at Different Stages of Development and in Different Functional States. *Acta Endocrinol.*, Supp. 130, 1968.

Soffer, L. J., Dorfman, R. I., and Gabrilove, J. L.: *The Human Adrenal Gland.* Philadelphia, Lea & Febiger, 1961.

Visser, H. K. A.: The Adrenal Cortex. *Arch. Dis. Childhood*, 41:2, 113, 1966.

Wilkins, L.: *The Diagnosis and Treatment of Endocrine Disorders in Childhood and Adolescence.* 3rd ed. Springfield, Ill., Charles C Thomas, 1965.

Adrenal Cortical Insufficiency

Blizzard, R. M., and Kyle, M.: Studies of the Adrenal Antigens and Antibodies in Addison's Disease. *J. Clin. Invest.*, 42: 1653, 1963.

Blizzard, R. M., and Gibbs, J. H.: Candidiasis: Studies Pertaining to Its Association with Endocrinopathies and Pernicious Anemia. *Pediatrics*, 42:231, 1968.

Boyd, J. F., and McDonald, A. M.: Adrenal Cortical Hypoplasia in Siblings. *Arch. Dis. Child.*, 35:561, 1960.

Camacho, A. M., Kowarski, A., Migeon, C. J., and Brough, A. J.: Congenital Adrenal Hyperplasia Due to a Deficiency of One of the Enzymes in the Biosynthesis of Pregnenolone. *J. Clin. Endocr.*, 28:153, 1968.

Clayton, B. E., Edwards, R. W. H., and Renwick, A. G. C.: Adrenal Function in Children. *Arch. Dis. Childhood*, 38:49, 1963.

David, R., Golan, S., and Drucker, W.: Familial Aldosterone Deficiency, Enzyme Defect, Diagnosis and Clinical Course. *Pediatrics*, 4:403, 1968.

Ehrlich, R. M.: Ectopic and Hypoplastic Pituitary with Adrenal Hypoplasia; Case Report. *J. Pediat.*, 51:377, 1957.

Green, W. L., and Ingbar, S. H.: Decreased Corticotropin Reserve as an Isolated Pituitary Defect. *Arch. Int. Med.*, 108: 945, 1961.

Hintz, R. L., Menking, M., and Sotos, J. F.: Familial Holoprosencephaly with Endocrine Dysgenesis. *J. Pediat.*, 72:81, 1968.

Hung, W., Migeon, C. J., and Parrott, R. H.: A Possible Autoimmune Basis for Addison's Disease in Three Siblings, One with Idiopathic Hypoparathyroidism, Pernicious Anemia and Superficial Moniliasis. *New England J. Med.*, 269:658, 1963.

Kerenyi, N.: Congenital Adrenal Hypoplasia. Report of a Case with Extreme Adrenal Hypoplasia and Neurohypophyseal Aplasia Drawing Attention to Certain Aspects of Etiology and Classification. *Arch. Path.*, 71:336, 1961.

Malloy, B. M., and Woodruff, C. W.: Addison's Disease in Three Six-Year-Old Boys. *Am. J. Dis. Child.*, 95:364, 1958.

Margaretten, W., and McAdams, A. J.: An Appraisal of Fulminant Meningococcemia, with Reference to the Shwartzman Phenomenon. *Am. J. Med.*, 25:868, 1958.

Migeon, C. J., Kenny, F. M., Hung, W., and Voorhess, M. L.: Study of Adrenal Function in Children with Meningitis. *Pediatrics*, 40:163, 1967.

Mitchell, R. G., and Rhaney, K.: Congenital Adrenal Hypoplasia in Siblings. *Lancet*, 1:488, 1959.

Raine, D. N., and Roy, J.: A Salt-Losing Syndrome in Infancy. *Arch. Dis. Childhood*, 37:548, 1962.

Sampson, P. A., Winstone, N. E., and Brooke, B. N.: Adrenal Function in Surgical Patients After Steroid Therapy. *Lancet*, 2:322, 1962.

Steiker, D. D., Bongiovanni, A. M., Eberlein, W. R., and Leboeuf, G.: Adrenocortical and Adrenocorticotropic Function in Children. *J. Pediat.*, 59:885, 1961.

Stempfel, R. S., and Engel, F. L.: A Congenital, Familial Syndrome of Adrenocortical Insufficiency Without Hypoaldosteronism. *J. Pediat.*, 57:443, 1960.

Turkington, R. W., and Stempfel, R. S.: Adrenocortical Atrophy and Diffuse Cerebral Sclerosis (Addison-Schilder's Disease). *J. Pediat.*, 69:406, 1966.

Adrenal Cortical Hyperfunction

Bacon, G. E., and Lowrey, G. H.: Feminizing Adrenal Tumor in a Six-Year-Old Boy. *J. Clin. Endocr.*, 25:1403, 1965.

Bongiovanni, A. M., and Root, A.: The Adrenogenital Syndrome. *New England J. Med.*, 268:1283, 1342, 1391, 1963.

Bongiovanni, A. M., Eberlein, W. R., Goldman, A. S., and New, M.: Disorders of Adrenal Steroid Biogenesis. *Recent Progr. Hormone Res.*, 23:375, 1967.

Brackett, N. C., Koppel, M., Randall, R. E., and Nixon, W. P.: Hyperplasia of the Juxtaglomerular Complex with Secondary Aldosteronism Without Hypertension (Bartter's Syndrome). *Am. J. Med.*, 44:803, 1968.

Burkinshaw, J. H., O'Brien, D., and Pendower, J. E. H.: Cushing's Syndrome Associated with an Islet-Cell Tumor of the Pancreas in a Boy Aged Two Years. *Arch. Dis. Childhood*, 42:525, 1967.

Fraumeni, J. F., Jr., and Miller, R. W.: Adrenocortical Neoplasms with Hemihypertrophy, Brain Tumors, and Other Disorders. *J. Pediat.*, 70:129, 1967.

Gabrilove, J. L., Sharma, D. C., Wotiz, H. H., and Dorfman, R. I.: Feminizing Adrenocortical Tumors in the Male. A Review of 52 Cases Including a Case Report. *Medicine*, 44:37, 1965.

Godard, C., Riondel, A. M., Veyrat, R., Megevand, A., and Muller, A. F.: Plasma Renin Activity and Aldosterone Secretion in Congenital Adrenal Hyperplasia. *Pediatrics*, 41:883, 1968.

Goldsmith, O., Solomon, D. H., and Horton, R.: Hypogonadism and Mineralocorticoid Excess. The 17-Hydroxylase Deficiency Syndrome. *New England J. Med.*, 277:673, 1967.

Grim, C. E., McBryde, A. C., Glenn, J. F., and Gunnells, J. C.: Childhood Primary Aldosteronism with Bilateral Adrenocortical Hyperplasia: Plasma Renin Activity as an Aid to Diagnosis. *J. Pediat.*, 71:377, 1967.

Hutter, A. M., and Kayhoe, D. E.: Adrenal Cortical Carcinoma. Clinical Features in 138 Patients. *Am. J. Med.*, 41:572, 1966.

Hutter, A. M., and Kayhoe, D. E.: Adrenal Cortical Carcinoma. Results of Treatment with o,p' DDD in 138 patients. *Am. J. Med.*, 41:581, 1966.

James, V. H. T., Landon, J., Wynn, V., and Greenwood, F. C.: A Fundamental Defect of Adreno-cortical Control in Cushing's Disease. *J. Endocr.*, 48:15, 1968.

Kenny, F. M., Hashaida, Y., Askari, A., Sieber, W. H., and Fetterman, G. H.: Virilizing Tumors of the Adrenal Cortex. *Am. J. Dis. Child.*, 115:445, 1968.

Klevit, H. D., Campbell, R. A., Blair, H. R., and Bongiovanni, A. M.: Cushing's Syndrome with Nodular Adrenal Hyperplasia in Infancy. *J. Pediat.*, 68:912, 1966.

Krieger, D. T., Krieger, H. P., and Soffer, L. J.: Cushing's Syndrome Associated with a Suprasellar Tumor. *Acta Endocr.*, 47:185, 1964.

Migeon, C. J., Green, O. C., and Eckert, J. P.: Study of Adrenocortical Function in Obesity. *Metabolism*, 12:718, 1963.

New, M. I., and Peterson, R. E.: Aldosterone in Childhood. *Advances in Ped.*, 15:111, 1968.

Nichols, T., Nugent, C. A., and Tyler, F. H.: Steroid Laboratory Tests in the Diagnosis of Cushing's Disease. *Am. J. Med.*, 45:116, 1968.

Schletter, F. E., Cliff, G. V., Meyer, R., and Streeten, D. H. P.: Cushing's Syndrome in Childhood: Report of Two Cases with Bilateral Hyperplasia, Showing Distinctive Clinical Features. *J. Clin. Endocr.*, 27:22, 1967.

Schteingart, D. E., and Conn, J. W.: Effects of Aminoglutethimide upon Adrenal Function and Cortisol Metabolism in Cushing's Syndrome. *J. Clin. Endocr.*, 27:1657, 1967.

Snaith, A. H.: A Case of Feminizing Adrenal Tumor in a Girl. *J. Clin. Endocrinol. & Metab.*, 18:318, 1958.

Pheochromocytoma and Other Neural Tumors

Carman, C. T., and Brashear, R. E.: Pheochromocytoma as an Inherited Abnormality. Report of the Tenth Affected Kindred and Review of the Literature. *New England J. Med.*, 263:419, 1960.

Cone, T. E., and Pearson, H. A.: Malignant Pheochromocytoma. Report of a Case in a 12-Year-Old Girl. *Pediatrics*, 32:531, 1963.

Hamilton, J. R., Radde, I. C., and Johnson, G.: Diarrhea Associated with Ganglioneuroma. New Findings Related to the Pathogenesis of Diarrhea. *Am. J. Med.*, 44:453, 1968.

Kogut, M. D., and Kaplan, S. A.: Systemic Manifestations of Neurogenic Tumors. *J. Pediat.*, 60:697, 1962.

Sarosi, G., and Doe, R. P.: Familial Occurrence of Parathyroid Adenomas, Pheochromocytoma, and Medullary Carcinoma of the Thyroid with Amyloid Stroma (Sipples Syndrome). *Ann. Int. Med.*, 68:1305, 1968.

Schimke, R. N., Hartman, W. H., Prout, T. E., and Rimoin, D. L.: Syndrome of Bilateral Pheochromocytoma, Medullary Thyroid Carcinoma and Multiple Neuromas. A Possible Regulatory Defect in the Differentiation of Chromaffin Tissue. *New England J. Med.*, 279:1, 1968.

Smith, A. A., and Dancis, J.: Catecholamine Release in Familial Dysautonomia. *New England J. Med.*, 277:61, 1967.

Stackpole, R. H., Melicow, M. M., and Uson, A. C.: Pheochromocytoma in Children. Report of 9 Cases and Review of the First 100 Published Cases with Follow-up Studies. *J. Pediat.*, 63:315, 1963.

Studnitz, W. von, Kaser, H., and Sjoerdsma, A.: Spectrum of Catechol Amine Biochemistry in Patients with Neuroblastoma. *New England J. Med.*, 269:232, 1963.

Voorhess, M. L.: Urinary Catecholamine Excretion by Healthy Children. I. Daily Excretion of Dopamine, Norepinephrine, Epinephrine and 3-Methoxy-4-Hydroxymandelic Acid. *Pediatrics*, 39:252, 1967.

Adrenal Calcification

Crocker, A. C., Vawter, G. F., Neuhauser, E. B. O., and Rosowsky, A.: Wolman's Disease: Three New Patients with Recently Described Lipidosis. *Pediatrics*, 35:627, 1965.

Hill, E. E., and Williams, J. A.: Massive Adrenal Haemorrhage in the Newborn. *Arch. Dis. Childhood*, 34:178, 1959.

Jarvis, J. L., and Seaman, W. B.: Idiopathic Adrenal Calcification in Infants and Children. *Am. J. Roentgenol.*, 82:510, 1959.

Stevenson, J., MacGregor, A. M., and Connelly, P.: Calcification of the Adrenal Glands in Young Children. A Report of Three Cases with a Review of the Literature. *Arch. Dis. Childhood*, 36:316, 1961.

DISORDERS OF THE GONADS

The endocrine function of the testes is attributed to the male sex hormone, testosterone, a product of the interstitial cells of Leydig. Little is known about the endocrine role of the testes during childhood; though such a function cannot be denied *a priori*, there is little proof to substantiate its existence. Signs of castration and testicular failure do not become manifest before puberty. Production of testicular androgens increases markedly by about 12 years of age, and initiates the rapid growth phase of the penis and the development of male secondary sex characters. Spermatogenesis begins about 2 or 3 years later. The Leydig cells are stimulated to produce their hormones by the pituitary luteinizing hormone (LH); spermatogenesis is influenced by the pituitary follicle-stimulating hormone (FSH).

The mature ovary produces mainly 2 types of hormones: estrogens and progesterone. Several natural estrogens have been isolated: estrone, estriol and estradiol-17β. The last is the most potent of the natural estrogens. Diethylstilbestrol is the most important synthetic compound with estrogenic effects. Estrogens stimulate growth of the uterus, vagina, mammary glands and other female secondary sex characters. Progesterone is a product primarily of the corpus luteum. It is reduced to pregnanediol and excreted in the urine as pregnanediol glucuronide. The female hormones are secreted in periodic cycles, which last in the human being about 28 days. During the first half of the cycle the follicle matures until ovulation occurs in the middle of the intermenstrual period. During this phase of the cycle the estrogens induce proliferation of the uterine mucosa and of the mammary duct system. The secretion of estrogens reaches a peak at the time of ovulation and continues at a lower level during the second (luteal) phase of the cycle. After ovulation a corpus luteum is formed, which produces progesterone. Progesterone inhibits further proliferation of the endometrium, induces secretory activity of its cells, and prepares it for nidation of the ovum. It also develops the alveolar system of the mammary gland. In the absence of a fertilized ovum the progestational uterine endometrium degenerates. The products of degeneration are expelled, with blood and uterine secretions, in the process of menstruation.

The onset of menstruation, the menarche, is observed most frequently between the ages of 12 and 13 years. There is, however, a wide range of physiologic variation between 10 and 16 years. Menarche beyond this range is not necessarily abnormal, but a thorough examination should be made to rule out pathologic processes. Irregularities of cycles are frequent during the first year or two after the menarche, and during this time ovulation does not usually occur. Cramps are associated with ovulatory cycles only.

The normal and pathologic activities of the sex glands are reflected to a certain extent by hormonal substances excreted in the urine. The excreted sex hormones also permit certain conclusions about the functions of the pituitary and adrenal glands. The gonadotropic follicle-stimulating hormone (FSH) is estimated by biologic methods; androgens (17-ketosteroids), by chemical methods; and estrogens, by either method. Sensitive radio-immunoassay methods now exist for the measurement of FSH and LH in plasma. There are also reliable methods for measuring urinary and plasma levels of testosterone.

The gonads are stimulated in both boys and girls by the anterior pituitary. This stimulation becomes manifest at puberty. Only minute amounts of FSH are secreted in both sexes before puberty. In girls FSH can be detected in the urine frequently by the eleventh year of life and usually at least a year before the first menses. In boys this hormone does not appear in measurable amounts before the age of 13 years. This difference is in keeping with the earlier somatic maturation of girls.

Boys as well as girls secrete small but fairly constant amounts of estrogens until the age of 7 years (Fig. 17-21); about that time the excretion of these substances begins to increase in both sexes, but there is little difference in their respective values until the age of 11 years. Then girls show an augmented rate of excretion of estrogens, while that of boys undergoes little change. At the same time cyclic changes of excretion appear in girls. A single determination of urinary estrogens does not represent a measure of a girl's average excretion, since the values vary widely during every cycle. These cyclic variations precede the appearance of secondary sex characters and the menarche.

The excretion levels of 17-ketosteroids in both

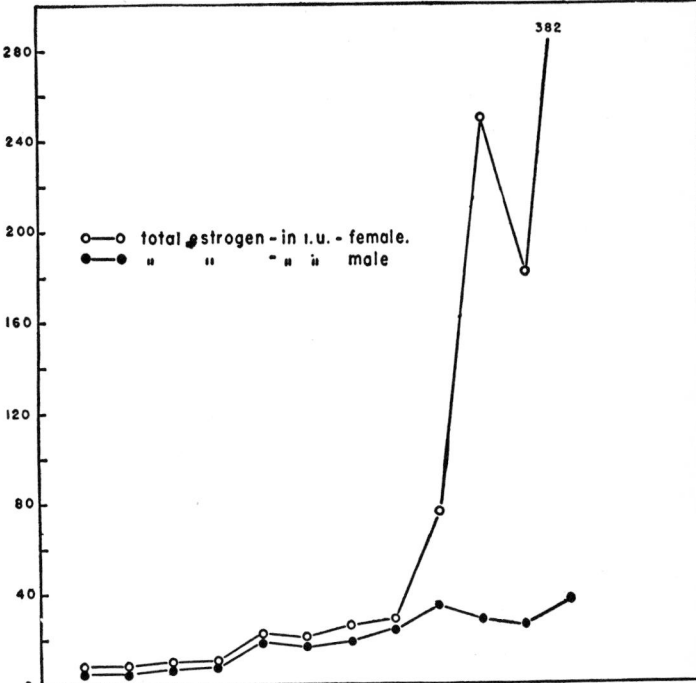

Figure 17-21. Excretion of estrogens at different ages. (Adapted from Nathanson, Towne and Aub: *Endocrinology*, Vol. 28.)

sexes during childhood and adolescence are indicated in Figure 17-22. During the first few days of life the daily urinary excretion of 17-ketosteroids may be as high as 2.5 mg. Thereafter amounts excreted are less than 0.5 mg. daily for the first year of life and remain under 1 mg. daily until about the age of 7 years. There is a decided rise between the ages of 10 and 18 years. There is no striking difference in the androgen excretion of boys and girls during childhood, but men show a higher excretion rate than women. The urinary 17-ketosteroids of the female are chiefly of adrenal origin; those of the male are of adrenal and testicular derivation.

The fact that boys and girls secrete about equal amounts of androgens and estrogens suggests that these hormones are not derived from the gonads in early childhood. It seems more likely that they are derived, at least in part, from the adrenal cortex. The greater output of sex hormones at

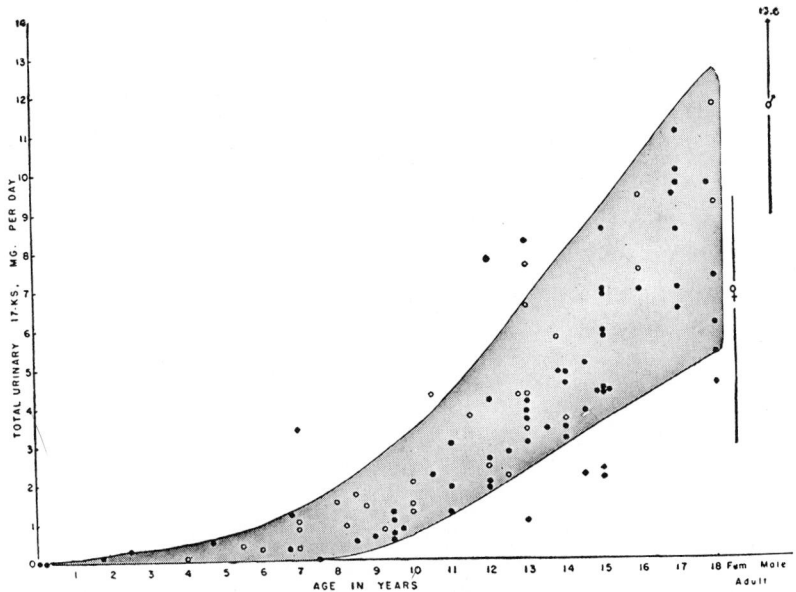

Figure 17-22. Excretion of 17-ketosteroids in normal persons. The black dots indicate values for boys; the circles, for girls. (Talbot and others: *Am. J. Dis. Child.*, Vol. 65.)

puberty parallels the development of the gonads and secondary sex characters so closely that it seems justified to attribute this increase to gonadal function. In various forms of hypogonadism urinary excretion of the sex hormones remains low. Under pathologic conditions high values of androgens and estrogens in the urine may be due to hyperfunction of the gonads or of the adrenal cortex.

Hypofunction of the Testes

The testes have an endocrine and a reproductive function; each is to some extent independent of the other. In some conditions, as in the adult with undescended testes, the interstitial cells may continue to function and secondary sex characters develop, although spermatogenesis is defective. On the other hand, normal spermatogenesis may occur when there is deficient production of androgen. Testicular hypofunction may be due to a primary defect of the testes (primary hypogonadism) or may be secondary to deficiency of pituitary gonadotropic hormone (secondary hypogonadism). Patients with primary hypogonadism have elevated urinary gonadotropin levels, and those with secondary hypogonadism have low or absent urinary gonadotropin levels. Thus hypogonadism may be divided into hypergonadotropic and hypogonadotropic syndromes. Clinical manifestations of hypogonadism develop only when the disorder involves both testes.

PRIMARY HYPOGONADISM

Etiology. In primary hypogonadism there is decreased production of androgen and impaired spermatogenesis. The clinical manifestations are most severe when all testicular tissue is lost as with traumatic or surgical castration or is never present as with congenital absence of both testes (anorchia or testicular agenesis). Anorchia includes only patients with a male phenotype and a normal XY chromosomal constitution. In this condition it is presumed that a noxious factor damaged the fetal testis of the chromosomally normal male some time after sexual differentiation had taken place. When testicular function fails before the seventh to fourteenth week of fetal life, normal male somatic differentiation does not take place, and an intersex results. Another cause for primary hypogonadism is atrophy of the testes following damage to their vascular supply, as may occur when there has been unskillful manipulation of the testes during surgical procedures for correction of cryptorchidism or as may result from bilateral torsion of the testes.

Acute orchitis in pubertal or adult males with mumps may also damage the testes; usually only the reproductive function of the testes is impaired, and the Leydig cells continue to function.

Estrogens and corticosteroids have been used to treat acute mumps orchitis, but their value has not been established. The routine immunization of all prepubertal males with mumps vaccine should prevent this complication.

Varying degrees of hypogonadism characterize Klinefelter's and Turner's syndromes in the male.

Clinical Manifestations. The clinical manifestations of hypogonadism are noted only at puberty or subsequently. Secondary sex characters fail to develop. Facial, pubic and axillary hair is scant or absent; there is neither acne nor regression of scalp hair, and the voice remains high-pitched. The penis and the scrotum remain infantile and may almost be obscured by pubic fat; the testes are small or absent. Fat accumulates in the region of the hips and buttocks and sometimes also in the breasts and on the abdomen. The epiphyses close late in life, resulting in long extremities. The span is several inches longer than the height, and the measurement from the symphysis pubis to the soles of the feet is much greater than from the symphysis pubis to the vertex. This clinical state is also known as *eunuchism*, and the proportions of the body are described as "eunuchoid."

PSEUDO-TURNER SYNDROME
("TURNER'S SYNDROME" IN THE MALE)

The term "male Turner's syndrome" has been applied to males who resemble females with Turner's syndrome in respect to certain anomalies which occur in both conditions. These boys have normal karyotypes. Moreover, this syndrome also occurs in girls with normal karyotypes. Such patients, both boys and girls, have been identified by a variety of designations, which include Turner phenotype with normal chromosomes, XY Turner phenotype (boys), XX Turner phenotype (girls), Ullrich-Turner syndrome, Ullrich's syndrome, familial Turner phenotype, and Noonan's syndrome. In order to emphasize the differences in phenotype, pathogenesis and genetics and at the same time point out the similarities to true Turner's syndrome, we favor the term "pseudo-Turner syndrome."

The most common abnormalities consist of short stature, webbing of the neck, pectus carinatum, cubitus valgus, congenital heart disease and a characteristic facies. Hypertelorism, epicanthus, an antimongoloid palpebral slant, ptosis, micrognathia and ear abnormalities are common. Other abnormalities such as clinodactyly, hernias and vertebral anomalies occur less frequently. The phenotype differs from true Turner's syndrome in the following respects: (1) Mental retardation is much more common. (2) The cardiac defect is most often pulmonary valvular or arterial stenosis, whereas coarctation of the aorta is rare; the reverse situation is seen in true Turner's syndrome. (3) There is a wide spectrum of gonadal defects varying from severe deficiency to apparently normal sexual development. Males frequently have cryptorchidism and small testes; they may be hypogonadal or normal. Females may have a normal or late puberty or fail to develop at all. The full spectrum of the syndrome has not been delineated, and it is probable that more than one discrete disorder is represented by these patients.

Males are chromatin-negative and have XY chromosomes; females are chromatin-positive and have normal XX chromosomes. Although the disorder usually occurs sporadically, affected siblings of the same and different sexes have been seen. At times parents, and particularly the mother of these children, exhibit some or many of the features of the syndrome. The mode of inheritance is not clear; X-linked dominant inheritance, an undetected deficiency or duplication of an autosome or sex chromosome, and multifactorial inheritance have all been suggested as possible mechanisms.

KLINEFELTER'S SYNDROME

Etiology. This common form of primary hypogonadism is due to an aberration of the sex chromosomes. Affected patients have two or more X and one or more Y chromosomes in at least some of their cells. Although the XXY complement is the most common chromosomal pattern, some persons with Klinefelter's syndrome have XXXY, XXXXY, XXYY, XXXYY and XXXXYY karyotypes, and some have such mosaic patterns as XX/XXY, XY/XXY, XY/XXXY, XXY/XXXY, XXY/XXXXY, XY/XXY/XXYY and XO/XY/XXY. It is noteworthy that despite the presence of up to 4 X chromosomes, the Y chromosome is male-determining. The chromosomal aberration can result from meiotic nondisjunction of an X chromosome during parental gametogenesis or mitotic nondisjunction in the zygote. Increased maternal age is a predisposing factor in meiotic nondisjunction and in the production of this syndrome. The incidence is approximately two per thousand liveborn males. In mentally defective populations the frequency is over 1 per cent. The occurrence of Klinefelter's and Down's syndromes in the same sibship suggests that there may be a predisposition to meiotic errors in some families. Klinefelter's syndrome and Down's syndrome have also

been noted in the same person. There is a higher than expected incidence of twinning among XXY patients.

A small percentage of males with clinical manifestations of Klinefelter's syndrome are sex-chromatin-negative and have a normal karyotype (XY); in such instances the patient should be carefully investigated for one of the other causes of hypogonadism.

Clinical Manifestations. The disorder usually becomes manifest in adolescence, when the small testes become evident, and gynecomastia commonly develops. Pubertal development may be delayed, and some degree of androgen deficiency is usually noted; some patients, however, may undergo almost normal masculinization. Azoospermia and infertility are usual, though rare instances of fertility are known. Twenty-five per cent of affected persons are mentally retarded to a moderate degree, and there is an increased frequency of antisocial behavior and delinquency. There also appears to be an increased incidence of pulmonary disease, varicose veins, cancer of the breast, and other disorders in affected adults.

When the number of X chromosomes exceeds two, the clinical manifestations are more severe; the degree of mental retardation and the impairment of masculinization in particular are related to the number of X chromosomes.

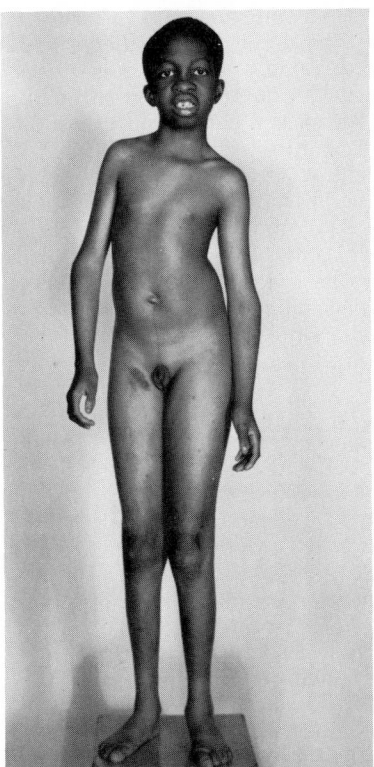

Figure 17-23. A 12-year-old boy with XXXY/XXXXY mosaicism, who has prognathism, epicanthal folds, scoliosis, very small testes, severe mental retardation, clinodactyly and radial-ulnar synostoses.

Persons with the XXXXY variant of Klinefelter's syndrome are sufficiently distinctive phenotypically to constitute a separate syndrome: they are severely retarded, and many have large malformed ears, a short neck and a typical facies with wide-set eyes which have a mild mongoloid slant, epicanthus, strabismus, a wide, flat upturned nose, and a large open mouth. The testes are small and may be undescended, the scrotum is hypoplastic, and the penis is very small. Defects suggestive of Down's syndrome, such as short incurved terminal fifth phalanges, single palmar creases, hypotonia and other skeletal abnormalities, including defects in the carrying angle of the elbows and restricted supination, are common. The most frequent radiographic abnormalities are radio-ulnar synostosis or dislocation, elongated radius, pseudo-epiphyses, scoliosis or kyphosis, coxa valga and retarded osseous age. Although most patients with such extensive changes have an XXXXY chromosome karyotype, they have also been observed with the following mosaic patterns: XXXY/XXXXY, XXXY/XXXXY/XXXXY and XXXY/XXXXY/XXXXYY.

Laboratory Data and Diagnosis. Patients with Klinefelter's syndrome are usually not recognized in childhood, since they appear normal until the age of puberty. They can be readily detected, however, by examination of buccal smears for sex chromatin. This test should be performed on all mentally retarded children, especially when they have other somatic anomalies. The number of X chromosomes can be deduced by the number of sex-chromatin bodies; there is one more X chromosome than the number of sex-chromatin bodies; thus XXXXY persons will have 3 sex-chromatin bodies. When cells are noted with variable numbers of sex-chromatin bodies, the karyotype is mosaic for X chromosomes.

Urinary gonadotropin levels are usually elevated by the time of puberty, but they may be normal, depending upon the amount of testicular androgen produced. Plasma testosterone levels in men with Klinefelter's syndrome are low or low normal.

Testicular biopsy before puberty may reveal only a deficiency or absence of germinal cells. After puberty the seminiferous tubular membranes are hyalinized, and there is adenomatous clumping of Leydig cells. Azoospermia is characteristic; only rarely is spermatogenesis sufficient to permit fertility.

Treatment. Substitution therapy with one of the testosterone preparations is indicated in all boys with primary hypogonadism regardless of causation. One of the esters of testosterone (enanthate, cyclopentylpropionate or phenylacetate) is injected intramuscularly in a dose of 200 mg. at intervals of 1 to 2 weeks until full sexual development is attained. Then 100 to 200 mg. may be administered every 3 to 5 weeks for maintenance. Plastic surgery is usually necessary to correct the gynecomastia when it is prominent enough to cause embarrassment.

REIFENSTEIN'S SYNDROME

This syndrome is characterized by hypospadias, diminished or absent virilization, azoospermia and infertility, normal or increased urinary gonadotropins and by varying degrees of gynecomastia. The phallus is normal in size, but cryptorchidism is common. Growth and development are normal until puberty, when hypogonadism becomes apparent. The testes are smaller than normal, but larger than those in patients with Klinefelter's syndrome. The mode of inheritance is either X-linked or autosomal dominant; the disorder can be suspected in prepubertal boys with similarly affected brothers, uncles, male cousins or other male relatives in the maternal line. Defective development of the external genitalia is thought to result from deficient secretion of androgen by the fetal testis.

OTHER CAUSES OF PRIMARY HYPOGONADISM

Testicular atrophy occurs in 80 per cent of males with *myotonic muscular dystrophy*; the atrophy involves primarily the seminiferous tubules; the Leydig cells are grossly normal, and gonadotropin levels are normal rather than elevated. *Germinal cell aplasia (del Castillo syndrome)* is a familial syndrome characterized by small testes, azoospermia and infertility. Leydig cells are normal, but there is complete absence of germinal epithelium in the seminiferous tubules. A *defect in testosterone synthesis* was found to be the cause for hypogonadism in a young man who had onset of gynecomastia and galactorrhea at 10 years of age. A maternal uncle had similar abnormalities.

XYY MALES

Males with the XYY sex chromosome constitution are usually normally developed physically and sexually; data on fertility, however, are scanty. The only characteristic physical trait observed has been height above average. The most important identifying feature may be the high incidence of aberrant behavior, which includes mild mental retardation, delinquency, school truancy, serious personality disorders and aggressive behavior. Some become involved in criminal activity at an early age; they exhibit little skill in crime, corrective training is usually unsuccessful, and the recidivist rate is high. Since most cases have been identified in penal institutions and in institutions for the criminally insane, the true incidence of these characteristics among all XYY males is unknown. Surveys of newborn infants indicate that the XYY syndrome may occur as frequently as one in 300 males.

In approximately a dozen XYY patients some degree of hypogonadism has been reported, including male pseudohermaphroditism with a female phenotype. The 2 Y chromosomes in this subgroup of patients may not be normal.

SECONDARY HYPOGONADISM

In secondary hypogonadism there is deficiency of follicle-stimulating hormone (FSH) or of luteinizing hormone (LH, ICSH) of the anterior pituitary. The testes are normal, but remain in the prepubertal state because of lack of stimulation by gonadotropic hormones. Affected persons can usually be categorized on etiologic bases.

Panhypopituitarism (Pituitary Dwarfism) (see p. 1174). Patients with panhypopituitary dwarfism have multiple deficiencies of pituitary hormones. The disorder may be caused by an organic lesion in or near the pituitary or may be idiopathic; the extent of testicular failure is roughly proportional to the completeness of the pituitary destruction or failure. The disorder is usually sporadic, but hypopituitary dwarfism may be familial. Signs and symptoms resulting from deficiency of other hormones of the pituitary gland are present. Since there is usually deficient production of growth hormone, eunuchoidal proportions do not develop, even though closure of the epiphyses is delayed.

Isolated Deficiency of Pituitary Gonadotropins. In this disorder the deficiency of gonadotropic function is a selective one, and other tropic hormones of the pituitary are not involved. The term "idiopathic eunuchoidism with low FSH" has also been applied to this syndrome, which is believed to be due to a congenital defect in the pituitary or hypothalamus. This form of hypogonadism may be familial and appears to be transmitted by an autosomal recessive gene, since both male and female siblings are affected.

Deficiency of Pituitary Gonadotropins with Anosmia (Kallmann's Syndrome). Persons with this syndrome fail to develop sexually, or exhibit only minimal development at puberty, and are short in stature. Inability to smell is present from early childhood, but it is usually not discovered except on direct questioning. There is impaired secretion of both pituitary FSH and LH, and urinary concentrations of gonadotropins are low. The anosmia is the result of agenesis of the olfactory lobes of the brain. Although no histologic lesion has been defined, it is presumed that the defect is in centers of the hypothalamus which produce gonadotropin-releasing hormones. The disorder is probably transmitted by a sex-linked dominant gene, since affected women have been detected, although sex-modified autosomal dominant transmission cannot be ruled out.

Isolated Deficiency of Luteinizing Hormone (The "Fertile Eunuch" Syndrome). This syndrome is characterized by varying degrees of androgen deficiency in the presence of normal-sized testes and active spermatogenesis. Absence or hypoplasia of the Leydig cells is demonstrated by testicular biopsy, but good response to administration of chorionic gonadotropin reveals the presence of normal Leydig cell precursors. Serum and urine FSH concentrations are normal, whereas those of LH are undetectable. The defect may be in the pituitary or in the hypothalamic-releasing hormone responsible for release of LH. Although fertility has occasionally been noted, evidence suggests that testicular androgen is necessary for completely normal spermatogenesis. The syndrome has been observed in brothers, suggesting a genetic origin in at least some instances.

Laurence-Moon-Biedl Syndrome. In its complete form this syndrome consists of obesity, polydactylism, retinitis pigmentosa, mental retardation, and hypogonadism. There is much variability in the expression of this syndrome, and gonadal function may be normal. Few of the hypogonadal subjects have been adequately studied, but deficiency of gonadotropic hormones has been found in a brother and a sister with this recessively inherited disorder. On occasion primary hypogonadism has also been observed.

Fröhlich's Syndrome

Lesions of the hypothalamus caused by craniopharyngiomas, tumors of the pituitary or other structures adjacent to the hypothalamus, trauma or encephalitis can cause a syndrome of obesity and sexual infantilism. Some of the patients also have diabetes insipidus and retardation of growth. Since obesity may occur in pituitary dwarfs, transitional forms are encountered in which the differential diagnosis between Fröhlich's syndrome and pituitary dwarfism becomes uncertain. It is assumed that the obesity is related to interference of hypothalamic function, whereas retardation of sexual development is explained by deficiency of pituitary gonadotropins. Other tropic hormone deficiencies are also common. The patient originally described by Fröhlich had a cyst in the region of the pituitary gland which caused headaches, vomiting, loss of vision, destruction of the dorsum sellae, obesity of the trunk, and retardation of sexual development. The term "Fröhlich's syndrome", if used at all, should be limited to children with this group of symptoms; it should *not* be used to describe boys who are otherwise normal and who only appear to have hypogenitalism, owing to the excessive fat in the genital areas.

Diagnosis. Physiologic delay of puberty is extremely difficult to differentiate from secondary hypogonadism before the patient is 19 or 20 years old. In normal boys with delayed sexual maturation there is a relatively late beginning of gonadotropin secretion. In both conditions urinary excretion of gonadotropins remains low after the usual age of puberty. The only way to differentiate the 2 conditions is by exogenous stimulation of testicular function followed by a period of observation after withdrawal of therapy.

Treatment. Administration of interstitial cell-stimulating hormone in the form of chorionic gonadotropin induces satisfactory development of secondary sex characters by stimulating the Leydig cells. The recommended dose is 4000 to 5000 I.U. 3 times weekly for approximately 6 months, followed by 2500 I.U. at like intervals for an additional 3 months. After discontinuation of therapy a period of observation for evidence of regression is necessary to establish the diagnosis. If puberty regresses, the patient has secondary hypogonadism, whereas, if puberty continues to progress, the patient has had physiologic delay of maturation. Several such courses may be necessary to exclude the diagnosis of physiologic delayed adolescence. When the diagnosis of secondary hypogonadism is established, maintenance therapy with androgen is initiated (see p. 1228).

Pseudoprecocity Resulting from Tumors of the Testes

Tumors of the testes which cause sexual pseudoprecocity are derived from the interstitial cells of Leydig. These cells are sparse before puberty, and tumors derived from them are more common in the adult. Fewer than 50 cases in children have been reported since the entity was described in 1895. The tumor has been observed in one of identical twins.

The first changes, enlargement of the penis and development of pubic hair, appear usually between the ages of 4 and 6 years. Later, but long before the usual age of puberty, axillary and facial hair appears. Hypertrichosis of the chest and extremities and acne may also be present. The boys grow rapidly; they gain in weight and appear muscular and strong. The voice becomes deep. Gynecomastia is occasionally seen. The blood pressure is usually within normal limits. The tumor of the testis as well as the enlarged prostate gland can be palpated. In one instance the tumor was located in the tunica vaginalis completely separate from the testis. Roentgenograms reveal advanced osseous development. The 17-ketosteroids in the urine are slightly or moderately increased.

Treatment consists in surgical removal of the testis which contains the tumor. Progression of virilization ceases after the tumor has been removed, and partial disappearance of the signs of precocity has been observed in some patients. If osseous maturation is advanced to the pubertal age range, however, the pseudoprecocity is replaced by true precocity. Hypothalamic maturation of gonadotropic function closely parallels osseous age. Leydig cell tumors are usually benign.

Gynecomastia

Gynecomastia, or unusual enlargement of mammary tissue in the male, is a common condition. It is seen most frequently as a variant of normal development in adolescent boys. It is thought to be due to secretion of estrogens, as well as androgens, by the pubertal testis. Spontaneous regression may occur within a few months; it rarely persists longer than 2 years. The gynecomastia may precede other signs of pubertal development, and it is not unusual for both breasts to enlarge at disproportionate rates, at different times, or for only one breast to be involved. Tenderness of the breast is frequent but transitory. No hormonal treatment is necessary. Surgical removal of the breast is rarely indicated; under unusual circumstances when enlargement is striking and causes serious emotional disturbance to the patient, removal may perhaps be justified. Both the boy and his family should be assured of the physiologic and transient nature of the phenomenon.

Gynecomastia may occur as a simple inherited disorder without significant hypogonadism *(familial gynecomastia)*; the mode of inheritance appears to be autosomal dominant. There are also a number of pathologic conditions with which gynecomastia is associated and which must be differentiated from the normally occurring gynecomastia in adolescent boys. It may be associated with interstitial cell tumors of the testis or with feminizing tumors of the adrenal. It occurs in patients with Klinefelter's syndrome, Reifenstein's syndrome, and with other types of testicular failure. It has also been observed in association with chorioepitheliomas, hepatic disease and paraplegia. Exposure to a very small amount of estrogens by inhalation, percutaneous absorption or ingestion, either accidentally or therapeutically administered, may cause gynecomastia; increased pigmentation of the nipple and areola should always suggest this cause. It is surprising that androgens such as testosterone as well as anabolic agents such as methandrostenolone may also cause gynecomastia.

An increased amount of fat in the mammary region of obese children is common and is referred to as *pseudogynecomastia.*

Hypofunction of the Ovaries

Hypofunction of the ovaries may be due to congenital failure of development or to postnatal destruction (primary hypogonadism) or to lack of stimulation by the pituitary (secondary hypogonadism). Many chronic diseases may result in the latter type.

PRIMARY HYPOGONADISM

Preadolescent Castration. Surgical removal of both ovaries results in primary hypogonadism. Fortunately removal of one ovary for lesions such as tumors or torsion has no adverse effect on sexual development. Roentgen therapy over the pelvic area may result in permanent ovarian deficiency; pelvic exposure to 1300 roentgens has resulted in permanent castration of an infant of 18 months of age.

The endocrine effects of preadolescent castration do not become manifest before puberty, when there is failure of sexual maturation. The external and internal genitalia remain infantile, the breasts do not develop, axillary and pubic hair is scanty, and there is no menarche. Such females grow tall, and the arms and legs are relatively long. Epiphyseal closure is delayed. Urinary estrogens are absent; urinary excretion of gonadotropins is elevated; that of 17-ketosteroids is usually normal.

TURNER'S SYNDROME
(Gonadal Dysgenesis)

In 1938 Turner described a syndrome consisting of sexual infantilism, webbed neck and cubitus valgus in adult females. It was subsequently demonstrated that such women have elevated levels of urinary gonadotropins and that the gonads consist of rudimentary elongated streaks. Histologically, the gonads contain no germinal elements, and consist of whorls of connective tissue suggestive of ovarian stroma.

Pathogenesis. In 1959 it was demonstrated that the majority of patients with gonadal dysgenesis have 45 chromosomes instead of the normal complement of forty-six. Only one X chromosome and no Y chromosome is present, and the sex-chromosome constitution is referred to as XO. Patients with this chromosomal abnormality are invariably sex-chromatin-negative and account for 60 to 80 per cent of females with gonadal dysgenesis. The X chromosome may be either paternal or maternal in origin. The aberration could arise from nondisjunction during oogenesis or spermatogenesis, or it could arise from nondisjunction during early mitosis. Unlike the situation in Klinefelter's syndrome, there is

no influence of maternal or paternal age on the occurrence of gonadal dysgenesis.

The XO disorder occurs in about one in 2500 live-born females and in about 5 per cent of aborted fetuses. Primordial germ cells were present in the gonadal ridges of the XO aborted fetuses studied up to 3 months of gestational age. Except as there are 2 XX chromosomes, these germ cells fail to mature into oocytes.

The majority of patients with Turner's syndrome who are sex-chromatin-positive are mosaics for the X chromosome; the most common karyotype is XO/XX, a disorder arising from mitotic nondisjunction. The remainder of the sex-chromatin-positive patients with gonadal dysgenesis have other types of mosaicism for the X chromosome, such as a normal X and an isochromosome for the long arm or a deletion of the short arm of the other X chromosome.

Clinical Manifestations. Patients with this disorder do not develop sexually at puberty. The breasts do not develop, the external genitalia remain infantile, and there is no menstruation.

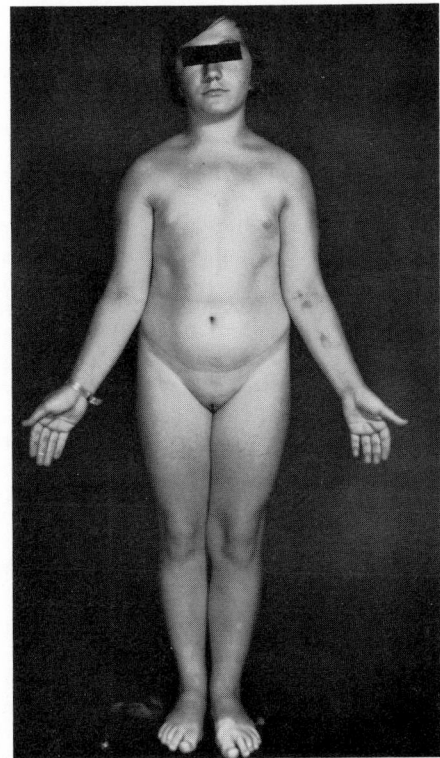

Figure 17-24. Turner's syndrome. Gonadal dysgenesis in a 15-year-old girl exhibiting failure of sexual maturation, short stature, cubitus valgus and a goiter. There is no webbing of the neck. Karyotype revealed XO/XX sex chromosome complement, and urinary gonadotropin was over 96 mouse units per 24 hours. PBI was 3.2 μg% and T₄ was 2.2 μg%. Biopsy of the thyroid revealed lymphocytic thyroiditis.

The diagnosis frequently can be suspected long before the age of puberty, because affected patients have a rather characteristic appearance and other associated defects. Infants may be significantly short at birth, and the height is usually below the third percentile thereafter. Rarely does the adult attain a height of more than 58 inches.

The clinical manifestations include a stocky build, an unusual facial appearance, webbing of the neck, a low posterior hairline, prominent ears, small mandible, epicanthal folds, broad chest with widely spaced nipples ("shield chest"), pigmented nevi, cubitus valgus and hyperconvex fingernails. In the young infant, instead of webbing of the neck there may be loose skin folds in the nape of the neck. Edema of the dorsum of the hands and feet, cardiac and renal anomalies, particularly coarctation of the aorta, horseshoe kidneys and skeletal defects are also common. Some of the defects are sufficiently serious to be lethal in infancy. A moderate degree of mental retardation is more common than in the general population.

There is some relation of the extent and type of malformations to the chromosomal constitution. Thus webbing of the neck, coarctation of the aorta and edema of the hands and feet are infrequent in the XO/XX mosaics, but common in XO persons. Short stature is a cardinal manifestation in both groups of patients. The child with XO/XX mosaicism occasionally exhibits some breast development and more rarely has irregular menstrual periods at puberty. Intermediate phenotypes may be seen in patients with deletions, isochromosomes, or rings of one of the X chromosomes, or in a wide variety of mosaics.

Laboratory Data. In patients over 10 to 13 years of age, urinary gonadotropins are elevated, and similar values have been found occasionally in prepubertal children. Urinary excretion of estrogens is low, and that of 17-ketosteroids is in the low normal range. Growth hormone secretion in response to insulin-induced hypoglycemia or to arginine infusion is normal.

Roentgenographic studies may reveal cardiovascular or renal abnormalities. The most common skeletal abnormalities are shortening of the fourth metatarsal and metacarpal bones, epiphyseal dysgenesis in the joints of the knee and elbow, inadequate osseous mineralization, scoliosis and spina bifida occulta.

The sex-chromatin pattern is usually negative, but it may be positive. Unusually large sex-chromatin bodies are seen in patients with an isochromosome of the X chromosome, and smaller than normal sex-chromatin bodies suggest a deletion of the short arm of one of the X chromosomes.

Patients with Turner's syndrome have a higher than expected incidence of chronic lymphocytic thyroiditis, and a high percentage of patients and other family members have significant titers of antibodies to thyroglobulin.

Diagnosis. All female infants and children with short stature should be suspected of having gonadal dysgenesis. A negative pattern of sex chromatin establishes the diagnosis; further confirmation is achieved by analysis of the chromosomes. A positive pattern of sex chromatin does not eliminate the possibility of gonadal dysgenesis, since patients who are mosaic for the X chromosome, such as XO/XX, may be sex chromatin-negative or chromatin-positive, depending upon the distribution of the 2 populations of cells in the buccal mucosa. Chromosomal analysis is indicated in sex-chromatin-positive girls who are suspected of having gonadal dysgenesis.

Treatment. Replacement therapy with estrogens is indicated for primary hypogonadism. This results in development and function of the secondary sex organs, which can simulate those of normal women. In the absence of ova and ovulation, however, reproduction is impossible, and the affected person remains sterile. Treatment may be started at 12 to 14 years of age. For the first 3 to 9 months 0.5 to 1.0 mg. of diethylstilbestrol is given daily; this results in mammary development and pigmentation of the areola. The uterus grows to adult size, and the vaginal epithelium shows signs of maturation. When these changes are apparent, cyclic treatment is begun. A recommended schedule of treatment consists of 1 mg. of diethylstilbestrol daily for 3 weeks. During the third week 10 to 20 mg. of a progestational compound such as medroxyprogesterone acetate is also administered daily by mouth. No treatment is given during the fourth week. Menstrual bleeding usually occurs after withdrawal of treatment. With adequate replacement therapy such children can lead completely normal lives except that they are sterile and may be limited by associated congenital anomalies.

PSEUDO-TURNER'S SYNDROME

Girls with a phenotype resembling those with Turner's syndrome, but with normal sex chromosomes, constitute a separate entity which is described on page 1226.

OTHER OVARIAN DEFECTS

An increasing number of young women are being found who have "streak" gonads. These structures may contain no or only occasional germ cells. No chromosomal abnormality is found, and urinary gonadotropins are increased. Some of these patients have been categorized as having pure gonadal dysgenesis. This disorder may be familial and may result from a mutant gene dealing with ovarian determiners on the X chromosome. Similar streak gonads ("ovarian hypoplasia") occur in girls with ataxia-telangiectasia and in some young women with autoimmune Addison's disease. The similarity of the "ovaries" in a variety of clinical conditions suggests that different pathogenetic mechanisms may interfere with normal gonadal development.

SECONDARY HYPOGONADISM

Hypofunction of the ovaries can result from failure to secrete normal levels of gonadotropins. This may be caused by a destructive lesion in or near the pituitary; such patients usually have other manifestations of pituitary deficiency. In some instances no organic lesion can be detected, and there may be no defect other than gonadotropin deficiency. Occasionally the defect is hereditary and may affect boys as well as girls (p. 1226).

It is difficult to separate such patients clinically from normal girls with delayed sexual maturation caused by delayed secretion of gonadotropic hormone.

The pituitary origin of the sexual immaturity in this group of patients is revealed by the absence of gonadotropic hormone in the urine. This hormone is found in excess in primary hypogonadism.

Treatment. Treatment consists of substitution therapy with estrogens. When the patient wishes to become pregnant, ovulation can be induced with human pituitary gonadotropin.

SEX CHROMOSOME ABNORMALITIES WITHOUT GONADAL DEFECTS

A variety of sex chromosomal abnormalities have been uncovered which are not associated with a defect in the gonads. These are of interest to the pediatrician primarily because mental retardation is a frequent finding in affected patients.

XXX Females. Females have been described who have 3 X chromosomes. Most have been detected through identification of 2 sex-chromatin bodies in cells from buccal smears. Surveys of live-born females at birth indicate that the frequency of the disorder is approximately one per 1000. The incidence is about four per 1000 institutionalized mentally retarded females. As in Klinefelter's syndrome and in gonadal dysgenesis, the XXX chromosome anomaly probably arises from nondisjunction during gametogenesis. No definite effect of parental age has been demonstrated.

No consistent clinical pattern has thus far evolved among the triple-X females. About 75 per cent of them have been mentally retarded, but this is a biased value, since most patients were found among institutionalized mental defectives. Menstrual irregularities, webbed neck and neurologic abnormalities have been found in only a few patients. Triple-X females who are otherwise apparently normal are being found with increasing frequency; many have normal fertility, and none of their offspring studied has had chromosomal abnormalities.

XXXX and XXXXX Females. Only a few females with 4 X or 5 X chromosomes have been described. The nuclei of cells from buccal smears contain 3 and 4 sex-chromatin bodies, respectively. All patients have been mentally retarded and some have findings suggestive of Down's syndrome. Epicanthic folds, incurved fifth finger, simian crease and patent ductus arteriosus have been noted in the penta-X syndrome.

Pseudoprecocity Due to Lesions of the Ovary

Most of the functioning lesions of the ovary in children are neoplasms, the majority of which synthesize estrogens; a few of them synthesize androgens. Infrequently a lesion produces both estrogens and androgens, or a given lesion may produce estrogenic manifestations in one patient and androgenic ones in another. Thus the rare Sertoli-Leydig cell tumor of the ovary has caused isosexual precocity in some girls and masculinization in others (p. 1462).

ESTROGENIC LESIONS OF THE OVARY

These lesions cause isosexual precocious sexual development, but account for only a small percentage of all instances of precocity.

Granulosa-Theca Cell Tumor. In childhood the most common neoplasm of the ovary with estrogenic manifestations is the granulosa-theca cell tumor. These tumors have variable proportions of granulosa and theca cells; in childhood the granulosa cell is dominant, and tumors which consist almost completely of theca cells (thecoma) are extremely rare. In spite of variable morphology, these tumors produce similar clinical manifestations because they actively synthesize estrogen. Which of the 2 cells is the site of estrogen synthesis is still unsettled.

The tumor has been observed in a newborn infant, but most often *clinical manifestations* do not appear until after 2 years of age. The breasts become enlarged, rounded and firm, and the nipples are prominent. Axillary and pubic hair appears, and total body growth is accelerated. The external genitalia resemble those of a normal girl at puberty, and the uterus is enlarged. A white vaginal discharge is followed by irregular or cyclic menstruation. Ovulation, however, does not occur;

the sexual development is of the pseudoprecocious variety.

A mass in the lower portion of the abdomen is readily palpable in most patients by the time sexual precocity is evident. The tumor may be small, however, and even escape detection by careful rectal and abdominal examination.

Association of these tumors with ascites and hydrothorax has been observed in children; it is more likely to occur with the thecoma. Such manifestations, known as *Meigs's syndrome*, should not be confused with metastases, and hence the primary tumor mistakenly considered inoperable.

Urinary estrogens may be markedly elevated or may be increased only to the usual level of normal adolescent girls. Vaginal smears reveal a significant estrogen effect. Urinary 17-keto-steroids are normal or only slightly elevated. Gonadotropin levels in the urine have on rare occasions been elevated to normal adult levels. This alteration is paradoxical, since usually the excessive production of estrogens by the tumor suppresses pituitary production of gonadotropins. Osseous development is moderately advanced.

A palpable abdominal tumor in association with sexual precocity in a girl suggests the *diagnosis* of a granulosa-theca cell tumor. When the tumor is not palpable and urinary estrogen levels are not markedly elevated, it is difficult to distinguish this disorder from idiopathic sexual precocity. Careful and repeated rectal and abdominal examinations, under anesthesia if necessary, may be required over a period of several years.

The tumor should be removed as soon as the diagnosis is established. The mortality rate is approximately 20 per cent; recurrences are known up to 25 years after removal of the tumor. Vaginal bleeding immediately after removal of the tumor is common. Signs of precocious puberty abate and may disappear within a few months after operation. The secretion of estrogens returns to normal postoperatively.

Luteoma. The cause for pseudoprecocity in 2 girls has been found to be a solid ovarian luteoma. The younger patient was 10 months of age.

Theca-Lutein Cyst. Ovarian cysts are common in childhood, but most are nonfunctioning and hence not feminizing. Ovarian cysts are also commonly encountered in the ovaries of children with constitutional sexual precocity. In such instances the cyst is a secondary event; it is not the cause of

sexual precocity, and removal of it does not alter the course of sexual precocity. By contrast, removal of a cyst has on rare occasions resulted in regression of sexual precocity. In such instances the theca-lutein cyst is believed to be functional and to be the cause of the sexual precocity. Patients with theca-lutein cysts have clinical manifestations similar to those of children with granulosa-theca cell tumors.

ANDROGENIC LESIONS OF THE OVARY

Virilizing ovarian tumors are rare in pre-pubertal girls; lipid cell tumors have been found as early as $2\frac{1}{2}$ years of age, and arrhenoblastomas as early as 4 years. The clinical features include hirsutism, clitoral enlargement and elevation of urinary 17-ketosteroids.

POLYCYSTIC OVARIES
(STEIN-LEVENTHAL SYNDROME)

This syndrome is characterized by amenorrhea, hirsutism, obesity and sterility. The ovaries are enlarged and covered by a condensation of collagen which gives the appearance of a "thickened capsule." Beneath this layer are many small follicular cysts. This disorder accounts for many more instances of virilism than do ovarian tumors. Since the disorder commonly begins at puberty or shortly thereafter, the diagnosis should be considered in adolescent girls with menstrual irregularities and hirsutism. In married women the most frequent complaint is infertility. The enlarged ovaries can often be detected by combined rectal and abdominal palpation. The cause of the disorder is unsettled, but evidence suggests that it is a defect in the neuroendocrine-homeostatic control of the ovary. Urinary 17-ketosteroid levels may be moderately elevated. Bilateral wedge resections of the ovaries frequently result in normal ovulatory menstrual cycles, but may be deferred until the patient wishes to become pregnant. For young girls, therapy with clomiphene citrate is probably preferable.

Hermaphroditism
(INTERSEXUALITY)

Hermaphroditism in man implies a discrepancy between the morphology of the gonads and of the external genitalia. Ambiguity of the external genitalia is frequent, but some hermaphrodites have normal external genitalia of one sex, whereas the gonads are of the opposite sex. Hermaphro-

ditism may be caused by an imbalance of the sex-chromosome constitution, by hormonal factors acting on the fetus, and by other, as yet undetermined, factors. In recent years the ability to establish the complement of the sex chromosomes of the individual has revealed many aberrations not necessarily associated with hermaphroditism. Thus patients with gonadal dysgenesis (XO) or Klinefelter's syndrome (XXY) cannot be considered hermaphrodites, although they are frequently referred to incorrectly as intersexes. The phenotype of the XO individual is female; the gonads are undifferentiated. The phenotype of the XXY individual is male, and the gonads are testes. Some individuals are completely normal in gonadal development, including fertility, but have an imbalance of the sex-chromosome complement. This is best exemplified by XXX females and XYY males.

Embryonic Sexual Differentiation. In normal differentiation all sexual structures are consistent with a normal complement of the sex chromosomes (XX or XY). The Y chromosome carries potent male-determining genes which induce testicular development even in persons with the XXXXY constitution. Two X chromosomes are required for the differentiation of the primitive gonad into an ovary. By the seventh week of intrauterine life the primordia for both the male and female genital ducts are present. Removal of the embryonic gonad (in either XX or XY fetuses) at this stage of development results in regression of the wolffian (mesonephric) duct and in the development of the female sex structures (müllerian duct derivatives and external genitalia). It is apparent that male differentiation requires the presence of normal fetal testes, whereas female differentiation does not require any gonad. Patients with male pseudohermaphroditism who have an XY karyotype, but female external genitalia with or without secondary sex structures, owe this discrepancy to absent or abnormal "secretion" of duct-organizing substance by the fetal testes. Testicular differentiation is directed by genetic information contained in the Y chromosome. Most hermaphroditic subjects who have testicular tissue have a Y chromosome. There are instances of true hermaphroditism (presence of testicular tissue) in which no Y chromosome was found. In these cases it is likely that mosaicism was not detected, or that the male-determining genes were transferred from the Y to the X chromosome.

Sex Chromatin. The sex-chromatin body (Barr body) is formed by one of the 2 X chromosomes in the female; hence it is characteristically present in normal females and absent in normal males. The X chromosome which forms the Barr body is the inactive X (Lyon hypothesis). Sex chromatin is typically located on the inner surface of the nuclear membrane and measures about 1 micron in diameter. Patients who have more than 2 X chromosomes have nuclei which contain more than 1 sex-chromatin body; in rare instances there may be 2, 3 or 4 sex-chromatin bodies per nucleus. There is a consistent relation between sex chromatin and the X chromosome; the number of sex-chromatin bodies is always one less than the number of X chromosomes.

In addition to the number of X chromosomes, one may secure other information from a study of the sex-chromatin pattern. Unusually small sex-chromatin bodies indicate deletion of a portion of an X chromosome, whereas larger than normal sex-chromatin bodies indicate an isochromosome of the long arm of the X chromosome. When 2 or more populations of cells which contain Barr bodies have differing numbers of such bodies, one may infer mosaicism involving the X chromosome.

Simple procedures are available for the study of sex chromatin by staining of easily available cells such as those of the buccal mucosa. These procedures have made possible the recognition of hermaphroditism and other anomalies of the sex chromosomes in early infancy.

FEMALE PSEUDOHERMAPHRODITISM

In the female pseudohermaphrodite whose gonads are ovaries, the external genitalia are ambiguous or completely masculinized. The female fetus is readily masculinized when exposed to androgens during intrauterine life; the most common cause is congenital adrenal hyperplasia (p. 1212). In rare instances a masculinizing tumor such as an arrhenoblastoma in the mother has been the cause of female pseudohermaphroditism in her infant.

Administration of various steroids to women during pregnancy can result in female pseudohermaphroditism. Testosterone and 17-methyltestosterone are potent androgens and have been reported as the masculinizing agents in some instances. The use of certain progestational compounds for the treatment of threatened abortion, however, has accounted for the greatest number of cases. Most of these progestins have been replaced by nonvirilizing ones, and this cause of female hermaphroditism has decreased. More difficult to explain has been the finding of female pseudohermaphroditism in infants born to mothers who had received only diethylstilbestrol during early pregnancy.

Female pseudohermaphroditism may occur in the absence of any identifiable masculinizing agent. In such instances the disorder is frequently associated with other abnormalities, particularly of the gastrointestinal and urinary tracts.

The appearance of infants with female pseudohermaphroditism at birth is the same as that described for congenital adrenal hyperplasia (p. 1214). The principal abnormalities are enlargement of the clitoris and labial fusion. Occasionally the fusion is complete and a penile urethra is present.

The sex-chromatin pattern is always positive, and the chromosomal constitution is that of a normal female (XX). A urethrovaginogram or endoscopic examination reveals a cervix and a uterus. Increased urinary excretion of 17-ketosteroids distinguishes the female pseudohermaphrodite with adrenal hyperplasia from the nonadrenal one. Repeated and careful inquiry about

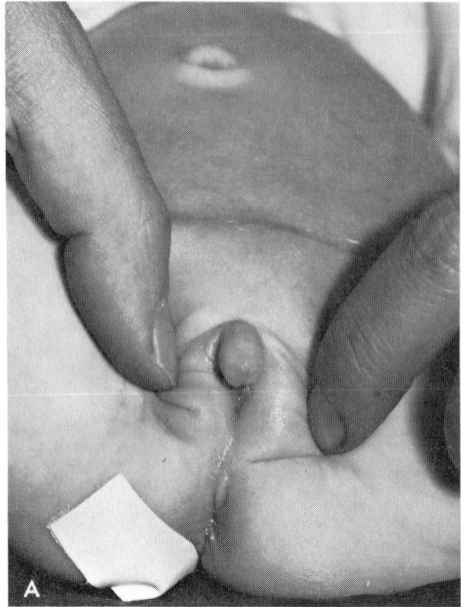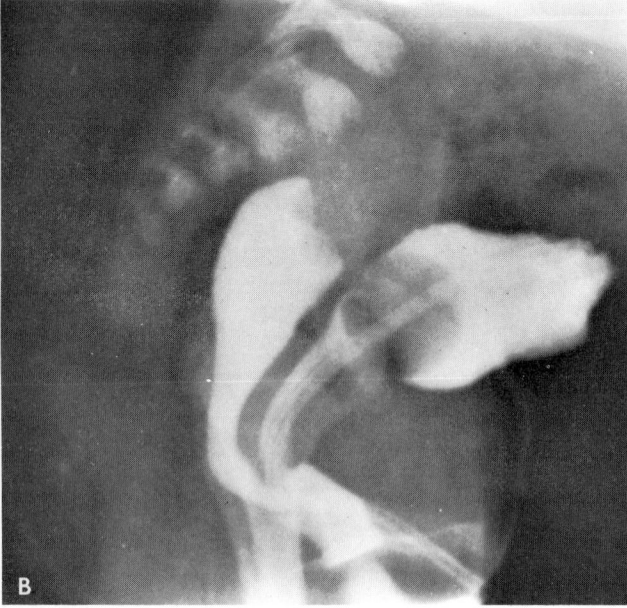

Figure 17-25. Female hermaphroditism. *A*, One-week-old infant with clitoral enlargement and labial fusion. Normal excretion of 17-ketosteroids and normal female karyotype. *B*, Contrast medium injected into the urogenital sinus visualized the vagina with indentation of the cervix as well as the urinary bladder. The mother had received progesterone during the first trimester of pregnancy; this agent is a rare cause of masculinization of the female fetus.

the prenatal administration of drugs is indicated in this latter group. These infants should always be reared as females; their potential for fertility is normal. If adrenal hyperplasia is excluded and no medications were administered during pregnancy, an exploratory laparotomy and gonadal biopsy are indicated to exclude the possibility of true hermaphroditism. When indicated, plastic procedures to correct the external genitalia are best performed between 18 months and 4 years of age.

MALE PSEUDOHERMAPHRODITISM

In the male pseudohermaphrodite the gonads are testes, but the external genitalia are ambiguous or completely feminized. These persons are almost always sex-chromatin-negative and with only doubtful exceptions have a Y chromosome. It is generally accepted that genetic material in the Y chromosome directs testicular differentiation. In the male pseudohermaphrodite the fetal testis has failed to bring about complete differentiation of the genital ducts and of the external genitalia. There is a wide variety of genital abnormalities, but several distinct clinical disorders have emerged from this heterogeneous category.

Testicular Feminizing Syndrome. This is a form of male pseudohermaphroditism in which chromosomal male patients are completely feminized. The external genitalia are those of a normal female. At puberty there is normal development of the breasts, and the habitus is female, though

sexual hair is often absent. Menstruation does not occur; the vagina ends blindly in a pouch, and the uterus is absent. The gonads are testes and consist largely of seminiferous tubules; they are located intra-abdominally or in the inguinal canal.

In adults, amenorrhea may be the only complaint, but prepubertal children with this disorder are often recognized because of inguinal masses which prove to be testes or because of an accidental finding of a testis during herniorrhaphy in an apparent female. Psychosexual orientation of such persons is entirely feminine, and the child should always be reared as a female.

The sex-chromatin pattern is negative, and the chromosomal constitution is that of a normal male (XY). The disorder is inherited, and the gene is transmitted by the female carrier; half of her sons are affected and reared as females, and half of her daughters are carriers. Some carrier females have had delayed menarche; a reduction in axillary and pubic hair has been observed in others. It is unsettled whether the trait is X-linked or a sex-modified autosomal dominant.

The testes of affected adult patients produce normal male levels of testosterone; the reason for absence of androgenic effects appears to be a defect in the action of testosterone at the peripheral cellular level. Failure of normal male differentiation during fetal life probably represents a similar defective response to testicular androgens during fetal life.

It is usually recommended that the testes be permitted to remain in order to permit normal feminization at puberty. When puberty is achieved, orchidectomy is indicated, since germinomas develop in one fifth of all patients. Replacement therapy with estrogens is then necessary.

Incomplete forms of this disorder occur in which there is some degree of masculinization, including enlargement of the phallus and labioscrotal fusion. Breast development occurs at puberty, but feminization is less complete. It is presumed that these patients have a lesser degree of insensitivity to androgens than those with the complete syndrome. The hereditary pattern is similar in both disorders.

Male Pseudohermaphroditism with XO/XY Mosaicism. The XO/XY syndrome may also be considered a variant of gonadal dysgenesis and has been termed *asymmetric* or *mixed gonadal dysgenesis*. The presence of some cells with a Y chromosome results in some virilization, and in most instances the genitalia are ambiguous. The phenotype, however, may be completely female or completely male. A vagina and an infantile uterus are usually present. There is usually one, but there may be 2 fallopian tubes. There is usually an undifferentiated "streak" on the side with the fallopian tube and a rudimentary testis on the opposite side, but bilateral "streaks" or bilateral rudimentary testes have also been observed. Absence of normal fetal testicular secretion in one or both testes results in persistence of müllerian structures. The local effect of the male duct evocator is demonstrated by the usual absence of the fallopian tube on the side with testicular tissue. Affected persons are always sex-chromatin-negative and may exhibit some of the features of patients with XO/XX mosaicism, particularly short stature. Androgen secretion is usually noted at puberty; the dysgenetic gonads often undergo neoplastic changes, resulting in gonadoblastomas (p. 1462).

Male Pseudohermaphroditism with XY Karyotype. Most male pseudohermaphrodites have a normal male karyotype (XY), but there is much variability of the external and internal genitalia within this group. There are varying degrees of phallic and müllerian development. Testes may be normal or rudimentary, or there may be only one. Defective function of the testis early in fetal life is postulated. Lack of male duct evocator from the fetal testes results in persistence of müllerian elements and failure of development of wolffian elements. Development of gonadoblastomas is relatively frequent.

Reifenstein's syndrome, a hereditary form of male pseudohermaphroditism, is discussed under primary hypogonadism (p. 1228).

Male Pseudohermaphroditism Due to Enzymatic Defects. Males with adrenal hyperplasia due to deficiency of *3-beta-hydroxysteroid dehydrogenase* are usually incompletely virilized (p. 1215). The testes may be undescended, and there is usually hypospadias. Failure of production of fetal testicular androgen accounts for these changes.

Lipoid adrenal hyperplasia is another cause for male pseudohermaphroditism. The few recognized males with this disorder have had a completely female phenotype. Affected infants have exhibited salt-losing manifestations early in life and have died in addisonian crisis (p. 1209). An affected male with a partial defect presented with ambiguity of the external genitalia and did not manifest hypoadrenalism until 7 months of age. The defect is a complete block in synthesis of steroid from cholesterol in the adrenals and in the testes. Absence of fetal testicular androgens results in failure of normal masculinization. Affected males are sex-chromatin-negative.

TRUE HERMAPHRODITISM

In true hermaphroditism both ovarian and testicular tissue are present either in the same or in opposite gonads. The clinical features may include any of those described for the other types of hermaphroditism. The phenotype may be male or female; usually there is ambiguity of the external genitalia.

The sex-chromatin pattern is most often positive, and most patients have an XX sex chromosome complement. The presence of testes in patients without a Y chromosome would appear contrary to current concepts that the Y chromosome is necessary for testicular development (see p. 1235 for possible explanations). True hermaphroditism has been observed in siblings, suggesting that recessive genes may be the cause in some instances.

Six examples of a special type of true hermaphroditism are known in which there is mosaicism not only of the sex chromosomes (XX/XY), but also of other characteristics, such as blood groups, serum proteins and skin pigmentation. The presence of both paternal alleles for some blood groups and of both maternal alleles for other blood groups is strong evidence for a double fertilization.

ANGELO M. DIGEORGE

REFERENCES

General

Grady, H. G., and Smith, D. E.: *The Ovary.* Baltimore, Williams & Wilkins Company, 1963.

Morris, J. M., and Scully, R. E.: *Endocrine Pathology of the Ovary.* St. Louis, C. V. Mosby Company, 1958.

Overzier, C.: *Intersexuality.* New York, Academic Press, 1963.

Williams, R. H.: *Textbook of Endocrinology.* 4th ed. Philadelphia, W. B. Saunders Company, 1968.

Hypofunction of Testes

Bowen, P., and others: Hereditary Male Pseudohermaphroditism with Hypogonadism, Hypospadias, and Gynecomastia (Reifenstein's syndrome). *Arch. Int. Med.,* 62:252, 1965.

Bruch, H.: The Frölich Syndrome; Report of the Original Case. *Am. J. Dis. Child.,* 58:1282, 1939.

Carakushansky, G., Neu, R. L., and Gardner, L. I.: XYY with Abnormal Genitalia. *Lancet,* 2:1144, 1968.

Court Brown, M. W.: Males with an XYY Sex Chromosome Complement. Review Article. *J. Med. Genet.,* 5:341, 1968.

De la Chapelle, A., and Hortling, H.: Cytogenetical and Clinical Observations in Male Hypogonadism. *Acta Endocr.*, 44:165, 1963.

Ewer, R. W.: Familial Monotropic Pituitary Gonadotropin Insufficiency. *J. Clin. Endocr.*, 28:783, 1968.

Faiman, C., Hoffman, D. L., Ryan, R. J., and Albert A.: The "Fertile Eunuch" Syndrome: Demonstration of Isolated Luteinizing Hormone Deficiency by Radioimmunoassay Technique. *Mayo Clin. Proc.*, 43:661, 1968.

Howard, R. P., Sniffen, R. C., Simmons, F. A., and Albright, F.: Testicular Deficiency: A Clinical and Pathologic Study. *J. Clin. Endocrinol. & Metab.*, 10:121, 1950.

Noonan, J. A.: Hypertelorism with Turner Phenotype. A New Syndrome with Associated Congenital Heart Disease. *Am. J. Dis. Child.*, 116:373, 1968.

Nora, J. J., and Sinha, A. K.: Direct Familial Transmission of the Turner Phenotype. *Am. J. Dis. Child.*, 116:343, 1968.

Nowakowski, H., and Lenz, W.: Genetic Aspects of Male Hypogonadism. *Recent. Progr. Hormone Res.*, 17:53, 1961.

Reinfrank, R. F., and Nichols, F. L.: Hypogonadotropic Hypogonadism in the Laurence-Moon Syndrome. *J. Clin. Endocr.*, 24:48, 1964.

Rimoin, D. L., Borgaankar, D. S., Asper, S. P., and Blizzard, R. M.: Chromatin-Negative Hypogonadism in Phenotypic Men. *Am. J. Med.*, 44:225, 1968.

Sparkes, R. S., Simpsen, R. W., and Paulsen, C. A.: Familial Hypogonadotropic Hypogonadism with Anosmia. *Arch. Int. Med.*, 121:534, 1968.

Volpe, R., Metzler, W. S., and Johnston, M. W.: Familial Hypogonadotropic Eunuchoidism with Cerebellar Ataxia. *J. Clin. Endocr.*, 23:107, 1963.

Wieland, R. G., Folk, R. L., Taylor, J. N., and Hamwi, G. T.: Studies of Male Hypogonadism. I. Androgen Metabolism in a Male with Gynecomastia and Galactorrhea. *J. Clin. Endocr.*, 27:763, 1967.

Zaleski, W. A., Houston, C. S., Pozsonyi, J., and Ying, K. L.: The XXXXY Chromosome Anomaly. Report of Three New Cases and Review of 30 Cases from the Literature. *Canad. M.A.J.*, 94:1143, 1966.

Pseudoprecocious Puberty Due to Tumor of the Testes

Camin, A. J., Dorfman, R. I., McDonald, J. H., and Rosenthal, I. M.: Interstitial Cell Tumor of the Testis in a Seven-Year-Old Child. *Am. J. Dis. Child.*, 100:389, 1960.

Engel, F. L., and others: Clinical, Morphological and Biochemical Studies on a Malignant Testicular Tumor. *J. Clin. Endocr.*, 24:528, 1964.

Martin, M. M., Canary, J. J., and Balsamo, P. A.: Virilizing Tumor of the Testis in One Twin. *J. Clin. Endocr.*, 22:345, 1962.

Savard, K., and others: Clinical, Morphological and Biochemical Studies of a Virilizing Tumor of the Testis. *J. Clin. Invest.*, 39:534, 1960.

Gynecomastia

Green, M.: Gynecomastia and Pseudoprecocious Puberty Following Diethylstilbestrol Exposure. *Am. J. Dis. Child.*, 95:637, 1958.

Laron, Z.: Breast Development Induced by Methandrostenolone (Dianabol). *J. Clin. Endocrinol. & Metab.*, 22:450, 1962.

Nydick, M., Bustos, J., Dale, J. H., Jr., and Rawson, R. W.: Gynecomastia in Adolescent Boys. *J.A.M.A.*, 178:449, 1961.

Wallach, E. E., and Garcia, C.: Familial Gynecomastia Without Hypogonadism: A Report of Three Cases in One Family. *J. Clin. Endocrinol.*, 22:1201, 1962.

Hypofunction of the Ovaries

Baikie, A. G., Garson, M., Weste, S., and Ferguson, J.: Numerical Abnormalities of the X Chromosome. *Lancet*, 1:398, 1966.

Brody, J., Fitzgerald, M. G., and Spiers, A. S. D.: A Female Child with Five X Chromosomes. *J. Pediat.*, 70:105, 1967.

Carneiro, L. J., Voorhess, M. L., Schlegel, R. J., and Gardner, L. I.: XX/XO Mosaicism in Nine Preadolescent Girls with Short Stature as Presenting Complaint. *Pediatrics*, 38:972, 1966.

Carr, D. H., Barr, M. L., and Plunkett, E. R.: An XXXX Sex Chromosome Complex in Two Mentally Defective Females. *Canad. M.A.J.*, 84:131, 1961.

Day, R. W., Larson, W., and Wright, S. W.: Clinical and Cyto-genic Studies on a Group of Females with XXX Sex Chromosome Complements. *J. Pediat.*, 64:24, 1964.

Lemli, L., and Smith, D. W.: The XO Syndrome: A Study of the Differentiated Phenotype in 25 Patients. *J. Pediat.*, 63:577, 1963.

Lindsten, J.: *The Nature and Origin of X Chromosome Aberrations in Turner's Syndrome. A Cytogenetical and Clinical Study of 57 Patients.* Stockholm, Almquist and Wiksell, 1963.

Maclean, N., Harnden, D. G., Court Brown, W. M., Bond, J., and Mantle, D. J.: Sex Chromosome Abnormalities in Newborn Babies. *Lancet*, 1:286, 1964.

Moore, K. L.: *The Sex Chromatin.* Philadelphia, W. B. Saunders Company, 1966.

Portmann, U. V., and McCullagh, E. P.: Developmental Defects Following Irradiation of the Ovaries in a Child. *J.A.M.A.*, 151:736, 1953.

Tumors of the Ovary

Ammann, A. J., Kaufman, S., and Gilbert, A.: Virilizing Ovarian Tumor in a 2½-Year-Old-Girl. *J. Pediat.*, 70:782, 1967.

Campbell, P. E., and Danks, D. M.: Pseudoprecocity in an Infant Due to a Luteoma of the Ovary. *Arch. Dis. Childhood*, 38:519, 1963.

Eberlein, W. R., Bongiovanni, A. M., Jones, I. T., and Yakovac, W. C.: Ovarian Tumors and Cysts Associated with Sexual Precocity. *J. Pediat.*, 57:484, 1960.

Faber, H. K.: Meigs' Syndrome with Thecomas of Both Ovaries in a 4-Year-Old Girl. *J. Pediat.*, 61:769, 1962.

Hermaphroditism

Alexander, D. S., and Ferguson-Smith, M. A.: Chromosomal Studies in Some Variants of Male Pseudohermaphrodites. *Pediatrics*, 28:758, 1961.

Bergada, C., Cleveland, W. W., Jones, H. W., Jr., and Wilkins, L.: Gonadal Histology in Patients with Male Pseudohermaphroditism and Atypical Gonadal Dysgenesis: Relation to Theories of Sex Differentiation. *Acta Endocr.*, 40:493, 1962.

Bongiovanni, A. M., DiGeorge, A. M., and Grumbach, M. M.: Masculinization of the Female Infant Associated with Estrogenic Therapy Alone During Gestation: Four Cases. *J. Clin. Endocrinol.*, 19:1004, 1959.

Corey, M. J., Miller, J. R., MacLean, J. R., and Chown, B.: A Case of XX/XY Mosaicism. *Am. J. Human Genetics*, 19:378, 1967.

Ferguson-Smith, M. A.: X-Y Chromosomal Interchange in the Aetiology of True Hermaphroditism and of XX Klinefelter's Syndrome. *Lancet*, 2:475, 1966.

Ferrier, P. E., and Kelley, V. C.: Influence of the Y Chromosome on Gonadal Differentiation: Asymmetrical Gonads in an XO/XY Mosaic. *J. Med. Genetics*, 4:288, 1967.

Gans, S. L., and Rubin, C. L.: Apparent Female Infants with Hernias and Testes. *Am. J. Dis. Child.*, 104:82, 1962.

Jeffcoate, S. L., Brooks, R. V., and Prunty, F. T. G.: Secretion of Androgens and Oestrogens in Testicular Feminization: Studies in Vivo and in Vitro in Two Cases. *Brit. J. Med.*, 1:208, 1968.

Jones, H. W., Ferguson-Smith, M. A., and Heller, R. H.: Pathologic and Cytogenetic Findings in True Hermaphroditism. *Obstet. & Gynec.*, 25:435, 1965.

Morris, J. M., and Mahesh, V. B.: Further Observations on the Syndrome, "Testicular Feminization." *Am. J. Obst. & Gynec.*, 87:731, 1963.

Rivarola, M. A., Saez, J. M., Meyer, W. J., Kenny, F. M., and Migeon, C. J.: Studies of Androgens in the Syndrome of Male Pseudohermaphroditism with Testicular Feminization. *J. Clin. Endocr.*, 27:371, 1967.

Robinson, A., Priest, R. E., and Bigler, P. C.: Male Pseudohermaphrodite with XY/XO Mosaicism and Bilateral Gonadoblastomas. *Lancet*, 1:11, 1964.

Rosenberg, H. S., Clayton, G. W., and Hsu, T. C.: Familial True Hermaphroditism. *J. Clin. Endocrinol. & Metab.*, 23:203, 1963.

Wilkins, L.: Abnormalities of Sex Differentiation, Classification, Diagnosis, Selection of Gender of Rearing and Treatment. *Pediatrics*, 26:846, 1960.

Wilkins, L., Jones, H. W., Jr., Holman, G., and Stempfel, R. S., Jr.: Masculinization of the Female Fetus Associated with Administration of Oral and Intramuscular Progestins During Gestation: Non-Adrenal Female Pseudohermaphroditism. *J. Clin. Endocrinol. & Metab.*, 18:559, 1958.

18.   The Genital Organs

MALE GENITAL ORGANS

EXAMINATION OF THE EXTERNAL GENITAL ORGANS

The external genitalia should be inspected for cleanliness, color, configuration, size, and symmetry or relation in position of one organ to another. Whether the penis is erectile, the opening from which urine flows, and the size of the external urethral meatus should also be noted. In instances of ambiguity, in order to determine the opening from which a child voids, it is sometimes necessary to probe suspected apertures with a sterile catheter.

Palpation of the testes is most successful when the examiner's hands and the examining room are warm. The location, size and consistency are determined. The examiner should attempt to "milk down" testes which are in the inguinal canal. If testes cannot be felt, one of the following maneuvers may result in their descent: the boy sits with his hips and knees in flexion and with his heels on the examining table, just in front of his buttocks; then he grunts. Examination is most effective when the child is not anticipating it; on occasion it may be wise to depend on the findings of a parent in the home. Examination while the child is bathing in a tub of warm water may be particularly revealing.

The skin of the external genitalia is normally more pigmented than that of other parts of the body. This increased pigmentation is particularly notable in Negro and Latin babies.

Swelling of the scrotum is common in the newborn. It is more severe in infants delivered from a breech presentation; after a few days the edema disappears.

The size of the penis varies. It may be erect when the urinary bladder is full. The foreskin of the newborn infant cannot be retracted. Testes are palpable in the normal newborn male and are frequently not equal in size. The prostate is not palpable.

ANOMALIES OF THE PENIS

Ambiguity of the External Genitalia. The external genitalia may be sufficiently ambiguous at birth to preclude the confident assignment of sex. The phallus may be larger than a clitoris, but smaller than a penis, and is often bound down by chordee. The urethra may open along the shaft of the phallus or on the perineum, or be part of a common outlet for the urethra and the vagina (urogenital sinus). Gonads may or may not be palpable. The male infant with hypospadias and undescended testes cannot be distinguished from the virilized female infant who has labioscrotal fusion and clitoral enlargement. A wide variety of factors may cause such genital abnormalities. In all instances investigation is required immediately after birth, prior to assignment of sex of rearing. Determination of sex-chromatin, chromosomal constitution and urinary excretion of 17-ketosteroids and pregnanetriol are indicated. In many instances exploratory laparotomy is needed to establish the true nature of the gonads. Reconstructive surgery may be deferred to a later date.

Anomalous development of the penis may vary from the clinically insignificant disorder of *torsion of the penis* to the catastrophic condition of penile agenesis. Total *absence of the penis* has been reported at least 28 times; it may occur as an isolated defect, but is frequently associated with other genitourinary and lower intestinal abnormalities. Duplications such as *double penis* or *bifid penis* are almost always associated with other defects, particularly with double bladder, exstrophy of cloaca and imperforate anus. Transposition of scrotum and penis *(retroscrotal penis)* is a rare and correctable defect.

A small penis is of concern to parents, but the size of the normal penis varies markedly, and true *micropenis* is uncommon. In most instances, growth during puberty results in a satisfactorily functional organ. The *penis of an obese boy* often appears pathologically small because it is partially covered by suprapubic fat. If the physician retracts the fat, he can readily demonstrate to parents and boy that the penis is of normal size. An unusually large penis is usually a manifestation of precocious puberty, but is infrequently brought to the attention of the physician until pubic hair has also made its appearance.

Hypospadias. In about one in 300 infants the urethral orifice is on the ventral surface of the penis. The opening may be at the junction of the glans and the shaft (subcoronal type), on the shaft, or on the perineum (penile, penoscrotal, scrotal and perineal types); there is usually chordee or ventral bowing of the penis, and often there is stenosis of the external urethral meatus. Cryptorchidism is an associated defect in approximately 15 per cent of patients. In such patients adequate investigation must exclude hermaphroditism or such disorders as the Smith-Lemli-Opitz syndrome.

Familial occurrence of this disorder is seen in Reifenstein's syndrome. Surgical correction of the chordee should usually be made by 2 years of age. Definitive urethroplasty should be performed before the boy enters school so that it will be possible for him to urinate in the standing position. Since the foreskin is used in the repair, boys with hypospadias should not be circumcised.

Epispadias. In this genital anomaly the opening of the urethra is on the dorsal surface of the penis. The condition occurs in about one in 30,000 infants. The urethral opening may be small and situated just behind the glans; in the more extreme varieties a fissure extends the entire length of the penis. This latter type frequently occurs in combination with exstrophy of the bladder. Treatment is surgical.

Other Anomalies. *Phimosis* is a narrowing of the preputial opening so that the prepuce cannot be retracted. Rarely there is no opening. The prepuce may be of normal length or elongated. When the opening of the prepuce is small, urination can be accomplished only by straining; the urine is passed in drops or in a small stream. If adhesions are not present, urine accumulates beneath the foreskin.

Treatment by retraction or stretching with forceps is often sufficient, or the preputial orifice may be widened by incision; in severe forms, circumcision is indicated. A redundant prepuce without phimosis is not an indication for circumcision.

In *paraphimosis* the prepuce, after retraction beyond the corona, cannot readily be replaced. The circulation in the glans is interrupted by the constriction; edema, bluish discoloration and even gangrene may ensue. Pain and dysuria are usually severe. The accident usually follows retraction of the prepuce by the patient or by mother or nurse when cleansing the penis. Cold compresses should be applied to reduce the swelling, and then an effort should be made to draw the foreskin forward into the normal position. The glans should be well oiled, steadily compressed, and the constricting prepuce pulled forward. If the paraphimosis cannot be corrected in this manner, incision of the constricting ring of skin may be required. If the foreskin is unduly narrow, circumcision should be performed after the inflammation has subsided.

A condition similar to that of paraphimosis may be produced if the patient ties a string around the penis or slips a ring or other object over it.

ABNORMALITIES OF THE TESTES

One testis (*monorchia*) or both (*anorchia*) may be absent (p. 1226). Artificial testes of silicone-rubber have been used as prostheses in such instances. It is estimated that when a testis is not palpable, there is a 3 per cent likelihood that it is congenitally absent. Supernumerary testes and fusion of the testes are rare abnormalities.

UNDESCENDED TESTES
(CRYPTORCHIDISM)

Maldescent of the testis is a common abnormality, but diagnosis of the condition may be difficult, and many aspects of its management are controversial. There are 2 types of undescended testes: those which are ectopic and those which are incompletely descended.

The *ectopic testis* is one which, having progressed down the inguinal canal and passed through the external ring, has been diverted to become lodged in the perineum, in the pubopenile area or in the femoral area. The testis which lies somewhere along the normal path of descent without ever having been in the scrotum is designated as *undescended, cryptorchid* or *incompletely descended*. Difficulty in diagnosis arises when a hyperactive cremaster muscle retracts the testis which has descended into the scrotum. Such *retractile testes* are intermittently in the scrotum; at other times they are in the inguinal canal or within the abdomen. It is usually possible to "milk" such testes into the scrotum, but other techniques of examination are often necessary to establish that the testis is retractile (see p. 1239). These mobile organs become less retractile with advancing years and will eventually reside in the scrotum. The condition is normal and requires only reassurance.

The testes are undescended in approximately 3 per cent of full-term and 30 per cent of premature infants at birth. Most such testes descend in the first weeks or months of life. Thereafter spontaneous descent rarely, if ever, occurs before puberty. A significant number of testes will be stimulated to descend at puberty by the testicular androgens secreted at that time. When the testes remain undescended past puberty, the seminiferous tubules do not develop and infertility results when the condition is bilateral, though androgen secretion is usually unimpaired. What percentage of cryptorchid testes will descend spontaneously and their ultimate functional status are unsettled questions.

During about the first 5 years of life the histologic appearance of the undescended testis is similar to that of its scrotal mate; thereafter the rate of development of the undescended testis begins to lag. The significance of such changes, particularly as to future potential for fertility, is unknown.

Undescended testes usually occur as an isolated defect, but significant abnormalities of the upper urinary tract have been found in about 13 per cent of patients with this defect. The undescended testis is often one of the characteristic defects of boys with syndromes known to occur in both sexes. Examples are the Smith-Lemli-Opitz syndrome, the Willi-Prader syndrome, the pseudo-Turner (male Turner) syndrome, the syndrome of absence of abdominal muscles, and others. Maldescent may occur as a manifestation of certain types of inherited hypogonadism such as Reifenstein's syndrome. In some instances, failure of normal descent is an indication that the testis is defective in other ways. It is often difficult to determine whether *testicular dysgenesis* which is observed histologically is congenital or a consequence of the maldescent. Another manifestation of the defective nature of cryptorchid testes is their proclivity for development of tumors. Tumors may develop even in testes which have undergone orchidopexy in the pubertal or postpubertal periods. It is not yet known whether orchidopexy before 5 years of age results in a decreased incidence of neoplastic formation.

There is general agreement that orchidopexy is the preferred method of treatment, when there is no reasonable doubt that the testis is incapable of descent. There are differences of opinion, however, concerning the advisability of initial therapy with gonadotropin to determine whether the testis can be caused to descend into the scrotum. In approximately 20 per cent of instances an undescended testis will descend with such therapy. When this is the case, it is assumed that descent would have occurred at puberty under the influence of endogenous gonadotropins.

Our current plan of therapy in the established case (see above) is to initiate gonadotropin therapy about 5 years of age. Chorionic gonadotropin is administered intramuscularly 5 times in individual doses of 4000 units on alternate days. If the testis descends, orchidopexy is not performed. If the testis does not descend, the gonadotropin therapy is not repeated, and orchidopexy is performed.

FAILURE OF DEVELOPMENT OF THE VAS DEFERENS

Failure of the vas deferens to develop may occur as an isolated congenital defect. The disorder is not recognized until adulthood, when the patient presents with infertility. Virility is unimpaired and spermatogenesis may occur, but there is lack of transport of spermatozoa from the testes; aspermia is found upon analysis of semen. Absence of the vas deferens may be suspected upon careful palpation of the testes and spermatic cords; the diagnosis is established by surgical exploration. Failure of development of the vas deferens accounts for the infertility of most adult males with cystic fibrosis; the cause for maldevelopment of the vas in this condition is unknown.

ACQUIRED DISEASE

Torsion of the Testis and Appendix Testis. Increased mobility of the testis may result in an axial twist with ensuing torsion of the spermatic cord and interference with its blood supply. Torsion of the spermatic cord almost always results in infarction and necrosis of the testis if it is not corrected within 24 hours of occurrence. The condition may be present at birth or may occur at any age; it is usually unilateral, but may be bilateral. The precipitating cause of the twisting is not known.

The *clinical manifestations* are variable. In the neonatal period there are often no symptoms, and the presenting evidence is reddish or bluish discoloration of the scrotum with enlargement and tenseness of the testis. It is not possible to transilluminate the mass. Systemic manifestations are rare in infants. Beyond infancy the boy may complain initially of a slight discomfort in the swollen testis; later there are intense pain, exquisite tenderness, lower abdominal pain, fever, nausea and vomiting. A prior history of trauma is not uncommon. When the torsion occurs in an undescended testis, diagnosis is more difficult. The disorder is frequently incorrectly diagnosed as epididymitis or orchitis, owing to the similarity in clinical manifestations; this results in delayed surgical exploration and in loss of the testis.

Treatment is immediate surgical exposure and untwisting of the torsion and fixation of the testis to the scrotal tissues. An abnormally mobile contralateral testis should be similarly fixed to scrotal tissues at the time of operation. The affected testis should be removed only when severe necrosis is apparent, since even when there is bluish-black discoloration some return of function may occur. When there is doubt as to the diagnosis, it is preferable to operate rather than delay, since orchitis is rare in childhood.

Torsion of one of the appendages of the testis also occurs, most often of the hydatid of Morgagni. The presenting symptom is acute onset of unilateral scrotal pain; the clinical course may be similar to that in torsion of the spermatic cord. Treatment consists in surgical removal of the necrotic appendix testis.

Balanoposthitis. Inflammation of the prepuce (posthitis) and glans (balanitis) is often associated with phimosis. It may follow injury by masturbation or other means, or it may occur as a complication of urethritis. Diphtheritic balanoposthitis is rare. The prepuce becomes red and edematous, and itches; the meatal orifice is narrowed, and there is a purulent secretion from the inflamed mucous membrane. There are dysuria and cystitis; hydronephrosis may be a complication in severe cases. Ordinarily the inflammation lasts but a few days. An appropriate antibiotic should be administered and cold compresses applied. Rarely, splitting of the foreskin or circumcision is necessary.

Stenosis of External Urethral Meatus. An abnormally small external urethral meatus is relatively common; occasionally it is responsible for obstructive uropathy.

The cause of the defect is not definitely established. Since circumcised infants often have urethral meatal ulcers in association with diaper rashes, and since small meatuses are seen with any frequency only in men circumcised in childhood, it is assumed that the strictures are secondary to ulcerations.

If a boy is found to have a small external ure-thral meatus, it is imperative that he be observed during micturition; a thin or weak stream due to a constricted meatus is an indication for an intra-venous pyelogram and for meatotomy.

CIRCUMCISION

Although circumcision is the operation most commonly performed on male infants in the United States, the medical indications for this procedure are not established. It has been noted that car-cinoma of the cervix is uncommon in Jewish women (circumcised husbands) and that carcinoma of the penis is rare among men who were circum-cised in infancy. A direct relationship is not proved.

The optimal time for circumcising the neonate is early on the first or after the seventh day of life. At these ages the available prothrombin is at the normal level. The operation should be performed by a physician. Circumcision is contraindicated in infants with anomalies of the external genitalia, since the foreskin may be needed for plastic surgery.

ANGELO M. DiGEORGE

REFERENCES

Altman, L. B., and Malament, M.: Carcinoma of the Testis Fol-lowing Orchidopexy. *J. Urol.,* 97:498, 1967.
Bender, L., Printz, L., and Presman, D.: Torsion of the Hydatid Testis: A Review of Thirteen Cases. *Pediatrics,* 42:531, 1968.
Benson, C. D., Mustard, W. T., Ravitch, M. M., Snyder, W. H., and Welch, K. J.: *Pediatric Surgery.* Chicago, Year Book Medical Publishers, Inc., 1962.
Felton, L. M.: Should Intravenous Pyelography Be a Routine Procedure for Children with Cryptorchidism or Hypo-spadias? *J. Urol.,* 81:335, 1959.
Gross, R. E., and Replogle, R. L.: Treatment of the Undescended Testis. *Postgrad. Med.,* 34:266, 1963.
Johnston, J. H.: The Undescended Testis. *Arch. Dis. Childhood,* 40:113, 1965.
Kaplan, E., and others: Reproductive Failure in Males with Cystic Fibrosis. *New England J. Med.,* 279:65, 1968.
Leape, L. L.: Torsion of the Testis. Invitation to Error. *J.A.M.A.,* 200:669, 1967.
Lilienfeld, A. M., and Graham, S.: Validity of Determining Cir-cumcision Status by Questionnaire as Related to Epidemio-logical Studies of Cancer of the Cervix. *J. Nat. Cancer Inst.,* 21:713, 1958.
Papadatos, C., and Moutsouris, C.: Bilateral Testicular Torsion in the Newborn. *J. Pediat.,* 71:249, 1967.
Richart, R., and Benirscke, K.: Penile Agenesis. Report of Case, Review of the World Literature, and Discussion of Pertinent Embryology. *Arch. Path.,* 70:252, 1960.
Salle, B., Hedinger, C., and Nicole, R.: Significance of Testic-ular Biopsies in Cryptorchidism in Children. *Acta Endocr.,* 58:67, 1968.
Weiss, C.: Ritual Circumcision. Comments on Current Practices in American Hospitals. *Clin. Pediat.,* 1:65, 1962.

FEMALE GENITAL ORGANS

The female reproductive system undergoes several periods of physiologic change before reaching maturity. Prerequisite to interpretation of the findings on pelvic examination in young females is an appreciation of the dynamics of hor-monal and morphologic interaction.

In *early intrauterine life* the secretion of the fetal gonad and not the maternal hormonal environment is responsible for differentiation and development of the genital system. Differentiation always tends to proceed along female lines in the absence of a male gonad. The embryonic testis is the only source of the nonsteroidal organizer sub-stance necessary to suppress the müllerian system and to stimulate development of the wolffian one. Thus the genitalia are phenotypically female if the fetal gonad is ovary, if the fetal gonads are absent (Turner's syndrome) or if the embryonic testis is deficient in production of testicular organizer sub-stance (male pseudohermaphroditism). In *late intrauterine life* high levels of female sex hormones normally produced by the fetoplacental unit induce feminizing changes in the breast and in the female genitalia. Exposure of the the female fetus to androgenic hormones does not cause suppression of the müllerian ducts as does testicular organizer substance. Under such a circumstance the internal genitalia tend to develop normally, but the ex-ternal genitalia undergo virilization, as with fetal congenital adrenal hyperplasia, maternal in-gestion of androgenic drugs or masculinizing tumors. In the *immature female* lack of estrogen greatly increases susceptibility of the external genitalia to infection and trauma and is respon-sible for most of the genital disorders in prepu-bertal girls, whereas during *adolescence* menstrual problems are most commonly due to imbalance in the estrogen-progesterone cycle. The levels of hor-mones found in normal female children are indi-cated in Table 18-1.

METHOD OF EXAMINATION

Pelvic examination can be performed at any age from infancy on. Anesthesia is rarely necessary; psychic implications have been overemphasized. The attitude and approach of the physician have much to do with the reactions of the child. Confi-dence, gentleness and reasonable speed are main assets. Inspection, including ample separation of the labia, and bimanual palpation which is per-formed rectally are the essentials. Endoscopy is included when conditions require inspection of the upper portion of the vagina and cervix. Firm pressure applied to the lateral aspects of the labia majora will expose the hymenal orifice with no dis-

TABLE 18-1. Average 24-Hour Urinary Excretion Rates of Sex-Related Hormones in Normal Females from Infancy to Maturity

	NEWBORN	1-6 YEARS	7 YEARS TO PUBERTY	MATURE ADULT
Total estrogens	1 mcg./24 hr. (first week)	0.5-1 mcg./24 hr.	1-8.5 mcg.	4-60 mcg./24 hr.
Pregnanediol	0-0.5 mg./24 hr.	0-0.5 mg./24 hr.	0.2-1 mg./24 hr.	0.5-7 mg./24 hr.
17-Ketosteroids	1 mg./24 hr. (first 3 wks= 1-2.5 mg.)	1 mg./24 hr.	5 mg./24 hr.	6-15 mg./24 hr.
17 Hydroxysteroids	0	0.5-3 mg./24 hr.	1.5-8 mg./24 hr.	3-12 mg./24 hr.
Pregnanetriol	0	0.06 mg./24 hr.	0.3-1.5 mg./24 hr.	1-2 mg./24 hr.
Pituitary gonadotropins	0	0	Less than 6 mouse uterine units/24 hrs.	6-50 M.U.U.

comfort, but the hymen itself is highly sensitive to touch. The posterior vaginal fornix is so short in the immature female that the cul-de-sac is almost nonexistent, and therefore the palpating finger cannot be advanced high enough vaginally to outline pelvic structures even under anesthesia. The uterus can be palpated and outlined and the adnexal structures explored more definitively by rectal examination. The uterus lies horizontally in midposition and is approximately 2.5 cm. in length during the prepubertal years; the cervix is proportionately much longer than the corpus. Under normal conditions the tubes and ovaries are not palpable.

A small plastic pipet with an aspirating bulb and tip somewhat longer than an average medicine dropper is easily inserted into the hymenal orifice for collection of vaginal secretions or discharge. A cotton swab moistened with saline solution may be used, but it is more traumatic if the aperture is small. Furthermore, contamination from the vulvar regions is less likely with the pipet. The aspirate is adequate for smear, culture, pH and cytologic examination. A vaginoscope, Kelly cystoscope or a tiny speculum is necessary for inspection of the vagina and cervix. Makeshift instruments, such as an otoscope or nasal speculum, are totally inadequate. The fearsome child may reject this portion of the examination. Her behavior or reaction to the earlier phases will indicate whether or not endoscopy can be done at this time. Otherwise, sedation or, exceptionally, anesthesia may be necessary.

DISORDERS OF THE FEMALE GENITAL ORGANS

Doubtful Sex and Anomalies of the External Genitalia. Problems involving sexual ambiguity of the newborn must be dealt with promptly and knowledgeably. Alarmed parents need to be informed convincingly that an accurate diagnosis can always be reached and that appropriate plans for the future can be made with confidence. Information derived from the family history, the preg-

nancy history, particularly in regard to maternal drug therapy, the physical examination of the newborn, a buccal smear and the 17-ketosteroid determination will provide a correct diagnosis in most cases of sexual ambiguity evident in the neonatal period. A positive buccal smear broadly differentiates nonadrenal virilization of the female due to maternal androgens and female pseudohermaphroditism due to adrenal hyperplasia from male pseudohermaphroditism with partial masculinization of the external genitalia. The urinary 17-ketosteroid values are elevated in adrenal hyperplasia and normal in nonadrenal virilization. The normal increase in fetal adrenal activity characteristic of later intrauterine life may persist for 2 or 3 weeks after birth. If the 17-ketosteroid values are not definitive in the neonatal period, an increase in pregnanetriol excretion in excess of 1 mg. per 24 hours confirms the diagnosis of adrenal hyperplasia. Exploratory laparotomy is necessary in rare instances when true hermaphroditism is suspected (see p. 1237).

Because of the close embryologic relations, developmental anomalies of the genital tract may be associated with or mistaken for anomalies of the urinary system. *Ectopic ureter* usually has its terminus just inside the vaginal vault. A cystic mass appearing at the introitus is more commonly an ectopic ureter with a blind terminus than a *vaginal or Gartner's duct cyst*. *Imperforate hymen* may also appear as a cystic bulging mass at the vaginal introitus, if it is distended with mucous secretions. Whether mucocele is associated or not, imperforate hymen is incised to allow for drainage as soon as the diagnosis is made. Complete *absence of vagina* is rare, often accompanied by rudimentary development of the uterus; operations for correction of this malformation should not be performed until after maturity. *Labial agglutination* resulting from irritation or inflammation of the labia minora is distinguished from the above-mentioned anomalies by the characteristic livid line of agglutination extending vertically down the center of the membrane. This condition is self-limited and disappears as puberty approaches and estrogen levels rise. The agglutination encourages pocketing of urine, irritation and infection. Application of an estrogenic cream induces cornification of the epithelium, and spontaneous separation will usually occur. Otherwise the edges can be easily separated with a small, well lubricated probe.

Noninfectious Vaginal Discharge. Vaginal discharge of a thick mucoid secretion from the estrogen-stimulated cervical glands is physiologic in the newborn. A small amount of bleeding due to endometrial shedding may accompany the discharge. This is transient and disappears within 2 weeks when gestational hormones have been metabolized and excreted.

Leukorrhea is also physiologic in young girls, beginning a year or more before the menarche when ovarian function starts and estrogen secretion is as yet unopposed by progesterone. Parental concern is the main problem. Fears should be allayed, but treatment otherwise avoided.

Vulvovaginitis. Almost any of the infectious or irritating agents may cause inflammation of the anestrogenic epithelium. Transfer of organisms from the upper respiratory tract, skin or the gastrointestinal tract occurs mainly when trauma such as friction or scratching is added to contamination.

Nonspecific infections with mixed bacterial cultures of the coliform-aerogenes group are most common. They tend to be low-grade, chronic, and difficult to eradicate permanently. They may be associated with foreign body or with pinworm infestations, in which case removal of the cause and local treatment are curative. Infections in which pure cultures of one of the gonococci, pneumococci, streptococci, staphylococci, proteus, Shigella or other organisms are found are generally more acute in onset and more responsive to treatment. A purulent discharge is common to all these organisms except the streptococcus, in which the discharge is more likely to be serosanguineous or frankly bloody.

Gonococcal infections require smear and culture for diagnosis. Intense redness and swelling of the vulva and vagina and thick purulent vaginal discharge are not in themselves pathognomonic. Upper genital tract infections are exceedingly rare.

Viral infections. Herpes simplex is most serious in the newborn (p. 634). No age group is immune to genital infection with this agent. Maternal herpes is a serious threat to the infant. Viremia which occurs in the neonate soon after the superficial lesions appear may seriously damage internal organs such as the liver and brain and may be fatal. Condylomata are seen occasionally in young girls. These are of viral origin and not venereal.

Monilial vaginitis occurs infrequently in the neonatal period when the estrogen-stimulated epithelium is rich in glycogen. The infection is rare in the prepubertal years except in children with diabetes mellitus or those receiving prolonged antibiotic therapy. *Trichomonal infestations* are seen infrequently before puberty.

Treatment. Hygienic measures, mild soaps rather than detergents, clean cotton panties, and local application of an estrogenic cream will clear most nonspecific infections in 10 to 12 days. Estrogens can be given orally to cornify the epithelium and increase local tissue resistance; suppositories are rarely necessary. Infections with specific organisms are treated in accordance with their in-vitro sensitivity to antibiotics. Procaine penicillin, 600,000 units on 3 successive days, is the most effective treatment for gonococcal infection, although post-treatment culture is a necessary step to detect a resistant strain of this organism. Monilial vaginitis responds to fungicidal ointments such as nystatin. Gentian violet as 1 per cent aqueous solution is effective but messy. Underlying diabetes should be kept in mind and blood sugar values determined. Metronidazole (Flagyl) is the most effective agent currently available for treatment of trichomonas infestation, but the oral preparation is applicable only to older girls weighing over 100 pounds. The local preparation should be used in smaller girls.

Lichen Sclerosus et Atrophicus. This disorder may involve the entire vulvar and perianal regions. The tissues appear white and thinned out, often excoriated by scratching. It is believed to be an inflammatory process, although the specific cause is not known. The gross appearance closely resembles leukoplakia, but differences are evident on biopsy. Lichen sclerosus et atrophicus is characterized by superficial hyperkeratosis, atrophy of the rest of the epidermis, loss of the rete pegs and a specific sclerotic change in connective tissue just beneath the epidermis. It is not neoplastic in behavior; it tends to disappear at puberty or shortly thereafter, and surgical management other than biopsy should be avoided. This restraint should be emphasized because local treatment with ointments containing estrogens, hydrocortisone or vitamins A and D may provide only minimal relief from pruritus, and repeated reassurance of the parents of its benign nature and self-limited course is necessary.

Vaginal Bleeding. Conditions commonly associated with this symptom in prepubertal girls include severe vaginitis, particularly a streptococcal type, foreign body, trauma, prolapsed urethra, precocious puberty, and neoplasm.

Traumatic injuries heal well with minimal scarring and do not interfere with future reproductive functions. *Injuries due to rape* require special handling. Secretions aspirated from the vagina and collected from the clothing should be examined immediately for gonococci, spermatozoa and for acid phosphatase, which is found in high concentration in semen. Administration of long-acting penicillin is advisable as prophylaxis against venereal disease.

Prolapse of the urethral mucosa appears as a mulberry mass protruding from and completely occluding the vagina. The mucosa becomes devitalized below the meatal margin and bleeds readily. Treatment is surgical excision at the line of demarcation.

Sarcoma botryoides (p. 1462), although rare, is so rapidly progressive that diagnosis by biopsy must be made without delay. Lesions may arise in multifocal sites along the course of the cervix and vagina with early involvement of all regional tissues by local invasion. Wide removal of pelvic organs has resulted in a few cures, but the prognosis is generally poor. Radiotherapy and chemotherapy are ineffectual.

Precocious puberty (p. 1180) as a cause for vaginal bleeding is accompanied by changes in secondary sex characteristics. Constitutional precocity is the most common type and accounts for approximately 90 per cent of the cases reported in girls between the ages of 2½ and 9 years. Central nervous system, ovarian, adrenal and thyroid disorders account for a small percentage of isosexual precocity in the female.

MENSTRUAL DISORDERS IN ADOLESCENCE

Normal menstruation is dependent upon the functional integrity of (1) the hypothalamus and its connections with higher centers, (2) the anterior pituitary, (3) the ovary, and (4) the uterus. The complexities of the processes involved in achieving full sexual maturation are such that menstrual irregularities are exceedingly common during the first few postmenarcheal years.

Delayed Menarche. In the United States the mean age at the menarche is 12.3 years, with a range of 9 to 17 years. Age differences for this event are attributed to general health and nutrition, heredity, climatic environment and psychosocial development. Whatever the stimulus, activation of the hypothalamus is clearly the force directly responsible for initiation of menstruation and ultimately for regulation of the fully mature ovulatory cycle. The anterior pituitary gland is capable of producing follicle-stimulating hormone (FSH) and luteinizing hormone (LH) in prepubertal girls, but secretion of pituitary gonadotropic hormones is inhibited until the hypothalamus stimulates release of humoral substances (releasing factors) from the median eminence. Ample laboratory and clinical evidence for these relations may be seen in destructive lesions of the hypothalamus which cause hastening of the onset of puberty, and in transplantation of the pituitary gland from prepubertal rats to adult hypophysectomized female hosts. Harris showed that the newborn or prepubertal pituitary under the influence of the adult hypothalamus was capable of supporting estrus, and in some cases pregnancies occurred.

Delay in the menarche beyond the sixteenth year warrants diagnostic survey. Exclusion of systemic, metabolic or anatomic defects is the first step. Obesity, malnutrition or psychosomatic disorders may play an important role. A buccal smear should be examined to determine nuclear sex. If any of the examinations suggest sexual aberration, further studies are indicated. The need for adequate evaluation before resorting to hormonal therapy is emphasized by findings in recent surveys in which modern cytogenetic and hormonal assays have been done. Such studies show that 40 per cent of the cases of primary amenorrhea extending into late adolescence are the result of genetic abnormalities. Of these, the most frequently encountered are various types of gonadal dysgenesis, the triple X or "superfemale" syndrome, isochromosomal abnormalities, testicular feminizing syndrome and, less frequently, true hermaphroditism.

Dysfunctional uterine bleeding. The symptoms characteristic of this disorder are irregular, protracted or excessive vaginal bleeding. It is due primarily to imbalance in secretion of the hormones that normally control menstrual function and variability in responsiveness of the target organs in adolescence. With rare exceptions the cycles are anovulatory. The hypothalamic-pituitary-gonadal-uterine axis may take as little as a few months or as long as 5 years to achieve reciprocal balance and full maturation. Ovulation occurs in only about 2 per cent of women during the first 6 months of menstrual activity and in only about 18 per cent by the end of the first year. Anovulatory cycles may be considered normal for the first 1 to 3 years after the menarche, irrespective of the chronologic age of the patient. This phase is known as the period of relative infertility.

Dysfunctional uterine bleeding is self-limited for the majority of adolescents. Complete physical and pelvic examinations are necessary to rule out systemic, metabolic and local organic causes, including pregnancy. Hypothyroidism accounts for only about 5 per cent of cases of menstrual dysfunction in adolescence, but, if present, treatment is usually curative. In contrast, if thyroid function is normal, empiric use of thyroid preparations is ineffectual and may be especially deleterious in this age group. Hematologic causes for dysfunctional uterine bleeding are rare, although excessive menstrual flow is occasionally the first symptom of thrombocytopenic purpura.

Treatment. If no organic causes are found, menstrual irregularities in adolescent girls should be treated expectantly with a high protein diet and vitamin and iron supplements. Bleeding sufficient to lower the hemoglobin or serum iron levels requires more active treatment. Since the cycles are anovulatory, the endometrium reflects persistent stimulation by estrogen and lack of progesterone. Administration of potent oral progestins such as medroxyprogesterone acetate during the last 5 to 7 days of the cycle is capable of inducing secretory changes in the endometrium. This in turn results in a more normal physiologic response to withdrawal of hormonal support and more controlled withdrawal bleeding. Treatment is repeated for 3 successive periods. The timing of administration of the progestational agent is extremely important. If given too early in the cycle, it will inhibit ovulation and delay the normal occurrence of menstruation. When maturation is complete and cycles are ovulatory, the menstrual irregularities are usually corrected.

Instances of severe bleeding present special problems. Control can usually be achieved by administration of large doses of progestational agents such as Provest, 10 to 30 mg. every 6 hours (medroxyprogesterone acetate, 10 mg., with ethynil estradiol, 0.05 mg.) until bleeding ceases. Dilatation and curettage may be necessary in some cases for control of hemorrhage, and in the minority of cases which fail to respond to conservative management.

Dysmenorrhea. Abdominal discomfort, cramping in nature, backache and leg ache associated with menstruation are extremely common complaints. The term *primary dysmenorrhea* is applied to these symptoms when they are severe enough to interfere with normal activity and when endometriosis, infection or other pelvic disease causing *secondary dysmenorrhea* is nonexistent. The specific cause of primary dysmenorrhea is unknown, although contributory factors are well recognized. The symptoms do not usually appear with the first few menstrual cycles. Instead they tend to be associated with ovulatory cycles, although this is not invariable. Vascular changes associated with menstrual flow provide the most convincing explanation for the local discomfort. Alternate vasoconstriction and vasodilatation of the vessels of the endometrial bed induce local ischemia, edema, necrosis and slough. Psychic factors, tension and anxiety can accentuate the local symptoms and may be entirely responsible for associated autonomic nervous system symptoms of nausea, vomiting, pallor, sweating and occasionally syncope when these appear. The pain is often misinterpreted as an indication of pelvic disease and as a portent of future reproductive difficulties.

Treatment. Pelvic examination is essential to exclude pelvic abnormalities. Reassurance, a straightforward explanation of the physiology of menstruation, encouragement of participation in all regular activities and good hygiene go a long way toward correction. Suppression of ovulation using estrogens or synthetic progestins for several months is usually effective. Psychotherapy may be necessary for severe problem cases, but surgical procedures are rarely warranted.

ELSIE R. CARRINGTON

REFERENCES

Bishop, P. M. F.: Intersexual States and Allied Conditions. *Brit. Med. J.*, 1:1255, 1966.

Bongiovanni, A. M.: The Adrenogenital Syndrome. *New England J. Med.*, 268:1283, 1342, 1391, 1963.

Capraro, V. J.: Sexual Assault of Female Children. Monograph on Pediatric and Adolescent Gynecology. *Ann. New York Acad. Sc.*, 142:817, 1967.

Carrington, E. R.: Laboratory Examination of the Pediatric Gynecologic Patient. *Ann. New York Acad. Sc.*, 142:623, 1967.

Ditkowsky, S. F., Falk, A. B., Baker, N., and Schaffner, M.: Lichen Sclerosus et Atrophicus in Childhood. A.M.A. *J. Dis. Child.*, 91:52, 1956.

Donovan, B. T., and Harris, G. W.: Neurohumoral Mechanisms in Reproduction. *Brit. Med. Bull.*, 11:93, 1955.

Federman, D. D.: Disorders of Sexual Development. *New England J. Med.*, 277:351, 1967.

Gray, L., and Kotcher, E.: Vaginitis in Childhood. *Am. J. Obst. & Gynec.*, 82:530, 1961.

Harris, G. W.: *Neural Control of the Pituitary Gland.* London, E. Arnold, Ltd., 1955.

Huffman, J. W.: *The Gynecology of Childhood and Adolescence.* Philadelphia, W. B. Saunders Company, 1968.

Jones, H. W., Jr., and Heller, R. H.: *Pediatric and Adolescent Gynecology.* Baltimore, Williams & Wilkins Company, 1966.

Lascano, E. F., Montes, L. F., and Mazzini, M. A.: Tissue Changes in Lichen Sclerosus et Atrophicus in Children Following Local Application of Oestrogens. *Brit. J. Dermatol.*, 76:496, 1964.

McArthur, J. W.: Functional Disorders of Menstruation in Adolescence. *New England J. Med.*, 249:361, 1953.

Philip, J., Sele, V, and Trolle, D.: Primary Amenorrhea: A Study of 101 Cases. *Fertility-Sterility*, 16:795, 1965.

Southam, A. L.: Disorders of Menstruation. *Clin. Obst. & Gynec.*, 9:779, 1966.

Southam, A. L., and Richart, R. M.: The Prognosis of Adolescents with Menstrual Abnormalities. *Tr. Am. A. Obst. Gynec.*, 76:43, 1965.

White, J. G.: Fulminating Infection with Herpes Simplex Virus in Premature and Newborn Infants. *New England J. Med.*, 269:455, 1963.

19.   Convulsive Disorders

Convulsive phenomena are common in children and occur with a wide variety of disorders of the central nervous system. Seizures may be classified according to (1) their cause or pathogenesis (see Table 19-1), (2) their clinical manifestations, (3) their electroencephalographic pattern.

Incidence. Consideration of the relative incidence of the various causative factors at different ages is frequently helpful in arriving at a correct diagnosis and in evaluating prognosis.

Convulsions are far more common during the first 2 years than at any other period of life. Intracranial birth injuries, including the effects of anoxia and hemorrhage and congenital defects of the brain, are the most frequent causes of convulsions in very young infants. In the latter part of infancy and in early childhood acute infections (extracranial and intracranial) are the most frequent causes. Far less frequent causes in infants are tetany, idiopathic epilepsy, hypoglycemia, brain tumors, renal insufficiency, poisoning, asphyxia, spontaneous intracranial hemorrhage and thrombosis, postnatal trauma and others listed in Table 19-1.

By midchildhood acute extracranial infections have become an infrequent cause of convulsions, whereas idiopathic epilepsy, first appearing as an important cause of convulsions about the third year of life, is the most common factor. Other causes in the postinfancy period are congenital defects of the brain, residual cerebral damage from earlier trauma, infection, lead poisoning, brain tumors, acute or chronic glomerulonephritis, certain degenerative diseases of the brain and drug ingestion.

ACUTE OR NONRECURRENT CONVULSIONS

Convulsions in the Newborn. A clinical seizure at any age is associated with a paroxysmal burst of electrical activity within the central nervous system. In the newborn infant the electrical activity of the cerebral hemispheres is poorly developed, but subcortical rhythms are present. Mass myoclonic movements have been said to occur in utero, but the tonic and clonic movements that characterize grand mal seizures are rarely apparent during the first several weeks of life. The low incidence of grand mal seizures reported during the neonatal period probably reflects both the poor development of the cerebral hemispheres and lack of uniformity in recognizing or classifying seizures or their equivalents. The electroencephalogram, though poorly developed in the newborn and technically difficult to obtain, may be the only objective means of detecting a seizure in many instances.

After an episode of acute anoxia, a convulsion in the newborn may take the form of a tonic spasm preceded by a few clonic jerks. The electroencephalogram becomes flattened. Focal seizures may be associated with irregular jerky movements and nystagmus or staring, pallor and hypotonia. Paroxysmal bursts of multiple spike and slow wave discharges appear on the electroencephalogram. In some instances the respirations become slow and irregular, with periods of apnea and a feeble cry. The neck becomes rigid, the pupils dilate, and the child drools. Alteration of the electroencephalogram may also occur in association with slight movements of the fingers, toes or eyelids, with a change in color or with chewing.

The presence of a seizure suggests a cerebral insult and should alert the physician to various causative factors, particularly those which can be altered favorably.

The prognosis for the newborn infant who has a seizure is best if the episode is early in onset, of brief duration, and associated with no other disease state. Tremors occurring during the first day of life seem to have the best prognosis, if the child's subsequent neonatal course is entirely normal. The outlook is poor if the heart rate is consistently slow or if symptoms of any kind persist for more than 72 hours. Although convulsions are rarely the only manifestation of a bacterial infection, this possibility cannot be excluded by examination alone.

Treatment and management of the newborn infant with seizures involve primarily adequate supportive care. This includes prevention of shock, maintenance of an adequate airway, and sedation appropriate to the infant's needs. Chloral hydrate and phenobarbital are the most widely used anticonvulsive agents.

Acute Convulsions in Infants and Children. The causes of acute convulsive attacks in children are extremely varied (Table 19-1). Any type of seizure may occur as a transient manifestation of acute disease involving the brain, but generalized

TABLE 19-1.   Etiologic Classification of Convulsive Disorders

I. Acute or nonrecurrent forms

"Febrile convulsions" (e.g. at onset of acute extracranial infections or in association with high environmental temperatures)

Intracranial infections (e.g. acute meningitis, encephalitis, sinus thrombophlebitis, cerebral abscess, tetanus, malaria, typhus fever)

Intracranial hemorrhage (e.g. from birth or other trauma, hemorrhagic disease, rupture of defective vessels, sickle cell disease)

Toxic:
1. Convulsant drugs (e.g. aminophylline, antihistamines, camphor, Darvon, Metrazol, phenothiazine, corticosteroids, strychnine and thujone)
2. Tetanus
3. Lead encephalopathy
4. Shigellosis, salmonellosis

Anoxic (e.g. sudden severe asphyxia, inhalation anesthesia)

Metabolic or nutritional (e.g. acute hypocalcemic tetany, alkalosis, therapeutic hypoglycemia, pyridoxine deficiency, phenylketonuria, glycinemia)

Acute cerebral edema (e.g. in acute glomerulonephritis or allergic edema of the brain)

Brain tumor

Miscellaneous (porphyria, systemic lupus erythematosus)

II. Chronic or recurrent forms

Epilepsy:
1. Idiopathic (primary, cryptogenic, essential or genuine epilepsy)
   (a) Hereditary or genetic type
   (b) Nongenetic or acquired idiopathic type (?)
2. Organic (secondary or symptomatic epilepsy — with residual brain damage from previous focal or diffuse injuries)
   (a) Post-traumatic (e.g. from direct laceration of brain tissue)
   (b) Posthemorrhagic (e.g. from injury at birth or later, from hemorrhagic diseases, pachymeningitis, rupture of miliary aneurysm)
   (c) Postanoxic (e.g. from severe asphyxia neonatorum)
   (d) Postinfectious (e.g. following encephalitis, meningitis, sinus thrombophlebitis or abscess)
   (e) Post-toxic (e.g. kernicterus, encephalopathy following lead, arsenic or other chronic poisoning)
   (f) Degenerative (e.g. "idiopathic atrophy," cerebromacular degeneration, encephalitis periaxialis diffusa, intracranial neurofibromatosis)
   (g) Congenital (e.g. cerebral aplasia, porencephaly, tuberous sclerosis, hydrocephalus, vascular anomalies such as the Sturge-Weber type and arteriovenous aneurysms)
   (h) Parasitic brain disease (cysticercosis, toxoplasmosis, syphilis)
   (i) Posthypoglycemic injury
3. Sensory (reading, touch, light, sound, music, self-induced)

Epilepsy-simulating states:

Narcolepsy and cataplexy

Hysteria ("psychogenic epilepsy")

Tetany:
1. Hypocalcemic (e.g. idiopathic, postoperative, neonatal, vitamin D deficiency, deficient intestinal absorption)
2. Of alkalosis (e.g. vomiting, administration of bicarbonate, hyperventilation)

Hypoglycemic states:
1. Hyperinsulinism (e.g. tumor or hyperplasia of islets of Langerhans)
2. Hypopituitarism (e.g. deficiency of adrenocorticotropic, thyrotropic and growth hormones)
3. Adrenal cortical insufficiency
4. Hepatic disorders (e.g. von Gierke's disease)
5. Miscellaneous (e.g. leucine-induced, idiopathic ketotic)

Uremia

"Cerebral" allergy

Cardiovascular dysfunction or syncopal attacks (e.g. simple fainting attacks, Stokes-Adams syndrome, hyperactive carotid sinus reflex)

Migraine

---

tonic and clonic convulsions similar to the grand mal attack of epilepsy are by far the most common. Practically all seizures resulting from extracranial disorders are of this type.

Approximately 6 to 8 per cent of all children have *febrile convulsions,* most of which occur after the first 6 months of life, but within the first 2 to 3 years. The incidence decreases up to 6 to 8 years, after which such seizures are rare. Males are more often affected than females, and there appears to be an increased susceptibility in some families.

Diagnosis. In the latter part of infancy and in the first few years of childhood most of the convulsions which occur merely represent an initial symptom of an acute febrile illness. A child who has had a convulsion should, however, be examined for the possibility of some other cause. Such disorders as tetany, lead encephalopathy, intracranial injury, hemorrhage or tumor, poisoning with a convulsant drug, hypoglycemia, asphyxia, cerebral sinus thrombosis (associated with cyanotic congenital heart disease or cachexia), acute nephritis and epilepsy should be considered. The age of the child should be taken into account in the consideration of causative factors (see above).

A carefully taken history of any previous attacks, of immediately preceding symptoms such as hyperirritability, fever, muscular cramps, headache, vomiting or dizziness, of a possible dietary deficiency, of poisoning of any kind, of cranial injury, of a hemorrhagic tendency, of exposure to infection or of a familial predisposition to seizures is invaluable for orientation.

A complete physical examination, including a thorough neurologic appraisal, is essential. Inspection of the eyegrounds may give the first clue to the nature of the primary illness by revealing an optic neuritis or choking of the disks. These may occur in the presence of an expanding intracranial lesion (tumor, cyst, hemorrhage or abscess), acute hydrocephalus or severe encephalitis. Such examination may also reveal the presence of retinal hemorrhages, suggesting intracranial bleeding from trauma or a blood dyscrasia. Albuminuric retinitis may furnish the first clue to the presence of subacute or chronic nephritis. There may be slight choking of the optic disks in acute nephritis with arterial hypertension. Chorioretinitis is suggestive of toxoplasmosis, but is not diagnostic of it. The reddish areas of degeneration in the macular region in cerebromacular degenerative disease and the choroidal tubercles of miliary tuberculosis are highly characteristic.

Determinations of serum calcium, blood sugar and urea nitrogen levels will aid in the diagnosis of hypocalcemic tetany, hypoglycemia and acute nephritis, respectively. Coexisting hypertension, albuminuria and cylindruria are evidences of nephritis. Roentgenograms may show the "lead line" of lead poisoning in the long bones, or thinning of the skull and separation of the sutures in the presence of an expanding intracranial lesion. Examination of the urine for coproporphyrin and for type III uroporphyrin (Watson test) may reveal evidence of lead intoxication or of acute intermittent porphyria.

If the primary disease is infectious, it should be ascertained whether the infection is extracranial (febrile or prefebrile convulsions) or intracranial. It is necessary to determine whether an intracranial infection is meningitis, encephalitis, abscess, sinus thrombophlebitis or tetanus. Certain other infectious diseases, such as typhus fever, shigellosis, salmonellosis and malaria, may occasionally cause convulsions; in some instances the convulsions are related to disturbances of water and electrolyte balance (see hyperelectrolytemia, p. 222).

Treatment. For the control of "febrile" convulsions which occasionally occur at the onset of acute extracranial infections a sedative dose of phenobarbital (3 mg. per kg.) and reduction of the elevated body temperature usually suffice.

If the convulsion is prolonged or if the child has a second convulsion before he recovers fully from the first, more vigorous anticonvulsant treatment is indicated (see p. 1254). Appropriate treatment for shock and for the primary condition must of course be provided.

Seizures secondary to electrolyte disturbances require special therapy (see p. 222). After other causes for seizures have been excluded as well as it is possible to do so, a clinical trial of pyridoxine may be indicated in young infants (see p. 174).

Prognosis. When a seizure results from some physical or metabolic disturbance, the prevention of recurrent convulsions is dependent upon the eradication or control of the underlying disease.

After a single febrile seizure the family can be reassured that the probability of chronic epilepsy is not great. The occurrence of more than one febrile seizure increases the probability of subsequent spontaneous nonfebrile convulsions. There is a relatively high probability that idiopathic epilepsy will develop in children who have more than 5 febrile convulsions in a 12-month period, single seizures which last for more than an hour, or persistent electroencephalographic abnormalities. (Note that the electroencephalogram of a child who has had a febrile convulsion may be abnormal as long as a week afterward.) Approximately 25 per cent of epileptic children have a history of febrile seizures.

Evidence seems to indicate that daily anticonvulsant therapy does not reduce the number or duration of febrile convulsions. Therefore, as long as the physician feels that a child has febrile convulsions, such therapy is not indicated. When convulsions recur with little or no evidence of infection, or if the electroencephalogram is significantly abnormal 2 weeks or more after the last seizure, a therapeutic trial of daily anticonvulsant therapy may be indicated.

An infant or young child who has had one or more febrile seizures is entitled to more prompt antipyretic measures, such as aspirin or tepid sponges, and *anti-infectious* therapy than might otherwise seem indicated. Some physicians give phenobarbital prophylactically to such infants during a febrile episode. If anti-infectious or anticonvulsant therapy is prescribed, the physician must observe the child closely for the possibility that such serious infections as meningitis may be masked.

CHRONIC OR RECURRENT CONVULSIONS

EPILEPSY

The terms *epilepsy* (from the Greek *epilépsia*, a seizure) and *recurrent convulsive disorder* can be used interchangeably. These terms designate a variable symptom complex characterized by recurrent, paroxysmal attacks of unconsciousness or impaired consciousness, usually with a succession of tonic or clonic muscular spasms or other abnormal behavior. If a cause of the patient's seizures cannot be found, he may be said to have *idiopathic* or *cryptogenic epilepsy*; if a cerebral abnormality is demonstrable, *organic* or *symptomatic epilepsy*.

Because many persons, from prejudice or ignorance, feel that a person with epilepsy will somehow fail to make an adequate social adjustment, some physicians are reluctant to use the term "epilepsy" in discussing the problem with parents. Although its use with a previous explanation of its meaning may be potentially harmful, an affected family should know the term and how it applies to them. This is part of the physician's responsibility as he educates the family toward living more comfortably with a chronic illness. There is considerable variation in a family's ability and desire to acquire information about a chronic illness. Too much information on a single visit is undesirable. Orientation should be a continuing process, especially during the early period of medical supervision.

Idiopathic Epilepsy. Although in the majority of instances the cause of recurrent seizures cannot be established, it would seem probable that some specific genetic defect in cerebral metabolism is responsible in many of the afflicted children.

Electroencephalographic tracings, particularly during sleep, show generalized abnormalities in 90 per cent of children with idiopathic seizures. Often there are focal electrical abnormalities on the electroencephalogram which migrate from one area to another as evidenced by variations in serial examinations. These are rarely associated with anatomic defects. Lennox pointed out that electroencephalographic abnormalities (cerebral dysrhythmias) are more likely to be found in parents and siblings of affected children than in the population at large. A hereditary factor is usually not clinically demonstrable, however.

Organic Epilepsy. A variety of genetically determined conditions (Table 19-1) are associated with seizures. These disorders have abnormalities demonstrable anatomically (congenital ectodermoses) or biochemically (phenylketonuria). In addition, convulsions may occur after cerebral damage acquired in the prenatal, natal or postnatal period. Neurologic examination of such children frequently shows a motor handicap of central nervous system origin (cerebral palsy) and mental retardation. These patients almost always have electroencephalographic abnormalities.

The recognition of genetically determined conditions is important for several reasons: (1) Cerebral damage in younger siblings of affected patients may be prevented in certain instances by prompt and effective therapy (leucine-induced hypoglycemia, phenylketonuria, kernicterus). (2) Indefinite signs and symptoms in siblings may be more readily recognized (tuberous sclerosis, cerebromacular degeneration, neurofibromatosis). (3) Identification of an organic cause of the seizures is important prognostically; in general, control of such seizures is less satisfactory and social adjustment of the child less adequate than in children with idiopathic seizures.

Clinical Manifestations. *Grand mal seizures.* These seizures may be preceded by a momentary aura, but fewer than a third of epileptic children can give a definite description of such an experience. In some instances a preliminary, localized spasm or twitching of muscles may precede a generalized seizure. This is often referred to as a "motor aura," or warning. Vague prodromal symptoms or signs, such as irritability, digestive disturbances, headache and mental dullness, may forewarn patients or their parents of impending motor seizures. The period intervening is usually short, but may be hours or even a day or two.

Grand mal seizures are generalized convulsions, usually with tonic and clonic phases of the muscular spasms. The onset of the paroxysm is abrupt, and the tonic spasm may occur simultaneously with loss of consciousness. The patient, if sitting or standing, falls to the ground. His face suddenly becomes pale, the pupils dilate, the conjunctivas become insensitive to touch, the eyeballs roll upward or to one side, the face is distorted, the glottis is closed, the head may be thrown backward or to one side, the abdominal and chest muscles are held rigidly, and the limbs are contracted irregularly or stiffen out. As the air is forced out of the lungs through the glottis by sudden contraction of the diaphragm and the intercostal muscles, a short, startling cry may be heard. The tongue may be severely bitten as a result of the rapid contraction of the jaw muscles. Micturition and less frequently defecation may follow the sudden forceful contraction of the abdominal muscles. As the tonic phase of the seizure continues, facial pallor is quickly followed by suffusion and this in turn by cyanosis, occasionally severe, owing to arrest of all respiratory movements. At the end of this phase, which usually lasts not more than 20 to 40 seconds, the clonic phase sets in, and lasts for variable periods of time.

The patient may awake from his postconvulsive sleep with a severe, generalized headache and in a state of confusion. He may go about in a semidazed or stuporous state in which he may perform more or less automatic acts without being able to recollect what he has experienced. These postparoxysmal or postictal reactions are interpreted as malfunctioning of neurons which have not yet recovered from the effects of the seizure. These may be so severe as to result in prolonged automatism, in transient paresis or, more rarely, in hemiplegia or other paralytic manifestations of focal injury or hemorrhage.

A grand mal seizure may occur at night *(nocturnal epilepsy)* without the patient's being aware of it. A bitten tongue or lip, headache, blood on his pillow or a bed wet with urine may be the only clue. Generalized motor seizures tend to be predominantly tonic during infancy, although the clonic feature is always present to some degree.

So-called secondary symptomatology, which pertains chiefly to personality traits such as egocentricity, shallowness, religiosity and chronic negativism and which is considered by some to be characteristic of epilepsy, is much less prominent in children than in adults. When such personality traits are manifest, they usually represent the patient's response, over a long time, to psychogenically injurious attitudes of other people toward him and his disability. These traits are not to be attributed to the disease itself or confused with the transient behavior disturbances of psychomotor attacks. Similar personality disturbances develop frequently for the same general reasons in children with any chronic handicapping condition.

Petit mal seizures. These seizures consist in a transient loss of consciousness. There may be such minor manifestations as an upward rolling of the eyes, moving of the lids, drooping or rhythmic nodding of the head, or slight quivering of the trunk and limb muscles. Clinical evidence of petit mal rarely appears before 3 years of age, and frequently disappears by the time of puberty. Girls are more often affected than boys. Intellectual development is rarely impaired in children who have only simple, staring petit mal seizures. Attacks of this type last less than 30 seconds and are most frequently described by parents or other associates of the child as "dizzy spells," "absences," "lapses" or "fainting turns." The patient rarely falls, but usually drops articles he may have in his hand or mouth. If the child, for example, is performing an act such as writing or reading at the onset, he will suddenly discontinue it, and then resume it when the seizure is ended. He may not be aware of having had a convulsion. Such seizures vary in frequency from 1 or 2 a month to as many as several hundred a day. After hyperventilation or exposure to a blinking light a child may have a typical episode. Individual petit mal seizures may, in rare instances, become progressively prolonged and gradually resemble a mild form of grand mal. Prolonged episodes of confusion, inappropriate action and loss of ability to speak or understand *(petit mal status)* are rare and can be distinguished from psychomotor sei-

zures only by an electroencephalogram during the attack.

PYKNOLEPSY (PYKNOEPILEPSY; "MYRIAD SPELLS"). Pyknolepsy is the designation used by Adie for a clinical state in which mild petit mal seizures suddenly appear in great numbers in otherwise normal children between the ages of 3 and 10 years. Such episodes recur over a period of months or years, then cease spontaneously and permanently without impairment of the victim's mentality. The electroencephalograms of such patients are typical of petit mal epilepsy. There is little justification for setting this condition apart as a separate clinical entity.

Psychomotor seizures. Psychomotor seizures are the most difficult to recognize and among the most difficult to control. They consist in purposeful but inappropriate motor acts, which are repetitive and often complicated. Most frequently a slight aura may manifest itself in a young child by a shrill cry or an attempt to run for help. Often the child is drowsy or sleeps for a short time after the spell. The seizure itself often consists in a gradual loss of postural tone. For example, the child may extend one arm and make a slow half-turn to one side while falling slowly to the ground. He often has vasomotor changes, such as circumoral pallor. After a 1- to 5-minute episode of unconsciousness the child may resume his normal activity or may sleep. There are usually no tonic or clonic movements. Fugue states or episodes of confusion, which may resemble petit mal, are rarely noted in children. A normal electroencephalogram, except at the time of psychomotor seizure, is not uncommon. Treatment is similar to that of grand mal seizures.

Focal seizures. These seizures may be sensory or motor in type *(jacksonian epilepsy)*, depending upon the location of the focal area of abnormal neuronal discharge. Focal seizures may occasionally occur in the absence of organic lesions. Localized sensory attacks which give rise to a variety of symptoms are rare in children. Unilateral motor or jacksonian attacks, though not infrequently preceded by a brief tonic phase, are typically clonic, indicating their origin in the motor cortex. The muscles most frequently involved in a jacksonian seizure are the ones most specialized for voluntary movements, as in the hand, face and tongue, less often those of the foot and trunk.

As might be expected from the relation of the areas of representation of the various muscle groups in the precentral gyrus, a focal motor seizure beginning in one member spreads or extends to others according to a fixed pattern, e.g. from thumb to fingers, to wrists, to arm, to face and then to the leg on the same side ("jacksonian march" of muscle spasms). When such an attack is of brief duration and remains localized to one area, consciousness may not be disturbed. When its spread is extensive and rapid, however, consciousness is lost, and a generalized convulsion follows, indistinguishable from a typical grand mal seizure.

Infantile myoclonic seizures. This convulsive seizure is also variously termed "infantile spasm," "lightning major" and "jackknife epilepsy." Unlike true petit mal seizures, these episodes occur before 2 years of age and involve more than a single group of muscles. The most common type of mass myoclonus is a sudden dropping of the head and flexion of the arms. The attack may be repeated several hundred times a day. The electroencephalographic changes consist of random high-voltage slow waves and spikes *(hypsarrhythmia)* and suggest a diffuse, disorganized state. It is one of the most characteristic encephalographic patterns and probably represents the response of the immature brain to a profound cerebral insult.

On the basis of age and developmental ability at the time of onset, an infant with myoclonic seizures may be placed in 1 of 2 groups. If his developmental level has never been normal or the seizures occur before 4 months of age, a congenital cerebral defect (Table 19-1) or other organic cause is most likely, and significant developmental retardation is to be expected. If the infant appeared to progress normally until 6 months of age or more before the hypsarrhythmia is detected, an unrecognized encephalitis or an underlying defect in cerebral metabolism may be responsible. The outlook is also unfavorable, but approximately 10 per cent of the infants in this group retain intellectual ability within the normal range.

Usually the infantile myoclonic seizures disappear spontaneously before the fourth year of life; other seizures may occur subsequently. Often the children in the second group have good motor ability, but poor adaptive and language abilities for their chronologic age. This has made the evaluation of treatment, such as with corticotropin, difficult.

A therapeutic trial with corticotropin, a corticosteroid or pyridoxine is indicated. In a number of instances such therapy, when started early, has appeared to be responsible for improvement in the clinical status and in the electroencephalographic pattern. At present, however, a cause-and-effect relation is speculative, since spontaneous improvement, though infrequent, does occur.

Myoclonic and akinetic seizures. Myoclonic jerks or involuntary muscular contractions may occur in conjunction with other manifestations of epilepsy, including loss of consciousness, or they may occur alone. A single group of muscles is usually affected. A patient may have a normal electroencephalogram while he is having myoclonic jerks involving one side or extremity. The origin of the seizure is presumed to be subcortical in such instances.

An akinetic seizure is associated with a sudden generalized loss of postural tone and therefore differs from single or repeated myoclonic jerks. These seizures in young children may resemble infantile myoclonic seizures and are sometimes called motor petit mal, jackknife or akinetic seizures. The electroencephalogram usually reveals a spike and wave pattern of less than 3 per second *(petit mal variant).*

Minor motor seizures are often a symptom of a degenerative disease, mental retardation or other central nervous system disorders and may be difficult to control.

Self-induced seizures. It is possible for some children to induce petit mal or grand mal seizures by overbreathing, by watching a blinking light, or by some other form of learned behavior. Self-induced seizures should be distinguished clinically from other types of convulsions because drug therapy alone is usually unsatisfactory. After a child has learned to draw attention to himself in this manner it is difficult to alter this defensive mechanism. Complex family problems probably underlie this kind of behavior, so that psychiatric consultation may be indicated.

Diagnosis. *Electroencephalography.* When there is clinical evidence of a convulsive disorder, an electroencephalogram should be obtained in practically all instances. An exception may be made in a child with an obvious clinical diagnosis of the staring type of petit mal seizure, since the characteristic 3-per-second spike and wave pattern is almost invariably present.

Three types of rhythms have been described in the electroencephalogram of the normal human adult. The most common one, the alpha rhythm, consists of regular sinusoidal waves occurring at frequencies of 8 to 12 per second, with a voltage of 20 to 60 microvolts when recorded from the scalp. The second most common is the beta rhythm; it is most prominent in the frontal cortex. It has a lower amplitude, and a frequency of 13 to 32 per second. The least common is the gamma rhythm, which arises from the frontal lobes and consists of a more rapid rate, 33 to 55 per second, with waves of extremely low voltage. Slower waves (theta, 5 to 7 per second, and delta, 1 to 4 per second) are not present in normal adults during the waking state.

The interpretation of the electroencephalograms of infants and children is more difficult than those of adults because of the presence of slow rhythms (3 to 8 per second) in normal children. Cortical rhythm is poorly developed in the newborn infant. As he matures, the electroencephalogram shows random 3- to 7-per-second waves and some low-voltage faster activity. Gradually the basic rhythm becomes more regular, and by 6 years of age the pattern is made up principally of 5- to 7-per-second waves, and by 10 years alpha waves, 8 to 12 per second, predominate. During childhood 14- and 6-per-second positive spikes (ctenoids) are commonly found in presumably healthy subjects. During adolescence some slow wave activity, 4 to 8 per second, is not uncommon and may be incorrectly interpreted if adult standards are used.

Sleep without the use of a hypnotic, hyperventilation for 2 minutes, Metrazol, artificially induced fever, the Pitressin test and flickering light serve to bring out latent abnormalities in the electroencephalogram and may on occasion pro-

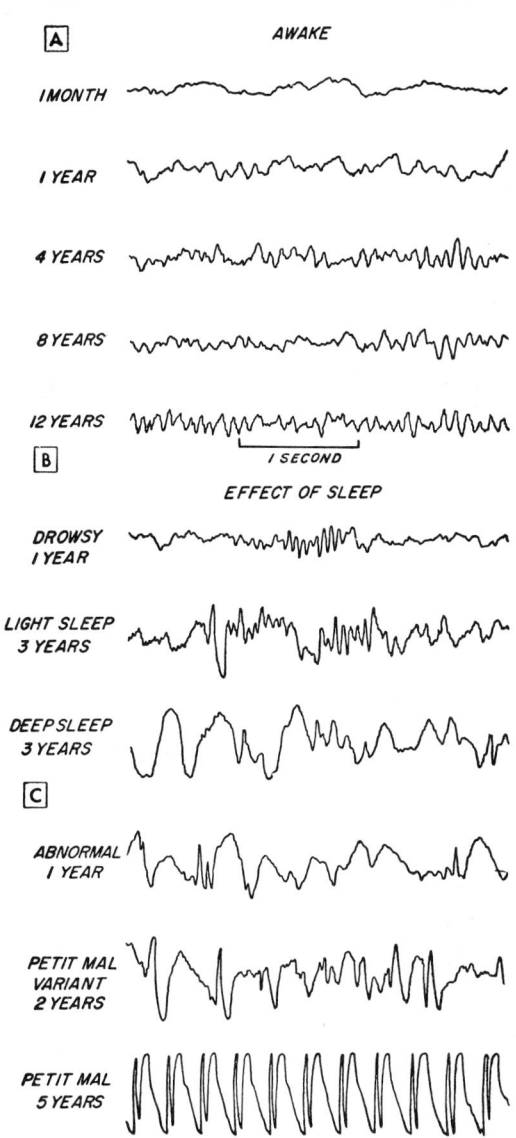

A

AWAKE

1 MONTH

1 YEAR

4 YEARS

8 YEARS

12 YEARS

1 SECOND

B

EFFECT OF SLEEP

DROWSY 1 YEAR

LIGHT SLEEP 3 YEARS

DEEP SLEEP 3 YEARS

C

ABNORMAL 1 YEAR

PETIT MAL VARIANT 2 YEARS

PETIT MAL 5 YEARS

Figure 19-1. Electroencephalograms of infants and children. *A*, Tracings from comparable areas of the scalp illustrating variations with age of electrical activity in the motor cortex; all were secured during a quiet phase just before sleep. *B*, The effects of sleep, variations of patterns in normal children; compare with tracings in *A* and *C. C*, Abnormal waves.

duce a seizure. Of these, sleep and hyperventilation are most frequently used in cooperative subjects.

ABNORMAL WAVES. Most patients with frequent *grand mal seizures* have definite abnormalities in their electroencephalograms in the intervals between seizures. These consist of random spike discharges, diffuse high-voltage slow waves or a pattern not consistent with the child's chronologic age. An electroencephalogram obtained during a grand mal seizure shows multiple high-voltage spike discharges. After the seizure

there are asymmetries between the 2 hemispheres and diffuse slowing.

Patients with seizures other than grand mal have a variety of electroencephalographic abnormalities. The most easily recognized one is that of *infantile myoclonic seizures* with its high-voltage, 1- to 2-per-second, spike and wave pattern, the so-called hypsarrhythmia (hyps = high and lofty). The record gives the impression of complete disorganization.

During *petit mal attacks* there is characteristically a 3-per-second spike and wave pattern.

A constant asymmetry of one area compared to its counterpart on the opposite side may be significant, especially if the electrical activity shows phase reversal of slow waves. Shifting foci are more common in children than in adults and indicate a functional disturbance rather than an anatomic lesion.

Absence of electrical activity over an area suggests a large lesion such as a subdural collection of fluid or an abscess. Serial electroencephalograms of children with hydrocephalus show a disturbance of function as the process progresses.

After cerebral insults such as trauma, encephalitis, cerebral thrombosis and prolonged seizures, electrical activity may be slow for a time and may be roughly correlated with the child's clinical course.

Metabolic disorders, such as hypoglycemia, hyperthyroidism and adrenal insufficiency, alter cortical activity; the clinical significance of these changes is not clear.

Various types of cerebral dysrhythmia may occur for short times between clinical seizures. The occurrence of abnormal discharges of short duration, such as a single wave and spike formation or a short series of spikes similar to those in grand mal seizures, without clinical manifestations has given rise to the designation of subclinical or larval seizures. These subclinical bursts may at times foretell the onset of clinical seizures.

Roentgenography. A roentgen examination of the skull is considered an essential part of the diagnostic appraisal in search for such abnormalities as intracranial calcifications, erosion of the base or increased densities, which may indicate reasons for seizures. A hammered-silver pattern of the cranium is present so commonly that by itself it is not considered abnormal. Routine pneumoencephalography in the epileptic child is not necessary, since space-filling lesions without localizing peripheral neurologic changes which justify surgical exploration are an uncommon cause of convulsions in children.

The decision as to additional laboratory examinations other than the routine urinalysis, blood cell count and tuberculin test should be based on leads obtained from the medical history, the physical examination and the clinical course. Examination of the cerebrospinal fluid need not be routine, but it may provide additional information when diagnostic considerations include lead poisoning, certain instances of mental deterioration and encephalitis.

When hypoglycemia (p. 1164), nephritis (p. 1130), lead poisoning (p. 1486), and tetany (p. 1260) are considered possible causes of convulsions, appropriate diagnostic steps are obviously indicated.

Treatment of Recurrent Convulsions. *Management of the individual seizure.* Practically all that should be done for a patient during an attack is to protect him from bodily injury. This necessitates constant supervision in severe cases. At the beginning of a major seizure, clothing about the neck should be loosened. The patient should then be turned on his side so that he does not aspirate his pooled secretions. He should be observed carefully for changes in color; administration of oxygen is indicated during prolonged convulsions. Any injury to the tongue and other tissues of the oral cavity during a convulsion is most apt to occur at the onset. Since subsequent injury is not very likely and because additional damage often results from crude efforts, the family should be counseled against placing a stick or other object between the teeth.

Status epilepticus. If a series of grand mal convulsions occurs before the patient has fully recovered, the prolonged seizure is termed status epilepticus. The intervals between individual convulsions may be so short that the seizures are virtually continuous. During status the muscular contractions may appear to be one-sided or to shift from one group of muscles to another. This does not constitute a true focal (jacksonian) seizure.

The most common cause of status epilepticus is discontinuance of previously continuous daily anticonvulsant medication; often this has occurred within less than 2 weeks.

Drug treatment consists in prompt administration of phenobarbital sodium intramuscularly (average doses, 60 mg. at 6 months of age to 120 mg. at 2 to 3 years, or 5 to 6 mg. per kg.; maximum single dose is 200 mg.). If the convulsion is not controlled within 15 minutes, the initial dose should be repeated. If the convulsion has been partially controlled by this time, half the initial dose should be given. Subsequent administrations may be necessary. The rhythmic contraction of a single group of muscles after a severe convulsion does not require additional therapy. Sedative therapy should be limited to a single agent. If the convulsions are not controlled by a total dose of phenobarbital of 15 mg. per kg. within 60 minutes, the possibility of some organic lesion such as encephalitis, metabolic disturbance or vascular accident should be considered. The administration of a small dose of phenobarbital (less than 2 to 3 mg. per kg.) to a child in status should be avoided, because it is likely to be inadequate and subsequent control may then be difficult.

The dangers of intravenously administered barbiturates and of inhalation anesthesia are similar to those of anesthetizing an excited child.

Such procedures are rarely necessary and, when indicated, should be performed by an experienced anesthesiologist. Laryngeal spasm and even sudden death may occur if treatment is too vigorous.

Recent experience with diazepam (Valium) (see p. 309) indicates that it is effective in the treatment of status epilepticus.

Each ampule of the preparation contains 10 mg. in 2 ml. of solution for intravenous administration. The solution should not be diluted and should be administered slowly (0.5 ml. per minute). The usual dose is 5 to 10 mg., and no more than 6 ml. (30 mg.) is recommended.

Within 1 minute the effect of the drug is usually apparent both clinically and in the electroencephalogram. The limbs become hypotonic, the rate of respiration decreases, the pupils first dilate and later decrease in size, and nystagmus often develops. Excessive salivation and hiccupping may occur. Although the child usually remains quiet, he will respond to painful stimuli. The corneal reflex may be diminished or absent. The effect of the drug lasts from $\frac{1}{2}$ to 3 hours, but drowsiness may be present in some children for as long as 18 hours.

The principal advantage of diazepam is the prompt control of the convulsion. The anxiety of parents, nurses and physicians which often complicates management is alleviated early. Disadvantages are that the underlying cause may be masked (e.g. infection, lead encephalopathy) and definitive therapy delayed. Sudden death, which has occurred after the intravenous administration of barbiturates for the treatment of grand mal status, has not yet been reported in children after the administration of diazepam. Its side effects, if any, are not yet fully known. Tolerance tends to occur after the administration of diazepam intravenously on 3 or 4 occasions, so that increasing amounts must be administered to achieve the same effect.

Administration of oxygen is indicated during prolonged convulsions, and administration of 5 per cent glucose in 0.45 per cent saline solution intravenously may shorten the recovery time.

A quiet and calm atmosphere, reassurance and avoidance of unnecessary annoyance to the patient are important factors in general management, especially during the recovery phase.

Continuous therapy of the epileptic child. The aims of treatment are to reduce the number of seizures, to encourage the child to function at a level commensurate with his natural endowment, and to promote his acceptance at home and in the community on the basis of his capabilities. The responsibilities of the physician include diagnostic and therapeutic services for the child, information and counsel for the parents, and guidance to the community and the school. The success of the physician at each level will often affect both the number of the seizures and the child's adjustment. There are a number of limiting factors, such as the duration and severity of symptoms, the kind of seizures, the presence of a genetic factor, the presence of complicating cerebral lesions, and the capacity of the patient and his family to cooperate.

If the patient or his family has been unduly frightened by laboratory studies, folk tales or by reading poorly selected medical information, additional explanations (education) by the physician will be necessary. Usually, however, the medical management is relatively easy after the diagnosis of an idiopathic convulsive disorder has been established.

Orientation of the child. The attitude of the child toward his disease generally reflects that of his parents. It is usually desirable for the child to be present during conferences with the parents. Even if the terms are vague, the child will sense the philosophy of the physician. If it combines realism with optimism, long-term benefits can be expected. Parents are often poorly equipped to explain a long-term illness to a child. By giving the parents and the child a chance to ask questions in each others' presence, many doubts and fears can be resolved. Attempts to disguise the existence of seizures are unwise and often harmful.

The questions of the child are apt to be related to activity in school, sports, and the like, or to the duration of therapy. Most children are pleased to find that their participation in regular activity is encouraged. The usual restrictions against riding a horse and against swimming except when attended by a responsible adult are readily accepted. Participation in competitive sports, in which injury to the child or others is possible, must be decided on an individual basis. Seizures during an athletic activity are rare in children who are otherwise well controlled.

The duration of therapy is not predictable. It is preferable to continue medication for a long time even if the dose of the drug is small. It is difficult for both the child and his parents to begin treatment again should seizures recur. A workable rule is to continue medication until the electroencephalogram is consistently normal; it can be repeated annually.

It is usually better to leave discussion about discontinuation of medication until the child has been without seizures for a year. To give the parent or the child an estimate is unwise because it will seem to them a form of penal sentence. Early in the course of treatment it is enough for the child to know that he may not always have to take medication. Later, if he can lead an otherwise normal life, he will be willing to accept this minor inconvenience.

After the diagnosis of an idiopathic convulsive disorder has been made, return visits to the physician every 2 to 4 weeks may be helpful. Additional questions, the possibility of additional history, information about environmental factors, physical findings and drug toxicity may be dealt with appropriately at these times.

Orientation of the adolescent. Although the behavioral changes of a boy or girl with a convulsive disorder during adolescence are similar to those of unaffected children, they are more likely to be brought to the attention of the physician. Unexplained tearfulness, hostility, clumsiness, inattention (particularly in school), forgetfulness, increased sibling rivalry, antiauthoritarianism, and overreaction (by adult standards) to petty annoyance are often part of normal adolescent behavior, but may in a boy or girl with a convulsive disorder be attributed to medication or to the disease. If the physician has previously discussed the increasing need for independence during adolescence, his reassurance after development of symptoms is more likely to be successful. It may be helpful to have the child's teachers and a psychologist work together toward finding a realistic educational placement.

The child with epilepsy wants to be "normal," to be independent, to be accepted and admired by his peers, and to achieve status symbols which are sometimes unrealistic. To achieve these goals, the adolescent with a convulsive disorder may wish to live the fantasy that there is nothing wrong with him and refuse or forget to take his medication. If a seizure occurs, his "forgetfulness," personality change (depression) and recurrent seizures may lead to unnecessary hospitalization and unjustified diagnostic procedures. These experiences may further delay the development of an independent, self-sufficient person. In some instances one or both parents may be reluctant to give up the control of the child. The patient who has had little opportunity to exercise judgment in activities of daily life is likely to use his handicap as a shield.

Orientation of the parents. Among the pertinent questions asked of the physician by the parents after the diagnosis of epilepsy has been established are these: Will punishment of the child cause a seizure? What of the child's future? Is his mental development likely to be retarded by the disease? Will mental deterioration occur? Will his life be shortened by it? Should he attend school? Should he marry and have children? As the physician helps the family to understand the general problem, the following points are fundamental.

1. The seizure is a symptom, and unless it is associated with clinical evidence of shock (peripheral vascular collapse) it will rarely produce irreversible damage to the central nervous system.

2. If the child gains attention directly or indirectly by having seizures, control by medication alone is likely to be difficult.

3. In most instances, avoidance of emphasis on the recurrence of seizures is helpful.

4. Restoration of confidence, in both the parents and the child, is important. The adults need to feel that they are competent and capable persons who meet their responsibilities appropriately.

5. If the child receives medication in the proper amount, therapy should in no way influence his mental ability or personality or cause him to become a drug addict.

6. It is best to rear the child in a normal fashion.

To reward or punish him differently only because he has seizures leads to behavioral difficulties.

7. The patient needs an environment which will allow him to compete successfully at his own level.

With some parents it is prudent for the physician to assume temporary responsibility for the child's management. He may say in effect to the parents, "You give the medication and handle the child in a normal fashion, and I will worry about the spells." As members of the family become more mature in their attitudes and less concerned, they will become more aware of important underlying difficulties. Commonly associated problems include unrecognized mental retardation, behavioral difficulties, inappropriate placement in school, and intrafamily conflicts.

Orientation of the community. If educational facilities appropriate to his needs are available, the child should attend school close to his own home and participate in activities to which he is naturally inclined. It is the duty of the physician, the nurse and the social worker who are acquainted with the problem to do everything possible to improve the attitude of the public toward the epileptic patient and his disease. Nearly every intelligent epileptic child sooner or later encounters attitudes toward him of pity and oversolicitousness or of disgust and horror. These are likely to be a source of constant anxiety unless he is able to acquire an adequate philosophy.

Drugs. Since the introduction of bromides for the treatment of epilepsy by Leacock in 1858, drug therapy has been the choice and usually the only form of treatment. The tendency to rely upon medication alone was encouraged by the introduction of phenobarbital in 1912. Subsequently dietotherapy came into use when it was discovered that fasting, the ketogenic diet and reduction of the water intake all tended to prevent epileptic seizures. Since the demonstration by Merritt and Putnam in 1938 that Dilantin (sodium diphenyl hydantoinate) was effective in the treatment of some patients not controlled by phenobarbital, the tendency to depend mainly upon drug therapy has again increased.

The successful management of the epileptic child requires determination of the most appropriate anticonvulsant drug or combination of drugs for him as well as the most appropriate dosages. To achieve this result, a systematic program for a trial of the various anticonvulsant drugs is necessary; a suggested schedule to determine an adequate therapeutic program is shown in Table 19-2. A change in the dose of a medication or from one medication to another should usually not be made more frequently than every 2 weeks.

PHENOBARBITAL, in tablet form, is the drug of choice for prolonged use in the average patient with grand mal epilepsy. Its virtues are its relative effectiveness, its comparative harmlessness in therapeutic doses for a prolonged time, its ease of administration and its low cost. Doses range from 8 mg. (⅛ grain) 1 to 3 times daily for an infant to 100 mg. (1½ grains) 1 to 3 times daily for an older child with a severe form of the disease. It may also be prescribed on a weight basis with an initial dose of 3 mg. per kg. per day in 2 divided doses, with gradual increases to the required maintenance dose. More than 6 mg. per kg. per day may result in drowsiness.

Occasionally a child will have an idiosyncrasy to phenobarbital. A maculopapular eruption on the skin and mucous membranes, excessive drowsiness and fever may be signs of sensitivity or overdosage. These soon disappear without permanent harm if the dose is reduced or if the drug is withdrawn. Rarely, and particularly when attacks are primarily petit mal, a patient appears to be made worse by phenobarbital and has petit mal variants or psychomotor attacks. In such an event Dilantin may also be administered. Rarely, it is necessary to discontinue medication, which should always be done gradually, and to substitute another drug.

MEBARAL. Mebaral (mephobarbital) is a barbiturate of value in some cases. The dose is approximately double that recommended for phenobarbital.

DILANTIN. The only drugs which rival the barbiturates in the control of grand mal seizures are certain hydantoin compounds, such as diphenylhydantoin sodium. U.S.P., also known as phenytoin sodium (Dilantin). They are administered to older children in capsules and to younger ones in tablet form crushed in a little food or fruit juice. Doses range from 25 mg. (½ tablet) 1 or 2 times daily in infants to 100 mg. (1½ grains) once or twice daily in older children. The drug may also be prescribed in an initial dose of 3 mg. per kg. per day in 2 doses, with gradual increases to the required maintenance dose. More than 8 mg. per kg. per day may result in toxic manifestations. The chief advantage of hydantoin compounds over the barbiturates is that they act as efficient anticonvulsants without producing excessive drowsiness. One of these should be given a trial, therefore, whenever grand mal seizures are not adequately controlled by phenobarbital alone in nondepressing doses. Replacement should be made gradually, however, since sudden changes may result in increased convulsive reactivity.

The occurrence of nonpainful, nonhemorrhagic hypertrophy of the gums usually follows the administration of Dilantin. It usually requires no special treatment other than good dental hygiene. If it becomes unattractive cosmetically, another drug should be substituted.

Ataxia and drowsiness may occur if the initial dose is too large, if the dose is increased too rapidly or if the total daily dose exceeds about 8 mg. per kg. per day. Serious toxic reactions such as nausea or vomiting, erythema or a morbilliform eruption, nervous manifestations such as tremor of the hands, ataxia, diplopia with nystagmus, paralytic manifestations and mild psychoses are uncommon. These disappear after reduction of the dose, usually to about two thirds of its former

TABLE 19-2. SUGGESTED SCHEDULE FOR A THERAPEUTIC PROGRAM IN EPILEPSY

Unless there is a specific contraindication, the administration of phenobarbital, 3 mg./kg./day, in 2 or 3 divided doses to every child with grand mal psychomotor, petit mal, infantile myoclonic or mixed seizures is the treatment of choice

Example: 20 kg. (44 lb.)⋀ 3 mg./kg. = 60 mg. daily; one 30-mg. tablet on arising and one at bedtime

GRAND MAL, PSYCHOMOTOR, AND MIXED SEIZURES

After 2 weeks if the seizures are not controlled, increase phenobarbital to 5 mg./kg./day in 2 or 3 divided doses. Unless status occurs, devote efforts to the improvement of environmental factors and avoid changes of medication

After another 2 weeks if seizures are not controlled, continue phenobarbital and add Dilantin, 2-3 mg./kg./day, in 1 or 2 divided doses

Example: 20 kg. (44 lbs.) × 3 mg./kg. = 60 mg.; one 30-mg. capsule on arising and one at bedtime

(Alternate) 20 kg. (44 lbs.) × 2.5 mg./kg. = 50 mg. or 1 tablet at bedtime

After the third 2 weeks, if grand mal or psychomotor seizures are not adequately controlled, continue phenobarbital, 5 mg./kg./day, and increase Dilantin to 5-6 mg./kg./day

After the fourth 2 weeks, Dilantin can again be increased to 7-8 mg./kg./day, but never to more than 300 mg. daily in the pediatric age range

PETIT MAL

Continue phenobarbital, 3 mg./kg./day, and if seizures are not controlled, add Zarontin, 250 mg. (1 capsule) daily. Each succeeding week, if petit mal seizures continue, add 1 capsule (250 mg.) of Zarontin to the daily dose (2 or 3 divided doses) until tolerance

is reached or spells disappear (not more than 6 capsules daily). If the petit mal spells are associated with a motor component which involves muscles below the neck, add Dilantin in doses of 2-3 mg./kg./day. Medications should be given together. The administration of medications twice daily (on arising and at bedtime) is most desirable because it is least likely to be forgotten and because other children may swallow tablets if they are left at an available site.

INFANTILE MYOCLONIC SEIZURES

If infantile myoclonic seizures have been of recent origin, the administration of corticotropin (ACTH-gel, 5-10 units daily for 2 weeks) is suggested in addition to phenobarbital, 3 mg./kg./day

If infantile myoclonic seizures continue or if the electroencephalogram continues to show a hypsarrhythmia, the corticotropin is discontinued, and pyridoxine, 10-15 mg./kg./day orally for 2 weeks, is prescribed in addition to phenobarbital, 3 mg./kg./day.

If there is no improvement either clinically or in the electroencephalogram, the phenobarbital is continued. Although there is no convincing evidence that steroid therapy is beneficial, it is our practice to administer corticotropin again, and to increase the amount by 5-10 units each week until 50 units daily is reached and maintained for 30 days. If 50 units of ACTH-gel for 30 days is not effective in changing the electroencephalogram to an apparently normal pattern, the administration of ACTH is reduced to 10 units weekly and discontinued within several weeks. A corticosteroid such as prednisone (Meticorten), 0.5 mg./kg./day, may be substituted for the corticotropin. If the patient does not respond to the administration of corticotropin or a corticosteroid, supportive care is continued. Although a variety of anticonvulsant medications has been suggested, phenobarbital, 3-5 mg./kg./day in 2 divided doses, seems to be most helpful

level. Dilantin should not be administered to infants and young children in the form of a suspension because most parents are not able to administer the small dose accurately.

TRIDIONE. Trimethadione (Tridione) (3,5,5-trimethyloxazolidine 2,4-dione) is an effective drug for the treatment of petit mal epilepsy in doses of 0.3 gm. (5 grains) 1 to 4 times daily. The drug may also be prescribed on a weight basis with an initial dose of 25 mg. per kg. per day in 2 to 4 doses, which may be gradually increased if necessary to 80 mg. per kg. per day. Tridione may increase the occurrence of grand mal attacks if they also exist, and the additional administration of a barbiturate or hydantoin is indicated. Excessive doses or prolonged use of Tridione may result in photophobia, hemeralopia (day blindness), drowsiness, nausea, skin eruptions or nephrosis. Such manifestations tend to disappear after withdrawal of the drug. Several fatalities from aplastic anemia have been reported in patients receiving Tridione regularly for several months. When it is given for more than a short time, periodic blood

cell counts should be obtained, and the drug discontinued if any abnormality is found.

PARADIONE. Paradione is less toxic than Tridione, but also less effective. The dosage is similar to that of Tridione.

ZARONTIN. Zarontin (ethosuximide) is probably a more useful agent for the treatment of petit mal seizures than is Tridione. Side effects have been reported to follow the administration of Zarontin, which usually disappear if the amount of medication is decreased. These effects include nausea, dizziness, drowsiness, rash and hiccups. The symptoms are unlikely to return if the drug is readministered, and the dose increased more gradually and maintained below the previously toxic level. The occurrence of a blood dyscrasia following the administration of Zarontin is unusual. A white blood cell and differential count should be obtained before starting therapy, after 1 month, and then every 3 to 6 months. Routine examination of the urine at these times is also desirable.

Because many children with petit mal seizures

can be controlled by phenobarbital alone, the administration of Zarontin is suggested only when necessary in addition to phenobarbital or Mebaral. Occasionally a child with more than one type of convulsion may have an increased number of seizures after Zarontin has been administered.

The recommended starting dose is one capsule (250 mg.) daily for a week. If necessary, the daily number of capsules is increased by 1 each week, until a total of 6 capsules daily is reached (2 capsules, 3 times daily). If the administration of the capsule is impractical in young children, the drug may be readily dissolved in 1 to 2 ounces of fluid, and its taste disguised by 8 to 10 drops of Sucaryl (cyclamate calcium), an artificial sweetener.

MYSOLINE. Mysoline (primidone) (5-phenyl-5-ethyl-hexahydropyrimidine-4:6-dione) is used in the treatment of grand mal and psychomotor seizures. It may be used alone or in combination with other drugs and does not depress hematopoietic activity. The chief side effects, drowsiness, ataxia and dermatitis, can be minimized by starting with small amounts (125 mg.) at bedtime and by increasing the dose slowly at 7- to 10-day intervals to a maximum dose of 250 mg., 3 times daily.

VALIUM (DIAZEPAM) (see p. 309). The administration of diazepam orally (1 to 10 mg. 3 times a day, as tolerated) for the treatment of convulsive disorders is under study. Preliminary indications are that some children, particularly those with petit mal who have been refractory to Zarontin and other agents, do respond favorably. In many instances tolerance occurs after 3 to 14 days of therapy. If the dosage is further increased, undesirable side effects may occur, such as drowsiness, ataxia and slurred speech.

Children who have seizures associated with degenerative disease of the central nervous system often tolerate diazepam well. The dosage schedule must be adjusted individually. We have found that the oral administration of diazepam with phenobarbital and Dilantin is a useful combination in some instances.

The ketogenic diet. Fasting causes cessation of grand mal seizures in a majority of epileptic children, the effect usually manifesting itself shortly after ketosis has appeared on the third day. A strongly ketogenic diet has a comparable anticonvulsive effect after ketosis has developed. Stringent restriction of the liquid intake, even when the diet is nonketogenic, results in cessation of grand mal seizures in most of those patients who respond favorably to fasting or the ketogenic diet. Establishment of a negative water balance, by restricting the intake or increasing the output, intensifies the anticonvulsive effects of the ketogenic regimen. Administration of alkaline salts in sufficient amount to neutralize the acidogenic effect of fasting or of the ketogenic diet abolishes the anticonvulsive action, whereas administration of inorganic acids or acid-forming salts fortifies or intensifies such action. The ketogenic diet has been used for petit mal and grand mal epilepsy.

The use of the ketogenic diet is limited because of the practical difficulties of adhering consistently to a restricted dietary intake and because of the possibility of attendant emotional disturbances. It may be helpful for children who have frequent seizures which are not controlled by moderate doses of one or more of the anticonvulsant drugs; in such instances the diet may often be used in conjunction with them. The child and his family must be willing and able to accept the dietary regimen without emotional conflict. Owing to the various difficulties of the diet, it is no longer widely used.

Prognosis. The prognosis of a convulsive disorder depends upon any coexisting mental retardation, physical handicaps, possible organic disease, and the adequacy of medical and environmental management.

The tendency to repeated seizures, with or without apparent organic cause, is found in some families, but the possibility of a convulsive disorder occurring in siblings or in offspring of affected persons is impossible to assess accurately. In a general discussion it may be helpful to stress that residual effects of a convulsion are rare, and to note the observation of Yannet that children who had parents with a history of a convulsive disorder were better adjusted and had fewer seizures than those children whose parents had not had seizures.

Although it is probable that a severe prolonged seizure of one or more hours may deplete available stores of glucose and interfere with oxygenation and thus cause secondary cerebral changes, there is reason to believe that the usual convulsive episode does not cause irreversible damage. Convulsions followed by permanent hemiplegia are probably more often the result of a vascular accident which occurred before the seizure than to injury during it. In such instances, there are likely to be recurrent convulsions which are more difficult to control than those of idiopathic epilepsy.

Epileptic patients who are otherwise normal seldom die or sustain serious injuries as a result of their disorder.

Seizures tend to become more numerous unless the course is modified by therapy. On the other hand, a number of patients with unquestioned idiopathic grand mal epilepsy appear to undergo spontaneous cessation of seizures after adequate treatment. Patients who are well controlled medically rarely have seizures during participation in athletic acitivities. The results of therapy are generally not satisfactory in infants and young children with infantile myoclonic seizures.

The prognosis for mental development in young epileptic patients or for mental deterioration in older patients was formerly gloomy, chiefly because opinion was based largely upon experiences with the more severe cases in public institutions. Collins and Lennox found the intelligence quotients of 100 children and 200 adults in private practice to average 109 with ranges of 52 to 153 for the former and of 47 to 139 for the latter. The intelligence quotients of those with evidence of cerebral damage before the first seizure averaged 10 points lower than of those with idiopathic epilepsy. The highest scores were found in those with essentially normal electroencephalograms and in those with typical petit mal activity, the lowest in those having both grand mal and psychomotor attacks. With proper treatment most epileptic patients with normal mentality can be expected to maintain it.

DISORDERS SIMULATING EPILEPSY

(Including So-Called Epileptic Equivalents)

Narcolepsy. Narcolepsy is a syndrome characterized by recurrent diurnal attacks of irrepressible sleep, usually precipitated by a sudden emotional change. It is rare in children and is said to be more frequent in boys than in girls.

Narcolepsy has been classified according to origin into "idiopathic" and "symptomatic" groups. Wilson further subdivided the latter group into 6 categories: (1) toxic-infective, e.g. postencephalitic, (2) circulatory, (3) post-traumatic, (4) endocrine, (5) neoplastic, and (6) psychopathologic.

The attacks resemble those of epilepsy in their brevity, in their abruptness of onset and in their paroxysmal and involuntary nature. The overpowering sleep of narcolepsy may come on suddenly while the patient is engaged in some activity such as talking, walking or driving. He then ceases what he is doing and falls "in a heap." The "sleep" is usually shallow, and the patient is easily aroused. The disturbance apparently has no relation to the physiologic need for sleep. Regular nocturnal sleep is normal. The patient exhibits mental alertness rather than somnolence after he has been aroused.

The disorder tends to be chronic, but spontaneous improvement and cure are more common than in epilepsy. The amphetamines have proved much more effective than ephedrine. Dosage for a child should be established on the basis of the minimal amount which will produce the desired effect.

Abdominal Epilepsy. Otherwise unexplained recurrent episodes of abdominal pain have on occassion been considered to be a manifestation of epilepsy. Some epileptic children with psychomotor or grand mal seizures do have abdominal pain just prior to the onset of a convulsion, but abdominal pain as the only overt manifestation of epilepsy must, if it does occur, be extremely rare. Recurrent abdominal pain associated with headache, but without nausea or vomiting, has also been attributed to migraine (see below). If abdominal epilepsy is to be accepted as a diagnostic designation, the criterion for its application in a given case should be quite restrictive. The following clinical pattern would probably be acceptable to most critical observers: recurrent episodes of abdominal pain, with or without associated headache, but without twitching or convulsive movements, somnolence as a postictal manifestation, an abnormal electroencephalogram, and relief from the attacks of abdominal pain with anticonvulsive therapy.

Breath-Holding. See page 83. These spells, comparatively common in early childhood, are sometimes associated with tonic and clonic movements.

Hysterical Fits. These can resemble true epileptic seizures in a superficial way. They are fairly easily distinguished by a number of characteristics. There is usually a typical neurotic background. Between attacks the patient may exhibit motor or sensory disturbances which do not follow the true neural patterns, and the gag reflex may be absent. Dilatation of the pupils and pallor of the skin and mucous membranes rarely accompany an attack. Loss of consciousness is superficial and variable. Sphincter control is not lost, and bodily injury from the seizure does not occur. Crying, moaning and disconnected talk throughout the attack, which may last half an hour or longer, are common. Hysterical patients, like other neurotic children with behavior problems, frequently show some abnormalities in the electroencephalogram. The treatment of hysterical seizures is that of the underlying psychogenic disorder.

Syncope. Syncopal attacks of various types due chiefly to transient cerebral anemia are frequently complicated by slight tonic and clonic convulsive reactions of short duration confined mostly to the face and arms. The most common form in early life is the *simple fainting spell*, which is brought on reflexly in certain children by a simple procedure such as removal of a sliver or insertion of a needle into the skin, or by a sudden fright while in a standing or sitting posture. The susceptibility to fainting appears to be related to defective reflex regulation of the vascular system, which manifests itself as a sudden relaxation of the visceral venous system with bradycardia and a fall in blood pressure. Placing the patient in a horizontal position or with the head tilted downward at a 45-degree angle will tend to shorten the period of unconsciousness. When it is necessary to subject a child known to faint easily to some painful test or treatment, it is advisable to have him lie on a table during the procedure. Vigorous crying before and during a procedure, such as taking a blood sample, tends to prevent fainting. In an older child active gripping of some object and voluntary contraction of the abdominal muscles have the same effect.

In the *Stokes-Adams syndrome*, which occurs in heart block (p. 1020), a short convulsive reaction often accompanies the syncopal attack. The seizure appears within 10 to 20 seconds after the onset of asystole. Similar syncopal attacks have been reported in patients as a result of *paroxysmal tachycardia*, and attacks occur fairly frequently after muscular effort in young children with certain congenital anomalies of the heart, such as the tetralogy of Fallot.

A *hyperactive carotid sinus reflex* manifests itself by episodes of unconsciousness with or without brief tonic and clonic convulsive attacks. This condition is extremely rare in both epileptic and nonepileptic patients. Pressure over the carotid sinuses in the anterior cervical region causes a slowing or temporary arrest of the pulse in persons subject to attacks. Associated with the asystole are symptoms of faintness, weakness, loss of consciousness and finally the convulsive reaction.

Apneic episodes during swimming, especially in competitive events, have, in rare instances, been responsible for sudden loss of consciousness and at times for clonic movements. Such attacks presumably have been observed most frequently in adolescent boys, and more often in association with the breast stroke than with other forms of swimming. Even expert underwater swimmers can, by forced hyperventilation before submerging, so deplete the body of carbon dioxide that hypoxia may produce unconsciousness before the respiratory center initiates a breath. Perhaps in somewhat the same way, an overwhelming desire to attain a competitive goal may dominate the urge to breathe. When respiration cannot be restarted by prompt artificial respiration, it is presumed that ventricular fibrillation has occurred.

Migraine (Hemicrania). (See also page 1274.) Migraine has long been regarded as being akin in some respects to epilepsy. The two frequently occur in the same family. Occasionally attacks of migraine are replaced by typical epileptic seizures. Its paroxysmal nature, its chronicity and its genetic features make migraine resemble idiopathic epilepsy. This has given rise to the unfortunate use of the designation "sensory epilepsy" for migraine. In true visual seizures of epileptic patients the eye symptoms are much shorter in duration than they are in migraine and are bilateral.

HENRY W. BAIRD

REFERENCES

Baird, H. W., and Borofsky, L. G.: Infantile Myoclonic Seizures. *J. Pediat.*, 50:332, 1957.

Baird, H. W., and Garfunkel, J. M.: Electroencephalographic Changes in Children with Artificially Induced Hyperthermia. *J. Pediat.*, 48:28, 1956.

Baird, H. W., and Pileggi, A. J.: Diminished Corneal Reflex After Diazepam. *Lancet*, 2:106, 1968.

Charlton, M. H., and Yahr, M. D.: Long Term Follow-up of Patients with Petit Mal. *Arch. Neurol.*, 16:595, 1967.

Crigler, J. F., and Cohen, R. B.: Hypoglycemia and Convulsions in Infancy. *New England J. Med.*, 266:1269, 1962.

Frame, B., and Carter, S.: Pseudohypoparathyroidism. *Neurology*, 5:297, 1955.

French, J. H., Grueter, B. B., Druckman, R., and O'Brien, D.: Pyridoxine and Infantile Myoclonic Seizures. *Neurology*, 15:101, 1965.

Holowach, J., Thurston, D. L., and O'Leary, J. L.: Petit Mal Epilepsy. *Pediatrics*, 30:893, 1962.

Lennox, W. G., and Lenox, M. A.: *Epilepsy and Related Disorders.* Boston, Little, Brown and Company, 1960.

Livingston, S.: Infantile Febrile Convulsions. *Develop. Med. Child. Neurol.*, 10:374, 1968.

Low, N. L.: Infantile Spasms with Mental Retardation. II. Treatment with Cortisone and Adrenocorticotropin. *Pediatrics*, 22:1165, 1958.

Merritt, H. H., and Putnam, T. J.: Sodium Diphenylhydantoinate in Treatment of Convulsive Disorders. *J.A.M.A.*, 111:1068, 1938.

Millichap, J. G.: *Febrile Convulsions.* New York, Macmillan Company, 1968.

Prensky, A. L., Raff, M. C., Moore, M. J., and Schwab, R. S.: Intravenous Diazepam in Treatment of Prolonged Seizure Activity. *New England J. Med.,* 276:779, 1967.

Prichard, J. S., Gauk, E. W., and Kidd, L.: Mechanism of Seizures Associated with Breath-Holding Spells. *New England J. Med.*, 268:1436, 1963.

Schwartz, I. H., and Lombroso, C. T.: 14 and 6/Second Positive Spiking (Ctenoids) in the EEG of Primary School Pupils. *J. Pediat.*, 72:678, 1968.

Zellweger, H., and Idriss, H.: Encephalopathy in Salmonella Infections. *Am. J. Dis. Child.*, 99:770, 1960.

TETANY

Tetany is a syndrome whose principal manifestations result from a state of increased neuromuscular irritability. Because it occurs in a number of unrelated conditions, the more important types are described elsewhere in appropriate sections. They are brought together here as an aid in the differential diagnosis of the various conditions in which tetany may be one of the manifestations.

Pathogenesis. The clinical forms of tetany can be divided into 2 groups: those caused by a decrease in serum calcium and those associated with alkalosis. The irritability of muscle is accentuated with increasing concentrations of sodium and potassium ions and with decreasing concentrations of calcium, magnesium and hydrogen ions. Ionic relations are normally maintained within physiologic limits by the mechanisms regulating (1) reabsorption and formation of bone, (2) renal excretion of calcium and phosphate, (3) gastrointestinal absorption of calcium, (4) distribution of calcium and phosphate in the body fluids and tissues, and (5) the intracellular and extracellular distribution and concentrations of sodium, potassium, and hydrogen ions.

Clinical laboratory methods determine the total calcium content of serum, which is composed of nondiffusible or protein-bound calcium (34 per cent) and diffusible calcium (66 per cent). Approximately 80 per cent of the nondiffusible calcium is bound to albumin and the remainder to globulin.

An increase in the concentration of hydrogen ions decreases the proportion of calcium bound to protein. About 80 per cent of the diffusible calcium is present in ionic form, and the rest is bound with phosphate, bicarbonate or citrate. The ionized fraction normally makes up about 54 per cent of the total serum calcium. Thus the amount of non-diffusible calcium depends upon the total concentration of protein in the blood, and the percentage of ionized calcium, which is the physiologically active fraction, may be increased or decreased, depending upon the level of serum protein. For example, in nephrosis, owing to low serum protein levels, the total serum calcium may be reduced below the usual tetany level without clinical manifestations because there remains an adequate concentration of ionized calcium. The serum protein level should be known for a proper evaluation of the total serum calcium.

Phosphate ion (inorganic phosphate) activity varies inversely with calcium ion activity. Total serum calcium is lowered by the intravenous injection of alkali or acid phosphate salts, although tetany occurs only after the administration of alkaline phosphate. The serum level of phosphate is influenced by parathyroid hormone, gonadal hormones, adrenocorticoglucogenic hormones, insulin and anterior pituitary growth hormone, and fluctuates directly with the blood sugar concentration. Thus in the evaluation of a patient it is desirable to obtain fasting phosphate levels.

The equilibrium between ionic calcium and phosphate activity in extracellular fluid and the exchangeable hydroxyapatite crystals in bone is reflected in the maintenance, within constant limits, of the product of total serum calcium (milligrams per 100 ml.) times total inorganic plasma phosphate (milligrams per 100 ml.). The product is 40 to 55 for growing children. The relation between these ions in the circulation and the exchangeable ones in the bone compartment has been postulated as one in which the body fluids are a supersaturated metastable solution of calcium and phosphate ions with respect to bone.

The calcium-phosphate ion product decreases with vitamin D deficiency. Although parathyroid hormone increases calcium ion activity in serum and can maintain it at higher levels than is possible with physiologic amounts of vitamin D, the product may be maintained within a constant range independently of the parathyroid gland. A higher product in growing children than in adults and in patients with acromegaly has suggested the influence of growth hormone of the anterior pituitary.

The mechanisms responsible for tetany which occurs as the result of alkalosis or during the correction of acidosis are not entirely understood. The symptoms of tetany can be eliminated by a decrease in blood pH without altering the level of serum calcium or phosphorus. Tetany has been observed in otherwise normal animals made alkalotic without lowering of the calcium ion concentration.

Animal studies have indicated that an increase in serum sodium concentration in association with potassium deficiency results in a decrease in calcium ion concentration. This effect could not be produced by manipulating either the sodium or potassium ions alone. This relation between these ions and neuromuscular irritability has been suggested as the explanation for tetany which occasionally occurs during correction of the acidosis of diarrhea.

A depressed magnesium concentration in conjunction with normal calcium and phosphorus blood levels and with hypocalcemia has been associated with tetany in a variety of clinical conditions. Tetany has been produced experimentally in animals by feeding them diets deficient in magnesium.

Clinical Forms. *Hypocalcemic tetany.* When the total concentration of serum calcium falls below 7 or 7.5 mg. per 100 ml., symptoms of tetany are likely to occur. In *tetany of the newborn* (p. 401) it is postulated that there is inadequate response of the parathyroid glands to the need for calcium homeostasis. The serum calcium level may be further lowered by too heavy initial feeding of cow's milk with its relatively high phosphorus content. Neonatal tetany in newborn infants of diabetic mothers has been reported. Neonatal tetany secondary to maternal hyperparathyroidism has also been observed. After the first 4 weeks of life vitamin D deficiency (p. 183) and celiac disease (p. 807) are the most frequent causes of hypocalcemic tetany. Infrequently in children hypoparathyroidism (p. 1201) is a factor. Tetany has occurred as the result of hypocalcemia in the late stages of renal insufficiency and during acute pancreatitis. A number of rare disorders are associated with hypocalcemia and potentially with tetany. These include the hypocalcemic form of vitamin D-resistant rickets (p. 1364), renal tubular lesions characterized by aminoaciduria, hypercalciuria or metabolic acidosis (p. 1147) and pseudohypoparathyroidism (p. 1203).

Hypomagnesemic tetany. Serum magnesium concentrations are normally somewhat lower in the first few postnatal days in comparison with later values, but tetany has not been attributed to such values (1.2 to 1.8 mEq. per liter in newborn, in contrast to 1.6 to 2.2 mEq. per liter subsequently). Abnormally low levels may result from exchange transfusions with citrated blood (see below) and at times are observed in infants of diabetic mothers (p. 402). Hypomagnesemic tetany (p. 226) with and without hypocalcemia has also been attributed to defective intestinal absorption in chronic diarrheal conditions and in the malabsorption syndromes, as well as in a variety of other conditions, which include hyperaldosteronism and primary hyperparathyroidism. Recently an infant has been described with primary hypomagnesemia and secondary hypocalcemia (Paunier et al.) which were responsible for tetany beginning within the first 2 months of life. Serum magnesium and calcium concentrations were 0.3 to 0.4 mEq. and

3.0 mEq. per liter, respectively. Therapy with calcium was not effective in controlling the convulsions, whereas oral or parenteral administration of magnesium prevented them and restored the serum magnesium as well as calcium values to normal. The child was still dependent on oral supplementation of magnesium to 3 years of age (the time of the published report).

Tetany of alkalosis. In *hyperventilation tetany* there is an excessive loss of plasma carbonic acid with a lesser loss of bicarbonate. The pH of the blood is elevated, and the carbon dioxide content is decreased, resulting in respiratory alkalosis. Overbreathing may be due to hysteria or high altitude or to irritation of the central nervous system by infectious or by toxic agents such as the salicylates.

Gastric tetany follows loss of chloride ions from excessive vomiting, acute gastric dilatation, repeated gastric lavage or gastric retention. It is occasionally observed in pyloric stenosis and in high intestinal obstruction. The chloride of the serum is reduced and the bicarbonate elevated. The carbon dioxide content and the pH of the blood are increased.

Bicarbonate tetany occasionally results from ingestion or intravenous administration of sodium bicarbonate. Both the carbon dioxide content and the pH of the blood are elevated. The danger of administration of bicarbonate in the presence of vomiting or renal insufficiency cannot be overemphasized.

Iatrogenic tetany. Hypocalcemia and hypomagnesemia may develop acutely as a consequence of an exchange transfusion when calcium or magnesium has not been given during the procedure.

During correction of the acidosis of diarrhea, neuromuscular irritability and signs of tetany may develop even when overcorrection has not resulted in alkalosis. This situation may be associated with low serum calcium concentration or with normal calcium levels in the presence of elevated sodium and depressed potassium concentrations.

Tetany as well as hypernatremia may occur in the newborn infant as a consequence of the treatment of asphyxia or hyaline membrane disease with sodium bicarbonate.

Clinical Manifestations. The symptoms of tetany are essentially the same, irrespective of the cause, and reflect a state of increased neuromuscular irritability. There are, of course, clinical manifestations peculiar to each of the various disturbances with which tetany is associated. The manifestations may be divided into 2 phases, latent and manifest.

Latent tetany. In the latent phase there are no spontaneous manifestations, but increased neuromuscular excitability may be elicited by the mechanical or electrical means described below. The diagnosis is confirmed in hypocalcemic tetany by a low serum calcium level.

CHVOSTEK'S SIGN. This is a unilateral contraction of reflex of the facial muscles about the mouth, nose and eye when the area in front of the auditory meatus, where the facial nerve approaches the surface, is tapped. The reflex cannot be obtained while the infant is crying. A positive Chvostek's sign is normal in the newborn infant and is obtained frequently in healthy children over 5 years of age, but in the age range of vitamin D-deficient tetany, 3 months to 3 years, it is strong presumptive evidence in favor of tetany.

PERONEAL SIGN. This is elicited by tapping the peroneal nerve just below the head of the fibula while the knee is relaxed and slightly flexed. A positive response consists in dorsal flexion and abduction of the foot.

TROUSSEAU'S SIGN. This is based on the production of carpal spasm. It is elicited by maintaining firm constriction of the upper arm for 2 or 3 minutes after the hand has become blanched. When the reaction is positive, the hand assumes the position of carpal spasm, which is described under Carpopedal Spasm.

ERB'S SIGN. This is obtained by measuring the amount of galvanic current required to elicit a muscular contraction and is based on the greater muscular irritability of the patient with tetany. It is the most sensitive of the various tests, but is now rarely used.

Manifest tetany. This phase is characterized by spontaneous muscular twitchings and spasms, laryngospasm and convulsions.

CARPOPEDAL SPASM. This is perhaps the most characteristic feature of tetany. The thumb is drawn into the cupped palm, the hands are abducted and the wrists flexed, and the fingers are flexed at the metacarpophalangeal joints, but extended at the more distal ones (Fig. 19-2). The foot is extended in the position of talipes equinus or equinovarus, the toes are flexed, and the sole is cupped (Fig. 19-3). Both the arms and the legs may be rigidly flexed and adducted.

LARYNGOSPASM. This is a relatively common manifestation and may be characterized simply by an inspiratory, high-pitched crowing sound, but in extremely severe cases there is such spasm that respirations may cease for an uncomfortable interval and the infant become quite cyanotic. Rarely intubation is required for relief, and occasionally an infant has died during such an attack.

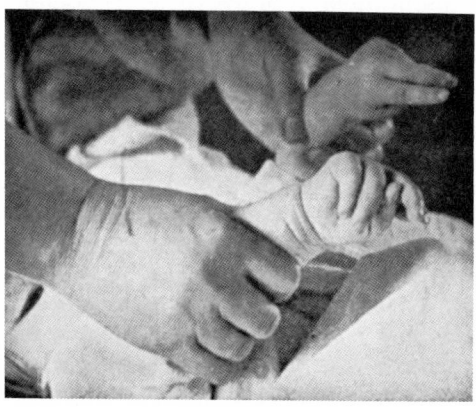

Figure 19-2. Carpal spasm in tetany.

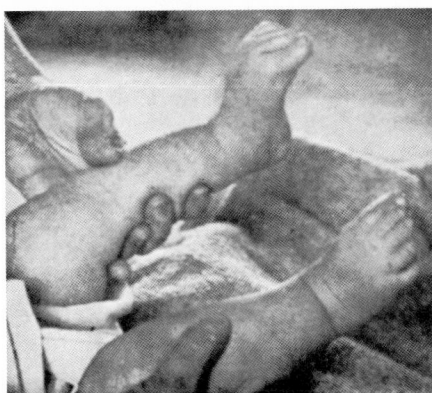

Figure 19-3. Pedal spasm.

CONVULSIONS. These do not differ from other generalized seizures, except as there may be carpopedal spasm.

Diagnosis. The diagnosis is based on the clinical manifestations and the laboratory data. Of the latter, the important measurements are the serum calcium level in hypocalcemic tetany and the pH of the blood in the tetany of alkalosis.

In the differential diagnosis other causes of convulsions and increased muscular irritability must be considered (p. 1248), as must other conditions which may be responsible for laryngospasm or stridor. *Congenital stridor* is eliminated as a possibility, since it is present from birth. The laryngospasm of *pertussis* has been confused with that of tetany. The characteristic cough of pertussis, with absence of other signs of tetany, should establish the diagnosis which, in many instances, may be confirmed bacteriologically. *Acute laryngeal infections* are characterized by fever and other evidences of infection. *Breath-holding spells* may be confused with tetany, but a history of previous episodes, the relation to fits of temper and the absence of other signs of tetany are differential factors.

Treatment. Treatment of the various hypocalcemic tetanies is considered under their respective headings. Primary attention should be directed to relieving the cause of the tetany. In hyperventilation tetany, rebreathing into a paper bag and inhalation of carbon dioxide are helpful procedures. Carefully controlled sedation is usually indicated to decrease the hyperpnea. In gastric tetany the underlying disturbance should be controlled, if possible, and generous amounts of physiologic saline solution should be administered parenterally. Acid salts such as ammonium chloride, calcium lactate, calcium gluconate or calcium chloride may be administered orally if vomiting is controlled.

WALDO E. NELSON

REFERENCES

Aub, J. C.: Diseases of the Parathyroid Glands; in R. L. Cecil, (Ed.): *Textbook of Medicine.* 8th ed. Philadelphia, W. B. Saunders Company, 1951.

Finberg, L.: Experimental Studies of the Mechanisms Producing Hypocalcemia in Hypernatremic States. *J. Clin. Invest.,* 36:434, 1957.

Howard, J. E.: Calcium Metabolism, Bones and Calcium Homeostasis; A Review of Certain Current Concepts. *J. Clin. Endocr. Metab.,* 17:1105, 1959.

Kramer, B., and Leibner, I. W.: Symposium on Endocrine and Metabolic Disorders; Tetany; Biochemical and Clinical Considerations. *M. Clin. N. Amer.,* 36:875, 1952.

McLean, F. C., and Hastings, A. B.: The State of Calcium in the Fluids of the Body; The Conditions Affecting the Ionization of Calcium. *J. Biol. Chem.,* 108:285, 1935.

Neuman, W. F. and Neuman, M. W.: *Chemical Dynamics of Bone Mineral.* Chicago, University of Chicago Press, 1958.

Paunier, L., Radde, I. C., Kooh, S. W., Conen, P. E., and Fraser, D.: Primary Hypomagnesemia with Secondary Hypocalcemia in an Infant. *Pediatrics,* 41:385, 1968.

Shelling, D. H.: *The Parathyroids in Health and in Disease.* St. Louis, C. V. Mosby Company, 1935.

Wong, H. B., and Teh, Y. F.: An Association Between Serum-Magnesium and Tremor and Convulsions in Infants and Children. *Lancet,* 2:18, 1968.

20. The Nervous System

DIAGNOSTIC STUDY OF NEUROLOGIC DISEASE

HISTORY AND PHYSICAL EXAMINATION

The physical examination in neurologic disease localizes the disease; the history suggests its nature. No other procedures can replace these two; carelessness, indifference or inadequacy in performing them ends in neglect of serious illness or in performance of unnecessary, painful or dangerous procedures. History and physical examination generally provide a reasonable differential neurologic diagnosis. Conclusions made before these are completed are usually erroneous.

History (see also p. 197). History-taking presents the opportunity to establish the beginning of friendly relations with the child and to observe his spontaneous behavior and activity, which suggest many of his physical signs.

Many neurologic ailments of childhood are present at birth or are acquired soon after; when such origins are possibilities, the family history and the record of pregnancy and labor must, if possible, be more detailed than with illnesses more clearly of recent onset. Repeated review of the history often brings out valuable information. The following outline may be expanded or reduced as circumstances indicate.

Family history. For parents, grandparents, aunts, uncles and cousins: present health or cause of death; symptoms similar to patient's; common neurologic symptoms, such as convulsions, visual or motor failure, disturbance of gait.

For the immediate sibship: date, parentage and outcome of each pregnancy; causes of deaths; present state of survivors; presence of symptoms similar to patient's.

Pregnancy. Difficulties in conception; duration as exactly as possible; onset and quality of fetal movements; data, duration, severity, treatment and effect if noted on fetal movement and heart rate, of maternal toxemias, illness or infections, injuries, radiation, exposure to drugs or toxins, vaginal bleeding and severe emotional stress.

Labor. Hour of onset and delivery; presentation; anesthesia and analgesia; operative procedures and indication for, if known; evidence of fetal distress.

Neonatal period. Birth weight; initial breathing and crying; cyanosis, asphyxia; resuscitative procedures, use of oxygen or incubator; signs of trauma; jaundice; duration and treatment of convulsions; infection; notable listlessness, vomiting, "jitteriness," stiffness or limpness.

Growth and development. Serial weights, heights and head measurements, if available; age at puberty; age of such developmental acquisitions as social smile, sitting alone, standing, walking, and the like; school progress. Compare with siblings.

Past health. Date and severity of each significant illness, injury or operation, with special note of high fevers, delirium, head trauma, convulsions, disturbances of gait, vision or hearing, and personality changes.

Present illness. List the symptoms with time of onset and further progression; try to document the way each came to attention. Summarize onset and principal features of each salient event of the illness chronologically.

Technique of Neurologic Examination. No rigid scheme of examination is necessary if the examiner remembers a few principles. No neurologic examination is complete without a general physical examination. A regular method of *recording* findings is essential for completeness and clarity. The physiologic and emotional condition of the child may affect his signs; fright, cold or embarrassment heightens reflexes and impairs fine motor performance; warmth, a full stomach, and sedatives diminish reflexes and alertness. At some time all clothing must be removed from the child; "much more is missed from not looking than from not knowing."

The neurologic examination includes (1) vital signs, (2) mental status, (3) gait, station and handedness, (4) cranial nerves and special senses, (5) motor system and reflexes, (6) sensory system, (7) coordinative system, (8) autonomic system, and (9) special findings.

The *vital signs* require no special comment. An estimate of the *mental status* in infants is based on alertness, response to examiners and quality of cry; in older children, from the playing of simple games, inquiries about siblings, pets, illness and the like, and by formal evaluation of the intelligence. *Gait, station and handedness* are determined by simple observations.

The *special senses* should be examined early, before fatigue impairs cooperation.

Vision. In the infant, or child with very low vision, the ability to follow a light or to avoid threatening movements is noted. If there is real doubt as to the presence of vision, demonstration of opticokinetic nystagmus is useful. A cylinder marked with alternating wide black and white stripes is rotated slowly before the child; if cortical vision is present, the eyes follow the stripes slowly, then jerk quickly back to midposition; this response appears normally within the first few weeks of life. Older children are tested with charts, or by having them pick up coins or bits of paper scattered on floor or table top; the latter procedure tests both fields and acuity.

To test *visual fields*, the child and the examiner stand about 3 feet apart and cover opposite eyes, and each fixes on the other's uncovered eye. The examiner brings his finger, or other test object, inward along radii of a circle, the center of which is on the axis of fixation, midway between examiner and child. The child states when he sees the object, the examiner's visual field serving as a check. The test object should be carried inward to the center, to detect central defects. With infants or young children, attention is held with a light or toy, and the hand moved in until the child notices it. The visual fields can usually be outlined by confrontation methods alone. Color fields and perimetry may be necessary for more exact work.

Ophthalmoscopy should be reserved till last with small children, who often struggle. Common errors are (1) overlooking early papilledema, the first signs of which are not blurring of the disk margins, but dilatation of retinal veins and obliteration of the optic cup; indistinct disk margins without the other signs usually represent refractive error or congenital peculiarity. (2) Mistaking optic neuritis or pseudoneuritis for papilledema; the appearances may be identical, but loss of acuity and color vision is marked with neuritis but is slight and appears late with papilledema. (3) Mistaking the normal grayish disk of infancy for optic atrophy.

Hearing. Startling or blinking at loud sounds is a test of hearing only at the lowest threshold, and may persist despite cortical deafness. Turning toward a sound or smiling at a parent's voice is a better sign of hearing. Children who can speak are asked to repeat aloud numbers whispered at their ears (see also p. 101).

Labyrinthine function. The child is held aloft, his face at a level with the examiner's, who turns round rapidly several times; after 3 or 4 turns the normal child shows definite nystagmus. To test 1 labyrinth, instill 5 to 10 cc. of ice water into the external ear with a soft catheter or syringe. Normally, nystagmus with the slow component to the stimulated side appears in about 40 seconds, and persists about 2 minutes. Lesions of the vestibular apparatus, the eighth nerve or brain stem diminish or obliterate the response; in decortication the slow phase alone is present, and the eyes deviate to the stimulated side.

Smell and taste. Tests of *olfaction*, with some familiar odor, and *taste*, with salt or sugar solutions applied to the tongue, are inapplicable to young children, and are done only when first, seventh or ninth nerve lesions are suspected.

Cranial nerves. To test the oculomotor group, the third, fourth and sixth nerves, observations are made for pupillary size, direct and consensual response to light and response to convergence, range of movement of eyes, ptosis and nystagmus. Tests of the facial group, the fifth and seventh nerves, include determinations of facial symmetry at rest and in movement (crying), equality of palpebral fissures, strength of lid closure, corneal reflexes, facial sensation to pin prick and light touch, and jaw movements. For the ninth, tenth, eleventh and twelfth nerves one should note the quality of voice, gag reflex, swallowing actions and the function of the trapezii and sternomastoids. Palatal asymmetries are not significant unless prominent or associated with diminished gag reflex. The tongue should be examined carefully for size, symmetry, movement and fibrillation.

The motor system. The child should be observed stripped at rest, and partially clothed in spontaneous and induced activity. He is asked to lie down, stand up, hop on one foot, walk, walk tandem, run and climb stairs; he is offered a toy, plays a game of catch, writes, or colors simple drawings. Note bodily proportions, spontaneity and symmetry of movements, handedness, evidence of generalized or localized weakness, steadiness of gait and presence and kind of involuntary movement. Look carefully for the following:

Physical status of muscles. *Atrophy* may be part of generalized wasting or may be due to disuse. If it is due to progressive motor neuron disease, it is accompanied by *fasciculations*, brief repetitive twitches, occurring at rest, increased by movement or percussion of the muscle. Completely denervated muscle *fibrillates*, producing a slow undulating movement, visible clinically only in the tongue. *Aplasia* or *hypoplasia* most frequently involves facial and extraocular muscles (Moebius' syndrome), but any muscle may be affected. Arrest of development with smallness of limbs, slight muscles, narrow nails and slender bones is seen in limbs paralyzed at an early age. *Hypertrophy* may be compensatory, as in the arms and shoulders of a patient with paralyzed legs, or result from constant overaction in choreo-athetosis. In *pseudohypertrophy*, size is increased by fatty infiltration, and the muscle is weak.

Disorders of tone. *Tonus* is the contraction in a muscle voluntarily relaxed. It is tested by inspection and palpation of the muscle and passive movement of joints. *Flaccidity*, the absence of tone, is seen in organically or physiologically denervated muscles. *Hypotonia* is a reduction of normal tone. *Spasticity* is an exaggeration of stretch reflexes, depending on impairment of central inhibition with maintenance of central facilitation of these reflexes. It expresses itself as diminished voluntary movement; the postures of the limbs indicate movements particularly impaired. It is characterized by (1) increased resistance to passive movement, giving way suddenly when overcome—"clasp knife" rigidity; (2) increased myotatic reflexes; (3) clonus. It is not produced by isolated lesions of the motor cortex, but rather by widespread damage to the motor system.

Rigidity implies increased tone and resistance,

not accentuated in any particular movement. The hypertonus may appear to abolish reflexes, but they are present and increased. When overcome, hypertonus may give way in a series of brief relaxations, producing the cogwheel phenomenon, or maintain a constant, plastic resistance.

INVOLUNTARY MOVEMENTS. *Myoclonic jerks* are brief contractions of whole muscles occurring irregularly and without pattern; massive myoclonus is a sudden jerk involving neck, shoulders and upper part of the trunk. *Myotonus* is sustained contraction following voluntary contraction or direct percussion of the muscle. *Tremors* are usually regular movements, principally flexion-extension, of segments of limbs, entire limbs or head and trunk; the rate varies from 3 to 10 per second. Tremor at rest, with limbs relaxed, suggests disease of the extrapyramidal system; intention tremor, or tremor on movement, indicates involvement of cerebello-rubro-thalamo-cortical circuits. *Athetosis* is an irregular wandering movement, most noted in fingers or toes. *Chorea*, often associated with athetosis, is a coarse, jerking, irregular movement involving large joints or segments of a limb. *Dystonia* is a slow, twisting movement of limbs or trunk, about the long axis of the segment involved. *Tics*, by contrast, are repetitive movements without organic dysfunction, which could be purposive, and can be stopped for a time by the patient.

MUSCULAR STRENGTH. The strength of muscles, and of particular movements, should be carefully tested. Certain patterns of weakness characterize special types of neurologic impairment. Pyramidal lesions weaken extension more than flexion in the arm, whereas the converse is true of the leg. In polyneuritis proximal muscle groups are usually weaker than distal ones in legs, the distal ones weaker than proximal ones in the arms. Most dystrophies weaken limb girdle, axial and proximal muscles much earlier than distal ones.

REFLEXES. The stimulus for the *myotatic* or *stretch* reflexes is deformation of nerve endings in the muscle of tendon; the reflexes are segmental, with afferent and efferent neural limbs, and a segmental center within the brain or cord. They are diminished or abolished by any process which (1) impairs nerve conduction, such as peripheral neuritis; (2) lowers the central excitatory state, such as spinal shock; (3) reduces reactivity of muscle, such as atrophy or metabolic disturbance. They are increased by processes which lower the central inhibitory state or reduce synaptic resistance, such as pyramidal tract lesions or tetanus.

The limb should be relaxed, and the muscle to be stimulated should be able to act at maximal mechanical advantage; usually this is a position of about half-flexion of the joint involved. The stimulus is a brisk tap on tendon or bony prominence, putting a muscle on stretch. The muscle itself should not be tapped; the contraction thus produced is not a myotatic reflex. Reflexes should not be considered absent until reinforcement has

been tried by causing muscular activity in another part of the body — having the older child squeeze the examiner's hand, or provoking the infant to tears.

The following myotatic reflexes, with their segmental arcs, are usually adequate:

REFLEX	CENTRAL ARC
Jaw jerk	Pons
Biceps jerk	C 5–6
Triceps jerk	C 6–7–8
Supinator jerk	C 5–6
Finger jerks (Hoffmann sign)	C 8–T 1
Knee jerk	L 3–L 4
Ankle jerk	S 1–S 2

The important superficial reflexes are the abdominal, anal, plantar and grasp reflexes.

Abdominal reflexes. Stroking away from the umbilicus, horizontally, upward or downward, with a blunt point causes contraction of the homolateral abdominal muscles, with some localizing significance depending on the level stimulated. A cerebral as well as spinal arc is present, and reduction of abdominal reflexes characterizes most acute pyramidal lesions, though they usually persist in hemiparesis of early and remote onset.

Anal reflex. Stroke the perianal skin with a pin; a prompt constriction of the anus follows, mediated through the lowermost sacral segments.

Plantar reflex. Stroke along the lateral margin of the sole, from the heel forward, ending medially at the base of the great toe. A reasonably firm stroke with key, fingernail or blunt pencil is best; the more lateral the stroke, the less the likelihood of avoidance reflexes. The foot should be warm, the leg in extension, and the initial strokes gentle. Three responses may occur: (1) The toes may plantar-flex; this is the response in all normal waking persons over 1 to 2 years of age. (2) The great toe may dorsiflex, with or without fanning of the other toes; the movement, unlike avoidance, is slow and maintained. This response, the only one properly called *Babinski's sign*, is evidence of structural or functional pyramidal tract deficit. A similar response occurs normally up to 1 to 2 years of age, and in sleep. (3) There may be no movement at all, as in spinal shock, deep anesthesia or coma or peripheral neuritis.

Grasp reflex. Stroking the palmar surface of the metacarpophalangeal joints toward the fingers brings out a sudden grasp reflex, followed by maintained contraction if the stimulus is continued. The reflex is normally present in infants under 4 months of age; at later ages it suggests frontal lobe lesions, though its localizing value is not absolute. When it is present, gentle stimulation of palmar and volar surfaces of fingers will often bring out groping movements of the hands as well.

The sensory system. Awareness of pin prick, the touch of a tuft of cotton, position of fingers and toes, and vibration are all that need ordinarily be tested. Sensory findings are less reliable than motor or reflex change, and minor aberrations, unless repeatable, should be disregarded. Sensation is best tested from a suspected toward a normal area, or from distal to proximal portion of limbs.

Coordinating system. Most disorders of coordination are apparent in spontaneous movement. Watch the child reach for a toy, build a block house, tear paper, "do his buttons," or open and close a safety pin. A small peg-board or chinese-checkers game may be used to advantage. Have him touch his nose and the examiner's finger alternately; move the target about, to prevent decomposition of movement and bring out ataxia. *Romberg's sign,* standing on either foot singly, and hopping on one foot, together with the heel-shin test, suffices for the legs.

Autonomic system. Color and temperature of the skin, mottling, edema and trophic sores should be looked for. Sweating, usually abolished below a transverse spinal cord lesion, may be demonstrated with the starch-iodine test (see below). A distended bladder should always be searched for; defects of sphincter function usually appear in the history.

Special findings. *Percussion* over the sphenion gives a flat note if the sutures are separated; this, *Macewen's sign,* is inapplicable to infants and unreliable in early sutural separation. In about 10 per cent of young children, *auscultation* over the vertex, temples or eyeballs discloses a bruit, systolic in time or accentuated in systole. Most head bruits are innocent; they are most common between 1 and 6 years of age, and are transmitted from the heart or due to angulation of basal vessels; some accompany anemia, hydrocephalus or increased intracranial pressure. Rarely they indicate vascular malformations. A significant bruit is usually loud and often lateralized. Hydranencephaly, extreme hydrocephalus and sometimes subdural hematoma or porencephaly can be demonstrated by *transillumination of the skull* of the infant; a strong flashlight with a sponge rubber cuff about the end and a completely dark room are necessary. Sweating tests, using starch powder over iodine rubbed on the skin, or an old-fashioned indelible pencil drawn from suspected to normal regions, aids in demonstrating spinal cord or autonomic lesions.

Examination of Newborn and Young Infants

The neurologic examination of newborn and young infants serves 2 purposes: first, the detection and localization of neurologic abnormalities; second, the assessment of the state of maturation of the nervous system. Individual responses or test procedures may be of great value and highly specific for one purpose, yet nonspecific and of little value for the other. A complete neurologic examination is time-consuming; the examiner should decide the purpose of his study, and adjust his

procedures to it, rather than attempt to follow an extensive and unvarying routine.

The infant should be in the optimal physiologic state to respond. He should be about 1½ to 2 hours from his last feeding, comfortably warm, unfettered by clothing or crib sides, and uninfluenced by sedative or stimulant drugs. For maturational estimations these conditions are obligatory. For the sick or damaged infant they often cannot be achieved.

The normal newborn infant can perform most basic functions characteristic of a more mature nervous system, though in limited or incomplete fashion. He blinks at a light, and the pupillary light reflex is present. He sees, can turn toward a light, and often shows a preference for red, though range of vision, color vision and binocular fusion are limited; he can exhibit opticokinetic nystagmus, and in some instances can demonstrate selective conditioned response to specific forms or shapes. The internal ear is functioning, since he can blink to a loud sound and show nystagmus on rotation. Taste is present, and he can yawn, sneeze, cough, belch or hiccup with evident satisfaction. He responds to pain by withdrawal and a cry of discomfort. In prone position he can lift his head, turn it from side to side, and make movements of quadrupedal progression.

The most important and constant evidence of neurologic abnormality in the infant is the absence of reflex patterns appropriate to age, or the persistence, reappearance or exaggeration of patterns either less mature or otherwise inappropriate to his age. The intrinsic reflex arcs and conducting systems through mesencephalic levels are intact and functioning at birth. Though the most readily tested reflexes are those of the brain stem and spinal cord, unmodified or only partially modified by suprasegmental control, the cerebral hemispheres exert some influence. The normal infant, for example, has visual responses which cannot be attributed to the brain stem alone; moreover, damage to cerebral hemispheres may present focal signs at birth, such as hemiparesis, which last only while the lesion is acute, disappearing in the early months, to reappear when normal functioning of the damaged areas should become manifest.

To determine the presence, absence or localization of neurologic abnormality, one relies on (1) general signs of alertness and responsiveness, such as rooting and sucking reflexes, turning of the head to light, blinking to light or to loud sound, and the amount of spontaneous activity; (2) signs demonstrating levels of neuromuscular tone and irritability, such as the Moro response or the resting posture; (3) localizing signs of which persistent asymmetries of spontaneous or evoked movements are perhaps most important. Particular attention is given to the ease, completeness and symmetry with which the tonic neck response and the myotatic reflexes are evoked. Lateralized hypertonicity may be shown by holding the baby by the ankles, head down, and releasing either leg alternately: the more hypertonic leg remains longer in extension. A thin gauze or nasal tissue dropped over the face stimulates movements to remove it, which may reveal asymmetry of tone or movement in the arms.

Assessment of maturational age by neurologic examination is difficult. Complicated schemata are available, but their accuracy is debatable. The basic principle is to search for reflex and volitional patterns inappropriate to chronologic age. Certain reflex responses closely related to gestational age are of considerable value in its estimation.

REFLEX	APPROXIMATE GESTATIONAL AGE AT TIME OF APPEARANCE
Pupillary response to light	29-31 weeks
Glabellar tap reflex	32-34 weeks
Traction response	33-36 weeks
Neck-righting reflex	36-37 weeks
Turning head and eyes to light	32-34 weeks

Some examiners place particular emphasis on tone in the estimation of maturational age and normality of the nervous system; the signs are hard to quantify, however, and the use of tone as an indicator of maturation requires great experience.

Postural Reflexes. Afferent impulses for the *tonic neck reflex* originate predominantly in neck muscles. With the infant supine, turn the head sharply to one side. The arm and the leg on the side to which the jaw is turned extend, or extensor tone increases; their fellows of the opposite side flex, or extensor tone decreases. In normal newborn infants these reflexes are incomplete, often more definite in leg than in arm; they tend to disappear during the first year, but partial responses may persist until the second or third year. Persistent asymmetry or complete and easy elicitation of the full response suggests a cerebral lesion.

Similar postural reflexes originate in the labyrinth *(otolith righting reflex)*. Tilting the body of the erect infant while his eyes are covered induces a reflex righting movement of the head, returning it to the erect position. When the head is turned, with the infant supine, the trunk rotates in the direction of head movement, the *neck-righting response*. (There may be a brief initial rotation in the direction opposite head movement, followed by strong rotation toward head direction.) Absence of this neck righting reflex is an early sign of spasticity. In the *Landau reflex* the child is held prone, horizontally; head and neck extend, shoulders draw back and hips extend, the entire body forming a convex arc upward. Gentle pressure on the head or gravity flexes the neck, and legs and arms drop with it, reversing the arc. The same response may be seen when the normal child is learning to sit; he balances his head

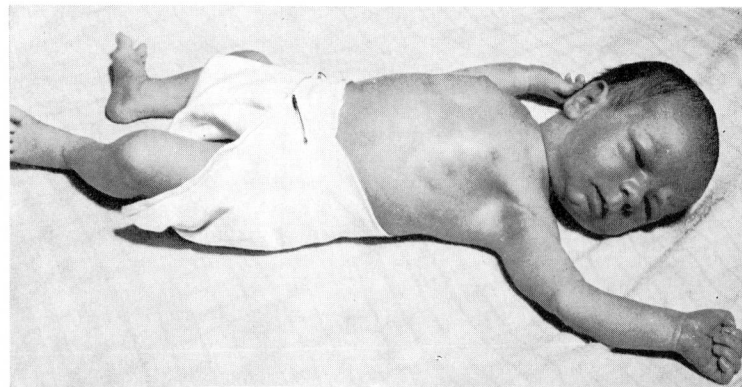

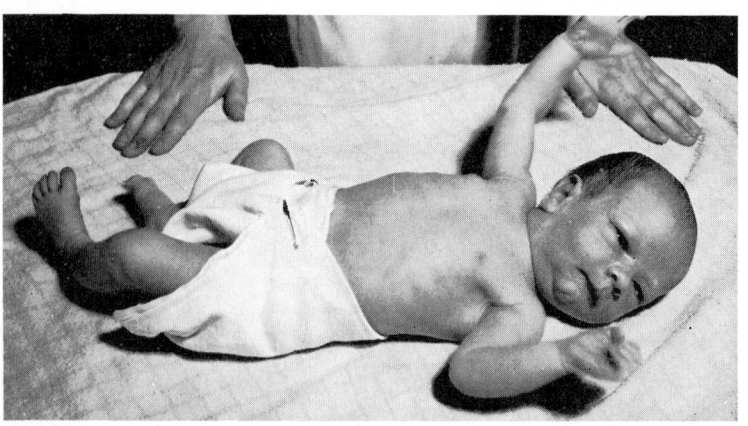

Figure 20-1. Upper photograph shows a spontaneous tonic neck reflex. Lower photograph shows the Moro reflex.

briefly, usually overextending slightly, then slumps forward with flexed neck and trunk, and arms dropping forward on the chest. When the spastic child attempts to sit, weakness of extension of trunk and neck forces him to slump forward, but pressure on the occiput produces overextension of neck and trunk, opisthotonos, exaggerated backward movement of shoulders and arms and extension of legs.

The *Moro reflex* is a generalized extension of trunk, and extension and abduction of limbs, followed by flexion and adduction; in some infants the hips and knees may be flexed throughout this maneuver. This reflex can be elicited by a hand clap or slap on the mattress while the infant is supine. Since the effective stimulus is not sound, but excitation of cervical and labyrinthine proprioceptors by movement, a better way is to support the supine infant with hands beneath head and shoulders, the trunk making an angle of about 30 degrees with the table. The head is then allowed to fall back 10 to 15 degrees, and the response appears at once. It is a good index of reflex irritability. Consistent absence of this reflex bilaterally suggests brain damage; lateralizing asymmetries indicate brain damage, fractures or obstetrical palsy. The reflex normally diminishes and disappears in the first few weeks of life.

Placing and Stepping Reflexes. Spontaneous limb movements of the newborn infant are either symmetrical or a part of quadrupedal progression. The prone newborn makes crawling movements; when held erect, with soles flat on the table top and trunk inclined forward, he takes regularly alternating steps, and, if the dorsum of the foot is drawn against the under edge of the table top, the foot is lifted and placed atop the table. The infant, supported about the trunk, feet touching the table top, should be lifted suddenly up and down; this normally produces a supporting extensor thrust of the legs. Persistent extension or scissoring of the legs *(DeLange's sign)* is abnormal, as is asymmetry in any of these responses.

Local Reflexes. Myotatic reflexes (e.g. triceps and patellar) are normally present, though extremely variable. Areflexia or persistent hyperactivity is abnormal; otherwise, only persistent asymmetry between the 2 sides is significant. The plantar response is usually extensor. Ankle jerks may appear to be absent because of fetal positioning of feet and laxness of the Achilles tendon. Abdominal reflexes are generally present, though sluggish and perhaps with prolonged latency. Strong grasp reflexes are present in hands and feet; that of the sole is commonly mistaken for a flexor plantar response. A brisk tap on the glabella results in a blink of the lids *(glabellar reflex)*; it must be distinguished from the generalized grimacing which premature infants often manifest. A corneal reflex is demonstrable. Stroking the lips produces sucking *(sucking reflex)*, and stimulating the side of the cheek or the upper or lower lip causes the infant to turn his mouth and

face to the stimulus, the *rooting reflex*, or *cardinal points response*. The skin is sensitive, and a light scratch along the paravertebral area causes an *incurvation reflex* of the trunk toward the stimulated side.

Chvostek's sign can often be elicited in the healthy newborn infant; it cannot be interpreted as evidence of disease.

Examination of the Hysterical Patient

Malingering is rare in childhood, but hysterical symptoms are fairly common; only very young children are exempt. Organic symptoms may coexist with, or be perpetuated as, hysterical ones. The diagnosis of hysteria depends anamnestically on demonstration of an appropriate emotional constitution and, almost always, a precipitating emotional crisis, sometimes clearly indicated by the kind of disability evoked. This portion of diagnosis, together with therapy, belongs in the domain of psychiatry. The role of the neurologist is to demonstrate the hysterical quality of the signs; he can best achieve this by physical examination without mechanical aids, hypnosis or narcosynthesis.

Hysterical symptoms, usually sudden in onset, tend to involve anatomic units or physiologic functions as a whole, and the victim shows a calm indifference inappropriate to his handicap. Common manifestations in childhood are (1) visual impairment or blindness, (2) paralysis of a limb or impairment of walking, (3) sensory loss or anesthesia, (4) loss of speech, (5) tremors or involuntary movements, (6) fits or disturbances of sensorium, (7) urinary retention.

Visual defect includes constriction of fields, amblyopia and amaurosis; hemianopsia and central scotomas are seldom if ever hysterical. Size of fields may change during perimetry, producing expanding, contracting or helical forms. If fixed in size, the field is very small and central and remains the same at whatever distance charted, a finding impossible for an organic constriction, owing to the divergence of the light rays subtended by the field. Impossible aberrations of color fields, e.g. red larger than blue, may be present. *Hysterical amblyopia* can generally be improved during examination by persuasion alone. In *hysterical amaurosis*, pupils and pupillary reflexes are normal and opticokinetic nystagmus is present, establishing the diagnosis. Photophobia, blepharospasm and convergence paralysis are common.

Hysterical paralysis may be paraplegic, monoplegic or hemiplegic. Normal reflexes and tone are preserved, and pathologic reflexes and the patterns of organic weakness are absent. The hemiparetic child may be tricked into movement by asking him to abduct or adduct both arms or both legs simultaneously; only conscious effort will keep a normal limb from moving, obvious voluntary contraction then keeping it still. In

Hoover's test the child elevates the normal leg strongly while the examiner keeps his hand beneath the heel of the paralyzed one; strong effort to raise the normal limb brings out downward pressure from a hysterically, but not an organically, paralyzed one. If partial movement is possible, the paretic limb regularly misses a mark set for it by about the same distance, whether a large or a small movement is required. Walking and standing are generally impaired together; both may be lost, though voluntary movement and coordination need not suffer (astasia-abasia).

Ataxia is usually greater in the trunk than in the limbs, and the stance is seldom wide-based; ataxia improves considerably if the child walks with 2 examiners ringing, but not touching, him with their arms.

Tremors are generally coarse, sometimes fairly rhythmic, but always reproducible by the examiner; they rarely cause difficulty in eating or dressing, except during observation.

Hysterical sensory loss, usually associated with paralysis, may be of glove or stocking type or involve a whole limb or one side of the body. It disregards neurologic boundaries and is usually absolute and to all modalities rather than incomplete or dissociated as in most organic illness. The level of sensory loss can be changed by shifting the point at which stimulation is begun; if one starts higher, the level is proportionately higher. Ask the child to close his eyes and say "Yes" when he feels a touch, "No" when he does not; hysterical children readily acquiesce and respond with "No" when the anesthetic area is touched. If one hand is involved, the *Japanese illusion* is useful: the child crosses his arms, palms opposed, clasps his fingers and brings the locked hands inward and upward. It is then very difficult for him to distinguish right from left; sensory stimulation or demand for movement produces gross inconsistencies.

Hysterical aphonia is seldom absolute; the child may not speak, but can whisper, sing or whistle; he may be mute with parents or physician, but speak to his fellows. Normal movements of tongue, palate and vocal cords are preserved. *Hysterical fits* are distinguished from epileptic ones by absence of tongue biting, incontinence, cyanosis or pallor, change in pupillary reflexes, Babinski sign and incidental injuries. In the *stupors* or *catatonias* which may follow them the eyes are actively closed; Bell's phenomenon is present when the lids are forcibly opened, and pupils are normally reactive. *Urinary retention* is seen almost exclusively in girls; it does not alter the cystometrogram unless secondary infection has occurred.

Examination of the Unconscious Patient

This should include the following:
Vital Signs.   Nature of pulse and respirations, color and responsiveness to stimuli. Record these at the beginning and the end of the examination to secure a time-lapsed record and an estimate of changes due to stimulus of examination.

Visuo-oculomotor System.   Position of eyes at rest, spontaneous movement and movement of eyes against passive movement of the head – a rough test for integrity of the vestibulo-ocular pathways. Note pupillary size, shape and reactivity to light and painful stimuli. Examine fundi carefully, but *do not dilate pupils*, since progressive pupillary dilatation is a valuable sign of increasing intracranial pressure.

Facial and Bulbar Functions.   Symmetry of movement of the face on breathing and on painful supraorbital pressure, corneal reflexes, presence of spontaneous swallowing movements and gag reflex.

Extremities.   Position at rest, the patient supine. Midbrain decerebration adducts, extends and internally rotates the arms, and extends and adducts the legs; tonic neck reflexes may appear spontaneously or be induced by turning the head. Note spontaneous and induced movements of limbs; hemiparetic limbs move less under both circumstances than normal ones; the leg in hemiplegia rotates externally at the hip, the oval outline of the thigh is transverse rather than vertical, and the foot points downward and outward. Raise the arms together and allow them to fall – a hemiplegic one falls more quickly and with less minor movements of adjustment than a normal one. Draw the legs up, knees flexed and soles flat, then release them suddenly – a hemiplegic leg falls outward, and the foot slips down on the sheet faster than a normal one. Check myotatic reflexes, which may be absent in recent hemiplegia, spinal shock or deep coma; asymmetries are more significant than generalized changes.

Sensation.   Stimulate fairly vigorously with a pin, especially on soles of feet and on hands. Cross the midline of the trunk and ascend either side with a series of pinpricks. Sensory impairment may be detected by a sudden twitch or an incomplete protective movement when one crosses from hyperesthetic to normally innervated skin.

Trophic and Circulatory Changes.   Note color, mottling and temperature of the skin. Fresh hemiplegias or transverse cord lesions cause warmth of the affected limbs from vasodilation. Palpate carefully for distended bladder.

Miscellaneous.   Signs include meningismus, nuchal rigidity, bruises, rashes, fractures, and odor of breath.

SPECIAL DIAGNOSTIC PROCEDURES

Special studies may be desirable for information and for the reason that abnormality demonstrated by a mechanical procedure often seems more comprehensible to the parent than that resting on clinical opinion. Some are harmless; others entail real hazard, which must be weighed carefully against the potential value of the information they may provide. Such special studies include (1) lumbar puncture, (2) subdural and ventricular punctures, (3) radiologic studies (plain films, pneumoencephalography, ventriculography, angiography, isotope scanning and myelography), (4) electroencephalography, (5) echoencephalography, (6) psychologic and psychometric studies, and (7) biopsy.

Lumbar Puncture. Carelessness and failure to pay attention to essential details often negate the potential value of the lumbar puncture. Contraindications include the possibilities of increased intracranial pressure due to space-taking lesions, local sepsis in the proposed puncture site, and in some instances a bleeding tendency. The equipment consists of no. 19 and 20 lumbar puncture needles, $1\frac{1}{2}$, 2 and $2\frac{1}{2}$ inches in length, well sharpened, short-bevelled and with smoothly fitting stylets, an Ayer type of glass manometer, procaine, hypodermic needles and syringes, a 3-way stopcock, collection tubes and the usual equipment for a minor, sterile procedure. Older children usually cooperate, younger ones need to be held; sedation is desirable, but volatile anesthetics should be avoided, since many raise intracranial pressure. The child lies with his back, widely prepared, absolutely vertical to the table, and knees, hips and neck flexed as little as necessary. A procaine infiltration is worthwhile, even in infants. The needle is introduced exactly in the midsagittal plane of the child's body, at the third, fourth or fifth lumbar interspace, its point slightly cephalad; it is advanced slowly, the stylet repeatedly withdrawn, until cerebrospinal fluid drips out. This slow approach avoids passing entirely through the theca. When fluid is dripping, the stopcock and manometer are attached, and the child is encouraged to relax by reassurance and appropriate distraction; a proper approach can accomplish much, even with infants. A resting pressure is recorded as soon as the fluid column stabilizes, oscillating freely. Jugular and abdominal compressions are done, if indicated, and appropriate quantities of cerebrospinal fluid are removed stepwise, in 1-ml. aliquots; the closing pressure is recorded, the needle removed, its track broken up by firm massage with the finger, and a small, dry sterile dressing placed over the site. Bed rest after the procedure is unnecessary, since post-puncture headache is rare in children; occasionally, stiff back and headache, with persistently low cerebrospinal fluid pressure, occur; these complications appear unrelated to technical errors of the procedure.

Proper examination of the cerebrospinal fluid is of great importance in differential diagnosis of central nervous system disease, though the values determined are few. One wishes to know (1) pressure, and freedom of oscillation, (2) color, (3) cellular constituents, (4) protein, (5) glucose and rarely chloride, (6) evidence of infection.

Pressure normally varies from about 60 to 180 mm. of fluid if the child is really relaxed; the mean is about 100 mm.; pressures in infancy are somewhat lower. Pressure must be read from a manometer; estimation by speed of flow is inaccurate. Compression of the abdomen raises cerebrospinal fluid pressure by about 10 to 20 per cent by raising the pressure in epidural veins and compressing the theca; pressure on the jugular vein raises cerebrospinal fluid pressure by 30 to 50 per cent by increasing the intracranial vascular compartment. If a block exists in the spinal theca, abdominal compression is effective, but jugular compression ineffective, in causing these rises, since intracranial changes cannot be communicated to the lumbar theca. Jugular compression is indicated when suspicion of a spinal block exists; in the face of increased intracranial pressure it can be dangerous by causing or worsening a cerebral hernia.

Color. Normal cerebrospinal fluid is as clear and colorless as distilled water; it should be compared to a tube of distilled water, held against a white background. High increase in protein gives a faint opalescence to a definite yellow tint; old hemorrhage produces definite xanthochromia; leukocytes above 100 per mm.[3] or so cause turbidity; and fresh blood, opalescence to pinkness or outright bloodiness. The bloody tap tends to clear on removal of successive quantities of fluid, xanthochromia after centrifugation is absent, and the proportion of erythrocytes to leukocytes is that of the child's peripheral blood. A differential count of red and white cells in the fluid, and an immediate red and white cell count on peripheral blood, may help to distinguish blood from a traumatic tap from endogenous blood.

Cells. The cerebrospinal fluid normally contains less than 5 leukocytes per mm.[3] More than 5 white blood cells, and polymorphonuclear or red cells in any number, are abnormal. Cells must be counted within 30 minutes, since sedimentation or breakdown soon occurs.

Protein. The quantity of protein varies with the location of the source of the fluid and with different laboratory methods. A quantitative total protein determination should always be obtained. Ventricular fluid contains 15 mg. of total protein per 100 ml. or less, cisternal fluid about the same or a trifle more, and lumbar fluid 15 to 40 mg., usually about 20 mg. per 100 ml. in children.

Glucose. The concentration is normally about one half to two thirds that of the blood sugar. The glucose level of the blood should be determined at the time of lumbar puncture.

Evidence of infection. Serologic tests for syphilis and colloidal gold or colloidal mastic and Treponema immobilization tests should be obtained when indicated. A cellular fluid should always be cultured for bacteria at the time of puncture and on warmed media; if meningitis is a possibility, even an acellular fluid should be cultured. Cultures for fungi and acid-fast bacilli should be obtained when indicated. All cellular fluids should be centrifuged, and a stained smear should be examined for a differential count of cells and for organisms. An estimation of the immune globulin profile or titers in serum or cerebrospinal fluid against viral agents may be helpful in chronic ("slow") viral infections. The levels of intracellular enzymes, particularly transaminases, dehydrogenases and creatine phosphokinase, are increased in certain degenerative or destructive diseases of the brain and should be determined when appropriate.

The cerebrospinal fluid of infants in the first few days or weeks of life is often xanthochromic, with protein as high as 80 to 100 mg. per 100 ml., and often has an excess of red and white blood cells. These findings are usually an expression of intracranial complications of birth, such as venous congestion or minor trauma, often without other symptoms or recognized residuals.

Cisternal Puncture. The only indication for cisternal puncture is unavailability of the lumbar route. Possible cerebellar herniation or the Arnold-Chiari defect is a contraindication. The child is placed either on his side, with the vertebral axis kept horizontal, or in the sitting position with his chin flexed on his chest. The spine of the axis is located, and a line joining the external auditory canal and glabella is determined. The needle is introduced immediately above the axial spine in the midline, inclining slightly upward from the auditory-glabellar plane until it touches the occipital bone; the approximate depth is noted; the needle is then withdrawn to the skin, but not through it, and reintroduced in planes successively closer to the auditory-glabellar one with the stylet withdrawn repeatedly until fluid drips out or the needle strikes the occiput again. The depth of the cistern from the surface varies from about 1.5 cm. in infants to 3 to 4 cm. in adults. The danger of fatal injury to the medulla or of hemorrhage is real; one should not attempt the procedure for the first time on a living child.

Subdural and Ventricular Punctures. These important diagnostic procedures are restricted to infants or children whose sutures are still open. It is occasionally possible to perform them on children up to age 3 years by forcing the needle through the suture, or using a small twist drill; this should be attempted only by experienced operators. The equipment is that for lumbar puncture. The child is entertained with a sugar or brandy nipple, his head shaved at least to the bregma or, better, entirely. A wide sterile preparation is made over the vault, and the head draped with a posterior drape towel. At the lateral angle of the anterior fontanel, as identified by palpation, a procaine skin wheal is raised. A short lumbar puncture needle is then introduced, perpendicular to the scalp surface, not less than 2.5 to 4 cm. lateral to the midline, firmly supported and not allowed to wobble. Scalp and skull once penetrated, the stylet is withdrawn. If subdural fluid is present, it usually drips out at once. More than 1 ml. of fluid, or fluid discolored by anything

other than proved fresh blood, is abnormal. If fluid is not encountered, the needle is passed inward about 1.5 cm., then withdrawn slowly, since occasionally membrane or outer clot of a hematoma may occlude it. Cell count, color estimation, protein concentration and culture are secured on any fluid obtained; both sides should be tapped, since four fifths of infantile subdural hematomas are bilateral. No more than 10 to 15 ml. of fluid should be removed at any time from either side, nor more than a total of 20 to 25 ml.; removal of 30 ml. or more may cause sudden intracranial decompression and shock. A sterile dressing is applied, and the track of this puncture avoided in succeeding ones.

Puncture of ventricles is accomplished in the same manner, except that the needle point is inclined forward toward the nasion. If freely entered, the ventricles are almost always enlarged. Phenolsulfonphthalein or Evans blue, 1 ml., may be injected, and patency of the foramina of Monro demonstrated by its recovery from the other ventricle; this is not always reliable, since fenestrae are sometimes present in the septum pellucidum. Rapid recovery of dye from the lumbar theca indicates a patent ventricular system; if there is no recovery in more than 20 minutes, there is almost always midline obstruction of the ventricular system or spinal block.

Radiologic Studies. *Plain films.* These should always precede any special radiologic study. Views of the skull, anteroposterior, posteroanterior, lateral and basal, are adequate for most neurologic studies. Films of the vertebral column in spinal cord disease, of the optic foramina, of bones and joints in metabolic disease and of the chest and abdomen may be indicated.

Pneumoencephalography. In this procedure, air or other gas such as helium or oxygen is introduced into the subarachnoid space, usually in the lumbar region, sometimes by cisternal puncture. By proper positioning, ventricles and subarachnoid spaces may be filled. The procedure usually requires general anesthesia; in so-called total replacement large volumes of cerebrospinal fluid (80 to 120 ml.) are replaced by air; in fractional replacement only 25 to 40 cc. of air are used. The former gives more complete filling, especially in the hands of the less skilled operator; the latter is more time-consuming and requires more skill and care in introducing the air and positioning the head. It is a much less severe procedure for the patient and better adapted to deliberate filling of specific parts of ventricular or subarachnoid systems.

Pneumoencephalography can be dangerous; the mortality rate attributable to the procedure is 0.2 to 0.3 per cent, usually in patients with a mass lesion; it is higher in young children and when too much air is used. Most patients have headache, irritability, fever and vomiting for a day or more afterward. Air accidentally entering the subdural space may cause subdural hematoma. The procedure causes pleocytosis and increased protein in the cerebrospinal fluid, sometimes with meningeal signs; cerebrospinal fluid studies should always precede it.

The pneumoencephalogram demonstrates shape, size, symmetry and position of the ventricular system and subarachnoid spaces. Its greatest value is in making visible localized static defects, atrophies and congenital malformations. A film taken 12 or 24 hours after the procedure may show porencephalic cysts and similar defects more clearly than the original films.

Ventriculography. When there is reasonable possibility of an expanding lesion or of increased intracranial pressure, ventriculography should be used. Here the gas is put directly into the ventricular system through the patent sutures of the infant or trephine holes in the older child. The mortality rate of the procedure is almost impossible to calculate, since the subjects often are seriously ill; it can be the direct cause of death in patients with high intracranial pressure by causing hemorrhage from subependymal veins. Visibility of the fourth ventricle and of the subarachnoid spaces is less satisfactory than with the pneumoencephalogram.

Angiography. A radiopaque substance is injected into a carotid, vertebral or brachial artery or into a dural sinus. General anesthesia and, especially in smaller children, surgical exposure of the vessel to be injected may be necessary. Angiography is the procedure of choice for vascular anomalies and lesions; it is also of value in localization of subdural hematoma and of avascular infarcted areas, as well as of tumors. It is not without danger. Hemiplegia, usually transient, occurs in as many as 4 per cent of cases. Convulsions, petechiae, transient loss of vision, occlusion of retinal arteries, thrombosis of the artery at the site of puncture, hematoma of the neck requiring tracheotomy, and even sudden death have been reported. For the delineation of vascular lesions the procedure is indispensable; for space-taking lesions its great advantage over gas-contrast studies is that it does not demand immediate operation if a mass is demonstrated. An intravenous pyelogram should be recorded after the arterial injection; unsuspected renal abnormalities have been detected in about 2 per cent of patients.

Isotope scanning procedures. In these the head is scanned with a scintillometer at intervals after injection of a short half-life isotope such as RIHSA (radioactive iodized human serum albumin), technetium or mercury. Both supratentorial and infratentorial masses may be demonstrated; vascular malformations may often be detected in an immediate scan. Infarcted areas will also take up the isotope; in general, circumscribed masses are better shown than infiltrative ones. Dubious areas of uptake should be considered seriously only if demonstrable on more than one projection. The possibilities and the difficulties of interpretation are not yet completely known. The procedure is much less traumatic and potentially dangerous than other contrast medium studies of the brain.

Myelography. Contrast radiography is also used in the localization of intraspinal masses; the common contrast medium is Pantopaque. Three to 6 ml. or more are introduced within the theca, either in the lumbar region or cisternally, and the flow of dye and irregularity or obstruction to the column observed fluoroscopically and on spot films taken on the tilting table. The dye should be removed.

The procedure is not especially dangerous, though in a few instances transverse myelitis, severe lesions of the cauda equina or obliterative arachnoiditis have seemed to follow it; if dye enters the cranium, a fatal, progressive obstructive hydrocephalus may ensue. Such accidents are thought to be due to contamination of equipment or dye with detergents or disinfectant solutions. Pleocytosis may follow the procedure, with an increase in cerebrospinal protein and with a mild fever for a day or so.

Electroencephalography (see also p. 1252). This procedure, having the advantage of being harmless and repeatable, can be relied upon too much in neurologic diagnosis. It is of value in establishing the presence of a central nervous system abnormality, and of assistance in the diagnosis of epilepsy, but the electroencephalogram alone is seldom the determining diagnostic factor. It sometimes localizes expanding lesions, but its accuracy is only about 60 per cent; it has prognostic value in following the course of encephalitis, encephalopathy or head injury. A great limitation is the variability of interpretation put on the same tracing by different observers. One should not commit himself irrevocably to a diagnosis whose sole support is an electroencephalogram.

Echoencephalography is of limited value in its current state of development, but may serve to identify major distortions of the ventricles in some instances.

Psychologic Studies. These are of great value. A careful psychologic evaluation often resolves the difficult differentiation of mental retardation from emotional disturbance. Too frequent repetition should be avoided, and the clinician should remember that such evaluations are not absolute measurements.

Biopsy. *Muscle biopsy* is innocuous and often indispensable in differentiating myopathic or myositic wasting from neural atrophy. A muscle showing clear, but not the most extreme, involvement should be selected, and skin biopsy included. If a neuronal storage disease is suspected, smears of the buffy coat may reveal intracytoplasmic lipid granules in lymphocytes. Similarly, autonomic neurons of the intrinsic bowel plexuses are readily obtained by wedge *biopsy of the posterior rectal wall* (not punch biopsy of the mucosa alone) and are often helpful in diagnosis. Renal or sural nerve biopsies will often demonstrate metachromatic material in tubular epithelium, myelin sheath or

Schwann cells in cases of metachromatic leuko-dystrophy. *Brain biopsy* is indicated for definitive diagnosis of a degenerative disease, which may be imperative for genetic counseling or otherwise dealing with needs of the family of the patient. It is often indispensable in study of the mechanisms of cerebral metabolic diseases. It is ordinarily justifiable only when the evidence is overwhelming of a progressive, untreatable condition; parents must understand the reasons for the procedure, the nature and value of the information to be gained, the probable lack of therapeutic benefit, and nature of possible complications, which are surprisingly few. The right temporal or frontal tip, or a wedge of cerebellum is removed through an osteoplastic craniotomy; punch or needle biopsies through trephine holes are more danger-ous and usually histologically worthless. Biopsy of muscle, nerve or brain should not be done un-less pathologists, chemists and enzymologists experienced with nervous and muscle tissue are available. Electron microscopy may help to de-lineate diseases not clearly identifiable with light microscopy.

Electromyography. This procedure aids in distinguishing between myopathies and neural wasting of muscle. Determination of conduction velocities in peripheral nerves is of assistance in the diagnosis of neuropathies. The procedure requires careful interpretation.

Chromosomal studies may be helpful, particu-larly in children with multiple handicaps.

SYMPTOMATOLOGY OF NEUROLOGIC DISEASE IN CHILDHOOD

Visual loss in infancy usually impairs ocular fixation and the conjugate movements of the eyes. Failure to focus or wandering movements of the eyes are the presenting features, and in later childhood these changes suggest early visual loss. In older children, holding of objects close to the eyes and mistaking of colors are the common symptoms. Poor vision in one eye, unless the eye deviates and strabismus develops, often goes un-suspected until a chance test of acuity reveals it. Vision may blur and fail from diplopia before strabismus is apparent. The child then tilts his head into positions in which diplopia is less, usually turning his face in the direction of action of the weak muscle, so that binocular vision is attained for objects directly ahead without its use. Head-tilting in association with a posterior fossa tumor may not be ocular in origin, but due to tonsillar herniation, meningeal irritation or stiff neck; the head then usually turns toward the side of the lesion.

Right halves of visual fields represent left halves of retinas, left optic tract and visual centers, and vice versa. A defect of the lateral or medial half of a visual field is termed a *hemianopsia*. *Homony-*

mous defects involve either the right or the left halves of the visual fields, and are caused by retrochiasmatic lesions. *Heteronymous hemian-opsia* is almost always bitemporal and is due to pressure on optic fibers decussating in the chiasm. Since fibers of the papillomacular bundle are more sensitive to pressure and toxins than the re-mainder of the nerve, early chiasmatic compres-sion and toxic states may cause *central scotomas.*

Hemianopsias lead to persistent ignoring or bumping into objects on one side and can be con-fused with lateralized cerebellar lesions, in which the child may constantly deviate to the side of his lesion. The child with tubular vision or a bi-temporal hemianopsia attends only to objects directly ahead. *Cortical blindness* is almost always accompanied by mental change or other signs of cortical deficit.

Impaired hearing (p. 101) has 2 principal symp-toms. The first is inattention to sounds unless they are very loud or productive of vibration transmissible through the body; the child will not react to a call when his back is turned, but will turn if one stamps on the floor. The second symp-tom, appearing with hearing loss in early child-hood, is failure of development of normal speech; in such cases hearing loss must be differentiated from mental retardation.

Vertiginous children, especially young ones, are unwilling to move; they wedge themselves, face down and eyes closed, in a corner of the crib or playpen.

Organic headache is due to distention and de-formation of pain-sensitive blood vessels and meninges. Meninges of the supratentorial region are supplied by the trigeminal nerve, those of the posterior fossa by upper cervical roots and the vagus. The pain from supratentorial lesions is usually bifrontal, that from infratentorial irri-tation, suboccipital. Organic headache is dull, throbbing or bursting; functional headache is more commonly manifest by a feeling of pressure. Though subjective descriptions are of less value in children than in adults, a headache lavishly described is usually not organic.

In young children the presence of headache is inferred from fretfulness and irritability, furrowed brow and sometimes ear-pulling or head-rolling. In older children the pattern of the headache is most important. Headache of increased intra-cranial pressure accompanies change of position, such as rising in the morning, stooping, straining or exercising; at first it is not constant; when it becomes so, lethargy and drowsiness usually ac-company it. Vascular headache, common in cyanotic heart disease, is due to increased cerebral oxygen demand and distention of blood vessels; it is regularly caused by activity and relieved by rest.

The distinctive feature of *migraine* is the repe-titive pattern of attacks. Prodromes and auras usually go unnoticed, though the mother may comment on a period of quiet before the child complains of headache and photophobia, becomes listless and, after an hour or so, is nauseated or vomits; vomiting relieves the headache, and after deep sleep the child wakens feeling as well as ever. Neurotic headache lasts for indefinite periods and fluctuates in relation to surrounding events; the child can often be distracted from his pain.

Vomiting as a neurologic symptom is distinctive only when it becomes projectile with severely increased intracranial pressure. In other cases it is the recurrence of vomiting, rather than its nature, which suggests the increased pressure.

With *cerebellar lesions* unsteady gait is usually the first symptom recognized. Ataxia of the extremities, impaired dexterity in writing, clumsiness, and (rarely) slurred ataxic speech may be noted later. Alert parents may note dysmetria, a tendency to overshoot or undershoot when reaching for objects, or decomposition of movements, each movement being broken into a series of lesser ones to control ataxia. Hypotonia reduces associated movement; e.g. an affected arm hangs limp and moves less as the child walks.

Nystagmus, the only ocular symptom of cerebellar disease per se, is noted by parents only if extreme and by children as blurring or dancing of objects. Expanding cerebellar lesions rarely cause spontaneous nystagmus, and then often in conjunction with a conjugate deviation. The nystagmus is slow and coarse when looking to the side of a lesion, fine and rapid when looking away from it. Skew deviations, the homolateral eye deviating downward and inward and the opposite one upward and outward, signify acute lesions. Vertigo makes the young child unwilling to move, but it may be mentioned spontaneously by the older one.

Lesions in the brain stem produce cranial nerve palsies early. Involvement of long motor pathways is more apparent than that of sensory pathways, and causes unsteady gait; sphincters are spared until late. Medullary lesions may cause vomiting without increased intracranial pressure; mesencephalic ones combine hemiplegia or tremor with oculomotor palsy. Interference with the reticular systems disturbs consciousness. This may vary from deep coma with bradycardia, bradypnea and hypertension in upper pontine and mesencephalic lesions to states of akinetic mutism, in which the patient appears awake, but does not speak or respond, or, in upper brain stem or thalamic lesions, to simple hypersomnolence.

Disorders of the cerebral hemispheres produce a variety of motor symptoms. Hemiparesis of cortical origin is not usually greatly spastic; if the deeper white matter or basal ganglia are involved, spasticity, rigidity or choreo-athetosis is present. The first symptom of motor impairment is disuse of affected limbs. In congenital lesions, disuse of the paretic hand causes apparent precocious handedness with the opposite member; when the child walks, he drags or circumducts the paretic leg. The older child uses the affected hand clumsily, shifts his handedness or limps. Growth arrest characterizes congenital or slowly progressive hemiparesis, especially if the lesion is parietal. Apraxia impresses parents only as clumsiness.

Sensory loss with cerebral lesions is almost always dissociated. For example, discrimination of shape and texture and of 2-point tactile stimulation suffers more than general cutaneous sensibility. The latter is reduced rather than lost, and the deficit is seldom mentioned. Simultaneous bilateral stimulation may reveal an otherwise unnoticed sensory loss, the child disregarding stimuli on the involved side. Specific sensory disorders, notably hemianopsias, and sensorimotor dysfunctions, particularly aphasias, may be present and aid in localization. Mental changes in the young child usually cause hyperirritability initially, less frequently lethargy. Older children become more emotionally labile, lose their powers of concentration and do poorly at school; lethargy and general restriction of interest come later. Seizures are the commonest symptom of irritative or discharging lesions; for practical purposes they limit the lesion to the cerebral hemispheres; they may be of any sort.

NEUROLOGIC LESIONS

STATIC AND DEVELOPMENTAL LESIONS

About two thirds of the neurologic disease of childhood is caused by lesions which are static. Progression occurs only in that (1) clinical manifestations become more apparent as the nervous system matures; (2) the primary defect impairs normal development of functionally related parts of the nervous system; and (3) complications, e.g. hydrocephalus or repeated seizures, may further damage the central nervous system.

Etiology. Such static lesions are caused by a variety of antenatal, perinatal and postnatal injuries to the nervous system. Antenatal damage often involves parts of the body other than the central nervous system; perinatal and postnatal lesions are more frequently limited to it. In the antenatal period the time and nature of the injury, together with genetic and environmental factors, affect the outcome for the fetus. Similar injuries may cause different maldevelopments, or widely differing agents may produce identical defects. *Antenatally*, genetic factors, chromosomal aberrations, hormonal or dietary disturbances, placental disease, maternal toxemia, age and parity of mother, age of father, intrauterine infection (particularly viral), hypoxia, toxic agents (including certain drugs) and radiation may all be factors. *Perinatally* acquired lesions are due principally to prematurity, hypoxia, trauma, hemorrhage, toxic states and infections. *Postnatal* lesions are mainly sequels of infection, trauma, metabolic disturbances, such as hyperelectrolytemia and hypoglycemia, and vascular disease. The effect of early dietary deficiency on maturation of myelin, and on total myelin and total cell mass, appears far greater than expected; infantile malnutrition or failure to thrive may prove a potent cause of static brain lesions.

The *incidence* of such static lesions is difficult to estimate, since accuracy of diagnosis and reporting vary tremendously. Further, the problem concerns a continuum of reproductive wastage; the loss due to abortion and stillbirth is seldom included. Approximately 60 per cent of all significant congenital defects involve the nervous system. About 6 per cent of all children at some time require special management for organic or functional illness referable to the central nervous system; about 1 per cent are handicapped by a static lesion of the brain.

Clinical Features and Pathology. Antenatal defects are often called maldevelopments. Many represent either failure of closure or cleftlike arrests of closure of the neural tube.

In *anencephaly* the trunk and limbs are normally formed, but the neck is short; cervical vertebrae are reduced in number; the cranial vault is largely absent; and a large spinal defect is often present. The brain is represented by a vascular mass in which optic nerves end blindly; the hypophysis is absent or hypoplastic, and the adrenals are very small. The cerebellum, brain stem and even the spinal cord may be involved (amyelia), though the muscles and sensory ganglia continue to develop. Sustained extrauterine life is impossible.

The forebrain alone may be defective in the *arrhinencephalies* (or *holoprosencephalies*), in which those centers which are ontogenetically part of the olfactory system are usually involved. In *cyclopia* the eye is single and central, with a proboscis-like nose below it; olfactory bulbs and tracts and optic nerves are absent, and the brain is represented by a single, solid mass anteriorly, with a saclike cavity posteriorly. In *cebocephaly* both eyes are present but microphthalmic, and the nose is flattened. Less extreme maldevelopments include absence or hypoplasia of olfactory tracts and bulbs, often with microphthalmos and small optic nerves. With all these defects the corpus callosum is necessarily absent or malformed, and other defects, such as microgyria, heterotopias of gray matter in both brain and meninges, porencephalies, and abnormalities of cellular arrangement, may occur together with cleft lip and cleft palate, cardiac malformations and peculiar feet and hands. The arrhinencephalies are common in chromosomal aberrations (Fig. 20-2), particularly in trisomy 13-15 and trisomy 18. The patients are usually profoundly retarded and spastic, though

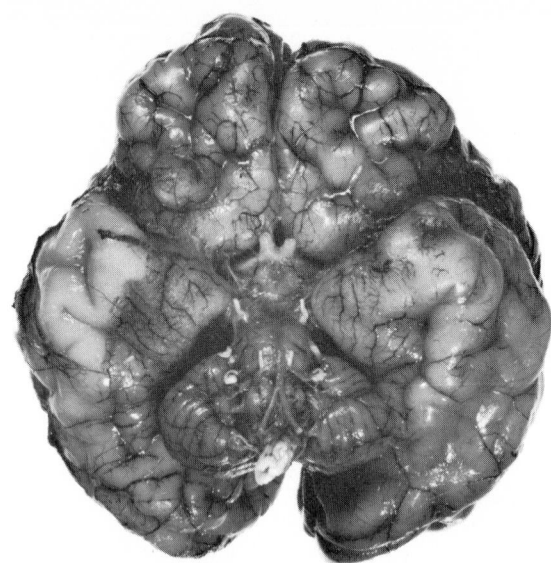

Figure 20-2. Arrhinencephaly as a malformation in trisomy 18. The olfactory tracts and bulbs are absent. The splenium and the body of the corpus callosum were also absent. Other congenital anomalies included a tracheo-esophageal fistula. Arrhinencephaly is more common with trisomy 13-15 than with trisomy 18. (Courtesy of Dr. James B. Arey.)

milder forms may be compatible with fairly normal life.

Agenesis of the corpus callosum, partial or complete, may occur as a more isolated defect, usually sporadic, though familial incidence occurs in rare instances. The pneumoencephalogram (Fig. 20-3) is diagnostic. Hydrocephalus, mental retardation, spasticity and seizures are frequent concomitants. They are due to associated defects and not primarily to absence of the corpus callosum; lipomas and meningiomas often develop at the site of the defect. Some patients may lead normal lives.

True porencephaly is a defect (cavity or cyst) of the cerebral hemisphere which is often bilateral and close to the midline. The defect extends from the ventricle to the pia without entering the subarachnoid space. It is distinguished from *false porencephaly*, single or multiple cavities which do not communicate with the ventricles and usually follow vascular damage at birth. Symptoms are hemiplegias, seizures or mental retardation.

Cranium bifidum is a herniation of meninges and sometimes of brain, protruding from a defect which is usually midline and posteriorly placed; it is covered by scalp. Similar hernias are sometimes just off the midline, presenting at the inner canthus of the eye, above the glabella or in the occipital region, or rarely into the sphenoidal sinus.

Growth of the skull is in large part dependent on growth of the brain; arrest of growth can result in *microcephaly*. In adult life the rather arbitrary upper limits for this condition are a skull circumference of 42 cm. or less and a brain weight of not

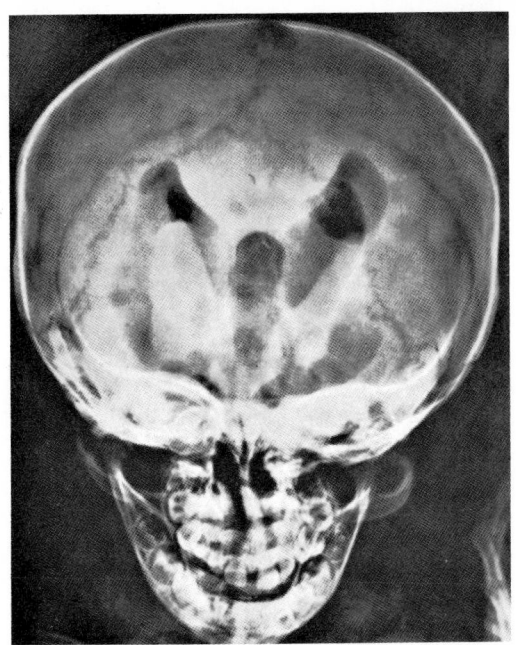

Figure 20-3. Agenesis of the corpus callosum. Ventricles are dilated, and the lateral ventricles widely separated.

more than 900 gm. A rare variety is *familial* and is transmitted as a recessive character. The ears and nose are large, the nose joining the receding brow without a bridge; the scalp is redundant and furrowed, and the cranial vault is abnormally small. The brain is agyric or microgyric; the cortex is often composed of alternating cellular and acellular bands. The patients may show surprisingly few neurologic signs other than generalized hypertonus. *Secondary* microcephaly occurs after a variety of injuries and infections and notably after maternal irradiation during early pregnancy. It is usually accompanied by overt neurologic signs. Severe mental retardation is present in both varieties.

True *megalencephalon* is rare, most large heads being due to hydrocephalus or space-taking lesions. In adult life the megalencephalic brain usually weighs 2000 gm. or more. The cortical gray matter is increased in amount; heterotopias and developmental defects are frequent; neurons are poorly differentiated, and glial cells are increased in number. Adrenal abnormalities and tuberous sclerosis are not infrequently associated. The patients are mentally retarded, usually epileptic and occasionally spastic. A pneumoencephalogram is necessary to distinguish megalencephalon from hydrocephalus, from space-occupying lesions or, rarely, from diffuse granulomatous or parasitic lesions.

The brains of many congenitally defective persons are not grossly or obviously deformed, beyond being small and having simple or irregular convolutional patterns, poor lamination of the cortex, poorly developed nerve cells and rather

scanty myelinization. The term *oligoencephalon* is used in such instances. The patients are moderately defective, and the specific neurologic manifestations are only slight. Family backgrounds are often characterized by mental deficiency, emotional instability and a sort of generalized socioeconomic inadequacy. Whether these deficiencies result simply from generally poor antenatal and postnatal environment or whether such patients should be regarded as biologic "runts" is uncertain.

In the posterior fossa 3 major defects occur. *Atresia of the aqueduct of Sylvius* (Fig. 20-4) is a congenital narrowing of the upper portion of the channel, which is sometimes forked or obstructed by a transverse septum. Secondary stenosis may follow ependymitis, intraventricular hemorrhage or birth trauma. Other developmental defects coexist, particularly meningomyelocele and heterotopias in the lateral ventricles. Symptomatically, the stricture causes obstructive hydrocephalus of the lateral and third ventricles, the posterior fossa remaining shallow.

The *Arnold-Chiari deformity* is a tonguelike projection of the cerebellum and choroid plexus extending with an elongated fourth ventricle into the cervical canal; the upper cervical spinal cord is kinked backward, and the cerebellar tonsils are drawn into and are adherent to the foramen magnum. Lumbosacral spina bifida and myelodysplasia are present in about half the cases, or there may be aqueductal stenosis and heterotopias. The defect appears between the sixteenth and twentieth fetal weeks and seems to be due to local overgrowth of the neural tube rather than to

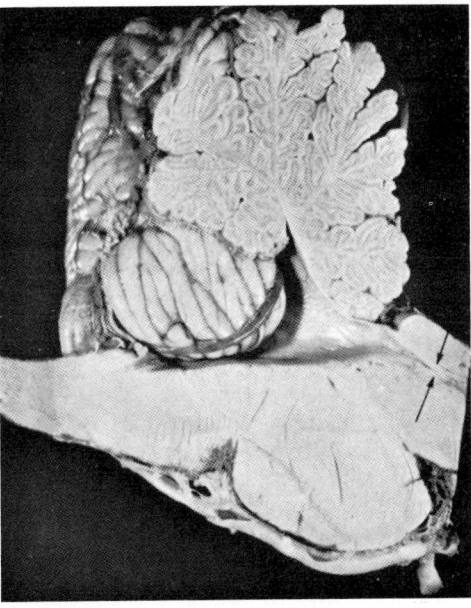

Figure 20-4. Congenital stenosis of aqueduct of Sylvius (arrows). Despite severe obstructive hydrocephalus, patient lived to sixth decade as a self-supporting person.

fixation and traction on the neuraxis by myelo-dysplasia. It causes obstructive hydrocephalus.

In *atresia of the foramina of Luschka and Magendie (Dandy-Walker deformity)* the fourth ventricle is ballooned out into a large cavity, above which lie the cerebellar vermis, the elevated lateral sinus and the torcular Herophili. Hydrocephalus is the common manifestation; demonstration of the elevated torcular by roentgenogram or sinography or, in the infant, simply by transillumination establishes the diagnosis.

Spinal Cord Lesions. In the spinal cord, defects are most frequent in the lumbosacral region, but may be cervical or thoracic. They include asymptomatic *spina bifida occulta* and *spina bifida with an associated lipoma or dermoid or with a meningocele or meningomyelocele*, a sac containing malformed cord and roots and covered by a thin, vascular membrane. The trunk and limbs below the level of the deformity are paralyzed, often underdeveloped and anesthetic, and bowel and bladder sphincters are nonfunctional (Fig. 20-5). *Dysrhaphia* is a duplication of parts of all of the cord. Complete duplication is *diplomyelia*; incomplete duplication, usually accompanied by vertebral defects and an osseous spur extending upward from the vertebral body separating the duplicated cords, constitutes *diastematomyelia*.

Congenital dermal sinuses are persistent, epithelium-lined defects extending from the skin toward or into neural structures. The "pilonidal" dimple in the sacral area is the commonest lesion in this category; dermal sinuses may be found anywhere along the vertebral column or in the occipital or frontal region of the skull. Externally, a tiny pore is often surrounded by hair or a portwine mark, and may exude a whitish secretion.

Cerebral Lesions. *Brain injury* of the *perinatal period* is due principally to metabolic and toxic disorders, trauma, hemorrhage and infections; vulnerability is accentuated by premature birth.

The commonest and most important metabolic disorder is *inadequate oxygenation*. Hypoxia is a part of almost all forms of birth injury to the brain (p. 378). Hypoglycemia, especially in infants of diabetic or toxemic mothers, is another metabolic cause.

The most important toxic state damaging the brain of the newborn is *hyperbilirubinemia*, which produces the syndrome of *kernicterus* (see pp. 395, 1060). In this condition excess bilirubin of the indirect type accumulates in the blood, owing to overproduction or limited capacity for conjugation with glucuronic acid; incompatibilities of blood type, immaturity of mechanisms of conjugation and excretion, neonatal sepsis, therapy with sulfisoxazole in the premature infant and excess administration of vitamin K are known causes. Permeability of the blood-brain barrier in the first few days of life permits bilirubin to reach nerve cells, which it damages, perhaps by inhibiting intracellular enzyme systems. Certain regions, particularly the corpus subthalamicum, hippo-

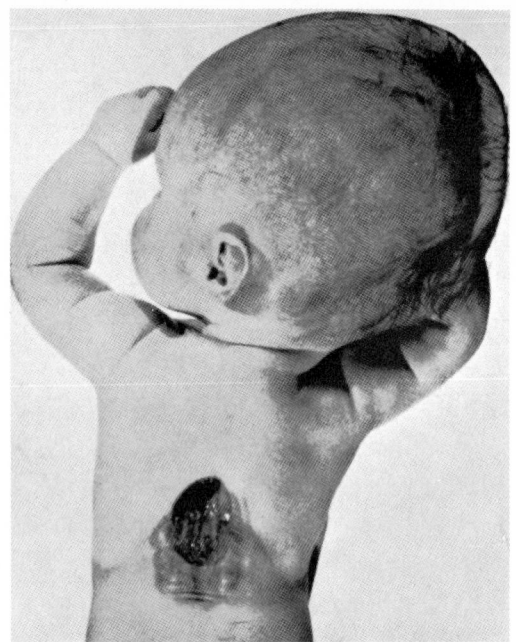

Figure 20-5. Thoracolumbar meningomyelocele, Arnold-Chiari defect and intrauterine hydrocephalus.

campus, striate bodies, thalamus, inferior olives, cerebellar nuclei and cranial nerve nuclei, are stained intensely yellow. This selectivity may depend on attainment of a specific state of maturation of neuronal enzyme systems; at any rate the cells commonly involved are all large and phylogenetically old. Previous damage to nerve cells, probably hypoxic, may be necessary for bilirubin staining to develop. Nonpigmented areas may also be damaged. Loss of neurons, reactive gliosis and atrophy of involved fiber systems are late findings.

The clinical symptoms of kernicterus usually appear from the second to the sixth day of life. Minimal cerebral damage may not be apparent at this time. Usually the infant either appears gravely ill, prostrated, with diminished Moro and tendon reflexes, failure to suck and respiratory distress, or he becomes opisthotonic, with bulging fontanel, twitching of face or limbs, shrill cry and convulsions. Rarely is there rigidity or involuntary movements. Many such infants die; the remainder, usually seriously damaged, appear to recover and for 2 or 3 months manifest few abnormalities. Later in the first year of life, opisthotonos and muscular rigidity return and irregular movements and convulsions occur. In the second year, opisthotonos and seizures abate, but involuntary movements, muscular rigidity and, in some infants, hypotonia increase steadily. By 3 years of age the complete neurologic syndrome is apparent. About 80 per cent of affected children have bilateral choreo-athetosis with involuntary mobile spasm. Pyramidal signs are rare in proportion to extrapyramidal ones, and hypotonia and ataxia distinguish a few. Seizures, mental deficiency, explosive dysarthric speech, high-tone hearing loss, squints and defective upward movement of the eyes are common. It is possible that Rh incompatibility without neonatal jaundice may result in hearing loss, mental limitation and learning disorders, though the relation is not proved. The hyperbilirubinemia of prematurity leads less frequently to kernicterus than does that of hemolytic disease. Only about 2 per cent of all premature infants exhibit the syndrome; in these the total bilirubin has generally exceeded 20 mg. per 100 ml.

Prematurity (p. 370) may be an expression or a cause of brain abnormality. At least one fifth of prematurely born infants later show signs of cerebral involvement. Some of this results from birth injury to the soft premature skull, hyperbilirubinemia, intraventricular hemorrhage or hypoxia, but the possibility of antenatal defects always exists.

Trauma (see also p. 373) of the perinatal period affects the brain more by deforming the skull and its contents than by impact force. Molding of the head and overriding of sutures tear small veins, sinuses or the tentorium, producing subarachnoid or subdural bleeding; large veins, sinuses or major arteries may be compressed and venous stasis, areas of hypoxia, and secondary hemorrhage produced. Direct compression of the skull by forceps or ischial spines can cause local ischemia or vascular damage.

Forced movements of the neck during delivery may compress or lacerate the vertebral arteries, tear cervical joint capsules, dura and nerve roots, and compress the spinal cord. Injuries of this sort are more common than is realized, since spinal cord symptoms in survivors are obscured by signs of associated cerebral damage. The premature infant is especially vulnerable.

Hemorrhage is a less common primary source of damage than was formerly thought; microscopic hemorrhage and slight xanthochromia of cerebrospinal fluid occur in perhaps one fifth of all newborn infants, but in themselves are not evidence of significant brain injury. Gross hemorrhage is now rare, but smaller petechial or perivascular hemorrhages following vascular compression or hypoxic damage to endothelium are common. Intraventricular hemorrhage, immediate or delayed, from the terminal veins is frequent in small premature infants (p. 366).

Infections include intrauterine and neonatal encephalitis and complications of neonatal sepsis. Toxoplasmosis (p. 745) and cytomegalic inclusion disease (p. 663) produce a severe encephalitis, the lesions of which may be calcified at birth (Fig. 20-6). Neonatal sepsis may cause hyperbilirubinemia, meningitis, venous or sinus thrombosis or toxemias severe enough to damage the brain.

It is difficult to relate any particular form of abnormal birth to any constant form of brain injury. Difficult labors with asphyxia pallida of the newborn seem associated with severe damage to the basal ganglia and thalamus; a peculiar

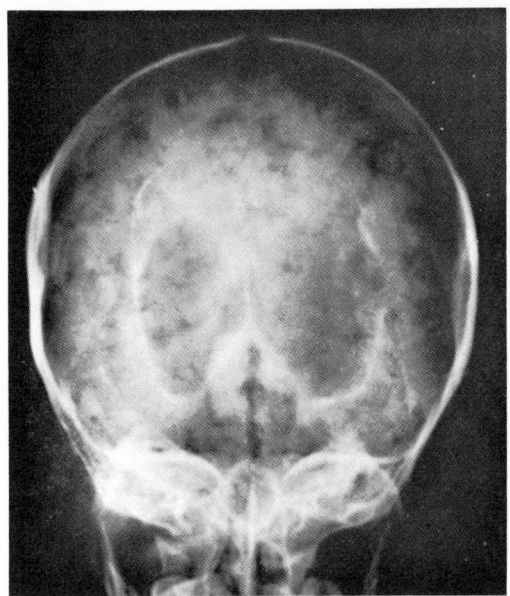

Figure 20-6. Calcified ependymitis and hydrocephalus following cytomegalic inclusion disease in the newborn.

marbled appearance, *status marmoratus*, is found in the basal ganglia, thalamus and sometimes the cortex. Clinically, there are usually combined pyramidal and extrapyramidal syndromes and mental retardation. Venous stasis, compression of the galenic vein and perhaps sudden fluctuations in intracranial pressure, when the head is delivered through a contracted pelvis or rapidly in breech delivery, may result in cystic degeneration of the white matter. Spastic diplegia is the usual result. Other than this, prediction of types of clinical abnormalities or of the pathologic lesions responsible for abnormalities recognized at birth can seldom be made.

Postnatal lesions are sequels of infections, principally meningitis and encephalitis, injuries, subdural hematomas, metabolic disturbances such as hyperelectrolytemia or embolic and inflammatory cerebral vascular disease. The cause and pathogenesis of postnatal lesions are usually clearer than those of prenatal or perinatal lesions. Special note, however, should be made of the infant or young child, said to be previously well, who begins to have seizures, goes into status epilepticus, and is left with unequivocal signs of brain injury. Perhaps 5 to 10 per cent of defective children have this history. It is often impossible to tell whether seizures, secondary to some intercurrent cause and complicated by hypoxia, hypoglycemia or other metabolic or vascular disturbances, injured a previously normal brain or whether these processes further damaged a brain of whose abnormality they were the first recognized manifestations. Subdural hematoma, with skull or other fractures, retinal hemorrhages and regressive behavior, will suggest the battered child syndrome (p. 1362).

Treatment. Prevention of static lesions is

obviously the goal. This demands far greater knowledge of etiology and pathogenesis than is presently available.

Some static lesions can be treated surgically. Aqueductal atresia and the Dandy-Walker or Arnold-Chiari defects produce obstructive hydrocephalus and are so managed (p. 1291). Simple cranium bifidum requires no treatment, but cranial meningocele or meningoencephalocele should be repaired by amputation of the sac and closure within the skull. Congenital dermal sinuses should be excised in toto as soon as discovered, since they offer a portal of entry for infection and entail constant risk of meningitis or brain abscess. Diastematomyelia and spinal meningocele, with or without lipoma or dermoid, are better left alone unless they are producing disorders of gait or sphincter control.

Myelodysplasia (spina bifida with meningomyelocele) offers one of the most serious problems. Operation can remove the sac, close the skin defect and lessen the nursing problem, but it does not improve the neurologic deficit. A life of paraplegia and incontinence, ending in the second or third decade with pyelonephritis and uremia, is the usual pattern. Since the Arnold-Chiari defect or aqueductal atresia is present in more than half the cases of myelodysplasia, obstructive hydrocephalus frequently develops, and early operation is blamed for its appearance. Good results cannot be expected from surgery in infants with severe paralysis of the legs, fecal and urinary incontinence, hydrocephalus, signs of severe retardation, or multiple congenital defects. With such infants the decision to operate is based as much on the possibility of easing the nursing problem by removing an open or thin-walled sac as on real therapeutic hopes.

In those children who offer a reasonable chance for effective life, operation on the sac should be done as early as possible after birth, even within hours, since there is some evidence for rapidly progressive damage to the malformed and partially exposed lower spinal cord. Hydrocephalus should be watched for carefully. Whatever the head size at birth, atresia of the aqueduct is almost certainly present if the infant has both meningomyelocele and lacunar skull; shunting procedures are then obligatory. Later in childhood, ileal-loop ureterostomies may aid in management of urinary incontinence. Results, even with orthopedic assistance, physiotherapy, efforts at bowel and bladder training, fluid restriction and low residue diets, are seldom very good. Perhaps the most tragic consequence is the feeling of isolation, of rejection by his fellows, and of limitation on almost every normal activity or goal which so many such children experience in adolescence.

Perinatal and postnatal static lesions are seldom treated surgically. If hydrocephalus appears, it is usually early, and the prognosis for surgical improvement is poor. Resection of scarred or atrophic areas or even hemispherectomy occasionally relieves otherwise intractable seizures, but should be considered only after intensive medical therapy has failed. Destructive operations on the brain or cord to relieve tremor, involuntary movements or spasticity have not often produced good results, though in selected cases they should be considered.

Most children with static lesions of the brain or cord present a variety of problems: mental limitation, neuromuscular handicaps, seizures, learning difficulties and problems of emotional and social adjustment. These are discussed in the treatment of the child with cerebral palsy (p. 1311).

ECTODERMAL DYSPLASIAS

These hereditary conditions, also known as phakomatoses, combine congenital lesions of the skin and nervous system with a wide variety of visceral and somatic abnormalities. Often inapparent at birth, they may appear as mixed and incomplete syndromes.

Tuberous sclerosis is inherited as a dominant trait. The widespread lesions include those (1) of the *skin*, fibroadenomas of sebaceous glands over the nose and cheeks (butterfly area), "shagreen" or leathery patches, *café-au-lait* and depigmented spots and subungual fibromas; (2) in the *viscera*, hemangiomas or mixed tumors of kidney, liver and spleen, multiple tiny mixed tumors of the lung associated with spontaneous pneumothorax, and rhabdomyoma of the heart, sometimes causing failure; (3) in the *eye*, nodular or cystic lesions; (4) in *bone*, osteoporosis, thickenings, osseous islands and cysts; (5) in the *brain*, cortical and subependymal nodules containing abnormal or neoplastic glia and neurons, which frequently calcify and are visible roentgenographically. The symptoms are seizures and usually mental deficiency. Renal failure, due to extensive sarcomatous degeneration of intrinsic tumors, is a late complication. Treatment is limited to symptomatic relief of the seizures.

Neurofibromatosis (von Recklinghausen's disease) is inherited as an autosomal dominant. The lesions are sharply outlined *café-au-lait* areas on the skin, cutaneous and subcutaneous neurofibromas which are often pedunculated, neurofibromas along craniospinal nerves and roots, osteitis fibrosa cystica disseminata without hyperparathyroidism, and often leading to fractures, and multiple central nervous system lesions. The last are mostly nodules similar to those of tuberous sclerosis, or are located in the aqueduct or central canal. Localized gigantism may occur, and neurofibromas may undergo sarcomatous degeneration; associated meningiomas are not uncommon. Four related syndromes are (1) glioma of the optic chiasm with extensive *café-au-lait* marks; (2) pheochromocytoma, 10 per cent of which are associated with *café-au-lait* patches or neurofibromas; (3) neurofibromatosis, cysts in the arachnoid, deepened middle cranial fossa, elevated sphenoidal wing and pulsating exophthalmos; (4) neurofibromatosis with generalized craniospinal nerve involvement and muscular wasting resembling interstitial hypertrophic polyneuritis. Treatment is limited to removal of locally troublesome neurofibromas, particularly those on nerve roots, which compress the brain stem or cord.

Encephalo-trigeminal angiomatosis (Sturge-Weber syndrome) is genetically not completely understood. The distinctive feature is a large telangiectasis or port-wine stain, trigeminal in distribution, involving skin, scalp, skull and meninges. It is most common in the ophthalmic division, but may extend downward over the face. The typical double-contoured opacities in the roentgenogram of the skull (Fig. 20-7) represent intracortical calcification and ferrugination secondary to circulatory slowing, and may appear within the first year of life. These usually appear first in the occipital lobe. Congenital glaucoma and buphthalmos on the affected side are due to nevi in the choroid; there is crossed hemiparesis and hemianopsia, the vault on the affected side is small, and the skull is thick. Telangiectasis, especially on the arm, may result in localized gigantism. The patients are often mentally defective and have lateralized seizures; subarachnoid hemorrhage occurs rarely. Local resection of the intracranial nevus or hemispherectomy may relieve seizures; glaucoma usually requires surgical treatment. Other treatment is symptomatic.

Von Hippel-Lindau disease comprises hemangioma of the retina, hemangiomatous cysts of the cerebellum and spinal cord and cysts of the kidney, pancreas, liver and testes. It is hereditary, but its mode of inheritance is not clear. The retinal lesions cause retinal detachment and blindness; they require coagulation. Cerebellar cysts symptomatically resemble other cerebellar tumors and, though sometimes multiple, are usually operable.

CONGENITAL VASCULAR LESIONS

These include saccular aneurysm, congenital arteriovenous fistulas, venous angiomas and telangiectases. Despite their congenital origin, clinical manifestations may appear at any time.

Saccular aneurysms in childhood arise from stumps of the arteries which normally disappear in fetal life, or from thin spots at major arterial bifurcations; they are frequently associated with coarctation of the aorta. Rarely they are acquired, either secondary to infection or to other local arterial disease. Three fourths of cerebral aneurysms are located anteriorly on the circle of Willis, one fourth posteriorly or on the basilar system. Almost all congenital aneurysms are on or close to the circle of Willis and the vertebrobasilar system; location of an aneurysm farther out on the cerebral arteries suggests an acquired lesion. The symptoms are (1) localized palsies due to pressure of the aneurysm (those of the third, the sixth and the ophthalmic division of the fifth cranial nerves being commonest) and (2) generalized manifestations due to rupture, subarachnoid hemorrhage and local damage to the brain. Incomplete rupture is common. There are sudden, severe headache, vomiting, loss of consciousness and convulsions; the clinical findings include nuchal rigidity, fever, flame-shaped or subhyaloid retinal hemorrhages, altered consciousness and bloody cerebrospinal fluid under increased pressure. The probability of a fatal outcome in such a bleeding episode is about 40 per cent. Persistent and recurrent slow bleeding tends to dissect into the brain and produce hemiplegia. Massive rupture is usually rapidly fatal.

Congenital arteriovenous fistulas are composed of one or several hypertrophied feeding arteries, a mass of communicating vessels often having aneurysmal dilatations, and a tangle of arterialized draining veins (Fig. 20-8). They may be anywhere in the brain or cord. Fistulas between the posterior cerebral arteries and the galenic system compress the aqueduct and may produce hydrocephalus; some form long tracts from the optic papilla to the midbrain. They usually become symptomatic in one of 3 ways: (1) migrainous headaches followed by lateralized seizures and, after several attacks, hemiparesis on the affected side; (2) evidences of subarachnoid hemorrhage or massive intracerebral bleeding which occurs without warning; and (3) increased intracranial pressure, due to enlargement of the malformation. Manifestations include (1) a cranial systolic bruit, best heard over the eyeball and diminished by carotid compression; (2) dilatation of scalp veins; and (3) sometimes polycythemia.

Venous angiomas on the surface of the cortex or in the subependymal area do not produce a bruit

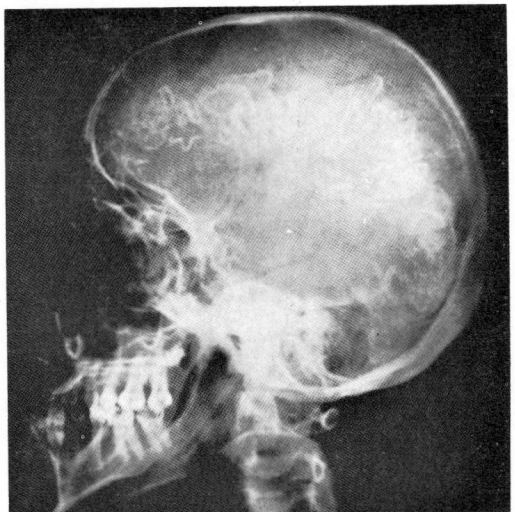

Figure 20-7. Unusually extensive calcification in Sturge-Weber disease.

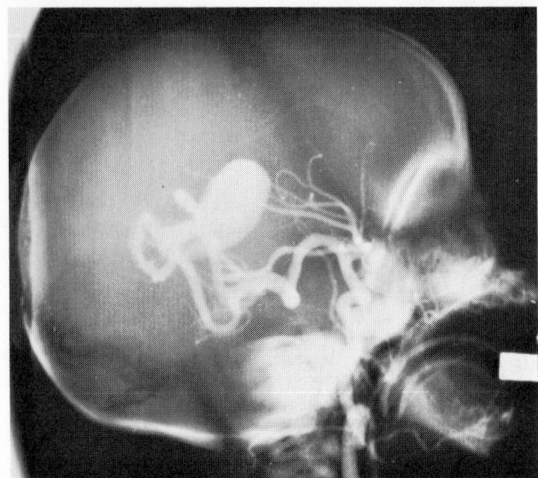

Figure 20-8. Intracranial arteriovenous fistula and aneurysm in a 2-week-old infant who presented with cardiac failure. Note the large feeding vessels.

and do not progress as do the arteriovenous fistulas. Their manifestations are usually focal seizures which appear early and are possibly due to thrombosis in the malformation. *Telangiectases* are most commonly found in the pons; thrombosis or rupture may occur.

The spinal cord may be involved by any of these malformations. Saccular aneurysm is rare, but if present may be associated with coarctation of the aorta. The manifestations are pain due to compression of the cord and subarachnoid hemorrhage. At times there is a cutaneous nevus over the cord defect.

Diagnosis. Spontaneous subarachnoid hemorrhage or intracranial bleeding always suggests such a vascular lesion. Prior to rupture, aneurysm may be suspected from otherwise unexplained unilateral ocular palsies; arteriovenous fistulas may be suspected if a bruit is associated with lateralized signs and headache. Polycythemia with arteriovenous fistula may be intense, and, if the bruit is transmitted to the heart, congenital heart disease may be suspected. Brain tumor is the principal differential consideration and must usually be excluded by angiography.

Treatment. Surgical removal of the vascular lesion, though ideal, is often impossible. Angiomatous malformations in a lobar tip or placed superficially on the nondominant hemisphere can sometimes be removed; microsurgical techniques increase the possibility. Most are centrally placed, with bilateral feeding vessels, and not surgically approachable. Small ones often go unsuspected until a fatal intracerebral hemorrhage occurs.

Saccular aneurysms, whether congenital or mycotic, should be approached surgically if feasible. If complicated by subarachnoid hemorrhage, the state of the patient determines operation; children who are awake or only slightly obtunded, and without localizing neurologic signs, are operated upon within the first day or so. Stuporous or comatose patients, with dilated pupils or severe

localized deficit, are managed at outset with bed rest, sedation as necessary, and steroids or hypothermia; should they survive until their condition improves, operation may be attempted. In general, right-sided aneurysms are more favorable than left-sided ones. In desperate situations, drainage of intracerebral hematomas may be justified.

EXPANDING LESIONS AND INCREASED INTRACRANIAL PRESSURE

The lesions to be discussed in this division, though of widely differing nature, all cause intracranial hypertension.

INCREASED INTRACRANIAL PRESSURE

Physiologic and Anatomic Considerations. The skull and vertebrae constitute a rigid case, vented to the outside only through the vascular system; they enclose the central nervous system and its membranes, a huge vascular bed, and cerebrospinal fluid under a pressure varying normally from 60 to 180 mm., with an average of about 100 mm. The pressure of the cerebrospinal fluid is equated with the intracranial pressure. Volume changes in any of the intracranial components are reflected in changed cerebrospinal fluid pressure, change in relative volumes of intracranial components, or both.

Cerebrospinal fluid is formed in the choroid plexuses of the 4 ventricles and in perivascular spaces of the brain and subarachnoid system by filtration and secretion. The process involves a 2-way exchange at least of water and certain ions between blood and cerebrospinal fluid. The volume of this exchange is large, far exceeding the net formation of cerebrospinal fluid, which varies from 45 to 130 ml. per day in the ventricles alone. Water, most monovalent electrolytes and protein are added to cerebrospinal fluid in the ventricular and subarachnoid spaces; water is added more rapidly in the subarachnoid space, as protein probably is, but sodium and chloride excretion is mainly in the ventricles. The fluid is moved through the ventricles into the subarachnoid space and finally to the great absorptive bed of the arachnoidal villi of the dural sinuses, cerebral veins, the spinal and some cranial nerve foramina.

Pressure and circulation of cerebrospinal fluid are the result of mechanical and vascular factors. Hydrostatic pressure alone accounts for about 50 mm. in the horizontal position; it falls in the head-up position and rises in the head-down position. The principal regulating factor is pressure in the cerebral vascular bed, the cerebrospinal fluid pressure rising or falling sharply with changes in arterial pressure, but accommodating smoothly to slow changes. Sudden changes in venous pressures cause similar fluctuations. Additions to or removal of cerebrospinal fluid, though reflected in an immediate fall or rise, are rapidly compensated by a decrease or increase in cerebral venous volume.

Maintained increased intracranial pressure without a space-taking lesion represents a primary abnormality of one of the space-taking components within the skull, followed by secondary changes in the others. Formation of cerebrospinal fluid itself may be increased with meningitis, papilloma of the choroid plexus, benign increased intracranial pressure and "toxic hydrocephalus." Obstruction to the flow of cerebrospinal fluid causes a rise in pressure, but formation of fluid persists until pressures in excess of 700 mm. are attained. Increase in arterial pressure does not result in a persistent intracranial hypertension unless it is extreme or paroxysmal; the total blood flow remains constant. Venous drainage outside the skull is so well provided with anastomoses that obstruction, unless close to the heart, causes little change in pressure; within the skull, sinus thrombosis, unless it is extensive or involves the posterior part of the superior sagittal sinus or torcular or the usually larger right lateral sinus, may have no persisting effect at all.

Space-occupying lesions increase intracranial pressure by their own bulk and by compression on the ventricular system with production of obstructive hydrocephalus. They are compensated for initially by reduction in cerebrospinal fluid volume, but ultimately the vascular component suffers and the total intracranial blood flow is reduced. A significant increase of tissue fluid in edema of the brain causes similar effects.

Clinical Features. Headache, the most common complaint, is due more to distortion of pain-sensitive meninges and basal blood vessels than to pressure itself. Blunting of intellect, forgetfulness and, in the young child, fretfulness and irritability are common. Low-pitched, roaring or buzzing tinnitus, giddiness, vomiting, diplopia and sometimes visual loss due to extreme papilledema are additional manifestations.

The patient may be dull and given to rubbing the face or nose. Young children often have separated sutures, a cracked-pot note on percussion and a nonlateralized bruit over the head. Focal neurologic signs, except for the nonlocalizing abducens palsy, are absent. Papilledema is almost the rule, unless extreme myopia or previous optic atrophy prevents it. It may be a relatively late manifestation in infants with readily expansile sutures. The retinal veins become distended, and pulsation diminishes; the disk reddens, and its polar and nasal margins blur, and the cup disappears. Extreme elevations, hemorrhages, arterial narrowing, exudates, retinal folds and pallor are late severe signs which may develop rapidly on pre-existent swelling. Visual acuity and the visual fields, except for enlarged blind spots and later concentric constrictions, are well preserved; these distinguish papilledema from optic neuritis. Alterations in consciousness, projectile vomiting, brady-cardia and bradypnea, systemic hypertension and seizures are late events brought about by brain stem distortion, ischemia and disturbed cerebral circulation.

Hernia Cerebri. The intracranial cavity is incompletely divided into compartments by dural and osseous septa. The posterior fossa communicates with the anterior and middle fossae through the tentorial incisure; inferiorly, it communicates with the spinal thecal space through the foramen magnum. Shifts of supratentorial contents can occur toward either side across the midline, but, if sufficiently great, cause herniation of brain through the tentorial notch. Shifts of infratentorial contents may herniate the cerebellar tonsils downward through the foramen magnum or the anterior lobe of the cerebellum upward through the notch. These shifts with resultant herniations of brain substance and pressure on neural and vascular structures are the basis for the signs and symptoms of severe increased intracranial pressure.

Increase of the supratentorial volume forces brain substance into the tentorial notch. Anteriorly the uncinate lobe and posteriorly the hippocampal gyrus are pushed downward to form a ring about the mesencephalon. The aqueduct and cerebrospinal fluid cisterns traversing the notch are compressed and obstruct the flow of fluid; the posterior cerebral arteries and the galenic veins are squeezed, causing hypoxia in the posterior thalamus and occipital lobes and venous congestion of the interior of the hemispheres. The sixth and third nerves are stretched and pinched, producing abducens, oculomotor or pupillary palsy. Finally, the brain stem is itself deformed, and hemorrhages occur into it. Acute anterior hernia of the uncinate lobe compresses the hypothalamus, damaging it by direct and vascular compression. Such brain stem hemorrhage and hypothalamic damage must in most cases be irreversible; small hernias need not be. It has been suggested that uncinate herniation during birth produces temporal lobe scarring which may later become epileptogenic.

Increase in the bulk of the posterior fossa contents forces cerebellar tonsils into the foramen magnum, causing meningeal irritation, nuchal rigidity and ultimately fatal medullary compression, or the anterior lobe may be forced upward through the tentorial notch, compressing the brain stem.

The development of shifts and hernias is affected by the rate of increase of intracranial pressure. Slowly increasing masses may, by reducing cerebrospinal fluid and vascular volume and producing local brain atrophy, cause little or no distortion or increased pressure. Slowly developing hernias may be well tolerated; at any time a sudden change in pressure, such as may follow a small hemorrhage into a pre-existing hematoma, the overhydration of an infant, an ill-advised lumbar puncture or even the increase in blood volume on coughing or straining, may convert a well tolerated hernia into a symptomatic or even a lethal one.

The cranial sutures of the infant and the young child are separable and provide some control of otherwise increasing pressure. Separation may explain sudden remissions in the history of expanding intracranial lesions of young children.

Treatment. Mildly or moderately increased pressure is an indication for immediate study, but not for immediate treatment. The best indicator of borderline cases is the degree of papilledema. If it is high grade with hemorrhages, arterial narrowing, pallor of disks, visual loss or recurrent transitory blurring or blacking out of vision, immediate intervention is necessary. Signs of herniation also call for prompt treatment. The procedures are all decompressions; most are surgical, and their choice depends on the specific lesion and the preference of the surgeon.

Chemical decompression. Hypertonic solutions such as 50 per cent glucose or sucrose, 10 per cent sodium chloride solution or salt-poor serum albumin will on intravenous injection cause immediate shrinkage of the brain through the osmotic effect on tissue fluid. The improvement is transitory and the procedure valuable *only for controlling herniation and reducing brain bulk at operation.* Such solutions should not be used to maintain patients with mass lesions, and they have no effect on edema of toxic or inflammatory origin. Solutions of urea (25 per cent) or mannitol (10 to 20 per cent), giving doses of these agents of 0.5 to 1.5 gm. per kg. per day, may have more prolonged effects, but even here usefulness is measured in hours, or a day or so at most. More prolonged control of cerebral edema may be obtained from dexamethasone, which is given in an initial dose of 2 to 4 mg., then 1 mg. every 6 hours; the mechanism of action is unknown. Acetazolamide is not constant in its effect; administered parenterally, it may increase the pressure.

Removal of cerebrospinal fluid. When intracranial pressure is high, the volume of cerebrospinal fluid adequate and the danger of herniation slight, repeated lumbar punctures reduce discomfort and may prevent progression of papilledema. The procedure is dangerous with mass lesions and often so with severe cerebral edema. Its greatest value is in "benign increased intracranial pressure."

When danger of herniation exists, ventricular puncture or closed constant ventricular drainage may be used as a semi-emergency procedure. These procedures require an adequate cerebrospinal fluid volume and hence are inapplicable for the small ventricles of a swollen brain. Tapping of ventricles under high pressure may produce disastrous hemorrhage from the subependymal veins or fatal upward herniation of the cerebellum in the presence of a posterior fossa lesion.

Surgical decompression. The ideal treatment is internal decompression by removal of the lesion. With inoperable lesions producing obstructive hydrocephalus, a suitable bypassing procedure, such as a variant of the Torkildsen tube, ventriculostomy or ventriculo-atrial shunting, is indicated. Generalized swelling or increased pressure, otherwise uncontrollable, requires extensive decompression by large fronto-temporo-parietal flaps. When severe herniation has occurred at the tentorial notch or foramen magnum, immediate decompression of the medulla or secretion of the free margins of the tentorium may be lifesaving.

BRAIN TUMOR

Neoplasms of the central nervous system make up a large portion of tumors in childhood. There is no general predilection for race or sex. Tumors are rare in infancy, but increase rapidly to a peak at the 5- to 6-year age level, probably owing to the increase in medulloblastoma at this age.

Pathology. Two factors, histologic structure and location, require particular consideration. About 75 per cent of intracranial tumors in childhood are gliomas, of which two thirds are astrocytomas and medulloblastomas. Ependymomas, brain stem gliomas and gliomas of the hemispheres constitute 15 per cent, and the remainder are craniopharyngiomas, meningiomas, sarcomas, pituitary adenomas, hamartomas, hemangiomas and dermoids. The acoustic neurinoma, meningioma and pituitary adenoma of adult life are rare, as are metastases from noncerebral neoplasms.

Sixty to 70 per cent of brain tumors in childhood are beneath the tentorium cerebri, the reverse of the pattern in the adult. Of the supratentorial tumors, more than half are in the midline. Thus the gravity of the problem in children is pointed up by the facts that about three fourths of all brain tumors are incapable of being completely removed, owing to their structural pattern; that about half of them are also difficult or impossible to remove, as a result of their location, and that others are so situated in relation to the brain stem or the ventricular system that functional embarrassment of these structures is frequent.

Clinical Manifestations. The general symptomatology of brain tumor in childhood is that of increased intracranial pressure. *Vomiting* is seldom absent. It usually occurs in the morning around breakfast time, often without nausea, the child returning at once to his meal; rarely it is pernicious. Only late in the course does projectile vomiting appear. *Headache* is less constant and occurs in only about 70 per cent of cases, perhaps in part because the child's descriptive powers are limited. Like vomiting, it is more frequent when the child rises from sleep. It is usually bifrontal or suboccipital; the latter may herald tonsillar herniation and be accompanied or followed by stiff neck. Persistently lateralized headache, especially if accompanied by percussion tenderness, is more suggestive of abscess than tumor. *Diplopia* is usually due to abducens palsy, the sixth nerve or nerves being stretched by intracranial deformity; such palsy has no localizing value. It accounts for most complaints of visual failure; papilledema usually produces little disturbance in acuity. *Enlargement of the head* is most frequent in children under 4 years. *Mental change* is usually a matter of lethargy, indifference or some irritability, giving way to drowsiness, stupor, coma and death. *Convulsions* are rare, generally indicating tumor of a cerebral hemisphere. In late stages of cerebellar tumor, "cerebellar fits" with head retraction, rigidity and extension of limbs and disturbances of pulse and respiration indicate intermittent decerebration, probably by vascular disturbance of the mesencephalon; these signs are of ominous portent.

Regional characteristics. The common *infratentorial tumors* are cerebellar medulloblastoma, cerebellar astrocytoma, brain stem glioma and ependymoma.

The *medulloblastoma*, most common of all brain tumors of childhood, has its peak incidence around 5 years of age and occurs twice as often in boys as in girls. The tumor usually originates in the posterior vermis; of all brain tumors, it most frequently spreads to the meninges of the brain and cord. The course is rapid, early morning vomiting and unsteadiness of gait being soon followed by enlargement of the head. Most children have papilledema and sutural separation; the gait disturbance is one of disequilibrium. Except for hypotonia, cerebellar signs are slight in the limbs. Fifth or seventh cranial nerve palsies and pyramidal signs are evidence of compression or invasion of the brain stem; nystagmus is common. Obstructive hydrocephalus is constant. Nuchal rigidity, cerebellar seizures and even cord signs are late events. Total removal is impossible; the best treatment is decompression and roentgen therapy. Survival is usually less than a year.

Cerebellar astrocytoma has a peak incidence around 8 years of age and a slight predilection for the female. The tumor usually begins close to the midline and is often cystic with a tough, gliosed wall enclosing a mural nodule and containing a yellow, protein-rich fluid. Occasionally the mass invades the cerebellar peduncles or brain stem. The course is slower, and lateralizing cerebellar signs, hypotonia, ataxia, diminished reflexes, rebound phenomenon and nystagmus are usually demonstrable. Headache and vomiting occur later and are less persistent manifestations than with medulloblastoma; papilledema is too often allowed to proceed to irreversible optic atrophy. Total surgical removal is usually possible, and cure is attainable. Roentgen therapy is not very effective and is indicated only when tumors have infiltrated too extensively to permit removal.

Brain stem gliomas account for 8 to 10 per cent of brain tumors in children; there is no sex dominance; the peak incidence is about the seventh year of age, but no age except perhaps infancy is exempt. The common syndrome is one of multiple cranial nerve palsies, particularly of the seventh,

sixth, ninth and tenth nerves and of the sensory portion of the fifth nerve combined with ataxia of the trunk, mild pyramidal signs usually without spasticity, little sensory loss and vomiting without other evidence of increased pressure. Cerebrospinal fluid pressure is elevated only late; the fluid is usually normal, but infrequently contains 5 to 20 lymphocytes and a slight excess of protein. Pneumoencephalography demonstrates backward and upward shift of the floor of the fourth ventricle in excess of 3.5 cm. behind the clivus, encroachment on pontine cisterns and some ventricular dilatation. Hypersomnia and hyperthermia are evidence of upward extension into the hypothalamic area. The tumor usually begins in the deep strata of the pons. Such tumors are inoperable, but the course may be slow, and roentgen therapy may permit a surprisingly long survival in fair condition.

Ependymoma has no sex or age predilection. The initial symptom is almost always vomiting followed by headache, unsteady gait, enlarging head and pyramidal and cerebellar signs. The clinical pattern is variable, since the tumor invades and exerts pressures in widely differing directions. Regression of symptoms is a frequent feature. Flecklike calcifications evident on the roentgenogram and internal hydrocephalus are common. The tumor is best treated by incomplete internal compression and roentgen therapy.

The common *supratentorial tumors* are those of the suprasellar and chiasmatic regions, of the thalamus and posterior third ventricle and of the hemispheres.

Tumors of the suprasellar and chiasmatic regions include craniopharyngioma and glioma of the optic chiasm. The *craniopharyngioma* can become symptomatic from the second year of life to as late as the eighth decade, but is chiefly a tumor of middle to late childhood. It is a solid tumor, at times with a cyst above it. The symptoms are those of increasing pressure due to distortion of the foramina of Monro and third ventricle, of compression of the optic chiasm, causing bitemporal field defects and later optic atrophy, and of pressure on the pituitary and hypothalamus, leading to retardation of growth and osseous development, fatigability, diabetes insipidus and disturbances of the sleep rhythm. Since the visual and the hypophyseo-hypothalamic changes advance slowly, headache and vomiting are the usual initial complaints. Growth retardation is not noted in very young children, and is common but not universal in older children or adolescents. Hypothalamic attacks of semistupor, fever, cardiac irregularities and miosis may occur. The child usually appears younger than his stated age, his head somewhat large. The roentgenogram of the skull reveals separated sutures, very often suprasellar calcification and some sellar deformity (Fig. 20-9). Hypoglycemia, a flat glucose tolerance curve, diabetes insipidus, a high eosinophil count, lowered excretion of 17-ketosteroids and hypotension

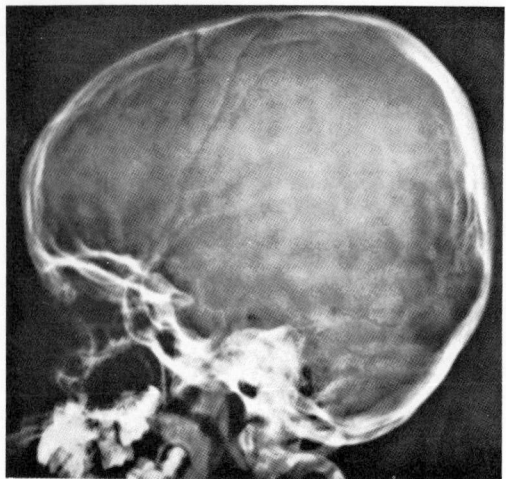

Figure 20-9. Craniopharyngioma in a boy 8 years of age. Note fluffy suprasellar calcification, enlarged sella turcica, digital markings of skull, and early sutural separation.

are common. Growth hormone excretion under stimulus of induced hypoglycemia is often reduced. The optic disks may be elevated, atrophic or normal. Surgical removal, once considered almost impossible, is now frequently achieved, largely owing to improved surgical technique and the use of preoperative and postoperative corticosteroids. Residua such as optic atrophy and damage to the hypothalamic-hypophyseal system remain troublesome. Diabetes insipidus is readily controlled with vasopressin, but deficiency in growth hormone remains a problem. More growth is possible than was once thought, however, even without growth hormone supplement. If total removal of the tumor is impossible, the cyst is drained, the cyst wall removed, and the solid portion controlled with roentgen therapy, often with success for years.

Glioma of the optic chiasm initially causes visual disturbances; later there are manifestations of increased pressure and of hypothalamic involvement. It is occasionally accompanied by cutaneous *café-au-lait* spots. Optic atrophy is more frequent than papilledema. Excavation beneath the anterior clinoids and an enlarged optic foramen are common roentgen findings. The tumor is generally inoperable beyond decompressive procedures; roentgen therapy is indicated.

Tumors of the posterior third ventricle are pinealomas, gliomas and hamartomas. All produce obstruction early in the course with signs of increased pressure. The pineal neoplasms compress the mesencephalon from above and cause pupillary dilatation and failure of upward conjugate gaze, the *syndrome of Parinaud.* They may produce precocious puberty in the male by pressure in the hypothalamic area. Gliomas in the thalamus or hypothalamus may cause similar hypothalamic disturbance, together with increased pressure and frequently hemiplegia. They are best treated by draining the ventricle with bypassing tubes and by radiation.

Tumors of the hemispheres are gliomas, ependymomas of the ventricle and sometimes sarcomas. Clinical manifestations are hemiplegia, seizures, those of increasing pressure and rarely choreic or dystonic movements. The tumors are frequently enormous.

Treatment. In general, treatment is unsatisfactory. Complete cure, for practical purposes, is restricted to the cystic cerebellar astrocytoma and some craniopharyngiomas, which affect only about 15 per cent of children with intracranial neoplasms. Death is hastened by intervention in about an equal percentage of instances. Even when complete cure is impossible, relief of symptoms and return to enjoyable life for months or years is often possible, and should never be denied a child. An attitude of nihilism breeds inadequate study and leads to death or permanent disability from treatable lesions. When there is a likelihood of an expanding lesion, diagnostic study should not cease until the lesion is located and the appropriate therapy decided.

Definitive study of such cases is a problem for experienced neurosurgeons and neurologists; the diagnostic procedures themselves are often major operations. The pediatrician performs 2 roles: (1) the vital one of suspecting the lesion and initiating study, and (2) the support and maintenance of a critically ill child. Careful correction of water and electrolyte disturbances, corticosteroid or corticotropin therapy during operations about the hypothalamus, supervision of hormonal replacement therapy, restoration of nutrition, and maintenance of the patient's and parents' morale are responsibilities he must share.

EXTRACEREBRAL ACCUMULATIONS OF FLUID

Subdural hematoma is an accumulation of blood, its degradation products and fluid within the subdural space. It may be acute, subacute or chronic and usually results from direct trauma to the head.

Chronic Subdural Hematoma of Infancy

Etiology. Direct or transmitted trauma to the head may produce bleeding into the subdural space. In the adult or older child a positive history of trauma is elicited in 80 per cent of cases; in infants the relation to trauma is less clear. Trauma at birth is considered a possible cause, but supportive evidence is inconclusive. The lesion is not especially common to premature infants, in whom the possibility of molding trauma to the head is great. Scurvy and purpuric states increase the hazard; in hemophilia subdural hematoma is less frequent than one would expect. Deliberate violence now appears to be the most common cause, especially to ill-cared for and unwanted children (see battered-child syndrome, p. 1362).

Epidemiology. More common in male than in female infants, the incidence rises sharply in the second month of life to a peak by about 4 months, followed by a rather sharp fall and virtual disappearance by 14 to 16 months of age.

Pathology. The subdural space is occupied by a sac which usually extends frontally and laterally over the hemispheres; it is bilateral in about 80 per cent of cases. The dural wall of the sac is thick, heavily vascularized and fused with the dura mater; the arachnoid wall is thinner, less vascularized and less firmly attached to the meninx. This sac contains a variable mixture of fresh and old blood and xanthochromic fluid. The brain beneath is compressed and its leptomeninx often thickened. In long-standing cases there is considerable atrophy of the underlying cortex.

Pathogenesis. At the time of trauma delicate bridging subdural veins, most numerous along the falx, are torn. Small hemorrhages occur in the subdural space. Originally insignificant in amount, the blood breaks down and imbibition of fluid occurs across the arachnoidal membrane. The breakdown products of blood stimulate the growth of connective tissue and capillaries, largely from the dura. As fluid increases the width of the subdural space, these capillaries are torn, further hemorrhage occurs, and the lesion enlarges. If unrelieved, the mass expands the skull, ultimately causing cerebral atrophy or death from compression and herniation. At any point the lesion may spontaneously arrest, only to be discovered as a calcified membrane over the brain in older patients. Further bleeding may occur into an already existing sac and may increase symptoms. The formation of such sacs occurs more readily over a previously atrophic brain, the *hematoma ex vacuo.*

In contrast to the foregoing theory of pathogenesis, continental and other authorities place more emphasis on inflammatory factors and regard most chronic subdural hematomas as hemorrhagic pachymeningitis with increased capillary permeability and effusion of blood cells and protein into the subdural space. An entirely satisfactory answer as to causation is not available.

Clinical Manifestations. The most characteristic ones are irritability and failure to thrive. There is a history of convulsions and vomiting in half the cases and of recurrent fever, drowsiness and birth or postnatal trauma in descending order. On admission, more than half the infants have fever; the reflexes are hyperactive. Mild hemiplegia is frequently overlooked. About half of the infants have bulging or tense fontanels, and the head is measurably enlarged, with a square, boxlike expansion of the vault in about one third. The scalp is tight and glossy, and the scalp veins are dilated. Retinal hemorrhages are a frequent late manifestation. Strabismus, pupillary inequality and ocular palsies are infrequent, but, if they occur suddenly during treatment or while the infant is under observation, may be an important clue to massive fresh subdural hemorrhage.

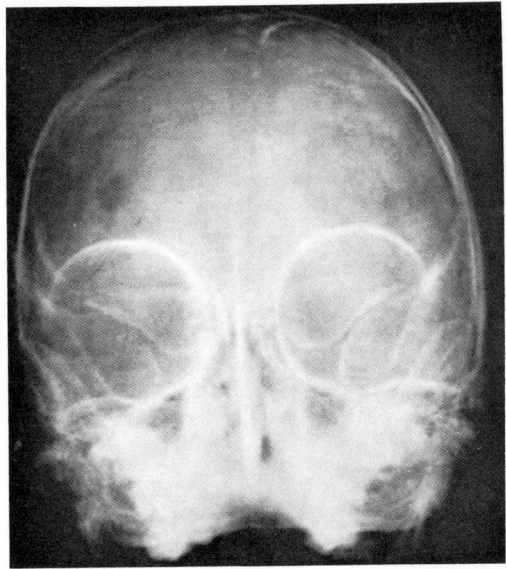

Figure 20-10. Calcified subdural membrane in a microcephalic idiot. Right subdural hematoma drained in infancy (note trephine), left side not explored. Calcified membrane discovered years later.

Laboratory Data. One third to one half of the infants have an anemia of blood loss and a low serum protein level. Sutural separation is demonstrable roentgenographically, but skull fractures are uncommon. Multiple fractures involving long bones, ribs or clavicles suggest the battered-child syndrome (p. 1362). The electroencephalogram may reveal reduction in voltage over very large hematomas; minor asymmetries, spikes or slowings are evidence only of brain injury. The cerebrospinal fluid is often under increased pressure and may contain red blood cells, a slight excess of white cells and increased protein. The definitive diagnostic procedure is a carefully performed subdural puncture (see p. 1272); fluid of any sort in excess of 1 to 2 ml., or with a protein content significantly higher than that of concomitantly obtained cerebrospinal fluid, is an abnormal finding. Arteriography is reliable, but not always available.

Differential Diagnosis. Subdural hematoma must be distinguished from hydrocephalus, chronic meningitis and brain tumor.

Treatment. Treatment for subdural hematoma at any age is by removal of the abnormal fluid with as much of any surrounding membrane as possible. In infants an immediate surgical approach results in a high fatality rate; reasonably good results can be expected from a regimen combining subdural drainage with later craniotomy.

No more than a total of 30 ml. of fluid should be removed at a time from the 2 sides. The infant's condition usually improves rapidly. With repeated taps (usually daily) the volume, red cells, xanthochromia and protein tend to decrease; occasionally the fluid disappears entirely. After 7 to 10 days of taps a frontoparietal burr hole is placed. If membranes are present, craniotomy is done and as much of the membrane and contents removed as possible. After recovery from the craniotomy the process is repeated on the other side. Even after craniotomy, fluid may continue to accumulate for a time, and drainage by needle may still be necessary, since all the membrane can seldom be removed. Occasionally a subdural-pleural shunt may be indicated. With this regimen, mortality may be kept well below 5 per cent, and complete recovery without mental or physical residuals attained in better than 50 per cent of the cases. The best prognostic sign is the condition of the brain at operation; if severe atrophy exists, the prognosis is poor.

Subdural Effusion

In the course of pyogenic meningitis, accumulations of protein-rich, xanthochromic, sometimes encapsulated, fluid occur in the subdural space. These are thought to be due to an effusion of fluid across an inflamed arachnoid or from thrombosed subdural veins into the subdural space; there the exudate stimulates encapsulation and grows by imbibition and capillary rupture, like a subdural hematoma.

The lesion can occur at any age and with any pathogen, though *Hemophilus influenzae* accounts for more than half, and with *Diplococcus pneumoniae*, for more than 90 per cent of cases. Peak age incidence is 3 to 10 months. Effusions should be suspected in any subacute or chronic pyogenic meningitis, and in acute meningitis when the fever fails to abate after 3 or 4 days of adequate therapy, when convulsions or neurologic signs appear, when cerebrospinal cultures remain positive or when the infant vomits or fails to thrive.

Effusions are treated like subdural hematomas. Membranes are much more delicate, and often absent, though the effusions may prove obstinate. Persistent effusions sometimes respond to subdural-atrial, subdural-pleural or subdural-peritoneal shunts.

Acute Subdural Hematoma, Subdural Hygroma and Chronic Subdural Hematoma in Older Children

Subdural bleeding can occur in severe head injury; if the condition of such a patient is worsening steadily, with deepening stupor and advancing hemiparesis, angiography or burr holes are indicated as an emergency measure, though the lesion found is most often brain swelling or intracerebral hematoma.

Subdural hygroma, in the strictest sense, is an accumulation of cerebrospinal fluid in the subdural space, to which it gains entrance through a valvelike rent in the arachnoid. It is always traumatic, and not clinically separable from epidural or subdural hematoma. It is rare, and many fluid accumulations so diagnosed are really effusions or leptomeningeal cysts containing fluid with an unusually low protein content.

Chronic subdural hematoma in older children is rare; the clinical syndrome is that of headache, mild hemiparesis and papilledema. At times there is vomiting or seizures. Visual field defects are rare; abducens palsy may appear. Angiography is often diagnostic and should be followed by craniotomy. If symptoms are not too severe, expectant therapy will sometimes be followed by disappearance of symptoms. This course is justifiable *only* under special circumstances, such as subdural hematoma in a hemophiliac.

Epidural Hematoma

This is an accumulation of blood between dura and bone. The cause is trauma; the lesion accounts for about 2 per cent of pediatric hospital admissions for head trauma. Half of the cases occur before 2 years of age. In the older child or adult the classic course is that of head trauma, the impact generally to the side of the head, with brief loss of consciousness followed by a lucid interval and then by deepening stupor, homolateral pupillary dilatation, contralateral hemiparesis, slowing pulse and respiration, rising blood pressure and death. The bleeding is arterial, usually as a result of a linear temporal fracture which lacerates the middle meningeal vessels. In the child under 2 years of age, loss of consciousness is less frequent, the fracture usually diastatic rather than linear, and the bleeding venous as well as arterial. The course is often slower, and the hematoma may become large enough to produce extensive blood loss, the symptoms being those of shock rather than increasing pressure and brain stem compression.

The common signs at any age are lacerations of the scalp, drowsiness, stupor and coma. Pupillary dilatation or advancing oculomotor palsy is almost always homolateral, rarely contralateral; hemiparesis is almost always contralateral, rarely homolateral. The temperature is often subnormal and the pulse pressure wide. In the early stages the pupillary and hemiparetic signs, as well as the slowing pulse and respiration, may be inconspicuous if the child is kept awake by examinations. Careful, quiet observation in a private room, with frequent recordings of pulse and respiration, is better than repeated vigorous examination.

This condition is a surgical emergency, and when its existence is considered likely, operation should not be delayed. Roentgenographic examination is valuable if the child's condition permits; other studies and especially lumbar puncture are best avoided. Since brisk hemorrhage is often encountered, a blood transfusion should be started before or be available during operation. Survival and functional recovery depend on early, successful evacuation of the clot and arrest of bleeding.

BRAIN ABSCESS

Focal sepsis in the brain in childhood generally occurs (1) by extension from infection in the mastoid, paranasal sinuses, scalp or skull; (2) metastatically from bronchopulmonary, pleural, cardiac or other remote sources; (3) as a complication of congenital cyanotic heart disease or pulmonary arteriovenous fistulas; or (4) rarely from penetrating wounds and craniotomy. In a small percentage of instances no source is found.

Infection from sources about the head is by direct extension or along thrombosed vessels and usually involves adjacent cerebral tissue. Hematogenous spread localizes at the junction of the cortex and white matter, with slight preference for the left hemisphere. A focus of septic encephalitis is established which may enlarge rapidly and produce paralysis, coma and death. More often the lesion becomes walled off, and an abscess forms. As it expands, there is edema of the surrounding area. Extension is toward the ventricle, and secondary abscesses in the wall are common. Rupture usually occurs into the ventricle. Some abscesses become sterile; the wall calcifies, and the lesion becomes static.

There are 3 stages. The *first stage* is characterized by focal encephalitis. The patient, already ill with a primary infection, has an elevation of temperature, is drowsy and complains of headache. He may have a convulsion, or there may be meningeal signs. Improvement occurs in a day or two, especially with antibiotic therapy. The *second stage*, during which the abscess is enlarging, is relatively quiet. For days or weeks the child is only vaguely ill, listless, occasionally feverish to 100 or 101°F., and complains of some headache, usually frontal. Neurologic signs are slight, unnoticed or absent. Eventually the tempo of illness increases, headache is worse and more localized, and a seizure often occurs. Focal signs appear, the optic disks blur, and the cranial sutures may separate. At any moment the child may pass into the *third stage*, with decompensated increased intracranial pressure and neurologic and cardiorespiratory signs of brain stem compression, or the abscess may rupture and be evidenced by high fever, meningeal signs, seizures and a decerebrate state.

Clinical signs depend on increased pressure and on the locus of the abscess. Drowsiness, headache, vomiting, sixth nerve palsies and papilledema are often manifestations. Since most abscesses are solitary and, with the exception of some otogenous ones, supratentorial, the common localizing signs are hemiparesis, visual field defects and aphasia. The frontal abscess is notably silent; lethargy and dullness are often the only evidence. A cerebellar abscess produces lateralized hypotonia, ataxia, adiadochokinesis, coarse nystagmus mainly toward the side of the abscess, and skew deviations. *Percussion tenderness over the abscess is one of the most valuable of all localizing signs.*

Leukocytosis, present during the first stage, is absent during the second one and becomes notable only with rupture of the abscess. Anemia of infection is usually present. Roentgenograms of the skull show only sutural separation or sellar demineralization; films of the chest, long bones, sinuses or mastoids may reveal an unsuspected infective focus. The cerebrospinal fluid in the first stage is marked by pleocytosis and elevated pressure, but the fluid is sterile; in the second stage, pressure and protein content are usually elevated, and there may be a few cells. In the third stage, pressure, protein and cells increase; high pleocytosis indicates leakage or rupture, in which case pathogens may be cultured from the fluid. The electroencephalogram is a valuable tool, since the large zone of edema often produces lateralized and sometimes sharply localized delta waves; serial electroencephalograms are of diagnostic value in the differential diagnosis.

At least 4 per cent of all patients with cyanotic heart disease or pulmonary arteriovenous fistulas suffer brain abscess. The cause is not clear. The abscesses do not arise from bacterial endocarditis, and a specific focus is rarely demonstrated. Relief of cyanosis by anastomotic procedures does not protect against cerebral abscess, which occurs in any form of cyanotic congenital heart disease. Clinically, diagnosis is difficult because a definite first stage is absent, and the symptoms of headache, irritability, recurrent fever and even sudden onset of localizing signs or hemiplegia are common in cyanotic heart disease. Only constant vigilance will detect the abscesses.

Treatment. Adequate antibiotic therapy probably often heals incipient abscesses during the first stage. An established abscess must be treated surgically. Since these children tolerate prolonged anesthesia poorly, repeated aspiration is the best means of treatment. Several methods are used. In one the abscess is tapped through a trephine hole and aspirated, and thorium dioxide or microdispersed barium sulfate is instilled to outline the cavity. Repeated aspirations are performed under roentgen guidance, and antibiotic therapy is continued until the abscess disappears. Alternatively, the initial treatment is the same, but after some days the abscess is resected in toto. Some surgeons prefer immediate resection in toto, without previous drainage. The author favors the first method because it is simple and seems less likely to leave neurologic residuals. Superiority of one method over the others, with respect to the later development of seizures, is not clearly established.

Mortality is about 25 per cent, which is far too high. Survivors have seizures in about 45 per cent of instances and hence should be maintained on anticonvulsant therapy for at least 5 years.

EPIDURAL AND SUBDURAL EMPYEMA

In the infected infant meningitic effusions form a subdural empyema. Most cases of epidural or subdural empyema develop by extension from infected paranasal sinuses or mastoid air cells, and occur in older children; a few follow scalp infections. A period of recurrent or persistent localized frontal or temporoparietal headache, usually with fever, is followed by sudden worsening, often with a seizure. Diagnostic findings are fever, peripheral leukocytosis, physical and roentgen signs of sinusitis or otitis, percussion tenderness over frontal or temporoparietal regions and pleocytosis of cerebrospinal fluid, which is marked with subdural and less with epidural lesions. At times there are papilledema and hemiparesis. The patient usually appears quite ill. Apical petrositis may produce homolateral abducens palsy, facial pain, and deafness, the *syndrome of Gradenigo*. Frontal osteomyelitis with swelling (*Pott's puffy tumor*) often accompanies extension from frontal sinuses.

The differential diagnosis includes intracranial abscess, cortical thrombophlebitis, which may be associated, and meningitis. Electroencephalograms and arteriography are often necessary. Treatment consists in administration of antibiotics, general supportive measures, and early, thorough surgical drainage of infected sinuses, air cells and empyema cavities. Careful search should be made for osteomyelitis. Drainage of the subdural space is difficult if pus has loculated or extended to the interhemispheric fissure.

INCREASED INTRACRANIAL PRESSURE WITHOUT MASS LESIONS

Dural Sinus Thrombosis

Occlusion of dural sinuses results from neighboring or remote infection, sometimes from polycythemia or hemoconcentration, anemia, blood dyscrasias, slowing of circulation, trauma or tumor invasion.

The signs and symptoms are (1) those of the primary condition, such as chills, fever, leukocytosis, otitis media and marasmic state; (2) neurologic ones stemming from the region of the brain affected by venous stasis, edema or infarction; and (3) manifestations of increased intracranial pressure. Any or all may be present; conversely, all may be absent and the occluded sinus discovered incidentally.

Superior Sagittal Sinus. The occlusion is most often nonseptic and occurs as a rule in dehydrated, marasmic, hypernatremic or toxic infants. The onset is abrupt; convulsions and single, or sometimes double, hemiplegia indicate extension of the thrombus into the superficial cortical veins. Stupor, head retraction, bulging fontanel, dilated scalp veins, papilledema and enlargement of the head are signs of obstruction of the sinus and of increased pressure. The cerebrospinal fluid often contains some red and white blood cells. The ventricles are initially compressed by congestion and

edema, but later enlarge, and the cortex atrophies. Incomplete occlusion in the middle third of the sinus with lateralizing neurologic signs and lesser increase of intracranial pressure is more common than complete occlusion and is less serious. This condition must be distinguished from the stupor, convulsions and rigidity of severe hypernatremia, which it may accompany.

Sinus Rectus and Galenic Vein. Occlusion here is either septic or nonseptic. Sudden onset of coma, generalized convulsions and high intracranial pressure are accompanied by initial flaccidity rapidly changing to decerebrate rigidity. The cerebrospinal fluid is grossly bloody, and the child soon dies.

Cavernous Sinus. Thrombosis of this sinus is almost always septic, being secondary to infections about the orbit, face, pharynx, sphenoidal sinus or the petrous apex. Chills, fever, headache and leukocytosis are accompanied by drowsiness, but rarely by seizures or stupor. Edema and chemosis of the eyelids, protrusion of the eyeball, thrombosis of retinal veins and later low-grade papilledema are associated with a decrease in vision and with extraocular palsies. Extension across the circular sinus to involve the other eye, meningeal signs and pleocytosis of the cerebrospinal fluid may occur; there is usually increased intracranial pressure.

Lateral Sinus Thrombosis. Evidence of otitis media, acute or chronic, is almost always present. The onset may be abrupt with septic fever, chills, leukocytosis and a positive blood culture, or it may be insidious with only signs of increasing intracranial pressure. If the onset is abrupt, contralateral facial weakness, sometimes contralateral seizures and rarely hemiparesis indicate spread of the thrombosis upward through the cortical veins across the hemisphere. Paralysis of the ninth, tenth and eleventh cranial nerves is due to thrombosis of the jugular vein, which may become palpable in the neck. There is headache, drowsiness and papilledema in about half of the cases. Differentiation from brain abscess may require ventriculography.

Treatment of Dural Sinus Thrombosis. Any infection must be appropriately and vigorously treated with antibiotics and surgical drainage when indicated. Anticoagulants to limit spread of the thrombosis are of doubtful value. Increased pressure, once the diagnosis is established, is best managed by repeated lumbar punctures, but if vision is threatened, subtemporal decompression may be used. Surgical removal of the thrombus is seldom done, since the clots recanalize rapidly.

Benign Increased Intracranial Pressure
(Toxic Hydrocephalus; Pseudotumor Cerebri; Quincke's or Serous Meningitis)

This term identifies a syndrome resulting from increased intracranial pressure and manifest by headache, papilledema, sixth nerve palsies, some-

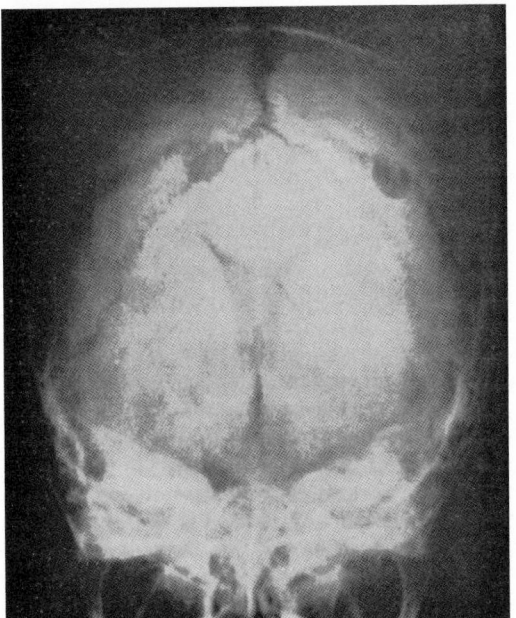

Figure 20-11. Benign increased intracranial pressure or pseudotumor in a boy 4 years of age. Sutures are separated, but ventricles are small and unshifted. Note trephine openings.

times vomiting and absence of other neurologic signs. Though most common in young adult women, it occurs in childhood. Some cases have been identified as "silent" lateral or longitudinal sinus thrombosis; others seem to follow various infections or slight head injuries, and the cause remains obscure. The definitive diagnostic procedure is ventriculography, which reveals small, symmetrical, unshifted ventricles (Fig. 20-11). Treatment is by repeated lumbar puncture, with surgical decompression if vision is threatened; attempts at chemical decompression, as with acetazolamide, have not been impressive. Elevated intracranial pressure may persist for months.

HYDROCEPHALUS

Hydrocephalus is an excess of cerebrospinal fluid within the ventricular and subarachnoid spaces. It is not synonymous with an enlarged head, since the latter may be due to megalencephalon or subdural fluid, while hydrocephalus may or may not notably enlarge the head. A simple increase in total intracranial fluid may be retained in the brain substance, as in pseudotumor cerebri, and produce increased pressure, but not hydrocephalus. *Communicating hydrocephalus* implies free communication between ventricles and spinal theca, and *obstructive hydrocephalus*, a block to such passage of fluid. The terms are misleading, since most hydrocephalus is due pathogenetically to some form of anatomic or physiologic obstruction between points of formation and absorption of cerebrospinal fluid. *Internal hydrocephalus* and *external hydrocephalus* indicate the site of greatest

enlargement of cerebrospinal fluid spaces, whether ventricular or subarachnoid.

A mechanical obstruction to the flow of cerebrospinal fluid somewhere between the points of formation and absorption is the commonest observed lesion, but many cases of "communicating" hydrocephalus are still inadequately explained. Such obstructing lesions include congenital atresia or forking of the aqueduct, the Arnold-Chiari and Dandy-Walker malformations, and perhaps failure of normal development of subarachnoid spaces. Hydrocephalus may also accompany other forms of cerebral malformations, such as agenesis of the corpus callosum, encephaloceles, porencephalies, and the like, though the location of the obstructive lesion is obscure. Inflammatory lesions, either meningitis or reaction to subarachnoid bleeding at birth or later, may lead to gliosis of the aqueduct or obliteration of subarachnoid spaces. Rarely meningeal deposits, lipid-laden phagocytes in gargoylism or metastases are responsible. Tumors, abscess, vascular malformations and cysts cause obstruction by compressing or occluding the ventricular system. Platybasia, developmental or due to such lesions as achondroplasia, may be responsible for obstruction. The incidence of hydrocephalus from all causes approaches 3 per 1000 births.

Accurate evaluation of the relative roles of overproduction or underabsorption of the cerebrospinal fluid in the human patient cannot be made. Occasionally, overproduction is due to a tumor of the choroid plexus. In occlusion of the dural sinuses (q.v.), which may impair absorption and cause increased intracranial pressure, the ventricles are small, and the excess of fluid is in the brain substances until provided with an egress through spinal drainage or trephine. An increased volume of cerebrospinal fluid with accompanying hydrocephalus is seen in both hypervitaminosis and hypovitaminosis A, and at least increased pressure in hypoparathyroidism. Intracranial pressure may be increased in infants receiving tetracyclines, but the state of the ventricles is not fully known.

Much of the pathogenesis is simple mechanics. The fluid system dilates above the point of obstruction; e.g. obstruction at Monro's foramina dilates one or both lateral ventricles; aqueductal lesions dilate the third and lateral ventricles; and obstruction at the fourth ventricular foramina or in the subarachnoid space enlarges all 4 ventricles. The actual ventricular enlargement seems due in part at least to the pumping action of the choroid plexuses, since it does not occur readily in their absence. The obstruction may be partial, intermittent or complete; the symptoms may be rapid or slow and steadily advancing or remittent. Atrophy of the choroid plexuses is a late event, and fluid continues to be formed in their absence. Fenestrations may develop in the septum pellucidum, in the membranous walls of ventricles or in other locations. Spontaneous bypassing of obstructed points also occurs.

Though hydrocephalus is sometimes recognized before birth, most cases become manifest in the first few weeks or months of life. The fontanels widen and are moderately tense, and the skull enlarges in all diameters. The brow bulges; the sclera becomes visible above the iris, owing rather to upper lid retraction than to pressure on the orbit; the scalp becomes shiny, and scalp veins dilate. Failure of upward gaze, strabismus, hyperactive reflexes, mild diplegia and optic atrophy are additional manifestations; papilledema in the infant is rare. Irritability, failure to thrive and a high-pitched cry are common. When the onset is later or the progress less rapid, the head may enlarge much more in one plane than in another, producing brachycephaly or scaphocephaly. The disproportion of the skull may help to locate the obstruction, a shallow posterior fossa suggesting aqueductal or third ventricular lesions.

If the brain is not seriously malformed, mental function remains surprisingly good; children with paper-thin cortex may have intelligence quotients within the normal range. Motor function is generally retarded, both by the weight of the head and by the actual neurologic impairment present.

Treatment. The intelligent management of the child in whom hydrocephalus is suspected demands initially that the diagnosis be established and that the existence of surgically treatable lesions such as subdural hematoma and resectable tumors or cysts be excluded. Secondly, in the hydrocephalic patient, any physical point of obstruction must be located by suitable radiographic constrast studies, and the advancement of the hydrocephalus established by serial head measurements, by worsening of the general condition, and by progression of physical signs. Head measurements alone are not entirely reliable, since ventricles sometimes enlarge considerably without concomitant increase in head size. Serial electroencephalograms and occasionally, in older children, psychometric evaluations may be helpful. Echoencephalography ("sonar scanning") may be helpful. Pneumoencephalograms or ventriculograms using a small amount of air are indispensable; large replacement air studies are unnecessary and not well tolerated. Angiography and dye studies using phenolsulfonphthalein may be of assistance; the latter, however, may mislead, since the dye may pass through secondary fenestrations.

Two therapeutic approaches have been attempted: (1) Reduction in the production of cerebrospinal fluid by choroid plexectomy, fluid restriction, blood letting, and the like; these procedures are ineffective and now generally abandoned. Acetazolamide, orally in large doses, has given inconsistent results. (2) Bypass of the point of obstruction by shunting the cerebrospinal fluid to normal or artificial locations for absorption or excretion. In older children with previously adequate subarachnoid systems, third ventricular or aqueductal obstruction may respond well to ventriculocisternostomy or to passage of a tube from a lateral ventricle to the cisterna magna. In young infants or when the subarachnoid system is obliterated or incompetent, the fluid may be conveyed (*a*) from the ventricular system to the lesser peritoneal or pleural spaces; this is ordinarily effective for a few weeks only. (*b*) From a lateral ventricle or, in cases of communicating hydrocephalus, from the spinal theca to a ureter, after nephrectomy. The ureteral shunt is often well maintained, even in infants, but it sacrifices one kidney. Loss of cerebrospinal fluid via the urine results in a negative electrolyte balance, and, especially in young children, 2 to 4 gm. of sodium or ammonium chloride must be given daily by mouth. Spinothecal ureterostomy is unaffected by growth; ventriculoureterostomies must be revised as the child grows. (*c*) From the ventricular system into the venous circulation, usually into the right atrium, by use of a polyethylene tube and valve to prevent reflux of blood. This is at present the most popular procedure; complications are principally (1) need for revision, which occurs in about 40 per cent of cases; (2) septicemia, with persistent bacterial growth in the valve. Whether septicemia is due to the valve acting solely as a foreign body or to its inadequate sterilization is not clear. It usually occurs soon after establishment of the shunt. The staphylococcus is the most common pathogen. Cure almost always requires removal of valve and tube; prolonged antibiotic therapy, as for subacute bacterial endocarditis, may occasionally sterilize the blood, but relapses are common, and subacute ventriculitis may develop and persist. (3) Multiple pulmonary thromboses with pulmonary hypertension and heart failure in later years. Whether the thromboses are produced by emboli originating from valve or tube or are due to effects of the cerebrospinal fluid directly on clotting mechanisms is unknown.

The indications for and contraindications to shunting operations are controversial. Spontaneous compensation, pleocytosis or increased spinal fluid protein and severe mental retardation are generally accepted contraindications. Age below 6 months and thinning of the cortex below 1 cm. are contraindications accepted by some, but should probably be ignored. The most difficult problems are those of associated congenital defects, most commonly meningomyeloceles and of borderline or uncertain intellectual potential.

The results of surgical treatment are not brilliant. Without operation, perhaps two thirds of all children with hydrocephalus of whatever cause will die at an early age. With operation, about two thirds of the children will survive, and the status of many of them will be improved. Of survivors, perhaps two fifths will have intelligence quotients below 70; about three fourths, below 90. Less than 5 per cent achieve an intelligence quotient of 110 or better. Even the most optimistic authorities do not claim that more than 15 to 20 per cent of treated patients will be normally competitive, both physically and intellectually.

Even the physically sound person of dull or

borderline intelligence faces many problems. The hydrocephalic is often additionally burdened by paraparesis, ataxia and incontinence if he had a meningomyelocele, and by seizures, poor vision and squints, and many more problems. The reoperation rate is high; the threat of infection is always present; late pulmonary complications are probably more common and severe than is recognized, and the habilitative period is prolonged and often physically, emotionally and financially exhausting to parents. The physician must not fail to weigh these considerations carefully in deciding his course.

HYDRANENCEPHALY

In this condition the cerebral cortex, except for the inferior temporal and mesial occipital lobes, is represented only by a membrane filled with clear fluid. The basal ganglia and thalamus are present, the cerebellum and brain stem are well preserved, but the aqueduct is generally obliterated. The size of the head at birth is normal. There are 2 theories of pathogenesis: (1) It may represent obstructive hydrocephalus in utero, the intrauterine pressure preventing enlargement of the head with resulting cortical atrophy. (2) The internal carotid arteries may be deficient or compressed, allowing only those parts of the brain supplied by the basilar artery to develop. Neither theory is proved, and the condition has been seen associated with cyto-

megalic inclusion disease. The infant is well formed, but obviously defective and blind, and may have poor temperature regulation. Diagnosis is readily established by transillumination of the head in a dark room (Fig. 20-12). There is no treatment.

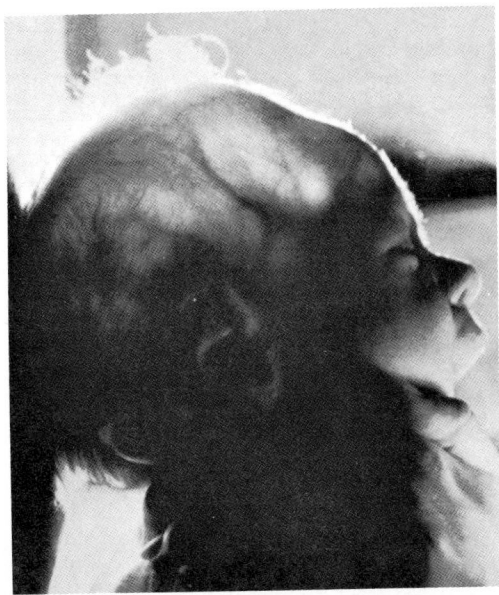

Figure 20-12. Hydranencephaly shown by transillumination.

DEGENERATIVE DISEASES

The outstanding characteristics of degenerative disorders of the central nervous system are progressive functional incapacitation and loss of nervous tissue. In only a few of these disorders is the cause understood. Clinical manifestations, though sometimes stereotyped and diagnostic, are often variable or lacking in specific features, so that a satisfactory classification is not possible. The following is one of convenience and strives to mention only the more generic and a few of the recently recognized forms:

I. **Storage diseases: lipidoses and leukodystrophies**
  A. Cerebromacular degenerations
    1. Infantile amaurotic family idiocy (Tay-Sachs disease)
    2. Late infantile and juvenile amaurotic family idiocy (syndromes of Bielschowsky, Spielmeyer-Vogt and Batten)
  B. Demyelinizing leukodystrophies
    1. Early infantile form (Krabbe's disease)
    2. Late infantile form (Greenfield's disease)
    3. Metachromatic form
  C. Other storage diseases
    1. Cerebral glycogenosis (glycogen storage disease, p. 440).
    2. Lipogranulomatosis (Farber-Uzman syndrome)
    3. Angiokeratoma corporis universale diffusum (Fabry's syndrome)

    4. Cerebral cholesterinosis
      a. Cerebral Hand-Schüller-Christian disease
      b. Familial cerebrotendinous xanthomatosis (van Bogaert, Scherer and Epstein syndrome)
II. **Demyelinizing encephalomyelopathies**
  A. Global demyelinization (Schilder's disease)
  B. Disseminated demyelinization (disseminated sclerosis)
  C. Neuromyelitis optica
III. **Metabolic errors**
  Hepatolenticular degeneration (Wilson's disease)
IV. **Degenerative diseases involving specific fiber tracts or neural groups**
  A. Spinocerebellar ataxia—Friedreich's disease and other spinocerebellar forms
  B. Pyramidal degeneration—familial progressive spastic paraplegia
  C. Basal ganglion or extrapyramidal diseases
    1. Dystonia musculorum deformans
    2. Huntington's chorea
  D. Lower motor neuron disease—the amyotonia congenita syndrome: Werdnig-Hoffmann disease (spinal muscular atrophy)
  E. Neuroradicular disease—peroneal muscular atrophy
  F. Leber's familial optic atrophy
V. **Degenerative diseases of uncertain classification**
  A. Ataxia-telangiectasia (syndrome of Louis-Bar, Boder and Sedgwick)
  B. Infantile subacute necrotizing encephalopathy (syndrome of Leigh, Wolf and Feigin)
  C. Acanthocytosis (syndrome of Bassen and Kornzweig)
  D. Heller's infantile dementia

(Continued on next page)

E. Cerebral degeneration with myoclonus
F. Spongy degeneration of white matter (Canavan's syndrome)
G. Congenital indifference to pain (syndrome of Ford and Wilkins)

STORAGE DISEASES: LIPIDOSES AND LEUKODYSTROPHIES

Lipidoses and leukodystrophies are primary disorders in the metabolism of sphingolipids. One or another of these compounds, accumulating in abnormal amounts in the brain, involves the cells of the gray matter in cerebromacular degenerations and the white matter with demyelinization and other disturbances in the leukodystrophies. Whether this deranged metabolism represents overproduction, underutilization or accumulation of products of degeneration is not known.

CEREBROMACULAR DEGENERATIONS

Infantile Amaurotic Family Idiocy (Tay-Sachs Disease). This disorder is the commonest of the cerebromacular degenerations. It is a disease of infancy, with arrest of development, progressive visual loss, spasticity, seizures, wasting, dementia and death. It is inherited as a recessive trait; it has occurred most commonly in eastern European Jewish families, but is not restricted to this ethnic group.

Apparently healthy at birth, the infant after about 5 to 6 months of age becomes apathetic, shows motor regression, and fails to fixate with his eyes. During the next several months he becomes a fat, flaccid, listless child, with hyperactive myotatic reflexes, increased response to sudden sounds, and obvious blindness. The classic macular cherry-red spots, which may be almost black in Negroes, with surrounding gray-white retina and optic atrophy, become apparent. Next is a stage of intense spasticity, with greatly heightened reflexes, extensor plantar responses, decerebrate posturing, increasing dementia and enlargement of the head. Unable to swallow and completely demented, he deteriorates despite all efforts, and usually dies by 3 to 4 years of age. If life is further prolonged, the ventricles may dilate and the head continues to enlarge.

Blood and cerebrospinal fluid determinations remain normal, but the lactic dehydrogenases and aldolases of the cerebrospinal fluid increase in the early stages and decrease toward normal in the chronic phase; the level of serum aldolases increases during active muscular wasting. Circulating lymphocytes may have lipid vacuoles in their cytoplasm.

Variations in the clinical pattern have been observed. These include a rare congenital form leading to death by a few weeks of age, an association with hepatosplenomegaly, and mixed forms having biochemical features of both lipidoses and leukodystrophies. The most important distinction is from Niemann-Pick disease, with which there may be similar macular and cerebral changes; later age at onset, anemia, foam cells, hepatosplenomegaly and the absence of cephalomegaly distinguish it.

The brain is firm and rather shrunken, especially the cerebellum. All surviving neurons, including peripheral ganglia, are ballooned with lipid, and there is a replacement gliosis. The lipid involved is ganglioside, and one of its constituents, neuraminic acid, is greatly increased. The metabolic defect may involve lack of one galactose molecule in the ganglioside.

Late Infantile and Juvenile Amaurotic Family Idiocy. Late infantile and juvenile forms of cerebromacular degeneration also occur. These are hereditary without racial predilection. The *late infantile form* begins in the second or third year of life, often with convulsions, followed by ataxia, dementia, spasticity and blindness. The optic disks atrophy, and the maculae become a reddish-brown. Death occurs within 3 to 5 years.

The *juvenile form, or Batten's disease,* transmitted as an autosomal recessive character, begins at later ages, commonly with visual failure and changes in the fundus, including optic atrophy, "pepper and salt" pigment deposits, gray-brown macular discoloration and loss of the foveal reflex. Mental changes may predominate at the onset, the child being labeled a behavior problem or psychotic for some time. Within 2 to 4 years, vision is gone or mostly so, and the illness proceeds with seizures, extrapyramidal and cerebellar disorders of gait, explosive laughing or crying, and finally extreme dementia, wasting, contractures and death. Rarely, the fundus may remain normal. The course is sometimes slow, patients surviving into the third decade. Distinction from retinitis pigmentosa and syphilitic optic atrophy is difficult in early stages; progressive deterioration and seizures exclude the first, and persistently negative serology excludes syphilis. If real doubt persists, and the family wishes information as a guide to future pregnancies, cortical or rectal biopsy is justified. Lipid vacuoles in lymphocytes of patients and parents are sometimes present, and anserine and carnosine may be present in the urine.

DEMYELINIZING LEUKODYSTROPHIES

Among the variety of conditions described as "diffuse sclerosis," some fairly clear entities have emerged. Genetic patterns of inheritance, usually recessive, are the rule, and all have certain clinical, histologic and biochemical features in common. Progressive dementia, gait disturbances, the evolution of a spastic quadriplegia, often with rigidity in terminal stages, visual loss due to optic atrophy or cortical blindness, or to both, convulsions, dysphagia, wasting and death constitute the clinical course; the patients are usually infants or young children, though older children are not exempt. Early disappearance of myelin, most notable in the corpus callosum and centrum semiovale, the accumulation of abnormal materials (mostly cerebrosides and glycolipids), disappearance of oligodendroglia and decided astrocytic scarring, together with absolute changes in cerebroside or cerebroside-sulfatide ratios in white matter, epitomize the histopathology and known biochemical abnormalities. In some, if not all, the metabolic defect is generalized, involving many viscera. A kinship with the lipidoses is probable, and cases pathologically and chemically intermediate between leukodystrophies and lipidoses are described.

The *infantile form,* or *Krabbe's disease,* begins in the first few months of life with fretfulness and apathy, then rigidity, seizures, vomiting, blindness, dysphagia and death within a year or so of onset. The white matter contains large globular bodies, possibly cerebrosides. The enzyme cerebroside sulfotransferase has been found to be deficient in brains of some patients.

In *Greenfield's disease,* onset is usually in the second year with ataxia and loss of myotatic reflexes, followed by speech impairment, visual loss, dementia and rigidity. Death occurs by about 3 years of age. The brain shows a rather selective destruction of later-myelinized fiber systems, with pronounced loss of oligodendroglia and deposits of material staining positively for glycolipid, and metachromatically with certain aniline dyes.

An even commoner *metachromatic form* may begin somewhat later, and the patients survive for 3 or 4 years. This begins with ataxia and gait disturbance, followed by mild dementia, optic atrophy, pyramidal signs, convulsions and death. Metachromatic material is present in other organs and can be demonstrated in urinary sediment, renal epithelium, and Schwann cells of peripheral nerves, making exact diagnosis during life a possibility. Sulfatide metabolism is deranged. A deficiency in Aryl sulfatase A has been observed in white blood cells and cultured fibroblasts in some patients.

There is no known treatment for these illnesses. Specific diagnosis is often dependent on a cerebral biopsy or postmortem examination. The most that one can conclude is that dementia, fundus changes, and seizures which precede outspoken neurologic signs usually indicate disease of the gray matter, whereas milder dementia with more pronounced physical signs and a later onset of seizures suggests primary involvement of white matter.

OTHER STORAGE DISEASES

Storage of glycogen or a glycolipid complex occurs in some types of glycogenosis or *glycogen storage disease,* most commonly in type II (p. 446). The affected infant begins, at a few weeks of age,

to regress in motor performance and alertness, becomes limp, has occasional cyanotic spells, and vomits. Tachycardia, cardiomegaly often without murmurs, and thick tongue are present. Death usually occurs in the first year, rarely as late as the third. Glycogen content of subcortical gray matter is increased several-fold. Cerebral and cerebellar cortices are spared for a time, but subcortical neurons, glia, and striated and cardiac muscle contain material staining for glycogen. The abnormal form of glycogen has not been identified. The electrocardiogram often shows high-voltage QRS complexes over the ventricles, and short P-R intervals. Differential diagnosis includes the amyotonia congenita syndrome, congenital heart disease, cretinism and mongolism.

In *lipogranulomatosis (Farber-Uzman syndrome)* the infant is well until a few weeks of age, when persistent stridor and periarticular swellings develop. The rheumatoid-like swellings, which are hyperesthetic, but without heat or redness, involve particularly the larger and more movable joints, as well as pressure points of the body. In later months mental and motor retardation without localizing signs of neurologic involvement become apparent. Flexion contractures develop, respiratory distress worsens, and the child dies in his second year. The hemogram is characterized by leukocytosis, granulocytosis and a normocytic, normochromic anemia; the blood chemical values and the urine are normal. Bones are demineralized, with extensive destruction and periarticular calcification of the larger joints.

The mesenchymal cells apparently elaborate mucopolysaccharides, and the nerve cells accumulate them in great excess. In mesenchymal tissues the response is formation of focal granulomatous lesions, in which lipid is secondarily deposited. Synovial and perichondrial tissues, epicardium, endocardium and valves of the heart, and liver all show yellowish plaques containing, in various stages, foci of mucopolysaccharide accumulation, granulomatous infiltrates, fatty accumulation in granulomas and finally scarring and hyalinization. In the nervous system, large neurons, glial cells and autonomic ganglion cells are ballooned out, presumably with mucopolysaccharides; gliosis and focal granulomas also are present. The inheritance, if any, is not known, nor is there any treatment beyond palliative measures.

Angiokeratoma corporis universale diffusum (Fabry's syndrome) is an X-linked disease whose manifestations are constant in the homozygous male, variable in the homozygous female. Symptoms begin as early as the sixth or seventh year of life, as remittent attacks of fever, lightning limb pains, and burning dysesthesias of extremities, intermittent proteinuria or hematuria, and abdominal pain resembling acute appendicitis or renal colic; ankle edema may occur. Small, keratinized macular or papular angiomatous skin lesions appear regularly in males, rarely in fe-

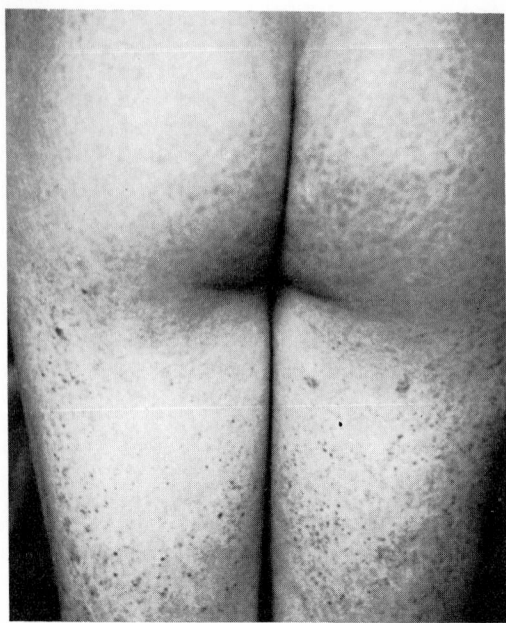

Figure 20-13. Skin lesions in angiokeratoma corporis universale diffusum. (Courtesy of Dr. D. Wise.)

males (Fig. 20-13). They occur initially on the scrotum, then about the umbilicus, girdle area, knees and elbows; they are often inconspicuous and require careful search. Both sexes may have dystrophies of corneal epithelium and irregular dilatations of retinal veins.

In early adult life the recurrent attacks cease, but renal function worsens, proteinuria and sometimes lipiduria are present, ankle edema is common, and skin lesions increase. Anhidrosis and other evidence of impaired vasomotor control appear. Death, due to renal failure, hypertension and cerebral vascular disease, commonly occurs in middle life.

All neurons of the autonomic nervous system, especially peripheral ganglia, dorsal motor vagal nuclei, hypothalamic autonomic nuclei and portions of the amygdaloid complex, show extensive intracellular lipid deposits. The lipid, probably a diaminophosphatide, is present in many other organs. The enzyme ceramide trihexoxidase has been demonstrated to be deficient in some patients. The diagnosis, if clinically in doubt, can be confirmed by rectal biopsy. Treatment is symptomatic.

Hand-Schüller-Christian disease (p. 1479) may involve the brain. Diabetes insipidus, a common feature, is due either to pressure on the hypothalamus and adjacent structures by granulomatous masses or to direct infiltration of these regions. More rarely, patchy areas of demyelination appear in the cerebrum and cerebellum.

In a possibly related condition, strongly familial, *cerebrotendinous xanthomatosis (syndrome of van Bogaert, Scherer and Epstein)*, the patients have xanthomas of tendons, xanthelasma, bilateral cataracts and a slowly progressive cerebellar syndrome, sometimes with myoclonus, sometimes with spasticity; they are either retarded from the outset or have a mild progressive dementia. The neurologic symptoms are due to masses of cholesterol crystals in the cerebellar white matter and cerebral peduncles.

DEMYELINIZING ENCEPHALOMYELOPATHIES

Encephalitis Periaxialis Diffusa (Global Demyelinization; Schilder's Disease). This is a progressive disease featured by bilateral spasticity, cortical blindness and deafness, optic atrophy or neuritis, dementia and death. The distinctive pathologic feature is massive destruction of myelin with production of neutral fats, largely confined to the cerebral hemispheres, with glial scarring and sometimes cavity formation. Arcuate fibers are spared, and neuronal changes are inconspicuous. The disease may be hereditary, but most cases are sporadic. The onset is at any age, but most commonly in later childhood. The child has often been vaguely ill, irritable or doing poorly in school for some months before the beginning of clear-cut symptoms. These usually are disorders of gait due to spasticity; often initially lateralized, they soon become bilateral. The onset may be almost apoplectic, with either optic neuritis or papilledema; in these circumstances the child is acutely ill, and there may be increased intracranial pressure and abducens palsies. Cortical blindness and deafness (sometimes the initial symptoms) or aphasia and apraxia signify extension into the occipital temporal and parietal lobes. Mental deterioration always ensues; convulsions may occur late or relatively early in the course. Optic atrophy is common, but cerebellar or spinal cord signs are unusual. Bronzing of the skin is a rare manifestation; the course varies from weeks to a few years. Addison's disease has been observed in some males with this disease.

Disseminated Sclerosis (Disseminated Demyelinization). This is a slowly progressive disorder in which recurrent attacks, usually interspersed with remissions, involve various parts of the central nervous system, principally the visual, cerebellar and spinal portions. The lesions are multiple plaques in which there is destruction of myelin, relative preservation of axons, phagocytosis of the products of myelin degeneration and finally glial scarring; wallerian degeneration is inconspicuous. The disease may start as (1) attacks of retrobulbar neuritis; (2) recurrent bouts of paraplegia; or (3) cerebellar disorders with disturbances of gait. Nystagmus, ataxia of speech, emotional lability with euphoria and sphincter disturbances are common. The course is long. During attacks and in cases of long standing, the proteins of the cerebrospinal fluid, particularly the gamma globulins, increase, and a paretic gold curve and mild pleocytosis are common. No single laboratory finding is diagnostic.

Disseminated sclerosis is rare in childhood. Most cases so diagnosed are perhaps better described as disseminated encephalomyelitis. In proved cases the common courses are as follows: (1) attacks of retrobulbar neuritis with sudden severe visual loss, central scotomas, loss of color vision and, rarely, swelling of the optic disks. Vision may return after several weeks or may remain permanently defective. In either case the disks become pale temporally. One or several such attacks may occur, and one or both eyes may be involved. During the course of these symptoms or after remissions of months or years, symptoms of spinal cord, cerebellar or cerebral disease appear, usually with weakness of the legs, urinary urgency, frequency or incontinence, cerebellar ataxia of a limb and at times hemiparesis. (2) In other instances the onset is characterized by manifestations of partial or fairly complete transverse myelitis; such attacks may occur repeatedly, often at or near the same site. In this clinical pattern retrobulbar neuritis may, though uncommonly, appear later.

Once the course of the illness is established, diagnosis is not difficult. The initial attack of retrobulbar neuritis cannot be distinguished from retrobulbar neuritis of other causes; some believe that all unexplained retrobulbar neuritis is disseminated sclerosis. In *Leber's hereditary optic atrophy* the central scotomas are usually larger, the loss of vision is less abrupt, and a familial history is usually present. Neuromyelitis optica, whether of spinal cord or optic nerve, may be indistinguishable. The leukodystrophies are not manifest by evidences of spinal cord lesions, and their course is steadily progressive. Disseminated encephalomyelitis is usually much more violent, the child much more ill, and signs of widespread lesions are apparent.

The prognosis is unfavorable, but long periods of remission are frequent, and the outlook is not hopeless. No specific treatment is available. Good nursing care, physiotherapy and especially careful attention to the bladder in acute involvement of the spinal cord are necessary.

Neuromyelitis Optica. Neuromyelitis optica is an illness combining visual loss due to optic neuritis with paraplegia due to transverse myelitis. The lesions typically are multiple foci of softening or necrosis in the optic nerves and chiasm and in the white and the gray matter of the brain and spinal cord. The disease occurs at any age. The onset may be with optic neuritis or transverse myelitis, or both. Fever and signs of systemic illness are generally present, especially in the myelitic type of onset. There is frequently pain and tenderness over the level of the cord lesion, and pain in the eyeball may precede optic neuritis. Polymorphonuclear cells are present in the cerebrospinal fluid. There may be complete destruction of several segments of the cord, and paralysis may ascend rapidly; such patients usually undergo severe muscular wasting. Cerebral signs, such as drowsiness, headache and convulsions, are rare.

Differential diagnosis is that of disseminated sclerosis (see above), which it closely resembles. The distinction may be largely artificial. There is no specific treatment, but since good recovery, for a time at least, is possible, the best of nursing care, tidal drainage of the bladder, respirators for respiratory paralysis, and physiotherapy early in the course are indicated.

DEGENERATIVE DISEASE ASSOCIATED WITH METABOLIC ERRORS

Hepatolenticular Degeneration (Wilson's Disease). This is an inborn metabolic error (see p. 418) affecting chiefly the brain, liver (see p. 842) and kidney; it is inherited as an autosomal recessive. The defect involves ceruloplasmin, the principal copper-containing plasma protein. Deficient synthesis, or possibly the synthesis of abnormal ceruloplasmins, disturbs copper metabolism and transport. Intestinal absorption, tissue deposition, chiefly in brain and liver, and urinary excretion of copper are increased, but total plasma copper and ceruloplasmin copper are reduced. Plasma ceruloplasmin is generally, though not invariably, reduced. A decided aminoaciduria and a negative phosphate balance are other important biochemical abnormalities. The outstanding anatomic lesions are a nodular cirrhosis of the liver, and discoloration, shrinkage or cavitation of the lenticular nuclei.

Familial incidence is common. Age at onset is probably determined by the time required for sufficient copper to accumulate in brain and liver to initiate symptoms; it may vary from 5 or 6 years to the fourth decade. The duration of the disease is usually several years.

In some instances the illness begins with obvious symptoms of liver disease, such as ascites, jaundice and hepatomegaly, which may go on steadily to neurologic involvement, or remit, to be followed much later by central nervous system symptoms. In other instances gradual evolvement of the neurologic disease calls attention to hepatic involvement which was either minimal or overlooked. On occasion the initial manifestations may simulate schizophrenia. If this possibility is not appreciated, it may result in needless therapy and institutionalization.

The common neurologic syndrome includes (1) indistinct, dysarthric speech, advancing dysarthria and mutism; (2) a fixed, unblinking stare with gaping mouth and drooling of saliva; (3) hypertonus and rigidity; (4) tremor at rest and in movement, usually beginning in hand or arm, but soon involving the whole body; (5) seizures (rarely), emotional lability and dementia. The onset at times seems rather abrupt, especially in children, with seizures and some lateralization of signs. Sensation remains intact, but reflexes are often increased, and Babinski's sign may appear. The characteristic *Kayser-Fleischer ring*, a golden brown discoloration in Descemet's membrane, beginning usually superiorly, but often overlooked, is the pathognomonic and most important physical sign. About 80 per cent of all cases ultimately develop osteoporosis and osteochondritis, involving especially the vertebrae, knees and ankles.

If hepatic symptoms preceded or are associated with the neurologic signs, little diagnostic difficulty can exist; if not, Wilson's disease must be distinguished from double athetosis, which is congenital and without resting tremor, from dystonia musculorum deformans, postencephalitic and other dystonic states, and occasionally from hysteria. The corneal ring, which should be looked for with the slit lamp, is unequivocal evidence. Aminoaciduria, high urinary and low plasma copper, abnormal liver function test results, and especially a plasma ceruloplasmin below 8 to 12 mg. per 100 ml. of plasma, are helpful laboratory tests.

Removal of copper by chelating agents such as BAL, versene and penicillamine gives partial and often poorly sustained relief. The most successful regimen combines a diet low in copper, orally administered potassium sulfide to increase fecal excretion of copper, and courses of penicillamine. Siblings and every patient with unexplained cirrhosis or jaundice should be examined carefully to detect early cases.

DEGENERATIVE DISEASES INVOLVING SPECIFIC FIBER TRACTS OR NEURAL GROUPS

SPINOCEREBELLAR ATAXIAS

Friedreich's Ataxia. Friedreich's ataxia is a degenerative disease of unknown cause transmitted by both dominant and recessive patterns. It is characterized by ataxia, loss of reflexes, pes cavus, kyphoscoliosis, cardiac abnormality, nystagmus, optic atrophy, and rarely retinitis pigmentosa. There is degeneration of the dorsal columns and spinocerebellar and pyramidal tracts, of some lemniscal systems, of the cerebellum and of the optic and auditory nerves.

The majority of affected persons become symptomatic before puberty, rarely as early as 3 years of age. Those with the recessive strain tend to have an earlier onset than those with the dominant pattern. The course varies from a few to many years, possibly even to a normal life span in incomplete forms; average duration of life is about 16 years. The first symptoms are either ataxia of gait or aching, cramping pains in the limbs. Then clumsiness of hands, truncal ataxia, dysarthria, kyphoscoliosis, nystagmus and optic atrophy appear. An early sign is pes cavus with hammer toe deformity, which, combined with absent reflexes, constitutes the commonest pattern of the incomplete forms. The deep reflexes disappear early; distal sensory loss, affecting stereognosis, position and vibratory sense, with little decrease in cutaneous sensation, is common. Ataxia is both cerebellar and spinal in type; the slapping, reeling gait and the compensatory movements of the trunk and limbs often suggest chorea. The intensity of the voice fluctuates, and the speech is nasal or explosive. Mental retardation is present in about 10 per cent of cases, and progressive dementia is a late event in about the same proportion.

Visceral symptomatology is of especial interest. Vomiting and other gastrointestinal disturbances occur, but most important are the cardiac symptoms. Tachycardia and loud murmurs are common. The electrocardiogram shows abnormalities of the S-T segment or inversion of the T wave in about half of the cases; the heart has a peculiar interstitial myocarditis and fibrosis. Death may be due to a cardiac arrhythmia or congestive failure.

The condition is to be distinguished from other spinocerebellar ataxias, from peroneal muscular atrophy, to which it may be related, from disseminated sclerosis, especially in older patients, and particularly from rheumatic heart disease with chorea. The last is a common diagnostic error, owing to the ataxic movements, heart murmur, leg pains and electrocardiographic abnormalities. The orthopedic defect and congestive failure should be treated symptomatically.

A number of other forms of hereditary ataxia have been described in children. Usually these are initially purely cerebellar in clinical pattern and later develop pyramidal signs; they may, however, combine ataxia with spasticity and hyperactive reflexes from the start. A positive family history, a slow course and frequently late visual failure and dementia are common. There is no treatment.

PYRAMIDAL DEGENERATION

Familial progressive spastic paraplegia is a hereditary degenerative disease, with destruction of Betz cells and pyramidal tract degeneration, most prominent farthest from the cortex. Its inheritance is variable, but it is usually recessive and sometimes sex-linked; males are more often affected than females. Symptoms usually begin in early childhood, first as stiffness and slowness in walking, then with steady development of a spastic paraplegia. The reflexes are increased, but Babinski's sign may appear late. The sensory systems, sphincters, arms and the intelligence are spared. Flexion deformities, arrest of growth of the lower limbs, and sometimes late dementia, blindness or other signs occur. The strong familial history usually distinguishes it, but in sporadic cases, tumor of the cord, vertebral disease and other degenerative or inflammatory lesions must be excluded by examination of the cerebrospinal fluid and by myelography. No curative treatment is known. Orthopedic measures may aid in relieving the handicap.

BASAL GANGLION OR EXTRAPYRAMIDAL DISEASES

Dystonia Musculorum Deformans. Torsion spasm and dystonic movements may occur in several disease processes, such as postencephalitic syndromes and Wilson's disease. There is, however, a fairly distinct clinical entity, dystonia musculorum deformans, in which the chief symptom is maintained torsion of limbs or trunk. The cause is unknown; the disease occurs commonly in eastern European Jewish families, the inheritance pattern being that of an autosomal dominant. Pathologically, there is loss of cells, especially of the large ones, in the basal ganglia.

The illness begins before puberty, usually by about 8 to 10 years of age, without sex predilection, but at times with a definite familial pattern. The first sign is a fixed posturing of one leg, with the foot extended and held in pes cavus with the toes flexed. Soon the thigh flexes and adducts, and the knee bends; then the other leg becomes involved, and the child walks on tiptoe. Extreme lumbar lordosis appears early. After some years the arms rotate internally, adduct, extend at the elbows and flex at the wrists. Finally, strong involuntary torsion movements appear, which are really a powerful exaggeration of the posturing of legs, trunk and arms; any movement, particularly walking, brings on fantastic writhing. These movements, absent in sleep, are greatly worsened by emotion, and may suggest hysteria, but psychotherapy is not helpful. Reflexes, sensation, sphincters, vision, speech, swallowing, and movements of the fingers are not impaired. The condition is distinguished from double athetosis, hepatolenticular degeneration and postencephalitic states by the bizarre picture described, the Jewish parentage, family history and the absence of hepatic involvement or of a history of encephalitis. The course is long, the disease ultimately confining the patient. There is no effective medical treatment; pallidotomy sometimes relieves the movements dramatically.

Huntington's Chorea. Huntington's chorea is a degenerative disease of genetic transmission (dominant) and is characterized by progressive choreic movements, dementia and death. The brain is atrophic, particularly the frontal lobes; the ventricles are enlarged, and there is a widespread, slow degeneration of neurons, greatest in the putamen and in the caudate nuclei. Unaffected members of the families have an unusually high incidence of psychopathic or psychotic behavior and suicide. The onset is usually in the fourth decade, but may occur as early as 6 years, with death by 10 years. The first symptom in the child may be an emotional disturbance, choreic movements, seizures or, perhaps most commonly, a progressive rigidity without definite involuntary movements. The choreic movements affect the face, trunk and arms at first, the large joints being more involved than the small ones. The movements initially are exaggerations of voluntary ones and tend to remain a crude parody of willed motions. Reflexes are normal or heightened; the cranial nerves at first are intact, but pseudobulbar palsy and swallowing difficulties finally appear. Progressive dementia, rigidity or the violence of the movements ultimately confines the patient.

Huntington's chorea is distinguished from Sydenham's chorea and congenital chorea principally by its progressive course, dementia and family history; the first and second are, of course, not initially apparent, and the third may be carefully concealed. Hepatolenticular degeneration is excluded by its corneal ring, hepatic involvement and tremor. There is no known treatment, though large doses of rauwolfia derivatives have been suggested for reduction of chorea.

LOWER MOTOR NEURON DISEASE

Werdnig-Hoffmann Disease. This disorder, identified by some as *spinal muscular atrophy*, is one of the conditions included in the amyotonia congenita syndrome (see below). It is characterized by progressive hypotonia and wasting of skeletal muscle in infancy and childhood as a result of degeneration of motor neurons. There is no evidence for consistent involvement of other parts of the nervous system, and the condition usually terminates fatally at an early age.

The cause is unknown. The essential lesion is progressive loss of motor neurons, with little reaction in the surrounding tissue (Fig. 20-14, C), beginning or most severe at the caudal end of the spinal cord, extending cranially and finally involving cranial nerve motor nuclei. The anterior roots are thin and pale (Fig. 20-14, B). The skeletal muscle shows atrophy or denervation as manifest by narrowed fibers, increased sarcolemmic nuclei, preserved cross striations and replacement by fibrous tissue (Fig. 20-14, A). Cerebellar defects and absence or underdevelopment of Betz cells in the motor cortex have been described.

The condition is familial in at least half the cases and may occur in successive generations; its inheritance is not clearly understood, though it is probably recessive, and sexes are equally affected. Fetal movements are often feeble or absent. The infant is born limp, flaccid and areflexic, but sensation, the cranial nerves, sphincter functions and intelligence are adequate. The infant lies in a froglike position and can be folded or doubled into almost any grotesque posture. The muscles are thin, soft and difficult to palpate; the only limb movements are feeble ones of the digits.

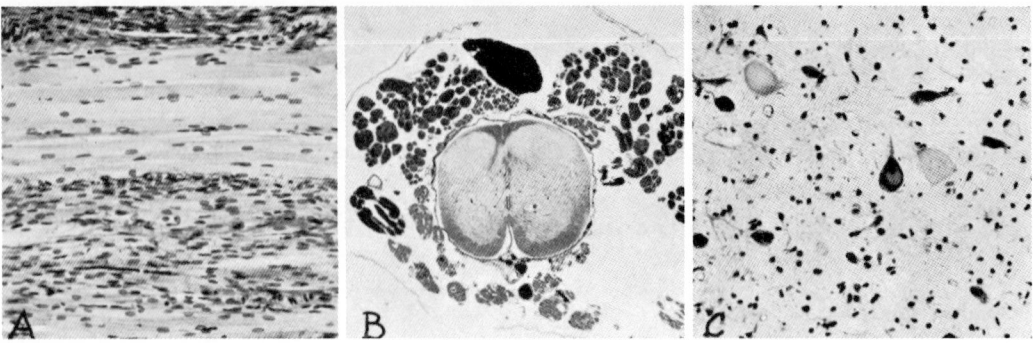

Figure 20-14. Werdnig-Hoffmann disease. *A*, Fascicular atrophy of muscle. *B*, Pallor of ventral roots. *C*, Degenerating motor neurons.

Side-to-side movements of the head are usually preserved. Paralysis of the intercostal muscles occurs before that of the diaphragm, resulting in sternocostal retractions and respiratory difficulty. Fibrillations of the tongue appear, sucking is lost, and the infant usually dies of respiratory infection by 8 to 12 months of age.

Variations in the time of onset or the rate of progression are common. Fetal movements may have been present, and the infant at birth appears to be normal, only to manifest the illness in the first few days or weeks. In other instances the symptoms may not appear for several months or even a year or two. In such instances the progress is slow, growth for a time outstrips degeneration, and the infant slowly makes some developmental progress; a few may live for years, some well beyond puberty. Respiratory infections are a constant hazard, and avoidance of gross spinal curvature and deformity is almost impossible.

Amyotonia Congenita Syndrome. Werdnig-Hoffmann disease is one of the many entities comprising the amyotonia congenita syndrome, which in actuality only implies extreme hypotonia in an infant. Other disorders include the following:

1. Diseases of the central nervous system or neuromotor unit—
   atonic diplegia
   Cerebral lipidoses
   Cerebral glycogenosis (glycogen storage disease) (p. 440)
   Kernicterus
   Neonatal poliomyelitis
   Infantile polyneuritis
   Spinal cord lesion—birth injury or congenital tumor
   Congenital or neonatal myasthenia gravis
   Congenital myopathies
   Polymyositis
2. Non-neurologic diseases
   Deficiency states such as rickets and scurvy
   Chronic infection
   Malnutrition
   Congenital defects, such as arachnodactyly
3. Benign congenital hypotonia

Differential diagnosis of the amyotonia congenita syndrome can be difficult. The diagnosis of *Werdnig-Hoffmann* disease depends on (1) a history of familial incidence and diminished or absent fetal movements; (2) the presence of extreme hypotonia and areflexia in an otherwise normal infant at or soon after birth, or develop-

ment of weakness and hypotonia in an infant or young child; (3) generally normal laboratory studies, except for muscle biopsy and perhaps electromyography. The infant with atonic diplegia may be exceedingly limp, but the reflexes are retained; there is often a history of abnormal pregnancy or labor, the infant makes powerful spontaneous movements at intervals, and signs of mental retardation soon become obvious. The cerebral degenerative diseases, lipidoses and cerebral glycogen storage disease may parallel Werdnig-Hoffmann disease in time of onset and general flaccidity, but the reflexes are retained and the progressive loss of vision and dementia are distinctive. A history of unusual neonatal jaundice and early athetoid movements suggests kernicterus as a sequel of hemolytic disease of the newborn. Neonatal poliomyelitis is best excluded by serologic studies, and infantile polyneuritis by an onset following intestinal or respiratory infection and by a maintained high cerebrospinal fluid protein level. Transient neonatal myasthenia affects only the infant of a myasthenic mother; as in congenital myasthenia, there is early involvement of ocular and bulbar muscles and a diagnostic response to Prostigmin. Congenital myopathies or polymyositis may require muscle biopsy to distinguish them.

The most important differential diagnosis is with the syndrome of *benign congenital hypotonia*, which at times is familial. This diagnosis should be made with caution; some patients so diagnosed have subsequently been found to have slowly progressive myopathies. Affected infants usually have moved well in utero; some tendon reflexes can always be obtained, and no other neurologic signs are present. Despite striking hypotonia and hypermobility of joints, the child occasionally makes strong movements. Sternocostal retraction and respiratory distress may occur, but evidence of progression or fibrillations of the tongue do not appear. Physical developmental achievements are delayed; few walk before 18 to 24 months of age, and many not until 3 to 5 years. Ultimately all are able to get about, and about half of them are quite normal by 8 or 9 years of age. In others the muscles remain feeble and may become contracted, but the joints always remain hypermobile. Muscle biopsy and electromyograms reveal no abnormalities. Treatment is limited to orthopedic assistance in the avoidance of contractures.

NEURORADICULAR DISEASE

Peroneal muscular atrophy (Charcot-Marie-Tooth disease) is a hereditary disease characterized by distal wasting, weakness and loss of reflexes in the extremities.

Pathologically, there is degeneration, apparently first in the motor nerves, then in the roots with some loss of motor cells. Similar changes appear later in the sensory nerves and dorsal root ganglia, and secondary degeneration extends up the dorsal columns. The muscles involved show atrophy of denervation.

The disease is transmitted genetically, but the pattern is not clear. Symptoms generally begin in late childhood or adolescence; progress is slow, and the disease is compatible with long life. Wasting, first of the extensors, everters and intrinsic muscles of the feet, produces dropped foot and equinovarus deformity; the peroneal, tibial and finally the calf muscles are involved, but wasting seldom goes much above the knee, thus producing the characteristic storklike leg. Loss of muscular strength parallels loss of bulk, and fasciculations may be present. The ankle reflexes disappear, but the patellar ones persist. Cramps and paresthesias may be present early, but sensory loss is slight, involving mostly positional and vibratory senses. Similarly, wasting and sensory and reflex losses later involve the forearms. Sphincters are not often affected; optic atrophy may occur late. The extremities are cyanotic, cold and mottled; after years, atrophy of bones and perforating ulcers of the feet appear. Incomplete forms, especially clawfoot with absent ankle jerk, are common.

The cerebrospinal fluid is usually unchanged, though the protein concentration may be increased. Conduction rates in peripheral nerves may be reduced, both in patients and in clinically unaffected members of the family. Familial incidence, slow course and absence of muscular tenderness distinguish it from chronic polyneuritis; absence of ataxia, nystagmus, widespread loss of reflexes and cardiac changes differentiate it from Friedreich's disease. Interstitial hypertrophic polyneuritis is characterized by miotic, fixed pupils, and palpable peripheral nerves, not present in peroneal atrophy. The disability is surprisingly slight in view of the wasting. Braces and fusion of ankle joints keep the patient ambulatory.

LEBER'S FAMILIAL OPTIC ATROPHY

Leber's disease is a hereditary degeneration of the retina and papillomacular bundle with serious loss of vision; at times there are associated neurologic symptoms. The ganglionic and, to a less extent, the inner nuclear layers of the retina are degenerated, and the axons and myelin sheaths of the papillomacular bundle are destroyed without inflammatory response, whereas the peripheral fibers are partially spared. There is transneuronal degeneration in the lateral geniculate bodies and in the optic radiation. The remainder of the brain is normal.

The condition is usually inherited as a sex-linked recessive, appearing in males, but dominant strains and occurrence in females are known. The onset is usually in the late teens, but may be in childhood or adult life. There is rapid loss of vision, which at times begins in one eye, but soon becomes bilateral. Large, absolute central scotomas and relative peripheral scotomas accompany mild swelling of the disks, which is replaced by pallor in a few weeks. The rest of the fundus is normal. Vision fails rapidly for a few weeks, then becomes stationary and remains so for years. Complete blindness is rare. Associated neurologic manifestations, such as epilepsy, ataxia, club feet, mental deficiency and sphincter involvement, are not uncommon. The family history, rate of onset, bilateral visual loss and large scotomas usually distinguish it from retrobulbar or optic neuritis. A suggested cause is a defect in cyanide metabolism with inability to convert cyanide to thiocyanate. There is no known treatment.

DEGENERATIVE DISEASES OF UNCERTAIN CLASSIFICATION

Ataxia-Telangiectasia (see also page 481). This autosomal recessive syndrome is characterized by (1) ataxia, apparent when the child begins to walk; (2) oculocutaneous telangiectases (Fig. 20-15) appearing at 4 to 6 years of age, first on the bulbar conjunctivas; (3) frequent otic and respiratory infections; (4) progressive course with mental deterioration; and (5) in many affected persons evidence of an immunologic disorder (see p. 482).

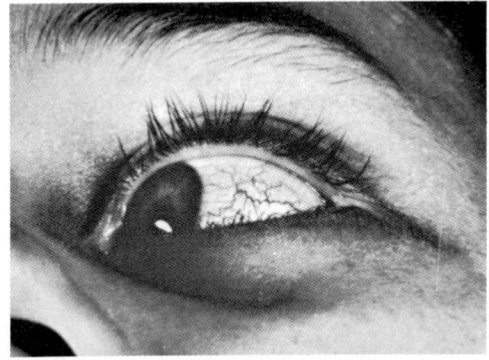

Figure 20-15. Ataxia-telangiectasia. Arterial telangiectasis on bulbar conjunctiva.

The ataxia is cerebellar in type, the myotatic reflexes are diminished or absent, but sensation is intact and plantar responses remain flexor. Later in the disease, choreo-athetoid movements, dysarthria, drooling and mutism develop. The telangiectases, primarily arterial, are often mistaken for conjunctivitis, but soon appear on ears, transnasal (butterfly) area of face, palate, sternum, antecubital and popliteal fossae and dorsa of extremities. Eye movements are jerky and irregular, with nystagmus and spasmodic blinking; these are worse on voluntary gaze than on reflex following. By adolescence, most patients are confined to a chair or bed and are moderately to markedly mentally retarded. Most die in their early teens, though some survive into the third decade. The conspicuous neuropathologic finding is cerebellar cortical degeneration with meningeal telangiectases. Treatment is symptomatic.

Infantile Subacute Necrotizing Encephalopathy (Leigh's Encephalomyelopathy). (See also page 440.) This progressive illness usually begins in early infancy; about half of the reported cases have been familial, present data suggesting an autosomal recessive inheritance. Some cases begin subacutely with feeding difficulties, poor weight gain, diarrhea, irritability and lethargy; others start with focal, myoclonic or generalized seizures. In both forms the child becomes limp, and bizarre movements of the eyes develop, along with ocular and other cranial nerve palsies, optic atrophy and either spasticity or hypotonia. Most laboratory findings are unremarkable, though elevated blood pyruvate and lactate levels have been reported. The electroencephalogram is abnormal, but no diagnostic pattern is described. In some instances patients have been retarded in motor and mental performance for months before the above-mentioned symptoms appear. The course varies from a few weeks to a few years.

The distinctive pathologic change is a symmetric patchy necrosis of gray matter, with relative preservation of neurons, and hyperplasia of endothelium. Such lesions are constant in the brain stem (Fig. 20-16) and may involve the spinal cord, striate bodies, cerebellum, cerebral cortex, optic tracts and cerebellar peduncles. There is some histologic resemblance to Wernicke's polioencephalitis, but mammillary bodies are unaffected. Treatment is symptomatic, but possible improvement has been reported with lipoic acid.

Acanthocytosis (Abeta-Lipoproteinemia). (See also pages 418 and 812.) This illness begins in infancy as a syndrome resembling celiac disease. Areflexia has been noted by the sixth year, but the child is usually clinically well until 8 to 10 years of age, when cerebellar tremor, ataxia and some involuntary movements appear, and worsen steadily. Proprioception is impaired, and a glove-and-stocking sensory loss develops. Increasing ataxia, muscular wasting, loss of vision due to atypical retinitis pigmentosa, and in some a

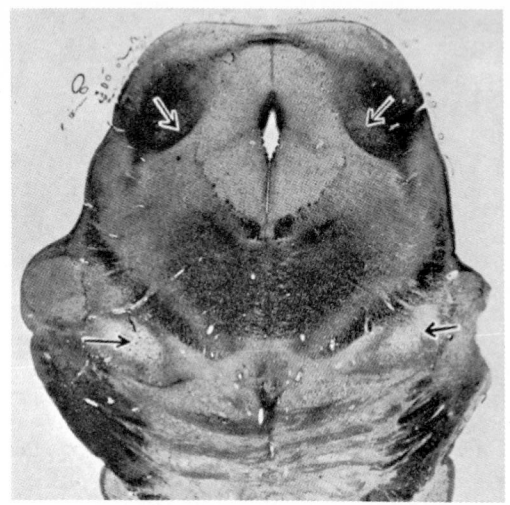

Figure 20-16. Infantile subacute disseminated necrotizing encephalopathy. Arrows indicate necroses in midbrain.

moderate dementia may render the patient bedfast by his late teens or early twenties. Gamma and beta globulins are decreased; total serum cholesterol is exceptionally low, and beta lipoproteins are absent. Acanthocytes, erythrocytes with thornlike projections in the peripheral blood, are a characteristic manifestation. The condition is presumed to be due to a rare autosomal recessive gene.

A variant form, in which beta-lipoproteins are normal and intestinal absorption is adequate, has recently been described. The neurologic symptoms vary from a syndrome resembling Friedreich's ataxia to one simulating Huntington's chorea.

Heller's Infantile Dementia. This singular illness is described as a progressive dementia without other signs of organic neurologic disease. Pathologic data are scanty; sclerotic, irregularly arranged cortical neurons, lipid deposits, meningeal fibrosis, degeneration of white matter and glial abnormalities have been described, but none is constant, nor has a definitive histopathologic pattern been described. The onset is in the second to fifth year of life. The child, previously well or perhaps after an infection, becomes irritable and disobedient, has temper tantrums, may manifest perverse behavior, and then begins to regress in speech and mentation. Within a year he is mute, pays no attention to speech, often has tics, is incontinent, and may have to be fed. All observers stress the intelligent expression said to persist despite extreme dementia. The patients survive many years.

This disorder should be regarded as a syndrome including diverse disease states. A few are progressive degenerative diseases; the majority are more probably due to static defects, or allied to the "brain-injury" syndrome

Cerebral Degeneration with Myoclonus. Myoclonic jerks are common to a number of disease states affecting nerve cells, including some epileptic states. In recent years the syndrome of infantile myoclonic seizures or hypsarrhythmia (p. 1252) has been recognized as a clinical entity. There are at least 2 other conditions in which myoclonus with or without generalized seizures is associated with signs of cortical, subcortical and cerebellar involvement and progressive degeneration. In the first the illness may begin in infancy with head-dropping spells and myoclonic jerks and progress steadily to ataxia, rigidity, cortical deafness, dementia, constant status epilepticus and blindness without optic atrophy. A juvenile form differs principally in that the course is slower, and the extrapyramidal and cerebellar signs are more obvious. The lesions consist of degeneration and neurosis, leading to status spongiosus and gliosis in outer cortical layers, basal nuclei, and the dentate and olivary nuclei.

The second form, *Unverricht's myoclonus epilepsy,* is a hereditary disease, probably recessive, characterized by convulsions, massive myoclonic jerks, ataxia or choreo-athetosis and dementia. Intracytoplasmic inclusion bodies in neurons and degeneration and gliosis of the outer cortical layers are characteristic pathologic features. The onset is prepubertal, and the first symptom is usually a convulsion. Minimal cerebellar ataxia or extrapyramidal signs and myoclonic jerks are usually present, but often overlooked. In succeeding years the child becomes irritable and regresses mentally. As dementia slowly increases, the convulsions disappear and are replaced by massive myoclonic jerks involving the shoulders, trunk and proximal parts of the limbs. They are so violent that they prevent walking, ultimately confine the patient and may conceal the evolution of cerebellar and extrapyramidal signs. No treatment is known other than the use of anticonvulsants for symptomatic relief.

Spongy Degeneration of White Matter. Symptoms of this disease, which is often familial and has been described mostly in Jews, are usually noted in the third to ninth month of life. They include progressive dementia, spasticity, cortical blindness and deafness, and sometimes seizures and enlarging head. Death usually occurs after 6 to 24 months, but a few children survive for years. Subarachnoid fluid is increased, and the brain is large and heavy. There is very little myelin in the cerebral white matter; in its place there is a mass of neuroglia and naked axons, which extend into the deeper layers of the cortex, converting it into a spongy zone. Lipid fractions of white matter are greatly reduced, resembling those of a premature infant.

Refsum's Syndrome. (See also page 1390.) Symptoms of this familial illness appear between 4 and 8 years of age and progress slowly; they include progressive nerve deafness, atypical retinitis pigmentosa with night blindness and miotic pupils, ichthyosis, ataxia and cerebellar symptoms, suppression and loss of myotatic reflexes, lightning, polyneuritic pains, pes cavus and mental deterioration. The important laboratory findings include increased cerebrospinal fluid protein without pleocytosis, and abnormalities of the QRS complex and Q-T interval on the electrocardiogram. The defect appears to be one of degradation of exogenously derived phytonic acid to carbon dioxide; phytonic acid is increased in the plasma. The mechanism may be interference with the function of fat-soluble vitamins.

Congenital Indifference to Pain. Congenital indifference to pain appears in at least 2 forms. In both forms it is noted early in life that the child pays little or no attention to ordinarily painful stimuli. These children are subject to unusually severe injuries from burns and other trauma, owing to their failure to break contact promptly with the traumatizing agent.

In one form the children may be mentally normal, though speech defects, learning disabilities and behavioral disorders are not infrequent. No physical or other abnormalities can be demonstrated, beyond the indifference to pain and the injuries consequent to it. In such children the handicap lessens as the child grows older, and the defect is thought by many to be an asymbolia for pain.

In the other form the children are mentally slow, if not frankly and severely retarded; the condition is often familial and is due to an intrauterine degeneration or congenital absence of sensory ganglion cells, from the trigeminal ganglion downward. The deep tendon reflexes are absent, and sweating disturbances may be present. Death due to hyperthermia has been reported.

The syndromes must be distinguished from syringomyelia, the stoicism of defective or disturbed children, and, in the second form, from familial dysautonomia (p. 1308). Treatment consists solely in protecting the child from trauma and from dehydration during illnesses.

NEUROLOGIC SYNDROMES PECULIAR TO CHILDHOOD

The following illnesses seem to be limited almost entirely to children. Syndromes rather than diseases, they are encountered frequently enough to deserve mention.

Spasmus Nutans (Nodding Spasms). This condition, found mainly in infants, is characterized by 3 cardinal symptoms: irregular movements of one or both eyes, head-nodding and deviations of the head. The cause is unknown. Vitamin A or D deficiency, wasting illness and in particular poor lighting of nurseries, which might delay development of optic fixation, have been suggested. The disease is more common in the low-income group, and symptoms usually begin in the winter, but convincing evidence for any causative factor is lacking.

The onset may be as early as a few weeks of age or as late as 3 years, but most often occurs between 4 and 12 months. There is no sex dominance; more than one sibling may be affected. Abnormal movements of the head or eye may be the first or the only symptoms. Head movement occurs in about 80 per cent of cases and perhaps is the most common initial symptom. It is slow, inconstant and irregular and occurs in any direction; it disappears during sleep or when the child lies down. Eye movements, which also occur in about 80 per cent of cases, usually begin in one eye and are almost always more pronounced in one than in the other. They are rapid, inconstant, irregular jerkings of small amplitude in any direction and without definite components. They disappear when the eyes are covered or the child sleeps, but are instigated or made worse by holding the head still. Deviations of the head, which occur in about one third of cases, are in any direction and do not lead to contractures; they may help the child to focus. Nonparalytic strabismus occurs at times; there are no other ocular or neurologic signs. The condition clears spontaneously, usually within several months. At times there are temporary exacerbations.

Congenital nystagmus is differentiated from spasmus nutans by the family history, earlier onset, compensatory head movements and failure to improve.

No treatment of spasmus nutans is necessary beyond ensuring adequate light and nutrition and reassuring the parents.

Acute Cerebellar Ataxia. Cerebellar syndromes after infections are not uncommon; measles and chickenpox are known precursors. Many cases of acute ataxia in childhood, however, have no apparent cause, and, since they are seldom fatal, the pathologic lesions are not known. The syndrome is commonest in young children who have begun to walk, usually between 1 and 4 years of age. There may be no history of previous illness, or only a slight cold. The onset is usually rather sudden. The child may vomit occasionally for a day or so; the principal feature is the evolution over a few hours to 3 or 4 days of a decided unsteadiness of gait; the child often refuses to walk or even to lift his head. Some irritability or change in personality is present, but convulsions, stupor or signs of systemic illness are usually absent. Physical signs include unsteadiness, wide-based gait, cerebellar ataxia, heightened or depressed reflexes, hypotonia and fugitive extensor plantar responses. Irregular or rapid jerking of the eyes, when the child attempts to fix his gaze, is common. The cerebrospinal fluid at the onset is normal or contains a few lymphocytes; after days or weeks the protein level may rise to 200 mg. per 100 ml. or more. Beyond a mild peripheral leu-

kocytosis and variable electroencephalographic abnormalities in about half the cases, no other laboratory data are abnormal. The unsteadiness and irritability may persist for weeks or months, but usually disappear completely; residual disability is rare.

Such cases must be differentiated from brain tumor, cerebral degenerative diseases, poliomyelitis and the early stages of polyneuritis. Absence of increased intracranial pressure and the course of the illness are the most valuable differential points. Tumor or degenerative disease inevitably advances, the former with signs of increased intracranial pressure, localizing signs or both. Facial diplegia, distal sensory loss and usually complete areflexia distinguish polyneuritis. There is a possibility that the condition represents cerebellar involvement by any of the various encephalitic viruses or perhaps by a variety of toxic agents. Clinically, classic cases have been proved to be due to ECHO, Coxsackie and poliomyelitis viruses. Treatment is entirely symptomatic.

ACUTE INFANTILE HEMIPLEGIA
(POLIO-ENCEPHALITIS OF MARIE-STRÜMPELL)

This syndrome of hemiplegia with lateralized seizures and usually severe neurologic residuals has a sudden onset. The cause is almost certainly manifold. Thrombosis on subintimal plaques in cerebral arteries, thrombosis of the carotid artery, embolism of unidentified source, intracerebral rupture of vascular anomalies and cortical thrombophlebitis are possibilities.

In the classic form the illness begins in a previously healthy child at 1 to 2 years of age with an apoplectic onset of seizures. These may be generalized, with greater severity on one side, or lateralized. Between seizures, the more severely affected limbs are flaccid and hemiplegic. The child is comatose and soon has fever and some leukocytosis. Meningeal signs are absent, and there are usually no changes in the cerebrospinal fluid at this time. The electroencephalogram shows principally voltage depression or absence over the affected hemisphere.

Coma persists for hours or days, but few children die. Cells appear in the cerebrospinal fluid after some days, probably as a reaction to necrotic tissue. Movement slowly returns to the affected side, first in the extremity last involved by seizures. Walking and talking, especially with right hemiplegias, must be learned again. The neurologic residuals include (1) hemiparesis, in about three quarters of the cases, with growth arrest and often choreo-athetoid movements of the affected side; (2) recurrent lateralized seizures, which may worsen the hemiparetic signs transitorily, in about two thirds; (3) intellectual disturbances in about three quarters, ranging from learning disorders to severe mental deficiency.

Hemianopsia is infrequent. Second attacks are almost unknown.

In the acute stage, pneumoencephalography may show swelling of the affected hemisphere and shift of the ventricles; later there is dilatation of the involved lateral ventricle and lateralized cortical atrophy. The skull grows asymmetrically, the vault on the affected side smaller, the bone thicker, the petrous ridge higher and the frontal sinus larger than those on the unaffected side.

This condition may be distinguished from meningitis, encephalitis and hemorrhagic encephalopathies by the tendency to lateralization of the signs and by normality of the cerebrospinal fluid in the early stage. Diseases with vascular changes such as the collagen diseases and homocystinuria can be distinguished by appropriate tests. Tumors and abscess lack such apoplectic onset and cause increased intracranial pressure. Occasionally severe and/or repeated convulsions may call attention to or worsen a hemiparesis of congenital origin, previously undetected, and cause some confusion.

In infants, usually under 1 year of age, hemiplegias and seizures occasionally occur during severe respiratory and intestinal infections. These infants are gravely ill; the signs are often bilateral, but more notable on one side. Pleocytosis of the cerebrospinal fluid appears early. These cases probably represent cortical thrombophlebitis or extensions of thrombosis from dural sinus occlusions into the cortical veins. In older children the onset may be slower with recurring attacks of numbness or weakness of an arm, leg or entire side over a period of hours or days before a persisting hemiplegia develops. Some have been proved to be due to thrombosis of the carotid artery.

Treatment. In the acute state, treatment consists in sedation or rectal anesthesia to control seizures, fluids, treatment of any infection, avoidance of secondary infection and possibly hypothermia. Since endarterectomy may improve the prognosis for carotid thrombosis, any atypical case should have arteriograms performed within the first few hours; if obstruction is found, immediate surgical removal of accessible clots should be attempted.

In chronic cases, physiotherapy and special schooling are necessary. Seizures are so frequently a residual that an anticonvulsant drug should be given routinely. Rarely, intractable seizures or behavior disorders at later ages may benefit by hemispherectomy.

CRANIOCEREBRAL AND SPINAL TRAUMA

The symptoms caused by a blow on the head are due mainly to differential movement of the brain and skull. Brief loss of consciousness is caused either by the effect of a sudden shift of intracranial contents on the hypothalamus and periaqueductal gray matter or by less-understood direct effects on nerve cells. At points where shifting of the brain brings it against the skull, multiple hemorrhagic foci or wedges of cortical necrosis appear; these lesions, with some swelling of the brain, may produce moderately prolonged unconsciousness and mild neurologic signs. Severe swelling of the brain or intracerebral hematoma compresses large vessels, damages widely distant parts of the brain and causes prolonged unconsciousness and localizing neurologic signs.

In open head injuries the skull and the dura are lacerated. The child is usually unconscious and in shock and has localizing signs. Such an injury is a grave surgical emergency, requiring immediate treatment of shock and debridement of the wound. Most head injuries of childhood are closed ones with or without fractures; operation is indicated for elevation of depressed bone, or when there is suspicion of epidural, subdural or intracerebral hematoma (p. 1288).

Mild Closed Injury. The usual history is that after a fall the child was unconscious for a few seconds, and then seemed pale and shaken or screamed lustily; 2 to 4 hours later he became irritable and drowsy and vomited, and his pulse rate was somewhat reduced. Neurologic signs are generally absent, though in rare instances transient blindness of a few hours' duration has been observed, especially with parieto-occipital trauma.

The management is careful, repeated observation of vital and neurologic signs to detect possible development of intracranial hypertension. A roentgenogram of the skull should be obtained, and the child put in a quiet room where pulse, respirations, blood pressure, state of consciousness, size and reactivity of pupils and appearance of any neurologic signs are recorded every half-hour for 4 hours. If no change occurs, observation of pulse, respirations and state of consciousness is continued at home, the child being wakened at least every 2 hours to make sure that he is not drifting into stupor. Recovery is usually complete in 12 to 24 hours.

Severe Closed Injury. The child is usually stuporous or unconscious, though seldom in deep shock. The presence of shock should lead to search for other injuries. A patent airway should be ensured at once, by intubation or tracheotomy if necessary, and shock should be treated. A sequential record is begun of vital signs, state of consciousness, pupillary size and reactions and such lateralizing neurologic signs as diminution of spontaneous or induced movement and appearance of Babinski's sign. Since such signs often fluctuate, it is the trend in one or another direction, rather than isolated observations, that is important. Rising blood pressure, slowing pulse and respiration and deepening stupor mean increasing intracranial pressure; if lateralized pupillary dilatation or motor signs appear, intracranial hematoma must be sought for.

Intravenous fluids should be given cautiously, glucose in 0.45 per cent saline solution being safest; oral or stomach tube feeding should be started as soon as possible. Fever, often due to the injury alone, responds to aspirin, sponging, and cooling by fans or air conditioners. Lumbar puncture is not generally advisable, but may help to control restlessness, for which paraldehyde rectally is also valuable. Opiates and mydriatics should not be used. Infection or suspicion of a basal fracture is an indication for antibiotic therapy.

Corticosteroids may be effective in combating brain swelling. Dexamethasone, 0.2 to 0.3 mg. per kg. per day, is in common use. Half the daily total is given as an initial dose, and the child is then maintained on divided doses every 4 to 6 hours. Controlled hypothermia, at 90 to 92°F., may have some benefit.

The presence or absence of *skull fracture* seldom changes the management. A linear fracture across a suture or a diastatic fracture in the infant increases the possibility of epidural hematoma. A depressed fracture in a newborn infant should be elevated as soon as discovered; in older children, elevation is deferred until edema subsides. A basal fracture is probably present if there is (1) bleeding from the nose, ears, pharynx or bilaterally into the orbits; (2) a peripheral facial palsy; or (3) escape of cerebrospinal fluid from the nose or ear. Antibiotics should be given to such patients, and the meningeal fistula closed surgically.

Post-traumatic syndromes include epilepsy, psychotic states and neuroses. Epilepsy follows closed head injury in about 3 per cent of cases, open head injury in as many as 50 per cent; it appears to be related to the site and nature of the injury, and is more frequent in patients with a family history of seizures. Its onset cannot be predicted by post-traumatic electroencephalographic abnormalities unless they become paroxysmal. The seizures are almost always controllable by drugs; the child recovering from an open injury or a severe closed one should be maintained on anticonvulsant therapy for at least a year.

Post-traumatic psychotic states are rarely persistent. Neuroses, headache, giddiness, fatigability, poor concentration and behavior disorders are not uncommon. Malingering, unless fostered by parents, is rare. Encouragement, reassurance and optimism on the part of the physician and parents are the best prevention and therapy.

Injury of the Spinal Cord. Much rarer but more crippling than head injury, spinal cord trauma is almost always associated with fracture or dislocation of vertebrae. In breech delivery excessive traction on the trunk before the aftercoming head is delivered is a cause of severe injury; a distinct snap may be heard. The lesion is a fusiform, central hemorrhagic necrosis in the lower cervical and upper thoracic portions; at times there is actual severance. The infant is paraplegic below the lesion, and there is urinary retention. Roentgenograms of the vertebral column usually show no lesion. Such an injury may be confused with congenital defects of the cord, with amyotonia congenita or congenital cord tumor. The mortality rate is high. In those who survive, recovery of function is insignificant, and arrest of growth occurs below the lesion. Only supportive treatment is possible.

In the older child, falls, blows or diving accidents are common causes of cord lesions; the usual sites are C 5–6 and T 12–L 1. Paraplegia is usually complete at first with sensory, motor and sphincter paralysis; tendon reflexes below the lesion are absent for some days. Fractures and dislocations are usually present. The child should be immobilized, from the moment of injury if possible, to prevent further injury; all movement of the vertebral column should be carefully avoided. Casts, hyperextension and traction are used for simple and compressed fractures; laminectomy is indicated only for comminuted fractures. High cervical lesions may require a respirator; tidal drainage of the bladder, maintained until voluntary or automatic control returns, and scrupulous care of the skin are essential. The return of function is usually poor. Paradoxical flexor plantar responses, appearing early, have bad prognostic significance.

DISEASES OF THE SPINAL CORD

The spinal cord suffers with the rest of the nervous system in most neurologic disease. A few conditions, however, require special mention. Nuclear aplasias and localized developmental defects may affect any motor nucleus, in which case the muscle supplied is small or absent. Nuclei for the anterior abdominal muscles and for parts of the pectoral muscle and, in the brain stem, the facial and abducens nuclei are common sites. Defective development of preganglionic autonomic centers or more widespread congenital malformations may be associated, as in the syndrome of bilateral congenital hydroureter and hydronephrosis, with absence of abdominal muscles and of motor nuclei and autonomic centers in the spinal cord.

In *syringomyelia* a tubelike cavity develops within the spinal cord. Originating in the lower cervical portion, it extends downward or upward.

A similar slitlike cavity in the lower brain stem is termed *syringobulbia*. The formation of the cavity destroys parts of the anterior and posterior horns, commissures and fiber tracts. The cause is unknown, but faulty fusion of alar and basal plates or trauma from repeated neck-bending may be contributing factors. Platybasia, dolichocephaly, sternal deformity, spina bifida, kyphoscoliosis and spinal cord tumors may coexist.

Symptoms rarely begin before the second or third decade. Weakness and wasting of the hands or arms, lack of cognizance of burns or other trauma to the arms and shoulders, shooting pains in the upper limbs, stiffness of gait and finally urinary urgency and frequency are common. The signs are wasting and loss of reflexes of the hands and forearms, spasticity and pyramidal signs in the legs and varying degrees of sensory loss over the involved dermatomes; incomplete syndromes are frequent. Syringobulbia produces lower cranial palsies, facial and corneal analgesia, and nystagmus.

The cavity, if under tension, may erode vertebral pedicles or cause spinal block. A spinal cord tumor must be excluded, for which laminectomy or a myelogram may be necessary. There is no satisfactory treatment; decompression of the cavity and roentgen therapy are thought to check its progress, which is usually slow and may arrest spontaneously.

Symptoms of *compressing lesions of the spinal cord* depend partly on the rate of development of pressure. Slowly advancing pressure produces spasticity, weakness and faulty gait with pyramidal signs; sensory loss and urinary urgency and incontinence come later. Rapidly advancing pressure causes sudden paraplegia, with urinary retention and areflexia. Other signs are stiff back or neck, radiating root pain which is worse after lying down or on coughing, percussion tenderness over the lesion and local muscular atrophy. Lesions of the cauda equina and conus produce overflow incontinence from the start.

Common causes of spinal compression are congenital vertebral defects, collapse of vertebral bodies from metastases or osteomyelitis or expanding lesions such as cysts, abscess or tumor. Intervertebral disk protrusion is rare in childhood; it follows direct trauma.

Intraspinal abscess is almost always epidural. It may be secondary to remote infection, to an infected dermal sinus, or develop by extension. In the commoner acute form, backache is followed rapidly by radicular pain, exquisite percussion tenderness over the site of the abscess, stiffness and weakness of legs, sphincter difficulties, and finally a complete paraplegia. The whole evolution takes from a few days to about a week. There is a chronic, granulomatous form, in which intermittent back pain and tenderness and a slow paraparesis may smolder on for months. The commonest site is the thoracic region. Treatment is immediate myelography and surgical drainage, combined with appropriate antibiotics. Results are excellent if drainage is accomplished before paralysis is severe. If paraplegia has developed, complete functional recovery is rare, and mortality may reach 40 per cent.

Primary intramedullary abscess is very rare; it is usually hematogenous in origin. Its signs and symptoms are those of any expanding intramedullary lesion. Treatment, by myelotomy and drainage, is fairly effective. Meticulous attention should be given to bladder, bowel, and paralyzed extremities to avoid infection, trophic sores, and contractures, since recovery may be protracted.

Spinal cord neoplasms, about one fifth as common as intracranial ones, include epidermoids, lipoma, teratoma, ependymoma, neurofibromas on nerve roots or centrally placed, and metastases usually from lymphomas or medulloblastomas. The symptoms are those of slow spinal cord compression with stiff back, root pain and localizing signs; the clinical course may be irregular and rapid. Papilledema is a rare and unexplained sign. Myelography will usually establish the diagnosis. All such lesions should be explored.

Cysts are either dermoids or epidural; the latter, in adolescent boys, may produce the syndrome of *kyphosis dorsalis juvenilis*.

Transverse myelopathy is a syndrome which may be part of a demyelinating disease or result from vascular occlusion or from rupture of vascular anomalies. It may occur in association with infections or immunizations, when it is probably due to vasculitis as a manifestation of hypersensitivity. The illness usually starts with fever, stiff neck and pains in the back or extremities; or, in case of rupture of a vascular anomaly, it may be abrupt without systemic signs. The signs of a transverse lesion of the cord evolve over hours to a few days. Cerebrospinal fluid protein is increased, pleocytosis may be present, but spinal block is rare. All degrees of severity may occur. Poliomyelitis is excluded by sensory loss and sphincter involvement; epidural abscess, by absence of spinal block. Recovery may be complete, or there may be residual paralysis. There is no specific treatment. Skilled nursing care is essential. Corticosteroid therapy has been used.

DISEASES OF THE AUTONOMIC NERVOUS SYSTEM

Symptoms of abnormal autonomic function are common to many neurologic diseases, but proved primary dysfunction of the autonomic system is rare. Congenital defects occur in Hirschsprung's disease, in which the intrinsic plexuses of the gastrointestinal tract are aplastic, and possibly in some congenital defects of the urinary tract; autonomic centers in the spinal cord, as well as in peripheral ganglia, may be defective.

Familial Dysautonomia (Riley-Day Syndrome). Familial dysautonomia occurs mostly in Jews. The constant features are defective or absent lacrimation and corneal sensory impairment leading to corneal ulceration; episodic hypertension and postural hypotension; blotchy skin and hyperhidrosis; generalized indifference to pain; mental and physical retardation; impaired temperature regulation and feeding problems in infancy. The children are small, emotionally unstable, hypotonic, hyporeflexic or areflexic and poorly coordinated. They swallow poorly, salivate excessively, drool, and have urinary frequency. Recurrent respiratory infection, often with wheezing, is common. Roentgenograms of the chest may reveal atelectasis, emphysema and pulmonary infiltrates resembling the appearance of fibrocystic pulmonary disease. These lesions are probably caused by bronchial hypersecretion and secondary obstruction rather than by primary infection.

General anesthesia is poorly tolerated and often complicated by cardiac arrest.

No adequate pathologic basis is known, though disseminated lesions in the reticular formation of the brain stem are described.

The diagnosis is a clinical one, based on the signs and symptoms described.

Treatment is limited to supportive therapy during hypertensive or vomiting crises, protection of the cornea, appropriate use of sedatives, ataractic drugs and antibiotics, and efforts to maintain a good emotional equilibrium. Some children may reach adult life.

The Diencephalic Syndrome. Infants and young children with tumors, usually astrocytomas in or near the diencephalon, sometimes have disturbances of nutrition and emotions, with few neurologic signs or symptoms of brain tumor. Profound emaciation, sometimes following a brief growth spurt, develops despite normal or ravenous appetite and adequate or even extraordinary caloric intake. For a time the children are hyperactive and euphoric. Pallor not due to anemia, hyperhidrosis and intermittent vomiting are often present, but enlarging head or neurologic signs beyond abnormal eye movements may be delayed. This clinical pattern is better regarded as an unusual presentation of brain tumor than as a specific syndrome, especially since it has occurred with tumors of the posterior fossa.

NEURITIS AND NEUROPATHIES

Degenerative changes in peripheral nerve, plexus or root have many causes. Mechanical injury usually involves single nerves or parts of plexuses; chemical, metabolic, toxic or infective substances are more likely to cause generalized damage. The pathology in most cases is similar, comprising breakdown of myelin sheath, proliferation of sheath cells, some invasion by phagocytes and often degenerative change or disruption of axons; true inflammatory changes are slight. In recovery, axons which remain intact are remyelinized, whereas the degenerated ones must proliferate from the proximal stump; regeneration is always more complete if physical continuity of the nerve trunk is maintained.

CHRONIC POLYNEURITIS

This is a syndrome with a clinical pattern like that of acute infective polyneuritis (p. 664), except that it may continue for several years. Occurring in infancy, it is frequently mistaken for Werdnig-

Hoffmann disease, from which it is distinguished by a high cerebrospinal fluid protein content, a mild sensory loss and protracted recovery over years.

Polyneuritis Due to Chemical, Metabolic and Toxic or Infective Agents. Polyneuritis due to heavy metals, such as lead and thallium, is rare in childhood and is usually accompanied by an encephalopathy which dominates the picture. Serum sickness following the injection of almost any foreign protein may cause a generalized polyneuritis or an isolated lesion of a peripheral nerve or plexus, usually of the fifth and sixth cervical roots. These lesions are independent of the site of the injection. Deficiency states, pellagra, porphyria, primary amyloidosis and certain drugs are also occasional causes. Muscular atrophy may be severe and permanent, though the prognosis is usually good.

Polyneuritic and sometimes mononeuritic manifestations occur in many infections of childhood, notably in scarlet fever, typhoid fever, dysentery and mumps. In diphtheria neuritic signs tend to appear in 3 stages: palato-pharyngo-laryngeal

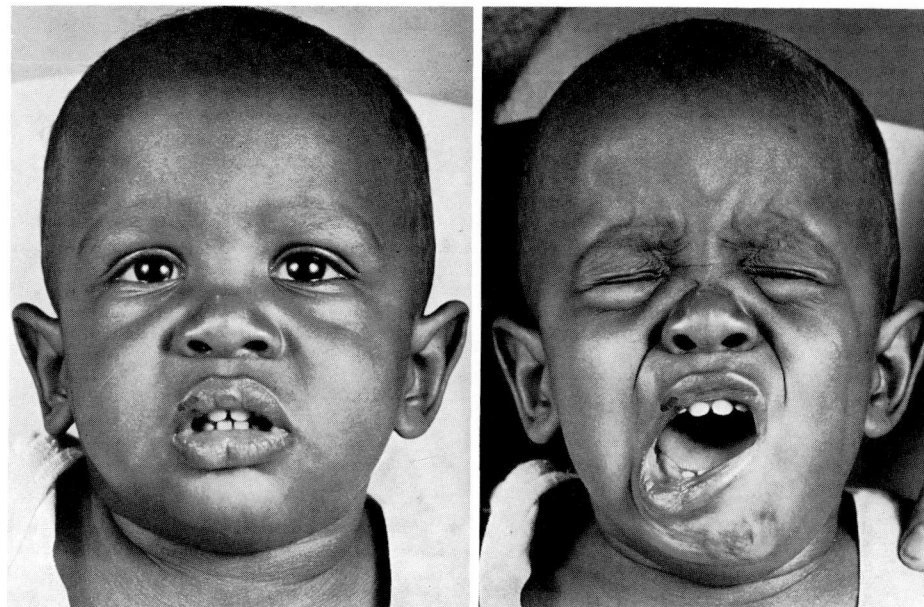

Figure 20-17. Congenital paralysis of left inferior angle of mouth. *A*, At rest, face is symmetrical. *B*, During crying the left labial angle does not depress, and *right* facial palsy may be misdiagnosed.

paralysis in the second week of the disease, paralysis of accommodation in the third week, and generalized polyneuritis in the second month. The last reaches its peak after 8 to 10 days and recedes slowly over several months.

Traumatic Neuritides. These are due to direct injury to nerve trunks or to transmitted injury through pressure, edema or scarring. Almost any nerve may be affected; the common groups are (1) obstetric palsies; (2) neonatal facial nerve palsy and Bell's palsy; (3) palsy due to pressure, laceration or to trauma from injection; (4) palsies due to neoplastic invasion.

Obstetric palsies. See page 376.

Neonatal facial nerve palsy. (See also page 377.) Congenital paralysis limited to the muscles of the angle of the mouth, apparently unrelated to birth trauma and perhaps due to intrauterine pressure on the ramus marginalis mandibulae, is sometimes present at birth. It may be confusing, since asymmetry is slight or absent with the face at rest, and sucking is unimpaired; during crying, depression of the normal side (Fig. 20-17) may cause misdiagnosis of paralysis of the intact side. No treatment is required beyond balancing the mouth by section of the intact ramus marginalis mandibulae should cosmetic reasons warrant it in later life.

Bell's palsy. Sudden peripheral facial palsy in childhood is identical with that in the adult, weakness being preceded frequently by otitis or exposure to cold; the side of the face is often numb or prickly for a day before paralysis ensues. Pathologically, swelling, congestion and constriction of the nerve in the facial canal are the principal findings.

Bell's palsy is sometimes confused with the early development of facial diplegia in polyneuritis, with bulbar poliomyelitis or other viral involvement of the facial nucleus or with herpetic lesions of the geniculate ganglion. True Bell's palsy is rare under 2 years of age; facial palsy in this age group should rouse suspicion of one of the foregoing or, more ominously, of tumor of the brain stem. Typical cases occur in severe hypertension.

More than 80 per cent of patients with Bell's palsy make a good recovery. When otitis media is present, it should be treated appropriately; no other treatment is indicated except protection of the cornea and perhaps adhesive strapping of the face to avoid stretching of facial muscles during recovery. Corticosteroids, started within the first 48 hours, are thought by some to reduce edema and improve recovery. Almost all patients maintain some slight asymmetry throughout life and may have persistent misregenerative movements: blinking the eye when the lips are smacked or twitching the corner of the mouth when the eyes are blinked.

Palsies due to pressure or laceration. Maintained pressure on a nerve trunk interrupts function and ultimately continuity of axons. A poorly placed cast or intravenous board, careless positioning of limbs in anesthetized children and pressure of knapsack straps are common causes. Recovery from such palsies is spontaneous and complete, usually requiring 1 to 4 months. Simple pressure palsies need only support of the involved limb in the position of rest and passive exercise. Lacerations or severances require careful surgical suture. Unless the laceration was a clean one, reparative surgery is best delayed 4 to 8 weeks, since the extent of destroyed nerve is usually greater than is originally apparent. Premature suture may end in ineffective regeneration and formation of a neuroma.

Palsies due to injection of serums and antibiotics deserve special attention. Sciatic and radial nerves are usually involved. Damage is due apparently to direct trauma and to pressure from secondary scarring, rather than to specific toxicity of the injected material. Complete wrist drop usually marks the radial palsy; in sciatic lesions the peroneal division suffers most, and foot drop and peroneal sensory loss are often the only signs. Sharp pain is instantaneous, but weakness may occasionally be delayed for some days; both are often overlooked in the young infant. A fair degree of recovery is the rule, but sciatic injuries in young infants usually arrest growth of the foot. Surgical dissection of scar from the nerve may be of some avail, though its beneficial effect is not proved. Newborn infants are especially vulnerable because of small size. Intramuscular injections in such patients should be restricted to the lateral aspect of the thigh.

Palsies due to tumors. Occasionally a primary tumor of peripheral nerve is responsible for a progressive monoparesis; fibromas or neurofibromas are most common. Treatment is by resection and anastomosis. More frequently, signs of isolated or multiple root or nerve lesions may be caused by malignancies, especially of pelvis and abdomen. Unexplained persistent weakness, pain, sensory or reflex loss, or wasting should provoke a thorough search.

Palsies of uncertain origin. In the newborn, transient radial palsy may accompany a patch of subcutaneous fat necrosis; the usual site is the lower, outer part of the upper arm; spontaneous recovery is the rule.

Sixth nerve palsies may appear after spinal anesthesia, or sometimes after otherwise uncomplicated lumbar puncture; recovery is rapid. A more interesting variety of abducens palsy has occasionally been seen in young children in small epidemics; the child usually has a history of a mild upper respiratory tract infection, followed in days or a few weeks by a sudden, often fairly complete paralysis of the sixth nerve. There is no other neurologic deficit, the child is not ill, the spinal fluid is normal, and beyond a modest lymphocytosis, all other findings are normal. Recovery occurs over weeks to a few months; the cause is unknown.

DAVID B. CLARK

REFERENCES

General

André-Thomas, Chesni, Y., and St. Anne Dargassies, S.: *The Neurological Examination of the Infant.* London, National Spastics Society, 1960.

Epstein, B., and Davidoff, L. M.: *An Atlas of Skull Roentgenograms.* Philadelphia, Lea & Febiger, 1953.

Ford, F. R.: *Diseases of the Nervous System in Infancy, Childhood and Adolescence.* 5th ed. Springfield, Ill., Charles C Thomas, 1966.

Greenfield, J. G.: *Neuropathology.* Baltimore, Williams & Wilkins Company, 1958.

Ingraham, F. D., and Matson, D. D.: *Neurosurgery of Infancy and Childhood.* Springfield, Ill., Charles C Thomas, 1962.

Martin, L. W., Landing, B. H., and Nakai, H.: Rectal Biopsy as an Aid in the Diagnosis of Diseases in Infants and Children. *J. Pediat.,* 62:197, 1963.

Monrad-Krohn, G. H.: *The Clinical Examination of the Nervous System.* 11th ed. New York, Paul B. Hoeber, Inc., 1958.

Nellhaus, G., and Chutorian, A.: Narcosis for Neuroradiologic Procedures in Children. *Arch. Neurol.,* 10:485, 1964.

Robertson, E. G.: *Pneumoencephalography.* Springfield, Ill., Charles C Thomas, 1957.

Robinson, R. J.: Assessment of Gestational Age by Neurological Examination. *Arch. Dis. Childhood,* 41:437, 1966.

Robinson, R. J., and Tizard, J. P. M.: The Central Nervous System in The New-Born. *Brit. Med. Bull.,* 22:49, 1966.

Walsh, F. B.: *Clinical Neuro-ophthalmology.* 2nd ed. Baltimore, Williams & Wilkins Company, 1957.

Static and Developmental Lesions, Ectodermal Dysplasias and Congenital Vascular Malformations

Alexander, G. L., and Norman, R. M.: *The Sturge-Weber Syndrome.* Bristol, J. Wright & Sons, Ltd., 1960.

Barry, A., Patten, B. H., and Stewart, B. H.: Possible Factors in the Arnold-Chiari Malformation. *J. Neurosurg.,* 14:285, 1957.

Benda, C. E.: *Developmental Disorders of Mentation and Cerebral Palsies.* New York, Grune & Stratton, Inc., 1952.

Bobath, K., and Bobath, B.: The Diagnosis of Cerebral Palsy in Infancy. *Arch. Dis. Childhood,* 31:408, 1956.

Crowe, F. W., Schull, W. J., and Neel, J. V.: *Clinical, Pathological and Genetic Study of Multiple Neurofibromatosis.* Springfield, Ill., Charles C Thomas, 1956.

Fishbein, M. (Ed.): *Birth Defects.* Philadelphia, J. B. Lippincott Company, 1963.

Hamby, W. B.: *Intracranial Aneurysms.* Springfield, Ill., Charles C Thomas, 1952.

Krabbe, K. H.: Facial and Meningeal Angiomatosis Associated with Calcifications of the Brain. A Clinical and Anatomopathological Contribution. *Arch. Neurol. & Psychiat.,* 32:737, 1934.

Lindenburg, R., and Swanson, P. D.: Infantile Hydranencephaly. A Report of Five Cases of Infarction of Both Cerebral Hemispheres in Infancy. *Brain,* 90:839, 1967.

Norman, R. M.: Malformations of the Nervous System, Birth Injury, and Diseases of Early Life; in J. G. Greenfield, and others: *Neuropathology.* Baltimore, Williams & Wilkins Company, 1958.

Sass-Kortsak, A. (Ed.): *Kernicterus.* Toronto, University of Toronto Press, 1961.

Terplan, K. L., and Cohen, M. M.: Cerebellar Changes in Association with "Partial" Trisomy 18. *Am. J. Dis. Child.,* 115:179, 1968.

Wolstenholme, G. E. W., and O'Connor, C. M. (Eds.): *Ciba Foundation Symposium on Congenital Malformations.* Boston, Little, Brown & Co., 1960.

Expanding Lesions and Increased Intracranial Pressure

Bailey, P., Buchanan, D. N., and Bucy, P. C.: *Intracranial Tumors of Infancy and Childhood.* Chicago, University of Chicago Press, 1939.

Bering, E. A.: Circulation of the Cerebrospinal Fluid. Demonstration of the Choroid Plexuses as the Generator of the Force for Flow of Fluid and Ventricular Enlargement. *J. Neurosurg.,* 19:405, 1962.

Fields, W. S., and Desmond, M. M. (Eds.): *Disorders of the Developing Nervous System.* Springfield, Ill., Charles C Thomas, 1961.

Foley, J.: Benign Forms of Intracranial Hypertension—"Toxic" and "Otitic" Hydrocephalus. *Brain,* 78:1, 1955.

Foley, J.: Physiology of Increased Intracranial Pressure; in D. Williams: *Modern Trends in Neurology.* New York, Paul B. Hoeber, Inc., 1957.

Ingraham, F. D., and Matson, D. D.: Subdural Hematoma in Infancy. *J. Pediat.,* 24:1, 1944.

Kenny, F. M., and others: Iatrogenic Hypopituitarism in Craniopharyngioma: Unexplained Catch-up Growth in Three Children. *J. Pediat.,* 72:766, 1968.

McKay, R. J., Jr., Ingraham, F. D., and Matson, D. D.: Subdural Fluid Complicating Bacterial Meningitis. *J.A.M.A.*, 152:387, 1953.

Nolsen, F. E., and Becker, D. P.: Control of Hydrocephalus by Valve-Regulated Shunt: Infections and Their Prevention. *Clinical Neurosurgery*, 14:256, 1967.

Noonan, J. A., and Ehmke, D. A.: Complications of Ventriculovenous Shunts for Control of Hydrocephalus: Report of Three Cases with Thromboemboli to the Lungs. *New England J. Med.*, 269:70, 1963.

Pennybacker, J.: Abscess of the Brain; in A. Feiling: *Modern Trends in Neurology*. London, Butterworth and Co., 1951.

Sweet, W. H.: Formation, Absorption, and Flow of Cerebrospinal Fluid; in D. Williams: *Modern Trends in Neurology*. New York, Paul B. Hoeber, Inc., 1957.

Degenerative Diseases

Abul-Haj, S. K., Martz, D. G., Douglas, W. F., and Geppert, L. J.: Farber's Disease. Report of a Case with Observations on Its Histogenesis and Notes on the Nature of the Stored Material. *J. Pediat.*, 61:221, 1962.

Aronson, S. M., Saifer, A., Kanof, A. A., and Volk, B.: Progress of Amaurotic Family Idiocy as Reflected by Serum and Cerebrospinal Fluid Changes. *Am. J. Med.*, 24:390, 1958.

Austin, J. H.: Recent Studies in the Metachromatic and Globoid Forms of Diffuse Sclerosis. *Res. Publ. Ass. Res. Nerv. Ment. Dis.*, 40:189, 1962.

Bell, J.: *Treasury of Human Inheritance*. Part I. Cambridge University Press, 1934.

Brandt, S.: *Werdnig-Hoffmann's Infantile Progressive Muscular Atrophy*. Copenhagen, E. Munksgaard, 1950.

Clayton, B. E., Dobbs, R. H., and Patrick, A. D.: Leigh's Subacute Necrotizing Encephalopathy: Clinical and Biochemical Study, with Special Reference to Therapy with Lipoate. *Arch. Dis. Childhood*, 42:467, 1967.

Critchley, E. M. R., Clark, D. B., and Wikler, A.: Acanthocytosis and Neurological Disorder Without A-Betalipoproteinemia. *Arch. Neurol.*, 18:134, 1968.

Farber, S., Cohen, J., and Uzman, L. L.: Lipogranulomatosis—A New Lipoglycoprotein Storage Disease. *J. Mount Sinai Hosp.*, 24:816, 1957.

Gall, J. C., Hayles, A. B., Siebert, R. G., and Kuth, H. M.: Multiple Sclerosis in Children. *Pediatrics*, 21:703, 1958.

Greenfield, J. G.: *The Spino-cerebellar Degenerations*. Springfield, Ill., Charles C Thomas, 1954.

Korey, S., and others: Studies in Tay-Sachs Disease. I. Methods. *J. Neuropath. Exp. Neurol.*, 22:2, 1963.

Lagos, J. C., and Gomez, M. R.: Tuberous Sclerosis: Reappraisal of a Clinical Entity. *Mayo Clin. Proc.*, 42:26, 1967.

Richter, R. B.: Infantile Subacute Necrotizing Encephalopathy with Predilection for the Brain Stem. *J. Neuropath. Exp. Neurol.*, 16:281, 1957.

Sedgwick, R. P., and Boder, E.: Progressive Ataxia in Childhood, with Particular Reference to Ataxia-Telangiectasia. *Neurology*, 10:705, 1960.

Steinberg, D., and others: Studies on the Metabolic Error in Refsum's Disease. *J. Clin. Invest.*, 46:313, 1967.

Svennerholm, L.: Chemical Structure of Normal Human Brain and Tay-Sachs Gangliosides. *Biochem. Biophys. Res. Commun.*, 9:436, 1962.

van Bogaert, L., Cumings, J. N., and Lowenthal, A.: *Cerebral Lipidoses. A Symposium.* Springfield, Ill., Charles C Thomas, 1957.

Walton, J. N.: The Limp Child. *J. Neurol., Neurosurg. & Psych.*, 20:144, 1957.

Wilson, J.: Leber's Hereditary Optic Atrophy. A Possible Defect of Cyanide Metabolism. *Clin. Sc.*, 29:505, 1965.

Zeman, W., and Dyken, P.: Dystonia Musculorum Deformans. *Psychiat. Neurol. Neurochir.*, 70:77, 1967.

Wise, D., Wallace, H. J., and Jellinek, E. H.: Angiokeratoma Corporis Universale Diffusum. A Clinical Study of Eight Affected Families. *Quart. J. Med.*, 31:177, 1962.

Neurologic Syndromes Peculiar to Childhood

Cottom, D. G.: Acute Cerebellar Ataxia. *Arch. Dis. Childhood*, 32:181, 1957.

Ford, F. R., and Schaffer, A. J.: The Etiology of Infantile (Acquired) Hemiplegia. *Arch. Neurol. & Psychiat.*, 18:323, 1927.

Craniocerebral and Spinal Trauma

Brock, S. (Ed.): *Injuries of the Skull, Brain, and Spinal Cord.* 4th ed. Baltimore, Williams & Wilkins Company, 1960.

Griffith, J. F., and Dodge, R. R.: Transient Blindness Following Head Injury in Children. *New England J. Med.*, 278:648, 1968.

Trauma of the Nervous System. *Proc. A. Res. Nerv. & Ment. Dis.*, 24:1945.

Diseases of the Spinal Cord and Autonomic Nervous System

Paine, R. S., and Byers, R. K.: Transverse Myelopathy in Childhood. *Am. J. Dis. Child.*, 85:151, 1953.

Richardson, F. L.: A Report of 16 Tumors of the Spinal Cord in Children; The Importance of Spinal Rigidity as an Early Sign of Disease. *J. Pediat.*, 57:42, 1960.

Riley, C. M., and Moore, R. H.: Familial Dysautonomia Differentiated From Related Disorders: Case Reports and Discussions of Current Concepts. *Pediatrics*, 37:435, 1966.

Russell, A.: A Diencephalic Syndrome of Emaciation in Infancy and Childhood. *Arch. Dis. Childhood*, 26:274, 1951.

Neuritis and Neuropathies

Gilles, F. H., and French, J. H.: Postinjection Sciatic Nerve Palsies in Infants and Children. *J. Pediat.*, 58:195, 1961.

Hoefnagel, R., and Penry, J. K.: Partial Facial Paralysis in Young Children. *New England J. Med.*, 262:1126, 1960.

Knox, D. L., Clark, D. B., and Schuster, F. F.: Benign VI Nerve Palsies in Children. *Pediatrics*, 40:560, 1967.

Lloyd, A. V. C., Jewitt, D. E., and Still, J. D. L.: Facial Paralysis in Children with Hypertension. *Arch. Dis. Childhood*, 41:292, 1966.

CEREBRAL PALSY

The term "cerebral palsy" designates a group of nonprogressive disorders resulting from malfunction of the motor centers and pathways of the brain, characterized by paralysis, weakness, incoordination or other aberrations of motor function which have their origin prenatally, during birth or before the central nervous system has reached relative maturity. Most persons with cerebral palsy have, in addition to the motor disability, other manifestations of organic brain damage such as seizures, mental retardation, and sensory and learning defects, and these are frequently complicated by behavior and emotional disorders. The pathologic and clinical findings are varied, resulting from a variety of cerebral defects; the degree of involvement depends on the extent and location of the central nervous system lesion and varies from a mild hemiplegia with no other neurologic defect to a totally incapacitating disorder producing dependency for life. The type of motor involvement in a given child varies with age and reaches a typical adult pattern as the damaged central nervous system matures. The problems also depend in part on the age at which interruption of development of the brain took place, and on the status of reflex patterns, and of motor, intellectual, language and social skills, if any, that may have been acquired before damage or injury occurred. Cerebral palsy is a nonfatal, noncurable condition that is frequently benefited by therapy and by training and education.

Cerebral palsy is one of the leading causes of crippling in children; the prevalence rate is estimated as 100 to 600 cases per 100,000 population, the majority of identifiable patients being under 21 years of age. The care and support of these children, who usually have multiple handicaps, present an important economic and social as well as a medical problem.

Cerebral palsy is classified by cause if known, by type (spastic, athetoid, ataxic), by anatomic distribution (such as hemiplegia or quadriplegia) and by functional state and intellectual ability.

Spasticity is characterized by the pathologic stretch reflex, increased activity of deep tendon reflexes, clonus, scissoring and contractures affecting the antigravity muscles. Among early signs are fixed posturing, often opisthotonos or maintained partial tonic neck responses. Sudden lifting of the child may produce scissoring of the legs. Tonic neck reflexes are too readily elicited or are asymmetric, and the trunk and the pelvis may fail to follow the head. Stepping and placing reflexes are absent or are done better with one foot than the other. Lifting the supine child with a hand under the occiput produces extension of the neck and retraction of the shoulders. In the prone position protective turning of the face does not occur, and the child remains nose down. Spasticity is frequently associated with prematurity or anoxia and is usually the result of damage or defect in the cortical motor area.

Athetosis is marked by involuntary incoordinate motion with varying degrees of muscle tension. Reflexes are usually normal. Initially the clinical manifestation may be one of hypotonia, and only during the second year may the fine wandering movements of the fingers, hands and feet become evident and develop into the typical pattern of athetosis. This type is frequently the aftermath of kernicterus in which there is damage to basal nuclei.

Ataxia is manifest by lack of coordination due to disturbances of the kinesthetic and balance senses. There may be associated hypotonia. The lesion is usually in the cerebellum.

Disturbance of muscle tone is almost always present. *Atonia* or *hypotonia* is characterized by soft, flabby muscles and may be associated with increase in activity of deep tendon reflexes. Loss of tone in the infant is frequently a precursor of other types of involvement.

On rare occasions, *tremors* of intentional or involuntary pattern may be manifest in children, but these are typically a late manifestation in older children and adults.

Mixed types are seen in children with more diffuse brain damage. Spasticity is the most frequent type and, together with athetosis, accounts for approximately three quarters of all cases. Sei-

zures occur at some stage of life in at least 25 per cent of all affected children. There is a significant visual problem in one fifth of affected persons, and many, especially those with athetosis, have a loss in hearing perception. At least half of the persons with cerebral palsy function at a significantly retarded level.

Diagnosis. Early diagnosis of brain injury is important to the child and his family, since many of the physical and psychologic complications can be decreased or avoided if parents are given help and guidance during the first year or two of the child's life.

When one manifestation of brain damage is recognized, others should be suspected. Children who have a history of any of the cerebral dysfunctions outlined above should be observed carefully for deviations from normal growth and development. The presence of any anomaly or of disturbances during the neonatal period such as feeding problems, irritability or drowsiness, cyanosis, jaundice, respiratory difficulties, abnormal muscle tone or seizures should lead to a careful evaluation of the central nervous system.

Severe cerebral damage or deficit is usually apparent early in life. That of a lesser degree should be suspected when there is a significant deviation from normal rates of growth and development or when there is persistence of infantile physiologic reflexes such as the Moro and the tonic neck ones beyond 6 to 8 months of age. The typical adult neurologic patterns may not develop during the first year or two of life even though the lesion is present from birth or earlier. Definite handedness apparent before 12 to 15 months of age suggests hemiparesis.

The *differential diagnosis* may include consideration of more acute conditions such as trauma to the brain or the peripheral nerves, poisoning, infection or tumor of the central nervous system, diastematomyelia, degenerative diseases, Sydenham's chorea, amyotonia congenita and muscular dystrophies. It must be remembered that, in children with motor dysfunction associated with organic brain damage, the other manifestations such as seizures, retardation, sensory and perceptual disorders and abnormal behavior are also frequently present.

Prognosis. Prognosis is dependent on a careful appraisal of all factors related to the child, his family and the community. With the knowledge that the basic defect cannot be cured, that associated or complicating conditions are usually present, that social, economic and psychologic factors are usually harder to control than the medical ones, the outlook for the group as a whole is not favorable for self-sufficiency or ability to compete effectively with peers. Only a small percentage of affected children achieve independence and a satisfying way of life. The goals should be much lower in the majority of cases, and only by observation of growth and maturation, by response to treatment and training and appreciation of the child's and the family's ability to use their own and the community's resources can a realistic goal be set. In general the child's intelligence is the best prognostic guide, so that use should be made of the best psychometric help available.

Treatment. The general features of management of a handicapped child are described elsewhere (p. 121); these include a realistic short- and long-term plan, assistance to the child in making full use of his residual assets, avoidance of secondary emotional problems, support and counseling for the family and use of available community resources. The goals must be reviewed periodically in the light of progress made, and therapy must be timed in accord with the child's developmental status. In general the aim of treatment should be to secure for the patient a happy childhood and a well adjusted adult life in which he performs well within the limits of his capabilities.

In the most seriously involved children, treatment may be largely supportive and aimed at prevention of complicating factors such as contractures, nutritional deficiencies, pressure sores, infections and emotional disturbances in all concerned.

If the child has motive enough to try to learn, efforts at developing muscle strength, balance and coordination, functional posture and skills in communication and self-help should be made. Since it is usually impossible to evaluate accurately the relative detrimental effect of several handicaps, all defects that lend themselves to correction should be treated. The total benefit of such efforts is frequently rewarding, although there are few well controlled clinical trials of any individual therapeutic regimen or combination of therapies to which such children are exposed.

The group that appears least seriously involved may not reach its full capability because of lack of attention to emotional factors that may be more handicapping than the motor defect itself.

More than anything else, the handicapped child and his parents need the continuing care of a physician who understands the needs of all children for growth and development and whose judgment is not blurred by too close contact with individual parts of the problem. The child with cerebral palsy has an injured brain whose performance is not that of the normal brain. Child and parents must not be allowed to succumb to a well meaning but tyrannical optimism aimed at improved performance of individual functions, but disregarding the limit set for the whole child by his organic handicap. The desired end-result of a happy adult, well adjusted and performing at his maximal ability, is best reached by early recognition of the extent of his handicap, and kindly but realistic direction toward attainable rather than unattainable goals. Acceptance by child, parents and physician of that part which cannot be altered should be achieved at least by the time of the early school years. *Planning for adult life on these terms accomplishes more for the child and his parents than all the mechanical de-vices, therapies and surgical procedures known to medicine.*

The specific treatments for various manifestations are discussed elsewhere.

The orthopedist is concerned with developing and maintaining good body mechanics. This is accomplished by bracing, by physical therapy and by surgery largely limited to tendon lengthening, to arthrodeses and to muscle transfers in older children.

Training resulting in functional improvement of body mechanics, muscular control, gait, use of hands, and in verbal communication can be effectively carried out by parents under the direction of physical, occupational and speech therapists. Success is proportionate to the degree of physical, mental and emotional involvement of the patient, to the therapist's understanding and use of physiologic approaches and to the integration of such therapies with a balanced home life and with other services for the child.

Physiotherapy, most of which can be carried out by the parent (after instruction), should be begun in infancy to avoid development of contractures and to stimulate control of movement. The joints involved—usually ankles, knees, hips, wrists and fingers—are manipulated against the direction of maximal contraction and are finally carried through a full range of movement. Short periods of therapy repeated at frequent intervals during the day are more effective than fewer long sessions; the procedure benefits the child physically and the parents emotionally. Active motions of functional use should be encouraged. Later, efforts at improving coordination by use of games, peg boards, training in sitting and standing in supportive chairs or at stand-up tables, and walking aids such as parallel bars, skis or crutches may be added as indicated under guidance of trained and imaginative therapists. A skilled therapist uses a variety of techniques to suit the needs and reactions of the child and is not restricted to a rigid pattern of exercises.

An insufficient number of therapists is available in many cerebral palsy clinics, so that the individual child often gets only scanty attention. Most of the procedures are relatively simple, and most of the equipment can be easily constructed by amateurs. Enthusiasm for clinic care should not overlook the powerful and much more available resources within the home. Parents should be trained and encouraged to carry out as much of the therapy as possible as a game leading to successes rather than as a frustrating ritual.

Neurosurgery may play a part in a small number of cases. Treatment of subdural collections of fluid, hydrocephalus, craniosynostosis, intracranial vascular anomalies or hemorrhage and acute trauma may play a part in modifying or preventing some of the conditions that lead to cerebral palsy. Procedures aimed at removing foci or at interruption of pathways in the brain to reduce uninhibited activity are under clinical investigation and in carefully selected cases appear to be effective.

Children with visual, auditory and dental problems are handled essentially as are other children with such problems, with appropriate modifications for their associated disabilities and limitations.

Many *drugs* having varied pharmacologic actions have been used, and others are under evaluation. None has satisfactory clinical effect on muscle tone without significant disadvantages. Various tranquilizers relieve secondary tension and may help at times to improve overall function. Anticonvulsive drugs should be used as indicated (see p. 1257).

Prevention. A review of the many causes of brain injury associated with hereditary defects, congenital anomalies, intrauterine damage, perinatal trauma and anoxia, and toxic and infectious agents reveals that many cases are preventable. The practicing physician can make a real contribution by carrying out and supporting delivery of known principles of primary and secondary preventive medicine.

JOHN B. BARTRAM

REFERENCES

Crothers, B., and Paine, R. S.: *The Natural History of Cerebral Palsy.* Cambridge, Harvard University Press, 1959.
Illingworth, R. S.: Diagnosis of Cerebral Palsy in the First Year of Life. *Dev. Med. Child Neurology,* 8:178, 1966.

21. Diseases of Muscle

Skeletal muscle makes up about 25 per cent of the body weight of the infant, and 40 per cent of that of the adult. Its special functions are maintenance of static and kinetic orientation of the body in space, effecting bodily responses involving movement, accomplishing the mechanical parts of such vital activities as respiration, and aiding in maintenance of heat production and exchange. It serves as a fairly rapidly alterable reservoir for intravascular fluid, tissue fluid, electrolytes and complex metabolites, and as a synthesizer of certain proteins.

Skeletal muscle of the trunk and limbs develops from the dorsomedial portion of the somites; that of the head and the neck arises in splanchnic mesoderm of the 5 branchial arches. Recognizable myoblasts join the dermatomes soon after the fourth week of embryonic life. Skeletal muscles develop before they receive innervation, and hence are not dependent on nerve impulses for initial differentiation, though maintenance of muscle in later life requires innervation.

The *functional element* of muscle is the muscle fiber, a giant multinucleated cell whose dimensions vary enormously; extremes are 16 or 17 microns in diameter and a few millimeters in length in extraocular muscles, as against 150 microns in diameter and 30 cm. in length in thigh muscles. The average diameter is about 40 to 50 microns. The *functional unit* is the *motor unit,* or number of muscle fibers innervated by one motor neuron; the unit varies from 5 or 10 fibers in extraocular muscles to 1500 or 1600 in the gastrocnemius. Each muscle fiber normally receives one motor nerve fiber, ending in a motor end-plate, and every muscle contains a number of specialized sensorimotor structures, the *muscle spindles.* These are small collections of muscle fibers in connective tissue capsules whose motor innervation is the gamma efferent fiber and whose sensory endings are complex. Specialized sensory endings also occur in tendons and connective tissue sheaths, and free endings, probably pain-sensitive, are described.

Since a muscle includes not only the muscle fiber, motor and sensory nerve endings, and nerve trunks and their sheaths, but also connective tissue, blood vessels and lymphatics, it is obvious that muscle can be involved in almost every disease process.

The causes of diseases of muscle are in many cases unknown, and terminology and classification correspondingly confusing and unsatisfactory. Aplasia, hypoplasia, atrophy and hypertrophy are self-explanatory; the last is troublesome in practice, since the bulk of a muscle may be increased by fatty or fibrous replacement, whereas the muscle fibers themselves have atrophied or degenerated, thus justifying the awkward term, "pseudohypertrophy." *Myo-edema* is a sharply defined, localized idiomuscular contraction produced by direct percussion of a muscle belly. It is seen in cachectic or emaciated states, and on inspection resembles a *myotonic contraction.* Here a similar ridge or indentation of contracted muscle persists for some seconds. *Myotonia* is a delayed relaxation of muscle after voluntary contraction or after electrical, mechanical or biochemical stimulation. *Fibrillations* are spontaneous contractions of denervated individual muscle fibers, appearing about the fifth day of denervation, and lasting until the fiber degenerates; they must be recorded electrically, since they cannot be seen except possibly in the tongue. *Fasciculations* are coarse twitches of one or several motor units, visible on inspection. They are a feature of motor neuron disease, but may also be seen as benign twitches during active contraction, and in some cachectic states. The term *myositis* implies the histopathology of inflammation at some time during the disease. *Dystrophies* are best regarded as primary metabolic disease, expressed principally by involvement of muscle. This categorization does not include a wide range of disease processes, some clearly metabolic in origin, some of unexplained origin, but marked by inflammatory or atrophic changes, which are best referred to noncommitally as *myopathies.*

METHODS OF STUDY

History. Since many disorders of muscle are genetic in origin, a careful search for similarly affected persons should be made not only among collateral relatives, but also among family members of preceding generations. Incomplete expression of familial myopathic or neuromyopathic syndromes is frequent, and "formes frustes" should also be inquired for.

Particular attention is paid to *weakness,* perhaps the most common symptom of muscular disease; it may be static, progressive in a given group of muscles, or extend into previously uninvolved muscles. Distribution of weakness is important, since dystrophies and some myopathies tend to involve proximal groups first; the reverse is more common in neurogenic weakness. *Pain,* aching or cramping, or frank *muscle cramp* should be inquired for, and its relation, as well as that of weakness, to exercise, diet and sleep investigated.

Systemic Symptoms. Fever, weight loss, anorexia, skin rashes, eruptions and change in texture often accompany myositis and myopathies. Dyspnea, orthopnea or mottling of extremities indicates extension to cardiac muscle or inadequate respiratory mechanisms, or both. A careful account of the first recognition of symptoms is important; most diseases of muscle are of much longer duration than parents appreciate.

Physical Examination. A careful general physical examination, with the child stripped, is essential. The child should walk about, lie down, roll over, stand up, climb stairs and grip the examiner forcibly. Particular attention should be paid to weakness and its distribution; to change in tendon reflexes, usually depressed or abolished by myopathies, dystrophies or myositides; to the bulk and consistency of muscles on palpation and to any pain so elicited, a feature of active myositis and some neuropathic weakness; to disorders of contraction, especially the maintained contraction of myotonia or the progressive weakness of myasthenia; and to fasciculations. Contractures of joints, due to fibrosis of muscles or ligaments, may indicate a pattern of weakness by their position or a congenital or familial illness by presence at birth. The skin should be examined for rashes, thickening or other chronic or acute inflammatory change, as well as for atrophy. Disorders of swallowing, tachycardia and cardiomegaly and impaired sphincter tone indicate involvement of involuntary muscle. The bones should be palpated carefully, since certain disorders of bone may present as muscle weakness.

Laboratory Data. Routine hemograms and urinalyses are usually of little help except for acute inflammatory processes, parasitic infection, and possibly for some collagen vascular diseases. The more chronic myositides, polymyositis and dystrophies rarely are associated with characteristic changes in blood cells or urine.

Any process which destroys muscle fairly rapidly may produce creatinuria and increase serum transaminases and aldolases, the latter especially because of their high concentration in muscle. Sharp reduction in muscle volume limits ability to store ingested creatine and is responsible for increased excretion of it in creatine tolerance tests. Porphyrinuria in porphyria with muscular wasting and myoglobinuria in paroxysmal or traumatic myoglobinuria are diagnostic. Pentosuria in dystrophies is inconsistent and unreliable. A few enzymatic abnormalities, such as the greatly increased phosphocreatine kinase in Duchenne dystrophy, are relatively specific and may be of value in detecting carrier states.

The *roentgenogram* is of value principally in demonstrating associated abnormalities and the calcification or ossification occurring in some myositides, e.g. after trauma; it may, however, confirm muscular wasting by relative reduction of muscle shadows.

Electromyography records muscle action potentials and thus indicates both the physiologic state of muscle and the activity of motor neurons. The test is not particularly disturbing; it is applicable even for small infants, readily repeatable and of value in following the course of illness. It will help to distinguish neurogenic from myogenic weakness, and peripheral neurogenic weakness from motor neuron involvement; it is of value in the diagnosis of myasthenic states. It requires cautious interpretation, however, and should not be the sole basis of a diagnosis.

Biopsy. Study of disease of muscle is rarely complete without this procedure. Moderately but clearly involved muscles (weaker ones in early cases, those retaining some power in long-standing cases) are selected for biopsy. Sites of previous electromyographic needle insertions should be avoided. A specimen of tissue at least 5 by 10 mm. carefully removed and fixed to avoid artifact is studied in longitudinal and cross sections with a variety of stains. Skilled interpretation is essential.

Biopsy will usually distinguish myopathic or dystrophic atrophy from neurogenic atrophy, identify myositis and sometimes its cause and demonstrate storage and collagen vascular diseases. Motor points may be located by stimulation, and motor endings studied by light or electron microscopy. Biochemical or enzymatic assay of excised muscle is a procedure of steadily increasing importance, especially in instances when there is some idea of the underlying process.

CONGENITAL DEFECTS OF MUSCLE

Congenital Absence. Almost any muscle may be congenitally absent, though with such inconstant phylogenetic residuals as the pyramidalis, absence is scarcely a defect. Absence of the pectoralis, particularly its sternocostal part (Fig. 21-1), is the most common, followed by absence of the trapezius, serratus anterior, quadratus femoris, omohyoideus, and semimembranosus. Usually unilateral, these defects are often genetic in origin. Association with other deformities is not infrequent, e.g. that of the pectoral muscle and mammary gland with syndactylism and microdactyly. Congenital absence of a pectoral muscle, the brachioradialis or biceps femoris may be associated with facioscapulohumeral or other muscular dystrophies.

Congenital absence of muscles of the abdominal wall, usually in males, mechanically weakens respiration, defecation and coughing; it is often associated with megaloureter and urinary tract infection. Congenital absence of the diaphragm may lead to collapse of the lung, or seriously impaired respiratory function at times of stress. In most instances, however, congenital absence of a muscle is not itself a serious handicap.

Congenital Ptosis. This may be unilateral or bilateral and varies from a slight droop to com-

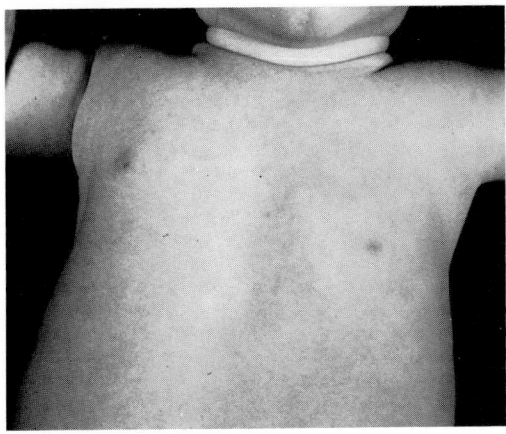

Figure 21-1. Congenital absence of left pectoral muscle. Note absence of anterior axillary fold and low placement of nipple.

plete ptosis. Often heredofamilial, it may be associated with cataract, polydactylism or syndactylism, epicanthus and other anomalies. The levator palpebrae superioris and sometimes the superior rectus are weak rather than absent; in about one fifth of cases, movement of the jaw in various directions causes elevation of the lid, the *Marcus-Gunn* or *jaw-winking phenomenon.* Improvement may be seen in the early months of life, but most often it does not occur, and the ptosis may require surgical correction. In the newborn infant, birth injury must be excluded as a diagnostic possibility; in later life, tumor, aneurysm, myasthenia and ocular dystrophy or myopathy must be considered.

Duane's Syndrome (Retraction Syndrome). In this condition one or both external recti are congenitally fibrosed. The visual axes are usually parallel in central position, but on attempted lateral gaze the adducting eye must pull back into the orbit before turning inward. The condition causes little or no disability, but recognition of the characteristic retraction may be delayed; consequently, unnecessary diagnostic studies may be made.

Congenital Facial Diplegia (Moebius' Syndrome). Congenital facial and ocular palsies often occur together or in combination with clubfoot or other malformations of the extremities, arthrogryposis, defects of ears, deafness and mental deficiency. Facial or facio-ocular palsies are occasionally hereditary, but most often sporadic. Facial muscles and external recti are most commonly involved. Expressive motions and sucking movements are impaired, and poor lid closure may result in exposure keratitis. Plastic surgery for squints and cosmetic defects may be necessary.

Other Cranial Nerve Defects. Unilateral *facial paralysis* is the most frequent of such defects. It is usually due to pressure of forceps or to pressure from bony prominences of the birth canal, but some lesions are developmental in origin and may be seen in successive generations. Rarely, facial paresis and vocal cord palsy are associated, and

very rarely an unexplained unilateral, nonprogressive atrophy of the tongue is encountered.

Torticollis (Wryneck). Tilting of the head may have many causes, congenital or acquired. Wryneck secondary to abnormality of the sternomastoid muscle is rarely familial, almost invariably unilateral, and affects the sexes equally; history of breech or otherwise difficult birth is common. A rather transient torticollis is noted soon after birth; about the second week a firm, circumscribed but not inflamed or discolored mass may appear in the sternomastoid muscle. In about two thirds of instances the torticollis disappears with little or no treatment, the mass subsides by the fifth to seventh month, and cure is complete. In other instances the torticollis and mass may seem to improve or disappear, but by 3 or 4 years of age, torticollis is more evident. The muscle is shortened and fibrous; the face is deformed; the ipsilateral eyebrow is slanted; the frontal bone is flattened, and there is an occipital bulge on this side. The contralateral frontal bone bulges, and the occiput is flattened (Fig. 21-2). The head tilts to the affected side, and the chin may turn slightly away. Cervical scoliosis, elongation of the mastoid process and rarely calcification in the muscle are present.

The tumor in infancy is whitish with proliferation of connective tissue and degeneration of muscle; later it becomes a fibrosed mass containing islands of normal muscle. Hemorrhage or hemosiderin is rarely found, so that a hematoma is an

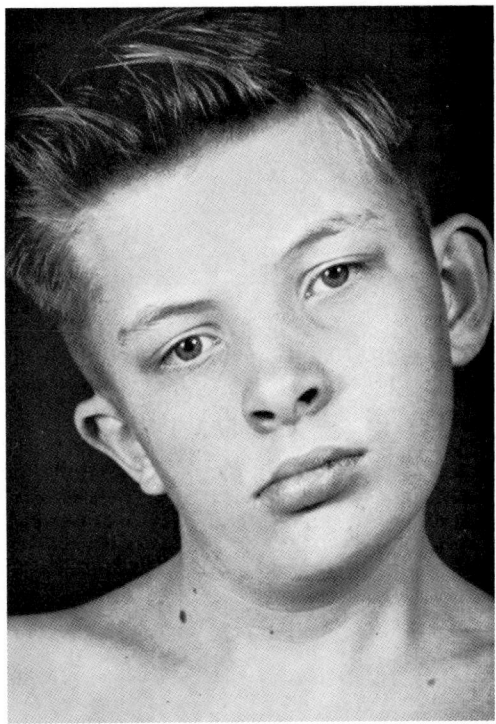

Figure 21-2. Congenital torticollis, untreated until age of 12 years. Note wryneck and deformity of face.

unlikely cause. Ischemia due to arterial compression and venous engorgement from pressure on cervical veins are more probable causes. Intra-uterine malposition is possible, especially when ipsilateral ear deformity or facial palsy is also present. The conditions must be distinguished in infancy from other defects, such as Sprengel's or Klippel-Feil deformity, cervical myelodysplasia and incorporation of the atlas into the occiput; in older children, from cervical adenitis, ocular head tilt, posterior fossa and spinal cord or vertebral tumors in the cervical area.

Treatment in the infant is by manipulation, best done with the baby supine: the neck is flexed forward and away from the side of the lesion, and the head is rotated toward it. Persistent or recurrent torticollis requires section of muscle to prevent osseous deformity. Treatment of acquired torticollis should be directed at elimination of the cause.

INFECTIOUS AND OTHER INFLAMMATORY DISEASES

INFECTIOUS MYOSITIS

Certain *viruses,* e.g. Coxsackie A, may invade muscle and cause damage. *Bacterial myositis* is usually caused by staphylococci or streptococci. A rare complication of septicemia, it commonly follows trauma or extends from an adjacent infection. Local and systemic signs of inflammation are present, and abscesses or phlegmon may form. The end-state is fibrosis, occasionally with contractures. Antibiotics and frequently surgical drainage are indicated.

Clostridial myositis (gas gangrene) follows deep puncture wounds or compound fractures. The onset of symptoms is often abrupt; constitutional signs and prostration are severe, and the spread of inflammation and crepitus is rapid. Trivalent antiserums, penicillin and immediate supportive measures are necessary; the mortality rate is high.

Tuberculous myositis and *actinomycotic myositis* almost always extend from adjacent sinus tracts, though miliary tuberculous myositis is recorded. Focal necrotizing myositis is common in *toxoplasmosis,* but is usually overlooked; a syndrome resembling acute polymyositis may occur. *Cysticercosis* and *trichinosis* cause myositis with local tenderness, fever and eosinophilia; focal calcifications are residuals. Trichinosis may cause transient ocular paresis.

Severe infections may produce hyaline, waxy or granular degeneration of muscle fibers without actual invasion by infectious agents. Typhoid fever and other enteric infections, influenza and leptospirosis are common causes; the rectus abdominis is the most frequently involved muscle. Rupture and hemorrhage are serious complications.

POLYMYOSITIS
(CHRONIC POLYMYOSITIS; MYOSITIS FIBROSA)

Muscular involvement with weakness and loss of reflexes, which is usually proximal in distribution and has histologic evidence of inflammation, may develop insidiously. There may be a skin rash, fever and other changes suggestive of a collagen vascular disease, or rarely the syndrome may occur in association with malignancy. The exact differentiation of polymyositis from dermatomyositis, and of either from other collagen vascular syndromes or from skin and muscle disease secondary to malignancy, is difficult and may be more apparent than real.

Clinical Manifestations. Even infants are not exempt, though onset before 2 or 3 years of age is rare, and cases in childhood are less frequent than in adulthood. Females are affected more frequently than males. At least 2 forms of the disease may be distinguished. In the first, cutaneous involvement is absent. The course is usually subacute or chronic; increasing weakness, the main symptom, involves limb girdles and trunk and produces disturbances of gait, stair-climbing and the like. It is out of proportion to accompanying wasting and decrease in reflex activity. Joint and muscle pain, fever and chills are rare except in acute cases. Pseudohypertrophy and bulbar weakness appear occasionally. The illness is generally protracted, and understandably misdiagnosed as muscular dystrophy.

In the second form the course is more rapid, and the early manifestations are frequently joint pains, fever or skin changes; there are transitory butterfly rashes, scaling or atrophy of skin and pinkish or violaceous discoloration. The muscular reflex and gait disturbances and occasional pseudohypertrophy resemble the pattern of the first form and may similarly be misdiagnosed.

Frank dermatomyositis (p. 526) with facial rashes, scaling or atrophy of skin, joint involvement and other evidence of a severe generalized illness may be accompanied by severe muscular weakness and wasting, impaired swallowing and respiratory difficulty. Malignancy, either carcinoma or lymphoma, may coexist. This may represent an extreme degree of polymyositis.

Acute cases occur in all 3 variants and have a bad prognosis. More chronic involvement of the first 2 forms may have long remissions or terminate in spontaneous cure.

Laboratory Data. Progressive anemia is common; less often there may be an elevated sedimentation rate, eosinophilia, leukocytosis or leukopenia. L.E. cells are rarely identified. Creatinuria is frequent, and occasionally there is albuminuria. The levels of serum gamma globulins, aldolases, transaminases and phosphorylases, including creatine phosphokinase, are usually raised. The cerebrospinal fluid is normal. Calcinosis and osteoporosis may be demonstrated radiographically; the electrocardiogram is generally normal. Biopsy will reveal degenerative changes and variation in sizes of muscle fibers, regeneration of fibers, inflammatory infiltrates and scarring. Electromyography is generally abnormal, with seesawing potentials and decided interference patterns.

Diagnosis. "Pure" polymyositis may be clinically indistinguishable from muscular dystrophy and may require muscle biopsy and electromyography to differentiate it. Variants with skin and joint manifestations or frank scleroderma may be misdiagnosed as disseminated lupus, rheumatic fever, trichinosis, scleroderma, polyarteritis, or even myelitis or neuritis.

Treatment. Corticosteroids or corticotropin is usually tried. Their effect on muscle disease is debatable, especially since spontaneous remission or cure may occur; results are probably better in adults than in children. General systemic measures, orthopedic procedures to alleviate weakness, a high protein diet and prompt attention to decubiti, infections and respiratory impairment are essential.

MYOSITIS OSSIFICANS PROGRESSIVA

This is a rare, progressive familial disease in which connective tissue of skeletal muscle, fasciae, tendons, ligaments and aponeuroses becomes edematous, proliferates, calcifies and ossifies.

Clinical Manifestations. The disease is familial and has occurred in homozygous twins. Three fourths of affected persons have other congenital abnormalities, which include, in descending frequency, microdactyly, especially of thumbs and great toes; curved, angled or ankylosed digits; webbed toes; polydactyly; deformed ears; absent teeth; and spina bifida. These defects are also common in relatives with normal muscles. Some pedigrees suggest transmission through males, who are affected 2 or 3 times as frequently as females.

Age at onset of connective tissue lesions varies, typical lesions having been noted at birth. In about three fourths of instances the onset is before the sixth year, but it may be delayed until after puberty. Death usually occurs from the second to the fourth decade, but survival to the seventh one is known.

Without apparent cause, or perhaps after slight trauma or trivial infection, doughy swellings develop over hours or days, usually on the back of the head, around the ears, or on the neck, shoulders or back. The lump may be hot and tender, feel cystic, or break down and drain grumous white material. The child at this time is irritable and mildly feverish. After a few weeks the lesion regresses and becomes indurated, pain subsides, and calcification and ossification develop in it. Some lesions may regress and then enlarge. Biopsy may provoke new lesions. The hands, forearms, hips and legs are not commonly involved, and the heart, diaphragm, sphincters and laryngeal muscles are spared. Involvement of the masseters may cause feeding difficulties. Ulti-

mately huge sheets of bone are formed over the trunk and neck, fusing the torso into a solid mass (Fig. 21-3) and leading to death usually from secondary heart disease and respiratory complications. Patients whose lesions appear before puberty generally remain sexually immature; postpubertal onset is compatible with fertility.

Laboratory Data. Demonstrable biochemical abnormalities are absent. There may be a mild anemia. Alkaline phosphatase is said to be increased in tissues obtained by biopsy from early lesions.

Histopathology. The initial lesion is swelling and proliferation of connective tissue with little inflammatory reaction. The tissue soon condenses to osteoid and then ossifies, sometimes with cartilage as an intermediate. Degenerating and regenerating muscle may be found within the osseous mass.

Differential Diagnosis. Myositis ossificans circumscripta or traumatic myositis ossificans may

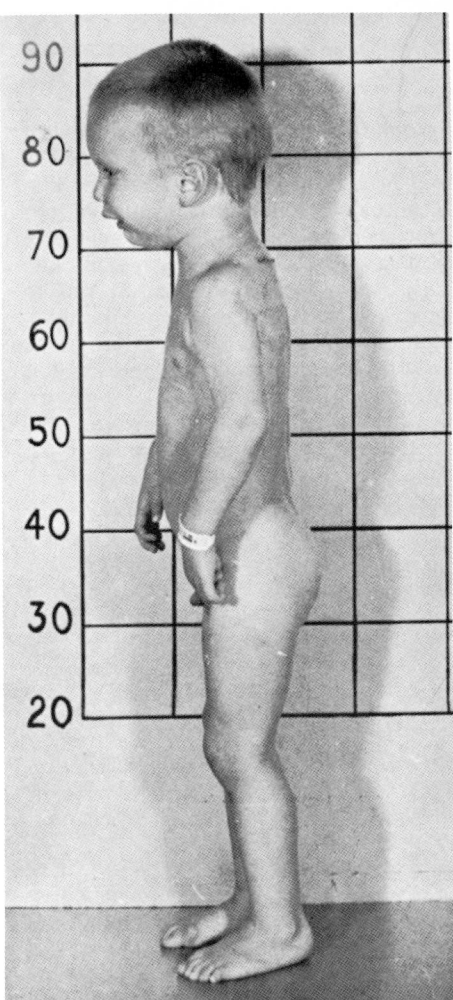

Figure 21-3. Myositis ossificans progressiva. No radiographically demonstrable calcification, but typical histologic changes. Note posture, and rigidity of neck and back.

occur at any age and is commonest in the anterior thigh or brachialis anticus. It clearly follows and is restricted to sites of trauma, and the roentgen shadow is feathery or circumscribed rather than sheetlike. Rheumatic fever has a predilection for joints, and ossification is absent. The Farber-Uzman syndrome occurs in young infants, and lesions are principally periarticular. Multiple exostoses are readily distinguished radiographically. The development of bone in pyogenic or granulomatous draining sinuses is rare; bacterial culture and biopsy are helpful.

Treatment. None is truly effective. Corticosteroids reduce fever and relieve irritability and may possibly have some effect on the lesions, though this is doubtful.

TOXIC AND METABOLIC MYOPATHIES

MYOPATHY DUE TO ENDOCRINE ABNORMALITIES

Thyroid. Muscular weakness and wasting with hyperthyroidism, though rarer in childhood than in adulthood, do occur, as do the ocular palsies of exophthalmic ophthalmoplegia. In cretinism and myxedema the muscles are sometimes weak, the reflexes diminished. In some instances the muscles appear large and firm, and myotonus is demonstrable by physical examination and by the electromyograph. The Cornelia de Lange syndrome and myotonia congenita are differential diagnostic considerations.

Parathyroid. Weakness, hypotonia and loss of reflexes in hyperparathyroidism may simulate muscular dystrophy or myasthenia and, with osteoporosis, contribute to severe deformities.

Adrenal Cortex. Muscular weakness appears in about four fifths of patients with hyperadrenocorticism. Similar weakness occurs less frequently during therapy with a variety of corticosteroid preparations. The muscles of the pelvic girdle are most severely involved; wasting is marked, but reflex activity is retained. Creatinuria is constant. Muscle fibers are vacuolated, but not otherwise much altered. Weakness may be extreme and, in the instances due to corticosteroid therapy, is in general proportional to the dose of the agent. Recovery can be expected with cessation of steroid therapy.

IDIOPATHIC MYOHEMOGLOBINURIA
(MEYER-BETZ DISEASE)

This is a rare genetic, probably recessive, disease, marked by sudden attacks of swelling, pain and paralysis of muscles and by myohemoglobinuria.

Clinical Manifestations. All age groups and both sexes are affected. Infection and exertion may precipitate attacks, which are characterized by fever, nausea, vomiting, and unevenly distributed swelling, pain and paralysis of muscles. The legs, arms and back, bulbar muscles, neck, chest and diaphragm tend to be involved in descending frequency. The urine becomes dark red or black, contains albumin and casts and gives a positive reaction for occult blood. Myohemoglobin may be identified spectroscopically. Attacks are recurrent, and may be mild or severe and even fatal, death being due to uremia or respiratory failure.

Pathology. Affected muscle fibers are swollen, vacuolated or liquefied, with little inflammatory reaction; cardiac or smooth muscle is not involved.

Laboratory Data. Distinction of myohemoglobin from occult blood or porphyrins in urine is the only important test.

Diagnosis. This includes acute or chronic nephritis, paroxysmal hemoglobinuria and acute porphyria. The disease should be thought of in any case of muscular pain and weakness associated with dark urine and unexplained by porphyria, occult blood or hemolytic disease.

Treatment. Treatment is symptomatic for the muscular discomfort. Renal tubular damage, as in hemoglobinuria, and respiratory paralysis are the serious threats and should be managed appropriately.

Myohemoglobinuria with severe muscle pain, weakness, and degeneration of muscle fibers may also appear in *crush injuries of muscle.* Care should be exercised in mobilizing such patients, since serious renal tubular damage might ensue.

THE MYASTHENIAS

Weakness of muscle and excessive fatigability on successive contractions, which is restored by rest, may occur in a variety of disease states. The neuromuscular syndromes of hyperthyroidism, malnutrition, polymyositis and dermatomyositis, myopathies accompanying malignancies, postinfectious polyneuritis, muscular dystrophies and even brain tumor and vascular disease of the brain stem may be responsible for such "myasthenic weakness." There may even be some response to anticholinesterase drugs.

In the primary disease state, known as *myasthenia gravis,* weakness and excessive fatigability are the principal symptoms, and response to anticholinesterase drugs is generally marked.

Etiology. The cause is not known. Best evidence indicates a block in neuromuscular transmission of competitive or acetylcholine inhibitory type. Whether this block is due to an abnormal response of end-plates to acetylcholine or to formation of abnormal acetylcholine or choline compounds is unknown.

Pathology. No change is constant or pathognomonic. Striated muscle may contain focal accumulations of lymphocytes (lymphorrhages) or plasma cells. Thymoma, present in 15 to 30 per cent of affected adults, is rare in childhood. Slight muscular atrophy is usually due to disuse. The serum in about 30 per cent of the cases contains a complement-fixing globulin which binds to the A bands of muscle and to the epithelial cells of the thymus; changes have also been described in motor endings and end-plates.

Laboratory Data. In general, the value of most laboratory tests is to exclude other associated conditions such as thymoma, hyperthyroidism and polymyositis. Ergometric demonstration of the progressive weakening of myasthenic muscles and electromyography, with and without neostigmine, may be helpful.

MYASTHENIA NEONATORUM

Clinical Manifestations. This is a transitory myasthenic response, affecting about 10 per cent of newborn infants of myasthenic mothers, and is more common in females. There is no apparent relation to the duration, severity or treatment of the maternal myasthenia; fetal movements are normal. Within 2 to 72 hours post partum, generalized weakness, gaping mouth or immobile face, ocular palsies, impaired sucking, dysphagia and respiratory distress are manifest. Response to anticholinesterase drugs is dramatic. The condition persists one to a few weeks; no unequivocal case of permanent myasthenia has been reported.

Maternal history, clinical findings and injection of neostigmine usually establish the **diagnosis**. If the maternal myasthenia is undiagnosed, birth injury, congenital defect, neonatal poliomyelitis, drug intoxication and the amyotonia syndrome may be suspected.

Treatment. A trial dose of neostigmine methyl sulfate (0.25 mg. intramuscularly) is used diagnostically. Subsequently, maintenance doses of neostigmine bromide (3.75 to 7.5 mg.) or pyridostigmine bromide (15 to 30 mg.) are given with each feeding; doses must then be adjusted to maintain effective respiration and swallowing without producing diarrhea, salivation or abdominal distress. Atropine is rarely necessary and may dangerously obscure signs of overdosage. Careful observation is essential; the myasthenic state may disappear rapidly, and the infant may slip undetected into a cholinergic crisis.

MYASTHENIA CONGENITA

This myasthenic state, which is present at birth, is persistent and often familial.

Clinical Manifestations. Whereas the mothers of these infants are rarely, if ever, myasthenic, familial incidence in sibships is high, and more distant members of kindreds may be affected; one of monovular twins may escape. Sex predilection is not marked. Fetal movements may be depressed. Symptoms at birth are chiefly ocular and bulbar: ptosis, external ophthalmoplegia, weak cry and dysphagia are common, whereas generalized weakness or respiratory distress is relatively rare. Congenital defects, mental retardation, amyotonia, Moebius' syndrome, muscular dystrophy, congenital ptosis and brain tumor should be considered in the differential diagnosis. Any infant or young child with unexplained ocular or bulbar weakness should have a test dose of neostigmine; the response in myasthenia congenita is clear-cut.

Treatment. Maintenance doses of oral neostigmine or pyridostigmine, adjusted to age and severity of symptoms, will generally improve strength and function, but complete relief of ocular palsies and complete remission are rarely attained. General management is that of myasthenia gravis juvenilis (see below).

MYASTHENIA GRAVIS JUVENILIS

In this condition, myasthenia is first apparent some time after infancy. In about 10 per cent of adults with myasthenia gravis the onset was during childhood; it is rare before 5 years of age, and the incidence increases steadily into adolescence. The ratio of females to males is about 6:1, and familial cases are known. Association with epilepsy and nonmyasthenic congenital ptosis is high.

Clinical Manifestations. The onset is only rarely abrupt; signs and symptoms usually appear over weeks or months and may be long unrecognized. Ptosis, unilateral or bilateral, is the most common sign. Ophthalmoplegias not referable to one nerve or muscle, difficulty in chewing or swallowing, nasal voice, and weakness of arms and legs are frequent manifestations. Increase of weakness on exercise or as the day progresses and improvement after rest or sleep are almost always noted. Worsening during infection or other stress is the rule; severe respiratory distress, requiring respirator or tracheotomy, occurs in about two fifths of patients. The pupils remain normal; myotatic reflexes are brisk except in severe states; sphincters are unimpaired, and sensation is intact. Thymoma in childhood is rare, but thyrotoxicosis, atypical muscular atrophy, emotional disturbances and migraine may coexist. The purely ocular forms have the best prognosis; bulbar weakness, generalized weakness and rapid progression are serious signs.

The high incidence of ocular and bulbar symptoms with normal pupils, fluctuating weakness and absence of signs of fixed neurologic deficit in conjunction with preservation of myotatic reflexes and sensation should permit early **diagnosis.** Hysteria, thyrotoxicosis, polyneuritis, muscular dystrophy and brain tumor, however, must be considered in the differential diagnosis. A careful history, observation of the clinical pattern and a neostigmine or edrophonium test are generally adequate for diagnostic purposes.

Treatment. The principal effective drugs are neostigmine bromide, neostigmine methyl sulfate, pyridostigmine bromide and edrophonium.

For the test observation a weak muscular movement, capable of rough quantification, is selected; this may be ptosis, facial movement on crying, or swallowing in the infant, or width of the palpebral opening, range of extraocular movements, and the like, in the older child. Atropine sulfate (0.01 mg. per kg., intramuscularly) is administered initially to avoid fasciculation, abdominal cramps and possible cardiac disturbances and is followed in 10 to 15 minutes by neostigmine methyl sulfate (0.04 mg. per kg., intramuscularly); the usual total dose for infants is 0.25 mg. and for older children 1.0 or 1.5 mg. Beginning 20 minutes after administration of the drug and continuing to 45 minutes, the range and fatigability of the muscular movements are checked repeatedly, and any observed improvement is measured, if possible, and recorded. Edrophonium IV (5 to 10 mg.) produces similar improvement, but the response is immediate, and the duration is very brief. The usual sources of error in testing are misinterpreting inconclusive responses and too small a dose of the testing drug. If myasthenia is seriously suspected, a negative result should not be accepted until the upper tolerable dose has been used. Rarely is typical myasthenia gravis unresponsive to adequate doses of these drugs.

For *maintenance therapy* exact dosage schedules are not possible, since requirements fluctuate among patients and from time to time for a given patient. Neostigmine methyl sulfate (intramuscularly) is generally restricted to diagnostic testing and to management of gravely ill patients. Pyridostigmine produces fewer autonomic side effects, and its response is more sustained than that of neostigmine; otherwise there is no preference. Initial oral doses for infants and small children are 3.75 to 7.5 mg. of neostigmine bromide to 15 to 20 mg. of pyridostigmine bromide with feedings; for older children, 7.5 mg. of neostigmine or 30 mg. of pyridostigmine are given as pills or syrup with meals. Atropine for maintenance therapy is unwise, since it obscures the symptoms of overdosage of the other drug. Each patient must be adjusted to his own optimal dosage. At best, only about half achieve really good control, and complete relief of diplopia is rare.

A thymoma, if present, should be removed. Opinions on *thymectomy* or *thymic irradiation* in the absence of a thymoma vary; a conservative view is to reserve them for severe cases which respond poorly to drugs, and for older children or adolescents in whom control is unusually difficult.

Myasthenic and Cholinergic Crises. Myasthenia gravis may worsen suddenly and seriously at times of stress. Parents should be warned, and respirator facilities should be available for transportation to a hospital if such is indicated. A myasthenic patient who requires minor surgery or has even a moderately severe infection should be hospitalized. When a crisis threatens, therapy with neostigmine methyl sulfate by intramuscular administration is more readily adjusted to the varying needs than is oral medication.

Excessive administration of anticholinesterase drugs can produce a state of weakness clinically similar to that of myasthenia, and often without previous increase in strength or pronounced cramp, diarrhea, salivation or sweating. The simplest procedure when there is doubt about the nature of the myasthenia, and if the weakness is not too severe, is to withhold further administration of the drug under careful observation; the strength will lessen in a myasthenic crisis and improve in a cholinergic one. A quicker diagnosis may be reached by giving 1 to 2 mg. of edrophonium IV, which will improve a myasthenic crisis, and will worsen a cholinergic weakness, but for so short a time as to permit it to be manageable.

THE MYOTONIAS

These diseases, clinically fairly distinct, share transmission in an autosomal dominant manner and the presence of myotonus. Predilection of the myotonus for the tongue and thenar eminences, progressive dystrophic wasting, gonadal and other endocrine abnormalities and mental change characterize myotonic dystrophy; generalized myotonus and hypertrophy of voluntary muscles are the hallmarks of myotonia congenita; and myotonus of the tongue and periodic flaccid weakness distinguish paramyotonia. Many patterns with overlapping features are known, and these 3 can be provisionally regarded as part of a larger myotonic syndrome. Adynamia episodica hereditaria may link them to periodic paralysis.

MYOTONIC DYSTROPHY
(STEINERT'S DISEASE)

This is a heredofamilial disorder, marked by myotonia, muscular wasting, cataract, gonadal and other endocrine abnormalities, mental deficiency, hyperostosis frontalis and cardiac abnormalities.

Pathology. In the muscle the subsarcolemmic nuclei proliferate and form long central chains; the sarcoplasm degenerates; ringed fibers and central condensation of myofibrils appear, and the sarcoplasm becomes vacuolated and is ultimately removed by phagocytes; there is variable fatty or fibrous replacement. Intramuscular motor nerve fibers may sprout, but otherwise there are no characteristic changes in the nervous system. Atrophy and hyalinization of spermatic tubules occur in adult males, but no constant changes are found in the ovaries or endometrium. Colloid goiter is the common change in the thyroid. Increase in basophils or other cells and increased colloid in the pituitary probably reflect end-organ failure. It has been suggested that the primary disorder is secretion of abnormally high levels of insulin, or of an abnormal insulin, the changes in the membranes of muscle cells being secondary; a hereditary disorder of immunoglobulin catabolism is another hypothesis.

Clinical Manifestations. The sexes are equally affected; twinning in affected sibships is 2 or 3 times as frequent as in unaffected kindreds.

In childhood only a drooping, immobile myopathic face and perhaps mental dullness may be obvious. Myotonus in the tongue and thenar eminences, worsened by cold, is almost constant, though easily overlooked; it is most readily demonstrated by posture of the hand on attempted relaxation of a strong grip. Speech is rather nasal. Deep reflexes initially may be intact, but diminish and disappear. Cataracts, almost universal, are either congenital opacification or a stellate form which advances from each pole, with subcapsular iridescent flecks and granules. Early weakness in facial and extraocular muscles is followed by characteristic temporal and sternomastoid wasting, weakness and wasting of the forearm extensors, the intrinsic muscles of the hands, the vasti, the quadriceps and the dorsiflexors of the feet; the last may require orthopedic correction. Frontal baldness, infertility, testicular atrophy, progressive mental deterioration, Reynaud's phenomenon, gastrointestinal disturbances and cardiac enlargement and failure are events of adolescence and adult life. Death occurs in the fourth or fifth decade.

Laboratory Data. The urinary concentrations of creatinine and especially of creatine are low; this is the reverse of most dystrophies. Urinary excretion of guanidoacetic acid is also low, and the synthesis of creatine deranged. In childhood, cardiac conduction defects, especially prolonged P-R intervals, are common. The emptying time of the gallbladder is increased. The presence of myotonus is confirmed by electromyography, and tissue obtained by biopsy will show the described changes. Hyperostosis frontalis interna and small pituitary fossae are said to be common. The urinary excretion of 17-ketosteroids is greatly diminished in the adult.

Diagnosis. In the child this is difficult only if one fails to think of the illness as a diagnostic possibility. Mental retardation with hypertonus, a muscular dystrophy or Moebius' syndrome may be considered, but the demonstration of myotonia, the distribution of muscular weakness, the wasting of the sternomastoids, cataracts and, above all, the family history establish the diagnosis.

Treatment. This is symptomatic. Quinine sulfate, 0.3 to 1.0 gm. daily, relieves myotonia, but side effects, such as tinnitus, are severe, and effective doses are usually poorly tolerated. Procainamide, 250 mg. 4 times daily, increased to tolerance (2 to 4 gm. for children and 6.0 gm. for adults), is effective, but insomnia, hallucinations and gastrointestinal distress are common. Potassium-binding resins have been claimed to be effective. Prednisone in doses of 5 to 15 mg. daily is also helpful, but causes hypercorticoidism. In view of the side effects of these drugs, the extent of the incapacity due to myotonia must be sufficient to warrant therapy.

Muscular weakness can be occasionally aided by orthopedic procedures or braces; and talipes, by tendon lengthening. Crutch eyeglasses are poorly tolerated; plastic procedures on the eyelids may be helpful. Good general care and avoidance of infection and fatigue are important.

MYOTONIA CONGENITA
(THOMSEN'S DISEASE)

This is a rare hereditary disease, characterized by myotonia and hypertrophy of most voluntary muscles, without evidence of progression or other abnormality.

Clinical Manifestations. Symptoms generally begin in childhood. The myotonia involves most of the voluntary muscles, but the hypertrophy is limited principally to those of the limbs and trunk, giving a herculean appearance. Myotonia is greatest on the initial muscular contraction and wears off on successive ones, so that an initially impaired movement can soon be performed fairly freely; contraction of other muscles follows a similar pattern. Excitement, chill and fatigue increase the myotonia, whereas ingestion of alcohol reduces it markedly. Impaired release of grip, falling on sudden movement, difficulty in chewing, tightness of respiratory movement and brief diplopia on sudden deviation of eyes are noted. Cataracts are not commonly associated. Mental illness and imbecility occur in some families; their relation to myotonia congenita is not clear. No other abnormality is characteristic, and the condition neither worsens greatly nor does it shorten life.

Histologically, the muscle fibers are hypertrophied with some centralization of nuclei; no other change is described.

The only laboratory finding of note is electrical evidence of myotonia.

The family history, early appearance and lack of progression of the myotonia and the hypertrophy distinguish it from myotonic dystrophy and from hypothyroidism with myotonia.

Treatment. The disease is annoying rather than disabling. Most patients learn to "warm up" before attempting major movements, and require no treatment. Quinine or procainamide, as for myotonic dystrophy, may be tried.

PARAMYOTONIA CONGENITA
(EULENBURG'S DISEASE)

This is a rare, hereditary, nonprogressive disease characterized by orofacial pharyngeal and distal myotonia and by periodic attacks of flaccid weakness brought on characteristically by cold exposure.

Clinical Manifestations. Symptoms are present from infancy. Brief exposure to cold elicits myotonia: the eyelids close, there is facial grimacing, and the hands are clenched, the fingers remaining flaccid. Cold food causes thickness of speech; in addition, a mild degree of weakness of the extremities may be noted. Warming relieves all symptoms. Prolonged exposure to cold may be followed by severe flaccid weakness of limbs, with abolition of deep reflexes and of faradic and galvanic responses of the muscles; this may last many hours. Neurologic and motor status apart from the attack is normal, though myotonia can be elicited mechanically in the tongue. The frequency and severity of attacks diminish with age.

No definite pathologic abnormalities have been described. Serum potassium levels are within the high normal range, but fluctuate rather widely.

Some consider this disorder to be allied to myotonia congenita, others to Gamstorp's adynamia episodica hereditaria. Episodic weakness, however, is not a feature of the first, nor is myotonia of the second.

In **management** of the patient, avoidance of chilling and the provision of frequent carbohydrate meals are recommended.

MUSCLE DISEASE WITH DISTURBED POTASSIUM LEVELS

Weakness or paralysis of skeletal muscle due to hyperkalemia or hypokalemia is well recognized in severe renal disease, or after excessive fluid therapy in treatment of diabetic acidosis or diarrhea. There are in addition at least 2 familial syndromes associated with striking and fairly constant changes in serum potassium levels, though one cannot assume that the primary defect is one of potassium metabolism.

ADYNAMIA EPISODICA HEREDITARIA
(GAMSTORP'S DISEASE)

This disease is inherited as an autosomal dominant and is characterized by periodic attacks of weakness of limbs and trunk. Attacks are provoked by rest, especially after exercise, hunger or cold; they may be slight or severe and brief or last for hours. There may be mild ocular, bulbar and respiratory symptoms. Myotonia is not present; deep reflexes may be retained or abolished. The attacks appear in early childhood, worsen through adolescence, and then gradually abate.

During attacks the serum potassium concentration is increased to as much as 7.0 mEq. per liter, but urinary excretion of potassium does not increase; during attacks there are high T waves in the electrocardiogram. Occasionally the changes of myotonic dystrophy may be seen in biopsy specimens.

This syndrome differs from paramyotonia in that myotonus is said to be absent, and the serum potassium level is constantly elevated during attacks, and possibly in the presence of histologic changes. Reports of cases in which both myotonus and an elevated serum potassium level were present suggest that they may be a single disease, and thus link the myotonias and the periodic paralyses.

FAMILIAL PERIODIC PARALYSIS

This is a rare hereditary disease, characterized by recurrent attacks of flaccid paralysis of limbs and trunk and sometimes of bulbar, respiratory and cardiac muscles. There is loss of deep reflexes and of electrical excitability during the attacks.

Vacuolization of muscle fibers is the only important pathologic change.

Clinical Manifestations. Most pedigrees indicate an autosomal dominant inheritance pattern with varying penetrance, which is more complete in males; sporadic cases are almost always in males. Autosomal and sex-linked recessive patterns have also been described.

The disease is more common and more severe in males, who are usually of athletic build and otherwise of robust health. Typical attacks commonly begin in childhood or adolescence and generally lessen in middle life. Hyperthyroidism, migraine and seizures may coexist and are often found in otherwise unaffected relatives. The attacks usually occur in sleep and are precipitated by (1) stresses, such as emotion, trauma, cold, infection or menstruation; (2) heavy ingestion of carbohydrates; (3) rest, especially after exercise; (4) drugs, especially epinephrine, corticotropin and corticosteroids. An inconstant prodrome of thirst, apprehension and tightness of muscles is followed by flaccid weakness which spreads centrally from the legs to the trunk and arms and usually spares the ocular and bulbar muscles and the diaphragm. Weakness may be hemiplegic or involve only a limb previously chilled. The muscles swell and are painful; paralysis is partial or complete with loss of reflexes and electrical responses. There may be headache, nausea, vomiting and constipation. Rarely there are cardiac arrhythmias, bradycardia, enlargement of the cardiac shadow and the murmur of mitral insufficiency. Attacks generally last for some hours and are ultimately fatal in about 10 per cent of patients, commonly by respiratory failure. After hours or a day or so, recovery begins with sweating and diuresis; strength returns in the reverse order in which it was lost. Pain and stiffness may persist for some days.

Some patients may experience but one attack. Others have brief attacks lasting only for minutes, with a feeling of weakness, but with few objective signs. Some find that exercise will abort brief or even threatened severe bouts, and that they can "walk themselves out of a spell." In later life there may be mild atrophy of muscles, or more rarely some hypertrophy, mainly in the calves, and only in patients who have had clear-cut attacks. In most patients the serum level of potassium is low during attacks, and oral or intravenous administration of potassium chloride relieves the weakness; in certain families, however, the level of serum potassium does not fall, and administration of potassium has no effect. A few are relieved by administration of sodium chloride.

Hemograms reveal only leukocytosis and eosinopenia during attacks and lymphocytosis and eosinophilia following them. There may be mild proteinuria or glycosuria. The electrocardiogram during attacks is characteristic of hypokalemia with inverted T waves, RS-T segment changes and U waves.

Treatment. Hyperkalemic paralysis responds rapidly to 0.2 to 0.3 ml. subcutaneously of a 1:1000 solution of epinephrine or to 10 to 20 ml. intravenously of 10 per cent calcium gluconate. For prevention, a high salt intake and frequent carbohydrate feedings are adequate; 5 to 15 mg. of dextroamphetamine daily, in a slowly absorbed form, may be useful.

Periodic paralysis with hypokalemia responds to potassium chloride in doses of 0.2 gm. per kg. orally. For prevention, administration of up to 10 gm. of potassium chloride daily may be effective, but in some instances it may increase the frequency or severity of attacks. Sodium restriction to less than 10 mg. daily with added potassium and intermittent diuresis may be more helpful, as may spironolactone, 100 to 200 mg. orally each day. If cardiac arrhythmias are present, infusions of 50 gm. of glucose, 50 mEq. of potassium and 10 units of insulin may be used; digitalis is contraindicated.

Avoidance of excessive exercise, chilling and heavy carbohydrate intake in the hypokalemic varieties, especially at night, is advisable. The attacks can be fatal; patients should be aware of the gravity of their illness and the need for medical supervision during attacks.

PROGRESSIVE MUSCULAR DYSTROPHIES

Muscular dystrophies make up the largest single group of muscle diseases in childhood. They are characterized by weakness and atrophy of the skeletal muscles with increasing disability and deformity as the disease progresses. Several clinical types are recognized, but muscular atrophy occurs in all forms; pseudohypertrophy

appears as an early and prominent sign in one form. Genetic patterns are varied and may be of a sex-linked, simple recessive or dominant type. Muscular dystrophy accompanied by pseudohypertrophy is usually transmitted by a sex-linked factor, and most cases of facioscapulohumeral dystrophy appear through a dominant genetic pattern. Manifestations of the disease are likely to occur early in life when it has been transmitted through sex-linked or simple recessive factors. In contrast, when a dominant mode of inheritance is involved, the onset occurs later in life. The disease occurs about 3 times as often in males as in females. Moreover, muscular dystrophy occurring in females is likely to be less severe and less rapidly progressive.

Pathology. There are no essential differences in the pathology of the various clinical types of the disease. On gross examination the muscles are pale and fibrous. In pseudohypertrophic muscles, fatty infiltration is responsible for producing a characteristic yellow color on gross section. True muscular hypertrophy is seldom if ever observed at necropsy. Microscopically, there are evidences of cellular degeneration. Muscle fibers vary in diameter, some appearing small and shrunken, others large and swollen. Accumulations of nuclei are found along the sacrolemmic sheath. There is fragmentation of fibrils and evidence of hyaline and granular degeneration. On cross section, muscle fibers will be seen to have lost their polygonal shape and are rounded or oval, individual fibers being widely separated from each other by fat, fibrous connective tissue and areolar tissue. Late in the disease connective tissue replaces most of the muscle mass, and only occasional, small, degenerative muscle fibers will be observed.

The myocardium may show similar changes, but usually the process affecting the cardiac muscle is less marked. Smooth muscle is unaffected. Changes in the anterior horn cells have been described, but are irregular in occurrence and cannot be considered responsible for the profound muscular atrophy. Decalcification and osseous atrophy are found in late stages. Thick, soft accumulations of subcutaneous fat often appear about the pelvic girdle and shoulders.

The disease is accompanied by excessive urinary excretion of creatine. Creatinine excretion, however, is decreased. There is, in addition, increased urinary excretion of glycocyamine, an intermediary compound in the biologic synthesis of creatine.

Clinical Forms. All clinical forms of muscular dystrophy may be considered variations of a single disease, differing only in the muscle groups affected, the age at onset and rate of progression. An individual patient may have characteristics of several forms. In deference to classic nomenclature, and since clinical manifestations greatly depend on the particular groups of muscles affected, the more important clinical forms of muscular dystrophy are described.

Pseudohypertrophic form (type of Duchenne).
This is the most common form in childhood. The
disease is transmitted by a sex-linked recessive
gene. The onset is usually before the fifth year of
life. Certain muscle groups are enlarged (see
below), presenting characteristic pseudohypertrophy. Atrophic changes are noted in other
muscles and follow in the muscles initially enlarged. The disease is progressive, few patients
living past the second decade.

The first signs may occasionally be noted in
infancy, the child finding it difficult to stand or
learn to walk. More often the child is observed
to have gradually increasing weakness of the legs.
A waddling gait results from weakness of the
gluteal muscles, and he walks with his feet
thrown widely apart. He may fall frequently.
Riding a tricycle or ascending stairs may become
impossible. The child may be unable to comb his
hair or raise his hands above his head because of
involvement of the muscles of the shoulder girdle.
Weakness of the shoulder muscles is manifested
by the manner in which the arms slip upwards
and through the examiner's hands when they are
placed in the axillas in an attempt to lift the child.

A characteristic feature is the patient's inability to rise readily to an upright position from
a sitting position on the floor (Fig. 21-4). The
patient turns on his side, flexes his knees and
hips, and with arms extended raises his trunk to
assume a position of kneeling. The feet are brought
forward and the legs extended at the knees. Then
by bringing the hands successively to the shins,
knees and thighs, he pushes his body to the upright position. This succession of movements is
generally considered pathognomonic of progressive muscular dystrophy.

In the upright position there is severe lordosis,
and the abdomen is thrust forward prominently.
The pelvis and sacrum tilt anteriorly, and there
is forward inclination of the lumbar vertebrae.
Winging of the scapulas may be noted.

Muscles are usually involved symmetrically.
Pseudohypertrophy is observed most frequently
in the infraspinatus, supraspinatus, deltoids and
triceps, and in the muscles of the calves. Macroglossia sometimes occurs. Atrophy is usually first
observed in the sternal portion of the pectoralis
major. As the disease progresses there is also
atrophy of the deltoid, triceps, biceps, gluteus and
the anterior thigh muscles. Atrophy begins near
tendinous ends, so that on contraction the muscle
stands out in bold relief. Late in the disease all
muscles of the legs, spine, pelvis and shoulder
girdle are atrophic. In some instances there are
large subcutaneous depositions of fat, which tend
to preserve body contours; in others the extreme
muscular atrophy results in an appearance of
inanition. Contractures and skeletal deformities
result.

Tendon reflexes may be normally active early
in the disease, but become hypoactive and later
disappear as the muscles become too weak to
respond to stimuli. The ankle reflexes, however,

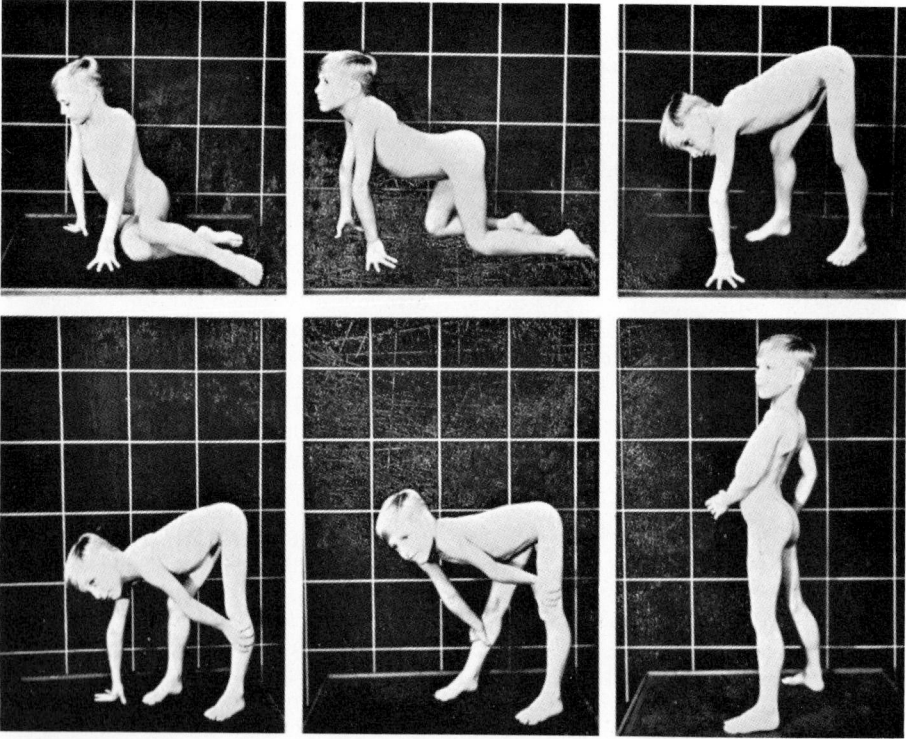

Figure 21-4. A child 7 years of age with pseudohypertrophic muscular dystrophy, showing characteristic manner
of rising from the floor. The last picture shows the standing position with the severe lordosis.

remain active. Superficial reflexes are unchanged. Fasciculation does not occur. Response to electrical stimulation is decreased, but the reaction of degeneration is not observed. Cramping pains in the abdomen and in the muscles of the legs are common. There may be mottling and cyanosis of the skin of the legs resulting from inadequate venous return, secondary to loss of muscle tone. In late stages of the disease, cardiomegaly and heart failure may be noted.

The children are usually surprisingly cheerful. At least one third are mentally retarded. Retardation cannot be attributed to limited schooling alone, though this may be a contributing factor; the retardation is not accompanied by specific learning disabilities, is rarely severe, and should not alter efforts to educate. Half to two thirds have electroencephalographic abnormalities, but clinical seizures seem no more frequent than in the general population.

A variant of this disorder is the hereditary *atrophic form of Leyden-Moebius*, which is not associated with pseudohypertrophy and apparently progresses more slowly.

Facioscapulohumeral form (type of Landouzy and Déjerine). In this type the onset usually occurs between the ages of 6 and 20 years. Hereditary transmission follows a dominant pattern. The muscles first affected are those of the face and the shoulder girdle. The first defect often noted is inability to raise the arms above the head. The face becomes expressionless and masklike, the patient being unable to close his eyelids, lift his eyebrows or wrinkle his forehead. The process progresses slowly and over a period of years spreads to muscles of the pelvis and legs.

Juvenile muscular atrophy (type of Erb). The onset of this type of the disease usually occurs in adolescence or early adult life. The muscles of the shoulder girdle are first affected, winging of the scapulas resulting because of atrophy of the serrati magni and the trapezii. There is difficulty in elevating the arms above the head.The muscles of the face are not involved. The disease is slowly progressive, the patient's condition often remaining unchanged for years.

Diagnosis. The clinical signs and characteristics of progressive muscular dystrophy which are important in differential diagnosis are the symmetrical and proximal distribution of muscular weakness, pseudohypertrophy, slow progression of the disorder, absence of sensory changes and the occurrence of the disease in other members of the family. In contrast, *polyneuritis* is associated with muscular weakness and atrophy of the extremities accompanied by pain, tenderness and sensory changes. Muscular weakness in *spinal muscular atrophy* is present at birth or appears early in infancy. *Progressive neural muscular atrophy* involves the distal muscles of the extremities and of the hands. It is also associated with fibrillary tremors and electrical changes of degeneration.

Many intracellular enzymes – aldolases, transaminases and dehydrogenases – are present in elevated concentrations in serum at various stages in these diseases; similarly, abnormal levels of magnesium, sodium and potassium are occasionally noted. These changes are unfortunately too variable and inconstant to be useful diagnostically. The most valuable serum enzyme measurement is that of creatine phosphokinase (CPK), which is constantly increased, not only in patients with active disease, but often in asymptomatic children or in asymptomatic female carriers of the Duchenne type.

Prognosis. The disease is progressive, death usually occurring within 5 to 10 years of the onset in the pseudohypertrophic form. Few patients survive adolescence. Intercurrent infection is the most common cause of death. Myocardial insufficiency may be the terminal event.

Treatment. There is no specific measure. Various diets, insulin combined with carbohydrate, amino acid hydrolysates, corticosteroids and digitalis, thyroid and a host of others have all been tried without success. Physiotherapy and avoidance of obesity, a common concomitant of inactivity and parental sympathy, keep the child ambulatory a little longer. Orthopedic procedures, braces, tendon lengthening, and the like, are useful in appropriate instances, usually to make physical care easier. Maintenance of the child's and the parents' morale is essential. The aim should be to keep the child ambulatory and in school as long as is possible, approximating a normal life as nearly as he can.

In later childhood, joint pains due to trauma to the laxly supported joints are troublesome and respond poorly to analgesics; if severe, they are indications for use of wheelchairs. Cardiomyopathy with failure is treated with digitalis and other appropriate measures.

Myopathies of Uncertain Causes and Classification. In recent years increasing numbers of families have been described in which signs, symptoms and electromyographic (EMG) and histologic changes suggestive of a dystrophic process have been combined with evidence of neural atrophy or of myotonia of various sorts. The place of these disorders is still too uncertain to warrant much discussion, beyond indicating the general incompleteness of present knowledge of neuromuscular disease.

Two conditions, apparently best classified as myopathies, are worthy of mention because they present as familial, chronic, nonprogressive muscular weakness.

Central core disease is familial, apparently inherited as an autosomal dominant with incomplete penetrance. In infancy, pronounced hypotonia arrests motor development, but by school age all patients can walk; weakness is greater proximally than distally, and may involve bulbar muscles. Wasting is not prominent, though urinary creatine is increased. Deep reflexes are normal or suppressed; the electromyogram is normal. The diagnostic feature is the presence of a central core in each muscle fiber, which stains intensely, but lacks oxidative enzymes. The course is benign, and treatment is not needed.

Nemaline myopathy is a similar nonprogressive congenital disorder, probably inherited as a recessive trait. It is characterized by hypotonia, very thin muscles, depressed reflexes, and very slow progression, if any. The diagnostic feature is the presence in affected muscle fibers of irregular, threadlike bands, apparently abnormal mitochondria, the change beginning in the Z bands. No treatment beyond physiotherapeutic support is necessary.

Hereditary juvenile muscular atrophy, the Kugelberg-Wehlander syndrome, has a more serious prognosis. The signs in childhood are those of a limb girdle dystrophy; in later years fasciculations, distal extension of weakness and loss of reflexes reveal its neurogenic nature. An electromyographic tracing or biopsy will usually reveal the neurogenic nature, even when the clinical pattern resembles a dystrophy. Inheritance is usually recessive.

DAVID B. CLARK

REFERENCES

General References

Adams, R. D., Denny-Brown, D., and Pearson, C. M.: *Diseases of Muscle*. 2nd ed. New York, Paul B. Hoeber, Inc., 1963.
Dreyfus, J. C., and Schapira, G.: *Biochemistry of Hereditary Myopathies*. Springfield, Ill., Charles C Thomas, 1962.
Greenfield, J. G., Shy, G. M., Alvord, E. C., and Berg, L.: *Atlas of Muscle Pathology in Neuromuscular Diseases*. London, E. & S. Livingstone, 1957.
Neuromuscular Disorders. *Res. Publ. Ass. Nerv. Ment. Dis.* 38. Baltimore, Williams & Wilkins Company, 1960.
Stanbury, J. B., Wyngaarden, J. B., and Frederickson, D. S.: *The Metabolic Basis of Inherited Disease*. 2nd ed. New York, McGraw-Hill Book Co., Inc., 1966.

Congenital Defects

Banker, B. Q., Victor, M., and Adams, R. D.: Arthrogryposis Multiplex Congenita Due to Congenital Muscular Dystrophy. *Brain*, 80:319, 1957.
Eagle, J. F., and Barrett, G. S.: Congenital Deficiency of Abdominal Musculature with Associated Genitourinary Abnormalities: A Syndrome Report of 9 Cases. *Pediatrics*, 6:721, 1950.
Evans, P. R.: Nuclear Agenesis—Moebius' Syndrome. The Congenital Facial Diplegia Syndrome. *Arch. Dis. Childhood*, 30:237, 1955.
Middleton, D. S.: Studies on Prenatal Lesions of Striated Muscle as a Cause of Congenital Deformity. Congenital Tibial Kyphosis, Congenital High Shoulder; Myodystrophia Foetalis Deformans. *Edinburgh M. J.*, 41:401, 1934.
Sheldon, W.: Amyoplasia Congenita. *Arch. Dis. Childhood*, 7:115, 1932.

Torticollis

Hulbert, K. F.: Torticollis. *J. Bone & Joint Surg.*, 32B:50, 1950.
Middleton, D. S.: The Pathology of Congenital Torticollis. *Brit. J. Surg.*, 18:188, 1930.

Progressive Myositis Ossificans

Eaton, W. L., Conkling, W. S., and Daeschner, C. W.: Early Myositis Ossificans Progressiva Occurring in Homozygotic Twins. *J. Pediat.*, 50:591, 1957.

Lockhart, J. D., and Burke, F. G.: Myositis Ossificans Progressiva. *Am. J. Dis. Child.*, 87:626, 1954.

Toxic and Metabolic Myopathies

Perkoff, G. T., Silber, R., Tyler, F. H., Cartwright, G. E., and Wintrobe, M. M.: Studies in Disorders of Muscle. XII. Myopathy Due to Administration of Therapeutic Amounts of Corticosteroids. *Am. J. Med.*, 26:891, 1959.
Schaar, F. E.: Paroxysmal Myoglobinuria. *Am. J. Dis. Child.*, 89:26, 1955.

Polymyositis

Walton, J. N., and Adams, R. D.: *Polymyositis*. Baltimore, Williams & Wilkins Company, 1958.
Wedgwood, R. J. P., Cook, C. D., and Cohen, J.: Dermatomyositis: Report of 26 Cases, with a Discussion of Endocrine Therapy in 13. *Pediatrics*, 12:447, 1953.

Myasthenia Gravis

Kibrick, S.: Myasthenia Gravis in the Newborn. *Pediatrics*, 14: 365, 1954.
MacRae, D. D.: Myasthenia Gravis in Early Childhood. *Pediatrics*, 13:511, 1954.
Millichap, J. G., and Dodge, P. R.: Diagnosis and Treatment of Myasthenia Gravis in Infancy, Childhood, and Adolescence. *Neurology*, 10:1007, 1960.
Schwab, R. S., and Prichard, J. S.: Myasthenia Gravis; in S. S. Gellis, and B. M. Kagan: *Current Pediatric Therapy*, 3. Philadelphia, W. B. Saunders Company, 1968, p. 597.
Strauss, A. J. L., and others: Immunofluorescence Demonstration of a Muscle Binding Complement Fixing Serum Globulin Fraction in Myasthenia Gravis. *Proc. Soc. Exper. Biol. & Med.*, 105:184, 1960.

The Myotonias and Periodic Paralyses

Caughey, J. E., and Myrianthopoulos, N. C.: *Dystrophia Myotonica and Related Disorders*. Springfield, Ill., Charles C Thomas, 1963.
Dodge, P. R., and others: Myotonic Dystrophy in Infancy and Childhood. *Pediatrics*, 35:3, 1965.
Drager, G. A., Hammill, J. F., and Shy, G. M.: Paramyotonia Congenita. *A.M.A. Arch. Neurol. & Psych.*, 80:1, 1958.
Estes, J. W., and others: Familial Myotonic Periodic Paralysis with Muscle Wasting. *Brain*, 91:295, 1968.
Gamstorp, I.: Adynamia Episodica Hereditaria. *Acta paediat., Supp.*, 108:126, 1956.
Geschwind, N., and Simpson, J. A.: Procaine Amide in Treatment of Myotonia. *Brain*, 78:81, 1955.
Huff, T. A., Horton, E. S., and Leibovitz, H. E.: Abnormal Insulin Secretion in Myotonic Dystrophy. *New England J. Med.*, 277:837, 1967.
Klein, R.: Periodic Paralysis; in S. S. Gellis, and B. M. Kagan: *Current Pediatric Therapy*, 3. Philadelphia, W. B. Saunders Company, 1968, p. 599.
Van der Meulen, J. P., Gilbert, G. J., and Kane, C. A.: Familial Hyperkalemic Paralysis with Myotonia. *New England J. Med.*, 264:1, 1961.

Muscular Dystrophies

Danowski, T. S., and others: Muscular Dystrophy. *A.M.A. J. Dis. Child.*, 91:326, 339, 346, 356, 429, 436, 442, 449, 1956.
Emery, A. E. H.: Clinical Manifestations in Two Carriers of Duchenne Muscular Dystrophy. *Lancet*, 1:1126, 1963.
Kugelberg, E., and Welander, L.: Heredo-Familial Juvenile Muscular Atrophy Simulating Muscular Dystrophy. *A.M.A. Arch. Neuro. Psychiat.*, 75:500, 1956.
Moore, W. F., Jr.: Cardiac Involvement in Progressive Muscular Dystrophy. *J. Pediat.*, 44:683, 1954.
Shy, G. M., and Magee, K. R.: A New Congenital Non-Progressive Myopathy. *Brain*, 79:610, 1956.
Shy, G. M., and others: Nemaline Myopathy—A New Congenital Myopathy. *Brain*, 86:793, 1963.
Swaimann, K. F., and Sandler, B.: The Use of Serum Creatine Phosphokinase and Other Enzymes in the Diagnosis of Progressive Muscular Dystrophy. *J. Pediat.*, 63:1116, 1963.
Zellweger, H., and Niedermeyer, E.: Central Nervous System Manifestations in Childhood Muscular Dystrophy (CMD). *Ann. Paediat.*, 205:25, 1965.

22. The Bones and Joints

The disturbances of the skeleton are divided here somewhat arbitrarily into 2 subsections: Skeletal Defects and Pediatric Orthopedics. In the first subsection are grouped various anatomic defects, many of which are genetically determined. Some develop in utero, some after birth. For the majority of them there is no therapy, but there are exceptions, e.g. the craniosynostoses, the funnel chest deformities associated with cardiorespiratory embarrassment, and basilar impression (platybasia) associated with compression of the brain stem.

The section entitled Pediatric Orthopedics includes the skeletal disturbances likely to be the joint concern of the pediatrician and the orthopedic surgeon. The remediable congenital dislocations and deformities are included in this division.

SKELETAL DEFECTS

Defects in Ossification of the Skull

ANENCEPHALY
(ACRANIA)
See page 1276.

CRANIOSYNOSTOSIS
(STENOCEPHALY)

Premature closure of one or more sutures of the skull results in deformity of the head and may cause damage to the brain and the eyes.

Etiology. Congenital craniosynostosis originates in embryonic life for unknown reasons and may be associated with other skeletal defects. In some instances it may be related to postnatal disorders such as rickets, hypophosphatasia and idiopathic hypercalcemia. Early recognition of the congenital synostoses is important, since some of these may be responsible for damage to the brain and in all instances there will be some degree of cranial deformity.

Pathology. In the normal newborn infant the bones of the cranium are separated, but soon after birth the definitive sutures are established. The edges of the flat bones are separated by fibrous tissue in which growth takes place perpendicular to the line of the suture. When a suture is obliterated, growth ceases and fibrous tissue disappears. Deformity results as growth of the vault is restricted at right angles to the involved suture and compensatory growth takes place in the regions where the sutures are open. The definitive sutures, such as the coronal, sagittal and lambdoid, begin to close after the thirtieth year.

Clinical Forms. When the *sagittal suture* is closed prematurely, the head becomes long and narrow *(scaphocephaly)*, and a bony ridge often marks the obliterated suture. Males are affected more often than females. Associated ocular or neurologic abnormalities are rarely related to the abnormality of the suture.

Closure of *one coronal suture* results in severe deformity *(oxycephaly)* with ipsilateral involvement of the face and the orbit. The roof of the orbit is depressed, exophthalmos develops, and there may be strabismus, nystagmus, papilledema, optic atrophy and loss of vision. The complications are more severe in those patients in whom *both coronal sutures* are obliterated or in whom other sutures are involved. Other malformations, such as cardiac anomalies, choanal atresia or defects of the elbow and knee joints, may also be present. Syndactylism is the most frequently associated anomaly (see below). A familial form of closure of the coronal sutures associated with hemolytic jaundice has been reported.

Acrocephalosyndactyly (Apert's syndrome) is a disorder consisting of pointing of the head anteriorly (acrocephaly), abnormalities of the sutures and syndactyly of the hands and sometimes of the feet. It has been observed in more than one generation and is thought to be transmitted on an autosomal dominant basis.

Acrocephalopolysyndactyly (Carpenter's syndrome) has certain similarities to Apert's syndrome and to the Laurence-Moon-Biedl syndrome (p. 1229). In addition to the acrocephaly, the syndrome is characterized by a peculiar facies, brachysyndactyly of the fingers, preaxial polydactyly, and syndactyly of the toes, hypogenitalism, obesity and mental retardation. It is transmitted on an autosomal recessive basis.

Craniofacial dysostosis (Crouzon's disease) is a syndrome characterized by acrocephaly, a beak-shaped nose, hypoplastic maxilla, short upper

1329

and protruding lower lips, hypertelorism, exoph-thalmos and external strabismus. This disorder is transmitted as a dominant hereditary trait with variable expressivity.

Differential Diagnosis. Oxycephaly must be distinguished from a familial form of high skulls in which premature closure of the sutures does not take place. In microcephaly the head is small, owing to failure of the brain to grow; there are no evidences of increased intracranial pressure. The vault is symmetrical. Although the anterior fontanel closes early, the sutures are not oblit-erated.

Roentgenograms of the skull in craniosynosto-sis reveal an abnormally shaped head and second-ary changes in the bones of the face and in the floor of the skull, depending on the suture or sutures involved. The involved suture may be obliterated or marked by a thin lucent line, but there is fre-quently thickening of bone along the suture and bony bridging (Fig. 22-1).

Prognosis. Closure of the sagittal suture is rarely associated with complications except for the cosmetic ones of a long narrow head. In other congenital forms of craniosynostosis there may be compression of the brain or cranial nerves which requires surgical treatment. In rare in-stances premature synostosis occurs as a hered-itary trait which results only in deformity of the skull without compression of the brain.

Treatment. When the lesion, e.g. coronal or multiple synostoses, is one which may result in significant cerebral or visual damage, surgical intervention in early infancy may lessen or avoid

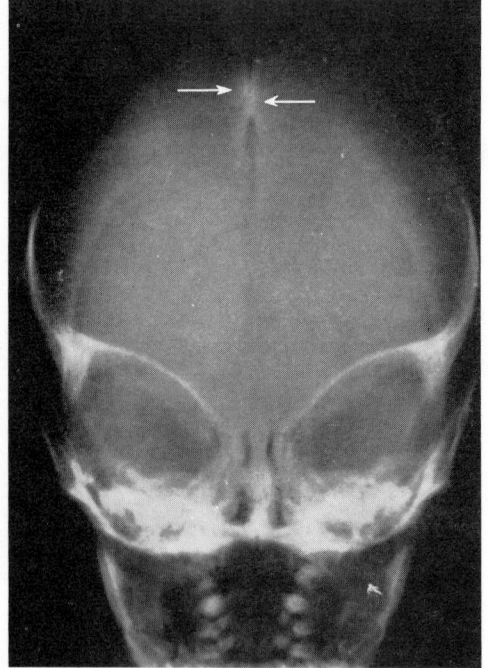

Figure 22-1. Craniosynostosis. The sagittal suture is narrow and bridged by bone (arrows). The skull was elongated in its anteroposterior dimension.

such damage. There is lack of evidence to support the decision to repair isolated sagittal synostosis except for cosmetic or psychologic reasons. Sur-gical treatment consists in linear craniectomy along the prematurely closed suture. Since there is rapid growth of the brain during the first 6 months of life, surgery will be most effective when performed soon after birth. Secondary closure of one or more of the cranial sutures occurs months after birth and only rarely requires surgical treat-ment.

BASILAR IMPRESSION
(Occipitalization of the Atlas; Platybasia)

This condition may be primary or secondary. In *primary* basilar impression, which is perhaps better designated as occipitalization or assimila-tion of the atlas, there is a congenital malforma-tion, with encroachment upon the upper cervical vertebral canal and posterior cranial fossa. The first and second occipital segments and the first and second cervical vertebrae may all be fused into one bony mass, similar to the fusion or failure of segmentation of the cervical vertebrae below the second one in the Klippel-Feil syndrome.

Secondary basilar impression occurs when disease has softened the cranial bones to such an extent that they no longer suffice to support the weight of the head. This may occur in rickets and certain forms of osteomalacia. The posterior cranial fossa is encroached upon as the cranial vertex approaches the occiput. Flattening of the base of the skull (platybasia or an increased basal angle) is at times associated with basilar impres-sion.

With either primary or secondary basilar im-pression the medulla may be kinked over the odontoid process of the second cervical vertebra, with resultant pressure upon the spinal tracts. Localized thickening of the dura at the cranio-vertebral junction is frequently associated with these bony anomalies and contributes to constric-tion of the brain stem.

The encroachment of the osseous structures upon the brain stem may be relieved in some in-stances by surgical means.

HYPERTELORISM

This condition, characterized by an abnormally large distance between the eyes and an apparent broadening of the root of the nose, is a symptom and not a disease entity. It is often associated with mental deficiency and may be combined with other congenital defects. Mild forms occur in other-wise normal children. The lesser wings of the sphenoid bone are overdeveloped, the greater wings relatively small. Hypertelorism can be transmitted through several generations. The diagnosis is made by determining the distance between the pupils, rather than by inspection alone. Epicanthic folds may result in an appearance similar to hypertelorism, but the interpupillary distance is normal.

PARIETAL FORAMINA

These are irregularly shaped congenital defects with well defined margins symmetrically placed on each side of the posterior third of the sagittal suture. They are palpable, but frequently their presence is discovered roentgenographically. They may be transmitted through several generations or occur sporadically and be found in otherwise normal persons. At times they are associated with other congenital defects of the skeleton, eye, central nervous system and heart. They must be distinguished from defects of the skull associated with meningoencephalocele or from defects caused by the reticuloendothelioses, infection, multiple myeloma or malignant metastases. Parietal foramina do not cause discomfort, and no treatment is indicated.

LACUNAR SKULL

This cranial anomaly is characterized by defects in the vault in the form of shallow depressions or deep cavitations extending to the outer surface and occurring mainly in the frontal or parietal areas. The thinned areas of bone are lined by dura and bordered by ridges of osseous tissue. The outer surface of the skull is smooth, but the inner table is rough, and on the irregular surface are many interlacing columns of bone surrounding oval depressions covered with a parchment-like membrane or a thin layer of bone. The roentgenographic appearance is diagnostic and shows diminution in the thickness of the skull bones and variations in their density as irregular patches of rarefaction, or lacunae, with interlacing ridges of increased density (Fig. 22-2). Differentiation must be made from the generalized "hammered-silver" or "digital impression" appearance of the skull bones which is observed on occasion without any apparent explanation for it and in other instances in association with increased intracranial pressure.

Meningocele is the most frequently associated defect. Lacunar skull can be detected in roentgenograms of about half of the infants with meningocele, particularly in those who have myelomeningocele or thoracic meningocele. When a meningocele is associated with a lacunar skull, progressive hydrocephalus is a frequent complication. As the cranium enlarges, the bony ridges become thin and the lacunae disappear.

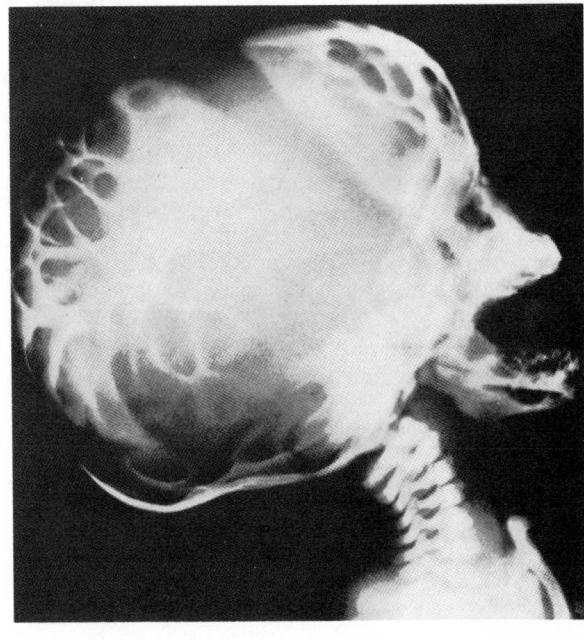

Figure 22-2. A typical example of lacunar skull (age, 18 days). Note the arborizing patterns of bony ridges which sharply delineate and separate rounded defects from one another. This patient had a large lumbosacral meningocele. (Vogt and Wyatt: *Radiology*, Vol. 36.)

Deformities of the Vertebrae, Scapulae and Sternum

Klippel-Feil Syndrome. In this syndrome there is a reduced number of cervical vertebrae, or there are multiple hemivertebrae fused into one osseous mass. Basilar impression, spina bifida, scoliosis, torticollis, Sprengel's deformity or other malformations may be associated. The neck is short, the hairline low. The motion of the neck is limited. In severe cases neurologic complications may develop.

Congenital Absence of Caudal Spine (Sacral Agenesis). Agenesis of the caudal vertebrae has been observed. The clinical picture varies with the degree of the deformity. If the first sacral vertebra is present, the bony ring of the pelvis is complete, and the weight of the trunk is transmitted normally. If the sacrum is completely missing and the iliac bones are in direct contact, the transverse diameter of the pelvis is diminished, the buttocks are flattened, and their cleft is short. Muscular atrophy of the legs is particularly notable below the knees. Dislocation of the hip, clubfoot, spina bifida, arthrogryposis, renal anomalies and fecal incontinence are additional manifestations. Roentgenograms reveal the extent of the skeletal anomaly. A syndrome of anomalies of the lower spine and of the lower extremities has been observed in children of diabetic mothers.

Sprengel's Deformity. In this congenital deformity (Fig. 22-3) one or both scapulae are in a high position with the lower angle turned toward the spine. Sometimes a bridge of bone unites the spine to the scapula (omovertebral bone). The arm on the affected side cannot be raised above a right angle with the body, and the head is inclined toward this side. Scoliosis is present. Sprengel's deformity may occur with the Klippel-Feil syndrome.

Deformities of the Sternum. The halves of the sternum may remain separated (*fissure of the sternum*). *Pigeon breast* consists in a prominence of the sternum and the cartilaginous parts of the ribs, with lateral depressions of the thorax. A short sternum is a common manifestation of trisomy 18.

Pectus Excavatum (Funnel Chest). Funnel chest, or indentation of the lower part of the sternum, may be rachitic in origin or the result of chronic obstruction to respiration. In most instances, however, the condition is congenital. The reason for the defect is not apparent in all instances, but in some it is due to a short central tendon of the diaphragm. The manubrium sterni is at the normal level, but the inferior parts are depressed, and the xiphoid may approach the vertebral bodies. The volume of the lung may be decreased, and the heart displaced to the left. There are often no symptoms, but respiration may be paradoxic, since contraction of the diaphragm exerts a pull on the xiphoid and the costal cartilages. The patient may appear round-shouldered, hollow-chested, thin and underdeveloped. The deformity may have untoward psychologic effects on the child. Surgical improvement may be attempted, for cosmetic reasons, if the deformity is severe or if compression causes pulmonary embarrassment.

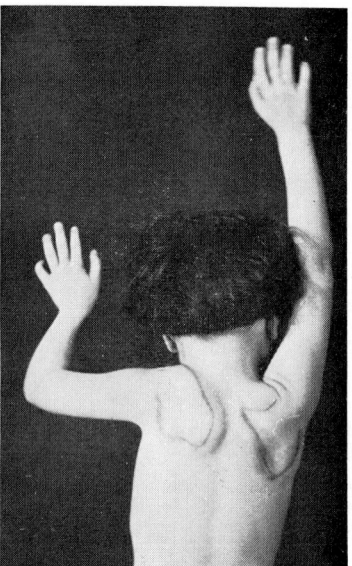

Figure 22-3. Sprengel's deformity, showing inability to raise the arm completely on the affected side.

Deformities of the Extremities

Severe deformities of the extremities are often not compatible with life because of associated malformations. Extensive defects of the limbs in surviving children were rarities until the epidemic of partial and total absence of limbs (reduction malformations) resulting from maternal ingestion of the drug thalidomide. Since rehabilitation of patients with such limb defects has become an important problem, knowledge of the terminology is necessary. Minor limb defects are frequent. They may be harmless variations of development or indicators of more serious anomalies of other organ systems.

Absence or extensive reductions of limbs present at birth are often called *congenital amputations*. This term should be reserved for secondary intrauterine destruction of limbs that were originally formed as normal anlagen. Limb defects due to primary inhibition of development or growth are better called *reduction malformations*. Such malformations frequently have terminal fingers or nails, indicating that no true amputation has occurred.

Amelia means absence of limbs. *Hemimelia* (absence of a portion) is commonly used for defects of the distal parts of the extremities such as absence of forearm and hand or lower leg and hand or lower leg and foot. *Phocomelia* signifies a great reduction in size of proximal parts of the limb, resulting in an approach of distal parts toward the trunk. In complete phocomelia the hand or foot seems to spring directly from the trunk (right side in Figure 22-4). *Acheiria* and *apodia* are terms for absence of a hand or foot; *adactylia* for absence of digits, and *aphalangia* for absence of phalanges. Individual bones may be absent. Absence of the humerus and ulna is rare; absence of the radius is usually associated with clubhand. Absence of the fibula is more frequently encountered than absence of the femur or tibia. As a rule, it is combined with pes valgus. Absence of the patella is indicated by a transverse fold of the skin in front of the knee joint during extension. It is often associated with iliac horns and deformity of the radial head.

Polydactyly (supernumerary fingers or toes) may be found in a single member of a sibship, but there are pedigrees in which polydactyly is inherited as a dominant trait. Polydactyly is sometimes associated with other malformations (see Chondro-ectodermal Dysplasia, p. 1337).

Syndactyly (Fig. 22-6), union of fingers or toes, may consist in fusion of the bones or webbing of the skin *(zygodactyly)*. Syndactyly most frequently involves the third and fourth fingers and the second and third toes. It is often seen in children with multiple malformations (acrocephalosyndactyly) and in children who otherwise are entirely normal. In the latter, syndactyly is often hereditary.

Split hand and split foot (lobster claw) are deep clefts in the anterior part of the hand or foot, and the fingers and toes have different degrees of syndactyly. The foot appears split in the area where the second or third toe should be. The parts

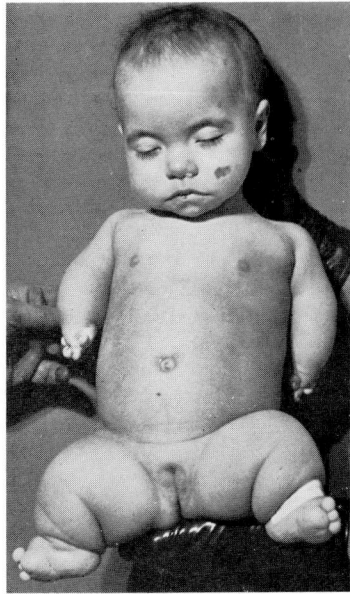

Figure 22-5. Partial phocomelia in an infant 11 months of age; picture taken at autopsy.

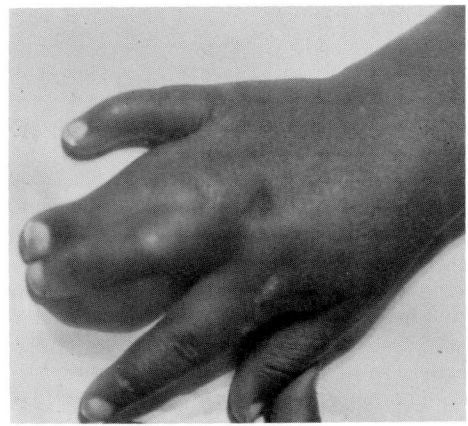

Figure 22-6. Syndactyly.

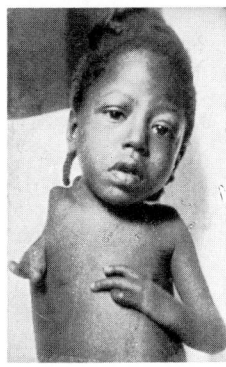

Figure 22-4. Phocomelia and partial adactylia in a girl 3½ years of age.

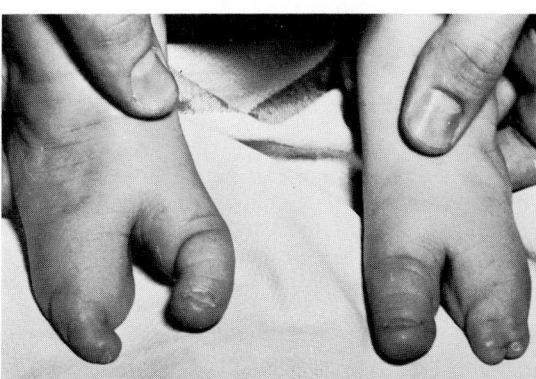

Figure 22-7. Split feet (lobster claws) in a child whose mother, maternal aunt and maternal grandfather had similar malformations.

of the foot which lie on either side of the cleft are fused into masses in which terminal digits can be recognized (Fig. 22-7). Many pedigrees are known in which this malformation is inherited as a dominant trait. *Brachydactyly,* abnormal shortness of the fingers and toes resulting from lack or reduction in size of a phalanx or metacarpal bone, may be genetically determined. It may be seen in pseudohypoparathyroidism, pseudo-pseudohypoparathyroidism and Turner's syndrome. *Clinodactyly*, incurving of the little finger, may be inherited as a dominant trait. It is also often seen in Down's syndrome. *Camptodactylia*, permanently flexed fingers, can be transmitted as a dominant trait; it also occurs in trisomies D and E (p. 332). *Macrodactylia* is a hypertrophy of one or several fingers and toes (Fig. 22-8). It may be a manifestation of neurofibromatosis.

A variety of skeletal defects, of which absence of thumbs and radii is common, occur at times in association with a congenital hypoplastic anemia (p. 1044), congenital heart disease, and other syndromes.

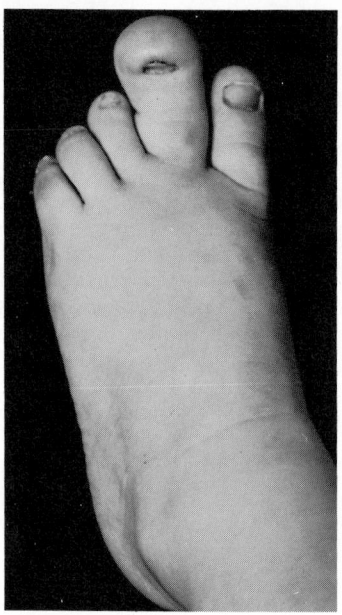

Figure 22-8.   Macrodactylia.

Generalized Skeletal Defects

ACHONDROPLASIA
(Chondrodystrophy)

Achondroplasia is a disorder of cartilage which begins in prenatal life and leads to a specific type of dwarfism. The long bones are most severely affected, so that disproportionate dwarfism becomes manifest with growth.

Etiology.   Genetic factors play a leading role, most pedigrees suggesting a dominant mode of transmission. Sporadic cases occur frequently; they should be attributed to new mutations. Advanced parental (probably paternal) age has been considered a possible factor. Males and females are equally affected.

Pathology.   The basic process is a disturbance of endochondral ossification caused by an inability of the epiphyseal plate to produce a sufficient amount of columnar cartilage. The result is deficient growth of bones of endochondral formation. The rows of columnar cartilage lack parallel arrangement and are of unequal length. The line of preparatory ossification is irregular. The bone trabeculae are short and thick and lack normal orderly arrangement. Sometimes a transverse vascular strip of connective tissue, which originates in the periosteum, grows between the epi-

physis and the diaphysis, thus adding another obstacle to longitudinal growth. If this strip affects only one side of the bone, bowing occurs with growth. Periosteal ossification is little affected, so that transverse growth of bone is not greatly disturbed. As a result, the bones appear thick.

The epiphyseal cartilage, which is underdeveloped in the longitudinal direction, may extend well beyond the shaft in the transverse direction, creating a mushroom-like enlargement. Hypoplasia of the cartilage may be seen in the transverse as well as in the longitudinal direction, in which case the enlargement of the metaphysis is less pronounced. Owing to insufficient cartilaginous growth, the base of the skull is short, but the bones of the cranial vault which are of membranous origin continue to grow. This disproportionate growth results in a typical profile characterized by a broad nose with a depressed bridge, and a bulging forehead.

Clinical Manifestations.   The chief characteristic of achondroplasia is the combination of short extremities with a head that is often somewhat enlarged (and in all instances seems even relatively larger than it is) and a trunk approximating normal size. The limbs are often curved, and their epiphyseal junctions enlarged and prominent. The proximal portions of the extremities are most severely affected; the hands, which are short and broad, may not reach the hips. The relatively large head exhibits a prominent forehead, flattening of the bridge of the nose, and a forward projection of the mandible; hydrocephalus is sometimes present. The chest is of normal length, but narrow in the anteroposterior dimension, and beading of the ribs and flaring of the costal margins are generally noticeable.

The thoracic kyphosis and the lumbar lordosis are usually accentuated. Protrusion of the abdomen and the gluteal region results in a characteristic posture. An umbilical hernia is common. The deformed pelvis may be an obstacle to delivery in women, often necessitating cesarean section. The gait is waddling. Extension of the joints may be impeded by the irregular shape of the epiphyses. The skin is loose and may form transverse folds and pads. The muscular development is good. The mentality is usually normal.

Diagnosis. The thickness of the bones and their irregular epiphyseal ends as seen in the roentgenogram make the diagnosis possible even in the newborn infant. The bones of the extremities are short and broad and have a mushroom-like broadening at the ends of the shafts. The

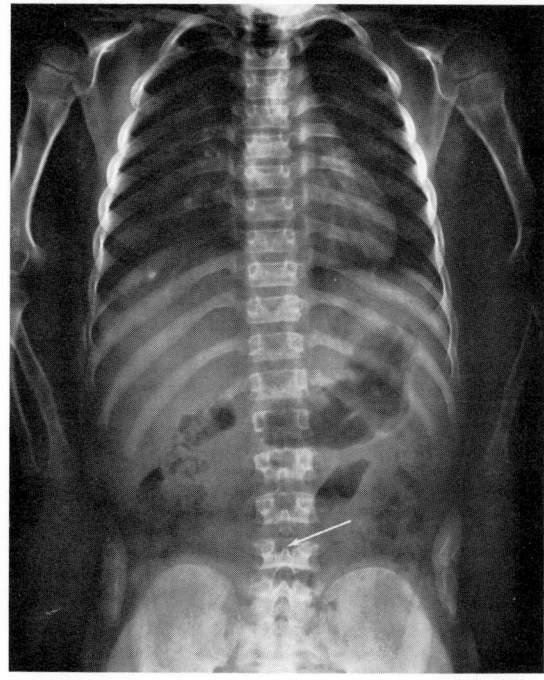

Figure 22-10. Achondroplasia. The length of the upper extremities may be compared with the length of the trunk. The small interpediculate distances of the lumbar vertebrae (arrow) and the narrow sacrum are evident.

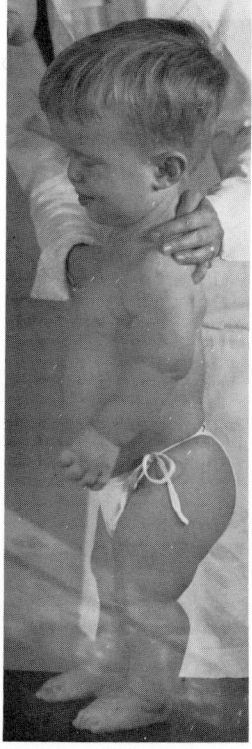

Figure 22-9. Achondroplasia in a child. Note the relatively large head, the saddle nose and brachycephaly, the short extremities and the lordosis with forward tilting of the pelvis.

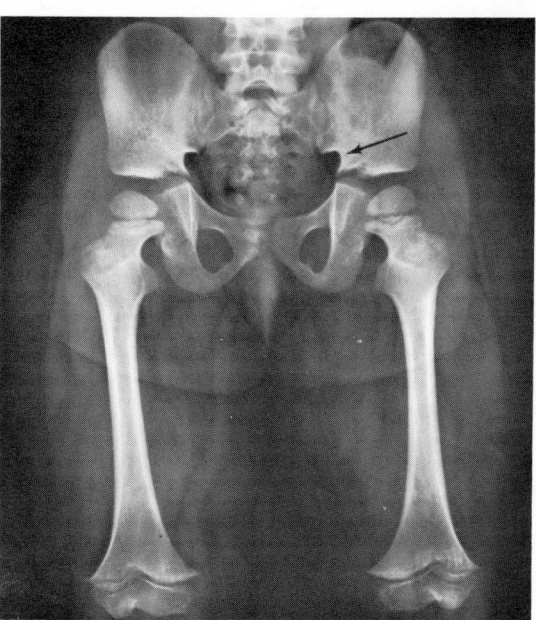

Figure 22-11. Achondroplasia. The sacrum articulates low on the ilia. The sciatic notch is small (arrow), and the roof of the acetabulum is broad and flat. Flaring of the distal end of the short femurs is evident.

fibula is often longer than the tibia. Curving may be seen in various places. At the epiphyseal ends of the shafts are such irregularities as cupping, fraying and spurs. The mineral content is good throughout the bones, and there are no periosteal changes. Ossification of the epiphyses and of the carpal and tarsal bones is not delayed, but their outlines are irregular. The metacarpal, metatarsal and phalangeal bones are also short and thick and have irregularities at their epiphyseal ends (Fig. 22-12). On the lateral view the base of the skull appears short. The bones of the vault bulge on all sides beyond the base.

The alterations of the bones of the pelvis and of the lumbar spine are important in diagnosis. The height of the iliac bones is diminished in the region of the acetabulum so that the acetabular roof is flat and broad, and the sciatic notch is small. There is a decrease in the interpediculate distances of the lumbar vertebrae as a manifestation of the small spinal canal. The vertebral bodies are usually of normal height, but occasionally a wedge-shaped vertebra is present. Herniation of intervertebral disks is common.

The serum values of calcium, phosphorus and alkaline phosphatase are normal.

The depressed bridge of the nose may suggest syphilis or cretinism. *Syphilis* can be ruled out by the roentgenogram and by serologic tests; normal mental development and normal serum concentration of protein-bound iodine rule out *cretinism.* A superficial examination of the roentgenograms may suggest *rickets;* however, the intensive calcification of the irregular epiphyses is characteristic of achondroplasia.

Other forms of micromelia can be distinguished by clinical examination or the roentgenogram. The legs of children with *osteogenesis imperfecta* or *osteopsathyrosis* may become shortened and deformed after repeated fractures, but the bones are long and slender. *Hypophosphatasia* resulting in congenital micromelia can be mistaken for achondroplasia in the neonatal period, but the deficiency of ossification and low serum phosphatase value establish the diagnosis.

Prognosis and Treatment. Many children with achondroplasia die in utero or soon after birth, particularly when born prematurely. Those who survive usually have good general health, and their mental development is satisfactory. Their height rarely exceeds 140 cm. (55 inches).

No specific treatment is known. Early orthopedic correction of developing deformities may improve the appearance.

OTHER CHONDRODYSPLASIAS

A variety of skeletal disorders which clinically resemble achondroplasia in some respects and the mucopolysaccharidoses in others have been observed in several generations of a kinship. These disorders, usually not noticeable at birth, manifest themselves during the first years of childhood and result in variable degrees of shortness of stature. Roentgenographically, the irregularities are most apparent in the epiphyses, but the diaphyses are not entirely spared.

DOMINANTLY INHERITED CHONDRODYSPLASIAS

The following four systemic skeletal disorders are inherited as dominant traits; there are many intermediate forms which are not readily classified.

Spondyloepiphyseal Dysplasia. This is a relatively recently described syndrome, which in the past was considered a variant of achondrodysplasia. It differs from the latter in several ways, but especially in that the infant appears to be normal at birth and the evidence of dwarfism is not apparent for several years. Other differences are the lack of involvement of the head and face and the more extensive changes in the epiphyses in spondyloepiphyseal dysplasia. The epiphyses are small, irregular and fragmented (Fig. 22-12). The vertebral bodies are somewhat flattened and have a tendency to be biconvex. By midchildhood the affected person has an outward appearance simulating that of achondrodysplasia with short extremities and lordosis; the head, however, though relatively large, is not abnormal.

Multiple Epiphyseal Dysplasia. A variety of terms have been used to describe irregularities of ossification which are largely limited to the epiphyses; differences evident at the moment appear to be largely in degree of involvement, but it is not unlikely that distinct entities may eventually be separated out from the general category. Roentgenographic changes in the epiphyses vary from stippling to an appearance of almost complete destruction. In the hips the roentgenographic appearance may resemble that of aseptic necrosis (Legge-Calvé-Perthes disease, p. 1356). The vertebral pattern is normal or nearly so. Shortness in stature is variable, and in later life arthritic changes are common.

Metaphyseal Dysostosis. The principal involvement is in the metaphyses of the long bones. Roentgenographically, the ends of the bones appear frayed, irregular and widened, resembling the osseous changes of rickets. The blood values of phosphorus, calcium and phosphatase, however, are within normal limits. The child is short in stature and bowlegged.

Dyschondrosteosis. In this disorder the forearms and the lower legs are principally affected, while the proximal portions of the skeleton appear to be normal or less involved (mesomelia). The radius is particularly bowed, often curving around the ulna. A bayonet-like volar displacement of the

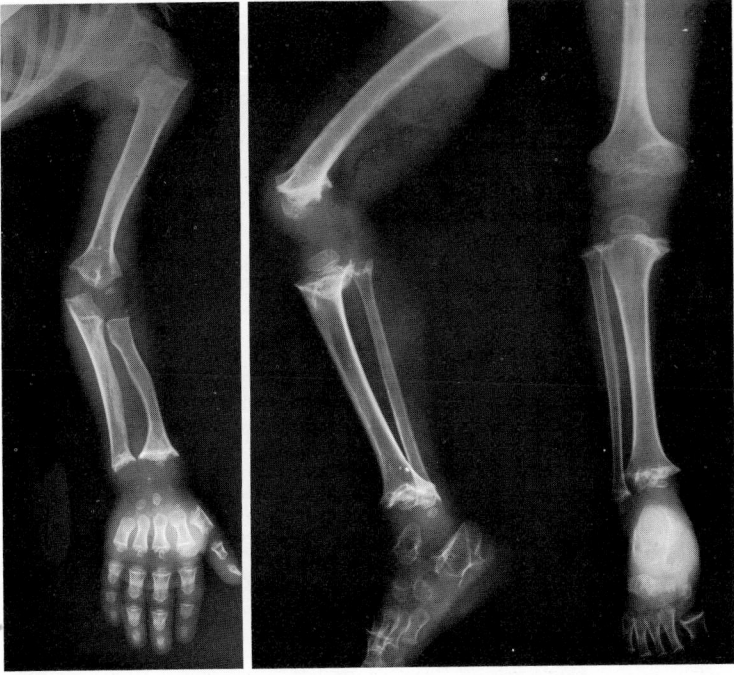

Figure 22-12. Spondyloepiphyseal dysplasia.

dorsum of the hand against the forearm is a prominent feature (Madelung's deformity).

RECESSIVELY INHERITED CHONDRODYSPLASIAS

Diastrophic Dwarfism. At birth the appearance is that of achondroplasia because of the shortness of the extremities, but there are characteristically clubfoot and often contractures of other joints, cleft palate, and ear deformities. During childhood, scoliosis, kyphosis and dislocations develop, and the clubfeet and flexion of knees and hips become more pronounced.

Chondro-Ectodermal Dysplasia (Ellis-Van Creveld Syndrome). The combination of chondrodysplasia, ectodermal dysplasia, polydactyly and congenital heart disease is a rare syndrome. The bones of the extremities are short and thick, and the terminal phalanges of the fingers and toes and the nails are dystrophic. The distal long bones are most severely affected. There is a sixth finger on the ulnar side of each hand. Dentition is defective, but the sweat glands and the skin are normal. Stillbirth or death in early infancy is common. This syndrome has been identified in the Amish of Lancaster County, Pennsylvania.

Asphyxiating Thoracic Dystrophy (Jeune's Syndrome). Asphyxiating thoracic dystrophy is a descriptive term applied to a dysplasia of the skeleton characterized by very short ribs, slight shortening of the long bones and peculiar cleftlike lesions in the acetabulum and in the metaphyses of the long bones. The skull and the spine appear to be normal. The thorax is small and relatively immobile, air exchange is limited, and the patient's course is complicated by repeated respiratory infections. This condition was first reported by Jeune in siblings; both males and females are affected.

Chondrodystrophia Calcificans Congenita. (Conradi's Disease). This rare form of chondrodysplasia has a typical roentgenographic appearance. The carpal and the tarsal bones are replaced by numerous small but distinctly calcified spots scattered about the affected areas. They represent deposits of calcium in cartilage. The epiphyses may be stippled with similar small calcium deposits. The limbs are often short, particularly in their proximal segments. Contractures are not rare, and cataracts are often present. Calcifications may also occur in the tracheal cartilages (Fig. 22-13) and be responsible for respiratory embarrassment. The severe form of this syndrome is transmitted on a recessive basis; a mild form of stippled epiphyses is dominantly transmitted.

MUCOPOLYSACCHARIDOSES

The mucopolysaccharidoses comprise a group of diseases which have in common a disorder in the metabolism of mucopolysaccharides and which are separated by genetic, clinical and biochemical

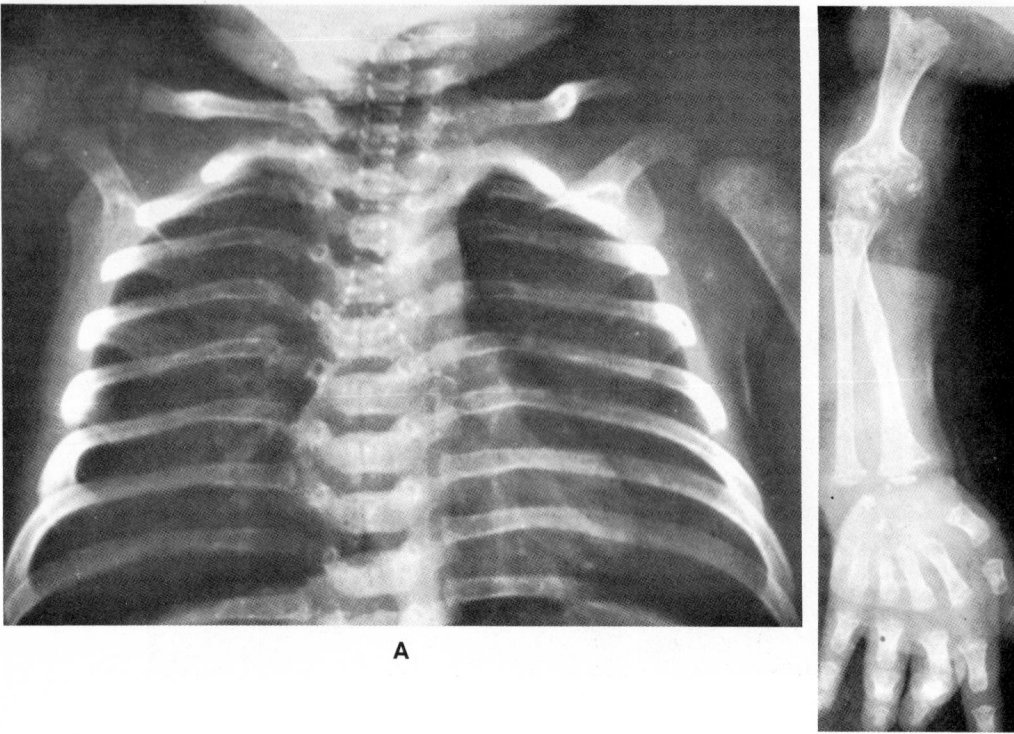

A

B

Figure 22-13. Chondrodystrophia calcificans congenita. *A*, Diffuse calcification of the laryngeal, tracheal and bronchial cartilages. In early infancy the infant had significant dyspnea, presumably due to the constricted tracheobronchial tree. *B*, Shortening of humerus. Numerous calcifications in the area of the elbow joint. Contractures of finger joints.

characteristics. Classification is still in flux; at present 6 subgroups are usually distinguished. Hurler's syndrome is the prototype of these disorders.

The mucopolysaccharides comprise much of the ground substance of connective tissue; they are present in mucous secretions; and one, heparin, is found in the circulation, where it exerts an anticoagulative effect. Chemically, they are long, linear polymers consisting of substituted glucose and galactose residues. They contain nitrogen in the form of glucosamine and galactosamine as well as carboxylic acid groups and sulfate molecules esterified to either one of the hydroxyl groups or bound to the amine groups.

The various compounds which are excreted, such as chondroitin A or B, hyaluronic acid, keratosulfate and heparatin sulfate, are all mucopolysaccharides whose structures are known. The acidic groups of the mucopolysaccharides react metachromatically with dyes such as toluidine blue. This reaction is used clinically in the detection of these disorders. Although some of the enzymology concerning these compounds is known, in none of the mucopolysaccharides has any specific enzyme dysfunction been implicated. Fibroblasts from patients with one of the mucopoly-

saccharidoses, when grown in tissue culture, stain metachromatically. The same is true of cells derived from heterozygotic individuals, and this technique may be used to screen for carriers of these disorders.

HURLER'S SYNDROME
(GARGOYLISM; DYSOSTOSIS MULTIPLEX; MPS-I)

This disorder is a metabolic disturbance which affects both skeleton and soft tissues. Although the metabolic disturbance is present at birth, most of the manifestations develop in postnatal life. The fully developed disease is characterized by cloudy corneas, hepatosplenomegaly, mental deficiency, skeletal changes and dwarfism. Both sexes may be affected. The disorder is genetically determined, being due to an autosomal recessive gene. The basic metabolic disturbance results in accumulation of an abnormal intracellular material which affects the cells and structure of many organs. The nature of the stored substances is inadequately defined, but they are thought to be acid mucopolysaccharides. Specifically, chondroitin sulfate B and heparatin sulfate are found in abnormal amounts in the urine.

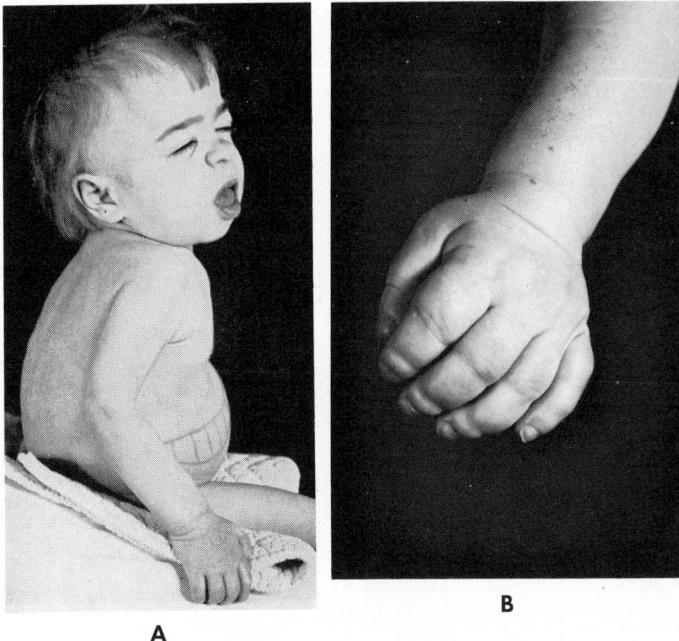

Figure 22-14. *A*, Hurler's syndrome in a child 2 years of age, showing heavy features, depressed nasal bridge, kyphosis and stunting of growth; also outline of the enlarged liver. Child had corneal opacity and was mentally deficient. *B*, Typical spadelike hand.

Clinical Manifestations. The skull is frequently malformed and may be scaphocephalic, oxycephalic or enlarged. Closure of the anterior fontanel may be delayed. The supraorbital ridges are prominent, and the bridge of the nose is depressed. A profuse nasal discharge is usually present because of the deformed pharynx, which is often blocked by lymphoid tissue. The tongue is enlarged, and the neck short. There is a kyphosis in the dorsolumbar region (Fig. 22-14, *A*). The heart is frequently enlarged, and a systolic murmur can be heard (p. 1031). Dyspnea occurs on slight exertion; cyanosis, in advanced stages. The abdomen is prominent; the spleen and liver are enlarged; and an umbilical hernia is frequently present. Externally, the sex organs appear normal, but sexual maturation does not occur. The joints have limited extensibility, particularly in the fingers. The appearance of the hands is characteristic (Fig. 22-14, *B*): the breadth is greater than the length, the fingers are maintained in a "clawing" position, and the fourth and fifth fingers are incurved. Coxa valga and genu valgum of a moderate degree may be present. The combination of the clawlike hands, the large head, the grotesque facies and deformed limbs accounts for the designation "gargoylism." The thickness of the skin contributes to the characteristic picture. Corneal opacities and mental retardation are prominent manifestations. In the white blood cells abnormal granulations *(Reilly bodies)* may be found. Increased amounts of mucopolysaccharides are present in the urine. A diagnostic spot test is available which is based on the detection of chondroitin sulfuric acid on paper chromatograms by toluidine blue.

Diagnosis. The stunted growth, the thickness of the skin and the mental retardation suggest cretinism, but the laboratory data and the roentgenographic changes are adequate for differentiation. Roentgenographically, the sella turcica is often found to be elongated and the mandibular condyles to be concave. The changes of the spinal column are best seen in the lateral view. The vertebral bodies are short in the sagittal direction, their anterior and posterior outlines appear concave, and the spinous processes are directed downward. The first or second lumbar vertebra is small and displaced backward, resulting in deformity of the spine (Fig. 22-15, *A*). The lower ribs are club-shaped. The humerus is long and thick, the ulna and radius, short and thick. Their epiphyseal ends and their epiphyses have irregular outlines. The metacarpal bones are bottle-shaped, the basal phalanges cylindrical (Fig. 22-15, *B*). The femur, tibia and fibula are moderately thickened, and their epiphyses are angular.

Prognosis and Treatment. The prognosis is unfavorable, since the patients remain retarded in mental and physical development. Orthopedic treatment may aid in correcting the deformity of the spine.

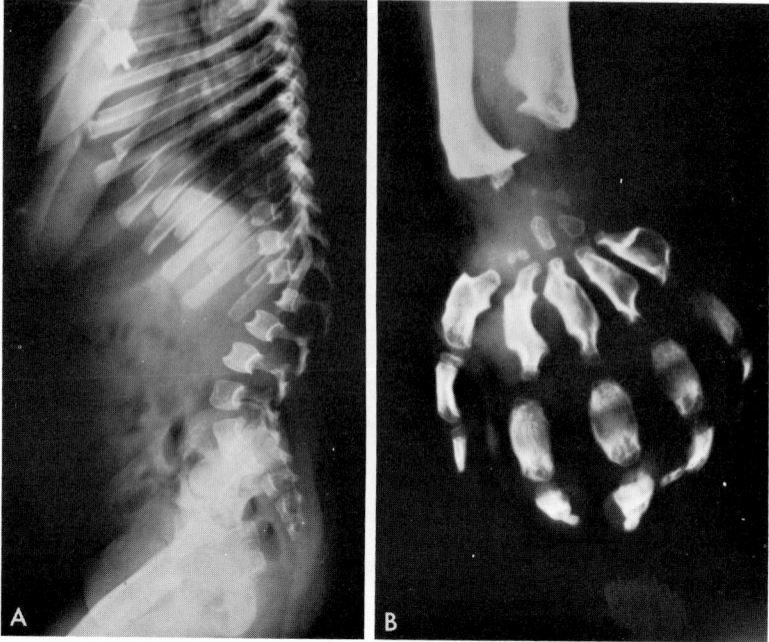

Figure 22-15. Hurler's syndrome. *A*, Lateral view of spinal column; *B*, hand.

HUNTER'S SYNDROME
(MPS-II)

This syndrome is characterized by a physical resemblance to Hurler's syndrome, but the disease is inherited as a sex-linked recessive. Mental deterioration is slower, and clouding of the cornea is rare. Progressive deafness is frequent. Chondroitin sulfate B and heparitin sulfate are found in the urine.

SANFILIPPO SYNDROME
(MPS-III)

This form is characterized by less severe somatic alterations, but mental retardation is profound. It is inherited as an autosomal recessive. Heparitin sulfate is found in the urine in large amounts.

MORQUIO'S DISEASE
(MPS-IV)

This chondrodystrophy is genetically determined. Consanguinity of the parents and also of the paternal grandparents was reported in the family described by Morquio. A recessive mode of transmission is suggested; in one unusual sibship the disorder was transmitted as a sex-linked

recessive trait (see p. 323). Sporadic cases have also been described. Abnormal amounts of keratosulfate may be found in the urine.

Clinical Manifestations. Development appears to be normal until the infant begins to walk. The face and the skull are only slightly affected; the neck is short (Fig. 22-16). In contrast to achondroplasia (p. 1334), the spine and the chest become severely deformed. Fusion of cervical vertebrae and platybasia may occur. The thorax is short and broad; the anteroposterior diameter is increased, and the sternum protrudes. There is an exaggerated thoracic kyphosis of the spine and scoliosis of a varying degree. The abdomen protrudes; genital development is normal. The relatively long arms extend to the knees. The hands and fingers are long and soft. Genu valgum and flat feet are present. The joints are enlarged; the muscles and ligaments are flaccid; the gait is waddling. The osseous manifestations are unlike those of the Hurler syndrome. The mentality is usually normal.

Diagnosis. There is an external resemblance to rickets, but the absence of hypophosphatemia and the roentgenographic appearance of the bones exclude rickets. In Morquio's disease basilar invagination and occipitalization may be present in addition to anomalous segmentation of the cervical vertebrae. The vertebrae are flattened, and their cranial and caudal surfaces are uneven. The shafts of the long bones are of normal length and shape. The outlines of their epiphyseal ends

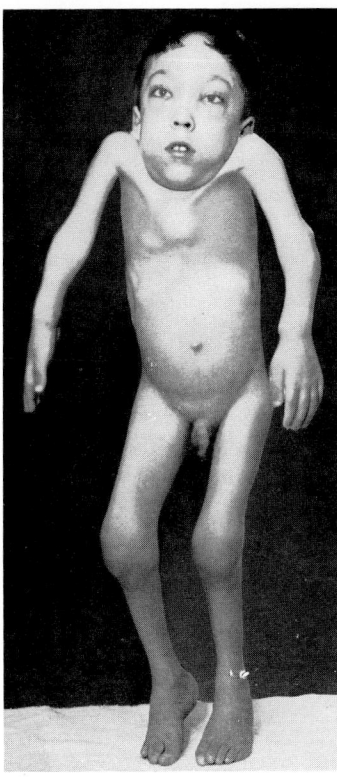

Figure 22-16. Morquio's disease.

are irregular, with flattening in some places and abnormal projections in others. The epiphyses are of irregular shape and sometimes fragmented. The ends of the metacarpal bones resemble those seen in typical achondroplasia.

Prognosis and Treatment. As far as physical development is concerned, the prognosis is unfavorable, since the deformities progress and become more pronounced. There is no specific treatment. Orthopedic treatment may prevent or correct the deformities to some extent.

SCHEIE'S SYNDROME
(MPS-V)

This form is characterized by physical changes resembling those of Hurler's syndrome, but intelligence is not impaired. Excessive amounts of chondroitin sulfate B are found in the urine.

POLYDYSTROPHIC DWARFISM
(MAROTEAUX-LAMY SYNDROME; MPS-VI)

The clinical manifestations, which include growth retardation, lumbar kyphosis, sternal protrusion and genu valgum, develop after 2 years of age. The facial features are coarse, and hepatosplenomegaly is present in most cases. There is no mental retardation. The patients excrete large amounts of chondroitin sulfate B.

OSTEOPETROSIS
(ALBERS-SCHÖNBERG DISEASE; MARBLE BONES)

Osteopetrosis is a rare disorder characterized by hard and brittle bones.

Etiology. In the majority of cases the mode of inheritance appears to be recessive; in some cases, dominant. Males and females are equally affected.

Pathology. The cortex of the bones, as well as the trabeculae, is thickened. Endochondral ossification is disturbed by lack of resorption of cartilaginous intercellular ground substance. Islands of this partly calcified ground substance, which under normal conditions is replaced by bone, persist and are found in the shafts of the bones. The trabeculae are unusually crowded and numerous. At the ends of the long bones, as well as in the scapulae and pelvic bones, zones of increased and decreased density alternate. The medullary cavity is reduced in volume, and the marrow may contain abnormal cells or fibrous tissue. The foramina for the cranial nerves are often constricted by an overgrowth of bone. The chemical composition of the bones is normal.

Clinical Manifestations. This condition probably always begins in utero, although clinical symptoms may be absent in infancy. Brittleness predisposes the bones to fracture, and roentgenograms taken on occasion of a fracture often reveal the underlying process for the first time. Although the fractures as a rule heal satisfactorily, deformities frequently develop. The head is square and somewhat enlarged, and deformities of the chest and spine may be present. Vision is usually disturbed early in life and diminishes progressively; the movements of the eyes may be impaired. Cataracts and optic atrophy may develop. There may be progressive deafness. The teeth develop abnormally and have a tendency to decay. The patient often has a hypochromic anemia and, in the final stage of the disease, a myelophthisic one. Hepatosplenomegaly and enlargement of the lymph nodes have been observed. Osteomyelitis is a frequent complication, particularly in the mandible or maxilla. General growth is retarded, and some of the patients are dwarfed. The mentality is normal, but chronic illness, blindness or deafness may interfere with its development.

Diagnosis. Roentgenographic demonstration of increased density of the entire skeleton is diagnostic. No distinction can be made between cortex and marrow. The bones of the base of the cranium are thick and dense; those of the vault are less

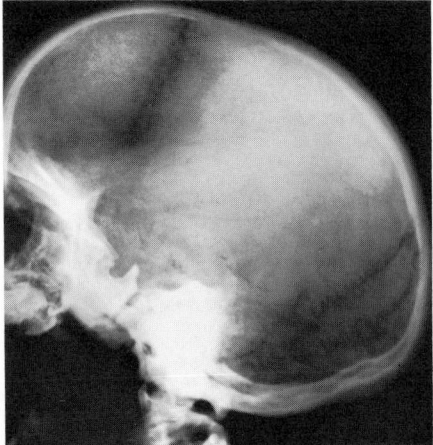

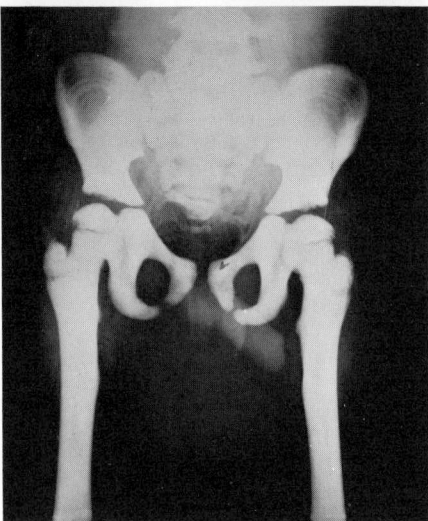

Figure 22-17. Osteopetrosis of skull, pelvis and femurs.

affected (Fig. 22-17). The long bones, particularly the femur and tibia, are club-shaped, and transverse bands are seen near their ends. Bandlike stratification may also be found in the os ilium and in the scapula. Skeletal maturation is normal.

Localized sclerotic processes as seen in *syphilis* and *sclerosing osteitis* are easily distinguished from osteopetrosis. A generalized *osteosclerosis* may result from fluorine poisoning, but in such cases calcification of muscles and ligaments is also often present. Cranial alterations in idiopathic hypercalcemia resemble those of osteopetrosis, as do those in craniometaphyseal dysplasia.

Prognosis and Treatment. The prognosis is unfavorable in the majority of cases observed during childhood. Accidental detection of osteopetrosis in a number of apparently healthy adults is evidence that the disorder may exist for a long time without causing significant symptoms.

There is no treatment. The complications are treated symptomatically.

PYKNODYSOSTOSIS

This is a form of osteosclerosis combined with delayed closure of the fontanels, separated cranial sutures and hypoplasia of the terminal phalanges. It may be confused with osteopetrosis, because the bones are denser than usual on the roentgenogram and they fracture with slight trauma.

OSTEOGENESIS IMPERFECTA

This disease is characterized by increased fragility of the bones, which are easily fractured by slight trauma. Patients with this disorder usually have blue scleras and flaccid ligaments; some of them become deaf later in life.

In severe cases, fractures occur in utero, and the infant is born with deformities *(osteogenesis imperfecta congenita)*. In other instances, fractures do not occur until several years after birth, and the tendency to fracture disappears after puberty *(osteopsathyrosis, osteogenesis imperfecta tarda)*. This latter form usually has a milder course, but often occurs repeatedly in the same family or sibship. Whether the 2 forms are identical is a matter of dispute.

Etiology. The disorder is determined before birth. Osteopsathyrosis is often transmitted as a dominant hereditary trait, but the different manifestations (blue scleras, fragility of the bones, deafness, and the like) may show intrafamilial variability (p. 322). The congenital form is usually not repeated in families, although rarely it may alternate with the late form (osteopsathyrosis). Recessive inheritance has been infrequently demonstrated.

Pathology. Osteogenesis imperfecta is a systemic disease whose manifestations are considered to be due to a defect of the mesenchyme and its derivatives (scleras, bones and ligaments).

The cortex is invariably diminished in thickness, owing to disturbed formation of periosteal bone. Inactivity of the patient contributes to the atrophy of the bones. Osteoblastic activity is defective. The generalized mesenchymal involvement in the congenital form of the disease is demonstrable in sections of the skin and scleras by a failure of the reticulum to differentiate into mature collagen. In some cases the abnormally thin scleras allow the underlying pigment to show through. In others increased transparency, but not thinness, of the sclera is observed. Occasionally cataract, coloboma and embryotoxon are asso-

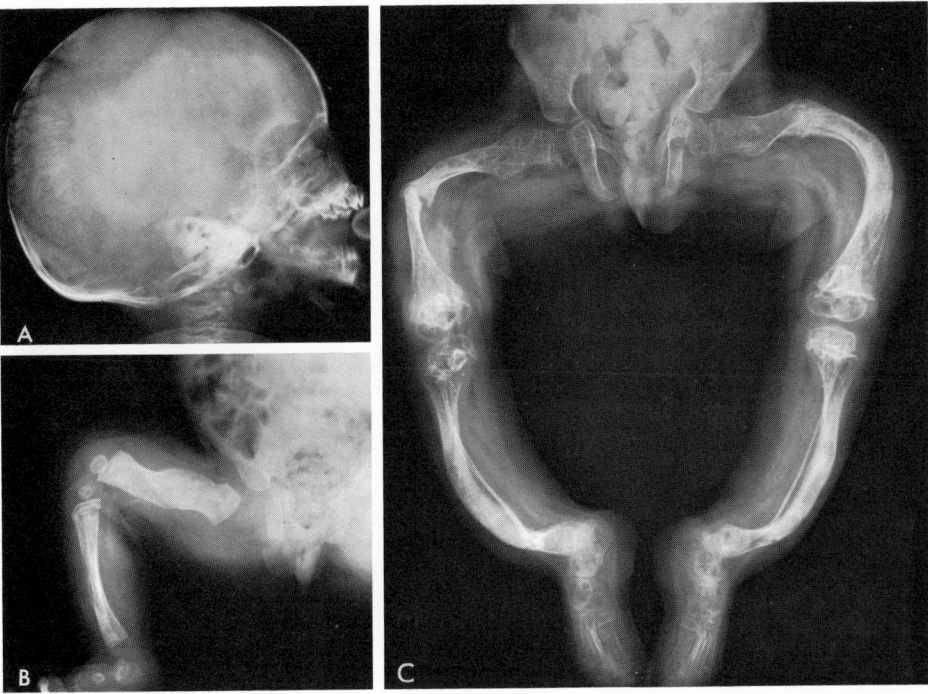

Figure 22-18. Osteogenesis imperfecta. *A*, Skull showing wormian bones. *B*, Roentgenogram of leg at birth. *C*, Roentgenogram of legs at 5 years of age.

ciated with this disorder. Deafness may be due to otosclerosis or labyrinthine disturbance.

Clinical Manifestations. In *osteogenesis imperfecta congenita* fractures may occur in utero, and the infant is born with deformities, since the bones generally heal in abnormal positions. Fractures may also occur during delivery. The skull has wide membranous spaces between the bones of the vault, and crackling is often felt on pressure. Many wormian bones are found within the occipital; parietal and temporal bones (Fig. 22-18). The eyes are often prominent, the scleras blue. Dental changes *(dentinogenesis imperfecta)* may be prominent. The neck is short. The chest and the spine are deformed in severe cases. Many children with the severe congenital form die soon after birth. In those who survive, fractures of the extremities may result from otherwise inconsequential trauma. Callus usually forms rapidly, and the process of healing is considered satisfactory. The callus, however, is often replaced by inferior bone which is prone to bend and fracture. Most of the fractures occur in the legs, where bizarre deformities develop.

Serum levels of calcium and phosphorus are within normal ranges.

In *osteopsathyrosis (osteogenesis imperfecta tarda)* the child appears normal at birth, and fractures usually do not occur until after the first year of life. There is great variation in the time of the first fracture. Occasionally osteopsathyrosis is so severe that it resembles the congenital form in the development of early and numerous fractures. In the majority of instances, however, only a moderate number of fractures occur, and the fragility ceases with puberty. The bones of the extremities are long and slender (Fig. 22-19); most of the fractures are in the legs. Healing takes place rapidly, but deformities may develop. As a rule all the affected members of a family can be recognized by their blue scleras. Only about two thirds of the members with blue scleras suffer from increased fragility of the bones, and only about one fourth from deafness. The flaccidity of the ligaments and muscles may result in repeated dislocations. Deafness is usually a late manifestation and is rare in children.

A clear distinction between osteogenesis imperfecta congenita and tarda cannot always be made, and intermediate forms may be encountered.

Diagnosis. In roentgenograms of the newborn infant the unbroken bones in *osteogenesis imperfecta congenita* are thin, but otherwise normal. The previously fractured bones appear irregularly thickened, curved or angulated; the epiphyseal ends are usually normal. The skull is characterized by thinness of the bones and by osseous islands, the wormian bones, which are separated from each other by numerous sutures of irregular

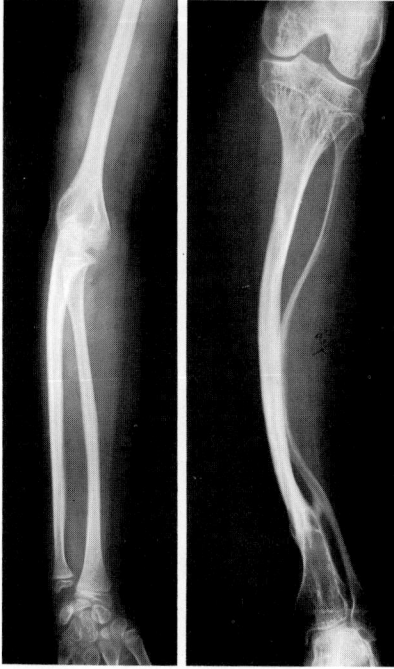

Figure 22-19. Osteopsathyrosis.

shape. The mineral content of the bones seems reduced, but the bone age corresponds to the child's chronologic age. As the child grows older and the processes of fracturing and healing con-

tinue, the shafts of the bones assume grotesque shapes.

In *osteopsathyrosis*, roentgenograms show the unbroken long bones to be slender and elongated. Their epiphyses are normal in appearance. Improper healing of fractures may result in deformities; demineralized areas are frequent.

The diagnosis of osteogenesis and of osteopsathyrosis is facilitated by the presence of blue scleras; and in osteopsathyrosis there is usually a family history. *Achondroplasia* and osteogenesis imperfecta result in micromelia, but otherwise the 2 disorders have little in common. In the former the bones are thick and short, and the epiphyseal ends irregular. *Hypophosphatasia* in the newborn may resemble osteogenesis imperfecta congenita, but is readily recognized (p. 1371) by the low serum phosphatase value and by the rachitic appearance of the bones.

Prognosis and Treatment. Many children with *osteogenesis imperfecta congenita* are stillborn or die soon after birth. Those who survive usually become severely deformed.

Children with the late form, *osteopsathyrosis*, may also become deformed, but the deformities can be lessened by orthopedic treatment. Frequently the patients can live fairly normal lives. The prospect of developing deafness and of transmitting the disorder to part of their offspring, however, must be considered in relation to the prognosis.

No effective treatment is known for osteogenesis imperfecta. Good nutrition and correct treatment for the fractures are essential.

Miscellaneous Disorders

CLEIDAL AND CLEIDOCRANIAL DYSOSTOSIS

This congenital syndrome is characterized by absence of the clavicles and often by delay of ossification of the skull. The defect is usually transmitted as a dominant trait; some cases are sporadic, and inheritance cannot be proved. The latter are regarded as new mutations. Males and females are equally affected. The defective bones are usually membranous in origin. The ends of the clavicles, which are often also missing, are derived from cartilage, however, and other bones of cartilaginous origin may also be affected.

Clinical Manifestations. The entire clavicle may be absent, or the sternal and acromial ends are present, but the connecting shaft is missing.

Sometimes the 2 ends are fairly well developed and joined by a narrow fibrous strip, thus simulating the appearance of a fractured clavicle on the roentgenogram.

In serious clavicular defect the shoulders can be approximated in front to a remarkable degree (Fig. 22-20). The muscles which are normally attached to the clavicle may also be defective. At birth, ossification of the calvarial bones is so delayed that the fontanels are excessively large and the sutures widely open. Large bosses develop in the frontal, parietal and occipital regions, and the skull assumes a globular shape, at times with a "hot cross bun" type of deformity, owing to depressions along the coronal and sagittal sutures. As the patient grows older, ossification of the calvarial bones progresses slowly, but the fontanels may remain open until adulthood. The

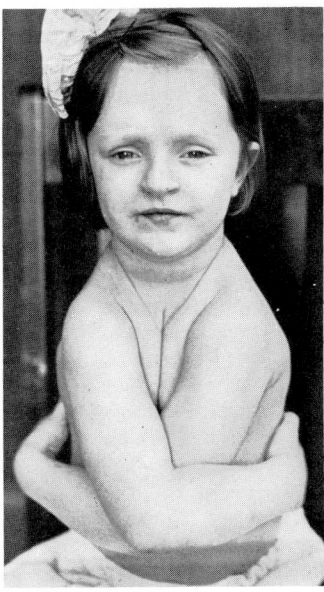

Figure 22-20. Cleidocranial dysostosis in a girl 5 years of age. (Cook: *Arch. Pediat.,* Vol. 51.)

a congenital anomaly which is frequently combined with luxation of the lens (Marfan's syndrome) and other malformations.

Etiology. The disorder is considered a general "mesodermal dystrophy." In many families the syndrome is inherited as a dominant trait. There are sporadic cases which are probably due to new mutations.

Clinical Manifestations. The patients tend to be tall and slender, and their extremities are long and thin (Fig. 22-21). The phalanges, metacarpals and metatarsals are unusually long; the fingers are often termed "spider fingers." The muscles are flaccid, so that the joints are hyperextensible except when the syndrome is combined with arthrogryposis. The skull is long and narrow, the palate high. The external ears are frequently deformed. Luxation of the lens may be combined with cataract, megalocornea, coloboma and other defects of the eye. Myopia, strabismus and nystagmus are frequently present. There may be scoliosis or kyphosis. Deformities of the chest and cardiovascular disease develop as the children grow older. Cardiac hypertrophy, valvular deformities, aortic cystic medionecrosis, aortic aneurysm (sometimes dissecting) and other anomalies have been found at autopsy. Imperfect

sutures frequently close with interposition of wormian bones. The facial bones are underdeveloped, and the sinuses may be absent. The palate is usually highly arched and, in some cases, cleft. The dentition is irregular. Congenital *cranial dysostosis* may occur without anomalies of the clavicle. Deformities of the vertebrae and of the bones of the fingers and toes and delayed ossification of the pubic bones have also been observed. In hereditary cases the cleidal and the cleidocranial forms have alternated in the same sibship. The patients are usually short of stature, but their mentality and general health may be unaffected.

Diagnosis. Roentgenograms reveal absence of all or part of the clavicles, and a lack of ossification of the cranial and pelvic bones, particularly of the pubic bones. The delayed ossification of the calvaria may suggest hydrocephalus or cretinism.

Prognosis and Treatment. The defects rarely cause discomfort or disability. Occasionally a clavicular fragment may press on nerves and cause pain; removal of the disturbing fragment is indicated.

ARACHNODACTYLY
(MARFAN'S SYNDROME;
DOLICHOSTENOMELIA)

Arachnodactyly, abnormal length of the extremities, particularly of the fingers and toes, is

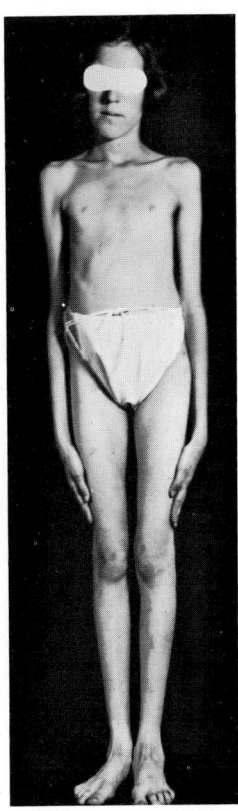

Figure 22-21. Arachnodactyly.

lobation of the lungs, renal ectopy, dislocation of the hips and other malformations are also occasionally associated with the syndrome. The mentality is normal in the majority of instances.

Prognosis and Treatment. Respiratory disease is common, but the prognosis depends chiefly upon the cardiac lesions. Some children reach maturity and transmit the disorder to some of their offspring.

Appropriate treatment of the deformities of the spine and of the eye defects is required.

Ectopia lentis and skeletal changes resembling arachnodactyly have been found associated with homocystinuria (p. 424), a metabolic disorder attributed to autosomal recessive inheritance.

MULTIPLE EXOSTOSES

(Osteochondroma; Diaphyseal
Aclasis; Dyschondroplasia;
Ecchondrosis ossificans)

In this disorder hard, irregular prominences appear in the region of the metaphyses of bones. The condition is hereditary in the majority of instances, a dominant mode of transmission being the rule. If a person appears to be "skipped" in a pedigree, roentgenographic examination may reveal small exostoses which have escaped external inspection. A sporadic instance may represent a new mutation, or the patient may belong to a family in which the disorder had not been noticed before. Males are affected more often than females.

Pathology. The exostoses consist of spongy bone covered by a layer of compact bone and a shell of hyaline cartilage. The excrescence enlarges by endochondral, periosteal and perichondral ossification. Exostoses develop only on parts of the skeleton previously cartilaginous. They develop from intraperiosteal or subcortical cartilaginous rests, whereas the enchondromas sometimes associated with them arise from cartilaginous islands situated in the spongiosa. Exostoses occur chiefly on the long bones, but occasionally the base of the skull, the vertebral column, the ribs, the scapulae and the pelvis are affected.

Clinical Manifestations. Although exostoses are frequently present at birth, they are usually not noticed before the second year of life, when osseous elevations become prominent near the ends of bones. Growth of the affected bones is retarded, and deformities may develop. The radius is often longer than the ulna and bends around the end of this bone, resulting in ulnar deviation of the entire hand. Genu valgum and pes planus frequently develop. The exostoses are usually bilateral and often symmetrical. Occasionally a large exostosis may interfere with movement of a joint or press on nerves or blood vessels.

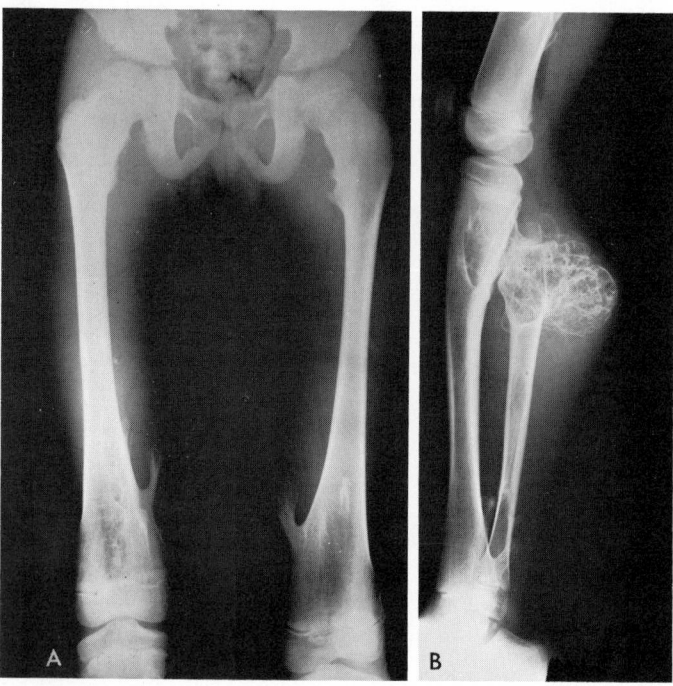

Figure 22-22. *A*, Exostoses of both femurs. *B*, Large exostosis or osteochondroma in the fibula of the same patient.

Diagnosis. On the roentgenogram, exostoses appear as small or large spurs (Fig. 22-22), which originate within the metaphysis and always grow away from the epiphysis. The structure of the entire metaphysis is abnormal; it is broad and may be irregularly ossified.

Prognosis and Treatment. Exostoses are not malignant; rarely they may be transformed into chondrosarcomas. Exostoses become quiescent when growth of the patient is complete. Surgical intervention may be required for limitation of movement or for the relief of pressure symptoms on nerves or blood vessels.

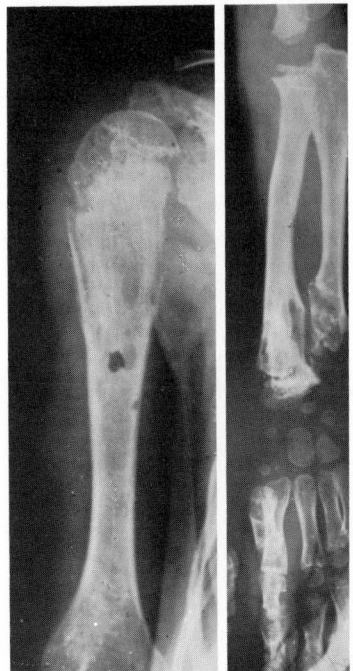

Figure 22-23. Humerus and forearm in Ollier's disease.

OLLIER'S DISEASE
(CHONDRODYSPLASIA; DYSCHONDROPLASIA)

This malformation of the ends of the shafts is characterized by the presence of nonossified cartilage in the metaphyses and adjacent diaphyses of long bones. The disorder is usually unilateral, but occasionally lesser changes of the same sort are found on the opposite side. Since facial asymmetry is often present, a relation to hemiatrophy seems probable. There is no evidence that this disorder is genetically determined.

Pathology. The cartilaginous islands consist of hyaline cartilage upon which bone is deposited. The cells are larger and more irregularly distributed than usual. The cartilage is calcified in parts of its periphery, but it does not ossify normally.

Clinical Manifestations. There is a gradual onset of symptoms during the first few years of life. It may be noticed that one limb is shorter than the other, or an external deformity may appear near a joint. In many instances the disease affects the arm and the leg of the same side, and the pelvic and facial bones may also be involved. There may be deformity, shortening of the limbs and limitation of movement. The process as such is not painful, but use of the deformed extremities may cause discomfort.

Diagnosis. The disorder is easily recognized when the lesions are unilateral. In the roentgenogram the upper end of the humerus, for example, appears thickened, the cortex of the diaphysis is defective, and linear areas of rarefaction are seen in the metaphysis and extending into the diaphysis. The distal ends of other long bones may have similar defects; the epiphyses are also affected (Fig. 22-23).

Isolated lesions may resemble those of *syphilis* or *leukemia,* but the unilateral involvement and absence of other diagnostic features of these diseases suffice for differentiation. Intrametaphyseal areas of rarefaction in bones with *multiple exos-*

toses may resemble Ollier's disease, but the bilateral occurrence of exostoses and their location on the external aspect of the bone permit differentiation.

Prognosis and Treatment. The process is not progressive, but shortening of affected bones becomes manifest as the rest of the body increases in size. Infrequently sarcoma has developed in an affected bone. Fractures may occur in the rarefied areas. Orthopedic treatment for the correction of malformations and the prevention of further deformities is indicated.

MELORHEOSTOSIS

This skeletal disorder is a form of hyperostosis which begins in infancy or childhood and progresses slowly on one side of the bones of a single extremity. Enlargement, swelling and curving of the fingers or toes, and pain and deformity of the proximal bones of the same limb are clinical manifestations. Roentgenograms reveal a characteristic hyperostosis limited to one side of the bone. Melorheostosis is probably a developmental disorder, but infection and disturbance of sympathetic vasomotor control have also been considered causative factors.

PROGRESSIVE DIAPHYSEAL DYSPLASIA
(ENGELMANN'S DISEASE)

This disorder is presumably a developmental anomaly. It is characterized by thickening of the cortices of the long bones and by neuromuscular dystrophy. The dystrophy is responsible for general wasting of muscles and a peculiar waddling gait. In some instances there is also thickening of the flat bones, including those of the skull.

Roentgenographically, there is thickening of the cortex of the diaphyses of the long bones with irregular narrowing of the medullary canal. The metaphyses and epiphyses are not involved, in contrast with osteopetrosis.

FIBROUS DYSPLASIA OF BONE
(OSTEITIS FIBROSA DISSEMINATA; POLYOSTOTIC FIBROUS DYSPLASIA; OSTEODYSTROPHIA FIBROSA)

Fibrous dysplasia may affect one or many bones of the skeleton. In polyostotic cases the distribution tends to be unilateral; if both sides are involved, one side is affected more than the other. Fibrous dysplasia is probably due to a develop-mental error of early embryonic life, but there is no proof that the disorder is hereditary. The lesion consists of a fibrous matrix studded with trabeculae of immature bone with varying degrees of calcification. Monostotic cases may be free of symptoms or show only a local swelling. Sometimes a fracture, pain or functional impairment leads to recognition of the disease. If several bones of a limb are affected, clinical complaints are more frequent, and bowing and fractures are common manifestations. Flat bones sometimes become distended into tumor-like masses, while long bones become shortened, curved and thickened. Roentgenographic changes include diffuse and cystlike lesions, sclerosis, evidence of fractures and abnormal outlines of the bones (Fig. 22-24). Sclerosis with thickening is the usual form of involvement of the bones of the orbit and face (Fig. 22-25). In the severest form of the disease several limbs may be involved, and the skull, vertebral column and pelvis may be included in the pathologic process. In such cases the osseous changes are often associated with brown pigmentation of the skin and with precocious osseous development and precocious puberty, which is seen more often in girls than in boys (McCune-Albright syndrome, p. 1182). The serum levels of calcium and phosphorus are normal, but the serum phosphatase is elevated. Fibrous dysplasia may also be associated with functioning arteriovenous fistulas, particularly in the extremities.

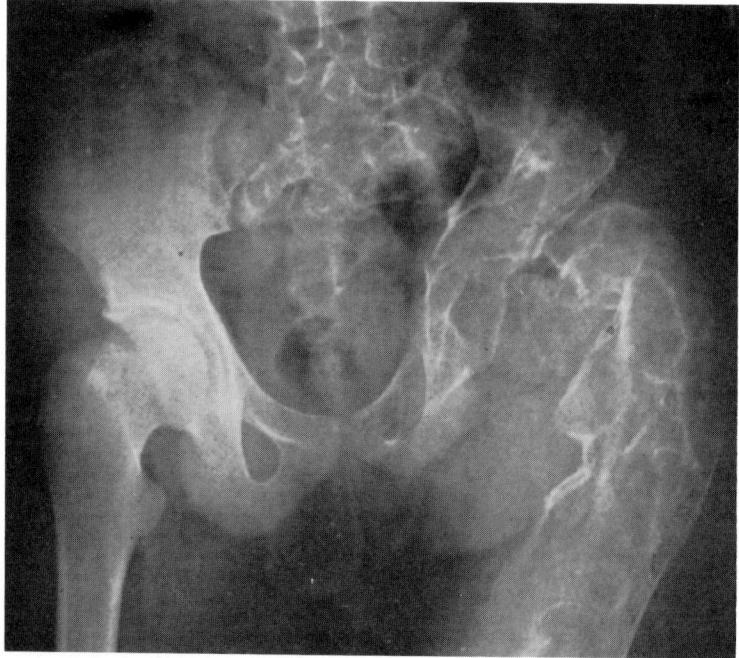

Figure 22-24.   Osteitis fibrosa disseminata. Roentgenogram showing extensive fibrous dysplasia of the sacrum, left ilium and femur. Note the irregular demineralization and expansion of the cortex. (Stauffer, Arbuckle and Aegerter: *J. Bone & Joint Surg.*, Vol. 23.)

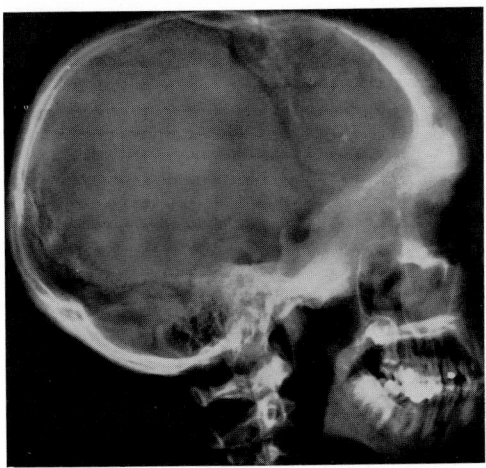

Figure 22-25. Fibrous dysplasia. The bones at the base of the skull are opaque and markedly thickened. The paranasal sinuses, except for the right maxillary sinus, are obliterated, and the left orbit is distorted. The patient is 17 years of age. (From E. Aegerter and J. A. Kirkpatrick, Jr.: *Orthopedic Diseases.* 3rd ed.)

ARTHROGRYPOSIS

The term "arthrogryposis" denotes congenital contraction of joints in flexion. It usually occurs alone, but may be associated with other malformations such as arachnodactyly and premature synostoses of the bones of the skull.

Pathology. The pathologic changes involve thick, inelastic articular capsules and atrophic muscle fibers with some fibrosis and fatty infiltration. Degeneration in the cells of the anterior horns of the spinal cord is found in typical arthrogryposis multiplex congenita.

Clinical Manifestations. *Arthrogryposis multiplex congenita* is the term used for a special form of this disorder in which there is a congenital stiffness of one or more joints associated with a hypoplasia of the attached muscles. It is the result of incomplete fibrous ankylosis. Dislocation of the hips and of other joints is common. Since ankylosis of some joints occurs in extension, the term "arthrogryposis" is not entirely justified, and *multiple congenital articular rigidities,* a name also used, is more adequate. The disorder has been attributed to prolonged intrauterine pressure, but the frequent association with such malformations as defects of the palate or vertebrae and absence of the sacrum and fibula indicates origin early in embryonic life before intrauterine pressure becomes a teratogenic factor.

The disorder appears sporadically, but 2 cases in the same family have been observed several times. The arms are rotated inward; the thighs, outward. The elbows and knees, which are described as cylindrical, are usually ankylosed in extension, although fixation of the knees in flexion also occurs. The wrists and fingers are flexed, and club feet are present. Certain muscle groups may be underdeveloped or absent *(amyoplasia congenita).* The skin appears thickened, and there may be dimples in the skin near the joints. Roentgenograms show only atrophy of the bones and small muscles.

Treatment. Treatment consists in massage, passive movements, gradual correction of deformities by splints and plaster casts, and orthopedic surgery.

HEMIHYPERTROPHY

In hemihypertrophy, a congenital malformation, one side of the body is larger than the other (Fig. 22-26).

Etiology. The most credible explanation of this malformation is a faulty cell division of the zygote resulting in 2 daughter cells of unequal size; it has been considered a form of incomplete twinning. Females are more often affected than males; the right side of the body more frequently than the left.

Clinical Manifestations. The difference in the 2 sides is usually greatest in the extremities, the genitalia and the trunk. Facial and palatal inequality may also be present. The paired internal organs are sometimes of unequal size. In true hemihypertrophy the bones of the larger side are longer and thicker than their corresponding

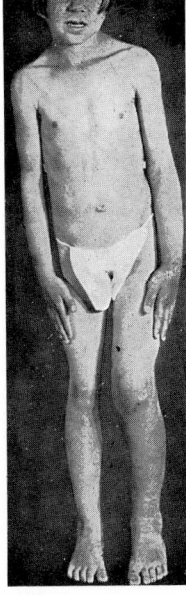

Figure 22-26. Hemihypertrophy in a girl 4 years of age. The hypertrophy was of the entire left side of the body, including the face, teeth and tongue.

ones. There may be a difference in maturation as seen roentgenographically in the centers of ossification. There may be associated malformations such as aniridia, polydactyly, hypospadias, cryptorchidism, nevi and hemangiomas. Instances of association with Wilms's tumor and adrenal or hepatic neoplasms have been reported. The mentality may be normal, but retarded development has been observed.

Differential Diagnosis. Differentiation from *hemiatrophy* may be difficult, but hemiatrophy is frequently associated with such neurologic lesions as paralysis and athetosis. A congenital arteriovenous fistula may result in overgrowth of one extremity, and a similar effect can be caused by a low-grade nondestructive infection near an epiphysis. In *Milroy's disease* the soft tissues only are involved. *Recklinghausen's neurofibromatosis* can result in hypertrophy of an entire limb.

Prognosis and Treatment. The differences in the 2 sides often become less as the child grows older. Treatment is symptomatic; orthopedic corrections should be instituted early in life.

HYPERTROPHIC PULMONARY OSTEOARTHROPATHY

This condition, sometimes termed "Marie-Bamberger disease" or "hippocratic fingers," occurs in association with chronic pulmonary conditions and with congenital cyanotic heart disease. The lesions are an ossifying periostitis, effusion into the joints, erosion of the cartilages and hypertrophy of the soft tissues. In mild cases there is only clubbing of the fingers, the nails being broad and curved both transversely and longitudinally. In well developed cases there is also enlargement of the ends of the long bones and of the hands and feet, with pain and swelling of the joints. Clubbing of the fingers does not appear until several weeks to a year or longer after development of the causative disease.

A hereditary type of clubbing of the fingers, not dependent upon circulatory or pulmonary disease, has been described.

JOSEF WARKANY
JOHN A. KIRKPATRICK, JR.

REFERENCES

Craniosynostosis

Hemple, D. J., Harris, L. E., Svien, H. J., and Holman, C. B.: Craniosynostosis Involving the Sagittal Suture Only; Guilt by Association? *J. Pediat.,* 58:342, 1961.

McLaurin, R. L., and Matson, D. D.: Importance of Early Surgical Treatment of Craniosynostosis. *Pediatrics,* 10:637, 1952.

Park, E. A., and Powers, G. F.: Acrocephaly and Scaphocephaly with Symmetrically Distributed Malformations of the Extremities. *Am. J. Dis. Child.,* 20:235, 1920.

Temtamy, S. A.: Carpenter's Syndrome: Acrocephalopolysyndactyly. *J. Pediat.,* 69:111, 1966.

Basilar Impression

Chamberlain, W. E.: Basilar Impression (Platybasia). *Yale J. Biol. & Med.,* 11:487, 1939.

Lacunar Skull

Vogt, E. C., and Wyatt, G. M.: Craniolacunia (Lückenschädel). *Radiology,* 36:147, 1941.

Malformations of the Extremities

Franty, C. H., and O'Rahilly, R.: Congenital Skeletal Limb Deficiencies. *J. Bone & Joint Surg.,* 43-A: 1202, 1961.

Klippel-Feil Syndrome

Shoul, M. I., and Ritvo, M.: Clinical and Roentgenological Manifestations of the Klippel-Feil Syndrome. *Am. J. Roentgenol.,* 68:369, 1952.

Congenital Absence of Caudal Spine

Blumel, J., Evans, E. B., and Eggers, G. W.: Partial and Complete Agenesis or Malformation of the Sacrum with Associated Anomalies; Etiologic and Clinical Study with Special Reference to Heredity; A Preliminary Report. *J. Bone & Joint Surg.,* 41-A: 497, 1959.

Achondroplasia

Caffey, J.: Achondroplasia; in I. McQuarrie (Ed.): *Brennemann's Practice of Pediatrics.* Hagerstown, Md., W. F. Prior Company, Inc., 1957, Vol. 4, Chap. 28.

Rischbieth, H.: Dwarfism; in *Treasury of Human Inheritance.* VII and VIII. Francis Galton Laboratory for National Eugenics, University of London, 1912.

Chondro-ectodermal Dysplasia

Ellis, R. W. B., and Van Creveld, S.: A Syndrome Characterized by Ectodermal Dysplasia, Polydactyly, Chondrodysplasia and Congenital Morbus Cordis. *Arch. Dis. Childhood,* 15: 65, 1940.

McKusick, V. A., Eldridge, R., Hostetler, J. A., et al.: Dwarfism in the Amish. II. *Bull. Johns Hopkins Hosp.,* 116:285, 1965.

Mucopolysaccharidoses

Hurler, G.: Ueber einen Typ multipler Abartungen, vorwiegend am Skelettsystem. *Ztschr. f. Kinderh.,* 24:220, 1919.

McKusick, V. A.: *Heritable Disorders of Connective Tissue.* 3rd ed. St. Louis, C. V. Mosby Company, 1966.

Morquio, L.: Sur une forme dè dystrophie osseuse familiale. *Arch. de méd. d. enf.,* 32:129, 1929.

Noorden, G. K., Zelliweger, H., and Ponsetti, I. V.: Ocular Findings in Morquio-Ulrich's Disease, with Report of Two Cases. *Arch. Ophthalmol.,* 64:585, 1960.

Strauss, L.: The Pathology of Gargoylism. Report of a Case and Review of the Literature. *Am. J. Path.,* 24:855, 1948.

Cleidal and Cleidocranial Dysostosis

Anspach, W. E., and Huepel, R. C.: Familial Cleidocranial Dysostosis (Cleidal Dysostosis); Preosseous and Dentinal Dystrophy. *Am. J. Dis. Child.,* 58:786, 1939.

Osteopetrosis

Clifton, W. M., and Frank, A.: Osteopetrosis (Marble Bones); in McQuarrie, I. (Ed.): *Brennemann's Practice of Pediatrics.* Hagerstown, Md., W. F. Prior Company, Inc., 1957, Vol. 4, Chap. 23, Section 2.

Elmore, S. M.: Pycnodysostosis: A Review. *J. Bone & Joint Surg.,* 49-A:153, 1967.

Osteogenesis Imperfecta

Follis, R. H.: Osteogenesis Imperfecta Congenita: A Connective Tissue Diathesis. *J. Pediat.,* 41:713, 1952.

Multiple Exostoses

Jaffe, H. L.: Hereditary Multiple Exostosis. *Arch. Path.,* 36:335, 1943.

Ollier's Disease

Ollier, M.: De la dyschondroplasie. *Bull. Soc. de chir. de Lyon,* 3:22, 1899.

Melorheostosis

Hall, G. S.: A Contribution to the Study of Melorheostosis: Unusual Bone Changes Associated with Tuberous Sclerosis. *Quart. J. Med.,* 12:77, 1943.

Progressive Diaphyseal Dysplasia

Neuhauser, E. B. D., Schwachman, H., Wittenborg, M., and Cohen, J.: Progressive Diaphyseal Dysplasia. *Radiology,* 51:11, 1948.

Mandibulofacial Dysostosis

Franceschetti, A., and Klein, D.: *The Mandibulofacial Dysostosis.* Copenhagen, Ejnar Munksgaard, 1949.

Arthrogryposis

Stern, W. G.: Arthrogryposis Multiplex Congenita. *J.A.M.A.,* 81:1507, 1923.

Hemihypertrophy

Miller, R. W., Fraumeni, J. F., and Manning, M. D.: Association of Wilms's tumor with Aniridia, Hemihypertrophy and

Other Congenital Malformations. *New England J. Med.,* 270:922, 1964.

Ward, J., and Lerner, H. H.: A Review of the Subject of Congenital Hemihypertrophy and a Complete Case Report. *J. Pediat.,* 31:403, 1947.

Osteitis Fibrosa Disseminata

Albright, F., Butler, A. M., Hampton, A. O., and Smith, P.: Syndrome Characterized by Osteitis Fibrosa Disseminata, Areas of Pigmentation and Endocrine Dysfunction, with Precocious Puberty in Females; Report of Five Cases. *New England J. Med.,* 216:727, 1937.

McCune, D. J., and Bruch, H.: Osteodystrophia Fibrosa; Report of a Case in Which Condition Was Combined with Precocious Puberty, Pathologic Pigmentation of Skin and Hyperthyroidism, with Review of Literature. *Am. J. Dis. Child.,* 54:806, 1937.

PEDIATRIC ORTHOPEDICS

RESPONSE OF BONE TO LOCAL AND GENERAL DISTURBANCES

Bones grow in length by new formation at the physis or growth plate and in width or diameter by appositional growth at the deepest layer of the periosteum. Neither growing nor mature bone is a solid substance of inert matter, but is a living tissue composed of constantly changing molecules and is responsive and changeable. "Tagged" calcium molecules in a particular bone at one examination may be in another bone at a subsequent examination or may have been excreted. Perhaps bone would remain relatively constant in its component molecules, and perhaps a certain calcium molecule deposited in bone would remain stationary for an indefinite time, if its environmental conditions were not changed. But bones are changing continuously, even in the normal person, and these changes are accentuated during infectious and metabolic diseases and starvation.

Traumatic, nutritional, metabolic, endocrine, neurologic, infectious, circulatory and mechanical factors all cause changes in the chemical and physical characteristics of bone. For example, increase in circulation, such as that caused by traumatic or hemangiomatous arteriovenous shunts or a local inflammation as rheumatoid arthritis, may cause increased growth in length. Some bone tumors retard growth. Interference with nerve supply to an extremity retards both linear and cross-sectional growth; complete inactivity causes atrophy and demineralization, and damage to a physis disrupts or causes total cessation of growth.

RELATION OF INTRAUTERINE POSITION TO ORTHOPEDIC DISTURBANCES

Congenital malformations are discussed on pages 1329-50.

Different etiologic factors can be responsible for identical structural defects in the fetus. For example, cleft palate in the rat may be genetic in origin or may be an environmental congenital defect resulting from infection, poisoning or vitamin deficiencies in the pregnant rat. It may also be that intrauterine posture can produce the same deformity. The *"position of comfort"* of the newborn with severe brachygnathia suggests this possibility. When the mandible is extremely small or posteriorly subluxated, it may be accompanied by cleft palate. The tongue, which is rarely, if ever, proportionately small, must be accommodated in the nasopharynx, since the mouth does not provide ample space for it.

Normally the fetus floats freely for the first half of the gestational period. After this time it begins to impinge on the uterine wall, and the mother translates these collisions as "feeling life." The fetus becomes increasingly restricted, and, when it changes position in relation to its mother, it is less able to alter its position.

In order to achieve maximal flexion, the fetus must have a minimum of tension in its stretched joint capsules.

The intrauterine position can be reconstructed after birth by "folding" the infant into his most comfortable position. Infants subjected to capsular stretch in the uterus are likely to be fretful in the unaccustomed position in which they find themselves after birth. When such an infant is "folded," his fretting may cease, and he may fall asleep in his "position of comfort."

"Positions of comfort" are of infinite variety. They include hands hyperflexed along the forearms or grooving the thorax, heads indented by an arm, feet pressed tightly against the tibias, and many others. Reconstruction of the "position of comfort" may possibly explain some instances of club feet, torticollis, dislocated elbows, and asymmetries, as well as other deformities.

After the first week of life the relaxation diminishes rapidly but selectively. Muscles and joint capsules which were not stretched or strained during fetal life retain considerable pliancy throughout infancy, whereas those affected by fetal position may be restricted in their range of motion. Perhaps the jaw which was pressed against the sternum cannot be opened wide, and the thighs of an infant whose hip joint capsule was stretched cannot be abducted. In other stretched joints this stiffness is present for only a few months, but in the jaw and in the hips it may last longer, in part because the muscles closing the mouth are stronger than those opening it, and those adducting the hip are stronger than those abducting it.

THE FOOT

Normal foot. The normal foot of the infant appears grossly abnormal if judged by adult standards. It is fatter and wider than that of the adult. Fat pads create a fullness which suggests flatfoot; it seldom has a distinct longitudinal arch and never a transverse one. This pattern is accentuated by the normally soft and pliable muscles. The line of the Achilles tendon may be moderately angulated laterally and the foot slightly everted.

Pronation (Flatfoot). The term *flatfoot* as applied to the infant most often indicates that the medial longitudinal arch does not *look* as high as the parents or physician would like to see it. Most often it is not an abnormality.

To decide whether the foot of a child is normal requires careful examination of its component parts and evaluation of its functional status. If the child with the suspected flatfoot will stand on his toes, a definite longitudinal arch will usually appear. Next the child is asked to stand on his heels with the front of the foot off the floor. If these maneuvers are successfully accomplished, there is high probability that the feet are within normal limits.

The joints are examined by checking their motions. The ankle joint moves in dorsiflexion and plantar flexion; the joints of the foot in eversion and inversion. After the physician has examined a few children with normal feet he will have learned the normal range of motion. The length of the heel cord must be tested with the knee straight and the foot inverted; then when the ankle is dorsiflexed, the lateral border of the foot should make an acute angle with the tibia of 80 degrees or less. A short heel cord is an abnormality and requires treatment.

The muscles which activate the joints are as follows: tibialis anticus, to produce dorsiflexion and inversion; tibialis posticus, to produce plantar flexion and inversion; peroneus tertius, to produce dorsiflexion and eversion; peroneus longus and brevis, to produce plantar flexion and eversion; and gastrocnemius and soleus, to produce plantar flexion. The child should carry out each of these motions actively, and the strength of the muscles should be tested. The range and strength of extension and flexion at the metatarsophalangeal

joints should be carefully examined, since the integrity of the anterior arch depends on the flexibility of these joints.

The dorsalis pedis and posterior tibial pulses are palpated, and the Achilles tendon and plantar reflexes tested. Sensation is checked on the dorsal and plantar surfaces.

If this systematic examination reveals no abnormalities, the feet are "normal," and no treatment for the "flatfoot" is required. Specifically, so-called orthopedic shoes with Thomas heels are not indicated.

Occasionally a child will complain of pain or fatigue in the feet after play, and neither the examination described nor a roentgenographic examination of the foot will reveal any abnormality. Foot strain is the usual cause of such complaints, and exercises to improve the tone of the muscles supporting the foot are indicated. The young child should be instructed to walk "tiptoe" for 5 to 10 minutes daily; the older one, to stand slightly pigeon-toed with the weight thrown on the lateral border of the foot for 5 to 10 minutes daily. Mechanical support for the arch is not required *and is contraindicated in the absence of abnormal findings.*

Pigeon Toe. Pigeon toe is a frequent complaint. There are 3 common causes for toeing-in. *Metatarsus adductus* consists in adduction of the forefoot with no deformity of the hindfoot. It is the most common of the congenital foot deformities and is frequently associated with congenital dysplasia of the hip. Treatment is required as early as possible and before the infant walks. The deformity is easily corrected by passive stretching, reverse shoe, or casts and wedging, depending on its severity. It rarely recurs.

The second most common cause of pigeon toe is *inward tibial torsion.* A line drawn from the anterior-superior iliac spine through the center of the patella normally intersects the second toe when the foot is held at a right angle to the tibia and when the forefoot is held neither abducted nor adducted. In tibial torsion this line intersects the fourth or fifth toe or a point lateral to the fifth one. Tibial torsion is always associated with a tibial bow. It requires no treatment such as braces, bars or shoe wedging, but is corrected as the extremity grows. Tibial torsion is frequently associated with metatarsus adductus; the latter should be corrected as described above. Some degree of pigeon toe will persist until growth has corrected the tibial torsion, when the toeing-in will be self-corrected. External rotation bars are unnecessary in the treatment of inward tibial torsion.

The third cause of pigeon toe is *inward femoral torsion.* For examination the child is placed supine, and the legs are inwardly rotated and then outwardly rotated at the hips. Normally, inward rotation is about 30 degrees and outward rotation 60 degrees. In inward femoral torsion the inward rotation will approach 90 degrees, the patellae will face each other, and outward rotation is practically nonexistent. No treatment is required;

correction usually does not occur with growth, but the patient develops an outward tibial torsion which compensates for the inward femoral torsion.

Clubfoot. The usual so-called congenital clubfoot is a secondary deformity of the foot and ankle. The most frequent deformity is that of *equinovarus,* in which the foot is in plantar flexion and deviates medially. More than 95 per cent of congenital club feet are of the equinovarus type. Next most frequent is the deformity of *calcaneovalgus,* in which the foot is dorsiflexed and deviated laterally. Many children are born with the positional abnormality of equinovarus or calcaneovalgus. If the foot can be passively brought into the opposite position, the infant does not have a clubfoot and requires only simple exercises for correction of the deformity. The primary type of congenital clubfoot is rare and results from absence of muscles or bones or of fusion of bones. *The foot which cannot be passively overcorrected is a clubfoot and requires orthopedic treatment.* Conservative treatment with casts and wedgings or the Denis Browne splint is preferred. Forcible manipulation and surgery are usually unnecessary.

Shoes. Before walking, it is unnecessary for an infant to wear shoes; while walking is limited to carpeted floors, the shoes should be the softest obtainable, usually of the moccasin type. Later, when the feet need protection against the pounding received on hard floors and pavements, somewhat thicker soles become desirable. These should be as pliable as possible, since stiff-soled shoes limit the range of foot motion and therefore impede development of the supporting muscles. It is essential that the shank be flexible, the leather soft and the last straight or swung in. The basic requirements for shoes during the growth period are adequate width and adequate length. The big toe should be a thumb's width from the end of the shoe in the weight-bearing position. The width of the shoe is determined in the weight-bearing position by the pinch test. The leather over the widest part of the forefoot should be sufficiently loose to pick up a small amount of leather by pinch. The so-called orthopedic shoe should be restricted to pathologic conditions. Under no circumstances should it be used for the normal foot.

THE LEG

Bowleg and Knock-Knees. In most instances bowleg and knock-knees cannot be explained on any pathologic basis. If such acquired lesions as rickets and such congenital abnormalities as achondroplasia can be ruled out, they should be considered to be developmental variants even though the apparent deformity is severe. It can be expected that they will be corrected by growth within the limits of the hereditary pattern. Wedges in the shoes have no effect on bowleg or knock-knee. Braces are used only in deformities in which the collateral ligaments of the knees are becoming stretched; they do not correct the deformity and are used only to prevent further relaxation of ligaments. A single anteroposterior roentgenogram of the knees should be obtained in patients with severe bowleg or knock-knee.

In developmental bowleg a record should be kept of measurements of the distance between the medial aspects of the knees when the medial malleoli are held against each other. In knock-knee the distances between the malleoli are measured when the medial aspects of the knees are held against each other. For either deformity serial tracings of the legs may be made on long sheets of paper.

Blount's disease, or tibia vara, is an acquired lesion of the proximal tibial metaphysis and epiphysis; it results in bowleg because of retardation of growth of this medial portion of the tibia. The cause is unknown. Roentgenographically, there is irregularity of the medial aspect of the tibial epiphyseal center and tibial metaphysis with the formation of a beaklike projection. Treatment may require bracing and frequently osteotomy, depending on the severity of the process and the degree of the deformity.

Congenital Genu Recurvatum. Hyperextension of the knee is not unusual in the newborn infant and may be the result of positioning in utero. It is usually corrected spontaneously within

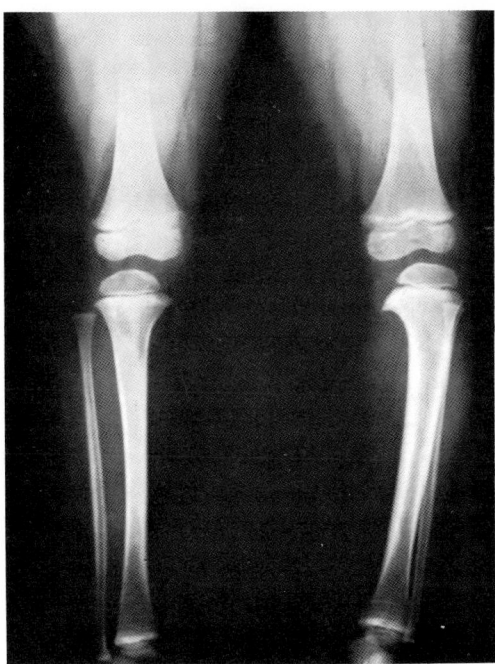

Figure 22-27. Blount's disease. The medial aspect of the proximal end of the left tibia is irregular and "beaked." There is also minimal involvement of medial aspects of the proximal tibial epiphyseal center. As a consequence of the proximal tibial deformity, there was abnormal weight bearing, which in turn was responsible for the thickening shown in the medial cortex of the left tibia. The right tibia is normal.

the first few months of life. Persistence for more than several months requires splinting in slight flexion to permit shortening of the posterior capsule of the knee joint.

THE HIP

CONGENITAL DYSPLASIA OF THE HIP

Congenital dysplasia of the hip is defined as abnormal development of the hip joint, the acetabulum, femoral head, capsule and other soft tissues. The head of the femur may be partially dislocated from the shallow acetabulum (congenital subluxation of the hip), or it may be completely dislocated (congenital dislocation of the hip).

The cause of congenital dysplasia of the hip is unknown. Abnormal development of the joint caused by fetal position or by genetic factors, and abnormal relaxation of the capsule and ligaments of the joint by hormonal factors have been suggested.

Congenital subluxation of the hip is much more frequent than congenital dislocation. In many infants with congenital subluxation, during the first week after birth the head of the femur may be made to dislocate from the acetabulum by Ortolani's maneuver: the child's hips are placed in the frog-leg position, flexed so that the thighs make a right angle with the trunk and abducted so that the legs are spread apart as far as possible. Then one thigh is adducted, while still flexed, and pressure is applied in the line of the femur in such a way as to push the head of the femur over the posterior lip of the acetabulum. As the head slips posteriorly, an unmistakable "click of exit" is felt. If the pressure in the line of the femur is then relieved and the hip is abducted, the head slips back into the acetabulum, and another click, "the click of entry," is felt. This maneuver provides the most accurate early evidence of congenital subluxation of the hip.

In congenital subluxation of the hip there may be no limitation of abduction in the first few weeks of life, but by 3 to 6 weeks, as secondary shortening of the adductor muscles occurs, abduction of the flexed hip will be limited (Fig. 22-28). When the normal infant is on his back with his hips flexed to a right angle with the trunk, the thighs can be abducted passively until the knees nearly reach the examining table. In unilateral dysplasia the limitation of abduction is obvious when the involved side is compared with the normal. When abduction of the hips which does not permit the knees to nearly touch the examining table is present, bilateral dysplasia must be suspected and roentgenograms obtained. *The hips should be flexed and abducted on every visit of the infant to the physician's office because limitation of abduction may appear even after the fourth or fifth month of age.*

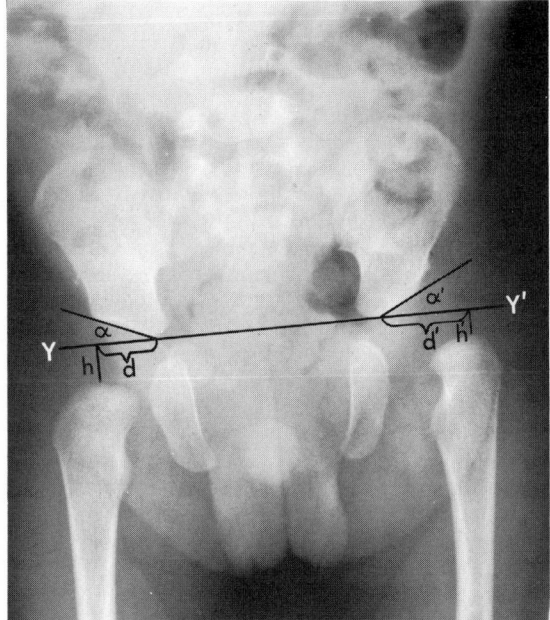

Figure 22-28. Hilgenreiner's method for identification of dysplasia of the hip prior to ossification of the capital femoral epiphysis. α' is greater than α, indicating greater obliquity of the acetabular roof. d' is greater than d, indicating lateral displacement of the femur. h is greater than h', indicating cephalic displacement of the femur. These relations indicate dysplasia of the hip on the right side.

Shortening of the leg is absent or minimal in congenital subluxation of the hip, and asymmetry of skin folds is of little or no value in diagnosis. An anteroposterior roentgenogram of the subluxated hip often shows: (1) An increased slope of the acetabular roof. Normally the angle which the roof of the acetabulum makes with a horizontal line drawn through the centers of the acetabular epiphyses is less than 40 degrees. (2) Slight lateral and cephalic displacement of the upper end of the femur. A true anteroposterior roentgenogram of the pelvis with the hips in a neutral position (not abducted or adducted, nor inwardly or outwardly rotated) is essential to appreciate differences between the two hips (see Fig. 22-28).

Coleman's criteria for the diagnosis of congenital dysplasia of the hip are (1) a positive Ortolani's sign, (2) an acetabular angle above 40 degrees, (3) lateral displacement of the upper end of the femur, or (4) persistent limitation of abduction of the flexed hip. Any one of these findings is an indication for treatment of the abnormal hip.

Treatment of congenital subluxation of the hip consists in maintenance of abduction of the hips until the hip is normal clinically and roentgenographically. In infants with a positive Ortolani's sign found during the first week after birth, simple double diapering is usually adequate to reconstruct the dysplastic hip. But if the Ortolani's sign persists past the third week or if limited abduction of the hip is found later, more adequate splinting is necessary. Usually the hip is normal by the third month if adequate treatment is begun in the first week of life.

In infants who have limitation of abduction, with or without a previously positive Ortolani's sign, abduction splinting applied by an orthopedist is necessary. The splint must be carefully applied so that forcible abduction is avoided; otherwise the vascular supply to the femoral capital epiphysis may be compromised.

In congenital dysplasia of the hip with subluxation, if treatment is not carried out, one of 3 things may occur: (1) The dysplastic hip may become normal because of the abduction produced by the diaper. (2) The hip may remain partially dislocated, the acetabulum shallow and the head of the femur slightly deformed. The patient usually has no symptoms until later in life, when degenerative changes may develop in the mechanically imperfect hip. (3) The partially dislocated (subluxated) hip may go on to complete dislocation, in which case the patient will have the signs of a congenital dysplasia of the hip with dislocation.

In congenital dysplasia of the hip with dislocation, the dislocation may be present at birth or may develop in an untreated, partially dislocated hip. The head of the femur is usually dislocated posterosuperiorly. It may be dislocated anteriorly, however, in which case the diagnosis is more difficult. In posterosuperior dislocation, abduction is limited. Ortolani's sign may be present in reverse. As the test is started, when the flexed hip is abducted, the head of the femur may slip back into the acetabulum, and a "click of entry" will be felt; then as the flexed hip is adducted, a "click of exit" will be felt. There is shortening of the leg, which is best demonstrated with the infant lying flat on his back and with his hips flexed to 90 degrees, a difference in the level of the knees indicating shortening of one thigh. Telescoping is present; alternating push and pull on the flexed thigh moves the head of the femur back and forth on the side of the ilium. Normally the femoral artery in the groin is palpated against the head of the femur; when the head is dislocated, the artery is not as easily palpated as on the normal side. The inguinal crease is deeper than on the normal side. The greater trochanter is palpated more cephalad than on the normal side. Straight-leg raising is greatly increased on the side with the dislocation. When the baby is turned face down on the examination table, the buttock on the involved side is flatter and wider than the normal one.

When the child can stand, if he stands on the abnormal leg, the pelvis drops on the normal side (Trendelenburg's sign). When he walks, his trunk dips when he puts weight on the involved leg, the so-called going-downstairs limp. Bilateral dislocation of the hip causes a "duck waddle" gait. Lumbar lordosis is increased when the child stands. If a line is drawn from the umbilicus to the ischial tuberosity (Nélaton's line), the trochanter will be palpated above the line.

If the head of the femur is dislocated anteriorly rather than posterosuperiorly, abduction of the flexed hip will be limited. The inguinal crease will not be as deep as on the normal side, and though shortening will be present, it will be minimal. Telescoping also will be much less than if the hip were dislocated posterosuperiorly. When the child starts to walk, although a limp will be present, it will not be very obvious, and the lumbar spine, instead of having increased lordosis, will be flattened.

The roentgenogram of the dislocated hip will demonstrate obvious dislocation; even in the early months of life before the capital epiphysis is ossified, the upper end of the femur does not point into the acetabulum.

Treatment of congenital dysplasia of the hip with dislocations is by closed reduction of the hip and maintenance of the reduction by adequate immobilization, usually in a hip spica cast. If diagnosis is delayed beyond 12 to 18 months, closed reduction may not be possible, and operative reduction will be necessary. The later the diagnosis is made and treatment started, the poorer the prognosis for a normal hip.

The emphasis in respect to congenital hip dysplasia should be on early diagnosis. The most important clinical findings are Ortolani's sign in the first week of life and limitation of abduction of the flexed hip thereafter. Since limitation of abduction may not appear early, it is essential that the physician abduct the flexed hips of the infant on every visit during the first year of life.

ACQUIRED DISEASES OF THE HIP

A variety of lesions of the hip, especially in their initial stage, may produce similar symptoms. These include trauma, acute and chronic infections, Perthes's disease and slipped epiphysis. The common presenting symptoms are those of *synovitis:* limp and pain in the hip, or, more often, pain referred to the knee.

Infection is usually manifest systemically by fever and signs of toxemia, as well as by such local signs as muscle spasm, tenderness, swelling and pain on attempted passive motion of the joint. Acute suppurative synovitis is not uncommon. Paracentesis should be done when infection is suspected.

Trauma is the most frequent cause of suddenly acquired limp and pain in the hip or knee *(synovitis of the hip)* which brings the child to the physician. Often the trauma has been so slight that it was overlooked or perhaps never known to the parents. A few hours later the joint is full of fluid and painful.

Examination may reveal limitation of motion, muscle spasm and swelling of the joint. Motion is tested in 3 planes: flexion and extension, abduction and adduction, and inward and outward rotation, and compared with that of the normal side. When limitation of motion is due to muscle spasm,

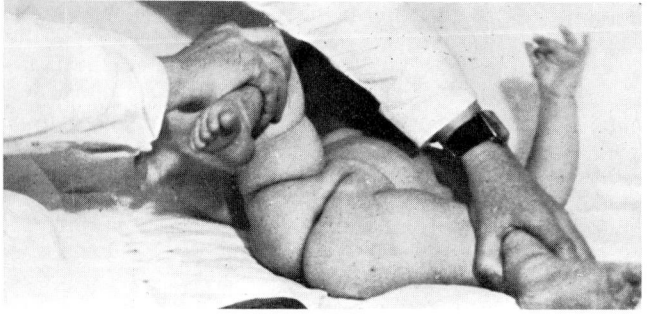

Figure 22-29. Limitation of abduction is an early sign of congenital dislocation of the hip. Note restriction in abduction of right leg.

the range of motion gradually increases as gentle pressure is maintained against the leg, and the muscle becomes fatigued. Swelling of the joint is demonstrated by placing the thumb over the femoral artery where it crosses the inguinal ligament and the other 4 fingers posteriorly over the buttock opposite the position of the thumb. In this way the joint with the soft tissue anterior and posterior to it is grasped between the thumb and fingers. When the hip joint is swollen, it will feel thicker than the normal one *(Gill's sign).*

It is impossible to distinguish the joint lesion of trauma from that of early Perthes's disease before roentgen changes have become manifest. If the roentgen examination is negative, the child should be put to bed for 3 or 4 days. If the spasm persists, the child should have Buck's traction on both legs for 3 weeks. If the signs of spasm have then disappeared, as they usually will have if

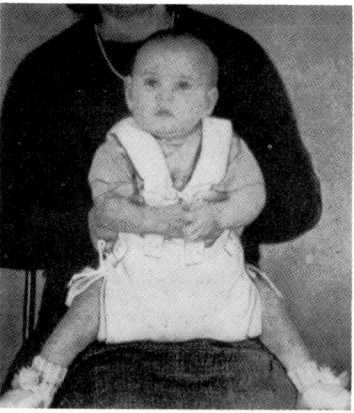

Figure 22-31. The Fredjka abduction splint for treatment of congenital dislocation of the hip. The splint is discontinued when roentgen and clinical studies demonstrate ossification of the acetabular roof and a stable hip joint. Use of the splint is usually required for several months. (Vernon L. Hart: *Congenital Dysplasia of the Hip Joint and Sequelae.* Springfield, Ill., Charles C Thomas.)

trauma has been the cause, he is allowed gradually increasing activity. If spasm persists, traction is continued for another 3 weeks, when the roentgen examination is repeated. The characteristic changes of Perthes's disease will usually have appeared by then.

Perthes's disease (Legg-Calvé-Perthes disease) is an aseptic necrosis of the capital femoral epiphysis causing signs and symptoms of synovitis as described above followed by characteristic roentgen changes.

The cause is unknown. Males between the ages of 4 and 10 years are most frequently affected; infrequently the disease is bilateral. Three stages are usually described, each lasting about 9 months to a year. The first stage is one of aseptic necrosis; roentgenographically, there may be no change during the first weeks, after which a relative opacity of the epiphysis becomes evident. The second stage consists in revascularization, and the epiphysis becomes mottled and fragmented (Fig. 22-32). In the third stage there is reossification, and serial films demonstrate gradual re-formation of the head of the femur. The principle of treatment is avoidance of weight bearing by any of several methods. The head of the femur tends to flatten and becomes mushroom-shaped, causing

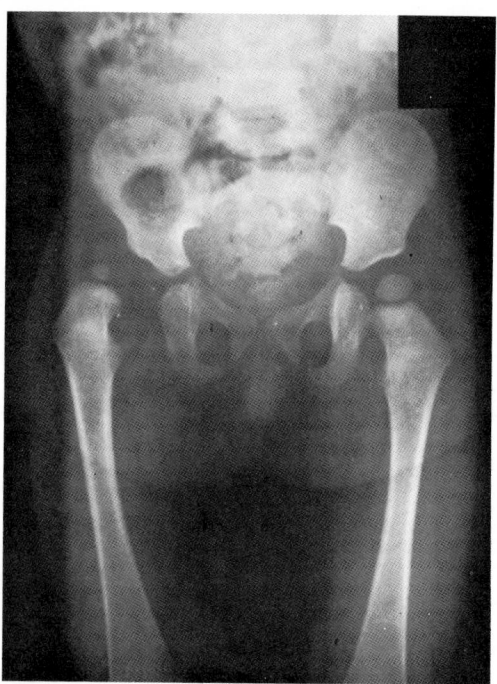

Figure 22-30. Untreated congenital dislocation of the right hip, demonstrating superior and lateral displacement of the underdeveloped femoral head and capital epiphysis, underdevelopment of the acetabulum and an increase in the slope of the acetabular roof.

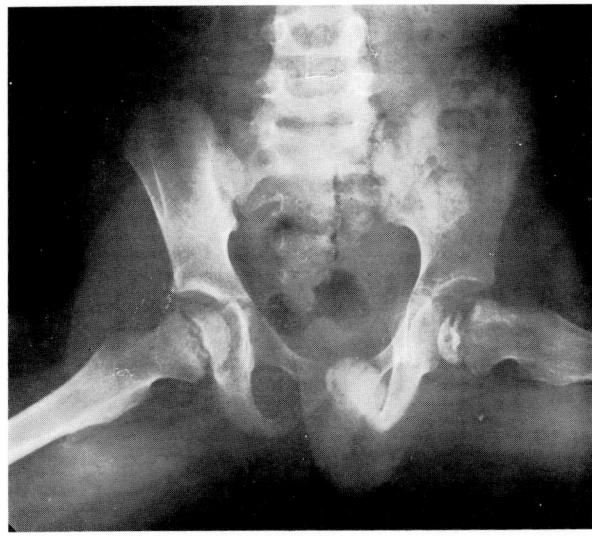

Figure 22-32. Legg-Calvé-Perthes disease of the left hip in a boy 6 years of age. The presenting complaints were limp and pain in the left knee. The lateral roentgenogram reveals sclerosis of the femoral capital epiphyseal center, which is also fragmented and flattened. The "joint space" is wider than normal. At this stage there is little deformity of the neck of the femur.

incongruity between head and acetabulum with degenerative changes later in life. The main prognostic factor as far as the eventual shape of the head of the femur is concerned is the age of the child at time of onset and the amount of involvement as shown roentgenographically.

Slipped epiphysis occurs typically in the adolescent. In its early stages it is characterized by the signs and symptoms of synovitis. The cause is unknown, but the condition occurs mostly in the "overlarge" child. The onset is insidious and characterized by pain in the knee, so that hip disease may not be suspected even though the child limps. Roentgen examination will reveal widening of the epiphyseal line or displacement posteriorly and inferiorly of the femoral capital epiphysis. This is shown on the lateral projection, but not always on the anterior-posterior one. The anterior bowing of the neck which occurs as the "slip" progresses makes subsequent therapy difficult, so that early diagnosis is of great importance.

The principle of treatment is arrest of the slipping, which can be attained by immobilization of the hip in a spica cast, or more surely by internal fixation of the epiphysis to the metaphysis of the neck of the femur.

THE SPINE

Spondylolisthesis. In this condition there is an anterior displacement of a lumbar vertebra, usually the fifth, associated with a bilateral defect in the *pars interarticularis*. The cause is unknown. In children under 10 years of age spondylolisthesis usually does not cause symptoms and is an incidental finding on a roentgenogram. If the vertebral body continues to be displaced forward as shown by serial roentgenograms, spinal fusion is indicated. Symptoms may appear in the adolescent child. Pain in the low-back area is occa-

sionally referred to the sciatic area, and there is an increasing lumbar lordosis. When such symptoms are present, a brace should be provided, and spinal fusion is indicated if the symptoms persist or if the slipping progresses. Frequently the earliest sign of nerve root irritation is spasm of the hamstring muscles with limited "straight-leg raising."

Scoliosis. Scoliosis is a lateral curvature of the spine. It is most commonly caused by a short leg and is overcorrectable by putting a lift under the short leg, or by bending toward the convex side

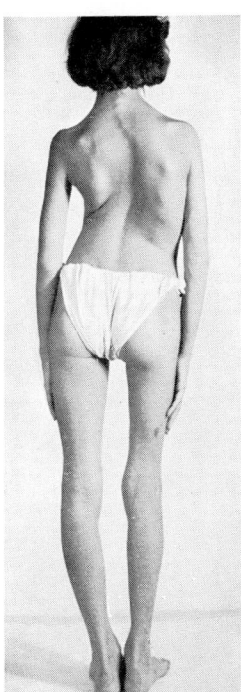

Figure 22-33. Scoliosis in a girl 10 years of age, showing the tilt of the pelvis and shoulders and the deformity of the thorax.

of the curve. Such a curve is termed a *functional scoliosis* and does not become structural. Functional scoliosis may also be caused by muscle spasm secondary to trauma.

A fixed scoliosis not overcorrectable by bending is termed a *structural scoliosis*. It may be caused by such lesions as hemivertebra, fusion of ribs, absence or paralysis of muscles, neurofibromatosis, or vertebral destruction by infection or tumor; most often it is idiopathic. Idiopathic scoliosis occurs most frequently in adolescent girls and requires treatment. The prognosis for excellent results of treatment has been greatly improved in recent years with the use of the Milwaukee brace, and with improved methods of mechanical correction of the curve followed by spinal fusion.

OSTEOCHONDROSIS

Several different entities were classified in the past as osteochondrosis because of a similarity in roentgen appearance. Aseptic necrosis of the capital femoral epiphysis *(Perthes' disease)* (see above), of a metatarsal head *(Freiberg's disease)*, of the tarsal navicular *(Köhler's disease)* are not uncommon and cause pain in the involved area and frequently limping and possibly subsequent deformity.

Scheuermann's disease of the spine, probably a developmental abnormality, causes kyphosis (round back) and frequently requires bracing to lessen pain and to prevent deformity. *Osgood-Schlatter disease* of the tibial tuberosity (Fig. 22-34), almost certainly caused by chronic trauma

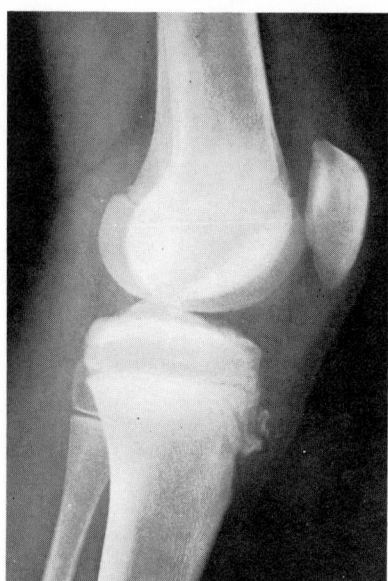

Figure 22-34. Osteochondrosis of tibial tubercle (Osgood-Schlatter disease) in a boy 13 years of age. Roentgenogram shows irregular ossification of tibial tubercle and associated thickening of infrapatellar tendon.

to the tibial tuberosity as a result of overuse of the quadriceps muscle, causes pain and swelling and should be treated by immobilizing the knee in a walking cast for 6 weeks. If not treated, it will usually persist until the epiphyseal line of the upper end of the tibia has closed. *Sever's disease* of the apophysis of the os calcis is analogous to Osgood-Schlatter disease and results from traction on the apophysis by the tendo Achillis. It, too, should be treated by immobilization for 6 weeks.

SUBLUXATION OF HEAD OF RADIUS

Subluxation of the head of the radius occurs frequently in children 2 to 5 years of age; it is rare after 9 years of age. The child has usually been forcibly jerked by the hand by a taller person while the elbow is in full extension; the subluxation occurs with an audible snap.

The symptoms are immediate but usually not persistent pain in the elbow, an inability to supinate the hand and a tendency to hold the arm in slight flexion. Palpation and roentgenograms of the elbow do not reveal any abnormality, and there is no edema. The diagnosis is confirmed by the easy reduction of the subluxation. This is accomplished by firmly grasping the hand of the affected arm and holding the elbow with the thumb of the other hand pressed against the head of the radius while forcibly supinating the forearm beyond the point of obstruction. The click of the return of the radial head to position is usually followed by immediate recovery of painless function.

INFECTIONS OF THE BONES AND JOINTS

ACUTE INFECTIOUS ARTHRITIS

This condition is most common in the first 6 months of life. It is usually preceded by an infection elsewhere in the body, often in the upper respiratory tract. The causative organism is usually one of the common pyogens, such as the staphylococcus, streptococcus, pneumococcus and, less commonly, the gonococcus, meningococcus, influenza bacillus, typhoid bacillus or one of the salmonella group of organisms. The shoulder, hip and other large joints are most commonly affected, but any joint may be involved. Pyogenic arthritis will result in rapid destruction of cartilage and porous ankylosis of the joint if diagnosis and treatment are delayed.

Clinical Manifestations. The onset is sudden with systemic symptoms of sepsis. Local swelling appears rapidly with muscular rigidity and intense pain on motion of the joint, and, if untreated, is followed quickly by suppuration. When the hip is affected, it may become dislocated with astonishing rapidity.

Differential Diagnosis. Acute suppurative arthritis must be differentiated from *acute osteomyelitis*. In acute suppurative arthritis even slight motion of the joint is painful, whereas in osteomyelitis the joint may be moved without pain if done carefully. In suppurative arthritis there is ring tenderness around the joint; in osteomyelitis the tenderness is localized to the metaphysis. In the hip the differentiation cannot be made. The roentgenogram may be of no value in early diagnosis. *Rheumatic fever* rarely occurs in infancy and often involves more than one joint; a prompt response to salicylate therapy is suggestive of rheumatic fever. When an acute pyogenic infection of a joint is suspected, the joint should be aspirated, and any material obtained cultured. A blood culture should also be obtained.

Treatment. The principle of treatment is immediate drainage of the joint. Emergency drainage can be obtained initially by paracentesis of the joint, but when, by smear or culture, the diagnosis of suppurative arthritis is established, surgical drainage of the joint should be done. Appropriate antibiotic therapy is also essential.

OSTEOMYELITIS

This disease occurs most often between 5 and 14 years of age and twice as frequently in boys as in girls. In infants under 2 years of age acute hematogenous osteomyelitis differs in many respects from that in older children.

Etiology and Predisposing Factors. The causative organism in the majority of instances is the hemolytic *Staphylococcus aureus*, though most of the other pathogenic bacteria may also be responsible. Primary lesions are often demonstrable and include furunculosis, impetigo, infected chickenpox and burns and vaccinations.

Pathology. Osteomyelitis begins as a hematogenous abscess in the metaphysis, and then, if uninterrupted, the abscess ruptures subperiosteally and spreads along the shaft of the bone *under the periosteum*. The infection then penetrates to the bone marrow. The separated periosteum forms a shell of new bone around the infected shaft. The pieces of dead bone are known as sequestra, and the new bone formed by the periosteum as the involucrum. Sinuses may form between the sequestra and the skin surface. In the hip the metaphyseal abscess ruptures into the joint and becomes a suppurative arthritis.

Clinical Manifestations. The onset is usually abrupt with fever, malaise, and pain with sharply localized tenderness in the bone *at the metaphysis*. Shortly thereafter, swelling and redness over the affected bone may be present. These signs appear earlier in infants than in older children. The patient is toxic and extremely weak and irritable.

When osteomyelitis follows an infection which has been treated with an antibacterial agent, the clinical course may be modified sufficiently so that the true nature of the lesion may not be suspected until it is well advanced. In addition, inadequate antibacterial therapy of an acute osteomyelitic infection may temporarily abolish the clinical manifestations, but permit the infection to continue in a suppressed state only to become evident days or weeks later.

Diagnosis. There is a leukocytosis of 15,000 to 25,000 cells or more, and the blood culture is usually positive. Roentgenographic examination does not reveal the process for at least 5 days in small children; in older children this period may be as long as 8 to 10 days. At this time there is rarefaction of the involved area, and soon there is evidence of the formation of involucrum.

Differential Diagnosis. Rheumatic fever, leukemia, primary or metastatic neoplasm, sprain, cellulitis, erysipelas and scurvy are likely to require differentiation. The presence of great toxicity and localized pain suggests osteomyelitis. Usually this is enough to distinguish the condition from *rheumatic fever*, but a history of involvement of other joints is indicative of the latter disease, as is the response to salicylates. *Scurvy* produces painful and tender swelling along the shaft of the bone, but roentgenograms of the long bones should be diagnostic. See also Acute Infectious Arthritis.

Prognosis. The mortality rate from acute pyogenic infections of the bones has decreased since the availability of specific antibacterial agents. The rate is lower in newborn infants than in older infants and children, as is the incidence of chronic and metastatic lesions. Both the course and prognosis depend on early institution of appropriate therapy and continuance of it for an adequate time.

Treatment. Acute osteomyelitis requires immediate treatment. When an acute pyogenic infection of a joint or bone is suspected, a blood culture should be obtained, and broad-spectrum antibacterial therapy should be started immediately. Immediate surgical drainage of the metaphysis is the local treatment of choice in the early stage of metaphysitis, although some clinicians prefer to wait 24 to 48 hours to evaluate the response to antibiotic therapy. When the abscess has ruptured into the subperiosteal space, chronic osteomyelitis is the inevitable sequel. Watching and waiting in such a situation is attended with considerable risk.

INFANTILE CORTICAL HYPEROSTOSIS

This lesion, also known as Caffey's disease, is a hyperplasia of subperiosteal bone (Fig. 22-35) over which there is soft tissue swelling and at times a brawny discoloration of the skin. Hyperostoses have been observed in the calvaria, mandible, clavicles, scapulas, ribs and the long bones of the extremities, including the metatarsals.

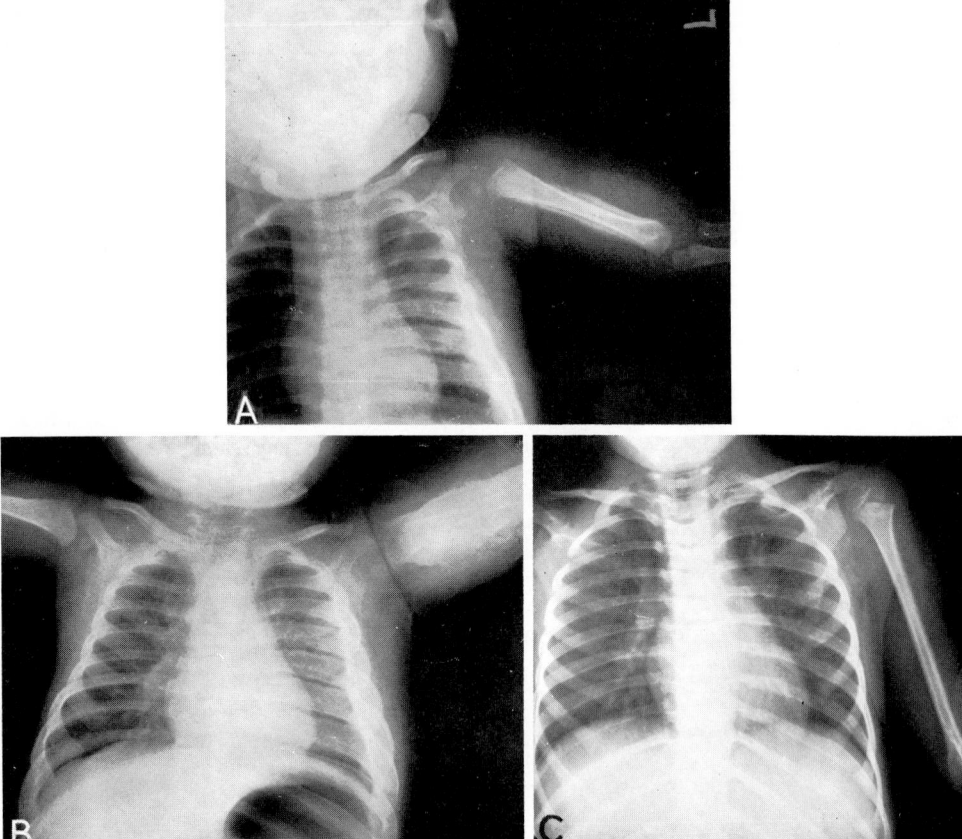

Figure 22-35. Infantile cortical hyperostosis. *A,* Subperiosteal calcification of left lower ribs and left humerus. No evidence of bone destruction. The infant was moderately ill with an upper respiratory tract infection and was somewhat listless. The only localized finding was a disinclination to use the left arm, but there was no paralysis of it. *B,* Increase in subperiosteal calcification of left ribs and humerus developed within 1 month. There is similar involvement of lower right ribs and of facial bones. Evidence of illness has mostly disappeared at the time this roentgenogram was made. *C,* One and a half years later there is no evidence of the cortical disturbance.

The mandible and clavicles appear to be most frequently affected. The clinical features vary considerably, but the symptoms are not severe as a rule. Fever, usually of a low degree, tenderness, hyperirritability, pseudoparalysis, dysphagia, pleurisy, anemia, increased sedimentation rate and elevated serum phosphatase level have been observed in variable combinations.

Duration of clinical activity has been observed for as long as 9 months. No treatment has been effective. Recovery has occurred in all reported instances. Residual deformity is infrequent; bridging of the bones of the forearms has been reported.

Hypervitaminosis A (p. 170) may simulate infantile cortical hyperostosis in certain respects. In hypervitaminosis A the ulnas and one or more metatarsals, other than the first, have been the bones most frequently involved; the mandibles and other flat bones are apparently not affected. This distribution plus a history of excessive ingestion of vitamin A serves to distinguish this entity.

TUBERCULOSIS

Tuberculous Lesions of the Bones and Joints. These lesions are hematogenous in origin, usually stemming from a pulmonary focus, which may not be demonstrable. There is usually only a single osseous lesion. The bones most frequently involved are the head of the femur (hip), the vertebrae and those of the fingers and toes.

Tuberculous Dactylitis. Dactylitis occurs most frequently in early childhood and involves one or more of the phalanges, the metacarpal bones or the corresponding bones of the feet. The medullary canal of the involved bone becomes caseous; the cortex, thinned and expanded; and the periosteum, thickened. The entire digit develops a spindle-shaped, hard, red swelling as the soft tissues are affected. The process is comparatively painless, but it lasts many months and may leave a permanent deformity. The differential diagnosis is chiefly from the dactylitis of congenital syphilis, which is more often multiple and symmetrical. Dactylitis may also occur in sickle cell anemia and in coccidioidomycosis.

The involved region should be put at rest with a splint or cast, and operation is indicated if an abscess develops.

TUBERCULOUS SPONDYLITIS
(POTT'S DISEASE)

This tuberculous osteitis originates in the body of one or more vertebrae, destroys the bone and spreads to all the tissues of the articulation. The spinous process and arches are unaffected. Kyphosis is most common in mid-dorsal lesions. Some scoliosis may accompany the kyphosis if the lesion is disproportionately unilateral.

The lower dorsal part of the spine is most likely to be involved, with the lumbar and the cervical segments next in order of frequency. Paraplegia may occur when the upper dorsal or cervical region is affected, but is rarely associated with involvement below the mid-dorsal region. *Psoas abscess* is a complication of caries in the lumbar vertebrae. A *cold abscess* in the cervical vertebrae may open into the pharynx (retropharyngeal abscess) or above the clavicle; one originating opposite the lower cervical or upper dorsal vertebrae may rupture into the pleura or penetrate to the scapula, but often it gravitates and points above Poupart's ligament.

Clinical Manifestations. Symptoms are insidious in onset, the earliest being irritability. Persistent or intermittent pain may occur over the distribution of the spinal nerves arising adjacent to the affected vertebrae. This pain is increased by pressure on the head, but not by pressure over the lesions. Muscular rigidity splints the back, and the child assumes a position which will best take the weight from the diseased spine and prevent jarring. He may avoid bending to reach an object on the floor, may walk stiffly or carefully on his toes, or may prefer to lie on his abdomen and to rest frequently across a chair or over his mother's lap. With cervical involvement the child may hold his head stiffly or support it with his hand.

Differential Diagnosis. *Rickets* produces kyphosis of greater length and uniformity, which is unaccompanied by rigidity and disappears when the patient is prone. *Nontuberculous scoliosis* is seldom accompanied by rigidity or pain. *Hip joint disease* may be suspected when lameness is the result of lumbar tuberculosis, but in the latter there is no limitation of movement of the hip except in the presence of psoas abscess, when extension will be limited. *Acute nontuberculous osteomyelitis of the vertebrae* can be distinguished by its greater toxicity, leukocytosis and fever. In addition, the roentgenographic findings are usually well established in a tuberculous lesion of the vertebrae when symptoms first become manifest, whereas they are not likely to be demonstrable during the first few days of an acute pyogenic osteomyelitis. The *Klippel-Feil* syndrome may be confused with tuberculosis of the cervical spine, but is readily distinguishable by roentgenogram.

Prognosis. The reparative process may not begin for 1 to 3 years, but in carefully treated cases recovery with ankylosis and little or no deformity can be expected in the majority of instances. Paraplegia often disappears completely.

Treatment. Traditionally, therapy consisted in continuous extension on a Bradford frame until there was no evidence of active infection, and then spinal fusion. Early surgical eradication of the tuberculous abscess in conjunction with specific antimicrobial therapy is now the accepted treatment.

TUBERCULOSIS OF THE HIP
(TUBERCULOUS COXITIS)

This is the most common tuberculous involvement of the joints. The disease may begin in the synovial membrane, but usually starts as an osteitis of the femoral epiphysis, followed by a tuberculous arthritis and finally by an abscess resulting in destruction of the femoral head.

Clinical Manifestations. Usually the first symptom is a slight lameness which is likely to be intermittent, occurring when the patient first gets out of bed and after exercise. It may disappear for days or weeks at a time. Pain may be present at this stage or may develop later and is usually referred to the knee or the inner side of the thigh. As destruction of the joint proceeds, the thigh is flexed and adducted, and the rotation which initially was outward becomes inward. Swelling about the hip increases, and an abscess may form from which pus may discharge anteriorly to the joint or be disseminated in other directions. Absorption of the head and neck of the femur may take place without evidence of suppuration.

Differential Diagnosis. Distinction must be made from *osteochondrosis of the femoral head* (Legg-Calvé-Perthes disease), which occurs in the same age group, but limits abduction to a greater extent than it does extension and whose roentgenographic changes do not extend beyond the femoral capitular epiphysis. In tuberculous coxitis the acetabulum may also be affected. The 2 conditions may be indistinguishable in the early stage, and the clinical course must be relied upon to differentiate them. A negative tuberculin reaction is of great value. The insidious onset of tuberculous coxitis serves to distinguish it from *rheumatic fever* and *acute arthritis.*

Prognosis. After abscess formation the disease may last 2 to 4 years or longer. When treatment is begun in the first few weeks of the disease, the inflammation may cease entirely before the joint itself is attacked, but in the majority of cases the joint is finally ankylosed.

Treatment. Treatment consists in bed rest, traction on the leg to reduce muscle spasm and specific antibacterial therapy (p. 606). Surgical eradication of the abscess may be considered in selected cases in conjunction with antibacterial therapy.

MULTIPLE TRAUMATIC SKELETAL LESIONS IN EARLY LIFE
(THE BATTERED-CHILD SYNDROME)

Traumatic lesions of the bones are relatively common in infants and small children, and often are not associated with clinical manifestations proportionate to their severity or at times even sufficient to call attention to them. Frequently they are recognized only by roentgen examination performed for some unrelated reason. In some instances the trauma is accidental and may or may not be known to the parents, and on occasion, when known, they may be hesitant to disclose it. In other instances the trauma is inflicted willfully by an adult, usually a parent, often in a burst of temper. Relatively frequently there are repeated assaults, and roentgen examination of the skeleton reveals multiple traumatic osseous lesions in different stages of healing. This clinical pattern has been termed the battered-child syndrome. It is recognized as a significant cause of failure to thrive, of disability and even of death. Nearly all the patients are under 3 years of age, and the majority are less than 1 year.

The skeletal lesions reflect the characteristics of growing bone. The periosteum is not firmly attached in infancy, is easily elevated by hemorrhage, and periosteal new bone formation is active. Epiphyseal separation and displacement are readily achieved. There may also be fractures of the metaphysis or diaphysis, at times with significant deformity. When there are multiple lesions, they are apt to be in varying stages of healing, indicative of repeated trauma and suggestive of a psychopathic situation within the home. Subdural hematomas frequently are found in association with the skeletal lesions and contribute to the failure of the infant to thrive.

At times the diagnosis is suggested by limitation of motion of an extremity, the failure to use it or pain on manipulation. Ecchymoses and other evidences of soft tissue injury are not as common as they are under similar circumstances in older children. The history is often not helpful, either because the parents are unaware of the accidents or because they choose not to disclose them. The differential diagnosis includes scurvy, congenital syphilis, cortical hyperostosis, osteogenesis imperfecta and neoplasm; if the injury is in the region of a joint, it may simulate suppurative arthritis.

In all instances the social and psychiatric aspects of the parent-child or caretaker-child relationship must be investigated and managed appropriately. It may be necessary to take legal action. When subsequent trauma seems probable, the child should be removed from the home. When it is evident that the trauma has been either accidental or due to a single burst of temper, one should take care that parents are not unfairly burdened with a sense of guilt. In many localities the attending physician is required to report to legal authorities any suspected instance of wilfully inflicted trauma.

JOHN LACHMAN
THEODORE LAMMOT

REFERENCES

Helfer, R. E., and Kempe, C. H. (Eds.): *The Battered Child.* Chicago, University of Chicago Press, 1968.
Staheli, L. T., Church, C. C., and Ward, B. H.: Infantile Cortical Hyperostosis (Caffey's Disease). *J.A.M.A.*, 203:384, 1968.

METABOLIC DISORDERS WITH OSSEOUS LESIONS

Differential diagnosis and management of metabolic bone disease depend upon clear understanding of the principles of osteogenesis. Essentials for the formation and maintenance of bone include an appropriate organic matrix (osteoid) and suitable concentrations of calcium and phosphorus in extracellular fluid. Most bones are endochondral, arising in cartilaginous models. Growth, mineralization, and systematic removal of cartilage are therefore determinants of skeletal form and composition.

Chondrocytes and osteoblasts synthesize cartilage and osteoid, respectively. The principal component of each of these matrices is collagen; small amounts of mucopolysaccharide, chiefly chondroitin sulfate, are also present. What determines calcification is not known. Neither epiphyseal cartilage nor osteoid can be distinguished chemically from tendon, fascia, or ear cartilage, none of which normally mineralizes.

The first perceptible mineral deposit in cartilage is amorphous tricalcium phosphate ($Ca_3(PO_4)_2$), which gradually accumulates hydroxyl ions to become crystalline hydroxyapatite. In osteoid, apatite crystals (and presumably their antecedent, tricalcium phosphate) are first seen in the light zones of the periodic bands characteristic of collagen fibers. During crystalline growth a close orientation with the underlying fibers persists. The fiber surface appears to create a microenvironment favorable to crystallization. Whether this involves adsorption, chelation or an enzyme-dependent reaction is presently obscure.

Alkaline phosphatase is abundant not only in areas of osteoid formation, but also wherever collagen synthesis is active, as in healing wounds. It is presently thought that this enzyme is more important in the production of matrix than in the increase of local concentration of phosphate by hydrolysis of phosphate esters.

Although apatite can be formed at very low concentrations of calcium and phosphate, mineralization of osteoid at a rate commensurate with normal bone growth requires an adequate supply of *both* ions. Howland and Kramer found that rickets ensued when the product of serum calcium and phosphorus (in milligrams per 100 ml.) was less than 30. Subnormal Ca × P products are usually due to hypophosphatemia, since calcium is closely regulated by the parathyroids.

Since the solubility of apatite varies inversely with pH, demineralization has been attributed to chronic acidosis. Respiratory acidosis does not affect bone, perhaps because the high concentration of bicarbonate in interstitial fluid decreases the solubility of calcium. In chronic renal insufficiency it is impossible to dissociate the effects of acidosis from those of other chemical disturbances. In diabetes mellitus and in acute renal failure the duration of acidosis is too brief to affect bone significantly. In untreated renal tubular acidosis, hyperphosphaturia is pronounced; this feature of the disease, rather than depression of pH, is probably responsible for osteomalacia.

Synthesis and destruction of osteoid are continuous throughout life. The amount of bone present at any given time is the resultant of these 2 processes, and the morphology of bone is determined by remodelling. Continuous removal of mineral from resorbing surfaces and redeposition of it in newly formed osteoid effect a slow redistribution of skeletal calcium and phosphate. Metabolic factors causing loss of calcium or phosphate from body fluids therefore lead to osteomalacia by compromising the mineralization of continuously synthesized osteoid. It is thus not necessary to postulate accelerated destruction to account for the appearance of bone lesions.

A direct osteolytic action of parathyroid hormone has been established, but the mechanism is not defined. This effect is presumably mediated through the osteoclasts, which increase in numbers and in apparent activity when the parathyroids are stimulated or when exogenous parathyroid hormone is given. Increases in local production of citrate may demineralize bone by chelating calcium; a decrease in local pH has also been postulated. Removal of osseous matrix accompanies demineralization. An increase in levels of mucopolysaccharide and hydroxyproline in urine follows administration of parathormone. Parathyroid hormone also has an indirect effect on bone through inhibition of renal tubular phos-

TABLE 22-1. SKELETAL EFFECTS OF METABOLIC DISORDERS

I. Disorders affecting formation or maintenance of bone matrix
  A. Nutritional
    Scurvy
    Protein deficiency
    Caloric deficiency
  B. Endocrine
    Hypothyroidism
    Hyperthyroidism
    Hyperadrenalism (Cushing's syndrome)
    Side effects of corticosteroid therapy
  C. Metabolic and genetic
    Osteoporosis of disuse
    Hypophosphatasia
    Hyperphosphatasia
    Osteogenesis imperfecta
    Gargoylism (and other mucopolysaccharidoses)
    Osteopetrosis
    Achondroplasia and other chondrodysplasias
II. Disorders affecting mineralization of bone matrix
  A. Nutritional
    Rickets due to vitamin D deficiency
    Malabsorptive states
      Celiac disease, cystic fibrosis, biliary atresia
  B. Endocrine
    Hypoparathyroidism
    Hyperparathyroidism
  C. Renal tubular dysfunction with losses of minerals
    Hypophosphatemic vitamin D-resistant rickets (renal hypophosphatemia)
    Hypocalcemic vitamin D-resistant rickets
    Fanconi's syndrome (renal hypophosphatemia with renal glycosuria and aminoaciduria)
    Lignac's syndrome (Fanconi's syndrome with cystinosis)
  D. Chronic metabolic acidosis
    Renal tubular acidosis
    Oculocerebrorenal syndrome (Lowe)
  E. Other
    Idiopathic hypercalciuria
III. Complex disorders of bone, affecting both matrix and mineralization
  A. Hyperparathyroidism
    Local osteolytic activity and hypophosphatemia
  B. Chronic renal failure
    Decreased calcium absorption and secondary hyperparathyroidism

phate reabsorption, which causes a decrease in the concentration of serum phosphorus.

The skeletal effects of metabolic disorders, considered in terms of these critical factors, are as shown in Table 22-1.

REFRACTORY RICKETS

Since vitamin D deficiency has become a rarity in the United States and many other countries, most rickets presently seen is of endogenous origin and is resistant to the usual intake of vitamin D

(400 to 1000 I.U. per day). Rickets refractory to vitamin D occurs in association with several complex disorders; these include the relatively common hypophosphatemic variety of vitamin D-resistant rickets and the rare hypocalcemic form, the Fanconi syndrome, cystinosis, renal tubular acidosis, Lowe's syndrome and renal osteodystrophy, each of which is described in this section. Rickets may also develop in the malabsorption syndromes if defective intestinal absorption of vitamin D is not compensated by the administration of relatively large doses in water-miscible preparations, or in extreme situations parenterally.

HYPOPHOSPHATEMIC VITAMIN D-RESISTANT RICKETS

In this clinical entity, rickets resistant to unusually large doses of vitamin D is the only obvious manifestation; this condition is commonly identified by the somewhat inadequate term "refractory rickets." It has also been categorized as "renal hypophosphatemia." It occurs in familial and sporadic forms, which are clinically and chemically indistinguishable.

Etiology. The theories of causation of refractory rickets attempt to explain the characteristic and apparently critical hypophosphatemia. Since cartilage from untreated patients will calcify in normal serum, and intravenous infusions of phosphate result in rapid mineralization of rachitic lesions in vivo, the osteoid appears to have its usual potential for apatite deposition. Serum calcium concentration is nearly always normal, but that of phosphorus is regularly low; the resulting $Ca \times P$ product is in the rachitic range (below 30).

Intestinal absorption of calcium is low before treatment and increases after very large doses of vitamin D. It has been postulated that the parathyroids, stimulated by calcium deficit, are continuously hyperactive, sustaining the serum level of calcium by withdrawing it from bone and by suppressing renal tubular reabsorption of phosphate. Phosphate clearance is increased even in the presence of hypophosphatemia, a finding consistent with compensatory hyperparathyroidism. When calcium is given intravenously, tubular reabsorption of phosphate increases promptly, as does the concentration of serum phosphorus. This effect, presumably due to parathyroid suppression, is interpreted as evidence that phosphaturia is a secondary phenomenon. There are several objections, however, to the theory of a primary intestinal absorptive defect: (1) since serum calcium in untreated patients is nearly always normal, there is no evident "feed-back" stimulus to the parathyroids; (2) although massive vitamin D therapy frequently causes hypercalcemia, the serum level of phosphorus usually remains low, and hyperphosphaturia persists; (3) the roentgenographic appearance of the bones

is not consistent with hyperparathyroidism; e.g. such changes as cysts, subperiosteal erosion and fraying of the terminal phalanges are absent; and (4) since tubular phosphate reabsorption can be increased by calcium infusion even in the absence of the parathyroids, this test is not diagnostic of hyperparathyroidism.

Refractory rickets was originally classified in the group of intrinsic renal tubular defects which includes nephrogenic diabetes insipidus, renal glycosuria, renal tubular acidosis, Fanconi's syndrome, Lowe's syndrome, cystinuria and glycinuria. The concept that hypophosphatemia depends on a primary incapacity of the tubules to reabsorb phosphate does not readily explain diminished intestinal absorption of calcium. If a tubular defect exists, it must be relative, since reabsorption of phosphate can be decreased by injection of parathyroid hormone and increased by infusion of calcium.

Epidemiology. Refractory rickets is often familial. Some family members without obvious disease may be found to have mild involvement on careful clinical and radiographic examination; others have hypophosphatemia without demonstrable osseous lesions. Roentgenography, however, is an insensitive indicator of bone composition, and too few chemical or histologic examinations have been made to conclude that apparently nonrachitic members of the kindreds studied have normal osseous structure and composition.

Genetic analysis indicates a sex-linked dominant mode of inheritance, with complete penetrance of hypophosphatemia, but irregular expressivity of overt osseous disease. Hypophosphatemic males have rachitic changes more often than their female counterparts; their serum phosphorus concentrations are likewise slightly lower. Whether persons with sporadic refractory rickets can transmit the disease to their offspring is unknown.

Clinical Manifestations. The general health of the child is unaffected, and the muscular hypotonia prominent in vitamin D-deficiency rickets is absent. Typical lateral bowing deformities of the legs appear during the second year; other rachitic stigmata such as frontal bossing, costochondral beading, enlarged wrists and dental defects are usually present, but easily missed. Sitting deformities (anterior bowing of the femora and tibiae) attest to the early onset of disease, but are rarely noticed by parents. Linear growth is retarded.

The roentgenographic appearance is indistinguishable from that of vitamin D-deficiency rickets. The serum phosphorus level is low and usually responds only partially to otherwise successful therapy. The serum calcium level is characteristically within the normal range. Rarely, however, it is low, and the untreated patient has tetany. Plasma electrolyte composition is otherwise normal. Alkaline phosphatase is elevated in active disease and decreases during successful

treatment. Aminoaciduria is an inconstant finding; it disappears after therapy in some instances,
as it does in deficiency rickets.

Diagnosis. Nonrachitic bowing is differentiated by roentgenography. In familial cases the
history may be diagnostic. If the intake of vitamin
D has been adequate and malabsorption is not
suggested by nutritional status and description
of stools, refractory rickets is probable. When the
primary disorder is renal tubular acidosis, Fanconi's syndrome or Lowe's syndrome, the general
health is severely affected. When rickets is the
sole manifestation, failure to respond to moderate
doses of vitamin D establishes the diagnosis of
refractory rickets.

When 1500 to 3000 I.U. of vitamin D are given
daily, a month is necessary to determine the
presence or absence of effect. This time can be
shortened by giving 600,000 I.U. in a single dose;
in simple vitamin D deficiency chemical improvement occurs within a few days and perceptible
roentgenographic changes within 2 weeks. Rarely
it may be necessary to repeat the dose after 2
weeks. This procedure requires close supervision,
preferably in the hospital, to avoid the dangers
of overdosage. If improvement occurs, the high
tissue level of vitamin D established suffices for
4 to 5 months, after which the usual supplement
may be instituted. Infection during the observation period may negate the test.

Treatment. Since resistance to vitamin D in
this disorder unfortunately does not protect
against its toxic effects, the large doses required
for healing may cause anorexia, hypercalcemia,
polyuria and renal damage. Therapy, therefore,
requires a compromise in determining a dose
which will promote maximal healing with min-

imal risk of renal damage. It is well to start with
25,000 I.U. per day, increasing by increments of
25,000 units at monthly intervals until healing
or toxicity is apparent. The dose is reduced to the
preceding level if serum calcium exceeds 11 mg.
per 100 ml. or if polyuria occurs. The Sulkowitch
test of urine is not very satisfactory as an indirect
indicator of hypercalcemia. Renal biopsies have
shown tubular calcification even in carefully controlled cases, indicating the desirability of conservatism in treatment. The aim should be to
prevent deformity rather than to achieve radiographic normality. The characteristic slowing of
linear growth is not impressively influenced by
therapy. As an adjunct, 1 to 2 gm. of phosphorus
should be given daily (as a mixture of sodium
monohydrogen and dihydrogen phosphate in a
molar ratio of 4:1) in divided doses. This regimen
may reduce the dose of vitamin D necessary for
healing. Even so, normal serum phosphorus concentration is not attained.

If deformities are pronounced before treatment
is begun, corrective osteotomy may be necessary;
mineralization should first be augmented by treatment. Administration of vitamin D should then
be discontinued 2 weeks before operation and
resumed only when the patient is ambulatory;
immobilization may otherwise cause dangerous
hypercalcemia.

HYPOCALCEMIC VITAMIN D-RESISTANT RICKETS
(PSEUDODEFICIENCY RICKETS)

This form of vitamin D-resistant rickets has
been separated out from the much more common

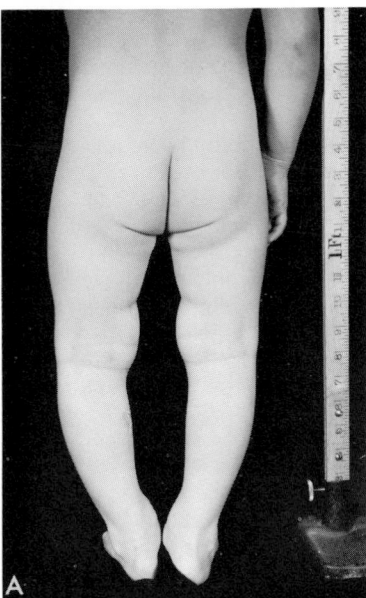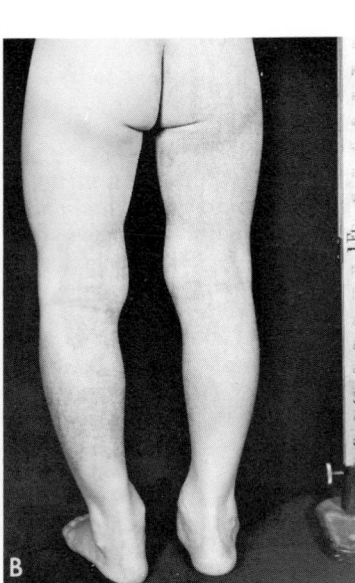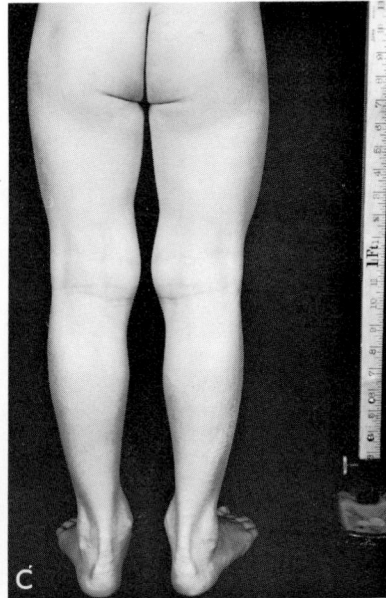

Figure 22-36. Refractory rickets. *A*, Untreated, age 3 years. *B*, Age 6 years, after vitamin D, 50,000 units per day
for 3 years. *C*, Age 7½ years, after corrective osteotomy of left tibia.

variety described above. Clinically, the two are similar in respect to the osseous changes in the untreated stage, which simulate those of rickets. Otherwise there are significant differences. In contrast to the low serum concentration of phosphate in the hypophosphatemic variety which is only partially corrected by administration of large doses of vitamin D, the concentration of phosphate in the hypocalcemic variety is within the normal range or nearly so and the concentration of calcium is abnormally low. Tetany can usually be demonstrated in its latent phase, and seizures may occur. Serum chloride and alkaline phosphatase values are high, and aminoaciduria is increased. The hypocalcemic form appears to be transmitted as an autosomal dominant pattern in contrast to the sex-linked inheritance of hypophosphatemic refractory rickets.

Treatment is similar to that described above. The daily dose of vitamin D should be adjusted so that the serum concentration of calcium is maintained at low to average values of the normal range. The osseous lesions disappear with such therapy, and in contrast to the situation in the hypophosphatemic form, growth in stature approximates normal expectancy. This feature suggests that stunting in hypophosphatemic rickets may be due to an inadequate supply of phosphorus for osseous metabolism.

FANCONI SYNDROME

(Refractory Rickets Associated with
Multiple Defects of the Renal Tubules;
de Toni-Debre-Fanconi Syndrome)

Aminoaciduria, renal glycosuria, hypophosphatemia and hyperphosphaturia characterize the Fanconi syndrome. Proteinuria, hyposthenuria and acidosis are often present; hypokalemia may occur in conjunction with acidosis. The disorder causes dwarfing and rickets resistant to vitamin D.

Etiology. The cause of the Fanconi syndrome is not clear. Both familial and sporadic cases occur. In some instances the syndrome accompanies other disorders, including heavy metal poisoning (lead, uranium, cadmium), Wilson's disease and multiple myeloma. It may occur in adults. A degradation product of outdated tetracycline can cause a reversible form of the disease.

Pathogenesis. The basic defect may be resistance to several effects of vitamin D, since large doses of vitamin D reduce fecal calcium, partially restore tubular transport of amino acids, glucose and phosphate, and improve acidosis and hypokalemia. Intestinal absorption of calcium, consistently low in simple refractory rickets, is not always depressed in multiple tubular dysfunction. As in simple refractory rickets, the chemical derangements of the Fanconi syndrome may occur without evident osseous involvement.

The characteristic histologic changes occur in the proximal tubules, which are shorter than normal and are connected to the glomeruli by an abnormally narrow segment ("swan's neck"). Vacuolization of distal tubular cells is a less specific finding, and may be due to depletion of potassium.

Changes in the plasma and urine in the Fanconi syndrome result from decreased tubular reabsorption of phosphate, glucose, amino acids and, in some instances, water. Urinary ammonia and titratable acidity are insufficient to prevent loss of fixed base. Hypophosphatemia and acidosis are both conducive to the development of rickets. Since acidosis is inconstant and its amelioration does not result in healing, its role in rachitogenesis is apparently minor.

Clinical Manifestations. Characteristically, the infant appears normal at birth; symptoms appear after the first 6 months of life, when growth failure, weakness, dehydration and fever may appear. Dehydration is often associated with polyuria and vomiting. Constipation is common.

The bony abnormalities of rickets appear despite adequate intake of vitamin D, and may dominate the clinical pattern if the systemic manifestations are mild. Linear growth is restricted. The skeletal changes may be those of renal osteodystrophy late in the course of the illness, when renal failure supervenes.

Laboratory Data. Serum analysis reveals low phosphorus and normal calcium values initially and, in some instances, hyperchloremic acidosis and hypokalemia. As renal function fails, the serum phosphorus level increases along with that of nonprotein nitrogen, and calcium may fall to tetanic levels. Alkaline phosphatase is elevated if active rickets is present. The urine contains glucose and excessive amounts of 10 or more amino acids; excretion of them may cease with renal failure. The pattern of excretion of amino acids may vary in different patients, but is consistent for the individual. Organic aciduria appears to reflect the same tubular defect which causes aminoaciduria.

Urinary ammonia and titratable acidity may be low, and excretion of bicarbonate high in proportion to the acidosis. Urinary pH may be relatively high. Proteinuria is inconstant.

Diagnosis. Since aminoaciduria, diminished tubular reabsorption of phosphate and elevated serum levels of alkaline phosphatase are present in other forms of rickets, they are not diagnostic. Demonstration of renal glycosuria in the presence of stunting and refractory rickets indicates multiple tubular dysfunction. Hyperchloremic acidosis and hypokalemia, if present, are corroborative. Glucose tolerance tests have caused severe and occasionally fatal shocklike reactions, probably by shifting potassium into cells during glycogen deposition in patients already hypokalemic.

Treatment. Rickets and osteomalacia respond to large doses of vitamin D (25,000 to 400,000 units daily). The dose should be individualized as suggested above for simple refractory rickets;

25,000 to 50,000 units per day is often sufficient. Hypercalcemia must be scrupulously avoided; additional calcium, however, may be required under unusual circumstances (see above). For correction of acidosis and hypokalemia a mixture of sodium and potassium citrate is appropriate. A liter of flavored syrup containing 100 gm. of each salt provides 2 mEq. of cation per ml. The dose is approximately 5 mEq. per kg. per day; it should be adjusted by periodic determinations of serum bicarbonate. Potassium should be included even if hypokalemia is not present, since sodium loading may otherwise cause depletion of potassium. In several instances renal tubular acidosis and glycosuria have responded to therapy with calciferol alone. Electrolyte supplementation should therefore be deferred until the effects of vitamin D have been observed for a few weeks. When renal failure supervenes, therapy must be re-evaluated in terms of the capacity to excrete sodium and potassium.

Although temporary improvement may be gratifying, most patients survive only a few years. The cause of death is usually chronic renal failure and uremia. When the disease begins in late childhood, the course may be more benign.

CYSTINOSIS
(LIGNAC'S SYNDROME; FANCONI SYNDROME
WITH CYSTINOSIS)

Cystinosis was first recognized at autopsy in 1903 and was established as a clinical entity by Lignac in 1924. This disorder is characterized by the clinical pattern of the Fanconi syndrome as described above combined with the presence of cystine crystals in various tissues of the body. Some investigators consider the Fanconi syndrome and cystinosis to be variants of the same disorder. Certainly some of the cases reported as Fanconi syndrome in the past may have had undetected deposition of cystine crystals. It is clear, however, that the Fanconi syndrome occurs without cystinosis.

The **pathogenesis** of cystinosis is unknown. It has been proposed that the renal defect may be due to the nephrotoxic activity of cystine. The deposition of cystine crystals in the tissues has been attributed to aberrant cystine metabolism, but an enzymatic defect has not been demonstrated.

The characteristic pathologic lesion is the deposition of cystine in the reticuloendothelial system, especially apparent in the liver, spleen, lymph nodes and bone marrow. Cystine deposits also occur in the renal tubular cells and in the cornea and conjunctiva. Changes in renal tubular morphology are similar to those described for the Fanconi syndrome. The crystals are most readily demonstrated in the cornea and in the bone marrow. The cornea may be normal on gross and ophthalmoscopic examination, but examination by slit-lamp biomicroscopy reveals a myriad of highly refractile bodies. Occasionally the crystals may be seen in the peripheral white blood cells, but more often they can be demonstrated in bone marrow aspirates, or in lymph node or renal tissue obtained by biopsy. Fixing or staining procedures which dissolve the cystine crystals should be avoided. Granular and circinate irregularities in the peripheral pigmentation of the retina may be seen funduscopically as early as 5 weeks of age. They antedate the appearance of perceptible crystals by several months.

The **clinical manifestations** and **laboratory findings** other than those of crystal deposition are similar to those described for the Fanconi syndrome. Photophobia and a preference or craving for meat and other protein foods may also be noted and should suggest cystinosis as a diagnostic possibility.

Treatment, in general, is the same as that for the Fanconi syndrome. The therapeutic use of penicillamine has been proposed; its efficiency is undetermined. Few children live beyond 8 years of age.

RICKETS ASSOCIATED WITH RENAL TUBULAR ACIDOSIS
(LIGHTWOOD'S SYNDROME; ALBRIGHT'S
SYNDROME)

This disorder is characterized by metabolic acidosis, hyperchloremia, inability to form an adequately acid urine, hypercalciuria and sometimes hypokalemia. There appear to be 2 distinct clinical types: the infantile form (Lightwood's syndrome) is self-limited; the persistent form of the disease has a later onset with rickets or osteomalacia.

Etiology. Hydrogen ion clearance is inadequate; i.e. the urine pH, though low at times, is always higher than is appropriate for the plasma bicarbonate. This results in excessive excretion of bicarbonate and increased tubular reabsorption of chloride. Associated losses of sodium and potassium may lead to acidosis and hypokalemia. Potassium deficit is probably the cause of hyposthenuria. Hypercalciuria, another aspect of fixed base loss, is readily reversed by administration of alkali; if it is allowed to persist, nephrocalcinosis and nephrolithiasis ensue. Susceptibility to these serious complications is increased by the absence of urinary citrate, a constituent which normally forms a soluble complex with calcium. Diminished tubular reabsorption of phosphate results in hypophosphatemia and rickets.

Although the chemical pattern of the disease can be simulated by giving carbonic anhydrase inhibitors, no deficiency of the enzyme has been established.

Clinical Manifestations. In infancy the principal manifestations are nonspecific and include anorexia, vomiting, constipation, apathy, irritability and weakness. Death may result from dehydration and acidosis. Rickets and nephrocalcinosis do not occur in the infantile form.

Later in childhood the presenting complaints may be similar, or may relate to growth retardation, bony deformities or pathologic fractures. Terminal renal insufficiency may result from nephrocalcinosis. Roentgenograms reveal rickets and, in later stages, nephrocalcinosis.

Epidemiology. Although familial cases occur, the mode of inheritance has not been defined.

Treatment. The mixture of sodium and potassium citrate recommended for the Fanconi syndrome (100 gm. of each per liter of vehicle) is satisfactory; the dose should be regulated by appropriate serum analyses. Calcium supplementation may be necessary during the initial period of rapid remineralization, but is not indicated thereafter. After acidosis has been corrected the vitamin D requirement is not elevated; conversely, even large doses are ineffectual in the presence of acidosis.

LOWE'S SYNDROME
(OCULOCEREBRORENAL DYSTROPHY)

This rare affliction is characterized by mental retardation, glaucoma, organic aciduria, aminoaciduria, and diminished renal production of ammonia. Hypotonia and areflexia appear in the latter half of the first year of life along with generalized hyperactivity. Cataracts are usually present. Febrile episodes are frequent, probably as a result of dehydration. Some patients have metabolic acidosis and rickets. Large doses of vitamin D are ineffectual unless calcium and sodium supplements are also provided.

The disease is inherited in a sex-linked partially dominant pattern; so far the fully manifest syndrome has been observed only in males. The female carrier may have lenticular opacities.

RENAL OSTEODYSTROPHY
(RENAL RICKETS)

Bone lesions resulting from chronic glomerular and tubular insufficiency were previously designated as renal rickets. This term, however, obscures the complex nature of the disorder and misrepresents the roentgenographic appearance.

Etiology. Renal hypoplasia, polycystic disease of the kidney, hydronephrosis, pyelonephritis and chronic glomerulonephritis are the commonest causes of reduction in effective renal mass. Acidosis and hyperphosphatemia result from tubular and glomerular hypofunction. Intestinal absorption of calcium is depressed. Extreme hypocalcemia is unusual, however, since the combination of acidosis and secondary hyperparathyroidism sustains a higher calcium concentration than would be predicted from the observed hyperphosphatemia. The $Ca \times P$ product is usually elevated and may exceed 100. Tetany is rare. Compensatory hyperparathyroidism may be detected by typical roentgenographic changes, by the microscopic appearance of bone in biopsy or necropsy material and by direct examination of the glands at autopsy. Such studies have made it clear that secondary hyperparathyroidism is variable in degree and that its role in the production of osteodystrophy may at times be minor.

Calcium deficiency and acidosis reduce the rate of mineralization in growing bone; hyperparathyroidism, when present, causes erosion and cyst formation. The microscopic appearance combines the features of osteomalacia (undermineralized osteoid) and osteitis fibrosa cystica (erosion of bone substance). Either may predominate. Areas of osteosclerosis also may occur, especially in the vertebral bodies; this phenomenon has not been explained.

Clinical Manifestations. Growth failure, anemia and general debility are the usual pre-

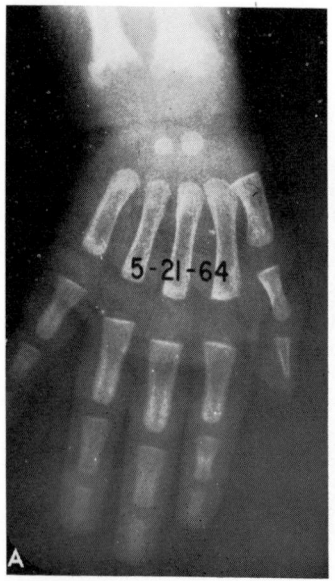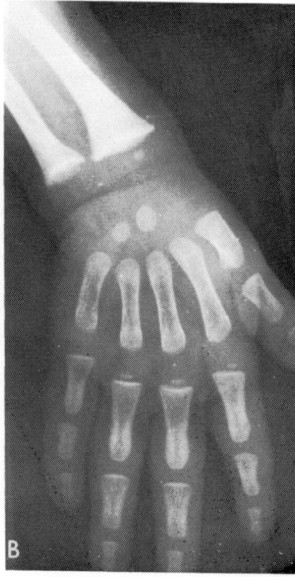

Figure 22-37. Renal osteodystrophy. *A*, Age 16 months. Calciferol, 400 units a day since early infancy. Serum: calcium, 9.5 mg. per 100 ml., phosphorus, 5 mg. per 100 ml.; pH, 7.35; blood urea nitrogen, 30. Intravenous pyelogram showed renal hypoplasia. *B*, Healing after 7 weeks of therapy with calciferol, 25,000 units a day. Hypercalcemia ensued after 3 months; 5000 units a day thereafter sustained healing without hypercalcemia.

senting complaints, preceding the appearance of bone deformities. In the patient presented in Figure 22-37 osteodystrophy was apparent within a year of the onset of uremia; in most instances the interval is longer. Skeletal involvement may create extremely severe functional and cosmetic handicaps, including bowing, knock-knee, frontal bossing and dental defects. Bone pain may be crippling. Roentgenograms reveal demineralization, coarsening of the trabecular pattern and usually subperiosteal rarefaction. When growth is minimal, the wide, clear epiphyseal zones of rickets are absent, being replaced by areas of ragged, chaotic erosion. Osteosclerosis of the axial skeleton may be seen. At autopsy the bones are generally soft, osteoclasts are abundant, and the proportion of ash to organic matrix is low. Azotemia is combined with the chemical changes in the serum mentioned above, and the concentration of alkaline phosphatase is increased. Hypertension, polyuria and isosthenuria are often present.

Diagnosis. This is seldom difficult. In primary hyperparathyroidism the foregoing clinical and chemical disorders may supervene when renal failure complicates the terminal stage, but this entity is extremely rare in childhood, fewer than 25 cases having been reported. No other condition is known to produce the combination of biochemical and morphologic changes described.

Treatment. Previously the therapeutic plan was based on restriction of dietary protein and phosphate and provision of supplementary alkali. Oral administration of aluminum hydroxide and a cation exchange resin to remove phosphate and potassium has also been recommended. These measures reduce azotemia and hyperphosphatemia; healing of bone lesions occasionally follows correction of metabolic acidosis, but results are seldom satisfactory. During the past several years the use of vitamin D in large doses has led to remarkable clinical and roentgenographic improvement in bone lesions and in suppression of secondary hyperparathyroidism. This regimen increases calcium absorption and promotes mineralization of bone by mechanisms presently obscure. The dose of vitamin D ranges from 25,000 to 250,000 units per day; after healing, 10,000 units per day may suffice. Good results ensue despite persistent acidosis, hyperphosphatemia and uremia. Close chemical and roentgenographic control is essential; as in refractory rickets, hypercalcemia is an indication of overdosage of vitamin D. Dihydrotachysterol is as effective as calciferol, the dose in milligrams being the same for each sterol. One milligram of calciferol (vitamin D_2) contains 40,000 units. Restriction of phosphate is apparently unnecessary and has in fact been found to exaggerate osteomalacia.

If correction of acidosis is desired, sodium citrate (10 mEq. per gm.) or sodium bicarbonate can be given, starting with 5 mEq. per kg. per day. Supplementary calcium should be provided, since tetany may otherwise ensue when the serum pH is increased in the presence of hyperphosphate-

mia. Calcium lactate (8 gm. = 1 gm. of calcium) may be given in fruit juice or ginger ale. It may be necessary to add potassium citrate in order to prevent hypokalemia.

Therapy must be individualized; the goal is a reasonably active and comfortable patient rather than a normal plasma electrolyte pattern.

IDIOPATHIC HYPERCALCEMIA

Osteosclerosis, best seen in the metaphyses, is the skeletal hallmark of this interesting disease. When the diaphyses are also involved, the long bones may mimic osteopetrosis.

In 1952 Lightwood described a syndrome comprising hypercalcemia and failure to thrive. The original patients appeared to have a relatively mild disorder, self-limited and reversible when administration of calcium and vitamin D was discontinued. Fanconi and Schlesinger then reported seriously affected infants, and a wide spectrum of severity was soon apparent. Hypercalcemia, "elfin" facies (combining prominent epicanthal folds, retroussé nose, long overhanging upper lip without Cupid's bow, wide mouth, receding chin and misshapen ears), mental retardation, hypertension and nephrocalcinosis characterize the disease in its most severe form. Irritability, anorexia, constipation and polyuria are nonspecific features presumably due to hypercalcemia. Hypercalcemic patients absorb a higher proportion of dietary calcium than normal infants.

Between 1953 and 1955 more than 200 cases were seen in Great Britain. At the same time fewer than 10 patients were reported in the United States. Dietary supplementation of vitamin D assured most British babies an intake of 2000 to 3000 units per day, or approximately 5 to 6 times the American average. When the British intake was reduced to 400 units per day, hypercalcemia promptly became a rarity. It has therefore been concluded that the disease represents chronic vitamin D intoxication resulting from variable individual tolerance of the sterol.

In 1961 Williams, Barrat-Bayes and Lowe described the association of supravalvular aortic stenosis, mental retardation and peculiar facies. By 1963, when several more reports of this syndrome had appeared, Black and Bonham-Carter recognized the facies as that of idiopathic hypercalcemia, and in reviewing autopsy material of the latter condition found descriptions of stenotic lesions of the aorta and renal arteries. Beuren and his associates noted similar facies and vascular lesions in German infants whose mothers had received several massive doses of vitamin D (500,000 units) during pregnancy. Friedman and Roberts then showed a high incidence of arterial stenoses in rabbits whose mothers had been given large doses of vitamin D (see pp. 1007-9).

It thus appears that vitamin D in excess of individual tolerance produces a variety of aberrations in form (vascular, facial, skeletal) and function (hypercalcemia, hypertension, growth retardation, mental retardation, and so forth). The nature and extent of the lesions produced and their reversibility depend on the time of exposure to the agent. Early severe damage may cause permanent morphologic changes which remain after recovery from hypercalcemia.

Treatment. Administration of vitamin D must be discontinued; this requires scrutiny of the whole diet to avoid unsuspected supplements in milk, cereals or other foods. A low calcium diet is achieved by substituting a meat-base formula for milk or use of decalcified milk (available in Great Britain as Locasol). Cortisone, 10 to 25 mg. per day (or equivalent amounts of predniso-lone), reduces intestinal absorption of calcium and has produced prompt improvement. Sodium ethylene diamine tetra-acetate administered par-enterally (sodium versenate) is rapidly effective but dangerous. Sodium sulfate (orally) has also been effective in reducing absorption of calcium, but it may cause hypernatremia. When hypercal-cemia has been corrected, the usual calcium intake can be gradually resumed. Most patients are soon able to maintain normal serum calcium concen-trations with vitamin D restriction, but they

remain sensitive to calciferol; in some instances exacerbations have followed exposure to sunlight. Osteosclerosis and facial deformities may be corrected by growth if the disease is recognized and treated early in infancy. Reversibility of vascular lesions has not been proved, and mental retardation is said to be permanent.

OSTEOPOROSIS IN MALNUTRITION

Caloric deficit can retard both skeletal growth and bone age. When dietary protein is especially deficient, as in kwashiorkor, both general and local rarefaction of bone may be seen in addition to delayed "bone age." The designation "osteo-porosis" implies that the fundamental defect lies in osteoid synthesis rather than in apatite forma-tion. This supposition has not been confirmed by chemical analyses. Osteoporosis attributed to protein deficit also occurs in Cushing's syndrome and in chronic hepatic diseases. In severely ill patients it may be difficult to separate the effects of malnutrition from those of inactivity, the latter resulting in *osteoporosis of disuse.*

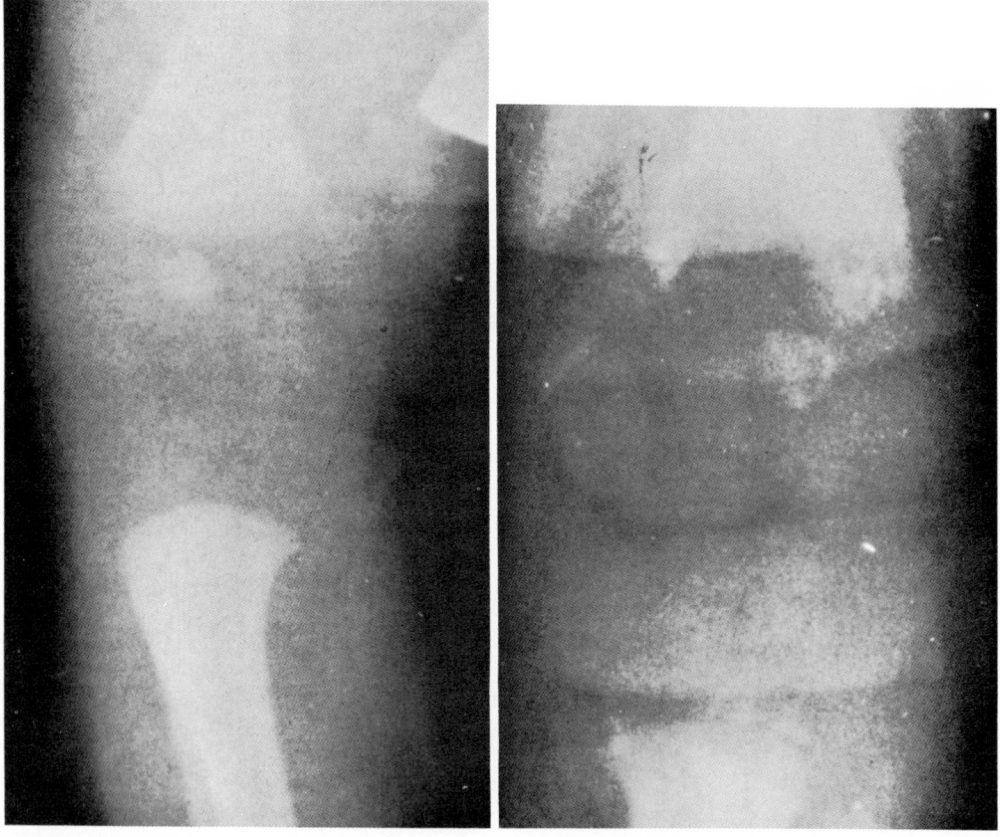

A   B

Figure 22-38. Evolution of osseous changes in hypophosphatasia. Roentgenograms of knee at 7 days *(A)* and at 4 months *(B)* of age. Serum alkaline phosphatase values 0.5 to 2.0 Bodansky units. (From T. M. Teree and L. Klein: Hyphophosphatasia: Clinical and Metabolic Studies. *J. Pediat.,* 72:41, 1968. Reproduced through the courtesy of C. V. Mosby Company.)

HYPOPHOSPHATASIA

(LOW PHOSPHATASE RICKETS)

Hypophosphatasia, first described by Rathbun in 1948, is characterized by abnormal mineralization of bone, diminished serum and tissue alkaline phosphatase activity and increased urinary excretion of phosphorylethanolamine and decreased excretion of hydroxyproline. The serum phosphorus level is normal, but calcium may be elevated in severely affected infants. Bone samples from patients do not mineralize in normal serum, indicating a defect in the synthesis of matrix. Teree and Klein also found that bronchial mucus was unusually viscid in infants who died after repeated episodes of pneumonia. The disorder appears to be inherited as a simple recessive trait. It is of interest that heterozygous relatives may be clinically well with serum phosphatase levels as low as those of affected infants.

The **clinical manifestations** vary widely in severity. They may be present at birth, appear in infancy, or remain inapparent until later.

Symptoms such as anorexia, irritability, vomiting, seizures, recurrent episodes of cyanosis, or pneumonia are seen in infants. In older children the initial signs may be orthopedic deformities such as genu valgum, growth failure or premature loss of deciduous teeth.

Roentgenograms of the bones reveal changes similar to those of rickets. There is disappearance of the zone of provisional calcification due to defective mineralization of osteoid tissue which may extend well into the diaphysis. In severely affected infants the skull is soft, and the fontanels and sutures appear large, owing to large areas of uncalcified osteoid. Paradoxically, cranial synostosis is common in survivors. In older children the osseous lesions are less notable.

When the disorder starts early in infancy, it is usually severe, and a fatal outcome is the rule. Less severely affected patients may have a normal life expectancy, and gradual improvement of the osseous lesions may occur. Vitamin D, even in large doses, has no therapeutic value and may be harmful by producing severe hypercalcemia. Cortisone has been reported to benefit some patients, but is usually ineffective.

HYPERPHOSPHATASIA

(HYPEROSTOSIS CORTICALIS DEFORMANS JUVENILIS)

The manifestations of this rare disease include pain in the bones, fever, hypochromic anemia and severe bowing deformities. The level of serum alkaline phosphatase is persistently elevated (130 King-Armstrong units in Swoboda's first case). There is cortical thickening of the bones and diminished density. The trabecular architecture is chaotic; osteoblasts are abundant. In one of the few examples thus far reported an osteoma arising from a rib was found in the chest. Symptomatic improvement without radiographic changes has been achieved with prednisolone.

WILLIAM H. BERGSTROM
LYTT I. GARDNER

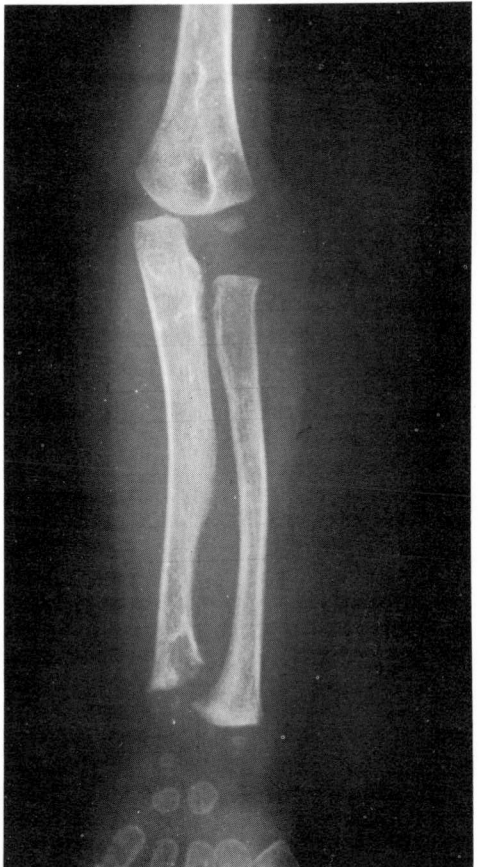

Figure 22-39. Hypophosphatasia. Infant at age of 19 months; Ca, 10.2 mg. per 100 ml.; P, 6.3 mg. per 100 ml.; alkaline phosphatase, 0.7 B-L units. Dwarfing and loss of teeth noted. Long bones show both diffuse and localized rarefaction.

REFERENCES

General

Fanconi, G.: Physiology and Pathology of Calcium and Phosphate Metabolism. *Advances in Pediatrics*, 12:307, 1962.

Fourman, P.: *Calcium Metabolism and the Bone.* Philadelphia, F. A. Davis Company, 1963.

Fraser, D., and Salter, R. B.: The Diagnosis and Management of the Various Types of Rickets. *Pediat. Clin. N. Amer.*, 5:417, 1958.

Stanbury, J. B., Wyngaarden, J. B., and Frederickson, D. S.: *The Metabolic Basis of Inherited Disease.* 2nd ed. New York, McGraw-Hill Book Company, Inc., 1966.

Osteogenesis

McLean, F. C., and Urist, M. R.: *Bone, Fundamentals of the Physiology of Skeletal Tissue.* Chicago, University of Chicago Press, 3rd ed., 1968.

Neuman, W. F., and Neuman, M. W.: *The Chemical Dynamics of Bone Mineral.* Chicago, University of Chicago Press, 1958.

Hypophosphatemic Vitamin D-Resistant Rickets

Harrison, H. E.: Mechanisms of Action of Vitamin D. *Pediatrics,* 14:285, 1954.

West, C. D., Blanton, J. C., Silverman, F. N., and Holland, N. H.: Use of Phosphate Salts as an Adjunct to Vitamin D in the Treatment of Hypophosphatemic Vitamin D Refractory Rickets. *J. Pediat.,* 64:469, 1964.

Winters, R. W., Graham, J. B., Williams, T. F., McFalls, V. W., and Burnett, C. H.: A Genetic Study of Familial Hypophosphatemia and Vitamin D-Resistant Rickets, with a Review of the Literature. *Medicine,* 37:97, 1958.

Hypocalcemic Vitamin D-Resistant Rickets

Prader, A., Illig, R., and Heierli, E.: Eine besondere Form der primären vitamin-D-resistenten Rachitis mit Hypocalcämie und autosomal-dominantem Erbgang: die hereditäre Pseudo-Mangelrachitis. *Helv. Paediat. Acta,* 16:452, 1961.

Soriano, J. R., Einhorn, A., Stark, H., and Edelmann, C. M., Jr.: Deficiency Type Rickets Due to Decreased Sensitivity to Vitamin D. *J. Pediat.,* 68:227, 1966.

Refractory Rickets with Multiple Tubular Dysfunction

Dent, C. E.: Rickets and Osteomalacia from Renal Tubular Defects. *J. Bone & Joint Surg.,* 34-B: 266, 1952.

Harrison, H. E.: The Fanconi Syndrome. *J. Chronic Dis.,* 7:346, 1958.

Leaf, A.: The Syndrome of Osteomalacia, Renal Glycosuria, Aminoaciduria, and Hyperphosphaturia (the Fanconi Syndrome); in Stanbury et al.: *Op. cit.*

Schneider, J. A., Wong, V., and Seegmiller, E.: The Early Diagnosis of Cystinosis. *J. Pediat.,* to be published.

Refractory Rickets with Renal Tubular Acidosis

Albright, F., Burnett, C. H., Parson, W., Reifenstein, E. C., Jr., and Roos, A.: Osteomalacia and Late Rickets. *Medicine,* 25:399, 1946.

Smith, L. H., Jr.: Renal Tubular Acidosis; in Stanbury et al.: *Op. cit.*

Refractory Rickets Associated with Lowe's Syndrome

Lowe, C. U., Terry, M., and MacLachlan, E. A.: Organic-Aciduria,

Decreased Renal Ammonia Production, Hydrophthalmos, and Mental Retardation: A Clinical Entity. *Am. J. Dis. Child.,* 83:164, 1952.

Renal Osteodystrophy

Burke, E. C., Stickler, G. B., and Rosevear, J. W.: Renal Osteodystrophy in Two Siblings. *Am. J. Dis. Child.,* 105:478, 1963.

Dent, C. E., Harper, C. M., and Philpot, G. R.: The Treatment of Renal-Glomerular Osteodystrophy. *Quart. J. Med.,* 30:1, 1961.

Fraser, D., and Salter, R. B.: *Op. cit.*

Stanbury, S. W., and Lumb, G. A.: Metabolic Studies of Renal Osteodystrophy. *Medicine,* 41:1, 1962.

Rickets in Steatorrhea

Parsons, L. G.: Celiac Disease: Rachford Memorial Lecture. *Am. J. Dis. Child.,* 43:1293, 1932.

Osteoporosis in Nutritional Deficiency

Teng, C. T., and others: Liver Diseases and Osteoporosis in Children. *J. Pediat.,* 59:684, 1961.

Jones, P. R. M., and Dean, R. F. A.: The Effects of Kwashiorkor on the Development of the Bones of the Knee. *J. Pediat.,* 54:176, 1959.

Talbot, N. B., Sobel, E. H., McArthur, J. W., and Crawford, J. D.: *Functional Endocrinology from Birth Through Adolescence.* Cambridge, Harvard Press, 1952.

Idiopathic Hypercalcemia

Smith, D. W., Blizzard, R. M., and Harrison, H. E.: Idiopathic Hypercalcemia. A Case Report with Assays of Vitamin D in the Serum. *Pediatrics,* 24:258, 1959.

Taussig, H. B.: Possible Injury to the Cardiovascular System from Vitamin D. *Ann. Int. Med.,* 65:1195, 1966.

Hypophosphatasia

Bartter, F. C.: Hypophosphatasia; in Stanbury et al.: *Op. cit.*

Teree, T. M., and Klein, L.: Hypophosphatasia, Clinical and Laboratory Studies. *J. Pediat.,* 72:41, 1968.

Hyperphosphatasia

Swoboda, W.: Hyperostosis Corticalis Deformans Juvenilis (Hyperphosphatasia). *Helv. Ped. Acta,* 13:292, 1958.

23. The Skin

The skin is a complex organ system in dynamic equilibrium with the internal milieu; it serves important physical, biochemical, physiologic and psychologic functions. Unlike most other organ systems, the skin must constantly respond to changes in both the external and the internal environment. An understanding of the anatomy, chemistry and physiology of the skin during its developmental phase will enhance the understanding of disorders in the infant and the child.

The skin of the infant differs in certain respects from that of the adult. The epidermis is thin, particularly the transitional and keratinous layers. The sebaceous and sudoriferous glands, which function transiently under the influence of maternal hormones during the neonatal period, are incompletely developed. Great differences in the reactivity of the infant's skin are reflected by the relatively high incidence of primary bacterial infections, by the ease of blister formation, by the absence of histamine-induced urticarial reaction and by immunologic incompetence.

DEVELOPMENT OF THE SKIN AND APPENDAGES DURING EMBRYONIC LIFE

The epidermis arises from the surface ectoderm, and the dermis and hypodermis develop from the mesoderm. The pluripotential cells of the epidermis later give rise to the sudoriferous glands (apocrine and eccrine sweat glands), the pilosebaceous complex and the nails. The pigmentary system is formed by pigment-producing cells (melanoblasts) which migrate from the neural crest into the differentiating embryonic skin. Pigmentary abnormalities may be due to variations in migration of melanocytes to the skin (blue nevus of Jadassohn, Mongolian spot, nevus of Ota) or in localization of melanocytes (melanocytic nevus, Peutz-Jeghers syndrome).

By the end of the first month of fetal development the epidermis consists of 2 layers of cells: a protective peritrichial outer layer (periderm) and an inner layer, the stratum germinativum, which contains the parent cells of the epidermis and the dermal appendages (pilosebaceous, sudoriferous and nail structures).

Angiogenesis occurs in the second month of fetal development as an extension of a subcutaneous vessel plexus.

The first evidence of epidermal melanogenesis is found early in the third fetal month as silver-staining dendritic cells appear adjacent to the basement membrane or within the 3-layered epidermis. By the fifth month these melanoblasts form a more complicated dendritic pattern, become intercalated among the epithelial cells of the basal and intermediate layers of the epidermis and begin to produce melanin. Melanogenesis proceeds at a high rate through the sixth and seventh months, the melanin produced being transferred through the surrounding epithelial cells by the dendrites; during the final fetal month the pattern of pigment distribution begun in the sixth and seventh months is intensified, culminating in the pigment pattern present at birth.

By the third fetal month the proliferating stratum germinativum extends into the dermis and differentiates into the epidermal ridges, the pilosebaceous apparatus and the sudoriferous glands. In congenital anhidrotic ectodermal defect, the sweat glands fail to develop. Beneath some of the clusters, epithelial and mesenchymal cells aggregate to form the hair follicle bulb and dermal papilla. Failure of development at this stage results in atrichia congenita. Functional pilary appendages appear from the third to the fourth month. Other clusters of epithelial cells extend deeper and form coils and tubules which, together with vascular elements of the underlying mesenchyme, form eccrine and apocrine glands. By the third month the posterior limiting sulcus of the nail bed is established as an invagination of the epidermis. The nail matrix produces hard keratin in a sequence analogous to that of the hair bulb.

After the fifth intrauterine month the periderm slowly disappears and is replaced by the stratum corneum. A number of congenital keratinizing abnormalities result from faulty development of epithelial cells at this stage (lamellar exfoliation, ichthyosis and congenital ichthyosiform erythroderma). In the last trimester of intrauterine life the newly formed stratum corneum is covered by vernix caseosa.

The components of the dermis arise from undifferentiated mesenchyme with the formation of a delicate argyrophilic reticulum by the fibroblasts during the third fetal month. Individual fibers of this newly formed reticulum increase in number and thickness to form collagen bundles. Alterations at this stage result in Ehlers-Danlos disease. The elastic fibers, whose origin is still uncertain, do not appear until about the sixth month. Fetal subcutaneous fat, which is highly cellular, becomes apparent at the third month of uterine life and persists into the neonatal period. Biochemical alteration of fetal fat may occur in the neonatal period, with unusual nonedematous hardening of the skin (subcutaneous fat necrosis, or sclerema neonatorum).

The epithelial cells of the epidermis are replenished from the basal layer (stratum germinativum). The cells of the stratum germinativum express their pluripotentiality after experimentally induced damage. A group of cells of the stratum germinativum are able on demand to reproduce appendageal structures, possibly excluding hair or normal prickle cells. As these epithelial cells arise from the stratum germinativum, they become displaced into the overlying prickle cell layer, where subsequently, in the more superficial layers, keratohyaline granules form in cytoplasm. Ultimately, all the internal structure of these epithelial cells is lost except the fibrous protein, keratin. The "turnover time" for this process is approximately 28 days.

The dermis and epidermis are strongly interdependent. An inflammatory reaction in the dermis leads to some alteration in epidermal layers. Scaling or blistering may occur. Scaling can be distinguished microscopically as hyperkeratosis (increase in the thickness of the stratum corneum, as with ichthyosis vulgaris), parakeratosis (abnormal keratinization with retention of pyknotic nuclei) or dyskeratosis (abnormal keratinization of individual epithelial cells). Abnormal keratinization may result from heritable alterations in function of the keratinocyte. A generalized form of hyperkeratosis (congenital ichthyosiform erythroderma) and a localized form (epithelial nevus and acrokeratosis verruciformis of Hopf) are inherited recessively; another generalized form (ichthyosis vulgaris) may be inherited either dominantly or recessively.

Blister formation may be categorized histologically as (1) spongiotic (increase in intercellular fluid, as seen in allergic contact dermatitis) (Fig. 23-1), (2) tension type (separation of the epidermis from the dermis at the basement membrane as seen in erythema multiforme) (Fig. 23-2) or (3) acantholytic (alteration of tonofibrils with dissolution of desmosomal attachments between cells as seen in some viral infections) (Fig. 23-3).

Altered physiology in the cutaneous system may be the result of cutaneous disease or may represent participation in a systemic disorder. The spectrum of skin changes is so variable that diagnostic confusion may result from the complexity of the clinical picture. Evaluation of the dynamics of the process through history and clinical appraisal helps to determine the type of primary pathology; these observations are correlated with histopathology.

The skin reflects generalized abnormalities or local disturbances in other organ systems through alteration of its metabolism; examples are the excessive secretion of sodium chloride by eccrine sweat glands in cystic fibrosis, the hyperpigmentation in Addison's disease or the abnormalities of hair in argininosuccinic aciduria. The skin may participate in such systemic diseases as the porphyrias, certain disturbances in lipid metabolism, the reticuloendothelioses, mast cell disease, neurofibromatosis of von Recklinghausen, Albright's

syndrome, tuberous sclerosis, various diseases of connective tissue, syphilis and other infections, and lymphomas. These are only a few of the situations in which diagnostic (macroscopic or microscopic) changes in the skin and its appendages may appear.

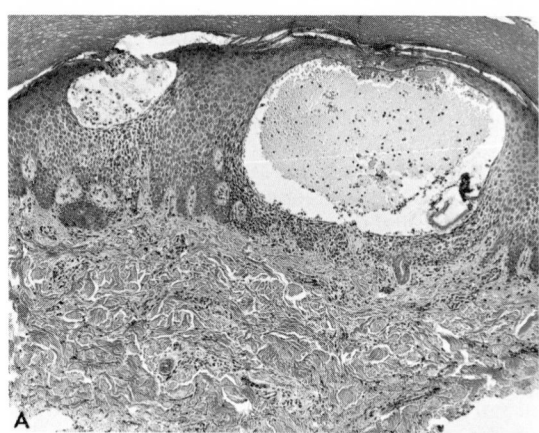

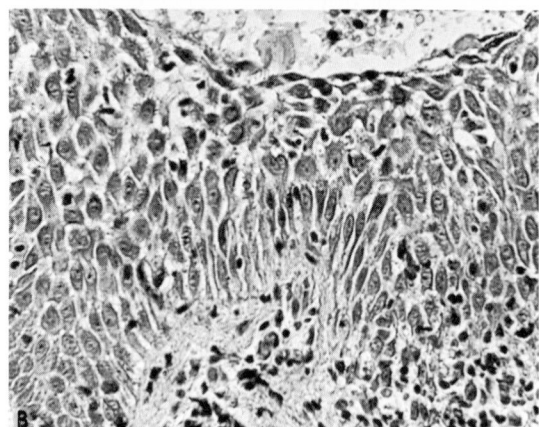

Figure 23-1. Spongiotic blister in lesion of allergic contact dermatitis. *A,* Intercellular edema and vesicle formation. × 50. *B,* "Stretching" of intercellular bridges by intercellular edema (spongiosis). × 250.

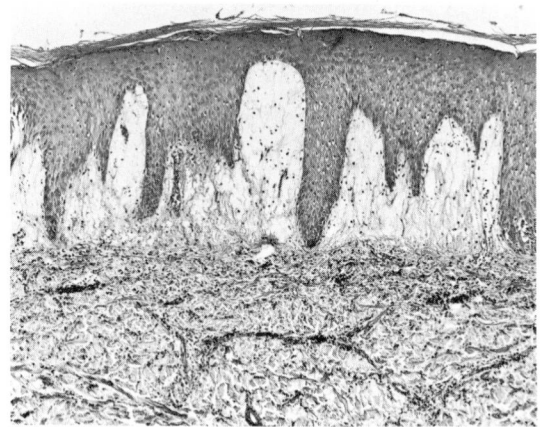

Figure 23-2. Tension type blister of erythema multiforme, demonstrating separation at dermal-epidermal junction. × 75.

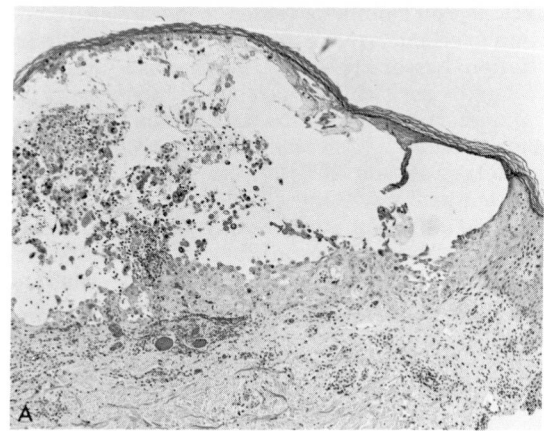

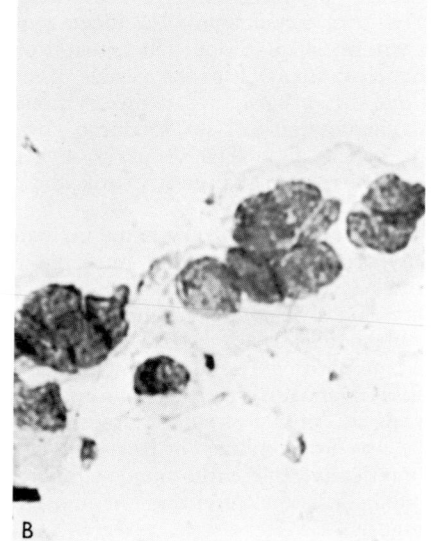

Figure 23-3. Acantholytic blister of herpetic infection. *A*, Loss of intercellular bridges and epithelial giant cells. *B*, Exfoliative cytology, showing diagnostic epithelial giant cells of varicella zoster or herpes infection. Giemsa stain.

Biopsy of the skin is accomplished easily with a 2- or 4-mm. punch after local anesthesia. Selection of a *representative early lesion* for biopsy is important. Suturing of the biopsy site is not essential, but results in a better cosmetic effect. Experienced evaluation of histologic sections of skin is important. Tumors will be familiar to most general pathologists, but the inflammatory diseases of skin occasionally present major diagnostic difficulty even to the dermal pathologist of wide experience.

THE SKIN OF THE INFANT

In late intrauterine life the stratum corneum is protected from maceration in the amniotic fluid by the vernix caseosa. Many other functions have been attributed to the vernix, including bacteriostasis, but none convincingly demonstrated. The vernix is a complete water and oil mixture containing sebum, peridermal cells, lanugo hairs and other debris. There is evidence that it has a high content of estrogenic substances. The extensive fetal deposits of vernix are rubbed off at the first bath, but some remains in the flexures, groin and axillae. Removal results in varying degrees of erythema that diminishes during the first days of life, with the appearance of a fine scaling desquamation.

TRANSIENT LESIONS

Traumatic ' Asphyxia (Compression Syndrome). Compression of the chest and abdomen during delivery may result in localized cyanosis of the head, and rarely of the neck and upper part of the trunk, which is not relieved by otherwise adequate oxygenation. Vascular damage in the involved areas produces petechiae and ecchymosis of the skin and subconjunctival hemorrhages. No therapy is required for the dermal involvement itself, nor are any residuals related to it.

Erythema Toxicum (Urticaria Neonatorum). Erythema toxicum is a transient eruption of unknown origin characterized by discrete erythematous areas 5 to 15 mm. in diameter with yellowish or whitish hivelike elevations in the center, resembling flea bites. The lesions appear suddenly in the first 2 days of life and disappear spontaneously by the ninth day. They are located predominantly on the trunk and buttocks. Infrequently, the lesions become pustular. Histopathologically, there is edema in the upper corium associated with a predominantly perivascular cellular infiltrate consisting mainly of eosinophilic leukocytes. Staphylococcal infection must be differentiated. No treatment is necessary.

Defluvium. Defluvium of the newborn is a physiologic form of diffuse loss of hair; it begins and is completed in the first 2 to 3 months of life in all infants. Loss of hair is first noted in the occipital and frontal areas; it may begin suddenly, progress rapidly and be completed in a few weeks, or it may be so gradual as to escape notice.

Milia Neonatorum. These are white, evanescent, pinhead-sized papules which occur on the face of the newborn infant and disappear within a few weeks. Histopathologically, they are keratin cysts filled with keratinous debris and are located superficially in the dermis. No treatment is required.

Acne Neonatorum. This syndrome represents a true acne vulgaris in a highly predisposed infant. The majority of these infants are males, who presumably have an abnormally high predisposition to severe acne vulgaris in adolescence. Milia-like whitish papules which persist may be the forerunners of this eruption. Typical acne lesions consisting of erythematous follicular papules and comedones usually appear on the cheeks by the third month of life. They rarely persist after the eighth month and subside spontaneously. The lesions are smaller, tend to be located more closely together than those of juvenile acne vulgaris and have a less severe perifollicular inflammation. Since the eruption is mild and self-limited, no treatment is indicated.

Perianal Dermatitis. Perianal dermatitis in the neonatal period (see Diaper Dermatitis) is a reaction to irritation of the skin of the anal area. It is characterized by an erythematous dermatitis and superficial erosion of the skin. The lesions will tend to disappear if diapers are removed promptly after a bowel movement. In some infants perianal dermatitis is related to gastrointestinal intoler-ance to cow's milk or other foods. In an infant whose perianal area is unusually susceptible to irritation, Lassar's paste may be used as a protective film after each change of diaper. In stubborn inflammatory reactions the application after each diaper change of an emollient base such as hydrophilic petrolatum U.S.P. 16 containing 0.5 to 1 per cent hydrocortisone (alcohol) is helpful.

Miliaria (Sweat Retention Syndrome; Prickly Heat). Miliaria is a transient inflammatory disease of the skin of infants caused by mechanical obstruction of the sweat ducts. In serial histopathologic sections, keratin plugs can be demonstrated at different levels of the sweat duct.

The clinical appearance of the skin lesions depends on the level of obstruction of the duct. Superficial plugging produces a blister with watery contents (*miliaria crystallina*). *Miliaria pustulosa* follows within 24 to 48 hours as a result of polymorphonuclear invasion of the vesicle of miliaria crystallina. In *miliaria rubra* an erythematous, papulovesicular lesion is produced by deep plugging of the duct. The eruption occurs most commonly on the cheeks, neck, trunk and diaper area.

In differential diagnosis, erythema toxicum, and yeast and pyogenic infections must be distinguished. They can be differentiated easily by the demonstration of eosinophils in erythema toxicum and of yeast or bacteria in the latter on direct microscopic examination of Giemsa-stained smears.

Effective management consists in preventing the lesions by control of the environmental temperature and by avoidance of excessive clothing. Symptomatically, the child may be made more comfortable by a cool environment and frequent cooling baths.

Blister-Producing Infections

Bacterial Infections. See also pages 405 and 1404.

Bullous response of the skin to staphylococcal and, occasionally, to streptococcal infection may occur in 2 different morphologic forms in the first few weeks of life (impetigo of the newborn and dermatitis exfoliativa).

Impetigo of the newborn (pemphigus neonatorum) generally starts between the fourth and tenth days of life. Easily ruptured bullous lesions appear on a slightly erythematous base on any part of the body, but most commonly on the face, hands and exposed areas. There is also a predilection for the diaper area in male infants. The blisters rupture and form crusts, and new bullae form; the entire cutaneous surface may become involved. Although constitutional symptoms are at first absent, septicemia may occur. The diagnosis can be established by a smear and culture of exudate.

Vigorous local and systemic antibiotic treatment should be started as soon as in-vitro testing of the antibiotic sensitivity of the causative agent has been initiated to guide any subsequent modification which may be indicated. Outbreaks of this type of infection in newborn nurseries can usually be traced to carriers among personnel. A prophylactic and treatment regimen should be followed as outlined in Staphylococcal Infection in the Neonatal Period (p. 406).

Toxic epidermal necrolysis (scalded-child syndrome; dermatitis exfoliativa neonatorum; Ritter's disease) has been described under a variety of names. This syndrome is an acute reaction of the skin, consisting in formation of flaccid bullae, a painful exfoliative erythroderma and a systemic reaction.

In infants, hemolytic staphylococci of several group 2 phage types have been isolated from "primary areas" of the disease, but cultures from the erythematous areas have been sterile. In older children the syndrome may be produced by drug hypersensitivity or by systemic viral infections

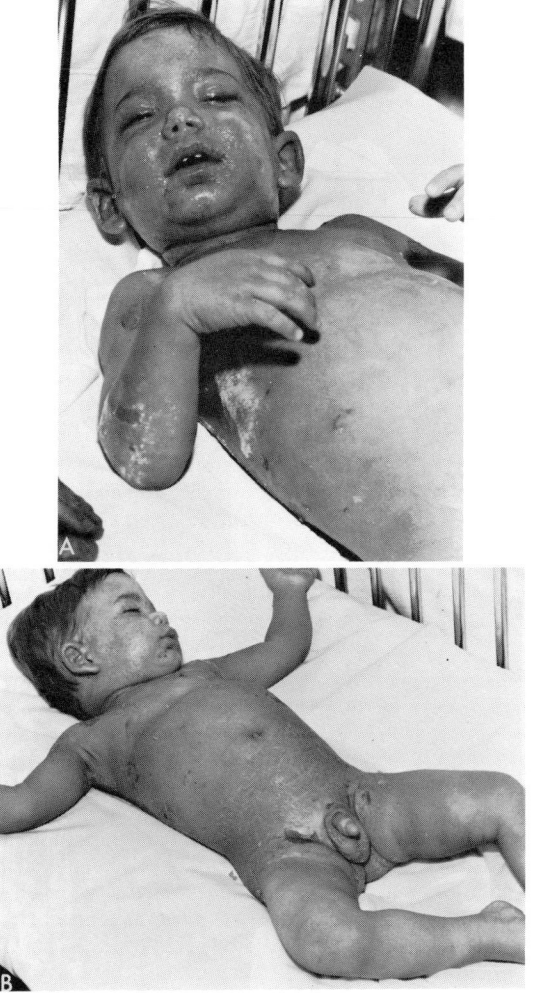

Figure 23-4. Toxic epidermal necrolysis of 36 hours' duration in a 9-month-old boy, caused by coagulase-positive *Staphylococcus aureus,* showing (*A*) periorificial weeping and crusting, and (*B*) generalized erythema and flaccid bullae formation.

such as measles, herpes simplex or cytomegalic inclusion disease. In biopsies of early lesions the histopathologic changes are indistinguishable from those of dermatitis exfoliativa neonatorum; they consist of reversal of staining properties of the stratum corneum and stratum malpighii with intraepidermal or subepidermal separation and a minimal dermal inflammatory reaction.

The skin changes usually start suddenly with perioral erythema and crusting and are followed by a tender, sensitive, generalized erythema within 24 to 48 hours (Fig. 23-4). A systemic reaction with temperature elevation (101 to 104°F.) and a moderate leukocytosis may be observed. The epidermis quickly becomes separated by fluid in poorly circumscribed areas of various sizes. These superficial blisters may be easily wiped off, and the erythematous skin in nonblistered areas may be removed by light rubbing (Nikolsky's sign), leaving a moist surface. Individual erythematous areas merge, giving the skin a scalded appearance. Denuded areas dry quickly, and within a few days the involved skin becomes dry and scaling; it returns to normal within 7 to 10 days. Involvement of mucous membrane is insignificant. Some infants may have one or more bullous lesions of impetigo, but others have no lesions prior to the appearance of generalized exfoliation (Fig. 23-25, p. 1385).

Refusal of feeding is invariably an early sign of systemic illness, and is followed by vomiting, prostration, abdominal distention and occasionally jaundice. Diarrhea with mucoid green stools may be associated with shock. A fatal course of illness may last less than 36 hours.

Though the appearance of toxic epidermal necrolysis is rather distinctive, several other diseases may have a superficial resemblance. Erythema multiforme in the newborn might be confused initially, but it does not have the rapid evolution or pain and does have a different histopathologic picture. The skin changes in boron poisoning may be similar in appearance, but are usually associated with neurologic disturbances and renal failure. Dystrophic epidermolysis bullosa may be ruled out by the appearance of blisters on sites of trauma, its slow progression and a completely different histopathologic pattern.

A semisynthetic penicillin should be administered initially, since penicillin-resistant organisms are frequently found. Incubator isolation is useful for the protection of the painful skin and for temperature and humidity control. The danger of absorption of toxic preparations through the damaged skin may be considerable; soap substitutes containing hexachlorophene should be avoided. The loosened areas of skin should be debrided, and the skin cleansed with a solution of benzalkonium chloride 1:10,000, followed by the application of an ointment containing bacitracin. Fluid and electrolyte balance must be maintained. Systemic administration of a corticosteroid may be indicated in older children when a drug causation is considered likely. During the scaling stage of regression an emollient ointment such as hydrophilic petrolatum U.S.P. 16 with 20 per cent distilled water is useful.

Spirochetal Infections. Vesiculobullous lesions, particularly on the palms and soles, may be seen in congenital syphilis. The presence of erythematous, infiltrated papular skin lesions, mucosal involvement, lymphadenopathy and hepatosplenomegaly suggests a treponemal infection (see p. 615).

Viral Infections. Infections caused by the viruses of herpes simplex, varicella or variola-vaccinia may produce vesiculobullous lesions in the newborn infant if the mother has the infection at the time of delivery and is in the phase of viremia. Infection may also occur in an infant who has no passively transferred antibodies if he has extraneous contact with the virus. The clinical appearance of the lesions is not dissimilar to that seen in any primary infection with the virus. A Giemsa-stained smear, skin biopsy and appropriate viral studies will establish the diagnosis.

Disturbances of Subcutaneous Tissue

Several disorders of the skin and subcutaneous tissue in infancy may cause confusion in differential diagnosis because in all of them the skin has a thickened or "fixed" feel on palpation. Of these, subcutaneous fat necrosis of the newborn is the most common; sclerema neonatorum and edema neonatorum are considerably less common, and scleroderma is rare.

Edema of the newborn (sclerema edematosum; scleredema) is a rare disorder of unknown cause seen in weak newborn and especially in premature infants; it is characterized by widespread pitting edema of the extremities and trunk and by pallor and lividity of the skin. Most infants so affected do not survive, but the edema may subside spontaneously if the general condition of the infant improves. Histopathologic examination reveals engorgement of the vessels in the corium with some perivascular infiltration and edema of the dermis and underlying muscles. In differential diagnosis sclerema and scleredema of Buschke must be differentiated. No specific therapy is known.

Subcutaneous fat necrosis of the newborn is an uncommon benign disorder occurring equally in both sexes and characterized by sharply circumscribed indurated lesions of the skin and underlying tissue of variable size which appear in the first few weeks of life in an otherwise healthy infant. Histopathologically, the earliest changes consist of endothelial swelling and a perivascular inflammatory infiltrate followed by necrosis of the subcutaneous fat and a dense granulomatous and inflammatory infiltrate containing foreign body type giant cells with needle-like crystals. The lesions generally appear near the end of the first week of life, but may appear as late as the sixth week. The onset is not associated with constitutional symptoms. Lesions vary in size from 1 or 2 up to 10 or more cm.; they are hard and plaque-like and do not pit on pressure. Although they may appear anywhere, they are located most commonly on the posterior portion of the trunk, buttocks, thighs, cheeks, arms and feet. The skin overlying the plaque may have a slightly livid discoloration. Small lesions may be freely movable over underlying structures. The borders of the lesions are sharply defined, and the plaques are slightly elevated above the normal skin. The hard plaque slowly softens after 6 to 8 weeks, and complete resolution usually occurs within several months. During the stage of resolution the mass may be misdiagnosed as an abscess. Calcification of some lesions may occur, but widespread calcification of such indurated areas would suggest hypercalcemia. No treatment is indicated, and under no circumstances should the mass be incised. The disease must be differentiated from nodular nonsuppurative panniculitis, which is usually associated with tender nodules in the skin and splenomegaly, and from lipogranulomatosis (Farber).

Sclerema neonatorum is an uncommon alteration of the subcutaneous fat in weak premature infants or in term infants with severe systemic, especially diarrheal, disease. It should be regarded as a physical sign and not as a disease entity. It is characterized by a rapidly spreading, waxy-appearing, cool, leathery change in the skin, with purplish mottling; the skin feels adherent to underlying structures. The histologic picture is similar to that of subcutaneous fat necrosis of the newborn, but usually has a less intense inflammatory infiltrate and fewer foreign body giant cells. The process frequently commences on the legs and gradually spreads in the course of a few days to involve the entire cutaneous surface. Immobility of the face produced by this castlike solidification of the subcutaneous tissue makes feeding difficult. Death usually occurs within a few days or weeks, though recovery has been reported. The process must be differentiated from edema neonatorum. Treatment, in general, is supportive and specifically is directed at the underlying disease.

PERMANENT LESIONS

Anatomic Abnormalities

Congenital aplasia of the skin is a localized developmental failure believed to be transmitted as a recessive trait or as an incomplete dominant and characterized by the presence of single or multiple atrophic or ulcerative lesions. Histopathologically, the hypoplastic dermis is covered by a single layer of epithelial cells. The dermal appendages are absent or hypoplastic, as is the subcutaneous fat. The lesions occur most commonly on the scalp as defects 2 to 3 cm. in diameter; they may be irregular in shape and cover larger areas. Treatment is generally unnecessary, spontaneous epithelialization being rapid. Application of a broad-spectrum antibiotic may prevent secondary bacterial infection.

Abnormalities of the Mucous Membranes.
Grooved tongue, or deep furrows on the surface of the tongue, is apparently inherited as a dominant characteristic. It is seen in approximately 0.5 per cent of the general population. In Down's syndrome it is acquired by friction of the tongue over the teeth in characteristic tongue-sucking.

Congenital fistula of the lip is a rare developmental abnormality probably transmitted as an autosomal dominant trait. The fistulous tracts are located symmetrically on either side of the midline of the transitional area of the mucous membranes of the lip. A clear mucoid fluid usually exudes from the mucous glands of the lip. The fistulous tracts should be excised.

Hypertrophied frenulum syndrome consists of an abnormally developed frenulum with a pseudocleft in the upper lip, tongue and palate, mental retardation, trembling and syndactyly. It is probably transmitted as a dominant autosomal trait.

Hereditary gingival fibromatosis is characterized by firm, enlarged gingival tissue over the crowns of permanent teeth. It usually becomes evident with the eruption of the permanent incisors. Hypertrichosis may be associated with the syndrome. It is probably transmitted as a dominant autosomal trait. Excision is usually associated with regrowth, whereas regression usually follows dental extraction.

Leukokeratosis is an asymptomatic, whitish thickening of the mucous membranes which is transmitted as an autosomal dominant trait in the white race. Irregular, thickened whitish plaques with a verrucoid surface appear most commonly in the mouth at birth or at any time up to adolescence. No treatment is necessary.

Fordyce's spots of the mucous membranes of the cheeks and lips are a common, asymptomatic developmental abnormality of ectopic sebaceous glands. They first appear in the preadolescent period and are characterized by discrete yellowish papules. They occur in approximately 50 per cent of children under 11 years of age. No treatment is necessary.

Transitory benign plaque of the mucous membrane of the mouth is a recurrent, asymptomatic alteration characterized by fleeting, sharply circumscribed, erythematous patches about 0.5 cm. in diameter which spread to form a ring with a yellowish-white border and then fade only to reform at a different spot. The tongue is the site of predilection, but the buccal, gingival and labial mucosa may be involved. No treatment is necessary.

Congenital Abnormalities of Hair. *Congenital alopecia* is an abnormality in the production of hair usually transmitted as a dominant trait, but occasionally as a recessive. It is characterized by complete absence of hair or poor growth of it on the scalp, and frequently of the eyebrows and eye-

lashes. Histopathologically, hair follicles are absent or hypoplastic, and sebaceous glands and arrectores pilorum muscles are hypoplastic.

In some families the infants are practically bald at birth, whereas in others the hair is normal, but later falls out and is replaced by a scanty growth. The abnormality has been associated with webbed fingers, cataracts and Friedreich's ataxia. It must be differentiated from the hidrotic and anhidrotic types of ectodermal dysplasia in children with scanty hair.

Monilethrix is characterized by constriction of the hair of the scalp at regular intervals, by fracture of the hair shafts and by follicular keratoses. It is inherited as a dominant trait. Histopathologically, under direct examination, the fusiform swelling of the hair which occurs at intervals of approximately 1 mm. is normal in appearance, but the medulla is absent; the cortex is diminished, and the cuticle is thickened at the constrictions. The pilar orifices contain hyperkeratotic plugs. In the differential diagnosis, pili torti, trichorrhexia nodosa, tinea capitis and trichotillomania must be considered. There is no treatment, although the frequency of fractures may be diminished by avoiding combing and brushing as much as possible.

Pili torti is characterized by twisting of the shaft of the hair on its axis and by increased fragility at the twisted sites. It is transmitted as an incomplete dominant trait.

The hair appears dry and lusterless, and areas of stubble appear where the hair has been broken off (Fig. 23-5). The cosmetic aspects are especially obvious in girls. There is no treatment, although the frequency of fractures may be diminished by avoidance of combing and brushing the hair as much as possible.

Pili annulati is a rare abnormality of the hair characterized by alternate pigmented and depigmented areas at intervals of approximately 1 mm. producing a ringed appearance. It is probably inherited as an irregular dominant trait. The abnormality is asymptomatic and does not require treatment.

Woolly hair is characterized by short, woolly, tightly curled hairs. It is transmitted as a simple autosomal dominant trait.

Congenital canities is characterized by depigmented patches of hair, usually present at birth. It is transmitted as an autosomal dominant trait or, in some families, as a sex-linked trait.

Waardenburg syndrome includes patchy depigmentation of the hair along with other developmental abnormalities (see p. 1435).

Nevi

Nevi are local anatomic alterations of the cellular or vascular components of the skin, with changes varying from aplasia to hyperplasia. Nevi are usually present at birth. Generally, these lesions are minor defects, but on occasion they are

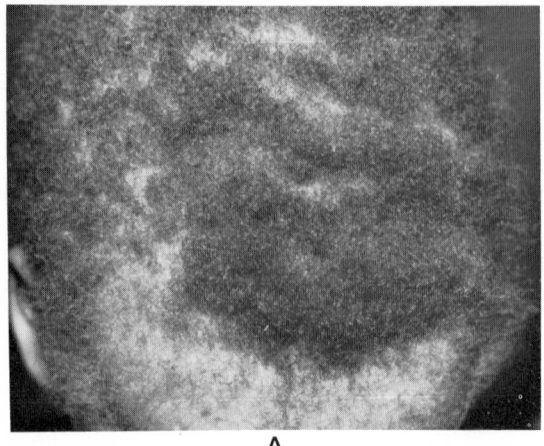

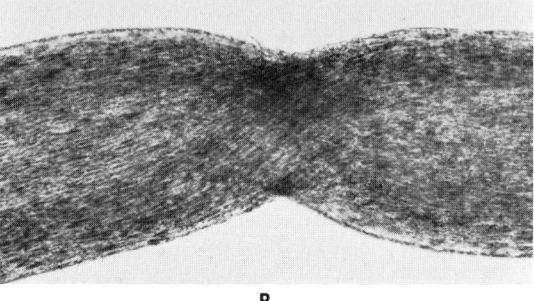

Figure 23-5. *A,* A 5-year-old Caucasian boy with short, "kinky" hairs; fracture of the hairs precluded hair cutting. *B,* Microscopic examination showing twisting of the hair shaft (KOH preparation). × 250.

so extensive (vascular nevi, pigmented nevi) that they cause cosmetic or functional problems.

Aplastic lesions, present at birth, include localized dermal defects in which an ulcer is present on delivery, which heals slowly with scarring. In these areas the dermis and epidermal appendages are absent. Adnexal structures may be absent, such as nails (anonychia congenita), hair (atrichia congenita), sudoriferous glands (anhidrotic ectodermal defect) or vessels (nevus anemicus).

Hyperplastic lesions may, depending upon the predominant component, be classified as melanocytic nevi, nevus cell nevi, epithelial (verrucous) nevi, sebaceous nevi, pilar (hairy) nevi, comedone nevi or vascular nevi.

Pigmented nevi, or *moles,* may be divided on morphologic and histologic features as follows: melanocytic, junctional, compound and intradermal nevi, and benign juvenile melanoma.

The *café-au-lait spot* of von Recklinghausen's disease is a MELANOCYTIC NEVUS in which there is not only an increase in melanogenesis, but also an increase in the number of melanocytes. The other nevi are composed of melanin-forming cells called nevus cells. The development of nevi is a dynamic process, the early macular lesions being of junctional type, later evolving into compound nevi with both junctional and dermal activity, and finally into mature nevi with only intradermal changes.

In some compound nevi in childhood there is rapid evolution, with the histologic appearance of active growth suggestive of neoplastic change, but these tumors are benign and are called benign juvenile melanoma.

Nevus cell nevi vary considerably in their morphology and degree of pigmentation; several different clinical types may be recognized: (1) macular lesions, (2) slightly elevated papules, (3) papillomatous lesions, (4) dome-shaped papules which may or may not be pigmented or contain hairs, and (5) pedunculated lesions. Less common forms of nevus cell nevi are the *halo nevus* and the *giant pigmented nevus* (bathing trunk nevus).

JUNCTIONAL NEVI are flat, sharply circumscribed, brown to black lesions found anywhere on the skin. Their special importance lies in the possibility that they may undergo melanomatous degeneration, although the risk is not serious; most persons have or have had one or more junctional nevi.

There is a variety of generalized pigmentary spots transmitted as a recessive trait which may be associated with electrocardiographic and other abnormalities. The histologic appearance of the lesions is that of lentigo, with features suggestive of junctional nevus. Surgical removal is indicated for cosmetic reasons or for such evidence of unusual activity as increase in the pigmented area, scaling, crusting or inflammation. Pathologic evaluation is mandatory; if malignancy is suspected, dermatologic pathologic consultation should be sought, owing to difficulties in evaluating the nature of these pigmented nevi.

Compound and intradermal nevi are extremely variable in their morphology and color. Most of the slightly elevated lesions, and some of the papillomatous lesions, are compound nevi; most of the papillomatous lesions and nearly all the dome-shaped and pedunculated lesions are intradermal nevi. They vary in color from flesh-colored or pink with little brownish pigment to brown or black. They vary in size from a few millimeters to extensive involvement, with a tendency toward the dermatome distribution of the giant pigmented nevus (bathing trunk nevus). In these giant nevi the involved area is pigmented, hairy and frequently verrucous. This variety of nevus is important because it tends to undergo melanomatous degeneration. The *halo nevus* is a variant of a compound or intradermal nevus, which is surrounded by depigmented cells. Over a period of several months, involution of the nevus occurs, leaving a depigmented patch which may also slowly disappear. This process often extends to other nevi simultaneously or successively. Treatment of small compound or intradermal nevi is indicated for cosmetic reasons, if they are in locations where they may be frequently irritated, or if there is suspicion of melanomatous degeneration. Excision is the treatment of choice. When cosmetic considerations are paramount, a shave excision gives an excellent cosmetic result; it is a safe procedure if controlled histologically. Because of its tendency to neoplastic degeneration, giant pigmented nevus should be removed, if feasible, by a plastic surgeon.

Benign juvenile melanoma occurs most frequently between the ages of 3 and 13 years. It is characterized by the appearance of a smooth, dome-shaped, circumscribed, firm, nonhairy, pink or purplish-red asymptomatic nodule, most frequently on the face, but it also occurs on the trunk and extremities. The tumors may vary in size from a few millimeters to several centimeters in diameter. Histologically, juvenile melanoma is a compound nevus, but because of the pleomorphism of the cells and the frequency of inflammatory infiltrate, the histologic picture closely resembles that of an invasive melanoma. In spite of this resemblance to melanoma, the experienced pathologist can usually make the distinction. In differential diagnosis, juvenile xanthogranuloma, granulomatous insect bite reaction, keloid, or a solitary nodule of urticaria pigmentosa are suggested. Since the natural history of these tumors is unknown and because they usually present a cosmetic problem, simple excision is recommended. Recurrences may be anticipated if the tumor is not completely removed.

The dermal localization of melanocytes may be responsible for the presence of bluish-gray to black pigmented lesions on the skin, as in Mongolian spot, the nevus of Ota and the blue nevus.

Mongolian spot results from delayed disappearance of dermal melanocytes, most commonly in the lumbosacral region. The pigmentation slowly fades with time.

The *nevus of Ota* is a usually unilateral, brown to slate-gray discoloration of the skin of the face, particularly in the periorbital region, temple, forehead and malar areas. There is often an associated bluish discoloration of the sclera, and occasionally of the conjunctiva, cornea or retina on the involved side. Like Mongolian spot, the lesion is made up of dermal melanocytes.

Blue nevus is a flat or dome-shaped blue-black lesion on the face or extremities made up of dermal melanocytes. It usually appears early in life, grows to 2 to 3 mm. in diameter, and then remains stationary in size. Its importance lies in the possible confusion with melanoma. Excisional biopsy is the treatment of choice.

In VERRUCOUS NEVI there is a brownish verrucoid overgrowth of epithelial cells distributed in a linear configuration. Occasionally, when they are located on exposed areas, treatment may be indicated. For treatment to be successful, destruction of the epithelial cells must be deep enough to produce scarring.

Nevus sebaceus of Jadassohn is a common organoid nevus present at birth and comprised of all elements of the skin. It is characterized by the presence on the hairy area of the scalp of round, linear or crescentic, well demarcated, yellowish to orange, flat or slightly raised patches devoid of normal hairs, though vellus hairs may be present. Because the nevus is made up of skin appendages

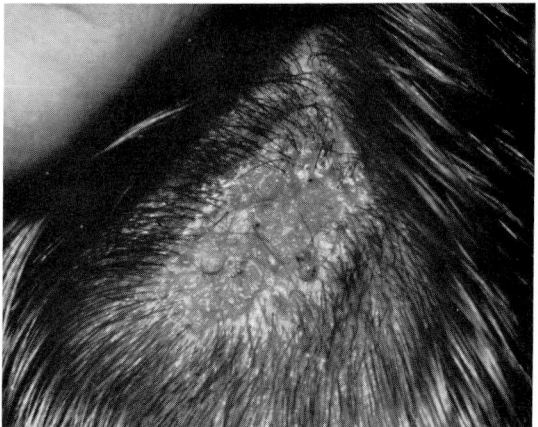

Figure 23-6. Nevus sebaceus of Jadassohn, showing verrucoid hyperplasia of the skin during adolescence.

that change with age, there is a characteristic overdevelopment of the normal constituents of the skin, and papillomatous changes occur on the surface of the nevus at puberty (Fig. 23-6). In some patients basal cell carcinoma or benign eccrine tumor (syringocystadenoma) may appear. Rarely, nevus sebaceus may be associated with developmental abnormalities of the eye or of the cardiovascular or nervous system. The cosmetic appearance of the bald patch and the possibility of secondary neoplastic degeneration make excision of the nevus the treatment of choice.

Pilar hyperplasia resulting in an unusual number of mature hairs in an abnormal location is seen in NEVUS PILOSUS. The hamartomas of the pilar structures have no importance except for their cosmetic appearance when they occur on exposed areas.

VASCULAR NEVI are the most common dermal tumors manifest at birth or during the neonatal period. They are generally benign tumors of the vasoformative mesenchyme, in which the dynamics of vessel formation may be observed ranging from benign hamartoma to frank malignancy (angiosarcoma). The benign vascular tumors may be divided clinically and pathologically into capillary types (nevus flammeus and nevus vasculosus), cavernous types, and mixed types, in which capillary and cavernous components are both present in the same tumor.

Nevus flammeus appears as a flat, irregular, erythematous patch of variable size present at birth; its significance depends mainly on its location. Lesions are especially common on the back of the neck and face, but may appear anywhere. The slightly erythematous patches present on the eyelids and in the glabellar area of the newborn infant, which undergo spontaneous resolution, should not be confused with the persistent patches of nevus flammeus.

Involvement of the skin in the distribution of the fifth cranial nerve has special significance because of the frequency of vascular abnormalities in the ipsilateral cerebral hemisphere (see p. 1281).

Many methods of treatment, including superficial roentgen therapy (Grenz), tattooing and cryotherapy, have produced indifferent results. When the lesions occur in exposed areas, the local application of an isotope of radium (thorium X) is a safe method of treatment which will produce some blanching of the lesion in approximately 50 per cent of instances. A cosmetically acceptable type of cover (Covermark) is recommended for use on lesions in exposed areas.

Nevus vasculosus (strawberry mark) is the most common of the vascular nevi; it is a sharply demarcated, erythematous, raised tumor which is usually present at birth or may appear during the first month of life. The earliest sign may be a blanched area in the skin preliminary to the appearance of the vascular nevus. Small vascular ectasias then arise within the pale zone, become raised, and finally develop the typical appearance of hemangioma. A blanched area around the small erythematous papule or larger vascular tumor is a useful prognostic sign, for it often marks the limits of future growth. During early infancy there is proliferation of endothelial cells and capillary proliferation, but when growth ceases, fibrosis replaces the capillaries, and shrinking of the tumor results. The tumors usually disappear spontaneously, but the growth pattern during the first 6 to 8 months of life is variable (Fig. 23-7).

Cavernous hemangioma consists of a subcuta-neous collection of vessels with normal, but bluish, overlying skin; nevus vasculosus may also be present (mixed vascular nevus). Histologically, there are in the lower dermis and subcutaneous tissue large, irregular vascular spaces filled with blood. In the mixed variety there are histologic changes of both the capillary nevus of the nevus vasculosus type and cavernous hemangioma. These tumors also tend to regress without treatment, but are more likely than nevus vasculosus to involute incompletely; in tumors in which there is arteriovenous shunting, involution does not occur. In rare instances a cavernous or mixed type hemangioma may undergo such tremendous increase in size as to interfere with function. An increase in volume of blood within the tumor can lead to severe anemia or thrombocytopenia due to sequestration of platelets. Treatment of these extensive hemangiomas has been frustrating; administration of prednisone (20 to 30 mg. each day) for 8 to 12 weeks may be helpful, or control may be obtained by intra-arterial infusion of nitrogen mustard. Both methods offer a more favorable outcome with fewer complications and long-term sequelae than does radiation therapy or injection of sclerosing agents.

Blue rubber bleb nevus is a variant of cavernous hemangioma in which there are innumerable bluish cavernous hemangiomas distributed over the skin surface. In addition to the cutaneous le-

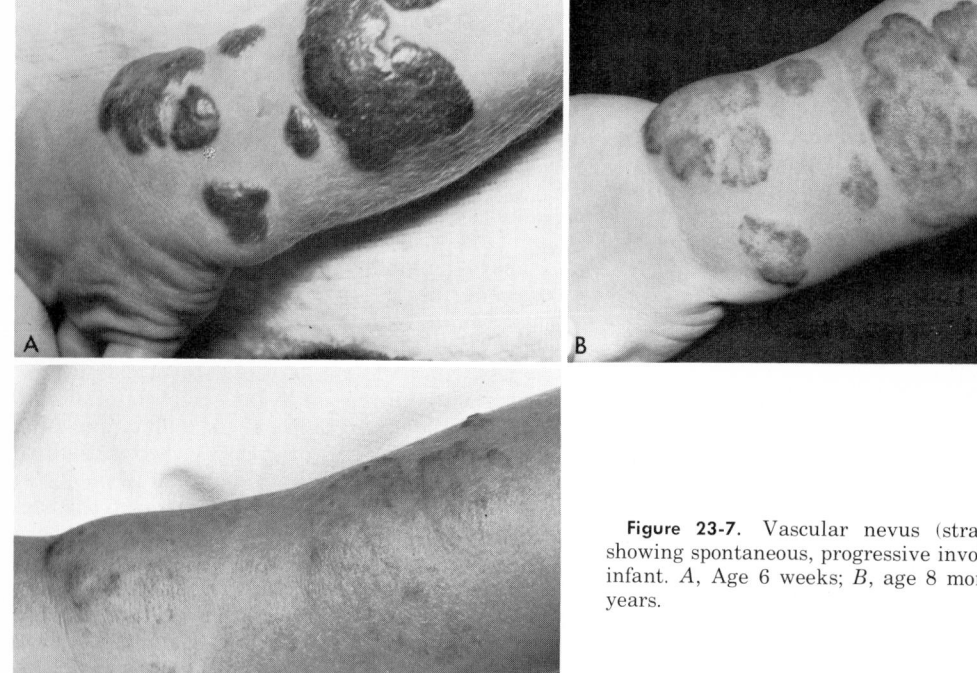

Figure 23-7. Vascular nevus (strawberry type), showing spontaneous, progressive involution in male infant. *A,* Age 6 weeks; *B,* age 8 months; *C,* age 2 years.

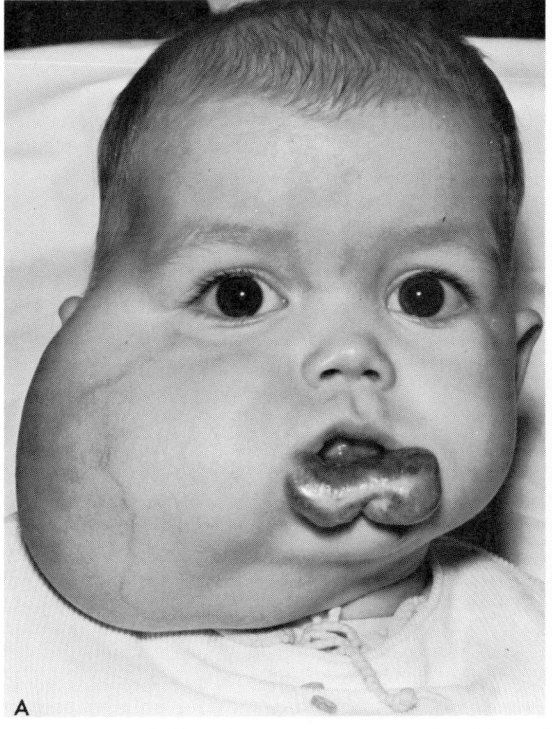
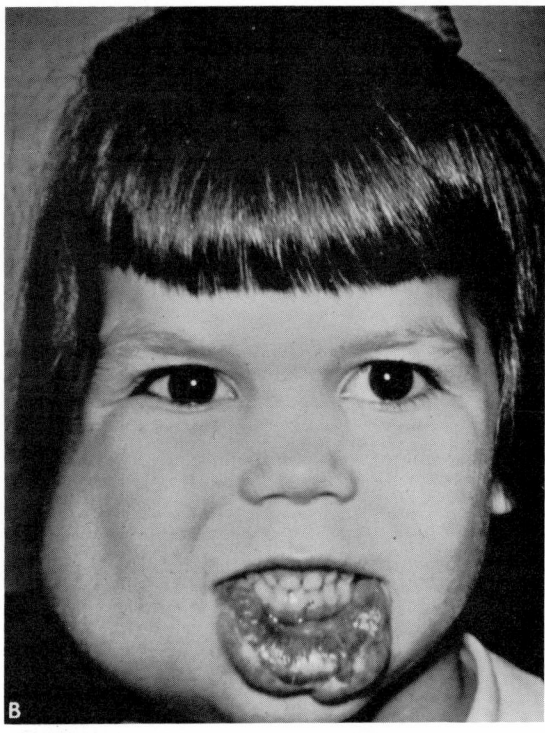

Figure 23-8. *A*, Vascular nevus (cavernous type) in an 8-month-old girl which progressed alarmingly in a 7-month period from a 3-cm. tumor in the right preauricular area; the increase in size was associated with progressive severe anemia. *B*, The tumor at age 4½ years, showing spontaneous regression, with scarring and eversion of the lower lip.

sions, there may be hemangioma in the intestinal tract and in other internal organs.

In *Maffucci's syndrome* the combination of cavernous hemangiomas and of dystrophy of cartilage causes bizarre deformities of the extremities.

Keratotic vascular nevus (verrucous hemangioma) is an uncommon persistent variant of a capillary or cavernous hemangioma in which epithelial hyperplasia occurs secondarily. Histologically, the typical lesions have a papillary surface with hyperkeratosis, parakeratosis, subepidermal dilated vessels, and capillary-like vessels in the dermis extending into subcutaneous tissue (Figs. 23-9, 23-9A). The deep dermal and subcutaneous vascular involvement precludes superficial removal of the lesion. The clinical picture varies from nonkeratotic, erythemato-violaceous, compressible retiform vascular lesions to hyperkeratotic patches which often become secondarily infected after trauma. Lesions are most common on the lower extremities either singly or in multiple patches with intervening areas of normal skin. These tumors do not regress spontaneously and become increasingly hyperkeratotic. If removal is indicated, it should be accomplished surgically.

Nevoid anomalies of the lymphatic vessels may be superficial *(lymphangioma circumscriptum)* or deep *(lymphangioma cavernosum)*. Histologically, the superficial variety is characterized by dilated lymph vessels in the upper portion of the dermis, which contain lymph fluid, lymphocytes, and occasionally erythrocytes. In the deep variety large lymph-filled cystic spaces are present in the lower dermis and the subcutaneous tissue.

The superficial variety appears clinically as groups of small, thick-walled vesicles, some of which may appear hemorrhagic, owing to the presence of erythrocytes. The treatment of both the superficial and cavernous lesions is excision when practical.

Another variety of purplish-black raised patch is the *angiokeratoma of Mibelli*, which may be distinguished from keratotic vascular nevi by the fact that it appears to be made up of confluent individual lesions. Histologically, this tumor differs from the keratotic vascular nevus in the presence of vascular channels within the epithelial layer itself as well as in the superficial portions of the dermis. Treatment is surgical removal when cosmetic considerations justify it.

Phlebectasia (venous cavernous angiectasia) is a rare abnormality of the vascular system, usually of an extremity; its cause is unknown. The process is slowly progressive, involving extensive portions of the superficial and deep vessels and producing skin tumors and alteration of growth of the involved extremity. Histopathologically, there is mixed venous and arterial proliferation with evidence of arteriovenous shunting in the dermis.

Single or multiple papules or tumors resembling cavernous hemangiomas may be present at birth; new tumors appear subsequently and are associated with enlargement of underlying vessels. Complications include alteration of bone growth,

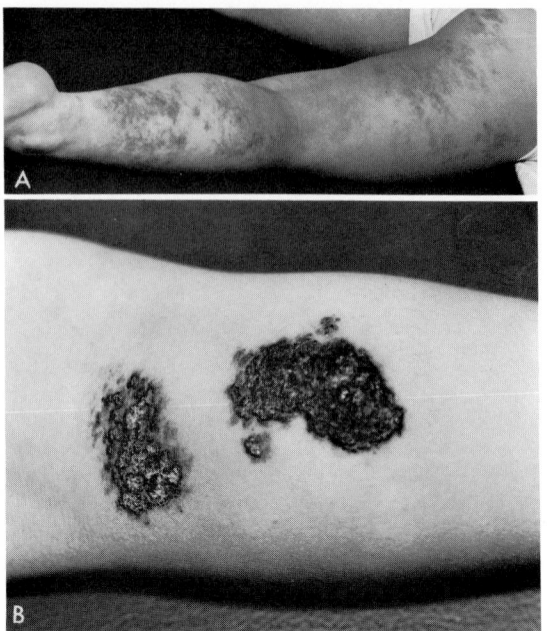

Figure 23-9. Keratotic vascular nevus. *A*, Early retiform vascular changes. *B*, Late keratotic changes superimposed on vessel abnormality.

muscular atrophy caused by vascular involvement, and increase in size of the extremity to such an extent as to limit function.

In differential diagnosis, hypertrophic angiectasis of Klippel-Trenaunay and simple cavernous hemangioma must be distinguished.

Treatment is surgical with wide excision and ligation of large vessels; recurrence is common.

Hypertrophic angiectasis of Klippel-Trenaunay (osteohypertrophic varicose nevus) is a rare mixed vascular abnormality of the vascular system of an extremity, with angiectasis of the vessels or arteriovenous shunting. It is present at birth and is associated with developmental enlargement of the underlying bone and soft tissue.

The skin of the enlarged extremity is warmer than that of the uninvolved limb; pulsations are frequently visible, and a palpable thrill and continuous bruit may be present. The skin may be thickened and rough with enlarged follicles and coarse hairs.

Function may be altered by extensive development of the lesion. No treatment is satisfactory.

Angiokeratoma corporis diffusum (Fabry) is an extremely rare, widespread vascular abnormality which involves the skin, cardiovascular, renal and pulmonary systems. Its cause is unknown; it appears before puberty in males. Histopathologically, the capillaries supplying the papillae are dilated, forming large vascular spaces filled with thrombi just below the epidermis. Similar changes are found in other organ systems. The skin lesions are purplish-black maculopapules varying in size from 1 to 2 mm. and located predominantly on the lower portion of the trunk and the thighs.

In differential diagnosis, hereditary hemorrhagic telangiectasia must be distinguished. There is no effective treatment.

Cerebellar ataxia-telangiectasia is a rare disease characterized by oculocutaneous telangiectasia, progressive cerebellar ataxia, peculiar eye movements and frequent sinopulmonary infections. It is transmitted as an autosomal recessive trait.

Histopathologically, there are telangiectatic vessels in the upper corium and in the cerebellum.

Ataxia is evident by 1 to 1½ years of age, and the telangiectasia appears by about the age of 5 years on the temporal and nasal sides of the bulbar conjunctiva and slowly progresses to involve the eyelid, malar areas, ears, chest, popliteal and antecubital fossae and dorsum of the hands.

In differential diagnosis familial hemorrhagic telangiectasia must be distinguished. Treatment of the skin lesions is not indicated.

Spider angioma (spider telangiectasis) occurs as a localized capillary dilatation of pre-existing blood vessels and is occasionally associated with the development of new vessels in the dermis. It is characterized by a slightly elevated red papule with fine radiating blood vessels which give the lesion a spider-like configuration. Spider angioma is barely visible initially, but gradually becomes more distinct and may present as a cosmetically disturbing red spot on the face or on the dorsa of the hands and fingers. Angiomas may be single or multiple. Treatment consists in destruction of the central dilated vessel with fine needle electrosurgery. If properly done, this procedure should not result in scarring.

Hereditary hemorrhagic telangiectasia is an uncommon familial disease characterized by numerous telangiectasias of the skin and mucous membranes (see also p. 842).

Histopathologically, the epidermis is normal, and in the papillary and subpapillary zones of the dermis are lakelike vascular dilatations. The vessels are made up of a single row of endothelial cells without muscular or elastic tissue.

The telangiectasias are nonpulsatile, spiderlike, bright red maculopapular lesions, 2 to 3 mm. in diameter. They occur initially on the mucous membranes and are most frequently manifest by nosebleeds in children; after maturity they appear on the skin.

In differential diagnosis, cerebellar ataxia-telangiectasia must be distinguished.

Cutis marmorata telangiectatica congenita is a rare transient abnormality of the superficial vessels of the dermis of unknown origin. It is present at birth or shortly after and produces a peculiar marbled appearance of the skin (Fig. 23-10). Histopathologically, there is a large number of capillaries in the dermis and subdermis, some with thick elastic fibers in their wall.

The skin changes consist of circumscribed, pinkish patches 2 to 4 cm. in diameter, bordered by a bluish discoloration; they produce a striking marmoraceous effect. The trunk and extremities

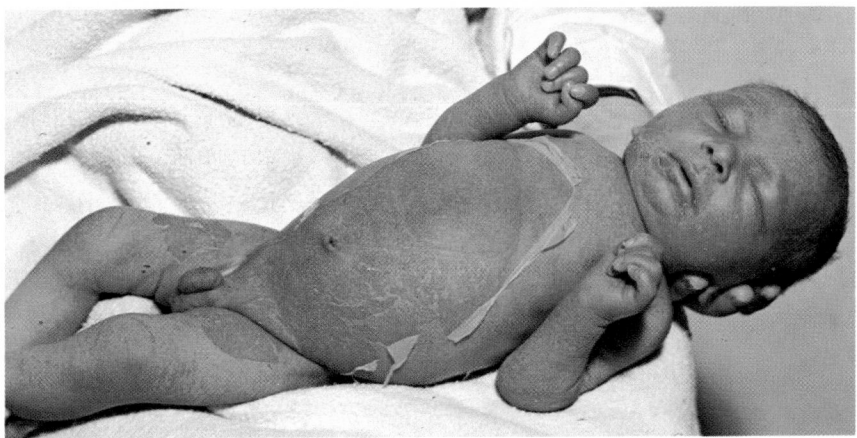

Figure 23-25. Dermatitis exfoliativa (Ritter's disease) in a newborn infant, showing erythema, edema and exfoliation at site of subcorneal blisters (see p. 1404).

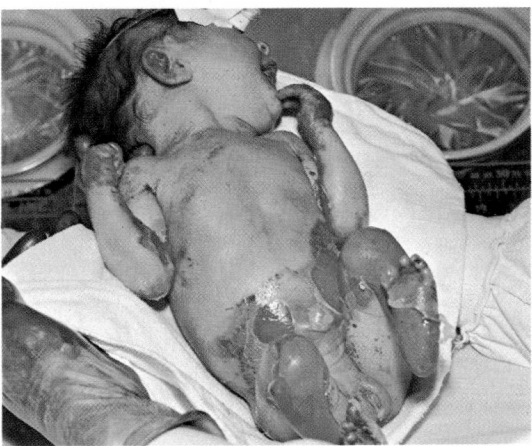

Figure 23-15. Epidermolysis bullosa. Dystrophic type in a newborn infant, showing large, flaccid blisters and denuded areas of skin (see p. 1393).

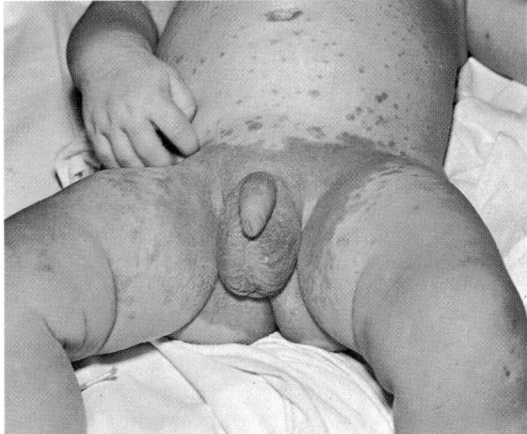

Figure 23-22A. Dermatitis with seborrheic distribution, which commenced in the genitocrural fold as diaper dermatitis and subsequently spread, producing a psoriasiform clinical picture (see p. 1402).

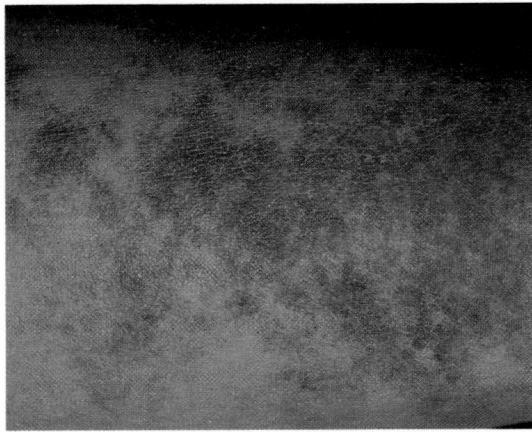

Figure 23-9A. Keratotic hemangioma.

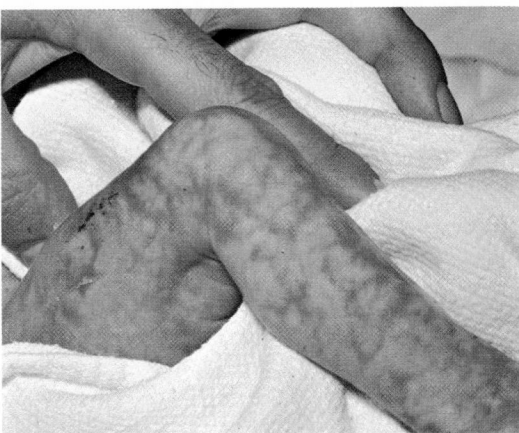

Figure 23-10. Cutis marmorata telangiectatica congenita in an infant, showing the characteristic reticular vascular pattern in the skin.

are usually involved in varying degrees, but the nose, lips, genitalia, palms and soles are uninvolved.

No treatment is necessary; the prominent vascular markings slowly regress over a period of years.

Tumors of the Skin

Tumors of the skin (see also p. 1465) are uncommon in infancy and childhood. Some benign tumors appear clinically and histologically aggressive in childhood, possibly as the result of growth stimulus during this period. In general, the neoplastic appearance diminishes with time, as in most hemangiomas and in benign juvenile melanoma, but malignant melanoma or angiosarcoma may rarely occur. Among the uncommon conditions which should be borne in mind are Gardner's syndrome, connective tissue tumors, pilomatrixoma, nevoid basal cell carcinoma syndrome, and basal cell carcinoma.

Gardner's syndrome (see p. 1448) is transmitted as an autosomal dominant trait and is characterized by cystic skin lesions, fibrous tissue tumors, multiple polyposis of the colon, osteomatosis and dental anomalies.

Nevoid basal cell carcinoma syndrome may appear early in childhood and is characterized by the appearance of multiple basal cell cancers, palmar and plantar pits, jaw cysts, ectopic calcification, and skeletal anomalies. It is transmitted as an autosomal dominant trait. Histologically, the skin tumors show the characteristic features of basal cell carcinoma. Clinically, they may be flesh-colored or pigmented pearly papules which appear during the first few years and continue to appear throughout life. There is a predilection for the face, head and neck, but many tumors occur also on the trunk, abdomen and extremities. They behave as neoplastic tumors, slowly increasing in size, and finally producing a classic rodent ulcer with bleeding and crusting. Asymptomatic pinhead-sized pits in the palms and soles are a hallmark of the syndrome, but they do not appear until after adolescence. When the tumors appear on the face, they must be differentiated from the periorbital eccrine sweat gland tumors and trichoepithelioma. Treatment of the tumors should be conservative, with electrocoagulation and curettage as the tumors arise. Treatment should be undertaken first in the critical areas around the eyelids.

Basal cell carcinoma is a neoplastic tumor rare in childhood, which may occur occasionally on the face or scalp. Basal cell epitheliomatous degeneration of pre-existing organoid lesions (nevus sebaceus of Jadassohn) is not uncommon. Histologically, there is basal cell proliferation and invasion of the dermis by basal cells in nests and cords, and with adenoid patterns. The tumor is characterized by a pearly-appearing papule with or without melanin pigment and prominent vascular markings. Pigmented lesions may resemble melanoma;

benign juvenile melanoma may also have a semitranslucent appearance and needs to be differentiated.

Connective Tissue Tumors. See Tumors of Soft Tissues (p. 1467).

Juvenile Xanthogranuloma (Nevoxanthoendothelioma). Juvenile xanthogranuloma is a transient, benign tumor of unknown origin which is seen in the first 2 years of life. The lesions are reddish-yellow to brown; they vary in size from papules to nodules and may appear singly, grouped or generalized. There is a predilection for the face, scalp and extremities. Involvement may rarely occur in other tissues such as the eye, pericardium, liver, lung or tonsils.

Histopathologically, the epiderm overlying the ill-defined infiltrated area is atrophic. The infiltrate may extend to the lower portion of the dermis and consists of lipophagic histiocytes, giant cells, and scattered foci of lymphocytes, plasma and eosinophilic cells. These changes represent a benign reactive process involving histiocytic cells which show xanthomatization.

In differential diagnosis the solitary tumors of urticaria pigmentosa and xanthoma should be considered.

Treatment is usually not necessary, but regression may be hastened by infiltration of the lesions with triamcinolone, injectable (5 mg. per cu. cm.).

Pyogenic Granuloma. Pyogenic granuloma is a rapidly growing vascular tumor which occurs at the site of an injury to the skin and bleeds profusely on slight trauma. The growth is bright red or purplish and may be crusted or moist. It may form a pedunculated or sessile tumor, up to a centimeter or so in diameter.

Histopathologically, it consists of newly formed capillaries; there are numerous microorganisms and an infiltrate consisting of mast and plasma cells and leukocytes, and, later, fibroplastic proliferation.

In differential diagnosis, hemangioma, hemangiosarcoma and melanoma must be distinguished.

Surgical excision is not indicated, since removal of the tumor electrosurgically with destruction of its vascular supply will prevent recurrence.

Juvenile Elastoma (Nevus Elasticus) is a nevus of elastic tissue with onset in childhood, which is transmitted as an autosomal dominant trait. Spotty, dense, sclerotic changes (osteopoikilosis) have been reported at the ends of the femora, tibiae and humeri.

Histologically, the elastic fibers in the subepidermal region are greatly increased in number and size, but otherwise normal. The skin changes consist of single or multiple, flat, yellowish plaques with a tendency to localization in the lumbosacral area. In differential diagnosis the connective tissue patches (shagreen) of epiloia need to be differentiated.

Adenoma sebaceum is the cutaneous expression of *tuberous sclerosis (epiloia)* (see p. 1280), which is characterized clinically by mental deficiency and epilepsy and transmitted as an autosomal dominant trait. Multiple benign tumors may be found in the brain and retina (gliomas), heart (rhabdomyomas) and the kidneys (angiomyolipomas). Histologically, the misnamed papules on the face consist of fibrosis, dilatation of capillaries and atrophy of the sebaceous glands. The skin changes are characterized by the presence of oval hypopigmented macules at birth and the later appearance of skin-colored or yellowish-red papules, located primarily on the medial aspects of the cheek and nose (Fig. 23-11); they are frequently associated with telangiectasia. Subungual fibromas frequently develop; thickened connective tissue patches (shagreen) appear by predilection in the lumbosacral area. The course of the disease is variable, depending on the extent of involvement; life span may be shortened. If the papules and patches of adenoma sebaceum are cosmetically disturbing, they can be satisfactorily removed by shaving off the lesions flush with the skin surface and lightly desiccating the base to control bleeding.

Cutaneous meningiomas are uncommon, benign, solitary tumors of the skin, probably derived from ectopic arachnoidal cells. The histologic appearance of the tumor is identical to that of intracranial meningiomas, with psammoma bodies scattered through the tumor. Clinically, a nondiagnostic, infiltrated, freely movable skin-colored patch is located on the scalp or trunk.

Calcifying epithelioma of Malherbe (pilomatrixoma) is a benign, freely movable subcutaneous nodule most commonly found on the face,

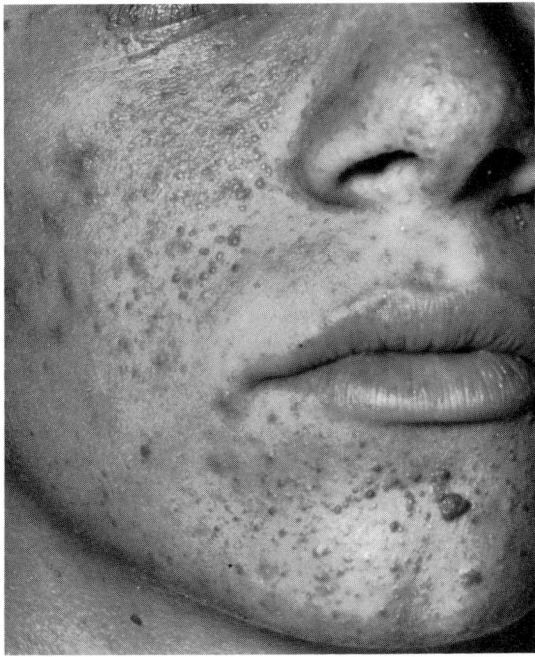

Figure 23-11. Adenoma sebaceum, showing scattered erythematous papules in a 12-year-old boy.

neck and arms. Histologically, there is a circumscribed mass of bands and sheets of epithelial cells in the dermis or in the subcutaneous fat tissue surrounded by compressed collagen. Keratin may be found in some areas; a high percentage of the tumors undergo calcification and ossification. It is generally accepted that this tumor arises from primitive epidermal germ cells which are differentiating toward hair matrix cells. It is usually single, but two or more may appear during infancy or early adolescence. They usually remain asymptomatic, but occasionally become inflamed. They are most frequently confused clinically with keratin cysts. Surgical excision is the treatment of choice.

Ectodermal Defects
(ECTODERMAL DYSPLASIA)

Congenital anhidrotic ectodermal defect is a hereditary developmental abnormality characterized by aplasia or hypoplasia of eccrine sweat, sebaceous and mucous glands, pilar structures and tooth buds.

Histopathologically, there is thinning of the epiderm and dermis. Eccrine sweat glands are absent or may be rudimentary. There is thinning of the epithelial layer in the respiratory mucous membranes and hypoplasia of the underlying mucous glands.

Affected infants appear normal at birth, but they do not perspire. In early infancy an otherwise unexplained fever which is directly related to high environmental temperature may provide a clue to early diagnosis. At this time confirmatory diagnostic evidence can be secured from a roentgenogram of the jaws, in which there are no or deficient dental structures.

Chronic rhinitis and pharyngitis are common. The hair of the scalp is very fine and sparse and grows slowly. Dentition is delayed or may be absent; when present, the incisors are widely spaced and the canines have a conical morphology. Characteristic alteration of the face occurs as early as 11 months and consists of prominent frontal bosses and a saddle-shaped nose. In differential diagnosis, congenital syphilis and chondroectodermal dysplasia must be distinguished.

Treatment is symptomatic.

Hidrotic ectodermal defect is transmitted as a dominant trait and is characterized by hypotrichosis, hyperpigmentation, dystrophic nails, and hyperkeratosis of palms and soles. Hair may be partially or completely absent at birth; when present, it is fine and easily fractured. The nails may be thin or thickened, striated, rough or completely absent. Palms and soles are hyperkeratotic, and there is hyperpigmentation on the extensor surfaces of the elbows, axillae, areolar area of the breasts, umbilicus and the interphalangeal joints.

In differential diagnosis the anhidrotic type of ectodermal defect must be distinguished.

Keratinizing Abnormalities

The hereditary keratinizing abnormalities (ichthyosis and the ichthyosiform dermatoses) may be considered to be the result of altered epithelial cell maturation. Normally, the basal cells reproduce at a steady rate, transit through the epidermis being characterized by the loss of nuclei and the formation of the keratinous layer. Disruption of the balance between cell proliferation and the elimination of keratin, through either increased production or decreased shedding, results in a thickened stratum corneum. The congenital keratodermas, relatively uncommon as a group, consist of a number of clinical entities which can be distinguished by genetic, clinical and histopathologic characteristics.

Ichthyosis vulgaris occurs in autosomal dominant and sex-linked forms.

Sex-linked ichthyosis vulgaris is the commonest form of ichthyosis in the first 3 months of life. The frequency is estimated at 1 in 6000 males. Genetic studies have indicated that the locus for X-linked ichthyosis and the locus for the Xg blood groups are probably closely placed on the short arm of the X chromosome. Skin changes resembling those of the "collodion baby" (see below) may be present at birth. Generalized scaling often commences in the first week of life, and though the process remains more or less generalized, the areas of involvement will vary with time. Children characteristically have thick scales on the scalp, with grayish, dirty-appearing hyperkeratotic changes on the sides of the face and neck, whereas in adults the abdomen, legs and the popliteal fossae are most frequently affected. The palms and soles are normal. The scales are typically large and grayish, and are shed episodically. The histologic features are striking hyperkeratosis, increased thickness of the stratum granulosum, prominent acanthosis and a perivascular inflammatory infiltrate in the dermis. The excessive proliferation of epithelial cells results in the excessive scaling. The characteristic skin change of the X-linked variety is the large scale, with prominent localization to the neck, but the hallmark of X-linked ichthyosis is the demonstration of deep corneal opacities by slit-lamp examination. There is striking improvement during warm weather.

Autosomal ichthyosis vulgaris is characterized by a family history of atopy, keratosis pilaris, and increased markings on the palmar and plantar skin. It is the most common variety of ichthyosis, but is seldom seen before the age of 3 months. This disease is inherited as a dominant trait. Frequency is difficult to determine because the manifestations may be so mild; a minimal estimate is on the order of 1 in 1000 persons. Atopic manifestations are observed in approximately 50 per cent of the patients, but this association does not seem to alter the clinical picture of ichthyosis. Involvement of the flexural surfaces is rare. The palmar surfaces of the hands and soles of the feet have increased markings. The scaling on the trunk is more prominent on the back than on the abdomen. Follicular keratoses are common, appearing primarily on the proximal lateral aspects of the arms and legs. The scales are small, fine and white, and there is striking diminution in the severity of scaling with increasing age. Warm weather has a beneficial effect. The histologic features are hyperkeratosis with a diminished or absent granular layer; cellular kinetics indicate a diminished rate of epithelial proliferation.

The skin can be kept in as good condition in winter as in summer by a technique of hydration followed by lubrication. The hydrophilic keratin is hydrated by soaking baths once or twice a day, which are followed by the application of a water-in-oil ointment (20 per cent distilled water in hydrophilic petrolatum) which impedes evaporation of absorbed water.

The ichthyosis-like dermatoses (congenital keratodermas) may be grouped according to the presence or absence of varying degrees of erythema at birth, the type of scale and the presence or absence of blisters. Brocq originally described congenital ichthyosiform erythroderma, which histologic and genetic studies have proved to be 2 separate entities. Included in the congenital keratodermas are the bullous and nonbullous types of Brocq's disease, which have been recently renamed *epidermolytic congenital ichthyosiform erythroderma*, and *psoriasiform erythroderma*; the category also contains lamellar ichthyosis and sex-linked ichthyosis. It has been concluded that the 2 forms of ichthyosis vulgaris congenita may be regarded as variant degrees of expression of ichthyosiform erythroderma.

"Harlequin fetus" is a descriptive term for the fetus with the most severe form of congenital ichthyosiform erythroderma. Death usually occurs before or shortly after birth. Until this rare condition is more clearly defined, however, the possibility that it may represent an extreme variant of bullous ichthyosiform erythroderma or of sex-linked ichthyosis cannot be excluded.

Congenital ichthyosiform erythroderma—nonbullous type of Brocq (psoriasiform erythroderma) is characterized by generalized lobster-red erythema and varying degrees of keratin accumulation at birth. A high frequency of parental consanguinity suggests autosomal recessive inheritance.

The principal clinical manifestations are hyperkeratosis and erythroderma. The skin at birth has a shiny red appearance; it becomes dry and begins to exfoliate large sheets of keratin within a few hours. Involvement of the skin around the eyes produces ectropion. The involvement of the fingers produces a clawlike appearance of the hands. The scalp is covered with a thick, yellowish seborrhea-like scale. The erythroderma and the profuse scale may persist or may diminish with time. There may be keratotic debris beneath the fingernails, and striations and stippling of the nails. Excessive proliferation of epithelial cells accounts for the accumulation of keratin. The histopathologic changes are psoriasiform, with hyperkeratosis and parakeratosis, acanthosis and frequent mitotic figures on the lower levels of the epidermis and a mild inflammatory infiltrate in the upper portion of the dermis. Sweat glands and ducts appear to be normal, except in the stratum corneum, where there is plugging of the poral orifices with keratinous debris. There are diminished sweating and intolerance to heat. Sweating is noted, however, in response to local injection of cholinergic drugs such as methacholine. Like psoriasis, this type of erythroderma responds to topical application of hydrocortisone and its analogues, as well as to systemic administration of folic acid antagonists. The use of drugs such as methotrexate to diminish turnover time of the epithelial cells is of interest, but does not seem to present a practical approach to an extremely chronic condition.

The main clinical features of the **bullous type of congenital ichthyosiform erythroderma** are hyperkeratosis and blisters, in addition to erythema at birth. The disease is inherited as an autosomal dominant trait. A thick, scaly mantle covers the skin at birth, but is shed almost immediately, leaving a raw surface. The skin gradually becomes dry and scaly again and assumes the changes characteristic of this disorder. The erythema is less vivid than in nonbullous congenital ichthyosiform erythroderma. It is most obvious on the face, neck, and body folds, but may be generalized. It may be most noticeable only when the thickened keratin is removed. The ichthyotic changes vary from slight dryness to dark brown, verrucoid elevated ridges (*ichthyosis hystrix*) resembling porcupine skin. The scalp is covered with thick, greasy, seborrhea-like scales. Hairs, nails, eyes, teeth and mucous membranes appear normal. The blisters appear spontaneously on any part of the body except the palms, soles and mucous membranes. Episodes of blister formation are frequently associated with secondary bacterial infection and may be accompanied by temperature elevation. Blisters are usually generalized, but may appear only in areas subjected to trauma. The palms and soles are usually slightly erythematous and scaly.

Histologically, there is a thickened, verrucous, loosely laminated, horny layer, with an accentuated granular layer and characteristic replacement of the cytoplasm by clear spaces. Through the electron microscope the "clear" spaces are seen to be large areas of perinuclear endoplasmic reticulum filled with ribosomes, keratinosomes and mitochondria. This pattern, together with increased mitoses, indicates increased cellular metabolism and an increased turnover time of the skin. In the dermis, blood vessels are slightly dilated and there is perivascular round cell infiltration. Intracellular and intercellular edema gives the epidermis a characteristic reticular pattern in histologic sections. Collections of coarse keratohyaline granules are seen beneath the stratum corneum.

The hydration and lubrication technique described above is useful in removing accumulated keratotic debris. Soaking baths twice a day for 15 to 20 minutes followed by the application of a water and oil base containing 2 per cent salicylic acid are useful. Smears and cultures should be taken from infected blisters and local or systemic antibacterial treatment instituted in accordance with in-vitro antibiotic testing of the isolated pathogen. Prevention of secondary bacterial infection may be accomplished by routine cleansing with a soap substitute containing hexachlorophene, and the application of a broad-spectrum antibiotic ointment on the broken blisters.

A milder variant of congenital ichthyosiform erythroderma is distinguished by the absence of blisters, but with the characteristic verrucoid hyperkeratotic lesions and erythema. The hyperkeratotic papules and ridges are localized to the flexural areas, with the remainder of the skin usually little involved. In some instances the changes may be generalized and indistinguishable from those of the bullous variety of the disease, except for the absence of blister formation. Treatment is the same as for the bullous variety, but secondary infection is not a problem.

Lamellar ichthyosis of the newborn ("collodion baby") is a rare congenital abnormality inherited as an autosomal recessive trait characterized by a collodion-like membrane which covers the entire cutaneous surface at birth (Fig. 23-12). The collodion-like membrane may be seen in infants whose later clinical course is typical of ichthyosiform erythroderma (nonbullous type), or sexlinked ichthyosis, or *the skin may clear completely and permanently by several months of age.* Typically, the infant is completely enveloped in a thin, dry, shining dermal layer, which is brownish-yellow and resembles a collodion coating. There are ectropion and eversion of the eyelids. The membrane cracks within a few hours, and thin sheets of scales peel off, leaving an erythematous base; the scales re-form, and the process is re-

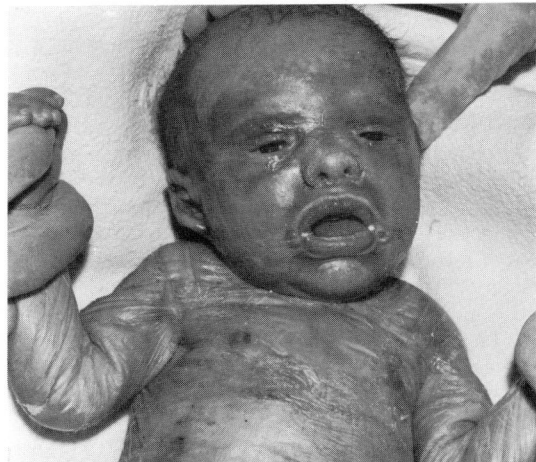

Figure 23-12. Collodion-like membrane in a newborn female infant who later had lamellar ichthyosis.

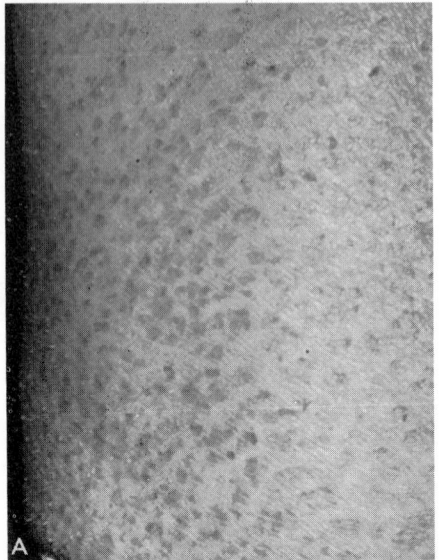

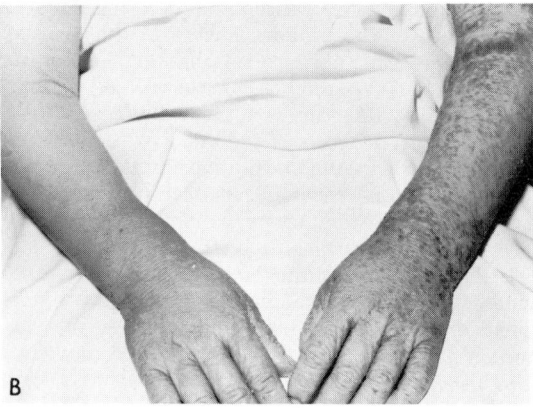

Figure 23-13. *A,* Lamellar ichthyosis in a 2½-year-old child who had a collodion type of covering and erythema at birth. Note the characteristic central adherence of the "potato chip" type of scale. *B,* Unilateral response to treatment with vitamin A acid ointment on the right, and absence of response on the left.

peated. If the ichthyotic scaling persists, it may be widespread or become localized to the flexural surfaces. The large, grayish-brown scales are adherent in the center with slightly raised edges (Fig. 23-13). Aggravation of the ichthyosis during warm weather has been reported.

Histologically, there is a dense, homogeneous, thickened keratin layer, with scattered parakeratotic nuclei. The epidermis is of normal thickness or moderately acanthotic with a distinct granular layer. Keratotic plugs are observed in the pilosebaceous orifices. There is a mild inflammatory infiltrate in the dermis. There is no histologic evidence of a persistent epitrichial layer.

Sjögren-Larsson syndrome. The Sjögren-Larsson syndrome is characterized by generalized ichthyosis and erythema involving the face and flexural surfaces of the palms and soles, in association with neurologic and ophthalmologic abnormalities. It is transmitted as an autosomal re-

cessive trait. Histologic changes in the skin consist of hyperkeratosis: a decreased or normal granular layer with acanthosis.

Heredopathia atactica polyneuritiformis (Refsum's syndrome) is a rare metabolic abnormality related to phytanic acid degradation. There is generalized ichthyosis, retinitis pigmentosa, peripheral neuropathy, progressive nerve deafness, and elevated levels of protein in cerebrospinal fluid. It is transmitted as an autosomal recessive trait.

Several other extremely rare inherited syndromes of ichthyosis are associated with epilepsy, dwarfism, infantilism, macrocytic anemia, polyneuritis or oligophrenia. There is also a sex-linked ichthyosis with hypogonadism in males.

Pachyonychia Congenita. This is a rare congenital disease transmitted as a dominant trait and characterized by remarkable thickening of the nails and by keratinizing abnormalities of the skin, hair and mucous membrane.

Histopathologically, the hyperkeratotic lesions have an intact stratum granulosum, parakeratosis and acanthosis; there are keratinous plugs in follicular and some eccrine orifices.

The nail changes are constantly present. A yellowish discoloration of the nails is noted during the neonatal period; later they become characteristically thickened. White patches resembling leukoplakia develop on the mucous membranes, and there are noninflammatory bullous lesions predominantly on the feet. Blisters become less frequent with time, but persistent keratotic patches appear, and follicular keratotic lesions also occur on the lateral, proximal aspects of the arms and legs. The growth abnormalities of the nails become so accentuated that the wearing of shoes is uncomfortable and manual dexterity is impaired. Less commonly, there may be involvement of the nasal mucosa, tympanic membrane or cornea. Epidermolysis bullosa may be considered in differential diagnosis because of blister formation and nail thickening, but the persistence of pustular patches at former sites of blisters and the leukokeratosis of mucous membranes serve as differentiating features. The nails should be removed and the nail matrix destroyed.

Other Defects in Keratinization. *Congenital ichthyosis of the palms and soles (keratosis palmaris et plantaris—tylosis of palms and soles)* is characterized by hyperkeratosis and by hyperhidrosis. It is usually transmitted as a dominant trait.

Histopathologically, there is excessive keratosis associated with hyperplasia of the prickle cell layer and with elongation of the papillae.

The skin of the palms and soles may appear normal at birth or become erythematous and scaly during the neonatal period. More commonly the thickening of the skin appears later in the first year of life and progresses with variable degrees of thickening of the palms, soles, and flexural surfaces of the fingers and toes. The changes stop abruptly at the lateral and medial borders of the hands and feet and at the flexural folds on the wrists.

Treatment is essentially the same as for ichthyosis; in addition, ointments or plasters containing a keratolytic agent (salicylic acid) are useful for severe hyperkeratosis.

Keratoderma of palms and soles and premature periodontoclasia (Papillon-Lefevre syndrome) is differentiated from other keratinizing abnormalities of the palms and soles by premature periodontoclasia and calcification of the dura. It is transmitted as an autosomal recessive trait. Histologically, there is acanthosis with a striking hyperkeratosis, and a perivascular inflammatory round cell infiltrate in a somewhat thinned dermis. The gingivae show a striking perivascular inflammatory infiltrate and edema, with destruction of the epithelial attachment and degeneration of the periodontal fibers.

The hyperkeratotic changes on the palms and soles usually appear around the fourth and fifth years of life concurrently with periodontal involvement of the deciduous dentition, but the skin changes may appear earlier. The palmar and plantar involvement is characterized by varying degrees of hyperkeratosis with sharp margination at the lateral borders. The hyperkeratosis is most frequently diffuse in the involved areas, but may also be patchy or punctate. As in ichthyosis, there may be exacerbation in the winter, with painful fissures. The development and eruption of deciduous teeth are normal, but with the appearance of hyperkeratosis the gingivae become red, swollen and boggy, and bleed easily. The formation of deep pockets of periodontal pus is accompanied by bad breath. The teeth rapidly become mobile and are shed by the fourth or fifth year of age. The mucous membranes then become normal, but the process is repeated when the permanent dentition erupts. When all the permanent teeth are lost, the gingivae return to normal and tolerate dentures well. Roentgenograms of the skull may show calcium deposits in the attachments of the tentorium and choroid plexus by the age of 4 or 5 years. No known treatment alters the course of the periodontoclasia. The hyperkeratotic lesions on the palms and soles are helped with the same technique of hydration and lubrication as described above for ichthyosis.

Mal de Meleda is a congenital symmetrical hyperkeratosis of palms, soles, elbows and knees, and dorsa of hands and feet. The disease is transmitted as a recessive trait; it is endemic on the island of Meleda in the Adriatic Sea.

Histopathologically, there is severe hyperkeratosis, as well as hyperplasia of the prickle cell layer with acanthosis. The stratum lucidum is increased, and the granular layer is prominent over the interpapillary portion of the prickle cell layer.

The first changes consist of erythema of the palms and soles within the first 2 years of life, followed by horny thickening which is characteristically surrounded by a dusky erythematous zone. This hyperkeratosis slowly spreads to involve the dorsa of the hands and feet, the extensor surfaces of forearms and legs and the elbows and knees. Hyperhidrosis and dystrophic changes of the nails also occur.

Treatment is not satisfactory, but is the same as for congenital ichthyosis of the palms and soles.

Acrokeratosis verruciformis of Hopf is a rare, localized epithelial nevus which is transmitted as a dominant trait. It is characterized by asymptomatic, symmetrical, flat wartlike papules 2 to 4 mm. in diameter located predominantly on the dorsa of the hands and feet. They may be present at birth or appear during infancy. Papules on the wrists, ankles, palms and soles, as well as ichthyotic changes of the skin, may also appear later, usually at puberty. The nails may be opaque and brittle with vertical, linear striations.

Histopathologically, there is thickening of the epidermis with hyperkeratosis and an accentuated granular layer with some parakeratosis. The dermis appears normal.

In differential diagnosis, juvenile flat warts must be considered. No treatment is known to be effective.

Lichen spinulosus is a rare keratinizing abnormality of unknown cause characterized by patches of horny spines involving primarily the hair follicles; there is a mild inflammatory reaction.

Histopathologically, there is widening of the orifices of the hair follicles and sweat ducts, which are filled with keratotic plugs. Keratotic accumulations occur independently of either pilar or sweat units. Sebaceous glands are atrophic or absent. There is an inflammatory infiltrate around the vessels in the dermis.

The skin lesions, which appear in crops, consist of slightly erythematous patches with spiny projections. The erythematous phase is transient, but the spiny papules persist. The eruption is usually asymptomatic.

In differential diagnosis, pityriasis rubra pilaris, keratosis pilaris, lichen scrofulosus and phrynoderma must be distinguished.

Treatment during the inflammatory phase consists in the application of an anti-inflammatory agent (0.5 per cent hydrocortisone) in an emollient base; in the keratotic phase a keratolytic agent (salicylic acid) in an emollient base is indicated.

Phrynoderma is a cutaneous expression of severe *vitamin A deficiency*, characterized by a dry, roughened skin with acuminate, follicular horny papules and dome-shaped keratotic papules. Skin lines are exaggerated, producing a wrinkled appearance. The eruption is usually generalized, but may appear in local areas of chronic trauma to the skin.

In differential diagnosis, pityriasis rubra pilaris, keratosis pilaris, lichen scrofulosus and lichen spinulosus must be distinguished.

Treatment consists in supplementation of vitamin A intake.

Pityriasis rubra pilaris is a rare, slightly inflammatory keratinizing abnormality which may be transmitted as an autosomal dominant trait. It is characterized by horny follicular, acuminate papules which coalesce into scaling patches. There are acquired and familial types; the latter appears in infancy or childhood.

Histopathologically, there is keratosis around the hair follicles and in the stratum corneum above the dermal papillae and plugging of the follicles; in the dermis there is perivascular and perifollicular and inflammatory infiltration.

The skin changes appear slowly; when established, they are usually symmetrical and include seborrheic scaling on the scalp, erythema of the face, hyperkeratosis of the palms and soles, and eventually circumscribed, scaling patches on the face, trunk and extremities. Follicular papules tend to persist on the proximal portion of the phalanges.

In differential diagnosis, phrynoderma, keratosis pilaris and lichen spinulosus should be distinguished.

The disease can be cleared with large doses of vitamin A by mouth, though there is no evidence of vitamin A deficiency. Local treatment consists of hydration and lubrication as in ichthyosis.

Pigmentary Abnormalities

Alteration of normal pigment of the skin may result from altered melanocyte physiology, from absorption of heavy metals (lead, bismuth), from ingestion of precursors of vitamin A (e.g. in carrots, squash, sweet potato or egg yolk) or of drugs, or from inborn errors of metabolism (ochronosis). Localized or generalized errors in melanogenesis may produce absence of or increase in pigment, as in albinism, partial albinism, Waardenburg's syndrome, Peutz-Jeghers syndrome, vitiligo, Albright's syndrome, incontinentia pigmenti, neurofibromatosis and pigmented nevi.

Albinism, partial albinism, Waardenburg's syndrome (p. 1435), Peutz-Jeghers syndrome (p. 1448), vitiligo, Albright's syndrome, incontinentia pigmenti and neurofibromatosis are genetic abnormalities of melanin production that may become manifest during the first 2 years of life.

Neurofibromatosis (von Recklinghausen's disease) (see p. 1280) characteristically presents as multiple *café-au-lait* patches of pigmentation. These sharply demarcated tan patches measuring 1 cm. or more may appear in the first weeks or months of life and are fully developed by 5 years of age. The more classic features of neurofibromatosis are often not present before puberty; six or more *café-au-lait* patches presume the diagnosis of neurofibromatosis. Such pigmented patches may provide a clue to the correct diagnosis in infants with glaucoma or skeletal anomalies at birth or shortly thereafter.

Albinism (see also p. 423) is a genetically transmitted relative or absolute incapability of melanocytes of the skin, hair and choroid to produce melanin.

Histopathologically, the skin is normal, although the melanocytes give a negative dopa reaction in absence of pigment, and dopa-positive cells are fewer when pigment is significantly decreased.

Absence of pigment produces a pinkish-white appearance of the skin at birth in the Caucasian, whereas in the nonwhite person freckle-like, pigmented macules are scattered over the skin. The hair is fine and white. The iris is pink in the Caucasian and pale blue in the nonwhite person. Ocular manifestations include photophobia, lacrimation and nystagmus, and less often retinitis pigmentosa, cataracts and color blindness. In one variation of albinism the melanocytes produce small amounts of pigment. In another variant the skin is considerably lighter than normal, but the iris is blue, and photophobia and nystagmus are absent.

Treatment consists in the prophylactic use of screening devices to protect against light and the avoidance of sunburn.

Partial albinism is transmitted as a dominant trait characterized by circumscribed areas of depigmentation in which the melanocytes give a negative dopa reaction. The patches of depigmentation are present at birth, and in most instances a white forelock is also present.

The Chediak-Higashi syndrome is a lethal variety of partial albinism transmitted as an autosomal recessive trait. It is characterized by photophobia, pale optic fundi, granular inclusions in leukocytes of blood and bone marrow, repeated pyogenic infections, and terminal hepatosplenomegaly.

Vitiligo may be an acquired disorder as well as a hereditary one. It is characterized by patchy, progressive loss of pigment due to a failure of the melanocytes to produce pigment. Histopathologically, the changes are indistinguishable from partial albinism. The halo nevus is a variant in which a depigmented area surrounds a pigmented nevus.

In differential diagnosis, piebaldness, postinflammatory depigmentation, leprosy and pinta must be distinguished.

Treatment is unsatisfactory.

Blister-Producing Abnormalities

For urticaria pigmentosa, see Mast Cell Disease (p. 1395).

Incontinentia pigmenti is an uncommon hereditary developmental defect appearing almost exclusively in females; it is probably transmitted as a sex-linked dominant. There are ectodermal abnormalities and occasionally mesodermal defects.

The histopathologic pattern varies with the stage of the disease. In the vesiculobullous stage there is intercellular edema with vesicle formation and a mixed inflammatory infiltrate in the dermis. In the hyperkeratotic stage there are proliferation of epithelial cells and hyperkeratosis. In the final

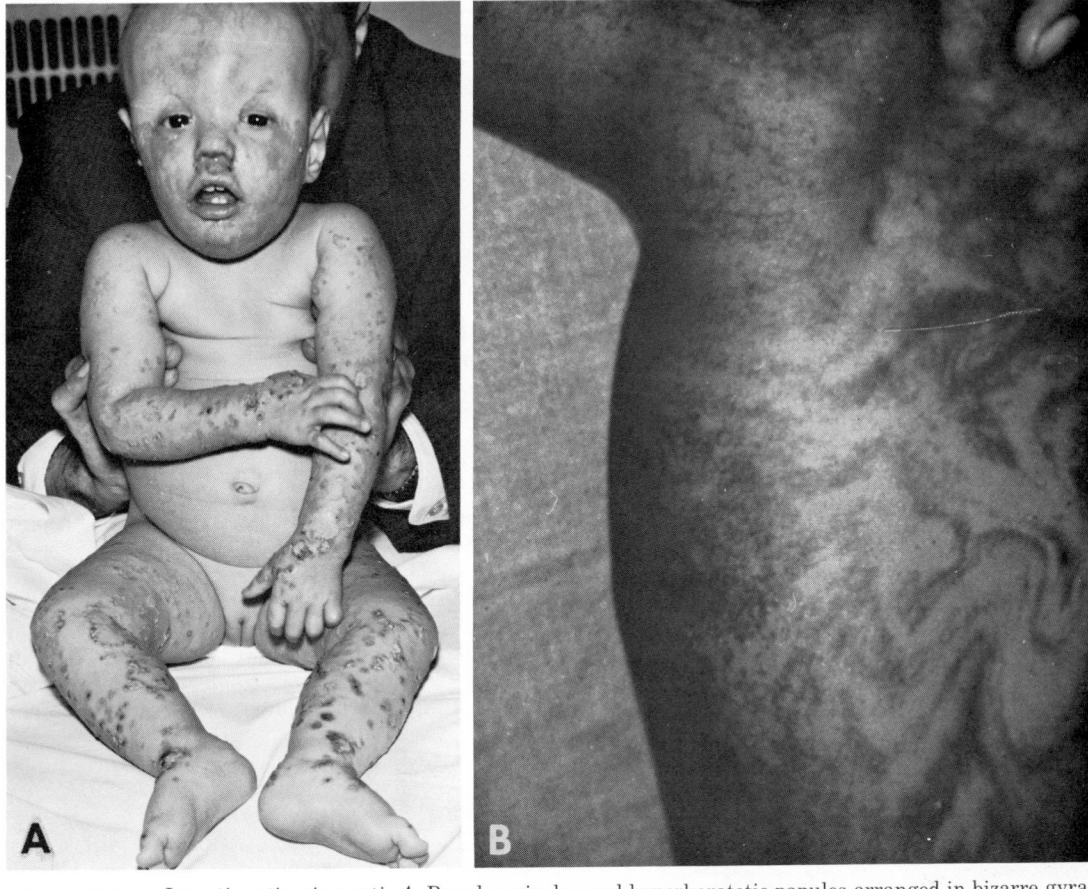

Figure 23-14. Incontinentia pigmenti. *A*, Papulovesicular and hyperkeratotic papules arranged in bizarre gyrate configuration in infant at 11 months of age; she had craniosynostosis and skin lesions at birth. A younger male sibling has similar skin changes and developmental defects. *B*, Final hyperpigmented stage.

stage the epidermis appears essentially normal except for the diminution of pigment in the lower epidermal layers and for large amounts of melanin in the melanophages in the upper portions of the dermis.

The skin changes are present at birth or appear shortly thereafter. The only evidence of the disease may be bizarre asymmetrical whorls or bands of macular brownish pigment on the extremities or trunk, or it may progress from an inflammatory reaction with blisters to a stage in which the vesicles are replaced by keratotic lesions (Fig. 23-14). The inflammatory or hyperkeratotic lesions ultimately disappear, leaving macular pigmentation at the site of previous activity. Abnormalities of the eyes, hair and teeth, epilepsy, mental deficiency and cardiac abnormalities have been associated.

During the inflammatory phase the morphologic changes may suggest an eczematous dermatitis (atopy), epidermolysis bullosa, dermatitis herpetiformis or bullous urticaria pigmentosa; melanocytic nevus must be considered in the pigmentary stage, and epithelial nevus in the keratotic stage.

No treatment is indicated except in the blister phase, when application of a broad-spectrum antibiotic is indicated to prevent secondary bacterial infection.

Epidermolysis bullosa is an uncommon blister-producing disease; it is usually present at birth and is characterized by the appearance of lesions at sites of slight trauma. On the basis of histologic, prognostic and genetic differences, the disease is classified into simple and dystrophic types; the latter are subdivided into dominant, recessive and lethal forms. Microscopic examination of the early stage of blisters reveals that the changes in the simplex type are at the level of the basal cell; in the lethal type, at the intermembrane space; and in the recessive dystrophic type, at the upper portion of the dermis.

The *simple form* is transmitted as an autosomal dominant trait. There is great variation in the degree of trauma required to produce blisters; lesions may follow the trauma of delivery or may not appear until late in infancy when the infant begins to crawl. The blister is superficial. Because early lesions are intraepidermal, there is no scarring.

The *dystrophic form* has varying degrees of severity. In some instances blister formation is at the epidermal-dermal junction. Scarring after healing is severe and is associated with contractures, adhesions between fingers, and loss of nails.

The dominant dystrophic form is intermediate in severity between the simple and recessive forms. The blisters are subepidermal and usually result in a thin scar. The mucous membranes may also be involved, and the nails may become atrophic or thickened and clawlike.

The recessive form is the most severe and destructive form compatible with life. It is frequently associated with other congenital defects. Blisters appear in the skin and mucous membranes spontaneously or after minimal trauma.

The lethal form is rare and except for its severity is not significantly different from the recessive type. Clear or hemorrhagic blisters are present at birth: they increase in number and rupture, leaving large denuded areas; buccal lesions are common (Fig. 23-15, p. 1385). Loss of fluid and secondary bacterial infection usually result in the neonatal period.

In differential diagnosis, acrodermatitis chronica enteropathica, incontinentia pigmenti, Ritter's disease and bullous syphiloderm need to be considered.

Treatment in all the variants is directed toward minimizing trauma. After blisters have appeared, efforts are directed toward preventing secondary bacterial infection (see p. 1404). Systemic administration of large doses of corticosteroids may diminish the frequency of blister production in the severe form.

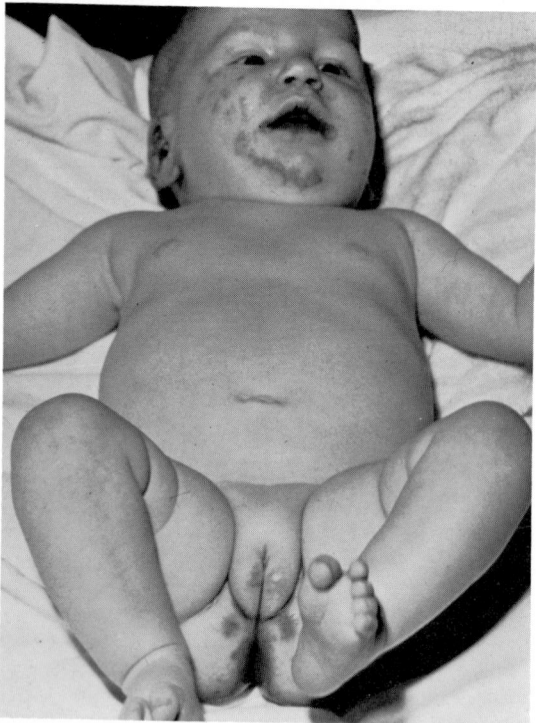

Figure 23-16. Acrodermatitis chronica enteropathica in a 4-month-old infant, showing the characteristic periorificial involvement. A male sibling had died with the disease.

Acrodermatitis chronica enteropathica is a chronic, often fatal disease of unknown origin, possibly transmitted as a recessive trait. It usually becomes manifest within the first 18 months of life. It is characterized by a vesiculo-pustulo-bullous eruption symmetrically arranged on the extremities and around the mouth and anal areas, by loss of hair and by diarrhea.

The blisters are located intraepidermally and contain polymorphonuclear leukocytes and eosinophils. There is a diffuse infiltrate in the papillary bodies and in the upper portion of the dermis with perivascular round cell infiltration in the mid-dermis. Chronic scaly lesions are characterized by acanthosis, hyperkeratosis and a dermal inflammatory infiltrate.

The blisters appear on normal skin and evolve to form eczematous patches; in a few weeks they become crusted and form erythematous psoriasiform plaques. Loss of hair occurs early; paronychial and dystrophic nail changes are usually present. The eruption may wax and wane, the gastrointestinal disturbance paralleling the skin changes, or the disease may become progressively more severe and the infant become apathetic and cachectic. Response to parenteral administration of fat suggests a basic defect of fatty acid metabolism.

Remissions may often be obtained by treatment with diiodohydroxyquinoline (Diodoquin) (see p. 277) daily for long periods of time. On occasion a child who fails to respond to this drug will respond to iodochlorhydroxyquinoline (Entero-Vioform). Secondary fungal and bacterial infections should be treated specifically.

Other Abnormalities

Lipoid Proteinosis. This is a rare metabolic disturbance transmitted as a recessive trait. A structureless hyaline material made up of a carbohydrate-protein complex is deposited in affected skin and mucous membranes as an extracellular mantle around vessels of the dermis and as a diffuse infiltrate in connective tissue. Lipids appear as the lesions become more advanced.

The skin lesions may be present at birth, but usually develop later. They characteristically consist of yellowish-white papules which may coalesce into plaques or nodules. Yellowish verrucoid lesions also occur on the extensor surface of the elbows, knees and hands. Subsequently there is extensive involvement of the mucous membrane of the tongue, lips, oral cavity, pharynx, larynx and rectal area. The infiltration of the vocal cords precludes speaking above a whisper as the child grows. Aplasia or hypoplasia of teeth is commonly associated.

In differential diagnosis the xanthomas may be distinguished by the woody feel of the tongue in this disorder.

The course of the disease is usually benign, and no treatment is necessary, but tracheotomy may be

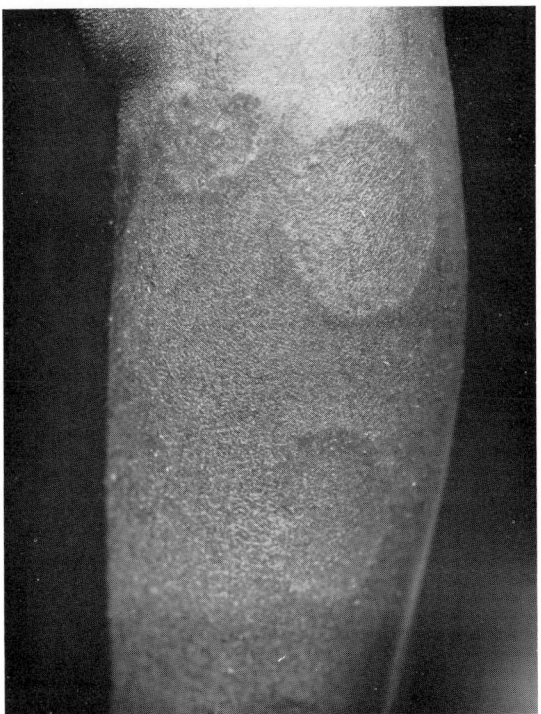

Figure 23-17. Granuloma annulare in a 5-year-old child, showing multiple, distinctive, annular lesions.

required for extensive infiltration of the vocal cords.

Lipogranulomatosis (Farber's Disease). Disseminated lipogranulomatosis is a rare form of the lipidoses which is manifest within the first few months of life. It follows a progressive course in which tenderness and swelling of the extremities are accompanied by dysphonia, a systemic reaction with temperature elevation, generalized joint involvement, nodules and infiltrated plaques in the skin, and cardiopulmonary and central nervous system involvement. The early skin lesions are slightly erythematous nodules which become ill-defined plaques with a predisposition for the extremities.

Granuloma Annulare. Granuloma annulare is a self-limited inflammatory process of unknown cause characterized by papules or nodules on the extremities. The primary lesion is a slightly erythematous or yellowish-red, waxy-appearing papule which slowly increases in size and clears in the center, or a group of papules may form a ring. Single lesions are the rule, but occasionally disseminated lesions appear on the extremities (Fig. 23-17).

Histopathologically, there is a distinctive area of coagulation necrosis in the upper portion of the dermis surrounded by a radially arranged infiltrate composed of epithelioid, lymphocytic, plasma and connective tissue cells.

In differential diagnosis the annular lesions of sarcoid (rare in children) and rheumatic nodules should be considered.

The disease is usually self-limited, and in many instances the lesions regress rapidly. In persistent lesions local application of triamcinolone in a 0.05 per cent cream under a plastic film or injection of it (5 mg. per ml.) into the lesion will produce prompt regression.

Mast Cell Disease (Urticaria Pigmentosa). Mast cell infiltration of the skin characterizes a chronic disease of unknown origin in which there are blisters, pigmented maculopapules, nodules or thickened skin (Fig. 23-18). It is usually present at birth or appears in the first 2 years of life. Mast cell disease may be classified as (1) *solitary mastocytoma*, (2) *urticaria pigmentosa* with or without blisters, (3) *diffuse mast cell infiltration* with systemic involvement. The histopathologic changes are distinctive and consist of an infiltrate of mast cells in the upper part of the dermis. The epidermis is usually normal in appearance except for some increase in melanin in the basal layer. In the bullous variety there are intracellular edema and vesicle formation.

Transient urticaria or blisters may appear at birth or shortly thereafter. Initially, urticarial lesions, blisters or orange-brown macules resembling a lipid deposit in the skin may be present, alone or in combination. In diffuse mast cell disease the entire skin is thickened, with a "parchment-like" yellow color and a fine, papular, "Scotch-grained" surface with exaggerated skin lines. Scratching in affected areas produces a wheal and flare (Darier's sign). The urticarial and blister-producing capabilities slowly decrease with approach of puberty. Cystic changes of the bone are present occasionally in urticaria pigmentosa, and widespread organ involvement is the rule in diffuse mastocytosis.

In differential diagnosis of solitary mastocytoma, juvenile xanthogranuloma and xanthoma must be distinguished; in the blistering form, dermatitis herpetiformis must be distinguished.

No treatment is known to be effective. In the vesiculobullous stage the local application of a broad-spectrum antibiotic may prevent secondary bacterial infection.

Cutis Hyperelastica and Cutis Laxa. The similarity in nomenclature and in some clinical features of these 2 diseases has caused considerable confusion. The essential alteration is in elastic tissue fibers in both diseases. The possibility of an associated alteration of collagen has not been completely excluded in either disease.

Cutis hyperelastica (Ehlers-Danlos syndrome) is a quantitative heritable abnormality of the elastic tissue transmitted as an incomplete dominant trait. It is usually present at birth and is characterized by hyperelasticity and fragility of the skin and hyperextensibility of the joints. Light microscopy and electron microscopy reveal a striking increase in the number of elastic fibers, but no morphologic abnormality of the fibers. Slight trauma produces in the fragile skin large lacerations which are impossible to suture and which

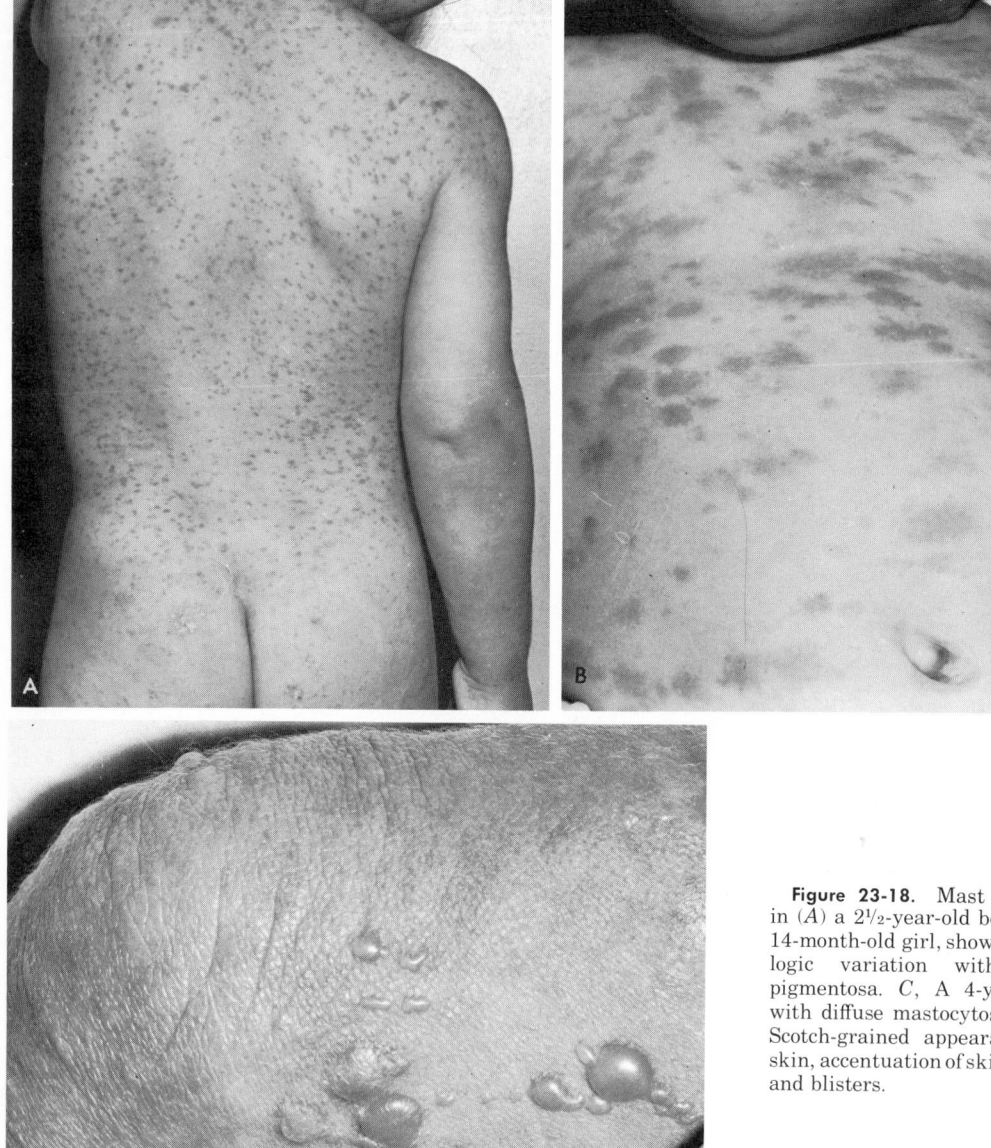

Figure 23-18. Mast cell disease in (*A*) a 2½-year-old boy and (*B*) a 14-month-old girl, showing morphologic variation with urticaria pigmentosa. *C*, A 4-year-old girl with diffuse mastocytosis, showing Scotch-grained appearance of the skin, accentuation of skin markings, and blisters.

heal with scars resembling cigarette paper. Minor trauma may also frequently produce large hematomas. Small nodules (pseudotumors) may be found on the skin at the sites of traumatic hemorrhage and consist of inflammatory infiltrate with foreign body giant cells or connective tissue proliferation with large numbers of vessels. Some nodules become calcified. The hemorrhagic tendency may suggest hemophilia, and the pseudotumors, neurofibromatosis, but the other classic features of the disease should make differentiation easy. Avoidance of trauma to the skin by protection of the lower portions of the legs and bony prominences

with foam rubber is useful. Closure of lacerations is impossible with single sutures and is difficult with mattress sutures, but can be accomplished by use of adhesive butterflies.

Cutis laxa (generalized elastolysis) is a generalized degenerative disease of elastic tissue fibers present at birth and inherited as a recessive trait. There are hypertrophy and laxity of the skin and underlying connective tissue which result in the skin hanging in folds and presenting a picture of premature senility. Histologic changes include a striking granular degeneration of elastic tissue fibers resulting in their complete disappearance in some areas. There is a striking increase in the acid mucopolysaccharide content of the dermis.

The skin is soft, doughy and inelastic, lies in folds on the face, neck, chest and abdomen, and droops over the eyelids and around the mouth. The pulmonary, genitourinary and gastrointestinal systems may be involved in the generalized elastic tissue alteration. When the disease is not limited to the skin, the systemic involvement may be incompatible with life. There is no known treatment for the basic defect, but appearance may be improved with plastic surgery.

LIPODYSTROPHY

Loss of subcutaneous fat results in 2 clinically distinct syndromes of unknown origin: partial and total lipodystrophy. Certain features are common to both.

Partial lipodystrophy is characterized by the symmetrical loss of fat from the face with or without disappearance of fat also from the arms, chest, abdomen and hips, but with normal distribution on the lower extremities. The ratio of affected females to males is approximately 4:1. The cause is unknown. The only histologic change observed is the absence of subcutaneous fat in affected areas, normal epidermis and dermis lying directly on fascia or muscle. The clinical onset is most often between 5 and 15 years of age, but may occur as early as the first year. There is an insidious loss of subcutaneous fat from the face without inflammatory reaction or symptoms. Slow progression may occur, with involvement of the neck, arms, chest and abdomen. Normal or even increased fat deposition may persist over the legs, but fat loss becomes complete on the face. These patients have a strikingly cadaverous appearance. Aside from the fat loss, the majority appear well, but renal disorders, disturbances of central nervous system function, hepatomegaly, hyperlipemia and disordered glucose metabolism have been associated. These features, which suggest total lipodystrophy, are more evident in the older patient. There is no known treatment for this disorder.

Total lipodystrophy is characterized by the complete loss of adipose tissue. It is regularly associated with liver disease and commonly with other variable features, including increased height, advanced bone maturation, hirsutism, pigmentation, prominence of muscles, abdominal protuberance, penile or clitoral enlargement, anatomic or functional disturbances of the central nervous system, neuropathy, cardiomegaly, insulin-resistant hyperglycemia, hyperlipemia and hypermetabolism. The ratio of affected females to males is 2:1. The disorder is transmitted as an autosomal recessive trait. The disease may be apparent at birth or may commence during childhood. The clinical appearance of the child is similar to that of patients with partial loss of fat, but because the condition is generalized, the striking contrast between affected and unaffected areas is absent, and the diagnosis may not be so apparent. Generalized pigmentation is common. Accentuated pigmentation in the axillary areas may be associated with the velvety verrucoid skin changes of acanthosis nigricans. A moderate degree of hirsuties may be present. Scalp hair may be abundant and may become curly concurrently with the loss of fat. An insulin-antagonizing and fat-mobilizing property has been found in the urine.

There is no known treatment for this disease.

LICHEN SCLEROSUS ET ATROPHICUS

Lichen sclerosus et atrophicus is a primary atrophic process of unknown origin which frequently involves the vulva, perineum, shoulders and lumbosacral areas. It has been reported in males, but occurs most frequently in females. Histologically, there is atrophy of the epidermal layer with edema and homogenization of the upper third of the dermis. The skin lesions consist of atrophic white maculopapules varying from 1 to 3 mm. in diameter with a small central horny plug. They are frequently grouped together to form patches, but the diagnostic discrete papules can be seen at the border of the lesion. Blisters may occasionally form on the patches. Pruritus is a common symptom, and painful fissures are often present in the perianal and vulvar lesions. The skin changes may persist for years or may regress spontaneously. The patches of confluent papules may resemble localized scleroderma (morphea). Relief of symptoms may be obtained by the use of a corticosteroid cream (1 per cent hydrocortisone). Topical estrogen creams are also useful in the genital area, but may produce side effects associated with percutaneous absorption.

SCLEREDEMA ADULTORUM

Scleredema (Buschke) is a disease of unknown origin, often appearing 4 to 6 weeks after a streptococcal infection, and characterized by progressive hardening of the trunk, face and upper extremities. The term "scleredema adultorum" is a misnomer, for there is no edema or sclerosis demonstrable histologically, and the disease occurs in children. The histologic changes consist of a mild, nonspecific inflammatory infiltrate and separation of collagen bundles in the lower two thirds of the dermis. Histochemical stains demonstrate an abundance of sulfated mucopolysaccharides (hyaluronic acid) in the empty spaces between the collagen bundles. Occasionally weakness, malaise or mild articular pain precedes the cutaneous changes. On casual examination the skin appears normal except for slight pallor. The face may have a masklike appearance. On palpation the skin is brawny, hard and nonpitting and cannot be easily moved over the underlying tissue. The changes fade off gradually into normal skin. Complete resolution of the disease may require months.

The clinical picture may suggest scleroderma, but the histopathologic changes permit differentiation. Treatment is difficult to evaluate because of the variable natural course of the disease. Infection should be eradicated, if present. Responses to corticosteroids have been unpredictable.

PITYRIASIS LICHENOIDES ET VARIOLIFORMIS ACUTA
(MUCHA-HABERMANN SYNDROME)

Mucha-Habermann syndrome is an asymptomatic inflammatory disease of the skin of unknown origin. In its more severe or acute form, papules, vesicles and papulonecrotic lesions appear in crops over a period of weeks or months. The lesions may resemble those of smallpox or varicella, but heal without scarring. In the milder form a few brownish-red papules appear in crops on the trunk and extremities and slowly resolve. In both instances new lesions recur with diminishing frequency as the disease disappears.

In the acute phase the histologic picture is essentially that of a lymphocytic vasculitis which damages the vessel wall and leads to necrosis of the overlying dermis and epidermis. The vasculitis differs from allergic vasculitis in the absence of neutrophils and in the fibrinoid deposits within and around the blood vessels. Varicella is most often confused clinically, but the short duration, contagiousness and constitutional symptoms of varicella serve to differentiate it. The multinucleated epithelial giant cells found at the base of a blister in varicella are diagnostic. Treatment is not necessary in most instances, owing to the self-limited nature of the disease. Corticosteroids may be useful in the severe form.

DIAPER DERMATITIS

Diaper dermatitis is a cutaneous reaction localized to the area ordinarily covered by the diaper. A variety of morphologic changes are produced by multiple causative factors. The histopathologic changes vary with the causative factor:

I. Predisposing factors
   A. Inheritance of a reactive skin that is easily irritated
   B. Inherited seborrheic diathesis with a propensity for irritation in the anal and genitocrural folds and vulnerability to secondary yeast and bacterial infections
   C. Atopic diathesis
   D. Systemic disease such as syphilis, acrodermatitis chronica enteropathica (Fig. 23-16) and Letterer-Siwe disease may produce a lowering of skin resistance
II. Activating factors
   A. Maceration caused by continuous contact with a wet diaper and increased by the moist heat produced by an impervious rubber or plastic cover

   B. Retention of sweat caused by keratotic plugging of orifices of eccrine glands, secondary to A
   C. Contact factors, allergic (e.g. sensitization to fluorochrome dyes in detergent soaps or to plastic diaper covers) and primary irritants (e.g. feces or ammonia in decomposed urine)
   D. Maternal factors such as failure to carry out instructions or being too assiduous in cleansing the affected areas
   E. Infection (e.g. yeast, bacterial, syphilitic, viral) (Fig. 23-19)
   F. Mechanical irritation in areas of friction or from pressure

Morphologic changes vary from diffuse erythema, in which the skin has a parchment-like appearance, to nodular infiltrated lesions, which may become vesicular, pustular or bullous.

Prevention consists in prompt changing of diapers after urination and in appropriate cleansing of the skin with each change of diaper, particularly after bowel movements, in elimination of an impervious diaper cover, covering with only 1 diaper, application of a protective paste (Lassar's paste), and in using diapers rinsed in a quaternary ammonium compound (Roccal 1:3000).

Treatment should be guided by a careful evaluation of the history of onset and of the morphology and localization of the lesions. Seborrheic lesions

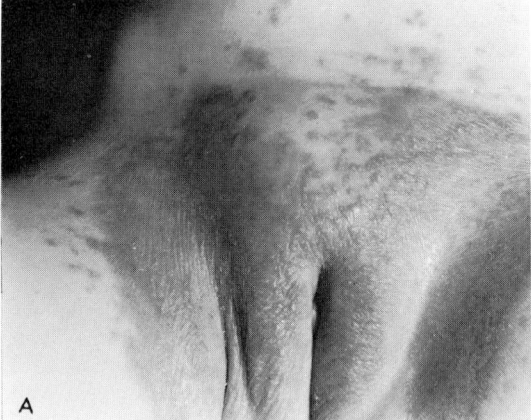

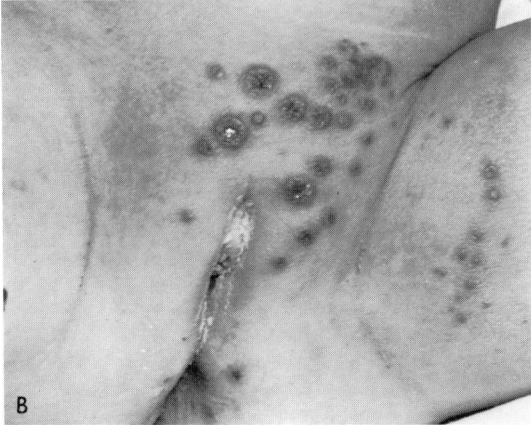

Figure 23-19. *A,* Diaper dermatitis caused by yeast infection, showing characteristic vesicular pustules; the organisms were demonstrated by direct microscopic examination (potassium hydroxide preparation). *B,* Staphylococcal infection in the diaper area secondary to sweat retention.

are treated with 0.5 per cent hydrocortisone ointment; yeast infections are sponged with benzalkonium chloride 1:3000 and then covered with Vioform cream alone or in combination with 0.5 per cent hydrocortisone or with nystatin (Mycostatin ointment); bacterial infections should be cleansed with a soap substitute containing hexachlorophene (pHisoHex), and a broad-spectrum antibiotic ointment such as neomycin, bacitracin or polymyxin should be applied. Contact dermatitis is treated with 0.5 per cent hydrocortisone ointment.

Exposure of the uncovered diaper area to dry heat, as from an electric light, is especially helpful and can be done to advantage during naps.

ALLERGIC DISORDERS

Cutaneous expressions of the hypersensitivity state include contact dermatitis, atopic dermatitis (p. 506), drug allergy, granulomatous vasculitis, allergy of infection (reactions to fungi, bacteria, viruses, protozoa) and allergy of infestation (parasites and insects).

Contact Dermatitis. Contact dermatitis is an acute inflammatory reaction of the skin which may be divided into 2 categories: (1) reactions which occur on first contact in all subjects and are usually produced by chemicals and (2) reactions which occur only in persons who have been previously sensitized. Contact dermatitis is the most common type of dermatitis in children from 2 to 12 years of age; atopic dermatitis is more common during infancy. The causative agents (excluding medications) in order of frequency are weeds and vines (usually poison ivy) (Fig. 23-20), the ether-soluble portion of airborne allergens, toys, cosmetics and chemicals in clothing and shoes.

Histopathologically, contact dermatitis is characterized by intercellular edema, exocytosis,

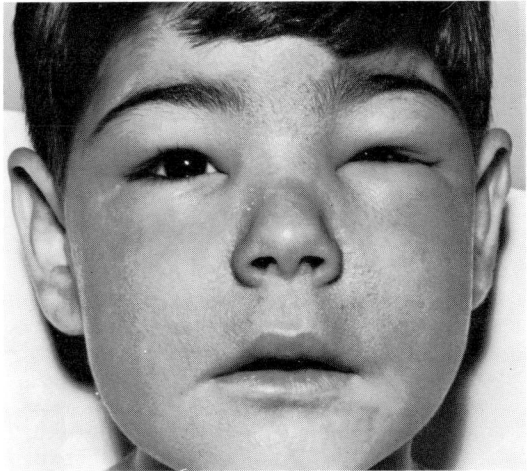

Figure 23-20. A 6-year-old boy with allergic contact dermatitis *(Rhus toxicodendron)* showing erythema, edema and vesicles 72 hours after contact.

and intraepidermal vesicle formation with a mild perivascular inflammatory infiltrate. A primary irritant reaction is differentiated from allergic reactions by the presence of polymorphonuclear leukocytes migrating through the epidermis and in the vesicles, whereas in the allergic reaction lymphocytes predominate. The skin response to a contact allergen depends on the level of sensitivity, varying from erythema with edema to blister formation. If additional contact is eliminated, the dermatitis is self-limited and regresses in approximately 2 weeks. In dermatitis produced by contact with weeds the eruption frequently appears in a linear streak at the site of brush contact. Characteristically, the eruption occurs on exposed areas, but the allergen may be carried to covered areas by the hands.

In differential diagnosis, nummular eczema and photosensitivity must be distinguished. Correlation of the history with responses to patch tests will frequently establish the causative allergen.

Treatment of all acute contact dermatitis is the same, irrespective of the cause. It consists in elimination of contact. Corticosteroids are the most effective agents for reducing the inflammatory reaction and lessening subjective reactions. Depending on the extent of involvement, they should be used locally or systemically. They are most effective when their administration is started prior to blister formation. For local treatment, 0.5 per cent hydrocortisone in a hydrophilic ointment is used. Systemic treatment is indicated only in children with widespread dermatitis; it may be given in full therapeutic doses for 5 to 7 days and stopped without fear of recurrence of the dermal lesions if contact with the allergen has been eliminated.

Prophylaxis is best accomplished by avoidance of contact. When poison ivy is the allergen, the child should be taught to recognize the vine. Thorough cleansing of the skin with soap and water within minutes of contact will prevent dermatitis. Hyposensitization may be tried by preseasonal treatment with the oral preparation of the ether-soluble fraction of *Rhus toxicodendron.* The antigen is administered daily by mouth in capsules in increasing doses and decreasing dilution, starting 2 to 3 months before expected contact.

Nummular Eczema. Nummular eczema is a common cutaneous reaction pattern characterized by the presence of round, papulovesicular patches. It is often an expression of atopic reactivity, but also occurs without family history of major hypersensitivity and without skin test evidence of atopic reactivity.

Histopathologically, the lesion is not diagnostic and consists of intercellular edema with slight endothelial swelling of the vessels in the dermis and a mild perivascular inflammatory infiltrate.

The individual patches are distinctively circinate, measuring from one to several centimeters in diameter. The lesions remain constant in size and location, occasionally clearing centrally. They are erythematous, palpably infiltrated, and ex-

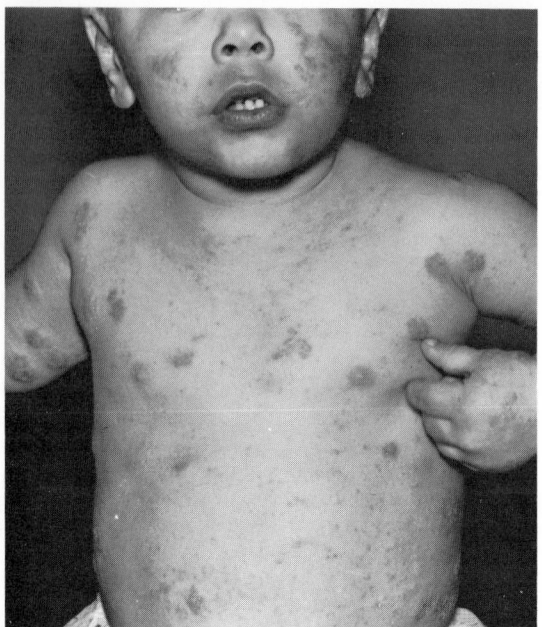

Figure 23-21. Nummular eczema in a 15-month-old child, showing scattered, pruritic, patchy, eczematous lesions.

tremely pruritic (Fig. 23-21). The primary lesions are papulovesicles, which later ooze and become crusted. The eruption often waxes and wanes; it tends to remain localized to hands and feet, but may be generalized. In differential diagnosis, tinea corporis, allergic contact dermatitis and pruritus hiemalis must be distinguished.

In treatment, allergic inhalants, ingestants and contact agents need to be regarded as causative possibilities and eliminated when indicated. Irrespective of the stage of the dermatitis, the most effective local treatment is the application of 0.5 to 1.0 per cent hydrocortisone (alcohol), 0.05 to 0.25 per cent triamcinolone cream; or 0.025 per cent 17-valerate of betamethasone in a cream base. The addition of 1 to 3 per cent iodochlorhydroxy-quinoline (Vioform) to the steroid cream may enhance its effectiveness. Antihistamines are of doubtful value, but some phenothiazines (such as Phenergan 6.25 to 12.5 mg. 3 to 4 times a day) may help control itching.

Drug Allergy. Drug allergy may be caused by diverse organic and inorganic substances which form conjugates with body protein and in this form act as allergens producing a reaction of hypersensitivity. Such reactions may occur in breast-fed infants from maternally administered drugs. The underlying factors which determine the capacity to become sensitized are unknown. Children who have inherited the atopic diathesis may be expected to have allergic reactions more frequently than others.

The histopathology of skin changes in drug allergy is not specific for individual drugs. Changes include endothelial swelling of the dermal blood vessels and a perivascular infiltrate of eosinophils,

histiocytes and lymphocytes. The epidermal changes may be minimal or profound with subepithelial blister formation. The morphology of the eruption varies greatly and may be that of practically any type characterized by sudden onset. Of the drugs used in pediatric practice, penicillin is most likely to produce an urticarial or erythema multiforme type of reaction; sulfonamides, novobiocin and barbiturates are apt to produce a maculopapular eruption; aspirin, angioneurotic edema of the face; phenothiazine derivatives and Declomycin, photosensitivity reactions (see below).

In diagnosis, biopsy is helpful in conjunction with basophile degranulation tests, the Schultz-Dale test utilizing monkey ileum, and lymphocyte transformation (p. 494).

The only satisfactory treatment is elimination of the drug; depending upon the severity of the reaction, this may be sufficient. The antihistaminic drugs are useful for relief of itching and for suppression of urticaria. Corticosteroids should be given in full therapeutic dosage for any severe generalized eruption. In widespread bullous involvement antibiotic therapy is indicated; previously administered ones, however, should not be selected. Local therapy in blistering reactions should include a wide-spectrum antibiotic ointment to prevent secondary bacterial infection.

ABNORMAL RESPONSES OF SKIN TO ULTRAVIOLET LIGHT

Exposure of the skin for a sufficient time to the ultraviolet portion of the spectrum (296 to 400 millimicrons) may produce a normal sunburn reaction or an abnormal cutaneous response. The normal response following exposure to sunlight consists of immediate pigmentation, produced mostly by the longer wavelengths of ultraviolet. After a latent period of about 8 hours the erythema of sunburn may appear, from wavelengths around 300 to 320 millimicrons, followed in several days by the pigmentation of delayed melanogenesis. After repeated exposures epidermal thickening, compacted stratum corneum and hyperpigmentation occur.

Abnormal cutaneous responses to ultraviolet (Table 23-2) are characterized by morphologic changes ranging from urticarial to eczematous reactions. These untoward cutaneous reactions may depend upon unknown factors (polymorphic light eruption), upon metabolic abnormalities (porphyrin, tryptophan), upon the ingestion or local application of photoactive agents such as phenothiazines, tetracyclines and halogenated salicylanilides, or upon specific reactivity to ultraviolet exposure in some diseases (lupus erythematosus).

Polymorphic Light Eruption. This is a recurrent erythematous dermatitis of unknown origin which appears on areas of the skin exposed to light in March or April in the north temperate zone and disappears spontaneously in August or September. The eruption is usually preceded by

TABLE 23-2. ABNORMAL RESPONSES OF SKIN TO ULTRAVIOLET LIGHT

I. Abnormal responses of skin to ultraviolet light
  A. Ultraviolet rays of wavelengths 280-320 mμ
    1. Recurrent summer eruptions
      a. Polymorphic light eruptions
      b. Hydroa vacciniforme
    2. Xeroderma pigmentosum
  B. Ultraviolet rays primarily of wavelengths longer than 320 mμ
    1. Erythropoietic protoporphyria
    2. Cockayne's syndrome
    3. Urticaria solare
    4. Hartnup's disease

II. Abnormal responses of skin to ultraviolet rays in conjunction with photoactive substances
  A. Substances administered systemically
    1. Sulfonamides
    2. Barbiturates
    3. Phenothiazine derivatives (chlorpromazine, Phenergan)
    4. Tetracyclines (Declomycin)
  B. Substances applied locally
    1. Furocoumarins (lime, parsley, parsnips, figs)
    2. Berloque (perfumes)
    3. Halogenated salicylanilides (soap)

III. Skin diseases flared by ultraviolet exposure
  A. Lupus erythematosus
  B. Pellagra

burning and itching shortly after exposure. Within hours pruritic, erythematous, urticaria-like papules appear on the exposed areas of the face, arms and hands. Subsequently the papules become confluent, forming relatively persistent plaques. Less commonly, eczematous patches with vesiculation appear as a morphologic variant. Tanning proceeds normally, and the skin returns to normal during the winter.

In differential diagnosis, lupus erythematosus, Hartnup disease and the porphyrias must be distinguished.

Therapy consists in the prophylactic use of sunscreens, such as 10 to 15 per cent PABA in hydrophilic ointment or red veterinary petrolatum with titanium dioxide (RVPaque). See Protective Effect (p. 1416). The antimalarial drugs such as chloroquin or Plaquenil are useful in treatment. Careful control is necessary because of the danger of drug toxicity. If the antimalarial drugs are used, ophthalmologic examination should precede treatment, and evaluation at 3-month intervals should be done, owing to the dangers of ocular toxicity.

The Porphyrias (see also p. 461). The porphyrias are a heterogeneous group of diseases characterized by the excretion either of porphyrins or of porphyrin precursors in the urine or stools.

Congenital porphyria is an extremely rare disorder of porphyrin metabolism characterized by blister formation on areas of skin exposed to light and the excretion of very large amounts of coproporphyrin and uroporphyrin. Hemolytic anemia and red teeth are usually present. Transmission is probably autosomal recessive.

Erythropoietic protoporphyria is a relatively uncommon abnormality of porphyrin metabolism characterized by photosensitivity in childhood, abnormal excretion of porphyrins in urine and slightly elevated fecal excretion of protoporphyrins. The skin changes include erythema, edema and itching of the exposed parts of the skin following brief exposure to sunlight. The reaction may be precipitated through window glass.

Hydroa aestivale and *hydroa vacciniforme* are photosensitive disturbances associated with erythropoietic protoporphyria. The aestivale variety consists of polymorphic skin lesions; the vacciniforme variety has been associated with blister formation and scarring. Histologically, the lesions resemble those of erythrocytic protoporphyria and consist of necrosis of the epidermis and adjacent dermis, with surrounding edema and a diffuse perivascular inflammatory infiltrate.

Treatment consists in avoidance of direct sunlight and the prophylactic use of sunscreens which eliminate all ultraviolet (benzophenones, Uval and RVP).

In **Hartnup disease** (p. 426) there is a photosensitive skin reaction during childhood, caused by an abnormality in tryptophan metabolism transmitted as an autosomal recessive trait. The clinical cutaneous picture resembles pellagra. Oral nicotinamide treatment is beneficial.

Cockayne's syndrome is characterized by the appearance of a photosensitive dermatitis, dwarfism, musculoskeletal anomalies, intracranial calcifications, hepatosplenomegaly, senile facies and ophthalmologic abnormalities. Neurologic defects appear during the second year of life. The photosensitivity of the skin is characterized by erythema, scaling and crusting, followed by hyperpigmentation and scarring.

In the differential diagnosis, progeria, Bloom's syndrome, Rothmund-Thomson syndrome, ataxia-telangiectasia and dyskeratosis congenita should be considered. Photosensitivity of the skin is a useful differential diagnostic point, for ultraviolet sensitivity is not found in progeria, is rare in dyskeratosis congenita, occurs occasionally in the Rothmund-Thomson syndrome, and is expected in Bloom's syndrome and ataxia-telangiectasia.

Bloom's syndrome is a heritable dermatosis characterized by telangiectatic erythema of the face, photosensitivity, small stature and a low birth weight after full-term gestation. The differential diagnosis includes such diseases as might be confused with Cockayne's syndrome.

Poikiloderma Congenita (Rothmund-Thomson Syndrome). Poikiloderma congenita is a rare hereditary dermatosis characterized by an initial inflammatory reaction followed by telangiectases, pigmentation and atrophy, and, in some instances, alteration of hair growth, juvenile cataracts, congenital bone defects, and photosensitivity. The syndrome is probably transmitted as a recessive trait.

Skin changes may be present at birth, but generally erythema and edema of the face appear before the sixth month of life. Soon the extensor and later the flexural surfaces of the extremities and the buttocks become involved. The process progresses slowly, and by the fifth year the erythematous phase subsides, leaving punctate areas of atrophy, telangiectasia and hyperpigmentation. Many patients have absent or sparse eyebrows and eyelashes as well as areas of alopecia or diminished hair on the scalp.

No treatment is known to be effective.

Xeroderma Pigmentosum (Malignant Freckles). This is a rare, hereditary skin disease which appears in the early years of life and is characterized by large freckles, areas of cutaneous atrophy, keratoses, photophobia and conjunctivitis. Eventual development of multiple skin cancers will lead to early death. The disease is inherited in a simple recessive manner. Relatives of affected children frequently have a tendency to intense freckling.

Histopathologically, atrophy alternating with acanthosis and hyperkeratosis are seen. There is much melanin deposition in the basal cell layer, basophilic degeneration of the collagen, disappearance of the elastic fibers and thinning of the dermis. The capillaries are relatively few, and large venules are common. The earliest symptom is avoidance of light because of photophobia. Erythema of the conjunctiva occurs on the first exposure of the infant to direct sunlight and recurs on subsequent exposures. Erythema followed by intense freckling of the exposed skin develops rapidly in areas exposed to direct sunlight. After a few months or years, telangiectases and atrophy appear in the freckled areas; warty, hard keratoses and multiple malignant skin tumors follow shortly. The tumors may be squamous cell carcinomas, sarcomas, basal cell carcinomas and even melanomas; death usually occurs in the adolescent years.

Therapy is nonspecific, consisting in protection from light and removal of malignant neoplasms when they appear. The prognosis is poor.

PAPULOSQUAMOUS ERUPTIONS

Pityriasis Rosea. Pityriasis rosea is an acute, self-limited disease probably infectious in origin. It is characterized by the appearance of pinkish, oval scaling lesions distributed mostly on the trunk. Histopathologically, there is a nonspecific dermatitic reaction consisting of intercellular edema, exocytosis, and a perivascular inflammatory infiltrate of lymphocytes, histiocytes and occasional polymorphonuclear leukocytes and plasma cells.

In the majority of instances the first sign is a solitary, erythematous papule on the trunk which enlarges peripherally and clears centrally (the herald lesion). Occasionally there is a mild prodrome of headache, malaise, pharyngitis and lymphadenitis. Within 5 to 14 days an erythem-

atous eruption similar to the original lesion except smaller, following the lines of skin cleavage, appears on the trunk and proximal portion of the arms and legs. In some instances the morphology of the eruption may be predominantly papulovesicular. The disease rarely occurs before 1 year of age.

In differential diagnosis the primary lesion must be differentiated from tinea corporis; the scaling lesion, from guttate psoriasis and seborrheic dermatitis; and the papulovesicular eruption, from nummular eczema.

Treatment is symptomatic in mild cases and consists of a local application of a cream containing solution of coal tar (10 per cent) and salicylic acid (2 per cent) or an anti-inflammatory cream of 0.5 per cent hydrocortisone. In addition, an erythema-producing dose of ultraviolet seems to have an ameliorating effect.

In children with severe pruritus and extensive eruption, administration of a corticosteroid orally for 5 to 7 days is justified.

Seborrheic Dermatitis. Seborrheic dermatitis is a chronic, recurrent inflammatory reaction of the skin transmitted genetically and characterized by a tendency to a dermatitic reaction in the scalp and intertriginous areas, vulnerability to secondary bacterial and yeast infections in the affected areas, and oily skin during adolescence.

Histopathologically, the lesion is not diagnostic; it consists of intermittent parakeratosis and variable acanthosis, intercellular edema, some inflammatory cells in the epidermis and mild perivascular inflammatory infiltrate in the dermis.

The most common expressions of seborrheic diathesis in infants and children in order of frequency are (1) "cradle cap," (2) intertriginous eruption beginning in the genitocrural fold of the diaper area (Figs. 23-22, 23-22A [p. 1385]), (3)

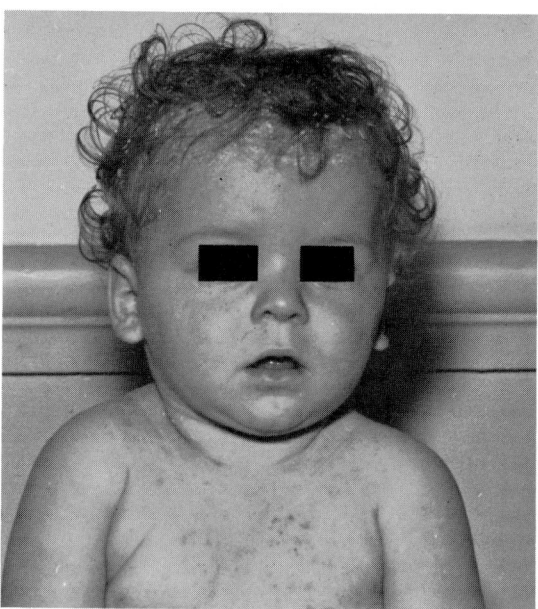

Figure 23-22. A 10-month-old boy with erythematous, papulosquamous eruption in a seborrheic distribution.

dermatitis in the auriculocephalic fold; (4) blepharitis, (5) otitis externa, (6) exfoliative erythroderma (Leiner's disease).

Cradle cap, common in infancy, varies considerably in severity. It is characterized by adherent, yellowish, scaling or crusted patches of plaques on the scalp; when it is extensive, the forehead may also be involved. Similar eruptions may also be located on the lid margins, external ears, genitocrural folds or postauricular areas. There may be mild inflammatory changes.

Leiner's disease is a severe expression of seborrheic dermatitis. It is characterized by the presence of an exfoliative, erythematous eruption which starts in any of the areas mentioned above and progresses to become generalized.

In differential diagnosis the following diseases should be distinguished: psoriasis, Letterer-Siwe disease and tinea capitis.

Treatment of the scalp consists of daily shampoos followed by application of a local preparation containing sulfur (2 per cent), salicylic acid or coal tar (5 to 10 per cent) alone or in combination (Pragmatar). The dermatitic reaction in the other areas responds promptly to the local application of 0.5 per cent hydrocortisone cream alone or in combination with 2 per cent sulfur.

Psoriasis. Psoriasis is a chronic, recurrent disease of unknown origin transmitted as an autosomal, irregular dominant trait and characterized by sharply circumscribed scaly patches. The histopathologic picture characteristically reveals parakeratosis, a diminished or absent granular layer, acanthosis, papillomatosis with thinned suprapapillary plate, mild perivascular infiltrate and microabscesses in the epidermis. On the other hand, morphologically characteristic skin lesions frequently have a nonspecific dermatitic reaction.

Psoriasis is not common in children under 6 years of age and, when compared to the adult disease, is usually atypical in its morphology and course. Often the only evidences of the disease are single or multiple sharply circumscribed, erythematous, scaling patches on the scalp or fine, pitted stippling of all or most of the nails without skin changes (Fig. 23-23, *A*). At times an erythematous papular eruption appears suddenly and becomes scaly within 7 to 14 days. In many instances the eruption is transient and clears completely, so that one only suspects that it is psoriasis; sooner or later the typical changes consisting of chronic circumscribed patches with a micaceous scale as seen in adults appear (Fig. 23-23, *B*).

The lesions must be differentiated from those of pityriasis rosea, seborrhea, secondary syphilis and drug eruptions; in addition, the scalp lesion must be distinguished from seborrhea and tinea capitis.

Response to treatment in young children is usually prompt with 5 to 10 per cent solution of coal tar and 2 per cent salicylic acid in hydrophilic ointment. Intertriginous involvement responds promptly to an anti-inflammatory cream (0.025 per cent triamcinolone) because of ease of percutaneous absorption in this anatomic area. Scalp lesions

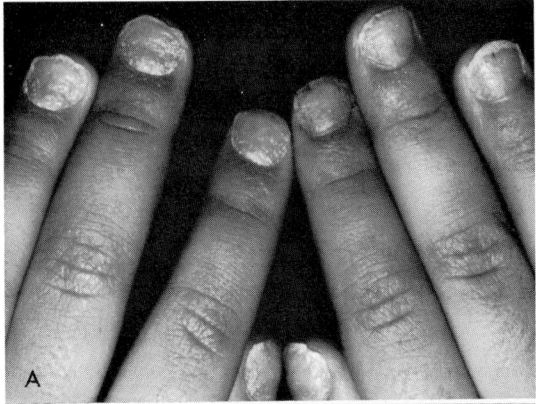

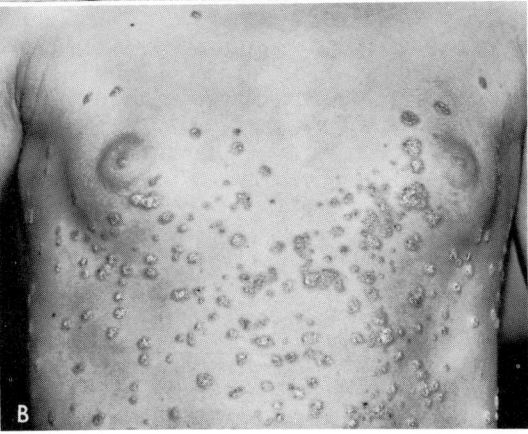

Figure 23-23. *A*, Psoriasis of the nails, showing characteristic pits in all nails. The skin was clear, but psoriatic skin lesions appeared later. *B*, Psoriasis of 3 weeks' duration in an 11-year-old child, showing erythematous, scaling papules.

may be treated with 2 to 4 per cent salicylic acid ointment or 10 per cent solution of coal tar in olive oil, or the 17-valerate of beta methasone (Valisone) in a cream base may be effective. Recalcitrant patches may be managed with 20 per cent oil of cade, 10 per cent sulfur and 5 per cent salicylic acid in petrolatum.

Pityriasis Alba. Pityriasis alba is a chronic, slightly inflammatory disease of unknown origin which is characterized by patchy scaling and hypopigmentation on the face.

Histopathologically, the changes are mild and consist of parakeratosis, acanthosis and spongiosis and a predominantly lymphocytic perivascular infiltrate in the upper corium.

There may be one or more sharply circumscribed, slightly erythematous, scaling hypopigmented patches on the cheeks, chin and forehead. Untreated lesions persist for many months; there are no symptoms.

Differential diagnosis includes vitiligo and postinflammatory depigmentation.

Regression can be produced by a variety of local therapeutic preparations such as 2 per cent salicylic acid in hydrophylic petrolatum, a broad-spectrum antibiotic such as Neosporin or perhaps

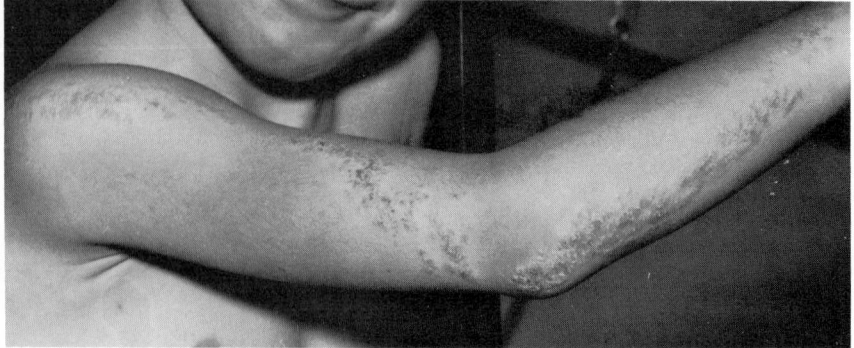

Figure 23-24. Lichen striatus in a 2½-year-old boy, showing the range of morphologic variation from lichenoid papules proximally to confluent eczematous patches distally.

most effectively by an anti-inflammatory agent (0.5 per cent hydrocortisone).

Lichen Striatus. Lichen striatus is an asymptomatic inflammatory eruption of unknown origin occurring principally in children. It is characterized by rapid appearance, usually on the extremities, of a nonsegmental linear papular eruption.

The histopathologic changes are not characteristic; there are perivascular inflammatory infiltrate, intercellular edema in the prickle layer and some hyperkeratosis.

Initially the eruption consists of discrete, erythematous, lichenoid papules in linear patterns. They rapidly coalesce to form a scaly dermatitic reaction (Fig. 23-24). The eruption usually regresses spontaneously, but occasionally may persist for a long time. Linear ectodermal nevus, the lesions of lichen planus, psoriasis and verruca occurring at sites of skin trauma as in a scratch should be differentiated.

Resolution of the lesion can be hastened by local application of 0.05 per cent triamcinolone cream beneath a plastic covering.

Lichen Nitidus. Lichen nitidus is an inflammatory disease of unknown origin characterized by an asymptomatic papular eruption on the flexor surfaces of the wrists, elbows, hands, genitalia or abdomen.

Histopathologically, the infiltrate consists of lymphocytes, epithelioid cells and occasional giant cells limited to papillary and subpapillary areas of the dermis. The papules are pinhead in size, slightly raised, slightly erythematous or waxy and semitranslucent, suggestive of deep-seated vesicles. They do not coalesce. Although the lesions usually remain localized, they may be widely distributed, and may occur along a scratch mark.

In differential diagnosis flat warts and lichen scrofulosus should be distinguished.

BACTERIAL INFECTIONS

The bacterial flora of the normal skin may be divided into 2 categories: transient organisms which may be cultured at one time or another, and resident organisms which multiply freely on the skin. The resident flora of children is different from that of adults and includes Sarcina, gram-positive facultative anaerobic bacilli which are mainly spore formers, Neisseria, and nonhemolytic streptococci. Establishment of the normal flora of the skin apparently begins about the fourth day of life. Colonization by staphylococci may begin in the first few hours after delivery.

The skin of infants and children differs from that of adults in its resistance and in its response to pathogenic staphylococci and streptococci. The high frequency of primary pyogenic infection of the skin in children reflects altered resistance, and the ease of blister production with pus-forming microorganisms indicates an altered response, which may be due to immaturity of the skin or to biochemical factors. The clinical patterns produced by infection of the skin with these microorganisms are extremely variable.

Primary pyodermas include dermatitis exfoliativa neonatorum (Ritter's disease, toxic epidermal necrolysis, see p. 1377, pemphigus neonatorum, impetigo, ecthyma, folliculitis, furunculosis (furuncles and carbuncles), eccrine sweat gland infections (periporitis), paronychial infections and erysipelas.

In *secondary pyodermas* bacterial infection may complicate a wide variety of pre-existing skin lesions, most frequently atopic dermatitis, allergic contact dermatitis and seborrheic dermatitis. The possibility of such infection must be continually in mind, for infected eczematized lesions may show only crusting, without purulent discharge, cellulitis, lymphangitis or lymphadenitis. The smear and culture of chronic eczematized lesions for bacteria are essential for management.

Impetigo contagiosa is a superficial infection of the skin caused by beta hemolytic streptococci, group A, or by coagulase-positive hemolytic *Staphylococcus aureus.* There are vesicular or pustular lesions which rapidly become exudative and crusted. Pathologically, the subcorneal blister in the epidermis is the same whether the infection is caused by streptococci or staphylococci. The stratum granulosum usually remains intact and forms the base of the blister. The blister fluid is filled with numerous polymorphonuclear leuko-

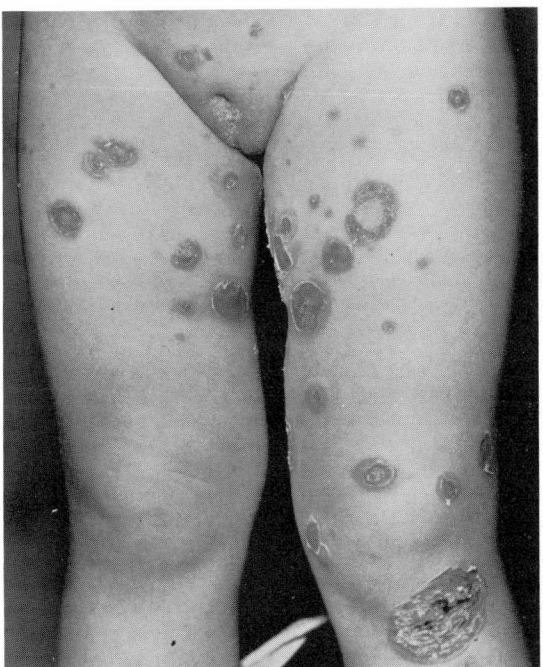

Figure 23-26. Impetigo, showing vesiculobullous lesions and crusting. Some lesions have cleared centrally and spread peripherally, simulating a ringworm infection.

cytes. There are perivascular inflammation and dilatation of the capillaries in the upper portion of the dermis.

The earliest skin changes consist of a blister with serum which rapidly becomes cloudy. The superficial location of the blisters makes them prone to early rupture, with the formation of yellowish, nonadherent crusts surrounded by erythema (Fig. 23-26). The individual lesions vary in size from a few millimeters to several centimeters. There is a tendency for central clearing and peripheral spreading, with the development of circles, arcs or serpiginous morphology. The infection occurs most commonly on the face, less frequently on the extremities and trunk. Removal of crusts leaves a weeping surface from which bacteria can be readily recovered; the disease is autoinoculable. The morphology does not differentiate between the causative organisms, but regional lymphadenopathy may be more frequent with streptococcal infection.

The yield of streptococci may be incorrectly low, unless precautions are taken in the diagnostic bacterial culture to offset the tendency of *Staphylococcus aureus* to overgrow and prevent identification of streptococci. The phage type of staphylococcus found in both pure and mixed impetigo is most commonly group 2 type 71. The earlier the lesion is cultured, the more likely streptococci are to be found, whereas staphylococci are most commonly isolated from older lesions. It is suggested that staphylococcus is often a secondary invader. The finding of an elevated ASO titer in patients with staphylococcal impetigo, but no history or culture of streptococci in the throat, strengthens this hypothesis.

Glomerular nephritis (see p. 1124) is a frequent complication of skin infection caused by group A streptococci. It most commonly follows impetigo, but may also follow secondarily infected eczematous dermatitis. The nephritogenic strains causing skin infection have different serotypes from those producing pharyngitis and nephritis. Nephritis following skin infection has its peak incidence in late summer and early fall, whereas nephritis and rheumatic fever following streptococcal pharyngitis occur chiefly in winter and spring. The incidence of positive streptococcal throat cultures is usually no higher in patients with either staphylococcal or streptococcal impetigo than in the general population. The incidence of nasal carriage of staphylococcus is high, however, in patients with staphylococcal impetigo, and in most instances the same phage type can be found in both nose and skin.

Since impetigo appears to be primarily a streptococcal infection which may be caused by nephritogenic strains of beta hemolytic streptococci, systemic antibiotic therapy is indicated. Penicillin is the drug of choice in streptococcal infections. Since over 50 per cent of the staphylococci recovered from skin infections are resistant to penicillin G, a semisynthetic penicillin may be preferred for treatment. Epidemics of bacterial infection complicated by nephritis sometimes occur which demand mass prophylaxis with penicillin. Local antibacterial treatment may control the infection if properly carried out. Crusts should be gently scrubbed off with cotton, using water and a soap substitute containing hexachlorophene. Then an antibiotic ointment containing bacitracin and neomycin is applied. To prevent autoinoculation, a soap substitute containing hexachlorophene is suggested for general cleansing, and the use of an ointment containing neomycin and bacitracin in the nares and beneath the fingernails is helpful.

Ecthyma is a superficial pyogenic infection of the skin caused by either staphylococci or streptococci, involving both the epidermis and dermis, and ultimately resulting in scarring. The pathologic changes differ from impetigo in the superficial ulceration of the epidermis and involvement of the dermis. The vessels in the epidermis are dilated at the periphery of the erosion and are frequently thrombosed near the center; beneath the degenerating epithelium the connective tissue may be necrotic and contain numerous polymorphonuclear leukocytes.

The primary lesion is a pustule which ruptures after several days. The patient is usually first seen with a crusted lesion; the crust is adherent peripherally and when removed leaves a small ulceration. The lesions may be multiple and vary in size from 0.5 to 2 cm. In the course of several weeks the lesions heal, leaving a scar with hyperpigmentation at the border. Lesions occur most frequently on the lower extremities below the knees. As with impetigo, the disease is infectious and autoinoculable. The patient should be investigated and treated as for impetigo. Usually, local treatment is all that is necessary in staphylococcal infection.

Bacterial infection of appendageal structures of the skin with staphylococci results in a variable clinical picture depending on the anatomic site of invasion and the depth of infection in eccrine sweat glands (periporitis and multiple sweat gland abscesses), in the pilosebaceous apparatus (folliculitis, furuncle, carbuncle) or in apocrine sweat glands (hidradenitis suppurativa). The main differences between the adnexal infections depend on the different anatomic distributions of the structures. Eccrine gland infections are seen most frequently during infancy; follicular infections occur at any age; apocrine sweat gland infections occur at puberty. The pathologic picture is similar and may vary from a periductal or perifollicular inflammatory process to dermal necrosis with abscess formation deep in the dermis or in the subcutaneous tissue.

Folliculitis is a superficial staphylococcal infection of the hair follicle. Usually there are multiple erythematous pustules centered about individual hair follicles. The individual infection is often self-limited and, if unscratched, dries up and forms a crust. Because of itching, lesions are scratched and the infection is disseminated.

A *furuncle* is a deeper staphylococcal infection of the hair follicle, producing an area of central necrosis. Furuncles are usually solitary, but may occur in successive crops (*furunculosis*). A *carbuncle* is a group of closely connected follicular infections with still deeper involvement of the hair follicles and penetration into the subcutaneous tissue. Deep follicular infection produces a red, extremely tender papule which becomes a pustule, with a central core which may be expressed 3 to 4 days after onset of the infection. Furuncles occur wherever there are hair follicles, but are most common on the buttocks, extremities and scalp. Infections in the central portion of the face constitute a threat to life because of the possibility of cavernous sinus thrombosis.

Hidradenitis suppurativa is an acute staphylococcal infection of the apocrine sweat glands, which are found on the female breast, in the inguinal regions and around the genitalia, in the axillae, and in the perianal region and buttocks. It is most common during the pubertal and postpubertal periods. Infection occurs most often in the axilla and is often mistaken for furunculosis. An erythematous, tender, solitary, deep-seated nodule appears that develops into an abscess, which may rupture spontaneously and resolve or become persistent. New nodules develop, and if lesions persist, a chronic, deep-seated infection with discharging sinuses and intercommunicating tracts and scar tissue develops.

Periporitis and *multiple sweat gland abscesses* are superficial and deep infections of the eccrine sweat glands which may occur in a few follicles or be generalized. The individual eccrine infections resemble those seen with folliculitis and furun-

culosis except that hairs cannot be found in the central portion of the inflammatory process. The severest form of infection is most commonly seen in infants under 1 year of age, in whom the infection may be progressive, old lesions regressing and new ones appearing as in chronic furunculosis.

Isolated lesions of the adnexa of the skin should be treated with intermittent hot surgical soaks until the lesions localize and drain. Local antibiotics are indicated, but systemic antibiotics are not usually necessary unless the infection occurs in the central area of the face. Surgical intervention is contraindicated because of the possibility of dissemination of the staphylococci and because scarring is increased. After localization of the infection the fluctuant area is opened or aspirated to allow drainage.

In recurrent infections a search for systemic causes such as abnormalities of immune mechanisms should be made, in addition to an epidemiologic survey of persons in the patient's environment. Prophylactic measures are indicated, as for impetigo, and an epidemiologic survey of the family should include nasopharyngeal cultures and phage typing of the staphylococci isolated. All members of an involved family should use a soap substitute containing hexachlorophene and rinse their hands with 70 per cent alcohol. An ointment containing neomycin and bacitracin may be used in the nostrils, under the fingernails and in the perianal area. There is no clear evidence that staphylococcal vaccines or toxoids are helpful. Patients should be advised to avoid sharing towels and washcloths with other members of the family.

Treatment of isolated infections is generally satisfactory, but widespread sweat gland infections with abscesses present special problems. In hidradenitis suppurativa, in addition to the routine management outlined above, the chronic sinus tracts should be marsupialized. In old scarred areas with multiple sinus tracts, block excision is necessary.

Pseudomonas Infections. In septicemia due to *Pseudomonas aeruginosa*, skin lesions consisting of yellowish-green pustules with a surrounding zone of erythema often appear suddenly. The pustules discharge a mucoid material with a characteristic fruity odor and subsequently become necrotic, leaving a punched-out ulcer which slowly enlarges. Occasionally, large necrotic lesions produced by an endotoxin of the organism will appear as the first cutaneous lesion.

Tuberculosis of the Skin. For erythema nodosum, see page 530.

Cutaneous tuberculosis is rare in the United States. The tubercle bacillus may invade the skin directly through an abrasion (primary infection), by continuity from an underlying tuberculous lesion such as that of a lymph node, or by hematogenous distribution. Cutaneous lesions such as tuberculides and erythema nodosum may also be produced by circulating toxins of the tubercle bacillus.

In *primary tuberculous lesions* tubercle bacilli invade the skin or mucous membrane through abrasions; the intact skin is not vulnerable. The resemblance of the primary lesion to a syphilitic chancre is at times striking. The common sites are the lip, nose, chin, extremities and genital region; there is an accompanying involvement of the regional lymph nodes to complete the primary complex. The initial lesion may occur as a dark red papule, a small crusted ulcer with an elevated border or as a small plaque. Tubercle bacilli may be found in the skin lesion and in the lymph nodes; the histologic findings are those of tuberculosis. Excision of the primary lesion and of the lymph nodes is indicated if they are in appropriate sites. Antibacterial therapy is indicated in all instances (see p. 606).

Lupus vulgaris frequently begins in childhood as numerous pinpoint- to pinhead-sized, grouped or disseminated, reddish, yellowish or brownish, flat papules. Gradually they enlarge to form tubercles or nodules which in turn coalesce into variously shaped and sized pustules. Although extension continues slowly, the older lesions may disappear, leaving a scaly, atrophic scar, or they may ulcerate, form crusts and eventually heal with a residual scar. The disease is chronic and may persist into adult life with considerable disfigurement.

Scrofuloderma begins in one or more lymph nodes or in bone and extends to the surface to involve the skin in a true tuberculous process. When lymph nodes are involved, they are initially swollen and painful, but later undergo caseation and suppuration and form sinuses which discharge a caseous, sanious pus. The resultant skin involvement appears as an oval or linear ulceration with violaceous, undermined edges and an uneven base with pale, flabby granulations. The surface may be crusted.

The lesions of *lichen scrofulosus* are pinhead-sized, firm, yellowish-brown or reddish nodules. The nodules coalesce into coin-sized patches and are situated chiefly on the trunk. They may be accompanied by slight itching. The course is chronic, although the prognosis is favorable.

Tuberculides are thought to be caused by the toxins of the tubercle bacillus, the most common lesion in children being the papulonecrotic tuberculide. The lesions, which appear in crops, are pea-sized or smaller, firm, bluish-red papules, crusted at the summit. When the crust is removed, there is a crater-like depression. Search should be made for the primary tuberculous focus, which is usually in the lungs.

Treatment of tuberculosis of the skin consists in improving the general health by means of fresh air, sunshine, vitamin D and an adequate diet. Antimicrobial therapy is indicated in all instances in children irrespective of apparent activity of other lesions (see p. 606).

Swimming Pool Granuloma. Swimming pool granuloma is a chronic infection of the skin caused by *Mycobacterium balnei*, an acid-fast rod antigenically related to *Mycobacterium tuberculosis*. This organism may grow in warm, nonchlorinated cement swimming pools, where it may gain entrance into traumatized skin.

Histopathologically, there is a nonspecific granulomatous infiltrate in which the organisms may be found. The skin lesions appear 3 to 6 weeks after a self-healing abrasion as brownish-red papules which coalesce to form a nodule, often on the elbows or knees. Later the nodule may become a crusted ulcer, which may persist for months. The nodules are usually but not invariably single. Regional lymphadenopathy is minimal or absent. In differential diagnosis, primary tuberculosis must be distinguished.

Prophylaxis consists in chlorination and in covering the cement surfaces of swimming pools with porcelain tile. The granulomas usually regress spontaneously within a few months; the organism is only moderately sensitive to streptomycin and is resistant to para-aminosalicylic acid and isoniazid.

FUNGUS INFECTIONS

The dermatomycoses are caused by highly specialized fungi, the dermatophytes. In their parasitic phase their growth is restricted to the keratinized structures. In children these organisms produce morphologically distinct diseases of the skin, mucous membranes and dermal appendages.

TINEA CAPITIS
(RINGWORM OF THE SCALP)

Etiology. Tinea capitis is caused by species of the genera Microsporum and Trichophyton. The source of infection varies: *M. audouini*, *T. tonsurans*, *T. violaceum*, *T. sulfureum* and *T. schoenleini* are transmitted from person to person; *M. canis*, *T. mentagrophytes* and *T. verrucosum* are contracted principally from animals; *M. gypseum* is acquired from soil. In the United States most epidemics are caused by *M. audouini*.

Clinical Manifestations. The clinical lesion varies from scaly, circumscribed patches resembling seborrhea to patchy, scaling areas of alopecia with broken hairs (Fig. 23-27). Generally the infection is asymptomatic, although a severe inflammatory reaction representing hypersensitivity of the host to the invading organism may occur (kerion). *Trichophyton schoenleini* infection produces a specific type of host response (favus) characterized by a peculiar mousey odor and cup-shaped, yellowish-brown crusts (scutula); it produces scarring and permanent alopecia.

Diagnosis. Examination of the scalp with a Wood's light which emits monochromatic ultraviolet (365 millimicrons) is a rapid, useful method for screening children with suspected infection. Only *M. audouini* and *M. canis* infections respond with typical greenish-white fluorescence. Hairs in-

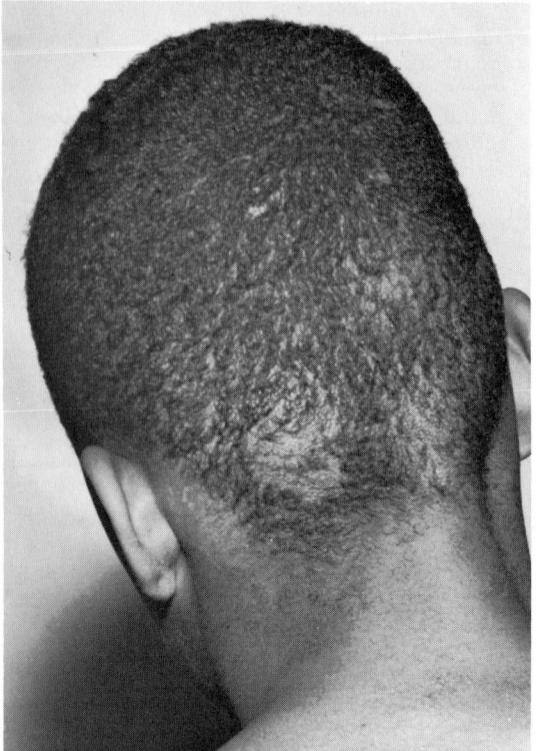

Figure 23-27. Tinea capitis, showing patchy scaling and loss of hair, but negative fluorescence under Wood's lamp. *Trichophyton sulfureum* was isolated on culture.

fected by *T. schoenleini* produce variable fluorescence, whereas other trichophyton infections are not fluorescent. Falsely positive or falsely negative fluorescence of hairs may result from the use of local medications. Direct microscopic examination of affected hairs in a 10 per cent solution of potassium hydroxide or in chlorolactophenol is necessary for positive diagnosis; culture is required for identification of species.

Alopecia areata, trichotillomania, monilethrix and loss of hair from inflammatory lesions must be considered in differential diagnosis.

Prevention. Transmission of infection from person to person (*M. audouini* and trichophyton species) is possible for the duration of the disease. Fortunately, there are significant host factors which do not permit easy infection of contacts.

Treatment. Oral administration of griseofulvin has revolutionized the treatment of infections of the scalp by all species of dermatophytes. A dose of 10 mg. per pound per day for 7 to 10 days results in cure in the majority of instances. Rarely a dose of 20 to 40 mg. per pound per day will be required.

Local therapy is probably not necessary, but the application of a strong antifungal ointment such as Whitfield's ointment, U.S.P. XV (12 per cent benzoic acid and 6 per cent salicylic acid), is advisable. Criteria for cure should include a negative direct microscopic examination and a negative culture. Fluorescence alone is unreliable as a crite-

rion of cure, since some of the fluorescence may be lasting even in the absence of demonstrable mycelia.

TINEA CORPORIS

Infection on the skin is caused by species of genera Trichophyton, Microsporum and Epidermophyton through close contact with infected animals or human beings. Generally the lesion is a round or oval, erythematous scaling patch which spreads peripherally and clears centrally. The spreading border is rather intensely inflamed and may become vesiculated.

A direct microscopic examination of scales from the periphery of a lesion will serve to differentiate the fungus infection from pityriasis rosea, nummular eczema, pityriasis alba, psoriasis and seborrheic dermatitis. The scalp should always be examined for evidence of infection when the glabrous skin is infected.

Treatment. The local treatment of choice is Whitfield's Ointment, U.S.P. XVI (6 per cent benzoic acid and 3 per cent salicylic acid). If local treatment fails, griseofulvin in a daily dose of 10 mg. per pound for 10 to 14 days in combination with local therapy will usually clear the infection.

TINEA CRURIS

Infection of the skin in the genitocrural region is rare in the preadolescent; it is most frequently caused by *E. floccosum* and *T. rubrum*. The response of the skin to the invading organism is similar to that to *T. corporis*, with central clearing and peripheral spreading. The infection remains localized, however, to the medial proximal aspect of the thigh and crural fold, but the skin of the scrotum may be involved. The intertriginous area should also be examined for evidence of infection. In differential diagnosis seborrheic psoriasis, seborrheic dermatitis and localized neurodermatitis should be considered.

The infection will in most instances respond promptly to an oil-in-water base (hydrophilic ointment, U.S.P. XVI) containing 2 per cent salicylic acid and 5 per cent benzoic acid.

TINEA PEDIS
(ATHLETE'S FOOT)

Infection of the intertriginous areas between the toes or on the plantar surface of the feet is usually caused by *E. floccosum, T. rubrum* and *T. interdigitale*.

Although infection occurs most frequently in adolescents and postadolescents, dermatophytic infections occasionally occur in preadolescent children. The lesions may vary from maceration and fissuring between the toes to patches with pinhead-sized vesicles on the plantar surface.

Candidiasis and nocardiosis (erythrasma) between the toes may produce lesions indistinguishable from those of tinea infections. A direct microscopic examination of scrapings will serve to differentiate them. Nocardial infected tissue will characteristically produce a coral-red fluorescence when examined under the Wood's lamp.

Local treatment of choice is Whitfield's Ointment, U.S.P. XVI. In chronic recurrent fungal infections between the toes, therapy with griseofulvin has not been very effective.

TINEA VERSICOLOR

Tinea versicolor is a benign, chronic superficial fungus infection caused by *Malassezia furfur*. It is a common infection world-wide in distribution, occurring most frequently in adults in temperate climates, but with frequency in younger age groups in the tropics. Pathologically, there are abundant short blunt mycelia and spores in the horny layer of the skin. The clinical picture is characterized by the occurrence of pigmented or hypopigmented maculopapular spots, patches or large confluent areas (Fig. 23-28), with an inapparent scale which may be easily demonstrated by light scratching. Infection occurs most frequently on the trunk, but may also appear on the neck, face, and proximal portions of the arms and legs. In infants there is a tendency to involve the face and diaper area. The epidemiology of the infection is not completely understood, but there is a familial tendency to susceptibility and also increased susceptibility in the presence of excessive glucocorticoid hormones (in Cushing's disease or iatrogenic hyperadrenal states). In differential diagnosis, localization of the infection to the face may suggest pityriasis alba, vitiligo or seborrheic dermatitis, from which it can usually be distinguished by the presence of organisms on the direct microscopic examination of a scale in potassium hydroxide. The use of almost any mild antifungal preparation is effective in the management of the infection, but recurrence is

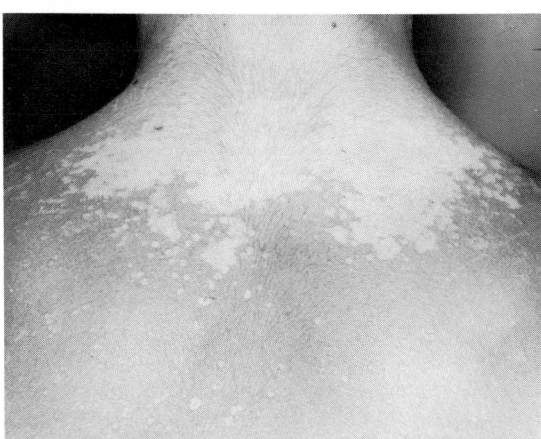

Figure 23-28. Tinea versicolor in an 11-year-old boy, showing discrete and confluent, hypopigmented areas. The patient's father had a similar infection.

common. A preparation of 2 per cent salicylic acid and 5 per cent benzoic acid in 70 per cent isopropyl alcohol or in hydrophilic ointment, U.S.P. XVI, applied once or twice daily is effective. A suspension of selenium sulfide (Selsun) applied in a thin layer after bathing is also effective, but this preparation should not be applied in the anogenital region because of the likelihood of irritation.

CANDIDIASIS

See also pages 763, 1202, 1209 and 1398.

A yeastlike fungus which can be recovered from the intestinal tract and mucous membranes of normal persons may cause infection of the mouth (thrush) (Fig. 23-29, *A*), nails (paronychia), vagina and intertriginous areas, and occasionally systemic infection. Oral thrush is a relatively common infection in newborn infants, including otherwise healthy ones. Subsequently moniliasis is practically nonexistent in healthy persons. These infections are usually caused by *Candida albicans*, but may be produced by *C. tropicalis, C. stellatoidea, C. parakrusei* and *C. guilliermondi*. In children with debilitating disease (hypoparathyroidism, hypoadrenalism, acrodermatitis chronica enteropathica, immunologic incompetence, Letterer-Siwe disease) such infections may be widespread and persistent.

Intertriginous moniliasis involving the genitocrural fold, gluteal fold, axillae and umbilicus is characterized by a sharply circumscribed, erythematous, moist surface with scattered, superficial satellite pustules. The infection is most frequently confused with a pyoderma because of the pustules, but organisms can be differentiated easily on direct microscopic examination or by culture on Sabouraud's medium. The infection can usually be cleared rapidly by sponging the area with 1:5000 benzalkonium chloride (U.S.P.) 3 times a day followed by local application of a cream containing nystatin (Mycolog) or amphotericin B (Fungizone).

Paronychial infection is characterized by erythema and swelling of the paronychial area and horizontal ridging of the nails after the infection has been established for several months (Fig. 23-29, *B*). It is seen most frequently on the thumbs of infants and children who are finger-suckers. Yeast paronychial infection must be differentiated from infection by staphylococci. The infection is best treated by soaking the involved fingers in 1:5000 benzalkonium chloride followed by application of 2 per cent salicylic acid in a 30 per cent alcohol solution. In order to cure the infection, the thumb should be protected to prevent sucking.

In widespread cutaneous infection accompanying underlying systemic disease, the infection does not remain localized to the intertriginous areas or mucous membranes, but spreads over the trunk, face, scalp and extremities (Fig. 23-29, *C*). The cutaneous lesions may be sharply demarcated or confluent, forming hyperkeratotic scaling

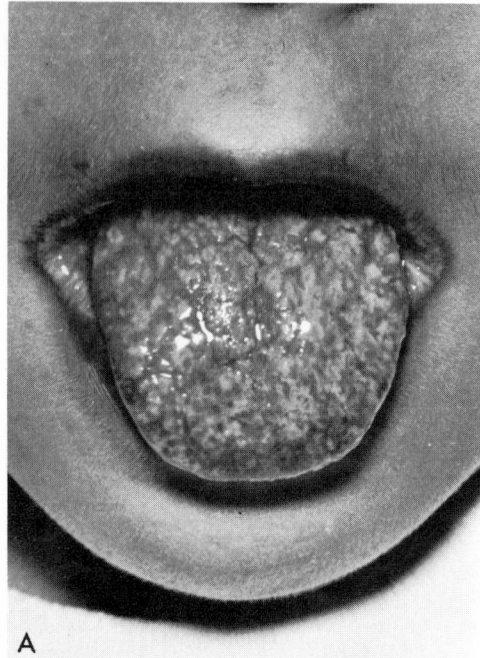

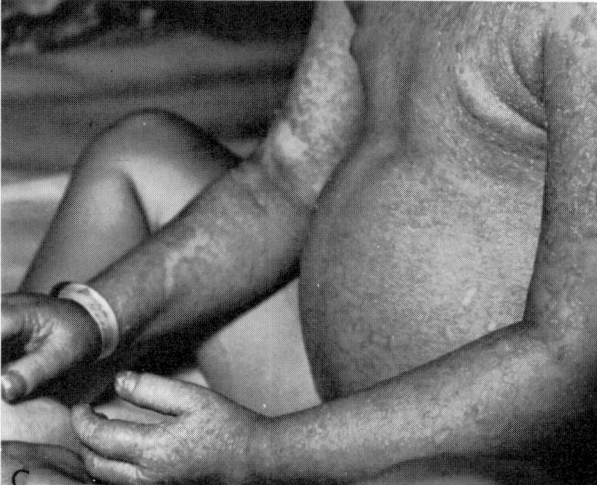

Figure 23-29. Candidiasis. *A*, Three-year-old boy with oral mucosal infection. *B*, Paronychial infection in 3-year-old boy who was a thumbsucker. *C*, Three-and-one-half-year-old girl with widespread skin, paronychial and mucosal infection associated with systemic disease.

patches which may resemble dermatophytic infections. Unless the underlying disease can be controlled, treatment of the cutaneous infection is not curative, but will diminish the severity of the infection. Local treatment with an antimonilial agent (amphotericin B or nystatin) is usually the most effective treatment.

Monilial granuloma is an unusual response to yeast organism infection which usually occurs in infancy or early childhood. In contrast to the usual superficial invasion of the skin, the inflammatory process extends into the corium. The oral mucosa, face, scalp, nails and paronychial areas are usually involved. The initial lesion is an inflammatory papule covered by an adherent, yellowish-brown crust surrounded by erythema. These papules become hornlike plaques which, on removal, leave bleeding granulation.

VIRAL INFECTIONS

Warts. Warts are small benign tumors of the skin or adjoining mucous membrane; they occur predominantly during the preschool and adolescent periods. They are caused by a specific viral agent, about 50 millimicrons in diameter, which grows within the nucleus of epithelial cells and produces hyperplasia. The elementary body is indistinguishable from that of polyoma virus morphologically, but there does not appear to be an antigenic relation. Although warts have been classified according to morphology and location of the tumor, they are apparently all produced by the same agent.

Histopathologically, there are acanthosis and hyperkeratosis; the proliferation of the prickle cell layer is accentuated in the central part of the tumor. With special staining for deoxyribonucleic acid and by diligent search, specific intranuclear inclusions can be found.

Common warts are raised circinate lesions with a pitted, keratinized surface and a semitranslucent base measuring 3 to 10 mm. in diameter. Thrombosed capillary tufts are frequently seen as black pinpoint spots. They are commonly situated on the fingers and dorsa of the hands, but may appear anywhere on the glabrous skin.

Plantar warts are, as the result of pressure, practically flat. They are often painful on weight bearing and may be inapparent because of an overlying callosity. If the callus is carefully pared away, the features of the common wart are observed. Early lesions may resemble deep-seated vesicles. Multiple warts are not uncommon and may be grouped to create a mosaic pattern.

Flat warts appear as small (1 to 6 mm.) flat, flesh-colored papules on the dorsa of the hands and on the face. They have a tendency to appear at the site of scratches in a linear distribution.

Filiform warts are single fine projections (5 to 10 mm. in length) with keratinized tips and a sessile base. Groups of these single projections are called *digitate warts.* These warts are uncommon in children.

Mucous membrane warts are usually multiple, frequently confluent, pinkish or flesh-colored nonkeratinizing, finger-like projections which occur in the moist areas around the anus, genitalia, mouth and, occasionally, the eye. These warts are common in the preschool period.

In differential diagnosis, plantar verruca must be distinguished from a foreign body reaction on the sole of the foot with overlying callosity or from a localized area of abnormal keratinization (inverted corn) with overlying callosity. Lichen planus, lichen nitidus and the papules of keratosis follicularis on the dorsum of the hands must be distinguished from flat warts.

Treatment of warts is not uniformly successful and depends upon local destruction, and at times apparently upon "suggestion." Treatment must be individualized according to the type and location of the wart and to the experience of the therapist. In preschool and adolescent age groups consideration must be given to the effect of painful, emotionally traumatic methods. Some type of therapeutic suggestion is sufficient to produce clearing in 30 to 50 per cent of infections. Cryotherapy (liquid nitrogen) and electrosurgery are locally destructive, nonscarring measures, and in experienced hands are effective in 75 to 85 per cent of instances. The local application of a mitotic poison (podophyllin) is the treatment of choice in mucous membrane lesions. The severe inflammatory reaction produced by 20 per cent podophyllin in compound tincture of benzoin on surrounding normal mucous membrane may be minimized by careful application.

Molluscum Contagiosum. Molluscum contagiosum is a small benign tumor of the skin which occurs predominantly in the preschool and adolescent periods. It is caused by a specific brick-shaped virus (300 by 220 millimicrons) which grows within the cytoplasm of epithelial cells.

Histopathologically, there is a localized proliferation of the prickle cells which pushes down into the dermis like an inverted mushroom. The molluscum cytoplasmic inclusion can be identified easily within the epithelial cells of the central portion of the tumor. The skin lesions are characteristically waxy papules varying in size from 2 to 10 mm. with a central umbilication; they may be found at any dermal site except on the palms and soles. Spontaneous resolution of papules often occurs in association with an inflammatory reaction which resembles a pustule.

In differential diagnosis flat warts, nonpigmented dermal type nevi, and xanthogranuloma must be distinguished. Expression of the molluscum body by squeezing the papule with opposing fingernails is diagnostic. Treatment is simple and effective: the molluscum body is shelled out by pricking the base with a scalpel (no. 11) or an acne stylet.

PARASITIC DISEASES

Parasitic infestation of human beings may be limited to the skin, or cutaneous lesions may be associated with systemic disease. The more common parasitic disorders are described in the section beginning on page 717.

Insect Bites. See also page 500.

The important role of some of the arthropods in transmission of disease has tended to minimize interest in the cutaneous reaction to the bites of insects. Local reactions may result from bites of many kinds of insects, including mosquitoes, fleas, lice, bedbugs and flies.

The skin reaction to the bite of an insect is due to hypersensitivity and is species-specific. There is little or no reaction in a nonsensitized person, whereas in the sensitized one there may be either an immediate or a delayed reaction or a combination of the two. The response of the sensitized skin to the bite is characterized by the immediate appearance of an evanescent, urticarial type of papule surrounded by an erythematous flare; pruritus is prominent. This reaction usually subsides within an hour and is followed within a few hours by a delayed, more persistent, erythematous, severely pruritic papule.

Papular Urticaria (Lichen Urticatus). This chronic, recurrent, pruritic, papulovesicular eruption is caused by sensitization to salivary polypeptides following the bite of fleas, lice, mites, mosquitoes or bedbugs (Fig. 23-30). The eruption associated with flea bites characteristically appears with a centrifugal distribution during the summer months. The bites from bedbugs are most commonly seen on the ankles, buttocks, knees and shoulders, but may appear on any part of the body.

Histopathologically, there are varying degrees of intercellular edema, including vesicle formation, vasodilatation, and perivascular infiltration by many eosinophils, histiocytes and lymphocytes in the middle and lower dermis. In chronic lesions there may be a lymphoma-like pattern.

The skin lesion is biphasic; the initial wheal is evanescent and is followed by an extremely pruritic inflammatory papule or papulovesicle. In the patient's effort to obtain relief from the itch, the papule is excoriated and frequently becomes secondarily infected. Most lesions are on the ex-

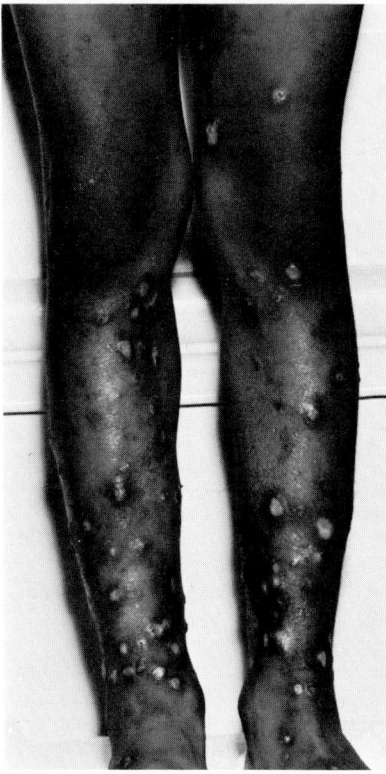

Figure 23-30. Papular urticaria caused by flea sensitivity, with secondary pyoderma (ecthyma).

tremities. In differential diagnosis, pyoderma, varicella, scabies and pediculosis must be distinguished.

Treatment depends on determination of the source of infestation. One should be aware of the longevity of lice in damp areas. Elimination of fleas from an animal's sleeping quarters can be attained by use of a spray containing DDT and rotenone. For satisfactory treatment, fleas or bedbugs must be eliminated from the environment. Carpets, cracks and crevices in the floor, overstuffed furniture, and bedding may be sprayed with 10 per cent DDT or other effective agents. It may be necessary to have the house fumigated by an experienced exterminator. A dog may be treated effectively with Tritox dip (Pitman Moore), and cats with a rotenone or pyrethrum powder. Repellants such as 6-12 or Off are useful in protecting the child from bites. Symptomatic relief can be accomplished by use of 0.5 to 1 per cent hydrocortisone cream, or its equivalent.

Pediculosis. Two species of lice produce infestation of the scalp, body and pubic area in man; only pediculosis of the scalp has practical significance in pediatric practice.

Pediculosis capitis is a chronic infestation of the scalp and hair and occasionally of the eyelids by *P. humanus* var. *capitis*. It feeds on blood and perishes within 2 to 3 days after removal from the host. As the eggs (nits) hatch, they become glued

to the hairs and reach maturity within 2 to 3 weeks.

The skin lesions at first are minimal, consisting of slight erythema and a purpuric spot at the site of feeding; repeated exposure results in sensitization, and an inflammatory papule appears at the site of each bite, followed by a severe pruritic reaction, secondary infection and occipital and posterior cervical lymphadenopathy. In all instances of pyoderma of the scalp, the possibility should be considered that pediculi are the initiating factor.

Treatment with a benzyl benzoate-DDT-benzocaine emulsion (Topocide) or gammabenzene hexachloride (Kwell) is effective. One application at night followed by shampoo in the morning is sufficient to produce a cure in most instances. Infection of the eyelids may be successfully treated with an ophthalmologic ointment containing 0.25 per cent physostigmine (Eserine Ointment). Examination of the remainder of the family for infestation is essential.

Scabies. This chronic infestation is caused by burrowing of the impregnated female mite (*Sarcoptes scabiei* var. *hominis*) into the skin. She lays a few eggs each day for several weeks in her burrow; the larvae developing from the ova emerge on the surface as adults; the female becomes impregnated and starts a new cycle. In this invasive process a burrow is formed which appears as a tiny, straight or tortuous linear elevation. As a result of the repetition of this process, sensitization with the production of symptoms occurs within a month or so after infestation. After this latent period a pruritic papulovesicular eruption appears, with a striking predisposition for the interdigital spaces, palms, flexural surfaces of the wrists, anterior axillary folds, waistline, areolar area of girls and penis of boys. In infants, vesiculobullous lesions are common and are frequent on the face and feet.

Histopathologically, the mite, ova and feces may be found in a burrow in the stratum corneum. After sensitization there is a mild inflammatory reaction with intracellular edema and vesicle formation in the prickle cell layer. There are vascular dilatation, perivascular infiltration and edema of the upper portion of the dermis.

Diagnosis may be difficult because the typical lesions are altered by excoriation or secondary infection; it is dependent upon demonstration of a mite from a burrow in the skin.

Treatment by the following plan is effective within 48 hours: A prolonged hot soaking bath is followed by 3 applications of a benzyl benzoate-DDT—benzocaine emulsion (Topocide) at intervals of 12 hours and by a second bath 12 hours after the last application. The medicine is applied to the face in infants with facial lesions, but otherwise to the entire skin surface from the neck down. Secondary bacterial infection should then be treated with a broad-spectrum antibiotic ointment, and 0.5 per cent hydrocortisone cream should be applied to counteract the irritative reaction.

ACNE VULGARIS

Acne is an inflammatory disease of the pilosebaceous glands produced by occlusion of the duct of the sebaceous gland in a predisposed person.

Approximately 85 per cent of preadolescent and adolescent children exhibit some manifestation of plugging of sebaceous glands, so that it may be considered one of the hallmarks of adolescence. The pilosebaceous system is probably conditioned by a genetic factor for the development of the acne process. A variety of factors, however, contribute to the production of acne: endocrine, dietary, emotional, traumatic and bacterial. Evidence of endocrine factors includes absence of acne in the eunuch, premenstrual exacerbation of acne in the female, appearance of acne in women with masculinizing tumors, and the production of acne in a predisposed person by injection of testosterone. The role of dietary factors is shown by the regularity with which the lesions flare up in many children after the ingestion of specific foods. The main dietary restrictions upon which most dermatologists agree are chocolate, nuts, seafood and cola drinks. Evidence that dietary restriction of fat or carbohydrate favorably affects the disease is lacking. Although sebaceous glands are apparently not under direct control of the nervous system, stress does appear to cause exacerbation of acne lesions. Mechanical factors such as manipulation and the use of occlusive cosmetics produce follicular blockage and may contribute to the acne process. The role of bacteria in the production of acne is unclear.

Tridimensional reconstruction of normal and acne-involved pilosebaceous structures indicates that the site of the earliest acne lesions is in the sebaceous duct before it joins the follicle neck. Subsequent upward extension of the keratotic plug obstructs the follicular orifice and produces the comedo. Breaks in the follicular epithelium permit intradermal leakage of the irritating follicular contents, which produce an inflammatory reaction. Scarring occurs when the entire pilosebaceous apparatus is destroyed and replaced by fibrous tissue. The clinical expressions of acne in the predisposed child vary from milia-like papules with comedones and erythematous follicular papules in the infant (acne neonatorum) and prepubertal child (juvenile acne) to papulopustular, nodular and nodulocystic lesions, the most severe form of the disease. Although acne tends to clear with maturity, the more severe the process, the less the probability of spontaneous clearing at an early age.

The purpose of treatment is to improve the cosmetic appearance by limiting the development of active lesions and by diminishing scarring. Local therapy includes ultraviolet radiation and the use of keratolytic and antiseborrheic agents; systemic therapy includes dietary control, the appropriate use of antibiotics and psychiatric support.

Local therapy is designed to alter sebaceous gland function and to produce controlled peeling of the stratum corneum by chemical (sulfur, salicylic acid or resorcinol), physiologic (ultraviolet) or mechanical (abrasives) means. An acceptable plan for local treatment is as follows:

1. Cleansing of the face with soap and water on arising, after school and at bedtime. A soap substitute containing sulfur and salicylic acid (Fostex) may be more effective than soap.

2. After each washing, application of a lotion containing sulfur and salicylic acid (Sulforcin, Fostril). The frequency of application depends upon the degree of dryness produced.

3. Ultraviolet (cold quartz or hot quartz) irradiation at weekly intervals to increase peeling of the stratum corneum.

4. Removal of comedones and pustular lesions with a comedo extractor. The stylet attached to the extractor is effective in securing drainage of nodulocystic lesions and produces less pain than a scalpel.

5. Roentgen therapy will suppress sebaceous gland activity, but it is mentioned only to condemn it. The beneficial effect is transient, and the hazards are significant.

6. Abrasive material incorporated in powder or soap is not necessary.

7. Removal of superficial pitted scars can be accomplished successfully by a variety of plastic planing procedures (sandpaper, stainless steel rotary brush, and shaving techniques). These procedures are not recommended during the active phase of the disease and not during adolescence.

In selected patients *systemic therapy* of resistant pustular, nodulocystic acne with antibiotics is justified; the tetracyclines are the drugs of choice in doses of 250 gm. 4 times a day for 4 days, 250 gm. 3 times a day for 3 days, and 250 gm. twice a day for a week, and then 250 gm. daily as indicated. Although estrogenic hormones will sometimes alter the course of resistant acne in the male, their use is not recommended in the adolescent child. In the girl with severe, uncontrollable premenstrual flare of her acne, treatment with oral estrogen (Premarin) in doses of 0.60 to 1.25 gm. per day beginning 7 to 10 days premenstrually and continued until the beginning of menstrual flow may be tried.

PSYCHOCUTANEOUS DISORDERS

Emotional factors are involved in diseases of the cutaneous system to varying degrees. They play a primary role in localized neurodermatitis, trichotillomania, and in some instances of chronic urticaria and alopecia areata; a secondary role in such widespread, chronic, disfiguring diseases of the skin as ichthyosis vulgaris, epidermolysis bullosa or congenital ichthyosiform erythroderma; and collaborative or potentiating roles in atopic dermatitis and psoriasis, wherein the basic problem may be accentuated by triggering emotional factors. Assessment of the role of emotions is an essential part of the dermatologic management of cutaneous problems. In every instance some psychologic guidance is needed, and in some cases psychiatric therapy may be required.

Localized Neurodermatitis. This chronic, extremely pruritic eruption is characterized by various-sized circumscribed patches in which the skin is thickened and the normal skin lines are exaggerated. It is seen infrequently in children. Histologically, there is hyperkeratosis with regular thickening of the epithelial layer. There is a mild inflammatory infiltrate in the upper portion of the dermis, and the picture may closely simulate the changes of chronic psoriasis.

Characteristically, the disorder begins with intermittent pruritus on the elbows, knees, ankles or less often at other sites without any skin changes.

As a result of persistent rubbing and scratching, the characteristic changes appear in the skin.

In differential diagnosis, psoriasis may cause confusion because of the appearance of lesions on elbows or knees. The lesions of localized neurodermatitis may be multiple, but usually only one is present.

When there is persistence or recurrence of localized neurodermatitis, the need for psychiatric help should be considered. In many instances, even though the emotional stress has disappeared, the lesions and pruritus persist, owing to changes in the skin. Local treatment is useful and consists in the application of a keratoplastic agent (2 to 10 per cent coal tar) in hydrophilic ointment or 0.05 per cent hydrocortisone cream. In addition, a hypnotic agent such as one of the phenothiazine drugs may be useful to control itching.

DISEASES OF THE HAIR

The loss of hair may be the result of any of the following factors: (1) congenital anatomic defects, (2) alteration of the hair growth cycle, (3) fracture of the hair by trauma, (4) epilation, (5) destruction of the hair follicle by dermal scarring.

I. Congenital anatomic defects (see p. 1379)
    Congenital alopecia
    Monilethrix
    Pili torti
    Pili annulati
II. Alteration of growth cycle
    Defluvium of the newborn (see p. 1375)
    Inflammation (second-degree thermal burn, kerion, alopecia areata, bacterial infection seborrhea)
    Fever
    Roentgen radiation (low dosage)
    Syphilis
    Drugs (thallium, folic acid antagonists, vitamin A toxicity)
    Endocrine (hypothyroidism)
    Systemic disease (dermatomyositis, systemic lupus erythematosus) (see p. 519)
III. Fracture of the hair shaft
    Trauma (hair twisting, compulsive brushing or combing)
IV. Epilation
    Trichotillomania
    Marginal alopecia
V. Scarring
    Congenital dermal defect
    Severe infection (bacteria, kerion)
    Third-degree thermal burn
    Roentgen radiation (high dosage)
    Discoid lupus erythematosus

ALOPECIA

Alopecia may be classified broadly as (1) scarring with permanent loss of hair and (2) nonscarring with transient loss of hair.

Marginal alopecia is a type of hair loss at the margins of the frontal, temporal and parietal areas of the scalp often caused by the continuous traction of the "pony tail" or tight hair braiding. The hair loss is typically symmetrical, triangular in shape, and anterior to and just above the ears. It may, of course, occur anywhere on the scalp, depending on the hairdo.

The process is usually reversible, but if the stress is continued for a long time, the hair follicles may atrophy, and the loss of hair may be permanent.

Alopecia areata is a nonscarring type of baldness in which single or multiple circumscribed patches of hair are suddenly lost from the scalp. Histologically, there is a perivascular, inflammatory infiltrate involving the vessels in the lower portion of the corium. The hair bulbs are reduced in size, and the shaft contains keratin. Initially, the skin has a slightly erythematous appearance, and there may be scattered broken hairs superficially resembling the stubble seen in trichotillomania. The scalp is primarily involved, but at times the eyebrows, eyelashes and hair on other parts of the body may be lost. The first patch is usually 2 or 3 cm. in diameter and may enlarge. Several areas of alopecia may appear simultaneously or consecutively and may become confluent. In rare instances all hair is lost within a few weeks. The alopecia may persist for many months, or there may be prompt regrowth followed by subsequent recurrences. There is a high incidence of emotional aberrations in affected children, and it has been suggested that alopecia areata is a psychocutaneous disturbance.

In differential diagnosis, trichotillomania, tinea capitis and discoid lupus erythematosus must be distinguished.

Treatment. Psychiatric guidance may be indicated. Systemic therapy with a corticosteroid will usually reverse the process, but the effect is usually transient, and the hair falls again when treatment is discontinued. A more practical method is the intralesional injection of triamcinolone (5 mg. per ml.) in single patches or the continuous application of 0.05 per cent triamcinolone beneath an impervious plastic film cap.

TRICHOTILLOMANIA

Trichotillomania is an emotional disorder in which the hair becomes the target of expression and is either pulled out or twisted off. The scalp is the most frequent site of involvement; less often the eyebrow and pubic hairs may be pulled out. There are usually no subjective symptoms, and the child frequently denies manipulating the hair. The hair loss is usually in a readily accessible area and results in one or more irregular patches of alopecia of variable size. (Fig. 23-31). The patchy alopecia is characterized by a "migrating" loss of hair, with an advancing border at one side and the stubble of regrowing hair at the other. The coarse stubble of regrowing hair in the area of involvement is the hallmark of this disturbance. Trichotillomania must be differentiated from alopecia areata, tinea capitis, and patchy hair loss in the occipital area caused by rubbing on the bed, and that seen in thumb-suckers who simultaneously manipulate the hair gently. Trichotillomania is an indication for psychiatric guidance.

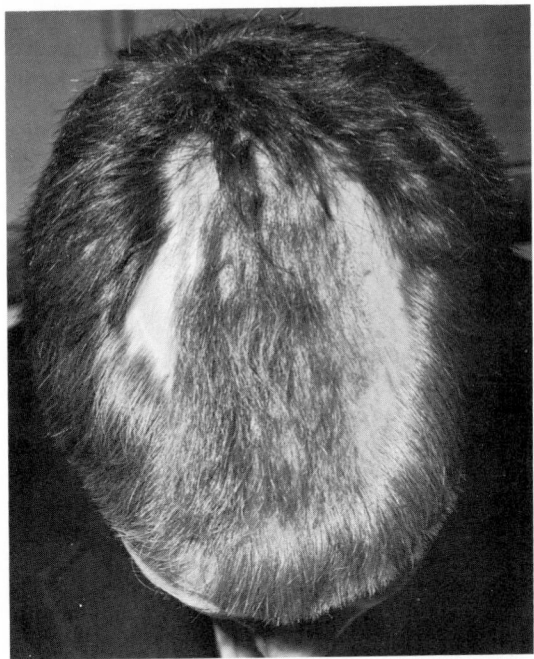

Figure 23-31. Trichotillomania in a 10-year-old child, showing typical "migrating" type of hair loss.

PHARMACOLOGIC BASIS FOR LOCAL THERAPY

The introduction of effective antibacterial, antifungal and anti-inflammatory agents and advances in formulation have revolutionized topical therapy. Such therapy should be planned to fit the problem at hand. The principal considerations are the choice of active ingredients, the vehicle, an esthetically acceptable preparation, and detailed instructions for use. In medications for local application, concentration of the active agent in the vehicle is a primary consideration, whereas total quantity of the drug applied is of no importance unless the drug is absorbed through the skin and is applied over large areas.

Absorption of drugs through the normal intact skin is negligible, but when the surface barrier membrane is damaged by a dermatitic process or denuded by scratching, absorption may be significant and produce systemic effects. Consideration of percutaneous absorption, therefore, is particularly important in pediatric practice. For example, boric acid powder when applied to inflamed skin can be absorbed and produce boron poisoning; ointments or powders containing mercury under similar circumstances can result in acrodynia. Application of corticosteroids topically over large surfaces of the skin has not produced undesirable side effects with the exception of those by alpha fluorohydrocortisone (Fluorinef). The covering of locally applied steroids by an occlusive plastic dressing

increases both absorption and the therapeutic response; this method of treatment, however, is usually not practical for infants and small children, owing to their resistance to being bandaged.

The following pharmacologic effects can be accomplished by the application of therapeutic agents to an abnormal skin surface:

Cleansing. Local treatment, to be effective, must be preceded by proper cleansing to remove crusts, scales and previously applied medication. This may be accomplished by scrubbing with cotton moistened with water and a soap substitute containing hexachlorophene.

Antipruritic Effect. Except for the local anesthetic agents, there is no medication administered locally or orally which is specifically effective in the relief of pruritus. Control of itching depends on reduction of the inflammatory reaction.

Anti-inflammatory effect is accomplished by vasoconstriction and by the antiexudative effect of hydrocortisone or one of its analogues. With vasoconstriction as a parameter of absorption, the acetate is the best absorbed of the analogues of corticosteroids. Triamcinolone, fluocinolone and the 17-valerate of betamethasone are the most effective steroids when applied locally. Their effect is enhanced by polyethylene film occlusion, but at the risk of adrenal cortical suppression, if used over a large area. Occasional dermal atrophy or striae may occur as complications of this type of treatment. When used intralesionally they may produce dermal atrophy and rarely calcium deposits in the atrophic area. The atrophy is usually reversible, but may be permanent.

Antibacterial Effect. Antibiotics should be selected which are not likely to be used systemically and which presumably have a low incidence of sensitization. An ointment containing bacitracin, neomycin and polymyxin meets these criteria and has broad-spectrum coverage. Owing to their sensitizing capacities, sulfonamides, penicillin, streptomycin and the furan derivatives should not be used topically.

Antifungal Effect. In tinea capitis the fungistatic effect of griseofulvin has revolutionized treatment. In superficial fungus infections of the skin, however, a modification of Whitfield's formulation is still preferred for treatment. In moniliasis, local applications of nystatin (Mycolog), amphotericin B (Fungizone), a quaternary ammonium compound (benzalkonium chloride 1:1000), or iodochlorhydroxyquinoline (Vioform) are highly effective. Although aqueous gentian violet 0.5 to 1 per cent is effective, it is far from esthetic.

Antiparasitic Effect. The combination of benzyl-benzoate, DDT and benzocaine in lotion form (Topocide) or gamma benzene hexachloride (Kwell) is effective for scabies and for pediculosis. Modern insect repellents such as 2-ethyl 1-3 hexanediol (6-12) are useful in the prevention of insect bites.

Emollient Effect. A dry, scaly skin results from decreased water-holding capacity of the keratinous layer. Lubrication may be obtained by soaking in plain water followed by the application of a greasy ointment to impede water loss. The technique of hydration and lubrication is useful in avoiding the drying of skin during cold weather.

Protective Effect. Protection from ultraviolet irradiation may be accomplished by incorporation of a mechanical barrier (titanium dioxide) and a chemical light screen (para-aminobenzoic acid) in an appropriate vehicle (A-Fil) or a screening preparation such as red veterinary petrolatum with titanium dioxide (RVPlus). Greasy ointments or pastes may also be used to protect the skin from excessive moisture in the diaper area.

Keratoplastic Effect. The distillation products of wood, coal and bituminous shales tend to diminish epithelial proliferation and hyperkeratosis and contribute to a return to normal keratinization. Coal tar is a complex mixture containing phenols, benzene, toluenes, naphthalene, creosote, anthracenes and fluorescent substances. Wood tars do not contain the anthracene compounds which are carcinogenic to the skin of mice, but they exert less of a keratoplastic effect. In spite of the carcinogenicity of coal tar for the skin of experimental animals, cancer has not been attributed to therapeutically applied coal tar products. Folliculitis and photosensitivity occur as undesirable side effects. Caution should be exercised in applying coal tar to areas exposed to light. The tars are generally used in ointment or cream vehicles in concentrations from 2 to 10 per cent, although undiluted tar may be used in certain instances.

Keratolytic Effect. Salicylic acid in concentrations of 2 to 5 per cent is the most frequently used agent to remove hyperkeratotic scales. It is useful in plaster form (40 per cent) for the removal of thickened keratotic lesions such as warts.

Antiseborrheic Effect. The chief antiseborrheic agent is sulfur; it is used principally for seborrheic dermatitis and acne vulgaris. The mechanism of its action is not understood. It is generally used in a precipitated or colloidal form which, on contact with the skin, is reduced to a sulfide.

Vehicles. The vehicle itself may have some therapeutic effect through its physical properties. In the past, pharmacologically active agents were applied to the skin in powders, lotions, emulsions, ointments or pastes or in solution on compresses or in baths. The formulations of the newer cream and ointment bases provide for a wide range of applicability and have largely replaced other types of vehicles.

Compresses and Baths. Wet dressings and baths have time-proved usefulness in the treatment of acute dermatitis, especially for the removal of crusts and scales. The antiexudative, anti-inflammatory, vasoconstrictive and antibacterial properties of potassium permanganate, Burow's solution and the like are minimal in comparison with those of the corticosteroid preparations and specific antibacterial agents.

Medicated baths containing emulsions of oils (cotton seed, mineral oil) or tars (coal or wood) alone or in combination are useful in the treatment of dry skin (Lubath, Alpha Keri) or in keratinizing abnormalities in which a keratoplastic effect (Zetar Emulsion) is desired.

Pastes. Ointment bases occlude the skin surface and impede the loss of water. Retention of water in the keratotic layer results in increased percutaneous absorption. The most occlusive ointment bases are mixtures of hydrocarbons (petrolatum) and mixtures of palmitic, stearic and oleic acid glycerides (lard). By definition, pastes contain 30 to 50 per cent solids in a greasy ointment base; they are now rarely used as vehicles. Owing to its physical properties, Lassar's paste, however, is an effective protective agent for the skin in the diaper area of the infant with readily irritated skin.

Some of the newer ointment vehicles have a greasy consistency and can be spread on the skin in a thin film. Care must be taken in choosing the proper vehicle to accomplish the therapeutic purpose.

Occlusiveness of the various ointment bases is directly related to their water miscibility. The following are listed in decreasing order in respect to their occlusive potential: petrolatum, lard, hydrophilic petrolatum, hydrophilic ointment, polyethylene glycol ointment. Owing to their effective occlusiveness, petrolatum, lard and hydrophilic petrolatum should not be used on acute inflammatory lesions.

There are many ointment vehicles available under different proprietary names; here only those contained in the United States Pharmacopeia are listed.

Hydrophilic ointment, U.S.P. XVI, oil-in-water emulsion, is a water-washable or vanishing cream type of base. It is relatively nonocclusive and may be used as a vehicle in acute dermatitic reactions. A semisolid emulsion can be obtained by adding 20 per cent distilled water; it can be used in place of a lotion on weeping dermatitic lesions.

Hydrophilic petrolatum, U.S.P. XVI, is a water-in-oil emulsion. It is the classic "cold cream" type base. Its cooling effect results from the evaporation of the aqueous phase after application to the skin.

Polyethylene glycol ointment, U.S.P. XVI, is a mixture of polymerized polyethylene glycols. It is water-soluble and is easily washed off.

CARROLL F. BURGOON, JR.

REFERENCES

Bain, G. O., and Shnitka, T. K.: Cutaneous Meningioma (Psammoma). *Arch. Derm.,* 74:590, 1956.

Balsaver, A. M., Butler, J. J., and Martin, R. G.: Congenital Fibrosarcoma. *Cancer,* 20:1607, 1967.

Burgoon, C. F., Jr., Graham, J. H., and McCaffree, D. L.: Mast Cell Disease: A Cutaneous Variant with Multisystem Involvement. *Arch. Derm.,* 98:590, 1968.

Cash, R., and Berger, C. K.: Acrodermatitis Enteropathica: Defective Metabolism of Unsaturated Fatty Acids. J. Pediat., 74:717, 1969.

Curth, H. O., and Warburton, D.: The Genetics of Incontinentia Pigmenti. *Arch. Derm.,* 92:229, 1965.

Fitzpatrick, T. B., and others: White Leaf-Shaped Macules. Earliest Visible Sign of Tuberous Sclerosis. *Arch. Derm.,* 98:1, 1968.

Fost, N. C., and Esterly, N. B.: Successful Treatment of Juvenile Hemangiomas with Prednisone. *J. Pediat.,* 72:351, 1968.

Gorlin, R. J., Sedano, H., and Anderson, B. E.: The Syndrome of Palmar-Plantar Hyperkeratosis and Premature Periodontal Destruction of the Teeth. A Clinical and Genetic Analysis of the Papillon-Lefevre Syndrome. *J. Pediat.,* 65:895, 1964.

Goslee, L., Clermont, V., Bernstein, J., and Woolley, P. V., Jr.: Superficial Connective Tissue Tumors in Early Infancy: A

Study of Fibromatosis and Lipoblastomatosis. *J. Pediat.,* 65:377, 1964.

Helwig, E. B., and Hackney, V. C.: Juvenile Xanthogranuloma (Nevoxantho-endothelioma). *Am. J. Path.,* 31:625, 1954.

Howell, J. B., Anderson, D. E., and McClendon, J. L.: Multiple Cutaneous Cancers in Children: The Nevoid Basal Cell Carcinoma Syndrome. *J. Pediat.,* 69:97, 1966.

Hughes, W. E., and Hammond, M. L.: Sclerema Neonatorum. *J. Pediat.,* 32:676, 1948.

Imperial, R., and Helwig, E. B.: Verrucous Hemangioma. A Clinicopathologic Study of 21 Cases. *Arch. Derm.,* 96:247, 1967.

Kellum, R. E., Ray, T. L., and Brown, G. R.: Sclerema Neonatorum. *Arch. Derm.,* 97:372, 1968.

Koph, A., and Andrade, R.: Benign Juvenile Melanoma; in *Year Book of Dermatology,* 1965-1966 Series. Chicago, Year Book Medical Publishers, Inc., 1966.

Lister, W. A.: Natural History of Strawberry Naevi. *Lancet,* 1:1429, 1938.

Marden, P. M., and Venters, H. D., Jr.: A New Neurocutaneous Syndrome. *Am. J. Dis. Child.,* 112:79, 1966.

Mehregan, H., and Pinkus, H.: Life History of Organoid Nevi, with Special Reference to Nevus Sebaceus of Jadassohn. *Arch. Derm.,* 91:574, 1965.

Rodriguez, H. A., and Ackerman, L. V.: Cellular Blue Nevus. *Cancer,* 21:393, 1968.

Rush, B. F., Jr.: Treatment of a Giant Cutaneous Hemangioma by Intra-arterial Injection of Nitrogen Mustard: Case Report. *Ann. Surg.,* 164:921, 1966.

Sagher, F., and Even-Paz, Z.: *Mastocytosis and the Mast Cell.* Chicago, Year Book Medical Publishers, Inc., 1967.

Sever, R. J., Frost, P., and Weinstein, G.: Eye Changes in Ichthyosis. *J.A.M.A.,* 206:2283, 1968.

Shaffer, B.: Pigmented Nevi. *Arch. Derm.,* 72:120, 1955.

Silver, H. K.: Rothmund-Thomson Syndrome: An Oculocutaneous Disorder. *Am. J. Dis. Child.,* 111:182, 1966.

Smith, A. D., and Waisman, M.: Connective Tissue Nevi; Familial Occurrence and Association with Osteopoikilosis. *Arch. Derm.,* 81:249, 1960.

Stegmaier, O. C., and Schneider, L. A.: Chediak-Higashi Syndrome. *Arch. Derm.,* 91:1, 1965.

Walther, R. J., Polansky, B. J., and Grotis, I. A.: Electrocardiographic abnormalities in a Family with Generalized Lentigo. *New England J. Med.,* 275:1220, 1966.

Weary, P. E., Graham, G. F., and Selden, R. F., Jr.: Subcutaneous Fat Necrosis of the Newborn. *South. M.J.,* 59:960, 1966.

Weary, P. E., Linthicum, A., Cawley, E. P., Coleman, C. C., Jr., and Graham, G. F.: Gardner's Syndrome: A Family Group Study and Review. *Arch. Derm.,* 90:20, 1964.

Webster, S. B., and others: Juvenile Xanthogranuloma with Extracutaneous Lesions. *Arch. Derm.,* 93:71, 1966.

Whitehouse, D.: Diagnostic Value of the Café-au-lait Spot in Children. *Arch. Dis. Childhood,* 41:316, 1966.

BURNS

Burns are among the most frequent accidental injuries of infants and children. Morbidity and mortality rates from these injuries exceed those from poisoning. Burns of infants and young children are incurred mostly in the home, whereas older children frequently sustain such injury elsewhere. In addition to open fires and hot liquids, other causes of burns include chemical agents, electricity, ultraviolet rays, roentgen rays and radioactive substances.

Permanent disfigurement and disability and immediate and delayed mortality depend upon the extent of the surface area involved and upon the depth to which the burn penetrates. Even small burns involving the skin over joints may produce contractures which seriously limit motion. Death during the acute phase results chiefly from peripheral vascular collapse. Plasma loss begins quickly

after the burn and persists at least 1 or 2 days. In third-degree burns considerable destruction of the red blood cells occurs immediately in addition to plasma loss. Moreover, during the first week after the burn, renal damage of the lower nephron type may exaggerate these changes. Death after the first few days results from local or intercurrent infection, especially septicemia, and from debilitation.

The **treatment** of burns involving small and superficial areas of the skin consists in cleansing the skin and applying sterile white petrolatum (U.S.P.) or an ointment with a local anesthetic. Boric acid ointment should never be used locally. Sedatives and analgesics may be necessary.

Since second- or third-degree burns involving 12 per cent or more of the body area usually require hospital treatment, it is important to have an approximate estimate of the area of the body surface involved. The extent of the burn may be estimated according to directions on page 230.

Because shock always occurs with extensive burns, measures to treat it should be instituted promptly. The patient should be given morphine parenterally and placed on a sterile sheet; the burned area should be covered with sterile towels until surgical care of the area can be undertaken. Blood from the patient should be obtained for hematocrit and hemoglobin determinations, as well as for typing and crossmatching for transfusion. Plasma should then be administered intravenously through a cannula until the results of these determinations are available.

Although there are no completely satisfactory formulas for calculation of the amounts of plasma, blood and electrolyte solutions to be administered, the method outlined on page 230 is a useful one. The amount of fluid calculated to be administered initially must be altered later in relation to subsequent laboratory determinations, urinary output and clinical appraisal of the patient. In all instances of shock whole blood is preferred over all other solutions. Plasma is preferred over colloidal solutions such as dextran. If plasma which has not been irradiated to kill the virus of infectious hepatitis must be used, gamma globulin should be administered as a prophylactic.

The foot of the bed should be elevated. Attempts to raise or reduce the patient's temperature are usually not indicated. Oxygen may be given to combat restlessness and cyanosis. Tetanus toxoid or antitoxin and gas gangrene antitoxin may be given, and therapy with antibacterial agents may be instituted while preparations for surgical care are being completed.

The pressure bandage method of Koch has gained favor when early treatment is possible. There is also wide use of topical applications of 0.5 per cent silver nitrate solution to produce an eschar which reduces exudation of fluids and decreases the likelihood of infection. An alternate plan of topical treatment is the local application of Sulfamylon to the burned areas in conjunction with careful débridement.

Wallace has treated burns by the open method, i.e. exposure to air, elevation of the burned area, immobilization and prophylactic antibacterial agents. No local irritants are applied, and dry heat, such as that provided by a cradle with an electric light, is avoided. This method is recommended for burns of the face or perineum.

The topical treatment of the burn is probably less important than the total supportive care available to the patient. Accordingly, treatment of patients with extensive burns is best carried out in hospitals with "burn centers," to which early transferral is recommended.

Early grafting of skin is indicated when possible for deep or extensive burns. Other types of reconstructive plastic surgery may be necessary.

After a severe burn adequate nutrition must be maintained. Protein intake is increased to balance the excessive loss of serum proteins in the burned areas. Emotional support is necessary to help children with extensive burns tolerate the long and often painful experiences of hospitalization and to face realistically the possibility of permanent disfigurement.

The importance of teaching children the hazards of fire cannot be overemphasized. Parents must exercise great care to keep hot objects beyond the reach of toddlers.

ROBERT H. HIGH

REFERENCES

Artz, C. P., and MacMillan, B. G.: Treatment of Burns of Difficult Areas. *Am. J. Surg.*, 91:517, 1956.

Blocker, T. G., Jr.: Local and General Treatment of Acute Extensive Burns. The Open-Air Regime. *Lancet*, 1:498, 1951.

Cope, O., and Moore, F. D.: The Redistribution of Body Water and the Fluid Therapy of the Burned Patient. *Ann. Surg.*, 126:1010, 1947.

Metcoff, J., and others: Losses and Physiologic Requirements for Water and Electrolytes After Extensive Burns in Children. *New England J. Med.*, 265:101, 1961.

Moncrief, J. A.: Management of Burns. *Surg. Sciences*, 3:175, 1966.

Wallace, A. B.: The Exposure Treatment of Burns. *Lancet*, 1:501, 1951.

24. Pediatric Ophthalmology

EYES OF THE NEWBORN INFANT

The eye and the brain achieve maximal postnatal growth rates during the first year and continue at a rapid but decelerating rate until the third year. Growth continues at a slower rate until puberty, after which additional growth is negligible. Various parts of the eye grow disproportionately at different times. In general, the structures of the anterior part of the eye grow proportionately less than those of the posterior portion.

At birth the eye is three quarters of adult size. The orbital margin is circular rather than oval. The diameter of the cornea is 10 mm. (it is 12 mm. in the adult). The sclera is thin, resulting in a bluish tint. The lacrimal gland is small, and is capable of producing tears at birth. The macula is completely developed shortly after birth; the fovea continues to be further differentiated for about 16 weeks. The angle of the anterior chamber contains mesodermal tissue, in some cases until the third postnatal month.

The infant sees at birth, but in a limited manner. The eyes remain closed most of the time in the early postnatal days and are sensitive to light. An optokinetic response has been recorded in infants ranging between 1½ hours and 5 days of age which was equivalent to approximately 20/670 on the usual Snellen chart. By the end of 2 weeks the infant is able to look at large objects, but does little or nothing in the way of following them with his gaze. By 4 or 5 weeks he can look at relatively small objects and by 8 to 10 weeks follow moving objects and turn his head away from bright light. There is a gradual increase in visual acuity, binocular vision, ocular motility, convergence and conjugate movements.

Characteristically in the fundus of the newborn infant, especially in the premature one, the nerve head has a grayish pallor, and there is absence of pigment and grayness in the periphery of the retina; the veins and arteries are more nearly alike in size and color than in the adult. Remnants of the hyaloid artery and of the pupillary membrane may occasionally be observed. Retinal hemorrhages have been observed in as many as 25 per cent of newborn infants, but they absorb promptly and only rarely leave any permanent effect.

EXAMINATION OF THE EYE

The infant or child with complaints referable to the eye is likely to have one or more of the following: (1) deformity; (2) injury; (3) redness, pain, watering or photosensitivity; (4) visual disturbance such as subnormal vision or double vision; or (5) reading disability.

General inspection of the eyes can be performed best in a room without direct or intense illumination. Simple toys which make a little noise are helpful in attracting the gaze in various directions to permit preliminary evaluation of muscular adequacy. A small flashlight is useful in detecting strabismus by observing the position of the corneal reflexes, while covering with the hand first one eye and then the other.

The **eyelids** are examined for crusts, ulceration of the margins and position of the lacrimal puncta. When pressure with the index finger over the lacrimal sac expresses mucopurulent material through the puncta, it is indicative of obstruction of the nasolacrimal duct and infection of the tear sac. The ability to open and close the lids should be tested. Ptosis is a common defect characterized by drooping of the eyelid; it is due to weakness of the levator muscle.

The **conjunctiva** is examined for color, smoothness, thickness, secretion, injection, follicles and papillae, and for the presence of a foreign body. The ability to evert the upper lid skillfully should be acquired. The child is asked to look down at his toes; the examiner then grasps the lashes with his right thumb and index finger; he pulls the lid downward and away from the globe, placing a probe, or his other index finger, at the upper level of the tarsal plate. The right fingers pull the eyelid upward and slightly outward, over the finger or probe. The lid is kept averted by holding the thumb against the brow and reminding the child to keep looking downward. Foreign bodies are usually found in the concavity just above the margin of the lid.

The **sclera** is examined for blueness which indicates thinness. The intraocular pressure can be estimated by palpation with both index fingers through the skin of the lid above the tarsus. It can be measured accurately with a tonometer or a special applanation tonometer during local (Pontocaine, Ophthaine, 0.5 per cent) or general anesthesia.

The **cornea** is examined for luster, ulceration, foreign body, blood vessels and scars. The diameter of the cornea should be appraised. Megalocornea is a benign condition to be differentiated from a large cornea; the latter is part of generalized enlargement of the globe in congenital glaucoma. Microcornea is often associated with other congenital anomalies. Keratoconus is not common in children except in Down's syndrome.

The **anterior chamber** is assessed for depth by estimating the distance between the cornea and the iris. Cellular activity may be observed with the aid of brilliant illumination and magnification such as is provided by a corneal microscope.

The **iris** should be examined for color, surface markings and for reaction to light and to accommodation. The last is tested by observing both pupils in equal light while the patient looks at a distant object and then at the examiner's finger. Adhesion of the iris to the cornea or the lens should be looked for.

The clarity of the **lens** can be examined by the ophthalmoscope with a plus 10 lens at a point 10 cm. from the patient's eye.

Examination of the Ocular Fundi. Dilatation of the pupil is essential for adequate examination of the fundus, especially in children who tend either to watch the ophthalmoscope light or to look around the room. Dilatation can be done quickly and effectively with 1 drop of 10 per cent phenylephrine (Neo-Synephrine) or 0.5 per cent Mydriacyl. Homatropine 5 per cent is also effective, but atropine is not safe for the newborn infant except in oil or ointment form, which prevents rapid absorption from the nasal mucous membrane. Cyclogyl (0.5 and 1.0 per cent) is an excellent cycloplegic agent. The lens and vitreous are examined for opacities. The nerve head is examined for shape, color, nature of its margins, type of cupping and evidence of edema. The macula should be examined routinely, but requires dilatation of the pupil. Some lesions of the macula in children are pathognomonic and aid in establishing the diagnosis in otherwise puzzling conditions. Each vein and artery should be followed from the disk to the periphery. Much more of the fundus can be seen if the child is directed to look up, down, right and left as the corresponding portions of the fundus are examined. One should not hesitate to examine children during general anesthesia or at least satisfactory sedation if the information desired is of sufficient importance. If the examination is made during anesthesia, it is essential to have forceps to steady and move the globe, which rolls upward during light anesthesia.

Visual Tests. Testing of visual acuity can be accomplished after 3 years of age by the use of a Snellen E chart, consisting of rows of the letter E in various sizes corresponding to the regular visual test chart. The E's have their "fingers" pointing upward, right, down and left. Cooperation is obtained more easily by having the child place his fingers on the chart itself, indicating the position of the "fingers" of a few of the E's; the chart is then moved 20 feet away, and the child is asked to continue to show which way the "fingers" point by extending his own fingers in the same direction. It is often helpful to have the parent instruct the child at home in the method of "playing the E" game. Other charts with familiar pictures of various sizes are useful for smaller children, but are less accurate.

Before the age of 2 years vision can be determined by the response of the child to a small toy or similar object of interest such as keys or his mother's bracelet. His ability to watch a light with each eye separately is a gross screening measure of visual acuity. Normal pupillary responses to light may be present in cerebral blindness. If the child loses interest or behaves badly when one eye is covered, but cooperates well when the other eye is tested, vision is probably reduced considerably in the first eye. In cases of strabismus, it is essential to determine which eye is preferred for visual fixation of the target or whether the eyes freely alternate.

The field of vision can be tested by the confrontation method until the child is old enough to cooperate in the use of a perimeter. With patience and a projection-type of perimeter, accurate visual fields can be elicited at a relatively early age.

Color blindness can be tested by use of colored wools or having a child trace numbers on an Ishihara or American Optical Color Chart with his finger. Defective color vision is not uncommon in the male, but is rare in the female. "Color ignorance" refers to inability to tell shades of color; this condition responds somewhat to education.

Children are frequently examined by the ophthalmologist because of *reading difficulties.* Recent surveys have shown a relatively high incidence of cerebral dysfunction, farsightedness, exophoria, fusional difficulties, convergence insufficiency, crossed dominance and inability to maintain binocular fixation in retarded readers.

Mothers suspect and inquire about mirror vision far more often than it occurs. It is probable that children often reverse letters on an experimental basis, just as they use toys in unexpected ways. This is a transient form of mirror vision; true mirror vision is rare. Children with reading disabilities may have difficulty in perceiving letters or words in their proper order. If a careful examination indicates no ocular problem in such children, they should be referred for remedial reading to qualified professional personnel. Every effort should be made to improve the ocular status prior to remedial reading (see p. 110).

Problems in visual perception are best handled first by an ophthalmologic examination to detect or exclude organic disease, and then in cooperation with the orthoptic technician, who will determine the degree of visual sensorimotor coordination.

Subnormal dark adaptation is difficult to test in young children. Vitamin A deficiency is the only causative condition amenable to treatment. Retinitis pigmentosa and choroideremia are characterized by night blindness with reduced peripheral vision.

Examination by the child's physician. Routine examinations of the eyes should include (1) the use of a Snellen E or letter chart (see above); (2) examination of motility of the eyes by checking rotations and the near-point of convergence and movements with the cover test described under Strabismus; and (3) examination of the media and fundi with an ophthalmoscope.

Visual screening tests of children in offices and in schools have proved to be effective. The Atlantic City eye test* can be done rapidly, provides adequate information, does not require a skilled examiner or extensive equipment and is readily interpreted. It tests visual acuity and muscle balance and provides a rough test for refractive error. After testing the visual acuity with the Snellen chart, a +1.75 lens is placed before each eye. If the child can then read the 20/20 line on the chart, he fails the test. Muscle balance is checked by the use of a green rectangle in which a red dot should be seen. If the red dot is outside the rectangle, the child has more than 1 prism diopter of hyperphoria or more than 4 prism diopters of esophoria or exophoria.

Examination by an ophthalmologist. Infants and children should be examined by an ophthalmologist whenever an ocular abnormality is noted. Children do *not* "grow out" of strabismus. The optimal schedule for examination by an ophthalmologist is (1) in the neonatal period; (2) before entering school (age 4 years); and (3) at intervals of 2 years beginning at puberty. In addition, examination is indicated whenever vision for either distance or nearness is defective; whenever strabismus is noted, since poor vision from disuse is usually not easily correctable after the sixth year of life; and at any sign or symptom of disease of the eye.

Cycloplegics traditionally include atropine, 0.5 to 1.0 per cent (in an ointment or oil rather than solution to lessen absorption from the nasal mucosa), and, in children over 12 years of age, homatropine, 4 per cent. Cyclogyl is now, however, the one of choice at all ages. It is almost as effective as atropine, acts more rapidly, and paralyzes accommodation for only 24 hours, as compared with 5 days for atropine and scopolamine.

REFRACTIVE ERRORS

Most children are born farsighted, about 5 per cent are nearsighted, and 20 per cent have practically no refractive error.

Hyperopia (Farsightedness). The hyperopic eye is shorter than normal, so that the focused image falls posterior to the retina. Hyperopia over 4 diopters is considered abnormal in children; in hyperopia of lesser degree the power of accommodation is sufficient to supplement the refracting power, but its constant use may cause fatigue and ocular discomfort. The total refractive error is determined under atropine or Cyclogyl cycloplegia. Refraction is indicated in children with

poor vision, lack of interest in reading or looking at picture books, headache, eye discomfort, strabismus, corneal disease, or inflammations of the lid. Proper lenses provide a correction adequate for distinct vision and prevention of fatigue.

Myopia (Nearsightedness). The myopic eye is longer than normal, so that the focused image falls anterior to the retina. There is poor vision for distant objects, and accommodation does not improve it. Proper lenses for full correction of the refractive error should be worn for best vision, and re-examination is ideally performed semiannually for the first few years and then annually. Children of myopic parents should be examined at an early age because of a hereditary tendency.

Astigmatism. In astigmatism there is a difference in the refractive power of the various corneal meridians of the eye, owing to a slight irregularity in the spherical shape of the eyeball. The child may appear to be a careless reader because a distorted image is obtained. Symptoms include headache, eye pain, fatigue, nervousness and conjunctival injection. Astigmatism may be combined with myopia or hyperopia; slight astigmatism is extremely common. Cylindric or spherocylindric lenses provide an optical correction for the defect. Slight degrees of astigmatism often do not require correction; moderate degrees usually require glasses for reading, movies, television, and so forth; severe degrees require that glasses be worn constantly.

Paralysis of accommodation may be due to diphtheritic paralysis of the ciliary muscle or to other neurologic conditions.

DISORDERS OF EYEBALL AND ADNEXA

Diseases of the *orbit* may be classified as developmental, inflammatory, vascular, traumatic, neoplastic, or secondary to a systemic defect. The eyeball responds to changes in orbital volume by appearing pushed forward (exophthalmos, proptosis), by being sunken (enophthalmos) or by being displaced vertically.

The method of examination involves inspection, palpation, auscultation and roentgenography. The use of retrobulbar air and contrast media may be of special help. The Hertel exophthalmometer is valuable in quantitating the degree of exophthalmos for comparison of serial measurements.

Developmental Abnormalities. Structural anomalies of the bony orbit, dermoid cysts, teratomas, encephalocele, and microphthalmos with cyst are included among the developmental abnormalities. Craniostenosis (p. 1329) may be responsible for deformities of the orbit, usually with loss of depth anteroposteriorly. Reduction in orbital volume may result in proptosis; exotropia, papilledema and optic atrophy are other possible sequelae.

Inflammation. Acute inflammatory orbital disease is usually secondary to inflammation in adjacent structures, except for penetrating orbital injuries. The most common sources of orbital infection are sinuses, teeth, eyelids and face. Edema of the lids and proptosis may occur in the child without definite orbital disease, particularly in paranasal sinus disease (ethmoiditis). Orbital cellulitis is usually associated with severe inflammation, proptosis, lid rigidity, and immobility of the eyeball. Allergic reactions about the lids may simulate orbital disease.

Chronic inflammatory disease of the orbit is relatively common; it is observed with chronic sinusitis, osteomyelitis, pseudotumors, tuberculosis and fungal and parasitic infections. *Cavernous sinus thrombosis* may occur as a rare sequel to orbital cellulitis. Severe pain, edema of the lid and conjunctiva, proptosis, immobility of the eye, papilledema, decreased vision and severe general toxicity are the principal manifestations of this complication.

Trauma. Traumatic injuries to the orbit may result from blunt or penetrating injuries; examination should include a search for retained foreign bodies. Blowout fractures of the floor of the orbit may be caused by a sharp blow. Routine roentgenograms frequently fail to demonstrate a fracture; laminograms may be required. All penetrating injuries to the orbit demand evaluation of the central nervous system to determine whether the brain has been injured by perforation of the posterior orbital wall. Orbital hemorrhage and infection are common with penetrating injuries and must be treated as emergencies.

Vascular Disease. Primary orbital vascular abnormalities are uncommon, as are varices, pulsating exophthalmos from carotid-cavernous sinus fistula and aneurysm. Hemangioma is the most common vascular tumor and can usually be removed surgically through a lateral orbitotomy.

Tumors. Rhabdomyosarcoma is the most common primary malignant orbital tumor in children. Glioma of the optic nerve is usually associated with von Recklinghausen's disease; it grows slowly, producing loss of vision with gradually increasing proptosis. Meningioma and carcinoma of the paranasal sinuses occur less commonly in children than adults. Dermoid cysts are benign encapsulated tumors which are relatively common in the region of the orbit. Their growth is slow in early life, but accelerated at puberty. Other benign orbital tumors include cholesteatoma, angioma, fibroma and neurofibroma.

Orbital Changes Secondary to Systemic Disease. Exophthalmos secondary to thyroid disease is uncommon in children. The Hand-Schüller-Christian syndrome includes exophthalmos. Proptosis secondary to orbital hemorrhage may be seen with blood dyscrasias and scurvy. Leukemia and neuroblastoma may produce proptosis through orbital hemorrhage and infiltration.

Congenital Ocular Abnormalities. Congenital defects of the eye occur in 2 primary ways:

(1) those which are presumably genetic in origin and interfere with embryonal development, e.g. microphthalmos, colobomata, cataract and dermoid tumor; or (2) those which are due to intrauterine inflammation, e.g. chorioretinopathies (toxoplasmosis and cytomegalic inclusion disease), corneal scars (syphilis) and cataract (German measles).

Colobomata characteristically arise from a failure of fusion of embryonic tissue. Failure of regression of vascular tissue is most commonly seen as a remnant of the hyaloid artery or a persistence of the tunica vasculosa lentis. *Congenital cataracts* develop at any time during the formation of the lens, which occurs about the sixth or seventh week of gestation. Congenital cataracts may be unilateral or bilateral, or in any stage of development from minimal involvement to complete opacification. *Microphthalmos* varies in degree, may involve one or both eyes, and may be accompanied by such conditions as cataract, aniridia, irideremia, colobomata, somatic abnormalities and meningoencephalocele. Microphthalmos is often determined by a recessive gene, but may appear as a dominant trait. When *aniridia* is not on a familial basis, but appears to be a new mutation, the concurrence of Wilms's tumor must be considered. Deficiencies in visual function are frequently associated with anatomic anomalies.

Congenital defects of the choroid and retina are visible ophthalmoscopically. Colobomata of the uveal structures may be located inferiorly or inferior-nasally. They may be unilateral or bilateral and may also involve the iris, choroid or optic nerve singularly or in combination. Central macular pigmentary lesions are often caused by toxoplasmosis and cytomegalic inclusion disease. Other congenital lesions of the choroid or retina include drusen, aneurysm, optic nerve malformation, medullated nerve fibers and macular degenerations. Persistence of the tunica vasculosa lentis or persistent hyperplastic vitreous must be differentiated from congenital cataract and retrolental fibroplasia.

EXTERNAL DISEASE OF THE EYE

Congenital Anomalies of the Lids. The most common congenital conditions of the lids are epicanthus and blepharoptosis. Blepharophimosis (small opening), dystrichiasis (misdirection or extra rows of lashes) and colobomata are occasionally seen.

Epicanthus is common and is produced by a fold of skin extending downward from the brow to the nose, obscuring the medial canthus. It is always bilateral and frequently produces an apparent asymmetry of the eyes suggesting strabismus. Epicanthus usually disappears as the nasal bridge develops and the face broadens.

Blepharoptosis results from a defect or a paresis

of the levator palpebral muscle. The condition is more commonly unilateral, but often bilateral. It may be familial. Sometimes it is associated with paresis of the superior rectus muscle. Surgical correction is frequently required by age 5 years and is accomplished by resecting the levator muscle.

Diseases of the Lids. The skin of the lids may be involved in a variety of conditions affecting the skin elsewhere in the body. Edema of the lids may be due to local or general disease. Allergy is a common cause. Infections of the skin, paranasal sinuses, orbit, tear sac or eyeball may produce edema. Hemorrhage into the lids results in ecchymosis and is of particular importance; when it appears 24 to 48 hours after a head injury, it suggests the possibility of basal skull fracture.

Emphysema of the lids usually denotes a fracture of the medial wall of the orbit (lamina papyracea), permitting communication with the nasal cavity (ethmoid sinus). The lids are swollen, and on palpation there is a sensation of crepitation.

Hordeolum (sty) is common in children and is nearly always due to staphylococcal infection. Vaccine appears at times to be helpful in treatment of persistent recurrences. *Acute chalazion* responds to anti-inflammatory measures, but if a lump remains after 2 months, excision of the granuloma is required. *Ectropion* is an outward turning of the lid margin, and *entropion* is an inward turning.

Benign neoplasms include papillomas, hemangiomas, dermoid cysts, nevi, lymphangioma and lipoma. Non-neoplastic growths which may be found on the lids are xanthoma, molluscum contagiosum and milium. These growths may be excised if they interfere with function or become unsightly. Malignant tumors of the lid are rare in children.

Blepharitis is an inflammation which principally involves the margins of the eyelids and the skin around the base of the cilia. Redness, scales, crusts and ulcerations may be present. The eyelashes are often matted by cellular debris and exudate and sometimes may cease to grow satisfactorily. Seborrhea is a common cause, alone or complicated by secondary infection. Treatment of seborrhea of the scalp and brows is important for improvement of the marginal blepharitis.

The Lacrimal Apparatus. Epiphora due to a congenital obstruction of the nasolacrimal duct is common. Dacryocystitis may result from obstruction of long standing. Pressure over the tear sac, combined with "drops" to control infection, is usually successful in opening the duct. Probing may be required, if conservative means fail, and is generally successful. In the event of repeated failures, however, a new opening from the tear sac to the nasal cavity may be required. Absence of the puncta or accessory puncta is rare.

The Conjunctiva. *Chemosis* is edema of the bulbar conjunctiva and results from trauma, local irritation, allergic reactions or trichinosis.

Hyperemia of the conjunctiva is caused by local irritations such as foreign bodies, dust, exposure to bright light, coryza or allergy. *Subconjunctival hemorrhage,* manifested by bright or dark red patches on the bulbar conjunctiva, may be the result of injury or inflammation. It may occasionally result from severe sneezing or coughing, or may be a manifestation of a blood dyscrasia.

Symblepharon is a cicatricial attachment of the conjunctiva of the lid to the eyeball; the lower lid is usually affected. It follows operation or injuries, especially burns from lye, acids or molten metals. It may interfere with motion of the eyeball and cause diplopia. The band should be separated and the raw surfaces kept from uniting during healing. Grafts of oral mucous membrane may be necessary.

Acute conjunctivitis, characterized by redness, chemosis and mucopurulent discharge, is common in children and particularly in newborn infants. The instillation into the eyes of prophylactic silver nitrate frequently produces in the newborn infant a chemical irritation, with a purulent discharge lasting 24 to 48 hours. Gonorrheal conjunctivitis of the newborn must be considered in differential diagnosis.

Gonorrheal conjunctivitis is manifested by an acute, copious, purulent discharge which begins within 3 to 5 days after birth. The conjunctiva becomes red and chemotic, and the lids are so swollen that separating them is very difficult. When there has been premature rupture of the membranes, infection may be present at birth. The term *ophthalmia neonatorum* applies to any acute conjunctivitis in the newborn infant. When smears and cultures indicate gonorrheal infection, therapy includes systemic penicillin and frequent local instillation of a chemotherapeutic agent.

Acute purulent conjunctivitis is more frequently caused by staphylococcus, streptococcus, pneumococcus, *Hemophilus influenzae* and Koch-Weeks bacilli, and usually responds promptly to antimicrobial therapy.

Vernal conjunctivitis is characterized by papillary hypertrophy of the palpebral conjunctiva and tends to occur principally in warm weather. Allergy plays a role in its origin. Symptoms include lacrimation, itching and photophobia. The upper palpebral conjunctivae contain hard, flattened papillae. In the bulbar form the conjunctiva adjacent to the limbus contains gelatinous elevations. The conjunctiva is congested and exhibits stringy, mucoid secretions which contain eosinophils. Vernal conjunctivitis responds to topical corticosteroid medication.

Inclusion blenorrhea is a viral infection transmitted in a variety of ways. The infant can be infected during birth by organisms in the maternal genital tract. During childhood, infection from contaminated swimming pools is relatively common. The neonatal lesion resembles gonococcal conjunctivitis at the outset, but it does not appear until 5 to 7 days after birth. These viral infections are effectively treated with a sulfonamide.

TABLE 24-1. DIFFERENTIAL DIAGNOSIS OF OCULAR INFLAMMATION IN CHILDREN

ACUTE CONJUNCTIVITIS	ACUTE UVEITIS	CONGENITAL GLAUCOMA	ACUTE KERATITIS
Common	Not common	Not common	Common, often secondary to trauma
Mucopurulent discharge	Lacrimation	Lacrimation	Lacrimation, but no discharge
Foreign body sensation	Pain and photophobia	Photophobia	Pain, photophobia and foreign body sensation
Conjunctival redness only	Redness at limbus	Minimal congestion	Perilimbal injection
Vision normal	Vision reduced	Vision poor	Vision reduced
Pupil normal	Pupil small, irregular	Pupil small	Pupil normal or smaller
Cornea clear	Cornea usually clear	Cornea hazy or quite cloudy	Cornea hazy or gray
Anterior chamber normal	Anterior chamber cloudy	Anterior chamber deep	Anterior chamber normal
Ocular tension normal	Ocular tension normal to low	Ocular tension elevated	Ocular tension normal

Epidemic keratoconjunctivitis is caused by adenovirus type 8 and is transmitted by direct contact. Initially there is a sensation of a foreign body beneath the lids and itching and burning. Edema and photophobia develop rapidly, and large oval follicles appear within the conjunctiva. There are frequently preauricular adenopathy and a pseudomembrane on the conjunctival surface. Blurring of vision results from subepithelial corneal infiltrates, which usually disappear, but have been known to reduce permanently the visual acuity.

Chronic catarrhal conjunctivitis can develop from repeated attacks of acute conjunctivitis and may be associated with chronic infections of the lids, chronic dacryocystitis, irritants, and viral warts at the lid margin. The conjunctiva is red and thickened, and there is a mild discharge. There is a scratchy, burning and heavy sensation about the lids. Determination and elimination of the cause are often difficult.

Vaccinia of the lids or conjunctiva may occur as a result of an accidental inoculation (p. 646). Single or multiple ulcers with gray necrotic material are characteristic. The great danger is corneal involvement, which can produce dense scarring and visual loss.

DISEASES OF THE CORNEA

The cornea has attained most of its growth at birth and therefore appears relatively large in comparison to other structures. The transverse diameter is 10 mm. at birth and attains adult size (12 mm.) during the first year of life. Any abnormal increase in size is an urgent cause for ophthalmologic consultation. Corneal haze or opacity accompanied by photophobia and lacrimation is a characteristic sign of congenital glaucoma. Corneal lesions may be classified as superficial or deep keratitis or as corneal ulcers where there is demonstrable loss of substance. Inflammatory lesions of the cornea appear as grayish infiltrations or opacities, accompanied by circumcorneal redness, pain, photophobia and lacrimation. Inflammatory lesions may be bacterial, viral or fungal and are frequently secondary to trauma.

Interstitial keratitis is a chronic cellular infiltration of the deeper layers of the cornea without ulceration. It is frequently associated with uveitis, corneal opacities and corneal vascularization. Congenital syphilis is the most frequent cause; tuberculosis and leprosy are less frequent ones. The lesion may be acute or chronic; in the acute form the cornea has a characteristic "salmon pink patch."

Phlyctenular keratoconjunctivitis appears as a small, gray, discrete, elevated lesion at the corneal limbus. Extreme photophobia and lacrimation make examination difficult. The lesion has been attributed to undernutrition and to tuberculosis.

Viral Keratitis. Dendritic keratitis, which may be caused by herpesvirus (p. 637), is the most troublesome of corneal viral infections. It is manifest as a dendritic, treelike staining figure on the cornea accompanied by photophobia and lacrimation. Not infrequently it follows trauma, especially if corticosteroid drops have been used for any length of time. Combined antibiotic-steroid eyedrops for ordinary external inflammatory disease of the eye are to be avoided unless there is a clear-cut indication for their use.

Corneal ulcers are always a cause for immediate concern and may result from traumatic lesions which become secondarily infected. Many organisms are capable of producing an infected ulcer, but the most troublesome is *Pseudomonas aeruginosa*. Fungi may be recovered from chronic corneal ulcers. Scarring or perforation due to corneal ulceration is an important cause of blindness throughout the world and is estimated to be responsible for 10 per cent of blindness in this country.

Vitamin A deficiency, abnormalities of the fifth cranial nerve and exposure can cause severe corneal changes. Trachoma, which is highly prevalent in North Africa and the Middle East, is probably the commonest cause of blindness in that area, producing severe corneal and conjunctival scarring, as well as lid deformities which lead to the rubbing of eyelashes against the eyeball.

THE PUPIL

In *Adie's syndrome* one pupil is myotonic and is larger than its mate; the Achilles and patellar reflexes are often absent. The slow contracture of the pupil in response to continuous direct light is characteristic. The pupil remains contracted for a long time after the light stimulation has been removed. The normal pupil fails to contract to 2.5 per cent Mecholyl, whereas the involved pupil does. The cause of the syndrome is not known. No treatment is required.

Horner's syndrome consists in unilateral miosis, apparent enophthalmos, narrow palpebral fissure and absence of facial sweating and represents a disturbance in the cervical sympathetic chain. The pupil fails to dilate with cocaine, but does dilate with epinephrine 1:1000, which ordinarily has no effect on the normal pupil.

Leukocoria (White Pupil). A white pupillary reflex in a child is indicative of a serious disorder; examination under general anesthesia is frequently indicated. The differential diagnosis includes cataract, retrolental fibroplasia, persistent primary hyperplastic vitreous, retinoblastoma, severe intraocular infection and exudative retinopathy (Coats's disease).

Retrolental fibroplasia occurs most commonly in premature infants treated with high concentrations of oxygen during the early days of life (see p. 386). When an infant has had excessive oxygen therapy in the early postnatal period, the eyes should be examined at frequent intervals for at least 3 months. The active stage of the disease is manifest by constriction of the arterioles followed by dilatation and tortuosity of the retinal vessels,

especially the veins. Ultimately, retinal detachment and scarring may occur.

Persistent primary hyperplastic vitreous results from failure of the embryonic hyaloid vascular system to regress normally. Elongated, finger-like ciliary processes visible through the dilated pupil are diagnostic.

Retinoblastoma is a malignant tumor of the retina. It is bilateral in about one third of the cases; in some instances it is hereditary and is transmitted in a dominant manner. It generally occurs by the age of 5 years. Strabismus may be an early sign, since vision is reduced when the lesion is central. Enucleation is indicated when the tumor is unilateral. If the tumor is bilateral, the less severely involved eye may be treated with radiation and triethylene melamine; the more involved eye should be excised.

Exudative retinopathy (Coats's disease) is an exudative process beneath the retina associated with recurrent hemorrhages and telangiectases. It is usually unilateral and results in detached retina with severe loss of vision.

DISORDERS OF THE LENS

Congenital cataracts are relatively common, but do not always cause significant visual disturbance. They are usually bilateral and often genetically determined. Maternal rubella (p. 630) is a common cause; galactosemia and hypocalcemia are less frequent ones. Cataracts may develop secondary to such intraocular diseases as uveitis, retinitis pigmentosa, retinal detachment or retrolental fibroplasia, or may represent the toxic effect of certain drugs and chemicals or the long-term administration of corticosteroids. Traumatic cataracts may develop from a direct blow or a penetrating injury. The lens opacity often becomes manifest rapidly and may be complicated by pain, inflammation and glaucoma.

Dislocation of the lens may be associated with arachnodactyly (Marfan's syndrome), Marchesani's syndrome, homocystinuria or trauma.

The opacities vary considerably in density and morphology. They can be observed through a +10 diopter lens with the ophthalmoscope held at a distance of approximately 10 cm. from the eye.

Other ocular abnormalities are frequently associated with congenital cataract such as microphthalmos, nystagmus, amblyopia, strabismus, corneal changes, aniridia, dislocation of the lens, and choroidal and retinal diseases. In addition, a high percentage of affected children may be mentally retarded or have associated disturbances of the cardiovascular, renal, skeletal or central nervous system, skin, muscles or endocrine glands.

The surgical results with congenital cataract are not as good as with the cataracts of adults. The high percentage of associated defects, including mental retardation and nystagmus, makes the prognosis guarded as to eventual visual function. In cases of maternal rubella, operation should be postponed until the age of 2 years, since activation of virus may occur if the operation is done earlier.

It is generally agreed that children with cataracts who have corrected vision of 20/50 or better should not be operated upon. If one eye is normal, a complete cataract in the other eye should be left alone until the patient is older. After the removal of a unilateral cataract binocular visual function is possible only with a contact lens or with a prosthetic lens placed within the eye.

In borderline cases with moderate involvement of both eyes, one must be guided by the child's ability to progress in schoolwork and to function socially. The ultimate decisions as to management must rest jointly with the ophthalmologist and the pediatrician.

GLAUCOMA

Infantile congenital glaucoma is characterized by increased intraocular pressure; it may be present at birth or become manifest in the first 3 years of life. It may be transmitted in an autosomal recessive manner. Congenital glaucoma may be associated with other congenital anomalies, which include aniridia (a vestigial root of iris remaining), pigmentary glaucoma (degeneration of pigment epithelium of iris), Axenfeld's syndrome (anomalous iris angle), Sturge-Weber syndrome, neurofibromatosis, Marfan's syndrome and Lowe's syndrome.

The earliest and most constant symptom is tearing, which must be differentiated from that due to congenital obstruction of the nasolacrimal duct. Corneal clouding associated with tears in Descemet's membrane is also an early sign. Photophobia may render ordinary examination difficult, since the avoidance of light is extreme. Increased intraocular pressure is the principal sign; accurate measurement must be made under general anesthesia. Cupping of the optic disk may occur early. Enlargement of the eye to a corneal diameter in excess of 12 mm. and a deep anterior chamber are significant. Repeated measurements of tension may be necessary to differentiate glaucoma from congenital megalocornea.

Treatment of infantile glaucoma is surgical, involving goniotomy and goniopuncture; the abnormally high insertion of the iris or membrane must be incised. Repeated goniotomies are frequently required, using a special lens to view the iris angle.

The operation should be performed as soon as the diagnosis is made; nearly 80 per cent of cases are evident by 3 months of age. The earlier the disease becomes manifest, the less favorable is the prognosis. Surgery leads to normal tension in about 75 per cent. Long-term visual results are not good despite normal tension.

STRABISMUS
(CAST; SQUINT; CROSS-EYE; WALLEYE; TROPIA; HETEROTROPIA)

Strabismus is an imbalance of the extraocular muscles. It is of considerable importance in pediatric practice, for it often results in functional loss of vision known as *amblyopia ex anopsia* (poor vision from disuse and absence of fusion). Owing to the cosmetic blemish, psychologic problems may arise. Parents should never be told to "wait and let the child outgrow crossed eyes."

Transient overconvergence or pseudostrabismus does occur, but the differential diagnosis should be the responsibility of the ophthalmologist. Infants with suspected strabismus should be referred to the ophthalmologist as soon as it is noticed. Strabismus may be congenital, and is familial in about 50 per cent of cases. Strabismus is frequently observed in cerebral palsy, in children born prematurely, and with many central nervous system abnormalities.

Few people have completely "normal" muscle balance (orthophoria); most have a tendency for the eyes to deviate in or out, up or down (heterophoria). A person with a *phoria* can keep his eyes straight by exerting effort to maintain fusion. A patient with a *tropia* frequently manifests an actual visible deviation, since the visual axes are not parallel. Some children have a phoria which at times becomes a tropia (or true deviation); this accounts for the parents' observation that the eyes are straight except under such circumstances as fatigue, illness, or for near or distant vision. Fusion may be possible in some fields of gaze, but impossible in others. For example, the child may see singly when he looks straight ahead or downward, but double when he looks upward. He therefore does all he can to avoid looking up.

Two conditions may give the appearance of strabismus when it is not there, or accentuate it when it is: epicanthal folds and the relative position of the eyeballs in the orbit. The latter represents a disparity between the anatomic axis and the visual axis.

Though there is wide variation in the manifestations of strabismus, there are general categories which are helpful to identify in planning the management of each case. *Paralytic (noncomitant) strabismus* is due to paralysis of a muscle. The eyes are straight except when they are moved in the direction of the paralyzed muscle. Double vision may be present in this case, or the child may in time learn to suppress the vision in the affected eye. Suppression in children under the age of 5 years frequently results in some degree of amblyopia. In *nonparalytic (comitant) strabismus,* which is the usual type, all the muscles are capable of rotating the eyeball as they should, but they do not work together. Both eyes are in the same relative position irrespective of the direction of gaze.

There are lateral, vertical and mixed lateral

and vertical types of strabismus. Paralysis of one of the vertically acting muscles may initiate the lateral imbalance. The child sees 2 images, one above the other and close together. He makes every attempt to avoid double vision. He may tilt his head, close one eye or allow one eye to deviate in or out in order to get the 2 images together or so far apart that they do not bother him. During this transient period of double vision the child may stumble, fall, overreach or otherwise appear awkward. He may be fussy and difficult to manage. This is the ideal time to start covering one eye. The procedure makes an alternator out of what would probably be a monocular squinter, and so promotes the development of good vision in each eye.

In *monocular* strabismus one eye deviates permanently, while the other eye is always being used. The deviating eye not used for definitive seeing fails to develop good central vision *(amblyopia ex anopsia)*. Amblyopia in this case implies that the eye is organically sound; the fundus appears normal. As previously noted, central vision is not fully developed at birth. The suppression of the image in the deviating eye will not permit central vision to develop normally. Peripheral vision, however, remains good. The nonstrabismic eye develops normally, and the child has no evidence of poor vision until this eye is covered; then the disparity in vision between the 2 eyes is striking. Patching of the good or fixating eye is essential. This must be done *constantly* for weeks or months, and care must be taken that the improved vision does not decrease when the patch is taken off.

Alternating strabismus is a condition in which either eye may be used for fixation while the other eye deviates. Since each eye is used part of the time for definitive seeing, vision is developed more or less equally in both eyes, and there may be no necessity for patching either eye. These children do not have double vision, since they suppress the image in the nonfixing eye. They do not, however, have binocular vision with depth perception, but they do not miss it since they have never had it. Operation is usually required, and generally the prognosis is good.

Accommodative strabismus depends upon the relation between convergence and accommodation, both of which are controlled by the third cranial nerve and are called upon to function at the same time. A high degree of hyperopia necessitates excessive accommodation, with accompanying overconvergence. Myopia is more likely to be associated with divergent strabismus. Accommodative esotropia may disappear during cycloplegia, and corrective lenses keep the eyes straight by relieving the stimulus for excessive accommodation-convergence. Good vision should be maintained in both eyes, but this is not automatically done in many cases. It is therefore sometimes necessary to use occlusion as well as glasses.

Strabismus and Cerebral Palsy. Children with cerebral palsy may have a variety of ocular palsies and as a result may have double vision in some directions of gaze. Esotropia is more common (46 per cent) than exotropia (8 per cent). It is desirable to remedy double vision as soon as possible, especially since many of these children have severe problems in locomotion and since improved cosmetic appearance may help in general social development. In cases of persistent esotropia with one eye deviating, patching the good eye to prevent amblyopia is indicated, although this may be rendered difficult by other problems. Children with cerebral palsy commonly have refractive errors, nystagmus, paralysis of conjugate gaze, blepharoptosis, cataracts, optic atrophy, defects of visual fields, aphasia and dyslexia, and such developmental ocular defects as microphthalmos, pupillary abnormalities, aniridia and colobomata.

Methods of Testing for Strabismus. In very young infants one can tell whether the eyes are straight by observing the position of the light reflexes on the corneas when a light is held before the face. Each reflex should be in the center of the pupillary space or at corresponding points in the 2 corneas, such as the corneoscleral junction nasally on one eye and temporally on the other.

For older children the screen or cover test is the best one; it is carried out by having the child look at or fixate a distant target while a narrow card is used to cover first one eye and then the other. Absolutely straight eyes *(orthophoria)* make no movement whatever when the card is moved. If crossing *(esotropia)* is present, each eye will move outward to fix on the light. If the eyes are divergent *(exotropia)*, each eye will jump inward to fix on the light. One watches only the eye which is just being uncovered. Measurement of the amount of deviation is obtained by holding prisms base-out or base-in before the eyes during the cover test. When the proper prism is found, no movement of either eye occurs.

The ocular rotations and the ability to converge should also be tested. The nearpoint of convergence is measured by bringing a small object of interest to the child slowly toward his nose. This nearpoint should be within 10 cm. of the base of the nose. When the rotations are tested, one should note the relative motility with both eyes opened and with each eye closed.

In using a light as a target of fixation it is useful to tell the child to "follow the light—don't let it get away." Simple toys, preferably those which move or create a gentle noise, are particularly useful in attracting the attention of young children. Sudden movements, loud noises and holding the child's head are to be avoided; rather the light or toy should be slowly moved from one position to another. Small children should sit on a parent's lap. Quiet observation of the youngster prior to examination frequently reveals considerable information. During the examination the

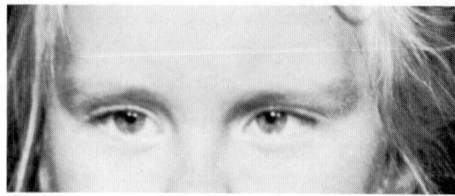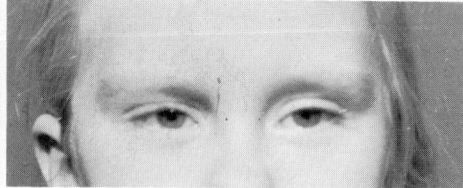

Figure 24-1. Alternating accommodative convergent strabismus with small deviation in which binocular vision was improved by orthoptic exercise techniques.

parent and office nurse should not talk or move about the room; a child's attention, once distracted, may not be regained at that session.

Treatment. *Parents should know that practically all deviating eyes can be straightened by corrective lenses, miotic therapy, orthoptics, surgery, or some combination of them, and that the straightening should be accomplished at the earliest possible time.*

Treatment of amblyopia ex anopsia should begin as soon as possible and must be carried out before the age of 6 years if vision is to be restored, and may be continued until the age of 10 years if necessary. A large number of children with strabismus have some degree of amblyopia; it has been estimated to occur in 5 per cent of the population. In a child with strabismus one may infer that amblyopia is present if one eye is invariably used for fixation of an object. At 1 year of age amblyopia may be eliminated within a few weeks by patching the good eye. The longer amblyopia persists, the more difficult it is to eradicate. Amblyopia should be prevented rather than treated. Good results are obtained in 80 per cent of children from 2 to 4 years of age, but in only 40 per cent of those from 4 to 7 years of age.

Glasses can correct only a portion of the deviation in accommodative esotropia. Successful correction of residual esotropia requires surgery. Not infrequently multiple surgical procedures are required, but the majority of uncomplicated cases of strabismus can be corrected with 2 procedures. The ophthalmic surgeon aims for functional results (single binocular vision), but in cases of refractory amblyopia must be satisfied with cosmetically straightened eyes.

Orthoptics and pleoptics. The techniques and training methods for adjusting binocular vision, visual perception and ocular motility are known as orthoptics. A series of complex instruments,

many of which are modifications of the major amblyoscope, are used for both diagnosis and therapy. Diagnostic orthoptic procedures have become established as a valuable aid to the ophthalmologist; there are, however, variations in opinion about the benefits to be obtained from orthoptic therapy. It is useful in children with intermittent divergence and in the postoperative management of children to assist in the development of fusional amplitude. In children with pure alternating strabismus of significant degree orthoptic treatment is usually unrewarding and may be a source of nervous fatigue.

A new method, pleoptics, has been developed for eccentric fixation (vision other than through the central macula), which may be effective in rehabilitating visual disturbances that heretofore had not been correctable in children of 8 years or older. Amblyopia is always present in cases of eccentric fixation.

Operative treatment is reserved for those children who do not respond to the wearing of glasses or to exercises. A high percentage of patients with strabismus, particularly convergent strabismus, eventually require operation. It is the only successful treatment for alternating strabismus. Monocular strabismus of even moderate degree should be operated upon as early as possible after treatment has overcome the amblyopia. Divergent strabismus offers less cosmetic blemish, and therefore surgical treatment is often delayed. Excellent results can usually be obtained, and binocular vision developed.

INJURIES

About one third of all blindness in children results from trauma, usually avoidable. Such

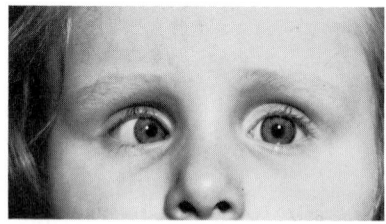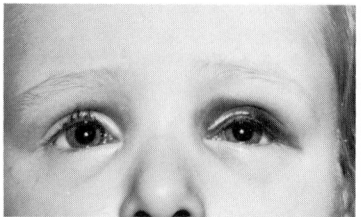

Figure 24-2. Alternating convergent strabismus corrected by surgery. Strabismus may be corrected by corrective lenses, orthoptic exercises or surgery or a combination of the 3 procedures. The early treatment of strabismus is emphasized, since best results are obtained when correction is undertaken before the age of 5 years.

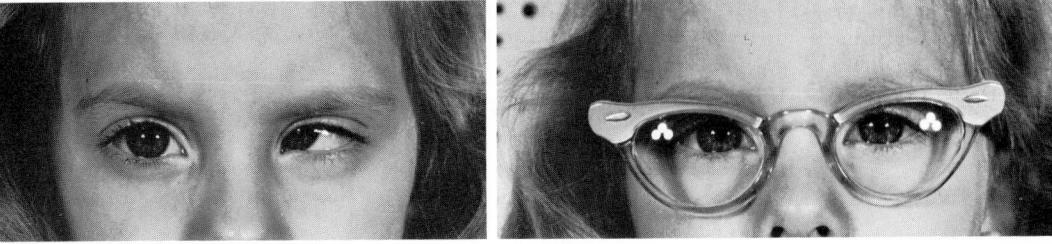

Figure 24-3. Accommodative convergent strabismus straightened by corrective lenses.

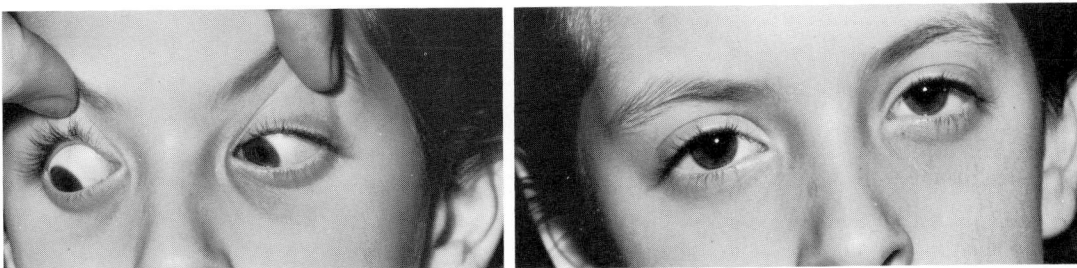

Figure 24-4. Right head tilt associated with paresis of left superior oblique muscle.

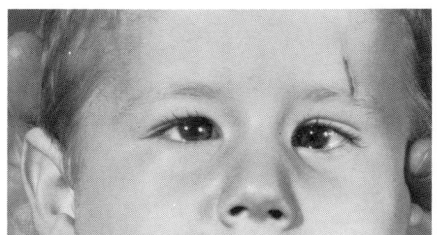

Figure 24-5. Congenital bilateral sixth and seventh cranial nerve palsy.

injuries are caused by air rifles, arrows, darts, stones and missile-throwing toys, sticks, sharp tools, explosives and strong chemicals. Small abrasions and superficial foreign bodies causing acute pain should prompt immediate consultation with a physician; unfortunately, some injuries do not produce pain, bleeding, sensitivity to light or blepharospasm, and often are ignored, e.g. intraocular foreign bodies, traumatic iritis, perforating wounds, dislocation of the lens and detachment of the retina. The end-results of injuries to the eye indicate that treatment should be the responsibility of the ophthalmologist from the outset.

Ecchymosis and edema are signs of injury to the *eyelids.* Ecchymosis (black eye) is usually of no great importance, except when the eyeball is involved. Blood from a basal skull fracture may appear under the bulbar conjunctiva a day or so after the injury.

Lacerations of the eyelid are generally more extensive than they appear externally. A small wound on the skin surface may not reflect the extent of the laceration of the tarsus. With any history of injury, prompt and complete examina-

tion of the lids, conjunctiva, cornea and sclera is necessary, even if general anesthesia is required. One or two sutures properly placed in the lid margin may obviate the necessity for extensive plastic repair at a later date, and even blindness may be avoided by prompt suturing of perforating wounds.

Slight *abrasions of the corneal surface* can be revealed by application of moistened fluorescein strips (sterile paper impregnated with fluorescein).

Large lacerations of the cornea and sclera require proper appositional suturing after excision of any free uveal tissue, vitreous or damaged lens tissue. Large wounds with escape of vitreous and with hemorrhage into the eye involve the choroid and retina. Detachment of the retina may occur. Frank infection is surprisingly infrequent. Emergency treatment should consist in instillation of a sterile atropine solution and application of a sterile pad. No ointment should be applied to the eyeball. After repair of the globe, atropine, a topical steroid-antibiotic solution and rest in bed are indicated until the true status of the eye can be determined.

Perforating wounds of the globe are always dangerous, even though the eye looks white and is not painful. Even small perforations may be complicated by *sympathetic ophthalmia.*

A *foreign body* on the cornea or conjunctiva is usually responsible for sudden onset of pain with tearing and congestion of the conjunctiva. Most foreign bodies can be located by examination with a good light and a magnifying lens. Irregularities on the corneal surface may indicate the location of the foreign body. If a foreign body is suspected, but not found, the eye should be examined roentgenographically. The instillation of 0.5 per cent tetracaine will facilitate examination as well as removal of the foreign body. It is wise to be certain that the anesthesia is complete and that the patient is relaxed enough to hold still. Foreign bodies which are not embedded may be removed by gently touching them with a moistened, cotton-tipped applicator. Embedded foreign bodies requiring instrumentation should be removed by an ophthalmologist.

Burns of the eye should be irrigated and covered with a bland oil or ointment and the eye bandaged. Initially, burns from acid appear to be more severe than those from alkali, but the latter are usually more serious. In powder burns the particles, when accessible, should be removed as soon as possible by copious irrigations. Tetracaine may be used to relieve the pain. Reparative operations may be necessary after the acute stage.

Ultraviolet burns of the cornea produce extensive loss of the cells of the corneal epithelium, causing pain, photophobia and blepharospasm. Treatment consists in dilatation of the pupil with homatropine, 5 per cent, and the frequent application of tetracaine ointment, 0.5 per cent. Both eyes should be kept closed until healing has taken place, which generally requires 24 to 48 hours.

INTERNAL DISEASES OF THE EYE

The *uveal tract* is the vascular inner coat of the eye composed of the iris, ciliary body and choroid. Iritis may occur alone or in conjunction with infection of its contiguous structure, the ciliary body, as iridocyclitis. Pain, photophobia and lacrimation are characteristic early symptoms.

All children with *acute anterior uveitis* deserve extensive investigation. The cause may be obscure, but the most common causes are rheumatoid arthritis, sarcoidosis and trauma; uveitis may also be secondary to a corneal lesion, such as an ulcer or herpetic keratitis.

Posterior uveitis is an inflammatory lesion of the choroid, but it invariably also involves the retina. The cause of posterior uveitis may also remain obscure, but the more common causes are toxoplasmosis, tuberculosis, syphilis, brucellosis, parasitic infestation and cytomegalic inclusion disease. Uveitis may also be a manifestation of septicemia.

Sympathetic ophthalmia is a rare inflammatory response of the normal eye following perforating trauma to the other eye in which there has been a prolapse of uveal tissue. It may occur weeks or even months after the accident. A hypersensitivity phenomenon involving uveal pigment is the most probable cause.

Endophthalmitis is usually a blood-borne infection; the initial manifestations may be retinitis and involvement of the vitreous and the uveal tract. It occurs with a variety of infections, such as meningitis, scarlet fever, measles and subacute bacterial endocarditis. It usually leads to blindness.

Panophthalmitis is an inflammation of all the structures of the eye and is frequently suppurative. It produces pain, severe congestion of the eyeball, eyelids and orbit, and loss of vision. Management includes symptomatic measures and systemic antibiotic therapy until it is safe to enucleate the globe.

Nevoxanthoendothelioma is a granulomatous lesion of the iris, which appears as a slightly raised yellowish mass. It is the most common cause of spontaneous bleeding in the anterior chamber of children. Blood in the anterior chamber may result in secondary glaucoma which may require surgery. The lesion responds to small doses of radiation.

RETINA

Defects of the choroid and retina can be plainly seen through a dilated pupil by means of an ophthalmoscope. The appearance of the choroid is determined to some degree by the density of the retinal pigment layer. In albinism and in the blond fundus, the choroidal vasculature is most prominent. In the darkly pigmented eye the choroidal vessels are less easily visible, except when sclerotic. Choroideremia, or absence of the choroid, is a rare, genetically determined defect. Colobomata involving the choroid and retina occur inferiorly and are usually associated with coloboma of the iris. Other congenital lesions of the choroid and retina include large "rock candy" drusen, aneurysms, malformations of the optic disk, medullated nerve fibers and hereditary macular degenerations.

There may be characteristic retinal changes with certain systemic diseases (see Medical Ophthalmology, p. 1432). In leukemia there may be hemorrhages with white centers, dilatation and tortuosity of the veins, and exudation. In rare instances in uncontrolled diabetic children the retinal vessels appear to be filled with cream (lipemia retinalis). In chronic nephritis and in hypertension there may be edema about the disk and adjacent retina accompanied by flame-shaped hemorrhages.

Chorioretinitis occurs with syphilis, tuberculosis, toxoplasmosis, cytomegalic inclusion disease, histoplasmosis, fungus infection, nematode infestation and septic infections. There is a reduction or loss of vision in the part of the field corresponding to the areas involved. These are at first yellowish with ill-defined margins; later there is organization, leaving atrophic areas which are whitish with pigmented margins. Vitreous opacities may be associated. The prognosis depends upon the location of the inflammation and the response to therapy. Treatment should include rest, injections of foreign protein, corticosteroids and whatever specific measures may be directed against the cause.

Retinal Detachment. Although a detached retina is more common in older persons, it may be observed in children, in whom there is frequently a history of trauma or a family history of retinal detachment or of other congenital ocular or systemic condition. Retinal detachment can be primary, with a retinal tear and liquefied vitreous behind the detached area, or it can be secondary, in which case the subretinal exudate originates from some disturbance in choroidal or retinal circulation. The secondary form of retinal detachment may be associated with uveitis, parasitic disease, hypertensive disease, collagen disease and diabetes mellitus. Retinal detachment is usually symptomless except for a decided loss in the visual field corresponding to the detached portion.

Juvenile retinoschisis is a sex-linked hereditary degenerative disease of the retina in which there is a splitting of the retina into 2 layers. The condition is bilateral and may be noted during infancy. The progress is slow, and visual loss may not result for many years. A retinal cyst must be considered in the differential diagnosis.

Retinal degenerations may be divided into central and peripheral forms. Changes are rarely present at birth, but may be noted during study of the child with "failure to thrive" or the child who ceases to develop normally. Retinal degenerations are associated with a number of the degenerative encephalopathies (p. 1293).

Cerebroretinal Lipidoses. See pages 453 and 1294.

Heredomacular Degeneration. A number of hereditary retinal macular dystrophies are characterized by bilateral degenerative changes in the macular area *without* degenerative changes in the central nervous system. They may appear at any age from infancy to adult life. A loss of central vision is the primary problem.

Peripheral Retinal Degeneration. Peripheral pigmentary degeneration occurs with a large group of diseases, which include Friedreich's ataxia and Laurence-Moon-Biedl syndrome. *Retinitis pigmentosa* and the closely related *retinitis punctata albescens* are classic examples of peripheral retinal degeneration. Night blindness is the first symptom; daytime vision and central vision remain good. Peripheral sight gradually deteriorates until the patient is reduced to "gun-barrel" vision.

Anomalies of the Optic Nerve. Some of the anomalies of the optic nerve may resemble papilledema and present difficult problems in differentiation. Pseudopapilledema is usually seen in hyperopic (farsighted) eyes. The disk margins are blurred and may be elevated. The physiologic cupping may be absent.

Medullated nerve fibers are a common finding at the disk margin; normally, they stop at the nerve head. These nerve fibers may extend as white, feathery patches from the disk onto the retina in any direction.

Drusen appear ophthalmoscopically as highly refractile, yellow, glistening, round bodies on or within the optic nerve head. They may give the disk an irregular, scalloped appearance.

The hyaloid vessels may persist as black, wavy lines from the disk, owing to failure of resorption during embryonic life.

Colobomata of the optic nerve, which result from inadequate closure of the fetal fissure, cause considerable distortion of the optic disk. Pits in the optic disk and choroidal pigment crescents at the disk margin also may be seen rather commonly; they do not impair visual function.

The Optic Nerve. Diagnosis of lesions of the optic nerve can be difficult, since many normal variations resemble organic changes. The optic disk of the infant may appear pale in comparison with that of an older child. Infants' eyes are difficult to examine, however, and one must be certain that pressure is not exerted on the eyeball which can produce blanching of the disk.

Pallor of the disk does not always signify optic atrophy. Optic atrophy implies functional loss of vision, which is not always easy to document. In the differentiation of the suspected "blind child" the electroretinogram is useful in differentiating cerebral from ocular blindness.

Papilledema (choked disk) in its fully developed form with marked elevation, hemorrhages at the disk margin and large distended veins is not difficult to recognize. Early papilledema, however, can easily be mistaken for structural blurring of the disk margins as well as for other congenital changes such as medullated nerve fibers and hyaline bodies. Choked disk is always a matter for concern; increased intracranial pressure of whatever cause must be the first consideration.

Optic neuritis is often bilateral in children. Rapid loss of central vision with or without papilledema is pathognomonic. Demyelinating diseases, inflammatory diseases of the eye or orbit, and encephalomyelitis must be considered in the causation of optic neuritis. When the inflammatory area occurs behind the disk, it is known as *retrobulbar neuritis,* and the disk may appear normal.

Optic atrophy is characterized by pallor of the disk, loss of disk substance, and loss of visual function. It may be primary, as in congenital optic atrophy, or secondary, following optic neuritis, long-standing papilledema, central nervous system degenerative disorders, congenital glaucoma or tumor of the optic nerve. Unilateral optic atrophy may be the first sign of glaucoma.

HYGIENE OF THE EYE

Proper illumination minimizes "eyestrain" and increases reading efficiency. There is no proof that poor lighting causes organic eye disease, but it definitely accelerates the onset of eye fatigue. Children should be encouraged to read in a good light (100 to 150 watts) which comes from behind and does not produce reflected glare. Fluorescent light, when it flickers, has been known to increase symptoms of discomfort and fatigue in some persons. Printed matter should be held at least 14 inches from the eye, and the print should not be too small. It is wise to have the book tilted to prevent reflection from glossy paper. Good posture while reading should be encouraged.

Television is not harmful to the eyes, though it frequently brings on symptoms of fatigue and "eyestrain." The child should sit at least 10 to 12 feet from the screen in a room which has some general illumination, and the picture should be sharply focused. The poor content of the programs is of more concern than is any possible deleterious effect on the eyes. Allowing a child to watch television while wearing a patch over one eye is sometimes effective in the treatment of amblyopia ex anopsia (see above).

There need be no restriction of children's reading because of refractive errors or muscular imbalance.

SIGHT-SAVING CLASSES AND SCHOOLS FOR BLIND CHILDREN

Sight-saving and training classes have been established in public and in private schools for children whose vision is reduced to such an extent that they cannot meet the requirements of the ordinary school curriculum. The training consists chiefly in following the regular school curriculum through books printed in large type on suitable contrast backgrounds so that ocular fatigue is minimized. Special attention is given to lighting and reading posture. With such a regimen children with limited but not complete loss of vision can be adequately educated. Books with large print are provided by the National Aid to the Visually Handicapped.* These promote self-help in partially sighted children.

The cooperative system for educating partially sighted children is recommended, rather than placing them in schools for the blind or in special schools where they are grouped with children with other handicaps, such as deafness or cerebral palsy. Even placement in segregated classes in public schools adds its stigma. The cooperative plan places the partially seeing children with the normally seeing children in regular classrooms. Projects requiring concentrated eye work by the partially sighted children are conducted in separate, specially equipped classrooms. The psychologic advantages of this plan are tremen-

dous, just as the term "semisighted" is preferable to "semiblind."

When vision has been reduced to 10/200 or less, it is almost impossible for the child to continue in sight-training classes, and he should then be enrolled in a school for the blind. Here he is taught one of the touch systems of reading. Emphasis is placed on the teaching of manual arts and the development of a sense of independence and self-sufficiency. Those schools in which the curriculum includes instruction for the parents as to how they may participate in the training of their visually handicapped child are the most effective ones.

Children who have never had vision do not miss it and may be content with their condition. They should be treated as normal children and neither pitied nor rejected. Parents often regard a blind infant with awe and must be helped to adjust to and manage the situation.

MEDICAL OPHTHALMOLOGY

Ocular findings are of interest and significance in a wide variety of medical conditions of children. The most important disorders include the following.

Hypertension. In the early stages there may be no observable ocular change. Generalized constriction and irregular narrowing of the arterioles are usually the first changes in the fundus. Other alterations include retinal edema, flame-shaped hemorrhages, "cotton-wool patches" and papilledema. These changes are reversible if the disease process can be eliminated in the early stages, but in hypertension of long standing the changes are irreversible and simulate those of arteriosclerotic disease. Hypertension in the child should alert the physician to renal disease, pheochromocytoma, collagen diseases and cardiovascular disorders, such as coarctation of the aorta.

Renal Retinopathy. Renal and other hypertensive retinopathies are often indistinguishable; pallor of the disk and macular star formations are more commonly associated with nephritis.

Cyanosis of the retina may occur with congenital heart diseases, chronic pulmonary insufficiency, or other disorders responsible for cyanosis. The conjunctival vessels may be congested and dark. The retinal veins are dark, tortuous and dilated, and the retina appears cyanotic at times with scattered hemorrhages.

Subacute Bacterial Endocarditis. Retinopathy is present in 40 per cent of cases during the course of the disease; the lesions include hemorrhages, Roth spots (white areas surrounded by hemorrhage), papilledema and, rarely, embolic occlusion of the central retinal artery.

Blood Disorders. *Primary and secondary anemias.* Retinopathy in the form of hemorrhages and "cotton-wool patches" generally occurs only when the red blood cell count drops to

---

*3201 Balboa St., San Francisco 21, Calif.

2 million or below. Vision will be affected if a hemorrhage is present in the macular area. The hemorrhages may be light and feathery or dense and preretinal.

Polycythemia vera. The retinal veins are dark, dilated and tortuous. Retinal hemorrhages, retinal edema and papilledema may be observed.

Hemorrhagic disorders. Retinal hemorrhages may be seen in any of the bleeding disorders. Spontaneous hemorrhages may be expected in those with thrombocytopenia.

Leukemia. The veins are characteristically dilated with sausage-shaped constrictions. Hemorrhagic exudates and white-centered hemorrhages are common during the severe stage. Exophthalmos occurs from orbital hemorrhage and leukemic infiltrations.

Diabetes Mellitus. The most common ocular complications of diabetes mellitus are in the fundi. Changes also occur in the iris, lens, optic nerve and extraocular muscles. Sudden changes in the refractive error may be the first sign of diabetes. The earliest retinal changes are punctate hemorrhages and capillary microaneurysms. The hemorrhages are characteristically small and round. Later the veins become dilated and somewhat tortuous. Small, yellow, waxy exudates appear, first in the macular area and later scattered over the posterior portion.

Contracture of the scar tissue at sites of hemorrhage may lead to irreversible changes and visual loss. From 60 to 75 per cent of juvenile diabetics suffer a severe retinopathy within 20 years or so. Minute, so-called snowflake cataracts are relatively common, and extensive opacification of the lens occurs occasionally. These changes may occur early in the disease.

Lipemia retinalis is a spectacular ophthalmoscopic finding during the uncontrolled phase of diabetes. The vessels appear as though the blood had been replaced by cream.

Genetically determined diseases with ocular manifestations are listed in Table 24-2.

Endocrine Diseases. Hyperthyroidism, hypoparathyroidism and hyperparathyroidism are discussed on pages 1197, 1201 and 1203.

TABLE 24-2. GENETICALLY DETERMINED DISEASES WITH OCULAR MANIFESTATIONS
(see also Morphologic Syndromes, p. 1509)

DISEASE	OCULAR MANIFESTATIONS	OTHER MANIFESTATIONS
Acrocephalosyndactyly (Apert's syndrome	Exophthalmos, exotropia, optic atrophy, ophthalmoplegia	Hypertelorism, acrocephalus, syndactyly
Albinism	1. In complete albinism: Iris is thin, pink or pale blue. A characteristic orange reflex from the pupil occurs when light rays penetrating the pigment-deficient membranes of the eye are reflected back to the observer's eye. Prominent choroidal vessels with poorly defined fovea. Nystagmus, head-nodding and frequently myopic astigmatism and strabismus. Marked photophobia. The eyelashes and eyebrows are white 2. In partial albinism: The iris may be pale gray; characteristic orange reflex may be present. The fundi are not pigmented; the choroidal vessels are prominent. May be nystagmus and a myopic refractive error	
Ataxia-telangiectasia.................	Prominent conjunctival vessels in medial and lateral canthal areas. Ocular motor apraxia	Ataxia, hypogammaglobulinemia, susceptibility to infection and lymphomatous diseases, mental retardation
Color blindness (complete monochromatism)	In total color blindness: photophobia, nystagmus, diminished vision	
Crouzon's disease	Exophthalmos, exotropia, optic atrophy	Craniofacial dysostosis, deafness, mental retardation

(Table Continues)

TABLE 24-2. *Continued*

DISEASE	OCULAR MANIFESTATIONS	OTHER MANIFESTATIONS
Cystic fibrosis	Dilated, tortuous retinal veins, retinal hemorrhages	Chronic pulmonary disease, intestinal malabsorption, excessive electrolytes in sweat
Cystinosis	Cystine crystals seen in cornea and conjunctiva with slit lamp. Peripheral retinal pigmentary degeneration	Small stature, aminoaciduria, renal failure
Down's syndrome (mongolism, trisomy 21)	Epicanthus, lateral upward slope of eyes, Brushfield's spots on iris, cataracts, keratoconus	Many characteristic features (see p. 331)
Ehlers-Danlos syndrome	Epicanthus, lacrimal apparatus defects, angioid streaks in retina	See page 1395
Galactosemia	Cataracts, bilateral	See page 437
Hallerman-Streiff	Microphthalmos, congenital cataracts, blue sclerae	Dwarfism, hypoplasia of mandible, hypotrichosis
Heterochromia of iris	May be transmitted in a dominant or recessive manner with Horner's syndrome (see also Waardenburg's syndrome)	
Hurler's syndrome	Haziness of corneas, glaucoma, chorioretinal changes	See page 1338
Incontinentia pigmenti	Strabismus, corneal opacities, cataract, persistent hyperplastic primary vitreous	Swirling patterns of skin pigmentation, skeletal malformation, seizures, retardation
Laurence-Moon-Biedl syndrome	Retinitis pigmentosa, optic atrophy, strabismus	Obesity, polydactyly, hypogenitalism, mental retardation
Marchesani's syndrome	Subluxated lenses, secondary glaucoma	Short stature, short digits, good musculature
Mandibulofacial dysostosis (Franceschetti's syndrome; Treacher-Collins syndrome)	Lid anomalies, antimongoloid slant, dystrichiasis	Hypoplasia of malar bone, low-set ears and ear anomalies, high-arched palate, malocclusion, deafness
Marfan's syndrome	Subluxated lenses	Arachnodactyly, kyphoscoliosis, laxity of joints, cardiovascular anomalies
Melanosis, congenital	Spotty hyperpigmentation of conjunctiva and sclera	
Neurofibromatosis (von Recklinghausen's disease)	Neurofibroma may involve any part of eye, especially the adnexa (lids)	See page 1280
Niemann-Pick disease	Brownish-red spot in macula	See page 455
Oculocerebrorenal syndrome (Lowe's syndrome)	Cataract, congenital glaucoma	See page 1368
Osteogenesis imperfecta	Blue sclerae	Osteitis fragilitas, otosclerosis, dwarfism, anomalies of skull. See page 1342

TABLE 24.2. *Continued*

DISEASE	OCULAR MANIFESTATIONS	OTHER MANIFESTATIONS
Pierre Robin syndrome	May be microphthalmos, retinal detachment, cataract, congenital glaucoma	Glossoptosis, cleft palate, micrognathia, respiratory difficulty
Pseudohypoparathyroidism	Bilateral cataracts, strabismus	See page 1203
Riley-Day syndrome (familial dysautonomia)	Deficiency of tears, corneal anesthesia, corneal ulcers and corneal scarring. Pupillary miosis with methacholine, 2.5%	See page 1308
Sickle cell anemia	Periphlebitis, retinal hemorrhages, "sea-fans," vascular occlusion. Conjunctival vessels, comma-shaped with sludging, occasional angioid streaks	See page 1056
Sturge-Weber syndrome	Congenital glaucoma, angiomatous formation in choroid, retinal detachment	See page 1281
Tay-Sachs disease	Cherry-red spot in macula, optic atrophy	See page 1294
Trisomy 13-15	Microphthalmos, corneal opacities, cataract, hypoplasia of optic nerve, anophthalmos, colobomata	See page 334
Trisomy 18	Ptosis, epicanthal folds, strabismus	See page 332
Tuberous sclerosis (Bourneville's disease	Characteristic yellow-white masses on retina	Adenoma sebaceum of face, *café-au-lait* spots, seizures, mental deficiency
Turner's syndrome (Bonnevie-Ullrich syndrome)	Paralytic strabismus, ptosis, epicanthus, colobomata, hypertelorism	See page 1231
Von Hippel-Lindau disease	Angiomatosis retinae, hemorrhages and exudates, retinal detachment	Angiomatosis of central nervous system and viscera
Waardenburg's syndrome	Blepharophimosis, heterochromia, lateral displacement of inner canthus and lower canaliculi	Congenital deafness, white forelock, prominent nasal root

TABLE 24-3. COMMON OCULAR THERAPEUTIC AGENTS*

Irrigating solution:
For ocular irrigation: physiologic saline solution

	GM. OR ML.
Astringent solution:	
Zinc sulfate	0.065
Epinephrine (1:1000)	4.00
Zephiran chloride (1:20,000)	30.00
One drop in each eye every 3 hours	
Local anesthetics:	
Proparacaine hydrochloride (Ophthaine) (Ophthetic)	0.5%
Tetracaine hydrochloride (Pontocaine)	0.5%
Cocaine hydrochloride	0.5%, 2%, 5%
Procaine hydrochloride	1%, 2%
Lidocaine hydrochloride (Xylocaine)	2%

(Table Continues)

TABLE 24-3. *Continued*

Parasympatholytic drugs (mydriatic or cycloplegic):
Homatropine hydrobromide... 5%
Tropicamide (Mydriacyl) .... 0.5% or 1%
Atropine sulfate (in ointment) .... 0.5% or 1%
Cyclopentolate hydrochloride (Cyclogyl) .... 0.5% or 1%

Parasympathomimetic drugs:
Pilocarpine hydrochloride .... 1 to 4% solution
Carbachol (Carcholin)
Echothiophate iodide (Phospholine Iodide)

Sympathomimetic drug:
Phenylephrine hydrochloride (Neo-Synephrine) .... 5% or 10%

Dyes:
Fluorescein sodium ophthalmic solution. (sterile paper strip or sterile solution
  in single-dose container) 2%

Antimicrobial and chemotherapeutic agents:
Sulfisoxazole (Gantrisin).. 4% solution and
                                                                                    ointment
Sodium sulfacetamide (Sod-Sulamyd) .... 10% or 15% solution
                                                                                    and ointment
Chloramphenicol (Chloromycetin) .... Prepared in oint-
                                                                                    ment or powder to
                                                                                    be reconstituted
Neomycin sulfate (Mycifradin) .... Ointment or solution
  Frequently combined with other drugs to widen the spectrum of activity, as in Neosporin, which contains
  neomycin, polymyxin and bacitracin

Adrenal corticosteroids:
Corticosteroids are frequently prescribed in combination with an antibiotic to reduce the inflammatory
  response. *Corticosteroids may be dangerous in herpes simplex keratitis, and their use in any condition
  for an extended time is not desirable except under the direction of an ophthalmologist.*
5-Iodo-2-deoxyuridine (I.D.U.):
This drug may be useful in the early epithelial stages of herpex simplex keratitis when begun early and
  used every hour.

---

*All the solutions listed are packaged in a sterile state in plastic squeeze bottles and are not readily contaminated.

Diseases related to Nutritional Deficiencies.
See Vitamin A Deficiency (p. 178), Hypervitaminosis A (p. 170), deficiencies of vitamin B (p. 171) and Scurvy (p. 175).
Diseases of Connective Tissue.   See page 511.

OPHTHALMIC PHARMACOLOGY

Table 24-3 is a list of ocular therapeutic agents in common use.

ROBISON D. HARLEY

REFERENCES

Adler, F. H.: *Textbook of Ophthalmology.* 7th ed. Philadelphia, W. B. Saunders Company, 1966.
Apt, L.: *Diagnostic Procedures in Pediatric Ophthalmology.* Boston, Little, Brown and Company, 1964.
Francois, J.: *Heredity in Ophthalmology.* St. Louis, C. V. Mosby Company, 1961.
Liebman, S., and Gellis, S.: *The Pediatrician's Ophthalmology.* St. Louis, C. V. Mosby Company, 1966.
Ophthalmic Staff of the Hospital for Sick Children: *The Eye in Childhood.* Chicago, Year Book Medical Publishers, Inc., 1967.

25. Neoplasms and Neoplastic-Like Lesions

Although less than 2 per cent of malignant neoplasms occur in children, cancer, including leukemia, is now the leading cause of death from disease in children beyond infancy in the United States. Between the ages of 1 and 14 years it is responsible for about 12 per cent of all deaths. Although the increasing importance of cancer as a cause of death in children is in large part related to the decline in death rates from infectious and other diseases, there is some evidence to indicate an absolute as well as a relative increase in its incidence.

The incidence of cancer among children is higher during the first 5 years of life than during either of the 2 ensuing quinquennia. The frequency of malignant neoplasms during the first 5 years of life probably reflects the embryonal nature of certain of the more common tumors encountered in this period, e.g. Wilms's tumor, neuroblastoma and possibly even acute leukemia. Such embryonal neoplasms tend to mimic structures normally present during active organogenesis and appear to be derived from cells which have never matured. They may be present at birth or may arise postnatally from cells which have not attained complete maturation.

The embryonal origin of certain neoplasms of early life is undoubtedly responsible for differences between these tumors and the more common malignant neoplasms encountered in adults. The rapidity of progress of many of the neoplasms of children as compared with those of adults is probably related to the growth characteristics of embryonic tissues. As a result of this rapid growth, the clinical manifestations of certain neoplasms in infants and children may be those of an acute infectious process, with few or none of the classic signs of malignancy encountered in adults. With the exception, however, of the 2 most common types of neoplasms encountered in early life, i.e. acute leukemia and tumors of the central nervous system, most malignant neoplasms in infants or children manifest themselves by the presence of an abnormal solid mass, which may attain a large size in a brief time. Characteristically, even large tumors are not associated with significant anemia, loss of weight or cachexia.

Benign tumors are far more common in early life than malignant ones, and many of them are hamartomas rather than true neoplasms.

Hamartomas are tumor-like, non-neoplastic malformations characterized by localized overgrowth of one or more tissues indigenous to the site in which they arise. They thus comprise such diverse lesions as hemangiomas and lymphangiomas, diffuse lipomatoses, osteochondromas, rhabdomyomas of the heart and the glial nodules in the central nervous system of persons with tuberous sclerosis. Some of them, notably the hemangiomas, may spontaneously regress and ultimately disappear. Although initially non-neoplastic, infrequently a malignant neoplasm may develop within a hamartoma, e.g. chondrosarcoma arising in an osteochondroma.

Malignant neoplasms of almost all types have been reported on one or more occasions during early life, but their common sites of origin differ sharply from those in adults. Thus the hematopoietic system, central and sympathetic nervous systems, including the eye and the adrenal, soft tissues, bone and kidney are the common sites of origin of malignant tumors in infants and children; the common epithelial tumors of adults, e.g. carcinoma of the skin, lung, stomach, breast and uterus, are rare in early life.

The natural course and the therapeutic response of tumors in infants and children cannot always be predicted accurately on the basis of experience with neoplasms in adults. Thus encapsulation of a neoplasm is often considered to be indicative of benignancy in adults, but in children Wilms's tumor and even the neuroblastoma are often initially encapsulated. Increased cellularity, invasion of adjoining tissues and the presence of mitotic figures are commonly associated with malignancy in adults, yet their occurrence in hemangiomas in infants is entirely compatible with a benign clinical course. Conversely, some "benign" tumors may, in early life, because of their location and continued growth, be responsible for death even in the absence of metastases, e.g. certain desmoids, juvenile nasopharyngeal angiofibromas or even mediastinal lymphangiomas.

Although the results of therapy are still far from satisfactory, when one compares the probability of cure of an infant with a Wilms's tumor or even a neuroblastoma with that of an adult with such a common malignant neoplasm as carcinoma of the lung or stomach, the results are certainly encouraging. Moreover, with few exceptions, rates of "cure" rather than simple "survival rates" can be determined for malignant neoplasms in infants and children; if, after removal of the tumor, metastases or recurrences have not taken place after a period of time equivalent to the age of the patient at the time of removal plus 9 months, their probability of doing so subsequently is only slight (Collin's law).

Every solid mass in an infant or child should be regarded as a malignant neoplasm until proved otherwise. Needless palpation of a suspected neoplasm should be avoided, and the mass should be removed as soon as is consistent with adequate clinical evaluation and preparation of the patient for operation; usually this period should not exceed 24 to 48 hours. As a general rule, treatment by other than surgical excision should not be instituted until an unequivocal diagnosis has been established by histologic study. With certain neoplasms, most notably the neuroblastoma, cures can sometimes be effected even in the presence of recognizable metastases. Observance of these principles should prevent a number of needless deaths from cancer in infants and children.

Although the *causes of neoplasms in early life* remain unknown, certain observations in recent years may provide clues to further understanding of some of the factors which may play a role in the development of neoplasms in infants and children.

The importance of therapeutic irradiation of the head, neck and chest in early life in the subsequent development of carcinoma (and less frequently adenoma) of the thyroid is now established. Although irradiation is not the sole factor responsible for the occurrence of such neoplasms, the incidence of carcinoma of the thyroid in persons receiving therapeutic irradiation to the thymus or to the head and chest for other benign conditions, e.g. acne vulgaris, in early life is approximately 100 times the expected incidence of this neoplasm. The carcinogenic effects of therapeutic irradiation in early life are further illustrated by the occurrence of osteosarcoma and other types of malignant neoplasms following curative radiotherapy of retinoblastomas. Benign tumors, in addition to adenomas of the thyroid, have also been observed following therapeutic irradiation, e.g. neurofibroma and, more frequently, osteochondroma. As many as 10 per cent of persons receiving therapeutic doses of irradiation for Wilms's tumor or neuroblastoma before the age of 3 years have osteochondromas after latent periods of about 2 to 10 years; less frequently a malignant mesenchymal neoplasm has followed such therapeutic irradiation.

Cancer mortality, predominantly leukemia, is about 40 per cent greater in children who have been irradiated in utero as the result of maternal abdominal or pelvic diagnostic roentgen studies than in the general population. The increased mortality from cancer in these children reaches its peak at ages 5 through 7 years.

Other factors also play a role in the development of malignant neoplasms in early life. For example, the incidence of leukemia in children with Down's syndrome is significantly higher than in their age peers. It should be noted, however, that some instances of a leukemoid reaction in infants with Down's syndrome which appear to be congenital leukemia disappear spontaneously.

The frequency of malignant lymphomas, e.g. lymphosarcoma, is increased in certain genetically determined defects with severe immunologic deficiency, e.g. ataxia-telangiectasia and the Wiskott-Aldrich syndrome. Malignant neoplasms, not of the lymphoreticular system, also occur with increased frequency in persons with certain congenital malformations which are apparently not genetically determined. Thus children with sporadic (rather than familial) aniridia have Wilms's tumors more frequently than do those in the general population. Hemihypertrophy is accompanied by an increase in the frequency not only of Wilms's tumor, but also of adrenal cortical carcinoma and hepatic neoplasms. Such isolated facts, many now apparently unrelated, should in the future provide further insight into the causes of a variety of neoplasms in early life.

Maternal Transmission of Neoplasms to the Fetus. Rarely a pregnant woman with far advanced neoplastic disease, especially malignant melanoma, may transmit the process to her offspring; to date such transmission has not been proved in the case of leukemia. Probably somewhat more frequently a maternal neoplasm metastasizes to the placenta without involvement of the fetus.

Placental chorioepithelioma may be responsible for widespread metastases in the fetus, which may not be recognized until after birth. The placental growth may invade the uterine wall and be responsible for a maternal neoplasm; in other instances it is apparently discharged from the uterine cavity without residual maternal disease.

TUMORS OF THE NOSE, SINUSES, PHARYNX, EAR AND ORAL CAVITY

Nasal polyps are the most common tumors in the nose and paranasal sinuses. The other lesions described below are rare, but are important in the differential diagnosis, since some of them may be confused clinically with nasal polyps and have a different prognosis. Embryonal rhabdomyosarcoma occurs in these areas in children with sufficient frequency to warrant consideration in the differential diagnosis of a tumor presenting in the upper air passages.

Nasal polyps are not true neoplasms, but are chronic, inflammatory pedunculated masses of edematous mucosa arising from the turbinates or accessory sinuses. Many of them are probably allergic in origin. Clinically, they contribute to chronic nasal obstruction and discharge, and at times to headache. The polyps appear as single or multiple, white to pale pink, relatively avascular, edematous masses. They are apt to recur after removal, unless the basis for their origin can be controlled.

Juvenile nasopharyngeal angiofibroma is a relatively rare neoplasm occurring almost entirely in males, usually between 10 and 20 years of age. The most frequent manifestations are those of nasal obstruction and epistaxis; the bleeding is usually intermittent and is sometimes alarmingly profuse, often necessitating nasal packing for its control. The tumor, which usually arises high on the lateral wall of the nasopharynx, may obstruct one or both posterior nasal orifices and often protrudes into the nasal cavity. Continued growth may be responsible for a variety of deformities, e.g. downward and forward displacement of the soft palate, replacement of the maxillary sinus and the subsequent development of a subcutaneous mass, or exophthalmos as a result of invasion of the orbit.

The tumor is nonencapsulated and has a sessile or slightly pedunculated base. It consists of a fibrous matrix and numerous vascular spaces of varying size and shape with walls of variable thickness. It is benign in that it does not metastasize, but recurrences following attempted removal are common. Severe hemorrhage may occur during removal or may develop postoperatively or after radiation therapy. Excision following adequate exposure is the treatment of choice; both transantral and transpalatine approaches have been advocated.

Olfactory neuroepithelial tumors (olfactory neuroblastomas) are rare malignant neoplasms; they originate in the olfactory mucous membrane high in the nasal fossa. Although they occur in children, they are predominantly a tumor of adult life. Unilateral nasal obstruction and epistaxis are the most common initial manifestations; in some instances there is a history of recurrent "nasal polyps." The neoplasm may be responsible for unilateral exophthalmos or swelling at the root of the nose. It may invade the paranasal sinuses, hard palate, intraorbital tissues, bones of the skull and the brain. Metastases may occur, sometimes after a period of several years, and involve especially the bones, lungs and cervical lymph nodes. The tumor is apt to be radiosensitive, but not radiocurable. It is probably best treated by a combination of surgery and irradiation, possibly with the addition of chemotherapeutic agents.

Histologically, the neoplasm is composed of sheets of undifferentiated cells with round or oval nuclei divided into incomplete lobules by slender vascular septa of connective tissue. Pseudorosettes similar to those in the classic neuroblastoma may be present, and some of the tumors contain true rosettes.

Teratomas may arise in the base of the skull, in the roof of the pharynx or in the hard or soft palate and project into the mouth, nose or cranial cavity. The more complex ones, in which both intracranial and extracranial masses are sometimes connected to each other through a defect in the basisphenoid, are present at birth; the infants seldom survive beyond the neonatal period. Some of the well differentiated teratomas projecting from the mouth contain structures resembling fetal parts and have been referred to as *epignathi*.

The less complex tumors, sometimes referred to as dermoids or *"hairy polyps,"* are often pedunculated structures composed of a central core of adipose tissue containing plaques of cartilage and mucous glands and covered by stratified squamous epithelium. The relation of these tumors to the complex teratomas is not clear. Nevertheless their histologic pattern, coupled with the fact that they

may arise laterally in the region of the tonsil, suggests that at least some of them may represent only malformations derived from the branchial arches and are not true neoplasms. More than half of them occur in infants under 1 year of age, in whom they may be responsible for respiratory distress and attacks of coughing and cyanosis. The tumor sometimes can be readily seen or may be detected in lateral roentgenograms of the nasopharynx as an osseous or soft tissue density depressing the soft palate. These less complex lesions usually occur in the absence of other malformations. If they are removed surgically, the prognosis is excellent.

Chordomas (p. 1475) of the base of the skull may project into the nasopharynx, or the initial manifestations may be those of an intracranial tumor. Owing to their location, surgical removal is difficult.

Osteoma. See page 1472.

Papillomas are rare benign epithelial tumors composed of irregular polypoid masses. They may be single or multiple; they arise from the nasal mucosa more often than from the paranasal sinuses. Clinically, they may be confused with nasal polyps. Repeated recurrences are common, and malignant transformation has been reported.

Adenomas are rare benign tumors arising from the glands of the mucous membrane of the nasal cavity and paranasal sinuses. They are most frequently located in the nasal cavity and ethmoidal region; those in the latter site may erode the cribriform plate. The symptoms are related to nasal obstruction or swelling, and nasal bleeding is common. Local recurrences are common, and the prognosis must be guarded because of the difficulty of complete removal.

Mixed tumors of salivary gland origin (p. 1441) may arise in the mucous membranes of the nose, paranasal sinuses or the palate. Palatal tumors commonly arise from the posterolateral portion of the hard palate and project into the floor of the nasal cavity and maxillary sinus. The symptoms are those of nasal obstruction. Difficulty in swallowing may be noted in association with palatal tumors. The tumors may be well circumscribed and erode the adjoining bone or may be poorly circumscribed invasive lesions. Clinical or pathologic differentiation of benign and malignant tumors may be difficult or impossible. Metastases are infrequent. Surgical removal is the treatment of choice, but some of these tumors, especially those in which the epithelial elements predominate, may respond to irradiation.

Carcinoma of the nasopharynx or of the *tonsil* may be a poorly differentiated epidermoid growth; it has been referred to as a transitional cell carcinoma or a lymphoepithelioma. A distinction between such neoplasms and lymphosarcomas arising in the lymphoid tissue of the nasopharynx may be difficult or even impossible. The primary neoplasm in the nasopharynx may be a diffuse, infiltrative, nonulcerated lesion; at times it may be so small that it is overlooked, and the initial manifestation may be metastases in the cervical lymph nodes. These tumors are radiosensitive, but the prognosis is grave.

Nasal glioma is a rare non-neoplastic lesion usually manifest at birth as a smooth, round, firm, nonpulsatile mass over the bridge of the nose. It is often located somewhat lateral to the midline and may extend to the inner canthus of one eye. The overlying skin is apt to be faintly red to purple, and the lesion has often been mistaken for a hemangioma. Infrequently the mass is intranasal and simulates a nasal polyp. Rarely both an intranasal and an extranasal mass are present; the two usually communicate through a defect in the nasal bone.

Nasal gliomas should be differentiated from encephaloceles, since removal of the latter may lead to meningitis. In contrast to encephaloceles, most nasal gliomas have no anatomic connection with the brain.

Congenital Macroglossia. See page 765.

Lymphangiomas of the tongue occur predominantly on the dorsum anteriorly. They vary from isolated, pinhead-sized cystic structures to diffuse lesions which infiltrate the entire tongue with resultant macroglossia, and even extend into surrounding structures such as the lips and cheeks. They may be present at birth or may not appear until adult life; more than one third of them are present before 6 years of age. Clinically, they are manifest by recurrent episodes of glossitis and swelling of the tongue, the surface of which is studded with irregular gray and pink nodules. Macroglossia may be so extreme as to preclude containment of the bulky tongue within the confines of the mouth. In the absence of symptoms no active therapy may be necessary, but in some patients local excision, wedge resection or hemiglossectomy may be indicated.

Hemangioma of the tongue may be localized or diffuse. It is a less frequent cause of macroglossia than is lymphangioma, from which it may be distinguished by its deep red color and tendency to bleed.

Neurofibroma may be responsible for unilateral macroglossia. It usually develops before the age of 3 years and is often associated with neurofibromas of the skin and *café-au-lait* spots. It is usually noncompressible and relatively avascular. Surgical excision may be difficult, since these neoplasms tend to be nonencapsulated and to extend to the floor of the mouth.

Multiple mucosal neuromas involving especially the lips, tongue, conjunctiva and eyelids may be the initial manifestation of a syndrome which includes pheochromocytoma, medullary carcinoma of the thyroid with amyloid and sometimes parathyroid adenomas and diffuse gastrointestinal ganglioneuromas. Histologically, the mucosal lesions may suggest plexiform neurofibromas or "amputation" neuromas. They may be present at birth or appear within the first few years of life. Both lips are usually diffusely enlarged, and there are often multiple pink, pedunculated lesions on the anterior aspect of the tongue. Nodules up to

several millimeters in diameter are often present on the eyelids, and medullated nerve fibers may traverse the cornea. An arachnodactyly habitus, diverticulosis and a dilated colon may also be present. Pheochromocytomas, more than one half of which are bilateral, usually do not appear until late childhood or adult life; this is also true of the carcinoma of the thyroid. Any child with multiple mucosal neuromas should therefore be followed up throughout adult life for the possible development of such endocrine tumors.

Granular Cell Myoblastoma. See page 1468.

Epulis is a term commonly used for any tumor-like growth of the gums, many of which are reactive rather than neoplastic. They are pedunculated or sessile growths which may recur after removal, but do not metastasize.

Congenital epulis is a soft, spherical mass most commonly located on the margin of the upper gum in the incisor region. It occurs almost exclusively in female infants and is usually noticed at birth or shortly afterwards. It is usually a solitary tumor, but sometimes 2 or 3 masses are present. Histologically, it consists of large polyhedral cells with lightly staining granular cytoplasm; scattered nests of paradental epithelium are sometimes present. It probably represents a non-neoplastic hamartomatous malformation.

The *lingual thyroid* is a mass in the region of the foramen cecum at the base of the tongue which must be differentiated from a thyroglossal duct cyst. It represents residual thyroid tissue along the course of the primitive thyroglossal duct; in some instances there may be complete failure of descent of the thyroid, in which case removal of the lingual thyroid is followed by hypothyroidism.

Rhabdomyosarcoma of the head and neck is primarily a disease of infancy and childhood; more than three fourths of affected persons are 12 years of age or less, one third of them being under 6 years; infrequently the tumor is present at birth. The orbit and the eyelid are the most common sites in the head and neck, and this tumor is the most common primary malignancy of the orbit in children. Orbital neoplasms usually present with unilateral proptosis, whereas those arising in the lids are apt to be responsible for a palpable, non-tender mass, which may be mistaken for a chalazion. Rhabdomyosarcomas arising in the nasopharynx, tongue, palate or elsewhere in the mouth, hypopharynx or maxillary sinus, as well as those originating in the region of the mandible, occiput or salivary gland, usually present as a mass or with signs and symptoms which lead to the detection of a mass; if the tumor grows freely into a cavity, the resultant mass often assumes a grape-like configuration (*sarcoma botryoides*). The neoplasm may also arise in the middle ear or mastoid and be responsible for "otitis media," a polypoid mass in the external auditory canal and a bloody discharge.

Most of these tumors are embryonal rhabdomyosarcomas; the alveolar and pleomorphic types are much less common. The lungs, lymph nodes and bones are the most frequent sites of metastases. The prognosis is extremely grave; less than 10 per cent of affected persons are alive 5 years after the diagnosis is established. The prognosis is somewhat better with orbital neoplasms; the 5-year survival rate is about 20 per cent. Treatment includes wide excision, irradiation and chemotherapy.

Retinal Anlage Tumor. See page 1473.

TUMORS OF THE MAJOR SALIVARY GLANDS

These tumors, uncommon in infants and children, arise more often in the parotid than in the submaxillary gland. The most common tumor of the major salivary glands in early life is the hemangioma of the parotid, a lesion which is almost confined to infants. *Other benign tumors* include mixed tumors, papillary cystadenoma lymphomatosum (Warthin tumor), fibromatoses, lipomas, myxomas, lymphangiomas, neurilemmomas and neurofibromas.

Malignant neoplasms are most often epithelial in origin, mucoepidermoid carcinoma being the most common type, and the undifferentiated carcinoma the second most frequent one. In the pediatric age period, adenocarcinomas, including adenoid cystic carcinoma and acinic cell carcinoma, as well as squamous cell carcinomas, have been observed almost entirely in older children and adolescents. Sarcoma of the major salivary glands is rare; embryonal rhabdomyosarcoma of the parotid has been observed in infancy (p. 1470).

Occasionally differentiation of a neoplasm from *chronic parotitis* may be difficult, but a history of repeated swelling of the gland, often bilateral, suggests the possibility of an inflammatory rather than a neoplastic process (p. 767); in such instances, if histologic diagnosis is deemed necessary, biopsy of the mass is preferable to total excision, since it is much less apt to be followed by paralysis of the facial nerve.

Mikulicz's disease, although predominantly a disease of adult women, may occur in childhood and may be responsible for painless enlargement of a salivary gland simulating a neoplastic process (p. 767).

Hemangioma of the parotid or, less frequently, of the submaxillary gland is the most common tumor of the salivary glands in early life. It usually manifests itself as a bluish preauricular swelling at or shortly after birth, sometimes with an associated hemangioma of the overlying skin. There may be an alarming increase in size during the first several months of life; subsequently there may be little or no growth. It seems probable that spontaneous regression of these tumors might take place, as is true of many of the rapidly growing hemangiomas of the skin, but proof of this is not available. Surgical excision is usually considered to be the treatment of choice; particular care must

be taken to avoid the facial nerve, which is more superficially located in the infant than in the adult. In spite of the cellularity and lack of encapsulation, these tumors are benign.

Mixed tumors of salivary glands are uncommon in children. The neoplasm may arise in the parotid or less frequently in the submaxillary gland. It usually presents as a round firm mass behind the ramus of the mandible. Recurrences are common after surgical excision, but metastases are almost nonexistent during childhood.

Mucoepidermoid carcinomas, although less common than mixed tumors, are the most frequent type of malignant neoplasm of the salivary glands in children. Most often the initial manifestations appear after the age of 5 years. The tumor arises in the parotid more often than in the submaxillary gland. Recurrence or persistent growth of the neoplasm after initial excision, as well as metastases to regional lymph nodes, occurs in 20 to 30 per cent of the children, but widespread metastases are rare. There is poor correlation between the histologic pattern of these neoplasms and biologic behavior.

Undifferentiated carcinoma is the second most frequent type of malignant neoplasm of the salivary glands in children. The tumor, which usually arises in the parotid, tends to be far more malignant than the mucoepidermoid carcinoma and to occur at an earlier age; it may be present at birth. It is apt to grow rapidly, to recur soon after removal and to metastasize to the regional lymph nodes and to the lungs.

Adenoid cystic carcinoma (cylindroma), a rare type of adenocarcinoma, is occasionally encountered in the parotid or submaxillary gland in older children. It is relatively slow-growing; it may recur years after excision and be responsible for distant metastases in adult life.

Acinic cell carcinoma, a specific type of adenocarcinoma which usually arises in the parotid gland, is rare in children. It is usually not encountered until late childhood or adolescence. It is a low-grade carcinoma which may recur repeatedly and, at least in adults, occasionally gives rise to widespread metastases.

TUMORS OF THE NECK

These are a heterogeneous group, some of which are true neoplasms and others hamartomatous malformations. Some of them are peculiar to this region, e.g. thyroglossal duct and branchial cleft cysts. Others, such as teratomas, neuroblastomas, rhabdomyosarcomas and lymphangiomas, occur not only in the neck, but also in a number of other sites. Owing to their location, complete removal of a cervical tumor is sometimes impossible, and even a non-neoplastic lesion such as a cystic lymphangioma or a diffuse neurofibroma rarely may be responsible for death. Of the malignant neoplasms, lymphomas, neuroblastomas and rhabdomyosarcomas are the most frequently encountered, and recognition of their occurrence in this region as primary rather than as metastatic neoplasms is of obvious importance in their management.

The occurrence of a single enlarged cervical lymph node or a group of persistently enlarged nodes presents a common diagnostic problem in infants and children. The differential diagnosis includes cervical lymphadenitis, including tuberculosis and cat-scratch disease, the reticuloendothelioses, malignant lymphoma, and metastatic malignant neoplasms such as carcinoma of the thyroid and neuroblastoma arising in the cervical region. The majority of such lesions will prove to be inflammatory rather than neoplastic, and a definitive diagnosis based on surgical excision and histologic examination should not be attempted until a reasonable length of time has elapsed. If, after 3 or 4 weeks, the lymphadenopathy has remained stationary or has increased, the nodes feel hard on palpation, the tuberculin reaction is negative and there is no recognizable source or history of a focus of infection to account for the enlarged nodes, excisional biopsy is indicated. This should be preceded by roentgenographic examination of the cervical region, since certain malignant neoplasms, notably the neuroblastoma, may have areas of calcification.

A *thyroglossal duct cyst* may be located anywhere from the base of the tongue at the foramen cecum to the isthmus of the thyroid gland along the course followed by this gland in its descent into the neck. Usually the duct atrophies; when it does not do so, a cystic swelling may appear superficially, usually in the midline of the neck just below the hyoid bone. The swelling usually develops as a painless, progressively enlarging and movable mass, and may appear at any age. The cyst moves upward when the tongue is protruded or during swallowing. It may become infected and may rupture spontaneously. Recurring inflammation or a discharging fistula causes the patient to seek medical attention. The discharge is intermittent and slight except when activated by infection.

The cyst and the entire tract, including the midportion of the body of the hyoid bone, must be completely excised to the base of the tongue. Incision and drainage are to be discouraged, since spontaneous resolution of the infection may occur. Surgical removal should be undertaken during a quiescent state.

The differential diagnosis of such a midline mass includes an epidermal inclusion cyst, commonly known as a dermoid, a lymph node which may be placed near enough to the midline to cause confusion, and the thyroglossal duct cyst. True differentiation can be made only after excision of the mass.

The *branchial cleft cyst* (lateral cervical cyst) is found in the neck anterior to the sternocleidomastoid muscle, but, in contrast to the thyroglossal duct cyst, not in the midline. The branchial cleft cyst represents a remnant of a right or left branch

of a branchial cleft. Although the cyst may not be recognized until adolescence, it or its anlage has been present since birth. It grows slowly, is ovalshaped and may become extremely large. It is usually smooth, fluctuant and moderately movable and may be attached to the skin. The cyst is sometimes mistakenly diagnosed as an abscess and incised.

The branchial cleft remnant may occur only as a sinus from which small amounts of mucus may be expressed. The course of the sinus, as with the cyst, is upward from above the lower third of the sternocleidomastoid muscle, traversing between the bifurcation of the carotid vessels to empty into the piriform sinus on either side. Any remnant of this pathway may persist. Total excision is the therapy of choice.

Adenomas of the thyroid are rare in children. They are encapsulated neoplasms which do not invade normal tissue or metastasize. They are usually solitary, but multiple adenomas may be present. The presenting complaint is that of a mass in the region of the thyroid without evidence of dysfunction of the gland. Any nodule in the thyroid should be removed and examined histologically; differentiation of benign adenoma and carcinoma, however, is not always possible.

Carcinoma of the Thyroid. See page 1198.

Congenital Goiter. See page 1189.

Teratomas of the neck may be located within or outside the thyroid. The neoplasms are usually present at birth and may be so large as to obstruct the airway. They consist of solid and cystic areas containing a variety of well differentiated tissues.

Cervical thymic masses may result from failure of the normal descent of the thymus on one side of the neck or from growth of a nodule of thymic tissue which has become separated from the main gland and has remained in the neck. A small nodule of thymic tissue near or even within the

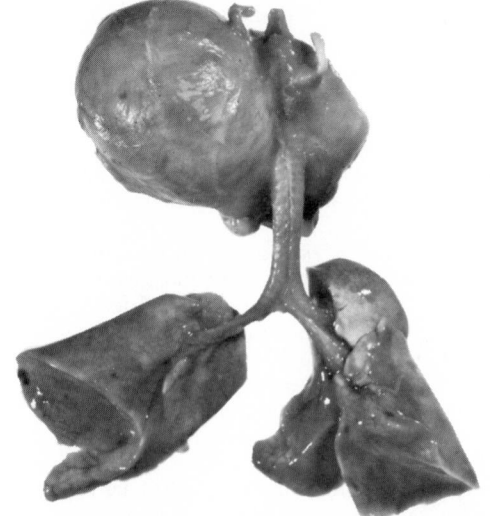

Figure 25-1. Teratoma arising from the region of the thyroid. The mass was responsible for obstruction of the airway and death at the age of 2 hours.

lower pole of the thyroid and separate from the remainder of the thymus is a common incidental finding at necropsy in infants. Infrequently an encapsulated mass removed from the anterior triangle of the neck of an infant as a cystic lymphangioma or branchial cyst will prove to be only normal thymic tissue.

Thymic cysts are rare lesions which may be located in the neck or in the anterior mediastinum or may extend into both regions. They are usually first detected in early childhood in the neck along a line extending from the angle of the jaw to the suprasternal notch. They are benign unilocular or more often multilocular cysts containing a cloudy or brown fluid in which there may be multiple yellow granules. Histologically, the cysts are lined by flattened, squamous, cuboidal or cylindrical epithelial cells, some of which may be ciliated. Distinct thymic tissue with Hassall's corpuscles is present in the wall. The lesion is non-neoplastic and is probably a developmental defect related to a branchial cyst.

Hygroma Colli. See page 1465.

Malignant lymphoma. See page 1093.

Cervical neuroblastoma. See page 1454.

Rhabdomyosarcoma of the head and neck. See page 1470.

TUMORS OF THE MEDIASTINUM

Mediastinal masses in infants and children are relatively common. If malignant lymphomas are excluded, most of which are accompanied by other manifestations in addition to those referable to the mediastinum, approximately three fourths of the mediastinal masses are neurogenic or teratomatous neoplasms or non-neoplastic cysts, e.g. duplications of the esophagus and neurenteric or bronchogenic cysts. Approximately 25 per cent of the mediastinal masses in infants and children are malignant as compared with 15 per cent of those in adults. Tumors arising in the anterior mediastinum are predominantly teratomas, whereas most of those originating in the posterior mediastinum are neurogenic neoplasms; masses confined to the mid-mediastinum are usually lymphomas or non-neoplastic cysts.

Approximately two thirds of the infants and children with a mediastinal mass are symptomatic; in the others the lesion is a chance finding on a roentgenogram of the chest. Cough, dyspnea, stridor and pain are the most frequent manifestations and are especially apt to occur with teratomas, malignant neoplasms of any type and with non-neoplastic cysts; vascular tumors and benign neurogenic ones are often unassociated with respiratory symptoms.

Mediastinal teratomas are located in the anterior mediastinum, usually in its superior aspect; rarely they arise within the pericardial sac and simulate a congenital cardiac lesion. Many are benign cystic neoplasms, commonly referred to as *dermoid cysts*. Since dermoid cysts appear to be merely cystic variants of the more solid teratomas, they need not be considered separate entities. Symptoms may not be apparent until adult life. Dyspnea, cyanosis and cough may be manifestations, and expectoration of hair and sebaceous material may occur if the tumor perforates into a bronchus. Infection of the cystic mass may produce symptoms simulating a pneumonic process. Rarely the neoplasm extends into the suprasternal or supraclavicular area. Compression of the superior vena cava causes dilation of the veins of the head, neck and upper part of the thorax. Roentgenographic examination reveals a circumscribed mass extending from the anterior mediastinum into one hemithorax; when teeth or skeletal elements are demonstrable roentgenographically, the nature of the mass is established.

The neoplasms may be composed of one or more cysts; less frequently they are predominantly solid tumors. The cysts contain sebaceous material, hair or mucoid material. Histologically, almost any type of tissue may be present, especially in the solid neoplasms. Malignant teratomas are usually solid or finely cystic tumors containing actively proliferating, poorly differentiated tissue in addition to more mature elements; the malignant element may be carcinomatous, or multiple tissues within the neoplasm may behave in a malignant manner. Mediastinal teratomas should be surgically removed.

Thymomas are extremely rare in children. In adults they sometimes accompany or precede the development of myasthenia gravis. This association has not been reported in children, in whom an association with aregenerative anemia has been recorded only once. Thymomas may be asymptomatic and discovered only roentgenographically, or they may be responsible for vague retrosternal pain, cough, dyspnea, or signs of compression of the superior vena cava. They are usually encapsulated and composed of an admixture of lymphoid and epithelial cells. True thymomas are usually benign; occasionally they infiltrate and implant on the pleura.

Thymic enlargement in children is more often caused by a *teratoma* arising within this organ than by a thymoma. By far the most common causes of a pathologically enlarged thymus, however, are leukemia, lymphosarcoma and Hodgkin's disease; in such cases there is usually but not invariably an accompanying enlargement of the mediastinal lymph nodes.

Thymolipoma is a rare tumor occurring predominantly in children 10 to 15 years of age. It may be responsible for cough, dyspnea and pain, or it may be discovered by chance on a roentgenogram of the chest. The tumor, which is benign and is apt to attain a large size, is located in the anterior portion of the mediastinum. It is encapsulated and composed of an admixture of fat and thymic tissue. A relation between thymolipomas and mediastinal lipomas has been suggested.

Angiomatous lymphoid hamartoma (benign lymphoid hamartoma) usually presents as a mass in the mid-mediastinum at the hilus of one lung. It may, however, arise in the anterior or posterior mediastinum, and about one fourth of the reported instances have been extrathoracic in location, e.g. in the neck, retroperitoneum, axilla, pectoralis or muscles of the upper extremity. The tumor occurs predominantly in young adults; about 10 per cent of affected persons are less than 15 years of age. Although almost always an asymptomatic mass, often of long duration, it is rarely associated with failure of growth, severe hypochromic anemia refractory to treatment with iron, hypergammaglobulinemia and low-grade fever; these manifestations disappear after removal of the mass. The tumor, which often reaches a rather large size, is well circumscribed or encapsulated. It is composed of lymphoid tissue devoid of normal sinusoids and containing evenly distributed follicles, the centers of which may bear a superficial resemblance to Hassall's corpuscles. The lesion has been confused with a thymoma, but it is probably not a true neoplasm. It is benign, and recurrences or metastases do not occur.

Lymphangioma of the mediastinum is usually associated with a cervical hygroma (p. 1465). Less frequently the tumor is confined to the mediastinum, where it may assume a bizarre shape and attain a large size in the absence of any clinical manifestations. The tumor is usually a multilocular cystic structure. It may arise anywhere in the mediastinum, but most frequently originates anteriorly. Chylothorax is an infrequent but serious complication.

Mediastinal hemangiomas are rare tumors occurring principally in infants and children. Although predominantly located in the anterior mediastinum, these tumors may arise posteriorly and involve the spinal cord with resultant neurologic manifestations. The patients may be asymptomatic or complain of pain or dyspnea. The diagnosis is rarely established prior to thoracotomy. The tumor, which is usually cavernous in type, is best treated surgically. Rarely it has been responsible for death in early infancy as a result of rupture into the pleural cavity.

Mediastinal lipomas usually rise in the anterior part of the mediastinum, often at the cardiophrenic angle. They may be unassociated with any clinical manifestations or may be responsible for pain and dyspnea. The tumors, although encapsulated, tend to grow extensively through the mediastinum and may reach an enormous size before giving rise to symptoms. They should be surgically excised.

Lipomas may also arise in the subpleural cavity, the cervical region or through an intercostal space. They may sometimes be identified by their radiolucency and may be suspected when there is extrathoracic extension of a mediastinal mass.

Fibromatosis of the mediastinum may be confined to this site or may occur in conjunction with similar changes in the cervical region or in the retroperitoneum. These are fibrous, infiltrative tumors which tend to grow slowly and almost never metastasize. They may encase the vena cava and be responsible for the superior vena cava syndrome.

Mesenchymomas are rare in the mediastinum, but both benign (p. 1468) and malignant (p. 1471) types have been observed in children. Even "benign" tumors composed of an admixture of mature mesenchymal elements may be so infiltrative as to be responsible for death.

Rhabdomyosarcoma (p. 1470) of the mediastinum is a rare, highly malignant neoplasm usually located in the anterior portion of the mediastinum.

Lymphoma. See page 1093.

Neuroblastoma. See page 1454.

Ganglioneuroma. See page 1456.

Neurilemmoma. See page 1469.

Neurofibroma. See page 1469.

Thymic cysts. See page 1443.

TUMORS OF THE HEART

Primary neoplasms of the heart are rare in all age groups. The majority are histologically benign, but their location may be responsible for death. Some of the neoplasms, e.g. myxomas, are apt to produce clinical manifestations at any age period in which they occur, but are usually encountered in adults. Others, such as fibromas, occur predominantly in infants and children, in whom they may be responsible for sudden death.

The diagnosis of a primary neoplasm of the heart is usually not suspected during life, death sometimes occurring suddenly with no previous symptoms of cardiovascular disease. In some instances, however, clinical manifestations referable to the cardiovascular system are present, and, through such studies as angiocardiography and coronary arteriography, the diagnosis may be established during life. Tumors such as myxomas of the atrium and intrapericardiac teratomas may be successfully treated surgically, and even intramural fibromas have been excised.

In addition to the lesions described below, a variety of other neoplasms or neoplastic-like lesions have been described in the heart of an infant or child on one or more occasions. *Lymphangioma* of the heart may occur as an isolated lesion or in association with an extracardiac hygroma. It may be a polypoid mass projecting from the epicardial surface or a diffuse infiltrative lesion with resultant thickening of the wall of the left ventricle by innumerable cystic spaces. Bleeding into a diffuse myocardial lymphangioma may be responsible for sudden death. Hemopericardium has occurred, even during the neonatal period, as a result of rupture of an epicardial hemangioma, and massive hemorrhagic pericardial effusion has occurred in an infant with juvenile xanthogranulomas involving the skin and the epicardium. Plexiform neurofibroma, intracardiac lipoma, epicardial cyst and epidermoid cysts arising in the atrial septum immediately above the tricuspid valve have been seen in infants and children. The relation of the epidermoid cyst to a benign or malignant intracardiac teratoma arising in a somewhat comparable location is not clear. Epidermoid cysts of the heart are probably distinct from the solitary cysts lined by ciliated epithelium, which are usually located in the left ventricle of adults; they may represent bronchogenic or esophageal cysts in the myocardium.

Primary malignant neoplasms of the heart in children are extremely rare, most of them being rhabdomyosarcomas; differentiation of primary from metastatic rhabdomyosarcoma of the heart may be difficult or impossible.

Rhabdomyomatous malformation of the heart (congenital rhabdomyoma) is not a true neoplasm and possibly represents a hamartomatous malformation. It is found predominantly in infants and children, about 60 per cent of affected persons being less than a year of age. It is often associated with tuberous sclerosis, some of the other manifestations of which may be present during the neonatal period. As a rule, however, the cerebral lesions so characteristic of tuberous sclerosis are not apparent in infants with rhabdomyomatous malformation of the heart who die during the first 2 or 3 months of life; of those who survive more than a few years, most will have other stigmata of tuberous sclerosis.

The myocardial lesions often are not responsible for any symptoms and are discovered incidentally at necropsy. Occasionally they are responsible for sudden death or for massive cardiomegaly and cardiac failure.

The cardiac lesions are usually multiple and are fairly well demarcated, yellowish-brown, firm, elastic nodules of varying size. Histologically, these are composed of tremendously enlarged cardiac muscle fibers which appear as empty, somewhat irregular tubes whose walls, although extremely thin, may still contain longitudinal and cross striations. A few granules of glycogen may be present within these otherwise empty, enlarged cardiac muscle fibers, but the bulk of their content is dissolved out by the usual fixatives, and there is some evidence to suggest that their enlargement and vacuolization may be caused by some substance other than glycogen. Many of the nuclei lie against the walls of the empty fibers, but some are centrally located with radially arranged cytoplasmic strands, producing the so-called spider cells.

Myxoma of the heart, the most common primary cardiac neoplasm in adults, is rare in children. It usually arises from the region of the fossa ovalis in the left atrium and projects as a polypoid, smooth or lobulated mass into the cavity of the atrium, where it may obstruct the mitral orifice. Rarely it extends through the foramen ovale and produces neoplastic masses in both atria.

The clinical manifestations are often bizarre and include the sudden onset of dyspnea, fainting spells or cyanosis. Adams-Stokes syndrome may occur, and the lesion may be responsible for sudden death. Embolic phenomena, especially cerebral ones, are common, and any embolic episode, systemic or less frequently pulmonic, should suggest the possibility of an atrial myxoma. The clinical manifestations may closely simulate those of rheumatic heart disease with mitral stenosis or insufficiency, but without any history of rheumatic fever. The sedimentation rate may be elevated, and some degree of anemia and leukocytosis are present in about one fourth of the patients. Splinter hemorrhages and other embolic phenomena may simulate bacterial endocarditis. Alterations in its nature or disappearance of the murmur with change of position or relief of symptoms following such a change suggests the possibility of an intracavitary tumor. As a rule the diagnosis of an intracavitary tumor can be established by demonstration of a filling defect, usually in the left atrium. Operation is the treatment of choice, and the patient can be cured.

Fibroma of the heart is a rare solitary tumor which is usually located in the wall of the left ventricle. It is sometimes associated with extracardiac anomalies and may be responsible for sudden death. The tumor is often several centimeters in diameter; it is a well circumscribed but nonencapsulated ovoid mass which grossly resembles a leiomyoma of the uterus. Histologically, it is composed of interweaving bundles of spindle-shaped fibroblasts associated with a variable amount of collagen and elastic fibers. Occasional foci of calcification may be present, and strands of cardiac muscle fibers are often incorporated within the tumor, especially in its peripheral portion.

Benign mesothelioma of the node of Tarawa is a rare, minute, primary tumor of the posterior part of the atrioventricular node. It may occur in children or adults and is always responsible for partial or complete heart block, sometimes accompanied by the Adams-Stokes syndrome. The tumor, which may be demonstrable only histologically, has been interpreted as a lymphangioendothelioma and as an epithelial hamartoma. Probably, however, it is derived from primitive epicardial (mesothelial) cells, which form cords and glandular-like spaces, some of the latter containing a colloid-like substance.

TUMORS OF THE LARYNX

Papillomas of the larynx (p. 903), though uncommon, are the only tumors which occur at this site with any degree of frequency. In infants subglottic hemangiomas, though rare, are important lesions which may be overlooked at laryngoscopy and even at necropsy. *Pseudosarcomas* (p. 1468) may occur in the larynx, trachea or bronchi, and their recognition as benign, non-neoplastic lesions is of obvious importance. In addition to these tumors and neurofibromas, isolated instances of lymphangioma, granular cell myoblastoma, fibrosarcoma, rhabdomyosarcoma and epidermoid carcinoma of the larynx have been reported in children; some have followed irradiation of laryngeal papillomas.

Hemangioma of the larynx is a rare tumor which affects girls more often than boys. Clinical manifestations are apparent during the first 6 months of life in approximately 90 per cent of affected infants, and inspiratory stridor is occasionally present at birth. Signs of high respiratory obstruction with stridor, wheezing and retractions may be intermittent and are sometimes misinterpreted as "croup." Since the tumor is characteristically subglottic, in contrast to the more common hemangioma on or above the vocal cords of adults, hoarseness is usually absent. Cutaneous hemangiomas are present in only about half of affected infants. Lateral roentgenograms often reveal a discrete tumor in the subglottic area. Laryngoscopically, the tumor characteristically appears as a soft, pink to bluish subglottic mass, but because of its diffuseness and the absence of distinct discoloration, the true nature of the mass may not be appreciated and may be interpreted simply as subglottic edema or stenosis. Even at postmortem examination the lesion may not be recognized macroscopically, and histologic examination of the subglottic region should be a routine procedure. Biopsy of the mass is contraindicated when the diagnosis is reasonably well established by history and laryngoscopic examination. The lesion is best treated by small amounts of irradiation with or without tracheotomy, depending upon the severity of the symptoms.

Neurofibromas of the larynx are rare. They are usually solitary lesions, only 10 to 20 per cent of them being accompanied by other stigmata of multiple neurofibromatosis. In infants and children, however, a number of them have been plexiform neurofibromas (p. 1469) and possibly have represented the initial manifestations of von Recklinghausen's disease. They are usually submucosal masses located at the level of the aryepiglottic folds and the ventricular bands. Clinical manifestations, which may begin in early infancy, are those of any slowly growing benign tumor of the larynx, e.g. hoarseness, stridor, cough and dyspnea. Recurrence following removal is rare.

TUMORS OF THE TRACHEA, BRONCHI AND LUNGS

Primary neoplasms of the trachea, bronchi or lung are rare in children, although pulmonary metastases from various sites are relatively common. Whenever a pulmonary tumor is demonstrated, every effort should be made to determine whether there is a primary extrapulmonary lesion. Removal of a suspected malignant neoplasm from any site should be preceded by roentgenographic examination of the chest in search for pulmonary metastases.

Papillomas of the trachea or bronchi are rare, and most of them are complications of laryngeal papillomas (p. 1445), the lesions tending to occur especially about a tracheostomy wound.

Tracheobronchial papillomatosis is a rare and usually late complication of laryngeal papillomas. The bronchial papillomas may occur with laryngeal papillomas or may follow them after many years. Rarely the papillomas are confined to the tracheobronchial tree and lungs, the larynx being spared. The papillary tumors grow slowly and extend into the alveolar spaces. The involved bronchi expand into cystic cavities containing bulky papillomatous masses which may contain columnar ciliated as well as squamous epithelium. The lesions, which have been erroneously interpreted as carcinoma, do not metastasize and are probably of multicentric origin rather than implants from an initial primary tumor. Clinically, they are characterized by recurrent hemoptysis; in a person with a preceding history of laryngeal papillomas such an occurrence should suggest the possibility of tracheobronchial papillomatosis. Roentgenographic examination reveals areas of nodular density and cavitation within the lungs and, with the history of hemoptysis, may lead to an erroneous diagnosis of tuberculosis. The cavities may become secondarily infected. Treatment should be conservative; if a symptomatic lesion must be excised, no more pulmonary parenchyma than is absolutely necessary should be removed.

Bronchogenic cysts are non-neoplastic lesions most frequently encountered in adults, in whom they are often asymptomatic. In the pediatric age period, and especially in infants, they are more apt to be associated with manifestations of bronchial obstruction, e.g. periodic episodes of dyspnea, wheezing, stridor, cough and cyanosis. These may begin early in life, even during the neonatal period, and are sometimes accompanied by recurrent attacks of pneumonia. The cyst, which only rarely communicates with the tracheobronchial tree, is typically located near the carina anterior to the esophagus, but may be lateral to the trachea at a somewhat higher level, in the wall of the esophagus or elsewhere in the mediastinum. It is characteristically manifest roentgenographically as a sharply circumscribed, dense, round or oval mass arising in the mid-mediastinum and displacing the esophagus posteriorly and laterally; only rarely is an air-fluid level present. Occasionally no mass has been detected roentgenographically, and failure to remove the cyst has proved lethal.

Bronchial adenoma is a low-grade carcinoma which presents as a firm, spherical tumor projecting into the lumen of the trachea or one of the larger bronchi. The tumor extends through the bronchial wall; the extrabronchial portion may be larger than the intraluminal one. Cough, wheezing and recurrent episodes of pneumonia, sometimes with hemoptysis, are the usual manifestations. Affected children are sometimes treated for bronchial asthma for years before the neoplasm is discovered. Bronchial obstruction and repeated infections may lead to bronchiectasis. Tracheal neoplasms may be unaccompanied by roentgenographic changes, but bronchial tumors, which are more common, are usually associated with emphysema, atelectasis or a pulmonary infiltrate in the area supplied by the affected bronchus. Histologically, the neoplasm may resemble a carcinoid (p. 1449) or, much less frequently, an adenoid cystic carcinoma (cylindroma) (p. 1441); rarely a polypoid tumor is a true adenoma composed of distinct glands lined by tall cylindrical epithelium and filled with mucus. The tumor should be surgically resected even if this requires lobectomy or pneumonectomy. Although in adults the cylindromatous neoplasm has proved to be more malignant than the carcinoid, metastases to regional lymph nodes have been observed in both types in children. In general the prognosis is good even if regional lymph nodes are involved.

Pulmonary arteriovenous fistulas (cavernous hemangiomas of the lung) are solitary or multiple lesions associated with telangiectases in other parts of the body in about half of the patients, and in more than half of the affected persons there is a family history of hemorrhagic telangiectasia (Rendu-Osler-Weber disease) (p. 842). The clinical manifestations are cyanosis, which may be present at birth or appear in early childhood, dyspnea, polycythemia and clubbing of the fingers and toes; repeated epistaxes are common. A systolic or continuous murmur may be audible over the lesion, and the diagnosis of congenital heart disease may be considered. Roentgenographically, the lesion is usually demonstrable as a homogeneous density of variable size and shape continuous with the hilar vascular shadows. The lesion should be excised.

Hamartomas of the lung in the pediatric age period are almost all cystic adenomatoid malformations (p. 912). The so-called chondromatous hamartoma found in adults is extremely rare in children. The chondromatous variety are usually small subpleural nodules composed predominantly of cartilage. Between the lobules of cartilage are clefts lined by bronchial epithelium and surrounded by loose connective tissue, fat and smooth muscle fibers.

Lymphangioma and *hemangioma* are rare types of hamartomas of the lung. Lymphangioma usually involves only a single lobe. Hemangioma of the lung is sometimes multicentric, involving both lungs.

Cystic Adenomatoid Malformation of the Lung. See page 912.

Fibrosarcoma of a bronchus is an extremely rare neoplasm which tends to occur in children and young adults; almost half of affected persons are less than 15 years of age. Cough, dyspnea, fever, and repeated episodes of atelectasis and lower respiratory tract infection are common. Metastases in the pediatric age period are almost nonexistent, and it seems probable that some of the reported instances are pseudosarcomas (p. 1468) which would have responded satisfactorily to local bronchoscopic excision (Fig. 25-2). If the diagnosis of fibrosarcoma is firmly established, however, lobectomy or pneumonectomy is indicated.

Leiomyomas, neurilemmomas or *neurofibromas* which arise in the pulmonary parenchyma are rare and usually asymptomatic lesions. Roentgenographically, any of these appears as a well circumscribed, spherical, homogeneous density. In contrast, intrabronchial leiomyomas and neurofibromas are responsible for cough, fever, atelectasis and recurrent lower respiratory tract infections. Lobectomy is the treatment of choice.

Leiomyosarcomas may arise in the trachea, bronchi or pulmonary parenchyma. These are usually responsible for symptoms such as cough and dyspnea, sometimes accompanied by pain in the chest. In children, in whom these neoplasms are extremely rare, there may be local extension into a pulmonary vein, but metastases rarely occur. Treatment is by excision, including lobectomy or pneumonectomy if necessary for complete removal of the mass.

Postinflammatory tumors of the lung are rare.

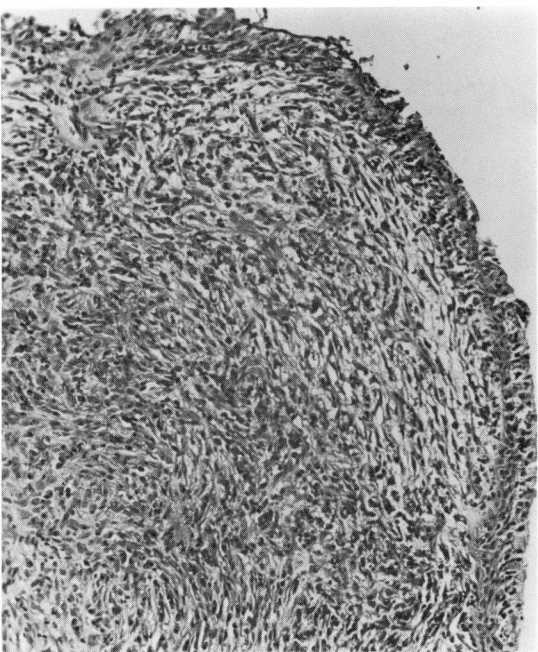

Figure 25-2. Pseudosarcoma of the left main bronchus from a boy 9 years old. Sheets of large, plump fibroblasts are haphazardly arranged in a small amount of myxoid ground substance. There is a sparse infiltrate of inflammatory cells. Eight years after bronchoscopic removal of the tumor the boy had no related clinical manifestations.

Symptoms are apt to be mild, e.g. a moderate cough. Hemoptysis, which is common in adults, is usually absent in children. There is usually a history of a preceding respiratory infection. Roentgenographically, the lesion is a solitary, sharply circumscribed, lobulated mass, infrequently with central cavitation. Histologically, the tumor is composed of spindle-shaped cells, often arranged in whorls or interlacing bundles, vascular channels, nests of foam cells and an infiltrate of inflammatory cells, predominantly plasma cells. The tumor is probably not a neoplasm, but is important because it may be confused clinically with tuberculosis or a true neoplasm. Pathologically, it may be erroneously interpreted as a neurofibroma or even a fibrosarcoma. The relation of these tumors with those described as *sclerosing hemangiomas* of the lung is not clear, but the two may well represent the same lesion.

Bronchogenic carcinoma is extremely rare in early life, but has been reported even in infants. The initial manifestations may be referable to the primary neoplasm, e.g. cough, dyspnea and pain in the chest, or to metastatic foci. The neoplasms may be large and bulky and may replace most of the affected lung, displace the mediastinum to the opposite side, obliterate the pleural space and even extend into the intercostal spaces; a primary focus within a bronchus is unusual. Metastases occur in lymph nodes, the opposite lung, bone and a variety of other sites; the brain, liver and adrenal are usually spared. Histologically undifferentiated, epidermoid and adenocarcinomas have been described.

TUMORS OF THE GASTROINTESTINAL TRACT

Tumors of the gastrointestinal tract may be symptomless or may be manifest by abdominal pain, intestinal obstruction (especially intussusception), hemorrhage, or rarely by a palpable mass. With the exception of the juvenile polyp, no tumor of the gastrointestinal tract can be considered common in children, but both benign and malignant neoplasms do occur.

Juvenile polyps are common tumors of the gastrointestinal tract in early life. They are much more common in the first than in the second decade, but are infrequent during the first year of life. The polyps are usually located in the rectum, less frequently in the sigmoid colon and uncommonly in the more proximal colon, the small intestine or the stomach. They are usually solitary, but occasionally several polyps may be scattered through the bowel, especially in the colon.

The common clinical manifestation is bleeding from the rectum, small amounts of bright red blood being passed with or after defecation. The continuous loss of even small amounts of blood over a period of several months may be responsible for hypochromic anemia. Abdominal pain may occur, but intussusception is infrequent. Occasionally the polyp prolapses through the anus and is spontaneously extruded.

These are benign tumors with an entirely different histologic pattern from the common polypoid lesion of the bowel in adults, from the polyps in multiple familial polyposis and from those in the Peutz-Jeghers syndrome. There is no evidence that the juvenile polyp undergoes malignant transformation; occasionally they may disappear spontaneously. Treatment consists in removal of a solitary polyp, usually at sigmoidoscopy. If additional polyps are demonstrated, they too should probably be removed, and certainly if they are responsible for symptoms. Some clinicians, however, have advocated observation when these additional polyps are not responsible for symptoms.

Multiple familial polyposis is a rare condition characterized by the presence of innumerable sessile and pedunculated tumors in the rectum and colon. It should not be confused with scattered juvenile polyps, which are benign and do not predispose to the development of carcinoma, nor with the Peutz-Jeghers syndrome, in which the polyps involve predominantly the small intestine. The disease is transmitted as a mendelian dominant trait with incomplete penetrance; approximately one third of the cases appear to be sporadic. The clinical manifestations are usually diarrhea and bleeding; they usually appear in the teen-age period. If untreated, these patients almost all develop carcinoma, many prior to 15 years of age. Treatment, therefore, consists in total colectomy.

Peutz-Jeghers syndrome is a rare condition inherited in a dominant manner and characterized by intestinal polyps and deposits of pigment especially in the lips and buccal mucosa, but sometimes also in the skin of the face and in the palmar and plantar surfaces of the fingers and toes. The polyps are usually multiple and may be located in the stomach, colon and rectum, small bowel or in all these sites. The clinical manifestations referable to the polyps are those of recurrent transient intussusception, gastrointestinal bleeding and hypochromic anemia. The polyps, which have been interpreted as hamartomas, contain glands lined by cells of all the types normally found in the affected part of the gastrointestinal tract. Cystic dilatation of the glands is common, and the polyps often contain strands of smooth muscle. The development of carcinoma, presumably from these polyps, is infrequent, but has occurred, especially in the duodenum. In general, treatment should be conservative with the removal of only those polyps which are responsible for symptoms.

Gardner's syndrome is inherited as an autosomal dominant trait and is characterized by the presence of multiple polyps of the colon and rectum, multiple osteomas involving especially the facial bones, multiple epidermoid cysts and the occurrence of fibromatous growths (desmoids) which tend to develop in incisional scars on the abdomen or in the mesentery after intestinal surgery. The polyps, which may not develop until adult life, are multiple but scattered, and do not carpet the colonic mucosa as is the case in multiple familial polyposis; they may, moreover, be associated with polyps elsewhere in the gastrointestinal tract. There is a striking tendency to malignant transformation of the colonic polyps. Intestinal manifestations are often preceded by one or more of the other stigmata of the syndrome, the presence of which should lead to a thorough investigation for the possibility of intestinal polyposis. The disease appears to be a distinct entity and not simply a variant of multiple familial polyposis.

Benign "lymphomas" of the rectum and anal canal are small polyploid lesions composed of aggregates of lymphocytes containing germinal centers. They are usually solitary, sessile lesions located in the lower third of the rectum. The lymphoid tissue comprising the mass usually does not extend beyond the submucosa and is covered by intact mucosa. The most frequent clinical manifestation is rectal bleeding. The lesions are not related to the malignant lymphomas, but are probably inflammatory in origin. Even though removal is incomplete, the incidence of recurrence is very low, and treatment should be nothing more than simple excision.

Occasionally a patient may have several benign lymphoid polyps, and in extremely rare instances innumerable sessile polyps composed of hyperplastic lymphoid elements may cover the mucosal surface of the colon and terminal ileum (*gastrointestinal pseudoleukemia*). The multiplicity of these lesions may lead to an erroneous diagnosis of multiple familial polyposis. Although there may be some degree of hepatosplenomegaly and lymphadenopathy associated with such multiple lesions, they are not followed by the development of leukemia and should be treated conservatively.

Lymphosarcoma is the most common malignant neoplasm of the gastrointestinal tract encountered in early life, its greatest incidence in childhood being from 3 to 8 years of age. Although usually arising in the small intestine, especially the ileum, it may originate in the colon, appendix or even the stomach. The presenting complaint is usually crampy abdominal pain often accompanied by vomiting and a palpable mass; the mass may be the neoplasm itself or an intussusception. Intestinal obstruction may be caused by narrowing of the lumen of the bowel by a diffuse infiltrative lesion or by intussusception. Morphologically, a considerable segment of the bowel may be diffusely infiltrated by neoplastic cells with resultant thickening of the wall and superficial ulceration of the mucosa, or a polypoid mass may project into the lumen of the bowel. Metastases may be widespread throughout the abdominal organs. The prognosis is grave, but not uniformly hopeless. Cures have been obtained by surgical removal of the affected segment of bowel and the regionally involved lymph nodes, in some instances supplemented by irradiation or chemotherapy.

Carcinoma of the colon is rare in children; it may occur as a complication of multiple familial polyposis (see above) or of prolonged chronic ulcerative colitis. The incidence of carcinoma appears to be greater in persons who have chronic ulcerative colitis in childhood than in those whose first manifestations are in adult life; occasionally malignancy may develop during childhood.

Rarely carcinoma of the colon occurs in infancy or childhood in the absence of known predisposing factors. It is more common in the rectum and distal colon than in the proximal large bowel. The symptoms are similar to those in adults. Abdominal pain, vomiting, constipation, loss of weight, and blood in the stools are the most common symptoms, and a mass is palpable in more than half of the affected children. In contrast to adults, in whom most of the neoplasms are fairly well differentiated adenocarcinomas, almost half of those in children are poorly differentiated neoplasms with signet ring cells. The prognosis is grave, but apparent cures have been effected, especially when the tumor is a well differentiated one.

Carcinoids (argentaffin tumors) occur in less than 0.2 per cent of appendices removed from children under 14 years of age. The tumor is usually located in the distal end of the appendix, where it presents as a firm, yellow mass arising deep in the mucosa, infiltrating the muscularis and often extending to the serosa. It is usually an incidental finding observed in an appendix removed because of a diagnosis of acute appendicitis or during laparotomy for some other reason. Infrequently, however, the mass may be located more proximally in the appendix and be responsible for obstruction of the lumen and acute appendicitis. Although appendiceal carcinoids are indistinguishable morphologically from malignant carcinoids arising elsewhere in the gastrointestinal tract, those arising in the appendix rarely metastasize. If, as is usually true, the tumor is less than 2 cm. in diameter and there are no grossly recognizable metastases, simple appendectomy is adequate treatment; this is true regardless of the location of the tumor in the appendix and regardless of histologic evidence of peritoneal involvement or lymphatic invasion.

Rarely a carcinoid may arise in a Meckel's diverticulum or in the ileum; in the ileum it is a rare cause of intussusception.

The *malignant carcinoid syndrome*, which consists of valvular disease of the right side of the heart, sudden flushing of the skin, an unusual type of patchy, changing cyanosis, frequent watery stools and "asthmatic attacks," may have its onset during childhood. It is caused by a carcinoid in the ileum, which has metastasized to such an extent as to be responsible for the presence of a large mass of neoplastic tissue within the body; the metastases usually involve the liver, but the syndrome has been observed in association with metastases confined to the mesenteric lymph nodes. The manifestations result from excessive amounts of serotonin (5-hydroxytryptamine) in the blood and tissues; the diagnosis can be confirmed by the demonstration of excessive amounts of its metabolite, 5-hydroxyindoleacetic acid, in the urine. Some of these patients survive for many months or even years in the presence of extensive inoperable metastatic disease.

Hemangiomas of the intestine are extremely rare, but have been observed in all age groups. They may be diffuse infiltrating lesions involving a segment of the bowel with resultant thickening of the wall and narrowing of the lumen or may be localized and project into the lumen. They are sometimes multiple and may be associated with hemangiomas elsewhere, e.g. in the stomach, liver and skin. The manifestations are those of intestinal obstruction, hemorrhage, pain or intussusception; only rarely is there a palpable mass.

Leiomyosarcomas have been observed in the stomach, small intestine and colon of children; their benign counterpart, the *leiomyoma*, has been reported as arising from these sites as well as from the esophagus and from a Meckel's diverticulum. Estimation of the biologic behavior of smooth muscle tumors based upon their histologic characteristics is extremely difficult, but with the exception of tumors arising in the stomach, recurrences or metastases from smooth muscle tumors of the gastrointestinal tract in children are rare. The neoplasms, regardless of their site of origin in the enteric canal, are usually firm, circumscribed but nonencapsulated tumors. Those arising in the stomach may be responsible for gross bleeding and a palpable mass, whereas those arising in the small intestine are apt to be manifest by signs of intestinal obstruction; tumors of the small bowel are rarely palpable, but they may serve as the lead point for an intussusception. Smooth muscle tumors of the large intestine may reach a large size and be responsible for obstruction and a palpable mass.

Teratoma of the stomach is an extremely rare benign lesion usually encountered in infants less than 1 year of age. In addition to a palpable mass, there may be severe anemia secondary to bleeding. The tumor may herniate into the thorax through the esophageal hiatus.

TUMORS OF THE LIVER

Metastatic neoplasms of the liver are more frequent than primary ones and may originate from a variety of tumors. Metastatic neoplasms within the liver are usually not responsible for any manifestations other than hepatomegaly, but in rare instances a clinical pattern simulating that of hepatic glycogenosis has been produced by extensive hepatic metastases from a neuroblastoma.

Primary neoplasms of the liver in infants and children, the majority of which are malignant, occur with sufficient frequency that they must be considered in the differential diagnosis of a mass in the upper part of the abdomen. Some of them can be successfully treated surgically.

Infantile hemangioendothelioma is the common vascular tumor of the liver in infants; cavernous hemangiomas similar to those encountered in adults are rare. The tumors are commonly multicentric within the liver, and extrahepatic hemangiomas are present in some instances. The multiplicity of the lesions and the active proliferation of vessels within them may suggest a malignant neoplasm, but they are probably simple vascular hamartomas rather than true neoplasms and are comparable to the cellular hemangiomas so common in the skin of infants.

Clinical manifestations are commonly present in the first weeks of life. An abdominal mass is often the only presenting complaint, but anemia and rarely ascites and jaundice may be present. In some instances cardiomegaly and congestive heart failure may lead to an erroneous diagnosis of congenital heart disease; cardiovascular manifestations have been attributed to arteriovenous shunts within the tumor. Fatal hemorrhage may occur spontaneously or after biopsy. The solitary tumors are probably best treated surgically. Multicentric tumors of the liver should be treated by irradiation, although spontaneous regression may occur in some instances.

Adenomas are rare, solitary circumscribed neoplasms composed of hepatic cells. There are no bile ducts or portal triads. There is no associated cirrhosis. The adenoma should be differentiated from the adenomatous hyperplastic nodules associated with hepatic damage. Differentiation from carcinoma may be difficult or impossible, and the diagnosis is often indefinite until sufficient time has elapsed to ensure that a recurrence is not likely. The tumor should be widely excised.

Focal nodular hyperplasia of the liver is a rare tumor whose exact nature is not known. It is probably not a true neoplasm. The initial complaint is usually related to abdominal enlargement or to a palpable mass; at times there is discomfort in the upper part of the abdomen.

The lesion, which is almost always a solitary one, may be pedunculated or located deep within the liver. It is sharply demarcated from the adjacent hepatic tissue; toward the center of the mass a stellate zone of connective tissue is present, from which bands of collagen radiate peripherally. The lesion is benign and does not warrant a radical surgical procedure. It should, however, be resected if this can be easily accomplished.

Mesenchymal hamartomas of the liver are cystic masses which are usually manifest during infancy. The presenting complaint is that of an upper abdominal mass which may increase rapidly in size, owing to the accumulation of fluid in it. The tumor is usually located near the lower margin of the right lobe of the liver to which it is sometimes attached by a pedicle. It may project into the pelvis and can often be outlined roentgenographically. The tumor can usually be identified grossly by its multicystic appearance. It is poorly demarcated from the adjoining hepatic parenchyma. Histologically, it consists of connective tissue containing cystic spaces, many of which may have no demonstrable lining cells. Small numbers of hepatic cells and bile ducts are present, especially about the periphery of the lesion. The tumor is benign, but should be excised.

Carcinoma of the liver in the pediatric age period occurs in 2 distinct forms: hepatoblastoma and hepatoma. They tend to occur at different ages and are distinct morphologically and probably pathogenetically. The prognosis, grave in both, may be somewhat better in the case of the hepatoblastoma. Both types are more common in males. Generalized demineralization of the skeleton occasionally occurs with each one, as may hyperlipemia. Isosexual precocious puberty in the male with elevated levels of urinary gonadotropins is a rare manifestation of carcinoma of the liver, usually a hepatoblastoma. Hepatomas occasionally appear to complicate other hepatic disease, such as neonatal hepatitis, galactosemia, glycogen storage disease, tyrosinosis or biliary cirrhosis secondary to atresia of the bile ducts. Hepatoblastomas appear to bear no such relation to pre-existing hepatic disease, but gonadotropin-producing ones have been associated with precocious puberty (p. 1184). Rupture of the neoplastic liver may be responsible for an acute abdominal crisis with either type of tumor.

Metastases from hepatoblastoma or hepatoma occur principally in the lungs, liver and abdominal lymph nodes. Cure of either type of tumor is rare, but has been effected by resection, including lobectomy.

Hepatoblastomas are more common in the pediatric age period than are hepatomas. They occur almost entirely in the first 3 years of life and may be present at birth. The initial manifestation is abdominal enlargement as the result of hepatomegaly; a distinct hepatic tumor may be palpable. Roentgenographic examination occasionally reveals mottled amorphous calcification within the tumor. Morphologically, the hepatic neoplasm is usually solitary, but at times it is accompanied by multiple smaller nodules of neoplastic tissue. Histologically, the tumor consists of discrete hepatic parenchymal cells resembling those of the fetal liver, but not arranged in the normal lobular pattern. Bile canaliculi may be present, and the neoplastic cells may contain glycogen and fat. Foci of extramedullary hematopoiesis are usually present. In addition, more primitive dark-staining cells arranged in sheets or ribbons, sometimes forming acini, rosettes or papillary structures, may be present, and in some there are also primitive mesenchymal elements with varying degrees of differentiation. Osteoid, bone, cartilage and islands of squamous epithelial cells with distinct keratinized pearls may be present.

Hepatomas tend to occur after 5 or 6 years of age. Progressive abdominal enlargement sometimes accompanied by a definite mass is common. A history of anorexia, nausea, loss of weight and intermittent abdominal pain is more frequent than with hepatoblastoma. Fetal alpha-l globulin iden-

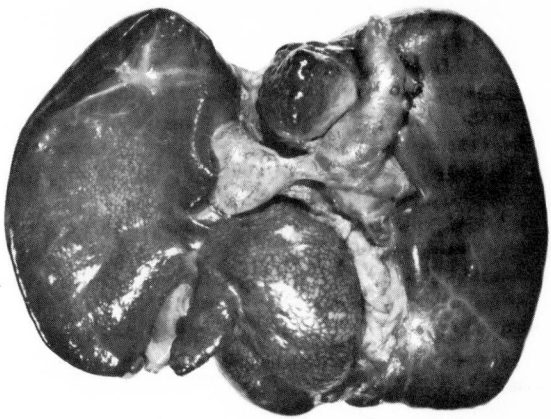

Figure 25-3. Multifocal hepatoma complicating giant cell hepatitis in a 2-year-old girl. There are multiple nodules of neoplastic tissue involving especially the left and quadrate lobes. The portal vein, which has been reflected upward, is distended with tumor (From J. B. Arey; *Pediat. Clin. N. Amer.* Vol. 10.)

tical with feto-protein of human fetuses is sometimes present in the serum and in various viscera of affected persons. The neoplasm may be solitary, or there may be multiple nodules. Histologically, the tumors are predominantly hepatocellular carcinomas similar to those encountered in adults; cholangiocarcinomas and mixed hepatic cell and cholangiocarcinomas are rare. The tumors consist of broad trabeculae of neoplastic cells containing variable amounts of fat, glycogen and bile. The trabeculae are separated from each other by sinusoids lined by endothelium.

Teratoma of the liver is a rare tumor, usually recognizable at or shortly after birth. It tends to have a bizarre lobated structure and contains a variety of tissues foreign to the liver and derived from multiple germ layers, e.g. skin, brain, bone, intestinal glands.

Mesenchymomas of the liver are composed of a mixture of mesodermal elements, i.e. angiomatous, fibrous and undifferentiated mesenchymal tissue. Epithelial elements are usually absent. Although those occurring in the liver usually appear to be malignant, some have been successfully resected.

Sarcoma of the liver is rare. The neoplasms are often undifferentiated and are classified with difficulty. Embryonal rhabdomyosarcomas may arise in the liver as well as within the common bile duct.

Ectopic adrenal tissue may occur beneath the hepatic capsule, and rarely benign or malignant adrenal cortical tumors may arise in the liver. The diagnosis of such an *adrenal rest tumor* within the liver probably should not be made unless evidences of adrenal cortical hyperfunction are present and the hormones are identified within the tumor.

TUMORS OF THE SPLEEN

Primary splenic tumors are rare in any age period, splenic enlargement usually being part of a systemic disease such as leukemia, hemolytic anemia, lipidosis or infection or the result of increased venous pressure (p. 1090).

Splenic cysts are rare. In children epidermoid cysts and pseudocysts are more frequent than parasitic ones resulting from echinococcal infection. *Pseudocysts* of the spleen are secondary to old trauma or infarction. Their walls are composed of fibrous or granulation tissue with no specific lining cells. Certain cysts that have been interpreted as pseudocysts, however, may well have been true or "neoplastic" ones, the lining cells of which were destroyed by trauma and hemorrhage.

Epidermoid cysts of the spleen, though rare, are the most common type of true cysts in the spleen in children (Fig. 25-4). They are usually large solitary cysts, sometimes with smaller satellite cysts about them. They contain clear or chocolate-colored fluid, that usually includes cholesterol. Their walls are trabeculated and consist of fibrous tissue lined in some areas by nonkeratinized squamous epithelial cells. Intercellular bridges are present, but there are no skin appendages. In some areas the lining cells are absent or resemble mesothelium. They occur predominantly in girls more than 5 years of age, in whom they are responsible for an asymptomatic mass in the left upper quadrant of the abdomen. Roentgenographic examination reveals a large, rounded, homogeneous density displacing the stomach to the right and the splenic flexure of the colon downward.

Hemangioma and *lymphangioma* are extremely rare causes of splenomegaly in children; they are usually incidental findings at autopsy in adults. Thrombocytopenia, purpura, anemia and a deficiency of fibrinogen have been observed in an infant with a giant hemangioma of the spleen.

Splenomas (*splenic hamartomas*) are rare, usually solitary, tumors most often found incidentally at autopsy in elderly adults. The tumors are solid, well circumscribed but not encapsulated

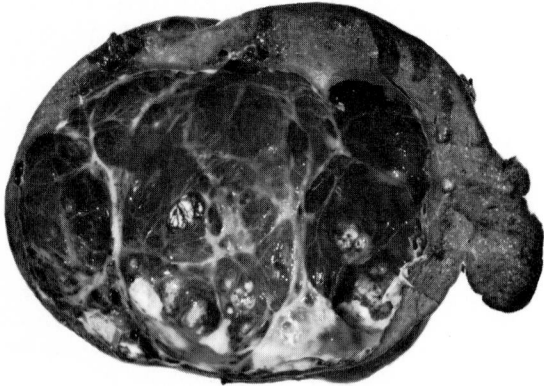

Figure 25-4. Epidermoid cyst of the spleen from a girl 8 years old. The spleen, which weighed 600 gm., has been hemisected. The cyst contained at least 335 cc. of turbid brown fluid. Its wall is trabeculated and is lined by cells which vary from cuboidal to flattened to squamous; intercellular bridges were present, but there was no keratinization.

structures within the splenic parenchyma, sometimes producing a bulge on the surface. They may differ from the surrounding spleen only by their consistency or paler color. Histologically, they are composed of lymphoid tissue, red pulp and sinusoids, often with considerable fibrosis. Tumors composed predominantly of lymphoid tissue may simulate malignant lymphoma, from which they may be differentiated by the presence of numerous sinusoids.

TUMORS OF THE PANCREAS

Carcinoma of the pancreas is extremely rare in early life. In 1964 Moyan et al. were able to collect only 15 examples of nonfunctioning pancreatic carcinoid in persons under 15 years of age, some of whom were infants. The manifestations include a palpable mass, diarrhea, anorexia and icterus. The tumor may involve the adjacent bowel and cause ulceration with gastrointestinal bleeding and severe anemia. In some instances there is a celiac-like syndrome. Metastases are especially apt to involve regional lymph nodes and the liver.

Tumors of the islets of Langerhans (p. 1167), whether functional (hypoglycemia) or nonfunctional, are predominantly lesions of adult life. Both types, however, have been observed in children. Severe, refractory diarrhea may be the sole manifestation.

Familial multiple endocrinopathy-peptic ulcer complex is a disorder characterized by the concomitant occurrence of hyperplasia or tumors of multiple endocrine glands, most frequently the parathyroids, pancreatic islets and pituitary; peptic ulcers are present in more than half of affected persons. The syndrome, which appears to be inherited as an autosomal dominant, usually manifests itself in the third and fourth decades of life, but evidence of endocrine dysfunction has been noted in some members of affected families before the age of 10 years. The endocrine tumors may or may not be functional, and any combination of glands may be affected, as a result of which the manifestations of the syndrome are protean. Within a family, however, the disorder often manifests itself in a fairly consistent manner.

Symptoms referable to a peptic ulcer are the initial ones in about one fourth of instances. In about one fifth the first manifestations are those of hypoglycemia. Altered parathyroid function, complaints referable to pituitary dysfunction or severe diarrhea and weight loss, probably related to pancreatic islet cell tumors, are less common initial manifestations. Hyperfunction may be limited to a single endocrine system for many years. Ultimately, however, hyperparathyroidism appears in about 85 per cent of affected persons; hyperplasia or adenomas involve multiple parathyroid glands in more than half of those with hyperparathyroidism. Multicentric tumors of the pancreatic islets composed of either alpha or beta cells are almost as frequent, and carcinoma of the islets is present in about one third of those with pancreatic involvement. Death from metastases, however, is rare. About one third of those with pancreatic involvement have evidence of hypoglycemia, but this is uncommonly the result of a carcinoma of the islets. Chromophobe adenomas and acidophilic hyperplasia or adenomas of the pituitary with acromegaly are present in more than half of affected persons.

Pseudocysts of the Pancreas. See page 868.

TUMORS OF THE KIDNEY

Wilms's tumor (nephroblastoma) is one of the most common abdominal neoplasms of early life. Approximately two thirds of these tumors appear before the age of 3 years; rarely are they noted at birth. Bilateral renal involvement is uncommon. (See relationship with aniridia and hemihypertrophy, page 1438.)

The presenting complaint is usually an abdominal mass; less frequently fever and abdominal pain are the initial manifestations. Physical examination reveals a firm, nontender mass which may extend down into the iliac fossa, but usually does not cross the midline. Hypertension may be present and is usually attributed to ischemia of the remaining renal tissue on the affected side. Hematuria is infrequent.

Roentgen examination reveals a soft tissue density which is apt to displace the intestine toward the opposite side. Calcification is rather infrequent and when present is apt to be dense and curvilinear, in contrast to the stippled appearance common with a neuroblastoma. Pyelography usually reveals distortion of the renal pelvis; in some instances the kidney on the affected side cannot be seen by intravenous pyelography. It should be emphasized that the pyelographic findings, even when typical, are not diagnostic of a Wilms's tumor, but are simply indicative of the presence of an intrarenal mass. Probably the most important reason for obtaining pyelograms is to demonstrate the presence and normality of the opposite nonaffected kidney.

Macroscopically, the neoplasm is encapsulated until a relatively late stage (Fig. 25-5), when it may invade the renal pelvis and ureter, renal veins or perirenal fat; extensive subcapsular hemorrhage is sometimes present. On section extensive necrosis is often apparent, especially in the larger tumors, and as a result much of the neoplasm may be soft and semiliquid. The renal pelvis is usually narrowed, elongated and distorted, and occasionally masses of neoplastic tissue project into its lumen.

The histologic pattern is variable. There are often broad sheets of undifferentiated mesenchymal cells within which are scattered epithelial-lined tubules. Bands of loose, more differentiated mesenchymal tissue often divide the more cellular

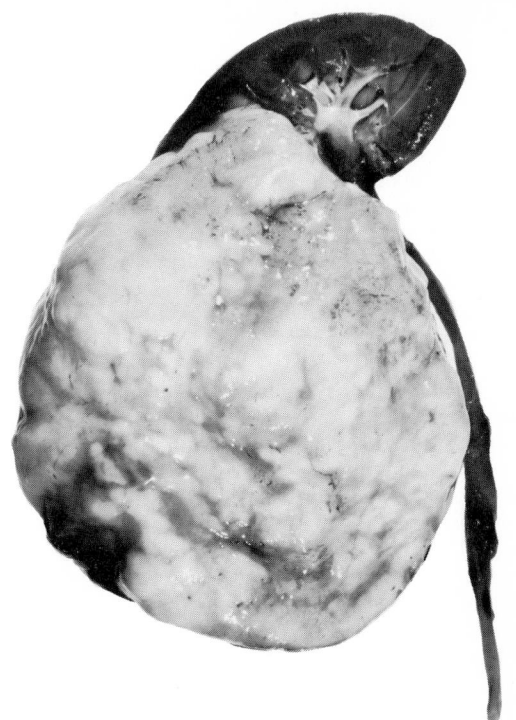

Figure 25-5. Wilms's tumor from a boy 15 months of age. A large intrarenal mass is present in the lower pole of the right kidney.

parts of the neoplasm into coarse lobules, and within these bands smooth and skeletal muscle fibers are often present; occasionally other elements such as abortive glomeruli, cartilage, bone or nests of squamous epithelium are present. Since all these elements are derived from mesenchymal tissue and are not indicative of an origin from multiple germ layers, these tumors should not be regarded as teratomas.

The basic treatment is prompt, radical nephrectomy. This should usually be performed within 24 to 48 hours after discovery of the mass. Undue palpation of the mass should be avoided. Preoperatively, roentgen films of the chest should be obtained, and the presence and normality of the opposite kidney should be established by pyelography. Blood should be available for use at operation. If a Wilms's tumor is strongly suspected, it is our practice to administer actinomycin D preoperatively and postoperatively. One fifth of the total dose is given immediately before operation; the remainder is given only after histologic confirmation of the nature of the neoplasm has been obtained, and is administered concomitantly with the course of postoperative irradiation.

The limits of the tumor are marked at operation by Cushing silver clips, in order to identify accurately the site to receive postoperative irradiation. Postoperative irradiation is used in our clinic. In infants less than 1 year of age, however, in whom a small, localized lesion can be shown histologically to have been completely removed, such therapy is probably not warranted.

The prognosis of Wilms's tumor is generally better for infants under 1 year of age than for older children, perhaps because of the earlier detection of the mass. There has, moreover, been a progressive improvement in the overall prognosis for children with this tumor. In 1 reported series apparent cures were obtained in 47 of 53 (89 per cent) of the patients with no demonstrable metastases on admission, and in 18 of 31 (58 per cent) of those with metastases who were treated. With rare exceptions, if a child with a Wilms's tumor is alive and well with no evidence of recurrent or metastatic disease 2 years after removal of the tumor, a cure has been effected.

Fibromyomatous hamartomas of the kidney are clinically and radiologically similar to Wilms's tumor. Macroscopically, the tumors do not have the areas of necrosis often present in Wilms's tumor, and the cut surfaces are firm, smooth and not lobulated, but have a whorl-like pattern similar to that of a uterine leiomyoma. Histologically, they consist of interweaving bundles of smooth muscle and fibroblastic tissue, embedded within which are nests of relatively normal-appearing renal tubules and glomeruli. There is no evidence to date that these tumors metastasize. They are probably benign lesions and should be treated by nephrectomy alone. It is possible that renal tumors recognized in the neonatal period and reported as Wilms's tumors belong in this category.

Renal cell carcinoma, the common malignant neoplasm of the kidney in adults, is extremely rare in childhood.

Lymphomas of the kidney are usually bilateral and associated with other evidences of *lymphosarcoma* or *leukemia.* Leukemic involvement of the kidney may take the form of nodular masses or of diffuse infiltration of both kidneys, the leukemic cells being most numerous in the cortices.

The extreme enlargement of the kidneys and the striking elongation of the pelves, infundibula and calices can be demonstrated roentgenographically. In spite of the extensive involvement of both kidneys, renal function is usually preserved. Regression of the renal enlargement usually occurs after relatively small doses of irradiation.

Angiolipoleiomyoma is a noncapsulated tumor which characteristically occurs in association with *tuberous sclerosis.* The tumors are usually multiple and involve both kidneys. They are present in about 40 per cent of children with tuberous sclerosis and in 75 per cent of those 15 years of age or older. Although clinical manifestations referable to the tumors have occurred as early as 15 years of age in conjunction with tuberous sclerosis, they are often only incidental findings at necropsy.

Angiolipoleiomyoma occurs infrequently in persons without other evidences of tuberous sclerosis; in such instances the tumor is usually a solitary one. It may hemorrhage into the substance of the tumor or into the perinephric tissue and be responsible for pain, and at times hematuria and a palpable mass.

The tumor, which is identical in persons with and without tuberous sclerosis, is composed of varying amounts of adult adipose tissue, smooth muscle and atypical vessels. They are probably hamartomas rather than true neoplasms, but in extremely rare instances in adults, metastases have been recorded.

Other renal lesions which have been encountered in persons with *tuberous sclerosis* include multiple small cysts lined by prominent cuboidal or columnar epithelium, multiple papillary adenomas, and glomerular inclusions of fat and of epithelial-like cells resembling those of the convoluted tubules.

Hemangioma of the kidney may be asymptomatic or may be responsible for painless hematuria or for bleeding associated with pain as a result of the passage of clots or of interstitial hemorrhage. Only about 5 per cent of these rare tumors occur in infants and children. The lesions may consist of solitary or multiple soft, dark red nodules, or there may be diffuse involvement of most of one kidney. The tumors, which are more often cavernous than capillary, are located anywhere in the kidney, e.g. in a calyx, the renal pelvis, the medulla or even the cortex. Occasionally they are large enough to be detected by urography. If responsible for symptoms, they are best treated surgically.

Lindau's disease is characterized by the presence of cysts or adenomas of the kidney, cysts of the pancreas, and hemangiomas of the retina, cerebellum, brain stem or spinal cord. A familial history may be elicited, some members of the family having only retinal angiomatosis (*von Hippel's disease*), some only angiomas of the central nervous system, and some the complete syndrome. Although visual impairment may develop during late childhood, manifestations referable to the central nervous system usually do not appear until adult life.

Teratoma of the kidney, in contrast to a Wilms's tumor, contains derivatives of all 3 germ layers. It is an extremely rare tumor which may occur in association with multiple congenital anomalies.

TUMORS OF THE ADRENAL

Neuroblastoma is one of the most common malignant neoplasms in infants and children. Although more than half of them arise from the adrenal or from the retroperitoneal sympathetic chain, the neoplasm may originate at any site along the sympathetic chain, e.g. in the posterior mediastinum, pelvis or cervical sympathetic ganglia; rarely multiple, apparently independent primary growths are present in several different sites. Neuroblastoma is primarily a disease of early life; about one fourth of the affected persons have their initial manifestations during the first year of life and three fourths of them before the age of 5 years. It is the most common malignant neoplasm to be identified at birth; metastases may already be present at this time.

The presenting manifestation of a neuroblastoma arising in the adrenal or in the neighboring sympathetic ganglia is usually an abdominal mass. It often crosses the midline, in contrast to a Wilms's tumor. Roentgen examination reveals a soft tissue mass which displaces the kidney on the affected side downward and laterally; focal areas of calcification are often present. Intravenous pyelography characteristically reveals displacement rather than distortion of the renal pelvis; occasionally, as with Wilms's tumor, the pelvis is not visible on the affected side.

Intrathoracic neuroblastomas are located in the posterior portion of the mediastinum at any level and may be responsible for cough, dyspnea and pain in the chest; in a number of instances, owing to extradural extensions of the mass, there are manifestations referable to compression of the spinal cord. *Pelvic neuroblastomas* usually produce a demonstrable mass which in some instances simulates a sacrococcygeal teratoma. They may be responsible for urinary or rectal obstruction. *Cervical neuroblastomas* usually do not reach a large size before being recognized. They are apt to present as a hard, lobulated mass involving the posterior triangle of the neck or extending both anterior and posterior to the sternocleidomastoid muscle. In some instances fine stippled areas of calcification within the mass are demonstrable roentgenographically.

Sometimes the presenting complaint of a patient with neuroblastoma is referable to metastases rather than to the primary neoplasm, e.g. massive hepatomegaly (especially in young infants), cervical or axillary lymphadenopathy or exophthalmos. Persistent pain and fever in association with osseous metastases may simulate rheumatic fever or rheumatoid arthritis.

Though the majority of patients with neuroblastoma have elevated levels of catecholamines or of one or more of their derivatives in the urine, only a few have such clinical signs of functional endocrine activity as hypertension, tachycardia, sweating and pallor. Diarrhea is uncommon. Measurements of the urinary excretion of catecholamines and of their metabolites, e.g. 3-methoxy-4-hydroxymandelic acid (VMA) and homovanillic acid (HVA), may be of diagnostic significance in any neoplasm of neural crest origin. Such determinations may also be helpful in the demonstration of residual, recurrent or metastatic disease.

Metastases of neuroblastoma occur by way of the lymphatic and blood streams; regional and distant lymph nodes, the skeletal system and the liver are the most frequent sites of metastatic spread. Pulmonary metastases occur in only about 10 per cent of patients. Osseous metastases are often bilateral; a unilateral lesion may lead to an erroneous diagnosis of a primary neoplasm of the bone. The roentgenographic changes in the skeleton are characterized by areas of destruction and proliferation of new bone which may closely simulate the appearance of Ewing's tumor or of skeletal involvement in leukemia. There may be extensive mottling of the cranial bones and separation of the sutures, owing to increased intracranial pressure secondary to metastases within the dura mater. Neoplastic cells are frequently demonstrable in smears of the bone marrow, even in the absence of roentgenographic changes in the bones themselves.

The neuroblastoma is initially an encapsulated neoplasm, but it soon infiltrates adjoining tissues and, if arising in the adrenal or neighboring sympathetic ganglia, may surround the aorta, inferior vena cava, ureter or renal pedicle and render complete surgical removal impossible. Areas of hemorrhage and necrosis are commonly present, as are minute flecks of calcium. Histologically, there may be varying degrees of differentiation toward mature ganglion cells or, less frequently, toward chromaffin cells. The least differentiated neoplasms may be misinterpreted as lymphosarcomas, but additional sections of the same tumor will usually reveal better differentiated areas of neoplastic cells embedded in a haphazard manner within a delicate fibrillary tissue or arranged as pseudorosettes. Less frequently immature or mature ganglion cells or even chromaffin cells may be present.

Treatment consists in extirpation of the primary neoplasm, even if it can be only incompletely removed. Currently, postoperative irradiation is being used, as are systemic antineoplastic agents such as vincristine sulfate and cyclophosphamide (Cytoxan). Cures may occur even in the presence of metastases, especially when they are confined to the liver. Cures following osseous metastases,

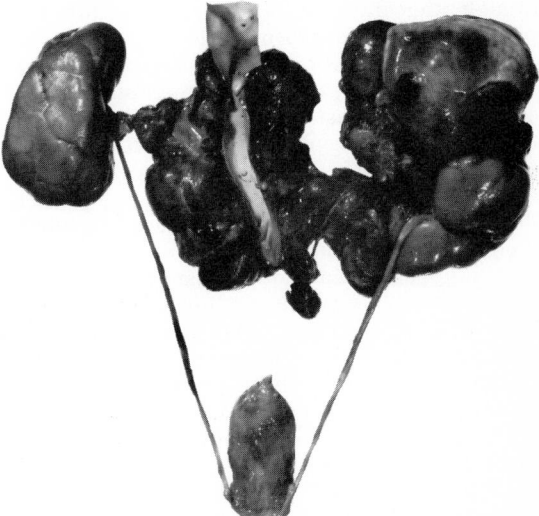

Figure 25-6. Posterior view of a neuroblastoma arising from the right adrenal and displacing the kidney laterally and downward. The tumor crosses the midline and surrounds the aorta and inferior vena cava. (From J. B. Arey: *Pediat. Clin. N. Amer.,* Vol. 10.)

though rare, have been recorded. Spontaneous cures of neuroblastoma are extremely rare; in some instances, destruction of the tumor appears to have been brought about by differentiation of the neuroblastic elements into mature ganglion cells with subsequent degeneration and necrosis of these cells.

The prognosis appears to be somewhat more favorable in children in whom the neoplasm is more highly differentiated and in those in whom the primary site is extra-abdominal. Survival, however, is more dependent upon age than upon either of these factors. The overall survival rate is about 35 per cent; in at least 1 series, however, it is as high as 76 per cent in infants under 1 year of age, in contrast to 18 per cent in older children. Survival for 2 years without evidence of recurrence or metastases is usually indicative of a cure.

Ganglioneuromas are benign tumors which arise from the sympathetic ganglia in the posterior mediastinum, retroperitoneum, pelvis or neck or from the adrenal. Rarely they arise in other sites such as the skin, tongue, pharynx or gastrointestinal tract; in the last site they may be diffuse rather than encapsulated and be accompanied by symmetric hypertrophy of the various layers of the affected intestinal segment. Although the majority of them are discovered before the age of 20 years, and most in the first decade, they tend to occur at a slightly older age than the neuroblastoma. Rarely they are associated with von Recklinghausen's disease. Neoplasms arising in the retroperitoneum or cervical region are apt to be responsible for a palpable mass, but many of the patients with posterior mediastinal ganglioneuromas are asymptomatic, and the tumors are found only by roentgenographic examination of the chest. In some instances dumbbell-shaped tumors extend through the intervertebral foramina into the spinal canal and are responsible for manifestations referable to compression of the spinal cord. Mature ganglioneuromas, as well as ganglioneuroblastomas and neuroblastomas, may be endocrinologically functioning neoplasms with resultant hypertension, tachycardia, fever, sweating, pallor and increased excretion of catecholamines (p. 1222). Chronic diarrhea with frequent watery, foulsmelling stools, failure to thrive, abdominal distention, hypokalemia and flushing of the skin accompany some neural tumors, especially those in which there is partial or complete differentiation toward ganglion cells. Urinary excretion of catecholamines and their metabolites is increased and falls to normal after removal of the neoplasm, and diarrhea ceases. The mechanism responsible for the diarrhea is not known.

The tumors are characteristically circumscribed and encapsulated, but may be so densely adherent to adjoining structures as to preclude complete removal. Histologically, they are composed of mature ganglion cells, occurring singly or in groups, and set in a matrix composed of large numbers of neurites with schwannian sheaths which occasionally are myelinated. Distinct palisading of the nuclei is sometimes present, making the pattern indistinguishable from that of a neurilemmoma (p. 1469).

Partially differentiated ganglioneuromas are composed of incompletely differentiated ganglion cells, with or without mature ganglion cells, but without truly undifferentiated neuroblastic elements. The prognosis appears to be somewhat better than with one composed of undifferentiated neuroblasts; metastases, however, may occur, in contrast to the fully differentiated ganglioneuroma.

Ganglioneuroblastomas are malignant neoplasms composed of undifferentiated neuroblasts and of partially or completely differentiated ganglion cells. Although the prognosis may be somewhat better than that of the pure neuroblastoma, metastases may occur.

Pheochromocytoma. See page 1220.

Adrenal cortical tumors. See page 1216.

RETROPERITONEAL TUMORS

Retroperitoneal neoplasms are associated with a palpable mass in about nine tenths of affected infants and children, and in most of them the mass or enlargement of the abdomen is the initial complaint. Infrequently no mass is palpable.

About half of abdominal masses which necessitate operative intervention in infants and children are derived from the kidney or adjacent structures; hydronephrosis, neuroblastoma and Wilms's tumor, in this order, are the most frequent ones. In the newborn infant a unilateral multicystic kidney is the most common abnormal mass. A variety of other benign and malignant tumors, however, must be included in the differential diagnosis. These include retroperitoneal teratoma, lymphosarcoma, ganglioneuroma, lipoma, liposarcoma, fibrosarcoma, rhabdomyosarcoma, benign and malignant mesenchymoma, hemangioma and hemangiopericytoma.

Retroperitoneal teratoma is the third most frequent type of retroperitoneal neoplasm (see above) in infants and children; it is somewhat more frequent in females than in males. They are often discovered in the first months of life, two thirds of them appearing in the first 2 years. The presenting complaint is usually abdominal enlargement and a palpable mass. The neoplasm usually arises high in the retroperitoneal region, close to the pancreas, kidney and root of the mesentery. It may present on either side of the abdomen or cross the midline. Roentgen examination often reveals spotty areas of mineralization or even distinct teeth or bones. Intravenous pyelography usually reveals displacement of the kidney and ureter on the affected side; mild hydronephrosis may be present as a result of ureteral compression. The recorded operative mortality rate is high, probably because of the large size and extensive attachments of many of these neoplasms to adjoining structures, but prompt removal is the treatment of choice. With rare exceptions these neoplasms are well differentiated and benign.

Occasionally a teratoma arising in the presacral region extends upward into the retroperitoneal tissue and presents as a mass in the pelvis or lower part of the abdomen, with or without an associated external mass in the sacrococcygeal region. Such neoplasms, which may be responsible for intestinal or urinary obstruction, are almost always attached to the coccyx or to the lowermost part of the sacrum. Although the incidence of malignancy appears to be higher in these than in the usual retroperitoneal teratomas, most of them are benign.

Retroperitoneal fetus in fetu (intraperitoneal teratoma) is a monozygotic twin included within its host during development. In contrast to the retroperitoneal teratomas, these are included within an amnion-like sac which projects into the peritoneal cavity and is attached by a pedicle to the upper retroperitoneal tissues near the origin of the superior mesenteric artery. The mass has a vertebral axis, indicative of the earlier primitive streak, often accompanied by an appropriate arrangement of other organs or limbs with respect to this axis.

Sacrococcygeal teratomas arise from the region of the coccyx or lowermost part of the sacrum. They are probably derived from the primordial, totipotential cells of the primitive knot (Hensen's node) which, during embryonic life, finally comes to rest in the region of the coccyx. These tumors are 3 or 4 times more frequent in girls than in boys, and there is a significant increase in the incidence of twinning in families of persons with sacrococcygeal teratomas. At least three fourths of the tumors are apparent at birth, usually presenting as a mass at the tip of the coccyx extending externally in the midline or into one or both buttocks. Large tumors, which may exceed the size of the infant's head, displace the coccyx posteriorly and the anus anteriorly. Occasionally the mass is responsible for urinary or intestinal obstruction, but, in contrast to large myelomeningoceles, they are not responsible for neurologic defects in the sphincters or extremities.

Rectal examination usually discloses a readily palpable mass posterior to the rectum, which is sometimes encircled by it. Roentgenographic examination usually reveals a soft tissue density in the pelvis, sometimes with displacement of the coccyx posteriorly. Areas of calcification or actual bone are demonstrable in about half of the tumors. In contrast to sacral chordomas, roentgenographic evidence of destruction of the sacrum is rare; when present, it is indicative of a malignant neoplasm. Occasionally spina bifida or lumbosacral anomalies are also present.

The differential diagnosis includes a meningocele or meningomyelocele; pressure on the sac will cause bulging of the fontanel, or, if this is closed, crying or straining should increase the tension within the mass. Neurogenic tumors, e.g. neuroblastoma and ganglioneuroma, may be clinically indistinguishable from a sacrococcygeal teratoma. Chordomas are rare in children; they are responsible for destruction of the sacrum and only rarely extend into the buttock. Myxopapillary ependymomas may present as a mass in the sacrococcygeal region. Cystic lymphangiomas and hemangiomas may simulate a sacrococcygeal teratoma, as may a duplication of the hind gut. Occasionally a sacrococcygeal teratoma presents as a red, inflamed mass or as a draining sinus and thus simulates an infected pilonidal sinus.

These neoplasms are connected to the lowermost part of the sacrum or to the coccyx, and the coccyx should always be removed with them; rarely the tumor extends into the vertebral canal. They are usually well circumscribed solid masses containing multiple cystic structures. Histologically, they contain a vast array of tissues; fat, neural elements, smooth and skeletal muscle, bone, cartilage and intestinal and bronchial elements are the most frequent ones. Teratomatous elements such as pancreatic islets or adrenocortical tissue are sometimes present, and rarely produce functional manifestations.

Most sacrococcygeal teratomas are benign, and cures are sometimes obtained even after one or more recurrences. Most of the tumors removed before 3 or 4 months of age consist only of mature or less often of immature fetal elements and are associated with an excellent prognosis. Tumors removed after 5 months of age, either because of their late appearance or because of delay in the institution of therapy, are more apt to contain embryonal carcinomatous elements; approximately two thirds of those treated in this age period are biologically malignant. Tumors detected after 5 years of age, as in adults, may be benign or malignant. Recurrences or metastases, if they occur, usually do so within 2 years after operation.

Tumors of the soft tissues of the retroperitoneum include benign and malignant tumors derived from adipose tissue or from multiple mesenchymal elements, fibromatoses, vascular tumors, lymphomas and malignant neoplasms derived from skeletal muscle. They may be bulky masses indistinguishable from the more common retroperitoneal neoplasms.

Myxopapillary ependymoma is a rare cause of a mass in the soft tissues overlying the sacrococcygeal region of a child; it may suggest a pilonidal cyst or sinus. Although the tumor may arise intraspinally and extend through the sacral foramen into the soft tissues, more frequently it appears to arise from heterotopic tissue overlying the sacrococcygeal region. The neoplasm is usually a lobulated, well circumscribed mass; it may, however, extend into the perirectal tissue and be attached to the sacrum. Excision is the treatment of choice. The patient should be followed up for many years because of the possibility of late recurrence.

Retroperitoneal lymphangiomas are large cystic tumors which may occur independently or in conjunction with similar tumors in the mesentery (p. 1465).

Retroperitoneal lipoma, liposarcoma, mesenchymoma, hemangioma, hemangiopericytoma, lymphoma and *rhabdomyosarcoma* are described elsewhere in this section.

TUMORS OF THE BLADDER AND PROSTATE

Neoplasms of the bladder or prostate are rare in infants and children. They are usually mesenchymal rather than epithelial, and most of them are malignant. Differentiation of a primary prostatic neoplasm from a neoplasm arising in the bladder may be impossible.

The initial clinical manifestations of a neoplasm of the bladder are apt to be intermittent pain, dysuria, enuresis and hematuria. Acute urinary retention may occur, or hydronephrosis and pyelonephritis may be responsible for uremia. Distortion of the rectum may be followed by tenesmus and obstruction. In girls the tumor sometimes protrudes through the urethral opening. Rectal examination usually reveals a soft or firm mass which may fill the vagina as well as the bladder.

Neoplasms of the prostate are usually not discovered until distortion of the rectal, ureteral or urethral passages has been responsible for obstruction.

Rhabdomyosarcoma (p. 1470) is the most common neoplasm to arise in the bladder or prostate in early life. Most of them appear before 5 years of age, and occasionally they are present at birth. Those arising in the prostate produce large, bulky, nodular masses which surround the prostate, base of the bladder and ureters, and compress the rectum. Neoplasms arising in the bladder usually involve the region of the trigone or posterior wall. They present as multiple soft, translucent, polypoid grapelike clusters, attached by a broad base, which protrude into the lumen of the bladder and invade its wall (sarcoma botryoides). Such a botryoid configuration is not assumed by neoplasms confined to the prostate and surrounding tissues, where they usually appear as bulky, nodular, somewhat gelatinous masses.

Histologically, the more solid masses are largely undifferentiated mesenchymal tissue. Only infrequently are cells observed in which cross striations can be identified; a clue to the rhabdomyoblastic origin may be provided by the presence of scattered round cells with sharply defined cell boundaries and bright acidophilic cytoplasm. The polypoid submucosal masses consist of myxomatous tissue containing scattered elongate and stellate cells, sometimes with a more compact zone of cells immediately beneath the epithelium.

Metastases usually occur relatively late, but the tumor is apt to spread locally and may soon fill nearly all the lower part of the abdomen. When metastases do occur, they are chiefly to the lungs and regional lymph nodes, but occasionally there are osseous metastases. Radical extirpation is the treatment of choice. This may be supplemented by irradiation or the administration of chemotherapeutic agents such as actinomycin D. The prognosis is extremely grave, and local recurrence or metastases usually follow therapy within about 4 months.

Leiomyomas as well as *leiomyosarcomas* may arise in the urinary bladder. In the prostate almost all the tumors of smooth muscle in children are malignant. *Leiomyosarcoma of the prostate* is apt to be a large tumor which extends locally so as to involve the adjoining structures and sometimes metastasizes. The prognosis for these as well as for the leiomyosarcomas of the bladder is very grave.

Rarely a *plexiform neurofibroma, hemangioma, lymphoma, neuroblastoma* or *pheochromocytoma* arises in the urinary bladder; the last may be associated with sustained hypertension and paroxysms characterized by an abrupt rise of blood pressure, headache, palpitation and nervousness. Low-grade *papillary transitional cell carcinomas* have been observed during the pediatric age period, and primary *ganglioneuroma of the bladder* has been responsible for clinical manifestations before the age of 20 years.

TUMORS OF THE TESTIS AND PARATESTICULAR STRUCTURES

Primary testicular neoplasms in infants and children are usually embryonal carcinomas or teratomas, each of which is probably of germ cell origin, being derived from undifferentiated, multipotent cells. Testicular tumors of nongerm cell origin, e.g. interstitial cell tumors and tumors of specialized gonadal stroma, as well as those derived from the supportive tissue of the testis, from the tunica and from the paratesticular tissues, are extremely rare; they include hemangiomas, sometimes of the scrotal septum, and rhabdomyosarcomas of the tunica or of the spermatic cord. An intrascrotal, extratesticular tumor resembling a pseudomucinous cystadenoma of the ovary has been described in an 11-year-old boy. We have seen a child with a papillary mesothelioma arising in a hernial sac and another with an epidermoid cyst of the tunica albuginea, located in the vicinity of the rete testis and sparing the testicular tissue itself. Somewhat comparable epidermoid cysts of the testis have been described in adults. Tumors of the epididymis are almost nonexistent in early life.

Malignant lymphoma may initially manifest itself as a testicular mass, often with subsequent involvement of the opposite testis. Most instances of lymphomatous involvement of the testis are accompanied by evidence of disseminated disease, especially by abdominal or pelvic masses. The testes may be secondarily involved by leukemic infiltrates.

TESTICULAR TUMORS OF GERM CELL ORIGIN

Testicular tumors in infants and children are usually of germ cell origin, i.e. embryonal carcinoma or teratoma, and occur predominantly during the first few years of life; the tumor may be apparent at birth. The presenting complaint is usually painless enlargement of the testis; occasionally this is accompanied by or is erroneously interpreted as a hydrocele. Infrequently the initial manifestation is an abdominal mass, the result of metastases from an unrecognized primary testicular tumor.

There are certain noteworthy differences between testicular neoplasms of infants and children and those of adults. Seminoma, the most common testicular neoplasm in adults, is rare in children, and chorioepithelioma must be extremely rare, if it occurs at all. As many as 10 per cent of testicular neoplasms in adults have been said to arise in undescended testes, but only infrequently is a testicular neoplasm in an infant or child associated with cryptorchidism. In general, the prognosis for infants and children with testicular neoplasms is considerably better than that for adults.

Embryonal carcinoma is the most common type of testicular neoplasm in early life. The majority occur during the first 2 years of life; the mass may be present at birth. Initially it may be mistakenly considered to be a hydrocele and in some instances has even been thought to transilluminate. It may grow rapidly, doubling in size within a few weeks.

The mass is usually ovoid, corresponding to the shape of the testis. As a rule the tunica albuginea is intact, and invasion of the epididymis is infrequent. On section the tumor is sharply circumscribed and usually replaces most of the testis; minute cysts and areas of hemorrhage may be present. Histologically, it consists of masses of undifferentiated cells with rather hyperchromatic nuclei. In areas with better differentiated tubules and papillary structures, there may be vacuoles of mucin confined to the basilar cytoplasm of the lining cells or located in their apical portions, giving them the appearance of goblet cells. Areas of poorly differentiated mesenchymal tissue and distinct epithelial-lined tubules simulating primitive neuroectoderm or mesonephric structures are sometimes present, but the neoplastic cells do not assume the degree of differentiation into recognizable fetal and adult structures which characterizes the classic teratoma.

Testicular adenocarcinoma with clear cells has been designated as a distinctive type of tumor of infants, unrelated to teratomas and possibly derived from immature testicular tubules; its embryonic nature has led to the designation *orchioblastoma*. There is, however, no convincing evidence that this tumor is distinct from the embryonal carcinoma, and areas with this same morphologic pattern are occasionally encountered in distinctly teratomatous neoplasms, e.g. sacrococcygeal teratoma. All these undifferentiated tumors might thus best be regarded as embryonal carcinomas.

Embryonal carcinoma of the testis is probably best treated by removal of the testis and spermatic cord and dissection of the retroperitoneal lymph nodes; if neoplastic tissue is identified in the lymph nodes, the entire periaortic chain should probably be irradiated. Metastases occur both to the retroperitoneal lymph nodes and by way of the bloodstream. The metastatic lesions resemble the primary tumor histologically. The prognosis for infants is certainly better than the primitive pattern of the tumor would suggest, and probably at least half of the patients should recover.

Most *testicular teratomas* of early life are discovered during the first few years of life, sometimes at birth; rarely there are bilateral tumors. The presenting complaint is usually that of painless enlargement of the testis. Growth of the tumor may not be as rapid as with an embryonal carcinoma, and the interval between the discovery of the mass and therapy thus tends to be somewhat longer. Macroscopically, these tumors are circumscribed and usually replace most of the testis. They vary from solid structures containing multiple minute cysts to grossly multicystic lesions; rarely they are composed of only a solitary cyst. Histologically, a wide variety of tissues are usually present, representative of all 3 germ layers. The cysts are commonly lined by epidermis, respiratory, neural and intestinal epithelium. Glial tissue is often abundant and may contain foci of necrosis and calcification. Structures resembling retina, the pigmented ciliary body, salivary gland and pancreas may be present in addition to lymphoid tissue, smooth muscle, cartilage, bone, adipose tissue and fibrous tissue. The more immature tissues may contain multiple mitoses, and occasional foci resemble embryonal carcinoma.

Testicular teratomas in early life, in contrast to those in adults, are usually benign. Even in the presence of immature elements, metastases to the retroperitoneal lymph nodes, lungs and liver are rare and occur principally in later childhood. Simple orchidectomy is probably the treatment of choice, especially for those discovered during the first year of life. In the presence of definite embryonal carcinomatous elements, however, retroperitoneal lymph node dissection is indicated.

TESTICULAR TUMORS OF NONGERM CELL ORIGIN

In any age group these are much less common than tumors of germ cell origin. They consist of a heterogeneous group of neoplasms, only two of which are specifically gonadal in origin: interstitial cell tumors and androblastomas.

Tumors of Specialized Gonadal Stroma (Testicular and Ovarian). The specialized stroma of the gonads, i.e. the endocrinologically active portion of the ovaries and testes, is derived from a common embryologic source, the mesoderm of the urogenital ridge. Tumors of this specialized stroma, whether located in testes or ovaries, are thus capable of reproducing all the endocrinologically active portion of the gonads of both sexes. They may contain Sertoli cells and their ovarian homologues, the granulosa cells, as well as Leydig cells and their ovarian counterparts, the theca cells. There may be varying degrees of luteinization of the specialized cells of the ovary.

A variety of endocrinologic disturbances may be associated with tumors of such specialized stroma, whether they are located in the testis or in the ovary. Attempts have been made to classify them on the basis of their endocrinologic function. Such a classification is unsatisfactory, however, since some of these tumors are inactive, whereas others may give rise to both androgenic and estrogenic substances; a morphologic classification is, in general, more applicable.

Interstitial (Leydig) Cell Tumor. See page 1230.

Androblastomas (Tumors of Specialized Gonadal Stroma; Gonadal Stromal Tumor; Sertoli Cell Tumor; Granulosa-Theca Cell Tumor of the Testis). These are rare tumors derived from the specialized stroma of the gonad and thus capable of reproducing the supporting tissues of the gonads of both sexes. They are characterized by a variety of histologic patterns ranging from an epithelial form having a close resemblance to normal Sertoli cell tubules or to granulosa cells to a form consisting largely of fibroblast-like cells. Elements resembling luteinized cells of the corpus luteum or interstitial cells of the testis may also be present. Although predominantly a tumor of adults, a significant number has occurred in infants less than 1 year of age, and the tumor may be present at birth. The presenting complaint is usually painless swelling of the testis, infrequently accompanied by gynecomastia. The hormonal mechanism responsible for the latter is not known. Although metastases have occurred in adults, only an isolated instance has been observed in a child.

The tumors vary considerably in size and are usually circumscribed, firm, gray-white to yellow, solitary masses confined to the testis; only rarely has the tumor invaded the epididymis. Histologically, some of the tumors are almost entirely epithelial, but most of them consist of varying admixtures of epithelial and fibrous elements. The epithelial components most frequently are arranged in a tubular manner simulating seminiferous tubules, the lumens of which may be filled with debris and eosinophilic precipitate. The cells, however, may be arranged in a cystlike pattern suggesting graafian follicles, or sheets and cords of small, cuboidal epithelial cells resembling those of

a granulosa cell tumor of the ovary may be present. In some instances there are nests of cells with abundant acidophilic cytoplasm which resemble luteinized cells or Leydig cells. The fibrous elements consist of bands of spindle-shaped cells with elongated nuclei and somewhat acidophilic cytoplasm interspersed between the tubular elements or scattered haphazardly through the tumor. Scattered mitotic figures are sometimes present. Little or none of the material stains positively with the periodic acid-Schiff technique, in contrast to the abundance of such deposits in embryonal carcinomas.

The tumors appear to recapitulate the structures formed by the specialized stroma of either the testis or ovary, and thus are the homologues of the ovarian arrhenoblastomas (p. 1462) and granulosa cell tumors (p. 1233). They do not contain cells characteristically believed to be of germ cell origin, in contrast to the gonadoblastoma (p. 1462), although cells closely resembling primitive germ cells are occasionally present within them.

Sertoli cell adenomas are benign tumors which frequently occur in the testes of persons with the testicular feminizing syndrome, in whom a variety of other testicular tumors may also be encountered, especially after puberty. Sertoli cell adenomas are sometimes bilateral. The individual lesion may be minimal or it may reach a large size and completely replace a gonad; in such a case it has been misinterpreted as a well differentiated Sertoli-Leydig cell tumor of the ovary. It is devoid of germ cells and consists of uniform tubules lined by Sertoli cells, with variable numbers of Leydig cells in the intertubular tissue. The tumors are benign and without demonstrable endocrine effects. They may represent hyperplasia of testicular tubules and be comparable to the smaller, nonneoplastic *tubular adenomas which are frequently found in cryptorchid testes* as minute, solitary or multiple discrete nodules composed of well differentiated Sertoli cells.

TUMORS OF THE OVARY

Although ovarian tumors are relatively infrequent during the pediatric age period, a variety of neoplasms and non-neoplastic cysts originating in or about the ovaries may be responsible for clinical manifestations. Teratomas, which comprise only 10 to 15 per cent of ovarian neoplasms in adults, are by far the most common tumor of the ovary in children. Non-neoplastic cysts, i.e. follicular, lutein or simple ovarian cysts, are second in frequency. Infrequently, a follicular or theca-lutein cyst of moderate to large size is apparently responsible for signs of precocious puberty (p. 1234). Much more often, however, precocious puberty resulting from ovarian disease is caused by a granulosa-theca cell tumor (p. 1233). Precocious puberty is only rarely caused by a malignant chorioepithelioma within an embryonal carcinoma or teratoma of the ovary. Pseudomucinous and serous cystadenomas and cystadenocarcinomas, the most common ovarian neoplasms of adults, are rare in children; when they do occur, they usually occur in older children.

Other primary ovarian neoplasms are rare in early life; they include dysgerminomas, embryonal carcinomas, thecomas, which are sometimes associated with Meigs's syndrome, fibromas, Sertoli-Leydig cell tumors and lipid cell tumors. Infrequently parovarian cysts and hydatids of Morgagni are responsible for clinical manifestations during childhood. Secondary involvement of the ovaries of children by neoplastic disease is usually from a lymphomatous process.

Clinical manifestations referable to an ovarian tumor in an infant or child are usually those of an acute attack or of recurrent episodes of abdominal pain. Nausea and vomiting are common, and the attack may closely simulate that of acute appendicitis. Such attacks usually result from *torsion of the ovarian pedicle*, which is more common in infants and children than in adults; it may occur with any type of ovarian mass and rarely may take place in an apparently normal ovary. Torsion of the ovarian pedicle may be followed by infarction and hemoperitoneum. In the absence of torsion an ovarian tumor usually presents as a mass in the lower part of the abdomen or as gradual enlargement of the abdomen. Rarely abdominal distention is present at birth as a result of rupture of an ovarian cyst. In the case of functional tumors the initial manifestations are apt to be those of sexual precocity or, much less frequently, of virilism or of a combination of these.

Teratoma of the ovary, the most common ovarian neoplasm of children, is usually benign. Most of them are cystic, the so-called dermoid cyst; solid or, more correctly, polycystic ovarian tumors are less common. Ovarian teratomas have been observed as early as 16 months of age. In addition to the clinical manifestations described above, there is rarely an associated hemolytic anemia which responds only to removal of the neoplasm. Roentgen examination frequently reveals areas of calcification in bone or teeth. Hydronephrosis and hydroureter secondary to obstruction by the mass are infrequent complications.

Macroscopically, an ovarian teratoma is usually a globular, unilocular cystic structure filled with sebaceous material and commonly contains hair. At one point in the wall a sessile mass often projects into the lumen. This mound of tissue is covered by thick squamous epithelium beneath which are numerous hair follicles, sebaceous glands, adipose tissue and sometimes bone and teeth. The remainder of the lining of the cyst is usually smooth, but is sometimes granular, shaggy and ulcerated, in which case the wall is apt to be thickened and fibrotic and contain areas of calcification.

Histologically, the tumors contain ectodermal elements, especially stratified squamous epithelium, abundant sebaceous glands and hair follicles and often sweat glands. Other tissue elements may include those of neural, osseous, muscular, fat and endodermal origins. The wall of the cyst may be ulcerated and reveal a chronic inflammatory reaction with numerous foamy macrophages and foreign body giant cells.

Much less frequently ovarian teratomas are predominantly solid structures with multiple small cysts containing hair, sebaceous material, and serous or mucoid fluid. Histologically, such tumors may be composed entirely of mature tissue, often with numerous neural elements, or they may contain varying amounts of embryonal tissue. Areas of embryonal carcinoma are sometimes present and render the prognosis more grave. Although solid ovarian teratomas have a greater potential for malignancy than does the usual cystic variety, they are not uniformly malignant. The prognosis is generally good in those in which the cells are well differentiated and in those in which there are only a few small foci of incompletely differentiated tissue. In several instances, children with multiple peritoneal implants composed of well differentiated neuroglial tissue have survived without evidence of recurrence for as long as 13 years.

Bilateral ovarian teratomas are infrequent in children in contrast to an incidence of over 10 per cent in adults.

The prognosis for children with cystic ovarian teratomas is good. Treatment should consist only of simple oophorectomy or, if possible, excision of the neoplasm, sparing any intact ovarian tissue on the affected side. Solid teratomas should be treated by salpingo-oophorectomy.

Dysgerminoma (germinoma), the ovarian counterpart of the testicular seminoma, occurs predominantly during the second and third decades of life, but as many as 7 per cent are found during the first decade. This neoplasm, which is believed to arise from primitive germ cells, is usually hormonally inactive; increased levels of follicle-stimulating hormone have been observed. The tumor is sometimes associated with genital hypoplasia or female pseudohermaphroditism; it has been observed with Turner's syndrome and rarely with precocious pseudopuberty. A cause and effect relation of these endocrine changes with the dysgerminoma has not been established. The tumor is bilateral in about one fourth of affected persons. It is a solid, rounded mass with a smooth or coarsely lobulated surface. On section multiple yellow patches of necrosis may be present. Histologically, its appearance is similar to that of the testicular seminoma. The neoplasm is malignant and may infiltrate locally within the pelvis and spread to the regional lymph nodes or to the viscera.

A tumor confined to one ovary in a child should probably be treated by unilateral salpingo-oophorectomy. With local spread, however, or in older persons in whom maintenance of reproductive ability is no longer important, the uterus, both fallopian tubes and ovaries and the iliac lymph nodes should be removed, and the area irradiated. The prognosis is somewhat graver than that for testicular seminoma. Although it has been considered to be more malignant in children than during the reproductive period, experience is too limited to warrant conclusions.

Embryonal carcinoma of the ovary is a rare neoplasm morphologically similar to the testicular tumor of this name. It is probably of germ cell origin and tends to occur in young persons. It is soft and friable, with multiple cystic spaces and areas of hemorrhage and necrosis, and is usually unilateral. Histologically, it is similar to the embryonal carcinomas of the testes. The prognosis is much graver than that of the testicular ones, and extirpation of the tumor, even when followed by irradiation, usually fails to effect a cure.

Tumors of Specialized Gonadal Stroma (Testicular and Ovarian). See page 1460.

Granulosa-Theca Cell Tumor. See page 1233.

Sertoli-Leydig cell tumors (arrhenoblastomas; testicular tubular adenomas of Pick; ovarian androblastomas) are rare neoplasms comparable to the testicular tumors of specialized gonadal stroma. They occur predominantly during the reproductive period and only rarely have been observed in children. Although characteristically they are masculinizing tumors, they may have no endocrine effects or may even be accompanied by estrogenic manifestations, e.g. isosexual precocious puberty. Aldosteronism with precocious puberty has been observed in a 9-year-old girl, and virilizing manifestations have been noted before 12 years of age.

The neoplasm is usually a slowly growing one involving only one ovary. It may be firm or soft, is frequently lobulated and occasionally is polycystic. Histologically, the pattern varies considerably. The well differentiated areas consist of distinct tubular structures lined by Sertoli cells, with or without Leydig cells in the intertubular tissue. Neoplasms exhibiting an intermediate degree of differentiation may assume a bewildering array of patterns. The Sertoli cells may be arranged as broad anastomosing trabeculae or as solid nests of cells; small cystic spaces resembling the Call-Exner bodies of the granulosa cell tumor are sometimes present. The intervening tissue consists of Leydig cells, spindle cells and hyalinized collagen. The least differentiated neoplasms may bear little or no resemblance to the foregoing patterns, but resemble a sarcoma or even a carcinoma. In contrast to the frequent absence of endocrinologic manifestations in persons with well differentiated tumors, masculinization is usually apparent in those with the less differentiated neoplasms.

Well differentiated Sertoli-Leydig cell tumors are usually benign, but recurrences or peritoneal metastases probably occur in at least 25 per cent of the less differentiated tumors. Treatment for an apparently localized tumor in a child may perhaps be limited to unilateral salpingo-oophorectomy. In older persons in whom maintenance of reproductive ability is no longer important, however, total hysterectomy with bilateral salpingo-oophorectomy is indicated.

Gynandroblastoma (sex cord-mesenchyme tumors of indeterminate or mixed cell type) is a rare ovarian tumor of specialized gonadal stroma which contains distinct cords or tubules of Sertoli cells as well as definite granulosa cell elements; varying numbers of Leydig cells, thecal cells and luteinized cells may also be present. It may be responsible for evidences of androgenic or estrogenic activity or both or may be simply responsible for a palpable mass. Gynandroblastomas are histologically and clinically benign.

Lipid cell tumors (adrenal rest tumors; masculinovoblastomas; Leydig [hilus] cell tumors; luteomas) are extremely rare ovarian tumors composed of nests of polyhedral cells with clear cytoplasm containing abundant lipid and resembling the cells of the adrenal cortex, Leydig cells or theca-lutein cells. Since morphologic differentiation of these cells may be impossible, the term "lipid cell tumor" is applied to the entire group.

Although there may be no endocrine effects, characteristically there is masculinization. In some instances in which the tumor has occurred before puberty there has been isosexual precocious puberty.

The neoplasm may reach a large size or may be so small that it is not detected upon physical examination. Metastases have been reported with both functioning and nonfunctioning tumors. In children the tumor should probably be removed by unilateral salpingo-oophorectomy.

NEOPLASMS ASSOCIATED WITH HERMAPHRODITISM

Gonadoblastomas are rare neoplasms occurring predominantly, if not exclusively, in the gonads of intersexes. A variety of other neoplasms may also occur in such gonads. The gonadoblastoma is composed of dysgerminoma cells, sometimes with an abundant lymphocytic infiltrate and a granulomatous reaction, in association with cells of specialized gonadal stroma, i.e. theca-lutein or Leydig cells and granulosa or Sertoli cells. There may be multiple foci of calcification. The neoplasms may be bilateral and, at least in adults, may metastasize. There may be evidence suggestive of associated hormonal effects; any dysgerminoma accompanied by endocrine disturbances should be carefully examined for the presence of cells of specialized gonadal stroma before the diagnosis of gonadoblastoma is excluded.

Sertoli Cell Adenomas. See page 1460.

TUMORS OF THE VAGINA AND UTERUS

Sarcoma botryoides is a descriptive term applied to a polypoid, grapelike malignant neoplasm of mesenchymal origin. In infants and children these are poorly differentiated neoplasms which do not invariably contain cells with distinct cross striations. Although the terminology is not entirely satisfactory, it seems best to regard these tumors in infants and children as *embryonal rhabdomyosarcomas* (p. 1470) which have assumed their grapelike or botryoid configuration as a consequence of their subepithelial origin and relatively unrestrained growth within a cavity.

Sarcoma botryoides is the most common tumor of the lower urogenital tract of infants and children. In girls it arises chiefly in the vagina and less often in the bladder, whereas in boys it usually arises in the bladder. Similar neoplasms occur in the common bile duct, anus, nasopharynx, oropharynx, middle ear and maxillary antrum.

Sarcoma botryoides of the vagina usually manifests itself during the first 4 years of life and occasionally is present at birth. The initial manifestation may be a bloody vaginal discharge, but as a rule the first complaint is a mass protruding from the vagina. The neoplasm arises from the vagina and may extend into the cervix, vulva or urethra as well as into the urinary bladder and pelvis; with extensive involvement it may be impossible to determine whether the primary site is in the vagina or bladder. The uterus is rarely, if ever, the primary site of the tumor. It may metastasize by way of the bloodstream and the lymphatics. The histologic appearance of the neoplasm is similar to that of its homologue in the urinary bladder (p. 1458).

The prognosis is extremely grave, but apparent cures have been effected. Treatment consists in resection of the uterus and vagina, leaving the ovaries; more extensive tumors may necessitate pelvic exenteration. Operative treatment should be supplemented by irradiation and chemotherapy.

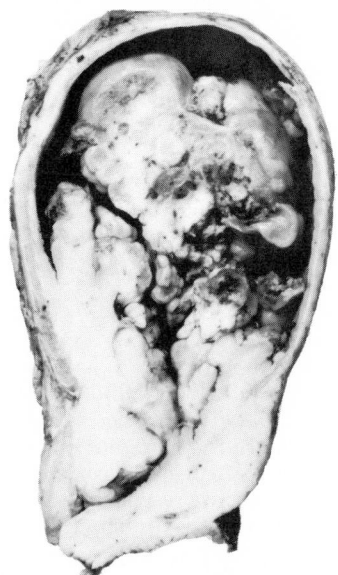

Figure 25-7. Sarcoma botryoides of the urinary bladder from a 3-year-old girl. Numerous gelatinous, grapelike masses protrude into the lumen.

Embryonal carcinoma of the vagina or cervix is a rare neoplasm which may simulate sarcoma botryoides and be responsible for vaginal bleeding or discharge, a friable polypoid mass, and urinary or intestinal complications as a result of local invasion. It may appear as early as 2 months of age, but more often between 1 and 2 years. Morphologically, it resembles its counterpart in the infantile testis or ovary. Early diagnosis and radical surgical extirpation probably offer the best possibility of cure, but the prognosis is extremely grave.

Carcinoma of the uterus, although extremely rare in the pediatric age period, has been observed in infants and children. Vaginal bleeding is usually the first manifestation. In most instances the neoplasm is an adenocarcinoma and arises from the cervix rather than from the body of the uterus. Metastases may occur by way of the bloodstream and lymphatics.

A benign *papilloma of the cervix* covered by columnar and squamous epithelium is an even rarer cause of vaginal bleeding in early life than is carcinoma of the uterus.

Hymenal polyps are benign, non-neoplastic, rounded tags or finger-like pedunculated lesions; they arise from the dorsal part of the hymen and protrude from the vulva. They are composed of a rather vascular stroma covered by well differentiated squamous epithelium. They are present in about 6 per cent of newborn female infants examined on the first or second day of life; they require no treatment, since they disappear spontaneously within a few weeks after birth.

Squamous cell *carcinoma of the vulva* has been observed in a girl 4 years of age; *carcinoma of the vagina*, in a girl not quite 15 years of age.

TUMORS OF VASCULAR ORIGIN

These are the most common tumors of early life. Most of them are probably hamartomas rather than true neoplasms, and most are benign. They may occur in any organ, but there are certain sites of predilection: the skin (p. 1381), skeletal muscle, subcutaneous tissues, liver (p. 1450), salivary gland (p. 1441), larynx and bone (p. 1473).

Capillary hemangiomas (nevus vasculosus; strawberry mark). See page 1382.

Cavernous hemangiomas are poorly circumscribed, blue or purple elevated tumors which tend to extend more deeply into the subcutaneous tissues than do the capillary hemangiomas. They consist of numerous cystic vascular spaces containing blood. Mixed forms of cavernous and capillary hemangiomas are common; in such lesions regression of the cavernous elements may be slower and less constant than that of the superficial capillary elements. Cavernous elements which do not regress spontaneously are probably best treated by surgical excision. Cavernous hemangiomas may occur in sites other than the skin, e.g. in bone, liver and the tongue. In skeletal muscles they manifest themselves by pain and a diffuse mass which decreases in size with elevation of the part; foci of calcification may be demonstrable by roentgenographic examination.

A *giant hemangioma*, usually of the skin or subcutaneous tissue, but infrequently a visceral one, may be accompanied by thrombocytopenia and bleeding; such a tumor should be treated by irradiation. *Diffuse hemangiomas* of an extremity may be associated with hypertrophy of the part and of the associated bone.

Nevus venosus (nevus flammeus, port-wine mark). See page 1381.

Cirsoid aneurysms (racemose hemangioma, congenital arteriovenous fistula) are rare lesions consisting of a pulsating mass of dilated tortuous arteries, veins and capillaries. Pulmonary arteriovenous fistulas are apt to be part of the Rendu-Osler-Weber disease.

Hereditary hemorrhagic telangiectasia (Rendu-Osler-Weber disease). See page 842.

Angiomas of the retina (von Hippel's disease) may be associated with cerebellar angiomas, cysts of the pancreas and adenomas of the kidney (Lindau's disease [p. 1281]).

Sturge-Weber syndrome. See page 1281.

Glomus tumor is a small, circumscribed red to blue tumor usually located in the dermis and subcutaneous tissue, especially of the extremities. Infrequently it arises in the ligaments, periosteum, phalanges or joint capsules. Only about 7 per cent of glomus tumors manifest themselves before 16 years of age, but the tumor may be present at birth. Multiple tumors are present in about one fourth of affected infants and children; pain is relatively uncommon in them. The tumors consist of congeries of capillaries sheathed by distinct cuboidal epithelial-like cells or pericytes. Infiltrative growth is more frequently associated with tumors which have their origin during childhood than in adulthood. The tumor is benign. It will not regress spontaneously and recurs if incompletely excised.

Kaposi's sarcoma, which involves predominantly males, is extremely rare in early life. Among the reported instances in infants and children almost half have occurred in African Negroes. The onset is characterized by the appearance of one or more bluish to red nodules of variable size in the skin, usually of the extremities, or by a maculopapular rash. Intractable edema of an extremity may precede or accompany the appearance of the lesions of the skin. In African Negro children the initial manifestation may be referable to involvement of lymph nodes, but otherwise visceral involvement is rare in early life.

Histologically, the lesions are characterized by anastomosing capillaries with endothelial proliferation, accompanied by an interstitial proliferation of fibroblasts; the latter may predominate and simulate a fibrosarcoma.

The course of the disease may be fulminant, especially in children, with the appearance of innumerable nodules in the skin and viscera, and death in less than 2 years. More frequently, however, the disease persists for many years.

Hemangiopericytomas are rare in all age groups, and only about 10 per cent are first manifest before 16 years of age. They are composed of capillaries surrounded by pericytes, but without the organoid pattern characteristic of the glomus tumor. Rarely there are multiple tumors. Clinically, the neoplasm rarely appears to be vascular; even in histologic sections reticulin stains may be necessary to identify the vascularity.

These tumors usually arise in the subcutaneous tissue, but occasionally in such sites as skeletal muscle, the retroperitoneum, tongue and brain. Differentiation of benign and malignant hemangiopericytomas may be difficult or impossible, but those present at birth are usually benign and those arising in deep sites such as the retroperitoneum and muscles of the thigh are apt to be malignant. They should be radically excised.

Low-grade angiosarcomas are rare neoplasms which usually arise in the soft tissues, sometimes within a diffuse hemangioma of an extremity or a tumor in bone. The lesion may be manifest at birth or not until late childhood. Histologically, it consists of anastomosing vascular channels lined by atypical-appearing endothelial cells; multiple papillary projections extend into the lumens of the vessels. Metastases may occur by way of the blood stream or to the regional lymph nodes; the better differentiated tumors can usually be cured by local excision.

Lymphangiomas, which are less common than hemangiomas, are also probably malformations (hamartomas) rather than true neoplasms. They are often present at birth. The most common locations are on the neck and extremities. The various types of lymphangioma may be associated with each other in a given tumor, and other mesodermal elements, including smooth muscle, adipose tissue, foci of lymphocytes and hemangiomatous areas, may also be present. The tumors are benign, but, because of their infiltrative tendency, recurrences after attempted surgical removal are common.

Lymphangioma of the tongue. See page 1440.

Simple lymphangiomas are rare, small, flat or verrucous lesions usually located on the face or neck. They consist of dilated lymphatic vessels in the superficial dermis.

Lymphangioma circumscriptum is a rare condition characterized by small groups of thick-walled vesicles in the skin. It may be present at birth or begin in infancy or childhood.

Diffuse lymphangiomas are poorly circumscribed tumors occurring in the skin, mucous membranes or muscles. They are usually congenital. In the tongue and lips they are responsible for macroglossia and macrocheilia, respectively. Diffuse lymphangioma of an extremity is responsible for one form of elephantiasis (*elephantiasis lymphangiectatica*). It may involve an entire extremity or only a portion, e.g. the fingers or foot; there may be associated hypertrophy of the bone in the affected area. Histologically, the dilated lymphatic channels may be obscured by abundant scar tissue. The more localized lesions should be treated by surgical excision, but recurrences are frequent. Treatment of the more diffuse lesions is apt to be unsatisfactory.

Cystic lymphangiomas (cystic hygromas) are most frequently encountered in the neck (*hygroma colli*) and in the axillae, but may also occur in the inguinal and retroperitoneal regions. In the cervical region they may extend into the mediastinum, and rarely mediastinal hygromas may occur in the absence of a cervical component (p. 1444). *Mesenteric cysts* are simply cystic lymphangiomas of the mesentery, and many omental cysts are lymphangiomas. *Sacral hygromas* may simulate lipomas or sacrococcygeal teratomas; they are sometimes connected with the spinal canal. Enlargement of cystic lymphangiomas may occur by enlargement of the individual cysts, by formation of new cysts or by hemorrhage into the cysts.

Hygroma colli is the most common type of cystic lymphangioma. It is usually demonstrable at birth as a soft, poorly defined mass, often in the posterior cervical triangle; many of the tumors can be transilluminated. Periodic fluctuations in the size of the mass are common; rapid increase in size is often associated with hemorrhage into the cystic spaces. The size of the cervical component of a cervicomediastinal hygroma is greatly influenced by crying or by the phase of respiration. The tumors

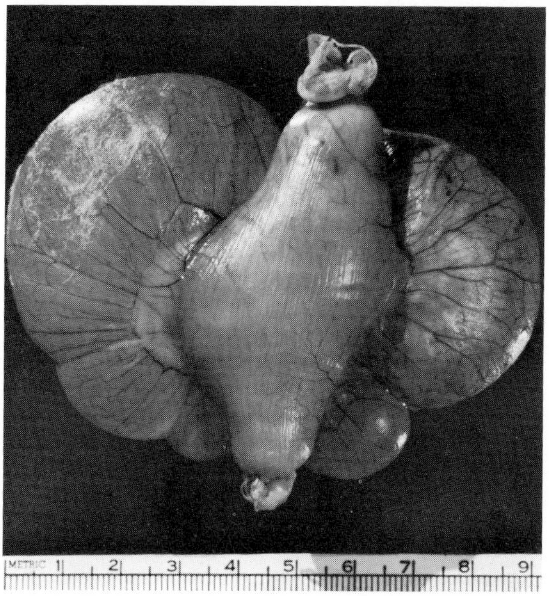

Figure 25-8. Cystic lymphangioma of the mesentery (mesenteric cyst) from a 4-year-old girl. The multilocular cystic mass extends on either side of the overlying bowel. Progressive painless abdominal enlargement, sometimes of several years' duration, is a common manifestation of a mesenteric cyst. In many instances no mass can be palpated and the presence of a fluid wave and shifting dullness may simulate ascites. (From J. B. Arey: *Pediat. Clin. N. Amer.*, Vol. 10.)

are often asymptomatic, but respiratory difficulty or difficulty in swallowing may occur.

The tumor may surround vessels and nerves, making surgical excision difficult. They are lobulated, thin-walled cystic structures which are usually multilocular; the cystic cavities may be independent of one another or may communicate freely. The contents usually consist of clear colorless fluid, but this may be xanthochromic or bloody.

Cystic lymphangiomas should be treated not only for cosmetic purposes, but also to prevent complications such as sudden enlargement of the mass as a result of hemorrhage into the lumens of the cyst, infection and mediastinal compression. Hygroma colli and hygromas of the mediastinum are best treated by surgical excision. In general the tumors are not susceptible to radiotherapy.

Angiomatosis is an uncommon disorder characterized by the presence of multiple hemangiomas or lymphangiomas in various sites, especially the bones, skin and subcutaneous tissues and the spleen. The lesions in the skin may be evident at birth or not until childhood or adolescence. Clinical manifestations are variable and are dependent upon the sites and extent of involvement. Massive chylous effusions, especially chylothorax, are relatively common. In some instances there may be a rash overlying the affected hemithorax, which waxes and wanes with the effusion. Multiple osteolytic defects in the bones are among the most common manifestations and may involve most of the bones, including those of the skull. Lesions of the skin and subcutaneous tissue may resemble cavernous hemangiomas or lymphangiomas. The prognosis is dependent upon the extent and sites of involvement; the lesions are often progressive, and, especially if chylous effusions are present, the outlook must be guarded.

TUMORS OF THE SKIN

Squamous cell and *basal cell carcinomas* are extremely rare in children, occurring especially in persons with xeroderma pigmentosum.

Multiple nevoid basal cell carcinoma syndrome is characterized by multiple lesions of the skin which are histologically indistinguishable from ordinary basal cell carcinomas, multiple cysts of the jaw, and a variety of osseous anomalies involving especially the ribs. Other less constant features include palmar dyskeratosis, mandibular prognathism, frontal bossing, mental retardation, dural calcification, scoliosis and ocular anomalies. Calcified ovarian fibromas and lymphangiomas of the mesentery have been observed in some affected adults. Shortening of the fourth metacarpals and absence of significant phosphorus diuresis after intravenous administration of parathyroid hormone have suggested a possible relation of this syndrome to *pseudohypoparathyroidism.*

Flesh-colored to pale brown, firm, painless papules may develop about the time of puberty, but may appear during infancy. They most frequently involve the skin of the nose, upper eyelids, cheeks, neck, trunk and arms; they may be suggestive of neurofibromatosis. Cysts in the jaw may appear as early as 7 or 8 years of age. They are often in juxta-position to the teeth, the roots of which may be destroyed. Even after thorough curettage, there is a tendency for the cysts to recur.

The disease is probably inherited as a mendelian dominant. All basal cell nevi should be completely removed.

Epidermoid cysts are spherical, benign tumors often located in the skin of the neck, face or scalp; they are probably derived from congenital ecto-dermal rests and are not true neoplasms. The wall of the cyst is lined by a thin layer of stratified squamous epithelium, and the lumen contains cor-nified debris; in some instances the epithelial lining is largely destroyed and is replaced by a foreign-body giant cell type of reaction. Skin ap-pendages are often present in the wall of the cyst.

Epidermoid cysts in the calvaria are demon-strable roentgenographically as sharply demar-cated defects surrounded by dense sclerotic bone.

Pigmented nevi in infants and children are usually clinically benign. They may be present at birth as large, rough, dark brown or black areas, as in the "bathing trunk" nevus. Smaller nevi may first be noted in infancy, childhood or even adult life at almost any site. They may be smooth or papillary, light brown to almost black, and may contain hair.

The histologic pattern of nevi in infants and children varies somewhat from that usually en-countered in adults. Benign nevi in children tend to be more cellular than those in adults, are more likely to have multinucleated cells and may contain mitotic figures. Failure to recognize these features may lead to an erroneous diagnosis of malignant melanoma.

Certain nevi reveal an even more striking his-tologic similarity to the malignant melanoma of adults and have been referred to as *epithelioid cell and spindle cell nevi (juvenile melanomas)*. They tend to be somewhat larger, purplish red rather than dark brown, hairless, and somewhat more elevated than the usual nevi in children. They are not usually clinically suspected of being nevi. They may recur if incompletely excised, but are benign lesions which should be treated by conservative surgical measures.

Owing to their frequency, removal of all nevi is not feasible. Those on the genitalia, palms of the hands and soles of the feet, as well as those in other sites which are subjected to repeated irritation, probably should be removed before puberty. The occurrence of increasing pigmentation, ulceration, rapid growth or a pigmented halo about a nevus is an indication for surgical excision of the growth with a wide margin of intact skin.

Balloon cell nevi contain a preponderance of large, pale, finely vacuolated cells. Although these cells may occur in nodular aggregates, they are usually diffusely distributed among the conven-tional nevus cells. Although balloon cells may be encountered in some malignant melanomas, their presence in an otherwise histologically benign nevus does not increase its malignant potential.

Malignant melanoma is rare before puberty, but may be present at birth. It may occur in association with xeroderma pigmentosum. About one fourth of the noncongenital, malignant melanomas in children have arisen in giant nevi. The risk of ma-lignancy developing in a giant nevus is probably relatively high; such melanomas in children are almost uniformly fatal; in contrast, the 3-year sur-vival rate, without recurrence, for other mela-nomas in children is about 25 per cent. Widespread malignant melanoma in the pregnant woman may metastasize to the placenta and fetus.

Blue nevi are usually smooth, firm, blue or bluish-black nodules occurring on the face, but-tocks or dorsum of the feet or hands. The lesion may resemble a Mongolian spot histologically, and cellular forms have been misinterpreted as malig-nant. Malignant transformation of a blue nevus, however, is rare.

Cutaneous leiomyomas are solitary or multiple small nodules in the skin, especially on the ex-tensor surfaces of the extremities. They are sometimes present from birth or early childhood. They may be tender and painful, but at times not for years after the tumor has been first noted. The tumors are circumscribed and consist of inter-lacing bands or cords of smooth muscle fibers. They may be quite vascular. The tumors are benign and should be excised.

Dermatofibrosarcoma protuberans is a slowly growing invasive tumor arising in the dermis. It begins as one or more hard, painless nodules which slowly coalesce, protrude from the skin and may ulcerate. The fibroblastic tissue within the neo-plasm tends to form irregular strands and whorls. The tumor may recur locally over a period of many years, but metastases are rare.

TUMORS OF SKIN APPENDAGE ORIGIN

The classification of neoplasms derived from skin appendages is not entirely uniform, and dif-ferentiation between neoplastic and non-neoplastic lesions may be difficult. The tumors tend to be clini-cally benign, although in some the histologic pattern may suggest a malignant neoplasm. Only a few of them will be discussed here.

Calcifying epitheliomas (pilomatrixomas) are relatively common, hard, sharply demarcated benign tumors of the skin which may arise at any site, especially in the face or arms. Clinically, they are usually confused with epidermoid cysts, and histologically they may be misinterpreted as carcinoma. They are probably derived from cells which are differentiating toward hair matrix cells.

Syringocystadenoma papilliferans is derived from the ducts of apocrine glands. It usually occurs as a single plaque, most frequently on the scalp; minute cysts are sometimes visible within the lesion. Histologically, it consists of numerous villus-like processes which project into the lumens of the dilated ducts.

Syringomas occur as hundreds of soft, slightly elevated, yellowish pinhead-sized nodules, especially about the eyelids, chest, abdomen and anterior aspects of the thighs. They occur predominantly in females and develop at puberty. Histologically, they consist of numerous small cystic ducts located in the dermis. These are benign lesions and are probably not true neoplasms.

Trichoepithelioma (epithelioma adenoides cysticum) also usually occurs in females at puberty. It is frequently familial. Multiple, small, discrete yellow to pink nodules appear on the face and occasionally on the upper part of the trunk. The tumor is derived from hair follicles and may contain areas closely simulating basal cell carcinoma; rarely a basal cell carcinoma may develop in adult life.

Cylindromas (turban tumors) are multiple benign growths which are often familial. They occur predominantly on the scalp of females, sometimes appearing in early childhood or at puberty. They usually appear initially on the forehead as smooth, firm, freely movable, painless nodules. They increase in number and size throughout life, so that ultimately the entire scalp may be covered by a lobulated mass of lesions. The origin of these tumors is not clear. They are nearly always benign and are best treated by surgical excision.

Nevus sebaceus is a circumscribed, slightly raised, firm yellow plaque usually occurring on the scalp or face and present at birth. It is composed of large numbers of sebaceous glands.

Adenoma Sebaceum. See pages 1280 and 1454.

TUMORS OF THE SOFT TISSUES

Neoplasms arising from muscle, fat and connective tissue comprise a miscellaneous but important group of tumors of early life. They may arise at almost any site and vary from benign neoplasms such as the lipoma to highly malignant sarcomas; the latter may be so undifferentiated as to preclude accurate determination of their cell of origin. They may occur at any age. The most frequent manifestation is a visible or palpable mass. Clinical differentiation of benign and malignant neoplasms is often impossible. Every solid mass should be considered malignant until proved otherwise by histologic examination of the excised mass.

Lipomas are benign rounded, encapsulated tumors composed of mature fat. They may be transilluminated and are radiolucent; rarely, calcific deposits are present. These tumors may reach an enormous size, and the rapid enlargement may suggest a malignant change. Malignancy developing within a pre-existing lipoma, however, is extremely rare.

Subcutaneous lipomas are rare in children. They are sometimes multiple and may be present at birth. They usually grow slowly but progressively and should be excised. A lipoma in the buttock may simulate a sacrococcygeal teratoma. Lipomas of the head, midline of the back or of the chest are sometimes connected by means of a pedicle with lipomas of the brain, spinal cord or mediastinum, respectively.

Retroperitoneal lipomas are rare; they may attain a huge size and be responsible for progressive abdominal enlargement. They usually arise in the perirenal region, but may arise from the mesentery. Roentgenographically, they are relatively radiolucent and may contain foci of calcification.

Lipoma of the parotid gland is encapsulated and is often attached to the deep lobe of the gland.

Hibernomas are rare benign tumors composed of brown fat, i.e. immature adipose tissue similar to that of the hibernating glands of animals. Although usually superficial, some are deeply located and may interfere with function sufficiently to be responsible for death.

Diffuse lipomatosis is probably a hamartomatous malformation rather than a true neoplasm. It consists of infiltrative, nonencapsulated masses of adult adipose tissue growing diffusely in the soft tissues. It may manifest itself at birth as enlargement of an extremity, sometimes accompanied by extensive deformities of adjoining bones. In other instances it may manifest itself as an ill-defined tumor, usually in skeletal muscle. Owing to their infiltrative nature, complete removal of these masses may be difficult or impossible, and recurrences are common, but the lesion is benign and does not metastasize.

Lipoblastomatosis refers to a rare tumor of the subcutaneous tissue of infants. It is believed to result from the continued proliferation of lipoblasts and of new lobules of adipose tissue in the postnatal period. The lobules contain adult fat cells as well as smaller, multivacuolated cells resembling fetal fat. In addition, spindle- and stellate-shaped cells lying in a myxoid ground substance may be present within the lobules and may be mistaken for a liposarcoma. Lipoblastomatosis is a benign tumor, but sometimes recurs repeatedly if incompletely excised.

Histiocytic tumors (fibrous xanthomas; histiocytomas; sclerosing hemangiomas) comprise a rather ill-defined group of neoplasms or neoplastic-like lesions, which usually involve the skin and subcutaneous tissue, synovia and tendon sheaths, and less frequently other sites, including skeletal muscle and lung. The tumor is painless, usually does not exceed 2 or 3 cm. in diameter, is well circumscribed, firm, and gray to yellow. It is composed predominantly of histiocytes and fibroblasts. Scattered lymphocytes and plasma cells, deposits of hemosiderin and multinucleated cells, including

Touton giant cells, may also be present. There are variable amounts of lipid in the cells. When the tumor consists almost entirely of histiocytes with a large amount of acidophilic cytoplasm, differentiation from the reticuloendothelioses may be difficult, if not impossible. When it is composed predominantly of fibroblasts, it may closely resemble, if not be identical with, a dermatofibrosarcoma protuberans.

These tumors are essentially benign, although they may recur if incompletely excised. A rare malignant variant has been described.

Giant cell tumors of tendon sheath origin (*benign synoviomas*) may represent one type of histiocytic tumor. These are small, firm tumors which arise from a tendon sheath or less often from an articular capsule. They are most frequent on the flexor surfaces of the fingers; less often they occur on the toes. They are benign, but may recur if incompletely removed. They are rare in children.

Pseudosarcomatous fasciitis is a rare lesion, probably inflammatory and not neoplastic, which is of importance principally because it may be misinterpreted as a malignant neoplasm. It occurs predominantly in the subcutaneous tissue, especially in an arm; less frequently it arises in such sites as skeletal muscle, breast or the tracheobronchial tree. The tumor, which may appear during infancy, usually grows rapidly and, at least in children, is apt to be painless. It usually does not exceed a few centimeters in diameter, is nonencapsulated and is apt to be adherent to the surrounding tissues. Histologically, it consists of a peculiar myxoid fibroblastic tissue with many capillaries and a variable number of inflammatory cells toward its periphery; these are usually predominantly lymphocytes and macrophages. The lesion invades the surrounding tissue and may contain considerable numbers of normal mitotic figures. Direct invasion of an adjoining lymph node is sometimes encountered, but metastases do not occur, and the lesion is usually cured by simple excision.

Myxomas are rare tumors in children. Although probably capable of arising in almost any site, they are located most frequently in the superficial soft tissues or in the bones, especially the maxilla. The tumor may be apparent at birth. These are nonencapsulated neoplasms which may recur and produce extensive destruction of the tissues in which they occur, but do not metastasize. Treatment is by wide excision.

Benign mesenchymomas (*mixed mesodermal tumors*) are rare tumors composed of an admixture of differentiated mesenchymal elements not ordinarily encountered in a single neoplasm. The tumors are usually solitary and well circumscribed, but occasionally infiltrate extensively and produce diffuse enlargement of a part. They occur predominantly in the skin, subcutaneous tissue and muscles of the extremities, but may arise in almost any site, including the mediastinum, retroperitoneum or viscera. They may be present at birth or appear during infancy or childhood. The tumors, many of which are probably hamartomas, may recur, but are essentially benign and do not metastasize.

Leiomyomas only rarely arise from the soft tissues of infants and children, but occur somewhat more frequently in the viscera, e.g. the bladder, lung, gastrointestinal tract and the kidney. They are well circumscribed tumors which should be excised.

Granular cell myoblastoma is a rare tumor in infants and children. It is usually solitary, but there may be multiple independent growths. In the pediatric age group, the site of origin is most commonly in the skin and subcutaneous tissue and the tongue, less frequently the vulva, muscles or even a bronchus. It is composed of large granular cells; the overlying epithelium of the skin or tongue characteristically reveals pseudoepitheliomatous hyperplasia. The cell of origin is not clearly established, but it may be neural rather than muscular. These tumors are benign in children.

Tumoral calcinosis is a rare disorder, distinct from calcinosis universalis or circumscripta. The onset is usually in the first or second decade. Siblings may be affected, and an association with pseudoxanthoma elasticum has been described. The serum calcium value is usually normal, but that of serum phosphate may be elevated. Clinically, there are large, nodular, periarticular deposits of calcium, especially about the hips, shoulders and elbows, and at times smaller deposits elsewhere. Histologically, the masses are composed of multicystic spaces filled with deposits of calcium and phosphorus and separated from each other by fibrous septa containing macrophages, multinucleated giant cells and chronic inflammatory cells. The general health of the affected persons is usually unimpaired. The cause of the disorder is unknown, but an inborn error of metabolism has been suggested.

Juvenile fibromatosis may be located in diverse anatomic sites, but most frequently in skeletal muscle, fascia (including that of the hands and feet) and subcutaneous tissue. Most of them are solitary, nonencapsulated, infiltrative lesions which grow rather slowly and are responsible for a palpable mass; in children, about 10 per cent are multiple. They almost never metastasize, but often recur if incompletely excised; infrequently they infiltrate so extensively as to necessitate mutilating operative procedures and may be responsible for death. In general they are composed of well differentiated fibroblastic tissue forming considerable amounts of collagen.

Desmoids are fibromatoses of the musculo-aponeurotic sheaths. Although their neoplastic nature is not universally accepted, their clinical behavior, with infiltration of surrounding tissue, continued growth and repeated recurrences, is certainly that of a neoplasm of low-grade malignancy. It does not, however, metastasize. These tumors are uncommon in early life, but may be present at birth.

They arise from such diverse sites as the abdominal wall, the shoulder girdle, thigh and neck. They are usually poorly circumscribed and may recur even after apparently complete excision. Treatment is by wide excision.

Fibromatosis of the plantar and palmar fascia, though rare, is of importance in children principally because it may be misinterpreted as fibrosarcoma and needless amputation performed.

Palmar fibromatosis is the basic lesion responsible for Dupuytren's contracture; this is extremely rare in children, and when it does occur in early life, is usually not associated with the presence of tumor-like nodules.

Fibromatosis of the plantar fascia is usually unassociated with contractures and manifests itself as single or multiple nodular swellings sometimes accompanied by pain. Rarely a nodule may be present in the sole of the foot at birth. These lesions are nonencapsulated firm masses only infrequently adherent to the overlying dermis. Histologically, they consist of closely packed, spindle-shaped cells in considerable amounts of mature collagen. As a rule few or no mitoses are present, but infrequently the nuclei are somewhat bizarre. Occasionally the pattern may simulate that of fibrosarcoma, but malignant neoplasms of fibroblastic origin are rare in this site. The lesion is benign, and if the diagnosis is established by biopsy and the patient is asymptomatic, no further treatment need be instituted. Recurrence may follow incomplete removal; if symptoms are present, the entire plantar fascia should be removed.

Juvenile aponeurotic fibroma is a rare tumor which occurs predominantly in infants and children and may be present at birth. Although usually arising in the palm, it may occur in the foot or presumably at any site among muscles and tendons. It presents as a firm, painless tumor not fixed to the overlying skin and not responsible for contractures. Although nonencapsulated and invasive, in older children it tends to be somewhat more compact and to be stippled with areas of calcification which are demonstrable roentgenographically. Histologically, it consists of numerous plump, oval nuclei of uniform appearance lying in a pink-staining matrix. All the cells appear to be oriented in one direction, in contrast to the interweaving pattern in other fibromatoses. The tumor is benign, but infiltrates fat and skeletal muscle and is apt to recur after limited excision. Localized removal and not amputation is the treatment of choice.

Digital fibromatoses generally first appear in early infancy as one or more firm masses on the lateral or dorsal surfaces of the fingers or toes. The tumors are often multiple. Histologically, the lesions are nonencapsulated and consist of interdigitating bands of fibrous connective tissue with abundant collagen. Mitotic figures are infrequent. The tumor should be removed by wide excision; amputation of the digit is indicated only for very advanced lesions.

Congenital generalized fibromatosis is an extremely rare condition characterized by the presence of multiple small, firm, spherical or ovoid tumors of the subcutaneous and muscular tissues as well as of the viscera and the osseous system. Numerous nodules are characteristically present at birth. The lesions vary from microscopic dimensions to several centimeters in diameter and may contain roentgenographically demonstrable foci of calcification. They are widely distributed over the body, possibly with some predilection for the shoulder girdle, arms, lower back, gluteal region and thighs. Some of the superficial tumors may resemble hemangiomas. Visceral involvement is characteristically widespread and may be responsible for varied manifestations, which include intestinal obstruction, diarrhea as a result of innumerable polypoid growths of the small and large intestines, and respiratory disturbances. Death often occurs during the neonatal period or early infancy. In a few instances in which the number of detectable nodules has been limited, survival has followed removal of them. Spontaneous regression of osseous defects as well as of multiple more superficial masses has been observed.

Fibrous hamartoma of infancy is an uncommon tumor of the skin and deep subcutaneous tissue which occurs almost exclusively in infants under 2 years of age and most frequently involves the region of the shoulder or an upper extremity. It may be present at birth and be adherent to the overlying skin. Histologically, it consists of septa of fibroblastic connective tissue, islands of cellular mesenchymal tissue with an organoid pattern and adipose tissue. It is a benign tumor which should be treated by simple excision.

TUMORS OF NERVE SHEATH ORIGIN

There is confusion about the nomenclature of tumors of nerve sheath origin and the relation of these tumors to neurofibromatosis. The neurilemmoma usually occurs as an isolated, encapsulated tumor, but occasionally there are associated stigmata of multiple neurofibromatosis. Neurofibromas are characteristically not well circumscribed or encapsulated and, though they also may occur as solitary growths, are much more commonly part of multiple neurofibromatosis.

Neuromas are not true neoplasms, but consist of proliferative masses of Schwann cells, axon fibers and connective tissue which develop at the proximal end of a severed nerve. They may be extremely painful.

Neurilemmomas (schwannoma, neurinoma) are benign, solitary, encapsulated tumors which arise from the peripheral, sympathetic or cranial nerves. The acoustic nerve is the commonest site of neurilemmoma rising from a cranial nerve. Peripherally located tumors are not likely to become as large as those in the posterior mediastinum or retroperitoneum. The tumor may be solid or partially cystic.

Neurofibromas may occur as solitary tumors, but

are often associated with multiple neurofibromatosis (p. 1280). The tumor may be firm or cystic. It is usually painless, but relatively large tumors in an enclosed space, e.g. the ulnar nerve at the elbow, may cause pain. *Plexiform neurofibromas* may first manifest themselves during infancy or more frequently during childhood. The affected nerves are elongated, tortuous and enlarged, appearing as a tangled mass of worms. They may occur as isolated lesions, but are often accompanied by other stigmata of multiple neurofibromatosis. Plexiform neurofibromas may be a part of *elephantiasis neuromatosa*, in which severe thickening of the part may be associated with hypertrophy of the bone. *Intraspinal neurofibromas* may occur singly or in association with multiple neurofibromatosis. The tumors may be entirely intraspinal or may penetrate an intervertebral foramen and produce a paravertebral mass.

Vascular neurofibromatosis may be responsible for coarctation of the abdominal aorta or aneurysm or stenosis of one or both renal arteries with resultant hypertension.

SARCOMAS OF SOFT TISSUES

These malignant mesenchymal neoplasms, situated in the connective tissue, muscle and fat of the nonparenchymatous tissues, probably comprise 10 to 20 per cent of malignant neoplasms in infants and children. They usually present as a mass which has grown rapidly; accelerated growth, however, does not occur with all such neoplasms and may also be manifest by benign tumors. Sarcomas may differentiate toward skeletal or smooth muscle or toward fat or fibrous tissues, but in highly undifferentiated neoplasms it may be impossible to determine the line of differentiation, if indeed it exists; infrequently there are several cell types, producing a mesenchymoma.

In general, treatment of sarcomas of soft tissues is by excision with removal of a substantial margin of surrounding normal tissue; the edges of the resected specimen should be examined histologically to determine the adequacy of removal. Inadequate removal of sarcomas of even low-grade malignancy, as well as of some benign tumors, is followed by recurrence. There is no convincing evidence that the malignancy of the recurrent tumor is increased. Sarcomas are usually radioresistant.

Rhabdomyosarcoma is the most common malignant neoplasm of soft tissues encountered in the pediatric age period. It occurs predominantly but not exclusively in males, the sites of predilection for its origin being the soft tissues of the extremities, the head and neck and the lower genitourinary tract. At least 3 different histologic types of rhabdomyosarcoma are described, but the distinction between them is not always clear, and some neoplasms contain morphologic features of more than one type.

Pleomorphic rhabdomyosarcoma is predominantly a lesion of the extremities of adults. It is a poorly demarcated, invasive neoplasm. *Alveolar rhabdomyosarcoma* tends to occur at a somewhat younger age than does the pleomorphic type. It may originate in the extremities, head and neck, genitourinary system or the trunk. It is characterized by alveoli lined by a single row of cells which are closely applied to their walls, with uninucleated and multinucleated cells lying free in the lumens. Such neoplasms may be misinterpreted as carcinoma, lymphoma, malignant melanoma or even neuroblastoma. *Embryonal rhabdomyosarcoma* occurs predominantly in infants and children and arises principally in the genitourinary tract, the pelvis and in the head and neck. It is apt to be poorly differentiated, containing stellate cells and long, thin, spindle-shaped cells with bright acidophilic cytoplasm. Cross striations are relatively infrequent.

Sarcoma botryoides is an embryonal rhabdomyosarcoma which, because of its location just beneath the mucous membrane of a hollow viscus or the serosal surface of a body cavity, assumes a grape-like or polypoid configuration. It may arise in the lower genitourinary tract, the head and neck or in the common bile duct. Ulceration of the overlying epithelium with secondary infection, coupled with the edematous appearance of the mass, may lead to an erroneous diagnosis of an inflammatory rather than a neoplastic lesion.

Rhabdomyosarcomas are apt to recur locally, and metastases are relatively frequent in regional lymph nodes and in the lungs and in bones. Prompt radical surgical extirpation is the treatment of choice, and, especially with the less differentiated tumors, the prognosis is improved by the use of irradiation and systemic antineoplastic agents. In general, however, the prognosis is very poor.

Fibrosarcomas may be present at birth. They are composed of spindle-shaped cells accompanied by reticulin fibers. It should be recognized that a variety of other cells, including lipoblasts and histiocytes, are capable of forming fibroblastic tissue and that neoplasms containing such tissue should not be considered fibrosarcomas. Low-grade fibrosarcomas may be difficult or impossible to differentiate from juvenile fibromatoses (p. 1468), and identification of the potential for metastasizing may be impossible. These tumors are locally invasive and should be widely excised with a generous margin of intact tissue. Since metastases occur in less than 10 per cent of instances, amputation should not be performed until attempts have been made to effect a cure by less radical means.

Neurofibrosarcomas (malignant schwannomas) may occur as solitary tumors or in conjunction with multiple neurofibromatosis. Children with such neoplasms usually have other stigmata of von Recklinghausen's disease, but only a minority of those with multiple neurofibromatosis have sarcomas during childhood. The incidence of sarcoma in persons with multiple neurofibromatosis is unknown, but probably is in the range of 5 to 15 per cent; in children it is much less. Not only malignant schwannoma, but also rhabdomyosarcoma and, at least in adults, liposarcoma and pleomorphic, unclassified sarcoma may occur in conjunction with multiple neurofibromatosis.

Synovial sarcomas are uncommon during childhood. They usually arise in the para-articular tissues, especially about the hand or knee. The initial manifestation may be localized pain or point tenderness or a palpable mass. Roentgenographic examination may disclose areas of calcification. Macroscopically, the neoplasm often appears encapsulated, but histologically there is commonly evidence of proximal extension along fascial planes. Recurrences are apt to follow incomplete excision, sometimes after an interval of several years. Metastases are chiefly to the lungs; involvement of the regional lymph nodes occurs in about one fourth of the patients. The prognosis is grave, but apparent cures have been effected by wide local excision and by amputation. Excision is probably preferable.

Clear-cell sarcomas of tendons and aponeuroses are rare neoplasms occurring principally in the region of the foot and knee and intimately bound to tendons or aponeuroses. They are usually small, slowly growing painless masses which are not fixed to the overlying skin. Histologically, they have a uniform pattern of nests of pale cells with an epithelioid appearance. Repeated local recurrence and eventual metastases are common, especially to the regional lymph nodes and the lung.

Liposarcomas are rare in early life; rarely the tumor is present at birth. They may grow rapidly, but metastases are extremely rare. The neoplasms are commonly found within muscles or superficially attached to them and occur in a variety of sites, including the extremities, neck, mediastinum, retroperitoneum and even the pharynx. They are locally invasive and may recur if incompletely excised. Treatment is by wide excision.

Malignant mesenchymomas contain 2 or more malignant mesenchymal elements; fibrosarcomatous tissue is not included as one of them. These are rare tumors, but may be present at birth. Although most of them arise in the skeletal soft tissues, they may occur in almost any site, including the mediastinum, retroperitoneum, liver, ileum, orbit, nasopharynx and spinal canal. Grossly, they often appear to be partially or completely encapsulated, but histologically they are usually found to be invasive. They are often variegated in structure, and the larger lesions are apt to contain multiple areas of necrosis. Histologically, a variety of malignant mesenchymal elements may be encountered, including those of the rhabdomyosarcoma, liposarcoma, chondrosarcoma, and the like. Metastases may occur by way of the lymphatic and blood streams. Apparent cures have been effected even in the presence of metastases to the regional lymph nodes, especially in infants. Most of the congenital neoplasms have behaved in a benign manner.

Leiomyosarcomas of the soft tissues are rare in the pediatric age period. Although some in children have behaved in a benign manner, others have recurred or metastasized. Recurrence sometimes takes place after an interval of several years. The tumors are infiltrative and should be widely excised.

Alveolar soft part sarcomas occur predominantly in the muscles of the extremities, and more commonly in girls than in boys. The tumor is usually a slowly growing one which may recur locally and may metastasize as long as 15 years after removal of the primary neoplasm. The histogenesis is unknown. Histologically, it is characterized by a pseudoalveolar arrangement of the neoplastic cells in relation to delicate endothelial-lined vascular channels and septa; the cells may contain crystalline deposits which stain positively with PAS after digestion with diastase. The tumor should be widely excised. These are indolent growths, and survival may be relatively long, even after metastases appear. The probability of cure, however, is slight.

Extraosseous chondrosarcoma and osteosarcoma are extremely rare, especially in children. They arise in the soft tissues, especially of the extremities, and are not attached to bone. Their behavior is similar to that of their counterparts in bone. They should be differentiated from mesenchymomas, approximately one fourth of which contain osteoid or bone, and from other neoplasms of soft tissues which may contain metaplastic bone, e.g. neurofibrosarcoma and synovial sarcoma. Of greater importance, however, is the differentiation of extraskeletal osteosarcoma from myositis ossificans circumscripta, a benign, reactive lesion which may closely simulate osteosarcoma.

NEOPLASMS OF BONE

A variety of benign and malignant neoplasms of bone have been described in children in addition to non-neoplastic lesions which clinically and roentgenographically simulate true neoplasms. Diagnosis and treatment of suspected neoplasms of bone require clinical, roentgenographic and *histologic* studies.

BENIGN NEOPLASMS AND NEOPLASTIC-LIKE LESIONS

Osteochondromas (osteocartilaginous exostoses) may be solitary or multiple. They are probably anomalies of development rather than true neoplasms. Multiple exostoses are discussed on page 1346. The solitary osteochondroma is one of the most common of the benign osseous tumors. It is most frequently located at or near the ends of the long bones, especially the lower end of the femur or upper end of the tibia, but may arise from any bone which is preformed in cartilage. It is usually manifest in childhood or adolescence by a bony protuberance; occasionally pain may result from a fracture through its stalk or from the development of an overlying bursitis. The tumor consists of a bony mass near the epiphysis which protrudes in the direction of the shaft and is covered by a cap of cartilage. Growth of the mass tends to cease at or before cessation of skeletal growth, when the cap of cartilage may disappear, leaving only the residual outgrowth of bone (osteoma). Malignant transformation of an osteochondroma usually does not occur until after cessation of skeletal growth and is more apt to occur with multiple exostoses; the resultant neoplasm may be a parosteal sarcoma, chondrosarcoma or even an osteosarcoma. About 5 per cent of patients with *multiple exostoses* can be expected to have malignant neoplasms from one or more sites. Surgical resection of the tumor should be performed whenever feasible as a prophylactic measure against malignancy.

Enchondromas are solitary benign cartilaginous tumors arising within the bones. They are probably hamartomas rather than true neoplasms. Skeletal *enchondromatosis* refers to the presence of such tumors in multiple sites; when the involvement is predominantly unilateral, the condition is referred to as *Ollier's disease* (p. 1347); when there are associated vascular malformations, it is referred to as *Maffucci's syndrome.*

Solitary enchondromas are usually located in cylindrical bones, especially in one of the short bones of the hands or feet. The initial symptoms are often pain and swelling following a pathologic fracture. Roentgenograms reveal a well circumscribed area of rarefaction within the bone, with or without expansion of it and attenuation of the overlying cortex; dense stippled foci representing areas of calcification are commonly present. There is usually no periosteal formation of new bone unless infraction of the cortex has occurred. Histologically, the tumors consist of lobules of atypical hyaline cartilage, the matrix of which may have undergone a myxomatous change. Malignant changes within an enchondroma may occur, but are not common. Treatment of solitary enchondroma consists in curettage, and the introduction of bone chips or a bone graft if necessary.

Benign chondroblastomas are rare tumors derived from young cartilage cells. They occur predominantly in adolescent males and characteristically involve the epiphyseal end of a long bone. The neoplasm is manifest by pain which is often referred to the neighboring joint. Roentgenographically, the lesion appears as a rarefied mottled focus arising in the epiphysis, but sometimes extending into the adjoining metaphysis; it tends to be encircled by a narrow line of increased density. Histologically, it consists of cellular areas of compact, round or polyhedral cells, deposits of hyaline cartilaginous matrix, focal areas of calcification, necrosis and hemorrhage. The presence of multinuclear giant cells may lead to an erroneous diagnosis of giant cell tumor. Treatment consists in curettage with instillation of bone chips.

Chondromyxoid fibroma is closely related to benign chondroblastoma. It is a rare benign tumor usually encountered in the metaphysis of one of the long bones of the extremities. The lesion appears as an eccentrically located, expansile, rarefied area in the metaphysis; the borders tend to be scalloped and well defined by a narrow band of opaque sclerotic bone. In small bones the roentgenographic appearance may be that of an expansile, pseudotrabeculated cyst occupying the entire width of the bone. Histologically, the tumor consists of lobulated masses of closely packed cells embedded in a myxoid matrix; the matrix may undergo extensive fibrosis, and in some areas recognizable cartilaginous matrix may be formed by the neoplastic cells. The tumor, though rare, is of importance because it may be confused with a malignant tumor, especially a chondrosarcoma. Curettage followed by instillation of bone chips usually suffices to cure the tumor, but recurrences may take place, and the tumor should be considered potentially malignant.

Osteomas are benign tumors of osseous tissue which arise in the bones of the face or skull and may project from the surface or extend into the orbit or paranasal sinuses. Their presence, if associated with multiple soft tissue tumors, should lead to a careful examination of the gastrointestinal tract for the presence of polyps, as a part of Gardner's syndrome (p. 1448).

Osteoid osteoma is most frequently located in the tibia or femur, but may occur in other bones. The predominant symptom is pain, often with localized tenderness; swelling and, rarely, slight local heat and redness may also be present. Roentgenograms may not demonstrate a distinctive lesion in the early stages. Characteristically, a small radiolucent area is surrounded by a zone of sclerotic bone which may extend well beyond the lesion and may obscure the area of radiolucency. In some instances the central nidus may be radiopaque and thus not be visible within the dense peripheral sclerotic bone.

The tumor consists of a central nidus of sharply circumscribed osteoid tissue with varying degrees of mineralization. The dense peripheral zone noted on the roentgenogram consists of reactive, non-neoplastic bone. The tumor is benign and can be cured by complete removal of the nidus; incomplete removal is followed by recurrence of symptoms.

Benign osteoblastoma (*osteogenic fibroma, giant osteoid osteoma, ossifying fibroma, fibrous osteoma*) is a rare neoplasm composed of a fibrous matrix with areas of osteoblastic activity, osteoid tissue and bone. It occurs predominantly in children and young adults and involves especially long bones, vertebrae and the maxilla and the mandible. Roentgenographically, it is a well circumscribed lesion which may expand and attenuate the cortex; its inner border tends to be limited by a zone of sclerotic bone. Although the lesion is clinically benign, its histologic features may simulate those of an osteosarcoma as well as of a variety of neoplastic and non-neoplastic lesions of bone. Complete clinical, roentgenographic and *histologic* findings must be carefully evaluated before accepting a diagnosis of benign osteoblastoma.

Nonosteogenic fibroma, a benign tumor whose neoplastic nature is in doubt, usually occurs near the end of the diaphysis of one of the long bones, especially in the leg. The lesion may be asymptomatic, or pain, sometimes interpreted as arthritis, may occur. Roentgenograms reveal a rarefied, trabeculated lesion with a sharply outlined margin of sclerotic bone; the lesion is usually eccentrically located within the bone. The tumor consists of bundles of spindle-shaped connective tissue cells with no attempt at the formation of bone. Abundant hemosiderin pigment, multinuclear giant cells, foam cells and collagen may be present. The lesion can be successfully treated by curettage, but often heals spontaneously.

Neurofibromas may involve the bones directly, with extensive destruction and deformity. *Multiple neurofibromatosis* may be associated with skeletal abnormalities such as scoliosis, pseudarthrosis, skeletal enlargement of part or of an entire extremity, or a defect in the wall of the orbit with unilateral pulsating exophthalmos.

Giant cell tumors are rare in childhood, since they characteristically occur in the ends of long bones after closure of the epiphyses. The majority of lesions interpreted as such are probably solitary unicameral cysts.

Hemangiomas may occur as primary osseous lesions or in association with hemangiomas in adjoining soft tissues. Primary osseous hemangiomas are located especially in the vertebrae, but occur in other sites. Roentgenographically, they may appear as pseudotrabeculated, cystic expansile lesions. In the skull a so-called sunray appearance may be noted on the roentgenogram. Hemangiomas may involve 2 or more adjoining vertebral bodies and produce a vertical striated appearance; collapse of the vertebrae with pressure on the spinal nerve rootlets may be responsible for symptoms.

Massive osteolysis (disappearing bone) occurs predominantly in otherwise healthy children and young adults; it is characterized by gradual absorption of one or more bones over a period of years. Almost any bone may be involved. The disease usually progresses until one or more of a group of bones have entirely or partially disappeared, after which the condition stabilizes. Rarely it results in death. The cause is unknown. Histologically, there is striking proliferation of thin-walled vessels in the bone and in the fibrous tissue which replaces it. The vascular channels usually contain red blood cells *(hemangiomatosis),* but sometimes appear to be lymphatics *(lymphangiomatosis).* The lesion differs from an ordinary hemangioma, which as a relatively localized process may destroy but does not completely dissolve bone. It is probably closely related to *angiomatosis* (p. 1465), but differs from classic instances of the latter in the absence of extraosseous lesions, in the unicentric nature of the osseous lesions and in the roentgenographic appearance of lysis of affected bone(s) rather than of multiple osteolytic defects.

Unicameral (solitary) cysts are common lesions in the metaphyses of long bones, especially in the upper ends of the tibia and the humerus and lower end of the femur. They rarely occur after closure of the epiphyseal line. The lesion is often symptomless until pain occurs after a pathologic fracture.

The lesion probably begins in the metaphysis, and growth of the bone displaces it away from the epiphyseal plate. It causes a central rarefaction of bone, often with a pseudotrabecular pattern; the defect is usually no wider than the adjacent metaphysis, although expansion of the shaft may occur. The cortex is attenuated and may be infracted. The roentgenographic appearance may be similar to that of such conditions as fibrous dysplasia, enchondroma or eosinophilic granuloma. In contrast to the giant cell tumor and benign chondroblastoma, it does not cross the epiphyseal plate.

The lesions are cystic and contain blood or fluid, which is often xanthochromic. The cyst is lined by a small amount of nonspecific vascular connective tissue containing deposits of hemosiderin, lipid-laden macrophages and multinucleated giant cells.

Treatment consists in curettage and packing with bone chips. Spontaneous healing may occur, especially after a pathologic fracture, but treatment is usually indicated.

Aneurysmal bone cysts are probably not true neoplasms. They may involve almost any bone, but especially the vertebrae. The presenting complaint is usually pain, at times associated with a palpable mass; neurologic manifestations may be present with lesions of the vertebrae. Roentgenographically, they appear as cystic expansile lesions which, especially in the long bones, tend to extend beyond the normal contour of the bone and produce a saccular, aneurysmal-like protrusion. Multiple incomplete septa are often visible within the radiolucent area. The expanded lesion is usually outlined by a thin shell of periosteal new bone, but rupture of this may occur with extension of the process into the adjoining soft tissues. Macroscopically, the cysts contain bloody fluid and soft, hemorrhagic or reddish brown tissue. Histologically, they consist of pools of blood separated by septa of connective tissue; giant cells, hemorrhages and newly formed bone may be present within the septa. Treatment is indicated because of the tendency of the lesion to progress; it consists in curettage. Even incomplete curettage may be followed by healing.

Melanotic neuroectodermal tumor of infancy (retinal anlage tumor) is a rare tumor which occurs in infants. A mass or swelling is usually present before the age of 6 months. The tumor arises predominantly in the maxilla, especially in the anterior portion, less frequently in the mandible and rarely in such sites as the scalp in the region of the anterior fontanel, in the subcutaneous tissue of the deltoid region, in the posterior mediastinum or in the epididymis. Roentgenographic examination reveals an expansile, rarefied lesion in the affected bone. Urinary excretion of VMA is sometimes elevated. The tumor is benign, although invasive. Recurrences following removal are rare.

Adenoameloblastoma is a benign, nonrecurrent lesion which occurs most frequently in girls in the second decade of life, usually in the maxilla in the region of an incisor or cuspid; it is *not* a variant of the ameloblastoma.

Myxomas. See page 1468.

Eosinophilic Granuloma. See page 1479.

Epidermoid Cyst. See page 1466.

MALIGNANT TUMORS OF BONE

By far the most frequent primary malignant tumors of bone are the osteosarcoma and Ewing's tumor, the majority of which occur between 10 and 25 years of age; males are affected more frequently than females. Osteosarcoma characteristically involves the metaphyseal end of a long bone, whereas Ewing's tumor involves the shaft, but roentgenographic differentiation of these neoplasms is not always possible. Of greater importance, however, is the fact that many, if not all, of the roentgenographic features of these tumors may be duplicated by non-neoplastic lesions of bone. Accordingly, treatment of lesions suspected of being malignant should not be instituted until an unequivocal diagnosis is established by histologic study of the tumor. Moreover, the pathologist is limited in his ability to establish a diagnosis on the basis of histologic studies alone. For example, an actively growing callus about a fracture may closely simulate the histologic appearance of an osteosarcoma, yet correlation of the material obtained at biopsy with the roentgenographic findings may clearly indicate the true non-neoplastic nature of the process. *Thus the pathologist must evaluate all pertinent clinical, roentgenographic and surgical data before he arrives at a diagnosis.*

Osteosarcoma (osteogenic sarcoma) is more common than Ewing's tumor. It usually begins at the lower end of the femur or the upper end of the tibia or humerus, but may arise at other sites. The presenting complaint is commonly that of pain and swelling of the affected part, which the patient may attribute to trauma.

Roentgenographic studies reveal varying degrees of destruction of bone and of new bone formation. Codman's triangle is a radiopacity at the end of the tumor where the periosteum has been elevated. Neither this finding nor the perpendicular striations of new bone in the subperiosteal neoplasm ("sunray appearance") are always present, nor are they pathognomonic of an osteosarcoma. The level of serum alkaline phosphatase may be elevated.

The neoplasm occupies the medullary cavity and penetrates the cortex to the subperiosteal zone; penetration of the periosteum into adjoining soft tissues may also occur. Histologically, the appearance is varied, but consists essentially of atypical mesenchymal cells with varying degrees of formation of collagen, typical or atypical osteoid tissue and true bone. Cartilaginous areas and areas of myxomatous tissue may be present. Osteosarcoma commonly metastasizes to the lungs, although other organs may also be involved; osseous metastases are rare. Amputation appears to offer the best possibility of cure, but the case fatality rate is high. In 1 series an exceptional 5-year survival rate of 19 per cent has been recorded.

Ewing's tumor may involve the same bones as does osteosarcoma; in addition, there is relatively frequent involvement of the flat bones and the ribs. The initial complaints are often similar to those associated with an osteosarcoma; fever and leukocytosis may occur with either tumor, but are more likely to be associated with Ewing's tumor.

Roentgenographically, there is a mottled area of rarefaction, often associated with increased density and periosteal formation of new bone (Fig. 25-9). The latter may be deposited in layers, resulting in an "onion-skin" appearance, but this finding is often absent and may appear in association with other osseous lesions. The roentgenographic appearance may closely simulate that of

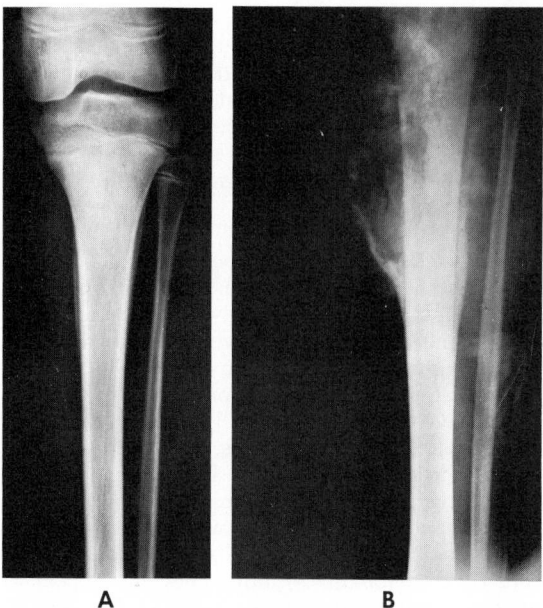

A   **B**

Figure 25-9. Roentgenograms of a Ewing's tumor of the tibia. *A,* The initial film revealed only slight periosteal proliferation. *B,* Roentgenogram taken 3 months later reveals cortical destruction and proliferation of new bone, the latter assuming a "sun-ray" appearance in some areas.

osteomyelitis, osteosarcoma, eosinophilic granuloma of bone or metastatic neuroblastoma.

Gross examination of an affected bone usually reveals more extensive neoplastic involvement than was demonstrable roentgenographically. Histologically, the tumor consists of sheets of uniform round or oval nuclei with little or no cytoplasm. The neoplastic cells do not form new bone. Extensive areas of hemorrhage and necrosis are commonly present. The histologic appearance may simulate that of a metastatic neuroblastoma, and every attempt should be made to exclude the presence of an extraosseous primary lesion.

Ewing's tumor usually involves a single bone when first recognized, but ultimately many bones may be affected. Metastases to the lungs are also common. Treatment currently consists in supervoltage irradiation of the entire bone and surrounding soft tissues rather than amputation; if the metaphysis is involved, the parts are extended so as to include the adjacent joint. Adjunctive chemotherapy is also indicated. With such techniques the 5-year survival rate should be in the vicinity of 25 per cent or possibly more.

Primary reticulum cell sarcoma of bone often arises in a long bone and may simulate Ewing's tumor both roentgenographically and histologically. Metastases to lymph nodes occur more frequently than in Ewing's tumor, and osseous metastases are infrequent. Irradiation is probably the treatment of choice. Although approximately 30 per cent can be cured, recurrences and metastases sometimes occur years after the initial treatment.

Chondrosarcoma is rare in children. It usually arises from the bones of the trunk or the upper ends of the humerus, femur or tibia. The clinical course is less rapid than that of osteosarcoma, and the prognosis, when amputation can be performed, is somewhat more favorable.

Primitive multipotential primary sarcoma of bone is rare in comparison to classic osteosarcoma and Ewing's tumor. It is most common in the second and third decades, but may occur as early as 2 years of age. It occurs about equally in the 2 sexes and may occur in long or flat bones, the most common site of origin being the femur. Histologically, it consists of sheets of undifferentiated cells interspersed among other neoplastic elements such as those of Ewing's sarcoma, osteosarcoma, chondrosarcoma and reticulum cell sarcoma. The predominant cell type is sometimes reflected in the roentgenogram. The presence of numerous pseudorosettes may suggest the diagnosis of metastatic neuroblastoma; other areas may simulate metastatic adenocarcinoma. Metastases occur not only to the lungs, but also to other bones; in a series of 25 patients there were only 5 survivors. The neoplasm is of importance because of the diagnostic problems it presents and because it affords some appreciation of the interrelations of various types of tumors which are usually considered to be distinct clinicopathologic entities, e.g. osteosarcoma, Ewing's tumor and chondrosarcoma.

Fibrosarcoma (p. 1470) may arise within the medullary cavity of a bone, commonly the lower end of the femur, or from the periosteum or adjoining connective tissue, and erode the adjacent bone. It differs from osteosarcoma in that there is no tendency to formation of even atypical osteoid or bone. Roentgenographically, the underlying bone may appear intact, or there may be areas of cortical destruction; the margins of the neoplasm are usually poorly defined. Treatment consists in wide surgical resection; amputation often is necessary. The 5-year survival rate is only about 30 per cent.

Multiple myelomas are extremely rare, if indeed they do occur in children. Roentgenographically, they may simulate metastatic neuroblastoma, Ewing's tumor, acute leukemia, multiple eosinophilic granulomas, Hand-Schüller-Christian or Letterer-Siwe disease.

Chordomas, or tumors derived from remnants of the notochord, are rare in children. Although not strictly neoplasms of bone, they invade and destroy bone at their site of development, usually the sacrococcygeal region or base of the skull. They are locally invasive tumors which usually cannot be successfully removed; metastases are unusual. Some chordomas in children have been reported as responding to irradiation.

Ameloblastomas (*adamantinoma*), which are epithelial tumors derived from remnants of the enamel organs, occur more frequently in the mandible than in the maxilla. Tumors arising in the maxilla may obliterate the antrum and bulge into the orbit, nasal cavity or mouth. Roentgenographically, they are usually expansile, well circumscribed lesions, but they may penetrate into adjoining tissues. Recurrences following curettage are frequent, and rarely metastases may occur. Craniopharyngiomas (p. 1285) may have the histologic appearance of an ameloblastoma, and tumors of similar appearance have been reported in the tibia, at least in adults.

JAMES B. AREY

REFERENCES

General

Marsden, H.B., and Steward, J. K. (Eds.): *Tumours in Children.* New York, Springer Verlag, 1968.

Miller, R. W.: Relation Between Cancer and Congenital Defects in Man. *New England J. Med.,* 275:87, 1966.

Willis, R. A.: *The Pathology of the Tumours of Children.* Springfield, Ill., Charles C Thomas, 1962.

Postradiation Neoplasia

Donohue, W. L., Jaffe, F. A., and Rewcastle, N. B.: Radiation-Induced neurofibromata. *Cancer,* 20:589, 1967.

Hagler, S., Rosenblum, P., and Rosenblum, A.: Carcinoma of the Thyroid in Children and Young Adults: Iatrogenic Relation to Previous Irradiation. *Pediatrics,* 38:77, 1966.

MacMahon, B., and Hutchison, G. B.: Prenatal X-ray and Childhood Cancer: A Review. *Acta Unio internat. contra cancrum,* 20:1172, 1964.

Tefft, M., Vawter, G. F., and Mitus, A.: Second Primary Neoplasms in Children. *Am. J. Roentgenol.,* 103:800, 1968.

Tumors of the Nose, Sinuses, Pharynx, Ear and Oral Cavity

Apostol, J. V., and Frazell, E. L.: Juvenile Nasopharyngeal Angiofibroma. A Clinical Study. *Cancer*, 18:869, 1965.

Gorlin, R. J., Sedano, H. O., Vickers, R. A., and Cervenka, J.: Multiple Mucosal Neuromas, Pheochromocytoma and Medullary Carcinoma of the Thyroid—A Syndrome. *Cancer*, 22:293, 1968.

Ringertz, N.: Pathology of Malignant Tumors Arising in the Nasal and Paranasal Cavities and Maxilla. *Acta oto-laryng.*, *Suppl.*, 27, 1938.

Yeh, S.: A Histological Classification of Carcinomas of the Nasopharynx, with a Critical Review as to the Existence of Lymphoepitheliomas. *Cancer*, 15:895, 1962.

Tumors of the Major Salivary Glands

Kauffman, S. L., and Stout, A. P.: Tumors of the Major Salivary Glands in Children. *Cancer*, 16:1317, 1963.

Wawro, N. W., Fredrickson, R. W., and Tennant, R.: Hemangioma of the Parotid Gland in the Newborn and in Infancy. *Cancer*, 8:595, 1955.

Tumors of the Head and Neck

Dito, W. R., and Batsakis, J. G.: Rhabdomyosarcoma of the Head and Neck. An Appraisal of the Biologic Behavior. *Arch. Surg.*, 84:582, 1962.

Tumors of the Mediastinum

Carey, L. S., Ellis, F. H., Jr., Good, C. A., and Woolner, L. B.: Neurogenic Tumors of the Mediastinum: A Clinicopathologic Study. *Am. J. Roentgenol.*, 84:189, 1960.

Heimburger, I. L., and Battersby, J. S.: Primary Mediastinal Tumors of Childhood. *J. Thoracic & Cardiovasc. Surg.*, 50:92, 1965.

Pachter, M. R., and Lattes, R.: Mesenchymal Tumors of the Mediastinum. *Cancer*, 16:74, 95, 108, 1963.

Taterman, A., and Amigo, A.: Thymoma Associated with Aregenerative and Aplastic Anemia in a Five-Year-Old Child. *Cancer*, 21:1212, 1968.

Tung, K. S. K., and McCormack, L. J.: Angiomatous Lymphoid Hamartoma. Report of Five Cases with a Review of the Literature. *Cancer*, 20:525, 1967.

Tumors of the Heart

Mahaim, I.: Les tumeurs et les polypes du coeur. Etude anatomoclinique. Paris, Masson et Cie, 1945, Chap. XV, p. 246-77.

Prichard, R. W.: Tumors of the Heart. Review of the Subject and Report of One Hundred and Fifty Cases. *A.M.A. Arch. Path.*, 51:98, 1951.

Simopoulos, A. P., and Breslow, A.: Tuberous Sclerosis in the Newborn. *Am. J. Dis. Child.*, 111:313, 1966.

Tumors of the Larynx

Ferguson, C. F., and Flake, C. G.: Subglottic Hemangioma as a Cause of Respiratory Obstruction in Infants. *Ann. Otol., Rhin. & Laryng.*, 70:1095, 1961.

Moore, R. L., and Lattes, R.: Papillomatosis of Larynx and Bronchi. Case Report with 34-Year Follow-up. *Cancer*, 12:117, 1959.

Norris, C. M., and Peale, A. R.: Sarcoma of the Larynx. *Ann. Otol., Rhin. & Laryng.*, 70:894, 1961.

Walsh, T. E., and Beamer, P. R.: Epidermoid Carcinoma of the Larynx Occurring in Two Children with Papilloma of the Larynx. *Laryngoscope*, 60:1110, 1950.

Tumors of the Trachea, Bronchi and Lungs

Anderson, A. E., Buechner, H. A., Yager, I., and Ziskind, M. M.: Bronchogenic Carcinoma in Young Men. *Am. J. Med.*, 16:404, 1954.

Condon, V. R., and Phillips, E. W.: Bronchial Adenoma in Children. A Review of the Literature and Report of Three Cases. *Am. J. Roentgenol.*, 88:543, 1962.

Giampalmo, A.: The Arteriovenous Angiomatosis of the Lung with Hypoxaemia. *Acta med. Scandinav.*, 139: Suppl. 248:1, 1950.

Guida, P. M., Fulcher, T., and Moore, S. W.: Leiomyoma of the Lung. Report of a Case. *J. Thoracic & Cardiovasc. Surg.*, 49:1058, 1965.

Iverson, L.: Bronchopulmonary Sarcoma. *J. Thoracic Surg.*, 27:130, 1954.

Umiker, W. O., and Iverson, L.: Postinflammatory "Tumors" of the Lung. Report of Four Cases Simulating Xanthoma, Fibroma, or Plasma Cell Tumor. *J. Thoracic Surg.*, 28:55, 1954.

Watts, W. R., and Hara, W. V.: Primary Fibrosarcoma of the Bronchus. *Am. Rev. Resp. Dis.*, 84:881, 1961.

Tumors of the Gastrointestinal Tract

Canby, J. P., and Mehlhop, F. H.: Ulcerative Colitis in Children. *Am. J. Gastroenterology*, 42:66, 1964.

Cornes, J. S., Wallace, M. H., and Morson, B. C.: Benign Lymphomas of the Rectum and Anal Canal: A Study of 100 Cases. *J. Path. & Bact.*, 82:371, 1961.

Duncan, B. R., Dohner, V. A., and Priest, J. H.: The Gardner Syndrome: Need for Early Diagnosis. *J. Pediat.*, 72:497, 1968.

Horn, R. C., Jr., Payne, W. A., and Fuie, G.: The Peutz-Jeghers Syndrome (Gastrointestinal Polyposis with Mucocutaneous Pigmentation): Report of a Case Terminating with Disseminated Gastrointestinal Cancer. *Arch. Path.*, 76:29, 1963.

Middelkamp, J. N., and Haffner, H.: Carcinoma of the Colon in Children. *Pediatrics*, 32:558, 1963.

Oeconomopoulos, C. T.: Argentaffin Cell Tumors (Carcinoids) of the Appendix in Children. *Pediatrics*, 27:134, 1961.

Roth, S. I., and Helwig, E. B.: Juvenile Polyps of the Colon and Rectum. *Cancer*, 16:468, 1963.

Tumors of the Liver

Edmondson, H. A.: Differential Diagnosis of Tumors and Tumor-Like Lesions of Liver in Infancy and Childhood. *A.M.A. Am. J. Dis. Child.*, 91:168, 1956.

Houštěk, J., Masopust, J., Kithier, K., and Rádl, J.: Hepatocellular Carcinoma in Association with a Specific Fetal a,-Globulin, Fetoprotein. *J. Pediat.*, 72:186, 1968.

Ishak, K. G., and Glunz, P. R.: Hepatoblastoma and Hepatocarcinoma in Infancy and Childhood. Report of 47 Cases. *Cancer*, 20:396, 1967.

Sutton, C. A., and Eller, J. L.: Mesenchymal Hamartoma of the Liver. *Cancer*, 22:29, 1968.

Tumors of the Spleen

Griscom, N. T.: Huge Splenic Cysts. *Am. J. Dis. Child.*, 109:224, 1965.

Wexler, L., and Abrams, H. L.: Hamartoma of the Spleen. Angiographic Observations. *Am. J. Roentgenol.*, 92:1150, 1964.

Tumors of the Pancreas

Ballard, H. S., Frame, B., and Hartsock, R. J.: Familial Multiple Endocrine Adenoma-Peptic Ulcer Complex. *Medicine*, 43:481, 1964.

Frantz, V. K.: Tumors of the Pancreas; in *Atlas of Tumor Pathology*. Washington, D.C., Armed Forces Institute of Pathology, 1959, Fascicles 27 and 28.

Moynau, R. W., Neerhout, R. C., and Johnson, T. S.: Pancreatic Carcinoma in Childhood. Case Report and Review. *J. Pediat.*, 65:711, 1964.

Wool, G., and Goldring, D.: Pseudocyst of the Pancreas. Report of Five Cases and Review of Literature. *J. Pediat.*, 70:586, 1967.

Tumors of the Kidney

Farber, S.: Chemotherapy in the Treatment of Leukemia and Wilms' Tumor. *J.A.M.A.*, 198:826, 1966.

Favera, B. E., Johnson, W., and Ito, J.: Renal Tumors in the Neonatal Period. *Cancer*, 22:845, 1968.

Fraumeni, J. F., Jr., and Glass, A. G.: Wilms' Tumor and Congenital Aniridia. *J.A.M.A.*, 206:825, 1968.

Fraumeni, J. F., Jr., Geiser, C. F., and Manning, M. D.: Wilms' Tumor and Congenital Hemihypertrophy: Report of Five New Cases and Review of Literature. *Pediatrics*, 40:886, 1967.

Garcia, M., Douglass, C., and Schlosser, J. V.: Classification and Prognosis in Wilms's Tumor. *Radiology*, 80:574, 1963.

Platt, B. B., and Linden, G.: Wilms's Tumor—A Comparison of 2 Criteria for Survival. *Cancer*, 17:1573, 1964.

Price, E. B., Jr., and Mostofi, F. K.: Symptomatic Angiomyolipoma of the Kidney. *Cancer*, 18:761, 1965.

Tumors of the Adrenal

Goldman, R. L., Winterling, A. N., and Winterling, C. C.: Maturation of Tumors of the Sympathetic Nervous System. Report of Long-Term Survival in 2 Patients, One with Disseminated Osseous Metastases, and Review of Cases from the Literature. *Cancer*, 18:1510, 1965.

Koop, C. E., and Hernandez, J. R.: Neuroblastoma: Experience with 100 Cases in Children. *Surgery*, 56:726, 1964.

Pinkel, D., and others: Survival of Children with Neuroblastoma Treated with Combination Chemotherapy. *J. Pediat.*, 73:928, 1968.

Studnitz, W. von, Kässer, H., and Sjoerdsma, A.: Spectrum of Catechol Amine Biochemistry in Patients with Neuroblastoma. *New England J. Med.*, 269:232, 1963.

Other Retroperitoneal Tumors

Anderson, M. S.: Myxopapillary Ependymomas Presenting in the Soft Tissue over the Sacrococcygeal Region. *Cancer*, 19:585, 1966.

Conklin, J., and Abell, M. R.: Germ Cell Neoplasms of Sacrococcygeal Region. *Cancer*, 20:2105, 1967.

Engel, R. M., Elkins, R. C., and Fletcher, B. D.: Retroperitoneal Teratoma. Review of the Literature and Presentation of an Unusual Case. *Cancer*, 22:1068, 1968.

Tumors of the Bladder and Prostate

Mostofi, F. K., and Morse, W. H.: Polypoid Rhabdomyosarcoma (Sarcoma Botryoides) of Bladder in Children. *J. Urol.*, 67:681, 1952.

Tumors of the Testis and Paratesticular Structures

Abell, M. R., and Holtz, F.: Testicular Neoplasms in Infants and Children. I. Tumors of Germ Cell Origin. *Cancer*, 16:965, 1963.

Holtz, F., and Abell, M. R.: Testicular Neoplasms in Infants and Children. II. Tumors of Non-germ Cell Origin. *Cancer*, 16:982, 1963.

ReMine, W. H., Woolmer, L. B., Judd, E. S., and Hopkins, D. M.: Testicular Teratoma in Infancy: Report of a Case with a 10-Year Follow Up. *Proc. Staff Meet., Mayo Clin.*, 36:661, 1961.

Rosvoll, R. V., and Woodard, J. R.: Malignant Sertoli Cell Tumor of the Testis. *Cancer*, 22:8, 1968.

Tumors of the Ovary

Ammann, A. J., Kaufman, S., and Gilbert, A.: Virilizing Ovarian Tumor in a 2½-Year-Old Girl. *J. Pediat.*, 70:782, 1967.

Borushek, S., Berger, I., Echt, C., and Gold, J. J.: Functioning Malignant Germ Cell Tumor of the Ovary in a 4½-Year-Old Girl. Case Report. *Cancer*, 18:1485, 1965.

Ehrlich, E. N., and others: Aldosteronism and Precocious Puberty Due to an Ovarian Androblastoma (Sertoli Cell Tumor). *J. Clin. Endocrinol.*, 23:358, 1963.

Garfinkel, B., and Rosenthal, A. H.: Teratomas and Follicular Cysts of the Ovary in Children. *Am. J. Obst. & Gynec.*, 83:101, 1962.

Neubecker, R. D., and Breen, J. L.: Embryonal Carcinoma of the Ovary. *Cancer*, 15:546, 1962.

Perry, R. W.: Ovarian Tumors in the Pediatric Patient. *Harper Hospital Bull.*, 19:209, 1961.

Tumors of the Vagina

Borglin, N. E., and Selander, P.: Hymenal Polyps in Newborn Infants. *Acta paediat., Suppl.*, 135:28, 1962.

Daniel, W. W., Koss, L. G., and Brunschwig, A.: Sarcoma Botryoides of the Vagina. *Cancer*, 12:74, 1959.

Vawter, G. F.: Carcinoma of the Vagina in Infancy. *Cancer*, 18:1479, 1965.

Tumors of Vascular Origin

Dutz, W., and Stout, A. P.: Kaposi's Sarcoma in Infants and Children. *Cancer*, 13:684, 1960.

Kauffman, S. L., and Stout, A. P.: Malignant Hemangioendothelioma in Infants and Children. *Cancer*, 14:1186, 1961.

Koblenzer, P. J., and Bukowski, M. J.: Angiomatosis (Hamartomatous Hemolymphangiomatosis). Report of a Case with Diffuse Involvement. *Pediatrics*, 28:65, 1961.

Kohout, E., and Stout, A. P.: The Glomus Tumor in Children. *Cancer*, 14:555, 1961.

Najman, E., Fabecic-Sabadi, V., and Temmer, B.: Lymphangioma in the Inguinal Region with Cystic Lymphangiomatosis of Bone. *J. Pediat.*, 71:561, 1967.

Tumors of the Skin and Skin Appendages

Forbis, R., Jr., and Helwig, E. B.: Pilomatrixoma (Calcifying Epithelioma). *Arch. Dermat.*, 83:606, 1961.

Gorlin, R. J., Vickers, R. A., Kelln, E., and Williamson, J. J.: The Multiple Basal-Cell Nevi Syndrome. *Cancer*, 18:89, 1965.

Skov-Jensen, T., Hastrup, J., and Lambrethsen, E.: Malignant Melanoma in Children. *Cancer*, 19:620, 1966.

Tumors of Soft Tissues

Dutz, W., and Stout, A. P.: The Myxoma in Childhood. *Cancer*, 14:629, 1961.

Enzinger, F. M.: Fibrous Hamartoma of Infancy. *Cancer*, 18:241, 1965.

Goslee, L., Clermont, V., Bernstein, J., and Wooley, P. V., Jr.: Superficial Connective Tissue Tumors in Early Infancy. A Study of Fibromatosis and Lipoblastomatosis. *J. Pediat.*, 65:377, 1964.

Kauffman, S. L., and Stout, A. P.: Lipoblastic Tumors of Children. *Cancer*, 12:912, 1959.

Moscovic, E. A., and Azar, H. A.: Multiple Granular Cell Tumors ("Myoblastomas"). Case Report with Electron Microscopic Observations and Review of the Literature. *Cancer*, 20:2032, 1967.

Najjar, S. S., Farah, F. S., Kurban, A. K., Melhem, R. E., and Khatchadourian, A. K.: Tumoral Calcinosis and Pseudoxanthoma Elasticum. *J. Pediat.*, 72:243, 1968.

Stout, A. P.: Juvenile Fibromatoses. *Cancer*, 7:953, 1954.

Stout, A. P.: Pseudosarcomatous Fasciitis in Children. *Cancer*, 14:1216, 1961.

Tumors of Nerve Sheath Origin

Cornell, S. H., and Kinkendall, W. M.: Neurofibromatosis of the Renal Artery. An Unusual Cause of Hypertension. *Radiology*, 88:24, 1967.

D'Agostino, A. N., Soule, E. H., and Miller, R. H.: Sarcomas of the Peripheral Nerves and Somatic Soft Tissues Associated with Multiple Neurofibromatosis (von Recklinghausen's Disease). *Cancer*, 16:1015, 1963.

Sarcomas of Soft Tissues

Botting, A. J., Soule, E. H., and Brown, A. L., Jr.: Smooth Muscle Tumors in Children. *Cancer*, 18:711, 1965.

Cadman, N. L., Soule, E. H., and Kelly, P. J.: Synovial Sarcoma. An Analysis of 134 Tumors. *Cancer* 18:613, 1965.

Enzinger, F. M.: Clear Cell Sarcoma of Tendons and Aponeuroses. An Analysis of 21 Cases. *Cancer*, 18:1163, 1965.

Horn, R. C., Jr., and Patton, R. B.: Rhabdomyosarcoma. *Clin. Orthopaedics*, 19:99, 1961.

Lieberman, P. H., Foote, F. W., Jr., Stewart, F. W., and Berg, J. W.: Alveolar Soft-Part Sarcoma. *J.A.M.A.*, 198:1047, 1966.

Nash, A., and Stout, A. P.: Malignant Mesenchymomas in Children, *Cancer*, 14:524, 1961.

Soule, E. H., Mahour, G. H., Mills, S. D., and Lynn, H. B.: Soft Tissue Sarcomas of Infants and Children: A Clinicopathologic Study of 135 Cases. *Mayo Clin. Proc.*, 43:313, 1968.

Tumors of Bone

Abrams, A. M., Melrose, R. J., and Howell, F. V.: Adenoameloblastoma. A Clinical Pathologic Study of Ten New Cases. *Cancer*, 22:175, 1968.

Aegerter, E., and Kirkpatrick, J. A., Jr.: *Orthopedic Diseases. Physiology, Pathology, Radiology.* 3rd ed. Philadelphia, W. B. Saunders Company, 1968.

Borello, E. D., and Gorlin, R. J.: Melanotic Neuroectodermal Tumor of Infancy—A Neoplasm of Neural Crest Origin. *Cancer*, 19:196, 1966.

Hustu, H. O., Holton, C., James, D., Jr., and Pinkel, D.: Treatment of Ewing's Sarcoma with Concurrent Radiotherapy and Chemotherapy. *J. Pediat.*, 73:249, 1968.

Hutter, R. V. P., Foote, F. W., Jr., Francis, K. C., and Sherman, R. S.: Primitive Multipotential Primary Sarcoma of Bone. *Cancer*, 19:1, 1966.

26. Unclassified Diseases

AMYLOIDOSIS

Amyloidosis is much less common in children than in adults. Its pathogenesis remains obscure. Electron microscopic, immunoelectrophoretic and biochemical studies suggest that amyloid consists of fine fibrils of protein produced by reticuloendothelial cells and deposited in a ground substance composed of abnormal mucopolysaccharides. When the deposition of amyloid is advanced, involved organs become enlarged, rubbery and pale. Liver, spleen, kidneys, adrenals, heart and gastrointestinal tract are the most frequent sites of deposition, but fibrils may be found in any organ, including the media and adventitia (sometimes the intima) of blood vessels. Several tests exist for recognition of amyloidosis, one of which involves the intravenous injection of Congo red; if 60 per cent or more of dye is removed rapidly from the circulation, the result is considered positive, but final diagnosis must rest on biopsy of involved tissue, in which such stains as Congo red produce with amyloid a green birefringence seen with the polarizing microscope.

Classifications of amyloidosis have been based on so-called types of amyloid, but the disorder is perhaps best categorized clinically as primary or secondary.

Amyloidosis not accompanying other diseases is logically, if perhaps temporarily, called *primary* and includes several rare heredofamilial disorders. *Familial amyloidosis with polyneuropathy* produces peripheral neuropathy, trophic skin lesions, especially of the lower extremities, vitreous opacities, and occasionally hepatosplenomegaly. Inheritance is dominant. The condition affects young adults and, only rarely, children. *Familial Mediterranean fever* is found primarily in ethnic groups originating from the Mediterranean area. It is included among the periodic diseases. Clinically there are bouts of fever and of abdominal or chest pain and recurrent joint pains; ultimately renal amyloidosis gives rise to proteinuria, the nephrotic syndrome and kidney failure. Inheritance is autosomal recessive. A history of family members having repeated laparotomies because of recurrent abdominal pain is not unusual. Rectal or gingival biopsy may permit a diagnosis of amyloidosis. Because amyloid may be found very early in association with familial Mediterranean fever, it is not felt to be a secondary phenomenon.

Other conditions in which amyloidosis may be "primary" include *heredofamilial urticaria, deafness and neuropathy, familial cutaneous amyloi-dosis* and *familial amyloid-producing thyroid carcinoma.*

Secondary amyloidosis was more common when antibiotic therapy was not available for such chronic diseases as osteomyelitis, bronchiectasis and tuberculosis. It has been reported also to complicate rheumatoid arthritis, ulcerative colitis and regional ileitis. It occurs in adults with multiple myeloma and Hodgkin's disease, but rarely in children with such disorders.

There is no treatment at present for the conditions associated with primary amyloidosis. Treatment of secondary amyloidosis depends on control of the basic disorder. It has been suggested that corticosteroids may augment amyloid formation, but this is not proved.

SYDNEY S. GELLIS

REFERENCES

Cohen, A. S.: Amyloidosis. *New England J. Med.,* 277:522, 528, 628, 1967.

Heller, H., Sohar, E., Gafni, J., and Heller, J.: Amyloidosis in Familial Mediterranean Fever: An Independent Genetically Determined Character. *Arch. Int. Med.,* 107:539, 1961.

Muckle, T. J., and Wells, M.: Urticaria, Deafness and Amyloidosis: New Heredo-familial Syndrome. *Quart. J. Med.,* 31: 235, 1962.

Sagher, F., and Shannon, J.: Amyloidosis Cutis: Familial Occurrence in Three Generations. *Arch. Derm.,* 87:171, 1963.

SARCOIDOSIS

Sarcoidosis, a disease of obscure origin, has been noted in children, although it is uncommon below the age of 10 years. The clinical patterns simulate those observed in adults. Pulmonary lesions, uveitis or iritis, skin lesions (commonly nodules) and generalized lymphadenopathy are the most frequent manifestations of sarcoidosis in children. Specific symptoms are related to the organs and tissues involved.

The pathologic abnormalities noted in sarcoidosis simulate those observed in chronic granulomatous diseases, especially tuberculosis. *Mycobacterium tuberculosis* has not been demonstrated in these lesions, and most patients with sarcoidosis do not have dermal reactions to tuberculin.

The *epidemiology* is obscure. Negroes are more commonly affected than white persons, and most patients, regardless of race, have come from rural communities in the southeastern United States.

Uveoparotid fever in children has been described with painless swelling of the parotid or salivary glands, fever, and uveitis. Disseminated sarcoi-

REFERENCES

Jasper, P. L., and Denny, F. W.: Sarcoidosis in Children. *J. Pediat.*, 73:499, 1968.
Kendig, E. L.: *Disorders of the Respiratory Tract in Children.* Philadelphia, W. B. Saunders Company, 1967, Chap. 52.
Longcope, W. T., and Freiman, D. G.: A Study of Sarcoidosis. *Medicine*, 31:1, 1952.
Proceedings of the International Conference on Sarcoidosis in *Am. Rev. Resp. Dis.*, 84:(part 2), 1961.
Siltzbach, L. E.: Sarcoidosis and Mycobacteria. *Am. Rev. Resp. Dis.*, 97:1, 1968.

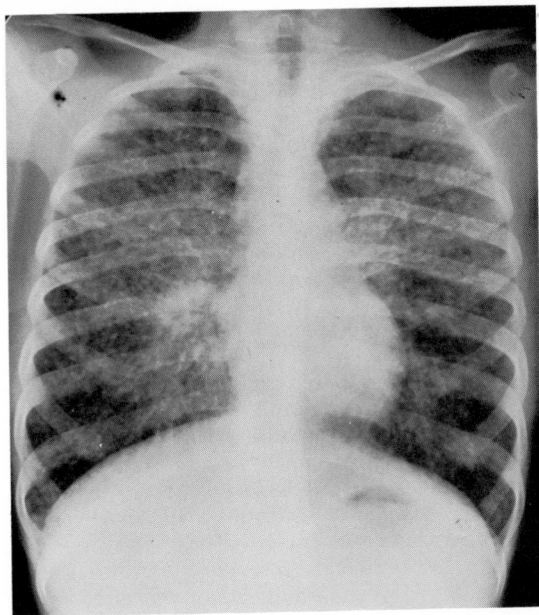

Figure 26-1. Sarcoidosis in a white girl 10 years of age. Note the widely disseminated peribronchial infiltrations and multiple small nodular densities, the overaeration of the lungs, and the hilar adenopathy.

dosis involving most of the viscera has also been reported. Pulmonary involvement in the adolescent or young adult is extremely variable in its extent and characteristics. Parenchymal infiltrates, miliary nodules and hilar and paratracheal lymphadenopathy have been observed singly or in combination.

Owing to the protean manifestations of sarcoidosis, the *differential diagnosis* is extremely broad. The diseases to be considered include tuberculosis, the various pulmonary mycoses and inflammatory ocular lesions such as phlyctenular conjunctivitis. Sarcoidosis is commonly associated with hyperproteinemia, hyperglobulinemia, hypercalcemia, hypercalciuria, leukopenia and eosinophilia. Multiple cystic lesions in the bones of the hands and feet have been noted in some patients. There are no specific diagnostic tests, although the Nickerson-Kveim test result, consisting in formation of a granuloma several weeks after intradermal injection of material from a sarcoid lesion, is positive in the majority of active adult cases. Biopsy of affected areas probably provides the most valuable diagnostic study.

Treatment is symptomatic and supportive. Corticosteroids suppress the acute manifestations of sarcoidosis, especially the inflammatory ocular lesions and the hypercalcemia.

The *prognosis* of sarcoidosis in children is not well established, but many show spontaneous recovery after a prolonged illness of several months' to several years' duration.

ROBERT H. HIGH

THE HISTIOCYSTOSIS SYNDROMES

(EOSINOPHILIC GRANULOMA OF BONE, HAND-SCHÜLLER-CHRISTIAN AND LETTERER-SIWE SYNDROMES, RETICULOENDOTHELIOSES)

The histiocytosis syndromes, identified by the foregoing diagnostic terms, present a wide spectrum of clinical patterns in which the underlying common denominator is the development of granulomatous lesions with histiocytic proliferation. The clinical expression appears to be a reactive phenomenon, the triggering mechanism for which is unknown, and may range from an isolated, slow-growing lesion, particularly in the medullary cavity of bone, to aggressive, widely disseminated disease with fatal outcome.

Separate diagnostic terms were originally suggested for the different forms of the disease. The defense for the "unitarian" concept derives from an inductive study of the histology of the various lesions, from the realization that many patients who eventually have generalized disease initially had only a localized lesion, and that an occasional patient will demonstrate a complete spectrum of clinical involvement.

Failure to identify the cause of the granulomatous process, or the true biologic setting for its development, has allowed the unsatisfactory nomenclature to persist. For the moment, therefore, it is reasonable to use the traditional terms, readily acknowledging their arbitrary nature. Hence "eosinophilic granuloma of bone" is applied to patients with bone lesions only; "Hand-Schüller-Christian syndrome" or "Schüller-Christian syndrome" to those with chronic, slowly advancing involvement resulting chiefly in symptoms from bone; and "Letterer-Siwe syndrome" to patients with a pattern of deeper, more rapid, visceral spread, often involving bones as well.

Etiology. Consideration of the cause of the histiocytosis syndromes must begin by acknowledging what the disease process *is not*. It is not hereditary or familial. It is not contagious and not transplantable to animals, and no microorganisms have been recovered from mature lesions by standard bacteriologic, fungal or viral isolation techniques. The process is not a true neoplasm, as shown by its potentiality for spontaneous resolution and its heterogeneous cellularity. Present knowledge allows one only to postulate that the granuloma lies in a borderland zone. It represents a response, perhaps because of a special reactivity in the susceptible patient, to a stimulus assumed to be exogenous, stopping short of the development of full malignancy. The role of the host in determining the final picture is suggested by the influence of age (younger patients tend to have more disseminated lesions), by the wide variation in the extent of involvement, and by the consistent predominance of males in each clinical group. In a few infants, skin lesions have been present even at birth.

Pathology. The microscopic picture of the lesions, whether in solitary foci or in disseminated disease, is that of a nodular or spreading infiltration, invariably containing numerous large histiocytes. Accompanying these characteristic cells may be variable numbers of other reactive elements, such as eosinophils, neutrophils and, less characteristically, lymphocytes and plasma cells. There is a tendency for the more rapidly developing and disseminated lesions to be more heavily histiocytic, whereas the isolated lesion in bone is notable for its high eosinophil population. An accurate prognosis cannot be made from the histology alone. The histiocyte may show giant cell formation, and may develop vacuolated cytoplasm. One can occasionally find masses of histiocytes which have become markedly lipidized, for obscure reasons, with greatly increased cholesterol content (especially in bone, dura, thymus and skin), but this does not imply any true relation to the constitutional lipidoses. In involuting phases the lesions are gradually replaced by fibrosis. Proliferative, destructive, xanthomatous and sclerosing features may coexist in the same lesion. In the severely affected child, tissues in all regions of the body may become involved, but marrow, skin, lymph nodes, lung, liver and meninges are the common sites. The pathologic diagnosis of these disorders is in part one of exclusion, and it is necessary to correlate the tissue findings with the clinical data before accepting the "idiopathic" nature of the granuloma being studied.

Clinical Manifestations. The assignment of a patient to a particular category among the histiocytosis syndromes is somewhat arbitrary. It is useful to note, however, that in the majority of affected children there is a natural progression for some months, followed by stabilization of their disease at a certain level. Most of the clinical disorders can be assigned to one of 5 general categories.

1. About half of the patients have *lesions only in bone*. From one to a dozen or so lytic defects may be present; the skull, legs, spine and pelvis are the areas most commonly involved. In this group the first symptoms typically occur at the age of 4 to 7 years, and consist of bone pain, local swelling or irritability. The process usually subsides within 1 to 2 years from the time of onset. Such children will ordinarily be classified as having "eosinophilic granuloma of bone."

2. A second, smaller group, if followed through the full course of the disease, will have *osseous lesions and minor additional involvement*, including anemia, limited eruptions on the skin or mucous membranes, and, infrequently, an invasive process in the pituitary-hypothalamic area which produces diabetes insipidus. This pattern is most common in the child whose illness begins at 2 to 3 years of age. The use of the term "Hand-Schüller-Christian syndrome" is appropriate here.

3. A third, more extensive form, which is relatively common, has *osseous lesions and moderate visceral involvement*. These children, who frequently manifest their illness at 1 to 2 years of age, may have papular skin lesions, a seborrhea-like eruption on the scalp and in the ear canals, stomatitis, pulmonary infiltrations, mild general adenopathy, some hepatomegaly, and invasion around the orbits, middle ears and pituitary area. The process usually continues to be active for several years and then may subside spontaneously. Some patients in this group die from complicating infections or from late effects of the intracranial involvement. Almost all these children, when first seen, have extension of the disease beyond the osseous lesions. The problems in nomenclature are demonstrated by such patients, who would be listed as having "Hand-Schüller-Christian syndrome" by some authors. The term "Letterer-Siwe syndrome" is also acceptable here, owing to its implication of a deeper penetration of the pathologic process.

4. The most serious clinical problem occurs in the infant who rapidly exhibits *major visceral involvement*. This pattern, also a common one, characteristically appears during the first year of life. Within a few months there may be significant hepatomegaly and splenomegaly, widespread pulmonary infiltration, adenopathy, marrow failure, fever and debilitating infection. Roentgenograms of the chest may reveal a granular appearance in the pulmonary parenchyma, or an extensive "miliary" type of infiltration. There is a variety of skin lesions, including a diffuse papular eruption of vesicular nature in the younger patient, a scaly and petechial dermatitis (especially on the forehead and trunk), and a moist, denuded involvement in intertriginous areas. An inflamed and pruritic eruption about the anal and vaginal orifices is common. In the mouth one may find gingival hypertrophy, inflammation, necrosis and retraction, with resultant loss of teeth. In some patients the osseous lesions are demonstrable on the roentgenogram, although they are usually not the source of the first symptoms; in others, osseous lesions as such are not evident, but in biopsy or autopsy studies a diffuse involvement of the medullary cavity may be demonstrated. A fatal outcome is to be expected when this picture becomes advanced, deaths being attributed to marrow failure, asphyxia or septicemia. The term "Letterer-Siwe syndrome" has been used for these patients.

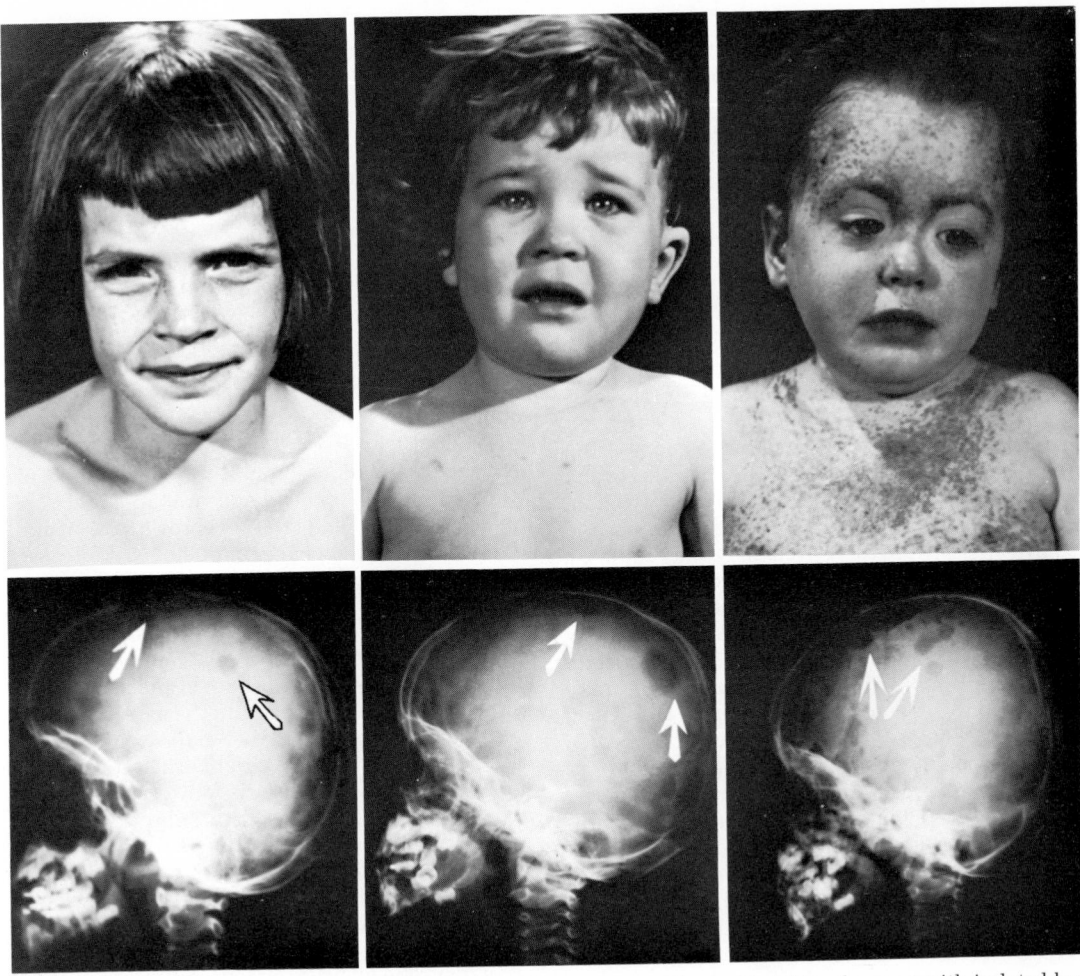

Figure 26-2. Common clinical patterns. *Girl on left* did not progress beyond brief involvement with isolated bone lesions which could be categorized as eosinophilic granuloma, had good recovery. *Girl in middle* had several dozen bone lesions, a papular skin eruption, scalp "seborrhea," stomatitis, vaginitis, pulmonary infiltration and diabetes insipidus. The diagnostic term "Hand-Schüller-Christian syndrome" is applicable here. Her disease responded well to chlorambucil therapy. *Girl on right* had extensive bone disease, plus a febrile course, anemia, severe skin eruption, generalized adenopathy, hepatosplenomegaly, pulmonary infiltration, and a fatal outcome in spite of ACTH therapy. This patient fits the category of Letterer-Siwe syndrome.

Early biopsies of bone lesions from all 3 patients showed a similar type of histiocytic granuloma.

5. Occasional patients have *atypical involvement*, with extreme progression in only one area, such as in the lungs, cervical lymph nodes or liver. Whenever the familiar osseous lesions are absent or not notable, a more thorough study of the histopathology is needed to rule out other diseases. For example, a number of syndromes of "familial reticuloendotheliosis" have been described which resemble the Letterer-Siwe syndrome superficially. In these syndromes there is characteristically significant involvement of the central nervous system, including pleocytosis of the spinal fluid, such hematologic abnormalities as leukopenia, lymphocytosis or eosinophilia, alteration of serum globulins, and a rapid, fatal course unaffected by corticosteroids or antitumor therapy.

Laboratory Data. There is no diagnostic serologic or immunologic test for these syndromes. Laboratory studies show only the nonspecific effects to be expected because of the organ or tissue involvement. Anemia is common, and leukocytosis may occur; the bone marrow is normal until the histiocytic proliferation has become widespread. Serum protein levels are usually normal, as are those of the serum lipids. The roentgenographic appearance of lesions in bones and lungs, although not completely specific, often provides the first clue to the nature of the disease, and allows the progress of the disease to be followed with some accuracy. Biopsy studies are mandatory.

Treatment. There is no specific treatment. A number of therapeutic measures suppress the granuloma, but appear to succeed only when favorable host factors are present simultaneously. Individual lesions of bone, troublesome skin eruptions and large lymph nodes are benefited by radiotherapy. This is especially useful for inducing rapid involution of bone lesions which threaten to produce pathologic fractures, as in the spine and femora. Relatively small doses (400 to 600 r at depth) usually suffice. If there is diabetes insipidus, early radiotherapy to the pituitary-hypothalamic area may eliminate interference with nerve tracts before irreversible nerve cell damage occurs. Pitressin replacement therapy is indicated as long as there is evidence of clinical deficit. Radiation therapy to visceral lesions, such as those in the lungs, liver and spleen, is not helpful. Antibacterial agents do not suppress the basic process.

At present, antitumor chemotherapy holds the greatest promise for eventual control of the granulomatous process; clinical investigations are under way in a number of medical centers. Corticosteroids provide useful support, but are not sufficient as the only medication. More definite suppressing action has been observed with the alkylating agents (nitrogen mustard, chlorambucil, cytoxan, and others). In the child with bone lesions and moderate visceral involvement they may induce a striking slowing of the clinical progression, and occasionally be considered lifesaving. Unfortunately, the patient who has early severe visceral spread of the disease seems to receive only temporary aid. Vinblastine and vincristine are additional medications of definite value. Folic acid antagonists have rarely produced favorable results. Although no single agent, or combination, has been discovered which consistently gives good results, the well planned use of presently available, partially successful drugs is to be encouraged. In addition, these patients receive great assistance from a program of general supportive care, which includes blood transfusions, antibiotic therapy, radiotherapy and orthopedic care as indicated.

ALLEN C. CROCKER

REFERENCES

Avery, M. E., McAfee, J. G., and Guild, H. G.: The Course and Prognosis of Reticuloendotheliosis (Eosinophilic Granuloma, Schüller-Christian Disease and Letterer-Siwe Disease); A Study of Forty Cases. *Am. J. Med.,* 22:636, 1957.

Beier, F. R., Thatcher, L. G., and Lahey, M. E.: Treatment of Reticuloendotheliosis with Vinblastine Sulfate: Preliminary Report. *J. Pediat.,* 63:1087, 1963.

Crocker, A. C.: The Reticuloendothelioses; in S. S. Gellis and B. M. Kagan (Eds.): *Current Pediatric Therapy 3.* Philadelphia, W. B. Saunders Company, 1968, p. 488.

Green, W. T., and Farber, S.: "Eosinophilic or Solitary Granuloma" of Bone. *J. Bone & Joint Surg.,* 24:499, 1942.

Mermann, A. C., and Dargeon, H. W.: The Management of Certain Nonlipid Reticulo-endothelioses. *Cancer,* 8:112, 1955.

Miller, D. R.: Familial Reticuloendotheliosis: Concurrence of Disease in Five Siblings. *Pediatrics,* 38:986, 1966.

Oberman, H. A.: A Clinicopathologic Study of 40 Cases and Review of the Literature on Eosinophilic Granuloma of Bone, Hand-Schüller-Christian Disease and Letterer-Siwe Disease. *Pediatrics,* 28:307, 1961.

PROGERIA
(PREMATURE SENILITY; HUTCHINSON-GILFORD SYNDROME)

Progeria is a rare type of dwarfism combined with premature senility. Children with progeria appear normal at birth, and their birth weight is usually within normal limits. The weight increases adequately during the first year of life, only to remain almost stationary during the remainder of the first decade; it may eventually reach that of a 2- or 3-year-old child during the second decade. The height increases slowly and may not exceed that of an average 4- or 5-year-old child during the first decade before growth stops completely.

The appearance is characteristic and has been described as that of premature old age and of a "plucked bird." The head appears large and is prematurely bald, and the eyebrows are usually absent. The eyes appear prominent, and the nose is beaked; the face is small in comparison with the skull, and the chin recedes. The chest is narrow, and the abdomen protrudes. The skin is atrophic, and brown pigmentations are common. The outstanding feature is the absence of subcutaneous fat in the face, on the chest and in the extremities. The veins are prominent; the nails show trophic changes, or they may be absent. The intelligence is not affected. Arteriosclerosis may occur as early as 5 years of age. Arthritis with enlargement of the joints and limitation of motion is common in older patients and has been reported in children as young as 6 years of age. Anginal attacks and hemiplegia have been reported in the first decade, and the most common cause of death is coronary occlusion. The average age at death is 16 years.

There are no characteristic changes in the blood. Aminoaciduria has been reported in one instance. Abnormally high levels of serum lipoprotein have also been reported. Roentgenograms show thinning and some decalcification of the long bones, coxa valga, a poorly developed mandible with crowding of the teeth and delay in primary dentition. The clavicles appear normal in infancy, but progressive osteolysis may result in their complete disappearance by 5 years of age.

The cause is obscure.

No treatment has proved effective.

ANGELO M. DIGEORGE

REFERENCES

Cooke, C. V.: The Rate of Growth in Progeria, with a Report of Two Cases. *J. Pediat.,* 42:26, 1953.

Thomson, J., and Forfar, J. O.: Progeria (Hutchinson-Gilford Syndrome). Report of a Case and Review of the Literature. *Arch. Dis. Childhood,* 25:224, 1950.

27. Radiation Injury

The possibility of untoward biologic effects of radiation is of special interest in relation to the child, for these effects may be most serious in growing tissues. By judicious limitation of roentgen procedures during childhood a margin of safety for unavoidable radiation exposure later in life can be preserved.

Ionizing radiation produces injury in the same manner regardless of the type of particle or ray emitted. The variation is quantitative rather than qualitative. Absorption of energy may cause molecules in the path of the radiations to become ionized. In attaining stability these molecules may form substances which alter, temporarily or perhaps permanently, biochemical processes within the cell or its environment. These effects upon cellular structures provide an explanation for the death of persons exposed to ionizing radiations, for the death of certain cancer cells treated with roentgen rays, for genetic mutations and for the production of cancer as a late effect of exposure to radiations.

Susceptibility of tissues to roentgen rays is, generally speaking, greater in the more rapidly mitosing and the more undifferentiated cells. Owing to an abundance of this type of tissue in the abdomen, a patient is more likely to have radiation sickness from roentgen therapy in this region than from comparable exposure elsewhere.

Dosage Factors. Radiation absorption increases with the volume of the child's body exposed, with prolongation of exposure or with an increase in amperage or voltage. Absorption decreases in relation to the effectiveness of filters used and with an increase in distance between the patient and the roentgen tube.

Adverse acute effects of roentgen rays are diminished when the total dose is administered in several exposures separated by sufficient time for recovery from the subclinical effects of each. Repeated exposures may produce pathologic effects not manifest until years later. Some of the chemical changes produced in cells by roentgen rays are irreversible, and may lie dormant until aging, infection, hormonal alterations or further exposure to toxic agents makes them manifest.

The young infant may be more susceptible to the effects of roentgen rays than is the adult. Moreover, even if there are no essential differences in susceptibility, his longer life span provides more time for such changes to develop.

The roentgen dosage from fluoroscopy generally exceeds that required for roentgenograms. A standard chest film, for example, involves about 0.05 roentgen, whereas chest fluoroscopy, using an old machine, might expose the child to 15 roentgens — a 300-fold difference. Contrary to general opinion, roentgen rays in low doses do not have a stimulative action on cells.

Early Effects of Irradiation. Exposure of the entire body to 100 roentgens usually produces illness in man. A dose of about 450 roentgens will cause death in 50 per cent of exposed persons. Higher doses can be tolerated if only a part of the body is exposed. Death results within hours to days when the entire body is exposed to the overwhelming dosage of an atomic bomb.

Symptoms of radiation sickness which vary with the exposure are malaise, fever, nausea, vomiting and diarrhea. Leukopenia develops rapidly, and in more severe instances thrombocytopenia may appear within a week. When the initial symptoms are not severe, they are followed by a temporary period of well-being. Epilation begins about 2 weeks after the exposure. The leukopenia increases susceptibility to infection, and the low platelet count predisposes to hemorrhage. When autopsy does not reveal the cause of death, one can only assume that the radiation injury was responsible for lethal "cytochemical changes." If the patient survives for 6 weeks, death is not likely from these effects of radiation.

Only a small percentage of deaths caused by an atomic explosion can be attributed to radiation effects alone; thermal and blast injuries account for most of them. Traumatic injuries do not heal effectively in persons with radiation sickness.

Therapy for radiation sickness resulting from exposure of the entire body is not very effective. Prophylactic administration of broad-spectrum antibiotics may diminish mortality. Transfusions of stored blood have not reduced the mortality in experimental animals or altered the bleeding diathesis. Transfusion of stored blood is therefore indicated only when the deficiency of red blood cells justifies it.

Late Effects of Irradiation. Within the decade following the detonations of the atomic bombs in Japan there was a significant rise in the incidence of leukemia in those who were within a radius of 1500 meters of the hypocenter (the spot on the ground immediately under the center of an air burst). The incidence of other hematologic abnormalities has not increased. Small lenticular opacities of the posterior capsule of the lens have developed in 85 per cent of those who epilated soon after the bomb explosion; the lesions are asympto-

1483

matic. Only 10 of the thousands of survivors have grade III or IV radiation-induced cataracts. Microcephaly with mental retardation has occurred in infants exposed in utero to atomic radiation. The incidence of these defects was dependent on dosage and gestational age, susceptibility being greatest among those whose mothers had last menstruated 7 to 15 weeks before the detonation of the bomb. There is no doubt that genetic damage occurred, but it could not be demonstrated in the 75,000 first-generation offspring examined.

Radiation-induced premature aging has been described in animals, characterized by early senescence and death in middle age from diseases that ordinarily beset the elderly members of the species. It has not been conclusively demonstrated in man.

That therapeutic doses of partial-body radiation may predispose to cancer is indicated by reports of a greater incidence of leukemia among adults treated for ankylosing spondylitis and of thyroid tumors among persons treated in early infancy for thymic enlargement. That repeated small doses of radiation to the entire body may predispose to leukemia is indicated by the increased occurrence of this disease among radiologists in the past.

Effects of exposure of parts of the body include temporary sterility, dermatitis, bone and skin tumors and developmental defects in the teeth. There are several reports of arrest in bone growth in children who received cancericidal doses of roentgen rays.

Radioisotopes. Radioisotopes provide approaches to diagnosis, therapy and investigative studies. Hazards are comparable to those of roentgen rays, but the total amount of radiation is much less because of the small doses used. Biologic effects continue until the radioisotopes are excreted or until they disintegrate.

Preventive Measures. It is presently estimated that the allowable occupational radiation exposure (whole-body) for man is 0.1 rem per week. This dose is based on exposure of the gonads, because all doses received by them are additive and presumably detrimental. The National Academy of Sciences has recommended for the *population at large* that the average cumulative gonadal exposure not exceed 10 rems per individual from conception to the age of 30 years; for the *individual* the cumulative dose should not exceed 50 rems.

The potentials for delayed somatic illnesses produced by partial-body radiation are not known, but it is thought that radiation changes within somatic cells are *incompletely* additive throughout life.

The child of today is likely to have repeated exposures to ionizing radiations, and there is a possibility that his tolerance may be dissipated. The pediatrician should limit as much as possible the exposure of his patients (and himself) to the emanations of roentgen-ray machines and radio-

isotopes, but should not refrain from using them for essential diagnostic and therapeutic procedures. When a roentgen examination is needed, a film study should be obtained initially whenever possible. Subsequent fluoroscopic examination can be made if it is still required.

The duration of fluoroscopy can be shortened if no conversation is conducted during the examination. The machine should be operated only while the physician can use his eyes most effectively, i.e. after he has adapted to the dark and while he is thinking only of the picture before him—*not while he is trying to interpret the findings.* The field under study must be kept as small as possible by reducing the shutter opening to a minimum. The machine should be operated with the most effective filter available, with the roentgen-ray tube at the greatest possible distance from the patient, and with the lowest amperage and kilovoltage permitting adequate examination. Electronic amplification of the fluoroscopic image, image intensification, permits fluoroscopy at very low levels of radiation. The method is particularly adaptable to the examination of children because the room need not be darkened. Thus the patient is more apt to be cooperative and the examination is shortened.

A pregnant woman should *not* enter a fluoroscopy or therapy room for fear of fetal injury.

Roentgen therapy should never be used except when the indications are unmistakable or the risk justified, as, for example, in the treatment of malignant tumors. Extreme care must be exercised to avoid unnecessary damage to osseous growth centers and tooth buds.

Roentgen ray machines should be checked at least once a year for leakage which might be a hazard to personnel. The physician should wear his lead apron and gloves whenever the machine is in operation and should not expose unshielded parts of his body to the radiation beam.

Robert W. Miller

REFERENCES

Bizzozero, O. J., Johnson, K. G., and Ciocco, A.: Radiation-Related Leukemia in Hiroshima and Nagasaki, 1946-1964. I. Distribution, Incidence and Appearance Time. *New England J. Med.*, 274:1095, 1966.

Hempelmann, L. H., Pifer, J. W., Burke, G. J., Terry, R., and Ames, W. R.: Neoplasms in Persons Treated with X-Rays in Infancy for Thymic Enlargement. A Report of the Third Follow-up Survey. *J. Nat. Cancer Inst.*, 38:317, 1967.

Miller, R. W.: Effects of Ionizing Radiation from the Atomic Bomb on Japanese Children. *Pediatrics*, 41:257, Suppl. 1968.

Neel, J. V.: *Changing Perspectives on the Genetic Effects of Radiation.* Springfield, Ill., Charles C Thomas, 1963.

Summary Reports of the Committees on the Biological Effects of Atomic Radiation. Washington, National Academy of Sciences, National Research Council, 1956.

Sutow, W. W., and Conard, R. A.: Effects of Ionizing Radiation in Children. *J. Pediat.*, 67:658, 1965.

Yamazaki, J. N.: A Review of the Literature on the Radiation Dosage Required to Cause Manifest Central Nervous System Disturbances from in Utero and Postnatal Exposure. *Pediatrics*, 37:877, Suppl. 1966.

28. Poisoning from Food, Metals, Chemicals and Drugs

FOOD POISONING

So-called food poisoning may be produced by (1) contamination of food by chemical poisons, (2) contamination by bacteria, and (3) chemical or toxic substances natural to certain plants or animals.

Contamination of food may occur at the source from insecticides, such as lead arsenate, or from preservatives or fungicides, such as formaldehyde or copper sulfate. Lead arsenate may be on fruits and vegetables in sufficient quantity to produce symptoms of acute or chronic poisoning. Foods may become contaminated after packaging. The container or its lining may dissolve in the food or enter into a chemical reaction with it. At times foods have been placed in containers previously used for mixing arsenic sprays or lead paints. Insect powders have been added to foods by mistake for baking powder or flour. Silverware cleaned with cyanide polish has produced poisoning. Ingestion of the flesh of cattle and fowl that have fed on fruits and vegetables heavily contaminated with arsenic may also cause poisoning.

Natural foodstuffs contain large numbers of toxic components, such as lathyrogens, pressor amines, azoglycosides and labile sulfur compounds. Of particular interest are the osteolathyrogens such as γ-glutamyl-β-aminopropionitrile, which is found in sweet pea (*Lathyrus odoratus*) seeds and induces skeletal deformities and aortic rupture, probably by interfering with normal maturation of collagen fibers. Neurolathyrism in man may be caused by β-N-oxalyl-L-α,β-diaminopropionic acid, a neurotoxin identified in *Lathyrus sativus* seeds. Histamine, tyramine, norepinephrine, serotonin and other pressure amines occur in foods such as bananas, pineapples, cheese and wine. Consumption of such foods by patients taking monoamino-oxidase-inhibiting drugs may produce serious hypertensive crises. Cycad nuts, widely used as human food in tropical and subtropical areas, contain methyl asoxymethanol, which is removed by bleaching in water.

Bacterial contamination of foods usually takes place between the time of preparation and the time of consumption. A large variety of organisms may produce poisoning. Two general types of bacterial toxins are known: the exotoxins freed into the external medium, which cause disease without association of living bacteria at the time of ingestion; and the endotoxins, which are formed within the bacterial cell after invasion of the host.

BOTULISM

Botulism is an often fatal intoxication due to the ingestion of food containing *Clostridium botulinum*, an anaerobic spore-former. The source of the infection is chiefly home-canned foods, especially underprocessed, nonacid meat, fish and vegetables. Six distinct serotypes A to F are known. A, B and E are of most concern to man; C and D produce disease in birds and certain animals; D may infect domestic cattle. E is found more commonly in foods of marine origin, particularly in the Baltic Sea and the Great Lakes of North America. The spores show varied heat resistance. The toxins are not heat-stable and can be completely destroyed by thorough cooking (80° C. for 10 minutes).

Symptoms. Some patients may have an acute digestive disturbance with nausea, vomiting and sometimes diarrhea, abdominal pain and distention, and difficulty in urinating. Central nervous system symptoms develop in 12 to 48 hours and are due to the curare-like action of the toxin on the motor end-plate. Decreased synthesis of acetylcholine, both in vivo and in vitro, has been observed with small amounts of A or B toxin. Acetylcholine and nicotine may still cause muscle contraction in botulinum poisoning, but fail to do so in curare poisoning. There may be a somewhat characteristic triad consisting in the absence of pupillary reflex, a peculiar dry, rough surface of the tongue, and progressive respiratory paralysis. Anorexia, weakness, dizziness, diplopia, ptosis of the eyelids, strabismus, and difficulty in breathing, swallowing and talking are common. Death may occur in 1 to 8 days. Diagnosis may be confirmed by serologic demonstration of toxin in the blood.

Treatment. In addition to lavage and catharsis, specific antitoxin, up to 50 ml., should be given intravenously as early as possible after testing for sensitization. Parenteral fluid therapy should be continued during the acute phase.

STAPHYLOCOCCAL AND OTHER BACTERIAL POISONING

Some strains of staphylococci produce heat-stable enterotoxins in pastry and other starchy foods, whereas other strains may develop a soluble heat-labile enterotoxin in such foods as salads, chicken, ham and beef in hash, or in gelatin, whipped cream and custards, especially when prepared in large quantities some time before consumption. These foods are particularly susceptible to becoming infected unless caution is taken in their preparation and refrigeration.

Symptoms. The symptoms of staphylococcal poisoning appear suddenly within 1 to 6 hours after the ingestion of contaminated food and include severe nausea and vomiting with retching, abdominal pain, acute prostration and diarrhea. There may be blood and mucus in the stools. The temperature may or may not be elevated. There is frequently sweating, hypotension and shock. The course of the poisoning is usually limited to 12 to 24 hours. Staphylococcal poisoning should always be suspected when an entire family or a large group of people become ill about the same time.

C. botulinum and *Staphylococcus aureus* are the only food poisoning organisms for which causative exotoxins have been unequivocally demonstrated, but several other species have been implicated in illnesses in which leukocytosis and elevated temperature are usually absent, and hence the disease differs from the known enteric infections. The spores of *C. perfringens* are heat-resistant, and may produce symptoms of mild malaise, abdominal pain and diarrhea, often without vomiting, 8 to 24 hours after ingestion. Food poisoning due to *Bacillus cereus* and pathogenic halophiles is similar to *C. perfringens* poisoning, but the food is usually heavily infected and the organisms are found in large numbers. Large populations, particularly in Japan, have been infected with uncooked fish containing large quantities of gram-negative pleomorphic rods originally called *Pseudomonas enteriditis*. Food poisoning from the enterococci such as *Streptococcus fecalis* has not been clearly established.

Treatment. If the patient is seen within the first few hours, a saline cathartic may be given. Food should be withheld until the diarrhea is controlled. The important measures, however, are supportive ones. Fluids should be administered intravenously to combat dehydration and shock as well as any acidosis.

LEAD POISONING

Lead poisoning is relatively common in infants and children. The residual effects of the toxic action of lead on the central nervous system are at times permanent and may even be progressive for years.

Infants and children may ingest lead in paint and plaster, particularly in older homes and from repainted cribs, furniture and window sills. They may also get lead from fruit covered with insecticides, lead nipple shields, face powders, lead soldiers and toys, and water from lead pipes. Childhood art products such as colored crayons, water colors, chalk or modeling clay labeled AP, CP or CS 130-46 contain less than 0.05 per cent lead, arsenic or other toxic materials and are considered "nontoxic"; however, industrial crayons and oil paints may well contain toxic pigments and dyes. Lead may also be inhaled from fumes as from the burning of storage batteries.

The likelihood of permanent damage to the central nervous system increases with the duration of exposure to lead. Pica is a common habit in infants and children with lead intoxication, and the child who has been treated for lead poisoning often continues to ingest lead if the opportunity is available. The physician should be certain that all sources of lead are eliminated from the home or should recommend a different environment.

The incidence of lead poisoning appears to be increasing in certain metropolitan areas in the eastern United States. Failure to repaint woodwork and walls permits flaking of old lead-containing paint to which small children have easy access. Elevated concentration of lead in the blood has been observed in 10 per cent of children having pica without symptoms of poisoning. Pica is particularly frequent among lower socioeconomic groups, and is also a manifestation of iron deficiency anemia in some children.

Lead enters the body through the gastrointestinal tract, skin or lungs. Except in acute poisoning, symptoms develop insidiously and may at times be intermittent. A single ingestion may produce no symptoms, but the same quantity distributed over a long time may be toxic. The slow absorption and gradual accumulation of lead within the blood and soft tissues produce the clinical features of progressive poisoning. In the gastrointestinal tract soluble lead salts are formed which are absorbed. Lead salts contained in dust may be absorbed from the respiratory tract, or from the intestines as a result of swallowed saliva containing dust. A large part of the absorbed lead enters the portal circulation and is excreted by the liver. Lead that reaches the systemic circulation is deposited in bone and in soft tissues, particularly in the liver, kidney, pancreas and brain. In the brain there is intense edema, widespread vascular damage, destruction of brain cells, and disintegration of the neuroglia. In the peripheral nerves the axon may be destroyed. Lead is slowly transferred from soft tissues to bone, where it is deposited as insoluble tertiary lead phosphate along with calcium. Factors which facilitate deposition of calcium favor the deposition of lead; decalcification is associated with release of lead from bone. The lead content in the dentin of deciduous teeth is essentially the same as in bone. Dentin from normal children contains an average of 1.5 mg. of lead per 100 gm. of tissue, while 11.6 mg. per 100 gm. has been found in children surviving lead poisoning, and 15.9 mg. per 100 gm. has been observed in fatal cases.

Lead in the scalp hair may be 2 to 5 times greater than in bone, 10 to 15 times greater than in blood, and 100 to 500 times greater than the concentration in the urine in healthy persons. Analysis of the hair is of value in confirming the diagnosis and in screening children. In chronic lead poisoning in children there is a good correlation between radiologic findings and other symptomatology.

The occurrence of symptoms depends upon the amount of lead in soft tissues and in the blood. Radiologic evidence of lead deposition in bones may be seen at blood levels of 0.05 to 0.08 mg. per 100 ml. Coproporphyrinuria may be noted at 0.08 to 0.11 mg. per 100 ml. or above. The amount of lead in the urine roughly parallels the amount in the blood and is thus an indication of the rate of transport to or from the tissues.

ACUTE LEAD POISONING

Symptoms. Acute lead poisoning is rare and occurs after the accidental ingestion of lead salts (lead acetate, lead carbonate) or the inhalation of lead fumes. Nausea, vomiting and abdominal pain follow. There may be acute paresthesia, pain and muscular weakness and occasionally a hemolytic crisis with anemia and hemoglobinuria. Renal damage is common. Death from shock may result in 2 to 3 days. Symptoms of chronic lead poisoning may follow recovery from acute poisoning.

Treatment. Gastric lavage followed by catharsis with magnesium sulfate, general supportive measures and treatment for shock are indicated. Absorbed lead should be mobilized into the bone as outlined under Chronic Lead Poisoning. Recovery is slow.

CHRONIC LEAD POISONING

Symptoms. The symptoms of chronic lead poisoning depend upon the rate and degree of transport of lead from intestine or bone to the soft tissues or blood. Symptoms may develop progressively from mild to the characteristically severe manifestations; or there may be, for months or even years, a sequence in which periods of mild symptoms alternate with symptom-free periods. In the infant or young child, owing to the extreme vulnerability of the central nervous system, a relatively short period of exposure may be followed by severe symptoms of encephalitis, even before anemia, colic, peripheral neuritis or other milder symptoms have developed. Or encephalitis may be precipitated in an otherwise quiescent case by release of lead from bones during an intercurrent acute infection or metabolic disturbance. Mild symptoms are weakness, irritability, loss of weight, vomiting, anemia, pallor out of proportion to the anemia, headache, abdominal pain or colic, loss of appetite (particularly for breakfast) and insomnia. Severe symptoms are muscular incoordination, peripheral motor paralysis of the most commonly used muscles (dorsiflexors of the feet or wrists), joint pains, hypertension, bradycardia or labile pulse rate, encephalopathy with separation of sutures, convulsions, and edema of the optic nerve. Encephalopathy is common in young children, whereas severe abdominal colic is more frequent in adults.

Diagnosis. The principal diagnostic features are basophilic stippling in the red blood cells, a lead line at the gums, roentgenographic evidence of increased densities at the ends of long bones (Fig. 28-1) and along margins of flat bones, an excessive concentration of lead in the urine or blood and excretion of coproporphyrin in the urine. Roentgenographic evidence is lacking in the presence of rickets. Evidence of ingestion of lead at the gums or in bones does not necessarily mean that clinical symptoms are due to lead toxicity; conversely, lead intoxication may be present in the absence of radiologic evidence in the bones.

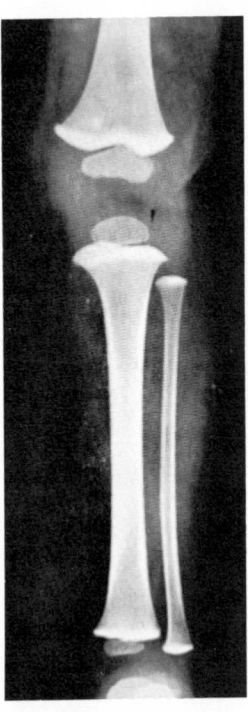

Figure 28-1. Lead poisoning. Long bones of a child 20 months of age, showing an increase in the thickness and density of the zones of provisional calcification. The child chewed paint from her crib and presented with anemia and irritability.

When there is encephalopathy, the cerebro-spinal fluid is under increased pressure and may contain a large amount of protein and a few lymphocytes, usually less than 100 per cu. mm.

Transient proteinuria and hematuria may be present. Glycosuria, fructosuria, hyperphosphaturia, hyperaminoaciduria and citraturia occur in the more severe cases. These abnormalities as well as histochemical evidence indicate the presence of proximal tubular damage in the kidney. These changes usually disappear within 2 months after treatment.

The range of values for excretion of lead in the urines of normal children and of those with symptoms of poisoning is great, and considerable overlapping exists. Normal children excrete an average of 15 micrograms per liter of urine (range 0 to 160), and children with manifestations of lead poisoning excrete an average of 146 micrograms per liter of urine (range 0 to 500). Confirmatory evidence in clinically suspect children may be obtained by measuring the amount of lead excreted after administration of a test dose of edathamil calcium disodium (75 mg. per kg. divided into 3 doses and given intramuscularly at 8-hour intervals). An excretion of lead of more than 500 micrograms per liter of urine after ingestion of the drug indicates excessive body content of lead-containing substances. The total urinary excretion of lead during a 24-hour period is more significant than the amount in a single specimen. The excretion of less than 50 micrograms per 24 hours can be considered normal. Excretion of more than 150 micrograms per day indicates unusual exposure to lead and may be associated with signs of toxicity. Circulatory failure and renal ischemia or damage in severe lead poisoning may inhibit urinary excretion of lead.

The concentration of lead in whole blood of children without a history of lead poisoning or pica has been found to range from 0.003 to 0.054 mg. per 100 ml. Symptoms may be present at blood concentrations of 0.1 mg. per 100 ml. Spectrographic examination of the blood may be of value.

A microcytic hypochromic anemia of moderate degree is a fairly constant feature of lead poisoning in children. Nutritional iron deficiency anemia may precede or be associated with the anemia of chronic lead poisoning, since the age incidence for both conditions is similar. Moderate anisocytosis and poikilocytosis are present. The reticulocyte count is above 2 per cent; the degree of reticulocytosis is not correlated with the extent of basophilic stippling. The plasma iron and percentage of saturation are low. Total iron-binding capacity may be low. Lead affects the surface of the red cell, increasing the mechanical fragility and reducing the half-life. The degree of hemolysis is slight; elevated blood bilirubin levels are seldom seen. The ribonucleoprotein of young erythrocytes appears to be injured, resulting in the precipitation of basophilic material with Wright's stain.

Thiol groups essential to oxidation of pyruvate may be inactivated by lead. It has been noted that an abnormal increase in blood pyruvate may follow administration of a glucose load.

Disturbance in the metabolism of porphyrin is a constant finding and may be demonstrated in acute poisoning in animals and is present in chronic poisoning in children. Lead causes complete inhibition of the synthesis of delta-aminolevulinic acid as well as of the synthesis of protoporphyrin from this acid. Coproporphyrin III, uroporphyrin I, porphobilinogen and delta-aminolevulinic acid are excreted in acutely poisoned rabbits. The urine and blood of chronically poisoned subjects contain increased amounts of porphobilinogen and delta-aminolevulinic acid. The free erythrocyte protoporphyrin may be elevated in certain cases. As evidence of a disturbance in porphyrin metabolism, red fluorescence may be seen in 75 to 100 per cent of red blood cells viewed in wet preparation under ultraviolet light. The porphyrinuria may be demonstrated in a simple qualitative test by shaking 10 ml. of urine, 2 drops each of glacial acetic acid and of 3 per cent hydrogen peroxide, and 2 ml. of ether in a 25-ml. glass-stoppered test tube and then viewing the degree of red fluorescence present in the ether phase under a Wood's lamp. Light blue to green fluorescence is normal, and slight red to deep red fluorescence indicates slight to decided increase in porphyrin concentration.*

Differential Diagnosis. Acute lead poisoning may simulate acute gastrointestinal disturbances with severe abdominal pain. Both the acute and chronic forms may simulate poliomyelitis, postdiphtheritic paralysis, localized neuritis or polyneuritis and rheumatic fever. In infants especially, lead encephalitis must be differentiated from other forms of encephalitis, brain tumor, brain abscess and meningitis, particularly tuberculous meningitis. The lead lines in the bones may be similar to those produced by bismuth and other heavy metals. When there is glycosuria associated

---

*The qualitative test described by Benson and Chisolm is more accurate than the one described above. It removes the interference of other fluorescent pigments and identifies patients with potentially dangerous blood lead concentrations (0.10 mg. per 100 gm. of blood or over). Five milliliters of urine, acidified to pH 4 (p-Hydrion test paper) with 2 or 3 drops of glacial acetic acid, are extracted carefully with 5 ml. of ether, avoiding emulsion formation. The ether extract is then removed, and 5 ml. of 1.5 normal hydrochloric acid are added to it and carefully shaken under pressure obtained by occluding the top of the tube with the thumb. The degree and type of fluorescence are observed in the lower hydrochloric acid layer, using a Wood's lamp (ultraviolet) held at a 45-degree angle. Comparison with known coproporphyrin standards may be made. A blue-violet color (less than 0.1 gamma per ml. of urine) is found when blood lead concentrations are within normal range (less than 0.06 mg. per 100 gm.). Faint blue-orange (1+), blue-orange (2+), orange-red (3+) and deep orange-red (4+) indicate 0.1, 0.2, 0.5, and above 0.5 gamma per ml., respectively, of coproporphyrin in the urine. Certain urine samples contain significant amounts of coproporphyrin in a nonfluorescent state, and the fluorescence observed in the hydrochloric acid layer can be intensified by adding exactly 0.25 ml. of 0.1 per cent iodine in 95 per cent alcohol weight by volume to the ether and hydrochloric acid mixture.

with encephalopathy, the possibility of diabetic acidosis must be eliminated.

Prognosis. The prognosis is generally poor. Approximately half of affected infants and small children have encephalitic manifestations, and among these the mortality rate is about 25 per cent. Of those who recover from the active encephalitic phase, at least one third have permanent neurologic or mental sequels. One long-term study has shown that of 20 children who had only mild evidences of lead poisoning during infancy, 19 were mentally retarded or manifested some specific defect in mental development 3 to 9 years later. Vascular nephrosclerosis as a residual of lead poisoning has been described.

Treatment. The primary aim of therapy is reduction of the concentration of lead in the blood and tissues by (1) prevention of continued absorption of lead from the intestines or other sources; (2) an increase in the excretion of lead, primarily through the urine. A secondary consideration, particularly important in the presence of encephalopathy, is the promotion of deposition of lead in the bones. Supportive treatment is of the utmost importance.

Prevention of absorption. All sources of lead must be removed from the environment. If oral fluids can be tolerated, relatively large amounts of milk should be given to form insoluble, poorly absorbed lead salts in the intestines.

Increase in excretion. Salts of ethylenediamine tetra-acetic acid (EDTA) form a nonionized chelate with lead which is nontoxic and is excreted in the urine. Decrease in the concentration of lead in the blood occurs rapidly after its administration. EDTA is usually administered by intravenous infusion. A test dose of 0.2 gm. diluted with 200 ml. of 5 per cent glucose in distilled water is administered intravenously over a one-hour period. Observation for such untoward reactions as rash, vomiting, tetany, lethargy or shock should be continued for 4 hours after completion of the test dose. If none appears, then 1 gm. dissolved in 200 ml. of 5 per cent glucose in distilled water is given intravenously. The amount and rate of administration of this solution depend upon the total dose to be given. The maximum dose for children should not exceed 1. gm. per 15 kg. per day. This amount is usually administered daily by intravenous drip for 5 days. The presence of continued signs and symptoms of lead intoxication or a rise in the blood concentration of lead may necessitate a second course of therapy after an interval of at least 2 days. The administration of calcium EDTA orally may be effective, but its actions are delayed when given by this route. *The use of EDTA by any route is contraindicated when lead is present in the intestines,* since it facilitates absorption of lead, and encephalitic symptoms may be precipitated. A roentgenogram of the abdomen to detect the presence of lead in the intestines should precede therapy with EDTA.

Penicillamine has also been used for deleading and may be given orally over a period of days in doses of 150 mg. twice a day for children up to 5 years of age, 300 mg. twice a day between 5 and 10 years of age, and 450 mg. twice a day over 10 years of age.

BAL (p. 1507) and EDTA may be used together. The following schedule is recommended: a first dose of BAL, 4 mg. per kg., is given intramuscularly; 4 hours later and every 4 hours thereafter for 5 days (in severe cases, 7 days) intramuscular injections of BAL, 4 mg. per kg., and calcium EDTA, 12.5 mg. per kg., are given at separate sites. An interval of 2 to 3 weeks should be allowed before repeating this schedule. Drug toxicity may be indicated by elevation in blood urea nitrogen, proteinuria, abnormalities in urinary sediment and hypercalcemia.

Increasing deposition of lead in the bones. Lead appears to be absorbed, transported, deposited and excreted similarly to calcium. A relatively high intake of calcium, phosphorus and vitamin D diminishes the solubility of lead in the blood and hastens its deposition in bone.

Disturbances of electrolyte equilibrium, often associated with acidosis, are common in lead poisoning. Correction of the disturbance is imperative, since the deposition of lead in the bones is inhibited in the presence of acidosis (see Parenteral Fluid Therapy, p. 217). Sodium citrate may be of value, not only in control of the acidosis, but because it forms with lead a soluble complex which is excreted in the urine; the administration of 1 to 2 gm. 3 times a day has been associated with decreases in the blood level of lead.

Infection also interferes with deposition of lead in the bones and should be controlled.

Treatment of lead colic. Lead colic may be controlled by the use of antispasmodics, such as atropine, but on occasion opiates may be necessary. Lead colic is also often benefited by administration of calcium salts; 10 ml. of a 10 per cent solution of calcium gluconate or 10 ml. of a 5 per cent solution of calcium chloride may be given slowly by the intravenous route.

Treatment of encephalopathy. The increased intracranial pressure and associated complications of encephalopathy require therapeutic measures in addition to those outlined above. The most careful observation and constant nursing care are required.

Convulsions are best controlled by phenobarbital administered intramuscularly (p. 1254). Care must be taken to avoid further depression of the damaged brain by excessive sedation.

The increased intracranial pressure due to cerebral edema may need repeated, careful lumbar punctures using a small-bore needle. Only small amounts of fluid should be removed at one time, owing to the extreme danger of brain-stem herniation; carefully performed, the procedure may be lifesaving. Surgical decompression by craniotomy may occasionally be necessary.

Oxygen should be administered for even mild evidences of respiratory depression.

Correction of fluid and electrolyte disturbances

is imperative, but must be carried out with caution. Excessive administration of water and electrolytes may increase the cerebral edema, as may dextrose in an electrolyte-free solution. Dextrose in hypotonic saline solution is the solution of choice; quantities of water and electrolytes are best gauged by the combination of clinical (hydration, adequate urinary output, blood pressure and evidences of increased intracranial pressure) and laboratory (carbon dioxide and pH, sodium, chloride and potassium) evaluation. Underhydration is safer than overhydration.

Urinary retention may require intermittent or continuous catheterization.

Central nervous system stimulants are rarely indicated. The severity of the involvement of the brain makes their use ineffective, and they may cause further damage.

Retreatment. The initial course of therapy may eradicate the clinical manifestations of poisoning even while lead remains in the bones. The residual lead is often liberated gradually and excreted without renewal of symptoms of toxicity, but this may not be the case, especially with intercurrent infection. The need for retreatment will be indicated by a significant rise in the concentration of lead in the blood or the return of manifestations of toxicity. Close observation for a long time is essential for prevention of additional damage to the central nervous system.

CHEMICAL AND DRUG POISONING

General Considerations. In the United States accidents and poisonings account for the largest number of deaths in the pediatric age group, more than the next 7 causes of fatalities combined.

Over 1400 fatal poisonings occur each year in persons of all ages; one third occur in children under the age of 15, and approximately four fifths of these are in children of 1 to 4 years. Nonfatal poisonings are estimated to be 100 to 150 times the number of reported fatalities. Poisoning is more frequent in boys than in girls under the age of 5 years. The frequency and causes of poisoning vary in different sections of the country and between rural and metropolitan populations. Fatal poisonings from petroleum products are most frequent in the Southern states and in the non-white population; lye poisoning also occurs mostly in the Southern states and in rural communities. The most frequent causes of poisoning in children under 5 years of age in frequency order are aspirin, soaps, detergents, cleansers, bleaches, vitamins, minerals—including iron—insecticides (excluding mothballs), plants, polishes and waxes, hormones, tranquilizers and other analgesics and antipyretics.

Since the establishment of the National Clearing House for Poison Control Centers, little change in the causes of poisoning from year to year has been noted. Seasonal variation in respect to aspirin, plants, petroleum products and pesticides remain about the same. There is a tendency for younger children to ingest common household products and older children to ingest medicines. The reduction in deaths under the age of 5 years since 1959 is in large part due to a decrease in number of deaths from aspirin and salicylate poisoning.

Prevention of Poisoning. The majority of cases of accidental poisoning in childhood are preventable. The responsibility for prevention lies not only with the parents, but also with the child's physician.

In the home, parents have a primary responsibility to keep medicines and poisons out of the reach of the naturally curious child. Highly poisonous substances should be locked in cabinets, and all medicines and poisonous chemicals should be properly discarded when they are no longer needed. Poisons should never be stored with foods. All medicines and chemicals should be kept in their original containers, which should be properly labeled. Two thirds of poisonings from household medications occur because the medicine was not returned to its usual storage place. The physician and the pharmacist, by meticulous attention to accurate prescription writing and compounding, may prevent many cases of poisoning. Prescriptions containing poisonous drugs should be written for small quantities sufficient only for the immediate medical need. Proprietary medicines should be properly labeled with instructions and precautions about administration to children. Particular attention to the dangers of medication in "candy" form is imperative, since it is responsible for as much as 87 per cent of the cases of aspirin poisoning. *Fatal* aspirin poisoning is, however, more often due to ingestion of tablets for adult use.

Parents fail to realize that a number of common household substances are poisonous; legislation requiring manufacturers to declare the presence and the nature of the hazardous ingredients on the labels of household products is essential. Caution must be taken in the storage of many household products such as bleaches, polishes and insecticides which, as a group, account for approximately half of the poisonings from household materials in both the United States and England. These substances are often stored in cabinets under sinks and are easily accessible to the young child. Poisonings are more frequent in families in which the mother is employed away from the home.

Safety instructions to parents should become a routine part of pediatric care when the infant is about 6 months of age (see p. 192).

Diagnosis of Poisoning. Acute poisoning may simulate many acute diseases such as peritonitis, intestinal obstruction, appendicitis, acute diarrheal disease, tetany, meningitis or encephalitis. When adequate evidence cannot be found for the symptoms of an acutely ill child, poisoning should be suspected, and gastric lavage should be considered. Symptoms occurring in several persons after ingestion of food from the same source are strongly suggestive of food poisoning.

The action of many poisons may be characteristic. Gastrointestinal disorders with vomiting, diarrhea and abdominal pain occur commonly in metallic, acid, alkali, veratrum and bacterial poisonings. Convulsions are characteristic of poisoning by central nervous system stimulants such as camphor, picrotoxin and strychnine and by poisons producing anoxia from methemoglobin formation. Central nervous system depressants, such as alcohol, atropine (initial effect is stimulation), chloral hydrate, barbiturates, opiates, chloroform and others causing anoxia may produce coma. Dilated pupils suggest poisoning from atropine, nicotine (late), cocaine and ephedrine. Pinpoint pupils may be due to opiates, physostigmine, muscarine and nicotine (initial). Caustic alkalis produce lesions of the mucous membranes of the mouth and skin. The odor of some poisons is characteristic; e.g. turpentine and eucalyptol may impart an odor of violets to the urine, arsenic or phosphorus the odor of garlic.

Mercury poisoning tends to cause pronounced proteinuria; poisoning by other metals, boric acid and phenol derivatives, a moderate proteinuria. Intense cyanosis and dyspnea suggest poisoning by carbon monoxide, cyanide, strychnine, aniline derivatives or botulism. Cherry-red mucous membranes are associated with carbon monoxide poisoning.

Methemoglobinemia. This is caused by many poisons and deserves special attention, since the resulting anoxia may lead to death or serious disturbance of vital functions. Nitrites, aniline derivatives, acetanilid, pyridium, dinitrophenol and potassium chlorate are the poisons which most commonly produce methemoglobinemia. (See also p. 1058.) Relatively small amounts of methemoglobin (15 per cent of the total hemoglobin) may produce recognizable cyanosis, which is usually more gray than blue and often not associated with dyspnea.

The symptoms of methemoglobinemia are those of anoxia and are related to the concentration of methemoglobin in the blood. A concentration of 15 per cent produces only cyanosis, particularly acrocyanosis; one of 20 per cent causes mild fatigue and cyanosis, and one of 30 to 40 per cent may produce weakness, tachycardia, nausea and generalized pains. Concentrations over 40 per cent cause weakness, tachycardia, confusion and coma, and death may occur.

Hypoglycemia. This may occur in a variety of chemical intoxications, and symptoms attributed to the drug action may in fact be due to severe hypoglycemia. Hypoglycemia has been noted in toxic hepatitis due to herbal poisoning, in acute alcohol intoxication, in salicylate intoxication and in organic phosphate poisoning.

Identification of the poisonous agent. Attempts should always be made to identify the poison. If the child is known to have ingested some household substance or drug, knowledge of its use may be of value in diagnosis. If the specific contents are not listed on the label, the container or bottle should be obtained and information about its contents sought from the prescribing druggist, poison control center or manufacturer. If this information is not available, the residual gastric contents should be analyzed. Emergency treatment should not be delayed until an analysis can be done, but the first emesis or initial lavage specimen and a specimen of urine should be saved for analysis. Analysis and the clinical picture may be complicated by the fact that many household products and prescriptions contain several potentially poisonous ingredients. Approximately 50 per cent of poisonings are due to such medications as salicylates (especially aspirin), laxatives, sedatives and cough preparations; cleaning, polishing and sanitizing agents such as bleaches, lyes, furniture polishes and cleaning fluids are responsible for at least 25 per cent, and petroleum products, including kerosene, produce 10 to 20 per cent.

General Treatment of Poisoning. The treatment of acute poisoning is always an emergency. Time cannot be taken initially to analyze the poison ingested, and most emergency treatment is, of necessity, symptomatic. Procedures generally to be followed and always to be considered are (1) removal of the poison, (2) administration of an antidote, and (3) general or specific supportive and symptomatic treatment. At times it is necessary to give a specific antidote before removal of the poison is attempted.

Removal of the poison. Poisons on the external surface of the body and in the nasal and oral cavities should be removed by copious irrigation with water. Acids should be neutralized with weak bases, and alkalis with weak acids. If toxic oils are present, organic solvents should be applied, and removed with a mild soap solution. Orally ingested poisons may be removed by inducing emesis or by gastric lavage. Certain drugs are absorbed in the intestines and resecreted back into the stomach for several days; for these intermittent gastric lavage with water may be helpful. Immediate induction of vomiting may be lifesaving and can be carried out by the parents before the physician's arrival. Emesis may be induced by administering 15 ml. of syrup of ipecac or strong salt solution or powdered mustard in lukewarm water followed by stimulation of the posterior pharynx with the finger. The child should be held with his head dependent to avoid aspiration. Ipecac syrup may be sold without prescription in 30-ml. amounts. A dose of 15 ml.

will induce vomiting in over 95 per cent of children if food is present in the stomach or if water has been given. At least 85 per cent of the gastric volume may be emptied in 10 to 30 minutes. A second dose of 15 ml. may be given if vomiting does not occur in 15 to 30 minutes. Other drug emetics are usually ineffective and may intensify the depressing action of some poisons. Emesis should never be induced in a comatose patient or after ingestion of caustic alkali or kerosene. Lavage is also not without danger. In corrosive poisoning the esophagus may be perforated; in strychnine ingestion the stimulation of a lavage tube may induce a fatal convulsion, and in kerosene poisoning, lavage, improperly done, may cause aspiration and pneumonia.

Gastric aspiration should be performed with caution. The child should be properly restrained, with his head slightly dependent and his face turned to one side. The gastric contents should be removed with a well lubricated, large-bore (28 French or larger) catheter, using an Ewald aspirating bulb. Small amounts of lavage solution (150 to 200 ml.) should be injected and aspirated as many times as necessary to remove all traces of the poison. Two to 4 liters of solution should be used. Water, weak salt and sodium bicarbonate solutions may be used until a more suitable solution is available.

Activated charcoal mixed with water will absorb large amounts of certain drugs such as strychnine, morphine and atropine, mercuric and arsenic compounds, pentobarbital and malathion. Tannic acid also precipitates alkaloid and metallic poisons, and strong tea may be used. Magnesium oxide suspensions are of value in mineral acid poisoning. Potassium permanganate 1:5000 solution will oxidize various organic poisons.

Administration of an antidote. Antidotes for poisons are of 2 types: (1) chemical agents which by direct combination render the poison innocuous or unabsorbable and (2) physiologic agents which counteract the effects of poisons after absorption. Specific chemical and physiologic antidotes are not available for all poisons.

Milk and egg white are more or less specific chemical antidotes for metallic poisons. Strong tea, tannic acid and dilute iodine solutions are effective against alkaloids.

Sodium formaldehyde sulfoxalate, if given immediately, is effective in the treatment of mercury poisoning. Nitrites and sodium thiosulfate have a specific action in cyanide poisoning. Methylene blue is indicated in methemoglobinemia, and ascorbic acid given intravenously may also be effective. Methylene blue is of questionable value in sulfhemoglobinemia and in large doses may produce further methemoglobin. Epinephrine, strychnine, picrotoxin and inhalations of oxygen and carbon dioxide may be indicated when central nervous system depression and anoxia are present. Stimulant and convulsive poisons demand sedation.

Gastric lavage may be followed by a large dose of a saline cathartic to hasten removal of poisons from the gastrointestinal tract. Catharsis is contraindicated in severe phosphorus poisoning when bloody diarrhea and desquamation of the intestinal mucosa are present. Magnesium sulfate may produce severe central nervous system depression because the rate of absorption of magnesium from the bowel may exceed the rate of excretion, particularly if there is oliguria or renal damage.

British anti-lewisite (BAL, 2,3-dimercaptopropanol) deserves special mention because of its remarkable effect on some metallic poisons. The toxic action of the metallic ions, particularly mercury and arsenic, is thought to be due to their chemical combination with important tissue sulfhydryl groups, with inactivation of essential enzyme systems. The administration of BAL can reverse the inhibiting action of antimony, bismuth, chromium, nickel, copper and zinc on the sulfhydryl enzymes. BAL is ineffective in poisoning caused by tellurium, thallium or vanadium. Under certain conditions it may augment the toxic effects of lead and may actually hasten death in poisoning due to cadmium and selenium.

Undesirable side effects are common with administration of BAL. These are lacrimation, salivation, nausea, vomiting, headache, pain in teeth, a burning sensation of the lips, mouth, throat and eyes, sweating, generalized muscular aching with tingling of the extremities, a sense of constriction in the chest, tachycardia, fever and agitation. Toxic symptoms begin within 10 to 15 minutes after injection and gradually subside within 1 to 2 hours. (For dosage schedule of BAL see Treatment of Arsenic and Mercury Poisoning, pp. 1495 and 1499.)

Certain metallic poisonings, particularly lead, mercury and iron, have responded to treatment with ethylenediamine tetra-acetic acid (EDTA), a synthetic polyamino acid. Various soluble salts of this compound, such as calcium disodium versenate, have the property of forming with divalent and trivalent metal ions virtually nonionized metal complexes (chelates). The chelate is less toxic than the ionized metal and is excreted in the urine. Increase in the excretion of lead and mercury results without increase in toxicity. Toxic reactions of chelating compounds have not been clearly defined.

An exchange transfusion may be of value in certain poisonings. Exchange transfusions should be considered for poisoning with methyl salicylate, boric acid, paranitraniline, chlorinated hydrocarbons, benzene, chlorate and bromate, copper sulfate, cyanide, dicoumarin, ferrous sulfate, naphthalene, phenol and thiocyanates. Hemodialysis is also of value when (1) the poison is distributed in an accessible body compartment and is diffusible through a cellophane membrane, and (2) the toxicity is related to the concentration of the poison in the blood. Hemodialysis may be of value in poisoning with barbiturates, salicylates, radioactive calcium, tritium, bromide, thiocyanate, ammonia and strontium. Little value would be expected when the poison is a protein-binding one.

Supportive therapy. Excessive manipulation of the child must be avoided at all times, and medications, particularly stimulants and sedatives, should be administered with caution. Overtreatment may cause more damage than the poison itself. General supportive therapy is frequently more effective than removal of the poison or administration of specific antidotes. The type of supportive therapy required is dependent upon the actions of the poison involved. All organ systems of the body may be affected by poisons, and toxicity of one system may seriously affect other vital functions; e.g. respiratory depression may be secondary to central nervous system intoxication.

The nervous system is exceptionally vulnerable to the toxic action of poisons, but the symptomatology is variable. Evidence of stimulation or depression is usually noted. Stimulation results in convulsions, restlessness, confusion and delirium. Sedation is frequently indicated, but must be administered with caution to avoid depression. Sedation also masks many signs and symptoms, making evaluation of the patient's condition difficult. Depression of the central nervous system is the most dangerous complication of poisoning. It is manifested by lethargy, stupor and coma. Central nervous system depression and coma may be primary, in which case the action of the poison is directly on the nervous system, or secondary as a result of shock, destruction of tissues, or of cardiac, hepatic or renal failure. Prompt, intensive therapy is mandatory and is directed toward stimulation of the central nervous system and support of other systems affected.

The respiratory system is affected by many poisons, and the patient must be observed for evidence of respiratory depression, obstruction, pulmonary edema and pneumonia. Tachypnea may result from central nervous system stimulation and produce respiratory alkalosis. Artificial respiration, administration of oxygen and maintenance of a patent airway may be imperative.

Involvement of the cardiovascular system is frequent. Peripheral circulatory collapse may occur and must be combated by intravenous administration of saline and glucose solution, plasma or blood and possibly sympathomimetic vasoconstricting agents. Cardiac failure may occur initially or later, and disturbances of the heart rate and rhythm require emergency treatment.

Some poisons cause intense gastrointestinal irritation with severe vomiting and diarrhea. Replacement of water and electrolyte loss by parenteral fluid therapy is imperative. Nausea, pain and abdominal distention may be severe. Poisons affect the kidney either by direct toxic action or by the production of shock with renal ischemia. The most important aspect of therapy is administration of appropriate amounts of fluids and electrolytes which will maintain homeostasis of the intracellular and extracellular fluid compartments. The extent of renal damage varies from mild involvement to acute tubular necrosis. If metabolic equilibrium is maintained by the judicious use of fluids containing electrolytes, glucose and protein, severe renal damage may be reversible. Hypertension from renal or peripheral vascular involvement is frequent. Urinary retention may also result from bladder atony or vesical neck spasm, and repeated catheterizations or the insertion of an indwelling catheter may be necessary.

The extent of liver involvement in poisoning varies from minimal damage to severe necrosis. Supportive therapy is primarily the provision of a diet adequate in protein and carbohydrate and low in fat, with vitamin supplementation. The extent of recovery is variable, but considerable regeneration of liver cells does occur. A serious manifestation of hepatic toxicity is depletion of prothrombin; vitamin K administration is indicated prophylactically.

Disturbance of fluid and electrolyte balance is associated with many poisonings. The types, amounts and methods of administration of fluids and electrolyte-containing solutions must be selected for the individual case. The following are general considerations:

1. Administration of total fluids in amounts adequate to meet the daily body requirements

2. Avoidance of water intoxication, hyperelectrolytemia or hypoelectrolytemia resulting from administration of inadequate or excessive amounts of water or electrolyte-containing solutions

3. Correction of any potassium or calcium imbalances

4. Maintenance of an adequate caloric and vitamin intake. For children oral feedings are preferable if they can be retained.

The control of body temperature is frequently impaired, and avoidance of hyperthermia or hypothermia is important. In barbital and opiate poisonings the depressant action of these drugs is intensified by hypothermia.

The child who is poisoned may be susceptible to infection, and use of antimicrobial agents should be considered, but not instituted routinely. Antibiotic therapy is indicated for the prevention of secondary bacterial infection in poisoning by kerosene and other hydrocarbons which produce chemical pneumonitis.

The child may often be in severe pain, which must be alleviated. In planning the management of the child who has been poisoned, the need for competent, continuous nursing care must never be overlooked.

CHEMICAL POISONING

In each case of poisoning efforts should be made to identify the toxic agent. The chemical constituents of many medicinal, household and chemical products are recorded on the labels, and this practice must become increasingly common. If the chemical composition is not recorded, it may be obtained from the manufacturer or text-books of toxicology. Information about new or unusual poisons and their pharmacologic action, as well as the composition of commercial products, is available through Poison Control Centers. Further information is available from the National Clearing House of Poison Information Centers, Department of Health, Education, and Welfare, Accident Prevention Division, Washington, D.C.

It is impossible to include in a pediatric text-book all known toxic chemical substances. In the following sections a number of potentially toxic chemical compounds are listed; included are general classes of chemicals (alphabetically arranged) with associated signs and symptoms of toxicity and recommended therapy. The List of Chemicals (p. 1502) includes individual chemi-cal compounds. Many chemicals are now assigned commercial or trade names, and, in general, these are used rather than the chemical nomen-clature. Synonyms are also listed.

1. **Abrin.** The toxic albumin found in jequirity beans *(Abrus precatorius).* Ricin is a related toxic albumin found in castor beans *(Ricinus communis).* The beautiful scarlet jequirity bean with a black "eye" at the hilus is used for necklaces, belts, bead bags, moccasins and slippers, rosaries, brooches, earrings and eyes for dolls and grotesque animal ornaments. One bean thoroughly chewed may cause fatal poisoning. Toxic material causes hemolysis of red blood cells at extreme dilutions. In acute poisoning, vomiting, diarrhea and circulatory collapse may occur. Symptoms may be delayed 1 to 3 days. Hemolysis, hemorrhages and edema of the gastrointestinal tract occur.

TREATMENT. Gastric lavage followed by catharsis, and treat-ment for shock are indicated and alkalinization of the urine if hemoglobinuria is present.

2. **Acids, Corrosives and Acid-Like Substances.** Cor-rosive acids produce irritation, blistering and destruction of mucous membranes within a few moments after ingestion. Le-sions may be brown or black except with nitric and picric acids, which produce yellow stains. Severe burning pain in the mouth, pharynx and abdomen followed by bloody vomiting and diarrhea may occur. Shock followed quickly by death occurs in approxi-mately half of the cases. Esophageal stricture occurs in the majority of patients who recover.

TREATMENT. Water, milk or beaten eggs should be given immediately and repeated to dilute any free acid. Gastric lavage is not without danger at any stage and probably should not be performed later than ½ hour after ingestion. Later, perforation of the esophagus may occur. For more detailed treatment see page 771.

3. **Alcohols and Glycols. *Methyl alcohol.*** The ingestion of 30 to 60 ml. may be fatal. The metabolic products, formic acid or formaldehyde, inhibit cellular metabolism, particularly retinal glycolysis and respiration. Toxic and degenerative changes occur in the liver, kidneys, heart and brain. Optic atrophy may follow recovery from acute poisoning. Ethyl alco-hol delays competitively the metabolism of methyl alcohol to formaldehyde, since it has a greater affinity for the involved enzyme systems. There may be a delay in onset of symptoms of several hours to as long as 2 days.

TREATMENT. Gastric lavage should be done promptly and repeated over a period of 24 to 48 hours, since methanol may continue to be resecreted into the stomach. Intravenous admini-stration of large amounts of alkali is indicated to combat severe acidosis due in part to organic acids, which may increase 20- to 40-fold in the urine. Potassium should be administered to cor-rect hypokalemia. Peritoneal dialysis can reduce the blood level of methanol to practically zero in 24 hours.

Ethyl alcohol. Signs and symptoms are primarily those of central nervous system depression. Fatalities occur at blood alcohol concentrations above 0.3 to 0.5 per cent.

	BLOOD CONCENTRATION
Mild intoxication	0.05–0.15%
Moderate intoxication	0.15–0.3 %
Severe intoxication	0.3 –0.5 %
Coma	Above 0.5 %
Fatal dose for an adult	300–400 ml.

TREATMENT is supportive.

Ethylene glycol, diethylene glycol. These substances are metabolized to oxalic acid (see Oxalates and Oxalic Acid). Cen-tral nervous system depression, shock and anuria may occur within a few hours, and respiratory failure and pulmonary edema occur within 24 hours.

TREATMENT. Lavage, catharsis and calcium gluconate.

4. **Aluminum and Zinc Salts.** Aluminum and zinc salts are used as astringents, deodorants and antiseptics. Symptoms include burning pain in the mouth and throat, vomiting, watery or bloody diarrhea, anuria, hepatic damage, collapse and con-vulsions.

TREATMENT. Immediate dilution with water or milk followed by repeated gastric lavage (see 2 and 49).

5. **Amphetamine, Privine, Ephedrine and Related Drugs.** Acute poisoning from ingestion, inhalation, injection or applica-tion to mucous membranes produces nausea, vomiting, chills, cyanosis, nervousness, irritability and fever. Blurred vision, mydriasis, altered ocular reflexes, spasms, convulsions, coma and respiratory failure may follow.

TREATMENT. Lavage and catharsis are indicated. Admini-stration of barbiturates may be followed by severe depression.

6. **Aniline, Dimethylaniline, Nitroaniline, Toluidine and Nitrobenzene, Acetophenetidin, Acetanilid.** These dyes are used in paints, paint removers, printing inks and cloth-marking inks and as solvents. Aniline poisoning of infants may occur from dye materials recently stamped on diapers or shirts. Para-nitraniline is found in some yellow and orange wax crayons. A roentgenogram of the abdomen may show the opaque pieces of crayon in the intestine. Intense methemoglobinemia is pro-duced by all these compounds. Symptoms include cyanosis, headache, shallow respiration, dizziness, hypotension, convul-sions and coma. Hemolytic anemia may occur later. Five to 20 gm. of acetanilid may be fatal; a single dose of 0.5 to 5.0 gm. pro-duces sweating, chills, gastric irritation, tinnitus, hypotension and circulatory collapse.

TREATMENT. Removal of poison from skin, repeated gastric lavage followed by catharsis. Oxygen, transfusion, exchange transfusion and methylene blue are of value.

7. **Antimony.** After ingestion, nausea, vomiting and severe diarrhea occur. Anemia, eosinophilia, hemoglobinuria and hematuria may be present.

TREATMENT. See 9.

8. *ANTU (Alphanaphthylthiourea).* ANTU produces pul-monary edema and pleural effusion in animals by its action on the pulmonary capillaries and by increasing lymph flow. It is thought to be relatively nonpoisonous to man; more than 1 pound of a 20 per cent mixture has been ingested without pro-ducing symptoms.

9. **Arsenic.** Arsenic poisoning may be acute, subacute or chronic. Arsenic compounds may be absorbed from the gastro-intestinal tract, lungs and skin. Arsenic inactivates sulfhydryl-containing enzymes and inhibits cellular respiration. It is stored in the tissues for a long time and is excreted slowly in the urine and feces. The more soluble salts may produce death quickly. In *acute poisoning,* symptoms usually occur within ½ to 1 hour after ingestion. If arsenic is ingested with a meal, there may be delay as long as 12 hours. Constriction of the thorax with dys-phagia, intense gastric pain and persistent and projectile vomit-ing of large amounts of "rice water" occur; a severe watery diarrhea, becoming bloody, is common. The loss of fluids leads to severe dehydration, oliguria, hematuria and albuminuria. Eventually shock develops with cardiovascular and respiratory failure, terminating in coma and convulsions.

Subacute or chronic poisoning. If the patient survives the acute phase, there may be residual symptoms such as multiple neuritis, myelitis and hypoplastic anemia. Alopecia, dermatitis, macular erythema and pigmentation of the skin may also occur. In chronic arsenic poisoning due to ingestion of small amounts of arsenic over a period of time the development of symptoms is insidious, with weakness, languor, anorexia, occasional nausea and vomiting, and constipation or diarrhea. Later, coryza, nasal and conjunctival congestion, edema of the lower eyelids, stomatitis, salivation and a garlic-like odor to the breath are present. The early symptoms may be followed by or associated with any of the residual signs of involvement of the nervous system, the liver or the hematopoietic and epithelial tissues that occur in patients surviving acute poisoning. Pigmentation, hyperkeratosis of the soles and palms and exfoliative dermatitis are sometimes striking.

TREATMENT. Even though symptoms of acute arsenic poisoning are present, intensive and repeated lavage is indicated. If the patient is seen early, repeated lavage with a freshly prepared mixture of ferric hydroxide and magnesium oxide is said to be of value. Intensive intravenous hydration therapy is necessary. Sedation and morphine for pain are advisable.

BAL should be given promptly. The recommended intramuscular dose is 2.5 to 5 mg. per kg.; the larger amount is approximately half of the toxic dose, so that undesirable side effects are frequent (see p. 1492 for toxic reactions). For mild arsenic reactions each subsequent injection should provide 2.5 mg. of BAL per kg. Four injections are given on the first day and 4 injections on the second day, two on the third day, and one injection on each of the following 10 days, or until recovery. For severe arsenic reactions each injection should provide 3 mg. per kg. On the first and second days 6 injections are given each day at intervals of 4 hours; on the third day 4 injections are given, and subsequently, until recovery, 2 injections are given daily. For reactions to gold, dosage schedules are essentially the same.

Treatment should also be directed toward support of the damaged nerve, liver and kidney tissues.

10. **Aspidium, Male Fern.** The oleoresin, used as a vermifuge, produces progressive vomiting, diarrhea, abdominal pain, headache, colored or blurred vision, tremors, collapse, convulsions and death in respiratory failure. If recovery occurs, jaundice and blindness may persist for weeks.

TREATMENT. Gastric lavage followed by catharsis and general supportive measures. Castor oil and other oily cathartics should be avoided.

11. **Asterol.** A commercial fungicidal agent used against tinea infections. It has been reported to produce generalized muscular contractions. The sensorium is clear. There may be rotatory nystagmus and mydriasis.

TREATMENT is supportive.

12. **Atropine.** Active alkaloid of a number of the Solanaceae, which include *Datura stramonium* (Jimson weed, thorn apple), *Hyoscyamus niger* (henbane), *Datura arborea* (angel's trumpet), *Solanum nigrum* (black or deadly nightshade), *Solanum pseudocapsicum* (Jerusalem cherry), *Solanum dulcamara* (true bittersweet) and *Dubosia* (cork woods in New South Wales and Queensland). Severe poisoning may occur in children from the therapeutic use of atropine, homatropine and scopolamine. Symptoms develop promptly after ingestion. Dryness and burning of the mouth, thirst and difficulty in swallowing and talking occur. The vision is blurred, and photophobia is prominent. The skin is dry, hot and flushed. A rash occurs over the face, neck and upper part of the trunk, and desquamation may follow. In infants and small children the temperature may rise as high as 107°F. The pupils are widely dilated; the pulse becomes weak and rapid, although no change may occur in infants; the blood pressure is elevated, and there may be palpitation, urinary urgency and difficult micturition. There may also be restlessness, excitability, confusion, weakness, muscular incoordination, giddiness and mild delirium, suggesting an acute psychosis. In infants the outstanding manifestations may be extreme abdominal distention, rapid respirations and distinct discomfort. Symptoms may persist for several hours or days, and the initial phase of excitement may be followed by depression with circulatory collapse, respiratory failure and death. Diagnosis is often difficult; the rash, fever, tachycardia and delirium may suggest the onset of scarlet fever. The subcutaneous injection of 3 to 10 mg. of acetylbetamethylcholine (Mecholyl) may be of diagnostic value. If salivation, sweating, lacrimation and intestinal hyperactivity do not occur after its injection, atropine poisoning may be present.

TREATMENT. Administration of water, milk or universal antidote should be followed by repeated gastric lavage and measures to reduce high fever. Short-acting barbiturates may control excitement and delirium.

13. **Barbiturates.** Five to 6 times the average hypnotic doses are toxic. The depressant action of barbiturates is due to an inhibition of the pyruvic-oxidase system. Symptoms vary with the rapidity of action and the duration of the effect of the various compounds, and include somnolence, stupor, contracted pupils, coma, fall in blood pressure, respiratory and circulatory depression and occasionally pulmonary edema. In some instances there is hyperexcitability and confusion.

TREATMENT. The intensity of therapy should be adjusted to the degree of depression. Careful evaluation of the reflex responses and the cardiocirculatory and respiratory states should be made before institution of therapy. Short-acting barbiturates may produce death within an hour. Long-acting barbiturates may have depressing effects for 4 or 5 days. Lavage, saline catharsis, establishment of an unimpeded airway, artificial respiration, and oxygen are indicated. Analeptics such as bemegride (Megimide), methylphenidate (Ritalin) and ethimivan (Emivan) are capable of causing arousal and return of consciousness in lightly narcotized patients, and in deeply narcotized patients who cannot be aroused they may produce a variable degree of elevation in reflex activity as well as help to maintain blood pressure. The repeated administration of picrotoxin intravenously in the comatose patient may avoid further respiratory failure and lessen the depth of coma, but does not produce arousal or return to consciousness. Intravenous glucose and saline solutions facilitate excretion of the drug and aid the liver in its detoxification. But, owing to the low ventilatory exchange, administration of large amounts of fluids too rapidly may lead to pulmonary edema. Maintenance of body temperature is of great importance.

14. **Barium Salts.** The carbonate, hydroxide and chloride salts are used as pesticides; the sulfide, in depilatories. The barium ion produces stimulation of all muscle cells. After ingestion, tightness of the muscles of the face and neck, vomiting and diarrhea, muscular tremors, weakness, difficulty in breathing, cardiac irregularity, convulsions and death, from cardiac or respiratory failure, occur.

TREATMENT. Ten milliliters of 10 per cent sodium sulfate should be injected slowly intravenously every 15 minutes until symptoms subside. Thirty grams of sodium sulfate in 250 ml. of water should be administered orally and repeated in 1 hour.

15. **Benzene Derivatives.** *Benzene.* Ingestion or inhalation of benzene fumes produces central nervous system depression. Principal clinical findings are coma and anemia. In mild poisoning, dizziness, weakness, euphoria, headache, nausea, vomiting, tightness in the chest and staggering occur. In severe poisoning visual blurring, tremors, shallow rapid respiration, paralysis, unconsciousness and convulsions ensue. Violent excitement or delirium may precede unconsciousness. Chronic poisoning from inhalation produces headache, anorexia, drowsiness, nervousness, pallor, anemia, petechiae and abnormal bleeding.

TREATMENT. Gastric lavage followed by catharsis. Great care should be taken to avoid aspiration. Epinephrine and ephedrine may induce ventricular fibrillation and should not be given.

Naphthalene. Common ingredient of moth repellents. Naphthalene produces hemolysis of red blood cells resulting in hemoglobinuria and hematuria. Liver necrosis may occur. Symptoms from acute poisoning following ingestion or inhalation are nausea, vomiting, diarrhea, oliguria, anemia, jaundice and pain on urination. Excitement, coma and convulsions may occur. Mental confusion and visual disturbances may occur after inhalation of fumes. Hemoglobinuria, albuminuria and casts may be present (p. 1055).

TREATMENT. Gastric lavage followed by catharsis. Blood transfusions for anemia and exchange transfusion may be of value.

Turpentine. One-half ounce may cause fatal poisoning. Turpentine produces severe abdominal burning, nausea and vomiting. Diarrhea, pain on urination, unconsciousness, shallow respiration, bronchopneumonia and convulsions occur. Anemia, hemoglobinuria, hematuria, albuminuria and glycosuria may be present.

TREATMENT. Lavage should be performed carefully to avoid aspiration. Mineral oil may allay gastric irritation. General supportive measures and exchange tranfusion are indicated.

16. Bismuth. Poisoning from injectable bismuth compounds is rare.

TREATMENT. See 9.

17. Boric Acid and Borate Salts. Boric acid may produce toxic symptoms when ingested or used as a wet dressing or as an ointment on large areas of injured skin, as in burns, diaper rashes or eczema. The mortality rate in infants is about 70 per cent. Excretion of boric acid from the body is slow, and cumulative action may occur. Symptoms include nausea, vomiting, abdominal pain and diarrhea. A maculapapular, urticarial or scarlatiniform rash occurs; the soles and palms are red. Desquamation follows in a few days. The mucous membranes are intensely congested. In infants signs of meningeal irritation may occur. Convulsions, delirium and coma follow. Albuminuria and azotemia may occur.

TREATMENT is symptomatic. Exchange transfusion or hemodialysis may be lifesaving.

18. Bromate. Potassium bromate is used as a neutralizer in hair permanents. Ingestion results in release of hydrogen bromate. Three ounces of the 3 per cent neutralizer solution may be fatal. Vomiting, diarrhea, abdominal pain, oliguria, lethargy, coma, convulsions and shock may occur.

TREATMENT. Gastric lavage followed by catharsis. Sodium thiosulfate solution is recommended: 100 to 500 ml. of a 1.0 per cent solution, intravenously. It acts to reduce the highly toxic bromate ion to bromide. Sodium thiosulfate, 1.0 per cent solution, may be used also for gavage, but it should not be left in the stomach, since highly toxic hydrogen sulfide may be formed with gastric acid.

19. Bromides. Bromides are depressant to the central nervous system. Delirium and hallucinations may occur.

TREATMENT. The chloride ion, particularly ammonium chloride, may expedite elimination of bromide; 5 to 8 gm. per day in divided doses is recommended for adults. Intake of fluids should be generous.

20. Cadmium. Cadmium may be dissolved from plated pitchers and ice trays by such acid-containing foods as citrus fruit juices. Symptoms are manifest within approximately ½ hour and include nausea, vomiting, cramps and occasionally diarrhea, accompanied by general weakness. Recovery is usually rapid, within less than 24 hours.

TREATMENT. General supportive and sedative therapy is indicated. Edathamil calcium disodium given orally for a week may reduce the elevated cadmium level in the blood in cases of chronic poisoning. BAL will increase the concentration of cadmium in the urine, producing destructive tubular changes, and should not be used.

21. Carbon Disulfide. Inhalation of fumes or ingestion of the liquid produces central nervous system depression, with coma and terminal convulsions. Recovery may be followed by permanent damage to the central nervous system or the peripheral nerves. Absence of corneal reflex is said to be highly characteristic of chronic poisoning. The blood may show moderate lymphocytosis, marked monocytosis, and occasionally eosinophilia.

TREATMENT is supportive.

22. Carbon Monoxide. The symptoms of carbon monoxide poisoning are predominantly those of anoxia of varying degrees, with severe headache, weakness, dizziness, dimness of vision, nausea, vomiting, collapse, coma, intermittent convulsions and failing respiration. The symptoms depend upon the concentration of carboxyhemoglobin in the blood. A cherry-red color is particularly noticeable on the lips and fingernails. Permanent residual damage to the central nervous system may occur if the anoxia is profound or prolonged.

Blood containing more than 40 per cent carboxyhemoglobin remains bright red after diluting 1 drop with 5 ml. of 1 per cent ammonium hydroxide and adding 10 mg. of sodium hydrosulfite. Normal blood becomes brown or brown-black. The addition of an equal volume of 10 per cent sodium hydroxide to normal blood, diluted 1:10 with water, will turn it dark green; whereas blood containing carbon monoxide retains a light-red color for several minutes. Two dark spectroscopic bands, between 500 and 600 millimicrons, are observed with 0.2 per cent dilution of normal blood as well as with carboxyhemoglobin; however, the addition of a few drops of ammonium sulfide will cause the 2 bands produced by normal oxyhemoglobin to fuse, while those produced by carboxyhemoglobin remain unchanged.

TREATMENT. Carbon monoxide can be removed almost completely from the blood in 30 minutes if oxygen in high concentration with not greater than 5 per cent carbon dioxide is administered. Controlled hypothermia has been effective in experimental animals; however, it is contraindicated if barbiturate poisoning is also present. Artificial respiration should be continued until normal breathing is resumed.

23. Chenopodium (Wormseed Oil). Ten to 12 drops of oil of chenopodium may produce toxic symptoms and death. The symptoms are dizziness, tinnitus, impaired vision, vomiting, profound depression and unconsciousness and, in more severe cases, diarrhea, muscular twitchings and convulsions. Glycosuria has been observed. If the patient survives the acute symptoms, deafness may be present for a few days to a month. Damage to the liver is manifested by jaundice; injury to the kidney by hematuria and albuminuria.

TREATMENT. Saline catharsis, stimulants, oxygen and copious amounts of oral and parenteral fluids are required.

24. Chlorobenzene Derivatives. A large number of chlorobenzene derivatives are found in household solvents, insecticides, fungicides, sprays, waxes, paint solvents and cleansers. The volatile halogenated hydrocarbons are very toxic. Chlorinated insecticides are less toxic and are usually only so by ingestion. They are fat-soluble and often are marketed in a hydrocarbon vehicle.

25. Chlorinated Insecticides. These consist of the *chlorobenzene derivatives:* DDT, TDE, DFDT, Methoxychlor, Dimite, DMC, Neotran, Ovotran, Dilan; *the chlorinated camphenes* such as toxaphene; and the *indan derivatives,* Chlordane, heptachlor, Aldrin, Dieldrin, Endrin and Diendrin. These are fat-soluble, highly stable insecticides used as dusts, wetting powders and solutions in organic solvents. Most toxic is Aldrin. Skin absorption of indan derivatives in organic solvents may be fatal within an hour. One to 3 gm. of these derivatives produces severe symptoms and may be fatal. Symptoms are stimulation of the central nervous system such as hyperexcitability, tremors, ataxia and convulsions beginning within 30 minutes to 6 hours. Central nervous system depression with respiratory failure ensues. Recovery is more likely if convulsions are delayed.

TREATMENT. Gastric lavage with large volumes of water followed by catharsis. The skin should be scrubbed with soap and water to remove contamination. Convulsions may be controlled with barbiturates, intramuscularly or intravenously. Stimulants should be avoided, and epinephrine is contraindicated.

26. Chromates. Chromate salts are highly irritating and destructive to tissues. After ingestion, dizziness, intense thirst, abdominal pain, vomiting, shock and oliguria or anuria occur. Chronic poisoning produces an eczematous dermatitis.

TREATMENT. Gastric lavage followed by catharsis and supportive fluid therapy.

27. Cleaning Solutions. Chemical constituents of various types: *automobile paint cleaners* (free alkali, alkali salts, detergents, soap); *brush cleaners* (aromatics, halogenated hydrocarbons, alcohols, paraffins); *carbon cleaners* (aromatics, halogenated hydrocarbons, alcohols, paraffins); *dry cleaners for clothes* (halogenated hydrocarbons, alcohols, paraffins); *glass and furniture cleaners* (ammonium hydroxide, methyl alcohol, sodium hydroxide, detergents, soap); *grease removers* (usually contain paraffins such as kerosene, hydrocarbons, gasoline or free alkali, alkali and salts, detergents, soap); *gun cleaners* (nitranilines); *metal cleaners* (nitric acid, sulfuric acid, cyanides); *silver polish* (silver nitrate, free alkali, alkali salts); *radiator (automobile) cleaning compounds* (free alkali, alkali salts, detergents, soap); *straw hat cleaners* (oxalic acid); *toilet and drain cleaners* (hydrochloric acid, sulfuric acid, sodium sulfate, sodium hydroxide, sodium carbonate); *typewriter cleaners* (aromatics, halogenated hydrocarbons, and paraffins).

28. Cocaine (Butacaine, Tetracaine, Metycaine, Nupercaine, etc.). Toxicity develops quickly after oral ingestion, hypodermic injection or local application of cocaine or its derivatives to mucous membranes. Symptoms are excitability, restlessness, confusion, delirium, hyperactive reflexes, rapid pulse, elevated blood pressure, widely dilated pupils and exophthalmos. Nausea and vomiting are due to central stimulation. Death is preceded by Cheyne-Stokes respiration and convulsions.

TREATMENT. See 73. The patient should be catheterized to prevent reabsorption of cocaine from the bladder.

29. Coniine. Toxic component of the parsley family. These include poison hemlock *(Conium maculatum)* and water hemlock *(Cicuta maculata* and other Cicuta species). Coniine produces peripheral muscular paralysis similar to that of curare. Increasing muscular weakness, paralysis and respiratory failure occur.

TREATMENT. Gastric lavage followed by catharsis, artificial respiration, and oxygen.

30. **Cosmetics.** *Deodorants* (aluminum salts); *depilatories* (barium or sodium sulfide); *freckle removers* (bichloride of mercury, bismuth, ammoniated mercury); *skin foods and creams* (mercury, salicylic acid); *hair sprays* (synthetic and natural resins). Inhalation produces diffuse pulmonary granulomatous lesions.

Some 70,000 cosmetic preparations are or have been marketed under individual names, and it is estimated that at least 1000 new cosmetics appear each month. Poison Control Centers may have details.

31. **Cough medicines** commonly contain antibiotics, antihistamines, chloroform, codeine, ephedrine sulfate and related compounds, opium derivatives and barbital derivatives.

32. **Cyanide.** Acute cyanide poisoning from ingestion of the salt or inhalation of hydrocyanic acid produces symptoms of giddiness, hyperpnea, headache, palpitation, cyanosis, unconsciousness and asphyxial convulsions resulting in death within a few seconds to minutes. Death may be delayed as long as 3 hours. The odor of oil of bitter almonds on the breath is diagnostic. Symptoms may be confused with those of nitrobenzene poisoning, which produces methemoglobinemia with cyanosis.

TREATMENT. Specific, prompt treatment is sometimes successful. Poisoning following inhalation of cyanide gas should be treated with amyl nitrite inhalation immediately and repeated every 5 minutes unless blood pressure falls. Clothing should be removed and the skin washed with soap and water. Artificial respiration and oxygen should be given. Ten milliliters of 3 per cent sodium nitrate solution should be administered intravenously at a rate of 2.5 to 5 ml. per minute; if the systolic blood pressure falls below 80 mm. Hg, it should be stopped. After administration of sodium nitrite, 50 ml. of a 25 per cent solution of sodium thiosulfate should be given intravenously at a rate of 2.5 ml. per minute. The sodium nitrite produces methemoglobin, which can combine with the cyanide ion to form cyanmethemoglobin. The sodium thiosulfate is injected slowly to convert the cyanide released by dissociation of cyanmethemoglobin to thiocyanate. One per cent solution of methylene blue intravenously may be of some value.

33. **Daphne (Daphnin).** In bright red berries and all parts of the plant. Ingestion of the plant produces abdominal pain, vomiting, bloody diarrhea, weakness, convulsions and renal damage.

34. **Darnel.** The seeds contain temuline. Flour may be contaminated with darnel, and bread made with such flour may produce vertigo, staggering, vomiting, visual disturbances, burning pain in the mouth, and prostration.

35. **Detergents.** *Cationic: Phemerol* (benzethonium chloride), *Zephiran* (benzalkonium chloride), *Diaparene* (benzethonium chloride) and *Ceepryn* chloride (cetyl pyridinium chloride) destroy bacteria and are used as skin cleansers, on surgical instruments, cooking equipment, sick room supplies and diapers. Ingestion of 1 to 3 gm. may be fatal. Symptoms are vomiting, collapse and coma with death within a few hours. *Ionic surfactants:* Sodium tripolyphosphate, fatty acid amides, tetrasodium pyrophosphate, sodium-o-phosphate, sodium silicate-sulfate or carbonate are alkaline and burn mucous membranes. Certain polyphosphates produce hypocalcemia.

TREATMENT. Gastric lavage should be done immediately and thoroughly, using ordinary soap solutions.

36. **Digitalis.** Poisoning occurs most commonly from medicinal preparations. Digitalis glucosides, however, are contained in a large number of plants. Symptoms of poisoning occur within $\frac{1}{2}$ to 6 hours after ingestion of large doses and are usually initiated by nausea and vomiting of reflex origin. Arrythmias and bradycardia may be present. Headache, drowsiness and coma have been described. Death occurs from ventricular fibrillation. Electrocardiographic changes are present in about 66 per cent of overt poisonings. Overdosage of digitalis during therapeutic administration of the drug produces first anorexia, followed soon by nausea and vomiting. These symptoms may become manifest over a period of several days; if large doses have been given, the vomiting may occur without preceding episodes of nausea. Excessive salivation and diarrhea may appear, often accompanied by abdominal discomfort and pain. Cardiac arrhythmias,

particularly extrasystoles of ventricular origin, and paroxysmal tachycardia may also occur. Bradycardia resulting from the direct action of digitalis on the sinoatrial pacemaker or the atrioventricular conduction system may follow. Death may occur from ventricular fibrillation. Headaches, fatigue, malaise, blurred vision, drowsiness and mental symptoms of confusion, disorientation and even convulsions may occur.

TREATMENT. When poisoning is due to accidental ingestion, prompt gastric lavage is indicated, but when it results from continued overdosage, lavage will not be helpful. Adequate fluids should be given to facilitate excretion, but diuretics may be dangerous, owing to excessive extraction of digitalis from the tissues. Absolute bed rest should be enforced until clinical and electrocardiographic evidence of toxicity to the heart has disappeared. Nothing more is indicated if the pulse is slow or even if there is a heart block, but when there is ventricular tachycardia, emergency treatment is required to avoid ventricular fibrillation.

The disturbance in rate and rhythm may be modified, at least transiently, by one or more of the following drugs: atropine, potassium salts, magnesium salts, procainamide, quinidine, and sodium salts of EDTA (ethylenediamine tetra-acetic acid). These are largely empiric attempts to control the mechanism of heart beat until the body can eliminate the glucoside. Potassium is probably most useful and may be given as potassium chloride, the dose to be monitored by blood levels and electrocardiograms.

Rarely, magnesium sulfate is useful; 5 to 10 ml. of a 10 per cent solution may be given intravenously for an immediate effect; it should be followed by oral administration of quinidine sulfate, 1 to 2 grains every 2 to 3 hours for 2 or 3 days. If the child is vomiting, intramuscular injection of quinidine is required.

37. **Dinitro-ortho-cresol.** Derivatives of phenol and cresol are used as insecticides and herbicides. They inhibit phosphate synthesis and result in increased cellular respiration. *Acute poisoning* from skin contamination, ingestion or inhalation produces fever, prostration, thirst, nausea and vomiting, excessive perspiration and difficulty in breathing. Later, anoxia, cyanosis, muscular tremors and coma occur. *Chronic poisoning* produces skin eruption, neuritis, hepatic and renal damage and injury to the bone marrow.

Urine which darkens rapidly on contact with air may contain dinitrophenol or 2-amino-4-nitrophenol.

TREATMENT. Thorough lavage with saturated bicarbonate solution should be done, followed by catharsis. Control of body temperature, oxygen and support of respiration are required. Intravenous glucose to support increased metabolic activity is advisable.

38. **Ergot.** Ergot is present in certain proprietary mixtures used as abortifacients. Rye flour may be contaminated with ergot fungus. Acute poisoning from ingestion, injection or application to mucous membranes produces vomiting, diarrhea, dizziness, unstable blood pressure, weak pulse, dyspnea, convulsions and loss of consciousness. The dose required to produce an abortion may cause death.

TREATMENT. Absorption may be delayed by giving water, milk or universal antidote; gastric lavage should follow. Saline catharsis is indicated. Sedation should be prescribed for convulsions.

39. **Esters, Aldehydes and Ethers.** *Dimethylsulfate* is caustic to mucous membranes of the eyes, nose, throat and lungs. Inhalation produces pulmonary edema. Symptoms of intense irritation and erythema of the eyes, severe lacrimation, and chemosis occur after inhalation, skin absorption or ingestion. Cough and edema of the tongue, lips, larynx and lungs follow. The corrosive action is similar to that of sulfuric acid; dimethylsulfate in the presence of water hydrolyzes to methyl alcohol and sulfuric acid.

TREATMENT. Copious washing of contaminated mucous membranes and skin surfaces.

Tri-ortho-cresyl-phosphate. The ortho form is toxic. The agent is used as a lubricant, fireproofer and plasticizer in coating plastics. Food may become contaminated. Symptoms are due to inhibition of cholinesterase, producing weakness and paralysis of distal muscles. Death from respiratory paralysis may occur. Symptoms may be delayed several weeks, and degenerative changes in the muscles and spinal cord may be observed at autopsy.

TREATMENT. Gastric lavage followed by saline cathartics and support of respiration are necessary.

Acetaldehyde, metaldehyde and paraldehyde. Paraldehyde

POISONS

and metaldehyde are thought to degrade to acetaldehyde in the body. Toxicity is related to limited oxidation of acetaldehyde. Acetaldehyde vapors cause severe irritation of mucous membranes, cough, pulmonary edema and narcosis. Ingestion causes nausea, vomiting, diarrhea, narcosis and respiratory failure. Paraldehyde produces deep and prolonged sleep, and metaldehyde causes nausea, severe vomiting, abdominal pain, muscular rigidity, convulsions, and death from respiratory failure.

TREATMENT. Copious washings of material from mucous membranes and gastric lavage, followed by saline catharsis. Artificial respiration is necessary.

40. **Favism.** Ingestion of *Vicia fava* (broad beans, horsebean) or inhalation of the dust of such beans may produce, particularly in children, symptoms of poisoning. The mechanism by which hemolysis is brought about is related to a defect in the glucose-6-phosphate dehydrogenase system of the erythrocytes (p. 1055).

TREATMENT. Severe hemolytic anemia may require transfusions.

41. **Fish Poisoning.** Several varieties of fish contain poisons within their bodies throughout the year. Others are poisonous only during the spawning season. Fish may also become contaminated with pathogenic or saprophytic organisms (Salmonella, typhoid, staphylococci). Fish poisoning (ichthyotoxism) may be due to eating of Tetraodontidae (puffers) or of the Diodontidae (porcupine fish). The Clupeidae (herring family), particularly *Clupea thrissa* and *venonosa,* and the Scarus (parrot fish) may also contain poisons. An alkaloid-like substance, fugin, present in puffers and certain other fish produces headaches, restlessness, salivation, vomiting, paralysis, cyanosis, and dilatation of the pupils. Death occurs from dyspnea and anoxia. Some varieties of sturgeon (Acipenseridae), pike (Esocidae) and barbel (species of Barbus) have poisons in their reproductive organs during their spawning season.

42. **Fluoride.** Fluoride salts and compounds are rapidly absorbed and slowly excreted. They are protoplasmic poisons inhibiting cellular enzyme action. Fluoride poisoning produces severe nausea and vomiting, diarrhea and collapse within a few hours. If patients are ill over a longer time, there are excessive salivation, dilated pupils, thready pulse, shallow unlabored respirations and weak heart tones. Cyanosis due to fluoromethemoglobinemia is not uncommon. Occasionally there is paralysis of the muscles of deglutition, carpopedal spasm and muscular spasm of the extremities.

TREATMENT. Immediate lavage with 1.0 per cent calcium chloride prevents absorption by forming insoluble calcium fluoride; if calcium chloride is not available, copious quantities of milk may be given after lavage with warm water. Intravenous calcium chloride or calcium gluconate may also be of value. Treatment is largely symptomatic and supportive. Exchange transfusion may be indicated.

43. **Fluoroacetate.** Fluoroacetate blocks aerobic metabolism at the citric acid level of the Krebs cycle. Very small doses may be fatal for children, and 300 mg. may be fatal for an adult. Symptoms are prompt, vomiting, apprehension, stupor and generalized convulsions occurring within 6 hours. Carpopedal spasm may be present. Respiratory and cardiac irregularity and failure may occur.

TREATMENT. Lavage and catharsis are indicated. Cardiac and central nervous system symptoms may be modified by administration of 0.1 to 0.5 ml. per kg. of acetate such as glycerol monoacetate injected intramuscularly at hourly intervals. An overdose of monoacetate may lead to nervous system depression and death. Calcium may be of value for tetanic manifestations. Digitalization for cardiac irregularities is of little value. Fluid therapy should be cautious because of cardiac and respiratory stress.

44. **Formaldehyde.** Formaldehyde is a general protoplasmic poison. It is a protein precipitant which preserves and hardens tissues. The gas is now infrequently used as a fumigant. Exposure to the gas produces intense conjunctivitis and irritation of the respiratory tract, often with resulting coryza, bronchitis and pneumonia. Ingestion of formaldehyde is followed by severe irritation of the mucosa of the mouth, throat and intestinal tract, intense abdominal pain, vomiting and diarrhea. Formaldehyde depresses the central nervous system, producing vertigo, depression and coma. Convulsions are rare. Oxidation of formaldehyde by the body produces formic acid and a resultant acidosis.

TREATMENT. Lavage should be carried out using 0.2 per cent

ammonia water (1 teaspoonful of strong ammonia water diluted with 1 pint of water), ammonium acetate (3 teaspoonfuls in 1 pint of water), egg whites or universal antidote. Ammonium salts convert formaldehyde to methenamine. The acidosis and impending shock must be treated, and respiratory stimulants may be indicated.

45. **Hydrocarbons (Kerosene, Solvent Distillate and Gasoline).** As the amount of these petroleum distillates ingested exceeds 10 ml., the toxicity increases tremendously. These agents produce over 200 deaths a year in children in the United States. Within 15 minutes to an hour after ingestion of most hydrocarbons, symptoms of nausea, vomiting, cough and central nervous system stimulation may occur. Kerosene produces a gastroenteritis; gasoline usually does not. The hydrocarbons are readily absorbed and are excreted by the lungs. Vertigo, fever, drowsiness and confusion result. Methemoglobin formation is common. Bronchitis or pneumonia from aspiration of hydrocarbons may develop within the first 24 hours or be delayed. Inhalation of gasoline produces intense burning sensation in the throat and lungs within a few minutes after exposure, and bronchopneumonia may develop rapidly.

TREATMENT. It is advisable not to induce vomiting in hydrocarbon poisoning, since the frequency of pulmonary complications is thought to be greater. Lavage carefully done is advisable, extreme caution being taken to avoid aspiration. The administration of mineral oil will reduce absorption of ingested kerosene. When only small amounts have been taken, saline cathartics are indicated, and lavage is usually not necessary. General supportive measures, oxygen, transfusion for methemoglobinemia, and carbon dioxide stimulation may prevent development of secondary bacterial pneumonia.

46. **Hydrocarbons (Halogenated).** *Carbon tetrachloride.* A nonflammable volatile solvent, used as a cleaner in floor waxes and in fire extinguishers. Ingestion of 3 to 5 ml. may be fatal. Exposure to an atmosphere containing 45 to 100 parts per million may produce symptoms. Symptoms occur quickly after inhalation or ingestion or from skin absorption. Signs of central nervous system depression, such as dizziness, confusion and unconsciousness, occur. Respiratory and cardiac irregularity and collapse occur. Recovery may be followed in a few days or up to 2 weeks by evidence of liver or kidney damage. Carbon tetrachloride probably does not act directly on the liver, but may release sympathetic neurohormones, which in turn cause constriction of liver sinusoids, producing anoxia of liver cells. Adrenergic blocking agents can prevent liver necrosis in poisoned animals.

TREATMENT. General supportive measures, artificial respiration and gastric lavage followed by catharsis. A high carbohydrate intake is advisable. A clinical trial with one of the adrenergic blocking agents may be desirable as soon as acute nervous system symptoms subside.

Methyl bromate, methyl chloride. These gases are used as refrigerants and fumigants. They may be present with carbon tetrachloride in fire extinguishers. Toxic tissue effects are similar to those of carbon tetrachloride except that bronchopneumonia and pulmonary edema are more common. The substances are metabolized to methyl alcohol and hydrobromic or hydrochloric acid in the body. Acute poisoning from inhalation, ingestion or skin absorption produces nausea, vomiting, vertigo, weakness, oliguria, drowsiness, hypotension, coma and convulsions. Pulmonary edema develops and progresses for several hours. In mild poisoning the symptoms may not develop for several hours. Vesiculation of the skin may be present where contact has occurred.

TREATMENT as for carbon tetrachloride with special measures for pulmonary edema.

Trichloroethane. This solvent may be present in rug, wall and clothing cleaners. Symptoms are severe depression of the central nervous system followed by evidence of myocardial, hepatic and renal injury. Recovery may be rapid after removal of the poison; late jaundice occurs rarely.

TREATMENT as for carbon tetrachloride.

Tetrachloroethane. Occasionally present in household cleaners, it is the most poisonous of the halogenated hydrocarbons. Death from acute poisoning may occur quickly and leave evidence of congestion of the lungs, kidneys, brain and gastrointestinal tract. Symptoms of acute poisoning are intense irritation of the eyes and nose, headache, nausea, cyanosis and central nervous system depression appearing over a period of 1 to

4 hours. After recovery, jaundice, anuria and uremia may be present.

TREATMENT as for carbon tetrachloride.

Ethylene chlorohydrin. Used as a cleaning solvent and also to speed the germination of seeds and potatoes. Ingestion results in pulmonary edema, vascular damage, direct toxic action on cardiac muscle and depression of the nervous system followed by damage to the liver and kidneys. Symptoms are those of respiratory and circulatory failure.

Chlorinated naphthalene and chlorinated diphenyl (Halowax, Arochlor). These substances are used as high-temperature dielectrics for electrical equipment. Chronic poisoning produces acneiform lesions, drowsiness, hepatic injury and coma.

TREATMENT as for carbon tetrachloride.

47. **Iodine.** The toxic effects of iodine are due largely to its corrosive action on the gastrointestinal tract. Iodine is highly reactive and combines readily with starch, proteins and fats in the digestive tract. Ingestion is followed by reflex vomiting, burning, abdominal pain and bloody diarrhea. Shock may result from fluid loss, and death may occur in 1 to 48 hours. The diagnosis is obvious from the brownish staining of the mucous membrane and the blue color of the vomitus or lavaged material.

TREATMENT. Lavage with soluble starch solutions or a combination of sodium thiosulfate (5 per cent) and albumen (egg white). Intravenous fluid is indicated to avert dehydration and shock.

48. **Iron (Ferrous Salts).** The oral ingestion of 2 to 4 gm. of soluble iron salts (ferrous sulfate, gluconate) may be fatal in 50 per cent of cases. The amount of iron exceeding the iron-binding capacity of the plasma and tissue proteins is very likely responsible for certain toxic manifestations. The serum iron concentration is helpful in diagnosis, but does not necessarily correlate with symptoms or prognosis.

The principal life-threatening pathophysiology consists of hemodynamic alterations producing shock and associated central nervous system depression. Early symptoms are due to gastrointestinal irritation and hemorrhagic necrosis of gastrointestinal mucosa, producing vomiting and shortly thereafter diarrhea, often bloody. Direct hepatic damage may occur. Pallor, drowsiness, lethargy and coma may develop as early as 15 to 30 minutes after ingestion or may be delayed for several hours. The hemodynamic alterations are due to the action of vasodepressor materials, most likely ferritin. Acidosis occurs, probably owing in part to accumulation of lactic and citric acids.

If coma and shock do not ensue, recovery is likely. Fatal cases are invariably among patients who are semicomatose or comatose and in shock. In animals respiratory failure due to metabolic acidosis appears to be the direct cause of death. Fibrous stricture of the pylorus may occur in patients who survive.

TREATMENT. Lavage with sodium bicarbonate may have 2 useful actions. Insoluble ferrous carbonate may be formed; but it may be more important that, at pH 6.0 or above, the chelating agent desferrioxamine has an equimolar binding capacity for iron.

Deferoxamine, a sideramine derived from Actinomycetes and composed of trihydroxamic acid, has proved to be of value in experimental animal toxicity and in acute poisoning in children. Theoretically, 100 mg. of deferoxamine combines with 9.3 mg. of trivalent iron and removes iron from transferrin, hemosiderin and ferritin. As deferoxamine complexes unabsorbed iron in the intestinal tract, the nontoxic complex may be readily absorbed, whereupon an increase in the serum iron concentration occurs. The complex is readily excreted in urine.

Because the pH of the gastric and duodenal secretions is acid, excess deferoxamine, 5 to 10 gm. in 200 ml. of water, should be given by gavage. The intravenous dose may vary between 500 and 1500 mg. (in 50 to 250 ml. of 5 per cent glucose); the amount required is related to the variable amount of free iron in the plasma and tissues. Administration should be slow, and the patient should be observed for restlessness, flushing, tachypnea, tachycardia, circumoral pallor and hypotension, since both deferoxamine and the iron-deferoxamine complex have a hypotensive action, probably mediated through release of histamine. Shock should be treated vigorously. The organic acidosis should be corrected, preferably with sodium bicarbonate rather than with sodium lactate.

The chelating agents, BAL (British anti-lewisite), EDTA (ethylenediamine tetra-acetic acid) and DTPA (diethylenetriaminepentacetic acid), can detoxify absorbed iron and remove it from the body by the renal route, but experience has shown that they have not significantly reduced mortality.

49. **Lye and Corrosive Alkalis.** Potassium hydroxide, sodium hydroxide, potassium carbonate, sodium carbonate, sodium phosphate and sodium silicate are corrosive alkalis. Ammonia and ammonium hydroxide may also produce corrosive tissue actions. These substances produce intense local irritation of the mouth, pharynx, esophagus and stomach. Perforation of the esophageal or gastric wall may occur within relatively few hours. Recovery is invariably associated with scarring of the esophagus and with stenosis unless proper precautions are taken. Ingestion of alkali produces severe pain, vomiting, diarrhea and collapse.

TREATMENT. Lavage with copious volumes of dilute vinegar, lemon juice or weak acids. Instillation of several ounces of olive oil or flour paste after lavage may be of value. Vomiting should not be induced in corrosive alkali poisoning. If an hour or more has elapsed since ingestion, lavage should be avoided, and only aspiration of the thick accumulated secretions from the pharynx should be performed. Small quantities of olive oil should be given at frequent intervals. A liquid diet and parenteral fluids are necessary, owing to the dysphagia. Stricture of the esophagus may at times be avoided by use of corticosteroids and early dilation (see p. 771).

50. **Meadow Saffron (Colchicum Autumnale).** Colchicine is present in the leaves and seeds, which may be eaten in salad. Symptoms occur 3 to 6 hours after ingestion, with abdominal discomfort and violent, uncontrollable vomiting and purging. Bloody diarrhea and collapse from exhaustion and dehydration follow.

TREATMENT. Lavage followed by saline catharsis. Dehydration and shock must be treated.

51. **Mercury.** Mercury, usually ingested by children in the form of mercury bichloride tablets, is a protein precipitant (see also Acrodynia, p. 1506). Mercury produces severe, painful lesions of an ashen-gray color on the mucous membranes of the mouth, throat, stomach and intestines. In the stomach it causes intense gastric pain and vomiting within a short time. The prognosis is improved if the interval between ingestion and vomiting is short and if there is extensive vomiting. If mercury reaches the small intestine, a severe, profuse, bloody diarrhea occurs. Mucosal shreds may be passed. Profound shock due to circulatory collapse soon follows. If the patient survives the acute phase, severe symptoms of systemic toxicity appear within a few hours and last for many days. Damage to the renal capillaries and tubules is responsible for the albuminuria, hematuria and excretion of casts. Diuresis sometimes occurs initially, owing to the faulty reabsorption of water by damaged renal tubules, but eventually there is oliguria and anuria. Widespread capillary hemorrhages and transudation of protein and fluid from the bloodstream result in circulatory failure and shock.

TREATMENT. Immediate and repeated lavage with raw egg white or milk provides protein for precipitation by the mercury. BAL is particularly effective. It should be given intramuscularly as promptly as possible, since experimentally it is less effective after extensive tissue damage has occurred. The initial dose should be 5 mg. per kg., followed in 1 to 2 hours by a dose of 2.5 mg. per kg. After 2 to 4 hours the latter dose should be repeated, and in severe cases a fourth one should be administered within the first 12 hours after the first injection. On the second day 2 injections may be given, each of 2.5 mg. per kg. On the third day only one dose of 2.5 mg. per kg. is necessary.

Sodium formaldehyde sulfoxalate is said to reduce soluble mercuric salts to the insoluble monovalent (mercurous) form; the stomach is lavaged with 250 ml. of a 5 per cent solution. From 100 to 250 ml., depending upon the age of the child, are then left in the stomach. This procedure is followed by intravenous administration of 50 to 200 ml. of a 10 per cent solution. Lavage with 10 ml. of 10 per cent sodium hypophosphite containing 2.5 ml. of hydrogen peroxide and diluted to 100 ml. is also of value. Sodium hyposulfite, chalk, freshly precipitated ferrous hydroxide, milk of magnesia or starch paste may also be used. After lavage, attention should be given to maintenance of a normal composition of the body fluids; one-half isotonic Ringer's or polyionic solutions should be given parenterally to maintain body fluids and to produce a copious diuresis in order to protect the kidneys from high concentrations of mercury. Such therapy should be continued unless edema and oliguria develop. Prognosis depends upon the amount of mercury taken, the interval

P O I S O N S

between ingestion and lavage, and the degree and duration of kidney damage. The immediate removal of ingested mercury is of utmost importance since absorption is rapid.

52. **Milk sickness**, or "trembles," occurs in animals from eating the rayless goldenrod or the white snakeroot, which contain toxic substances (tremetol). In man the ingestion of milk products or the flesh of poisoned animals produces nausea, vomiting and constipation. The tongue becomes dark red and tremulous; the cheeks are flushed and the lips red. Abdominal pain and muscular weakness may occur. Deaths have been reported.

53. **Monk's Hood Root (Wolfsbane) and Larkspur.** The fresh leaves and roots of these plants contain aconite. Absorption occurs readily and may result in instantaneous death, probably from paralysis of the heart. Symptoms are tingling in the mouth, stomach and skin (most important diagnostic feature), excessive salivation, nausea, vomiting and diarrhea. The pulse is slow and feeble, and there are dyspnea, weakness, impaired speech, unconsciousness and convulsions. Death usually follows in 2 to 6 hours.

TREATMENT. Prompt lavage with potassium permanganate, 1:1000, should be followed by saline catharsis; artificial respiration, oxygen and cardiac and respiratory stimulants should be used when indicated.

54. **Mountain Laurel (Andromedotoxin).** Ingestion of young shoots and leaves produces salivation, lacrimation and nasal discharge. Vomiting, convulsions, slowing of pulse, lowering of blood pressure, and paralysis may occur.

TREATMENT. See 77.

55. **Mushroom.** *Amanita muscaria (Mycetismus nervosus, fly amanita).* This plant contains muscarine and produces severe gastrointestinal symptoms soon after ingestion, followed shortly by profuse perspiration, salivation, miosis, delirium, hallucinations, convulsions and coma. The pharmacologic action of muscarine on smooth muscle and glands is similar to that of acetylcholine. Mild degrees of intoxication occur, and there may be individual susceptibility.

TREATMENT. Lavage followed by saline catharsis is imperative. Atropine given hypodermically is of value.

Amanita phalloides (Mycetismus choleriformis, death cup, destroying angel). This plant, which is extremely toxic, contains several toxins not completely identified; the mortality rate in human poisoning is 60 to 100 per cent. Symptoms may be delayed 6 to 15 hours after ingestion, when there are sudden, severe abdominal cramps followed by vomiting and diarrhea, with mucous and bloody stools. The intoxication is prolonged, and jaundice develops in 2 to 3 days, indicating severe degenerative changes in the liver. The kidney is involved, and direct toxic action on the heart may result in cardiac failure and death within 5 to 8 days.

TREATMENT. Immediate lavage, enemas and saline catharsis are indicated. Dehydration and shock must be treated. The degree of toxic tissue changes may be ameliorated by large amounts of glucose, plasma and blood intravenously.

56. **Nicotine.** The toxicity and rapidity of action of nicotine are comparable to those of cyanide. The local caustic action produces nausea, salivation, abdominal pain, vomiting and diarrhea. After absorption there are headache, dizziness, visual and hearing disturbances, mental confusion and intense weakness, and death may follow within a few minutes. Respiratory stimulation, elevated blood pressure and slow pulse are also early manifestations. Later there are pinpoint pupils and a curare-like action on the skeletal and respiratory muscles. Respiratory and circulatory failure is followed by convulsions and death.

TREATMENT. Lavage with tannic acid, strong coffee or tea for ingested poison. Nicotine on the skin should be thoroughly washed off. Owing to the rapid destruction of nicotine in the body, death can be averted if primary attention is directed toward prevention of respiratory failure. Artificial respiration and oxygen should be continued until normal breathing is resumed or the heart has stopped. Epinephrine, caffeine, and the like, are not ordinarily indicated unless respiratory failure develops.

57. **Nitrites.** Medications such as bismuth subnitrite, amyl nitrite, sodium nitrite or spirit of glyceryl trinitrate may be taken accidentally by children. Therapeutic use of bismuth subnitrite may result in formation of nitrites by bacterial decomposition in the intestines. Cyanosis in infants due to poisoning with water containing nitrates has been described. Water seeping from barnyards heavily laden with bacteria and dissolved nitrogenous materials may become increasingly purified by passage through the soil, but certain soil bacteria oxidize the

ammonia and other nitrogenous compounds to nitrates. The solution of nitrates, free of coli organisms, may enter subsurface channels leading directly into wells used for drinking purposes. Ingestion of such water in milk formulas may result in conversion of the nitrates to nitrites by gastrointestinal organisms. Flushing of the skin, fall in blood pressure, severe methemoglobinemia, cyanosis and dyspnea develop. Syncope and respiratory failure may occur.

TREATMENT. Lavage should be followed by saline catharsis, particularly in bismuth subnitrite poisoning. When syncope occurs, epinephrine and other vasopressor agents should be avoided. A deep Trendelenburg position of the body and passive movements of extremities may facilitate return of venous blood to the heart. Transfusions and oxygen may be indicated for the methemoglobinemia, and methylene blue is of value.

58. **Nutmeg.** One teaspoonful of powdered nutmeg may produce severe toxic symptoms. Narcosis with periods of delirium and excitability may occur within 1 to 6 hours.

59. **Oils.** Most of the nonvolatile hydrocarbon oils are nontoxic. Ingestion, however, may be associated with vomiting and aspiration into the lungs. Pulmonary complications are more intense with vegetable and animal oils.

TREATMENT. Emetics should not be given. Lavage should be done with care, avoiding emesis.

60. **Opiates.** Several natural alkaloids of opium, particularly morphine and codeine, and some synthetic narcotics cause toxic effects in infants and children. Poisoning occurs as a result of excessive therapeutic administration or from accidental ingestion. Manifestations of opiate poisoning are those of central nervous system depression. Somnolence, coma and respiratory depression, often severe, may be noted. Pinpoint pupils occur, but are not diagnostic of opiate poisoning.

TREATMENT. Prompt, vigorous treatment is mandatory and should be directed to the prevention of anoxia and further respiratory depression. Oxygen and artificial respiration may be indicated, and the airway must be kept patent.

Two specific opiate antagonists are available: N-allylnormorphine (Nalline) and L-3 hydroxy-N-allylmorphinan tartrate (Lorfan). Both drugs have specific antagonistic actions against all opiates, natural and synthetic. They are ineffective against other central nervous system depressants such as phenobarbital, and, in fact, will produce the toxic effects of opiates if used in situations other than opiate poisoning. The drugs should be administered intravenously as rapidly as possible. See page 272 and package inserts for dosages.

61. **Oxalates and Oxalic Acid.** Local irritation is produced by ingested oxalic acid. Both the acid and its salts are rapidly absorbed, and death occurs quickly. Absorbed oxalate combines with the ionized calcium of the blood, producing hypocalcemia leading to muscular twitchings, laryngospasm, tetany and convulsions. The heart stops beating in diastole. If recovery from the acute phase occurs, renal tubular necrosis may follow.

TREATMENT. Lavage with 0.1 per cent potassium permanganate should be followed by a 5 per cent calcium chloride, chalk or lime solution. Calcium gluconate or calcium chloride intravenously is of value if signs of tetany are present.

62. **Phenols (Carbolic Acid, Cresol, Creosote, Creolin, Lysol, Resorcinol and Pyrogallol).** Phenol may produce symptoms leading to death within a few minutes, dependent upon the surface from which the substance is absorbed. Death (lethal dose is 8 to 15 gm.) usually occurs within 24 hours from respiratory failure. Initial symptoms are severe, painful local corrosion of mucous membranes and severe vomiting. Widespread capillary damage, medullary depression and shock occur quickly. Fleeting excitement may occur, followed by unconsciousness. Other symptoms are low blood pressure, cold sweat, hypothermia, oliguria, albuminuria and hemoglobinuria.

TREATMENT. The drug must be removed promptly before absorption occurs. Lavage with olive oil or other vegetable oils provides a solvent for the phenol. Neither alcohol nor mineral oil should be used; alcohol facilitates absorption, and mineral oil is a poor solvent for phenol. After lavage several ounces of olive oil should be left in the stomach. Copious parenteral fluid administration should be instituted to protect the kidneys. The acidosis responds promptly to intravenous administration of sodium bicarbonate or sixth-normal sodium lactate. Artificial respiration should be performed when respiratory failure occurs.

63. **Phenolphthalein.** Phenolphthalein is present in many candy cathartics (Analax, Ex-lax, Phenolax and cathartic chewing gum). Children have been known to eat more than a box of

the tablets. Apparently, large amounts of phenolphthalein can be ingested without serious results. The range of toxic doses is not known. Severe toxic reactions may be manifest in hypersusceptible persons. A violent cathartic action results several hours later. A bright red skin eruption and swelling of the eyelids may occur. High fever, meningismus, hemiplegia, albuminuria, oliguria, and respiratory and cardiac failure have been attributed to phenolphthalein poisoning.

TREATMENT. General supportive treatment is indicated. If violent catharsis is present, and dehydration and acidosis ensue, parenteral fluid therapy should be administered. Diagnosis may be established easily by the development of a pink color in lavaged material, stool or urine on the addition of alkali.

64. **Phenothiazines (prochlorperazine [Compazine], promazine [Sparine], perphenazine [Trilafon] and others).** The major toxic symptoms are motor: dystonia (incoordinated spasmodic movements producing torticollis, retrocollis, opisthotonos, trismus and oculogyric crises); dyskinesia (rhythmic movements of jaws, tongue, swaying and rocking of the body); akathisia (inability to sit still); rigidity; and tremor. Large doses may produce seizures, and patients with brain damage are particularly susceptible. Permanent neurologic damage has been noted in patients with previous evidence of brain damage.

TREATMENT. Lavage. Diphenhydramine hydrochloride (Benadryl) may be effective in treatment of extrapyramidal symptoms.

65. **Phosphorus, Inorganic.** Red phosphorus is nonabsorbable and therefore nonpoisonous. Yellow phosphorus is highly poisonous, producing severe tissue destruction. Yellow or white phosphorus is used in rodent and insect poisons, in fireworks and in the manufacture of fertilizer. Zinc phosphide used in rat poisons releases phosphine on contact with water. Symptoms of acute poisoning occur within 1 to 2 hours. Nausea, vomiting, diarrhea, and a garlic odor of the breath and excreta may be noted. Coma may occur within 24 to 48 hours. If recovery from the acute phase occurs, symptoms may return in 2 days with nausea, vomiting, diarrhea, large tender liver, jaundice, shock, oliguria and multiple hemorrhages. Phosphorus causes second-to third-degree burns on contact with the skin.

TREATMENT. Acute poisoning should be treated by gastric lavage with large amounts of 0.2 per cent copper sulfate. Potassium permanganate, 1:1000, or 2 per cent hydrogen peroxide tends to convert elemental phosphorus to harmless oxidation products. Phosphorus is soluble in mineral oil; therefore the instillation of 100 to 200 cc. of mineral oil after lavage may facilitate its elimination. Supportive measures include treatment for dehydration, acidosis and shock, and subsequently a high carbohydrate diet and amino acids, orally or parenterally, to protect the liver from serious injury. When there has been liver damage, such treatment should be continued until there is evidence that function has returned.

66. **Phosphorus, Organic.** Phosphate ester insecticides should never be used in homes. All are anticholinesterase compounds. There are 3 main types of organic phosphate insecticides; the nitrophenyl thiophosphates, the alkyl pyrophosphates, and the phosphoramides. They vary in distribution in tissues and in duration of action. The phosphoramide compounds have no cerebral action, acting entirely by peripheral inhibition of cholinesterase. The alkyl pyrophosphates are rapidly hydrolyzed in the body to nontoxic metabolites. The thiophosphates are more stable and are detoxified slowly. Potentiation may occur between 2 organophosphates, ethyl-P-nitrophenyl benzenthionophosphonate (EPN) and malathion, belnav and malathion, or guthion and dipterex. Accidents are possible when small amounts of potentiating compounds are present in the daily diet. Moreover, certain drugs of the phenothiazine type potentiate the toxic effect of organophosphates. The importance of long-term consumption of pesticide-contaminated foods is not known.

Most of these compounds are several times more toxic than nicotine. One drop of parathion in the eye may be fatal. Malathion is probably the least toxic. One gram, however, may be fatal. Symptoms are prompt within 30 minutes, and may continue for 24 to 48 hours. They include increased secretions (such as sweat, saliva, tears, and bronchial fluids), nausea, vomiting, diarrhea, miosis, blurred vision, bronchiolar spasms and pulmonary edema. Ataxia, vertigo, tremors, muscular weakness, fibrillation, fasciculation, finger and mouth twitching, muscular paralysis, cyanosis, dyspnea, chest constriction, stupor, coma and convulsions may also occur.

TREATMENT. Artificial respiration to maintain ventilatory exchange is indicated. Wash all insecticide off the skin and mucous membranes. Atropine is helpful, but its action is limited to neutralization of the excess acetylcholine accumulated as a result of decreased cholinesterase activity. In severe poisoning, atropine should be given intravenously and should be repeated at 5 to 10-minute intervals until signs of atropinization occur. The specific cholinesterase reactivator, 2-pyridine aldoxime methiodide (2-PAM), should be given. Doses of 1 gm. intravenously have been found to be effective in adults. 2-Pyridine aldoxime ethanesulfonate (P2S) has been shown to be equally effective as 2-PAM iodide and has the advantage of being water-soluble. Reflexes are restored within 20 minutes. Morphine, barbiturates and respiratory depressants should be avoided.

67. **Rotenone (Derris Root, Cubeb).** An insecticide frequently mixed with pyrethrum powder. The lethal dose is probably large. Solutions or powder may be absorbed from the lungs or gastrointestinal tract. Symptoms are predominantly respiratory. There is an acceleration in the respiratory rate followed by a decrease; death occurs from respiratory failure. Evidence of gastric irritation such as nausea and vomiting may occur. Symptoms occur promptly within a few minutes to an hour.

TREATMENT. Lavage, catharsis and supportive measures.

68. **Salicylates (Methyl Salicylate, Salicylic Acid, Sodium Salicylate, Acetylsalicylic Acid and a Variety of Proprietary Ointments and Medications Containing Either Salicylic Acid or Salicylates).** Prolonged excessive or accidental ingestion of salicylates may result in severe poisoning. Absorption may occur from the mouth, gastrointestinal tract and the skin. The peak action occurs about 4 hours after a single toxic dose and may last longer than 18 hours. Rarely, effects of poisoning may persist for 10 days. Methyl salicylate and salicylic acid produce symptoms rapidly. Both cause severe gastrointestinal irritation with nausea and vomiting. Local painful lesions are caused by the caustic action of the acid. Intoxication may occur from the use of salicylic acid powder or ointment on large, open, weeping skin lesions. The toxic dose is usually in excess of 0.15 gm. per kg.

Initial symptoms are respiratory. Respiratory stimulation occurs via the vagus. There is an increase in the respiratory minute volume without necessarily an increase in rate, leading to a decrease in the pCO_2. The resulting respiratory alkalosis leads to cerebral symptoms of apathy, confusion, coma and an increase in cerebrospinal fluid pressure. Renal compensation follows, producing an increase in bicarbonate in the urine, a decrease in urine chloride, with corresponding rise in plasma chloride and a decrease in serum base. Renal compensation thus leads to loss of base from the body, predominantly sodium. In addition, salicylates appear to disturb the metabolism of carbohydrate. An unusually striking and persistent ketosis is associated with or soon follows early symptoms of toxicity. The ketoacidosis produces further base depletion through the kidney, and a true metabolic acidosis may be superimposed upon the respiratory alkalosis. Thus diagnosis of the electrolyte disorder cannot be made merely by determination of the carbon dioxide content of the blood. Measurement of the pH of the blood is of value, when correlated with other findings. Salicylates have an inhibiting effect on the formation of prothrombin by the liver, leading to purpuric manifestations. Dehydration in uncomplicated salicylate poisoning in a well child is usually not striking; salicylate poisoning often occurs, however, in children who are ill, and the dehydration produced may be moderate to severe. Vertigo, tinnitus, deafness, visual blurring, anorexia, vomiting, sweating, pallor or flushing, cyanosis, tetany, numbness and tingling of the face, lips and extremities, and bleeding from any area of the body may occur. Laboratory findings of diagnostic value are acetonuria and a falsely positive test result for diacetic acid with ferric chloride. Diacetic acid produces with ferric chloride a burgundy color in urine, whereas salicylates produce a violet to a deep purple color. Boiling of acidified urine will volatilize the diacetic acid, producing a negative ferric chloride test result in the absence of salicylate. Later evidences of toxicity may consist of erythematous, scarlatiniform, pruritic, eczematous or desquamative skin lesions. Salicylates may also impair coagulation (see p. 185).

TREATMENT. See page 217.

69. **Santonin.** The high solubility of santonin in bile and alkaline solutions causes rapid absorption from the upper intestine and leads to rapid development of toxic symptoms. An unknown product is formed which, when excreted, is an aid in

P O I S O N S

diagnosis, since it produces a yellow color in acid urine and a pink color in alkaline urine. Toxic symptoms are manifested initially by transitory blue vision and later by yellow vision. Other symptoms include headache, vomiting and confusion; with large doses there may be abdominal pain, diarrhea and bloody urine. The skin is cold and clammy and covered with perspiration. A fall in body temperature, a skin rash, tremors, cardiac and respiratory depression and convulsions develop.

TREATMENT. Immediate lavage should be followed by saline catharsis. Intramuscularly administered barbiturates may be used for convulsions.

70. **Shellfish.** Most shellfish poisoning in the United States is due to contamination by staphylococci or to allergic sensitivity. In some localities during certain seasons (summer and fall) mussels and clams may contain powerful neurotoxins. The origin of the poison is thought to be a dinoflagellate in the bodies of the clams. The poison is not destroyed by heating. Three general types of involvement occur: (1) gastroenteritis with nausea, vomiting and diarrhea; (2) nervous symptoms, diffuse erythema, urticaria, angina and dyspnea; and (3) a paralytic form in which symptoms simulate those of curare poisoning with respiratory paralysis.

71. **Sodium Hypochlorite.** Bleaching solutions contain sodium hypochlorite, 3 to 6 per cent in water. Their action is similar to that of sodium hydroxide in high concentrations. Acid secretions in the stomach release irritating hypochlorous acid. Fifteen to 30 ml. orally may be fatal for children. Inhalation of hypochlorous acid fumes produces pulmonary irritation, coughing and choking, and pulmonary edema. Ingestion causes irritation and corrosion of mucous membranes. Edema of the pharynx and larynx may be intense.

TREATMENT. Lavage with sodium bicarbonate solution repeatedly. Administration of a saline cathartic is advisable. Acid antidotes should never be used.

72. **Solanine (Solanism).** Symptoms of poisoning may follow ingestion of sprouted potatoes containing an alkaloid, solanine, found in or near the peel. Species of solanum (black nightshade, bittersweet) also contain the poison. Vomiting, diarrhea, colicky pains, headaches, depression, pain in the rectum, suppression of urine, and collapse occur within a few hours. Hallucinations and coma are sometimes present.

73. **Strychnine.** Strychnine is a powerful central nervous system stimulant. It produces little local gastrointestinal reaction, and the first symptoms are those of nervous system stimulation. At first a stiffness of the face and neck muscles occurs, followed by hyperactive reflexes of all muscles, and later by muscular twitchings and spinal convulsions. A characteristic position of the body occurs due to the action of the stronger groups of muscles. The back is arched in a position of opisthotonos; the legs are adducted and extended, and the feet turned in; the fists are clenched and the facial muscles are tightly contracted, producing risus sardonicus; there is exophthalmos and mydriasis. Involvement of the muscles of respiration produces respiratory arrest with resultant cyanosis. The patient usually remains conscious and is in severe pain. After such a convulsion, which lasts a minute or more, there is a period of relaxation with depression and, in some instances, unconsciousness due to apnea and anoxemia. In 10 to 15 minutes another spinal convulsion occurs. Medullary paralysis, due to excessive stimulation or anoxemia, follows the second to fifth convulsion.

TREATMENT. Lavage should not be done during convulsive attacks. Recurrence of convulsions must be prevented. Large doses of short-acting barbiturates should be given intravenously and repeated if necessary; sodium phenobarbital and amytal are effective. The dose should be sufficient to prevent or stop convulsions and keep the patient asleep, but not to depress respiration or blood pressure. Anesthesia may be temporarily necessary until a barbiturate can be given. All types of stimuli should be avoided. Lavage with 2 per cent tannic acid or strong tea may be performed when the patient is asleep.

74. **Thallium.** Thallium acetate has been administered orally to produce depilation in the treatment of ringworm of the scalp and locally as a depilatory for cosmetic purposes, but owing to the danger of serious toxic effects such use is to be condemned. The initial acute gastrointestinal symptoms, which usually result from accidental ingestion, occur 12 to 24 hours after ingestion. There is severe, paroxysmal abdominal pain with vomiting and diarrhea. Hemorrhage, desquamation of the mucosa, and eosinophilia may be present. The late effects of acute or chronic poisoning are predominantly on the nervous

system. Peripheral neuritis with paralysis, optic atrophy and cerebral symptoms occur. Alopecia is common, and attributed to a toxic effect on the sympathetic nervous system.

TREATMENT. Essentially the same as for arsenic (9), but BAL is of limited value.

75. **Thiocyanate Insecticides.** These agents induce coma, cyanosis, dyspnea and tonic convulsions. Respiratory difficulty may occur.

TREATMENT. Skin contamination should be removed by scrubbing with soap and water. Gastric lavage with tap water and saline catharsis are advisable. Renal and hepatic injury may occur later.

76. **Veratrine.** An alkaloid obtained from *V. cevadilla* (sabadilla), a false hellebore plant. Cevadine is crystallized veratrine. Sabadilla dusts and spray and extracts of sabadilla are used as insecticides and pediculicides. Ingestion produces violent vomiting and diarrhea, intense burning and generalized muscular weakness. Muscular and autonomic nervous system reactions are similar to those from pyrethrum and nicotine.

TREATMENT. See 56.

77. **Veratrum.** Veratrum and Zygadenus are found in hellebore *(Veratrum album, viride* or *californicum). Zygadenus venenosus,* the death camass, contains similar nitrogenous compounds. Ingestion of these plants produces nausea, severe vomiting, diarrhea, muscular weakness, visual disturbances, bradycardia and low blood pressure. Very large doses may produce hypotension.

TREATMENT. Gastric lavage followed by saline catharsis. Atropine is of value to block the fall of blood pressure and the bradycardia.

78. **Warfarin (Dicoumarin) (3-Alpha-acetonyl benzyl-4-hydroxycoumarin).** A rodenticide found in Dethmor, Rax Powder, D-con and other products. Available in 1:200 concentration in cornstarch and used as a rat bait in 1:400 concentration in corn meal. The dicumarol action inhibits prothrombin formation, but it is 40 times more potent than dicumarol. Absorption is slow and irregular; 24 to 48 hours may elapse before any effect is noted. Elimination is slow. The action is chiefly on the synthesis of prothrombin with a gradual depression of prothrombin levels in the blood leading to spontaneous hemorrhages. The action may persist for 10 days.

TREATMENT. Gastric lavage and catharsis should be instituted. Vitamin K in large doses should be given intravenously. Whole blood transfusions may also be needed.

79. **Zinc Stearate Powder.** A severe irritation of the respiratory mucous membranes is produced by aspiration with resulting congestion, hyperemia, edema, and obstruction of bronchioles with mucus. Bronchopneumonia is common in infants who survive the first day or two. Choking, coughing, cyanosis and signs of suffocation tend to develop immediately.

TREATMENT. Aspiration of the powder and accumulated secretions by bronchoscopy is worthy of trial, but it is not likely to be effective because of the adhesive quality of the powder. Administration of oxygen is important, and there may be an added advantage in giving it in combination with helium. Powders containing zinc stearate should *never* be used for infants and small children.

LIST OF CHEMICALS

The following list includes individual chemical compounds, alphabetically arranged, with an appended numeral referring to the class (see above with which they are associated; e.g. Chloroethane (46) is referred to Hydrocarbons (Halogenated).

Abrin, 1
Acetaldehyde (ethyl aldehyde), 39
Acetanilid (N-phenylacetamide), 6
Acetic acid, concentrated, 2
Acetoarsenite (Paris green), 9
Acetone, 3
Acetophenetidin (phenacetin), 6
Acetylene tetrachloride (tetrachloroethane), 46
Acetylsalicylic acid (aspirin), 68
Acid. See particular acid.

POISONS

POISONS

JOHN A. ANDERSON

REFERENCES

Arena, J. M.: *Poisoning: Chemistry, Symptoms and Treatment.* Springfield, Ill., Charles C Thomas, 1963.

Chisholm, J. J. Jr., The Use of Chelating Agents in the Treatment of Acute and Chronic Lead Intoxication in Childhood. *J. Pediat.*, 73:1, 1968.

Chisholm, J. J., Jr., and Kaplan, E.: Lead Poisoning in Childhood—Comprehensive Management and Prevention. *J. Pediat.*, 73:942, 1968.

Coffin, R., Phillips, J. L., Staples, W. L., and Spector, S.: Treatment of Lead Encephalopathy in Children. *J. Pediat.* 69: 198, 1966.

Gleason, M., Gosselin, R., and Hodge, H.: *Clinical Toxicology of Commercial Products.* 2nd ed. Baltimore, Williams & Wilkins Company, 1963.

Goodman, L. S., and Gilman, A.: *The Pharmacological Basis of Therapeutics.* 3rd ed., New York, Macmillan Company, 1965.

ACRODYNIA

(PINK DISEASE; SWIFT'S DISEASE; FEER'S DISEASE; ERYTHREDEMA; DERMATOPOLYNEURITIS)

Acrodynia (the term, derived from the Greek, denotes painful extremities) is a syndrome consisting of many unusual symptoms which in the well established case are so distinctive that there is practically no differential diagnosis. There are few clinical conditions in which extreme and persistent misery is such a prominent part of the clinical picture.

History. As early as 1903 Selter of Solingen described this disease and called it a trophodermatosis. Feer of Zurich, whose name is attached to the disease in Europe, did not know that such a clinical entity existed until the early 1920's, when he described his interpretation of it as "Vegetative Neurose des Kleinkindes." The condition had been recognized in Australia as early as 1890 as "pink disease," but it was not until 1914 that Swift's paper brought it into focus as a distinct clinical entity under the name "erythredema." The disease had been observed and commented upon as early as 1915 in Oregon, but there was nothing in British or American literature on the condition until 2 physicians in the United States independently published articles describing it in 1920.

Etiology and Epidemiology. Acrodynia is principally a disease of infancy and early childhood. In the United States it has become uncommon, as it apparently has in other parts of the world where it once was relatively common, especially in England and Australia.

From the studies of Warkany and Hubbard and of others, it now seems that most and perhaps all cases of acrodynia represent the clinical response to repeated ingestion of or contact with mercury. Whether this response is the result of chronic poisoning or is an unusual reaction modified by other factors is not clear. Since only a fraction of the infants and children exposed to mercury for periods of time apparently adequate for the development of acrodynia acquire the disease, the latter possibility would seem the more likely.

The frequency with which unusual amounts of mercury are demonstrated in urine would seem to be highest in areas where mercurial medications are or have been widely prescribed. In the southern United States and in England, teething powders and lotions have been a principal source of mercury, whereas in France and Switzerland, vermifuges have been a more common source. Other reported sources of mercury include calomel, mercurial ointments, diaper rinses, paint and wallpaper. The possibility of accidental ingestion, of course, exists.

Pathology. No consistent or characteristic pathologic changes have been observed. Many of the changes can be explained on the basis of a chronic disease in association with a state of semistarvation with resultant degeneration of nervous tissue.

Clinical Manifestations. The natural course of acrodynia is prolonged, extending from several months to a year. There are all grades of severity. The child becomes listless; he is no longer interested in play and is restless and irritable. Generalized, inconstant rashes which are protean recur from time to time. Early the tips of the fingers and toes acquire a pinkish color, and later the hands and feet become a dusky pink which shades off at the wrists and ankles; they are cold and clammy. These changes in the extremities are the most distinctive features of the syndrome, being different from those of any other disease occurring in children, and are responsible for the term "pink disease." Frequently the cheeks and the tip of the nose acquire a scarlet color.

As the disease becomes established, the sweat glands are enormously dilated and enlarged, and perspiration is profuse; at times the infant may be drenched, necessitating frequent changes of clothing. A severe pyoderma may develop. There is desquamation of the soles and palms, which, though usually superficial, may be severe and recur during the course of the disease. The fingers and toes appear edematous; the swelling is due to hyperplasia and hyperkeratosis of the skin. An outstanding symptom is excruciating pain in the hands and feet. Children will rub their hands together for hours, and older children will complain of a severe burning sensation.

The nails become dark and frequently drop off. Occasionally gangrene of the toes and fingers develops, and trophic ulcers may result from the constant rubbing of the hands and feet. The hair tends to fall out and is often pulled out by the child.

In more than 60 per cent of the cases there is photophobia without evidence of local inflammation of the eyes. The children shield their eyes or bury their faces in their pillows. The lax ligaments and hypotonia permit the children to assume unusual positions (Fig. 28-2), and they often lie for hours with their heads between their legs. The so-called salaam position is frequently assumed, often with constant rubbing motions of the hands and feet, owing to the pain and itching.

In extreme cases the teeth may be lost; necrosis of the jaw bones frequently follows. Initially the gums appear normal except for a slightly deeper red color; later they become inflamed and swollen. Salivation then becomes pronounced, and the saliva often flows from the mouth in a constant

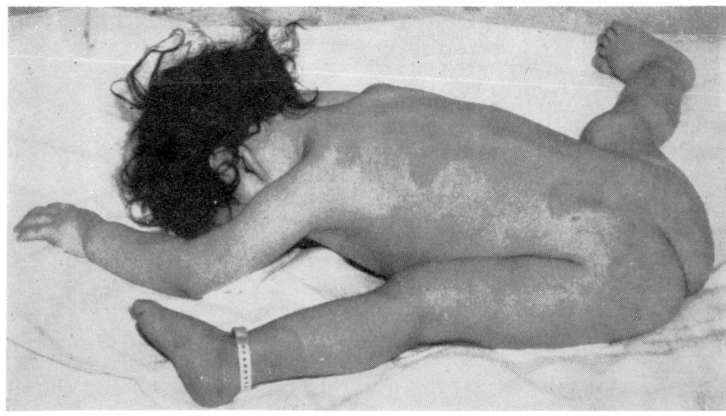

Figure 28-2. Extreme hypotonia and photophobia in an infant with acrodynia. This bizarre position may be maintained for hours.

stream. Anorexia is prominent, but because of the excessive perspiration large quantities of water are consumed. There may be diarrhea, and prolapse of the rectum is a frequent complication. The blood pressure and pulse rate may be increased significantly. Fever is usually not present unless there is some complication as a urinary tract infection or bronchopneumonia.

Nervous symptoms are an important part of the syndrome. Early in the disease the tendon reflexes may be normal or increased, but later they disappear. There is not a true motor paralysis, but because of the soft, flabby musculature the child has no desire to walk. Many of the symptoms and signs suggest involvement of the vasomotor mechanism. The severe pain prevents normal sleep. There is no time when a child with acrodynia appears happy or comfortable; he does not play or smile, but appears dejected and melancholic, a picture of abject misery.

Laboratory Data. There are no characteristic morphologic changes of the blood or significant changes in the cerebrospinal fluid. There may be albuminuria, but the only characteristic urinary finding is the presence of mercury.

Prophylaxis. There is little or no need for mercurial medications in pediatric practice, and they should be avoided whenever possible. It is most important that one be alert for possible contacts with mercury in various household and industrial preparations.

Treatment. There is probably no more difficult problem in pediatrics than the management of an infant with severe acrodynia. The extreme restlessness, irritability and pain are not readily allayed. Barbiturates are usually not as effective as paraldehyde administered rectally in olive oil (5 to 10 ml.). Symptomatic relief has also been reported from the use of Priscoline in doses of 12.5 mg. at intervals of 4 to 6 hours.

BAL (British anti-lewisite; 2,3-dimercaptopropanol) has been used therapeutically, apparently with good effect in some instances and especially when administration was begun early in the disease. The recommended plan of treatment is 3 mg. per kg. every 4 hours for 48 hours, then every 6 hours for 24 hours, followed by administration at intervals of 12 hours for 7 days. The drug is administered intramuscularly in a 10 per cent solution. Toxic effects of BAL have been observed (p. 1492).

Penicillamine (N-acetyl-II l-penicillamine) has been used with apparent beneficial effect in chronic mercury poisoning, including acrodynia, and has the advantage over BAL that it is administered orally.

The diet should contain generous amounts of proteins, minerals and vitamins. Frequently anorexia is so great that feeding must be by gavage.

Owing to the profuse sweating, thirst is usually prominent, and, in contrast to the frequent refusal to eat, the child will usually take relatively large quantities of fluids. Deficits of electrolytes should be taken into account in the planning of parenteral fluid therapy. So far as possible, fluid intake should be oral rather than parenteral.

The child should be kept as clean as possible to minimize the chances of secondary pyogenic skin infections. Frequent alcohol rubs may aid in this respect in addition to being soothing. The clothing should be light, preferably of cotton, and should be changed frequently when perspiration is profuse.

It is obvious that the family must be made aware of the nature of the illness and of its prolonged course if they are to be expected to play their part successfully.

J. B. BILDERBACK

REFERENCES

Bilderback, J. B.: Group of Cases of Unknown Etiology and Diagnosis. *Northwest Med.,* 19:263, 1920.

Bilderback, J. B.: Acrodynia, *J.A.M.A.,* 84:495, 1925.

Bilderback, J. B.: Acrodynia, Swift's Disease. *Northwest Med.,* 31:161, 1932.

Bivings, L.: Acrodynia: A Summary of BAL Therapy Reports and a Case Report of Calomel Disease. *J. Pediat.,* 34:322, 1949.

Byfield, A. H.: A Polyneuritic Syndrome Resembling Pellagra-Acrodynia (?) Seen in Very Young Children: Report of Cases. *Am. J. Dis. Child.,* 20:347, 1920.

Editorial: New Source of Mercury Poisoning. *New England J. Med.,* 269:926, 1963.

Fanconi, G., and Botsjtejn, A.: Die feersche Krankheit (Akrodynia) und Quecksilbermedikation. *Helvet. paediat. Acta,* 3:264, 1948.

Feer, E.: Die spezifische vegetative Neuropathie des Kleinkindes (kindliche Akrodynia). *Schweiz. med. Wchnschr.,* 65:977, 1935.

Hirschman, S. Z., Feingold, M., and Boylen, G.: Mercury in House Paint as a Cause of Acrodynia. Effect of Therapy with N-acetyl, L-Penicillamine. *New England J. Med.,* 269:889, 1963.

Peterson, J. C., and Laughmiller, R.: Acrodynia: Treatment with Adrenolytic Drugs. *Acta pediat.,* 43:517, 1954.

Smith, A. D. M., and Miller, J. W.: Treatment of Inorganic Mercury Poisoning with N-Acetyl-D, L-Penicillamine. *Lancet,* 1:640, 1961.

Swift, H.: Erythroedema; in *Transactions of the Tenth Session, Australasian Medical Congress,* Auckland, New Zealand, 1914, p. 547.

Warkany, J.: Acrodynia—Postmortem of a Disease. *Amer. J. Dis. Child.,* 112:147, 1966.

Warkany, J., and Hubbard, D. M.: Adverse Mercurial Reactions in Form of Acrodynia and Related Conditions. *Lancet,* 1: 829, 1948.

Weston, W.: Acrodynia. *Arch. Pediat.,* 37:513, 1920.

29. Appendix

MORPHOLOGIC SYNDROMES

Multiple physical defects may be the consequence of a *single primary* error in morphogenesis. An example is the combination of meningomyelocele, clubfoot and hydrocephalus; the *primary* defect in this situation is incomplete closure of the neural tube. *Multiple primary* major or minor defects of one or more systems also occur, and some of these are listed as syndromes in the following table.

KEY TO USE OF TABULAR LISTING OF SYNDROMES

The formulation of the following tabular listing of morphologic syndromes is based on the concept that individual defects are rarely pathognomonic, but that identification of two or more anomalies may provide a diagnostic core pattern for a particular syndrome. Thus for each syndrome a core pattern of two or more clinically detectable abnormalities has been selected which is highly suggestive or even diagnostic of that syndrome *as contrasted to all other recognized conditions.* For example, webbed neck is not included under XO (Turner's) syndrome because it is not one of the more frequent features, and simian crease was not included in any of the core patterns because it is a feature of many syndromes and therefore is of limited value in differential diagnosis. For each disorder, in addition to the core pattern of defects, small stature and mental deficiency are listed if they are part of the syndrome; the etiology and genetic pattern are listed if they are known; a representative reference (literature) is added as a source of more complete information, and the page reference to description in this text is noted. Below the number of each syndrome in the left hand column of the table the numbers in parentheses indicate the listed syndromes which merit especial consideration in the differential diagnosis.

The grouping of syndromes is based on the systems involved, the type of abnormality and, in the case of chromosomal aberrations, the etiology. Within each group the order of presentation is determined principally by clinical similarities.

The groups in order of listing are as follows:

I. Bone and connective tissue dysplasias
    A. Connective tissue disorders
    B. Mucopolysaccharidoses
    C. Osteochondrodystrophies
II. Chromosomal imbalance syndromes
III. Miscellaneous patterns of malformation
    A. Predominantly facial defects
    B. Unusually small stature with associated defects
    C. Senile-like appearance with associated defects
    D. Joint dysplasia with associated defects
    E. Broad thumb with associated defects
    F. Deafness with associated defects
    G. Neurologic disorders with associated defects
    H. Muscular disorders with associated defects
    I. Hematopoetic disorders with associated defects
    J. Other disorders
IV. Hamartoses
V. Ectodermal dysplasias

The reader is cautioned that the core patterns were selected as leads to aid in the diagnosis of each syndrome, rather than to describe it, and that not all patients with a given disorder will have all the anomalies of the core pattern. Nor are all syndromes of multiple defects included in these tables; the author has listed only those which appear to be well defined syndromes of *multiple primary* defects. The reader is further cautioned that vague or partial similarity is insufficient for a diagnosis. The table is only a guide; specific diagnosis must rest on careful correlation of the patient's signs with the total picture of the syndrome as derived from study of the appropriate references. Genetic counsel should be rendered only after a careful assessment of the family history; many patients with a single altered gene have a fresh mutation which does not increase the risk that the parents will have another affected child. For example, about 85 per cent of children with achondroplasia, an autosomal dominant disorder, are born of normal parents.

ALPHABETICAL LISTING

SYNDROMES

BONE AND CONNECTIVE TISSUE DYSPLASIAS: A. CONNECTIVE TISSUE DISORDERS

The CONNECTIVE TISSUE disorders are so categorized because the basic problem appears to be in fibrous tissue and its derivatives. Relative laxity of joints, bluish sclerae, and inguinal hernias are rather nonspecific and may be found as features of syndromes 1 through 4. Abnormality in blood vessels may lead to serious vascular disease in conditions 1 through 3 and 5.

SYNDROME	DIAGNOSTIC MANIFESTATIONS				MENTAL DEFIC.	SHORT STATURE	GENETIC TRANS-MISSION	REFER-ENCE
	FACIAL	LIMBS	OTHER					
1. Marfan's syndrome (2)*†	Subluxation of lens	Arachnodactyly	Aortic dilatation				Aut. Dom.	3
2. Homocystinuria (1)*†	Subluxation of lens, malar flush	Osteoporosis	Venous thromboses		+/−		Aut. Rec.	3
3. Ehlers-Danlos syndrome†		Hyperextensible joints	Hyperextensible skin, poor wound healing with thin scar, subcutaneous nodules				Aut. Dom.	3
4. Osteogenesis imperfecta†	Bluish sclerae, odontogenesis imperfecta	Fragile bone	+/− Deafness			+/−	Aut. Dom.; rare Aut. Rec.	3
5. Pseudoxanthoma elasticum	Angioid retinal streaks	Thickened yellowish skin in flexural areas	Arterial medial degeneration with hemorrhagic tendency				Aut. Rec.	3
6. Fibrodysplasia ossificans progressiva (myositis ossificans)†		Short hallux +/− short thumb	Fibrous dysplasia in muscle and subcutaneous tissues leading to mineralization			+/−	Aut. Dom.	3

1512

BONE AND CONNECTIVE TISSUE DYSPLASIAS: B. MUCOPOLYSACCHARIDOSES

The MUCOPOLYSACCHARIDOSES are categorized together on the basis of excess tissue storage and urinary excretion of mucopolysaccharides. Clinically, all tend to produce some coarsening of the facial features. Other manifestations are broadening and altered configuration of bone, joint limitation, corneal opacity, hepatosplenomegaly, mental deterioration and cardiovascular changes—all features of the prototype, Hurler's syndrome. The age of onset may be a helpful clinical clue in these disorders. With the exception of generalized gangliosidosis, these disorders become clinically manifest *after* birth.

SYNDROME	DIAGNOSTIC MANIFESTATIONS			MENTAL DEFIC.	SHORT STATURE	GENETIC TRANSMISSION	REFERENCE
	FACIAL	SKELETAL	OTHER				
7. Generalized gangliosidosis (familial neurovisceral lipidosis)†	Coarse facies, hypertrophy of alveolar ridges at birth	Kyphosis in early infancy	Renal dysfunction	?+	+	Aut. Rec.	42
8. Hurler's syndrome (MPS type I) (9, 10)*†	Coarse facies; cloudy cornea, early	Stiff joints by 1 yr.; kyphosis by 1-2 yr.	Valvular heart disease	+	+ Onset, 6-18 mo.	Aut. Rec.	3
9. Hunter's syndrome (MPS type II) (8, 10)*†	Coarse facies; clear cornea	Stiff joints; kyphosis, rare	Deafness develops	+	+ Onset, 2-4 yr.	X-Linked Rec.	3
10. Maroteaux-Lamy syndrome (MPS type VI) (8, 9)*†	Mildly coarse facies; cloudy cornea, early	Stiff joints, kyphosis			+ Onset, 1-3 yr.	Aut. Rec.	3
11. Morquio's disease (MPS type IV) (15, 19, 20)*†	Mildly coarse facies; cloudy cornea, usually after 5 yr.	Mildly stiff joints; vertebrae become flattened; severe kyphosis			+ Onset, 1-3 yr.	Aut. Rec.	3

*The numbers in parentheses refer to syndromes listed in this table which merit special consideration in the differential diagnosis.
†Syndrome is described in text; see index for location.

BONE AND CONNECTIVE TISSUE DYSPLASIAS: B. MUCOPOLYSACCHARIDOSES *(Continued)*

SYNDROME	DIAGNOSTIC MANIFESTATIONS			MENTAL DEFIC.	SHORT STATURE	GENETIC TRANS-MISSION	REFER-ENCE
	FACIAL	SKELETAL	OTHER				
12. Sanfilippo syndrome (MPS type III) (13)*†	Mildly coarse facies; clear cornea	Mildly stiff joints, no kyphosis		+		Aut. Rec.	3
13. Scheie syndrome (MPS type V) (12)*†	Broad mouth; cloudy cornea	Stiff joints by 5-8 yr.; no kyphosis				Aut. Rec.	3

BONE AND CONNECTIVE TISSUE DYSPLASIAS: C. OSTEOCHONDRODYSTROPHIES

SYNDROME	DIAGNOSTIC MANIFESTATIONS			MENTAL DEFIC.	SHORT STATURE	GENETIC TRANS-MISSION	REFER-ENCE
	CRANIOFACIAL	LIMBS	OTHER				
14. Achondroplasia (15-19, 21)*†	Low nasal bridge +/− macrocephaly	Short limbs, short hands and feet, limited elbow extension	Caudal narrowing of spinal canal, short ileum with sacroiliac notch		+	Aut. Dom.	3, 4
15. Metatropic dwarfism (14, 19, 21)*	Normal facies	Short limb, small epiphyses, metaphyseal flare	Severe early kyphoscoliosis, flattened vertebrae		+	? Aut. Rec.	29
16. Diastrophic dwarfism (14, 15, 21)*†	Hypertrophied or cystic auricular cartilage, cleft palate	Short limbs, short 1st metacarpal, joint limitations with clubfoot			+	Aut. Rec.	3
17. Ellis-van Creveld syndrome (chondroectodermal dysplasia) (18)*†	Neonatal teeth, hypoplasia of teeth	Short distal limbs, polydactyly, nail hypoplasia	Small thorax, cardiac defect		+	Aut. Rec.	3

# Syndrome	Facies	Clinical/radiographic features	Additional features			Inheritance	No.
18. Thoracic asphyxiant dystrophy (14, 17, 19)*†	Normal facies	Short limbs, short hands, +/− polydactyly	Constricted small thorax +/− renal disease		+	Aut. Rec.	21
19. Spondyloepiphyseal dysplasia (pseudoachondroplasia) (14, 15, 16, 18, 21)*†	Normal facies	Postnatal onset of short limbs, irregular epiphyses and metaphyses, limited elbow extension	Short trunk, lumbar lordosis		+	Aut. Dom.	3
20. X-linked spondyloepiphyseal dysplasia (11)*	Normal facies	Onset of epiphyseal irregularity at 5-10 years	Short trunk due to flattening of vertebrae		+ (late)	X-linked Rec.	3
21. Multiple epiphyseal dysplasia†	Normal facies	Short fingers, epiphyseal hypoplasia, metaphyseal flaring	Joint limitation, eventual osteoarthritis of hip		+	Aut. Dom.	3
22. Metaphyseal dysostosis dominant type (23)*†	Normal facies	Bowlegs; irregular, wide metaphyses	Variable limitation of fingers in full extension		+	Aut. Dom.	4
23. Cartilage-hair hypoplasia (22)*†	Fine, sparse hair, normal facies	Mild bowing of legs; wide, slightly irregular metaphyses	+/− Intestinal malabsorption		+	Aut. Rec.	3
24. Multiple exostoses†	Normal facies	Diaphyseal outgrowths leading to limb deformities	+/− Short metacarpals		+/−	Aut. Dom.	3
25. Conradi's disease; chondrodystrophia calcificans congenita†	Flattened nasal bridge, cataracts	Short proximal long bones, joint contractures	Calcific stippling in developing cartilage	+/−	+	Aut. Rec.	4

*The numbers in parentheses refer to syndromes listed in this table which merit special consideration in the differential diagnosis.
†Syndrome is described in text; see index for location.

SYNDROMES

BONE AND CONNECTIVE TISSUE DYSPLASIAS: C. OSTEOCHONDRODYSTROPHIES *(Continued)*

SYNDROME	DIAGNOSTIC MANIFESTATIONS			MENTAL DEFIC.	SHORT STATURE	GENETIC TRANS-MISSION	REFER-ENCE
	CRANIOFACIAL	LIMBS	OTHER				
26. **Hypophosphatasia**⋇	Delayed closure of fontanels +/− cranio-synostosis, early loss of deciduous teeth	Bowing of legs, poor irregular mineraliza-tion, especially at metaphyses			+	Aut. Rec.	4
OSTEOPETROSES:							
27. **Cranio-metaphyseal dysplasia of Pyle**	Broad flat nasal bridge, thick calvaria with cranial nerve com-pression	Enlarging, splayed metaphyseal ends of long bones, knock knee			+/−	Aut. Rec.	3
28. **Osteopetrosis, severe (Albers-Schönberg dis-ease) (29)**⋇†	Thick calvaria with cranial nerve com-pression +/− macrocephaly	Dense, thick, fragile bones	Secondary pancytopenia, splenomegaly		+/−	Aut. Rec.	3
29. **Osteopetrosis, mild (28)**	Dense calvaria	Moderately dense bone liable to fracture, +/− osteomyelitis				Aut. Dom.	3
30. **Pyknodysostosis of Maroteaux and Lamy (31, 32)**⋇†	Tooth anomalies, delayed closure of fontanels, facial bone hypoplasia	Osteosclerosis, shorten-ing of distal phalanges			+	Aut. Rec.	3
31. **Pyknodysostosis of Stanesco (30)**⋇	Brachycephaly with thin cranium, facial bone hypoplasia	Osteosclerosis, relatively short upper arms			+	Aut. Dom.	46

32. Cleidocranial dysostosis (30)*†	Delayed closure of fontanels with frontal bossing, late eruption of teeth	Defect of outer clavicle		+	Aut. Dom.	4
CRANIOSYNOSTOSES:						
33. Apert's syndrome (acrocephalosyndactyly) (34)*†	Craniosynostosis, irregular midfacial hypoplasia, and hypertelorism	Syndactyly, broad distal thumb and toe	+		Aut. Dom.	2
34. Carpenter's syndrome (33, 98)*†	Craniosynostosis, midfacial hypoplasia, lateral displacement of inner canthi	Polydactyly, syndactyly; Obesity	+	+/−	Aut. Rec.	49
35. Crouzon's disease (craniofacial dysostosis)*†	Proptosis with shallow orbits, maxillary hypoplasia, craniosynostosis				Aut. Dom.	2
OTHER SKELETAL DYSPLASIAS:						
36. Aminopterin-induced syndrome	Cranial dysplasia with broad nasal bridge, low-set ears		?	+		32
37. Nail-patella syndrome	Patella hypoplasia, nail hypoplasia	Iliac horns, scoliosis			Aut. Dom.	28

*The numbers in parentheses refer to syndromes listed in this table which merit special consideration in the differential diagnosis.
†Syndrome is described in text; see index for location.

SYNDROMES

BONE AND CONNECTIVE TISSUE DYSPLASIAS: C. OSTEOCHONDRODYSTROPHIES *(Continued)*

SYNDROME	DIAGNOSTIC MANIFESTATIONS			MENTAL DEFIC.	SHORT STATURE	GENETIC TRANS-MISSION	REFER-ENCE
	CRANIOFACIAL	LIMBS	OTHER				
OTHER SKELETAL DYSPLASIAS (Continued)							
38. Dyschondrosteosis of Leri-Weill†		Short forearms with Madelung deformity, +/– short lower leg			+	Aut. Dom.	4
39. Albright's hereditary osteodystrophy (pseudohypopara-thyroidism) (44, 41)*	Rounded facies	Short metacarpal bones, especially 4th	Obesity, hypocalcemia and/or extraskeletal mineralization	+	+	? X-Linked Dom.	4
40. Brachydactyly type E (39, 41)*		Brachydactyly, short 3rd and 5th metacarpals			+	Aut. Dom.	30
41. Marchesani's syndrome (39, 40)*†	Small spherical lens	Brachydactyly			+	Aut. Rec.	4

CHROMOSOMAL IMBALANCE SYNDROMES:

The following CHROMOSOMAL ABNORMALITIES give rise to particular patterns of multiple defects which allow for clinical recognition. They are grouped together to aid the clinician in deciding which patients clearly merit chromosomal study for confirmatory diagnosis and genetic counsel.

SYNDROME	DIAGNOSTIC MANIFESTATIONS			MENTAL DEFIC.	SHORT STATURE	CHROM.	REFER-ENCE
	CRANIOFACIAL	LIMBS	OTHER				
42. Down's syndrome (mongolism) (43, 44, 83)*†	Upward slant to palpebral fissures, flat facies	Short hands, clinodactyly of 5th finger	Hypotonia	+	+/–	21 Tri-somy	4

No. & Syndrome							
43. **Penta-X** (42, 44, 83)*†	Upward slant to palpebral fissures	Small hands, clinodactyly of 5th finger	+	+	Patent ductus arteriosus	+	XXXXX 11
44. **XXXXY** (42, 82, 98)*†	Inner epicanthic fold and/or upslanting of palpebral fissures	Limited elbow pronation, low dermal ridge count on fingertips (mostly low arches)	+	+	Hypogenitalism	+	XXXXY 4
45. **18 Trisomy** (46, 99)*†	Microstomia, short palpebral fissure	Clenched hand, 2nd finger over 3rd; low arches on fingertips	+	+	Short sternum	+	18 Trisomy 4
46. **13 (D_1) Trisomy** (45, 48, 70)*†	Defects of eye, nose, lip and forebrain of holoprosencephaly type	Polydactyly, narrow hyperconvex fingernails	+	+	Skin defects, posterior scalp	+	13 Trisomy 45
47. **Schmid-Fraccaro syndrome (cat-eye syndrome)**	Hypertelorism with slight downslanting of palpebral fissures, coloboma of iris and/or preauricular fistula		+/−		Anal atresia	+/−	Unusually small extra acrocentric chrom. 41
48. **Chromosome No. 4 short-arm deletion syndrome (46)***†	Ocular hypertelorism +/− prominent glabella, low-set simple ear with preauricular dimple, +/− cleft lip and palate		+	+	+/− Midline scalp defects	+	# 4 p- 22
49. **Cri du chat syndrome**†	Epicanthic folds and/or slanting palpebral fissures, microcephaly with round facial contour		+	+	Catlike cry in infancy	+	# 5 p- 4
50. **Chromosome No. 18 long-arm deletion syndrome***	Midfacial hypoplasia, atretic or narrow ear canal	High frequency of whorl digital pattern	+	+		+	# 18 q- 25

*The numbers in parentheses refer to syndromes listed in this table which merit special consideration in the differential diagnosis.
†Syndrome is described in text; see index for location.

SYNDROMES

1519

CHROMOSOMAL IMBALANCE SYNDROMES (Continued)

SYNDROME	DIAGNOSTIC MANIFESTATIONS			MENTAL DEFIC.	SHORT STATURE	GENETIC TRANSMISSION	REFERENCE
	CRANIOFACIAL	LIMBS	OTHER				
51. Chromosome No. 21 long-arm deletion syndrome	Downslanting palpebral fissures, large malformed external ears, micrognathia			+	+	# 21 q-	6
52. XO (Turner's) syndrome (97)*†	Heart-shaped facies, prominent ears	Congenital lymphedema or its residua	Broad chest with widely spaced nipples, low posterior hairline	+/-	+	XO	2, 4

MISCELLANEOUS PATTERNS OF MALFORMATION

A. PREDOMINANTLY FACIAL DEFECTS: [35]*

SYNDROME	DIAGNOSTIC MANIFESTATIONS			MENTAL DEFIC.	SHORT STATURE	GENETIC TRANSMISSION	REFERENCE
	CRANIOFACIAL	LIMBS	OTHER				
53. Treacher-Collins syndrome (mandibulofacial dysostosis) (54)*†	Malar and mandibular hypoplasia, down-slanting palpebral fissures	Defect of lower eyelid	Malformation of external ear			Aut. Dom.	2
54. Goldenhar's syndrome (53)*	Malar hypoplasia	Epibulbar dermoid and/or lipodermoid +/- other eye defect	Malformed ear with pre-auricular tags			Unknown ? Aut. Rec.	2
55. Pierre Robin syndrome†	Micrognathia	Glossoptosis	Cleft palate			?	2

B. UNUSUALLY SMALL STATURE WITH ASSOCIATED DEFECTS: [7 to 11, 16, 17, 23, 36, 39, 41, 45, 48 to 52, 74, 99, 103]

Syndrome						Inheritance	No.
56. Lower lip fistula and cleft lip (67)*	Lower lip fistulas (pits)	Cleft lip and/or cleft palate				Aut. Dom.	2
57. Familial blepharophimosis	Lateral displacement of inner canthi	Inverted inner canthal fold	Ptosis of eyelids			Aut. Dom.	26
58. Silver's syndrome†	Triangular hypoplastic facies with downturning mouth	Skeletal asymmetry, clinodactyly of 5th finger			+	?	4
59. Bloom's syndrome	Cutaneous photosensitivity, telangiectatic erythema, malar hypoplasia		Chromosomal breakage in vitro		+	Aut. Rec.	4
60. Seckel's syndrome	Facial hypoplasia, prominent nose, microcephaly	Multiple minor joint and skeletal abnormalities		+	+	Aut. Rec.	4
61. Cornelia de Lange syndrome	Synophrys (continuous eyebrows), thin downturning upper lip	Small or malformed hands and feet, proximal thumb	Hirsutism	+	+	?	4
62. Hallerman-Streiff syndrome (63)*†	Microphthalmia and cataracts, small pinched nose, micrognathia	Thin skin over nose, hypotrichosis			+	? Aut. Dom.	4

*The numbers in parentheses refer to syndromes listed in this table which merit special consideration in the differential diagnosis.
†Syndrome is described in text; see index for location.

SYNDROMES

MISCELLANEOUS PATTERNS OF MALFORMATION *(Continued)*

C. SENILE-LIKE APPEARANCE WITH ASSOCIATED DEFECTS: [62]

	FACIAL	CUTANEOUS	OTHER	MENTAL DEFIC.	SHORT STATURE	GENETIC TRANSMISSION	REFERENCE
63. Progeria (62, 64)*†	Facial bone hypoplasia	Alopecia, thin skin with atrophy of subcutaneous adipose	Straight femoral neck, short distal phalanges, premature atherosclerosis		+	?	4
64. Cockayne's syndrome (63)*	Retinal degeneration	Hypotrichosis, photosensitivity, thin skin, diminished subcutaneous adipose	Impaired hearing	+	+	Aut. Rec.	4
65. Rothmund-Thomson syndrome (poikiloderma congenita) (115)*†	Development of cataracts	Development of poikiloderma	Other features of ectodermal dysplasia		+/−	Aut. Rec.	1, 2

D. JOINT DYSPLASIA WITH ASSOCIATED DEFECTS: [8-13, 14-16, 19, 21, 22, 25, 44, 45, 58, 87, 88, 94, 95, 99]

	CRANIOFACIAL	LIMBS	OTHER	MENTAL DEFIC.	SHORT STATURE	GENETIC TRANSMISSION	REFERENCE
66. Familial dwarfism with stiff joints (68)*	Hyperopia	Stiff joints			+	Aut. Dom.	33
67. Popliteal web syndrome (56)*	Lower lip pits, cleft palate	Popliteal web				? Aut. Rec. or Aut. Dom.	20

	CRANIOFACIAL	LIMBS	OTHER				
68. Stickler's progressive arthro-ophthalmopathy (66)*	Progressive myopia, retinal detachment	Joint limitation from childhood	Sensorineural deafness			Aut. Dom.	48
69. Larsen's syndrome	Flat facies	Multiple joint dislocations, short metacarpals				?	27

E. BROAD THUMB WITH ASSOCIATED DEFECTS: [33, 34]

	CRANIOFACIAL	LIMBS	OTHER				
70. Rubinstein-Taybi syndrome (46, 71, 72)*	Slanting palpebral fissures, maxillary hypoplasia, microcephaly	Broad thumbs and toes		+	+	?	4
71. Leri's pleonosteosis (70, 72)*	Upward slant to palpebral fissures	Broad thumb in valgus position, joint limitation with partial flexion of fingers				Aut. Dom.	3
72. Taybi's oto-palato-digital syndrome (70, 71)*	Cleft soft palate, microstomia	Broad distal digits, "tree-frog-like"	Deafness, conductive	+/−	+	? X-linked	14
73. Mohr's syndrome	Cleft tongue	Partial duplication of hallux	Deafness, conductive	+/−		? Aut. Rec.	38

F. DEAFNESS WITH ASSOCIATED DEFECTS: [9, 10, 27, 28, 46, 53, 54, 72, 73, 108, 119-122]

	CRANIOFACIAL	LIMBS	OTHER				
74. Rubella syndrome†	Cataract		Deafness, patent ductus arteriosus	+/−	+/−		4

*The numbers in parentheses refer to syndromes listed in this table which merit special consideration in the differential diagnosis.
†Syndrome is described in text; see index for location.

MISCELLANEOUS PATTERNS OF MALFORMATION (Continued)

F. DEAFNESS WITH ASSOCIATED DEFECTS: (Continued)

	CRANIOFACIAL	LIMBS	OTHER	MENTAL DEFIC.	SHORT STATURE	GENETIC TRANSMISSION	REFERENCE
75. Waardenburg's syndrome†	Lateral displacement of inner canthi and puncta		Partial albinism; white forelock, heterochromia of iris, vitiligo, +/− deafness			Aut. Dom.	2
76. Forney's syndrome		Fusion of some carpal and tarsal bones	Deafness (stapes defect), mitral insufficiency		+	? Aut. Dom.	4

G. NEUROLOGIC DISORDERS OTHER THAN MENTAL DEFICIENCY, WITH ASSOCIATED DEFECTS: [27, 28, 42, 45, 46, 105, 107, 111, 112, 116]

	NEUROLOGIC	OTHER	MENTAL DEFIC.	SHORT STATURE	GENETIC TRANSMISSION	REFERENCE
77. Ataxia-telangiectasia†	Development of ataxia	Telangiectasia, frequent upper respiratory tract infections		+	Aut. Rec.	4
78. Biemond's syndrome	Ataxia	Short 4th metacarpal			Aut. Dom.	10
79. Marinesco-Sjögren syndrome	Cerebellar ataxia, hypotonia	Cataracts, sparse hair	+	+	Aut. Rec.	34
80. Sjögren-Larsson syndrome	Spasticity, especially of legs	Ichthyosis	+	+	Aut. Rec.	2
81. Menkes's syndrome	Progressive cerebral deterioration with seizures	Twisted, fractured stubby hair	+	+	X-Linked Rec.	4

H. MUSCULAR DISORDERS WITH ASSOCIATED DEFECTS: [6, 42, 44, 45]

	CRANIOFACIAL	LIMB AND OTHER	MUSCLE DYSFUNCTION				
82. Prader-Willi syndrome (44, 98)*†	+/− Upward slant to palpebral fissures	Small hands and feet, obesity from late infancy, hypogenital-ism, diabetes mellitus	Hypotonia, especially in early infancy	+	+	?	4
83. Cerebro-hepato-renal syndrome (42, 84)*	High forehead, flat facies	Hepatomegaly, death in early infancy	Hypotonia	?+	+	? Aut. Rec.	35
84. Lowe's syndrome (oculo-cerebro-renal syndrome) (83)*†	Cataract	Renal tubular dysfunction	Hypotonia	+	+	X-Linked Rec.	36
85. Myotonic dystrophy of Steinert (86)*	Cataract	Hypogonadism	Myotonia with muscle atrophy	+/−		Aut. Dom.	12
86. Rieger's syndrome (85)*	Hypodontia, iris dysplasia		Myotonic dystrophy	+/−		Aut. Dom.	2
87. Freeman-Sheldon "whistling face" syndrome (88)*	Hypoplastic alae nasi	Club feet	Masklike "whistling face"	+/−	+/−	? Aut. Dom.	2
88. Schwartz's syndrome (87)*	Blepharophimosis	Joint limitation	Myotonia		+	? Aut. Rec.	5
89. Abdominal muscle deficiency syndrome		Renal and urinary tract dysplasia, cryptor-chidism	Abdominal muscle hypoplasia			?	18

*The numbers in parentheses refer to syndromes listed in this table which merit special consideration in the differential diagnosis.
†Syndrome is described in text; see index for location.

SYNDROMES

MISCELLANEOUS PATTERNS OF MALFORMATION (Continued)

H. MUSCULAR DISORDERS WITH ASSOCIATED DEFECTS (Continued)

	CRANIOFACIAL	LIMB AND OTHER	MUSCLE DYSFUNCTION	MENTAL DEFIC.	SHORT STATURE	GENETIC TRANS-MISSION	REFER-ENCE
90. Poland's syndrome	Unilateral syndactyly of hand	+/− Unilateral hypoplasia to absence of nipple	Unilateral absence of pectoralis minor			?	13

I. HEMATOPOETIC DISORDERS WITH ASSOCIATED DEFECTS: [28, 59, 74, 117]

	CRANIOFACIAL	LIMBS	OTHER	MENTAL DEFIC.	SHORT STATURE	GENETIC TRANS-MISSION	REFER-ENCE
91. Fanconi's syndrome of pancytopenia and multiple defects (92, 117)*†		Hypoplastic thumb and/or radius	Hyperpigmentation, development of pancytopenia	+/−	+	? Aut. Rec.	4
92. Radial aplasia-thrombocytopenia syndrome (91)*†		Radial aplasia	Thrombocytopenia with megakaryocytopenia, +/− cardiac defect			Aut. Rec.	44

J. OTHER DISORDERS:

	CRANIOFACIAL	LIMBS	OTHER	MENTAL DEFIC.	SHORT STATURE	GENETIC TRANS-MISSION	REFER-ENCE
93. Oro-facial-digital syndrome (94)*	Hypoplasia of alae nasi, oral frenula and clefts	Digital asymmetry		+/−		Dom. ? Lethal in male	2
94. Mieten's syndrome (93)*	Narrow nose, corneal opacity	Flexion contracture of elbow		+	+	? Aut. Rec.	31
95. Oculo-dento-digital syndrome	Narrow nose, microphthalmos, +/− glaucoma, enamel hypoplasia	Camptodactyly of 5th fingers				? Aut. Rec.	19

Syndrome						Inheritance	No.
96. **Holt-Oram syndrome (cardiac-limb syndrome)**		Upper limb defect, especially of thumb and radius	Cardiac septal defect, narrow shoulders			Aut. Dom.	17
97. **Turner-like syndrome (male Turner's syndrome, Noonan's syndrome, pseudo-Turner's syndrome) (52)*†**	Webbing of posterior neck		Pectus excavatum, cryptorchidism, pulmonic stenosis	+/−	+	?	4
98. **Laurence-Moon-Biedl syndrome (34, 44, 82)*†**	Retinal pigmentation	Polydactyly	Obesity	+	+/−	Aut. Rec.	9
99. **Smith-Lemli-Opitz syndrome (45)***	Anteverted nostrils and/or ptosis of eyelid	Syndactyly 2nd - 3rd toes	Hypospadias, cryptorchidism	+	+	? Aut. Rec.	4
100. **Fraser's syndrome**	Cryptophthalmos (lids fused), defect of auricle		Genital anomaly	+		? Aut. Rec.	16
101. **Cerebral gigantism†**		Large hands and feet	Large size in early life, poor coordination	+/−		?	24
102. **Hypercalcemia, peculiar facies, supravalvular aortic stenosis†**	Full lips, small nose with anteverted nostrils		+/− Hypercalcemia in infancy, supravalvular aortic stenosis	+	+	?	4

*The numbers in parentheses refer to syndromes listed in this table which merit special consideration in the differential diagnosis.
†Syndrome is described in text; see index for location.

SYNDROMES

MISCELLANEOUS PATTERNS OF MALFORMATION *(Continued)*

J. OTHER DISORDERS: *(Continued)*

	CRANIOFACIAL	LIMBS	OTHER	MENTAL DEFIC.	SHORT STATURE	GENETIC TRANS-MISSION	REFER-ENCE
103. Leprechaunism (Donohue's syndrome)	Full lips		Adipose deficiency, extreme growth deficiency with large hands and feet, enlarged phallus, hirsutism, especially face	?	+	Aut. Rec.	4
104. Berardinelli's lipodystrophy			Tall stature and muscle hypertrophy, phallic hypertrophy, lipoatrophy, hepatomegaly and hyperlipemia	+/−		Aut. Rec.	43

HAMARTOSES

The HAMARTOSES are a group of diseases in which there is an organizational defect leading to abnormal admixture of tissues, often with a tumor-like excess of one or more tissues. Included are hemangiomas, melanomas, including altered skin pigmentation, fibromas, lipomas, adenomas, and some strange admixtures which create nosological confusion such as the "adenoma sebaceum"—which are not derived from sebaceous glands—in tuberous sclerosis. Certain hamartomatous lesions are liable to grow locally or metastasize, a low-risk phenomenon in some of these diseases such as the Peutz-Jeghers syndrome, but a major risk in others such as Gardner's syndrome. Altered morphogenesis other than hamartoma occurs in some of these conditions, notably the altered facies of the basal cell nevus syndrome and syndactyly in Goltz's syndrome.

DIAGNOSTIC MANIFESTATIONS

SYNDROME	CRANIOFACIAL	SKELETAL	OTHER	MENTAL DEFIC.	SHORT STATURE	GENETIC TRANS-MISSION	REFER-ENCE
105. Sturge-Weber syndrome†	Flat hemangioma of face, most commonly trigeminal in distribution		Hemangiomas of meninges with seizures	+/−		?	2

Syndrome					Inheritance	
106. Maffucci's syndrome		Enchondromatosis	Cavernous hemangiomas		?	7
107. Von Hippel-Lindau syndrome†	Retinal angiomas		Cerebellar hemangioblastoma		Aut. Dom.	1
108. Riley's syndrome†	Macrocephaly, pseudopapilledema		Cutaneous hemangiomas		? Aut. Dom.	37
109. Gardner's syndrome (110)*†		Osteomas	Polyposis of colon, fibromatous growths in scars, epidermal cysts		Aut. Dom.	50
110. Peutz-Jeghers syndrome (109)*†	Mucocutaneous spotty pigmentation, especially lips		Intestinal polyposis		Aut. Dom.	1, 2
111. Tuberous sclerosis (adenoma sebaceum)*†	Hamartomatous pink to brownish facial skin nodules	+/− Bone lesions	Seizures	+/−	Aut. Dom.	1, 2
112. Neurofibromatosis†		+/− Bone lesions	Neurofibromata, café-au-lait spots		Aut. Dom.	1, 2
113. Basal cell nevus syndrome†	Broad facies	Rib anomalies	Basal cell cutaneous nevi	+	Aut. Dom.	2
114. McCune-Albright syndrome†		Polyostotic fibrous dysplasia	Irregular skin pigmentation, sexual precocity, female		?	2

*The numbers in parentheses refer to syndromes listed in this table which merit special consideration in the differential diagnosis.
†Syndrome is described in text; see index for location.

SYNDROMES

HAMARTOSES *(Continued)*

SYNDROME	DIAGNOSTIC MANIFESTATIONS			MENTAL DEFIC.	SHORT STATURE	GENETIC TRANSMISSION	REFERENCE
	CRANIOFACIAL	SKELETAL	OTHER				
115. Goltz's syndrome (focal dermal hypoplasia), mainly female (65)*	Dental anomalies	Cutaneous syndactyly	Poikiloderma with focal dermal hypoplasia		+/-	Dom.	23
116. Incontinentia pigmenti, mainly in female†	+/- Dental defect		Irregular skin pigmentation in fleck, whorl or spidery form, +/- patchy alopecia	+/-		Dom.	1, 2
117. Dyskeratosis congenita syndrome (91)*		Nail dystrophy	Hyperpigmentation, leukoplakia, development of pancytopenia, +/- hemangiomas		+/-	? Aut. Rec.	1, 2

ECTODERMAL DYSPLASIAS

The ECTODERMAL DYSPLASIAS, so categorized because the abnormal tissues were predominantly derived from embryonic ectoderm, include hypoplasia of skin and its derivatives plus defects of nails, teeth and lens or sensorineural deafness. The most common type is anhidrotic ectodermal dysplasia. The other types are called hidrotic ectodermal dysplasias since they do not have serious defects in sweating.

SYNDROME	DIAGNOSTIC MANIFESTATIONS			MENTAL DEFIC.	SHORT STATURE	GENETIC TRANSMISSION	REFERENCE
	FACIAL	NAILS	OTHER				
118. Anhidrotic ectodermal dysplasia†	Peg-shaped teeth, partial anodontia, midfacial hypoplasia		Hypoplasia to aplasia of sweat glands, hyperthermia, alopecia			X-Linked	2

HIDROTIC ECTODERMAL DYSPLASIAS (see p. 1387)

119. Marshall type	Cataract, midfacial hypoplasia		Deafness		Aut. Dom.	2
120. Robinson type (121)*	Peg-shaped teeth	Hypoplastic nails	Deafness		Aut. Dom.	4
121. Feinmesser type (120)*		Rudimentary nails	Deafness		? Aut. Rec.	15
122. Pili torti and deafness			Deafness; hair twisted, fine, and short		? Aut. Rec.	39
123. Enamel hypoplasia and curly hair	Enamel hypoplasia	+/− Nail dystrophy	Hair thick and curly		Aut. Dom.	40
124. Clouston type		Nail dystrophy	Dyskeratotic thick palms and soles	+/−	Aut. Dom.	47
125. Basan type		Thin, fragile nails	Smooth palms and soles		Aut. Dom.	8

*The numbers in parentheses refer to syndromes listed in this table which merit special consideration in the differential diagnosis.
†Syndrome is described in text; see index for location.

DAVID W. SMITH

SYNDROMES

REFERENCES

General

1. Butterworth, T., and Strean, L. P.: *Clinical Genodermatology.* Baltimore, Williams & Wilkins Company, 1962.
2. Gorlin, R. J., and Pindborg, J. J.: *Syndromes of the Head and Neck.* New York, McGraw-Hill Book Company, Inc., 1964.
3. McKusick, V. A.: *Heritable Disorders of Connective Tissue.* 3rd ed. St. Louis, C. V. Mosby Company, 1966.
4. Smith, D. W.: The Compendium on Shortness of Stature. *J. Pediat.,* 70:463, 1967.

Specific Disorders (as numbered in the table)

5. Aberfeld, D. C., Hinterbuchner, L. P., and Schneider, M.: Myotonia, Dwarfism, Diffuse Bone Disease and Unusual Ocular and Facial Abnormalities (a New Syndrome). *Brain,* 88:313, 1965.
6. Al-Aish, M. S., and others: Autosomal Monosomy in Man. *New England J. Med.,* 277:777, 1967.
7. Anderson, I. F.: Maffuci's Syndrome. Report of a Case with a Review of the Literature. *S. Afr. Med. J.,* 39:1066, 1965.
8. Basan, M.: Ektodermale Dysplasie. Fehlendes Papillarmuster, Nagelveränderungen und Vierfingerfurche. *Arch. klin. exp. Derm.,* 222:546, 1965.
9. Bell, J.: The Laurence-Moon Syndrome; in L. S. Penrose (Ed.): *The Treasury of Human Inheritance.* London, Cambridge University Press, 1958, Vol. 5, Part 3.
10. Biemond, A.: Brachydactylie, nystagmus en cerebellaire ataxie als familiair syndroom. *Nederl. T. Geneesk.,* 78:1423, 1934.
11. Brody, J., Fitzgerald, M. G., and Spiers, A. S.: A Female Child with Five X Chromosomes. *J. Pediat.,* 70:105, 1967.
12. Caughey, J. E., and Myrianthopoulos, N. C.: *Dystrophia Myotonica and Related Disorders.* Springfield, Ill., Charles C Thomas, 1963.
13. Clarkson, P.: Poland's Syndactyly. *Guy's Hosp. Rep.,* 111:335, 1962.
14. Dudding, B. A., Gorlin, R. J., and Langer, L. O.: The Otopalato-digital Syndrome. A New Symptom-Complex Consisting of Deafness, Dwarfism, Cleft Palate, Characteristic Facies, and a Generalized Bone Dysplasia. *Am. J. Dis. Child.,* 113:214, 1967.
15. Feinmesser, M., and Zelig, S.: Congenital Deafness Associated with Onychodystrophy. *Arch. Otolaryng.,* 74:507, 1961.
16. François, J.: Syndrome malformatif avec cryptophthalmie. (Note préliminaire.) *Ophthalmologica,* 150:215, 1965.
17. Gall, J. C., Stern, A. M., Cohen, M. M., Adams, M. S., and Davidson, R. T.: Holt-Oram Syndrome: Clinical and Genetic Study of a Large Family. *Am. J. Hum. Genet.,* 18:187, 1966.
18. Gellis, S. S., and Feingold, M.: Congenital Absence of Abdominal Musculature (Prune Belly). *Am. J. Dis. Child.,* 109:571, 1965.
19. Gorlin, R. J., Meskin, L. H., and St. Geme, J. W.: Oculodento-digital Dysplasia. *J. Pediat.,* 63:69, 1963.
20. Hecht, F., and Jarvinen, J. M.: Heritable Dysmorphic Syndrome with Normal Intelligence. *J. Pediat.,* 70:927, 1967.
21. Herdman, R. C., and Langer, L. O.: Thoracic Asphyxiant Dystrophy and Renal Disease. *Am. J. Dis. Child.,* 116:192, 1968.
22. Hirschorn, K., Cooper, H. L., and Firschein, I. L.: Deletion of Short Arms of Chromosome 4-5 in a Child with Defects of Midline Fusion. *Humangenetik,* 1:479, 1965.
23. Holden, J. D., and Akers, W. A.: Golt's Syndrome: Focal Dermal Hypoplasia. A Combined Mesoectodermal Dysplasia. *Am. J. Dis. Child.,* 114:292, 1967.
24. Hook, E. B., and Reynolds, J. W.: Cerebral Gigantism: Endocrinological and Clinical Observations of Six Patients, Including a Congenital Giant, Concordant Monozygotic Twins, and a Child Who Achieved Adult Gigantic Size. *J. Pediat.,* 70:900, 1967.
25. Insley, J.: Syndrome Associated with Deficiency of Part of the Long Arm of Chromosome No. 18. *Arch. Dis. Childhood,* 42:140, 1967.
26. Johnson, C. C.: Surgical Repair of the Syndrome of Epicanthus Inversus, Blepharophimosis and Ptosis. *Arch. Ophthal.,* 71:510, 1964.
27. Larsen, L. J., Schottstaedt, E. R., and Bost, F. C.: Multiple Congenital Dislocations Associated with Characteristic Facial Abnormality. *J. Pediat.,* 37:574, 1950.
28. Lucas, G. L., and Opitz, J. M.: The Nail-Patella Syndrome. Clinical and Genetic Aspects of 5 Kindreds with 38 Affected Family Members, *J. Pediat.,* 68:273, 1966.
29. Maroteaux, V. P., Spranger, J., and Wiedemann, H. R.: Der metatropische Zwergwuchs. *Arch. f. Kinderheilk.,* 173:212, 1966.
30. McKusick, V. A., and Milch, R. A.: The Clinical Behavior of Genetic Disease: Selected Aspects. *Clin. Orthop.,* 33:22, 1964.
31. Mietens, C., and Weber, H.: A Syndrome Characterized by Corneal Opacity, Nystagmus, Flexion Contracture of the Elbows, Growth Failure, and Mental Retardation. *J. Pediat.,* 69:624, 1966.
32. Milunsky, A., Graef, J. W., and Gaynor, M. F., Jr.: Methotrexate Induced Congenital Malformations, with a Review of the Literature. *J. Pediat.,* 72:790, 1968.
33. Moore, W. T., and Federman, D. D.: Familial Dwarfism and "Stiff Joints." Report of a Kindred. *Arch. Int. Med.,* 115:398, 1965.
34. Norwood, W. F., Jr.: Marinesco-Sjögren Syndrome. *J. Pediat.,* 64:478, 1964.
35. Passarge, E., and McAdams, A. J.: Cerebro-hepato-renal Syndrome. *J. Pediat.,* 71:691, 1967.
36. Richards, W., Donnell, G. N., Wilson, W. A., Stowens, D., and Perry, T.: The Oculo-cerebro-renal Syndrome of Lowe. *Am. J. Dis. Child.,* 109:185, 1965.
37. Riley, H. D., and Smith, W. R.: Macrocephaly, Pseudopapilledema and Multiple Hemangiomata. A Previously Undescribed Heredofamilial Syndrome. *Pediatrics,* 26:293, 1960.
38. Rimoin, D. L., and Edgerton, M. T.: Genetic and Clinical Heterogeneity in the Oral-Facial-Digital Syndrome. *J. Pediat.,* 71:94, 1967.
39. Robinson, G. C., and Johnston, M. M.: Pili Torti and Sensory Neural Deafness. *J. Pediat.,* 70:621, 1967.
40. Robinson, G. C., Miller, J. R., and Worth, H. M.: Hereditary Enamel Hypoplasia: Its Association with Characteristic Hair Structure. *Pediatrics,* 37:498, 1966.
41. Schachenmann, G., and others: Chromosomes in Coloboma and Anal Atresia. *Lancet,* 2:290, 1965.
42. Scott, C. R., Laganoff, D., and Trump, B. F.: Familial Neurovisceral Lipidosis. *J. Pediat.,* 71:357, 1967.
43. Senior, B., and Gellis, S. S.: The Syndromes of Total Lipodystrophy and of Partial Lipodystrophy. *Pediatrics,* 33:593, 1964.
44. Shaw, S., and Oliver, R. A. M.: Congenital Hypoplastic Thrombocytopenia and Skeletal Deformities in Siblings. *Blood,* 14:374, 1959.
45. Smith, D. W.: Autosomal Abnormalities. *Am. J. Obst. & Gynec.,* 90(Suppl.):1055, 1964.
46. Stanesco, V., and others: Syndrome héreditaire dominant, etc. *Rev. franç. Endocr. Clin.,* 4:219, 1963.
47. Stevenson, G. H.: A Family with Inherited Ectodermal Dystrophy. *Canad. M.A.J.,* 53:226, 1945.
48. Stickler, G. B., and Pugh, D. G.: Hereditary Progressive Arthro-ophthalmopathy. *Mayo Clin. Proc.,* 42:495, 1967.
49. Temtamy, S. A.: Carpenter's Syndrome: Acrocephalopolysyndactyly. An Autosomal Recessive Syndrome. *J. Pediat.,* 69:111, 1966.
50. Weary, P. E., Linthicum, A., Cawley, E. P., Coleman, C. C., and Graham, G. F.: Gardner's Syndrome. A Family Group Study and Review. *Arch. Derm.,* 90:20, 1964.

S
Y
N
D
R
O
M
E
S

NORMAL BLOOD VALUES

TABLE 29-1. CHEMICAL CONSTITUENTS OF BLOOD

ACID-BASE CONSTITUENTS

Total fixed cations (Na + K + Ca + Mg)   (serum)...................150–155 mEq./liter
   By methods of Hald and Sunderman, normal
   values tend to be lower..143–150 mEq./liter
Sodium*   (serum)...................136–143 mEq./liter
Potassium*   (serum)...................4.1–5.6 mEq./liter
Calcium*   (serum)...................10–12 mg./100 ml.
     5–6 mEq./liter
Calcium,* diffusible (ionized Ca)   (serum)...................5–5.5 mg./100 ml.
Magnesium*   (serum)...................2–3 mg./100 ml.
   In the newborn a value as low as 1.3 mEq./liter   1.65–2.5 mEq./liter
   would be considered normal
Chlorides* (Cl)   (serum)...................98–106 mEq./liter
   At birth and during early infancy the plasma
   (serum) chloride is 6–10 m.Eq./liter higher than
   that of older infants and children..585–620 mg./100 ml.

Phosphorus, inorganic, as P   (serum)...................4.0–6.5 mg./100 ml.
   Slightly higher in the newborn (in infants, up
   to 8 mg./100 ml. considered normal)..1.29–2.1 mM./liter
$HPO_4^{--}/H_2PO_4^-$ (average valence 1.8 at pH 7.4)............................2.3–3.8 mEq./liter
Serum protein cation-binding power   (serum)...................15.5–18.0 mEq./liter
Bicarbonate cation-binding power   (serum)...................19–30 mEq./liter
   The above two constitute a major portion of the
   buffer base (Hastings and Singer) of serum
Standard bicarbonate (Astrup)†   (plasma)...................21–25 mEq./liter
Buffer base [BB]$_b$ (blood) ....46–52 mEq./liter
Base excess [BE]$_b$ (blood) ....–2.3 to +2.3 mEq./liter
Sulfates, inorganic, as SO_4^{--} (serum)...................0.5–1.0 mEq./liter
     2.5–5.0 mg./100 ml.
Sulfates, ethereal   (serum)...................0.1–1.0 mg./100 ml.
Sulfur, neutral   (serum)...................1.7–3.5 mg./100 ml.
Lactic acid   (serum)...................10–20 mg./100 ml.
pH at 38° C.   (blood, plasma or
     serum).................7.3–7.45

   The sample must be protected against loss of
CO_2 and determination made as soon as possible. Arterial blood in a resting person is about
0.03 pH unit higher than venous blood.

pH at 38° C.   (serum from arterial
     blood)

(Data from Cassels and Morse)
   1.5– 3.4 years..7.30–7.40
   3.5– 5.4 years..7.35–7.43
   5.5–12.4 years...7.37–7.43
   12.5–17.4 years...7.35–7.41

---

* In human red blood cells an average concentration of sodium would be about 21 mEq./liter of red blood cells; of potassium about 86 mEq./liter.
   The level of calcium in serum is influenced by the concentration of serum protein because part of the calcium is associated with or bound to the protein. Practically all the calcium in blood is in the plasma.
   The chloride concentration of whole blood depends largely on the cell volume, since the erythrocyte contains approximately half as much chloride as serum.
   † Concentration of bicarbonate in plasma which is separated from the cells with the hemoglobin completely oxygenated, at a $pCO_2 = 40$ mm. Hg and at a temperature of 38° C.

APPENDIX

TABLE 29-1. *(Continued)*

ACID BASE CONSTITUENTS

Carbon dioxide content	(serum from venous blood) ....45–70 vol. per cent
	20.3–31.5 mM./liter

The CO_2 content is lower at birth and rises slightly during the first 4 days of life

Carbon dioxide content	(whole venous blood) 40–60 vol. per cent
	18–27 mM./liter
Carbon dioxide content	(arterial blood)
(Data from Cassels and Morse)	
1.5– 3.4 years..15.5–20.5 mM./liter
3.5– 6.4 years..18.7–21.2 mM./liter
6.5–11.4 years..19.3–21.6 mM./liter
11.5–14.4 years..19.9–22.2 mM./liter
14.5–17.4 years..20.4–22.4 mM./liter
Carbon dioxide tension	(arterial blood)
(Data from Cassels and Morse)	
1.5– 6.4 years..33.5–41.1 mm. Hg
6.5–12.4 years..35.4–40.6 mm. Hg
12.5–17.4 years..38.3–44.4 mm. Hg
Oxygen tension P_{O_2}	(arterial blood).........85–100 mm. Hg
Oxygen capacity*	(whole blood)...........19–22 vol. per cent
Oxygen saturation	(whole venous blood) 60–85 per cent
Blood of newborn ....30–80 per cent
Hemoglobin	
At birth	(whole blood)...........17–20 gm./100 ml.
3 months..10.5–12 gm./100 ml.
1 year..11–12.5 gm./100 ml.
5 years..12–13 gm./100 ml.
10 years..13–14 gm./100 ml.
Above 10 years ....14–16 gm./100 ml.
Methemoglobin	(whole blood)...........0.0–0.3 gm./100 ml.
Premature infants at higher level ....(0.4)
Carbon monoxide hemoglobin	(whole blood)...........up to 5% of total hemoglobin
Haptoglobin	(serum)..................40–170 mg. % as hemoglobin-binding capacity
Water	(whole blood)...........79–81 gm./100 ml.
	(serum)..................91–92 gm./100 ml.
	(red blood cells)........64–65 gm./100 ml.

* The oxygen capacity and iron content of blood are directly related to the hemoglobin content of the blood (1.335 ml. O_2/gm. of hemoglobin).

CARBOHYDRATES, LIPIDS AND PIGMENTS

Sugar, fasting	
(Somogyi-Nelson)	(blood) ....60–90 mg./100 ml.
Under fasting conditions capillary or arterial blood and venous blood are nearly the same	
Sugar, fasting arterial (Folin-Wu)	(blood) ....80–120 mg./100 ml.
fasting venous (Folin-Wu)	(blood) ....70–100 mg./100 ml.
Lactic acid. See *Acid-Base Constituents*	
Pyruvic acid, fasting	(blood) ....0.7–1.2 mg./100 ml.
Citric acid	(blood) ....1.3–2.3 mg./100 ml.
Citric acid	(plasma)..................1.6–2.7 mg./100 ml.
α-Ketoglutaric acid	(blood) ....8–10 mg./100 ml.
Acetone bodies (as acetone)	(serum)..................1–6 mg./100 ml.
Total cholesterol (over 6 yr.)	(serum)..................150–250 mg./100 ml.
Infants..70–125 mg./100 ml.
Newborn..50–100 mg./100 ml.
Cholesterol esters..125–180 mg./100 ml.
17-Hydroxycorticosteroids	(plasma)..................10–13.5 microgm./100 ml.
Total lipids	
(Rafsted) 2–14 years	(serum)..................490–1000 mg./100 ml.
3 days–1 year..240–800 mg./100 ml.

TABLE 29-1. *(Continued)*

CARBOHYDRATES, LIPIDS AND PIGMENTS

3 days–10 days		430–760 mg./100 ml.
Newborn		170–450 mg./100 ml.
Free fatty acids	(serum)	230–380 microgm./ml.
More variable in young children		
Phosphatides (lipid P × 25)	(plasma)	
Children		180–295 mg./100 ml.
Up to 1 year		100–275 mg./100 ml.
Newborn		75–170 mg./100 ml.
Bilirubin (total)	(serum)	0.2–0.8 mg./100 ml.
Higher in newborn		1.0 or more
Conjugated bilirubin (direct)		0–0.3 mg./100 ml.
Icterus index		4–6 units

PROTEINS

Total protein (from nitrogen determination) (serum)................6.5–7.5 gm./100 ml.
  At birth the protein is slightly lower
Albumin* [globulins precipitated by Na_2SO_4-Na_2SO_3
  mixture (20.8% Na_2SO_4 + 7.0% Na_2SO_3)] (serum)................3.9–4.5 gm./100 ml.
Globulins (by difference) ....2.3–3.5 gm./100 ml.
  A/G ratio ....1.2–1.9 gm./100 ml.
Protein values vary slightly with age. The follow-
  ing values for plasma are adapted from the
  paper of Metcoff and Stare (*New England J.
  Med.*, 1947)
Total protein (plasma)
  Premature infant ....4.55 ± 0.59 gm./100 ml.
  Full-term infant ....5.11–5.70 gm./100 ml.
  Birth to 1 year ....6.10 ± 0.29 gm./100 ml.
  1–4 years ....6.94 ± 0.47 gm./100 ml.
  5–12 years ....7.30 ± 0.59 gm./100 ml.
  12 years and above ....7.16 gm./100 ml.
Albumin (plasma) (globulin precipitation by 22% Na_2SO_4; Howe)
  Premature infant ....3.55 ± 0.65 gm./100 ml.
  Full-term infant ....3.76–3.79 gm./100 ml.
  Birth to 1 year ....4.97 ± 0.73 gm./100 ml.
  1–4 years ....4.59–4.83 gm./100 ml.
  5–12 years ....5.0 ± 0.78 gm./100 ml.
  12–15 years ....4.72 gm./100 ml.
Globulin (plasma)
  Premature infant ....1.01 ± 0.45 gm./100 ml.
  Full-term infant ....1.34–1.66 gm./100 ml.
  Birth to 1 year ....1.38 ± 0.68 gm./100 ml.
  1–4 years ....2.03 ± 0.34 gm./100 ml.
  5–12 years ....2.4 ± 0.74 gm./100 ml.
  12–15 years ....2.49 gm./100 ml.
Fibrinogen (plasma)................0.2–0.4 gm./100 ml.
Gamma globulin ....10–15% of total protein
                              0.7–1.2 gm./100 ml.
  At birth values approximate adult levels, owing to passive transfer from the mother; during the ensuing weeks
  there is a decrease, the "low point" being reached between the second and fourth months. After this there is a
  gradual increase to the "adult level" by about the second year of life.
Ceruloplasmin (serum)................16–33 mg./100 ml.
Mucoprotein (serum)................45–105 mg./100 ml.
Mucoprotein tyrosine (serum)................2–4.5 mg./100 ml.
Serum protein partition by paper electrophoresis (Durrum)
  % of total protein
  Albumin 50–60%
  α_1-globulin 5–8%
  α_2-globulin 8–13%
  β-globulin 11–17%
  γ-globulin 15–25%

---

*When the globulin is precipitated with the Na_2SO_4-Na_2SO_3 mixture, the albumin values agree with those obtained by electrophoresis.

TABLE 29-1. *(Continued)*

NITROGEN CONSTITUENTS

Nonprotein nitrogen	(whole blood)............25–40 mg./100 ml.	
(Tungstic acid filtrate; zinc hydroxide filtrates give lower values because more small molecule nitrogenous compounds are precipitated)	(plasma)..................18–30 mg./100 ml.	
Urea nitrogen	(whole blood)...........7–15 mg./100 ml.	
	(plasma)..................10–17 mg./100 ml.	
Creatinine	(serum)...................0.4–1.2 mg./100 ml.	
Absorption by Lloyd's reagent	(whole blood)...........0.5–2.0 mg./100 ml.	
Creatine + creatinine	(whole blood)...........5–8 mg./100 ml.	
Concentration of creatine is low in plasma		
Uric acid	(serum)...................2–6 mg./100 ml.	
At birth the uric acid concentration of the blood of the infant is identical with that of the mother		
Ammonia	(whole blood)...........0.1–0.3 mg./100 ml.	
Amino acid nitrogen	(plasma)..................3.5–5.5 mg./100 ml.	
Serum gives slightly lower value than plasma		
Phenylalanine	(serum)...................0.7–4.0 mg./100 ml.	
Proline (fasting)	(plasma)..................13.8–32.5 microgm./liter	
Glutamine	(plasma)..................6–12 mg./100 ml.	
Citrulline	(plasma)..................0.3–1 mg./100 ml.	

ENZYMES

Amylase	(plasma or serum).....70–200 Somogyi units
	6–33 Close-Street units
Aldolase	(serum)...................0.15–0.8 units (micromoles of fructose diphosphate split/per ml. serum/hour)
Alkaline phosphatase	
Infants	(serum)...................5–10 Bodansky units
Children (2–15 years)...3–13 Bodansky units	
The values by the Shinowara Jones and Reinhardt method are about ⅓ higher, owing to incubation at pH 9.3 instead of 8.6	
Infants...4–14 Bessey-Lowry-Brock units (substrate p-nitrophenol-phosphate) (Sigma units)	
Children ....3.4–9 B.L.B. units	
Children ....10–20 King-Armstrong units (Substrate disodium phenyl-phosphate)	
Infants...3.8–11 Klein-Babson-Reed units	
Children ....2–15 (Substrate buffered sodium phenolphthalein phosphate); 1 unit of activity liberates 1.0 mg. phenolphthalein in 30 minutes at 37° C.	
Phosphatase, acid	(serum)...................1–5 King-Armstrong units
Creatine phosphokinase (CPK)	(serum)...................to −0.72 milliunits (Bergmeyer)
Lactic acid dehydrogenase (Snodgrass method)	(serum)...................30–120 units
Copper oxidase (Ravin method) (ceruloplasmin)	(serum)...................0.14–0.57 O.D. units
Lipase	(serum)...................< 1 unit/ml. Sigma-Tietz unit (ml. of 0.05 N NaOH to neutralize free fatty acid during 6-hr. incubation period)
Transaminase (children)	(serum-glutamate-oxalacetate)
SGO, spectrophotometric method ....4–40 units (higher in infants)	
Serum glutamate pyruvate ....1–45 units	

MISCELLANEOUS

Ascorbic acid	(serum)...................0.4–1.5 mg./100 ml.
Vitamin A	(serum)...................15–60 microgm./100 ml.
Carotenoids	(serum)...................40–400 microgm./100 ml.
Iron...0.04–0.18 mg./100 ml.	

TABLE 29-1. *(Continued)*

MISCELLANEOUS

Iron-binding capacity	(serum)	0.187–0.65 mg./100 ml.
Transferrin	(serum)	0.2–0.3 gm./100 ml.
Copper	(serum)	0.08–0.235 mg./100 ml.
Lead	(serum)	0.001–0.003 mg./100 ml.
Lead	(blood)	0.01–0.06 mg./100 ml.
Bromine	(serum)	0.7–1 microgm./100 ml.
Iodine, protein-bound	(serum)	0.003–0.008 mg./100 ml.
Iodine, butanol extractable		0.003–0.0065 mg./100 ml.
Potassium	(erythrocytes)	86–104 mEq./liter of red blood cells
Thiamine	(blood)	5.5–9.5 microgm./100 ml.
Tocopherols	(serum)	0.6–1.2 mg./100 ml.

Lower in the newborn

PHYSICAL MEASUREMENTS

Specific gravity (whole blood) 1.048–1.05
Newborn infants: falls rapidly during first 2
weeks and continues to decrease until second
or third year (plasma) 1.025–1.03
Prothrombin time (Quick) (plasma) 12–15 seconds
This determination should always be controlled by a determination on a normal blood,
since the activity of the thromboplastin preparations may vary greatly

Bleeding time 1–3 minutes
Coagulation time (test tube method) 3–9 minutes
Cephalin flocculation (serum) 0–1+ units
During first 6 months of life this test may be
negative in the presence of liver disease
Thymol turbidity (serum) 0–4 Maclagan units
Zinc sulfate turbidity (serum) 2–8 Maclagan units
Viscosity, compared to water as unity (whole blood) 4.5–5.5
(serum) 1.7–2.1

Corrected erythrocyte sedimentation rate
(Rourke-Ernstene) 0.1–0.35 mm./min.
Cutler method 2–10 mm./hr.
The rate is slower in the neonatal period
Freezing point depression (serum) −0.535°–(−0.555°) C.
Osmolality (plasma) 270–285 milliosmoles/liter plasma water
Refractive index, 20° C. 1.3485–1.3505

Whole blood specific gravity (newborn): 1.06–1.085

NORMAL CEREBROSPINAL FLUID VALUES

TABLE 29-2.

Amount in the newborn	Up to 5 ml.
Increases with age to adult figure	100–150 ml.
Initial pressure	70–200 mm. H_2O
Cell count	
Under 1 year	Up to 10 cells/mm.³
1–4 years	Up to 8 cells/mm.³
5 years to puberty	0–5 cells/mm.³
Specific gravity	1.005–1.009
Freezing point depression	−0.56–(−0.60)°C.
Refractive index at 20°C.	1.33554
pH 38°C. (protected against loss of CO_2)	7.33–7.42
Fluid exposed to air becomes alkaline	
Carbon dioxide-combining power	40–70 vol. per cent
	18–31 m.Eq./liter
Chloride	
7 days–3 months	108.8–122.5 mEq./liter
4–12 months	112.7–128.5 mEq./liter
13 months–12 years	116.8–130.5 mEq./liter
Cholesterol	Trace–0.22 mg./100 ml.
Glucose, 6 months–10 years	71–90 mg./100 ml.
over 10 years	50–80 mg./100 ml.
The glucose level is less than, and varies proportionally with, the rise and fall of the plasma glucose level	
Total fixed cations	About 155 mEq./liter
Sodium	130–165 mEq./liter
Potassium	2.8–4.1 mEq./liter
Calcium	4.5–5.5 mg./100 ml.
Magnesium	2.8–3.3 mg./100 ml.
Phosphorus, inorganic	1.5–3.0 mg./100 ml.
3 mg. first day of life	
Lactic acid	Trace
Fluid on standing may increase in concentration with disappearance of glucose	
Protein	15–40 mg./100 ml.
The ventricular fluid contains much less protein than does lumbar fluid. Fluid from the cisterna magna contains more protein than that from the ventricle and less than that from lumbar region. The range is greater in the newborn and during the first month of life (20–120 mg./100 ml.)	
Albumin	80% of total protein
Globulin	20% of total protein
Fibrinogen	None
Pandy reaction	No precipitate
Urea nitrogen	7–15 mg./100 ml.
Nonprotein nitrogen	8.5–20 mg./100 ml.
Creatinine	0.45–1.9 mg./100 ml.
Uric acid	0.3–1.5 mg./100 ml.
Amino acid nitrogen	1.5–3 mg./100 ml.
Ammonia nitrogen	0–0.015 mg./100 ml.
Bilirubin	None
Iodine	Trace
Transaminase (GOT)	2–20 units (about ½ the value of SGOT)
Colloidal gold number (Wuth and Faupel)	0000000000
Dilutions 1–10 to 1–5120 with 0.4% NaCl solution	

CONVERSION TABLES

TABLE 29-3. METHOD FOR CONVERSION OF
MILLIGRAMS TO MILLIEQUIVALENTS PER LITER

mg. = milligrams
gm. = grams
ml. = milliliter
1 ml. = 1.000027 cc.
mEq./liter (milliequivalents per liter) =

$$\frac{\text{mg. per liter}}{\text{equivalent weight}}$$

$$\text{equivalent weight} = \frac{\text{atomic weight}}{\text{valence of element}}$$

For example: A sample of blood serum contains 10 mg.
of Ca in 100 ml. The valence of Ca is 2, and the atomic
weight is 40. The equivalent weight of Ca is therefore
40 ÷ 2, or 20. The milliequivalents of Ca per liter are
10 × 10 ÷ 20, or 5 milliequivalents per liter.

$$\text{mM./liter (millimoles per liter)} = \frac{\text{mg./liter}}{\text{molecular weight}}$$

Vol. % (volumes per cent) = mM./liter × 2.24 for a gas
whose properties approach that of an ideal gas, such
as oxygen or nitrogen.

For carbon dioxide the factor is 2.226.

TABLE 29-4. FACTORS FOR CONVERSION OF
CONCENTRATION EXPRESSED IN MILLEQUIVALENTS
PER LITER TO MILLIGRAMS PER 100 MILLILITERS,
AND VICE VERSA, FOR COMMON IONS THAT
OCCUR IN PHYSIOLOGIC SOLUTIONS.

ELEMENT OR RADICAL	mEQ. PER LITER	MG. PER 100 ML.	MG. PER 100 ML.	mEQ. PER LITER
Sodium	1	2.30	1	0.4348
Potassium	1	3.91	1	0.2558
Calcium	1	2.005	1	0.4988
Magnesium	1	1.215	1	0.8230
Chloride	1	3.55	1	0.2817
Bicarbonate (HCO₃)	1	6.1	1	0.1639
Phosphorus valence 1	1	3.10	1	0.3226
Phosphorus valence 1.8	1	1.72	1	0.5814
Sulfur valence 2	1	1.60	1	0.625

Example: To convert milliequivalents of magnesium
per liter to milligrams per 100 milliliters, multiply by
the factor 1.215.

To convert milligrams of potassium per 100 milliliters
to milliequivalents per liter, multiply by the factor
0.2558.

TABLE 29-5. Milliequivalents and Milligrams of Cations and Anions Present in a Millimole of Salts Commonly Used in Physiologic Solutions

SALT	MM. PER LITER	MG. PER LITER	CATION	ANION	mEq. CATION PER LITER	MG. CATION PER LITER	mEq. ANION PER LITER	MG. ANION PER LITER
Sodium chloride (NaCl)............	1	58.5	Na^+	Cl^-	1	23.0	1	35.5
Potassium chloride (KCl)...........	1	74.6	K^+	Cl^-	1	39.1	1	35.5
Sodium bicarbonate ($NaHCO_3$).....	1	84.0	Na^+	HCO_3^-	1	23.0	1	61.0
Sodium lactate ($CH_3CHOHCOONa$).	1	112.0	Na^+	Lactate$^-$	1	23.0	1	89.0
Potassium phosphate (K_2HPO_4) dibasic......................	1	174.2	K^+	HPO_4^{--}	2	78.2	1	96.0
Potassium phosphate (KH_2PO_4) monobasic....................	1	136.1	K^+	$H_2PO_4^-$	1	39.1	1	97.0
Calcium chloride anhydrous ($CaCl_2$).	1	111.0	Ca^{++}	Cl^-	2	40.0	2	71.0
Calcium chloride dihydrate ($CaCl_2.2H_2O$).................	1	147.0	Ca^{++}	Cl^-	2	40.0	2	71.0
Magnesium chloride anhydrous ($MgCl_2$).................	1	95.2	Mg^{++}	Cl^-	2	24.3	2	71.0
Magnesium chloride hexahydrate ($MgCl_2.6H_2O$).............	1	203.3	Mg^{++}	Cl^-	2	24.3	2	71.0
Ammonium chloride (NH_4Cl).......	1	53.5	NH_4^+	Cl^-	1	18.0	1	35.5

Milliosmolal and Milliosmolar Solutions. The total osmotic pressure of a solution is dependent on the number of particles in the solution, regardless of their charge, size or shape. In an ideal solution one mole of an ideal substance, assumed to be a nonelectrolyte, dissolved in a kilogram of water will lower the freezing point of the solvent (water) $-1.8557°$ C. Such a solution would have 1 osmole in a kilogram of water. One milliosmole is equal to one-thousandth of an osmole. The osmometer used in the clinical laboratory measures the freezing point by determining the resistance of a glass-enclosed metallic probe at the freezing point of the specimen. The electrical resistance is proportional to the temperature. In this instrument the osmolality of serum, urine or other biological fluids is determined by comparing their freezing points with that of a carefully prepared sodium chloride solution of known osmotic pressure. The lowering of the freezing point is proportional to the mole fraction (gram-mole of solute per kg. of solvent), and gives the milliosmolal concentration, which is slightly different from the milliosmolar concentration, which represents milliosmoles of solute per liter of water. For dilute solutions these 2 values approach each other and are often used without distinction. Osmolality should be the preferred term, because that is what is measured by the osmometer.

In studying osmotic pressure relations in solution it is useful to express the concentration in terms of ionic concentrations. The term "milliosmolar" is used instead of millimolar to show the additive osmotic effect of the ions.

For example: A millimolar solution of glucose (180 mg. per liter) is also a milliosmolar solution (1 milliosmole per liter), because there is no increase in the number of active particles through ionization. A millimolar solution of sodium chloride (58.5 mg. per liter) contains 1 chemical milliequivalent of sodium ions and 1 milliequivalent of chloride ions. The milliosmolar concentration is 2 milliosmoles per liter, because 1 chemical milliequivalent of sodium or chloride ions is equal to 1 milliosmole of sodium or chloride ions, respectively. This is true for all univalent ions. The chemical milliequivalence of a divalent ion is twice the milliosmolar value. In a millimolar solution of calcium chloride ($CaCl_2$) there are 2 chemical milliequivalents of calcium ions, but only 1 milliosmole of calcium ions. The millimolar solution of calcium chloride contains 2 chemical milliequivalents of chloride ions or 2 milliosmoles of chloride ions per liter. A millimolar solution of calcium chloride contains 3 milliosmoles per liter, because it ionizes into 1 calcium ion and 2 chloride ions.

In blood serum containing 10 mg. of calcium per 100 ml., there are 5 chemical milliequivalents of

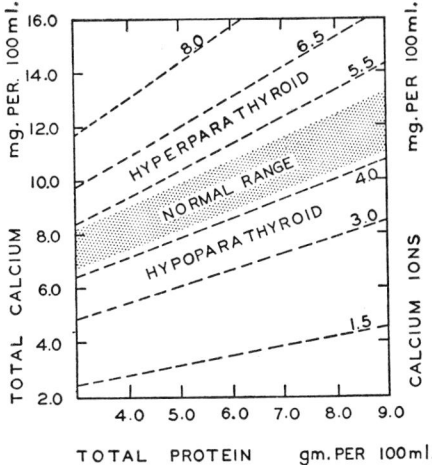

Figure 29-1. Nomogram for estimation of serum ionized calcium from total calcium and total protein values. Modified by Lytt I. Gardner from the McLean-Hastings data (*J. Biol. Chem.*, Vol. 108).

calcium per liter, but only 2.5 milliosmoles of calcium per liter. The average normal total ionic concentration of blood serum is 290 milliosmoles; cation concentration 151, anion concentration 139. In blood serum the portion of milliosmoles accounted for by glucose or urea (3 to 6 milliosmoles) is small compared to the osmolal effect of the electrolytes. The osmotic pressure of the blood serum of infants and children is comparable to that of adults.

HOWARD W. ROBINSON

SODIUM AND POTASSIUM CONTENTS OF ORAL FLUIDS*

TABLE 29-6.

FLUID	MEQ./1000 GM.	
	Na	K
Apple juice (sweet cider, bottled)...	1.7	26
Ginger ale.....................	3.5	0.15
Grape juice (Concord, sweetened, bottled).....................	0.4	31
Grapefruit juice (sweetened, canned).	0.2	38.5
Milk, whole....................	21.7	36
Orange juice (unsweetened, canned).	0.2	48.8
Pepsi-cola.....................	6.5	0.77
Pineapple juice (unsweetened, canned).....................	0.2	36
Root beer.....................	3.5	0.13
Tomato juice (canned, salt added)..	100	59
Water (New Haven, Conn.).......	0.13	0.03

*Calculated from C. E. Bills, F. G. McDonald, W. Niedermeier and M. G. Schwartz: Sodium and Potassium in Foods and Waters. Determination by the Flame Photometer. *J. Am. Dietetic A.*, 25:304, 1949. Prepared by R. E. Cooke.

FOOD VALUES

TABLE 29-7. Food Composition Table for Short Method of Dietary Analysis

FOOD AND APPROXIMATE MEASURE	WEIGHT, GM.	FOOD ENERGY, CAL.	PROTEIN, GM.	FAT, GM.	CARBOHYDRATE, GM.	CALCIUM, MG.	IRON, MG.	VITAMIN A VALUE, I.U.	THIAMINE, MG.	RIBOFLAVIN, MG.	NIACIN, MG.	ASCORBIC ACID, MG.
Milk, cheese, cream; related products												
Cheese: blue, cheddar (1 cu. in. 17 gm.).												
cheddar process (1 oz.). Swiss (1 oz.)	30	105	6	9	1	165	0.2	345	0.01	0.12	Trace	0
cottage (from skim) creamed (½ c.)	115	120	16	5	3	105	0.4	190	0.04	0.28	0.1	0
cream: half-and-half (cream and milk) (2 tbsp.)	30	40	1	4	2	30	Trace	145	0.01	0.04	Trace	Trace
For light whipping add 1 pat butter												
Milk: whole (3.5% fat) (1 c.)	245	160	9	9	12	285	0.1	350	0.08	0.42	0.1	2
fluid, nonfat (skim) and buttermilk (from skim)	245	90	9	Trace	13	300	Trace	—	0.10	0.44	0.2	2
milk beverage (1 c.): cocoa, chocolate drink made with skim milk. For malted milk add 4 tbsp. half-and-half (270 gm.)	245	210	8	8	26	280	0.6	300	0.09	0.43	0.3	Trace
milk desserts, custard (1 c.) 248 gm., ice cream (8 fl. oz.) 142 gm.		290	8	17	29	210	0.4	785	0.07	0.34	0.1	1
cornstarch pudding (248 gm.), ice milk (1 c.) 187 gm.		280	9	10	40	290	0.1	390	0.08	0.41	0.3	2
White sauce, med (½ c.)	130	215	5	16	12	150	0.2	610	0.06	0.22	0.3	Trace
Egg: 1 large	50	80	6	6	Trace	25	1.2	590	0.06	0.15	Trace	0
Meat, poultry, fish, shellfish, related products												
Beef, lamb, veal: lean and fat, cooked, inc. corned beef (3 oz.) (all cuts)	85	245	22	16	0	10	2.9	25	0.06	0.19	4.2	0
lean only, cooked; dried beef (2+ oz.) (all cuts)	65	140	20	5	0	10	2.4	10	0.05	0.16	3.4	0
Beef, relatively fat, such as steak and rib, cooked (3 oz.)	85	350	18	30	0	10	2.4	60	0.05	0.14	3.5	0
Liver: beef, fried (2 oz.)	55	130	15	6	3	5	5.0	30,280	0.15	2.37	9.4	15
Pork, lean and fat, cooked (3 oz.) (all cuts)	85	325	20	24	0	10	2.6	0	0.62	0.20	4.2	0
lean only, cooked (2+ oz.) (all cuts)	60	150	18	8	0	5	2.2	0	0.57	0.19	3.2	0
ham, light cure, lean and fat, roasted (3 oz.)	85	245	18	19	0	10	2.2	0	0.40	0.16	3.1	0
Luncheon meats: bologna (2 sl.), pork sausage, cooked (2 oz.), frankfurter (1), bacon, broiled or fried crisp (3 sl.)		185	9	16	—	5	1.3	—	0.21	0.12	1.7	0
Poultry												
chicken: flesh only, broiled (3 oz.)	85	115	20	3	0	10	1.4	80	0.05	0.16	7.4	0
fried (2+ oz.)	75	170	24	6	1	10	1.6	85	0.05	0.23	8.3	0
turkey, light and dark, roasted (3 oz.)	85	160	27	5	0	—	1.5	—	0.03	0.15	6.5	0
Fish and shellfish												
salmon (3 oz.) (canned)	85	130	17	5	0	165	0.7	60	0.03	0.16	6.8	0
fish sticks, breaded, cooked (3-4)	75	130	13	7	5	10	0.3	—	0.03	0.05	1.2	0
mackerel, halibut, cooked	85	175	19	10	0	10	0.8	515	0.08	0.15	6.8	0
bluefish, haddock, herring, perch, shad, cooked (tuna canned in oil, 20 gm.)	85	160	19	8	2	20	1.0	60	0.06	0.11	4.4	0

Food, approximate measure, and weight (gm.)	Food energy (cal.)	Protein (gm.)	Fat (gm.)	Carbohydrate (gm.)	Calcium (mg.)	Iron (mg.)	Vitamin A (I.U.)	Thiamine (mg.)	Riboflavin (mg.)	Niacin (mg.)	Ascorbic acid (mg.)
clams, canned: crab meat, canned; lobster; oyster, raw; scallop; shrimp, canned 85	75	14	1	2	65	2.5	65	0.10	0.08	1.5	0
Mature dry beans and peas, nuts, peanuts, related products											
Beans: white with pork and tomato, canned (1 c.) 260	320	16	7	50	140	4.7	340	0.20	0.08	1.5	5
red (128 gm.), cowpeas (125 gm.), cooked (½ c.) 125	125	8	—	25	35	2.5	5	0.13	0.06	0.7	—
Nuts: almonds (12), cashews (8), peanuts (1 tbsp.), peanut butter (1 tbsp.), pecans (12), English walnuts (2 tbsp.), coconut (¼ c.) 15	95	3	8	4	15	0.5	5	0.05	0.04	0.9	—
Vegetables and vegetable products											
Asparagus, cooked, cut spears (⅔ c.) 115	25	3	Trace	4	25	0.7	1055	0.19	0.20	1.6	30
Beans: green (½ c.) cooked 60 gm.; canned 120 gm.	15	1	Trace	3	30	0.4	340	0.04	0.06	0.3	8
Lima, immature, cooked (⅔ c.) 100	90	6	1	16	40	2.0	225	0.14	0.08	1.0	14
Broccoli spears, cooked (⅔ c.) 85	25	3	Trace	4	90	0.8	2500	0.09	0.20	0.8	90
Brussels sprouts, cooked (⅔ c.)	30	3	Trace	5	30	1.0	450	0.07	0.12	0.7	75
Cabbage (110 gm.); cauliflower, cooked (80 gm.); and sauerkraut, canned (150 mg.) (reduced ascorbic acid value by one-third for kraut) (⅔ c.) 95	20	1	Trace	4	35	0.5	80	0.05	0.05	0.3	37
Carrots, cooked (⅔ c.)	30	1	Trace	7	30	0.6	10,145	0.05	0.05	0.5	6
Corn, 1 ear, cooked (140 gm.); canned (130 gm.) (½ c.)	75	2	Trace	18	5	0.4	315	0.06	0.06	1.1	6
Leafy greens: collards (125 gm.), dandelions (120 gm.), kale (75 gm.), mustard (95 gm.), spinach (120 gm.), turnip (100 gm. cooked, 150 gm. canned) (⅔ c. cooked and canned) (reduce ascorbic acid one-half for canned) 80	30	3	Trace	5	175	1.8	8570	0.11	0.18	0.8	45
Peas, green (½ c.)	60	4	1	10	20	1.4	430	0.22	0.09	1.8	16
Potatoes, baked, boiled (100 gm.), 10 pc. French fried (55 gm.) (for fried, add 1 tbsp. cooking oil) 85	85	3	Trace	30	10	0.7	Trace	0.08	0.04	1.5	16
Pumpkin, canned (½ c.) 115	40	1	1	9	30	0.5	7295	0.03	0.06	0.6	6
Squash, winter, canned (½ c.) 100	65	2	1	16	30	0.8	4305	0.05	0.14	0.7	14
Sweet potato, canned (½ c.) 110	120	2	—	27	25	0.8	8500	0.05	0.05	0.7	15
Tomato, 1 raw, ⅔ c. canned, ⅔ c. juice 150	35	2	Trace	7	14	0.8	1350	0.10	0.06	1.0	29
Tomato catsup (2 tbsp.) 35	30	1	Trace	8	10	0.2	480	0.04	0.02	0.6	6
Other, cooked (beets, mushrooms, onions, turnips) (½ c.) 95	25	1	—	5	20	0.5	15	0.02	0.10	0.7	7
Other commonly served raw, cabbage (½ c., 50 gm.), celery (3 sm. stalks, 40 gm.), cucumber (¼ med., 50 gm.), green pepper (½, 30 gm.), radishes (5, 40 gm.) 25	10	Trace	Trace	2	15	0.3	100	0.03	0.03	0.2	20
carrots, raw (½ carrot) 25	10	Trace	Trace	2	10	0.2	2750	0.02	0.02	0.2	2
lettuce leaves (2 lg.) 50	10	1	Trace	2	34	0.7	950	0.03	0.04	0.2	9
Fruits and fruit products											
Cantaloupe (½ med.) 385	60	1	Trace	14	25	0.8	6540	0.08	0.06	1.2	63
Citrus and strawberries: orange (1), grapefruit (½), juice (½ c.), strawberries (½ c.), lemon (1), tangerine (1) 60	50	1	—	13	25	0.4	165	0.08	0.03	0.3	55
Yellow, fresh: apricots (3), peach (2 med.); canned fruit and juice (½ c.) or dried, cooked, unsweetened: apricot, peaches (½ c.) 85	85	—	—	22	10	1.1	1005	0.01	0.05	1.0	5

TABLE 29-7. (Continued)

FOOD AND APPROXIMATE MEASURE	WEIGHT, GM.	FOOD ENERGY, CAL.	PRO-TEIN, GM.	FAT, GM.	CARBO-HY-DRATE, GM.	CAL-CIUM, MG.	IRON, MG.	VITA-MIN A VALUE, I.U.	THIA-MINE, MG.	RIBO-FLAVIN, MG.	NIACIN, MG.	ASCOR-BIC ACID, MG.
Other, dried: dates, pitted (4), figs (2), raisins (¼ c.)	40	120	1	—	31	35	1.4	20	0.04	0.04	0.5	—
Other, fresh: apple (1), banana (1), figs (3), pear (1)		80	—	—	21	15	0.5	140	0.04	0.03	0.2	6
Fruit pie: to 1 serving fruit add 1 tbsp. flour, 2 tbsp. sugar, 1 tbsp. fat												
Grain products												
Enriched and whole grain: bread (1 sl., 23 gm.), biscuit (½), cooked cereals (½ c.), prepared cereals (1 oz.) Graham crackers (2 lg.), macaroni, noodles, spaghetti (½ c., cooked), pancake (1, 27 gm.), roll (½), waffle (½, 38 gm.)		65	2	1	16	20	0.6	10	0.09	0.05	0.7	—
Unenriched: bread (1 sl., 23 gm.), cooked cereal (½ c.), macaroni, noodles, spaghetti (½ c.), popcorn (½ c.), pretzel sticks, small (15), roll (½)		65	2	1	16	10	0.3	5	0.02	0.02	0.3	—
Desserts												
Cake, plain (1 pc.), doughnut (1). For iced cake or doughnut add value for sugar (1 tbsp.). For chocolate cake add chocolate (30 gm.)	45	145	2	5	24	30	0.4	65	0.02	0.05	0.2	—
Cookies, plain (1)	25	120	1	5	18	10	0.2	20	0.01	0.01	0.1	—
Pie crust, single crust (⅐ shell)	20	95	1	6	8	3	0.3	0	0.04	0.03	0.3	—
Flour, white, enriched (1 tbsp.)	7	25	1	Trace	5	1	0.2	0	0.03	0.02	0.2	0
Fats and Oils												
Butter, margarine (1 pat, ½ tbsp.)	7	50	Trace	6	Trace	1	0	230	—	—	—	0
Fats and oils, cooking (1 tbsp.)	14	125	0	14	0	0	0	0	0	0	0	0
Salad dressings, mayonnaise type (1 tbsp.)	15	80	Trace	9	1	2	0.1	45	Trace	Trace	Trace	0
Sugars, sweets												
Candy, plain (½ oz.), jam and jelly (1 tbsp.), syrup (1 tbsp.), gelatin dessert, plain (½ c.), beverages, carbonated (1 c.)		60	0	0	14	3	0.1	Trace	Trace	Trace	Trace	Trace
Chocolate fudge (1 oz.), chocolate syrup (3 tbsp.)		125	1	2	30	15	0.6	10	Trace	0.02	0.1	Trace
Molasses (1 tbsp.), caramel (½ oz.)		40	Trace	Trace	8	20	0.3	Trace	Trace	Trace	Trace	Trace
Sugar (1 tbsp.)	12	45	0	0	12	0	Trace	0	0	0	0	0
Miscellaneous												
Chocolate, bitter (1 oz.)	30	145	3	15	8	20	1.9	20	0.01	0.07	0.4	0
Sherbet (½ c.)	96	130	1	1	30	15	Trace	55	0.01	0.03	Trace	2
Soups: bean, pea (green) (1 c.)		150	7	4	22	50	1.6	495	0.09	0.06	1.0	4
noodle, beef, chicken (1 c.)		65	4	2	7	10	0.7	50	0.03	0.04	0.9	Trace
clam chowder, minestrone, tomato, vegetable (1 c.)		90	3	2	14	25	0.9	1880	0.05	0.04	1.1	3

From E. D. Wilson, K. H. Fisher and M. E. Fuqua: *Principles of Nutrition.* 2nd ed. New York, John Wiley & Sons, Inc., 1965, pp. 528-33.

TABLE 29-8. Nutritive Value of Baby Foods (per 100 Grams Edible Portion-About 7 Tablespoons)

FOOD	ENERGY CALORIES	PROTEIN GM.	FAT GM.	CARBO-HYDRATE GM.	CALCIUM MG.	IRON MG.	VITAMIN A VALUE I.U.	THIAMINE MG.	RIBO-FLAVIN MG.	NIACIN MG.	ASCORBIC ACID MG.
Cereals, precooked, dry and other products											
Barley, added nutrients	348	13.4	1.2	73.6	736	53.2	(0)	3.71	1.20	32.2	0
High protein, added nutrients	357	35.2	3.7	48.1	815	63.1	—	3.67	1.15	24.0	0
Mixed, added nutrients	368	15.2	2.9	70.6	820	56.4	—	3.15	1.35	22.3	0
Oatmeal, added nutrients	375	16.5	5.5	66.0	757	48.2	(0)	2.58	1.05	21.3	0
Rice, added nutrients	371	6.6	1.6	80.0	858	50.2	(0)	2.56	1.24	19.7	0
Dinners, canned											
Cereal, vegetable, meat mixtures (approx. 2–4% protein).											
Beef noodle dinner	48	2.8	1.1	6.8	12	0.5	620	0.02	0.05	0.5	2
Cereal, egg yolk and bacon	82	2.9	4.9	6.6	29	0.8	520	0.05	0.06	0.4	—
Chicken noodle dinner	49	2.1	1.3	7.2	27	0.3	800	0.03	0.06	0.4	1
Macaroni, tomatoes, meat and cereal	67	2.6	2.0	9.6	21	0.5	500	0.14	0.12	1.0	1
Split peas, vegetables and ham or bacon	80	4.0	2.1	11.2	29	0.7	600	0.08	0.05	0.5	1
Vegetables and bacon, with cereal	68	1.7	2.9	8.7	17	0.6	2200	0.07	0.05	0.6	1
Vegetables and beef, with cereal	56	2.7	1.6	7.6	17	0.8	2800	0.03	0.04	0.9	1
Vegetables and chicken, with cereal	52	2.1	1.4	7.7	33	0.4	1000	0.03	0.04	0.5	Trace
Vegetables and ham, with cereal	64	2.8	2.2	8.3	25	0.3	1000	0.08	0.05	0.5	3
Vegetables and lamb, with cereal	58	2.2	2.0	7.7	23	0.7	2200	0.03	0.05	0.7	1
Vegetables and liver, with cereal	47	3.1	0.4	7.8	17	2.7	4700	0.04	0.37	1.6	3
Vegetables and liver, with bacon and cereal	57	2.4	1.9	7.5	11	2.6	4600	0.03	0.33	1.3	2
Vegetables and turkey, with cereal	44	2.1	0.8	7.2	22	0.3	400	0.01	0.03	0.4	1
Meat or poultry (approx. 6–8% protein)											
Beef with vegetables	87	7.4	3.7	6.0	13	1.2	1100	0.07	0.17	1.6	2
Chicken with vegetables	100	7.4	4.6	7.2	22	0.9	1000	0.09	0.15	1.6	2
Turkey with vegetables	86	6.7	3.2	7.6	38	0.6	1000	0.13	0.13	1.8	2
Veal with vegetables	63	7.1	1.6	5.1	11	0.8	800	0.08	0.15	2.0	2
Fruits and fruit products with or without thickening, canned											
Applesauce	72	0.2	0.2	18.6	4	0.4	40	0.01	0.02	0.1	Trace

TABLE 29-8. (Continued)

FOOD	ENERGY CALORIES	PROTEIN GM.	FAT GM.	CARBO-HYDRATE GM.	CALCIUM MG.	IRON MG.	VITAMIN A VALUE I.U.	THIAMINE MG.	RIBO-FLAVIN MG.	NIACIN MG.	ASCORBIC ACID MG.
Applesauce and apricots	86	0.3	0.1	22.6	4	0.3	600	0.01	0.02	0.1	2
Bananas (with tapioca or cornstarch, added ascorbic acid), strained	84	0.4	0.2	21.6	13	0.2	70	0.02	0.02	0.2	35
Bananas and pineapple (with tapioca or cornstarch)	80	0.4	0.1	20.7	20	0.2	30	0.01	0.01	0.1	2
Fruit dessert with tapioca (apricot, pineapple or orange)	84	0.3	0.3	21.5	15	0.4	450	0.02	0.01	0.2	4
Peaches	81	0.6	0.2	20.7	6	0.3	500	0.01	0.02	0.7	3
Pears	66	0.3	0.1	17.1	7	0.2	30	0.02	0.02	0.2	2
Pears and pineapple	69	0.4	0.2	17.6	7	0.2	20	0.03	0.02	0.2	2
Plums with tapioca, strained	94	0.4	0.2	24.3	5	0.4	250	0.01	0.02	0.2	2
Prunes with tapioca	86	0.3	0.2	22.4	7	0.9	400	0.02	0.06	0.4	4
Meats, poultry and eggs; canned:											
Beef:											
Strained	99	14.7	4.0	(0)	8	2.0	—	0.01	0.16	3.5	0
Junior	118	19.3	3.9	(0)	8	2.5	—	0.02	0.20	4.3	0
Chicken	127	13.7	7.6	(0)	—	1.9	—	0.02	0.16	3.5	0
Egg yolks, strained	210	10.0	18.4	0.2	81	3.0	1900	0.12	0.22	Trace	Trace
Lamb:											
Strained	107	14.6	4.9	(0)	9	2.1	—	0.02	0.17	3.3	—
Junior	121	17.5	5.1	(0)	13	2.7	—	0.02	0.21	4.1	—
Liver, strained	97	14.1	3.4	1.5	6	5.6	24,000	0.05	2.00	7.6	10
Liver and bacon, strained	123	13.7	6.6	1.3	6	4.2	22,000	0.05	1.99	7.8	7
Pork:											
Strained	118	15.4	5.8	(0)	8	1.5	—	0.19	0.20	2.7	—
Junior	134	18.6	6.0	(0)	8	1.2	—	0.23	0.23	2.8	—
Veal:											
Strained	91	15.5	2.7	(0)	10	1.7	—	0.03	0.20	4.3	—
Junior	107	18.8	3.0	(0)	8	1.6	—	0.03	0.22	6.0	—
Vegetables, canned:											
Beans, green	22	1.4	0.1	5.1	33	1.1	400	0.02	0.06	0.3	3
Beets, strained	37	1.4	0.1	8.3	18	0.7	20	0.02	0.03	0.1	3
Carrots	29	0.7	0.1	6.8	23	0.5	13,000	0.02	0.03	0.4	3
Mixed vegetables, including vegetable soup	37	1.6	0.3	8.5	22	0.9	4700	0.05	0.04	0.6	2
Peas, strained	54	4.2	0.2	9.3	11	1.2	500	0.08	0.09	1.2	10
Spinach, creamed	43	2.3	0.7	7.5	64	0.6	5000	0.02	0.13	0.3	6
Squash	25	0.7	0.1	6.2	24	0.4	2400	0.02	0.04	0.3	8
Sweet potatoes	67	1.0	0.2	15.5	16	0.4	4900	0.04	0.03	0.4	8
Tomato soup, strained	54	1.9	0.1	13.5	24	0.4	1000	0.05	0.12	0.7	3

From C. H. Robinson: Normal and Therapeutic Nutrition. 13th ed. New York, Macmillan Company, 1967.

METHOD FOR DIET CALCULATION*

The following is a convenient method for calculation of diabetic and other quantitative diets which can be used by the average practitioner. It is sufficiently accurate for clinical use. The principle is based on the classification of foods on the basis of the approximate equality of their carbohydrate, protein and fat contents, so-called food equivalents (see Table 29-10).

The steps for determining the diet for a given child are as follows:

1. Determine dietary prescription.

(For diabetic diet, see p. 1159)

Example below based on diabetic diet of C, 200; P, 70; F, 80.

2. List number of servings from each list of food exchanges in Table 29-10, which are considered essential for the basic needs of the child; tabulate amounts of carbohydrate, protein and fat for each list and total each element separately.

3. Subtract amounts of carbohydrate, protein and fat in (2) from amount of each specified for the prescribed diet.

	CARBOHYDRATE GM.	PROTEIN GM.	FAT GM.
Prescribed diet	200	70	80
Basic diet	166	69	75
Deficit	34	1	5

4. Make up deficits of carbohydrate, protein and fat in preliminary diet list (step 2) by adding appropriate number of servings from any of the lists of food exchanges (Table 29-10), based on child's dietary habits and desires.

Example:

LIST	SERVING	CARBOHYDRATE GM.	PROTEIN GM.	FAT GM.
3	3	30	0	0
4	1	5	2	0
6	1	0	0	5
		35	2	5
Basic diet		166	69	75
Final prescription		201	71	80

Example:

LIST	FOOD	NO. OF SERVINGS	CARBOHYDRATE GM.	PROTEIN GM.	FAT GM.
1	Milk	4 cups (1 qt.)	48	32	40
2A	Vegetables	As desired	0	0	0
2B	Vegetables	4	28	8	0
3	Fruit	3	30	0	0
4	Bread	4	60	8	0
5	Meat	3	0	21	15
6	Fat	4	0	0	20
			166	69	75

*Adapted from E. K. Caso and F. J. Stare: Simplified Method for Calculating Diabetic Diets. *J.A.M.A.*, 133: 169, 1947.

TABLE 29-9. COMPOSITION OF FOOD EXCHANGES

LIST	FOOD	MEASURES	Gm.	C	P	F	Cal.
1	Milk exchanges	½ pint	240	12	8	10	170
2A	Vegetable exchanges	As desired	—	—	—	—	—
2B	Vegetable exchanges	½ cup	100	7	2	—	36
3	Fruit exchanges	Varies	—	10	–	—	40
4	Bread exchanges	Varies	—	15	2	—	68
5	Meat exchanges	1 oz.	30	—	7	5	73
6	Fat exchanges	1 tsp.	5	—	–	5	45

TABLE 29-10. FOOD EXCHANGES

LIST 1. MILK EXCHANGES (carbohydrate, 12 gm.; protein, 8 gm.; fat, 10 gm.; calories, 170)

	MEASURE	GM.
Milk, whole*	1 cup	240
Milk, evaporated	½ cup	120
Milk, powdered*	¼ cup	35
Buttermilk*	1 cup	240

* Add 2 fat exchanges if fat-free.

LIST 2. VEGETABLE EXCHANGES

A. These vegetables may be used as desired in ordinary amounts. Carbohydrates and calories negligible.

Asparagus		Lettuce
Broccoli		Mushrooms
Brussels sprouts	Beet greens	Okra
Cabbage	Chard	Peppers
Cauliflower	Collard	Radishes
Celery	Dandelion	Rhubarb
Chicory	Kale	Sauerkraut
Cucumbers	Mustard	String beans, young
Escarole	Spinach	Summer squash
Eggplant	Turnip greens	Tomatoes

B. Vegetables: 1 serving equals ½ cup equals 100 gm. (carbohydrate, 7 gm.; protein, 2 gm.; calories, 36)

Beets	Peas, green	Squash, winter
Carrots	Pumpkin	Turnip
Onions	Rutabaga	

LIST 3. FRUIT EXCHANGES (carbohydrate, 10 gm.; calories, 40)

	MEASURE	GM.
Apple	1 sm. (2″ diam.)	80
Applesauce	½ cup	100
Apricots, fresh	2 medium	100
Apricots, dried	4 halves	20
Banana	½ small	50
Berries: straw., rasp., black	1 cup	150
Blueberries	⅔ cup	100
Cantaloupe	¼ (6″ diam.)	200
Cherries	10 large	75
Dates	2	15
Figs, fresh	2 large	50
Figs, dried	1 small	15
Grapefruit	½ small	125
Grapefruit juice	½ cup	100
Grapes	12	75
Grape juice	¼ cup	60
Honeydew melon	⅛ (7″ diam.)	150
Mango	½ small	70
Orange	1 small	100
Orange juice	½ cup	100
Papaya	½ medium	100
Peach	1 medium	100
Pear	1 small	100
Pineapple	½ cup	80
Pineapple juice	⅓ cup	80
Plums	2 medium	100
Prunes, dried	2 medium	25
Raisins	2 tbsp.	15
Tangerine	1 large	100
Watermelon	1 cup	175

LIST 4. BREAD EXCHANGES (carbohydrate, 15 gm.; protein, 2 gm.; calories, 68)

	MEASURE	GM.
Bread	1 slice	25
Biscuit, roll	1 (2″ diam.)	35
Muffin	1 (2″ diam.)	35
Cornbread	1 (1½″ cube)	35
Flour	2½ tbsp.	20
Cereal, cooked	½ cup	100
Cereal, dry (flake and puffed)	¾ cup	20
Rice, grits, cooked	½ cup	100
Spaghetti, noodles, etc., cooked	½ cup	100
Crackers, graham (2½″ sq.)	2	20
Oyster	20 (½ cup)	20
Saltines (2″ sq.)	5	20
Soda (2½″ sq.)	3	20
Round, thin (1½″ diam.)	6–8	20
Vegetables		
Beans and peas, dried, cooked	½ cup	90
(lima, navy, split peas, cowpeas, etc.)		
Baked beans, no pork	¼ cup	50
Corn	⅓ cup	80
Parsnips	⅔ cup	125
Potatoes, white, baked, boiled	1 (2″ diam.)	100
Potatoes, white, mashed	½ cup	100
Potatoes, sweet, or yams	¼ cup	50
Sponge cake, plain	1 (1½″ cube)	25
Ice cream (omit 2 fat exchanges)	½ cup	70

LIST 5. MEAT EXCHANGES (protein, 7 gm.; fat, 5 gm.; calories, 73)

	MEASURE	GM.
Meat and poultry (med. fat)	1 oz.	30
(beef, lamb, pork, liver, chicken, etc.)		
Cold cuts (4½″ sq., ⅛″ thick)	1 slice	45
Frankfurter	1 (8–9/lb.)	50
Fish: cod, mackerel, etc.	1 oz.	30
Salmon, tuna, crab	¼ cup	30
Oysters, shrimp, clams	5 small	45
Sardines	3 medium	30
Cheese, cheddar, American	1 oz.	30
Cottage	¼ cup	45
Egg	1	50
Peanut butter*	2 tbsp.	30

* Limit use or adjust carbohydrate.

LIST 6. FAT EXCHANGES (fat, 5 gm.; calories, 45)

	MEASURE	GM.
Butter or margarine	1 tsp.	5
Bacon, crisp	1 slice	10
Cream, light, 20%	2 tbsp.	30
Cream, heavy, 40%	1 tbsp.	15
Cream cheese	1 tbsp.	15
French dressing	1 tbsp.	15
Mayonnaise	1 tsp.	5
Oil or cooking fat	1 tsp.	5
Nuts	6 small	10
Olives	5 small	50
Avocado	⅛ (4″ diam.)	25

ELIMINATION DIETS (ROWE) FOR THE STUDY AND CONTROL OF FOOD ALLERGY

These diets may be modified by eliminating foods which elicit large dermal reactions or are disliked by the patient or disagree with him. They may be used before or after the failure of "test-negative diets."

The cereal-free diets exclude all cereals as well as milk, egg and other allergenic foods. Fruit-free elimination diets also exclude tomato and uncooked vegetables and fruits. The preliminary use of diet 4 is rarely satisfactory.

A minimal diet of lamb, white potato, tapioca cooked with pear and sugar, carrots, peas, pears, salt and sugar is a practical and simple one.

The patient should be given a list of allowed foods with menus and recipes and never a list of foods to avoid. Strict adherence to the diet is imperative. Allergens of foods remain in the body for more than a few days, so that dietary change must not be made until there has been an opportunity to evaluate the preceding one. The handling and odors of eliminated foods must also be avoided. Synthetic vitamins should be given as supplements to the diet.

The time necessary to maintain the elimination diets depends on the frequency with which symptoms have been manifest. Thus relief for 1 week from symptoms occurring daily, for 2 weeks from symptoms recurring every 2 to 3 days, for 3 weeks from weekly recurring symptoms, and for 3 months from symptoms recurring every 3 to 6 weeks indicates that causative allergenic foods have been eliminated.

After relief has been assured, individual foods can be added, excluding any which reproduce symptoms. Each food should be taken daily for 3 to 5 days before trying another. Symptoms may recur in a few minutes, hours or days according to the degree of allergy that exists.

REFERENCES

Rowe, A. H.: *Elimination Diets and the Patients' Allergies.* Philadelphia, Lea & Febiger, 1944.

Rowe, A. H.: Elimination Diets (Rowe) for the Study and Control of Food Allergy. *Quart. Rev. Allergy,* 4:227, 1950.

Rowe, A. H.: *The Elimination Diets (Rowe).* 5th Revision. Berkeley, California, Sather Gate Book Shop, 1958.

TABLE 29-11. ELIMINATION DIETS

DIET 1	DIET 2	DIET 3	DIET 4
Rice	Corn, rye	Tapioca	Milk
Rice biscuit	Corn pone	White potato	Tapioca
Rice bread	Corn, rye muffin	Breads made of any combina-	Cane
Tapioca	Rye bread, Ry-Krisp	tion of soy, lima, potato	sugar
Lettuce, chard	Beets, squash	starch, and tapioca flours	
Spinach, carrot	Asparagus, artichoke	Tomato	
Sweet potato or yam	Chicken (no hens)	Carrot	
Lamb	Bacon	Lima beans	
Lemon, grapefruit	Pineapple	String beans	
Pears	Peach, apricot	Peas	
Cane sugar	Prune	Beef	
Sesame oil, olive oil*	Cane or beet sugar	Bacon	
Salt	Mazola oil	Lemon	
Gelatin, plain or flavored with	Sesame oil	Grapefruit	
lime or lemon	Salt	Peach	
Maple syrup or syrup made with	Gelatin, plain or flavored with	Apricot	
cane sugar flavored with maple	pineapple	Cane sugar	
Royal baking powder	Karo corn syrup	Soy bean oil	
Baking soda	White vinegar	Gelatin, plain	
Cream of tartar	Royal baking powder	Salt	
Vanilla extract	Baking soda	Syrup made with cane sugar	
Lemon extract	Cream of tartar	Cream of tartar	
	Vanilla extract	Corn starch-free baking powder	

Straight lines enclose foods in the cereal-free elimination diets.

* Allergy to olive oil may occur with or without allergy to olive pollen. Mazola oil may be used if corn allergy is not present.

CONVERSION TABLES OF APOTHECARY'S MEASURES TO METRIC EQUIVALENTS

TABLE 29-12.

WEIGHTS

Apothecary		Metric	
	Approximate		More Nearly Accurate
1 grain............................ 60 mg.	0.06 gm.	0.06479 gm.	
2 grains........................... 120 mg.	0.12 gm.		
3 grains........................... 180 mg.	0.2 gm.		
5 grains........................... 300 mg.	0.3 gm.		
15 grains..........................1000 mg.	1.0 gm.		
60 grains or 1 dram............................	4.0 gm.	3.888	gm.
240 grains or 4 drams, ½ oz......................	15.0 gm.		
480 grains or 8 drams, 1 oz......................	30.0 gm.	31.103	gm.
		31.103	gm. (Troy)
		28.350	gm. (Avoir.)
12 oz. or 1 pound.....................360.0 gm.		373.24177 gm.	
12 oz. or 1 pound.....................360.0 gm.		373.24177 gm. (Troy)	
16 oz. or 1 pound.....................480.0 gm.		453.592	gm. (Avoir.)
¾ grain.............................. 45	mg.		
½ grain.............................. 30	mg.		
⅜ grain.............................. 23	mg.		
¼ grain.............................. 15	mg.		
⅙ grain.............................. 10	mg.		
⅛ grain.............................. 8	mg.		
⅒ grain.............................. 6	mg.		
1/16 grain.............................. 4	mg.		
1/32 grain.............................. 2	mg.		
1/64 grain.............................. 1	mg.		
1/100 grain.............................. 0.6	mg.		
1/250 grain.............................. 0.25	mg.		
1/300 grain.............................. 0.2	mg.		
1/1000 grain.............................. 0.06	mg.		

LIQUID MEASURES

1 minim...........................	0.06 ml...........................		0.06161 ml.
3 minims...........................	0.2 ml.		
15 minims...........................	1.0 ml...........................		0.92415 ml.*
60 minims, 1 fl. dram...................	4.0 ml.		3.6967 ml.
480 minims 1 fl. oz...............	30.0 ml...........................		29.5737 ml.
16 fl. oz. or 1 pt........	500.0 ml...........................		473.179 ml.
32 fl. oz. or 1 qt........	1000.0 ml...........................		946.358 ml.

* 1 ml. is equal to 16.23 minims.
Quantity of drug prescribed in grams per 2 ounces (60 ml.) gives dose in grains per dram.

EQUIVALENT TEMPERATURE READINGS

TABLE 29-13.

CENTIGRADE DEGREES	FAHRENHEIT DEGREES	CENTIGRADE DEGREES	FAHRENHEIT DEGREES
0...........................	32.0	40...........................	104.0
21...........................	69.8	41...........................	105.8
27...........................	80.6	42...........................	107.6
30...........................	86.0	43...........................	109.4
35...........................	95.0	100...........................	212.0
36...........................	96.8		
37...........................	98.6		
38...........................	100.4		
39	102.2		

To convert Centigrade readings to Fahrenheit, multiply by 1.8 and add 32. To convert Fahrenheit readings to Centigrade, subtract 32 and divide by 1.8.

THE DENVER DEVELOPMENTAL SCREENING TEST

The Denver Developmental Screening Test (DDST) offers a simple and effective way of assessing the developmental status of children during the first six years of life. Abbreviated instructions follow:

The Denver Developmental Screening Test (DDST), a device for detecting developmental delays in infancy and the preschool years, has been standardized on a large cross section of the Denver child population. The test is administered with ease and speed and lends itself to serial evaluations on the same test sheet.

Test Materials: Skein of red wool; box of raisins; rattle with a narrow handle; Abbott aspirin bottle (Abbott — 50 children's, aluminum); bell; tennis ball; test form; pencil; 8 one-inch cubical counting blocks.

General Instructions: The mother should be told that this is a developmental screening device to obtain an estimate of the child's level of development and that it is not expected that the child will be able to perform each of the test items. This test relies on observations of what the child can do and on report by a parent who knows the child. Direct observation should be used whenever possible. Since the test requires active participation by the child, every effort should be made to put the child at ease. The younger child may be tested while sitting on the mother's lap. This should be done in such a way that he can comfortably reach the test materials on the table. The test should be administered before any frightening or painful procedures. One may start by laying out one or two test materials in front of the child while asking the mother whether he performs some of the personal-social items. It is best to administer the first few test items well below the child's age level in order to assure him an initial successful experience. To avoid distractions it is best to remove all test materials from the table except for the one that is being administered.

Steps in Administering the Test:

1. Draw a vertical line on the examination sheet through the four sectors (Gross Motor, Fine Motor-Adaptive, Language and Personal-Social) to represent the child's chronologic age. Place the date of the examination at the top of the age line. For premature children, subtract the number of months premature from the chronologic age.

2. The items to be administered are those through which the child's chronologic age line passes, unless there are obvious deviations. In each sector one should establish the area in which the child passes all the items and the point at which he fails all the items.

3. In the event that a child refuses to do some of the items requested by the examiner, it is suggested that the parent administer the item, provided she does so in the prescribed manner.

4. If a child passes an item, a large letter "P" is written on the bar at the 50% passing point. "F" designates a failure, and "R" designates a refusal.

5. Note how the child adjusted to the examination, i.e., his cooperation, attention span, self-confidence, and how he related to his mother, the examiner and the test materials.

6. Ask the parent if the child's performance was typical of his performance at other times.

7. To retest the child on the same form, use a different color pencil for the scoring and age line.

8. Instructions for administering footnoted items are on the back of the test form.

Interpretations: The test items are placed into four categories: Gross Motor; Fine Motor-Adaptive; Language; and Personal-Social. Each of the test items is designated by a bar which is so located under the age scale as to indicate clearly the ages at which 25%, 50%, 75% and 90% of the standardization population could perform the particular test item. The left end of the bar designates the age at which 25% of the standardization population could perform the item; the hatch mark at the top of the bar 50%; the left end of the shaded area 75%, and the right end of the bar the age at which 90% of the standardization population could perform the item. (See below.)

Failure to perform an item passed by 90% of children of the same age should be considered a "delay." Such a failure may be emphasized by coloring the right end of the bar of the failed item. Two or more "delays" in one sector constitute an abnormal performance. If in any sector only a single delay occurs, or if in that sector no item is passed which the age line intersects, then the performance is considered questionable. Developmental delays may be due to:

(25%)   (50%)   (75%)   (90%)

//////////////// 13 ← ───── Footnote #
//////////////////////////

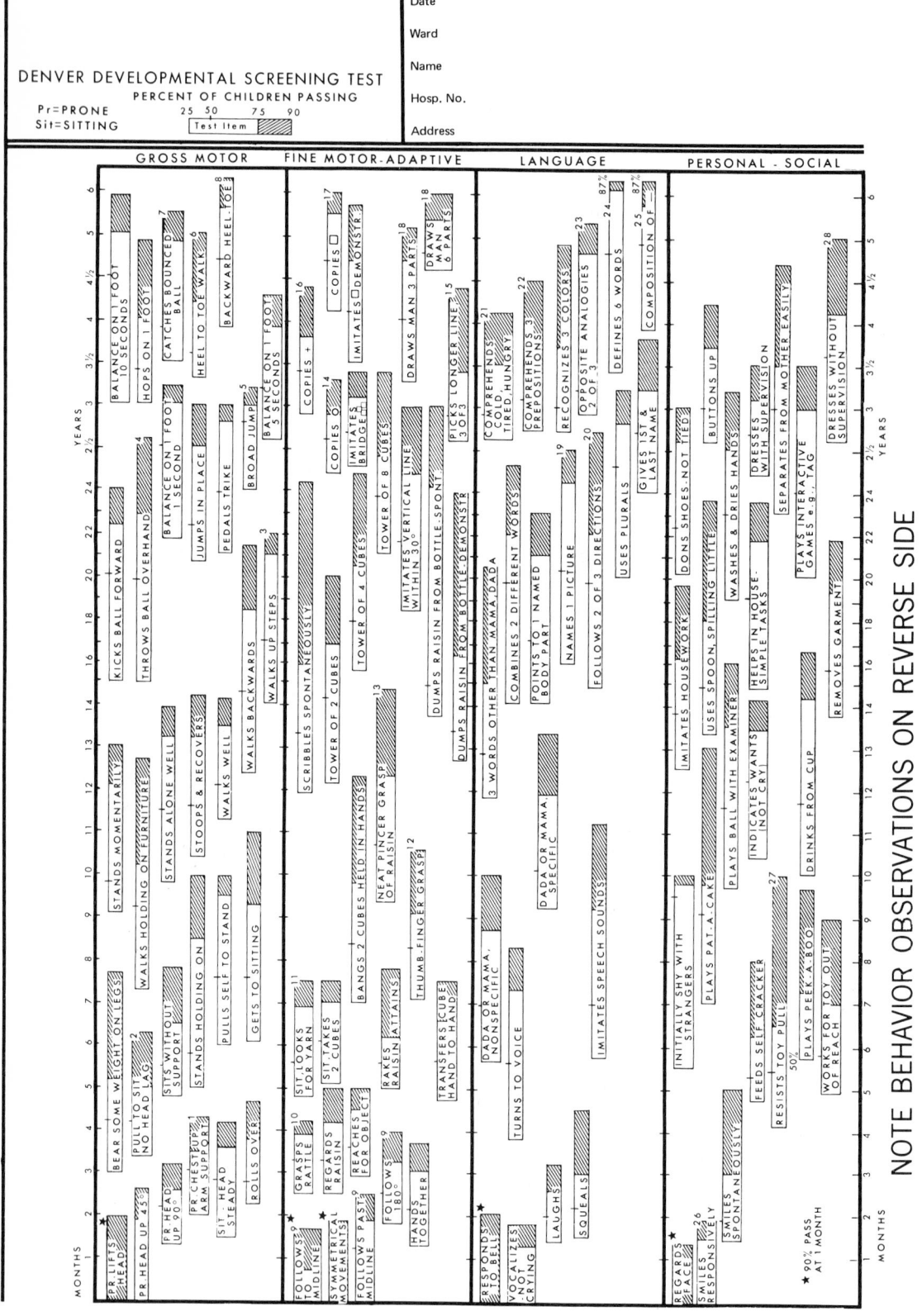

NOTE BEHAVIOR OBSERVATIONS ON REVERSE SIDE

DIRECTIONS

Date

Ward

Name

Hosp. No.

Address

1. Infant, when prone, lifts chest off table with support of forearms and/or hands.
2. Examiner grasps child's hands, pulls him from supine to sitting, child has no head lag.
3. Child may use wall or rail only, not person, may not crawl.
4. Child throws ball overhand 3 feet to within examiner's reach.
5. Child performs standing broad jump over width of test sheet.
6. Ask child to walk forward, ⬤⬤⬤⬤➡ heel within 1 inch of toe.
7. Examiner bounces ball to child, child must catch with hands (2 of 3 trials).
8. Ask child to walk backwards, ⬅⬤⬤⬤⬤ toe within 1 inch of heel.
9. Examiner moves yarn in arc from side to side 1 foot above baby's head. Note if eyes follow 90° to midline (past midline; 180°).
10. Infant grasps rattle when touched to his finger tips.
11. Child looks after yarn dropped from sight over table's edge.
12. Child grasps raisin between thumb and index finger.
13. Child performs overhand grasp of raisin with tips of thumb and index finger.

14. Copy: Pass any enclosed form. Do not demonstrate. Do not name form.

15. "Which line is longer?" (Not bigger.) Turn paper upside down, repeat (Pass 3 of 3).

16. Pass crossing lines, any angle.

17. Have child copy first. If fail, demonstrate. Pass figure with 4 square corners.

18. When scoring, symmetrical parts count as one (2 arms or 2 eyes count as one part only).
19. Point to picture and have child name it.

20. Examiner asks child to: "Give block to Mommie, put block on table, put block on floor" (2 of 3). Caution: Examiner not to gesture with head or eyes.
21. Child answers 2 of 3 questions: "What do you do when you are cold? hungry? tired?"
22. Examiner asks child to: "Put block on table, under table, in front of chair, behind chair." Caution: Examiner not to gesture with head or eyes.
23. Examiner asks child: "Fire is hot, ice is____. Mother is a woman, dad is a____. A horse is big, a mouse is____." (Pass if 2 of 3 are correct.)
24. Ask child to define 6: ball; lake; desk; house; banana; curtain; hedge; pavement. Pass if defined in terms of use, structure, composition or classification.
25. Examiner asks: "What is a spoon made of? a shoe made of? a door made of?" (No other objects may be substituted.) Must pass all 3.
26. Examiner attempts to elicit a smile by: smiling, talking or waving to infant, do not touch, baby smiles responsively in 2 or 3 attempts.
27. When child is playing with toy, pull it away from him. Pass if he resists.
28. Child need not be able to tie shoes or button in the back.

W. K. Frankenburg, M.D. and J. B. Dodds, Ph.D., Univ. of Colo. Medical Center, Denver, Colo.

DATE AND BEHAVIORAL OBSERVATIONS

(how child feels at time of the evaluation, relation to examiner, attention span, verbal behavior, self-confidence, etc.):

1. the unwillingness of the child to use his ability
   (a) owing to temporary factors, such as fatigue, illness, hospitalization, separation from the parent, fear, etc.
   (b) general unwillingness to do most things that are asked of him — such a condition may be just as detrimental as an inability to perform
2. an inability to perform the item due to
   (a) general retardation
   (b) pathologic factors such as deafness or neurological impairment
   (c) familial pattern of slow development in one or more areas

If unexplained developmental delays are noted and are a valid reflection of a child's abilities, he should be rescreened a month later. If the delays persist he should be further evaluated with more detailed diagnostic studies.

Caution: The DDST is *not* an intelligence test. It is intended as a screening instrument for use in clinical practice to note whether the development of a particular child is within the normal range.

These abbreviated instructions are amplified in the manual which accompanies the test kit.

The test form and footnoted instructions are given on pages 1552 and 1553. The form is copyrighted; forms and kits are available on request to physicians and medical students in the United States and Canada, through Mead Johnson Laboratories, Evansville, Indiana 47721, and Mead Johnson Laboratories, Ltd., 95 Saint Clair Avenue West, Toronto 7, Ontario. Kits also may be purchased through LADOCA Project and Publishing Foundation, Inc., East 51st Avenue and Lincoln Street, Denver, Colorado 80216.

We are indebted to the authors for permission to include the test in this volume.

REFERENCE

Frankenburg, W. K., and Dodds, J. B.: The Denver Developmental Screening Test. *J. Pediat.,* 71:181, 1967.

INDEX

Note: In this index the expression "re" has been used to mean "in relation to." Thus "Addison's disease re adrenal calcification" is the equivalent of "Addison's disease in relation to adrenal calcification."

The expression "vs." denotes "differential diagnosis." Thus "Asthma vs. bronchiolitis" is the equivalent of "Asthma, differential diagnosis from bronchiolitis."

1555